The 5-Minute Clinical Consult

2012

20TH EDITION

The 5-Minute Clinical Consult

2012

20TH EDITION

Editor-in-Chief

Frank J. Domino, MD
Professor
Clerkship Director
Department of Family Medicine and Community Health
The University of Massachusetts Medical School
Worcester, Massachusetts

Associate Editors

Robert A. Baldor, MD
Professor
Department of Family Medicine and Community Health
The University of Massachusetts Medical School;
Vice-Chairman
Department of Family Medicine and Community Health
UMass Memorial Health Care
Worcester, Massachusetts

Jeremy Golding, MD
Professor of Family Medicine and of Obstetrics and
    Gynecology
The University of Massachusetts Medical School
Quality Officer - Department of Family Medicine and
    Community Health
UMass Memorial Health Care - Hahnemann Family
    Health Center
Worcester, Massachusetts

Jill A. Grimes, MD
Clinical Instructor
Department of Family Medicine
University of Massachusetts Medical School
Worcester, Massachusetts;
Private Practice
West Lake Family Practice
Austin, Texas

Julie Scott Taylor, MD, MSc
Associate Professor of Family Medicine
Director of Clinical Curriculum
Alpert Medical School of Brown University
Providence, Rhode Island

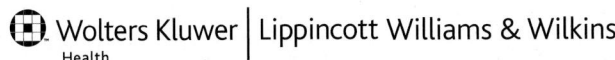
Wolters Kluwer | Lippincott Williams & Wilkins
Health
Philadelphia · Baltimore · New York · London
Buenos Aires · Hong Kong · Sydney · Tokyo

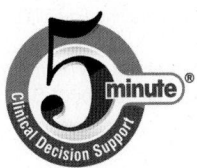

Acquisitions Editor: Avé McCracken
Product Manager: Michelle LaPlante
Vendor Manager: Bridgett Dougherty
Senior Manufacturing Manager: Benjamin Rivera
Marketing Manager: Kimberly Schonberger
Design Coordinator: Teresa Mallon
Production Service: Aptara, Inc.

Printed in China

Library of Congress Cataloging-in-Publication Data

ISBN 13: 978-1-4511-0303-8
ISBN:10: 1-451-1030-34

Care has been taken to confirm the accuracy of the information presented and to describe generally
accepted practices. However, the authors, editors, and publisher are not responsible for errors or omissions
or for any consequences from application of the information in this book and make no warranty, expressed
or implied, with respect to the currency, completeness, or accuracy of the contents of the publication.
Application of the information in a particular situation remains the professional responsibility of the
practitioner.

The authors, editors, and publisher have exerted every effort to ensure that drug selection and dosage
set forth in this text are in accordance with current recommendations and practice at the time of publication.
However, in view of ongoing research, changes in government regulations, and the constant flow of
information relating to drug therapy and drug reactions, the reader is urged to check the package insert
for each drug for any change in indications and dosage and for added warnings and precautions. This is
particularly important when the recommended agent is a new or infrequently employed drug.

Some drugs and medical devices presented in the publication have Food and Drug Administration (FDA)
clearance for limited use in restricted research settings. It is the responsibility of the health care provider to
ascertain the FDA status of each drug or device planned for use in their clinical practice.

To purchase additional copies of this book, call our customer service department at (800) 638-3030 or fax
orders to (301) 223-2320. International customers should call (301) 223-2300.

Visit Lippincott Williams & Wilkins on the Internet: at LWW.com. Lippincott Williams & Wilkins customer
service representatives are available from 8:30 am to 6 pm, EST.

10 9 8 7 6 5 4 3 2 1

"I'm just a tugboat, putting the big ships out to sea."
This is how my father viewed his role as a college professor and administrator. His greatest pride came not from his own accomplishments, but from seeing his students excel both in the academic realm and (more importantly) out in the real world. I believe my Dad embodied the spirit of all great teachers, regardless of their discipline, as he challenged his pupils to think critically, creatively and ethically, and then to act judiciously on those decisions.

I'd like to dedicate this edition to my father, Dr. William Litzinger, and all the wonderful teachers who continue to inspire their students. I am privileged that our editorial team is not only made up of such leaders, but led by my wonderful mentor, dear friend, and Professor of Medicine, Dr. Frank Domino. His generous offer to allow his associate editors a chance to dedicate our book is vintage Dr. Domino, as he continues to lift up those around him. To Frank—a sincere thank you.

Many of our authors are professors at medical schools spanning across our country and beyond, and I challenge all of our authors to recognize their topic is an extension of medical education, bringing current, evidence-based diagnostic and treatment guidelines outside the classroom and into our "real world" practices. Each author has the opportunity to be that effective teacher who directly impacts patient care across the globe. Again, I dedicate this book to each of you.

Finally, perhaps my greatest teachers in life are my husband, Drew, and our beautiful daughters, Brittany and Nicole. I am delighted my husband joins our team of authors this year, sharing his extensive clinical experience and medical wisdom from an anesthesia perspective. Every day I learn something new from each member of our family. Your love, support, patience and encouragement allow me to continue to dedicate my time and energy to this wonderful mission.

–JILL A. GRIMES, MD

PREFACE

I don't know what your destiny will be, but one thing I know: the only ones among you who will be really happy are those who will have sought and found how to serve.

— Albert Schweitzer

All who participate in healthcare delivery, serve. If you are holding this book or looking at a screen, as a clinician, administrator or policy maker, you do so to help someone live a little better. This resource provides knowledge, but it is just one instrument in the toolbox of service. Adding skill, insight, and intuition makes you a master in your service.

I am honored to welcome you to the 2012 edition of the **5-Minute Clinical Consult.** Our editorial team has again collaborated with hundreds of authors to bring you this comprehensive and current resource whose mission is to assist in your service to your patients.

Using your feedback, we present this highly organized content and newly added features in print and online:

- Better and faster search functionality providing you with answers in **30 seconds or less**
- Current evidence-based designations highlighted in each topic's text
- A revised and updated Health Maintenance section
- More than 900 topics
- 200+ diagnostic and treatment algorithms linked to topics for quick diagnosis and treatment planning
- Video library for procedures and treatment
- Drug database from Facts & Comparisons including monographs, images, monthly updates and more
- More than 1,350 patient handouts in English and Spanish from The American Academy of Family Physicians linked directly from content
- Full-color images

- Updates that include new topics, videos, images, etc.
- Mobile version for quick reference on your Smartphone
- And more

Evidence based health care is the integration of the best medical information with the values of the patient **and your** skill as a clinician. We have improved our content and visibility of the best evidence, so you can focus on how to apply it.

The Health Maintenance recommendations included here have been updated through December 2010, based on the U.S. Preventive Services Task Force, and has been organized by age into *1-page* summaries.

Please check out the online and mobile versions at www.5minuteconsult.com. Your access is included in your purchase, allowing you to quickly reference the 5-Minute wherever needed. Included are over **900 topics** on the web via an easy-to-use interface. This new feature includes easy maneuverability between topics, algorithms, images, video procedures, and more as well as extra topics not in the book (including a pediatric section).

The algorithms section in the front of the book has been again expanded and includes both **diagnostic *and treatment* algorithms.** Our goal here is to provide you with a graphic method to evaluate an abnormal finding and how to prioritize treatment. I urge you to look through this section and recognize its utility.

Welcome to the 2012 edition of Lippincott Williams & Wilkins' 5-Minute Clinical Consult. The editorial team and I greatly value your observations and thoughts, so please drop me an email and share your thoughts, suggestions, and constructive criticism at 5MinConsultFeedback@lww.com.

Frank J. Domino, MD
Professor
University of Massachusetts Medical School
Worcester, Massachusetts
January 9, 2011

WHAT IS EVIDENCE BASED MEDICINE AND WHY IS THIS NEW?

Remember when we used to treat every otitis media with antibiotics? These recommendations came about because we applied logical reasoning to observational studies. If bacteria cause an acute otitis media, then antibiotics should help it resolve sooner, with less morbidity. Yet, when rigorously studied (via a systematic review), we found little benefit to this intervention.

The underlying premise of evidence-based medicine (EBM) is the evaluation of medical interventions, and the literature that supports those interventions, in a systematic fashion. EBM hopes to encourage treatments proven to be effective and safe. And when insufficient data exists, it hopes to inform you, on how to safely proceed.

EBM uses as endpoints of real patient outcomes; morbidity, mortality and risk. It focuses less on intermediate outcomes (bone density), and more on patient conditions (hip fractures).

Implementing EBM *requires* 3 components: the best medical evidence, the skill and experience of the provider, and the values of the patients. Should this patient be screened for prostate cancer? It depends on what is known about the test, on what you know of its benefits and harms, your ability to communicate that information, and that patient's informed choice.

"All this in 15 minutes" you ask? This is not an easy task. My goal is to provide you with the tools to assist in this process.

This book hopes to address the first EBM component; providing you access the best information in a quick format. While not every test or treatment has this level of detail, many of the included interventions here use systematic review literature support.

The language of medical statistics is useful to interpreting the concepts of EBM. Below is a list of these terms, with examples to help take the confusion and mystery out of their use.

POPULATION INFORMATION

These terms are designed to help you and epidemiologists look at the "community" as a whole, and determine how frequently disease occurs:

Prevalence: *Proportion of people* in a population who have a disease
"In the US, "0.3% (3 in 1,000) people over the age 50 have colon cancer"
Incidence: How many *new cases of a disease* occur in a population during an interval of time; for example, "the estimated incidence of colon cancer in the US is 104,000 in 2005"

TESTING INFORMATION

We often hear the words *Sensitivity* and *Specificity* and cringe. They are, at a minimum, very confusing. These terms are characteristics of a test, but they tell us little about the lab result we are holding in our hands. Rather, it is the *Predicative Value* that helps us interpret test results.

ML is a 53-year-old woman who you saw for a Health Maintenance visit; you ordered a *screening* mammogram and the report demonstrates an irregular area of microcalcifications. She is waiting in your office to receive her test results; what can you tell her?

Sensitivity (Sn): percent of People with Disease who test positive; for mammography, the Sensitivity is 71–96%.
Specificity (Sp): percent of People without Disease who test negative; for mammography, the Specificity is 94–97%.

Does this help in your discussion with ML? No, because these tests refer to characteristics of people who are known to have disease (sensitivity) or those that are known not to have (specificity) disease. What you have is an abnormal test result. To better explain this result to ML, you need to know the Positive Predictive Value.

Positive Predictive Value (PPV): Percent of **Positive** Test Results that are truly positive; the PPV for a woman 50–59 ~22%. Only 22% of abnormal screening mammograms in this group truly identified cancer. The other 78% are false positives.
Negative Predictive Value (NPV): Percent of negative test results that are truly negative.

You can tell ML only 1 out of 5 abnormal mammograms correctly identify cancer; the 4 are false positives, but the only way to know which mammogram is correct is to do further testing.

You may both find some comfort knowing the chance she has cancer is so low.

The PPV and NPV tests are population dependent, while the Sensitivity and Specificity are characteristics of the test, and have little to do with the patient in front of you. So when you receive an abnormal lab result, especially a screening test like mammography or PSA value, understand their limits based upon their PPV and NPV.

TREATMENT INFORMATION

In discerning the statistics of randomized, controlled trials of interventions, first consider an example. The Scandinavian Simvastatin Survival Study (4S): (*Lancet.* 1994;344(8934):1383–1389) found using simvastatin in patients at high risk for heart disease for 5 years resulted in deaths in 8% of patients vs. 12% of those on placebo; this results in a Relative Risk of 0.70, a Relative Risk Reduction of 33%, and a Number Needed to Treat of 25.

There are two ways of considering the benefits of an intervention with respect to a given outcome. The Absolute Risk Reduction (ARR) is the difference in the percent of people with the condition before and after the intervention. Thus, if the incidence of MI was 12% for the placebo group and 8% for the simvastatin group, the ARR is 4% (12−8% = 4%).

The Relative Risk Reduction (RRR) reflects the improvement in the outcome as a percentage of the original rate and is commonly used to exaggerate the benefit of an intervention. Thus if the risk of MI were reduced by simvastatin from 12% to 8% then the RRR would be 33% (4%/12% = 33%). 33% may appear better than 4%, the 4% that reflects the true outcome.

ARR is usually a better measure of *clinical* significance of an intervention. For instance, in one study, the treatment of mild hypertension was been shown to have a RRR of 40% over 5 years (40% fewer strokes in the treated group). However, the ARR was only 1.3%. Because mild hypertension is not strongly associated with strokes, aggressive treatment of mild hypertension yields only a small clinical benefit. Don't confuse Relative Risk Reduction with Relative Risk.

Absolute (or Attributable) Risk (AR): The percent of people in the placebo or intervention group who reach an end point; in the simvastatin study, the absolute risk of death was 8%

Relative Risk (RR): The risk of disease of those treated or exposed to some intervention (i.e., simvastatin) divided by those in the placebo group or who were untreated.

—If RR <1.0, it reduces risk—the smaller the number, the greater the risk reduction.

—If RR >1.0, it increases the risk—the greater the number, the greater the risk increase.

Relative Risk Reduction (RRR): The relative decrease in risk of an end point compared to the percent of that endpoint in the placebo group.

If you are still confused, just remember the RRR is an over estimation of the actual effect.

Number Needed to Treat (NNT): This is the number of people who need to be treated by an intervention to prevent one adverse outcome. A "good" NNT can be a large number (>100) if risk of serious outcome is great. If the risk of an outcome is not that dangerous, then lower (<25) NNTs are preferred.

The NNT should be compared to a similar statistic, the Number Needed to Harm (NNH). This is the number of people who have to be given treatment before one excess side effect or harm occurs. When the NNT is compared to the NNH, you and the patient can judge whether the benefit of the intervention is great enough to outweigh the risk of harm.

REFERENCES

To help you interpret diagnostic and treatment recommendations within the *5-Minute Clinical Consult*, we have graded the best information within the text, and highlighted this content.

An "A" grade means the reference is from the highest-quality resource, like a systematic review. A *systematic review* is a summary of the medical literature on a given topic that uses strict, explicit methods to perform a thorough search of the literature and then provides a critical appraisal of individual studies, concluding in a recommendation. The most prestigious collection of systematic reviews is from the Cochrane Collaboration (www.cochrane.org).

A "B" grade means the data referenced comes from high-quality randomized controlled trials performed to minimize bias in their outcome. Bias is anything that interferes with the truth; in the medical literature, it is often unintentional, but is much more common than we appreciate. In short, always assume some degree of bias exists in any research endeavor.

A "C" grade implies the reference used does not meet the A or B requirements; they are often treatments recommended by consensus groups (like the American Cancer Society). In some cases, they may be the standards of care. But implicit in a group's recommendation is the bias of the author or the group that supports the reference. For example, the American Urological Society's recommendation around screening for prostate cancer may be motivated by their need for funding rather than patient outcomes. Compare this to the highly valid recommendations of the U.S. Preventive Services Task Force (www.ahrq.gov), the organization that determines which health maintenance interventions are reasonable, and does so with the least bias.

BIAS

Bias is anything interferes with the truth. There are many types of bias that should be considered by the publishers of medical information. Below describes a number of bias types which often affects our care without us knowing it is present.

Publication bias occurs when research is not published; this is often when a study finds data that does *not* support an intervention. The motivation to publish information that "didn't work" is low. It is estimated that up to 40% of all medical research never gets published. So when you read of an intervention that "works," wonder if other studies were done that didn't show benefit and went unpublished.

Comparator bias occurs when research compares an intervention to placebo, when placebo isn't the standard of care. Knowing a new antibiotic is more effective than placebo for treating acute otitis media is not helpful if you typically use amoxicillin.

Why not release research comparing the new drug to the standard of care? Often, the research has been done, and the new drug proved no better. If this study does not get published, you have an example of Publication Bias.

Selection bias involves either using a tool that doesn't discriminate between populations selected or just reporting a just subset of study participants from a study. Either will result in the data being skewed because it can only be applied to small subset of people.

Attrition bias and the concept of intention to treat. Attrition bias is when researchers do not fully acknowledge and address how a study deals with participants who do not adhere to the research protocol or drop out completely. Intention to Treat Analysis hopes to diminish Attrition Bias by statistically considering the non-adhering or dropped out patients as unsuccessfully benefiting from the intervention.

Commercial (funder) bias involves who paid for the research being done, and do they have a vested interest in the outcome. Despite its size and scope, the recent *Jupiter* trial on treating low risk adults with a statin has been called into question as the company who funded the study makes the brand name drug used in the study and the lead author is part owner of the unique test employed in the trial. The data may be accurate, but until this is studied by less vested interests, some feel its outcome cannot be clinically applied.

I hope this brief introduction to EBM has been informative, clear, and helpful. If any of the information above seems unclear, or if you have a question, please drop me an email at 5MinConsultFeedback@lww.com

ACKNOWLEDGMENTS

This 20th edition of the *5-Minute Clinical Consult*, powered by its content, and supported by its ever-updated and improved interfaces, continues to be the most clinically useful tool in your health care box. From the diagnostic and treatment algorithms, through the knowledge components of each topic, and including the appendices like the Health Maintenance section, one cannot find a better collect of clinically useful content.

A book and Web site of this magnitude requires an equally broad effort from its supporting team. I wish to thank the dedication and tireless efforts of the team: Point-of-Care Editor, Ave McCracken; Senior Managing Editor, Michelle LaPlante; Kim Schonberger, Marketing Manager; Lisa McAllister, Director, Electronic Product Strategy; and Jennifer Gibson, Content Technology. They have given of themselves far beyond their call of duty, and I am deeply indebted to their effort. For the vision of making the 5-Minute the leading resource in health care around the world, my sincerest thanks to Diane Harnish, who brought us together. Lastly, my sincerest thanks for the gifts of Arlene and Marion.

This 2012 edition is the direct result of the dedication and insights of our Associate Editors. I wish to thank Drs. Robert Baldor, Jeremy Golding, Jill Grimes, and Julie Scott Taylor for their insights, hard work, and overwhelming commitment to the *5-Minute Clinical Consult*.

I wish to especially thank my wife, Sylvia, and my daughter, Molly, who have given greatly for this book.

The challenge of completing a book covering this broad a spectrum of medicine requires insights and skills far beyond my own.

Many thanks to my mentors Bob Baldor and Mark Quirk who are an enormous support—always there to encourage, reassure, and impart wisdom.

Many in the academic and health care worlds are due thanks for support, insight, and friendship: Daniel Lasser, Alan Chuman, Michele Pugnaire, Karen Rayla, Isabel Feliciano, Phil Fournier, Erik Garcia, Jeff Stovall, Jim Comes, Len Levin, Judy Norberg, J. Herb Stevenson, Mick Godkin, Zainab Nawab, Sanjiv Chopra, Susan Gauquier, Vasilios (Bill) Chrisostomidis, James (Jay) Broadhurst, Danuta Antkowiak, Atreyi Chakrabarti, Kerry Morse, Mark Powicki, Steve Messineo, and the faculty and students of the University of Massachusetts Medical School.

Medicine is a challenge I have fortunately not had to meet alone. Thanks to my parents, Frank and Angela (Jean); my brother John and his family, Marylou, Cate, and Jane; Frank, Mary Anne, Diane, and David Christian; the Diana and Hymie Lipschitz family; and the Bob and Ruth Pabreza family; they are responsible for who I am and my success in life.

I am blessed with the best of friends; without them, I would not be a physician. Thanks to Bob Bacic, Ron Jautz, Richard Onorato, John Horcher, Auguste Turnier, Bob Smith, Paul Saivetz, Antoinette and (Gary) Francis, Bob and Nancy Gallinaro, Drew and Jill Grimes, Louay Toma, Laurie, Alan, Daniel, Jenny and Matt Bugos, Alan Ehrlich, Teri and Andy Jennings, Mark Steenbergen, John and Kathleen Polanowicz, Phil Pettine, Mark Shelton, Steve Bennett, Vicki Triolo, Michael Bernatchez, and Milo.

—FRANK J. DOMINO, MD

CONTRIBUTING AUTHORS

Jose Abad, MD
University of California, Davis
Sacramento, California

Dawn Abbott, MD
Department of Internal Medicine
Rhode Island Hospital
Providence, Rhode Island

Cheryl Abel, PharmD
Assistant Professor of Pharmacy Practice
Massachusetts College of Pharmacy and
    Health Sciences
Manchester, New Hampshire

George Abraham, MD, MPH
Associate Professor
Department of Medicine
University of Massachusetts Medical
    School;
Associate Program Director
Department of Internal Medicine
Saint Vincent Hospital
Worcester, Massachusetts

Luis K. Abrishamian, MD
Department of Emergency Medicine
University of Southern California
    Medical Center
Los Angeles, California

Abdulrazak Abyad, MD, PhD, MBA, MPH, AGSF, AFCHSE
Director, Abyad Medical Center & Middle
    East Longevity Institute
Tripoli, Lebanon

Amos O. Adelowo, MD, MPH
Department of Obstetrics and
    Gynecology
University of Massachusetts Memorial
    Hospital
Worcester, Massachusetts

Ronald Adler, MD
Assistant Professor
Department of Family and Community
    Health
University of Massachusetts Medical
    School
Worcester, Massachusetts

Nitin Aggarwal, MD
Warren Alpert Medical School of Brown
    University
Providence, Rhode Island

Maria I. Aguilar, MD
Assistant Professor of Neurology
Department of Neurology
Mayo Clinic College of Medicine;
Consultant, Department of
    Neurology
Mayo Clinic Hospital
Phoenix, Arizona

Augusto Aguirre, MD
Department of Pathology
Corpath, Inc.
Columbus, Ohio

Francisco Aguirre, MD
Department of Pathology
Corpath, Inc.
Columbus, Ohio

Jaspal S. Ahluwalia, MD, MPH
Preventive Medicine
Walter Reed Army Institute of
    Research
Silver Spring, Maryland

Mazen J. AlBeldawi, MD
Department of Internal Medicine
Cleveland Clinic Foundation
Cleveland, Ohio

Antoin M. Alexander, MD
Associate Program Director
Staff Family Physician
Department of Family Medicine
David Grant Medical Center
Travis AFB, California

Fozia A. Ali, MD
Department of Family Medicine
University of Texas Health Science Center,
    San Antonio
University Hospital
San Antonio, Texas

Satya Allaparthi, MD
Fellow, Robotic Laparoscopic
    Urology
University of Massachusetts Medical
    School
Worcester, Massachusetts

Andrew Allegretti, MD
Department of Internal Medicine
Harvard Medical School
Massachusetts General Hospital
Boston, Massachusetts

Richard W. Allinson, MD
Associate Professor
Department of Ophthalmology
The Texas A&M University System,
    Health Sciences Center
College Station, Texas;
Senior Staff Physician
Department of Ophthalmology
Scott & White Clinic
Waco, Texas

Ginger Allister, MD
University of Massachusetts Medical
    School
Worcester, Massachusetts

Brian Alverson, MD
Assistant Professor
Department of Pediatrics
Warren Alpert School of Medicine
Brown University;
Head of Pediatric Hospitalist
    Section
Department of Pediatrics
Rhode Island Hospital
Providence, Rhode Island

James G. Anderson, MD
University of Massachusetts Medical
    School
Worcester, Massachusetts

Jeffrey Scott Anderson, MD
Department of Psychiatry
Vanderbilt University
Nashville, Tennessee

Nadeem Anwar, MD
Assistant Professor of Medicine
University of Massachusetts Medical
    School
Worcester, Massachusetts

Armin Arasheben, MD
Department of Family Medicine
State University of New York Upstate
    Medical Center;
Department of Medical Education
St. Joseph's Hospital
Syracuse, New York

Steffani Araya, MD
University of Massachusetts Medical
    School
Worcester, Massachusetts

Ivan A. Arenas, MD, PhD
Department of Internal Medicine
Framingham Union Hospital
MetroWest Medical Center
Framingham, Massachusetts

Paul Arguin, MD
Medical Epidemiologist
Centers for Disease Control and Prevention
Atlanta, Georgia

James J. Arnold, DO
Faculty
Department of Family Medicine
David Grant (USAF) Medical Center
Travis Air Force Base, California

Patricia K. Aronson, MD
Assistant Professor
Generalist Division
Department of Obstetrics and Gynecology
University of Massachusetts Memorial
   Medical Center
Worcester, Massachusetts

Elias Arous, MD
Associate Chief Medical Officer
Chief, Surgery
UMass Memorial Medical Center;
Professor of Surgery
University of Massachusetts Medical School
Worcester, Massachusetts

Melissa E. Arthur, LCSW, MA
Assistant Professor
Department of Family Medicine
SUNY Upstate Medical University;
Director, Behavioral Science
Family Medicine Residency
St. Joseph's Hospital
Syracuse, New York

Swati B. Avashia, MD
Clinical Assistant Professor
Department of Family Medicine
University of Texas Southwestern
Austin, Texas

Mouhanad Ayach, MD
University of Massachusetts
Fitchburg Family Medicine
Fitchburg, Massachusetts

Jennifer L. Ayres, PhD
Clinical Psychologist
University of Texas Southwestern Medical
   Center Austin
Austin, Texas

Stephen J. Bacak, DO, MPH

Elisabeth L. Backer, MD
Clinical Associate Professor
Department of Family Medicine
University of Nebraska Medical Center
Omaha, Nebraska

Yolanda Backus, MD
Family Practice
Rockville, Maryland

Elizabeth Bade, MD
Clinical Assistant Professor
Department of Family Medicine
University of Wisconsin School of Medicine
   and Public Health
Madison, Wisconsin;
Chief
Department of Family Medicine
Aurora Sinai Medical Center
Milwaukee, Wisconsin

Faisal Badri, MD
Consultant and Head of General
   Surgery Unit
Department of Surgery
Rashid Hospital and RH Trauma Center
Dubai, United Arab Emirates

Justin M. Bailey, MD
Assistant Professor
Department of Family Medicine
Uniformed Services University of Health
   Sciences
Bethesda, Maryland;
Faculty
Department of Medicine Residency
David Grant Medical Center
Travis Air Force Base, California

Sangeetha Balasubramanian, MD
Fellow
Department of Rheumatology
University of Massachusetts Medical
   School
Worcester, Massachusetts

Robert A. Baldor, MD
Professor
Family Medicine and Community
   Health
University of Massachusetts Medical
   School;
Vice-Chairman
Family Medicine and Community Health
University of Massachusetts Memorial
   Health Care
Worcester, Massachusetts

Jerry Balikian, MD
Professor
Departments of Medicine and Radiology
University of Massachusetts Medical
   School
Worcester, Massachusetts

Brent J. Barber, MD
Assistant Professor of Clinical Pediatrics
   (Cardiology)
Director, UMC Pediatric Cardiac Services
University of Arizona College of Medicine
Tucson, Arizona

David M. Barclay, III, MD, MPH, FAAFP
Associate Professor
Associate Chair
Undergraduate Education Department of
   Family and Community Medicine
Temple University School of Medicine
Philadelphia, Pennsylvania

Daniel J. Barker, MD
University of Massachusetts Medical
   School
Worcester, Massachusetts

Katharine Barnard, MD
Assistant Professor
Department of Family Medicine
University of Massachusetts Medical
   School;
Plumley Village Health Services
University of Massachusetts Memorial
   Medical Center
Worcester, Massachusetts

Timothy J. Barreiro, DO
Associate Professor of Medicine
Department of Internal Medicine
Ohio University College of Osteopathic
   Medicine;
Section Chief, Critical Care Medicine
Section of Pulmonary and Critical Care
Humility of Mary Health System,
   St. Elizabeth Hospital
Youngstown, Ohio

Michael C. Barros, PharmD, BCPS
Ambulatory Care Pharmacy Resident
Department of Pharmacy
Providence Veterans Affairs Medical
   Center
Providence, Rhode Island

Adam Barta, MD
Assistant Professor
Department of Family Medicine
University of Texas Southwestern,
   Austin
Austin, Texas

Kay A. Bauman, MD, MPH
Clinical Professor
Department of Family Medicine and
   Community Health
John A. Burns School of Medicine
University of Hawaii at Manoa
Honolulu, Hawaii

Francesca L. Beaudoin, MS, MD
Assistant Professor
Department of Emergency Medicine
Warren Alpert Medical School of Brown
    University;
Attending Physician
Department of Emergency Medicine
Rhode Island Hospital
Providence, Rhode Island

Armando Bedoya, MD
Warren Alpert Medical School at Brown
    University
Providence, Rhode Island

Petra Belady, MD
Department of Obstetrics and Gynecology
University of Massachusetts Medical
    School
Worcester, Massachusetts

Paul Belliveau, PharmD, RPh
Associate Professor of Pharmacy
    Practice
Massachusetts College of Pharmacy
    and Health Sciences
Worcester, Massachusetts;
Clinical Pharmacist
Pharmacy
Concord Hospital
Concord, New Hampshire

Daniel E. Belz, MD
Department of Family Medicine
University of Nebraska Medical Center
Omaha, Nebraska

Elise R. Bender, MD
University of Massachusetts Medical
    School
Worcester, Massachusetts

Sheldon Benjamin, MD
Director, Psychiatry Residency Training
Director, Neuropsychiatry
University of Massachusetts Medical
    School
Worcester Massachusetts

Andrew Bentley, MS
Clinical Herbalist
Private Practice
Lexington Complementary and Integrative
    Therapies
Lexington, Kentucky

Jamie Berkes, MD
Instructor, Hepatology
Department of Medicine
University of Illinois at Chicago Medical
    Center
Chicago, Illinois

Robert E. Berry, Jr., MD
Associate Professor Obstetrics and
    Gynecology
Obstetrics and Gynecology Residency
    Program Director
University of Massachusetts Medical School
UMass Memorial Medical Center
Worcester, Massachusetts

Bryan Beutel, MD
The Warren Alpert Medical School of
    Brown University
Providence, Rhode Island

Jacob L. Bidwell, MD
Assistant Professor of Family Medicine
University of Wisconsin Medical School
Milwaukee, Wisconsin

Dale E. Bieber, MD
Associate Professor
Department of Medicine
University of Iowa
Iowa City, Iowa

Garreth C Biegun, MD
House Staff Officer in Emergency Medicine
Warren Alpert Medical School
Brown University;
Resident Physician
Department of Emergency Medicine
Rhode Island Hospital, Lifespan Health
    System
Providence, Rhode Island

Kenneth M. Bielak, MD
Sports Medicine Fellowship
University Tennessee-Knoxville
Knoxville, Tennessee

Jhilam Biswas, MD
University of Massachusetts Medical
    School
Worcester, Massachusetts

Melissa Phillips Black, MD
Instructor of Clinical Medicine
Internal Medicine, Geriatrics Division
Emory University School of Medicine
Atlanta, Georgia

Robert M. Black, MD
Clinical Professor of Medicine
Department of Renal Medicine
UMass Medical School;
Chief, Division of Renal Medicine
St. Vincent Hospital & Fallon Clinic
Worcester, Massachusetts

Timothy L. Black, MD
Pediatric Surgeon
Department of Pediatric Surgery
Cook Children's Medical Center
Fort Worth, Texas

Joseph Blazuk, MD
University of Massachusetts Medical School
Worcester, Massachusetts

Kimberly Bombaci, MD
University of Massachusetts Medical School
Worcester, Massachusetts

Naomi F. Botkin, MD
Assistant Professor
Division of Cardiovascular Medicine
University of Massachusetts
    Medical School and Memorial Center
Worcester, Massachusetts

Jaclyn Boulais, MD
University of Massachusetts Medical School
Worcester, Massachusetts

Katherine Boyle, MD
University of Massachusetts School of
    Medicine
Worcester, Massachusetts

Doreen Brettler, MD
Department of Hematology/Oncology
University of Massachusetts Medical School
Worcester, Massachusetts

Ivan J. Briones, MD
University of Massachusetts School of
    Medicine
Worcester, Massachusetts

Juan-Pablo Brito-Campana, MD
Department of Endocrinology
Mayo Clinic
Rochester, Minnesota

Ekaterina Brodski-Quigley, MD
UMass Memorial Medical Center
Worcester, Massachusetts

Theodore R. Brown, DO, MPH
Preventive Medicine Officer
Headquarters, U.S. Central Command
Departments of Family, Preventive, and
    Occupational and Environmental
    Medicine
MacDill Air Force Base, Florida

Patricia Bruno, DO
Assistant Professor
Director of Inpatient Services;
Department of Family Medicine
University of Connecticut School
    of Medicine
Saint Francis Hospital and Medical Center
Hartford, Connecticut

Karen Bryant, MD
Hospitalist Program
Concord Hospital
Concord, New Hampshire

Kathleen Bryant, MS, APRN, BC
Family Nurse Practitioner
Montpelier Health Center
Central Vermont Medical Center
Montpelier, Vermont

Rebecca Burch, MD
UMass Memorial Medical Group
Worcester, Massachusetts

K. John Burhan, MD
Instructor
Department of Family Medicine
Creighton University School of Medicine
Omaha, Nebraska

John R. Burk, MD
Adjunct Professor
Integrative Physiology
University of North Texas Health
    Science Center;
Owner/Partner
Texas Pulmonary & Critical Care
    Consultants, PA
Fort Worth, Texas

Kristin Burke, MD
University of Massachusetts Medical School
Worcester, Massachusetts

Leah A. Burnett, MD
Department of General Surgery
University of Pittsburgh Medical Center /
    Mercy Hospital
Pittsburgh, Pennsylvania

Harold J. Bursztajn, MD
Associate Clinical Professor
Department of Psychiatry
Harvard Medical School;
Associate Clinical Professor
Department of Psychiatry
Beth Israel Deaconess Medical Center
Boston, Massachusetts

David E. Burtner, MD
Vice Chairman and Professor
Department of Family and Community
    Medicine
Mercer University School of Medicine
Macon, Georgia

Nancy Byatt, DO, MBA
Associate Professor
Department of Psychiatry
University of Massachusetts Medical School;
Attending Psychiatrist
Psychosomatic Medicine and Emergency
    Mental Health
Department of Psychiatry
University of Massachusetts Medical Center
Worcester, Massachusetts

Adriana Cabrera, PharmD
Assistant Professor of Pharmacy Practice
Massachusetts College of Pharmacy and
    Health Science;
Consulting Pharmacist
Department of Family Medicine
Family Health Center of Worcester
Worcester, Massachusetts

David Cachia, MD
Department of Neurology
University of Massachusetts Medical
    School
Worcester, Massachusetts

Marie Ellen Caggiano, MD, MPH
Assistant Professor
Department of Family Medicine and
    Community Health
University of Massachusetts Medical
    School;
Physician
Hahnemann Family Health Center
Worcester, Massachusetts

Mitchell A. Cahan, MD
Assistant Professor
Department of Surgery
University of Massachusetts Medical
    School;
Director of Acute Care Surgery
Department of Surgery
UMass Memorial Medical Center
Worcester, Massachusetts

Kristy M. Cahill, MD
University of Massachusetts Medical
    School
Worcester, Massachusetts

Katherine M. Callaghan, MD
Department of Obstetrics and Gynecology
University of Massachusetts Medical
    School
Worcester, Massachusetts

Jennifer A. Caragol, MD
Assistant Professor
Department of Family and Community
    Medicine
University of Kentucky
Lexington, Kentucky

Paloma F. Cariello, MD
Department of Infectious Diseases
University of Massachusetts Medical
    School
Worcester, Massachusetts

Stephanie Carinci, MD
Central Florida Neurologic Consultants
Deland, Florida

David Carne, MD
Department of General Surgery
Northeast Ohio University College of
    Medicine
Rootstown, Ohio;
Department of General Surgery
Akron General Medical Center
Akron, Ohio

Stephanie Carreiro, MD
Department of Emergency Medicine
Brown University;
Rhode Island Hospital
Providence, Rhode Island

Laurie A. Carrier, MD
Clinical Instructor
Department of Family and Community
    Medicine
Northwestern University Feinberg School
    of Medicine
Family Physician and Psychiatrist
Heartland International Health Center
Chicago, Illinois

Mary Cataletto, MD
Associate Professor of Clinical Pediatrics
Department of Pediatrics
SUNY Stony Brook
Stony Brook, New York;
Associate Director
Pediatric Pulmonology
Winthrop University Hospital
Mineola, New York

Jan Cerny, MD, PhD
Assistant Professor of Medicine
Department of Medicine
Division of Hematology and Oncology
University of Massachusetts Medical
    School;
UMass Memorial Medical Center
Worcester, Massachusetts

Olga M. Céron, MD
Retina/Vitreous Specialist
Staff Physician
Massachusetts Eye Research and Surgery
    Institution (MERSI)
Cambridge, Massachusetts

Teresa V. Chan, MD
Assistant Professor
Department of Otolaryngology—Head and
    Neck Surgery
University of Texas—Southwestern
    Medical Center
Dallas, Texas

Allen Chang, MD
University of Massachusetts Medical
    School
Worcester, Massachusetts

Felix B. Chang, MD
Assistant Professor
Department of Family Medicine and
    Community Health
University of Massachusetts School of
    Medicine;
Inpatient Service Director
UMass Fitchburg Family Medicine
    Residency Program
UMass Memorial Health Alliance Hospital
Leominster, Massachusetts

Phillip Chang, MBBS
Visiting Medical Officer
Department of Otolaryngology
St. Vincent's Hospital
Sydney, Australia

Denisse Tafur Chang, MD
Universidad de Especialidades Espiritu
    Santo
Guayaquil, Ecuador

Jason Chao, MD, MS
Professor
Department of Family Medicine
Case Western Reserve University;
Department of Family
    Medicine
University Hospitals Case Medical
    Center
Cleveland, Ohio

**Arabinda Chatterjee, MD, FRCS, MS,
D. Urology**
Assistant Professor
Department of Family and Community
    Medicine
University of Massachusetts
    Medical Center
Worcester, Massachusetts;
Family Physician
Department of Family Medicine
Day Kimball Hospital
Putnam, Connecticut
William Backus Hospital
Norwich, Connecticut

Arka Chatterjee, MD
Department of Internal Medicine
University of Louisville School of
    Medicine
Louisville, Kentucky

Shaila V. Chauhan, MD
Assistant Professor of Obstetrics and
    Gynecology
Division of Reproductive Endocrinology
University of Massachusetts Medical
    School
Worcester, Massachusetts

Michael K. Chen, MD
Department of Family Medicine
University Hospitals Case Medical Center
Cleveland, Ohio

Stephanie Yu-hsuan Chen, MD
University of Massachusetts Medical
    School
Worcester, Massachusetts

Josue Chery, MD
University of Massachusetts School of
    Medicine
Worcester, Massachusetts

Vasilios Chrisostomidis, DO
Assistant Professor
Department of Family Medicine
University of Massachusetts Medical
    School
Worcester, Massachusetts

Atul R. Chugh, MD
Chief Fellow
Division of Cardiovascular Medicine
University of Louisville
Louisville, Kentucky

S. Lindsey Clarke, MD
Associate Professor
Department of Family Medicine
Medical University of South Carolina
Area Health Education Consortium
Charleston, South Carolina;
Director of Predoctoral Education
Montgomery Center for Family Medicine
Self Regional Healthcare
Greenwood, South Carolina

Deborah S. Clements, MD
Associate Program Director
Associate Professor
Department of Family Medicine
University of Kansas Medical Center
Kansas City, Kansas

Lisa Clemons, MD
Assistant Professor
Department of Family Medicine
University of Texas Southwestern—Austin;
Brackenridge Hospital
Austin, Texas

Kara M. Coassolo, MD
Attending Physician, Maternal Fetal
    Medicine
Department of Obstetrics and Gynecology
Lehigh Valley Health Network
Allentown, Pennsylvania

Cameron J. Codd, DO
Department of Obstetrics and Gynecology
Akron General Medical Center
Akron, Ohio

Naida Cole, MD
Alpert Medical School of Brown University
Providence, Rhode Island

Irene C. Coletsos, MD
University of Massachusetts Medical School
Worcester, Massachusetts

Dana M. Collaguazo, MD
Assistant Professor
Department of Emergency Medicine
The University of Iowa
Iowa City, Iowa

Jason Conforti, MD
University of Massachusetts Medical School
Worcester, Massachusetts

Nathan T. Connell, MD
House Staff Officer in Medicine
Department of Medicine
Brown University;
Rhode Island and The Miriam Hospitals
Providence, Rhode Island

Caitlin M. Connolly, MD
University of Massachusetts Medical
    School
Worcester, Massachusetts

Brynna Connor, MD
Department of Family Practice
University of Texas Southwestern-Austin
Austin, Texas

Kyle V. Contini, MD
Department of Family Medicine
Creighton University School of Medicine
Omaha, Nebraska

Maryann Cooper, PharmD
Assistant Professor of Pharmacy Practice
Hematology/Oncology
Massachusetts College of Pharmacy and
    Health Sciences
Manchester, New Hampshire
Worcester, Massachusetts

Michael Cooper, MD
University of Massachusetts Medical
    School
Worcester, Massachusetts

Macario C. Corpuz, Jr., MD
Assistant Professor
Department of Family Medicine and
    Community Health
University of Massachusetts Medical
    School;
Medical Staff
Department of Family Medicine
University of Massachusetts Memorial
    Hospital
Worcester, Massachusetts

Alan J. Cropp, MD
Professor of Medicine
Department of Internal Medicine
Northeastern Ohio Universities College
 of Medicine and Pharmacy
Rootstown, Ohio;
Medical Staff
Department of Internal Medicine
St. Elizabeth Hospital Health Center
Youngstown, Ohio

Katie Crowder, MD

Sandra Cuellar, PharmD, BCOP
Clinical Assistant Professor
Department of Pharmacy Practice
University of Illinois at Chicago College
 of Pharmacy;
Clinical Oncology Pharmacist
Department of Pharmacy Practice
University of Illinois at Chicago Medical
 Center
Chicago, Illinois

Hongyi Cui, MD, PhD
Assistant Professor of Surgery
Department of General and Laparoscopic
 Surgery
University of Massachusetts Medical School;
Associate Director, Acute Care Surgery
Department of Surgery
University of Massachusetts Memorial
 Medical Center
Worcester, Massachusetts

Paul T. Cullen, MD
Clinical Associate Professor
Department of Family Medicine
University of Pittsburgh
Pittsburgh, Pennsylvania;
Residency Program Director
Department of Family Medicine
Washington Hospital
Washington, Pennsylvania

James F. Cunagin, MD
Senior Clinical Instructor and Director of
 Behavioral Science, Department of
 Family Medicine
Senior Clinical Instructor, Department of
 Psychiatry
University Hospitals Case Medical Center
Case Western Reserve University School
 of Medicine
Cleveland, Ohio

Carol Curtin, MSW, LICSW
Research Assistant Professor
Department of Family Medicine and
 Community Health
E.K. Shriver Center
University of Massachusetts Medical School
Waltham, Massachusetts

Jennifer S. Daly, MD
Professor
Department of Medicine
University of Massachusetts Medical
 School;
Clinical Chief
Division of Infectious Diseases and
 Immunology
University of Massachusetts Memorial
 Health Center
Worcester, Massachusetts

Gaurav Dang, MD
Department of Family Practice
Summa Barberton Hospital
Barberton, Ohio

Akhil Das, MD
Assistant Professor of Urology
Department of Urology
Thomas Jefferson University;
Attending Physician
Department of Urology
Thomas Jefferson University Hospital
Philadelphia, Pennsylvania

Janice E. Daugherty, MD
Associate Professor
Department of Family Medicine
The Brody School of Medicine at East
 Carolina University;
Patient Care Privileges
PIH County Memorial Hospital
Greenville, North Carolina

Raul Davaro, MD
Associate Professor
Department of Medicine
University of Massachusetts
Worcester, Massachusetts

Autumn Davidson, MD
University of Massachusetts Medical
 School
Worcester, Massachusetts

Jessica Davidson, MD
University of Massachusetts Medical
 School
Worcester, Massachusetts

Marin Dawson-Caswell, DO
Assistant Professor
Department of Family Medicine
Louisiana State University Health Sciences
 Center
New Orleans, Louisiana

Lauren Michal de Leon, MD
Warren Alpert Medical School at Brown
 University
Providence, Rhode Island

Robert De Marco, MD
Professor and Immediate Past Chairman
Department of Internal Medicine
Northeastern Ohio Universities College of
 Medicine;
St. Elizabeth Health Center
Rootstown, Ohio

Peerawut Deeprasertkul, MD
Department of Internal Medicine
Metrowest Medical Center
Framingham, Massachusetts

Meaghan Delaney, MD
University of Massachusetts Medical
 School
Worcester, Massachusetts

Sophia L. Delano, MD
University of Massachusetts Medical
 School
Worcester, Massachusetts

Konstantinos E. Deligiannidis, MD, MPH
Assistant Clinical Professor
Department of Family Medicine and
 Community Health
University of Massachusetts Medical
 School;
UMass Memorial Health Care
Worcester, Massachusetts

Deborah DeMarco, MD
Associate Dean, GME
Professor of Medicine
Division of Rheumatology
University of Massachusetts Medical
 School
Worcester, Massachusetts

Penelope Dennehy, MD
Director, Division of Pediatric Infectious
 Diseases
Professor of Pediatrics
Hasbro Children's Hospital
The Pediatric Division of Rhode Island
 Hospital
Providence, Rhode Island

Amar Deshpande, MD
University of Miami Miller School of
 Medicine
Miami, Florida

Alicia R. Desilets, PharmD
Assistant Professor of Pharmacy
 Practice
Department of Pharmacy Practice
Massachusetts College of Pharmacy and
 Health Sciences
Manchester, New Hampshire

Richard F. DeSouza, MD
Department of Medicine
Brown University - Rhode Island Hospital
Providence, Rhode Island

Adam W. DeTora, MD
Department of Pediatrics
University of Massachusetts Medical School
Worcester, Massachusetts

Mathew J. Devine, DO
Senior Instructor
Department of Family Medicine
University of Rochester;
Associate Medical Director
Department of Family Medicine
Highland Family Medicine
Rochester, New York

Suneel Dhand, MD
Attending Physician
Department of Medicine
Fallon Clinic/Saint Vincent Hospital
Worcester, Massachusetts

David Dildine, MD
University Massachusetts Medical School
Worcester, Massachusetts

Rino H. Dizon, MD
Department of Family Medicine
David Grant Medical Center
Travis Air Force Base, California

Frank J. Domino, MD
Professor
Clerkship Director
Department of Family Medicine and
    Community Health
University of Massachusetts Medical School
Worcester, Massachusetts

David J. Donahue, MD
Medical Director
Department of Pediatric Neurosurgery
Cook Children's Medical Center;
Surgical Director
Pediatric Epilepsy Program
Cook Children's Medical Center
Fort Worth, Texas

Ryan Dono, MD
University of Massachusetts School of
    Medicine
Worcester, Massachusetts

Susan E. Donohue, MD
Assistant Professor
Department of Medicine
University of Massachusetts Medical School
Commonwealth Hematology and
    Oncology, PC
Worcester, Massachusetts

Anna Doubeni, MD
Assistant Professor
Family Medicine and Community Health
University of Massachusetts Medical
    School
Worcester, Massachusetts

Cary D. Douglass, MD
President
West Lake Family Practice, P.A.
West Lake Hills, Texas

Abigail Drucker, MD
Department of Obstetrics and Gynecology
Creighton University Medical Center
Omaha, Nebraska

Kaelen C. Dunican, PharmD, RPh
Assistant Professor
Department of Pharmacy Practice
Massachusetts College of Pharmacy and
    Health Sciences
Worcester, Massachusetts

Nedim Durakovic, MD
Alpert Medical School of Brown University
Providence, Rhode Island

Cheryl Durand, PharmD, RPh
Assistant Professor of Pharmacy
    Practice
Massachusetts College of Pharmacy and
    Health Sciences
Manchester, New Hampshire

William J. Durbin, MD
Professor, Residency Director
Department of Pediatric Infectious Disease
University of Massachusetts Medical
    School;
Chair, Department of Pediatric Infectious
    Disease
UMass Memorial Healthcare
Worcester, Massachusetts

Matthew J. Dykhuizen, MD
University of Massachusetts Medical
    School
Worcester, Massachusetts

Gerry Edwards, MD
Assistant Professor
Department of Family Medicine
State University of New York—Upstate
    Medical University;
Faculty Family Medicine Residency
St. Joseph's Hospital Health Center
Syracuse, New York

Shannon Ehleringer, DO
Department of Family Medicine
David Grant Medical Center
Travis Air Force Base, California

Alan M. Ehrlich, MD
Assistant Clinical Professor
Department of Family Practice
University of Massachusetts Medical
    School
Worcester, Massachusetts

William G. Elder, Jr., PhD
Associate Professor
Department of Family and Community
    Medicine
University of Kentucky College of
    Medicine;
University of Kentucky Chandler
    Medical Center
Lexington, Kentucky

Amy Ellingson-Itzin, MD
Department of Obstetrics and Gynecology
University of Massachusetts Medical
    School;
UMass Memorial Medical Center
Worcester, Massachusetts

Pamela I. Ellsworth, MD
Associate Professor of Urology/Surgery
Department of Surgery
The Warren Alpert School of Medicine at
    Brown University;
Pediatric Urologist
Department of Surgery
Hasbro Children's Hospital
Providence, Rhode Island

Kevin Engelhardt, MD
Department of Pediatrics
University of Arizona College of Medicine
Tucson, Arizona

Michael Engels, MD
University of Massachusetts School of
    Medicine
Worcester, Massachusetts

Joseph K. Erbe, MD
Staff Physician
Department of Family Medicine
David Grant Medical Center
Travis Air Force Base
Fairfield, California

Rasai L. Ernst, MD
Department of Family Medicine
University Hospitals Case Medical Center
Cleveland, Ohio

Martin A. Espinosa Ginic, MD
House Staff
Department of Graduate Medical
    Education
University of Louisville
University of Louisville Hospital
Louisville, Kentucky

Janelle M. Evans, MD
Department of Obstetrics and Gynecology
University of Massachusetts Medical
    School
Worcester, Massachusetts

Kristyn Fagerberg, MD
West Lake Family Practice
Austin, Texas

Ashley Falk, MD
Family Practice
Offutt Air Force Base, Nebraska

Nathan P. Falk, MD
Physician
Department of Family Medicine
University of Nebraska Medical Center
Omaha, Nebraska

Pang-Yen Fan, MD
Associate Professor of Medicine
Division of Renal Medicine
University of Massachusetts Medical
    School
Worcester, Massachusetts

Rhonda A. Faulkner, PhD
Director, Behavioral Medicine
Department of Family Medicine
University of Illinois College of Medicine at
    Saint Joseph Hospital
Chicago, Illinois

Neil J. Feldman, DPM
Central Massachusetts Podiatry, PC
Worcester, Massachusetts

Edward Feller, MD
Clinical Professor of Medicine
Adjust Professor of Community Health
Department of Gastroenterology, Public
    Health
Warren Alpert Medical School of Brown
    University
Providence, Rhode Island

Warren J. Ferguson, MD
Associate Professor
Department of Family Medicine and
    Community Health
University of Massachusetts Medical
    School;
Vice Chair
Department of Family Medicine and
    Community Health
UMass Memorial Medical Center
Worcester, Massachusetts

Lauren Ferrara, MD
New York Medical College
Valhalla, New York

Shawn M. Ferullo, MD
Assistant Professor
Department of Family Medicine
Boston University;
Assistant Director, Sports Medicine
Department of Family Medicine
Boston Medical Center
Boston, Massachusetts

Jo Ellen Feugate, MD, PhD
Department of Medicine
Arizona Arthritis Center
University of Arizona
Tucson, Arizona

Scott A. Fields, MD
Professor and Vice Chair
Department of Family Medicine
Oregon Health and Science
    University
Portland, Oregon

Stanley Fineman, MD
Associate Clinical Professor
Department of Pediatrics
Emory University School of Medicine
Atlanta, Georgia

Jonathon M. Firnhaber, MD
Clinical Assistant Professor
Department of Family Medicine
East Carolina University
Greenville, North Carolina

David Fish, MD
University of Massachusetts Medical
    School
Worcester, Massachusetts

Timothy P. Fitzgibbons, MD
Fellow
Department of Cardiology
University of Massachusetts Medical
    School
Worcester, Massachusetts

Jonathan M. Flacker, MD
Assistant Professor
Department of Medicine
Emory University;
Medical Director, Emory Clinic at Wesley
    Woods
Geriatrics
Wesley Woods Health Center
Atlanta, Georgia

Michael P. Flaherty, MD, PhD
Assistant Professor
Division of Cardiovascular Medicine
University of Louisville
Louisville, Kentucky

Sarah B. Fleisig, MD
Warren Alpert Medical School
Brown University
Providence, Rhode Island

Joseph A. Florence, MD
Professor/Director, Division of
    Programs
Department of Family Medicine
East Tennessee State University
    Quillen College
Johnson City, Tennessee

Terence R. Flotte, MD
Dean of the Medical School
Department of Pediatrics
University of Massachusetts Medical
    School;
Professor
Department of Pediatrics
University of Massachusetts Memorial
    Health Center
Worcester, Massachusetts

Mary K. Flynn, MD
Department of Family Medicine and
    Community Health
University of Massachusetts
    Medical School
Worcester, Massachusetts

Jay Gar-Yee Fong, MD
Assistant Professor
Department of Pediatric Gastroenterology
University of Massachusetts School of
    Medicine and Medical Center
Worcester, Massachusetts

Tiffany M. Forti, MD, MPH
Department of Obstetrics and
    Gynecology
University of Massachusetts Medical
    School;
UMass Memorial Healthcare
Worcester, Massachusetts

Grant C. Fowler, MD
Professor and Vice Chair
Department of Family and Community
    Medicine
University of Texas Medical School at
    Houston;
Assistant Chief
Department of Family Medicine
Memorial Hermann Hospital
Houston, Texas

Robert L. Frachtman, MD
Austin Gastroenterology, PA
Austin, Texas

Jennifer E. Frank, MD
Assistant Professor
Department of Family Medicine
University of Wisconsin
Madison, Wisconsin

Samuel Frank, MD
Assistant Professor of Neurology
Boston University School of Medicine
Boston, Massachusetts

Nancy J. Freeman, MD
Clinical Associate Professor of Medicine
Warren Alpert School of Medicine at
    Brown University;
Chief, Hematology/Oncology
Providence VA Medical Center
Providence, Rhode Island

Rebecca A. Frye, DO
Faculty
Department of Family Medicine
David Grant Medical Center
Travis Air Force Base, California

Matthew J. Furman, MD
Department of Surgery
University of Massachusetts Medical
    Center
Worcester, Massachusetts

Richard Gacek, MD
Director, Otology/Neurotology
UMass Memorial Medical Center;
Professor of Otolaryngology, University
    of Massachusetts Medical School
Worcester, Massachusetts

Heidi L. Gaddey, MD
Department of Family Medicine
David Grant Medical Center
Travis Air Force Base, California

J. Scott Gaertner, MD
West Lake Family Practice
Austin, Texas

Tyeese Gaines Reid, DO, MA
Emergency Medicine Resident
Yale-New Haven Hospital
New Haven, Connecticut

Stephanie Galica, MD
University of Massachusetts Medical
    School
Worcester, Massachusetts

Eric P. Gall, MD
Professor of Clinical Medicine
    (Rheumatology)
Interim Director of the Arthritis Center
    of Excellence
University of Arizona

Sumanth Gandra, MD, MPH
Infectious Disease Fellow
University of Massachusetts Medical
    School
Worcester, Massachusetts

Jennifer Gao, MD
Department of Internal Medicine
Alpert Medical School, Brown University
Providence, Rhode Island

Andrew Gara, MD
University of Massachusetts Medical School
Worcester, Massachusetts

Erik J. Garcia, MD
Assistant Professor
Department of Family and Community
    Medicine
UMass Memorial Medical Center
Worcester, Massachusetts

Juan Antonio Garcia, MD
Assistant Professor
Department of Family Medicine
University of Calgary
University of Calgary Medical Centre
    Sunridge
Calgary, Alberta
Canada

Luis T. Garcia, MD
Clinical Instructor
Department of Family Medicine
University of Illinois—Chicago campus;
Chairman and Program Director
Department of Family Medicine
Saint Joseph Hospital
Chicago, Illinois

Amit Garg, MD
Director, Residency Program
Department of Dermatology
Boston University School of Medicine;
Assistant Professor
Department of Dermatology
Boston Medical Center
Boston, Massachusetts

Christopher Garofalo, MD
Active Staff
Department of Family Practice
Sturdy Memorial Hospital
Attleboro, Massachusetts

William T. Garrison, PhD
Professor
Department of Pediatrics
University of Massachusetts Medical School;
Division Director
Developmental and Behavioral Pediatrics
UMass Memorial Healthcare
Worcester, Massachusetts

Gail Gazelle, MD
Assistant Clinical Professor of Medicine
Department of Medicine
Harvard Medical School;
Position Member
Division of General Medicine
Brigham and Women's Hospital
Boston, Massachusetts

Renata Gazzi, MD
Clinical Faculty
Department of Family Medicine
University of Illinois at Chicago;
Clinical Faculty/Attending Physician
Department of Family Medicine
Saint Joseph Hospital
Chicago, Illinois

Gerald Gehr, MD
Assistant Professor of Medicine
Dartmouth Medical School
Hanover, New Hampshire;
Hematology/Oncology Program
Dartmouth-Hitchcock Manchester
Norris Cotton Cancer Center Manchester
Manchester, New Hampshire

John J. Gentile, DMD
Department of Dental Medicine
University of Massachusetts Medical
    School
Worcester, Massachusetts

Thomas Germano, MD
Assistant Clinical Professor
Department of Emergency Medicine
Warren Alpert Medical School at Brown
    University;
Attending Physician
Rhode Island Hospital
Providence, Rhode Island

Jeff Ray Gibson, Jr., MD
Assistant Professor
Department of Anesthesiology
The Texas A&M University Health
    Sciences Center College of Medicine;
Senior Staff Anesthesiologist
Department of Anesthesiology
Scott & White Memorial Hospital
Temple, Texas

Timothy Gibson, MD
Assistant Professor
Department of Pediatrics
University of Massachusetts Medical
    School;
Chief
Hanshaw Hospitalist Service
Department of Pediatrics
UMass Memorial Children's Medical
    Center
Worcester, Massachusetts

Javed M. Gilani, MD
Clinical Professor
Department of Internal Medicine
Drexel University
Philadelphia, Pennsylvania;
Christiana Care Health System
Wilmington, Delaware

David B. Gilchrist, MD
Assistant Professor
Department of Family Medicine
University of Massachusetts Medical School
University of Massachusetts Memorial
    Hospital
Worcester, Massachusetts

Neil A. Gilchrist, PharmD
Adjunct Assistant Professor
Department of Pharmacy Practice
Massachusetts College of Pharmacy and
    Health Sciences;
Clinical Pharmacy Specialist
Department of Pharmacy
UMass Memorial Medical Center
Worcester, Massachusetts

Cheryl L. Gilmartin, PharmD
Clinical Assistant Professor
Department of Pharmacy Practice
College of Pharmacy
University of Illinois;
Clinical Pharmacist
Section of Nephrology
University of Illinois
Chicago, Illinois

John W. Gittinger, Jr., MD
Professor of Ophthalmology and Neurology
Department of Ophthalmology
Boston University School of Medicine;
Residency Program Director
Division of Ophthalmology
Boston Medical Center
Boston, Massachusetts

Alfred Chege Gitu, MD
Faculty Physician
Department of Family Medicine
Greenwood Family Medicine Residency
    Program;
Self Regional Healthcare
Greenwood, South Carolina

Richard H. Glew, MD
Professor Medicine, Molecular Genetics,
    and Microbiology
Department of Medicine
University of Massachusetts Medical School
Infectious Disease Consultant
Department of Medicine
University of Massachusetts Medical Center
Worcester, Massachusetts

Luke Godwin, MD
The Warren Alpert Medical School of
    Brown University
Providence, Rhode Island

Jeremy Golding, MD
Professor of Family Medicine and of
    Obstetrics and Gynecology
The University of Massachusetts Medical
    School
Quality Officer—Department of Family
    Medicine and Community Health
UMass Memorial Health Care—
    Hahnemann Family Health Center
Worcester, Massachusetts

Michael Golding, MD
Senior Attending
New Hanover Hospital
Medical Director, Psych Support Inc.
Raleigh, North Carolina

Walter K. Goljan, MD
Department of Internal Medicine
UMass Memorial Medical Center
Worcester, Massachusetts

Leonard G. Gomella, MD
The Bernard W. Godwin Professor of
    Prostate Cancer Chairman
Associate Director of Clinical Affairs
Department of Urology
Jefferson Medical College
Philadelphia, Pennsylvania

Christian D. Gonzalez, MD
Assistant Professor
Department of Anesthesiology
University of Massachusetts Medical
    School;
Director, Pain Medicine
Department of Anesthesiology
Worcester, Massachusetts

Herbert P. Goodheart, MD
Assistant Clinical Professor
Department of Dermatology
Mount Sinai College of Medicine
New York, New York

Jeffrey L. Goodie, PhD
Assistant Professor
Department of Family Medicine
Uniformed Services University of the
    Health Sciences
Bethesda, Maryland

Mark D. Goodman, MD
Associate Professor and Interim Chairman
Department of Family Medicine
Creighton University School of Medicine
Omaha, Nebraska

Ilya Gorbachinsky, MD
Wake Forest University Baptist Medical
    Center
Winston-Salem, North Carolina

Paul R. Gordon, MD, MPH
Associate Professor
Department of Family and Community
    Medicine
University of Arizona—College of
    Medicine
Tucson, Arizona

Yelena Gorfinkel, MD
Boston Medical Center
Boston, Massachusetts

Parag Goyal, MD
New York Presbyterian Hospital-Weill
    Cornell Medical Center
New York, New York

Heath A. Grames, PhD
Assistant Professor and Program Director
for the Family Therapy Program
Department of Child and Family Studies
The University of Southern Mississippi
Hattiesburg, Mississippi

Chris Graves, MD
House Staff, Orthopaedics
University of Iowa Carver College of
    Medicine
Iowa City, Iowa

Caron J. Gray, MD
Associate Professor
Department of Obstetrics and Gynecology
Creighton University School of Medicine;
Chief of the Medical Staff
Creighton University Medical Center
Omaha, Nebraska

Michael Gray, MD
University of Massachusetts Medical
    School
Worcester, Massachusetts

Darius Greenbacher, MD
Assistant Professor of Emergency
    Medicine
Tufts University School of Medicine
Boston, Massachusetts

Ellen Greenblatt, BSC, MDCM
Associate Professor
Department of Obstetrics and Gynecology
University of Toronto;
Medical Director
Centre for Fertility and Reproductive
    Health
Mount Sinai Hospital
Toronto, Ontario
Canada

Jennifer J. Greene Welch, MD
Assistant Professor
Department of Pediatrics
Alpert Medical School Brown University;
Attending Physician
Division of Pediatric Hematology/
    Oncology
Department of Pediatrics
Hasbro Children's Hospital
Providence, Rhode Island

Ronald A. Greenfield, MD
Professor of Medicine and Chief
Infectious Diseases Section
Department of Medicine
University of Oklahoma Health Sciences
    Center;
VA Medical Center
Oklahoma City, Oklahoma

Pamela Lynn Grimaldi, DO
Assistant Professor
Department of Family Medicine and
    Community Health
University of Massachusetts Medical
    School;
Staff, Physician
Department of Family Medicine
University of Massachusetts Memorial
    Hospital
Worcester, Massachusetts

Drew Grimes, MD
Capital Anesthesiology Associates
Austin, Texas

Jill A. Grimes, MD
Clinical Instructor
Department of Family Medicine
University of Massachusetts Medical
    School
Worcester, Massachusetts;
Private Practice
West Lake Family Practice
Austin, Texas

Daria I. Grisanzio, PharmD, RPh
Adjunct Instructor
Department of Pharmacy Practice
Massachusetts College of Pharmacy and
    Health Sciences;
Clinical Research Fellow
Clinical Pharmacology Study Group
Worcester, Massachusetts

Joseph Grisanzio, MD
Consultant
Department of Medicine
Morton Hospital and Medical Center
Taunton, Massachusetts

Shanin Gross, DO
Assistant Professor, Attending Physician
Department of Family and Community
    Medicine
Penn State College of Medicine
Hershey Medical Center
Hershey, Pennsylvania

Marc Grossman, MD

Neil Grossman, MD
Department of Pediatrics
University of Massachusetts Medical
    School
Worcester, Massachusetts

Christopher Gudas, MD
University of Massachusetts Medical
    School
Worcester, Massachusetts

John A. Guisto, MD
Clinical Professor
Department of Emergency Medicine
University of Arizona College of Medicine;
Medical Director
Department of Emergency Medicine
University Medical Center
Tucson, Arizona

Adarsh K. Gupta, DO, MS
Assistant Professor
Department of Family Medicine
University of Medicine and Dentistry New
    Jersey-School of Osteopathic Medicine;
Attending Physician
Department of Family Medicine
Kennedy Memorial Hospital
Stratford, New Jersey

Gregory D. Gutke, MD, MPH
Physician Epidemiologist
Clinical Informatics Branch
Air Force Medical Support Agency
Brooks City-Base, Texas;
Physician Provider
Department of Occupational Health
Brooke Army Medical Center
Fort Sam Houston, Texas

Michael S. Guy, MD
Department of Obstetrics and
    Gynecology
Akron General Medical Center
Akron, Ohio

Krista Hachey, MD
The Warren Alpert Medical School of
    Brown University
Providence, Rhode Island

Mazen Hadid, MD

Laura Hagopian, MD
University of Massachusetts Medical
    School
Worcester, Massachusetts

Jessica Hahn, MD
University of Massachusetts Medical
    School
Worcester, Massachusetts

Diane M. Haleem, PhD, RN
Chair and Associate Professor of Nursing
    and Public Administration
Marywood University
Scranton, Pennsylvania

Jessica E. Haley, MD
Department of Pediatrics
University of Arizona;
University Medical Center
Tucson, Arizona

Thomas J. Hansen, MD
Associate Dean for Medical Education
Assistant Professor
Department of Family Medicine
Creighton University
Omaha, Nebraska

Allison Hargreaves, MD
University of Massachusetts Medical
    School
Worcester, Massachusetts

Natasha Harrison, MD
Department of Family Medicine
University of Pennsylvania School of
    Medicine
Philadelphia, Pennsylvania

Linda H. Hatch, MD

Fern R. Hauck, MD, MS
Associate Professor
Departments of Family Medicine and
    Public Health Sciences
University of Virginia School of Medicine
Charlottesville, Virginia

Beverly N. Hay, MD
Assistant Professor of Pediatrics
Department of Pediatrics
University of Massachusetts Medical
    School;
Chief, Division of Genetics
Department of Pediatrics
University of Massachusetts Memorial
    Health Care
Worcester, Massachusetts

Rajneesh S. Hazarika, MD, MS
Assistant Professor
Department of Family Medicine and
    Community Health
University of Massachusetts Medical
    School
Worcester, Massachusetts;
Physician
Department of Family Medicine
Health Alliance Hospital
Leominster, Massachusetts

Daithi S. Heffernan, MD
Department of Surgery
Division of Trauma and Surgical Critical
    Care
Alpert Medical School of Brown
    University;
Rhode Island Hospital
Providence, Rhode Island

Russell C. Hendershot, DO, MS
Associate Professor of Family Medicine
Chair of Family Medicine
Edward Via Virginia College of Osteopathic
    Medicine
Blacksburg, Virginia

Scott T. Henderson, MD
Assistant Director
Student Health Center
University of Missouri
Columbia, Missouri

Kerry Hensley, MD
University of Massachusetts Medical
    School
Worcester, Massachusetts

Benjamin Hilliker, MD
University of Massachusetts Medical
    School
Worcester, Massachusetts

Nadine T. Himelfarb, MD
Department of Emergency Medicine
The Warren Alpert Medical School of
    Brown University;
Rhode Island Hospital
Providence, Rhode Island

W. Jeff Hinton, PhD
Associate Professor
Director of Clinical Training for the Family
    Therapy Program
Department of Child and Family Studies
The University of Southern Mississippi
Hattiesburg, Mississippi

Vu Ho, MD
Boston Medical Center
Boston, Massachusetts

N. Wilson Holland, MD
Assistant Professor
Department of Medicine
Emory University School of Medicine;
Fellowship Program Director
Division of Geriatric Medicine
Staff Physician, Geriatrics and Extended
    Care
VA Medical Center
Atlanta, Georgia

David M. Holmes, MD
Clinical Associate Professor
Department of Family Medicine
State University of New York at Buffalo
Buffalo, New York

Michael P. Hopkins, MD, MEd
Professor and Chair
Northeastern Ohio University College of
    Medicine
Department of Obstetrics and Gynecology
Rootstown, Ohio;
Director
Department of Obstetrics and Gynecology
Aultman Health Foundation
Canton, Ohio

Mark C. Horattas, MD
Professor of Surgery
Department of Surgery
Northeastern Ohio Universities College
    of Medicine
Rootstown, Ohio;
Chief of Endocrine Surgery
Department of Surgery
Akron General Medical Center
Akron, Ohio

Evan R. Horton, PharmD
Assistant Professor of Pharmacy Practice
Massachusetts College of Pharmacy and
    Health Sciences
Worcester, Massachusetts;
Clinical Specialist
Department of Pharmacy (Pediatrics)
Baystate Medical Center
Springfield, Massachusetts

Kim House, MD
Medical Director
Atlanta Eagle's Nest—A Community Living
    Center
Decatur, Georgia

Elizabeth E. Houser, MD
Staff Urologist
Department of Urology
Seton Family of Hospitals
St. David's Family of Hospitals
Westlake Hospital
Austin, Texas

Jay U. Howington, MD
Associate Clinical Professor
Department of Surgery and Radiology
Mercer University School of Medicine;
Medical Director, Stroke Program
Memorial Health University Medical Center
Savannah, Georgia

Dennis E. Hughes, DO
Staff Attending Physician
Department of Emergency Medicine
Skaggs Regional Medical Center
Branson, Missouri

Karen A. Hulbert, MD
Assistant Professor
Department of Family and Community
    Medicine
Medical College of Wisconsin
Milwaukee, Wisconsin

Kam Hunter, MD
Clinical Educator, Family Medicine
Banner Health
Phoenix, Arizona

Caitlin Hurley, MD
University of Massachusetts Medical
    School
Worcester, Massachusetts

John C. Huscher, MD
Assistant Professor
Department of Family Medicine
University of Nebraska Medical Center
Omaha, Nebraska;
Staff Physician
Hospitalist
Faith Regional Health Services
Norfolk, Nebraska

Lawrence M. Hwang, MD
Assistant Clinical Professor
Department of Family Medicine
University of California Los Angeles
Los Angeles, California;
University of California Los Angeles Santa
    Monica and Orthopedic Hospital
Santa Monica, California

Robert J. Hyde, MD
Clinical Faculty
Department of Emergency Medicine
Christiana Care Health System
Newark, Delaware

Luis Idrovo Freire, MD
Neurologist
Hospital Ntra Sra del Rosario
Neurosonology Lab—Neurology Dept
Madrid Spain

Sabrina A. Indyk, MD
Department of Family Medicine
Resurrection Medical Center
Chicago, Illinois

Pablo I. Hernandez Itriago, MD
Medical Director
South End Community Health Center
    (SECHC)
Boston, Massachusetts

Mark Iverson, MD

Christine K. Jacobs, MD
Associate Professor
Department of Family and Community
    Medicine
St. Louis University School of Medicine
St. Louis, Missouri

Deepa Jagadeesh, MD, MPH
Hematology/Oncology Fellow
Department of Medicine—
    Hematology/Oncology
University of Massachusetts Medical
    School
Worcester, Massachusetts

Catherine Janes, MD
Assistant Professor
Attending Physician
Department of Pediatrics, Division of
    Pediatric Emergency Medicine
University of Massachusetts School of
    Medicine
University of Massachusetts Memorial
    Medical Center
Worcester, Massachusetts

Courtney I. Jarvis, PharmD
Associate Professor
Department of Pharmacy Practice
Massachusetts College of Pharmacy and
    Health Sciences
Worcester, Massachusetts;
Clinical Pharmacy Pharmacist
Department of Family Medicine
UMass Memorial Medical Center
Barre, Massachusetts

Joselyn Jedick, DO
Department of Family Medicine
Banner Good Samaritan Hospital
Phoenix, Arizona

Nathaniel J. Jellinek, MD
Clinical Assistant Professor
Department of Dermatology
Warren Alpert Medical School at Brown
    University
Providence, Rhode Island;
Dermatology Professionals, Inc.
East Greenwich, Rhode Island

Eric L. Jenison, MD
Professor
Department of Obstetrics and
    Gynecology
Northeastern Ohio Universities College of
    Medicine and Pharmacy
Rootstown, Ohio;
Chairman and Program Director
Department of Obstetrics and
    Gynecology
Akron General Medical Center
Akron, Ohio

John Jenkins, MD

Myrlene Jeudy, MD
University of Massachusetts Medical
    School
Worcester, Massachusetts

Adeliza S. Jimenez, MD
Department of Family and Community
    Medicine
University of Texas Health Science
    Center at San Antonio
San Antonio, Texas

Stacy Jones, MD

Maurice F. Joyce, III, MD
Department of General Surgery
Lahey Clinic
Burlington, Massachusetts

Patrick W. Joyner, MD
Department of Orthopaedic
    Surgery
Duke University Medical Center
Durham, North Carolina

Marc Jeffrey Kahn, MD
Professor of Medicine
Department of Medicine
Tulane University School of
    Medicine
New Orleans, Louisiana

Monica Kaitz, MD
Warren Alpert Medical School of Brown
    University
Providence, Rhode Island

Bharati Kalasapudi, MD
Warren Alpert Medical School of Brown
    University
Providence, Rhode Island

Abir O. Kanaan, PharmD, RPh
Assistant Professor
Department of Pharmacy Practice
Massachusetts College of Pharmacy and
    Health Sciences—Worcester/
    Manchester;
Clinical Specialist, Worcester Medical
    Center
Coronary Intensive Care Unit
Co-Director, Pharmacy Medication Safety
    Fellowship—Saint Vincent Hospital
Pharmacy Department
Worcester, Massachusetts

Packrisamy Kannan, MD
Senior Lecturer in Surgery
Department of Surgery
Dubai Medical College for Girls;
Senior Specialist Surgeon
Department of Surgery
Rashid Hospital & RH Trauma Center
Dubai, United Arab Emirates

Mark Kaplan, MD
Clinical Associate Professor of
    Orthopedics and Physical
    Rehabilitation
University of Massachusetts Medical
    School
Worcester, Massachusetts

Paul E. Kaplan, MD
President
Capitol Clinical Neuroscience
Folsom, California

Margo L. Kaplan-Gill, MD
Associate Professor
Department of Family Medicine
UMass Memorial Medical Center;
Family Health Center of Worcester
Worcester, Massachusetts

Rahul Kapur, MD, CAQSM
Assistant Director, Primary Care Sports
    Medicine Fellowship
Assistant Professor, Family Medicine and
    Sports Medicine
Department of Family Medicine and
    Community Health &
University of Pennsylvania Sports Medicine
    Center
University of Pennsylvania Health System
Philadelphia, Pennsylvania

Ioannis Karakis, MD
Department of Neurology
Boston University Medical Center
Boston, Massachusetts

Kristy Kedian Brown, DO
Associate Professor
Family Medicine
University of Massachusetts Medical
   School;
Faculty
Family of Medicine
University of Massachusetts Memorial
   Hospital
Worcester, Massachusetts

Molly P. Keegan, MD
Department of Emergency
   Medicine
University of Southern California
   Medical Center
Los Angeles, California

Rick Kellerman, MD
Professor and Chair
Department of Family and Community
   Medicine
University of Kansas School of
   Medicine–Wichita
Wichita, Kansas

Brandi Kelly, PharmD
MedTrak Services
Overland Park, Kansas

John J. Kelly, MD
Associate Professor
Department of Surgery
University of Massachusetts Medical
   School;
Chief
Department of Surgery
University of Massachusetts Memorial
   Medical Center
Worcester, Massachusetts

Kristen Kelly, MD
Department of Obstetrics and
   Gynecology
University of Massachusetts Medical
   School
Worcester, Massachusetts

Bevin Kenney, MD
Instructor in Medicine
Department of Internal Medicine
Harvard Medical School;
Brigham & Women's Hospital
Boston, Massachusetts

Robert M. Kershner, MD, MS
Eye Physician and Surgeon, Refractive and
   Cataract Surgery
Professor III, Microbiology, Anatomy
   and Physiology
Palm Beach State College
Palm Beach Gardens, Florida;
Clinical Professor of Ophthalmology
University of Utah School of Medicine
John A. Moran Eye Center
Salt Lake City, Utah;
Adjunct Professor Health Administration
Kaplan University
Ft. Lauderdale, Florida;
Ik Ho Visiting Professor of Ophthalmology
Chinese University of Hong Kong
Founder and Director Emeritus of Cataract
   and Refractive Surgery and Anterior
   Segment Fellowship Program
Eye Laser Center
Tucson, Arizona

Martin Kerzer, MD
Clinical Assistant Professor
Department of Family Medicine
Brown Alpert Medical School
Providence, Rhode Island;
Associates in Primary Care Medicine
Warwick, Rhode Island

Kerri Keslow, MD
Department of Family Medicine
Santa Monica-UCLA Medical Center and
   Orthopaedic Hospital
Santa Monica, California

Farah Y. Khan, MD
Department of Family Medicine
University of Texas Southwestern Medical
   School
Austin, Texas

Omar A. Khan, MD, MHS
Clinical Assistant Professor
Departments of Family Medicine and
   Public Health
University of Pennsylvania
Drexel University
Philadelphia;
Clinical Assistant Professor
University of Vermont
Burlington, Vermont

Saira Khan, MD
UT Health Science Center at San Antonio
Department of Family and Community
   Medicine
San Antonio, Texas

Salwa Khan, MD, MHS
Pediatric Hospitalist
Department of Pediatrics
Children's Hospital of Philadelphia
Philadelphia, Pennsylvania

Birgit N. Khandalavala, MD
Assistant Professor, Family Medicine
Creighton University
Omaha, Nebraska

Shefali B. Khandwala, DO
Assistant Clinical Professor
Department of Family Medicine
University of California at Irvine Medical
   Center
Orange, California

Morteza Khodaee, MD, MPH
Assistant Professor
Department of Family Medicine
University of Colorado Denver School of
   Medicine
Denver, Colorado

George E. Kikano, MD
Chair and Dorothy Jones Weatherhead
   Professor
Department of Family Medicine
Case Western Reserve University
University Hospitals of Cleveland
Cleveland, Ohio

Sam Seung Yeol Kim, MBBS, Mmed
Associate Clinical Lecturer
Department of Medicine
University of Sydney;
Surgical Resident
Department of Surgery
Westmead Hospital
Westmead, Sydney, Australia

Walter M. Kim, MD, PhD
University of Massachusetts Medical
   School
Worcester, Massachusetts

Scott E. Kinkade, MD, MSPH
Assistant Professor
Department of Family and Community
   Medicine
University of Texas Southwestern
   Medical Center at Dallas Southwestern
   Medical School;
Dallas, Texas

Rebecca G. Kinney, MD
Department of Family Medicine
Family Medicine Residency
   of Idaho
Boise, Idaho

George P. Kinzfogl, III, MD
Clinical Instructor
Department of Cardiology
Harvard Medical School
Boston, Massachusetts;
Heart Center of MetroWest
Framingham, Massachusetts

Jeffery T. Kirchner, DO
Clinical Associate Professor
Department of Family and Community
  Medicine
Temple University School of Medicine
Philadelphia, Pennsylvania;
Associate Director, Family Medicine
  Residency Program
Department of Family and Community
  Medicine
Lancaster General Hospital
Lancaster, Pennsylvania

Jason Kittler, MD, PhD, JD
Berkshire Medical Group
Pittsfield, Massachusetts

Michael Klein, MD
Warren Alpert Medical School
Brown University
Providence, Rhode Island

Michael S. Kleinman, DO
Department of Neurology
Boston University
Boston, Massachusetts

Dagmar Klinger, MD
Assistant Professor
Department of Medicine
University of Massachusetts Medical
  School;
Nephrologist
Department of Medicine
UMass Medical Center
Worcester, Massachusetts

Joshua T. Kluetz, DO
Family Medicine Residency
Resurrection Medical Center
Chicago, Illinois

William J. Knaus, II, MD
Department of Surgery
University of Texas Southwestern;
Department of Surgery
Parkland Hospital
Dallas, Texas

Teresa Knight, MD
Women's Health Specialists of St. Louis
Creve Coeur, Missouri

Ajar Kochar, MD
The Warren Alpert Medical School at
  Brown University
Providence, Rhode Island

Benjamin Kohnen, MD
David Grant Medical Center
Travis Air Force Base, California

Anjali Koka, MD
Department of Anesthesia, Critical Care
  and Pain Management
Massachusetts General Hospital
Boston, Massachusetts

Scott Kopec, MD
Department of Pulmonary Medicine
University of Massachusetts
  Medical Center
Worcester, Massachusetts

Galina Korsunsky, MD
MetroWest Medical Center
Framingham, Massachusetts

Anya S. Koutras, MD
Associate Professor
Department of Family Medicine
University of Vermont College of Medicine;
Faculty Attending
Department of Family Medicine
Fletcher Allen Health Care
University of Vermont
Burlington, Vermont

Michael S. Krathen, MD
Department of Dermatology
Boston University School of Medicine;
Department of Dermatology
Boston Medical Center
Boston, Massachusetts

Allison Kreiner, MD
Resident
Department of Obstetrics and Gynecology
Akron General Medical Center
Akron, Ohio

David W. Kruse, MD
Assistant Clinical Professor
Department of Orthopaedic Surgery
University of California, Irvine
Irvine, California

Rebecca Kruse-Jarres, MD, MPH
Assistant Professor
Department of Medicine
Tulane University
New Orleans, Louisiana

Eric J. Kujawski, DO
Sports Medicine Fellow
Department of Family Medicine
University of Tennessee
Knoxville, Tennessee

Santosh Kumar, MBBS
Department of Family Medicine
Freighton University Medical Center
Omaha, Nebraska

Tara N. Kumaraswami, MD
Department of Obstetrics and
  Gynecology
University of Massachusetts Medical
  School
Worcester, Massachusetts

Alphonsus K. Kung, MD
Department of Family Medicine and
  Community Health
University of Massachusetts Medical
  School
Worcester, Massachusetts

Jason M. Kurland, MD
Fellow, Department of Nephrology
Rhode Island Hospital/Brown
  University
Providence, Rhode Island

Daniel B. Kurtz, PhD
Assistant Professor
Department of Biology
Utica College
Utica, New York

Dylan C. Kwait, MD
Department of Radiology
Maimonides Medical Center
Brooklyn, New York

Chris G. Kyriakedes, DO
Professor, Emergency Medicine
Northeast Ohio Universities College
  of Medicine and Pharmacy
Rootstown, Ohio;
Attending Physician
Department of Emergency Medicine
Akron General Medical Center
Akron, Ohio

Mildred LaFontaine, MD
Department of Neurology
Concord Hospital
Concord, New Hampshire

Amara Lai, MD
Department of Family Medicine
Banner Good Samaritan
Phoenix, Arizona

Katherine Lang, MD
University of Massachusetts School of
  Medicine
Worcester, Massachusetts

Eduardo Lara-Torre, MD
Associate Professor
Department of Obstetrics and Gynecology
Virginia Tech-Cariolion School of Medicine;
Associate Residency Program Director
Department of Obstetrics and Gynecology
Carilion Clinic
Roanoke, Virginia

Lars C. Larsen, MD
Professor
Associate Dean for Academic and
    Faculty Development
Department of Family Medicine
The Brody School of Medicine at East
    Carolina University
Greenville, North Carolina

Austin Larson, MD
Department of Pediatrics
The Children's Hospital
Aurrora, Colorado

Richard A. Larson, MD
Professor
Department of Medicine, Section of
    Hematology/Oncology
The University of Chicago
Chicago, Illinois

Bonnie W. Lau, MD, PhD
The Warren Alpert Medical School of
    Brown University
Providence, Rhode Island

Margo Lauterbach, MD
Staff Psychiatrist
Neuropsychiatry Program
Sheppard Pratt Health System
Baltimore, Maryland

Ann Lavers, MD

Justin P. Lavin, Jr., MD
Professor
Department of Obstetrics and Gynecology
Northeastern Ohio College of Medicine
Rootstown, Ohio;
Vice Chairman, Chief of Maternal Fetal
    Medicine
Department of Obstetrics and Gynecology
Akron General Medical Center
Akron, Ohio

Alexis Lawrence, MD
University of Massachusetts Medical
    School
Worcester, Massachusetts

Jay Lawrence, MD
University of Massachusetts Medical
    School
Worcester, Massachusetts

Antonella M. Leary, MD
Assistant Professor
Department of Obstetrics and
    Gynecology
UMass Memorial Medical Center
Worcester, Massachusetts

Daniel J. Lee, MD
Assistant Professor
Department of Otology and Laryngology
Harvard Medical School;
Division of Otology and Neurotology
Department of Otolaryngology
Massachusetts Eye and Ear Infirmary
Boston, Massachusetts

Daniel T. Lee, MD
Associate Clinical Professor
Department of Family Medicine
David Geffen School of Medicine at UCLA
Los Angeles, California;
Staff Attending
Department of Family Practice
Santa Monica–UCLA Medical Center
    and Orthopaedic Hospital
Santa Monica, California

Justin A. Lee, MD
Department of Family Medicine
University of Colorado Health Sciences
    Center
Denver, Colorado

Juyong Lee, MD, PhD
Physician
Department of Internal Medicine
MetroWest Medical Center
Framingham, Massachusetts

Paul J. Lee, MD
Assistant Professor
Pediatrics
SUNY Stony Brook School of Medicine
Stony Brook, New York;
Attending Pediatrician
Pediatric Infectious Diseases
Winthrop-University Hospital
Mineola, New York

Matthew R. Leibowitz, MD
Assistant Clinical Professor
Department of Medicine
David Geffen School of Medicine at UCLA;
Attending Physician
Department of Infectious Diseases
UCLA Medical Center
Los Angeles, California

Meg Lekander, MD
Assistant Instructor in Family Medicine
Warren Alpert School of Medicine of
    Brown University
Providence, Rhode Island

Sergio A. Leon, MD
Rheumatology Fellow
Division of Rheumatology
University of Massachusetts Medical
    School
Worcester, Massachusetts

Andrew Leone, MD
Department of Urology
Brown Alpert Medical School;
Rhode Island Hospital
Providence, Rhode Island

Maya Leventer-Roberts, MD, MPH
Department of Pediatrics
Mount Sinai School of Medicine
Mount Sinai Kravis Children's Hospital
New York, New York

John M. Levey, MD
Clinical Chief, GI Division
Department of Digestive Disease
University of Massachusetts Medical
    School
Worcester, Massachusetts

Nikki Levin, MD, PhD
Associate Professor of Medicine
Division of Dermatology
University of Massachusetts Medical
    School
UMass Memorial Medical Center
Worcester, Massachusetts

Gary I. Levine, MD
Associate Professor
Department of Family Medicine
Brody School of Medicine
East Carolina University
Greenville, North Carolina

James H. Lewis, MD
Professor of Medicine
Division of Gastroenterology
Georgetown University Medical Center
Washington, District of Columbia

Desiree Lie, MD
Health Sciences Clinical Professor
Director, Research and Faculty
    Development
University of California, Irvine
Irvine, California

Brian K. Linn, MD
Medical Staff
Department of Family Medicine
North Arkansas Regional Medical Center
Harrison, Arkansas

Vasileios-Arsenios Lioutas, MD
Department of Neurology
Boston University Medical Center
Boston, Massachusetts

Janice A. Litza, MD
Assistant Professor
Department of Family Medicine
University of Wisconsin School of Medicine
    and Public Health
Madison, Wisconsin;
Aurora University of Wisconsin Medical
    Group
Aurora Healthcare
Milwaukee, Wisconsin

Kimberly E. Liu, MD, FRCSC
Assistant Professor
Department of Obstetrics and
    Gynecology
University of Toronto;
Staff Physician
Mount Sinai Hospital
Toronto, Ontario
Canada

Nancy Y. Liu, MD
Associate Professor of Clinical
    Medicine
Department of Medicine
University of Massachusetts Medical
    School
Worcester, Massachusetts

Samantha R. Llanos, PharmD, RPh
Adjunct Assistant Professor
Massachusetts College of Pharmacy
Worcester, Massachusetts

John Paul Lock, MD
Assistant Professor
Department of Medicine
University of Massachusetts School of
    Medicine
Worcester, Massachusetts

Madaiah Lokeshwari, MD
Hospitalist
Department of Medicine
Heywood Hospital
Gardner, Massachusetts

Rich Londo, MD
Assistant Professor of Clinical Family
    Medicine
Department of Family and Community
    Medicine
University of Illinois College of
    Medicine-Rockford
Rockford, Illinois

David Longstroth, MD
Contra Costa Health Services
Martinez, California

Claudia M. Lora, MD
Visiting Instructor
Department of Medicine
University of Illinois at Chicago;
Faculty
Department of Medicine
University of Illinois Medical Center
Chicago, Illinois

Claudine Lott, MD
University of Massachusetts Medical
    School
Worcester, Massachusetts

Jane K. Louie, MD
Attending Physician
Neurological Services, PC
MetroWest Medical Center
Framingham, Massachusetts

Zhen Lu, MD
Attending Physician
South Bay Family Medical Group;
Attending Physician
Torrance Memorial Medical Center
Torrance, California

Brock D. Lutz, MD
Partner
East Texas Infectious Disease Consultants
Tyler, Texas

Ann M. Lynch, PharmD, RPh
Assistant Professor
Department of Pharmacy Practice
University of Massachusetts College of
    Pharmacy Health Science
Worcester, Massachusetts

Paul E. Lyons, MD
Professor and Associate Chair
Department of Family and Community
    Medicine
Temple University School of Medicine
Philadelphia, Pennsylvania

Jonathan MacClements, MD
Director of Medical Education/DIO
Associate Professor and Chair/Program
    Director of the Family Medicine
    Department
Certificate of Knowledge American Society
    of Travelers' Health and Tropical
    Medicine
University of Texas Health Center at Tyler
Tyler, Texas

David C. Mackenzie, MD
Clinical Instructor
Department of Emergency Medicine
Brown University;
Rhode Island Hospital
Providence, Rhode Island

Heather Mackey-Fowler, MD
Assistant Professor
Department of Family Medicine and
    Community Health
University of Massachusetts Medical
    School;
Primary Care Physician
Department of Family Medicine
St. Vincent Medical Group
Worcester, Massachusetts

Theodore G. MacKinney, MD, MPH
Assistant Professor
Department of General Internal
    Medicine
Medical College of Wisconsin;
Staff Physician
Department of Internal Medicine
Froedtert Memorial Lutheran Hospital
Milwaukee, Wisconsin

Douglas W. MacPherson, MD,
    MSc(CTM)
Associate Professor
Department of Pathology and Molecular
    Medicine
McMaster University
Hamilton, Ontario, Canada;
President, Migration Health Consultants,
    Inc.
Cheltenham, Ontario, Canada

Tracy Madsen, MD
Department of Emergency Medicine
Brown University
Rhode Island Hospital
Providence, Rhode Island

Katherine M. Mahon, MD
Department of Family Medicine and
    Community Health
University of Pennsylvania Health
    System Presbyterian Medical Center
Philadelphia, Pennsylvania

Anne M. Mahoney, MD
Boston University School of Medicine
Boston, Massachusetts

Patrick Mailloux, DO
Assistant Professor of Medicine
Tufts University School of Medicine;
Associate Program Director
Critical Care Medicine Fellowship
Baystate Medical Center
Springfield, Massachusetts

Barbara A. Majeroni, MD
Clinical Professor
Department of Family Medicine
University of Buffalo, SUNY;
Attending Physician
Department of Family Medicine
Erie County Medical Center
Buffalo, New York

M. Keenan Mak, MD
Creighton University School of Medicine
Omaha, Nebraska

Dominique Malacàrne, MD
The Warren Alpert Medical School
Brown University
Providence, Rhode Island

Maricarmen Malagon-Rogers, MD
Associate Professor
Department of Family Medicine
University of Tennessee Graduate School
   of Medicine;
Director, Pediatric Nephrology
Department of Pediatrics
University of Tennessee Medical Center,
   Knoxville
Knoxville, Tennessee

Melanie J.S. Malec, MD
Fellow
Department of Family Medicine
Case Western Reserve University;
University Hospitals Case Medical
   Center
Cleveland, Ohio

Samir Malkani, MD
Associate Professor of Clinical
   Medicine
Division of Diabetes
University of Massachusetts Medical
   School
Worcester, Massachusetts

Ronald L. Malm, DO
Assistant Professor
University of Wyoming;
Family Practice Residency Program
Cheyenne, Wyoming

Michael A. Malone, MD
Assistant Professor
Department of Family Medicine
Pennsylvania State College of
   Medicine;
Staff
Department of Family Medicine
Pennsylvania State Milton S. Hershey
   Medical Center
Hershey, Pennsylvania

Joshua M.V. Mammen, MD, PhD
Assistant Professor
Department of Surgery
University of Kansas
Kansas City, Kansas

Lee A. Mancini, MD, CSCS, CSN
Assistant Professor
Department of Family Medicine and
   Community Health
University of Massachusetts Medical
   School;
Sports Medicine Physician
Department of Family Medicine and
   Community Health
University of Massachusetts Medical
   Center
Worcester, Massachusetts

Daniel Mandell, MD
University of Massachusetts Medical
   School
Worcester, Massachusetts

Jeffrey Manning, MD

Mark J. Manning, DO, Med
Assistant Professor
Department of Obstetrics and
   Gynecology
University of Massachusetts Medical
   School;
UMass Memorial Medical Center
Worcester, Massachusetts

Mariann Manno, MD
Associate Professor
Departments of Pediatrics and Emergency
   Medicine
University of Massachusetts Memorial
   Medical Center;
Division Director
Department of Pediatrics
University of Massachusetts Memorial
   Children's Medical Center
Worcester, Massachusetts

Katherine A. Mansalis, MD
Department of Family Medicine
David Grant Medical Center
Travis Air Force Base, California

Aaron S. Mansfield, MD
Clinician-Investigator/Fellow
Department of Medicine/Division of
   Hematology
Department of Oncology
Mayo Clinic
Rochester, Minnesota

Eric Mao, MD
Warren Alpert Medical School at Brown
   University
Providence, Rhode Island

Murat Mardirossian, MD
Department of Family Medicine
University of California, Irvine
UC Irvine Douglas Hospital
Orange, California

Geoffrey M. Margo, MD, PhD
Clinical Associate Professor
Department of Psychiatry
University of Pennsylvania Health
   System;
Director, Consultation/Liaison Psychiatry
Department of Psychiatry
Pennsylvania Hospital
Philadelphia, Pennsylvania

Katherine L. Margo, MD
Assistant Professor
Department of Family Medicine and
   Community Health
University of Pennsylvania School of
   Medicine;
Faculty
Department of Family Medicine and
   Community Health
Presbyterian Hospital
Philadelphia, Pennsylvania

Kathy Mariani, MD
Assistant Professor
Center for Health & Well Being
The University of Vermont
Burlington, Vermont

Robert A. Marlow, MD, MA
Professor of Clinical Family Medicine
Department of Family and Community
   Medicine
University of Arizona College of
   Medicine
Tucson and Phoenix, Arizona;
Associate Director/Director of
   Research
Family Medicine Residency Program
Scottsdale Healthcare
Scottsdale, Arizona

William L. Marshall, MD
Associate Professor
Department of Medicine
University of Massachusetts Medical
   School;
Attending Physician
Department of Medicine
University of Massachusetts/Memorial
   Medical Center
Worcester, Massachusetts

Michelle T. Martin, PharmD
Clinical Assistant Professor
Department of Pharmacy
   Practice
University of Illinois at Chicago;
Clinical Pharmacist
Ambulatory Care Pharmacy
University of Illinois Medical Center
   at Chicago
Chicago, Illinois

Stephen A. Martin, MD, EdM
Instructor
Department of Family Medicine and
   Community Health
University of Massachusetts
   Medical School
Worcester, Massachusetts

A. Raquel Mateo-Bibeau, MD
Infectious Disease Specialist
Department of Medicine
John F. Kennedy Medicine Center
St. Mary's Medical Center
Atlantis, Florida

Donnah Mathews, MD
Assistant Professor
Department of Medicine
Alpert School of Brown University;
Attending Physician
Department of General Internal
   Medicine
Rhode Island Hospital
Providence, Rhode Island

Michele L. Matthews, PharmD
Assistant Professor
Department of Pharmacy Practice
Massachusetts College of Pharmacy
   Health Sciences
Boston, Massachusetts;
Clinical Pharmacy Specialist
Pain Management Center
Brigham & Women's Hospital
Chestnut Hill, Massachusetts

Jason Matuszak, MD
Department of Family Medicine
University of Buffalo;
Chief of Sports Medicine
Department of Sports Medicine
Excelsior Orthopaedics
Amherst, New York

Karen L. Maughan, MD
Associate Professor
Attending Faculty
Department of Family Medicine
University of Virginia
Charlottesville, Virginia

George Maxted, MD
Assistant Clinical Professor
Department of Family Medicine and
   Community Health
UMass Memorial Health Care
Worcester, Massachusetts

Aimee Mayo Nilsen, PharmD
Assistant Adjunct Faculty
Massachusetts College of Pharmacy and
   Health Sciences
Genzyme Corporation
Worcester, Massachusetts

Beth Mazyck, MD
Clinical Associate Professor
Department of Family Medicine and
   Community Health
University of Massachusetts
   Medical School
Worcester, Massachusetts;
Vice President of Medical Services
Community Health Connections, Inc.
Family Health Center
Fitchburg, Massachusetts

Elizabeth McAninch, MD
Physician
Department of Internal Medicine
University of Miami;
Jackson Memorial Hospital
Miami, Florida

Frank J. McCabe, MD
Clinical Instructor
Department of Ophthalmology
Tufts Medical Center
Boston, Massachusetts

Margaret McCormick, MS, RN
Clinical Assistant Professor
Department of Nursing
Towson University
Towson, Maryland

Timothy R. McCurry, MD
Clinical Assistant Professor
Department of Family Medicine
Stritch School of Medicine
Loyola University
Maywood, Illinois;
Program Director
Family Medicine Residency
Resurrection Medical Center
Chicago, Illinois

Elizabeth Colman McKeen, MD
Department of Pediatrics
Harvard University;
Massachusetts General Hospital
   for Children
Boston, Massachusetts

Patricia McQuilkin, MD
Assistant Professor
Department of Pediatrics
University of Massachusetts Medical
   School
Worcester, Massachusetts

Gary Mark McWilliams, MD
Executive VP Chief Ambulatory
   Services Officer
Ambulatory Operations
University Health System
San Antonio, Texas

Colleen F. Medeiros, PharmD, BCPS
Department of Internal Medicine
Boston Medical Center
Boston, Massachusetts

Eva Medvedova, MD
Fellow, Hematology and Oncology Fellow
Department of Medicine
University of Massachusetts Medical School
Worcester, Massachusetts

Erika Mello, MD
University of Massachusetts Medical School
Worcester, Massachusetts

Hannah Melnitsky, MD
University of Massachusetts Medical School
Worcester, Massachusetts

Timothy Menz, MD
University of Massachusetts Medical School
Worcester, Massachusetts

Tracy O. Middleton, DO
Chair, Family Medicine
Midwestern University
Arizona College of Osteopathic Medicine
Glendale, Arizona

James P. Miller, MD
Medical Director
Department of Pediatric Surgery
Cook Children's Medical Center
Fort Worth, Texas

Nathan Miller, MD, CAPT, MC
Department of Family Medicine
David Grant (USAF) Medical Center
Travis Air Force Base, California

Sandra Miller, MD
Assistant Director
Family Medicine Residency
Banner Good Samaritan Medical Center
Phoenix, Arizona

Jonathan Min, MD
University of Massachusetts Medical
   School
Worcester, Massachusetts

Jeffrey F. Minteer, MD
Clinical Associate Professor
Department of Family Medicine
University of Pittsburgh
Pittsburgh, Pennsylvania;
Program Director, Family Medicine
    Residency
Washington Hospital
Washington, Pennsylvania

Mark H. Mirabelli, MD
Assistant Professor
Department of Orthopaedics and Family
    Medicine
University of Rochester
Rochester, New York

Anna Mirk, MD
Instructor
Department of Geriatrics, Extended Care
    and Rehabilitation
Atlanta VA Medical Center
Decatur, Georgia

Ann Mitchell, MD
Associate Professor of Clinical Neurology
Department of Neurology
University of Massachusetts Memorial
    Medical Center
Worcester, Massachusetts

Jack H. Mitstifer, MD
Assistant Professor of Clinical Emergency
    Medicine
Department of Emergency Medicine
Northeastern Ohio Universities College of
    Medicine and Pharmacy
Rootstown, Ohio;
Chairman
Department of Emergency Medicine
Akron General Medical Center
Akron, Ohio

Vinod P. Mitta, MD
University of Southern California Keck
    School of Medicine
Los Angeles, California

Bryan K. Moffett, MD
Assistant Professor
Department of Internal Medicine
University of Louisville School of
    Medicine;
Hospitalist, Internal Medicine
University of Louisville
Louisville, Kentucky

Aaron Moore, DO
University of Massachusetts Medical
    School
Worcester, Massachusetts

Tiffany A. Moore Simas, MD, MPH, Med
Assistant Professor
Department of Obstetrics and Gynecology
University of Massachusetts Medical
    School;
Full-Time Generalist
    Obstetrician-Gynecologist
Department of Obstetrics and
    Gynecology
University of Massachusetts Medical
    Center—Memorial Campus
Worcester, Massachusetts

Wayne Morgan, MD
Combined Child/Adult Psychiatry
Department of Psychiatry
University of Massachusetts Medical
    School
Worcester, Massachusetts

Richard A. Moriarty, MD
Professor of Clinical Pediatrics
Department of Pediatrics
UMass Medical School;
Pediatric Infectious Disease Consultant
Department of Pediatrics
UMass Memorial Health Care
Worcester, Massachusetts

Anna K. Morin, PharmD
Associate Professor
Department of Pharmacy Practice
Massachusetts College of Pharmacy
    and Health Sciences;
Clinical Pharmacist
Department of Pharmacy Services
Worcester State Hospital
Worcester, Massachusetts

Peter Morse, MD
University of Massachusetts School of
    Medicine
Worcester, Massachusetts

Mohammad Ansar Mughal, MD
Eastern New Mexico Family Medicine
Roswell, New Mexico

Christian Müller, PhD
Assistant Professor
Department of Pediatrics
University of Massachusetts Medical
    School
Worchester, Massachusetts

Herbert L. Muncie, Jr., MD
Professor
Director of Student Education
Department of Family Medicine
Louisiana State University School of
    Medicine
New Orleans, Louisiana

Mallika Mundkur, MD
University of Massachusetts Medical
    School
Worcester, Massachusetts

Amanda Murchison, MD
Assistant Professor
Department of Obstetrics and Gynecology
Virginia Tech-Carilion School of Medicine;
Assistant Residency Program Director
Department of Obstetrics and Gynecology
Carilion Clinic
Roanoke, Virginia

Lawrence Murphy, MD
University of Massachusetts Medical
    School
Worcester, Massachusetts

Eleftherios Mylonakis, MD
Associate Professor of Medicine
Division of Infectious Diseases
Harvard Medical School
Massachusetts General Hospital
Boston, Massachusetts

**Shashidhara Nanjundaswamy, MD,
MBBS, MRCP, DM**
Assistant Professor
Department of Neurology
University of Massachusetts Medical
    School;
Neurologist
Neurology
University of Massachusetts Memorial
    Health Care
Worcester, Massachusetts

Johra Nasreen, MD
Department of Family Medicine
University Hospital
University of Texas Health Science Center
San Antonio, Texas

David M. Navel, MD
Department of Family Medicine
David Grant Medical Center
Travis Air Force Base, California

Beverly L. Nazarian, MD
Clinical Associate Professor of Pediatrics
Department of Pediatrics
University of Massachusetts Medical
    School;
Pediatrician
Pediatric Primary Care
University of Massachusetts Medical
    Center
Worcester, Massachusetts

James G. Nee, MD
Clinical Faculty
Department of Family Medicine
University of Illinois–Chicago;
Clinical Faculty–Attending
Department of Family Medicine
Resurrection Healthcare–St. Joseph
Hospital
Chicago, Illinois

Donald A.F. Nelson, MD
Director of Medical Informatics
Cedar Rapids Medical Education
Foundation;
Active Medical Staff
Department of Family Medicine
St. Luke's Hospital
Cedar Rapids, Iowa

Elizabeth Ann Nelson, MD
Senior Associate Dean, Medicine-General
Medicine
Baylor College of Medicine
Houston, Texas

Carla M. Nester, MD
Assistant Professor
Department of Medicine and Pediatrics
Division of Adult and Pediatric Nephrology
The University of Iowa Hospitals and Clinics
Iowa City, Iowa

Kristyn Newhall, MD
University of Massachusetts School of
Medicine
Worcester, Massachusetts

Constance Nichols, MD
Clinical Associate Professor of Emergency
Medicine
Director of Medical Informatics
University of Massachusetts Medical
School
Worcester, Massachusetts

David L. Nickerson, PharmD
Department of Community Pharmacy
Practice
Massachusetts College of Pharmacy and
Health Sciences
Worcester, Massachusetts

Prachaya Nitichaikulvatana, MD
Fellow, Department of Rheumatology
University of Massachusetts Medical
School
Worcester, Massachusetts

Laura L. Novak, MD
Associate Director
Barberton Family Practice Residency
Summa Barberton Hospital
Barberton, Ohio

Sean P. O'Reilly, MD
Assistant Professor of Medicine
Pulmonary, Allergy and Critical Care
Medicine
University of Massachusetts Medical
School;
UMass Memorial Healthcare
Worcester, Massachusetts

Kelly O'Callahan, MD
Instructor
Department of Medicine
University of Massachusetts Medical
School;
Physician
Department of Gastroenterology
St. Vincent's Hospital
Worcester, Massachusetts

**Jacqueline L. Olin, MS, PharmD,
BCPS, CPP**
Associate Professor of Pharmacy
Wingate University School of Pharmacy
Wingate, North Carolina

Ken S. Ota, DO
Department of Family Medicine
Banner Good Samaritan Medical Center
Phoenix, Arizona

Balakumar Pandian, MD
Assistant Professor
Internal Medicine & Pediatrics
University of Texas Southwestern;
Hospitalist
Department of Internal Medicine
Brackenridge Hospital
Austin, Texas

Kathleen Pangia, MD
University of Pennsylvania
Philadelphia, Pennsylvania

Debra Papa, MD
Assistant Professor of Obstetrics and
Gynecology
UMass Memorial Health Care
University of Massachusetts Medical
School
Worcester, Massachusetts

Jon S. Parham, DO, MPH
Associate Professor
Department of Family Medicine
University of Tennessee, Graduate School
of Medicine;
Active Staff
Department of Family Medicine
University of Tennessee Medical Center
Knoxville, Tennessee

Douglas S. Parks, MD
Associate Professor
Family Practice Residency
University of Wyoming;
Chair
Department of Family Practice
Cheyenne Regional Medical Center
Cheyenne, Wyoming

Aleema Patel, MD
The Warren Alpert Medical School
Brown University
Providence, Rhode Island

Birju B. Patel, MD
Assistant Professor of Medicine
Emory University School of Medicine
Division of Geriatrics and Gerontology;
Department of Medicine
Atlanta VA Medical Center
Decatur, Georgia

Krunal Patel, MD
University of Massachusetts Medical School
Worcester, Massachusetts

Neepa Patel, MD
Department of Neurology
Boston Medical Center
Boston, Massachusetts

Nihal Patel, MD
University of Massachusetts Medical School
Worcester, Massachusetts

Nilay Patel, MD
Warren Alpert Medical School of Brown
University
Providence, Rhode Island

Payal S. Patel, DO
Pediatric Hospitalist
Department of Pediatrics
Edward Hospital
Naperville, Illinois

Sagar C. Patel, MD
Warren Alpert Medical School of Brown
University
Providence, Rhode Island

Elizabeth W. Patton, MD
Department of Obstetrics and Gynecology
Northwestern University
Prentice Women's Hospital
Chicago, Illinois

Rashmi V. Patwardhan, MD
Clinical Professor
Department of Medicine
University of Massachusetts Medical School;
Director Outpatient Clinic,
Gastroenterology Division
Department of Medicine
University of Massachusetts Memorial
Medical Center
Worcester, Massachusetts

Vilas Patwardhan, MD
Department of Internal Medicine
Massachusetts General Hospital
Boston, Massachusetts

Laura Paulin, MD, MHS
Montefiore Medical Center of the Albert
    Einstein College of Medicine
Bronx, New York

Ernest Pedapati, MD
Cincinnati Children's Hospital
Cincinnati, Ohio

Rade N. Pejic, MD
Assistant Professor of Family Medicine
Tulane University;
Lead Physician of Multi-Specialty Clinic
Department of Family Medicine
Tulane Medical Center
New Orleans, Louisiana

Elizabeth B. Pelkofski, MD
Department of Obstetrics and Gynecology
University of Massachusetts
Worcester, Massachusetts

Amy Pelletier, DO
Department of Pediatrics
Baystate Medical Center
Springfield, Massachusetts

Randall S. Pellish, MD
Assistant Professor of Medicine
Division of Gastroenterology
University of Massachusetts Medical School
University of Massachusetts Memorial
    Medical Center
Worcester, Massachusetts

Lisa Pelunis-Messier, PharmD
Adjunct Faculty Member
Department of Pharmacy
Clinical Pharmacy Research Services
Massachusetts College of Pharmacy
Worcester, Massachusetts

Douglas A. Pepple, MD
Department of Family Medicine
University of Illinois at Chicago;
University of Illinois at Chicago Medical
    Center
Chicago, Illinois

Ruben Peralta, MD
Director of Trauma and Critical Care
    Fellowship Program
Department of Surgery
Hamad Medical Corporation
Department of Medical Education;
Senior Consultant, Surgery, Trauma
    and Care
Department of Surgery
Hamad General Hospital
Doha, Qatar
United Arab Emirates

Adam B. Pesaturo, PharmD, BCPS
Critical Care Pharmacist
Department of Pharmacy Services
Baystate Medical Center
Springfield, Massachusetts

Kimberly A. Pesaturo, PharmD
Assistant Professor
Department of Pharmacy Practice
Massachusetts College of Pharmacy and
    Health Sciences;
Clinical Specialist-Pediatrics
Department of Pharmacy
University of Massachusetts Memorial
    Medical Center
Worcester, Massachusetts

Bobby X. Peters, MD
Assistant Professor
Department of Emergency
    Medicine
University of Iowa
Iowa City, Iowa

Nicole D. Pilevsky, MD
Private Practice
Obstetrics and Gynecology
Howard County General Hospital
Columbia, Maryland

Jochebed A. Pink, MD
University of Massachusetts Medical
    School
Worcester, Massachusetts

Barbara R. Pober, MD
Geneticist
Children's Hospital Boston
Boston, Massachusetts

Gregory A. Poland, MD
Mary Lowell Leary Professor of
    Medicine
Department of General Internal
    Medicine
College of Medicine, Mayo Clinic;
Director
Mayo Vaccine Research Group
Mayo Clinic
Rochester, Minnesota

Phyllis Pollak, MD
Associate Clinical Professor
Department of Pediatrics
University of Massachusetts Medical
    School;
Consultant
Department of Pediatrics
University of Massachusetts Medical
    Center
Worcester, Massachusetts

David A. Pope, MD
Private Practice
Mayo Health System
Janesville, Minnesota

Stacy E. Potts, MD
Assistant Clinical Professor
Department of Family Medicine and
    Community Health
University of Massachusetts;
Family Physician
Department of Family Medicine and
    Community Health
University of Massachusetts Memorial
    Health Care
Worcester, Massachusetts

Thomas Price, MD
Assistant Professor
Division of Geriatric Medicine and
    Gerontology
Emory University;
Chief, Department of Medicine
Wesley Woods Geriatric Hospital
Atlanta, Georgia

William A. Primack, MD
Professor of Medicine and Pediatrics
University of North Carolina Kidney
    Center
University of North Carolina School of
    Medicine
Chapel Hill, North Carolina

Kimberly Pringle, MD
Department of Emergency Medicine
Rhode Island Hospital and
Hasbro Children's Hospital
Providence, Rhode Island

**Barbara Provo, MSN, APNP,
CWOCN, FNP-BC**
Coordinator
Wound and Ostomy Program
Froedtert Hospital
Milwaukee, Wisconsin

George Gunter A. Pujalte, MD
Clinical Lecturer
Department of Family Medicine
University of Michigan
University of Michigan Medical Center
Ann Arbor, Michigan

Elise H. Pyun, MD
Clinical Associate Professor
Department of Medicine
University of Massachusetts Medical
    School;
Rheumatology Attending
Department of Medicine
University of Massachusetts Medical
    Center
Worcester, Massachusetts

Juan Qiu, MD, PhD
Assistant Professor
Department of Family and Community
   Medicine
Pennsylvania State University College
   of Medicine;
Attending Physician
Department of Family Medicine
Mount Nittany Medical Center
State College, Pennsylvania

Jonna M. Quinn, DO
Aultman Hospital
Canton, Ohio

Naureen B. Rafiq, MBBS, MD
Instructor, Family Medicine
Creighton University Medical Center
Omaha, Nebraska

Mhd Basheer Rahmoun, MD
Assistant Professor, Adjunct
Department of Pharmacy Practice
Massachusetts College of Pharmacy and
   Health Sciences;
Clinical Research Fellow
Clinical Pharmacology Study Group
Worcester, Massachusetts

Jyoti Ramakrishna, MD
Assistant Professor
Department of Pediatrics
University of Massachusetts Medical
   School
University of Massachusetts Memorial
   Healthcare
Worcester, Massachusetts

Manju Ramchandani, MD
Private Practice
Mt. Vernon Family Health Center
Mt. Vernon, Illinois

Neha Raukar, MD
Assistant Professor of Emergency
   Medicine
Department of Bio-Med Emergency
   Medicine
Brown Alpert Medical School at Brown
   University
Providence, Rhode Island

Tejesh S. Reddy, MBBS
Department of Family Medicine
Creighton University
Omaha, Nebraska

**Derek M. Richardson, Capt USAF AMC
60 MDOS/SGOF**
Department of Family Practice
David Grant Medical Center
Travis Air Force Base, California

Tara J. Rizvi, MD
Assistant Professor
Department of Allergy, Immunology and
   Rheumatology
Baylor College of Medicine;
Attending Physician
Department of Rheumatology
Ben Taub General Hospital
Houston, Texas

Teresa M. Robb, MD
Clinical Instructor
Department of Obstetrics & Gynecology
Jefferson Medical College of Thomas
   Jefferson University;
Attending Physician
Department of Obstetrics & Gynecology
Albert Einstein Medical Center
Philadelphia, Pennsylvania

Michele Roberts, MD, PhD
Diplomate American Board of Pathology
   (AP/CP)
Diplomate American Board of Medical
   Genetics
Paxton, Massachusetts

Leslie Robinson-Bostom, MD
Associate Professor of Dermatology
Warren Alpert Medical School of Brown
   University
Providence, Rhode Island

Ann M. Rodden, DO, MS
Assistant Professor
Department of Family Medicine
Medical University of South Carolina
Charleston, South Carolina

Karla M. Rodriguez, MD
Department of Psychiatry
UMass Medical Center
Worcester, Massachusetts

Jennifer L. Rogers, MD
Aultman Hospital
Canton, Ohio

Lewis C. Rose, MD
Associate Professor
Department of Family and Community
   Medicine
University of Texas Health Sciences
   Center at San Antonio;
Active Medical Staff
Department of Family Medicine
University Hospital
San Antonio, Texas

Montiel T. Rosenthal, MD
Assistant Clinical Professor
Director of Maternity Services
Department of Family Medicine
University of Cincinnati;
Director of Prenatal Clinic
Department of Family Medicine
The Christ Hospital
Cincinnati, Ohio

Steven E. Roskos, MD
Associate Professor
Department of Family Medicine
Michigan State University
College of Human Medicine
East Lansing, Michigan

Julie L. Roth, MD
Assistant Professor
Department of Neurology
The Warren Alpert Medical School of
   Brown University
Providence, Rhode Island

Michael Rousse, MD, MPH
Hospitalist Director
Department of Medicine
Northeastern Vermont Regional Hospital
St. Johnsbury, Vermont

Paul G. Rubinstein, MD
Hematology/Oncology Fellow
Department of Medicine: Section of
   Hematology/Oncology
University of Illinois at Chicago
   Medical Center
Chicago, Illinois

Stephanie Ruest, MD
University of Massachusetts Medical
   School
Worcester, Massachusetts

Beth Ryder, MD
Assistant Professor of Surgery
Warren Alpert Medical School at Brown
   University
Providence, Rhode Island

Roland Saavedra, MD
Department of Family Medicine and
   Community Health
University of Massachusetts School of
   Medicine
Worcester, Massachusetts;

Aman D. Sabharwal, MD
Clinical Assistant Professor
Department of Medicine
Florida International University
College of Medicine;
Chief Utilization Officer
Jackson Health System
Miami, Florida

Anup Kumar Sabharwal, MD
Assistant Professor in Clinical Medicine
 Endocrinology, Diabetes, and
 Metabolism
University of Miami
Miller School of Medicine
Miami, Florida

Stanley Sagov, MD
Assistant Professor
Department of Family Medicine
University of Massachusetts
Worcester, Massachusetts;
Chief of Family Medicine
Department of Medicine
Mount Auburn Hospital
Cambridge, Massachusetts

Karen I. Salomon-Escoto, MD
Assistant Professor
Department of Medicine
University of Massachusetts Medical
 School
Worcester, Massachusetts

Ricardo A. Samson, MD
Professor
Department of Pediatrics
The University of Arizona;
Chief
Section of Pediatric Cardiology
University Medical Center
Tucson, Arizona

Arthur B. Sanders, MD, MHA
Professor
Department of Emergency Medicine
University of Arizona;
Attending Physician
University Medical Center
Tucson, Arizona

Darshak Sanghavi, MD
Departments of Pediatrics and Cardiology
University of Massachusetts Medical
 School
Worcester, Massachusetts

Ann Saunders, MD
University of Massachusetts Medical
 School
Worcester, Massachusetts

Jennifer L. Savitski, MD
Clinical Instructor
Department of Obstetrics and Gynecology
Northeastern Ohio University College of
 Medicine
Rootstown, Ohio;
Assistant Residency Program Director
Department of Obstetrics and Gynecology
Akron General Medical Center
Akron, Ohio

Shailendra K. Saxena, MD
Assistant Professor, Family Medicine
Creighton University School of Medicine
Omaha, Nebraska

Dalia Sbat, PharmD
Adjunct Faculty
Department of Pharmaceutical Science
Massachusetts College of Pharmacy and
 Health Sciences
Worcester, Massachusetts;
Pharmacist
Walgreens Pharmacy
Shrewsbury, Massachusetts

Stephanie Scandale, MD
Assistant Clinical Professor
Department of Family Medicine
University of California, Los Angeles;
University of California, Los Angeles Santa
 Monica Hospital
Santa Monica, California

Fred Schiffman, MD
Vice Chairman, Department of Medicine
Sigal Family Professor of Humanistic
 Medicine
Clinical Director, Comprehensive Cancer
 Center
Professor of Medicine
Alpert Medical School of Brown University
The Miriam Hospital
Providence, Rhode Island

Eric Schmidt, MD
Clinical Associate Professor of Emergency
 Medicine
Co-Director, Undergraduate Medical
 Education
Department of Emergency Medicine
University of Massachusetts Medical
 School
Worcester, Massachusetts

Lisa M. Schroeder, MD
Assistant Director
Family Practice Residency Program
Summa Barberton Hospital
Barberton, Ohio

Alexandra Schultes, MD
Associate Professor
Department of Family Practice
University of Massachusetts
Worcester, Massachusetts

Bradford Schwartz, MD
University of Massachusetts Medical
 School
Worcester, Massachusetts

Deanna M. Scinto, PharmD
Adjunct Assistant Professor
Department of Pharmacy Practice
Massachusetts College of
 Pharmacy—Worcester
Worcester, Massachusetts

Christopher J. Scola, MD
Departments of Medicine and
 Rheumatology
Hartford Hospital
Hartford, Connecticut

Stephen M. Scott, MD, MPH
Assistant Professor
Department of Family and Community
 Medicine
Baylor College of Medicine
Houston, Texas

Gail Scully, MD, MPH
Assistant Professor
Department of Medicine
Division of Infectious Disease and
 Immunology
University of Massachusetts Medical
 School
Worcester, Massachusetts

David P. Sealy, MD
Clinical Professor
Department of Family Medicine
Director, Sports Medicine Fellowship
Department of Sports Medicine
Medical University South Carolina
Greenwood, South Carolina

Jose Oscar Seda, MD
Department of Family Medicine
University of Texas Health Science
 Center
San Antonio, Texas

Sheila M. Seed, PharmD, MPH
Associate Professor
Department of Pharmacy Practice
Massachusetts College of Pharmacy and
 Health Sciences
Worcester, Massachusetts

Patricia Seymour, MD
Department of Family Medicine and
 Community Health
University of Massachusetts Medical
 School
Worcester, Massachusetts

Amy Shah, MD
Department of Psychiatry
University of Cincinnati;
The University Hospital
Cincinnati, Ohio

Binay K. Shah, MD
Department of Hematology
St. Joseph Regional Medical Center
SJRMC Cancer Center
Lewiston, Idaho

Dhvani Shah, MD
Alpert Medical School
Brown University
Providence, Rhode Island

Archit Sharma, MD
Department of Family Medicine
Creighton University Medical Center
Omaha, Nebraska

Mohammed Shahsabebi, MD
Department of Community and Family
    Medicine
Duke University Medical Center
Durham, North Carolina

Sanjeev K. Sharma, MD
Associate Professor, Family Medicine
Creighton University School of Medicine
Omaha, Nebraska

Sujata Sharma, MD
Department of Family Medicine
Resurrection Medical Center
Chicago, Illinois

Douglas Shemin, MD
Associate Professor
Department of Medicine
Brown University School of Medicine;
Interim Director
Division of Kidney Diseases
Rhode Island Hospital
Providence, Rhode Island

David S. Shepro, MD
Assistant Professor
Department of Medicine
University of Massachusetts Medical
    School
Commonwealth Hematology and
    Oncology, PC
Worcester, Massachusetts

Awais Siddiki, MD
Department of Internal Medicine
University of Massachusetts Medical
    School
Worcester, Massachusetts

Aamir Siddiqi, MD
Associate Director
St. Luke's Family Medicine Residency
Aurora Health Care;
Vice President Medical Staff
Aurora Sinai Medical Center
Milwaukee, Wisconsin

Najmul H. Siddiqui, MBBS, MD
Department of Family Practice
Creighton University Medical Center
Omaha, Nebraska

Hugh J. Silk, MD
Assistant Professor
Department of Family Medicine and
    Community Health
University of Massachusetts Medical
    School;
Staff
Department of Family Medicine and
    Community Health
University of Massachusetts Memorial
    Medical Center
Worcester, Massachusetts

Matthew A. Silva, PharmD, RPh, BCPS
Assistant Professor
Pharmacy Practice
Massachusetts College of Pharmacy and
    Health Sciences;
Clinical Pharmacist
Department of Family Medicine/Pharmacy
Family Health Center of Worcester
Worcester, Massachusetts

B. Brent Simmons, MD
Assistant Professor
Department of Family Medicine
Drexel University-College of Medicine
Philadelphia, Pennsylvania

Linda Sinclair, MD
University of Massachusetts Medical
    School
Worcester, Massachusetts

Jaspreet Singh, DO

Manoj Singh, MD
Assistant Professor
Department of Family Medicine
University of Cincinnati;
Attending Physician
Department of Family Medicine
The Christ Hospital
Cincinnati, Ohio

Patrick Smallwood, MD
Assistant Professor of Psychiatry
Department of Psychiatry
University of Massachusetts Medical
    School;
Attending Psychiatrist/Medical Director
    of Psychosomatic Medicine and
    Emergency Mental Health
Department of Psychiatry
University of Massachusetts Medical
    Center
Worcester, Massachusetts

Robert A. Smith, DO
Colonel, Medical Corps
Deputy Commander for Clinical Service
U.S. Army Medical Department Activity
Heidelberg Germany

Stanley G. Smith, MA, MB, FCFP
Professor Emeritus
Department of Family Medicine
University of Western Ontario
London, Ontario, Canada

John C. Smulian, MD, MPH
Vice Chair and Chief of Maternal Fetal
    Medicine
Department of Obstetrics and
    Gynecology
Lehigh Valley Health Network
Allentown, Pennsylvania

Nancy J. Snapp, MD, MPH
Physician
Department of Family Medicine
International Community Health
    Services
Seattle, Washington

Michael Snyder, MD
Professor
Department of Medicine—Hematology/
    Oncology, Pathology
University of Massachusetts Medical
    School
Worcester, Massachusetts

Augustine J. Sohn, MD, MPH
Assistant Professor
Department of Clinical Family Medicine
Department of Family Medicine
University of Illinois at Chicago;
Attending Physician
Department of Family Medicine
University of Illinois Hospital
Chicago, Illinois

Weily Soong, MD
Clinical Associate Professor
Department of Pediatric Allergy and
    Immunology
University of Alabama School of
    Medicine;
Managing Partner
Alabama Allergy and Asthma Center
Birmingham, Alabama

Mia D. Sorcinelli, MD
Attending Physician
Department of Family Medicine
Lawrence General Hospital
Lawrence, Massachusetts

John Spangler, MD, MPH
Associate Professor
Department of Family and Community
　Medicine
Wake Forest University School of
　Medicine
Winston-Salem, North Carolina

Mikayla Spangler, PharmD, BCPS
Assistant Professor
Creighton University School of Pharmacy
　and Health Professions
Clinical Pharmacist, Creighton Family
　Healthcare
Omaha, Nebraska

Joshua J. Spooner, PharmD, MS
Director of Clinical and Outcomes Services
Advanced Concepts Institute
University of the Sciences in Philadelphia
Philadelphia, Pennsylvania

Kellie A. Sprague, MD
Assistant Professor
Division of Hematology-Oncology
Tufts University School of Medicine;
Assistant Director
Bone Marrow Transplant Program
Division of Hematology-Oncology
Tufts Medical Center
Boston, Massachusetts

Dana Sprute, MD, MPH
Assistant Professor
University of Texas Southwestern
　Medical Center;
Assistant Clinical Professor
University of Texas Medical Branch
Austin, Texas

Michelle St. Fleur, MD
University of Massachusetts Medical
　School
Worcester, Massachusetts

Joan M. Stachnik, PharmD, BCPS
Clinical Assistant Professor
Drug Information Group
Department of Pharmacy Practice
College of Pharmacy
University of Illinois Medical Center at
　Chicago
Chicago, Illinois

Michael S. Stalvey, MD
Assistant Professor, Pediatric
　Endocrinology
University of Massachusetts Medical
　School
Department of Pediatrics
Gene Therapy Center
Worcester, Massachusetts

Oscar Starobin, MD
Department of Cardiology
University of Massachusetts Medical
　Center
Worcester, Massachusetts

Mark Steenbergen, DO
Private Practice, Family Practice
Poughkeepsie, New York

Gillian S. Stephens, MD, MSc
Assistant Professor
Department of Family and Community
　Medicine
Saint Louis University
Saint Louis, Missouri

Debora B. Sternaman, PharmD
Regional Medical Scientist
Department of Medical Affairs
Boehringer Ingelheim
Georgetown, Texas

Edward C. Sternaman, II, MD
Hospitalist
Department of Internal Medicine
Seton Williamson
Round Rock, Texas

J. Herbert Stevenson, MD
Director, Sports Medicine Fellowship
Department of Family and Community
　Medicine
University of Massachusetts Medical
　School;
Director, Sports Medicine
Department of Family and Community
　Medicine
University of Massachusetts Memorial
　Medical Center
Worcester, Massachusetts

Sheila O. Stille, DMD, MAGD
Assistant Professor
Department of Family Medicine and
　Community Health
University of Massachusetts Medical
　School;
Program Director, General Practice
　Residency in Dentistry
Department of Family Medicine and
　Community Health
University of Massachusetts Memorial
Worcester, Massachusetts

Jeffrey G. Stovall, MD
Associate Professor
Department of Psychiatry
Vanderbilt University School of Medicine;
Residency Training Director, Adult
　Psychiatry
Vanderbilt Psychiatric Hospital
Nashville, Tennessee

Charles Strom, MD
University of Massachusetts School
　of Medicine
Worcester, Massachusetts

Ryung Suh, MD, MPP, MBA, MPH
Assistant Professor
Health Systems Administration
Georgetown University
Washington, District of Columbia;
Command Surgeon and Occupational
　Health Division Chief
Defense Threat Reduction Agency
Fort Belvoir, Virginia

James J. Sullivan, Jr., MD, USN
Emergency Medicine Department
University of Massachusetts Medical
　School
Worcester, Massachusetts

Karyn M. Sullivan, PharmD, MPH
Associate Professor
Department of Pharmacy Practice
Massachusetts College of Pharmacy and
　Health Sciences;
Clinical Pharmacist
Department of Pharmacy
St. Vincent Hospital
Worcester, Massachusetts

Laura Sullivan Eurich, MD
University of Massachusetts School of
　Medicine
Worcester, Massachusetts

Anna Svircev, DO, MPH
Department of Family Medicine
University of Colorado
Denver, Colorado

Sheela Swaminatha, MD
Department of Neurology
Georgetown University;
Department of Neurology
Georgetown University/DC Veterans
　Administration
Washington, DC

Sana Syed, MD
Department of Neurology
Boston Medical Center
Boston, Massachusetts

Vassiliki P. Syriopoulou, MD
Professor of Pediatrics
First Department of Pediatrics
Athens University;
Chief of Infectious Diseases
First Department of Pediatrics
Aghia Sophia Children's Hospital
Athens, Greece

Alfonso J. Tafur, MD
Assistant Professor of Medicine
Department of Cardiovascular–Vascular
 Medicine
Mayo Clinic
Rochester, Minnesota

Chris Tang, MD
Occupational Medicine
Care on Site
Long Beach, California

Nikki D.Y. Tang, MD
Warren Alpert School of Medicine at Brown
 University
Providence, Rhode Island

Dawn S. Tasillo, MD
Associate Clerkship Director
Department of Obstetrics and
 Gynecology
University of Massachusetts Medical
 School;
Assistant Professor
UMass Memorial Medical Center
Worcester, Massachusetts

Erica Tavares, PharmD, RPh
Clinical Pharmacist
Department of Pharmacy
UMass Memorial Medical Center
Worcester, Massachusetts

Julie Scott Taylor, MD, MSc
Associate Professor of Family
 Medicine
Director of Clinical Curriculum
Alpert Medical School of Brown
 University
Providence, Rhode Island

Peter Than, MD
Alpert Medical School, Brown
 University
Providence, Rhode Island

Richard J. Thomas, MD, MPH
Associate Professor
Department of Preventive Medicine and
 Biometrics
Uniformed Services University of the
 Health Sciences;
Acting Department Head
Department of Occupational Medicine
National Naval Medical Center
Bethesda, Maryland

Margaret E. Thompson, MD
Associate Professor
Department of Family Practice
Michigan State University College of
 Human Medicine
Grand Rapids, Michigan

Michelle A. Tinitigan, MD
Clinical Assistant Professor
Department of Family and Community
 Medicine
University of California-San Francisco
San Francisco, California

Rochelle J. Tinitigan, MD
Department of Family and Community
 Medicine
University of Texas Health Science Center
 at San Antonio
San Antonio, Texas

Moshe S. Torem, MD, DLFAPA
Professor of Psychiatry
Department of Psychiatry
Northeastern Ohio Universities College of
 Medicine
Rootstown, Ohio;
Chief of Integrative Medicine
Department of Medicine
Akron General Medical Center
Akron, Ohio

William A. Tosches, MD
Associate Clinical Professor of Neurology
 and Medicine
Department of Neurology
University of Massachusetts Medical
 School
Worcester, Massachusetts;
Chief of Neurology Service
Milford Regional Medical Center
Milford, Massachusetts

Alyssa H. Tran, DO
Department of Family and Community
 Medicine
University of Texas Health Science
 Center
University Hospital
San Antonio, Texas

Natasha A. Travis, MD
Assistant Professor of Medicine
Department of General Internal
 Medicine
Medical College of Wisconsin
Froedtert Hospital
Milwaukee, Wisconsin

Michelle Trivedi, MD
University of Massachusetts Medical
 School
Worcester, Massachusetts

Zoltan Trizna, MD, PhD
Private Practice, Dermatology
Austin, Texas

Katherine Tromp, PharmD
Assistant Professor
Department of Pharmacy Practice
Lake Erie College of Osteopathic Medicine
LECOM-Bradenton School of Pharmacy
Bradenton, Florida

Richard E. Trowbridge, MD
David Grant Medical Center
Travis AFB, California

Caroline Tschibelu, MD
Department of Emergency Medicine
Alpert Medical School at Brown University
Providence, Rhode Island

Kristin A. Tuiskula, PharmD
Assistant Professor
Pharmacy Practice
Massachusetts College of Pharmacy and
 Health Sciences
Worcester, Massachusetts

Katharine Tumilty, MD
University of Massachusetts Medical
 School
Worcester, Massachusetts

Auguste Turnier, MD
Internist/Gastroenterologist, Private
 Practice
Haddonfield, New Jersey

Lawrence E. Udom, MD, MPH
Department of Psychiatry/Family Medicine
University of Cincinnati, University Hospital
Cincinnati, Ohio

Katherine Upchurch, MD
Clinical Professor
Department of Medicine
University of Massachusetts Medical
 School;
Clinical Chief
Division of Rheumatology
UMass Memorial Medical Center
Worcester, Massachusetts

Eric Ursprung, MD
University of Massachusetts Medical
 School
Worcester, Massachusetts

Richard P. Usatine, MD
Professor
Department of Family and Community
 Medicine
University of Texas Health Science Center
 at San Antonio
San Antonio, Texas

Santiago O. Valdes, MD
Assistant Professor
Department of Pediatrics
University of Arizona
Tucson, Arizona

Anthony Valdini, MD
Director of Research
Director of the Faculty Development
  Fellowship
Director of Faculty Development
Greater Lawrence Family Health Center
Lawrence, Massachusetts

Ron Van Ness-Otunnu, MD
House Staff Officer
Department of Emergency Medicine
Warren Alpert Medical School of Brown
  University;
Rhode Island Hospital
Providence, Rhode Island

Adam Vasconcellos, MD
Alpert Medical School, Brown University
Providence, Rhode Island

Jake D. Veigel, MD
University of Massachusetts Primary Care
  Sports Medicine Fellowship
University of Massachusetts Medical
  School
Fitchburg, Massachusetts

Colleen Veloski, MD
Associate Professor
Department of Endocrinology
Temple University School of
  Medicine
Philadelphia, Pennsylvania

Richard Viken, MD
Professor
Department of Family Medicine
University of Texas Health Science Center
  at Tyler
Tyler, Texas

Siva Vithananthan, MD
University Surgical Associates Inc.
Providence, Rhode Island

Rishi Vohora, DO
Dept of Cardiology
University of Massachusetts Medical
  Center
Worcester, Massachusetts

Kenton I. Voorhees, MD
Associate Professor and Vice Chair,
  Education
Department of Family Medicine
University of Colorado Denver School of
  Medicine
Aurora, Colorado

Yongkasem Vorasettakarnkij, MD, MSc
Instructor, Department of Medicine
Faculty of Medicine
Chulalongkorn University
Bangkok, Thailand;
Program in Cardiovascular MR
Martinos Center for Biomedical Imaging
Massachusetts General Hospital
Charlestown, Massachusetts

Kimberle Vore, MD
Clinical Assistant Professor of Family
  Medicine
Department of Family Medicine
Penn State College of Medicine
Hershey, Pennsylvania;
Clinical Instructor
Department of Family Medicine
The Washington Hospital
Washington, Pennsylvania

John B. Waits, MD
Associate Professor/Program Director-
  Tuscaloosa Family Medicine Residency
Department of Family Medicine/Obstetrics
  and Gynecology
University of Alabama School of Medicine;
Physician
Department of Family Medicine/Obstetrics
DCH Regional Medical Center
Tuscaloosa, Alabama

Noah S. Walman, MD
Department of Family Medicine
University of Illinois at Chicago College of
  Medicine
Chicago, Illinois

Anne M. Walsh, PA-C, MMSc
Clinical Instructor
Department of Family Medicine
Keck School of Medicine
University of Southern California
Los Angeles, California

William V. Walsh, MD
Assistant Professor of Medicine
Division of Hematology Oncology
University of Massachusetts Medical
  School;
UMass Memorial Medical Center
Worcester, Massachusetts

Erik E. Wang, MD
Department of Emergency Medicine
Brown University;
Rhode Island Hospital
Providence, Rhode Island

Otis Warren, MD
Department of Emergency Medicine
Warren Alpert School of Medicine
Brown University
Providence, Rhode Island

Donald E. Watenpaugh, PhD
Adjunct Professor
Department of Integrative Physiology
University of North Texas Health
  Science Center
Fort Worth, Texas

Ramothea L. Webster, MD, PhD
Department of Family Medicine
SUNY Downstate Medical Center
Lutheran Medical Center
Brooklyn, New York

Kathryn W. Weibrecht, MD
Clinical Instructor
Department of Emergency Medicine
UMass Memorial Health Center
Worcester, Massachusetts

Patrice Weiss, MD
Professor
Department of Obstetrics and Gynecology
Virginia Tech-Carilion School of Medicine;
Residency Program Director and
  Vice-Chair
Department of Obstetrics and
  Gynecology
Carilion Clinic
Roanoke, Virginia

Nathan Weldon, MD
Department of Family Medicine
University of California, Irvine
Irvine, California

Andrew J. Westwood, MD
Department of Neurology
Boston Medical Center
Boston, Massachusetts

Chris Wheelock, MD
Faculty Southwest Washington Family
  Medicine
Clinical Instructor of Family Medicine
University of Washington
Vancouver, Washington

Brett White, MD
Assistant Professor
Department of Family Medicine
Oregon Health and Science University
Portland, Oregon

Christopher C. White, MD, JD
Assistant Professor
Department of Psychiatry and Family
    Medicine
University of Cincinnati College of
    Medicine;
Medical Director, Psychiatric Consultation
Department of Psychiatry & Behavioral
    Neuroscience
University Hospital
Cincinnati, Ohio

Susan White, MD
Assistant Professor
Program Director, School of PA Studies
Manchester/Worcester Massachusetts
    College of Pharmacy & Health Sciences
Manchester New Hampshire

Michelle Whitehurst-Cook, MD
Associate Professor of Family Medicine
Associate Dean for Admissions
VCU School of Medicine
Richmond, Virginia

Kristine Willett, PharmD
Assistant Professor
Pharmacy Practice
Massachusetts College of Pharmacy and
    Health Sciences
Manchester, New Hampshire

Alan L. Williams, MD
Adjunct Professor of Family Medicine
Department of Family Medicine
Uniformed Services University of the
    Health Sciences
Bethesda, Maryland

Faren H. Williams, MD
Chief Physical Medicine and Rehabilitation
Clinical Professor
University of Massachusetts School of
    Medicine
Worcester, Massachusetts

**Pamela M. Williams, MD, Lt Col,
USAF, MC**
Assistant Professor
Department of Family Medicine
Uniformed Services University of the
    Health Sciences
Bethesda, Maryland

Alan Williamson, MD
Department of Family Medicine/Sports
    Medicine
David Grant USAF Medical Center
Travis Air Force Base, California

Jessica Lenore Wilson, MD
University of Illinois at Chicago College
    of Medicine
Chicago, Illinois

Robyn D. Wing, MD
Department of Pediatrics
University of Massachusetts Medical
    School
Worcester, Massachusetts

Christopher M. Wise, MD
W. Robert Irby Professor of Medicine
Department of Internal Medicine
Division of Rheumatology
Virginia Commonwealth University Medical
    College of Virginia
Richmond, Virginia

Jeffrey D. Wolfrey, MD
Clinical Professor
Department of Family and Community
    Medicine
University of Arizona College of Medicine
Tucson, Arizona;
Residency Director
Department of Family Medicine
Banner Good Samaritan Medical Center
Phoenix, Arizona

Zerlina Wong, MD
The Warren Alpert Medical School of
    Brown University
Providence, Rhode Island

Kyle D. Wood, MD
Department of Urology
Wake Forest University Baptist Medical
    Center
Winston Salem, North Carolina

Fae G. Wooding, PharmD
Assistant Professor of Pharmacy Practice
Massachusetts College of Pharmacy and
    Health Sciences
Worcester, Massachusetts

Frances Y. Wu, MD
Clinical Assistant Professor
Department of Family Medicine
UMDNJ-New Jersey Medical School
Newark, New Jersey;
Assistant Director
Department of Family Practice
Somerset Medical Center
Somerville, New Jersey

Frederick Wu, MD
Assistant Professor
Department of Veterans Affairs, Atlanta
    Medical Center
Emory University School of Medicine
Decatur, Georgia

Congjun Yao, MD
Department of Family Medicine
University of Texas Health Science Center
    at San Antonio
San Antonio, Texas

Julie Yeh, MD, MPH
Assistant Professor
Department of Family, Community, &
    Preventive Medicine
Drexel University College of Medicine;
Medical Staff
Department of Family, Community, and
    Preventive Medicine
Hahnemann University Hospital
Philadelphia, Pennsylvania

Gary Yen, MD
Clinical Lecturer
Department of Family Medicine
University of Michigan
Ann Arbor, Michigan

Robert A. Yood, MD
Clinical Professor of Medicine
Department of Medicine
University of Massachusetts Medical
    School;
Chief
Division of Rheumatology
Fallon Clinic
Worcester, Massachusetts

James L. Young, MD, PhD
Program in Molecular Medicine
University of Massachusetts Medical
    School
Worcester, Massachusetts

Edward L. Yourtee, MD
Southern New Hampshire Internal
    Medicine Associates
Derry, New Hampshire

Leanne Zakrzewski, MD
Department of Family Medicine
University of California, Los Angeles,
    David Geffen School of Medicine
Los Angeles, California

Ali Zarrabi, MD
The Warren Alpert Medical School of
    Brown University
Providence, Rhode Island

John K. Zawacki, MD
Professor of Medicine
Department of Medicine
Division of Gastroenterology
University of Massachusetts
    Medical School;
UMass Memorial Health Care
Worcester, Massachusetts

William Zawatski, MD
University of Massachusetts Medical
   School
Worcester, Massachusetts

Katrina Darlene Zedan, MSPAS, PA-C
Department of Acute Care/Family
   Medicine
University of Texas Health Science
   Center—San Antonio
San Antonio, Texas

Liang Zhao, MD
University of Massachusetts Medical
   School
Worcester, Massachusetts

Peter J. Ziemkowski, MD
Assistant Professor
Department of Family Medicine
Michigan State University
East Lansing, Michigan;
Clerkship Director
Family Medicine Residency Program
MSU/Kalamazoo Center for Medical
   Studies
Kalamazoo, Michigan

Susan Ziglar, MD
Assistant Professor
School of Pharmacy
Wingate University
Wingate, North Carolina

Richard Kent Zimmerman, MD, MPH
Professor
Department of Family Medicine
University of Pittsburgh
Pittsburgh, Pennsylvania

Jill N. Zink, MD
Department of Surgery
Akron General Medical Center
Akron, Ohio

Gennine M. Zinner, RNCS, ANP
Clinical Instructor
Department of Nursing
MGH Institute of Health Professions
Boston, Massachusetts

Anthony M. Zizza, III, MD
University of Massachusetts Medical
   School
Worcester, Massachusetts

Deborah E. Zuckerman, MD
Clinical Instructor
Department of Ophthalmology
Tufts University School of Medicine
Boston, Massachusetts;
Active Staff Physician
Department of Ophthalmology
Winchester Hospital
Winchester, Massachusetts

Susan L. Zweizig, MD
Associate Professor
Division of Gynecologic Oncology
Department of Obstetrics and Gynecology
University of Massachusetts Medical
   Center
Worcester, Massachusetts

CONTENTS

xlvi · · · **Contents**

5minuteconsult.com

U.S. Preventive Services Task Force Recommendations

This section is designed to be a quick reference to the best screening and prevention recommendations from the least biased sources. They are the United States Preventive Services Task Force (USPSTF), the U.S. Centers for Disease Control (CDC), the American Academy of Pediatrics, and the American Academy of Family Physicians. Each intervention receives an evidence-based grading set by the USPSTF. They are:

2005 TASK FORCE RATINGS
Strength of Recommendations

The U.S. Preventive Services Task Force (USPSTF) grades its recommendations according to one of five classifications (A, B, C, D, I) reflecting the strength of evidence and magnitude of *net benefit* (benefits minus harms).

A. The USPSTF strongly recommends clinicians provide [the service] to eligible patients. The USPSTF found good evidence that [the service] improves important health outcomes and concludes that benefits substantially outweigh harms.

B. The USPSTF recommends clinicians provide [this service] to eligible patients. The USPSTF found at least fair evidence that [the service] improves important health outcomes and concludes that benefits outweigh harms.

C. The USPSTF makes no recommendation for or against routine provision of [the service]. The USPSTF found at least fair evidence [the service] can improve health outcomes but concludes the balance of benefits and harms is too close to justify a general recommendation.

D. The USPSTF recommends against routinely providing [the service] to asymptomatic patients. The USPSTF found at least fair evidence that [the service] is ineffective or that harms outweigh benefits.

I. The USPSTF concludes the evidence is insufficient to recommend for or against routinely providing [the service]. Evidence the [service] is effective is lacking, of poor quality, or conflicting and the net benefit cannot be determined.

In 2008, the USPSTF updated their rating system for *all new recommendations*; they are:

GRADE DEFINITIONS AFTER MAY 2007
What the Grades Mean and Suggestions for Practice

The U.S. Preventive Services Task Force (USPSTF) has updated its definitions of the grades it assigns to recommendations and now includes "suggestions for practice" associated with each grade. The USPSTF has also defined levels of certainty regarding net benefit. These definitions apply to USPSTF recommendations voted on after May 2007.

Grade	Definition	Suggestions for Practice
A	The USPSTF recommends the service. There is high certainty that the net benefit is substantial.	Offer or provide this service.
B	The USPSTF recommends the service. There is high certainty that the net benefit is moderate or there is moderate certainty that the net benefit is moderate to substantial.	Offer or provide this service.
C	The USPSTF recommends against routinely providing the service. There may be considerations that support providing the service in an individual patient. There is at least moderate certainty that the net benefit is small.	Offer or provide this service only if other considerations support the offering or providing the service in an individual patient.
D	The USPSTF recommends against the service. There is moderate or high certainty that the service has no net benefit or that the harms outweigh the benefits.	Discourage the use of this service.
I Statement	The USPSTF concludes that the current evidence is insufficient to assess the balance of benefits and harms of the service. Evidence is lacking, of poor quality, or conflicting, and the balance of benefits and harms cannot be determined.	Read the clinical considerations section of USPSTF Recommendation Statement. If the service is offered, patients should understand the uncertainty about the balance of benefits and harms.

Levels of Certainty Regarding Net Benefit

Level of Certainty*	Description
High	The available evidence usually includes consistent results from well-designed, well-conducted studies in representative primary care populations. These studies assess the effects of the preventive service on health outcomes. This conclusion is therefore unlikely to be strongly affected by the results of future studies.
Moderate	The available evidence is sufficient to determine the effects of the preventive service on health outcomes, but confidence in the estimate is constrained by such factors as: • The number, size, or quality of individual studies. • Inconsistency of findings across individual studies. • Limited generalizability of findings to routine primary care practice. • Lack of coherence in the chain of evidence. As more information becomes available, the magnitude or direction of the observed effect could change, and this change may be large enough to alter the conclusion.
Low	The available evidence is insufficient to assess effects on health outcomes. Evidence is insufficient because of: • The limited number or size of studies. • Important flaws in study design or methods. • Inconsistency of findings across individual studies. • Gaps in the chain of evidence. • Findings not generalizable to routine primary care practice. • Lack of information on important health outcomes. More information may allow estimation of effects on health outcomes.

*The USPSTF defines certainty as "likelihood that the USPSTF assessment of the net benefit of a preventive service is correct." The net benefit is defined as benefit minus harm of the preventive service as implemented in a general, primary care population. The USPSTF assigns a certainty level based on the nature of the overall evidence available to assess the net benefit of a preventive service.
Current as of May 2008

These recommendations should be tailored to patients' preferences. For example, screening for carcinoma of the prostate receives an "I" recommendation, yet many providers (and their patients) are concerned. Use of a detailed *Informed Consent* discussion for prostate cancer screening empowers the patient and the clinician to use these recommendations in a patient-centered manner.

Absent are in these recommendations "vested interests." Many disease specific groups (American Cancer Society, the American Heart Association, National Osteoporosis Foundation, etc.) suggest interventions that serve *their* goals, but do not always have a strong evidence base (i.e. PSA testing for Prostate Cancer, Bone Mineral Density before age 65, etc.). The USPSTF provides the least biased evaluations.

—Frank J. Domino, MD
Editor-in-Chief

HEALTH MAINTENANCE: BIRTH TO 10 YEARS

(http://www.ahrq.gov/clinic/cps3dix.htm)

Leading causes of death:

- Perinatal infections
- Congenital anomalies
- Sudden infant death syndrome (SIDS)
- Accidents (drowning, abuse)
- Motor vehicle accidents

Recommended counseling, testing or interventions:

Height, weight, growth chart	
Immunizations (*http://www.cdc.gov/nip/* or *www.immunizationed.org*)	(DPaT, IPV, Hib, hepatitis A, hepatitis B, MMR, pneumococcal, rotavirus, varicella, influenza 6 mo–18 years)
Counseling:	Injury prevention: –Car seats –Seat belts –Bicycle helmets –Smoke & carbon monoxide detector –Window/stair guards –Firearm storage
Breast fed infants	400 IU vitamin D started before 2 months
Congenital hypothyroidism	At birth
Dental caries in preschool children	Oral fluoride supplementation for children older than 6 months whose primary water source is deficient in fluoride –6 months–3 years 0.25 mg, –3–6 years 0.5 mg, –6–16 years 1.0 mg/day
Diet	Low Saturated Fat diet & Physical Exercise
Hearing screening	At birth
Lead screening	High risk: Minority, urban residency, low SES, house built before 1950, recent immigration
Obesity	Screen children >/= 6 years for obesity and offer/refer to comprehensive, intensive behavioral interventions to promote improvement in weight status
Substance abuse prevention	Tobacco, alcohol counseling
Tuberculosis screening	High risk: Urban residency, Low SES, recent immigration or exposure to recent immigrant
Vision screening: strabismus, amblyopia, visual acuity	For first 5 years of life

Insufficient to recommend for or against:

Dysplasia of the hip	By physical examination

Leading causes of death:

- Motor vehicle accidents
- Unintentional injuries
- Homicide
- Suicide
- Malignant neoplasms

Immunizations:
(http://www.cdc.gov/vaccines/ or www.immunizationed.org)

Tetanus-diphtheria-pertussis (Tdap), meningococcal (MCV4), human papilloma virus (females), varicella (2 total for those without immunity), influenza

Disease	Recommended intervention (A or B grade)
General	Height, weight, BMI, blood pressure, injury prevention (seat belts, firearms), low saturated fat diet, physical exercise
Alcohol & substance abuse screening	*
Breast & ovarian cancer by BRCA mutation	If high risk: Ashkenazi, or two 1° relatives with breast or ovarian cancer at <50 years of age
Cervical cancer screening	3 years after first intercourse or age 21
Chlamydia, gonorrhea and syphilis screening	If high risk: Sexually active, pregnancy, IV drug use
Depression	In clinical practices that have systems in place to assure accurate diagnosis, effective treatment, and followup.
Diabetes mellitus (non fasting glucose)	if BP >135/80
Domestic/family violence	If sexually active
HIV screening	If high risk: Sexually active, pregnancy, IV drug use
Hepatitis B	If high risk: Sexually active, pregnancy, IV drug use
Lipid disorders	20 to 35 if they are at increased risk for coronary heart disease (family history of premature CHD, diabetes, etc.)
Tuberculosis screening	If high risk: Travel, immigrant, alcohol abuse, IV drug use
Obesity (counseling for obese patients)	Screen children >/= 6 years for obesity and offer/refer to comprehensive, intensive behavioral interventions to promote improvement in weight status.
Folic acid for women	all women planning or capable of pregnancy take a daily supplement of 0.4 to 0.8 mg (400 to 800 μg) of folic acid
Tobacco cessation	Ask all adults about tobacco use and provide tobacco cessation interventions for those who use tobacco
Suicide screening	Depression*

*Additional screening

Alcohol abuse	"Risky"/"hazardous" alcohol use: >7 drinks per week or more than 3 drinks on any on occasion for women, and >14 drinks per week or more than 4 drinks on any one occasion for men. OR
	Screen: "on any occasion during the last 3 months, have had more than 5 alcohol drinks" or
	CAGE: Tried to CUT down, been ANGERED by questions about your drinking, felt GUILTY about your drinking, had an EYE OPENER (drink in the morning)
Domestic violence	Screen all at risk patients (all women, especially when pregnant) "Do you feel safe in your present relationship?" "Have you been hit, kicked, punched or otherwise hurt in the last year?"
Substance abuse	Question about drug use and related problems should be considered in all adolescent and adult.
Suicide	Risk factors include history of mood or other mental disorder, substance abuse, history of "deliberate self-harm"

Against (D grade)

Coronary heart disease via ECG, ETT, etc.
Hemochromatosis
Scoliosis screening
Testicular cancer

(http://www.ahrq.gov/clinic/cps3dix.htm)

Leading causes of death

Accidental overdose (narcotics, etc.)

Motor vehicle accidents

Cardiovascular disease

Malignant neoplasm

HIV

Immunizations *(http://www.cdc.gov/nip/ or http://www.immunizationed.org/)*

Tetanus	Tdap every 10 years or just at age 50 (if completed primary series)
Influenza	All adults

Disease	Recommended intervention (A or B grade)
General	Height, weight, BMI, blood pressure, injury prevention (seat belts, firearms), low saturated fat diet, physical exercise
Alcohol and substance abuse	*
Breast and ovarian cancer by genetic testing	Refer for genetic counseling if: Ashkenazi heritage, or two 1st degree relatives with breast or ovarian cancer at <50 years of age
Breast cancer screening by Mammography	Mammography starting at age >/= 40; repeat every 1–2 years
Cervical cancer screening	Begin 3 years after first intercourse
Coronary heart disease	Evidence is insufficient to recommend using nontraditional risk factors (high-sensitivity C-reactive protein (hs-CRP), ankle-brachial index (ABI), leukocyte count, fasting blood glucose level, periodontal disease, carotid intima-media thickness (carotid IMT), coronary artery calcification (CAC) score on electron-beam computed tomography (EBCT), homocysteine level, and lipoprotein(a) level) to screen asymptomatic men and women with no history of CHD to prevent CHD events
Depression	In clinical practices that have systems in place to assure accurate diagnosis, effective treatment, and follow up.
Diabetes mellitus, type II (if BP >135/80)	Random serum glucose if sustained blood pressure (either treated or untreated) greater than 135/80 mm Hg
Domestic/family violence	If sexually active
Diet/obesity	Intensive behavioral dietary counseling for patients with known risk factors for cardiovascular and diet-related chronic disease
Chlamydia, gonorrhea, syphilis testing	All adults who are at increased risk (sexually active, IV drug use, etc.)
HIV screening	All adults who are at increased risk (sexually active, IV drug use, etc.)
Hepatitis B	All pregnant women and those with multiple sexual partners, IV drug use, etc.
Lipid disorders	Men: 35 and older for lipid disorders & 20 to 35 if they are at increased risk for coronary heart disease (family history of premature CHD, diabetes, etc.)
	Women: 45 and older for lipid disorders & 20 to 35 if they are at increased risk for coronary heart disease (family history of premature CHD, diabetes, etc.)
Suicide screening	If depressed*
Tobacco abuse	Ask all adults about tobacco use and provide tobacco cessation interventions for those who use tobacco
Tuberculosis screening	If high risk: Travel, immigrant, alcohol abuse, IV drug use

*Additional screening

Alcohol abuse	"Risky"/"hazardous" alcohol use: >7 drinks per week or more than 3 drinks on any on occasion for women, and >14 drinks per week or more than 4 drinks on any one occasion for men. OR Screen: "on any occasion during the last 3 months, have had more than 5 alcohol drinks" or CAGE: tried to CUT down, been ANGERED by questions about your drinking, felt GUILTY about your drinking, had an EYE OPENER (drink in the morning)
Domestic violence	Screen all at risk patients (all women, especially when pregnant) "Do you feel safe in your present relationship?" "Have you been hit, kicked, punched or otherwise hurt in the last year?"
Substance abuse	Questioning about drug use and related problems should be considered in all adolescent and adult.
Suicide	Risk factors include history of mood or other mental disorder, substance abuse, history of "deliberate self-harm"

Recommends against

Aspirin	The USPSTF recommends against the use of aspirin for stroke prevention in women younger than 55 years and for myocardial infarction prevention in men younger than 45 years.

Leading Causes of Death

Cardiovascular Disease

Malignant Neoplasm

Accidents

Cirrhosis

Immunizations *(http://www.cdc.gov/nip/ or http://www.immunizationed.org/)*

Tetanus	Tdap every 10 years or just at age 50 (if completed primary series)
Influenza	All adults

Disease / Recommended intervention (A or B grade)

Disease	Recommended intervention (A or B grade)
General	Height, weight, BMI, blood pressure, injury prevention (seat belts, firearms), low saturated fat diet, physical exercise
Alcohol and substance abuse	*Insufficient for population; screen at risk
Aspirin	Recommends use of aspirin for men age 45 to 79 and women age 55 to 79 years when potential benefit due to a reduction in myocardial infarctions outweighs the potential harm due to an increase in gastrointestinal hemorrhage.
Breast and ovarian cancer by genetic testing	Refer for genetic counseling if: Ashkenazi heritage, or two 1st degree relatives with breast or ovarian cancer at <50 years of age
Breast cancer screening by mammography	Mammography starting at Age >/= 50; repeat every 1–2 years
Cervical cancer screening	Begin 3 years after first intercourse
Chlamydia, gonorrhea, syphilis testing	All adults who are at increased risk (sexually active, IV drug use, etc.)
Colon cancer	Start at age 50–75 by fecal occult blood testing, sigmoidoscopy, or colonoscopy
Coronary heart disease	Evidence is insufficient to recommend using nontraditional risk factors (high-sensitivity C-reactive protein (hs-CRP), ankle-brachial index (ABI), leukocyte count, fasting blood glucose level, periodontal disease, carotid intima-media thickness (carotid IMT), coronary artery calcification (CAC) score on electron-beam computed tomography (EBCT), homocysteine level, and lipoprotein(a) level) to screen asymptomatic men and women with no history of CHD to prevent CHD events
Depression	In clinical practices that have systems in place to assure accurate diagnosis, effective treatment, and follow up.
Diabetes mellitus, type II if BP > 135/80	Random serum glucose if sustained blood pressure (either treated or untreated) greater than 135/80 mm Hg
Domestic/family violence	*If sexually active
Diet/obesity	Intensive behavioral dietary counseling for patients with known risk factors for cardiovascular and diet-related chronic disease
HIV screening	All adults who are at increased risk (sexually active, IV drug use, etc.)
Hepatitis B	All pregnant women and those with multiple sexual partners, IV drug use, etc.
Lipid disorders	All Adults over 45 should be screened
Suicide screening	If depressed*
Tobacco abuse	Ask all adults about tobacco use and provide tobacco cessation interventions for those who use tobacco
Tuberculosis screening	If high risk: Travel, immigrant, alcohol abuse, IV drug use

*Additional screening

Alcohol abuse	"Risky"/"hazardous" alcohol use: >7 drinks per week or more than 3 drinks on any on occasion for women, and >14 drinks per week or more than 4 drinks on any one occasion for men. OR Screen: "on any occasion during the last 3 months, have had more than 5 alcohol drinks" or CAGE: Tried to CUT down, been ANGERED by questions about your drinking, felt GUILTY about your drinking, had an EYE OPENER (drink in the morning)
Domestic violence	Screen all at risk patients (all women, especially when pregnant) "Do you feel safe in your present relationship?" "Have you been hit, kicked, punched or otherwise hurt in the last year?"
Substance abuse	Questioning about drug use and related problems should be considered in all adolescent and adult.
Suicide	Risk factors include history of mood or other mental disorder, substance abuse, history of "deliberate self-harm"

HEALTH MAINTENANCE 65 YEARS AND ABOVE

(http://www.ahrq.gov/clinic/cps3dix.htm)

Leading causes of death

Cardiovascular disease

Malignant neoplasm

Stoke

COPD

Dementia

Immunizations *(http://www.cdc.gov/nip/ or http://www.immunizationed.org/)*

Tetanus	Tdap every 10 years or just at age 50 (if completed primary series)
Influenza	All adults

Disease	Recommended Intervention (A or B Grade)
General	Height, weight, BMI, blood pressure, injury prevention (seat belts, firearms), low saturated fat diet, physical exercise
Alcohol and substance abuse	*Insufficient for population; screen at risk
Aspirin	Recommends use of aspirin for men age 45 to 79 and women age 55 to 79 years when potential benefit due to a reduction in myocardial infarctions outweighs the potential harm due to an increase in gastrointestinal hemorrhage.
Breast and ovarian cancer by genetic testing	Refer for genetic counseling if: Ashkenazi heritage, or two 1st degree relatives with breast or ovarian cancer at <50 years of age
Breast cancer screening by mammography	Mammography through Age 75; repeat every 1–2 years; after age 75, at discretion
Cervical cancer screening	May cease to screen if had adequate recent screening and are not at high risk
Chlamydia, gonorrhea, syphilis testing	All adults who are at increased risk (sexually active, IV drug use, etc.)
Colon cancer	Start at age 50–75 by fecal occult blood testing, sigmoidoscopy, or colonoscopy
Coronary Heart Disease	Evidence is insufficient to recommend using nontraditional risk factors (high-sensitivity C-reactive protein (hs-CRP), ankle-brachial index (ABI), leukocyte count, fasting blood glucose level, periodontal disease, carotid intima-media thickness (carotid IMT), coronary artery calcification (CAC) score on electron-beam computed tomography (EBCT), homocysteine level, and lipoprotein(a) level) to screen asymptomatic men and women with no history of CHD to prevent CHD events
Depression	In clinical practices that have systems in place to assure accurate diagnosis, effective treatment, and follow up.
Diabetes mellitus, type II if BP >135/80	Random serum glucose if sustained blood pressure (either treated or untreated) greater than 135/80 mm Hg
Domestic/family violence	*If sexually active
Diet/obesity	Intensive behavioral dietary counseling for patients with known risk factors for cardiovascular and diet-related chronic disease
HIV screening	All adults who are at increased risk (sexually active, IV drug use, etc.)
Hepatitis B	All pregnant women and those with multiple sexual partners, IV drug use, etc.
Lipid disorders	All adults over 45 should be screened
Suicide screening	If depressed*
Tobacco abuse	Ask all adults about tobacco use and provide tobacco cessation interventions for those who use tobacco
Tuberculosis screening	If high risk: Travel, immigrant, alcohol abuse, IV drug use

*Additional screening

Alcohol abuse	"Risky"/"hazardous" alcohol use: >7 drinks per week or more than 3 drinks on any on occasion for women, and >14 drinks per week or more than 4 drinks on any one occasion for men. OR Screen: "on any occasion during the last 3 months, have had more than 5 alcohol drinks" or CAGE: tried to CUT down, been ANGERED by questions about your drinking, felt GUILTY about your drinking, had an EYE OPENER (drink in the morning)
Domestic violence	Screen all at risk patients (all women, especially when pregnant) "Do you feel safe in your present relationship?" "Have you been hit, kicked, punched or otherwise hurt in the last year?"
Substance abuse	Questioning about drug use and related problems should be considered in all adolescent and adult.
Suicide	Risk factors include history of mood or other mental disorder, substance abuse, history of "deliberate self-harm"

Diagnosis and Treatment: An Algorithmic Approach

This section contains flowcharts (or algorithms) to help the reader in the diagnosis of clinical signs and symptoms, and treatment of a variety of clinical problems. They are organized by the presenting sign, symptom or diagnosis.

These algorithms were designed to be used as a quick reference and adjunct to the reader's clinical knowledge and impression. They are not an exhaustive review of the management of a problem, nor are they meant to be a complete list of diseases.

ABDOMINAL PAIN, CHRONIC

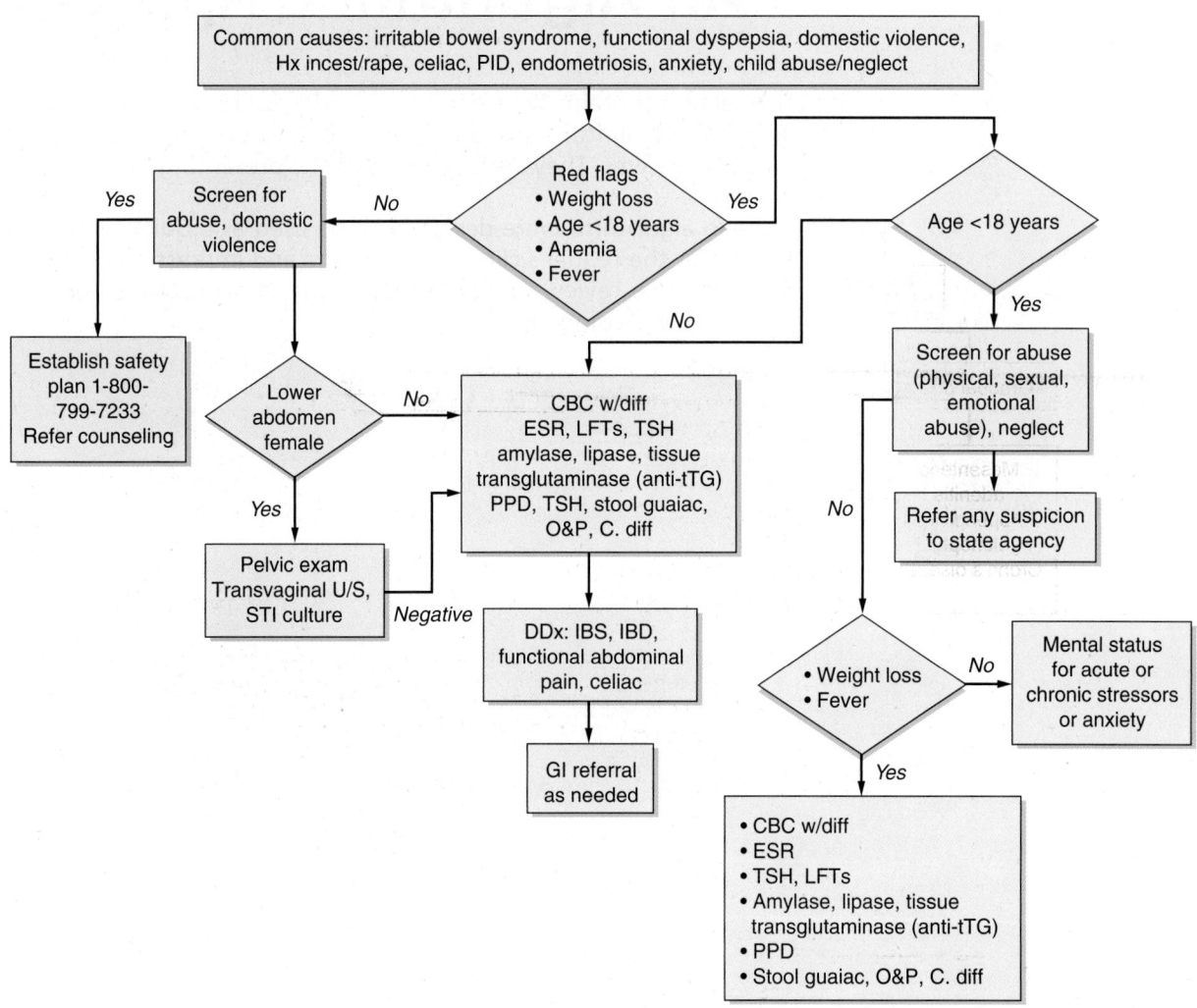

Common causes: irritable bowel syndrome, functional dyspepsia, domestic violence, Hx incest/rape, celiac, PID, endometriosis, anxiety, child abuse/neglect

Red flags
- Weight loss
- Age <18 years
- Anemia
- Fever

Yes → Screen for abuse, domestic violence → Yes → Establish safety plan 1-800-799-7233 Refer counseling

Lower abdomen female

No → CBC w/diff ESR, LFTs, TSH amylase, lipase, tissue transglutaminase (anti-tTG) PPD, TSH, stool guaiac, O&P, C. diff

Yes → Pelvic exam Transvaginal U/S, STI culture → Negative

DDx: IBS, IBD, functional abdominal pain, celiac

GI referral as needed

Age <18 years

Yes → Screen for abuse (physical, sexual, emotional abuse), neglect → Refer any suspicion to state agency

No

- Weight loss
- Fever

No → Mental status for acute or chronic stressors or anxiety

Yes →
- CBC w/diff
- ESR
- TSH, LFTs
- Amylase, lipase, tissue transglutaminase (anti-tTG)
- PPD
- Stool guaiac, O&P, C. diff

Josue Chery, MD

ABDOMINAL PAIN, LOWER

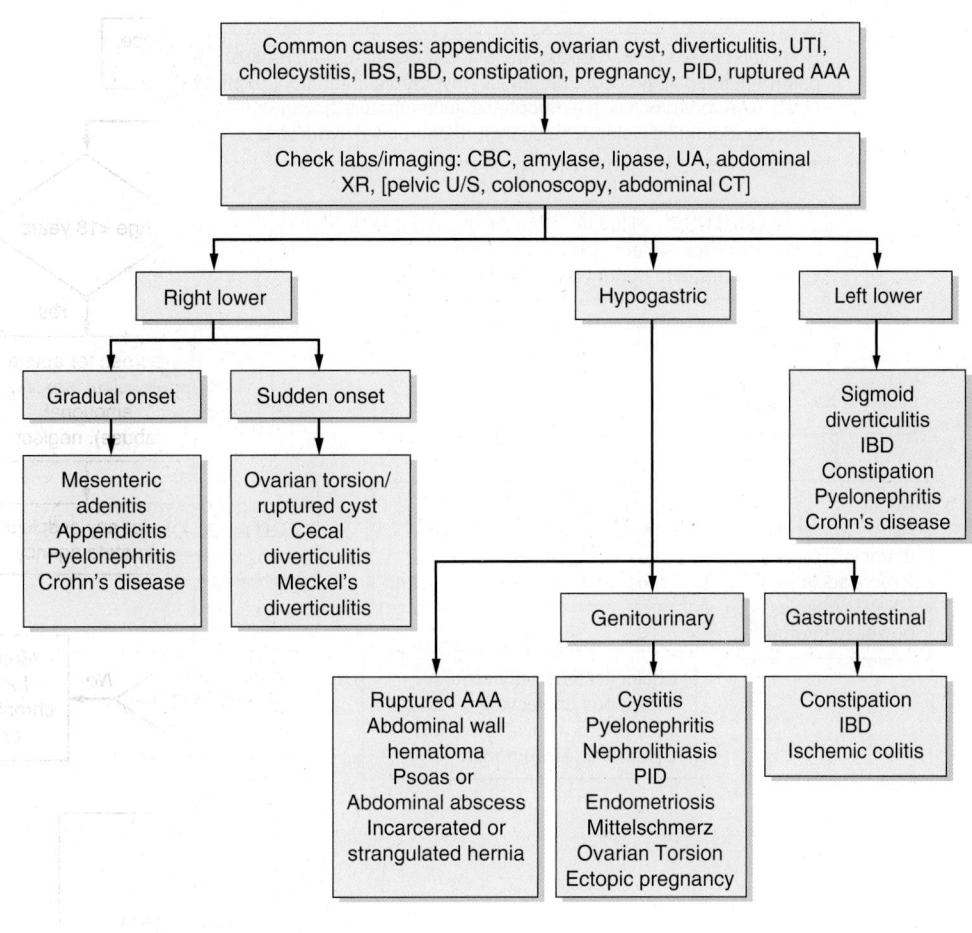

Common causes: appendicitis, ovarian cyst, diverticulitis, UTI, cholecystitis, IBS, IBD, constipation, pregnancy, PID, ruptured AAA

Check labs/imaging: CBC, amylase, lipase, UA, abdominal XR, [pelvic U/S, colonoscopy, abdominal CT]

Right lower

Hypogastric

Left lower

Sigmoid diverticulitis
IBD
Constipation
Pyelonephritis
Crohn's disease

Gradual onset

Sudden onset

Mesenteric adenitis
Appendicitis
Pyelonephritis
Crohn's disease

Ovarian torsion/ ruptured cyst
Cecal diverticulitis
Meckel's diverticulitis

Genitourinary

Gastrointestinal

Ruptured AAA
Abdominal wall hematoma
Psoas or Abdominal abscess
Incarcerated or strangulated hernia

Cystitis
Pyelonephritis
Nephrolithiasis
PID
Endometriosis
Mittelschmerz
Ovarian Torsion
Ectopic pregnancy

Constipation
IBD
Ischemic colitis

Nilay Patel, MD and Siva Vithananthan, MD

Scand J Gastroenterol. 1999;231(Suppl):3–8.

ABDOMINAL PAIN, UPPER

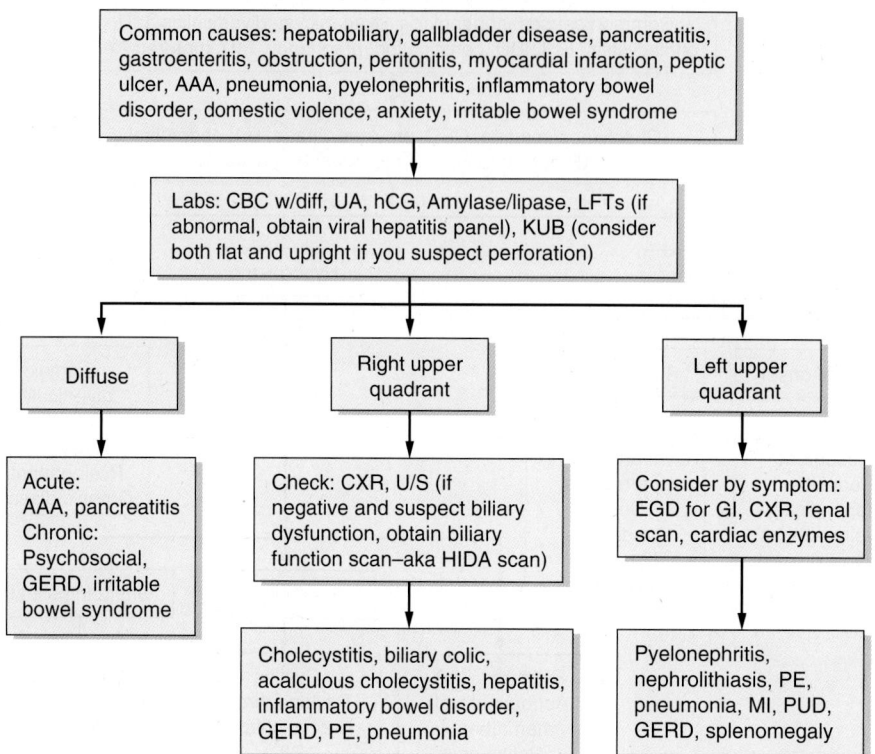

Common causes: hepatobiliary, gallbladder disease, pancreatitis, gastroenteritis, obstruction, peritonitis, myocardial infarction, peptic ulcer, AAA, pneumonia, pyelonephritis, inflammatory bowel disorder, domestic violence, anxiety, irritable bowel syndrome

Labs: CBC w/diff, UA, hCG, Amylase/lipase, LFTs (if abnormal, obtain viral hepatitis panel), KUB (consider both flat and upright if you suspect perforation)

Diffuse

Right upper quadrant

Left upper quadrant

Acute:
AAA, pancreatitis
Chronic:
Psychosocial, GERD, irritable bowel syndrome

Check: CXR, U/S (if negative and suspect biliary dysfunction, obtain biliary function scan–aka HIDA scan)

Consider by symptom: EGD for GI, CXR, renal scan, cardiac enzymes

Cholecystitis, biliary colic, acalculous cholecystitis, hepatitis, inflammatory bowel disorder, GERD, PE, pneumonia

Pyelonephritis, nephrolithiasis, PE, pneumonia, MI, PUD, GERD, splenomegaly

Nilay Patel, MD and Siva Vithananthan, MD

Scand J Gastroenterol. 1999;231(Suppl):3–8.

ABDOMINAL RIGIDITY

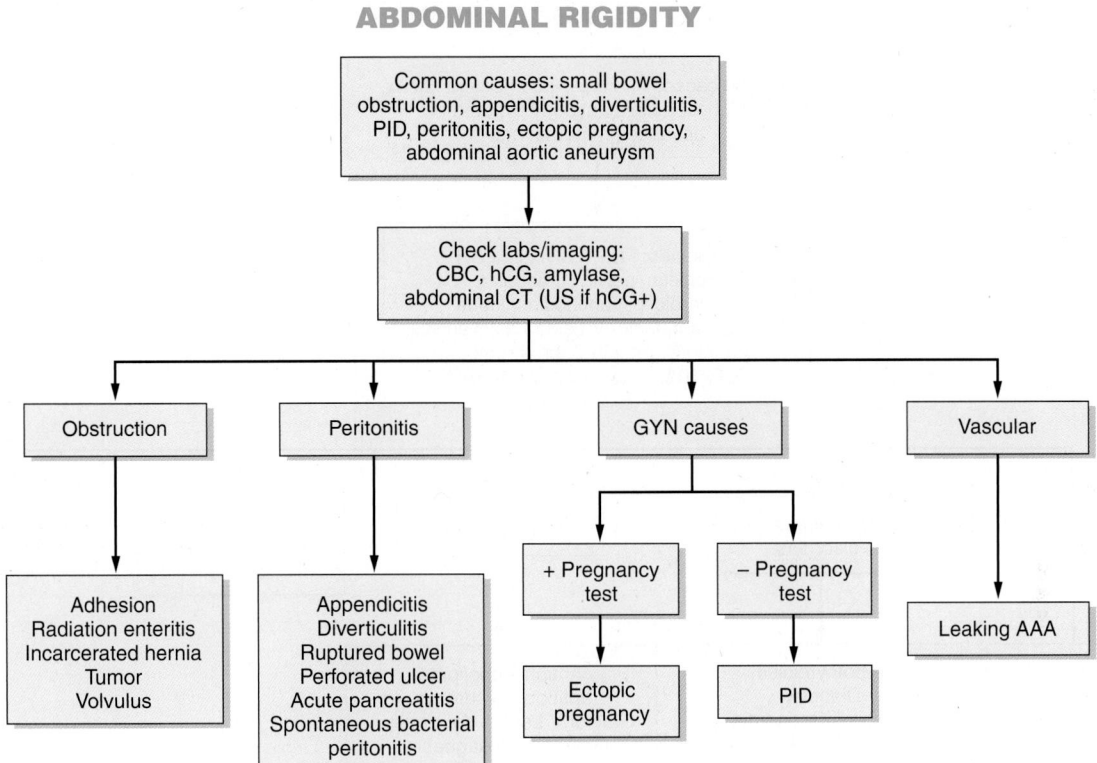

Robert A. Baldor, MD and Alan M. Ehrlich, MD

Med Clin North Am. 2008;92(3):599–625, viii–ix.

ABORTION, RECURRENT

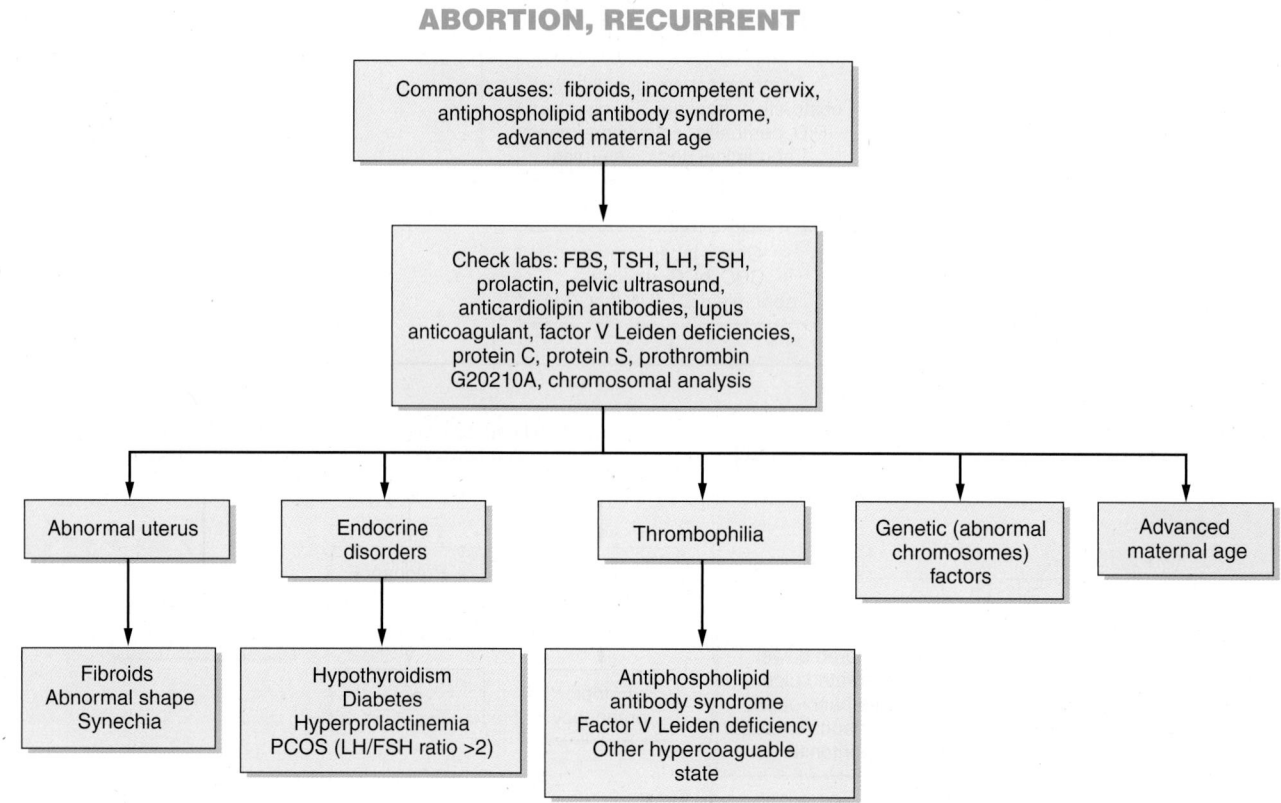

Common causes: fibroids, incompetent cervix, antiphospholipid antibody syndrome, advanced maternal age

Check labs: FBS, TSH, LH, FSH, prolactin, pelvic ultrasound, anticardiolipin antibodies, lupus anticoagulant, factor V Leiden deficiencies, protein C, protein S, prothrombin G20210A, chromosomal analysis

- Abnormal uterus
  - Fibroids
    Abnormal shape
    Synechia
- Endocrine disorders
  - Hypothyroidism
    Diabetes
    Hyperprolactinemia
    PCOS (LH/FSH ratio >2)
- Thrombophilia
  - Antiphospholipid antibody syndrome
    Factor V Leiden deficiency
    Other hypercoaguable state
- Genetic (abnormal chromosomes) factors
- Advanced maternal age

Robert A. Baldor, MD and Alan M. Ehrlich, MD

J Obstet Gynaecol Res. 2009;35(4):609–22.

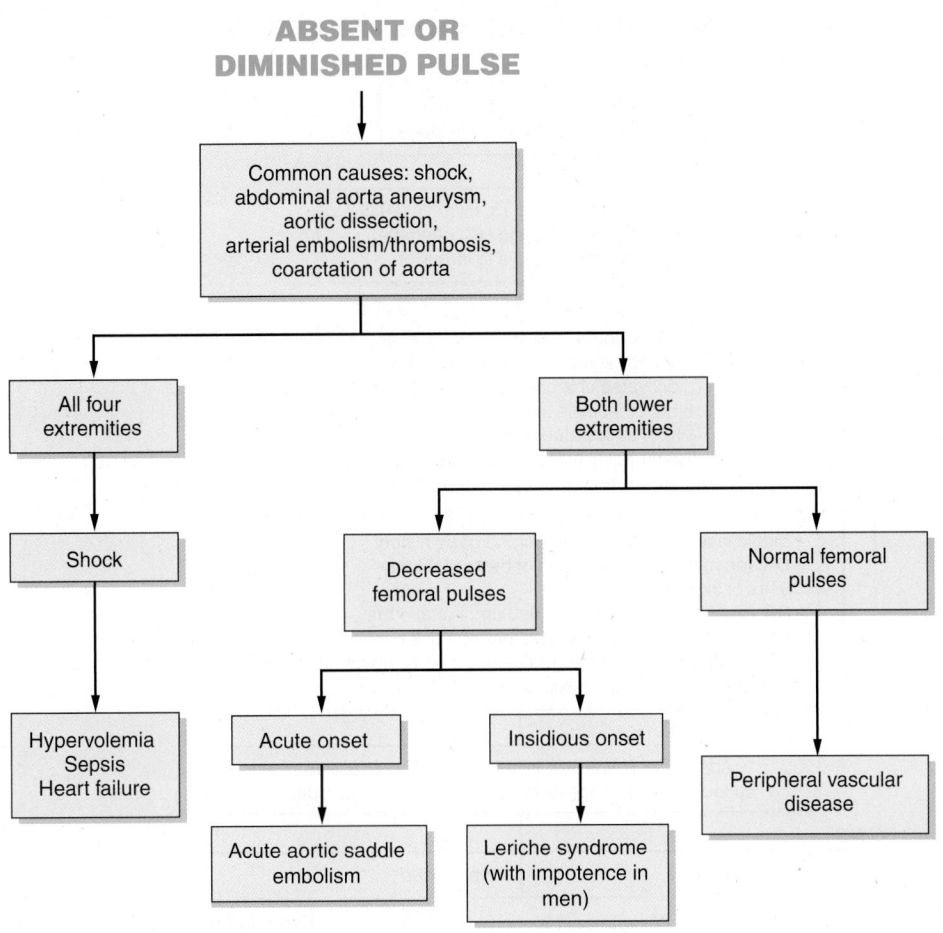

Robert A. Baldor, MD and Alan M. Ehrlich, MD

Semin Vasc Surg. 2009;22(1):10–6.

ACETAMINOPHEN POISONING, TREATMENT

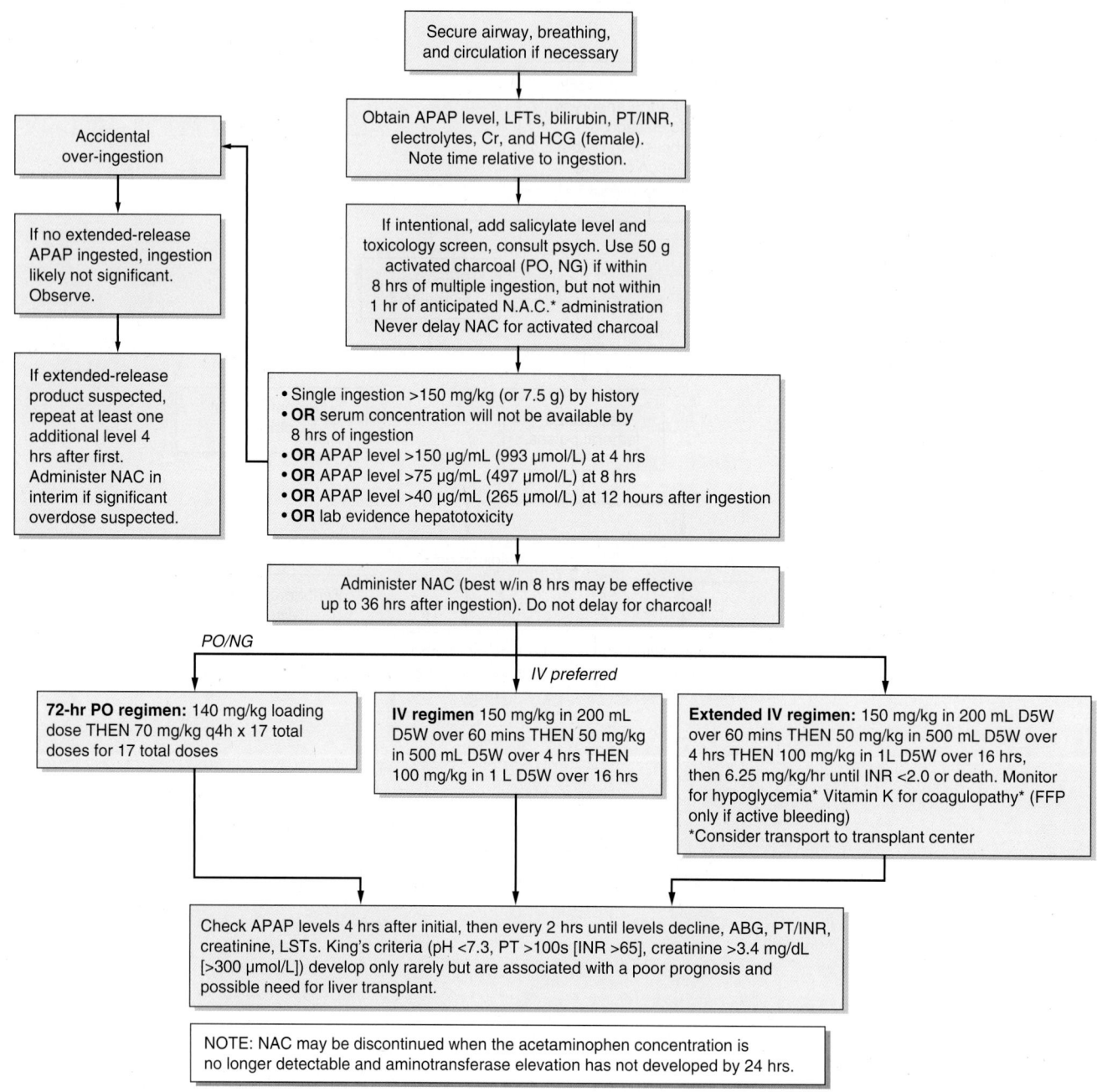

Secure airway, breathing, and circulation if necessary

Obtain APAP level, LFTs, bilirubin, PT/INR, electrolytes, Cr, and HCG (female). Note time relative to ingestion.

If intentional, add salicylate level and toxicology screen, consult psych. Use 50 g activated charcoal (PO, NG) if within 8 hrs of multiple ingestion, but not within 1 hr of anticipated N.A.C.* administration Never delay NAC for activated charcoal

Accidental over-ingestion

If no extended-release APAP ingested, ingestion likely not significant. Observe.

If extended-release product suspected, repeat at least one additional level 4 hrs after first. Administer NAC in interim if significant overdose suspected.

- Single ingestion >150 mg/kg (or 7.5 g) by history
- **OR** serum concentration will not be available by 8 hrs of ingestion
- **OR** APAP level >150 µg/mL (993 µmol/L) at 4 hrs
- **OR** APAP level >75 µg/mL (497 µmol/L) at 8 hrs
- **OR** APAP level >40 µg/mL (265 µmol/L) at 12 hours after ingestion
- **OR** lab evidence hepatotoxicity

Administer NAC (best w/in 8 hrs may be effective up to 36 hrs after ingestion). Do not delay for charcoal!

PO/NG

IV preferred

72-hr PO regimen: 140 mg/kg loading dose THEN 70 mg/kg q4h x 17 total doses for 17 total doses

IV regimen 150 mg/kg in 200 mL D5W over 60 mins THEN 50 mg/kg in 500 mL D5W over 4 hrs THEN 100 mg/kg in 1 L D5W over 16 hrs

Extended IV regimen: 150 mg/kg in 200 mL D5W over 60 mins THEN 50 mg/kg in 500 mL D5W over 4 hrs THEN 100 mg/kg in 1L D5W over 16 hrs, then 6.25 mg/kg/hr until INR <2.0 or death. Monitor for hypoglycemia* Vitamin K for coagulopathy* (FFP only if active bleeding) *Consider transport to transplant center

Check APAP levels 4 hrs after initial, then every 2 hrs until levels decline, ABG, PT/INR, creatinine, LSTs. King's criteria (pH <7.3, PT >100s [INR >65], creatinine >3.4 mg/dL [>300 µmol/L]) develop only rarely but are associated with a poor prognosis and possible need for liver transplant.

NOTE: NAC may be discontinued when the acetaminophen concentration is no longer detectable and aminotransferase elevation has not developed by 24 hrs.

*APAP = Acetaminophen NAC = N-acetylcysteine

John Jenkins, MD

Med J Aust. 2008;188(5):296–301.

ACID PHOSPHATASE ELEVATION

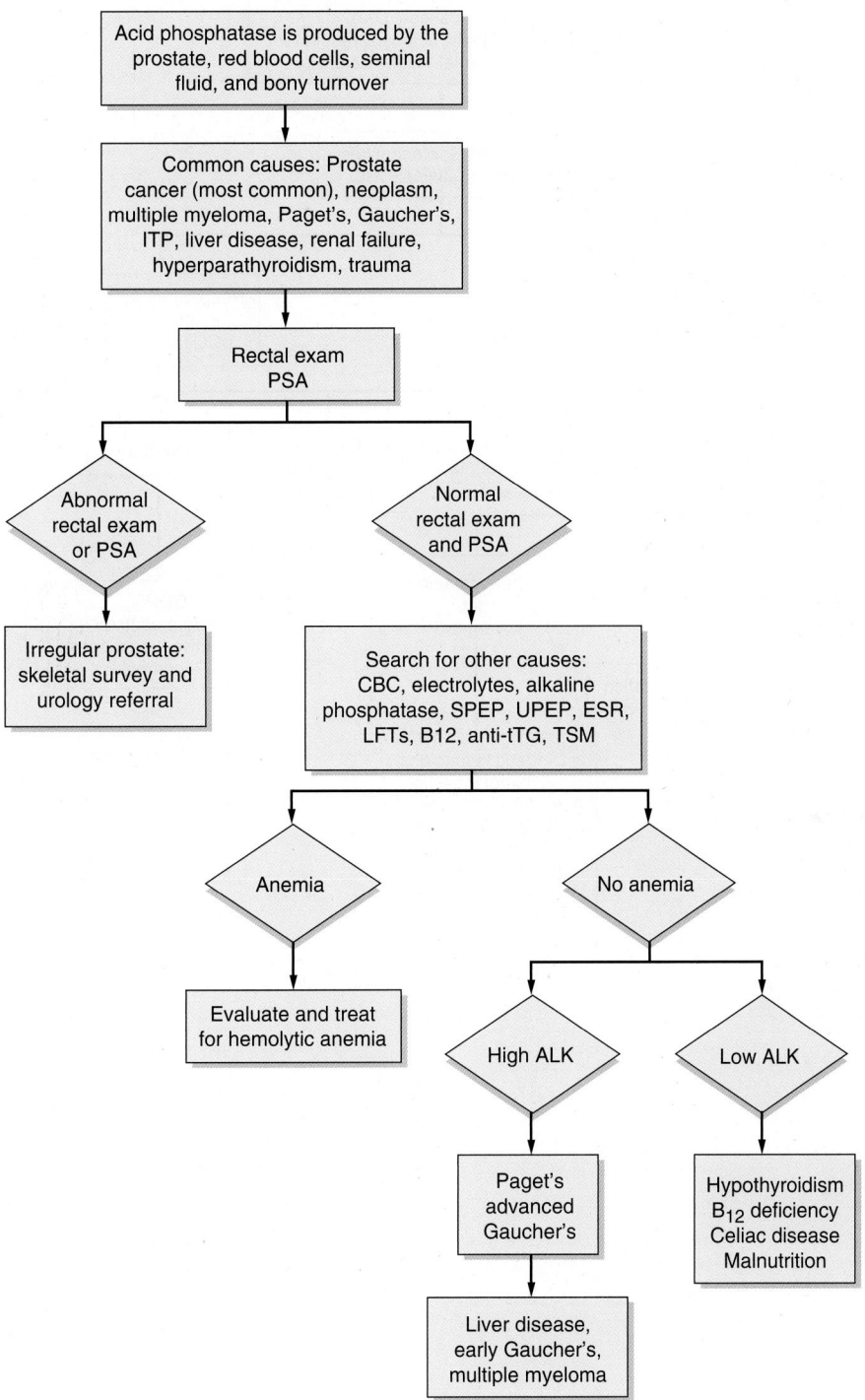

Laura Hagopian, MD and Michael Snyder, MD

ACIDOSIS

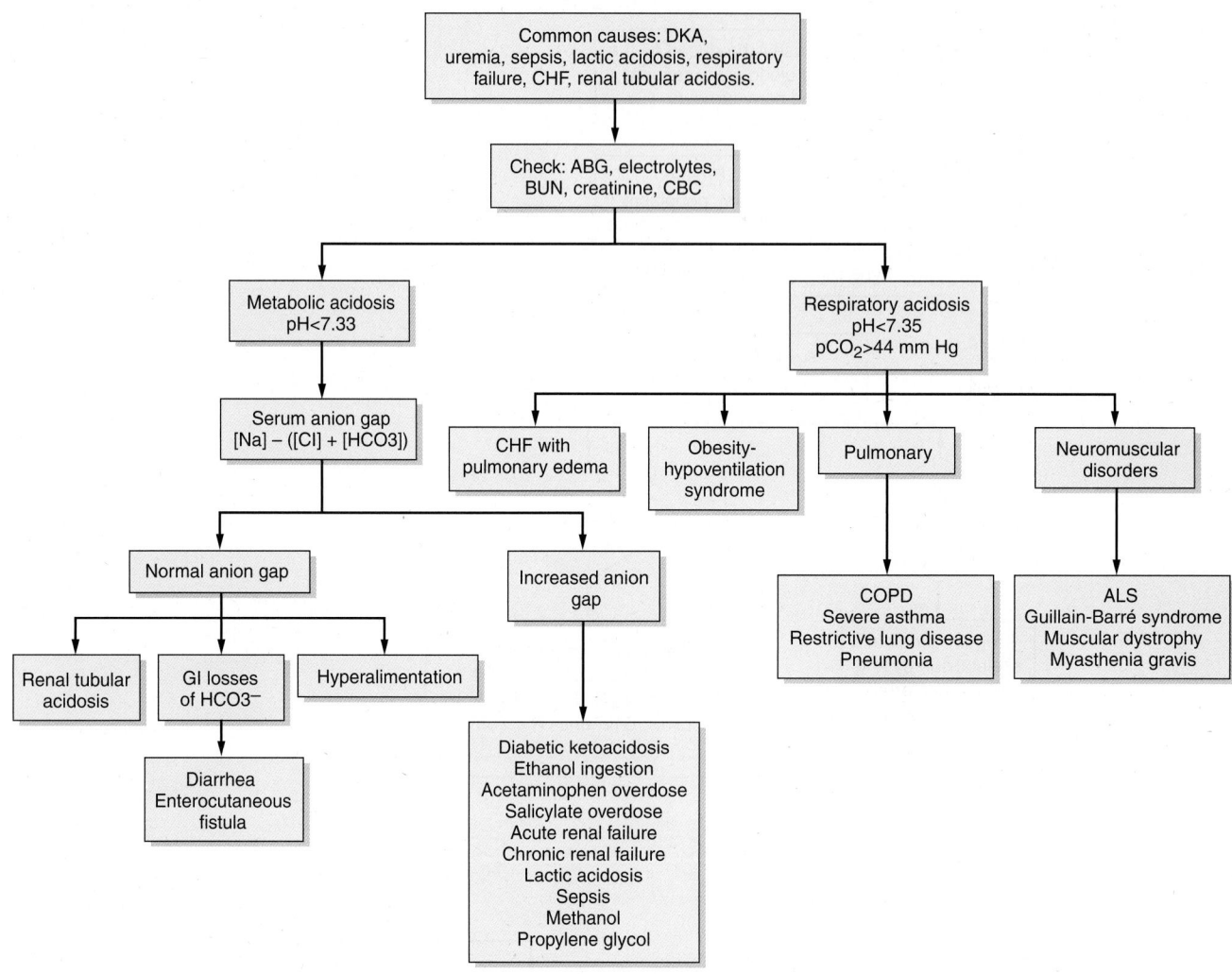

Common causes: DKA, uremia, sepsis, lactic acidosis, respiratory failure, CHF, renal tubular acidosis.

Check: ABG, electrolytes, BUN, creatinine, CBC

Metabolic acidosis
pH<7.33

Respiratory acidosis
pH<7.35
pCO_2>44 mm Hg

Serum anion gap
[Na] − ([Cl] + [HCO3])

CHF with pulmonary edema

Obesity-hypoventilation syndrome

Pulmonary

Neuromuscular disorders

Normal anion gap

Increased anion gap

COPD
Severe asthma
Restrictive lung disease
Pneumonia

ALS
Guillain-Barré syndrome
Muscular dystrophy
Myasthenia gravis

Renal tubular acidosis

GI losses of HCO3−

Hyperalimentation

Diarrhea
Enterocutaneous fistula

Diabetic ketoacidosis
Ethanol ingestion
Acetaminophen overdose
Salicylate overdose
Acute renal failure
Chronic renal failure
Lactic acidosis
Sepsis
Methanol
Propylene glycol

Robert A. Baldor, MD and Alan M. Ehrlich, MD

Diabetes Care. 2009;32(7):1335–43.

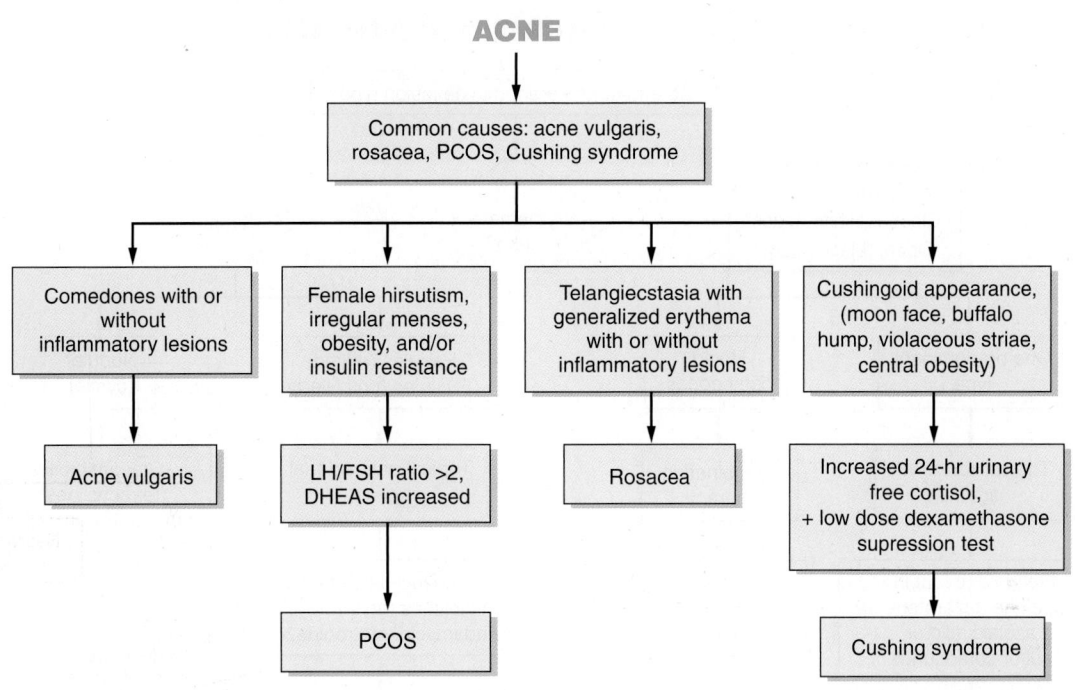

ACNE

Common causes: acne vulgaris, rosacea, PCOS, Cushing syndrome

Comedones with or without inflammatory lesions → Acne vulgaris

Female hirsutism, irregular menses, obesity, and/or insulin resistance → LH/FSH ratio >2, DHEAS increased → PCOS

Telangiecstasia with generalized erythema with or without inflammatory lesions → Rosacea

Cushingoid appearance, (moon face, buffalo hump, violaceous striae, central obesity) → Increased 24-hr urinary free cortisol, + low dose dexamethasone supression test → Cushing syndrome

Robert A. Baldor, MD and Alan M. Ehrlich, MD

Dermatol Clin. 2009;27(4):459–71, vi.

ACNE VULGARIS, TREATMENT

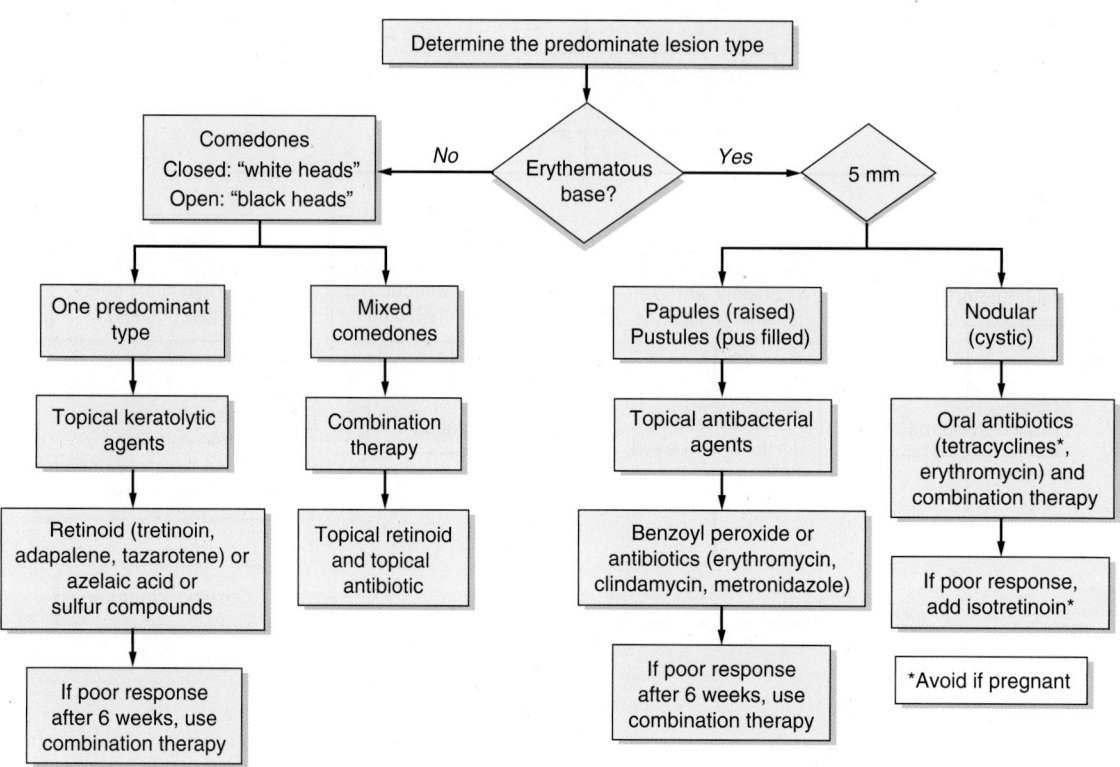

Robert A. Baldor

Treat Guidel Med Lett. 2008;6(75):75–82.

ADRENOCORTICAL INSUFFICIENCY

Common causes: corticosteroid withdrawal, TB, HIV infection, malignancy, pituitary disorders

↓

Recent corticosteroid use

→ Yes
→ No

Yes:
Corticosteroid withdrawal

No:
Check: HIV test, PPD, RPR, ACTH CT of adrenals, brain MRI

- Infections
  - TB
  - HIV infection
  - Syphilis
  - Fungal infection

- Metastatic disease
  - Lung
  - Breast
  - Colon
  - Lymphoma

- Adrenal abnormality
  - Meningococcemia
  - Sepsis
  - Thrombotic disorders

- Pituitary ACTH deficiency
  - Tumor
  - Aneurysm
  - Infarction
  - Sheehan syndrome

Robert A. Baldor, MD and Alan M. Ehrlich, MD

Ann Intern Med. 2003;139(3):194–204.

ALCOHOL WITHDRAWAL, TREATMENT

History: Duration and quantity of alcohol intake, time since last drink, previous episodes of alcohol withdrawal, concurrent substance use, pre-existing medical and psychiatric conditions, prior detoxification admissions, prior seizure activity, living situation, social supports, stressors, triggers, etc.

Physical: VS (fever, tachycardia, tachypnea, hypertension), **CIWA** (see below), MSE (arousal, orientation, hallucinations), HEENT (diaphoresis, scleral icterus), CV (arrythmias, M/R/G), eval s/sx liver failure (ascites, varices, caput madusae, asterixis, palmar erythema), neuro (nystagmus, tremor, seizure activity)

Include assessment of conditions likely to *complicate*, *exacerbate* or *precipitate* alcohol withdrawal: arrhythmias, CHF, CAD, dehydration, GI bleeding, infections, liver disease, pancreatitis, neurologic deficits

Clinical Institute Withdrawal Assessment of Alcohol Scale

– Nausea and vomiting 0–7; (7 constant nausea, frequent dry heaves/vomiting)
– Tremor 0–7; (7-severe, even with arms not extended)
– Paroxysmal sweats 0–7; (7-drenching sweats)
– Anxiety 0–7; (7-acute panic state)
– Agitation 0–7; (7-constantly thrashing about or pacing)
– Tactile disturbances 0–7; (4–7 for hallucinations, 1–3 for pruritus or paresthesias)
– Auditory disturbances 0–7; (4–7 for hallucinations, 1–3 for increased sensitivity)
– Visual disturbances 0–7; (4–7 for hallucinations, 1–3 for increased sensitivity)
– Headache, fullness in head 0–7
– Orientation and clouding of sensorium 0–4:
    o cannot do serial additions or is uncertain about date
    o disoriented to date but within 2 calendar days
    o disoriented to date by > 2 days
    o disoriented to place or person

Mild withdrawal; CIWA 0–7 (onset 5–8 hours after cessation or significant decrease in consumption): Anxiety, restlessness, agitation, mild nausea, decreased appetite, sleep disturbance, facial sweating, mild tremulousness, fluctuating tachycardia and hypertension, possible mild cognitive impairment

May be monitored as outpatient, *unless* pregnant, history of seizure d/o or withdrawal seizures, chronic or acute comorbid illness requiring inpatient observation, lack of ability to follow-up

– Admit to inpatient detox program for monitoring
– Vital signs q4h; CIWA q1–3h

Moderate withdrawal; CIWA 8–14 (onset 24–72 hours after cessation): marked restlessness and agitation, moderate tremulousness with constant eye movement, diaphoresis, nausea, vomiting, anorexia, diarrhea

– Admit to inpatient detox program
– Private room if possible
– Vital signs q4h
– CIWA q1–3h
– Institute seizure precautions
– IVF

Diazepam 20 mg PO q1–2h until CIWA<8, **OR**
Diazepam 2–5 mg IV/min-maximum 10–20 mg q1h
If severe liver disease, severe asthma or respiratory failure, elderly, debilitated, or low serum albumin:
Lorazepam SL, PO 1–2 mg q2–4h PRN

Long-acting benzodiazepines (diazepam) have rapid onset of action, and provide smooth treatment course with fewer breakthrough symptoms.
Short-acting (lorazepam) may have lower risk when there is concern about prolonged sedation, e.g., elderly patients or those with severe hepatic insufficiency.

Severe withdrawal/delirium tremens; CIWA >15 (onset 72–96 hours after alcohol cessation): Marked tremulousness, fever, drenching sweats, severe hypertension and tachycardia, delirium

– Admit to ICU for inpatient detox
– VS q30
– CIWA q1h
– NPO, IVF
– Lateral decubitus position, restrain if necessary
– Glucose, Na, K, PO4, Mg replacement as needed

Diazepam 5–20 mg IV q10 min until calm, then q1hr to maintain light somnolence for duration of delirium
If severe liver disease, severe asthma or respiratory failure, elderly, debilitated, or low serum albumin:
Lorazepam 1–4 mg IV q10 min until calm, then q1h to maintain light somnolence for duration of delirium

Labs: Tox screen/BAL to assess need for and timing of withdrawal regimen; electrolytes, phos, Mg with severe withdrawal [B12 and folate repleted regardless of levels], amylase/lipase if sx pancreatitis, PT, PTT if suspect liver failure; CBC if suspect infection
Imaging: Head CT if history of trauma or mental status changes out of range expected for degree of withdrawal. Seizure workup if no history of withdrawal siezures. Head CT and EEG if focal neurologic signs or prolonged post-ictal state

– **Thiamine** 100 mg IM/IV/PO q24h x 5 days; up to 1000 mg/day if oculogyric crisis

– **Sympatholytic adjunctive therapy:** Atenolol 50–100 mg q24
Beta blockers and clonidine may be used only in conjunction with benzodiazepines since *may mask symptoms of alcohol withdrawal and articially lower CIWA score*, reduce peripheral signs and symptoms of alcohol withdrawal but have not been shown to prevent or treat delirium or seizures

– **Phenothiazines for hallucinosis:** Haloperidol 2–5 mg IM/PO q1–4h max 5 mg/day used only in conjunction with benzodinzepines. May lower seizure threshold, use with extreme caution.

Discharge Planning:
– CIWA scores<8–10 for 24 hours
– Begin 1:1 or group therapy
– Discharge to treatment center, day program, home
– Facilitate entry into Alcoholics Anonymous
– Do not discharge with benzodiazepine rx
– Nutrition consult
– Social work consult

Alexis Lawrence, MD and Warren J. Ferguson, MD

N Engl J Med. 2003;348:1786.

ALDOSTERONISM

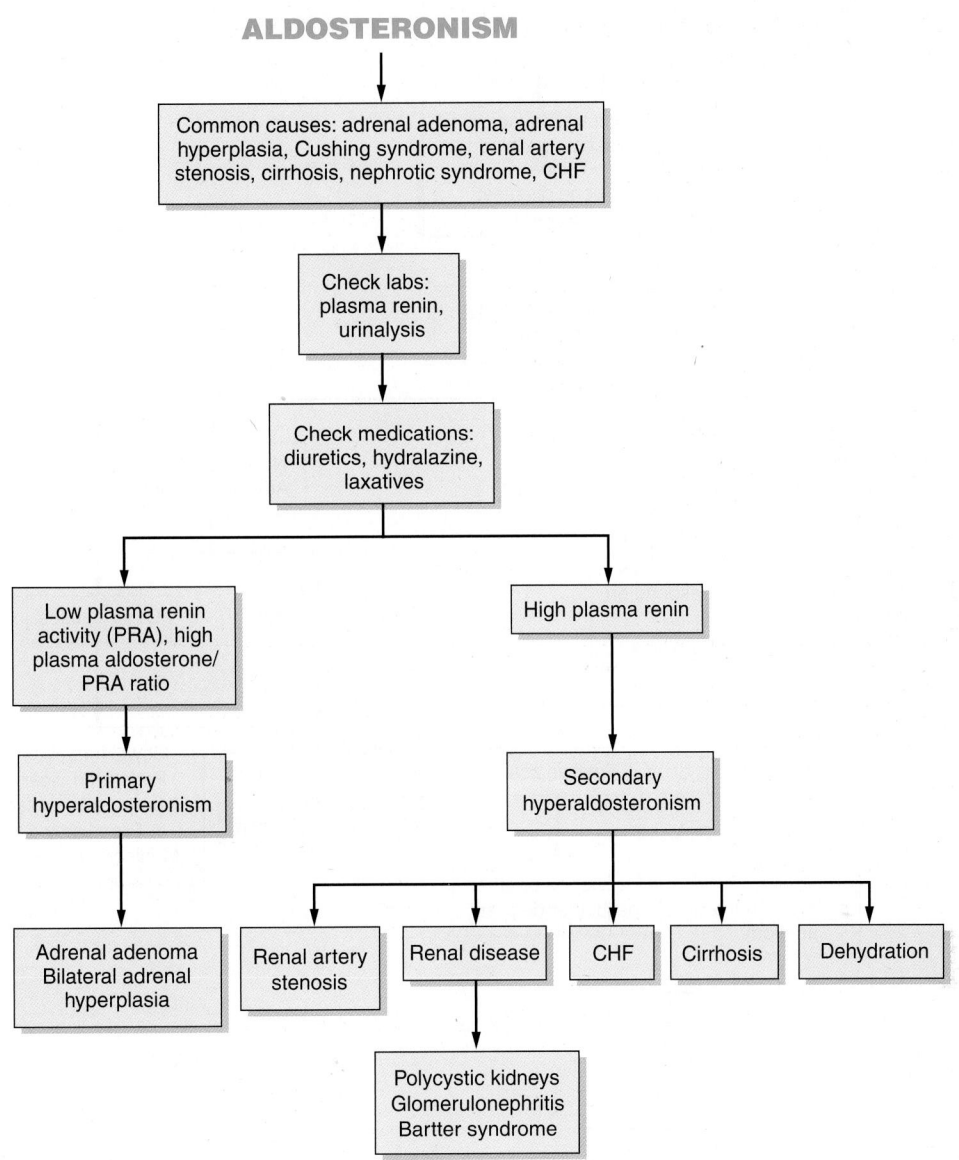

Robert A. Baldor, MD and Alan M. Ehrlich, MD

Cardiology. 1985;72(Suppl. 1):57–63.

ALKALINE PHOSPHATASE ELEVATION

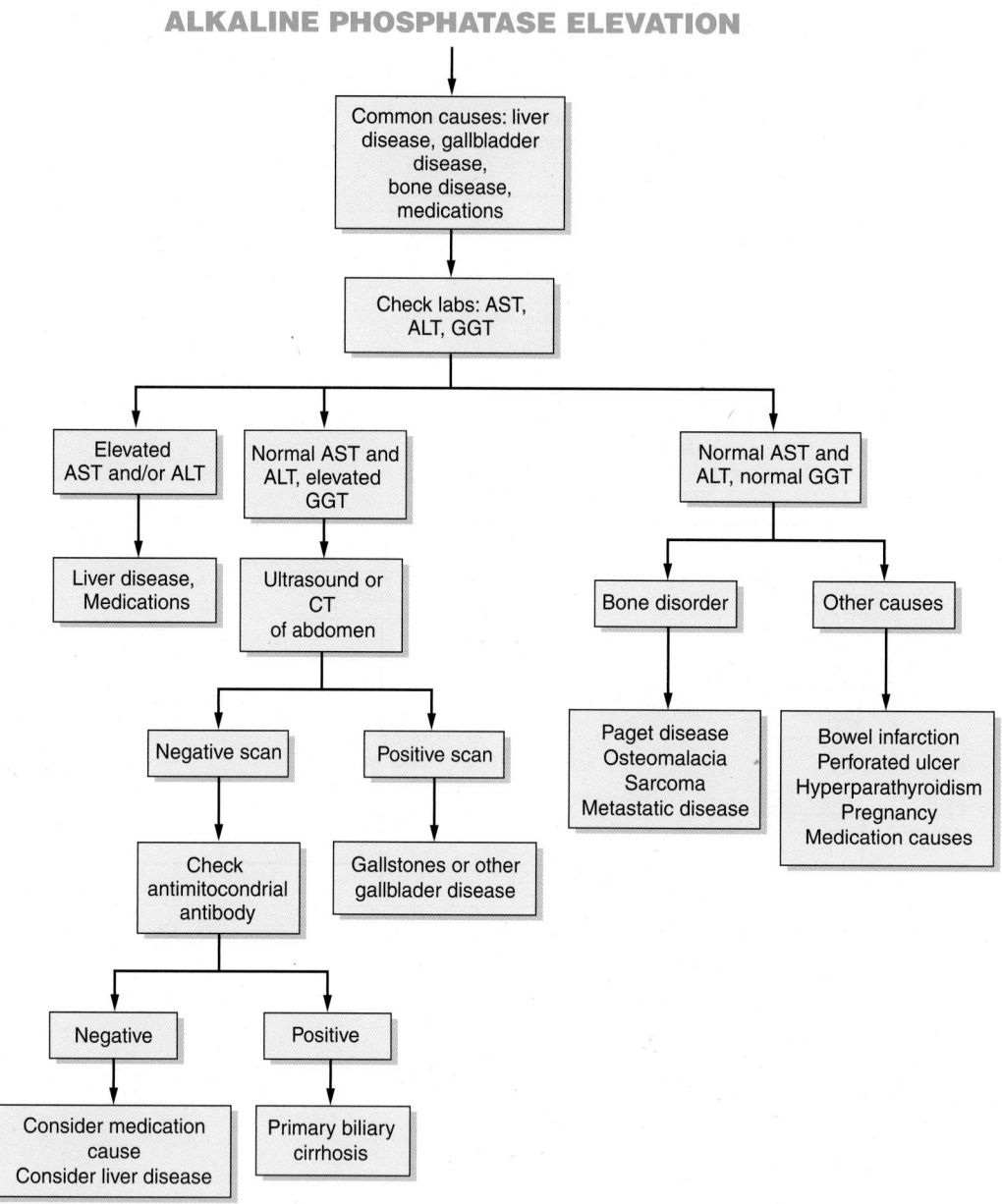

Robert A. Baldor, MD and Alan M. Ehrlich, MD

J Fam Pract. 2001;50(6).

ALKALOSIS

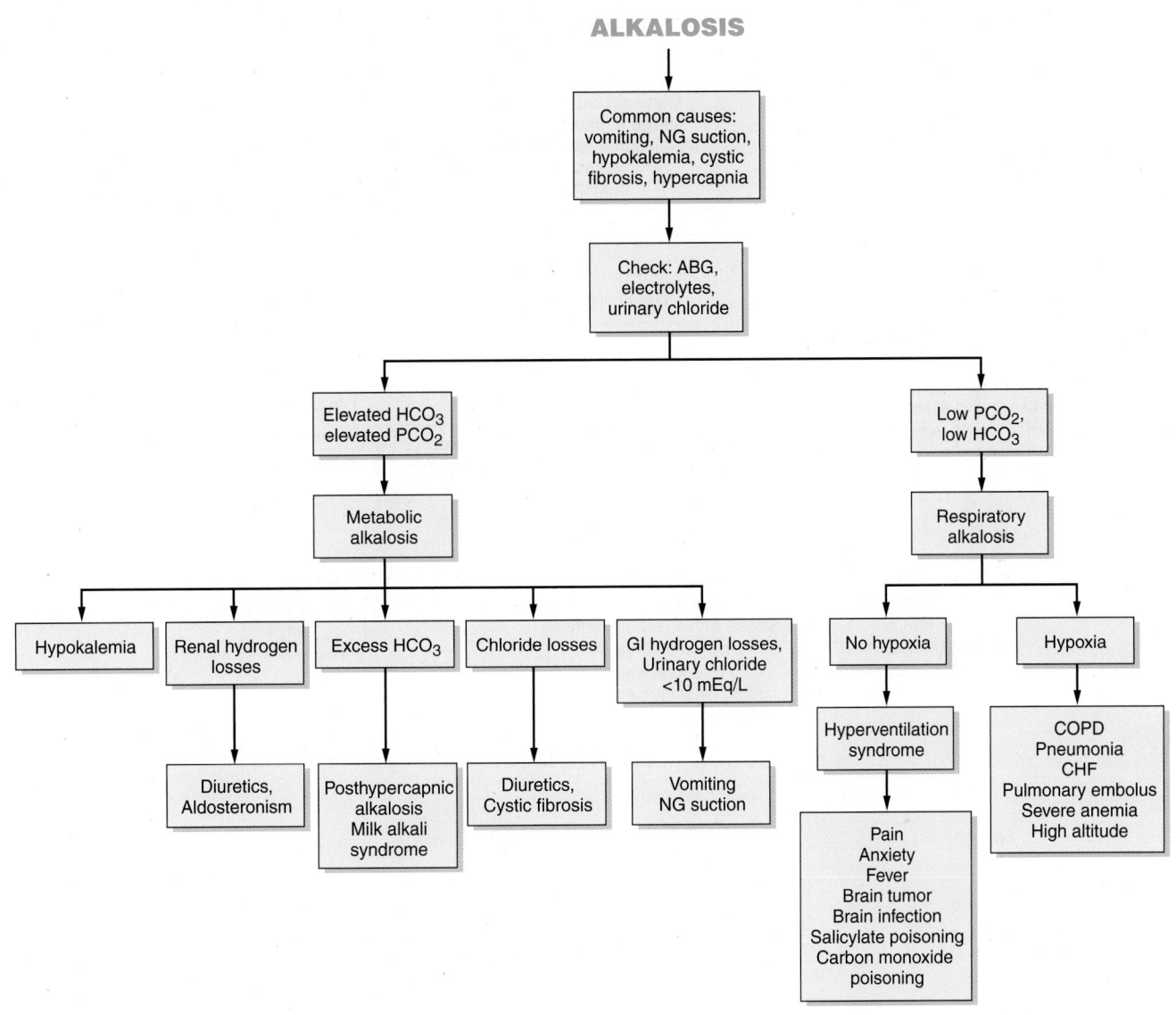

Robert A. Baldor, MD and Alan M. Ehrlich, MD

Nutr Clin Pract. 2008;23(2):122–7.

ALOPECIA

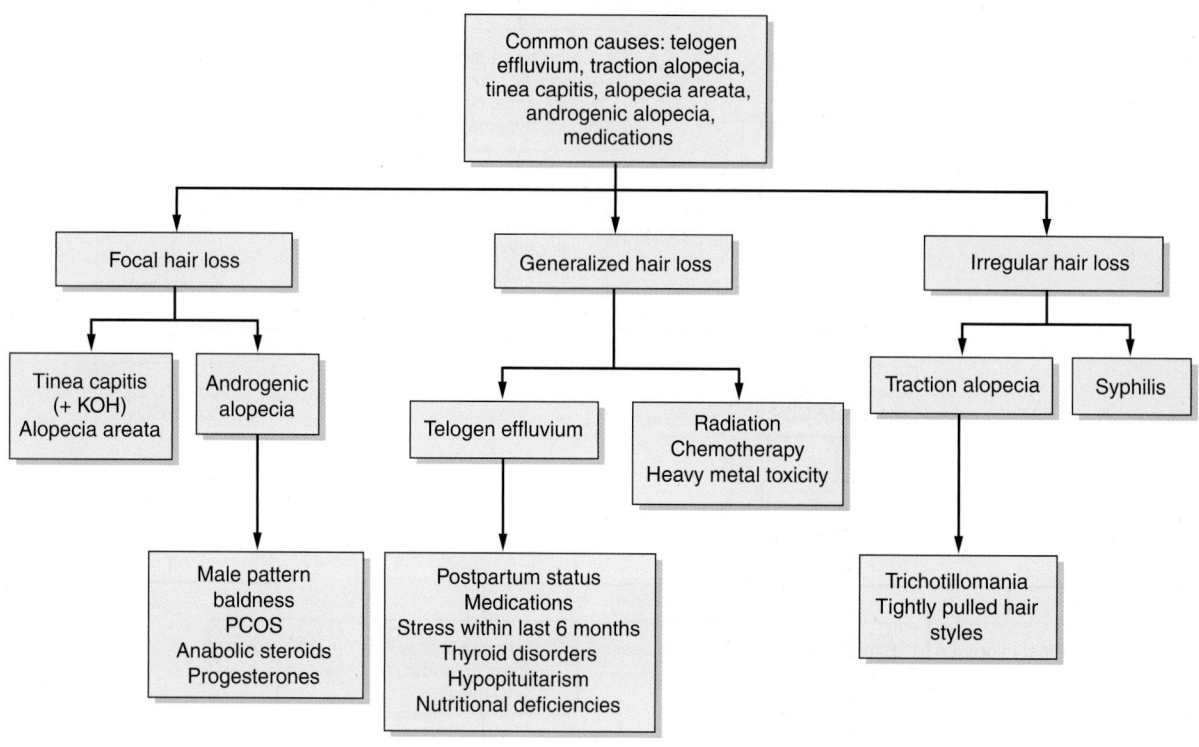

Robert A. Baldor, MD and Alan M. Ehrlich, MD

Am Fam Physician. 2009;80(4):356–62.

AMENORRHEA, PRIMARY
(ABSENCE OF MENARCHE BY AGE 16)

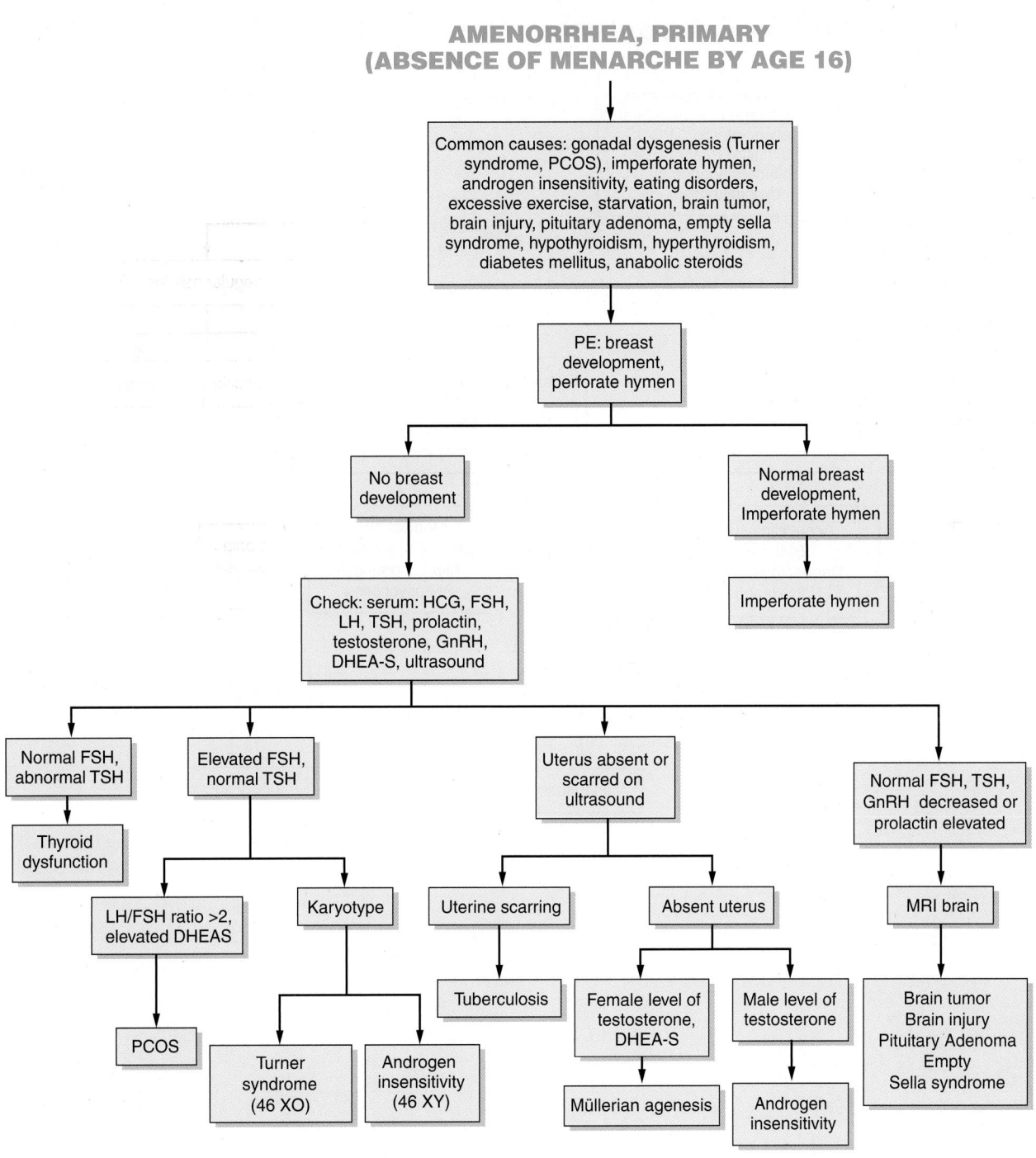

Robert A. Baldor, MD and Alan M. Ehrlich, MD

Am Fam Physician. 2006;73:1374–82.

AMENORRHEA, SECONDARY

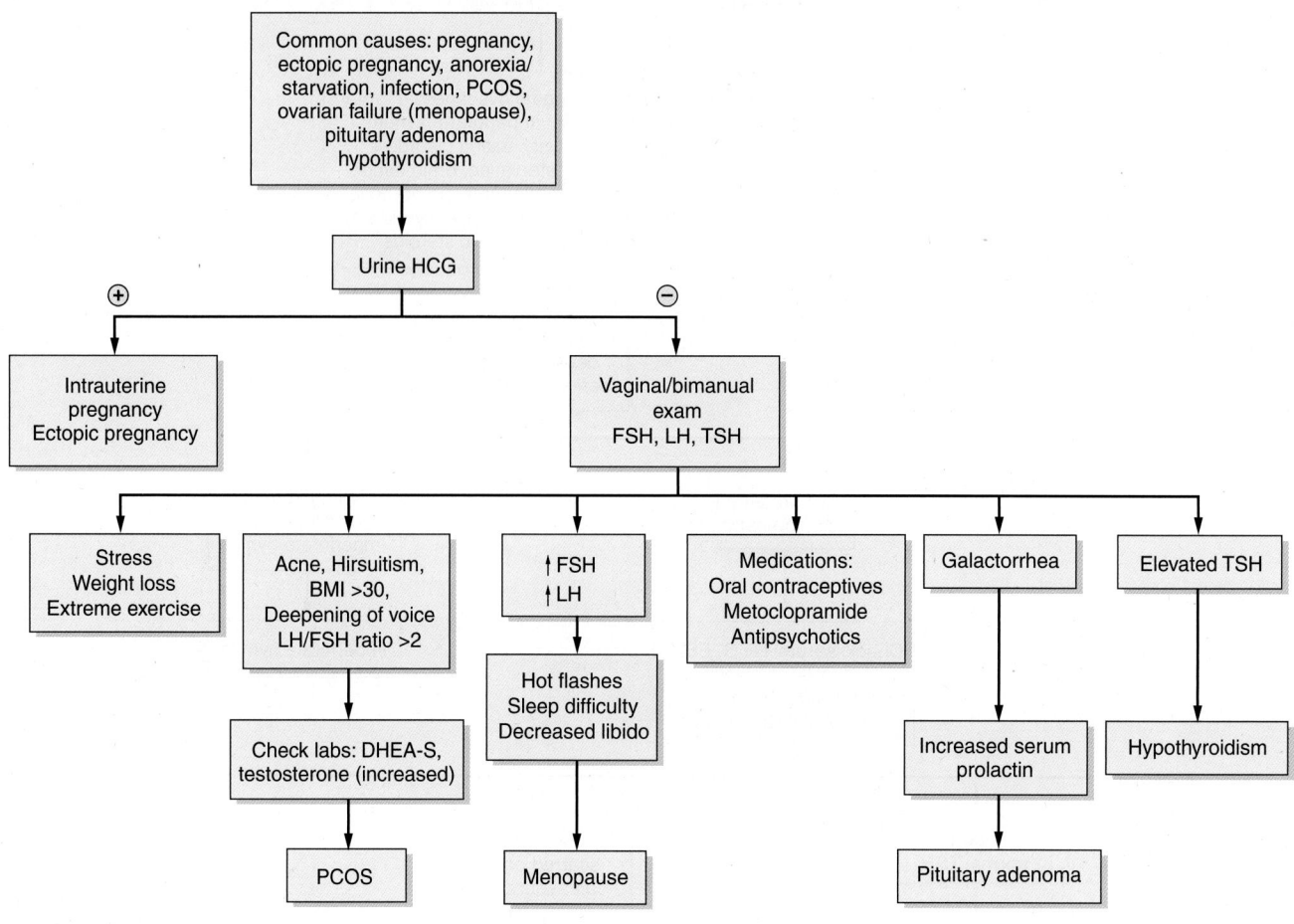

Robert A. Baldor, MD and Alan M. Ehrlich, MD

Am Fam Physician. 2006;73:1374–82.

AMNESIA

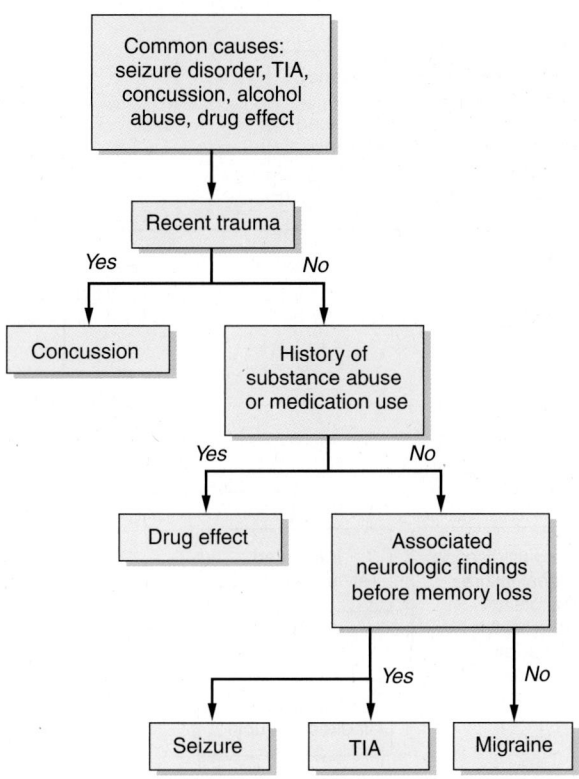

Robert A. Baldor, MD and Alan M. Ehrlich, MD

Ann Intern Med. 2007;146(6):397–405.

ANEMIA

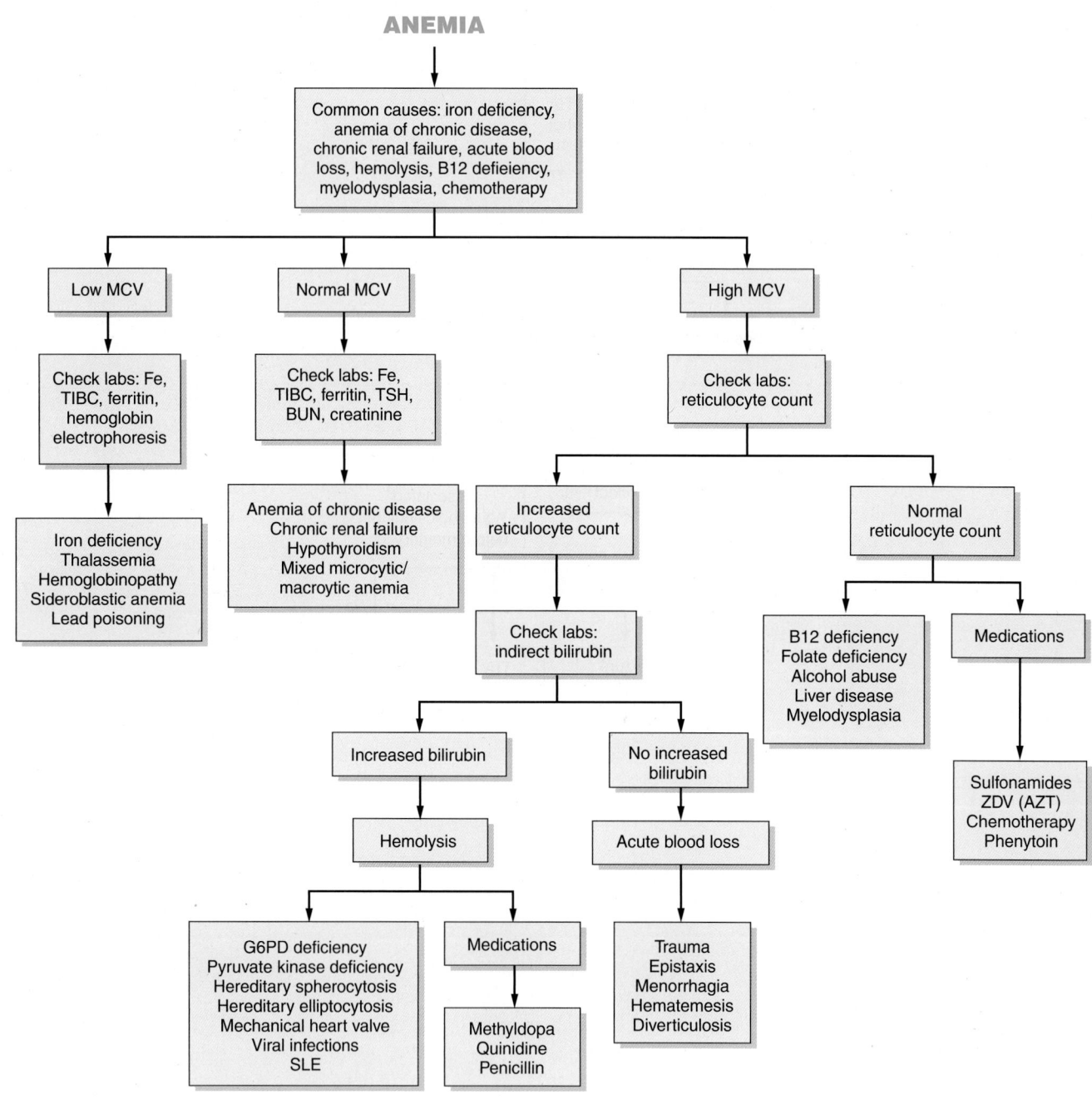

Common causes: iron deficiency, anemia of chronic disease, chronic renal failure, acute blood loss, hemolysis, B12 defieiency, myelodysplasia, chemotherapy

Low MCV

Check labs: Fe, TIBC, ferritin, hemoglobin electrophoresis

Iron deficiency
Thalassemia
Hemoglobinopathy
Sideroblastic anemia
Lead poisoning

Normal MCV

Check labs: Fe, TIBC, ferritin, TSH, BUN, creatinine

Anemia of chronic disease
Chronic renal failure
Hypothyroidism
Mixed microcytic/
macroytic anemia

High MCV

Check labs: reticulocyte count

Increased reticulocyte count

Check labs: indirect bilirubin

Increased bilirubin

Hemolysis

G6PD deficiency
Pyruvate kinase deficiency
Hereditary spherocytosis
Hereditary elliptocytosis
Mechanical heart valve
Viral infections
SLE

Medications

Methyldopa
Quinidine
Penicillin

No increased bilirubin

Acute blood loss

Trauma
Epistaxis
Menorrhagia
Hematemesis
Diverticulosis

Normal reticulocyte count

B12 deficiency
Folate deficiency
Alcohol abuse
Liver disease
Myelodysplasia

Medications

Sulfonamides
ZDV (AZT)
Chemotherapy
Phenytoin

Robert A. Baldor, MD and Alan M. Ehrlich, MD

Am Fam Physician. 2000;62:1565–72.

ANOREXIA

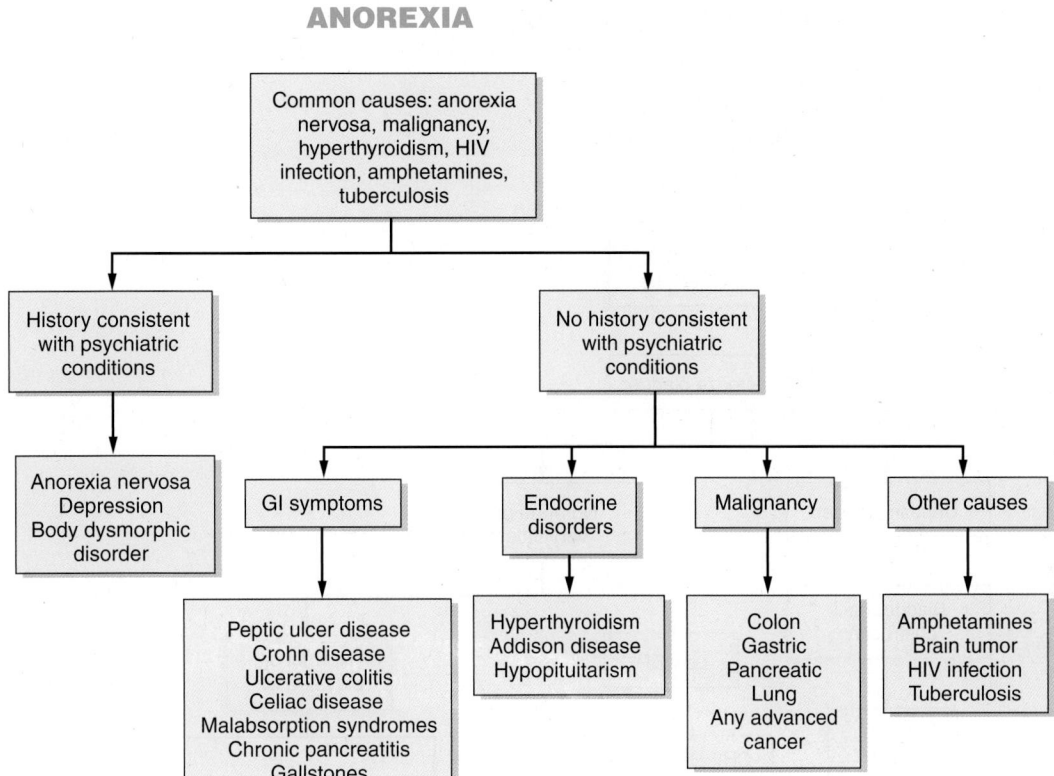

Robert A. Baldor, MD and Alan M. Ehrlich, MD

Am Fam Physician. 2003;67:297–304, 311–2.

ANURIA OR OLIGOURIA

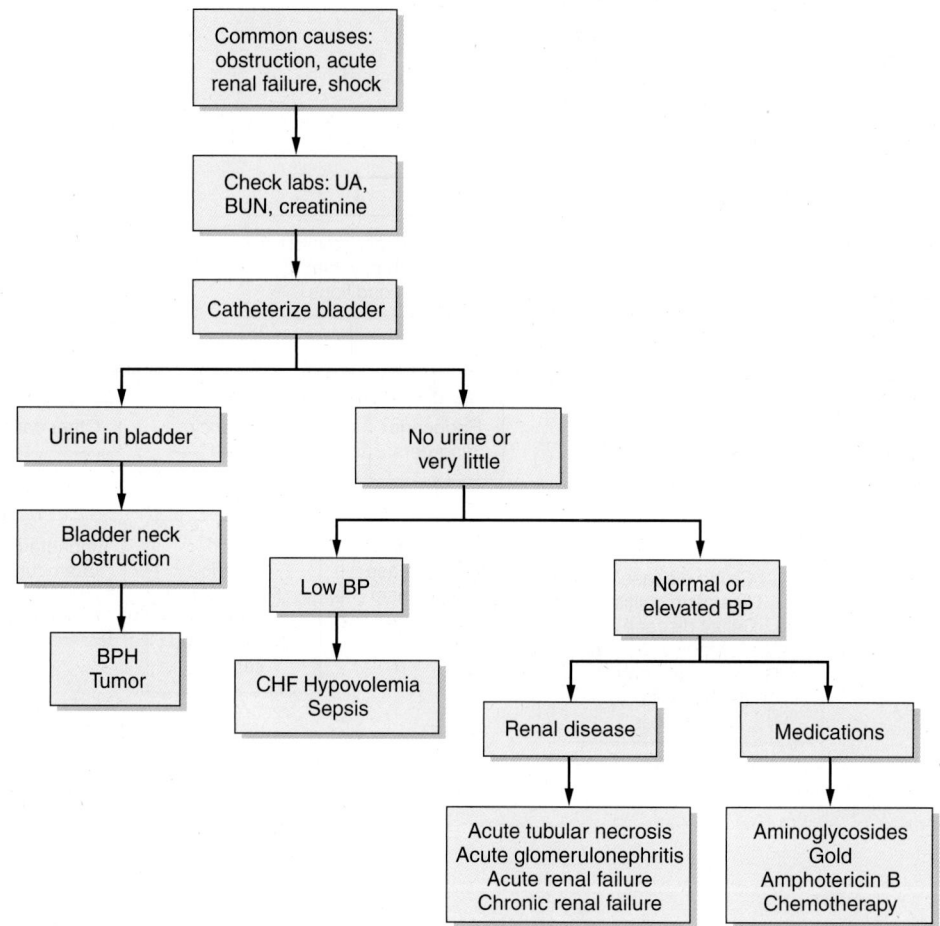

Robert A. Baldor, MD and Alan M. Ehrlich, MD

Am Fam Physician. 2000;61:2077–88.

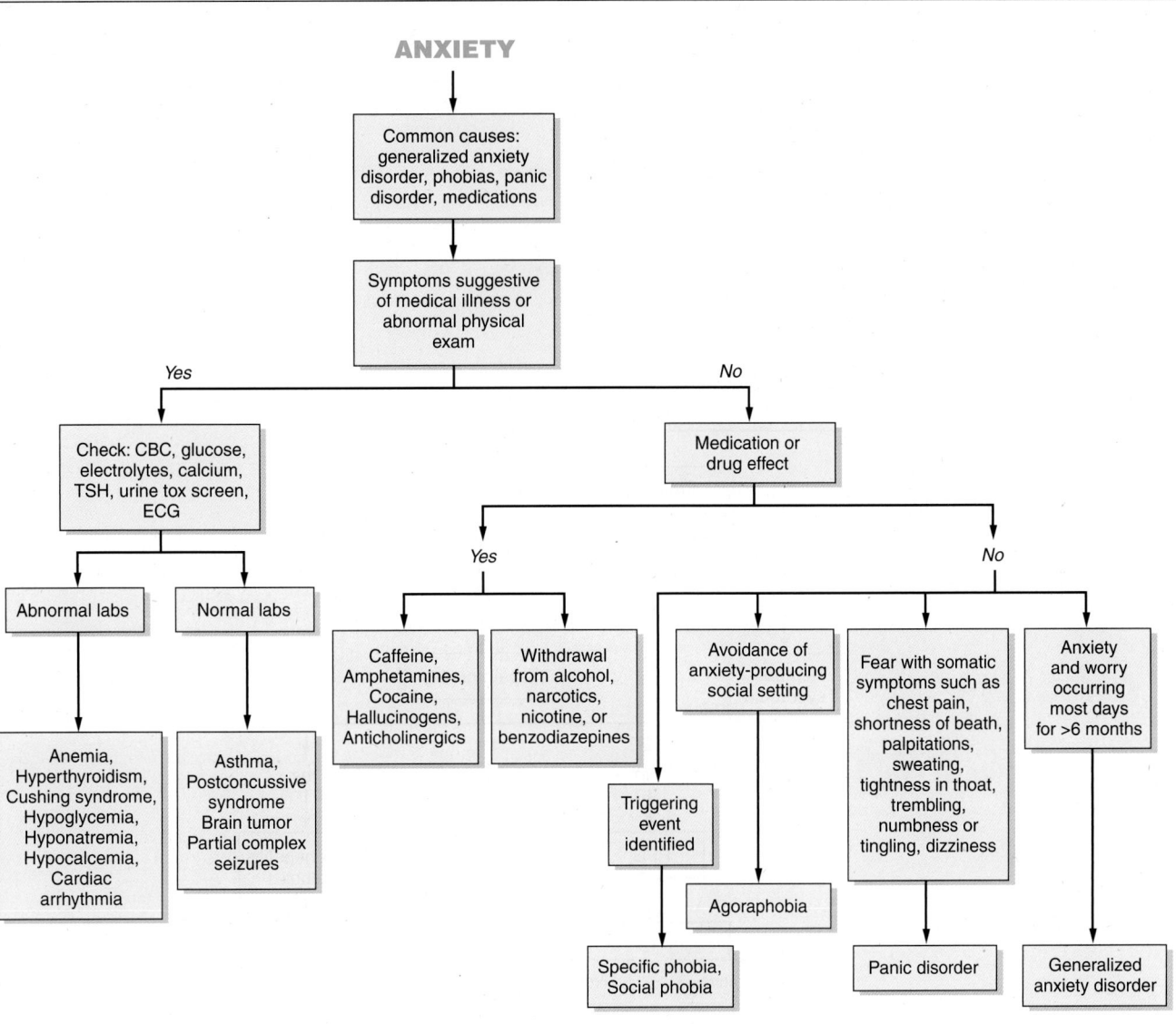

ANXIETY

Robert A. Baldor, MD and Alan M. Ehrlich, MD

Am J Psychiatry. 1999;156:1677–85.

ASCITES

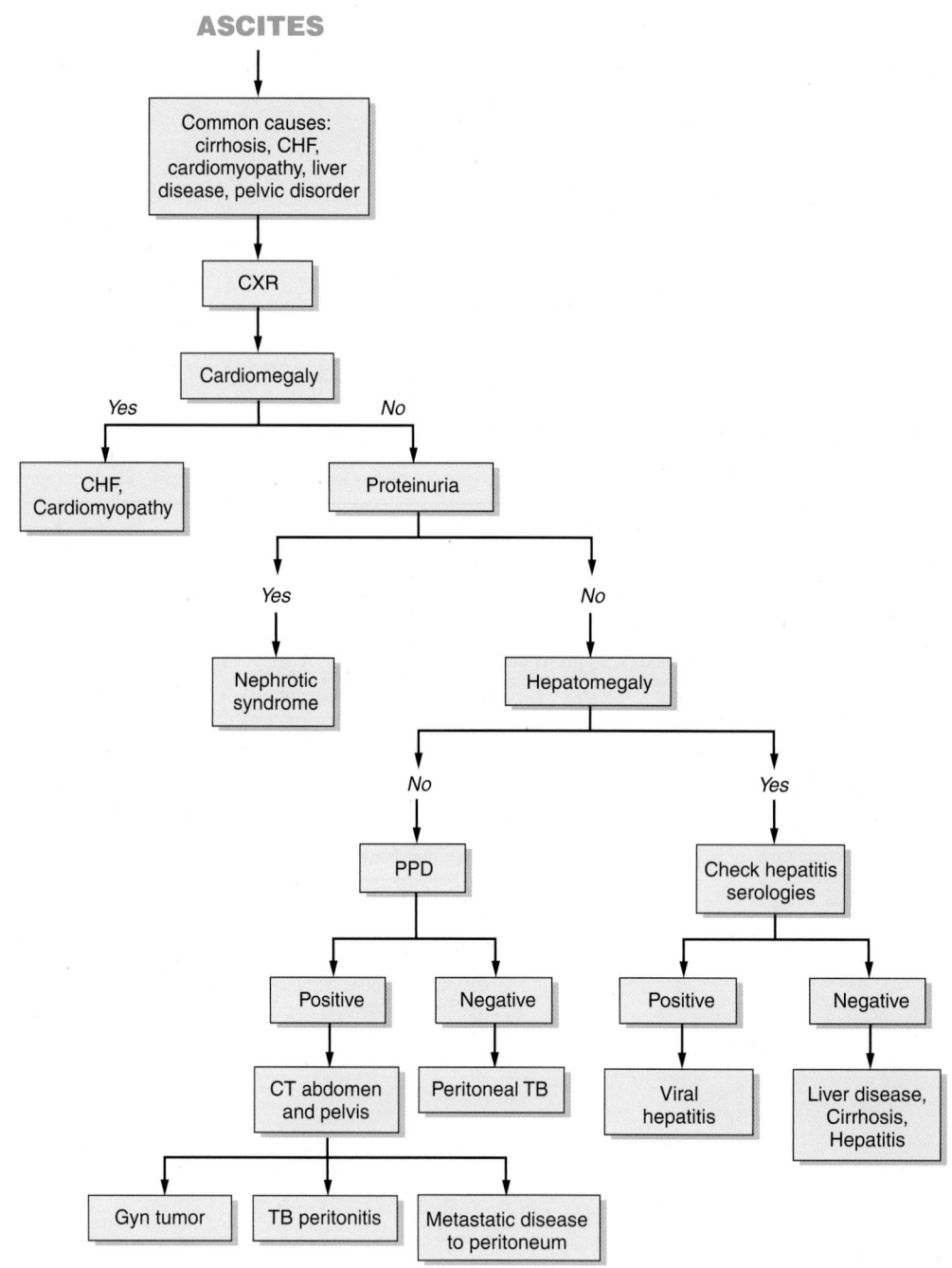

Robert A. Baldor, MD and Alan M. Ehrlich, MD

Am Fam Physician. 2006;74:767–76.

AST ELEVATION

Common causes: hemolysis, liver disease, myocardial infarction, CHF, acute renal failure, biliary obstruction, pancreatitis, muscle disorders, medications

↓

Check: LFTs, consider CBC, BUN, creatinine, hepatitis serologies, CPK, amylase, CXR, ultrasound/CT of abdomen

| Jaundice | Chest pain or dyspnea | Abdominal pain Elevated amylase | Edema | Muscle disorder | Liver toxicity |

| Liver disease Biliary obstruction Hemolysis Viral hepatitis | Myocardial infarction CHF | Pancreatitis | CHF Acute renal failure | | Alcohol Medications |

Robert A. Baldor, MD and Alan M. Ehrlich, MD

Am Fam Physician. 2005;71:1105–10.

ASTHMA EXACERBATION, PEDIATRIC ACUTE

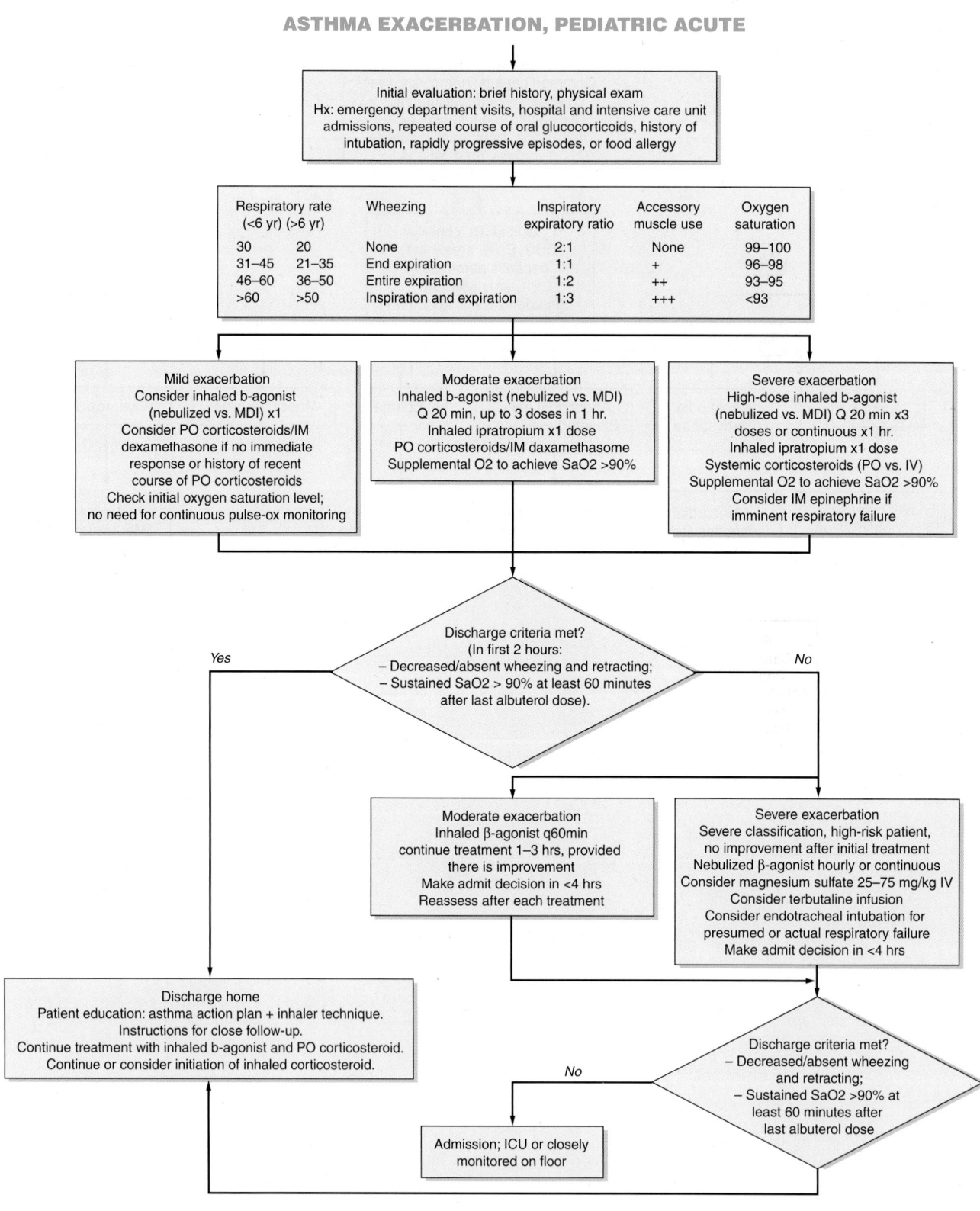

Initial evaluation: brief history, physical exam
Hx: emergency department visits, hospital and intensive care unit admissions, repeated course of oral glucocorticoids, history of intubation, rapidly progressive episodes, or food allergy

Respiratory rate (<6 yr) (>6 yr)	Wheezing	Inspiratory expiratory ratio	Accessory muscle use	Oxygen saturation
30 20	None	2:1	None	99–100
31–45 21–35	End expiration	1:1	+	96–98
46–60 36–50	Entire expiration	1:2	++	93–95
>60 >50	Inspiration and expiration	1:3	+++	<93

Mild exacerbation
Consider inhaled b-agonist (nebulized vs. MDI) x1
Consider PO corticosteroids/IM dexamethasone if no immediate response or history of recent course of PO corticosteroids
Check initial oxygen saturation level; no need for continuous pulse-ox monitoring

Moderate exacerbation
Inhaled b-agonist (nebulized vs. MDI) Q 20 min, up to 3 doses in 1 hr.
Inhaled ipratropium x1 dose
PO corticosteroids/IM daxamethasome
Supplemental O2 to achieve SaO2 >90%

Severe exacerbation
High-dose inhaled b-agonist (nebulized vs. MDI) Q 20 min x3 doses or continuous x1 hr.
Inhaled ipratropium x1 dose
Systemic corticosteroids (PO vs. IV)
Supplemental O2 to achieve SaO2 >90%
Consider IM epinephrine if imminent respiratory failure

Discharge criteria met?
(In first 2 hours:
– Decreased/absent wheezing and retracting;
– Sustained SaO2 > 90% at least 60 minutes after last albuterol dose).

Yes   No

Moderate exacerbation
Inhaled β-agonist q60min
continue treatment 1–3 hrs, provided there is improvement
Make admit decision in <4 hrs
Reassess after each treatment

Severe exacerbation
Severe classification, high-risk patient, no improvement after initial treatment
Nebulized β-agonist hourly or continuous
Consider magnesium sulfate 25–75 mg/kg IV
Consider terbutaline infusion
Consider endotracheal intubation for presumed or actual respiratory failure
Make admit decision in <4 hrs

Discharge home
Patient education: asthma action plan + inhaler technique.
Instructions for close follow-up.
Continue treatment with inhaled b-agonist and PO corticosteroid.
Continue or consider initiation of inhaled corticosteroid.

Discharge criteria met?
– Decreased/absent wheezing and retracting;
– Sustained SaO2 >90% at least 60 minutes after last albuterol dose

No

Admission; ICU or closely monitored on floor

Catherine Janes, MD

Am Fam Physician. 2005;71:1959–68.

ATAXIA

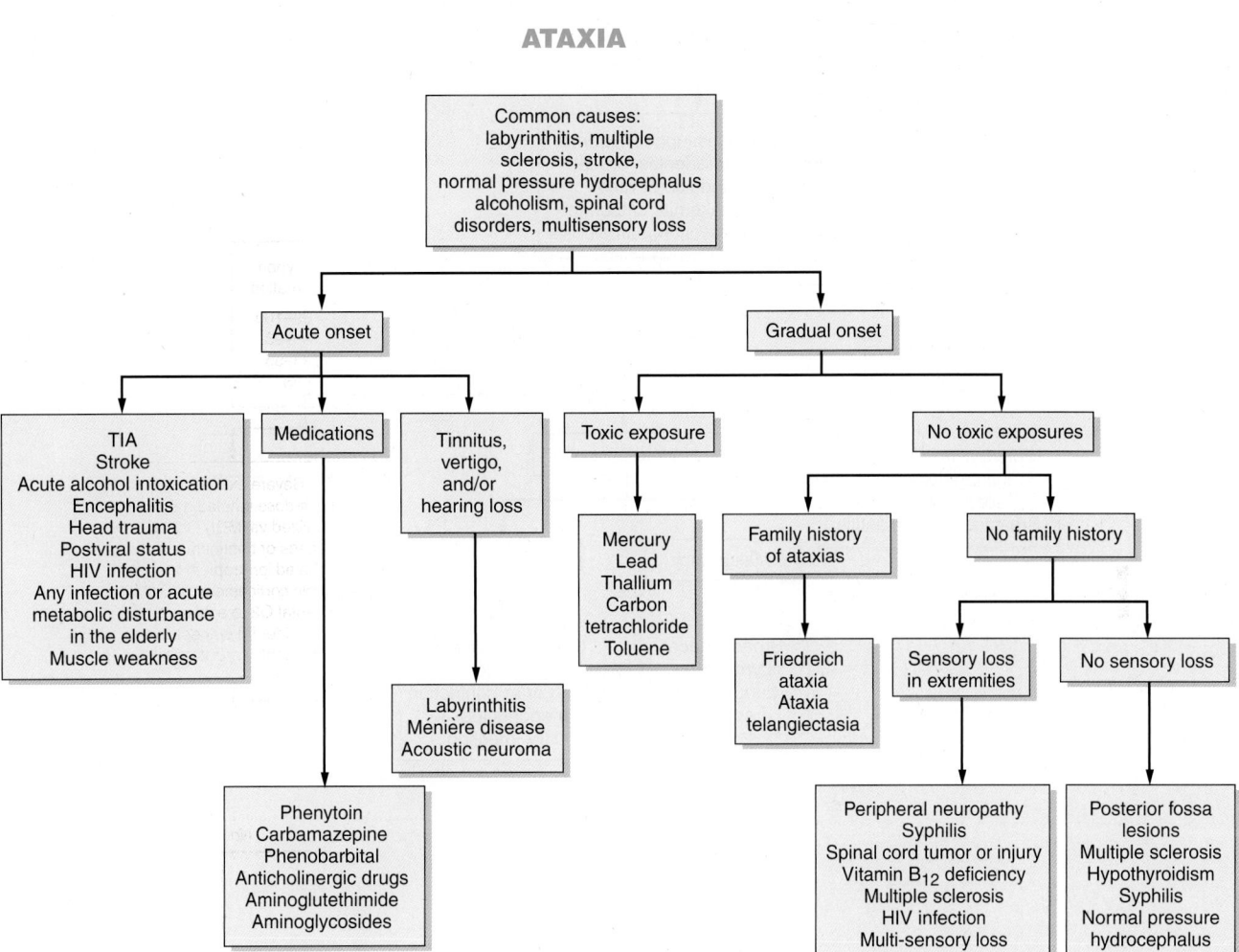

Robert A. Baldor, MD and Alan M. Ehrlich, MD

Arch Neurol. 2008;65(10):1296–303.

AXILLARY MASS

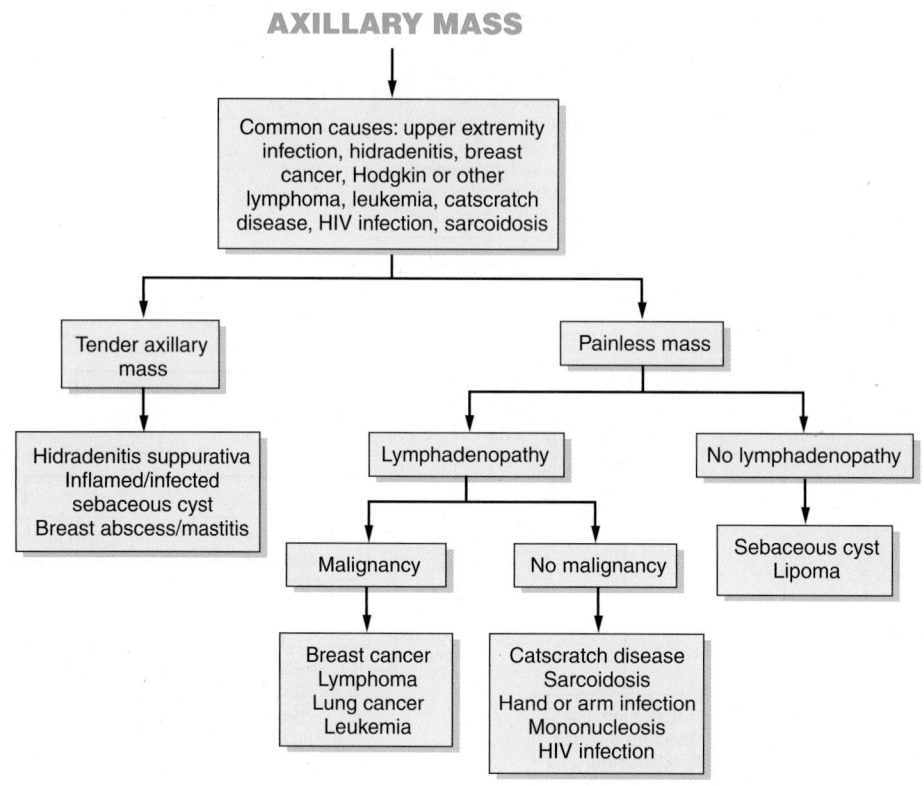

Common causes: upper extremity
infection, hidradenitis, breast
cancer, Hodgkin or other
lymphoma, leukemia, catscratch
disease, HIV infection, sarcoidosis

Tender axillary mass

Painless mass

Hidradenitis suppurativa
Inflamed/infected
sebaceous cyst
Breast abscess/mastitis

Lymphadenopathy

No lymphadenopathy

Malignancy

No malignancy

Sebaceous cyst
Lipoma

Breast cancer
Lymphoma
Lung cancer
Leukemia

Catscratch disease
Sarcoidosis
Hand or arm infection
Mononucleosis
HIV infection

Robert A. Baldor, MD and Alan M. Ehrlich, MD

Ann Surg Oncol. 2000;7:411–5.

BABINSKI SIGN POSITIVE

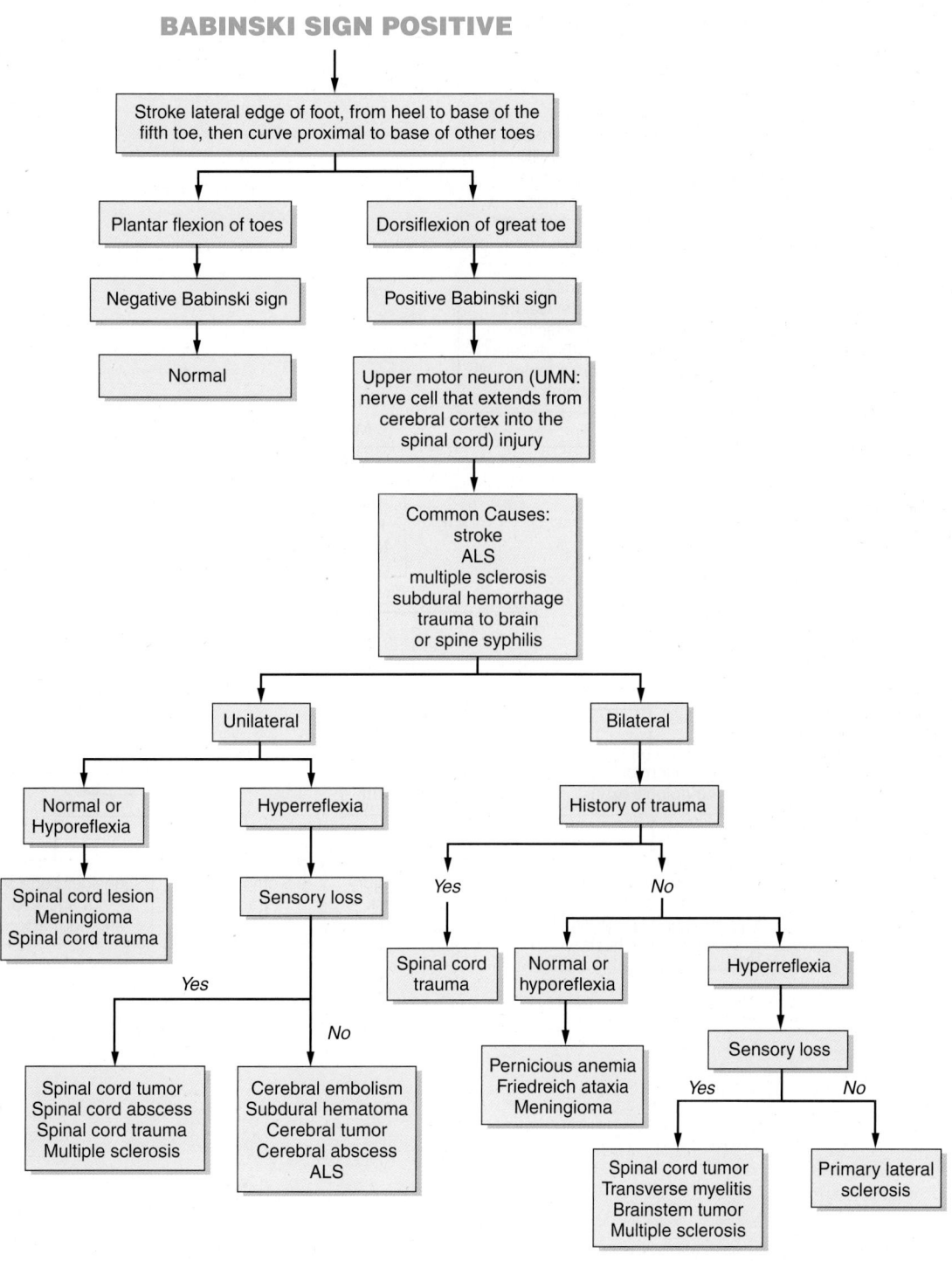

Robert A. Baldor, MD and Alan M. Ehrlich, MD

J Neurol Neurosurg Psychiatry. 2002;73(4):360–2.

BACK PAIN, ACUTE

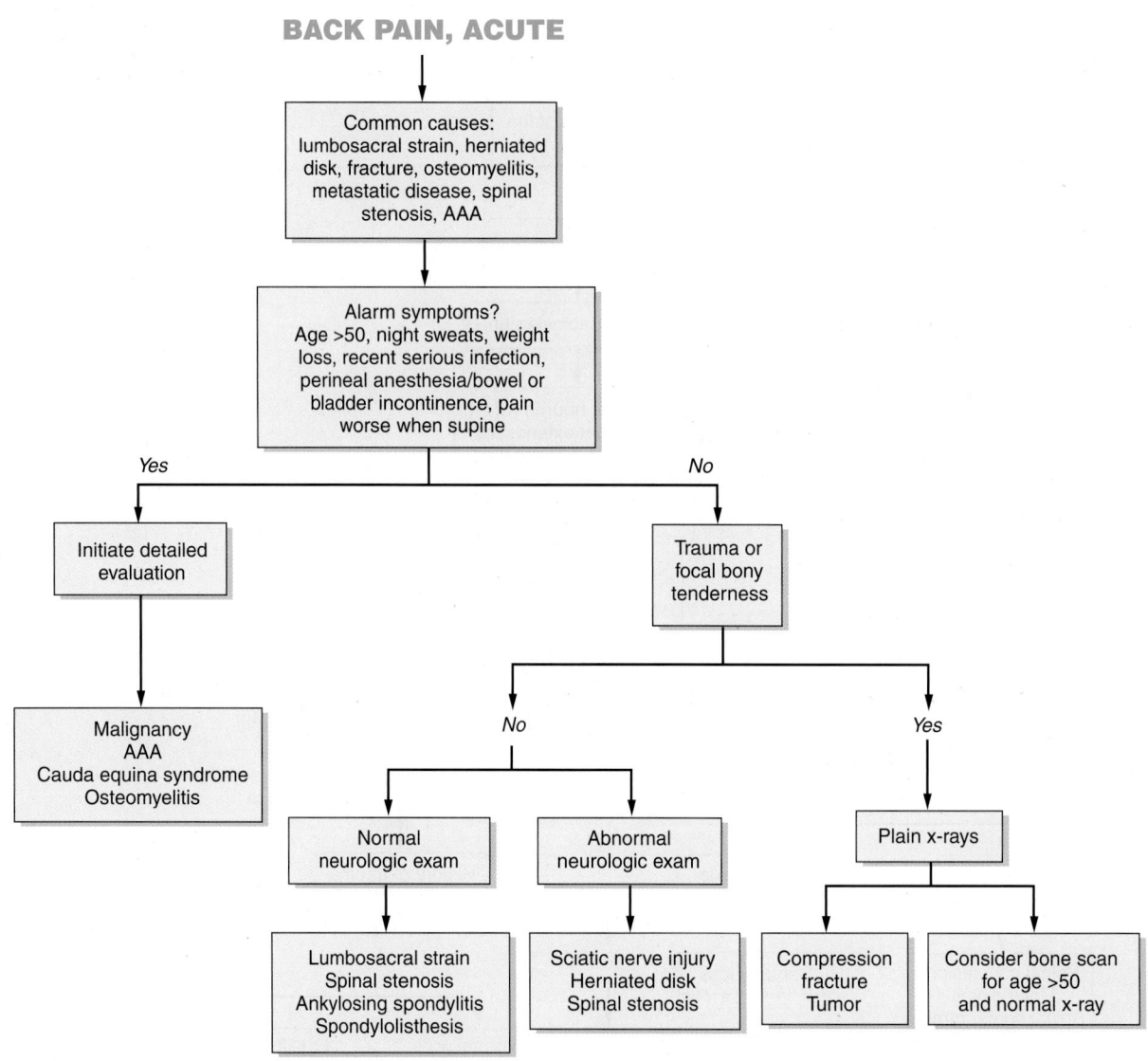

Common causes:
lumbosacral strain, herniated
disk, fracture, osteomyelitis,
metastatic disease, spinal
stenosis, AAA

Alarm symptoms?
Age >50, night sweats, weight
loss, recent serious infection,
perineal anesthesia/bowel or
bladder incontinence, pain
worse when supine

Yes

No

Initiate detailed
evaluation

Trauma or
focal bony
tenderness

Malignancy
AAA
Cauda equina syndrome
Osteomyelitis

No

Yes

Normal
neurologic exam

Abnormal
neurologic exam

Plain x-rays

Lumbosacral strain
Spinal stenosis
Ankylosing spondylitis
Spondylolisthesis

Sciatic nerve injury
Herniated disk
Spinal stenosis

Compression
fracture
Tumor

Consider bone scan
for age >50
and normal x-ray

Robert A. Baldor, MD and Alan M. Ehrlich, MD

Am Fam Physician. 2007;75:1181–8.

BLEEDING GUMS

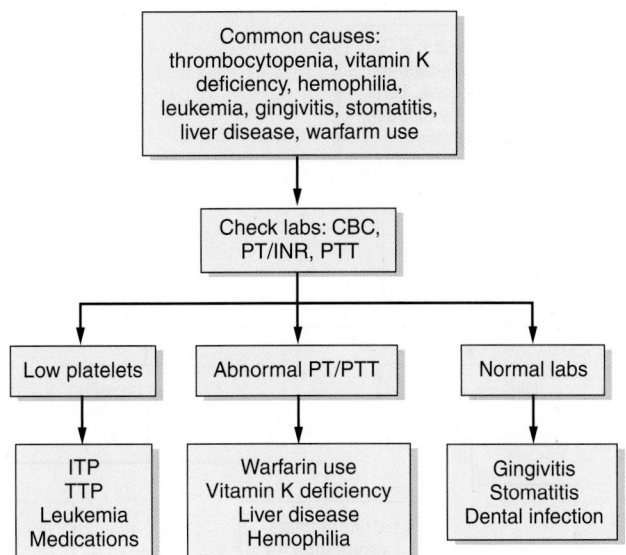

Robert A. Baldor, MD and Alan M. Ehrlich, MD

Compend Contin Educ Dent. 1999;20(10):936–40.

BLEEDING URETHRAL

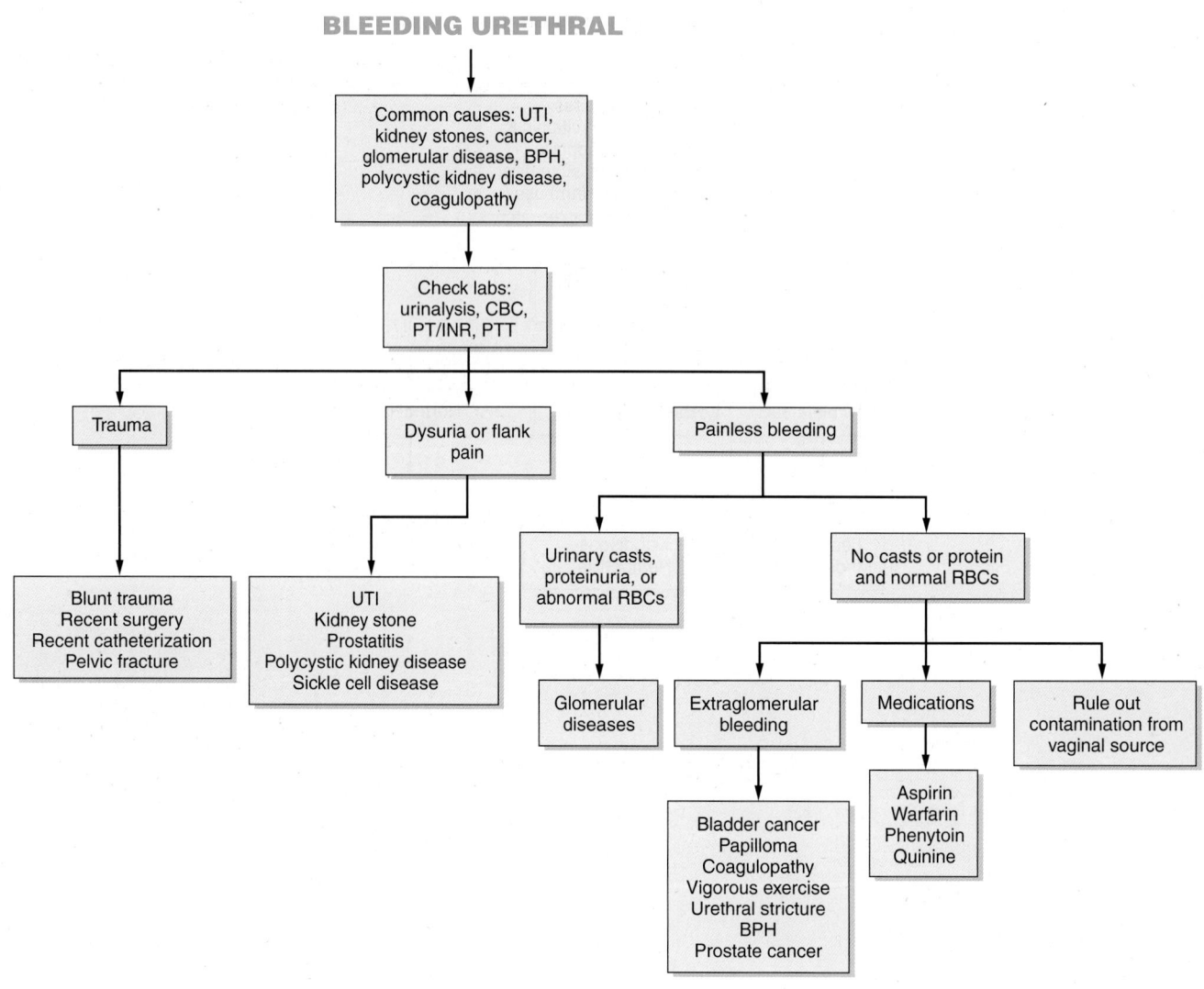

Robert A. Baldor, MD and Alan M. Ehrlich, MD

Am Fam Physician. 2001;63:1145–54.

BREAST DISCHARGE

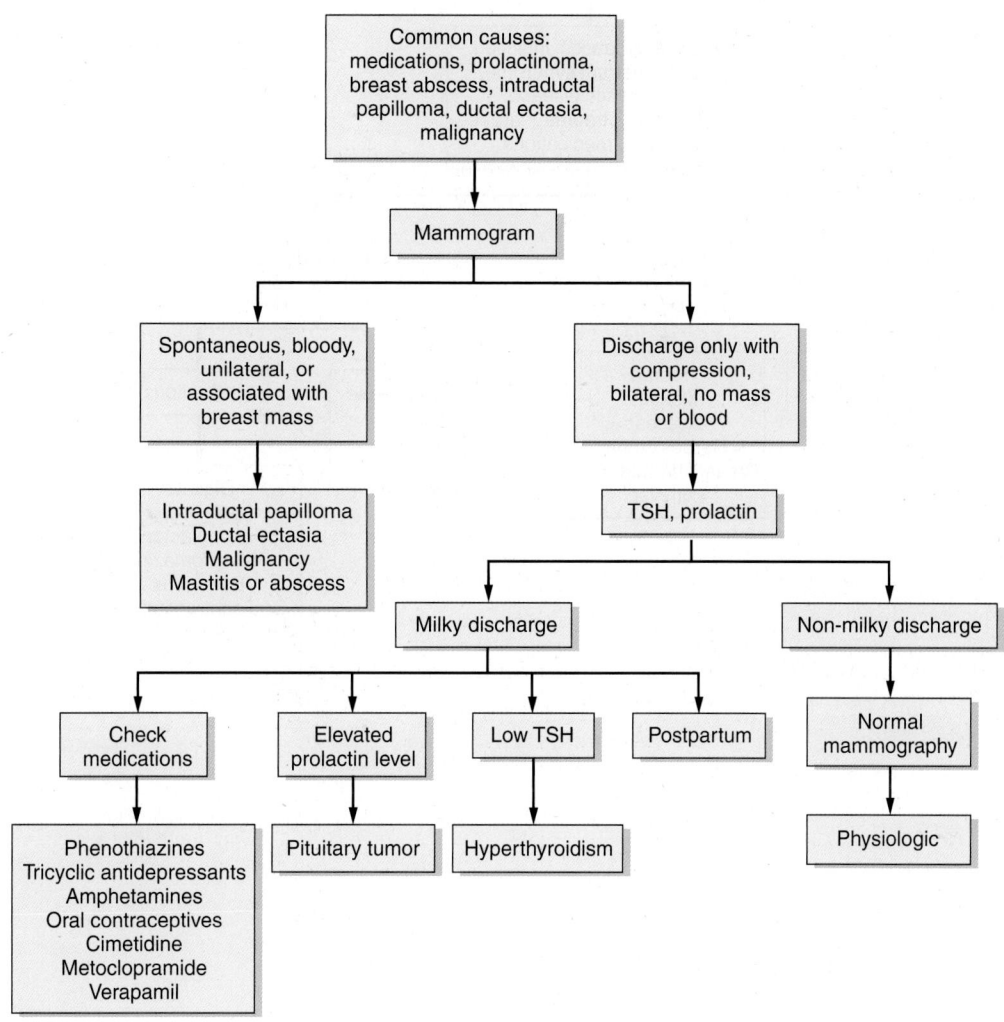

Robert A. Baldor, MD and Alan M. Ehrlich, MD

Breast J. 2009;15(3):230–5.

BREAST PAIN

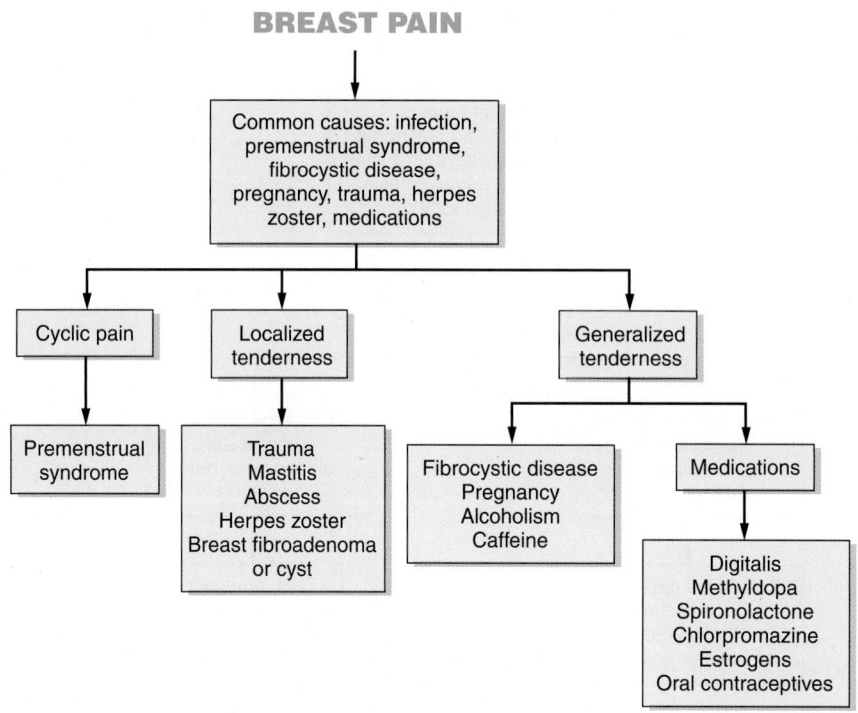

Robert A. Baldor, MD and Alan M. Ehrlich, MD

Obstet Gynecol Clin North Am. 2008;35(2):285–303.

CARDIAC ARRHYTHMIAS

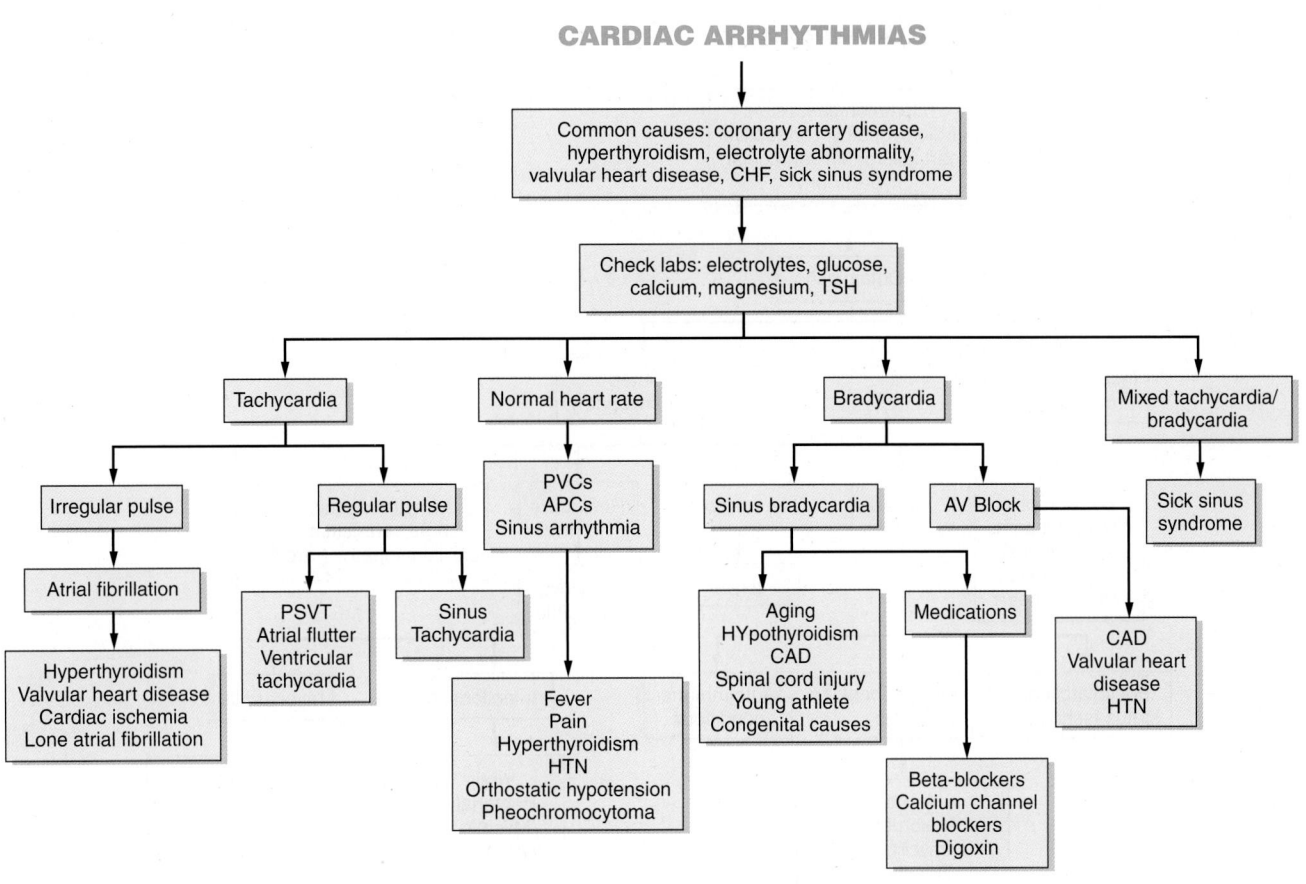

Robert A. Baldor, MD and Alan M. Ehrlich, MD

Am Fam Physician. 2005;743–50, 755–9.

CARDIOMEGALY

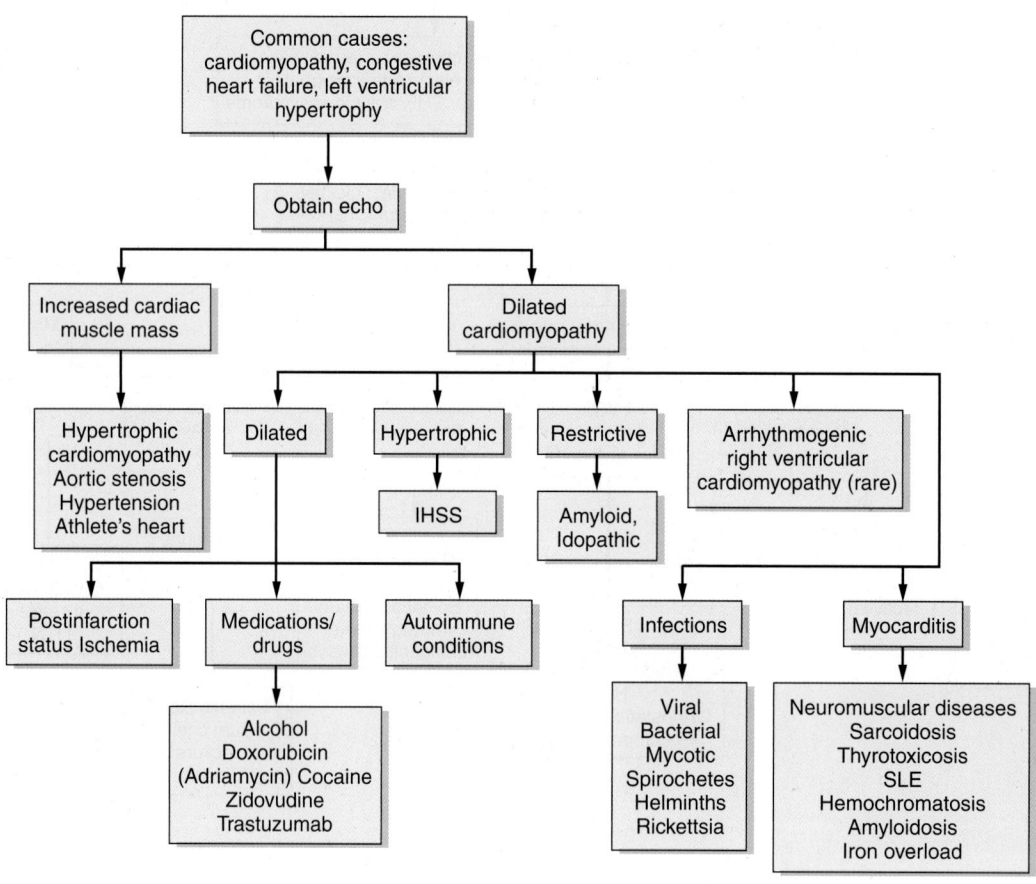

Robert A. Baldor, MD and Alan M. Ehrlich, MD

Eur J Echocardiogr. 2009;10(8):iii15–21.

CARPAL TUNNEL SYNDROME

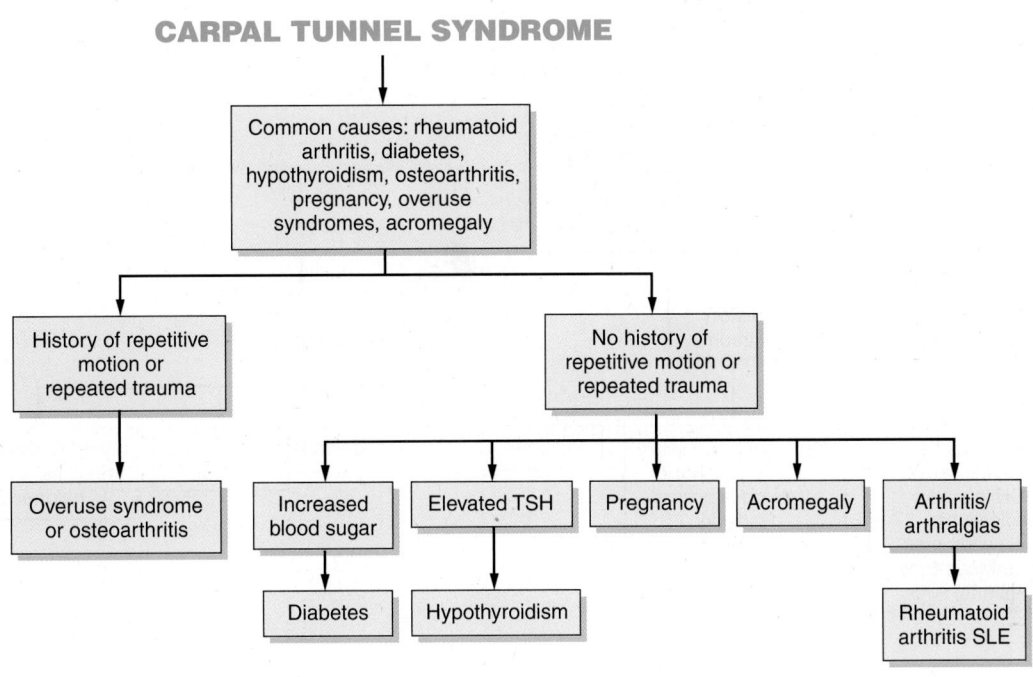

Robert A. Baldor, MD and Alan M. Ehrlich, MD

BMJ. 2007;335(7615):343–6.

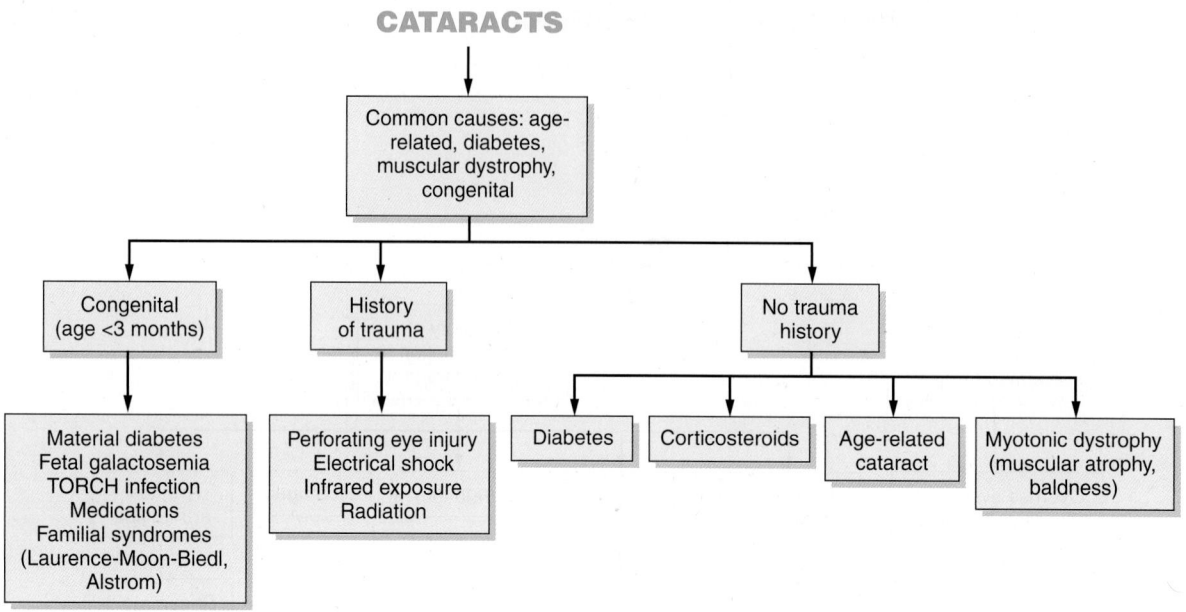

CATARACTS

Common causes: age-related, diabetes, muscular dystrophy, congenital

Congenital (age <3 months)
- Material diabetes
- Fetal galactosemia
- TORCH infection
- Medications
- Familial syndromes (Laurence-Moon-Biedl, Alstrom)

History of trauma
- Perforating eye injury
- Electrical shock
- Infrared exposure
- Radiation

No trauma history
- Diabetes
- Corticosteroids
- Age-related cataract
- Myotonic dystrophy (muscular atrophy, baldness)

Robert A. Baldor, MD and Alan M. Ehrlich, MD

Ophth. 2010;117(8):1471–8.

CERVICAL BRUIT

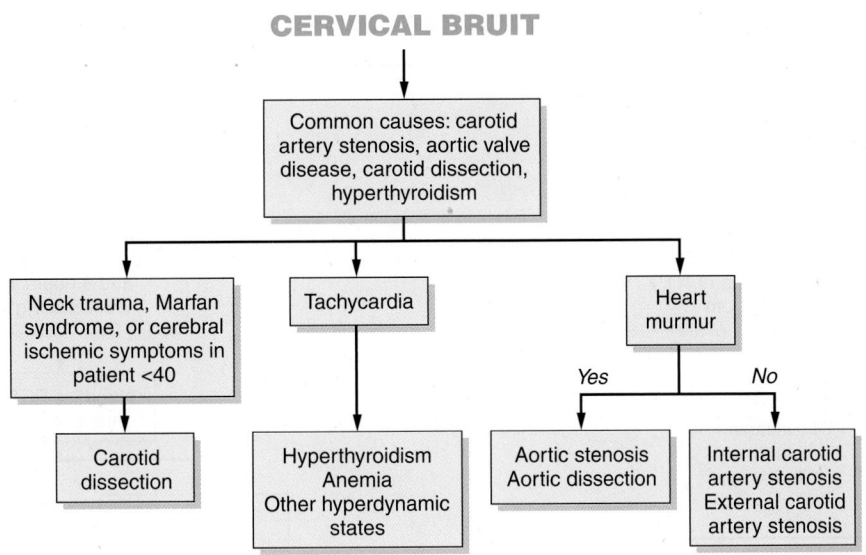

Robert A. Baldor, MD and Alan M. Ehrlich, MD

http://www.ncbi.nlm.nih.gov/bookshelf/br.fcgi?book=cm&part=A593

CHEST PAIN/ACUTE CORONARY SYNDROME

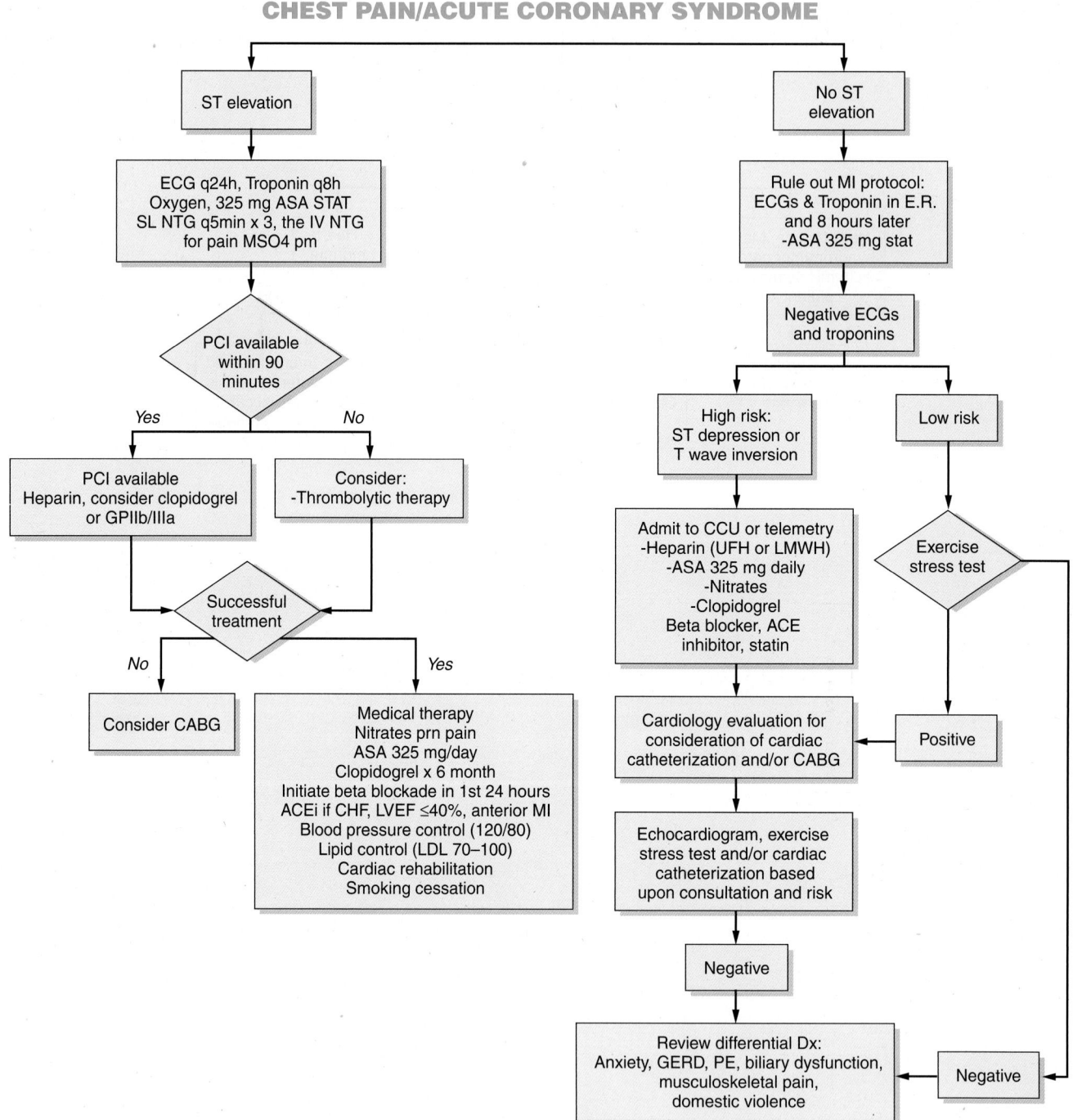

ST elevation

ECG q24h, Troponin q8h
Oxygen, 325 mg ASA STAT
SL NTG q5min x 3, the IV NTG
for pain MSO4 pm

PCI available
within 90
minutes

Yes   *No*

PCI available
Heparin, consider clopidogrel
or GPIIb/IIIa

Consider:
-Thrombolytic therapy

Successful
treatment

No   *Yes*

Consider CABG

Medical therapy
Nitrates prn pain
ASA 325 mg/day
Clopidogrel x 6 month
Initiate beta blockade in 1st 24 hours
ACEi if CHF, LVEF ≤40%, anterior MI
Blood pressure control (120/80)
Lipid control (LDL 70–100)
Cardiac rehabilitation
Smoking cessation

**No ST
elevation**

Rule out MI protocol:
ECGs & Troponin in E.R.
and 8 hours later
-ASA 325 mg stat

Negative ECGs
and troponins

High risk:
ST depression or
T wave inversion

Low risk

Admit to CCU or telemetry
-Heparin (UFH or LMWH)
-ASA 325 mg daily
-Nitrates
-Clopidogrel
Beta blocker, ACE
inhibitor, statin

Exercise
stress test

Cardiology evaluation for
consideration of cardiac
catheterization and/or CABG

Positive

Echocardiogram, exercise
stress test and/or cardiac
catheterization based
upon consultation and risk

Negative

Review differential Dx:
Anxiety, GERD, PE, biliary dysfunction,
musculoskeletal pain,
domestic violence

Negative

Allen Chang, MD and Naomi F. Botkin, MD

Circulation. 2005;112(22 Suppl):III55–72.

CHRONIC OBSTRUCTIVE PULMONARY DISEASE (COPD), DIAGNOSIS AND TREATMENT

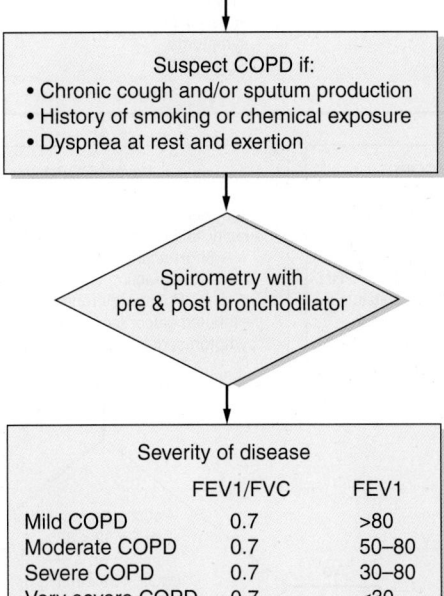

Suspect COPD if:
- Chronic cough and/or sputum production
- History of smoking or chemical exposure
- Dyspnea at rest and exertion

Spirometry with pre & post bronchodilator

Severity of disease

	FEV1/FVC	FEV1
Mild COPD	0.7	>80
Moderate COPD	0.7	50–80
Severe COPD	0.7	30–80
Very severe COPD	0.7	<30

Functional dyspnea scale

0   Not troubled with breathlessness except with strenuous exercise.
1   Troubled by shortness of breath when hurrying or walking up a slight hill.
2   Walks slower than people of same age due to breathlessness or has to stop for breath when walking at own pace on the level.
3   Stops for breath after walking ~100 m or after a few minutes on the level.
4   Too breathless to leave the house or breathless when dressing or undressing.

Diagnosis confirmed, initiate preventative measures:
Influenza vaccine (yearly), pneumococcal vaccine (every 5 years)

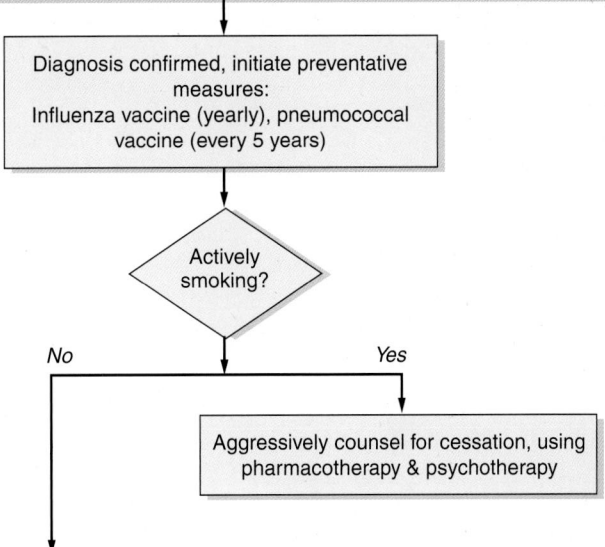

Actively smoking?

No   *Yes*

Aggressively counsel for cessation, using pharmacotherapy & psychotherapy

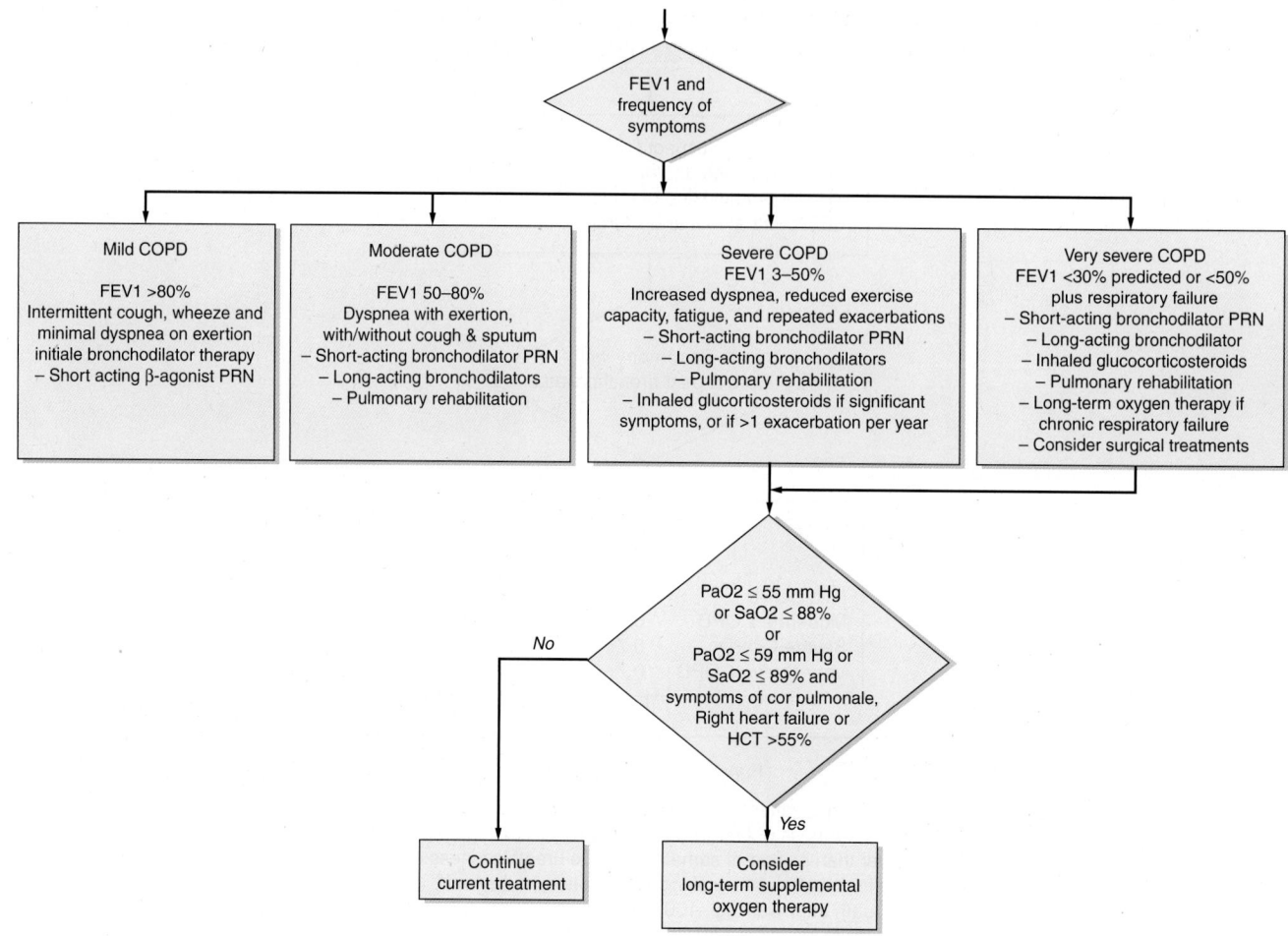

Laura Paulin, MD, MHS and Scott Kopec, MD

National Guidelines Clearinghouse. Global Initiative for Chronic Obstructive Lung Disease (GOLD); 2008.

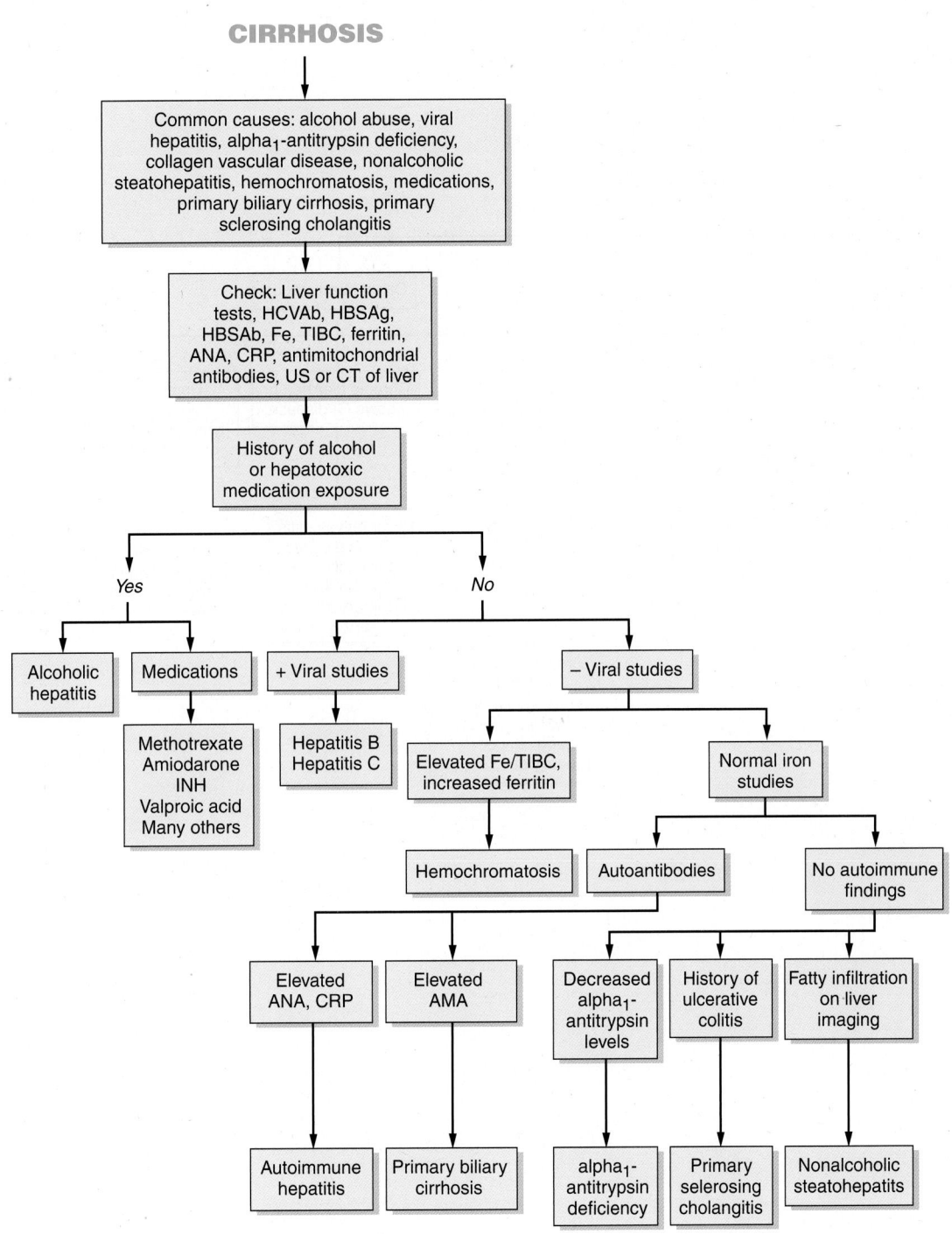

CIRRHOSIS

Common causes: alcohol abuse, viral hepatitis, alpha$_1$-antitrypsin deficiency, collagen vascular disease, nonalcoholic steatohepatitis, hemochromatosis, medications, primary biliary cirrhosis, primary sclerosing cholangitis

Check: Liver function tests, HCVAb, HBSAg, HBSAb, Fe, TIBC, ferritin, ANA, CRP, antimitochondrial antibodies, US or CT of liver

History of alcohol or hepatotoxic medication exposure

Yes

Alcoholic hepatitis

Medications

Methotrexate
Amiodarone
INH
Valproic acid
Many others

No

+ Viral studies

Hepatitis B
Hepatitis C

− Viral studies

Elevated Fe/TIBC, increased ferritin

Hemochromatosis

Normal iron studies

Autoantibodies

No autoimmune findings

Elevated ANA, CRP

Elevated AMA

Decreased alpha$_1$-antitrypsin levels

History of ulcerative colitis

Fatty infiltration on liver imaging

Autoimmune hepatitis

Primary biliary cirrhosis

alpha$_1$-antitrypsin deficiency

Primary selerosing cholangitis

Nonalcoholic steatohepatits

Robert A. Baldor, MD and Alan M. Ehrlich, MD

Med Clin North Am. 2009;93(4).

CLUBBING

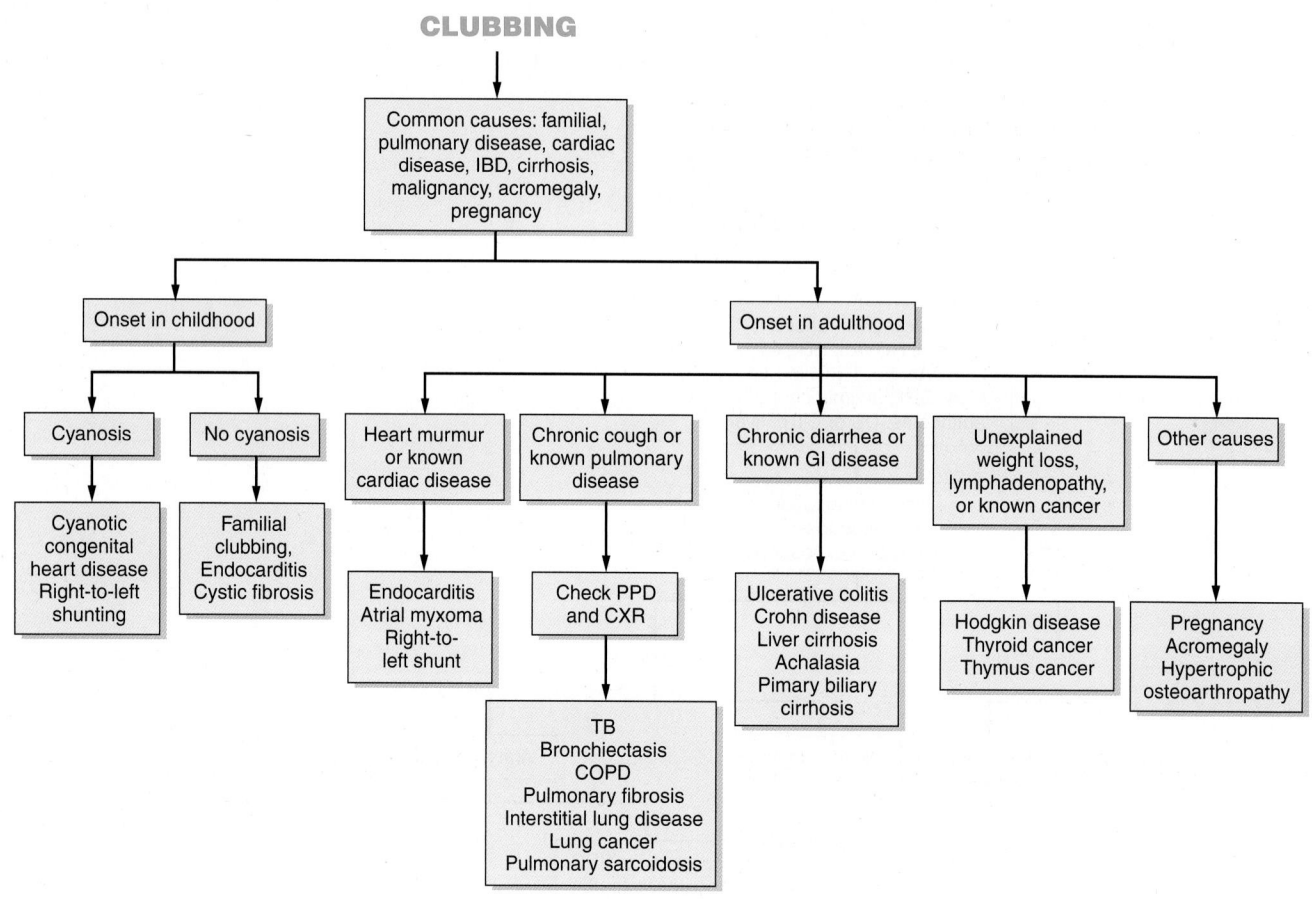

Common causes: familial, pulmonary disease, cardiac disease, IBD, cirrhosis, malignancy, acromegaly, pregnancy

Onset in childhood

Cyanosis
Cyanotic congenital heart disease Right-to-left shunting

No cyanosis
Familial clubbing, Endocarditis Cystic fibrosis

Onset in adulthood

Heart murmur or known cardiac disease
Endocarditis Atrial myxoma Right-to-left shunt

Chronic cough or known pulmonary disease
Check PPD and CXR

TB
Bronchiectasis
COPD
Pulmonary fibrosis
Interstitial lung disease
Lung cancer
Pulmonary sarcoidosis

Chronic diarrhea or known GI disease
Ulcerative colitis
Crohn disease
Liver cirrhosis
Achalasia
Pimary biliary cirrhosis

Unexplained weight loss, lymphadenopathy, or known cancer
Hodgkin disease
Thyroid cancer
Thymus cancer

Other causes
Pregnancy
Acromegaly
Hypertrophic osteoarthropathy

Robert A. Baldor, MD and Alan M. Ehrlich, MD

Clin Dermatol. 2008;26(3):296–305.

COMA

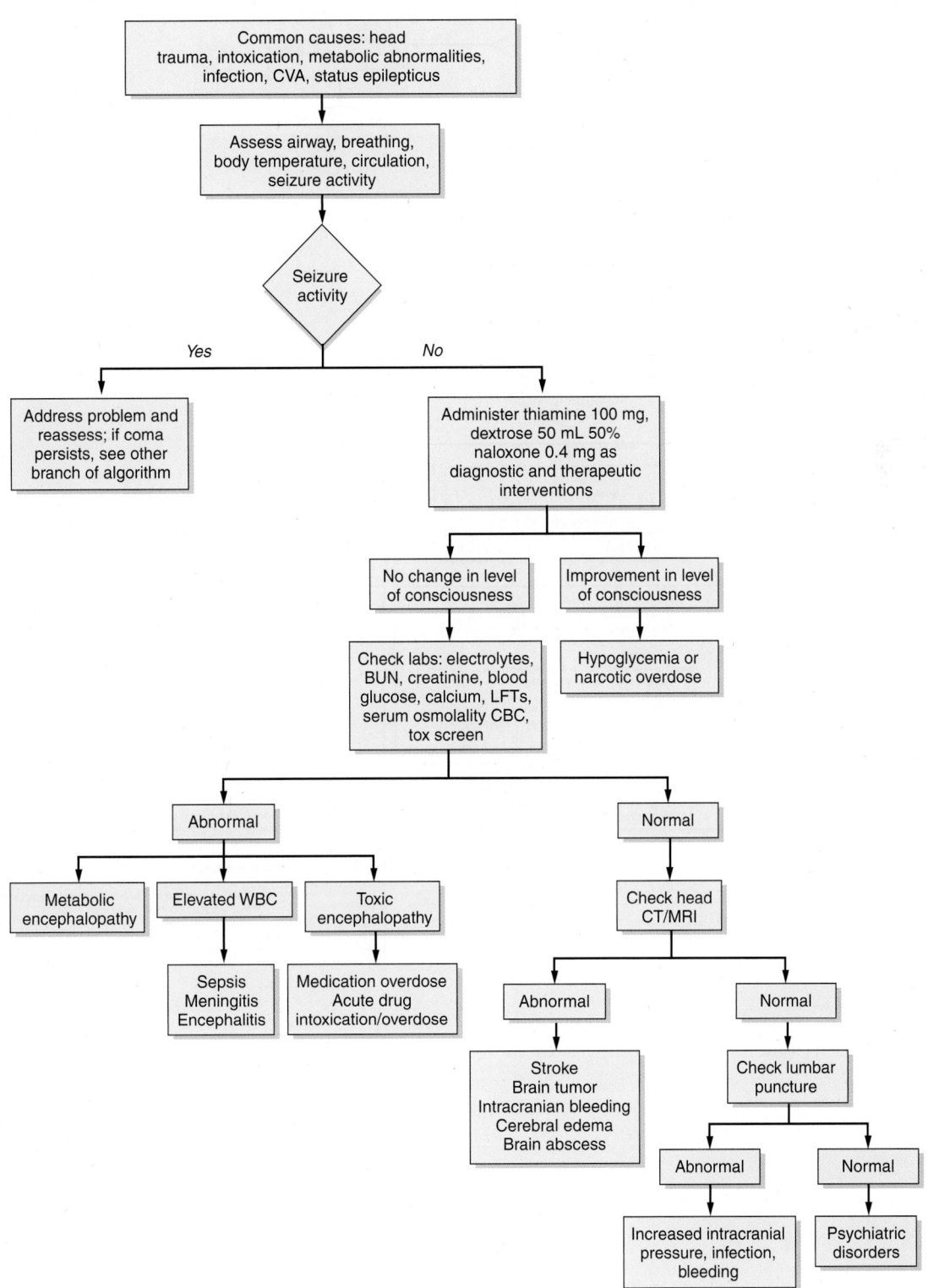

Robert A. Baldor, MD and Alan M. Ehrlich, MD

Neurol Clin. 2008;26(2).

CONCUSSION, SIMPLE EVALUATION AND MANAGEMENT (SPORTS)

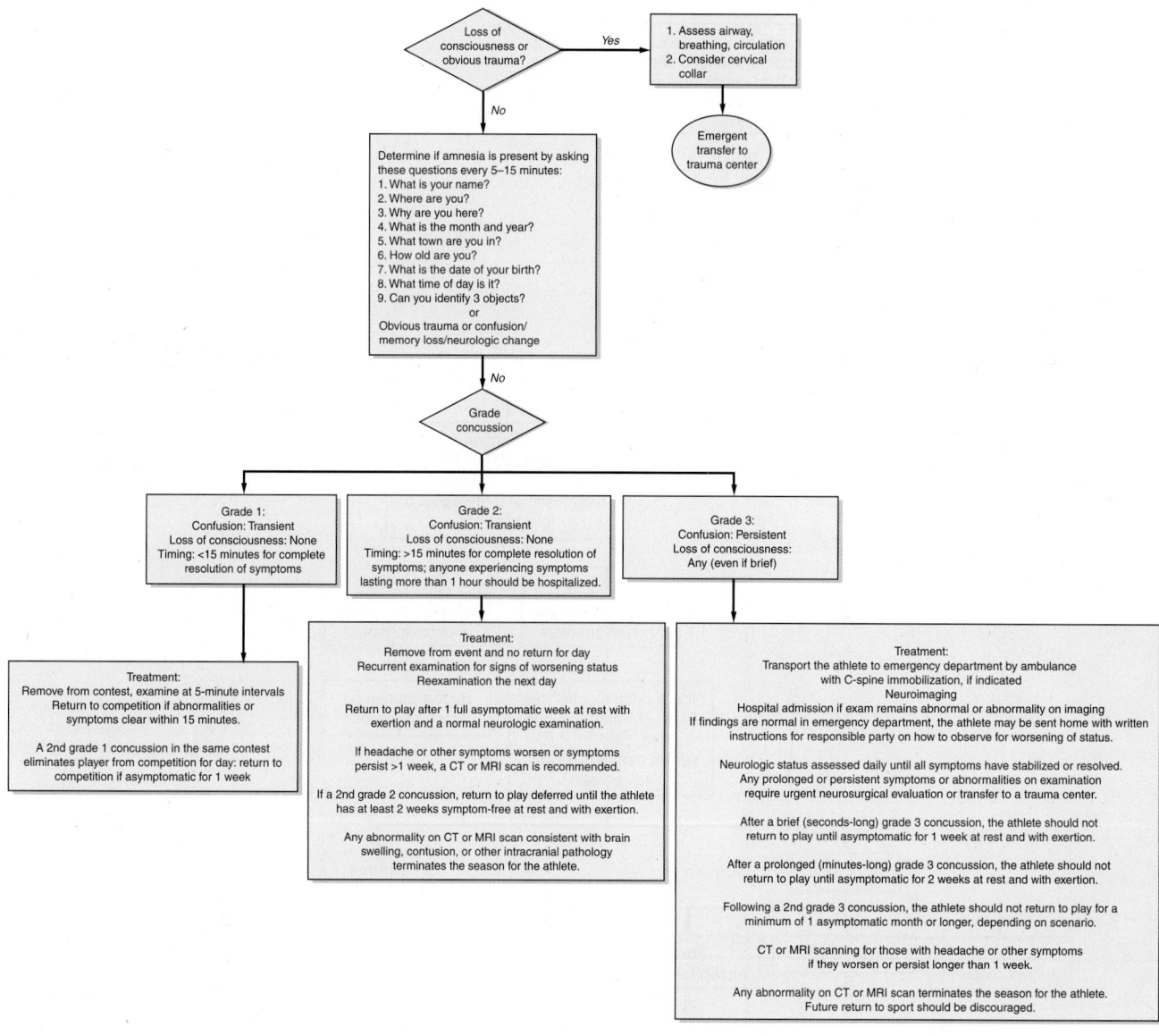

Armin Arasheben, MD and Jason Matuszak, MD

Br J Sports Med. 2005;39:691.

CONGESTIVE HEART FAILURE: DIAGNOSIS AND TREATMENT

Common causes: Ischemia, myocardial infarction, cardiomyopathy, aortic stenosis, aortic insufficiency, atrial fibrillation, thyrotoxicosis, HIV infection, medications

Check: ECG, CPK, troponin, echo

+ECG, CPK, and/or troponin

Normal valves

Abnormal valves

Acute myocardial infarction

History of HTN, alcohol abuse, HIV infection, or cardiotoxic drugs (e.g., doxorubicin, trastuzumab)

+ Stress test

Atrial fibrillation

Nonspecific viral cardiomyopathy

Oxygen
MSO$_4$
Loop diuretic
Nitroglycerin
ACE inhibitor

Ischemic cardiomyopathy

Cardiomyopathy secondary to underlying illness

Decreased ejection fraction secondary to decreased diastolic filling

Aortic stenosis
Mitral regurgitation
Aortic insufficiency

Correct underlying disorder

Symptoms resolved — Yes → Follow clinically

No

Classify based upon symptoms

No

Candidate for valve replacement

Yes

Surgical evaluation

NYHA I	NYHA II	NYHA III	NYHA IV
No limitation of physical activity. Ordinary physical activity does not cause undue fatigue, palpitation, or dyspnea (shortness of breath).	Slight limitation of physical activity. Comfortable at rest, but ordinary physical activity results in fatigue, palpitation, or dyspnea.	Marked limitation of physical activity. Comfortable at rest, but less than ordinary activity causes fatigue, palpitation, or dyspnea.	Unable to carry out any physical activity without discomfort. Symptoms of cardiac insufficiency at rest. If any physical activity is undertaken, discomfort is increased.
Beta blocker ACE inhibitor Cardiac rehabilitation	Beta blocker ACE inhibitor Loop diuretic (IV if acute) Cardiac rehab	Beta blocker ACE inhibitor Loop diuretic (IV if acute) Potassium Sparing diuretics Digoxin (pm for symptom control) Cardiac rehab	Beta blocker ACE inhibitor Loop diuretic (IV if acute) Potassium Sparing diuretics Digoxin (pm for symptom control) Cardiac rehab

AICD, automated implanted cardiac defribrillator; NYHA, New York Heart Association classification

Robert A. Baldor, MD and Alan M. Ehrlich, MD

Joint ACC/AHA Guideline for Diagnosis and Management of Chronic Heart Failure in the Adult at guidelines.gov.

COUGH, CHRONIC

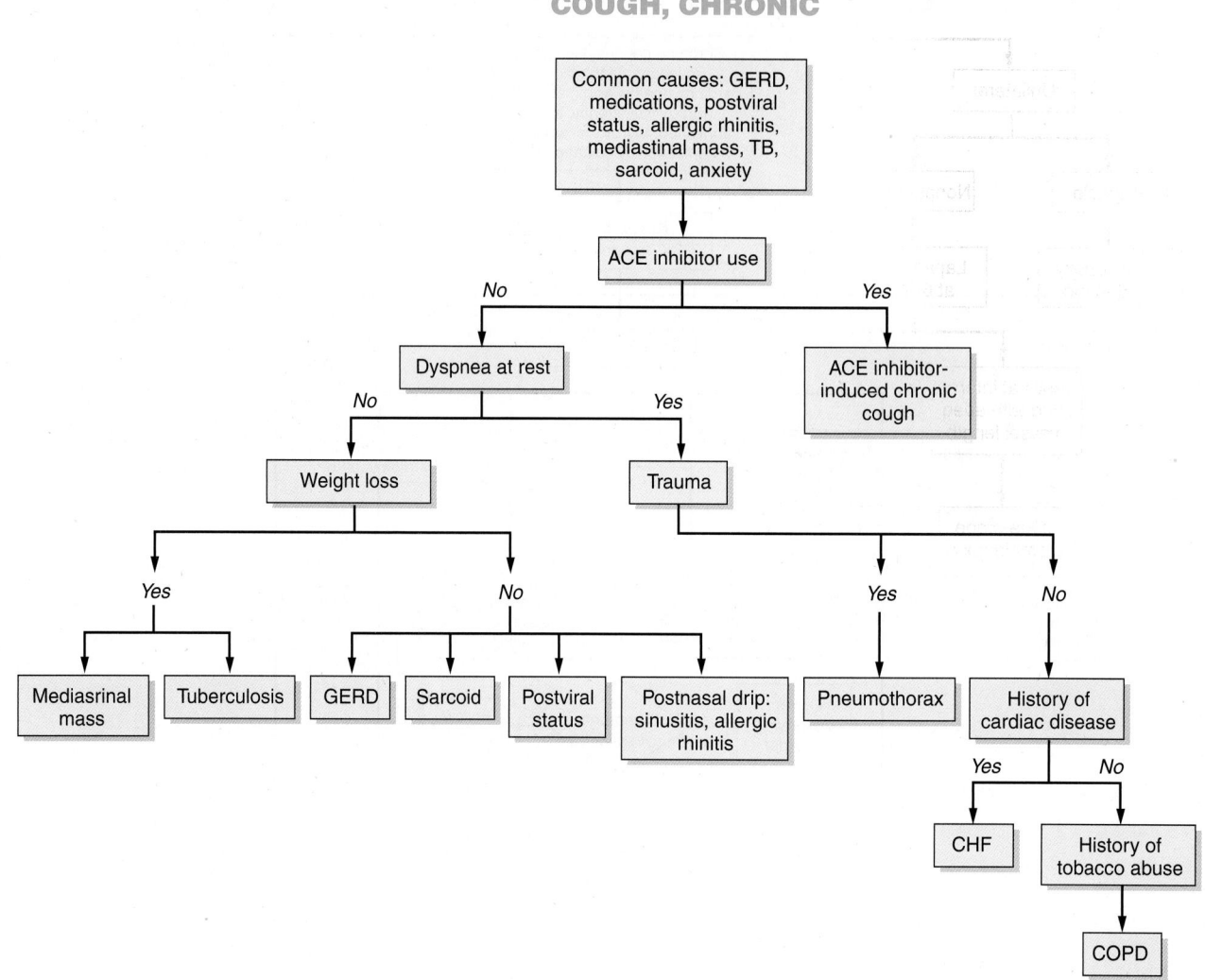

Robert A. Baldor, MD and Alan M. Ehrlich, MD

ACCP Guideline Chronic Cough Chest. 2006;129(1 Suppl):220S–1S.

CRYPTORCHIDISM (Undescended Testes)

```
                                CRYPTORCHIDISM (Undescended Testes)
          ┌──────────────────────────────┬──────────────────────────────────────────┐
     Unilateral                       Bilateral                          Bilateral-
                                                                         Nonpalpable
                                                                         After birth
   ┌──────────┬──────────┐       ┌──────────┬──────────┐                     │
Palpable   Nonpalpable         Palpable  One palpable/                 HCG Stim test
                                          one nonpalpable
   │           │                  │           │                    ┌──────────┴──────────┐
Orchidopexy  Laparoscopy      Orchidopexy  Orchidopexy for      Positive          Negative
at 6–9 mo    at 6–9 mo        at 6–9 mo    palpable UDT,        response          response
                                           laparoscopy for
         ┌───────┴───────┐                 nonpalpable UDT         │                 │
    Testis at         High intra-          at 6–9 mo          Laparoscopy and    Anorchia: will
    internal          abdominal testis                       Rx as for          require future
    ring with         and/or short                           unilateral         endocrine
    adeq vessel       vessels                                 nonpalpable UDT    therapy
    length                                                    at 6–9 mo
         │                 │
    One-stage         Fowler Stephens
    orchidepxy        orchidopexy,
                      single or two-
                      stage
```

Robert A. Baldor, MD and Alan M. Ehrlich, MD

Am Fam Physician. 2000;62:2037–44, 2047–8.

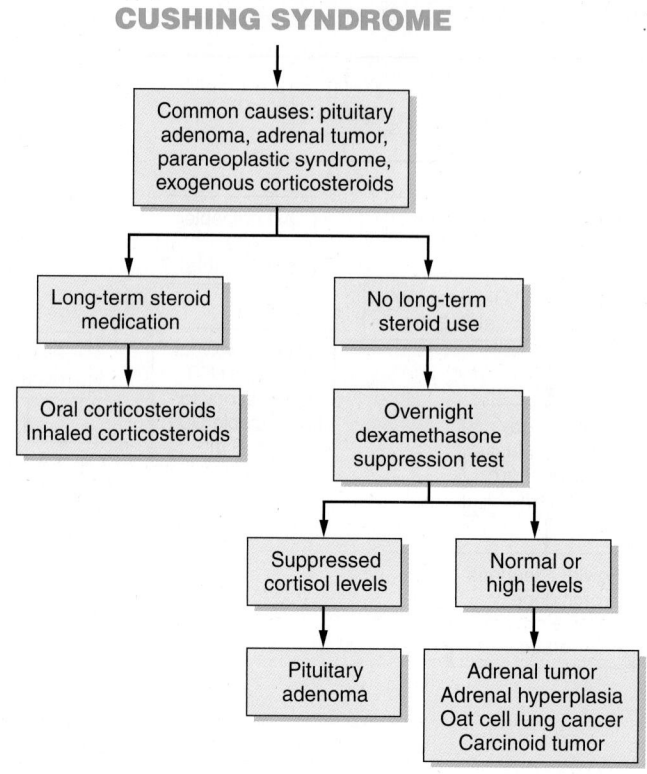

CUSHING SYNDROME

Common causes: pituitary adenoma, adrenal tumor, paraneoplastic syndrome, exogenous corticosteroids

Long-term steroid medication

No long-term steroid use

Oral corticosteroids
Inhaled corticosteroids

Overnight dexamethasone suppression test

Suppressed cortisol levels

Normal or high levels

Pituitary adenoma

Adrenal tumor
Adrenal hyperplasia
Oat cell lung cancer
Carcinoid tumor

Robert A. Baldor, MD and Alan M. Ehrlich, MD

J Clin Endocrinol Metabol. 2009;94(9).

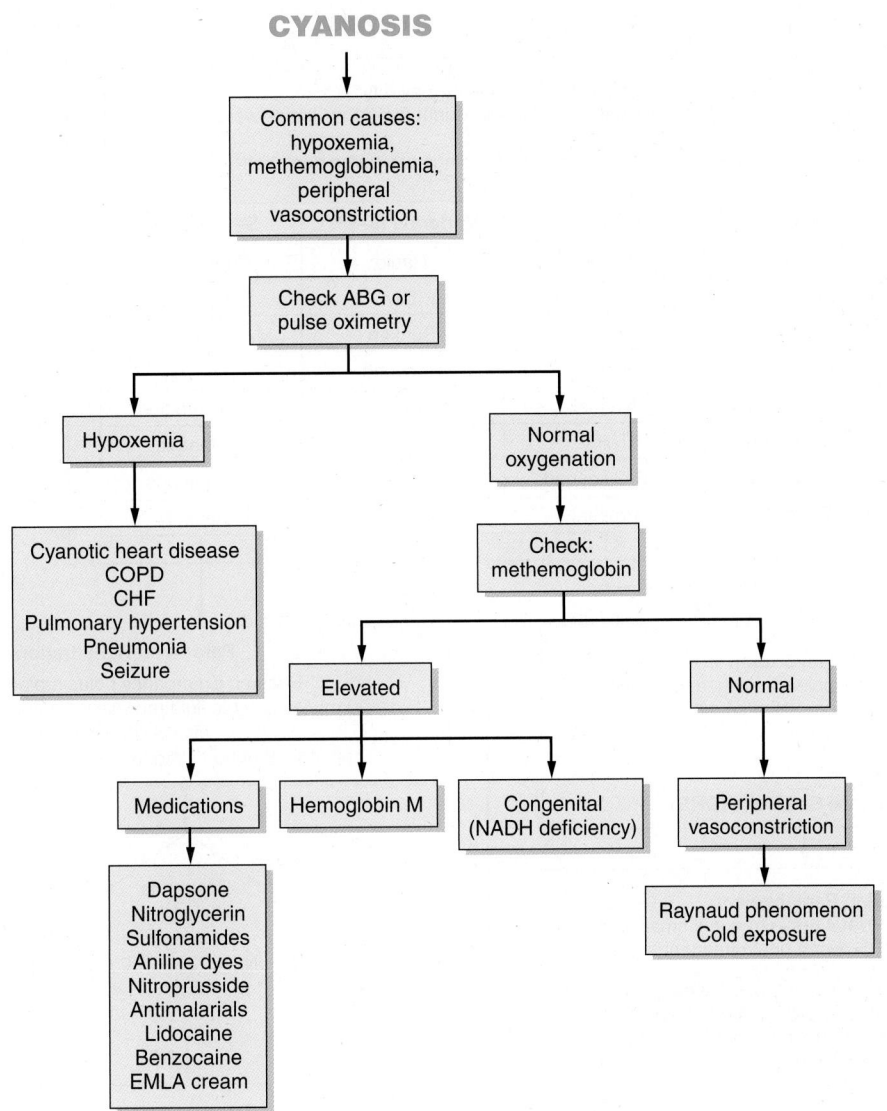

CYANOSIS

Common causes: hypoxemia, methemoglobinemia, peripheral vasoconstriction

Check ABG or pulse oximetry

Hypoxemia → Cyanotic heart disease / COPD / CHF / Pulmonary hypertension / Pneumonia / Seizure

Normal oxygenation → Check: methemoglobin

Elevated → Medications / Hemoglobin M / Congenital (NADH deficiency)

Medications → Dapsone / Nitroglycerin / Sulfonamides / Aniline dyes / Nitroprusside / Antimalarials / Lidocaine / Benzocaine / EMLA cream

Normal → Peripheral vasoconstriction → Raynaud phenomenon / Cold exposure

Robert A. Baldor, MD and Alan M. Ehrlich, MD

Am J Roent. 2005;189:241–7.

DEHYDRATION, PEDIATRIC

Determine Dehydration Severity:

% Dehydration = [Pre-illness weight (kg) – illness weight (kg)]/ Pre-illness weight (kg) x 100%

or

Clinical Assessment: Physical findings of volume depletion

Finding	Mild (3–5%)	Moderate (6–9%)	Severe (10%)
Pulse rate	Full, normal	Rapid	Rapid, weak
Buccal mucosa	Slightly dry	Dry	Parched
Eyes	Normal	Sunken	Markedly sunken
Skin turgor	Normal	Reduced	Tenting
Skin	Normal	Cool	Cool, mottled
Systemic signs	↑Thirst	Irritable	Lethargic
Capillary refill	>1.5–2 seconds	2–3 seconds	>3 seconds
Tears	Present	Decreased	Absent

Oral Rehydration

(contraindications: Intractable vomiting, acute abdomen, severe gastric distention, >10 mL/kg/hr stool loss)

Oral Replace Solutions (ORS)

Deficit Replacement

Mild: 50 mL/kg ORS over 4 hrs in frequent small amounts
Moderate: 100 mL/kg ORS over 4 hrs in frequent small amounts

If continued, excessive stool output or severe, persistent vomiting and inadequate rehydration with ORS, consider parenteral treatment

Maintenance

ORS by age	ORS by weight per hour
Infants: 1 oz/hr	<10 kg: 4 mL/kg ORS
Toddlers: 2 oz/hr	11–20 kg: 40 mL + 2 mL/kg (per kg 11–20)
Older child: 3 oz/hr	>20 kg: 60 mL + 1 mL/kg (per kg >20)

Ongoing Losses

For every loose stool: 10 mL/kg ORS

For every emesis episode: 2 mL/kg ORS

Parenteral Rehydration

Phase I: Emergency bolus replacement
–20 mL/kg isotonic fluid (normal saline or lactated ringer) over 5–10 minutes
–Repeat up to total of 60 mL/kg; reassess etiology if no improvement

Responds to fluid bolus and serum Na = 130 – 150 mEq/L

Yes

No

Treat for hypo- or hypernatremia

Phase II: Maintenance

a) 100 mL/kg for 1st 10 kg, then
50 mL/kg for next 10 kg, then
25 mL/kg for each kg >20 kg.
b) Give 1st half over 8 hours, 2nd half over next 16 hours.

Stephanie Galica, MD

Am Fam Physician. 2009;80(7):692–6.

DELAYED PUBERTY

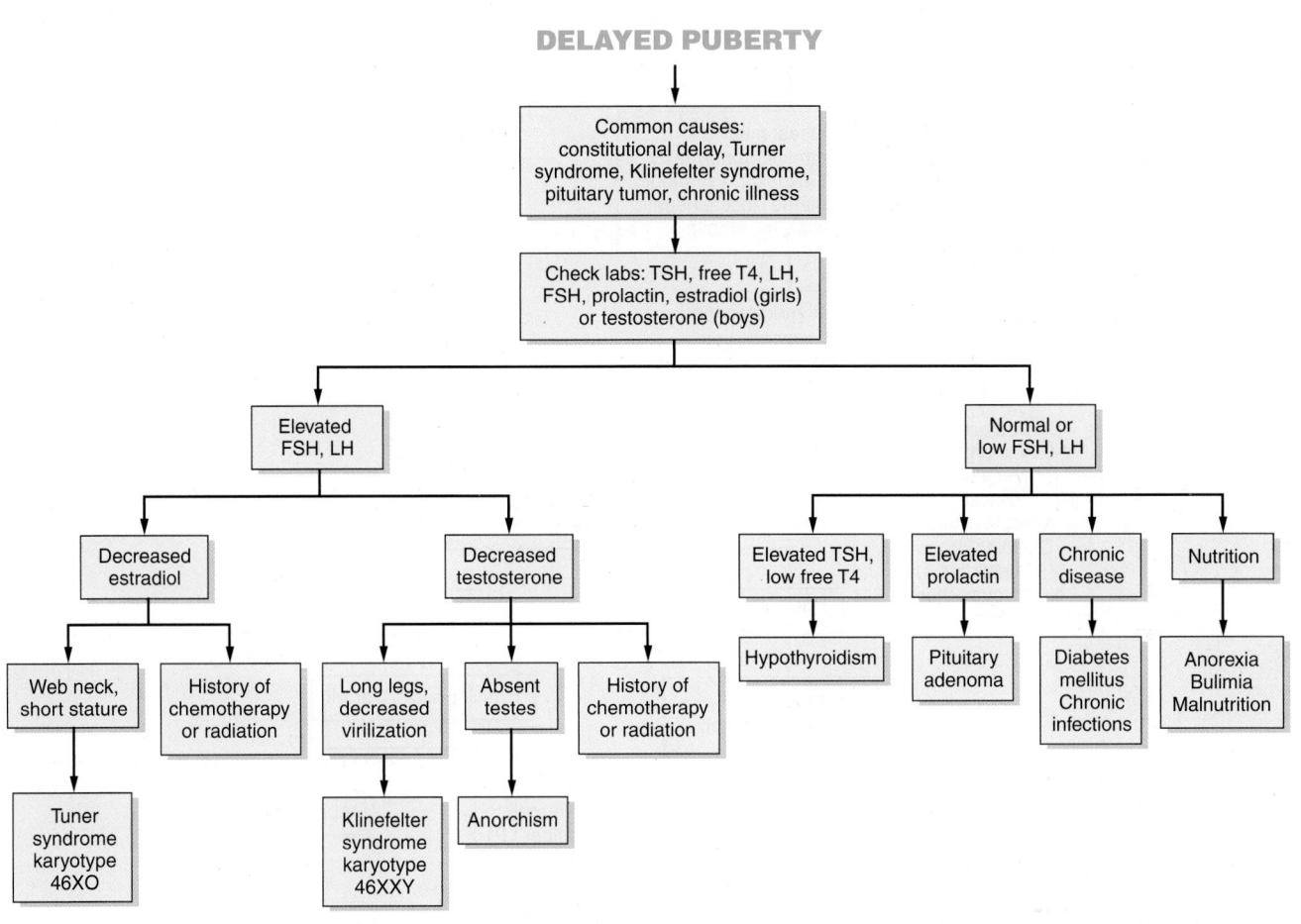

Robert A. Baldor, MD and Alan M. Ehrlich, MD

Am Fam Physician. 1999;60:209–24.

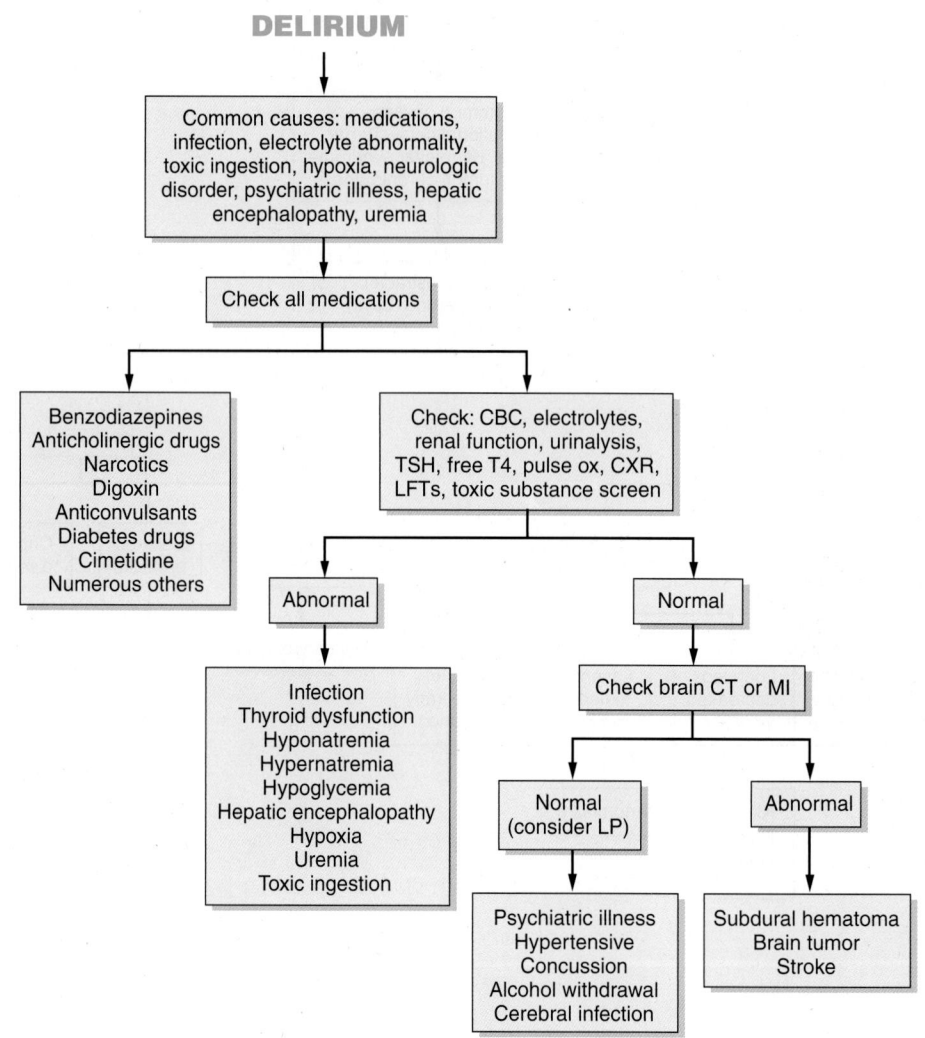

DELIRIUM

Common causes: medications, infection, electrolyte abnormality, toxic ingestion, hypoxia, neurologic disorder, psychiatric illness, hepatic encephalopathy, uremia

Check all medications

Benzodiazepines
Anticholinergic drugs
Narcotics
Digoxin
Anticonvulsants
Diabetes drugs
Cimetidine
Numerous others

Check: CBC, electrolytes, renal function, urinalysis, TSH, free T4, pulse ox, CXR, LFTs, toxic substance screen

Abnormal

Normal

Infection
Thyroid dysfunction
Hyponatremia
Hypernatremia
Hypoglycemia
Hepatic encephalopathy
Hypoxia
Uremia
Toxic ingestion

Check brain CT or MI

Normal
(consider LP)

Abnormal

Psychiatric illness
Hypertensive
Concussion
Alcohol withdrawal
Cerebral infection

Subdural hematoma
Brain tumor
Stroke

Robert A. Baldor, MD and Alan M. Ehrlich, MD

Am Fam Physician. 2003;67:1027–34.

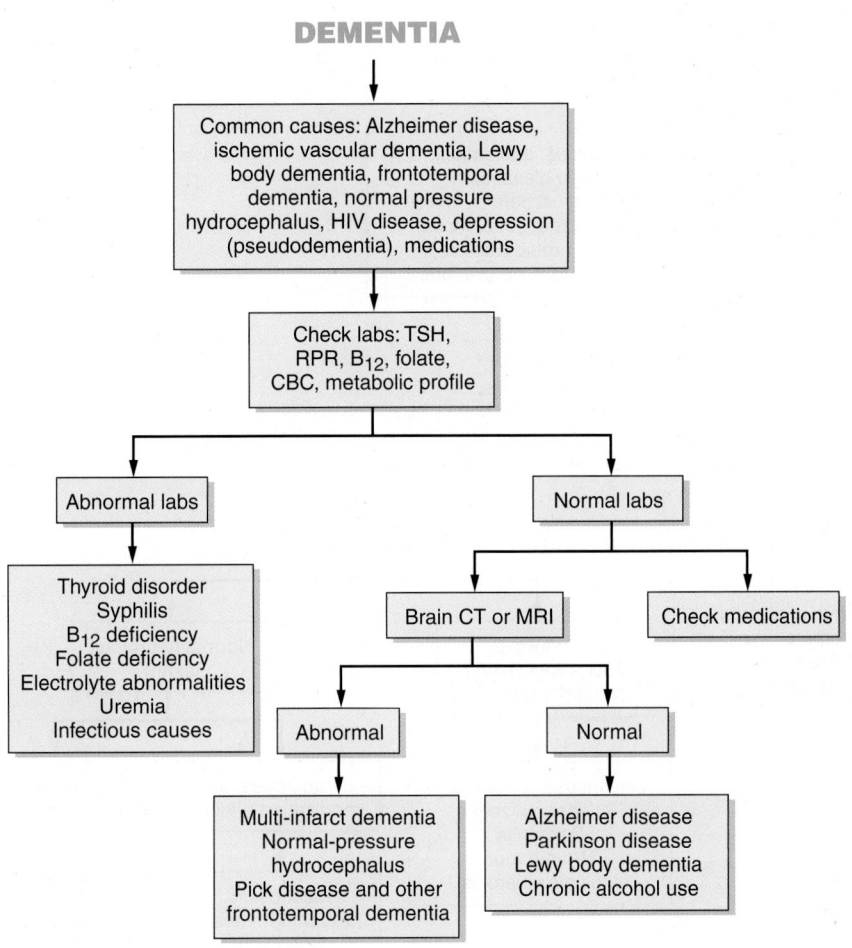

DEMENTIA

Common causes: Alzheimer disease, ischemic vascular dementia, Lewy body dementia, frontotemporal dementia, normal pressure hydrocephalus, HIV disease, depression (pseudodementia), medications

Check labs: TSH, RPR, B_{12}, folate, CBC, metabolic profile

Abnormal labs

Normal labs

Thyroid disorder
Syphilis
B_{12} deficiency
Folate deficiency
Electrolyte abnormalities
Uremia
Infectious causes

Brain CT or MRI

Check medications

Abnormal

Normal

Multi-infarct dementia
Normal-pressure hydrocephalus
Pick disease and other frontotemporal dementia

Alzheimer disease
Parkinson disease
Lewy body dementia
Chronic alcohol use

Robert A. Baldor, MD and Alan M. Ehrlich, MD

Neurology. 2001;56(9):1143–53.

DEPRESSED MOOD RESULTING FROM MEDICAL ILLNESS

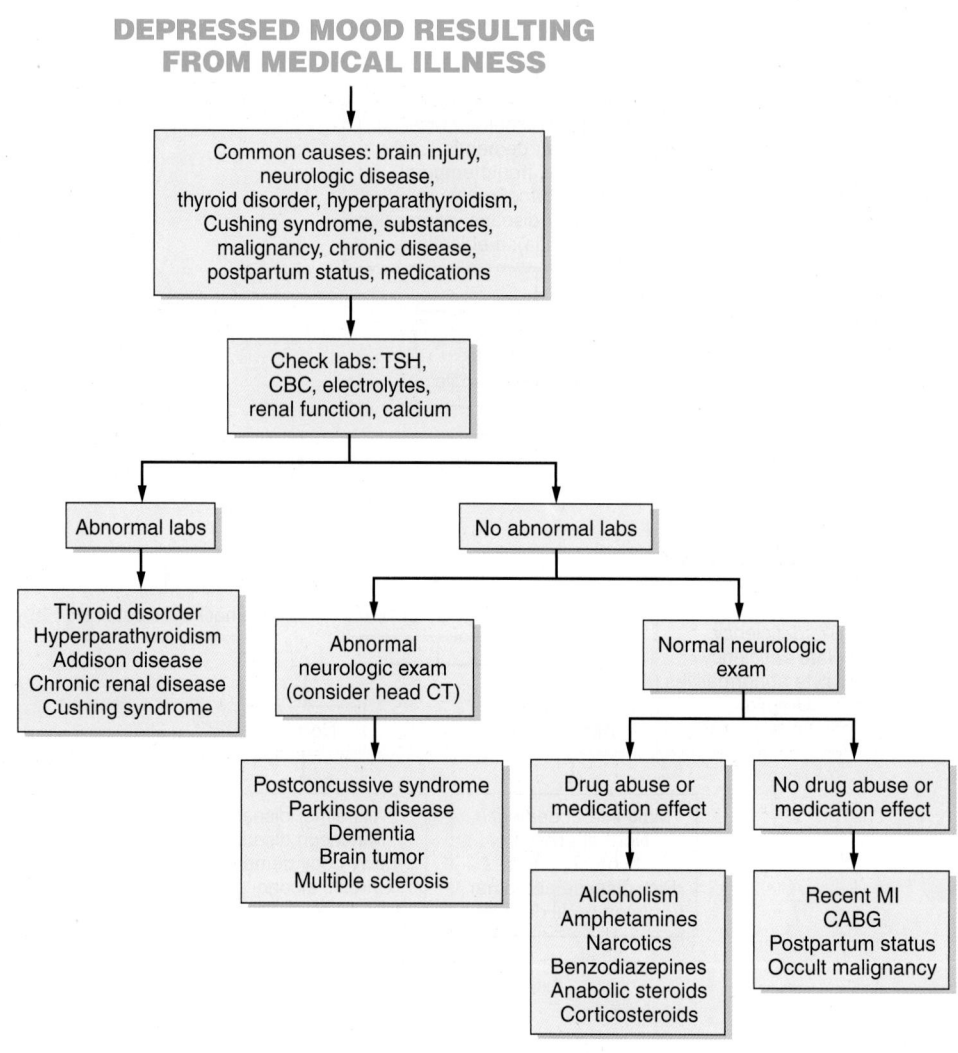

Common causes: brain injury, neurologic disease, thyroid disorder, hyperparathyroidism, Cushing syndrome, substances, malignancy, chronic disease, postpartum status, medications

Check labs: TSH, CBC, electrolytes, renal function, calcium

Abnormal labs
- Thyroid disorder
- Hyperparathyroidism
- Addison disease
- Chronic renal disease
- Cushing syndrome

No abnormal labs

Abnormal neurologic exam (consider head CT)
- Postconcussive syndrome
- Parkinson disease
- Dementia
- Brain tumor
- Multiple sclerosis

Normal neurologic exam

Drug abuse or medication effect
- Alcoholism
- Amphetamines
- Narcotics
- Benzodiazepines
- Anabolic steroids
- Corticosteroids

No drug abuse or medication effect
- Recent MI
- CABG
- Postpartum status
- Occult malignancy

Robert A. Baldor, MD and Alan M. Ehrlich, MD

Phys Sportsmed. 2009;37(2):141–5.

DEPRESSIVE EPISODE, MAJOR

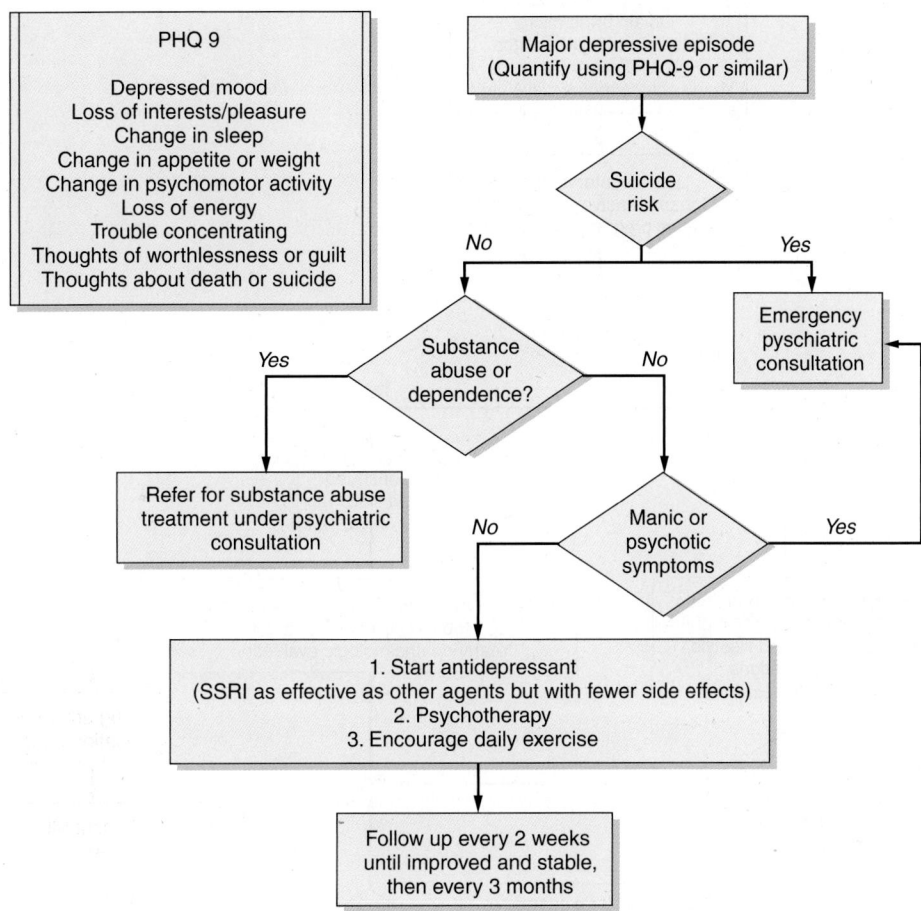

PHQ 9

Depressed mood
Loss of interests/pleasure
Change in sleep
Change in appetite or weight
Change in psychomotor activity
Loss of energy
Trouble concentrating
Thoughts of worthlessness or guilt
Thoughts about death or suicide

Major depressive episode
(Quantify using PHQ-9 or similar)

Suicide risk

No   Yes

Emergency pyschiatric consultation

Substance abuse or dependence?

Yes   No

Refer for substance abuse treatment under psychiatric consultation

Manic or psychotic symptoms

No   Yes

1. Start antidepressant
(SSRI as effective as other agents but with fewer side effects)
2. Psychotherapy
3. Encourage daily exercise

Follow up every 2 weeks until improved and stable, then every 3 months

James F. Cunagin, MD

Depression. University of Michigan Health System; 2005 Oct. 20 at National Guidelines Clearinghouse.

DIABETES MELLITUS, TYPE 2

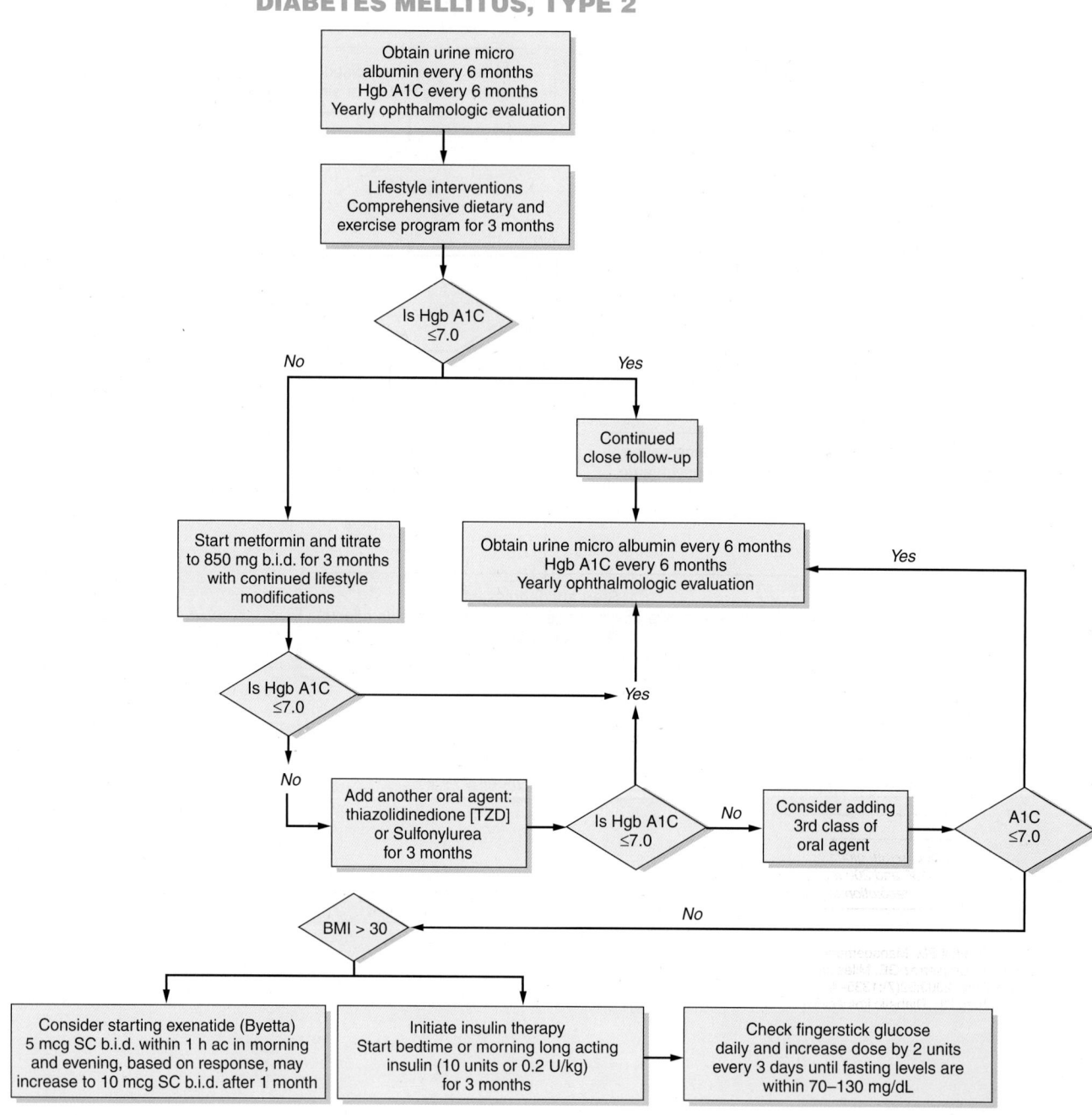

Frank J. Domino, MD

Am Fam Physician. 2003;67(5).

DIABETIC KETOACIDOSIS (DKA), TREATMENT

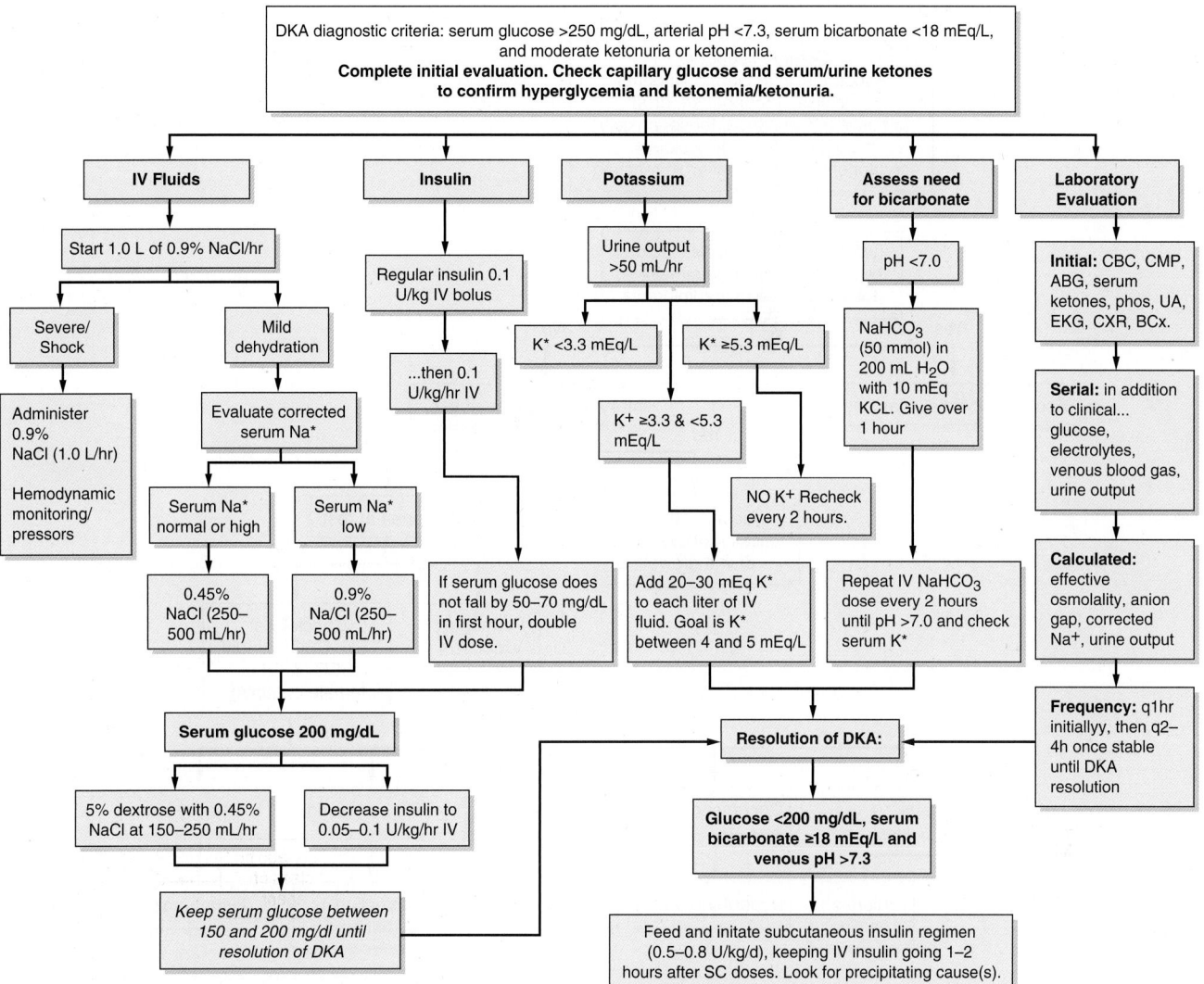

DKA diagnostic criteria: serum glucose >250 mg/dL, arterial pH <7.3, serum bicarbonate <18 mEq/L, and moderate ketonuria or ketonemia.
Complete initial evaluation. Check capillary glucose and serum/urine ketones to confirm hyperglycemia and ketonemia/ketonuria.

IV Fluids

Start 1.0 L of 0.9% NaCl/hr

Severe/ Shock

Administer 0.9% NaCl (1.0 L/hr)

Hemodynamic monitoring/ pressors

Mild dehydration

Evaluate corrected serum Na*

Serum Na* normal or high

Serum Na* low

0.45% NaCl (250–500 mL/hr)

0.9% Na/Cl (250–500 mL/hr)

Serum glucose 200 mg/dL

5% dextrose with 0.45% NaCl at 150–250 mL/hr

Decrease insulin to 0.05–0.1 U/kg/hr IV

Keep serum glucose between 150 and 200 mg/dl until resolution of DKA

Insulin

Regular insulin 0.1 U/kg IV bolus

...then 0.1 U/kg/hr IV

If serum glucose does not fall by 50–70 mg/dL in first hour, double IV dose.

Potassium

Urine output >50 mL/hr

K* <3.3 mEq/L

K* ≥5.3 mEq/L

K+ ≥3.3 & <5.3 mEq/L

NO K+ Recheck every 2 hours.

Add 20–30 mEq K* to each liter of IV fluid. Goal is K* between 4 and 5 mEq/L

Assess need for bicarbonate

pH <7.0

NaHCO3 (50 mmol) in 200 mL H2O with 10 mEq KCL. Give over 1 hour

Repeat IV NaHCO3 dose every 2 hours until pH >7.0 and check serum K*

Laboratory Evaluation

Initial: CBC, CMP, ABG, serum ketones, phos, UA, EKG, CXR, BCx.

Serial: in addition to clinical... glucose, electrolytes, venous blood gas, urine output

Calculated: effective osmolality, anion gap, corrected Na+, urine output

Frequency: q1hr initiallyy, then q2–4h once stable until DKA resolution

Resolution of DKA:

Glucose <200 mg/dL, serum bicarbonate ≥18 mEq/L and venous pH >7.3

Feed and initate subcutaneous insulin regimen (0.5–0.8 U/kg/d), keeping IV insulin going 1–2 hours after SC doses. Look for precipitating cause(s).

Kitabchi AE, Wall BM. Management of diabetic ketoacidosis. *Am Fam Physician.* 1999;60(2):455–64.
Kitabchi AE, Umpierrez GE, Miles JM, Fisher JN. Hyperglycemic crises in adult patients with diabetes. *Diabetes Care.* 2009;32(7):1335–43.
Trachetenbarg DE. Diabetic ketoacidosis. *Am Fam Physician.* 2005;71(9):1705–14.

John B. Waits, MD

LMAJ. 2003;168(7):859–6.

DIAPHORESIS

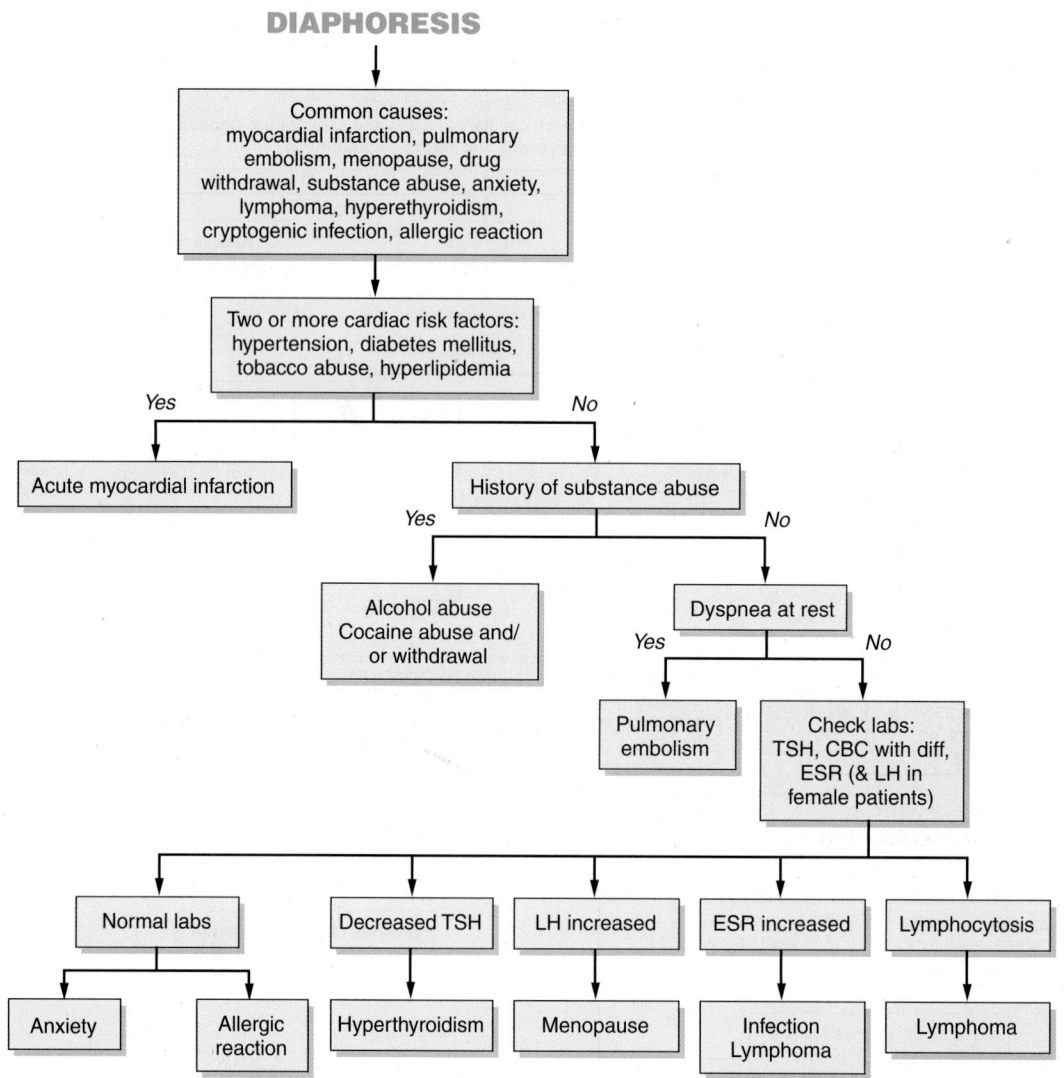

Robert A. Baldor, MD and Alan M. Ehrlich, MD

Depression University of Michigan Health System; 2005 Oct. 20 at National Guidelines Clearinghouse.

DIARRHEA, CHRONIC

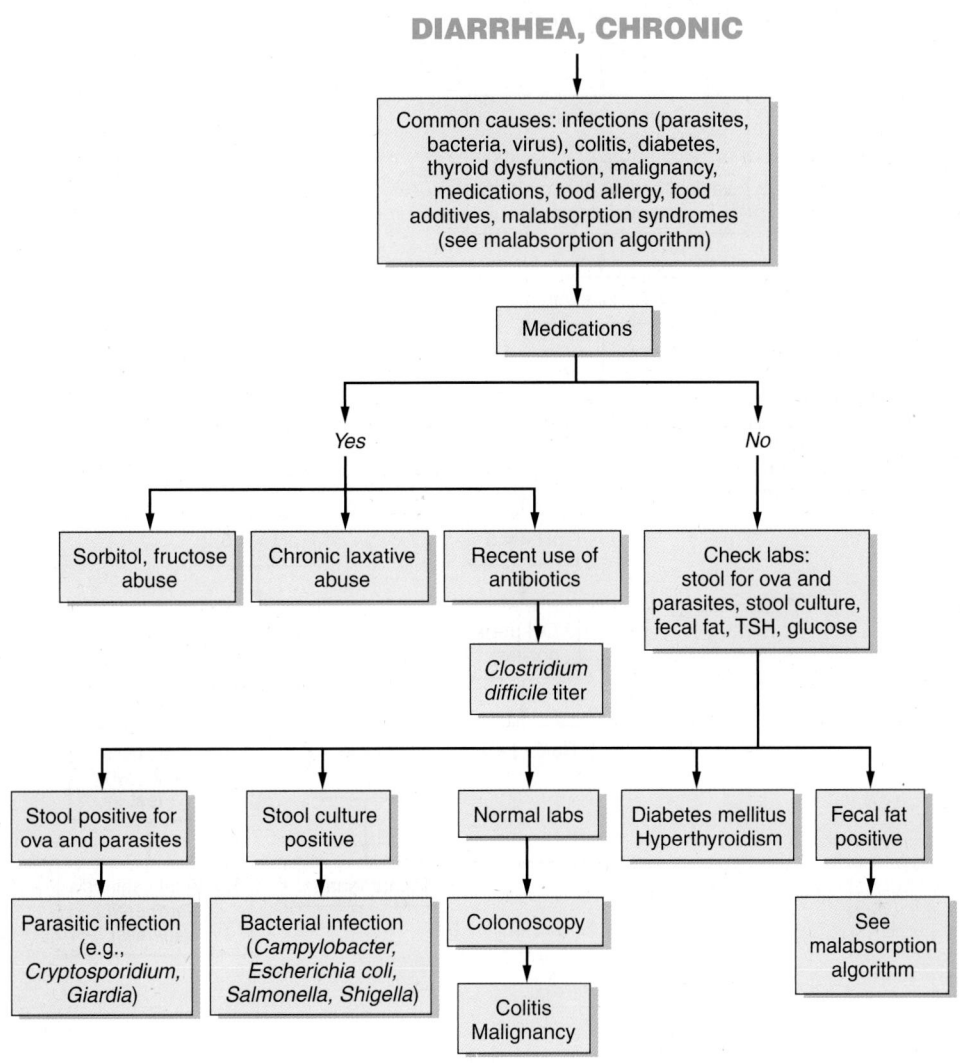

Common causes: infections (parasites, bacteria, virus), colitis, diabetes, thyroid dysfunction, malignancy, medications, food allergy, food additives, malabsorption syndromes (see malabsorption algorithm)

Medications

Yes

No

Sorbitol, fructose abuse

Chronic laxative abuse

Recent use of antibiotics

Check labs: stool for ova and parasites, stool culture, fecal fat, TSH, glucose

Clostridium difficile titer

Stool positive for ova and parasites

Stool culture positive

Normal labs

Diabetes mellitus Hyperthyroidism

Fecal fat positive

Parasitic infection (e.g., *Cryptosporidium*, *Giardia*)

Bacterial infection (*Campylobacter*, *Escherichia coli*, *Salmonella*, *Shigella*)

Colonoscopy

See malabsorption algorithm

Colitis Malignancy

Robert A. Baldor, MD and Alan M. Ehrlich, MD

Institute for Clinical Systems Improvement (ICSI); 2009 May. 114 p. at National Guidelines Clearinghouse.

DISCHARGE, VAGINAL

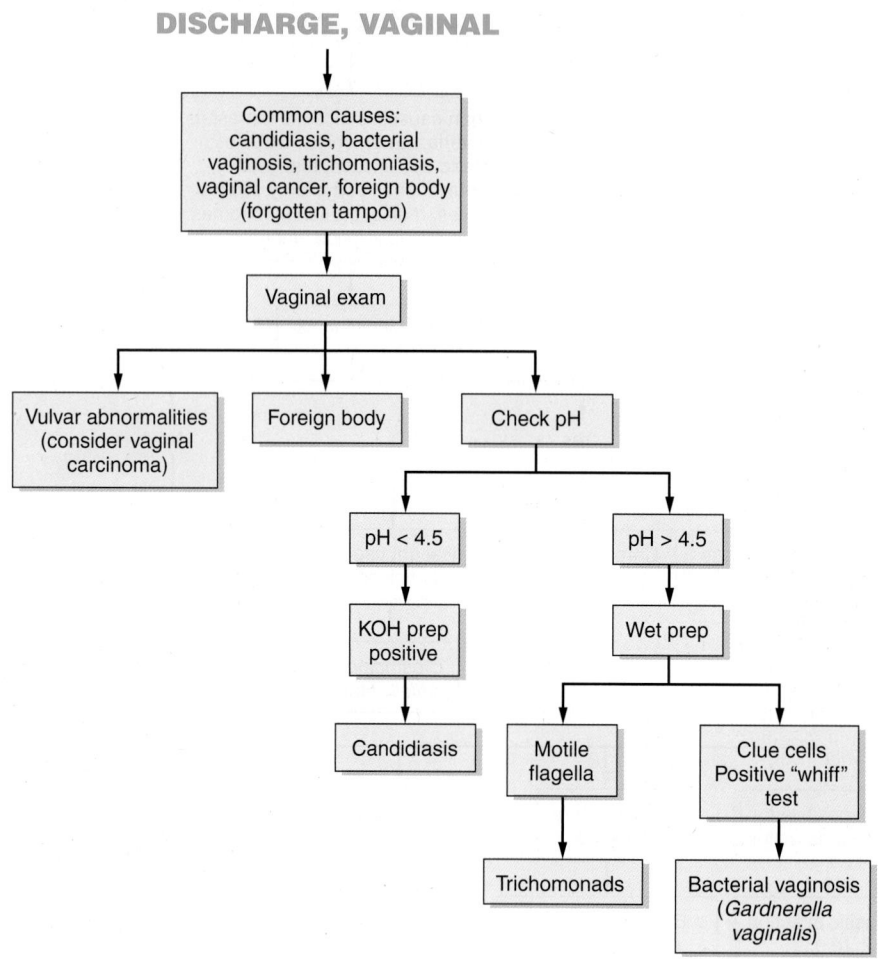

Robert A. Baldor, MD and Alan M. Ehrlich, MD

Primary Care Clin Office Pract. 2009;36(1).

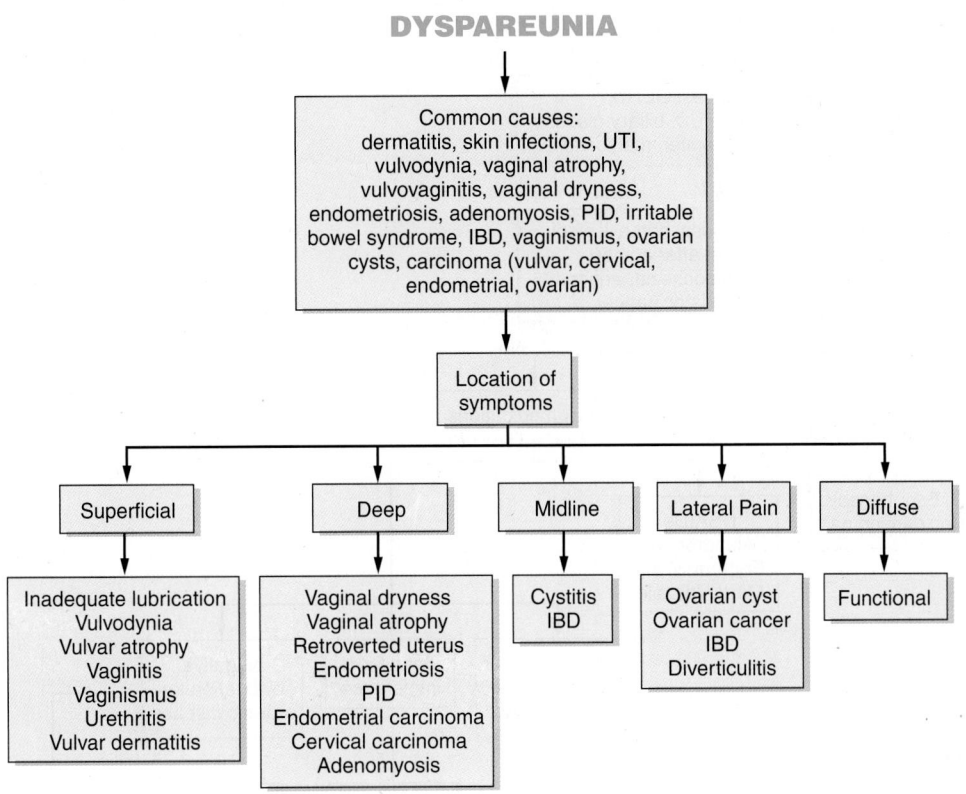

DYSPAREUNIA

Common causes:
dermatitis, skin infections, UTI, vulvodynia, vaginal atrophy, vulvovaginitis, vaginal dryness, endometriosis, adenomyosis, PID, irritable bowel syndrome, IBD, vaginismus, ovarian cysts, carcinoma (vulvar, cervical, endometrial, ovarian)

Location of symptoms

Superficial
Inadequate lubrication
Vulvodynia
Vulvar atrophy
Vaginitis
Vaginismus
Urethritis
Vulvar dermatitis

Deep
Vaginal dryness
Vaginal atrophy
Retroverted uterus
Endometriosis
PID
Endometrial carcinoma
Cervical carcinoma
Adenomyosis

Midline
Cystitis
IBD

Lateral Pain
Ovarian cyst
Ovarian cancer
IBD
Diverticulitis

Diffuse
Functional

Robert A. Baldor, MD and Alan M. Ehrlich, MD

Obstet Gynecol Clin. 2006;33(4).

DYSPEPSIA

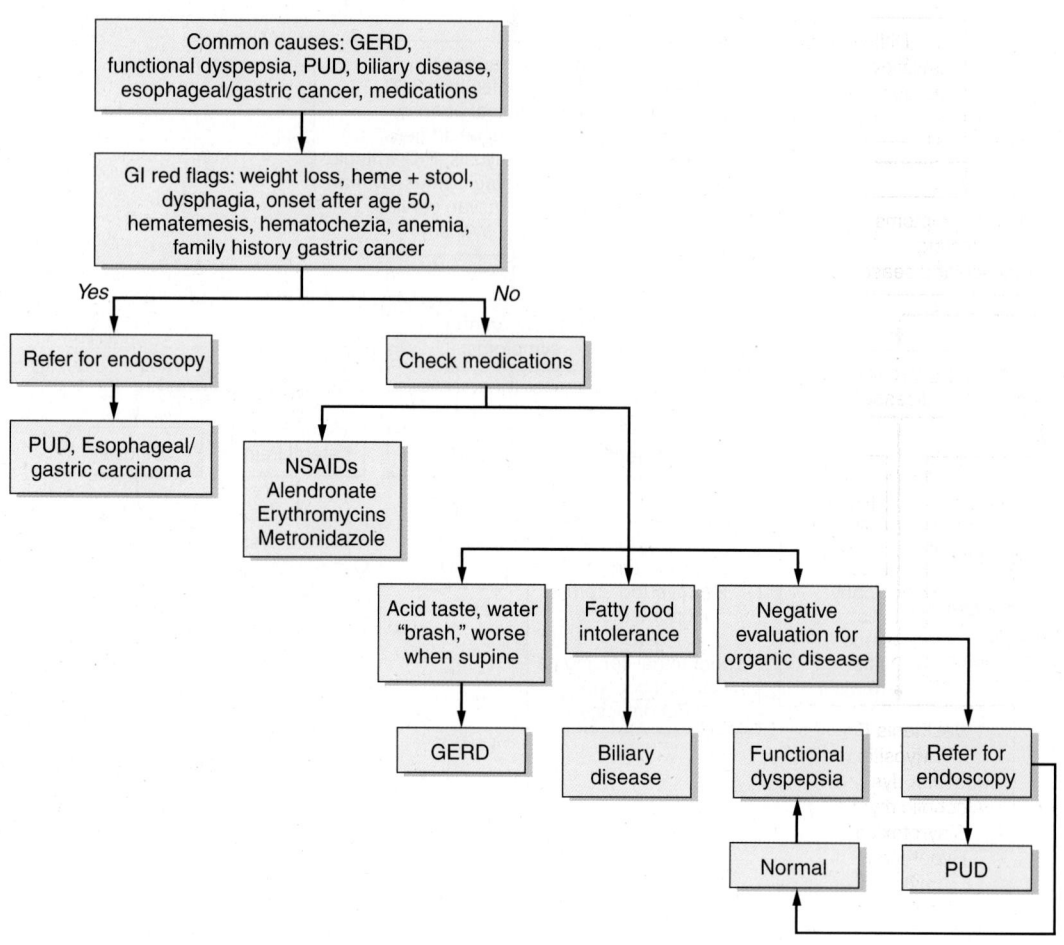

Robert A. Baldor, MD and Alan M. Ehrlich, MD

J Fam Pract. 2009;58(7 Suppl Short):S1–1.

DYSPHAGIA

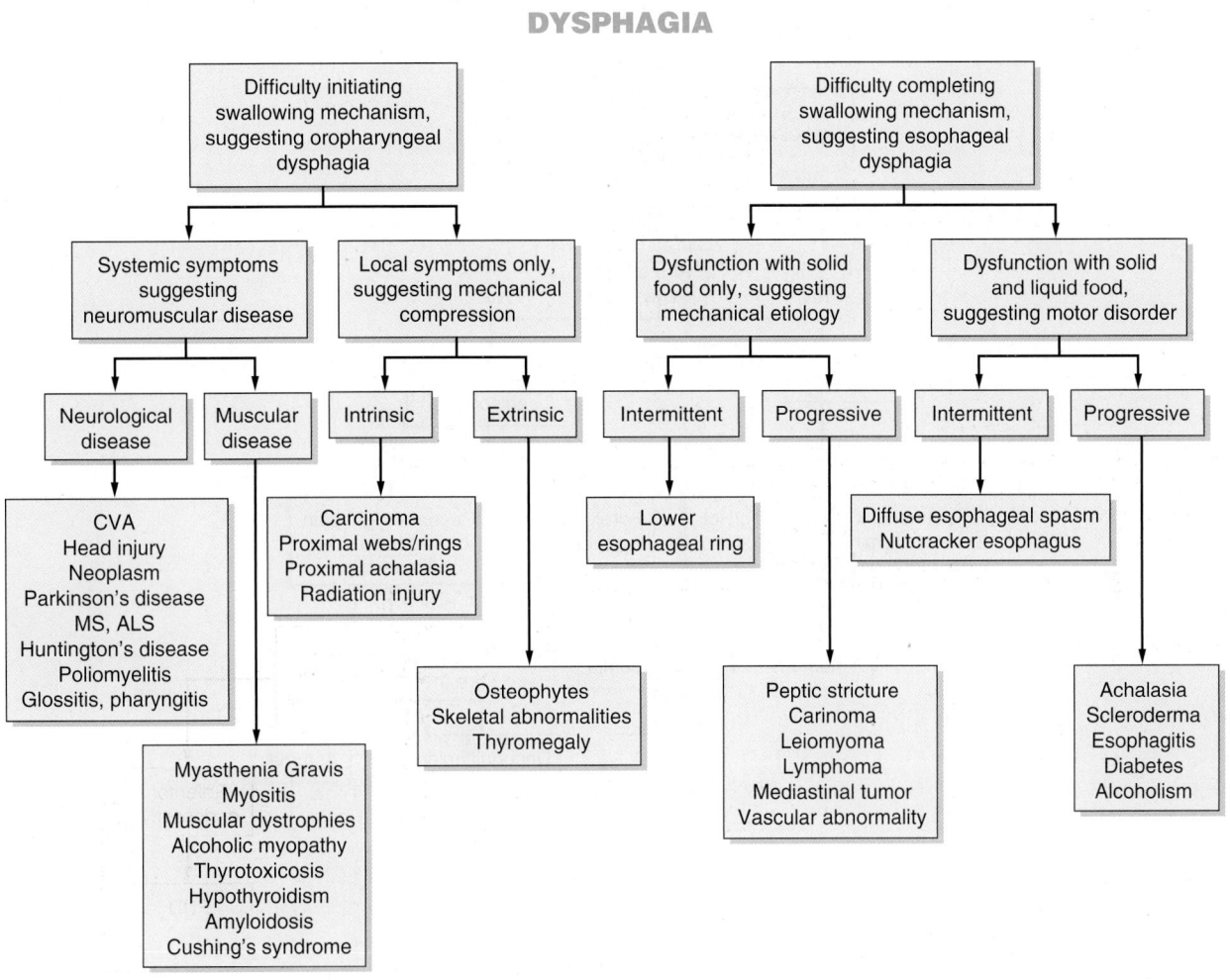

Difficulty initiating swallowing mechanism, suggesting oropharyngeal dysphagia

- Systemic symptoms suggesting neuromuscular disease
  - Neurological disease
    - CVA
      Head injury
      Neoplasm
      Parkinson's disease
      MS, ALS
      Huntington's disease
      Poliomyelitis
      Glossitis, pharyngitis
  - Muscular disease
    - Myasthenia Gravis
      Myositis
      Muscular dystrophies
      Alcoholic myopathy
      Thyrotoxicosis
      Hypothyroidism
      Amyloidosis
      Cushing's syndrome
- Local symptoms only, suggesting mechanical compression
  - Intrinsic
    - Carcinoma
      Proximal webs/rings
      Proximal achalasia
      Radiation injury
  - Extrinsic
    - Osteophytes
      Skeletal abnormalities
      Thyromegaly

Difficulty completing swallowing mechanism, suggesting esophageal dysphagia

- Dysfunction with solid food only, suggesting mechanical etiology
  - Intermittent
    - Lower esophageal ring
  - Progressive
    - Peptic stricture
      Carinoma
      Leiomyoma
      Lymphoma
      Mediastinal tumor
      Vascular abnormality
- Dysfunction with solid and liquid food, suggesting motor disorder
  - Intermittent
    - Diffuse esophageal spasm
      Nutcracker esophagus
  - Progressive
    - Achalasia
      Scleroderma
      Esophagitis
      Diabetes
      Alcoholism

Parag Goyal, MD

Gastroenterol Clin North Am. 2003;32(2):553–75.

DYSPNEA

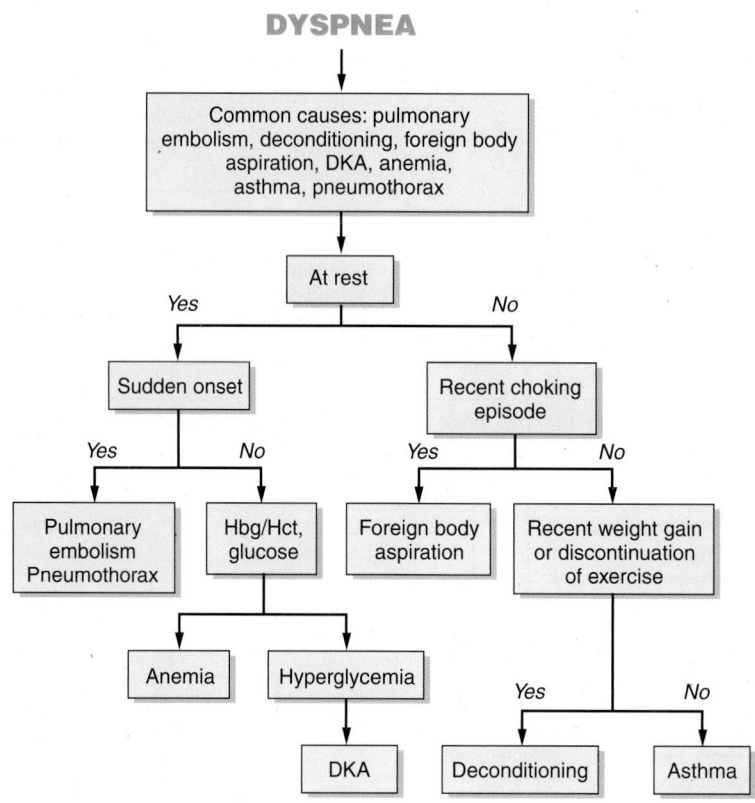

Robert A. Baldor, MD and Alan M. Ehrlich, MD

Diagnostic evaluation of dyspnea. *Am Fam Physician.* Feb 15, 1998.

DYSURIA

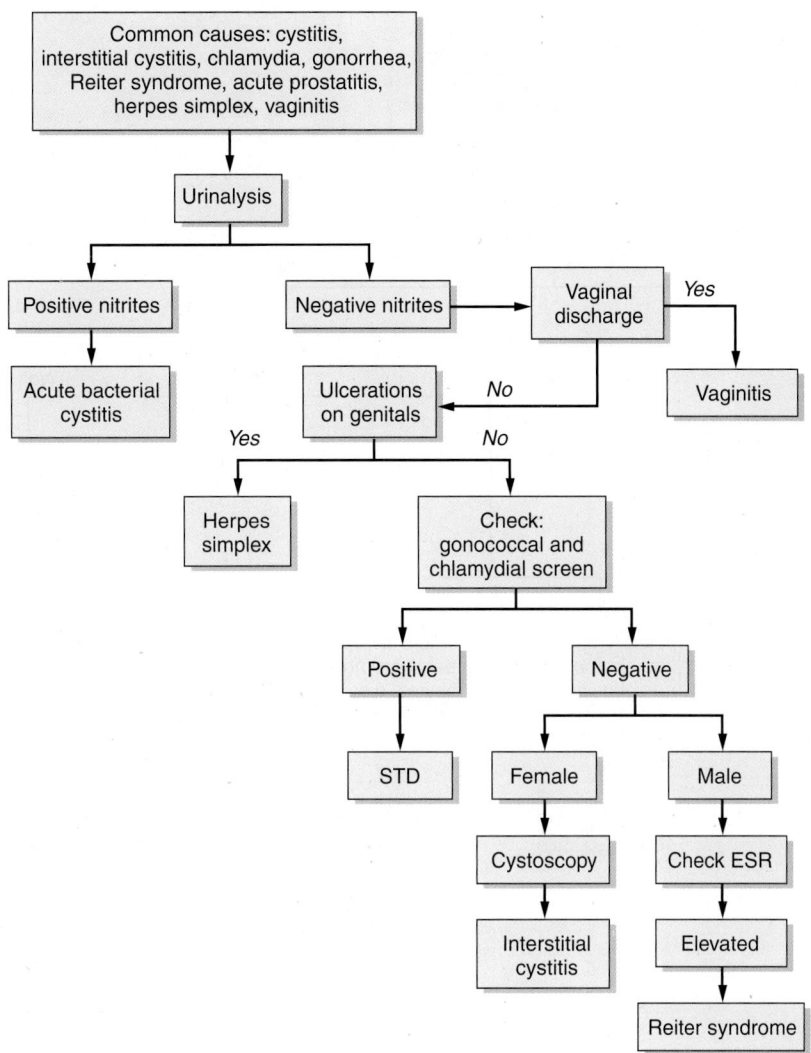

Robert A. Baldor, MD and Alan M. Ehrlich, MD

Am Fam Physician. 2002;65:1589–97.

EAR PAIN

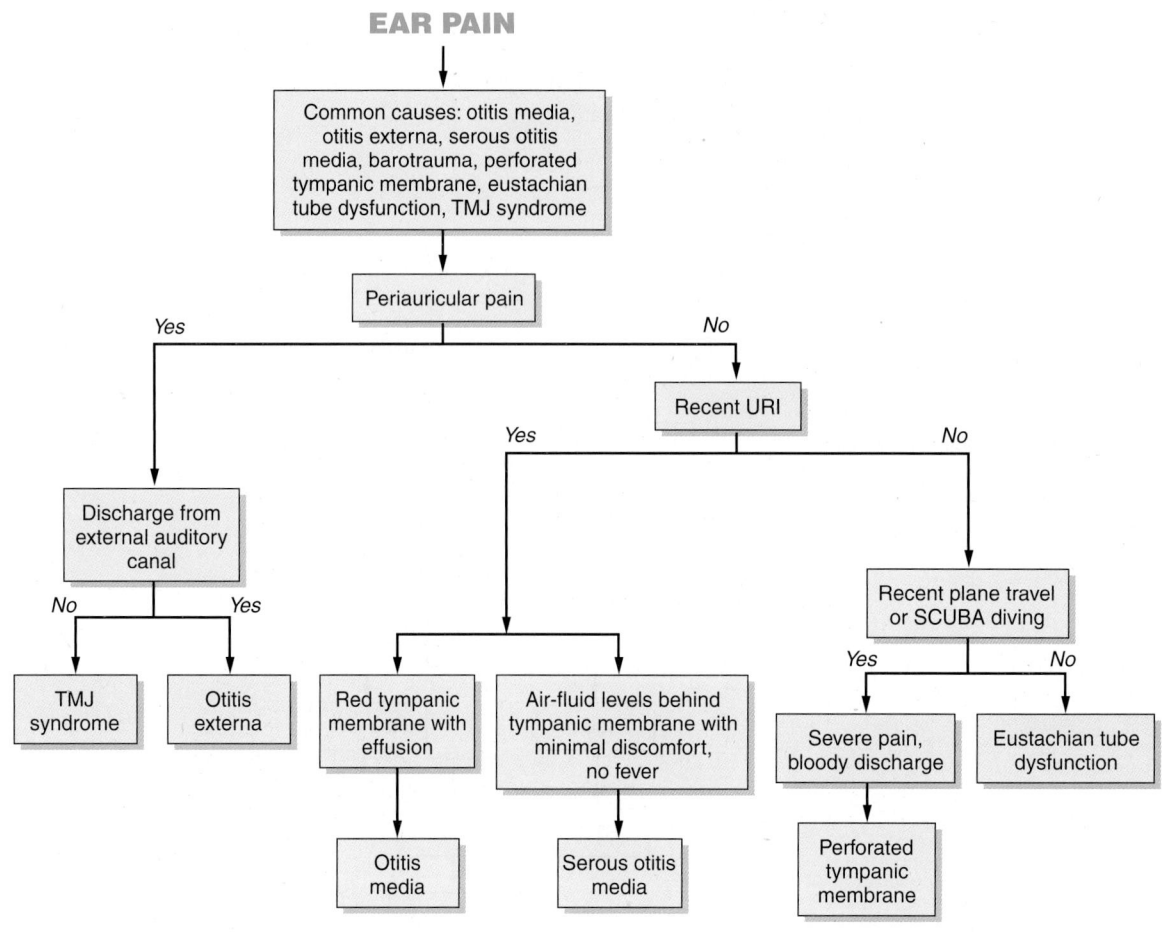

Robert A. Baldor, MD and Alan M. Ehrlich, MD

Am Fam Physician. 2008;77(5).

ECCHYMOSIS

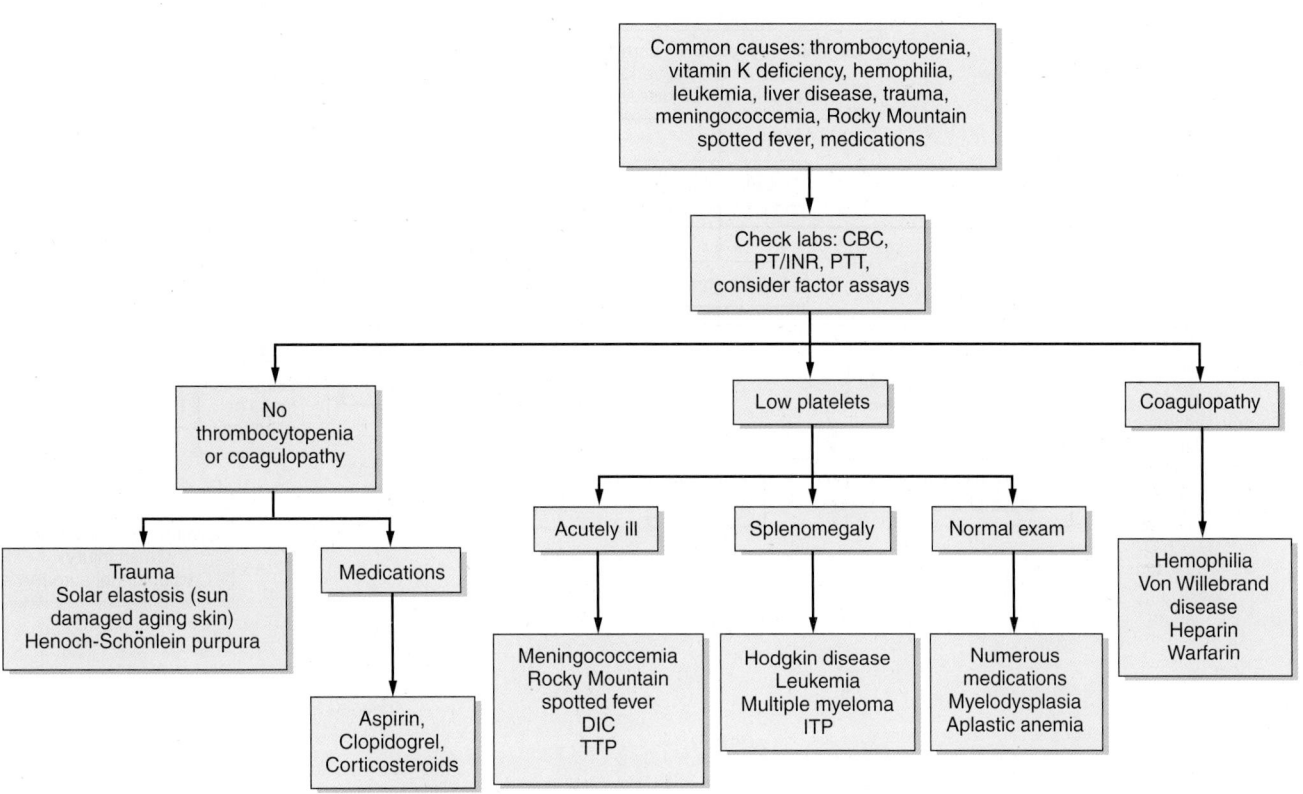

Robert A. Baldor, MD and Alan M. Ehrlich, MD

Arch Dermatol. 2010;146(1):94–5.

EDEMA, FOCAL

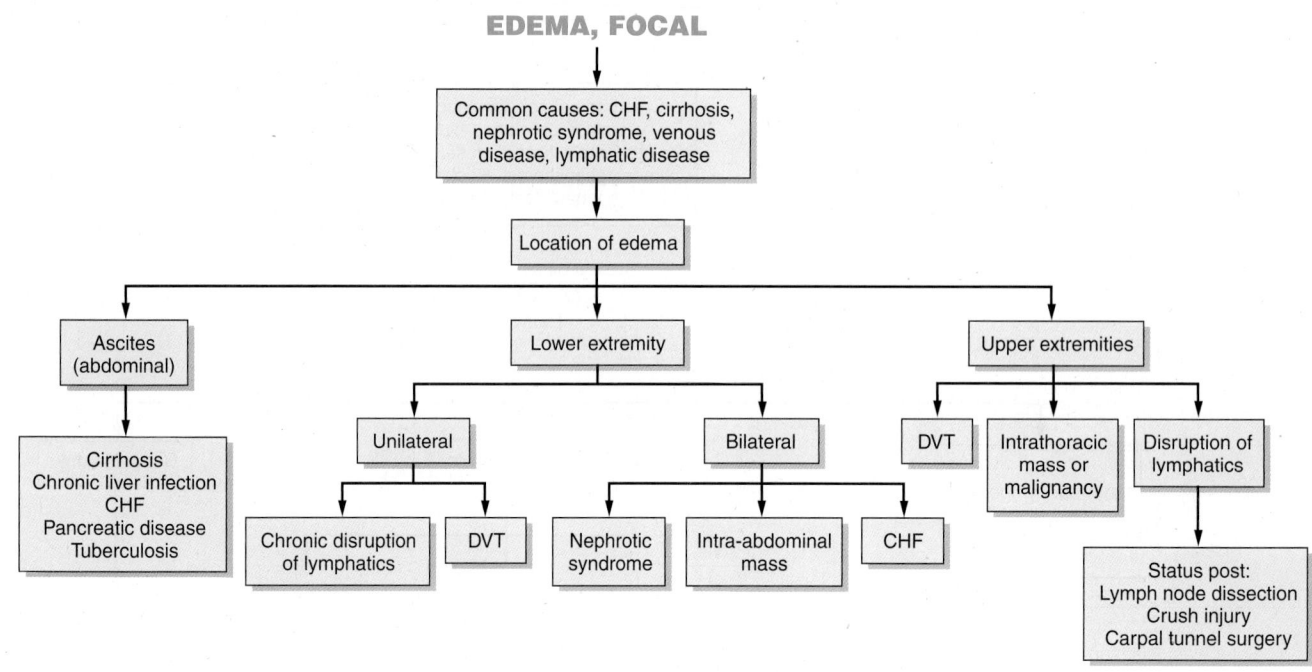

Robert A. Baldor, MD and Alan M. Ehrlich, MD

Am J Med. 2002;113(7):580–6.

ENURESIS

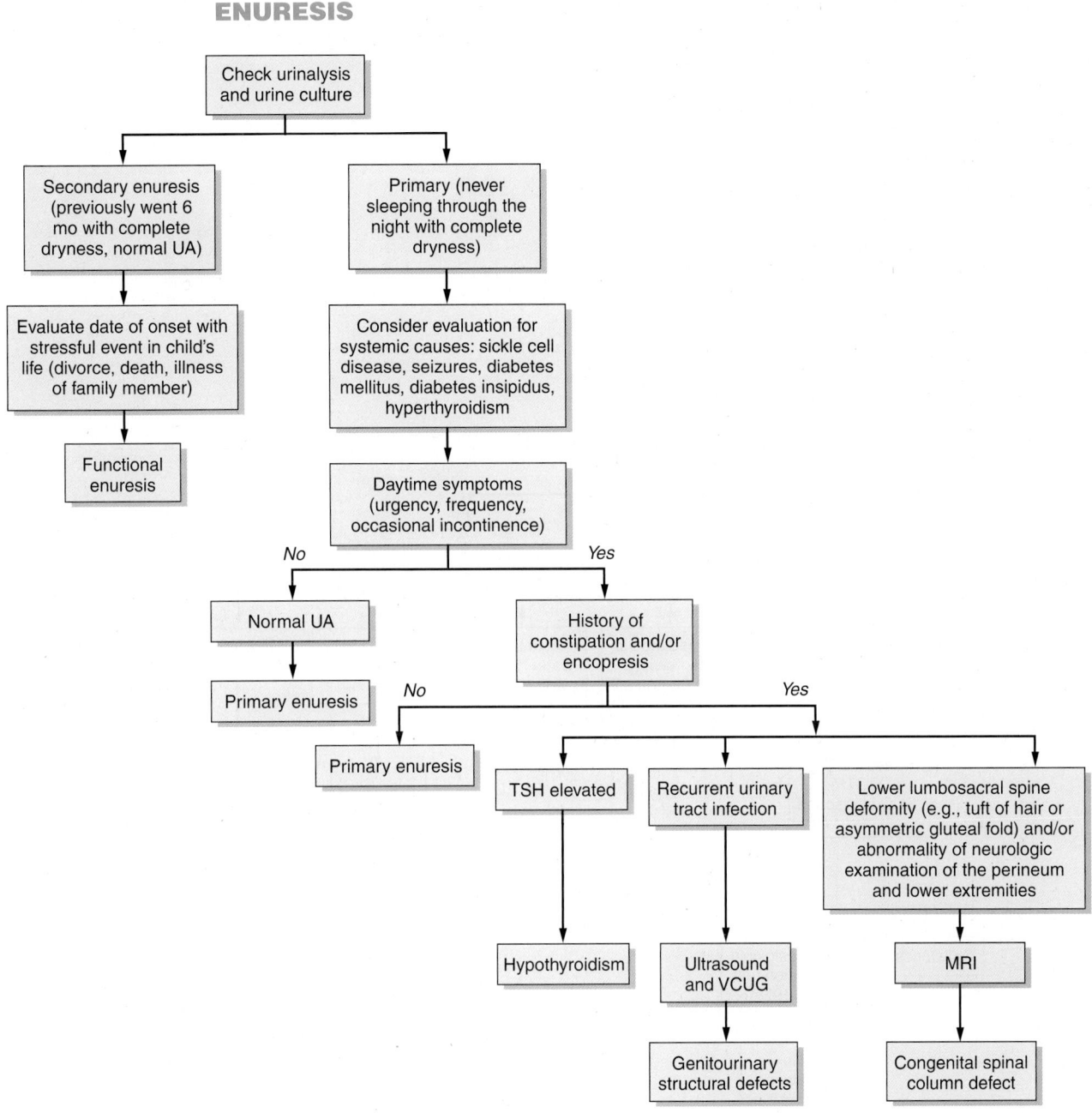

Robert A. Baldor, MD and Alan M. Ehrlich, MD

J Am Acad Child Adolesc Psychiatry. 2004;43(1).

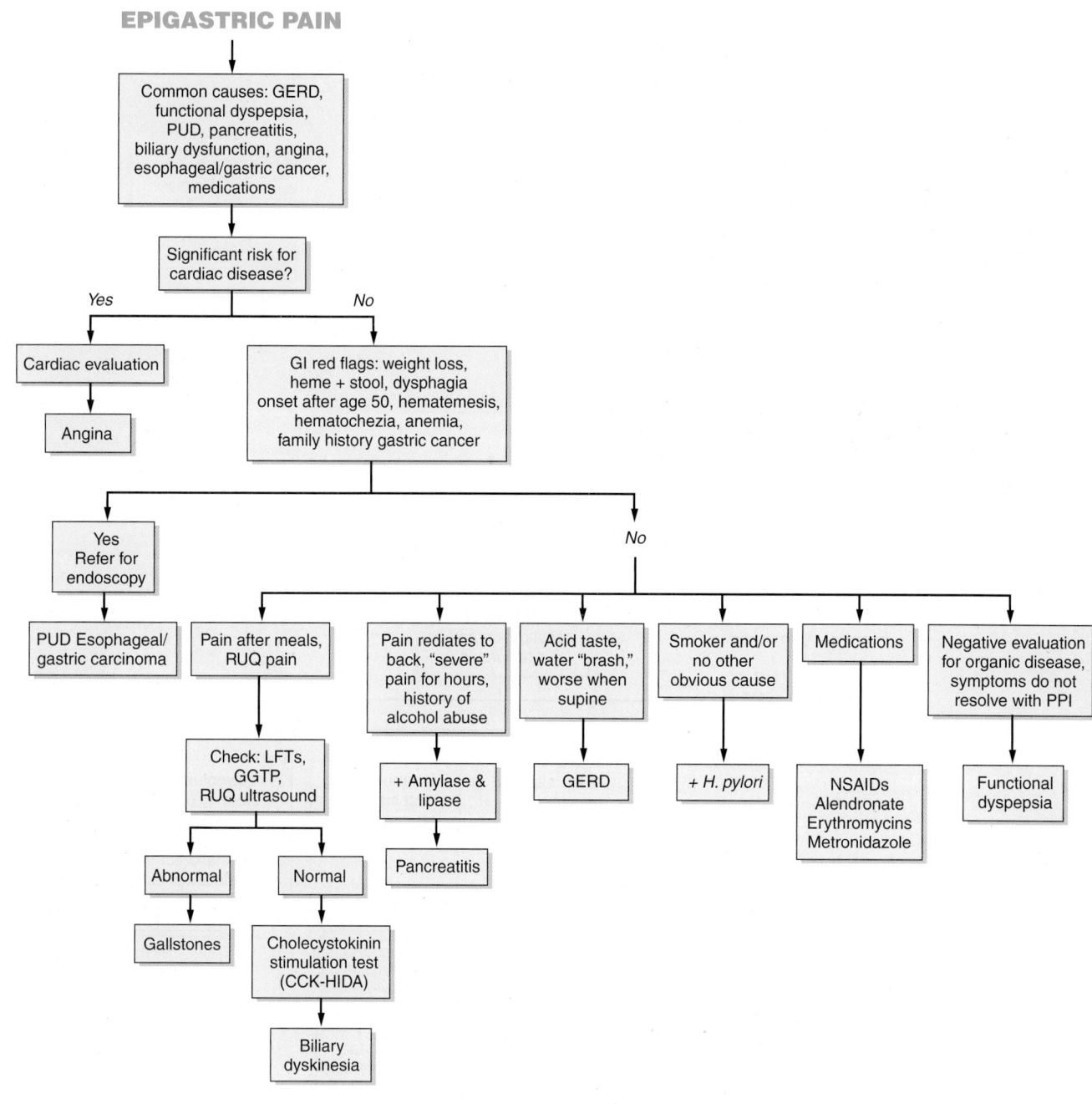

EPIGASTRIC PAIN

Common causes: GERD, functional dyspepsia, PUD, pancreatitis, biliary dysfunction, angina, esophageal/gastric cancer, medications

Significant risk for cardiac disease?

Yes → Cardiac evaluation → Angina

No → GI red flags: weight loss, heme + stool, dysphagia onset after age 50, hematemesis, hematochezia, anemia, family history gastric cancer

Yes Refer for endoscopy → PUD Esophageal/gastric carcinoma

No

Pain after meals, RUQ pain → Check: LFTs, GGTP, RUQ ultrasound → Abnormal → Gallstones / Normal → Cholecystokinin stimulation test (CCK-HIDA) → Biliary dyskinesia

Pain rediates to back, "severe" pain for hours, history of alcohol abuse → + Amylase & lipase → Pancreatitis

Acid taste, water "brash," worse when supine → GERD

Smoker and/or no other obvious cause → + H. pylori

Medications → NSAIDs Alendronate Erythromycins Metronidazole

Negative evaluation for organic disease, symptoms do not resolve with PPI → Functional dyspepsia

Robert A. Baldor, MD and Alan M. Ehrlich, MD

Curr Gastroenterol Rep. 2009;11(4):288–94.

EYE PAIN

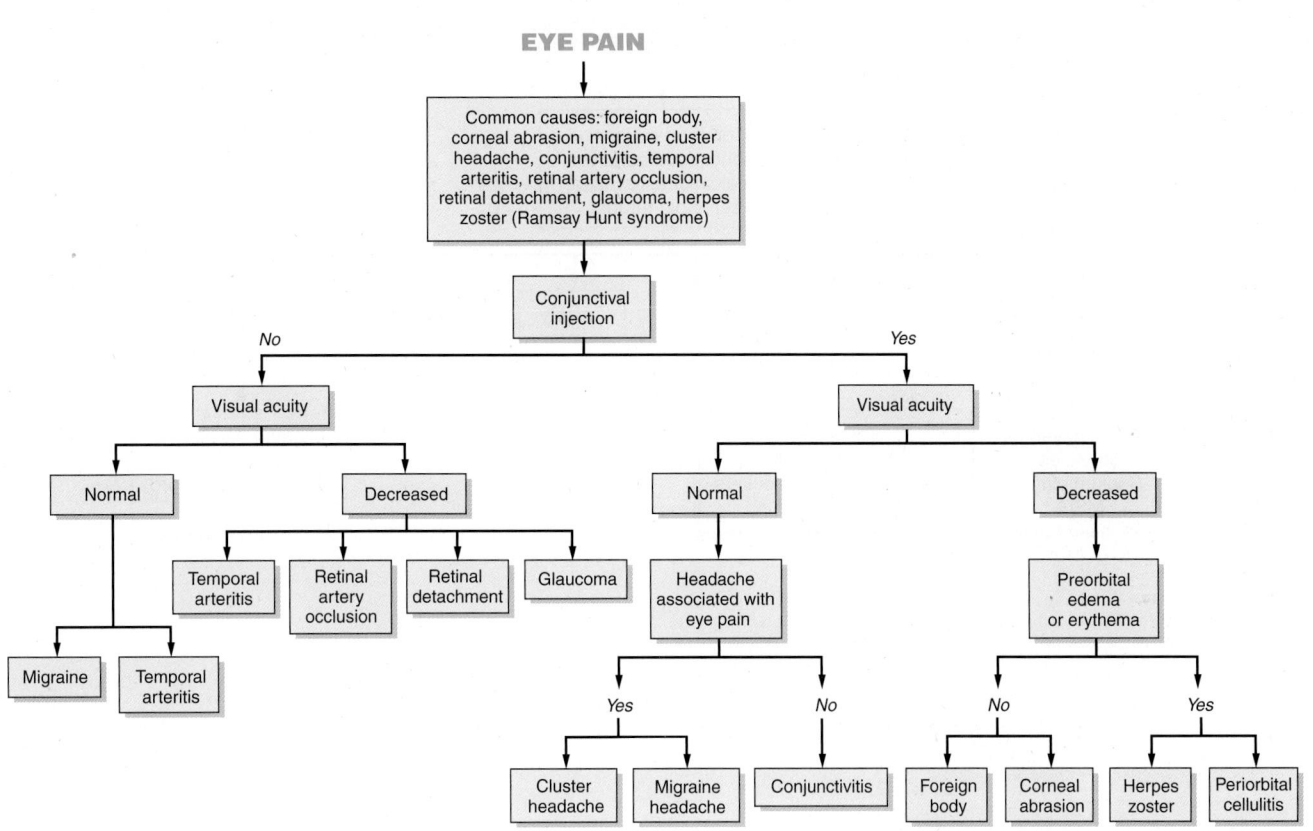

Common causes: foreign body, corneal abrasion, migraine, cluster headache, conjunctivitis, temporal arteritis, retinal artery occlusion, retinal detachment, glaucoma, herpes zoster (Ramsay Hunt syndrome)

Conjunctival injection

No → Visual acuity

- Normal
  - Migraine
  - Temporal arteritis
- Decreased
  - Temporal arteritis
  - Retinal artery occlusion
  - Retinal detachment
  - Glaucoma

Yes → Visual acuity

- Normal
  - Headache associated with eye pain
    - **Yes**
      - Cluster headache
      - Migraine headache
    - **No**
      - Conjunctivitis
- Decreased
  - Preorbital edema or erythema
    - **No**
      - Foreign body
      - Corneal abrasion
    - **Yes**
      - Herpes zoster
      - Periorbital cellulitis

Robert A. Baldor, MD and Alan M. Ehrlich, MD

Curr Pain Headache Rep. 2008;12(4):296–304.

FACIAL FLUSHING

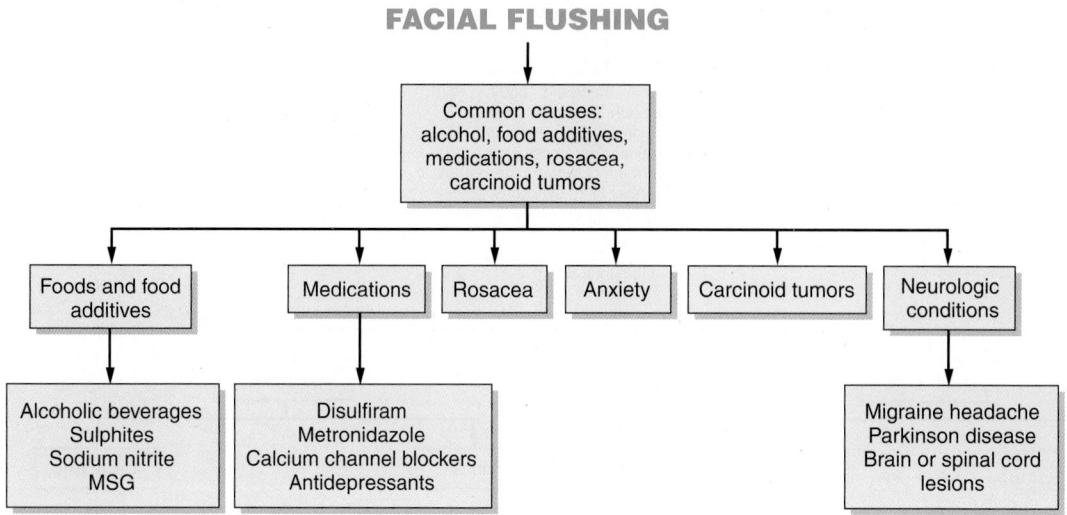

Robert A. Baldor, MD and Alan M. Ehrlich, MD

PLoS Med. 2009;6(3):e50.

FACIAL PARALYSIS

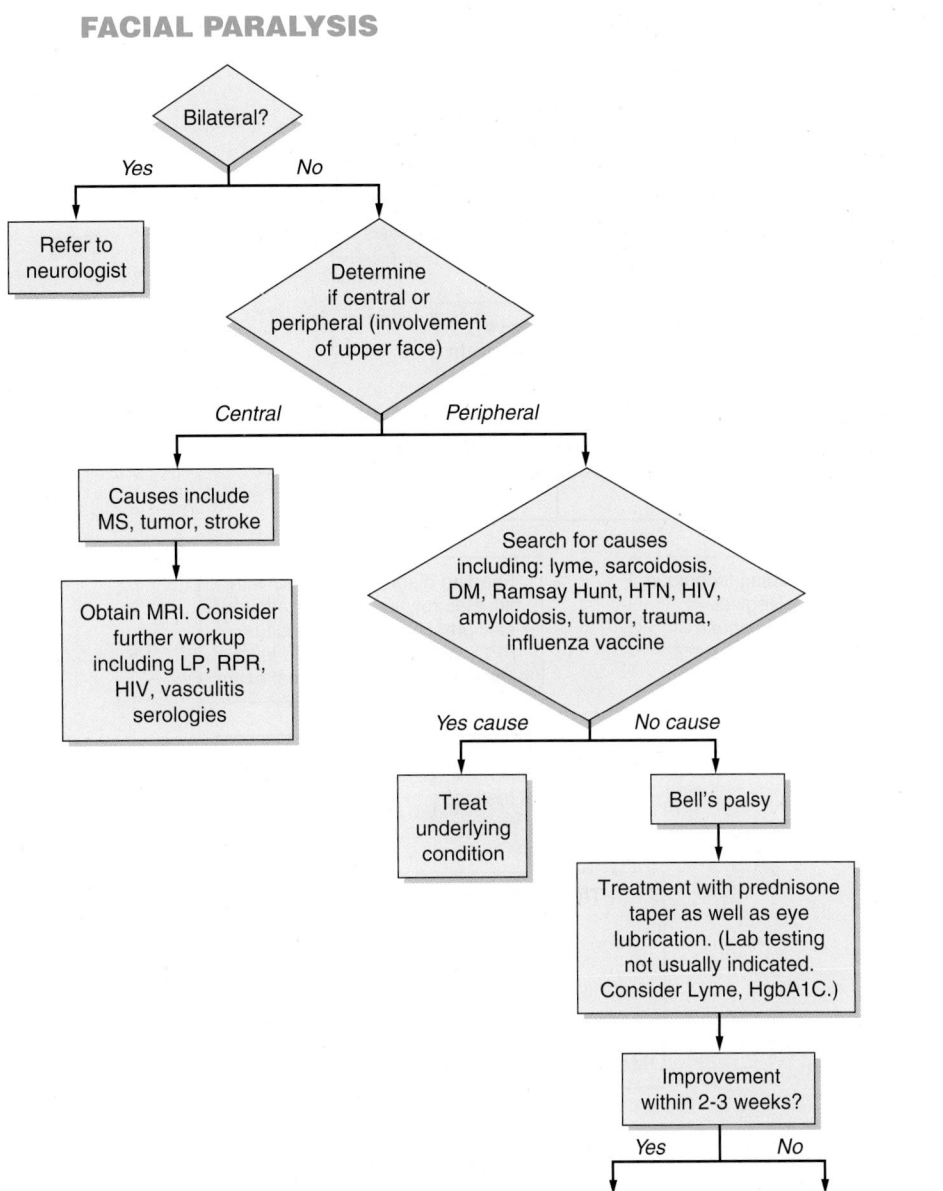

Laura Hagopian, MD and William A. Tosches, MD

Rev Med Intern. 2009;30(9):769–75.

FAILURE TO THRIVE

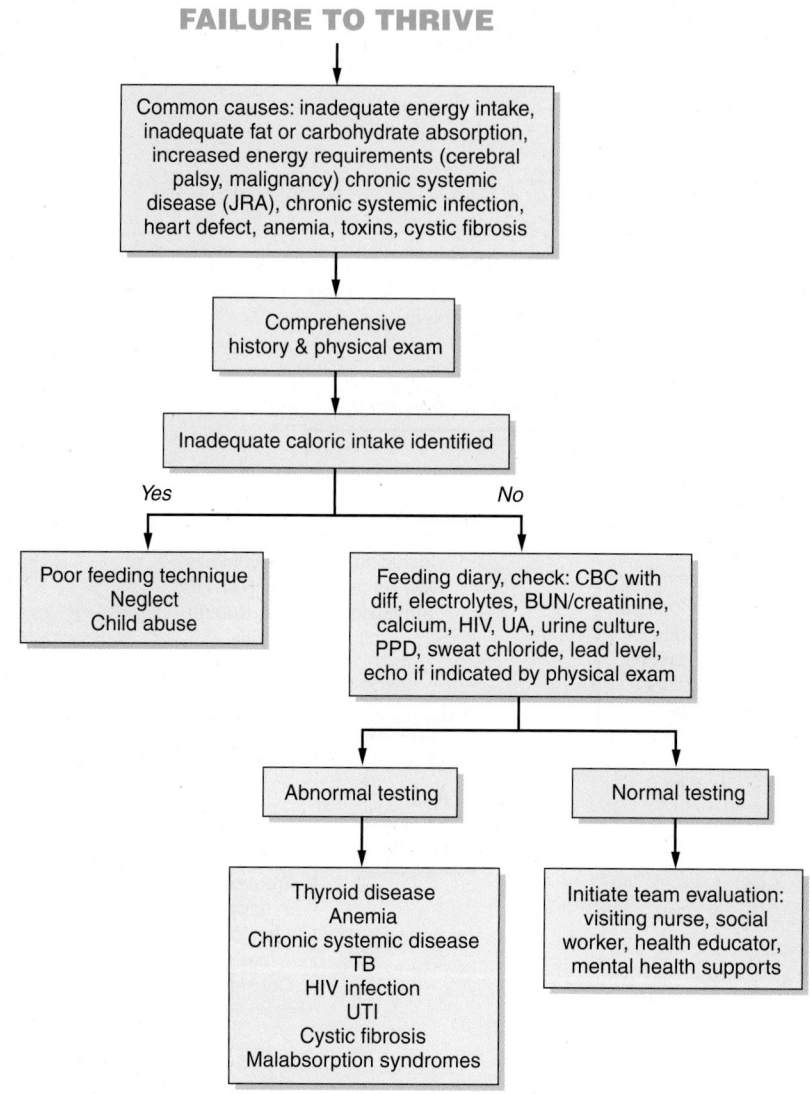

```
                    ↓
┌─────────────────────────────────────────┐
│ Common causes: inadequate energy intake, │
│ inadequate fat or carbohydrate absorption,│
│ increased energy requirements (cerebral   │
│ palsy, malignancy) chronic systemic       │
│ disease (JRA), chronic systemic infection,│
│ heart defect, anemia, toxins, cystic fibrosis│
└─────────────────────────────────────────┘
                    ↓
        ┌─────────────────────┐
        │ Comprehensive       │
        │ history & physical exam│
        └─────────────────────┘
                    ↓
      ┌───────────────────────────────┐
      │ Inadequate caloric intake identified│
      └───────────────────────────────┘
       Yes                      No
```

Poor feeding technique
Neglect
Child abuse

Feeding diary, check: CBC with diff, electrolytes, BUN/creatinine, calcium, HIV, UA, urine culture, PPD, sweat chloride, lead level, echo if indicated by physical exam

Abnormal testing   **Normal testing**

Thyroid disease
Anemia
Chronic systemic disease
TB
HIV infection
UTI
Cystic fibrosis
Malabsorption syndromes

Initiate team evaluation:
visiting nurse, social
worker, health educator,
mental health supports

Robert A. Baldor, MD and Alan M. Ehrlich, MD

Eur J Pediatr. 2009;168(7):839–45. Epub 2008 Oct 16.

FATIGUE

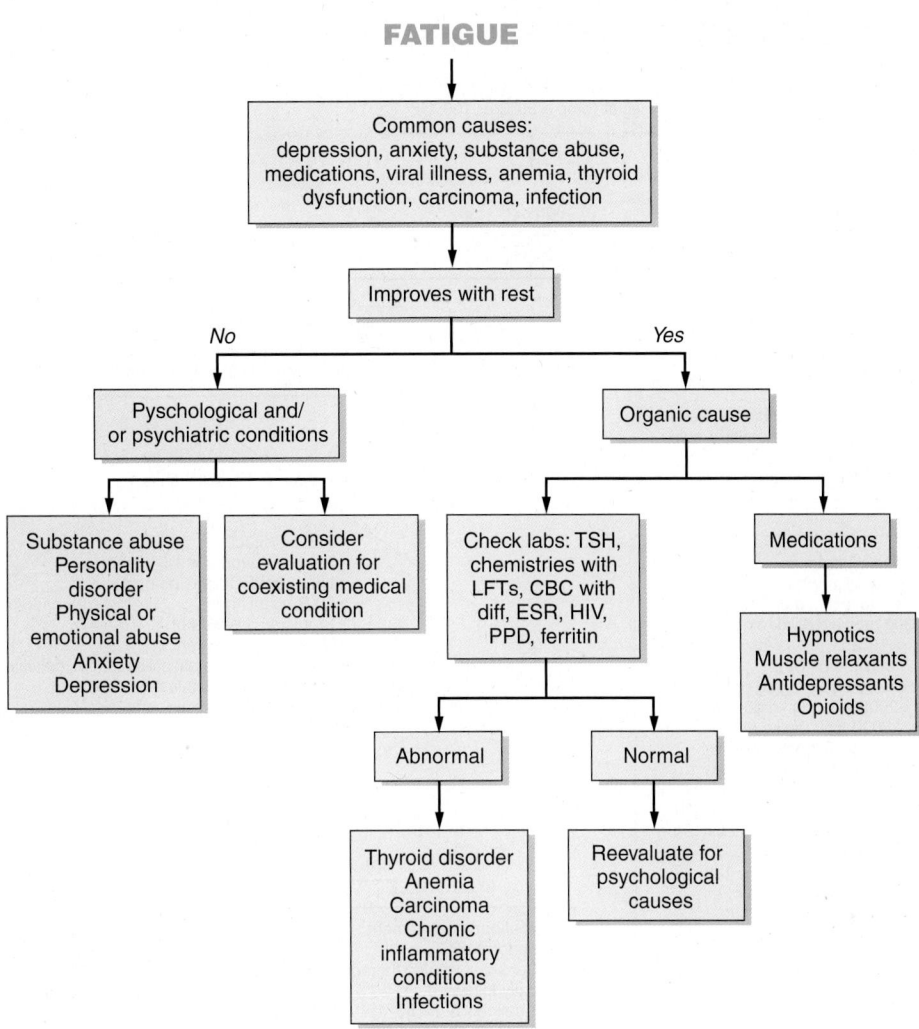

Common causes:
depression, anxiety, substance abuse, medications, viral illness, anemia, thyroid dysfunction, carcinoma, infection

Improves with rest

No → Pyschological and/ or psychiatric conditions

Yes → Organic cause

Pyschological and/or psychiatric conditions:

Substance abuse
Personality disorder
Physical or emotional abuse
Anxiety
Depression

Consider evaluation for coexisting medical condition

Organic cause:

Check labs: TSH, chemistries with LFTs, CBC with diff, ESR, HIV, PPD, ferritin

Medications → Hypnotics Muscle relaxants Antidepressants Opioids

Abnormal → Thyroid disorder Anemia Carcinoma Chronic inflammatory conditions Infections

Normal → Reevaluate for psychological causes

Robert A. Baldor, MD and Alan M. Ehrlich, MD

CMAJ. 2009;181(10):683–7. Epub 2009 Oct 26.

FEVER IN THE FIRST 3 MONTHS OF LIFE

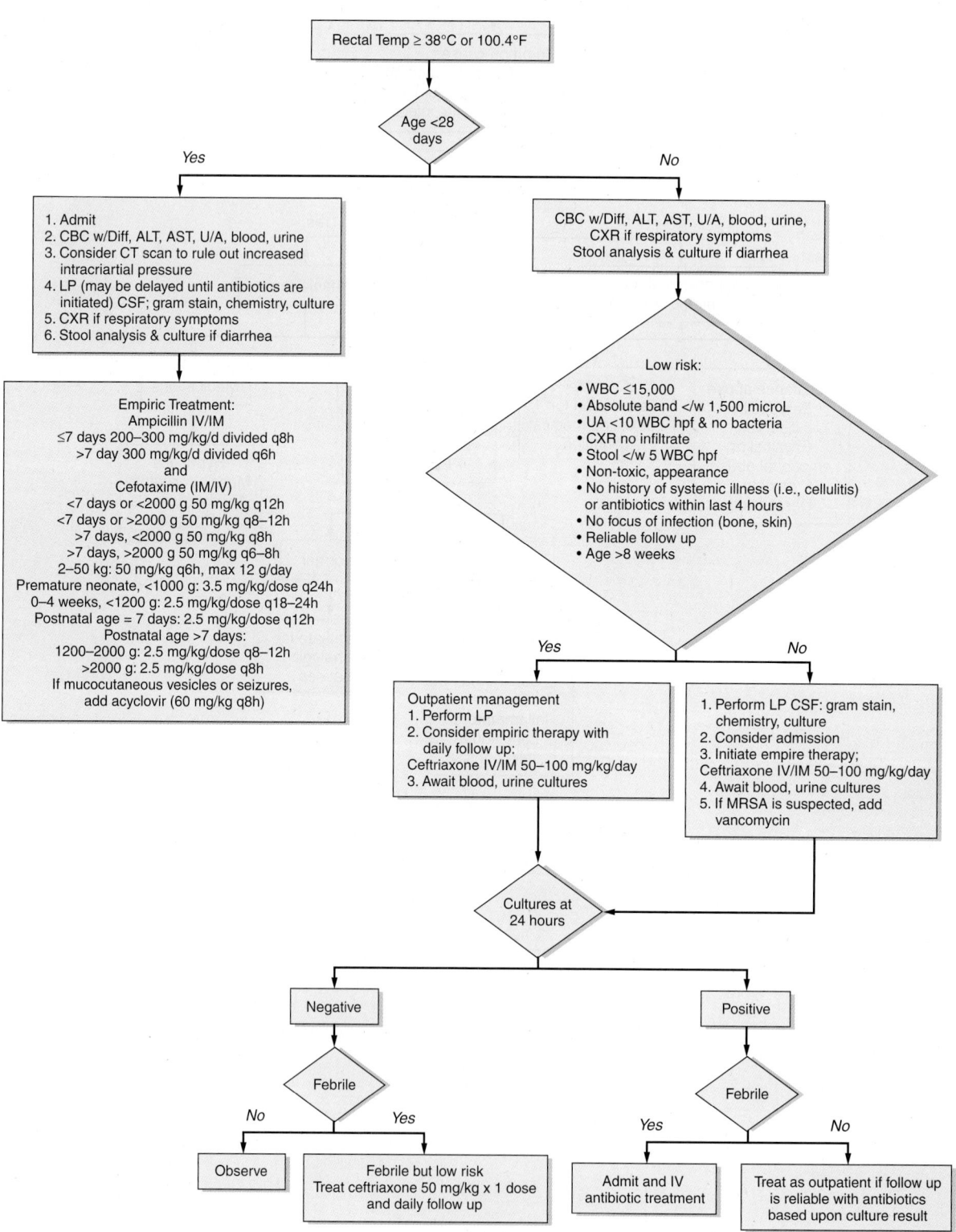

Katharine Tumilty, MD, William J. Durbin, MD, and Mariann Manno, MD

Ann Emerg Med. 2003;42(4):530–45.

FEVER OF UNKNOWN ORIGIN (FUO)

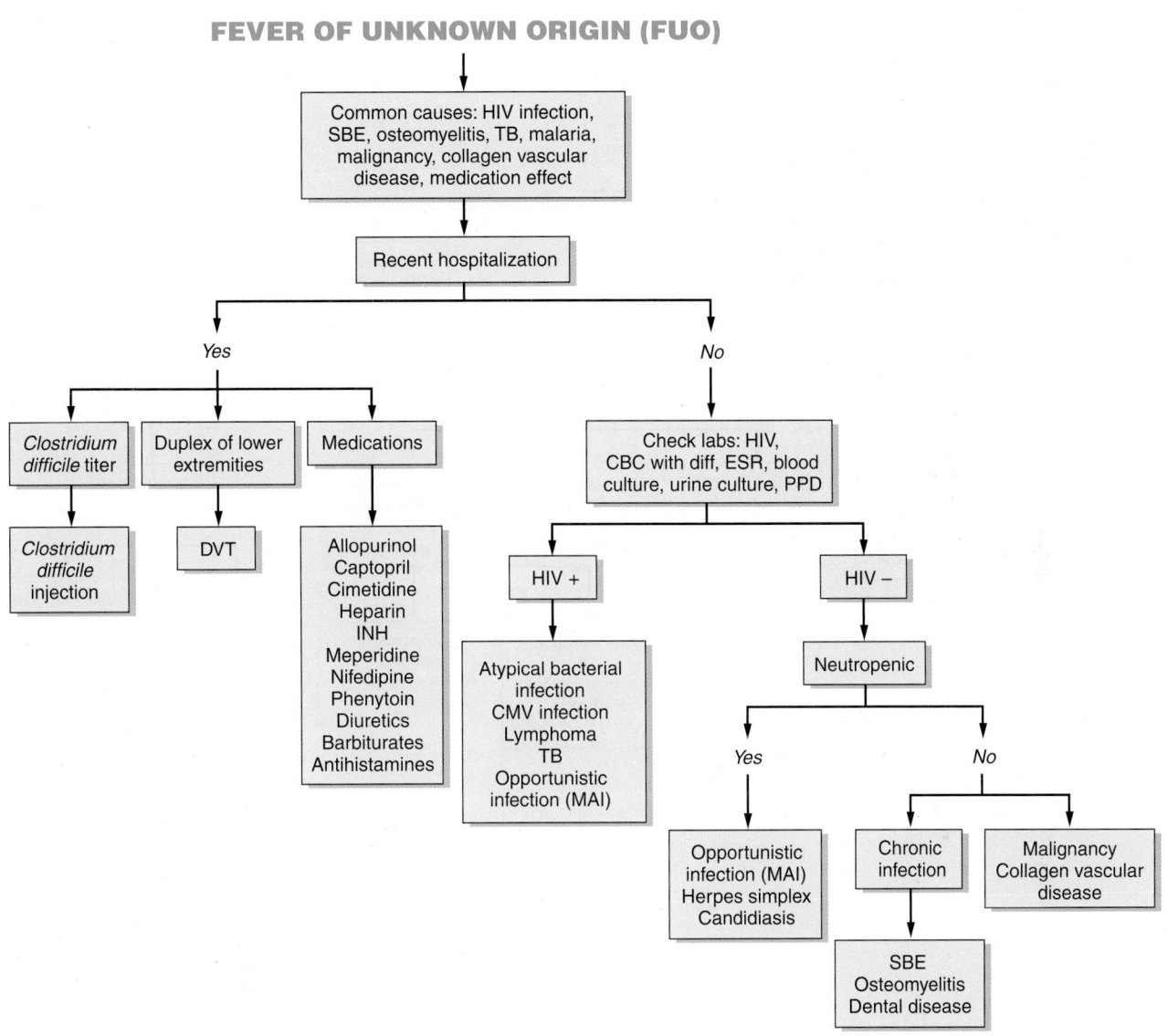

Robert A. Baldor, MD and Alan M. Ehrlich, MD

Pediatr Infect Dis J. 2009 Nov 25.

FEVER, ACUTE

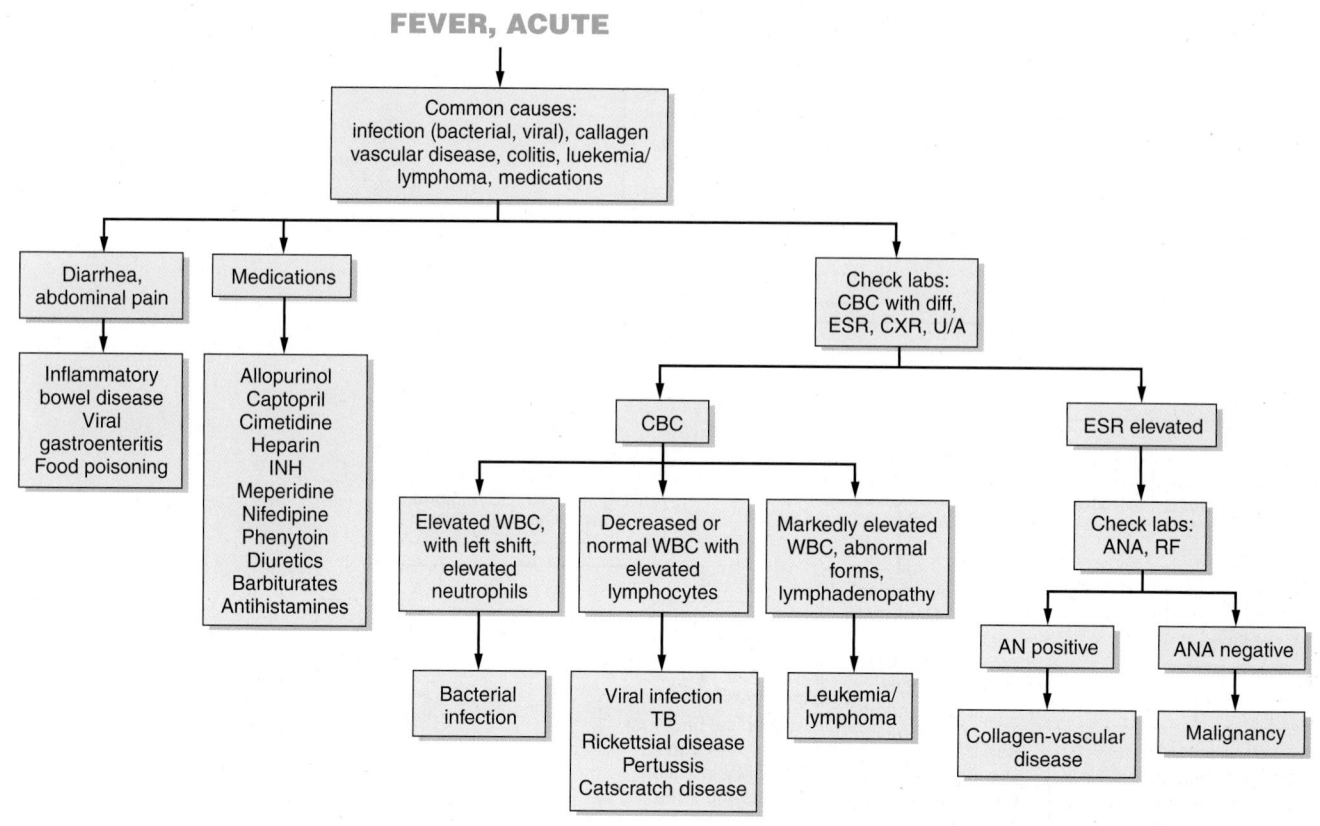

Common causes:
infection (bacterial, viral), callagen vascular disease, colitis, luekemia/lymphoma, medications

Diarrhea, abdominal pain
- Inflammatory bowel disease
- Viral gastroenteritis
- Food poisoning

Medications
- Allopurinol
- Captopril
- Cimetidine
- Heparin
- INH
- Meperidine
- Nifedipine
- Phenytoin
- Diuretics
- Barbiturates
- Antihistamines

Check labs: CBC with diff, ESR, CXR, U/A

CBC

- Elevated WBC, with left shift, elevated neutrophils → Bacterial infection
- Decreased or normal WBC with elevated lymphocytes → Viral infection, TB, Rickettsial disease, Pertussis, Catscratch disease
- Markedly elevated WBC, abnormal forms, lymphadenopathy → Leukemia/lymphoma

ESR elevated

Check labs: ANA, RF

- AN positive → Collagen-vascular disease
- ANA negative → Malignancy

Robert A. Baldor, MD and Alan M. Ehrlich, MD

Crit Care Med. 2010;38(2):457–63.

FOOT PAIN

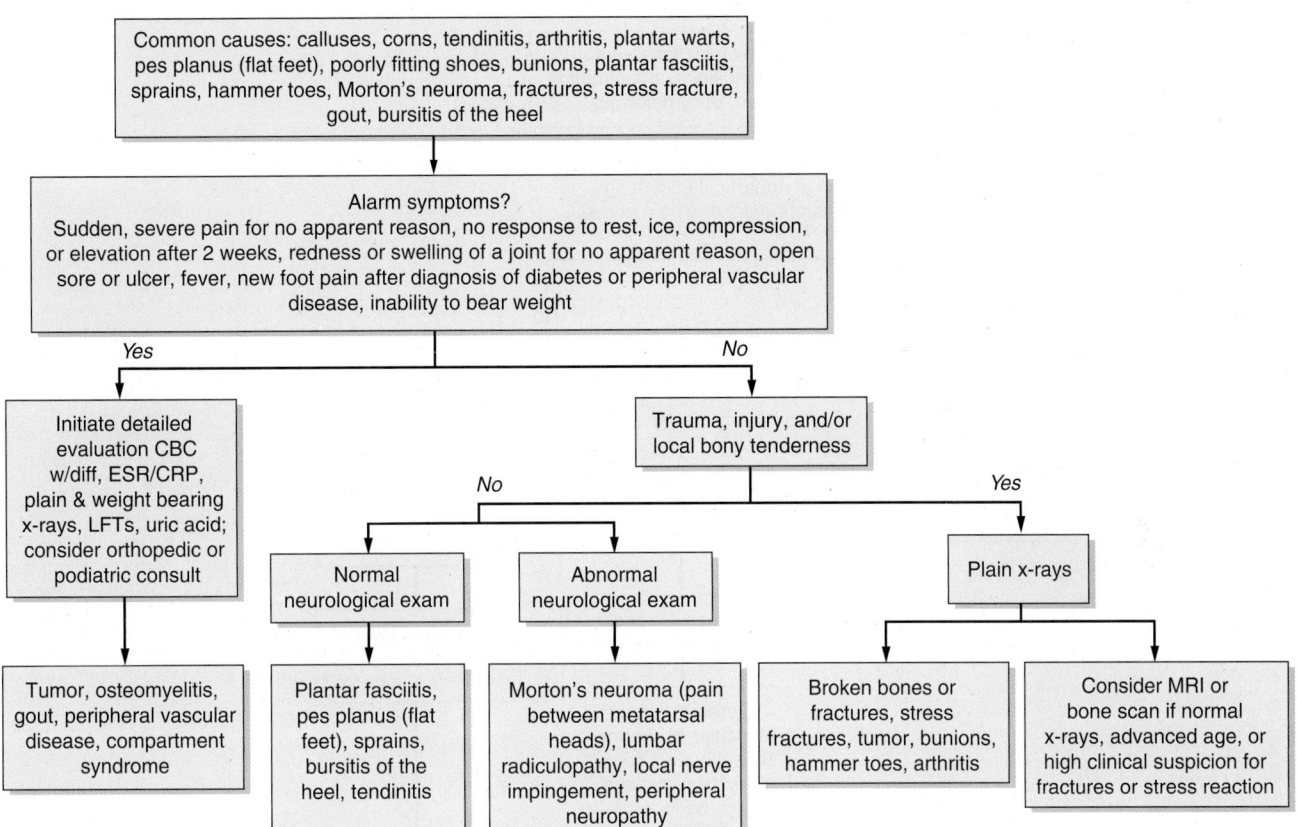

Common causes: calluses, corns, tendinitis, arthritis, plantar warts, pes planus (flat feet), poorly fitting shoes, bunions, plantar fasciitis, sprains, hammer toes, Morton's neuroma, fractures, stress fracture, gout, bursitis of the heel

Alarm symptoms?
Sudden, severe pain for no apparent reason, no response to rest, ice, compression, or elevation after 2 weeks, redness or swelling of a joint for no apparent reason, open sore or ulcer, fever, new foot pain after diagnosis of diabetes or peripheral vascular disease, inability to bear weight

Yes

No

Initiate detailed evaluation CBC w/diff, ESR/CRP, plain & weight bearing x-rays, LFTs, uric acid; consider orthopedic or podiatric consult

Trauma, injury, and/or local bony tenderness

No

Yes

Normal neurological exam

Abnormal neurological exam

Plain x-rays

Tumor, osteomyelitis, gout, peripheral vascular disease, compartment syndrome

Plantar fasciitis, pes planus (flat feet), sprains, bursitis of the heel, tendinitis

Morton's neuroma (pain between metatarsal heads), lumbar radiculopathy, local nerve impingement, peripheral neuropathy

Broken bones or fractures, stress fractures, tumor, bunions, hammer toes, arthritis

Consider MRI or bone scan if normal x-rays, advanced age, or high clinical suspicion for fractures or stress reaction

George Gunter A. Pujalte, MD

BMJ. 2003;326(7386):417.

GAIT DISTURBANCE

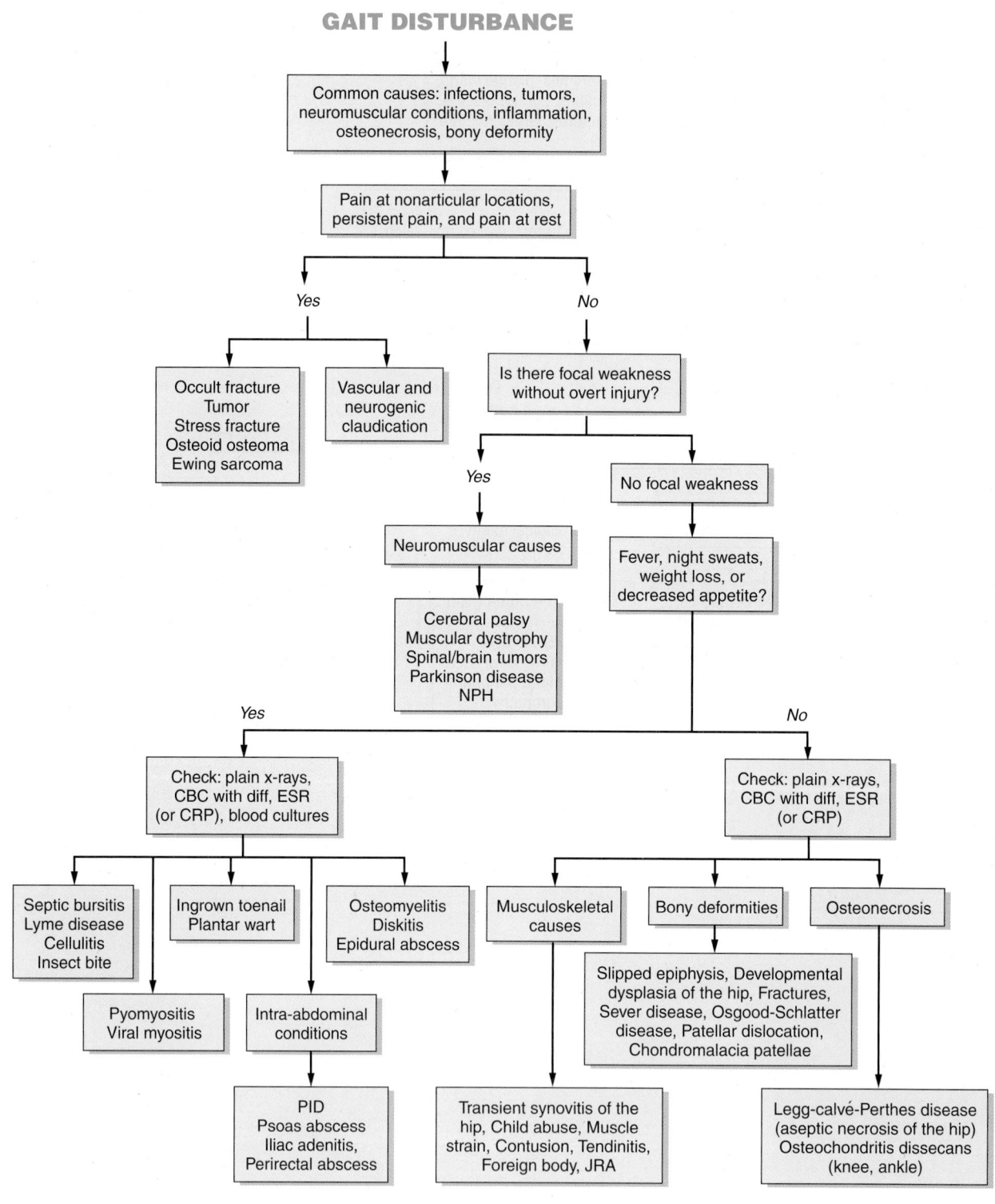

Robert A. Baldor, MD and Alan M. Ehrlich, MD

Stroke. 2009;40(12):3816–20.

GASTROESOPHAGEAL REFLUX DISEASE (GERD), TREATMENT

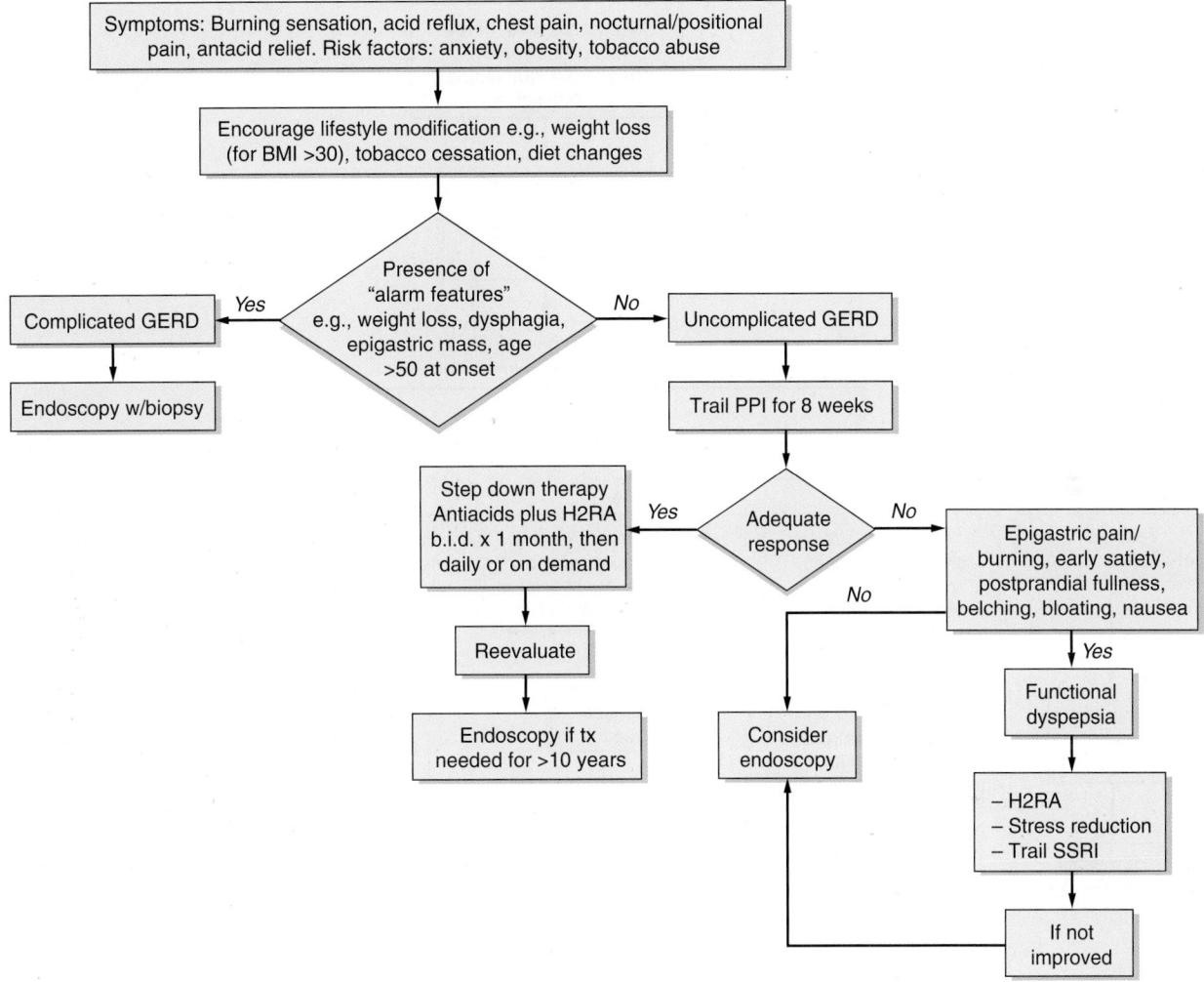

Richard E. Trowbridge, MD and Rebecca A. Frye, DO

Am J Med. 2010;123(7):583–92.

GENITAL ULCERS

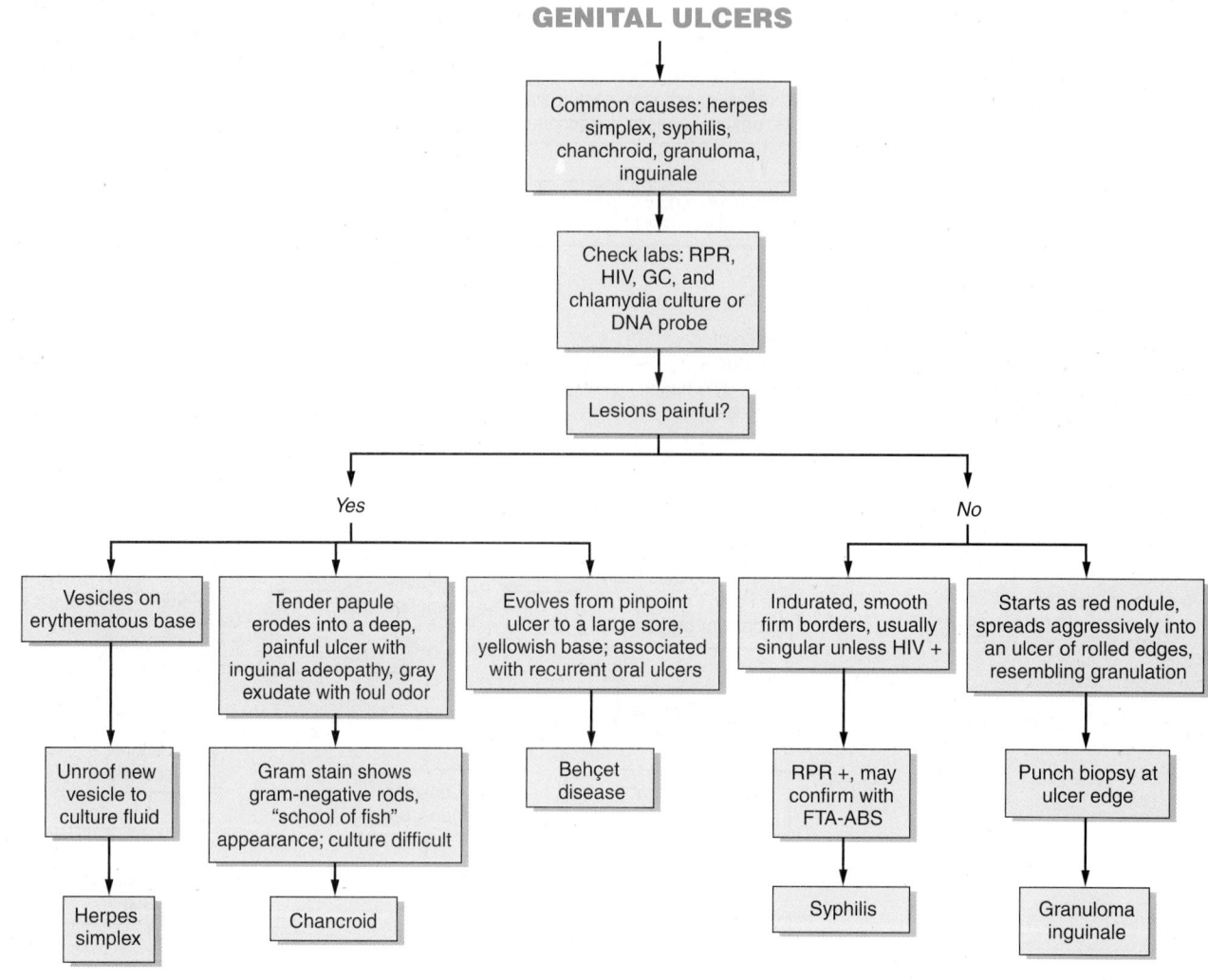

Common causes: herpes simplex, syphilis, chanchroid, granuloma, inguinale

Check labs: RPR, HIV, GC, and chlamydia culture or DNA probe

Lesions painful?

Yes

- Vesicles on erythematous base → Unroof new vesicle to culture fluid → **Herpes simplex**
- Tender papule erodes into a deep, painful ulcer with inguinal adeopathy, gray exudate with foul odor → Gram stain shows gram-negative rods, "school of fish" appearance; culture difficult → **Chancroid**
- Evolves from pinpoint ulcer to a large sore, yellowish base; associated with recurrent oral ulcers → **Behçet disease**

No

- Indurated, smooth firm borders, usually singular unless HIV + → RPR +, may confirm with FTA-ABS → **Syphilis**
- Starts as red nodule, spreads aggressively into an ulcer of rolled edges, resembling granulation → Punch biopsy at ulcer edge → **Granuloma inguinale**

Robert A. Baldor, MD and Alan M. Ehrlich, MD

Sex Transm Dis. 2008;35(6):545–9.

GLUCOSURIA

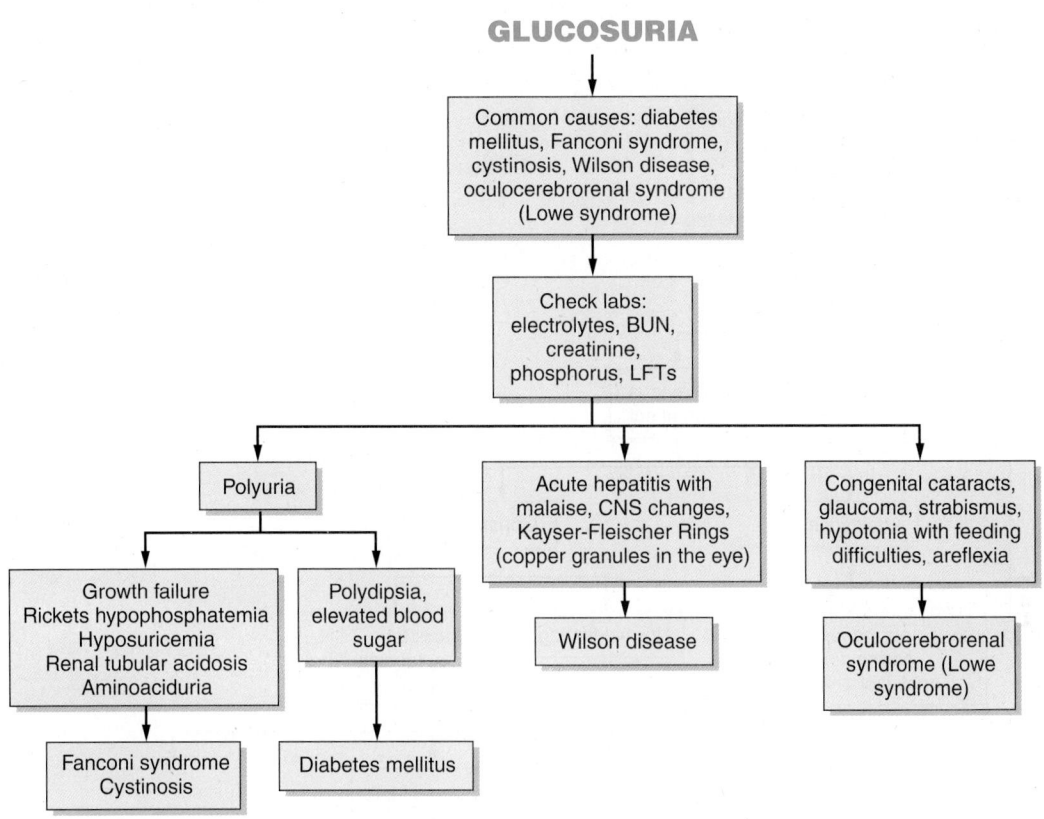

Robert A. Baldor, MD and Alan M. Ehrlich, MD

Scand J Clin Lab Invest. 2009;69(6):662–72.

GYNECOMASTIA

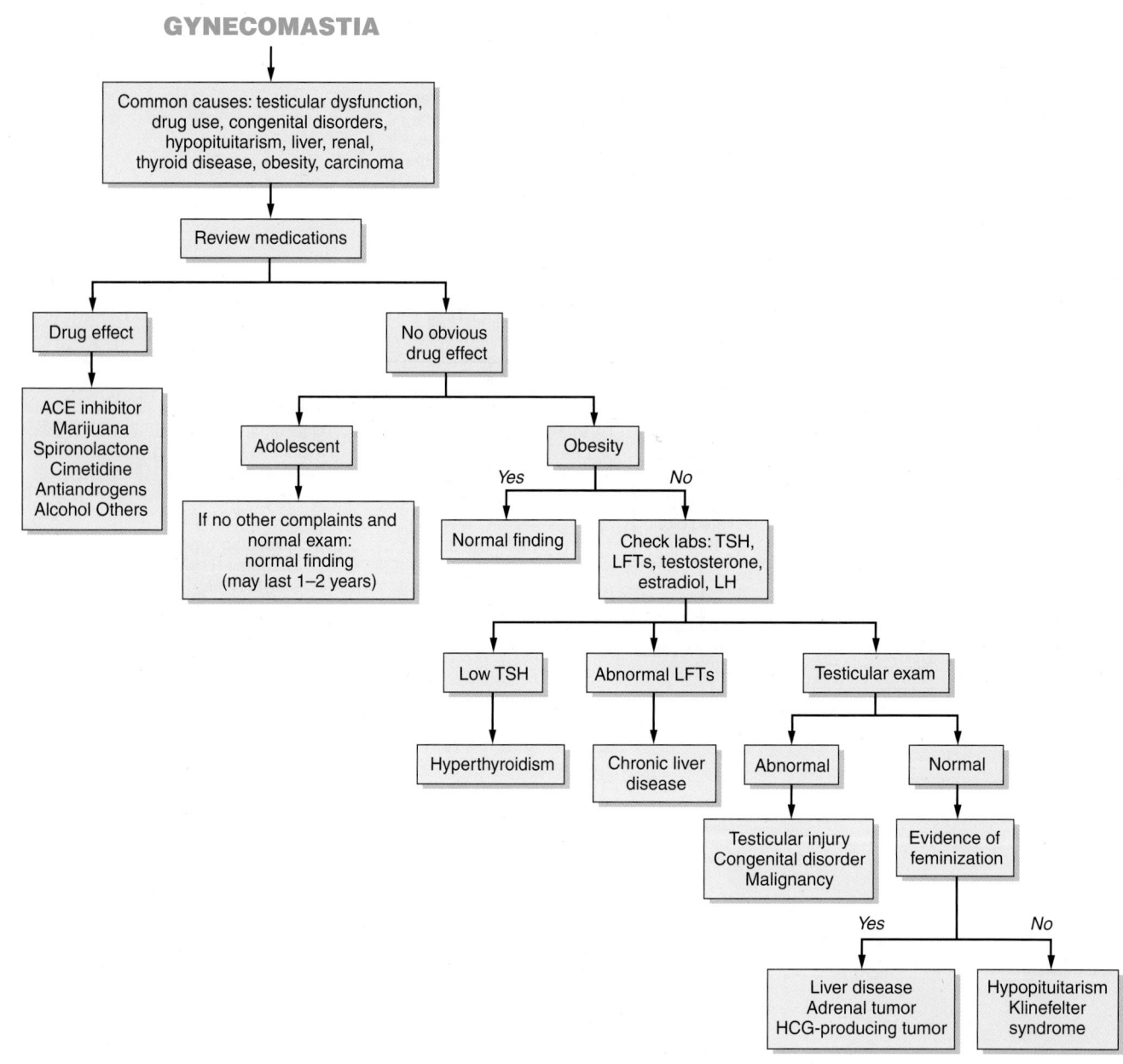

Robert A. Baldor, MD and Alan M. Ehrlich, MD

J Clin Endocrinol Metab. 2009;94(8):2975–8. Epub 2009 May 26.

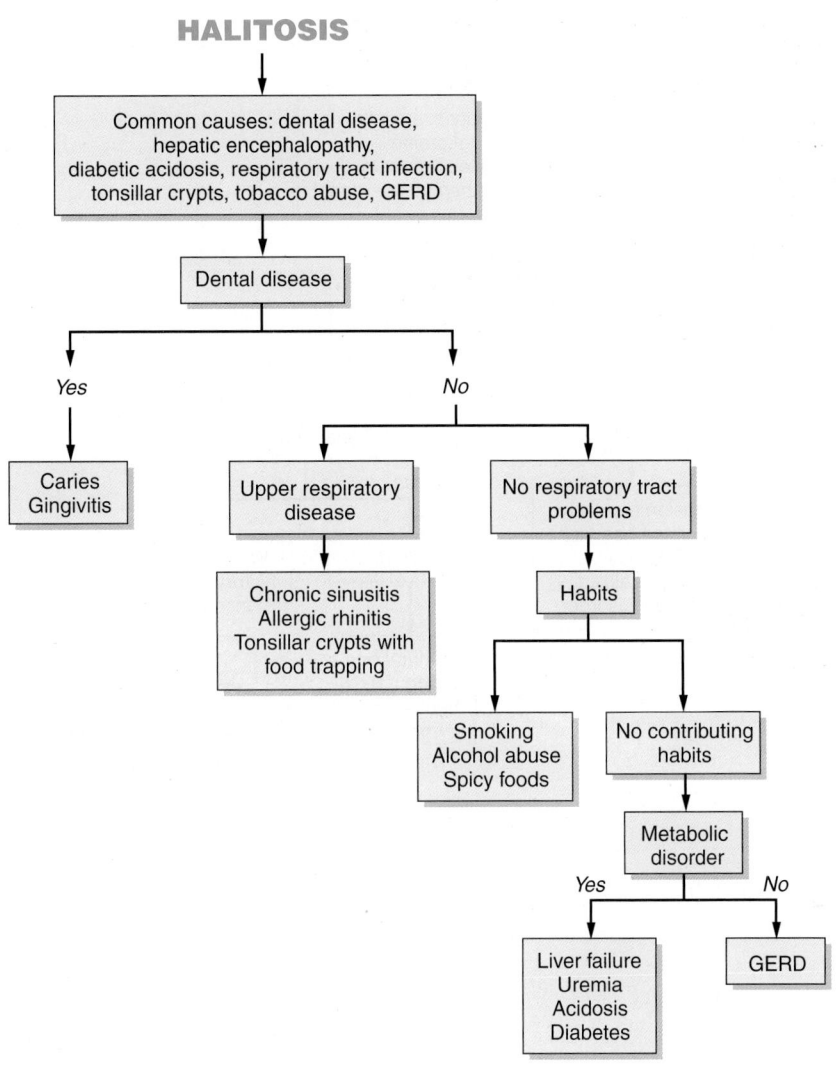

HALITOSIS

Common causes: dental disease,
hepatic encephalopathy,
diabetic acidosis, respiratory tract infection,
tonsillar crypts, tobacco abuse, GERD

Dental disease

Yes

No

Caries
Gingivitis

Upper respiratory
disease

No respiratory tract
problems

Chronic sinusitis
Allergic rhinitis
Tonsillar crypts with
food trapping

Habits

Smoking
Alcohol abuse
Spicy foods

No contributing
habits

Metabolic
disorder

Yes

No

Liver failure
Uremia
Acidosis
Diabetes

GERD

Robert A. Baldor, MD and Alan M. Ehrlich, MD

Oral Surg Oral Med Oral Pathol Oral Radiol Endod. 2008;106(3):384–8. Epub 2008 Jul 7.

HEADACHE, CHRONIC

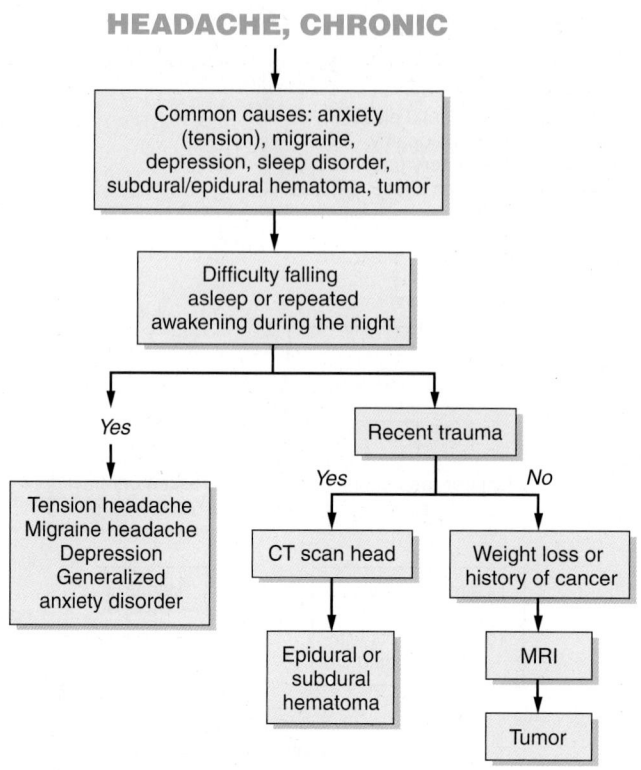

Robert A. Baldor, MD and Alan M. Ehrlich, MD

Acta Neurochir Suppl. 2010;107:65–9.

HEART MURMUR

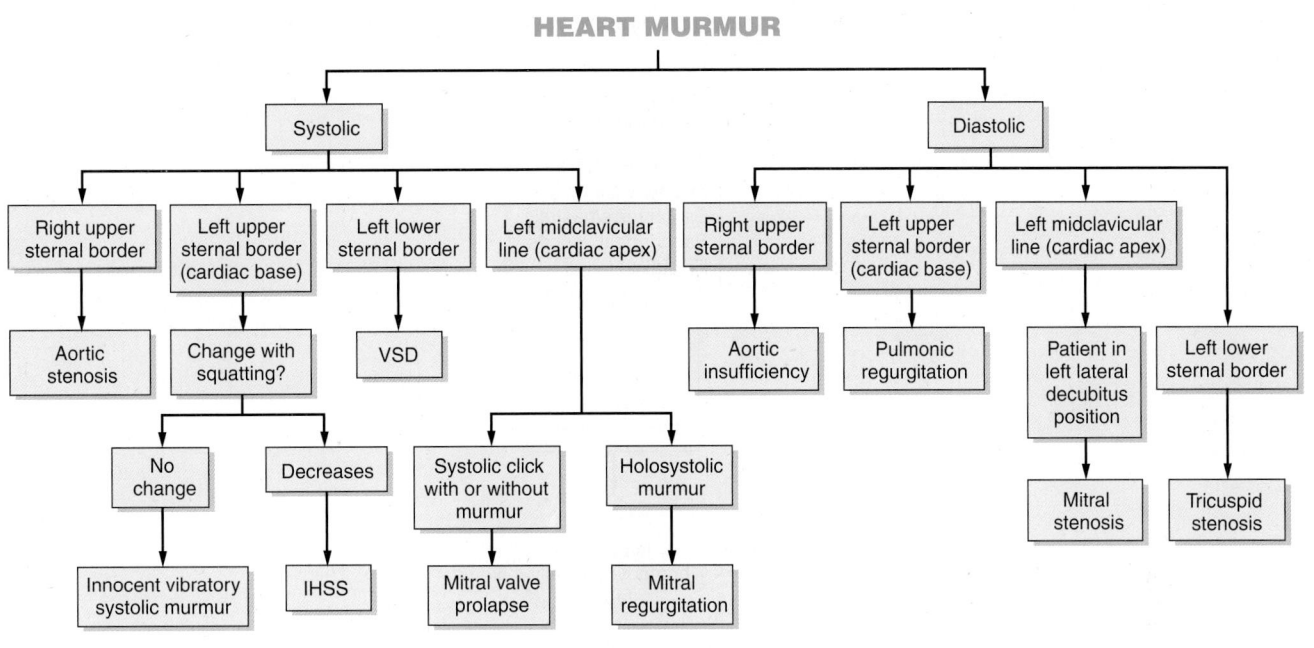

Robert A. Baldor, MD and Alan M. Ehrlich, MD

Pediatr Int. 2008;50(2):145–9.

HEMATEMESIS (BLEEDING, UPPER GI)

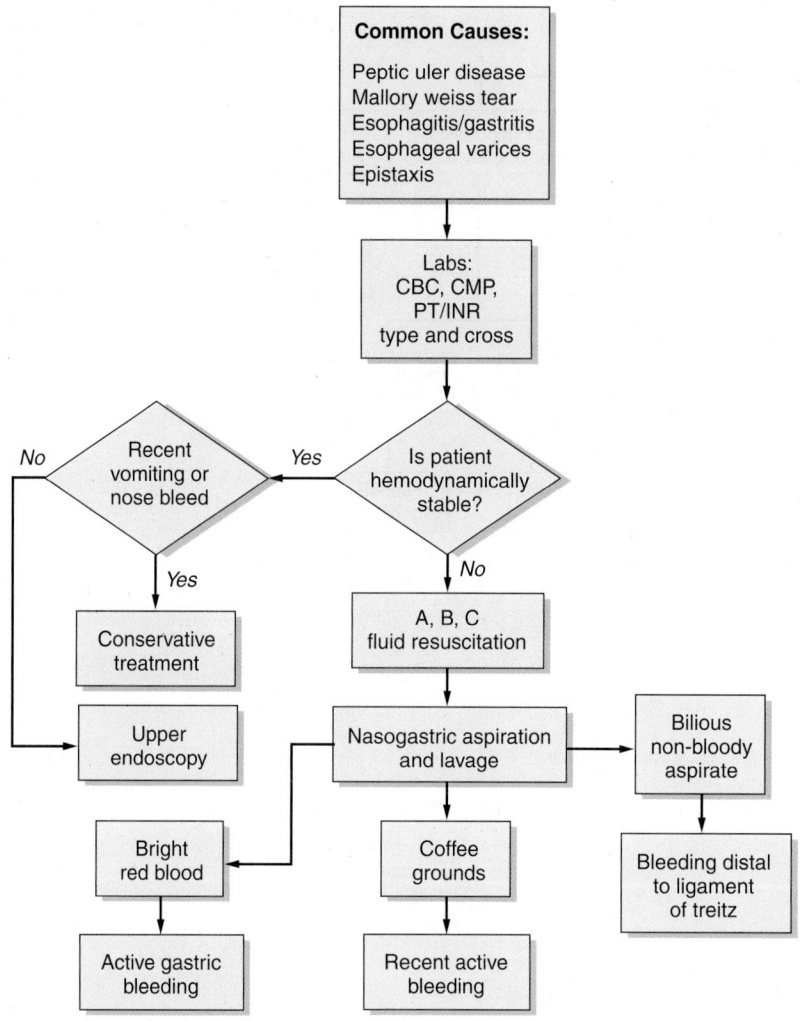

Sanjeev K. Sharma, MD and Kyle V. Contini, MD

Can J Gastroenterol. 2004;18(10):605–9.

HEMATURIA

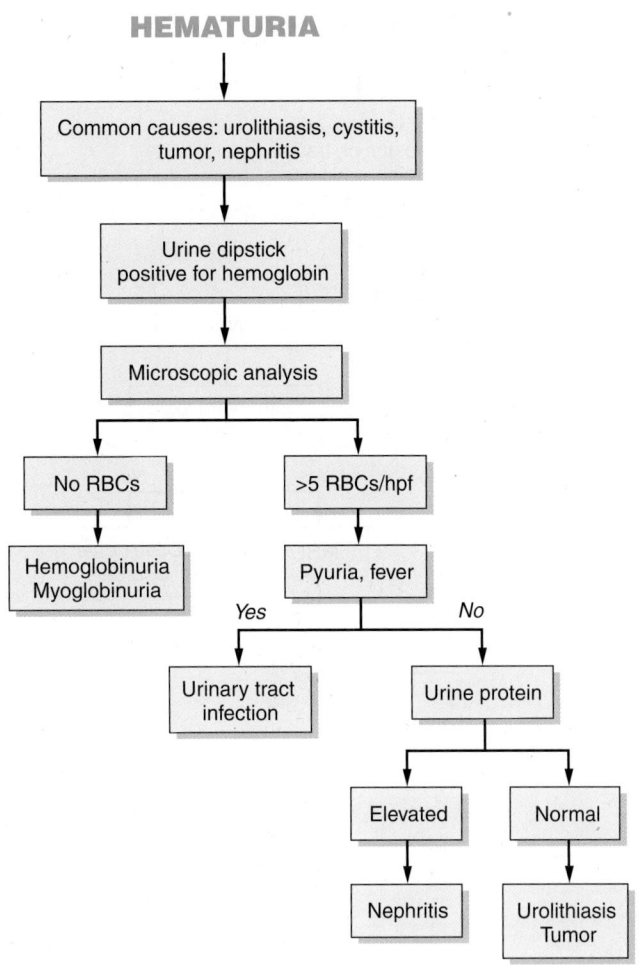

Common causes: urolithiasis, cystitis, tumor, nephritis

↓

Urine dipstick positive for hemoglobin

↓

Microscopic analysis

- No RBCs → Hemoglobinuria Myoglobinuria
- >5 RBCs/hpf → Pyuria, fever
  - *Yes* → Urinary tract infection
  - *No* → Urine protein
    - Elevated → Nephritis
    - Normal → Urolithiasis Tumor

Robert A. Baldor, MD and Alan M. Ehrlich, MD

Med Clin North Am. 2004;88(2):329–43.

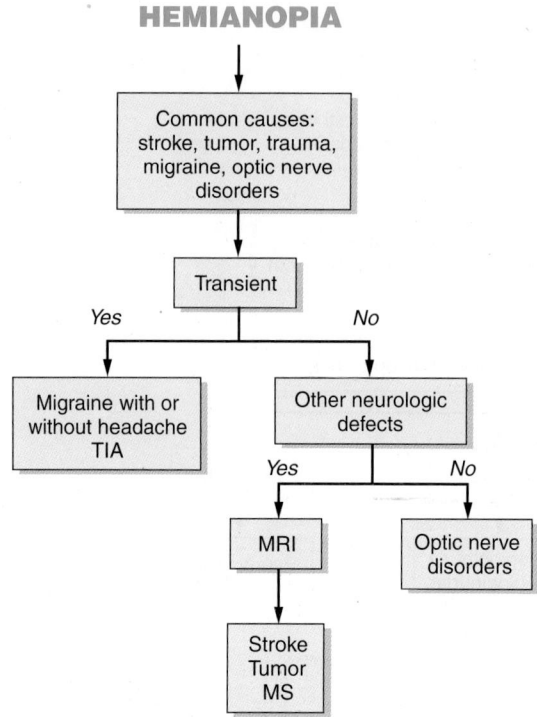

HEMIANOPIA

Common causes: stroke, tumor, trauma, migraine, optic nerve disorders

Transient

Yes — Migraine with or without headache TIA

No — Other neurologic defects

Yes — MRI — Stroke Tumor MS

No — Optic nerve disorders

Robert A. Baldor, MD and Alan M. Ehrlich, MD

Stroke. 2010;41(2):e88–90.

HICCUPS, PERSISTENT

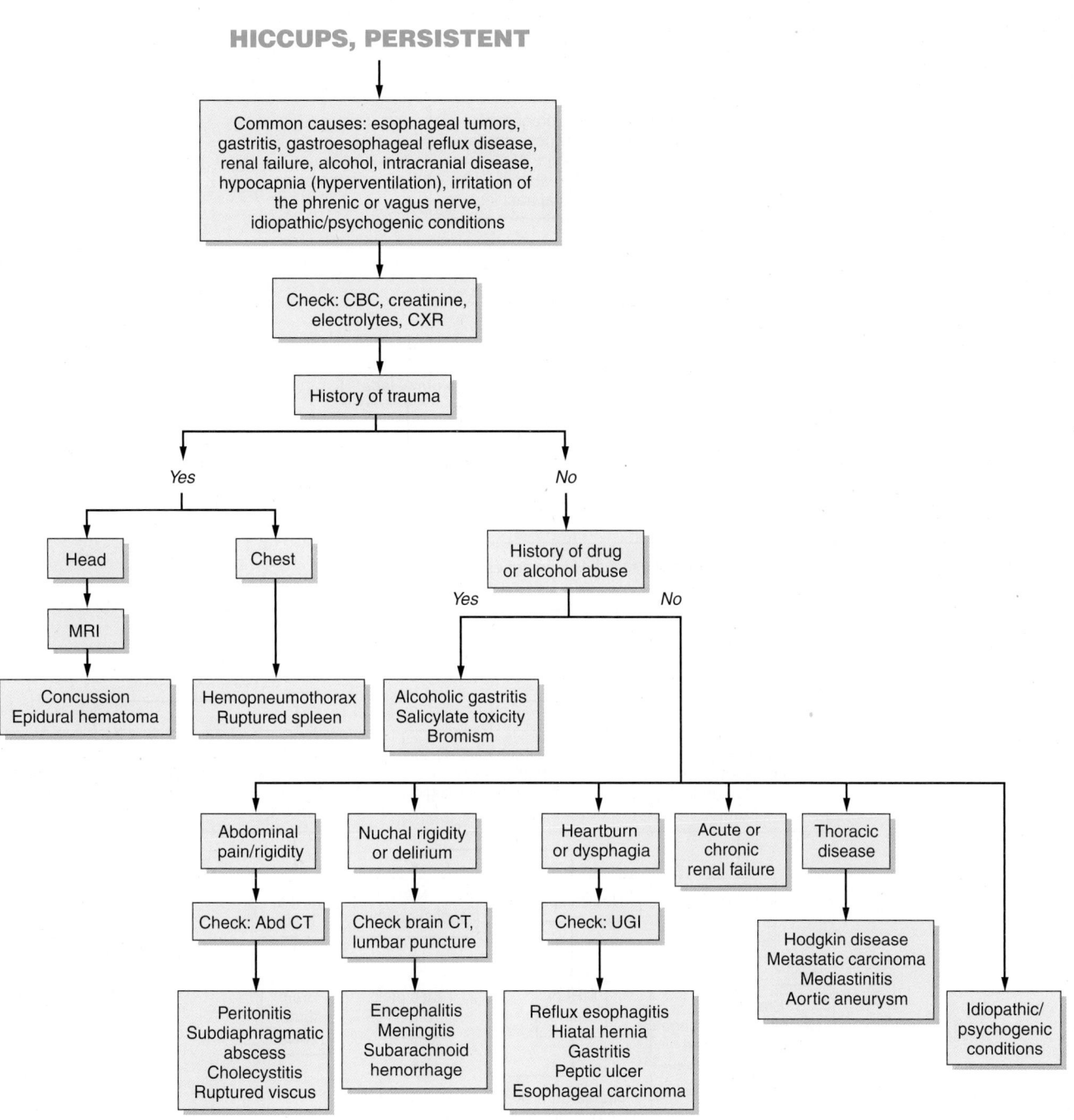

Common causes: esophageal tumors, gastritis, gastroesophageal reflux disease, renal failure, alcohol, intracranial disease, hypocapnia (hyperventilation), irritation of the phrenic or vagus nerve, idiopathic/psychogenic conditions

Check: CBC, creatinine, electrolytes, CXR

History of trauma

Yes →
- Head → MRI → Concussion / Epidural hematoma
- Chest → Hemopneumothorax / Ruptured spleen

No → History of drug or alcohol abuse

Yes → Alcoholic gastritis / Salicylate toxicity / Bromism

No →
- Abdominal pain/rigidity → Check: Abd CT → Peritonitis / Subdiaphragmatic abscess / Cholecystitis / Ruptured viscus
- Nuchal rigidity or delirium → Check brain CT, lumbar puncture → Encephalitis / Meningitis / Subarachnoid hemorrhage
- Heartburn or dysphagia → Check: UGI → Reflux esophagitis / Hiatal hernia / Gastritis / Peptic ulcer / Esophageal carcinoma
- Acute or chronic renal failure
- Thoracic disease → Hodgkin disease / Metastatic carcinoma / Mediastinitis / Aortic aneurysm
- Idiopathic/psychogenic conditions

Robert A. Baldor, MD and Alan M. Ehrlich, MD

J Support Oncol. 2009;7(4):122–7, 130.

HYPERACTIVE REFLEXES

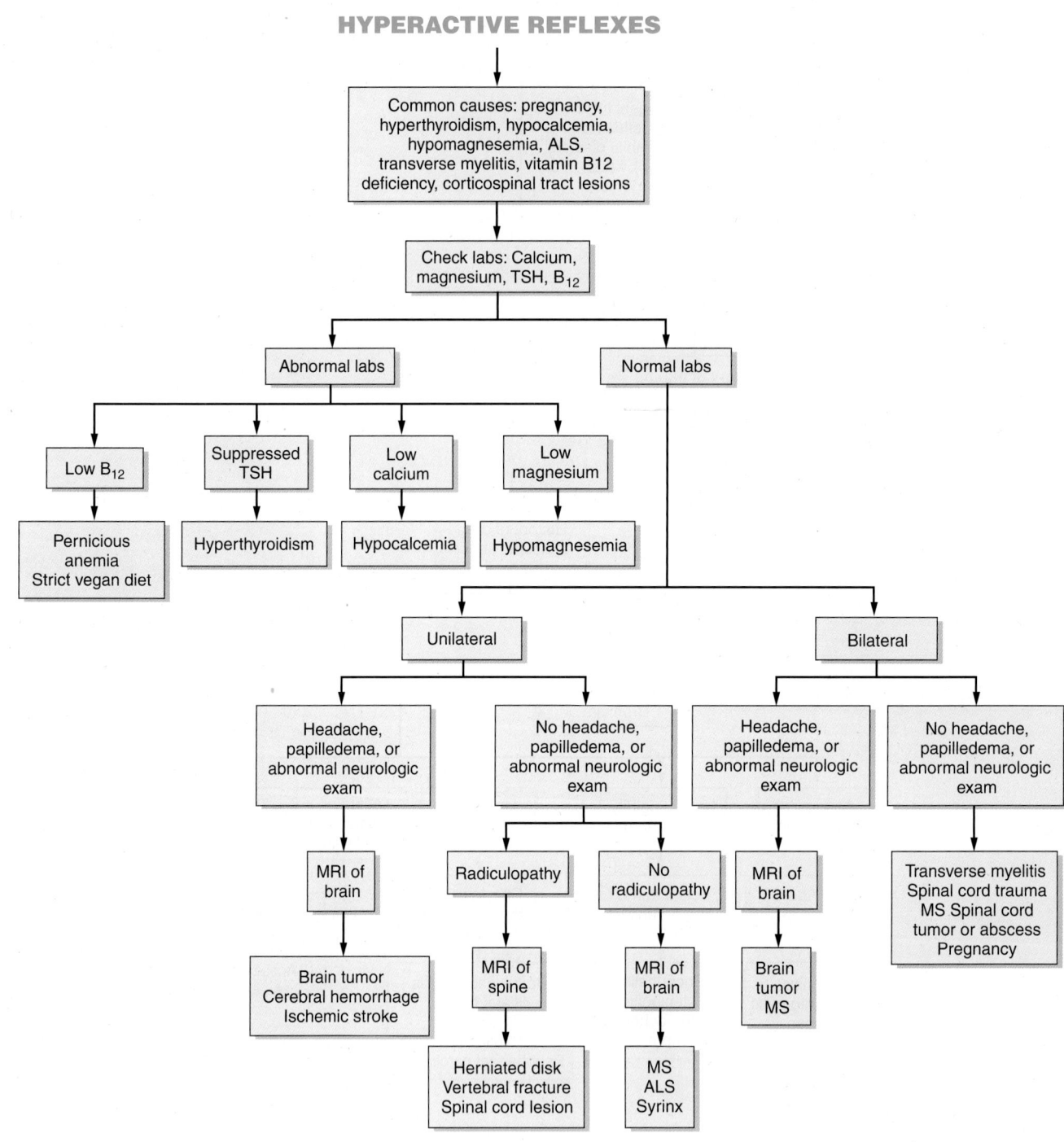

Common causes: pregnancy, hyperthyroidism, hypocalcemia, hypomagnesemia, ALS, transverse myelitis, vitamin B12 deficiency, corticospinal tract lesions

Check labs: Calcium, magnesium, TSH, B_{12}

Abnormal labs — **Normal labs**

Low B_{12} → Pernicious anemia / Strict vegan diet

Suppressed TSH → Hyperthyroidism

Low calcium → Hypocalcemia

Low magnesium → Hypomagnesemia

Unilateral / **Bilateral**

Headache, papilledema, or abnormal neurologic exam → MRI of brain → Brain tumor / Cerebral hemorrhage / Ischemic stroke

No headache, papilledema, or abnormal neurologic exam

- Radiculopathy → MRI of spine → Herniated disk / Vertebral fracture / Spinal cord lesion
- No radiculopathy → MRI of brain → MS / ALS / Syrinx

Headache, papilledema, or abnormal neurologic exam → MRI of brain → Brain tumor / MS

No headache, papilledema, or abnormal neurologic exam → Transverse myelitis / Spinal cord trauma / MS Spinal cord tumor or abscess / Pregnancy

Robert A. Baldor, MD and Alan M. Ehrlich, MD

Dev Med Child Neurol. 2009;51(2):128–35. Epub 2008 Oct 17.

HYPERBILIRUBINEMIA

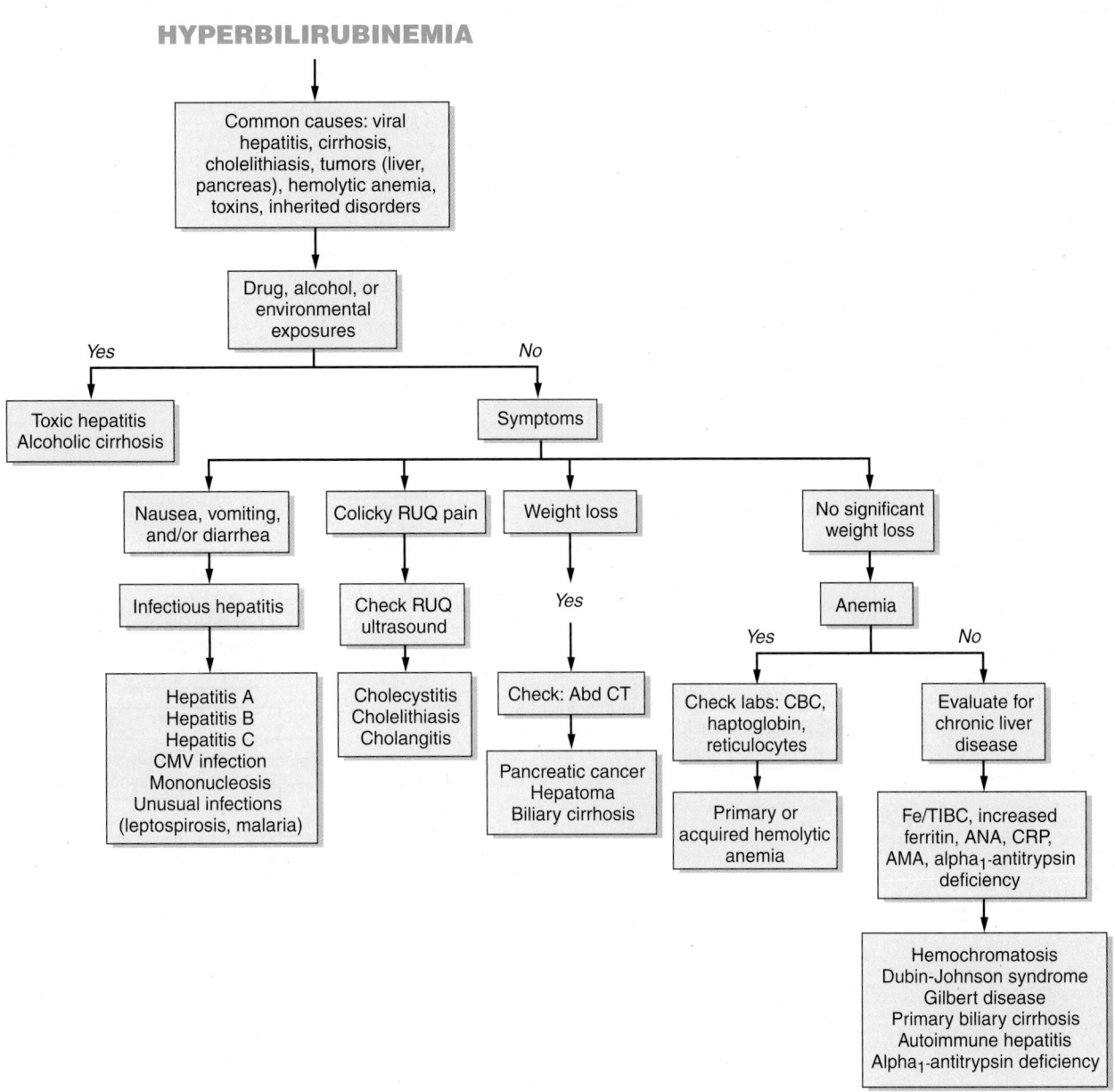

Robert A. Baldor, MD and Alan M. Ehrlich, MD

Am J Surg. 2009;198(2):193–8. Epub 2009 Mar 23.

HYPERCALCEMIA

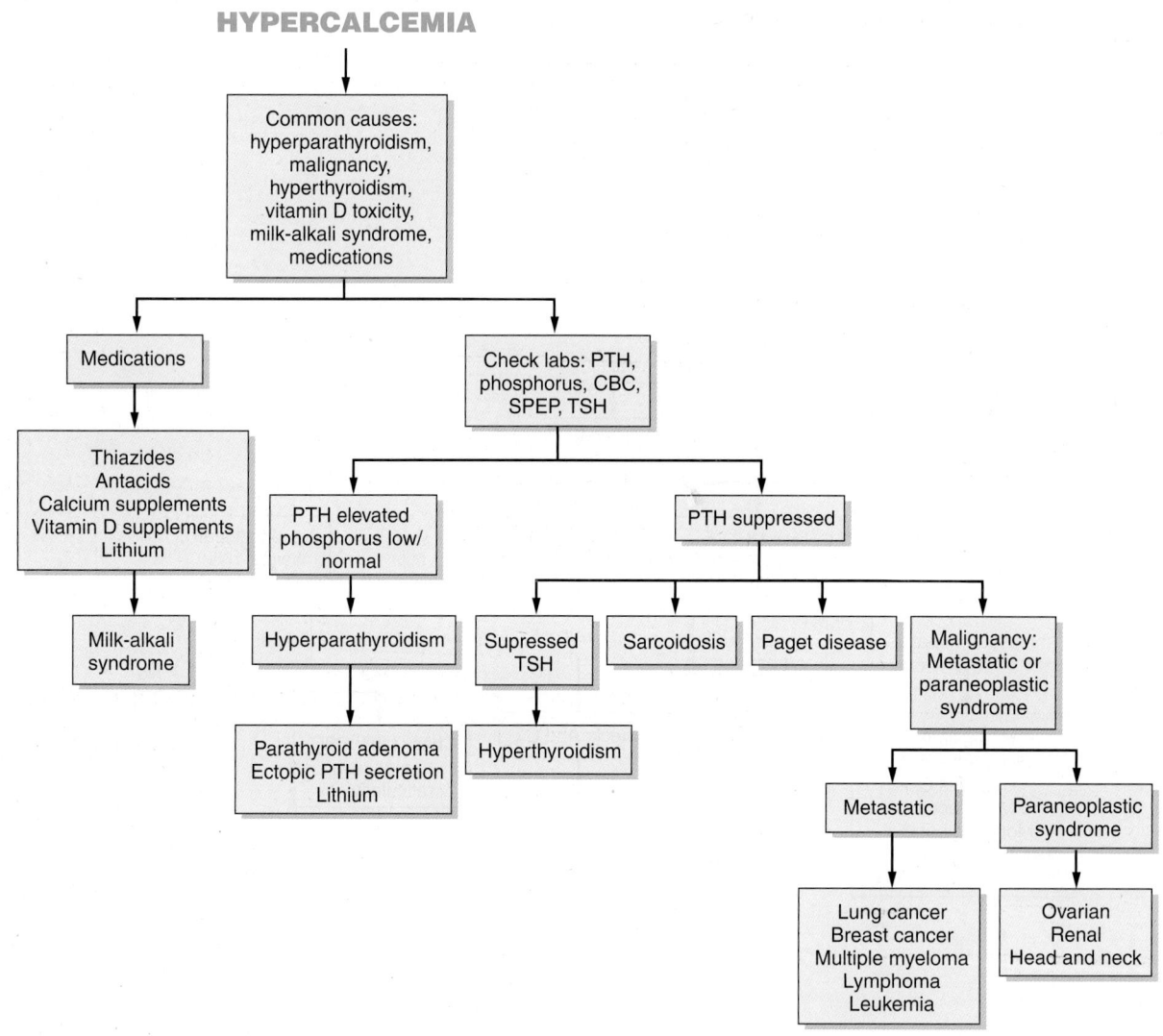

Robert A. Baldor, MD and Alan M. Ehrlich, MD

Iran J Kid. 2009;54(4):19–37.

HYPERCHOLESTEROLEMIA

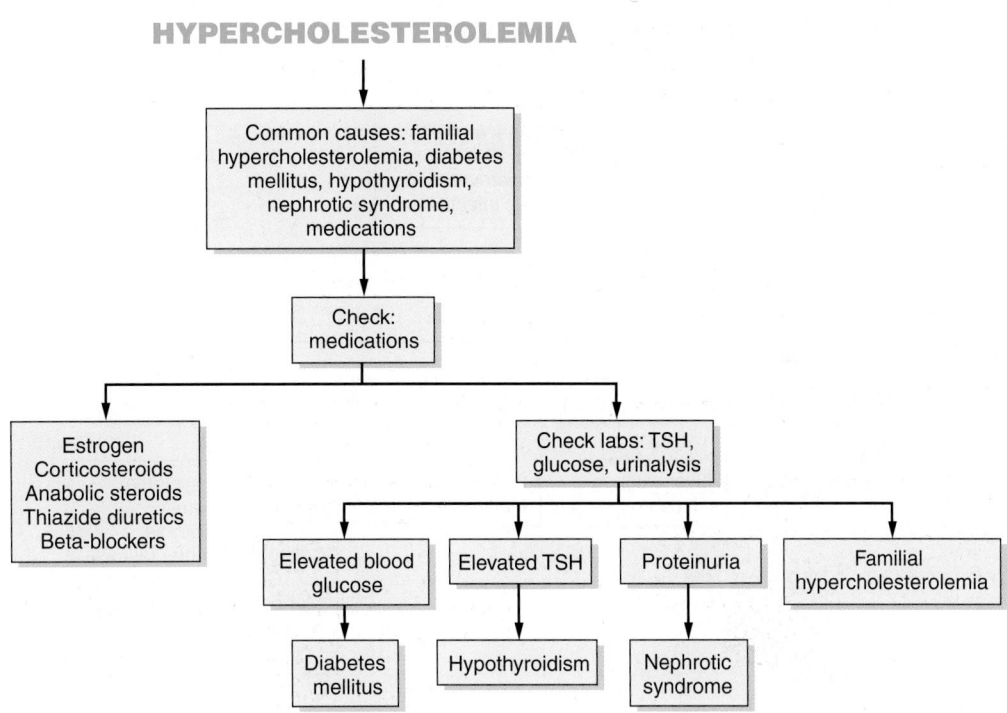

Robert A. Baldor, MD and Alan M. Ehrlich, MD

Curr Med Res Opin. 2009;25(2):431−47.

HYPERGAMMAGLOBULINEMIA

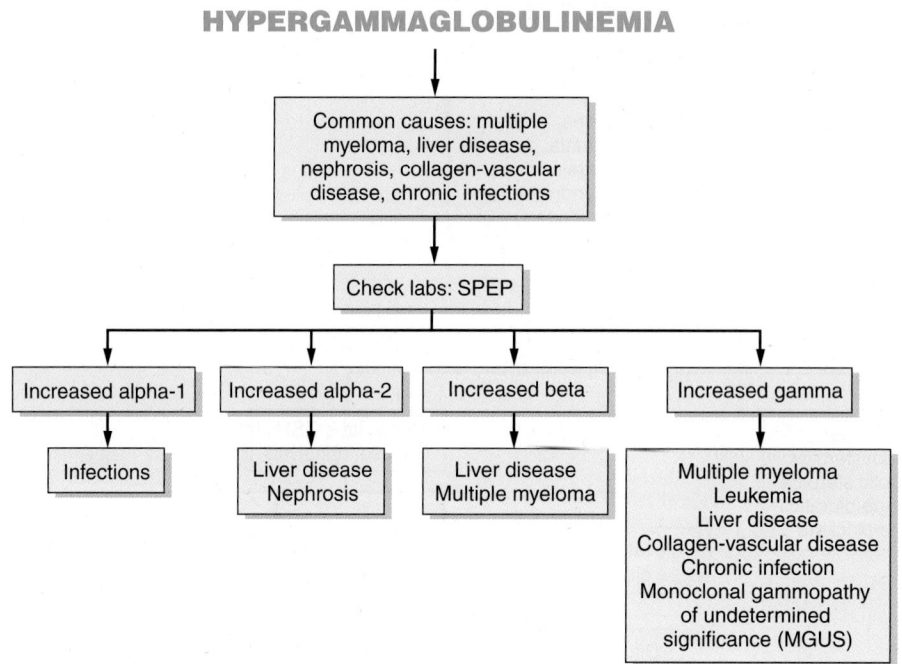

Robert A. Baldor, MD and Alan M. Ehrlich, MD

Medicine (Baltimore). 2009;88(5):284–93.

HYPERGLYCEMIA

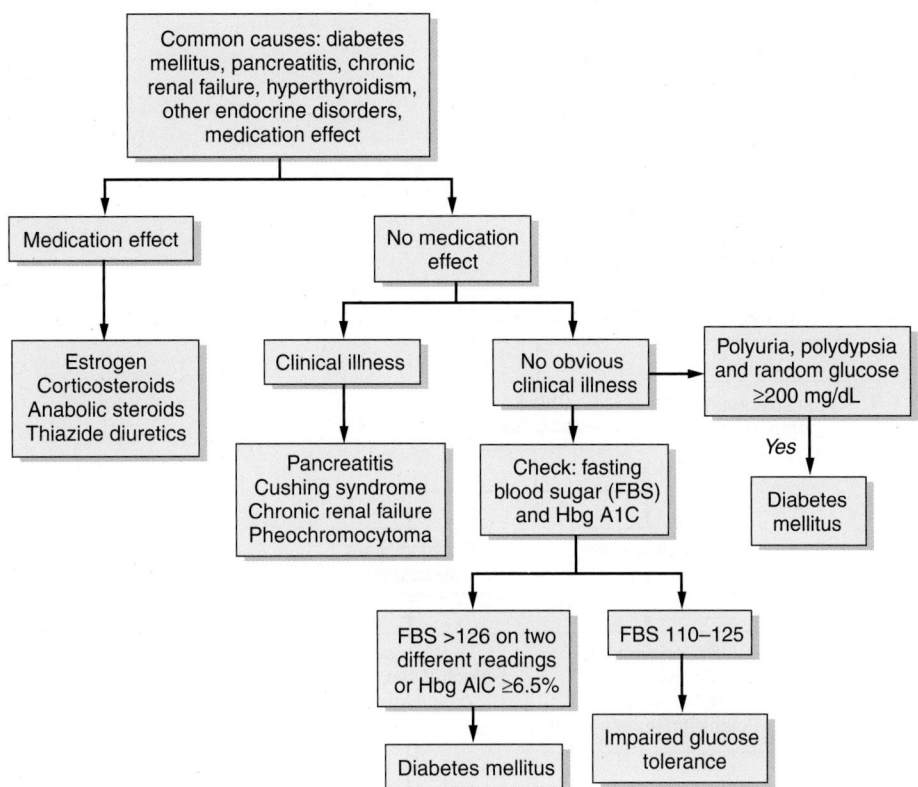

Robert A. Baldor, MD and Alan M. Ehrlich, MD

Crit Care Med. 2009;37(5):1769–76.

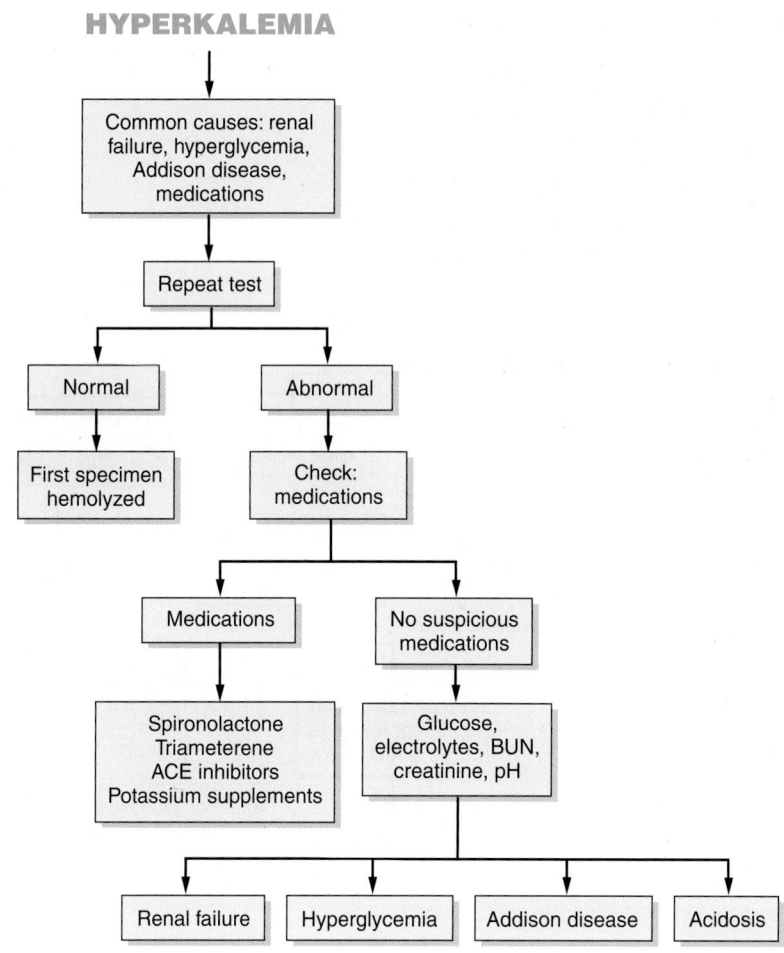

HYPERKALEMIA

Common causes: renal failure, hyperglycemia, Addison disease, medications

Repeat test

Normal

First specimen hemolyzed

Abnormal

Check: medications

Medications

No suspicious medications

Spironolactone
Triameterene
ACE inhibitors
Potassium supplements

Glucose, electrolytes, BUN, creatinine, pH

Renal failure

Hyperglycemia

Addison disease

Acidosis

Robert A. Baldor, MD and Alan M. Ehrlich, MD

J Gen Intern Med. 2010.

HYPERLIPIDEMIA

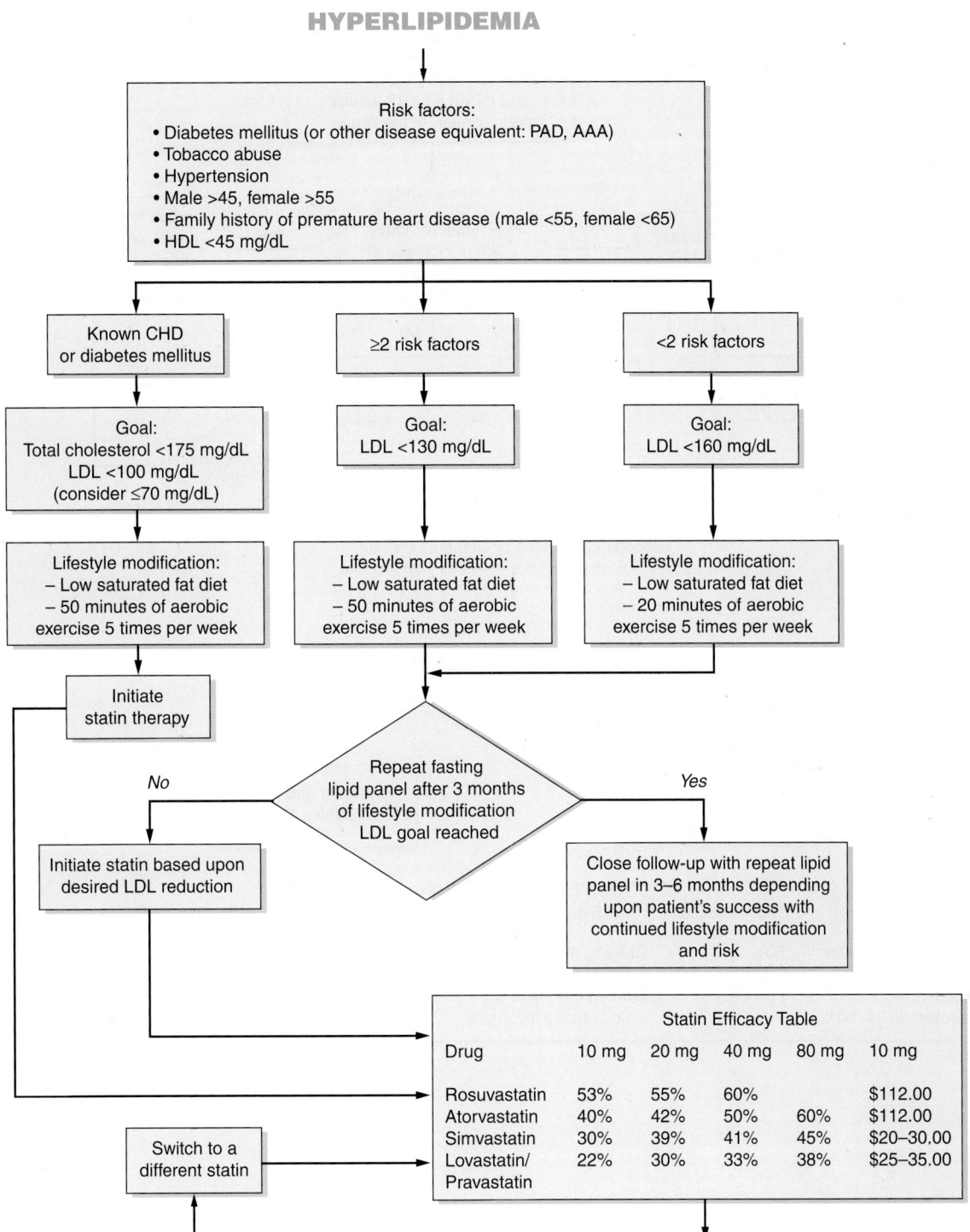

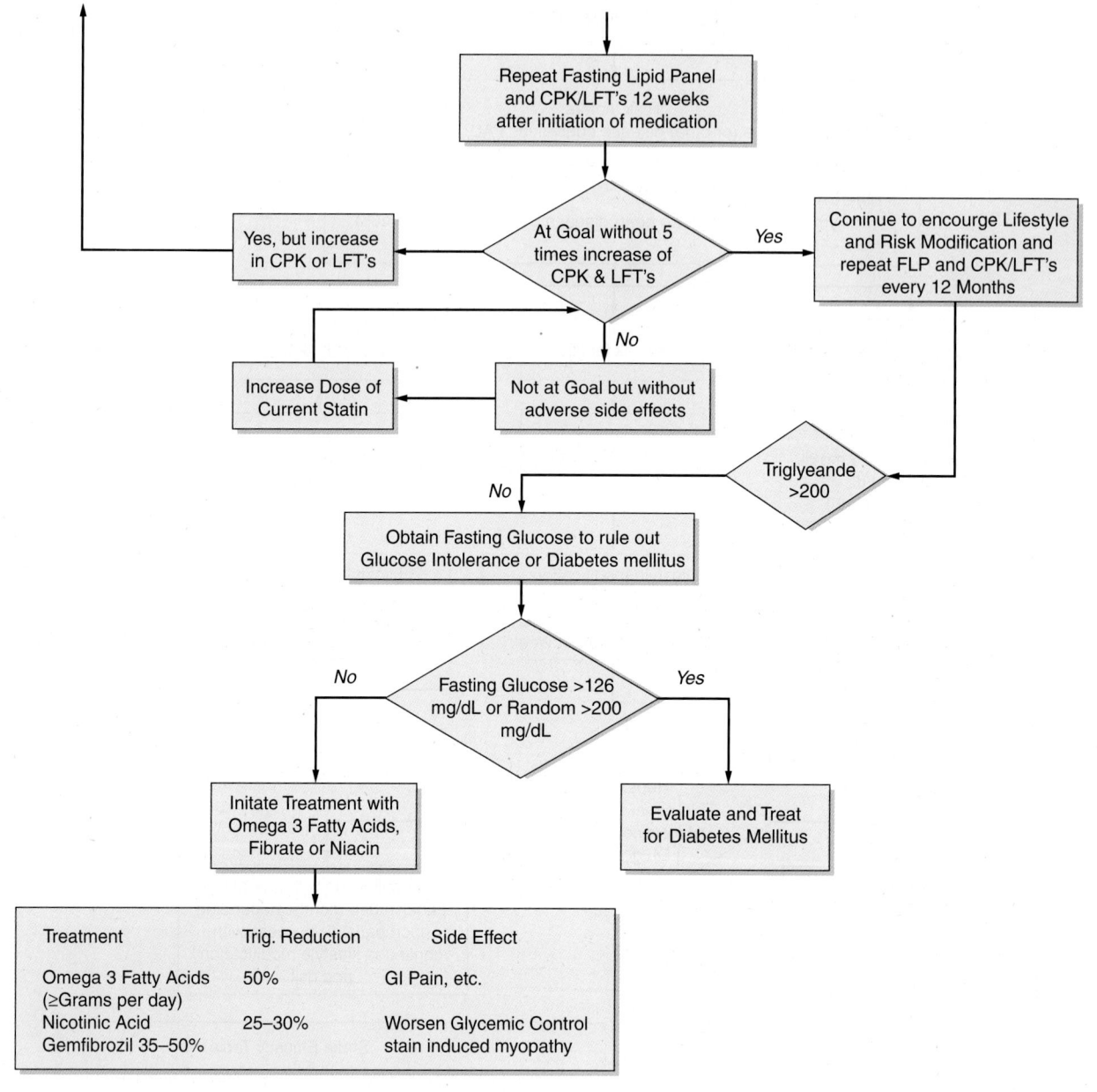

```
                    ┌─────────────────────────┐
                    │  Repeat Fasting Lipid Panel │
                    │  and CPK/LFT's 12 weeks  │
                    │  after initiation of medication │
                    └─────────────────────────┘
```

Repeat Fasting Lipid Panel and CPK/LFT's 12 weeks after initiation of medication

At Goal without 5 times increase of CPK & LFT's

Yes, but increase in CPK or LFT's

Yes → Coninue to encourge Lifestyle and Risk Modification and repeat FLP and CPK/LFT's every 12 Months

No

Increase Dose of Current Statin ← Not at Goal but without adverse side effects

Triglyeande >200

No → Obtain Fasting Glucose to rule out Glucose Intolerance or Diabetes mellitus

Fasting Glucose >126 mg/dL or Random >200 mg/dL

No → Initate Treatment with Omega 3 Fatty Acids, Fibrate or Niacin

Yes → Evaluate and Treat for Diabetes Mellitus

Treatment	Trig. Reduction	Side Effect
Omega 3 Fatty Acids (≥Grams per day)	50%	GI Pain, etc.
Nicotinic Acid	25–30%	Worsen Glycemic Control
Gemfibrozil	35–50%	stain induced myopathy

Rade N. Pejic, MD

Adv Ther. 2010;27(6):348–64.

HYPERNATREMIA

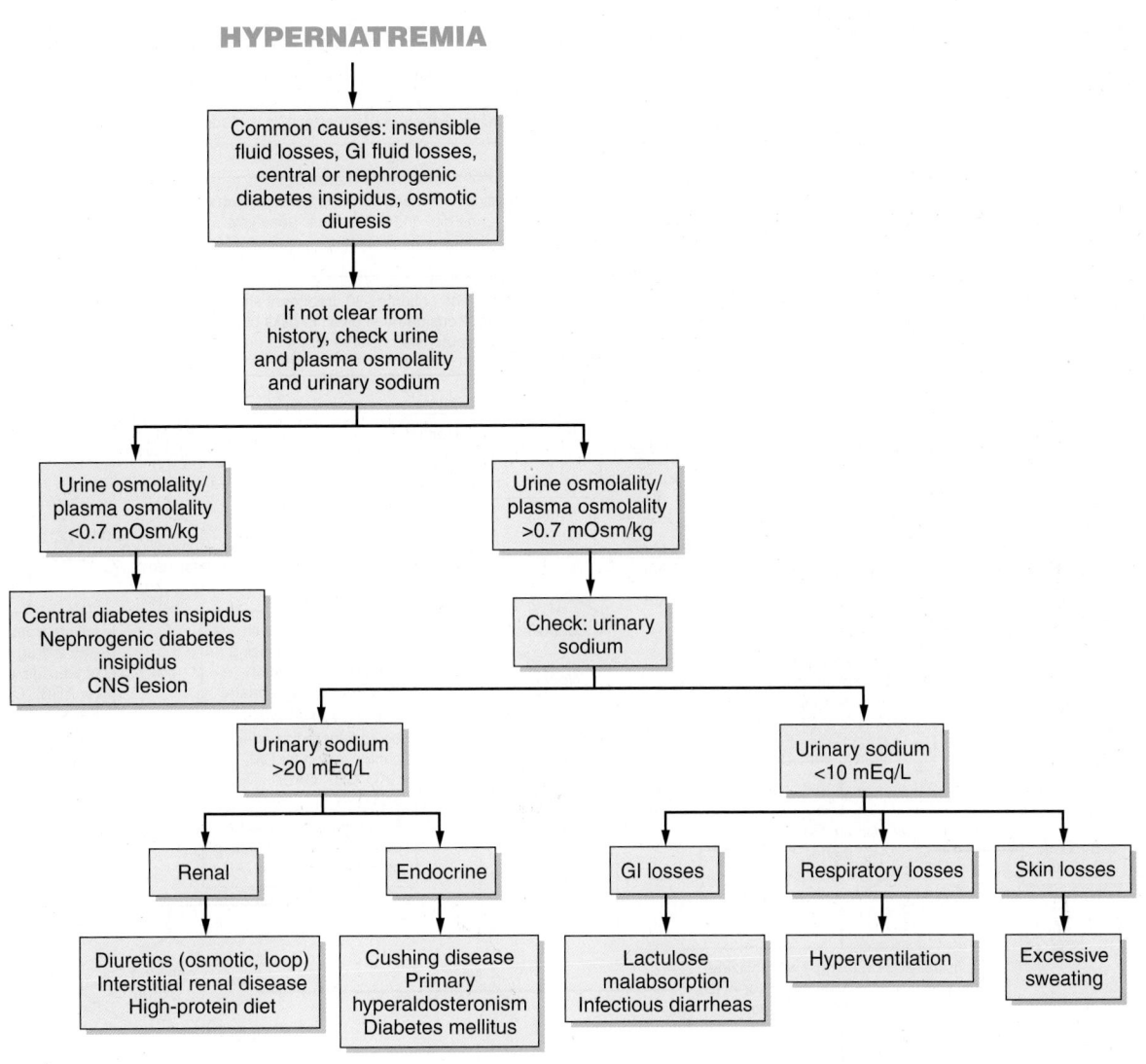

Robert A. Baldor, MD and Alan M. Ehrlich, MD

N Engl J Med. 2000;342(20):1493–9.

HYPERTENSION AND ELEVATED BLOOD PRESSURE, TREATMENT

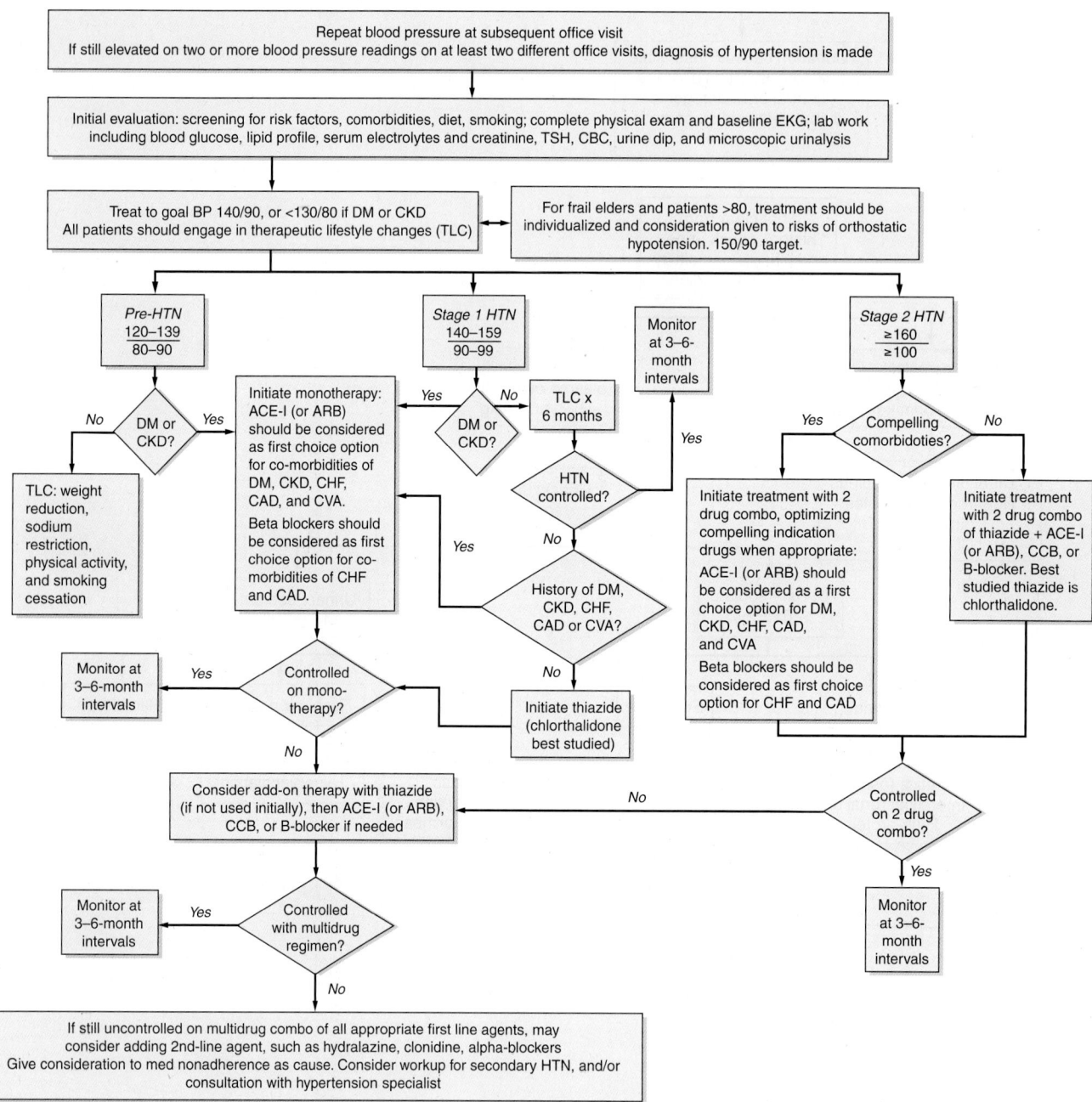

B. Brent Simmons, MD

Hypertension. 2003;42:1206.

HYPERTRIGLYCERIDEMIA

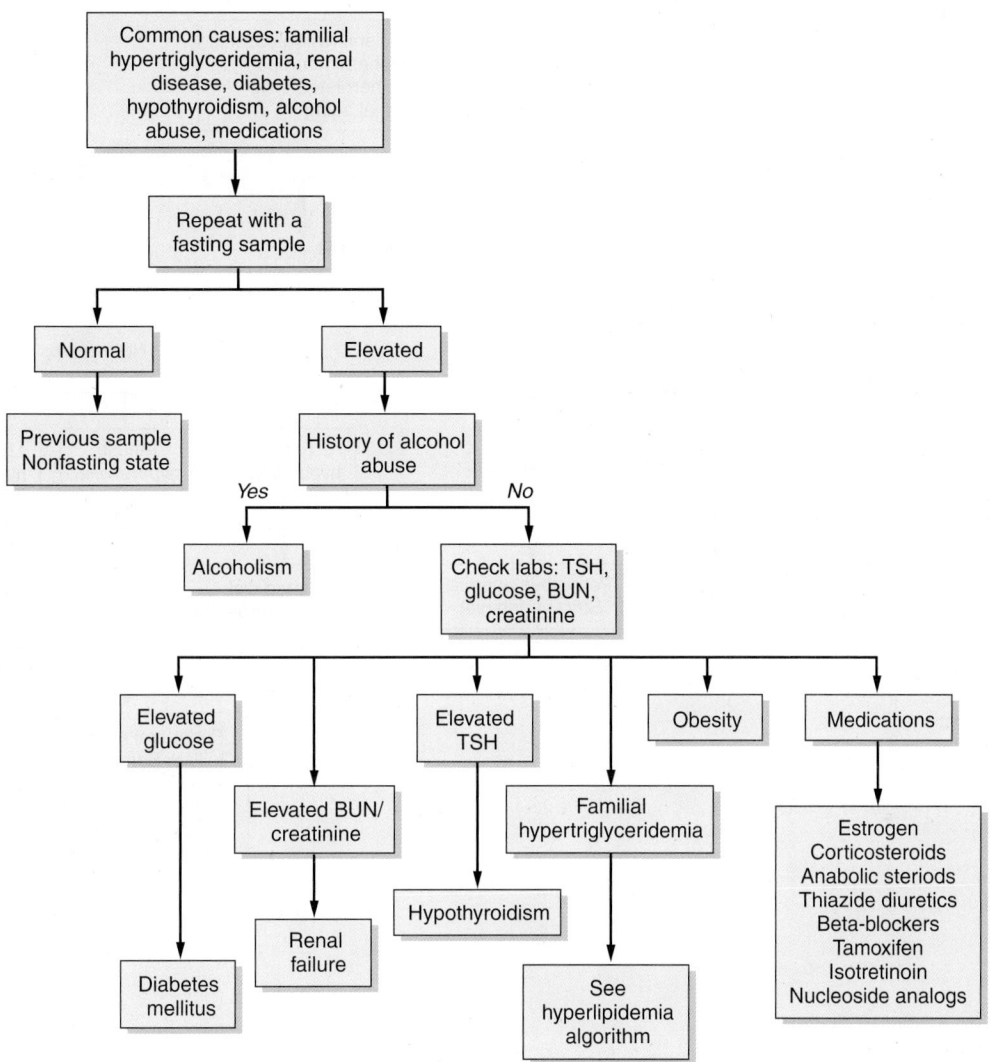

Robert A. Baldor, MD and Alan M. Ehrlich, MD

Am J Cardiol. 2001;87:1174.

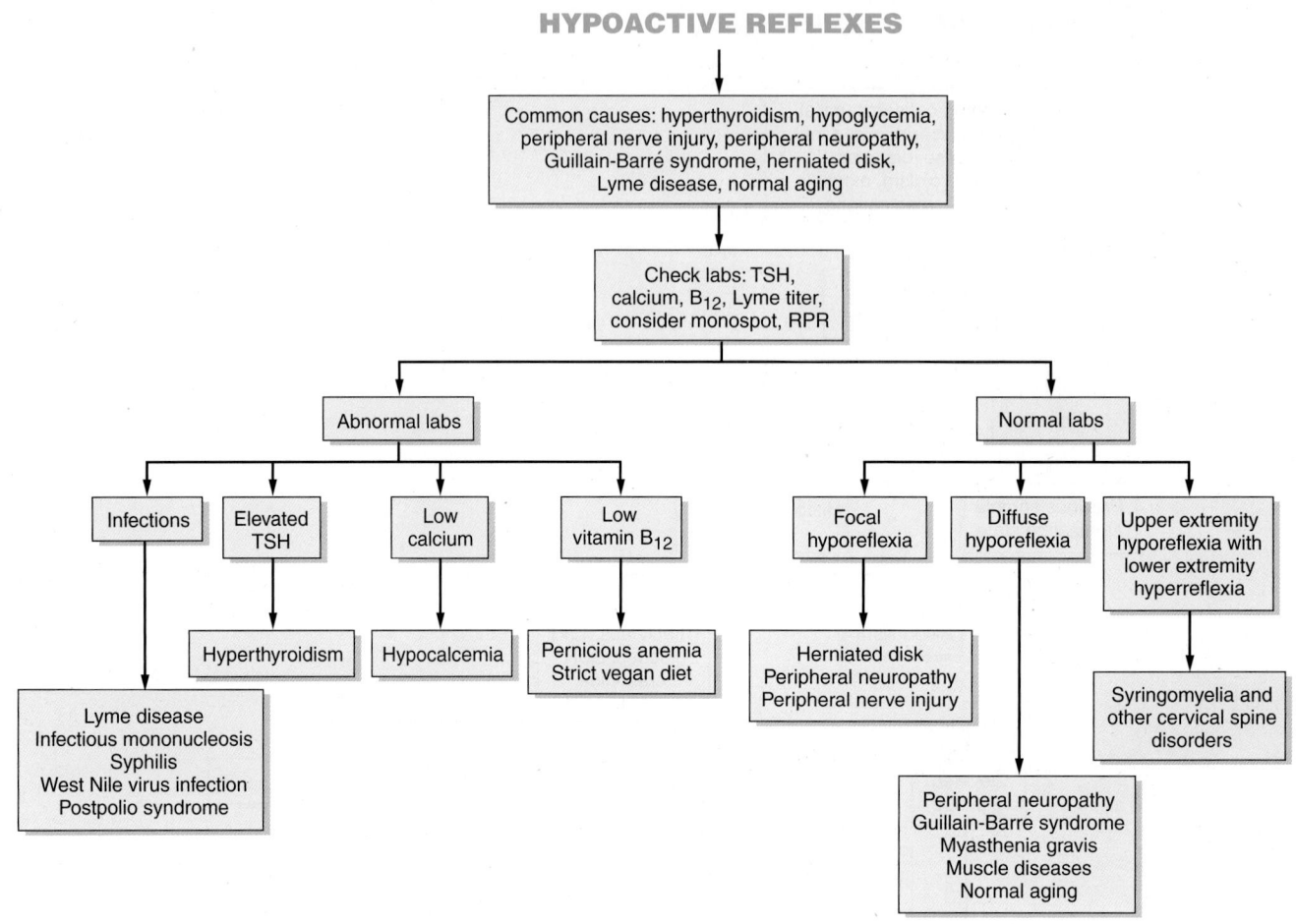

HYPOACTIVE REFLEXES

Common causes: hyperthyroidism, hypoglycemia, peripheral nerve injury, peripheral neuropathy, Guillain-Barré syndrome, herniated disk, Lyme disease, normal aging

Check labs: TSH, calcium, B$_{12}$, Lyme titer, consider monospot, RPR

Abnormal labs

Infections

Elevated TSH

Low calcium

Low vitamin B$_{12}$

Hyperthyroidism

Hypocalcemia

Pernicious anemia
Strict vegan diet

Lyme disease
Infectious mononucleosis
Syphilis
West Nile virus infection
Postpolio syndrome

Normal labs

Focal hyporeflexia

Diffuse hyporeflexia

Upper extremity hyporeflexia with lower extremity hyperreflexia

Herniated disk
Peripheral neuropathy
Peripheral nerve injury

Syringomyelia and other cervical spine disorders

Peripheral neuropathy
Guillain-Barré syndrome
Myasthenia gravis
Muscle diseases
Normal aging

Robert A. Baldor, MD and Alan M. Ehrlich, MD

Med Clin North Am. 2009;93(2):317–42, vii–viii.

HYPOALBUMINEMIA

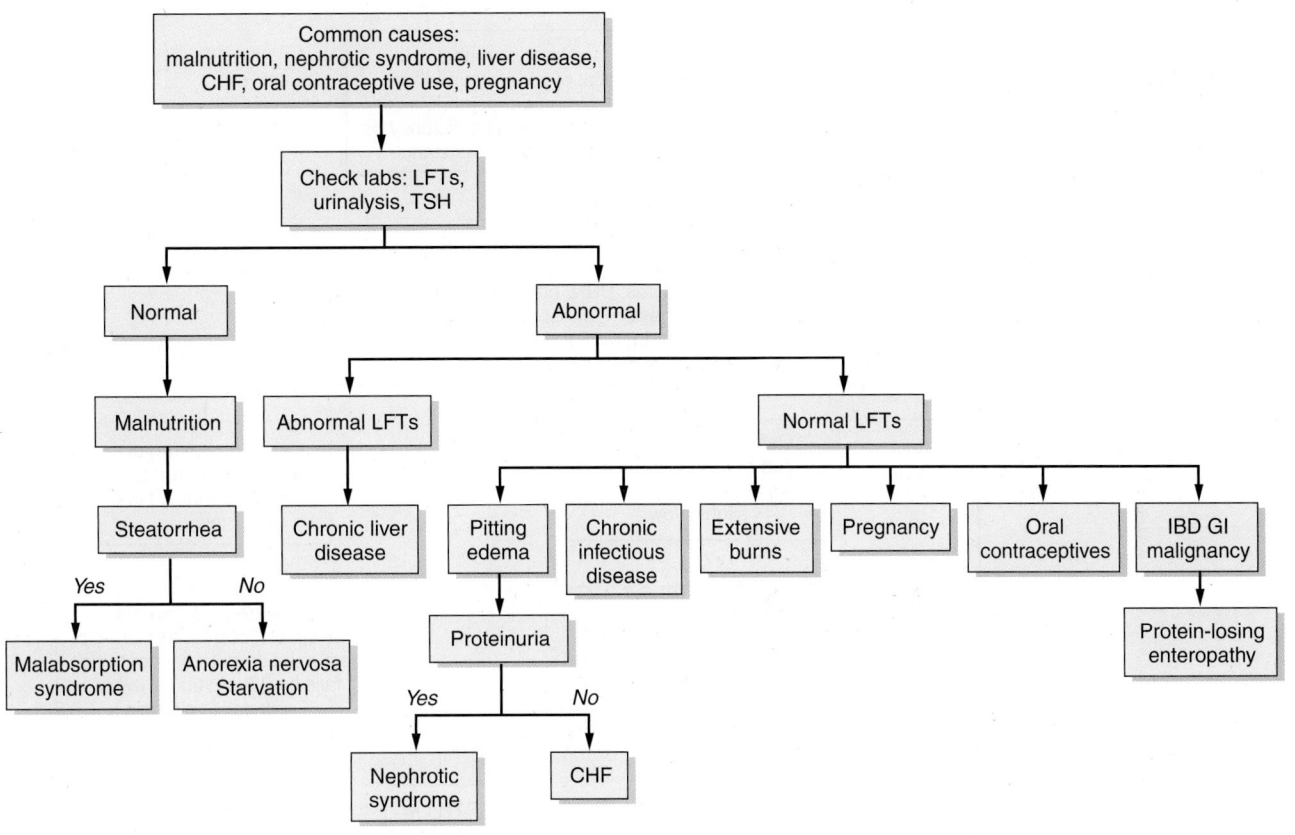

Robert A. Baldor, MD and Alan M. Ehrlich, MD

Am Fam Physician. 2009;80(10):1129–34.

HYPOCALCEMIA

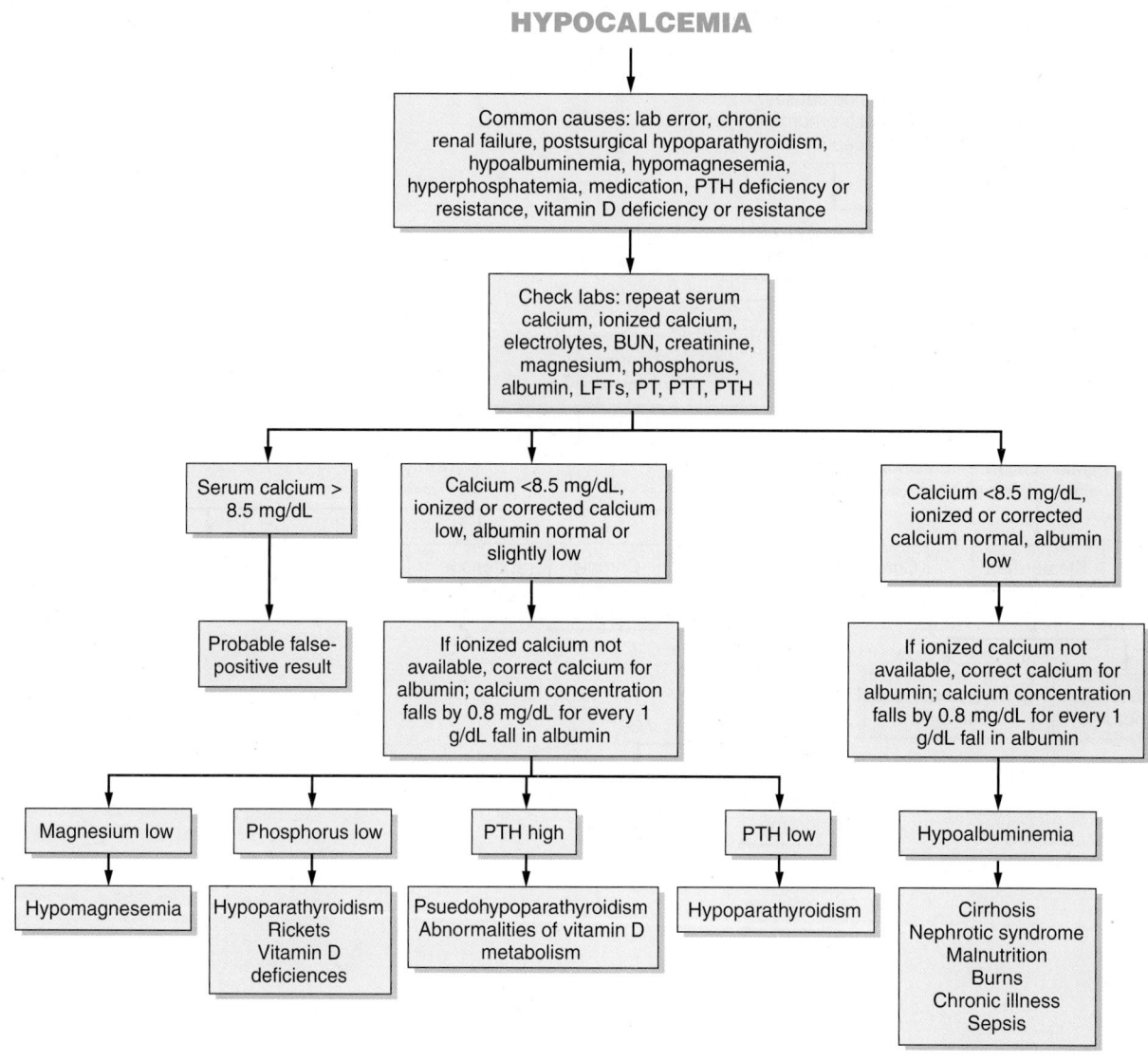

Robert A. Baldor, MD and Alan M. Ehrlich, MD

J Fam Pract. 2008;57(10):677–9.

HYPOGLYCEMIA

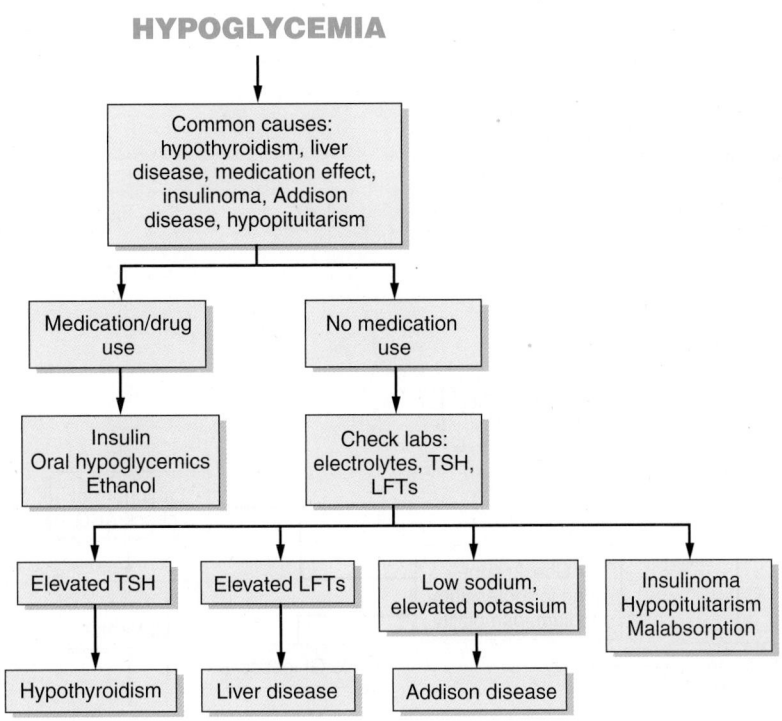

Robert A. Baldor, MD and Alan M. Ehrlich, MD

J Clin Endocrinol Metab. 2009;94(3):741–5. Epub 2008 Dec 16.

HYPOKALEMIA

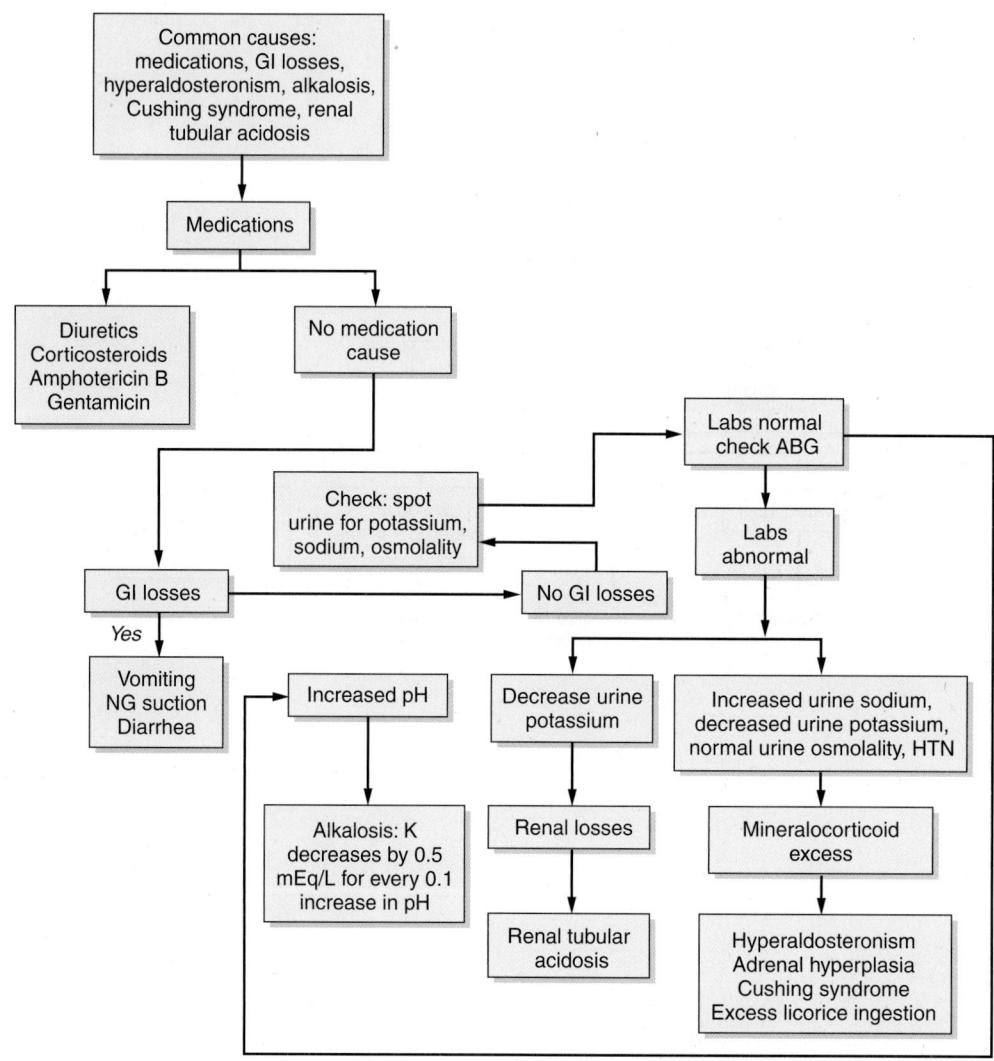

Robert A. Baldor, MD and Alan M. Ehrlich, MD

Ann Intern Med. 2009;150(9):619–25.

HYPONATREMIA

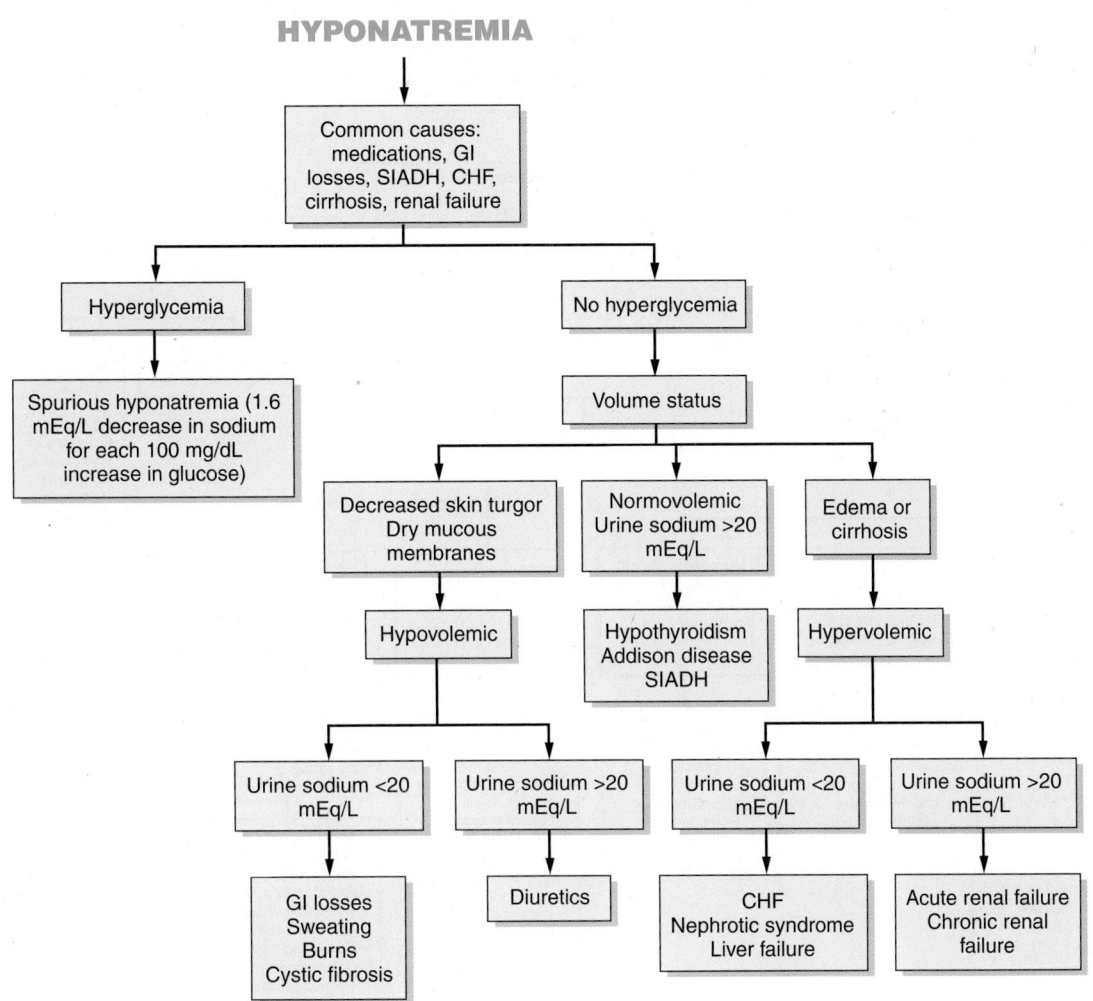

Robert A. Baldor, MD and Alan M. Ehrlich, MD

Am J Med. 2007;120(8):653–8.

HYPOTENSION

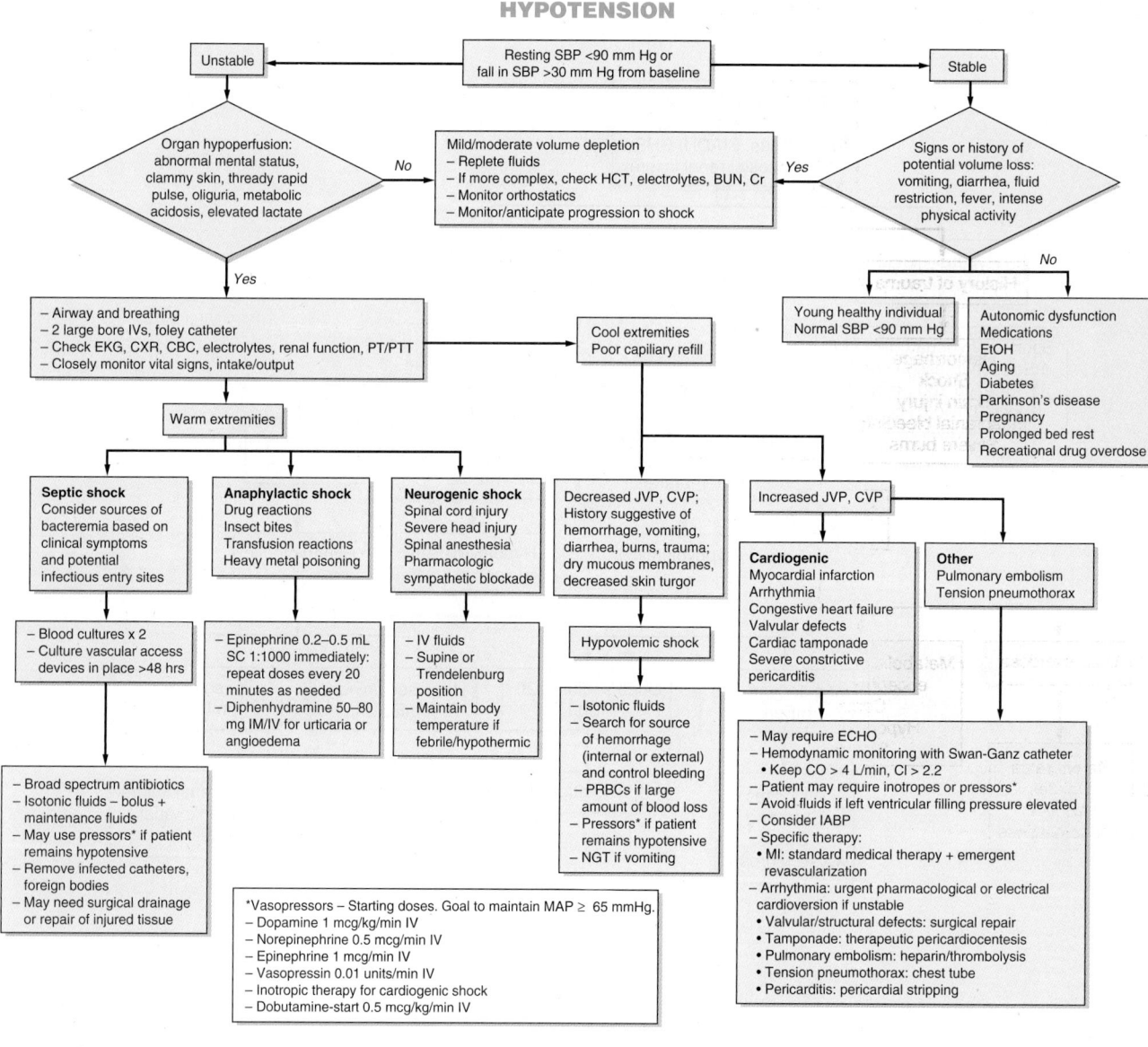

Martin A. Espinosa Ginic, MD and Bryan K. Moffett, MD

Arch Phys Med Rehabil. 2009;90(5):876–85.

HYPOTHERMIA

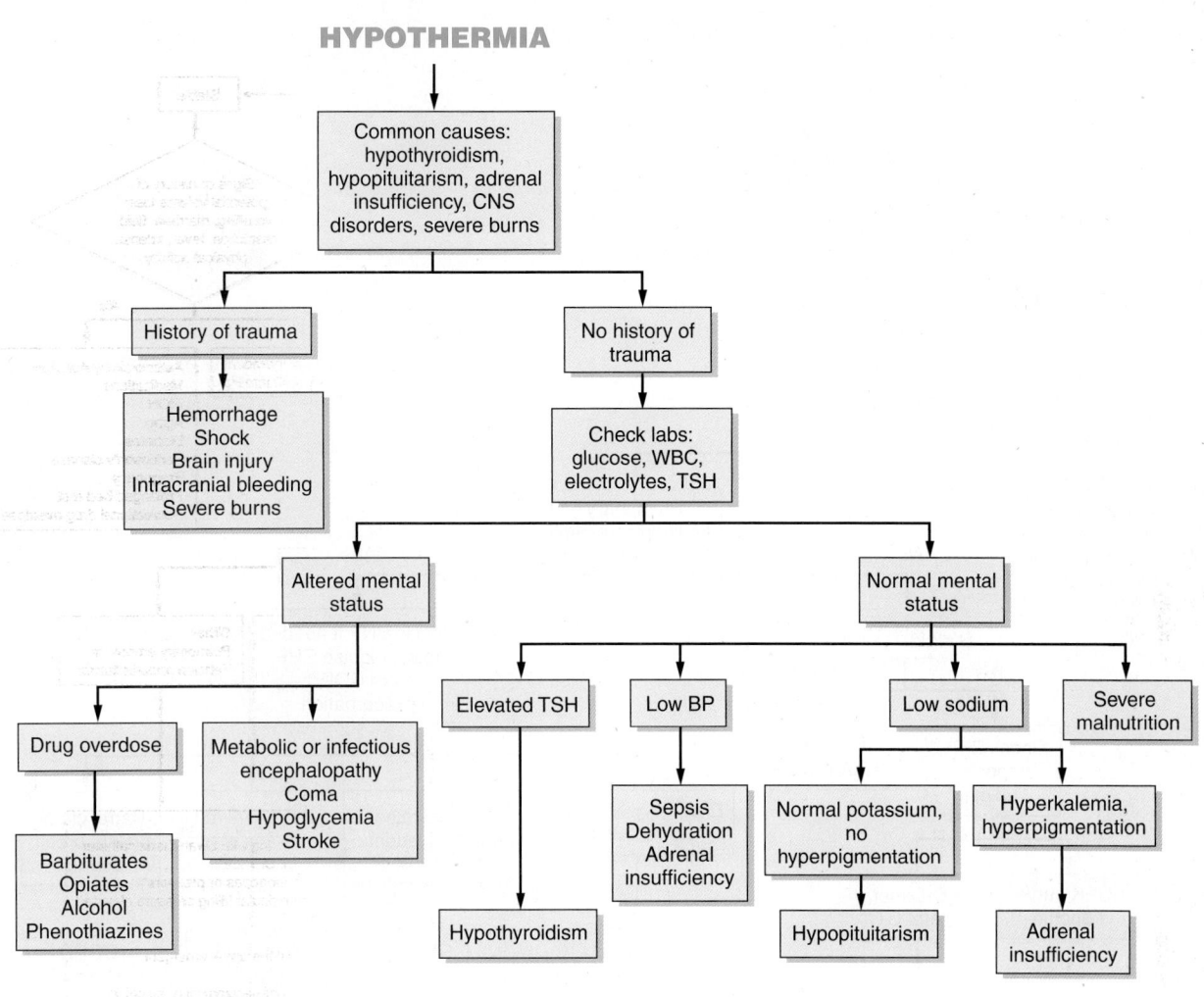

Robert A. Baldor, MD and Alan M. Ehrlich, MD

Am J Med. 2006;119(4):297–301.

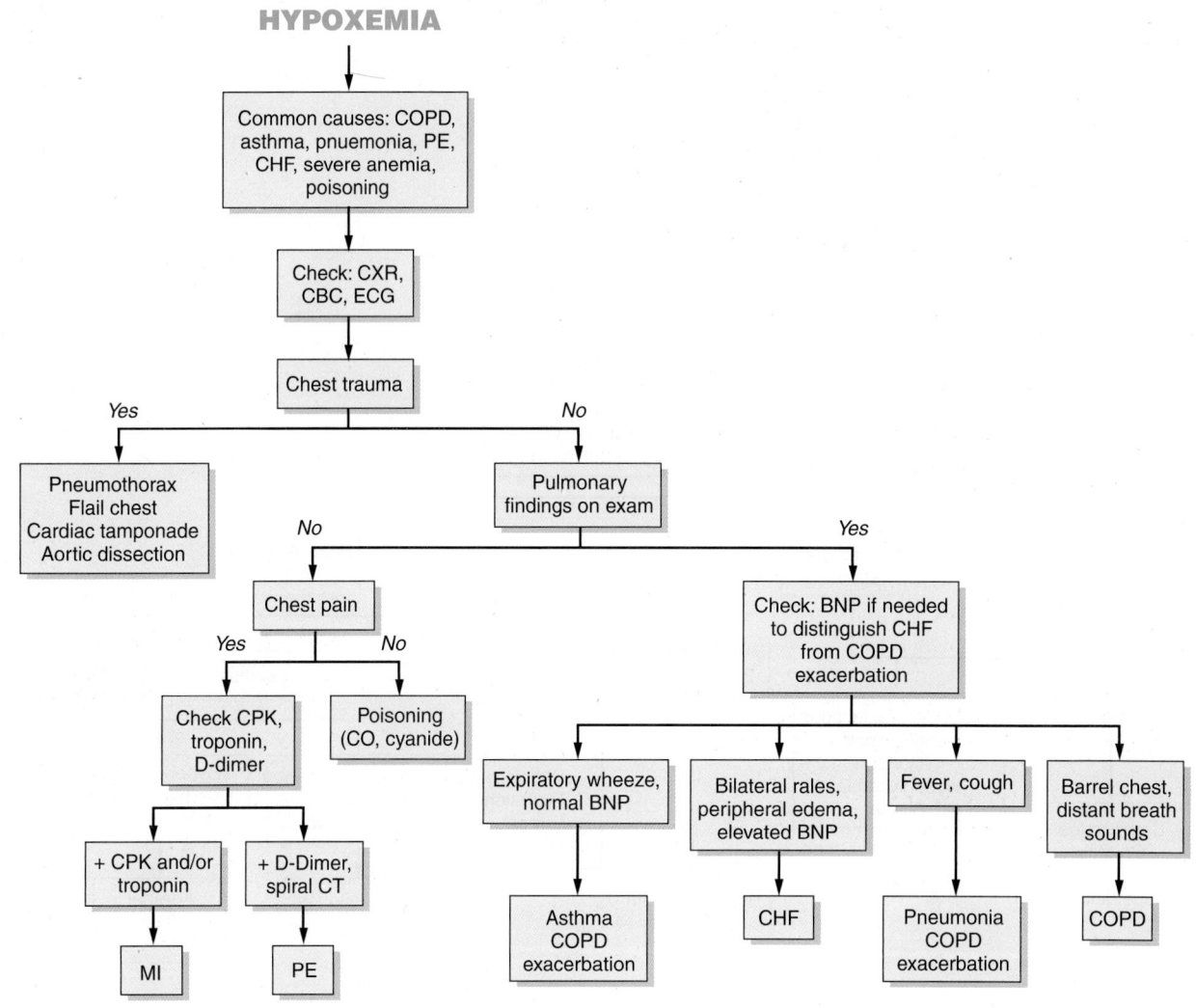

HYPOXEMIA

Common causes: COPD, asthma, pnuemonia, PE, CHF, severe anemia, poisoning

Check: CXR, CBC, ECG

Chest trauma

Yes → Pneumothorax, Flail chest, Cardiac tamponade, Aortic dissection

No → Pulmonary findings on exam

Pulmonary findings on exam — *No* → Chest pain

Chest pain — *Yes* → Check CPK, troponin, D-dimer

Chest pain — *No* → Poisoning (CO, cyanide)

Check CPK, troponin, D-dimer → + CPK and/or troponin → MI

Check CPK, troponin, D-dimer → + D-Dimer, spiral CT → PE

Pulmonary findings on exam — *Yes* → Check: BNP if needed to distinguish CHF from COPD exacerbation

Expiratory wheeze, normal BNP → Asthma COPD exacerbation

Bilateral rales, peripheral edema, elevated BNP → CHF

Fever, cough → Pneumonia COPD exacerbation

Barrel chest, distant breath sounds → COPD

Robert A. Baldor, MD and Alan M. Ehrlich, MD

Lancet. 2009;374(9691):721–32.

INFERTILITY

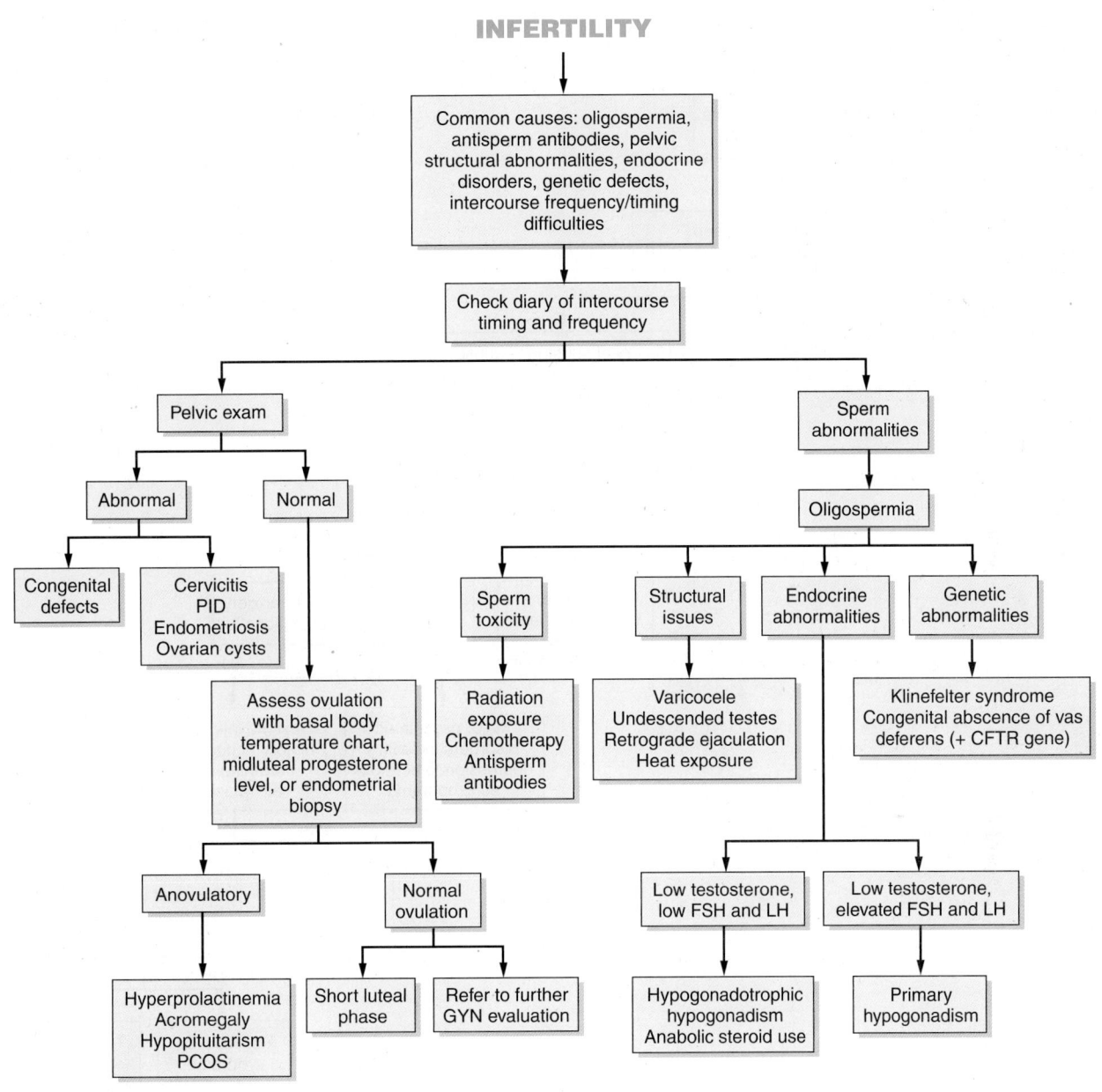

Common causes: oligospermia, antisperm antibodies, pelvic structural abnormalities, endocrine disorders, genetic defects, intercourse frequency/timing difficulties

Check diary of intercourse timing and frequency

Pelvic exam

- Abnormal
  - Congenital defects
  - Cervicitis PID Endometriosis Ovarian cysts
- Normal
  - Assess ovulation with basal body temperature chart, midluteal progesterone level, or endometrial biopsy
    - Anovulatory
      - Hyperprolactinemia Acromegaly Hypopituitarism PCOS
    - Normal ovulation
      - Short luteal phase
      - Refer to further GYN evaluation

Sperm abnormalities

- Oligospermia
  - Sperm toxicity
    - Radiation exposure Chemotherapy Antisperm antibodies
  - Structural issues
    - Varicocele Undescended testes Retrograde ejaculation Heat exposure
  - Endocrine abnormalities
    - Low testosterone, low FSH and LH
      - Hypogonadotrophic hypogonadism Anabolic steroid use
    - Low testosterone, elevated FSH and LH
      - Primary hypogonadism
  - Genetic abnormalities
    - Klinefelter syndrome Congenital abscence of vas deferens (+ CFTR gene)

Robert A. Baldor, MD and Alan M. Ehrlich, MD

Med Clin North Am. 2008;92(5):1163–92, xi.

INSOMNIA, CHRONIC

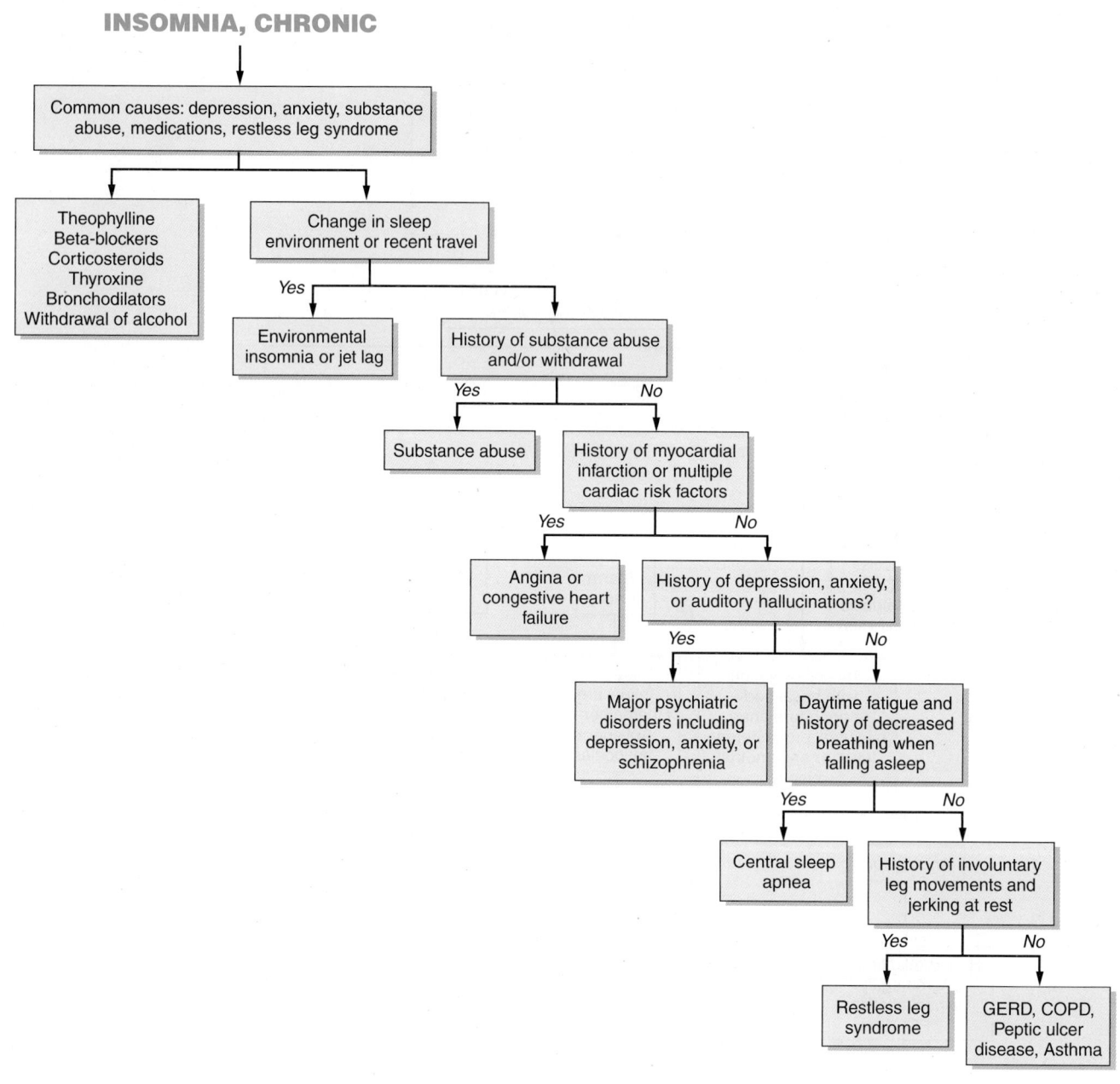

Robert A. Baldor, MD and Alan M. Ehrlich, MD

Am Fam Physician. 2007;76(4):517–26.

INTESTINAL OBSTRUCTION

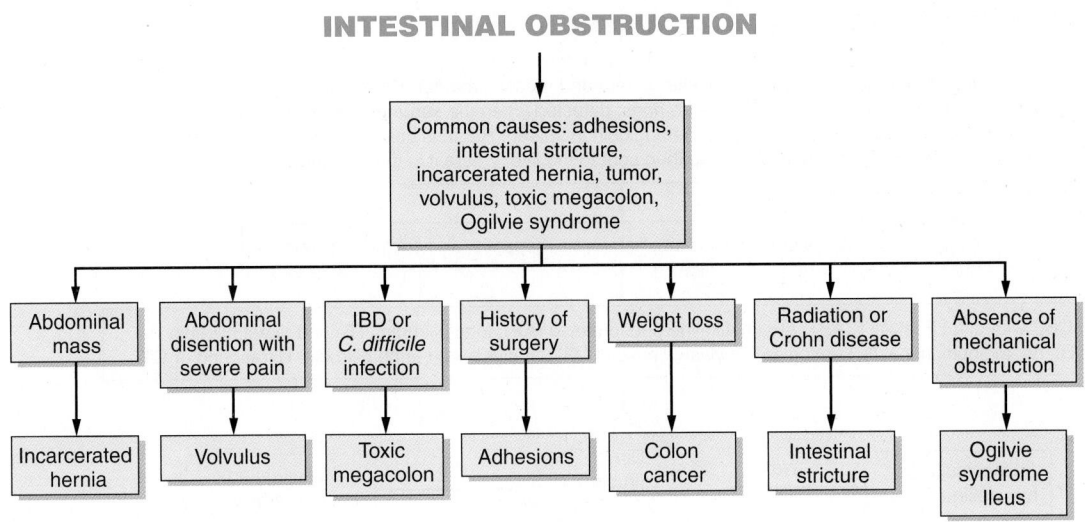

Robert A. Baldor, MD and Alan M. Ehrlich, MD

Med Clin North Am. 2008;92(3):575–97, viii.

JAUNDICE

Jaundice: A yellow discoloration of skin, sclera and mucous membranes by bilirubin, a bile pigment formed by the breakdown of heme rings; detected when the serum bilirubin level >3 mg/dL. Bilirubin results from the breakdown of hemoglobin in spleen. Heme is converted to unconjugated bilirubin, bound to albumin and then sent to the liver where it is then conjugated.

Common causes: Gilbert's syndrome, hemolysis, hepatitis, and choledocholithiasis

CBC with diff, LFTs: ALT, AST, serum alkaline phosphatase (AP), total bilirubin (TB) and direct bilirubin (DB), haptoglobin, hepatitis serologies, amylase, lipase, hCG, urinalysis with urine bilirubin. Ultrasound or CT

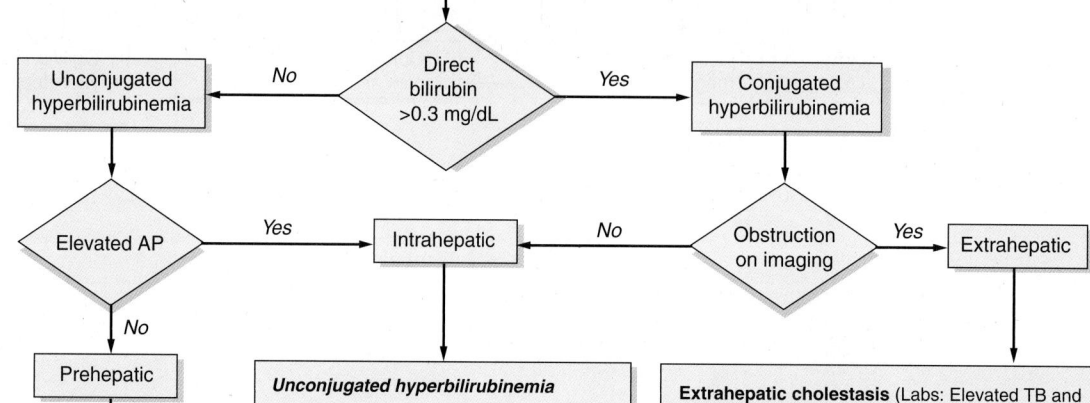

Unconjugated hyperbilirubinemia ← *No* — Direct bilirubin >0.3 mg/dL — *Yes* → Conjugated hyperbilirubinemia

Elevated AP — *Yes* → Intrahepatic ← *No* — Obstruction on imaging — *Yes* → Extrahepatic

Elevated AP — *No* → Prehepatic

Prehepatic

- **Hemolytic anemia**
- **Reabsorption of large hematoma**

Labs: Anemia, possible reticulocytosis, mild TB elevation (5 mg/dL), increased indirect bilirubin, normal DB levels and negative urine bilirubin. All other LTs are normal.

Unconjugated hyperbilirubinemia

Enzyme defects:

○ **Gilbert's syndrome:** Mild defect in UDP glucuronosyltransferase (UGT, responsible for conjugation of bilirubin)
○ **Crigler-Najjar syndromes:** More severe defect in UGT, usually presents during infancy
• *Conjugated hyperbilirubinemia*
○ **Dublin-Johnson syndrome:** Defective secretion of conjugated bilirubin
○ **Rotor's syndrome**

Both Conjugated & Unconjugated Hepatocellular injury:

○ **Hepatitis:** Viral, alcohol, or autoimmune insult leading to inflammation which impedes or prevents transport/secretion of conjugated bilirubin
○ **Medication/drug:** Acetaminophen
○ **Cirrhosis**
○ **Congestive heart failure:** Hypoxia/anoxia of hepatocytes leads to cellular injury.

○ **Intrahepatic cholestasis:** (Elevated LTs, primarily AP. US shows normal sized bile duct(s).)

○ **Medication/drug induced**
○ **Total parenteral nutrition (TPN)**
○ **Sepsis**
○ **Sarcoidosis**
○ **Pregnancy**

Extrahepatic cholestasis (Labs: Elevated TB and DB, elevated AP and positive urine bilirubin. US shows dilated bile duct(s).

- Choledocholithiasis
- Chronic pancreatitis alcohol
- **Cholangitis:** Fever, pain and jaundice, altered mental status, sepsis
- **Biliary structure:** History of surgical/invasive procedure
- Primary biliary cirrhosis
- Primary sclerosing cholangitis
- **Biliary tract tumor/cholangiocarcinoma:** Hepatomegaly, weight loss, abdominal pain
- **Pancreatic tumor:** Painless jaundice, palpable gallbladder (rare)

Krunal Patel, MD and John K. Zawacki, MD

Am Fam Physician. 2004;60(2):200–305.

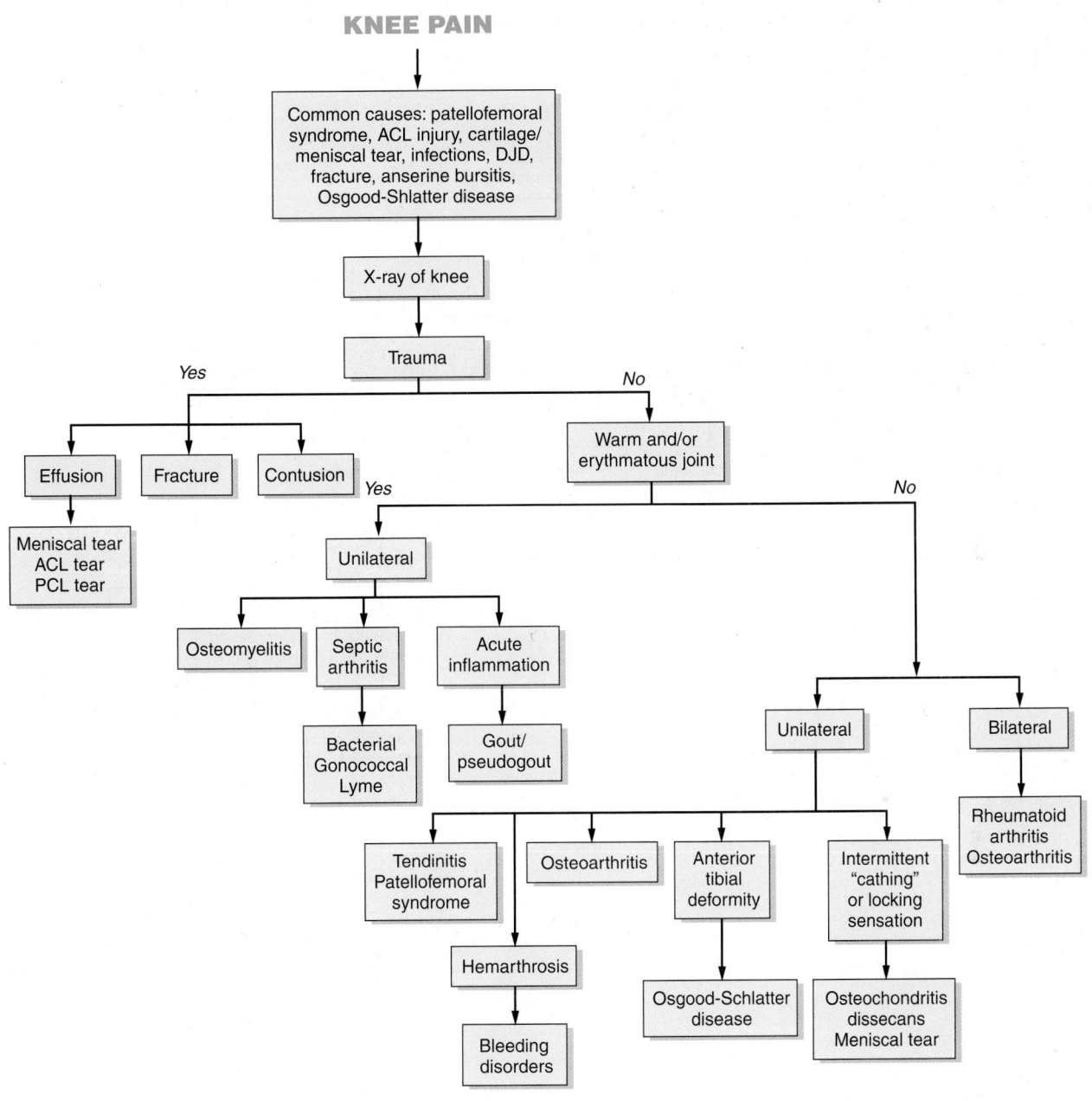

KNEE PAIN

Common causes: patellofemoral syndrome, ACL injury, cartilage/meniscal tear, infections, DJD, fracture, anserine bursitis, Osgood-Shlatter disease

X-ray of knee

Trauma

Yes

Effusion → Meniscal tear, ACL tear, PCL tear

Fracture

Contusion

No

Warm and/or erythmatous joint

Yes

Unilateral

Osteomyelitis

Septic arthritis → Bacterial, Gonococcal, Lyme

Acute inflammation → Gout/pseudogout

No

Unilateral

Tendinitis Patellofemoral syndrome → Hemarthrosis → Bleeding disorders

Osteoarthritis

Anterior tibial deformity → Osgood-Schlatter disease

Intermittent "cathing" or locking sensation → Osteochondritis dissecans Meniscal tear

Bilateral → Rheumatoid arthritis Osteoarthritis

Robert A. Baldor, MD and Alan M. Ehrlich, MD

J Fam Pract. 2008;57(2):116–8.

LACTOSE DEHYDROGENASE ELEVATION

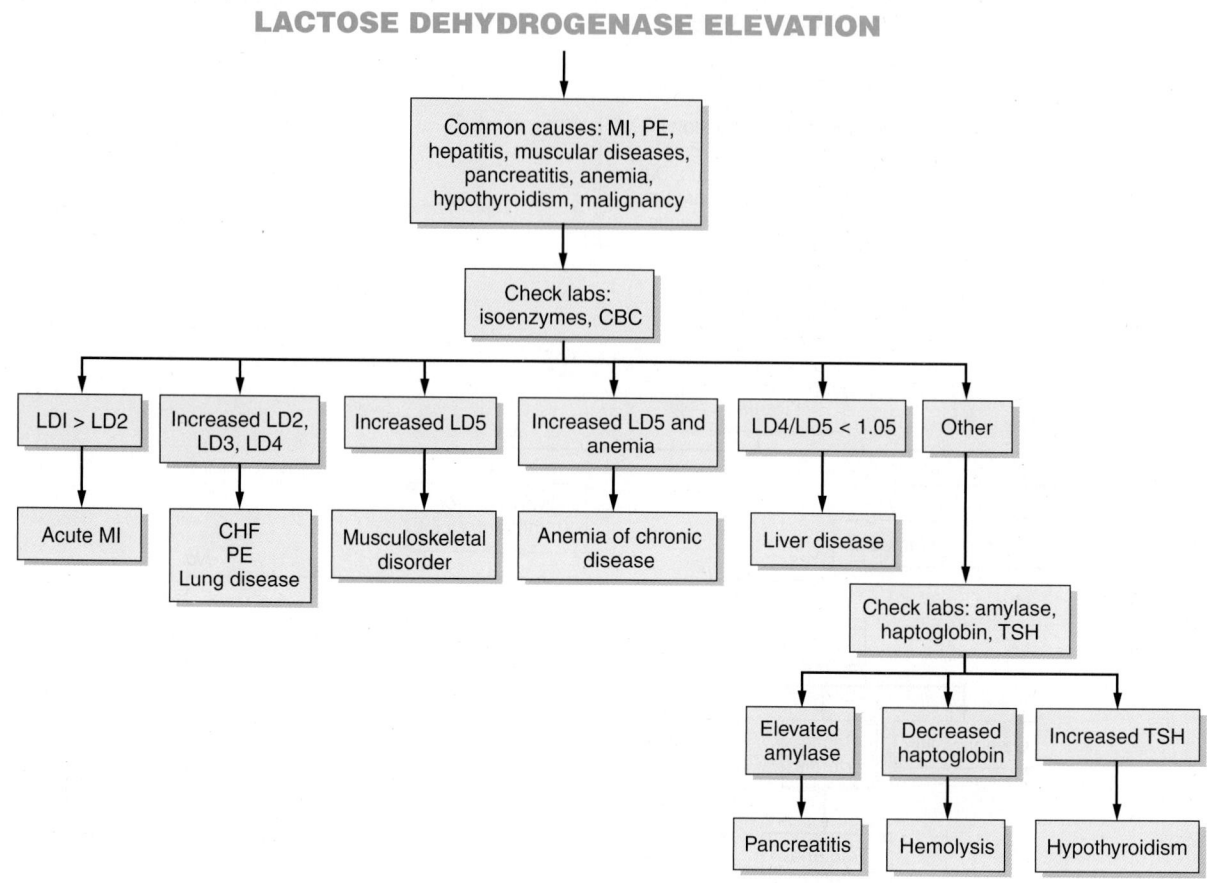

Robert A. Baldor, MD and Alan M. Ehrlich, MD

Ann Int Med. 1991;115(12):931–5.

LEG ULCER

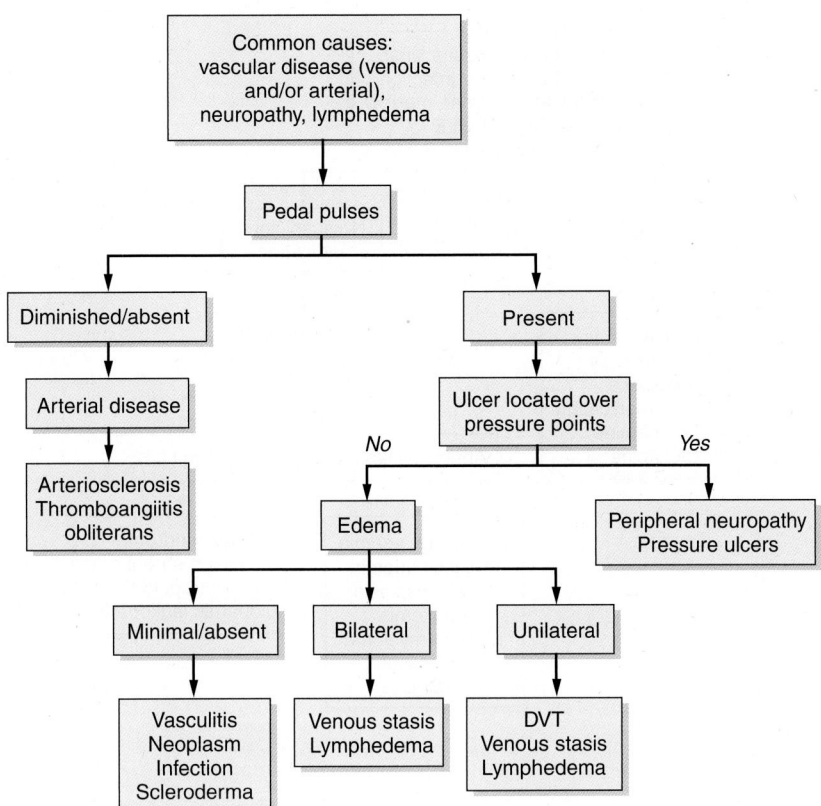

Robert A. Baldor, MD and Alan M. Ehrlich, MD

Surg Clin North Am. 2007;87(5):1149–77, x.

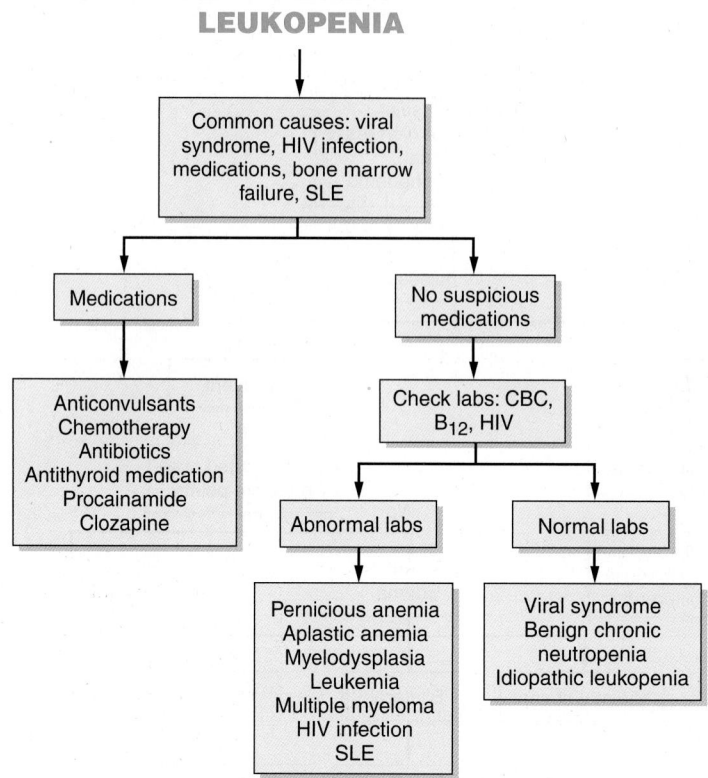

LEUKOPENIA

Common causes: viral syndrome, HIV infection, medications, bone marrow failure, SLE

Medications

No suspicious medications

Anticonvulsants
Chemotherapy
Antibiotics
Antithyroid medication
Procainamide
Clozapine

Check labs: CBC, B_{12}, HIV

Abnormal labs

Normal labs

Pernicious anemia
Aplastic anemia
Myelodysplasia
Leukemia
Multiple myeloma
HIV infection
SLE

Viral syndrome
Benign chronic neutropenia
Idiopathic leukopenia

Robert A. Baldor, MD and Alan M. Ehrlich, MD

Mayo Clin Proc. 2005;80(7):923–36.

LOW BACK PAIN, ACUTE

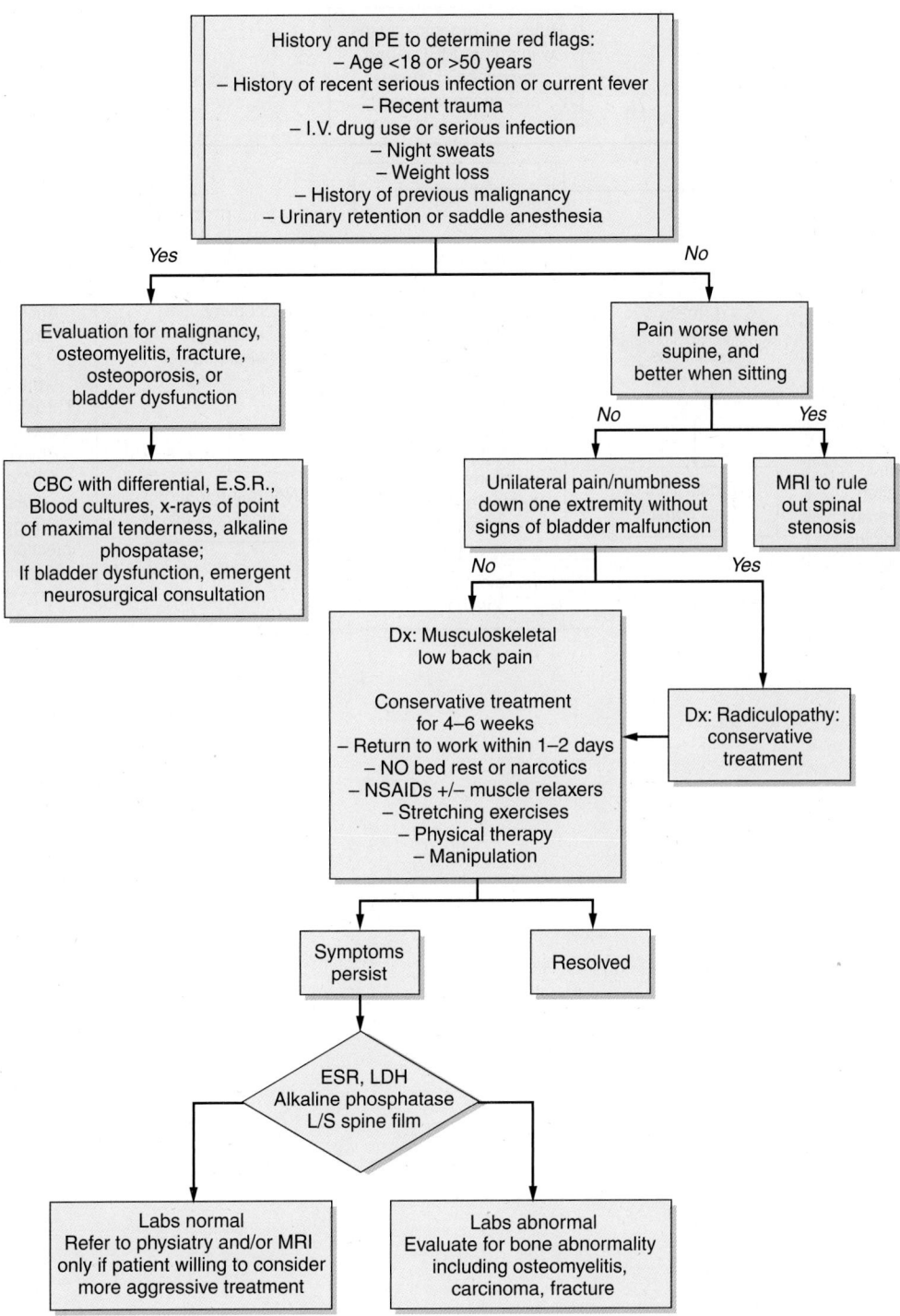

History and PE to determine red flags:
– Age <18 or >50 years
– History of recent serious infection or current fever
– Recent trauma
– I.V. drug use or serious infection
– Night sweats
– Weight loss
– History of previous malignancy
– Urinary retention or saddle anesthesia

Yes / **No**

Evaluation for malignancy, osteomyelitis, fracture, osteoporosis, or bladder dysfunction

Pain worse when supine, and better when sitting

No / **Yes**

CBC with differential, E.S.R., Blood cultures, x-rays of point of maximal tenderness, alkaline phospatase;
If bladder dysfunction, emergent neurosurgical consultation

Unilateral pain/numbness down one extremity without signs of bladder malfunction

MRI to rule out spinal stenosis

No / **Yes**

Dx: Musculoskeletal low back pain

Conservative treatment for 4–6 weeks
– Return to work within 1–2 days
– NO bed rest or narcotics
– NSAIDs +/– muscle relaxers
– Stretching exercises
– Physical therapy
– Manipulation

Dx: Radiculopathy: conservative treatment

Symptoms persist

Resolved

ESR, LDH
Alkaline phosphatase
L/S spine film

Labs normal
Refer to physiatry and/or MRI only if patient willing to consider more aggressive treatment

Labs abnormal
Evaluate for bone abnormality including osteomyelitis, carcinoma, fracture

Patricia Bruno, MD

Med Clin North Am. 2009;93(2):477–501, x.

LOW BACK PAIN, CHRONIC

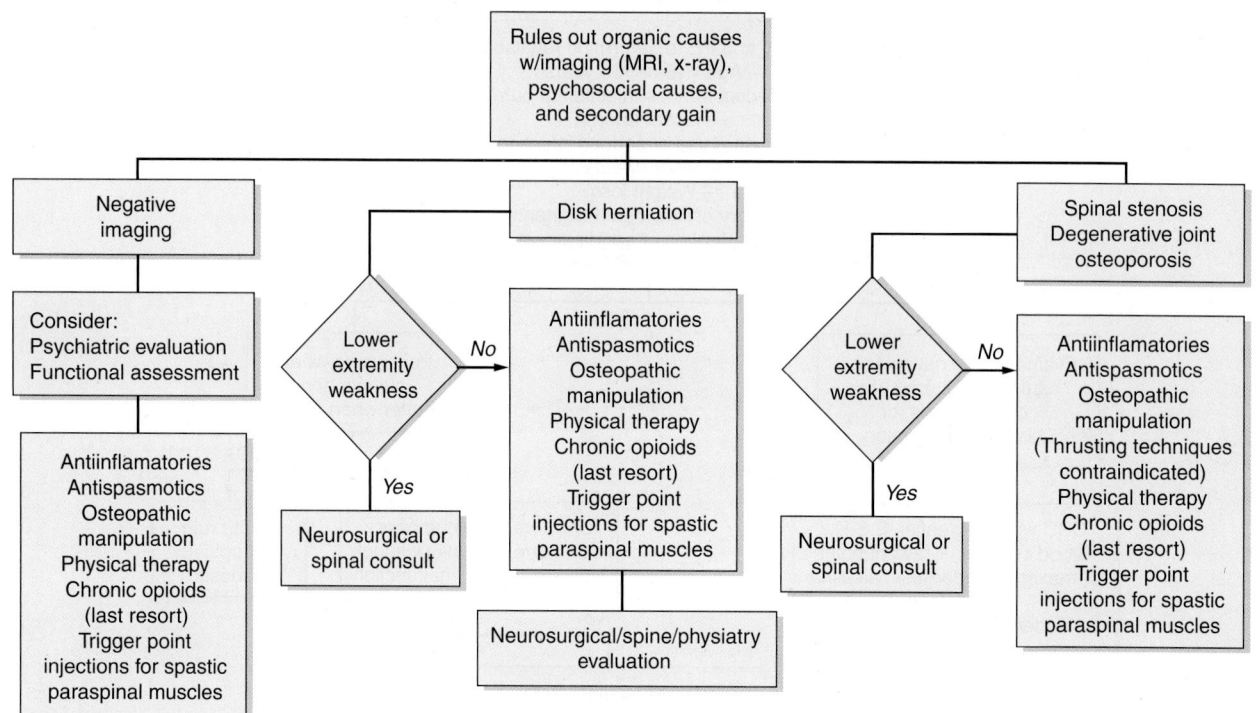

Patricia Bruno, MD

Spine. 2009;34(7):718–24.

LYMPHADENOPATHY

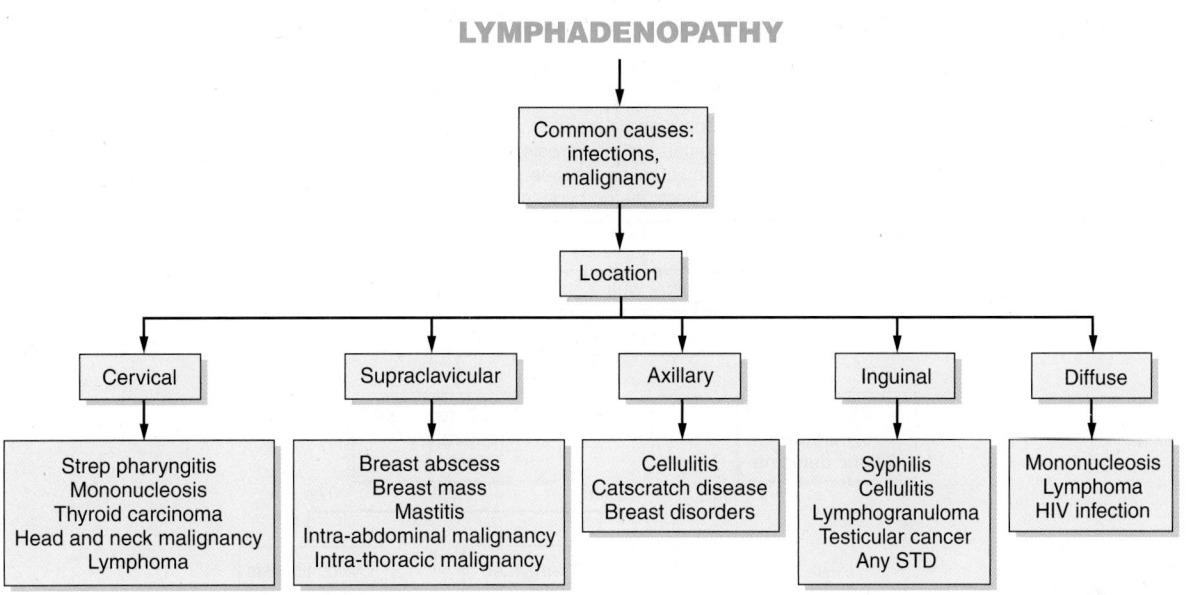

Robert A. Baldor, MD and Alan M. Ehrlich, MD

Radiol Clin North Am. 2008;46(2):175–98, vii.

MALABSORPTION SYNDROME

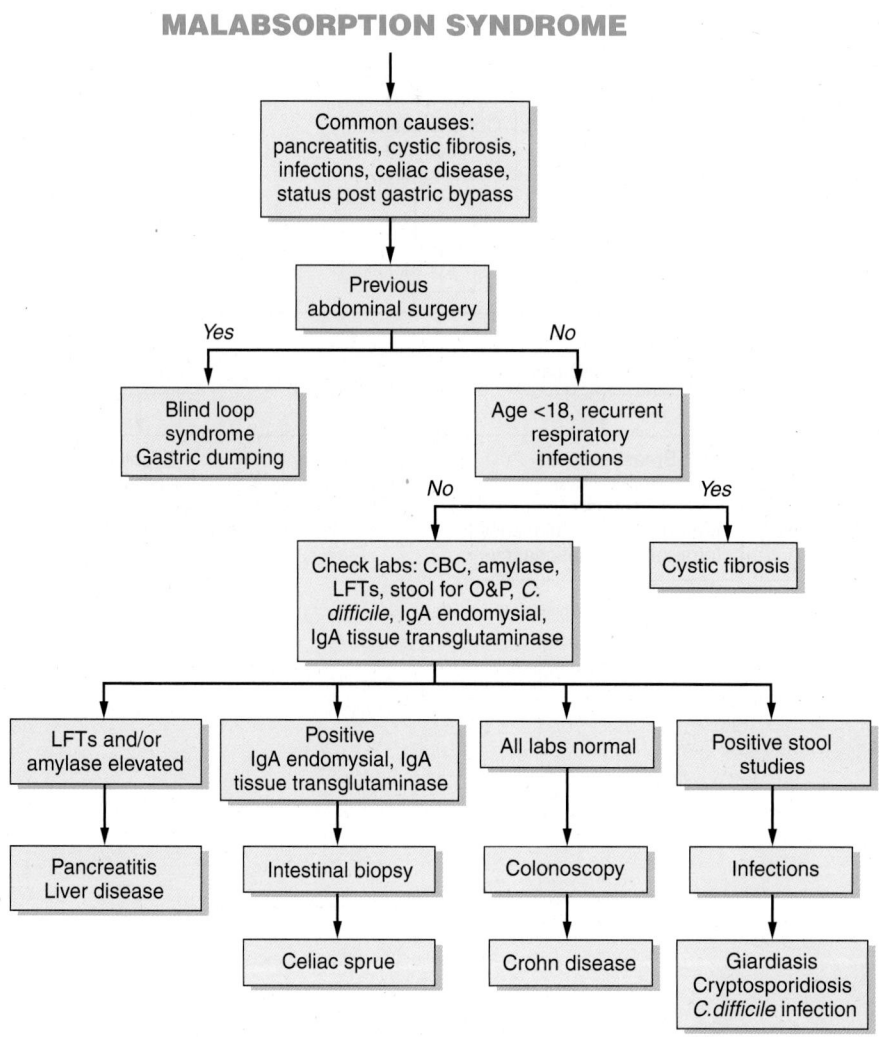

Robert A. Baldor, MD and Alan M. Ehrlich, MD

Pediatr Clin North Am. 2009;56(5):1105–21.

MENORRHAGIA (EXCESSIVE BLEEDING)

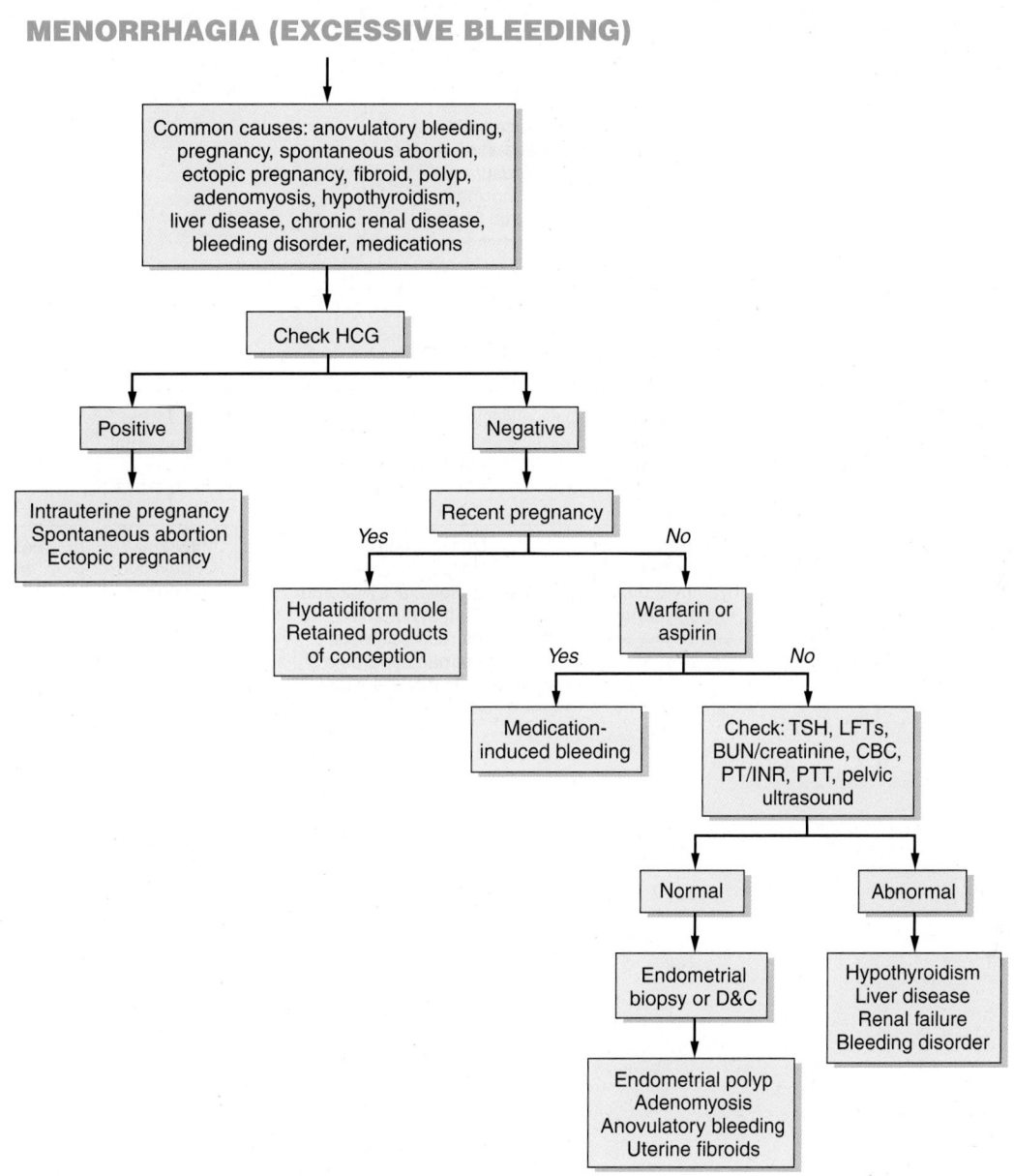

Robert A. Baldor, MD and Alan M. Ehrlich, MD

Am Fam Physician. 2004;69(8):1915–26.

MENTAL RETARDATION

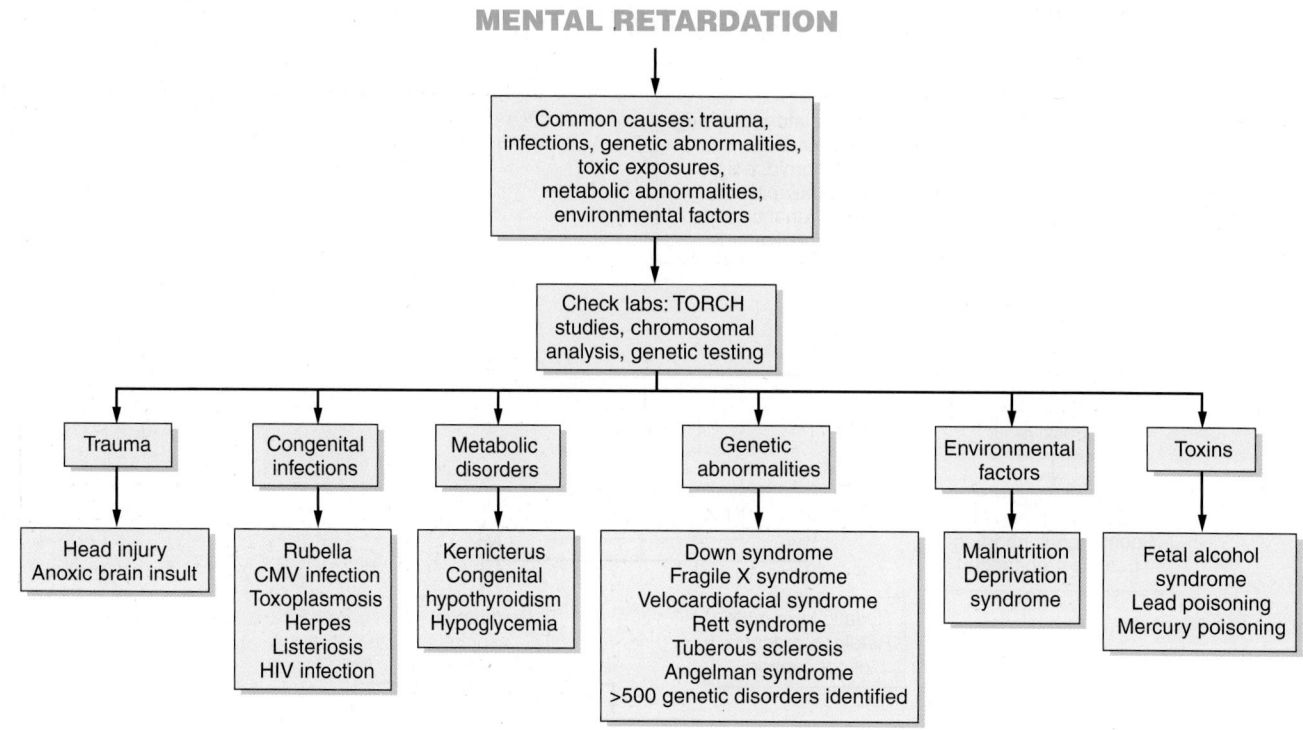

Common causes: trauma, infections, genetic abnormalities, toxic exposures, metabolic abnormalities, environmental factors

Check labs: TORCH studies, chromosomal analysis, genetic testing

Trauma
Head injury
Anoxic brain insult

Congenital infections
Rubella
CMV infection
Toxoplasmosis
Herpes
Listeriosis
HIV infection

Metabolic disorders
Kernicterus
Congenital hypothyroidism
Hypoglycemia

Genetic abnormalities
Down syndrome
Fragile X syndrome
Velocardiofacial syndrome
Rett syndrome
Tuberous sclerosis
Angelman syndrome
>500 genetic disorders identified

Environmental factors
Malnutrition
Deprivation syndrome

Toxins
Fetal alcohol syndrome
Lead poisoning
Mercury poisoning

Robert A. Baldor, MD and Alan M. Ehrlich, MD

Pediatr Clin North Am. 2008;55(5):1071–84, xi.

METORRHAGIA (INTERMENSTRUAL BLEEDING)

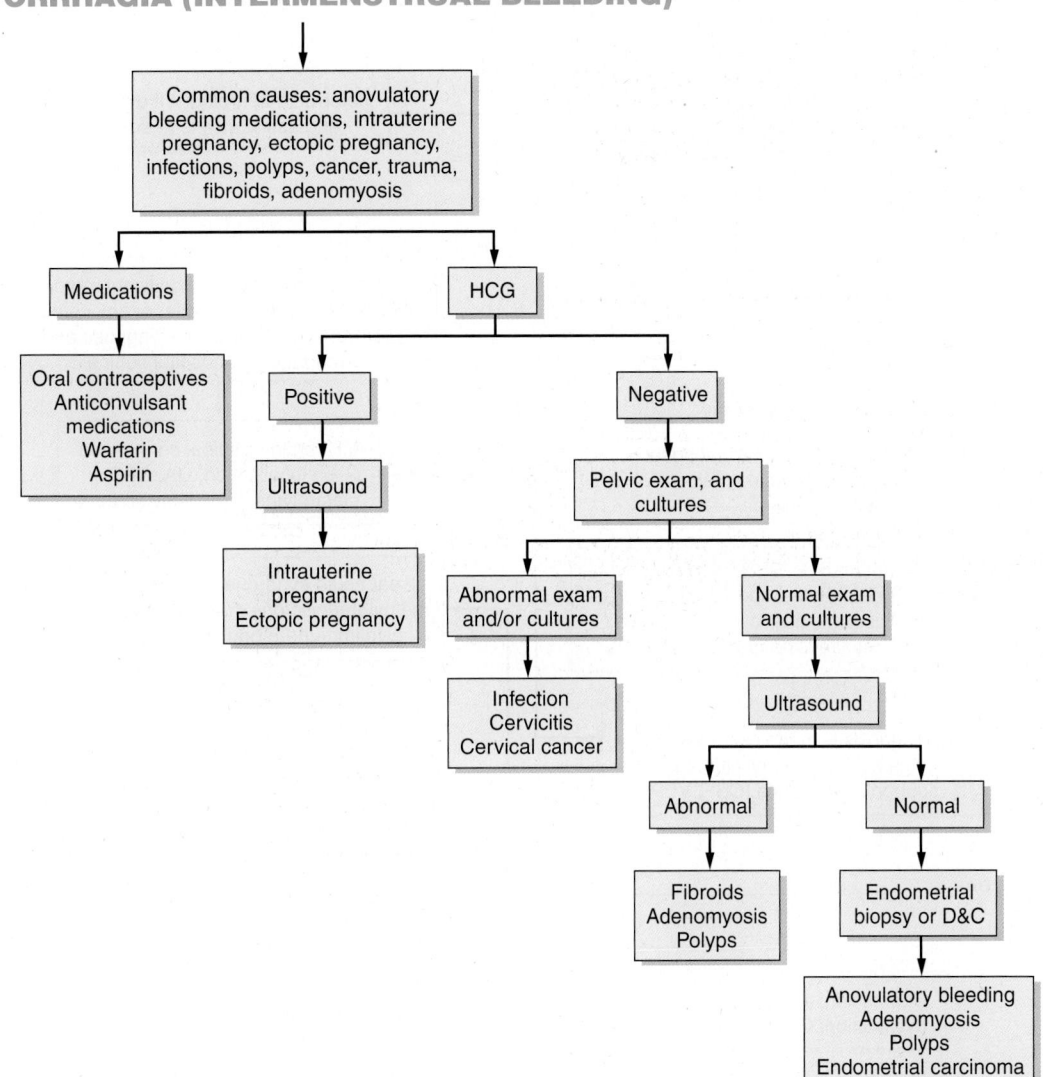

Robert A. Baldor, MD and Alan M. Ehrlich, MD

Am Fam Physician. 2004;69(8):1915–26.

MULTIPLE SCLEROSIS, TREATMENT

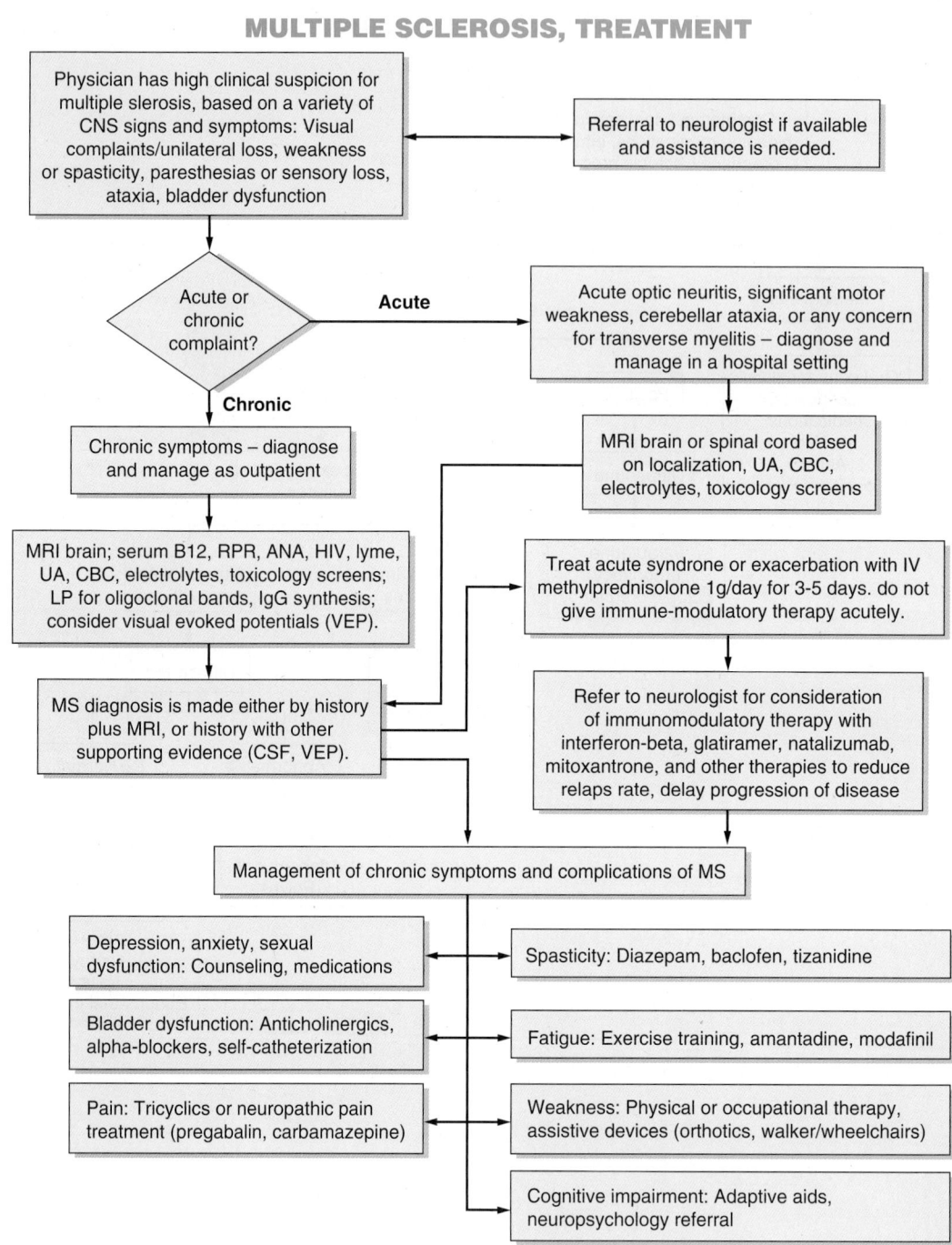

Physician has high clinical suspicion for multiple slerosis, based on a variety of CNS signs and symptoms: Visual complaints/unilateral loss, weakness or spasticity, paresthesias or sensory loss, ataxia, bladder dysfunction

Referral to neurologist if available and assistance is needed.

Acute or chronic complaint?

Acute

Acute optic neuritis, significant motor weakness, cerebellar ataxia, or any concern for transverse myelitis – diagnose and manage in a hospital setting

Chronic

Chronic symptoms – diagnose and manage as outpatient

MRI brain or spinal cord based on localization, UA, CBC, electrolytes, toxicology screens

MRI brain; serum B12, RPR, ANA, HIV, lyme, UA, CBC, electrolytes, toxicology screens; LP for oligoclonal bands, IgG synthesis; consider visual evoked potentials (VEP).

Treat acute syndrone or exacerbation with IV methylprednisolone 1g/day for 3-5 days. do not give immune-modulatory therapy acutely.

MS diagnosis is made either by history plus MRI, or history with other supporting evidence (CSF, VEP).

Refer to neurologist for consideration of immunomodulatory therapy with interferon-beta, glatiramer, natalizumab, mitoxantrone, and other therapies to reduce relaps rate, delay progression of disease

Management of chronic symptoms and complications of MS

Depression, anxiety, sexual dysfunction: Counseling, medications

Spasticity: Diazepam, baclofen, tizanidine

Bladder dysfunction: Anticholinergics, alpha-blockers, self-catheterization

Fatigue: Exercise training, amantadine, modafinil

Pain: Tricyclics or neuropathic pain treatment (pregabalin, carbamazepine)

Weakness: Physical or occupational therapy, assistive devices (orthotics, walker/wheelchairs)

Cognitive impairment: Adaptive aids, neuropsychology referral

Julie L. Roth, MD

Ann Neurol. 2005;58:840–6.

MUSCULAR ATROPHY

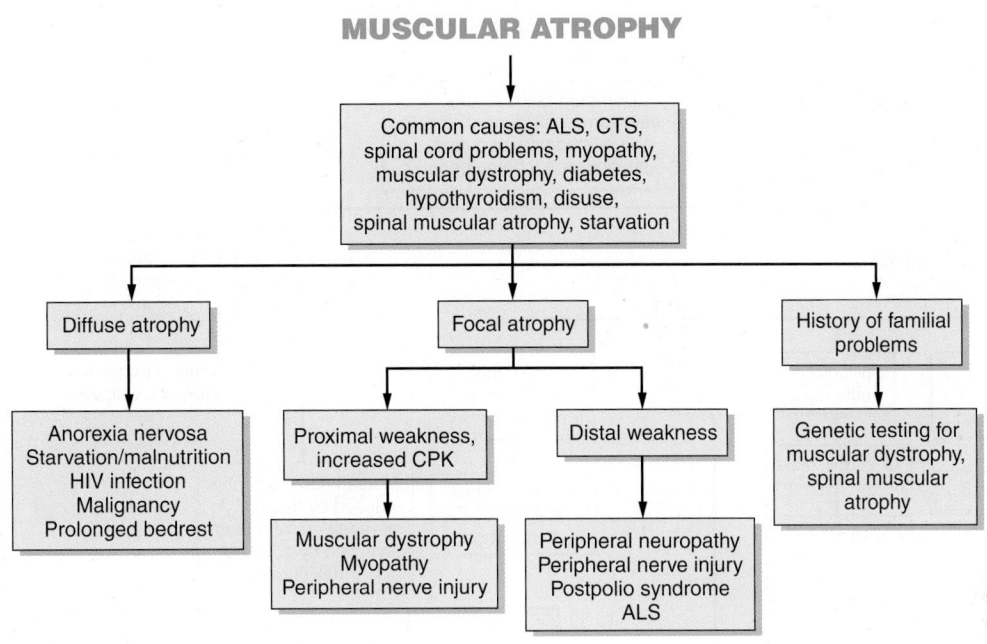

Robert A. Baldor, MD and Alan M. Ehrlich, MD

Lancet. 2007;369(9578):2031–41.

NAIL ABNORMALITIES

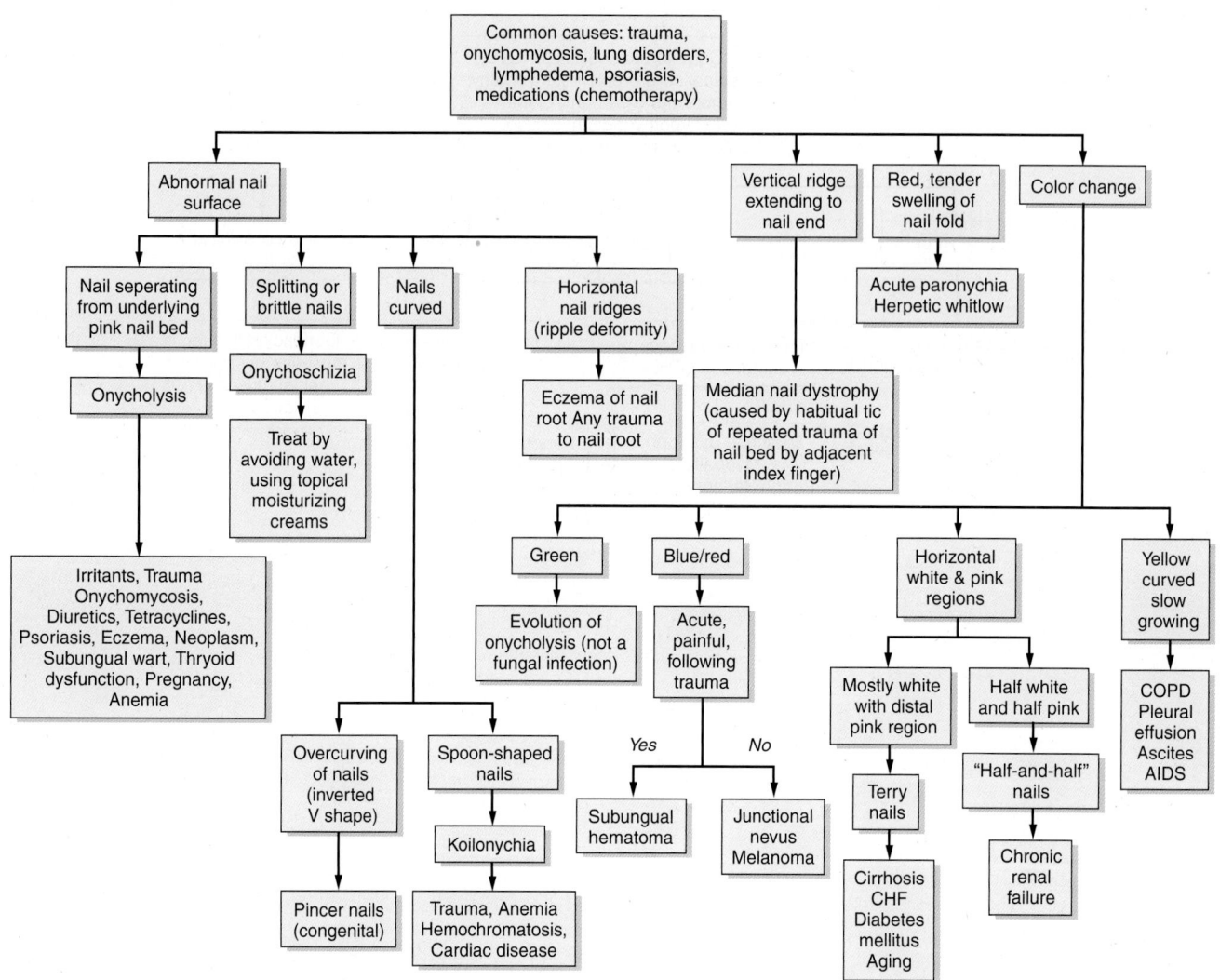

Robert A. Baldor, MD and Alan M. Ehrlich, MD

Am Fam Physician. 2004;69(6):1417–24.

NASAL DISCHARGE, CHRONIC

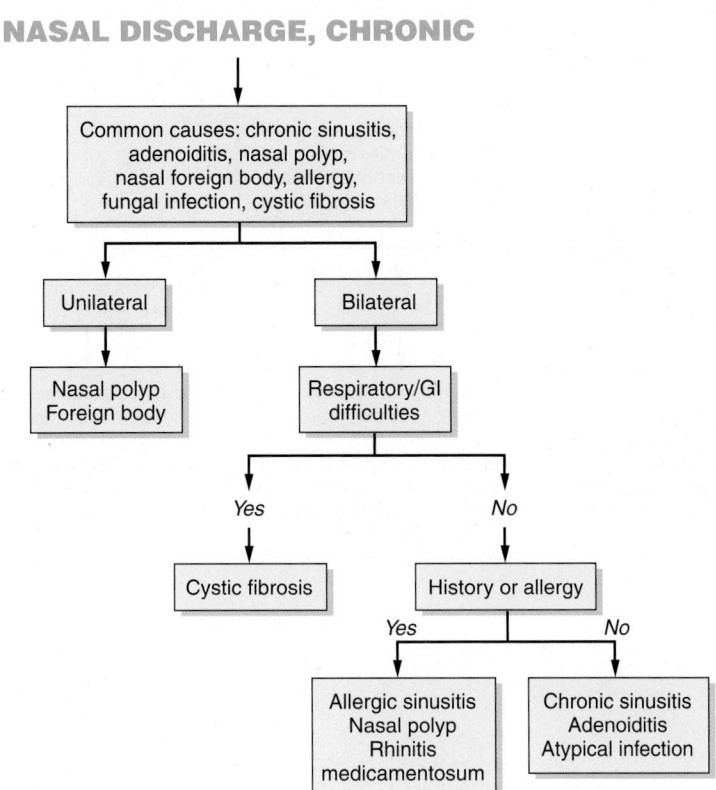

Robert A. Baldor, MD and Alan M. Ehrlich, MD

Postgrad Med. 2009;121(6):121–39.

NECK SWELLING

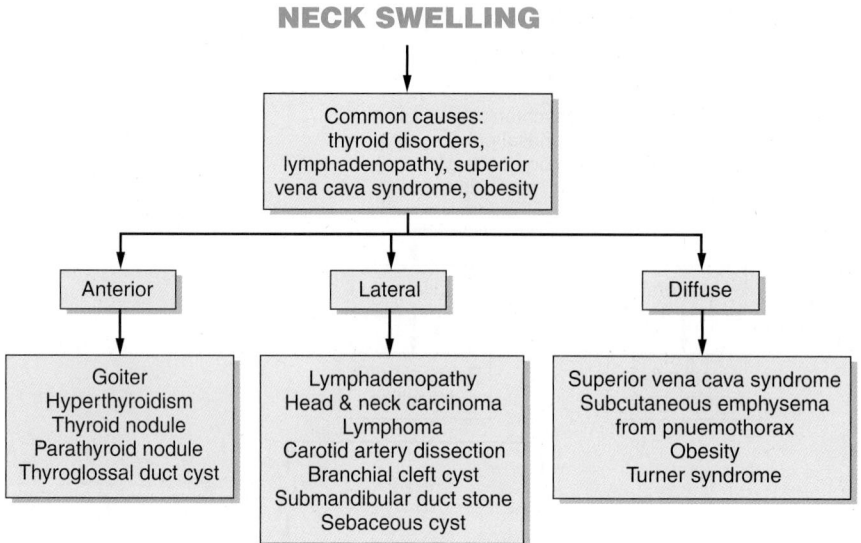

Common causes:
thyroid disorders,
lymphadenopathy, superior
vena cava syndrome, obesity

Anterior

Goiter
Hyperthyroidism
Thyroid nodule
Parathyroid nodule
Thyroglossal duct cyst

Lateral

Lymphadenopathy
Head & neck carcinoma
Lymphoma
Carotid artery dissection
Branchial cleft cyst
Submandibular duct stone
Sebaceous cyst

Diffuse

Superior vena cava syndrome
Subcutaneous emphysema
from pnuemothorax
Obesity
Turner syndrome

Robert A. Baldor, MD and Alan M. Ehrlich, MD

Am Fam Physician. 1995;51(8):1904–12.

NEPHROTIC SYNDROME

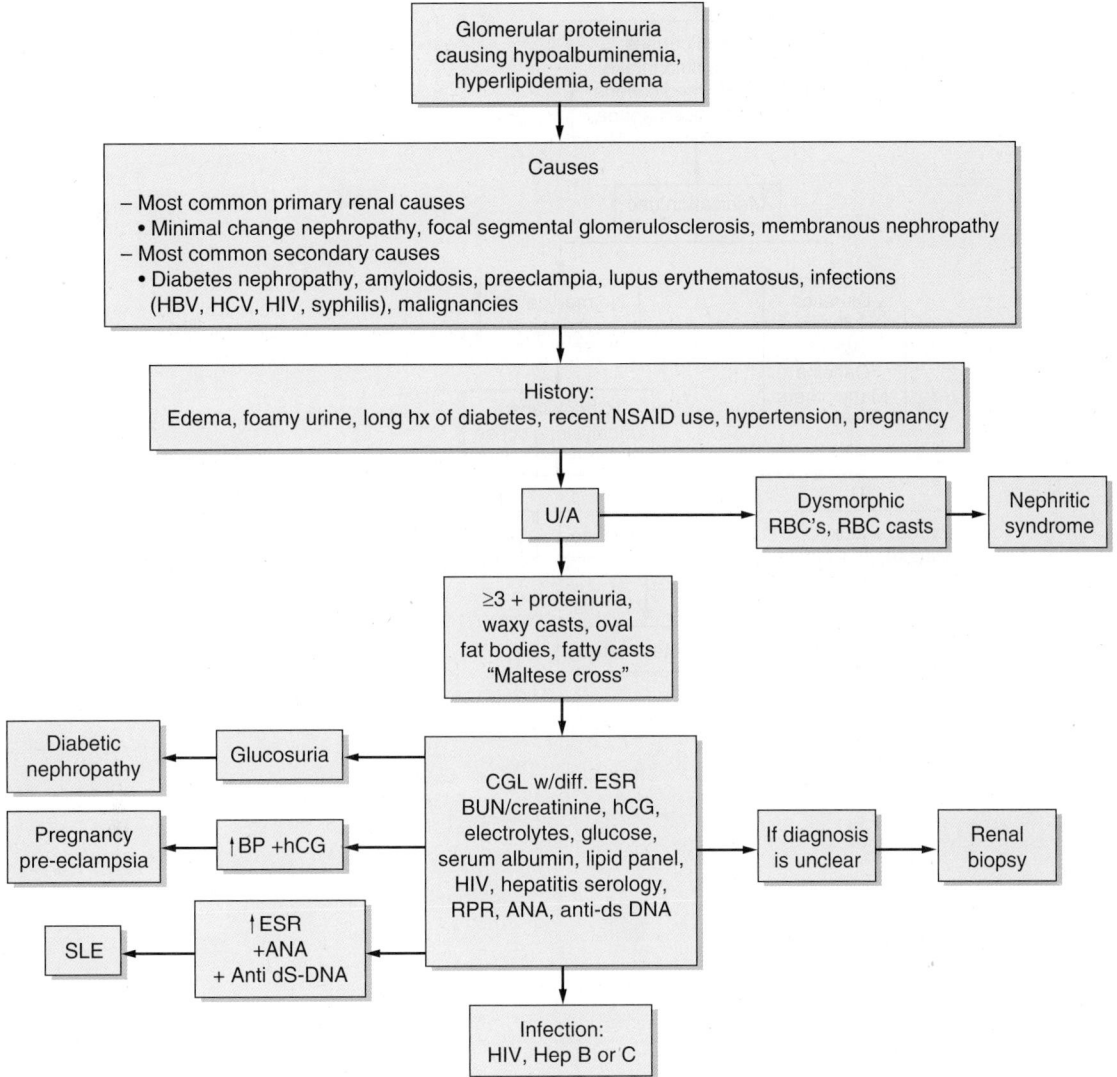

Jonathan Min, MD and Robert M. Black, MD

Cleve Clin J Med. 2006;73(2):161–7.

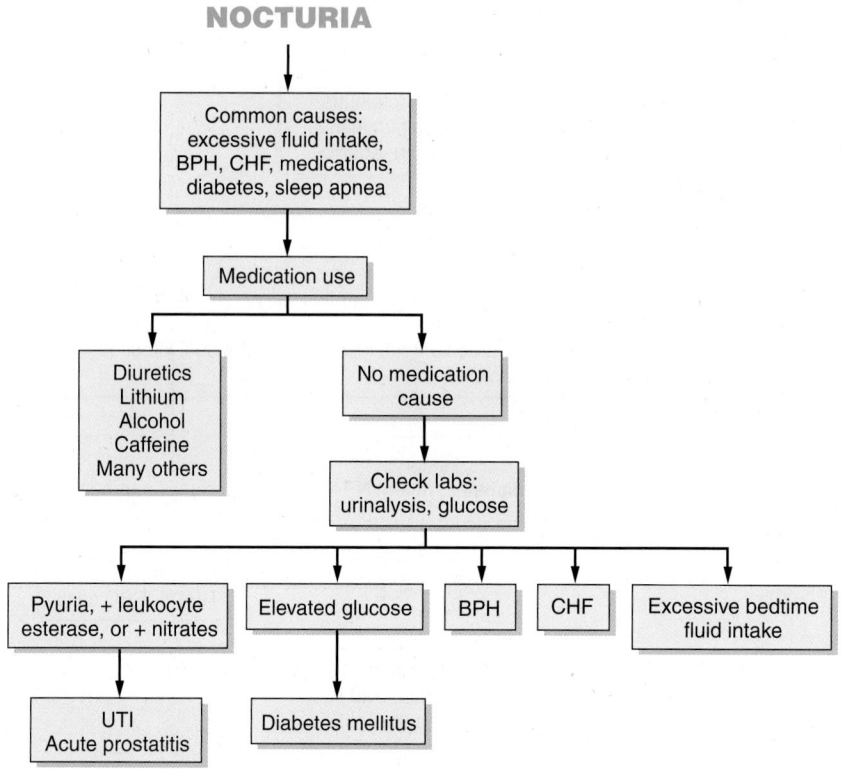

NOCTURIA

Common causes:
excessive fluid intake,
BPH, CHF, medications,
diabetes, sleep apnea

Medication use

Diuretics
Lithium
Alcohol
Caffeine
Many others

No medication
cause

Check labs:
urinalysis, glucose

Pyuria, + leukocyte
esterase, or + nitrates

Elevated glucose

BPH

CHF

Excessive bedtime
fluid intake

UTI
Acute prostatitis

Diabetes mellitus

Robert A. Baldor, MD and Alan M. Ehrlich, MD

BMJ. 2004;328(7447):1063–6.

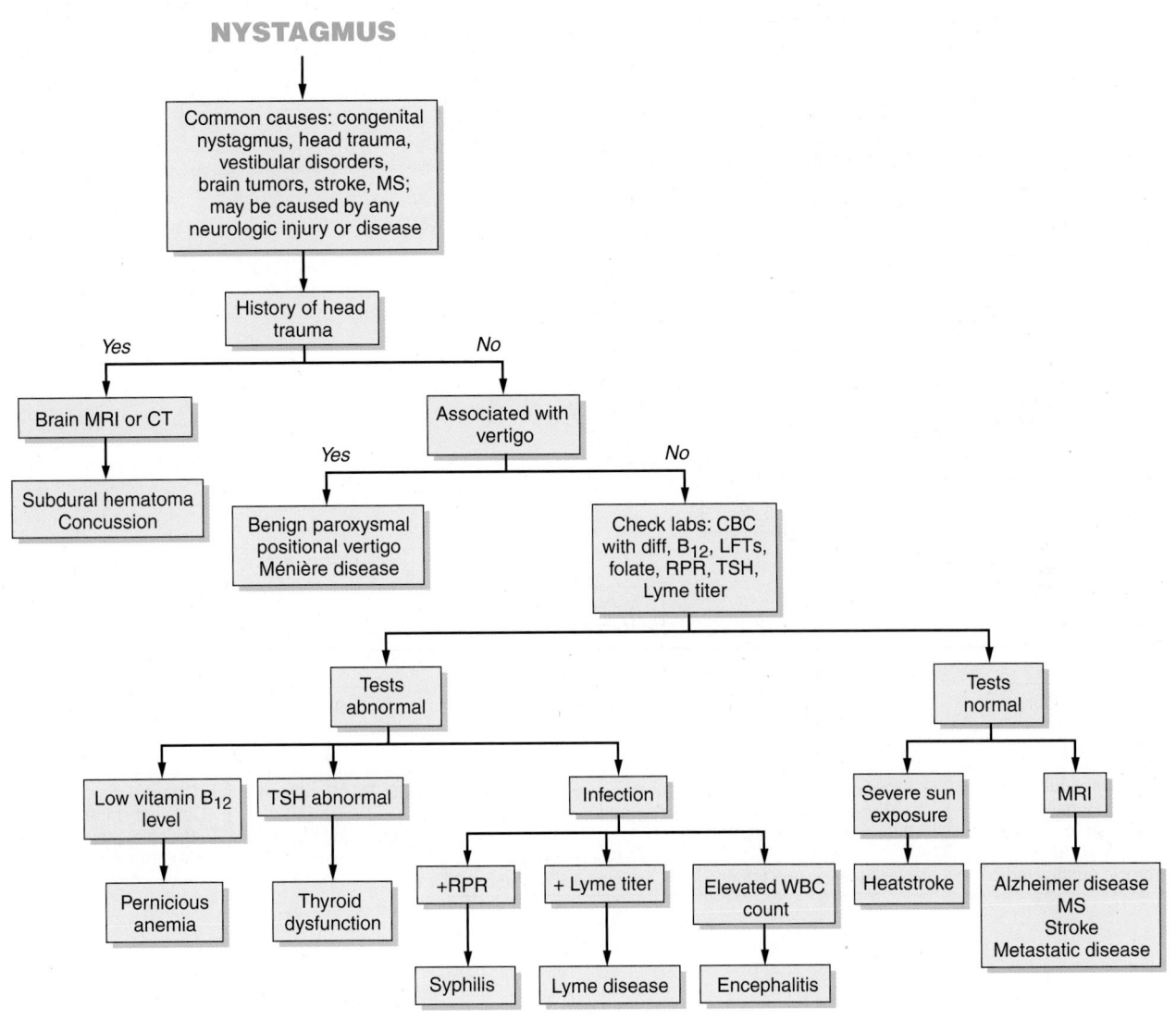

NYSTAGMUS

Common causes: congenital nystagmus, head trauma, vestibular disorders, brain tumors, stroke, MS; may be caused by any neurologic injury or disease

History of head trauma

Yes → Brain MRI or CT → Subdural hematoma / Concussion

No → Associated with vertigo

Yes → Benign paroxysmal positional vertigo / Ménière disease

No → Check labs: CBC with diff, B_{12}, LFTs, folate, RPR, TSH, Lyme titer

Tests abnormal:
- Low vitamin B_{12} level → Pernicious anemia
- TSH abnormal → Thyroid dysfunction
- Infection:
  - +RPR → Syphilis
  - + Lyme titer → Lyme disease
  - Elevated WBC count → Encephalitis

Tests normal:
- Severe sun exposure → Heatstroke
- MRI → Alzheimer disease / MS / Stroke / Metastatic disease

Robert A. Baldor, MD and Alan M. Ehrlich, MD

Med Clin North Am. 2009;93(2):263–71, vii.

PAIN IN UPPER EXTREMITY

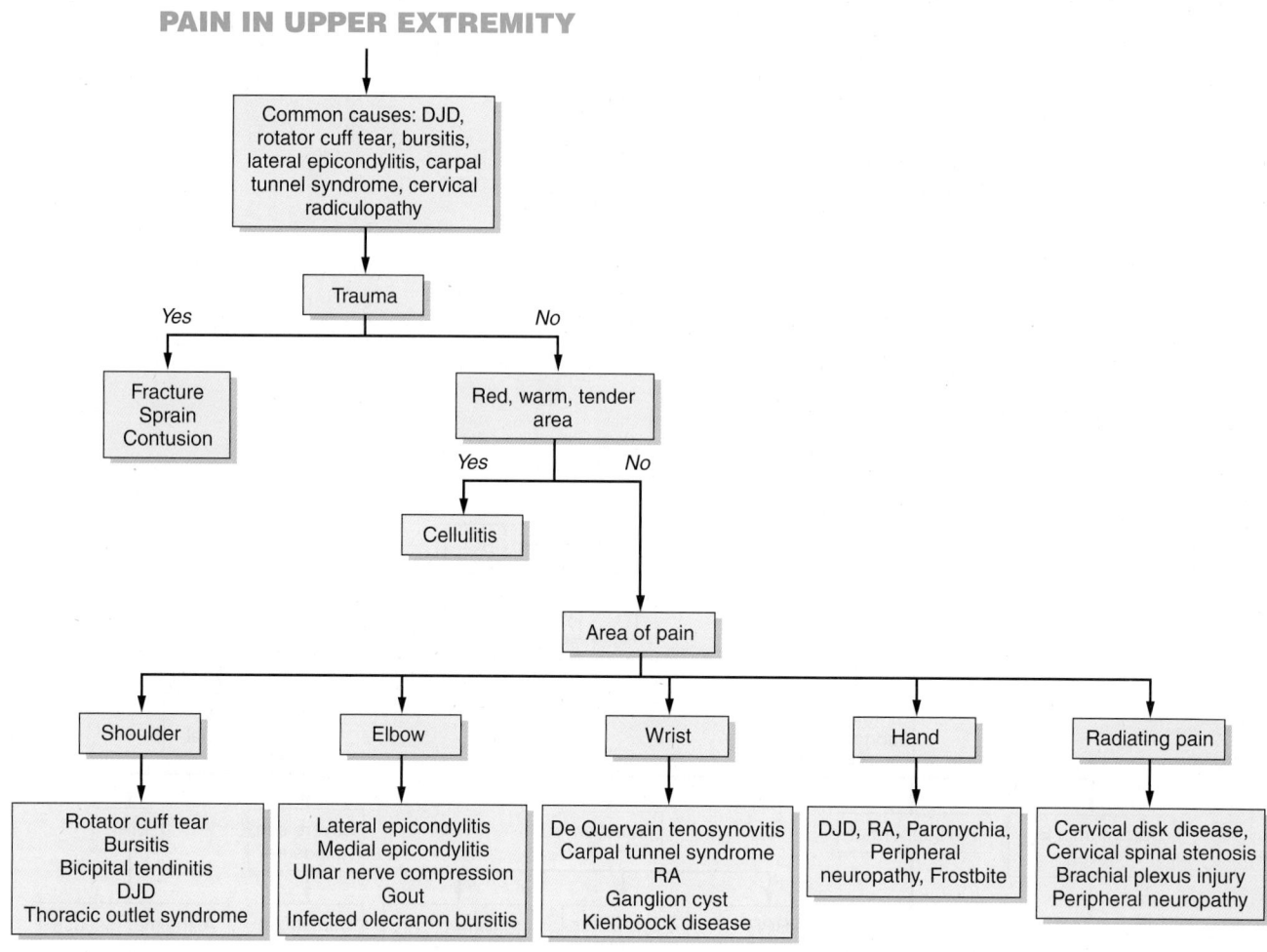

Common causes: DJD, rotator cuff tear, bursitis, lateral epicondylitis, carpal tunnel syndrome, cervical radiculopathy

Trauma

Yes → Fracture / Sprain / Contusion

No → Red, warm, tender area

   Yes → Cellulitis

   No → Area of pain

Shoulder
- Rotator cuff tear
- Bursitis
- Bicipital tendinitis
- DJD
- Thoracic outlet syndrome

Elbow
- Lateral epicondylitis
- Medial epicondylitis
- Ulnar nerve compression
- Gout
- Infected olecranon bursitis

Wrist
- De Quervain tenosynovitis
- Carpal tunnel syndrome
- RA
- Ganglion cyst
- Kienböock disease

Hand
- DJD, RA, Paronychia, Peripheral neuropathy, Frostbite

Radiating pain
- Cervical disk disease,
- Cervical spinal stenosis
- Brachial plexus injury
- Peripheral neuropathy

Robert A. Baldor, MD and Alan M. Ehrlich, MD

N Engl J Med. 2008;358(20):2138–47.

PALLOR, GENERALIZED

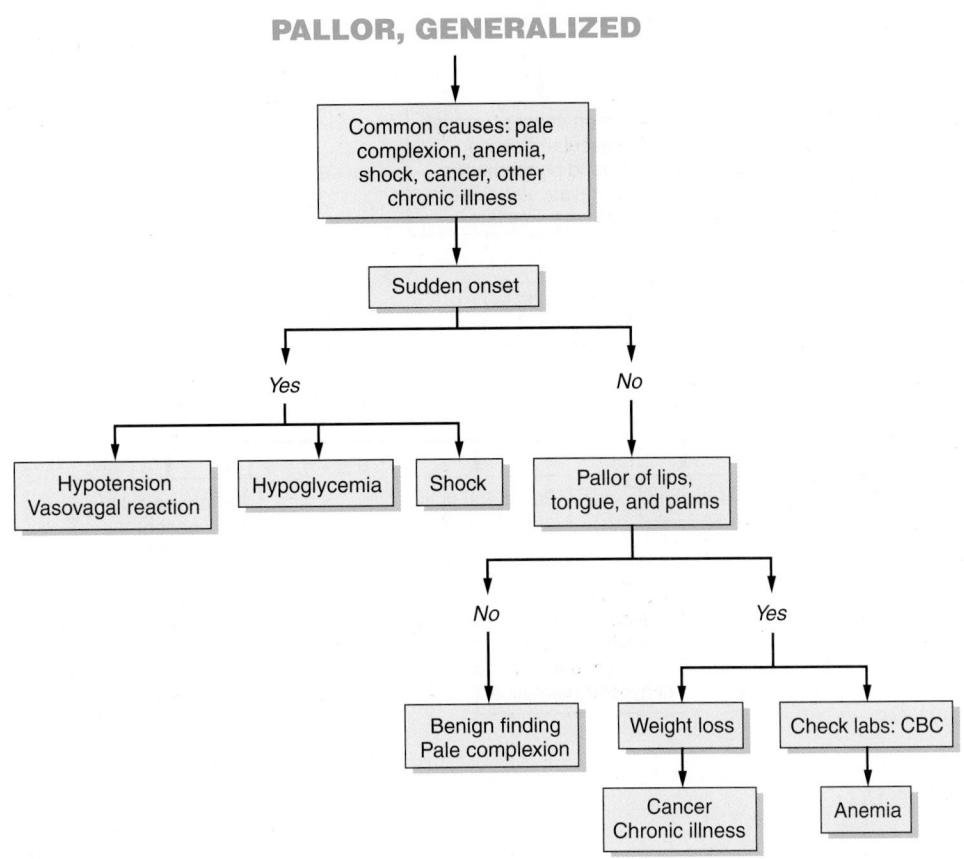

Robert A. Baldor, MD and Alan M. Ehrlich, MD

Am Fam Physician. 2007;75(5):671–8.

PALLOR, LOCALIZED

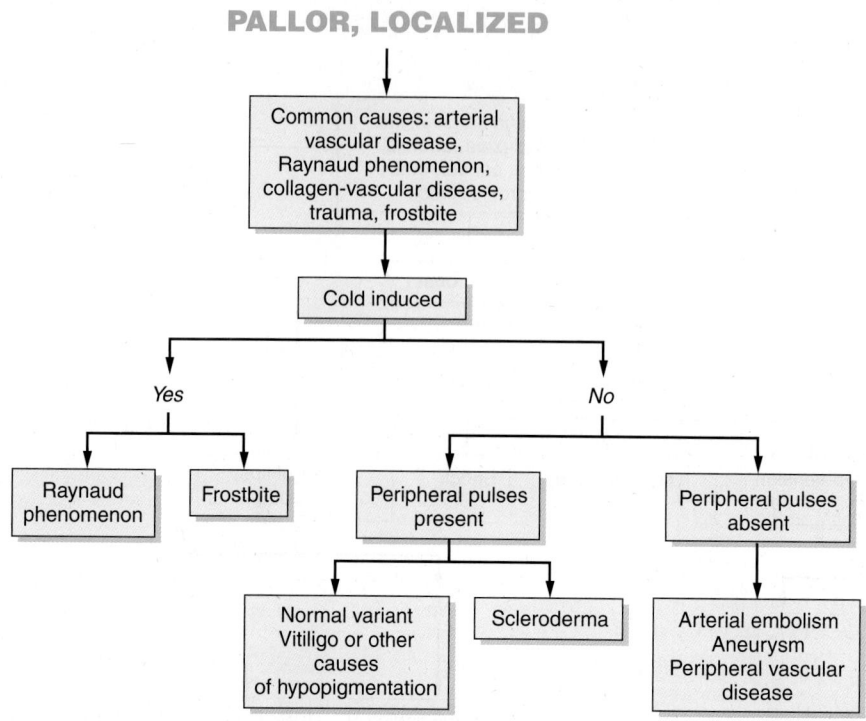

Common causes: arterial vascular disease, Raynaud phenomenon, collagen-vascular disease, trauma, frostbite

Cold induced

Yes → Raynaud phenomenon | Frostbite

No → Peripheral pulses present | Peripheral pulses absent

Peripheral pulses present → Normal variant Vitiligo or other causes of hypopigmentation | Scleroderma

Peripheral pulses absent → Arterial embolism Aneurysm Peripheral vascular disease

Robert A. Baldor, MD and Alan M. Ehrlich, MD

South Med J. 2009;102(11):1141–9.

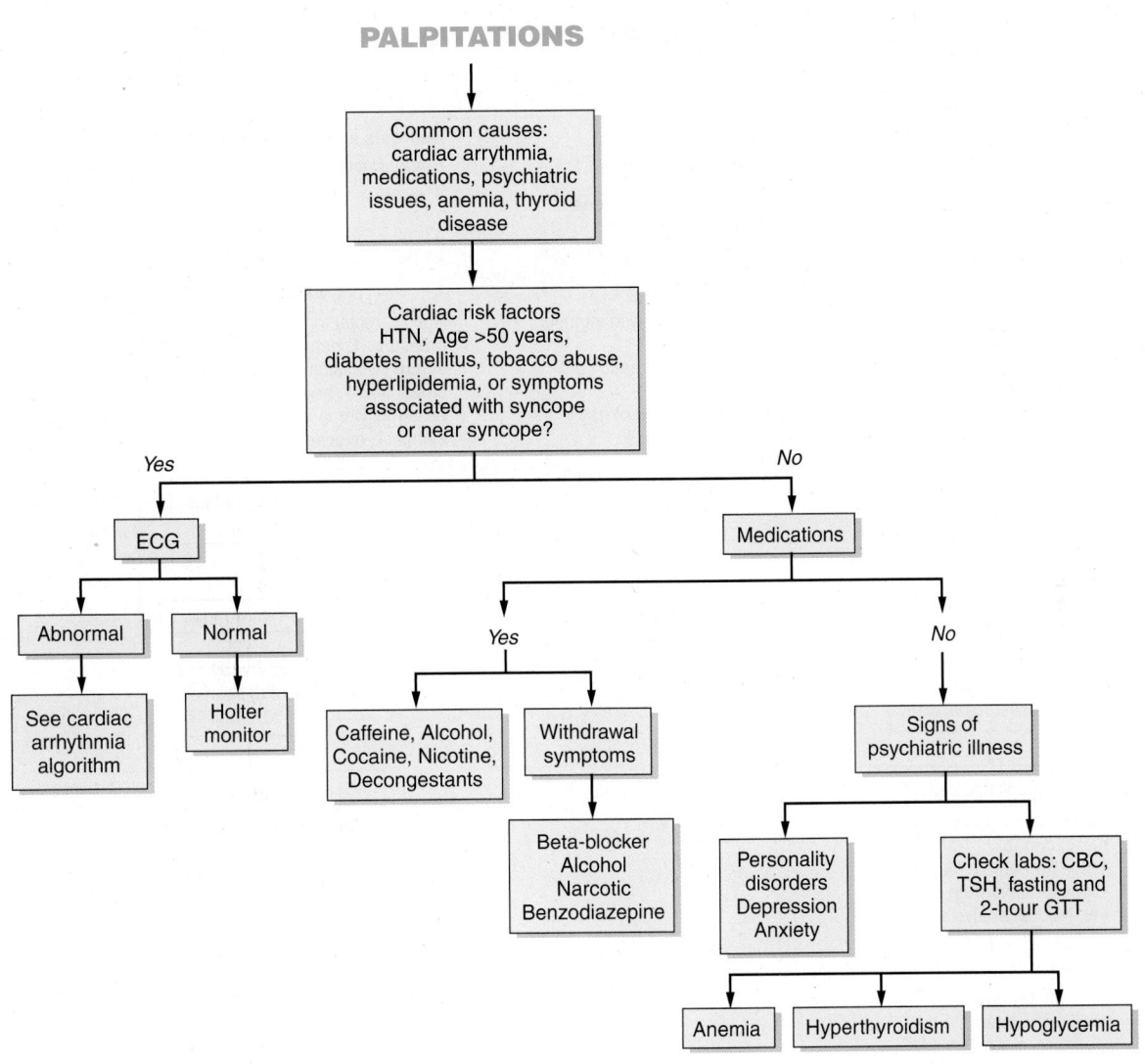

PALPITATIONS

Common causes:
cardiac arrythmia,
medications, psychiatric
issues, anemia, thyroid
disease

Cardiac risk factors
HTN, Age >50 years,
diabetes mellitus, tobacco abuse,
hyperlipidemia, or symptoms
associated with syncope
or near syncope?

Yes

ECG

Abnormal

Normal

See cardiac
arrythmia
algorithm

Holter
monitor

No

Medications

Yes

Caffeine, Alcohol,
Cocaine, Nicotine,
Decongestants

Withdrawal
symptoms

Beta-blocker
Alcohol
Narcotic
Benzodiazepine

No

Signs of
psychiatric illness

Personality
disorders
Depression
Anxiety

Check labs: CBC,
TSH, fasting and
2-hour GTT

Anemia

Hyperthyroidism

Hypoglycemia

Robert A. Baldor, MD and Alan M. Ehrlich, MD

NEJM. 338(19):1369–73.

PANCREATITIS, ACUTE

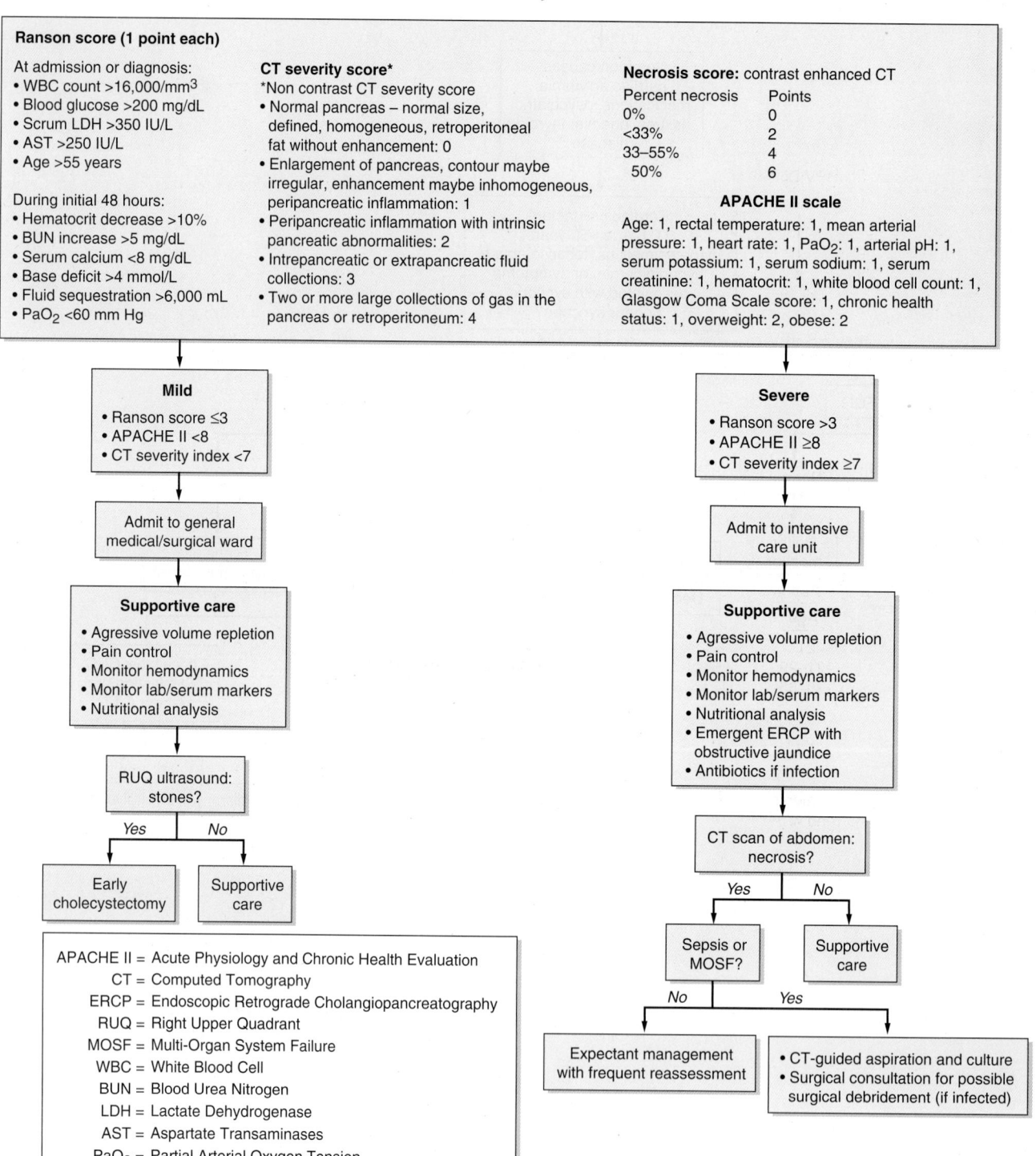

Ranson score (1 point each)

At admission or diagnosis:
- WBC count >16,000/mm^3
- Blood glucose >200 mg/dL
- Scrum LDH >350 IU/L
- AST >250 IU/L
- Age >55 years

During initial 48 hours:
- Hematocrit decrease >10%
- BUN increase >5 mg/dL
- Serum calcium <8 mg/dL
- Base deficit >4 mmol/L
- Fluid sequestration >6,000 mL
- PaO$_2$ <60 mm Hg

CT severity score*
*Non contrast CT severity score
- Normal pancreas – normal size, defined, homogeneous, retroperitoneal fat without enhancement: 0
- Enlargement of pancreas, contour maybe irregular, enhancement maybe inhomogeneous, peripancreatic inflammation: 1
- Peripancreatic inflammation with intrinsic pancreatic abnormalities: 2
- Intrepancreatic or extrapancreatic fluid collections: 3
- Two or more large collections of gas in the pancreas or retroperitoneum: 4

Necrosis score: contrast enhanced CT

Percent necrosis	Points
0%	0
<33%	2
33–55%	4
50%	6

APACHE II scale

Age: 1, rectal temperature: 1, mean arterial pressure: 1, heart rate: 1, PaO$_2$: 1, arterial pH: 1, serum potassium: 1, serum sodium: 1, serum creatinine: 1, hematocrit: 1, white blood cell count: 1, Glasgow Coma Scale score: 1, chronic health status: 1, overweight: 2, obese: 2

Mild
- Ranson score ≤3
- APACHE II <8
- CT severity index <7

↓

Admit to general medical/surgical ward

↓

Supportive care
- Agressive volume repletion
- Pain control
- Monitor hemodynamics
- Monitor lab/serum markers
- Nutritional analysis

↓

RUQ ultrasound: stones?

— *Yes* → Early cholecystectomy
— *No* → Supportive care

Severe
- Ranson score >3
- APACHE II ≥8
- CT severity index ≥7

↓

Admit to intensive care unit

↓

Supportive care
- Agressive volume repletion
- Pain control
- Monitor hemodynamics
- Monitor lab/serum markers
- Nutritional analysis
- Emergent ERCP with obstructive jaundice
- Antibiotics if infection

↓

CT scan of abdomen: necrosis?

— *Yes* → Sepsis or MOSF?
— *No* → Supportive care

Sepsis or MOSF?
— *No* → Expectant management with frequent reassessment
— *Yes* →
- CT-guided aspiration and culture
- Surgical consultation for possible surgical debridement (if infected)

APACHE II = Acute Physiology and Chronic Health Evaluation
CT = Computed Tomography
ERCP = Endoscopic Retrograde Cholangiopancreatography
RUQ = Right Upper Quadrant
MOSF = Multi-Organ System Failure
WBC = White Blood Cell
BUN = Blood Urea Nitrogen
LDH = Lactate Dehydrogenase
AST = Aspartate Transaminases
PaO$_2$ = Partial Arterial Oxygen Tension

Maurice F. Joyce, III, MD and Mitchell A. Cahan, MD

PAP (ABNORMAL), >21 YEARS OF AGE*

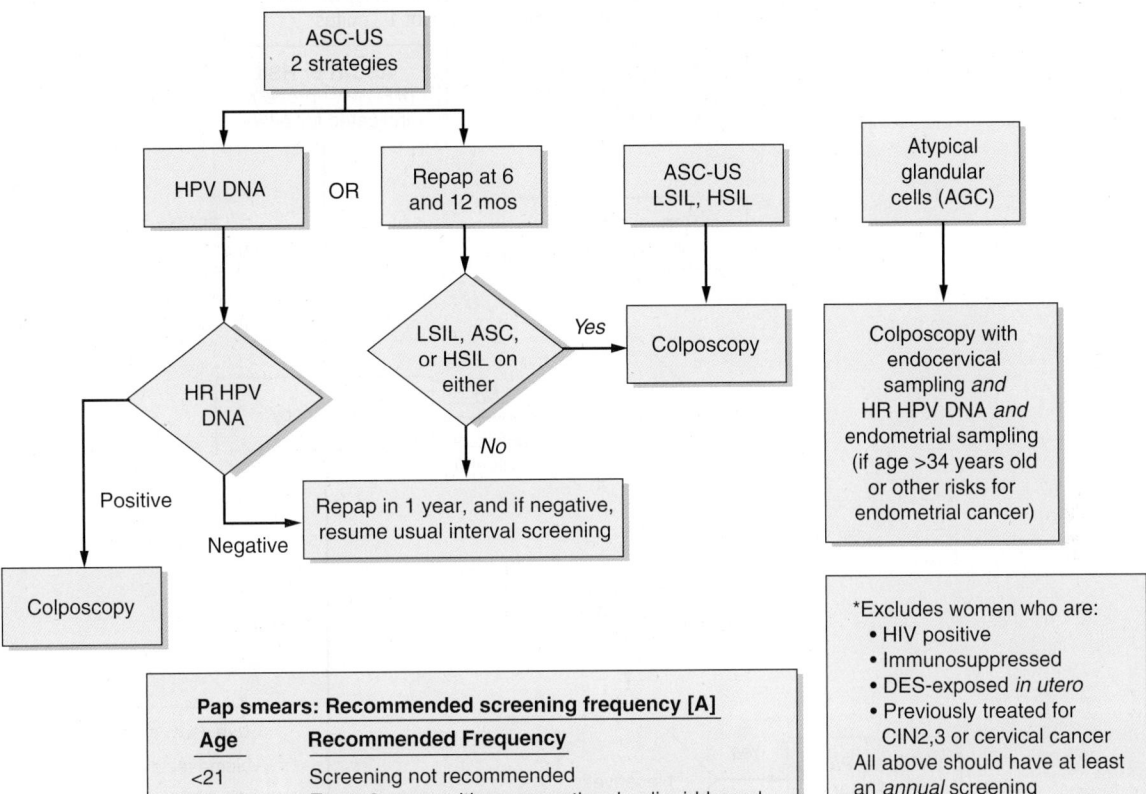

Pap smears: Recommended screening frequency [A]

Age	Recommended Frequency
<21	Screening not recommended
21–29	Every 2 years, either conventional or liquid-based
30–65	Every 3 years if either • Previous 3 paps (every 1–2 years) all normal *or* • Cytology negative and HR HPV DNA negative
>65	Discontinue screening if 3 previous paps normal and no abnormal results in past 10 years

Women of any age who had total hysterectomy for benign disease (and w/o history of high-grade CIN) do *not* require Pap smears

*Excludes women who are:
• HIV positive
• Immunosuppressed
• DES-exposed *in utero*
• Previously treated for CIN2,3 or cervical cancer
All above should have at least an *annual* screening

HR HPV DNA = probe for high-risk HPV strains

Jeremy Golding, MD

ACOG Practice Bulletin Number 109, December 2009.

PAP (ABNORMAL), ADOLESCENTS

Note: Pap no longer recommended for most women
<21 years of age regardless of age of 1st coitus

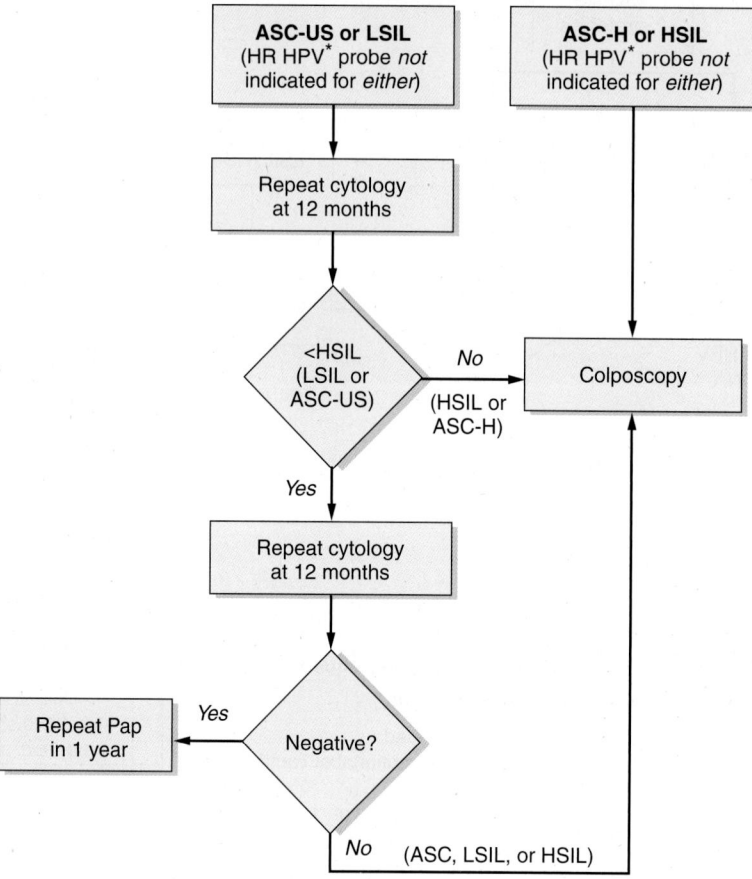

HR HPV DNA = probe for high-risk HPV strains

Jeremy Golding, MD

ACOG Practice Bulletin Number 109, December 2009.

PAP, USE OF HPV DNA TESTING IN WOMEN OVER 30*

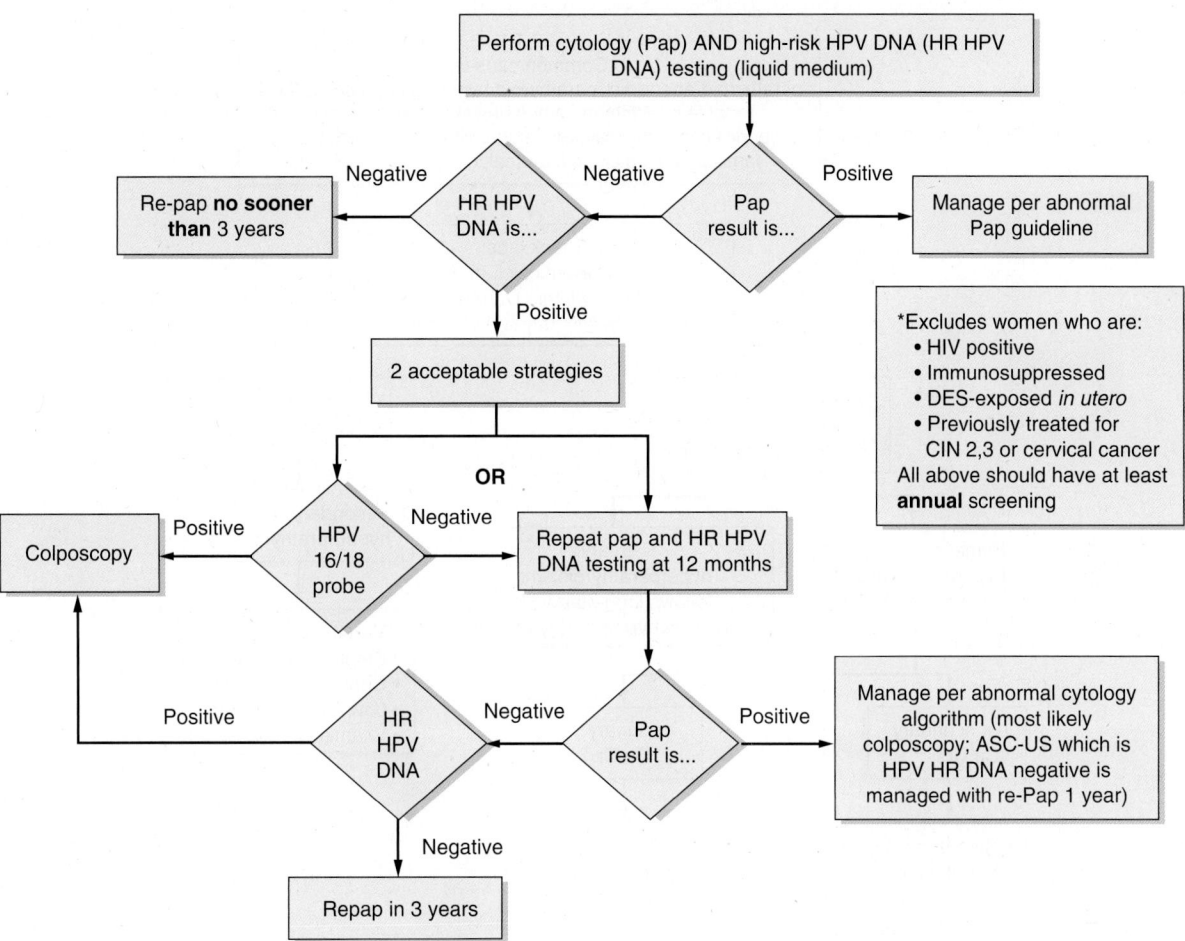

Perform cytology (Pap) AND high-risk HPV DNA (HR HPV DNA) testing (liquid medium)

HR HPV DNA is...
Negative → Re-pap **no sooner than** 3 years
Positive → 2 acceptable strategies

Pap result is...
Negative → HR HPV DNA is...
Positive → Manage per abnormal Pap guideline

2 acceptable strategies
OR

HPV 16/18 probe
Positive → Colposcopy
Negative → Repeat pap and HR HPV DNA testing at 12 months

Repeat pap and HR HPV DNA testing at 12 months

Pap result is...
Positive → Manage per abnormal cytology algorithm (most likely colposcopy; ASC-US which is HPV HR DNA negative is managed with re-Pap 1 year)
Negative → HR HPV DNA

HR HPV DNA
Positive → Colposcopy
Negative → Repap in 3 years

*Excludes women who are:
• HIV positive
• Immunosuppressed
• DES-exposed *in utero*
• Previously treated for CIN 2,3 or cervical cancer
All above should have at least **annual** screening

Jeremy Golding, MD

ACOG Practice Bulletin Number 109, December 2009.

PARATHYROID HORMONE, ELEVATED SERUM

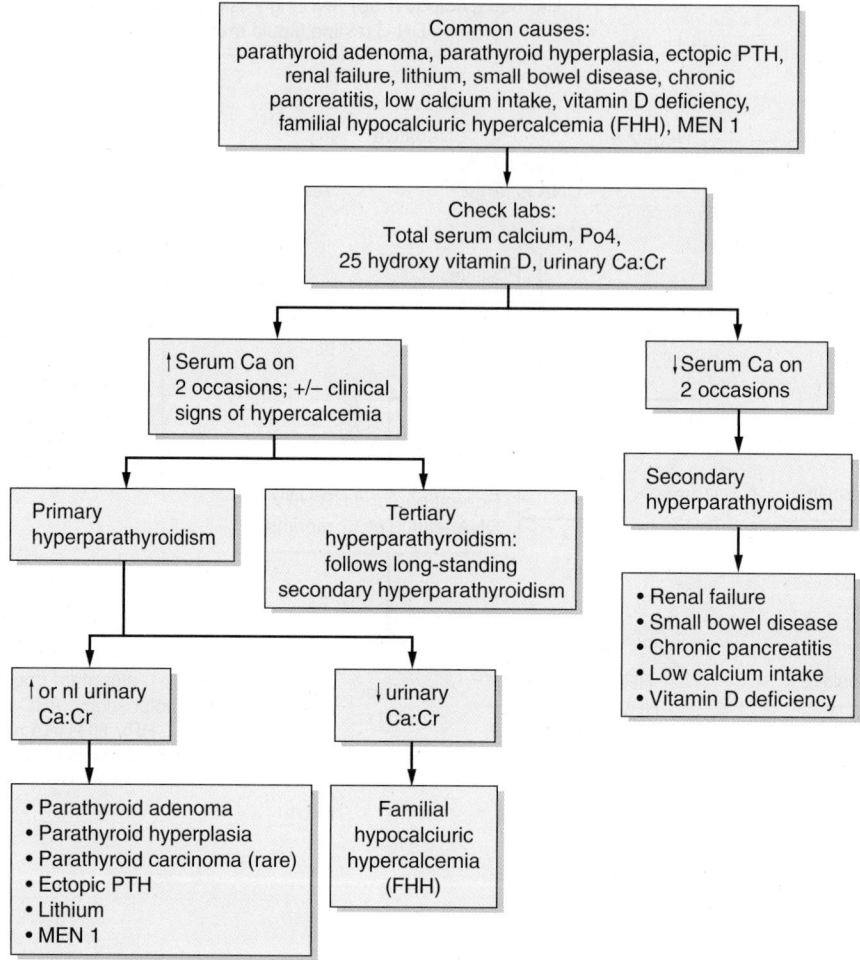

Common causes:
parathyroid adenoma, parathyroid hyperplasia, ectopic PTH, renal failure, lithium, small bowel disease, chronic pancreatitis, low calcium intake, vitamin D deficiency, familial hypocalciuric hypercalcemia (FHH), MEN 1

Check labs:
Total serum calcium, Po4, 25 hydroxy vitamin D, urinary Ca:Cr

↑Serum Ca on 2 occasions; +/– clinical signs of hypercalcemia

↓Serum Ca on 2 occasions

Primary hyperparathyroidism

Tertiary hyperparathyroidism: follows long-standing secondary hyperparathyroidism

Secondary hyperparathyroidism

- Renal failure
- Small bowel disease
- Chronic pancreatitis
- Low calcium intake
- Vitamin D deficiency

↑ or nl urinary Ca:Cr

↓ urinary Ca:Cr

- Parathyroid adenoma
- Parathyroid hyperplasia
- Parathyroid carcinoma (rare)
- Ectopic PTH
- Lithium
- MEN 1

Familial hypocalciuric hypercalcemia (FHH)

Andrew Gara, MD and Auguste Turnier, MD

JAMA. 2005;294(21):2700.

PELVIC PAIN

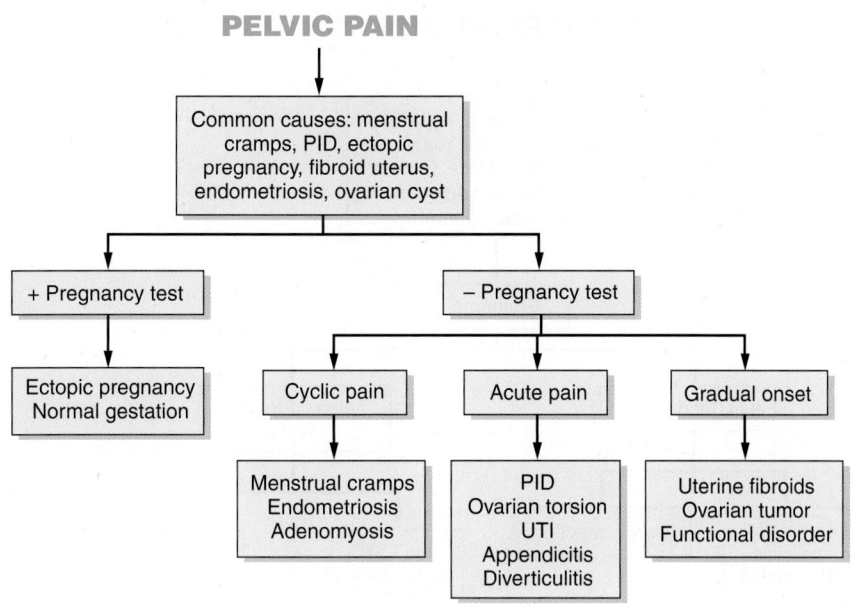

Robert A. Baldor, MD and Alan M. Ehrlich, MD

Am Fam Physician. 2008;77(11):1535–42.

PERIORBITAL EDEMA

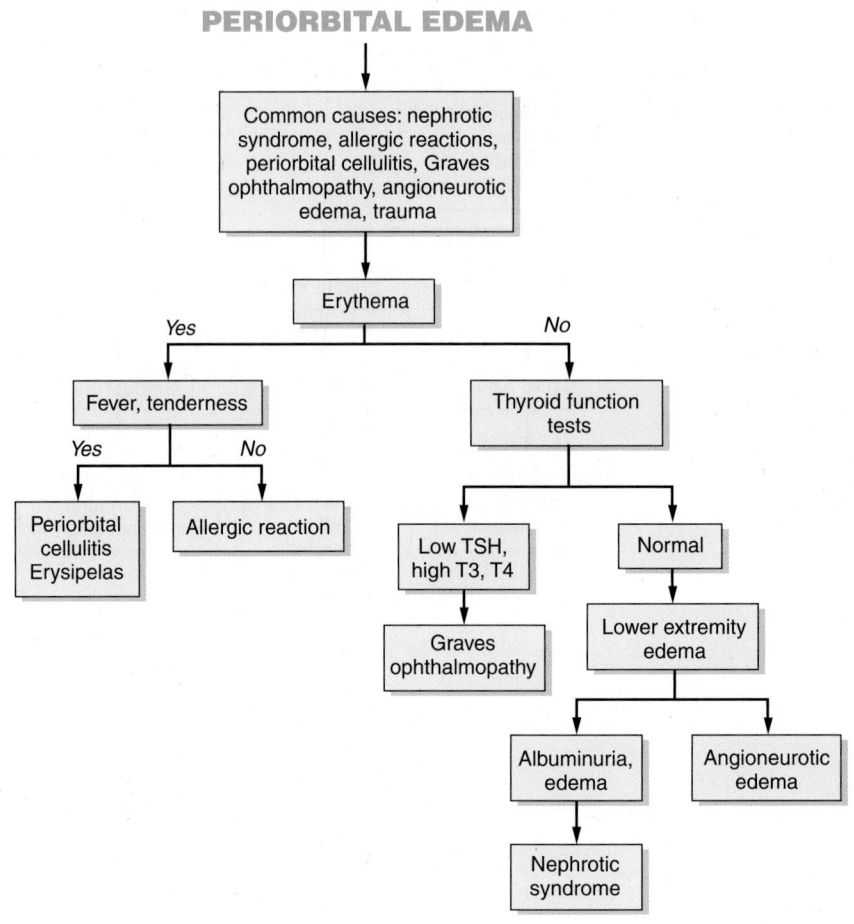

Robert A. Baldor, MD and Alan M. Ehrlich, MD

Infect Dis Clin North Am. 2007;21(2):393–408.

PLEURAL EFFUSION

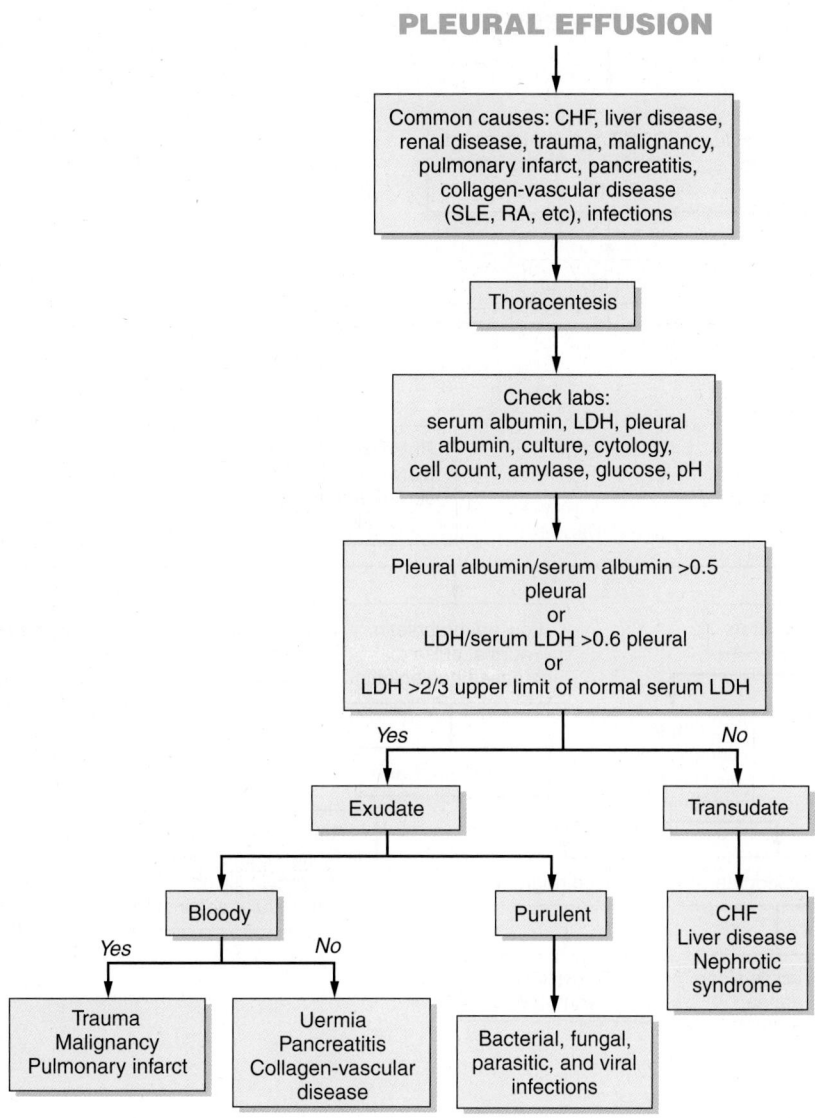

Common causes: CHF, liver disease, renal disease, trauma, malignancy, pulmonary infarct, pancreatitis, collagen-vascular disease (SLE, RA, etc), infections

Thoracentesis

Check labs: serum albumin, LDH, pleural albumin, culture, cytology, cell count, amylase, glucose, pH

Pleural albumin/serum albumin >0.5 pleural
or
LDH/serum LDH >0.6 pleural
or
LDH >2/3 upper limit of normal serum LDH

Yes — Exudate

No — Transudate

Exudate → Bloody / Purulent

Bloody: *Yes* — Trauma, Malignancy, Pulmonary infarct

Bloody: *No* — Uermia, Pancreatitis, Collagen-vascular disease

Purulent — Bacterial, fungal, parasitic, and viral infections

Transudate — CHF, Liver disease, Nephrotic syndrome

Robert A. Baldor, MD and Alan M. Ehrlich, MD

Am Fam Physician. 2006;73:1211–20.

POLYCYTHEMIA

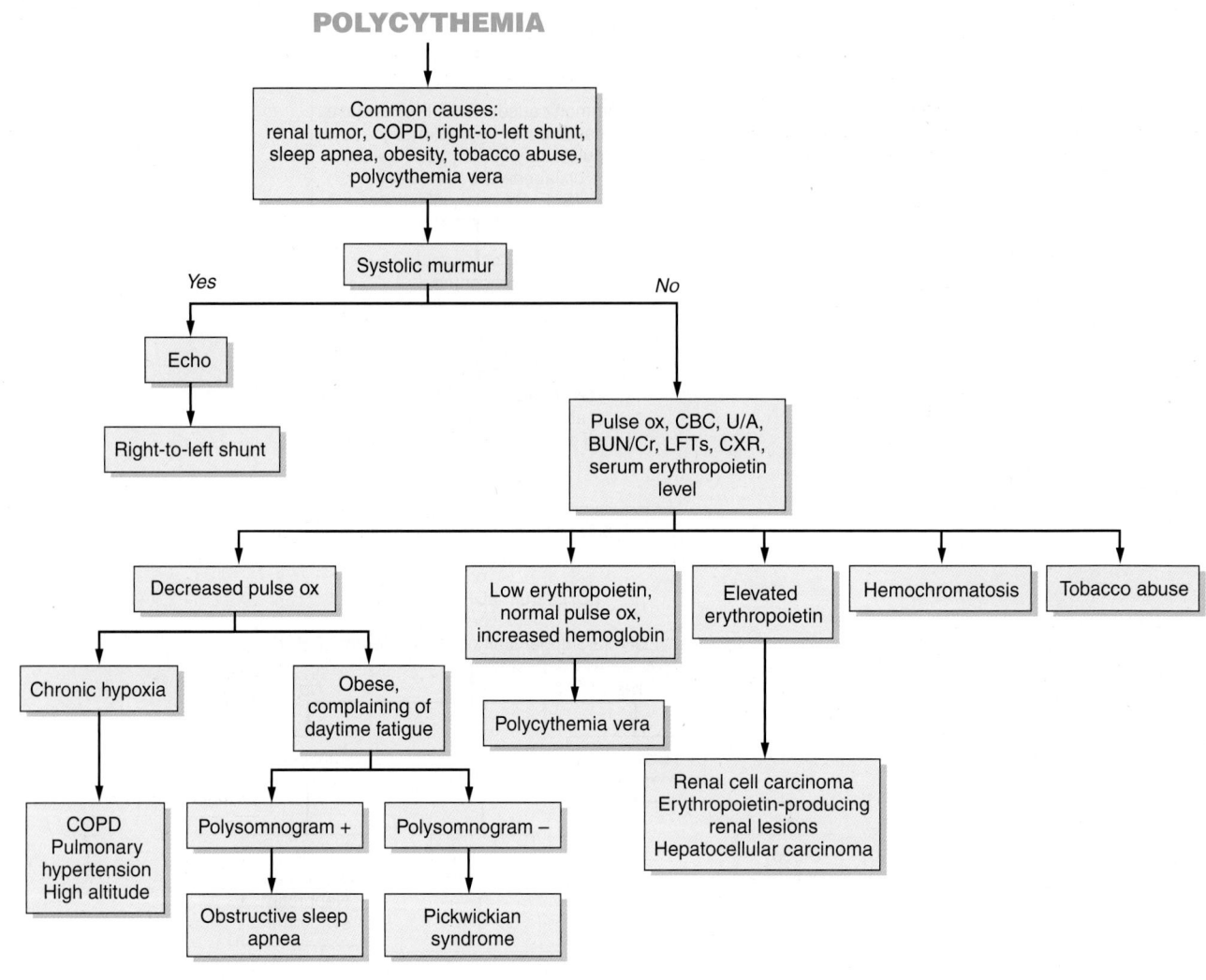

Robert A. Baldor, MD and Alan M. Ehrlich, MD

Mayo Clin Proc. 2005;80(7):923–36.

POLYDIPSIA

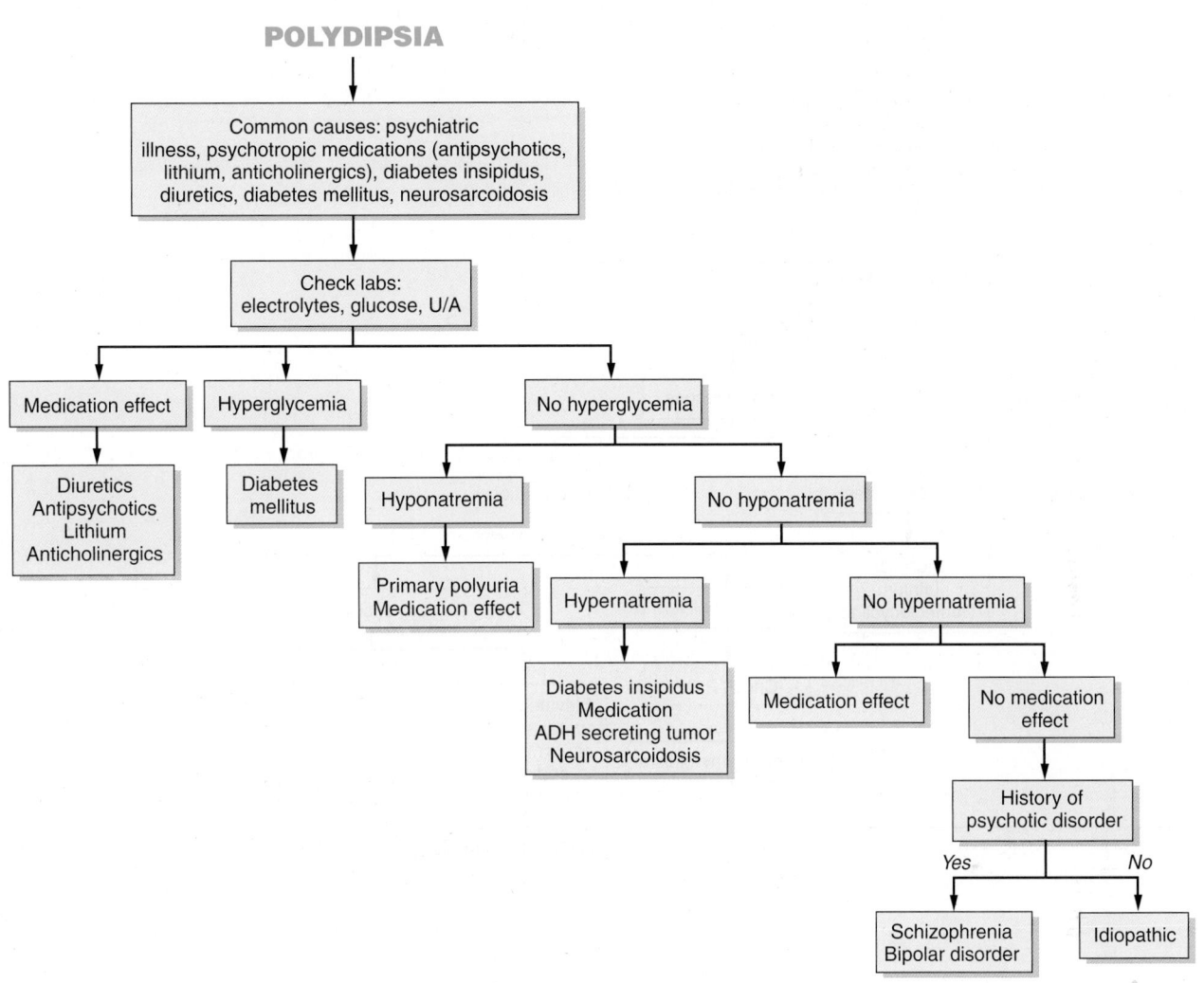

Common causes: psychiatric
illness, psychotropic medications (antipsychotics,
lithium, anticholinergics), diabetes insipidus,
diuretics, diabetes mellitus, neurosarcoidosis

Check labs:
electrolytes, glucose, U/A

Medication effect

Diuretics
Antipsychotics
Lithium
Anticholinergics

Hyperglycemia

Diabetes
mellitus

No hyperglycemia

Hyponatremia

Primary polyuria
Medication effect

No hyponatremia

Hypernatremia

Diabetes insipidus
Medication
ADH secreting tumor
Neurosarcoidosis

No hypernatremia

Medication effect

No medication
effect

History of
psychotic disorder

Yes   *No*

Schizophrenia
Bipolar disorder

Idiopathic

Robert A. Baldor, MD and Alan M. Ehrlich, MD

Nat Clin Proc Nephrol. 2007;3(7):374–82.

POLYURIA

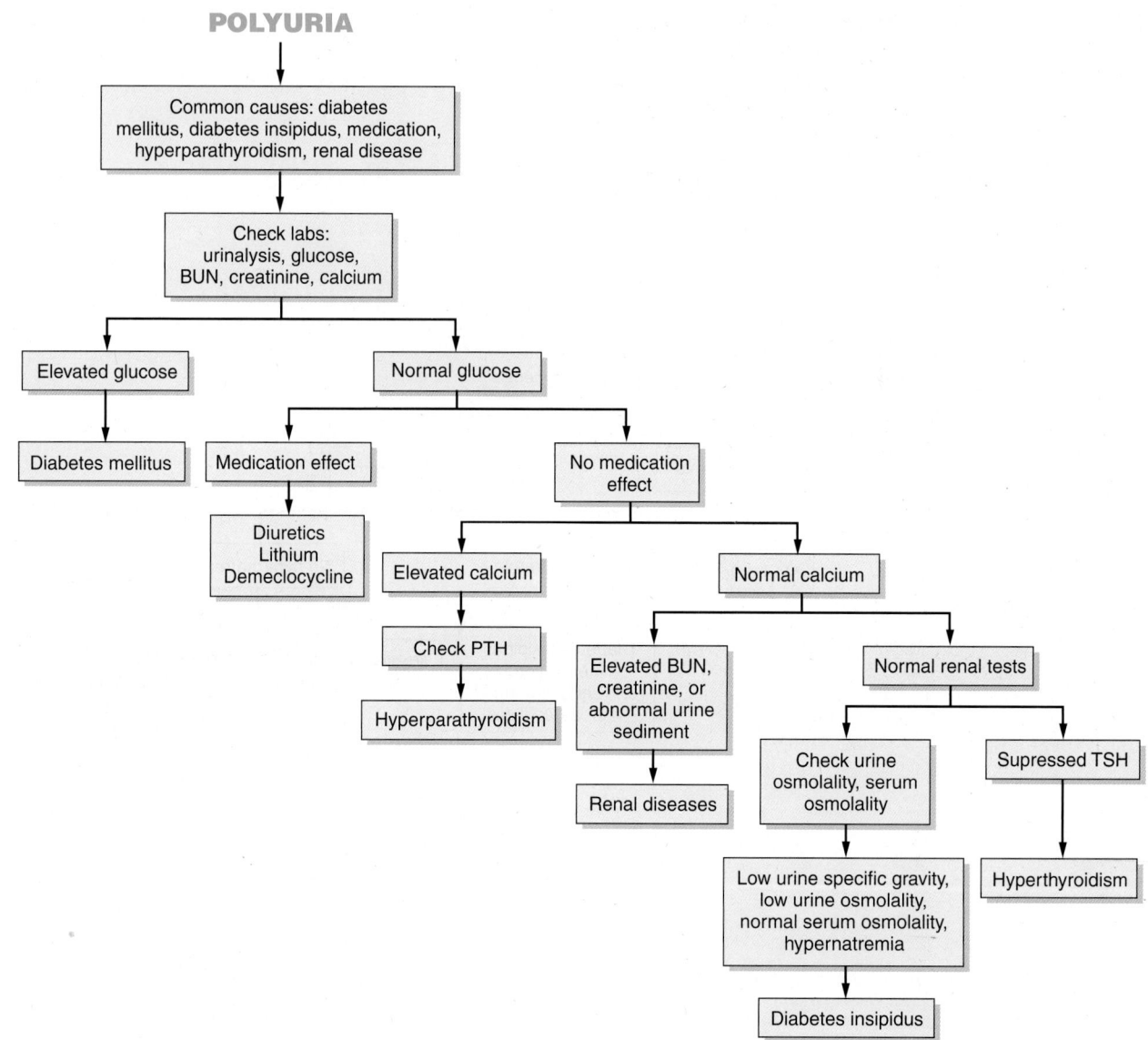

Common causes: diabetes mellitus, diabetes insipidus, medication, hyperparathyroidism, renal disease

Check labs: urinalysis, glucose, BUN, creatinine, calcium

Elevated glucose → Diabetes mellitus

Normal glucose

Medication effect → Diuretics, Lithium, Demeclocycline

No medication effect

Elevated calcium → Check PTH → Hyperparathyroidism

Normal calcium

Elevated BUN, creatinine, or abnormal urine sediment → Renal diseases

Normal renal tests

Check urine osmolality, serum osmolality → Low urine specific gravity, low urine osmolality, normal serum osmolality, hypernatremia → Diabetes insipidus

Supressed TSH → Hyperthyroidism

Robert A. Baldor, MD and Alan M. Ehrlich, MD

POPLITEAL MASS

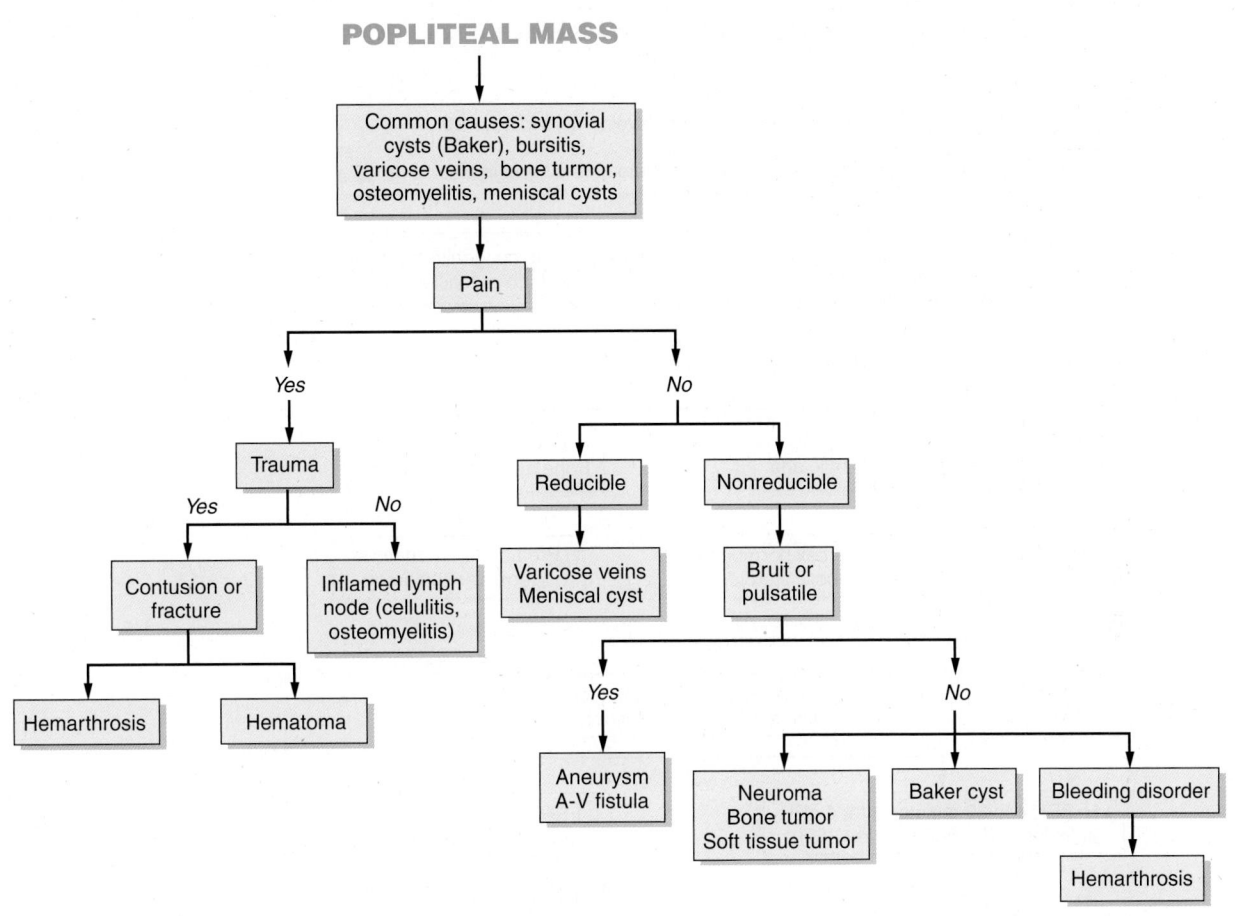

Robert A. Baldor, MD and Alan M. Ehrlich, MD

Am Fam Physician. 2003;68:917–22.

PRECOCIOUS PUBERTY

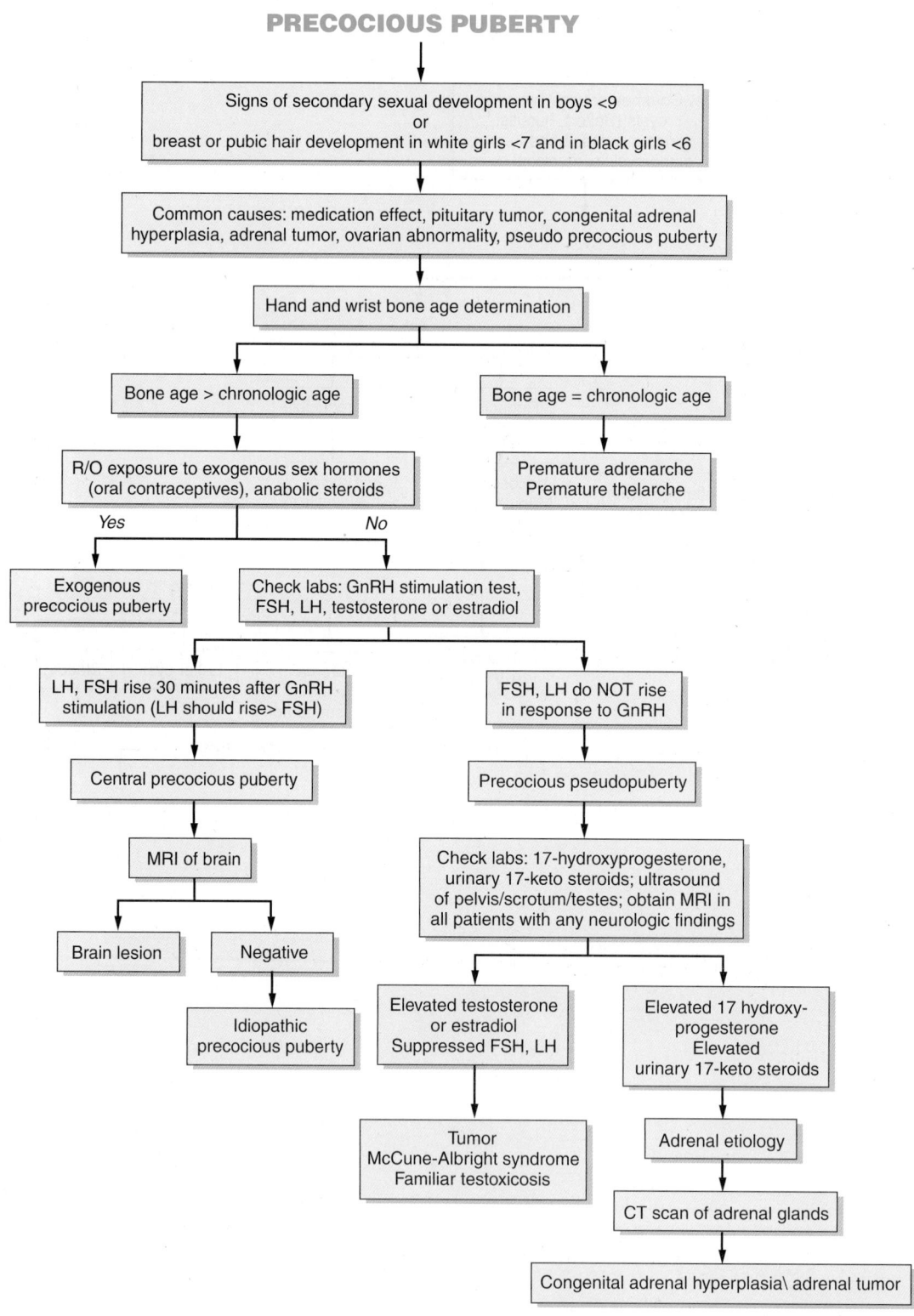

Signs of secondary sexual development in boys <9
or
breast or pubic hair development in white girls <7 and in black girls <6

Common causes: medication effect, pituitary tumor, congenital adrenal hyperplasia, adrenal tumor, ovarian abnormality, pseudo precocious puberty

Hand and wrist bone age determination

Bone age > chronologic age

Bone age = chronologic age

R/O exposure to exogenous sex hormones (oral contraceptives), anabolic steroids

Premature adrenarche
Premature thelarche

Yes

No

Exogenous precocious puberty

Check labs: GnRH stimulation test, FSH, LH, testosterone or estradiol

LH, FSH rise 30 minutes after GnRH stimulation (LH should rise> FSH)

FSH, LH do NOT rise in response to GnRH

Central precocious puberty

Precocious pseudopuberty

MRI of brain

Check labs: 17-hydroxyprogesterone, urinary 17-keto steroids; ultrasound of pelvis/scrotum/testes; obtain MRI in all patients with any neurologic findings

Brain lesion

Negative

Idiopathic precocious puberty

Elevated testosterone or estradiol
Suppressed FSH, LH

Elevated 17 hydroxy-progesterone
Elevated urinary 17-keto steroids

Tumor
McCune-Albright syndrome
Familiar testoxicosis

Adrenal etiology

CT scan of adrenal glands

Congenital adrenal hyperplasia\ adrenal tumor

Robert A. Baldor, MD and Alan M. Ehrlich, MD

Am Fam Physician. 2008;78(5):597–04.

PREOPERATIVE EVALUATION OF NONCARDIAC SURGICAL PATIENT

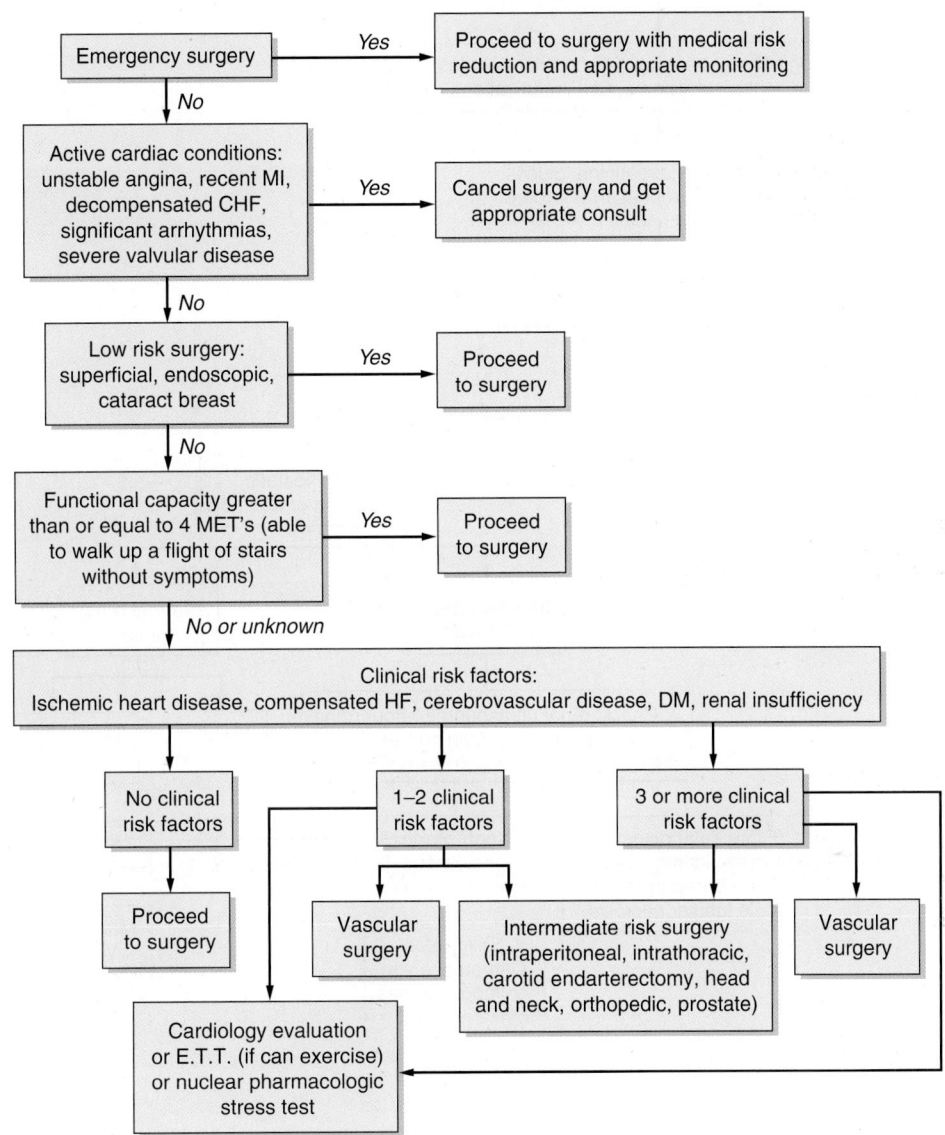

Drew Grimes, MD and Stacy Jones, MD

Circulation. 2007;116(17):e418–99.

PROTEINURIA

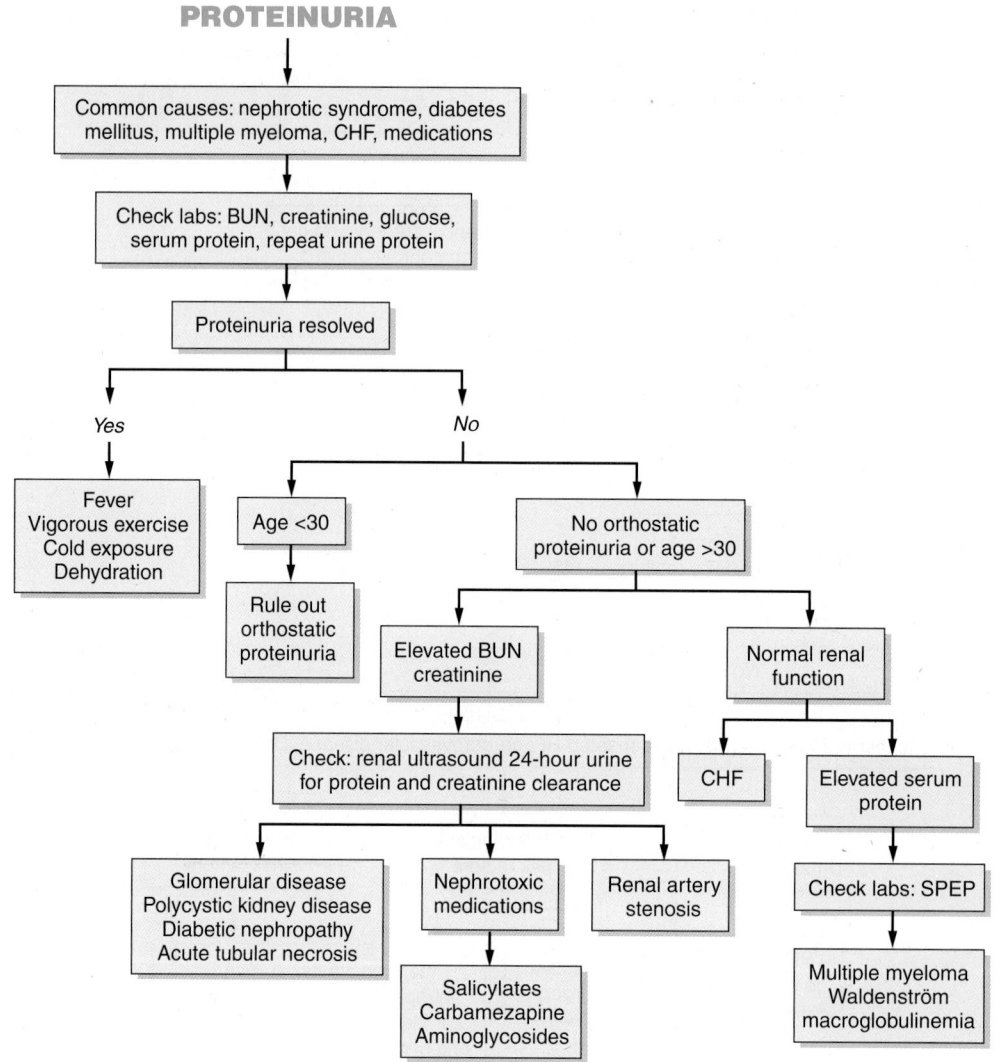

Common causes: nephrotic syndrome, diabetes mellitus, multiple myeloma, CHF, medications

Check labs: BUN, creatinine, glucose, serum protein, repeat urine protein

Proteinuria resolved

Yes

Fever
Vigorous exercise
Cold exposure
Dehydration

No

Age <30

Rule out orthostatic proteinuria

No orthostatic proteinuria or age >30

Elevated BUN creatinine

Check: renal ultrasound 24-hour urine for protein and creatinine clearance

Glomerular disease
Polycystic kidney disease
Diabetic nephropathy
Acute tubular necrosis

Nephrotoxic medications

Salicylates
Carbamezapine
Aminoglycosides

Renal artery stenosis

Normal renal function

CHF

Elevated serum protein

Check labs: SPEP

Multiple myeloma
Waldenström macroglobulinemia

Robert A. Baldor, MD and Alan M. Ehrlich, MD

Am Fam Physician. 2000;62:1333–40.

PULMONARY EMBOLISM, DIAGNOSIS

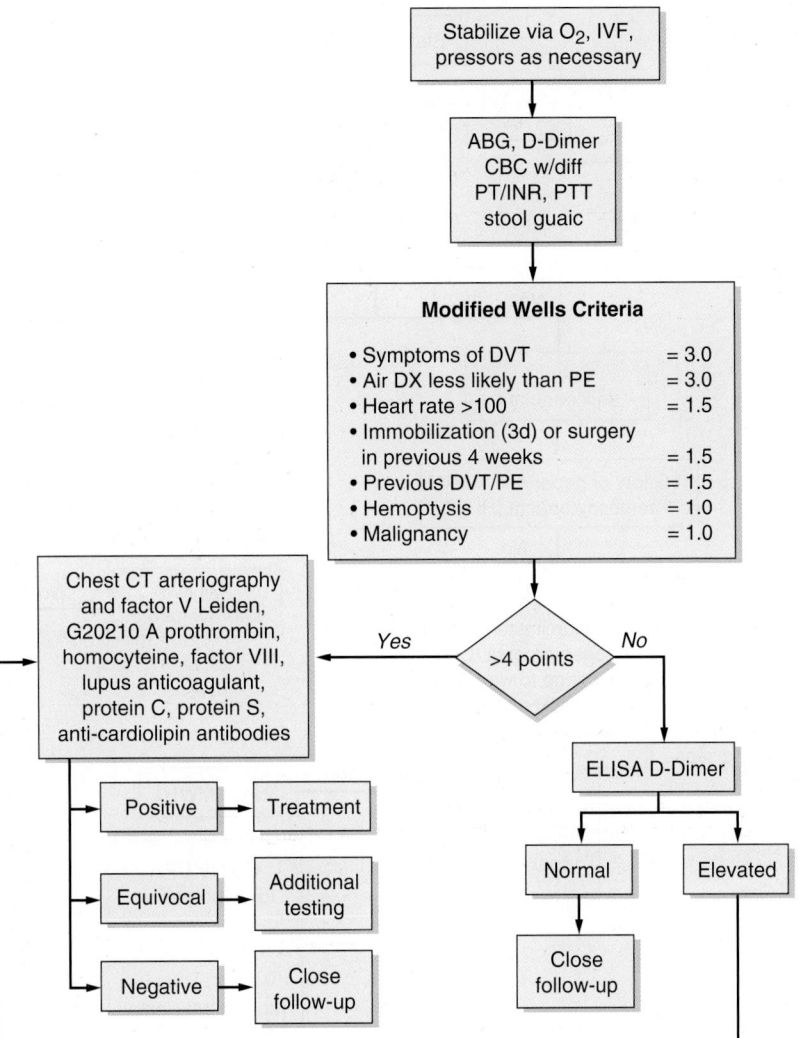

Parag Goyal, MD

Radiol Clin North Am. 2010;48(1):31−50.

PULMONARY EMBOLISM, TREATMENT

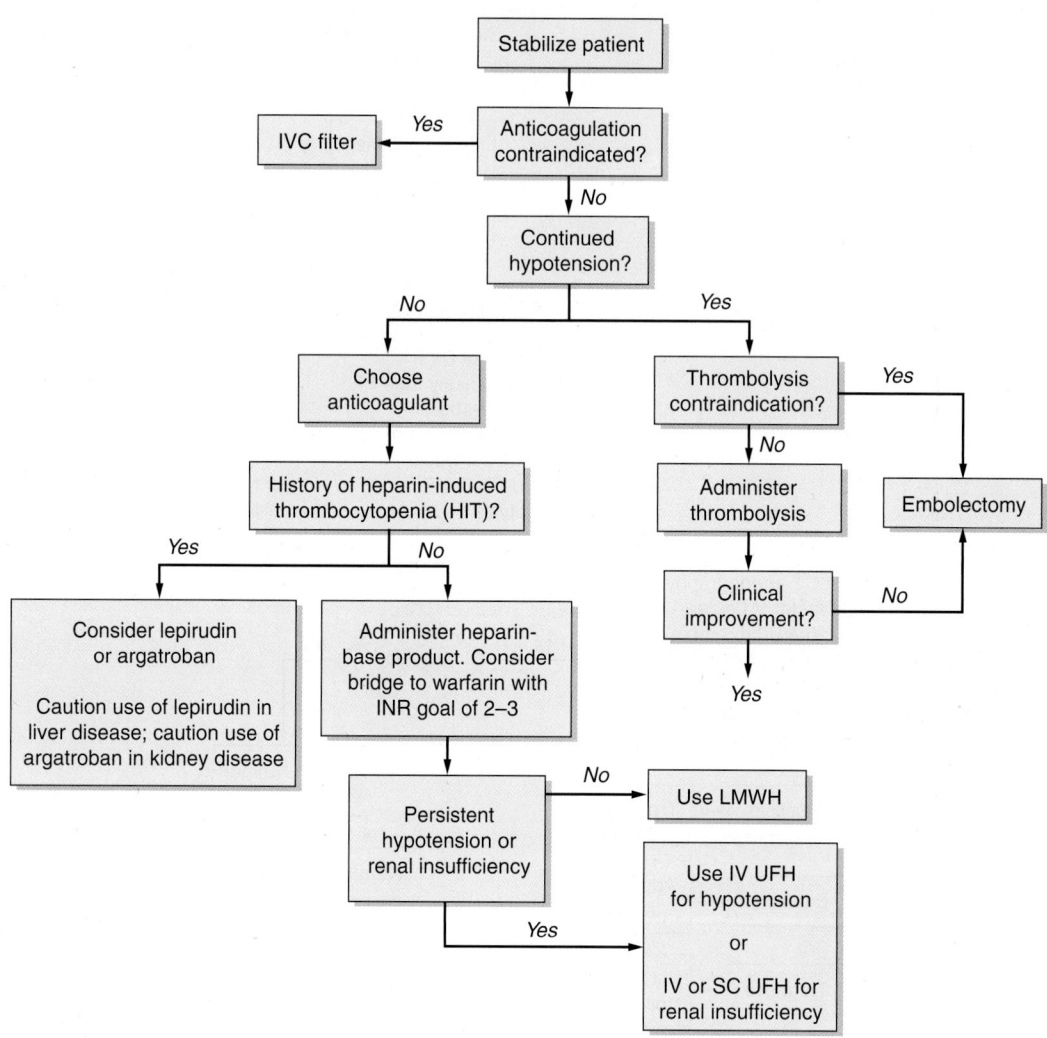

Parag Goyal, MD

NEJM. 2008;358(10):1037–52.

PUPIL ABNORMALITIES

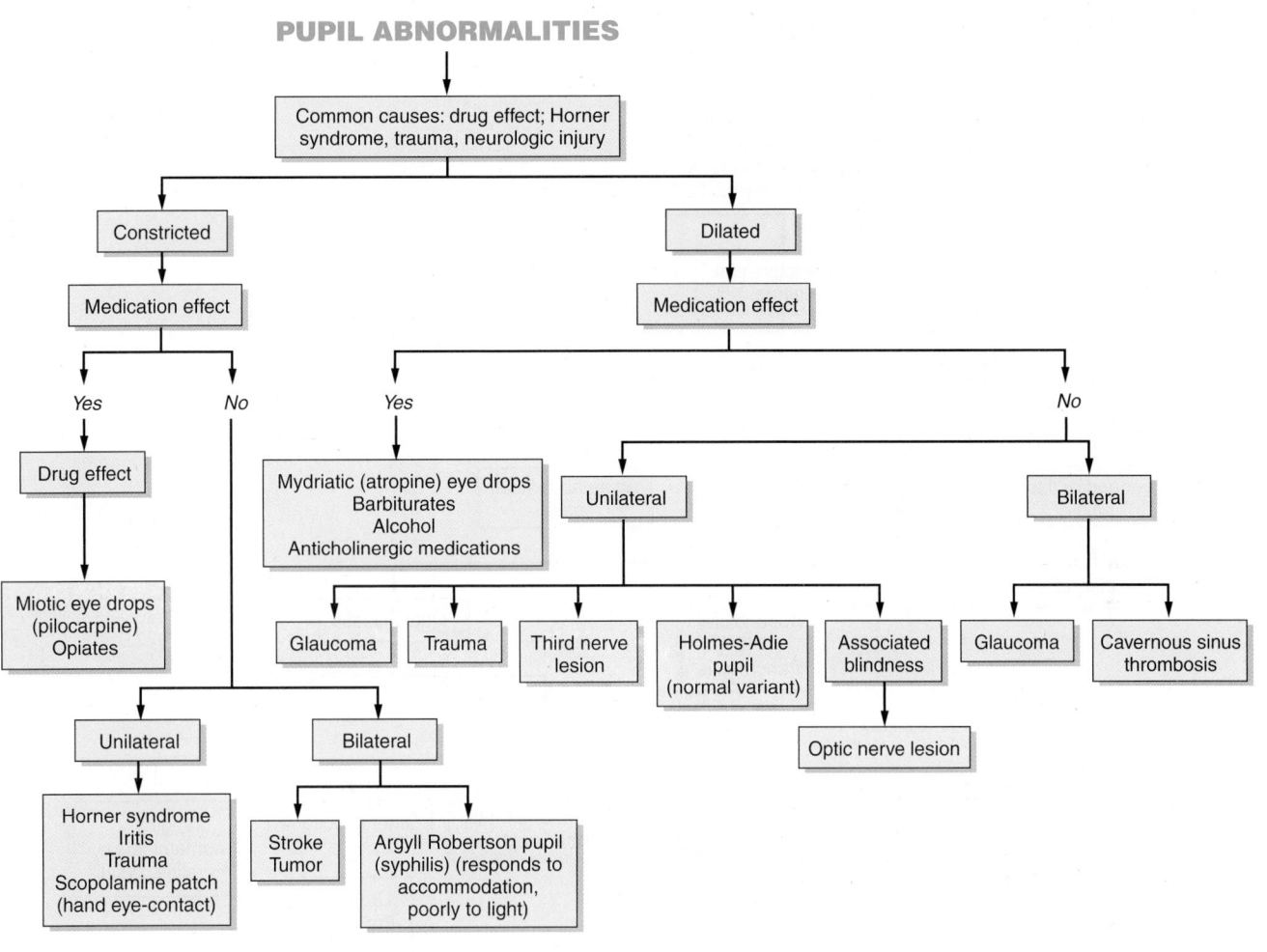

Robert A. Baldor, MD and Alan M. Ehrlich, MD

Vision Res. 2005;45(19):2549–63.

PYURIA

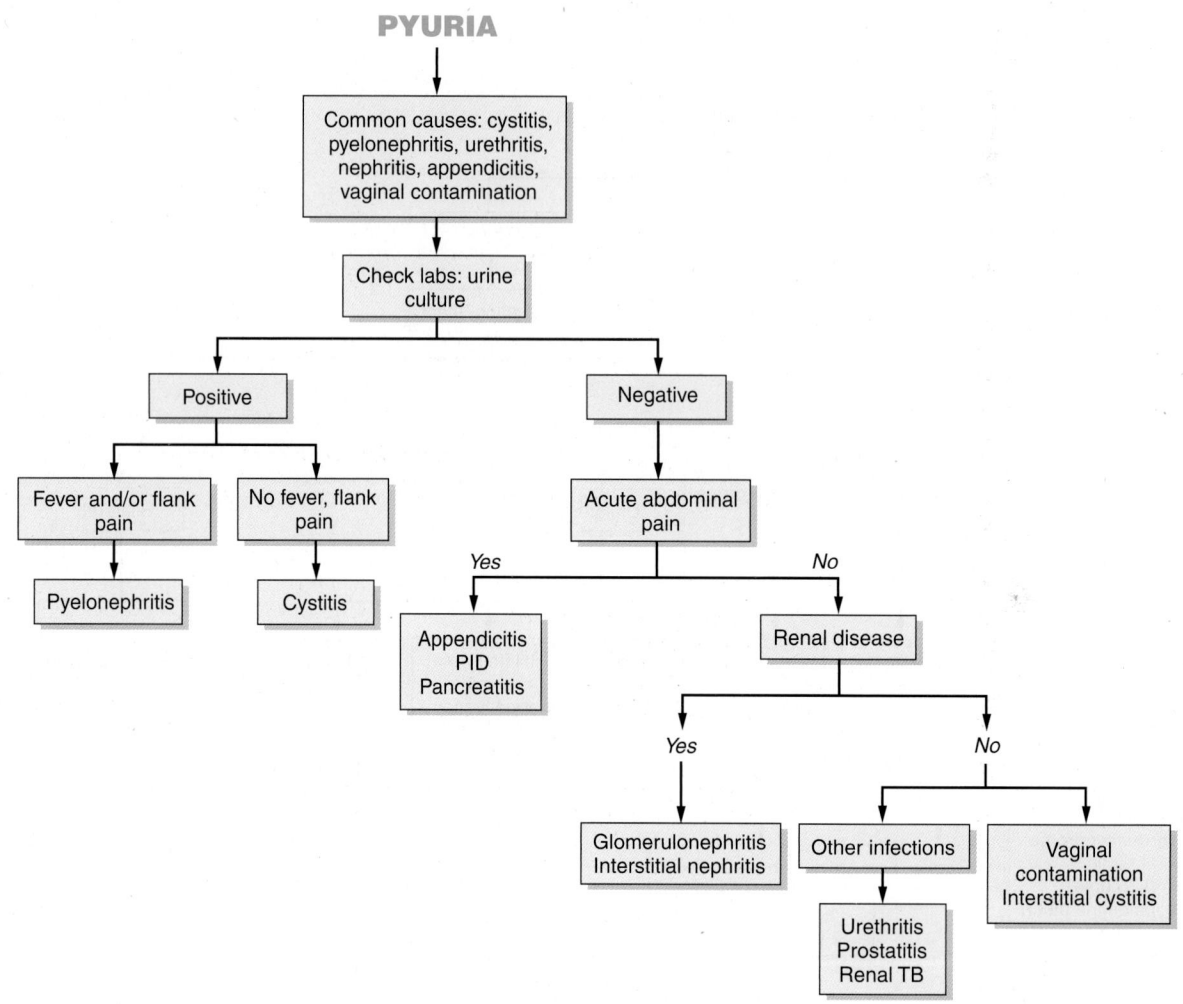

Robert A. Baldor, MD and Alan M. Ehrlich, MD

Am Fam Physician. 2005;71:1153–62.

RADIOPAQUE LESION OF LUNG

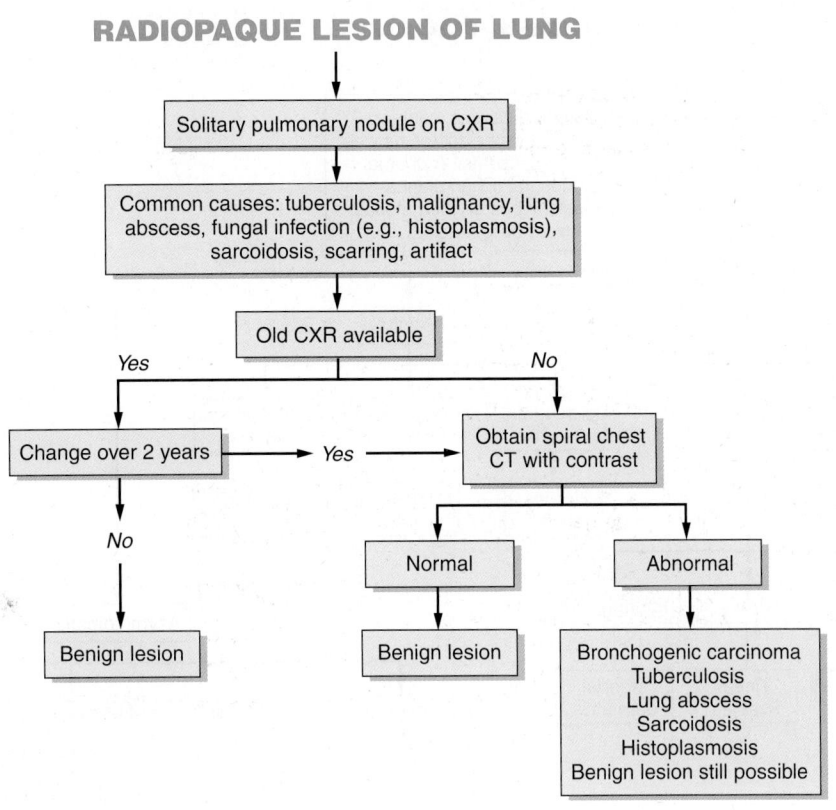

Robert A. Baldor, MD and Alan M. Ehrlich, MD

NEJM. 348(25):2535–42.

RASH, FOCAL

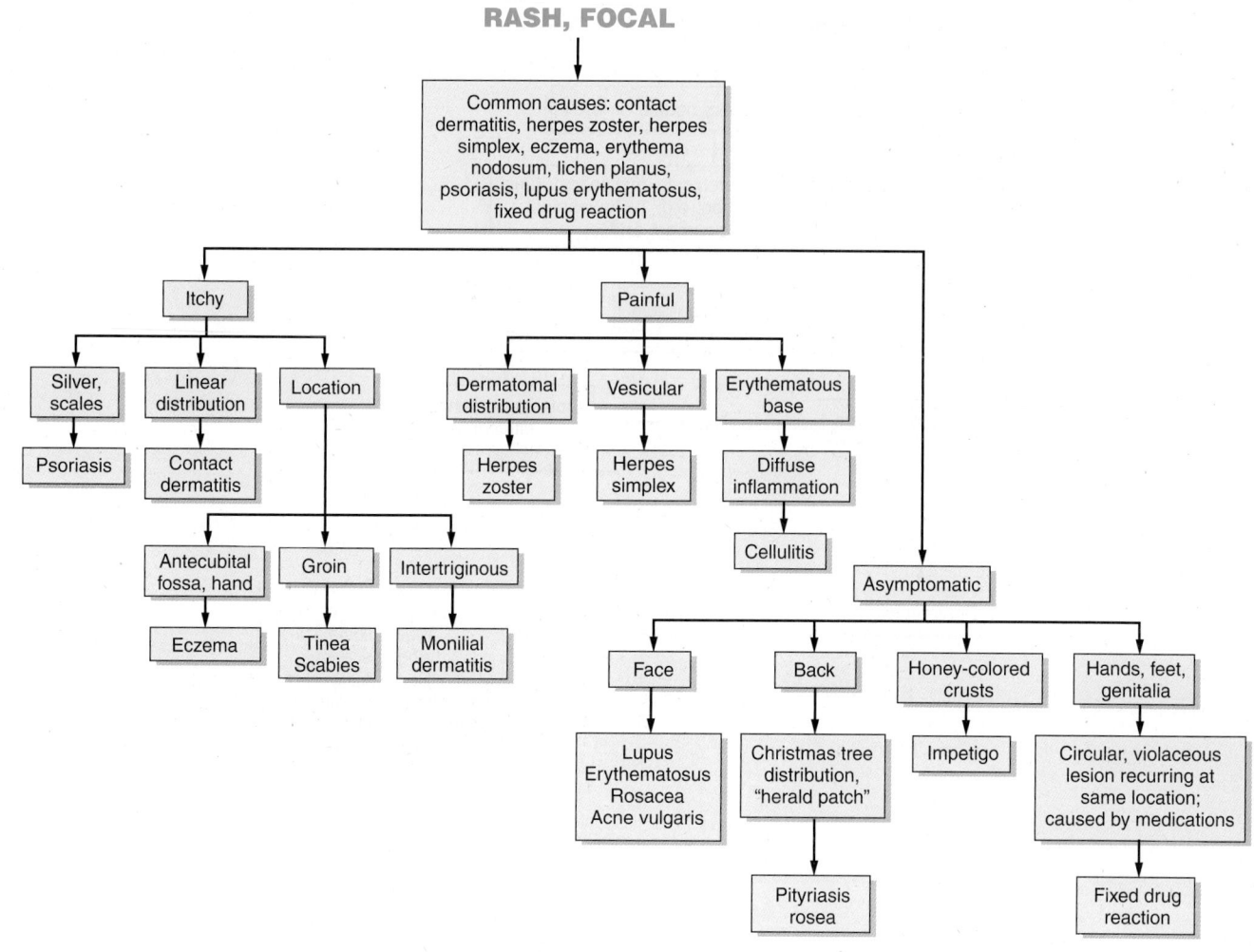

Common causes: contact dermatitis, herpes zoster, herpes simplex, eczema, erythema nodosum, lichen planus, psoriasis, lupus erythematosus, fixed drug reaction

Itchy
- Silver, scales → Psoriasis
- Linear distribution → Contact dermatitis
- Location
  - Antecubital fossa, hand → Eczema
  - Groin → Tinea Scabies
  - Intertriginous → Monilial dermatitis

Painful
- Dermatomal distribution → Herpes zoster
- Vesicular → Herpes simplex
- Erythematous base → Diffuse inflammation → Cellulitis

Asymptomatic
- Face → Lupus Erythematosus, Rosacea, Acne vulgaris
- Back → Christmas tree distribution, "herald patch" → Pityriasis rosea
- Honey-colored crusts → Impetigo
- Hands, feet, genitalia → Circular, violaceous lesion recurring at same location; caused by medications → Fixed drug reaction

Robert A. Baldor, MD and Alan M. Ehrlich, MD

Arch Dermatol. 2001;137(1):25–9.

RAYNAUD PHENOMENON

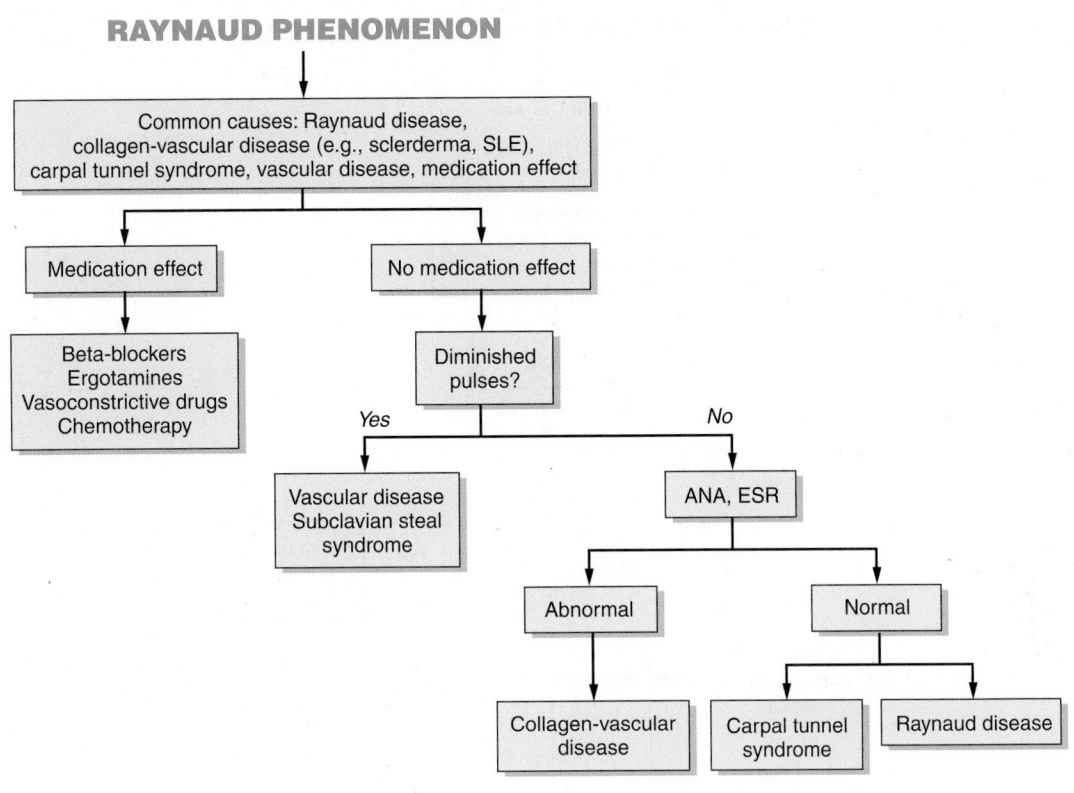

Common causes: Raynaud disease, collagen-vascular disease (e.g., sclerderma, SLE), carpal tunnel syndrome, vascular disease, medication effect

- Medication effect → Beta-blockers, Ergotamines, Vasoconstrictive drugs, Chemotherapy
- No medication effect → Diminished pulses?
  - Yes → Vascular disease, Subclavian steal syndrome
  - No → ANA, ESR
    - Abnormal → Collagen-vascular disease
    - Normal → Carpal tunnel syndrome; Raynaud disease

Robert A. Baldor, MD and Alan M. Ehrlich, MD

JFP. 2005 (54:6).

RECTAL BLEEDING AND HEMATOCHEZIA

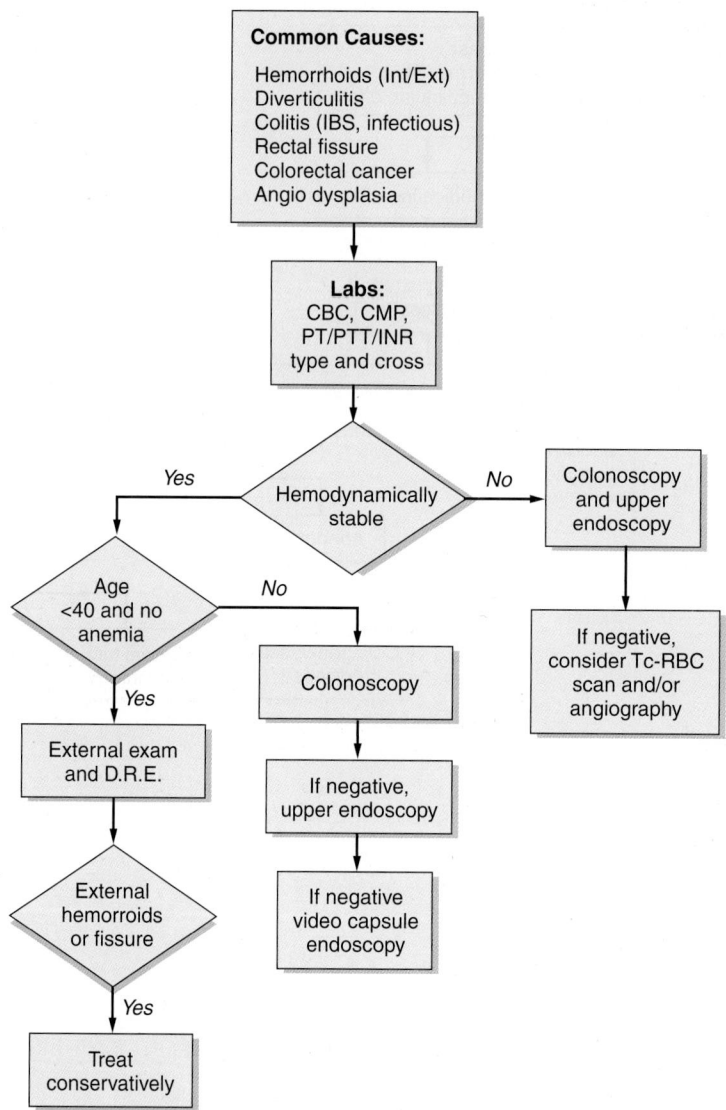

Common Causes:

Hemorrhoids (Int/Ext)
Diverticulitis
Colitis (IBS, infectious)
Rectal fissure
Colorectal cancer
Angio dysplasia

Labs:
CBC, CMP,
PT/PTT/INR
type and cross

Hemodynamically stable

Yes — Age <40 and no anemia

No — Colonoscopy and upper endoscopy

If negative, consider Tc-RBC scan and/or angiography

No — Colonoscopy

If negative, upper endoscopy

If negative video capsule endoscopy

Yes — External exam and D.R.E.

External hemorroids or fissure

Yes — Treat conservatively

Mohammad Ansar Mughal, MD

Dis Colon Rectum. 2005;48(11):2010–24.

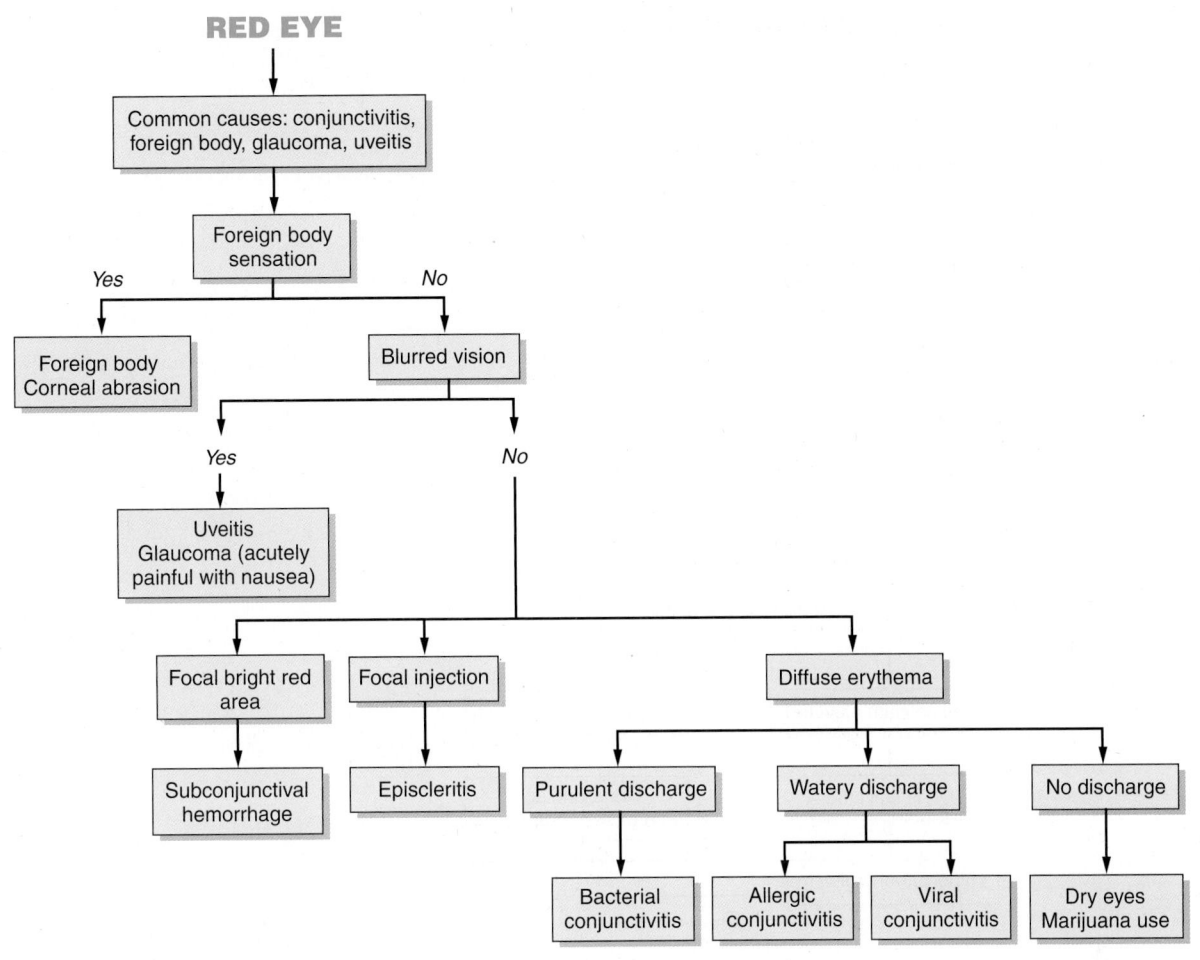

Robert A. Baldor, MD and Alan M. Ehrlich, MD

NEJM. 2000;343(5):345–51.

RENAL CALCULI

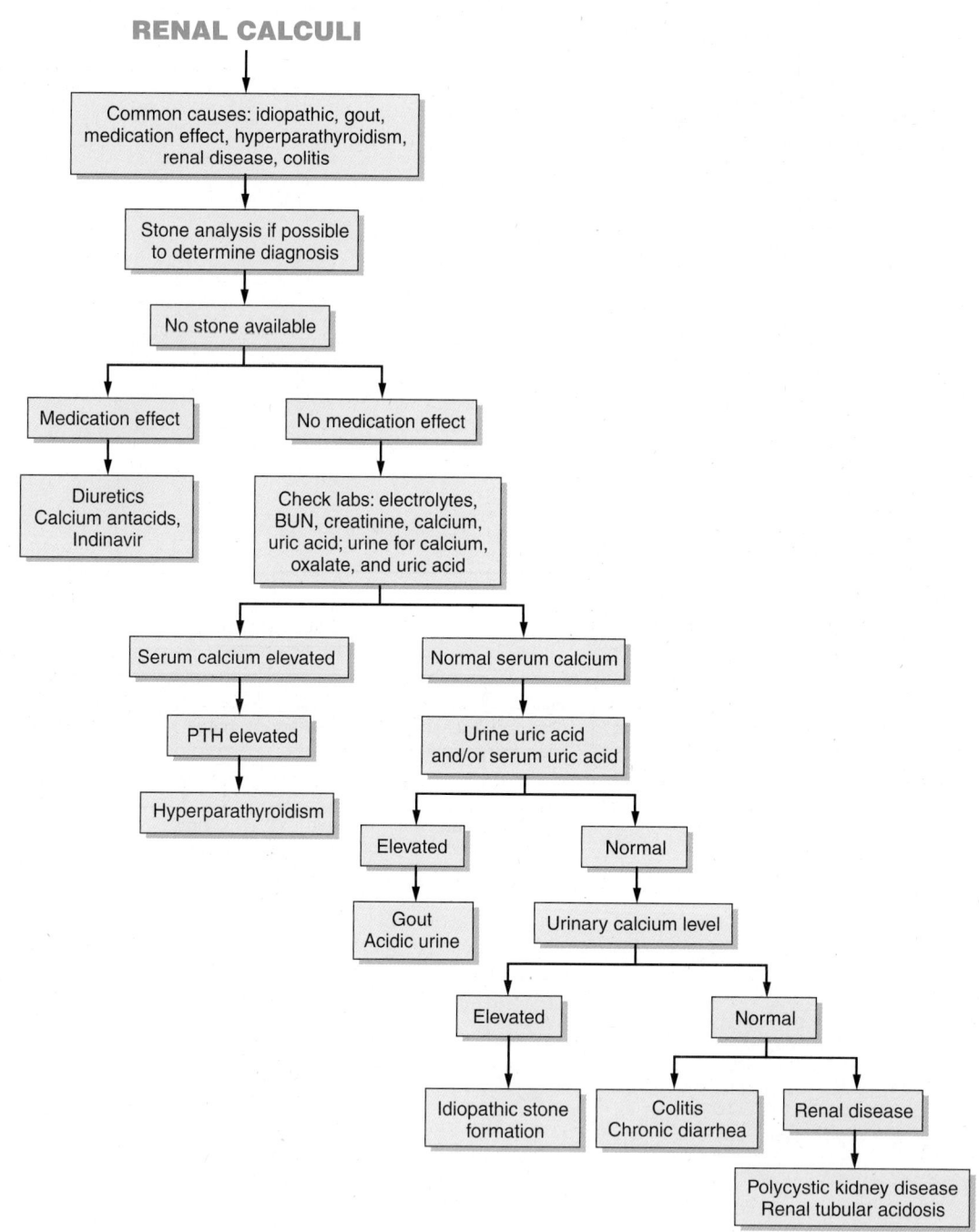

Robert A. Baldor, MD and Alan M. Ehrlich, MD

Prim Care. 2008;35(2):369–91.

RENAL FAILURE, ACUTE

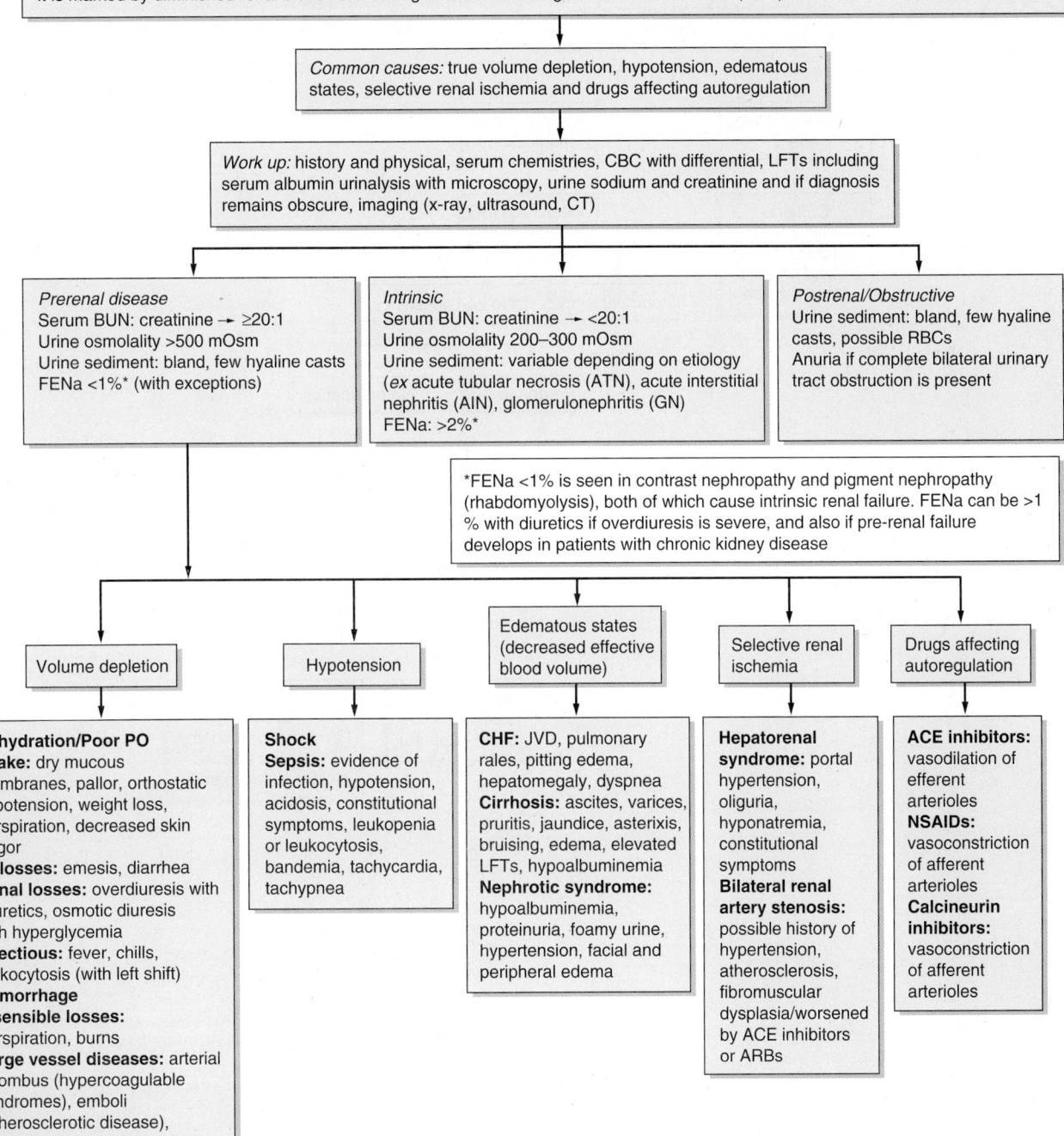

Acute kidney injury (AKI, previously called acute renal failure) is an acute loss of kidney function over days to weeks resulting in an inability to excrete nitrogenous wastes and creatinine. Patients are often asymptomatic, and are recognized by an increase in serum creatinine level (>0.5 mg/dL from baseline). Prerenal disease (PD) is one category of AKI where the injury occurs outside the nephron; it is marked by diminished renal blood flow leading to a decrease in glomerular filtration rate (GFR).

Common causes: true volume depletion, hypotension, edematous states, selective renal ischemia and drugs affecting autoregulation

Work up: history and physical, serum chemistries, CBC with differential, LFTs including serum albumin urinalysis with microscopy, urine sodium and creatinine and if diagnosis remains obscure, imaging (x-ray, ultrasound, CT)

Prerenal disease
Serum BUN: creatinine → ≥20:1
Urine osmolality >500 mOsm
Urine sediment: bland, few hyaline casts
FENa <1%* (with exceptions)

Intrinsic
Serum BUN: creatinine → <20:1
Urine osmolality 200–300 mOsm
Urine sediment: variable depending on etiology (*ex* acute tubular necrosis (ATN), acute interstitial nephritis (AIN), glomerulonephritis (GN)
FENa: >2%*

Postrenal/Obstructive
Urine sediment: bland, few hyaline casts, possible RBCs
Anuria if complete bilateral urinary tract obstruction is present

*FENa <1% is seen in contrast nephropathy and pigment nephropathy (rhabdomyolysis), both of which cause intrinsic renal failure. FENa can be >1% with diuretics if overdiuresis is severe, and also if pre-renal failure develops in patients with chronic kidney disease

Volume depletion

Hypotension

Edematous states (decreased effective blood volume)

Selective renal ischemia

Drugs affecting autoregulation

Dehydration/Poor PO intake: dry mucous membranes, pallor, orthostatic hypotension, weight loss, perspiration, decreased skin turgor
GI losses: emesis, diarrhea
Renal losses: overdiuresis with Diuretics, osmotic diuresis with hyperglycemia
Infectious: fever, chills, leukocytosis (with left shift)
Hemorrhage
Insensible losses: perspiration, burns
Large vessel diseases: arterial thrombus (hypercoagulable syndromes), emboli (atherosclerotic disease), aortic dissection (connective tissue disease, trauma)

Shock
Sepsis: evidence of infection, hypotension, acidosis, constitutional symptoms, leukopenia or leukocytosis, bandemia, tachycardia, tachypnea

CHF: JVD, pulmonary rales, pitting edema, hepatomegaly, dyspnea
Cirrhosis: ascites, varices, pruritis, jaundice, asterixis, bruising, edema, elevated LFTs, hypoalbuminemia
Nephrotic syndrome: hypoalbuminemia, proteinuria, foamy urine, hypertension, facial and peripheral edema

Hepatorenal syndrome: portal hypertension, oliguria, hyponatremia, constitutional symptoms
Bilateral renal artery stenosis: possible history of hypertension, atherosclerosis, fibromuscular dysplasia/worsened by ACE inhibitors or ARBs

ACE inhibitors: vasodilation of efferent arterioles
NSAIDs: vasoconstriction of afferent arterioles
Calcineurin inhibitors: vasoconstriction of afferent arterioles

Krunal Patel, MD and Dagmar Klinger, MD

Am Fam Physician. 2005;72(9):1739–47.

RESTLESS LEG SYNDROME (RLS)

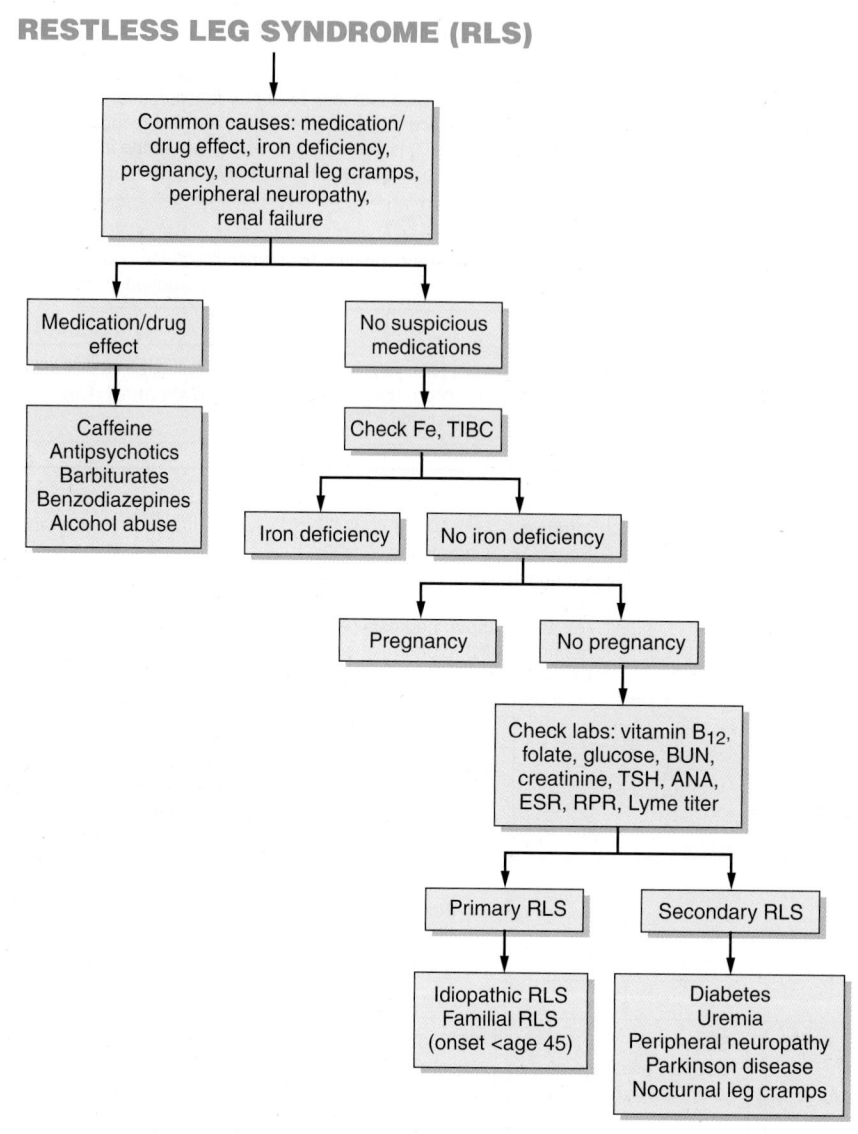

Robert A. Baldor, MD and Alan M. Ehrlich, MD

Am Fam Physician. 2000;62:108–14.

SEIZURE, NEW ONSET

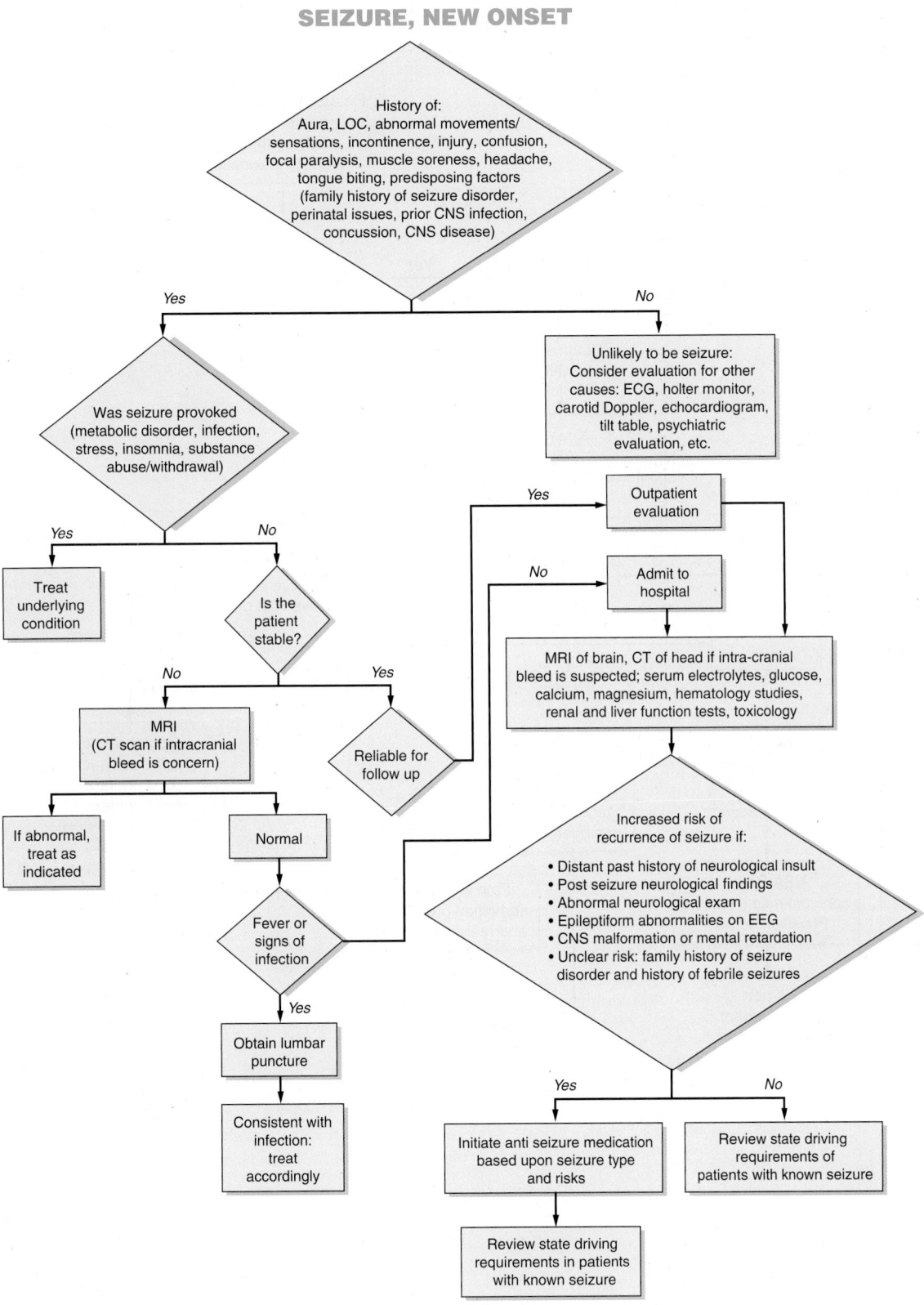

Neepa Patel, MD and Ioannis Karakis, MD

N Engl J Med. 2003;349:1257.

SHOULDER PAIN

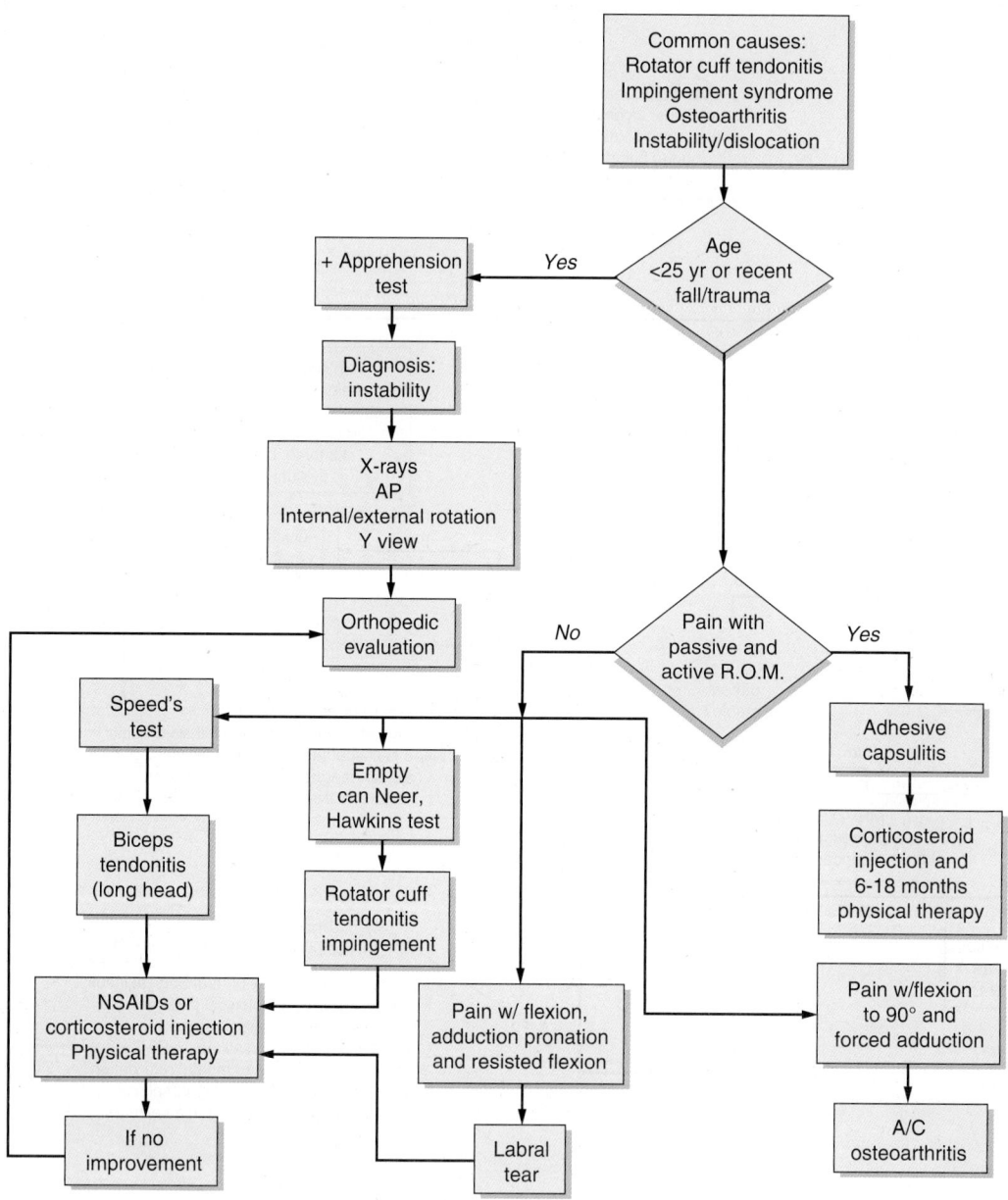

David W. Kruse, MD and Murat Mardirossian, MD

Am Fam Physician. 2000;61:3079–89.

SICKLE CELL ANEMIA, ACUTE COMPLICATIONS

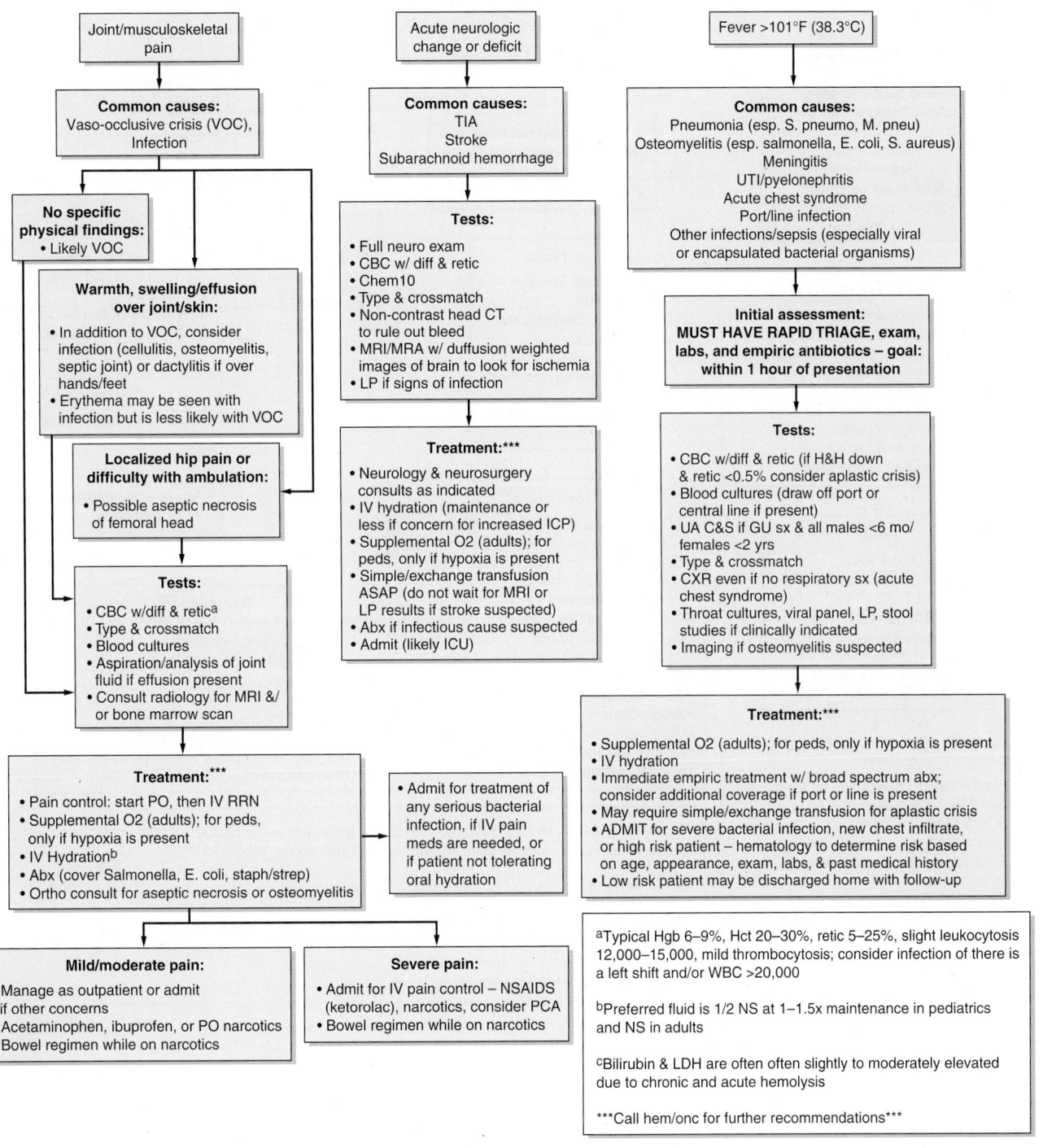

Joint/musculoskeletal pain

Common causes:
Vaso-occlusive crisis (VOC), Infection

No specific physical findings:
• Likely VOC

Warmth, swelling/effusion over joint/skin:
• In addition to VOC, consider infection (cellulitis, osteomyelitis, septic joint) or dactylitis if over hands/feet
• Erythema may be seen with infection but is less likely with VOC

Localized hip pain or difficulty with ambulation:
• Possible aseptic necrosis of femoral head

Tests:
• CBC w/diff & retic[a]
• Type & crossmatch
• Blood cultures
• Aspiration/analysis of joint fluid if effusion present
• Consult radiology for MRI &/ or bone marrow scan

Treatment:***
• Pain control: start PO, then IV RRN
• Supplemental O2 (adults); for peds, only if hypoxia is present
• IV Hydration[b]
• Abx (cover Salmonella, E. coli, staph/strep)
• Ortho consult for aseptic necrosis or osteomyelitis

Mild/moderate pain:
• Manage as outpatient or admit if other concerns
• Acetaminophen, ibuprofen, or PO narcotics
• Bowel regimen while on narcotics

Severe pain:
• Admit for IV pain control – NSAIDS (ketorolac), narcotics, consider PCA
• Bowel regimen while on narcotics

Acute neurologic change or deficit

Common causes:
TIA
Stroke
Subarachnoid hemorrhage

Tests:
• Full neuro exam
• CBC w/ diff & retic
• Chem10
• Type & crossmatch
• Non-contrast head CT to rule out bleed
• MRI/MRA w/ duffusion weighted images of brain to look for ischemia
• LP if signs of infection

Treatment:***
• Neurology & neurosurgery consults as indicated
• IV hydration (maintenance or less if concern for increased ICP)
• Supplemental O2 (adults); for peds, only if hypoxia is present
• Simple/exchange transfusion ASAP (do not wait for MRI or LP results if stroke suspected)
• Abx if infectious cause suspected
• Admit (likely ICU)

• Admit for treatment of any serious bacterial infection, if IV pain meds are needed, or if patient not tolerating oral hydration

Fever >101°F (38.3°C)

Common causes:
Pneumonia (esp. S. pneumo, M. pneu)
Osteomyelitis (esp. salmonella, E. coli, S. aureus)
Meningitis
UTI/pyelonephritis
Acute chest syndrome
Port/line infection
Other infections/sepsis (especially viral or encapsulated bacterial organisms)

Initial assessment:
MUST HAVE RAPID TRIAGE, exam, labs, and empiric antibiotics – goal: within 1 hour of presentation

Tests:
• CBC w/diff & retic (if H&H down & retic <0.5% consider aplastic crisis)
• Blood cultures (draw off port or central line if present)
• UA C&S if GU sx & all males <6 mo/ females <2 yrs
• Type & crossmatch
• CXR even if no respiratory sx (acute chest syndrome)
• Throat cultures, viral panel, LP, stool studies if clinically indicated
• Imaging if osteomyelitis suspected

Treatment:***
• Supplemental O2 (adults); for peds, only if hypoxia is present
• IV hydration
• Immediate empiric treatment w/ broad spectrum abx; consider additional coverage if port or line is present
• May require simple/exchange transfusion for aplastic crisis
• ADMIT for severe bacterial infection, new chest infiltrate, or high risk patient – hematology to determine risk based on age, appearance, exam, labs, & past medical history
• Low risk patient may be discharged home with follow-up

[a]Typical Hgb 6–9%, Hct 20–30%, retic 5–25%, slight leukocytosis 12,000–15,000, mild thrombocytosis; consider infection of there is a left shift and/or WBC >20,000

[b]Preferred fluid is 1/2 NS at 1–1.5x maintenance in pediatrics and NS in adults

[c]Bilirubin & LDH are often often slightly to moderately elevated due to chronic and acute hemolysis

Call hem/onc for further recommendations

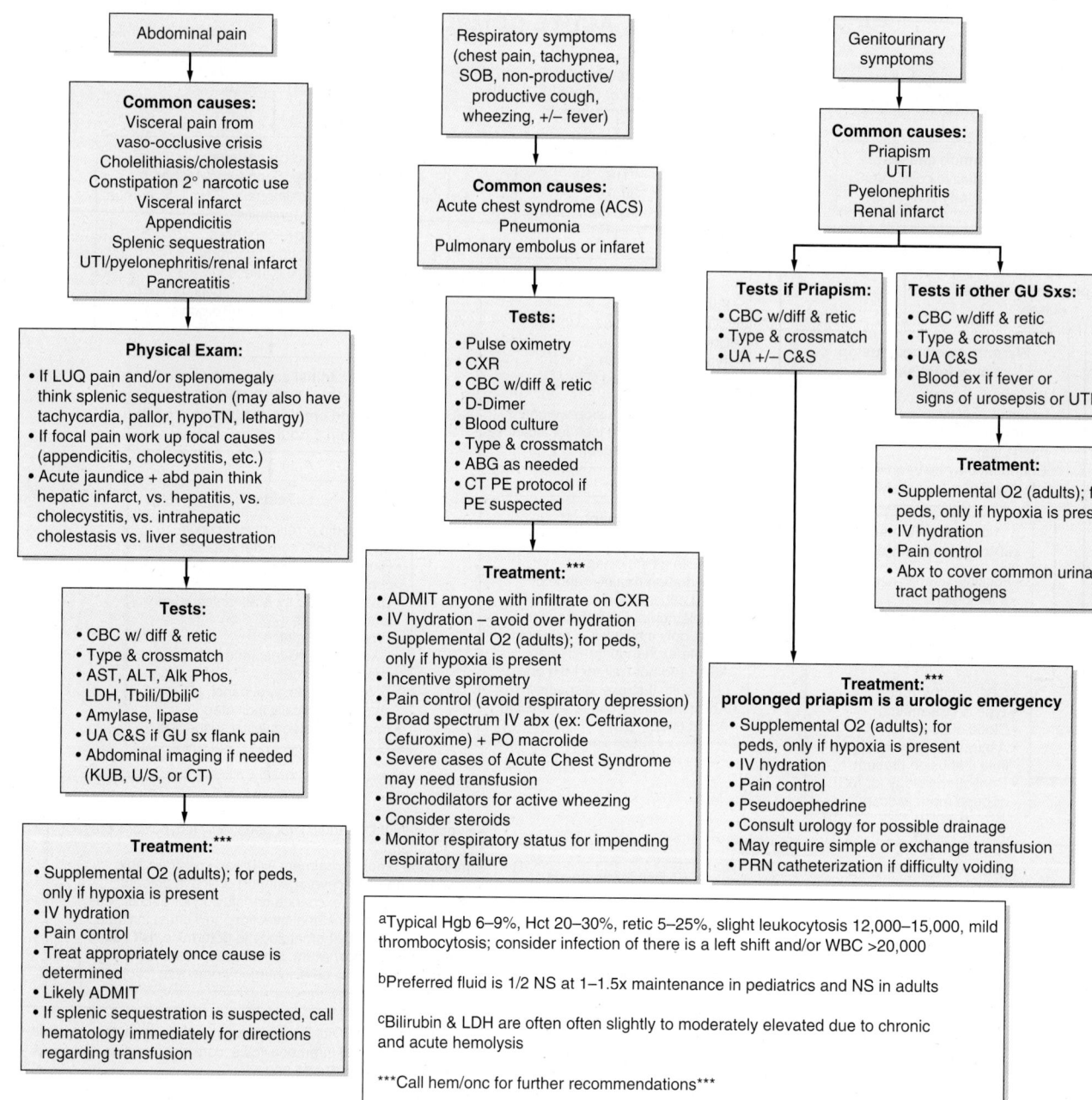

Abdominal pain

Common causes:
Visceral pain from vaso-occlusive crisis
Cholelithiasis/cholestasis
Constipation 2° narcotic use
Visceral infarct
Appendicitis
Splenic sequestration
UTI/pyelonephritis/renal infarct
Pancreatitis

Physical Exam:
- If LUQ pain and/or splenomegaly think splenic sequestration (may also have tachycardia, pallor, hypoTN, lethargy)
- If focal pain work up focal causes (appendicitis, cholecystitis, etc.)
- Acute jaundice + abd pain think hepatic infarct, vs. hepatitis, vs. cholecystitis vs. intrahepatic cholestasis vs. liver sequestration

Tests:
- CBC w/ diff & retic
- Type & crossmatch
- AST, ALT, Alk Phos, LDH, Tbili/Dbili[c]
- Amylase, lipase
- UA C&S if GU sx flank pain
- Abdominal imaging if needed (KUB, U/S, or CT)

Treatment:[***]
- Supplemental O2 (adults); for peds, only if hypoxia is present
- IV hydration
- Pain control
- Treat appropriately once cause is determined
- Likely ADMIT
- If splenic sequestration is suspected, call hematology immediately for directions regarding transfusion

Respiratory symptoms (chest pain, tachypnea, SOB, non-productive/productive cough, wheezing, +/− fever)

Common causes:
Acute chest syndrome (ACS)
Pneumonia
Pulmonary embolus or infaret

Tests:
- Pulse oximetry
- CXR
- CBC w/diff & retic
- D-Dimer
- Blood culture
- Type & crossmatch
- ABG as needed
- CT PE protocol if PE suspected

Treatment:[***]
- ADMIT anyone with infiltrate on CXR
- IV hydration – avoid over hydration
- Supplemental O2 (adults); for peds, only if hypoxia is present
- Incentive spirometry
- Pain control (avoid respiratory depression)
- Broad spectrum IV abx (ex: Ceftriaxone, Cefuroxime) + PO macrolide
- Severe cases of Acute Chest Syndrome may need transfusion
- Brochodilators for active wheezing
- Consider steroids
- Monitor respiratory status for impending respiratory failure

Genitourinary symptoms

Common causes:
Priapism
UTI
Pyelonephritis
Renal infarct

Tests if Priapism:
- CBC w/diff & retic
- Type & crossmatch
- UA +/− C&S

Tests if other GU Sxs:
- CBC w/diff & retic
- Type & crossmatch
- UA C&S
- Blood ex if fever or signs of urosepsis or UTI

Treatment:
- Supplemental O2 (adults); for peds, only if hypoxia is present
- IV hydration
- Pain control
- Abx to cover common urinary tract pathogens

Treatment:[***]
prolonged priapism is a urologic emergency
- Supplemental O2 (adults); for peds, only if hypoxia is present
- IV hydration
- Pain control
- Pseudoephedrine
- Consult urology for possible drainage
- May require simple or exchange transfusion
- PRN catheterization if difficulty voiding

[a]Typical Hgb 6–9%, Hct 20–30%, retic 5–25%, slight leukocytosis 12,000–15,000, mild thrombocytosis; consider infection of there is a left shift and/or WBC >20,000

[b]Preferred fluid is 1/2 NS at 1–1.5x maintenance in pediatrics and NS in adults

[c]Bilirubin & LDH are often often slightly to moderately elevated due to chronic and acute hemolysis

Call hem/onc for further recommendations

Stephanie Ruest, MD, Neil Grossman, MD and Doreen Brettler, MD

http://www.nepscc.org/index.html.

STROKE

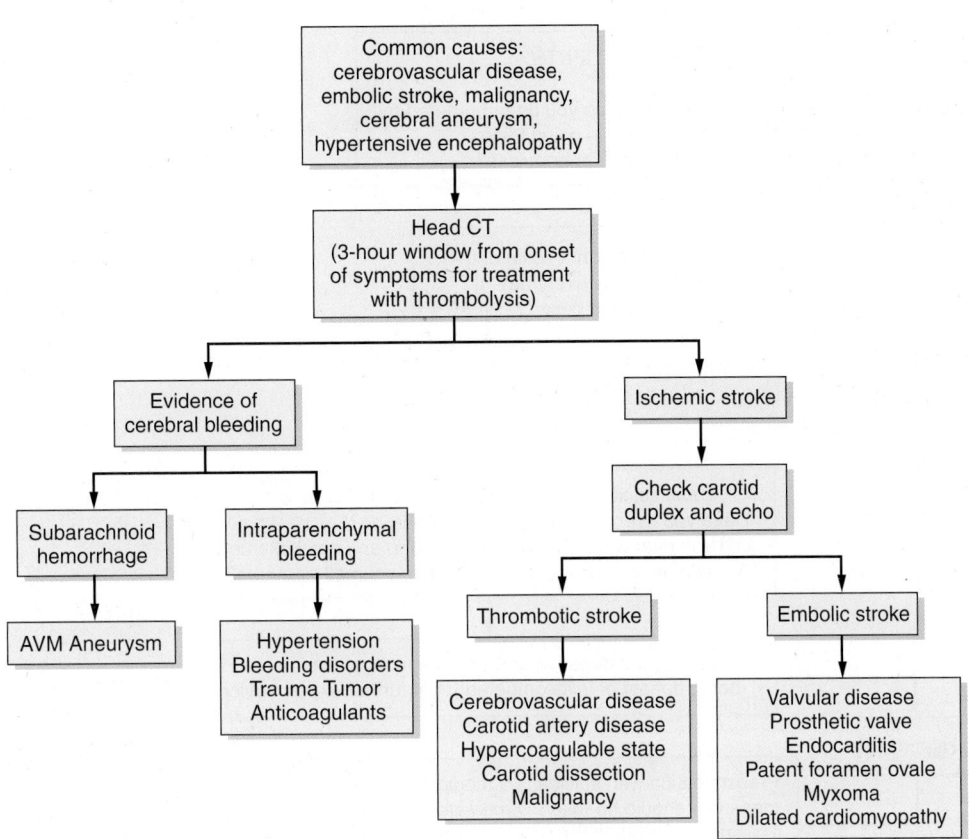

Robert A. Baldor, MD and Alan M. Ehrlich, MD

Stroke. 2007;38:1655–711.

SUICIDE, EVALUATING RISK FOR

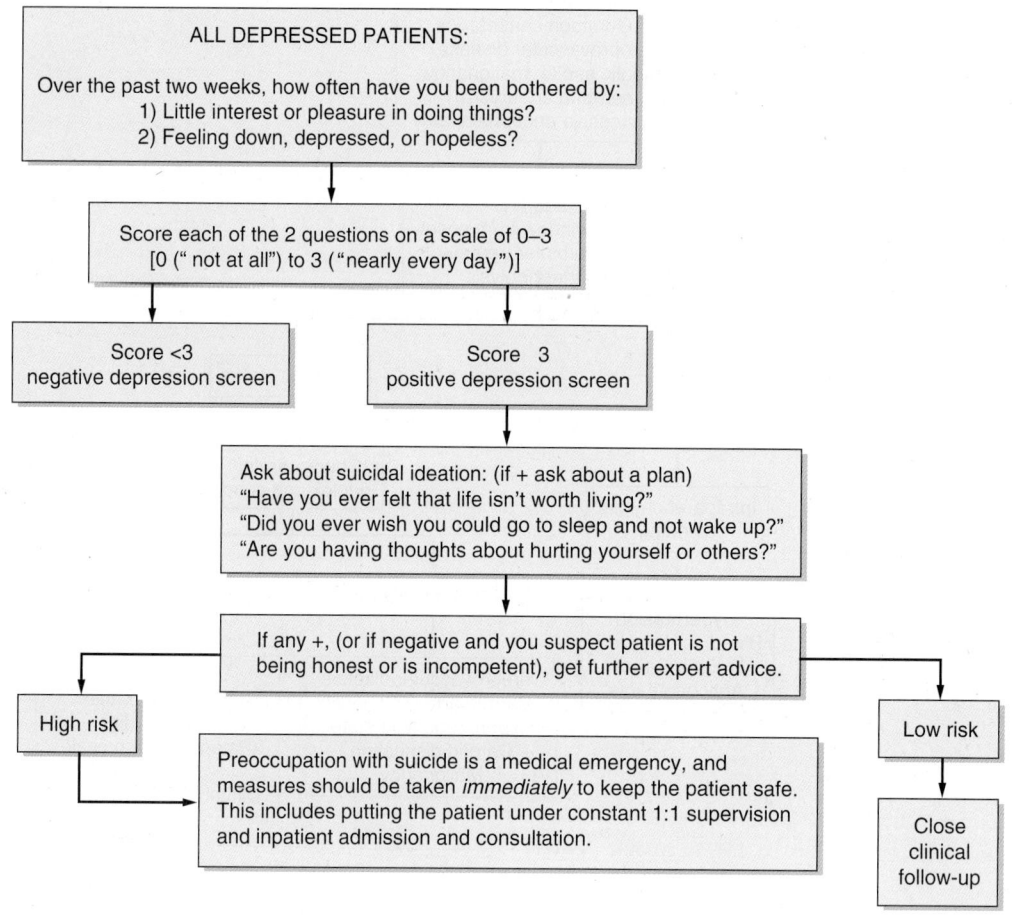

ALL DEPRESSED PATIENTS:

Over the past two weeks, how often have you been bothered by:
1) Little interest or pleasure in doing things?
2) Feeling down, depressed, or hopeless?

Score each of the 2 questions on a scale of 0–3
[0 (" not at all") to 3 ("nearly every day")]

Score <3
negative depression screen

Score 3
positive depression screen

Ask about suicidal ideation: (if + ask about a plan)
"Have you ever felt that life isn't worth living?"
"Did you ever wish you could go to sleep and not wake up?"
"Are you having thoughts about hurting yourself or others?"

If any +, (or if negative and you suspect patient is not
being honest or is incompetent), get further expert advice.

High risk

Preoccupation with suicide is a medical emergency, and
measures should be taken *immediately* to keep the patient safe.
This includes putting the patient under constant 1:1 supervision
and inpatient admission and consultation.

Low risk

Close
clinical
follow-up

Irene C. Coletsos, MD and Harold J. Bursztajn, MD

Am J Psych. 2007;164:1035–43.

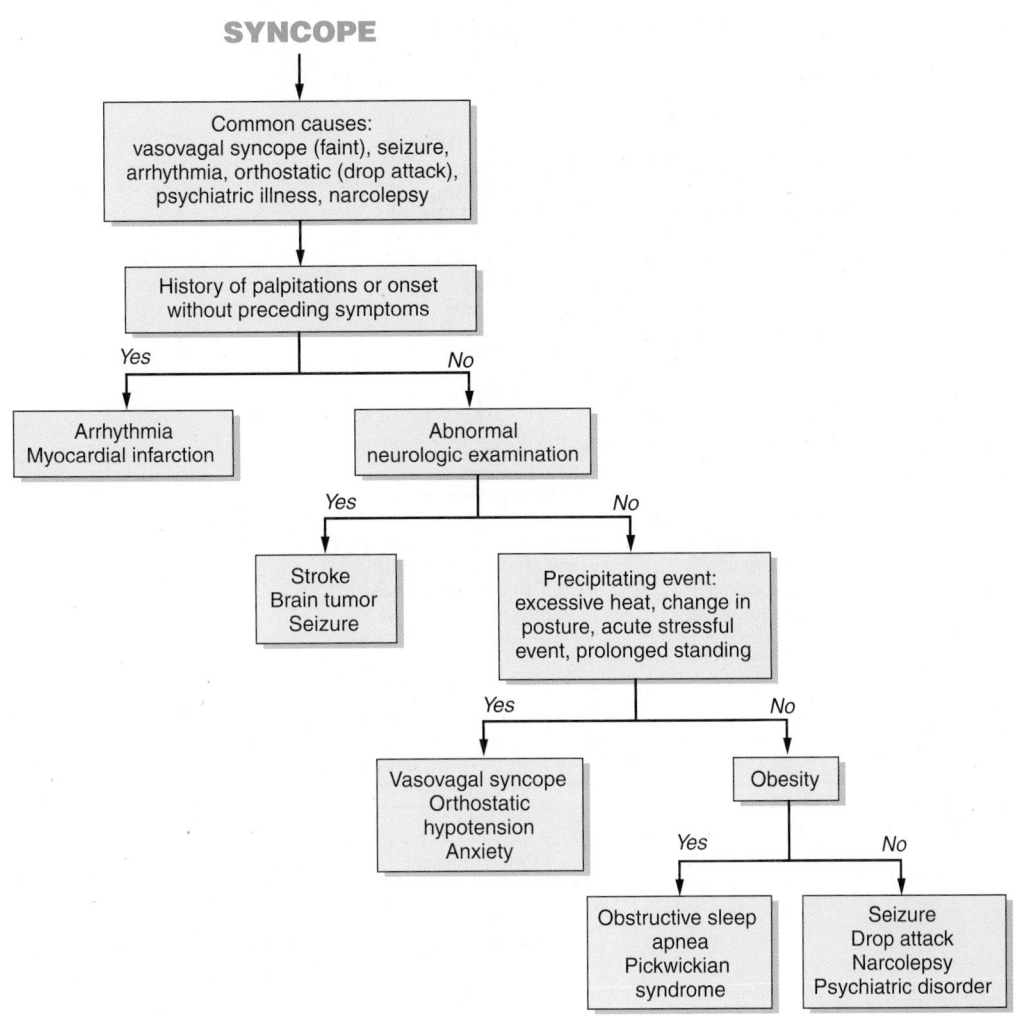

SYNCOPE

Common causes:
vasovagal syncope (faint), seizure,
arrhythmia, orthostatic (drop attack),
psychiatric illness, narcolepsy

History of palpitations or onset
without preceding symptoms

Yes

Arrhythmia
Myocardial infarction

No

Abnormal
neurologic examination

Yes

Stroke
Brain tumor
Seizure

No

Precipitating event:
excessive heat, change in
posture, acute stressful
event, prolonged standing

Yes

Vasovagal syncope
Orthostatic
hypotension
Anxiety

No

Obesity

Yes

Obstructive sleep
apnea
Pickwickian
syndrome

No

Seizure
Drop attack
Narcolepsy
Psychiatric disorder

Robert A. Baldor, MD and Alan M. Ehrlich, MD

Med Clin North Am. 1995;79(5):1153–70.

THROMBOCYTOPENIA

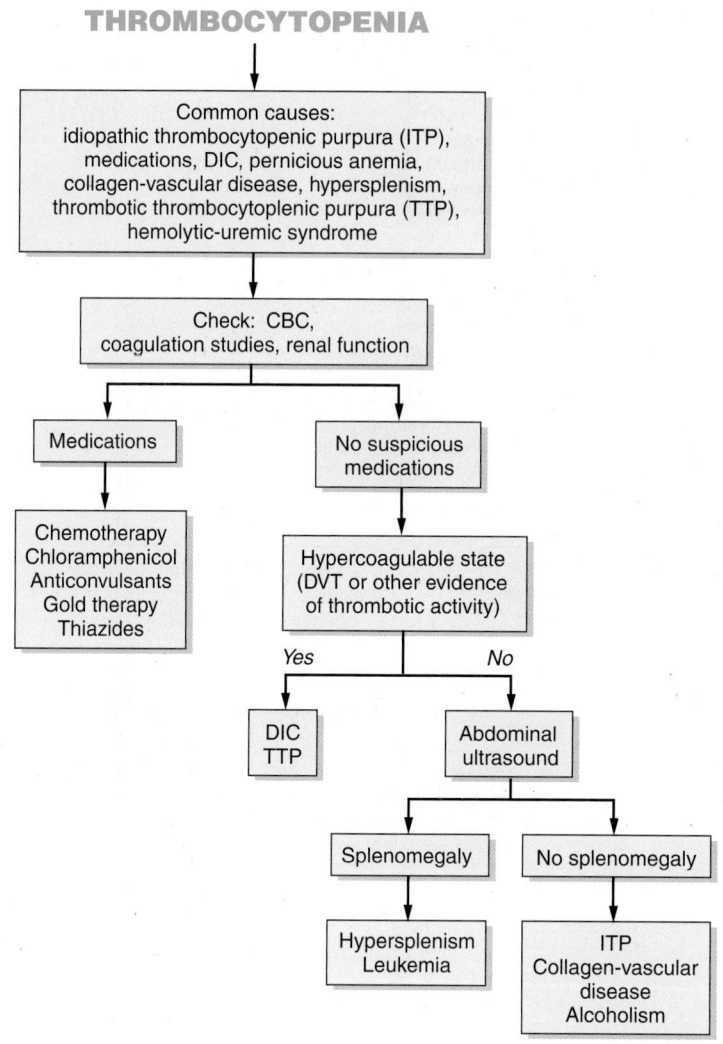

Common causes:
idiopathic thrombocytopenic purpura (ITP),
medications, DIC, pernicious anemia,
collagen-vascular disease, hypersplenism,
thrombotic thrombocytoplenic purpura (TTP),
hemolytic-uremic syndrome

Check: CBC,
coagulation studies, renal function

Medications

No suspicious
medications

Chemotherapy
Chloramphenicol
Anticonvulsants
Gold therapy
Thiazides

Hypercoagulable state
(DVT or other evidence
of thrombotic activity)

Yes   No

DIC
TTP

Abdominal
ultrasound

Splenomegaly

No splenomegaly

Hypersplenism
Leukemia

ITP
Collagen-vascular
disease
Alcoholism

Robert A. Baldor, MD and Alan M. Ehrlich, MD

Blood. 2005;106(7):2244–51.

TRANSIENT ISCHEMIC ATTACK AND TRANSIENT NEUROLOGIC DEFICIT

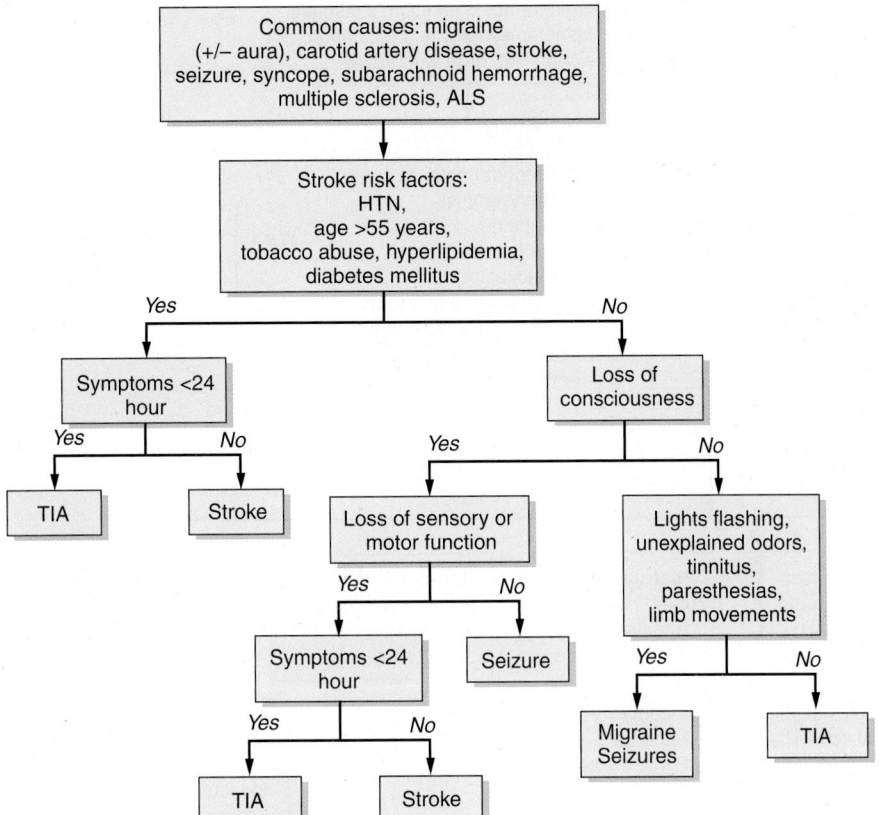

Robert A. Baldor, MD and Alan M. Ehrlich, MD

Am Fam Physician. 2004;69:1665–74, 1679–81.

TREMOR

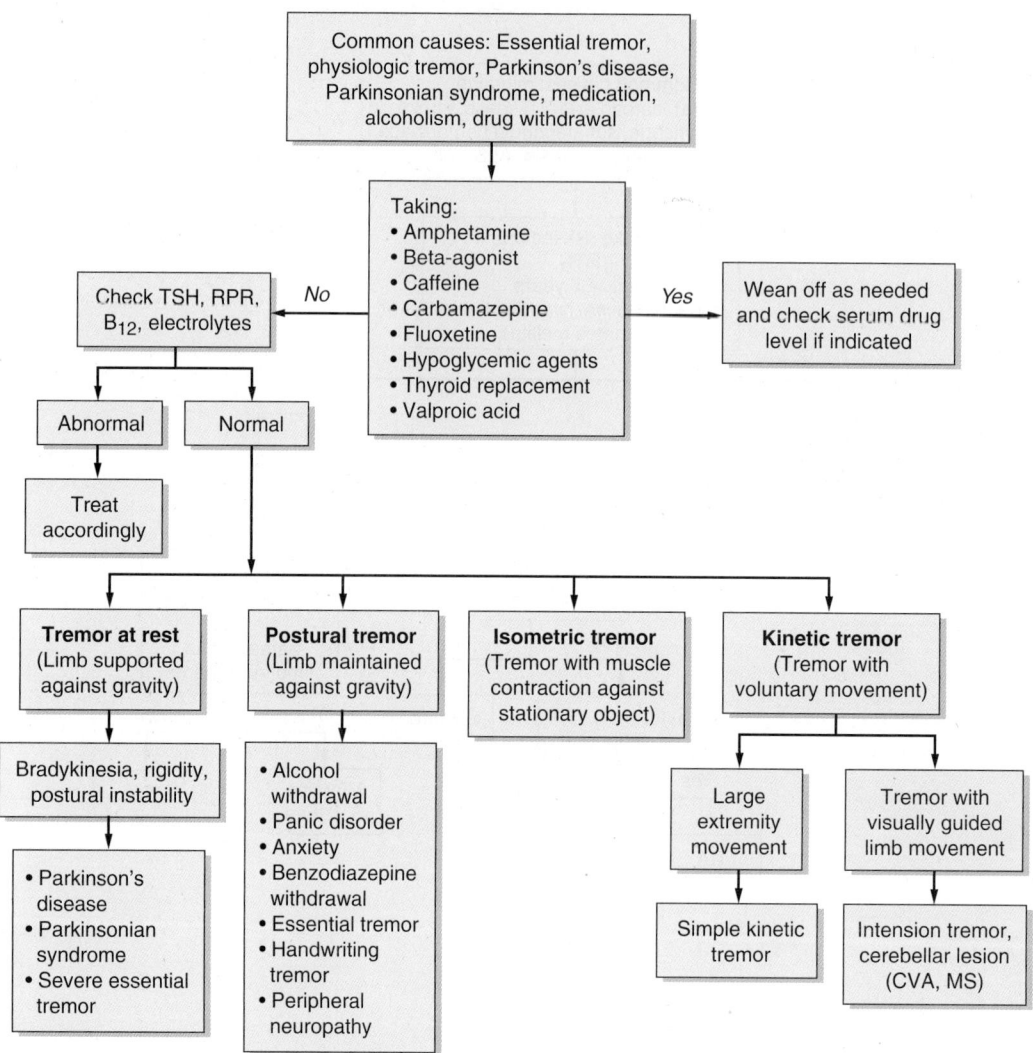

Common causes: Essential tremor, physiologic tremor, Parkinson's disease, Parkinsonian syndrome, medication, alcoholism, drug withdrawal

Taking:
- Amphetamine
- Beta-agonist
- Caffeine
- Carbamazepine
- Fluoxetine
- Hypoglycemic agents
- Thyroid replacement
- Valproic acid

Yes → Wean off as needed and check serum drug level if indicated

No → Check TSH, RPR, B_{12}, electrolytes

Abnormal → Treat accordingly

Normal

Tremor at rest (Limb supported against gravity)

Bradykinesia, rigidity, postural instability
- Parkinson's disease
- Parkinsonian syndrome
- Severe essential tremor

Postural tremor (Limb maintained against gravity)
- Alcohol withdrawal
- Panic disorder
- Anxiety
- Benzodiazepine withdrawal
- Essential tremor
- Handwriting tremor
- Peripheral neuropathy

Isometric tremor (Tremor with muscle contraction against stationary object)

Kinetic tremor (Tremor with voluntary movement)

Large extremity movement → Simple kinetic tremor

Tremor with visually guided limb movement → Intension tremor, cerebellar lesion (CVA, MS)

Andrew J. Westwood, MD

Am Fam Physician. 2003;68(8):1545–52.

UREMIA

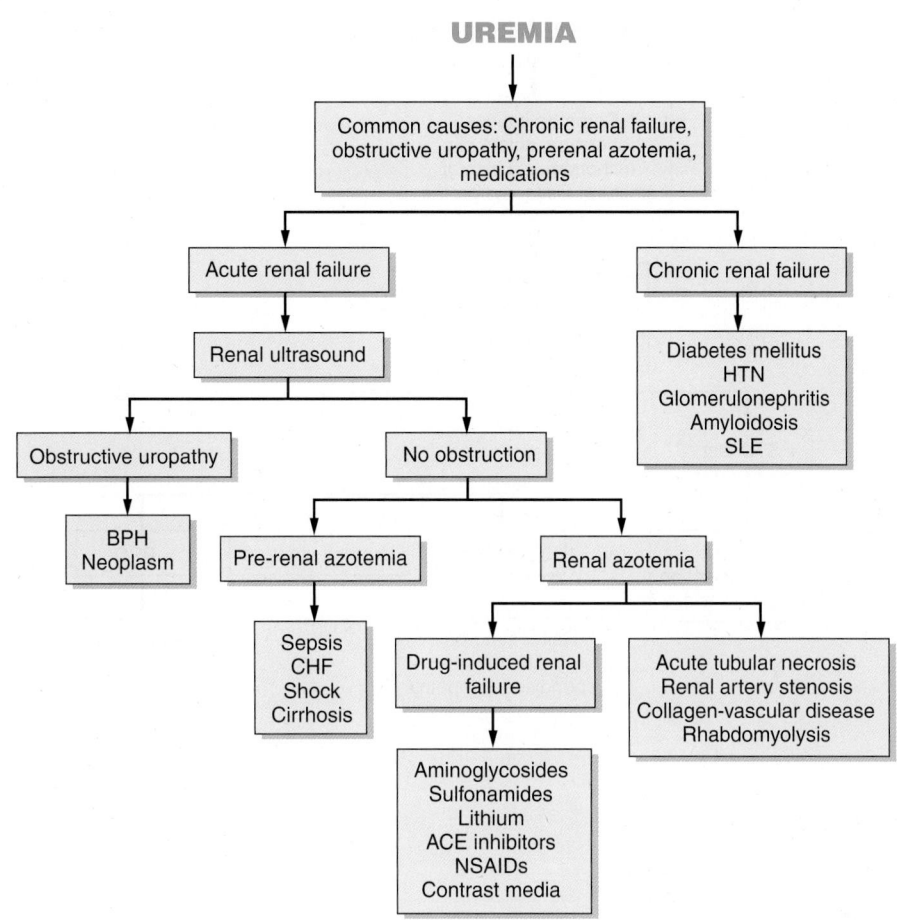

Common causes: Chronic renal failure, obstructive uropathy, prerenal azotemia, medications

Acute renal failure

Chronic renal failure

Diabetes mellitus
HTN
Glomerulonephritis
Amyloidosis
SLE

Renal ultrasound

Obstructive uropathy

No obstruction

BPH
Neoplasm

Pre-renal azotemia

Renal azotemia

Sepsis
CHF
Shock
Cirrhosis

Drug-induced renal failure

Acute tubular necrosis
Renal artery stenosis
Collagen-vascular disease
Rhabdomyolysis

Aminoglycosides
Sulfonamides
Lithium
ACE inhibitors
NSAIDs
Contrast media

Robert A. Baldor, MD and Alan M. Ehrlich, MD

Diagnosis and management of adults with chronic kidney disease.
Michigan Quality Improvement Consortium - Professional Association.
2006 Nov (revised 2008 Nov). 1 page. NGC:007054.

URETHRAL DISCHARGE

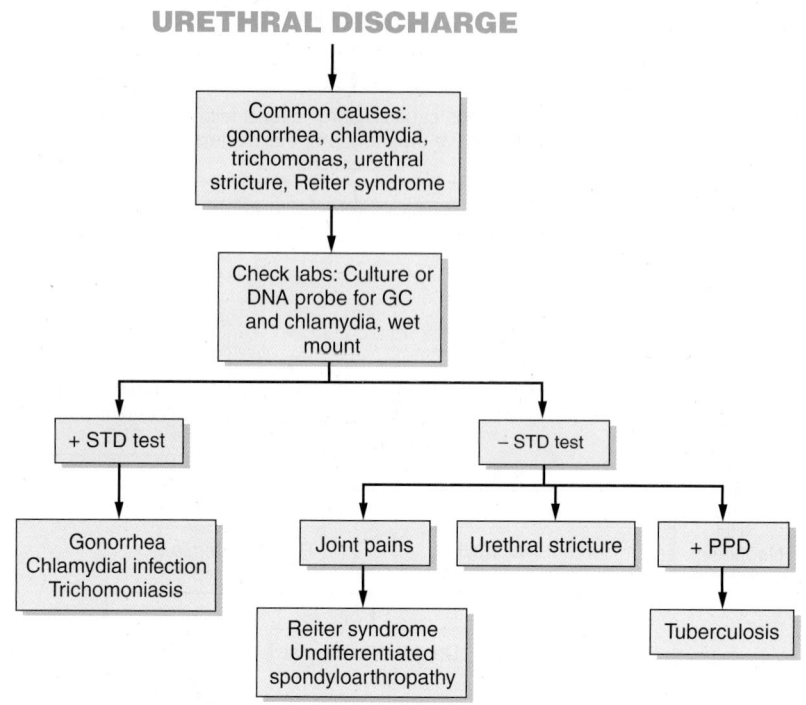

Robert A. Baldor, MD and Alan M. Ehrlich, MD

Sex Transm Infect. 1998;74(Suppl 1):S29–33.

VAGINAL BLEEDING DYSFUNCTIONAL

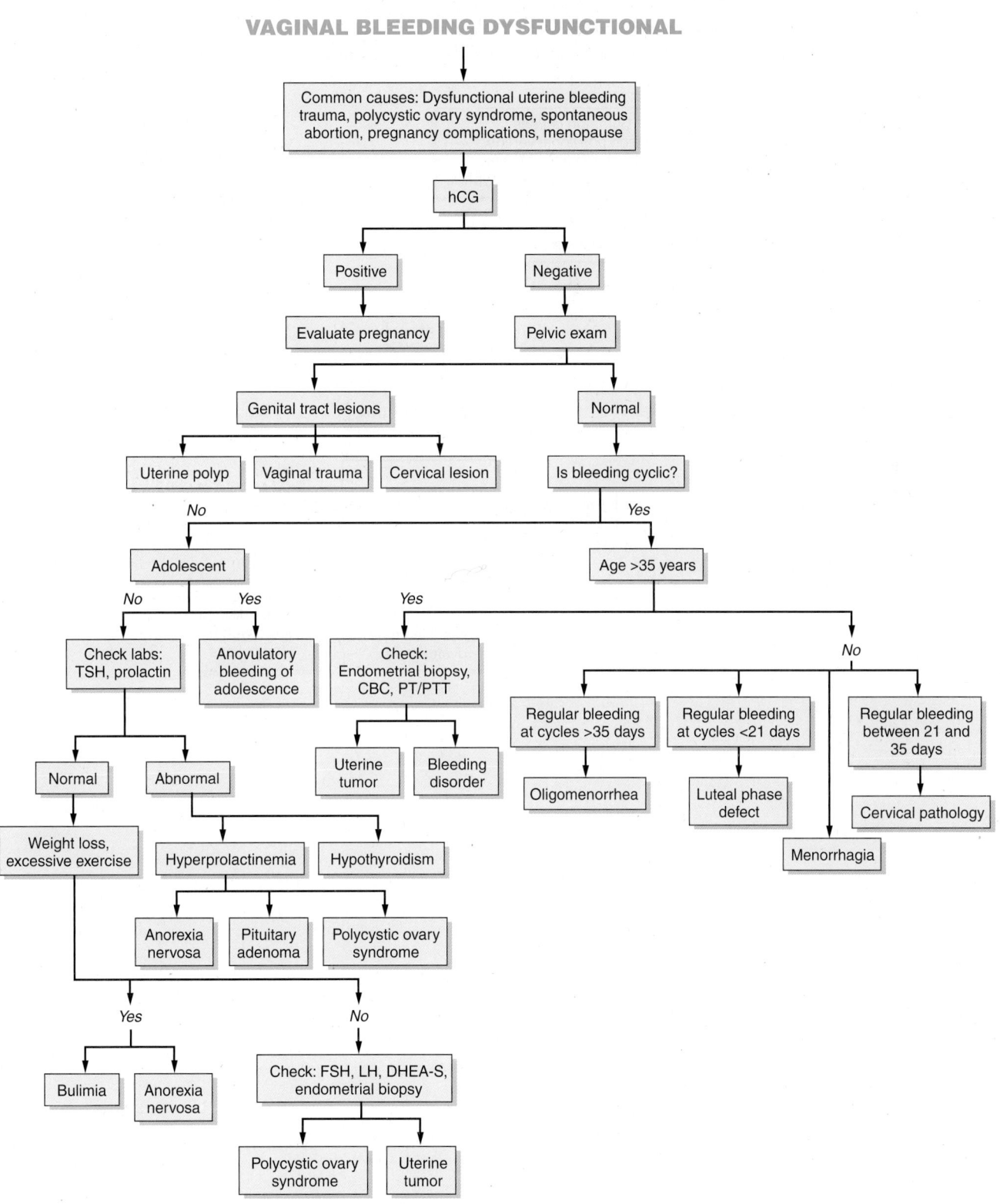

Robert A. Baldor, MD and Alan M. Ehrlich, MD

Am Fam Physician. 2004;69:1915–26;1931–3.

VERTIGO (SYMPTOM OF MOVEMENT DUE TO ACUTE VESTIBULAR DYSFUNCTION)

```
                    ↓
        ┌─────────────────────────────┐
        │      Common causes:         │
        │   benign positional vertigo,│
        │   acutel abyrinthitis, Ménière│
        │ disease, medications, neurosyphilis│
        └─────────────────────────────┘
                    ↓
              ┌───────────┐
              │ Nystagmus │
              └───────────┘
              ┌─────┴──────────────────┐
              ↓                        ↓
        ┌───────────┐          ┌──────────────┐
        │ Sustained │          │ Brief or none│
        └───────────┘          └──────────────┘
              ↓                        ↓
       ┌──────────────┐     ┌─────────────────────────┐
       │ Central lesion│     │   Vertigo is brief or   │
       └──────────────┘     │ + Dix-Hallpike maneuver │
                            └─────────────────────────┘
                          Yes                      No
                           ↓                        ↓
                 ┌──────────────────┐        ┌───────────┐
                 │ Benign positional│        │ Recent URI│
                 │     vertigo      │        └───────────┘
                 └──────────────────┘      Yes            No
                                            ↓              ↓
                              ┌──────────────────────┐ ┌──────────────┐
                              │ Vestibular neuronitis│ │    Stroke    │
                              │  (acute labyrinthitis)│ │Ménière disease│
                              │   Eustachian tube    │ │ Neurosyphilis│
                              │     dysfunction      │ │  Medications │
                              └──────────────────────┘ └──────────────┘
```

Robert A. Baldor, MD and Alan M. Ehrlich, MD

Am Fam Physician. 2006;73:244–51, 255.

WEIGHT LOSS

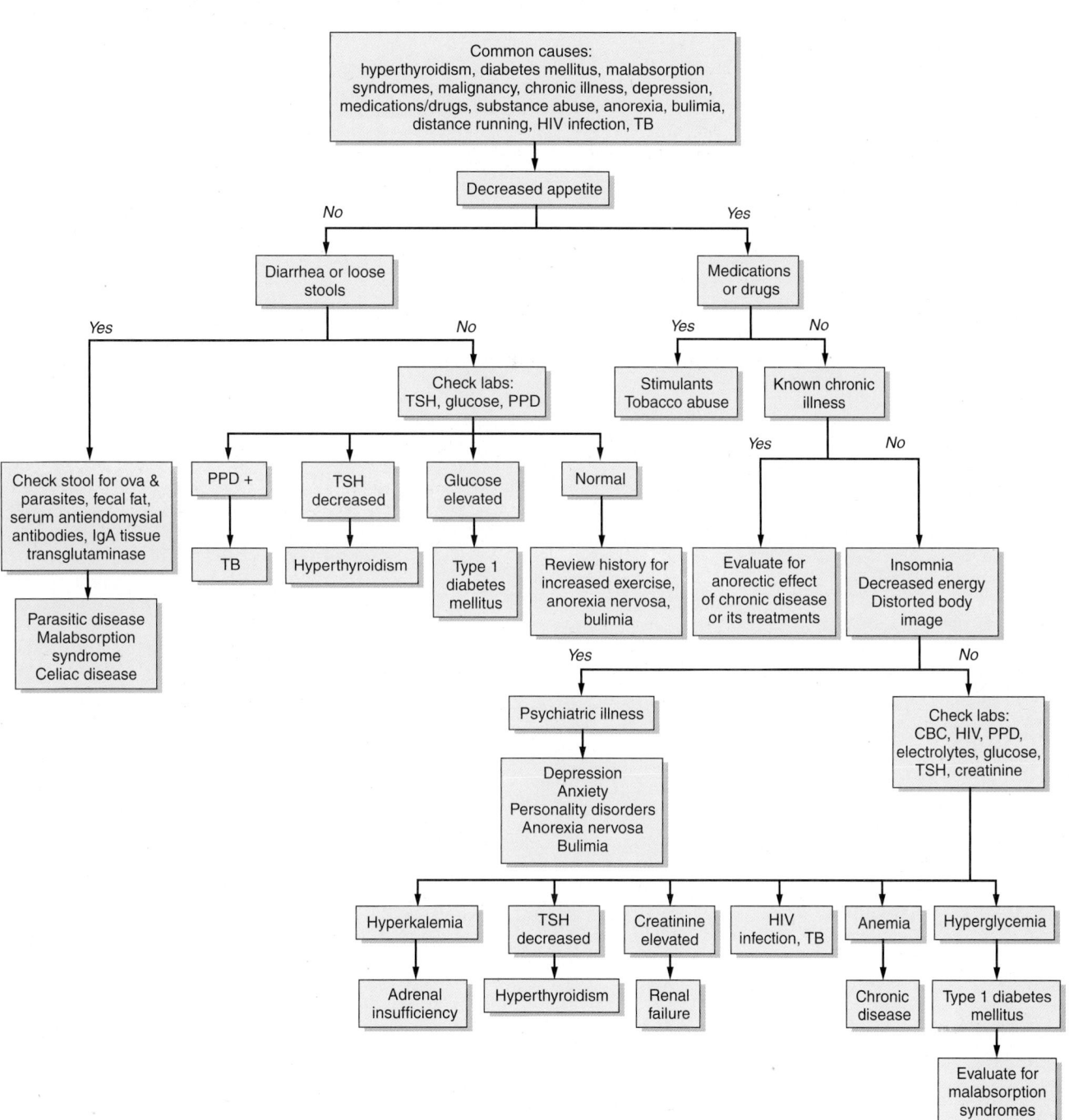

Robert A. Baldor, MD and Alan M. Ehrlich, MD

Am Fam Physician. 2002;65:640–51.

The 5-Minute Clinical Consult

2012

20TH EDITION

ABNORMAL PAP AND CERVICAL DYSPLASIA

Jeremy Golding, MD
Patricia Seymour, MD

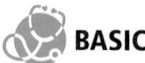

BASICS

DESCRIPTION
Cervical dysplasia: Precancerous epithelial changes in the transformation zone of the uterine cervix almost always associated with human papillomavirus (HPV) infections:

- Mild dysplasia (cervical intraepithelial neoplasia [CIN] I): Cellular changes are limited to the lower 1/3 of the squamous epithelium.
- Moderate dysplasia (CIN II): Cellular changes are limited to the lower 2/3 of the squamous epithelium.
- Severe dysplasia (CIN III or carcinoma in situ): Cellular changes involve the full thickness of the squamous epithelium.
- Pap smear:
  – Screening test for cervical cellular pathology. In many laboratories, automated cervical screening complements the Pap smear or supersedes it.
  – Abnormal cervical smear results can range from benign cellular changes to suggestion of invasive cancer.
- System(s) affected: Reproductive

ALERT
Cervical cancer arises from HPV, which is a sexually acquired disease. Good evidence that screening for cervical cancer with Pap smears reduces incidence of and mortality from cervical cancer (1)[A].

Geriatric Considerations
Natural progression of cervical dysplasia involves acquisition of HPV at or after first coitus with a small percentage of lesions progressing. See guidelines below.

Pregnancy Considerations
- Squamous intraepithelial lesions can progress during pregnancy, but often regress postpartum.
- Colposcopy only to rule out invasive cancer in high-risk women (2)

EPIDEMIOLOGY
- Predominant age: Can occur at any age
- Incidence of CIN III peaks between ages 25 and 29; invasive disease peaks 15 years later.

Incidence
- Low-grade squamous intraepithelial lesion ranges from 2–3% of all Pap smears.
- High-grade squamous intraepithelial lesion and invasive cancer present on 1% of Pap smears.
- Other reactive, reparative, and ASC-US (atypical squamous cells of undetermined significance) results are difficult to assess because of the lack of reporting mechanisms.

Prevalence
26.8% of women are HPV-positive.

RISK FACTORS
- Cigarette smoking
- Possible deficiency of antioxidants
- Early age at first coitus
- Multiple sexual partners
- Some correlation to low socioeconomic level
- Intercourse with a high-risk male partner
- HPV infection
- Immunosuppression

GENERAL PREVENTION
- HPV immunization of girls and women prior to first intercourse (e.g., Gardasil) 3 doses (0, 2, 6 months) (3)[C] reduces dysplasia due to covered and related HPV strains; long-term effect on cancer as yet uncertain. Role of immunization of boys and men not yet established.
- Delay first intercourse beyond early adolescence
- Monogamous relationship for both partners
- Smoking cessation
- Adequate antioxidant-rich food intake has been associated with decreased risk
- Obtain routine Pap smears (see guidelines below)
- Use barrier methods of birth control if in nonmonogamous relationship (likely decreases but does not eliminate HPV transmission)
- Screening guidelines:
  – Screening indicated for woman beginning at age 21
  – Frequency of screening recommendations vary:
    ○ United States Preventive Services Task Force: Every 3 years
    ○ American Cancer Society/American Congress of Obstetricians and Gynecologists: Every 2 years until age 30 then every 3 years if normal
    ○ May be beneficial to do combined cellular screening (Pap) and high-risk HPV test in women >age 30. If normal cytology and high-risk HPV negative, screening should be repeated in no less than 3 years. If cytology is normal but HPV is positive, repeat BOTH cytology and HPV in 1 year, and if HPV remains positive (or if abnormal cytology), proceed to colposcopy (2,4).
- Screen until age 65–70. May discontinue if 3 or more consecutive, satisfactory normal or negative smears, no abnormal smears in past 10 years, or until total hysterectomy for benign conditions (1,5)

PATHOPHYSIOLOGY
- HPV DNA is found in virtually all cervical carcinomas and precursor lesions worldwide.
- HPV viral types 16, 18, 31, 35, 45, 51, 52, 56, and 58 are common high-risk or oncogenic virus types for cervical cancer.
- HPV viral types 6, 11, 42, 43, and 44 are considered common low-risk types, and may cause genital warts.

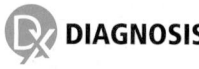

DIAGNOSIS

Frequently no symptoms

HISTORY
- Occasionally vaginal discharge related to sexually transmitted disease
- Rarely vaginal bleeding

PHYSICAL EXAM
Pelvic exam occasionally reveals external HPV lesions.

DIAGNOSTIC TESTS & INTERPRETATION
- ThinPrep is a fluid-based collection and thin-layer preparation for cervical cancer screening.
- Sensitivity of a single Pap smear for HSIL ~70%; specificity of ~90%

Lab
- Bethesda system for reporting Pap/cervical smear results (*cytologic grading*) (6)
- Specimen adequacy
- Presence of endocervical cells:
  – Negative for intraepithelial lesion or malignancy
  – Epithelial cell abnormalities:
    ○ ASC: Atypical squamous cells
    ○ ASC-US: ASC of undetermined significance
    ○ ASC-H: Atypical cells cannot exclude high-grade squamous intraepithelial lesion (SIL)
    ○ LSIL: Low-grade SIL (combines mild dysplasia (CIN I) with HPV)
    ○ HSIL: High-grade SIL (combines CIN II and III)
    ○ Squamous cell carcinoma
    ○ Glandular cells
    ○ AGC: Atypical glandular cells
    ○ AGCs of undetermined significance
    ○ Atypical glandular cells, favor neoplasia
    ○ Endocervical adenocarcinoma in situ
    ○ Adenocarcinoma

Diagnostic Procedures/Surgery
- Colposcopy with or without biopsy recommended for the following (2) (and see algorithms):
  – Initial Pap smear with LSIL (exception for adolescent, although screening of adolescents no longer recommended), HSIL; ASCUS that is + for high-risk HPV types on (reflex) HPV hybrid capture 2 test.
  – ASC-US present on 2 Pap smears 6 months apart if HPV testing not available
  – ASC-H needs colposcopic evaluation.
  – Any abnormal or suspicious lesion of the cervix or vagina that is visualized by the eye
  – Atypical glandular cells (mandate colposcopy and uterine sampling)
- HPV viral typing:
  – Hybrid capture 2 test has 2 viral type probes: a low-risk probe and a high-risk probe.
  – High-risk (HR) probe can be used to identify patients with ASC-US who need colposcopy follow-up.

– HPV typing may be used in combination with Pap smear for women ≥30.

  ○ Low-risk women with negative cytology and who are negative for high-risk HPV may be followed every 3 years.

  ○ Women with negative cytology but positive (HR) probe may be approached with 1 of 2 strategies (optimal strategy uncertain): Repeat Pap and HPV in 1 year. If either Pap abnormal or HPV HR positive, then colposcopy. Order an HPV 16/18-specific probe on cytology fluid. If either probe for 16 or 18 is positive, evidence suggests the risk of a high-grade lesion is still similar to the risk for ASCUS/HPV+, and colposcopy is recommended. If HPV 16 and 18 are negative with a negative Pap and a high-risk HPV screen positive, the risk of a high-grade lesion is about 15-fold less, and repeat Pap plus HPV screen in 1 year is recommended. At 1 year, if either the Pap or the HPV test is NOT negative, then colposcopy is recommended.

– Little utility for low-risk viral type screening

• Loop electrosurgical excision procedure (LEEP):
  – "See and treat" for HSIL in nonadolescent age groups acceptable, but not for adolescents (as they should no longer be screened).

• Cone biopsy

• Cervicography: Photographic evaluation of cervix

Pathological Findings

• Atypical squamous or columnar cells
• Coarse nuclear material
• Increased nuclear diameter
• Koilocytosis (HPV hallmark)

DIFFERENTIAL DIAGNOSIS

• Acute or chronic cervicitis
• Cervical squamous intraepithelial neoplasia
• Cervical glandular neoplasia
• Invasive cervical malignancy
• Uterine malignancy (rare)

TREATMENT

Evidence-based management algorithms guide Pap smear and post-colposcopic diagnostics and therapeutics (2,4).

MEDICATION

• Infective/reactive Pap smear:
  – Metronidazole 250 mg t.i.d. p.o. for 7 days
• Condyloma acuminatum:
  – Cryotherapy
  – Podophyllin topically q1–2wk
  – Trichloroacetic acid, applied topically by a physician and covered for 5–6 days

ADDITIONAL TREATMENT

General Measures

• Office evaluation and observation
• Promote smoking cessation.
• Promote protected intercourse.

SURGERY/OTHER PROCEDURES

• LSILs and HSILs and carcinoma in situ can be treated with outpatient surgery:
  – Cryotherapy, laser ablation, LEEP/large loop excision of transition zone, or cold-knife conization all effective, but requiring different training and with different side effects for patient
• If cervical malignancy, see Cervical Malignancy.

ONGOING CARE

FOLLOW-UP RECOMMENDATIONS

• LSIL/CIN1: Observation with Pap smear repeated every 6 months or high-risk HPV testing every year is appropriate for young women with LSIL, especially with confirmed CIN I.
• HPV-related CIN I typically resolves within 2–3 years.
• LSIL persisting beyond 2–3 years in a young woman is indication for colposcopy

DIET

Promote increased intake of antioxidant-rich foods.

PATIENT EDUCATION

• Promote HPV immunization.
• Promote smoking cessation.
• Promote protected intercourse.
• Promote regular Pap smears according to recognized guidelines.
• Reschedule follow-up consultation for any abnormality.

PROGNOSIS

• Generally excellent
• <50% of persistent infective, reactive, reparative, or ASC-US Pap/cervical smears will have more advanced lesions.
• Only a small percentage of LSILs will progress to more advanced lesion (80% or more of adolescent and young adult CIN I resolves in 2–3 years).
• Lesions discovered early are amenable to treatment, with excellent results and few recurrences.

COMPLICATIONS

• Minor abnormalities on Pap/cervical smears can mask more advanced lesions.
• HSIL does progress to invasive cancer. Best estimate of risk of CIN III progression to invasive cervical cancer is >50% (7).
• Aggressive cervical surgery may be associated with cervical stenosis, cervical incompetence, and scarring affecting cervical dilatation in labor.

REFERENCES

1. Guide to Clinical Preventive Services: Report of the US Preventive Services Task Force 2003. Accessed 4/22/2009 at www.ahrq.gov/clinic/3rduspstf/cervcan/cervcanrr.htm
2. Wright TC Jr, et al. 2006 Consensus Guidelines for the management of women with abnormal cervical cancer screening tests. *AJOG* 2007;346–56. Accessed 4/22/2009 at http://www.asccp.org/consensus.shtml.
3. Markowitz LE, Dunne EF, Saraiya M et al. Quadrivalent Human Papillomavirus Vaccine: Recommendations of the Advisory Committee on Immunization Practices (ACIP). *MMWR Recomm Rep*. 2007;56:1–24.
4. ICSI. Management of abnormal pap smear 2008. Accessed 4/22/2009 at http://guidelines.gov/summary/summary.aspx?doc_id=13311&nbr=006755&string=ICSI+AND+abnormal+AND+pap
5. Saslow D, Runowicz CD, Solomon D et al. American Cancer Society guideline for the early detection of cervical neoplasia and cancer. *CA Cancer J Clin*. 2002;52:342–62.
6. Solomon D, Davey D, Kurman R et al. The 2001 Bethesda System: terminology for reporting results of cervical cytology. *JAMA*. 2002;287:2114–9.
7. McCredie MR, Sharples KJ, Paul C et al. Natural history of cervical neoplasia and risk of invasive cancer in women with cervical intraepithelial neoplasia 3: a retrospective cohort study. *The Lancet Oncology* 2008;5(9):425–434.

ADDITIONAL READING

Dunne EF, Unger ER, Sternberg M et al. Prevalence of HPV infection among females in the United States. *JAMA*. 2007;297:813–9.

See Also (Topic, Algorithm, Electronic Media Element)

Cervical Malignancy; Condyloma Acuminata; Failure to Thrive; Trichomoniasis; Vulvovaginitis, Prepubescent Algorithm: Abnormal Pap Smear in Adolescents, Pap smear in Women age 20–30, Pap Smear in Women >30 years of age

CODES

ICD9

• 622.10 Dysplasia of cervix, unspecified
• 622.11 Mild dysplasia of cervix
• 622.12 Moderate dysplasia of cervix

CLINICAL PEARLS

• A connection exists between HPV infection and abnormal Pap smears. HPV was defined as a "carcinogen" by World Health Organization in 1996. HPV is present in virtually all cervical cancers (99.7%).
• No evidence suggests that offering HPV immunization increases the likelihood of early sexual intercourse and acquisition of sexually transmitted infections.
• Preliminary data suggest that vaccine is much less effective for prevention of cervical dysplasia if offered after women are infected with HPV, and no effect on regression of existing CIN has been seen thus far in trials. Vaccine should therefore be offered prior to onset of any sexual activity (even nonintercourse activity) for maximum effectiveness.

ABORTION, SPONTANEOUS (MISCARRIAGE)

Elizabeth W. Patton, MD
Patricia K. Aronson, MD

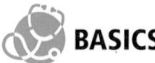 **BASICS**

DESCRIPTION
- Separation of products of conception from the uterus prior to the potential for fetal survival outside the uterus
- Spontaneous abortion (SAb):
  - Expulsion or extraction from the uterus of an embryo or fetus weighing ≤500 g
- Threatened abortion:
  - Vaginal bleeding early in pregnancy without dilatation of the cervix, rupture of the membranes, or expulsion of products of conception
- Inevitable abortion:
  - Cervical dilatation, rupture of membranes, or expulsion of products in the presence of vaginal bleeding
- Complete abortion:
  - Entire contents of uterus expelled; common before 12 weeks' gestation
- Incomplete abortion:
  - Abortion with retained products of conception, generally placental tissue; more common after 12 weeks' gestation
- Missed abortion:
  - In utero death of embryo/fetus prior to 20 weeks' gestation; products of conception retained
- Induced abortion:
  - Evacuation of uterine contents or products of conception medically or surgically
- Septic abortion:
  - Common complication of illegally performed induced abortions; a spontaneous or therapeutic abortion complicated by pelvic infection
- Habitual spontaneous abortion:
  - 2 or more consecutive pregnancy losses at <15 weeks' gestation
- Synonym(s): Miscarriage; Habitual abortion; Recurrent abortion; Involuntary pregnancy loss

EPIDEMIOLOGY
Predominant age: Increases with advancing age, especially >35 years; at age 40, the loss rate is twice that of age 20

Prevalence
- ~8–20% of all clinically recognized pregnancies end in spontaneous abortion, 80% of these in the first 12 weeks.
- When both clinical and biochemical (B-HCG detected) pregnancies are considered, up to 50% of pregnancies end in spontaneous abortion.

RISK FACTORS
Most cases of spontaneous abortion occur in patients without identifiable risk factors; however, risk factors listed in order of importance include:
- Chromosomal abnormalities
- Advancing maternal age
- Uterine abnormalities
- Maternal chronic disease (diabetes mellitus, polycystic ovarian syndrome, systemic lupus erythematosus, hypertension, antiphospholipid antibodies, thyroid disease, renal disease)
- Other possible contributing factors include smoking, alcohol, infection, and luteal phase defect, although conclusive data are currently lacking.

Genetics
~50–65% of 1st-trimester spontaneous abortions have significant chromosomal anomalies, with 1/2 of these being autosomal trisomies and the remainder being triploidy, tetraploidy, or 45X monosomies.

GENERAL PREVENTION
- Progestogens: Currently, there is no evidence that routine use of oral or IM progestogens prevents miscarriage in early to mid-pregnancy. However, there is some evidence that women with a history of recurrent miscarriage may benefit from this type of treatment (1)[A].
- Immunotherapy: No current evidence to support use of immunotherapy in patients with a history of recurrent miscarriage (2)[A]

ETIOLOGY
- Chromosomal anomalies
- Congenital anomalies
- Trauma
- Maternal factors: Uterine abnormalities, infection (toxoplasma, other viruses, rubella, cytomegalovirus, herpesvirus), maternal endocrine disorders, hypercoagulable state

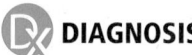 **DIAGNOSIS**

HISTORY
- Consider any reproductive-age woman with vaginal bleeding to be pregnant until proven otherwise.
- Vaginal bleeding:
  - Characteristics (amount, color, consistency, associated symptoms), onset (abrupt or gradual), duration, intensity/quantity, and exacerbating/precipitating factors
- Abdominal pain/uterine cramping
- Rupture of membranes
- Passage of products of conception
- Prenatal course: Toxic or infectious exposures, family or personal history of genetic abnormalities, past history of ectopic pregnancy or spontaneous abortion, endocrine disease, autoimmune disorder, bleeding/clotting disorder

PHYSICAL EXAM
- Any pregnant woman with vaginal bleeding needs immediate evaluation.
- Estimate hemodynamic stability:
  - Obtain orthostatic vital signs.
- Abdominal exam for tenderness (SAb), guarding, rebound, bowel sounds (peritoneal signs more likely seen with ectopic pregnancy)
- Pelvic exam for cervical dilation, blood, products of conception, uterine size/tenderness

DIAGNOSTIC TESTS & INTERPRETATION
Lab
Initial lab tests
- Urine human chorionic gonadotropin (HCG)
- Complete blood count
- Rh type
- Cultures: Gonorrhea/chlamydia
- Serial serum HCG measurements can assess viability of the pregnancy. Serum HCG should rise at least 67% every 48 hours in early pregnancy.

Pregnancy Considerations
HCG levels are particularly useful in cases where an intrauterine pregnancy (IUP) has not been documented by ultrasound.

Follow-Up & Special Considerations
- In the case of vaginal bleeding with no documented IUP, follow serum HCG levels weekly to zero to ensure complete expulsion of all products of conception.
- If levels plateau, suspect ectopic pregnancy or retained products of conception.

Imaging
Initial approach
- Ultrasound (US) exam to evaluate fetal viability and to rule out ectopic pregnancy:
  - HCG >2,000 U/L necessary to detect IUP via transvaginal US (TVUS), >6,500 U/L for abdominal ultrasound
- TVUS criteria for nonviable intrauterine gestation include 5-mm fetal pole without cardiac activity or 16-mm gestational sac without a fetal pole.

Follow-Up & Special Considerations
- If initial HCG level does not permit documentation of IUP by TVUS, follow serum HCG in 48 hrs to ensure appropriate rise.
- Follow HGC and repeat US once HCG at a level commensurate with visualization on US (see above).
- Provide patient with ectopic precautions in interim.

Diagnostic Procedures/Surgery
- Fetal heart tones can be auscultated with Doppler starting between 10–12 weeks' gestation from last menstrual period for a viable pregnancy.
- 90–96% of pregnancies with fetal cardiac activity and vaginal bleeding at 7–11 weeks' gestation result in continued pregnancy.

Pathological Findings
Products of conception, placental villi

DIFFERENTIAL DIAGNOSIS
- Ectopic pregnancy: Potentially life-threatening; must be ruled out with US in any woman of childbearing age with abdominal pain and vaginal bleeding
- Cervical polyps, neoplasias, and/or inflammatory conditions can cause vaginal bleeding.
- Hydatidiform mole pregnancy
- HCG-secreting ovarian tumor
- Physiologic bleeding in normal pregnancy (implantation bleeding)

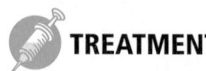 **TREATMENT**

MEDICATION
- Long-term conception rate and pregnancy outcomes are similar for women who undergo medical or surgical evacuation.
- Postinfection rates lower with medical vs surgical management

First Line
- Misoprostol: Most common agent for inducing passage of tissue in missed or incomplete abortion:
  - Not approved by Food and Drug Administration for treatment of early pregnancy failure
  - Efficacy: Complete expulsion of products of conception in 71% by day 3, 84% by day 8
  - Efficacy depends on route of administration, gestational age of pregnancy, and dose
  - Recommended dose 800 μg vaginally (3)[A]; alternate regimens exist including World Health Organization regimen of 800 μg vaginally or 600 μg sublingually q.3 hours for up to 3 doses; multidose regimens and oral dosing may result in increased side effects
- Common adverse effects include abdominal pain/cramping, nausea, and diarrhea. Pain increases at higher doses, but manageable with analgesia. No increase in nausea/diarrhea with higher dose.
- Recommended for stable patients who decline surgery but do not want to wait for spontaneous passage of products of conception

Second Line
Rh-negative patients should be given Rh immune globulin following spontaneous abortion (4)[C].

ADDITIONAL TREATMENT
General Measures
Explore any 1st-trimester vaginal bleeding.

Issues for Referral
Patients should be monitored for up to 1 year for the development of psychosomatic symptoms such as depression and anxiety (5)[A].

COMPLEMENTARY AND ALTERNATIVE MEDICINE
Vitamin supplementation does not appear to prevent miscarriage (6)[A].

SURGERY/OTHER PROCEDURES
- Uterine aspiration (dilation and curettage or via vacuum aspiration) is the conventional treatment.
- Indications: Septic abortion, heavy bleeding, hypotension, patient choice
- Risks: Anesthesia, uterine perforation, intrauterine adhesions, cervical trauma, infection that may lead to infertility or increased risk of ectopic pregnancy
- Surgical intervention leads to fewer days of vaginal bleeding, with a lower risk of incomplete abortion and heavy bleeding. It does carry a higher risk of infection (7)[A].
- Vacuum aspiration may be less painful than dilatation and curettage (D & C), and does not require general anesthesia (8)[B].
- Data from induced abortions suggests that antibiotic prophylaxis with doxycycline 100 mg b.i.d. substantially reduces postprocedure infection risk; however, data for incomplete abortions treated surgically is inconclusive (9)[A].
- For patients who desire contraception after completion of a spontaneous abortion, immediate insertion of an intrauterine device is acceptable and safe (10)[A].

IN-PATIENT CONSIDERATIONS
Initial Stabilization
If patient with orthostatic vital signs, initiate resuscitation with IV fluids and/or blood products if needed

IV Fluids
Hemodynamically unstable patients may require IV fluids and/or blood products to maintain blood pressure.

 ## ONGOING CARE

FOLLOW-UP RECOMMENDATIONS
All patients should be seen in 2–6 weeks to monitor for resolution of bleeding, reestablishment of menses, review of contraception plan, and psychosomatic symptoms.

Patient Monitoring
- Identification of products of conception within material expelled from the uterus or D & C specimen (important to distinguish villi and sac from decidua)
- If abortion is complete, observe the patient for further bleeding.
- Pelvic rest until 2 weeks after evacuation
- If spontaneous abortion occurs in setting of previously documented IUP and abortion is completed with resumption of normal menses, it is not necessary to check or follow serum HCG to 0.

DIET
n.p.o. if patient to undergo dilation and curettage

PATIENT EDUCATION
Patient pamphlet (no. AP090) available from the American College of Obstetricians and Gynecologists 409 12th St., SW, Washington, DC 20090-6290; (800) 762-2264 or online at http://www.acog.org

PROGNOSIS
- If bleeding ceases, prognosis is excellent.
- Habitual abortion:
  - Prognosis depends on etiology.
  - Prognosis is still excellent, with up to 70% rate of success with subsequent pregnancy.

COMPLICATIONS
- Potential complications of D & C include uterine perforation, bleeding, adhesions, cervical trauma, infection that may lead to infertility, or increased risk of ectopic pregnancy.
- Retained products of conception
- Psychological morbidity, including depression, anxiety, feelings of guilt

REFERENCES

1. Haas DM, Ramsey PS. Progestogen for preventing miscarriage. *Cochrane Database Syst Rev.* 2008; CD003511.
2. Porter TF, LaCoursiere Y, Scott JR. Immunotherapy for recurrent miscarriage. *Cochrane Database Syst Rev.* 2006;CD000112.
3. Neilson JP, Hickey M, Vazquez J. Medical treatment for early fetal death (less than 24 weeks). *Cochrane Database Syst Rev.* 2006;3: CD002253.
4. Prevention of Rho(D) alloimmunization. American College of Obstetricians and Gynecologists Practice Bulletin No 4. American College of Obstetricians and Gynecologists, Washington, DC: 1999.
5. Lok IH, Neugebauer R. Psychological morbidity following miscarriage. *Best Pract Res Clin Obstet Gynaecol.* 2007;21:229–47.
6. Rumbold A, Middleton P, Crowther CA. Vitamin supplementation for preventing miscarriage. *Cochrane Database Syst Rev.* 2005;CD004073.
7. Nanda K, Peloggia A, Grimes D et al. Expectant care versus surgical treatment for miscarriage. *Cochrane Database Syst Rev.* 2006;CD003518.
8. Forna F, et al. Surgical procedures to evacuate incomplete miscarriage. *Cochrane Database Sys Rev.* 2001;1:CD001993.
9. May W, Gülmezoglu AM, Ba-Thike K et al. Antibiotics for incomplete abortion. *Cochrane Database Syst Rev.* 2007;CD001779.
10. Grimes DA, Lopez LM, Schulz KF, Van Vliet HA, Stanwood NL et al. Immediate post-partum insertion of intrauterine devices. *Cochrane Database Syst Rev.* 2010;5:CD003036.

ADDITIONAL READING
- Harwood B, et al. Quality of life and acceptability of medical vs. surgical management of early pregnancy. *Br J Obstet and Gynaec.* 2008;115(4):501–8.
- Tam WH, Tsui MH, Lok IH et al. Long-term reproductive outcome subsequent to medical versus surgical treatment for miscarriage. *Hum Reprod.* 2005;20:3355–9.
- Zhang J, Gilles JM, Barnhart K, Creinin MD, Westhoff C, Frederick MM, National Institute of Child Health Human Development (NICHD) Management of Early Pregnancy Failure Trial et al. A comparison of medical management with misoprostol and surgical management for early pregnancy failure. *N Engl J Med.* 2005;353:761–9.

 ### See Also (Topic, Algorithm, Electronic Media Element)

Ectopic Pregnancy
Algorithm: Abortion, Recurrent

 ## CODES

ICD9
- 632 Missed abortion
- 634.90 Spontaneous abortion, unspecified, without mention of complication
- 640.03 Threatened abortion, antepartum

CLINICAL PEARLS
- Any reproductive-age woman or pregnant woman with abdominal pain and vaginal bleeding must be evaluated. Ectopic pregnancy must be ruled out, and hemodynamic stability must be ensured.
- Patient preference should determine whether management is medical, expectant, or surgical, as all options have similar long-term outcomes.
- Assessment of psychological symptoms after spontaneous abortion should be an integral part of follow-up visits, with counseling, medication, and referral as appropriate.
- Patients and their partners should be reassured that there are no known interventions to prevent spontaneous abortion, and should be provided with appropriate medical explanations to reduce anxiety and guilt.

ABRUPTIO PLACENTAE

Mark J. Manning, DO, Med
Amy Ellingson-Itzin, MD

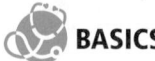 **BASICS**

DESCRIPTION
- Premature separation of an otherwise normally implanted placenta
- Grades:
  - Grade 1: Minimal or no bleeding; detected as retroplacental clot after delivery of viable fetus. Mild uterine irritability (40% of cases).
  - Grade 2: Viable fetus with bleeding and tender, irritable uterus. Mild-to-moderate bleeding; fibrinogen level decreased (45% of cases).
  - Grade 3: Type A with dead fetus and no coagulopathy; type B with dead fetus and coagulopathy (Types A and B = 15% of all cases)

EPIDEMIOLOGY
Incidence
- 0.5–1.2% of all deliveries:
  - Placental abruption is the most common cause of serious vaginal bleeding in late pregnancy (1).
- 15% if 1 prior abruption
- 25% if 2 or more prior abruptions
- 80% of cases occur prior to onset of delivery.
- Peaks at 24–26 weeks, then decreases with increasing gestation
- Rising in the US from 0.8% 1979–1981 to 1.2% 1999–2001

RISK FACTORS
- Prior abruption: Increases 15–20-fold (2)
- Increasing maternal age and parity
- Advanced maternal age
- Maternal smoking: dose–response relationship (2)
- Cocaine use and abuse
- Factor V Leiden and other thrombophilic disorders
- Hypertensive disorders
- Uterine anomalies
- Multiple-gestation pregnancies (3)[B]
- 1st- or 2nd-trimester bleeding
- Preeclampsia: Mild and severe
- Increased risk if hypertension and parity >3
- Preterm rupture of membranes (4)[B]
- Hydramnios
- Severe small-for-gestational-age birth
- Blunt trauma/motor vehicle accident

Genetics
- Genetic predisposition may be the cause of abruption in women with no other inciting factor discovered.
- Placental growth is primarily under control of paternally inherited fetal genes.

GENERAL PREVENTION
Eliminate risk factors when possible: Quit smoking and cocaine use, control hypertension, use seat belts, etc.

PATHOPHYSIOLOGY
Exact cause is unknown: Appears to be the final common clinical event secondary to a variety of causes

ETIOLOGY
- Acute:
  - Trauma of variable amounts, especially blunt abdominal trauma in which external signs of trauma may be incongruent with fetal injury
  - Sudden decompression of overdistended uterus, as in hydramnios or twin gestation
  - Vasospasm secondary to cocaine use
- Chronic (majority of cases):
  - Hypertensive disorders and growth restriction associated with chronic process
  - Early bleeding in pregnancy releases thrombin, which is a potent uterotonic agent

COMMONLY ASSOCIATED CONDITIONS
- Preeclampsia and other forms of hypertension in pregnancy
- Uteroplacental insufficiency
- Postpartum hemorrhage
- Disseminated intravascular coagulation (DIC)
- Rupture of membranes

 DIAGNOSIS

HISTORY
- Classic triad of vaginal bleeding, abdominal pain, and contractions
- Abruption in prior pregnancy
- Early trimester bleeding
- Recent trauma
- Cocaine or tobacco use
- Back pain
- Frequent or tetanic contractions
- May present in active labor

PHYSICAL EXAM
- Vital signs: Tachycardia, hypotension:
  - Because blood volumes increase in pregnancy, volume lost may exceed 30% before signs of shock or hypovolemia occur.
- Uterine tenderness, hypertonia, or high-frequency contractions
- Vaginal bleeding (not always present):
  - Clinical signs of shock may occur with little vaginal bleeding.
- Fetal distress or demise
- Idiopathic preterm labor with or without fetal distress

DIAGNOSTIC TESTS & INTERPRETATION
Lab
Initial lab tests
- Blood type, Rh, cross-match for possible transfusion:
  - RHoD immune globulin administered <12 weeks prior may affect antibody test.
- Complete blood count with platelet count
- Prothrombin time (PT)/partial thromboplastin time (PTT)
- Kleihauer-Betke test checks for evidence of fetal blood in maternal circulation; >30 mL fetal blood indicative of large fetal blood loss:
  - 300 μg dose of RhoGAM will cover up to 30 mL whole fetal blood in maternal circulation

- Bedside clot test: Red-top tube of maternal blood with poor or nonclotting blood after 7–10 minutes indicates coagulopathy.

Follow-Up & Special Considerations
- DIC can result from a large abruption. Best to stabilize patient without waiting for DIC labs. This is typically a clinical diagnosis.
- Can send PT/PTT, fibrinogen levels at clinician discretion when stable or following resolution of DIC:
  - Fibrinogen levels climb to 350–550 mg/dL in 3rd trimester and must fall to 100–150 mg/dL before PTT will rise.
  - Fibrin split or degradation products are elevated in pregnancy and are not specific in assessing DIC.

Imaging
Initial approach
- Placental abruption is a clinical diagnosis.
- Ultrasound can help to make the diagnosis, but has low sensitivity and is only helpful in cases of a large abruption.

Follow-Up & Special Considerations
Ultrasound: Appearance depends on size and location of the bleed:
- With acute bleed, nothing may be seen.
- Will fail to detect at least 50% of abruptions
- Retroplacental clot is diagnostic of abruption (2):
  - If incidental abruption is found in a patient at term, delivery is reasonable.
  - A preterm patient with an incidental abruption may be managed conservatively if stable.

Diagnostic Procedures/Surgery
- Tocometer often shows elevated baseline pressure and frequent low-amplitude contractions.
- External fetal monitoring may show recurrent late decelerations, variable decelerations, sinusoidal fetal heart tracing, bradycardia, or decreased variability—all indicative of fetal stress.

Pathological Findings
- Placental examination after delivery may show a retroplacental clot, pathologic signs of early separation/inflammation
- Normocytic normochromic anemia with acute bleeding
- Elevated PT/PTT, fibrinogen levels <100–150 mg/dL (1.0–1.5 g/L), platelets 20,000–50,000/μL if DIC is active
- Positive Kleihauer-Betke reaction if fetal–maternal transfusion has occurred
- Positive antibody if RhoD isosensitization has occurred

DIFFERENTIAL DIAGNOSIS
- Placenta previa or vasa previa (1)
- Uterine rupture
- Bloody show associated with labor
- Cervical and vaginal infections (e.g., chlamydia or gonorrhea with bloody, friable cervix)
- Other painful abdominal conditions (e.g., appendicitis, pyelonephritis)
- Fibroid degeneration
- Ovarian pathology: Torsed ovary, ruptured cyst

TREATMENT

MEDICATION

First Line
- Tocolytics are generally contraindicated in presence of abruption:
  - Tocolytics, such as nifedipine or terbutaline, may be used in mild noncompromising preterm abruption (specific cases only, such as for fetal lung maturity)
- RhoD immune globulin for RhoD-negative mother if undelivered or indicated after delivery if Kleihauer-Betke is positive
- Fluid resuscitation as required for signs of shock

Second Line
- Transfuse packed red blood cells (PRBC) or other factors to stabilize patient as needed.
- Steroids for fetal lung maturation, if fetus is viable

ADDITIONAL TREATMENT

Issues for Referral
- If preterm and hemodynamically stable, refer to tertiary care center.
- Alert anesthesia if delivery via cesarean section is likely.

SURGERY/OTHER PROCEDURES
- May need cesarean delivery after maternal stabilization if fetus is viable, remote from delivery, and nonreassuring fetal heart tracing is present.
- Postpartum hemorrhage/DIC may be treated medically or with uterine packing, embolization, or hysterectomy.

IN-PATIENT CONSIDERATIONS

Initial Stabilization
- History and physical exam with medical history, allergies, prior ultrasounds (present gestation), and time of last meal
- Management depends on presentation, gestational age, and degree of maternal and fetal compromise:
  - In general, severe abruption is best managed by delivery of fetus.
  - Grade 1: Usual labor protocol
  - Grade 2: Rapid delivery, most often by cesarean delivery (if mother stable)
  - Grade 3: Vaginal delivery preferable if mother stable
- In trauma (2)[B], monitor in the inpatient setting for at least 4 hours for evidence of fetal insult, abruption, fetal–maternal transfusion. If contractions or preterm labor occur, patient should be monitored for at least 24 hours. Risk factors for contractions with trauma include:
  - Gestational age >35 weeks
  - Assaults and pedestrian/vehicular collisions, even without direct abdominal trauma
  - Ejections from vehicle or lack of restraints
- Early aggressive restoration of maternal physiology to protect fetus and maternal organs from hypoperfusion/DIC
- Stabilize vitals
- Bedrest with external fetal and labor monitoring, if fetus is viable
- Large-bore, 16- to 18-gauge IV crystalloid infusion to maintain volume

- Transfusions of whole blood and PRBCs as necessary
- Fresh frozen plasma and platelet transfusions for coagulopathy, with cryoprecipitate and fibrinogen given if indicated
- Follow hemoglobin/hematocrit and coagulation status.
- Consider internal monitoring of fetus if patient is in active labor.
- Role of amniotomy to prevent amniotic fluid embolism is debatable, but may speed delivery
- Positioning on left side may enhance venous return and cardiac output
- Oxygen as needed

Admission Criteria
Patients with suspected placental abruption should be admitted for workup until deemed clinically stable and ready for discharge/outpatient follow-up or delivered for medical indication.

IV Fluids
Saline or Ringer's lactate to restore maternal vascular volume

Nursing
- Bed rest until status defined
- Frequent vital sign monitoring
- Record fluid ins and outs

Discharge Criteria
- 2nd trimester suspected abruption may be managed on outpatient basis if hemodynamically stable
- Viable patients may be discharged if maternal/fetal status is stable.

 ONGOING CARE

FOLLOW-UP RECOMMENDATIONS
- Monthly growth ultrasonograms for those patients where conservative management is possible.
- Serial ultrasounds may also be used to follow regression or progression of abruption (2).

Patient Monitoring
Severe cases or unstable patients may require critical care unit admission.

DIET
n.p.o. until status is defined and possibility of immediate cesarean delivery ruled out

PATIENT EDUCATION
- Call physician or proceed to hospital whenever patient experiences vaginal bleeding or if severe uterine or back pain or decreased fetal movement occurs.
- Wear seat belts while in automobile.
- Discontinue use of cocaine, tobacco
- Visit Mayo Health: http://mayohealth.org

PROGNOSIS
- 0.5–1% fetal mortality and 30–50% perinatal mortality:
  - 1/2 of perinatal deaths due to preterm delivery
- With trauma and abruption, 1% maternal and 30–70% fetal mortality

COMPLICATIONS
- Maternal complications include anemia, stroke, myocardial infarction, DIC, and Sheehan's syndrome, and may include maternal death with severe hemorrhage.

- Surgical interventions and transfusion carry their own morbidity/mortality.
- Amniotic fluid embolism is rare, but may present with severe respiratory distress.

REFERENCES
1. Sakornbut E, Leeman L, Fontaine P. Late pregnancy bleeding. *Am Fam Physician*. 2007;75:1199–206.
2. Ananth CV, Getahun D, Peltier MR et al. Placental abruption in term and preterm gestations: evidence for heterogeneity in clinical pathways. *Obstet Gynecol*. 2006;107:785–92.
3. Salihu HM, Bekan B, Aliyu MH et al. Perinatal mortality associated with abruptio placenta in singletons and multiples. *Am J Obstet Gynecol*. 2005;193:198–203.
4. Ananth CV, Oyelese Y, Srinivas N et al. Preterm premature rupture of membranes, intrauterine infection, and oligohydramnios: risk factors for placental abruption. *Obstet Gynecol*. 2004;104:71–7.

ADDITIONAL READING
- *Creasy & Resnik's Maternal-Fetal Medicine, Principles and Practice*, 6th ed. Saunders Elsevier. 2009;731–737.
- Getahun D, et al. Acute and chronic respiratory diseases in pregnancy: Associations with placenta abruption. *Am J Obst Gynecol* 2006;195(4):1180–4.
- Oyelese Y, et al. Placental abruption. *Obst Gynecol* 2006;108:1005–16.
- Pressman EV. Imaging of the Placenta. *Ultrsound Clinics*. Volume 3, Issue 1. January 2008.
- Yang Q, Wen SW, Oppenheimer L et al. Association of caesarean delivery for first birth with placenta praevia and placental abruption in second pregnancy. *BJOG*. 2007;114:609–13.

 CODES

ICD9
641.23 Premature separation of placenta, antepartum

CLINICAL PEARLS
- Placental abruption is the most common cause of serious vaginal bleeding in late pregnancy.
- Abruption is a clinical diagnosis. The classic triad is vaginal bleeding, abdominal pain, and contractions. Ultrasound can help to make the diagnosis, but has low sensitivity and is only helpful in cases of a large abruption.
- Because blood volumes increase in pregnancy, volume lost may exceed 30% before signs of shock or hypovolemia occur.
- Individualize management on a case-by-case basis, depending upon maternal and fetal considerations.

ACETAMINOPHEN POISONING

Lars C. Larsen, MD

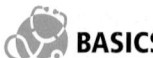 **BASICS**

DESCRIPTION
- A disorder characterized by hepatic necrosis following large ingestions of acetaminophen. Symptoms may vary from initial nausea, vomiting, diaphoresis, and malaise to jaundice, confusion, somnolence, coma, and death. The clinical hallmark is the onset of symptoms within 24 hours of ingestion of acetaminophen-only or combination products.
- Acetaminophen poisoning is most often encountered following large single ingestions of acetaminophen-containing medications. Usual toxic doses are above 10 g in adults and 150 mg/kg in children. However, poisoning also occurs after acute and chronic ingestions of lesser amounts in susceptible individuals, including those who regularly abuse alcohol, are chronically malnourished, or take medications that affect hepatic metabolism of acetaminophen.
- Therapeutic adult doses are 0.5–1 g q4–6h, up to a maximum of 4 g/d. Therapeutic pediatric doses are 10–20 mg/kg q4–6h.
- System(s) affected: Gastrointestinal; Cardiovascular; Renal/Urologic:
  – Multisystem organ failure can occur.
- Synonym(s): Paracetamol poisoning

Geriatric Considerations
Hepatic damage may be increased if taking hepatotoxic medications chronically.

Pediatric Considerations
Hepatic damage at toxic acetaminophen levels is decreased in children <6 years.

Pregnancy Considerations
- Increased incidence of spontaneous abortion, especially with overdose at early gestational age
- Incidence of spontaneous abortion or fetal death appears to be increased when N-acetylcysteine (NAC) treatment is delayed.
- The optimal route for administration of NAC in pregnant patients remains debatable, although IV NAC may offer greater bioavailability.

EPIDEMIOLOGY
- Predominant age: Children and adults
- Predominant sex: No reported association

Incidence
- More than 50,000 calls placed to poison control centers in 2007 related to possible acetaminophen overdoses.
- 74 deaths in 2006, none in children <6 years of age

Prevalence
Approximately 29% of single exposures are in children <6 years.

RISK FACTORS
- Age >6 years
- Concurrent poisoning with other substances
- Psychiatric illness
- Previous toxic ingestions or suicide attempts
- Regular ingestion of large amounts of alcohol

GENERAL PREVENTION
Parent/caregiver education essential:
- Education during well-child exams regarding poisoning prevention
- Emergency telephone numbers

ETIOLOGY
- Accidental or intentional ingestion of acetaminophen or combination medications containing acetaminophen
- Approximately 96% of ingested acetaminophen is metabolized in the liver with only 2% to 4% excreted unchanged in the urine. When taken in therapeutic doses, 90–95% of hepatic metabolism occurs via glucuronidation and sulfation and results in the formation of benign metabolites. 5–10% of hepatic metabolism is by oxidation through the cytochrome P_{450} enzyme system (CYP 3A4 and CYP 2E1) and results in the formation of the toxic metabolite N-acetyl-p-benzoquinoneimne (NAPQI). NAPQI is rapidly conjugated with glutathione to form a nontoxic metabolite. The metabolites are excreted in the urine along with the small amount of unchanged drug. Hepatocellular damage typically occurs when toxic doses of acetaminophen result in saturation of the glucuronidation and sulfation pathways with subsequent production of excessive amounts of NAPQI. Available glutathione stores become depleted, NAPQI accumulates, and hepatocellular damage occurs.

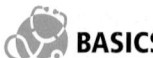 **DIAGNOSIS**

- Signs and symptoms develop over the 1st 24 hours following large ingestions, and may last as long as 8 days.
- May develop gradually following long-term ingestion of near maximal-therapeutic amounts of acetaminophen. Such patients may present in stages 1–3, without a history of ingestion of the usual toxic doses.
- Severe symptoms indicate large ingestions or coingestants:
  – Stage 1: 1st 24 hours after time of ingestion:
    ○ Nausea
    ○ Vomiting
    ○ Diaphoresis
  – Stage 2: 24–48 hours:
    ○ Right upper quadrant pain
    ○ Typically less nausea, vomiting, diaphoresis, and malaise than in stage 1
  – Stage 3: 72–96 hours:
    ○ Nausea, vomiting, malaise reappear
    ○ Severe poisonings may result in jaundice, confusion, somnolence, and coma.
  – Stage 4: 7–8 days:
    ○ Resolution of clinical signs in survivors
- Fulminant hepatic failure occurs in <1% of adults and is very rare in children <6 years of age.
- Patients with an unexplained rise in liver function tests (LFTs) with negative acetaminophen levels may be overdose patients presenting in stage 3.

HISTORY
Ingestion or suspected ingestion of acetaminophen-containing product

DIAGNOSTIC TESTS & INTERPRETATION
Lab
- Plasma acetaminophen levels should be drawn on all patients 4 hours or more after ingestion (levels prior to 4 hours not helpful).
- At least 1 additional acetaminophen level drawn 4–6 hours after the 1st level is recommended if the ingested acetaminophen is an extended-release product (e.g., Tylenol Extended Relief) or is not known to be an immediate-release product.
- If the 2nd level is higher than the 1st level or is close to the "possible risk" level on the Rumack-Matthew nomogram, it may be prudent to obtain additional acetaminophen levels every 2 hours until the levels stabilize or decline.
- If coingestants include drugs that slow gastrointestinal (GI) motility, an acetaminophen level drawn 4–6 hours after the 2nd level may detect a late increase in serum acetaminophen concentration.
- Screens for suspected coingestants (aspirin, iron, and others) may be positive (especially when suicide attempt is a possibility).
- With toxic ingestions, aspartate transaminase (AST; serum glutamic-oxaloacetic transaminase), alanine transaminase (ALT; serum glutamic-pyruvic transaminase), and bilirubin levels begin to rise in stage 2 and peak in stage 3. In severe poisonings, the PT/INR will parallel these changes and should be monitored.
- AST levels >1,000 IU/L are consistent with the diagnosis, and levels of 20,000 IU/L are not uncommon.
- Laboratory abnormalities usually resolve by stage 4.
- Renal function abnormalities are common in patients with hepatotoxicity.
- Evidence of damage to the pancreas and heart may present following severe poisonings.
- Drugs that may alter lab results: None with clinically significant cross-reactivity with plasma acetaminophen assay
- Disorders that may alter lab results: Diseases or toxic substances that damage the liver, particularly alcohol.

Initial lab tests
- Acetaminophen serum concentration: 4 hours after ingestion and again per comments above (see General)
- AST, ALT (rise in first 72 hours, then slowly decline), prothrombin time (PT)/international normalized ration (INR), bilirubin, LDH
- Electrolytes, glucose, blood urea nitrogen (BUN), creatinine
- Pregnancy screen in females (urine or serum)
- Urinalysis
- Consider arterial blood gas if pH disturbance suspected on clinical or lab grounds.

Follow-Up & Special Considerations
- Repeat 4 hours after ingestion and possibly every 2 hours thereafter if long-acting product is ingested or acetaminophen ingested with other agents that slow GI passage.
- Arterial blood gas after hydration if pH is acidotic

Imaging
No specific imaging required

Pathological Findings
Centrilobular hepatic necrosis

DIFFERENTIAL DIAGNOSIS
- Consider presence of coingestants, especially alcohol and aspirin.
- Other ingested toxins that produce severe acute hepatic injury, including the mushroom *Amanita phalloides* and products containing yellow phosphorus or carbon tetrachloride

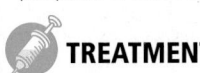

TREATMENT
- Contact a regional poison control center for management recommendations. In the US, a local poison control center can be reached by calling (800) 222-1222.
- NAC should be given when plasma acetaminophen concentrations measured 4 hours or more after ingestion are in the "possible risk" or higher levels on the Rumack-Matthew nomogram. This corresponds to acetaminophen levels >150 μg/mL (993 μmol/L), >75 μg/mL (497 μmol/L), and >37 μg/mL (244 μmol/L) at 4, 8, and 12 hours after ingestion, respectively. See http://www.ars-informatica.ca/toxicity_nomogram.php?calc=acetamin or http://www.merck.com/mmpe/sec21/ch326/ch326c.html
- NAC should be started within 8 hours of ingestion for best chance of hepatic protection. Patients presenting near 8 hours should empirically receive NAC while waiting for labs.
- All patients with acetaminophen liver injury (even after 8 hours) should receive NAC.
- NAC therapy may be effective up to 36 hours or more after ingestion.
- Single dose activated charcoal can be used (especially in cases of coingestants) (1,2)[C],(3)[A] but not within 1 hour of administration of the antidote NAC. Never delay NAC for activated charcoal.
- NAC should be initiated within 8 hours of ingestion whenever possible.
- Ipecac and gastric lavage are no longer recommended for routine use at home or in health care facilities (4)[C].

MEDICATION
First Line
- Acetylcysteine (NAC, Mucomyst) should be initiated within 8 hours of ingestion whenever possible; single dose activated charcoal may be given 1 hour after oral NAC. NEVER delay oral NAC for activated charcoal.
- Acetylcysteine may be given p.o. or IV, depending on situation and availability: IV is often preferred, particularly if activated charcoal is given:
  – Currently, IV is the recommended form of administration:
    ○ Oral loading dose of 140 mg/kg, followed by 70 mg/kg q4h for 17 additional doses. IV loading dose of Acetadote 150 mg/kg over 15 to 60 minutes followed by an infusion of 50 mg/kg over 4 hours (12.5 mg/kg/hour); this is followed by an infusion of 100 mg/kg over the next 16 hours (6.25 mg/kg/hour).
- Contraindications: Medication allergies
- Precautions:
  – Oral NAC may cause significant nausea and vomiting due to its sulfur content; consider IV administration or by nasogastric tube.

– Nausea can be treated with metoclopramide (Reglan), 0.5–1 mg/kg IV, or ondansetron (Zofran), 0.15 mg/kg IV (for age >4 years, usually 4 mg/dose).
– IV NAC (Acetadote) may cause anaphylactoid reactions, including rash, bronchospasm, pruritus, angioedema, tachycardia, or hypotension (higher rates seen in asthmatics and those with atopic history) (5,6)[C].
- Reactions usually occur with loading dose. Slow or temporarily stop the infusion; may concurrently treat with antihistamines.
- Significant possible interactions: Activated charcoal given within 1 hour of oral NAC may adsorb the NAC, limiting its effectiveness.
- Activated charcoal: 1 g/kg p.o. for initial dose; preferably not within 1 hour of NAC administration. Additional concurrent use during NAC therapy is controversial.

Second Line
Oral racemethionine (methionine)

ADDITIONAL TREATMENT
Issues for Referral
- Psychiatric and psychological evaluation in emergency room and close follow-up for all after intentional ingestions
- Consider child abuse reporting if neglect led to overdose.

IN-PATIENT CONSIDERATIONS
Initial Stabilization
Aggressive age- and weight-appropriate IV hydration

Admission Criteria
- Toxic and intentional ingestions
- Any reported ingestion with increased LFTs, acidosis on arterial blood gas (ABG), elevated creatinine, etc.

ONGOING CARE

FOLLOW-UP RECOMMENDATIONS
- All patients should be evaluated at a health care facility.
- Patients with evidence of organ failure, increased LFTs, or coagulopathy should be evaluated for transfer to a site capable of liver transplant.
- Outpatient for nontoxic accidental ingestions
- Activity may be restricted if significant hepatic damage.

Patient Monitoring
Inquire as to possible ingestion by others (i.e., suicide pacts).

DIET
No special diet, except with severe hepatic damage

PATIENT EDUCATION
- Patients should be counseled to avoid Tylenol if already using combination product containing acetaminophen.
- Education of parents/caregivers during well-child visits
- Anticipatory guidance for caregivers, family, and cohabitants of potentially suicidal patients
- Patient brochure (item no. 1515), *Child safety: keeping your home safe for your baby*. American Academy of Family Physicians: www.familydoctor.org or http://familydoctor.org/online/famdocen/home/healthy/safety/kids-family/027.html
- Education of patients taking long-term acetaminophen therapy

PROGNOSIS
- Complete recovery with early therapy
- <1% of adult patients develop hepatic failure. King criteria (pH <7.3, PT >100 s [INR >65], creatinine >3.4 mg/dL [>300 μmol/L]) are associated with a poor prognosis and possible need for liver transplant (7)[C].
- Hepatic failure is very rare in children <6 years of age.

COMPLICATIONS
Rare following recovery from acute poisoning

REFERENCES
1. Gaudreault P. Activated charcoal revisited. *Clin Ped Emerg Med*. 2005;6:76–80.
2. Heard K. Gastrointestinal decontamination. *Med Clin North Am*. 2005;89:1067–78.
3. Brok J, Buckley N, Glud C. Interventions for paracetamol (acetaminophen) overdoses. *The Cochrane Database of Systematic Reviews* 2006 volume 1.
4. American Academy of Pediatrics Committee on Injury, Violence, and Poison Prevention. Poison treatment in the home. American Academy of Pediatrics Committee on Injury, Violence, and Poison Prevention. *Pediatrics*. 2003;112:1182–5.
5. Acetylcysteine (Acetadote) for acetaminophen overdosage. *Med Lett*. 2005;47:70–1.
6. Culley CM, Krenzelok EP. A clinical and pharmacoeconomic justification for intravenous acetylcysteine: a US perspective. *Toxicol Rev*. 2005;24:131–43.
7. O'Grady JG, Alexander GJ, Hayllar KM et al. Early indicators of prognosis in fulminant hepatic failure. *Gastroenterology*. 1989;97:439–45.

 CODES

ICD9
965.4 Poisoning by aromatic analgesics, not elsewhere classified

CLINICAL PEARLS
- Contact a regional poison control center for management recommendations. In the US, a local poison control center can be reached by calling (800) 222-1222.
- NAC should be given when plasma acetaminophen concentrations measured 4 hours or more after ingestion are in the "possible risk" or higher levels on the Rumack-Matthew nomogram. This corresponds to acetaminophen levels >150 μg/mL (993 μmol/L), >75 μg/mL (497 μmol/L), and >40 μg/mL (265 μmol/L) at 4, 8, and 12 hours after ingestion, respectively.
- NAC should be started within 8 hours of ingestion for best chance of hepatic protection. Patients presenting near 8 hours should empirically receive NAC while waiting for labs.
- All patients with acetaminophen liver injury (even after 8 hours) should receive NAC.

ACL INJURY
J. Herbert Stevenson, MD

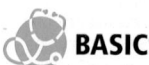

BASICS

DESCRIPTION
- The anterior cruciate ligament (ACL) is one of the major stabilizers of the knee. It prevents excessive anterior translation and internal rotation of the tibia on the femur. During dynamic movement, the ACL and PCL work together to stabilize the knee.
- ACL injuries are common and can occur through noncontact or contact mechanisms. >70% of ACL injuries are caused by noncontact forces (1,2).
- Partial tears of the ACL can occur, but complete tears are far more common.
- Female athletes are at 2–5 times higher risk of ACL tear, particularly in soccer, basketball, and skiing (2).
- ACL injury is associated with early onset of knee osteoarthritis, regardless of surgical or nonsurgical treatment (3,4)[B].

EPIDEMIOLOGY
Incidence
- 250,000 ACL injuries annually in the US (1)
- Female athletes incidence 2- to 5-fold > male athletes (2)
- Greater incidence of noncontact ACL injuries in sports requiring cutting, pivoting, and rapid deceleration, such as basketball and soccer.

Prevalence
- Young athletes aged 15–25 years sustain >50% of all ACL injuries (5).
- >2/3 of patients with complete ACL tear have associated menisci and/or articular cartilage injury (1).

Geriatric Considerations
Management is based on anticipated activity level, associated injuries, coexisting medical conditions, and acute versus long-standing ACL deficiency.

Pediatric Considerations
- Must be concerned about physeal injuries in the skeletally immature
- The incidence of ACL tears in patients with open physes has increased in recent years.
- ACL injury rates increase for both boys and girls beginning at age 11 years.

RISK FACTORS
- No single risk factor correlates directly with higher ACL injury rates in female athletes. Likely multifactorial etiology:
  - Sex hormones:
    - Increased rate may be due to monthly hormonal fluctuations.
    - No conclusive evidence linking a menstrual cycle phase
  - Anatomical gender differences:
    - Increased Q angle, increased genu valgum, narrower femoral notch size, smaller ACL
    - Neuromuscular imbalances (increased quadriceps activation, decreased hamstring activity during landings)
  - Movement patterns (sudden deceleration, change of direction cutting movements, landing from a jump in hyperextension)

Genetics
Familial tendency has been identified.

GENERAL PREVENTION
- Neuromuscular training with proprioceptive, plyometric, and strength exercises may reduce ACL injuries in female athletes (1,2,6)[B].
- No evidence that prophylactic knee bracing prevents ACL injuries (5)[C]
- Educate the patient about possible risk factors for ACL injury and provide instruction on neuromuscular training exercises.

ETIOLOGY
- Noncontact mechanisms (torsional or hyperextension forces)
- Direct trauma (player, object on playing field)

COMMONLY ASSOCIATED CONDITIONS
- Meniscal tear
- Collateral ligament tear
- PCL tear
- Tibia or femur fractures
- Osteochondral injury
- Loose bodies
- Early-onset degenerative joint disease

DIAGNOSIS

HISTORY
May recall mechanism:
- Noncontact:
  - Sudden deceleration
  - Cutting, sudden change in direction
  - Landing from a jump in extension
  - Combination of mechanisms
- Contact with player, object
- May recall sudden pop or snap
- Sudden pain and giving way
- Marked effusion/hemarthrosis within 4–12 hours

PHYSICAL EXAM
- Pain
- Effusion
- Decreased range of motion (ROM)
- Joint instability
- Giving way
- Difficulty bearing weight
- Inspect for malalignment (fracture, dislocation)
- Palpate for effusion
- Evaluate extensor mechanism integrity
- Evaluate ROM:
  - Deficits may be secondary to pain, effusion, mechanical blocks (meniscal tear, loose body, torn ACL stump).

DIAGNOSTIC TESTS & INTERPRETATION
- Lachman test: Most sensitive and highly specific diagnostic test for ACL injury, especially in acute setting (7)[A]:
  - Knee placed in 20–30° flexion. Tibia is pulled forward while femur is stabilized with opposite hand. Increased anterior translation compared with uninjured knee indicates injury. Lack of a solid endpoint indicates rupture.
- Pivot shift test: Lower sensitivity, but more specific for ACL tear than Lachman test (7)[B]:

  - Knee placed in extension. Knee is flexed while applying a valgus and internal rotation stress. A positive test is subluxation at 20–40° of flexion.
- Anterior drawer test:
  - Low sensitivity for ACL integrity, especially in acute setting (7)[A]
- Posterior drawer test assesses PCL integrity.
- McMurray test assesses for meniscal tears.
- Valgus/varus stress test for MCL/LCL integrity

Imaging
- Radiographs to rule out associated bony injury
- AP, lateral, and tunnel views:
  - Segond fracture: Avulsion fracture of the lateral capsular margin of the tibia
  - Tibial eminence avulsion fracture
  - Fracture of proximal tibia or distal femur
  - Osteochondral injuries
- MRI is the gold standard for imaging ligamentous and intra-articular structures; MRI will reveal associated bone bruises.

Diagnostic Procedures/Surgery
Surgical management should be considered in the active population, young or old.

DIFFERENTIAL DIAGNOSIS
- Fracture
- Meniscal injury
- Patellar dislocation/subluxation
- Tendon disruption
- PCL injury
- Collateral ligament injury

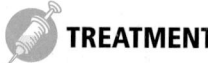

TREATMENT

MEDICATION
First Line
- NSAIDs:
  - Acute ligament sprains (8)[C]:
    - Ibuprofen: 200–800 mg t.i.d.
    - Naproxen: 375–500 mg b.i.d.
    - Indomethacin: 25–50 mg t.i.d.
- Acetaminophen
- Narcotics for severe pain (e.g., acetaminophen-hydrocodone)
- Contraindications/Precautions/Interactions: Refer to the manufacturer's profile of each drug.

ADDITIONAL TREATMENT
General Measures
- Acute injury: PRICEMM therapy: Protection, Relative rest, Ice, Compression, Elevation, Medications, Modalities
- Crutches may be indicated until patient is able to ambulate without pain.
- Knee immobilizer or brace may be used initially for comfort.
- Aspiration of large effusion may be indicated to alleviate pain and increase ROM.

Issues for Referral
Surgical management should be considered in the active population.

Additional Therapies
- Physical therapy is recommended if an athlete chooses nonsurgical or surgical treatment. Nonsurgical PT is focused on restoring ROM, strength, and proprioception.
- Preoperative phase:
  – Increase ROM, minimize inflammation.
- Early postoperative phase: Weeks 2–4:
  – ROM full extension is the most important goal. Rehabilitation begins immediately.
  – Progress to full weight bearing.
- Intermediate postoperative phase: Weeks 4–12:
  – ROM: Full flexion, hyperextension
  – Quadriceps and hamstring strengthening proprioceptive training, normalize gait
- Late postop phase: 2–3 months postop:
  – Straight-line running
  – Increased speed, duration over 6–8 weeks
  – Progress to cutting and sport-specific drills.
  – Strength and proprioceptive training

SURGERY/OTHER PROCEDURES
- Surgical versus conservative management depends on patient's activity level, age, associated injuries, and presence of OA.
- Insufficient evidence for ACL reconstructive surgery versus conservative management in the skeletally immature patient (9)[A]
- Insufficient evidence from randomized trials comparing surgical versus nonoperative management of ACL injuries in adults based on studies in the 1980s (10)[A]
- Reconstruction techniques:
  – Bone-patella tendon-bone autograft
  – Hamstring autograft
  – Allograft tendon
- No consistent significant differences in outcome between patellar tendon and hamstring tendon autografts (11)[A]
- Concomitant meniscal tears are repaired at the time of ACL reconstruction.

IN-PATIENT CONSIDERATIONS
Initial Stabilization
Outpatient

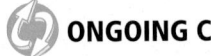

ONGOING CARE

FOLLOW-UP RECOMMENDATIONS
- ROM exercises to regain full flexion and extension
- Advance activity as tolerated

Patient Monitoring
Assess functional status, rehabilitative exercise compliance, and pain control at follow-up visit.

PROGNOSIS
- Athletes typically are out of competitive play for 6–9 months after injury to undergo ACL reconstructive surgery and rehabilitation.
- High prevalence of OA, even in those with early ACL reconstruction (3,4)[B].
- Delay of surgical reconstruction of torn ACL raises risk of secondary meniscal injury.

COMPLICATIONS
- Instability
- Secondary meniscal and articular cartilage injury
- Early-onset degenerative arthritis
- Surgical risks:
  – Infection, PE, subsequent ACL graft rupture, laxity due to failure of graft remodeling

REFERENCES
1. Silvers HJ, Mandelbaum BR. Prevention of anterior cruciate ligament injury in the female athlete. *Br J Sports Med*. 2007;41 Suppl 1:i52–9.
2. Renstrom P et al. Non-contact ACL injuries in female athletes: an International Olympic Committee current concepts statement. *Br J Sports Med*. 2008;42:394–412.
3. Fithian DC, Paxton EW, Stone ML et al. Prospective trial of a treatment algorithm for the management of the anterior cruciate ligament-injured knee. *Am J Sports Med*. 2005;33:335–46.
4. Lohmander LS et al. Long term consequences of anterior cruciate ligament and meniscus injuries. *Am J Sports Med*. 2007;35:1756–69.
5. Griffin LY, Albohm MJ, Arendt EA et al. Understanding and preventing noncontact anterior cruciate ligament injuries: a review of the Hunt Valley II meeting, January 2005. *Am J Sports Med*. 2006;34:1512–32.
6. Hewett TE, Ford KR, Myer GD. Anterior cruciate ligament injuries in female athletes: Part 2, a meta-analysis of neuromuscular interventions aimed at injury prevention. *Am J Sports Med*. 2006;34:490–8.
7. Jackson JL, O'Malley PG, Kroenke K. Evaluation of acute knee pain in primary care. *Ann Intern Med*. 2003;129:575–88.
8. Mehallo CJ, Drezner JA, Bytomski JR. Practical management: Nonsteroidal anti-inflammatory drug use in athletic injuries. *Clin J Sports Med*. 2006;16:170–4.
9. Mohtadi N, Grant J. Managing anterior cruciate ligament deficiency in the skeletally immature individual: A systematic review of the literature. *Clin J Sports Med*. 2006;16:457–64.
10. Linko E, Harilainen A, Malmivaara A, Seitsalo S. Surgical versus conservative interventions for anterior cruciate ligament rupture in adults. *The Cochrane Database of Systematic Reviews* 2005 Issue 4.
11. Spindler KP, Kuhn JE, Freedman KB et al. Anterior cruciate ligament reconstruction autograft choice: bone-tendon-bone versus hamstring: does it really matter? A systematic review. *Am J Sports Med*. 2004;32:1986–95.

ADDITIONAL READING
Cascio BM, Culp L, Cosgarea AJ. Return to play after anterior cruciate ligament reconstruction. *Clin Sports Med*. 2004;23:395–408, ix.

 See Also (Topic, Algorithm, Electronic Media Element)

Algorithm: Knee pain

 CODES

ICD9
844.2 Sprain of cruciate ligament of knee

CLINICAL PEARLS
- Lachman test: Most sensitive and highly specific diagnostic test for ACL injury, especially in acute setting (7)[A]
- Pivot shift test: Less sensitive but more specific for ACL tear than the Lachman test (7)[B]
- Anterior drawer test: Low sensitivity for ACL integrity, especially in acute setting (7)[A]
- 2/3 of complete ACL tears have associated meniscal or articular injuries.

ACNE ROSACEA

Adarsh K. Gupta, DO, MS

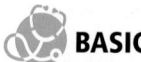 **BASICS**

DESCRIPTION
- Rosacea is a chronic condition characterized by recurrent episodes of facial flushing, erythema (due to dilatation of small blood vessels in the face), papules, pustules, and telangiectasia (due to increased reactivity of capillaries) in a symmetrical, facial distribution. Sometimes associated with ocular symptoms (ocular rosacea).
- System(s) affected: Skin/Exocrine
- Synonym(s): Rosacea

Geriatric Considerations
- Uncommon >60 years of age
- Effects of aging might increase the side effects associated with oral isotretinoin (at present, data is insufficient due to lack of clinical studies in elderly patients aged 65 and above).

EPIDEMIOLOGY
Prevalence
- Predominant age: 30–50 years
- Predominant sex: Female > Male. However, male will often progress to later stages.

RISK FACTORS
- Exposure to cold, heat, hot drinks
- Environmental trigger factors: Sun, wind, cold

Genetics
People of Northern European and Celtic background commonly afflicted

GENERAL PREVENTION
No preventive measures known

ETIOLOGY
- No proven cause
- Possibilities include:
  - Thyroid and gonadal disturbance
  - Alcohol, coffee, tea, spiced food overindulgence (unproven)
  - Demodex follicular parasite (suspected)
  - Exposure to cold, heat, hot drinks
  - Emotional stress
  - Dysfunction of the gastrointestinal tract

COMMONLY ASSOCIATED CONDITIONS
- Seborrheic dermatitis of scalp and eyelids
- Keratitis with photophobia, lacrimation, visual disturbance
- Corneal lesions
- Blepharitis
- Uveitis

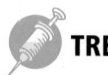 **DIAGNOSIS**

HISTORY
- Usually have a history of episodic flushing with increases in skin temperature in response to heat stimulus in mouth (hot liquids), spicy foods, alcohol, sun (solar elastosis). Acne may have preceded the onset of rosacea by years; nevertheless, rosacea usually arises de novo without any preceding history of acne or seborrhea.
- Excessive facial warmth and redness is the predominant presenting complaint. Itching is generally absent.

PHYSICAL EXAM
- Rosacea has typical stages of evolution:
  - The rosacea diathesis: Episodic erythema, "flushing and blushing"
  - Stage I: Persistent erythema with telangiectases
  - Stage II: Persistent erythema, telangiectases, papules, tiny pustules
  - Stage III: Persistent deep erythema, dense telangiectases, papules, pustules, nodules; rarely persistent "solid" edema of the central part of the face (phymatous)
- Facial erythema, particularly on cheeks, nose, and chin. At times, entire face may be involved.
- Inflammatory papules are prominent, and there may be pustules and telangiectasia.
- Comedones are absent (unlike acne).
- Women usually have lesions on the chin and cheeks, whereas nose is commonly involved in men.
- Ocular findings (mild dryness and irritation with blepharitis, conjunctival injection, burning, stinging, tearing, eyelid inflammation, swelling, and redness) are present in 50% of patients.

DIAGNOSTIC TESTS & INTERPRETATION
Diagnosis is based on physical exam findings.

Pathological Findings
- Inflammation around hypertrophied sebaceous glands, producing papules, pustules, and cysts
- Absence of comedones and blocked ducts
- Vascular dilation and dermal lymphocytic infiltrate

DIFFERENTIAL DIAGNOSIS
- Drug eruptions (iodides and bromides)
- Granulomas of the skin
- Cutaneous lupus erythematosus
- Carcinoid syndrome
- Deep fungal infection
- Acne vulgaris
- Seborrheic dermatitis
- Steroid rosacea (abuse)
- Systemic lupus erythematosus

TREATMENT

MEDICATION
First Line

- Azelaic acid (Finacea) with oral doxycycline is very effective as initial therapy and then Azelaic acid topical alone is effective for maintenance (3,4)[A].

Precautions: Tetracycline may cause photosensitivity; sunscreen is recommended.
Significant possible interactions:
- Tetracycline: Avoid concurrent administration with antacids, dairy products, or iron.
- Broad-spectrum antibiotics: May reduce the effectiveness of oral contraceptives; barrier method is recommended.

Pediatric Considerations
- Tetracycline: Not for use in children <8 years

Pregnancy Considerations
Tetracycline: Not for use during pregnancy
- Isotretinoin: Teratogenic; not for use during pregnancy or in women of reproductive age who are not using reliable contraception

Second Line

- Topical erythromycin
- Topical clindamycin lotion preferred
- Possible utility of calcineurin inhibitors (tacrolimus 0.1%; pimecrolimus 0.1%)
- Permethrin 5% cream (5)[A] similar efficacy compared to metronidazole
- Topical steroids should not be used, as they may aggravate rosacea.
- For severe cases, isotretinoin p.o. for 4 months

ADDITIONAL TREATMENT

General Measures

- Use of mild, nondrying soap is recommended; local skin irritants should be avoided.
- Reassurance that rosacea is completely unrelated to poor hygiene
- Treat psychological stress if present
- Avoid oil-based cosmetics:
  – Others are acceptable and may help women tolerate the symptoms.
- Electrodesiccation or chemical sclerosis of permanently dilated blood vessels
- Possible evolving laser therapy
- Support physical fitness

SURGERY/OTHER PROCEDURES

Laser treatment is an option for progressive telangiectasias or rhinophyma.

 ONGOING CARE

FOLLOW-UP RECOMMENDATIONS

Outpatient treatment

Patient Monitoring

- Occasional and as needed
- Close follow-up for women using isotretinoin

DIET

Avoid alcohol, excessive sun exposure, and hot drinks of any type.

PROGNOSIS

- Slowly progressive
- Subsides spontaneously (sometimes)

COMPLICATIONS

- Rhinophyma (dilated follicles and thickened bulbous skin on nose), especially in men
- Conjunctivitis
- Blepharitis
- Keratitis
- Visual deterioration

REFERENCES

1. Zuuren EJ, et al. Interventions for rosacea (Cochrane review). In: *The Cochrane Library* 2007 Issue 1. Chichester, UK: John Wiley and Sons, Ltd.
2. Del Rosso JQ, Webster GF, Jackson M et al. Two randomized phase III clinical trials evaluating anti-inflammatory dose doxycycline (40-mg doxycycline, USP capsules) administered once daily for treatment of rosacea. *J Am Acad Dermatol*. 2007;56:791–802.
3. Thiboutot DM, Fleischer AB, Del Rosso JQ, Rich P et al. A multicenter study of topical azelaic acid 15% gel in combination with oral doxycycline as initial therapy and azelaic acid 15% gel as maintenance monotherapy. *J Drugs Dermatol*. 2009;8:639–48.
4. Liu RH, Smith MK, Basta SA et al. Azelaic acid in the treatment of papulopustular rosacea: a systematic review of randomized controlled trials. *Arch Dermatol*. 2006;142:1047–52.

5. Koçak M, Ya?li S, Vahapo?lu G et al. Permethrin 5% cream versus metronidazole 0.75% gel for the treatment of papulopustular rosacea. A randomized double-blind placebo-controlled study. *Dermatology*. 2002;205:265–70.

ADDITIONAL READING

 See Also (Topic, Algorithm, Electronic Media Element)

Acne Vulgaris; Blepharitis; Dermatitis, Seborrheic; Lupus Erythematosus, Discoid; Uveitis
Algorithm: Acne

 CODES

ICD9
695.3 Rosacea

CLINICAL PEARLS

- Rosacea usually arises de novo without any preceding history of acne or seborrhea.
- Rosacea may cause chronic eye symptoms, including blepharitis.
- Avoid alcohol, sun exposure, and hot drinks.
- Medication treatment resembles that of acne vulgaris with oral and topical antibiotics.

ACNE VULGARIS

Gary I. Levine, MD

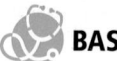 **BASICS**

DESCRIPTION
- Acne vulgaris is a disorder of the pilosebaceous units. It is a chronic inflammatory dermatosis notable for open/closed comedones and inflammatory lesions, including papules, pustules, or nodules.
- System(s) affected: Skin/Exocrine

Geriatric Considerations
Favre-Racouchot syndrome:
- Comedones on face and head due to sun exposure

Pregnancy Considerations
- May result in a flare or remission of acne
- Erythromycin can be used in pregnancy; use topical agents when possible.
- Isotretinoin is a teratogenic; Class X
- Avoid topical tretinoin, although no good evidence exists that its use is teratogenic.
- Contraindicated: Isotretinoin, tazarotene, tetracycline, doxycycline, minocycline

Pediatric Considerations
- Neonatal acne
- Infantile acne: Increased risk for severe teenage acne vulgaris
- Rare in ages 1–7 years:
  - Check for hyperandrogenemia of adrenal or ovarian origin.
  - Do not use tetracyclines <8 years of age

EPIDEMIOLOGY
- Predominant age: Early to late puberty, may persist into 4th decade
- Predominant sex:
  - Male > Female (adolescence)
  - Female > Male (adult)

Prevalence
- 17–50 million cases in the US
- Nearly 80–95% of adolescents affected. A smaller percentage will seek medical advice.
- 8% of adults aged 25–34 years, 3% of those aged 35–44 years

RISK FACTORS
- Increased endogenous androgenic effect
- Oily cosmetics: Cleansing creams, moisturizers, and oil-based foundations; pomade
- Rubbing or occluding skin surface (e.g., sports equipment such as helmets and shoulder pads), telephone, or hands against the skin
- Polyvinyl chloride, chlorinated hydrocarbons, cutting oil, tars
- Numerous drugs including androgenic steroids (e.g., steroid abuse, some birth control pills)
- Endocrine disorders: Polycystic ovarian syndrome, Cushing syndrome, congenital adrenal hyperplasia, androgen-secreting tumors, acromegaly
- Stress

Genetics
- Familial association in 50%
- If a family history exists, the acne may be more severe and occur earlier.

PATHOPHYSIOLOGY
- Immune changes and inflammatory responses may predate hyperkeratinization

- Androgens (testosterone and dehydroepiandrosterone [DHEA]) stimulate sebum production and proliferation of keratinocytes in hair follicles.
- Keratin plug obstructs follicle os, causing sebum accumulation and follicular distention.
- *Propionibacterium acnes*, an anaerobe, colonizes and proliferates in the plugged follicle.
- *P. acnes* promotes chemotactic factors and proinflammatory mediators, causing inflammation of follicle and dermis.

COMMONLY ASSOCIATED CONDITIONS
- Acne fulminans
- Pyoderma faciale
- Acne conglobata
- Hidradenitis suppurativa
- Pomade acne
- SAPHO syndrome: Synovitis, acne, pustulosis, hyperostosis, osteitis
- PAPA syndrome: Pyogenic sterile arthritis, pyoderma gangrenosum, cystic acne
- Behçet syndrome
- Apert syndrome
- Dark-skinned patients: 50% keloidal scarring and 50% acne hyperpigmented macules

 DIAGNOSIS

HISTORY
Ask duration, medications, cleansing products, stress, smoking, exposures, family history. Factors influencing symptomatology:
- Males later onset, greater severity
- Females may worsen prior to menses

PHYSICAL EXAM
- Closed comedones (whiteheads)
- Open comedones (blackheads)
- Nodules or papules
- Pustules ("cysts")
- Scars: Ice pick, rolling, boxcar, atrophic macules, hypertrophic, depressed, sinus tracts
- Grading system (American Academy of Dermatology, 1990):
  - *Mild*: Few papules/pustules; no nodules
  - *Moderate*: Some papules/pustules; few nodules
  - *Severe*: Numerous papules/pustules; many nodules
  - *Very severe*: Acne conglobata, acne fulminans, acne inversa
- Most common areas affected are: Face, chest, back, and upper arms (areas of greatest concentration of sebaceous glands)

DIAGNOSTIC TESTS & INTERPRETATION
Lab
Labs only indicated if there are additional signs of androgen excess; if so: Free testosterone, dehydroepiandrosterone sulfate (DHEA-S), luteinizing hormone, and follicle-stimulating hormone (1)[A]

DIFFERENTIAL DIAGNOSIS
- Folliculitis: Gram negative and gram positive
- Acne (rosacea, cosmetica, steroid-induced)
- Perioral dermatitis
- Chloracne
- Pseudofolliculitis barbae

- Drug eruption
- Verruca vulgaris and plana
- Keratosis pilaris
- Molluscum contagiosum
- Facial angiofibromas
- Sarcoidosis

 TREATMENT

- Topical retinoid plus a topical antimicrobial agent 1st-line treatment
- Topical retinoid plus antibiotic (topical or p.o.) is better than either alone (2,3)[A]
- Topical retinoids 1st-line agents for maintenance. Avoid antibiotics for maintenance.
- Comedonal acne (grade 1): Keratolytic agent (2,3)[A]
- Mild inflammatory acne (grade 2): Benzoyl peroxide +/− topical antibiotic. Keratolytic if needed (3,4)[A].
- Moderate inflammatory acne (grade 3): Add systemic antibiotic to grade 2 regimen.
- Severe inflammatory acne (grade 4): As in grade 3, or isotretinoin (2,3)[A]
- Recommended vehicle type:
  - Cream: Dry or sensitive skin
  - Gel or solution: Oily skin, humid weather
  - Lotion: Hair-bearing areas
- Mild soap daily to control oiliness; avoid abrasives
- Avoid drying agents with keratinolytic agents.
- Use of a gentle cleanser and noncomedogenic moisturizer helps decrease irritation from keratinolytic agents.
- Oil-free, noncomedogenic sunscreens
- Stress management if acne flares with stress

MEDICATION
Keratinolytic agents (side effects include dryness, erythema, scaling, and photosensitivity; start with lower strength; increase as tolerated) (1,2)[A]:
- Tretinoin (Retin-A, Retin A micro, Avita): Apply at bedtime; wash skin and let skin dry 30 minutes before topical application:
  - Retin-A Micro and Avita are less irritating, less phototoxicity
  - May cause an initial flare of lesions. May be eased by 14-day course of oral antibiotics.
- Adapalene (Differin): 0.1%, Apply topically at night:
  - Effective; less irritation than tretinoin or tazarotene (2,4)[A]
  - May be combined with benzoyl peroxide
- Tazarotene (Tazorac): Apply at bedtime:
  - Most effective and most irritating
  - Teratogenic
- Azelaic acid (Azelex, Finevin): 20% topically, b.i.d.:
  - Keratinolytic, antibacterial, anti-inflammatory
  - Reduces postinflammatory hyperpigmentation in dark-skinned individuals
  - Side effects: Erythema, dryness, scaling, hypopigmentation
  - Less effective in clinical use than in studies
- Salicylic acid: Less effective than tretinoin
- Alpha-hydroxy acids: Available over-the-counter

- Topical antibiotics and anti-inflammatories (2)[A]:
  – Topical benzoyl peroxide:
    ○ Bactericidal through direct toxic effect
    ○ No *P. acnes* resistance noted
    ○ 2.5% as effective as stronger preparations
    ○ When used with tretinoin, apply benzoyl peroxide in morning and tretinoin at night
    ○ Side effects: Irritation; may bleach clothes
- Topical antibiotics (1,2)[A]:
  – Erythromycin 2%
  – Clindamycin 1%
  – Metronidazole gel or cream: Apply once daily.
  – Azelaic acid (Azelex, Finevin): 20% cream: Enhanced effect and decreased risk of resistance when used with zinc and benzoyl peroxide
  – Benzoyl peroxide-erythromycin (Benzamycin): Especially effective with azelaic acid
  – Benzoyl peroxide-clindamycin (BenzaClin, DUAC, Clindoxyl): Effective combined (4)[A]
  – Sodium sulfacetamide (Sulfacet-R, Novacet, Klaron): Useful in acne with seborrheic dermatitis or rosacea
- Oral antibiotics (1,2)[A]:
  – Tetracycline: 500–2,000 mg/d b.i.d.–q.i.d.; high dose initially, taper in 6 months, as tolerated. Side effects: Photosensitivity, esophagitis:
    ○ Avoid use with antacids, iron
  – Minocycline 50–200 mg/d, q.i.d.–b.i.d. Side effects: Photosensitivity, urticaria, gray-blue skin, vertigo, autoimmune hepatitis, pseudotumor cerebri, lupuslike syndrome. May be more effective than tetracycline (1)[A].
  – Doxycycline 50–200 mg/d, given b.i.d.–q.i.d.; side effects include photosensitivity
  – Erythromycin: 500–1,000 mg/d; given b.i.d.–q.i.d.; decreasing effectiveness as a result of increasing *P. acnes* resistance
  – Trimethoprim-sulfamethoxazole (Bactrim DS, Septra DS); 1 daily or b.i.d.
- Oral retinoids:
  – Isotretinoin (Accutane) (1,2)[A]: 0.5–2.0 mg/kg/d b.i.d.; 60–90% cure rate; usually given for 12–20 weeks; maximum cumulative dose = 120–150 mg/kg; 20% of patients relapse and require retreatment:
    ○ Side effects: Numerous (see package insert). Highly teratogenic.
    ○ Avoid tetracyclines or vitamin A preparations during isotretinoin therapy.
    ○ Monitor for pregnancy, complete blood count, lipids, and liver function tests at baseline and every month.
    ○ Should be registered member of manufacturer's iPLEDGE program

Pregnancy Considerations
- Isotretinoin is a teratogenic; Class X
- Medications for women only:
  – Oral contraceptives (1,2)[A]:
    ○ Norgestimate/ethinyl estradiol (Orth Tricyclen), norethindrone acetate/ethinyl estradiol (Estrostep), drospirenone/ethinyl estradiol (Yaz, Yasmin) are approved by Food and Drug Administration.
    ○ Levonorgestrel/ethinyl estradiol (Alesse) is also effective.
  – Spironolactone (Aldactone); 25–200 mg/d; antiandrogen; reduces sebum production
  – Flutamide (Eulexin) 250–500 mg/d; potentially hepatotoxic

ADDITIONAL TREATMENT
Acne hyperpigmented macules:
- Topical hydroquinones (1.5–10%)
- Azelaic acid (20%) topically
- Topical retinoids as above
- Corticosteroids: Low dose, suppresses adrenal androgens (1)[B]
- Dapsone 5% gel (Aczone): Topical, anti-inflammatory use in patients >12 years

Issues for Referral
Consider referral/consultation to dermatologist:
- Refractory lesions despite appropriate therapy
- Consideration of isotretinoin therapy
- Management of acne scars

Additional Therapies
- Light-based treatments
  – UVA/UVB, blue light, blue/red light, pulse dye laser, KTP laser, infrared laser
  – Photodynamic therapy for 30–60 minutes with 5-aminolevulinic acid × 3 sessions is effective for inflammatory lesions:
    ○ Greatest utility when used as adjunct to medications or in patient who can't tolerate medications
  – More data needed to define role of light-based therapies in treating acne

COMPLEMENTARY AND ALTERNATIVE MEDICINE
- Zinc gluconate 30 mg/d may reduce inflammatory lesions (2)[B]:
  – Topical zinc is ineffective.
- Topical tree oil is effective, but has slow onset (1)[B].

SURGERY/OTHER PROCEDURES
- Comedo extraction after incising the layer of epithelium over comedo (1)[C]
- Incision and drainage for abscesses
- Inject large cystic lesions with 0.05–0.3 mL triamcinolone (Kenalog 2–5 mg/mL); use 30-g needle to inject and slightly distend cyst (1)[C].
- Acne scar treatment: Retinoids, steroid injections, cryosurgery, electrodessication, microdermabrasion, dermabrasion, chemical peels, laser resurfacing, grafting, subcutaneous incision, punch excision, punch elevation, subcision, tissue augmentation injections

 ## ONGOING CARE

FOLLOW-UP RECOMMENDATIONS
Use oral or topical antibiotics for 3 months; stop if inflammatory lesions resolve. Can switch abruptly from oral to topical without taper. Do not use topical and oral together.

Patient Monitoring
- Pretreatment and monthly lipids, liver function tests, and pregnancy tests when on isotretinoin
- Consider antibiotic resistance (60% overall) or gram-negative folliculitis if treatment fails.

DIET
Special diets do not diminish acne (1)[B].

PATIENT EDUCATION
- There may be a worsening of acne during 1st 2 weeks of treatment.
- Treatment takes a minimum of 4 weeks to show results.

- Topical agents can cause redness and drying of the skin.
- Picking at or popping lesions may increase inflammation and scarring.

PROGNOSIS
Gradual improvement over time (usually within 8–12 weeks after beginning therapy)

COMPLICATIONS
- Acne conglobata: Severe confluent inflammatory acne with systemic symptoms
- Facial and psychological scarring
- Gram-negative folliculitis: Superinfection due to long-term oral antibiotic use; treatment with ampicillin, trimethoprim-sulfa, or isotretinoin

REFERENCES
1. Strauss JS, Krowchuk DP, Leyden JJ et al. Guidelines of care for acne vulgaris management. *J Am Acad Dermatol*. 2007;56:651–63.
2. Feldman S, Careccia RE, Barham KL et al. Diagnosis and treatment of acne. *Am Fam Physician*. 2004;69:2123–30.
3. Webster G. Mechanism-based treatment of acne vulgaris: The value of combination therapy. *J Drugs and Dermatol*. 2005;4(3):281–8.
4. Haider A, Shaw JC. Treatment of acne vulgaris. *JAMA*. 2004;292:726–35.

ADDITIONAL READING
- Heymann WR. Oral contraceptives for the treatment of acne vulgaris. *J Am Acad Dermatol*. 2007;56:1056–7.
- Thibadout D, et al. New insights into the management of acne: An update from the Global Alliance to Improve Outcomes in Acne Group. *Journal of the American Academy of Dermatology*. 2009;60(5 supp1).

 See Also (Topic, Algorithm, Electronic Media Element)

Acne Rosacea
Algorithm: Acne

CODES

ICD9
706.1 Other acne

CLINICAL PEARLS
- Expect worsening for the 1st 2 weeks. Full results take 8–12 weeks.
- Decrease topical frequency from b.i.d. to every day or every day to every other day for irritation; may also use a moisturizing soap and a moisturizer before treatment application.
- Acne resolves with age for most individuals, although 8% of 30-year-olds and 3% of 40-year-olds may have persistent lesions.
- Acne often appears more significant to adolescent than to doctor; may be "entry ticket" for other advice.

ACOUSTIC NEUROMA

Sam Seung Yeol Kim, MBBS, Mmed
Phillip Chang, MBBS

BASICS

DESCRIPTION

- Slow-growing benign tumor, most often arising from the vestibular division of 8th cranial nerve
- Originates from Schwann cells of the nerve sheath ("schwannoma")
- Usually arises in the internal auditory canal near the cerebellopontine angle
- Often has extracanalicular portion into the cerebellopontine angle, but may also stay purely intracanalicular
- Most are unilateral; bilateral only seen in neurofibromatosis type II

EPIDEMIOLOGY

- 6–10% of all intracranial tumors
- 80–90% of cerebellopontine angle tumors
- 95% of cases are unilateral.
- Present most commonly in the 5th–6th decade
- Female predominance
- Bilateral acoustic neuroma occurring in neurofibromatosis II present before age 30

Incidence

- 1/100,000 per year
- Asymptomatic lesions may be more common.

Prevalence

3,000 diagnosed annually in the US

RISK FACTORS

- Pregnancy and epilepsy may increase risk (1).
- Smoking may decrease the risk (1).

Genetics

- Unknown for unilateral acoustic neuroma (AN)
- Neurofibromatosis type II: Bilateral ANs:
  – Autosomal dominant
  – Gene located on chromosome 22q1

PATHOPHYSIOLOGY

- Exerts pressure on the surrounding structures
- Compression of acoustic and facial nerve when located within internal acoustic canal
- Compression of brainstem, 4th ventricle, and trigeminal nerve when tumor at the cerebellar pontine angle

ETIOLOGY

Unknown

COMMONLY ASSOCIATED CONDITIONS

- Neurofibromatosis type II
- Pregnancy may accelerate the growth of the tumor.

DIAGNOSIS

HISTORY

- Common:
  – Sensorineural hearing loss (unilateral), often progressive
  – Loss of speech discrimination
  – Tinnitus
  – Balance problems are common, but vertigo is less common.
- Less common:
  – Weakness/loss of facial muscle functions
  – Headache with hydrocephalus and increased intracranial pressure
  – Trigeminal nerve involvement when tumor is large and compressing on cranial nerve (CN) V
  – Ataxia due to cerebellar or brainstem compression from very large tumor

PHYSICAL EXAM

- Examination with otoscope to exclude other causes of hearing loss (e.g., middle ear effusion, infection, wax, cholesteatoma, or tympanic membrane rupture)
- Detailed neurologic exam concentrating on the cranial nerves
- Weber and Rinne tests to confirm sensorineural hearing loss
- Evaluation of the contralateral ear in patients <30 years; suspect neurofibromatosis type II

DIAGNOSTIC TESTS & INTERPRETATION

Lab

Initial lab tests

- Pure-tone and speech audiometry (asymmetrical, high-frequency sensorineural hearing loss)
- Speech discrimination
- Stacked auditory brainstem response (ABR): 95% sensitivity and 88% specificity (2). Can detect tumors <1 cm.
- Standard ABR: Can only detect tumors >1 cm

Imaging

Initial approach

- Magnetic resonance imaging (MRI) with gadolinium (gold standard):
  – 100% specificity
  – Detects tumors starting at 2 mm
  – Tumor has marked enhancement with gadolinium
- Noncontrast T2-weighted fast spin-echo MRI:
  – 98% specificity
  – Cheaper than MRI with gadolinium
- Computed tomography (CT):
  – Detect tumors as small as 1 cm
  – Up to 37% false-negatives
  – Provides good information of surrounding bony structures of the tumor

Pathological Findings

- Well-demarcated and encapsulated mass attached to neural structures without direct invasion
- Can be dense or cystic
- Microscopic: Densely packed spindle cells (Schwann cells) mixed in with myxoid and collagenous matrix:
  – Zones of alternatively dense and sparse areas of Antoni A and B

DIFFERENTIAL DIAGNOSIS

- Cerebellopontine lesions:
  – Meningioma
  – Glioma
  – Facial nerve schwannoma
  – Epidermoid
  – Hemangioma
  – Arachnoid cyst
- Sensorineural hearing loss:
  – Ménière disease
  – Ototoxicity
  – Presbycusis
  – Cerebellar pathology

TREATMENT

MEDICATION

Chemotherapy has not yet been explored sufficiently.

ADDITIONAL TREATMENT

General Measures

- Conservative management is suitable for elderly patients with contraindications to surgery and radiotherapy.
- Up to 57% of acoustic neuromas may show zero growth or shrinkage (3)[B].
- Up to 70% of extracanalicular tumors may never have growth rate exceeding 2 mm per year (4)[B].
- Growth rate of enlarging acoustic neuromas decreases over time:
  – From 4.9 mm/yr in the 1st year of detected growth to 0.75 mm in 4th year.
- Up to 20% of patients may eventually fail conservative management and require intervention.
- More likely to preserve hearing than radiotherapy or surgery (5)[C]
- 69% of patients with 100% speech discrimination at diagnosis have maintained good hearing even after 10 years of observation (6)[B]

Issues for Referral

- Yearly MRI follow-up for slow-growing tumors
- If an asymptomatic tumor becomes symptomatic, this is often indication for intervention.

Additional Therapies
Stereotactic radiosurgery:
- Gamma knife single-dose stereotactic radiosurgery:
  - Performed on an outpatient basis
  - Alternative for those with smaller tumor (<3 cm) or contraindications to microsurgery
  - No discernible significant difference between growth patterns of untreated tumors and those treated radiosurgically (7)[A]
  - Lower-dose radiation has lower complication rates, but evidence is insufficient on whether as effective as high-dose radiation in tumor control (8)[A]
  - Higher-dose radiation significantly influences hearing preservation rates (9)[C]
  - Complications include trigeminal and/or facial nerve neuropathy from radiation damage.
- Fractionated stereotactic radiosurgery:
  - Conformal radiation delivers a higher dose of radiation within the tumor and less damage to surrounding healthy tissue.
  - Requires multiple treatments and the total dose of radiation is higher compared to the single-dose radiation
  - Suitable for all sizes of tumor

SURGERY/OTHER PROCEDURES
- Recommended definitive treatment (10)[A]
- Lowest rate of recurrence, with up to 97.5% complete tumor removal (10)[A]
- Intraoperative facial nerve monitoring is generally used.
- 3 standard approaches, all using operating microscopes:
  - Retromastoid/retrosigmoid: For any size, especially tumor located mostly outside the internal auditory canal and adjacent to the brainstem. May require retraction of cerebellum.
  - Middle cranial fossa: For small tumors with aim of preserving hearing. Involves retraction of temporal lobe and has higher risk of facial nerve injury.
  - Translabyrinthine: For larger tumors. Hearing not preserved. Completely exposes the distal internal auditory canal and has more favorable facial nerve results.
- Endoscopic approach used in some centers
- Surgical complications:
  - Hearing loss
  - Cerebrospinal fluid leakage
  - Facial nerve injury
  - Headache
  - Meningitis

 ONGOING CARE

FOLLOW-UP RECOMMENDATIONS
MRI and audiometric follow-up for those treated by radiotherapy and conservative management

COMPLICATIONS
Due to pressure effect of a large tumor:
- Cranial nerve compression
- Hydrocephalus
- Brainstem compression
- Cerebellar tonsil herniation

REFERENCES
1. Schoemaker MJ, Swerdlow AJ, Auvinen A et al. Medical history, cigarette smoking and risk of acoustic neuroma: an international case-control study. *Int J Cancer*. 2007;120:103–10.
2. Don M, Kwong B, Tanaka C et al. The stacked ABR: a sensitive and specific screening tool for detecting small acoustic tumors. *Audiol Neurootol*. 2005;10:274–90.
3. Smouha EE, Yoo M, Mohr K et al. Conservative management of acoustic neuroma: a meta-analysis and proposed treatment algorithm. *Laryngoscope*. 2005;115:450–4.
4. Stangerup SE, Caye-Thomasen P, Tos M et al. The natural history of vestibular schwannoma. *Otol Neurotol*. 2006;27:547–52.
5. Lin VY, Stewart C, Grebenyuk J et al. Unilateral acoustic neuromas: long-term hearing results in patients managed with fractionated stereotactic radiotherapy, hearing preservation surgery, and expectantly. *Laryngoscope*. 2005;115:292–6.
6. Stangerup SE, Thomsen J, Tos M, Cayé-Thomasen P et al. Long-term hearing preservation in vestibular schwannoma. *Otol. Neurotol*. 2010;31:271–5.
7. Battaglia A, Mastrodimos B, Cueva R. Comparison of growth patterns of acoustic neuromas with and without radiosurgery. *Otol Neurotol*. 2006;27:705–12.
8. Weil RS, et al. Optimal dose of stereotactic radiosurgery for acoustic neuromas: A systematic review. *Brit J Neurosurg* 2006:195–202.
9. Combs SE, Welzel T, Schulz-Ertner D, Huber PE, Debus J et al. Differences in clinical results after LINAC-based single-dose radiosurgery versus fractionated stereotactic radiotherapy for patients with vestibular schwannomas. *Int. J. Radiat. Oncol. Biol. Phys.* 2010;76:193–200.
10. Kaylie DM, Horgan MJ, Delashaw JB et al. A meta-analysis comparing outcomes of microsurgery and gamma knife radiosurgery. *Laryngoscope*. 2000;110:1850–6.

 CODES

ICD9
- 225.1 Benign neoplasm of cranial nerves
- 237.70 Neurofibromatosis, unspecified
- 237.71 Neurofibromatosis, type 1, von recklinghausen's disease

CLINICAL PEARLS

A bone-anchored hearing aid can restore hearing for those patients with sensorineural hearing loss that may be present before or after the surgery.

ADOPTION, INTERNATIONAL
Maya Leventer-Roberts, MD, MPH

BASICS

DESCRIPTION
Adoption of children from foreign countries into the US has tripled in the past 15 years, and the demographics of those children and their homelands have also shifted significantly during that time. The diverse birth countries, disease exposures, and unknown health histories of these children make them a population that requires special attention (1).

EPIDEMIOLOGY
Incidence
- More than 20,000 international adoptions by US families every year
- >90% are from Asia, Central and South America, and Eastern Europe, with growing numbers from Africa and the Middle East

RISK FACTORS
- Unknown birth history, past medical history, and vaccination status
- Possible exposure to toxins and/or inadequate nutrition in utero
- Exposures to infectious diseases not commonly seen in the US
- Previous living conditions:
  – Overcrowding
  – Institutionalization (orphanages)
  – Environmental toxins
- History of neglect, deprivation, or abuse

GENERAL PREVENTION
- Required to be examined by a US State Department physician in their native country before immigration to the US (2)
- Should be examined by US physician within 3 weeks of arrival
- A follow-up visit 4–6 weeks after their post-adoption appointment is recommended.
- All internationally adopted children should be routinely screened for hearing, vision, growth, and developmental delays.

COMMONLY ASSOCIATED CONDITIONS
- Infectious diseases, including (2,3):
  – Hepatitis B
  – Intestinal parasites
  – Tuberculosis
  – Syphilis
- Emotional or behavioral problems
- Developmental delay
- Fetal alcohol syndrome
- Feeding difficulties
- Anemia
- Congenital conditions, including:
  – Cleft lip/palate
  – Orthopedic deformities
- Prematurity or low birth weight
- Malnutrition, rickets
- Inadequate immunizations
- Lead poisoning
- Sensorineural and conductive hearing loss
- Strabismus, blindness

DIAGNOSIS

HISTORY
- Immunization records and titers (most helpful when dates of administration are included) (4)
- Birth/prenatal history
- Known family history of birth parents
- Prenatal and perinatal disease or toxin exposures
- Documented history of emotional or nutritional deprivation, or physical or sexual abuse
- Duration of time, if any, spent in orphanage. (Studies have suggested every 3–5 months spent in orphanage is associated with 1 month delay in developmental milestones, although quality of care can vary widely.)
- Growth charts when available: Failure to gain weight appropriately (or weight loss) is earliest sign of malnutrition, followed by slowed linear growth, and finally lagging head circumference (brain growth).
- Development, behavior, attachment, parent stress, and parent-child interactions should also be routinely monitored.

PHYSICAL EXAM
- Age-appropriate complete physical exam, particular attention to growth, evaluation for microcephaly (red flag for fetal alcohol syndrome, genetic disorders, or perinatal brain injury), vision, and hearing
- Evaluate for signs of dental decay and refer for prompt treatment
- Developmental assessment, especially for those with unknown date of birth
- Skin exam for signs of scabies, pediculosis, and tinea

DIAGNOSTIC TESTS & INTERPRETATION
- Developmental screening: Denver II Test ($\pm$) PEDS parent questionnaire or other validated developmental screening tools at each visit to screen for potential developmental delay and to assess improvement, decline, and need for additional services
- Age-appropriate hearing screening
- Age-appropriate vision screening

Lab
Initial lab tests
- Obtain (5):
  – Hepatitis B (HBsAg, HBsAb, anti-HBc)
  – Hepatitis C
  – HIV
  – Rapid plasma reagin (RPR)
  – Tuberculin skin test
  – 3 stool specimens for ova and parasites, and single specimen for *Giardia lamblia* and *Cryptosporidium parvum* antigens
  – Complete blood count (CBC)
  – Lead
  – Thyroid-stimulating hormone (TSH)
  – Ca^{++}, PO_4, alkaline phosphate, and 25 vitamin D level (if signs of rickets)
  – Urinalysis
- >6 months old: Measure titers for antibodies to diphtheria and tetanus toxoids and poliovirus (regardless of immunization documentation).
- >12 months old: Measure titers for antibodies to diphtheria, tetanus toxoids, poliovirus, measles, mumps, rubella, and varicella (regardless of immunization documentation).

Follow-Up & Special Considerations
Follow-up testing (5):
- Hep B: Repeat at 6 months.
- Hep C: Required in children from China, Russia, Eastern Europe, and Southeast Asia (decision to test children from other countries depends on history and prevalence of infection)
- HIV: Transplacentally acquired maternal antibody may be present in uninfected infants up to 18 months, so will need to retest those with an initial positive result.
- Tuberculosis (TB): Positive test should NOT be attributed to BCG vaccine, and must be investigated further. Give preventive therapy if known exposures. Consider repeat testing at 6 months because poor nutrition may result in false-negative (anergic) skin test.
- Gastrointestinal tract signs or symptoms occurring years after immigration: Test for intestinal parasites.
- If anemia is detected with a normal lead level, may consider G6PD deficiency in appropriate countries of origin (Africa, Asia, Mediterranean, Middle Eastern), and can test with rapid fluorescent spot test.
- Developmental screening: Repeat at each visit and follow progress. 50–90% of all internationally adopted children are delayed upon adoption; however, most of them have normal cognition at long-term follow-up.
- Social history screening: Behavioral concerns may first present during adolescence, even for children were adopted in infancy. (6)

TREATMENT

MEDICATION
- Immunizations per Centers for Disease Control and Prevention schedule with catch-up as needed: http://www.cdc.gov/vaccines/recs/schedules/
- It is recommended that if the child does not have records, or has records that do not comply with the US or World Health Organization guidelines, then he or she should be treated as unimmunized and started on an appropriate catch-up immunization schedule.

ADDITIONAL TREATMENT
General Measures
- Regular diet for children who arrive malnourished should result in rapid weight gain to appropriate weight for height (or length).
- Monitor linear growth; American growth chart might not be applicable to all children.
- If developmental delay is diagnosed, consider early services (such as early intervention) or referral to developmental specialist, depending on the nature and severity of the delay.
- Recommend local support groups for parents.
- Attention to parental interactions: Post-adoption depression may occur.

Issues for Referral
- Many internationally adopted children show sensory-seeking behaviors early on that are sometimes thought to be related to the sensory-depriving orphanage experience of their past. These behaviors typically improve or abate without treatment, but may benefit from work with occupational therapy if the behaviors are significant. Out of context, they may appear quite similar to autistic-like features on exam (hand-flapping,

rocking, etc.), but as long as the child is otherwise developing normally (socially, emotionally), should not raise significant levels of concern (2).

- If a child continues to have disruptive behaviors, or would rather self-soothe than seek nurturing human interaction, he or she warrants a complete and thorough developmental evaluation with a specialist (developmental/behavioral pediatrician or pediatric psychiatrist).
- Persistent behavioral issues in the parent-child interactions should also be evaluated by a pediatric psychologist or psychiatrist.
- Concerns about vision should be referred to pediatric ophthalmology for more extensive vision workup.
- Concerns about hearing should be referred to audiology and/or ENT for more extensive workup for conductive vs sensorineural hearing loss.
- Recommend pediatric dental evaluation by 12 months, sooner if signs of dental pathology.

 ONGOING CARE

FOLLOW-UP RECOMMENDATIONS
Patient Monitoring
- Regular well child visits, particularly within first months of entry into the US
- Close monitoring of developmental milestones, behavior, and individual attachment

DIET
- Regular diet
- Weight catch-up will occur with a normal diet, barring other medical conditions, and eating habits should normalize using parenting methods discussed below.

PATIENT EDUCATION
- Eating: The recommended approach is to allow access to as much healthy food as the child wants, as often as he or she wants it, so that the child can learn the important self-regulatory behaviors of eating that may not have been learned in an institution (hunger, satiety) and can build trust with the parent(s) who feed him or her.
- Toileting: While some children may simply not be trained yet, others may have accidents in their new home because of regression. Time and positive reinforcement, avoiding punishment, will resolve this issue as the child becomes comfortable with his or her new surroundings.
- Sleeping: Children must learn to trust their new home and parents, and thus this is not a time for aggressive sleep rules (i.e., ferberization). Parents should be present, physically and emotionally, just enough to let the child know he or she is safe, establish a bedtime ritual upon arrival, and then should gently reinforce this ritual.
- Language: As the child experiences a myriad of changes, it may be helpful for the adoptive family to have learned some key phrases in the child's native language for the first few weeks post-adoption. Depending on the child's age and language proficiency, an interpreter may also be useful in the home and at medical appointments until English becomes more comfortably understood and familiar (2).
- Adopted children may experience grieving of lost family, relationships, and culture, which is normal and expected behavior.

- At 3–4 years old, adopted children will begin to recognize physical differences between themselves and adoptive family if they are of differing racial origin.
- Children and families should be encouraged to learn about the heritage and culture of the birth countries or ethnic groups.
- Relationships with others of the same racial or ethnic group may be very helpful to the adopted child.

PROGNOSIS
Long-term issues include (7,8):
- Children who experienced early neglect, deprivation, or loss prior to adoption are more likely to have developmental delay or behavioral or attachment problems.
- These issues decrease with time the child has spent within the adoptive family, although those with significant histories of deprivation are at risk for difficulties that may persist for life.
- Although most adopted children are healthy, as a group they have been found to have higher rates of moderate to severe physical and mental health problems, hearing and visual impairment, learning disability, developmental delay, or special health care needs when compared with biologic children of the same parents.
- Developmental delay, in particular, is reportedly found to be 2–3 times more likely in an internationally adopted child than in his or her nonadopted peers. However, recent studies show marked catch-up development reported after living in adoptive homes, with many children achieving normal-range development later in life (depending on length of time spent in an institution prior to adoption).
- Fortunately, international adoption pairs some of the most vulnerable, potentially high-risk children with the lowest-risk parents (usually financially stable, well-educated, with relatively extremely low divorce rates).
- Most families have found the process of international adoption deeply rewarding, while acknowledging the potential challenges.

REFERENCES

1. Dawood F, Serwint JR. International adoption. *Pediatr Rev.* 2008;29:292–4.
2. Schulte EE, Springer SH. Health care in the first year after international adoption. *Pediatr Clin North Am.* 2005;52:1331–49, vii.
3. Johnson DE. Long-term medical issues in international adoptees. *Pediatr Ann.* 2000;29: 234–41.
4. American Academy of Pediatrics Committee on Early Childhood, Adoption & Dependent Care: Initial medical evaluation of an adopted child. *Pediatrics.* 1991;88:642–4.
5. American Academy of Pediatrics. Medical evaluation of internationally adopted children for infectious diseases. In: Pickering LK ed. *Red Book: 2006 Report of the Committee on Infectious Diseases – 27th Ed.*

6. Hawk B, McCall RB et al. CBCL behavior problems of post-institutionalized international adoptees. *Clin Child Fam Psychol Rev.* 2010;13:199-211
7. Van Ijzendoorn MH, Bakermans-Kranenburg MJ, Juffer F. Plasticity of Growth in Height, Weight, and Head Circumference: Meta-analytic Evidence of Massive Catch-up After International Adoption. *J Dev Behav Pediatr.* 2007;28:334–43.
8. Weitzman C, Albers L. Long-term developmental, behavioral, and attachment outcomes after international adoption. *Pediatr Clin North Am.* 2005;52:1395–419, viii.

ADDITIONAL READING
- Borchers D, American Academy of Pediatrics Committee on Early Childhood, Adoption, and Dependent Care. Families and adoption: the pediatrician's role in supporting communication. *Pediatrics.* 2003;112:1437–41.
- http://www.travel.state.gov/pdf/Prospective_Adoptive_Parents_Guide.pdf.

 CODES

ICD9
V70.3 Other general medical examination for administrative purposes

CLINICAL PEARLS
- Initial labs:
  – Hepatitis B (HBsAg, HBsAb, anti-HBc), hepatitis C IgG, HIV, RPR, CBC, TSH, lead, Ca, PO4, 25 OH vitamin D
  – Tuberculin skin test
  – 3 stool specimens for ova and parasites, and single specimen for *Giardia lamblia* and *Cryptosporidium parvum* antigens
  – Urinalysis
- >6 months old: Measure antibodies to diphtheria and tetanus toxoids and poliovirus (regardless of immunization documentation).
- >12 months old: Measure antibodies to diphtheria, tetanus toxoids, poliovirus, measles, mumps, rubella, and varicella (regardless of immunization documentation).
- Many internationally adopted children show sensory-seeking behaviors early on that are sometimes thought to be related to the sensory-depriving orphanage experience of their past. These behaviors typically improve or abate without treatment, but may benefit from work with occupational therapy if the behaviors are significant. Out of context, they may appear quite similar to autistic-like features on exam (hand-flapping, rocking, etc.), but as long as the child is otherwise developing normally (socially, emotionally), they should not raise significant levels of concern.

ALCOHOL ABUSE AND DEPENDENCE

Gennine M. Zinner, RNCS, ANP

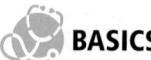 **BASICS**

DESCRIPTION

- Any pattern of alcohol use causing significant physical, mental, or social dysfunction; key features are tolerance, withdrawal, and persistent use despite problems
- Alcohol abuse: Maladaptive pattern of alcohol use manifested by 1 (or more) of:
  - Failure to fulfill obligations at work, school, or home
  - Recurrent use in hazardous situations
  - Recurrent alcohol-related legal problems
  - Continued use despite related social or interpersonal problems
- Alcohol dependence: Maladaptive pattern of use manifested by 3 (or more) of the following:
  - Tolerance
  - Withdrawal
  - Using more than intended
  - Persistent desire or attempts to cut down/stop
  - Significant amount of time obtaining, using, or recovering from alcohol
  - Social, occupational, or recreational activities sacrificed for alcohol use
  - Continued use despite physical or psychological problems
- National Institute on Alcohol Abuse and Alcoholism criteria for "at-risk" drinking: Men >14 drinks a week or >4 per occasion. Women: >7 drinks a week or >3 per occasion.
- System(s) affected: Nervous; Gastrointestinal
- Synonym(s): Alcoholism; Alcohol abuse; Alcohol dependence

Geriatric Considerations
- Common and underdiagnosed in elderly; less likely to report problem. May exacerbate normal age-related cognitive deficits and disabilities.
- Multiple drug interactions
- Signs and symptoms may be different or attributed to chronic medical problem or dementia.
- Assessment tools may be inappropriate.

Pediatric Considerations
- Children of alcoholics at high risk
- In 2004, 28% of persons 12–20 years reported use in past month, 1 in 5 binge drink; binge drinkers are 7 times more likely to report illicit drug use.
- Negative effect on maturation and development
- Early drinkers are 4 times more likely to develop a problem than those who begin >21.
- Depression, suicidal or disorderly behavior; family disruption; violence or destruction of property; poor school or work performance; sexual promiscuity; social immaturity; lack of interests; isolation; moodiness

Pregnancy Considerations
- Alcohol is teratogenic, especially during the 1st trimester; women should abstain during conception and throughout pregnancy.
- 10–50% of children born to women who are heavy drinkers will have fetal alcohol syndrome.
- Women experience harmful effects at lower levels and are less likely to report problems.

EPIDEMIOLOGY
- Predominant age: 18–25, but all ages affected
- Predominant sex: Male > Female (3:1)

Prevalence
- Lifetime prevalence: 13.6%
- 20% in primary care setting
- 48.2% of 21-year-olds in the US reported binge drinking in 2004.

RISK FACTORS
- Family history
- Depression (40% with comorbid alcohol abuse)
- Anxiety
- Other substance abuse
- Tobacco
- Male gender
- Low socioeconomic status
- Unemployment
- Peer/social approval
- Family dysfunction or childhood trauma
- Posttraumatic stress disorder
- Antisocial personality disorder
- Bipolar disorder
- Eating disorders
- Criminal involvement

Genetics
50–60% of risk is genetic.

GENERAL PREVENTION
Counsel with family history and risk factors

PATHOPHYSIOLOGY
Alcohol is a central nervous system depressant, facilitating γ-aminobutyric acid (GABA) inhibition and blocking N-methyl-d-aspartate receptors.

ETIOLOGY
Multifactorial: Genetic, environment, psychosocial

COMMONLY ASSOCIATED CONDITIONS
- Cardiomyopathy
- Atrial fibrillation
- Hypertension
- Peptic ulcer disease/gastritis
- Cirrhosis
- Fatty liver
- Cholelithiasis
- Hepatitis
- Diabetes mellitus
- Pancreatitis
- Malnutrition
- Upper gastrointestinal (GI) malignancies
- Peripheral neuropathy
- Seizures
- Abuse
- Violence
- Trauma (falls, motor vehicle accidents [MVAs])
- Severe psychiatric disorders (depression, bipolar, schizophrenia): >50% of patients with these disorders have a comorbid substance abuse problem.

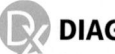 **DIAGNOSIS**

HISTORY
- Behavioral issues:
  - Anxiety, depression, insomnia
  - Psychological and social dysfunction, marital problems
  - Social isolation/withdrawal
  - Domestic violence
  - Alcohol-related legal problems
  - Repeated attempts to stop/reduce
  - Loss of interest in nondrinking activities
  - Employment problems (tardiness, absenteeism, decreased productivity, interpersonal problems, frequent job loss)
  - Blackouts
  - Complaints about alcohol-related behavior
  - Frequent trauma, MVAs, emergency department visits
- Physical symptoms:
  - Anorexia
  - Nausea, vomiting
  - Abdominal pain
  - Palpitations
  - Headache
  - Impotence
  - Menstrual irregularities
  - Infertility

PHYSICAL EXAM
- Physical exam may be completely normal
- General: Fever, agitation, diaphoresis
- Head/eyes/ears/nose/throat: Plethoric face, rhinophyma, poor oral hygiene, oropharyngeal malignancies
- Cardiovascular: Hypertension, dilated cardiomyopathy, tachycardia
- Respiratory: Aspiration pneumonia
- GI: Stigmata of chronic liver disease, peptic ulcer disease, pancreatitis, esophageal malignancies, esophageal varices
- Genitourinary: Testicular atrophy
- Musculoskeletal: Poorly healed fractures, myopathy, osteopenia, bone marrow suppression
- Neurologic: Tremors, cognitive deficits (e.g., memory impairment), peripheral neuropathy, Wernicke-Korsakoff syndrome
- Endocrine/metabolic: Hyperlipidemias, cushingoid appearance, gynecomastia
- Dermatologic: Burns (e.g., cigarettes), bruises, poor hygiene, palmar erythema, spider telangiectasias, caput medusa, jaundice

DIAGNOSTIC TESTS & INTERPRETATION
- CAGE Questionnaire: (Cut down, Annoyed, Guilty, and Eye opener): More than 2 "yes" answers is 74–89% sensitive, 79–95% specific for alcohol use disorder; less sensitive for white women, college students, elderly. Not an appropriate tool for less severe forms of alcohol abuse (1)[A].
- Alcohol Use Disorders Identification Test: 10 items, if >4: 70–92% sensitive (2)[A]
- Single Question for Screening: "How many times in the last year have you had X or more drinks in one day" (X = 5 for men, 4 for women); sensitive screen for unhealthy alcohol use; 81.8% sensitive, 79% specific for alcohol use disorders (3)

Lab

- Blood alcohol concentration:
  - >100 mg/dL in outpatient setting
  - >150 mg/dL without obvious signs of intoxication
  - >300 mg/dL at any time
- Serum levels increased in chronic abuse:
  - AST/ALT ratio >2.0
  - γ-Glutamyl transferase (GGT)
  - Carbohydrate-deficient transferrin
  - Elevated mean corpuscular volume
  - Prothrombin time
  - Uric acid
  - Triglycerides
  - Cholesterol (total)
- Often decreased:
  - Calcium, magnesium, potassium, phosphorus
  - Blood urea nitrogen
  - Hemoglobin, hematocrit
  - Platelet count
  - Serum protein, albumin
  - Thiamine, folate

Imaging

- Radiograph: Multiple old rib fractures
- Computed tomography scan, magnetic resonance imaging of brain: Cortical atrophy, lesions in thalamic nucleus and basal forebrain
- Abdominal ultrasound: Ascites, periportal fibrosis, fatty infiltration, inflammation

Pathological Findings

- Liver: Inflammation or fatty infiltration (alcoholic hepatitis), periportal fibrosis (alcoholic cirrhosis occurs in only 10–20% of alcoholics)
- Gastric mucosa: Inflammation, ulceration
- Pancreas: Inflammation, liquefaction necrosis
- Heart: Dilated cardiomyopathy
- Immune system: Decreased granulocytes
- Endocrine organs: Elevated cortisol levels, testicular atrophy, decreased female hormones
- Brain: Cortical atrophy, enlarged ventricles

DIFFERENTIAL DIAGNOSIS

- Other substance use disorders
- Depression
- Dementia
- Cerebellar ataxia
- Cerebrovascular accident (CVA)
- Benign essential tremor
- Seizure disorder
- Hypoglycemia
- Diabetic ketoacidosis
- Viral hepatitis

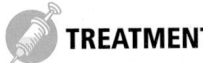 TREATMENT

For management of acute withdrawal, please see Alcohol Withdrawal.

MEDICATION

First Line

- Adjuncts to withdrawal regimens:
  - Naltrexone 50–100 mg/d p.o. or 380 mg IM once every 4 weeks: Opiate antagonist reduces craving and likelihood of relapse (IM route may enhance compliance and thus efficacy) (4,5)[A]
  - Acamprosate (Campral) 666 mg p.o. t.i.d. beginning after completion of withdrawal; reduces relapse risk (4)[A]
  - Topiramate (Topamax) 25–300 mg/d p.o. or divided b.i.d.; enhances abstinence (4)[B]

- Supplements to all:
  - Thiamine 100 mg/d (1st dose IV prior to glucose to avoid Wernicke encephalopathy)
  - Folic acid 1 mg/d
  - Multivitamin daily
- Contraindications:
  - Naltrexone: Pregnancy, acute hepatitis, hepatic failure
  - Monitor liver function tests.
- Precautions: Organic pain, organic brain syndromes
- Significant possible interactions: Alcohol, sedatives, hypnotics, naltrexone, and narcotics

 ALERT

Treat acute symptoms if in alcohol withdrawal.

Second Line

- Disulfiram 250–500 mg/d p.o.: Unproven efficacy; may provide psychologic deterrent
- Selective serotonin reuptake inhibitors may be beneficial if comorbid depression exists.

ADDITIONAL TREATMENT

General Measures

- Brief interventions by primary care clinicians are effective for problem drinking (6)[A].
- Involve family, if feasible.
- Treat comorbid problems (sleep, anxiety, etc.); use caution if prescribing medications with cross-tolerance to alcohol (benzodiazepine).
- Group programs and/or 12-step programs may have benefit in helping patients accept treatment.

Issues for Referral

Addiction specialist, 12-step or long-term program, psychiatrist

IN-PATIENT CONSIDERATIONS

Assess medical and psychiatric condition.

Initial Stabilization

- Correct electrolyte imbalances, acidosis, hypovolemia (treat if in alcohol withdrawal)
- Thiamine 100 mg IM, followed by orally 100 mg, and folic acid 1 mg/day
- Benzodiazepines used to lower risk of alcohol withdrawal, seizures

 ONGOING CARE

FOLLOW-UP RECOMMENDATIONS

Patient Monitoring

- Outpatient detoxification: Daily visits
- Early outpatient rehabilitation: Weekly visits
- Detoxification alone is not sufficient.

PATIENT EDUCATION

- American Council on Alcoholism: (800) 527-5344 or http://www.aca-usa.org (treatment facility locator, educational information)
- National Clearinghouse for Alcohol and Drug Information: (800) 729-6686 or http://www.health.org
- Center for Substance Abuse Treatment: (800) 662-HELP or http://www.csat.samhsa.gov
- Alcoholics Anonymous: http://www.aa.org
- Rational Recovery: http://www.rational.org
- Secular Organizations for Sobriety: www.cfiwest.org/sos/index.htm
- http://www.alcoholanswers.org/list: An evidence-based Web site for those seeking credible information on alcohol dependence and online support forums.

PROGNOSIS

- Chronic relapsing disease; mortality rate > twice general population, death 10–15 years earlier
- Abstinence benefits survival, mental health, family, employment
- 12-step programs, cognitive behavior, and motivational therapies are effective during 1st year following treatment (2)[B].

COMPLICATIONS

- Cirrhosis (women sooner than men)
- GI malignancies
- Neuropathy
- Dementia
- Wernicke-Korsakoff syndrome
- CVA
- Ketoacidosis
- Infection
- Adult respiratory distress syndrome
- Depression
- Suicide
- Trauma

REFERENCES

1. Dhalla S, Kopec JA. The CAGE questionnaire for alcohol misuse: a review of reliability and validity studies. *Clin Invest Med*. 2007;30:33–41.
2. Enoch MA, et al. Problem drinking and alcoholism: Diagnosis and treatment. *Am Fam Phys* 2002;65:441–8.
3. Smith PC, Schmidt SM, Allensworth-Davies D et al. Primary Care Validation of a Single-Question Alcohol Screening Test. *J Gen Intern Med*. 2009;
4. Williams SH. Medications for treating alcohol dependence. *Am Fam Phys*. 2005;72(pt 9):1775–80.
5. Pettinati HM, Gastfriend DR, Dong Q et al. Effect of Extended-Release Naltrexone (XR-NTX) on Quality of Life in Alcohol-Dependent Patients. *Alcohol Clin Exp Res*. 2008.
6. Asplund CA, Aaronson JW, Aaronson HE. 3 regimens for alcohol withdrawal and detoxification. *J Fam Pract*. 2004;53:545–54.

ADDITIONAL READING

 See Also (Topic, Algorithm, Electronic Media Element)

Substance Use Disorders; Alcohol Withdrawal

CODES

ICD9

- 303.90 Other and unspecified alcohol dependence, unspecified drinking behavior
- 305.00 Nondependent alcohol abuse, unspecified drinking behavior

CLINICAL PEARLS

Clinicians should avoid assumptions and adopt an "addiction-oriented" practice style, asking a few basic questions regarding substance use of all patients.

ALCOHOL WITHDRAWAL

Ryan Dono, MD
Erik J. Garcia, MD

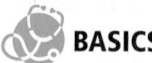 ## BASICS

DESCRIPTION
Alcohol withdrawal syndrome (AWS) is a spectrum of symptoms that results from abrupt cessation of alcohol in a dependent patient. Symptoms can begin within 5 hours of last drink and persist for 5–10 days, ranging in severity.

EPIDEMIOLOGY
Each year, 8.2 million Americans meet diagnostic criteria for alcohol dependence. It is more prevalent among men, whites, Native Americans, younger and unmarried adults, and those with lower socioeconomic status. Only 24.1% of those with alcohol dependence are ever treated.

RISK FACTORS
- Older age
- High tolerance, prolonged use, high quantities
- Previous alcohol withdrawal episodes, detoxifications, alcohol withdrawal seizures, and delirium tremens
- Symptoms of withdrawal in the presence of high blood alcohol level
- Serious medical problems
- Concomitant benzodiazepine dependence

Geriatric Considerations
- Geriatric populations dependent on alcohol are more susceptible to symptoms of alcohol withdrawal and often have chronic comorbid conditions placing them at higher risk of complications from withdrawal.

Pregnancy Considerations
- Hospitalization or inpatient detoxification is usually required for medical treatment and monitoring of acute alcohol withdrawal.

Genetics
There is some evidence for a genetic basis of alcohol dependence.

GENERAL PREVENTION
- The US Preventative Services Task Force recommends routine screening for alcohol misuse for all adults (1)[B].
- Screening for alcohol abuse during the office visit and appropriate follow-up with the CAGE or similar questionnaire:
  - Feeling the need to **C**ut down
  - **A**nnoyed by criticism about alcohol use
  - **G**uilt about drinking/behaviors while intoxicated
  - "**E**ye opener" to quell withdrawal symptoms
  - Useful to detect problematic alcohol use, positive screen is ≥2 "yes" responses
- 10-question AUDIT screening test is also useful to identify problem drinking.

PATHOPHYSIOLOGY
- Consumption of alcohol potentiates the effect of the inhibitory neurotransmitter GABA. With chronic alcohol ingestion, this repeated stimulation down-regulates the inhibitory effects of GABA.
- Concurrently, alcohol ingestion inhibits the stimulatory effect of glutamate on the central nervous system with chronic alcohol use up-regulating excitatory NMDA glutamate receptors.
- When alcohol is abruptly stopped, the combined effect of a down-regulated inhibitory neurotransmitter system (GABA-modulated) and up-regulated excitatory neurotransmitter system (glutamate-modulated)—no longer suppressed by alcohol—results in brain hyperexcitability; clinically seen as AWS.

COMMONLY ASSOCIATED CONDITIONS
- General: Poor nutrition, hyponatremia, hypomagnesemia, hypokalemia, low thiamine, dehydration
- Gastrointestinal: Hepatitis, cirrhosis, varices, GI bleed
- Heme: Splenomegaly, thrombocytopenia, macrocytic anemia
- Cardiovascular: Cardiomyopathy, hypertension, atrial fibrillation, other arrhythmias
- CNS: Trauma, seizure disorder, generalized atrophy, Wernicke-Korsakoff syndrome
- PNS: Neuropathy, myopathy
- Psychiatric: Depression, posttraumatic stress disorder, bipolar disease, polysubstance abuse

 ## DIAGNOSIS

- The *Diagnostic and Statistical Manual (4th ed. - TR)* can be used to assess symptoms of AWS. AWS may be diagnosed when ≥2 of the following symptoms present within a few hours to several days after the cessation or reduction of heavy and prolonged alcohol ingestion:
  - Autonomic hyperactivity (sweating, tachycardia)
  - Increased hand tremor
  - Insomnia
  - Psychomotor agitation
  - Anxiety
  - Nausea
  - Vomiting
  - Grand mal seizures
  - Transient (visual, auditory, or tactile) hallucinations or illusions
  - These should cause clinically significant distress or impair functioning and not be secondary to an underlying medical condition or mental disorder.
  - There are 3 stages to AWS.
- Stage 1 (Minor withdrawal; onset 5–8 hours after cessation):
  - Mild anxiety, restlessness, and agitation
  - Mild nausea/GI upset and decreased appetite
  - Sleep disturbance
  - Sweating
  - Mild tremulousness
  - Fluctuating tachycardia and hypertension
- Stage 2 (Major withdrawal; onset 24–72 hours after cessation):
  - Marked restlessness and agitation
  - Moderate tremulousness with constant eye movements
  - Diaphoresis
  - Nausea, vomiting, diarrhea, anorexia
  - Marked tachycardia and hypertension
  - Alcoholic hallucinosis (auditory, tactile, or visual); may have mild confusion but can be reoriented
- Stage 3 (Delirium tremens; onset 72–96 hours after cessation):
  - Fever
  - Severe hypertension, tachycardia
  - Delirium
  - Drenching sweats
  - Marked tremors

- Alcohol withdrawal– associated seizures are often brief, generalized tonic-clonic seizures and can occur 6–48 hours after last drink.

HISTORY
Essential historical information should be:
- Duration and quantity of alcohol intake
- Time since last drink
- Previous episodes/symptoms of alcohol withdrawal
- Prior detox admissions
- Concurrent substance use
- Pre-existing medical and psychiatric conditions
- Prior seizure activity
- Social history: Living situation, social support, stressors, triggers, etc.

PHYSICAL EXAM
Should include assessment of conditions likely to complicate or that are exacerbated by AWS:
- Cardiovascular: Arrhythmias, congestive heart failure, coronary artery disease
- Gastrointestinal: GI bleed, liver disease, pancreatitis
- Neuro: Oculomotor dysfunction, gait ataxia, neuropathy
- Psych: Orientation, memory
- General: Hand tremor, infections

DIAGNOSTIC TESTS & INTERPRETATION
Lab
Initial lab tests
- Blood alcohol level
- Urine drug screen
- Complete blood count (CBC)
- Electrolytes
- Blood glucose
- Magnesium
- Liver function tests
- Renal function tests

Imaging
Initial approach
Low threshold for CNS imaging in any patient with acute mental status changes, given high incidence of traumatic brain injury.

DIFFERENTIAL DIAGNOSIS
- Cocaine, amphetamine intoxication
- Neuroleptic malignant syndrome
- Anticholinergic drug toxicity
- Liver failure
- CNS infection or hemorrhage
- Opioid withdrawal
- Mania, psychosis
- Thyroid crisis (2)[C]

 ## TREATMENT

- The goal of treatment is to reduce the likelihood of adverse clinically significant events (i.e., seizures, DTs, cardiovascular events). This is done mainly with benzodiazepines that reduce withdrawal intensity and raise the seizure threshold.
  - Medical and psychiatric causes, along with withdrawal from other psychotropic substances, must be excluded first.
  - The patient should be provided a quiet, protective environment.

- The Clinical Institute Withdrawal Assessment for Alcohol Scale, Revised (CIWA-Ar) is useful for determining medication dosing and frequency of evaluation for AWS. The CIWA-Ar scale numerically rates the severity of 10 symptoms on a scale from 1–7, 1 being without the symptom and 7 the max score.
- The 10 symptoms in the CIWA-Ar scale are:
  – Nausea and vomiting
  – Tremor
  – Paroxysmal sweats
  – Anxiety
  – Agitation
  – Tactile disturbances
  – Auditory disturbances
  – Visual disturbances
  – Headache or fullness in head
  – Orientation and clouding of sensorium
- Frequent reevaluation with CIWA-Ar is crucial.

MEDICATION
First Line
- Benzodiazepine (BZD) monotherapy remains the treatment of choice, and has been found to be effective against placebo (3)[A]:
  – Long-acting BZDs (e.g., diazepam, chlordiazepoxide) are more effective at preventing seizures and delirium.
  – Short-acting BZDs (e.g., lorazepam, oxazepam) preferable when severe hepatic insufficiency may impair metabolism; also preferable in elderly to limit oversedation (4)[A].
- BZD amounts will vary from patient to patient. Medication can be given in symptom-triggered or fixed-schedule regimens. Symptom-triggered regimens have been found to require less BZD amounts and reduce hospitalization times, but require persistent observation (4)[A].
- Example symptom-triggered regimen: Start with chlordiazepoxide 50–100 mg IV, repeat CIWA-Ar every hour and if score is ≥8, give additional dose of chlordiazepoxide 50 mg IV. Continue to reevaluate with CIWA-Ar hourly until adequate sedation achieved (score <8). May substitute chlordiazepoxide with respective doses of diazepam, lorazepam, or oxazepam (4)[C].

Second Line
- β-blockers (e.g., atenolol) and α2 agonists (e.g., clonidine) help to control hypertension and tachycardia, and can be used in conjunction with BZDs (2)[C]. These should not be used as a monotherapy, due to their inability to prevent DTs and seizures.
- Antiepileptic agents such as carbamazepine (Tegretol) have not shown clear benefit over BZDs (5)[B].
- Thiamine 100 mg/d for at least 3 days:
  – Note that IV glucose administered before treatment with thiamine may precipitate Wernicke's encephalopathy.
- If patient exhibits significant agitation and alcoholic hallucinosis, an antipsychotic (haloperidol) can be used, but this requires close observation, as it lowers the seizure threshold (2)[C].

ADDITIONAL TREATMENT
Additional Therapies
Peripheral neuropathy and cerebellar dysfunction merit physical therapy evaluation.

IN-PATIENT CONSIDERATIONS
- Individuals in stages 1 and 2 of alcohol withdrawal can be treated safely in the outpatient setting unless medical comorbidities require inpatient observation. However, a reliable and supportive social environment should be in place with frequent, consistent follow-up.
- Individuals in or approaching stage 3 should always be treated as inpatients.

Admission Criteria
- CIWA score >15, or severe withdrawal
- Concurrent acute or chronic illness requiring inpatient treatment and monitoring
- Poor ability to follow up or no reliable social support
- Pregnancy
- Seizure disorder or history of severe alcohol-related seizures
- Suicide risk
- Concurrent benzodiazepine dependence
- High risk for severe withdrawal or delirium tremens
- >40 years old
- Prolonged heavy drinking >8 years
- Consumes >1 pint of alcohol or 12 beers per day
- Random blood alcohol level >200 mg/dL
- Elevated MCV, blood urea nitrogen
- Cirrhosis, liver failure

IV Fluids
IV hydration is required in withdrawal due to losses from autonomic hyperactivity.

Discharge Criteria
CIWA scores of <10 on 3 consecutive determinations

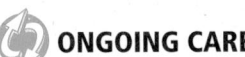 ONGOING CARE

FOLLOW-UP RECOMMENDATIONS
Arrangements for aftercare include discharge to a treatment facility (i.e., sober house or residential program), outpatient substance abuse counseling, peer support groups (Alcoholics Anonymous), the use of adjuvant treatment such as acamprosate (Campral), naltrexone (ReVia, Depade, Vivitrol), or topiramate (Topamax).

Patient Monitoring
Frequent patient follow-up is recommended to monitor for relapse.

PATIENT EDUCATION
- Alcoholics Anonymous at www.aa.org
- SMART Recovery (Self-Management and Recovery Training) at www.smartrecovery.org (not spiritually based)
- National Institute on Alcohol Abuse and Alcoholism at www.niaaa.nih.gov
- FamilyDoctor.Org: Alcoholism (Spanish resources available)

PROGNOSIS
Current mortality from severe withdrawal (delirium tremens) is 1–5%.

COMPLICATIONS
Complications may occur more frequently in individuals who have prior episodes of withdrawal or concomitant illnesses.

REFERENCES

1. Rockville MD. Screening and Behavioral Counseling Interventions in Primary Care to Reduce Alcohol Misuse, Topic Page. *USPSTF* April 2004.
2. Bayard M, et al. Alcohol withdrawal syndrome. *Am Fam Phys*. 2004;69:1443.
3. Ntais C, Pakos E, Kyzas P, Ioannidis JP et al. Benzodiazepines for alcohol withdrawal. *Cochrane Database Syst Rev*. 2005;CD005063.
4. Mayo-Smith MF. Pharmacological Management of Alcohol Withdrawal: A Meta-Analysis and Evidence-Based Practice Guideline. *JAMA* 1997;278:144–151.
5. Polycarpou A, Papanikolaou P, Ioannidis JP et al. Anticonvulsants for alcohol withdrawal. *Cochrane Database Syst Rev*. 2005;CD005064.

ADDITIONAL READING
- Blondell RD. Ambulatory detoxification of patients with alcohol dependence. *Am Fam Phys*. 2005;71: 495–502, 509–10.
- Daeppen JB, Gache P, Landry U et al. Symptom-triggered vs fixed-schedule doses of benzodiazepine for alcohol withdrawal: a randomized treatment trial. *Arch Intern Med*. 2002;162:1117–21.
- Kosten TR, O'Connor PG. Management of drug and alcohol withdrawal. *N Engl J Med*. 2003;348: 1786–95.
- Lohr RH. Treatment of alcohol withdrawal in hospitalized patients. *Mayo Clin Proc*. 1995;70: 777–82.
- Mayo-Smith MF, Beecher LH, Fischer TL et al. Management of alcohol withdrawal delirium. An evidence-based practice guideline. *Arch Intern Med*. 2004;164:1405–12.
- Reoux JP, Miller K. Routine hospital alcohol detoxification practice compared to symptom triggered management with an Objective Withdrawal Scale (CIWA-Ar). *Am J Addict*. 2000;9:135–44.

 See Also (Topic, Algorithm, Electronic Media Element)

Substance Use Disorders

 CODES

ICD9
- 291.0 Alcohol withdrawal delirium
- 291.81 Alcohol withdrawal
- 303.90 Other and unspecified alcohol dependence, unspecified drinking behavior

CLINICAL PEARLS
- Kindling phenomenon: Postulated that long-term exposure to alcohol affects neurons resulting in increased alcohol craving and progressively worse withdrawal episodes
- The CIWA-Ar is a useful tool for managing symptoms and treatment of alcohol withdrawal.
- Be sure to administer thiamine before patient receives glucose, so as not to precipitate Wernicke's encephalopathy.
- Frequent outpatient follow-up is recommended to monitor for relapse.

ALDOSTERONISM, PRIMARY

Amara Lai, MD

BASICS

DESCRIPTION
- Aldosterone secretion independent of the renin-angiotensin system, usually caused by:
  - a unilateral aldosterone-producing adenoma, treated with unilateral adrenalectomy, *or*
  - bilateral adrenal hyperplasia, treated with aldosterone antagonists
- Clinically manifested by hypertension, hypokalemia, normal or mildly elevated sodium, and metabolic alkalosis
- Systems affected: Endocrine/Metabolic
- Synonyms: Conn syndrome, hyperaldosterism, aldosteronoma

Pregnancy Considerations
Can be associated with toxemia during pregnancy or persistent HTN following delivery. Treat HTN with agents safe during pregnancy; avoid spironolactone and ACE inhibitors.

EPIDEMIOLOGY
Prevalence
- Uncommon in the general population
- Approximately 5–10% of hypertensive patients
- 11.3% prevalence reported in a study of patients with resistant hypertension (1)
  - Resistant hypertension was defined as blood pressure >140/90 mm Hg despite 3 antihypertensive agents, including a diuretic.
- 14% prevalence reported in a study of patients with both type 2 diabetes and resistant hypertension (2)
  - Resistant hypertension was defined as blood pressure >140/90 mm Hg despite ≥3 antihypertensive agents.

RISK FACTORS
Genetics
Familial hyperaldosteronism is categorized as either glucocorticoid-remediable (autosomal dominant) or type II, and it is a rare finding.

PATHOPHYSIOLOGY
- Aldosterone secretion independent of renin-angiotensin stimulation
- Negative feedback loop suppresses renin.
- Increased aldosterone results in retention of sodium and excretion of potassium and hydrogen ions in the distal renal tubules.

ETIOLOGY
- Aldosterone-producing adenoma, APA (85% unilateral, <5% bilateral)
- Idiopathic bilateral adrenal hyperplasia (10–40%)
- Less common causes include unilateral hyperplasia, aldosterone-producing adrenocortical carcinoma, aldosterone-producing ovarian tumor, or familial hyperaldosteronism including glucocorticoid-remediable hyperaldosteronism.

COMMONLY ASSOCIATED CONDITIONS
Hypertension, especially treatment-resistant or severe

DIAGNOSIS

HISTORY
- Usually asymptomatic
- Can be associated with headaches, muscle weakness, fatigue, cramping, polyuria (hypokalemic nephropathy), nocturia, polydipsia, paresthesias, or tetany

PHYSICAL EXAM
- Hypertension
- Edema (uncommon)
- Fundoscopy: Benign or grade 1–2 hypertensive retinopathy
- Forceful and sustained apical impulse consistent with left ventricular hypertrophy, or cardiac arrhythmias (complications of primary aldosteronism)

DIAGNOSTIC TESTS & INTERPRETATION
Lab
- Patients should be screened for primary aldosteronism with laboratory testing if they are at higher risk (3)[C].
- Higher risk is variably defined as:
  - Hypertension (BP >140/90) resistant to treatment with 3 antihypertensive agents
  - Hypertension with hypokalemia
  - Hypertension in the presence of an adrenal incidentaloma
  - Hypertension that meets Joint National Commission criteria as stage 2 (BP >160/100)

Initial lab tests
- Serum aldosterone and plasma renin activity to determine the aldosterone-renin ratio (ARR) is recommended (3)[C], but no consensus cutoff value has been established at the time of this writing.
  - ARR values are affected by posture, time of day, and acute salt loading.
  - In one study, morning values obtained after 30 minutes in the seated position, in the absence of salt loading, suggest a cutoff value of 23.6 (using conventional units of ng/dL and ng/ml°h), which conveys a sensitivity of 96.8 [95% CI 83.2–99.5], specificity of 94.1 [95% CI 71.2–99.0], and positive LR of 16.45) (4)[B].
  - It is suggested that the most sensitive testing is performed in the morning, after 2 hours of upright posture, and being seated for 5–15 minutes, on patients with unrestricted dietary salt intake before testing, and the most commonly used cutoff with this method is 30 (using conventional units of ng/dL and ng/ml°h) (3)[C].
- Basic metabolic panel to determine serum sodium, potassium, chloride, and bicarbonate levels
  - Sodium may be high-normal or elevated.
  - Hypokalemia, although "classic," may be present in a minority of patients.
    - Reported as low as 9–37% (5)
  - Chloride-resistant metabolic alkalosis
- Urine analysis may reveal dilute urine.
- Urine potassium may demonstrate inappropriate kaliuresis, usually >30 mmol/L.

ALERT
Lab results may be altered by malignant HTN or certain drugs, such as diuretics, ACE inhibitors, and aldosterone antagonists.

Follow-Up & Special Considerations
- Patients with a positive ARR screen should undergo confirmatory testing with one of the following (3)[C]:
  - Oral sodium loading test
    - Sodium intake of >200 mmol per day (~6 g per day) for 3 days
    - 24-hour urine aldosterone is measured from the morning of day 3 to the morning of day 4
    - Elevated urinary aldosterone (>12 mcg per 24 hours) make primary aldosteronism highly likely
    - Notes and precautions: Patients should receive adequate slow-release KCl supplementation to maintain plasma potassium in the normal range. This test should not be performed in patients with severe uncontrolled HTN, renal insufficiency, cardiac insufficiency, cardiac arrhythmia, or severe hypokalemia. There are currently two methods available for measuring the urinary aldosterone, with the HPLC-tandem mass spectrometry preferred over the RIA.
  - Saline infusion test
  - Fludrocortisone suppression test
  - Captopril challenge test
- Confirmed cases should then undergo CT scan and adrenal vein sampling (AVS) for subtype classification (3)[C].

Imaging
Initial approach
Adrenal CT with fine cuts for subtype testing and to exclude large masses that may represent adrenocortical carcinoma (3)[C]

Diagnostic Procedures/Surgery
Adrenal vein sampling should be performed to lateralize an aldosteronoma (6)[A],(7)[B].
- Post-ACTH stimulation values are the most accurate measurement for AVS lateralization (7)[B].

Pathological Findings
- Aldosteronoma usually solitary, benign
- Bilateral adrenal (zona glomerulosa) hyperplasia
- Aldosterone-producing adrenocortical carcinoma, rare

DIFFERENTIAL DIAGNOSIS
- Diuretic use
- Renovascular HTN
- Malignant HTN
- Pheochromocytoma
- Dexamethasone-suppressible hyperaldosteronism
- Congenital adrenal hyperplasia
- High-dose glucocorticoid therapy
- Exogenous mineralocorticoid
- Bartter syndrome
- Licorice (glycyrrhizinic acid) ingestion
- Edema secondary to other conditions (CHF, nephrotic syndrome, liver failure)

TREATMENT

- Treat hypertension and electrolyte abnormalities, particularly hypokalemia, if present.
- Unilateral laparoscopic adrenalectomy is the definitive treatment for patients with documented unilateral APA or hyperplasia.
- Medical management with aldosterone antagonists is the treatment of choice for bilateral hyperplasia.

MEDICATION

First Line

Aldosterone antagonist: spironolactone (Aldactone), or eplerenone (Inspra) as an alternative

Second Line

- Other potassium-sparing diuretics: amiloride (Midamor) or triamterene (Dyrenium)
- Antihypertensive agents: Calcium channel antagonist, ACE inhibitor, angiotensin-II receptor antagonist, beta-blocker, or low-dose thiazide diuretic
- Contraindications: Potassium-sparing agent and ACE inhibitors in renal failure, hyperkalemia, and pregnancy
- Precautions: Monitor serum potassium closely after any adjustment in potassium replacement or potassium-sparing agent
- Significant possible interactions: Lithium with diuretics, NSAIDs with diuretics, and ACE inhibitors with diuretics

ADDITIONAL TREATMENT

Issues for Referral

- Endocrinology for confirmatory testing of an ARR suggestive of primary aldosteronism
- Interventional radiology to perform AVS
- General surgery to perform unilateral laparoscopic adrenalectomy in patients with confirmed unilateral APA or hyperplasia

SURGERY/OTHER PROCEDURES

The treatment of choice for patients with unilateral APA or hyperplasia is laparoscopic adrenalectomy.

IN-PATIENT CONSIDERATIONS

Initial Stabilization

Control of any HTN

Admission Criteria

- Hypertensive urgency/emergency
- Refractory HTN
- Severe hypokalemia
- Cardiovascular events

IV Fluids

As needed

Nursing

Careful monitoring of BP

Discharge Criteria

When hemodynamically stable

ONGOING CARE

FOLLOW-UP RECOMMENDATIONS

Follow BP and potassium

Patient Monitoring

- BP checks
- Serum potassium check
- 24-hour urine aldosterone following surgery

DIET

Low-sodium, high-potassium

PATIENT EDUCATION

- HTN teaching
- Medication management

PROGNOSIS

- Hypertension and hypokalemia can usually be controlled by doses of 25 to 100 mg spironolactone every 8 hours.
  - Chronic therapy in men may be limited by side effects of gynecomastia, decreased libido, and impotence.
- Surgical adrenalectomy resulted in hypertension cure or improvement in 77% of patients with unilateral adenoma (8).
- There is no further increased risk of complications of primary aldosteronism (see below) after treatment with either surgery or medical management (9,10).

COMPLICATIONS

- Increased GFR and albuminuria in untreated primary aldosteronism compared with essential hypertension (9)
- Increased prevalence of cardiovascular events in untreated primary aldosteronism compared with essential hypertension (35% vs 11%, OR 4.61) (10)[B]
- Left ventricular hypertrophy
- Cardiac arrhythmias if hypokalemia is severe

REFERENCES

1. Douma S, et al. Prevalence of primary hyperaldosteronism in resistent hypertension: a retrospective observational study. *Lancet*. 2008; 371:1921–1926.
2. Umpierrez GE, et al. Primary aldosteronism in diabetic subjects with resistant hypertension. *Diabetes Care*. 2007;30(7):1699.
3. Funder JW, et al. Case Detection, Diagnosis, and Treatment of Patients with Primary Aldosteronism: An Endocrine Society Clinical Practice Guideline. *J Clin Endocrinol Metab*. 2008;93(9):3266–3281.
4. Sau-Cheung Tiu et al. The Use of Aldosterone-Renin Ratio as a Diagnostic Test for Primary Hyperaldosteronism and Its Test Characteristics under Different Conditions of Blood Sampling. *J Clin Endorinol Metab*. 2005; 90(1):72–78.
5. Mulatero P, et al. Increased diagnosis of primary aldosteronism, including surgically correctable forms, in centers from 5 continents. *J Clin Endocrinol Metab*. 2004;89:045.
6. Kempers et al. Systematic Review: Diagnostic Procedures to Differentiate Unilateral from Bilateral Adrenal Abnormality in Primary Aldosteronism. *Ann Intern Med*. 2009;151(5): 329–337.
7. Mathur A, et al. Consequences of Adrenal Venous Sampling in Primary Hyperaldosteronism and Predictors of Unilateral Adrenal Disease. *Journal of the American College of Surgeons*. 2010.
8. Letavernier E, et al. Blood Pressure Outcome of Adrenalectomy in Patients with Primary Hyperaldosteronism with or without Unilateral Adenoma. *J Hypertens*. 2009;27(3):656–657.
9. Sechi LA, et al. Long-term renal outcomes in patients with primary aldosteronism. *JAMA*. 2006;295(22):2638–2645.
10. Catena C, et al. Cardiovascular outcomes in patients with primary aldosteronism after treatment. *Arch Intern Med*. 2008;168(1):80–85.

ADDITIONAL READING

Mansmann G, Lau J, Balk E et al. The clinically inapparent adrenal mass: update in diagnosis and management. *Endocr Rev*. 2004;25:309–40.

 See Also (Topic, Algorithm, Electronic Media Element)

Algorithm: Aldosteronism

 CODES

ICD9

255.10 Hyperaldosteronism, unspecified

CLINICAL PEARLS

- Patients with drug-resistant HTN, HTN plus hypokalemia, HTN plus adrenal incidentaloma, or stage 2 HTN are at increased risk for primary aldosteronism.
- Patients at increased risk should have testing with serum aldosterone and plasma renin activity, and the ARR should be calculated.
- Suggestive ARR values (in general, at least 20–30 in conventional units) should be referred for confirmatory testing.
- Confirmed primary aldosteronism warrants an adrenal CT and AVS for lateralization.
- Unilateral adrenalectomy is the treatment of choice for unilateral APA or hyperplasia; spironolactone for the treatment of bilateral hyperplasia.

ALOPECIA
Ann M. Rodden, DO, MS

BASICS

DESCRIPTION
- Alopecia: Absence of hair from any areas where it normally exists:
  - Anagen hairs: Growing hairs
  - Telogen hairs: Dead, "resting" hairs
- Androgenic alopecia (male- or female-pattern hair loss): Hair loss along with miniaturization of hair follicles:
  - In men: Frontal recession, then vertex affected; over time, only has lateral and occipital hair
  - In women: Thinning across the crown, with frontal hair initially in place but later may be lost
- Alopecia areata: Patchy, nonscarring hair loss:
  - Alopecia totalis: Hair loss of the entire scalp
  - Alopecia universalis: Loss of all body hair
- Telogen effluvium: Diffuse hair loss that (usually) results in temporarily decreased hair density but not complete baldness:
  - Abnormal hair cycling leads to excessive loss of hairs in telogen phase.
  - Usually occurs 3 months after the trigger occurs
- Anagen effluvium: Diffuse shedding of hairs, including growing hairs, that may progress to complete baldness:
  - Growth arrest of hair in anagen phase and sheds
  - Begins days to weeks after inciting incident
- Cicatricial alopecia (scarring alopecia): Slick, smooth scalp without any evidence of follicular openings for hair
- Traction alopecia: Patchy, initially nonscarring hair loss usually due to physical stressors on hair:
  - Trichotillomania: Hair loss due to the person pulling hair out
- Tinea capitis: Patches of hair broken off close to the scalp, with or without associated inflammation, caused by fungal infection

Pediatric Considerations
Tinea capitis is more common among children.

Pregnancy Considerations
Telogen gravidarum: Hair loss 2 to 4 months after childbirth

EPIDEMIOLOGY
- Age:
  - Androgenic alopecia: May begin after puberty and increases in prevalence over time
- Predominant sex: Male > Female

Incidence
Alopecia areata: 0.1–0.2% incidence in all races

Prevalence
- Androgenic alopecia:
  - Men: 15% of adolescent males:
    - 50% of white men over 50 years old
  - Women: 6% under age of 50:
    - 38% of postmenopausal women
- Alopecia areata:
  - 1.7% of US population

RISK FACTORS
- Physiologic or psychologic stress
- Pregnancy
- Poor nutrition
- Use of certain medications/chemotherapy
- Tight living quarters
- Sharing hair products/supplies

Genetics
- Family history of early hair loss
- Polygenic inheritance of androgenic alopecia

GENERAL PREVENTION
- For traction alopecia: Minimize braids, coloring, bleaching, waving of hair, or hair styles that pull hair.
- For tinea capitis: Avoid sharing hats, combs, hairbrushes, hair ornaments, and pillows.

PATHOPHYSIOLOGY
- All hair follicles pass through stages of anagen and telogen.
- When many are in the telogen phase at one time, the hair loss becomes noticeable.
- Activity of hair follicles may diminish due to trauma, medications, or disease.

ETIOLOGY
- Androgenic alopecia:
  - Genetically predisposed
  - Polycystic ovarian syndrome
  - Adrenal hyperplasia
  - Pituitary hyperplasia
  - Drugs (testosterone, progesterone, danazol, adrenocorticosteroids, anabolic steroids)
- Alopecia areata (autoimmune process):
  - Autoimmune thyroiditis
- Telogen effluvium:
  - In most cases, no specific etiology is found.
  - Postpartum
  - Adding or changing medications (oral contraceptives, anticoagulants, anticonvulsants, selective serotonin reuptake inhibitors, retinoids, β-blockers, angiotensin-converting enzyme inhibitors, colchicine, cholesterol-lowering medications, cimetidine, levodopa, bromocriptine, chemotherapeutic agents, interferon, others)
  - Stress: Physical (fever, trauma, surgery) or psychologic
  - Chronic illness (systemic lupus erythematosus [SLE], syphilis, systemic amyloidosis, hepatic failure, chronic renal failure, inflammatory bowel disease, dermatomyositis, human immunodeficiency virus, lymphoproliferative disorders)
  - Hormonal (hypo-/hyperthyroid, pituitary dysfunction)
  - Malnutrition (iron deficiency, zinc deficiency, caloric restriction/eating disorder)
  - Malabsorption (celiac disease, pancreatic disease)
  - Inflammatory skin disorders (psoriasis, seborrheic dermatitis, allergic contact dermatitis)
- Anagen effluvium:
  - Chemotherapy is most common trigger
  - Radiation to the area
  - Drugs (chemotherapeutic agents, allopurinol, colchicine)
  - Poisoning (mercury, thallium, bismuth, arsenic, gold, boric acid)
  - Severe protein malnutrition
- Cicatricial alopecia:
  - Physical agents/trauma (burns, freezing, radiation)
  - Congenital (aplasia cutis congenital, Conradi-Hunermann chondropysplasia punctata)
  - Lymphocytic (central centrifugal cicatricial alopecia, cutaneous discoid lupus erythematous, lichen planopilaris)
  - Neutrophilic (folliculitis decalvans, dissecting folliculitis)
  - Acne keloidosis
  - Infection (zoster, kerion, folliculitis)
  - Metastatic or primary neoplasm
- Traction alopecia:
  - Trichotillomania (direct self-pulling of the hair, obsessive-compulsive behavior)
  - Tight rollers or braids
- Tinea capitis (*Microsporum, Trichophyton*)

COMMONLY ASSOCIATED CONDITIONS
Alopecia areata:
- Down syndrome
- Autoimmune thyroiditis
- Vitiligo
- Diabetes

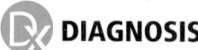

DIAGNOSIS

HISTORY
- Duration of hair loss
- Episodic or continuous
- Pattern of hair loss
- Medications
- Chronic disease, recent illness, surgeries, pregnancy
- Changes in health/medication in past 2–3 months
- Psychological stress
- Dietary history and weight changes
- Menstrual history
- Family history of hair loss or autoimmune disorders
- Radiation or exposure to heavy metals
- Pruritus (in tinea capitis)

PHYSICAL EXAM
- Pattern of hair loss:
  - Is hair loss generalized or local?
  - If local, is it symmetrical at the vertex and/or the hairline at the forehead?
- Scalp scaling, inflammation (in tinea capitis)
- Changes in the hair:
  - Hair-pull test: Pinch 25–50 hairs between thumb and forefinger, and exert slow, gentle traction while sliding fingers up:
    - Normal: 1–2 dislodge
    - Abnormal: ≥6 hairs dislodged (in effluvium, alopecia areata)
  - Broken hairs (tinea capitis, traction alopecia)
  - Broken-off hair at the borders of the patch that are easily removable (in alopecia areata)
  - Hair loss in circular pattern (in alopecia areata, tinea capitis)
- Clinical signs of thyroid disease, lupus, or other diseases
- Clinical signs of virilization: Acne, hirsutism, acanthosis nigrans, truncal obesity (in androgenic alopecia)

DIAGNOSTIC TESTS & INTERPRETATION
Lab
- Thyroid-stimulating hormone and free thyroxine (fT_4) (hypo- or hyperthyroidism)
- Complete blood count (anemia)
- Comprehensive metabolic panel (liver and renal disease)
- Free testosterone and dehydroepiandrosterone sulfate (hyperandrogenism)
- Serum ferritin and total iron-binding capacity (iron deficiency)

- Serum zinc (deficiency)
- Rapid plasma reagin test (syphilis)
- Prolactin (pituitary hyperplasia)
- ANA (SLE)

Diagnostic Procedures/Surgery

- Light hair-pull test:
  - Pull on 25–50 hairs and ≥6 hairs dislodge is consistent with shedding (effluvium, alopecia areata)
- Direct microscopic exam of the hair shaft:
  - Anagen hairs: Elongated and possibly pigmented bulb with gelatinous root sheath
  - Exclamation point hairs: At periphery of lesion and has club-shaped root with thinner proximal shaft that distally becomes normal in size (alopecia areata)
- Daily hair counts: Collect hair in dated envelopes:
  - More than 100 hairs per day is consistent with effluvium
- Ultraviolet light fluorescence and potassium hydroxide prep (to rule out tinea capitis)

Pathological Findings

Scalp biopsy with routine microscopy will aid in the diagnosis.

DIFFERENTIAL DIAGNOSIS

Search for type of alopecia and then for reversible causes.

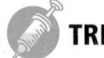 **TREATMENT**

MEDICATION

- Androgenic alopecia:
  - Minoxidil (Rogaine) 2% topical solution (1 mL b.i.d.) for women, 5% topical solution (1 mL b.i.d.) or foam (daily) for men (1)[A]
  - Finasteride (Propecia), 1 mg/day p.o. for men (1)[A]
  - Spironolactone (Aldactone) 100–200 mg/day in women who are hyperandrogenic (off-label) (1)[C]:
    - Diuretic with antiandrogen action
  - Oral contraception pills with low levels of androgenic affect in women (Yasmin, Ortho-TriCyclen, Ortho-Cyclen, Ortho-Evra, Mircette) (off-label) (2)[C]
  - Ketoconazole 2% shampoo with minoxidil 2% (1)[C]
- Alopecia areata:
  - Intralesional steroids: triamcinolone 2.5–10 mg/mL (3,4)[C]
    - First line in adults if <50% scalp involved
    - Repeat every 4–6 weeks
    - 0.5-inch, 30-gauge needle and inject 0.1 mL at each point at 1-cm intervals
    - If no improvement in 6 months, stop treatment
  - If >50% scalp involved, refer to dermatologist (3)
  - Topical midpotent corticosteroids for children (3)[C]
  - Systemic glucocorticoids: May induce regrowth, but alopecia recurs after cessation of medication and risks may outweigh benefits for long-term use (3,4)[C]
- Telogen effluvium: Remove offending medication (5)[C].
- Tinea capitis: See appropriate section on tinea.
- Side effects/precautions:
  - Topical minoxidil:
    - Irritant dermatitis or contact allergic dermatitis
    - Hypertrichosis
    - Exacerbation of angina (rare)

- Intralesional steroids:
  - Local burning/stinging/pruritis/skin atrophy
- Spironolactone:
  - Menstrual cycle abnormalities
  - Postural hypotension
  - Electrolyte imbalance (hyperkalemia)
- Finasteride:
  - Caution in known liver disease
  - Sexual side effects
  - Monitor prostate-specific antigen (PSA): Will decrease PSA level by 50%

Pregnancy Considerations

Finasteride not indicated for use in women; pregnancy Category X. Women should not handle crushed or broken pills during childbearing years.

ADDITIONAL TREATMENT

General Measures

- Trial off medication that may have triggered the hair loss may resolve issue. If unsure it was the medication, may repeat trial with medication to determine if hair loss occurs again (if patient is willing).
- Traction alopecia:
  - Only with discontinuation of the hair pulling will the disorder resolve.
  - Psychologic or psychiatric intervention may be necessary.
  - Successful therapeutic approaches have included medications, behavior modification, and hypnosis.

COMPLEMENTARY AND ALTERNATIVE MEDICINE

Androgenic alopecia:

- Low-energy laser light: HairMax LaserComb (1)[C]: Safe alternative, but lacking research

SURGERY/OTHER PROCEDURES

- Hair transplantation
- Wigs/hairpieces
- Androgenic alopecia:
  - Surgical (hair transplantation, scalp reduction, transposition flap, and soft tissue expansion)
  - Medical tattooing of eyebrows
- Cicatricial alopecia:
  - The only effective treatment is surgical (graft transplantation, flap transplantation, or excision of the scarred area).

 ONGOING CARE

DIET

If nutritional deficit noted, supplementation may be necessary.

PATIENT EDUCATION

National Alopecia Areata Foundation: www.naaf.org

PROGNOSIS

- Androgenic alopecia:
  - Prognosis depends on treatment
- Alopecia areata:
  - Usually regrows within 1 year even without treatment
  - Recurrence common
  - 10% have severe, chronic form
- Telogen effluvium:
  - Maximum shedding 3 months after the inciting event (medication, stress, nutritional deficiency) and recovery following correction of the cause
  - Usually subsides in 3–6 months
  - Rarely permanent baldness
  - Chronic effluvium uncommon

- Anagen effluvium:
  - Shedding begins days to a few weeks after the inciting event, with recovery following correction of the cause.
  - Rarely permanent baldness
- Cicatricial alopecia:
  - Hair follicles permanently damaged
- Traction alopecia:
  - Depends on behavior modification
- Tinea capitis:
  - Usually complete recovery

REFERENCES

1. Rogers NE, Avram MR. Medical treatments for male and female pattern hair loss. *J Am Acad Dermatol.* 2008;59:547–66; quiz 567–8.
2. Goh C, Zippin JH et al. Androgenetic alopecia: diagnosis and treatment with a focus on recent genetic implications. *J Drugs Dermatol.* 2009;8: 185–92.
3. Alkhalifah A, Alsantali A, Wang E, McElwee KJ, Shapiro J et al. Alopecia areata update: part II. Treatment. *J Am Acad Dermatol.* 2010;62:-
4. Mounsey AL, Reed SW et al. Diagnosing and treating hair loss. *Am Fam Physician.* 2009;80: 356–62.
5. Harrison S, Bergfeld W. Diffuse hair loss: its triggers and management. *Cleve Clin J Med.* 2009;76: 361–7.

ADDITIONAL READING

 See Also (Topic, Algorithm, Electronic Media Element)

Tinea (Capitis, Corporis, Cruris); Syphilis; Systemic Lupus Erythematosus; Polycystic Ovarian Syndrome; Lichen Planus; Hyperthyroidism
Algorithm: Alopecia

CODES

ICD9

- 704.00 Alopecia, unspecified
- 704.01 Alopecia areata
- 704.02 Telogen effluvium

CLINICAL PEARLS

- History and physical examination findings will usually determine type of alopecia.
- Treatment of underlying medical condition or removal of triggering medication in many types of alopecia will reinstate hair growth without the need of further interventions.
- Educating the patient about the nature of the condition and expectations is key to patient care.

ALTITUDE ILLNESS

Robert J. Hyde, MD

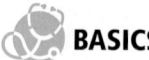 **BASICS**

DESCRIPTION
Altitude illness is a spectrum of medical problems ranging from mild discomfort to fatal illness that may occur on ascent to higher altitude [elevations >1,500 m (4,921 feet)]. It is divided into 3 categories: High, 1,500–3,500 m; very high, 3,500–5,500 m; and extreme, 5,500–8,850 m (1). It can affect anyone, including the most experienced and fit individual. For most, it is an unpleasant but self-limiting syndrome that will not require physician intervention.
- Acute mountain sickness (AMS): Symptoms associated with a physiologic response to a hypobaric, hypoxic environment. Onset occurs within 24 hours of arrival at altitude, often within 1–4 hours. Neurologic symptoms are predominant and range from mild-to-moderate headache and malaise to severe impairment.
- High-altitude pulmonary edema (HAPE): Noncardiogenic pulmonary edema. Onset 1–4 days at altitude. Rare <8,000 feet (2,438 m).
- High-altitude cerebral edema (HACE): A potentially fatal neurologic syndrome; considered the end stage of AMS. Onset within 3–5 days at elevation as low as 9,022 feet (2,750 m), but may be more abrupt at higher altitudes. Death results from brain herniation.
- System(s) affected: Nervous/Pulmonary
- Synonym(s): Mountain sickness

Geriatric Considerations
- Risk does not increase with age.
- Age alone should not preclude travel to high altitude; allow extra time to acclimate.
- Preexisting medical problems made worse are referred to as altitude-exacerbated conditions.

Pediatric Considerations
- Altitude illness seems to have the same incidence in children as in adults, but diagnosis may be delayed in younger children.
- Any child who experiences behavioral symptoms after recent ascent should be presumed to be suffering from altitude illness.

Pregnancy Considerations
- The risk during pregnancy is unknown.
- No evidence that exposure to high altitude (1,500–3,500 m) poses a risk to a pregnancy
- It may be prudent to advise a low-altitude dwelling for any pregnant woman experiencing complications.

EPIDEMIOLOGY
Most epidemiologic studies are limited to relatively homogenous populations of men.

Incidence
- AMS: 10–90% globally
- HAPE/HACE: 0.01–1% of sojourner ascents at typical mountain resorts, although incidence increases with rapid and higher ascents (2).

RISK FACTORS
- Rapid rate of ascent
- Maximum altitude attained
- Increased duration at high altitude
- Failure to acclimatize at lower altitude
- Higher altitude during sleep cycle
- Prior history of altitude illness
- Cardiac congenital abnormalities

GENERAL PREVENTION
- General guidelines:
  - Preacclimatization affords some protection against altitude illness.
  - Staged or graded ascent (rest every 600–1,200 m) and a slow ascent rate (maximum 600 m/d) should allow adequate time for acclimatization.
  - Sleeping elevation: "Climb high and sleep low" is a prudent practice for anyone going above 3,500 m.
  - Avoid heavy exertion for the 1st 1–3 days.
  - Avoid respiratory depressants such as alcohol and soporifics.
  - Preascent physical conditioning is not preventive.
- Drug prophylaxis:
  - Acetazolamide and dexamethasone (see below)
  - For HAPE only:
    - Consider nifedipine and beta agonists (see Treatment section).

PATHOPHYSIOLOGY
- Not completely understood
- Hypobaric hypoxia and hypoxemia are the pathophysiologic precursors to altitude illness.
- Symptoms of AMS may be the result of cerebral swelling, either through vasodilatation induced by hypoxia or through cerebral edema.
- Other mechanisms include impaired cerebral autoregulation, release of vasogenic mediators, and alteration of the blood–brain barrier.
- HAPE is a noncardiogenic pulmonary edema characterized by exaggerated pulmonary hypertension leading to vascular leakage through overperfusion, stress failure, or both.

ETIOLOGY
Individuals with a prior episode of HAPE have an increased risk of recurrence (3).

 DIAGNOSIS

HISTORY
- AMS, mild-to-moderate symptoms:
  - Headache, plus at least 1 of the following:
    - Anorexia
    - Nausea or vomiting
    - Dizziness or lightheadedness
    - Insomnia
- AMS, severe symptoms:
  - Increased headache
  - Irritability
  - Marked fatigue
  - Dyspnea with exertion
  - Nausea and vomiting
  - HAPE (Lake Louise diagnostic criteria):
    - At least 2 of the following symptoms: Dyspnea at rest, cough, weakness, decreased exercise performance, chest tightness, congestion
    - AND at least 2 of the following signs: Crackles or wheezing in at least 1 lung field, central cyanosis, tachycardia, tachypnea. (Note: Fatigue may be pulmonary edema.)
  - HACE symptoms: Mental status changes (irrational behavior, lethargy, obtundation, coma)

PHYSICAL EXAM
- HAPE:
  - Lung crackles or wheezing
  - Central cyanosis
  - Tachycardia
  - Tachypnea
- HACE:
  - Abnormal mental status exam (behavioral change, lethargy, obtundation, coma)
  - Truncal ataxia
  - Papilledema, retinal hemorrhage, cranial nerve palsies
  - Focal neurologic deficits (rare)

DIAGNOSTIC TESTS & INTERPRETATION
Electrocardiogram may show sinus tachycardia or right-sided heart strain.

Lab
- AMS: Laboratory studies are nonspecific and rarely required for diagnosis.
- HAPE: Severe hypoxemia demonstrated with oximetry or blood gas analysis.

Imaging
No radiographic feature is specific to HAPE.

DIFFERENTIAL DIAGNOSIS
Onset of symptoms >3 days at a given altitude, the absence of headache, or the lack of rapid response to oxygen or descent suggest other diagnoses.

- AMS/HACE:
  - Subarachnoid hemorrhage, central nervous system (CNS) mass, cerebrovascular accident
  - Migraine headache
  - Dehydration
  - Ingestion of toxins, drugs, or alcohol
  - Carbon monoxide exposure
  - CNS infection
  - Acute psychosis
- HAPE:
  - Pneumonia
  - Cardiogenic pulmonary edema
  - Spontaneous pneumothorax
  - Pulmonary embolism
  - Asthma
  - Bronchitis
  - Myocardial infarction
  - Hyperventilation syndrome

 TREATMENT

MEDICATION
First Line
- Oxygen: 2–15 L/min to maintain SaO_2 >90% until symptoms improve
- Acetazolamide: (If patient has a history of problems at altitude and/or plans to ascend >500 m/d). Dosage is usually 125–500 mg p.o. b.i.d. starting 2 days before ascent and continued for 3 days at maximum altitude. Patients with a drug allergy to sulfonamides should avoid acetazolamide.
  - Prevention of AMS: 125–500 mg p.o. b.i.d. starting 1 day before ascent and continued for 2 days at maximum altitude
  - Treatment of AMS: 125–500 mg p.o. b.i.d. until symptoms resolve
- Dexamethasone: May significantly reduce the incidence and severity of AMS. Dosage is 2–4 mg p.o. q6h, begun the day of ascent, continued for 3 days at the higher altitude, and then tapered over 5 days. Adverse side effects are rare:
  - Prevention of AMS: 2 mg p.o. q6h or 4 mg p.o. q12h, starting 1 day before ascent and discontinued cautiously after 2 days at maximum altitude
  - Treatment of AMS: 4 mg p.o./IV/IM q6h
  - Treatment of HACE: 8 mg p.o./IV/IM initially, then 4 mg q6h
- Nifedipine (reduces pulmonary arterial pressure):
  - Prevention of HAPE: 20–30 mg extended-release p.o. b.i.d. starting 1 day prior to ascent and continued for 2 days at maximum altitude
  - Treatment of HAPE: 10 mg, then 20–30 mg extended-release p.o. b.i.d.
- Salmeterol:
  - Prevention and possible treatment of HAPE: 125 μg inhaled b.i.d. starting 1 day before ascent and continued for 2 days at maximum altitude
- Nonsteroidal anti-inflammatory drugs:
  - Prevention and treatment of headache
  - Aspirin 325 mg p.o. q4h for total 3 doses
  - Ibuprofen 400–600 mg p.o.
  - Prevention of AMS: Dose unknown. Begin 1–5 days before ascent.

- Antiemetics:
  - Prochlorperazine 10 mg p.o./IM q6–8h
  - Promethazine 25–50 mg p.o./IM/p.r. q6h

Second Line
Furosemide: Consider for treatment of AMS or HACE, 20–80 mg p.o./IV q12h for a total of 2 doses. Currently out of favor; not recommended for prophylaxis; not established for use in HAPE.

ADDITIONAL TREATMENT
General Measures
- Therapy must be tailored to fit disease severity.
- Early recognition is critical.
- Stop ascent, acclimatize at the same altitude, and/or descend if symptoms do not improve over 24 hours. Definitive treatment is to descend to a lower altitude. Dramatic improvement accompanies even modest reductions in altitude.
- Oxygen helps relieve symptoms. Give continuously by cannula or mask initially, and then titrate to SaO_2 >90%.
- AMS:
  - Acetazolamide is effective in reducing mild-to-moderate symptoms of AMS, but the optimum dosage is unknown. Consider 125–500 mg p.o. b.i.d. until symptoms resolve.
  - Dexamethasone may also be effective in treating moderate AMS. Consider 4 mg p.o./IM/IV q6h
  - Analgesics and antiemetics as needed for symptomatic relief
- HAPE:
  - Oxygen therapy
  - Minimize exertion and keep patient warm.
  - Immediate descent or evacuation to a lower altitude
  - Portable hyperbaric therapy (2–15 psi), such as the Gamow bag or Chamberlite, is an effective and practical alternative when descent is not possible.
  - Consider nifedipine 10 mg p.o., then 20–30 mg extended-release p.o. b.i.d.
- HACE:
  - Immediate descent
  - Supplemental oxygen (highest flow available; maintain SaO_2 >90%)
  - Dexamethasone 8 mg IV/IM/p.o. initially, then 4 mg q6h
  - Hyperbaric therapy if unable to descend

IN-PATIENT CONSIDERATIONS
Initial Stabilization
Outpatient treatment for mild cases

 ONGOING CARE

FOLLOW-UP RECOMMENDATIONS
Patient Monitoring
- For mild cases, no follow-up is needed.
- For more severe cases, follow until symptoms subside.

PATIENT EDUCATION
Patients should be counseled about the risks of high-altitude travel and how to recognize high-altitude illnesses.

PROGNOSIS
Most cases of mild-to-moderate AMS are self-limiting and do not require physician intervention. Patients may resume ascent once symptoms subside. HAPE and HACE respond well to descent, evacuation, and/or pharmacologic treatment if identified early.

COMPLICATIONS
Patient may experience high-altitude retinal hemorrhage, which can cause visual changes, but is usually asymptomatic.

REFERENCES
1. Gallagher SA, Hackett PH. High-altitude illness. *Emerg Med Clin North Am.* 2004;22:329–55, viii.
2. Maloney JP, Broeckel U. Epidemiology, risk factors, and genetics of high-altitude-related pulmonary disease. *Clin Chest Med.* 2005;26:395–404, v
3. Basnyat B, Murdoch DR. High-altitude illness. *Lancet.* 2003;361:1967–74.

ADDITIONAL READING
- Barry PW, Pollard AJ. Altitude illness. *BMJ.* 2003;326:915–9.
- Dumont L, Mardirosoff C, Tramèr MR. Efficacy and harm of pharmacological prevention of acute mountain sickness: quantitative systematic review. *BMJ.* 2000;321:267–72.
- Hackett PH, Roach RC. High-altitude illness. *N Engl J Med.* 2001;345:107–14.
- Luks AM, Swenson ER. Medication and dosage considerations in the prophylaxis and treatment of high-altitude illness. *Chest.* 2008;133:744–55.
- Rodway GW, Hoffman LA, Sanders MH. High-altitude-related disorders–Part I: Pathophysiology, differential diagnosis, and treatment. *Heart Lung.* 2003;32:353–9.
- Rodway GW, et al. High altitude–related disorders: Part II. Prevention, special populations and chronic medical conditions. *Heart Lung.* 2003;33(1):3–12.

 CODES

ICD9
993.2 Other and unspecified effects of high altitude

CLINICAL PEARLS
- Slow ascent and timely descent are important tenets in the prevention and treatment of high-altitude illnesses, respectively.
- High-flow oxygen, followed by oxygen titrated to maintain SaO_2 >90%, is the first-line treatment for all patients with more than mild illness.

ALVEOLAR PULMONARY PROTEINOSIS

Caitlin M. Connolly, MD
Jerry Balikian, MD

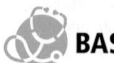

BASICS

DESCRIPTION
- Pulmonary alveolar proteinosis (PAP) is a rare disease characterized by accumulation of lipoproteinaceous (surfactantlike) material in the alveolar spaces, leading to impaired gas exchange. There are 3 recognized categories of PAP (1).
- Congenital PAP (2% of cases):
  - Congenital PAP results from several rare gene mutations (2).
- Secondary PAP (<10% cases):
  - Secondary PAP is associated with environmental exposures, immunodeficiency disorders, and hematologic disorders and malignancies (1).
- Primary or idiopathic PAP (90% of cases):
  - Primary PAP, which is discussed here, has recently been found to be associated with antigranulocyte-macrophage colony-stimulating-factor (GM-CSF) autoantibodies (2).
- Whole lung lavage, the standard treatment for PAP, has improved prognosis (94% 5-year survival) (3).
- Systems affected: Pulmonary

EPIDEMIOLOGY
- Seen worldwide with median age of onset at 39 years old (4)
- 2-3:1 Male:Female incidence; however, may be confounded by greater male smoking, a known association (3)

Incidence
Estimated 0.36 per million annually (5)

Prevalence
Estimated 3.7 per million (5)

RISK FACTORS
- Association between tobacco smoke exposure and primary PAP (3)
- Exposure to environmental dusts, specifically silica, aluminum, cement, titanium dioxide, nitrogen dioxide, and insulation fibers, has been associated with secondary PAP (2).

Genetics
- No genetic predilection in primary or secondary PAP.
- Congenital PAP mostly transmitted in autosomal recessive pattern (1)

Pediatric Considerations
- Congenital PAP leads to neonatal respiratory distress syndrome not responsive to surfactant or corticosteroids. Caused by mutation in surfactant protein B or C genes, or GM-CSF receptor beta or alpha chain abnormalities (2). Lung transplant is primary therapy, but prognosis is poor (1)[C].

GENERAL PREVENTION
No specific measure for prevention; avoid tobacco smoke exposure

PATHOPHYSIOLOGY
Primary PAP has recently been found to be associated with neutralizing anti-GM-CSF autoantibodies causing impaired functioning of alveolar macrophages, resulting in disruption in surfactant homeostasis (6). Surfactant accumulates in alveoli due to reduced clearance.

ETIOLOGY
Primary PAP: Autoimmune

COMMONLY ASSOCIATED CONDITIONS
No conditions commonly associated with primary PAP

DIAGNOSIS

HISTORY
- Diagnosis often delayed due to nonspecific presentation
- Occupational and exposure history to exclude secondary PAP
- Symptoms:
  - Progressive dyspnea with insidious onset (most common presentation)
  - Nonproductive cough (75%):
    - Less common
  - Fatigue
  - Weight loss
  - Low-grade fever (prominent fever should prompt search for complicating infection); hemoptysis or chest pain (<20%)

PHYSICAL EXAM
Often unremarkable:
- Fine crackles (50%)
- Clubbing or cyanosis (<20%)

DIAGNOSTIC TESTS & INTERPRETATION
Lab
Initial lab tests
- Complete blood count, liver and renal function tests to exclude systemic disorders
- Nonspecific:
  - Mild-moderate elevation in serum lactate dehydrogenase (LDH) (82%)
  - Serum levels of carcinoembryonic antigen, cytokeratin 19, and mucin KL-2 can be elevated.
  - Serum levels of surfactant protein-A, -B, and -D can be elevated.
  - Assay for anti-GM-CSF antibodies available at some centers (not commercially available) (2)

Follow-Up & Special Considerations
Serial serum LDH level can correlate with disease activity.

Imaging
Initial approach
- Chest x-ray: Bilateral, symmetric, central lung opacities (often appears worse than clinical symptoms)
- Chest computed tomography (CT): "Crazy-paving" patchy ground-glass opacities with network of thickened reticular lines in a geographic pattern (7) is characteristic of PAP but not specific.

Follow-Up & Special Considerations
Posttherapeutic brachioalveolar lavage (see Treatment), CT shows ground-glass opacities resolve, but thickened septal lines can persist (7).

Diagnostic Procedures/Surgery
Pulmonary function tests:
- Severe reduction of carbon monoxide diffusing capacity
- Restrictive ventilatory defect
- Arterial blood gas: Hypoxemia
- Bronchoalveolar lavage: Milky fluid with large, foamy alveolar macrophages and large, acellular eosinophilic bodies that stain with periodic acid-Schiff

Pathological Findings
Open-lung biopsy is gold standard for diagnosis, but not always required. Can have false negative due to mosaic pattern leading to sampling error (6)[C]:
- Normal alveolar architecture. Alveoli filled with granular, eosinophilic material that stains with periodic acid-Schiff (6)[C].

DIFFERENTIAL DIAGNOSIS
Primary PAP is diagnosis of exclusion; must exclude causes of secondary PAP:
- Differential for material in alveolar space includes pneumonia, cardiogenic pulmonary edema, acute respiratory distress syndrome, sarcoidosis, alveolar hemorrhage, hypersensitivity pneumonitis, bronchiolitis obliterans organizing pneumonia, bronchoalveolar carcinoma

TREATMENT

MEDICATION
No specific medication

First Line
- Whole lung lavage is the standard treatment for symptomatic PAP; however, there are no randomized controlled trials on any treatment for PAP yet available (2)[C]:
  - Whole lung lavage is performed under general anesthesia with a dual-lumen endotracheal tube while ventilating the other lung.
  - Large volumes of saline are flushed until returning fluid becomes clear.

- About 70% of patients with PAP become symptomatic enough to require whole lung lavage within 5 years of diagnosis.
- Most patients experience a return to normal exercise capacity after lavage; however, a subset of patients do not respond for unknown reason.
- Median duration of freedom from symptoms is 15 months, with many patients requiring repeat lavage (2)[C].
- Patients with secondary PAP should have underlying disorder treated, or should avoid exposure to inciting environmental agent. Whole lung lavage can also be used for symptomatic secondary PAP (4)[C].

ADDITIONAL TREATMENT
General Measures
Supportive measures such as supplemental oxygen, bronchodilators, antibiotics for infection, smoking cessation, and treatment of concurrent diseases that impair respiratory function can improve dyspnea temporarily. Respiratory support should be given when appropriate:

- Steroids should be avoided when possible due to interference with surfactant maturation and secretion (1)[C].
- Pulmonary rehabilitation may be helpful (1)[C].

Issues for Referral
Patients with symptomatic PAP should be referred to centers performing whole lung lavage, with anesthesiologists skilled in management of double-lumen catheters (4)[C].

Additional Therapies
Clinical trials examining the usefulness of GM-CSF therapy in treating primary PAP are currently ongoing. Initial trials appear to show that high doses of exogenous GM-CSF can overcome anti-GM-CSF neutralizing antibodies. Trials are studying dosage routes of subcutaneous injection for a systemic approach vs nebulized treatment for a localized approach. These trials are still in the initial stages, and whole lung lavage remains standard therapy (8)[C]:

- There is no role for GM-CSF therapy in secondary or congenital PAP, as they are not related to anti-GM-CSF antibodies.

SURGERY/OTHER PROCEDURES
Lung transplantation has been used in congenital PAP and for PAP that is not responsive to whole lung lavage (1)[C].

ONGOING CARE

FOLLOW-UP RECOMMENDATIONS
Patient Monitoring
Respiratory infections are a common complication of PAP, especially with atypical organisms such as *Norcardia*. Any sign of infection should lead to thorough search for organism, including bronchial washings and/or bronchoalveolar lavage (1).

PATIENT EDUCATION
The American Lung Association at http://www.lungusa.org/

PROGNOSIS
Prognosis for those who do not undergo whole lung lavage is 85% 5-year survival compared to 94% 5-year survival for those who do undergo therapeutic lavage (4). PAP can result in death from respiratory distress (80%) or infection (20%) (1):

- Congenital PAP has an especially poor prognosis.

COMPLICATIONS
Complications from PAP include respiratory failure and increased susceptibility to infection, especially *Norcardia* species:

- Whole lung lavage complications: Hypoxemia, pneumonia, sepsis, adult respiratory distress syndrome, pneumothorax (1)

REFERENCES

1. Ioachimescu OC, Kavuru MS et al. Pulmonary alveolar proteinosis. *Chron Respir Dis*. 2006;3: 149–59.
2. Huizar I, Kavuru MS et al. Alveolar proteinosis syndrome: pathogenesis, diagnosis, and management. *Curr Opin Pulm Med*. 2009;15: 491–8.
3. Presneill JJ, Nakata K, Inoue Y, Seymour JF et al. Pulmonary alveolar proteinosis. *Clin. Chest Med* 2004;25:593–613, viii.
4. Juvet SC, Hwang D, Waddell TK, Downey GP et al. Rare lung disease II: pulmonary alveolar proteinosis. *Can Respir J*. 2008;15:203–10.
5. Seymour JF, Presneill JJ et al. Pulmonary alveolar proteinosis: progress in the first 44 years. *Am J Respir Crit Care Med*. 2002;166:215–35.
6. Trapnell BC, Whitsett JA, Nakata K et al. Pulmonary alveolar proteinosis. *N Engl J Med*. 2003;349: 2527–39.
7. Frazier AA, Franks TJ, Cooke EO, Mohammed TL, Pugatch RD, Galvin JR et al. From the archives of the AFIP: pulmonary alveolar proteinosis. *Radiographics*. 2008;28:883–99; quiz 915.
8. Greenhill SR, Kotton DN et al. Pulmonary alveolar proteinosis: a bench-to-bedside story of granulocyte-macrophage colony-stimulating factor dysfunction. *Chest*. 2009;136:571–7.

ADDITIONAL READING

- Chung MJ, Lee KS, Franquet T, et al. Metabolic lung disease: imaging and histopathologic findings. *Eur J Radiol*. 2005;54:233–45.
- Wang BM, Stern EJ, Schmidt RA, Pierson DJ, et al. Diagnosing pulmonary alveolar proteinosis. A review and an update. *Chest*. 1997;111:460–6.

CODES

ICD9
516.0 Pulmonary alveolar proteinosis

CLINICAL PEARLS

- Pulmonary alveolar proteinosis is a rare disease characterized by accumulation of surfactantlike material in the alveolar spaces leading to impaired gas exchange.
- Nonspecific respiratory symptoms and physical exam findings often delay diagnosis.
- Chest CT finding of "crazy paving" is characteristic, but not specific.
- Whole lung lavage is standard therapy for symptomatic patients. 5-year survival is 94% with treatment.

ALZHEIMER DISEASE

Jill A. Grimes, MD
Linda H. Hatch, MD

 BASICS

DESCRIPTION

- Most common cause of dementia in the elderly
- Degenerative neurologic disease with progressive cognitive and behavioral impairment
- Usual course: Progressive and chronic
- System(s) affected: Nervous
- Synonym(s): Presenile dementia; senile dementia of the Alzheimer type

Geriatric Considerations
Asymptomatic screening is not recommended.

EPIDEMIOLOGY

- Predominant age: >60 years
- Predominant sex: Female > Male (slightly)

Incidence
40% of those >85 years of age are affected, which is 1,100/100,000 population.

Prevalence
5.3 million in US

RISK FACTORS

- Aging
- Low education level
- Down syndrome
- Positive family history
- Inheritance of the E4 allele of apolipoprotein E gene on chromosome 19 (E4 is much less of a risk factor for African Americans and Hispanics)
- Cardiovascular and carotid artery disease
- Smoking (2- to 4-fold increase) (1)

Genetics
Positive family history in 50% of the cases, but 90% of Alzheimer disease (AD) cases are sporadic.

GENERAL PREVENTION

- Studies show that nonsteroidal anti-inflammatory drugs (NSAIDs), estrogen, and vitamin E do NOT delay AD (2)[A].
- Hormone-replacement therapy (HRT) is not recommended (3)[A].
- Intellectual challenge (puzzles) and regular physical exercise may offer preventive benefit.
- Control vascular risks factors (e.g., hypertension). Statins and lowering cholesterol may retard pathogenesis of AD (4)[A].
- Ginkgo biloba may be beneficial in treatment for cognition, but not activities of daily living (5).
- Participation in physical activities and omega-3 fatty acids may help to prevent or delay cognitive decline (6).
- Ultrasound may help to identify asymptomatic patients at increased risk with chronic brain hypoperfusion secondary to cardiovascular or carotid artery pathology (7).

ETIOLOGY

- Unknown, but toxic β-amyloid deposits in neuritic plaques and arterial walls appear critical to pathogenesis.
- β-Amyloid precursor gene localized to chromosome 21

COMMONLY ASSOCIATED CONDITIONS

- Down syndrome
- Depression

 DIAGNOSIS

HISTORY

- Include family members in interview (for accuracy and for behavioral assessment)
- Progressive and disruptive memory loss
- Depression, anhedonia, or apathy
- Intellectual decline; difficulty with calculations; multiple missed appointments
- Loss of interest, social withdrawal
- Date or time confusion
- Occupational dysfunction or personality change
- Restlessness and sleep disturbances

PHYSICAL EXAM

- Neurologic exam to rule out other causes
- Folstein Mini Mental Status Exam (MMSE): Copyrighted, but available (http://www.aafp.org/afp/20010215/703.html)
- No focal neurologic signs
- Short-term memory loss
- Acalculia (e.g., cannot balance checkbook)
- Agnosia: Inability to recognize objects
- Apraxia: Inability to carry out movements
- Confabulation
- Delusions
- Impaired abstraction
- Decreased attention to hygiene
- Visuospatial distortion
- Late signs: Psychotic features; mutism

DIAGNOSTIC TESTS & INTERPRETATION
Neuropsychologic testing (if clinical picture is confusing or to help determine level of independence for skills such as balancing checkbooks, driving, or managing medicines)

Lab
To help rule out other causes of dementia

Initial lab tests
- Complete blood count, erythrocyte sedimentation rate
- Chemistry panel
- Thyroid-stimulating hormone
- Folate and B$_{12}$ levels
- VDRL or RPR
- HIV antibody (selected cases)

Follow-Up & Special Considerations
For genetic testing for E4 allele of apolipoprotein, discuss with genetic counselor (2)[A].

Imaging
Initial approach
- Controversy exists; consider MRI or CT scan if:
  - cognitive decline is recent; history of stroke; or focal neurologic signs
- Evidence is not sufficient to include resting electroencephalogram in routine clinical practice (8).

Follow-Up & Special Considerations
- CT scan/MRI: Moderate cortical atrophy, ventricular enlargement
- MRI: Hippocampal volumetry; positron-emission tomography (PFT) and single-photon-emission computed tomography not indicated
- Medicare pays for PET to distinguish AD from frontotemporal dementia.

Pathological Findings
- Gross: Diffuse cerebral atrophy in hippocampus, amygdala, and some subcortical nuclei
- Micro:
  - Neuritic senile plaques
  - Neurofibrillary tangles
  - Pyramidal cell loss
  - Decreased cholinergic innervation (other neurotransmitters variably decreased)
  - Degeneration of locus ceruleus and basal forebrain nuclei of Meynert; amyloid angiopathy

DIFFERENTIAL DIAGNOSIS

- Vascular dementia, multi-infarct dementia
- Lewy body disease
- Dementia associated with Parkinson disease
- Normal-pressure hydrocephalus
- Creutzfeldt-Jakob disease
- End-stage multiple sclerosis
- Brain tumor: Primary or metastatic
- Subdural hematoma
- Progressive multifocal leukoencephalopathy
- Metabolic dementia (hypothyroidism)
- Drug reactions, alcoholism, other addictions
- Dementia pugilistica
- Depression
- Toxicity from liver and kidney failure
- Vitamin and other nutritional deficiencies
- Vasculitis
- Neurosyphilis

TREATMENT

MEDICATION
Memory enhancement and slowing progression of disease:

- Cholinesterase inhibitors (9)[A] (Equally effective; all have largely GI side effects):
  - Best in mild to moderate disease (Folstein MMSE scores 10–24); drugs *may* be effective in Lewy body dementia.
  - Donepezil (Aricept): Start at 5 mg p.o. daily; may increase to 10 mg daily after 1 month
    - Comes in tablets or orally disintegrating tabs
    - Generic available
    - Caution with digoxin or beta-blockers (can cause 3* heart block)
    - Aricept 23 mg tablet approved in 2010
  - Rivastigmine (Exelon): Start tabs at 1.5 mg p.o. b.i.d., increase by 1.5 mg b.i.d. every 2 weeks; maintenance 6-12 mg total daily
    - Capsule, solution, or patch (patch greatly reduces side effects)
    - Indicated for both AD and Parkinson dementia
  - Galantamine (Razadyne): Start 4 mg b.i.d. for 4 weeks, then increase by 4 mg b.i.d. every month with goal 16–24 mg daily dose
    - Tablets, solution, and extended release capsule (ER has daily dosing)
- NMDA receptor antagonists (for moderate to severe AD; MMSE 5–14)
  - Monotherapy or in combination with acetylcholinesterase inhibitors
  - Memantine (Namenda): Start at 5 mg daily, with starter pack titrating to target dose of 10 mg b.i.d. after 4 weeks
  - Often improves behavioral issues

First Line

- Behavioral techniques and environmental modification help more than medications for wandering, restlessness, uncooperativeness, hoarding, and irritability.
- For depression (occurs in 1/3 of patients), use selective serotonin reuptake inhibitors (SSRIs).
- Insomnia:
  - Trazodone 25–100 mg at bedtime, zolpidem (Ambien) 5 mg at bedtime, zaleplon (Sonata) 5–10 mg at bedtime, ramelteon (Rozerem) 8 mg at bedtime
  - Avoid diphenhydramine in elderly males, which can cause urinary retention.
- Moderate anxiety/restlessness: Consider low-dose, short-acting benzodiazepines, buspirone, or SSRIs, but efficacy unproven.
- Severe aggressive agitation (especially if psychotic features present):
  - Memantine (Namenda) (9)[A]: 1st of new class of NMDA receptor antagonists; can be used as monotherapy or in combination with acetylcholinesterase inhibitors to enhance or preserve memory; shows efficacy in severe disease (Folstein MMSE score 5–14). Start at 5 mg daily, titrating to target dose of 10 mg b.i.d. after 4 weeks. Often improves behavioral issues.
  - Risperidone (Risperdal) 0.25–1.0 mg b.i.d., olanzapine 2.5 mg/d b.i.d.; other newer atypical antipsychotic agents may be preferred owing to fewer side effects (10)[A], but all are likely to increase mortality. Minimize use.
  - Carbamazepine (Tegretol) 100 mg b.i.d.–t.i.d., propranolol (Inderal) 10–40 mg b.i.d.–t.i.d., trazodone 200 mg daily, and valproic acid 250–1,500 mg daily
- Contraindications:
  - Avoid anticholinergic drugs, such as tricyclic antidepressants and antihistamines.
  - Ginkgo biloba: Avoid anticoagulants and aspirin.
- Precautions:
  - Benzodiazepines may produce paradoxical excitation or daytime drowsiness.
  - Triazolam (Halcion) can produce confusion, memory loss, and psychotic behavior.
  - Atypical antipsychotic agents are associated with hyperglycemia, ketoacidosis, increased stroke risk, and increased mortality in elders and dementia patients.
  - Cholinesterase inhibitors provide only modest benefit for 1–2 years, after which decline continues at somewhat lesser rate than placebo. Number needed to treat (NNT) = 7. No deterioration over 6–12 months is evidence of efficacy (9)[A].
- Significant possible interactions:
  - Antipsychotics: Lithium may induce extrapyramidal symptoms, disorientation.
  - Benzodiazepines may increase serum phenytoin concentration; cimetidine may increase benzodiazepine concentration.
  - Donepezil (Aricept): Use with caution with anticholinergic medication or in patients with sick sinus syndrome or a history of peptic ulcers.
  - Paroxetine causes increased donepezil levels.

Second Line

Conflicting efficacy for selegiline 5 mg b.i.d., vitamin E 1,000 mg b.i.d., or NSAIDs in slowing the progression of the disease (2)[A].

ADDITIONAL TREATMENT
General Measures
- Outpatient, day care, assisted living, skilled nursing facility
- Optimize treatment of associated comorbidities.
- Analyze environment for safety and security and avoid sudden changes in environment.
- Assess needs of spouse/caregiver.
- Advance directives planning

Issues for Referral
- Assess DRIVING SAFETY (vision, spatial relations, hearing, judgement)
  - http://www.nhtsa.gov/people/injury/olddrive/Driving%20Safely%20Aging%20Web/
- Visiting nurse or social worker
- Physical, occupational, or speech therapist
- Lawyer (living will, power of attorney)
- Support groups for patient and family

Additional Therapies
- Exercise to reduce restlessness
- Continued cognitive challenge

COMPLEMENTARY AND ALTERNATIVE MEDICINE
- Ginkgo biloba extracts (120 mg a day) show conflicting efficacy in treatment of AD but may be beneficial (5).
- Coenzyme Q_{10}, huperzine not effective
- Occupational therapy, music therapy (10)[B], aroma therapy (10)[B], pet therapy (10)[B]

 ## ONGOING CARE

FOLLOW-UP RECOMMENDATIONS
Patient Monitoring
- Schedule regular follow-up (every 3 months) to assess medical complications, provide support for family, and assess need for placement.
- Serial mental status testing is potentially helpful, but bedside tests (Folstein MMSE) offer wide variability and lack of sensitivity.

PATIENT EDUCATION
- Printed patient and family information: Alzheimer Association, 919 N. Michigan Ave., Suite 1000, Chicago, IL; (800) 272-3900; http://www.alz.org/
- Explain progressive nature of the disease and start advance directives planning as early as possible.
- Prenatal testing is available for the *PSEN1* mutation (which causes 30–70% of early-onset familial AD).

PROGNOSIS
Poor: Average survival from diagnosis is 4–6 years (diagnosis is often delayed).

COMPLICATIONS
- Behavioral: Hostility, agitation, wandering, uncooperative
- Metabolic: Infection, dehydration, drug toxicity, malnutrition
- Falls
- "Sundowning" (increase full-spectrum lights in evenings/winter)
- Depression (1/3 of patients)
- Suicide: Especially in early stages

REFERENCES

1. Cataldo JK, Prochaska JJ, Glantz SA, et al. Cigarette smoking is a risk factor for Alzheimer's Disease: an analysis controlling for tobacco industry affiliation. *J Alzheimers Dis*. 2010;19:465–480.
2. Patterson C, Feightner JW, Garcia A et al. Diagnosis and treatment of dementia: 1. Risk assessment and primary prevention of Alzheimer disease. *CMAJ*. 2008;178:548–56.
3. Hogervorst E, et al. Hormone replacement therapy for cognitive function in postmenopausal women. *Cochrane Database Syst Rev*. 2006;4:CD003799.
4. Scott, H Denman. Laake, Knut. Statins for the prevention of Alzheimer's disease and dementia. [Systematic Review] Cochrane Dementia and Cognitive Improvement Group. *Cochrane Database of Systematic Reviews*. 1, 2009.
5. Weinmann S, Roll S, Schwarzbach C, et al. Effects of Ginkgo biloba in dementia: systematic review and meta-analysis. *BMC Geriatr*. 2010;10:14.
6. Daviglus ML, Bell CC, Berrittini W, et al. NIH State-of-the-Science Conference: Preventing Alzheimer's Disease and Cognitive Decline. 2010.
7. de la Torre JC. Vascular risk factor detection and control may prevent Alzheimer's disease. *Ageing Res Rev*. 2010;10.
8. Jelic V, Kowalski J, et al. Evidence-based evaluation of diagnostic accuracy of resting EEG in dementia and mild cognitive impairment. *Clin EEG Neurosci*. 2009;40:129–42.
9. Raina P, Santaguida P, Ismaila A et al. Effectiveness of cholinesterase inhibitors and memantine for treating dementia: evidence review for a clinical practice guideline. *Ann Intern Med*. 2008;148:379–97.
10. Sink KM, Holden KF, Yaffe K. Pharmacological treatment of neuropsychiatric symptoms of dementia: a review of the evidence. *JAMA*. 2005;293:596–608.

See Also (Topic, Algorithm, Electronic Media Element)
Substance Use Disorders; Hypothyroidism, Adult; Depression

 ## CODES

ICD9
- 290.0 Senile dementia, uncomplicated
- 290.10 Presenile dementia, uncomplicated
- 331.0 Alzheimer's disease

CLINICAL PEARLS

- Daily intellectual stimulation, such as puzzles, and moderate physical exercise may help prevent AD.
- Imaging studies have low yield in patients with a history typical of AD.
- Encourage families to join a chapter of the Alzheimer Association and to pursue advanced directive planning early in the course of the disease.
- Atypical antipsychotic medications increase mortality.

AMBLYOPIA

Robert M. Kershner, MD, MS

 BASICS

DESCRIPTION
A reduction in visual acuity resulting from abnormal visual development in the absence of a structural or pathologic abnormality of the eye, which cannot be corrected by eyeglasses or contact lenses. The lesion is typically unilateral, although it may be bilateral:
- System(s) affected: Nervous
- Synonym(s): Lazy eye

Pediatric Considerations
More commonly seen in the pediatric age group early in life. The mean age at presentation is 3–6 years old.

EPIDEMIOLOGY
- Predominant age: The onset may be present from birth or in early childhood. The condition may go undiagnosed and be detected at any age.
- Predominant gender: Male = Female

Prevalence
~2–2.5% in the general population

RISK FACTORS
Preexisting refractive error, such as myopia, hyperopia, or astigmatism. More common with occlusion of the visual pathway. Conditions that cause anisometropia (refractive difference between the eyes) or obstruction to clear vision, i.e., cataract, corneal abnormalities, can lead to permanent amblyopia.

Genetics
Increased incidence in children with 1 parent with a history of amblyopia

PATHOPHYSIOLOGY
- Strabismic amblyopia is a loss of visual acuity in an individual with misalignment of the visual axis in 1 eye, due to suppression of the images from an eye that turns out or in.
- Anisometropic amblyopia is present when 1 eye has a significantly different refractive error from the fellow eye, leading to visual blurring and suppression of the image from that eye.
- Refractive amblyopia is due to uncorrected high refractive error, resulting in visual blurring in either or both eyes.

- Deprivation amblyopia (amblyopia ex anopsia) is due to relatively complete visual deprivation in 1 eye, which may be caused by a congenital abnormality such as a corneal scar or cataract.
- Deficiency amblyopia is also known as nutritional optic neuropathy or tobacco–alcohol amblyopia. Deficiencies of vitamin B_1 or B_{12} or riboflavin may be responsible.
- Amblyopia can only occur early in life. When the brain detects unequal images, for any reason, it is forced to ignore one. The ability of a brain to suppress the unwanted image can only occur when the development of neuroadaptive responses is in a critical "plastic" period, usually the first several years of life. If amblyopia has not developed after that period has passed, the individual will be unable to "suppress" the unwanted image and diplopia or double vision will result.

ETIOLOGY
Strabismus causes disparate retinal images whereby one eye sees the object of regard in the fovea and the other in a different part of the retina. Inability to fuse the 2 images results in the brain ignoring the less preferred image (this does not necessarily need to be the less clear image). Refractive errors such as anisometropia (a difference in refractive error between the 2 eyes) can cause the 2 retinal images to be of unequal clarity. An obstruction to the visual axis, such as cataracts, also causes unequal clarity of the retinal image. The result of one eye seeing better than the other is the interruption of development of fine visual perception, which can contribute to the development of amblyopia. Individuals with amblyopia do not have normal degrees of stereo vision and often complain of not appreciating 3D images.

 DIAGNOSIS

HISTORY
- Squinting one eye in bright light is the most common symptom, hence the alternative term for strabismus, "squint."
- Rubbing the eyes
- Sitting close to television or computer screen
- Problems in sports
- Preference for front-row seating
- Covering or closing an eye
- Eye turns in or out, wandering eye
- Poor vision in one eye without apparent explanation or a diagnosable organic cause
- Poor vision that does not correct with glasses

PHYSICAL EXAM
- Ophthalmologic exam to screen for unequal refractive error, outward or inward turning of the eye (strabismic amblyopia), obstruction to the visual pathway. Vision testing of the eye under monocular conditions can reveal dissimilarities.
- All children should have complete visual exams prior to starting school, with each eye tested individually. Children from families with a known history of amblyopia or strabismus should have dilated exams performed by an ophthalmologist.
- The corneal light reflex test (shining a light into the child's eyes and noting the location of the light in relation to the pupil) may be used to assess ocular alignment in young children. An abnormal test should prompt referral to an ophthalmologist.
- When a dilated examination is not possible, evaluation of the "red reflex" such as that seen with flash photography may indicate an obstruction of vision that would warrant prompt evaluation by an ophthalmologist.
- Any of the above conditions indicate prompt evaluation and referral. In a young child the earlier the diagnosis, the better the therapeutic outcome. Children with cataract may require cataract surgery, and unequal refractive errors need to be promptly treated with glasses or contact lenses to improve sight before amblyopia sets in.

DIFFERENTIAL DIAGNOSIS
The diagnosis of amblyopia can be confused with an organic lesion causing decreased visual acuity, and this must always be excluded before the diagnosis of amblyopia is considered. Intraocular tumors, glaucoma, and congenital abnormalities can result in and be mistaken for amblyopia.

 TREATMENT

ADDITIONAL TREATMENT
General Measures
- Correction of the underlying disorder should be instituted promptly as the condition may become irreversible if the child is more than 4–6 years of age.
- Patching of the stronger eye to encourage visual development of the amblyopic eye is warranted. There may be resistance of the child to the wearing of a patch, which may lessen benefit. Various patching regimens have been studied (from 2–23 hours of patching per day for 4–6 months, and alternate patching). Close follow-up is necessary. Should the "good" eye be patched excessively, the risk of development of amblyopia in that eye increases.
- An alternative therapy to patching is pharmacologic blurring, usually achieved with atropine eye drops. Similar efficacy is achieved compared to patching, with improved compliance. The risk associated with systemic effects from the antimuscarinic effects of the drug cannot be ignored (1)[A].

- Corrective lenses should be prescribed for refractive errors.
- Correction of anatomic obstructions, including cataracts or ptosis, may improve vision and minimize recurrence.
- Amblyopia never corrects itself spontaneously and will always require treatment. Children do not outgrow amblyopia.
- Deficiency amblyopia: Balanced diet, vitamins, and avoidance of alcohol and tobacco

Issues for Referral
Obstruction of vision in the infant or toddler is a potential medical emergency. Failure to refer can result in irreversible loss of vision in an otherwise healthy eye.

COMPLEMENTARY AND ALTERNATIVE MEDICINE
None. There are no effective homeopathic remedies for amblyopia. Vision training can be an effective adjunct only if the underlying organic causes are addressed and patching therapy instituted.

SURGERY/OTHER PROCEDURES
Surgical correction of an abnormal eye position, or intraocular obstruction may be required.

ONGOING CARE

FOLLOW-UP RECOMMENDATIONS
All children diagnosed with amblyopia need to be followed for years to prevent recurrence.

Patient Monitoring
Once the diagnosis of amblyopia is made, the patient must be seen frequently until complete resolution of the problem occurs.

PATIENT EDUCATION
Advise all parents to have children's eyes examined prior to starting school.

PROGNOSIS
- A treatable condition in most cases if the diagnosis is made early:
  – Patching therapy, pharmacologic blurring, eyeglasses, and surgical correction of abnormal eye positions can result in near-normal vision when instituted early.
  – Visual development occurs during the first several years of life, and amblyopia therapy can be effective until 12 years of age.
- The risk of recurrence is 24% after 1 year; reinstitution of treatment is warranted.

COMPLICATIONS
Failure to institute early therapy may result in permanent unilateral visual loss. Unilateral amblyopia causes an increased risk of severe visual impairment due to loss of vision in the nonamblyopic eye. Psychosocial complications include difficulty in schooling, work, or physical activity, and an increased risk of depression and anxiety.

REFERENCES

1. Kushner BJ. Atropine vs patching for treatment of amblyopia in children. *JAMA*. 2002;287(16): 2145–6.
2. Levi DM, Li RW. Perceptual Learning as a potential treatment for amblyopia: a mini-review. *Vision Res*. 2009.

ADDITIONAL READING

- Li T, Shotton K et al. Conventional occlusion versus pharmacologic penalization for amblyopia. *Cochrane Database Syst Rev*. 2009;CD006460.
- Schmucker C, Grosselfinger R, Riemsma R et al. Diagnostic accuracy of vision screening tests for the detection of amblyopia and its risk factors: a systematic review. *Graefes Arch Clin Exp Ophthalmol*. 2009.

- Schmucker C, Kleijnen J, Grosselfinger R, Riemsma R, Antes G, Lange S, Lagrèze W et al. Effectiveness of early in comparison to late(r) treatment in children with amblyopia or its risk factors: a systematic review. *Ophthalmic Epidemiol*. 2010;17:7–17.
- Teed RG, Bui CM, Morrison DG, Estes RL, Donahue SP et al. Amblyopia therapy in children identified by photoscreening. *Ophthalmology*. 2010;117: 159–62.

See Also (Topic, Algorithm, Electronic Media Element)
Refractive Errors; Strabismus

CODES

ICD9
- 368.00 Amblyopia, unspecified
- 368.01 Strabismic amblyopia
- 368.02 Deprivation amblyopia

CLINICAL PEARLS

- Amblyopia typically presents between the ages of 3 and 6 years, but it needs to be diagnosed earlier if treatment is to be effective. It is never too early to refer if an inequality in visual appearance of the eyes or function is suspected.
- Due to increased incidence in families where there is a history of amblyopia, all related children should be screened by an ophthalmologist.
- Perceptual learning appears to be beneficial in older youth and adults diagnosed late with amblyopia (2)[A].

AMEBIASIS

Najmul H. Siddiqui, MBBS, MD
Naureen B. Rafiq, MBBS, MD

 BASICS

DESCRIPTION
- Amebiasis is caused by *Entamoeba histolytica*, an intestinal protozoan found worldwide.
- Most common in developing countries, immigrants from or travelers to endemic regions, those who perform anal sex, and immunocompromised individuals.
- Most infected patients are asymptomatic or have minimal gastrointestinal symptoms (about 90%).
  - Severe infection (i.e., amebic colitis), can occur in very young patients, pregnant women, patients on steroid therapy, and malnourished individuals (1,2).
- Infection is spread by the feco-oral route and caused by the ingestion of *E. histolytica* cysts (infective form) in contaminated food (garden vegetables), fecally contaminated soil, or water. It is then followed by excystation in the terminal ileum or colon to form highly motile trophozoites (invasive form). The trophozoites then encyst and are excreted in the feces or invade the intestinal mucosal barrier and spread hematogenously via the portal circulation to the liver or other distant organs. The excreted cysts reach the environment to complete the cycle.
- Amebiasis is primarily an infection of the colon but extraintestinal (liver, kidney, bladder, skin, lung, brain, male or female genitalia) disease can occur. Amebic liver abscess is the most common complication of invasive amebiasis. It can develop during the acute attack or 1–3 months later.
- May play a substantial role in the clinical initiation and relapses of inflammatory bowel disease (3).
- The genus *Entamoeba* contains many species, including *E. histolytica*, *E. dispar*, *E. moshkovskii*, *E. polecki*, *E. coli* and *E. hartmanni*. Only *E. histolytica* has been clearly associated with disease; the others are considered nonpathogenic (4).
- System(s) affected: GI; Nervous; Renal/Urologic; Reproductive; Skin/Exocrine
- Synonym(s): Amebic colitis; Amebic dysentery

Geriatric Considerations
More severe in elderly

Pediatric Considerations
More severe in neonates

Pregnancy Considerations
More severe in pregnancy

EPIDEMIOLOGY
- Infection can affect patients of all ages.
- Amebic colitis affects both sexes equally (1).
- Amebic liver abscess incidence greater in men than women for unknown reasons.

Pediatric Considerations
Very young children seem to be predisposed to fulminant colitis.

Prevalence
- The overall prevalence of amebiasis in the United States is approximately 4% and approximately 10% of the world's population.
- Entamoeba infection is as high as 50% in areas of Central and South America, Africa, and Asia.

RISK FACTORS
- Low socioeconomic status
- Institutional living
- Male homosexuality
- Immunocompromised
- Invasive disease is more common in certain geographic locations, including some parts of Mexico, South Africa, and India.

GENERAL PREVENTION
- Eradication of fecal contamination of food and water through improved sanitation, hygiene, and water treatment.
- Individuals traveling to endemic areas should be advised on proper food and water handling. Water should be boiled for more than 1 minute and uncooked vegetables washed with a detergent soap or soaked in acetic acid or vinegar for 10–15 minutes before consumption.
- Avoiding sexual practices that involve fecal–oral contact with potential contamination of infective cysts
- Treatment of patients and close contacts, since reinfection is common
- Amebiasis does not confer lifelong immunity and thus individuals with previous infection are as susceptible to reinfection as other members of the population (2).

PATHOPHYSIOLOGY
- Invasion to the colonic mucosa is mediated by a galactose/N-acetylgalactosamine (GAL/GalNAc)-specific lectin, able to activate lytic and apoptotic pathways, and direct inhibition of the complement system by the trophozoite.
- Extraintestinal disease can result from hepatobiliary and/or hematogenous spread.

ETIOLOGY
Infection results from ingestion of *E. histolytica* cysts in contaminated food, water, or by direct fecal–oral transmission.

DIAGNOSIS

HISTORY
- Noninvasive infection (symptoms are often nonspecific):
  - Asymptomatic
  - Mild diarrhea
  - Abdominal discomfort
- Invasive infection (amebic colitis):
  - Gradual onset of bloody diarrhea
  - Abdominal pain
  - Fever (10–30%)
  - Weight loss and anorexia
  - Fulminant colitis with severe bloody diarrhea, worsening abdominal pain with peritonitis and fever. Risk factors include malnutrition, pregnancy, steroid use, and very young age.

- Extraintestinal infection:
  - Amebic liver abscess:
    - Fever (up to 90%), right upper quadrant (RUQ) pain <10 days duration
    - Subacute presentation is associated with mild fever, weight loss, and anorexia
    - Cough can occur. Jaundice not common.
    - Up to 70% can present without colitis.
    - Symptoms may start years after exposure.
  - Pleuropulmonary amebiasis: Pleuritic chest pain, cough, and respiratory distress after rupture of amebic liver abscess through the diaphragm
  - Cerebral amebiasis: Headache, nausea, vomiting, and rapid mental status change with rapid progression

PHYSICAL EXAM
- Amebic colitis:
  - Diffuse abdominal tenderness (12–85%)
  - Fever (10–30%)
  - Weight loss (40%)
  - Heme-positive stools (70–100%)
- Amebic liver abscess:
  - Fever (85–90%)
  - RUQ tenderness (85–90%)
  - Hepatomegaly (30–50%)
  - Weight loss (30–50%)

DIAGNOSTIC TESTS & INTERPRETATION
Lab
Initial lab tests
- Microscopic stool examination for trophozoites from a single sample is only 33–50% sensitive. Serial stool sampling × 3 in no more than 10 days increase detection to 85–95% but with poor specificity as it cannot differentiate *E. histolytica* from nonpathogenic *E. dispar* and *E. moshkovskii* (1).
- ELISA to detect *E. histolytic*-specific antigens, with an overall sensitivity of 71–100% and specificity of 93–100%. Antigen testing from serum and liver aspirate in amebic liver abscess yields a sensitivity of 96% and 100%, respectively.
- Serology assays are available for diagnosis measuring the presence of serum antilectin antibodies (IgG), with a sensitivity of 97.9% and specificity of 94.8% in *E. histolytica* infection with amebic liver abscess.
- Polymerase chain reaction (PCR) techniques are more sensitive for detection of *E. histolytica* in fecal or liver aspirate samples, but are not routinely available in clinical laboratories.
- In bladder infections: Amoebae and/or cysts in urine
- Liver enzymes, alkaline phosphatase (80%), and erythrocyte sedimentation rate may be elevated, and anemia and leucocytosis without eosinophilia (80%) may be present in amebic liver abscess.

Follow-Up & Special Considerations
Follow-up stool examination after completion of therapy to ensure intestinal eradication.

Imaging
Initial approach
Ultrasonography and computed tomography (CT) scanning are sensitive but nonspecific for amebic liver abscess. Usually solitary lesions in the right hepatic lobe (70–80%).

Diagnostic Procedures/Surgery
- Ultrasound or CT-guided needle aspiration for suspected amebic abscess with studies of aspirate
- Colonoscopy with biopsy can be performed in highly suspicious cases with negative stool and antigen testing. It is contraindicated in fulminant colitis due to increased perforation risk.

Pathological Findings
- Colon biopsy:
  - Amebic invasion through the mucosa and into submucosa is the hallmark of amebic colitis, which gives the classical flask-shaped ulcers.
  - Periodic acid–Schiff-stained trophozoites in magenta color
  - Neutrophils at the periphery
- Liver biopsy:
  - Necrosis surrounded by a rim of trophozoites
- Liver aspirate:
  - Red-brown material (anchovy paste)

DIFFERENTIAL DIAGNOSIS
- Other infectious causes of colitis:
  - Shigellosis
  - Campylobacter infection
  - Pseudomembranous colitis
  - Occasionally salmonellosis or *Yersinia* infection
  - Viral hepatitis
- Noninfectious causes of colitis:
  - Ulcerative colitis
  - Crohn colitis
  - Ischemic colitis in elderly
  - Hepatocellular adenoma
- Hepatic amebiasis must be distinguished from pyogenic liver abscess or superinfection of amebic abscess.

 ## TREATMENT

- Mostly treated as an outpatient but fulminant colitis with hypovolemia and complicated liver abscess require inpatient management.
- Asymptomatic *E. histolytica* infection should be treated with luminal agent (iodoquinol, paromomycin) alone to eradicate infection as invasive infection may develop and also continuous shedding of cyst transmits infection through feco-oral route.
- *E. dispar* and *E. moshkovskii* infections do not require treatment as they are nonpathogenic strains (2,4).

MEDICATION
First Line
- Noninvasive infection: Treat with luminal agents only.
  - Paromomycin: Adult: 500 mg PO t.i.d. for 10 days; Pediatric: Administer as in adults
- Invasive infection: Treat with nitroimidazole (metronidazole/tinidazole) followed by luminal agent.
  - Metronidazole: Adult: 500–750 mg t.i.d PO for 10 days, Pediatric: 35–50 mg/kg PO divided tid for 10 days. It is then followed by a 20-day course of diiodohydroxyquin to eliminate intestinal carriage.
  - Tinidazole: 2 g/d for 3 days with food for intestinal infection and 2 g/d for 3–5 days for liver abscess; better tolerated than metronidazole (5)[A]

- Contraindications:
  - Known allergy to given medication
  - Diiodohydroxyquin should be used with caution in patients with thyroid disease. It is contraindicated in renal and hepatic patients and may cause optic nerve and peripheral neuropathy.
- Precautions:
  - None of the agents has been proven safe during pregnancy, but pregnant women with invasive disease should still be treated.
- Significant possible interactions:
  - Metronidazole and tinidazole: Disulfiram reaction with concomitant use of ethanol.

Pregnancy Considerations
- Most agents are avoided in pregnancy (especially 1st trimester) because of concerns of teratogenicity, but invasive disease must still be treated.
  - Paromomycin is sometimes recommended for noninvasive disease because it is not absorbed.
- Infectious disease consultation should be obtained.

Second Line
- Luminal agent for noninvasive infection:
  - Diloxanide: Adult: 500 mg PO tid for 10 days; Pediatric: <2 years not recommended; >2 years 20 mg/kg PO divided tid for 10 days
  - Diiodohydroxyquin (also called iodoquinol): Adult: 650 mg tid PO for 20 days (if available); Pediatric: 10–13 mg/kg PO tid for 20 days
- Invasive infection:
  - Dehydroemetine (as effective as metronidazole, but cardiotoxic): 1–1.5 mg/kg IM for 5 days
  - Chloroquine (less effective): 600 mg base/day PO for 2 days, then 200 mg/day PO for 2–3 weeks (pediatric dose: 10 mg/kg/day up to maximum of 300 mg/d)
  - Treatment for invasive infection should be followed by a luminal agent.

ADDITIONAL TREATMENT
General Measures
- Fluids and nutrition
- Electrolyte management

SURGERY/OTHER PROCEDURES
- Surgery may be necessary in severe amebic colitis, peritonitis, and perforated viscus.
- Surgical drainage of uncomplicated amebic liver abscess should be avoided.

 ## ONGOING CARE

FOLLOW-UP RECOMMENDATIONS
Patient Monitoring
- Patient signs and symptoms should be monitored.
- Stool studies should be repeated after the completion of therapy to ensure eradication since no regimen is completely effective.

DIET
As tolerated

PATIENT EDUCATION
Maintain good hygiene and avoid situations of re-exposure.

PROGNOSIS
- Untreated invasive amebiasis is frequently fatal.
- With treatment, improvement usually occurs within a few days.
- Some patients with amebic colitis have irritable bowel symptoms for weeks after successful treatment.
- Relapses possible

COMPLICATIONS
- Amebic colitis:
  - Fulminant or necrotizing colitis
  - Toxic megacolon
  - Ameboma
  - Rectovaginal fistula
- Amebic liver abscess:
  - Rupture to intraperitoneal, intrathoracic, or intrapericardial spaces with secondary bacterial infection
  - Direct extension to pleura or pericardium
  - Hematogenous dissemination and formation of brain abscess

REFERENCES
1. Fotedar R, Stark D, Beebe N et al. Laboratory diagnostic techniques for entamoeba species. *Clin Microbiol Rev.* 2007;20:511–32.
2. Stanley SL. Amoebiasis. *Lancet.* 2003;361: 1025–34.
3. Yamamoto-Furusho JK, Torijano-Carrera E et al. Intestinal protozoa infections among patients with ulcerative colitis: prevalence and impact on clinical disease course. *Digestion.* 2010;82:18–23.
4. Haque R, Huston CD, Hughes M et al. Amebiasis. *N Engl J Med.* 2003;348:1565–73.
5. Gonzales ML, Dans LF, Martinez EG. Antiamoebic drugs for treating amoebic colitis. *Cochrane Database Syst Rev.* 2009:CD006085.

ADDITIONAL READING
- Haque R, Kabir M, Noor Z, Rahman SM, Mondal D, Alam F, Rahman I, Al Mahmood A, Ahmed N, Petri WA et al. Diagnosis of amebic liver abscess and amebic colitis by detection of Entamoeba histolytica DNA in blood, urine, and saliva by a real-time PCR assay. *J Clin Microbiol.* 2010;48:2798–801.
- Stark D, van Hal S, Marriott D, Ellis J, Harkness J et al. Irritable bowel syndrome: a review on the role of intestinal protozoa and the importance of their detection and diagnosis. *Int J Parasitol.* 2007;37: 11–20.

See Also (Topic, Algorithm, Electronic Media Element)
Diarrhea, Acute; Diarrhea, Chronic

 ## CODES

ICD9
- 006.0 Acute amebic dysentery without mention of abscess
- 006.3 Amebic liver abscess
- 006.4 Amebic lung abscess

CLINICAL PEARLS
- Most infected patients are asymptomatic or have minimal diarrheal symptoms.
- Untreated invasive disease is frequently fatal and treated cases may get relapses.
- Irritable bowel symptoms may persist for weeks despite successful treatment of infection.
- Nonpathogenic strains of Entamoeba species do not require treatment.

AMENORRHEA

Heidi L. Gaddey, MD

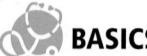

BASICS

DESCRIPTION
- Primary amenorrhea:
  - No menses by age 13–14 with absence of secondary sexual characteristics or
  - No menses by age 15–16 with normal secondary characteristics
- Secondary amenorrhea: Absence of menses for 3 months in a woman with previously normal menstruation or 6 months in a woman with a history of irregular cycles
- System(s) affected: Endocrine/metabolic; Reproductive

Pregnancy Considerations
Pregnancy is by far the most common cause of secondary amenorrhea.

EPIDEMIOLOGY
Prevalence
- Primary amenorrhea: <1% of female population
- Secondary amenorrhea: 3–5% of female population
- No evidence for race and ethnicity affecting prevalence
- Secondary amenorrhea more common than primary

RISK FACTORS
- Obesity
- Overtraining
- Eating disorders
- Malnutrition
- Anovulatory disorders
- Psychosocial crisis

Genetics
No known genetic pattern

GENERAL PREVENTION
Maintenance of proper body mass index (BMI) and healthy lifestyle with respect to food and exercise

PATHOPHYSIOLOGY
- Pathophysiology varies, depending on etiology.
- Primary amenorrhea should be evaluated in context of presence or absence of secondary sexual characteristics.
- Can result from dysfunction in hypothalamic–pituitary–gonadal axis, anatomic abnormalities, or other endocrine gland disorder

ETIOLOGY
- Primary amenorrhea:
  - Hypothalamic-pituitary abnormalities:
    ○ Constitutional delay of puberty
    ○ Isolated GnRH deficiency
    ○ Eating disorder
    ○ Stress/exercise
    ○ Central lesions (tumors, hypophysitis, granulomas)
    ○ Hyperprolactinemia
  - Gonadal abnormalities:
    ○ Chromosomal abnormalities (androgen insensitivity syndrome)
    ○ Euchromosomal gonadal agenesis or dysgenesis (Turner syndrome, Swyer syndrome, and pure gonadal dysgenesis)
    ○ Ovarian resistance syndrome
    ○ Abnormal gonadotropin function
    ○ Autoimmune gonadal failure
    ○ Idiopathic gonadal failure

- Anatomic abnormalities:
  ○ Imperforate hymen
  ○ Transverse vaginal septum
  ○ Congenital absence of the cervix
  ○ Müllerian agenesis
- Secondary amenorrhea:
  - Pregnancy
  - Thyroid disease
  - Hyperprolactinemia (altered metabolism, ectopic production, breastfeeding/stimulation, hypothyroidism, medications, empty sella syndrome, pituitary adenoma)
  - After pregnancy, thyroid disease, and hyperprolactinemia are ruled out, other causes classified as:
    ○ Normogonadotropic amenorrhea: Hyperandrogenic anovulation (acromegaly, androgen secreting tumors, Cushing's disease, exogenous androgens, nonclassical congenital adrenal hyperplasia, PCOS); outflow tract obstruction (Asherman's syndrome, cervical stenosis, fibroids or polyps)
    ○ Hypergonadotropic hypogonadism. Postmenopausal ovarian failure; premature ovarian failure (autoimmune, chemotherapy, galactosemia, genetic, 17-hydroxylase deficiency, idiopathic, mumps oophoritis, pelvic radiation)
    ○ Hypogonadotropic hypogonadism (eating disorders, CNS tumors, chronic illness, cranial radiation, excessive weight loss/exercise/malnutrition, hypothalamic or pituitary destruction, Sheehan's syndrome)

COMMONLY ASSOCIATED CONDITIONS
- Premature ovarian failure may be associated with autoimmune abnormalities (autoimmune thyroiditis, type 1 diabetes).
- Polycystic ovarian syndrome associated with insulin-resistance and obesity

DIAGNOSIS

HISTORY
- Careful review of systems, including recent weight changes, symptoms of early pregnancy or menopause, virilizing changes, cyclic pelvic pain, galactorrhea, headaches, vision changes, fatigue, palpitations
- Growth and pubertal development history, including age of breast development, pubertal growth spurt, and adrenarche
- History of chronic illness, trauma, surgery, medications, prior chemotherapy or radiation
- Psychiatric history
- Social history, including diet and exercise history, drug abuse, and sexual history

PHYSICAL EXAM
- General appearance
- Vital signs, including height and weight, BMI: Hypotension, bradycardia, hypothermia (anorexia nervosa)
- HEENT exam: Evidence of dental erosions, trauma to palate (bulimia), visual field defect, fundoscopic changes, cranial nerve findings (prolactinoma), webbed neck (Turner syndrome), thyromegaly
- Skin exam: Evidence of androgen excess (acne, hirsutism), acanthosis nigricans (PCOS)

- Breast: State of development, evidence of galactorrhea (prolactinoma)
- Pelvic exam: Presence or absence of pubic hair (if sparse: Androgen insensitivity or deficiency); clitoromegaly (androgen excess); distention or bulging of external vagina (imperforate hymen); thin, pale vaginal mucosa without rugae (estrogen deficiency and ovarian failure); presence of cervical mucus (evidence for estrogen production); blind vaginal pouch (müllerian agenesis, androgen insensitivity syndrome); ovarian enlargement (tumors, PCOS, autoimmune oophoritis)

DIAGNOSTIC TESTS & INTERPRETATION
Lab
Initial lab tests
- Primary amenorrhea:
  - Serum prolactin (PRL) and thyroid stimulating hormone (TSH)
  - If no secondary sexual characteristics, measure serum follicle stimulating hormone (FSH) and luteinizing hormone (LH):
    ○ FSH/LH <5 IU per L suggests primary hypothalamic or pituitary etiology
    ○ FSH >20 and LH >40 IU per L suggests gonadal failure and karyotype analysis should be performed
  - If secondary sexual characteristics present, evaluate for anatomic abnormalities. If uterus absent or abnormal, perform karyotype analysis.
- Secondary amenorrhea:
  - Exclude pregnancy with HCG
  - Serum TSH: Elevated in hypothyroidism, decreased in hyperthyroidism
  - Serum chemistry, complete blood count (CBC), urinalysis to rule out underlying disease
  - Serum prolactin (PRL):
    ○ >100 ng per mL suggests empty sella syndrome or pituitary adenoma. Perform MRI for evaluation.
    ○ < 100 ng per mL, evaluate for other etiologies of which medications are most common
- If PRL and TSH are normal, perform progestin challenge (see Treatment):
  - If withdrawal bleed: Normogonadotropic amenorrhea related to hyperandrogenic chronic anovulation most commonly PCOS
  - If no withdrawal bleed: Follow up with estradiol priming (see Diagnostic Procedures/Other and Treatment) and repeat progestin challenge:
    ○ If no bleed: Consider outflow tract obstruction.
    ○ If bleed occurs: Check FSH/LH: Elevated in hypergonadotropic hypogonadism, decreased in pituitary tumors or hypogonadotropic hypogonadism
- If virilizing signs and significant acne present, measure free testosterone, DHEA-S, and 17-OH progesterone levels.

Follow-Up & Special Considerations
- Women <30 with ovarian failure (see below) should have karyotype analysis and be investigated for premutations of FMR1 gene (fragile X syndrome) and for adrenal antibodies.
- If absence of uterus or foreshortened vagina, karyotype analysis should also be performed.

Imaging
* Imaging is not generally indicated as a 1st-line approach for amenorrhea.
* Ultrasound may show ovarian cysts (PCOS), presence or absence of uterus, and endometrial thickness.
* Magnetic resonance imaging (MRI) of the pelvis can clarify any uterine or vaginal anomalies suggested by ultrasound, or if pediatric patient is unable to tolerate transvaginal ultrasound probe.
* MRI of the sella turcica if prolactinoma suspected (elevated serum prolactin >100), and consider with functional hypothalamic amenorrhea (other adenomas)

Follow-Up & Special Considerations
* Laparoscopy: Diagnosis of the streak ovaries of Turner syndrome or PCOS (not often done)
* Hysterosalpingogram: To rule out Asherman syndrome and other etiologies of outflow obstruction

Diagnostic Procedures/Surgery
If suspect constitutional delay: Obtain bone age. If hypothalamic amenorrhea from functional suppression: Consider dual-energy x-ray absorptiometry (DEXA) scan to assess for bone loss.

DIFFERENTIAL DIAGNOSIS
Includes all causes listed in Etiology

TREATMENT
MEDICATION
* Progesterone challenge and replacement: Medroxyprogesterone (Provera) 10 mg/d for 10 days will result in withdrawal bleed if hypothalamic–pituitary–gonadal axis intact
* Estrogen replacement: Cycling with a combination oral contraceptive (containing 35 or 50 mcg of estrogen) or conjugated estrogen (Premarin) 0.625 mg for 25 days with progesterone added as above for the last 10 days will result in a withdrawal bleed if the uterus and lower genital tract are normal.
* Use of hormonal therapies will not correct underlying problem. Other drugs might be required to treat specific conditions (e.g., bromocriptine for hyperprolactinemia).
* Use of hormonal replacement therapy is NOT recommended for long-term management of amenorrhea in older women (1)[A]:
  – It may be safe for symptom management in young women (1)[C].
  – Give to maintain secondary sex characteristics, prevent osteoporosis in adolescents and young women
* Combination estrogen/progesterone contraceptives (oral contraceptive pills [OCPs], patch, ring) replace estrogen and prevent pregnancy:
  – They also have a positive effect on bone mineral density in oligo-/amenorrheic women (2)[B].
  – Can decrease hirsutism in PCOS
* Calcium supplementation 1,500 mg/d if cause is hypoestrogenism
* Because PCOS is related to insulin resistance, metformin (Glucophage) has been used (often starting at 500 mg b.i.d.) in an effort to correct metabolic abnormalities, improve ovulation (3)[A], and restore normal menstrual patterns (3)[B].

* Contraindications to estrogen administration:
  – Pregnancy, thromboembolic disease, previous myocardial infarct or cerebrovascular accident, estrogen-dependent malignancy, severe hepatic impairment or disease
* Precautions:
  – Patients who are amenorrheic and wish to become pregnant should not be given hormone replacement therapy, but should receive treatment for infertility based on the specific cause.

ADDITIONAL TREATMENT
General Measures
* Definitive treatment depends on determining the cause of the amenorrhea.
* May not be necessary to treat all cases, especially if just temporary amenorrhea

Issues for Referral
Many causes of amenorrhea require referral to specialists in ob/gyn, endocrine, surgery, and/or psychiatry.

SURGERY/OTHER PROCEDURES
* Hymenectomy, done as a day surgery, required for those whose primary amenorrhea is due to imperforate hymen
* Lysis of adhesions in Asherman syndrome has been shown to be effective in restoring menstrual regularity and fertility.
* In patients with karyotype XY, gonads must be removed due to increased risk of gonadal tumors.
* Patients with müllerian agenesis and other congenital anatomical abnormalities of the vagina can undergo surgery to create a functioning vagina.

ONGOING CARE
FOLLOW-UP RECOMMENDATIONS
If overtraining is suspected, activity level should be reduced by 25–50%.

Patient Monitoring
* Depends on the cause and treatment chosen
* If hormonal replacement is used, discontinuation after 6 months is advised to assess spontaneous resumption of menses.

DIET
* Correct overweight or underweight by dietary management and behavior modification.
* If PCOS is the etiology, weight loss diet will help restore ovulation.

PATIENT EDUCATION
* Patient education consists of fully informing the patient of your findings, including the presence or absence of pregnancy, and of the underlying cause.
* Specific educational resources can be utilized as necessary (e.g., prenatal classes and menopause support groups).
* Specific information should be given about the expected duration of amenorrhea (temporary or permanent), effect on fertility, and the long-term sequelae of untreated amenorrhea (e.g., osteoporosis, vaginal dryness).
* Appropriate contraceptive advice should be given, as fertility returns before menses.
* Additional support may be needed if the amenorrhea is associated with a reduction in, or loss of, fertility.
* Society for Menstrual Cycle Research, 10559 N. 104th Place, Scottsdale, AZ 85258, (602) 451-9731.

PROGNOSIS
* Reflects the underlying cause
* In secondary amenorrhea from functional suppression of hypothalamic–pituitary–ovarian axis (stress, disordered eating, exercise), 1 study demonstrated 83% reversal rate in presence of obvious contributing factor

COMPLICATIONS
* Estrogen-deficiency symptoms (e.g., hot flashes, vaginal dryness)
* Osteoporosis in prolonged hypoestrogenic amenorrhea
* Increased risk of endometrial cancer in patients whose amenorrhea is secondary to anovulation with estrogen excess (obesity, PCOS)

REFERENCES
1. Farquhar CM, Marjoribanks J, Lethaby A et al. Long term hormone therapy for perimenopausal and postmenopausal women. *Cochrane Database Syst Rev.* 2005:CD004143.
2. Liu SL, Lebrun CM. Effect of oral contraceptives and hormone replacement therapy on bone mineral density in premenopausal and perimenopausal women: a systematic review. *Br J Sports Med.* 2006;40:11–24.
3. Andy C, Flake D, French L. Clinical inquiries. Do insulin-sensitizing drugs increase ovulation rates for women with PCOS? *J Fam Pract.* 2005;54:156, 159–60.

See Also (Topic, Algorithm, Electronic Media Element)
Diabetes Mellitus, Type 1; Diabetes Mellitus, Type 2; Hyperthyroidism; Hypothyroidism, Adult; Osteoporosis
Algorithms: Amenorrhea, Primary; Amenorrhea, Secondary; Delayed Puberty

CODES
ICD9
626.0 Absence of menstruation

CLINICAL PEARLS
* There are both physiological and pathological causes of amenorrhea.
* Pregnancy is the most common cause of secondary amenorrhea.
* Among certain women with amenorrhea, a progestin challenge is a useful diagnostic tool.
* Use of hormonal replacement therapy is NOT recommended for long-term management of amenorrhea in older women.

AMNESTIC DISORDER

Jessica Lenore Wilson, MD
Noah S. Walman, MD

BASICS

- Memory is an arbitrary term that encompasses:
  - Knowledge of facts (*semantic* memory)
  - Knowledge of previous self-experiences (*episodic* memory)
  - Exercise of a learned skill (*procedural* memory)
  - Temporary knowledge for immediate use (*working* memory)
- Coded for by various regions of the brain, with significant involvement of the:
  - Medial temporal lobe, including:
    o Amygdaloid nucleus
    o Hippocampus
    o Parahippocampal region
  - Thalamus, especially the dorsomedial nuclei
  - Hypothalamus
  - Basal forebrain
- Amnestic disorder is a blanket statement to describe a deficit in any of these various memory types.

DESCRIPTION

- A single disease process can manifest with abnormalities in more than one memory system.
- For example, Alzheimer disease sufferers have a notable deficit in semantic memory, but can also have working memory deficits.
- Amnestic disorder, amnestic syndrome, or simply amnesia comes from the Greek for forgetfulness.
- Indicates a loss of, or gap in, one's memory, usually due to brain injury, shock, fatigue, repression, or illness
- Can be categorized based on amnesia for:
  - Events prior to the causative event, as in *retrograde*
  - Events after the causative event, as in *anterograde*
  - Information related to all senses and past experiences, as in *global* amnesia
- Unless otherwise stated, this topic will deal in particular with transient global amnesia (TGA).

EPIDEMIOLOGY

- Incidence and prevalence of amnesia is in direct proportion to the epidemiology of the primary cause.
- In transient global amnesia, incidence is greater among individuals over the age of 50.

Incidence

- In 1 study (1) in Rochester, Minnesota, TGA was found to be 5.2 cases per 100,000.
- The study further estimated 23.5 cases per 100,000 per year among 50+-year-olds.
- TGA recurrence rate is low, 4–5% in this study.

RISK FACTORS

- Evidence for and against established risk factors (1)
- Not a symptom of arteriosclerosis
- No higher risk of heart or cerebrovascular disease

Genetics

Recent evidence supports the possibility of a genetic predisposition (2).

PATHOPHYSIOLOGY

- Transient global amnesia is well studied, but not fully understood.
- Thought to have various mechanisms
- Findings from positron emission tomography, diffusion-weighted imaging magnetic resonance imaging (MRI), single photon emission computed tomography, and MR spectroscopy have demonstrated involvement of known memory-related structures in patients with TGA.
- Some theorize spreading depression of cortical electrical activity; that is, a wave of cellular depolarization and subsequent cellular edema.
- Others suggest that TGA is the result of:
  - Migraines
  - Venous congestion of the brain
  - Jugular valvular insufficiency

ETIOLOGY

- In general, metabolic or structural changes that cause an imbalance in the memory-related regions of the brain can cause an amnestic disorder
- Common causes include:
  - Thiamine deficiency
  - Hypothalamic tumors
  - Vertebrobasilar ischemia
- Less common are:
  - Neurodegenerative dementias such as Alzheimer disease
  - Bilateral damage to the medial temporal lobes
  - Head trauma
  - Chronic alcoholism
  - Nutritional disorders
  - In the case of dissociative amnesia, extreme psychological trauma causes the deficit.

- Transient global amnesia has been associated with:
  - Physical exertion
  - Emotional stress
  - Pain
  - Exposure to cold water
  - Sex
  - Valsalva maneuver

COMMONLY ASSOCIATED CONDITIONS

- Some relationship has been found between migraines and transient global amnesia.
- TGA patients were found to have a higher frequency of psychiatric disease relative to transient ischemic attack controls in 1 study.

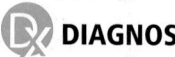

DIAGNOSIS

HISTORY

- In TGA, patients have confusion and global amnesia, usually for 6–12 hours.
- Retrograde, and to a lesser extent anterograde, memory deficits
- Complete resolution
- Social history and family history are important.
- TGA in women is associated with an emotional precipitating event, a history of anxiety, and a pathological personality.
- TGA in men occurs more after a physical precipitating event.
- There is a history of headaches among younger patients.
- No association with vascular risk factors

PHYSICAL EXAM

- If there are no focal abnormalities on exam, then transient global ischemia can be diagnosed.
- Loss of memory for recent events
- Difficulty with retaining new information
- If neurological exam demonstrates more than memory dysfunction, other differential diagnoses should be further explored.

DIAGNOSTIC TESTS & INTERPRETATION
- TGA is largely a clinical diagnosis.
- Physical exam largely unremarkable

Lab
Initial lab tests
- Complete blood count with differential
- Basic metabolic profile
- Prothrombin time/partial thromboplastin time to rule out hypercoagulable state

Imaging
Initial approach
MRI and/or computed tomography to rule out stroke

Diagnostic Procedures/Surgery
- Electroencephalogram if seizure is suspected
- Electrocardiogram if cardiac etiology is suspected

DIFFERENTIAL DIAGNOSIS
- Basilar artery thrombosis
- Cardioembolic stroke
- Complex partial seizures
- Epilepsy of frontal or temporal lobe
- Lacunar syndromes
- Migraine variants
- Posterior cerebral artery stroke
- Syncope

TREATMENT

- Supportive care for TGA
- Reassurance that recurrence of TGA is low (3)
- If there is an underlying disease process present (i.e., Alzheimer disease, herpes encephalitis), it should be treated.

ONGOING CARE

Schedule at least 1 follow-up visit to a neurologist in a patient diagnosed with transient global amnesia.

DIET
No restrictions on diet

PROGNOSIS
TGA is a benign condition, with low risk of recurrence (3).

REFERENCES
1. Miller JW, Petersen RC, Metter EJ et al. Transient global amnesia: clinical characteristics and prognosis. *Neurology*. 1987;37:733–7.
2. Segers-van Rijn J, de Brujin SF et al. Transient global amnesia: a genetic disorder? *Eur. Neurol.* 2010;63:186-7
3. Hinge HH, Jensen TS, Kjaer M et al. The prognosis of transient global amnesia. Results of a multicenter study. *Arch Neurol*. 1986;43:673–6.

ADDITIONAL READING
- Agosti C et al. Recurrency in transient global amnesia: a retrospective study. *Eur J Neurol*. 2006;13(9):986–9.
- Budson A et al. Memory Dysfunction. *N Engl J Med*. 2005;352:7.
- Greer DM, Schaefer PW, Schwamm LH. Unilateral temporal lobe stroke causing ischemic transient global amnesia: role for diffusion-weighted imaging in the initial evaluation. *J Neuroimaging*. 2001;11:317–9.
- Jenkins KG, Kapur N, Kopelman MD. Retrograde amnesia and malingering. *Curr Opin Neurol*. 2009.
- Piñol-Ripoll G, de la Puerta González-Miró I, Martínez L et al. [A study of the risk factors in transient global amnesia and its differentiation from a transient ischemic attack.] *Rev Neurol*. 2005;41:513–6.
- Quinette P, Guillery-Girard B, Dayan J et al. What does transient global amnesia really mean? Review of the literature and thorough study of 142 cases. *Brain*. 2006.
- Sellal F. Transient amnesia in the elderly. *Psychol Neuropsychiatr Vieil*. 2006;4(1):31–8.
- Shekhar R. Transient global amnesia—a review. *Int J Clin Pract*. 2008.
- Zorzon M et al. Transient global amnesia and transient ischemic attack. Natural history, vascular risk factors, and associated conditions. *Stroke*. 1995;26(9):1536–42.

See Also (Topic, Algorithm, Electronic Media Element)
Algorithm: Amnesia

 # CODES

ICD9
- 291.1 Alcohol-induced persisting amnestic disorder
- 292.83 Drug-induced persisting amnestic disorder
- 294.8 Other persistent mental disorders due to conditions classified elsewhere

CLINICAL PEARLS
- Any patient with possible TGA should be ruled out for stroke, especially if stroke risk factors are present.
- In a patient diagnosed with TGA, reassurance and a follow-up appointment with a neurologist are appropriate management.
- Other than memory problems, the neurological exam of a TGA patient is most often normal.

AMYLOIDOSIS

Tara J. Rizvi, MD

BASICS

DESCRIPTION
- A group of diseases characterized by extracellular deposition of insoluble protein fibrils in organs and tissues
- Classification is based on the nature of precursor plasma proteins that form fibril deposits (1):
  - Primary (AL): Plasma cell dyscrasia; deposition of protein derived from immunoglobulin light chain fragments
  - Secondary or reactive (AA): Complicates chronic infections or inflammatory diseases; deposition of serum amyloid A(SAA) protein
  - Heritable or familial (AF): Many different types of variant plasma proteins form amyloid deposits beginning in midlife; most common form is caused by mutations of transthyretin (ATTR)
  - Dialysis-related: Deposition of fibrils derived from β_2-microglobulin; predilection for osteoarticular structures
  - Senile systemic amyloidosis: Deposition of otherwise normal (wild-type) transthyretin in myocardium and other sites seen in elderly
  - Organ-specific amyloidosis: Deposition isolated to 1 organ, resulting in specific syndromes; most common is Alzheimer disease caused by cerebral amyloid plaques:
    - Localized amyloidosis: Results from local amyloid deposits in tracheobronchial tree, urinary tract, or skin, which are also derived from monoclonal light chains, but not due to underlying systemic plasma cell disorder

EPIDEMIOLOGY
Incidence
- AL: 1,275–3,200 new cases annually in US (2):
  - Easily missed, so incidence may be higher
- AA: Rare; occurs in <5% of patients with chronic inflammatory diseases, most commonly with rheumatoid arthritis (RA)

Prevalence
- AF: Rare, <1 per 100,000 population
- AL: Most common type in North America, 4.5 per 100,000 population (2)
  - Predominant age: 60–70
  - Predominant sex: Male > Female (2:1)
- AA is more prevalent in:
  - Japan, Finland, developing countries due to less adequate treatment of inflammatory and infectious diseases
  - Turkey, Middle East in association with familial Mediterranean fever (FMF)

RISK FACTORS
Depends on type of systemic amyloidosis:
- Age (senile systemic/Alzheimer)
- Heredity (AF/AA)
- Underlying plasma cell dyscrasia (AL)
- Untreated chronic inflammatory diseases (AA)
- Untreated chronic infections (AA)
- Long-term hemodialysis

Genetics
- Only familial amyloidosis can be inherited; usually autosomal-dominant inheritance.
- Three types of genetic abnormalities have been identified in amyloidogenic proteins: Polymorphisms, variant molecules, and genetically determined post-translational modifications.

GENERAL PREVENTION
Early detection and treatment of underlying disorders, such as plasma cell dyscrasias, chronic inflammatory conditions, chronic infections

PATHOPHYSIOLOGY
- Fibrillogenesis results from disorder of protein folding; cofactors may significantly modulate this.
- Soluble precursor proteins undergo transformation to a β-pleated fibrillar configuration.
- Amyloid fibrils thus formed are insoluble polymers composed of LMW subunits of a variety of proteins, many of which circulate as plasma constituents:
  - In AL, monoclonal Ig light chain deposits are predominantly composed of λ chains.
  - In AA, IL-1, IL-6, and TNF associated with chronic inflammation induce serum amyloid A protein (SAA), an acute-phase reactant.
- Fibril deposition in extracellular matrix results in damage to the structure and function of the tissues involved.

ETIOLOGY
Cause of amyloid production and its deposition in tissues is unknown.

COMMONLY ASSOCIATED CONDITIONS
- Primary amyloidosis (AL):
  - Multiple myeloma
  - Non-Hodgkin lymphoma
  - Rarely Waldenström macroglobulinemia
- Secondary amyloidosis (AA) (1):
  - Chronic inflammatory arthritides:
    - Most commonly seen in adult and juvenile RA
    - Spondyloarthropathies: Ankylosing spondylitis, psoriatic arthritis
    - Rarely in SLE, Sjögren, and vasculitides
  - Periodic fever syndromes:
    - FMF
    - TRAPS syndrome
    - Muckle–Wells syndrome
  - Chronic infections:
    - Bronchiectasis, tuberculosis, osteomyelitis
    - Pressure sores, UTIs, other infections seen in complications of paraplegia
  - Crohn disease
  - Due to IVDA
  - Neoplasms, particularly renal cell CA
  - Castleman disease

DIAGNOSIS

HISTORY
- Careful family history to assess for familial amyloidosis: ATTR can present as syndromes of:
  - Familial amyloidotic polyneuropathy
  - Familial amyloidotic cardiomyopathy
- Suspect secondary AA amyloidosis with a history of long-standing inflammatory disease, uncontrolled for >5 years
- Symptoms are determined by the organ or system involved, and can often be obscured by the underlying disease:
  - Renal and cardiac involvement are most common.
  - Primary (AL) can affect all organs except CNS.
  - Heritable (ATTR) can present similar to AL, but with more peripheral and autonomic neuropathic symptoms and less renal involvement.
  - Secondary AA: Mostly kidney, liver involved
- Symptom manifestations are nonspecific:
  - Initial: Fatigue, malaise, weight loss
  - Other: Nephrotic syndrome, CHF, dyspnea, abdominal pain, diarrhea, early satiety (due to autonomic neuropathy), malabsorption, carpal tunnel syndrome, arthralgias, arthritis, myalgias, symptoms due to hypothyroidism

PHYSICAL EXAM
- Renal involvement is most common and can present as asymptomatic proteinuria or nephrotic syndrome, particularly in AL-type amyloidosis. Microscopic hematuria is more prominent in AA type.
- Cardiac involvement is common and may present as restrictive cardiomyopathy resulting in diastolic dysfunction, conduction abnormalities.
- Autonomic neuropathy: Postural hypotension
- Peripheral neuropathy: Carpal tunnel syndrome
- Hepatic amyloid deposition can lead to hepatomegaly but rarely jaundice
- GI amyloid may cause esophageal motility abnormalities, gastric atony, small and large intestinal motility abnormalities, malabsorption, bleeding, or pseudo-obstruction
- Thyromegaly due to infiltration of thyroid
- Amyloid arthropathy may mimic RA: Symmetrical polyarthritis, periarticular soft tissue swelling.
- Due to infiltration of soft tissue by amyloid:
  - Macroglossia: Pathognomonic for primary AL; occurs in 20%; and is characterized by a large, stiff tongue, frequently rimmed by teeth indentation
  - Shoulder pad sign
  - Nail dystrophy, alopecia
  - Hoarse, weak voice (vocal cord infiltration)
- Vascular infiltration can lead to raccoon eyes or spontaneous purpura with minimal trauma such as sneezing.
- Rarely, bleeding diathesis may occur with factor X deficiency.

DIAGNOSTIC TESTS & INTERPRETATION
Lab
Initial lab tests
- CBC, electrolytes, creatinine, calcium, U/A, TSH
- Assess for proteinuria, Bence-Jones proteins, renal insufficiency, anemia, hypothyroidism

Follow-Up & Special Considerations
- Primary AL: Serum and urine protein electrophoresis with immunofixation for monoclonal protein spike
- Secondary AA: Tests to assess underlying inflammatory disease:
  - ESR, CRP, RF, anti-CCP, ANA
  - Gene testing for FMF, TRAPS
- Familial (ATTR): Abnormal transthyretin protein may be isolated

Imaging
Initial approach
- Echocardiogram: Thickening of interventricular septum and ventricular walls, restrictive pattern
- Consider renal U/S, bone scan as appropriate

Follow-Up & Special Considerations
Radiolabeled serum amyloid P component (SAP) scintigraphy: Quantitatively monitors accumulation of amyloid deposits. This is available only at specialized centers in Europe.

Diagnostic Procedures/Surgery
- Confirmation of diagnosis requires presence of amyloid deposits on biopsy.
- Less invasive and 1st-line: Abdominal fat pad aspirate, rectal, bone marrow, or skin biopsy
- If negative, biopsy of affected organs have higher sensitivity: Kidney, liver, sural nerve.

Pathological Findings
- Light microscopy: Demonstration of amyloid deposits as amorphous, nodular hyaline material
- Fibrils bind to Congo red, leading to apple green birefringence under polarized light, and thioflavin T, producing intense yellow-green fluorescence.
- Electron microscopy: Fibrils are rigid, linear, nonbranching; measure 7.5–10 nm in width (3)[B].
- Bone marrow biopsy in AL may show clonal excess of plasma cells (λ or κ).

DIFFERENTIAL DIAGNOSIS
- Distinguish different forms of amyloidosis from each other after biopsy by immunofluorescence, or immunohistochemical staining for SAA protein, TTR, κ/λ light chains.
- Particularly distinguish AL from genetic, senile, and localized amyloidosis, since management and prognosis vary considerably.

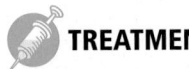

TREATMENT
MEDICATION
First Line
- Primary AL (4,5)[A]:
  - High-dose melphalan followed by hemopoietic cell transplant (HCT): Improves quality of life and even results in remission in some cases
  - Melphalan and high-dose dexamethasone for patients who cannot tolerate HCT
  - Precautions with melphalan: Bone marrow suppression, cytopenias, infections
- Secondary AA:
  - Control of underlying inflammatory disease: Consider anticytokine therapy for autoimmune diseases (6)[A]
  - Colchicine for familial Mediterranean fever (3)[A]

Second Line
Primary AL (5)[B]:
- Lenalidomide with dexamethasone (7)[B]:
  - Precautions: Neutropenia, thrombocytopenia, rash, fatigue
- Bortezomib with dexamethasone

ADDITIONAL TREATMENT
General Measures
- Secondary AA: Treat underlying cause
- Familial (ATTR): Liver transplant
- Hemodialysis-related amyloidosis: Change to peritoneal dialysis

Issues for Referral
- Refer to specialized amyloidosis centers if diagnosis is unclear and/or for treatment failures.
- Consider referral to rheumatology, hematology, cardiology, and other specialties based on underlying disease association.

Additional Therapies
Investigational:
- Eprodisate for secondary AA (8)[B]:
  - Interferes with AA amyloid protein interaction with glycosaminoglycans, disrupting fibril formation
  - Shown to decrease the rate of deterioration in renal function (5)[A]
- Diflunisal for familial amyloidosis (5)[C]

SURGERY/OTHER PROCEDURES
For localized amyloidosis of lip, skin, nasopharynx, or urinary tract, removal or excision at site of occurrence may be sufficient.

IN-PATIENT CONSIDERATIONS
Admission Criteria
- Acute nephrotic syndrome/renal failure
- Cardiomyopathy/acute CHF
- Hepatic failure, pseudo-obstruction

 ONGOING CARE

FOLLOW-UP RECOMMENDATIONS
Patient Monitoring
- Routine monitoring of renal function
- Monitor adverse effects of medications.
- AA: Maintenance of low serum amyloid A protein levels correlates to better outcome (1)[B].
- AL: Prognostic indicators to follow are: NT-pro-BNP, cardiac troponin T and I, serum-free light chains.

DIET
- Low-protein, low-salt diet for patients with renal disease
- Low-salt, cardiac diet for CHF patients

PATIENT EDUCATION
- The Amyloidosis Support Network: http://www.amyloidosis.org
- Amyloid Research Group of Indiana University: http://www.iupui.edu/~amyloid/

PROGNOSIS
- In general, older patients do less well.
- Primary AL: Median survival is 1–2 years after diagnosis (2):
  - Cardiac involvement: 6 months
  - Renal involvement: 21 months
- Secondary AA: Based on underlying disease:
  - Mean survival = 133 months (1)
- ATTR: 5–15 years, based on precursor protein
- Senile (cardiac) amyloidosis: Survival is better than AL amyloid.

REFERENCES
1. Lachmann HJ, Goodman HJ, Gilbertson JA et al. Natural history and outcome in systemic AA amyloidosis. *N Engl J Med*. 2007;356:2361–71.
2. Falk RH, Comenzo RL, Skinner M. The systemic amyloidoses. *N Engl J Med*. 1997;337:898–909.
3. Rajkumar SV, Gertz MA. Advances in the treatment of amyloidosis. *N Engl J Med*. 2007;356:2413–5.
4. Jaccard A, Moreau P, Leblond V et al. High-dose melphalan versus melphalan plus dexamethasone for AL amyloidosis. *N Engl J Med*. 2007;357:1083–93.
5. Dember LM. Modern Treatment of Amyloidosis: Unresolved Questions. *J Am Soc Nephrol*. 2008.
6. Keersmaekers T, Claes K, Kuypers DR et al. Long-term efficacy of infliximab treatment for AA-amyloidosis secondary to chronic inflammatory arthritis. *Ann Rheum Dis*. 2009;68:759–61.
7. Sanchorawala V, Wright DG, Rosenzweig M et al. Lenalidomide and dexamethasone in the treatment of AL amyloidosis: results of a phase II trial. *Blood*. 2006.
8. Dember LM, Hawkins PN, Hazenberg BP et al. Eprodisate for the treatment of renal disease in AA amyloidosis. *N Engl J Med*. 2007;356:2349–60.

See Also (Topic, Algorithm, Electronic Media Element)
Multiple Myeloma

CODES

ICD9
277.30 Amyloidosis, unspecified

CLINICAL PEARLS
- Consider amyloidosis in patients with multiple myeloma, RA, JRA, familial Mediterranean fever, and other long-standing chronic inflammatory conditions.
- Biopsy for definitive diagnosis: Congo red stain demonstrates apple green birefringence under polarized light.
- Differentiate specific type based on immunohistochemical staining.
- Remember that treatment varies vastly depending on type of amyloidosis.

AMYOTROPHIC LATERAL SCLEROSIS

Mhd Basheer Rahmoun, MD
Dalia Sbat, PharmD

BASICS

Amyotrophic Lateral Sclerosis (ALS) is a degenerative disease that affects the upper and lower motor neurons (UMN and LMN).

DESCRIPTION
- Sporadic ALS is the most common form of the disease. It includes a number of overlapping syndromes, such as pseudobulbar palsy, progressive bulbar palsy, progressive muscular atrophy, and primary lateral sclerosis.
- Familial ALS is an autosomal-dominant or -recessive disease, which is clinically similar to sporadic ALS but probably represents a distinct entity pathologically and biochemically.
- Guam ALS and Parkinson-dementia complex is an ALS-like syndrome often, but not always, associated with Parkinson syndrome and dementia, which is prevalent among the Chamorro Indians of Guam and rare in the US.
- System(s) affected: Nervous
- Synonym(s): Motor neuron disease, MND, Lou Gehrig's disease, ALS

Pediatric Considerations
- Infantile and juvenile spinal muscular atrophies are conditions distinct from ALS, both clinically and pathologically.
- Symptoms of ALS may inappropriately be attributed to age.

Pregnancy Considerations
- Uncommon among affected individuals
- Pregnancy would be unwise in any individual suffering from a disease with poor prognosis.
- If pregnancy did occur, the only foreseeable difficulties would be related to weakness.

EPIDEMIOLOGY
Incidence
In Europe and North America, between 1.47 and 2.7 per 100,000/year

Prevalence
- Estimated prevalence rates range between 2.7 and 7.4 per 100,000.
- Predominant age: Uncommon before age 40
- Predominant sex: Male > Female in sporadic ALS:
  - After 65: Male = Female

RISK FACTORS
- Family history
- Age >40
- Smoking (in women) (1)[A]

Genetics
- Familial ALS (10% of cases) can be autosomal-dominant or -recessive; X-linked cases have been reported.
- Gene locus has been localized to the long arm of chromosome 21 and encodes the superoxide dismutase (SOD1) enzyme in 20% of familial ALS cases
- Mutation in the gene encoding fused in sarcoma (FUS) was identified in familial ALS type 6 (2).
- Mutations in the angiogenin gene (ANG) have been recently discovered to be associated with sporadic ALS (3,4).

- Mutations in TARDP region encoding TAR DNA-binding protein TDP-43 have also been identified in familial and sporadic ALS (5).

GENERAL PREVENTION
Genetic counselling is advised if there is a family history of ALS.

PATHOPHYSIOLOGY
Degeneration of the upper and lower motor neurons with their respective axons and with gliosis replacing lost neurons

ETIOLOGY
- Sporadic: Cause is unknown, but elevated levels of glutamate have been found in serum and cerebrospinal fluid (CSF).
- Familial ALS: A genetically transmitted degenerative disease
- Guam ALS and Parkinson-dementia complex: Possible relationship to ingestion of the cycad nut or to some other environmental toxin

DIAGNOSIS

Diagnosis can be established according to Revised El Escorial World Federation of Neurology criteria
- The presence of:
  - Evidence of LMN degeneration by clinical, electrophysiological, or neuropathologic examination
  - Evidence of UMN degeneration by clinical examination
  - Progressive spread of symptoms or signs within a region or to other regions, as determined by history or examination
- The absence of:
  - Electrophysiological and pathological evidence of other disease processes that might explain the signs of LMN and/or UMN degeneration
  - Neuroimaging evidence of other disease processes that might explain the observed clinical and electrophysiological signs

HISTORY
ALS is suggested when symptoms are consistent with UMN and LMN dysfunction that worsen over time. Symptoms include:
- Loss of muscle strength and coordination
- Difficulty opening and closing the jaw, drooling
- Voice change, hoarseness
- Muscle cramps, difficulty breathing, difficulty swallowing, paralysis

PHYSICAL EXAM
Variable combinations of:
- Unexplained weight loss
- Limb weakness with variable symmetry and distribution
- Gait disorder (steppage-waddling)
- Slurring of speech
- Inability to control affect (inappropriate laughing, crying, yawning)
- Focal atrophy of muscle groups (initially in a myotomal distribution)
- Fasciculations (other than calves)
- Hyper-reflexia (including jaw jerk—Hoffman's sign)
- Babinski sign, present in 50% of patients
- Spasticity

- Sialorrhea
- Spares cognitive, oculomotor, sensory, and autonomic functions

DIAGNOSTIC TESTS & INTERPRETATION
Lab
No simple reliable laboratory test is available that confirms the diagnosis.
Initial lab tests
- Elevated levels of glutamate in CSF and serum
- Anti-monosialoganglioside autoantibodies in low titer commonly found (of unclear significance)
- Possibly reduced levels of nerve growth factor

Imaging
Initial approach
MRI: To exclude other possible diagnoses in the evaluation of suspected ALS:
- MRI is usually normal in ALS, although increased signal in the corticospinal tracts on T2-weighted and FLAIR images and hypointensity of the motor cortex on T2-weighted images has been reported (6).

Diagnostic Procedures/Surgery
- Electromyography: Denervation potentials (fibrillations-positive sharp waves) and often doublets are associated with prominent fasciculations, which suggest anterior horn cell dysfunction. Voluntary motor unit potentials have increased amplitude, long duration, and/or polyphasic pattern. The recruitment pattern is reduced for the force generated, and individual motor units have a high rate of discharge (7).
- Nerve conduction studies: Sensory and motor NCS are most often normal in ALS, although compound motor action potential (CMAP) amplitudes may be reduced in severely atrophic and denervated muscles (7).
- Motor unit number estimation is a nerve conduction–based method that assesses the number of viable motor axons innervating small hand or foot muscles. In ALS, it drops prior to the onset of clinical weakness (8).
- Muscle biopsy: Not a routine part of the diagnostic evaluation of ALS, but may be performed if myopathy is suspected on clinical, electrodiagnostic, or serologic grounds:
  - Muscle biopsy will show groups of shrunken angulated muscle fibers (grouped atrophy) amid other groups of fibers with a uniform fiber type (fiber type grouping).

Pathological Findings
- Loss of Betz cells in the motor cortex
- Atrophic or absent anterior horn cells of spinal cord
- Atrophic or absent neurons within the motor nuclei of the medulla and pons
- Degeneration of the lateral columns of the spinal cord
- Atrophy of the ventral roots
- Grouped atrophy of muscle (motor units)

DIFFERENTIAL DIAGNOSIS
- Multifocal motor neuropathy
- Cervical radiculomyelopathy
- Cervical spondylosis
- Lead intoxication
- Spinal muscular atrophy (adult form)
- Primary lateral sclerosis
- Familial spastic paraparesis

- Benign fasciculations
- Lyme disease
- Spinal multiple sclerosis
- Tropical spastic paraparesis
- Myasthenia gravis

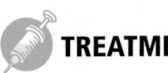 **TREATMENT**

MEDICATION
Riluzole 50 mg PO b.i.d.: The only FDA-approved drug for ALS. It produces a slight prolongation in life expectancy by decreasing the release of glutamate (9,10), and it slows the disease progression.

ALERT
Riluzole withhold should be considered for patients developing fatigue.

ADDITIONAL TREATMENT
These drugs may be used to relieve severe spasticity:
- Baclofen 5 mg PO t.i.d. initially, followed by gradual increase of 5 mg per day every 4–7 days; not to exceed 80 mg per day divided q.i.d.
- Tizanidine 4–8 mg PO every 8 hours p.r.n.; not to exceed 36 mg per day

General Measures
- Outpatient may ultimately need nursing home placement or hospice.
- Supportive care is necessary for complicating emergencies (aspiration, respiratory failure). Use of a respirator is a major ethical dilemma. Consideration should be given to those with selective respiratory dysfunction.
- Discussion of advance directives, focusing on patient's specific values about which interventions to be used, is critical to meeting the patient's needs.
- Prosthetic devices

Issues for Referral
- Multidisciplinary clinic referral to optimize health care delivery, prolong survival, and enhance quality of life
- Early exam by a neurologist can confirm diagnosis of ALS.
- Tracheostomy or G-tube placement may be performed by surgeon or gastroenterologist.
- Pulmonologist and respiratory therapist for ventilator assistance and management of intercurrent infections and tracheostomy

COMPLEMENTARY AND ALTERNATIVE MEDICINE
- Research offering therapy with stem cells is evolving, providing a new approach in cellular replacement and support for patients (11,12)[A].
- Therapeutic trials of the efficacy of antioxidants (vitamin E and vitamin C and β-carotene), nerve growth factor, gabapentin, Myotrophin, and thyrotropin-releasing hormone, and creatine have been undertaken. Reports are not encouraging (13)[A].

SURGERY/OTHER PROCEDURES
- Treatment for refractory sialorrhea
  – Botulinum toxin B
  – Low-dose radiation therapy to the salivary glands
- Percutaneous endoscopic gastrostomy (PEG) tube should be considered with early signs of malnutrition to stabilize weight and prolong survival.
- Noninvasive ventilation (NIV) can lengthen survival and improve quality of life.

- Elective tracheostomy should be considered in patients with early signs of respiratory difficulty.

 ONGOING CARE

FOLLOW-UP RECOMMENDATIONS
Patients should be involved in regular exercise and a physical therapy program.

Patient Monitoring
- Initially every 3 months; frequency to be increased as needed for symptomatic therapy
- Patients with a presumed diagnosis of ALS should have neuroimaging and electrodiagnostic studies.

DIET
- Evaluate swallowing to quantify any dysphagia.
- Modify the patient's diet to prevent aspiration.
- Consider a gastrostomy tube when patient cannot swallow fluids or soft foods (14).

PATIENT EDUCATION
Printed material for patients (and reference lists for physicians) available from:
- The Muscular Dystrophy Association: (520) 529-2000; (800) 572-1717; http://www.mdausa.org
- The ALS Association: (800) 782-4747; http://www.alsa.org
- Families of Spinal Muscular Atrophy: http://www.fsma.org

PROGNOSIS
- ALS usually results in death within 5 years.
- Patients who predominantly manifest progressive muscular atrophy have a better prognosis.
- There have been reports of spontaneous arrest of the disease.

COMPLICATIONS
- Aspiration pneumonia
- Pulmonary embolism
- Nutritional deficiency
- Complications from wheelchair-bound or bedridden states, including decubitus ulcers and skin infections

REFERENCES

1. Alonso A, Logroscino G, Hernán MA et al. Smoking and the risk of amyotrophic lateral sclerosis: a systematic review and meta-analysis. *Journal of Neurology, Neurosurgery, and Psychiatry*. 2010;
2. Vance C, Rogelj B, Hortobágyi T et al. Mutations in FUS, an RNA processing protein, cause familial amyotrophic lateral sclerosis type 6. *Science*. 2009;323:1208–11.
3. Conforti FL et al. A novel Angiogenin gene mutation in a sporadic patient with amyotrophic lateral sclerosis from southern Italy. *Neuromuscul Disord*. 2008;18:68.
4. Paubel A, Violette J, Amy M et al. Mutations of the ANG gene in French patients with sporadic amyotrophic lateral sclerosis. *Arch Neurol*. 2008; 65:1333–6.
5. Sreedharan J, Blair IP, Tripathi VB et al. TDP-43 mutations in familial and sporadic amyotrophic lateral sclerosis. *Science*. 2008;319:1668–72.
6. Oba H, Araki T, Ohtomo K et al. Amyotrophic lateral sclerosis: T2 shortening in motor cortex at MR imaging. *Radiology*. 1993;189:843–6.
7. Daube JR. Electrodiagnostic studies in amyotrophic lateral sclerosis and other motor neuron disorders. *Muscle Nerve*. 2000;23: 1488–502.
8. Olney RK, et al. Motor unit number estimation (MUNE): How may it contribute to the diagnosis of ALS? *Neurol Neurosurg Psychiatry*. 2000; 1(Suppl 2):S41–4.
9. Bensimon G, Lacomblez L, Meininger V. A controlled trial of riluzole in amyotrophic lateral sclerosis. ALS/Riluzole Study Group. *N Engl J Med*. 1994;330:585–91.
10. Riluzole for amyotrophic lateral sclerosis. *Med Lett*. 1995;37:113.
11. Lunn JS, Hefferan MP, Marsala M et al. Stem cells: comprehensive treatments for amyotrophic lateral sclerosis in conjunction with growth factor delivery. *Growth Factors*. 2009;1.
12. Kim SU, de Vellis J. Stem cell-based cell therapy in neurological diseases: A review. *J Neurosci Res*. 2009.
13. Pastula DM, Moore DH, Bedlack RS et al. Creatine for amyotrophic lateral sclerosis/motor neuron disease. *Cochrane Database Syst Rev*. 2010;6: CD005225.
14. Andersen PM, Borasio GD, Dengler R et al. Good practice in the management of amyotrophic lateral sclerosis: clinical guidelines. An evidence-based review with good practice points. EALSC Working Group. *Amyotroph Lateral Scler*. 2007; 8:195–213.

ADDITIONAL READING

- Miller RG, Jackson CE, Kasarskis EJ, et al. Practice parameter update: The care of the patient with amyotrophic lateral sclerosis: drug, nutritional, and respiratory therapies (an evidence-based review): report of the Quality Standards Subcommittee of the American Academy of Neurology *Neurology*. 2009;73(15):1218–26.
- Practice parameter update: The care of the patient with amyotrophic lateral sclerosis: multidisciplinary care, symptom management, and cognitive/behavioral impairment (an evidence-based review): report of the Quality Standards Subcommittee of the American Academy of Neurology. *Neurology*. 2009;73(15):1227–33.

 CODES

ICD9
335.20 Amyotrophic lateral sclerosis

CLINICAL PEARLS

- ALS is an upper and lower motor neuron disease.
- Diagnosis is made by history, physical exam, EMG, and NCS.
- Riluzole is the only available treatment that might increase survival.

ANAEROBIC AND NECROTIZING INFECTIONS

Ruben Peralta, MD
Packrisamy Kannan, MD

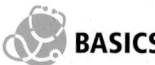 **BASICS**

DESCRIPTION
- Necrotizing infections of the skin and fascia are called necrotizing cellulitis and necrotizing fasciitis (NF), respectively.
- Necrotizing fasciitis is a rapidly spreading and potentially fatal soft tissue infection located in the fascia, with secondary necrosis of the subcutaneous tissue. Organisms spread from the subcutaneous tissue along the deep fascial planes, presumably facilitated by bacterial enzymes and toxins.
- Type I necrotizing fasciitis is a mixed infection caused by the synergistic effect of both aerobic and anaerobic bacteria; type II necrotizing fasciitis is a monomicrobial infection caused by group A β-hemolytic streptococci (Streptococcus pyogenes).
- Gas gangrene is a subset of necrotizing infection usually caused by the Clostridium sp. with gas formation within the tissue (type III), and type IV is commonly due to fungal infections.
- Necrotizing skin and soft tissue infections are associated with extensive tissue destruction, systemic toxicity, and loss of limb, and are potentially fatal.
- Synonym(s): Fournier gangrene; Cullen ulcer; Meleney ulcer; Flesh-eating infections

EPIDEMIOLOGY
- Predominant age: Any age
- Predominant sex: Male = Female

Incidence
Incidence of necrotizing fasciitis: 500–1,500 cases annually in the US (1)[B]

RISK FACTORS
Can occur in young, previously healthy persons without predisposing or precipitating risk factors. However, some cases are associated with the following:
- Predisposing risk factors:
  – Advanced age
  – Obesity
  – Malnutrition
  – Diabetes mellitus
  – Immune suppression (e.g., HIV, malignancies, alcoholism, steroid exposure)
  – Peripheral vascular disease
  – Inadequate tissue perfusion
- Precipitating risk factors:
  – Intravenous drug abuse
  – Trauma
  – Burns
  – Skin ulceration
  – Herpes zoster
- Prior surgical procedures
- Risk factors with patient undergoing surgical procedures includes:
  – Prior operations
  – Duration of operation
  – Hypoalbuminemia
  – History of chronic obstructive pulmonary disease

GENERAL PREVENTION
- Avoid tight orthopedic casts.
- Routine surgical principles for surgical procedures and skin closure (2)

ETIOLOGY
Most commonly due to polymicrobial infection, including both aerobic and anaerobic bacteria. Bacteria extend from subcutaneous tissue and proliferate along fascial planes. Bacterial toxins and surface proteins facilitate this process and can cause systemic toxicity with serious consequences (such as septic shock).

 DIAGNOSIS

HISTORY
- Symptoms of malaise, anorexia, and fever progress rapidly over hours; rare cases with slower evolution over days.
- Some cases arise from previous trauma or infection (surgical wound from open or laparoscopic procedure, ulcers, burns, IV drug injection site, abscess).
- In >20%, a precipitant is never identified.
- Given the significant risk of delayed diagnosis, keep high index of suspicion if suggestive history but no clear risk factors (1)[B].

PHYSICAL EXAM
- The diagnosis of necrotizing fasciitis is made clinically. A high index of suspicion is necessary to make the diagnosis (1)[B].
- Not uncommonly, patients report pain out of proportion to physical exam.
- Fever, often low-grade early in the disease
- Tachycardia
- Hypotension
- Diaphoresis
- Foul odor
- Rapidly spreading skin lesions
- Skin changes, including localized erythema or discoloration, bullae, vesicles, ulceration, necrosis, edema
- Crepitus
- Bacterial toxins may trigger an inflammatory response leading to multiorgan failure or sepsis; in some advanced cases, this may be the presenting concern and necrotizing infection may not be immediately apparent.

DIAGNOSTIC TESTS & INTERPRETATION
Lab
- Hyponatremia, leukocytosis, anemia, hypocalcemia, acidosis, prolonged prothrombin time, elevated creatine kinase and serum glucose level
- Elevated liver function tests may result from release of bacterial toxins.
- Renal dysfunction may occur secondary to hypotension and myoglobinuria.
- Cultures and sensitivities are not diagnostic, but may be used to narrow initial broad-spectrum antibiotic treatment.

- Commonly associated pathogens:
  – Gram-positive anaerobes:
    ○ Cocci: Group A streptococci, Peptostreptococcus (anaerobic Streptococcus), or Staphylococcus aureus
    ○ Bacilli: Clostridium perfringens and other clostridia
  – Gram-negative aerobes: Bacilli: Escherichia coli, Klebsiella pneumoniae, Enterobacter, Proteus
- Gram-negative anaerobes: Bacilli: Bacteroides fragilis (usually with other gram-negative bacilli)
- Recently reported in salt water contaminated with Vibrio species (3)
- In the Far East, the Laboratory Risk Indicator for Necrotizing Fasciitis scoring system has been useful and incorporated in the clinical practice of some centers (4).

ALERT
Antibiotics given before cultures are performed may alter lab results.

Imaging
- Plain radiographs may show subcutaneous air (a rare finding that is specific but not sensitive).
- Computed tomography may reveal soft tissue swelling and presence of gas in tissues.

Pathological Findings
- Only frozen-section biopsy of the fascia is diagnostic. However, treatment should not be delayed while awaiting biopsy.
- Soft tissue necrosis, with polymorphonuclear cells and vascular thrombosis

DIFFERENTIAL DIAGNOSIS
Other soft tissue infection, including abscess and postsurgical wound infection

 TREATMENT

MEDICATION
- Precautions: Without surgical debridement, antibiotics will not be effective (see General Measures).
- Important: Do not delay antibiotic treatment, even if smear, cultures, and tests are negative.
- Start with a broad-spectrum antibiotic regimen, then tailor antibiotics to organisms identified by blood and wound cultures and organism sensitivities (5)[B].
- Initial broad-spectrum coverage should include penicillin to cover Streptococcus and clindamycin, which works synergistically with penicillin when large bacterial load is present and also binds group A streptococci toxin.
- Aminoglycosides will cover enteric gram-negative organisms.
- Metronidazole is an alternative to clindamycin for treatment of anaerobic organisms.
- Retrospective studies suggest there may be a survival benefit with the use of IV immunoglobulin (IVIG) therapy. IVIG works by binding toxins and superantigens, which suppresses proinflammatory mediators (6)[B].

- Unlike *C. perfringens* and group A β-hemolytic streptococci, the *Aeromonas* sp. are uniformly resistant to penicillin-G, but are reported to be highly sensitive to 3rd-generation cephalosporins.

ADDITIONAL TREATMENT
General Measures
- Prompt and wide surgical debridement is the cornerstone of treatment.
- Infectious disease consultation, if available
- Hyperbaric oxygen (HBO) is used as an adjunct to antimicrobial agents and aggressive surgical debridement. No survival benefit has been found.
- The results of studies on the use of HBO therapy in NF are inconsistent (7).
- Do not delay surgical intervention for HBO.
- IV fluids with electrolyte repletion, if indicated
- Prophylaxis for tetanus

SURGERY/OTHER PROCEDURES
- Necrotizing soft tissue infections are a surgical emergency. Patients should be taken to the operating room as soon as the diagnosis is made or when there is high clinical suspicion.
- All necrotic tissue should be resected. Dissection should be carried out along all involved fascial planes. Adequate debridement should take priority over preservation of tissue.
- Limb amputation may be necessary because of extensive fascial and subcutaneous soft tissue necrosis and overwhelming systemic toxicity.
- Adequate surgical treatment can rarely be accomplished with a single operation. Repeated daily debridement may be necessary. Debridement should continue until all necrotic tissue is removed (8)[C].
- Negative-pressure suction dressing (i.e., vacuum assisted closure dressing) may be utilized to improve wound care and assist with postoperative fluid management.
- Reconstruction can be undertaken once systemic sepsis has been controlled and all nonviable tissue has been removed.

IN-PATIENT CONSIDERATIONS
Nursing
- Following surgical debridement, patients often require intensive care unit (ICU) level of care.
- Close contacts of patients and health care workers do not require chemoprophylaxis with antibiotics (9)[B].

ONGOING CARE

FOLLOW-UP RECOMMENDATIONS
Patient Monitoring
- May require ICU-level critical care
- Diligence required to recognize spreading gangrene that would require repeated debridement
- As clinically indicated; may include following cultures, electrolytes, drug levels

DIET
Depends on clinical scenario; ranges from n.p.o. to diet as tolerated

PROGNOSIS
- Mortality for necrotizing fasciitis ranges from 16–45%, and 1 publication has shown a decreased trend from nearly 28% in 1994 to 14% in 2002 (10).
- Increased mortality associated with age >60 years, male, IV drug abuse, malnutrition, significant medical comorbidities (e.g., cardiac or pulmonary disease), carcinoma, presence of bacteremia. Recent study suggests that Fournier's gangrene in females has an increased risk for mortality due in part to more aggressive inflammatory manifestations in the retroperitoneum and abdominal cavity (11).
- Independent predictors of mortality include:
  – Admission white blood cell count >30,000
  – Creatinine level >2 mg/dL within 48 hours of admission
  – Presence of clostridial infection
  – Presence of heart disease
- Independent predictors of limb loss include:
  – Shock (systolic pressure <90 mm) on admission
  – Clostridial infection
  – Presence of heart disease

COMPLICATIONS
- Tissue and functional losses
- Amputation
- Septic shock
- Death
- Physiologic derangement, as estimated by the Acute Physiology and Chronic Health Evaluation II score, is predictive of death (12)[B].

REFERENCES

1. Anaya DA, Dellinger EP. Necrotizing soft-tissue infection: diagnosis and management. *Clin Infect Dis*. 2007;44:705–10.
2. Kirby JP, Mazuski JE. Prevention of surgical site infection. *Surg Clin North Am*. 2009;89:365–89.
3. Tsai YH, Huang TJ, Hsu RW et al. Necrotizing soft-tissue infections and primary sepsis caused by Vibrio vulnificus and Vibrio cholerae non-O1. *J Trauma*. 2009;66:899–905.
4. Su YC, Chen HW, Hong YC, Chen CT, Hsiao CT, Chen IC et al. Laboratory risk indicator for necrotizing fasciitis score and the outcomes. *ANZ J Surg*. 2008;78:968-72
5. Dellinger RP, Carlet JM, Masur H et al. Surviving Sepsis Campaign guidelines for management of severe sepsis and septic shock. *Crit Care Med*. 2004;32:858–73.
6. Norrby-Telund A, et al. Group A streptococcal toxic syndrome and necrotizing fasciitis. *Curr Treat Opt Infect Dis*. 2003;5:419–29.
7. Jallali N, Withey S, Butler PE. Hyperbaric oxygen as adjuvant therapy in the management of necrotizing fasciitis. *Am J Surg*. 2005;189:462–6.
8. Marshall JC, Maier RV, Jimenez M et al. Source control in the management of severe sepsis and septic shock: an evidence-based review. *Crit Care Med*. 2004;32:S513–26.
9. Smith A. Invasive group A streptococcal disease: Should close contacts routinely receive antibiotic prophylaxis? *Lancet Inf Dis*. 2005;5:494–500.
10. Anaya DA, McMahon K, Nathens AB et al. Predictors of mortality and limb loss in necrotizing soft tissue infections. *Arch Surg*. 2005;140:151–7; discussion 158.
11. Czymek R, Frank P, Limmer S, Schmidt A, Jungbluth T, Roblick U, Bürk C, Bruch HP, Kujath P et al. Fournier's gangrene: is the female gender a risk factor? *Langenbecks Arch Surg*. 2010;395:173–80.
12. Gunter OL, Guillamondegui OD, May AK et al. Outcome of necrotizing skin and soft tissue infections. *Surg Infect (Larchmt)*. 2008;9:443–50.
13. Malangoni MA. Timing is everything. *Ann Surg*. 2009;250:17–8.
14. Steinberg JP, Braun BI, Hellinger WC et al. Timing of antimicrobial prophylaxis and the risk of surgical site infections: results from the Trial to Reduce Antimicrobial Prophylaxis Errors. *Ann Surg*. 2009;250:10–6.

ADDITIONAL READING
- de Lissovoy G, Fraeman K, Hutchins V et al. Surgical site infection: incidence and impact on hospital utilization and treatment costs. *Am J Infect Control*. 2009;37:387–97.
- Morgan MS et al. Diagnosis and management of necrotising fasciitis: a multiparametric approach. *The Journal of hospital infection*. 2010.

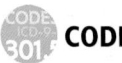 CODES

ICD9
- 041.84 Other specified bacterial infections in conditions classified elsewhere and of unspecified site, other anaerobes
- 728.86 Necrotizing fasciitis
- 785.4 Gangrene

CLINICAL PEARLS
- A necrotizing infection is a potentially life-threatening condition consisting of a soft tissue infection with rapidly progressive, widespread fascial necrosis.
- The symptom most commonly associated with necrotizing soft tissue infection is pain out of proportion to the physical exam.
- Necrotizing fasciitis may be an infection of 1 species of bacteria or may be polymicrobial.
- Prompt diagnosis and treatment are essential (13).
- Surgical debridement and antibiotic therapy are the primary treatment options.
- Be aware of antibiotic-resistant organisms (13,14).

ANAL FISSURE

Michael Rousse, MD, MPH

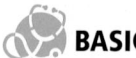 **BASICS**

DESCRIPTION
Anal fissure is a benign anorectal disease characterized by a knifelike tearing sensation on defecation. An anal fissure is a tear in the lining of the anal canal distal to the dentate line, most commonly in the posterior midline.

EPIDEMIOLOGY
Very common anorectal condition often confused with hemorrhoids

Incidence
Exact incidence is unknown. Patients often treat with home remedies and do not seek medical care.

ALERT
- Common in infants 6–24 months; not common in children; suspect abuse or trauma. Elderly are spared owing to lower resting pressure in the anal canal.
- Predominant sex: Male = Female, but women are more likely to get anterior midline tears (25% vs 8%).

Prevalence
- 80% of infants, usually self-limited
- 20% of adults, the majority of whom do not seek medical advice, have symptoms referable to the anorectum.

RISK FACTORS
Constipation, passage of hard or large-caliber stool, high resting tone of internal anal sphincter (prolonged sitting), trauma (anal sex), inflammatory bowel disease (Crohn's disease), syphilis, tuberculosis

Genetics
None known

GENERAL PREVENTION
Avoid constipation and prolonged sitting on toilet.

PATHOPHYSIOLOGY
High resting pressure within the anal canal can lead to ischemia of the anodermal tissues resulting in splitting of the tissues with passage of stool. Exposed internal sphincter muscle spasms causing the knifelike pain.

ETIOLOGY
Splitting of susceptible anodermal tissue

COMMONLY ASSOCIATED CONDITIONS
Constipation, Crohn's disease, tuberculosis, leukemia, and HIV

 DIAGNOSIS

HISTORY
Severe rectal pain, often with and following defecation, but can be continuous; some will see bright red blood on the stool or when wiping. Occasionally, itch or perianal irritation is the presenting sign.

PHYSICAL EXAM
Gentle spreading of the buttocks will reveal a tear in the anodermal tissue, typically posterior midline, occasionally anterior midline, rarely eccentric to midline. Minimal swelling or bleeding. Hypertrophic papillae (*sentinel tag*) is seen in chronic fissure.

DIAGNOSTIC TESTS & INTERPRETATION
Diagnostic Procedures/Surgery
- Avoid anoscopy or endoscopy initially unless necessary for other diagnoses.
- Some patients may require exam under anesthesia to diagnose properly.

DIFFERENTIAL DIAGNOSIS
- Thrombosed external hemorrhoid: Swollen, painful mass; no fissure
- Perirectal abscess: Sinus tract with purulent drainage rather than a fissure
- Pruritus ani: Shallow excoriations rather than a fissure

 TREATMENT

The goal of treatment is to avoid repeated tearing of the anal mucosa with resultant spasm of the internal anal sphincter.

MEDICATION
First Line
- Stool softeners (docusate)
- Fiber supplements (psyllium)
- Topical analgesics (2% lidocaine gel)
- Warm sitz baths

Second Line
- Topical nitroglycerin ointment 2% diluted to 0.2% applied q.i.d., marginally but significantly better than placebo in healing (48.6% vs 37%), late recurrence was common (50%) (1)[A]; effect is to reduce resting anal pressure through the release of nitric oxide (2)[B]
- Calcium channel blockers (e.g., nifedipine, diltiazem), oral or topical; no better than nitrates but with fewer side effects (1)[A]; effect is to relax the internal sphincter muscle, thereby reducing the resting anal pressure (3)[B]
- Botulinum toxin 4 mL injected into the internal sphincter muscle; no better than topical nitrates but with fewer side effects (1)[A]; effect is to inhibit the release of acetylcholine from nerve endings to inhibit muscle spasm (3)[B]

ADDITIONAL TREATMENT

General Measures

Wash area with warm water; high-fiber diet; avoid constipation

Issues for Referral

• Late recurrence is common (50%).
• Medical therapy usually is tried for 90–120 days before referral (4)[B].

SURGERY/OTHER PROCEDURES

• Reserved for failure of medical therapy; involves division of the internal sphincter muscle
• Lateral internal sphincterectomy appears to be the surgical procedure of choice (5)[B].
• Risk for fecal incontinence: 45% short term, 6–8% long term (3)[C]
• Anal stretching/dilation: Unlikely to benefit (2)[C]

 ONGOING CARE

DIET

High fiber

PATIENT EDUCATION

Avoid prolonged sitting during bowel movements; drink plenty of fluids; avoid constipation

PROGNOSIS

Medical therapy is less likely to be successful for chronic anal fissures; 40% failure rate (6)[A],(7)[B].

COMPLICATIONS

Fecal incontinence and incontinence to flatus; primarily associated with surgery (8)[B]

REFERENCES

1. Nelson RL. Non surgical therapy for anal fissure. *Cochrane Database of Systematic Reviews* 2006, Issue 4. Art. No.: CD003431. DOI:10.1002/14651858.CD003431.pub2.
2. Madoff RD, Fleshman JW. AGA Technical Review on the Diagnosis and Care of Patients with Anal Fissure. *Gastroenterology* 2003;124:235–245.
3. Breen E, Bleday R. *Anal Fissures*, Up To Date 18.1, updated Jan 29, 2010.
4. Essani R, Sarkisyan G, Beart RW, Ault G, Vukasin P, Kaiser AM et al. Cost-saving effect of treatment algorithm for chronic anal fissure: a prospective analysis. *J Gastrointest Surg.* 2005;9:-
5. Mousavi SR, Sharifi M, Mehdikhah Z et al. A comparison between the results of fissurectomy and lateral internal sphincterotomy in the surgical management of chronic anal fissure. *J Gastrointest Surg.* 2009;13:1279–82.
6. Shao WJ, Li GC, Zhang ZK et al. Systematic review and meta-analysis of randomized controlled trials comparing botulinum toxin injection with lateral internal sphincterotomy for chronic anal fissure. *Int J Colorectal Dis.* 2009;24:995–1000.
7. Mente BB, Irkörücü O, Akin M, Leventolu S, Tatliciolu E et al. Comparison of botulinum toxin injection and lateral internal sphincterotomy for the treatment of chronic anal fissure. *Dis Colon Rectum.* 2003;46:232–7.
8. Sileri P, Stolfi VM, Franceschilli L, Grande M, Di Giorgio A, D'Ugo S, Attina' G, D'Eletto M, Gaspari AL et al. Conservative and surgical treatment of chronic anal fissure: prospective longer term results. *J Gastrointest Surg.* 2010;14:773–80.

 CODES

ICD9

565.0 Anal fissure

CLINICAL PEARLS

• Best chance to prevent recurrence is to avoid prolonged sitting on toilet and avoid constipation.
• No medical therapy approaches the cure rate of surgery.

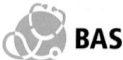

ANAPHYLAXIS

Bobby X. Peters, MD

BASICS

DESCRIPTION
- An IgE-mediated, acute systemic reaction following antigen exposure in a sensitized person
- A non–IgE-mediated idiopathic anaphylactoid reaction also may occur. Anaphylactoid reactions are clinically indistinguishable from anaphylaxis and are treated in the same manner.
- System(s) affected: Cardiovascular; Endocrine/Metabolic; Gastrointestinal; Hematologic/Lymphatic/Immunologic; Pulmonary; and Skin/Exocrine
- Synonym(s): Anaphylactoid reactions

EPIDEMIOLOGY
- Predominant age: All ages
- Predominant sex: Male = Female

Incidence
- Up to 40,000 cases of idiopathic anaphylaxis with no identifiable cause occur each year.
- Drug-induced anaphylaxis occurs in 1/2,700 hospitalized patients.
- Anaphylaxis deaths: 0.3–0.7/100,000 per year
- Food allergic reactions constitute 1/3 to 1/2 of all anaphylactic reactions worldwide.
- Anaphylaxis may occur secondary to allergy skin testing.
- Asthmatics are more prone to anaphylaxis than nonasthmatics. Female asthmatics are at greater risk of anaphylaxis than their male counterparts.

RISK FACTORS
- Previous anaphylaxis
- History of atopy or asthma

Genetics
Genetic predisposition for sensitization to antigens

GENERAL PREVENTION
- Avoid inducing drugs and foods.
- Carry a prefilled epinephrine syringe. Keep a syringe at home, work/school, and in vehicle, although syringe should be protected from temperature extremes.
- Avoid areas where insect exposure is likely. Avoid wearing insect attractants (e.g., perfumes, colored clothing); avoid bare feet outdoors.
- Carry or wear a medical alert ID about the anaphylaxis-causing substance or event.
- When radiologic contrast is unavoidable, use of low osmolar contrast agents (e.g., iothalamate) reduces the risk of contrast reactions to 3.1%:
  – Only 0.22% were considered severe.
  – Stop beta blockers before administering contrast materials.
  – Pretreat with diphenhydramine (50 mg IV) and a steroid (e.g., methylprednisolone 60 mg IV q6h) until procedure. Start methylprednisolone the day before the procedure is scheduled.
  – Those with frequent (>6 per year) episodes of idiopathic anaphylaxis should be treated prophylactically with prednisone (40–60 mg/d in a single morning dose), hydroxyzine (25 mg tid), and albuterol (2 mg PO tid). The prednisone should be rapidly tapered to an every-other-day regimen.

ALERT
- Have a latex-free kit (gloves, etc.) available for the treatment of latex-allergic patients. Some latex-allergic patients will react to tropical fruits, such as kiwi, bananas, avocados, and chestnuts.
- Avoid beta-blockers.

ETIOLOGY
- IgE-mediated mast cell degranulation
- Complement activation (C3a, C4a, C5a) by antigen–antibody complexes that contain complement-fixing antibodies
- Other non–IgE-dependent anaphylaxis-like syndromes may be caused by modulators of arachidonic acid metabolism, sulfiting agents, exercise-induced anaphylaxis, and idiopathic recurrent anaphylaxis.
- Some important causes of anaphylaxis are:
  – Antimicrobials (e.g., penicillin)
  – Blood products (especially in IgA deficiency)
  – Iodinated contrast media
  – Ethylene oxide gas (dialysis tubing, other sterilized products)
  – Exercise
  – Foods (commonly, peanuts, nuts, fish, crustaceans, mollusks, cow's milk, eggs, and soy)
  – Immunotherapy
  – Insect stings (e.g., honeybees, wasps, kissing bugs, and deer flies)
  – Latex rubber (gloves, catheters)
  – Macromolecules (e.g., chymopapain, insulin, dextran, glucocorticoid, and protamine)
  – Vaccines

COMMONLY ASSOCIATED CONDITIONS
- Asthma
- Atopy

DIAGNOSIS

HISTORY
Rapid progression within minutes to hours of the signs and symptoms of anaphylaxis, with or without an obvious trigger, including but not limited to: Cutaneous symptoms (90% of cases), respiratory symptoms (70%), gastrointestinal symptoms (40%), and cardiovascular symptoms (35%)

PHYSICAL EXAM
- Pruritus, flushing, urticaria, angioedema
- Dyspnea, cough, rhonchi
- Rhinorrhea, bronchorrhea, wheezing, stridor
- Difficulty swallowing
- Nausea, vomiting, diarrhea, cramps, bloating
- Tachycardia, hypotension, shock, syncope
- Malaise, shivering
- Mydriasis

DIAGNOSTIC TESTS & INTERPRETATION
Lab
- Hypoxemia, hypercarbia, acidosis
- Acidosis may cause apparent hyperkalemia by moving potassium extracellularly
- Elevated serum tryptase, a mast cell enzyme for allergic and anaphylactic reactions (1)[B]
- Drugs that may alter lab results: Epinephrine and albuterol may cause apparent hypokalemia by shifting K+ intracellularly.

DIFFERENTIAL DIAGNOSIS
- Anaphylactoid reactions:
  – May occur after the 1st contact with substance such as polymyxin, pentamidine, radiographic contrast media, and aspirin
- Carcinoid syndrome
- Globus hystericus:
  – May mimic pharyngeal edema
- Hereditary angioedema:
  – C1q esterase deficiency with painless, pruritus-free angioedema without urticaria, flushing, or wheezing
- Pheochromocytoma:
  – Paradoxically, because of beta-2 stimulation, some patients have hypotensive attacks accompanied by tachycardia.
  – Urticaria, angioedema, and wheezing are absent.
- Pseudoanaphylactic reaction:
  – After injection of procaine penicillin
    ○ Is a drug effect of procaine and not a penicillin allergy
- Scombroid poisoning:
  – From ingestion of dark meat fish (e.g., tuna, mackerel, and mahi-mahi)
  – Histamine-like mediator: Symptoms include flushing, sweating, nausea, vomiting, diarrhea, headache, palpitations, dizziness, rash, swelling of face and tongue, respiratory distress, and vasodilatory shock.
- Serum sickness:
  – Occurs several days after exposure
- Systemic mastocytosis:
  – Benign or malignant overgrowth of mast cells
  – Urticaria pigmentosa seen in the benign form and the presence of reddish-brown macular–papular cutaneous lesions, which urticate after trauma (Darier sign)
- Vasovagal reactions:
  – Bradycardia and hypotension without tachycardia, flushing, urticaria, angioedema, pruritus, and wheezing
- Pulmonary embolism, foreign body aspiration, and arrhythmia

TREATMENT

MEDICATION

First Line

- Epinephrine:
  - Less severe reaction: 0.3–0.5 mg (0.01 mg/kg in children) = (0.3–0.5 mL of a 1:1,000 solution, 0.01 mL/kg in children), SQ q20–30min as needed, up to 3 doses
  - Life-threatening reactions: 0.5 mg (5 mL of a 1:10,000 solution) (for children: 0.05–0.1 mL/kg per dose) given intravenously, slowly: q5–10min as needed. If IV access is not possible, endotracheal or intraosseous may be effective.
- Diphenhydramine: (SOR Grade A) an H_1 blocker: 25–50 mg intravenously (IM or PO:) q6h for 72 hours (children 1.25 mg/kg to 25 mg)
- Cimetidine: an H_2 blocker: 300 mg IV over 3–5 minutes (children 5–10 mg/kg per dose) and then 400 mg PO bid is helpful and may be more effective than diphenhydramine.
- Corticosteroids: No immediate effect and unclear if they prevent recurrence:
  - Hydrocortisone sodium succinate: 250–500 mg IV q4–6h (4–8 mg/kg for children)
  - Prednisone: 1 mg/kg in children, up to 60 mg
  - Methylprednisolone: 60–125 mg IV in adults (1–2 mg/kg in children)
- Bronchodilator, if persistent bronchospasm:
  - Inhaled beta-2 agonists. Continuous nebulized albuterol of 10 mg/hour or 2.5 mg q15–20min is safe, effective, and preferable to aminophylline as a first line.
- Laryngeal edema:
  - Epinephrine: 5 mL 1:1,000 by nebulizer is more effective than racemic epinephrine and is usually available.
- Persistent hypotension:
  - Dopamine: 200 mg in 500 mL of dextrose in water given by infusion pump; titrate to BP (3–20 mcg/kg/min)
  - Glucagon: May be beneficial for resistant hypotension caused by concurrent beta blockade therapy; 50 mcg/kg IV bolus over 1 min, or alternatively, give as continuous infusion at 5–15 mcg/min
- Normal saline or Ringer's lactate: As necessary to maintain tissue perfusion
- Oral antihistamines and steroids for 72 hours

Geriatric Considerations

Epinephrine may induce myocardial ischemia in those with cardiac disease, but is the drug of choice. Be alert for anticholinergic and CNS side effects after giving diphenhydramine or cimetidine.

Pediatric Considerations

Epinephrine could reduce the placental blood flow, but may save the life of the mother and fetus. It also increases risk of congenital malformation.

Second Line

- Several reports of tranexamic acid: 1,000 mg IV or sigma-aminocaproic acid for refractory anaphylaxis
- These drugs are not standard care; use only in patients who do not respond to other therapy.
- Aminophylline: 5–6 mg/kg IV in 100 cc D_5W over 20 min, then maintenance at 1 mg/kg/h drip

- Anti-IgE monoclonal antibody may have a role in long-term management of food-induced anaphylaxis.
- Venom immunotherapy has been effective in the prevention of sting anaphylaxis, but with a high side-effect risk (2)[A].

ADDITIONAL TREATMENT

General Measures

- Treatment depends on severity
- Maintain a patent airway:
  - Endotracheal intubation and assisted ventilation may be necessary.
  - Possibly tracheostomy or needle cricothyrotomy in children <12 years
- Oxygen
- IV fluids (normal saline/lactated Ringer's)

Issues for Referral

- Allergist referral if anaphylaxis cause unclear
- Patients with anaphylaxis from insect stings benefit from desensitization immunotherapy.

IN-PATIENT CONSIDERATIONS

Admission Criteria

Moderate–severe anaphylaxis, admit for observation.

Discharge Criteria

Outpatient: Patients with cutaneous angioedema, urticaria, and minimal bronchospasm may be released when symptoms and signs have cleared.

ONGOING CARE

FOLLOW-UP RECOMMENDATIONS

Bedrest until anaphylaxis clears and patient is hemodynamically stable

DIET

NPO until acute symptoms are controlled

PATIENT EDUCATION

- Asthma and Allergy Foundation of America, 1717 Massachusetts Avenue, Suite 305, Washington, DC 20036; (800)-7-ASTHMA or American Allergy Association, P.O. Box 7273, Menlo Park, CA 94026, (415) 322-1663
- Medic-Alert–type tags (Medic-Alert Foundation, Turlock, CA 95381-1009)
- Avoid beta-blockers, if possible.
- Instruct patient in the use of the bee sting kit.

PROGNOSIS

- Good prognosis if treated immediately; worse outcome with a delay of >30 minutes in administration of epinephrine.
- Of those with idiopathic anaphylaxis, 60% are free of anaphylactic episodes at 2.5 years; most others are steroid-free.

COMPLICATIONS

- Hypoxemia
- Cardiac arrest
- Death

REFERENCES

1. Brown SG, Blackman KE, Heddle RJ. Can serum mast cell tryptase help diagnose anaphylaxis? *EMA*. 2004;2:120–4.
2. Brown SG, Wiese MD, Blackman KE, Heddle RJ. Ant venom immunotherapy: A double-blind, placebo-controlled, crossover trial. *Lancet*. 2003;(361)9362:1001–6.

ADDITIONAL READING

- Arias K, Waserman S, Jordana M. Management of food-induced anaphylaxis: unsolved challenges. *Curr Clin Pharmacol* 2009;4(2):113–25.
- González-Pérez A, Aponte Z, Vidaurre CF, Rodríguez LA et al. Anaphylaxis epidemiology in patients with and without asthma: A United Kingdom database review. *The Journal of allergy and clinical immunology*. 2010;
- Pitsios C, Dimitriou A, Stefanaki EC, Kontou-Fili K et al. Anaphylaxis during skin testing with food allergens in children. *Eur J Pediatr*. 2010;169: 613–5.
- Sheikh A, Shehata YA, Brown SGA, Simons FER. Adrenaline (epinephrine) for the treatment of anaphylaxis with and without shock. *Cochrane Database of Systematic Reviews* 2008, Issue 4. Art. No.: CD006312. DOI:10.1002/14651858. CD006312.pub2.
- Sheikh A, ten Broek VM, Brown SGA, Simons FER. H1-antihistamines for the treatment of anaphylaxis with and without shock. *Cochrane Database of Systematic Reviews* 2007, Issue 1. Art. No.: CD006160. DOI:10.1002/14651858. CD006160.pub2.
- Tanus T, Mines D, Atkins PC et al. Serum tryptase in idiopathic anaphylaxis: a case report and review of the literature. *Ann Emerg Med*. 1994;24:104–7.
- Wittbrodt ET, Spinler A. Prevention of anaphylactoid reactions in high-risk patients receiving radiographic contrast media. *Ann Pharmacother*. 1994;28: 236–41.

See Also (Topic, Algorithm, Electronic Media Element)

Food Allergy; Insect Bites; Stings

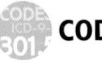 CODES

ICD9

- 989.5 Toxic effect of venom
- 995.0 Other anaphylactic shock, not elsewhere classified
- 995.60 Anaphylactic shock due to unspecified food

CLINICAL PEARLS

- Allergy to one species of legume (e.g., peanuts) or one type of seafood (e.g., shrimp) doesn't mean allergy to all products in that category. Skin testing is prudent.
- MMR vaccine can be safely administered to those with a history of egg allergy; most egg allergies are related to the albumin.
- Penicillin-allergic patients can generally tolerate 2nd- and 3rd-generation cephalosporins as well as monobactams (e.g., aztreonam). Generally, they will be allergic to carbapenems (e.g., imipenem) and 1st-generation cephalosporins.
- IgA-deficient patients should have washed red blood cells for transfusion.
- Those allergic to seafood are not allergic to iodine-based radiocontrast. Shellfish allergy is protein related.

ANEMIA, APLASTIC

Kerri Keslow, MD
Daniel T. Lee, MD

 BASICS

DESCRIPTION
- Aplastic anemia is defined as pancytopenia in the setting of a hypocellular bone marrow without the presence of infiltrates or fibrosis. There are two forms: Acquired (much more common) and congenital.
- Acquired aplastic anemia has an insidious onset and is caused by an exogenous insult triggering an autoimmune reaction. This form is usually responsive to immunosuppressive agents.
- The congenital forms are rare and occur mostly in childhood. The exception is an atypical presentation of Fanconi syndrome later in adult life, into the 30s for males and up to age 48 years in females.
- The identification of specific mutations in genes of the telomere complex in patients with acquired aplastic anemia has blurred the distinction between the congenital and acquired forms.
- System(s) affected: Heme/Lymphatic/Immunologic
- Synonym(s): Hypoplastic anemia; panmyelophthisis; refractory anemia; aleukia hemorrhagica; toxic paralytic anemia

ALERT
- Early intervention for aplastic anemia greatly improves the chances of treatment success.
- Hematopoietic growth factors should not be used without close supervision in newly diagnosed patients.

Geriatric Considerations
The elderly are often exposed to large numbers of drugs and, therefore, may be more susceptible to acquired aplastic anemia.

Pediatric Considerations
- Congenital forms of aplastic anemia require different treatment regimens than the acquired forms.
- Acquired aplastic anemia is seen in children exposed to ionizing radiation or treated with cytotoxic chemotherapeutic agents.

Pregnancy Considerations
- Pregnancy appears to be a real but rare cause of aplastic anemia. Symptoms may resolve after delivery and have been shown to disappear with pregnancy termination.
- Complications in pregnant patients appear to be more likely with low platelet counts and paroxysmal nocturnal hemoglobinuria-associated aplastic anemia.

EPIDEMIOLOGY
- Predominant age: Biphasic 15–25 (more common) and over 60
- Predominant sex: Male = Female

Incidence
- 2–3 new cases per million per year in Europe and North America
- The incidence is 3-fold higher in Thailand and China, when compared to the Western world.

RISK FACTORS
- Treatment with high-dose radiation or chemotherapy
- Exposure to toxic chemicals
- Use of certain medications
- Certain blood diseases, autoimmune disorders, and serious infections
- Tumors of thymus (red cell aplasia)
- Pregnancy, rarely

Genetics
- Telomerase mutations have been found in a small number of patients with acquired and congenital forms. These mutations render carriers more susceptible to environmental insults.
- Mutations in genes called TERC and TERT were found in pedigrees of adults with acquired aplastic anemia who lacked the physical abnormalities or a family history typical of inherited forms of bone marrow failure. These genes encode for the RNA component of telomerase.
- HLA-DR2 is twice as frequent as in the normal population.

GENERAL PREVENTION
- Avoid possible toxic industrial agents.
- Use safety measures when working with radiation.

PATHOPHYSIOLOGY
- The immune hypothesis describes immune suppression through the activation of T cells with associated cytokine production leading to the destruction or injury of the hematopoietic stem cells. This leads to a hypocellular bone marrow in the absence of marrow fibrosis.
- The activation of T cells likely occurs because of both genetic and environmental factors. Exposure to specific environmental precipitants, diverse host genetic risk factors, and individual differences in the characteristics of the immune response likely account for variations in its clinical manifestations and patterns of responsiveness to treatment.
- Telomerase deficiency leads to short telomeres and a quantitative reduction in marrow progenitors and likely a qualitative deficiency in the repair capacity of hematopoietic tissue.
- Reduction of natural killer T cells in the bone marrow

ETIOLOGY
- Idiopathic (~70% of the cases)
- Drugs: Phenylbutazone, chloramphenicol, sulfonamides, gold, cytotoxic drugs, antiepileptics (felbamate, carbamazepine, valproic acid, phenytoin)
- Viral: HIV, Epstein-Barr virus (EBV), nontypeable postinfectious hepatitis (not A, B, or C), parvovirus B19 (mostly in the immunocompromised), atypical mycobacterium
- Toxic exposure (benzene, pesticides, arsenic)
- Radiation exposure
- Immune disorders (systemic lupus erythematosus, eosinophilic fascitis, graft-vs-host disease)
- Pregnancy (rare)
- Congenital (Fanconi anemia, dyskeratosis congenita, Shwachman-Diamond syndrome, amegakaryocytic thrombocytopenia)

 DIAGNOSIS

HISTORY
- Detailed solvent and radiation history, as well as family, environmental, travel, and infectious disease history
- Patients are often asymptomatic but may complain of frequent infections, fatigue, or bleeding.

PHYSICAL EXAM
- Mucosal hemorrhage, petechiae
- Pallor
- Fever
- Hemorrhage, menorrhagia, occult stool blood, melena, epistaxis
- Dyspnea
- Palpitations
- Progressive weakness
- Retinal flame hemorrhages
- Systolic ejection murmur
- Weight loss
- Signs of congenital aplastic anemia:
  – Short stature
  – Microcephaly
  – Nail dystrophy
  – Abnormal thumbs
  – Oral leukoplakia
  – Hyperpigmentation (café au lait spots) or hypopigmentation

DIAGNOSTIC TESTS & INTERPRETATION
Screening tests to exclude other etiologies:
- Complete blood count (CBC) and reticulocyte count
- Blood smear exam
- Cytogenetic studies of peripheral lymphocytes if <35 to exclude Fanconi anemia
- Liver function test
- Viral serology: Hepatitis A, B, C; EBV; cytomegalovirus (CMV); HIV
- Vitamin B_{12} and folate levels
- Autoantibody screening ANA and anti-DNA
- Flow cytometry or Ham test for paroxysmal nocturnal hemoglobinuria
- Fetal hemoglobin in children
- Red cell adenosine deaminase (pure red cell aplasia)
- Cytogenetic analysis of bone marrow

Lab
- CBC: Pancytopenia, anemia (usually normocytic), leucopenia, neutropenia, thrombocytopenia
- Decreased absolute number of reticulocytes
- Increased serum iron secondary to transfusion
- Normal total iron binding capacity (TIBC)
- High mean corpuscular volume (MCV) >104
- CD 34+ cells decreased in blood and marrow
- Urinalysis: Hematuria
- Abnormal liver function tests (hepatitis)
- Increased fetal hemoglobin (Fanconi)
- Increased chromosomal breaks under specialized conditions (Fanconi)
- Molecular determination of abnormal gene (Fanconi)

Imaging
- Computed tomography (CT) of thymus region if thymoma-associated red blood cell (RBC) aplasia suspected
- Radiographs of radius and thumbs (congenital anemia)
- Renal ultrasound (to rule out congenital anemia or malignant hematologic disorder)
- Chest x-ray to exclude infections such as mycobacterial

Diagnostic Procedures/Surgery
Bone marrow aspiration

Pathological Findings
- Normochromic RBC
- Bone marrow:
  - Decreased cellularity (<10%): No fibrosis, no malignant cells seen
  - Decreased megakaryocytes
  - Decreased myelocytes
  - Decreased erythroid precursors
  - Prominent fat spaces and marrow stroma

DIFFERENTIAL DIAGNOSIS
Includes other causes of bone marrow failure and pancytopenia:

- Marrow replacement:
  - Acute lymphoblastic leukemia
  - Lymphoma
  - Hairy cell leukemia (increased reticulin and infiltration of hairy cells)
  - Large granular lymphocyte leukemia
  - Fibrosis
- Megaloblastic hematopoiesis:
  - Folate deficiency
  - Vitamin B_{12} deficiency
- Paroxysmal nocturnal hemoglobinuria, hemolytic anemia (dark urine), pancytopenia venous thrombosis (classically hepatic veins)
- Systemic lupus erythematosus
- Prolonged starvation or anorexia nervosa (bone marrow is gelatinous with loss of fat cells and increased ground substance)
- Transient erythroblastopenia of childhood
- Overwhelming infection:
  - HIV with myelodysplasia
  - Viral hemophagocytic syndrome

 TREATMENT

Early treatment increases the chance of success. Two major treatment pathways: Immunosuppressive therapy and hematopoietic stem cell transplantation. Treatment decisions are based on the age of the patient, the severity of the disease, and the availability of an HLA-matched sibling donor for transplantation.

MEDICATION
Immunosuppressive therapy:

- 1st-line treatment is a combination of antithymocyte globulin (ATG) plus cyclosporine. ATG lyses lymphocytes, and cyclosporin blocks T cell function.
- Antithymocyte globulin (ATG):
  - A horse serum containing polyclonal antibodies against human T cells
  - Treatment for patients >40 and patients without a compatible donor. Consider in patients 30–40.
  - May be used as a single agent, but is more common in combination with cyclosporine

- Cyclosporine following initial ATG therapy for minimum of 6 months:
  - Monitor through blood levels. Normal values for assays vary.
- Granulocyte colony-stimulating factor (G-CSF):
  - Used in conjunction with ATG and cyclosporine
  - Shows faster neutrophil recovery, but survival is not improved
  - Treatment is costly and is disputed in two randomized trials.
- Note: Relapses may occur after the initial response to the immunosuppressive therapy if cyclosporine is discontinued too early.

ADDITIONAL TREATMENT
General Measures
- Supportive measures: RBC and platelet transfusions. Use only CMV-negative blood initially if patient is candidate for hematopoietic stem cell transplantation.
- Antibiotics, antifungals, antivirals when appropriate
- Oxygen therapy for severe anemia
- Good oral hygiene
- Control menorrhagia with norethisterone.
- Avoid causative agents/isolation if necessary.
- Human leukocyte antigen (HLA) testing on all patients and their immediate families
- Transfusion support (judiciously prescribed RBCs for severe anemia, consider leukocyte-depleted units; platelets for severe thrombocytopenia; white blood cells [WBCs]):
  - Transfuse when platelet count is $<10 \times 10^9$ or if $<20 \times 10^9$ with fever
- Immunosuppressive therapy (antithymocyte globulin [ATG] and cyclosporine) if no suitable donor

SURGERY/OTHER PROCEDURES
- Hematopoietic stem cell transplantation for patients with severe aplastic anemia and an HLA-identical donor, <30 years old. Consider in patients 30–40 in good general medical condition.
- Patients >45 have higher rates of graft-vs-host disease and graft rejection compared with children.
- Unrelated donor transplants, if other therapy fails and/or <16 without HLA-matched sibling
- Thymectomy for thymoma

IN-PATIENT CONSIDERATIONS
Initial Stabilization
Referral to an institution that has experience in treating these patients is recommended.

Nursing
If neutropenic, use antiseptic mouthwash such as chlorhexidine and give food low in bacterial content.

 ONGOING CARE

FOLLOW-UP RECOMMENDATIONS
Activity: Isolation procedures if neutropenic

Patient Monitoring
Close monitoring for all treatments is recommended. Drugs and other forms of treatment have numerous and severe side effects.

DIET
If neutropenic, give food low in bacterial content.

PATIENT EDUCATION
Printed patient information available from Aplastic Anemia & MDS International Foundation, Inc., 800-747-2828. Web: www.aamds.org/aplastic

PROGNOSIS
- Hematopoietic stem cell transplantation with HLA-matched sibling:
  - Age <16, 91%
  - Age >16, 70–80%
- Immunosuppressive therapy using ATG and cyclosporine: Overall survival of 75%; 90% among responders at 5 years.

COMPLICATIONS
- Infection (fungal, sepsis)
- Graft-vs-host disease in bone marrow transplant recipients (acute 18%; chronic 26%)
- Side effects of immunosuppressant medications
- Hemorrhage
- Transfusion hemosiderosis
- Transfusion hepatitis
- Heart failure
- Development of secondary cancer: Leukemia or myelodysplasia (15–19% risk at 6–10 years)
- Refractory pancytopenia

ADDITIONAL READING

- Bacigalupo A, Passweg J. Diagnosis and Treatment of Acquired Aplastic Anemia. *Hematol Oncol Clin N Am.* 2009;23:159–70.
- Guinan EC. Acquired Aplastic Anemia in Childhood. *Hematol Oncol Clin N Am.* 2009;23:171–91.
- Rosenfeld S, Follman D, Nunez O, et al. Antithymocyte Globulin and Cyclosporine for Severe Aplastic Anemia: Association Between Hematologic Response and Long-term Outcome. *JAMA.* 2003; 289(9):1130–35.
- Scheinberg P, Wu CO, Nunez O, Young NS. Long-Term Outcome of Pediatric Patients with Severe Aplastic Anemia Treated with Antithymocyte Globulin and Cyclosporine. *J Pediatr.* 2008;153: 814–19.
- Young NS. Pathophysiologic Mechanisms in Acquired Aplastic Anemia. *Hematology.* 2006(1): 72–7.

See Also (Topic, Algorithm, Electronic Media Element)
Leukemia, Hairy Cell; Myelodysplastic Syndromes (MDS); Systemic Lupus Erythematosus
Algorithm: Anemia

CODES

ICD9
- 284.01 Constitutional red blood cell aplasia
- 284.89 Other specified aplastic anemias
- 284.9 Aplastic anemia, unspecified

CLINICAL PEARLS

- Acquired aplastic anemia has an insidious onset and is caused by an exogenous insult triggering an autoimmune reaction. This form is usually responsive to immunosuppressive agents.
- Immunosuppressive therapy using ATG and cyclosporine: Overall survival of 75%; 90% among responders at 5 years.

ANEMIA, AUTOIMMUNE HEMOLYTIC

Nathan T. Connell, MD

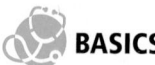 **BASICS**

DESCRIPTION
- Acquired anemia induced by antibodies binding to red blood cell (RBC) membrane antigens
- Three main types defined by maximal binding temperature of the autoantibodies:
  - Warm-reacting [37°C (98.6°F)] IgG antibody
  - Cold-reacting [0–4°C (32–39.2°F)] IgM antibody
  - Mixed type: Both warm-reacting IgG and cold-reacting C3 antibodies
- Drug-induced: Mostly warm-reacting IgG antibodies
- System(s) affected: Hematopoietic/Lymphatic/Immunologic

EPIDEMIOLOGY
Incidence
- Predominant age: <50 years
- Predominant sex: Female > Male
- Estimated incidence is 1/80,000 population per year (1).

RISK FACTORS
- Malignancy
- Autoimmune disorders
- Infection
- Medications
- Prior blood transfusion
- Prior hematopoietic cell transplant

Genetics
No known genetic predisposition

PATHOPHYSIOLOGY
- Warm autoimmune hemolytic anemia (AIHA): IgG attaches to erythrocytes, which are then ingested by macrophages of the spleen.
- Cold AIHA:
  - IgM binds erythrocyte surface temporarily, which then activates complement, causing deposition of C3 on cell surface. Erythrocytes then are ingested by macrophages of the liver.
  - Rarely, complete complement cascade is activated, with membrane attack complex insertion causing intravascular hemolysis.
- Mixed-antibody AIHA: Both warm IgG and cold C3 involved
- Drug-induced:
  - Hapten-induced: Drug attaches to erythrocyte membrane, inducing IgG production.
  - Immune complex: Drug–IgM immune complex binds erythrocyte membrane, activating complement.
  - Autoantibody: Drug induces production of anti-RBC IgG.

ETIOLOGY
- Warm antibody (48–70% cases):
  - Primary cause: Idiopathic
  - Secondary causes:
    - Lymphoproliferative disorders (chronic lymphocytic leukemia, Hodgkin disease, non-Hodgkin lymphoma)
    - Autoimmune disorders
    - Viral infection (especially in children)
- Cold antibody:
  - Cold agglutinin syndrome (CAS) (16–32%):
    - Acute: Infection (mycoplasma, mononucleosis, viral)
    - Chronic: Lymphoproliferative disorders (lymphoma) (2)
  - Paroxysmal cold hemoglobinuria: Infection
- Mixed type:
  - Idiopathic
  - Secondary to lymphoproliferative or autoimmune disorders
- Drug-induced:
  - Penicillin: Hapten-induced
  - Quinine: Immune complex
  - α-Methyldopa: Autoantibody-induced

COMMONLY ASSOCIATED CONDITIONS
- Evans syndrome (AIHA and idiopathic thrombocytopenic purpura)
- Systemic lupus erythematosus
- Chronic lymphocytic leukemia (CLL): AIHA is the most common autoimmune condition associated with CLL and occurs in 5–37% of patients with CLL (2,3).
- Diffuse lymphomas

 DIAGNOSIS

HISTORY
- Weakness/fatigue
- Exertional dyspnea
- Dizziness
- Palpitations
- Malaise
- Association with cold (CAS)

PHYSICAL EXAM
- Pallor
- Jaundice
- Splenomegaly
- Hepatomegaly
- Tachycardia
- Flow murmur
- Blue-gray discoloration of acral surfaces (CAS)

DIAGNOSTIC TESTS & INTERPRETATION
Lab
Initial lab tests
- Direct Coombs [direct antiglobulin test (DAT)]: Positive test indicates presence of antibodies or complement on RBC surface.
- Complete blood count:
  - Anemia (normocytic, normochromic); may be sudden and life-threatening
  - Mild to moderate increase in mean corpuscular volume depending on level of reticulocytosis
  - Increased mean cell hemoglobin concentration
  - Spherocytosis
  - Poikilocytosis
  - Anisocytosis
  - Rouleaux
  - Reticulocytosis
  - Nucleated RBCs
  - Large polychromatophilic reticulocytes
- Hyperbilirubinemia (unconjugated)
- Decreased haptoglobin
- Elevated lactate dehydrogenase
- Hemoglobinemia
- Serology:
  - IgG antibody (warm, mixed, drug-induced, paroxysmal hemoglobinuria)
  - IgM antibody (cold)
- Urinalysis: Hemoglobinuria, hemosiderinuria

Pathological Findings
- Peripheral blood smear: Spherocytes, schistocytes
- Bone marrow biopsy: Bone marrow hyperplasia, increased marrow hemosiderin

DIFFERENTIAL DIAGNOSIS
- Other hemolytic anemias
- Evans syndrome
- Microangiopathic hemolytic disorders
- Aplastic anemia
- Megaloblastic anemia

 TREATMENT

MEDICATION
First Line
- Warm antibody:
  - Glucocorticoids: Prednisone 1 mg/kg/d PO in divided doses:
    - 70–80% patients improve within 3 weeks.
    - Taper gradually to 20 mg/d over 2 weeks.
    - May require maintenance dose of 10 mg every other day (4,5)
  - Precautions: Significant side effects with long-term use
- Cold antibody:
  - Malignancy-induced: Chemotherapy
  - Rituximab for cold AIHA owing to chronic lymphoproliferative disorders (3,4,5)[C]
- Mixed antibody: Prednisone as in warm AIHA

Second Line

* Warm antibody:
  – Immunosuppressive drugs: Recommended for patients who fail splenectomy, relapse after splenectomy, cannot tolerate corticosteroids, and nonsurgical candidates:
    ○ Cyclophosphamide 50 mg/kg/d × 4 days, followed by GCSF for those with refractory anemia (6)[C]
    ○ Precautions: Monitor for marrow suppression.
    ○ Azathioprine (Imuran) 1–2 mg/kg/d within 2 weeks of starting steroids if not responding (7)[C]
    ○ Cyclosporine 5–10 mg/kg/d in 2 divided doses
    ○ Rituximab (anti-CD20 monoclonal antibody) 375 mg/m^2 once weekly × 2–4 weeks for children and refractory cases (8)
    ○ Mycophenolate mofetil 500–1,000 mg/d in 2 divided doses; increase to 1–2 g daily (6)[C].
  – Other medical therapies for refractory cases:
    ○ Danazol 600–800 mg/d PO
    ○ Intravenous immunoglobulin (IVIG) (4)[C]
* Mixed antibody: Immunosuppressives if refractory to steroids and splenectomy

ADDITIONAL TREATMENT
General Measures

* Warm antibody:
  – Folic acid supplementation
  – Mild and moderate: See "Medication."
  – Severe:
    ○ Plasmapheresis as a temporizing measure for refractory or life-threatening anemia (4)[C]
    ○ Packed RBC transfusion for life-threatening anemia; difficult to cross-match; need special blood bank techniques; in emergency, use most compatible cross-match (6)[C].
* Cold antibody:
  – Cold agglutinin syndrome:
    ○ Avoid cold; maintain high temperatures indoors; wear additional clothing outdoors
    ○ Folic acid supplementation
    ○ Plasmapheresis as a temporizing measure for refractory or life-threatening anemia (9)[C]
    ○ Packed RBC transfusion for life-threatening anemia (6)[C]
* Paroxysmal cold hemoglobinuria: Supportive care
* Mixed: Steroids, splenectomy, and immunosuppressives as in warm AIHA
* Drug-induced:
  – Stop the offending drug.
  – Plasmapheresis/exchange transfusion for severe life-threatening cases

Issues for Referral

It is recommended that treatment be in consultation with an experienced hematologist.

SURGERY/OTHER PROCEDURES

* Warm antibody: Splenectomy is the preferred 2nd-line treatment for warm AIHA for those who have failed steroids.
  – 50% initial response rate
  – Patients may require low-dose maintenance prednisone <15 mg daily.
  – After splenectomy: Vaccinate against encapsulated organisms such as *Pneumonococcus* and *Meningococcus* (6)[A]. Patients who have had splenectomy are at increased risk for overwhelming postsplenectomy infection and should receive empirical antibiotics if they develop fever.
* Cold antibody: Surgery not recommended (3,9)
* Mixed antibody: Splenectomy

IN-PATIENT CONSIDERATIONS
Initial Stabilization

If patients start to develop symptoms related to the anemia (i.e., tachycardia, hypotension, chest pain, dyspnea), transfusion may be required.

Admission Criteria

Patients requiring plasmapheresis should be monitored in an ICU setting.

IV Fluids

Use only warmed IV fluids and blood products for cold AIHA in order to prevent further exacerbation of the condition.

 ONGOING CARE

FOLLOW-UP RECOMMENDATIONS
Patient Monitoring

* Monitor carefully if a transfusion is essential.
* Use only warm IV fluids and blood products for cold AIHA.
* Avoid hypothermic surgical procedures for cold AIHA.
* Patients are at increased risk for venous thromboembolism, especially those with systemic lupus erythematosus. Consider prophylactic anticoagulation for patients at highest risk (i.e., those with other risk factors for venous thromboembolism, including immobilization, surgery, or concomitant malignancy) (10).

DIET

No special diet

PROGNOSIS

* Good with appropriate treatment
* Determined by course of the primary disease if secondary to an underlying disorder

COMPLICATIONS

* Shock (severe anemia)
* Venous thromboembolism
* Thrombocytopenic purpura (Evans syndrome)
* Lymphoproliferative disorders in warm AIHA
* Postsplenectomy sepsis syndrome

REFERENCES

1. Garratty G et al. Drug-induced immune hemolytic anemia. *Hematology Am Soc Hematol Educ Program*. 2009;73–9.
2. Zent CS, Ding W, Reinalda MS, Schwager SM, Hoyer JD, Bowen DA, Jelinek DF, Tschumper RC, Call TG, Shanafelt TD, Kay NE, Slager SL et al. Autoimmune cytopenia in chronic lymphocytic leukemia/small lymphocytic lymphoma: changes in clinical presentation and prognosis. *Leuk. Lymphoma*. 2009;50:1261–8.
3. Petz LD. Cold antibody autoimmune hemolytic anemias. *Blood Rev*. 2008;22:1–15.
4. Gehrs BC, Friedberg RC. Autoimmune hemolytic anemia. *Amer J Hematol*. 2002;69:258–71.
5. Dearden C et al. Disease-specific complications of chronic lymphocytic leukemia. *Hematology Am Soc Hematol Educ Program*. 2008;450–6.
6. King KE, Ness PM. Treatment of autoimmune hemolytic anemia. *Sem in Hematology*. 2005; 42:131–6.
7. Pruss A, Salama A, Ahrens N et al. Immune hemolysis-serological and clinical aspects. *Clin Exp Med*. 2003;3:55–64.
8. Bussone G, Ribeiro E, Dechartres A, Viallard JF, Bonnotte B, Fain O, Godeau B, Michel M et al. Efficacy and safety of rituximab in adults' warm antibody autoimmune haemolytic anemia: retrospective analysis of 27 cases. *Am J Hematol*. 2009;84:153–7.
9. Gertz MA et al. Management of cold haemolytic syndrome. *Br J Haematol*. 2007;138:422–9
10. Hoffman PC et al. Immune hemolytic anemia–selected topics. *Hematology Am Soc Hematol Educ Program*. 2006;13–8.

See Also (Topic, Algorithm, Electronic Media Element)

Lymphoma, Non-Hodgkin's; Leukemia; Systemic Lupus Erythematosus (SLE)
Algorithm: Anemia

 CODES

ICD9
283.0 Autoimmune hemolytic anemias

CLINICAL PEARLS

* Initial workup of suspected hemolytic anemia includes complete blood count, DAT, fractionated bilirubin, haptoglobin, lactate dehydrogenase, and urinalysis.
* It is important to distinguish between cold and warm antibody autoimmune hemolytic anemia because treatments are different.
* Have a low threshold to hospitalize patients or step up level of care to an ICU if indicated.
* Consultation with an experienced hematologist is recommended, especially for severe cases.

ANEMIA, CHRONIC DISEASE

Cheryl L. Gilmartin, PharmD
Claudia M. Lora, MD

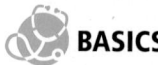 **BASICS**

DESCRIPTION
Anemia of chronic disease (ACD) is a normocytic, normochromic, hypoproliferative anemia associated with infectious, neoplastic, and inflammatory processes. The chronic immune activation accompanying these processes results in the production of inflammatory cytokines, which in turn create an anemic state by interfering with iron homeostasis and impairing erythropoiesis. ACD is the 2nd most common type of anemia and is the most common anemia found in hospitalized patients (1).

EPIDEMIOLOGY
Incidence
Incidence of anemia in cancer: 53.7% (2)

Prevalence
The estimated reports of ACD prevalence for individual conditions varies widely in the literature.

PATHOPHYSIOLOGY
Inflammatory cytokines (e.g., TNF-α, IFN-γ, IL-6) released by cells of the immune system in the setting of malignant, autoimmune, or infectious disease are the major mediators of anemia in ACD. They exert their effects in 3 main ways:

- Disrupted iron homeostasis:
  - Chronic inflammation, infection, malignancy → ↑ IFN-γ, LPS, TNF-α → ↑ iron uptake by and ↓ iron release from reticuloendothelial system (RES) cells → ↓ iron availability for heme biosynthesis and RBC production in the bone marrow
  - Chronic inflammation, infection, malignancy → ↑ IL-6, LPS → ↑ hepatocyte production of hepcidin, a major negative iron regulator → ↓ iron absorption in duodenum and ↓ iron release from RES cells → ↓ iron availability for RBC production
- Impaired erythropoiesis:
  - ↑ IFN-γ, TNF-α, IL-1 → down-regulation of erythropoietin (EPO) receptors on erythroid precursors, cytokine-induced apoptosis of erythroid precursors, ↓ hematopoietic growth factors in the marrow → impaired function, proliferation, and differentiation of erythroid cells → ↓ RBC production
  - ↑ IFN-γ, TNF-α, IL-1 → ↓ synthesis and diminished effect of EPO → ↓ RBC production
- RBC destruction:
  - ↑ TNF-α, IL-1 → ↑ phagocytosis of RBCs by RES cells → ↓ RBC half-life
  - ↑ IFN-γ, TNF-α, IL-1 → ↑ free radical formation → ↑ RBC destruction

ETIOLOGY
Inflammatory cytokines (e.g., TNF-α, IFN-γ, IL-6) released by cells of the immune system in the setting of infectious, inflammatory, or neoplastic diseases cause anemia by interfering with iron metabolism and RBC production.

COMMONLY ASSOCIATED CONDITIONS
- Autoimmune disease:
  - Rheumatoid arthritis
  - Systemic lupus erythematosus
  - Inflammatory bowel disease
  - Sarcoidosis
  - Vasculitis
- Infectious disease:
  - HIV and other viral infections
  - Chronic or subacute bacterial, fungal, parasitic infection
- Neoplastic disease:
  - Both solid and hematologic tumors
  - Chronic kidney disease
  - Chronic rejection post solid-organ transplantation

 DIAGNOSIS

HISTORY
History or symptoms of an acute or chronic inflammatory, infectious, or neoplastic process and no clinical evidence for occult bleeding

PHYSICAL EXAM
Findings related to the underlying disease

DIAGNOSTIC TESTS & INTERPRETATION
Lab
Initial lab tests
- Hemoglobin: Mild (Hgb <10–12 g/dL) or moderate (Hgb 8–10 g/dL) or severe (Hgb <8 g/dL) anemia
- Reticulocyte production index: Inappropriately low or normal, <2%
- Absolute reticulocyte count: Low, <25,000/μL
- MCV: Normal, 80–100 fL (in the absence of coexistent additional cause of anemia)
- Peripheral smear: No evidence of other hematologic disorders
- Serum iron: Low (M: <65 μg/dL, F: <50 μg/dL)
- Transferrin or TIBC: Low
- Ferritin: Normal (M: 215–365 mg/dL, F: 250–380 mg/dL) or high in the absence of coexisting iron deficiency
- Soluble transferrin receptor: Normal
- Ratio of soluble transferrin receptor: Log ferritin <1
- Elevated levels ESR, CRP, fibrinogen, cytokines
- Rule out other causes of anemia with appropriate tests if doubt as to diagnosis. Additional tests might include TSH, Hgb electrophoresis, B$_{12}$ and folate levels, direct and indirect Coombs tests, bone marrow aspiration.

DIFFERENTIAL DIAGNOSIS
- Iron deficiency anemia
- Thalassemia
- Myelodysplastic syndromes
- Hyperthyroidism or hypothyroidism
- Hypopituitarism
- Hyperparathyroidism

 TREATMENT

- Treat the underlying disease. (1).
- The erythropoietic stimulating agents (ESA), recombinant erythropoietin (rEPO), and darbepoetin (DARB) decrease the need for transfusions, increase hemoglobin levels in chronic kidney failure, and may improve quality of life in patients with CKD. According to the Food and Drug Administration, therapy should be initiated when hemoglobin levels (Hgb) are <10 g/dL and TSAT >20% (3). The National Kidney Foundation Kidney Disease Outcomes Quality Initiatives (KDOQI) recommend individual evaluation of the benefit of ESA utilization and maintaining the Hgb between 11–12 g/dL patients TSAT >20% and ferritin >100 ng/mL in nondialysis CKD patients and >200 ng/mL in dialysis-treated CKD patients (4)[A].
- rEPO also increases Hgb levels in patients with ACD from HIV and chronic renal failure (5)[A].
- DARB has a simpler dosing schedule than rEPO (6).
- Iron therapy given prior to or concurrently with ESA improves response to ESA. IV iron is recommended for dialysis-treated CKD patients. Iron indices should be evaluated prior to and during ESA use (4).
- Target Hgb levels in patients treated with ESA should not exceed 12 g/dL because of the increased risk of thromboembolic events at higher levels.
- Treatment with ESA should be reserved for symptomatic chemotherapy-induced anemia (CIA) in cancer treatment without curative intent. Treatment should be discontinued when chemotherapy is complete or if a rise in Hgb is not achieved within 8–9 weeks (7)[A].
- ESA therapy in patients with cancer has been associated with increased risk of venous thromboembolism and mortality (8).
- Iron studies and therapy for iron-deficient asymptomatic CIA cancer treatment without curative intent are recommended for absolute iron deficiency (7).

MEDICATION
- Epoetin α:
  - CKD start at 50–100 U/kg IV or SC 3 times a week (TIW). ESA dosage should be adjusted according to the patient's Hgb level and response (4,9,10).
  - Cancer patients on chemotherapy start at 150 U/kg SC TIW or 40,000 U SC weekly; if no rise in Hgb >1 g/dL in 4 weeks, may increase to 300 U/kg TIW or 60,000 U SC weekly, respectively (7). Decrease dose by 25–50% if a rise in Hgb >1 g/dL in 2 weeks.

- Darbepoetin α:
  - CKD start at 0.45 μg/kg IV or SC weekly; alternative for CKD not on dialysis 0.75 μg/kg SC every 2 weeks. Dose adjustments are made similar to epoetin α (3,4).
  - Cancer patients on chemotherapy start with 2.25 μg/kg weekly or 500 μg/kg every 3 weeks SC. If HgB rise $\leq$1 g/dL in 4 weeks, increase to 4.5 μg/kg SC weekly (7). Decrease dose by 25–50% if a rise in Hgb >1 g/dL in 2 weeks.

ALERT
With EPO/DARB use:
- CKD: Increased risk for death and serious cardiovascular events when dosed to Hgb $\geq$13 g/dL
- Cancer-related anemia and CIA with curative intent: ESA are not indicated. ESA therapy is only indicated in CIA without curative intent. Dose adjustments should be made to maintain the lowest Hgb to avoid transfusion.
- The FDA has included ESA therapy in CIA without curative intent in the Risk Evaluation and Mitigation Strategy (REMS) to assess the risk vs benefit for ESA use in this indication. To utilize ESA therapy physicians need to enroll in the **A**ssisting **P**roviders and cancer **P**atients with **R**isk **I**nformation for the **S**afe use of **E**SAs (APPRISE). Enrollment in the ESA Oncology APPRISE Program may be found at www.esa-apprise.com or by calling 1-866-284-8089.

ADDITIONAL TREATMENT
General Measures
- Most patients with ACD have a mild, asymptomatic anemia. However, if anemia becomes severe (Hgb <8 g/dL) and patients symptomatic, transfusion with PRBCs may become necessary, especially with a concurrent bleeding complication.
- Long-term transfusion therapy is not recommended in ACD patients with chronic kidney disease (1).

ONGOING CARE

FOLLOW-UP RECOMMENDATIONS
To minimize the risks of thromboembolic events, the lowest dose needed to avoid RBC transfusion should be utilized (3,7,9,10).

Patient Monitoring
Hgb or hematocrit levels should be followed, especially during therapy with ESA, when they should be checked biweekly until a stable dose, then monthly.

PROGNOSIS
Although ACD is chronic, it is usually not progressive.

COMPLICATIONS
- Anemia is associated with a worse prognosis in cardiovascular, chronic renal, and neoplastic disease (1).
- Treating anemia in these conditions improves quality of life (1) but may not improve length of life (and may shorten in some circumstances).

REFERENCES
1. Weiss G. Anemia of chronic disease. *N Engl J Med*. 2005;52:1011–23.
2. Ludwig H, Van Belle S, Barrett-Lee P et al. The European Cancer Anaemia Survey (ECAS): a large, multinational, prospective survey defining the prevalence, incidence, and treatment of anaemia in cancer patients. *Eur J Cancer*. 2004;40: 2293–306.
3. Product Information: ARANESP(R) injection, darbepoetin alfa injection. Amgen, Inc, Thousand Oaks, CA, 2007.
4. KDOQI, National Kidney Foundation. KDOQI Clinical Practice Guidelines and Clinical Practice Recommendations for Anemia in Chronic Kidney Disease. *Am J Kidney Dis*. 2006;47:S11–145.
5. Volberding P. Consensus statement: anemia in HIV infection–current trends, treatment options, and practice strategies. Anemia in HIV Working Group. *Clin Ther*. 2000;22:1004–1020; discussion 1003.
6. Vanrenterghem Y, Bárány P, Mann JF et al. Randomized trial of darbepoetin alfa for treatment of renal anemia at a reduced dose frequency compared with rHuEPO in dialysis patients. *Kidney Int*. 2002;62:2167–75.
7. National Comprehensive Cancer Network (NCCN.org). Jenkintown: NCCN Clinical Practice Guidelines in Oncology. Cancer- and Chemotherapy-Induced Anemia. V.2.2010. Accessed May 12, 2010 Fort Washington, PA: National Comprehensive Cancer Network; 2010, at http://www.nccn.org/professionals/physician_gls/PDF/anemia.pdf.
8. Bennett CL, Silver SM, Djulbegovic B et al. Venous thromboembolism and mortality associated with recombinant erythropoietin and darbepoetin administration for the treatment of cancer-associated anemia. *JAMA*. 2008;299:914–24.
9. Product Information: PROCRIT(R) injection, epoetin alfa injection. Ortho Biotech Products, LP, Raritan, NJ, 2005.
10. Product Information: EPOGEN(R) injection, epoetin alfa injection. Amgen, Inc, Thousand Oaks, CA, 2007.

ADDITIONAL READING
Nissenson AR, Swan SK, Lindberg JS et al. Randomized, controlled trial of darbepoetin alfa for the treatment of anemia in hemodialysis patients. *Am J Kidney Dis*. 2002;40:110–8.

See Also (Topic, Algorithm, Electronic Media Element)
Algorithm: Anemia

CODES

ICD9
- 285.21 Anemia in chronic kidney disease
- 285.22 Anemia in neoplastic disease
- 285.29 Anemia of other chronic disease

CLINICAL PEARLS
- ACD and iron-deficiency anemia (IDA) may coexist. The following parameters can generally distinguish them:
  - ACD-normocytic, $\downarrow$ or normal transferrin, $\uparrow$ or normal ferritin, normal soluble transferrin receptor levels (sTfR), ratio sTfR:log ferritin <1.
  - IDA-microcytic, $\uparrow$ transferrin, $\downarrow$ ferritin, $\uparrow$ sTfR levels, ratio sTfR:log ferritin >2.
- Anemia in ACD is usually symptomatic, although anemia is often mild or moderate. Patients with ACD always have an underlying disease, such as RA or chronic renal failure. These diseases will usually limit the patient's mobility, exercise capacity, or energy level, and typical symptoms of anemia (e.g., exertional dyspnea, fatigue, weakness) are attributed to the underlying disease.
- Iron sequestration and anemia may be an adaptive response when inflammation, infection, or neoplasia are present. When iron is hoarded in RES cells in ACD, rapidly proliferating micro-organisms or tumor cells do not have access to it, thereby limiting their growth. These rapidly proliferating cells also have increased oxygen demand, which is more difficult to meet in an anemic state.

ANEMIA, IRON DEFICIENCY

Pablo I. Hernandez Itriago, MD
Matthew A. Silva, PharmD, RPh, BCPS

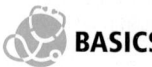 **BASICS**

DESCRIPTION
- A deficiency in red blood cells, hemoglobin, or blood volume due to decreased iron stores
- Onset may be acute with rapid blood loss or chronic with poor diet or slow blood loss.
- System(s) affected: Hemic/Lymphatic/Immunologic
- Synonym(s): Anemia of chronic blood loss; Hypochromic; Microcytic anemia; Chlorosis

Geriatric Considerations
60% of anemias in people >65 years

Pediatric Considerations
Frequent problem in infants whose major source of nutrition is unfortified cow's milk and/or juices

Pregnancy Considerations
Common during pregnancy unless iron supplements are included in the diet

EPIDEMIOLOGY
- Iron deficiency anemia (IDA) is the most common cause of anemia in the US.
- Predominant age: All ages, but especially toddlers and menstruating women
- Predominant sex: Female > Male
- More likely in the poor and in underimmunized children

Incidence
- Adults: Men 2%, women 15–20% annually
- Infants and toddlers: 3–5% annually
- Pregnant patients: 20%

Prevalence
- Infants and children <12: 4–7% (1)
- Males: 2–5% (1)
- Females: 9–16% (18–50% in menstruant blood donors) (1,2)

RISK FACTORS
- Female
- Frequent blood donor
- Pregnancy

GENERAL PREVENTION
- Screen asymptomatic pregnant women (3)[B].
- Supplementation in asymptomatic children 6–12 months if at increased risk for IDA (3)[B]

PATHOPHYSIOLOGY
Depletion of iron stores leads to decrease in reticulocyte count and decrease in production of hemoglobin.

ETIOLOGY
- Blood loss (e.g., menses, gastrointestinal [GI] bleeding, trauma)
- Poor iron intake
- Poor iron absorption (e.g., atrophic gastritis, postgastrectomy, celiac disease)
- Increased demand for iron (e.g., infancy, adolescence, and pregnancy)

COMMONLY ASSOCIATED CONDITIONS
- Hookworm infestation
- Pregnancy
- Gastric or colon carcinoma
- Hypermetrorrhagia

 DIAGNOSIS

HISTORY
- Asymptomatic in most cases
- Weakness/fatigue
- Exertional dyspnea
- Palpitations
- Malaise
- Dizziness
- Headaches, inability to concentrate, irritability, listlessness
- Pica

PHYSICAL EXAM
- Pallor
- Cheilosis
- Tachycardia
- Tachypnea
- Koilonychia (spoon-shaped, brittle nails)

DIAGNOSTIC TESTS & INTERPRETATION
Lab
Initial lab tests
- Hemoglobin: <13 g in men and <12 g in women (4). Patients with higher premorbid hemoglobin (such as patients with chronic hypoxemia, smokers, living in high altitude) may be anemic at higher hemoglobin levels.
- Mean corpuscular volume (MCV): <80 fL
- Ferritin: <45 ng per mL. It is the best noninvasive test in adults, but may miss some deficient patients (e.g., cirrhosis), because ferritin is an acute-phase reactant.
- Transferrin saturation: <9 percent
- Total iron-binding capacity (TIBS): Increased
- Complete blood count (CBC) with differential, peripheral smear, reticulocyte count, and index. A peripheral smear usually shows hypochromia and microcytosis, but may be normal, and reticulocyte production index is low.
- Fe/total iron binding capacity (transferrin ratio) is usually not recommended, because it is less sensitive and less specific than ferritin.
- Stainable iron in bone marrow aspiration is the gold standard.
- Consider testing for G6PD deficiency: Assay at least 6 weeks after last drop in hemoglobin.
- Rule out thalassemia:
  – Review prior CBCs for persisting mild anemia and marked micro-ovalocytosis, elevated hemoglobin A2 or hemoglobin F, family history, and especially high or high normal red blood cell (RBC) count
  – A low RBC count in chronic bleeding helps to distinguish it from thalassemia trait where the count is high or high-normal
  – Microcytosis with ovalocytosis and anemia unresponsive to iron suggests the thalassemia trait.

- MCV may be normal in mild anemia or hidden by the population of larger cells (e.g., reticulocytes or macrocytes). Red cell distribution width (RDW) will be increased if a mixed population of cells is present (e.g., mixed iron deficiency anemia and B12 deficiency)
- An empiric trial of iron at 3 mg/kg/d may be the best way to diagnose decreased iron stores in infants and children; reticulocytes become elevated in 7–10 days or hemoglobin increases >1.0 g/dL weekly, indicating Fe deficiency.
- Drugs that may alter lab results: Iron supplements or multivitamin–mineral preparations that contain iron
- Disorders that may alter lab results:
  – Elevated ferritin: Acute or chronic liver disease, Hodgkin disease, acute leukemia, solid tumors, fever, acute inflammation, renal dialysis
  – Elevated hemoglobin: Smoking, chronic hypoxemia, long-term residency at high altitude
  – Stool guaiac (2)[C]; if high index of suspicion of GI bleed, GI endoscopy. Under appropriate circumstances, stool for ova and parasites.
  – Rule out poor reutilization: Trial of iron, bone marrow aspiration, and iron stain
  – Rule out colorectal cancer and gastric carcinoma, especially in the elderly.

Diagnostic Procedures/Surgery
GI endoscopy to discover occult bleeding sites

Pathological Findings
- Absent marrow iron stores
- Marrow: Hyperplastic, micronormoblastic

DIFFERENTIAL DIAGNOSIS
- Gastritis
- Peptic ulcer disease
- GI bleeding
- Gastrointestinal carcinomas
- Defective iron utilization (e.g., thalassemia trait, sideroblastosis, G6PD deficiency)
- Defective iron reutilization (e.g., infection, inflammation, cancer, other chronic diseases)
- Hypoproliferation (e.g., decreased erythropoietin from hypothyroidism, renal failure)

 TREATMENT

MEDICATION
- Ferrous sulfate 325 mg t.i.d. on an empty stomach 1 hour before meals provides 180 mg of elemental iron per day:
  – Reduce dose as needed for GI symptoms, which affect 15% of patients on standard iron therapy, or the dose can be taken with meals, which may reduce the delivery of iron by 50%. Constipation will occur in approximately 1 in 4 patients using various iron formulations (5).
  – Drugs that increase gastric pH (e.g., proton pump inhibitors [PPIs], H_2 antagonists) also reduce iron absorption (6).
  – Individuals with moderate anemia (Hg = 10 g/dL) need only a total of 1,500–2,000 mg of elemental iron replacement; reducing the iron per dose as much as necessary to abate adverse effects will make parenteral iron therapy unnecessary in almost all cases.

– Special oral iron formulations and compounds are expensive and reduce symptoms only to the degree that they reduce the delivery of iron.

- Liquid iron preparations are useful for children, with a recommended dose of 3 mg/kg/d; can also be used in adults when tablets are not absorbed or low tolerance requires a dose reduction.
- Foods and beverages containing ascorbic acid (vitamin C) enhance iron absorption when taken simultaneously with the iron.
- Continued bleeding and untreated hypothyroidism are causes for "failure to respond" to iron.
- Consider parenteral iron for patients with an Hgb <6 g/dL, malabsorption, if higher oral doses and use of vitamin C fail:
  – Anaphylaxis to parenteral iron therapy has occurred; ferric gluconate or iron sucrose may be safer alternatives to iron dextran (7,8)[B]
  – Iron sucrose 200 mg IV × 5 doses over 2 weeks, or 500 mg IV q2 weeks × 2 doses (less experience with this regimen). Total dose is 1000 mg, then re-evaluate. 1 ml = 20 mg elemental iron. 100 mg IV × 10 weekly doses in hemodialysis-dependent patients.
- Contraindications:
  – Antacids concomitantly
  – Dairy products concomitantly
  – Tetracycline concomitantly
- Significant possible interactions:
  – Allopurinol
  – Antacids
  – Penicillamine
  – Quinolones
  – Tetracyclines
  – Vitamin E
- Precautions:
  – Iron preparations may cause black bowel movements and constipation.
  – Iron overdose is highly toxic; patients should be instructed to keep tablets and liquids out of the reach of small children.

ADDITIONAL TREATMENT
General Measures
- Search for the cause and correct it.
- Occult GI malignancy should be suspected in all older individuals with iron deficiency.
- Avoid transfusions except in rare cases.

Issues for Referral
- Pregnant women with an Hgb <9 g/dL or failure to respond to a 4–6-week trial or oral iron therapy
- Nonpregnant women or other patients with an Hgb <6 g/dL

IN-PATIENT CONSIDERATIONS
Initial Stabilization
Outpatient

 ## ONGOING CARE

FOLLOW-UP RECOMMENDATIONS
Patient Monitoring
- Regularly after Hgb returns to normal (in order to detect recurrences)
- Hgb increases 1 g/dL every 2–3 weeks.
- Iron stores may take up to 4 weeks to correct after Hgb returns to normal.

DIET
- Do not consume milk, other dairy products, antacids, quinolones, or tetracycline within 2 hours of iron supplement ingestion.
- Limit tea, coffee, and caffeinated beverages.
- Limit milk to 16 ounces per day (adults).
- Emphasize protein and iron-containing foods (meat, beans, and leafy green vegetables).
- Taking iron with orange juice or ascorbic acid increases absorption but decreases GI tolerability.
- Increase fluid and dietary fiber to decrease likelihood of constipation during iron replacement therapy.

PATIENT EDUCATION
National Heart, Lung & Blood Institute, Communications & Public Information Branch, National Institutes of Health, Building 31, Room 41-21, 9000 Rockville Pike, Bethesda, MD 20892; (301) 251-1222.

PROGNOSIS
- Can be resolved with iron therapy if the underlying cause can be discovered and appropriately treated
- Treat subclinical hypothyroidism and iron deficiency anemia together when these conditions co-exist. Failure to treat hypothyroidism results in poor response to iron therapy (9)[B].

COMPLICATIONS
- Neglecting to identify hidden bleeding points, particularly a bleeding malignancy
- Maternal iron deficiency negatively affects mother–child interactions. Iron supplementation protects against these negative effects (10).

REFERENCES

1. Iron Deficiency—United States, 1999–2000. *MMWR Morb Mortal Wkly Rep.* 2002;51:897–9.
2. Dubois RW, Goodnough LT, Ershler WB et al. Identification, diagnosis, and management of anemia in adult ambulatory patients treated by primary care physicians: evidence-based and consensus recommendations. *Curr Med Res Opin.* 2006;22:385–95.
3. U.S. Preventative Services Task Force (USPSTF). Screening for iron deficiency anemia—including iron supplementation for children and pregnant women. Rockville (MD): Agency for Healthcare Research and Quality (AHRQ); 2006. 12p.
4. Worldwide prevalence of anaemia 1993–2005: WHO global database on anaemia/Edited by Bruno de Benoist, Erin McLean, Ines Egli and Mary Cogswell.
5. Melamed N, Ben-Haroush A, Kaplan B et al. Iron supplementation in pregnancy–does the preparation matter? *Arch Gynecol Obstet.* 2007; 276:601–4.
6. Killip S, Bennett JM, Chambers MD. Iron deficiency anemia. *Am Fam Physician.* 2007;75:671–8.
7. Chertow GM, Mason PD, Vaage-Nilsen O et al. On the relative safety of parenteral iron formulations. *Nephrol Dial Transplant.* 2004;19:1571–5.
8. Chertow GM, Mason PD, Vaage-Nilsen O et al. Update on adverse drug events associated with parenteral iron. *Nephrol Dial Transplant.* 2006; 21:378–82.
9. Cinemre H, Bilir C, Gokosmanoglu F, Bahcebasi T et al. Hematologic effects of levothyroxine in iron-deficient subclinical hypothyroid patients: a randomized, double-blind, controlled study. *J. Clin. Endocrinol. Metab.* 2009;94:151–6
10. Murray-Kolb LE, Beard JL. Iron deficiency and child and maternal health. *Am J Clin Nutr.* 2009.

ADDITIONAL READING

- Andrews NC. Disorders of iron metabolism. *N Engl J Med.* 1999;341:1986–95.
- Auerbach M, Ballard H, Glaspy J. Clinical update: intravenous iron for anaemia. *Lancet.* 2007;369: 1502–4.
- Baker WF. Iron deficiency anemia in pregnancy, obstetrics and gynecology. *Hematol Oncol Clin North Am.* 2000;64(4):231–6.
- Iron Deficiency – United States, 1999–2000. *MMWR Morb Mortal Wkly Rep.* 2002;51(40): 897–9.
- Provan D, Weatherall D. Red cells II: acquired anaemias and polycythaemia. *Lancet.* 2000;355: 1260–8.
- Recommendations to prevent and control iron deficiency in the United States. *MMWR Morb Mortal Wkly Rep.* 1998;47(RR-3):1–36.
- Steensma DP, Tefferi A. Anemia in the elderly: How should we define it, when does it matter, and what can be done? [Review]. *Mayo Clinic Proc.* 2007; 82(8):958–66.
- Tefferi A, Hanson CA, Inwards DJ. How to interpret and pursue an abnormal complete blood cell count in adults. *Mayo Clin Proc.* 2005;80:923–36.

See Also (Topic, Algorithm, Electronic Media Element)
Algorithm: Anemia

 ## CODES

ICD9
280.9 Iron deficiency anemia, unspecified

CLINICAL PEARLS
- Iron deficiency anemia is the most common type of anemia in the US.
- Blood loss and reduced iron stores due to malabsorption or poor utilization are major factors for iron deficiency anemia.
- Premenopausal women and children are at the greatest risk for iron deficiency anemia.
- Oral iron supplementation is the standard treatment option for patients with IDA.

ANEMIA, SICKLE CELL

Diane M. Haleem, PhD, RN
William V. Walsh, MD

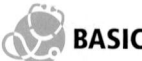

BASICS

DESCRIPTION
- Chronic hemoglobinopathy marked by moderately severe chronic hemolytic anemia, periodic acute episodes of painful "crises," and increased susceptibility to intercurrent infections. Hereditary, generally manifesting in 1st year of life.
- Sickle cells are abnormally shaped, fragile red blood cells. Increased red cell destruction causes an inability to maintain adequate hemoglobin levels and results in fatigue.
- The heterozygous condition (Hb A/S), sickle cell trait, is usually asymptomatic without anemia.
- System(s) affected: Hematologic; Lymphatic/Immunologic; Musculoskeletal
- Synonym(s): Sickle cell disease; Hb S disease

Pediatric Considerations
- Sequestration crises and hand–foot syndrome seen typically in infants/young children
- Adolescence/young adulthood:
  - Frequency of complications and organ/tissue damage increases with age (except for strokes, which occur mostly in childhood).
  - Psychological complications: Body image and sexual identity problems; interrupted schooling, career; restriction of activities; stigma of disease; low self-esteem
- Consider periodic transcranial Doppler ultrasound in all children ages 2–16.

Pregnancy Considerations
- Usually complicated and hazardous, especially 3rd trimester and delivery:
  - Fetal survival is >90% if the fetus reaches the 3rd trimester.
- Increased risk of pain rises, toxemia, infection, pulmonary infarction, phlebitis
- Fetal mortality 35–40%
- Partial exchange transfusion in 3rd trimester may reduce maternal morbidity and fetal mortality, but this is controversial.
- Chronic transfusions have been effective in diminishing pain episodes in pregnant women.

EPIDEMIOLOGY
Prevalence
- Almost 90,000 Americans have sickle cell disease and >2 million carry the trait. ~1/500 African Americans and 1/1,000 Hispanics have homozygous sickle cell anemia. Each year in the United States, about 1 in 400 African American infants are born with sickle cell disease.
- 10% of African Americans have sickle trait.
- To a lesser extent, people from the Middle East, Mediterranean area, and aboriginal tribes in India may be affected.

RISK FACTORS
- For vaso-occlusive crisis ("painful crisis"): Pain results from tissue ischemia and necrosis: Hypoxia, dehydration, fever, infection, acidosis, cold, anesthesia, strenuous physical exercise, smoking
- For aplastic crisis (suppression of RBC production): Severe infections, human parvovirus B19 infection, folic acid deficiency

- Hyperhemolytic crisis (accelerated hemolysis) (existence is controversial): Acute bacterial infections, exposure to oxidant drugs

Genetics
Autosomal recessive, mostly in African Americans. Homozygous presence of a variant hemoglobin, Hb S, or sickle hemoglobin (genotype SS). Heterozygous condition Hb AS.

GENERAL PREVENTION
- General: Genetic counseling
- Prevention of crises:
  - Avoid hypoxia, dehydration, cold, infection, fever, acidosis, and anesthesia.
  - Guidelines for prompt management of fever, infections, pain, and specific complications should be reviewed at each visit.
  - Stress importance of keeping well hydrated.
  - Avoid alcohol and smoking.
  - Avoid high-altitude areas. Traveling to a high-altitude area may trigger a crisis because of lower partial pressure of oxygen.
- Teach early recognition of possible complications, especially priapism.
- Stress importance of minimizing trauma; care using aseptic technique is imperative.

PATHOPHYSIOLOGY
Sickle cells express very late antigen (VLA)-4 on the surface. VLA-4 interacts with the endothelial cell adhesive molecule, vascular cell adhesive molecule (VCAM)-1. VCAM-1 is upregulated by hypoxia and inhibited by nitric oxide. Hypoxia also decreases nitric oxide production, thereby adding to the adhesion of sickle cells to the vascular endothelium. Nitric oxide is a vasodilator (1).

ETIOLOGY
- At molecular level: Substitution of valine for glutamic acid in the 6th amino acid position of the hemoglobin β-chain. As a result of the mutation, red blood cells (RBCs) change from biconcave to sickle shape when deoxygenated.
- At cellular level: Sickle RBCs are inflexible, which causes increased blood viscosity, stasis, mechanical obstruction of small arterioles and capillaries, and ischemia. Sickle RBCs are fragile, leading to hemolysis.
- At clinical level: Chronic anemia; crises:
  - Vaso-occlusive crisis ("painful crisis"): Pain results from tissue ischemia and necrosis. Progressive organ failure and tissue damage from repeated vaso-occlusive episodes.
  - Hand–foot syndrome: When vessel occlusion and ischemia affects small blood vessels in hands or feet, pain and swelling can result.
  - Aplastic crisis: Suppression of RBC production by severe infection or by parvoviral (and other viral) suppression of RBC production
  - Hyperhemolytic crisis: Accelerated hemolysis; increased RBC fragility/shortened lifespan
  - Sequestration crisis: Splenic sequestration of blood (only in infants/young children—occasionally seen in adults with sickle variants) causing acute anemia and acute splenic enlargement
- Susceptibility to infection: Impaired/absent splenic function; defect in the alternate pathway of complement activation

COMMONLY ASSOCIATED CONDITIONS
The psychosocial effects can result in low self-esteem, depression, and dependency.

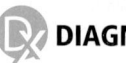

DIAGNOSIS

A chronic hemolytic anemia. Increased infection risk, (ex: pneumococcal sepsis and Salmonella osteomyelitis), with functional asplenia by ~5–6 years of age, and delayed physical/sexual maturation. Diagnosis now often made by newborn screening programs.

HISTORY
- >6 months of age, earliest symptoms are irritability and painful swelling of the hands and feet (hand–foot syndrome).
- Often asymptomatic in early months of life due to presence of fetal hemoglobin.
- Painful crises in bones, joints, abdomen, back, and viscera (account for 90% of all hospital admissions)
- Acute chest syndrome: Tachycardia, fever, bilateral infiltrates caused by decrease in hemoglobin and pulmonary infarction

PHYSICAL EXAM
- Fever, pale skin and nail beds, mild jaundice
- Acute chest syndrome: Tachycardia, fever, bilateral infiltrates caused by decrease in hemoglobin and pulmonary infarction

DIAGNOSTIC TESTS & INTERPRETATION
Lab
- Hb electrophoresis (diagnostic test of choice). Sickle cell anemia (FS pattern):
  - 80–100% Hb S, variable amounts of Hb F and no Hb A
  - Sickle cell trait (FS pattern): 20–40% Hb S, 60–80% Hb A1, minimal Hb F
- Screening tests: Sickledex test
- Hemoglobin ~8 g/dL (1.24 mmol/L); RBC indices usually normal, but mean corpuscular volume (MCV) <75/m^3 (<75 fL), reticulocytosis of 10–20%
- Leukocytosis; bands in absence of infection, and thrombocytosis
- Peripheral smear: Sickled RBCs, nucleated RBCs, Howell-Jolly bodies
- Serum bilirubin mildly elevated (2–4 mg/dL [34–68/mmol/L]); fecal/urinary urobilinogen high
- Erythrocyte sedimentation rate (ESR) low
- Serum lactate dehydrogenase (LDH) elevated, haptoglobin absent or very low

Imaging
Need for imaging depends upon clinical circumstances:
- Bone scan to rule out osteomyelitis
- Computed tomography (CT)/magnetic resonance imaging (MRI) to rule out cerebrovascular accident (CVA)
- Chest x-ray (CXR): May show enlarged heart; diffuse alveolar infiltrates in acute chest syndrome
- Transcranial Doppler: Start at age 2; repeat yearly (2,3)[B]. Transcranial Doppler ultrasound identifies children age 2-16 at higher risk of stroke. Those at increased risk may be treated with regular red blood cell transfusion to reduce risk of stroke.
- Electrocardiogram (ECG) to detect pulmonary hypertension (3)[C]

Pathological Findings
- In moderate-to-severe cases, hyposplenism due to autosplenectomy is common.
- Hypoxia/infarction in multiple organs

DIFFERENTIAL DIAGNOSIS
- Anemia: Other hemoglobinopathies
- Painful crises: Other causes of acute pain in bones, joints, and abdomen

TREATMENT
MEDICATION
First Line
- Supplemental oxygen
- Painful crises (mild, outpatient):
  – Non-narcotic analgesics (ibuprofen, tramadol) (2,3)[C]
- Painful crises (severe, hospitalized) (2,3)[B]:
  – Parenteral narcotics (e.g., morphine on fixed schedule); patient-controlled analgesia (PCA) pump may be useful.
- Prevention of painful crisis:
  – Hydroxyurea in adult patients with ≥3 crises/year. Start with 15 mg/kg/d single daily dose; titrate upward every 12 weeks if blood counts satisfactory:
    ○ Increase in 5 mg/kg increments to maximum of 35 mg/kg/d. Reduces crisis and chest syndrome 50%; long-term safety unknown.
    ○ Contraindicated in pregnancy (4)[A]
  – Inhaled nitric oxide, arginine butyrate (may enhance availability of nitric oxide), and combination of erythropoietin with hydroxyurea (4)[B]
- For infections prior to culture results (3), prescribe an antibiotic(s) that covers *S. pneumoniae*, *H. influenzae*, *Mycoplasma pneumoniae*, and *Chlamydia pneumoniae*—for example, ceftriaxone and azithromycin. If osteomyelitis, cover for *Staphylococcus aureus* and *Salmonella*—for example, ciprofloxacin. If the patient has an apparent pneumonia not promptly responding to antibiotics, consider diagnosis of acute chest syndrome and consider simple transfusions or exchange transfusion.
- Prophylactic penicillin is indicated in all infants and children starting at 2 months (2,4)[A]: 2–6 months of age: 62.5 mg b.i.d. 6 months–3 years: 125 mg b.i.d. 3–5 years: 250 mg b.i.d. If no pneumococcal infections and no splenectomy, stop at 6 years; if high risk remains, continue until puberty. Alternative penicillin, benzathine IM 300,000 U/mo, ages 4 months–3 years, then 600,000 U/mo for 3–5 years. Rising pneumococcal resistance to penicillin may change future recommendations.
- Precautions: Avoid high-dose estrogen oral contraceptives; consider Depo-Provera.

Second Line
- Other nonsteroidal anti-inflammatory drugs (NSAIDs)
- Folic acid supplements (2,3)[C]: 0–6 months: 0.1 mg/d; 6–12 months: 0.25 mg/d; 1–2 years: 0.5 mg/d; >2 years of age 1 mg/d

ADDITIONAL TREATMENT
- Blood transfusions carry risk of iron overload, resulting in damage to heart, liver, and other organs. Consider chelation with Deferasirox, an oral agent, if transfusion therapy is necessary. This medication can be used in people older than 2.

- Transfusion needed with aplastic crises, severe complications (i.e., CVA), prophylactically before surgery, and as part of treatment for acute chest syndrome. However, there is a dearth of randomized trials in this area.

General Measures
- Infections/fever: Treat with antibiotics.
- Minimize factors that enhance sickling.
- Painful crises: Hydration, analgesics; oxygen regardless of whether the patient is hypoxic
- Transfusion needed with aplastic crises, severe complications (i.e., CVA), before surgery, and as treatment for acute chest syndrome
- Retinal evaluation starting at school age to detect proliferative sickle retinopathy
- Occupational therapy, cognitive and behavioral therapies, support groups
- Special immunizations (2,3)[B]:
  – Influenza vaccine yearly starting at age 2
  – Heptavalent conjugated pneumococcal vaccine at 2, 4, 6 months; booster at 15 months, 2 years, 5 years
  – 23-valent pneumococcal vaccine at 2 years; booster at age 5; always separate this by 8 weeks from heptavalent vaccine
- Meningococcal vaccine >2 years of age

Additional Therapies
Physical therapy to include heat, massage, and exercise

COMPLEMENTARY AND ALTERNATIVE MEDICINE
Nicosan: This is an herbal treatment in early trials in the US. Nicosan has been used to prevent sickle crises in Nigeria.

SURGERY/OTHER PROCEDURES
Gene therapy experimental. Approaches under consideration: Replacement with a normal gene and attempts to inactivate Hgb S while reactivating Hgb F (fetal hemoglobin)

IN-PATIENT CONSIDERATIONS
Admission Criteria
Severe pain, suspected infection or sepsis
IV Fluids
The preferred maintenance IV fluid is 1/2 NS, as NS may theoretically increase the risk of sickling.
Nursing
- Psychosocial support
- Education about disease

 ONGOING CARE

FOLLOW-UP RECOMMENDATIONS
Bed rest with crises

Patient Monitoring
- Treat infections early. Parents and patients should be instructed that a temperature of ≥101°F (38.3°C) requires immediate medical attention.
- For patients who receive chronic transfusions, monitor for hepatitis and hemosiderosis.
- Begin periodic eye evaluations at age 5 to detect proliferative sickle retinopathy (2,3)[C].

DIET
Folic acid supplementation, avoid alcohol (leads to dehydration), maintain hydration

PATIENT EDUCATION
Sicklecellkids.org—Education Web site for children with sickle cell anemia: http://www.sicklecelldisease.org
American Sickle Cell Anemia Association: http://www.ascaa.org

PROGNOSIS
- In 2nd decade of life, fewer crises, but complications are more frequent. Median age of death is 42 for men and 48 for women. Common causes are infections, thrombosis, pulmonary emboli, pulmonary hypertension, and renal failure.
- Children become anemic in infancy and begin to have sickle cell crises at 1–2 years of age; some children die in their 1st year.

COMPLICATIONS
- Alloimmunization, bone infarct, aseptic necrosis of femoral head
- Cerebrovascular accidents (peak age 6–7), decreased intelligence, even without stroke
- Cholelithiasis/abnormal liver function
- Chronic leg ulcers, poor wound healing
- Impotence, priapism, hematuria/hyposthenuria, renal concentrating and acidifying defects
- Retinopathy, splenic infarction (by 10 years of age)
- Acute chest syndrome (infection/infarction) leading to chronic pulmonary disease
- Infections (pneumonia, osteomyelitis, meningitis, pyelonephritis); sepsis (leading cause of morbidity and mortality)
- Hemosiderosis (secondary to multiple transfusions). Substance abuse related to chronic pain.

REFERENCES
1. Marti-Carvajal AJ, Conterno LO, Kinght-Madden JM. Antibiotics for treating acute chest syndrome in people with sickle cell disease. *Cochrane Database of Systematic Reviews* 2007, Issue 2.
2. Section on Hematology/Oncology Committee on Genetics, American Academy of Pediatrics. Health supervision for children with sickle cell disease. *Pediatrics*. 2002;109:526–35.
3. National Institutes of Health. *The management of sickle cell disease*, 4th ed. 2002. NH Publ No. 02-2117.
4. Bonds DR. Three decades of innovation in the management of sickle cell disease: the road to understanding the sickle cell disease clinical phenotype. *Blood Rev.* 2005;19:99–110.

See Also (Topic, Algorithm, Electronic Media Element)
Algorithm: Anemia

 CODES

ICD9
- 282.60 Sickle cell disease, unspecified
- 282.61 Hb SS disease without crisis
- 282.62 Hb SS disease with crisis

ANEMIA, SIDEROBLASTIC

Ekaterina Brodski-Quigley, MD

BASICS

DESCRIPTION
A subgroup of myelodysplastic syndromes, characterized by the presence of ringed sideroblasts in the bone marrow and impaired erythropoiesis. Peripheral blood smear may show micro-, macro-, or normocytic red blood cells (RBCs). Severity and course may range from severely progressive to indolent asymptomatic anemia; may be congenital or acquired (acquired is most prevalent in older males).

EPIDEMIOLOGY
- As a group, sideroblastic anemias (SAs) are uncommon, and specific incidence/prevalence is ill defined.
- Acquired forms are more common than hereditary forms (1) and usually occur in older adults; present in 25–30% of alcoholics with anemia, most commonly with folate and B_6 deficiency.
- Several hundred X-linked cases described
- Hereditary forms vary in severity, usually manifesting in childhood.

RISK FACTORS
- Male gender (X-linked SA)
- Family history of hereditary SA
- Chronic alcohol abuse
- Gastric bypass surgery (1 case report) (2)
- Family history of mitochondrial disorders (3,4)

Genetics
- Congenital form, usually X-linked:
  – Defect in aminolevulinic acid synthase (ALAS-2 mutation), the 1st and rate-limiting enzyme in heme biosynthesis
  – With congenital ataxia: hABC7 gene mutations (mitochondrial transport protein)
- Rarely autosomal-dominant or -recessive; gene(s) unknown
- Mitochondrial cytopathy:
  – Heterogeneous, involve deletions in mtDNA (4)
  – Unpredictable maternal inheritance
- See Etiology

GENERAL PREVENTION
Pyridoxine prophylaxis with INH therapy or as maintenance in congenital forms

PATHOPHYSIOLOGY
- Impaired heme biosynthesis within mitochondria
- Ineffective erythropoiesis despite abundance of iron in the body
- Increased gastrointestinal (GI) absorption of iron (Fe overload)
- Enhanced apoptosis in bone marrow
- Possibly, reactive oxygen species play a role.

ETIOLOGY
- Drugs and toxins:
  – Ethanol (related to associated folate and B_6 deficiency)
  – INH
  – Pyrazinamide
  – Chloramphenicol
  – Cycloserine
  – Azathioprine
  – D-penicillamine
  – Zinc toxicity (Cu deficiency)
- Nutritional deficiencies:
  – Pyridoxine deficiency
  – Copper deficiency:
    ○ Postgastrectomy
    ○ Prolonged parenteral nutrition
    ○ Prolonged zinc supplementation
- Hypothermia
- Acquired idiopathic sideroblastic anemia (AISA):
  – Pure sideroblastic anemia (PSA):
    ○ Only the erythroid line affected
  – Refractory anemia with ringed sideroblasts (RARS):
    ○ Myelodysplasia, other cell lines also affected
  – Associated with hematologic malignancies, myeloproliferative disorders
- Other:
  – X-linked
  – Autosomal dominant, recessive, maternal inheritance
  – Mitochondrial cytopathy:
    ○ Wolfram syndrome
    ○ Pearson syndrome
    ○ Kearns-Sayre syndrome (3)
- Disproportionately male, sporadic, mild to severe; kindreds too small to analyze inheritance

COMMONLY ASSOCIATED CONDITIONS
- Alcoholism
- According to mutation, e.g., severe congenital ataxia (hABC7 mutation), pancreatic dysfunction (Pearson syndrome)
- Iron overload or secondary hemochromatosis from transfused blood products
- Rarely, coexisting iron deficiency masks SA.
- Transformation into leukemia rare, 1–2%

DIAGNOSIS

- Often an incidental finding
- Moderate to severe anemia:
  – Fatigue
  – Dizziness or dyspnea
  – Diminished exercise tolerance
  – More symptomatic in older patients with comorbid conditions
- Specific to cause:
  – Pyridoxine deficiency (peripheral neuropathy, dermatitis)
  – Alcoholism
- Manifestations of iron overload

HISTORY
- Toxin, alcohol, or drug exposures
- Family history of anemia or myopathy, especially in men

PHYSICAL EXAM
- No pathognomonic physical findings
- Pallor
- Mild to moderate hepatosplenomegaly at diagnosis in 1/3–1/2 of patients with AISA

DIAGNOSTIC TESTS & INTERPRETATION
Lab
- Complete blood count (CBC):
  – Low mean corpuscular hemoglobin (MCH) and low mean corpuscular hemoglobin concentration (MCHC)
  – Low, normal or high MCV
  – Red cell distribution width (RDW) and hemoglobin (Hgb) highly variable
  – Siderocytes in peripheral smear (occasional)
  – White blood cell (WBC) normal; may be reduced if hypersplenism, myelodysplasia
  – Platelets normal; may be reduced if hypersplenism, myelodysplasia
  – Low reticulocyte count
- Iron studies:
  – Ferritin increased
  – Transferrin saturation increased
  – Serum transferrin decreased
  – Reticuloendothelial iron increased
  – Total iron binding capacity (TIBC) normal
- Erythrogram of peripheral blood is predictive of bone marrow changes.
- Serum copper, ceruloplasmin, serum zinc if suspected as cause
- Liver enzyme derangements possible, depending on cause (EtOH, cirrhosis, Fe overload)
- Folate and B_{12} levels if EtOH-related malnutrition suspected

- Molecular studies identify specific mutations causing hereditary SA syndromes.
- Myelodysplasia: Morphologic and cytogenetic evaluation required for prognosis

Diagnostic Procedures/Surgery
- Bone marrow biopsy confirms diagnosis.
- Liver biopsy is best; test to assess degree of iron overload.
- See Pathological Findings

Pathological Findings
- Bone marrow exam is the key diagnostic modality (1)[C]:
  - Normoblastic erythroid hyperplasia
  - Perls Prussian blue iron stain: Ringed sideroblasts, >10% of erythroblasts with increased number of abnormally large granules ringing the nucleus
  - Electron microscopy: Iron-overloaded mitochondria within erythroblasts
  - Iron-laden macrophages
- Liver biopsy:
  - Iron deposition as in hereditary hemochromatosis
- Micronodular cirrhosis by 3rd, 4th decade

DIFFERENTIAL DIAGNOSIS
- Thalassemias
- Iron deficiency anemia
- Folate or B_{12} deficiency
- Anemia of chronic disease
- Myelodysplastic syndromes
- Lead toxicity with anemia
- Marrow dysplasia secondary to viral or drug toxicity (should be transient)

 TREATMENT

MEDICATION
First Line
- Trial of pyridoxine is indicated because it has few drawbacks and is very beneficial in responsive cases (1)[B]:
  - Pyridoxine 50–100 mg p.o. daily
  - Maintenance: Minimum dose to maintain acceptable Hgb
  - Supplement folate to compensate for increased erythropoiesis if effective.
  - Response likely if SA caused by alcohol abuse, pyridoxine antagonists, or some forms of hereditary X-linked SA
- Chelation therapy for iron overload (1)[B]
- Deferoxamine 40 mg/kg daily in continuous 12–24-hour daily infusions:
  - Limit ascorbate intake to 200 mg daily.
  - Auditory/visual toxicity very rare
- Deferasirox is an oral once-daily iron chelator:
  - No long-term safety data
  - Main complications skin rash, GI upset
- Goal is to maintain serum ferritin <500 μg/L

Second Line
- Myelodysplasia: PSA and RARS
- Treatment considerations as above, although no expected response to pyridoxine
- Some respond to combination of erythropoietin (EPO) and granulocyte colony-stimulating factor (G-CSF) (1)[C].
- Chemotherapeutic agents may have a role.

ADDITIONAL TREATMENT
General Measures
- Treatment is largely supportive:
  - Pyridoxine supplementation improves symptoms in responsive cases (1)[B].
  - Eliminate toxins and causative drugs.
  - Periodic transfusion: Maintain acceptable Hgb to alleviate symptoms and allow normal growth and development (children) (1)[B].
  - Prevent end-organ damage from severe iron overload (1)[B]:
    - Phlebotomy preferred modality if anemia is mild or moderate
- Iron chelation in patients with more severe anemia or requiring more transfusions

Issues for Referral
- Hematology consultation is helpful for diagnosis and management, particularly if no reversible cause is identified.
- Genetic counseling is important for patients with heritable cause of SA.

Additional Therapies
Allogeneic stem cell transplantation has been successful in a few cases in younger patients with myelodysplastic syndromes.

SURGERY/OTHER PROCEDURES
Splenectomy is contraindicated due to frequent postoperative thromboembolic complications.

IN-PATIENT CONSIDERATIONS
Admission Criteria
Generally managed in outpatient settings except for treatment of complications such as congestive heart failure (CHF), dysrhythmias

IV Fluids
RBC transfusion when necessary

 ONGOING CARE

FOLLOW-UP RECOMMENDATIONS
Patient Monitoring
- Yearly ferritin and transferrin saturation to monitor for Fe overload
- Follow response to treatment: Reticulocytosis within 2 weeks, improved Hgb within 1–2 months of response to pyridoxine, and correction of nutritional deficiency or withdrawal of reversible cause

DIET
Address relevant nutritional deficiencies. Address alcohol intake.

PROGNOSIS
- 2 methods of classification of myelodysplastic syndromes: French-American-British (FAB) and World Health Organization (WHO) (5)
- 75% of X-linked SA with ALAS-2 mutations are pyridoxine-responsive.
- Prognosis is better if iron overload is prevented.
- Acquired idiopathic SA:
  - RARS: Median survival 3–6 years, <10% progression to leukemia
  - When only the erythroid line is affected (PSA), course as in age-matched controls, transformation to leukemia not observed
- If SA follows treatment for malignancy, leukemic transformation is common.

COMPLICATIONS
- Iron overload causing organ damage:
  - Cardiac arrhythmia or CHF
  - Hepatic dysfunction
- Transfusion complications

REFERENCES
1. Alcindor T, Bridges KR. Sideroblastic anaemias. Br J Haematol. 2002;116:733–43.
2. Almhanna K, Khan P, Schaldenbrand M et al. Sideroblastic anemia after bariatric surgery. Am J Hematol. 2006;81:155–6.
3. Casas K, et al. Mitochondrial myopathy and sideroblastic anemia. Am J Med Genetics. 2004; 125A:201–4.
4. Matthes T, et al. Different pathophysiological mechanisms of intramitochondrial iron accumulation in acquired and congenital sideroblastic anemia caused by mitochondrial DNA deletion. Eur J Haematol. 2006;77:169–174.
5. Müller-Berndorff H, Haas PS, Kunzmann R et al. Comparison of five prognostic scoring systems, the French-American-British (FAB) and World Health Organization (WHO) classifications in patients with myelodysplastic syndromes: Results of a single-center analysis. Ann Hematol. 2006;85:502–13.

ADDITIONAL READING
Rovó A, Stüssi G, Meyer-Monard S et al. Sideroblastic changes of the bone marrow can be predicted by the erythrogram of peripheral blood. Int J Lab Hematol. 2009.

See Also (Topic, Algorithm, Electronic Media Element)
Algorithms: Anemia, Sideroblastic; Anemia

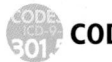 **CODES**

ICD9
285.0 Sideroblastic anemia

ANEURYSM OF THE ABDOMINAL AORTA

James J. Sullivan, Jr., MD, USN
Michael Gray, MD

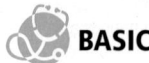

BASICS

DESCRIPTION
- An infrarenal aorta 3 cm in diameter or larger is considered aneurysmal.
- Types:
  - Fusiform aneurysm: Involves the whole circumference or wall of the artery
  - Saccular aneurysm: Does not involve the full circumference, often appears as an asymmetrical bleb or blister on the side of the aorta. Clinical presentation relates to aneurysm location, size, type, and comorbid factors affecting the patient. The majority are asymptomatic. May present with rupture, embolism, or thrombosis. Treatment and indications for surgical repair dictated by risk of rupture, risk of surgical repair, and estimated patient life expectancy.
- System(s) affected: Cardiovascular; Neurologic; Heme/Lymphatic/Immunologic
- Synonym(s): Aortic aneurysms; AAA

Geriatric Considerations
Incidence of AAA, risk of rupture, and operative morbidity and mortality all rise with age.

Pediatric Considerations
AAA in children is rare and may be associated with umbilical artery catheters, connective tissue diseases, arteritides, or congenital abnormalities.

EPIDEMIOLOGY
- Frequency increases >50 years of age
- Predominant sex: Male > Female (5:1)

Incidence
- >15,000 deaths per year in US
- 10th leading cause of death in men 65–75

Prevalence
- Depends on risk factors associated with AAA
- Prevalence of AAAs 2.9–4.9 cm in diameter ranges from 1.3% for men aged 45–54 to up to 12.5% for men aged 75–84 years of age. Data for women are 0% and 5.2%, respectively (1); however, when detected, women presented at an older age and were more likely to present with a ruptured AAA. Female sex is an independent risk factor for death from AAA .

RISK FACTORS
Older age, male, white, family history, smoking, hypertension (HTN), hyperlipidemia, peripheral vascular disease, peripheral aneurysms, chronic obstructive peripheral disease (COPD)

Genetics
- Familial aggregations exist: Aneurysms may develop at an earlier age.
- The frequency of AAA in 1st-degree relatives is 15–19% compared with 1–3% in unrelated patients.
- Marfan syndrome
- Ehlers-Danlos syndrome
- Polycystic kidney disease
- Tuberous sclerosis

GENERAL PREVENTION
- Address cardiovascular disease risk factors.
- Follow screening guidelines.

PATHOPHYSIOLOGY
- Vascular inflammatory degenerative disease with major role of matrix metalloproteinases and inflammatory markers that result in aortic medial degeneration (1)
- Gradual and/or sporadic expansion of aneurysm and accumulation of mural thrombus
- Aneurysms tend to expand over time. (Laplace law: T (wall tension) = pressure × radius. Wall tension directly related to blood pressure and the radius of the artery.) When wall tension exceeds wall tensile strength, rupture occurs.
- Average small AAA (<5.5 cm) grows at a rate of 2.6–3.2 mm/year. Larger aneurysms grew at a faster rate, as did increased tobacco use, but otherwise no identifiable risk factors to assess which small AAAs will advance to require further intervention (2).

ETIOLOGY
- Degenerative: Atherosclerotic (80%)
- Rare causes: Inflammatory diseases; trauma; connective tissue disorders; infection (Brucella, Salmonella, staph, tuberculosis)

COMMONLY ASSOCIATED CONDITIONS
- HTN, myocardial infarction (MI), heart failure, carotid artery, and/or lower extremity peripheral arterial disease
- Screening for thoracic aneurysm should also be considered.

DIAGNOSIS

Screening: Recommended 1-time ultrasound for AAA in men 65–75 years of age who have ever smoked. Men >60 years old who are siblings or offspring of patients with AAA should undergo physical exam and ultrasound screening (1)[B]. US Preventative Services Task Force has recommended against routine screening for women (3):

- Most often asymptomatic: Discovered during exams for other complaints
- Symptomatic: Embolization, thrombosis, vague abdominal or back pain, syncope, lower extremity paralysis
- Rupture

ALERT
- The triad of shock, pulsatile mass, and abdominal pain always suggests rupture of AAA:
  - Shock may be absent if rupture is contained.
  - Palpable pulsatile mass may be absent in up to 50% of the patients with rupture.
  - Pain may radiate to the back, groin, flank, buttocks, or legs.
- Unusual presentations:
  - Primary aortoenteric fistula: Erosion/rupture of AAA into duodenum
  - Aortocaval fistula: Erosion/rupture of AAA into vena cava or left renal vein: 3–6%
  - Inflammatory aneurysm: Encasement by thick inflammatory rind; can cause chronic abdominal pain, weight loss, and elevated erythrocyte sedimentation rate. Surrounding viscera densely adherent.

HISTORY
Abdominal or back pain; AAA risk factors

PHYSICAL EXAM
- Pulsatile supraumbilical mass
- Vague abdominal tenderness: May radiate to the back or flank
- Encroachment by aneurysm:
  - Vertebral body erosion; gastric outlet obstruction; ureteral obstruction
  - Lower extremity ischemia secondary to embolization of mural thrombus
- Rupture leads to tachycardia, hypotension, evidence of shock and anemia, and possible flank contusion (Grey-Turner sign).
- Scrotal sign of Bryant: Painless scrotal ecchymosis a rare manifestation of ruptured AAA.

DIAGNOSTIC TESTS & INTERPRETATION
Lab
Initial lab tests
If rupturing AAA being considered: Complete blood chemistry, chemistries, coags, type and cross, electrocardiogram

Follow-Up & Special Considerations
Evaluation for coronary artery disease is appropriate prior to elective AAA repair (i.e., cardiac clearance).

Imaging
Initial approach
- Ultrasonography: Simplest and least expensive diagnostic procedure
- Multiple studies have demonstrated high sensitivity (94–100%) and specificity (98–100%) of ultrasonographic diagnosis of AAA by emergency physicians.
- Although effective in detecting AAA, it is a poor test to show leakage or rupture if bleeding is into the retroperitoneal space.
- Screening: Ultrasound screening for detection of AAA in male patients, ages 65–75, who have ever smoked and men >60 who are siblings or offspring of patients with AAA
- Surveillance of known asymptomatic aneurysm:
  - <3 cm: No further testing
  - 3–4 cm: Screen annually
  - 4–4.5 cm: Screen every 6 months
  - >4.5 cm: Refer to vascular specialist
- Computed tomography (CT) scans are the preferred pre-op study (caution w/IV contrast in renal failure).
- Magnetic resonance imaging/magnetic resonance angiography can also visualize AAA, but is often not plausible in emergent situations.
- Aortography: Does not define outer dimensions of aneurysm
- Abdominal x-rays can be diagnostic if calcifications exist; not a diagnostic tool of choice
- Indications for vascular imaging:
  - Associated renovascular hypertension
  - Symptoms of visceral angina
  - Significant iliofemoral occlusive disease
  - Peripheral aneurysms
- Horseshoe or pelvic kidney

Diagnostic Procedures/Surgery

ALERT
Use clinical judgment: Patients with known AAA having abdominal or back pain symptoms may be rupturing despite a negative CT scan.

DIFFERENTIAL DIAGNOSIS
- Other abdominal masses
- Other causes of abdominal or back pain (e.g., peptic ulcer disease, renal colic, diverticulitis, appendicitis, incarcerated hernia, gastrointestinal hemorrhage, arthritis, metastatic disease)

TREATMENT

- Emergent treatment in unstable or symptomatic patients is immediate vascular surgery consultation, adequate IV access and resuscitation, type and cross for multiple units, and rapid bedside ultrasound.
- Less acute treatment of AAA and prevention of rupture is elective repair and risk factor modification.

MEDICATION
- Beta-blockers may be initiated to reduce the rate of aneurysm expansion (1)[B].
- Beta-blockers should be used perioperatively in absence of contraindications (1)[A].
- Early studies suggest that statins may be beneficial both perioperatively and to inhibit further expansion.
- Doxycycline, and aspirin may also inhibit expansion, but further studies are needed. Early animal studies indicate a possible role for ACE-I/ARBs, mast cell stabilizers, prostaglandin inhibitors, and novel gene therapy, but no human studies yet (1,2).

ADDITIONAL TREATMENT
General Measures
- Treat atherosclerotic risk factors
- Medical optimization of cardiac, renal, and pulmonary conditions; smoking cessation

SURGERY/OTHER PROCEDURES
Current recommendations (4)[C]:
- Elective:
  - 5.5-cm diameter is the threshold for repair in "average" patient.
  - Younger, low-risk patients with long life expectancy may prefer early repair.
  - Women or AAA with high risk of rupture: Consider elective repair at 4.5–5 cm
  - Consider delayed repair in high-risk patients.
- High risk of rupture:
  - Expansion >0.6 cm/yr
  - Smoking/COPD severe/steroids
  - Family history multiple relatives
  - Hypertension poorly controlled
  - Shape nonfusiform
- High-risk patients for elective repair:
  - Risk factors for open repair include age >70 years, COPD, CRI, suprarenal clamp site with 1-year mortality if 0 risk factors present of 1.2% and 67% for all 4 risk factors present.
  - Other risk factors include inactive/poor stamina, congestive heart failure, significant coronary artery disease, liver disease, and family history of AAA.

- Emergent/symptomatic repair:
  - Traditionally has been open repair; however, candidates with appropriate anatomy can have endovascular repair, with an estimated mortality of 32% for endovascular vs 44% open.
- Open repair vs endovascular repair (EVAR):
  - Open repair indicated in patients who are good or average surgical candidates (1)[B].
  - EVAR for patients at high risk of complication based on cardiopulmonary or other comorbid illness: Periodic long-term surveillance indicated to monitor for endoleak, status of aneurysmal sac, and need for further intervention (1)[B]

IN-PATIENT CONSIDERATIONS
Risk of abdominal compartment syndrome after repair 4–12%; usually associated with large fluid resuscitation

ONGOING CARE

FOLLOW-UP RECOMMENDATIONS
See surveillance recommendations

Patient Monitoring
Blood pressure and fasting lipid values: Control as would for atherosclerotic disease (1)[C]

DIET
Low-fat, low-salt, and low-caffeine diet

PATIENT EDUCATION
Smoking cessation (1)[B], aerobic exercise

PROGNOSIS
- Annual risk of rupture (5):
  - <4 cm diameter: ~0%
  - 4–4.9 cm: ~1%
  - 5–5.9 cm: ~11%
  - 6–6.9 cm: ~26%
  - >7 cm: ~32%
- Patients with AAAs measuring 5.5 cm or larger should undergo repair (1)[B], as should all patients with symptomatic AAA (1)[C].
- Only ~18% of patients with ruptured AAA survive.
- Although there is a 5:1 ratio of AAA between males and females, women have a higher mortality and morbidity associated with AAA, regardless of open or endovascular repair (6).

COMPLICATIONS
- Nonoperative:
  - Rupture, dissection, thromboembolization
- Elective operative (conventional):
  - Death 2–8%
  - All cardiac 10–12% (MI 2–8%)
- Pulmonary 5–10%; renal 5–7%; wound infection >5%; colon ischemia 1%; spinal cord ischemia <1%

REFERENCES

1. Hirsch AT, et al. ACC/AHA 2005 Practice Guidelines for Management of Patients With Peripheral Arterial Disease: A Collaborative Report. *Circulation*. 2006;113:e563–e601.
2. Baxter BT, et al. Medical management of small abdominal aortic aneurysms. *Circulation*. 2008;117(14):1883–9.
3. U.S. Preventive Services Task Force. Screening for Abdominal Aortic Aneurysm. *Ann Intern Med*. 2005;142:198–202.
4. Brewster DC, Cronenwett JL, Hallett JW et al. Guidelines for the treatment of abdominal aortic aneurysms. Report of a subcommittee of the Joint Council of the American Association for Vascular Surgery and Society for Vascular Surgery. *J Vasc Surg*. 2003;37:1106–17.
5. Lederle FA, Johnson GR, Wilson SE et al. Rupture rate of large abdominal aortic aneurysms in patients refusing or unfit for elective repair. *JAMA*. 2002;287:2968–72.
6. Abedi NN, Davenport DL, Xenos E et al. Gender and 30-day outcome in patients undergoing endovascular aneurysm repair (EVAR): An analysis using the ACS NSQIP dataset. *J Vasc Surg*. 2009.

ADDITIONAL READING

- Fleming C, Whitlock EP, Beil TL et al. Screening for abdominal aortic aneurysm: a best-evidence systematic review for the U.S. Preventive Services Task Force. *Ann Intern Med*. 2005;142:203–11.
- Hamerlynck JV, Legemate DA, Hooft L et al. [From the Cochrane Library: ultrasonographic screening for abdominal aortic aneurysm in men aged 65 years and older: low risk of fatal aneurysm rupture] *Ned Tijdschr Geneeskd*. 2008;152:747–9.

See Also (Topic, Algorithm, Electronic Media Element)
Aortic Dissection; Thoracic Aneurysms; Ehlers-Danlos; Giant Cell Arteritis; Marfan Syndrome; Polyarteritis Nodosa; Turner Syndrome

CODES

ICD9
- 441.3 Abdominal aneurysm, ruptured
- 441.4 Abdominal aneurysm without mention of rupture

CLINICAL PEARLS
- Major risk factors: Smoking, HTN, hyperlipidemia, family history, male gender, age
- Triad of hypotension/shock, pulsatile abdominal mass, and abdominal/back pain always suggests rupture, which requires emergent evaluation for surgery.
- 5.5 cm is the threshold diameter for elective surgical treatment (with some exceptions).
- Ultrasound is the procedure of choice for screening and initial diagnosis.

ANGINA PECTORIS, STABLE

Balakumar Pandian, MD

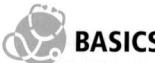 **BASICS**

DESCRIPTION
* Predictable and reproducible chest discomfort that occurs in a consistent pattern at a certain level of exertion or emotional stress and is relieved with rest or sublingual nitroglycerin
* Definitions:
  – Typical angina: A sense of choking or of pressure or heaviness deep to the precordium, frequently radiating to the jaw, arms, or epigastrium; usually brought on by exertion or anxiety and relieved by rest. Discomfort may be described with a clenched fist over the sternum (Levine sign).
  – Anginal equivalent: Occasionally, patients with angina will present without chest discomfort, but with nonspecific symptoms such as dyspnea, fatigue, belching, nausea, lightheadedness, indigestion
* Unstable angina: Anginal symptoms that are new or are changed in character to become more frequent, more severe, or both. Considered an acute coronary syndrome in the same continuum as non-ST segment elevation myocardial infarction (NSTEMI).
* System(s) affected: Cardiovascular

Geriatric Considerations
Elderly patients may present with atypical anginal symptoms. Maintain a high degree of suspicion during evaluation. They may also be very sensitive to the side effects of medications.

Pregnancy Considerations
Other diagnoses should be excluded and the patient managed closely by an obstetrician or family physician and cardiologist; the metabolic demands of pregnancy can exacerbate symptoms and directly interfere with treatment.

EPIDEMIOLOGY
* Predominant age: Most common in middle age and older men, postmenopausal women
* Predominant sex: Male > Female

Incidence
~500,000 new cases of stable angina occur yearly in the United States.

Prevalence
More than 10 million people in the United States suffer from angina.

RISK FACTORS
Risk factors for coronary artery disease include:
* Family history of premature CAD in 1st-degree relatives (in male relatives <55 yrs old or female relatives <65 yrs old)
* Obesity
* Hypercholesterolemia
* Elevated blood pressure
* Cigarette smoking
* Diabetes mellitus
* Male gender
* Advanced age

GENERAL PREVENTION
* Stop smoking.
* Low-fat/low-cholesterol diet
* Regular aerobic exercise program
* Weight loss (goal BMI <25)
* Blood pressure control (goal BP <140/90)
* Antilipidemics if indicated by current ATP guidelines or a risk-based approach
* Optimize glycemic control in those with diabetes mellitus.

PATHOPHYSIOLOGY
* Anginal symptoms occur during times of myocardial ischemia caused by a mismatch between coronary artery perfusion and myocardial oxygen demand. Sensory nerves from the heart travel up the sympathetic chain and enter the spinal cord at levels C7-T4, causing diffuse referred pain/discomfort in the associated dermatomes.
* Atherosclerotic narrowing of the coronary arteries (stenosis of >70%) is the most common pathology. Angina may occur in those with significant aortic valve disease or hypertrophic cardiomyopathy, even with normal coronary arteries.

ETIOLOGY
* Atherosclerosis of the coronary arteries (most common)
* Aortic stenosis
* Hypertrophic cardiomyopathy
* Aortic insufficiency
* Primary pulmonary HTN

COMMONLY ASSOCIATED CONDITIONS
* Hypercholesterolemia
* Peripheral vascular disease
* Hypertension
* Overweight
* Diabetes mellitus

Dx **DIAGNOSIS**

* Predictable and reproducible anginal symptoms lasting 3–15 minutes brought on by exertion, emotional stress, meals, cold air, or smoking; symptoms relieved by rest or nitrates
* Careful history is important in eliciting symptoms of angina as listed above.
* Dyspnea on exertion may present as the only symptom.
* Atypical symptoms more likely in women, elderly, and diabetic patients.
* Canadian Cardiovascular Society grading of chronic stable angina severity:
  – Class 1: Ordinary physical activity does not cause angina; angina with strenuous or rapid or prolonged exertion
  – Class 2: Slight limitation of ordinary activity (walking rapidly or >2 blocks, climbing >1 flight of stairs, emotional stress)
  – Class 3: Marked limitation of ordinary physical activity.
  – Class 4: Inability to carry on any physical activity without discomfort. Angina may occur at rest.

HISTORY
* Quality of any previous anginal episodes and pattern over time
* Underlying history of heart disease or valvular disease
* Family history of myocardial infarction, CAD, sudden death

PHYSICAL EXAM
* Measure vital signs such as blood pressure, heart rate, respiratory rate, and oxygen saturation.
* Cardiac exam may reveal dysrhythmias, heart murmurs indicative of valvular disease, signs of ventricular hypertrophy, gallops, or signs of congestive heart failure.
* Vascular exam may show signs of peripheral vascular disease (diminished pulses, bruits, abdominal aneurysm)
* Pulmonary exam may reveal signs of obstructive or restrictive diseases, pulmonary edema
* May see signs of dyslipidemia (xanthomas, xantholesma)
* Normal physical exam should not exclude cardiac causes of anginal symptoms.

DIAGNOSTIC TESTS & INTERPRETATION
* ECG:
  – May show evidence of prior myocardial infarction. However, ECG is frequently unremarkable when asymptomatic. May show signs of myocardial ischemia during symptomatic episodes.
  – Bundle branch block, Wolff Parkinson White syndrome, or intraventricular conduction delay may make stress ECG interpretation unreliable.
* Stress testing (exercise testing preferable):
  – Exercise testing for those who can physically exercise (≥5 METS):
    ○ Standard exercise ECG for those with normal baseline ECG
    ○ Exercise stress testing with echocardiography or perfusion imaging for those with abnormal baseline ECG or in premenopausal women
  – In patients who cannot tolerate exercise, pharmacologic stress testing with adenosine, regadenoson, or dipyridamole. Dobutamine preferred if asthma or heart block (2° or 3°).
* Coronary angiography is the gold standard for confirmation and delineation of coronary disease and direction of interventional therapy or surgery.

Lab
* Total cholesterol and low-density lipoprotein (LDL) may be elevated and high-density lipoprotein (HDL) cholesterol may be reduced.
* CRP: Most useful for those individuals at intermediate risk of developing coronary artery disease (10–20% over 10 years by Framingham risk criteria) in whom an elevated CRP may suggest an increased likelihood of benefit from statin therapy

Initial lab tests
Hematocrit, fasting lipid profile, fasting blood sugar, basic metabolic panel

Imaging
* Consider echocardiogram if valvular disease or hypertrophic cardiomyopathy is suspected.
* Stress imaging with echocardiogram or perfusion imaging (see section on stress testing)
* Consider chest radiography if signs of pulmonary disease

DIFFERENTIAL DIAGNOSIS
- Pulmonary disease
- Deconditioning

TREATMENT
MEDICATION
First Line
- Anti-ischemic (anti-anginal) medications:
  – Beta blockers decrease heart rate, blood pressure, and myocardial contractility:
    ○ Atenolol (25–100 mg/d), metoprolol (25–100 mg b.i.d.)
    ○ Adjust doses according to clinical response. Aim to maintain resting heart rate of 50–60 beats per minute.
    ○ Side effects may include fatigue, exercise intolerance, erectile dysfunction, bradycardia, or heart block.
    ○ Contraindications include decompensated CHF, severe bradycardia, advanced AV block, or severe lung disease.
  – Nitrates dilate systemic veins and arteries (including coronary vessels) and cause decreased afterload and increased myocardial flow:
    ○ Sublingual nitroglycerin 0.4 mg SL. For acute anginal episodes. Repeat 2–3 times over a 10–15 minute period; if no relief, immediate medical attention must be sought.
    ○ Long–acting nitrates: Should be used with a drug–free interval of 8–12 hours to prevent tolerance. Side effects such as headaches and hypotension tend to clear with continued usage.
    ○ Concurrent use of phosphodiesterase inhibitors for erectile dysfunction (e.g. sildenafil, vardenafil, tadalafil) may cause life-threatening hypotension and are contraindicated.
  – Calcium channel blockers (CCB) cause arterial vasodilation, decrease myocardial oxygen demand, and improve coronary blood flow. Only long-acting CCBs should be used:
    ○ Dihydropyridine CCBs such as nifedipine (30–90 mg/d), amlodipine (5–10 mg/d), or felodipine (2.5–10 mg/d) cause more vasodilation. Nondihydropyridine CCBs such as diltiazem (120–480 mg/d) or verapamil (120–480 mg/d). Amlodipine preferred in patients with low ejection fraction.
    ○ Side effects include constipation and peripheral edema. The nondihydropyridine CCBs may also cause bradycardia, heart block, and precipitate heart failure in those with severe systolic dysfunction.
  – Ranolazine (500–1000 mg b.i.d.) likely works by improving left ventricular function, although the exact mechanisms are unclear:
    ○ Use as adjunctive therapy in those who are still symptomatic on optimal doses of β-blockers, nitrates, or amlodipine
    ○ Side effects may include nausea, constipation, dizziness, and headache.
    ○ Contraindications include combination with nondihydropyridine calcium channel blockers, prolonged QT, and medications that inhibit cytochrome P-450 system.

- Vasculoprotective therapies:
  – Antiplatelet therapy is indicated in all patients:
    ○ Aspirin (81–325 mg/d) is preferred
    ○ Clopidogrel (75 mg/d) may be used in patients with contraindications to aspirin.
    ○ Combination of aspirin and clopidogrel is indicated for those with stent placement to reduce rate of stent thrombosis (1 month for bare metal stents and $\geq$12 months for drug eluting stents)
  – Statins (e.g., simvastatin, atorvastatin, pravastatin, lovastatin) for hypercholesterolemia:
    ○ Most beneficial as secondary prevention in those with CAD. Decrease incidence of symptomatic CAD and reduce both myocardial infarction and death from MI.
    ○ LDL target <100 mg/dL for established CAD. Consider target <70 in high-risk patients.
    ○ Current ATP guidelines support using lipid-lowering drugs for those with suspected or documented CAD.
    ○ Side effects may include elevated transaminases, myalgias. May rarely cause myositis or rhabdomyolysis. Monitor labs with any changes in medication doses.
  – ACE inhibitors have been shown to reduce both cardiovascular death and MI. Indicated in patients with CAD or other vascular disease (1)[B], particularly in those with diabetes or left ventricular (LV) systolic dysfunction (1)[A]:
    ○ Angiotensin receptor blockers may be used in patients intolerant of ACE inhibitors.

ADDITIONAL TREATMENT
General Measures
Lifestyle modifications are very important:
- Blood pressure control
- Smoking cessation
- Minimize emotional stress
- Weight reduction in obese patients (2)[C]
- Daily physical activity (30–60 minutes) (3)[C]
- Annual influenza vaccination (3)[C]

COMPLEMENTARY AND ALTERNATIVE MEDICINE
Relaxation/stress reduction therapy may help reduce anginal episodes.

SURGERY/OTHER PROCEDURES
- Revascularization therapies: Consider if optimal medication management is inadequate in controlling symptoms:
  – Percutaneous coronary intervention (PCI):
    ○ Balloon angioplasty
    ○ Stent placement (with drug eluting or bare metal stent)
  – Coronary artery bypass grafting (CABG)
- For refractory angina (4):
  – Spinal cord stimulation
  – Enhanced external counterpulsation
  – Myocardial laser revascularization therapy

IN-PATIENT CONSIDERATIONS
Admission Criteria
Inpatient evaluation is warranted in any patient with new changes in their angina symptoms.

ONGOING CARE
FOLLOW-UP RECOMMENDATIONS
Lifestyle modifications should be stressed at every visit.

Patient Monitoring
Changes in severity or frequency of anginal symptoms need further evaluation.

DIET
Low-fat, low-cholesterol, low-salt diet

PROGNOSIS
Variable; depends on severity of symptoms, the extent of CAD, and LV function

COMPLICATIONS
- Unstable angina or myocardial infarction
- Arrhythmia
- Cardiac arrest
- Congestive heart failure (CHF)

REFERENCES
1. Yusuf S, Sleight P, Pogue J, Bosch J, Davies R, Dagenais G et al. Effects of an angiotensin-converting-enzyme inhibitor, ramipril, on cardiovascular events in high-risk patients. The Heart Outcomes Prevention Evaluation Study Investigators. *N Engl J Med*. 2000;342:145–53.
2. Gibbons RJ, et al. Committee on the Management of patients with chronic stable angina. ACC/AHA 2002 guideline update for the management of patients with chronic stable angina—summary article: a report of the American College of Cardiology/American Heart Association Task Force on Practice Guidelines. *Circulation*. 2003;107: 149–58.
3. Fraker TD, Fihn SD writing on behalf of the 2002 Chronic Stable Angina Writing Committee. 2007 Chronic Angina Focused Update of the ACC/AHA 2002 Guidelines for the Management of Patients with Chronic Stable Angina. *Circulation*. 2007; 116:2762–2772.
4. Khan SN, Dutka DP. A systematic approach to refractory angina. *Current Opinion in Supportive and Palliative Care*. 2008;2:247–251.

See Also (Topic, Algorithm, Electronic Media Element)
Algorithms: Chest Pain; Chest Pain/Acute Coronary Syndrome

CODES

ICD9
413.9 Other and unspecified angina pectoris

CLINICAL PEARLS
- Careful history taking is important in diagnosis, especially in the elderly.
- Maximize antianginal therapy by combining β blockers, CCB, and nitrates in those still symptomatic with monotherapy.
- Exercise testing may be useful diagnostically and to assess effectiveness of antianginal therapy.

ANGIOEDEMA

Michelle T. Martin, PharmD
Jamie Berkes, MD

 BASICS

DESCRIPTION

- Angioedema (AE) is an acute, localized swelling of skin, mucosa, and submucosa caused by extravasation of fluid into the affected tissues.
- Often resolves in hours to days but can be life-threatening if the upper airway is involved
- Usually involves the face, tongue, larynx, GI tract, and extremities
- Causes:
  - Idiopathic
  - Medications such as angiotensin-converting enzyme (ACE) inhibitors
  - Allergens such as foods, latex, or venom
  - Physical elements such as vibration or cold
- Hereditary AE (HAE) and acquired AE (AAE) are diseases of the complement cascade that result in recurrent episodes of AE of the skin, upper airway, and GI tract.
- System(s) affected: Skin/Exocrine
- Synonym(s): Angioneurotic edema; Quincke edema

EPIDEMIOLOGY

- Predominant age:
  - Allergen, medication, or other triggers can affect all ages.
  - HAE: Infancy to 2nd decade of life
  - AAE: Typically patients in 4th decade of life
- Predominant gender: Male = Female (except type III HAE affects more women than men)

Incidence

25% of ACE inhibitor–induced AE cases will occur within the 1st month of taking the medication; however, they are not limited to this period.

Prevalence

- AE occurs in about 15% of the population over a lifetime.
- AE: 0.1–2.2% of patients receiving ACE inhibitors: African Americans have a 4–5 times greater risk of ACE inhibitor–induced AE than Caucasians.
- HAE: 1:10,000–50,000 population in US

RISK FACTORS

- Consuming medications and foods that can cause allergic reactions
- Preexisting diagnosis of HAE or AAE

Genetics

- HAE types I and II are autosomal dominant, whereas type III is dominant X-linked.
- HAE occurs in 25% of patients as a result of spontaneous genetic mutations.

GENERAL PREVENTION

- Avoid known triggers.
- Avoid ACE inhibitors in patients with a history of AE.
- Do not use ACE inhibitors in patients with C1 esterase inhibitor (C1 INH) deficiency.

PATHOPHYSIOLOGY

- Type 1 hypersensitivity reaction
- Increase in vascular permeability secondary to IgE-mediated mast cell–stimulated histamine release or from activation of the complement system and an elevation in bradykinin (HAE)

- Attacks of HAE are triggered by prolonged mechanical pressure, cold, heat, trauma, emotional stress, menses, illness, and inflammation.
  - Type I HAE is the most common form, caused by decreased production of C1 esterase inhibitor (C1 INH), and has autosomal-dominant inheritance.
  - Type II HAE has functionally impaired C1 INH and autosomal-dominant inheritance.
  - Type III HAE involves an X-linked factor XII gene mutation (often estrogen-dependent, associated with estrogen administration).
- AAE is a rare condition.
  - Type I is associated with lymphoproliferative diseases or paraneoplastic diseases.
  - Type II is due to autoimmune disorders (anti-C1 INH antibody).
  - Affected patients have circulating antibodies directed either against specific immunoglobulins expressed on B cells (type I) or against C1 INH (type II).

ETIOLOGY

- Idiopathic
- Medication-induced:
  - ACE inhibitors cause 10–25% of AE cases, mostly occurring within the first 3–4 weeks of use of the medication. However, onset may be delayed years.
  - Angiotensin-receptor blockers (ARBs) also can cause AE, but more rarely than ACE inhibitors.
- Allergic triggers:
  - Food allergens such as shellfish, nuts, eggs, milk, wheat, soy
  - Medications such as aspirin, nonsteroidal anti-inflammatory drugs (NSAIDs), antibiotics, narcotics, and oral contraceptives
- Physically induced: Cold, heat, pressure, vibration, trauma, emotional stress, ultraviolet light
- Hereditary or acquired C1 INH deficiency
- Thyroid autoimmune disease–associated AE

COMMONLY ASSOCIATED CONDITIONS

- Quincke disease (AE of the uvula)
- Urticaria

 DIAGNOSIS

HISTORY

- Identify potential triggers, including medication history, recent exposure to allergens, physical elements, or trauma (1)[C].
- In comparison with urticaria, AE typically is nonpruritic, but it can cause a burning sensation.
- Obtain family medical history.

PHYSICAL EXAM

- Acute onset of asymmetric localized swelling, usually of the face (eyelids, lips, ears, nose) and less often of the extremities or genitalia
- GI tract involvement may manifest as intermittent unexplained abdominal pain.

ALERT

10–35% of patients present with severe respiratory compromise requiring endotracheal intubation.

DIAGNOSTIC TESTS & INTERPRETATION

Lab

Initial lab tests

- If AE with urticaria and/or anaphylaxis, check for allergen-specific IgE to verify suspected trigger. Serum tryptase is elevated during acute AE (1)[C].
- Without a clear etiology and recurrence in AE and urticaria, check complete blood count (CBC) and erythrocyte sedimentation rate (ESR).
  - Macrocytosis implies a pernicious anemia.
  - Eosinophilia may imply atopy or, rarely, a parasitic infection.
  - Elevated ESR may imply systemic disorders (1)[C].
- In recurrent AE without a clear etiology and without urticaria, consider ordering serum C4 level determination.
  - Low serum C4 is a sensitive but nonspecific screening test for hereditary and acquired C1 INH deficiency.
  - If C4 is normal, determine C1 INH level and function, and recheck C4 during an acute attack.
  - If C4 level and C1 INH level and function are still normal, consider other causes (i.e., medications or HAE type III) for AE (2)[C].
  - If C4 level, C1 INH level, and C1 INH function are low, this indicates HAE type I.
  - HAE type II is characterized by low C4 and low C1 INH function, but C1 INH level can be normal or elevated (2)[C].
  - C1q is decreased in AAE but normal in all types of HAE (2)[C].

Follow-Up & Special Considerations

If C4 and C1q are low (as in AAE), neoplastic and autoimmune workup is warranted. CBC, a peripheral smear, protein electrophoresis, immunophenotyping of lymphocytes, and imaging studies are often undertaken to rule out hematologic malignancies or cancer (2)[C].

Imaging

Initial approach

- Abdominal radiographs and CT scan can demonstrate GI angioedema or ileus.
- C1 INH deficiency may occur in association with internal malignancy, so angioedema rarely can be a paraneoplastic disease. Imaging (CT scan, radiography, etc) then would be done as part of a neoplastic workup for patients with AAE.

Diagnostic Procedures/Surgery

Skin biopsy (may be nonspecific)

Pathological Findings

- Edema of deep dermis and subcutaneous tissue
- Variable perivascular and interstitial infiltrate

DIFFERENTIAL DIAGNOSIS

- Urticaria (with AE in 40–50% of patients)
- Allergic contact dermatitis
- Connective-tissue disease: Lupus, dermatomyositis
- Anaphylaxis
- Cellulitis, erysipelas
- Lymphedema
- Diffuse subcutaneous infiltrative process

TREATMENT

MEDICATION

First Line

- Acute allergic AE (with airway compromise):
  - Epinephrine 1:1,000, 0.3 mL IV or SC (1)[C]
  - Glucocorticoids (hydrocortisone 200 mg IV or Solu-Medrol 40 mg IV) (1)[C]
  - Diphenhydramine 50 mg IV
  - If medication-induced, stop the causative agent.
- Idiopathic recurrent AE:
  - 1st-generation antihistamines for acute AE (cause drowsiness)
  - Older children and adults: Hydroxyzine (Vistaril 5 mg/5 mL, 25-mg tablets) 10–25 mg t.i.d., or diphenhydramine (Benadryl) 25–50 mg q6h (3)[C]
  - Children <6 years of age: Diphenhydramine 12.5 mg (elixir) q6–8h (5 mg/kg/d) (3)[C]
  - 2nd-generation H_1 blockers: Fexofenadine (Allegra) 180 mg/d b.i.d., loratadine (Claritin) 10 mg/d, cetirizine (Zyrtec) 10 mg/d, desloratadine (Clarinex) 5 mg/d (3)[C]; use with caution in pregnancy and in the elderly.
- HAE chronic prophylaxis:
  - A nanofiltered plasma-derived C1 INH concentrate (Cinryze) is dosed at 1,000 units/10 mL IV at a rate of 1 mL/min (for 10 min) q3–7d (4)[B].
  - Attenuated androgens increase hepatic production of C1 INH: Danazol 50–200 mg/d or stanozolol 2–4 mg/d; danazol maximum dose 600 mg/d; use lowest effective dose. Side effects include headache, weight gain, liver dysfunction, hirsutism, and menstrual disturbances. Monitor CBC, liver function tests (LFTs), fasting lipid profile (FLP), and urinalysis every 6 months. Danazol is not to be used in children, during first 2 trimesters of pregnancy, during lactation, and in patients with prostate cancer (2)[C].
- HAE short-term prophylaxis:
  - Minor procedures (dental work): If C1 INH is available, no prophylaxis; otherwise: danazol 10 mg/kg/d (maximum 600 mg/d) or tranexamic acid [not approved by the Food and Drug Administration (FDA) in US] 75 mg/kg/d divided b.i.d. or t.i.d. × 4–5 days prior to and 2–4 days after event (2)[C]
  - Major procedures (including intubation): C1 INH 1 h prior with an additional dose on hand during procedure or 1–4 units fresh-frozen plasma (FFP) 1 day prior (for an adult)
- Acute HAE treatment:
  - C1 INH concentrate IV, dosed at 1,000 units if <50 kg; 1,500 units if 50–100 kg; 2,000 units if >100 kg (2)[C]; a pasteurized human plasma–derived C1 INH concentrate (Berinert P), dosed at 20 units/kg (available in 500 units/10 mL, to be infused at a maximum rate of 4 mL/min IV. Worsening of HAE pain was reported as the most severe adverse event (4,5)[B].
  - Kalbitor (Ecallantide), a kallikrein inhibitor, is dosed in patients ≥16 years old at 30 mg SC with 3 separate 10 mg/mL injections in the abdomen, thigh, or upper arm, and a 2nd 30-mg dose may be repeated within 24 h if needed. Injection-site rotation is not necessary but must be 2 in away from site of the attack. Anaphylaxis is a potential adverse event (4)[B].
  - Antihistamines and glucocorticoids typically do not benefit HAE patients.

- New therapies are in phase 3 clinical trials for HAE treatment:
  - A bradykinin receptor-2 antagonist (icatibant), dosed SC, was not approved by the FDA for use in the US in April 2008 and is currently undergoing further clinical trials. It was approved in the European Union under the trade name Firazyr (4)[C].
  - Other C1 INH replacement therapies, including a recombinant C1 INH isolated from the milk of transgenic rabbits (Rhucin), dosed IV (6)[C]
  - Cinryze is awaiting FDA approval for use during acute attacks (4)[C].
- Acute AAE treatment:
  - C1 INH concentrate and FFP
  - Treatment of underlying lymphoproliferative disease is often curative in AAE type I.
  - Immunosuppressive therapy to suppress antibody production
  - Clinical trials underway with recombinant human C1 INH (Rhucin) (4)[C]

Second Line

- HAE chronic prophylaxis: If patient cannot tolerate attenuated androgens, antifibrinolytic agents (plasmin inhibitors), such as tranexamic acid (not FDA approved in US) and ϵ-aminocaproic acid could be used. They are less effective than attenuated androgens and have many side effects. On rare occasions, they have been linked to (but not proven to cause) thrombophlebitis, embolism, or myositis (6).
- Acute HAE: FFP if C1 INH concentrate is not available, but it can potentially worsen attack (6).
- Idiopathic AE: Doxepin (Sinequan) may be effective for AE (10–25 mg at bedtime).
- H2RA: Ranitidine (Zantac) 150 mg/d b.i.d.

ADDITIONAL TREATMENT

General Measures

Intubation if airway is threatened

SURGERY/OTHER PROCEDURES

Tracheostomy if progressive laryngeal edema prevents endotracheal intubation

IN-PATIENT CONSIDERATIONS

Initial Stabilization

Ensure patent airway. If anaphylaxis, epinephrine (1:1,000) SC 0.3–0.5 mg q10–15min

IV Fluids

Given if needed to stabilize patient

ONGOING CARE

FOLLOW-UP RECOMMENDATIONS

Patient Monitoring

- Diagnostic workup if symptoms are severe, persistent, or recurrent
- Protect airway if mouth, tongue, or throat is involved.

DIET

Avoid known dietary allergens.

PATIENT EDUCATION

Educate on avoidance of triggers (i.e., food, medication, other physical stimuli), types of treatment, when to seek emergency care, and wearing Medic Alert bracelet.

PROGNOSIS

- AE symptoms often resolve in hours to 2–3 days. If airway is compromised, AE can be life-threatening.
- Patients with HAE have an average of 20 attacks/year; each may last 3–5 days. Prophylaxis can decrease the frequency of events and number of missed days of school or work.

COMPLICATIONS

Anaphylaxis

REFERENCES

1. Temiño VM, Peebles RS. The spectrum and treatment of angioedema. *Am J Med*. 2008;121:282–6.
2. Bowen T, Cicardi M, Farkas H et al. Canadian 2003 International Consensus Algorithm For the Diagnosis, Therapy, and Management of Hereditary Angioedema. *J Allergy Clin Immunol*. 2004;114:629–37.
3. Frigas E, Park M. Idiopathic recurrent angioedema. *Immunol Allergy Clin North Am*. 2006;26:739–51.
4. Levy JH, Freiberger DJ, Roback J et al. Hereditary angioedema: current and emerging treatment options. *Anesth Analg*. 2010;110:1271–80.
5. Craig TJ, Levy RJ, Wasserman RL, Bewtra AK, Hurewitz D, Obtuowicz K, Reshef A, Ritchie B, Moldovan D, Shirov T, Grivcheva-Panovska V, Kiessling PC, Keinecke HO, Bernstein JA et al. Efficacy of human C1 esterase inhibitor concentrate compared with placebo in acute hereditary angioedema attacks. *J Allergy Clin Immunol*. 2009;124:801–8.
6. Craig T, Riedl M, Dykewicz MS, Gower RG, Baker J, Edelman FJ, Hurewitz D, Jacobs J, Kalfus I et al. When is prophylaxis for hereditary angioedema necessary? *Ann Allergy Asthma Immunol*. 2009;102:366–72.

See Also (Topic, Algorithm, Electronic Media Element)

Urticaria; Anaphylaxis

CODES

ICD9

995.1 Angioneurotic edema, not elsewhere classified

CLINICAL PEARLS

- Trigger identification and avoidance are key in the prevention of AE.
- New AE treatments are in development.
- Patients with a history of allergies and angioedema should be prescribed an epinephrine autoinjector.

ANKLE FRACTURES

Francesca L. Beaudoin, MS, MD
Kimberly Pringle, MD

 BASICS

- Bones: Tibia, fibula, talus
  - Mortise: Tibial plafond (horizontal surface of the tibia), medial malleolus, and lateral malleolus.
- Ligaments:
  - Syndesmotic ligaments: tibia-fibular ligaments
  - Lateral collateral ligaments: Posterior tibiofibular, calcaneofibular, lateral talocalcaneal, anterior talofibular
  - Medial collateral ligaments; "Deltoid ligament": Posterior tibiotalar, tibiocalcaneal, anterior tibiotalar, tibionavicular

DESCRIPTION
- Fractures involving the distal fibula (lateral malleolus) and/or distal tibia (medial malleolus and plafond)
- Two common classification systems useful for describing fractures, but neither address ankle stability or reliably describe prognosis (1)[B].
- Danis-Weber system (level of fibular fracture):
  - Type A: Below the level of syndesmosis (of tibiofibular joint); usually stable
  - Type B: At syndesmosis; usually stable
  - Type C: Above syndesmosis; usually unstable
    - Maisonneuve fracture: Proximal fracture of fibula from external rotation; partial or complete disruption of syndesmosis
- Lauge Hansen (theorized the type of fracture based on foot position and applied force):
  - Pronation-abduction rotation: Injury to medial malleolus or deltoid, injury to syndesmotic ligaments, fracture of the fibula
  - Pronation-external rotation: Transverse fracture of medial malleolus or deltoid ligament, rupture of anterior tibiofibular ligament, oblique/spiral fracture of fibula, tibiofibular ligament rupture
  - Supination-adduction: Transverse avulsion fracture of fibula below the level of the joint
    - Associated with osteochondral fractures of talus
  - Supination-external rotation: Oblique fracture at the level of the syndesmosis
- The most basic nomenclature refers to the number of fractures: Unimalleolar, bimalleolar, trimalleolar
- Pilon fracture: Fracture of the talar dome and the tibial plafond; usually axial loading mechanism; unstable

Pediatric Considerations
- Different injury pattern in children
- Injuries more likely to affect the growth plate
- Salter-Harris classification of fractures

EPIDEMIOLOGY
- Predominant ages: Even age distribution
- Predominant sex:
  - Age <50: Male > Female
  - Age >50: Female > Male
- Unimalleolar (fibular fractures) = 60–70%; bimalleolar = 15–20%; trimalleolar = 7–12%

Incidence
- 1–2 cases per 1,000 people per year
- Highest incidence in elderly women (2)[B]

RISK FACTORS
- Increased body mass index
- History of smoking or osteoporosis

GENERAL PREVENTION
- Proper shoe wear (i.e., flat, supportive shoes)
- Avoid, or use caution for, activities on uneven or slick surfaces.
- Avoid physical activity when fatigued.

PATHOPHYSIOLOGY
- The location and pattern of injury depend on foot position and the direction of force applied.
- Most commonly the foot is plantar flexed and inverted, and the force is external rotation.
- Axial loading can cause a tibial plafond or pilon fracture, an intra-articular fracture of the distal tibia where it articulates with the talus.

ETIOLOGY
- Fall or twisting injury to the ankle
- Alcohol involved in 1/3 injuries
- Slippery surfaces involved in 1/3 cases

COMMONLY ASSOCIATED CONDITIONS
- Ligamentous injury (sprains)
- Syndesmosis injury
- Ankle or subtalar dislocation
- Fractures of metatarsals, talus, or calcaneus
- Osteochondral fractures
- Posterior ankle impingement (Os trigonum)
- Peroneal tendon dislocation
- Compartment syndrome (rare)
- Neurovascular injury (rare)
- Other axial loading or shearing injuries:
  - Vertebral compression fractures
  - Contralateral pelvic fractures

DIAGNOSIS

HISTORY
- Location of pain
- Timing/Mechanism of injury
- Weight-bearing status at scene of injury
- Past history of ankle injuries or surgery
- Comorbidities (diabetes, coagulopathy)

Geriatric Considerations
- Assess for safety and fall risk
- More likely to require higher level of care

PHYSICAL EXAM
- Pain, swelling, and ecchymosis
- Inability to bear weight
- Possible deformity
- Find point of maximal tenderness
- Skin integrity: tenting, lacerations, or blistering
- Neurovascular status: Motor/Sensory exam of Foot/Ankle; Check dorsalis pedis and posterior tibial pulses
- Capillary refill

- Evaluate for compartment syndrome:
  - Swelling and pain with passive extension
- Palpate ankle, foot, leg, and knee
- Examine for other associated injuries (i.e., Pilon fractures: vertebral injuries, contralateral tibial plateau)

DIAGNOSTIC TESTS & INTERPRETATION
Imaging
- Plain radiographs are the standard
- Ottawa Ankle Rules (OAR) has a sensitivity 96.4–99.6% in adults (3)[B]:
  - X-rays indicated when malleolar pain AND:
    - Bone tenderness at the posterior edge or tip of the medial malleolus, or
    - Bone tenderness at the posterior edge or tip of the lateral malleolus, or
    - Inability to bear weight both immediately and in the emergency department, or
    - Pain at navicular or along 5th metatarsal
  - If OAR criteria not met but symptoms persist beyond 48–72 hours, obtain films
  - OAR performs well in children (missing ~1% of fractures) (3), but some experts have proposed alternate rules.
  - OAR are not valid in intoxicated patients, patients with multiple injuries, or sensory deficits (diabetics with neuropathy).
- Three standard views:
  - AP
  - Lateral: Instability depicted by talar dome and distal tibia incongruity
  - Mortise (15–25° internal rotation view): Look for parallel lines between joint spaces, and space between the medial malleolus and talus should not exceed 4 mm.
- CT useful for pilon fractures or fractures with intra-articular involvement; can find subtle injuries (i.e., stress fracture)
  - Newer 3-D reconstruction technology shows relationships between ligaments and bones.
- MRI sometimes used to explore Salter-Harris fractures or ligamentous injuries.

Diagnostic Procedures/Surgery
- Arthroscopy is an option in cases of persistent pain or suspicion of any cartilaginous lesions.
- Surgery is definitive in cases of instability (see Treatment).

DIFFERENTIAL DIAGNOSIS
- Stress fracture
- Ankle sprain
- Osteochondral fracture
- Talus fracture
- 5th metatarsal fracture
- Calcaneus fracture

TREATMENT

Medication, joint support, consultation, surgical repair, physical therapy

MEDICATION
In general, ankle fractures are painful, particularly in the 1st 5–7 days following an injury. As the swelling decreases, so does the pain.

First Line
- Acetaminophen 1,000 mg QID
- NSAIDs
- Opioid analgesics

Second Line
Nonopioid analgesics (i.e., tramadol)

ADDITIONAL TREATMENT
General Measures
- Assess the extent of all injuries
- Immobilization:
  - If there is a suspected open fracture, remove any debris from the wound, place a moist (Betadine) dressing over the wound
  - Noncircular cast; Short leg posterior splint stirrup
  - Jones compression bandage
  - Crutches
  - For suspected open fractures tetanus booster, broad-spectrum cephalosporin and aminoglycoside Penicillin G for farm injuries at risk for *Clostridium perfringens*
  - Do not reduce the fracture or dislocation unless neurovascular compromise is apparent.
- Ice and elevate the extremity.

Issues for Referral
- Send to Emergency Department for surgical evaluation:
  - Neurovascular compromise
  - Tenting of skin/open fracture
  - Displaced fracture of malleoli
  - Intra-articular fracture
  - Bi- or trimalleolar
  - Pilon fracture
  - Unstable fracture
  - Signs of compartment syndrome
  - Instability
  - Pediatric Salter types III, IV, V
  - Maisonneuve fracture
- All other fractures orthopaedic follow-up within 1 week and be non-weight bearing EXCEPT:
  - Isolated avulsion fractures of the tip of the lateral malleolus may be weight bearing as tolerated.
  - Pediatric Salter I, II of the distal fibula

SURGERY/OTHER PROCEDURES
- Surgical options:
  - Open reduction internal fixation
  - External fixation for comminuted distal tibia fractures
- Timing of surgery:
  - Within 6–8 hours for emergent cases (i.e., open fractures)
  - After swelling decreased in all other cases (preferably not >1 week)
- Length of recovery:
  - In general, 6–8 weeks for healing
  - 6–8 weeks in a cast or splint (longer if fracture involves both medial and lateral malleoli)
  - 2–4 months for syndesmotic injury
  - Orthopedist may allow range of motion after 4 weeks and place in removable cast boot (fracture pattern and surgeon dependent)

- Circular cast or protective boot
  - Isolated nondisplaced medial malleolar: non-weight bearing 3 weeks + 6–8 weeks in a cast
  - Posterior malleolar with no instability: 6-week cast
  - Bimalleolar: Surgery vs. cast; orthopedic follow-up

IN-PATIENT CONSIDERATIONS
Admission Criteria
Admit to the hospital if:
- Patient will require emergency surgery (e.g., open fracture, neurovascular injury, compartment syndrome)
- Cannot maintain non-weight bearing status and requires physical therapy consultation
- Concern of mechanism of injury (i.e., syncope, MI, head injury)

Nursing
- Apply ice
- Instruct patient to keep leg elevated.

Discharge Criteria
When patient has completed the following:
- Able to ambulate with walker/crutches
- Medical workup (if needed) is completed
- Appropriate orthopedic follow-up is arranged
- Elderly patients may require a short stay in a rehabilitation facility.

ONGOING CARE

FOLLOW-UP RECOMMENDATIONS
If the fracture does not require emergent orthopedic consultation, most ankle fractures require an orthopedic consultation within 1 week and close follow-up.

Patient Monitoring
- Orthopedic follow-up:
  - Serial x-rays should be performed weekly for 4 weeks if there is any question about stability.
  - Otherwise, x-rays should be performed at 2 weeks, 4 weeks, and 8 weeks or until the fracture is healed .
- Physical therapy: once begins healing
  - Encourage toe and knee motion as soon as possible.
  - Start ankle ROM.
  - Physical therapy for strength and proprioception critical for full recovery.

DIET
NPO if surgery is being considered

PATIENT EDUCATION
- It may take the bone 6–12 weeks to heal.
- Ice and elevate the affected leg for 2–3 weeks following the injury to decrease swelling.
- Prevent splint/cast from getting wet.
- Use crutches/cane as instructed.
- Call physician if:
  - Swelling increases
  - Toes become numb or painful
  - Burning pain under the cast
  - Pain increases and is not helped by elevation and pain medication

PROGNOSIS
- Good results can be achieved in many ankle fractures without surgery, provided the ankle mortise is maintained (4)[B].
- Long term, 30% of patients may develop ankle arthritis; timing is unpredictable.
- Effusion or pain can persist for up to 1 year.

COMPLICATIONS
Nonoperative and operative:
- Displacement of the fracture
- Malunion or nonunion
- Skin breakdown or necrosis (early)
- DVT (rarely pulmonary embolism)
- Complex regional pain syndrome
- Infection (osteomyelitis)
- Loss of fixation (post-op)
- Osteoarthritis (late)

REFERENCES
1. Michelson JD, et al. Clinical Utility of a Stability-Based Ankle Fracture Classification System. *J Orthop Trauma* 2007;21:301–307.
2. Court-Brown CM, McBirnie J, Wilson G. Adult ankle fractures–an increasing problem? *Acta Orthop Scand*. 1998;69:43–7.
3. Bachmann LM, Kolb E, Koller MT, Steurer J, ter Riet G, et al. Accuracy of Ottawa ankle rules to exclude fractures of the ankle and mid-foot: systematic review. *BMJ*. 2003;326:417.
4. Michelson JD. Ankle fractures resulting from rotational injuries. *J Am Acad Orthop Surg*. 2003;11:403–12.

ADDITIONAL READING
- Bucholz RW, Heckman JD, eds. *Rockwood and Green's Fractures in Adults* 5th ed. Philadelphia: Lippincott Williams & Wilkins Publishers; 2001.
- StiellI G, Greenberg GH, McKnight RD, et al. Decision rules for the use of radiography in acute ankle injuries: Refinement and prospective validation. *JAMA*. 1993;269:1127–32.

CODES

ICD9
- 824.0 Fracture of medial malleolus, closed
- 824.8 Unspecified fracture of ankle, closed
- 824.9 Unspecified fracture of ankle, open

CLINICAL PEARLS
- OAR have a near 100% sensitivity in adults for identifying ankle fractures.
- Ankle fractures mandating immediate surgical consultation include: Signs of compartment syndrome, neurovascular compromise, or skin compromise (open or tenting).

ANKYLOSING SPONDYLITIS

Sangeetha Balasubramanian, MD
Nancy Y. Liu, MD

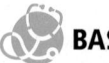 **BASICS**

DESCRIPTION

- Ankylosing spondylitis (AS) is a chronic inflammatory seronegative arthritis affecting mainly the axial skeleton and sacroiliac (SI) joints, but hips and shoulders may also be involved.
- System(s) affected: Musculoskeletal; Eyes; Cardiac; Neurological; Pulmonary
- Synonym: Marie-Strümpell disease

EPIDEMIOLOGY

- Predominant age: Onset usually in early 20s, rarely occurs after age 40
- Predominant sex: Male > Female (2–3:1)

Incidence
Age- and gender-adjusted rate of 6.3–7.3 per 100,000 person-years

Prevalence
0.1–1% in US

RISK FACTORS

- HLA-B27 (but only 1–8% of HLA-B27–positive adults have AS)
- Positive family history: A HLA-B27–positive child of a parent with AS has 10–30% risk of developing the disease.

Genetics
90–95% of Caucasian patients with AS are HLA-B27–positive.

PATHOPHYSIOLOGY
Inflammation at the insertion of tendons (enthesitis), ligaments and fasciae to bone, causing inflammation, erosion, and new bone formation

ETIOLOGY
Interaction between genetic factors and unknown trigger(s)

COMMONLY ASSOCIATED CONDITIONS

- Uveitis/iritis (up to 40%)
- Aortitis
- Cardiac conduction defects
- Spondylitis and sacroiliitis also seen in psoriatic arthritis, reactive arthritis, and arthropathy associated with inflammatory bowel disease

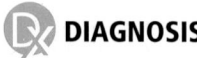 **DIAGNOSIS**

HISTORY

- Insidious onset of back pain
- Duration >3 months
- Morning stiffness in spine lasting more than 1 hour
- Frequent awakenings at night secondary to back pain
- Increased pain and stiffness with rest and improvement with activity
- Alternating buttock pain common symptom
- Constitutional symptoms (fatigue, weight loss, low-grade fever)

PHYSICAL EXAM

- Sacroiliac joint tenderness, loss of lumbar lordosis, and cervical spine rotation
- Diminished range of motion in the lumbar spine in all 3 planes of motion
- Modified Wright-Schober test for lumbar spine flexion is abnormal or <5 cm:
  - Mark the patient's back over the L5 spinous process (or at dimples of Venus) and measure 10 cm above and 5 cm below this point. Have the patient bend forward. The normal exam is at least 5 cm of expansion between these two marks.
- Thoracocervical kyphosis (rarely occurs before 10 years of symptoms)
- Chest pain with inspiration due to enthesitis at costochondral junction and chest wall expansion
- Measurement of respiratory excursion of chest wall:
  - Normal is >5 cm of maximal respiratory excursion of chest wall measured at 4th intercostal space
  - <2.5 cm is virtually diagnostic of ankylosing spondylitis.
- Aortic regurgitation murmur (1%)
- Acute anterior uveitis (usually unilateral on initial presentation but can recur on contralateral side)
- Achilles tendonitis
- Plantar fasciitis
- Peripheral oligoarthritis rare; seen mostly with psoriatic arthropathy, reactive arthritis, and arthropathy associated with inflammatory bowel disease
- Cauda equina syndrome is rare but well recognized late in the disease.

DIAGNOSTIC TESTS & INTERPRETATION

Lab

- Since up to 10% of Caucasian population and 4% of African American population is HLA-B27–positive, gene testing is not recommended as part of initial evaluation.
- Erythrocyte sedimentation rate (ESR) and c-reactive protein (CRP) may be mildly elevated or normal; if high, correlate poorly with disease activity and prognosis
- Absent rheumatoid factor
- Mild normochromic anemia (15%)
- Synovial fluid: mild leukocytosis

Imaging

- SI joints: Preferred position for imaging the SI joints with plain films is oblique projection:
  - X-ray changes may not be apparent for up to 10 years after disease onset. Magnetic resonance imaging (MRI) is more sensitive in documenting changes; increased signal from the bone and bone marrow suggesting osteitis and edema.
  - Sequential plain radiographic changes with time: Widening, erosions, sclerosis on both sides of joint not extending >1 cm from articular surface and finally ankylosis of sacroiliac joint

- Spine:
  - Early plain radiograph changes include "shiny corners" due to osteitis and sclerosis at site of annulus fibrosus attachments to the corners of vertebral bodies and "squaring" due to erosion and remodelling of vertebral body; contrast enhanced MRI imaging is more sensitive in revealing these early changes
  - Late changes include ossification of annulus fibrosis resulting in bony bridging between vertebral bodies (syndesmophytes) to give the classic "bamboo spine" appearance; ankylosis of apophyseal joints, ossification of spinal ligaments, and/or spondylodiscitis also occurs
- Peripheral joints:
  - Rare; asymmetric involvement of joints of lower extremities
  - Pericapsular ossification, sclerosis, loss of joint space, and erosions may occur.

Diagnostic Procedures/Surgery

- Electrocardiogram: Conduction defects
- Dual energy x-ray absorptiometry scan may reveal osteopenia/osteoporosis.

Pathological Findings

- Erosive changes coupled with new bone formation at the attachment of the tendons and ligaments to the bone, resulting in ossification of periarticular soft tissues
- Synovial hypertrophy and pannus formation, mononuclear cell infiltrate into subsynovium and subchondral bone marrow inflammation in the SI joint with erosions is followed by granulation tissue formation, and finally, obliteration of joint space by fusion of joint and sclerosis of para-articular bone

DIFFERENTIAL DIAGNOSIS

- Osteoarthritis of the axial spine
- Diffuse idiopathic skeletal hypertrophy (DISH)
- Psoriatic arthritis
- Reactive arthritis
- Spondylitis associated with inflammatory bowel disease
- Osteitis condensans illi: Benign sclerotic changes in the iliac portion of the SI joint found in women after pregnancies
- Infectious arthritis or discitis, especially unilateral sacroiliitis: Tuberculosis, brucellosis, bacterial (in IV drug users)

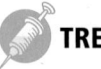 **TREATMENT**

Aggressive physical therapy, with referral to a physical therapist for daily home exercises, as well as group programs, is the most important nonpharmacological management.

MEDICATION

First Line

- Anti-inflammatory drugs:
  - Nonsteroidal anti-inflammatory drugs (NSAIDs) provide rapid and dramatic symptomatic relief, which can be virtually diagnostic of AS. NSAIDs chosen empirically but most importantly, in high doses
  - Injection of intra-articular corticosteroids into SI joints and esthesias can provide relief, but systemic corticosteroids are usually ineffective.

- Precautions:
  - All patients on long-term NSAIDs should have their hepatic and renal function monitored.
  - NSAIDs may aggravate peptic ulcer disease or cause gastritis; such patients and all patients >60 years of age should receive prophylactic proton pump inhibitors (PPIs) or misoprostol while on NSAIDs.
  - NSAIDs should be used with caution in patients with a bleeding diathesis or patients requiring anticoagulants
  - Please refer to complete package insert with each drug for complete information on the individual drug.

Second Line
- Disease-modifying agents:
  - Used in those patients who have persistently high disease activity, fail, or become intolerant of NSAIDs
  - Biologic disease-modifying agents: Anti-TNF-α-blocking agents that are approved by FDA for AS include: Etanercept (recombinant TNF receptor fusion protein) (1)[A], infliximab (chimeric monoclonal IgG1 antibody to TNF-α) (2)[A], adalimumab (fully humanized IgG1 monoclonal antibody to TNF-α) (3), and golimumab (human IgG1 kappa monoclonal antibody to TNF-α) (4).
  - Pamidronate may also help function and decrease disease activity.
  - Nonbiologic disease-modifying antirheumatic drugs such as methotrexate and sulfasalazine are ineffective for axial disease; sulfasalazine may be effective for peripheral arthritis.
- Precautions:
  - Anti-TNFs increase the risk for all infections.
  - It is imperative to screen for latent tuberculosis before initiation of treatment.
  - Screening for hepatitis B is also required.
  - Monitoring for reactivation of tuberculosis in all patients and invasive fungal infections like histoplasmosis, especially with travel to or residence in endemic areas
  - Please refer to complete package insert with each drug for complete information on individual drugs.

ADDITIONAL TREATMENT
General Measures
- Posture training and range-of-motion exercises for spine are essential.
- Firm bed, sleep in supine position without a pillow
- Breathing exercises 2–3 times a day
- Smoking cessation

Issues for Referral
Confirmation of diagnosis before initiating any type of second-line therapy

Additional Therapies
May need treatment with antiresorptive medications if osteopenia or osteoporosis is present

SURGERY/OTHER PROCEDURES
- Crucial to evaluate for c-spine ankylosis/instability before intubation
- Total hip replacement should be considered to restore mobility and to control pain.
- Vertebral osteotomy can improve posture for those patients with severe cervical or thoracolumbar flexion

ONGOING CARE

FOLLOW-UP RECOMMENDATIONS
- Maintaining physical activity and posture is critical in preventing disability.
- Swimming, tai chi, walking, and maintenance of active lifestyle are recommended.
- Avoid trauma/contact sports.
- Appropriate work ergonomics

Patient Monitoring
- Visits every 6–12 months to monitor posture and range of motion
- Counsel about risk of spinal fracture.

PATIENT EDUCATION
- Arthritis Foundation: http://www.arthritis.org
- Spondylitis Association of America: http://www.spondylitis.org

PROGNOSIS
- Extent and rapidity of progression of ankylosis are highly variable.
- Progressive limitation of spinal mobility necessitates lifestyle modification.

COMPLICATIONS
- Spine:
  - Spinal fusion causing kyphosis
  - Cervical spine fracture carries high mortality rate but fracture can occur at any level of ankylosed spine
  - C1–C2 subluxation
  - Cauda equina syndrome (rare)
- Pulmonary:
  - Restrictive lung disease
  - Upper lobe fibrosis (rare)
- Cardiac:
  - Conduction defects at atrioventricular (AV) node
  - Aortic insufficiency
  - Aortitis
  - Pericarditis extremely rare
- Uveitis and cataracts
- Renal:
  - IgA nephropathy
  - Amyloidosis (<1%)
- GI: Microscopic, subclinical ileal, and colonic mucosal ulcerations in up to 50% of patients, mostly asymptomatic

REFERENCES

1. Davis JC, van der Heijde DM, Braun J et al. Sustained durability and tolerability of etanercept in ankylosing spondylitis for 96 weeks. *Ann Rheum Dis.* 2005;64:1557–62.
2. Baraliakos X, Listing J, Brandt J et al. Radiographic progression in patients with ankylosing spondylitis after 4 yrs of treatment with the anti-TNF-alpha antibody infliximab. *Rheumatology (Oxford).* 2007;46:1450–3.
3. Haibel H, Rudwaleit M, Brandt HC et al. Adalimumab reduces spinal symptoms in active ankylosing spondylitis: clinical and magnetic resonance imaging results of a fifty-two-week open-label trial. *Arthritis Rheum.* 2006;54:678–81.
4. Inman RD, Davis JC, Heijde DV et al. Efficacy and safety of golimumab in patients with ankylosing spondylitis: Results of a randomized, double-blind, placebo-controlled, phase III trial. *Arthritis Rheum.* 2008;58:3402–12.
5. Sieper J, Rudwaleit M. Early referral recommendations for ankylosing spondylitis (including pre-radiographic and radiographic forms) in primary care. *Ann Rheum Dis.* 2005;64:659–63.

ADDITIONAL READING

- van der Heijde D, Maksymowych WP et al. Spondyloarthritis: state of the art and future perspectives. *Ann Rheum Dis.* 2010;69:949–54.
- Zochling J, van der Heijde D, Burgos-Vargas R, Collantes E, Davis JC, Dijkmans B, Dougados M, Géher P, Inman RD, Khan MA, Kvien TK, Leirisalo-Repo M, Olivieri I, Pavelka K, Sieper J, Stucki G, Sturrock RD, van der Linden S, Wendling D, Böhm H, van Royen BJ, Braun J, 'Assessment in AS' international working group, European League Against Rheumatism et al. ASAS/EULAR recommendations for the management of ankylosing spondylitis. *Ann Rheum Dis.* 2006;65:442–52.

See Also (Topic, Algorithm, Electronic Media Element)
Arthritis, Psoriatic; Arthritis, Rheumatoid; Crohn Disease; Reiter Syndrome; Ulcerative Colitis

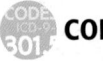 CODES

ICD9
720.0 Ankylosing spondylitis

CLINICAL PEARLS

- HLA-B27 antigen exists in 8–10% of Caucasians and 4% of African Americans in the general US population.
- Diagnosis is based on history of inflammatory back pain and morning stiffness for more than an hour, alternating buttock pain, and evidence of limitation of chest wall expansion and spinal movements in all planes; evidence of sacroiliitis and response to NSAIDs (5).
- HLA-B27 testing is an expensive and unnecessary test when clinical diagnosis is clear, but may help support the diagnosis when clinical features are less definitive.
- Plain radiography may fail to reveal changes of sacroiliitis or axial changes for up to 10 years.
- MRI is sensitive for detecting early changes of sacroiliitis or enthesitis in the axial spine.
- Physical therapy to maintain posture and mobility remains the most important nonpharmacological intervention.
- NSAIDs and TNF-α blockers are the mainstay of treatment and improve symptoms and function, but unfortunately, there is no current evidence that the latter treatment prevents bony ankylosis.

ANORECTAL ABSCESS

Timothy L. Black, MD

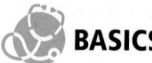 **BASICS**

DESCRIPTION
- Localized induration and fluctuance due to inflammation of the soft tissue near the rectum or anus
- 80% are perianal; the remainder are intrasphincteric or supralevator.
- System(s) affected: Gastrointestinal; Skin/Exocrine

Geriatric Considerations
A high pelvirectal abscess may cause minimal symptoms, such as lower abdominal pain and fever.

Pediatric Considerations
Common in 1st year of life

EPIDEMIOLOGY
- Predominant age: All ages (most common in infants) (1)[C]
- Predominant sex: Male > Female (4:1)

Incidence
Common

RISK FACTORS
- Inciting trauma:
  - Injections for internal hemorrhoids
  - Enema tip abrasions
  - Puncture wounds from eggshells or fish bones
  - Foreign objects
  - Prolapsed hemorrhoid
- Inflammatory bowel disease
- Chronic granulomatous disease (especially Crohn disease)
- Immunodeficiency disorders
- Hematologic malignancies (5–8% of these patients will have abscess at some time)
- Diabetes
- Chronic medical immunosuppression

GENERAL PREVENTION
- Avoid constipation.
- Avoid rectal thermometers, enemas, or suppositories whenever possible in immunocompromised patients.

ETIOLOGY
- Bacterial invasion of the anal glands found in the intersphincteric space, which may begin with an abrasion or tear in lining of anal canal, rectum, or perianal skin
- Organisms (usually mixed):
  - *Escherichia coli*
  - *Proteus vulgaris*
  - *Streptococci*
  - *Staphylococci* (especially methicillin-resistant variety)
  - *Bacteroides*
  - *Pseudomonas aeruginosa*

COMMONLY ASSOCIATED CONDITIONS
- Crohn disease
- Other inflammatory disease (e.g., appendicitis, salpingitis, diverticulitis)
- Possible perianal hidradenitis suppurativa or HIV infection in patients with recurring perianal or ischiorectal abscesses
- Anal fistula should be considered in patients with recurrent perianal abscesses in same location

 DIAGNOSIS

HISTORY
- Pain on defecation
- Pain with sitting
- Spontaneous foul-smelling drainage

PHYSICAL EXAM
- Perirectal swelling for superficial abscesses
- Perirectal redness
- Perirectal tenderness
- Perirectal throbbing pain
- Fever and other toxic symptoms with deep abscesses
- If abscess is not accompanied by external swelling, digital rectal exam will reveal a swollen tender mass.
- Digital rectal examination is mandatory.

DIAGNOSTIC TESTS & INTERPRETATION
Lab
Complete blood count: Leukocytosis

Follow-Up & Special Considerations
Culture and sensitivity testing of purulent fluid may be important in guiding antibiotic treatment (especially in high or extensive abscess).

Imaging
- Barium enema (rarely needed)
- Computed tomography scan of pelvis and perineum indicated if horseshoe or ischiorectal abscess suspected (2)[C]

Diagnostic Procedures/Surgery
Only indicated if diagnosis in doubt:
- Sigmoidoscopy: Rule out unusual causes
- Proctoscopy: Redness, induration of anus; tender mass

Pathological Findings
- Inflammation of anal mucosa
- Pus
- Inflammatory tissue
- Possible fistula tract

DIFFERENTIAL DIAGNOSIS
- Carcinoma
- Retrorectal tumors
- Crohn disease
- Primary lesions of syphilis
- Tuberculous ulceration
- Thrombosed hemorrhoid

 TREATMENT

MEDICATION
- Antibiotics (gram-negative and anaerobic coverage; based on culture results)
- Stool-softening laxatives

ADDITIONAL TREATMENT
General Measures
- Outpatient surgery with oral antibiotics (although in some cases antibiotics may not be necessary) (3)[B]
- Inpatient surgery with IV antibiotics for supralevator abscess or toxicity (2)[C]

SURGERY/OTHER PROCEDURES
- Perianal abscess:
  - Incise and drain abscess (3)[B].
  - Local anesthetic frequently appropriate with small abscesses
  - Pack wound with iodoform gauze (24–48 hours).

- Ischiorectal abscess:
  - Incise and drain abscess (3)[B].
  - General anesthetic usually required
  - Pack wound with iodoform gauze or similar packing (removed gradually over several days).
  - Fistulectomy may be done at the same time in selected cases.
- Supralevator abscess:
  - Incise and drain abscess into lower rectum or anal canal (2)[C].
  - General anesthesia required
- Treatment of anorectal fistula at time of abscess drainage may be performed (4)[C],(5):
  - Recurrent abscess risk lower when fistula treated at same procedure
  - Incontinence risk higher when fistula treated as delayed procedure
  - Recommended in cases of subcutaneous, intersphincteric, or low trans-sphincteric fistula
- After surgery:
  - Sitz baths every 2–4 hours
  - Heating pad, heat lamp, or warm compress as needed for pain
  - Encourage moving legs as soon as possible
  - Prevent constipation.

IN-PATIENT CONSIDERATIONS
Admission Criteria
- Fever
- Systemic toxicity
- Most supralevator abscesses

 ONGOING CARE

FOLLOW-UP RECOMMENDATIONS
Resume work and normal activity as soon as possible.

Patient Monitoring
Routine postoperative care with attention to wound healing, which should progress from the inside out

DIET
Increase fiber and fluid intake.

PATIENT EDUCATION
- Provide sitz bath instructions.
- Provide diet instructions.
- Provide dressing change instructions.
- Stress length of time to heal.
- Stress physical cleanliness.
- Watch for possible development of fistula-in-ano.
- Stress stool regularity; avoid constipation.

PROGNOSIS
- Slow healing depending on extent of disease and concurrent illnesses; complete healing by 6 months if no complications
- Healing in infants may be complete in 1–3 weeks.
- Drainage alone results in cure rate of 50% or more.

COMPLICATIONS
- Possible anorectal fistula (in 25% of patients) (1,2)[C]
- Possible rectovaginal fistula
- Fecal incontinence due to rupture through sphincter muscle
- Recurrence of abscess if underlying cause not corrected
- Necrotizing infection with rapid progression, sepsis, and death (2)[C]

REFERENCES

1. Ziegler M, Azizkhan R, Weber T, et al., eds. *Operative Pediatric Surgery*. New York: McGraw-Hill, 2003.
2. Townsend C, Beauchamp RD, Evers BM, et al., eds. *Sabiston Textbook of Surgery*, 17 ed. Philadelphia: Elsevier Saunders, 2006.
3. Whiteford MH, Kilkenny J, Hyman N et al. Practice parameters for the treatment of perianal abscess and fistula-in-ano (revised). *Dis Colon Rectum*. 2005;48:1337–42.
4. Oliver I et al. Randomized clinical trial comparing simple drainage of anorectal abscess with and without fistula track treatment. *Int J Colorectal Dis*. 2003;18:107–10.
5. Malik AI, Nelson RL, Tou S. Incision and drainage of perianal abscess with or without treatment of anal fistula (Protocol). *Cochrane Database of Systematic Reviews*. 2007, Issue 4. Art. No.: CD006827. DOI: 10.1002/14651858.CD006827.

ADDITIONAL READING

Schubert MC, Sridhar S, Schade RR, Wexner SD et al. What every gastroenterologist needs to know about common anorectal disorders. *World J Gastroenterol*. 2009;15:3201–9.

See Also (Topic, Algorithm, Electronic Media Element)
Anorectal Fistula

 CODES

ICD9
566 Abscess of anal and rectal regions

CLINICAL PEARLS

- Anorectal abscess should be treated as soon as possible after diagnosis.
- Any patient who has systemic signs of infection requires hospital admission for treatment. Most infants and children do not require admission.
- Incision and drainage with packing is the treatment of choice for perianal abscesses, and may be done under local anesthesia. Ischiorectal and supralevator abscesses usually require drainage under general anesthesia.

ANORECTAL FISTULA

Timothy L. Black, MD

 BASICS

DESCRIPTION

Inflammatory tract with 1 opening in the anal canal and another in perianal skin. Fistulas occur spontaneously or secondary to perirectal abscess. Most fistulas originate in the anal crypts at the anorectal junction:

- Goodsall rule:
  - If external opening is anterior to an imaginary line drawn horizontally through anal canal, fistula usually runs directly into anal canal. Positive predictive value is ~70%.
  - If external opening is posterior to line, fistula usually curves to posterior midline of anal canal. PPV is ~40%.
  - In children, tract is usually straight.
- Classification (1)[C]:
  - Intersphincteric: Fistula is confined to the intersphincteric plane (most common).
  - Trans-sphincteric: Fistula connects intersphincteric plane with ischiorectal fossa by perforating the external sphincter.
  - Suprasphincteric: Fistula connects intersphincteric plane with ischiorectal fossa but loops over external sphincter.
  - Extrasphincteric: Fistula connects rectum to perineal skin but passes external to sphincter.
- System(s) affected: Gastrointestinal; Skin/Exocrine
- Synonym(s): Fistula-in-ano; Anal fistula

Geriatric Considerations
Constipation is a common complication.

Pediatric Considerations
- Most common in infants
- More frequent in males

EPIDEMIOLOGY
- Predominant age: All ages
- Predominant sex: Male > Female

Incidence
Common

RISK FACTORS
- Injection of internal hemorrhoids, puncture wound from eggshells or fish bones, foreign objects, enema tip injuries
- Ruptured anal hematoma
- Prolapsed internal hemorrhoid
- Acute appendicitis, salpingitis, diverticulitis
- Inflammatory bowel disease (chronic ulcerative colitis, Crohn disease)
- Previous perirectal abscess
- Radiation treatment to perineum/pelvis
- Trauma, either internal or external
- Carcinoma

GENERAL PREVENTION
Prevention or prompt treatment of anorectal abscess

ETIOLOGY
- Erosion of anal canal
- Extension from infection from a tear in lining of anal canal
- Infecting organism is commonly *E. coli* (other enteric pathogens may also contribute to infection)

COMMONLY ASSOCIATED CONDITIONS
- Possibly associated with penetrating injury, intestinal tuberculosis, ulcerative colitis
- Hidradenitis suppurativa
- Crohn disease

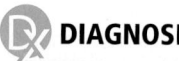 **DIAGNOSIS**

HISTORY
- History of perianal drainage
- History of perianal pain
- History of perianal abscesses in 26–37% (may be higher in recurrent abscesses) (2)[A]

PHYSICAL EXAM
- Constant or intermittent drainage or discharge (drainage may be purulent, bloody, or fecal)
- Firm, tender perianal mass
- External anal sphincter pain during and after defecation
- Spasm of external anal sphincter during and after defecation
- Anal bleeding
- Discoloration of skin surrounding fistula
- Fistulous opening frequently granulose or scarred
- Possible fever (uncommon)
- Perineal or perianal draining orifice
- Recurrent perianal abscesses in identical location
- Small palpable lesion sometimes identified on rectal exam at level of anal crypts

DIAGNOSTIC TESTS & INTERPRETATION
Lab
- Complete blood count (usually not indicated)
- Serologic testing using perinuclear antineutrophil cytoplasmic antibody and antisaccharomyces cerevisiae antibody if inflammatory bowel disease (i.e., Crohn disease) suspected
- Consider rapid plasma reagin for recurrent fistulas in sexually active patients to rule out syphilis

Imaging
- Lower gastrointestinal series if inflammatory bowel disease suspected
- Pelvic magnetic resonance imaging or endorectal ultrasound may be useful in complex or recurrent fistulas.

Diagnostic Procedures/Surgery
- Proctoscopy or sigmoidoscopy
- Colonoscopy and esophagogastroduodenoscopy if Crohn disease suspected
- Probe inserted into tract to determine its course (be careful not to create an artificial opening); best done at time of surgery
- Injection of dilute methylene blue into abscess cavity at time of surgery may be helpful in demonstrating fistula (1)[C]

Pathological Findings
- Fistulous tract may be simple or multiple
- Fistulous tract has primary opening in anal crypt; secondary opening in anal skin, para-anal skin, perineal skin, or in rectal mucous membrane
- Anal sinus: Opens in anal crypt
- Termination of sinus is blind and located in para-anal or pararectal tissue.

DIFFERENTIAL DIAGNOSIS
- Pilonidal sinus
- Perianal abscess
- Urethroperineal fistulas
- Ischiorectal abscess
- Submucous or high muscular abscess
- Pelvirectal abscess (rare)
- Rule out: Crohn disease, carcinoma, retrorectal tumors

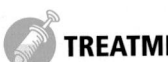 **TREATMENT**

MEDICATION
- Broad-spectrum antibiotic if active infection:
  - Cephalexin (Keflex)
  - Cefadroxil (Duricef)
  - Ampicillin-sulbactam (Unasyn)
  - Amoxicillin-clavulanate (Augmentin)
  - Cefoxitin or piperacillin/tazobactam (Zosyn) for IV use
- Stool-softening laxative

ADDITIONAL TREATMENT
General Measures
- Appropriate health care: Outpatient surgery
- Sitz baths 3–4 times per day until definitive surgery

SURGERY/OTHER PROCEDURES
- Fistulotomy:
  - Surgical incision of entire length of fistula (unroofing) (3)[A]
  - Mucosal tract should be cauterized or curetted.
  - Consider fistulotomy at time of initial abscess drainage if fistula tract can be identified.
  - Sphincterotomy
- Fistulectomy:
  - Complete excision of tract (rarely indicated because of extensive tissue loss)
  - Sphincterotomy
- Consider Seton stitch placement (especially for suprasphincteric or trans-sphincteric fistulas) (3)[A].
- Endorectal advancement flap closure for complex fistulas (3)[A]
- General anesthesia or regional anesthesia usually required (usually done as outpatient procedure in children)
- Consider use of fibrin glue in selected cases of anal fistulas (3)[A],(4)[C].
- Fistulas in Crohn disease (3)[A],(5)[B]:
  - Asymptomatic fistulas may not need treatment.
  - Simple fistulas treated with unroofing
  - Complex fistulas treated with advancement flap or long-term Setons
  - Fibrin glue may be of benefit in patients with complex fistulae or Crohn disease (2)[A].
  - May require a diverting stoma
  - Occasional patients may require proctectomy.
  - Aggressive treatment of Crohn disease
- Postoperative: Sitz baths several times per day
- Avoid constipation.

 ONGOING CARE

FOLLOW-UP RECOMMENDATIONS
Resume work and normal activity as soon as possible.

Patient Monitoring
Frequent follow-up examinations following surgery to ensure complete healing and assess continence

DIET
Clear liquid diet until gastrointestinal function returns

PROGNOSIS
- Surgical results usually excellent
- Postoperative healing:
  - 4–5 weeks for perianal fistulas
  - 12–16 weeks for deeper fistulas
  - Less than 1/3 of patients with Crohn disease who have active proctitis demonstrate significant healing following surgical intervention (5)[B].
- Postoperative healing may occur within 2–3 weeks in children.
- Recurrence rates 2–9% in simple fistulas (3)[A]
- Healing may be significantly delayed in patients with Crohn disease.

COMPLICATIONS
- Constipation (urge to defecate may be suppressed due to pain)
- Rectovaginal fistula
- Partial incontinence of fecal material if sphincter is divided
- Delayed wound healing
- Low-grade carcinoma may develop in long-standing fistulas.
- Recurrent anorectal fistula if fistula is incompletely opened or excised
- Chronic intermittent infections
- Sepsis (rarely)

REFERENCES

1. Townsend C, Beauchamp RD, Evers BM, et al., eds. *Sabiston Textbook of Surgery*, 17th ed. Philadelphia: Elsevier Saunders; 2006.
2. Malik AI, Nelson RL et al. Surgical management of anal fistulae: a systematic review. *Colorectal Dis.* 2008;10:420–30.
3. Whiteford MH, Kilkenny J, Hyman N et al. Practice parameters for the treatment of perianal abscess and fistula-in-ano (revised). *Dis Colon Rectum.* 2005;48:1337–42.
4. Hammond TM, Grahn MF, Lunniss PJ. Fibrin glue in the management of anal fistulae. *Colorectal Dis.* 2004;6:308–19.
5. Lewis RT, Maron DJ et al. Anorectal Crohn's disease. *Surg Clin North Am.* 2010;90:83–97, Table of Contents

See Also (Topic, Algorithm, Electronic Media Element)
Anorectal Abscess; Crohn Disease

 CODES

ICD9
565.1 Anal fistula

CLINICAL PEARLS
- Suspect anorectal fistula when patient complains of constant or intermittent perianal drainage or discharge (drainage may be purulent, bloody, or fecal).
- Surgery is the definitive treatment and usually produces excellent results.
- Antibiotics should be reserved for acute infection.

ANOREXIA NERVOSA

Pamela M. Williams, MD, Lt Col, USAF, MC
Jeffrey L. Goodie, PhD

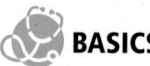 ## BASICS

DESCRIPTION
- Refusal to maintain normal body weight, with associated fear of weight gain, body-image disturbance, and amenorrhea
- Restricting and binge eating/purging subtypes
- System(s) affected: Cardiovascular; Endocrine; Metabolic; GI; Nervous; Reproductive

EPIDEMIOLOGY
- Predominant age: 13–20 years
- Predominant sex: Female > Male (20:1)
- Global distribution

Incidence
8–19 women, 2 men per 100,000 population per year

Prevalence
- 0.9% in women
- 0.3% in men (higher in gay and bisexual men)

RISK FACTORS
- Female gender
- Body dissatisfaction
- Perfectionism, obsessionality, rigidity
- Negative self-evaluation
- Academic and other achievement pressure
- Severe life stressors
- Participation in sports or artistic activities that emphasize leanness or involve subjective scoring: Ballet, running, wrestling, figure skating, gymnastics, cheerleading, weight lifting
- Type I diabetes mellitus
- Family history of substance abuse, affective disorders, or eating disorder

Genetics
- Underlying genetic vulnerability likely but not well understood
- 1st-degree female relative with eating disorder increases risk 6- to 10-fold.

GENERAL PREVENTION
Prevention programs can reduce risk factors and future onset of eating disorders (1)[C].
- Target adolescents and young women 15 years of age or older.
- Encourage realistic and healthy weight-management strategies and attitudes.
- Decrease body dissatisfaction.
- Promote self-esteem.
- Reduce focus on thin as ideal.
- Moderate overly high self-expectations.
- Decrease anxiety/depressive symptoms.
- Improve stress management.

PATHOPHYSIOLOGY
- Complex relationship between biologic, psychological, and social factors that results in an unrealistic perception of fatness
- Subsequent malnutrition leads to disorder of multiple organs.

ETIOLOGY
- Serotonin neuronal systems are implicated.
- Multifactorial with psychological, biologic, genetic, environmental, and social factors

COMMONLY ASSOCIATED CONDITIONS
- Mood disorder
- Social phobia, obsessive-compulsive disorder
- Substance abuse disorder
- High rates of cluster C personality disorders

 ## DIAGNOSIS

- (DSM-IV-TR) criteria:
  - Refusal to maintain body weight at or above a minimally normal weight for age and height
  - Intense fear of gaining weight even though underweight
  - A disturbance in the way body weight/shape is experienced; undue influence of body on self-evaluation or denial of seriousness of low body weight
  - Specific types:
    ○ Restricting type: Not engaged in binge eating or purging behaviors
    ○ Binge eating/purging type: Regularly engages in binge eating or purging behaviors (see bulimia information related to these behaviors)
- Psychological self-report screening tools:
  - Eating Attitudes Test (EAT)
  - Eating Disorder Inventory (EDI)
  - Eating Disorder Screen for Primary Care (ESP)
  - SCOFF (sick, control, one, fat, food) questionnaire

HISTORY
- Patient unlikely to self-identify problem; corroborate with family or friends.
- Ascertain fear of weight gain and/or distorted body image.
- Onset may be insidious or stress-related.
- Report feeling fat even when emaciated
- Preoccupation with body size, weight control
- Elaborate food preparation and eating rituals
- Extensive exercise
- Amenorrhea (primary or secondary) .
- Weakness, fatigue, cognitive impairment
- Cold intolerance
- Constipation, bloating, early satiety
- Growth arrest, delayed puberty
- Decreased bone density, fractures

PHYSICAL EXAM
- Often normal
- Vital signs: Hypothermia, bradycardia, orthostatic hypotension, body weight <85% of expected
- Cardiac: Dysrhythmias, midsystolic click of mitral valve prolapse
- Skin/extremities: Dry skin; lanugo hair on extremities, face, and trunk; hair loss; edema
- Neurologic and abdominal exams: To rule out other causes of weight loss and vomiting

DIAGNOSTIC TESTS & INTERPRETATION
Lab
- No specific test for anorexia nervosa (AN)
- Most findings are related directly to starvation and/or dehydration.
- All findings may be within normal limits.

Initial lab tests
- Low serum leuteinizing hormone, follicle-stimulating hormone; low serum testosterone in males
- Thyroid function tests: Low thyroid-stimulating hormone with normal T_3/T_4
- Liver function tests: Abnormal liver enzymes
- Chem 7: Altered blood urea nitrogen, creatinine clearance; electrolyte disturbances
- Hypoglycemia, hypercholesterolemia, hypercortisolemia, hypophosphatemia
- Low sedimentation rate
- Complete blood count: Anemia, leukopenia, thrombocytopenia
- 12-lead electrocardiogram to assess for prolonged QT interval

Imaging
Dual-energy x-ray absorptiometry (DEXA) of bone only if underweight for >6 months to assess for diminished bone density

Pathological Findings
- Osteoporosis/osteopenia, pathologic fractures
- Sick euthyroid syndrome
- Cardiac impairment

DIFFERENTIAL DIAGNOSIS
- Hyperthyroidism, adrenal insufficiency
- Inflammatory bowel disease, malabsorption
- Immunodeficiency, chronic infections
- Diabetes
- CNS lesion
- Bulimia; body dysmorphic disorder
- Depressive disorders with loss of appetite
- Anxiety disorder, food phobia
- Conversion disorder, schizophrenic disorder

ALERT
AN may exist concurrently with chronic medical disorders such as diabetes and cystic fibrosis.

TREATMENT

- Most patients should be treated as outpatients using an interdisciplinary team (2,3)[C].
- Behavioral therapies (e.g., cognitive-behavioral, interpersonal, or family therapy) should be offered (2,4,5,6)[C].
- Pharmacotherapy should not be used as the sole treatment modality (2,3,7)[C].

MEDICATION
First Line
- No medications are available that effectively treat patients with AN, but pharmacotherapy may be used as an adjuvant to cognitive-behavioral therapies (2,3,6,7)[C].
- Selective serotonin reuptake inhibitors (SSRIs) may
  - Help to prevent relapse after weight gain
  - Treat comorbid depression or obsessive-compulsive disorder (2,3,6,7)[C].
- Studies using atypical antipsychotics are underway.
- Attend to black-box warnings concerning antidepressants, and conduct appropriate informed consent if prescribed.

Second Line
- Management of osteopenia:
  - Primary treatment is weight gain (3)[C].
  - Elemental calcium 1,200–1,500 mg/d plus MVI containing 800 IU of vitamin D (3)[C]
  - No indication for bisphosphonates in AN (3)[C]
  - Weak evidence for use of hormone-replacement therapy (3)[C]
- Psyllium (Metamucil) preparations (1 T) to prevent constipation

ADDITIONAL TREATMENT
General Measures
- Initial treatment goal geared to weight restoration; most managed as outpatients
- Outpatient treatment:
  - Interdisciplinary team (primary care physician, mental health provider, nutritionist) (2,3)[C]
  - Average weekly weight gain goal: 0.5–1.0 kg (2,3)[C], with stepwise increase in calories
  - Cognitive-behavioral therapy, interpersonal psychotherapy, family-based therapy (2,4,5,6)[C]
  - Focus on health, not weight gain alone.
  - Build trust, treatment alliance.
  - Involve patient in establishing diet and exercise goals.
  - Challenge fear of uncontrolled weight gain; help the patient to recognize feelings that lead to disordered eating.
  - In chronic cases, goal may be to achieve a safe weight rather than a healthy weight.
- Inpatient treatment:
  - If possible, admit to specialized eating disorders unit (3)[C].
  - Assess risk for refeeding syndrome (weight loss >10% in 2–3 months; current weight <70% ideal body weight).
  - Monitor vital signs, electrolytes, cardiac function, edema, weight gain.
  - Initial bed rest with supervised meals may be necessary.
  - Stepwise increase in activity
  - Tube feeding or total parental nutrition is used only as a last resort.
  - Supportive symptomatic care as needed

Issues for Referral
Patients with AN require an interdisciplinary team (primary care physician, mental health provider, nutritionist).

IN-PATIENT CONSIDERATIONS
Admission Criteria
- Suggested physiologic values: Heart rate <40 beats/min, blood pressure <90/60 mm Hg, symptomatic hypoglycemia, potassium <3 mmol/L, temperature <97.0°F (36.1°C), dehydration, other cardiovascular abnormalities, weight <75% of expected, rapid weight loss, lack of improvement while in outpatient therapy
- Suggested psychological indications: Poor motivation/insight, lack of cooperation with outpatient treatment, inability to eat, need for nasogastric feeding, suicidal intent or plan, severe coexisting psychiatric disease, problematic family environment

Pediatric Considerations
- Children often present with nausea, abdominal pain, fullness, and inability to swallow.
- Additional indications for hospitalization: Heart rate <50 beats/min, orthostatic blood pressure, hypokalemia or hypophosphatemia, rapid weight loss even if weight not <75% below normal

Geriatric Considerations
Late-onset AN (>50 years of age) may be long-term disease or triggered by death of loved one, marital discord, or divorce.

Discharge Criteria
Lower relapse rate when discharged at expected healthy weight

 ONGOING CARE

FOLLOW-UP RECOMMENDATIONS
- Close follow-up until patient demonstrates forward progress in care plan
- Focus on enjoyable activities rather than goal-oriented ones.
- Emphasize importance of moderate activity for health, not thinness.

Patient Monitoring
- Level of exercise activity
- Weigh weekly until stable, then monthly.
- Depression, self-esteem, suicidal ideation

DIET
- Importance of adherence to prescribed diet
- Goal is stabilization at a healthy weight on a balanced diet with normal eating pattern.
- Diminished ruminations about calories, weight; increased enjoyment

PATIENT EDUCATION
- Provide patients and families with information on the diagnosis and its natural history, health risks, and treatment strategies.
- The National Alliance on Mental Illness has information at www.nami.org/helpline/anorexia.htm
- Also: familydoctor.org

PROGNOSIS
- Prognosis: ~50% recover; 30% improve; 20% are chronically ill.
- Mortality: 5%

COMPLICATIONS
- Refeeding syndrome
- Cardiac arrhythmia, cardiac arrest
- Cardiomyopathy, congestive heart failure
- Delayed gastric emptying, necrotizing colitis
- Seizures, Wernicke encephalopathy, peripheral neuropathy, cognitive deficits
- Osteopenia, osteoporosis

Pregnancy Considerations
- Fertility may be affected.
- Behaviors may persist, decrease, or recur in pregnancy and postpartum interval.
- Increased risk for preterm labor, operative delivery, and infants with low birth weight, smaller head circumference, and/or microcephaly; anemia; genitourinary infections; and labor induction; should be managed as high risk

REFERENCES

1. Stice E, Shaw H, Marti CN. A meta-analytic review of eating disorder prevention programs: encouraging findings. *Annu Rev Clin Psychol.* 2007;3:207–31.
2. NICE. Eating disorders—core interventions in the treatment and management of anorexia nervosa, bulimia nervosa and related eating disorders. NICE Clinical Guideline no 9. London: NICE, 2004 (accessed May 8, 2010).
3. American Psychiatric Association. Practice Guideline for the Treatment of Patients with Eating Disorders. 3rd ed. 2006 (accessed May 8, 2010).
4. Hay P, Bacaltchuk J, Claudino A, Ben-Tovim D, et al. Individual psychotherapy in the outpatient treatment of adults with anorexia. *Cochrane Database Syst Rev.* 2003 Issue 4:CD003909.
5. Fisher CA, Hetrick SE, Rushford N et al. Family therapy for anorexia nervosa. *Cochrane Database Syst Rev.* 2010;4:CD004780.
6. Bulik CM, Berkman ND, Brownley KA, Sedway JA, Lohr KN et al. Anorexia nervosa treatment: a systematic review of randomized controlled trials. *Int J Eat Disord.* 2007;40:310–20.
7. Claudino A, Hay P, Lima M, et al. Antidepressants for anorexia nervosa. *Cochrane Database Syst Rev.* 2006 Issue 1:CD04365.

ADDITIONAL READING
American Psychiatric Association. *Diagnostic and Statistical Manual of Mental Disorders DSM-IV-TR,* 4/e. American Psychiatric Publishing, Inc, 2000.

See Also (Topic, Algorithm, Electronic Media Element)
Amenorrhea; Osteoporosis; Bulimia Nervosa
Algorithm: Weight Loss

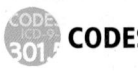 **CODES**

ICD9
307.1 Anorexia nervosa

CLINICAL PEARLS
- Particularly among young women with a risk factor, asking, "Are you satisfied with your eating patterns?" and/or "Do you worry that you have lost control over how you eat?" may help to screen those with an eating problem.
- In AN, there is a sustained and determined pursuit of weight loss resulting in a body weight <85% of expected.
- To care for a patient with AN, an interdisciplinary team that includes a medical provider, a dietician, and a behavioral health professional is the most accepted approach.

ANTHRAX

Gregory D. Gutke, MD, MPH
Richard J. Thomas, MD, MPH

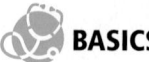 **BASICS**

DESCRIPTION
- Anthrax is a highly infectious disease of animals, especially ruminants (hooved animals such as cows, goats, and sheep) that is caused by the bacteria *Bacillus anthracis*. Cutaneous (95% of US cases), inhalational, and GI forms can be transmitted to humans by contact with the animals or their products (typically hair or hides).
- Synonym(s) for cutaneous anthrax: Charbon; Malignant pustule; Siberian ulcer; Malignant edema; Splenic fever; Milzbrand
- Synonym(s) for inhalational anthrax: Ragpicker disease; Woolsorter disease

EPIDEMIOLOGY
- Total of 235 anthrax cases (224 cutaneous and 11 inhalational) occurred in the US between 1955 and 1994, resulting in 20 fatalities.
- Cutaneous: 95% of cases in the US; cases of cutaneous anthrax without occupational risk should raise concern for bioterrorism.
  - ~5–20% of untreated cases result in death; case fatality rate is <1% with antibiotic therapy.
- GI: Very rare in the US (no documented case in the 20th century).
- Inhalational anthrax is very rare in US; must be considered a bioterrorist event in US until proven otherwise (the last US occupational case occurred in 1976):
  - Death results in 99% of untreated cases and in 45–80% of patients with severe symptoms who are treated in a state-of-the-art facility.
- Anthrax is most common in agricultural regions, where it occurs in animals. These regions include the Middle East, Asia, Southern and Eastern Europe, Africa, South and Central America, and the Caribbean.

RISK FACTORS
- Contact with infected animals or their products
- Bioterrorist event

GENERAL PREVENTION
- Anthrax vaccine protects against all forms of anthrax and is as safe as other vaccines, according to the FDA, CDC, and the National Academy of Sciences.
- A 2009 review by the Cochrane Infectious Disease Group concluded that the anthrax vaccine is effective in reducing the risk of contracting anthrax and has a low rate of adverse effects (1)[A]
- Anthrax vaccine should be effective against all known strains of *B. anthracis* as well as against any strains that might be bioengineered by terrorists or others.

- Vaccine schedule and route changed in late 2008: Route is now intramuscular (previously subcutaneous) and schedule is decreased from 6 doses down to 5 doses (0 and 4 weeks, and 6, 12, and 18 months) plus annual boosters. Intramuscular versus subcutaneous injection greatly reduces the incidence of injection-site adverse events (2):
  - Anthrax vaccine adsorbed (trade name BioThrax) is FDA approved for ages 18 through 65 and is pregnancy category D.
  - If you get behind schedule, do not start the series over; begin where you left off (delays do not reduce the resulting protection).
  - Individuals are not considered protected until they have completed the full vaccination series.
  - The most common (>10%) local (injection-site) adverse reactions observed in clinical studies were tenderness, pain, erythema, and arm motion limitation. The most common (>5%) systemic adverse reactions were muscle aches, fatigue and headache.
  - The Advisory Committee on Immunization Practices recommends vaccination for the following groups:
    - Persons who work directly with the organism in the laboratory
    - Persons who work with imported animal hides or furs in areas where standards are insufficient to prevent exposure to anthrax spores
    - Persons who handle potentially infected animal products in high-incidence areas
    - Military personnel deployed to areas with high risk for exposure to organisms (when used as a biologic warfare weapon)
    - Pregnant women should be vaccinated for anthrax only if absolutely necessary.
- Patients with a likely inhalational exposure history but no symptoms are candidates for postexposure prophylaxis with either ciprofloxacin 500 mg PO b.i.d. or doxycycline 100 mg PO b.i.d. for 60 days. Levofloxacin is also FDA approved for patients age 18 or older. CDC guidelines state patients should also receive 3 doses of Anthrax vaccine (0, 2 weeks, 4 weeks), but since BioThrax is not licensed for post-exposure prophylaxis or for a 3-dose series this would need to be conducted under an Investigational New Drug application. Prophylactic medications are not indicated for prevention of cutaneous anthrax.

PATHOPHYSIOLOGY
- *B. anthracis* is a spore-forming, gram-positive bacterium found in the soil worldwide. The word *anthracis* is derived from a Greek word meaning "coal," which is used to describe the cutaneous form of the disease that leads to a characteristic black lesion.
- *B. anthracis* has 3 known virulence factors: An antiphagocytic capsule and 2 protein toxins (known as edema factor and lethal factor):
  - The capsule provides resistance to phagocytosis.
  - Lethal factor and edema factor are named for the effects they induce when injected into experimental animals.
  - A protein called *protective antigen* binds to the host cell's surface; when cleaved by a protease on the cell surface it creates a site to which the lethal factor and edema factor can bind; protective antigen is required for the action of the 2 protein toxins.

- *B. anthracis* spores introduced into the host are ingested at the exposed site by macrophages and then germinate into vegetative forms that produce the virulence factors.

ETIOLOGY
- Cutaneous: Occurs when *B. anthracis* enters the skin through a cut or abrasion during the handling of animal products (such as meat, wool, or hides infected with *B. anthracis*)
- GI: Ingestion of bacillus-contaminated meat
- Inhalational: Inhalation of aerosolized *B. anthracis* spores

 DIAGNOSIS

- Cutaneous: Incubation period is usually immediate up to 1 day. Begins as a pruritic spot, followed by a red-brown papule that enlarges with peripheral erythema, vesiculation, and induration, followed by black eschar formation within 7–10 days of the initial lesion:
  - The papule, blister, and eschar are painless, and cutaneous symptoms may be accompanied by fever, malaise, and headache.
  - A black eschar with massive edema is nearly pathognomonic for cutaneous anthrax.
- GI: Incubation period is usually 1–7 days. Presents as 1 of 2 distinct syndromes—oropharyngeal and abdominal:
  - Oropharyngeal syndrome presentation can include fever, edema, ulcer, severe sore throat, and lymphadenopathy, resulting in marked unilateral or bilateral neck swelling.
  - Abdominal syndrome may present with fever, malaise, hematemesis, anorexia, severe abdominal pain, and hematochezia or melena. 2–4 days after onset of symptoms, pain begins to subside and ascites develops, with shock and death within just a few days.
- Inhalational: Incubation period is usually less than one week, but may be up to 60 days. Biphasic presentation, with initial phase featuring nonspecific influenzalike symptoms such as low-grade fever, chills, headache, nonproductive cough, diaphoresis, malaise, chest discomfort, nausea, vomiting, diarrhea, and abdominal pain:
  - This initial phase is followed by a 2nd fulminant phase that begins 1–5 days after onset of the initial phase symptoms. Signs and symptoms of the fulminant phase include abrupt onset of high fever, severe dyspnea, hypoxia, hypotension, and death within 24–36 hours.

HISTORY
- Cutaneous: Crucial clinical clues are rapid evolution of symptoms, lack of pain, occasional massive edema, and the near pathognomonic black eschar. Incubation period is usually immediate but may last up to 1 day.
- GI: Incubation period usually 1–7 days; 2–4 days after onset of symptoms, ascites develop as abdominal pain decreases. Shock and death occur within 2–5 days after onset of symptoms.

- Inhalational: Incubation period is usually <1 week but may be as long as 2 months. 2nd portion of the biphasic presentation begins 1–5 days after onset of initial symptoms. There may be a 1- to 3-day period of improvement after the 1st phase and before the 2nd phase begins. Shock and death occur within 24–36 hours after onset of the 2nd phase.

PHYSICAL EXAM
- Cutaneous: Red-brown papule, vesicles, or black eschar
- GI: Acute abdomen with rebound tenderness may occur. Ascites present later in course.
- Inhalational: Rhonchi may be present.

DIAGNOSTIC TESTS & INTERPRETATION
Lab
Gram stain and culture. Obtain specimens for culture before initiating antimicrobial therapy. *B anthracis* is easily isolated from blood cultures in <24 hours. A presumptive diagnosis can be made if gram-positive rods are present that are nonmotile, nonhemolytic, and encapsulated (usually seen with India ink). If antibiotics have been given for >24 hours, perform immunohistochemical staining and/or PCR.

Imaging
- Inhalational: Widened mediastinum on chest X-ray may be present; pleural effusions frequently present; infiltrates are rare.
- GI: Mesenteric adenopathy on computed tomography scan is likely.

DIFFERENTIAL DIAGNOSIS
- Skin cellulitis
- Brown recluse spider bite
- Cat-scratch disease
- Rat bite fever
- Rickettsial spotted fever
- Carbuncle
- Cowpox
- Bullous erysipelas
- Tularemia vasculitides
- Ecthyma gangrenosum
- Orf (a transmissible viral disease of goats and sheep)

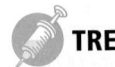 **TREATMENT**

MEDICATION
First Line
- Cutaneous: Ciprofloxacin 500 mg PO b.i.d. or doxycycline 100 mg PO b.i.d. for 7–10 days for localized or uncomplicated cases of naturally acquired cutaneous anthrax. Treat for 7–10 days with IV instead for severe cases of naturally acquired cutaneous anthrax with signs of systemic involvement, extensive edema, or lesions of the head and neck.
  – If cutaneous case is localized or uncomplicated but is bioterrorism-related, the patient must be treated for 60 days with PO ciprofloxacin or doxycycline since they are at risk for inhalational anthrax.
  – Patients with bioterrorism-related cutaneous anthrax who show signs of systemic involvement, massive edema, or lesions on the head or neck should be treated per inhalational anthrax recommendation (below) (3,4)[C].

- Inhalational and GI: Intravenous ciprofloxacin 400 mg q12h (1st line) or doxycycline 100 mg q12h (2nd line) and 1 or 2 additional antimicrobials such as rifampin, vancomycin, penicillin, ampicillin, chloramphenicol, imipenem, clindamycin, and clarithromycin
  – May switch to PO when clinically appropriate.
  – Must complete 60-day course (combined PO and IV) (3)[C].
  – Early and aggressive pleural fluid drainage is recommended for all inhalational anthrax patients (4)[C].

Second Line
Patients being treated for anthrax may also benefit from vaccination as part of their regimen (5)[C].

ADDITIONAL TREATMENT
General Measures
- Inhalational and GI anthrax are not known to spread from person to person, so communicability concerns are not an issue during management of the patient.
- Although cutaneous anthrax is also considered noncontagious, avoidance of contact with the wound or wound drainage seems prudent.

 ONGOING CARE

FOLLOW-UP RECOMMENDATIONS
Patient Monitoring
Must monitor patient for 60 days to ensure completion of the treatment course

PROGNOSIS
- Cutaneous: Death in 5–20% of untreated cases, but the case fatality rate is <1% with antibiotic therapy
- GI: Mortality rates as high as 50% reported
- Inhalational: Death in 45–80% of patients with severe symptoms who are treated in a state-of-the-art facility; case fatality rate approaches 99% in untreated cases.

REFERENCES

1. Donegan S, Bellamy R, Gamble CL. Vaccines for preventing anthrax. *Cochrane Database of Systematic Reviews* 2009, Issue 2. Art. No.: CD006403. DOI:10.1002/14651858.CD006403. pub2.
2. Marano N, Plikaytis BD, Martin SW et al. Effects of a reduced dose schedule and intramuscular administration of anthrax vaccine adsorbed on immunogenicity and safety at 7 months: a randomized trial. *JAMA*. 2008;300:1532–43.
3. Centers for Disease Control and Prevention. Update: Investigation of bioterrorism-related anthrax and interim guidelines for exposure management and antimicrobial therapy, October 2001. *MMWR Morb Mortal Wkly Rep*. 2001;50: 909–19.
4. Stern EJ, Uhde KB, Shadomy SV et al. Conference report on public health and clinical guidelines for anthrax. *Emerg Infect Dis*. 2008;14.
5. Centers for Disease Control and Prevention. Use of anthrax vaccine in the US, ACIP Recommendations. *MMWR Recommendations & Reports*. 2000; 49(RR-15):1–20.

ADDITIONAL READING
- Centers for Disease Control and Prevention, Emergency Preparedness and Response. http://www.bt.cdc.gov/agent/anthrax/
- Durning SJ, Roy MJ. Anthrax. In: Roy MJ, ed. *Physician's guide to terrorist attack*. Totowa, NJ: Humana, 2003.
- Schwartz MN. Recognition and management of anthrax—an update. *N Engl J Med*. 2001;345:1621–1626.
- The anthrax vaccine immunization program. http://www.anthrax.mil

 CODES

ICD9
- 022.0 Cutaneous anthrax
- 022.1 Pulmonary anthrax
- 022.2 Gastrointestinal anthrax

CLINICAL PEARLS
- Anthrax vaccine (only recommended for high-risk groups) protects against all forms of anthrax and is as safe as other vaccines, according to the FDA, CDC, and the National Academy of Sciences.
- Inhalational anthrax is very rare in US; must be considered a bioterrorist event until proven otherwise (last U.S. occupational case occurred in 1976).
  – Death results in 99% of untreated cases and in 45–80% of patients with severe symptoms who are treated in a state-of-the-art facility.
- Widened mediastinum on chest X-ray may be present; pleural effusions frequently present; infiltrates are rare.

ANTIPHOSPHOLIPID ANTIBODY SYNDROME

Shefali B. Khandwala, DO
Desiree Lie, MD

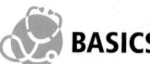

BASICS

DESCRIPTION

Antiphospholipid antibody syndrome (APS) is an autoimmune thrombotic syndrome characterized by the presence of antiphospholipid antibodies (APAs) in association with either recurrent venous or arterial thromboembolic events or repeated fetal loss. The antiphospholipid antibodies are directed against phospholipid-binding plasma proteins and cause an increased risk of clot formation.

- Types:
  - Primary (50%): Occurs in patients without clinical evidence of another autoimmune disease
  - Secondary: Occurs in association with another disease, most commonly systemic lupus erythematosus (SLE)
  - Catastrophic APS (<1%):
    ○ Differs from primary and secondary types in the caliber of vessels affected. Venous or arterial thrombosis of large vessels is less common, and patients present with acute thrombotic microangiopathy, the kidneys being the most commonly affected organ.
    ○ DIC, which does not occur in primary or secondary forms, is seen in up to 25% of patients with the catastrophic type
    ○ Has a high mortality, approaching 50% even with treatment
- Synonym(s): Hughes syndrome

Geriatric Considerations
Atherosclerosis and cancer are more frequent causes of thrombosis than is APS.

Pregnancy Considerations
- Increased frequency of recurrent fetal loss
- Increased risk of premature delivery due to pregnancy-related hypertension and uteroplacental insufficiency

EPIDEMIOLOGY
- No specific age or race predilection
- Equal frequency occurs among males and females for both primary and secondary forms in young pre-pubertal patients
- Female predilection for both primary and secondary forms because of the inclusion of pregnancy-related events in the classification criteria and because of the female predominance in autoimmune diseases such as SLE, respectively.

Incidence
- 15% of women with recurrent pregnancy loss have APS
- 5–21% of all patients with DVT have APS

Prevalence
APAs are present in 1–15% of the general population and in up to 70% of those with SLE. Of those with SLE who have APAs, 50–70% may develop this syndrome.

RISK FACTORS
The following may increase the likelihood of thrombosis in patients with APAs:
- Smoking
- Oral contraceptive use
- Surgery
- Immobilization
- Pregnancy

Genetics
Increased risk in relatives of individuals with APS, however, no specific genetic patterns isolated

GENERAL PREVENTION
- Modification of secondary risk factors for atherosclerosis includes control of HTN, diabetes, hyperlipidemia, and smoking cessation
- Avoidance of oral contraceptives in patients with known APA

PATHOPHYSIOLOGY
APAs may promote thrombosis in any organ by the following hypotheses:
- Increased platelet adhesion and aggregation due to interactions of the antibodies with platelet membrane phospholipids
- Oxidant-mediated injury of vascular endothelium
- Interference with the phospholipid-binding proteins involved in the regulation of coagulation

ETIOLOGY
- Mechanism by which APAs become generated is speculative, but may occur as a result of autoimmunity, as a response to inner membrane antigens exposed on apoptotic cells, or from cross-reactivity to exogenous antigens from infectious organisms
- The presence of APAs alone may not generate thrombosis, but the occurrence of a "second hit" via environmental factors or comorbidities may be required for activation

COMMONLY ASSOCIATED CONDITIONS
- SLE (most common rheumatic disease associated with APAs)
- Thrombotic thrombocytopenic purpura (TTP)
- Hemolytic-uremic syndrome (HUS)
- Malignant hypertension
- Acute renal failure
- Nephrotic syndrome
- HELLP syndrome (hemolysis, elevated liver enzymes, and low platelet count in association with pregnancy)
- DVT/pulmonary embolus (PE)
- Valvular disease
- Sneddon syndrome (APS variant syndrome in which livedo reticularis is associated with HTN and stroke)
- Malignant neoplasms
- Multiple bacterial, viral, and parasitic infections may result in transient increases in APAs
- Certain medications may be associated with APA production, including phenothiazines, hydralazine, procainamide, and phenytoin, but usually do not result in thrombotic events

DIAGNOSIS

- Sapporo criteria, revised 2006 (1):
- The presence of at least 1 of the following clinical criteria:
  - Vascular thrombosis:
    ○ ≥1 clinical episodes of arterial, venous, or small vessel thrombosis, occurring within any tissue or organ, confirmed by imaging studies, Doppler studies, or histopathology
  - Complications of pregnancy:

○ ≥1 unexplained deaths of morphologically normal fetuses at or after the 10th week of gestation OR
○ ≥1 premature births of morphologically normal neonates at or before the 34th week of pregnancy due to severe preeclampsia, eclampsia, or placental insufficiency OR
○ ≥3 unexplained consecutive spontaneous abortions before the 10th week of pregnancy, unexplained by maternal or paternal chromosomal abnormalities or maternal anatomic or hormonal causes
- AND the presence of at least 1 of the following laboratory criteria on ≥2 occasions at least 12 weeks apart:
  - Lupus anticoagulant antibodies detected in the blood
  - Anticardiolipin IgG or IgM antibodies present at moderate or high levels in the blood via a standardized ELISA
  - Anti-B$_2$ glycoprotein-I IgG or IgM antibodies in blood at a titer >99th percentile via a standardized ELISA
  - Valid lab findings should occur no more than 5 years prior to clinical manifestations

HISTORY
- Personal history of thrombosis (DVT, PE, stroke)
- Obstetric history (especially pregnancy losses)
- Bleeding (from thrombocytopenia)
- Family history of rheumatologic illness
- Vaso-occlusive events can occur in any organ system, so perform thorough review of systems

PHYSICAL EXAM
- DVT of the legs (most common manifestation of APS)
- Skin exam may include findings of livedo reticularis (lacy, erythematous rash in net-like pattern, typically on wrists and knees), purpuric lesions, or ulcerations
- Insufficiency murmur of aortic or mitral valve
- Diverse neurologic symptoms: paresthesias, weakness, tremors, cognitive deficits, stroke/TIA

DIAGNOSTIC TESTS & INTERPRETATION
- May result in false-positive VDRL/RPR
- The risk of thrombosis may increase with the level of APA detected and the number of APA types present in one individual
- The clinical significance of other autoantibodies, including those directed against prothrombin, annexin V, phosphatidylserine, and phosphatidylinositol, remains unclear

Lab
"Lupus anticoagulant" (LA) is a misnomer since it results in an increased risk of thrombus, not an anticoagulant effect. The antibodies cause an increase in the aPTT in vitro, although they are associated with hypercoagulable state in vivo.

Initial lab tests
- Clotting test for lupus anticoagulant
- ELISA test for anticardiolipin antibodies
- ELISA test for anti-β_2 glycoprotein-I antibodies
- CBC to determine if thrombocytopenia (platelet count usually 50,000–140,000/μL) or hemolytic anemia are present

Follow-Up & Special Considerations
LAs cannot be detected in patients treated with unfractionated heparin, but may be detected in

patients on low molecular weight heparin or warfarin within therapeutic ranges

Imaging
- Doppler ultrasonography of lower extremities to look for DVT
- If PE suspected, CT angiography or other diagnostic modalities
- Echocardiography may be helpful in some cases with cardiac involvement
- MRI may demonstrate CNS involvement, with high-intensity lesions suggestive of a vasculopathy
- Arteriography in patients with arterial thrombotic events

Diagnostic Procedures/Surgery
Biopsy of the affected organ system may be necessary in select cases to distinguish the vasculopathy of this syndrome from a vasculitis

Pathological Findings
- Usual finding is microangiopathic process with bland thrombosis and with minimal vascular or perivascular inflammation:
  - Acute changes: Capillary congestion and noninflammatory fibrin thrombi
  - Chronic changes: Ischemic hypoperfusion
- Atrophy and fibrosis

DIFFERENTIAL DIAGNOSIS
- Conditions that cause thrombotic microangiopathy, such as hemolytic-uremic syndrome or TTP
- Thrombophilic conditions, such as:
  - Deficiency of protein C, protein S
  - Deficiency of antithrombin III
  - Mutation of factor V Leiden
  - Prothrombin gene mutation
  - Neoplastic and myeloproliferative disorders
  - Hyperviscosity syndromes
- Embolic disease secondary to atrial fibrillation, marked LV dysfunction, endocarditis, cholesterol emboli
- Heparin-induced thrombocytopenia
- Homocystinemia
- Atherosclerosis

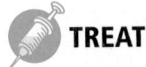 ## TREATMENT

MEDICATION
Asymptomatic individuals with APAs and no other underlying illness are unlikely to benefit from low-dose ASA in the absence of other risk factors (2)[A]

First Line
- In symptomatic non-pregnant individuals with APS:
  - Initial therapy with both unfractionated or LMW heparin and warfarin, then continuing on only warfarin once therapeutic

  - Warfarin treatment of moderate intensity (to achieve INR between 2.0–3.0) significantly reduces the rate of recurrent thrombosis after an initial thromboembolic event (2)[A]

  - Warfarin treatment may require higher intensity (to achieve INR 3.0–4.0) in patients with an initial arterial thromboembolic event or recurrent venous thromboembolic event despite anticoagulation, although further evidence-based studies are required to establish such a recommendation
  - Lifelong treatment is recommended, although this remains heavily debated

- In patients with noncardioembolic stroke and a single APA result without other indications for anticoagulation, moderate intensity warfarin OR ASA (325 mg daily) may be administered (3)[A]
  - Consider adding dipyridamole extended-release (200 mg twice daily) to aspirin (30 to 325 mg daily) as the combination has been shown to be superior to aspirin alone (4)[A]
  - Clopidogrel (75 mg daily) alone may be used as an equivalent alternative to the combination of aspirin and dipyridamole (5)[A]

- In pregnant individuals with APS:
  - For women with no prior history of thrombosis and ≥2 early pregnancy losses or ≥1 late pregnancy loss, consider ASA (81 mg daily) with attempted conception and add low-dose unfractionated heparin 5,000–10,000 units SC b.i.d. or LMWH (enoxaparin 40 mg sc daily) when a viable intrauterine pregnancy is documented (3)[A]
  - Treatment should continue until at least the third trimester (rate of fetal loss may exceed 90% in untreated patients, while therapies such as aspirin and heparin can reduce the rate to 25%) and consider through delivery and for a few weeks postpartum (6)[B]

- For the catastrophic form, recommendation for aggressive therapy with steroids, anticoagulation, and plasma exchange (+/− IVIG)

SURGERY/OTHER PROCEDURES
Patients with thrombosis may require thrombectomy or an IVC filter for those with lower extremity DVT for whom anticoagulation is contraindicated

IN-PATIENT CONSIDERATIONS
Patients with APS-related events should be considered for inpatient treatment in the following situations:
- Massive DVT, symptomatic PE, high risk of bleeding on anticoagulation therapy, comorbid conditions

 ## ONGOING CARE

FOLLOW-UP RECOMMENDATIONS
Patient Monitoring
Warfarin therapy is lifelong; patients need monitoring to maintain INR of 2.0–3.0. Pregnant patients on prolonged heparin (esp UFH) should be closely monitored for heparin-induced thrombocytopenia (HIT).

DIET
- Those on anticoagulation should maintain a consistent diet of foods containing vitamin K and avoid foods with anticoagulant properties
- Healthy diet to prevent obesity and dyslipidemia to decrease risk of atherothrombosis

PATIENT EDUCATION
Avoid use of oral hormonal contraceptives.

PROGNOSIS
- Pulmonary HTN, neurologic involvement, myocardial ischemia, nephropathy, gangrene of extremities, and catastrophic APS are associated with a worse prognosis
- Most patients experience recurrences months or years after the initial event.
- Mortality rate is ~50% in patients presenting with the catastrophic type, and death is due to multiorgan system failure.

COMPLICATIONS
Discontinuation of warfarin results in increased risk of thrombosis (even death), particularly in the 1st 6 months after stopping treatment.

REFERENCES

1. Miyakis S, Lockshin MD, Atsumi T et al. International consensus statement on an update of the classification criteria for definite antiphospholipid syndrome (APS). *J Thromb Haemost.* 2006;4:295–306.
2. Erkan D, Lockshin MD. New approaches for managing antiphospholipid syndrome. *Nat Clin Pract Rheumatol.* 2009;5:160–70.
3. Lim W, Crowther MA, Eikelboom JW. Management of antiphospholipid antibody syndrome: a systematic review. *JAMA.* 2006;295:1050–7.
4. ESPRIT Study Group, Halkes PH, van Gijn J, Kappelle LJ, Koudstaal PJ, Algra A et al. Aspirin plus dipyridamole versus aspirin alone after cerebral ischaemia of arterial origin (ESPRIT): randomised controlled trial. *Lancet.* 2006;367:1665–73.
5. Sacco RL, Diener HC, Yusuf S, et al. Aspirin and extended-release dipyridamole versus clopidogrel for recurrent stroke. *N Engl J Med.* 2008;359: 1238–51.
6. Ziakas PD, Pavlou M, Voulgarelis M et al. Heparin treatment in antiphospholipid syndrome with recurrent pregnancy loss: a systematic review and meta-analysis. *Obstet Gynecol.* 2010;115: 1256–62.

ADDITIONAL READING

- Derksen, RHWM and PG de Groot. Towards evidence-based treatment of thrombotic antiphospholipid syndrome. *Lupus.* 2010;19: 470–474.
- Giannakopoulos B, Krilis SA, et al. How I treat the antiphospholipid syndrome. *Blood.* 2009;114: 2020–30.

CODES

ICD9
- 289.81 Primary hypercoagulable state
- 289.82 Secondary hypercoagulable state

CLINICAL PEARLS

- APS can be of either the primary form or the secondary form associated with another underlying illness
- The diagnosis of APS requires both clinical and laboratory criteria
- Thrombosis is the most common clinical manifestation of APS; most common site of venous thrombosis are DVTS and the most common site of arterial thrombosis is the brain
- Treatment is usually with lifelong moderate-intensity warfarin, but may vary, depending on the underlying condition
- Patients with APS and recurrent fetal loss should be considered for combination heparin and ASA treatment during pregnancy

ANTITHROMBIN DEFICIENCY

Marc Jeffrey Kahn, MD
Rebecca Kruse-Jarres, MD, MPH

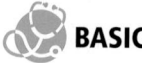 BASICS

DESCRIPTION

Antithrombin is a protease that inhibits thrombin by forming an irreversible thrombin-antithrombin complex. Antithrombin can also inhibit factors Xa, IXa, and XIa. This process is catalyzed by the presence of heparin. Patients deficient in antithrombin have an increased incidence of venous thrombosis, including deep vein thrombosis (DVT) of the lower extremity. Arterial thrombosis is much less common in patients deficient in antithrombin:

- System(s) affected: Cardiovascular; Nervous; Pulmonary; Reproductive; Hemic/Lymphatic/Immunologic
- Synonym(s): Antithrombin III deficiency

EPIDEMIOLOGY

- Predominant age: Mean age of 1st thrombosis is in 2nd decade.
- Predominant sex: Male = Female

Incidence

4% of patients with thrombophilia

Prevalence

0.16% of normal individuals

RISK FACTORS

- Oral contraceptives, pregnancy, and the use of hormone replacement therapy (HRT) increase the risk of venous thrombosis in patients with antithrombin deficiency.
- Patients with antithrombin deficiency and another prothrombotic state, such as factor V Leiden or the prothrombin 20210 mutation, have increased rates of thrombosis.
- Heterozygotes have an odds ratio of venous thrombosis of 10–20.

Pregnancy Considerations

Increases thrombotic risk in patients with antithrombin deficiency

Genetics

Autosomal dominant

GENERAL PREVENTION

Patients with antithrombin deficiency without a history of thrombosis do not require prophylactic treatment.

PATHOPHYSIOLOGY

- Type I deficiency is characterized by low levels of antigen. Type II deficiency is found when the antithrombin molecule is dysfunctional.
- Type II deficiencies are due to mutations in either the active center of antithrombin that binds the target enzyme or the heparin-binding site.

- No patients homozygous for defects in the active center have been described, suggesting that this is a lethal condition. Patients heterozygous for mutations in the heparin-binding site rarely have thrombotic episodes.

ETIOLOGY

Many mutations in the antithrombin gene have been identified.

COMMONLY ASSOCIATED CONDITIONS

Venous thromboembolism

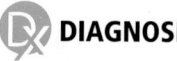 DIAGNOSIS

HISTORY

- Previous thrombosis
- Family history of thrombosis
- Family history of antithrombin deficiency

PHYSICAL EXAM

Deep or superficial venous thrombosis

DIAGNOSTIC TESTS & INTERPRETATION

Lab

Initial lab tests

- Specific testing depends on the clinical setting, and standard coagulation tests should be obtained as necessary in the setting of thrombosis and to rule out other coagulopathies such as protein C and S deficiencies (see Differential Diagnosis).
- Testing should be done off heparin.
- Two tests useful in the workup of antithrombin deficiency include:
  – Antithrombin-heparin cofactor assay, which measures the ability of heparin to bind to antithrombin, which neutralizes the action of thrombin and factor Xa. This is an indirect measure of factor Xa inhibition.
  – Antithrombin activity assay
- Drugs that may alter lab results: Heparin, estrogen, and asparaginase can lower antithrombin levels.

Follow-Up & Special Considerations

- The role of family screening for antithrombin deficiency is unclear, because most patients with this mutation do not have thrombosis. Screening may be considered for women considering using oral contraceptives or for pregnant women with a family history of factor protein S deficiency (1)[C].
- Antithrombin levels are low in:
  – DIC
  – Sepsis
  – Burns
  – Severe trauma
  – Acute thrombosis
  – Pregnancy
  – Liver disease
- Antithrombin levels could be elevated by oral contraceptive pills

Imaging

Initial approach

- Ultrasound to diagnose DVT if clinically indicated
- Spiral computed tomography (CT) or V/Q scan to diagnose pulmonary embolism (PE) if clinically indicated

Follow-Up & Special Considerations

- Ultrasound may not show DVT acutely; repeat in 1–2 days if strong suspicion.
- V/Q scan may be difficult to interpret in patients with other lung disease.

Pathological Findings

Venous thrombosis

DIFFERENTIAL DIAGNOSIS

- Factor V Leiden
- Protein C deficiency
- Protein S deficiency
- Dysfibrinogenemia
- Dysplasminogenemia
- Homocystinemia
- Prothrombin 20210 mutation
- Elevated factor VIII levels

 TREATMENT

MEDICATION

First Line

- Patients with antithrombin deficiency and a 1st thrombosis should be anticoagulated initially with unfractionated heparin followed by oral anticoagulation with warfarin (1)[A].
- After the INR is 2–3, heparin can be stopped after 5 total days of therapy (1)[A].
- Oral anticoagulant following the initial administration of heparin. Warfarin (Coumadin) 5 mg/d p.o. and adjusted to INR of 2–3. Patients should be maintained on warfarin for at least 6 months (1)[A].
- Recurrent thrombosis requires indefinite anticoagulation (1)[A].

- Contraindications:
  – Active bleeding precludes anticoagulation; risk of bleeding is a relative contraindication to long-term anticoagulation.
- Precautions:
  – Observe patient for signs of embolization, further thrombosis, or bleeding.
  – Avoid IM injections.
  – Periodically check stool and urine for occult blood, and monitor complete blood counts, including platelets.
  – Heparin-thrombocytopenia and/or paradoxical thrombosis with thrombocytopenia

- Significant possible interactions:
  – Agents that intensify the response to oral anticoagulants: Alcohol, allopurinol, amiodarone, anabolic steroids, androgens, many antimicrobials, cimetidine, chloral hydrate, disulfiram, all nonsteroidal anti-inflammatory drugs (NSAIDs), sulfinpyrazone, tamoxifen, thyroid hormone, vitamin E, ranitidine, salicylates, acetaminophen
  – Agents that diminish the response to oral anticoagulants: Aminoglutethimide, antacids, barbiturates, carbamazepine, cholestyramine, diuretics, griseofulvin, rifampin, oral contraceptives

Second Line
- Argatroban 0.4–0.5 μg/kg/min. Case reports describing the use of the direct thrombin inhibitor in patients with antithrombin deficiency have been published (2)[C].
- Antithrombin III (ATnativ, Thrombate III) 50–100 IU/min IV titrated to antithrombin level desired. Precise role in therapy remains unclear (1)[C].
- LMWH is difficult to manage in this population (1)[C].

ADDITIONAL TREATMENT
General Measures
Routine anticoagulation for asymptomatic patients with antithrombin deficiency is not recommended (1)[A].

Issues for Referral
- Recurrent thrombosis on anticoagulation
- Difficulty anticoagulating
- Genetic counseling

Additional Therapies
- Patients with severe antithrombin deficiency may require plasma replacement of thrombin in order for heparin to be effective (3)[C].
- Compression stockings for prevention

SURGERY/OTHER PROCEDURES
Thrombectomy may be indicated in complicated cases.

IN-PATIENT CONSIDERATIONS
Initial Stabilization
Heparin initial bolus of 80 U/kg followed by infusion of 18 U/kg/hour. Frequent monitoring of the partial thromboplastin time (PTT) is important, as nearly 50 percent of patients deficient in antithrombin require more than 40,000 U of heparin daily to adequately prolong PTT (1)[C].

Admission Criteria
Complicated thrombosis, such as pulmonary embolus

Discharge Criteria
Stable on anticoagulation

 ## ONGOING CARE
FOLLOW-UP RECOMMENDATIONS
Patient Monitoring
Warfarin use requires periodic INR measurements (monthly after initial stabilization) with a goal of 2–3 (1)[A].

DIET
Foods high in vitamin K may interfere with anticoagulation on warfarin. Consider nutrition consultation.

PATIENT EDUCATION
- Patients should be educated about:
  – Use of oral anticoagulant therapy
  – Avoidance of NSAIDs while on warfarin
- The role of family screening is unclear, as most patients with this mutation do not have thrombosis. In a patient with a family history of factor V Leiden, consider screening during pregnancy or if considering oral contraceptive use.

PROGNOSIS
- The odds ratio of thrombosis in a patient with antithrombin deficiency is much higher than in patients with other thrombophilic conditions. The recurrence rate is similarly high.
- There is no difference in clinical severity between patients with type I defects and type II mutations.
- Overall, prognosis is good, if appropriately anticoagulated.

COMPLICATIONS
Recurrent thrombosis (requires indefinite anticoagulation)

REFERENCES
1. Vinazzer H. Hereditary and acquired antithrombin deficiency. *Semin Thromb Hemost*. 1999;25: 257–63.
2. Dager WE, Gosselin RC, Owings JT. Argatroban therapy for antithrombin deficiency and mesenteric thrombosis: case report and review of the literature. *Pharmacotherapy*. 2004;24:659–63.
3. Maclean PS, Tait RC. Hereditary and acquired antithrombin deficiency: epidemiology, pathogenesis and treatment options. *Drugs*. 2007;67: 1429–40.

ADDITIONAL READING
- Bates SM, Greer IA, Pabinger I et al. Venous thromboembolism, thrombophilia, antithrombotic therapy, and pregnancy: American College of Chest Physicians Evidence-Based Clinical Practice Guidelines (8th Edition). *Chest*. 2008;133: 844S–86S.
- Kottke-Marchant K, Duncan A. Antithrombin deficiency: issues in laboratory diagnosis. *Arch Pathol Lab Med*. 2002;126:1326–36.
- Vossen CY, et al. Risk of a first venous thrombotic event in carriers of a familial thrombotic defect. The European Prospective Cohort on Thrombophilia (EPCOT). *J Thromb Heamost*. 2005;3:459–64.

See Also (Topic, Algorithm, Electronic Media Element)
Thrombosis, Deep Vein (DVT)

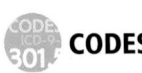 ## CODES

ICD9
289.81 Primary hypercoagulable state

CLINICAL PEARLS
- Antithrombin levels will be low on heparin and during acute thrombosis.
- Diagnosis can be difficult, and conditions causing low levels of antithrombin III, such as pregnancy, liver disease, sepsis, and DIC must be ruled out.
- Both antepartum and postpartum prophylaxis for pregnant women with no prior history of venous thromboembolism but antithrombin deficiency is indicated.

ANXIETY

Mary K. Flynn, MD
Margo L. Kaplan-Gill, MD

BASICS

DESCRIPTION
- The *Diagnostic and Statistical Manual of the American Psychological Association*, Revised Fourth Edition (DSM-IV-R) recognizes generalized anxiety disorder (GAD) as a persistent, excessive, and difficult-to-control anxiety with significant symptoms of motor tension, autonomic hyperactivity, and/or disturbances of sleep or concentration lasting >6 months.
- System(s) affected: Nervous (resulting in increased sympathetic tone and increased catecholamine release)

EPIDEMIOLOGY
Prevalence
- 12-month prevalence rate: 3.1%
- Lifetime prevalence rate: 5.7%
- Onset can occur any time in life, from adolescence to adulthood.
- Predominant age: Median age of onset in US is 31 years.
- Predominant sex: Female > Male (2:1)

RISK FACTORS
- Caucasian race
- Adverse life events, including medical illness, disability, and unemployment
- Family history
- Lack of social support
- Increase in stress
- Lesbian/bisexual women at increased risk above heterosexual women; no increased risk found for homosexual/bisexual men
- Depression

Genetics
- GAD and major depression are strongly linked in heritability studies.
- A variant of the serotonin transporter gene (*5HT1A*) may contribute to both conditions; other genes (such as that for glutamic acid decarboxylase) also may play a role.

GENERAL PREVENTION
Regular exercise is associated with decreased anxiety and depression.

ETIOLOGY
Mediated by abnormalities of neurotransmitter systems [i.e., serotonin, norepinephrine, and γ-aminobutyric acid (GABA)]

COMMONLY ASSOCIATED CONDITIONS
- Major depressive disorder (>60%), dysthymia, bipolar disorder
- Alcohol/drug abuse (37.6%/27.6%)
- Cigarette smoking in adolescence
- Panic disorder
- Agoraphobia, simple phobia
- Social anxiety disorder

DIAGNOSIS

HISTORY
History and evaluation should carefully identify GAD versus other anxiety disorders. In GAD:
- Symptoms (excessive anxiety and worry) must occur more often than not for at least 6 months.
- 3 (or more) additional criteria are required for diagnosis of GAD. Only 1 is required in children:
  - Restlessness or feeling keyed up or on edge
  - Easily fatigued
  - Difficulty concentrating or mind going blank
  - Irritability
  - Muscle tension
  - Sleep disturbances (difficulty falling or staying asleep)
  - Difficulty controlling worry
- Persistent worry must cause significant distress or impairment in social, occupational, or other areas of functioning.
- Focus of anxiety and worry is not consistent with or limited to the occurrence of other types of psychiatric disorders and is not directly related to posttraumatic stress disorder (PTSD).
- All other causes of anxiety and worry have been ruled out (see "Differential Diagnosis") (1).
- Tremor
- Patient may report symptoms of dyspnea, palpitations, diaphoresis, nausea, or diarrhea.

PHYSICAL EXAM
No specific physical findings, but patient may be noted to be irritable or easily startled and may have bitten nails, a tremor, or clammy hands.

DIAGNOSTIC TESTS & INTERPRETATION
Lab
Initial lab tests
Laboratory tests are normal. Initial tests should include
- Thyroid-stimulating hormone
- Complete blood count
- Bone morphogenetic protein
- Electrocardiogram
- See "Differential Diagnosis" for other conditions to rule out.

Diagnostic Procedures/Surgery
Psychological testing:
- GAD-2: 2-question self-reporting scale [22% positive predictive value (PPV)/78% negative predictive value (NPV)] (2)
- GAD-7: 5 additional questions; provides more detailed information for treatment (29% PPV/71% NPV); a positive GAD-2 or GAD-7 also may be indicative of panic disorder (GAD-7: 29% PPV/71% NPV).
- Hamilton's Anxiety Scale (HAM-A)
- Anxiety Disorders Interview Schedule (ADIS)

DIFFERENTIAL DIAGNOSIS
- Cardiovascular: Ischemic heart disease, valvular heart disease, cardiomyopathies, myocarditis, arrhythmias, mitral valve prolapse, congestive heart failure, myocardial infarction
- Respiratory: Asthma, chronic obstructive pulmonary disease, pulmonary embolism, pneumonia
- CNS: Stroke, seizures, dementia, migraine, vestibular dysfunction, encephalitis, neoplasms

- Metabolic and hormonal: Hyper- or hypothyroidism, pheochromocytoma, adrenal insufficiency, Cushing syndrome, hypokalemia, hypoglycemia, hyperparathyroidism
- Nutritional: Thiamine, pyridoxine, or folate deficiency; iron-deficiency anemia
- Drug-induced anxiety: Alcohol, sympathomimetics (cocaine, amphetamine, caffeine), corticosteroids, herbals (ginseng)
- Withdrawal: Alcohol, sedative-hypnotics
- Psychiatric: Other disorders (e.g., panic disorder, obsessive-compulsive disorder, PTSD, social phobia, adjustment disorder, and somatization disorder)

TREATMENT

MEDICATION
Antidepressants take longer to have effect but outperform benzodiazepines in the long term.
- Selective serotonin reuptake inhibitors (SSRIs) (2,3):
  - Escitalopram (Lexapro): Initially 10 mg/d; may titrate to a maximum of 20 mg/d
  - Paroxetine (Paxil): Initially 10–20 mg/d; may titrate to a maximum of 50 mg/d (no added benefit above 20 mg/d)
  - Sertraline (Zoloft): Initially 25 mg/d; may titrate to a maximum of 200 mg/d
- Selective-norepinephrine reuptake inhibitors (SNRIs) (2,3):
  - Duloxetine (Cymbalta): Initially 30 mg/d; may titrate to a maximum of 120 mg/d
  - Venlafaxine XR (Effexor XR): Initially 37.5–75 mg; may titrate up by 75 mg every 4 days to a maximum of 225 mg/d
- Tricyclic antidepressants (TCAs): Imipramine (Tofranil): Initially 25–50 mg/d; maximum of 300 mg/d, 100 mg/d in the elderly (2,3)[A]
- Azapirones: Buspirone (BuSpar): 15 mg/d divided b.i.d. to t.i.d. initially; maximum of 60 mg/d divided b.i.d. to t.i.d. (2,3)[A]

Second Line
- Hydroxyzine: Initially 50 mg q6h; maximum of 400 mg/d
- Benzodiazepines (short-term use) (2,3)[A]:
  - Alprazolam (Xanax): 0.25–0.5 mg b.i.d. to t.i.d.; may increase by 0.25 mg to 4 mg/d
  - Clonazepam (Klonopin): 0.25 mg b.i.d.; may increase to 4 mg/d divided b.i.d.
  - Diazepam (Valium): 2–5 mg b.i.d. to q.i.d.; may increase to a maximum of 40 mg/d
  - Lorazepam (Ativan): 0.5 mg b.i.d. to t.i.d.; may increase to 6 mg/d divided t.i.d.
- Hydroxyzine (Vistaril, Atarax): CNS depressant, antihistamine, anticholinergic; decreased risk of dependence compared with benzodiazepines: Usual dose: 50–100 mg PO q.i.d.
- Pregabalin (Lyrica) and quetiapine (Seroquel) have shown preliminary promise as treatments, but further investigation is needed into their safety and efficacy.

Geriatric Considerations
Avoid TCAs and long-acting benzodiazepines.

Pediatric Considerations
- Black box warning (SSRIs): Antidepressants increase the risk of suicidal thinking and behavior in children, adolescents, and young adults.

- Anxiety often comorbidly exists with attention deficit–hyperreactivity disorder (ADHD).

Pregnancy Considerations
- Buspirone: Category B: Secreted in breast milk; inadequate studies to assess risk
- Benzodiazepines: Category D: May cause lethargy and weight loss in nursing infants; avoid breast-feeding if the mother is taking chronically or in high doses.
- SSRIs: If possible, taper and discontinue. After 20 weeks' gestation, there is increased risk of pulmonary hypertension; mild transient neonatal syndrome of CNS; and motor, respiratory, and GI signs.
  - Paroxetine: Category D, conflicting evidence regarding the risk of congenital cardiac defects and other congenital anomalies
  - Other SSRIs are category C.
- Hydroxyzine: Category C: Case reports of neonatal withdrawal exist.

ALERT
Precautions:
- Benzodiazepines: Advanced age (>65 years), hepatic insufficiency, respiratory disease/sleep apnea, renal insufficiency, suicidal tendency, contraindicated with narrow-angle glaucoma, precaution with open-angle glaucoma; sudden discontinuation increases the risk of seizures, especially with alprazolam. Long-term use has small potential for tolerance and dependence; use with caution in patients with history of substance abuse.
- Buspirone: Hepatic and/or renal dysfunction; monoamine oxidase inhibitor (MAOI) treatment
- TCAs: Advanced age, glaucoma, benign prostate hypertrophy, hyperthyroidism, cardiovascular disease, liver disease, urinary retention, MAOI treatment

ADDITIONAL TREATMENT
Additional Therapies
Psychological:
- Cognitive-behavioral therapy (CBT): Has shown comparable benefit to medical management; also may improve comorbid conditions such as depression
- Mindfulness-based cognitive therapy and stress-reduction studies have been limited. 2010 meta-analysis showed promise in reducing acute symptoms of anxiety in individuals diagnosed with anxiety disorders and in other populations with high anxiety (i.e., the chronically ill) (4).
- Relaxation training: Historically, treatment of choice for GAD but limited evidence for objective benefit
- Psychodynamic psychotherapy: Treatment is focused on patient discovering and verbalizing unconscious content of the psyche.

General Measures
- All patients with GAD are at increased risk for suicidal ideation and attempts; risk increases with comorbid conditions.
- Identify and treat coexisting substance abuse and other psychiatric conditions.

Issues for Referral
Concomitant depression with GAD should prompt a psychiatric evaluation in light of increased suicide risk.

COMPLEMENTARY AND ALTERNATIVE MEDICINE
- Yoga and meditation may be helpful; additional studies are needed, but few adverse effects are known.
- Kava: Evidence for benefit over placebo in mild to moderate anxiety, but significant concern exists regarding potential for hepatotoxicity.
  - May consider for short-term use (up to 24 weeks) (5,6)
  - Studied doses 70–240 mg/d; up to 330 mg/d appears to be safe (7).
  - Must avoid concomitant use of alcohol or other medications metabolized via the liver (CYP 450 inhibitor)
  - Other adverse effects include dermatopathy (usually reversible), ataxia, hearing loss, and loss of appetite; dermatopathy is seen in doses much higher than recommended here.
- St. John's wort: Case reports of benefit in adults, but little evidence for use with anxiety in randomized, controlled trials
  - Drug interactions: CYP 450 3A4, 1A2, or 2E1 inducer; may activate P-glycoprotein
  - In combination with SSRI or buspirone, may lead to serotonin syndrome; otherwise, benign side-effect profile (rare photosensitivity or triggering of mania)
- Passionflower, valerian: Little evidence to support use; benign side-effect profile
- Inositol: Evidence for efficacy in panic disorder and obsessive-compulsive disorder; not studied in GAD

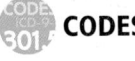 ONGOING CARE

FOLLOW-UP RECOMMENDATIONS
Patient Monitoring
- Continue to monitor for development of comorbid conditions.
- Monitor mental status on benzodiazepines, and avoid drug dependence.
- Monitor blood pressure, heart rate, and anticholinergic side effects of TCAs.
- Monitor all patients for suicidal ideation, but especially those on SSRIs, SNRIs, and imipramine.

DIET
- Limit caffeine intake.
- Avoid alcohol (drug interactions, high rate of abuse, potential for increased anxiety).

PATIENT EDUCATION
- Regular exercise may be beneficial for both anxiety and comorbid conditions.
- Continue with meditation, CBT, and other therapies that provide relief.
- Additional patient information is available at:
  - www.familydoctor.org
  - The National Institute of Mental Health (NIMH) Web site: www.nimh.nih.gov/health/publications/index.shtml

PROGNOSIS
- GAD is a chronic disease, with many patients experiencing continued symptoms or relapse.
- Successful treatment is possible but must be carried out over the long term.
- Relapse is more likely with the discontinuation of medications, particularly in the first year of treatment and during periods of increased stress.

REFERENCES
1. American Psychiatric Association. *Diagnostic and Statistical Manual of Mental Disorders*, 4e. Washington, DC: American Psychiatric Association, 2000:429–84.
2. Kavan MG, Elsasser GN, Barone EJ. Generalized Anxiety Disorder: Practical Assessment and Management. *Am Fam Physician*. 2009;79:785–91.
3. Davidson JR. First-line pharmacotherapy approaches for generalized anxiety disorder. *J Clin Psychiatry*. 2009;70(Suppl 2):25–31.
4. Hofmann SG, Sawyer AT, Witt AA, Oh D et al. The effect of mindfulness-based therapy on anxiety and depression: A meta-analytic review. *J Consult Clin Psychol*. 2010;78:169–83.
5. Saeed SA, Bloch RM, Antonacci DJ. Herbal and dietary supplements for treatment of anxiety disorders. *Am Fam Physician*. 2007;76:549–56.
6. Pittler MH, Ernst E. Kava extract for treating anxiety. *Cochrane Database Syst Rev*. 2003:CD003383.
7. Ernst E. The risk-benefit profile of commonly used herbal therapies: Ginkgo, St. John's Wort, Ginseng, Echinacea, Saw Palmetto, and Kava. *Ann Intern Med*. 2002;136:42–53.

ADDITIONAL READING
- Gorman JM. Treating generalized anxiety disorder. *J Clin Psychiatry*. 2003;64(Suppl 2):24–9.
- Shearer SL. Recent Advances in the Understanding and Treatment of Anxiety Disorders. *Prim Care*. 2007;34:475–504.
- Ströhle A. Physical activity, exercise, depression and anxiety disorders. *J Neural Transm*. 2008.
- Weisberg RB. Overview of generalized anxiety disorder: epidemiology, presentation, and course. *J Clin Psychiatry*. 2009;70(Suppl 2):4–9.

See Also (Topic, Algorithm, Electronic Media Element)
Algorithms: Depression, Adult; Anxiety

CODES

ICD9
- 300.00 Anxiety state, unspecified
- 300.02 Generalized anxiety disorder
- 300.09 Other anxiety states

CLINICAL PEARLS
- GAD is a chronic disease with a relapsing and remitting course for many patients; long-term treatment is required.
- Psychiatric comorbidities, especially depression, are extremely common with GAD.
- Patients are at increased risk for suicidality and should be screened accordingly.
- Antidepressants are the treatment of choice, although they require up to 4 weeks for full effect.
- Benzodiazepines may be used to relieve anxiety initially; they should be tapered and then withdrawn to avoid dependence and tolerance.
- CBT is comparable with medical management; mindfulness meditation and other techniques have shown initial promise.

AORTIC DISSECTION

Mia D. Sorcinelli, MD

 BASICS

DESCRIPTION
Intimal tear in the aorta resulting in hematoma formation. Accumulating blood in false lumen of arterial wall leads to propagation of dissection (1):
- Stanford classification (most widely used):
  - Type A: Involves ascending aorta and aortic arch regardless of site of intimal tear
  - Type B: Involves descending aorta
- DeBakey classification (based on origin site):
  - Type 1: Originates in ascending aorta, propagates at least as far as aortic arch
  - Type 2: Involves only ascending aorta
  - Type 3: Originates in descending aorta, may propagate proximately or distally
- Svensson:
  - Class 1: Classic dissection with true and false lumen
  - Class 2: Intramural hematoma or hemorrhage
  - Class 3: Subtle dissection without hematoma
  - Class 4: Atherosclerotic plaque rupture and ulceration
  - Class 5: Iatrogenic
- Synonym: Dissecting aneurysm

EPIDEMIOLOGY
- Predominant age varies with cause
- Type A dissection average age 60
- Type B dissection patients generally older
- Patients with Marfan syndrome have mean age 36
- Approximately 2/3 of patients are male
- Studies indicate peak time of day between 8 and 9 AM
- Some studies also report slightly higher incidence in winter months

Incidence
About 3 cases per 100,000 people per year

Prevalence
United States:
- Diagnosed in 1 in 10,000 patients admitted to hospital
- Found in 1:350 patients at autopsy
- Numbers may be slightly higher due to unexplained deaths at home or in hospital without autopsy

RISK FACTORS
- Most common associated factors:
  - Hypertension (about 70% of patients)
  - Old age
  - Atherosclerosis
  - Previous cardiovascular surgery, particularly repair of aneurysm or dissection
- Collagen abnormalities:
  - Marfan syndrome
  - Ehlers-Danlos syndrome
- Recreational drug use:
  - Smoking
  - Cocaine
- Inflammatory vasculitis:
  - Takayasu arteritis
  - Giant cell arteritis
- Chest trauma
- Turner syndrome
- Bicuspid aortic valve

- Uncommonly seen in infants following infection
- Also seen in infants during balloon dilation of aortic coarctation
- Reports of dissection in patients with untreated coarctation of the aorta

Genetics
Up to 20% of patients with thoracic aneurysm or dissection were found to have first-degree relatives with aneurysm or dissection. Studies have found the TGFBR1 and TGFBR2 genes are related to aneurysm and dissection in isolated cases and in patients with Marfan's syndrome. Other research has found ACTA2 gene mutations to be involved in isolated and familial dissections and aneurysms.

GENERAL PREVENTION
- Rigorous medical management of precipitating risk factors such as hypertension
- Surveillance of aortic root and replacement when appropriate in patients with collagen disorders (e.g., Marfan, Ehlers-Danlos)

PATHOPHYSIOLOGY
In most cases, dissection develops in the absence of aneurysm, but the false lumen that can be created during dissection can later expand to form an aneurysm. In patients with inherited connective tissue disease, abnormal and/or deficient proteins lead to weakening of vessel walls. Bicuspid aortic valves may also lead to an acquired dysfunction of vascular walls and smooth muscle cells. Histological investigation of postmortem and biopsy specimens reveal cystic medial necrosis, especially in those patients with known preexisting aneurysm

ETIOLOGY
Although the exact sequence of events is controversial, aortic dissection is likely the result of multiple pathological processes. Stress on the aortic wall from hypertension, intimal damage with subsequent tear, rupture or ulceration of atherosclerotic plaques, and involvement of vasa vasorum and intramural hematoma may be contributory.

COMMONLY ASSOCIATED CONDITIONS
See Risk Factors

 DIAGNOSIS

HISTORY
- High level of clinical suspicion is key to correct and prompt diagnosis
- Typical patient is a hypertensive man aged 60–80
- Positive family history raises index of suspicion
- Subjective complaints (2):
  - 85% of patients report abrupt onset of pain
  - Pain was more often described as sharp, less often as tearing or ripping
  - 90% of patients stated that the pain was "severe" or "worst ever"
  - Patients with type A dissections more often report chest pain
  - Patients with type B dissections more often report back and abdominal pain
  - Symptoms overlap between type A and type B dissections

PHYSICAL EXAM
- Hypotension and shock are more common with type A dissection.
- Hypertension is more common with type B dissection.
- Syncope or cerebrovascular accident symptoms
- Any pulse deficit
- Auscultation of aortic regurgitation
- Signs of congestive heart failure
- Limb ischemia
- Acute myocardial infarction/angina
- Spinal cord syndromes/deficits (3)
- Features of tamponade

DIAGNOSTIC TESTS & INTERPRETATION
- Important to use easily available testing to assist in prompt diagnosis
- Blood testing, EKG, chest x-ray, CT scans, and echocardiograms can all assist in diagnosis.
- A normal EKG and chest x-ray cannot be used to rule out the diagnosis if clinical suspicion is high.
- EKG may show (2):
  - Normal findings in up to 1/3 of patients
  - Nonspecific ST-T changes (about 40%)
  - Left ventricular hypertrophy (about 25%)
  - Ischemic changes (about 15%)
  - Acute MI (about 3%)
  - Old MI with Q waves (about 7%)

Lab
Possible novel markers for aortic dissection include a combination of D-dimer, elastin fragments, and smooth-muscle myosin heavy-chain protein. Presently, none of these tests are used routinely as diagnostic tools, and several authors debate the use of D-dimer alone, with research being inconclusive as to its sensitivity and specificity.

Imaging
- Chest X-ray may show:
  - Normal findings in about 15% of patients
  - Widening of the mediastinum (about 60%)
  - Abnormal aortic outline (about 50%)
  - Abnormal cardiac silhouette (about 25%)
  - Calcified or displaced aorta (about 15%)
  - Pleural effusion (about 19%)
- Studies suggest that CT scan with IV contrast, transesophageal echocardiography, and MRI imaging all provide around 95% sensitivity and specificity for diagnosis:
  - MRI may be better for patients where clinical suspicion and pretest probability for aortic dissection are already high.
  - CT scan may be better to rule out dissection in those patients where clinical suspicion and pretest probability are both low.
  - Transesophageal echocardiography can be done at the bedside of an unstable patient in 15–20 minutes, and can offer additional information about heart function (4).
  - In reality, the ready availability and speed with which CT scans can be performed in many hospitals may outweigh the above considerations.
- Both MRI and CT scans can be used by clinicians to assess the extent, size, and location of the dissection, as well as involvement of the branches off the aorta, although some sources suggest MRI as the preferred modality for precise anatomic definition.

Diagnostic Procedures/Surgery
Contrast angiography can be used specifically as a diagnostic tool, especially when visceral perfusion defects are suspected. Angiography may also be used as entry point into endovascular treatment of dissection.

Pathological Findings
* ~60% of intimal tears occur in the proximal ascending aorta. Remainder are between origin of left subclavian artery and ligamentum arteriosum, descending aorta (20%), aortic arch (10%), and abdominal aorta.
* Although medial necrosis is found in aging aortas, it is more extensive in patients who develop aortic dissection.
* Cystic medial necrosis is seen in patients with defects in elastin and connective tissue organization (e.g., Marfan, Ehlers-Danlos).
* Death usually is due to rupture and tamponade.

DIFFERENTIAL DIAGNOSIS
Myocardial infarction, pericarditis, pericardial tamponade not from aortic dissection, angina or atherosclerotic embolism, pulmonary embolism, pneumonia, pleurisy, acute pancreatitis or cholecystitis, penetrating duodenal ulcer, Mallory-Weiss tear or esophageal rupture, mediastinal pathology, musculoskeletal pain

TREATMENT

Due to the acute nature of aortic dissection, there are no randomized controlled trials related to treatment and management.

MEDICATION
For uncomplicated dissection of descending aorta (Stanford B), medical therapy is indicated.

First Line
The cornerstone of medical management is blood pressure control using beta blockers, including propranolol, metoprolol, labetalol, and esmolol

Second Line
* For patients with severe asthma, calcium-channel blockers may be used
* If hypertension is refractory to initial therapies, nitroprusside can be considered, but the patient should be evaluated for possible surgical intervention at that time

ADDITIONAL TREATMENT
General Measures
* Patients should be monitored in intensive care units
* Arterial BP monitoring is preferred, particularly in less stable patients
* Pain control should involve the use of morphine
* If surgical repair of aneurysm is indicated, do not delay repair to evaluate for CAD and valvular dysfunction
* Prompt correction of hypotension, along with identification of the cause, are essential
* Hemodynamically unstable patients will likely require intubation and mechanical ventilation

SURGERY/OTHER PROCEDURES
* Stanford A type dissection:
  – Surgery is the treatment of choice for dissections of the ascending aorta (80% treated surgically) to prevent aortic rupture and cardiac tamponade, while relieving any aortic regurgitation that may be present (2).

– Patients who are inappropriate surgical candidates (comorbid medical conditions, patient choice, very advanced age) have an in-hospital mortality of 50% after 30 days.
  – Surgical correction aims to resect ascending aorta and arch, and replace them with a graft.
  – Other procedures, including repair/replacement of aortic valves and coronary arteries, may be indicated depending on the extent of the dissection.
  – Many different surgical options exist and depend on the extent of dissection.
* Stanford B type dissection:
  – Surgical resection of aorta for type B generally associated with worse outcomes than medical management.
  – Surgical indications for Stanford B include (2):
    ○ Continued aortic expansion
    ○ Impending aortic rupture
    ○ Occlusion of major aortic branch to renal, mesenteric, or iliac arteries
    ○ Persistent and recurrent chest pain
    ○ Periaortic or mediastinal hematoma
* Poor prognostic factors for surgical success:
  – Age >70 years
  – Abrupt-onset chest pain
  – Hypotension, shock, or tamponade at presentation
  – Renal failure
  – Pulse deficit
  – Abnormal ECG, ST segment elevation
  – History of aortic valve replacement
  – Renal and/or visceral ischemia
* Stenting of complicated type B dissections seems to be a reasonable and safe alternative to surgical management, although further follow-up is needed

IN-PATIENT CONSIDERATIONS
Initial Stabilization
* Admit to ICU
* Intubate hemodynamically unstable patients
* Control BP:
  – Systolic 100–120 mm Hg
  – IV beta blocker to achieve HR 60
  – Determine etiology of hypotension:
    ○ Blood loss
    ○ Tamponade
    ○ Heart failure
* Pain control

Admission Criteria
Low threshold for admission in presence of thoracic or abdominal pain, radiographic corroboration, or pulse deficit.

ONGOING CARE

FOLLOW-UP RECOMMENDATIONS
Patient Monitoring
* Maintain systolic BP at 120 mm Hg (16 kPa) or below, as tolerated
* Routine chest films and/or chest CT may be helpful for patient treated medically long term.
* During follow-up, pay careful attention to signs and symptoms of aortic insufficiency, chest or back pain, and development of saccular aneurysms as displayed on chest films.

DIET
NPO until surgical evaluation is complete and patient classified as medical therapy only.

PATIENT EDUCATION
Depending on etiology, emphasis must be placed on risk factors and prevention of recurrence:
* Smoking cessation
* Blood pressure control with beta blockers
* Diabetic control

PROGNOSIS
* Hospital survival estimate, treated medically and surgically: 70% (2)
* Data for Type A dissections treated surgically show a 90% survival rate at 3 years (5).
* Survival at 10 years similar for medically and surgically treated patients.
* Redissection risk:
  – 5 years: 13%
  – 10 years: 23%

COMPLICATIONS
Redissection, localized saccular aneurysm, cardiac tamponade, aortic valvular insufficiency, progressive aortic enlargement. Stent placement risks include paraplegia, stroke, embolization, side-branch occlusion, infection

REFERENCES

1. Golledge J, Eagle KA. Acute aortic dissection. *Lancet.* 2008;372:55–66.
2. Hagan PG, Nienaber CA, Isselbacher EM et al. The International Registry of Acute Aortic Dissection (IRAD): new insights into an old disease. *JAMA.* 2000;283:897–903.
3. Gaul C, Dietrich W, Friedrich I et al. Neurological symptoms in type A aortic dissections. *Stroke.* 2007;38:292–7.
4. Nair HC et al. Transesophageal echocardiography evaluation of thoracic aorta. *Ann Card Anaesth.* 2010;13:186.
5. Tsai TT, Evangelista A, Nienaber CA, Trimarchi S, Sechtem U, Fattori R, Myrmel T, Pape L, Cooper JV, Smith DE, Fang J, Isselbacher E, Eagle KA, International Registry of Acute Aortic Dissection (IRAD) et al. Long-term survival in patients presenting with type A acute aortic dissection: insights from the International Registry of Acute Aortic Dissection (IRAD). *Circulation.* 2006;114:1350–6.

See Also (Topic, Algorithm, Electronic Media Element)
Hypertension; Ehlers-Danlos Syndrome; Marfan Syndrome

CODES

ICD9
* 441.00 Dissection of aorta, unspecified site
* 441.01 Dissection of aorta, thoracic

CLINICAL PEARLS

* 90% of patients with aortic dissection report acute pain, more often sharp than tearing, and located in the chest, abdomen, or back
* Maintain a high level of suspicion and act quickly if the diagnosis of aortic dissection is suspected.
* Survival at 10 years similar for medically and surgically treated patients.

AORTIC VALVULAR STENOSIS

Ajar Kochar, MD
Dawn Abbott, MD

 BASICS

DESCRIPTION
Aortic stenosis (AS) is a narrowing of the aortic valve area that causes an obstruction to left ventricular outflow. The disease has a long asymptomatic latency period, but development of severe obstruction or onset of symptoms such as syncope and angina as associated with a high mortality rate if surgical intervention is not accomplished promptly.

EPIDEMIOLOGY
- Most common valvular disease in developed countries
- >50% of patients with isolated aortic stenosis also have a congenitally malformed valve (1).
- Predominant age:
  - <30 years: Congenital
  - 30–70 years: Congenital or rheumatic fever
  - >70 years: Degenerative calcification of aortic valve

Prevalence
- 1.3% at 65–74 years old, 2.4% at 75–84 years old, 4% at >84 years old (1)
- Bicuspid aortic valve: 1–2% of population (1)

RISK FACTORS
- Congenital (1):
  - Bicuspid valve
    ○ Most commonly in men
    ○ AS occurs at younger age
    ○ Associated with coarctation of aorta
  - Unicommissural valve
- Acquired (1):
  - Rheumatic fever
  - Degenerative (CAD-related RF): Hypercholesterolemia [elevated LDL, lipoprotein (a)], smoking, male gender, age, hypertension, diabetes mellitus

PATHOPHYSIOLOGY
- Progressive stiffening of aortic valve results in LV outflow obstruction
- Obstruction causes increased afterload and decreased forward flow.
- Increased afterload is compensated for by development of concentric left ventricular hypertrophy (LVH).
- LVH preserves ejection fraction but adversely affects heart functioning:
  - LVH impairs coronary blood flow reserve by compression of coronary arteries and reduced capillary ingrowth into hypertrophied muscle.
  - LVH results in diastolic dysfunction by reducing ventricular compliance.
- Diastolic dysfunction mandates stronger left atrial (LA) contraction to augment pre-load and maintain stroke volume. Loss of LA contraction by atrial fibrillation (AFib) can induce acute deterioration.
- Angina: Myocardial demand is elevated due to increased left ventricular pressure. Myocardial supply is compromised due to LVH.
- Syncope (exertional): Ventricular contraction cannot augment cardiac output enough to match increase demands of exercise due to the fixed obstruction to LV outflow.

- Heart Failure: Eventually LVH cannot compensate for increasing afterload resulting in high LV Pressure and Volume which is accompanied with a rise in LA and Pulmonary pressures

ETIOLOGY
- Calcific aortic stenosis (2): Initiating insult is mechanical stress to valve leaflets:
  - Note bicuspid valves are at higher risk for shear stress
  - Early lesions: Subendothelial accumulation of oxidized LDL and macrophages and T-lymphocytes (inflammatory response)
  - Disease progression: Fibroblasts undergo transformation into osteoblasts. Protein production of osteopontin, osteocalcitonin, and BMP-2, which modulate calcification of leaflets
- Congenital: Unicuspid valve. Tricuspid valve with fusion of commissures, hypoplastic annulus
- Rheumatic Fever: Fusion of commissures and scarring

COMMONLY ASSOCIATED CONDITIONS
- Coronary artery disease (50% of patients)
- Hypertension (40% of patients) Results in "double-loaded" left ventricle (dual source of obstruction from AS and hypertension)
- Aortic regurgitation (common in calcified bicuspid valves and rheumatic disease)
- Mitral valve disease: 95% of patients with AS from rheumatic fever also have mitral valve disease.
- LV dysfunction and CHF
- Atrial fibrillation associated with CHF
- Acquired von Willebrand disease: Impaired platelet function and decreased vWF results in bleeding (ecchymosis and epistaxis) in 20% of AS patients. Severity of coagulopathy is directly related to severity of AS.
- Rarely: Calcific embolization to systemic organs

 DIAGNOSIS

HISTORY
- Primary symptoms: Angina, syncope, and heart failure (3). Angina is most frequent symptom. Syncope is often exertional. Heart failure symptoms include: Fatigue, exertional dyspnea, orthopnea, paroxysmal nocturnal dyspnea, shortness of breath
- Palpitations
- Neurologic events (transient ischemic attack or cerebrovascular accident) owing to embolization
- Geriatric patients may have subtle symptoms such as fatigue and exertional dyspnea
- Note: Symptoms do not always correlate with valve area (severity of AS) but most commonly occur when AV area is <1.0 cm^2

PHYSICAL EXAM
- Auscultation (3):
  - Harsh, systolic crescendo-decrescendo murmur (grade 4/6):
    ○ Best heard at 2nd right sternal border
    ○ Radiates into carotid arteries
    ○ Peak of murmur correlates with severity of stenosis: Earlier peaking murmur suggests less severe narrowing

- High-pitched diastolic blow, suggests associated aortic regurgitation
- Paradoxically split S2 or absent A2
- Note: Normally split S2 reliably excludes severe AS
- S4
- Other associated signs: (3) Thrill (denotes more severe narrowing); Parvus et Tardus: Carotid upstrokes decreased in volume, delayed in rate. LV heave

DIAGNOSTIC TESTS & INTERPRETATION
Lab
BNP may be elevated (no cutoffs exist) (1). Values altered by obesity, pulmonary hypertension, renal disease

Imaging
Initial approach
- Chest x-ray (CXR) (1)
  - May be normal in compensated, isolated valvular aortic stenosis.
  - Boot-shaped heart reflective of concentric hypertrophy
  - Post-stenotic dilatation of ascending aorta
  - Calcification of aortic valve (seen on lateral PA CXR)
- Electrocardiogram (ECG):
  - Often normal ECG (ECG is non-diagnostic)
  - LV hypertrophy
  - Left atrial enlargement
  - Nonspecific ST and T-wave abnormalities
- Echo Indications:
  - Initial workup:
    ○ Doppler echocardiogram is mainstay of diagnosis
    ○ Severity of AS
    ○ Assess left ventricular wall thickness, size, function.
  - In known AS and changing signs/symptoms
  - In known AS and pregnancy due to hemodynamic changes of pregnancy
- Echo findings:
  - Aortic valve morphology, thickening, calcifications
  - Decreased aortic valve excursion
  - Aortic valve area
  - LV hypertrophy
  - LV ejection fraction
  - Chamber dimensions will often be normal.
  - Wall-motion abnormalities suggesting coronary artery disease (CAD)
  - Evaluate for concomitant mitral valve disease.
- Doppler echo adds information on:
  - Transvalvular gradient
  - Valve area
  - Diastolic function
  - Associated aortic regurgitation
- Aortic stenosis severity based on echo values (assumes normal cardiac output):
  - Normal: Area: 3–4 cm Gradient: 0 mm Hg Jet Vel. <2.5 m/s
  - Mild: Area: 1.5–2 cm Gradient: <25 mm Hg Jet Vel. 2.5–2.9 m/s
  - Mod: Area: 1–1.5 cm Gradient: 25–40 mm Hg Jet Vel. 3–4 m/s
  - Severe: Area: <1 cm Gradient: >40 mm Hg Jet Vel. >4 m/s

- Patients with severe AS and low cardiac output may have a relatively low transvalvular pressure gradient (i.e., mean gradient less than 30 mm Hg)

Diagnostic Procedures/Surgery
- Exercise stress testing:
  - Asymptomatic patients (4)[B]: Helpful to uncover subtle symptoms or changes, abnormal blood pressure (increase less than 20 mm Hg), and EKG changes (ST depressions). 1/3 of patients develop symptoms with exercise testing – STOP testing at this point.
  - Symptomatic patients (4)[B]: DO NOT perform exercise stress testing as may induce hypotension or ventricular tachycardia
  - CHF patients (4)[B]: Dobutamine stress echocardiography is reasonable to evaluate patients with low-flow/low-gradient AS and LV dysfunction.
- Cardiac catheterization: Perform Prior to AVR in patients with suspected CAD (4)[B]. Determines need for Coronary Artery Bypass Graft (CABG). If unambiguous diagnosis of AS, only perform coronary angiography.
- Perform as diagnostic adjunct:
  - Catheterization is gold standard for diagnosis
  - Use if noninvasive testing is inconclusive.
  - Use if discrepancy in severity of symptoms and findings on echo
  - Perform complete right and left heart catheterization.
  - Measure: Transvalvular flow, transvalvular pressure gradient, and effective valve area
  - Hemodynamic measurements with infusion of dobutamine can be useful for evaluation of patients with low-flow/low-gradient AS and LV dysfunction

Pathological Findings
- Aortic valve: nodular calcification on valve cusps (initially at bases), cusp rigidity, cusp thickening, and fibrosis
- LV hypertrophy
- Myocardial interstitial fibrosis
- 50% incidence of concomitant CAD

DIFFERENTIAL DIAGNOSIS
- Mitral regurgitation: Either primary or secondary to underlying coronary artery disease or dilated cardiomyopathy. Usually an apical, high-frequency, pansystolic murmur, often radiating to axilla.
- Hypertrophic obstructive cardiomyopathy: Also systolic crescendo-decrescendo murmur, but best heard at left sternal border and may radiate into axilla. Murmur intensity increases by changing from squatting to standing and/or by Valsalva maneuver.
- Discrete fixed subaortic stenosis 50–65% have associated cardiac deformity (PDA, VSD, coarctation of aorta)
- Aortic supravalvular stenosis Williams syndrome, homozygous familial hypercholesterolemia

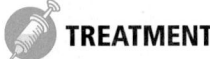

TREATMENT

MEDICATION
- NO medical therapy for severe or symptomatic aortic stenosis
- Prevention: Currently no recommended medical therapy. Statins may have a role if initiated during mild disease. Antibiotic prophylaxis against recurrent rheumatic fever is indicated for patients with rheumatic AS (Penicillin G 1,200,000 U IM every 4 weeks, duration varies with age and history of

carditis). Antibiotic prophylaxis is no longer indicated for prevention of infective endocarditis (4).
- Complications: Decompensated heart failure responds rapidly to IV nitroprusside (dose titrated to MAP of 60–70); can be used as bridge therapy until surgery.
- Co-morbidities: Hypertension: ACE inhibitors, start with low dose and increase cautiously. Be cautious of vasodilators which may cause hypotension

ADDITIONAL TREATMENT
Percutaneous balloon aortic valvotomy or valvuloplasty (BAV)
- Percutaneous prosthetic valve implantation is under development and improves outcomes in patients that are not candidates for surgery. Poor surgical candidates: Advanced age, left ventricular dysfunction, numerous comorbidities
- In young adults and others without significantly calcified aortic valves and no AR, BAV is indicated in the following patients:
  - Symptoms of angina, syncope, dyspnea on exertion, and peak-to-peak gradients at catheterization greater than 50 mm Hg.
  - Asymptomatic adolescents or young adults who demonstrate ST or T-wave abnormalities in the left precordial leads on ECG at rest or with exercise and a peak-to-peak catheter gradient greater than 60 mm Hg (4)[C].
  - Asymptomatic adolescent or young adult with AS and a peak-to-peak gradient on catheterization greater than 50 mm Hg when the patient is interested in playing competitive sports or becoming pregnant (4)[C].
- In older adults with rheumatic or degenerative AS, BAV may be considered as a bridge to surgery in hemodynamically unstable adults with AS, adults at high risk for AVR, or when AVR cannot be performed secondary to significant comorbidities (4)[C].

SURGERY/OTHER PROCEDURES
Indications for aortic valve replacement (AVR):
- Symptomatic and severe AS (4)[B] should be performed rapidly due to high risk of sudden cardiac death
- Asymptomatic, severe AS and
  - Requires aortic root surgery or other valvular surgery (4)[C]
  - Requires coronary artery bypass grafting (CABG) (4)[C]
  - Ejection fraction (EF) (<50%) (4)[C]
  - Positive exercise stress testing findings (4)[C]
  - Risk of rapid progression (moderate-severe calcification, age, CAD) (4)[C]
- Asymptomatic, extremely severe AS (4)[C]: Aortic valve area <0.6 cm, gradient >60 mm Hg, or jet velocity >5 m/s
- Moderate stenosis and undergoing CABG or valvular surgery (4)[B]
- Mild AS and CABG and high risk of rapid progression (4)[C]. Note if AV Area >1.5 cm and gradient <15 mm Hg no benefit from AVR

ONGOING CARE

FOLLOW-UP RECOMMENDATIONS
- Advise patient to immediately report symptoms referable to AS.
- Asymptomatic patients: Yearly history and physical (4)[C]

- Serial echo: Recommendation (4)[B]: Yearly for severe AS, every 1–2 years for moderate AS, every 3–5 years for mild AS

PATIENT EDUCATION
Physical activity limitations:
- Asymptomatic mild AS: No restrictions, competitive sports are okay
- Asymptomatic moderate-to-severe AS: Avoid competitive sports that have high muscle demand. Milder exercise can be done safely. Consider exercise stress test prior to starting exercise program.

PROGNOSIS
- 25% mortality/year in symptomatic patients who do not undergo valve replacement; Average survival is 2–3 years without AVR surgery
- Median survival in symptomatic AS (3): Heart failure: 2 years syncope: 3 years angina: 5 years
- After aortic valve replacement, a patient's lifespan returns to near that of an unselected population
- Peri-surgical mortality AVR surgery has 4% mortality; AVR + CABG has 6.8% mortality
- Adverse postoperative prognostic factors: Age, HF NYHA III/IV, cerebrovascular disease, renal dysfunction, CAD

REFERENCES
1. Carabello BA, Paulus WJ et al. Aortic stenosis. *Lancet*. 2009;373:956–66
2. Otto CM et al. Calcific aortic stenosis–time to look more closely at the valve. *N Engl J Med*. 2008;359:1395–8.
3. Grimard BH, Larson JM et al. Aortic stenosis: diagnosis and treatment. *Am Fam Physician*. 2008;78:717–24.
4. Bonow RO, et al. ACC/AHA 2006 guidelines for the management of patients with valvular heart disease: a report of the American College of Cardiology/American Heart Association Task Force on Practice Guidelines *Circulation*. 2006;114:e84–231.

CODES

ICD9
- 395.0 Rheumatic aortic stenosis
- 424.1 Aortic valve disorders
- 746.3 Congenital stenosis of aortic valve

CLINICAL PEARLS
- Aortic stenosis is diagnosed on physical exam by a systolic crescendo-decrescendo murmur, and delayed and diminished pulses.
- Symptomatic AS most commonly presents as angina, syncope, and heart failure.
- Symptomatic AS has a very poor prognosis unless treated with surgical intervention.

APPENDICITIS, ACUTE

Francesca L. Beaudoin, MS, MD
Erik E. Wang, MD

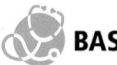

BASICS

DESCRIPTION
- Acute inflammation of the vermiform appendix, first described by Reginald Fitz in 1886
- Arising from the base of the cecum in right lower quadrant (RLQ); can be localized anterior, posterior, medial, lateral to the cecum, as well as in the pelvis
- Vascular supply by appendicular artery, a branch of the ileocolic artery
- Most common cause of the acute surgical abdomen

EPIDEMIOLOGY
- Predominant age: 10–30 years:
  - Rare in infancy
- Predominant sex: Slight male predominance:
  - Ages 10–30: Male > Female (3:2)
  - Age >30: Male = Female

Incidence
- 1 case per 1,000 people per year
- Lifetime incidence 1 in every 15 persons (7%)

Pregnancy Considerations
- Most common extrauterine surgical emergency
- 1 in 2,000 pregnancies

RISK FACTORS
- Adolescent males
- Familial tendency
- Intra-abdominal tumors

Genetics
1st-degree relative with history of appendicitis increases risk, although no direct genetic link has been found

PATHOPHYSIOLOGY
The initial event inciting appendicitis is thought to be obstruction of the appendiceal lumen. This leads to distention, ischemia, and bacterial overgrowth. Without intervention, most cases of appendicitis will lead to perforation and subsequently abscess formation or generalized peritonitis.

ETIOLOGY
Causes of obstruction:
- Fecaliths (most common)
- Lymphoid tissue hyperplasia (in children)
- Inspissated barium
- Vegetable, fruit seeds
- Other foreign bodies
- Intestinal worms (ascarids)
- Strictures, fibrosis
- Neoplasms

DIAGNOSIS

Diagnosis of acute appendicitis relies on the clinical integration of history, physical exam, and often laboratories and imaging. Scoring systems, including the Alvarado Score and the Pediatric Appendicitis Score, have been developed to help predict the likelihood of acute appendicitis, although diagnosis is still considered a clinical decision.

HISTORY
- The classic history is vague periumbilical pain, followed by anorexia/nausea/vomiting. Over the next 4–48 hours, pain then migrates to the right lower quadrant.
- Only 50% of patients present with this classic history.
- Pain before vomiting (~100% sensitive)
- Abdominal pain (~100%)
- Anorexia (~100%)
- Nausea (90%)
- Vomiting (75%)
- Pain migration (50%)
- Obstipation
- Atypical symptoms and pain with retrocecal and pelvic appendix

PHYSICAL EXAM
- Fever; temp >100.4°F (can be absent)
- Tachycardia
- RLQ tenderness
- Maximal tenderness at McBurney's point
- Voluntary and involuntary guarding
- Cutaneous hyperesthesia at T10–12
- Rovsing sign: RLQ pain with palpation of left lower quadrant
- Psoas sign: Pain with right thigh extension (retrocecal appendix)
- Obturator sign: Pain with internal rotation of flexed right thigh (pelvic appendix)
- Local and suprapubic pain on rectal exam (pelvic appendix)
- Pelvic and rectal exams necessary to explore other pathology (pelvic inflammatory disease, prostatitis, etc.)
- Serial exams can be useful in indeterminate cases.

Pediatric Considerations
- Decreased diagnostic accuracy
- Higher fever, more vomiting

Pregnancy Considerations
- Difficult diagnosis
- Appendix displaced by gravid uterus

Geriatric Considerations
Decreased diagnostic accuracy, atypical presentations

DIAGNOSTIC TESTS & INTERPRETATION
Lab
- Leukocytosis: white blood cells (WBC) >10,000/mm^3 (70%)
- Polymorphonuclear predominance or "left shift" (>90%)
- hCG (if negative, rules out ectopic pregnancy)
- Urinalysis:
  - Elevated specific gravity
  - Hematuria, pyuria (~30%)
- C-reactive protein:
  - Nonspecific inflammatory marker
  - When paired with an elevated WBC can increase the likelihood of appendicitis
- Drugs that may alter lab results:
  - Antibiotics
  - Steroids

Imaging
- Used in cases of suspected appendicitis when the diagnosis is not clear

- Helpful to detect complications (abscess)
- Computed tomography (CT) scan: Sensitivity ~91–98%; specificity 95–99%; imaging modality of choice.
- CT scan with IV contrast alone provides equivalent information to CT scan with rectal or oral contrast (1)[A].
- Ultrasound: Viable alternative in pregnant patients, children, and in women with suspected gynecologic pathology (2)[B]. Sensitivity ~86%; specificity ~81%. An initial ultrasound and, if negative, a CT scan has been shown to be an effective workup strategy for all patients (3)[B].
- Plain films: Little utility, nonspecific findings, may visualize fecalith
- Magnetic resonance imaging: May be helpful in pregnant patients
- Radioisotope-labeled WBC scans: May be used in patients with indeterminate CT scans and suspected appendicitis as an alternative to observation or surgery

Diagnostic Procedures/Surgery
Diagnostic laparoscopy useful in equivocal cases, especially in fertile women (1)[A]

Pathological Findings
- Acute appendiceal inflammation
- Local vascular congestion
- Obstruction
- Gangrene
- Perforation with abscess (15–30%)
- Fecalith

DIFFERENTIAL DIAGNOSIS
- Gastrointestinal:
  - Gastroenteritis
  - Inflammatory bowel disease
  - Diverticulitis
  - Ileitis
  - Cholecystitis
  - Pancreatitis
  - Intussusception
  - Volvulus
- Gynecologic:
  - Pelvic inflammatory disease
  - Ectopic pregnancy
  - Ovarian cyst, ovarian torsion
  - Endometriosis
  - Ruptured graafian follicle
- Urologic:
  - Testicular torsion, epididymitis
  - Kidney stones
  - Prostatitis, cystitis, pyelonephritis
- Systemic:
  - Diabetic ketoacidosis
  - Henoch Schönlein purpura
  - Sickle cell crisis
  - Porphyria

- Other:
  – Acute mesenteric lymphadenitis
  – No organic pathologic condition
  – Hernias
  – Psoas abscess
  – Rectus sheath hematoma
  – Epiploic appendagitis
  – Pneumonia (basilar)

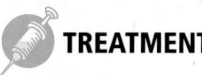

TREATMENT

MEDICATION
First Line
- Uncomplicated acute appendicitis: Perioperative dose of broad-spectrum antibiotic (4)[A]:
  – Cefoxitin (Mefoxin); cefotetan (Cefotan)
- Gangrenous or perforating appendicitis:
  – Broadened antibiotic coverage for aerobic and anaerobic enteric pathogens
  – Fluoroquinolone and metronidazole typical
  – Adjust dosage and choice of antibiotic based on intraoperative cultures.
  – Continue antibiotics for 7 days postoperatively or until patient becomes afebrile with normal white blood cell count.

Second Line
- Ampicillin-sulbactam (Unasyn)
- Ticarcillin-clavulanate (Timentin)
- Piperacillin-tazobactam (Zosyn)

ADDITIONAL TREATMENT
General Measures
Surgery (appendectomy) is still the standard of care. However, nonoperative management with antibiotics has been studied as an alternative. Some literature suggests that antibiotic therapy alone may be initially as successful as appendectomy, but this approach carries recurrent appendicitis rates of 14–20% in the first year (5). The possibility of recurrence or progression to perforation must be weighed against the potential complications of surgery.

Issues for Referral
All cases of appendicitis require emergent surgical consultation.

SURGERY/OTHER PROCEDURES
- Inpatient surgery is appropriate measure
- Patients presenting within 72 hours of onset:
  – Immediate appendectomy; laparoscopic favored unless perforation (6)[A]
  – Drainage of abscess, if present
- Patients who present late (>4–5 days after symptom onset) may be treated initially with antibiotics, bowel rest, and drainage of any abscess. Later (4–10 weeks) appendectomy can then be performed in this subgroup only.

IN-PATIENT CONSIDERATIONS
Admission Criteria
All patients with appendicitis should be admitted.

IV Fluids
- Fluid resuscitation with NS or LR
- Correct fluid and electrolyte deficits

Nursing
Preoperative preparation

Discharge Criteria
Tolerating p.o.; return of bowel function; afebrile; normal WBC

ONGOING CARE

FOLLOW-UP RECOMMENDATIONS
- Return to work is usually possible 1–2 weeks following most uncomplicated appendicitis.
- Restrict activity for 4–6 weeks after surgery: No heavy lifting (>10 lbs) or strenuous physical activity.

Patient Monitoring
Routine visits at 2 and 6 weeks after surgery

DIET
n.p.o. before surgery

PATIENT EDUCATION
Contact physician for postoperative development of:
- Anorexia
- Nausea
- Vomiting
- Abdominal pain
- Fever
- Chills

PROGNOSIS
- Generally uncomplicated course in young adults with unruptured appendicitis
- Factors increasing morbidity and mortality:
  – Extremes of age
  – Appendiceal rupture
- Morbidity rates:
  – Nonperforated appendicitis: 3%
  – Perforated appendicitis: 47%
- Mortality rates:
  – Unruptured appendicitis: 0.1%
  – Ruptured appendicitis: 3%
  – Patients >60 years of age: 50% of deaths from appendicitis
  – Older patients with ruptured appendix: 15%

Pediatric Considerations
- Rupture earlier
- Rupture rate: 15–50%

Pregnancy Considerations
Fetal mortality rate: 2–8.5%

Geriatric Considerations
Rupture rate: 67–90%

COMPLICATIONS
- Wound infection
- Intra-abdominal abscess; lower rate with antibiotic prophylaxis (1)[A]
- Intestinal fistulas
- Intestinal obstruction
- Incisional hernia
- Liver abscess (rare)
- Paralytic ileus
- Pyelophlebitis

REFERENCES

1. Mun S, Ernst RD, Chen K et al. Rapid CT diagnosis of acute appendicitis with IV contrast material. *Emerg Radiol*. 2006;12:99–102.
2. Old JL, Dusing RW, Yap W et al. Imaging for suspected appendicitis. *Am Fam Physician*. 2005;71:71–8.
3. Poortman P, Oostvogel HJ, Bosma E, Lohle PN, Cuesta MA, de Lange-de Klerk ES, Hamming JF et al. Improving diagnosis of acute appendicitis: results of a diagnostic pathway with standard use of ultrasonography followed by selective use of CT. *J Am Coll Surg*. 2009;208:434–41.
4. Andersen BR, Kallehaue FL, Andersen HK. Antibiotics versus placebo for prevention of postoperative infection after appendectomy. *Cochrane Database Syst Rev*. 2006;(1).
5. Hansson J, Körner U, Khorram-Manesh A et al. Randomized clinical trial of antibiotic therapy versus appendectomy as primary treatment of acute appendicitis in unselected patients. *Br J Surg*. 2009;96:473–81.
6. Sauerland S, Lefering R, Neugebauer EAM. Laparoscopic versus open surgery for suspected appendicitis. *Cochrane Database Syst Rev*. 2006;(1).

ADDITIONAL READING

- Anderson SW, Soto JA, Lucey BC, Ozonoff A, Jordan JD, Ratevosian J, Ulrich AS, Rathlev NK, Mitchell PM, Rebholz C, Feldman JA, Rhea JT et al. Abdominal 64-MDCT for suspected appendicitis: the use of oral and IV contrast material versus IV contrast material only. *AJR Am J Roentgenol*. 2009;193:1282–8.
- Hlibczuk V, Dattaro JA, Jin Z, Falzon L, Brown MD et al. Diagnostic accuracy of noncontrast computed tomography for appendicitis in adults: a systematic review. *Ann Emerg Med*. 2010;55:51–59.e1.
- Gaitini D, Beck-Razi N, Mor-Yosef D, Fischer D, Ben Itzhak O, Krausz MM, Engel A et al. Diagnosing acute appendicitis in adults: accuracy of color Doppler sonography and MDCT compared with surgery and clinical follow-up. *AJR Am J Roentgenol*. 2008;190:1300–6.

See Also (Topic, Algorithm, Electronic Media Element)
Algorithm: Abdominal Rigidity

CODES

ICD9
- 540.0 Acute appendicitis with generalized peritonitis
- 540.9 Acute appendicitis without mention of peritonitis
- 541 Appendicitis, unqualified

CLINICAL PEARLS

- Classic history of anorexia with periumbilical pain localizing to RLQ is the cornerstone of diagnosis for acute appendicitis.
- Diagnosis is much more challenging in children, pregnant patients, and the elderly due to varying symptoms and signs.
- CT of abdomen and pelvis is the diagnostic test of choice, although ultrasound in experienced hands has good sensitivity and avoids radiation exposure.
- Acute appendicitis is the most common surgical emergency during pregnancy.

ARTERIAL GAS EMBOLISM

Naida Cole, MD
Neha Raukar, MD

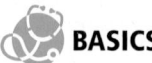 **BASICS**

DESCRIPTION
- Arterial gas embolism (AGE) is an uncommon, potentially fatal event caused by the entry of gas either directly into the arteries of the systemic circulation or indirectly into the pulmonary veins.
- Emboli can travel to any artery but the most serious consequences occur when they affect the cerebral or coronary circulation, as a result of the inherent vulnerability of the brain and heart to hypoxia.

EPIDEMIOLOGY
- Predominant age: Young adult
- Predominant sex: Male > Female

Incidence
Among divers, the incidence of AGE is <0.1%, but it is the cause of 18% of diving fatalities (based on Divers Alert Network America Report) (1).

RISK FACTORS
- Scuba diving is the most common cause of AGE. Arterial gas embolism is the most serious and rapidly fatal of all scuba diving injuries and is second only to drowning as the leading cause of death associated with sport diving. Two mechanisms may lead to arterial gas embolism:
  - Rapid ascent may lead to decompression sickness (the evolution of bubbles in blood or tissues from dissolved inert gas).
  - Breath holding during ascent may lead to pulmonary barotrauma and subsequent arterial gas emboli.
- Any right-to-left cardiac shunt is a risk factor for paradoxical embolism. These shunts include a patent foramen ovale, pulmonary arteriovenous malformation, or a septal defect. Divers with a patent foramen ovale have a greater than 4-fold increase in decompression illness events and sustain twice as many ischemic brain lesions than in divers without this condition.
- Diagnostic or therapeutic medical procedures can also introduce air directly into the arterial system. AGE most commonly occurs during radiologic procedures, cardiac bypass or coronary artery bypass graft surgery, and neurosurgical procedures.

GENERAL PREVENTION
- Scuba diving:
  - Adhere strictly to diver safety protocols.
  - Do not dive when dehydrated, after recent alcohol use, or with a dive injury or medical condition until evaluated and approved by a physician knowledgeable in diving medicine.
  - Avoid fatigue and hypothermia when diving and avoid rapid ascent with breath-holding.
  - Do not fly or travel to altitudes >700 feet within 24 hours of the last dive.

- Medical:
  - Minimize airway pressures in mechanically ventilated patients to prevent pulmonary barotrauma.
  - Avoid hypovolemia and low blood pressures in high-risk procedures.
  - Occlude the hub of the central venous catheter and ask patient to Valsalva/breath-hold during insertion and removal of a central venous catheter.
  - When flushing any arterial line, take extreme care to avoid air entering the fluid used to flush the line.
  - Place patient in Trendelenburg position when performing any procedure entering a large vein, in case of right to left shunt.

PATHOPHYSIOLOGY
- Two conditions must be present for AGE to occur:
  - Direct communication between arterial circulation and a source of gas
  - Pressure gradient favoring entry of gas into the arterial vessel (normally, arterial pressures exceed atmospheric pressure)
- Scuba diving:
  - AGE in divers occurs due to pulmonary barotrauma. Air in the lungs expands upon rapid ascent as predicted by Boyle's Law. This leads to overdistention and alveolar rupture. If the vascular parenchyma is also damaged, air can enter the arterial system and travel systemically.
- Medical:
  - AGE in the medical setting occurs when arterial blood is exposed to a pressure gradient that favors the flow of air from the atmosphere to the vasculature. This can be a result of pulmonary barotrauma (ventilator associated) or through direct introduction (surgery or central line placement).
  - AGE may also be the result of a paradoxical embolism.
- Emboli travel to all organs and if not absorbed, will eventually occlude end-arteries. Ischemic damage is most severe in brain and coronary arteries. Two separate mechanisms of damage exist (2):
  - Decreased perfusion leads to hypoxia and cell death (if bubble is large and cannot be quickly absorbed)
  - Local inflammatory response to the bubble leads to cytotoxic edema
    - Cerebral arterial gas embolism: Air bubbles occlude vasculature → unequal distribution of blood in brain → hyperemia and ischemia with focal deficits and increased ICP. In addition, bubbles irritate vascular wall → breakdown of blood-brain barrier → edema, increased ICP

ETIOLOGY
- Decompression illness
  - Pulmonary barotrauma: Pulmonary overpressurization causes alveolar rupture, which allows for gas to enter the pulmonary veins and then travel to the systemic circulation.

- Rapid changes in pressure will cause the nitrogen in the bloodstream to come out of solution and create bubbles in the vascular system. These bubbles then travel systemically until they are lodged and cause ischemic damage. This is due to rapid ascent as seen in divers, aviators, or astronauts participating in "space walks."
- Ventilator-associated barotrauma
- Paradoxical embolism
- Diagnostic or therapeutic procedures, most commonly:
  - Cardiac surgery with extracorporeal bypass
  - Craniotomy with the patient in a seated position
  - Cesarean section

COMMONLY ASSOCIATED CONDITIONS
- Pulmonary barotrauma causing arterial gas embolism can lead to:
  - Pneumomediastinum
  - Subcutaneous emphysema
  - Pneumopericardium
  - Pneumothorax
  - Pneumoperitoneum
- Coronary arterial gas embolism leads to:
  - Temporary ischemia of myocardium
  - Labile blood pressure
  - Arrhythmias
  - Cardiac failure and/or arrest
- Cerebral arterial gas embolism leads to:
  - Focal or diffuse neurologic signs
  - Altered mental status, coma

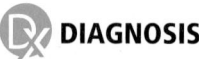 **DIAGNOSIS**

HISTORY
Rapid onset (usually within minutes) of new neurologic, cardiac, renal, or mucocutaneous symptoms after completion of a scuba dive or during or after a surgical procedure.

- Nonspecific symptoms
  - Nausea
  - Pain (e.g., joint pain "the bends")
  - Malaise
- Neurologic symptoms
  - Headache
  - Dizziness
  - Paresthesias
  - Weakness
  - Tinnitus
  - Visual disturbances, e.g., hemianopsia
- Cardiac symptoms
  - Chest pain
  - Palpitations

PHYSICAL EXAM
- Cerebral arterial gas embolism signs and symptoms
  - Altered mental status
  - Aphasia
  - Minor motor weakness
  - Paralysis
  - Seizures
  - Asymmetric pupils
  - Focal sensory deficits
  - Air in retinal vessels on ophthalmoscopic exam

- Coronary arterial gas embolism signs and symptoms
  – Arrhythmias
  – Arrest
- Renal arterial gas embolism signs and symptoms
  – Hematuria
  – Proteinuria
  – Elevated blood urea nitrogen (BUN)/creatinine
  – Elevated serum creatinine
- Mucocutaneous signs and symptoms
  – Cutis marmorata (cyanotic marbling of the skin)
  – Focal area of pallor in the tongue

DIAGNOSTIC TESTS & INTERPRETATION
Lab
No tests are diagnostic for arterial gas embolism. Clinical evaluation is preferred.

Initial lab tests
- Urinalysis and basic metabolic profile (to check for renal involvement)
- Hb/Hct (to check for hemoconcentration; poor specificity)
- Troponin (for myocardial ischemia)

Imaging
- CXR (to rule out pneumothorax)
- ECG (for signs of myocardial infarct)
- CT scan: Changes are often very subtle, air may be visible (poor sensitivity)
- MRI: Sometimes can show increased volume of water in injured tissue (poor sensitivity)
- TTE or TEE: May show evidence of intracardiac shunt, or visible air embolism

DIFFERENTIAL DIAGNOSIS
- Decompression sickness
- Cerebral infarct
- Intracerebral bleed
- Coronary artery spasm
- Myocardial infarction due to acute coronary syndrome
- DVT/Pulmonary embolism

TREATMENT

- Immediate measures:
  – Lifesaving treatment and stabilization must take precedence: CPR, if required; clear the airway and prevent aspiration; intubate if somnolent or comatose.
  – Ventilate with highest possible concentration of oxygen.
  – Transfer to a hyperbaric oxygen chamber for recompression immediately.
- When air transport is required, helicopter transport should be at an altitude <1,000 feet, and fixed-wing transfer should be limited to an aircraft that can maintain cabin pressure at 1 atm.

MEDICATION
Medication is used as an adjunct to 1st-line treatment; hyperbaric oxygen therapy (HBOT).

First Line
No medication is considered 1st-line treatment for arterial gas embolism.

Second Line
- Aspirin
- Adjunctive therapy with glucocorticoids, lidocaine, heparin, barbiturates or indomethacin: Efficacy unclear

ADDITIONAL TREATMENT
General Measures
- Place the patient supine. Placing the patient in the Trendelenburg position to capture the gas at the apex of the heart is considered controversial as this maneuver also increases intracranial pressure.
- Maintain hydration with IV fluids.
- Hyperbaric 100% oxygen recompression (3):
  – HBOT is treatment of choice for arterial gas embolism regardless of the cause; transport patient immediately to a hyperbaric chamber. There is no evidence that therapy >6 hours after insult has a negative impact on outcome.
  – Optimal strategy has yet to be determined; however, the most common regimen consists of 2.8 atm (284kPa) maximum pressure, with 100% oxygen for 4 hours 45 minutes.
  – Proposed mechanism of HBOT:
    ○ HBOT decreases bubble size (↑ambient pressure, so ↓volume and ↑surface area:volume ratio, therefore producing faster diffusion of nitrogen from the bubble).
    ○ Systemic hyperoxia creates a diffusion gradient favoring oxygen diffusion into bubble, and nitrogen out of bubble.
    ○ HBOT may prevent cerebral edema by causing vasoconstriction with ↓neutrophil influx and ↓vascular permeability, thereby supporting the blood-brain barrier.
  – For assistance and advice on locating the nearest treatment chamber in your area, call Divers Alert Network (DAN) at any hour (919) 684-9111. Worldwide contact information available at http://www.diversalertnetwork.org.

IN-PATIENT CONSIDERATIONS
IV Fluids
Goal: to achieve normovolemia. Colloids preferred in order to dilute any hemoconcentration.

ONGOING CARE

FOLLOW-UP RECOMMENDATIONS
None until after treatment

Patient Monitoring
Complete neurologic assessment at 1, 3, 6, and 12 months

DIET
Nothing to be consumed until after treatment

PATIENT EDUCATION
- Divers Alert Network: http://www.diversalertnetwork.org
- Medical emergencies: call Divers Alert Network/Duke University Medical Center hotline 24 hours a day, 7 days a week at +1-919-684-9111 or +1-919-684-4DAN (-4326) for collect calls.

PROGNOSIS
Complete recovery occurs in 91% of patients with decompression illness undergoing HBOT; residual deficits despite repeated HBOT occur in 67% (according to study of US military in Okinawa).

COMPLICATIONS
- Long-term serious neurologic impairments
- Death

REFERENCES
1. Vann RD, Denoble PJ, Dovenbarger JA. *2005 Report on Decompression Illness, Diving Fatalities and Project Dive Explorations*. 2003 Data Durham: Diving Alert Network. 2005:1–142.
2. van Hulst RA, Klein J, Lachmann B et al. Gas embolism: pathophysiology and treatment. *Clin Physiol Funct Imaging*. 2003;23:237–46.
3. Bennett MH, Lehm JP, Mitchell SJ, Wasiak J et al. Recompression and adjunctive therapy for decompression illness: a systematic review of randomized controlled trials. *Anesth Analg*. 2010;111:757–62.

ADDITIONAL READING
- Blanc P, Boussuges A, Henriette K, Sainty JM, Deleflie M et al. Iatrogenic cerebral air embolism: importance of an early hyperbaric oxygenation. *Intensive Care Med*. 2002;28:559–63.
- Muth CM, Shank ES et al. Gas embolism. *N Engl J Med*. 2000;342:476–82.
- Neuman TS et al. Arterial gas embolism and decompression sickness. *News Physiol Sci*. 2002;17:77–81.

See Also (Topic, Algorithm, Electronic Media Element)
Air Embolism

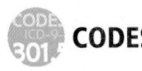 CODES

ICD9
958.0 Air embolism as an early complication of trauma

CLINICAL PEARLS
ALERT
- Any diver who has new symptom(s) or sign(s) after recently completing a self-contained underwater breathing apparatus (SCUBA) dive of any type, to any depth, for any period of time, should be considered for a dive-related injury.
- AGE should be considered in any patient undergoing central venous cannulation or invasive surgery, especially neurosurgical or radiological procedures, who suffer acute symptoms.
- Anesthesia and/or analgesics alter the symptomatology and may complicate evaluation of the patient's clinical status. Delayed recovery from general anesthesia may be a clue to cerebral arterial embolism.

ARTERIOSCLEROTIC HEART DISEASE

Felix B. Chang, MD
Jeremy Golding, MD

BASICS

The term *coronary artery disease* (CAD) is generally used to refer to a pathologic process affecting the coronary arteries (usually atherosclerosis).

DESCRIPTION
Arterio (athero) sclerosis progressively blocks coronary arteries and their branches.

EPIDEMIOLOGY
- Leading cause of death in the US and Europe
- Predominant sex: Male > Female
- Predominant age for peak clinical manifestations:
  – Men: 50–60 years
  – Women: 60–70 years
- In postmenopausal women, the risk for incident coronary disease is tripled compared with premenopausal women.
- Mortality from coronary heart disease (CHD) has fallen over the past four decades

Incidence
- Framingham data suggest that the age-adjusted annual incidence for men aged 35–64 is 12 per 1,000 per year, and for women, 5 per 1,000 per year. For men >65, the incidence is 27 per 1,000 per year, and for women, 16 per 1,000 per year.
- For persons aged 40 years, the lifetime risk of developing CHD is 49% in men and 32% in women. For those reaching age 70 years, the lifetime risk is 35% in men and 24% in women.

Prevalence
The 2010 Heart Disease and Stroke Statistics update of the American Heart Association reported that 17.6 million persons in the US have CHD, including 8.5 million with myocardial infarction (MI) and 10.2 million with angina pectoris.

RISK FACTORS
- Primary risk factors:
  – Diabetes mellitus
  – Male age >45; female >55
  – Family history of premature CHD (1st-degree relative: Male <55 years; female <65 years)
  – Blood pressure >140/90
  – Active cigarette abuse
  – High-density lipoprotein (HDL) cholesterol <40 mg/dL (HDL >60 mg/dL is a protective factor)
  – Elevated low-density lipoprotein (LDL) cholesterol
  – ESRD
- Secondary risk factors:
  – Obesity
  – Mild renal insufficiency
  – Estrogen deficiency
  – Inflammation
  – Depression and stress

Genetics
Family history is an independent risk factor.

GENERAL PREVENTION
- Lifestyle changes are indicated when lifestyle-related factors (obesity, physical inactivity, increased triglycerides, decreased HDL, or metabolic syndrome are present), regardless of LDL.
- HDL has antiatherogenic properties.

ETIOLOGY
- Atherosclerosis, inflammation, including autoimmunity
- Embolism compromising coronary arteries
- Subintimal atheromas in large and medium vessels

COMMONLY ASSOCIATED CONDITIONS
Cerebrovascular disease (ischemic stroke); peripheral arterial disease (claudication); aortic atherosclerosis (abdominal aortic aneurysm); metabolic syndrome

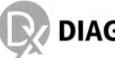

DIAGNOSIS

- Clinical manifestations:
  – Substernal chest pain, diaphoresis, palpitations
  – Exertional dyspnea
  – Orthopnea
  – Paroxysmal nocturnal dyspnea
  – Cardiac arrhythmias
  – Cardiomegaly
  – Pedal edema/fluid overload

Advanced obstructive CHD can exist with minimal or no symptoms, and can progress rapidly.

PHYSICAL EXAM
Focus on stigmata of vascular disease and manifestations of heart failure.

DIAGNOSTIC TESTS & INTERPRETATION
- ECG: Variable; may be normal or may see ST-segment elevation/depression and/or T-wave inversion, or Q waves from old infarction. 10–20% of acute MI have initially normal ECG.
- Exercise ECG testing is the most commonly used noninvasive test because it is simple and inexpensive, but sensitivity no better than 60–70%. Specificity is much higher.
- Stress testing (exercise, pharmacologic), with or without radionuclide or ECG imaging
- Echocardiography using either exercise or pharmacologic (dobutamine or dipyridamole) stress.
- Radionuclide myocardial perfusion imaging using either exercise or pharmacologic stress improves sensitivity somewhat (70–80%).
- Positron emission tomography
- Coronary artery calcium as measured by electron beam and multidetector row computed tomography and histologic, ultrasonographic, and angiographic measures of coronary disease.
- Cardiac computed tomography angiography is an emerging technique for examining coronary anatomy noninvasively.

Lab
- Fasting lipid profile.
- hs-CRP may be useful as an independent marker of prognosis in patients with stable CHD or in ACS.

Follow-Up & Special Considerations
- Specific changes in diet may reduce serum CRP.
- Hormone replacement therapy raises serum CRP in postmenopausal women.

Imaging
- Angiography: Narrowed coronary arteries
- Echocardiography: Possible wall-motion abnormalities

Pathological Findings
- Focal thickening of the intima with an increase in smooth muscle cells and extracellular matrix

- Accumulation of intracellular lipid deposits or extracellular lipids or both, which produce the fatty streak
- Development of fibrous plaques
- Advanced lesions become revascularized from both the luminal and medial aspects.

TREATMENT

The use of aspirin for primary prevention is controversial because of the difficulty determining benefits and risk for a given individual. Benefits in terms of reduction in risk of stroke and MI must be balanced against risk of hemorrhage:
- AHA: For men with >10%, 10-year risk of symptomatic CHD (Framingham risk score) (AHA) (1), consider 75–160 mg aspirin per day. A risk calculator is available online at http://hp2010. nhlbihin.net/atpiii/calculator.asp
- Low-risk diabetics (those aged <50 years with 1 or fewer additional risk factors) may not benefit from aspirin (AHA/ADA) for primary prevention.
- For high-risk women, aspirin (75–160 mg/dl) should be used unless contraindicated (AHA) (2)[A]. If intolerant of aspirin, clopidogrel should be substituted (2)[B].
- Women aged ≥65 years: Consider aspirin therapy (81 mg daily or 100 mg every other day) if blood pressure is controlled and benefit for ischemic stroke and MI prevention likely to outweigh risk of gastrointestinal bleeding and hemorrhagic stroke (2)[B]. Stroke risk calculator available at http:// www.westernstroke.org/personalstrokerisk1.xls
- Consider in most diabetics aged >50 years with one or more additional risk factors (cigarette smoking, hypertension, obesity, albuminuria, hyperlipidemia, or family history of CHD) (3)[C]. Recent trials failed to show a significant reduction in CVD end points (4).
- The 2009 USPTF statement on the use of aspirin for the prevention of cardiovascular disease:
  – In women aged 55–79 years, when the potential benefit of a reduction in ischemic stroke outweighs the risk of an increase in gastrointestinal hemorrhage (5).
  – In men aged 45–79, when the potential benefit of a reduction in the rate of MI outweighs the risk of an increase in gastrointestinal hemorrhage (6). This occurs with 10-year MI risk of 10–20% in patients with average risk of GI bleeding.
- Aspirin is recommended for secondary prevention of CVD after acute MI and unstable angina, occlusive stroke, transient ischemic attack, stable angina, and coronary artery bypass surgery to reduce risk of MI, stroke and vascular death (7)[A].
- In secondary prevention, the absolute benefit is large compared to the absolute risk of major bleeding.
- Statins:
- Primary prevention: Benefit depends more on overall risk than cholesterol levels
- Statins may reduce incidence of cardiovascular death, myocardial infarction and stroke in patients without cardiovascular disease, but number needed to treat is high and use is increasingly controversial, especially since it is not clear that statins decrease overall death in primary prevention (8)[B].

- WHO Cooperative Trial (clofibrate), Lipid Research Clinics Coronary Primary Prevention Trial (cholestyramine), and the Helsinki Heart Study (gemfibrozil) did not demonstrate a reduction in coronary mortality.
- The ASCOT-LLA trial (atorvastatin) did not show statistically significant reductions in cardiovascular mortality.

Secondary Prevention:

- Statins reduce mortality and myocardial infarction in adults with coronary heart disease (7) (SOR)[A].
- Lipid-lowering therapy (primarily with statins) is recommended for most patients with diabetes (SOR) (3)[A].

MEDICATION
First Line
- For established CAD: Aspirin/ASA: 75–160 mg/day; clopidogrel 75 mg PO daily, if ASA is contraindicated.
- Angiotensin-converting enzyme (ACE) inhibitors in all with increased risk factors, diabetes mellitus (DM), or known CAD
- Beta blockers for post-MI patients
- Cholesterol-lowering agents:
  - Data for mortality reduction best for HMG-CoA reductase inhibitor statins. Atorvastatin (10–80 mg PO once daily), initial dose 10–20 mg/d; fluvastatin (20–80 mg/d), initial dose 20–40 mg/dL; lovastatin (10–80 mg/d), initial dose 10–20 mg/dL; pravastatin (maintenance 10–80 mg/d), initial dose 40 mg/dL; simvastatin (20–40 mg once daily), maintenance 5–80 mg/dL; rosuvastatin (5–40 mg once daily), initial dose 10–20 mg/dL
  - Statins also have anti-inflammatory and immunomodulatory effects, and effects on vascular tone and thrombogenicity.
  - Average reduction % in LDL is dose-dependent: Atorvastatin 35–60%, fluvastatin 22–35%, lovastatin 21–42%; pravastatin 22–37%, rosuvastatin 45–63%, simvastatin 26–47%.
- Fish oil and other γ-3 acid ethyl esters: 3 standard fish oil capsules daily supply approximately 1 g of EPA + DHA.
- To increase HDL cholesterol (no proven benefit):
  - Niacin: 2–6 g/d in divided doses
  - Gemfibrozil: 600 mg 2 b.i.d.
  - Fenofibrate: 67–200 mg/d
  - Probucol: 500 mg 2 b.i.d.
  - Colesevelam: 3.75–4.375 g/d
- Average reduction % in triglyceride from baseline:
  - Bile acid sequestrant: Cholestyramine 11–28%; colesevelam (no effect); colestipol 12–15%
  - Fibric acid: Fenofibrate 28.9%; gemfibrozil 31%; niacin E 16–31%, niacin IR 18%
  - Statin: Baseline TG levels >250 mg/dl 35–45%; baseline TG levels <250 mg/dl >25%
- Average increase % in HDL from baseline:
  - Bile-acid sequestrant: Cholestyramine 4–8%; colesevelam 3–8%; colestipol, no effect
  - Ezetimibe 3.5%
  - Fibric acid: fenofibrate 1%; gemfibrozil 6%
  - Niacin ER 20–40%; Niacin IR 17%
  - Statins: 5–10%

Second Line
Antiplatelet activity: Ticlopidine, dipyridamole, clopidogrel

ADDITIONAL TREATMENT
General Measures
- Known CHD or CHD-risk equivalent (10-year risk >20%) has a LDL-C goal <100 mg/dL
- Prevention of further disease progression:
  - Smoking cessation, treatment of hypercholesterolemia (diet, drugs); increase HDL (diet, exercise); control of BP (<140/90; if DM or renal disease, <130/80); diabetes mellitus, exercise 30–40 minutes 5 times/week, moderate alcohol consumption, stress reduction, treatment of depression, diet changes, weight loss (body mass index <25).

 ## ONGOING CARE
FOLLOW-UP RECOMMENDATIONS
For patients with type 2 diabetes taking statins, routine monitoring of liver function test or muscle enzymes is not recommended.

Patient Monitoring
- Monitor lipid panel.
- Preventive programs (weight loss, smoking cessation, diabetes nutritional education)

DIET
- Low fat: 20–30 g/d, and eliminate or reduce trans fats
- Weight loss diet if obesity a problem
- Increase soluble fiber and plant stanols.
- Reduce consumption of red meat; increase fish, olive oil, and nuts.
- Individuals who consume a healthy diet have significantly lower risks of CVD, including both CHD and stroke:
  - High intake of fruits and vegetables
  - High fiber intake, including cereals
  - Low glycemic index and low glycemic load
  - Monounsaturated fats rather than trans fatty acids or saturated fats
  - Limited intake of red or processed meats
  - Omega-3 fatty acids (from fish, fish oil supplements, or plant sources)

PATIENT EDUCATION
American Heart Association, 7320 Greenville Avenue, Dallas, TX 75231, (214) 373-6300.

PROGNOSIS
- In population studies, for every 10% reduction in serum cholesterol, CHD was reduced by 15%; and total mortality risk, by 11%
- The incidence of a MI is increased 6-fold in women and 3-fold in men who smoke at least 20 cigarettes per day.
- Current smoking was associated with a 50% increase in the progression of atherosclerosis versus nonsmokers.

COMPLICATIONS
- MI
- Ventricular fibrillation
- CHF
- Angina pectoris
- Sudden cardiac death

REFERENCES

1. AHA Guidelines for Primary Prevention of Cardiovascular Disease and Stroke: 2002 Update: Consensus Panel Guide to Comprehensive Risk Reduction for Adult Patients Without Coronary of Other Atherosclerotic Vascular Diseases. American Heart Association Science Advisory and Coordinated Committee. *Circulation*. 2002;106(3): 388–91.
2. Evidence-based guidelines for cardiovascular disease prevention in women: 2007 update. *Circulation*. 2007;115(11):1481–501.
3. Standards of Medical Care in diabetes. *Diabetes Care*. 2010;33(Suppl 1):S11–S61.
4. Belch J, MaqcCuish A, et al. The prevention of progression of arterial disease and diabetes (POPADAD) trial: factorial randomized placebo controlled trial of aspirin and antioxidants in patients with diabetes and asymptomatic peripheral arterial disease. *BMJ*. 2008;337:1840.
5. Aspirin for the prevention of cardiovascular disease: U.S. Preventive Services Tasks Force recommendation statement. *Ann Intern Med*. 2009;150(6):396–404.
6. Wolff T, Miller T, Ko S. Aspirin for the primary prevention of cardiovascular events: an update of the evidence for the U.S. Preventive Services Task Force. *Ann Intern Med*. 2009;150(6):405–10.
7. Becker RC, Meade T, et al. The primary and secondary prevention of coronary artery disease: American College of Chest Physicians Evidence-Based Clinical Practice Guidelines (8th Edition). *Chest*. 2008;133:776S.
8. Primary prevention of cardiovascular mortality and events with statin treatments: a network meta-analysis involving more than 65,000 patients. *J Am Coll Cardiol*. 2008;52(22):1469–81.

ADDITIONAL READING

- Aspirin for the prevention of cardiovascular disease. U.S. Preventive Services Task Force recommendation statement. *Ann Intern Med*. 2009;150(6):396–404.
- Framingham risk estimates: http://www.nhlbi.nih.gov/guidelines/cholesterol/index.htm

See Also (Topic, Algorithm, Electronic Media Element)
Angina; Atherosclerosis; Myocardial Infarction, ST-Segment Elevation (STEMI)
Algorithm: Chest_Pain/Acute Coronary Syndrome

CODES

ICD9
414.00 Coronary atherosclerosis of unspecified type of vessel, native or graft

CLINICAL PEARLS

- Net benefit of aspirin increases with increasing cardiovascular risk.
- Insufficient evidence to recommend for or against aspirin for low-risk patients.
- Aspirin significantly reduced the relative risk of subsequent vascular events (nonfatal MI, nonfatal stroke, and vascular death) by approximately 22%.
- The CHD death rate increases at higher plasma concentrations of total and LDL-cholesterol, and statins for patients with known CAD reduce morbidity and mortality.

ARTERITIS, TEMPORAL

Jo Ellen Feugate, MD, PhD
Eric P. Gall, MD

BASICS

DESCRIPTION
Also known as giant cell arteritis. A large vessel vasculitis affecting the elderly. Primarily involves the cranial branches of the carotid arteries and can cause visual loss.

EPIDEMIOLOGY
- Disease of the elderly, almost never seen in persons <50 years. Incidence increases with age
- Female > Male (2:1)

Incidence
More common in Northern Europe, esp. Scandinavia (20 per 100,000 per year) vs Southern Europe (10 per 100,000 per year). In the US, incidence in a largely white Minnesota cohort was 19 per 100,000 per year. It is likely less for the US as a whole. Temporal arteritis is very rare in populations of non-European ancestry.

RISK FACTORS
- Increasing age
- Polymyalgia rheumatica
- Atherosclerosis and smoking in women but not men

Genetics
- Some family clusters have been documented.
- HLA-DR4 and HLA-DRB1 are associated with temporal arteritis.

ETIOLOGY
Unclear, involves cell-mediated immune response and Il-6 production

COMMONLY ASSOCIATED CONDITIONS
Polymyalgia rheumatica

DIAGNOSIS

HISTORY
Usually gradual in onset but may be abrupt
- New or changed headache (usually unilateral temporal but may be generalized)
- Scalp and facial tenderness
- Jaw and tongue claudication with chewing (most specific symptom for temporal arteritis)

- Visual changes
  - Amaurosis fugax
  - Diplopia
  - Scotoma
  - Blindness
- Nonproductive cough
- Arm claudication
- Constitutional symptoms
  - Fever
  - Weight loss
  - Fatigue
  - Polymyalgia rheumatica (stiffness and aching in shoulder and hip girdles). Present in 50%.

PHYSICAL EXAM
- Prominent, tender, or pulseless temporal artery
- Scalp tenderness
- Cranial nerve palsies
- Visual field defect
- Abnormal retinal exam (cotton wool spots, pale edematous retina)
- Proximal muscle tenderness but no weakness

DIAGNOSTIC TESTS & INTERPRETATION
Lab
- ESR/CRP; usually very elevated (ESR >50). <10% have a normal ESR. If both ESR and CRP are normal, consider alternative diagnoses.
- Normocytic, normochromic anemia; usually mild
- Elevated acute phase reactants (platelets, LFTs, albumin)

Imaging
- Ultrasonography of the temporal artery can be up to 88% sensitive and 97% specific for diagnosing temporal arteritis but is quite operator dependent. It does not replace biopsy for definitive diagnosis. (1)
- MRI/MRA in patients with arm claudication or other evidence of aortic branch involvement. It also should be considered, esp. in patients with an aortic insufficiency murmur, to evaluate for presence of aortic aneurysm.

Diagnostic Procedures/Surgery
Temporal artery biopsy: The gold standard for the diagnosis of temporal arteritis
- Treatment prior to biopsy is unlikely to affect the biopsy results, but biopsy should be done within 2 weeks of commencing treatment.
- A segment >2 cm long is needed as there are often skip lesions.

- Serial sections should be done.
- Routine biopsy of both temporal arteries is not necessary; however, if the first biopsy is negative and clinical suspicion remains high, a contralateral biopsy could be considered.

Pathological Findings
Inflammatory infiltrate (either mononuclear cells or granulomas with giant multinucleated cells) seen in the intima and media of large vessels with resultant disruption of the internal elastic lamina. Lesions may be isolated (e.g., skip lesions).

DIFFERENTIAL DIAGNOSIS
- CNS vasculitis
- Embolic disease
- Temporomandibular joint syndrome
- Space-occupying lesion or other cause for new headache in the elderly
- Retinal disease
- CVA

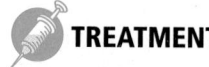
TREATMENT

MEDICATION
First Line
Prednisone:

- Due to the risk of irreversible vision loss, treatment with high-dose steroids should be started on strong clinical suspicion of temporal arteritis, prior to the temporal biopsy being done. The initial dose of prednisone is 60 mg/day [B]. Steroids should not be in the form of alternate day therapy, as this is more likely to lead to a relapse of vasculitis.
- Pulsed dose intravenous methylprednisolone (1 g/day for 3 days) may be of benefit to patients who present with recent onset of visual symptoms (2)[C]. This is followed by prednisone 60 mg/day as above.
- At 6–8 weeks, prednisone can be tapered by 5 mg every 2 weeks to a dose of 25 mg/day. Then the taper is slowed to 2.5 mg every 2 weeks to a dose 10 mg/day. After that, the prednisone is very gradually weaned by 1 mg every 3–6 months. Dose reduction should be considered only in the absence of clinical symptoms, signs and laboratory abnormalities suggestive of active disease. Many patients may require a slower taper.
- Consider low-dose aspirin for all patients with giant cell arteritis (3)[C]
- Patients on corticosteroids should be on bone protection therapy unless they have contraindications

Second Line
Methotrexate (10–15 mg/week) has a modest effect in temporal arteritis and could be considered in patients who have not responded to glucocorticoids or who have significant side effects from steroids (4)[B].

 ## ONGOING CARE

FOLLOW-UP RECOMMENDATIONS
- Follow up in clinic at least monthly initially. When stable and steroids are being tapered, every 3 months.
- Disease relapse should be suspected in patients with new headaches, visual changes, fever, myalgias. A rise in ESR/CRP is usually seen with relapse. An increase in steroids by 10 mg/day is usually significant to control a relapse.

Patient Monitoring
- Check ESR/CRP with each visit to monitor disease activity.
- Consider yearly CXR (to evaluate for aortic aneurysm) and biannual DEXA scans.

DIET
Calcium and vitamin D supplementation

PATIENT EDUCATION
- Consequences of discontinuing steroids abruptly (adrenal suppression, disease relapse)
- Risks of long-term steroid use
- Importance of reporting new headaches and vision changes to provider immediately

PROGNOSIS
- Prior vision loss is unlikely to be recovered, but treatment resolves the other symptoms and prevents future vision loss and stroke.
- Average disease duration 3–4 years but may be up to 10 years.

COMPLICATIONS
- Sequelae of long-term steroid use (osteoporosis, diabetes, thinned skin, weight gain)
- Blindness
- Stroke
- Aortic aneurysm/dissection

REFERENCES
1. Karassa FB, Matsagas MI, Schmidt WA, Ioannidis JP et al. Meta-analysis: test performance of ultrasonography for giant-cell arteritis. *Ann Intern Med*. 2005;142:359–69.
2. Hayreh SS, Zimmerman B, Kardon RH et al. Visual improvement with corticosteroid therapy in giant cell arteritis. Report of a large study and review of literature. *Acta Ophthalmol Scand*. 2002;80: 355–67.
3. Lee MS, Smith SD, Galor A et al. Antiplatelet and anticoagulant therapy in patients with giant cell arteritis. *Arthritis Rheum*. 2006;54:3306–9.
4. Mahr AD, Jover JA, Spiera RF, Hernández-García C, Fernández-Gutiérrez B, Lavalley MP, Merkel PA et al. Adjunctive methotrexate for treatment of giant cell arteritis: an individual patient data meta-analysis. *Arthritis Rheum*. 2007;56:2789–97.

ADDITIONAL READING
- Hunder GG, Bloch DA, Michel BA et al. The American College of Rheumatology 1990 criteria for the classification of giant cell arteritis. *Arthritis Rheum*. 1990;33:1122–8.
- Mukhtyar C, Guillevin L, Cid MC, Dasgupta B, de Groot K, Gross W, Hauser T, Hellmich B, Jayne D, Kallenberg CG, Merkel PA, Raspe H, Salvarani C, Scott DG, Stegeman C, Watts R, Westman K, Witter J, Yazici H, Luqmani R, European Vasculitis Study Group et al. EULAR recommendations for the management of large vessel vasculitis. *Ann Rheum Dis*. 2009;68:318–23.

See Also (Topic, Algorithm, Electronic Media Element)
Depression; Fibromyalgia; Headache, Cluster; Headache, Tension; Polymyalgia Rheumatica; Polymyositis/Dermatomyositis

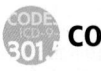 ## CODES

ICD9
446.5 Giant cell arteritis

CLINICAL PEARLS
- Due to the risk of irreversible vision loss, treatment with high-dose steroids (prednisone 60 mg/day) should be started immediately in patients suspected of temporal artery.
- Temporal artery biopsy is the gold standard for diagnosis. Temporal artery biopsy is not likely to be affected by a few weeks of treatment.
- Treatment consists of a very slow steroid taper. Bone protection therapy and low dose aspirin should be considered.

ARTHRITIS, INFECTIOUS, BACTERIAL

Christopher J. Scola, MD
Raul Davaro, MD

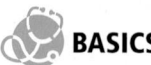

BASICS

DESCRIPTION
- Invasion of joints by pyogenic microorganisms. One of the curable causes of arthritis. May be part of systemic infection/disease.
- System(s) affected: Musculoskeletal
- Synonym(s): Suppurative arthritis; Septic arthritis; Pyarthrosis; Pyogenic arthritis; Bacterial arthritis

EPIDEMIOLOGY
- Predominant age:
  - Neisserial: Especially 15–40 years of age; can occur at any age
  - Nonneisserial (approximate):
    - Years <2: 60% *Staphylococcus*, 20% *Streptococcus*, 10% gram-negative rods, <5% miscellaneous
    - Years 2–14: 60% *Staphylococcus*, 30% *Streptococcus*, 5% *Haemophilus*, 5% other gram-negative rods, 5% miscellaneous
    - Adult: 60% *Staphylococcus*, 25% *Streptococcus*, <1% *Haemophilus*, and 15% other gram-negative rods
- Predominant gender:
  - Neisserial: Female > Male (4:1)
  - Nonneisserial: Male > Female (2:1)

Prevalence
- Neisserial:
  - Responsible for 50% of infectious arthritis
  - 0.6% of women with gonorrhea
  - 0.1% of men with gonorrhea
  - Arthritis occurs in 7% of individuals with *Neisseria meningitidis*
- Nonneisserial: Half as frequent as neisserial

RISK FACTORS
- Sexual exposure: Neisserial
- Inflammatory arthritis, e.g., rheumatoid arthritis
- Concurrent extra-articular infection
- Prior arthritis in affected joint
- Trauma
- Joint puncture or surgery
- Prosthetic joint (1)[A]
- Prior corticosteroid or immunosuppressive therapy
- Serious chronic systemic illness (e.g., diabetes, liver disease, malignancy, immunodeficiency)
- Defective phagocytic mechanisms (e.g., chronic granulomatous disease)
- Injection drug use
- Sickle cell anemia
- Complement deficiency
- Systemic infection; infection elsewhere
- Immunodeficiency; immunosuppression
- Dental procedures; poor dental/gingival hygiene
- Advanced age >80 years

GENERAL PREVENTION
- Prompt treatment of skin and soft tissue infections
- Condoms and limiting number of sexual partners for sexually transmitted disease protection

ETIOLOGY
- Hematogenous invasion (80–90%)
- Contiguous spread (10–15%)
- Direct penetration of microorganisms secondary to trauma or joint infection (5%)

COMMONLY ASSOCIATED CONDITIONS
- Serious chronic illness (e.g., rheumatoid arthritis, diabetes, liver disease, malignancy, primary immunodeficiency, complement deficiencies)
- Immunosuppressive therapy (disease-modifying antirheumatic drugs [DMARDs] agents, glucocorticoids, chemotherapy)
- Systemic infection associated with bacteremia, especially endocarditis

DIAGNOSIS

HISTORY
- Nongonococcal:
  - Predominantly monoarticular (90%)
- Fever: In 90% during course of infection
- Malaise
- Back pain: Subacute bacterial endocarditis
- Neisserial:
  - Bacteremic phase: Migratory polyarthritis, tenosynovitis, high fever, chills, pustules
  - Localized phase: Usually monoarticular with low-grade fever

PHYSICAL EXAM
- Limited or loss of joint use/motion
- Joint effusion, tenderness
- Joint warmth and redness: Present intenosynovitis; pustular skin lesions common for neisserial infection
- Hip and shoulder involvement may reveal severe pain on range of motion with less obvious joint swelling on exam.

DIAGNOSTIC TESTS & INTERPRETATION
Lab
Initial lab tests
- Synovial fluid (2)[A]:
  - Arthrocentesis prior to starting antibiotics increases diagnostic yield
  - Synovial fluid is usually cloudy with >50,000 white blood cells (WBC)/HPF.
    - Caveat: To be valid, cell count must be performed within 1 hour of obtaining specimen.
    - WBC count alone is not sufficient to rule in or rule out septic arthritis (3)[A]
  - Polymorphonuclear leukocytes usually predominate in synovial fluid, >90%.
  - Crystals (e.g., urate or calcium pyrophosphate) do not exclude infectious arthritis.
  - Joint fluid: For Gram stain (positive in 50%); culture (positive in 50–70%); usually negative in neisserial

- Cervical culture or urethral culture highest diagnostic yield for disseminated gonococcal infection in young adults

Pediatric Considerations
- There is no single lab test that can distinguish septic arthritis from transient synovitis (4)[A].
- The combination of fever, non-weight bearing, C-reactive protein >20 or erythrocyte sedimentation rate >40, and a white cell count >12 is suspicious of septic arthritis (4)[B].

Follow-Up & Special Considerations
- Bedside culture is recommended to enhance isolation of fastidious organisms.
- All cultures should be maintained and observed for 3 days to 2 weeks (2,5)[A].
- Neisserial infection generally requires use of special media (e.g., chocolate or Thayer Martin).
- Drugs that may alter lab results: Antibiotics

Imaging
Initial approach
- X-ray (5)[A]:
  - Soft tissue swelling
  - Juxta-articular osteoporosis
  - Radiolucent area (gas) in a joint space from gas-forming organisms (Caveat: May be normal as a "vacuum phenomenon")
  - Effacement of obturator fat pad (with hip involvement)
  - X-ray changes usually a late phenomenon
  - Rarefaction of subchondral bone may occur
  - Joint-space loss (secondary to cartilage destruction) may occur in 4–10 days.
  - Erosions
  - Joint destruction with ankylosis may occur.

- Other imaging techniques:
  - Technetium joint scans: Reveal distribution of inflammation; sensitive, not specific
  - Gallium WBC scan, indium scans: Reveal inflammation as well as infection
  - Computed tomography: To identify sequestration
  - Magnetic resonance imaging: Effusion, perhaps early cartilage damage, osteomyelitis

Diagnostic Procedures/Surgery
Arthrocentesis with Gram stain and culture: Positive in 50–70% (6)[A]:
- Shoulder or hip joints may require image-guided aspiration.
- Must always be done when possibility of infectious arthritis is considered
- Arthrocentesis should be performed prior to initiation of antibiotics whenever possible. Arthrocentesis approach must avoid contaminated tissue (e.g., overlying cellulitis) when possible.

Pathological Findings
Synovial biopsy will reveal polymorphonuclear leukocytes and possibly the causative organism, if synovial fluid and blood cultures are negative.

DIFFERENTIAL DIAGNOSIS
- Gout
- Pseudogout (calcium pyrophosphate deposition disease)
- Spondyloarthropathy (Reiter syndrome, psoriatic arthritis, ankylosing spondylitis, arthritis of inflammatory bowel disease)
- Juvenile rheumatoid arthritis
- Foreign-body synovitis
- Rheumatoid arthritis
- Rheumatic fever
- Cellulitis
- Palindromic rheumatism
- Neuropathic arthropathy
- Lyme arthritis
- Granulomatous arthritis

TREATMENT
MEDICATION
First Line
- Neisserial (5)[A]:
  – Ceftriaxone 1 g IM or IV every day for 14 days (and at least 7 days after symptoms resolve)
  – Fluoroquinolone for 14 days; caveat resistance
  – Concomitant treatment for *Chlamydia*
- Nonneisserial (5)[A]:
  – Gram-positive cocci in clusters: Empiric therapy: Vancomycin or linezolid IV. If methicillin-sensitive *Staphylococcus aureus* (MSSA), nafcillin or cefazolin IV
  – Gram-positive cocci in chains: Ceftriaxone
  – Gram-negative bacilli: Neonates: Cefotaxime, and gentamicin; ages 6 months to 4 years: 3rd-generation cephalosporin; adult: 3rd-generation cephalosporin plus gentamicin. No bacteria seen on smear: Vancomycin or linezolid plus 3rd-generation cephalosporin.
- Precautions:
  – Observe for allergic reactions
- Significant possible interactions:
  – Broad-spectrum antibiotics: May reduce effectiveness of oral contraceptives; barrier method recommended

Second Line
Fluoroquinolones (e.g., ciprofloxacin)

ADDITIONAL TREATMENT
General Measures
- Hospitalization for parenteral therapy
- Outpatient treatment rarely possible for extremely compliant patient with known organism
- Repeat (once) arthrocentesis if fluid reaccumulates. Next step is arthroscopic debridement and irrigation.
- Avoid anti-inflammatory therapy to allow assessment of therapeutic response to antibiotic.

- If joint prosthesis is present in an infection, orthopedic surgery, to include possible removal of the prosthesis, must be considered.
- Continue treatment for 1–2 weeks after total resolution of all signs of inflammation, for a total of 4–6 weeks for most organisms, except Neisserial (2–3 weeks).
- Intra-articular antibiotics are not required.

Issues for Referral
Infectious disease and orthopedic consults strongly advised to supplement rheumatologist

SURGERY/OTHER PROCEDURES
- Arthroscopy indicated if fluid accumulated is loculated and/or not amenable to needle drainage
- Surgical drainage typically is required for shoulder or hip involvement.

ONGOING CARE
FOLLOW-UP RECOMMENDATIONS
Patient Monitoring
- Repeat arthrocentesis (once) if fluid reaccumulates to verify sterilization of joint and reversion of inflammatory signs to normal.
- If no improvement within 24 hours, re-evaluate and consider arthroscopy.
- CBC, liver and kidney function, and urinalysis twice a week while on antibiotics (with creatinine when gentamicin used)
- Aminoglycoside levels
- Follow-up 1 week and 1 month after stopping antibiotics to detect any relapse.

PROGNOSIS
- Early treatment should allow cure.
- Delayed recognition/treatment complicated by morbidity and mortality

COMPLICATIONS
- Death (9–33% in elderly)
- Limited joint range of motion
- Secondary osteoarthritis
- Flail or fused or dislocated joint
- Septic necrosis
- Sinus formation
- Ankylosis
- Osteomyelitis
- Postinfectious synovitis
- Shortening of limb (in children)

REFERENCES
1. Zimmerli W, Trampuz A, Ochsner PE. Prosthetic-joint infections. *N Engl J Med*. 2004;351:1645–54.
2. Mathews CJ, Weston VC, Jones A, et al. Bacterial septic arthritis in adults. *Lancet*. 2010;375(9717):846–55.
3. O'Malley A, Svinos H et al. Towards evidence based emergency medicine: Best BETs from the Manchester Royal Infirmary. BET 3: Is the white cell count of the joint aspirate sufficiently sensitive/specific to rule in/out septic arthritis? *Emerg Med J*. 2009;26:435–7.
4. Taekema HC, Landham PR, Maconochie I et al. Towards evidence based medicine for paediatricians. Distinguishing between transient synovitis and septic arthritis in the limping child: how useful are clinical prediction tools? *Arch Dis Child*. 2009;94:167–8.
5. Margaretten ME, Kohlwes J, Moore D et al. Does this adult patient have septic arthritis? *JAMA*. 2007;297:1478–88.
6. Khachatourians AG, Patzakis MJ, Roidis N et al. Laboratory monitoring in pediatric acute osteomyelitis and septic arthritis. *Clin Orthop Relat Res*. 2003;186–94.

ADDITIONAL READING
- Mathews CJ, Coakley G. Septic arthritis: current diagnostic and therapeutic algorithm. *Curr Opin Rheumatol*. 2008;20:457–62.
- Ross JJ, Hu LT. Bacterial and Lyme arthritis. *Curr Infect Dis Rep* 2004;5:380–7.

CODES
ICD9
- 040.89 Other specified bacterial diseases
- 711.40 Arthropathy, site unspecified, associated with other bacterial diseases

CLINICAL PEARLS
- Neisseria is the most common cause of septic arthritis in young adults.
- Acute onset of joint pain with redness and warmth is typical of nonneisserial infection.
- Crystalline process can mimic septic arthritis.
- Aspiration of joint prior to the initiation of antibiotics will optimize diagnostic yield.
- Synovial fluid appears inflammatory and is typically purulent.

ARTHRITIS, INFECTIOUS, GRANULOMATOUS

Christopher J. Scola, MD
Raul Davaro, MD

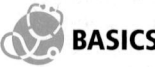 **BASICS**

DESCRIPTION
- Invasion of joints by microorganisms; may be part of systemic infection/disease
- One of the few curable causes of arthritis
- System(s) affected: Musculoskeletal
- Synonym(s): Fungal arthritis; Mycobacterial arthritis; Subacute bacterial arthritis

EPIDEMIOLOGY
- 1–3% of patients with tuberculosis (TB) infections
- 10–30% of extrapulmonary TB will present with musculoskeletal involvement
- Predominant age: Broad range
- Predominant gender:
  - Male > Female (*Brucella* and mycobacterial).
  - Female > Male (fungal).

Prevalence
1 in 3 million population

Pediatric Considerations
Infrequent in pediatric population

RISK FACTORS
- Acquired immune-deficiency disease (AIDS)
- Concurrent extraarticular infection
- Chronic inflammatory arthritis, such as rheumatoid arthritis (RA)
- Trauma, especially penetrating
- Prosthetic joint
- Prior antibiotic, corticosteroid, or immunosuppressive therapy
- Serious chronic systemic illness (e.g., diabetes mellitus, liver disease, malignancy, primary immunodeficiency)
- Defective phagocytic mechanisms (e.g., chronic granulomatous disease)
- Injection drug use
- Exposure (e.g., brucellosis, unpasteurized milk, farmers, butchers, veterinarians)
- Travel/habitat history
- Gardening (sporotrichosis)
- Aquatic exposure (e.g., fish hook puncture)

ETIOLOGY
- Hematogenous invasion is most common.
- Contiguous spread
- Direct penetration via trauma
- Fungal infections may disseminate from primary pulmonary involvement, particularly in immunocompromised hosts.

COMMONLY ASSOCIATED CONDITIONS
- Systemic infection
- Infection elsewhere
- Immunodeficiency/immunosuppression (e.g., from HIV/AIDS, lymphoma, transplantation, medications)

 DIAGNOSIS

HISTORY
- Predominantly monarticular (90%)
- Fungal may present as a migratory polyarthritis, particularly with C. *immitis* and H. *capsulatum* owing to hypersensitivity reaction (1,2).
- Flare of arthritis in a single joint with preexisting joint disease
- Fever in 50% at some time during infection
- Fever of unknown origin (FUO) can be an early sign of brucellosis.
- Cutaneous lesions are seen with B. *dermatitidis* and S. *schenckii*.
- Back pain, especially in TB and brucellosis
- Sternal or rib involvement can occur with TB.
- Prosthetic joint infections owing to fungal infection can occur months to years after initial surgery (1).
- Prosthetic joint can present with subacute onset of pain and swelling.
- Fretfulness, in children

PHYSICAL EXAM
- Joint-line tenderness
- Joint effusion
- Synovial thickening (doughy consistency); may have only minimal tenderness
- Limited joint use/motion, especially in children
- Overlying warmth, redness; present in fewer than 50%
- Fungal joint infections can form draining sinus tracts.
- Spinal tenderness with TB (Pott disease) and with brucellosis
- Gibbous deformity with TB
- Tenosynovitis
- Dactylitis
- Erythema nodosum (H. *capsulatum* and TB) (2)
- Nodular skin lesions with mycobacterium and fungal
- Iritis (with mycobacterial arthritis)
- Brucellosis:
  - Hepatosplenomegaly
  - Lymphadenopathy

DIAGNOSTIC TESTS & INTERPRETATION
Lab
Initial lab tests
- Arthrocentesis (3,4,5)[A]
- Bacterial: For Gram stain, silver, and acid-fast stain and culture, cell count and differential, glucose
- Mycobacterial: Acid-fast smear (positive in 20%), culture (positive in 80%); polymerase chain reaction (PCR)
- To be done in all patients when possibility of infectious arthritis is considered
- Synovial fluid usually cloudy with >20,000 white blood cell count (WBCs)/high-power field (HPF) but may have fewer WBCs present or over 100,000/mm^3
- Synovial fluid analysis, including wet-mount prep, typically positive in B. *dermatidis* (1)
- Polymorphonuclear leukocytes usually predominate in synovial fluid, although granulomatous and viral arthritis may have a mononuclear cell predominance.
- Approach must avoid contaminated tissue during arthrocentesis (e.g., overlying cellulitis)
- Synovial membrane: Biopsy and culture
- Blood, urine, sputum cultures
- Fungal blood cultures or serologies (6)[C]
- All cultures should be held for 2 weeks; acid-fast cultures for 6 weeks.
- Drug susceptibility testing is recommended.
- The presence of crystals in the synovial fluid (e.g., urate or calcium pyrophosphate) does not exclude infectious arthritis.
- PCR for specific microorganisms
- Serum testing (i.e., cryptococcal antigen, *Brucella* antibody >1:160)
- PCR DNA analysis for TB
- Positive fungal tissue culture should not be disregarded as contaminated.

Imaging
Initial approach
- Radiographs (1,4,5,7)[A]
- X-ray changes usually a late phenomenon
- Soft tissue swelling
- Rarefaction of subchondral bone
- Joint-space loss
- Erosions
- Joint destruction with ankylosis
- Subchondral erosion with preservation of joint space strongly suggests granulomatous infection.
- CT scan to identify sequestration
- MRI: T$_2$-weighted signals increase in affected soft tissue and bone (4,8)[A].

Diagnostic Procedures/Surgery
Synovial biopsy or synovectomy is often needed to diagnose specific pathogen.

Pathological Findings
Synovial biopsy may reveal granulomata and possibly the causative organism on microscopy or culture.

DIFFERENTIAL DIAGNOSIS
- Gout
- Pseudogout (calcium pyrophosphate deposition disease)
- Spondyloarthropathy (Reiter syndrome, psoriatic arthritis, ankylosing spondylitis, arthritis of inflammatory bowel disease)
- Juvenile RA
- Foreign-body synovitis (e.g., plant thorn synovitis)
- RA
- Pigmented villonodular synovitis (PVNS)
- Palindromic rheumatism
- Neuropathic arthropathy
- Lyme arthritis
- Sarcoidosis
- Pyogenic arthritis

TREATMENT
MEDICATION
First Line
- Medications based on sensitivity of organisms
- Mycobacterial infection (4,5,7,9)[A]:
  – Use 4-drug combination initially: isoniazid, rifampin, pyrazinamide, and ethambutol.
  – Continue therapy for 9–24 months.
- *Brucella:* Tetracycline plus streptomycin (or gentamicin or trimethoprim-sulfamethoxazole or rifampin)
- Fungal infection (5):
  – Choice of medication depends on organism.
  – Amphotericin B preparations
  – Azoles
- Contraindications: Tetracycline not for use in pregnancy or children <8 years
- Precautions:
  – Observe for allergic reactions/serum sickness.
  – Tetracycline may cause photosensitivity; sunscreen is recommended.
- Significant possible interactions:
  – Tetracycline: Avoid concurrent administration with antacids, dairy products, or iron
  – Azoles: Multiple drug interactions

Second Line
Fungal:
- Azoles: Fluconazole, itraconazole

ADDITIONAL TREATMENT
General Measures
- Appropriate care:
  – Fungal: Initial hospitalization for parenteral therapy
  – Mycobacterial: Outpatient, once diagnosed
  – *Brucella:* Outpatient, once diagnosed

- Repeat arthrocentesis if fluid reaccumulates.
- Infection associated with prosthetic joints may be difficult to eradicate without removal.
- For *Brucella* or fungal infections, continue treatment for 1–2 weeks after total resolution of all signs of inflammation and 6–8 weeks if joint was diseased previously (e.g., arthritis).
- Antimicrobic therapy requires a long program (i.e., in TB, fungal infection, brucellosis).
- Intraarticular antibiotics are not indicated.
- Infectious disease and rheumatology consultation helpful

SURGERY/OTHER PROCEDURES
- Arthrotomy is indicated only if fluid accumulated is loculated and/or not amenable to needle drainage.
- Prosthetic joints will require removal of hardware.
- Root joints, such as shoulder and hips, will require surgical intervention.

ONGOING CARE
FOLLOW-UP RECOMMENDATIONS
Patient Monitoring
- Verify sterilization of joint and reversion of inflammatory signs to normal.
- Treatment of mycobacterial arthritis requires monthly complete blood count, assessment of liver and kidney toxicity, and urinalysis.
- Essential to follow up frequently after stopping antibiotics to detect relapse.

PATIENT EDUCATION
Arthritis Foundation, 1314 Spring Street, NW Atlanta, GA 30309, (404) 872-7100.

PROGNOSIS
- Early initiation of treatment should allow cure.
- Delayed recognition/treatment is complicated by increased morbidity and mortality.

COMPLICATIONS
- Limited joint range of motion
- Flail or fused joint
- Carpal tunnel syndrome
- Septic necrosis
- Sinus formation
- Ankylosis
- Osteomyelitis
- Shortening of limb (in children)

REFERENCES

1. Kohli R, Hadley S. Fungal arthritis and osteomyelitis. *Infectious Dis Clin N Am*. 2005;19:831–51.
2. Kroot EJ, Hazes JM, Colin EM et al. Poncet's disease: reactive arthritis accompanying tuberculosis. Two case reports and a review of the literature. *Rheumatology (Oxford)*. 2006.
3. Rothschild BM, Martin L. *Skeletal Impact of Disease Pathology*. Albuquerque, NM: New Mexico Museum of Natural History, 2006.
4. Fukushima M, Kakinuma K, Hayashi H et al. Detection and identification of Mycobacterium species isolates by DNA microarray. *J Clin Microbiol*. 2003;41:2605–15.
5. Hus C-Y, Shih TT-F. Tuberculous infection of the wrists: MRI features. *Am J Roentgenol*. 2004;183: 623–8.
6. Costa RO, de Mesquita KC, Damasco PS, Bernardes-Engemann AR, Dias CM, Silva IC, Lopes-Bezerra LM et al. Infectious arthritis as the single manifestation of sporotrichosis: serology from serum and synovial fluid samples as an aid to diagnosis. *Rev Iberoam Micol*. 2008;25:54–6.
7. Papagelopoulos PJ, Papadopoulos ECh, Mavrogenis AF et al. Tuberculous sacroiliitis. A case report and review of the literature. *Eur Spine J*. 2005;14: 683–8.
8. Leigh Moore S, Rafii M. Advanced imaging of tuberculosis arthritis. *Semin Musculoskelet Radiol*. 2003;7:143–53.
9. Yilmaz E, Parlak M, Akalin H et al. Brucellar spondylitis: review of 25 cases. *J Clin Rheumatol*. 2004;10:300–7.

ADDITIONAL READING

Sawlani V, Chandra T, Mishra RN et al. MRI features of tuberculosis of peripheral joints. *Clin Radiol*. 2003;58:755–62.

CODES

ICD9
- 711.00 Pyogenic arthritis, site unspecified
- 711.40 Arthropathy, site unspecified, associated with other bacterial diseases
- 711.50 Arthropathy, site unspecified, associated with other viral diseases

CLINICAL PEARLS

- Fungal infection of joint may present with synovial thickening and tenderness, but intense erythema and pain may not be present.
- Brucellosis can present initially as an FUO picture.
- TB can involve the spine, resulting in deformity.
- Synovial biopsy or synovectomy is often needed to diagnose specific pathogen.

ARTHRITIS, JUVENILE IDIOPATHIC

Caitlin Hurley, MD
Timothy Gibson, MD

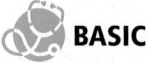 **BASICS**

DESCRIPTION

- Most common chronic rheumatic illness in children and a significant cause of short- and long-term disability
- General characteristics:
  - Age of onset <16 years
  - Signs of arthritis: Joint swelling, limitation of motion, pain, heat, or tenderness
  - >6 weeks of symptoms
- 7 subtypes exist, according to the International League of Associations for Rheumatology, determined by clinical characteristics seen in 1st 6 months of illness:
  - Systemic: Occurs in 10–20% of affected children; usually characterized by febrile onset and evanescent rash with multiple physical and laboratory abnormalities
  - Polyarticular RF (+): Occurs in 5–10% of affected children; multiple (≥5) joint involvement; large and small joints affected. RF positive 2x on tests at least 3 months apart
  - Polyarticular RhF (−) : Occurs in 30% of affected children; ≥5 joint involvement, large and small joints affected; RF negative
  - Oligoarticular: Occurs in 40–50% of affected children; involvement of ≤4 joints, usually larger joints, especially of lower extremities; risk for chronic uveitis in young girls and axial skeletal involvement in older boys
  - Psoriatic arthritis: Occurs in 2–15% of affected children. Arthritis with psoriasis or arthritis with at least 2 of following: dactylitis, nail pitting or onycholysis, psoriasis in 1st-degree relative.
  - Enthesitis arthritis: Occurs in 1–7% of affected children. Includes ankylosing spondylitis and inflammatory bowel disease–related arthritis. Peripheral and axial involvement.
  - Undifferentiated arthritis: Arthritis that does not fulfill above categories or fills 2 or more categories
- System(s) affected: Hematologic/Lymphatic/Immunologic; Musculoskeletal
- Synonym(s): Juvenile chronic arthritis; Juvenile arthritis; Juvenile rheumatoid arthritis (JRA); Still disease

EPIDEMIOLOGY

- Predominant age: 1–4 years and 9–14 years old
- Predominant sex:
  - Poly/oligoarticular: Female > Male
  - Systemic: Female = Male
  - Enthesitis: Male > Female

Incidence
1–22 per 100,000 children <16 years per year

Prevalence
8–150 per 100,000 children <16 years

Pediatric Considerations
Behavioral and compliance problems frequent in toddlers and teenagers

Pregnancy Considerations
Unpredictable effect on disease activity

RISK FACTORS

- Rheumatoid factor (RF) positivity increases risk for severe arthritis in polyarticular juvenile idiopathic arthritis (JIA).
- Antinuclear antibody (ANA) positivity increases risk for uveitis in oligo-JIA and poly-JIA.

Genetics
- Certain HLA class I and II alleles
- HLA-A2 in early-onset oligoarthritis in girls
- HLA-DRB1*11 confers increased risk of systemic and oligo-JIA.
- HLA-B27 risk of enthesitis-related arthritis
- HLA-DR4 associated with RF (+) polyarticular disease

GENERAL PREVENTION
No known preventive measures

ETIOLOGY
Multifactorial, including:
- Immunodysregulation
- Genetic predisposition
- Environmental triggers, possibly infectious:
  - Rubella or parvovirus B19 (1)
  - Heat shock proteins (1)
- Immunoglobulin or complement deficiency

COMMONLY ASSOCIATED CONDITIONS
- Other autoimmune disorders
- Chronic anterior uveitis (iridocyclitis)
- Nutritional impairment
- Growth disturbances (1)

 DIAGNOSIS

Clinical diagnostic criteria: Age of onset <16 years and >6 weeks duration of objective arthritis in ≥1 joints, defined as swelling or limitation of motion of a joint accompanied by heat, pain, or tenderness

HISTORY
- Arthralgias, fever, fatigue, malaise, myalgias, weight loss, morning stiffness, rash, limp in patients with lower extremity involvement
- Arthritis for at least 6 weeks

PHYSICAL EXAM
- Arthritis: Swelling, effusion, limitation of motion, tenderness, pain on motion, warmth
- Rash, rheumatoid nodules, lymphadenopathy, hepato- or splenomegaly, enthesitis, dactylitis

DIAGNOSTIC TESTS & INTERPRETATION
Lab
Initial lab tests
- Complete blood count (CBC):
  - Leukocyte count normal or markedly elevated (systemic), lymphopenia
  - Reactive thrombocytosis
  - Anemia
- Joint-fluid aspiration and analysis helpful in excluding infection
- Inflammatory markers: Erythrocyte sedimentation rate and C-reactive protein may be elevated
- ANA positive (>1:80): 40% (polyarticular or oligoarticular): Increased risk of uveitis
- RF positive: 2–10% (usually polyarticular): Poor prognosis
- HLA-B27 positive: Enthesitis-related arthritis

Follow-Up & Special Considerations
- In polyarticular RF-positive variant, positivity should be confirmed at least twice, 3 months apart (2).
- RF and ANA may be present in mixed connective tissue disease.

Imaging
Diagnostic radiography, magnetic resonance (MR) imaging, ultrasonography, and computed tomography all play an important role in diagnosing or monitoring juvenile idiopathic arthritis (JIA); no one modality has evidence for superior diagnostic value (3)[A].

Initial approach
- Radiograph of affected joint(s)
- Early radiographic changes: Soft tissue swelling, periosteal reaction, juxta-articular demineralization
- Later changes include joint-space loss, articular surface erosions, subchondral cyst formation, sclerosis, joint fusion
- Electrocardiogram (pericarditis)
- Radionuclide scans (infection, malignancy)
- MRI can assess synovial hypertrophy, cartilage degeneration, and clinical responsiveness to treatment in peripheral joints in JIA (4)[B].

Follow-Up & Special Considerations
In interpreting results of dual energy x-ray photon absorptiometry scans, it is important to use pediatric, not adult, controls as normative data.

Diagnostic Procedures/Surgery
- Synovial biopsy occasionally indicated
- Arthrocentesis

Pathological Findings
Synovium shows hyperplasia of synovial cells, hyperemia, and infiltration of small lymphocytes and mononuclear cells.

DIFFERENTIAL DIAGNOSIS
- Other rheumatic diseases:
  - Systemic lupus erythematosus, dermatomyositis, mixed connective tissue disease, sarcoidosis
- Musculoskeletal:
  - Legg-Calve-Perthes, toxic synovitis, growing pains
- Infectious:
  - Septic arthritis, osteomyelitis, Lyme disease
- Reactive arthritis:
  - Postinfectious, rheumatic fever, Reiter's syndrome
- Inflammatory bowel disease:
  - Crohn's disease and ulcerative colitis
- Hemoglobinopathies
- Malignancy:
  - Leukemia, bone tumors, neuroblastoma
- Vasculitis
- Kawasaki disease

 TREATMENT

MEDICATION
First Line
- Nonsteroidal anti-inflammatory drugs (NSAIDs) are adequate in ~50% of patients, symptoms often improve within days, full efficacy 2–3 months
- Drugs for children include:
  - Ibuprofen (Motrin, Advil, Nuprin): 30–40 mg/kg/d, divided q.i.d., max 800 mg t.i.d.
  - Naproxen (Naprosyn, Aleve): 10–20 mg/kg/d divided b.i.d., max dose of 500 mg b.i.d.

- Tolmetin sodium: 15–30 mg/kg/d; t.i.d. or q.i.d., max dose 600 mg t.i.d.
  - Diclofenac 2–3 mg/kg, divided t.i.d., max of 50 mg t.i.d.
  - Indomethacin 3 mg/kg/d, max of 200 mg/d
- Contraindications to NSAIDs: Known allergies
- Precautions: May worsen bleeding diatheses; use caution with all NSAIDs in renal insufficiency and hypovolemic states
- Significant possible interactions: NSAIDs may lower serum levels of digitalis and anticonvulsants and blunt the effect of loop diuretics. NSAIDs may increase serum methotrexate levels.
- Intra-articular long-acting corticosteroids especially for oligo-JIA. Immediately effective, local treatment. Improve synovitis, joint damage, contractures, and prevent leg length discrepancy (2)[B]:
  - Triamcinolone hexacetonide
- Glucocorticoids: Only in patients with extreme pain and functional limitation, while waiting for a 2nd-line agent to show some effect

Second Line
- 30–40% of patients will require addition of disease-modifying antirheumatic drugs (DMARDs), including methotrexate, sulfasalazine, leflunomide, and tumor necrosis factor antagonists (etanercept, infliximab, adalimumab). Newer biologic therapies including IL-1 and IL-6 receptor antagonists currently under investigation
- Methotrexate: Standard dose 8–12.5 mg/m^2/wk p.o. or SC. 10 mg/m^2/wk is most frequently used (2)[B]:
  - Plateau of efficacy reached with 15 mg/m^2/wk; further increase in dosage is not associated with therapeutic benefit (5)
- Sulfasalazine: Oligoarticular and HLA B27 spondyloarthritis
- Leflunomide: Not Food and Drug Administration approved for JIA
- Etanercept (Enbrel) 0.4 mg/kg, max of 25 mg, given SC twice weekly (2)[B]
- Infliximab 3–6 mg/kg q6–8 weeks
- Adalimumab 40 mg SC every 2 weeks (6)[B]
- Tocilizumab IL-6 antibody demonstrating efficacy in phase III open label trials, ongoing studies to evaluate efficacy and appropriate dosing regimen (2)
- Anakinra IL-1 receptor antibody under investigation with phase II and III clinical trials for systemic JIA (2)
- Alternative drugs:
  - Other NSAIDs and salicylates: Avoid salicylate therapy during serious viral illness, especially influenza or varicella, secondary to risk of Reye syndrome
- Analgesics for pain control, including narcotics

ADDITIONAL TREATMENT
General Measures
- Treatment goal: Control active disease and extra-articular manifestations to maintain musculoskeletal function as normal as possible.
- Outpatient care except for initial diagnostic workup of systemic JIA disease and complications for all subtypes
- All patients require regular (every 3–4 months for oligo-JIA and in ANA-positive patients) ophthalmic exams to uncover asymptomatic eye disease, at least for 1st 3 years.

- Moist heat, sleeping bag, or electric blanket to relieve morning stiffness
- Splints for contractures

Issues for Referral
- In general, a pediatric rheumatologist is best suited to manage juvenile idiopathic arthritis.
- Orthopedic surgeon: Need for surgery (joint replacement)
- Ophthalmologist: Uveitis
- Physical therapist for joint protection, to maintain range of motion, improve muscle strength, prevent deformities
- Occupational therapist to maintain and improve the normal life function
- Psychologists for coping

Additional Therapies
Physical therapy including daily home exercise program and orthotics for support

SURGERY/OTHER PROCEDURES
- Total hip and/or knee replacement may be needed for severe disease.
- Soft tissue release, if splinting, traction unsuccessful
- Limb length or angular deformity corrections
- Synovectomy is rarely performed.

IN-PATIENT CONSIDERATIONS
Admission Criteria
- Patient loses ambulatory ability
- Signs/symptoms of pericarditis
- Persistent fever

Discharge Criteria
Resolution of fever and swelling or serositis

 ## ONGOING CARE

FOLLOW-UP RECOMMENDATIONS
Patient Monitoring
Determined by medication:
- NSAIDs: Periodic complete blood count (CBC), urinalysis, liver function tests (LFTs), renal function tests
- Aspirin and/or other salicylates: Transaminase and salicylate levels, weekly for 1st month, then every 3–4 months
- Methotrexate: Monthly LFTs, CBC, blood urea nitrogen, creatinine

DIET
Regular diet with special attention to adequate calcium, iron, protein, and caloric intake

PATIENT EDUCATION
- Ongoing education of patients and families with attention to:
  - Psychosocial needs
  - School issues, educational needs
  - Behavioral strategies for dealing with pain and noncompliance
  - Use of health care resources
- Printed and audiovisual information available from local arthritis foundation

PROGNOSIS
- 50–60% ultimately remit, but functional ability depends on adequacy of long-term therapy (disease control, maintaining muscle and joint function).
- Poorest prognosis in patients with RF + poly-JIA or patients with systemic JIA

COMPLICATIONS
- Blindness, band keratopathy, glaucoma
- Short stature
- Micrognathia if temporomandibular joint involvement
- Debilitating joint disease
- Disseminated intravascular coagulation; hemolytic anemia
- Patient on NSAIDs: Peptic ulcer, GI hemorrhage, central nervous system reactions, renal disease, leukopenia
- Patient on DMARD: Bone marrow suppression, hepatitis, renal disease, dermatitis, mouth ulcers, retinal toxicity (antimalarials, rare)
- Patients on tumor necrosis factor antagonists: Higher risk of infection
- Osteoporosis
- Macrophage activation syndrome:
  - Decreased blood cell precursors secondary to histiocyte degradation of marrow

REFERENCES
1. Weiss JE, Ilowite NT. Juvenile Idiopathic Arthritis. *Rheum Dis Clin N Am.* 2007;33:441–70.
2. Kahn P et al. Juvenile idiopathic arthritis–current and future therapies. *Bulletin of the NYU hospital for joint diseases.* 2009;67:291–302.
3. McKay GM, Cox LA, Long BW et al. Imaging juvenile idiopathic arthritis: assessing the modalities. *Radiol Technol.* 2010;81:318–27.
4. Miller E, Uleryk E, Doria AS. Evidence-based outcomes of studies addressing diagnostic accuracy of MRI of juvenile idiopathic arthritis. *AJR Am J Roentgenol.* 2009;192:1209–18.
5. Takken T, van der Net J, Helders P. Methotrexate for treating juvenile idiopathic arthritis. *The Cochrane Database of Systematic Reveiws.* 2009, Issue 1.
6. Lovell DJ, et al. Adalimumbab with or without Methotrexate in Juvenile Rheumatoid Arthritis. *New Engl J Med.* 2008;359(8):810–20.

CODES

ICD9
- 714.30 Chronic or unspecified polyarticular juvenile rheumatoid arthritis
- 714.31 Acute polyarticular juvenile rheumatoid arthritis
- 714.32 Pauciarticular juvenile rheumatoid arthritis

CLINICAL PEARLS
- Consult pediatric rheumatologist
- High-titer RF correlates with severity
- ANA confers risk of uveitis
- No specific biomarker or test
- Diagnosis is one of exclusion

ARTHRITIS, OSTEO

Sergio A. Leon, MD
Jill A. Grimes, MD

 BASICS

DESCRIPTION
- Most common form of joint disease
- Involves progressive loss of articular cartilage and reactive changes at joint margins and in subchondral bone
- Primary:
  - Idiopathic: Divided into subsets depending on clinical features (i.e., localized, generalized, erosive)
- Secondary:
  - Posttraumatic
  - Childhood anatomic abnormalities (e.g., congenital hip dysplasia)
  - Inheritable metabolic disorders (e.g., Wilson disease, alkaptonuria, hemochromatosis)
  - Neuropathic arthropathy (Charcot joints)
  - Hemophilic arthropathy
  - Endocrinopathies: Acromegalic arthropathy, hyperparathyroidism, hypothyroidism
  - Paget disease
  - Noninfectious inflammatory arthritis (e.g., rheumatoid arthritis [RA], spondyloarthropathies)
  - Gout, calcium pyrophosphate deposition disease (pseudogout)
  - Septic or tuberculous arthritis
- System(s) affected: Musculoskeletal
- Synonym(s): Osteoarthrosis; Degenerative joint disease

EPIDEMIOLOGY
Predominant age:
- Symptomatic disease: >40 years old
- Leading cause of disability in those >65 years old
- Radiographic evidence (estimates): 33% to almost 90% in those >65 years old
- Predominant sex: Male = Female

Prevalence
- ~60 million patients
- Increases with age, almost universal >65 (by x-ray study but not clinically)

RISK FACTORS
- Increasing age: >50 years old
- Obesity (weight-bearing joints)
- Prolonged occupational or sports stress
- Injury to a joint from trauma, infection, or preexisting inflammatory arthritis
- Female gender (i.e., knee and hand osteoarthritis [OA])

Genetics
- OA has strong genetic factors, although they may be site- and gender-specific (i.e., hand OA in women).
- Up to 65% of OA may occur on a genetic basis.
- The genetic contribution may involve a combination of effects on structure (collagen), cartilage, or bone metabolism or inflammation.
- Failure of chondrocytes to maintain the balance between degradation and synthesis of extracellular matrix

ETIOLOGY
Biomechanical, biochemical, inflammatory, and immunologic factors all implicated in pathogenesis

 DIAGNOSIS

HISTORY
- Slowly developing joint pain
- Pain that follows use of a joint
- Stiffness of <15 minutes duration (especially morning and after sitting)

PHYSICAL EXAM
- Joint bony enlargement (e.g., Heberden nodules of distal interphalangeal joints)
- Decreased range of motion with pain at the end of the range
- Tenderness usually absent; may occur along joint margin associated with synovitis
- Crepitation as late sign
- Weakness and wasting of the muscles acting on the joint
- Local pain and stiffness with OA of spine, with radicular pain (if compression of nerve roots present)

DIAGNOSTIC TESTS & INTERPRETATION
Lab
Initial lab tests
Usually not helpful in diagnosis (sedimentation rate not increased)

Follow-Up & Special Considerations
- May be useful in monitoring treatment with NSAIDs (renal insufficiency and GI bleeding)
- In secondary OA, underlying disorder may have abnormal lab results, e.g., hemochromatosis (abnormal iron studies).

Imaging
Initial approach
- X-ray films usually normal early
- Later often show:
  - Narrowed, asymmetric joint space
  - Osteophyte formation
  - Subchondral bony sclerosis
  - Cyst formation
- Erosions may occur on surface of distal and proximal interphalangeal joints when OA is associated with inflammation (erosive OA).

Diagnostic Procedures/Surgery
- Joint aspiration:
  - May be helpful in distinguishing from chronic inflammatory arthritis
  - OA: Cell count usually <500 cells/mm^3, predominantly mononuclear
  - Inflammatory: Cell count usually >2,000 cells/mm^3, predominantly neutrophils
- Calcium pyrophosphate dihydrate and/or apatite crystals may be seen in effusions.

Pathological Findings
- Characterized macroscopically by patchy cartilage damage and bony hypertrophy
- Histological phases:
  - Edema of the extracellular matrix and cartilage microcracks
  - Fissuring and pitting of the subchondral bone
  - Erosion and osteocartilaginous loose bodies
- Subchondral bone trabecular microfractures and sclerosis with osteophyte formation
- Degradation response produced by release of proteolytic enzymes, collagenolytic enzymes, prostaglandins, and immune responses

DIFFERENTIAL DIAGNOSIS
- Distinguish from other types of arthritis by:
  - Absence of systemic findings
  - Minimal articular inflammation
  - Distribution of involved joints (e.g., distal and proximal interphalangeal joints, not wrist and metacarpophalangeal joints)
- In spine, distinguish from osteoporosis, metastatic disease, multiple myeloma, or other bone diseases.

TREATMENT

MEDICATION
- Management of pain and inflammation:
  - Acetaminophen up to 1,000 mg q.i.d. Good evidence as most effective for pain relief in OA of knee or hip (1)[A].
  - A number of studies, mainly of knee osteoarthritis, have shown short-term (<4 weeks) benefits from topical NSAID gels, creams, and ointments when compared to placebo. Topical NSAIDs should be a core treatment for knee and hand OA.
  - If acetaminophen or topical NSAIDs are insufficient, then the addition or substitution by an oral NSAID/COX-2 inhibitor should be considered. They should be used at the lowest effective dose for the shortest possible period. Prolonged use is associated with renal insufficiency, hypertension (HTN), leg edema, and GI bleeding.
  - May use nonacetylated salicylates (e.g., salsalate, choline-magnesium salicylate) or low-dose ibuprofen ≤1,600 mg/d.
  - Topical NSAIDs and capsaicin can be effective as adjunctives and alternatives to oral analgesic/anti-inflammatory agents in knee OA (1)[A].
  - Other NSAIDs have similar efficacy.
- Contraindications:
  - All oral NSAIDs/COX-2 inhibitors have analgesic effects of a similar magnitude but vary in their potential GI and cardio-renal toxicity; therefore, the choice of agent and dose should take into account individual patient risk factors.
  - NSAIDs are contraindicated in patients with renal disease, CHF, HTN, active peptic ulcer disease, and previous hypersensitivity to an NSAID or aspirin (asthma, nasal polyps, hypotension, urticaria/angioedema).
  - Combinations of NSAIDs are contraindicated due to risk of adverse reactions.
  - Avoid concomitant use of aspirin with NSAIDs.
  - In patients with increased cardiovascular risk, the combination of a nonselective NSAID, low-dose aspirin, and a proton-pump inhibitor (PPI) is preferred treatment.
  - Oral or parenteral corticosteroids are contraindicated.

- Precautions:
  - If oral NSAID/COX-2 inhibitor is necessary for a patient aged >65 or a patient <65 with any increased GI risk factors, offer a PPI.
  - Significant possible interactions:
    - NSAIDs reduce effectiveness of ACE inhibitors and diuretics.
    - Aspirin and NSAIDs (except COX-2 inhibitors) may increase effects of anticoagulants.
    - Increased hypoglycemic effects of oral hypoglycemics with aspirin
    - Salicylates reduce effectiveness of spironolactone (Aldactone) and uricosurics.
    - Corticosteroids and some antacids increase salicylate excretion, whereas ascorbic acid and ammonium chloride reduce salicylate excretion and may cause toxicity.

Pregnancy Considerations
- ASA and NSAIDs: Some risk to fetus during 1st and 3rd trimesters of pregnancy
- Compatible with breastfeeding

Second Line
- A number of studies, mainly of knee OA, have shown short-term (<4 weeks) benefits from topical NSAID gels, creams, and ointments when compared to placebo. Topical NSAIDs should be a core treatment for knee and hand OA (2)[B].
- Topical capsaicin should be considered as an adjunct therapy for knee and hand OA; may cause local burning.
- Rubefacients are not recommended.
- Opioid analgesics (e.g., codeine, oxycodone, propoxyphene): Evidence supporting their use in OA is extremely poor and should be restricted for treatment of acute episodes of pain.
- Judiciously use intra-articular injections of corticosteroids for selected acute flare-ups of joints (no more than 3/year up to a maximum of 12 injections per joint). If used excessively, can accelerate joint deterioration.
- Intra-articular viscosupplementation with hyaluronic acid preparations into a painful knee may provide relief of pain and improve function at earlier stages, though not statistically significant over injections with saline (placebo) (3)[B]. Definitive evidence is lacking in other joints. However, there are few randomized head-to-head comparisons of different products.

ADDITIONAL TREATMENT
General Measures
- Reassure patient of absence of generalized systemic disease, but recognize potential disability.
- Weight reduction if obese and fitness program, including physical therapy (1)[A]
- Walking aids instruction and proper footwear (1)[A]
- Heat (e.g., local, tub baths) or cold applications
- Physical therapy to maintain or regain joint motion and muscle strength. Quadriceps-strengthening exercises can relieve knee pain and disability.
- Protect joints from overuse (e.g., cane, crutches, walker).
- Assessment for bracing, joint supports, or insoles in those with biomechanical joint pain or instability

Additional Therapies
Address psychosocial factors: Self-efficacy, coping skills, prevent, treat anxiety and depression, and improve social support

COMPLEMENTARY AND ALTERNATIVE MEDICINE
- Nutritional supplements such as glucosamine and chondroitin sulfate may symptomatically benefit some patients and have low toxicity, but studies lack standardized case definition and outcome assessments. *If no response is apparent within 6 months, treatment should be discontinued.*
- A 2010 meta-analysis shows glucosamine, chondroitin, and their combination do not reduce joint pain or have an impact on narrowing of joint space compared with placebo (4)[A].
- TENS units and acupuncture may be beneficial (1)[A].

SURGERY/OTHER PROCEDURES
May be indicated in advanced disease (e.g., osteotomy, debridement, removal of loose bodies, joint replacement, fusion)

ONGOING CARE
FOLLOW-UP RECOMMENDATIONS
As active as tolerated

Patient Monitoring
- Follow range of motion and functional status at regular intervals.
- Watch for GI blood loss and follow cardiac, renal, and mental status in older patients on NSAIDs or aspirin.
- Periodic complete blood count, renal function tests, stool for occult blood

PATIENT EDUCATION
- American College of Rheumatology patient education overviews: http://www.rheumatology.org/public/factsheets/index.asp?aud=pat
- American Academy of Family Physicians Foundation: http://www.familydoctor.org.
- Arthritis Foundation: http://www.arthritis.org

PROGNOSIS
- Disease tends to be progressive
- Early in course, pain relieved by rest; later, pain may occur at rest and at night.
- Joint effusions may occur, especially in knees.
- Joint enlargement occurs later in course due to bony enlargement.
- Osteophyte (spur) formation, especially at joint margins, as disease progresses
- Advanced stage with full-thickness loss of cartilage down to bone

COMPLICATIONS
- One of the leading causes of pain and disability
- Decompensated CHF, GI bleeding, decreased renal function on NSAIDs or aspirin
- Hypoglycemic reactions (rare) in diabetic patients taking oral hypoglycemic agents:
  - Infection or accelerated cartilage loss with intra-articular corticosteroids

REFERENCES
1. Zhang W, Moskowitz RW, Nuki G, Abramson S, Altman RD, Arden N, Bierma-Zeinstra S, Brandt KD, Croft P, Doherty M, Dougados M, Hochberg M, Hunter DJ, Kwoh K, Lohmander LS, Tugwell P et al. OARSI recommendations for the management of hip and knee osteoarthritis, Part II: OARSI evidence-based, expert consensus guidelines. *Osteoarthr Cartil.* 2008;16:137–62.
2. Altman R, Barkin RL. Topical therapy for osteoarthritis: clinical and pharmacologic perspectives. *Postgrad Med.* 2009;121:139–47.
3. Kul-Panza E, Berker N et al. Is hyaluronate sodium effective in the management of knee osteoarthritis? A placebo-controlled double-blind study. *Minerva Med.* 2010;101:63–72
4. Wandel S, Jüni P, Tendal B, Nüesch E, Villiger PM, Welton NJ, Reichenbach S, Trelle S et al. Effects of glucosamine, chondroitin, or placebo in patients with osteoarthritis of hip or knee: network meta-analysis. *BMJ (Clinical research ed.).* 2010;341:c4675.

ADDITIONAL READING
- Harvey WF, Hunter DJ et al. Pharmacologic intervention for osteoarthritis in older adults. *Clin Geriatr Med.* 2010;26:503–15.
- Hunter DJ, Lo GH. The management of osteoarthritis: an overview and call to appropriate conservative treatment. *Med Clin North Am.* 2009;93:127–43.
- Lane NE. Clinical practice. Osteoarthritis of the hip. *N Engl J Med.* 2007;357:1413–21.
- National Institute for Health and Clinical Excellence. *Osteoarthritis: national clinical guideline for care and management in adults.* London: NICE, 2008. http://www.nice.org.uk/CG059.
- Walsh NE, Hurley MV. Evidence based guidelines and current practice for physiotherapy management of knee osteoarthritis. *Musculoskeletal Care.* 2008.

CODES
ICD9
- 715.10 Osteoarthrosis, localized, primary, involving unspecified site
- 715.20 Osteoarthrosis, localized, secondary, involving unspecified site
- 715.90 Osteoarthrosis, unspecified whether generalized or localized, involving unspecified site

CLINICAL PEARLS
- Morning stiffness lasts <15 minutes (vs an hour in rheumatoid arthritis)
- Distal predominance in hands
- Limit intra-articular steroid injections to 3 per year.

ARTHRITIS, PSORIATIC

Michael S. Krathen, MD
Amit Garg, MD

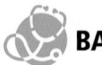 **BASICS**

Psoriatic arthritis (PsA) is a chronic destructive seronegative arthropathy seen most commonly in patients with long-standing psoriasis.

DESCRIPTION

- PsA is a seronegative spondyloarthropathy characterized by inflammatory arthritis and enthesitis.
- 5 patterns of arthritis in PsA include
  - Asymmetric oligoarthritis: Usually involves large joints
  - Distal interphalangeal (DIP) joint predominant: Often associated with nail psoriasis
  - Symmetric polyarthritis: May be indistinguishable from rheumatoid arthritis (RA)
  - Spondyloarthritis: Asymmetric and discontinuous, unlike ankylosing spondylitis (AS)
  - Arthritis mutilans: Destructive, resorptive arthritis; produces so-called opera-glass or telescoping digit
- Although psoriasis generally is present, it may be limited in extent.
  - Course of arthritis and extent of psoriasis do not appear to correlate.
  - Other extraarticular features, such as iritis, are less common.
  - Damaging joint disease may occur in 40–57%. Characteristic radiologic changes include joint erosions that begin marginally and move centrally ("pencil-in-cup deformity") and periostitis.
- Rheumatoid factor (RF) and cyclic citrullinated peptide (anti-CCP) antibody are usually negative. HLA-B27 may be positive.

EPIDEMIOLOGY

- Peak onset age: 35–40 years
- Predominant gender: Female = Male
- Polyarthritis is more common in women.
- Spondylitis in up to 25%, more common in males
- Psoriasis precedes arthritis in the majority by an average of 12 years. Arthritis may precede psoriasis in up to 15%, and this occurs more often in children. Arthritis and psoriasis also may present simultaneously.
- Psoriasis occurs in 2–3% of the US population; 6–42% of these individuals develop PsA (1).

Prevalence
Prevalence: 1–2/1,000 population (1)

RISK FACTORS
- Psoriasis
- Family history of PsA

Genetics
- 30–40% concordance in identical twins
- HLA-B27 in 15–50% with PsA (spondylitis pattern) vs 90% in AS
- Other HLA associations in psoriatic arthritis: HLA-B7, HLA-B38, HLA-B39, HLA-Cw6

GENERAL PREVENTION
There are no currently available prevention strategies. It is unknown if early systemic treatment of psoriasis prevents the onset of PsA.

PATHOPHYSIOLOGY
- CD4+/CD8+ T cells; tumor necrosis factor α (TNF-α); interleukins 1 (IL-1), 6, 8, and 10; and matrix metalloproteases present in synovial fluid (1)
- Osteoclast precursor cell upregulation

ETIOLOGY
Unknown. Probably multifactorial: Immunologic, genetic, environmental factors

COMMONLY ASSOCIATED CONDITIONS
Psoriasis

 DIAGNOSIS

- Establishing a history of inflammatory arthritis, dactylitis, or enthesitis in a patient with existing psoriasis is usually adequate to establish the diagnosis. Nonetheless, differentiation from other inflammatory arthropathies such as RA can be difficult.
- The CASPAR criteria (2) comprise a validated instrument that may be used to screen patients for the presence of PsA. The sensitivity and specificity of the CASPAR criteria are 91.4% and 98.7%, respectively. To establish the presence of PsA, a patient must have inflammatory articular disease (joint, spine, or entheseal) with $\geq$3 points from the following five categories: (1) evidence of current psoriasis, a personal history of psoriasis, or family history of psoriasis (2 points), (2) typical psoriatic nail dystrophy, including onycholysis, pitting, and hyperkeratosis (1 point), (3) a negative rheumatoid factor, preferentially analyzed by enzyme-linked immunosorbent assay (1 point), (4) current dactylitis or a history of dactylitis (1 point), and (5) radiologic evidence of new bone formation (excluding osteophyte formation) on plain radiographs of the hand or foot (1 point).

HISTORY
- Long-standing (most often) psoriasis
- Morning stiffness of hands, feet, or low back for >45 minutes
- Discomfort or pain of involved joints
- Swelling or redness of peripheral joints
- Low back or buttock pain
- Ankle or heel pain
- Dactylitis, or uniform swelling of an entire digit

PHYSICAL EXAM
- Affected peripheral joints may have overlying erythema, warmth, and swelling.
  - Synovitis
  - Dactylitis
  - Swelling of tendons (e.g., Achilles tendon) and tenderness at insertion sites (e.g., calcaneus)
  - Limited range of motion of axial skeleton
  - Pain with stress on the sacroiliac joint
- Well-demarcated pink to red erythematous plaques with a white silvery scale; common locations include scalp, ears, trunk, buttocks, elbows and forearms, knees and legs, and palms and soles.
- Nails may be dystrophic with pits, oil spots, crumbling, leukonychia, and red lunulae.

DIAGNOSTIC TESTS & INTERPRETATION
History and physical examination may provide adequate data to establish the diagnosis of PsA. Plain radiographs may demonstrate characteristic changes and aid in the diagnosis of PsA. Imaging allows assessment of current damage, disease progression, and response to therapy.

Lab
There is no specific blood test for PsA. Autoantibodies associated with RA or systemic lupus erythematosus, for example, generally are not found.

Initial lab tests
- Serum RF is usually negative.
- Anti-CCP is usually negative.
- Antinuclear antibodies are usually negative.
- Acute-phase reactants (erythrocyte sedimentation rate and C-reactive protein) may be elevated.
- HLA-B27 is noted in 50–70% with axial disease and <15% with peripheral disease.

Imaging
Juxtaarticular new bone formation (periostitis) and marginal joint erosions that may progress centrally to form the "pencil-in-cup" erosions are the most characteristic plain radiographic features.

Initial approach
Baseline plain radiographs of affected joints

Follow-Up & Special Considerations
Follow-up radiographs; interval based on severity

Diagnostic Procedures/Surgery
Diagnosis is clinical.

Pathological Findings
Diagnosis is clinical, and biopsy of either skin or synovium is not usually required.

DIFFERENTIAL DIAGNOSIS
- Reactive arthritis
- Psoriasis and RA
- Psoriasis and osteoarthritis
- Psoriasis and polyarticular gout
- Psoriasis and AS

TREATMENT

- Treatment algorithms in PsA are based on severity of joint symptoms, extent of structural damage, and extent and severity of psoriasis (3)[A].
- It is essential that the psychological burden of skin disease not be underestimated or discounted.
- Nonsteroidal anti-inflammatory drugs (NSAIDs) may be considered for control of symptoms. Intraarticular glucocorticoid injections may be given judiciously to control symptoms for persistent mono- or oligoarthritis.
- All patients with severe or moderate peripheral arthritis should be started on disease-modifying antirheumatic drugs (DMARDs). DMARDs have the potential to reduce or prevent joint damage and preserve joint integrity and function.
- DMARDs recommended as 1st-line therapy are sulfasalazine, leflunomide, methotrexate, and cyclosporine. No evidence supports the use of combination DMARD therapy.
- Patients who fail to respond to at least 1 standard DMARD drug should be considered for anti-TNF-α therapy. Patients with poor prognosis could be considered for anti-TNF-α therapy even if they have not failed a standard DMARD.

MEDICATION
First Line
NSAIDs (4)[A]

Second Line
- Sulfasalazine (4)[A]
- Methotrexate (4)[B]
- Cyclosporine (4)[B]
- Azathioprine (4)[B]

- TNF-α inhibitors:
  – Adalimumab (4)[A]
  – Etanercept (4)[A]
  – Infliximab (4)[A]

- IL-12/23 inhibitor: Ustekinumab (5)[A]

ALERT
Anti-TNF agents should not be used in the setting of active infection, including patients with tuberculosis and hepatitis B infection, with concurrent live vaccinations, with New York Heart Association (NYHA) class III–IV congestive heart failure, with malignancy, or with history of demyelinating disease.

Pregnancy Considerations
- Avoid teratogenic medications (e.g., methotrexate, gold, antimalarials, sulfasalazine, acitretin) during pregnancy.
- Adalimumab, etanercept, and infliximab are currently listed as category B medications.

ADDITIONAL TREATMENT
General Measures
Physical therapy may be beneficial in all stages of disease.

Issues for Referral
- Rheumatology
- Dermatology

SURGERY/OTHER PROCEDURES
Joint fusion or replacement for advanced destruction

 ONGOING CARE

FOLLOW-UP RECOMMENDATIONS
Epidemiologic evidence suggests a relationship between psoriasis, the metabolic syndrome, myocardial infarction, and stroke. Periodic measurement of blood pressure, fasting lipids and glucose, cholesterol, and body mass index is recommended (6).

PATIENT EDUCATION
- Stress noncontagious nature of condition
- For a listing of sources for patient education materials favorably reviewed on this topic, physicians may contact:
  – American Academy of Family Physicians Foundation, P.O. Box 8418, Kansas City, MO 64114, (800) 274-2237, ext. 4400. Also see http://www.familydoctor.org.
  – National Psoriasis Foundation, 6600 SW 92nd Ave., Suite 300, Portland, OR 97223-7195. Also see http://www.psoriasis.org/about/psa.
  – Arthritis Foundation, 1314 Spring Street N.W., Atlanta, GA 30309, (404) 872-7100 or http://www.arthritis.org/conditions/diseasecenter/psoriatic_arthritis.asp.

PROGNOSIS
- Course: Insidious and chronic joint disease and recurring and remitting chronic skin disease
- More favorable than for RA (except for patients who develop arthritis mutilans)

COMPLICATIONS
- Chronicity
- Disability
- Psychosocial impact of psoriasis

REFERENCES

1. Gottlieb A, et al. Guidelines of care for management of psoriatic arthritis. *JAAD.* 2008;58: 851–64.
2. Taylor W, Gladman D, Helliwell P, Marchesoni A, Mease P, Mielants H; CASPAR Study Group. Classification criteria for psoriatic arthritis: development of new criteria from a large international study. *Arthritis Rheum.* 2006;54(8): 2665–73.
3. Menter A, et al. American Academy of Dermatology. Links Guidelines of care for the management of psoriasis and psoriatic arthritis. Section 3. Guidelines of care for the management and treatment of psoriasis with topical therapies. *J Am Acad Dermatol.* 2009;60(4):643–59.
4. Kavanaugh AF, Ritchlin CT, GRAPPA Treatment Guideline Committee. Systematic review of treatments for psoriatic arthritis: an evidence based approach and basis for treatment guidelines. *J Rheumatol.* 2006;33:1417–21.
5. Gottlieb A, Menter A, Mendelsohn A, Shen YK, Li S, Guzzo C, Fretzin S, Kunynetz R, Kavanaugh A et al. Ustekinumab, a human interleukin 12/23 monoclonal antibody, for psoriatic arthritis: randomised, double-blind, placebo-controlled, crossover trial. *Lancet.* 2009;373:633–40.
6. Gottlieb AB, Dann F et al. Comorbidities in patients with psoriasis. *Am J Med.* 2009;122:1150.e1–9.
7. Prey S, Paul C, Bronsard V, Puzenat E, Gourraud PA, Aractingi S, Aubin F, Bagot M, Cribier B, Joly P, Jullien D, Maitre ML, Richard-Lallemand MA, Ortonne JP et al. Assessment of risk of psoriatic arthritis in patients with plaque psoriasis: a systematic review of the literature. *J Eur Acad Dermatol Venereol.* 2010;24(Suppl 2):31–5.

ADDITIONAL READING

Ritchlin CT, Kavanaugh A, Gladman DD et al. Treatment recommendations for psoriatic arthritis. *Ann Rheum Dis.* 2008.

CODES

ICD9
696.0 Psoriatic arthropathy

CLINICAL PEARLS

- Severity of psoriasis may correlate with the likelihood of developing arthritis; however, severity of psoriasis does not correlate with severity of arthritis; 24% of psoriasis patients develop PsA (7)[A].
- Often overlooked locations of psoriasis include scalp, ears, umbilicus, and gluteal cleft.
- Other conditions may mimic or coexist with PsA: Osteoarthritis and polyarticular gout.
- The polyarticular pattern of PsA may mimic RA; however, the presence of enthesitis and recognition of psoriasis characterize PsA.
- Axial skeleton in PsA is asymmetric and discontinuous, in contrast to axial involvement in AS.

ARTHRITIS, RHEUMATOID (RA)

Sergio A. Leon, MD

BASICS

DESCRIPTION
- RA is a chronic systemic inflammatory disease (typically joint-involving) of unknown cause.
- Articular inflammation may be remitting, but if continued, may result in joint damage and disability.
- Characteristic extra-articular manifestations include rheumatoid nodules, vasculitis, neuropathy, scleritis, pericarditis, and splenomegaly.
- System(s) affected: Musculoskeletal; Skin; Hematologic; Lymphatic; Immunologic; Muscular; Renal; Cardiovascular; Neurologic; Pulmonary

Geriatric Considerations
- Increased contribution/interaction of age-related comorbidities; pericarditis, septic arthritis, Sjögren syndrome are more common
- Less tolerance to drugs; increased incidence of hydroxychloroquine-associated maculopathy, D-penicillamine rash, and sulfasalazine-induced nausea/vomiting

Pregnancy Considerations
- Use effective contraception with disease-modifying antirheumatic drugs (DMARDs). Modify regimen with pregnancy or breast-feeding.
- Labor/delivery pose no serious problems, unless severe mechanical joint disease.
- >75% improve during pregnancy, but relapse in 6 months. 1st episodes may occur in pregnancy.

EPIDEMIOLOGY
Incidence
- Predominant age: 3rd–6th decades
- Predominant sex:
  – Female > Male (2–3:1; overall incidence and prevalence of articular manifestations)
  – Male > Female (systemic disease)

Prevalence
- US population: 0.5–1.5%
- Native Americans: >3.5–5.3%

RISK FACTORS
- HLA genes contribute to 30–50% genetic risk.
- Family history
- Native American ethnicity

Genetics
- 1st-degree relatives have 1.5-fold higher risk than the general population of developing RA.
- Twin studies show heritability of 60%.
- Seropositive RA aggregates in families.
- HLA-DR4+ person has increased relative risk of 4–5 x.

PATHOPHYSIOLOGY
Antibody-complement complex results in intra-articular inflammation

ETIOLOGY
- Genetic factors
- Host factors: Hormonal, immunologic, obesity
- Environmental: Socioeconomic, smoking

COMMONLY ASSOCIATED CONDITIONS
- Sjögren syndrome, Felty syndrome, Amyloidosis
- Increased incidence of infections, lymphomas, renal and cardiovascular disease

DIAGNOSIS

PHYSICAL EXAM
Evaluate specific joints and extra-articular involvement

DIAGNOSTIC TESTS & INTERPRETATION
Lab
Initial lab tests
- Hematocrit: Mild anemia (of chronic disease)
- ESR: Usually elevated
- C-reactive protein: Unspecific, direct measure of impact of IL-6 on liver cells
- Rheumatoid factor (RF): >1:80 in 70–80% of patients with RA (most commonly IgM Ab):
  – Poor screening tool
  – Disorders that may yield false-positive RF results: Sjögren syndrome, mixed cryoglobulinemia, parasitic infections (e.g., malaria), liver disease, endocarditis, acute viral infections.
- Anticyclic citrullinated peptide antibodies (Anti-CCP antibodies) are highly specific and present early. Linked to erosive RA.
- Antinuclear antibody: Present in 20–30%
- Electrolytes, creatinine, liver function, urinalysis to assess comorbid states

Follow-Up & Special Considerations
RF is not useful for monitoring course of illness

Imaging
Initial approach
- Radiographic abnormalities are very useful in the diagnosis and treatment.
- Periarticular osteopenia is the earliest change.
- More typical findings are juxta-articular bone erosions and symmetrical joint space narrowing.
- CT/MRI and ultrasound are useful in specific situations such as cervical-spine symptoms or detection of early joint erosions.
- Bone scan if suspected aseptic necrosis

Follow-Up & Special Considerations
Radiographs of the hands, wrists, and feet can be repeated to follow disease progression.

Diagnostic Procedures/Surgery
Synovial fluid:
- No pathognomonic findings
- Yellowish-white, turbid, poor viscosity
- WBC increased (3,500–50,000)
- Protein: ~4.2 g/dL (42 g/L)
- Serum-synovial glucose difference ≥30 mg/dL (≥1.67 mmol/L)

Pathological Findings
Synovial tissue is expanded by the recruitment and retention of inflammatory cells, with formation of villous projections and pannus that invades and destroys cartilage and bone.

DIFFERENTIAL DIAGNOSIS
- Other systemic connective tissue diseases: Sjögren syndrome, systemic lupus erythematosus, systemic sclerosis, adult Still disease, mixed
- Psoriatic arthritis
- Viral-induced arthritis: Parvovirus B19, hepatitis C (with cryoglobulinemia)
- Occult malignancy
- Vasculitis: Behçet syndrome
- Seronegative polyarthritis
- Erosive osteoarthritis
- Chronic infections: Lyme disease

TREATMENT

Goals: Controlling disease activity, relieving pain, maintaining or improving function, preventing or correcting impairments, and promoting self-management

MEDICATION
Disease-Modifying Anti-Rheumatic Drugs (DMARDs) are usually administered in combination following four general strategies: sequential monotherapy, step-up therapy, induction therapy or individualized targeted 'tight' control.

First Line
- Nonbiologic DMARDs:
  – Start DMARDs within 2 months of diagnosis if patient has ongoing active disease despite appropriate dose of aspirin or other NSAIDs.
  – Precautions: Offer proton pump inhibitors (PPIs) for chronic NSAID therapy; avoid NSAID combination.
  – Due to their greater convenience, lower toxicity profiles, and quicker onset of action, the initial therapy is a nonbiologic DMARD: Methotrexate, sulfasalazine, or leflunomide have shown evidence of comparable efficacy. Hydroxychloroquine is a less potent agent.
  – Combination DMARDs may be more effective than individual drugs.

– Bridging and/or low-dose corticosteroids, NSAIDs, and simple analgesics are often required to maximize symptoms management.

– Prednisone: 5–15 mg/d for severe disease or to minimize disease activity. Use only for short periods, or intermittently. Low-dose prednisolone is more effective than NSAIDs (1)[A].

– Methotrexate (MTX) (Rheumatrex): 7.5–25 mg per week PO. The DMARD with most predictable benefit. Many significant side effects, but the addition of folate reduces toxicity. 3–6-month trial. Monitor CBC, renal, and liver function every 8–12 weeks. Contraindicated in renal disease

– Sulfasalazine (SSZ): 500 mg/d, increase to 2 g/d over 1 month; max: 2–3 g/d; 6-month trial (2)[A]. Monitor CBC, liver enzymes every 8–12 weeks. Screen for G6PD deficiency.

– Leflunomide (Arava): Dose: 10–20 mg/d. Modifies T-cell function to decrease autoimmune activity, reduce structural damage. Response rate similar to SSZ and MTX. GI side effects and potentially teratogenic (3)[A]. Contraindicated in pregnancy.

– Antimalarials: Hydroxychloroquine (HCQ) (Plaquenil) 400 mg qhs for 2–3 months, then 200 mg at bedtime; 6-month trial usual (4)[A]. Usually to treat milder forms or in combination with other DMARDs. Yearly ophthalmologic exam. Adjust dose in renal insufficiency.

- Biological DMARDs:

– Tumor necrosis factor (TNF) inhibitors: IV infliximab (Remicade), SC adalimumab (Humira), and SC etanercept (Enbrel). No evidence to suggest that one is superior to another. The combination with MTX appears to be the most effective regimen. Optimal dosage and duration of treatment unclear. Low toxicity. Costly. Check PPD prior to treatment and periodic CBC. Risk of lymphoma, CHF.

– Anakinra (Kineret), an IL-1 receptor antagonist. Injection site reaction, neutropenia, bacterial infections. Fewer clinical benefits than TNF inhibitors.

– Abatacept (Orencia) and rituximab (Rituxan) are approved for active moderate to severe RA with inadequate response to other DMARDs or failed anti-TNF agent.

– Two long-acting anti-TNF agents, Certolizumab pegol (Cimzia) and golimumab (Simponi), have been also approved in moderate-to-severe disease.

- Other older nonbiologic DMARDs have been virtually abandoned in developed countries for the treatment of RA:

– Minocycline: In active mild/moderate disease.

– Auranofin (Ridaura): 6–10 mg/d PO. Slow onset of action. Poor GI tolerability.

– Injectable gold (Aurolate): Seldom used because of frequent toxicity

– D-Penicillamine: 250–1000 mg/d. Has dose-related side effects. Close monitoring.

– Protein A immunoadsorption (Prosorba): Removes antibodies. Costly.

– Cyclosporine: Inhibition of T-cell response. Incremental benefit combined with MTX.

– Azathioprine: Because of toxicity, reserved for persons not responsive to other DMARDs.

Second Line

- Intra-articular steroids: If disease is well controlled except for a single joint or two, after establishing that the joint is not infected
- Hyaluronate (Hyalgan): Hyaluronic acid substitute. For pain relief; exact role in RA unclear.

ADDITIONAL TREATMENT

Interdisciplinary care and management is necessary to minimize the consequences of loss of function, joint damage, maladaptive coping, and social isolation.

General Measures

- Complete remission of disease activity should be the ultimate goal
- Early, aggressive treatment is desirable to prevent structural damage and disability.
- Key elements include periodical evaluation of disease activity and extent of synovitis.
- Arthritis self-management education is a proven effective intervention in RA.

SURGERY/OTHER PROCEDURES

Surgical treatment, including synovectomy, tendon reconstruction, joint fusion, and joint replacement are powerful treatment modalities to prevent disability in advanced RA.

 ONGOING CARE

The goals of comprehensive, interdisciplinary care are to stop the disease process, reduce pain, manage symptoms such as fatigue and stiffness, preserve joint integrity and function, and maintain social and occupational roles and quality of life.

FOLLOW-UP RECOMMENDATIONS

- Encourage full activity, but avoid heavy work or exercise during active phases.
- Emphasize exercise, mobility, and reduction of joint stress.
- Promote general health care and psychosocial functional status.

Patient Monitoring

- Address risk factors and evaluate for osteoporosis, a major comorbidity that can result from the disease itself or corticosteroids.
- Cardiovascular disease is the number one cause of death. Evaluate and manage CV risk factors, use low-dose aspirin as preventive.

DIET

No specific diet recommended

PATIENT EDUCATION

- American College of Rheumatology patient education overviews: www.rheumatology.org/public/factsheets/index.asp?aud=pat
- American Academy of Family Physicians Foundation: www.familydoctor.org.
- Arthritis Foundation: www.arthritis.org

PROGNOSIS

- Poor prognostic findings:
  – Persistent moderate-to-severe disease
  – Inheritance of shared epitope
  – Early or advanced age at disease onset
- 50% cannot function in primary job within 10 years of onset.

COMPLICATIONS

Extra-articular involvement: Pulmonary disease, vasculitis, pericarditis, nephropathy, nerve entrapment, muscle atrophy, eye disease, Felty syndrome, chronic anemia

REFERENCES

1. Gotzsche PC, Johansen HK. Short-term low-dose corticosteroids vs. placebo and NSAIDs in rheumatoid arthritis. *Cochrane Database Syst Rev.* 2006:1.
2. Suarez-Almazor ME, et al. Sulfasalazine for treating rheumatoid arthritis. *Cochrane Database Syst Rev.* 2006:1.
3. Osiri M, et al. Leflunomide for treating rheumatoid arthritis. *Cochrane Database Syst Rev.* 2006:1.
4. Suarez-Almazor ME, et al. Antimalarials for treating rheumatoid arthritis. *Cochrane Database Syst Rev.* 2006:1.

ADDITIONAL READING

- Aletaha D, Neogi T, Silman AJ et al. 2010 rheumatoid arthritis classification criteria: an American College of Rheumatology/European League Against Rheumatism collaborative initiative. *Ann Rheum Dis.* 2010;69:1580–8.
- Mertens M, Singh JA. Anakinra for Rheumatoid Arthritis: A Systematic Review. *J Rheumatol.* 2009.

 CODES

ICD9
- 714.0 Rheumatoid arthritis
- 714.1 Felty's syndrome
- 714.2 Other rheumatoid arthritis with visceral or systemic involvement

CLINICAL PEARLS

- Females have more articular disease and males have more systemic presentations.
- Morning stiffness with symmetrical joint involvement of wrists, proximal interphalangeal and metacarpophalangeal joints.
- Start DMARDs early if patient still having symptoms despite adequate doses of NSAIDS or aspirin and use combination of DMARDs.

ASBESTOSIS

Ruben Peralta, MD

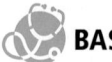 **BASICS**

DESCRIPTION
- Slowly progressive lung disease caused by inhalation of dust from fibrous silicate asbestos used in insulation, cement, and other building and construction materials
- Nodular interstitial fibrotic lung disease caused by cascade of inflammatory responses to inhaled asbestos fibers:
  – Pleural fibrosis, pleural plaques, and interstitial fibrosis develop.
  – Lung cancer risk is increased.
- Synonym(s): Asbestos pneumoconiosis

EPIDEMIOLOGY
- In the US, an estimated 1.3 million people who work in maintenance and construction are at risk for exposure (1).
- In a very large part of the world, data on mesothelioma are not available (2).
- Predominant age: Middle age (40–75 years)
- Predominant sex: Male > Female, owing to exposure pattern

RISK FACTORS
- Professional exposures most common in construction workers; those who mine, mill, or remove asbestos; ship builders; textile workers; railroad workers.
- Office workers, teachers, and students in buildings with asbestos in place have exposure significantly lower than those of construction workers.
- Dose-response phenomenon: Higher amounts of asbestos exposure are associated with higher risk of asbestosis (3,4,5).
- Cigarette smoking markedly increases risk of radiographic changes and eventual lung cancer risk:
  – Likely mechanism: Decreased clearance of asbestos fibers

Genetics
- Genetic polymorphisms have been implicated (6,7,8,9,10).
- Familial mesothelioma has been reported (11).

GENERAL PREVENTION
- In the US, asbestos is federally regulated by the Occupational Health and Safety Administration.
- Primary responsibility of employers is to provide safe work environment (3,12,13,14,15)
- Exposure control: Substitution of safer materials or adoption of control technologies
- During high-exposure periods, such as building repair, use fit-tested personal respirators for workers.
- To limit exposure to others in their household, those who work with asbestos should leave their clothing at work, if possible. Work clothes should be washed and stored separately from other clothing.

ETIOLOGY
- Asbestos fibers are inhaled. Macrophages engulf the fibers and release inflammatory mediators. Inflammatory mediators cause fibroblast proliferation, leading to fibrosis and remodeling of interstitial lung tissue, including intra-alveolar fibrosis and loss of alveolar capillary units (16).
- Disease continues to slowly progress over the course of years, even if exposure is not ongoing (14,17,18).
- Symptoms may be related to impaired gas exchange and/or a pattern of restrictive lung disease.

COMMONLY ASSOCIATED CONDITIONS
In addition to asbestosis, inhalation of asbestos is associated with several lung problems (11,18,19,20,21,22), including:
- Benign plaques
- Benign pleural effusions
- Lung cancer
- Malignant mesothelioma

 DIAGNOSIS

HISTORY
- Credible history of exposure (usually occupational) to asbestos fibers (3,4,5,17,23,24):
  – Ask about intensity and duration of exposure.
  – Aircraft or electrical maintenance
  – Shipyard workers
  – Those exposed to cement or building materials
  – Asbestos mining
  – People exposed to asbestos when it is disrupted during building maintenance
  – Family members of those who work with asbestos
- In addition to job type and activities and length of exposure, ask patients whether there was visible dust in air or on surfaces, visible dust in sputum, personal protective equipment used, and whether the workplace was cleaned during or after a shift (25).
- Common symptoms include:
  – Dyspnea upon exertion
  – Nonproductive cough (26,27,28)
- Delay from exposure to detection typically becomes clinically apparent 10–15 years after exposure.

PHYSICAL EXAM
- Insidious onset
- Progressive dyspnea is the most common symptom.
- Dry cough
- Progressive exercise intolerance
- Pleuritic chest pain
- Inspiratory crackles (may be best heard laterally)
- Wheeze with forced exhalation
- Digital clubbing and cyanosis in advanced disease
- Right-sided heart failure

DIAGNOSTIC TESTS & INTERPRETATION
Pulmonary function test:
- Not diagnostically specific
- Mainly restrictive pattern unless a smoker (29)
- Decreased total lung capacity and vital capacity
- Reduction in diffusing capacity to carbon monoxide (25)[B]
- Useful for following level of impairment

Lab
No pathognomonic lab findings

Imaging
- Chest x-ray (CXR) (sensitivity 90%, specificity 93%):
  – Most common findings are bilateral pleural thickening and circumscribed calcified pleural plaques
  – Pleural plaques usually posterior-lateral, may also involve diaphragm (30)
  – As disease progresses, small, irregular, linear opacities with a fine reticular pattern are seen
  – Less common: Rounded atelectasis (Blesovsky syndrome) when fibrosis of visceral pleura extends into parenchyma (31)
- Classification scheme available through International Labour Office (at http://www.ilo.org)
- High-resolution computed tomography (CT) may increase sensitivity to near 100%:
  – Improves detection of interstitial fibrosis
  – May show honeycombing in later stages of the disease
- Gallium scan with higher uptake even if the CXR and CT are normal

Pathological Findings
- Lung biopsy or bronchoalveolar lavage (BAL) can reveal asbestos fibers or asbestos bodies (25):
  – May help diagnostically in cases with history of minimal exposure or with atypical clinical or radiographic features
  – Transbronchial biopsy is less reliable than BAL or open-lung biopsy in establishing diagnosis.
- Pleural plaques are found in parietal pleura; made up of collagen bundles with rare inflammatory cells. Pleural thickening involves the visceral pleura (30).
- Asbestos bodies may be seen with iron staining in intra-alveolar macrophages.

DIFFERENTIAL DIAGNOSIS
Other pneumoconioses:
- Idiopathic pulmonary fibrosis
- Hypersensitivity pneumonitis
- Sarcoidosis
- Other pneumoconiosis, including mixed exposures

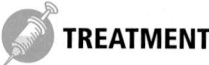 **TREATMENT**

MEDICATION
First Line
- No specific pharmacologic treatment
- Oxygen
- Bronchodilators for pulmonary toilet

Second Line
- Antibiotics for respiratory infections
- Diuretics if cor pulmonale develops

ADDITIONAL TREATMENT
General Measures
- As of now, there is no effective treatment to reverse the course of the disease.
- Clinical approach is directed at amelioration of symptoms, elimination of progression, and reduction of risk of associated disorders.
- Withdrawal from exposure (30)[B]:
  – Workers with no symptoms and only radiographic changes may make an informed choice to continue employment using maximum environmental and personal protection.
- Smoking cessation:
  – Cigarette smokers have more radiographic signs of disease and have a significantly increased risk for lung cancer.
- Pneumococcal and influenza vaccines (28)[B]
- Chest physiotherapy as needed
- Home oxygen as needed

Issues for Referral
All new cases must be reported to health authorities.

ONGOING CARE

Follow World Health Organization (WHO) recommendations for regular health screening of exposed workers (32):

- CXR film at baseline
- For workers with <10 years since 1st exposure: CXR every 3–5 years
- >10 years: CXR every 1–2 years
- >20 years: CXR annually
- All workers: Annual respiratory symptom questionnaire, physical exam, and spirometry (alternatively can be done on CXR schedule)

FOLLOW-UP RECOMMENDATIONS
Patient Monitoring
- CXR
- Occasional pulmonary function tests
- Prompt treatment of infections

DIET
High-calorie, high-protein with advanced disease

PATIENT EDUCATION
- Smoking cessation counseling as needed
- In the US, asbestos has been federally regulated by the Occupational Health and Safety Administration since 1972: http://www.osha.gov.
- Printed patient information available from National Cancer Institute: http://www.cancer.gov/cancertopics/factsheet/Risk/asbestos
- Agency for Toxic Substances and Disease Registry: http://www.atsdr.cdc.gov

PROGNOSIS
- Severity depends on duration and intensity of exposure.
- Lung disease is irreversible.
- Increased risk for lung cancer (synergistic increase with cigarette smoking) and mesothelioma (25)[B]

COMPLICATIONS
- Mesothelioma:
  – Related to dose, time elapsed from exposure (usually 25–40 years after exposure)
  – Risk is higher with exposure to amphibole fibers rather than chrysotile fibers.
  – Pleural effusion in 80–95% (31)[B]
  – Insidious but progressive. Median survival for mesothelioma is 8–18 months (33)[B].
- Lung cancer risk is associated with asbestos exposure, whether asbestosis is present or not; synergistically increased risk in asbestos workers who smoke (13).
- Gastrointestinal cancer risk may also be increased with asbestos exposure.

REFERENCES

1. American Thoracic Society. Diagnosis and initial management of nonmalignant diseases related to asbestos. *Am J Respir Crit Care Med*. 2004;170: 691–715.
2. Bianchi C, Bianchi T. Malignant mesothelioma: global incidence and relationship with asbestos. *Ind Health*. 2007;45:379–87.
3. Lin RT, Takahashi K, Karjalainen A et al. Ecological association between asbestos-related diseases and historical asbestos consumption: an international analysis. *Lancet*. 2007;369:844–9.
4. Bhattacharya K, Dopp E, Kakkar P et al. Biomarkers in risk assessment of asbestos exposure. *Mutat Res*. 2005;579:6–21.
5. Chow S, Campbell C, Sandrini A et al. Exhaled breath condensate biomarkers in asbestos-related lung disorders. *Respir Med*. 2009.
6. Horská A, Kazimírová A, Barancoková M et al. Genetic predisposition and health effect of occupational exposure to asbestos. *Neuro Endocrinol Lett*. 2006;27(Suppl 2):100–3.
7. Franko A, Dolzan V, Arneri N et al. The Influence of Genetic Polymorphisms of GSTP1 on the Development of Asbestosis. *J Occup Environ Med*. 2008;50:7–12.
8. Helmig S, Belwe A, Schneider J. Association of Transforming Growth Factor beta1 Gene Polymorphisms and Asbestos-Induced Fibrosis and Tumors. *J Investig Med*. 2009.
9. Franko A, Dodic-Fikfak M, Arneri N et al. Manganese and extracellular superoxide dismutase polymorphisms and risk for asbestosis. *J Biomed Biotechnol*. 2009;2009:493083.
10. Neri M, Ugolini D, Dianzani I et al. Genetic susceptibility to malignant pleural mesothelioma and other asbestos-associated diseases. *Mutat Res*. 2008;659:126–36.
11. You B, Blandin S, Gérinière L et al. [Family mesotheliomas: genetic interaction with environmental carcinogenic exposure?] *Bull Cancer*. 2007;94:705–10.
12. Mueller TB. Tomorrow's causation standards for yesterday's wonder material: Reiter v. Acands, Inc. and Maryland's changing asbestos litigation. *J Contemp Health Law Policy*. 2009;25:437–61.
13. Dement J, Welch L, Haile E et al. Mortality among sheet metal workers participating in a medical screening program. *Am J Ind Med*. 2009.
14. Centers for Disease Control and Prevention (CDC). Asbestosis-related years of potential life lost before age 65 years—United States, 1968–2005. *MMWR Morb Mortal Wkly Rep*. 2008;57:1321–5.
15. Gehanno JF, Takahashi K, Darmoni S et al. Citation classics in occupational medicine journals. *Scand J Work Environ Health*. 2007;33:245–51.
16. Tercelj M, Salobir B, Simcic S et al. Chitotriosidase activity in sarcoidosis and some other pulmonary diseases. *Scand J Clin Lab Invest*. 2009;1–4.
17. Kurumatani N, Kumagai S. Mapping the risk of mesothelioma due to neighborhood asbestos exposure. *Am J Respir Crit Care Med*. 2008.
18. Mastrangelo G, Ballarin MN, Bellini E et al. Asbestos exposure and benign asbestos diseases in 772 formerly exposed workers: Dose-response relationships. *Am J Ind Med*. 2009.
19. Wagner GR. The fallout from asbestos. *Lancet*. 2007;369:973–4.
20. Wagner JC. The discovery of the association between blue asbestos and mesotheliomas and the aftermath. *Br J Ind Med*. 1991;48:399–403.
21. Wagner GR. Asbestosis and silicosis. *Lancet*. 1997;349:1311–5.
22. Toyokuni S. Mechanisms of asbestos-induced carcinogenesis. *Nagoya J Med Sci*. 2009;71:1–10.
23. Hansell A. Airborne environmental exposure to asbestos. *Am J Respir Crit Care Med*. 2008;178: 556–7.
24. Banks DE, Shi R, McLarty J et al. American College of Chest Physicians consensus statement on the respiratory health effects of asbestos. Results of a Delphi study. *Chest*. 2009;135:1619–27.
25. Costabel U, Uzaslan E, Guzman J. Bronchoalveolar lavage in drug-induced lung disease. *Clin Chest Med*. 2004;25:25–35.
26. Reid A, Berry G, de Klerk N et al. Age and sex differences in malignant mesothelioma after residential exposure to blue asbestos (crocidolite). *Chest*. 2007;131:376–82.
27. Wilson D, Takahashi K, Pan G et al. Respiratory symptoms among residents of a heavy-industry province in China: prevalence and risk factors. *Respir Med*. 2008.
28. O'Reilly KM, Mclaughlin AM, Beckett WS et al. Asbestos-related lung disease. *Am Fam Physician*. 2007;75:683–8.
29. Abejie BA, Wang X, Kales SN, Christiani DC et al. Patterns of pulmonary dysfunction in asbestos workers: a cross-sectional study. *J Occup Med Toxicol*. 2010;5:12.
30. Huggins JT, Sahn SA. Causes and management of pleural fibrosis. *Respirology*. 2004;9:441–7.
31. Cugell DW, Kamp DW. Asbestos and the pleura: a review. *Chest*. 2004;125:1103–17.
32. Welch LS, Haile E. Asbestos-related disease among sheet metal workers 1986–2004: Radiographic changes over time. *Am J Ind Med*. 2009.
33. Martino D, Pass HI. Integration of multimodality approaches in the management of malignant pleural mesothelioma. *Clin Lung Cancer*. 2004; 5:290–8.

ADDITIONAL READING

- Antonescu-Turcu AL, Schapira RM et al. Parenchymal and airway diseases caused by asbestos. *Curr Opin Pulm Med*. 2010;16:155–61
- Brody AR et al. Asbestos and lung disease. *Am J Respir Cell Mol Biol*. 2010;42:131–2.
- Kamp DW et al. Asbestos-induced lung diseases: an update. *Transl Res*. 2009;153:143–52.

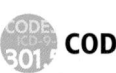 **CODES**

ICD9
- 501 Asbestosis
- 515 Postinflammatory pulmonary fibrosis

CLINICAL PEARLS

- Associations between asbestos and all histologic subtypes of lung cancer have been observed.
- Higher amounts of asbestos exposure are associated with higher risk of asbestosis.
- Smoking cessation is particularly important because cigarette smokers have more radiographic signs of asbestosis and are at a synergistically increased risk for lung cancer.
- For those who work with asbestos, to limit exposure to others in their household, clothing should be left at work, if possible, or should be washed and stored separately from other clothing.

ASCITES

Anne M. Walsh, PA-C, MMSc
Auguste Turnier, MD

BASICS

DESCRIPTION
Pathologic accumulation of fluid in the abdominal cavity; may occur in any condition that causes generalized edema.

EPIDEMIOLOGY
- Children: Nephrotic syndrome and malignancy most common
- Adults: Cirrhosis, heart failure, nephrotic syndrome, peritonitis most common

RISK FACTORS
Those associated with possible causes

ETIOLOGY
- Peritoneal infection and inflammation:
  - Tuberculosis
  - Fungal disease
  - Bacterial infection (foreign body, fistula)
  - Perforated viscus
  - Granulomatous peritonitis (e.g., sarcoidosis)
  - Parasitic infection
- Metabolic diseases:
  - Cirrhosis
  - Prehepatic and posthepatic portal hypertension
  - Myxedema
  - Nephrogenous
  - Dialysis-related
  - Protein malnutrition (hypoalbuminemia <2 g/dL)
- Cardiac congestion:
  - CHF
  - Constrictive pericarditis
  - Tricuspid stenosis or insufficiency
- Trauma:
  - Pancreatic or biliary fistula
  - Lymphatic tear (chylous ascites)
  - Hemoperitoneum (trauma, ectopic pregnancy, tumor)
- Malignancy:
  - Peritoneal seeding: ovarian, colon, pancreas, others
  - Primary peritoneal carcinoma
  - Leukemia, lymphoma
- Mixed (more than one of the above causes, e.g., cirrhosis and cancer)
- Acute liver failure

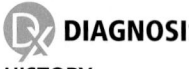

DIAGNOSIS

HISTORY
- Abdominal pain
- Anorexia
- Nausea
- Early satiety
- Heartburn
- Flatulence
- Flank pain
- Weight gain
- Shortness of breath
- Dyspnea/orthopnea
- Edema

PHYSICAL EXAM
- Abdominal distention
- Bulging flanks
- Weight gain
- Abdominal fluid wave
- Shifting dullness or "puddle sign" (dullness over dependent abdomen)
- Penile/scrotal edema
- Umbilical/inguinal herniae
- Pleural effusion
- Pedal edema
- Rales
- Tachycardia
- Palmar erythema, spider angiomata in cirrhosis

DIAGNOSTIC TESTS & INTERPRETATION
Lab
Ascitic fluid should be sampled in all new-onset, new-to-treat, or hospitalized cases (1)[B].

- Obtain in all:
  - Total cell count
    - Polymorphonuclear leukocytes: ≥ 250 mm^3 suggests infection (even if culture is negative) requiring antibiotics
  - Albumin in both serum and ascites: Calculate serum-to-ascites albumin gradient (SAAG):
    - <1.1 g indicates exudate (i.e., inflammatory, biliary/pancreatic, carcinomatosis)
    - ≥ 1.1 g indicates transudate/portal hypertension
  - Protein: >2 g (some sources cite 2.5 g) indicates exudate
- Of use in specific circumstances:
  - Culture if infection suspected (fever, abdominal pain, hypotension, etc.)
  - Amylase, triglycerides, glucose
  - Lactate dehydrogenase
  - Acid-fast or fungal cultures/smears
  - Cytology only if exudate
- Blood tests:
  - BUN/creatinine
  - Electrolytes
- Urine tests:
  - Sodium levels in single sample:
    - <10 mEq/L (<10 mmol/L) diuretic response unlikely
    - >10–70 mEq/L (>10–70 mmol/L) diuretic response likely
    - >70 mEq/L (>70 mmol/L) diuretics unnecessary
- Other labs as indicated by underlying condition (liver enzymes, tumor markers, etc.)

Imaging
- Abdominal ultrasound highly sensitive
- CT scan to rule out intra-abdominal pathology
- MRI best for evaluation of liver disease and presence of hepatoma

Diagnostic Procedures/Surgery
- Diagnostic paracentesis
- Diagnostic laparoscopy

Pathological Findings
- Peritoneal biopsy may reveal tuberculosis or malignancy; of no value in other types of fluid
- Cytology may reveal malignant cells:
  - Typically adenocarcinoma (ovary, breast, GI tract)
  - Rarely primary peritoneal carcinoma

DIFFERENTIAL DIAGNOSIS
- Obesity
- Bowel obstruction
- Pregnancy in reproductive-age female
- If transudate, likely causes include:
  - Congestive heart failure
  - Constrictive pericarditis
  - Cirrhosis
  - Nephrotic syndrome
  - Protein malnutrition/hypoalbuminemia
- If exudate, likely causes include:
  - Neoplasm
  - Tuberculosis
  - Pancreatitis
  - Myxedema
  - Biliary pathology
  - Budd-Chiari syndrome

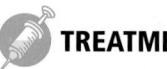

TREATMENT

Outpatient or inpatient, depending on physical condition
For all patients:

- Sodium restriction required (1)[A]:
  - 2 g/day until renal excretion improves, usually required 3–6 months
- Water restriction only necessary if serum sodium <120 mEq/L
- Persistent elevation of creatinine >2.5 mg/dL should lead to decreasing diuretic doses and therapeutic paracentesis
- Daily record of weight to monitor gains and losses

MEDICATION

ALERT
Carefully approach to diuresis as too aggressive treatment can induce hepatorenal syndrome. Monitor creatinine and electrolytes closely.

First Line
- Diuretics needed in nearly all patients:
  - Spironolactone 100–300 mg daily p.o. in single dose best for cirrhotic ascites; typical initial dose is 100–200 mg given in AM
  - Furosemide 20–120 mg daily p.o. best for all other etiologies; typical initial dose is 40 mg given in AM
  - May use spironolactone and furosemide together
  - Dose should be sufficient to obtain net sodium loss in urine
  - Discontinue NSAIDs except 81 mg dose of aspirin.
  - Follow body weight daily. If there is a <2-pound loss in the next 4 days, increase either spironolactone by 100 mg or furosemide by 40 mg. If the 2-pound weight loss continues in the next 4 days, continue with the same dose. Emphasize sodium restriction.
  - Spot sodium in mEq/L × estimated urine output (1 L if no information) should equal estimated dietary sodium. Increase diuretics daily until this goal is attained. Measure serum electrolytes before each dose change.

- Precautions:
  - In hospital or in rapid diuresis, observe creatinine and electrolytes closely. NSAIDs may worsen or initiate oliguria or azotemia.
  - Spironolactone or amiloride may increase potassium; monitoring necessary after 1st week of therapy and at least monthly thereafter.
  - Observe patients closely for signs of volume depletion, encephalopathy, and renal insufficiency.
- Significant possible interactions: Avoid concomitant potassium supplements if spironolactone used alone

Second Line
Alternative diuretics unlikely to success if combinations of spironolactone and furosemide fail or result in increased BUN/creatinine:

- Most commonly used in cases of GI intolerance or allergic reactions
- Alternatives to spironolactone: Amiloride up to 10 mg/day; triamterene up to 200 mg/day in divided doses
- Alternatives to furosemide: Torsemide up to 100 mg/day; ethacrynic acid 50 mg IV (may be effective when oral drugs cannot be used)

ADDITIONAL TREATMENT
General Measures
- For ascites with edema:
  - Salt restriction and diuretics usually effective
  - Maximum weight loss of 5 lb/day
  - Draw weekly serum electrolytes during rapid weight loss.
- For ascites without edema:
  - Dietary restrictions and diuretics as above
  - Maximum weight loss of 2 lb/day
- Refractory ascites:
  - Confirm patient compliance with adequate sodium restriction (most common cause)
- Diuretic-intractable ascites: worse despite max doses spironolactone (300 mg/day) and furosemide (160–200 mg/day) and sodium restriction OR progressive rise in creatinine to 2.0:
  - Paracentesis 5–10 L per session:
    - Complications: Infection, hemodynamic collapse, renal failure
    - Replace albumin IV for all removals >5 L at rate of 8 g albumin for each liter removed
  - Continue diuretics at 1/2 previous dose.

Issues for Referral
Referral for evaluation to liver transplant center in patients with cirrhosis and ascites may be appropriate. (2)[B]

COMPLEMENTARY AND ALTERNATIVE MEDICINE
Caution patients to avoid herbs and other supplements unless approved by health care provider (risk drug interactions, hepatotoxicity, coagulopathy).

SURGERY/OTHER PROCEDURES
- Transjugular intrahepatic portosystemic shunt (TIPS) (2)[A]:
  - TIPS is a transjugular conduit from the liver to the hepatic vein used for intractable ascites; placed by interventional radiologists under fluoroscopy.
    - At time of placement, measure portal pressure; should drop ≥20 mm Hg or to <12 mm Hg, and ascites should be readily controlled with diuretics. Conduct yearly ultrasonographic study to confirm functional shunt.

- Dilation/replacement may be required after >2 years.
- Encephalopathy is a known complication; however, no difference in mortality compared to paracentesis. (1)
- Surgical portacaval shunt: An 8–10 mm mesenteric caval shunt often is effective:
  - Significant operative mortality, morbidity, encephalopathy; most experts prefer TIPS, rarely used in the US due to its greater risks than TIPS (2)[C]
- When recurrent pleural effusion is present in patient with chronic ascites, fusing of pleural surfaces is sometimes used. Alternative is TIPS.
- Liver transplant referral should be considered in patients with decompensated liver disease, whether or not ascites is present/controlled.

 ## ONGOING CARE

FOLLOW-UP RECOMMENDATIONS
Bed rest only if heart failure and/or prominent leg edema.

Patient Monitoring
- Daily body weight
- Closely follow creatinine and electrolytes when initiating diuresis and 1 week after change in dose/type of diuretic
- Mental status to assess for encephalopathy

DIET
Consultation with dietician helpful:
- Sodium restriction, 2 g/day, monitored
- Adequate nutrition
- Fluid restriction (1–1.5 L/day) only if dilutional hyponatremia (Na <120 mEq/L)
- Complete abstinence from alcohol if liver disease

PROGNOSIS
- Varies depending on underlying cause
- Rarely life-threatening in itself, but may be a sign of life-threatening disease (e.g., cancer, end-stage liver disease):
  - Conservative therapy usually successful if cause is reversible or treatable (e.g., infection)

COMPLICATIONS
- Spontaneous bacterial peritonitis (SBP):
  - Ascitic fluid cell count ≥250, polymorphonuclear leukocytes, fever, clinical deterioration. Treat with 3rd-generation cephalosporin or comparable antibiotic; combined antibiotic treatment plus IV albumin results in improved survival in some patients (3)[B].
  - Lifetime antibiotic prophylaxis with norfloxacin or TMP/SMX is indicated in some patients who survive an episode of SBP (1)[A].
  - No antibiotic prophylaxis is necessary for patients with cirrhotic ascites and no GI bleeding as there is concern of developing resistant pathogens and transplant complication (1)[B]
  - GI bleeding and cirrhosis: IV ceftriaxone for 7 days to prevent bacterial infection (1)[A]
- Overly aggressive diuresis may lead to hypokalemia, worsening encephalopathy; intravascular volume depletion may lead to azotemia, renal failure, and death as a result of hepatorenal syndrome.
- Hepatorenal syndrome:
  - Acute renal failure secondary to decreased intravascular volume in ascites

- May be induced by aggressive diuresis or paracentesis
- Urine volume <500 mL/day, decreasing urine sodium, rising blood urea nitrogen, and creatinine >1.5 mg/dL:
  - Full discussion of hepatorenal syndrome, see Hepatorenal Syndrome
  - Stop all diuretics; IV fluid challenge of 1.5 L plasma expander after 1 day if no improvement.
  - Vasopressors (e.g., terlipressin IV every 4–6 hours) may resolve renal failure in 50% of patients (3)[B]
- Hydrothorax: Always on right side; cell and lab properties same as ascites. Treat ascites vigorously; if hydrothorax does not disappear, consider TIPS. Chest tube rarely helpful in acute setting.

REFERENCES
1. Runyon BA, Practice Guidelines Committee, American Association for the Study of Liver Diseases (AASLD). Management of adult patients with ascites due to cirrhosis. *Hepatology.* 2009;49:2087–2107.
2. Saab S, Nieto JM, Lewis SK, Runyon BA. TIPS versus paracentesis for cirrhotic patients with refractory ascites. *Cochrane Database of Systematic Reviews* 2006, Issue 4. Art. No.: CD004889. DOI: 10.1002/14651858.CD004889.pub2.
3. Talwalkar JA, Kamath PS. Influence of recent advances in medical management on clinical outcomes of cirrhosis. *Mayo Clin Proc.* 2005; 80:1501–8.

ADDITIONAL READING
Rössle M, Gerbes AL et al. TIPS for the treatment of refractory ascites, hepatorenal syndrome and hepatic hydrothorax: a critical update. *Gut.* 2010;59: 988–1000.

See Also (Topic, Algorithm, Electronic Media Element)
Cirrhosis of the Liver; Congestive Heart Failure; Nephrotic Syndrome; Hepatorenal Syndrome
Algorithm: Cirrhosis

CODES

ICD9
- 789.51 Malignant ascites
- 789.59 Other ascites

CLINICAL PEARLS
- Diuretics are used for clinically significant ascites; spironolactone, alone or in combination with furosemide are highly effective treatments.
- Ultrasound is highly sensitive to detect ascites, but use CT to rule out intra-abdominal pathology and MRI if evaluating liver disease.
- Most common cause of "refractory ascites" is patient noncompliance with dietary sodium restriction.

ASTHMA

Fozia A. Ali, MD

BASICS

DESCRIPTION
- Chronic, reversible inflammatory airway disease
- Four major classifications of asthma severity used primarily to initiate therapy (1,2):
  - Intermittent: Symptoms ≤ 2 days/week, night-time awakenings $\leq 2\times$/month, short-acting β-agonist use ≤ 2 days/week, no interference with normal activity, and normal FEV1 between exacerbations with FEV1 (predicted) >80% and FEV1/FVC >85%
  - Mild persistent: Symptoms >2 days/week but not daily, night-time awakenings 1–4$\times$/month, short-acting β-agonist use >2 days/week but not daily, minor limitations in normal activity, and FEV1 (predicted) >80% and FEV1/FVC >80%
  - Moderate persistent: Daily symptoms, night-time awakenings 3–4$\times$/month or $\geq 1\times$/week but not nightly, depending on age, daily use of short-acting β-agonist, some limitation in normal activity, and FEV1 (predicted) 60–80% and FEV1/FVC 75–80%
  - Severe persistent: Symptoms throughout the day, night-time awakenings >1$\times$/week, short-acting β-agonist use several times a day, extremely limited normal activity, and FEV1 (predicted) <60% and FEV1/FVC <75%

EPIDEMIOLOGY
Prevalence
- One of the most common chronic diseases of childhood, affecting 6 million children
- In children, more common in boys than girls
- In adults, more common in women than men

Pregnancy Considerations
- In the US, 3.7–8.4% of pregnant women are affected. Maternal asthma complicates approximately 4–8% of all pregnancies.
- Prevalence of asthma in seniors (>age 65) is 5.3%

RISK FACTORS
- Host factors: Genetic predisposition, gender, race, body mass index
- Environmental exposures: Viral infections, airborne allergens, tobacco smoke, etc.
- Patients with food allergies and asthma are at increased risk for fatal anaphylaxis from those foods.

Genetics
- Inheritable component with complex genetics
- Active area of research: Treatments may be directed to specific genotypes.

GENERAL PREVENTION
- Eliminate or modify exposure to asthma triggers.
- Consider allergen immunotherapy when indicated.
- Treat comorbidities such as allergic rhinitis.
- Annual influenza vaccine (inactivated influenza vaccine) is recommended for all patients <6 months (3).
- Patients at risk for anaphylaxis should carry an EpiPen.

PATHOPHYSIOLOGY
- Inflammatory cell infiltration, sub-basement fibrosis, mucus hypersecretion, epithelial injury, smooth muscle hypertrophy, angiogenesis
- Remodeling of airways may occur (1).

ETIOLOGY
Host and environmental factors

COMMONLY ASSOCIATED CONDITIONS
- Atopy: Eczema, allergic conjunctivitis, allergic rhinitis
- Obesity (associated with higher asthma rates)
- Sinusitis
- Gastroesophageal reflux disease (GERD)
- Obstructive sleep apnea (OSA)
- Allergic bronchopulmonary aspergillosis (rare)
- Stress/depression

DIAGNOSIS

It is important to classify asthma severity.

HISTORY
Symptoms include:
- Cough (particularly if worse at night)
- Wheeze
- Chest tightness
- Difficulty breathing

PHYSICAL EXAM
- May be normal
- Focus on:
  - General appearance: Signs of respiratory distress such as use of accessory muscles
  - Upper respiratory tract: Rhinitis, nasal polyps, swollen nasal turbinates
  - Lower respiratory tract: Wheezing, prolonged expiratory phase
  - Skin: Eczema

DIAGNOSTIC TESTS & INTERPRETATION
Lab
Initial lab tests
- Spirometry: Does not rule out disease
- Peak expiratory flow rates are inappropriate for diagnosis.

Follow-Up & Special Considerations
- Bronchoprovocation (methacholine, histamine, cold air, or exercise) is only definitive diagnostic test.
- Asthma Action Plan: Patients monitor their own symptoms and/or peak flow measurements.

Imaging
Initial approach
Chest x-ray is used to exclude alternative diagnoses and to evaluate patients for complicating cardiopulmonary processes.

Diagnostic Procedures/Surgery
- Allergy skin testing may be considered to evaluate atopic triggers.
- Sweat testing if diagnosis of cystic fibrosis.
- Arterial blood gases is indicated for patients with respiratory distress and hypoxia.

Pathological Findings
Inflammatory cell infiltration, edema, goblet cell hyperplasia, smooth muscle hyperplasia, thickened basement membrane

DIFFERENTIAL DIAGNOSIS
- In children:
  - Upper airway diseases (allergic rhinitis or sinusitis)
  - Large airway obstruction (foreign-body aspiration, vocal cord dysfunction, vascular ring or laryngeal web, laryngotracheomalacia, lymph nodes or tumor)
  - Small airway obstruction (viral bronchiolitis, cystic fibrosis, bronchopulmonary dysplasia, heart disease)
  - Other causes (recurrent cough *not* due to asthma, aspiration/GERD)
- In adults:
  - Chronic obstructive pulmonary disease, congestive heart failure, pulmonary embolism, benign or malignant tumor, pulmonary infiltration with eosinophilia, drugs such as an angiotensin-converting enzyme inhibitor, vocal cord dysfunction

TREATMENT

MEDICATION
First Line
Short-acting β-agonist (SABA) for quick relief of acute symptoms and for prevention of exercise-induced bronchospasm

ALERT
- Delivery of SABA and other inhaled agents via "spacer" or holding chamber (AeroChamber, OptiChamber, others) provides increased efficacy with decreased side effects when compared to nebulized delivery. Reserve nebulized delivery of medication for those unable to use spacer (infants, those intubated, etc.).
- All short-acting agents are pregnancy Category C.
- Specific medicines include albuterol, levalbuterol (Xopenex), metaproterenol (Alupent) Pirbuterol (Maxair) (4)
- Anticholinergic agent:
  - Ipratropium bromide: Used in combination with SABA for added benefit in emergency situations
- Systemic corticosteroids can be used:
  - In moderate-to-severe asthma as adjunct
  - In patients with all but the mildest of acute asthma exacerbations (5)[A]
  - Steroids should be prescribed for up to 7 days in adults and for 3–5 days in children with no need for tapering.
  - Use corticosteroid doses of prednisolone 1–2 mg/kg/day or equivalent.

Second Line
For long-term control (4):
- Inhaled corticosteroids (ICS):
  - Preferred long-term controller therapy for children and adults with persistent asthma and persistent asthma during pregnancy

Pregnancy Considerations
- Most ICS agents are pregnancy Category C, except Budesonide which is category B.
- Long-acting β_2-agonists (LABA):
  - Should *not* be used as monotherapy
  - Salbutamol or formoterol
- Combination products, including a LABA and ICS, are available and offer additional control over ICS alone; preferred in moderate persistent asthma.
- Leukotriene receptor agonists: Alternative, not preferred for mild persistent asthma:
  - Montelukast or
  - Zafirlukast (patients ≥ 7 years)

- Lipoxygenase pathway inhibitor: Alternative not preferred for adjunctive treatment in adults
  – Zileuton (patients $\geq$12 years)
- Theophylline alternative not preferred as adjunctive therapy with inhaled corticosteroids
- Cromolyn sodium and nedocromil are alternatives, but not a preferred option
- Immunomodulators:
  – Omalizumab: Adjunctive not preferred therapy for patients $\geq$12 years with allergies and severe persistent asthma

ADDITIONAL TREATMENT
General Measures
- Identify triggers and control exposures.
- Identify patients at risk for reactions to aspirin and nonsteroidal anti-inflammatory drugs (NSAIDs), and avoid exposure.

Issues for Referral
Referral to an asthma specialist (either a pulmonologist or an allergist) should be considered:
- Diagnosis unclear
- Additional asthma education needed
- Comorbidities: Rhinitis, GERD, sinusitis, OSA
- Specialized testing (bronchoprovocation, skin testing, etc.)
- Specialized treatments (e.g., immunotherapy, anti-IgE therapy)
- Moderate-to-severe persistent asthma in adults
- Moderate-to-persistent asthma in children
- Not well controlled or very poorly controlled asthma: Multiple emergency room visits, for asthma

Additional Therapies
- Allergen immunotherapy
- Omalizumab (Xolair): Anti-IgE therapy

COMPLEMENTARY AND ALTERNATIVE MEDICINE
Patients should be cautioned regarding the potential for harmful ingredients and for interactions with recommended asthma medications.

IN-PATIENT CONSIDERATIONS
Initial Stabilization
- Supplemental oxygen to correct hypoxemia
- Repeated doses or continuous administration of SABA (1)[A]
- Ipratropium bromide may be used in the emergency room, but is not recommended for inpatient treatment (1)[B].
- Systemic corticosteroids for moderate or severe exacerbations or poor response to SABA (1)[A]
- Adjunctive therapy with $MgSO_4$ or Heliox may be considered in severe cases, but not routinely (1,6)[B].

Admission Criteria
No single measure is predictive:
- Dyspnea
- Hypoxia
- Poor or no response to SABA
- PEFR or FEV_1 <40%
- Decision for admission should be based on duration and severity of symptoms, severity of airflow obstruction, response to emergency department treatment, course and severity of prior exacerbations, access to medical care and medication, and adequacy of home condition. (1)

IV Fluids
- Avoid aggressive hydration in older children and adults.
- Monitor electrolytes.

Nursing
- Careful respiratory monitoring, including vital signs, pulse oximetry, response and duration of response to SABA, and, when possible, an objective measure of lung function such as PEF or FEV1
- Asthma education

Discharge Criteria
- Minimal or absent asthma symptoms
- Hypoxia has resolved
- FEV1 or PEF $\geq$70% predicted or personal best
- Bronchodilator response sustained $\geq$60 minutes

 ## ONGOING CARE

FOLLOW-UP RECOMMENDATIONS
Smoking cessation counseling or elimination of secondhand smoke, if applicable

Patient Monitoring
- Quality-of-life measures: Impact on activities, sleep, emergency visits, hospitalizations, etc.
- Pharmacotherapy: Efficacy, compliance, side effects, technique
- Lung function: Peak flow is an inexpensive and easily available monitoring device once the diagnosis of asthma has been established.

DIET
Food allergies and sulfites (in food and wine) can precipitate symptoms for some patients. GERD precautions may be helpful with both symptomatic reflux and in those who are asymptomatic for reflux but with poorly controlled or nocturnal asthma.

PATIENT EDUCATION
- Patients' technique for using inhaled medications should be reviewed at every visit.
- American Academy of Allergy, Asthma & Immunology: 1-800-822-2762 or http://www.aaaai.org
- American Lung Association: http://www.lungusa.org
- Food Allergy & Anaphylaxis Network: http://www.foodallergy.org
- Asthma and Allergy Foundation of America: 1-800-727-8462 or http:www.aafa.org

PROGNOSIS
- Risk factors for persistent asthma (in children <3 years of age with $\geq$4 episodes of wheezing in preceding year): Either history of asthma in $\geq$1 parent or documented atopic dermatitis or aeroallergen sensitivity
- Alternatively, $\geq$2 of the following will also place these children at increased risk:
  – Food sensitivity
  – $\geq$4% peripheral eosinophilia
  – Wheezing episodes unrelated to upper respiratory tract infections
- Asthma worsens in 1/3 of women during pregnancy and improves in another 1/3.

COMPLICATIONS
- Atelectasis
- Pneumonia
- Air leak syndromes: Pneumomediastinum, pneumothorax
- Medication-specific side effects/adverse effects/interactions
- Respiratory failure
- Death: Approximately 50% of asthma deaths occur in the elderly (age >65 years), and mortality is increasing in that population (7).

REFERENCES
1. National Asthma Education and Prevention Program Expert Panel Report 3, Guidelines for the Diagnosis and Management of Asthma. No. 08-5846 Washington DC: NIH, Oct 2007.
2. Reddel HK, Taylor DR, Bateman ED et al. An official American Thoracic Society/European Respiratory Society statement: asthma control and exacerbations: standardizing endpoints for clinical asthma trials and clinical practice. *Am J Respir Crit Care Med*. 2009;180:59–99.
3. Centers for Disease Control and Prevention, Recommended adult immunization schedule – United States 2009 *MMWR*. 2008;57(53).
4. Fanta CH. Asthma. *N Engl J Med*. 2009;360: 1002–14.
5. Doherty S. Prescribe systemic corticosteroids in acute asthma. *BMJ*. 2009;338:b1234.
6. McGarvey JM, Pollack CV. Heliox in airway management. *Emerg Med Clin North Am*. 2008;26:905–20, viii.
7. Stupka E, deShazo R. Asthma in seniors: Part 1 evidence for underdiagnosis, undertreatment and increasing morbidity and mortality. *Am J Med*. 2009;122(1):6–11.

ADDITIONAL READING
- Busse, WW, NHLBI: NAEPP asthma & Pregnancy Working Group. NAEPP Expert Panel report: Managing asthma during pregnancy: Recommendations for pharmacologic treatment - 2004 update, *J Allergy Clin Immunol*. 2005;115:34–46.
- Dombrowski M, ACOG Practice Bulletin, Clinical Management Guidelines for Obstetrician-Gynecologists. *Asthma in Pregnancy*. 2008;111(2 Part 1): 457–64.
- Global Strategy for Asthma Management and prevention, 2006. At: http://www.ginasthma.org

See Also (Topic, Algorithm, Electronic Media Element)
http://www.ala.org
Algorithm: Asthma Exacerbation, Pediatric Acute

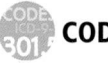 ## CODES

ICD9
- 493.00 Extrinsic asthma, unspecified
- 493.90 Asthma, unspecified
- 493.92 Asthma, unspecified, with (acute) exacerbation

CLINICAL PEARLS
- Asthma is a chronic, reversible inflammatory airway disease whose exacerbations are characterized by reversible bronchoconstriction, airway hyper-responsiveness, and airway edema.
- Short-acting β-agonist (SABA) is the most effective rescue therapy for acute asthma symptoms.
- Inhaled corticosteroids (ICS) are the preferred long-term control therapy for patients of all ages.
- Peak flow is an inexpensive and easily available monitoring device once the diagnosis of asthma has been established.

ATHEROSCLEROSIS
Manoj Singh, MD

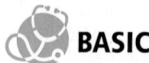 **BASICS**

DESCRIPTION
Atherosclerosis is the common form of arteriosclerosis in which deposits of yellowish plaques (atheromas) containing cholesterol, lipid material, and lipophages are formed within the intima and inner media of large and medium-sized arteries.

Geriatric Considerations
- Atherosclerosis happens to all who live long enough.
- Effects and complications can be minimized and/or delayed by avoiding all risk factors possible.

Pediatric Considerations
Fatty streaks and deposits in the intima of the aortas of all children begin as early as 3 years of age.

EPIDEMIOLOGY
- Incidence/prevalence in the US:
  - Common, but declining steadily
  - The effects on the brain, heart, kidneys, extremities, and other vital organs form the leading cause of morbidity and mortality in the US and most Western countries.
  - Complications of atherosclerosis account for 1/2 of all deaths and 1/3 of the deaths in persons 35–65 years of age.
- Predominant age: 35 and older
- Predominant sex: Male > Female

RISK FACTORS
- Modifiable:
  - Hypertension
  - Tobacco smoking
  - Diabetes mellitus (risk factor for death or myocardial infarction [MI] considered equivalent to established coronary heart disease [CHD])
  - Obesity
  - Physical inactivity
  - Decreased high-density lipoprotein (HDL) cholesterol
  - Increased low-density lipoprotein (LDL) cholesterol
  - Comorbidities that may increase risk:
    - Hypothyroidism
    - Elevated homocysteine levels
    - High testosterone levels in women
    - Low testosterone levels in men
- Nonmodifiable:
  - Male gender
  - Increasing age
- Family history of *premature* atherosclerosis

Genetics
There is a probable genetic link; many risk factors for atherosclerosis (lipid metabolism, hypertension, and diabetes) are clearly inheritable. Inheritance is polygenic.

GENERAL PREVENTION
Treat or control modifiable risk factors.

ETIOLOGY
- Biochemical, physiologic, environmental factors that lead to inflammation, thickening, and occlusion of the lumen of arteries
- Aging (some degree of atherosclerosis is universal)
- 1 or more of the risk factors listed under Risk Factors

COMMONLY ASSOCIATED CONDITIONS
- Essential hypertension
- Coronary arteriosclerosis
- Heart failure (congestive heart failure [CHF])
- Cerebrovascular accident
- Atrial arrhythmias
- Ventricular arrhythmias
- Renal failure, chronic
- Aortic dissection
- Thrombosis and embolism, arterial
- Atherosclerotic occlusive disease

 DIAGNOSIS

- Characteristically silent until atheromas produce:
  - Stenosis
  - Thrombosis
  - Aneurysm
  - Embolus
- For lists of possible symptoms, see the following topics:
  - Essential hypertension
  - Coronary arteriosclerosis
  - CHF
  - Cerebrovascular accident
  - Atrial arrhythmias
  - Renal failure, chronic
  - Dissecting aneurysm
  - Thrombosis and embolism, arterial

DIAGNOSTIC TESTS & INTERPRETATION
Lab
- Associated with elevated serum cholesterol
- Elevated LDL and low HDL
- Inflammation plays an as-yet incompletely defined role.

Imaging
Extensively calcified atherosclerotic plaques may be identified in major blood vessels on radiography.

Diagnostic Procedures/Surgery
- Arterial Doppler studies (carotid, renal)
- Angiography
- Ankle–brachial index

Pathological Findings
- Early changes (simple), potentially reversible:
  - Accumulation of lipid-laden cells in the intimal layer of the artery (usually monocytes/macrophages from circulating blood)
  - Lipid streaks in aorta and coronary arteries

- Late changes (complicated) usually reversible:
  - Atheromatous plaques with necrosis, fibrosis, calcification
  - Weakening of elastic lamellae
  - Neovascularization
  - Arterial obstruction
  - Thrombosis
- Oxidized low-density lipoprotein induces vascular smooth-muscle cell apoptosis and cell death.
- Alteration of endothelial function involving mostly nitrous oxide pathways promotes platelet adhesion and aggregation, local clotting, and vascular growth, and alters vascular tone.
- Decrease in elastin with aging along with collagen degeneration and increased intima-media thickness of arterial wall

 TREATMENT

MEDICATION
First Line
HMG-CoA reductase inhibitors (statins) have multiple effects in addition to lipid-lowering effects (they improve endothelial function, enhance the stability of atherosclerotic plaque, decrease oxidative stress and inflammation, and inhibit thrombogenic response). It is likely that these so-called pleiotropic effects of statins are clinically important, perhaps even more so than their absolute lipid-lowering effect.

Second Line
- Bile acid sequestrants
- Fibric acid derivatives
- Ezetimibe (lowers LDL effectively, but no outcomes data currently support use)
- Niacin

ADDITIONAL TREATMENT
General Measures
Treat hypertension, hypothyroidism (if present), and diabetes.

COMPLEMENTARY AND ALTERNATIVE MEDICINE
Good evidence exists showing the following do not lower atherosclerotic risk:
- Omega-3 fatty acids (1)
- Vitamin E (2)
- Lowering homocysteine levels (3)
- Chelation therapy (4)
- Anticoagulation (5)
- Garlic (6)
- No evidence that testosterone treatment is beneficial for aortic atherosclerosis (7)

SURGERY/OTHER PROCEDURES

- Angioplasty (8)[A]
- Stent (9)[A]
- Carotid endarterectomy: For symptomatic patients, NNT 15 if severe (>70%) blockage, NNT 21 if blockage less severe (50–69%) (10)[A]
- Rotational atherectomy (in selected cases where angioplasty and stent may be ineffective) (11)[C]

IN-PATIENT CONSIDERATIONS
Initial Stabilization
- Outpatient until complications occur
- Emphasis on prevention

 ## ONGOING CARE

FOLLOW-UP RECOMMENDATIONS
Encourage physical fitness, as this may prevent progression (12)[B].

DIET
American Heart Association Dietary recommendations are controversial and have not been proven effective at lowering atherosclerotic risk:

- Initial diet, step 1:
  - Total fat: <30% of total calories; saturated fat: <10%
  - Carbohydrates: 50–60% of total calories
  - Protein: 10–20% of total calories
  - Cholesterol: <300 mg/d
  - Total calories: Amount required to achieve and maintain desirable weight
  - Sodium: 1,650–2,400 mg
  - Alcohol: <30 g
- Initial diet, step 2:
  - Total fat: <30% of total calories; saturated fat: <7%
  - Carbohydrates: 50–60% of total calories
  - Protein: 10–20% of total calories
  - Cholesterol: <200 mg/d
  - Total calories: Amount required to achieve and maintain desirable weight
  - Sodium: 1,650–2,400 mg
- Alcohol: <30 g
- A "Mediterranean" diet consisting of a low-salt, low red-meat diet with liberal amounts of fresh fruit and vegetables and whole grains, and regular consumption of fish, olive oil, and nuts is likely to be beneficial in preventing and treating atherosclerosis. Moderate consumption of red wine may also be of benefit.

PATIENT EDUCATION
- Crucial parts of preventing and treating atherosclerosis involve nutrition, fitness, and smoking cessation, and treating modifiable risk factors.
- Extensive educational materials are available from many agencies (e.g., American Heart Association, US Government Printing Office, National Cholesterol Education Program). Use these to help teach patients how to avoid or eliminate risk factors.

PROGNOSIS
Modifying risk factors has greatly decreased mortality rates in the last decade.

COMPLICATIONS
- Coronary artery disease
- Renal failure
- Cerebrovascular accidents
- Dissecting or ruptured aneurysms
- CHF
- Arterial thrombosis
- Gangrene
- Cardiac arrhythmias
- Sudden death

REFERENCES

1. Sommerfield T, Price J, Hiatt WR. Omega-3 fatty acids for intermittent claudication. *Cochrane Database of Systematic Reviews* 2007, Issue 4. Art. No.: CD003833. DOI:10.1002/14651858. CD003833.pub3.
2. Kleijnen J, Mackerras D. Vitamin E for intermittent claudication. *Cochrane Database of Systematic Reviews* 1998, Issue 1. Art. No.: CD000987. DOI:10.1002/14651858.CD000987.
3. Hansrani M, Stansby GP. Homocysteine lowering interventions for peripheral arterial disease and bypass grafts. *Cochrane Database of Systematic Reviews* 2002, Issue 3. Art. No.: CD003285. DOI:10.1002/14651858.CD003285.
4. Dans AL, Tan FN, Villarruz-Sulit EC. Chelation therapy for atherosclerotic cardiovascular disease. *Cochrane Database of Systematic Reviews* 2002, Issue 4. Art. No.: CD002785. DOI:10.1002/14651858.CD002785.
5. Cosmi B, Conti E, Coccheri S. Anticoagulants (heparin, low molecular weight heparin and oral anticoagulants) for intermittent claudication. *Cochrane Database of Systematic Reviews* 2001, Issue 2. Art. No.: CD001999. DOI:10.1002/14651858.CD001999.
6. Jepson RG, Kleijnen J, Leng GC. Garlic for peripheral arterial occlusive disease. *Cochrane Database of Systematic Reviews* 1997, Issue 2. Art. No.: CD000095. DOI:10.1002/14651858.CD000095.
7. Price J, Leng GC. Steroid sex hormones for lower limb atherosclerosis. *Cochrane Database of Systematic Reviews* 2001, Issue 3. Art. No.: CD000188. DOI:10.1002/14651858.CD000188.
8. Fowkes G, Gillespie IN. Angioplasty (versus non surgical management) for intermittent claudication. *Cochrane Database of Systematic Reviews* 1998, Issue 2. Art. No.: CD000017. DOI:10.1002/14651858.CD000017.
9. Bachoo P, Thorpe PA, Maxwell H, Welch K. Endovascular stents for intermittent claudication. *Cochrane Database of Systematic Reviews* 2010, Issue 1. Art. No.: CD003228. DOI:10.1002/14651858.CD003228.pub2.
10. Cina C, Clase C, Haynes RB. Carotid endarterectomy for symptomatic carotid stenosis. *Cochrane Database of Systematic Reviews* 1999, Issue 3. Art. No.: CD001081. DOI:10.1002/14651858.CD001081.
11. Villanueva E, Wasiak J, Petherick E. Percutaneous transluminal rotational atherectomy for coronary artery disease. *Cochrane Database of Systematic Reviews* 2003, Issue 4. Art. No.: CD003334. DOI:10.1002/14651858/CD003334.
12. Nordstrom CK, Dwyer KM, Merz CN et al. Leisure time physical activity and early atherosclerosis: the Los Angeles Atherosclerosis Study. *Am J Med.* 2003;115:19–25.

See Also (Topic, Algorithm, Electronic Media Element)
Aortic Dissection; Arterial Embolus and Thrombosis; Atherosclerotic Occlusive Disease; Congestive Heart Failure; Hypertension, Essential; Renal Failure, Chronic; Stroke
Algorithm: Chest Pain/Acute Coronary Syndrome

 ## CODES

ICD9
440.9 Generalized and unspecified atherosclerosis

CLINICAL PEARLS

- Atherosclerosis is a generalized condition, affecting multiple organ systems.
- It is very likely that improvement in diet and exercise, control of hypertension, and elimination of risk factors like smoking can effectively stave off or at least delay the development of this condition.
- Statins control atherosclerosis via multiple mechanisms in addition to their lipid-lowering effects.

BASICS

This topic covers both atrial fibrillation (Afib) and atrial flutter (Aflut).

DESCRIPTION
- Afib: Continuous or paroxysmal arrhythmia characterized by chaotic atrial electrical activity and an irregularly irregular ventricular response
- In some patients, ventricular response is rapid (>110 bpm), because AV node is bombarded with nearly continuous atrial electrical impulses.
- Aflut: Continuous or paroxysmal arrhythmia with regular atrial electrical activity, typical atrial rate 250–350, manifested as sawtooth flutter waves on ECG. A 2:1 or 4:1 conduction through the AV node to the ventricle is common, so the ventricular response is frequently regular at a rate of 150 or 75 bpm.
- Clinical pattern:
  - Persistent: Sustained >7 days, usually requiring pharmacologic or DC cardioversion to restore sinus rhythm
  - Paroxysmal (PAF): Self-terminating episodes, usually <7 days
  - Permanent: Sinus rhythm cannot be restored; cardioversion has failed or has not been attempted.

EPIDEMIOLOGY
- Incidence/prevalence increases with age.
- Predominant gender: Male > Female

Incidence
- Afib: Age <40, <0.1%/year; >80, >1.5%/year, less for atrial flutter
- Lifetime risk: 25% for those ≥40 years

Prevalence
- Estimated 0.4–1% of general population <60
- ~2–5%, 7th decade; 5–10%, 8th decade

RISK FACTORS
In US, hypertension/coronary disease most common. See Etiology.

Genetics
Familial forms rare, but do exist. Multiple culprit genes have been identified.

GENERAL PREVENTION
Ethanol may trigger AF in some; so-called "holiday heart syndrome." Adequate HTN control may prevent development of AF due to hypertensive heart disease.

PATHOPHYSIOLOGY
- In patients with PAF and no/minimal structural heart disease, triggering premature atrial beats and/or bursts of tachycardia emanate from the pulmonary venous ostia or other sites.
- In patients with persistent/permanent AF and significant structural heart disease, multiple reentrant wavelets within atria may be the cause.

ETIOLOGY
- Cardiac: Hypertensive heart disease, valvular/rheumatic disease, CAD, acute MI, cardiomyopathy, CHF, pericarditis, infiltrative heart disease, sick sinus syndrome
- Pulmonary: Pulmonary embolism, COPD, pneumonia
- Ingestion: (e.g., ethanol in holiday heart), digoxin toxicity (AFlut)

- Endocrine: Hyperthyroidism
- Postoperative (e.g., cardiothoracic surgery)
- Idiopathic: Including lone AF (<60 without clinical or electrocardiogram [EKG] evidence of cardiopulmonary disease, including HTN)

COMMONLY ASSOCIATED CONDITIONS
- Sick sinus syndrome.
- Afib and Aflut are frequently associated with each other. Aflut tends to be a more unstable rhythm and tends to not last as long.

 DIAGNOSIS

HISTORY
- Symptoms vary from none–mild (palpitations, lightheadedness, fatigue, poor exercise capacity) to severe (angina, dyspnea, syncope). Symptoms frequently more serious in patients with structural heart disease.
- In patients with Wolff-Parkinson-White syndrome and other types of bypass tracts, Afib may lead to an extremely rapid ventricular rate that may swiftly degenerate into ventricular fibrillation.

PHYSICAL EXAM
- Afib: Irregularly irregular pulse, frequently tachycardic
- Aflut: Regular pulse, frequently tachycardic

DIAGNOSTIC TESTS & INTERPRETATION
- Afib: EKG is diagnostic; low-amplitude fibrillatory waves without discrete P waves; irregularly irregular pattern of QRS complexes
- Aflut: Sawtooth P-waves are the classic sign. Narrow complex QRS. Frequent tachycardia.
- Holter monitor and event monitor helpful in diagnosing PAF and monitoring for recurrence.

Lab
Initial lab tests
TSH, CMP, cardiac enzymes, PT/INR (if anticoagulation is contemplated), consider digoxin level (if appropriate) and CBC

Follow-Up & Special Considerations
Occasional Holter monitoring and/or exercise stress testing to assess for adequacy of rate control

Imaging
- Chest x-ray (CXR) for cardiopulmonary disease
- EKG for structural heart disease, signs of ischemia, heart blocks, and other arrhythmias
- Spiral chest computed tomography (CT) (or other tests such as D-dimer, ventilation-perfusion scan, or pulmonary angiography) if pulmonary embolus possible etiology for new-onset disease
- Transesophageal echocardiogram to detect left atrial appendage thrombus if cardioversion planned

Diagnostic Procedures/Surgery
Electrophysiologic studies should be considered in patients with recurrent Aflut to map the source of the arrhythmia for possible ablation.

Pathological Findings
- Atrial dilatation and fibrosis
- Atrial injury (chronic or acute)
- Atrial thrombus, especially in atrial appendage
- Sclerosis/fibrosis of sinoatrial node
- Coronary artery disease, valvular/rheumatic disease, cardiomyopathy, pulmonary embolus
- Tachycardia-induced cardiomyopathy

DIFFERENTIAL DIAGNOSIS
- Multifocal atrial tachycardia
- Sinus tachycardia with frequent atrial premature beats
- Atrial flutter/atrial fibrillation

 TREATMENT

MEDICATION
- Anticoagulation guidelines (same for Afib and Aflut):
  - Unless contraindicated, patients with AF with any high-risk factors for stroke (prior transient ischemic attack (TIA)/cerebrovascular accident (CVA)/thromboembolism, mitral stenosis, prosthetic valve) should receive warfarin to maintain INR of 2.0–3.0. Patients with mechanical valves should maintain INR >2.5.
  - CHADS2 score: Patients with ≥2 moderate risk factors (**C**HF, **H**TN, **A**ge >75 and/or **D**M), should receive warfarin (INR 2.0–3.0) unless contraindicated.
  - Patients with 1 moderate risk factor should be treated with warfarin (INR 2.0–3.0) or aspirin (81–325 mg/d). Discuss with patient risks and benefits.
  - Patients at low risk of thromboembolic complications or in whom warfarin is contraindicated should receive aspirin (81–325 mg/d) or clopidogrel.
  - Anticoagulation recommendations are independent of AF pattern (paroxysmal, persistent, permanent).
- So-called "rate control" and "rhythm control" strategies have approximately equivalent outcomes in terms of mortality. Rhythm control tends to have more adverse reactions.
- Control of ventricular rate:
  - Nondihydropyridine calcium channel blockers:
    - Diltiazem (Cardizem)
    - Class contraindications: Hypotension, documented sensitivity, 2nd- or 3rd-degree AV block, severe CHF, sick sinus syndrome
    - Precautions: Use caution with CHF, left ventricular (LV) dysfunction, liver or kidney disease. Adverse reactions: Hypotension, CHF, peripheral edema, AV block.
    - Interactions: May increase digoxin levels; with amiodarone or beta-blockers, may severely decrease cardiac output, trigger complete heart block
  - Beta-blockers:
    - Metoprolol (Lopressor)
    - Contraindications: Hypotension, documented sensitivity, 2nd- or 3rd-degree AV block, severe CHF, sick sinus syndrome
    - Precautions: Use caution with CHF, LV dysfunction, kidney disease, asthma
    - Interactions: Bradycardia with digoxin; with amiodarone or calcium channel blockers, may severely decrease cardiac output or trigger complete heart block
    - Adverse reactions: Hypotension, CHF, peripheral edema, AV block

- Digoxin (Lanoxin):
  - Indicated for CHF, hypotension
  - Contraindications: Documented sensitivity, sick sinus syndrome, hypertrophic cardiomyopathy
  - Precautions: Use caution with electrolyte abnormalities (especially hypokalemia, hypercalcemia), impaired renal function, thyroid disease, acute myocardial infarction (MI), AV block
  - Interactions: Unpredictable effects with many antiarrhythmics; additive bradycardia with calcium channel blockers, beta-blockers
  - Adverse reactions: AV block, bradycardia, mental disturbances, nausea
  - Rate control usually achieved in 4 hours (1).
- Conversion to/maintenance of sinus rhythm:
  - DC cardioversion
  - Caution: Antiarrhythmic therapy for chemical cardioversion and maintenance of sinus rhythm following cardioversion may be proarrhythmic.
  - Ibutilide, an IV type III agent, for chemical cardioversion of AF and flutter of short duration (<90 days)
  - If duration of AF is >24–48 hours or unknown, treat with warfarin for ≥3 weeks before cardioversion. Or, once anticoagulation is established, perform transesophageal EKG. If no atrial thrombus, may cardiovert. Anticoagulation should be continued for ≥4 weeks following cardioversion.
  - Long-term, perhaps indefinite, anticoagulation should be considered in patients with thromboembolic risk factors with chronic or recurrent AF.
- Chronic oral antiarrhythmic therapy to suppress AF recurrences:
  - Type IA (procainamide, disopyramide, quinidine): Generally not used
  - Type IC (flecainide, propafenone) in patients with structurally normal hearts or mild hypertensive heart disease. Concomitant use of β-blocker recommended.
  - Type III (sotalol, amiodarone, dofetilide)
- Contraindications:
  - Type IC drugs are contraindicated in patients with coronary artery disease, cardiomyopathy, and significant LVH.
  - Type IA and III drugs should not be used in patients with torsade de pointes history or long QT. The risk of torsade de pointes increases with the extent of QT interval prolongation (the QTc), so these medications should be used with great caution, if at all, in patients on medications that prolong the QT.
- Precautions: Avoid hypokalemia and hypomagnesemia.
- With type IC drugs, stress testing to exclude exercise-induced arrhythmia or QRS widening
- With amiodarone, careful surveillance for hepatic, thyroid, pulmonary, skin, ophthalmologic adverse effects
- In many patients, adequate medical therapy of AF will cause bradycardia, necessitating a permanent pacemaker.
- According to a recent Cochrane Review, several class IA, IC, and III drugs are effective in maintaining sinus rhythm but increase adverse events, including pro-arrhythmia, and disopyramide and quinidine are associated with increased mortality. Any benefit on clinically relevant outcomes (embolisms, heart failure, mortality) remains to be established (1).

ADDITIONAL TREATMENT
Issues for Referral
AF refractory to medical therapy (unable to achieve adequate rate control or significant bradycardia) should be considered for more definitive therapy such as pacemaker +/−AV node ablation. Antiarrhythmic therapy should be prescribed by experienced practitioners.

SURGERY/OTHER PROCEDURES
- Current guidelines reserve catheter ablation in Afib to highly symptomatic patients who have failed at least 1 course of antiarrhythmic drug therapy [C]. It is the treatment of choice for patients who are in chronic Aflut, with a number needed to treat (NNT) of 2.2 to prevent rehospitalization, vs antiarrhythmics.
- Catheter ablation success rates vary with the type of Afb (paroxysmal > persistent > permanent) and the presence of structural heart disease, particularly left atrial enlargement. May require ≥2 ablation procedures to achieve clinical success.
- Cardiac surgery (e.g., the maze procedure or minimally invasive epicardial procedures) may be considered in severely symptomatic, medically refractory patients.
- Permanent dual-chamber pacing may reduce incidence of new-onset AF and reduce frequency of PAF episodes in patients with sick sinus syndrome.

IN-PATIENT CONSIDERATIONS
Initial Stabilization
Acute therapy for hemodynamically compromised patients:
- Heparin for anticoagulation (not generally necessary; may just initiate warfarin without "bridge" therapy)
- IV β- or calcium channel blocker for control of ventricular rate if blood pressure (BP) adequate
- Urgent cardioversion if hemodynamically unstable:
  - DC cardioversion is best treatment (2)[C].
  - Begin with dose of 50 J (with biphasic defibrillator) or 200 J (with monophasic defibrillator) and increase as needed (2)[C].
  - Atrial overdrive pacing also effective

Admission Criteria
- Inpatient if:
  - Significant symptoms
  - Extremely rapid ventricular rate
  - Initiating antiarrhythmic therapy
  - AF triggered by acute process (acute myocardial infarction, congestive heart failure [CHF], pulmonary embolus)
  - High risk for stroke (rheumatic heart disease, prior TIA/stroke)
- Outpatient management for low-risk patients with controlled ventricular rates

Discharge Criteria
Adequate rate or rhythm control without symptoms. Long-term plan for anticoagulation established.

 ## ONGOING CARE

There continues to be debate about whether rate or rhythm control is best for treating patients with chronic Afib/Aflut. Mortality is the same for both. Risk of stroke is higher for electrical cardioversion, but there are some measures of symptom control and quality of life that appear to be improved. Pharmacologic cardioversion is associated with more adverse events and hospitalization in elderly patients. Take into account the patient with their associated health conditions when deciding what path to take (3,4).

FOLLOW-UP RECOMMENDATIONS
Patient Monitoring
- Monitor warfarin levels.
- EKG to monitor QTc interval if on antiarrhythmic therapy

DIET
Avoid potential triggers: Ethanol, caffeine, nicotine

PROGNOSIS
Warfarin anticoagulation reduces annual embolic stroke rate from ~5% to 1–2%. Aspirin reduces risk to 3–4% annually. AF increases risk of morbidity and mortality, but prognosis is a function of underlying heart disease.

COMPLICATIONS
- Embolic stroke
- Peripheral arterial embolization
- Bleeding with anticoagulation
- Tachycardia-induced cardiomyopathy with prolonged periods of inadequate rate control

REFERENCES
1. Lafuente-Lafuente C, Mouly S, Longas-Tejero MA, Bergmann JF et al. Antiarrhythmics for maintaining sinus rhythm after cardioversion of atrial fibrillation. *Cochrane Database Syst Rev.* 2007;CD005049.
2. Fuster, Rydén LE, Cannom DS, et al. ACC/AHA/ESC 2006 guidelines for the management of patients with atrial fibrillation. *Circulation.* 2006;114: e257–354.
3. Mead GE, Elder AT, Flapan AD, Kelman A et al. Electrical cardioversion for atrial fibrillation and flutter. *Cochrane Database Syst Rev.* 2005; CD002903.
4. Cordina J, Mead G et al. Pharmacological cardioversion for atrial fibrillation and flutter. *Cochrane Database Syst Rev.* 2005;CD003713.

 ## CODES

ICD9
- 427.31 Atrial fibrillation
- 427.32 Atrial flutter

CLINICAL PEARLS
- There continues to be debate about whether rate or rhythm control is best for treating patients with chronic Afib/Aflut. Mortality is the same for both. When in doubt and in absence of other contraindications, rate control appears to have the best outcome data.
- AF with rapid ventricular rates may be the initial presentation of tachy/brady syndrome with underlying sinus node dysfunction, particularly in the elderly. Exercise caution when initiating AV nodal-blocking agents in the elderly patient with rapid AF.

ATRIAL FLUTTER

Michael K. Chen, MD

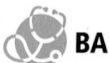 **BASICS**

DESCRIPTION

Atrial flutter (A. flutter) is a cardiac arrhythmia resulting in a (usually) narrow QRS rhythm, often tachycardia with an atrial rate of 250–350 beats per minute:

- "Saw-toothed" P-waves are classic.
- Ventricular rate is dependent upon AV node conduction (see Pathophysiology).
- System(s) affected: Cardiac

EPIDEMIOLOGY

Incidence

- Age: 5 per 100,000 person-years in people <50 years of age. 587 per 100,000 person-years in people >80 years of age.
- Sex: Male > Female (2.5:1)

RISK FACTORS

- Heart disease (e.g., left ventricular [LV] dysfunction), LV hypertrophy, hypertension [HTN], valvular heart disease (especially rheumatic), coronary artery disease, acute myocardial infarction [MI], atrial fibrillation [A. fib], pericarditis, history of congenital heart disease, recent cardiac surgery, atrial scarring
- Pulmonary disease (e.g., chronic obstructive pulmonary disease [COPD], pulmonary embolism, pneumonia)
- Hyperthyroidism
- Obesity

Genetics

Although several genes have been identified that may predispose to A. fib, there is no definite association of these genes with A. flutter.

GENERAL PREVENTION

Risk factor avoidance

PATHOPHYSIOLOGY

Most commonly caused by a rapid re-entrant circuit around the tricuspid valve (specifically, the cavotricuspid isthmus):

- AV node conduction is variable:
  - 2:1 most common (~150 bpm); 3:1, 4:1 possible, 1:1 more rare (>~200 bpm)
  - Variable conduction ratios can cause irregularly irregular pulse, mimicking A. fib.

ETIOLOGY

- Most cases associated with a predisposing factor (see Risk Factors)
- Lone A. flutter; no predisposing factor:
  - 1.7% of patients with A. flutter
- Digitalis toxicity; rare cause

COMMONLY ASSOCIATED CONDITIONS

- See Risk Factors.
- Atrial fibrillation patients frequently go in and out of atrial flutter.

 DIAGNOSIS

HISTORY

- Common:
  - Palpitations, shortness of breath, fatigue, lightheadedness
- Less common:
  - Chest pain, near-syncope
  - Insidious onset with fatigue or worsening of a chronic cardiac/pulmonary disease
- Rare:
  - Syncope
  - Symptoms/signs of acute embolic stroke

PHYSICAL EXAM

- Common: Often normal exam
  - Tachycardia: May be regular or irregularly irregular
  - Mild dyspnea
  - Evidence of a predisposing factor
- Less common:
  - Moderate dyspnea
  - CHF: More common in elderly or with prior history
- Rarely, hemodynamic compromise occurs:
  - Hypotension
  - Severe dyspnea or respiratory failure
  - Hypoxia with cyanosis or pallor
  - Decreased level of consciousness

DIAGNOSTIC TESTS & INTERPRETATION

Lab

Initial lab tests

Complete blood count (CBC), BMP, cardiac enzymes, thyroid-stimulating hormone (TSH), digoxin level (as indicated), prothrombin time (PT)/international normalized ratio (INR) (if anticoagulated or anticoagulation being considered)

Imaging

Initial approach

- Chest x-ray to evaluate for acute cardiopulmonary disease
- Electrocardiogram (ECG) to evaluate for signs of ischemia, heart blocks, intervals, and for diagnosis of atrial flutter

Follow-Up & Special Considerations

- For new-onset atrial flutter, transthoracic echocardiogram is helpful in assessing atrial size, ejection fraction, valvular function, and evaluating right-sided pressures (acute pulmonary embolism).
- Transesophageal echocardiogram may be necessary if thrombus suspected before cardioversion.

Diagnostic Procedures/Surgery

When clinically indicated:

- Holter monitor: If symptoms are concerning but rhythm not present at time of evaluation
- Electrophysiologic studies should be considered in patients with recurrent A. flutter to map the source of the arrhythmia for possible ablation.

DIFFERENTIAL DIAGNOSIS

- Paroxysmal supraventricular tachycardia
- Sinus tachycardia
- Junctional tachycardia
- Multifocal atrial tachycardia (MAT)
- Wolff-Parkinson-White syndrome

 TREATMENT

MEDICATION

First Line

- Rate-control agents useful in the initial management, but generally not efficacious in controlling chronic or recurrent arrhythmia (1)[C]
- Nondihydropyridine calcium channel blockers:
  - Diltiazem (Cardizem):
    ○ Initial dose: 0.25 mg/kg IV × 1, may give 0.35 mg/kg IV × 1 after 15 min if needed
    ○ Maintenance: 5–15 mg/h IV up to 24 hours
  - Verapamil (Isoptin, Calan, Verelan):
    ○ As efficacious as diltiazem; increased hypotension (1)
  - Class contraindications: Hypotension, documented sensitivity, 2nd- or 3rd-degree AV block, severe CHF, sick sinus syndrome
  - Precautions: Use caution with CHF, left ventricular (LV) dysfunction, liver or kidney disease
  - Interactions: May increase digoxin levels; with amiodarone or beta-blockers, may severely decrease cardiac output, trigger complete heart block
  - Adverse reactions: Hypotension, CHF, peripheral edema, AV block
- Beta-blockers:
  - Metoprolol (Lopressor):
    ○ Initial: 5 mg IV, repeat q5min; max, 15 mg
    ○ Maintenance: 5–15 mg IV q3–6h
  - Esmolol (Brevibloc):
    ○ Initial dose: 500 mcg/kg IV over 1 minute, repeat q4min to total of 3 doses if needed
    ○ Maintenance: 50 mcg/kg/min, increased by 50 mcg/kg/min q4min p.r.n.; max of 200 mcg/kg/min
    ○ Half-life ~8 min; good choice for patients at risk for complications
  - Contraindications: Hypotension, documented sensitivity, 2nd- or 3rd-degree AV block, severe CHF, sick sinus syndrome
  - Precautions: Use caution with CHF, LV dysfunction, kidney disease, or asthma.
  - Interactions: Bradycardia with digoxin; with amiodarone or calcium channel blockers may severely decrease cardiac output or trigger complete heart block
  - Adverse reactions: Hypotension, CHF, peripheral edema, AV block
- Digoxin (Lanoxin):
  - Indicated for CHF, hypotension
  - Initial dose: 0.75–1.25 mg p.o. or 0.5–1 mg IV divided 50% initially, then 25% × 2 q6–12h
  - Maintenance: 0.125–0.5 mg/d p.o. or 0.1–0.4 mg/d IV
  - Therapeutic level: 0.8–2 ng/mL
  - Contraindications: Documented sensitivity, sick sinus syndrome, hypertrophic cardiomyopathy
  - Precautions: Use caution with electrolyte abnormalities (especially hypokalemia, hypercalcemia), impaired renal function, thyroid disease, acute myocardial infarction (MI), and AV block.

– Interactions: Unpredictable effects with many antiarrhythmics; additive bradycardia with calcium channel blockers, beta-blockers
– Adverse reactions: AV block, bradycardia, mental disturbances, nausea
– Rate control usually achieved in 4 hours (1).

Second Line

- Pharmacologic cardioversion is 2nd-line to electrical cardioversion in restoring sinus rhythm.
- Pure class III antiarrhythmics:
  – Ibutilide (Corvert) IV:
    ○ Initial dose: <60 kg, 0.01 mg/kg over 10 minutes; 60 kg, 1 mg over 10 minutes; may repeat in 10 minutes p.r.n.
  – Dofetilide (Tikosyn) Oral:
    ○ Dosing: Dependent on QTc interval and creatinine clearance; see package insert
  – Contraindications: Documented sensitivity, QTc >440 ms, use of a class I or III antiarrhythmic within 4 hours, structural heart disease, sinus node disease
  – Precautions: Correct hypokalemia and hypomagnesium prior to use; use caution in AV block, CHF, QT prolongation, renal/hepatic disease, and elderly patients.
  – Interactions: Many antiarrhythmics have unpredictable effects with digoxin; additive bradycardia with calcium channel blockers and beta-blockers.
  – Adverse reactions: Polymorphic VT/torsades de pointes (1.5–3%), AV block, QT prolongation, CHF, renal failure, allergy, hypotension, HTN, headache (4%)
  – Efficacy = 60–70% (1)

ADDITIONAL TREATMENT
General Measures

- Identify and treat underlying causes first.
- A. flutter often self-resolves within days:
  – Watchful waiting may be appropriate in hemodynamically stable patients, particularly with a reversible predisposing cause and normal left atrial size.
- Restoration of normal sinus rhythm is generally the goal of therapy (1)[C]:
  – Self-limited A. flutter related to an underlying cause rarely requires chronic therapy (1)[C].
  – >50% of patients with chronic or recurrent A. flutter experience recurrence within 1 year of successful cardioversion (2).

Issues for Referral
Cardiology referral recommended for refractory cases and for ablation.

Additional Therapies

- Anticoagulation for cardioversion: If >48 hrs duration, recommend warfarin anticoagulation (INR 2–3) 3 weeks before and 4 weeks after cardioversion (3)[B].
- If immediate cardioversion needed for hemodynamic instability in A. flutter >48 hrs or unknown, bridge with heparin (regular or LMWH) until warfarin therapeutic. Treat for 4 weeks. None needed for <48 hrs (3)[C].
- If TEE (–) for thrombus, no prior anticoagulation needed, but heparin bridge to 3–4 weeks of warfarin therapy (2)[B]. If (+) then treat as if >48 hrs. Longer post-cardioversion AC (3)[C].

SURGERY/OTHER PROCEDURES
Catheter ablation is the treatment of choice for patients with recurrent or chronic A. flutter (1)[A]. 80% remain in sinus rhythm at 21 months compared to 36% with antiarrhythmics (1). To prevent rehospitalization with ablation compared to antiarrhythmics, NNT is 2.2 (1). Catheter ablation results in improved symptoms and improved quality of life (1).

IN-PATIENT CONSIDERATIONS
Initial Stabilization
1st priority is to determine stability of patient:

- Hemodynamically stable:
  – Consider calcium channel blocker or beta-blocker for rate control (1)[C].
- Hemodynamically unstable (see Physical Exam: Hemodynamic compromise):
  – DC cardioversion is best treatment (1)[C].
  – Begin with dose of 50 J (with biphasic defibrillator) or 200 J (with monophasic defibrillator) and increase as needed (1)[C].
  – Atrial overdrive pacing also effective (1)[C]

Admission Criteria

- Most patients with 1st diagnosis of persistent A. flutter require admission for cardiac monitoring.
- All patients who cannot be rate-controlled in the outpatient setting should be admitted.
- Patients with hemodynamic compromise may require intensive care unit (ICU) admission.

IV Fluids

- If hemodynamic unstable, use fluid boluses to maintain blood pressure (BP).
- Caution in LV dysfunction: Avoid CHF.
- If n.p.o., use appropriate maintenance fluid.

Nursing
Strict I/O

Discharge Criteria
Patients can be discharged if rate-controlled, but typically they are when back in NSR.

 ONGOING CARE

FOLLOW-UP RECOMMENDATIONS
Patient Monitoring
Telemetry

DIET
n.p.o. until rate controlled

COMPLICATIONS

- Incidence of embolization with A. flutter is similar to that of A. fib: 1.7–7% (1).
- Hemodynamic instability, CHF

REFERENCES

1. Blomström-Lundqvist C, Scheinman MM, Aliot EM et al. ACC/AHA/ESC guidelines for the management of patients with supraventricular arrhythmias–executive summary. a report of the American college of cardiology/American heart association task force on practice guidelines and the European society of cardiology committee for practice guidelines (writing committee to develop guidelines for the management of patients with supraventricular arrhythmias) developed in collaboration with NASPE-Heart Rhythm Society. *J Am Coll Cardiol*. 2003;42:1493–531.
2. Crijns HJ, Van Gelder IC, Tieleman RG et al. Long-term outcome of electrical cardioversion in patients with chronic atrial flutter. *Heart*. 1997; 77:56–61.
3. Fuster V, Ryden L, et al. ACC/AHA/ESC Guidelines for the management of Patients with Atrial Fibrillation. *Circulation*. 2006;114:257–354.

ADDITIONAL READING

Scholten MF, Thornton AS, Mekel JM et al. Anticoagulation in atrial fibrillation and flutter. *Europace*. 2005;7:492–9.

See Also (Topic, Algorithm, Electronic Media Element)
Atrial Fibrillation

 CODES

ICD9
427.32 Atrial flutter

CLINICAL PEARLS

- Atrial flutter is an unstable rhythm and will sometimes spontaneously resolve.
- Goals of care should be stabilization and rate control.
- Catheter ablation is the treatment of choice for recurrent or chronic atrial flutter.

ATRIAL SEPTAL DEFECT (ASD)

Jonathan Min, MD
Darshak Sanghavi, MD

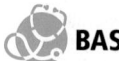 **BASICS**

DESCRIPTION
- Congenital defect or opening in the atrial septum allowing flow of blood between the 2 atria
- Shunting:
  - Typically left to right; occurs in late ventricular systole and early diastole
  - Degree depends on size of the defect and relative compliance (pressures) of the 2 ventricles
  - There can be minimal right-to-left shunting in early ventricular systole, especially during inspiration.
- Asymptomatic early in life. Exertional dyspnea or fatigue. Late cyanotic shunt.
- Types by location in the interatrial septum:
  - 75%: Ostium secundum defect occurs in the fossa ovalis region; most common and most amenable to percutaneous device closure
  - 10%: Sinus venosus defect occurs in the superior-posterior atrial septum near the orifice of the superior vena cava; usually associated with partial anomalous right upper pulmonary venous return
  - 15%: Ostium primum occurs in the inferior portion of the atrial septum, often associated with cleft mitral valve and failure of endocardial cushion development. Ostium primum also seen with incomplete persistent common atrioventricular canal.
- Definitive diagnosis is by transthoracic echocardiography:
  - Symptomatic patients or patients with a high degree of shunt flow should undergo closure to reduce subsequent morbidity (right ventricular dysfunction and failure, atrial tachyarrhythmias, or stroke) and mortality. The risk of arrhythmias may not be decreased unless the atrial septal defect (ASD) is detected and corrected during childhood.
  - Surgery is the only option for ostium primum and sinus venosus defects.
  - Percutaneous closure is an alternative to surgical repair for patients with secundum ASD.
- System(s) affected: Cardiovascular; Pulmonary

Pediatric Considerations
- Most cases of ASD are detected in the pediatric population and corrected at that time.
- Infants/children may just be small for their age, even in the absence of other symptoms.

EPIDEMIOLOGY
Incidence
- Predominant age: Newborn, but may be diagnosed at any age
- Predominant sex: Female > Male (2:1)
- No race predilection
- 4 per 10,000 births, or 1,574 cases per year, based on reporting on 11 US states 1999–2001 (1)

Prevalence
- Accounts for 10% of congenital heart defects, and accounts for 25–30% of congenital heart defects detected in adulthood
- Prevalence of asymptomatic patent foramen ovale in cohort of 2,291 adult patients undergoing cardiothoracic surgery—17.3% (2)[B]

RISK FACTORS
- Other congenital heart defects
- Family history
- Thalidomide, alcohol

Genetics
- 5% chromosomal abnormalities
- Ostium primum in Down syndrome

PATHOPHYSIOLOGY
- Flow across ASD based on relative compliance of left and right ventricles; therefore, usually left-to-right shunt because of higher left-sided pressures
- Symptoms typically occur due to right ventricular and pulmonary vascular volume overload, sometimes with resultant pulmonary hypertension.

COMMONLY ASSOCIATED CONDITIONS
- ASDs often may occur in the setting of other complex cardiac structural defects.
- Important to exclude anomalous pulmonary venous return
- Occasionally can indicate underlying genetic syndromes:
  - Holt-Oram syndrome: Secundum defect with bony abnormalities of forearms + hands
  - Ellis-von-Creveld syndrome: Chondroectodermal dysplasia + ASD
  - VACTERL:
    - V = vertebral abnormalities
    - A = anorectal malformation
    - C = congenital cardiac defects
    - T = tracheoesophageal fistula/esophageal atresia
    - R = renal–urinary defects
    - L = limb defects

 DIAGNOSIS

HISTORY
- Easy fatigability, dyspnea on exertion, heart failure (late), palpitations, frequent respiratory tract infections
- Stroke due to paradoxical emboli
- Can be initially asymptomatic
- Symptoms can include (but not limited to) easy fatigability, dyspnea on exertion, right heart failure (later during course of disease), palpitations, and frequent respiratory tract infections.
- Other symptoms include stroke or unexplained end-organ infarcts due to paradoxical emboli.

PHYSICAL EXAM
Signs vary according to extent of shunting:
- Prominent precordial bulge
- Right ventricular lift
- Palpable pulmonary artery pulse
- Fixed, widely split S2
- Pulmonic flow murmur: Systolic ejection murmur
- Low-pitched diastolic murmur at left lower sternal border
- Cyanosis and clubbing (with severe pulmonary hypertension: Eisenmenger syndrome, jugular venous distention, edema)

- Key physical finding: *Fixed widely split S2*
- May have systolic ejection murmur (pulmonic flow murmur)
- Prominent precordial lift
- Low-pitched diastolic murmur at left lower sternal border

DIAGNOSTIC TESTS & INTERPRETATION
Lab
Oximetry: Cyanosis may suggest Eisenmenger syndrome (right-to-left shunting)

Initial lab tests
Electrocardiogram (ECG) findings:
- General findings for secundum ASDs:
  - Right axis deviation
  - Right atrial enlargement
  - Right ventricular conduction delay
  - Q wave in lead V1
  - Mild PR prolongation
- ECG findings for specific types of ASD:
  - Sinus venosus: Leftward axis, inverted P wave in lead III
  - Ostium primum: Leftward axis

Imaging
Initial approach
- Chest x-ray: Varying degrees of cardiac enlargement, increased pulmonary vascular workings, right ventricle and pulmonary artery enlargement
- Echocardiography: Type and size of ASD, pulmonary arterial and right ventricular dilatation and anterior systolic (paradoxical) septal motion

Follow-Up & Special Considerations
- Cardiac catheterization (indicated in select patients) demonstrates right ventricle enlargement and location of the shunt or if pulmonary hypertension is suspected.
- Left ventricular angiography: Identifies prolapse of the mitral valve and allows assessment of the magnitude of the mitral regurgitation that might be present
- Transesophageal echocardiography might be required to define ASD morphology and to locate the pulmonary veins.

Follow-Up & Special Considerations
- Cardiac catheterization can be diagnostic (to assess anatomy, shunt fraction, and pulmonary vascular resistance) and therapeutic (for device closure).
- Transesophageal echocardiography might be required to define ASD morphology and to locate the pulmonary veins, often as adjunct to percutaneous closure.

Diagnostic Procedures/Surgery
- Echocardiography is the preferred noninvasive modality, unless patient body habitus prohibits adequate imaging.
  - A saline-contrast ("bubble") study is needed only for diagnosis of patent foramen ovale (PFO), rather than hemodynamically significant ASD
- Cardiac magnetic resonance allows excellent imaging and quantitation of shunt fraction.
- Ultrafast computed tomography scans can also define ASDs, but with significant radiation exposure.

Pathological Findings
- Gross defect in atrial septum
- Dilated right atrium, right ventricle
- Enlarged pulmonary artery

DIFFERENTIAL DIAGNOSIS
- Other congenital heart disease
- Right bundle branch block (for widely split S2)

TREATMENT

MEDICATION

First Line
- Consider catheter or surgical closure of the significant ASD if pulmonary hypertension is not present.
- May require antiarrhythmic medications for atrial fibrillation or supraventricular tachycardia
- Respiratory tract infections should be treated promptly.
- Proper treatment of heart failure

Second Line
- There are no data to support antibiotic prophylaxis against infective endocarditis; however, when a device or patch is placed, prophylaxis is recommended until complete neoendothelialization of the foreign material occurs (usually 6 months).
- To prevent thrombus formation after device deployment, aspirin 325 mg daily for 6 months and clopidogrel 75 mg for a month

ADDITIONAL TREATMENT

General Measures
75% of small ASDs (less than 8 mm) will close spontaneously by 18 months of age; however, close follow-up is warranted (3)[B]. Likelihood of spontaneous closure mainly dictated by diameter of defect: >10 mm at time of diagnosis—unlikely spontaneous closure (4)[B].

Issues for Referral
Appropriate health care: Referral to a cardiologist for evaluation

SURGERY/OTHER PROCEDURES
- Closure via percutaneous transcatheter device or surgery (particularly when the pulmonary systemic flow ratio is ≥1.5:1 or evidence of right heart enlargement)
- Percutaneous transcatheter device closure of secundum atrial septal defects and patent foramen ovale is now considered a standard and low-risk procedure that has largely replaced the surgical approach (5)[A].
- Secundum ASDs that are suitable for percutaneous closure should be 35 mm or less in stretched balloon diameter and should have a sufficient rim of surrounding atrial tissue.
- In children, closure is usually delayed until preschool age (2–4 years), except for symptomatic defects (poor growth or exercise intolerance).
- In general, PFOs are treated differently from ASDs with significant shunt burden, and the benefits of PFO closure are unclear. Consultation with a neurologist and cardiologist may be considered prior to device closure. Closure in adult patients with stroke reduces the risk of further neurologic events (6)[B]:
  – PFO diagnosed intraoperatively not associated with any increase in risk of complications; closure at that time, however, increases risk of postoperative stroke vs unrepaired (7)[B].
  – Some evidence suggests possible symptomatic migraine relief following patent foramen ovale closure (8)[B], although this remains controversial and unproven.

ONGOING CARE

FOLLOW-UP RECOMMENDATIONS
Echocardiography follow-up

Patient Monitoring
- In otherwise asymptomatic healthy children, follow until defect has closed or become negligible in size.
- Appropriate evaluation and management for atrial tachyarrhythmias in patients with long-term follow-up
- If ASD repaired as an adult, periodic long-term follow-up indicated
- ASDs repaired in childhood generally do not have late complications.
- Female patients with unrepaired ASD and Eisenmenger syndrome: Pregnancy not recommended due to increased risk of maternal and fetal mortality

DIET
Cardiac diet in patients with symptoms of cardiac failure, ascites, or edema

PATIENT EDUCATION
For patient education materials on this topic, contact American Heart Association, 7320 Greenville Avenue, Dallas, TX 75231, (214) 373-6300.

PROGNOSIS
- ASD closure in asymptomatic or minimally symptomatic adults reduces morbidity but not mortality (9)[A].
- ASD closure before age 25 in symptomatic adults improves morbidity and likely reduces mortality, and some benefits may occur even in older patients. However, if ASD repair is deferred until after adolescence, the long-term risk of future atrial arrhythmias may not be decreased.
- 50% mortality by age 50 in untreated symptomatic patients with large defects

COMPLICATIONS
- Congestive heart failure
- Late-onset arrhythmias 10–20 years after surgery (5%)
- Stroke
- Pulmonary hypertension
- Eisenmenger syndrome
- Infective endocarditis (ostium primum defects > ostium secundum defects)
- Perioperative atrial tachyarrhythmias occurred in 10–13% of patients.
- Device embolization (1%), cardiac perforation, thrombus formation, endocarditis, supraventricular arrhythmias postpercutaneous closure

REFERENCES
1. Improved National Prevalence for 18 Selected Major Birth Defects – United States, 1999–2001. *MMWR.* 2006;54(51–54):1301.
2. Hart SA, Krasuski RA et al. Incidence of asymptomatic patent foramen ovale according to age. *Ann Intern Med.* 2009;150:431–2.
3. McMahon CJ, Feltes TF, Fraley JK et al. Natural history of growth of secundum atrial septal defects and implications for transcatheter closure. *Heart.* 2002;87:256–9.
4. Hanslik A, Pospisil U, Salzer-Muhar U, Greber-Platzer S, Male C et al. Predictors of spontaneous closure of isolated secundum atrial septal defect in children: a longitudinal study. *Pediatrics.* 2006; 118:1560–5.
5. Holzer R, Hijazi ZM. Interventional approach to congenital heart disease. *Curr Opin Cardiol.* 2004;19:84–90.
6. Onorato E, Melzi G, Casilli F et al. Patent foramen ovale with paradoxical embolism: mid-term results of transcatheter closure in 256 patients. *J Interv Cardiol.* 2003;16:43–50.
7. Krasuski RA, Hart SA, Allen D, Qureshi A, Pettersson G, Houghtaling PL, Batizy LH, Blackstone E et al. Prevalence and repair of intraoperatively diagnosed patent foramen ovale and association with perioperative outcomes and long-term survival. *JAMA.* 2009;302:290–7.
8. Morandi E, Anzola GP, Angeli S et al. Transcatheter closure of patent foramen ovale: a new migraine treatment? *J Interv Cardiol.* 2003;16:39–42.
9. Attie F, Rosas M, Granados N et al. Surgical treatment for secundum atrial septal defects in patients >40 years old. A randomized clinical trial. *J Am Coll Cardiol.* 2001;38:2035–42.

ADDITIONAL READING
Lindsey J, Hillis L. Clinical update: atrial septal defect in adults. http://www.thelancet.com Vol 369 April 14, 2007.

See Also (Topic, Algorithm, Electronic Media Element)
Aortic Valvular Stenosis; Coarctation of the Aorta; Patent Ductus Arteriosus; Pulmonic Valvular Stenosis; Tetralogy of Fallot; Ventricular Septal Defect

CODES

ICD9
- 745.5 Ostium secundum, type atrial septal defect
- 745.60 Endocardial cushion defect, unspecified type
- 745.61 Ostium primum defect

CLINICAL PEARLS
- ASD is often missed due to subtle clinical presentation.
- Ideally, hemodynamically significant ASDs should be closed in early childhood, though some benefit from closure also is present in older patients.
- Many ASDs can be treated by catheter-directed percutaneous closure, rather than open-heart surgery.
- Routine endocarditis prophylaxis is not recommended for isolated ASDs.
- PFOs, unlike large ASDs, are very common and generally require no treatment in asymptomatic people.

ATTENTION DEFICIT/HYPERACTIVITY DISORDER

Laura L. Novak, MD

BASICS

DESCRIPTION
- Attention deficit hyperactivity disorder (ADHD) is a behavior problem characterized by a short attention span, distractibility, low frustration tolerance, impulsivity, and hyperactivity.
- ADHD is divided into 3 subsets: predominantly hyperactivity-impulsive, predominantly inattentive, or both.
- System affected: Nervous
- Synonym(s): Attention deficit disorder; Hyperactivity

EPIDEMIOLOGY
- Predominant age: Onset <7 years old; lasts into adolescence and adulthood; 50% meet diagnostic criteria by age 4 years.
- Predominant sex: Male > Female (5:1); predominantly inattentive type may be more common in girls.

Incidence
5% of school-aged children

RISK FACTORS
- Family history
- Comorbid conditions (associated with, but not caused by):
  - Learning disabilities
  - Mood disorders
  - Oppositional defiant disorder
  - Conduct disorder

Genetics
Familial pattern

GENERAL PREVENTION
- Children are at risk for abuse, depression, and social isolation.
- Parents need regular support and advice.
- Parents should establish contact with teacher each school year.

COMMONLY ASSOCIATED CONDITIONS
See Risk Factors

DIAGNOSIS

- American Academy of Pediatrics (AAP) guidelines recommend using the *DSM-IV* criteria to establish the diagnosis.
- Children undergoing extreme stress (divorce, illness, homelessness, abuse) may demonstrate ADHD behaviors secondary to stress. This can be assessed using the American Academy of Child and Adolescent Psychiatry (AACAP) screening tool, if needed.
- If diagnostic behaviors are noted in only one setting, explore the stressors in that setting.
- The diagnostic behaviors are more noticeable in tasks that require concentration or boredom tolerance than in free play or office situations.
- *DSM-IV* criteria: 6 or more inattention criteria and/or 6 or more hyperactivity/impulsivity criteria. Symptoms must begin by age 7 years, be present for >6 months, and be noticed in 2 settings (e.g., home and school). Teachers and caretakers should fill out assessments in addition to parents.

- Inattention:
  - Careless mistakes in tasks
  - Difficulty in sustaining attention
  - Does not seem to listen
  - Does not follow through or finish tasks
  - Difficulty in organizing tasks
  - Avoids tasks that require sustained mental effort
  - Loses things
  - Easily distracted
  - Forgetful
- Hyperactivity/impulsivity:
  - Fidgets
  - Difficulty in remaining seated
  - Runs or climbs excessively
  - Difficulty in playing quietly
  - Acts as if "driven by a motor"
  - Talks excessively
  - Blurts out answers before question is complete
  - Has difficulty in awaiting turn
  - Interrupts others

HISTORY
- Birth and development history
- Comprehensive psychosocial evaluation of home environment
- School performance history

DIAGNOSTIC TESTS & INTERPRETATION
Behavioral testing:
- Behavior rating scales (Connors, others) should be completed by parents and teachers. They are repeated after therapy is started to gauge differences (*DSM-IV* criteria can be used).
- An ADHD toolkit with forms is available from www.nichq.org/adhd.html
- Testing for learning disability (e.g., dyslexia) through the school

Lab
Rarely needed; check lead level if high risk

Diagnostic Procedures/Surgery
- Electroencephalogram not needed unless symptoms are highly suggestive of seizure disorder (e.g., absence seizures).
- Patients with a personal or family history of congenital heart disease or sudden death should be screened with an electrocardiogram (EKG) and possible cardiology consultation before beginning stimulant medication (1).

Pathological Findings
Motor tics can be present (e.g., cough, noises, twitching).

DIFFERENTIAL DIAGNOSIS
- Activity level appropriate for age
- Hearing or vision disorder
- Lead poisoning
- Medication reaction (decongestant, antihistamine, theophylline, phenobarbital)
- Dysfunctional family situation
- Learning disability (e.g., dyslexia)
- Pervasive developmental delay (autism)
- Asperger syndrome: High-functioning autism
- Oppositional/defiant disorder (see *DSM-IV*)
- Conduct disorder (see *DSM-IV*)
- Tourette syndrome: Motor and verbal tics
- Absence seizures (attention deficit only)

TREATMENT

MEDICATION
First Line
The 2001 AAP guideline recommends (1)[C] the use of stimulant medications as 1st-line in treatment. A 2nd type of stimulant should be tried if the 1st treatment fails.

> **ALERT**
> The Food and Drug Administration (FDA) has considered applying a "black box" warning to stimulants based on some reported cases of sudden death seen in patients using stimulant medications. It recommends that patients with a personal or family history of congenital heart disease or sudden death be screened with an EKG and possible cardiology consultation before beginning stimulant medication.

- Stimulant:
  - Methylphenidate (Ritalin, Concerta, Metadate CD, Ritalin LA, others):
    - Short-acting: Ritalin 5–20 mg in the morning, at noon, and at 4 p.m.; maximum dose, 60 mg/d
    - Long-acting: Concerta 18, 36, 54 mg in the morning; Metadate CD 40 mg in the morning; Ritalin LA 20, 30, 40 mg in the morning
    - Methylphenidate patch (Daytrana): Apply to hip for up to 9 hours daily. Begin at 10 mg and titrate upward weekly as needed. Available as 10, 15, 20, and 30 mg.
  - Amphetamines:
    - Adderall: 2.5–20 mg q4–6h
    - Adderall XR: 5–30 mg every morning; ≥6 years
- Precautions:
  - If not responding, check compliance and consider another diagnosis (1)[C].
  - Some children experience withdrawal (tearfulness, agitation) after a missed dose or when medication wears off.
  - Stimulants are drugs of abuse and should be monitored carefully.
  - Drug holidays should be given only if family/peer relationships are not harmed.
- Significant possible interactions:
  - Stimulants may increase levels of anticonvulsants, selective serotonin reuptake inhibitors (SSRIs), tricyclics, and warfarin.

Pregnancy Considerations
Medications used in ADHD are Category C: Caution in pregnancy.

Second Line
- Nonstimulant:
  - Atomoxetine carries a "black box" warning regarding potential exacerbation of suicidality (similar to selective serotonin reuptake inhibitors). Because of this, the manufacturer recommends weekly visits for 4 sessions, then every-other-week visits for 4 sessions, then every-12-weeks visits. Atomoxetine has also been associated with hepatic injury in a small number of cases, and the manufacturer recommends checking liver enzymes if symptoms (jaundice, fatigue, malaise) develop.

– Atomoxetine (Strattera): Selective norepinephrine reuptake inhibitor; 0.5–2 mg/kg/d every morning (10 mg, 18 mg, 25 mg, 40 mg, 60 mg). Maximum dose, 1.4 mg/kg/d or 100 mg/d, whichever is less:
  ○ Slower onset of efficacy; gastrointestinal side effects and sedation. Not addictive.
– Atomoxetine interacts with paroxetine (Paxil), fluoxetine (Prozac), and quinidine.
- Other nonstimulant drugs (e.g., clonidine, tricyclic antidepressants, SSRIs): Owing to the mixed efficacy and high side effects of these drugs, they are not recommended for use without a consultant.

ADDITIONAL TREATMENT
- Medication alone or combined with behavioral therapy produced better results than behavioral therapy alone.
- Behavioral therapy may be useful in cases where parents object to medication (2).

General Measures
- Parent/school/patient education (2)
- Work closely with teacher.
- Avoid unproven therapies.

COMPLEMENTARY AND ALTERNATIVE MEDICINE
- Surveys have shown that parents of children with ADHD use herbals and complementary treatments frequently (20–60%) (3,4).
- Many herbals have been assessed for efficacy, but studies are small and brief and, therefore, difficult to translate into clinical recommendations.
- Dietary and nutritional supplements have also been assessed:
  – Omega-3 fatty acids (found in fish oil and some supplements) showed improvement in rating scales in 2 double-blind, placebo-controlled studies of 116 and 130 patients.
- Rapid eye training and biofeedback have contradictory results and can be costly.

ONGOING CARE

The "toolkit for physicians" may be useful: http://www.nichq.org/adhd.html

FOLLOW-UP RECOMMENDATIONS
Patient Monitoring
- Parent/teacher rating scales initially, 2 weeks after an intervention such as starting medication, and regularly
- Office visits to monitor side effects and efficacy: Endpoints are improved grades, improved rating scales, acceptable family interactions, and improved peer interactions.
- Monitor growth (especially weight gain) and blood pressure.

DIET
"Insufficient evidence exists to suggest that dietary interventions improve the symptoms of ADHD in children" (5).

PATIENT EDUCATION
- Key points for parents:
  – 50% of children with ADHD have 1 parent with ADHD; modify education sessions with parents accordingly.
  – Behavioral interventions such as token systems may be helpful (1)[A].
  – Find things child is good at and emphasize these.
  – Reinforce good behavior (with rewards and attention).
  – Make eye contact with each request.
  – Give one task at a time.
  – Stop behavior before it escalates.
  – Some families benefit from "parent training" and family therapy.
  – Coordinate homework with teachers using daily assignment notebook.
  – Refer to advocacy and support groups.
- Schools are required by law to provide necessary testing and Individualized Educational Plans (IEPs) or 504 plans to accommodate the child's educational needs
- Support groups:
  – Children and Adults with Attention Deficit Disorder (CHADD): chadd.org; 800-233-4050
  – Attention Deficit Disorder Warehouse: addwarehouse.com; 800-233-9273
  – Learning Disabilities Association (LDA): LDAlearning.com
  – National Information Center for Children and Youth with Disabilities: www.nichcy.org

PROGNOSIS
- May last into adulthood
- The hyperactivity component may become easier to control with increasing age.
- Encourage career choices that allow autonomy and mobility.
- With treatment, there is no increased incidence of delinquency unless other comorbid features exist (e.g., conduct disorder).
- Encourage parents to subtract 2 years from their child's chronological age when allowing privileges (e.g., treat a 16-year-old like a 14-year-old, delay driving until age 18).

COMPLICATIONS
- Untreated ADHD can lead to failing school, parental abuse, social isolation, and poor self-esteem.
- Some children experience withdrawal (tearfulness, agitation) after a missed medication dose or when medication wears off.
- If appetite is poor as a side effect of stimulant medication, offer small frequent meals.

REFERENCES

1. American Academy of Pediatrics. Subcommittee on Attention-Deficit/Hyperactivity Disorder and Committee on Quality Improvement. Clinical practice guideline: treatment of the school-aged child with attention-deficit/hyperactivity disorder. *Pediatrics*. 2001;108:1033–44.
2. Laforett DR, Murray DW, Kollins SH. Psychosocial treatments for preschool-aged children with Attention-Deficit Hyperactivity Disorder. *Dev Disabil Res Rev*. 2008;14:300–10.
3. Sawni A. Attention-deficit/hyperactivity disorder and complementary/alternative medicine. *Adolesc Med State Art Rev*. 2008;19:313–26, xi.
4. Weber W, Newmark S. Complementary and alternative medical therapies for attention-deficit/hyperactivity disorder and autism. *Pediatr Clin North Am*. 2007;54:983–1006; xii.
5. Sinn N. Nutritional and dietary influences on attention deficit hyperactivity disorder. *Nutr Rev*. 2008;66:558–68.

ADDITIONAL READING

- *American Psychiatric Association. Diagnostic and Statistical Manual of Mental Disorders*. 4th ed. Revised. Washington, DC: American Psychiatric Association, 2000.
- Barkley RA. *ADHD: A Handbook for Diagnosis and Treatment*. 2nd ed. New York: Guilford Press, 1998.
- Brown RT, Amler RW, Freeman WS, et al. Treatment of attention deficit/hyperactivity disorder: Overview of the evidence. *Pediatrics*. 2005;115(6): e749–e757.
- Ghuman JK, Arnold LE, Anthony BJ. Psychopharmacological and other treatments in preschool children with attention-deficit/hyperactivity disorder: Current Evidence and Practice. *J Child Adolesc Psychopharmacol*. 2008.
- Pliszka S, AACAP Work Group on Quality Issues. Practice parameter for the assessment and treatment of children and adolescents with attention-deficit/hyperactivity disorder. *J Am Acad Child Adolesc Psychiatry*. 2007;46:894–921.
- Rader R, McCauley L, Callen EC. Current strategies in the diagnosis and treatment of childhood attention-deficit/hyperactivity disorder. *Am Fam Physician*. 2009;79:657–65.
- Rappley, MD. attention deficit-hyperactivity disorder. *N Engl J Med*. 2005;352(2):165–73.
- Rostain AL. Attention-deficit/hyperactivity disorder in adults: evidence-based recommendations for management. *Postgrad Med*. 2008;120:27–38.
- Soileau EJ. Medications for adolescents with attention-deficit/hyperactivity disorder. *Adolesc Med State Art Rev*. 2008;19:254–67, viii–ix.

 CODES

ICD9
- 314.00 Attention deficit disorder of childhood without mention of hyperactivity
- 314.01 Attention deficit disorder of childhood with hyperactivity

CLINICAL PEARLS

- Children undergoing extreme stress (divorce, illness, homelessness, abuse) may demonstrate ADHD behaviors secondary to stress.
- 50% of ADHD children have a parent with ADHD.
- AAP recommends the use of stimulant medications as the 1st-line treatment.

AUTISM SPECTRUM DISORDERS

Macario C. Corpuz, Jr., MD
Alphonsus K. Kung, MD

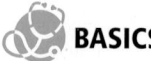

BASICS

DESCRIPTION
Group of neurodevelopmental disorders of early childhood

- Includes autistic disorder, Rett disorder, childhood disintegrative disorder, Asperger disorder, and pervasive developmental disorder not otherwise specified (PDD-NOS)
- Autistic disorder includes classic autism and childhood autism.
- Rett disorder involves mutations in the MECP2 gene. Mostly in females with initial normal development until approximately 18 months of age with microcephaly and dementia.
- Childhood disintegrative disorder: Regression after at least 2 years of normal development
- Asperger disorder: Better development with mechanics of verbal expression, higher levels of cognition and interest in social activity
- PDD-NOS: Meet some, but not all of DSM-IV-TR criteria for autistic disorder
- Characterized by:
  - Impairment of effective social skills
  - Absent or impaired communication skills
  - Repetitive and/or stereotyped behaviors and interests, especially in inanimate objects
  - System(s) affected: Nervous

EPIDEMIOLOGY
- Predominant age: Onset in early childhood
- Predominant sex: Male > Female (4:1) except for Rett disorder

Pediatric Considerations
Symptom onset seen in children <3 years (except for childhood disintegrative disorder)

Prevalence
Estimated 1/100 to 1/500 children

RISK FACTORS
Siblings with autism have shown to have a 5× greater risk of developing autism. Prevalence ranging from 2% to 8%.

Pregnancy Considerations
Siblings with autism have shown to have a 5× greater risk of developing autism. Prevalence ranging from 2% to 8%.

Genetics
- High concordance in monozygotic twins
- Increased recurrence risk (3–7%) in subsequent siblings

GENERAL PREVENTION
- Early screening for early treatment = better prognosis.
- Some ASDs such as Rett disorder are known to be caused by genetic mutations.

PATHOPHYSIOLOGY
Pathophysiology is incompletely understood.

ETIOLOGY
- No single cause has been identified.
- General consensus: A genetic abnormality leads to altered neurologic development.
- Research continues to investigate the links between heredity, genetics, and medical problems.

- No documented scientific evidence exists that proves vaccines or thimerosal cause ASDs.

COMMONLY ASSOCIATED CONDITIONS
- Mental retardation
- Attention deficit/hyperactivity disorder (ADHD)
- Phenylketonuria (PKU), tuberous sclerosis, fragile X syndrome, Angelman syndrome, and fetal alcohol syndrome (rare)
- Anxiety
- Depression
- Obsessive behavior
- Seizures (increased risk if severe mental retardation)

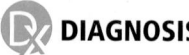

DIAGNOSIS

HISTORY
- Impairment in social interaction:
  - Impairment in nonverbal behaviors such as eye-to-eye gaze, facial expression
  - Unable to develop peer relationships
  - Does not smile nor share emotions
  - Loss of social or emotional reciprocity
- Communication impairment:
  - Delay or lack of development in language skills
  - Inability to initiate or sustain conversation
  - Stereotyped and repetitive use of language
  - Preoccupation with parts of toys or body parts
- Repetitive and stereotyped patterns of behavior:
  - Excessively lines up toys or other objects
  - Unusually attached to 1 particular toy or object
  - Repetitive odd movements (toe walking, hand flapping)
  - Adherence to specific routines or rituals
- Asperger disorder does not have clinically significant delays in cognitive development, language acquisitions, nor learning/adaptive skills.
- Rett disorder is predominantly in females without macrocephaly.
- Childhood disintegrative disorder with normal development until 2 years of age
- PDD-NOS does not meet DSM-IV-TR criteria for autism.
- Prenatal, neonatal, and developmental history
- Seizure disorder
- Family history of autism, genetic disorders, learning disabilities, psychiatric illness, neurological disorders, genetic disorders, or mental retardation

PHYSICAL EXAM
- Macrocephaly in 25% (except in Rett syndrome); head circumference growth peaks at age 6 months and begins to decline by 1 year.
- Dysmorphic features consistent with genetic disorder (fragile X syndrome)
- Hypotonia can occur in autism, but neurological deficit is a sign that imaging may be needed.
- Wood lamp skin exam to rule out tuberous sclerosis

DIAGNOSTIC TESTS & INTERPRETATION
- Checklist for Autism in Toddlers (CHAT) to screen for ASDs at 18 months of age. (To order: http://www.nas.org.uk/nas/jsp/polopoly.jsp.)
- The Pervasive Developmental Disorders Screening Test-II (PDDST-II) to screen for ASDs beginning at 18 months
- Modified Checklist for Autism in Toddlers (M-CHAT) to screen for ASDs at 16–30 months

- Social Communication Questionnaire (SCQ) (formerly Autism Screening Questionnaire)—used with children age 4 years and older—the gold-standard diagnostic interview used in research studies

Lab
- Lead screening
- PKU screening
- Karyotype and DNA analysis (fragile X, PKU, tuberous sclerosis, and others)
- Metabolic testing if signs of:
  - Lethargy, limited endurance
  - Hypotonia
  - Recurrent vomiting and dehydration
  - Developmental regression
  - Unusual habits
  - Specific food intolerance

Follow-Up & Special Considerations
- Hearing tests: Audiometry and BAERS
- Comprehensive speech and language evaluation
- Evaluation by multidisciplinary team: Includes a psychiatrist, neurologist, psychologist, speech therapist, and other autism specialists
- Intellectual level needs to be established and monitored, as it is one of the best measures of prognosis.
- Test used to follow autism are:
  - Autism Behavior Checklist (ABC)
  - Gilliam Autism Rating Scale (GARS)
  - Childhood Autism Rating Scale (CARS)
  - Autism Diagnosis Interview-Revised (ADI-R)
  - Autism Diagnostic Observation Schedule-Generic (ADOS-G) Imaging

Imaging
Initial approach
Magnetic resonance imaging (MRI) useful only if focal neurologic symptoms

Diagnostic Procedures/Surgery
Electroencephalogram (EEG) only if history of seizures or spells

DIFFERENTIAL DIAGNOSIS
Other mental and central nervous system (CNS) disorders:
- Obsessive-compulsive disorder
- Elective mutism
- Language disorder/hearing impairment
- Intellectual disability/global developmental delay
- Stereotyped movement disorder
- Severe early deprivation/reactive attachment disorder
- Anxiety disorder
- Developmental language disorder

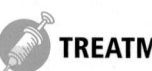

TREATMENT

MEDICATION
Medical causes of autistic-like behavior should be excluded with behavioral management maximized prior to considering medication with symptom-specific therapy, as pharmacological therapy data are scant.

First Line
- No true 1st-line medical therapy
- Stimulant medications (such as methylphenidate): Efficacious in treating concomitant symptoms of attention deficit disorder, such as impulsiveness,

hyperactivity, and inattention; however, the magnitude of response is less than in typically developing children, and adverse effects are more frequent.

- Selective serotonin reuptake inhibitors (SSRIs) have shown some help in reducing ritualistic behavior and improving mood and language skills. Initial choice for anxiety and depressive mood. Also administered for dysregulated mood (1).
- Risperidone (an atypical antipsychotic) has been shown to be effective for short-term treatment of tantrums, aggression, and self-injurious behavior. Improvements in stereotyped behavior, hyperactivity, irritability, repetitious behaviors, and social withdrawal have also been noted (2)[A]. Precautions: Causes weight gain as an adverse effect. Associated with sedation, dry mouth, agitation enuresis, dyspepsia, diarrhea, constipation, and tremor.

Second Line
Vitamin B6 and magnesium with inconclusive evidence in improving speech and language (3,4)[C].

ADDITIONAL TREATMENT
General Measures
- Comprehensive structured educational programming of a sustained and intensive design, most commonly applied behavioral analysis therapy
- Core features of a successful education program:
  – High staff–student ratio 1:2 or less
  – Individualized programming
  – Specialized teacher training with ongoing evaluation of teachers and programs
  – 25 hours a week minimum of specialized services
  – A structured routine environment that emphasizes attention, imitation, communication, socialization, and play interactions
  – Functional analysis of behavioral problems
  – Transition planning and involvement of the family
- Currently no cure for ASDs. Early diagnosis and initiation of multidisciplinary intervention help enhance functioning in later life.
- Early intervention for ages 3 and under
- School-based special education for older children
- Find alternative methods of communication: Sign language; picture exchange communication system

Issues for Referral
- Refer early to:
  – Early learning for evaluation of behavior and language
  – Genetic counseling
  – Audiology
- Consider referrals to psychiatry, ophthalmology, otolaryngology, neurology, and nutrition
- Refer family members to parent support groups and respite programs

COMPLEMENTARY AND ALTERNATIVE MEDICINE
- Music therapy has been shown to improve communication skills in autistic patients with limited data (5)[B].
- Auditory integration training is used for autistic children with sound sensitivity (6)[B].
- Osteopathic manipulative therapy (OMT) has been shown to improve sensory and motor performance with neurological problems, including autism. Treatment that starts before the age of 2 years showed the greatest effect (7)[C].

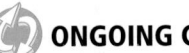 ONGOING CARE

FOLLOW-UP RECOMMENDATIONS
Patient Monitoring
- Constant by caregivers
- Reevaluation every 6–12 months by physician for seizures, sleep and nutritional problems, and prescribed medical management
- Intellectual and language testing every 2 years in childhood

DIET
Gluten- and casein-free diets show some reduction in autistic traits; however, large-scale, good-quality randomized controlled trials are needed (8).

PATIENT EDUCATION
- Autism Society of America: http://www.autismsociety.org.
- The Centers for Disease Control and Prevention, Autism Info. Center: http://www.cdc.gov/ncbddd/autism/index.htm
- The Centers for Disease Control and Prevention, "Learn the Signs. Act Early": http://www.cdc.gov/ncbddd/autism/actearly
- First Signs: http://www.firstsigns.org
- Autism Speaks: http://www.autismsspeaks.org/index2.php
- Supplemental security income: http://www.socialsecurity.gov/ssi/index.htm
- Autism and vaccines: http://www.aap.org/immunization/families/faq/VaccineStudies.pdf

PROGNOSIS
- Those who begin treatment at a young age (2–4 years) have significantly better outcomes.
- Prognosis is closely related to initial intellectual abilities, with only 20% functioning above the mentally retarded level.
- Communicative language development before 5 years is also associated with a better outcome.
- The general expected course is for a lifelong need for supervised structured care.

COMPLICATIONS
- Increasing incidents of seizure disorders in up to 1 in 4 children.
- Increased risk for physical and sexual abuse
- If pica, increased risk of lead poisoning
- Limited variety of food consumed due to dietary obsessions
- Increased risk for gastrointestinal symptoms, including weight abnormalities and abnormal stool patterns

REFERENCES

1. Selective serotonin reuptake inhibitors (SSRIs) for autism spectrum disorders (ASD). Williams, Katrina. Wheeler, Danielle M. Silove, Natalie. Hazell, Philip. *Cochrane Developmental, Psychosocial and Learning Problems Group Cochrane Database of Systematic Reviews*. 8, 2010.
2. Risperdone for autistic spectrum disorder. Jesner, Ora S. Aref-Adib, Mehrnoosh. Coren, Esther. *Cochrane Developmental, Psychosocial and Learning Problems Group Cochrane Database of Systematic Reviews*. 1, 2009.
3. Vitamin B6 for cognition. Malouf, Reem. Grimley Evans, John. *Cochrane Dementia and Cognitive Improvement Group Cochrane Database of Systematic Reviews*. 1, 2009.
4. Combined vitamin B6-magnesium treatment in autism spectrum disorder. Nye, Chad. Brice, Alejandro. *Cochrane Developmental, Psychosocial and Learning Problems Group Cochrane Database of Systematic Reviews*. 1, 2009.
5. Music therapy for autistic spectrum disorder. Gold, Christian. Wigram, Tony. Elefant, Cochavit. *Cochrane Developmental, Psychosocial and Learning Problems Group Cochrane Database of Systematic. Reviews*. 1, 2009.
6. Auditory integration training and other sound therapies for autism spectrum disorders. Sinha, Yashwant. Silove, Natalie. Wheeler, Danielle M. Williams, Katrina J. *Cochrane Developmental, Psychosocial and Learning Problems Group Cochrane Database of Systematic Reviews*. 1, 2009.
7. Frymann VM, Carney RE, Springall P. Effect of osteopathic medical management on neurologic development in children. *J Am Osteopath Assoc*. 1992;92:729–44.
8. Gluten- and casein-free diets for autistic spectrum disorder. Millward, Claire. Ferriter, Michael. Calver, Sarah J. Connell-Jones, Graham G. *Cochrane Developmental, Psychosocial and Learning Problems Group Cochrane Database of Systematic Reviews*. 1, 2009.

See Also (Topic, Algorithm, Electronic Media Element)
Algorithm: Mental Retardation

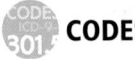 CODES

ICD9
- 299.00 Infantile autism, current or active state
- 299.10 Disintegrative psychosis, current or active state
- 299.80 Other specified early childhood psychoses, current or active state

CLINICAL PEARLS

ALARM mnemonic from the American Academy of Pediatrics (AAP):
- Autism spectrum disorder is prevalent (screen ALL children between 18–24 months).
- Listen to parents when they feel something is wrong.
- Act early: Screen all children who fall behind in language and social developmental milestones (use early learning to help with evaluation).
- Refer to multidisciplinary teams (speech and language evaluation, genetic screening, social support groups).
- Monitor support for patient and families.

AUTONOMIC DYSREFLEXIA

Shashidhara Nanjundaswamy, MD, MBBS, MRCP, DM
Madaiah Lokeshwari, MD

BASICS

DESCRIPTION
A medical emergency characterized by a sudden, dangerously elevated blood pressure (BP) due to a massive sympathetic/catecholamine surge in patients with spinal cord injury (SCI) above the level of T6 in response to a noxious stimulus below the level of injury.

EPIDEMIOLOGY
Incidence
- 16% of children and adolescents with SCI
- 50–90% of adults with SCI above level of T6; more common with complete SCI; rarely seen with lesions down to T10.
- Occurs 4 times more frequently in men:
  - Can occur as early as 2 months and as late as 12 years after the SCI
  - Occurs most often in the 1st year after SCI
  - Frequency varies from daily to once in a few years.

Pediatric Considerations
- Because of lower incidence of SCI in children, autonomic dysreflexia (AD) is often unrecognized or inappropriately treated.
- Recommendations include giving the nationally standardized guidelines to the child's primary care physician and school, along with the child's baseline BP and a description of AD (1)[A].

Pregnancy Considerations
- Occurs during labor in 2/3 of pregnancies in patients with SCI at or above T6 level.
- AD can occur in antepartum, intrapartum, and postpartum periods. AD should be recognized and treated early by all health care providers dealing with pregnant women to minimize the risk of intracranial bleeding and death.

RISK FACTORS
Spinal cord lesion at or above level T5–6, rarely as low as T10:
- Any unpleasant stimulus below the lesion can cause AD.
- Bladder distention (most common cause):
  - Urinary retention/blocked catheter
  - Detrusor sphincter dyssynergia
  - Urinary tract infection
  - Urinary calculi
  - Instrumentation
  - Cystoscopy
  - Urodynamics
  - Bladder irrigation
- Fecal impaction (2nd most common cause):
  - Bowel impaction
  - Anal fissure
  - Rectal digital disimpaction
  - Rectal exam
  - Enema administration

- Other:
  - Ingrown toe nails
  - Painful stimulus of any etiology
  - All causes of acute abdomen
  - Burns
  - Labor
  - Sexual intercourse
  - Pressure sore
  - Testicular torsion
  - Fracture dislocation
  - Heterotopic ossification
  - Pregnancy
  - Electroejaculation for sperm retrieval

GENERAL PREVENTION
- Good bladder and bowel care
- Use lubricant for catheter insertion or fecal digital disimpaction.
- Lubricants for instrumentation
- Use of local anesthetics for procedures below the level of SCI even if patient does not feel pain.

PATHOPHYSIOLOGY
- In AD, a disconnect occurs between the sympathetic and parasympathetic nervous systems.
- AD does not occur during the spinal shock phase. It occurs once the spinal shock phase is over and the spinal reflexes start returning. Any noxious stimulus below the level of SCI creates a volley of impulses that are transmitted via the intact peripheral nerves through the spinothalamic and posterior columns to the sympathetic neurons in the intermediolateral cell column of the thoracic spinal cord. Inhibitory responses from the cerebral vasomotor centers, although increased, are blocked by the SCI. The unopposed sympathetic outflow (as the parasympathetic outflow cannot reach below the level of SCI) causes massive release of neurotransmitters norepinephrine, dopamine-b-hydroxylase, dopamine, which result in piloerection, skin pallor, and severe vasoconstriction of the arterial vasculature, thus resulting in sudden elevation of BP and vasodilatation above the level of injury.
- Baroreceptors located in the cerebral vessels, carotid sinus, and aorta detect the rising BP and attempt to trigger visceral and peripheral vasodilatation, but the impulses cannot pass through the damaged spinal cord. The parasympathetic response is limited to vagal slowing of the heart rate and vasodilatation, flushing, nasal congestion, and diaphoresis above the level of spinal cord injury.
- SCI below the T6 level very rarely causes AD as the intact splanchnic innervation allows compensatory dilatation of the splanchnic vascular bed.

ETIOLOGY
SCI above the T5–6 level

DIAGNOSIS

AD is a clinical diagnosis and hence all personnel dealing with SCI patients should be aware of the clinical symptomatology/presentation.

HISTORY
- Pounding headache (due to elevated BP and vasodilatation of pain-sensitive intracranial vasculature)
- Piloerection (goose bumps above the level of lesion), less often below the level
- Profuse sweating above the level of lesion could be the 1st sign.
- Flushing above the level of lesion
- Nasal congestion
- Chest pain
- Palpitations
- Dyspnea due to neurogenic pulmonary edema
- Nausea and malaise secondary to parasympathetic/vagal stimulation
- Blurred vision
- Mydriasis
- Rarely, absent symptoms
- Triad of bitemporal throbbing headache, head and neck sweating, and systolic hypertension.

PHYSICAL EXAM
- BP 20–40 mm Hg above range for the patient
- BP 15–20 mm Hg above baseline in adolescents
- BP 15 mm Hg above baseline in children
- Normal BP for a quadriplegic could be 90/60 mm Hg, hence even 120/80 mm Hg could indicate AD.
- Mild increase in BP initially and if untreated
- Further elevation to 200/100 or higher when it becomes a life-threatening medical emergency
- Systolic BP as high as 250–300 mm Hg and diastolic pressure as high as 200–220 mm Hg have been reported.
- Reflex bradycardia secondary to vagal stimulation, usually a relative bradycardia with heart rate in the normal range
- Piloerection
- Tachycardia, rarely
- Profuse sweating above the level of the lesion
- Flushing, red skin above the level due to vasodilatation
- Nasal congestion
- Cold, pale skin due to vasoconstriction below the level of the injury
- Blotchy skin above the level of the lesion
- Blurred vision
- Retinal hemorrhages
- Minimal or no symptoms despite an elevated BP (silent AD)
- Rarely, seizures

DIAGNOSTIC TESTS & INTERPRETATION
No diagnostic lab test or imaging makes the diagnosis of AD. Clinical suspicion and physical exam are paramount in making a diagnosis of this rare, potentially reversible life-threatening condition.

Imaging
Head CT scan if patient complains of worst headache of his life or is in altered sensorium or has new focal neurologic deficits, as abrupt increase in BP could cause cerebral hemorrhage

DIFFERENTIAL DIAGNOSIS
- Spinal cord plaque above T6 in multiple sclerosis
- Coexisting catecholamine-secreting tumor in SCI patients (symptoms similar to AD related to catecholamines released from the tumor)
- Eclampsia

 # TREATMENT

Nonpharmacologic treatment must be tried immediately: Removing noxious stimuli, sitting patient up, and loosening clothing.

MEDICATION
Antihypertensive agents with rapid onset and short duration of action, while sorting out the etiology or if the SBP is >150 mm Hg. BP should be lowered without causing hypotension, prior to checking for fecal impaction or digital stimulation. BPs above 140 mm Hg in an adolescent, 130 mm Hg in children 6–12 years old, or 120 mm Hg in children <5 years old will necessitate initiation of medications (2,3)[A].

First Line
- Nifedipine immediate-release form, 10-mg cap initially; bite and swallow is the mainstay of therapy (3)[A].

  - However, severe hypotension can be caused by the short-acting form of nifedipine.
  - This hypotension can be avoided by using a pin or needle to puncture the nifedipine capsule and administering the liquid medication 1 drop at a time to titrate to effectiveness.
  - The dose of nifedipine can be repeated in 15 minutes if needed. Care should be exercised to avoid hypotension, especially in older patients, and with coronary artery as well as cerebrovascular disease.

- Nitrates: Sublingual 0.4-mg spray; second most commonly used drug in patients with SCI (2)[B]

- 2% nitroglycerine ointment, 0.5- to 1-inch strip to chest wall (above the level of the lesion) and titrate as needed; this is safer but slower.
- Nitroglycerine: 0.15- to 0.6-mg tab SL
- Nitrates are contraindicated if patient has taken any phosphodiesterase inhibitors such as sildenafil (Viagra), vardenafil (Levitra) within the past 24 hours or tadalafil (Cialis) within the previous 48 hours.

Second Line
- Prazosin 0.5–1 mg PO q8h prn for prophylaxis of AD (3)[A]
- Captopril 25 mg PO sublingually during AD (2)[B]
- Terazosin (3)[A]
- Clonidine: 0.1–0.3 mg PO q 8h to a maximum of 0.8 mg

ADDITIONAL TREATMENT
Issues for Referral
Pregnant women with a SCI at T6 or above with features of AD should be referred to an obstetrician if:
- Life-threatening AD
- 1st episode of AD
- AD in the 3rd trimester

- Vaginal bleeding or suspected labor
- Persistent symptoms despite treatment
- Choice of antihypertensive therapy

Additional Therapies
- Physical therapy
- Therapists should be aware of AD, its manifestations, and general measures of treatment.
- When AD suspected, patient should be supported to sit upright.
- If stretching exercise evoked the episode of AD, it should be stopped.

SURGERY/OTHER PROCEDURES
Transurethral sphincterotomy for chronic form of AD that is related to detrusor sphincter dyssynergia and overdistention of bladder

IN-PATIENT CONSIDERATIONS
Initial Stabilization
- Treatment should be initiated as quickly as possible.
- Most important step is removal of the causative noxious stimulus:
  - Patient should be helped to sit upright as venous pooling helps reduce the BP.
  - Loosen any constrictive clothing or devices.
  - Pressure relief should be tried.
  - Check the urinary catheter to make sure it is not kinked and is draining.
  - Irrigate a blocked catheter to reestablish drainage and irrigate bladder with 60 mL of 2% lidocaine. If unsuccessful, remove the catheter, insert 2% lidocaine jelly into the urethra; 30 minutes later insert a new catheter.
  - Do not allow bag to get full.
  - Gentle rectal exam using lidocaine jelly, as rectal exam of a spastic anal sphincter can aggravate AD.
  - Rectal disimpaction if constipated, using lidocaine jelly (unless procedure started AD)
  - If BP is significantly elevated, it may need to be lowered before checking for fecal impaction or digital stimulation.

Admission Criteria
- Poor response to treatment
- Undetermined precipitant of AD
- Obstetrical complications
- Transfer to ICU if antihypertensive measures fail, for IV hypotensive agents, including nitroprusside, 0.5 mcg/min IV (contraindicated with previous sildenafil use) and possibly spinal anesthesia.
- Epidural anesthesia in pregnant woman with AD during labor (4)

Nursing
Monitor BP frequently, every 5 minutes until normal, and then every 30 minutes for 4 hours, as BP tends to fluctuate during AD.

Discharge Criteria
- BP and pulse back to patient's norm
- Asymptomatic, no signs of cardiac failure or raised intracranial pressure
- Etiology of the AD is ascertained.

 # ONGOING CARE

FOLLOW-UP RECOMMENDATIONS
- Detailed medical evaluation if recurrent AD
- Patient and family education regarding early recognition of AD and its prevention
- For recurrent AD, consider the alpha blocker prazosin.

Patient Monitoring
Monitor symptoms and BP for at least 2 hours after resolution of AD because of risk of developing hypotension.

PATIENT EDUCATION
- Most important strategy is to prevent AD.
- All patients prone to develop AD should be counseled about the causes, manifestations, prevention, and treatment of AD.
- Optimal bladder and bowel care
- Patients should carry a Medic Alert bracelet informing of their risk of developing AD.
- Patients should carry AD emergency medical card summarizing the causes of AD and its treatment.
- Educate all health professionals who deal with SCI patients.

PROGNOSIS
Life-threatening if unrecognized and untreated due to massive elevation in BP

COMPLICATIONS
- Retinal, cerebral, and subarachnoid hemorrhage
- Myocardial infarction
- Seizures
- Cardiac arrest secondary to vagal overreactivity and death.

REFERENCES
1. McGinnis KB, Vogel LC, McDonald CM et al. Recognition and management of autonomic dysreflexia in pediatric spinal cord injury. *J Spinal Cord Med.* 2004;27(Suppl 1):S61–74.
2. Consortium for Spinal Cord Medicine. *Acute management of autonomic dysreflexia*, 2nd ed. Clinical Practice Guidelines, 2001.
3. Krassioukov A, Warburton DE, Teasell R, Eng JJ, Spinal Cord Injury Rehabilitation Evidence Research Team et al. A systematic review of the management of autonomic dysreflexia after spinal cord injury. *Arch Phys Med Rehabil.* 2009;90:682–95.
4. Pereira L. Obstetric management of the patient with spinal cord injury. *Obstet Gynecol Surv.* 2003;58:678–87.

ADDITIONAL READING
- Gall A, Turner-Stokes L, Guideline Development Group. Chronic spinal cord injury: management of patients in acute hospital settings. *Clin Med.* 2008;8:70–4.
- Weaver LC, Marsh DR, Gris D, Brown A, Dekaban GA et al. Autonomic dysreflexia after spinal cord injury: central mechanisms and strategies for prevention. *Prog Brain Res.* 2006;152:245–63.

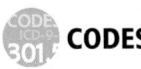 # CODES

ICD9
337.3 Autonomic dysreflexia

CLINICAL PEARLS
- AD is a potentially life-threatening but reversible disorder, so early recognition and prevention is vital.
- Normal BP for a quadriplegic could be 90/60 mm Hg; hence even 120/80 mm Hg could indicate AD.

AVIAN FLU

Sheila M. Seed, PharmD, MPH
Walter K. Goljan, MD

 BASICS

DESCRIPTION
- Avian influenza A subtype H5N1 is a highly pathogenic and aggressive form of influenza.
- Presents with influenzalike symptoms, with lower respiratory tract symptoms (limited upper respiratory tract symptoms)
- High mortality rate in elderly and very young

EPIDEMIOLOGY
Incidence
- More than 490 confirmed human cases (60% fatality rate); primarily in Asia
- Predominate age: All age groups

Prevalence
Rare

RISK FACTORS
- Direct contact with H5N1 virus
- Contact with infected poultry
- Close contact with infected person
- Travel to affected country within 10 days of symptom onset

GENERAL PREVENTION
- Consider with any patient with influenzalike symptoms who has had close contact with H5N1 or ill poultry
- 2007: Food and Drug Administration approved a vaccine for adults 18–65. Currently only available from the government.
- Chemoprophylaxis with antivirals should be considered if H5N1 is circulating in the community.
- Ongoing environmental screening is more accessible now with availability of avian fecal testing (1)[B].

ETIOLOGY
- Infected poultry (domesticated ducks, turkeys, chickens)
- Low incidence of human-to-human transmission in household clusters and health care workers
- Incubation period: 7 days (range 2–3 days)

COMMONLY ASSOCIATED CONDITIONS
Severe respiratory distress (common in severe cases)

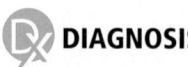 DIAGNOSIS

- Primary phase (2,3)[A]:
  - Influenzalike symptoms with lower respiratory tract symptoms
  - Temp >100.4°F (38°C)
  - Cough
  - Sore throat
  - Shortness of breath
  - Diarrhea (watery without blood)
  - Pleuritic pain
  - Bleeding of nose and gums
  - Conjunctivitis (rare)

- Secondary acute phase:
  - Severe respiratory distress
  - Pneumonia not responsive to antibiotics
  - Multiorgan dysfunction

- Respiratory (2,3)[A]:
  - Respiratory distress
  - Tachypnea
  - Inspiratory crackles

HISTORY
- Known close contact with suspected or confirmed case
- Close contact with infected poultry
- Travel within 10 days in high-risk area

DIAGNOSTIC TESTS & INTERPRETATION
Lab
Initial lab tests
- Complete blood count (CBC) with differential
- Liver profile
- Chemical profile
- Blood culture

- Lab abnormalities (2,4)[A]:
  - Leukopenia (mainly lymphopenia)
  - Thrombocytopenia (mild-to-moderate)
  - Elevated aminotransferases (slight-to-moderate)
  - Decreased leukocyte, platelet, and lymphocyte counts are associated with increased risk of death.

Imaging
Initial approach

Chest x-ray (CXR): Consolidation bilateral and multifocal (2,3)[A]:
- After 7 days: Patchy lobar and interstitial infiltrates
- Pleural effusions with cavitation (less common)

Follow-Up & Special Considerations
- Admit to negative-pressure room; if not available, cohort with other confirmed cases.
- Supplemental oxygen is essential to keep SaO_2 >90% (3)[A].

Diagnostic Procedures/Surgery
Lab confirmation of H5N1 virus is done case-by-case and requires 1 of the following (2,5)[A]:
- Positive influenza A/H5 (Asian lineage) virus real-time reverse transcription polymerase chain reaction (PCR) (Laboratory Response Network labs)
- Positive immunofluorescence test for antigen with use of monoclonal antibody against H5
- Positive isolation of H5N1 virus
- 4-fold rise in H5-specific antibody titer in paired serum samples

DIFFERENTIAL DIAGNOSIS
- Acute respiratory syndrome
- Influenza
- Pneumonia
- Severe acute respiratory syndrome

 TREATMENT

All patients should receive neuraminidase inhibitors as soon as possible pending results of diagnostic lab tests (within 24–48 hours after exposure).

MEDICATION
ALERT
The use of amantadine (Symmetrel) and rimantadine (Flumadine) is not considered beneficial unless access to newer agents is unavailable. Vaccine is available only through US Strategic National Stockpile to be distributed by public health officials.

First Line
- Treatment of mild-to-moderate cases (2,3)[C]: Oseltamivir (Tamiflu) 75 mg p.o. b.i.d. for 5 days
- Treatment of severe cases (2,3)[C]: Oseltamivir (Tamiflu) 150 mg b.i.d. for 7–10 days
- Postexposure prophylaxis (2,3)[C]: Oseltamivir (Tamiflu) 75 mg p.o. once a day for 7–10 days
- Adverse effects: Neuropsychiatric events (hallucinations, delirium, and abnormal behavior) have been reported. Monitor for abnormal behavior. Nausea, vomiting, diarrhea, abdominal pain, insomnia, bronchitis, vertigo.
- Drug interactions: Not metabolized by CYP 450; drug interactions with drugs metabolized by this system are unlikely. Does not affect metabolism of acetaminophen.
- Higher doses may be considered case-by-case if present with pneumonic illness.
- Monitor for resistance; some H5N1 viruses isolated show resistance to oseltamivir.

Pediatric Considerations
- Pediatric treatment is weight-based. Safety and efficacy not established for children <1 year of age (2,3)[C]:
  - Oseltamivir 30 mg p.o. b.i.d. for 5 days ≤15 kg
  - Oseltamivir 45 mg p.o. b.i.d. for 5 days >15–23 kg
  - Oseltamivir 60 mg p.o. b.i.d. for 5 days >23–40 kg
  - Oseltamivir 75 mg p.o. b.i.d. for 5 days >40 kg
- Postexposure prophylaxis (2,3)[C]:
  - Dosing is weight-based as above but administered once daily for 7–10 days.

Geriatric Considerations
- Renal impairment (2,3)[C]:
  – Creatinine clearance 10–30 mL/min
    ○ Treatment: Oseltamivir 75 mg/d p.o.
    ○ Postexposure prophylaxis: Oseltamivir 75 mg p.o. every other day or 30 mg p.o. daily
- Hepatic impairment (2,4)[C]:
  – No dosage adjustment needed

Pregnancy Considerations
- Oseltamivir is Category C
- Use with caution only if potential benefits outweigh possible risk
- Unknown if distributed in breast milk

Second Line
- Zanamivir (Relenza) is considered 2nd-line agent. Not recommended for patients with underlying respiratory disease (asthma, chronic obstructive pulmonary disease) (3)[C].
- Treatment (ages 13 to ≥65 years):
  – Zanamivir 10 mg (2 inhalations) b.i.d. for 5 days
- Postexposure prophylaxis (ages 13 to ≥65):
  – Zanamivir 10 mg (2 inhalations) once daily for 7–10 days.
- Adverse effects:
  – Hypersensitivity reactions: Bronchospasms and allergiclike reactions have occurred.
  – Diarrhea, nausea, vomiting, headache, dizziness, sinusitis, cough, throat infections
  – Some adverse effects due to lactose in powder of inhaler
- Drug interactions: Not metabolized by CYP 450; drug interactions with drugs metabolized by this system are unlikely.

Pediatric Considerations
- Zanamivir is not licensed for use in children <7 years of age for treatment and <5 years for prophylaxis (3)[C]
- Treatment (7–13 years of age): Zanamivir 10 mg (2 inhalations) b.i.d. for 5 days
- Prophylaxis (5–13 years of age): Zanamivir 10 mg (2 inhalations) once daily 7–10 days

Geriatric Considerations
No dosage adjustment for renal or hepatic impairment (3)[C]

Pregnancy Considerations
- Zanamivir is Category C
- Use with caution only if potential benefits outweigh possible risk
- Unknown if distributed in breast milk
- Other medications (2,4)[C]:
  – Broad-spectrum antibiotics: Follow hospital protocols for community-acquired pneumonia.
- High-dose corticosteroids use associated with increased mortality.
- Immunomodulating drugs: No clear evidence of benefits, not recommended

ADDITIONAL TREATMENT
General Measures
Ventilatory support within 48 hours (2,6)[B]

IN-PATIENT CONSIDERATIONS
Initial Stabilization
- Broad-spectrum antibiotics, antiviral agents, with or without corticosteroids until lab confirmation of H5N1 virus (3)[A]
- Ventilatory support within 48 hours (2,6)[B]

Admission Criteria
If known H5N1 activity in the community, or if patient has traveled to country with H5N1 activity, admit if patient presents with:
- Severe acute respiratory illness
- Serious unexplained illness (encephalopathy or diarrhea)

Nursing
- Use standard and droplet precautions.
- N-95 masks

Discharge Criteria
- If discharged early, family requires education of proper hand hygiene and infection-control measures (surgical mask).
- Postexposure prophylaxis given to family members

 ## ONGOING CARE

FOLLOW-UP RECOMMENDATIONS
Patient Monitoring
Clinical deterioration is rapid.

PATIENT EDUCATION
Hand hygiene, cough etiquette

PROGNOSIS
Mortality rate is high. Median time to death was 9 days (range 6–17 days) with or without treatment.

COMPLICATIONS
- Multiorgan failure, acute (2,4,5,6)[C]
- Renal dysfunction
- Cardiac compromise
- Cardiac dilatation, supraventricular
- Tachyarrhythmias
- Ventilator-associated pneumonia
- Pulmonary hemorrhage
- Pneumothorax
- Pancytopenia
- Reye syndrome
- Sepsis syndrome without documented bacteremia

REFERENCES

1. Pannwitz G, Wolf C, Harder T. Active surveillance for avian influenza virus infection in wild birds by analysis of avian fecal samples from the environment. *J Wildl Dis*. 2009;45:512–8.
2. Beigel JH, et al. Avian influenza A (H5N1) infections in humans. *N Engl J Med*. 2005;350:1374–1385.
3. World Health Organization. WHO Interim Guidelines for Avian Influenza Case Management. 2007. Accessed 4/12/2010 at http://www.searo.who.int/LinkFiles/Publication_CD-167-Interim-guidelines-AI.pdf.
4. World Health Organization. Clinical management of human infection with avian influenza A (H5N1) virus. August 15, 2007. Accessed 4/11/2010 at http://who.int/csr/disease/avian_influenza/guidelines/Clinical Management07.pdf.
5. Tran TH, Nguyen TL, Nguyen TD et al. Avian influenza A (H5N1) in 10 patients in Vietnam. *N Engl J Med*. 2004;350:1179–88.
6. Chotpitayasunondh T, Ungchusak K, Hanshaoworakul W et al. Human disease from influenza A (H5N1), Thailand, 2004. *Emerg Infect Dis*. 2005;11:201–9.

ADDITIONAL READING

Centers for Disease Control and Prevention CDC: Key facts about Avian Influenza (Bird Flu) and Avian Influenza (H5N1) Virus. Accessed 4/11/2010 at http://www.cdc.gov/flu/avian/gen-info/facts.

 ## CODES

ICD9
- 488.01 Influenza due to identified avian influenza virus with pneumonia
- 488.02 Influenza due to identified avian influenza virus with other respiratory manifestations
- 488.09 Influenza due to identified avian influenza virus with other manifestations

CLINICAL PEARLS

- Consider avian influenza in the differential diagnosis for patients presenting with acute febrile respiratory illness and recent travel to high-risk areas (especially Asia) or who have spent time on poultry farms.
- Oseltamivir is considered 1st-line antiviral treatment: May need double usual dosage in patients with pneumonia.
- Perform: CBC, CXR, rapid tests for Ag detection, nasopharyngeal swabs for PCR, blood cultures, AST/ALT/CD4.

BABESIOSIS

Eleftherios Mylonakis, MD
Vassiliki P. Syriopoulou, MD

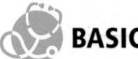 **BASICS**

DESCRIPTION
- Tickborne hemolytic disease that is caused by intraerythrocytic protozoan parasites of the genus *Babesia*
- Rarely reported outside the US:
  - Sporadic cases have been reported from a number of countries, including France, Italy, the former Yugoslavia, the United Kingdom, Ireland, the former Soviet Union, and Mexico.
  - In US, infections have been reported in many states, but most endemic areas are islands off the coast of Massachusetts (including Nantucket and Martha's Vineyard), New York (including Long Island, Shelter Island, and Fire Island), and in Connecticut. In these areas, asymptomatic human infection seems to be common.
- Incubation period of babesiosis varies from 5–33 days. Most patients do not recall recent tick exposure. After an infected blood transfusion, the incubation period can be up to 9 weeks.
- System(s) affected: Cardiovascular; Gastrointestinal; Hemic/Lymphatic/Immunologic; Musculoskeletal; Nervous; Pulmonary; Renal/Urologic

Geriatric Considerations
Morbidity and mortality are higher in patients >65.

EPIDEMIOLOGY
Predominant age: All ages; most patients present in their 40s or 50s.

Incidence
- Between 1968 and 1993, >450 *Babesia* infections were confirmed in US by blood smears or serologic testing. Prevalence is difficult to estimate because of lack of surveillance and because infections are often asymptomatic (1).
- In a recent 1-year seroconversion study of patients in New York State who were at high risk for tickborne diseases, antibodies to *B. microti* were seen in 7 of 671 participants (1%).

RISK FACTORS
- Exposure to endemic areas
- Transfusion-associated babesiosis and transplacental/perinatal transmission have been reported.
- High-level parasitemia is more common in asplenic patients. Such patients have been treated successfully with exchange transfusion in addition to drugs.

GENERAL PREVENTION
- Avoid endemic regions during the peak transmission months of May–September (especially relevant for asplenic or immunocompromised persons, in whom babesiosis can be a devastating illness).
- Using insect repellant is advised during outdoor activities, especially in wooded or grassy areas:
  - Products with 10–35% N-diethyl-meta-toluamide (DEET) will provide adequate protection under most conditions.
- Early removal of ticks is important; the tick must remain attached for at least 24 hours before the transmission of *B. microti* occurs. Daily self-examination is recommended for persons who engage in outdoor activities in endemic areas.
- Pets must be examined for ticks because they may carry ticks into the home.

ETIOLOGY
- *B. microti* (in US) and *B. divergens* and *B. bovis* (in Europe) cause most infections in humans. Recently, 1 case of *B. divergens* was reported in US.
- A previously unknown species of *Babesia* (WA-1) was isolated from an immunocompetent man in Washington State who had clinical babesiosis. Researchers also described another probable new *Babesia* species (MO1) associated with the 1st reported case of babesiosis acquired in Missouri. MO1 is probably distinct from *B. divergens*, but the two share morphologic, antigenic, and genetic characteristics.
- Ixodid (or hard-bodied) ticks, in particular, *Ixodes dammini* (*Ixodes scapularis*) and *I. ricinus*, are the vectors of the parasite.

COMMONLY ASSOCIATED CONDITIONS
- Coinfection with *Borrelia burgdorferi* and *B. microti* is relatively common in endemic areas.
- Coinfection with *Ehrlichia* sp. may also be seen. 3 species of *Ehrlichia* have been described that infect humans: *E. chaffeensis*, *E. phagocytophila*, and *E. ewingii*:
  - Typically, patients have a nonspecific febrile illness.
  - Rash is uncommon with human granulocytic ehrlichiosis, but common with human monocytic ehrlichiosis.
  - Laboratory findings often include leukopenia, thrombocytopenia, and increases in serum hepatic enzyme activities (2).

 DIAGNOSIS

HISTORY
- High fever [up to 40°C (104°F)]
- Chills
- Diaphoresis
- Gastrointestinal (anorexia, nausea, abdominal pain, vomiting, diarrhea)
- Generalized weakness
- Fatigue
- Myalgia
- Respiratory (cough, shortness of breath)
- Headache

PHYSICAL EXAM
- Hepatomegaly and splenomegaly or evidence of shock
- Rash (uncommon)
- Central nervous system involvement includes headache, photophobia, neck and back stiffness, altered sensorium, emotional lability
- Jaundice and dark urine may develop later in course of illness.

DIAGNOSTIC TESTS & INTERPRETATION
Lab
Initial lab tests
- Mild-to-severe hemolytic anemia (common nonspecific finding)
- Normal-to-slightly depressed leukocyte count (common nonspecific finding)
- Typical morphologic picture on the blood smear
- A Wright- or Giemsa-stained peripheral blood smear is most commonly used to demonstrate the presence of intraerythrocytic parasites.
- Rarely, tetrads of merozoites are visible.
- Serologic evaluation with the indirect immunofluorescent antibody test with use of *B. microti* antigen is available in a few laboratories:
  - The cut-off titer for determination of a positive result varies with the particular laboratory protocol used, but in most laboratories, titers of >1:64 are considered consistent with *B. microti* infection.
  - 10–20-fold higher titers can be observed in the acute setting, with a gradual decline over weeks to months:
    - The correlation between the level of the titer and the severity of symptoms is poor.
- Detection of B. microti by PCR is more sensitive and equally specific for the diagnosis of acute cases, in comparison with direct smear examination and hamster inoculation. PCR-based methods may also be indicated for monitoring of the infection.

Follow-Up & Special Considerations
Monitoring the degree of intraerythrocytic parasitemia can help guide treatment.

Diagnostic Procedures/Surgery
Based on typical morphologic picture on the blood smear in conjunction with epidemiologic information

DIFFERENTIAL DIAGNOSIS
- Bacterial sepsis
- Hepatitis
- Lyme disease
- Ehrlichiosis
- Leishmaniasis
- Malaria

TREATMENT

MEDICATION

First Line
Atovaquone (Mepron): Suspension 750 mg b.i.d. plus azithromycin (Zithromax) 500–1,000 mg/d (3)[B]

Second Line
- Combination of quinine sulfate (Quinamm): 650 mg orally t.i.d. and clindamycin (Cleocin) 600 mg orally t.i.d., or 1.2 g parenterally b.i.d. for 7–10 days is the most commonly used treatment. (Pediatric: Dosage is 20–40 mg/kg/d for quinine and 25 mg/kg/d for clindamycin.)
- Several other drugs have been evaluated, including tetracycline, primaquine, sulfadiazine (Microsulfon), and pyrimethamine (Fansidar). Results have varied. Pentamidine (Pentam) has proved to be moderately effective in diminishing symptoms and decreasing parasitemia.
- Precautions: Clindamycin can lead to *Clostridium difficile*-associated diarrhea.

ADDITIONAL TREATMENT

General Measures
- In areas endemic for Lyme disease and ehrlichiosis, it may be advisable to add doxycycline (Vibramycin) 100 mg b.i.d. p.o. in the management of patients with babesiosis until serologic testing is completed.
- Note that some resistance is emerging to standard treatment in patients with severe immunocompromise (4).

Issues for Referral
Exchange transfusion, together with antibabesial chemotherapy, may be necessary in critically ill patients. This treatment is usually reserved for patients who are extremely ill (blood parasitemia >10%, massive hemolysis, and asplenia).

ONGOING CARE

FOLLOW-UP RECOMMENDATIONS
- When left untreated, silent babesial infection may persist for months or even years.
- 139 hospitalized cases in New York State between 1982 and 1993:
  – 9 patients (6.5%) died.
  – 25% of the patients were admitted to the intensive care unit.
  – 25% of the patients required hospitalization for >14 days.
- Alkaline phosphatase levels >125 U/L, white blood cell counts $>5 \times 10^9$/L, history of cardiac abnormality, history of splenectomy, presence of heart murmur, and parasitemia values of 4% or higher were associated with disease severity.

Patient Monitoring
Monitor for complications (congestive heart failure [CHF], etc.) and follow parasitemia as needed.

COMPLICATIONS
- CHF
- Disseminated intravascular coagulation
- Acute respiratory distress syndrome (can occur even a few days after the onset of effective antimicrobial treatment)
- Renal failure and myocardial infarction also have been associated with severe babesiosis.

REFERENCES

1. Persing DH, Herwaldt BL, Glaser C, et al. Infection with a babesia-like organism in northern California. *N Engl J Med*. 1995;332:298–303.
2. Mylonakis E. When to suspect and how to monitor babesiosis. *Am Fam Physician*. 2001;63:1969–74.
3. Krause PJ, Lepore T, Sikand VK, et al. Atovaquone and azithromycin for the treatment of babesiosis. *N Engl J Med*. 2000;343:1454–8.
4. Wormser GP, Prasad A, Neuhaus E, Joshi S, Nowakowski J, Nelson J, Mittleman A, Aguero-Rosenfeld M, Topal J, Krause PJ et al. Emergence of resistance to azithromycin-atovaquone in immunocompromised patients with Babesia microti infection. *Clin Infect Dis*. 2010;50:381–6.

ADDITIONAL READING

- Beattie JF, Michelson ML, Holman PJ. Acute babesiosis caused by Babesia divergens in a resident of Kentucky. *N Engl J Med*. 2002;347:697–8.
- Berman KH, Blue DE, Smith DS, et al. Fatal case of babesiosis in postliver transplant patient. *Transplantation*. 2009;87:452–3.

- Gelfand JA. Babesia species. In: Mandell GL, et al., eds. *Mandell, Douglas, and Bennett's Principles and Practice of Infectious Diseases*, 6th ed. New York: Churchill Livingstone, 2005:3209–15.
- Gubernot DM, Lucey CT, Lee KC, et al. Babesia Infection through Blood Transfusions: Reports Received by the US Food and Drug Administration, 1997-2007. *Clin Infect Dis*. 2008.
- Gutman JD, Kotton CN, Kratz A. Case records of the Massachusetts General Hospital. Weekly clinicopathological exercises. Case 29-2003. A 60-year-old man with fever, rigors, and sweats. *N Engl J Med*. 2003;349:1168–75.
- Krause PJ, Gewurz BE, Hill D, et al. Persistent and relapsing babesiosis in immunocompromised patients. *Clin Infect Dis*. 2008;46:370–6.
- Wormser GP, Dattwyler RJ, Shapiro ED, et al. The clinical assessment, treatment, and prevention of lyme disease, human granulocytic anaplasmosis, and babesiosis: clinical practice guidelines by the Infectious Diseases Society of America. *Clin Infect Dis*. 2006;43:1089–134.

CODES

ICD9
088.82 Babesiosis

CLINICAL PEARLS
- High-level parasitemia is more common in asplenic patients.
- 1st-line treatment is atovaquone plus azithromycin.
- Coinfection with *B. burgdorferi* is relatively common in endemic areas. Coinfection with *Ehrlichia* species may also be seen. In areas endemic for Lyme disease and ehrlichiosis, it may be advisable to add doxycycline in the management of patients with babesiosis until serologic testing is completed.
- When left untreated, silent babesial infection may persist for months or even years.
- Tick must remain in place for 24 hours to transmit infection, so daily self-screening of skin is protective.

BACK PAIN, LOW
Christopher Garofalo, MD

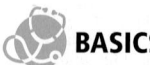 **BASICS**

DESCRIPTION
- Mechanical low back pain (LBP) is generally a benign and self-limiting condition responsive to conservative measures that include maintaining activity while using short-term pharmacologic therapy.
- Patients typically present with pain, muscle tension, or stiffness at the posterior belt line with occasional referred pain to the buttocks and/or posterior thighs; symptoms are often the result of the mechanical stresses and functional demands placed on the low back area by everyday activities.
- For most patients, pain is of short duration, and complete recovery is expected within 6 weeks.
- The primary goal is to rule out red-flag symptoms that may be indicative of possible underlying spinal pathology or nerve root problems; when such symptoms are absent, the patient is considered to have nonspecific LBP.
- System(s) affected: Musculoskeletal; Nervous
- Synonym(s): Low back syndrome; Lumbar strain/sprain; Lumbago

Geriatric Considerations
Tumors, degenerative conditions, fractures, and stenosis are common.

Pediatric Considerations
The presence of LBP is considered a red-flag symptom. A thorough workup is imperative.

Pregnancy Considerations
Pregnancy is commonly associated with LBP and/or sciatica; treatment is conservative.

EPIDEMIOLOGY
Incidence
- 90% of Americans experience mechanical LBP some time in their life.
- LBP is one of the most common primary-care complaints.
- Repetitive episodes are common.
- Predominant age: ≥25 years
- Predominant sex: Male = Female

RISK FACTORS
- Age
- Activity (e.g., heavy lifting, bending, twisting)
- Smoking
- Obesity
- Vibration (e.g., driving motor vehicles)
- Sedentary lifestyle
- Psychosocial factors such as increased stress, anxiety, or depressed mood

GENERAL PREVENTION
- Maintaining physical fitness
- Weight loss
- Smoking cessation
- Stress reduction
- Avoidance of aggravating tasks (e.g., heavy lifting, bending, twisting, sudden unexpected movements, or any combination of these tasks)

ETIOLOGY
- Normal aging process of musculoskeletal system aggravates an acute event.
- Degenerative joint disease of LS spine
- In primary-care setting, <15% of LBP patients have identifiable underlying disease.

COMMONLY ASSOCIATED CONDITIONS
- Deconditioning, obesity
- Psychosocial disease
- Compression fracture

 DIAGNOSIS

HISTORY
- Onset of pain begins either suddenly after injury or gradually over the next 24 h.
- Occasional radiation of pain to buttocks and/or posterior thighs stopping at knees
- Pain pattern is referred rather than radicular.
- Back pain is worse than leg pain.
- Pain is aggravated by back motion, sitting, standing, lifting, bending, and twisting.
- Pain is relieved by rest.
- Bowel and bladder function are preserved.
- Psychosocial stressors at work and/or home may be present.
- Medical history and previous injuries should be noted.
- Red flags (possible etiology):
  - Age >50 years or <20 years (neoplastic)
  - History of cancer (carcinoma recurrence)
  - Night sweats or weight loss (neoplasm, rheumatologic)
  - Incontinence or saddle anesthesia (nerve compromise/cauda equina syndrome)
  - Recent bacterial infection (infectious)
  - Pain worse when supine (rheumatologic, nerve compromise)
  - History of trauma (fracture)

PHYSICAL EXAM
- Observation reveals preferred posture, facial expressions, and pain behaviors.
- Normal motor, sensory, and reflex examinations
- Decreased lumbar range of motion, paraspinous musculature tenderness, and spasm
- Nerve root stretch tests are often negative.
- Straight-leg raise (causing spinal motion) may increase LBP, but not leg pain.

DIAGNOSTIC TESTS & INTERPRETATION
Lab
Initial lab tests
- Not typically indicated on initial presentation (1)
- For those with red flags, pain that worsens, persists for >6 weeks, and/or is recalcitrant to conservative treatment measures, consider the following:
  - CBC with differential
  - Erythrocyte sedimentation rate (ESR)
  - Alkaline and acid phosphatase
  - Serum calcium
  - Serum protein electrophoresis
- Special tests: System-directed investigation

Imaging
Initial approach
- Plain radiographs:
  - Not recommended in the absence of red flags (2)[B]
  - Indicated for persistent symptoms (>6 weeks), age >50 years, systemic symptoms, presence of neurologic deficits or trauma, history of cancer, use of immunosuppressants, IV drug abuse, or if abnormalities such as ankylosing spondylitis are suspected
  - Anteroposterior, lateral, spot lateral of L5–S1, and oblique films are included in routine lumbosacral series.
- Bone scan (scintigraphy): Technetium-99m-labeled phosphorus to rule out fractures, infections, or metastases

Diagnostic Procedures/Surgery
MRI and CT scan indicated only for persistent symptoms, neurologic deficits, and/or suspected infection or malignancy:
- MRI is useful for visualization of soft tissue.
- CT scan is useful for visualization of bony anatomy.

DIFFERENTIAL DIAGNOSIS
- Structural:
  - Lumbar strain/sprain
  - Herniated lumbar intervertebral disk
  - Degenerative disk disease
  - Degenerative segmental instability
  - Spinal stenosis
  - Spondylolisthesis
  - Congenital disease: Severe kyphosis, severe scoliosis
  - Fractures
- Inflammatory:
  - Ankylosing spondylitis and related inflammatory spondylopathies
  - Infection: Vertebral osteomyelitis
  - Rheumatoid arthritis
- Neoplastic:
  - Primary tumors
  - Metastases
- Referred pain:
  - Orthopedic: Osteoarthritis of hip
  - Sacroiliac joint disease
  - GI: Duodenal ulcer, chronic pancreatitis, cholecystitis, irritable bowel syndrome, diverticulitis
  - Genitourinary: Pyelonephritis, nephrolithiasis, prostatism
  - Gynecologic: Pregnancy, endometriosis, ovarian cystic disease, pelvic inflammatory disease
  - Cardiovascular: Abdominal aortic aneurysm, vascular claudication

TREATMENT

MEDICATION

First Line

- Nonsteroidal anti-inflammatory drugs (NSAIDs):
  - Agents are considered equally effective (3)[A]:
    ○ Ibuprofen: 800 mg PO q6h × 10 days, then as needed (maximum 3,200 mg/d)
    ○ Naproxen: 500 mg PO b.i.d. × 10 days, then as needed (maximum 1,500 mg/d)
  - Adverse reactions: Fluid retention, rash, GI discomfort, dizziness, GI bleeding, acute renal failure
  - Contraindications: Treatment of perioperative pain in the setting of coronary artery bypass grafting (CABG); aspirin allergy
  - Precautions: High risk of cardiovascular event, high risk of GI bleeding, history of ulcer disease, elderly, renal disease
  - Possible interactions: Antiplatelets, ACE inhibitors, lithium, low-molecular-weight heparin
- COX-2 inhibitors are as effective as traditional NSAIDs and have fewer side effects (3)[A]. Precautions: Patients with cardiovascular concerns
- Muscle relaxants:
  - Use with caution (avoid alcohol, no driving or operating heavy machinery); comparative efficacy to NSAIDs is unknown (4)[A]:
    ○ Cyclobenzaprine (Flexeril): 10 mg PO at bedtime or q8h (maximum 60 mg/d)
    ○ Carisoprodol (Soma): 350 mg PO t.i.d. and at bedtime
    ○ Metaxalone (Skelaxin): 800 mg PO t.i.d.–q.i.d.
  - Adverse reactions: Sedation, N/V, dizziness
  - Contraindications:
    ○ Cyclobenzaprine: Arrhythmias, congestive heart failure, hyperthyroidism, concomitant monoamine oxidase inhibitors
    ○ Carisoprodol: Acute intermittent porphyria
    ○ Metaxalone: Anemia, renal or hepatic impairment
  - Precautions: Concomitant use of CNS depressants; history of substance abuse
  - Possible interactions: CNS depressants

Second Line

Short-acting combination opioid analgesic products should be considered only for moderate–severe pain not controlled with NSAIDs and/or muscle relaxants alone (5)[B].

ALERT

Use of narcotics in acute LBP may increase risk of progression to chronic LBP.

ADDITIONAL TREATMENT

General Measures

- Outpatient management is appropriate.
- Activity modification as appropriate
- Short-term nonopioid analgesics at fixed time intervals: NSAIDs and/or muscle relaxants
- Avoid short-acting combination opioid analgesic products (e.g., Vicodin); associated with inducing chronic LBP.
- Use of opioid analgesics does not improve return-to-work status.

Issues for Referral

Refer patients with progressive motor and sensory symptoms and/or evidence of infection, tumor, or fracture to a neurosurgeon or ER for further evaluation.

Additional Therapies

There is strong evidence that an intensive individual education session is as effective as other interventions in short- and long-term return to work (6)[A].

COMPLEMENTARY AND ALTERNATIVE MEDICINE

- Chiropractic manipulation (5)[B]
- Devil's claw, white willow bark, and capsaicin have demonstrated efficacy versus placebo for acute episodes of chronic LBP (7)[B].

IN-PATIENT CONSIDERATIONS

Admission Criteria

Limit to patients who require surgical procedures for underlying causes.

ONGOING CARE

FOLLOW-UP RECOMMENDATIONS

- Bed rest is *not* recommended (5)[A].
- Restricted activities for 3–6 weeks.
- Back-specific exercises should be avoided.
- Activities of daily living should be resumed as soon as possible (5)[A].

Patient Monitoring

- Estimated duration of care is 1–6 weeks.
  - Schedule follow-up at 2–4 weeks.
  - Assess the following at each follow-up visit: Pain, functional status, and medication-related adverse effects.
- Reevaluate for possible underlying causes if relief does not occur.
- Patients should be encouraged to maintain normal levels of activity.
- Consider ongoing physical therapy.

DIET

Weight reduction, if appropriate

PATIENT EDUCATION

Advise the patient to stay active, use medication as prescribed, and discuss adverse drug effects.

PROGNOSIS

- Usually self-limiting; recovery is expected within 6 weeks in 90% of patients (4).
- Symptoms can recur in 50–80% of patients within the 1st year.
- Adverse psychosocial factors to resolving back pain:
  - Pending litigation or compensation
  - Prolonged use of habit-forming medications or alcohol
  - Poor coping strategies, depressed or hostile patient
  - Job dissatisfaction

COMPLICATIONS

- Chronic LBP
- Persistent psychosocial impairment

REFERENCES

1. Chou R, Qaseem A, Snow V, et al. Diagnosis and treatment of low back pain: a joint clinical practice guideline from the American College of Physicians and the American Pain Society. *Ann Intern Med*. 2007;147:478–91.
2. Jarvik JG, Deyo RA. Diagnostic evaluation of low back pain with emphasis on imaging. *Ann Intern Med*. 2002;137:586–97.
3. Roelofs PDDM, Deyo RA, Koes BW et al. Non-steroidal antiinflammatory drugs for low back pain. *Cochrane Database of Systematic Reviews*. 2008; 1:CD000396. DOI:10.1002/14651858. CD000396.pub3.
4. van Tulder MW, Touray T, Furlan AD et al. Muscle relaxants for non-specific low back pain. *Cochrane Database of Syst Rev*. 2006;(3).
5. Koes BW, van Tulder MW, Thomas S. Diagnosis and treatment of low back pain. *BMJ*. 2006;332: 1430–4.
6. Engers AJ, Jellema P, Wensing M et al. Individual patient education for low back pain. *Cochrane Database of Systematic Reviews*. 2008(1): CD004057. DOI:10.1002/14651858. CD004057.pub3.
7. Gagnier JJ, van Tulder MW, Berman B, et al. Herbal medicine for low back pain. *Cochrane Database Syst Rev*. 2006;19(2).

See Also (Topic, Algorithm, Electronic Media Element)

Lumbar (intervertebral) disk disorders
Algorithm: Low Back Pain, Acute

CODES

ICD9
724.2 Lumbago

CLINICAL PEARLS

- Red flags include age <20 years or >55 years, nonmechanical pain, night sweats and/or weight loss, temperature >38°C, history of cancer, history of trauma, presence of neurologic deficits, and pain worse when supine.
- Bed rest is not recommended; patients are encouraged to maintain activity.
- NSAIDs are beneficial and should be considered as 1st-line therapy.

BAKER CYST
Chris Wheelock, MD

 BASICS

DESCRIPTION
- A fluid-filled synovial sac arising in the popliteal fossa
- Distention of the gastrocnemial-semimembranous bursa
- Can be unilateral or bilateral
- Primary cysts are a distention of the bursa arising independently without an intra-articular disorder
- Secondary cysts occur if a communication exists between the bursa and knee joint, allowing articular fluid to fill the cyst. Pathologic joint processes can also be transmitted in this manner.
- Associated with synovial inflammation
- Synonym: Popliteal cyst

EPIDEMIOLOGY
Incidence
- Bimodal distribution: Children ages 4–7, and adults increasing with age
- Primary cysts usually seen in children under 15 years of age
- Secondary cysts seen in the adult population

Prevalence
- Varies by study
- Studies report a prevalence of 19–47% in symptomatic knees, 2–5% in asymptomatic knees
- In children, 6.3% in symptomatic knees, 2.4% in asymptomatic knees

RISK FACTORS
- Osteoarthritis of knee (most common) (1)[B]
- Rheumatoid arthritis
- Meniscal degeneration or tear
- Advancing age
- Ligamentous insufficiency

PATHOPHYSIOLOGY
- Extension or herniation of synovial membrane of the knee joint capsule or connection of normal bursa with the joint capsule
- May be the result of increased intra-articular pressure

- Commonly seen with knee effusions
- Direct trauma to the bursa likely the primary cause in children since there is no communication between the bursa and the joint in children
- A valve-like mechanism allowing one-way passage of fluid from the joint to the bursal connection has been described.

ETIOLOGY
Associated intra-articular pathological findings include:
- Meniscal tears, posterior horn
- ACL insufficiency
- Degenerative articular cartilage lesions
- Rheumatoid arthritis
- Osteoarthritis
- Osteochondritis
- Other potential factors: Infectious arthritis, polyarthritis, villonodular synovitis, and connective tissue diseases

COMMONLY ASSOCIATED CONDITIONS
Any condition causing knee joint effusion

 DIAGNOSIS

HISTORY
- Painless mass arising in the popliteal fossa
- Most cysts are asymptomatic
- Painful if cyst ruptures
- May report restricted range of motion or tightness with knee flexion
- Large cysts may cause entrapment neuropathy of the tibial nerve.
- Vascular compression, most commonly of the popliteal vein, may produce claudication or thrombophlebitis.
- Activity will alter the cyst size.

PHYSICAL EXAM
- Examine in full extension and 90° of flexion
- Foucher sign: Mass increases with extension and disappears with flexion.
- Most commonly found in medial aspect of popliteal fossa lateral to the head of the gastrocnemius and medial to the neurovascular bundle.
- Mass may be fluctuant or tender.
- Transillumination can distinguish cyst from solid mass.
- Ruptured cyst typically painful with associated swelling over calf and medial malleolus, pseudothrombophlebitis

DIAGNOSTIC TESTS & INTERPRETATION
Lab
Initial lab tests
- CBC, sedimentation rate if suspicious of septic arthritis
- Send aspirate for cell count to determine nature of effusion: Infectious, inflammatory, or mechanical.

Follow-Up & Special Considerations
In children, consider observation before invasive testing.

Imaging
Initial approach

- Ultrasound confirms presence and size; with Doppler can differentiate Baker cysts from popliteal vessel aneurysms or soft tissue tumors (2)[B].
- MRI is useful to assess for causal derangements of internal joint structures.
- Radiographs may show soft tissue density posteriorly.
- Arthrography may demonstrate communication with joint capsule, or rupture.
- CT–arthrography together is superior in visualizing cystic details and can help separate lipomas, aneurysms, and malignancies from cysts.

DIFFERENTIAL DIAGNOSIS

- Infection/abscess
- Lipoma
- Liposarcoma
- Fibroma
- Fibrosarcoma
- Hematoma
- Deep venous thrombosis
- Vascular tumor
- Popliteal vein varices
- Xanthoma
- Aneurysm (rare)
- Ganglion cyst
- Any condition causing synovitis
- Thrombophlebitis
- Muscular herniation (rare, related to trauma)

 TREATMENT

MEDICATION

- Once etiology is identified from cellular fluid examination, treat the underlying condition
- Analgesics, NSAIDS for symptomatic relief

ADDITIONAL TREATMENT

General Measures

- No treatment if cyst is asymptomatic
- Compressive wrap or sleeve may be used for comfort

Additional Therapies

- Physical therapy improves knee range of motion and strength, particularly with coexisting pathology
- Temporary relief with needle aspiration, recurrence common
- Improvement in joint range of motion, knee pain, swelling, accompanied reduction in bursa size has been shown after intra-articular or intracystic corticosteroid injection (2)[B]
- Sclerotherapy injections of ethanol or dextrose/sodium morrhuate shown to have good results in studies with small sample sizes (3)[B]

 SURGERY/OTHER PROCEDURES

- Consider excision when symptoms persist despite treatment or no etiology is found.
- Recurrence after standard surgery is common and is highest when chondral lesions are present (4)[B].
- A modified surgical technique in children has been proven effective without recurrence (5)[B].
- Excision via arthroscopy or open procedure often requires concomitant treatment of underlying pathology (6)[B].

 ONGOING CARE

PROGNOSIS

- Variable
- Many cysts remain asymptomatic.
- Some will regress or resolve with treatment of underlying etiology
- In children, most resolve without treatment.

COMPLICATIONS

- Compartment syndrome in ruptured cyst
- Thrombophlebitis from compression of the popliteal vein
- Infection of popliteal cyst
- Hemorrhage into cyst if on anticoagulants

REFERENCES

1. Chatzopoulos D, Moralidis E, Markou P, et al. Baker's cysts in knees with chronic osteoarthritic pain: a clinical, ultrasonographic, radiographic and scintigraphic evaluation. *Rheumatol Int.* 2008 Jun 27.
2. Acebes JC, Sanchez-Pernaute O, Diaz-Oca A, et al. Ultrasonographic Assessment of Baker's Cysts after Intra-articular Corticosteroid Injection in Knee Osteoarthritis. *J Clin Ultrasound.* 2006;34:113–7.
3. Centeno CJ, Schultz J, Freeman M, et al. Sclerotherapy of Baker's Cyst with Imaging Confirmation of Resolution. *Pain Physician.* 2008;11:257–61.
4. Rupp S, Seil R, et al. Popliteal cysts in adults: Prevalence, associated intraarticular lesions, and results after arthroscopic treatment. *Am Sport Med.* 2002;30(1):112–5.
5. Chen J-C, Cheng-Chang L, Lu Y-M, et al. A modified surgical method for treating Baker's cyst in children. *The Knee.* 2008;15:9–14.
6. Handy JR. Popliteal cysts in adults: A review. *Semin Arthritis Rheu.* 2001;31(2):108–18.

ADDITIONAL READING

- Fritschy D, Fasel J, Imbert J, et al. The popliteal cyst. *Knee Surg Sports Traumatol Arthosc.* 2006;14: 623–8.
- Marra MD, Crema MD, Chung M, et al. MRI features of cystic lesions around the knee. *The Knee.* 2008 Jun 16.
- Seil R, Rupp S, et al. Prevalence of popliteal cysts in children: A sonographic study and review of the literature. *Arch Ortho Traum Su.* 1999;119:73–5.
- Van Rhijn L, Jansen E, Pruijs H. Long term follow up of conservatively treated popliteal cysts in children. *Journal of Pediatric Orthopedics Part B.* 2000;9: 62–64.

See Also (Topic, Algorithm, Electronic Media Element)

Algorithm: Knee Pain

CODES

ICD9
727.51 Synovial cyst of popliteal space

CLINICAL PEARLS

- In children, it is acceptable to wait and observe.
- Treat underlying cause.
- Pain and swelling over the medial malleolus is classic for cyst rupture, also known as pseudothrombophlebitis.

BALANITIS

James P. Miller, MD
Timothy L. Black, MD

 BASICS

DESCRIPTION
- Balanitis is an inflammation of the glans penis.
- Posthitis is an inflammation of the foreskin.
- Balanitis xerotica obliterans (BXO) is lichen sclerosis of the glans penis (uncommon).
- System(s) affected: Reproductive; Skin/Exocrine

Geriatric Considerations
Condom catheters can predispose to balanitis.

Pediatric Considerations
Oral antibiotics predispose male infants to *Candida balanitis*.

EPIDEMIOLOGY
- Predominant age: Adult
- Predominant gender: Male only

RISK FACTORS
- Presence of foreskin
- Morbid obesity
- Poor hygiene
- Diabetes
- Nursing home environment

GENERAL PREVENTION
- Proper hygiene and avoidance of allergens
- Circumcision

ETIOLOGY
- Allergic reaction (condom latex, contraceptive jelly)
- Infections (*C. albicans, Borrelia vincentii*, streptococci, *Trichomonas*)
- Fixed-drug eruption (sulfa, tetracycline)
- Plasma cell infiltration (Zoon balanitis)
- Autodigestion by activated pancreatic transplant exocrine enzymes

 DIAGNOSIS

HISTORY
- Pain
- Drainage
- Dysuria

PHYSICAL EXAM
- Erythema
- Edema
- Discharge
- Ulceration
- Plaque

DIAGNOSTIC TESTS & INTERPRETATION
Lab
- Microbiology culture
- Wet mount
- Serology for syphilis
- Serum glucose

Initial lab tests
- Gram stain
- Wet prep

Diagnostic Procedures/Surgery
Biopsy, if persistent

Pathological Findings
Plasma cells infiltration with Zoon balanitis

DIFFERENTIAL DIAGNOSIS
- Leukoplakia
- Lichen planus
- Psoriasis
- Reiter syndrome
- Lichen sclerosus et atrophicus
- Erythroplasia of Queyrat
- Balanitis xerotica obliterans (BXO)

 TREATMENT

MEDICATION
- Antifungal:
  - Clotrimazole (Lotrimin), 1% b.i.d.
  - Nystatin (Mycostatin), b.i.d.–q.i.d.
  - Fluconazole, 150-mg single dose (1)[B]

- Antibacterial:
  - Bacitracin, q.i.d.
  - Neomycin-polymyxin B-bacitracin (Neosporin), q.i.d.
  - If cellulitis, cephalosporin or sulfa drug PO or parenteral:
    ○ Dermatitis: Topical steroids q.i.d.
    ○ Zoon balanitis: Topical steroids q.i.d.
- BXO:
  - 0.05% betamethasone b.i.d. (2)[B]
  - 0.1% tacrolimus b.i.d. (3)[C]

ADDITIONAL TREATMENT
General Measures
- Appropriate health care: Outpatient
- Warm compresses or sitz baths
- Local hygiene

Issues for Referral
Recurrent infections or development of meatal stenosis

SURGERY/OTHER PROCEDURES
Consider circumcision as preventive measure.

IN-PATIENT CONSIDERATIONS
Admission Criteria
- Uncontrolled diabetes
- Sepsis

Nursing
Appropriate hygiene if condom catheters are used

Discharge Criteria
Resolution of problem

ONGOING CARE
FOLLOW-UP RECOMMENDATIONS
Patient Monitoring
- Every 1–2 weeks until etiology has been established
- Persistent balanitis may require biopsy to rule out malignancy or BXO.

DIET
Weight reduction, if obese

PATIENT EDUCATION
- Need for appropriate hygiene
- Avoidance of known allergens

PROGNOSIS
Should resolve with appropriate treatment

COMPLICATIONS
- Meatal stenosis
- Premalignant changes from chronic irritation
- Urinary tract infections

REFERENCES

1. Stary A, Soeltz-Szoets J, Ziegler C, et al. Comparison of the efficacy and safety of oral fluconazole and topical clotrimazole in patients with candida balanitis. *Genitourin Med*. 1996;72:98–102.
2. Kiss A, Csontai A, Pirót L, et al. The response of balanitis xerotica obliterans to local steroid application compared with placebo in children. *J Urol*. 2001;165:219–20.
3. Pandher BS, Rustin MH, Kaisary AV. Treatment of balanitis xerotica obliterans with topical tacrolimus. *J Urol*. 2003;170:923.

See Also (Topic, Algorithm, Electronic Media Element)
Reiter Syndrome

CODES

ICD9
- 112.2 Candidiasis of other urogenital sites
- 607.1 Balanoposthitis

CLINICAL PEARLS

- With recurrent infections and a plaque, a biopsy should be done to rule out BXO or malignancy.
- If there is a true phimosis that interferes with appropriate hygiene, treatment of the phimosis with steroids or circumcision should be performed to help with hygiene.

BAROTRAUMA OF THE MIDDLE EAR, SINUSES, AND LUNG

Michele Roberts, MD, PhD
Jeremy Golding, MD

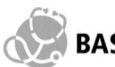 BASICS

DESCRIPTION

- Physical damage to tissue lining an enclosed body cavity resulting from an imbalance between ambient pressure and pressure within the cavity.
- Cavities at greatest risk for barotrauma include the middle ear (otic barotrauma), paranasal sinuses (sinus barotrauma), and lungs (pulmonary barotrauma).
- Otic and sinus barotrauma are associated with rapid or extreme changes in environmental pressure, as might result from air travel, mountain climbing, or scuba diving, especially in the presence of nasal congestion or eustachian tube dysfunction of any etiology:
  - Pressure changes with failure of eustachian tube to equilibrate pressure may distort the tympanic membrane (TM), causing discomfort and injury.
  - Rupture of round or oval membrane may cause inner ear barotrauma, vertigo, and sensorineural hearing loss.
- Pulmonary barotrauma:
  - An iatrogenic complication of mechanical ventilation
  - Also a complication of scuba diving
- Dental barotrauma is seen occasionally in scuba divers in whom small pockets of air trapped in dental work can cause rupture of teeth
- System(s) affected: Ear/Nose/Throat (ENT); Pulmonary
- Synonym(s): Dysbarism; aerotitis; otitic barotrauma; middle ear barotrauma

ALERT
- Dizziness and sensorineural hearing loss warrant immediate ENT referral for inner ear involvement.
- Valsalva maneuver can spread nasopharyngeal infection into the middle ear.
- Vertigo and hearing loss may cause disorientation.

EPIDEMIOLOGY
- Predominant age: All ages
- Predominant sex: Male = Female

Incidence
- Pulmonary barotrauma is the 2nd leading cause of death among divers.
- Otic barotrauma is common in air travel, especially among flight personnel.
- Pulmonary barotrauma is noted in 3% of mechanically ventilated patients.

Pediatric Considerations
- Children have difficulty opening the eustachian tube and have frequent upper respiratory infections. This combination results in higher risk for otic or sinus barotraumas at small pressure changes, as compared with adults.
- Mechanical ventilation of neonates is associated with barotrauma contributing to bronchopulmonary dysplasia.

Pregnancy Considerations
Increased nasal congestion in pregnancy increases risk of barotitis media.

RISK FACTORS
- Otic or sinus:
  - Participation in high-risk activities without adequate pressure equilibration:
    - Scuba diving, especially with rapid ascent or breath-holding
    - Airplane flight (especially high performance)
    - Sky diving
    - High-altitude travel or elevator rides
    - Underwater employment
    - High-impact sports: Boxing, soccer, water skiing
  - Upper respiratory infection: Sinusitis, rhinitis, tonsillitis, adenoiditis, otitis media
  - Nasal congestion or allergic rhinitis
  - Any cause of eustachian tube dysfunction
  - Exposure to blasting
  - Pregnancy (associated nasal congestion)
  - Anatomic obstruction in the nasopharynx:
    - Deviated nasal septum
    - Nasal polyps
    - Congenital anomalies, including cleft palate
  - Trauma to ear
- Pulmonary:
  - Iatrogenic:
    - Mechanical ventilation, especially in the presence of asthma, chronic interstitial lung disease, acute respiratory distress syndrome
    - Hyperbaric oxygen therapy
  - Scuba diving or other underwater activities
  - Air travel in people with preexisting pulmonary pathology

GENERAL PREVENTION
- Pulmonary barotrauma:
  - Judicious use of mechanical ventilation and hyperbaric oxygen therapy
  - In scuba diving, avoidance of breath-holding during ascent
- Otic barotrauma:
  - Avoidance of altitude changes or scuba diving when at risk for eustachian tube dysfunction
  - Treatment of upper respiratory congestion
- Equilibration of pressure by Valsalva, yawning, swallowing, drinking, chewing gum

ETIOLOGY
- For any gas at a constant temperature, the volume of the gas varies inversely with the pressure. When gas is trapped in a confined space such as the middle ear, paranasal sinus, or lungs, a sudden decrease in ambient pressure causes expansion of the gas within the cavity.
- Otalgia and hearing loss occur as a result of stretching and deformation of the TM.
- Sudden pressure differential between middle and inner ear may lead to rupture of round or oval window and consequent labyrinthine fistula and leakage of perilymph. Damage to inner ear may be permanent.
- When transalveolar pressure disrupts the structural integrity of the alveolus, the alveolar wall ruptures, leading to interstitial emphysema, followed by pneumothorax, pneumomediastinum.

 DIAGNOSIS

- Otic (middle ear) barotrauma:
  - Otalgia, sensation of fullness or pressure in ear
  - Conductive hearing loss
  - Vertigo secondary to cold water entering middle ear
  - Transient facial paralysis
  - With TM rupture, discharge of fluid from ear
  - Abnormality of TM
- All patients with middle ear barotrauma should be evaluated for inner ear barotrauma:
  - Sensorineural hearing loss
  - Tinnitus
  - Vertigo
  - Disorientation
- Sinus barotrauma: Facial pain, sensation of fullness or pressure
- Pulmonary barotrauma:
  - Chest pain, dyspnea
  - Hypoxia, hypotension

HISTORY
- Otic barotrauma: History of high-risk activity
- Pulmonary barotrauma: Scuba diving, mechanical ventilation, air travel with preexisting lung disease

PHYSICAL EXAM
- Otic barotrauma:
  - Otoscopic exam
  - Assess patient's balance and hearing.
  - Palpate eustachian tube for tenderness.
- Pulmonary barotrauma:
  - Auscultation, percussion
- Assessment of respiratory distress

DIAGNOSTIC TESTS & INTERPRETATION
Lab
Initial lab tests
Pulmonary: Arterial blood gas

Imaging
Initial approach
- Otic or sinus: Imaging to rule out nasopharyngeal tumor or sinusitis, if indicated
- Pulmonary:
  - Chest radiograph
  - Chest computed tomography (CT) if chest x-ray (CXR) not informative
- Ultrasound

Diagnostic Procedures/Surgery
- Otic barotrauma:
  - Tympanometry
  - Audiometry: Conductive (middle ear) vs sensorineural (inner ear) hearing loss
  - Surgical exploration to rule out inner ear involvement if suspected
- Pulmonary barotrauma: Chest tube insertion if indicated for pneumothorax.

Pathological Findings
- TM retraction or bulging:
  - Teed 0: No visible damage
  - Teed 1: Congestion around umbo (2 psi)
  - Teed 2: Congestion of entire TM (2–3 psi)
  - Teed 3: Hemorrhage into middle ear
  - Teed 4: Extensive middle ear hemorrhage; TM may rupture
  - Teed 5: Entire middle ear filled with deoxygenated blood
- Inner ear involvement with rupture of the round or oval windows, perilymphatic fistula, and leakage of perilymph into the middle ear
- Pulmonary barotrauma:
  - Alveolar rupture may progress to interstitial emphysema, pneumoperitoneum, pneumothorax

DIFFERENTIAL DIAGNOSIS
- Acute and chronic otitis media
- Otitis externa
- Temporomandibular joint syndrome
- Pulmonary: Other causes of decompensation on mechanical ventilation

 ## TREATMENT

MEDICATION
- Treatment of predisposing conditions, upper respiratory congestion prior to air travel:
  - Oral decongestants
  - Nasal decongestants
  - Antihistamines
- Antibiotics are not indicated for middle ear effusion secondary to barotrauma.
- Analgesics for pain control
- Tinnitus can be treated with high-dose steroids if given within 3 weeks of onset (1)[C].

ADDITIONAL TREATMENT
General Measures
- Prevention/avoidance is best: Avoid flying or diving when risk factors are present.
- Autoinflate the eustachian tube during pressure changes:
  - Valsalva method (2)[B] during ascent and descent in air travel
  - Infants: Breast-feeding or sucking on pacifier or bottle
  - ≥4 years: Chewing gum
  - ≥8 years: Blowing up a balloon
  - Adults: Chewing gum, sucking hard candy, swallowing, or yawning
- Nasal balloon (2)[B]
- For inner ear barotrauma:
  - Bed rest with head elevated to avoid leakage of perilymph
  - Tympanotomy and repair of round or oval window may be necessary.
- Treatment of pneumothorax:
  - Removal of air from pleural space
- Adjustment of iatrogenic cause (adjustment of mechanical ventilation)

Issues for Referral
- Refer to otolaryngology if inner ear is exposed, perilymphatic fistula, or sensorineural hearing loss.
- Chest tube placement

SURGERY/OTHER PROCEDURES
- If necessary, myringotomy or tympanoplasty
- Tympanotomy and repair of round or oval window may be necessary in inner ear barotrauma.
- Tube thoracostomy for persistent pneumothorax

IN-PATIENT CONSIDERATIONS
Admission Criteria
- Patients with complicating emergencies (e.g., incapacitating pain requiring myringotomy, large tympanic perforation requiring tympanoplasty)
- Inner ear barotrauma with hearing loss
- Management of pneumothorax

 ## ONGOING CARE

FOLLOW-UP RECOMMENDATIONS
- No flying or diving until complete resolution of all signs and symptoms, and Valsalva succeeds in equalizing pressure.
- Complete bed rest for inner ear barotrauma
- No high-risk activities or air travel until pneumothorax is completely resolved.

Patient Monitoring
- Otoscopic exams until symptoms clear
- In severe cases, audiograms

PATIENT EDUCATION
- Teach Valsalva maneuver.
- Educate on how to create allergy-free environment.
- American Academy of Pediatrics Travel Safety Tips: http://www.aap.org
- Divers Alert Network of Duke University Medical Center information line: (919) 684-2948

PROGNOSIS
- Mild barotitis media may resolve spontaneously.
- Tympanic rupture: Recovery within weeks–months
- Hearing loss may be permanent in barotitis externa.
- Prognosis of pulmonary barotrauma depends on underlying pathology.

COMPLICATIONS
- Permanent hearing loss
- Ruptured TM
- Chronic tinnitus, vertigo
- Fluid exudate in middle ear
- Perilymphatic fistula
- Sensorineural hearing loss

REFERENCES
1. Duplessis C, Hoffer M. Tinnitus in an active duty navy diver: a review of inner ear barotrauma, tinnitus, and its treatment. *Undersea Hyperbaric Med.* 2006;33(4):223–30.
2. Stangerup SE, et al. Point prevalence of barotitis and its prevention and treatment with nasal balloon inflation: a prospective, controlled study. *Otol Neurol.* 2004;25(2):89–94.

ADDITIONAL READING
- Mirza S, Richardson H. Otic barotrauma from air travel. *J Laryngol Otol.* 2005;119:366–70.
- Plötz FB, Slutsky AS, van Vught AJ, et al. Ventilator-induced lung injury and multiple system organ failure: a critical review of facts and hypotheses. *Intensive Care Med.* 2004;30:1865–72.

See Also (Topic, Algorithm, Electronic Media Element)
Algorithm: Ear Pain

 ## CODES

ICD9
- 993.0 Barotrauma, otitic
- 993.1 Barotrauma, sinus

CLINICAL PEARLS
- Small children can equalize eustachian tube pressure by sucking on bottles or pacifiers. Crying also serves as autoinflation.
- Pulmonary barotrauma is the 2nd leading cause of death among divers.
- Otic barotrauma is common in air travel, especially among flight personnel.
- Pulmonary barotrauma is noted in 3% of mechanically ventilated patients.

BARTONELLA INFECTIONS

Michael K. Chen, MD

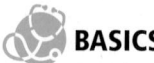

BASICS

DESCRIPTION
- Fastidious intracellular anaerobic gram-negative bacilli:
  - At least 20 distinct species, 8 known to cause disease in humans
  - *Bartonella henselae* and *B. quintana* ("trench fever") most common in North America
- Infections manifest in 2 broad categories:
  - Localized skin lesions and prominent regional lymphadenitis (cat scratch disease [CSD])
  - Bacteremia with localized vascular lesions in various organs and potential for persistent disseminated infection
- System(s) affected: Cardiovascular; Gastrointestinal; Heme/Lymphatic/Immunologic; Musculoskeletal; Nervous; Pulmonary; Skin/Exocrine; Ocular; Renal (rare)
- Synonym(s): Bartonellosis

EPIDEMIOLOGY
Incidence
- Carrion disease: 12.7/100 person-years in endemic areas
- CSD: Estimated 9.3/100,000 in US (~25,000 cases annually)
- Endocarditis: Estimated 3–4% of cases, up to 1/3 of "culture-negative" cases
- Others: Unknown

Prevalence
- Worldwide
- Seroprevalence studies of *B. henselae* suggest many childhood infections are asymptomatic.
- Seroprevalence studies of domestic cats show 25–51%.
- Studies of *B. quintana* in homeless populations suggest seroprevalence of 10%.

RISK FACTORS
- Vector exposure with cutaneous inoculation:
  - *B. henselae*: Domestic cat (especially scratch/bite from kitten), transmitted horizontally from cat fleas
  - *B. bacilliformis*: *Lutzomyia* sandflies, limited to Andean South America, cause of carrion disease
  - *B. quintana*: Human body louse, typically in alcoholic, homeless men
- Cell-mediated immune dysfunction (particularly in bacillary angiomatosis/bacillary peliosis):
  - HIV infection, especially with CD4+ lymphocyte count <100/mcL
  - Chronic steroid, immunosuppressant, or alcohol use

Genetics
No known genetic predisposition

GENERAL PREVENTION
Vector avoidance

PATHOPHYSIOLOGY
- Erythrocyte and endothelial cell invasion
- In immune-competent hosts, progresses to granulomatous and suppurative disease mainly in lymph nodes
- In immune-compromised hosts, leads to angiogenesis with mixed inflammatory cell infiltrate

DIAGNOSIS

HISTORY
- Carrion disease (aka bartonellosis); usually has 2 distinctive stages:
  - Oroya fever (acute bacteremia): In severe cases, abrupt onset 3 weeks after inoculation. Profound anemia, many complications, may be fatal.
  - Verruga peruana: Crops of nodular angiomatous skin lesions months after Oroya fever; mucosal and internal lesions also; involute in months to years
  - Asymptomatic persistent bacteremia: <15% of untreated Oroya fever survivors
- Typical cat scratch disease (up to 90% of cases):
  - Days after inoculation 2–3-mm nontender papules develop at the trauma site; progress to reddened then crusted vesicles
  - Tender regional adenopathy 1–8 weeks postinoculation; fever, malaise, headache
  - Usually involves nodes of upper extremities, neck, head, or groin; suppuration of nodes common, but only 10% require drainage
  - Resolution in 2–4 months for majority
- A typical cat scratch disease:
  - Parinaud oculoglandular syndrome: Unilateral granulomatous conjunctivitis and preauricular lymphadenitis
  - Neuroretinitis: Abrupt, painless unilateral vision loss; macular star exudate, papilledema; self-limited, full recovery
  - Encephalopathy: Rapid progression from headache to lethargy, coma, and seizure
  - Other manifestations self-limited, sequelae rare: Granulomatous hepatitis/splenitis, osteolysis, atypical pneumonitis, fever of unknown origin, mononucleosis-type syndrome, others
- Bacteremia (short-term mortality uncommon):
  - *B. quintana* (urban trench fever, Wolhynia fever, shinbone fever, quintan fever): Incubation days–weeks; sudden onset of fever, headache, leg pain; self-limited illness may be brief (4–5 days), prolonged (2–6 weeks), most commonly paroxysmal (3–5 episodes of 5 days duration). Insidious course in HIV.
  - *B. henselae*: If HIV-infected, insidious onset of fatigue, malaise, aches, weight loss, recurring fevers, headache; localizing findings uncommon. If HIV-uninfected, abrupt onset of fever (may persist or relapse), myalgias, arthralgias, headache; localizing findings unusual; may persist without symptoms.

- Endocarditis: Fever, dyspnea, murmur, embolic phenomena; aortic valve involvement most common
- Bacillary angiomatosis: Mostly immunocompromised hosts (e.g., HIV-infected); involves skin (crops of subcutaneous or dermal nodules and/or skin-colored to purple papules; may ulcerate with serous or bloody drainage and crusting), regional lymph nodes, internal organs
- Bacillary peliosis: Involves liver and spleen in immunosuppressed persons; can involve lymph nodes; nonspecific clinical manifestations
- Neurologic syndromes in HIV: Cognitive dysfunction, behavioral disturbances; may be mistaken for dementia, psychiatric disease
- Pseudomalignancy: Increasing numbers of reports in literature; sometimes confused with lymphoma, case reports of breast nodules

PHYSICAL EXAM
See History.

DIAGNOSTIC TESTS & INTERPRETATION
Lab
- Nonspecific typical lab findings
- Skin testing reagents: Not recommended
- Giemsa-stained blood smear may show *B. bacilliformis* adherent to erythrocytes.
- Non-*bacilliformis* species:
  - Indirect fluorescent antibody (IFA) and enzyme immunoassay tests are available:
    - Interpretation complicated by variable correlation between titers and disease stage, lack of uniformity among serologic tests, and cross-reactivity among *Bartonella* species and other bacteria (1)[C]
    - In general, IFA IgG titers <1:64 suggest no current infection and >1:256 suggest active or recent infection. Immune-compromised patients may not develop adequate titers.

ALERT
- Advise lab if *Bartonella* infection is suspected so that blood, tissue, and cerebrospinal fluid cultures are prepared with appropriate media under optimal conditions; prolonged incubation required.
- Polymerase chain reaction (PCR) of valve tissue can aid diagnosis of endocarditis; otherwise, less helpful clinically.
- Antibiotics may result in false-negative culture.

Imaging
Initial approach
Ultrasound, computed tomography, transesophageal echocardiogram (as indicated)

Diagnostic Procedures/Surgery
Biopsy of lymph nodes for histology and culture. Consider biopsy of involved organs.

Pathological Findings

- Verruga peruana: Neovascular proliferation; bacteria uncommonly are identified.
- CSD: Granulomas, stellate necrosis, mixed inflammatory infiltrates; bacilli in tissue may be demonstrable by silver impregnation stains (e.g., Warthin-Starry).
- Endocarditis: Warthin-Starry-stained bacilli may be seen in vegetations.
- Bacillary angiomatosis:
  - Lobular proliferations of small blood vessels are seen, containing cuboidal endothelial cells interspersed with inflammatory cells, mostly neutrophils.
  - Warthin-Starry stain or electron microscopy may show clusters of bacilli.
- Bacillary peliosis: Blood-filled cystic structures. Warthin-Starry stain may show surrounding clumps of bacilli.

DIFFERENTIAL DIAGNOSIS

- Typical CSD: Sporotrichosis, histoplasmosis, plague, tularemia, brucellosis, mycobacteria, staphylococci, streptococci, other agents associated with injection drug use; lymphoma; metastatic malignancy
- Atypical CSD: Non-*bacilliformis* bacteremia syndromes:
  - Immunocompromised: *Cryptococcus neoformans*, *Histoplasma capsulatum*, *Coccidioides immitis*, *Mycobacterium avium*-complex
  - Arthropod exposure: Rickettsial infections, tularemia, plague, babesiosis, borreliosis
  - Cat/dog scratch/bite: Pasteurella
  - Influenza, infectious mononucleosis, hepatitis
- Endocarditis: Other slow-growing bacteria (*Haemophilus, Actinobacillus, Cardiobacterium, Eikenella, Kingella, Coxiella*)
- Bacillary angiomatosis/bacillary peliosis: Kaposi's sarcoma, pyogenic granuloma, hemangioma
- Neurologic syndrome in HIV: Tertiary syphilis, cryptococcal meningitis, toxoplasmosis, progressive multifocal leukoencephalopathy, alcohol or drug abuse

TREATMENT

MEDICATION

- Antibiotic choice depends on clinical situation; much data are secondary to case studies, as opposed to randomized controlled trial (RCT) data.
- Oroya fever: Chloramphenicol 500 mg (pediatric dose 50–75 mg/kg/d) p.o./IV q.i.d. + B-lactam (IV: PCN G 3 million U q4h (40K units/kg q4h for peds)/p.o.: PCN V recommended 500 mg q.i.d. or 20 mg/kg q.i.d. for peds) for 14 days (2)[B]
- Verruga peruana: Rifampin 10/mg/kg/d (not to exceed 600 mg/d in children) for 10–14 days (2)[B]
- Typical CSD: No clear benefit, although oral azithromycin may speed resolution of extensive lymphadenopathy: Adults and children >45.5 kg: 500 mg on day 1; 250 mg daily on days 2–5; children ≤4 5.5 kg: 10 mg/kg on day 1; 5 mg/kg daily on days 2–5 (2)[A]

- Retinitis: Doxycycline 100 mg p.o. b.i.d. (in peds <8 y/o, consider erythromycin 20 mg/kg/d to max daily dose of 2 g/d) + rifampin 300 mg p.o. b.i.d. for 4–6 weeks (2)[B]. Some data show that retinitis is self-limited, so some authors suggest no antibiotics are needed.
- Trench fever or chronic *B. quintana* bacteremia: Doxycycline 200 mg p.o. daily for 4 weeks + gentamicin 3 mg/kg IV daily for 2 weeks (2)[A]
- Bacillary angiomatosis/peliosis: Erythromycin 500 mg (pediatric dose 40 mg/kg/d to maximum daily dose of 2 g/d) p.o. q.i.d. or doxycycline 100 mg p.o. b.i.d. for 3 months (4 months for peliosis); consider longer course if immunocompromised (2)[B].
- Endocarditis (culture-positive): Gentamicin 1 mg/kg IV t.i.d. for 2 weeks + doxycycline 100 mg p.o. b.i.d. for 6 weeks (2)[B]. Add ceftriaxone 2 g IV/IM daily for 6 weeks for culture-negative.

ADDITIONAL TREATMENT

Issues for Referral
Cardiac surgery if endocarditis

SURGERY/OTHER PROCEDURES
Valve replacement if indicated in endocarditis

IN-PATIENT CONSIDERATIONS

Initial Stabilization
ABCs, high degree of clinical suspicion, and awareness of local infection risk. Blood transfusions if symptomatic severe anemia.

Admission Criteria
Consider admission for patients who are immune-compromised, hemodynamically unstable, or may not have access to appropriate antibiotics.

Discharge Criteria
Patients may be discharged when stable on p.o. antibiotics or receiving IV antibiotics through a peripherally inserted central catheter line.

ONGOING CARE

FOLLOW-UP RECOMMENDATIONS

Patient Monitoring
Immune-compromised patients at increased risk for relapse. Extended periods of antibiotics recommended.

DIET
No diet modifications needed

PATIENT EDUCATION
Vector avoidance information

PROGNOSIS
- CSD: Spontaneous resolution usually in 2–4 months without specific therapy
- Other syndromes: With proper treatment, full resolution; if relapse, consider long-term suppressive antibiotics after retreatment
- Oroya fever: If untreated >40% mortality

COMPLICATIONS
Disseminated disease can present with specific organ-related findings such as focal seizures or renal microabscesses (3,4)[C]

REFERENCES

1. Vermeulen MJ, Verbakel H, Notermans DW et al. Evaluation of sensitivity, specificity and cross-reactivity in Bartonella henselae serology. *J Med Microbiol*. 2010;59:743–5.
2. Rolain JM, Brouqui P, Koehler JE et al. Recommendations for treatment of human infections caused by Bartonella species. *Antimicrob Agents Chemother*. 2004;48:1921–33.
3. Salehi N, Custodio H, Rathore MH et al. Renal microabscesses due to Bartonella infection. *Pediatr Infect Dis J*. 2010;29:472–3.
4. Farooque P, Khurana DS, Melvin JJ et al. Persistent focal seizures after cat scratch encephalopathy. *Pediatr. Neurol*. 2010;42:215–8.

 ## CODES

ICD9
- 041.84 Other specified bacterial infections in conditions classified elsewhere and of unspecified site, other anaerobes
- 078.3 Cat-scratch disease
- 083.1 Trench fever

CLINICAL PEARLS

- Bartonella infection and its various clinical manifestations can be difficult to identify, unless there is a high degree of clinical suspicion and awareness of local infection risks.
- CSD will resolve by itself in most immune-competent patients. Systemic lymphadenopathy will resolve faster with azithromycin.
- Immune-compromised patients are at increased risk for developing occult infections, but tend to have more dramatic response to antibiotics.

BARTTER'S SYNDROME

Maricarmen Malagon-Rogers, MD

 BASICS

- Bartter's syndrome and Bartter's-like syndrome are a group of rare autosomal, recessive, salt-wasting nephropathies characterized by polyuria, hypokalemia, metabolic alkalosis, and normotension with hyperreninemic-hyperaldosteronism (1).
- Traditionally they have been divided into two main disorders according to where the defect is located in the renal tubule, but since genetic classification has been available there are more subtypes (2).
- Bartter (Furosemide type) with 5 subtypes and Gitelman (Thiazide type) with 2 subtypes and combinations of the two.

DESCRIPTION
Bartter's disorders have diverse genetic origins, with a common pathological mechanism of a severe reduction in salt reabsorption by the thick ascending limb of Henle (TAL) and/or the distal convoluted tubule (DCT).

EPIDEMIOLOGY
Prevalence
Gitelman's prevalence is calculated at 1:40000. Heterozygote state in Caucasians: 1% (3)

RISK FACTORS
Consanguinity

Genetics
Autosomic recessive

PATHOPHYSIOLOGY
- Bartter type is caused by inactivating mutations in one of several genes encoding membrane proteins in charge of transporting Na, Cl, K, and sometimes Ca in the loop of Henle where 25% of the filtered solute load is reabsorbed. This causes large urinary losses of Na, Cl, K, Mg, and Ca. It resembles the effect of large doses of furosemide, which results in hypovolemia with activation of the renin aldosterone system without any hypertension. According to which transporter is compromised, the disease will be more or less severe and it will start sooner or later. When it starts in utero it causes polyhydramnios because of fetal polyuria. There is also secondary stimulation of prostaglandin E2 (PGE2) production with worsening of salt losses (2).

- In the Gitelman type the inactivating mutations are in the distal convoluted tube where 5% of the filtered Na is reabsorbed. It resembles the effect of thiazides and causes urinary losses of Na, Cl, K, and Mg, but not Ca. It is clinically less severe (2).

ETIOLOGY
- The inactivating mutations in Bartter syndrome are in type I. The Na^+-K-$2Cl^-$ cotransporter (*SLC12A1* encoding NKCC2), in type II the apical inward-rectifying potassium channel (*KCNJ1* encoding ROMK), in type III the basolateral chloride channel (*ClCNK* encoding ClC-Kb), and in type IV the *BSND*, a protein that acts as an essential activator β-subunit for ClC-Ka and ClC-Kb chloride channels. Type V is a gain-of-function mutations in the extracellular calcium ion-sensing receptor (CaSR) that cause a variant with hypocalcemia (12).
- In Gitelman the inactivating mutations are in the *SLC12A3* gene encoding the thiazide sensitive Na-Cl cotransporter, or NCCT (23).

COMMONLY ASSOCIATED CONDITIONS
- Polyhydramnios, prematurity
- Nephrocalcinosis, rickets, growth retardation
- Hyperprostaglandin levels
- Sensorineural deafness, mental retardation in type IV
- Cardiac problems (4)
- Gallstones (5)
- Constipation

 DIAGNOSIS

HISTORY
- Polyuria and polydipsia are always present. History of episodes of dehydration.
- In types I, II, IV, and V the presentation is usually prenatal with polyhydramnios, prematurity, and postnatally there is failure to thrive, dehydration, muscle weakness, seizures, tetany, and paresthesias. This type has been called Neonatal Bartter of In Bartter there is always hypercalciuria with normomagnesemia. Nephrocalcinosis is present in type I and II. Type II can show hyperkalemia at birth and less hypokalemia than the other subtypes.
- Type III is variable and can present later in early childhood with no nephrocalcinosis.
- Gitelman usually presents later with muscle weakness and hypokalemia, hypomagnesemia, and hypocalciuria.

PHYSICAL EXAM
- Premature AGE, normotension, and failure to thrive later on
- Dysmorphic features, including triangular facies, protruding ears, large eyes, and drooping mouth.
- Tetany, hypotonia.

DIAGNOSTIC TESTS & INTERPRETATION
Lab
- Hypokalemia of <2.5 mEq/L with metabolic alkalosis is almost universal. Only in type II hypokalemia may not be as severe and it may even have hyperkalemia in the newborn period.
- Prenatal testing of amniotic fluid may be diagnostic (6).

Initial lab tests

- Na, K, Cl, tCO2, Ca, and Mg in serum and in urine. There will be hypokalemia with elevated tCO2 and normomagnesemia with hyperkaluria, hyperchloruria, and hypercalciuria in Bartter, while in Gitelman there will be hypomagnesemia and decreased urinary calcium.
- Renin and aldosterone will always be elevated and Prostaglandin E2 will be elevated in Bartter but not in Gitelman.

Follow-Up & Special Considerations

- Electrolytes need to be followed very frequently until they stabilize and then monthly. Urinary random Ca/Cr should be followed at least twice a year.
- Creatinine and BUN should be followed because there can be renal failure mainly from nephrocalcinosis (7).
- Cardiac studies are indicated (4).

Imaging

Renal ultrasound is indicated always in Bartter because of the presence of nephrocalcinosis. It should be done about every 2 years.

Pathological Findings

Renal biopsy shows hyperplasia of the juxtaglomerular apparatus.

DIFFERENTIAL DIAGNOSIS

- Chronic diuretic abuse
- Chronic vomiting

TREATMENT

- The main goal in the neonatal period is to keep patients hydrated with correction of hypokalemia.
- In Gitelman, correction of hypomagnesemia is also important.

MEDICATION

Non-steroidal antiinflammatory drugs (NSAIDs) should be used in Bartter's (8).

First Line

- Bartter: NSAIDs, potassium and sodium supplementation, spironolactone
- Gitelman: Potassium and magnesium supplementation. NSAIDs are not useful.

Second Line

H2 blockers or proton-pump inhibitors when using NSAIDs

ONGOING CARE

DIET

High in salt, potassium, and water

PROGNOSIS

Good in general. With adequate management patients can grow normally (8).

COMPLICATIONS

Nephrocalcinosis, gastric ulcers, chronic kidney disease (1)

REFERENCES

1. Chadha V, Alon US et al. Hereditary renal tubular disorders. *Semin Nephrol*. 2009;29:399–411.
2. Seyberth HW et al. An improved terminology and classification of Bartter-like syndromes. *Nature clinical practice. Nephrology*. 2008;4:560–7.
3. Knoers NV, Levtchenko EN et al. Gitelman syndrome. *Orphanet J Rare Dis*. 2008;3:22.
4. Scognamiglio R, Calò LA, Negut C et al. Myocardial perfusion defects in Bartter and Gitelman syndromes. *Eur J Clin Invest*. 2008;38:888–95.
5. Shin JI, Lee JS et al. Comment on: Bartter syndrome and cholelithiasis in an infant: is this a mere coincidence? (*Eur J Pediatr* 2008;167(1):109–110). *Eur J Pediatr*. 2009;168.
6. Garnier A, Dreux S, Vargas-Poussou R et al. Bartter syndrome prenatal diagnosis based on amniotic fluid biochemical analysis. *Pediatr Res*. 2010;67: 300–3.
7. Lin CM, Tsai JD, Lo YF et al. Chronic renal failure in a boy with classic Bartter's syndrome due to a novel mutation in CLCNKB coding for the chloride channel. *Eur J Pediatr*. 2009;168:1129–33.
8. Puricelli E, Bettinelli A, Borsa N et al. Long-term follow-up of patients with Bartter syndrome type I and II. *Nephrol Dial Transplant*. 2010;25: 2976–81.

ADDITIONAL READING

- Brochard K, Boyer O, Blanchard A et al. Phenotype-genotype correlation in antenatal and neonatal variants of Bartter syndrome. *Nephrol Dial Transplant*. 2009;24:1455–64.
- Nozu K, Iijima K, Kanda K et al. The pharmacological characteristics of molecular-based inherited salt-losing tubulopathies. *J Clin Endocrinol Metabol*. 2010.

CODES

ICD9

255.13 Bartter's syndrome

CLINICAL PEARLS

Bartter's and Bartter's-like syndromes are autosomic recessive hypokalemic salt-losing nephropathies that mimic diuretic effects.

BASAL CELL CARCINOMA

Aleema Patel, MD
Leslie Robinson-Bostom, MD

BASICS

Incidence in US: ~1,000,000 cases/year and is increasing about 10% each year

DESCRIPTION
Basal cell carcinoma (BCC) is the most common cancer, originating from the basal cell layer of the skin appendages:
- Rarely metastasizes, but capable of local tissue destruction

Geriatric Considerations
- Greater frequency in geriatric patients (ages 55–75 have 100 times incidence of age <20)
- The incidence is rapidly increasing in 20–40-year-olds.

Pediatric Considerations
Rare in children, but childhood sun exposure is important in adult disease.

EPIDEMIOLOGY
Worldwide, the most common form of cancer.

Incidence
- Incidence in US: 1,000,000 cases/year and is increasing about 10% each year
- Predominant age: Generally >40, but incidence is increasing in younger populations
- Predominant sex: Male > Female (although incidence is increasing in females)
- Lifetime risk of white North Americans: 30%

RISK FACTORS
- Chronic sun exposure (UV radiation)
- Most common in the following phenotypes:
  - Light complexion: Skin type I (burns but does not tan) and skin type II (usually burns, sometimes tans)
  - Red or blond hair
  - Blue or green eyes
- Tendency to sunburn
- Male sex, although increasing risk in women due to lifestyle changes such as tanning beds
- History of nonmelanoma skin cancer:
  - After initial diagnosis of skin cancer, 35% risk of new nonmelanoma skin cancer at 3 years and 50% at 5 years.
- Family history of skin cancer
- 3–4 decades after chronic arsenic exposure
- 2 decades after therapeutic radiation
- Chronic immunosuppression: Transplant recipients (10 times higher incidence), patients with HIV or lymphomas

Genetics
Several genetic conditions increase the risk of developing BCC:
- Albinism (recessive alleles)
- Xeroderma pigmentosum (autosomal recessive)
- Bazex syndrome (rare, x-linked dominant)
- Nevoid basal cell carcinoma syndrome/Gorlin syndrome (rare, autosomal dominant)
- Cytochrome P-450 CYP2D6 and glutathione S-transferase detoxifying enzyme gene mutations (especially in truncal basal cell carcinoma, marked by clusters of basal cell carcinomas and a younger age of onset)

GENERAL PREVENTION
- Use broad-spectrum sunscreens of at least SPF 30 daily and reapply after swimming or sweating.
- Avoid overexposure to the sun by seeking shade between 10 a.m. and 4 p.m. as well as wearing wide-brimmed hats and long-sleeved shirts.
- Avoid tanning and sunburns (including tanning salons).

PATHOPHYSIOLOGY
- UV-induced inflammation and cyclooxygenase activation in skin
- Mutation of PTCH1 (patched homolog 1), a tumor-suppressor gene that inhibits the hedgehog signaling pathway
- Mutation of the SMO (smoothened homolog) gene, which is also involved in the hedgehog signaling pathway
- UV-induced mutations of the TP53 (tumor protein 53), a tumor-suppressor gene
- Activation of BCL2, an antiapoptosis proto-oncogene

COMMONLY ASSOCIATED CONDITIONS
- Cosmetic disfigurement since head and neck most often affected
- Loss of vision with orbital involvement
- Loss of nerve function due to perineural spread or extensive and deep invasion
- Ulcerating neoplasms are prone to infections.

DIAGNOSIS

HISTORY
Exposure to risk factors, family history

PHYSICAL EXAM
- 80% on face and neck, 20% on trunk and lower limbs (mostly women) (1)[B]
- Nodular: Most common (60%); presents as pinkish, pearly papule, plaque, or nodule often with telangiectatic vessels, ulceration, and a rolled periphery usually on face:
  - Pigmented: Presents as a translucent papule with "floating pigment"; more commonly seen in darker skin types
- Superficial: (30%); light red, scaly papule or plaque with atrophic center, ringed by translucent micropapules, usually on trunk or extremities; more common in men
- Morpheaform: (5–10%); firm, smooth, flesh-colored, scarlike papule or plaque with ill-defined borders

DIAGNOSTIC TESTS & INTERPRETATION
Diagnostic Procedures/Surgery
- Clinical diagnosis and histological subtype are confirmed through skin biopsy and pathological examination.
- Shave biopsy is typically sufficient; however, punch biopsy is more useful to assess depth of tumor and perineural invasion.
- If a genetic disorder is suspected, additional tests may be needed to confirm it.

Pathological Findings
- Nodular BCC:
  - Extending from the epidermis are nodular aggregates of basaloid cells.
  - Tumor cells are uniform; rarely have mitotic figures; and have large, oval, hyperchromatic nuclei with little cytoplasm, surrounded by a peripheral palisade.
  - Early lesions are usually connected to the epidermis, unlike late lesions.
  - Increased mucin in dermal stroma:
    - Cleft formation (retraction artifact) common between BCC "nests" and stroma due to mucin shrinkage during fixation and staining.
- Superficial BCC:
  - Appear as buds of basaloid cells attached to undersurface of epidermis
  - Peripheral palisading

- Morpheoform BCC:
  - Thin cords and strands of basaloid cells, embedded in dense, fibrous, "scarlike" stroma
  - Less peripheral palisading and retraction, greater subclinical involvement
- Infiltrating BCC:
  - Like morpheoform BCC, but no "scarlike" stroma and thicker, more spiky, irregular strands
  - Less peripheral palisading and retraction, greater subclinical involvement
- Micronodular BCC:
  - Small, nodular aggregates of tumor cells
  - Less retraction artifact and higher subclinical involvement than nodular BCC

DIFFERENTIAL DIAGNOSIS

- Sebaceous hyperplasia
- Epidermal inclusion cyst
- Intradermal nevi (pigmented and nonpigmented)
- Molluscum contagiosum
- Squamous cell carcinoma
- Nummular dermatitis
- Psoriasis
- Melanoma (pigmented lesions)
- Atypical fibroxanthoma
- Rare adnexal neoplasms

 TREATMENT

MEDICATION

- May be especially useful in those who cannot tolerate surgical procedures and in those who refuse to have surgery
- 5-fluorouracil cream inhibits thymidylate synthetase, interrupting DNA synthesis for superficial lesions in low-risk areas; primary treatment only 5% applied b.i.d. for 3–10 weeks
- Imiquimod (Aldara) cream approved for treatment of low-risk superficial BCC; daily dosing for 6–12 weeks; 90% histologic cure

ADDITIONAL TREATMENT

- Radiation therapy:
  - Useful for patients who cannot or will not undergo surgery
  - Used following surgery, particularly if margins of tumor were not cleared
  - Cure rate is approximately 90%.
  - Tumors that recur in areas previously treated with radiation are harder to treat, and the area is more difficult to reconstruct.
- Photodynamic therapy (PDT) (2)[A]:
  - 5-aminolevulinic acid, a photosensitizer, is activated by specific wavelengths of light, creating singlet oxygen radicals that destroy local tissue (no damage to surrounding or deep tissues).
  - Useful in areas where tissue preservation is cosmetically or functionally important

SURGERY/OTHER PROCEDURES

- Generally 1st choice; specific treatment selection varies with extent and location of lesion as well as tumor border demarcation (3)[A]
- High-risk areas:
  - Inner canthus, nasolabial sulcus, philtrum, preauricular area, retroauricular sulcus, lip, temple
- Curettage and electrodesiccation:
  - If nodular lesion <1 cm, in low-risk area, not deeply invasive
- Excision:
  - Useful for lesions in high-risk areas
  - Not as dependent on lesion size
- Cryosurgery:
  - Reserved for small lesions in low-risk areas
  - May want pre- and post-treatment biopsies
- Mohs surgery:
  - Preferred microsurgically controlled surgical treatment for lesions in high-risk areas, recurrent lesions, and lesions exhibiting an aggressive growth pattern
  - Requires referral to appropriately trained dermatologic surgeon

IN-PATIENT CONSIDERATIONS

Outpatient unless extensive lesion

 ONGOING CARE

FOLLOW-UP RECOMMENDATIONS

- Avoid sun exposure.
- Oral retinoids may prevent the development of new basal cell carcinomas in patients with Gorlin syndrome, renal transplant patients, and patients with severe actinic damage.

Patient Monitoring

- Every month for 3 months, then twice yearly for 5 years; yearly thereafter
- Increased risk of other skin cancers (4)[C]

PATIENT EDUCATION

- Teach patient appropriate sun-avoidance techniques, sunscreens, etc.
- Monthly self skin exam
- Educate patients concerning adequate calcium and vitamin D intake.

PROGNOSIS

- Proper treatment yields 90–95% cure.
- Most recurrences happen within 5 years.
- Development of new BCCs: Patients (36%) will develop a new lesion within 5 years.

COMPLICATIONS

- Local recurrence and spread
- Usually, recurrences will appear within 5 years.
- Metastasis: Rare (<0.1%), but metastatic disease usually fatal within 8 months

REFERENCES

1. Wong CS, Strange RC, Lear JT. Basal cell carcinoma. *BMJ*. 2003;327:794–8.
2. Soler AM, Angell-Petersen E, Warloe T, et al. Photodynamic therapy of superficial basal cell carcinoma with 5-aminolevulinic acid with dimethylsulfoxide and ethylendiaminetetraacetic acid: a comparison of two light sources. *Photochem Photobiol*. 2000;71:724–9.
3. Bath FJ, Bong J, Perkins W, et al. Interventions for basal cell carcinoma of the skin. *Cochrane Database Syst Rev*. 2003;CD003412.
4. Friedman GD, Tekawa IS. Association of basal cell skin cancers with other cancers (United States). *Cancer Causes Control*. 2000;11:891–7.

 CODES

ICD9

- 173.0 Other malignant neoplasm of skin of lip
- 173.1 Other malignant neoplasm of skin of eyelid, including canthus
- 173.2 Other malignant neoplasm of skin of ear and external auditory canal

CLINICAL PEARLS

- Use diagnostic keys above to differentiate between BCC and cutaneous squamous cell carcinoma (SCC). SCC arises from actinic keratosis in 60% of cases and generally presents as an asymptomatic hyperkeratotic lesion. If unsure, biopsy or refer to a specialist.
- Some hyperpigmented BCCs may appear similar to melanoma. Remember the ABCDEs of melanoma recognition: *A*symmetry, *B*order irregularities, *C*olor variability, *D*iameter >6 mm, *E*nlargement. If unsure, refer to a specialist.
- The USPSTF concludes there is insufficient evidence to recommend for or against routine total body skin exams for melanoma, BCC, or SCC. Exams should be based on risk factors, including exposures and family and prior medical history. All patients may receive education about risks and self-exam.

BEHAVIORAL PROBLEMS, PEDIATRIC

Elizabeth Bade, MD

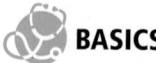 **BASICS**

DESCRIPTION

Behavior that disrupts ≥1 areas of psychosocial functioning but not seriously enough to receive an official DSM-IV diagnosis; most commonly reported behavioral problems are

- Noncompliance: Purposeful refusal (active/passive) to do what is requested by parent or other adult authority figure
- Temper tantrums: Loss of internal control believed to be provoked by overtiredness, physical discomfort, or fear that leads the child to exhibit behaviors such as crying, whining, breath holding, or in extreme cases, acts of aggression
- Sleep disorders: Sleep patterns that are distressing to parents, child, or physician; this can be further broken down into 2 categories based on polysomnograph:
  - Primary sleep disorders have abnormal polysomnograph. Examples include sleepwalking and night terrors.
  - Secondary sleep disorders have normal polysomnograph and are the most common sleep disorders. Examples include night awakenings and bedtime resistance.
- Nocturnal enuresis: Enuresis that occurs only at night in children >5 years of age with no medical problems
  - Primary: Nocturnal enuresis in a child who has never been dry at night
  - Secondary: Nocturnal enuresis in a child who has been dry at night for at least 6 months

EPIDEMIOLOGY

- Noncompliance: More common in children <1 year of age, especially as they develop autonomy; boys have a modestly greater likelihood of being noncompliant. Noncompliant behavior decreases with age.
- Temper tantrums: 70% of 18- to 24-month-old children; 75.3% of 3- to 5-year-old children; in children with severe tantrums, 52% have other non-tantrum-related behavioral/emotional problems (1).
- Sleep disorders (secondary): 25% of children between 1 and 5 years of age and 20–30% of infants, toddlers, and preschoolers
- Nocturnal enuresis:
  - At least 20% of children in the 1st grade wet the bed occasionally, and 4% wet 2 or more times per week; more common in boys than in girls (2):
    ◦ Enuresis in boys aged 7 and 10 years is 9% and 7%, respectively.
    ◦ Enuresis in girls aged 7 and 10 years is 6% and 3%, respectively.

RISK FACTORS
Genetics

- Genetic components contribute to the pathogenesis of primary nocturnal enuresis. One locus was assigned to chromosome 13q (3).
- Major genes are involved in a large proportion of enuresis families. Linkage results suggest that such a gene is located on chromosome 12q.
- Nocturnal enuresis is a genetic and heterogeneous disorder. The associations between genotype and phenotype are complex and are susceptible to environmental influences (4).

 DIAGNOSIS

HISTORY

- Noncompliance: Complete history taken from parents and teachers; direct observation of child or child–parent interaction:
  - Criteria: Is problematic for at least some adults in child's life, leading to stressful/difficult interactions for minimum period of 6 months
  - Reduces child's ability to take part in structured activities
  - Creates stressful interactions and relationships with compliant children
  - Disrupts academic progress; places child at risk for physical injury
- Temper tantrums: History with focus on development, family depression, or violence:
  - Criteria: May consist of stiffening limbs and arching back, dropping to the floor, shouting, screaming, crying, pushing/pulling, stamping, hitting, kicking, throwing, or running away (1)
  - Screening for depression with the Preschool Feelings Checklist (5)
- Sleep disorders: Screening questions about sleep during well-child visit; complete history, including questions about snoring (6)
- Nocturnal enuresis: Complete history specifically asking about urine output/fluid intake/bowel movements; consider asking parent to keep a voiding diary.

PHYSICAL EXAM

- Nocturnal enuresis: Physical exam should focus on abdomen, spine, genitalia, and perineum, followed by a neurologic exam. Specifically, evaluate for
  - Abdomen: Enlarged bladder, kidneys, or fecal masses
  - Spine: Dimpling or tufts of hair on sacrum
  - Genital urinary exam:
    ◦ Males: Meatal stenosis, hypospadias, epispadias, phimosis
    ◦ Females: Vulvitis, vaginitis, labial adhesions, ureterocele at introitus; wide vaginal orifice with scar or healed laceration may be evidence of abuse.
- Rectal exam: Tone and constipation
- Neurologic exam: Focused on the lower extremities

DIAGNOSTIC TESTS & INTERPRETATION
Lab
Initial lab tests
For nocturnal enuresis: Urinalysis and urine culture

Follow-Up & Special Considerations
Sleep studies should be performed in children if there is a history of snoring and daytime attention-deficit hyperactivity disorder (ADHD)–type symptoms.

Diagnostic Procedures/Surgery
- General screening tools: Child Behavioral Checklist
- Pediatric Symptom Checklist (www. brightfutures. org/mentalhealth/pdf/professionals/ped_symptom_chklst.pdf)
- NICHQ Vanderbilt Assessment (ADHD screen; www.myadhd.com/vanderbiltparent6175.html)

Pathological Findings
Certain tantrum behaviors are more likely to be indicative of a serious illness such as major depression or other DSM-IV diagnosable disorders such as ADHD, oppositional defiant disorder (ODD), etc. These behaviors include (5)

- Self-injurious behaviors
- Slow recovery time from tantrums
- More tantrums in the home than outside the home
- More aggressive behaviors toward others, including oral aggression

 TREATMENT

- General: Educate parent about the specific behavioral problem (2).
- Noncompliance: In the case of extreme child disobedience, consider parent training programs. Child may need to be screened for ADHD, ODD, or conduct disorder (CD).
- Temper tantrums: Remind parent(s) that this is a normal aspect of childhood.
  - If tantrum is set off by external factors such as hunger or overtiredness, then correct.
  - Other methods for dealing with a tantrum include 1 of the following:
    ◦ Ignoring the tantrum
    ◦ Removing the child and placing him or her in time-out (1 minute for each year of age)
    ◦ Holding child/restraining child until he or she calms down
    ◦ Giving child clear, firm, and consistent instructions as well as enough time to obey
- Sleep disorders: Aside from parent education, other interventions include
  - Extinction: Child goes to bed at designated time, and cries/tantrums are ignored while monitoring child for safety.
  - Graduated extinction: Parent ignores cries/tantrums for specified period. Parent can check at a fixed time or check at increasing intervals.
  - Studies show that parent education and extinction are the most effective approaches (6).

- Nocturnal enuresis:
  - Bedwetting alarm: Continue for at least 2–3 months.
  - Little evidence from clinical trials, but good empirical evidence for behavioral training, including positive reinforcement (small reward for each dry night), or responsibility training (if old enough, child is responsible for changing or washing sheets), encouraging daily bowel movements, and frequent bladder emptying during the day (2).
  - If behavioral therapy fails: Desmopressin if child >6 years of age.
  - If behavioral and medical therapy fail, then refer to a specialist.

MEDICATION
Most pediatric behavioral issues respond well to nonpharmacologic therapy.

- Sleep disorders:
  - For certain delayed sleep onset disorders, after behavioral methods are exhausted, melatonin at low doses can be tried while behavior modification is continued (7). However, this is not approved by the Food and Drug Administration (FDA) for pediatric patients.
  - Melatonin has been used in pediatric patients in doses of 0.5–10 mg PO given at night.
- Nocturnal enuresis (also see topic Enuresis):
  - If behavioral therapy fails: Desmopressin is the only medicine approved as 1st-line therapy if child >6 years of age.
    - As of 2007, the FDA recommends against use of intranasal formulations in children owing to reports of severe hyponatremia resulting in seizures and death in children using intranasal formulations of desmopressin.
    - Oral desmopressin (DDAVP): Dose-dependent; begin with 0.2-mg tablet taken at bedtime on empty stomach; may titrate to 0.6 mg
    - Maximally effective in 1 hour; cleared within 9 hours
    - Give nightly for 6 months; then stop for 2 weeks for test of dryness.
    - Suspend dose in children who experience acute condition affecting fluid/electrolyte balances (i.e., fever, vomiting, diarrhea, vigorous exercise).
    - Potential risks include water intoxication with hyponatremia.
    - 10–60% success; safe even when used for >12 months; high relapse rate after discontinuation without a structured withdrawal program

ADDITIONAL TREATMENT
Issues for Referral
A patient who exhibits self-injurious behaviors, slow recovery time from tantrums, more tantrums in the home than outside the home, or more aggressive behaviors toward others (including oral aggression) may require referral to a neurodevelopmental or psychiatric specialist.

COMPLEMENTARY AND ALTERNATIVE MEDICINE
- The EPA portion of omega-3 fatty acids has been shown to be useful in treating depression and mood disorders in the pediatric population (8). For patients >8 years of age, 1 g of fish oil is recommended daily, <8 years old, 700 mg/d is recommended.
- For irritability, there is some limited evidence for calcium at 400–800 mg/d and magnesium at 200–400 mg/d, B complex vitamins at 50 mg/d, vitamin C at 1,000 mg/d if younger than 8 years of age and 500 mg/d if over 8 years of age (8)[C].

 ## ONGOING CARE

DIET
- Nutrition is very important in behavioral issues. Avoiding high-sugar foods and providing balanced, whole meals has been shown to decrease aggressive and noncompliant behaviors in children.
- Eliminate caffeine and increase protein.

PATIENT EDUCATION
- A few examples of parent training programs are
  - The Oregon Social Learning Center program: www.oslc.org
  - Forehand and McMahon program: Helping the Noncompliant Child (ages 3–8 years): www.strengtheningfamilies.org/html/programs_1999/02_HNCC.html
  - The BASIC program by Webster-Stratton: www.incredibleyears.com
- Also check local community organizations for parenting classes.

REFERENCES

1. Potegal M, Davidson RJ. Temper tantrums in young children: 1. Behavioral composition. *J Dev Behav Pediatr*. 2003;24:140–7.
2. Robson WL. Clinical practice. Evaluation and management of enuresis. *N Engl J Med*. 2009; 360:1429–36.
3. Arnell H, Hjälmås K, Jägervall M, et al. The genetics of primary nocturnal enuresis: inheritance and suggestion of a second major gene on chromosome 12q. *J Med Genet*. 1997;34:360–5.
4. von Gontard A, Schaumburg H, Hollmann E, et al. The genetics of enuresis: a review. *J Urol*. 2001;166:2438–43.
5. Belden AC, Thomson NR, Luby JL. Temper tantrums in healthy versus depressed and disruptive preschoolers: defining tantrum behaviors associated with clinical problems. *J Pediatr*. 2008;152:117–22.
6. Mindell JA, Kuhn B, Lewin DS, et al. Behavioral treatment of bedtime problems and night wakings in infants and young children. *Sleep*. 2006;29: 1263–76.
7. Gringras P. When to use drugs to help sleep. *Arch Dis Child*. 2008.
8. Shannon S et al. Integrative approaches to pediatric mood disorders. *Altern Ther Health Med*. 2009; 15(5):48–53.

ADDITIONAL READING

- Albrecht SJ, Dore DJ, Naugle AE. Common behavioral dilemmas of the school-aged child. *Pediatr Clin North Am*. 2003;50:841–57.
- Brown P, Schnall JG, Hallgren JD. When (and how) should you evaluate a child for obstructive sleep apnea? *J Fam Pract*. 2007;56:317–20.
- Caldwell PHY, et al. Bedwetting and toileting problems in children. *JAMA*. 2005;182:190–5.
- Kalb LM, Loeber R. Child disobedience and noncompliance: a review. *Pediatrics*. 2003;111: 641–52.
- Luby JL, Heffelfinger A, Koenig-McNaught AL, et al. The Preschool Feelings Checklist: a brief and sensitive screening measure for depression in young children. *J Am Acad Child Adolesc Psychiatry*. 2004;43:708–17.
- Miller JW. Screening children for developmental behavioral problems: principles for the practitioner. *Prim Care Clin Office Pract*. 2007;34:177–201.
- Thiedke CC. Sleep disorders and sleep problems in childhood. *Am Fam Physician*. 2001;63:277–84.

See Also (Topic, Algorithm, Electronic Media Element)
Enuresis

CODES

ICD9
- V40.3 Other behavioral problems
- 312.9 Unspecified disturbance of conduct

CLINICAL PEARLS

- Most commonly reported pediatric behavioral problems are noncompliance, temper tantrums, sleep disorders, and nocturnal enuresis.
- Well-child visits provide opportunities to systematically screen for these common conditions.
- Parental education is a key component of treatment.
- Nutrition is an important factor in behavior disorders and should be screened at the well-child visit.

BEHÇET SYNDROME

Prachaya Nitichaikulvatana, MD
Sangeetha Balasubramanian, MD

 BASICS

DESCRIPTION
- Multisystem, chronic disease characterized by oral and genital mucocutaneous ulcerations, skin rashes, arthritis, thrombophlebitis, uveitis, colitis, and neurologic symptoms
- Rare in US and northern Europe, endemic in Japan, Middle East, and Mediterranean region (along "Silk Route")
- Rare in pediatric and geriatric populations
- Synonym(s): Mucocutaneous ocular syndrome; Franceschetti-Valero syndrome

Pregnancy Considerations
- Thalidomide for treatment contraindicated in pregnancy
- Possible increase in thrombosis and fetal demise

EPIDEMIOLOGY
- Predominant age: 3rd–4th decades
- Predominant gender: Male = Female, with males affected more severely and more in the Middle East

Prevalence
- 1/100,000 population in US
- In other countries, per 100,000:
  – Japan: 10
  – Iran: 16–100
  – Northern Europe: 0.3
  – Saudi Arabia: 20

RISK FACTORS
HLA-B51-positive

Genetics
One report in a mother and newborn

ETIOLOGY
Unknown: Classified as systemic vasculitis; associated with HLA-B51; possible immune response to ubiquitous heat-shock protein; possible infectious causes: herpes simplex virus (HSV), *Streptococcus*; report associated with HIV infection; possible environmental toxin: heavy metals, pesticides, possibly English walnuts or ginkgo nuts

COMMONLY ASSOCIATED CONDITIONS
- Amyloid
- Myelodysplastic syndrome and trisomy 8

 DIAGNOSIS

HISTORY
- GI: Recurrent painful stomatitis or aphthous ulcers (nearly all cases); at least 3 crops in 12 months; spontaneous healing without scar, abdominal pain, melena
- Genital: Recurrent, painful ulcers with scarring
- Musculoskeletal: Myositis (rare), morning stiffness (1/3 of patients), arthralgias
- Ocular: Painful, red eyes
- Neurologic: Headache, weakness, numbness, cranial nerve palsy, seizures

PHYSICAL EXAM
- GI: Painful, shallow, or deep oral ulcers with central yellowish necrotic base and punched-out, clean margin; commonly on tongue, lips, buccal mucosa, and gingivae; ulceration in terminal ileum, cecum, ascending colon
- Genital: Painful, scarring ulcers
- Dermal: Papulopustular (acneiform) lesions, erythema nodosum, pyoderma
- Musculoskeletal: Self-limited, nonerosive arthritis mostly mono- or oligoarthritis predominantly affecting lower extremities, rarely polyarthritis
- Ocular: Anterior uveitis with hypopyon, iridocyclitis, chorioretinitis, retinal vasculitis, vitreous hemorrhage, papilledema, secondary glaucoma, optic atrophy
- Thrombophlebitis: Peripheral, pulmonary, cerebral, Budd-Chiari syndrome
- Neurologic: Parenchymal involvement, common in brain stem; cranial nerve palsy, hemiplegia, intracranial hypertension, meningoencephalitis and recurrent meningitis, confusional state (1)
- Pulmonary infiltrates, possibly related to thrombosis, noncavitating mass lesion
- Vascular: Peripheral gangrene, aneurysms
- Renal: Glomerulonephritis, epididymitis (rare)

DIAGNOSTIC TESTS & INTERPRETATION
- Pathergy phenomenon: Hallmark of this condition: Nonspecific cutaneous hypersensitivity reaction—formation of sterile pustules and/or papules along sites of puncture or needle track
- Normal to mildly elevated erythrocyte sedimentation (ESR) and C-reactive protein (CRP)

- Circulating immune complexes detected by Raji cell and C1q solid-phase assays and elevated interleukin 1 (IL-1), IL-8, and tumor necrosis factor α (TNF-α), but not clinically useful
- Hypergammaglobulinemia
- Depression of plasma antithrombin III levels with active disease
- Increased fibrinolytic activity during attacks; demyelinating antibodies in neurologic Behçet syndrome
- Anticardiolipin antibodies (rare), lupus anticoagulants
- Antiendothelial antibodies

Lab
Initial lab tests
- ESR and CRP
- If elevated or high clinical suspicion, order additional tests noted earlier.

Follow-Up & Special Considerations
- Periodic ophthalmologic examinations
- A careful history and examination, with attention to the vascular and neurologic systems

Diagnostic Procedures/Surgery
- Careful history and physical examination, with frequent reevaluations
- Synovial fluid: Inflammatory effusion
- Arteriography: For aneurysms or thrombosis

Pathological Findings
- May be no recognizable changes; neutrophilic perivascular infiltration ± fibrinoid necrosis
- Picture of leukocytoclastic vasculitis in older lesions
- Neutrophilic dermatitis (Sweet syndrome) (rarely)

DIFFERENTIAL DIAGNOSIS
- Reactive arthritis and other forms of seronegative spondyloarthropathy
- Inflammatory bowel disease (Crohn disease and ulcerative colitis)
- Syphilis and other venereal diseases
- Multiple sclerosis
- Aphthous stomatitis
- Herpes simplex
- Stevens-Johnson syndrome
- Other systemic vasculitides
- Relapsing polychondritis (MAGIC syndrome)
- Coxsackievirus and echovirus infection
- Mollaret meningitis
- Sarcoidosis

TREATMENT
MEDICATION
First Line
- Colchicine: 0.6 mg b.i.d. for mucocutaneous and joint symptoms
- Topical steroids for ocular and genital lesions Prednisone: 1 mg/kg for severe involvement, especially central nervous system
- Dapsone: 50–150 mg/d (2)[B]
- Azathioprine: 2–3 mg/kg/d PO
- Methotrexate: Use lowest possible dose; perhaps 7.5 mg per week. Monitor LFT.
- Cyclosporine: 1–4 mg/kg, but monitor liver function, creatinine, magnesium, and lipids every 2 weeks for 3 months, then every month
- Sulfasalazine 2–6 g/day for GI involvement
- Resistant cases may require:
  – Tacrolimus (FK 506) 0.09–0.15 mg/kg/d
  – Thalidomide 100 mg/d or 300 mg/d (3)[A]: Regulated prescription, teratogenic, refer to manufacturer's literature
  – Interferon alpha for severe ocular and mucocutaneous syndrome (4)[A] and GI manifestations
  – Anticoagulants for patients with anticardiolipin antibodies: Warfarin (Coumadin) to establish PT international normalized ratio 3.0 to 3.5
  – Precautions:
    ○ Absorption of drugs such as amitriptyline, diazepam, carbamazepine, phenytoin, and acetaminophen may be reduced in Behçet syndrome

Second Line
- Levamisole: 100–150 mg 2 days per week
- Chlorambucil: But concern with respect to toxicity, especially its malignant potential
- Cyclophosphamide: 2–2.5 mg/kg/day PO for severe cutaneous, arterial, pulmonary vasculitic or aneurysmal manifestations, risk of hemorrhagic cystitis with drug
- Tumor necrosis factor inhibitors: Infliximab (5)[A] etanercept (6)[A]
- Stem cell transplantation
- Anti-CD52 antibody
- Topical sucralfate suspension (7)[A]

ADDITIONAL TREATMENT
Issues for Referral
Ophthalmologic, neurological, gastrointestinal, vascular surgery referrals as appropriate

IN-PATIENT CONSIDERATIONS
Initial Stabilization
- Usually outpatient
- Inpatient usually required for neurologic complication or GI perforation

ONGOING CARE
FOLLOW-UP RECOMMENDATIONS
Patient Monitoring
Depends on severity of system involvement and medication monitoring

DIET
No special diet

PATIENT EDUCATION
American Behçet Association, 421 21st Avenue SW, Rochester, MN 55902; (507) 281-3059

PROGNOSIS
- Normal life expectancy, except with neurologic involvement, ruptured aneurysms, and catastrophic GI involvement
- Remissions and exacerbations of disease activity, with severity abating with time

COMPLICATIONS
- Death
- Blindness (most serious morbidity)
- Paralysis
- Embolism/thrombosis [pulmonary, vena cava, peripheral, intracardiac (rare)]
- Aneurysms
- Amyloidosis
- Thrombotic events, especially when anticardiolipin antibodies present
- Intestinal perforation

REFERENCES
1. Al-Araji A, Kidd DP et al. Neuro-Behçet's disease: epidemiology, clinical characteristics, and management. *Lancet Neurol*. 2009;8:192–204.
2. Lin P, Liang G et al. Behçet disease: recommendation for clinical management of mucocutaneous lesions. *J Clin Rheumatol*. 2006;12:282–6.
3. Hamuryudan V, Mat C, Saip S, Ozyazgan Y, Siva A, Yurdakul S, Zwingenberger K, Yazici H et al. Thalidomide in the treatment of the mucocutaneous lesions of the Behçet syndrome. A randomized, double-blind, placebo-controlled trial. *Ann Intern Med*. 1998;128:443–50.
4. Alpsoy E, Durusoy C, Yilmaz E, Ozgurel Y, Ermis O, Yazar S, Basaran E et al. Interferon alfa-2a in the treatment of Behçet disease: a randomized placebo-controlled and double-blind study. *Arch Dermatol*. 2002;138:467–71.
5. Tugal-Tutkun I, Mudun A, Urgancioglu M, Kamali S, Kasapoglu E, Inanc M, Gül A et al. Efficacy of infliximab in the treatment of uveitis that is resistant to treatment with the combination of azathioprine, cyclosporine, and corticosteroids in Behçet's disease: an open-label trial. *Arthritis Rheum*. 2005;52:2478–84.
6. Melikoglu M, Fresko I, Mat C, Ozyazgan Y, Gogus F, Yurdakul S, Hamuryudan V, Yazici H et al. Short-term trial of etanercept in Behçet's disease: a double blind, placebo controlled study. *J Rheumatol*. 2005;32:98–105.
7. Alpsoy E, Er H, Durusoy C, Yilmaz E et al. The use of sucralfate suspension in the treatment of oral and genital ulceration of Behçet disease: a randomized, placebo-controlled, double-blind study. *Arch Dermatol*. 1999;135:529–32.

ADDITIONAL READING
Alpsoy E, Akman A et al. Behçet's disease: an algorithmic approach to its treatment. *Arch Dermatol Res*. 2009;301:693–702.

CLINICAL PEARLS
- Nonsuperficial oral or genital ulcers suggest Behçet syndrome rather than reactive arthritis (previously called *Reiter syndrome*). The combination of oral and genital ulcers is especially suggestive.
- The pathergy phenomenon (a cutaneous hypersensitivity reaction—formation of sterile pustules and/or papules along sites of puncture or needle track) is helpful if present but is insufficiently sensitive to rule out Behçet syndrome if absent.
- Colchicine is the 1st-line of therapy for Behçet syndrome.
- IgG, IgM, and IgA assays for anticardiolipin antibody tests are indicated for vascular complications in Behçet syndrome.

BELL PALSY

Dylan C. Kwait, MD

 BASICS

DESCRIPTION
A peripheral lower motor neuron facial palsy, usually unilateral, which arises secondary to inflammation and subsequent swelling and compression of the 7th (facial) cranial nerve and the associated vasa nervorum.

EPIDEMIOLOGY
- Affects 0.02% of the population annually (1)[B]:
  - Most patients recover, but as many as 30% are left with facial disfigurement and pain (2)[B]
- Accounts for 60–75% of all cases of unilateral facial paralysis (3)[A]
- Predominant age:
  - Median age of onset is 40 years, but affects all ages (4)[A]
- Predominant sex: Male = Female (4)[A]

Incidence
- US: 20–30 cases per 100,000 people per year (4)[A]
- Lowest in children ≤10 years of age; highest in people ≥70 (4)[A]
- Higher among pregnant women (3)[A]
- Occurs with equal frequency on the left and right sides of the face (4)[A]

Prevalence
Affects 40,000 Americans every year (5)[A]

RISK FACTORS
- Pregnancy
- Diabetes mellitus
- Age >30
- Exposure to cold temperatures
- Upper respiratory infection (e.g., coryza, influenza)

Genetics
A genetic predisposition may be associated with Bell palsy, but it is unclear which factors are inherited.

ETIOLOGY
- Results from damage to the 7th (facial) cranial nerve
- Inflammation of the 7th nerve causes swelling and subsequent compression of both the nerve and the associated vasa nervorum
- May arise secondary to reactivation of latent herpes virus (HSV type 1 and herpes zoster virus) in cranial nerve ganglia (3)[A]
- May arise secondary to ischemia from arteriosclerosis associated with diabetes mellitus (4)[A]

COMMONLY ASSOCIATED CONDITIONS
- Herpes simplex virus
- Lyme disease
- Diabetes mellitus
- Hypertension
- Herpes zoster virus
- Ramsay-Hunt syndrome
- Sjögren syndrome
- Sarcoidosis
- Eclampsia
- Amyloidosis

DIAGNOSIS

HISTORY
- Time course of the illness (rapid onset)
- Any predisposing factors (e.g., recent viral infection, trauma, new medications, hypertension, diabetes mellitus)
- Presence of hyperacusis or history of recurrent Bell palsy (both associated with poor prognosis)
- Any associated rash (suggestive of herpes zoster, Lyme disease, or sarcoid)
- Weakness on affected side of face, often sudden in onset
- Pain in or behind the ear in 50% of cases (may precede the palsy in 25% of cases) (4)[A]
- Subjective numbness on the ipsilateral side of the face
- Alteration of taste on the ipsilateral anterior 2/3 of the tongue (chorda tympani branch of the facial nerve)
- Hyperacusis (nerve to the stapedius muscle)
- Decreased tear production

PHYSICAL EXAM
- Neurologic:
  - Determine if the weakness is due to a problem in either the central or peripheral nervous systems
  - Flaccid paralysis of muscles on the affected side, *including the forehead:*
    - Impaired ability to raise the ipsilateral eyebrow
    - Impaired closure of the ipsilateral eye
    - Bell phenomenon: Upward diversion of the eye with attempted closure of the lid
    - Impaired ability to smile, grin, or purse the lips
  - Patients may complain of numbness, but on sensory testing, no deficit is present
  - Examine for involvement of other cranial nerves
- HEENT:
  - Carefully examine head, neck, and oropharynx to exclude masses
  - Perform pneumatic otoscopic exam
- Skin:
  - Examine for erythema migrans (Lyme disease) and vesicular rash (herpes zoster virus)

DIAGNOSTIC TESTS & INTERPRETATION
Lab
Initial lab tests
- Lyme titer and IgM, IgG, and IgA for *B. burgdorferi*
- Salivary PCR for HSV1 or herpes zoster virus (these tests are largely reserved for research purposes) (3)[A]
- IgM, IgG, and IgA titers for varicella zoster virus, cytomegalovirus, rubella, hepatitis A, hepatitis B, and hepatitis C
- ESR
- Blood glucose level
- CBC
- RPR test
- HIV test

Follow-Up & Special Considerations
CSF analysis:
- Not routinely indicated
- CSF protein is elevated in 1/3 of cases
- CSF cells show mild elevation in 10% of cases with a mononuclear cell predominance.

Imaging
Initial approach
- Facial radiographs:
  - Rule out fractures.
- CT:
  - Rule out fractures.
  - Rule out stroke.
- Brain MRI:
  - Not routinely indicated
  - Rule out central pontine, temporal bone, and parotid neoplasms (4)[A].

Diagnostic Procedures/Surgery
- EMG:
  - Nerve conduction on affected and nonaffected sides can be compared to determine extent of nerve injury.
- Electroneurography:
  - Evoked potentials of affected and nonaffected sides can be compared.

Pathological Findings
Invasive diagnostic procedures are not indicated because biopsy could further damage the 7th cranial nerve.

DIFFERENTIAL DIAGNOSIS
- Infectious:
  - Lyme disease
  - Herpes zoster (Ramsay-Hunt syndrome)
  - Acute or chronic otitis media
  - Malignant otitis externa
  - Osteomyelitis of the skull base
  - Infectious mononucleosis
  - Leprosy
- Trauma:
  - Temporal bone fracture
  - Mandibular bone fracture
- Neoplastic (onset of palsy is usually slow and progressive, and accompanied by additional cranial nerve deficits and/or headache) (3)[A]:
  - Tumors of the parotid gland
  - Cholesteatoma
  - Skull-base tumor
  - Carcinomatous meningitis
  - Leukemic meningitis
- Cerebrovascular:
  - Brainstem stroke involving anteroinferior cerebellar artery
  - Aneurysm involving carotid, vertebral, or basilar arteries
- Other:
  - Multiple sclerosis
  - Myasthenia gravis (should be considered in cases of recurrent or bilateral facial palsy) (4)[A]
  - Guillain-Barré syndrome (may also present with bilateral facial palsy) (4)[A]
  - Sjögren syndrome
  - Sarcoidosis
  - Amyloidosis
  - Melkersson-Rosenthal syndrome
  - Polyneuritis

TREATMENT

MEDICATION

- Debate had existed over whether pharmacologic intervention with anti-inflammatory and/or antiviral agents is any more beneficial than watchful waiting for the treatment and prevention of long-term effects.
- Recent randomized control trials demonstrate definitively that corticosteroids decrease inflammation and limit nerve damage, thereby reducing the number of patients with residual facial weakness (6)[A].
- Evidence now shows that antivirals targeting herpes simplex are no more effective than placebo at producing full recovery (7)[A].
  - Antivirals are also less likely to produce full recovery than corticosteroids (1)[B].
  - A combination of valacyclovir and steroids provides minimal added benefit over steroid use alone (1)[B].
- Corticosteroids:
  - Prednisone (8)[B]: Total from 410 mg over 10 days to 760 mg PO over 16 days, tapering dose (adults only)
    - Treatment should begin immediately after onset, and should not be instituted if symptoms have been present for >7 days.
    - May reduce edema around the 7th cranial nerve.
  - Prednisolone (9)[B]: Total of 500 mg over 10 days, 25 mg PO b.i.d.:
    - Prednisolone alone may be an effective treatment.
    - Should be instituted within 72 hours of symptom onset
- Antivirals in combination with corticosteroids:
  - Valacyclovir (1)[B]: 1000 mg × 5 days plus prednisone 60 mg/day × 5 days then 30 mg/day × 3 days then 10 mg/day × 2 days
- Contraindications:
  - Documented hypersensitivity
  - Preexisting infections, including TB and systemic mycosis
- Precautions: Use with discretion in pregnancy, peptic ulcer disease, and diabetes
- Significant possible interactions: Measles-mumps rubella, oral polio virus vaccine, and other live vaccines

Pregnancy Considerations
Steroids should be used cautiously in pregnancy; consult with an obstetrician.

ADDITIONAL TREATMENT
General Measures
- Artificial tears should be used to lubricate the cornea.
- The ipsilateral eye should be patched and taped shut at night to avoid drying and infection.

Issues for Referral
Patients may need to be referred to an ENT specialist or a neurologist.

Additional Therapies
- Physical therapy: No evidence of significant benefit or harm, but there is a possibility that facial exercises may reduce time to recover and/or sequelae (10)[A].
- Electrostimulation has limited evidence of effect; more studies needed (11)[B].

SURGERY/OTHER PROCEDURES
- Surgical treatment of Bell palsy remains controversial and is reserved for intractable cases (3)[A].
- The 7th cranial nerve is surgically decompressed at the entrance to the meatal foramen where the labyrinthine segment and geniculate ganglion reside (4)[A].
- Decompression surgery should not be performed >14 days after the onset of paralysis because severe degeneration of the facial nerve is likely irreversible after 2–3 weeks (4)[A].

 ONGOING CARE

FOLLOW-UP RECOMMENDATIONS
Patient Monitoring
- Patients should start treatment immediately and be followed for 12 months.
- Patients who do not recover complete facial nerve function should be referred to an ophthalmologist for tarsorrhaphy.

DIET
No restrictions

PROGNOSIS
- Most achieve complete spontaneous recovery within 2 weeks (5)[A]
- 85% of untreated patients will experience the 1st signs of recovery within 3 weeks of onset (8)[C].
- Over 80% recover within 3 months (5)[A].
- 16% are left with a partial palsy, motor synkinesis, and autonomic synkinesis (3)[A].
- 5% experience severe sequelae, and a small number of patients experience permanent facial weakness and dysfunction (3)[A].
- Poor prognostic factors include:
  - Age >60 years
  - Complete facial weakness
  - HTN
  - Ramsay-Hunt syndrome
- Absence of recovery at 3 weeks

COMPLICATIONS
- Corneal abrasion or ulceration
- Steroid-induced psychological disturbances; avascular necrosis of the hips, knees, and/or shoulders
- Steroid use can unmask subclinical infection (e.g., TB)

REFERENCES

1. Worster A, Keim SM, Sahsi R, Pancioli AM, Best Evidence in Emergency Medicine (BEEM) Group et al. Do either corticosteroids or antiviral agents reduce the risk of long-term facial paresis in patients with new-onset Bell's palsy? *J Emerg Med*. 2010;38:518–23.
2. De Diego-Sastre JI, Prim-Espada MP, Fernández García F. [The epidemiology of Bell's palsy] *Rev Neurol*. 2005;41:287–90.
3. Holland NJ, et al. Recent developments in Bell's palsy. *Br Med J*. 2004;329:553–7.
4. Gilden DH. Clinical practice. Bell's Palsy. *N Engl J Med*. 2004;351:1323–31.
5. Holten KB. How should we manage Bell's palsy? *J Fam Pract*. 2004;53:797–8.
6. Salinas RA, Alvarez G, Daly F, Ferreira J et al. Corticosteroids for Bell's palsy (idiopathic facial paralysis). *Cochrane Database Syst Rev*. 2010; 3:CD001942.
7. Lockhart P, Daly F, Pitkethly M, Comerford N, Sullivan F et al. Antiviral treatment for Bell's palsy (idiopathic facial paralysis). *Cochrane Database Syst Rev*. 2009;CD001869.
8. Peitersen E. The natural history of Bell's palsy. *Am J Otol*. 1982;4(2):107–11.
9. Madhok V, Falk G, Fahey T, et al. Prescribe prednisolone alone for Bell's palsy diagnosed within 72 hours of symptom onset. *BMJ*. 2009;338:b255.
10. Teixeira LJ, et al. Physical therapy for Bell's palsy (idiopathic facial paralysis). *Cochrane Database Syst Rev*. 2008;16(3):CD006283.
11. Alakram P, Puckree T et al. Effects of electrical stimulation on House-Brackmann scores in early Bell's palsy. *Physiother Theory Pract*. 2010; 26:160–6.

See Also (Topic, Algorithm, Electronic Media Element)
Amyloidosis; Herpes Simplex; Herpes Zoster; Sarcoidosis; Amyloidosis; Lyme Disease; Diabetes Mellitus Type 1; Diabetes Mellitus Type 2; Ramsay-Hunt Syndrome; Sjögren Syndrome; Melkersson-Rosenthal Syndrome

 CODES

ICD9
351.0 Bell's palsy

CLINICAL PEARLS
- Steroids must be initiated immediately after onset of symptoms.
- Look closely at the voluntary movement on the upper part of the face on the affected side; in Bell palsy, all of the muscles are involved (weak or paralyzed), whereas in a stroke, the upper muscles are spared (due to bilateral innervation).
- Remember to protect the affected eye with lubrication and taping.
- In areas with endemic Lyme disease, Bell palsy should be considered to be Lyme disease until proven otherwise.

BIPOLAR I DISORDER

Laurie A. Carrier, MD

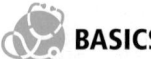 **BASICS**

DESCRIPTION
- Bipolar I (BP-I) is a mood disorder characterized by at least 1 manic or mixed episode, often alternating with episodes of major depression, that causes marked impairment and/or hospitalization.
- Symptoms are not caused by a substance (e.g., drug), a general medical condition, or a medication.

Geriatric Considerations
New onset in older patients (>50 years of age) requires a workup for organic or chemically induced pathology.

Pediatric Considerations
There is overlap with symptoms of attention-deficit hyperactivity disorder (ADHD) and oppositional defiant disorder (ODD). Children and adolescents experience more rapid cycling and mixed states. Depression often presents as irritable mood.

Pregnancy Considerations
- Potential teratogenic effects of commonly used medications (e.g., lithium, valproic acid)
- Symptoms may be exacerbated in the postpartum period.

EPIDEMIOLOGY
- Most common onset is between 15 and 30 years of age.
- More common in single and divorced persons
- Less common in college graduates
- Higher than average incidence in higher socioeconomic groups

Prevalence
- 1.0–1.6% lifetime prevalence
- Equal among men and women (manic episodes more common in men; depressive episodes more common in women)
- Women are more likely to be rapid cyclers (4 or more mood episodes per year)
- Equal among races; however, clinicians tend to misdiagnose schizophrenia in African-American patients with BP-I.

RISK FACTORS
Genetics, major life stressors (especially loss of parent or spouse), or substance abuse

Genetics
- Monozygotic twin concordance 40–70%
- Dizygotic twin concordance 5–25%
- 50% of patients have at least one parent with a mood disorder.
- 1st-degree relatives of people with BP-I are approximately 7× more likely to develop BP-I than the general population.

GENERAL PREVENTION
Treatment adherence and education can help to prevent relapses.

PATHOPHYSIOLOGY
Dysregulation of biogenic amines or neurotransmitters (particularly serotonin, norepinephrine, and dopamine). MRI findings suggest abnormalities in prefrontal cortical areas, striatum, and amygdala that predate illness onset (1).

ETIOLOGY
Genetic predisposition and major life stressors can trigger initial and subsequent episodes.

COMMONLY ASSOCIATED CONDITIONS
Substance abuse (60%), ADHD, anxiety disorders, and eating disorders

 DIAGNOSIS

- The diagnosis of BP-I requires at least 1 manic or mixed episode (simultaneous mania and depression). Although a depressive episode is not necessary for the diagnosis, 80–90% of people with BP-I also experience depression.
- Manic episode, DSM-IV-TR criteria:
  - Distinct period of abnormally and persistently elevated, expansive, or irritable mood lasting at least 1 week (or any duration if hospitalization is necessary)
  - During the period of mood disturbance, 3 or more of the "DIG FAST" symptoms must persist (4 if the mood is only irritable) and must be present to a significant degree:
    ○ *D*istractibility (attention too easily drawn to unimportant or irrelevant external stimuli)
    ○ *I*nsomnia, decreased need for sleep (e.g., feels rested after only 3 hours of sleep)
    ○ *G*randiosity or inflated self-esteem
    ○ *F*light of ideas or subjective experience that thoughts are racing
    ○ *A*gitation or increase in goal-directed activity (socially, at work or school, or sexually)
    ○ *S*peech pressured/more talkative than usual
    ○ *T*aking risks: Excessive involvement in pleasurable activities that have a high potential for painful consequences (e.g., financial or sexual)
- Major depressive episode: See "Bipolar II Disorder" for DSM-IV-TR criteria (*Note*: A depressive episode is not necessary for the diagnosis of BP-I.)
- Mixed episode: Criteria are met for both a manic and major depressive episode nearly every day during at least a 1-week period, and the mood disturbance causes significant impairment in functioning.
- Signs and symptoms more likely in bipolar than in unipolar depression (2): Agitation/restlessness, suicidal ideation/planning, increased frequency of depressive episodes, melancholia, psychomotor retardation, younger age of onset, hyperphagia, hypersomnia, family history of bipolar disorder, subsyndromal hypomanic symptoms (particularly increased goal-directed activity)

HISTORY
- Collateral information makes diagnostics more complete and is often necessary for a clear history.
- History: Safety concerns (e.g., Suicide/homicide ideation? Safety plan? Psychosis present?); Physical well-being (e.g., Number of hours of sleep? Appetite? Substance abuse?); Personal history (e.g., Told life of the party? Talkative? Speeding? Spending sprees or donations? Credit-card or gambling debt? Promiscuous? Other risk-taking behavior? Legal trouble? Religious infatuation?)

PHYSICAL EXAM
- Mental status exam in acute mania:
  - General appearance: Bright clothing, excessive makeup, disorganized or discombobulated, psychomotor agitation
  - Speech: Pressured, difficult to interrupt
  - Mood/affect: Euphoria, irritability/expansive, labile
  - Thought process: Flight of ideas (streams of thought occur to patient at rapid rate), easily distracted
  - Thought content: Grandiosity, paranoia, hyperreligious
  - Perceptual abnormalities: 3/4 of manic patients experience delusions, grandiose or paranoid
  - Suicidal/homicidal ideation: Irritability or delusions may lead to aggression toward self or others; suicidal ideation is common with mixed episode.
  - Insight/judgment: Poor/impaired
- See "Bipolar II Disorder" for an example of a mental status exam in depression.
- With mixed episodes, patients may exhibit a combination of manic and depressive mental states.

DIAGNOSTIC TESTS & INTERPRETATION
- BP-I is a clinical diagnosis.
- Mood Disorder Questionnaire is a self-assessment screen for bipolar disorders (sensitivity 73%, specificity 90%) (3).
- Patient Health Questionnaire-9 helps to determine the presence and severity of a depressive episode.

Lab
- Thyroid-stimulating hormone (TSH), complete blood count (CBC), CMP, liver function tests (LFTs), antinuclear antibody, RPR, human immunodeficiency virus, erythrocyte sedimentation rate, UDS
- Drug/alcohol screen with each presentation
- Dementia workup if new onset in seniors (e.g., TSH, RPR, vitamin B_{12}, brain imaging)

Imaging
Consider brain imaging (CT scan, MRI) with initial onset of mania to rule out organic cause (e.g., tumor, infection, or stroke), especially with onset in elderly and if psychosis is present.

Diagnostic Procedures/Surgery
Consider electroencephalogram if presentation suggests temporal lobe epilepsy (hyperreligiosity, hypergraphia).

DIFFERENTIAL DIAGNOSIS
- Other psychiatric considerations: Unipolar depression ± psychotic features, schizophrenia, schizoaffective disorder, personality disorders (particularly antisocial, borderline, histrionic, and narcissistic), attention-deficit disorder ± hyperactivity, substance-induced mood disorder
- Medical considerations: Epilepsy (e.g., temporal lobe), brain tumor, infection (e.g., AIDS, syphilis), stroke, endocrine (e.g., thyroid disease), multiple sclerosis
- In children, consider ADHD and ODD

 TREATMENT

- Ensure safety
- Medication management
- Psychotherapy (e.g., cognitive-behavioral therapy, social rhythm therapy)
- Stress reduction
- Patient and family education

MEDICATION
First Line
- Treatment may consist of 1–4 of the following mood stabilizers or other psychotropic medications. When combining these agents, consider adding different classes (e.g., an atypical antipsychotic and/or an antiseizure medication and/or lithium).
- Lithium (Lithobid, Eskalith, generic): *Dosing:* 600–1,200 mg/day divided bid–qid; start 600 mg PO tid in acute mania, and titrate based on blood levels. *Warning:* Use caution in kidney and heart disease; use can lead to diabetes insipidus, thyroid disease. Use caution in sodium-depleted patients (e.g., those using diuretics or ACE inhibitors); dehydration can lead to toxicity (seizures, encephalopathy, arrhythmias). Pregnancy category D (Ebstein anomaly). *Monitor:* Check electrocardiogram (ECG) >40 years, TSH, blood urea nitrogen, creatine, lytes at baseline and every 6 months; check level 5 days after initiation or dose change, then every 1–2 weeks ×3, then every 2–3 months (Goal: 0.8–1.2 mmol/L).
- Antiseizure medications:
  - Divalproex sodium, valproic acid (Depakote, Depakene, generic): *Dosing:* Start 250–500 mg bid–tid; maximum 60 mg/kg/day. *Black box warnings:* Hepatotoxicity, pancreatitis, thrombocytopenia, pregnancy category D (neural tube defects). *Monitor:* CBC, LFTs at baseline and every 6 months; check VPA level 5 days after initiation and dose changes (Goal: 50–125 μg/mL).
  - Carbamazepine (Carbatrol, Equetro, Tegretol, generic): *Dosing:* 800–1,200 mg/day PO divided bid–qid; start 100–200 mg PO bid and titrate to lowest effective dose. *Warning:* Do not use with tricyclic acid or within 14 days of a monoamine oxidase inhibitor. Use caution with kidney/heart disease; risk of aplastic anemia/agranulocytosis, enzyme inducer; pregnancy category D. *Monitor:* CBC, LFTs at baseline and every 3–6 months; check level 4–5 days after initiation and dose changes (Goal: 4–12 μg/mL).
  - Lamotrigine (Lamictal): *Dosing:* 200 mg/day; start 25 mg/day × 2 weeks, then 50 mg/day × 2 weeks, then 100 mg/day × 1 week (*Note:* Use different dosing if adjunct to valproate). *Warning:* Titrate slowly (risk of Stevens-Johnson syndrome); use caution with kidney/liver/heart disease; pregnancy category C.
  - Oxcarbmazepine (Trileptal), gabapentin (Neurontin), and topiramate (Topamax) are also used in BP-I but are not approved by the Food and Drug Administration (FDA).
- Atypical antipsychotics (AAs):
  - Side effects of AAs: Orthostatic hypotension, metabolic side effects (glucose and lipid dysregulation, weight gain), tardive dyskinesia, NMS, prolactinemia (except Abilify), increased risk of death in elderly with dementia-related psychosis, pregnancy category C
  - Monitor: LFTs, lipids, glucose at baseline, 3 months, and annually; check for EPS with AIMS and assess weight (with abdominal circumference) at baseline, at 4, 8, and 12 weeks, and then every 3–6 months; monitor for orthostatic hypotension 3–5 days after starting or changing dose.
  - Aripiprazole (Abilify): *Dosing:* 15 mg/day, max. 30 mg/day; less likely to cause metabolic side effects
  - Olanzapine (Zyprexa, Zydis): *Dosing:* 5–20 mg/day; most likely to cause metabolic side effects (weight gain, diabetes)
  - Symbyax (olanzapine + fluoxetine): *Dosing:* 6/25 mg, FDA approved for BP depression
  - Quetiapine (Seroquel): *Dosing:* In mania, 200–400 mg bid; in bipolar depression, 50–300 mg qhs. *Caution:* Cataracts
  - Risperidone (Risperdal): *Dosing:* 1–6 mg/day divided qid–bid. Generic and every 2 weeks IM preparations available
  - Ziprasidone (Geodon): *Dosing:* 40–80 mg bid; less likely to cause metabolic side effects. *Caution:* QTc prolongation (>500 ms) has been a/w use (0.06%). Consider ECG at baseline.

Second Line
- Antidepressants (in addition to mood stabilizers)
- Benzodiazepines (for acute agitation with mania, associated anxiety)
- Sleep medications

ADDITIONAL TREATMENT
General Measures
- Psychotherapy (e.g., cognitive-behavioral therapy, social rhythm therapy) in conjunction with medications is key (4).
- Regular exercise, a healthy diet, and sobriety have been shown to help prevent worsening of symptoms.

Issues for Referral
Comfort level of doctor, stability of patient, patients benefit from a multidisciplinary team, including a primary care physician and a psychiatrist.

Additional Therapies
- Electroconvulsive therapy can be helpful in acute mania and depression.
- Light therapy for seasonal component to depressive episodes (use with caution because it can precipitate manic episode)

COMPLEMENTARY AND ALTERNATIVE MEDICINE
Omega-3 fatty acids may help.

IN-PATIENT CONSIDERATIONS
Admit if acutely dangerous to self or others.

Admission Criteria
To admit a patient (>18 years of age) to a psychiatric unit involuntarily, the patient must have a psychiatric diagnosis (e.g., BP-I) or present a danger to him- or herself or others, or their mental disease must be inhibiting them from obtaining their basic needs (e.g., food, clothing, etc.).

Nursing
Alert staff to potentially dangerous or agitated patients. Acute suicidal threats need continuous observation.

Discharge Criteria
Determined by safety

 ## ONGOING CARE

FOLLOW-UP RECOMMENDATIONS
- Regularly scheduled visits support adherence with treatment.
- Frequent communication among primary care doctor, psychiatrist, and therapist

Patient Monitoring
Mood charts are helpful to monitor symptoms.

PATIENT EDUCATION
National Alliance on Mental Illness (NAMI): http://www.nami.org/

PROGNOSIS
- Frequency and severity of episodes are related to medication adherence, consistency with therapy, amount of sleep, and support systems.
- 40–50% of patients experience another manic episode within 2 years of the 1st episode.
- 25–50% attempt suicide, and 15% die.
- Substance abuse, unemployment, psychosis, depression, and male sex are associated with a worse prognosis.

REFERENCES
1. Fornito A, Yücel M, Wood SJ, et al. Anterior cingulate cortex abnormalities associated with a first psychotic episode in bipolar disorder. *Br J Psychiatry.* 2009;194:426–33.
2. Perlis RH, Brown E, Baker RW, et al. Clinical features of bipolar depression versus major depressive disorder in large multicenter trials. *Am J Psychiatry.* 2006;163:225–31.
3. Hirschfeld RM, Holzer C, Calabrese JR, et al. Validity of the mood disorder questionnaire: a general population study. *Am J Psychiatry.* 2003;160:178–80.
4. Depp CA, Moore DJ, Patterson TL, et al. Psychosocial interventions and medication adherence in bipolar disorder. *Dialogues Clin Neurosci.* 2008;10:239–50.

ADDITIONAL READING
- American Psychiatric Association. Practice guideline for the treatment of patients with bipolar disorder (revision). *Am J Psychiatry.* 2002;159:1–50.
- McAllister-Williams RH. Relapse prevention in bipolar disorder: a critical review of current guidelines. *Psychopharmacol.* 2006;20(2 Suppl):12–6.

See Also (Topic, Algorithm, Electronic Media Element)
Algorithm: Depression, Adult

 ## CODES

ICD9
- 296.40 Bipolar affective disorder, manic, unspecified degree
- 296.50 Bipolar affective disorder, depressed, unspecified degree
- 296.7 Bipolar I disorder, most recent episode (or current) unspecified

CLINICAL PEARLS
- Bipolar I is characterized by at least 1 manic or mixed episode, often alternating with episodes of major depression, that causes marked impairment.
- 25–50% of BP-I patients attempt suicide, and 15% die by suicide.
- There is no way to prevent the onset of BP-I, but treatment adherence and education can help to prevent further episodes.

BIPOLAR II DISORDER

Laurie A. Carrier, MD

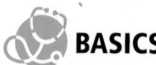

BASICS

DESCRIPTION
Bipolar II (BP-2) is a mood disorder characterized by at least 1 episode of major depression and at least 1 episode of hypomania, a milder form of mania.

Geriatric Considerations
New onset in older patients (>50) requires a workup for organic or chemically induced pathology.

Pediatric Considerations
- Large overlap with symptoms of attention deficit hyperactivity disorder (ADHD) and oppositional defiant disorder (ODD)
- Depression often presents as irritable mood.

Pregnancy Considerations
- Counsel women of childbearing age about potentially teratogenic effects of commonly used medications (e.g., lithium, valproic acid).
- Symptoms may be exacerbated in the postpartum period.

EPIDEMIOLOGY
More common in women

Prevalence
0.5–1.1% lifetime prevalence

RISK FACTORS
Genetics
Heritability estimate: >77%

GENERAL PREVENTION
There is no way to prevent the onset of BP-2, but treatment adherence and education can help to prevent further episodes.

PATHOPHYSIOLOGY
Dysregulation of biogenic amines or neurotransmitters (particularly serotonin, norepinephrine, and dopamine)

ETIOLOGY
- Genetics
- Major life stressors (especially loss of parent or spouse)

COMMONLY ASSOCIATED CONDITIONS
Substance abuse or dependence, ADHD, anxiety disorders, and eating disorders

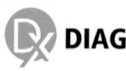

DIAGNOSIS

- DSM-IV-TR criteria: Patient must experience at least 1 hypomanic episode and at least 1 major depressive episode. The symptoms have caused *some* distress or impairment in social, occupational, or other areas of functioning. There can be no history of full manic or mixed episodes.
- Hypomania is a distinct period of persistently elevated, expansive, or irritable mood, different from usual nondepressed mood, lasting at least 4 days:
  - The episode must include at least 3 of the "DIG FAST" symptoms below (4 if the mood is only irritable):
    - **D**istractibility
    - **I**nsomnia, decreased need for sleep
    - **G**randiosity or inflated self-esteem
    - **F**light of ideas or subjective experience that thoughts are racing
    - **A**gitation or increase in goal-directed activity (socially, at work or school, or sexually)
    - **S**peech pressured/more talkative than usual
    - **T**aking risks: Excessive involvement in pleasurable activities that have high potential for painful consequences (e.g., sexual or financial)
  - The symptoms are not severe enough to cause *marked* impairment in functioning or hospitalization, and there is no associated psychosis as with BP-1.
- Major depression:
  - Depressed mood or diminished interest and 4 or more of the "SIG E CAPS" symptoms are present during the same 2-week period:
    - **S**leep disturbance (e.g., trouble falling asleep, early morning awakening)
    - **I**nterest: Loss or anhedonia
    - **G**uilt (or feelings of worthlessness)
    - **E**nergy, loss of
    - **C**oncentration, loss of
    - **A**ppetite changes, increase or decrease
    - **P**sychomotor changes (retardation or agitation)
    - **S**uicidal/homicidal thoughts
  - BP-2 with rapid cycling is diagnosed when a patient experiences at least 4 episodes of a mood disturbance in a 12-month period (either major depression or hypomania).
- Signs, symptoms, and history seen more often in BP-2 than in unipolar depression (1):
  - Agitation, hyperphagia, hypersomnia, melancholia, psychomotor retardation, suicidal ideation/planning, increased frequency of depressive episodes, younger age of onset, family history of bipolar disorder, subsyndromal hypomanic symptoms (especially overactivity) (2)
- Note: If symptoms have *ever* met criteria for a full manic episode or hospitalization was necessary secondary to manic/mixed symptoms or psychosis was present, then the diagnosis changes to bipolar I disorder (BP-1).

HISTORY
Collateral information makes diagnostics more complete and is often necessary for a clear history.

PHYSICAL EXAM
- Mental status exam in hypomania:
  - General appearance: Usually appropriately dressed, with psychomotor agitation
  - Speech: May be pressured, talkative, difficult to interrupt
  - Mood/affect: Euphoria, irritability/congruent or expansive
  - Thought process: May be easily distracted, difficulty concentrating on 1 task
  - Thought content: Usually positive with "big" plans
  - Perceptual abnormalities: None
  - Suicidal/homicidal ideation: Low incidence of homicidal or suicidal ideation
  - Insight/judgment: Usually stable/may be impaired by their distractibility
- Mental status exam in acute depression:
  - General appearance: Unkempt, psychomotor retardation, poor eye contact
  - Speech: Low, soft, monotone
  - Mood/affect: Sad, depressed/congruent, flat
  - Thought process: Ruminating thoughts, generalized slowing
  - Thought content: Preoccupied with negative or nihilistic ideas
  - Perceptual abnormalities: 15% of depressed patients experience hallucinations or delusions.
  - Suicidal/homicidal ideation: Suicidal ideation is very common.
  - Insight/judgment: Often impaired

DIAGNOSTIC TESTS & INTERPRETATION
- BP-2 is a clinical diagnosis.
- Mood disorder questionnaire, self-assessment screen for BP, sensitivity 73%, specificity 90% (3)
- Hypomania checklist-32 distinguishes between BP-2 and unipolar depression (sensitivity 80%, specificity 51%) (4)
- Patient health questionnaire-9 helps to determine the presence and severity of depression.

Lab
- Rule out organic causes of mood disorder during initial episode.
- Drug/alcohol screen is prudent with each presentation.
- Dementia workup if new onset in seniors (e.g., thyroid-stimulating hormone [TSH], rapid plasma reagin [RPR], B$_{12}$, brain imaging).

Initial lab tests
With initial presentation: Consider complete blood count (CBC), chem 7, TSH, liver function tests (LFTs), antinuclear antibody, RPR, HIV, erythrocyte sedimentation rate

Imaging
Consider brain imaging (computed tomography, magnetic resonance imaging) with initial onset of hypomania to rule out organic cause (e.g., tumor, infection, stroke), especially with onset in elderly.

DIFFERENTIAL DIAGNOSIS
- Other psychiatric considerations:
  - Bipolar 1 disorder, unipolar depression, personality disorders (particularly borderline, antisocial, and narcissistic), attention deficit disorder +/− hyperactivity, substance-induced mood disorder
- Medical considerations:
  - Epilepsy (e.g., temporal lobe), brain tumor, infection (e.g., AIDS, syphilis), stroke, endocrine (e.g., thyroid disease), multiple sclerosis
- In children, consider ADHD and ODD.

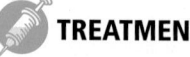

TREATMENT

- Ensure safety
- Medication management
- Psychotherapy (e.g., cognitive behavioral therapy [CBT], social rhythm therapy)
- Stress reduction
- Patient and family education

MEDICATION
- Less research has been conducted on the appropriate treatment of BP-2, but current consensus is to treat with the same medications as BP-1.
- Antidepressant medications must be used with caution during depressive episodes, as they may precipitate hypomanic episodes (less common than with BP-1).

First Line

- American Psychological Association guidelines state lithium or lamotrigine as first-line treatment for bipolar depression.
- Treatment may consist of 1–4. When combining mood stabilizers, consider adding different classes (e.g., an atypical antipsychotic and/or an antiseizure medication and/or lithium).
- Lithium (Lithobid, Eskalith, generic): Dosing 600–1200 mg/day divided b.i.d.–q.i.d., titrate based on blood levels:
  – Selected warnings: Caution in kidney or heart disease; use can lead to diabetes insipidus, thyroid disease; caution sodium-depleted patients (diuretics, angiotensin-converting enzyme inhibitors); dehydration can lead to toxicity, which may cause seizures, encephalopathic syndrome, arrhythmias, pregnancy category D (Ebstein anomaly with 1st trimester use)
  – Monitor: Check electrocardiogram (EKG) >40 y, TSH, blood urea nitrogen, creatinine, lytes at baseline and q6 months; check level 5 days after initiation or dose change, then q1–2 wk × 3, then q2–3 mo (goal: 0.8–1.2 mmol/L)
- Antiseizure medications:
  – Valproic acid, divalproex sodium (Depakene, Depakote, generic): Dosing: Start 250–500 mg b.i.d.–t.i.d., max 60 mg/kg/day. Selected warnings: Hepatotoxicity, pancreatitis, thrombocytopenia, pregnancy category D (neural tube defects). Monitor: CBC, LFTs at baseline and q6 mo; check valproic acid level 5 days after initiation and dose changes (goal: 50–125 mcg/mL).
  – Carbamazepine (Carbatrol, Equetro, Tegretol, generic): Dosing: 800–1200 mg/day p.o. div b.i.d.–q.i.d., start 100–200 mg p.o. b.i.d. and titrate to lowest effective dose. Selected warnings: Do not use with tricyclic antidepressants or within 14 d of monoamine oxidase inhibitor; caution with kidney or heart disease, may cause aplastic anemia/agranulocytosis, pregnancy category D. Monitor: CBC, LFTs at baseline and q3–6 mo; check level 4–5d after initiation and dose changes (goal: 4–12 mcg/mL).
  – Lamotrigine (Lamictal): Dosing: 200 mg a day, start 25 mg × 2 wk, then 50 mg × 2 wk, then 100 mg × 1 wk (Note: Different dosing if adjunct to valproate). Selected warnings: Titrate slowly (risk of Stevens-Johnson syndrome); caution with kidney, liver, or heart impairment; pregnancy category C. Monitor: Patient to monitor for rash.
  – Oxcarbmazepine (Trileptal), gabapentin (Neurontin), and topiramate (Topamax) are also used in BP but are not Food and Drug Administration (FDA)-approved.
- Atypical antipsychotics (AAs):
  – Side effects of AAs: Orthostatic hypotension, negative metabolic side effects (effect glucose and lipid regulation, weight gain), tardive dyskinesia, neuroleptic malignant syndrome, prolactinemia (except Abilify), increased risk of mortality in elderly with dementia-related psychosis, pregnancy category C
  – Monitor: LFTs, lipids, glucose at baseline, 3 months and annually; check for extrapyramidal symptoms with AIMS and assess weight (with abdominal circumference) at baseline, then 4, 8, and 12 weeks, then q3–6 m; monitor for orthostatic hypotension 3–5 days after starting or changing dose

– Aripiprazole (Abilify) Dosing: 15 mg/day, max 30 mg/day, less likely to cause metabolic side effects
– Olanzapine (Zyprexa, Zydis): Dosing: 5–20 mg/day, most likely AA to cause metabolic side effects (weight gain, diabetes mellitus)
– Symbyax (olanzapine + fluoxetine): Dosing: 6/25 mg, FDA-approved for bipolar depression
– Quetiapine (Seroquel): Dosing: Hypomania 200–400 mg b.i.d. Depression 50–300 mg q.h.s. Caution: Cataracts, sedation.
– Risperidone (Risperdal): Dosing: 1–6 mg/day every day-b.i.d. Generic and q2 wk IM preparations available.
– Ziprasidone (Geodon): Dosing: 40–80 mg b.i.d. Less likely to cause metabolic side effects, Warnings: QTc prolongation (>500 msec) has been associated with use (0.06%), consider EKG at baseline.

Second Line

- Antidepressants (in addition to mood stabilizers)
- Benzodiazepines (for acute agitation, anxiety)
- Sleep medications

ADDITIONAL TREATMENT

General Measures

- Psychotherapy (e.g., CBT, social rhythm therapy) in conjunction with medications is key.
- Regular exercise, a healthy diet, and sobriety have shown to help prevent worsening of symptoms.

Issues for Referral

- Experience and comfort level of physician
- Stability of patient
- Patients may benefit from care by a multidisciplinary team, including a primary care physician and a psychiatrist.

Additional Therapies

- Electroconvulsive therapy with severe depression (may precipitate hypomania)
- Light therapy if there is seasonal component to depressive episodes (may precipitate hypomania)

IN-PATIENT CONSIDERATIONS

If hypomanic symptoms are severe enough to necessitate hospitalization, the patient automatically meets criteria for mania and BP-1.

Initial Stabilization

- Medications for stabilization with acute depression
- Safety plan reviewed and safe environment assured

Admission Criteria

To admit a patient (>18) to a psychiatric unit involuntarily, they must have a psychiatric diagnosis (e.g., major depression) and present a danger to themselves or others, or their mental disease must be inhibiting them from providing their basic needs (e.g., food, clothing, and/or shelter).

Nursing

Acute suicidal threats need closer observation.

Discharge Criteria

Determined by safety

ONGOING CARE

FOLLOW-UP RECOMMENDATIONS

- Regularly scheduled visits support treatment adherence.
- Frequent communication between primary care doctor, psychiatrist, and therapist ensures comprehensive care.

Patient Monitoring

Mood charts are helpful adjuncts to care.

PATIENT EDUCATION

- Support groups for patients and families
- National Alliance on Mental Illness: http://www.nami.org/

PROGNOSIS

- Frequency and severity of problematic episodes are related to medication adherence, consistency with psychotherapy, sleep, support systems, regularity of daily activities, and social history.
- Substance abuse, unemployment, persistent depression, and male sex are associated with a worse prognosis.
- Although data are limited, evidence indicates that patients with BP-2 may be at greater risk of both attempting and completing suicide than with BP-1 and unipolar depression.

REFERENCES

1. Perlis RH, Brown E, Baker RW, et al. Clinical features of bipolar depression versus major depressive disorder in large multicenter trials. *Am J Psychiatry*. 2006;163:225–31.
2. Benazzi F. A prediction rule for diagnosing hypomania. *Prog Neuropsychopharmacol Biol Psychiatry*. 2009;33:317–22.
3. Hirshfeld RM. Validation of the Mood Disorder Questionnaire. *Bipolar Depression Bulletin*. 2004.
4. Angst J, Adolfsson R, Benazzi F, et al. The HCL-32: towards a self-assessment tool for hypomanic symptoms in outpatients. *J Affect Disord*. 2005; 88:217–33.

ADDITIONAL READING

- Benazzi F. Bipolar disorder–focus on bipolar II disorder and mixed depression. *Lancet*. 2007; 369:935–45.
- Benazzi F. Bipolar II disorder: epidemiology, diagnosis and management. *CNS Drugs*. 2007; 21:727–40.
- Edvardsen J, Torgersen S, Røysamb E, et al. Heritability of bipolar spectrum disorders. Unity or heterogeneity? *J Affect Disord*. 2007.

See Also (Topic, Algorithm, Electronic Media Element)

Algorithm: Depression, Adult

 CODES

ICD9
296.89 Other manic-depressive psychosis

CLINICAL PEARLS

- BP-2 is characterized by at least 1 episode of major depression and 1 episode of hypomania.
- Patients are often resistant to treatment during a hypomanic episode, as they enjoy the elevated mood and productivity.
- Evidence indicates that patients with BP-2 may be at greater risk of both attempting and completing suicide than with BP-1 and unipolar depression.

BITES

Jennifer S. Daly, MD

 BASICS

DESCRIPTION
- Animal bites to humans from dogs (85–90%), cats (5–10%), rodents (2–3%), humans (2–3%), and other animals, including snakes
- System(s) affected: Potentially any

Geriatric Considerations
Increased risk of infection if patient is >50.

Pediatric Considerations
Young children are more likely to have severe bites.

EPIDEMIOLOGY
- Predominant age: All ages, but children > adults
- Predominant gender: Dog bites: Male > Female; cat bites: Female > Male

Incidence
- 4–5 million dog bites per year in US
- Account for 1% of all emergency room visits
- 20% of bites will require medical attention, 10,000 will require hospital admission, and an average of 19 victims will die from the bites annually (1).

Prevalence
50% of all Americans are bitten during their lifetime.

RISK FACTORS
- Male dogs are more likely to bite.
- Clenched-fist human bites are frequently associated with the use of alcohol.
- Patients presenting >8 hours following the bite are at greater risk of infection.

GENERAL PREVENTION
- Instruct children and adults about animal hazards and strongly enforce animal control laws.
- Educate dog owners.

PATHOPHYSIOLOGY
- Animal bites can cause tears, punctures, scratches, avulsions, or crush injuries.
- Contamination of wound with flora from the mouth of the biting animal or from the broken skin of the victim can lead to infection.

ETIOLOGY
- Most bite wounds are from a domestic pet known to the victim.
- 89% of cat bites are provoked.
- Pit bull terriers, German shepherds, Rottweilers, and mixed breeds are most commonly associated with bites.
- Human bites are often the result of 1 person striking another in the mouth with a clenched fist. They can also occur incidentally in the case of paronychia due to nail biting or thumb sucking or "love nips" to the face, breasts, or genital areas.

 DIAGNOSIS

HISTORY
Obtain detailed history of the incident (provoked or unprovoked), the type of animal and vaccine status, the site of the bite, and the geographic setting.

PHYSICAL EXAM
- Dog bites (85–90% of bites):
  - Hands and face most common site of injury in adults and children, respectively
  - More likely to have associated crush injury
- Cat bites (5–10% of bites):
  - Predominantly involve the hands, followed by lower extremities, face, and trunk
  - Twice as likely to lead to infection as dog bites (due to puncture nature of wounds), with higher risk of osteomyelitis, tenosynovitis, and septic arthritis
- Human bites (2–3% of bites):
  - Intentional bite: Semicircular or oval area of erythema and bruising, with or without break in skin
  - Clenched-fist injury: Small wounds over the metacarpophalangeal joints from striking the fist against another's teeth
- Signs of wound infection include fever, erythema, swelling, tenderness, purulent drainage, lymphangitis

Pediatric Considerations
If human bite mark on child has intercanine distance >3 cm, bite probably came from an adult and should raise concerns about child abuse.

DIAGNOSTIC TESTS & INTERPRETATION
Lab
Initial lab tests
- Drainage from infected wounds should be Gram-stained and cultured:
  - If wound fails to heal, add cultures for atypical pathogens and ask lab to keep cultures for 7–10 days (some pathogens are slow-growing).
- 85% of bite wounds will yield a positive culture, with an average of 5 pathogens.
- Blood cultures should be obtained if bacteremia suspected (e.g., fever)

Follow-Up & Special Considerations
Previous antibiotic therapy may alter culture results.

Imaging
Initial approach
- If bite wound is near a bone or joint, a plain radiograph is needed to check for bone injury and to use for comparison later if osteomyelitis is subsequently suspected.
- Radiographs are needed to check for fractures in clenched-fist injuries.

Follow-Up & Special Considerations
Subsequent suspicion of osteomyelitis warrants comparison plain radiograph or magnetic resonance imaging (MRI).

Diagnostic Procedures/Surgery
Surgical exploration may be needed to ascertain extent of injuries, especially in serious hand wounds.

Pathological Findings
- Dog bites:
  - *Pasteurella* sp. is present in 50% of bites.
  - Also found: *Viridans streptococci, Staphylococcus aureus, Staphylococcus intermedius, Bacteroides, Capnocytophaga canimorsus, Fusobacterium*
- Cat bites:
  - *Pasteurella* sp. is present in 75% of bites.
  - Also found: *Streptococcus* spp. (including *Streptococcus pyogenes*), *Staphylococcus* spp. (including methicillin-resistant *Staphylococcus aureus* [MRSA]), *Fusobacterium* spp., *Bacteroides* spp., *Porphyromonas* spp., *Moraxella* spp.
- Human bites:
  - *Streptococcus* species, *S. aureus, Eikenella corrodens*, and various anaerobic bacteria (e.g., *Fusobacterium, Peptostreptococcus, Prevotella*, and *Porphyromonas* spp.)
  - Although rare, case reports have suggested transmission of viruses such as hepatitis, HIV, and herpes simplex (2)[C].
- Reptile bites:
  - In addition to snake venom tissue necrosis: *P. aeruginosa, Proteus* spp., *Salmonella, Bacteroides fragilis*, and *Clostridium* spp.
- Rodent bites:
  - *Streptobacillus moniliformis* or *Spirillum minor*, which cause rat-bite fever

ALERT
Asplenic patients and those with underlying hepatic disease are at risk of bacteremia and fatal sepsis after dog bites infected with *Capnocytophaga canimorsus* (gram-negative rod).

TREATMENT

MEDICATION
- Consider need for antirabies therapy: Rabies immune globulin and human diploid cell rabies vaccine for those bitten by wild animals (in US, primary vector is bat bite), rabid pets, or unvaccinated pets, or if animal cannot be quarantined for 10 days (3)[A].
- Tetanus toxoid for those previously immunized, but >5 years since their last dose and tetanus immune globulin and tetanus vaccination in patients without a full primary series of immunizations (4)[A]
- A patient negative for anti-HBs antibodies and bitten by an HBsAg-positive individual should receive both hepatitis B immune globulin (HBIG) and hepatitis B vaccine.
- HIV postexposure prophylaxis is generally not recommended for human bites, given the extremely low risk for transmission.
- Prophylactic antibiotics are only recommended for human bites and all penetrating animal bites to the hand (5,6)[A].
- For prophylaxis and for empiric treatment of established infection, amoxicillin-clavulanate is 1st line (3)[B]:
  - Adults: 500 mg p.o. t.i.d. or 875 mg p.o. b.i.d.
  - Children: <3 months: 30 mg/kg/d p.o. q12h; ≥3 months and <40 kg: 45 mg/kg/d q12h; >40 kg, use adult dosing

– Duration of therapy: Prophylaxis: 3–5 days; treatment: cellulitis/skin abscess: 5–10 days; bacteremia: 10–14 days. Antibiotic and duration of therapy should be adjusted based on culture results and clinical improvement:
  - Adults: Clindamycin (300 mg p.o. q.i.d.) plus either TMP-SMX (1 DS tablet p.o. b.i.d.–t.i.d.) or ciprofloxacin (500 mg p.o. b.i.d.) (3)[B]; moxifloxacin (Avelox) 400 mg q24h × 7–21 days
  - Children: Clindamycin (5–10 mg/kg IV [to a maximum of 600 mg] followed by 10–30 mg/kg/d in 3–4 divided doses to a maximum of 300 mg per dose) plus trimethoprim-sulfamethoxazole (8–10 mg/kg of trimethoprim) or cefoxitin IM/IV until culture results obtained

Pregnancy Considerations
- Penicillin-allergic pregnant women:
  – Azithromycin 250–500 mg p.o. every day (3)[B]
- Observe closely and note potential increased risk of failure.

ALERT
- 1st-generation cephalosporins (e.g., cephalexin), penicillinase-resistant penicillins (e.g., dicloxacillin), macrolides (e.g., erythromycin), and clindamycin (when not administered with another agent) lack activity against *P. multocida* (dog/cat bites) and *Eikenella corrodens* (human bites), and should be avoided (3)[B].
- Consider community-acquired MRSA as possible pathogen (from human skin or colonized pet). If high suspicion, doxycycline or trimethoprim-sulfamethoxazole provide good coverage (4)[A].
- Adverse reaction: Amoxicillin-clavulanate should be given with food to decrease gastrointestinal (GI) side effects.
- Precautions: Dose antibiotics by body weight and renal function.
- Significant possible interactions: Antibiotics may decrease efficacy of oral contraceptives.

ADDITIONAL TREATMENT
General Measures
- Elevation of the injured extremity to prevent swelling
- Contact the local health department regarding the prevalence of rabies in the species of animal involved (highest in bats).
- Snake bite: If venomous, patient needs rapid transport to facility capable of definitive evaluation. If envenomation has occurred, patient should receive antivenom. Be sure patient is stable for transport; consider measuring and/or treating coagulation and renal status along with any anaphylactic reactions before transport.

Issues for Referral
Deep wounds to the hand and face should be referred to a hand surgeon or plastic surgeon, respectively.

SURGERY/OTHER PROCEDURES
- Copious irrigation of the wound with normal saline via a catheter tip is needed to reduce risk of infection.
- Devitalized tissue needs debridement.
- Debridement of puncture wounds is not advised.

- Primary closure can be considered if the wound is clean after irrigation and bite is <12 hours old, and in bites to the face (cosmesis) (7)[B].
- Infected wounds and those at risk of infection (cat bites, human bites, bites to the hand, crush injuries, presentation >12 hours from injury) should be left open (8)[B].
- Delayed primary closure in 3–5 days is an option for infected wounds.
- Splint hand if it is injured.
- Large, gaping wounds should be reapproximated with widely spaced sutures or Steri-Strips.

IN-PATIENT CONSIDERATIONS
Initial Stabilization
ABCs for associated trauma or severe infection

Admission Criteria
- Patients with deep or severe wound infections, systemic infections requiring IV antibiotics, those requiring surgery, and the immunocompromised
- If hospitalized with established infection (animal or human bite):
  – Adults: Ampicillin/sulbactam 1.5–3 g IV q6h or piperacillin/tazobactam 3.375 g q6h or 4.5 g IV q8h or ticarcillin/clavulanate 3.1 g IV q4–6h (3)[B]
  – Children: Ampicillin/sulbactam 100–200 mg/kg/d IV given in 4 divided doses to maximum of 3 g per dose

Discharge Criteria
Pending clinical improvement

 ONGOING CARE

FOLLOW-UP RECOMMENDATIONS
Patient Monitoring
- Patient should be rechecked in 24–48 hours if not infected at time of 1st encounter (9)[B].
- Daily follow-up is warranted for infections.
- Subsequent revisions of empiric antibiotic therapy should be based on the culture results and the clinical response.

PATIENT EDUCATION
- Educate parents at well-child checks about how to avoid animal bites.
- AAFP: http://familydoctor.org/online/famdocen/home/healthy/safety/kids-family/668.html

PROGNOSIS
Wounds should steadily improve and close over by 7–10 days.

COMPLICATIONS
- Septic arthritis
- Osteomyelitis
- Extensive soft tissue injuries with scarring
- Hemorrhage
- Gas gangrene
- Sepsis
- Meningitis
- Endocarditis
- Post-traumatic stress disorder
- Death

REFERENCES
1. Langley RL. Human fatalities resulting from dog attacks in the United States, 1979–2005. *Wilderness Environ Med*. 2009 Spring;20(1):19–25.
2. Bartholomew CF, Jones AM. Human bites: a rare risk factor for HIV transmission. *AIDS*. 2006;20:631–2.
3. Stevens DL, Bisno AL, Chambers HF, et al. Practice guidelines for the diagnosis and management of skin and soft-tissue infections. *Clin Infect Dis*. 2005;41:1373–406.
4. Oehler RL, Velez AP, Mizrachi M, et al. Bite-related and septic syndromes caused by cats and dogs. *Lancet Infect Dis*. 2009;9:439–47.
5. Medeiros I, et al. Antibiotic prophylaxis for mammalian bites. *Cochrane Database Syst Rev*. 2008;2:CD001738.
6. Rittner AV, Fitzpatrick K, Corfield A. Best evidence topic report. Are antibiotics indicated following human bites? *Emerg Med J*. 2005;22:654.
7. Stefanopoulos PK, Tarantzopoulou AD. Facial bite wounds: management update. *Int J Oral Maxillofac Surg*. 2005;34:464–72.
8. Benson LS, Edwards SL, Schiff AP, et al. Dog and cat bites to the hand: treatment and cost assessment. *J Hand Surg [Am]*. 2006;31:468–73.
9. Okonkwo U, et al. Animal bites: Practical tips for effective management. *J Emerg Nursing*. 2008;34(3):225–6.

ADDITIONAL READING
Daly JS, et al. Bites and stings of terrestrial and aquatic life. In Fitzpatrick TB, Eisen AZ, Wolff K, et al. (eds). *Dermatology in General Medicine*, 6th ed. New York: McGraw Hill, 2008.

See Also (Topic, Algorithm, Electronic Media Element)
Cellulitis; Rabies; Snake Envenomations; Bartonella Infections

 CODES

ICD9
- 879.8 Open wound(s) (multiple) of unspecified site(s), without mention of complication
- 879.9 Open wound(s) (multiple) of unspecified site(s), complicated

CLINICAL PEARLS
- Wound cleansing, debridement, and culture are essential. Most wounds should be left open.
- Prophylaxis is recommended for human bites and bites to the hand.
- Consider rabies and tetanus vaccination.
- Patients bitten by animals or humans require close follow-up to monitor for infection.

BLADDER CANCER

Margaret E. Thompson, MD

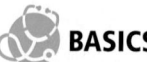

BASICS

DESCRIPTION
- Primary malignant neoplasms arising in the urinary bladder
- Most common type is transitional cell carcinoma (90%)
- Other types include adenocarcinoma, small cell carcinoma, squamous cell carcinoma
- Rhabdomyosarcoma of the bladder may occur in children.

EPIDEMIOLOGY
Incidence
- Increases with age (median age at diagnosis is 73 years)
- More common in Caucasians than in Asians or African Americans
- Male > Female (4:1)
- 37.2 per 100,000 men per year (1)
- 9.2 per 100,000 women per year (1)
- 21.1 per 100,000 men and women per year (1)

Prevalence
As of January 1, 2007, 535,236 cases in US (1)

RISK FACTORS
- Smoking is the single greatest risk factor (increases risk 4-fold) (2).
- Other risk factors:
  - Occupational carcinogens in dye, rubber, paint, plastics, metal, and automotive exhaust
  - Schistosomiasis in Mediterranean (squamous cell) cancer
  - History of pelvic irradiation
  - Chronic lower urinary tract infection (UTI)
  - Chronic indwelling urinary catheter
  - Cyclophosphamide exposure
  - High-fat diet
  - Chronic low fluid intake
  - Slight increase in risk with prostate cancer

ALERT
Any patient who smokes and presents with microscopic or gross hematuria, or irritative voiding symptoms such as urgency and frequency not clearly due to UTI, should be evaluated by cystoscopy for the presence of a bladder neoplasm.

Genetics
Hereditary transmission is unlikely, although transitional cell carcinoma pathophysiology is related to oncogenes.

GENERAL PREVENTION
Avoid smoking and other risk factors.

PATHOPHYSIOLOGY
- 70–80% is superficial (in lamina propria or mucosa):
  - Usually highly differentiated with long survival
  - Initial event seems to be activation of an oncogene on chromosome 9 in superficial cancers
- 20% of tumors are invasive (deeper than lamina propria) at presentation:
  - Tend to be high-grade with worse prognosis
  - Associated with other chromosome deletions

ETIOLOGY
Unknown, other than related to risk factors

DIAGNOSIS

HISTORY
- Hematuria
- Urinary symptoms (frequency, urgency)
- Abdominal or pelvic pain in advanced disease
- Exposures (see Risk Factors)

PHYSICAL EXAM
- Normal in early cases
- Pelvic or abdominal mass in advanced disease
- Wasting in systemic disease

DIAGNOSTIC TESTS & INTERPRETATION
Lab
Initial lab tests
- Urinalysis is the initial test in patients presenting with gross hematuria or urinary symptoms such as frequency, urgency, and dysuria.
- Macroscopic hematuria (55% sensitivity, positive predictive value [PPV] 0.22 for urologic cancer) (3)[C]

Follow-Up & Special Considerations
- Urine cytology 54% sensitivity overall (lower in less advanced tumors), 94% specific (4)[A]
- Other urine markers:
  - NMP22: 67% sensitive, 78% specific (4)[A]
  - Bladder tumor-associated antigen stat: 70% sensitive, 75% specific (4)[A]
  - Fluorescent in situ hybridization assay: 69% sensitive, 78% specific (PPV 27.1, negative predictive value 95.3) for all tumors, more sensitive and specific for higher grade (5)[B]
- Bottom line: None of the urine markers are sensitive enough to rule out bladder cancer on its own.
- Liver function tests, alkaline phosphatase if metastasis suspected

Imaging
Initial approach
- Done for staging and evaluating extent of disease, but not for diagnosis itself:
  - Computed tomography (CT) urogram replacing IV to image upper tracts if there is suspicion of disease there
  - Diffusion-weighted magnetic resonance (MR) imaging and multidimensional CT scan are undergoing study for use in diagnosis and staging of bladder tumors.
  - For invasive disease, metastatic workup should include chest x-ray.
  - Bone scan should be performed if the patient has bone pain or if alkaline phosphatase is elevated (6)[B].
- Urologic CT scan (abdomen, pelvis, with and without contrast) or MRI 40–98% accurate, with MRI slightly more accurate (6)[B], is recommended if metastasis is suspected.

Diagnostic Procedures/Surgery
- Cystoscopy with biopsy is the gold standard for diagnosis, but 1 study showed that 33% of patients had residual tumor after transurethral resection of superficial tumor (TURBT) (6)[B].
- TURBT with bladder washings: Sensitivity of cytology on bladder washings for carcinoma in situ is nearly 100%.

Pathological Findings
- Characterized as superficial or invasive
- 70–80% present as superficial lesion
- Superficial lesions:
  - Carcinoma in situ: Flat lesion, high grade
  - Ta: Noninvasive papillary carcinoma
  - T1: Extends into submucosa, lamina propria
- Invasive cancer:
  - T2: Invasion into muscle:
    - pT2a: Invasion into superficial muscle
    - pT2b: Invasion into deep muscle
  - T3: Invasion into perivesical fat:
    - pT3a: Microscopic
    - pT3b: Macroscopic
  - T4: Invasion into adjacent organs:
    - aT4a: Invades prostate, uterus, or vagina
    - aT4b: Invades abdominal or pelvic wall
  - N1–N3: Invades lymph nodes
- M: Metastasis to bone or soft tissue

DIFFERENTIAL DIAGNOSIS
- Other urinary tract neoplasms
- UTI
- Prostatism
- Bladder instability
- Interstitial cystitis
- Urolithiasis
- Interstitial nephritis
- Papillary urothelial hyperplasia

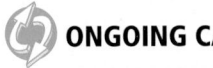 **TREATMENT**

For superficial bladder cancer, the treatment is generally removal via cystoscopic surgery. For muscle-invasive cancer, a radical cystectomy is preferred.

MEDICATION
First Line
- There is insufficient evidence to show that cisplatin-based neoadjuvant chemotherapy in patients with locally advanced bladder cancer improves survival (7)[A].
- Intravesical bacillus Calmette-Guérin (BCG) after TURBT in high-grade lesions has been shown to decrease recurrence in Ta and T1 tumors (8)[A].

Second Line
Chemotherapy is the 1st-line treatment for metastatic bladder cancer: Methotrexate-vinblastine-doxorubicin-cisplatin (MVAC) is the preferred regimen.

ADDITIONAL TREATMENT
Issues for Referral
Patients with microscopic or gross hematuria not otherwise explained or resolving should be referred to a urologist for cystoscopy.

Additional Therapies
Radiotherapy:
- In US, used for patients with muscle-invasive cancer who are not surgical candidates
- Preoperative (radical cystectomy) radiotherapy also an option
- Treatment of choice for muscle-invasive cancer in some European and Canadian centers:
  – 65–70 Gy over 6–7 weeks is standard

SURGERY/OTHER PROCEDURES
- Surgery is definitive therapy for superficial and invasive cancer:
  – Superficial cancer: TURBT sometimes followed by intravesical therapy
- Invasive cancer:
  – Radical cystectomy for invasive disease that is confined to the bladder is more effective than radical radiotherapy (9)[A]. Urine is diverted via an ileal loop with ostomy or neobladder constructed with intestine.

IN-PATIENT CONSIDERATIONS
Admission Criteria
Need for surgery or intensive therapy

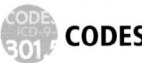 **ONGOING CARE**

FOLLOW-UP RECOMMENDATIONS
- Superficial cancers:
  – Urine cytology alone has not been shown to be sufficient for follow-up.
  – Cystoscopy every 3 months for 18–24 months, every 6 months for the next 2 years, then annually
- Follow-up for invasive cancers depends on the approach to treatment.
- Patients treated with BCG require lifelong follow-up.

DIET
Continue adequate fluid intake.

PATIENT EDUCATION
Smoking cessation

PROGNOSIS
- 5-year relative survival rates:
  – Localized: 93.7%
  – Regional metastasis: 46.0%
  – Distant metastasis: 6.2%
- Superficial bladder cancer:
  – BCG treatment prevents recurrence vs TURBT alone; difference 30%, NNT 3.3 (9)[A]
  – BCG prevents progression vs TURBT alone, difference 8%
- Invasive cancer:
  – T2 disease: Radical cystectomy results in 60–75% 5-year survival.
  – T3 or T4 disease: Radical cystectomy results in 20–40% 5-year survival.
  – Neoadjuvant chemotherapy with cystectomy has led to varying degrees of increased survival.
  – Radiation with chemotherapy has led to varying degrees of increased survival.
- Metastatic cancer:
  – MVAC resulted in mean survival of 12.5 months.

COMPLICATIONS
- Superficial bladder cancer:
  – Local symptoms:
    ○ Dysuria, frequency, nocturia, pain, passing debris in urine
    ○ Bacterial cystitis
    ○ Perforation
  – General symptoms:
    ○ Flulike symptoms
    ○ Systemic infection
- Invasive cancer:
  – Symptoms related to definitive treatment, including incontinence, bleeding
  – Patients with neobladder at risk for azotemia and metabolic acidosis

REFERENCES

1. Altekruse SF, Kosary CL, Krapcho M, et al. (eds). *SEER Cancer Statistics Review, 1975–2007*, National Cancer Institute. Bethesda, MD, http://seer.cancer.gov/csr/1975_2007/, based on November 2009 SEER data submission, posted to the SEER web site, 2010.
2. Kaplan M, Cologlu M. Bladder Tumors. In *Essential Evidence Plus*, John Wiley and Sons, Ltd, 2009, http://www.essentialevidenceplus.com/content/eee/480, accessed 4/26/10.
3. Buntinx F, Wauters H. The diagnostic value of macroscopic haematuria in diagnosing urological cancers: a meta-analysis. *Fam Pract*. 1997;14: 63–8.
4. Glas AS, Roos D, Deutekom M, et al. Tumor markers in the diagnosis of primary bladder cancer. A systematic review. *J Urol*. 2003;169: 1975–82.
5. Sarosdy MF, Kahn PR, Ziffer MD, et al. Use of a multitarget fluorescence in situ hybridization assay to diagnose bladder cancer in patients with hematuria. *J Urol*. 2006;176:44–7.
6. Kirkali Z, Chan T, Manoharan M, et al. Bladder cancer: epidemiology, staging and grading, and diagnosis. *Urology*. 2005;66:4–34.
7. Advanced Bladder Cancer Meta-analysis Collaboration. Neoadjuvant Cisplatin for advanced bladder cancer (Cochrane Review). In *the Cochrane Library Issue* 1, 2009. Chichester, UK: John Wiley and Sons, Ltd.
8. Shelley M, Court JB, Kynaston H, et al. Intravesical Bacillus Calmette-Guerin in Ta and T1 bladder cancer (Cochrane Review). In: *The Cochrane Library*, Issue 3, 2010. Chichester, UK: John Wiley and Sons, Ltd.
9. Shelley MD, et al. Surgery versus radiotherapy for muscle invasive bladder cancer (Cochrane Review). In: *The Cochrane Library*, Issue 4, 2005. Chichester, UK: John Wiley and Sons, Ltd.
10. U.S. Preventive Services Task Force. Screening for bladder cancer in adults: Recommendation statement. Rockville, MD: Agency for Healthcare Research and Quality; 2004.

ADDITIONAL READING

Vale C. Neoadjuvant chemotherapy for invasive bladder cancer (Cochrane Review). In: *The Cochrane Library* Issue 1, 2007. Chichester, UK: John Wiley and Sons, Ltd.

See Also (Topic, Algorithm, Electronic Media Element)
Hematuria
Algorithm: Hematuria

CODES

ICD9
188.9 Malignant neoplasm of bladder, part unspecified

CLINICAL PEARLS
- Gross hematuria in smokers should be evaluated with complete urologic workup.
- The United States Preventive Services Task Force recommends against routine screening for bladder cancer (10)[A].

BLADDER INJURY

Kyle D. Wood, MD
Ilya Gorbachinsky, MD

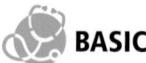

BASICS

DESCRIPTION
- Bladder injury can be the result of:
  - Blunt or penetrating trauma
  - Bladder rupture secondary to a full bladder or blunt injury
  - Surgical complication (iatrogenic injury)
- Classified as either intraperitoneal or extraperitoneal rupture
- Bladder contusion is injury to the mucosa or muscularis without full-thickness loss; without urine extravasation
- Often associated with ureter/urethral injury and/or other non-urological injuries

EPIDEMIOLOGY
Incidence
- ~0.5% of civilian trauma patients (1)
- 12% of civilian injuries in Iraq, mostly due to gunshot wounds (2)
- Blunt trauma with bladder injury is associated with other injuries 94% of the time (3); pelvic fracture being the most common followed by lower abdominal impact in the presence of a full bladder (4).
- During pelvic surgery, it is the most commonly damaged organ (5).

Pediatric Considerations
Children are more prone to rupture and are more likely to have intraperitoneal ruptures than adults (1).

RISK FACTORS
- High-energy mechanism (fall, motor vehicle accident [MVA])
- Pelvic fracture
- Penetrating wound
- Prior bladder/pelvic surgery
- Pelvic radiotherapy

GENERAL PREVENTION
Seat belts:
- Voiding prior to automobile travel

PATHOPHYSIOLOGY
- Bladder is often protected by its deep location in the bony pelvis.
- Contusion: Damage sustained to bladder mucosa and muscularis without loss of wall continuity (5)
- Intraperitoneal rupture: Increases in intravesical pressure can lead to rupture at the most weak and mobile portion, the bladder dome (6,7)
- Extraperitoneal rupture: Disruption of bony pelvis can tear bladder at fascial attachments while this or other bony protrusions can perforate the bladder (6).

Pediatric Considerations
Children <6 years old are more prone to bladder injury as the organ still lacks protection from the pubic symphysis (7).

ETIOLOGY
- The cause of injury is usually high-energy trauma (motor vehicle accidents, falls).
- Rupture due to increased pressure in nondistensible (full) bladder
- Laceration due to bone fragment or penetrating object (knife, bullet)
- Surgical complications: Gynecologic, general surgery, and urologic operations are the most common reported causes of iatrogenic bladder injury, in decreasing order of frequency (8).

ALERT
Rare instances of intravesical vascular graft erosion have recently been reported up to 8 years post-op (9).

COMMONLY ASSOCIATED CONDITIONS
- Pelvic fracture
- Urethral injury; almost exclusively males

DIAGNOSIS

HISTORY
- Isolated bladder injury is rare. Typically, patient has other serious injuries.
- High mechanism deceleration injury (fall, MVA)
- Penetrating trauma
- Recent abdominal/pelvic surgery
- Urinary retention
- Preexisting bladder outlet obstruction
- Anatomical abnormalities
- Inability to void or oliguria
- Pain in the genital area or abdomen

PHYSICAL EXAM
- Abdominal exam: Suprapubic tenderness to palpation, guarding, distention, decreased bowel sounds, bruising
- Genitourinary exam: Blood at meatus, gross hematuria, clots in the urine, scrotal/urethral hematoma, free floating or high riding prostate, unstable pelvis

ALERT
Peritonitis is unusual in bladder injury.

DIAGNOSTIC TESTS & INTERPRETATION
Lab
Initial lab tests
- Immediate catheterization will likely demonstrate gross hematuria (3).
- Urinalysis will demonstrate blood.
- Basic metabolic panel: Serum blood urea nitrogen (BUN), creatinine, chloride, and potassium levels may be elevated and sodium and bicarbonate may be decreased in intraperitoneal ruptures secondary to peritoneal absorption. An increase in BUN/creatinine ratio may also be observed (5).
- Serum labs are unchanged in extraperitoneal ruptures (6).

Follow-Up & Special Considerations
If blood at the meatus or if the catheter does not pass easily, consider urethral injury and need for retrograde urethrography.

Imaging
Initial approach
- 2 types of imaging are acceptable:
  - Plain film cystography: Fill bladder until patient has sense of discomfort or fill with 350 mL. Use 3-film technique capturing before filling, when full, and after drainage.
    - Contusion: No extravasation but may see distortion of bladder outline with contrast.
    - Intraperitoneal: Contrast may be seen in cul-de-sac and paracolic gutters. Bowel loops may also be outlined.
    - Extraperitoneal: Flame-shaped perivesical stranding of contrast (5)
  - CT cystography: High-resolution computed tomography (CT) cystogram is also acceptable. CT or radiology with only excreted contrast is not sensitive (6). Dilute contrast material.
- Absolute indication for immediate cystography: Gross hematuria with pelvic fracture as 29% of these patients will have a bladder injury (10).
- Relative indications: Gross hematuria without pelvic fracture, microhematuria with pelvic fracture, isolated microscopic hematuria (10)

ALERT
During plain film cystography, a post-void view is mandatory as contrast in the bladder may mask extravasation. This is not required with CT cystogram.

Follow-Up & Special Considerations
- Retrograde urethrography must be performed before placing a Foley catheter when urethral injury is suspected.
- Other signs of bladder injury can include free intraperitoneal fluid on CT scan or ultrasound

Pathological Findings
- Perivesicular hematoma
- Perforation at dome of bladder (in trigone, near urachus)
- Jagged tear in bladder
- Intraoperative clues (11)
  - Appearance of Foley catheter/balloon or urine in the operative field
  - Presence of gas in catheter bag (during laparoscopy)

DIFFERENTIAL DIAGNOSIS
- Isolated urethral injury
- Isolated pelvic fracture
- Isolated ureteral injury
- Other visceral rupture

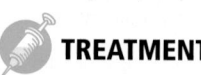

TREATMENT

- Contusion: Observation or 20–22 French Foley catheter for 10–14 days (6)[B]
- Intraperitoneal rupture: Immediate surgical repair (6)[C]
  - Often intraoperative damage falls under this heading and can also be treated immediately.
- Extraperitoneal rupture: 20–22 French Foley catheter for 10–14 days (6)

MEDICATION
- Analgesics
- Antibiotics
- Antispasmodics

First Line
- Narcotic pain control (i.e., morphine, hydromorphone); titrate to effect
- Broad-spectrum antibiotics like ciprofloxacin 500 mg b.i.d.
- Oxybutynin 5–10 mg t.i.d. for spasm

Second Line
- Broad-spectrum antibiotics
- Antispasmodics (i.e., flavoxate)

ALERT
There is concern about fluoroquinolones causing damage to cartilage in children.

ADDITIONAL TREATMENT
- If uncomplicated extraperitoneal bladder rupture:
  – Can be treated with urethral catheter alone (use large bore catheter [22 French])
  – Exception: In pediatric patients, consider placing a suprapubic catheter as small catheters through urethra will clot and larger catheters through urethra risk future urethral stricture
  – Catheter should remain in place for 2 weeks. Cystography is necessary prior to removal of catheter.
  – Antibiotics should be given on day of injury and continued for 3 days after catheter removal.
- If a complicated extraperitoneal bladder rupture:
  – Needs to be treated with open repair
  – Complicated rupture is considered when there is coexisting bladder neck injury, vaginal injury, or rectal injury. Also if open pelvic fracture, or bone fragments are present.
  – Consider open repair if patient is scheduled for exploratory laparotomy or internal fixation of pelvic fracture (prevents urine leak on hardware).
- If an intraperitoneal bladder rupture or penetrating injury:
  – Urgent operative management is necessary.
  – Cystography should be repeated 7–10 days after surgery.
  – Antibiotics are needed for 3 days .
  – No need for suprapubic catheter as urethral catheter is sufficient, except in pediatric population (3)
- During pelvic surgery, iatrogenic full thickness defects are likely to be intraperitoneal, so can fix immediately with 2-layer (mucosa and muscularis) closure via absorbable suture
  – Prior to repair, be sure to confirm that ureters were not damaged concomitantly either with IV indigo carmine administration and visulation of blue dye expulsion from the ureteral orifices (UO) or by confirming easy placement of ureteral catheters through the UO (11).

General Measures
- Place Foley catheter
- Pain control
- Antibiotics
- Antispasmodics (Ditropan)
- Obtain imaging diagnosis

Issues for Referral
A urologist or trauma surgeon should be involved with all bladder injury management.

SURGERY/OTHER PROCEDURES
- Urgent surgery is indicated for intraperitoneal or bladder neck rupture
- Extraperitoneal rupture is usually manageable with 10–14 days of catheter drainage (20–22 French).

IN-PATIENT CONSIDERATIONS
Initial Stabilization
- Cervical spine precautions
- Stabilize hemodynamics
- Stabilize pelvis
- Follow advanced trauma life support protocols

Admission Criteria
All bladder injuries require admission for monitoring renal function and hemodynamic stability.

IV Fluids
Lactated Ringer's for initial resuscitation, unless contraindicated (i.e., concomitant head injury)

Nursing
- Foley to gravity
- Hourly urine output recorded

Discharge Criteria
- Stable for transfer to rehabilitation or home if can perform activities of daily living
- Extraperitoneal ruptures controlled with indwelling Foley catheter if rupture not healed
- Able to void if no catheter in place
- No evidence of infection
- Pain controlled

 ## ONGOING CARE

FOLLOW-UP RECOMMENDATIONS
Patient Monitoring
- Hourly urine output
- Hemodynamic monitoring
- Progressive abdominal distention

DIET
No restrictions

PATIENT EDUCATION
- Regular lifestyle is expected
- Use of seat belts
- No special instructions needed

PROGNOSIS
Full return to normal function

COMPLICATIONS
- Infection
- Urine leak and/or urinoma
- Abscess formation
- Peritonitis or sepsis
- Bladder calculi
- Vesicocutaneous or other fistulas
- Stricture is a rare complication
- Death; usually from other injuries

REFERENCES

1. Inaba K, McKenney M, Munera F, et al. Cystogram follow-up in the management of traumatic bladder disruption. *J Trauma.* 2006;60:23–8.
2. Ramani AP, Ryndin I, Veetil RT, et al. Novel technique for removal of misdirected laparoscopic Weck clips. *Urology.* 2007;70:168–9.
3. Parry NG, Rozycki GS, Feliciano DV, Tremblay LN, Cava RA, Voeltz Z, Carney J et al. Traumatic rupture of the urinary bladder: is the suprapubic tube necessary? *J Trauma.* 2003;54:431–6.
4. Tezval H, Tezval M, von Klot C, Herrmann TR, Dresing K, Jonas U, Burchardt M et al. Urinary tract injuries in patients with multiple trauma. *World J Urol.* 2007;25:177–84.
5. Gomez RG, Ceballos L, Coburn M, Corriere JN, Dixon CM, Lobel B, McAninch J et al. Consensus statement on bladder injuries. *BJU Int.* 2004;94:27–32.
6. Corriere JN, Sandler CM. Diagnosis and management of bladder injuries. *Urol Clin North Am.* 2006;33:67–71, vi.
7. Kessler DO, Francis DL, Esernio-Jenssen D et al. Bladder rupture after minor accidental trauma: case reports and a review of the literature. *Pediatr Emerg Care.* 2010;26:43–5.
8. Armenakas NA, Pareek G, Fracchia JA et al. Iatrogenic bladder perforations: longterm followup of 65 patients. *J Am Coll Surg.* 2004;198:78–82.
9. Nakamura LY, Ferrigni RG, Stone WM, Fowl RJ et al. Urinary bladder injuries during vascular surgery. *J Vasc Surg.* 2010;52:453–5.
10. Morey AF, Iverson AJ, Swan A, Harmon WJ, Spore SS, Bhayani S, Brandes SB et al. Bladder rupture after blunt trauma: guidelines for diagnostic imaging. *J Trauma.* 2001;51:683–6.
11. Sharp HT, Swenson C et al. Hollow viscus injury during surgery. *Obstet Gynecol Clin North Am.* 2010;37:461–7.

ADDITIONAL READING
- ATLS Protocol from the Committee on Trauma of the American College of Surgeons, http://www.facs.org/trauma/atls/.
- Eastern Association for the Surgery of Trauma, Management of Genitourinary Trauma, 2004, http://www.east.org/tpg/GUmgmt.pdf.

See Also (Topic, Algorithm, Electronic Media Element)
Algorithm: Hematuria

 ## CODES

ICD9
- 596.6 Rupture of bladder, nontraumatic
- 596.9 Unspecified disorder of bladder
- 867.0 Injury to bladder and urethra without mention of open wound into cavity

CLINICAL PEARLS
- Foley should remain in place for 10–14 days. After this point, 85% of patients have healed all injuries.
- A cystogram must be performed before Foley removal to verify no extravasation of fluid. If extravasation continues, recheck every 3–5 days.
- An intraoperative consult to urology is indicated if an inadvertent bladder perforation occurs during another procedure. If urology is not available, the bladder must be examined intravesically, generally by increasing the size of the wound and searching for another occult injury. Do not delay repair.
- Repair bladder injuries in 2 layers with absorbable suture and place a Foley catheter.

BLEPHARITIS

Joshua J. Spooner, PharmD, MS
A. Raquel Mateo-Bibeau, MD

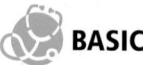 **BASICS**

DESCRIPTION
- An inflammatory reaction of the eyelid margin:
  - Usually occurs as seborrheic or staphylococcal blepharitis
  - Multiple types may coexist.
- System(s) affected: Skin/Exocrine
- Synonym(s): Granulated eyelids

EPIDEMIOLOGY
Incidence
- One of the most common ocular disorders
- Predominant age: Adult
- Predominant sex: Male = Female

RISK FACTORS
- Seborrheic dermatitis
- Contact dermatitis
- Herpes simplex dermatitis
- Varicella-zoster dermatitis
- Acne rosacea
- Diabetes mellitus
- Immunocompromised state (e.g., AIDS, chemotherapy)
- Isotretinoin use
- Dry eye syndromes

ETIOLOGY
- Seborrheic:
  - Accelerated shedding of skin cells with associated sebaceous gland dysfunction
  - *Malassezia furfur* (formerly *Pityrosporum ovale*) yeasts often colonize.
- Staphylococcal:
  - Superinfection of Zeis glands of lid margin and meibomian glands posterior to lashes with *Staphylococcus aureus*
  - Usually part of mixed blepharitis
- Meibomian gland dysfunction: Obstruction and inflammation of the meibomian glands; associated with acne rosacea, acne vulgaris, and oral retinoid therapy
- Other types of blepharitis:
  - Ulcerative blepharitis: More severe blepharitis with small marginal ulceration and destruction of the hair follicles
  - Contact dermatitis/blepharitis:
    - Develops from type IV hypersensitivity; common causes include ocular medications, topical anesthetics, antivirals, and cosmetics.
    - May occur with secondary *Staphylococcus* infection.

- Eczematoid blepharitis:
  - Caused by hypersensitivity reaction to exotoxins and antigens from local flora
  - Strong association with eczema, asthma
  - Staphylococcal infection common
- Angular blepharitis: Often caused by *Staphylococcus* or *Moraxella* infection.

COMMONLY ASSOCIATED CONDITIONS
See Risk Factors and Differential Diagnosis.

 DIAGNOSIS

HISTORY
- Duration of symptoms
- Unilateral or bilateral presentation
- Note any exacerbating conditions (e.g., smoke, allergens, wind, contact lenses, etc.).
- Symptoms related to systemic diseases
- Current and recent medication use
- Recent exposure to infected individuals
- Frequently reported in all types of blepharitis:
  - Burning
  - Itching
  - Eyelid erythema
  - Conjunctival infection (red eyes)
  - Lacrimation, tearing
  - Tear deficiency
  - Foreign-body sensation
  - Photophobia (light sensitivity)
  - Impaired vision

PHYSICAL EXAM
- Test of visual acuity
- External exam (skin and eyelids):
  - Staphylococcal:
    - Recurrent stye (external or internal hordeolum)
    - Missing, broken, or misdirected eyelashes (trichiasis)
    - Eyelid deposits: Matted, hard scales; collarettes (ringlike formation around the lash shaft)
    - Ulcerations at base of eyelashes (rare)
    - Eyelid scarring may occur
  - Seborrheic blepharitis:
    - Eyelid deposits: Dry flakes, oily or greasy secretions on lid margins and/or lashes
    - Associated dandruff of scalp, eyebrows
  - Meibomian gland dysfunction:
    - Eyelash misdirection may occur with long-standing disease
    - Eyelid deposits: Fatty deposits; may be foamy
    - Eyelid margin thickening
    - Plugged meibomian gland orifices
    - Chalazion (sometimes multiple)
    - Eyelid scarring with long-term disease
  - Mixed blepharitis: Signs and symptoms of >1 type of blepharitis may be present.

DIAGNOSTIC TESTS & INTERPRETATION
Lab
Follow-Up & Special Considerations
- Cultures in atypical blepharitis
- Biopsy in atypical cases for carcinoma

Imaging
Initial approach
Slit-lamp biomicroscopy:
- Examine tear film, eyelid margins, eyelashes, tarsal and bulbar conjunctivae, and cornea.
- Reveals loss of lashes (madarosis), whitening of the lashes (poliosis), trichiasis, crusting, eyelid margin ulcers, and lid irregularities

DIFFERENTIAL DIAGNOSIS
Masquerade syndrome:
- Persistent inflammation and thickening of eyelid margin may indicate squamous cell, basal cell, or sebaceous cell carcinoma masquerading as blepharitis. These carcinomas also may mimic styes or chalazia.
- Sebaceous carcinoma of the eyelid has a 22% fatality rate. Up to 1/2 of these potentially fatal sebaceous cell carcinomas may resemble benign inflammatory diseases, particularly chalazia and chronic blepharoconjunctivitis.
- Consider this in all cases of recurrent, persistent, or atypical chalazion; chronic unilateral unresponsive blepharoconjunctivitis; diffuse or nodular tumors of the eyelid; orbital mass developing after removal of an eyelid or caruncular tumor; and any tumor developing in a person with a history of ocular radiotherapy (1)[C].

 TREATMENT

MEDICATION
First Line
- Topical treatment to lid, if *Staphylococcus* likely: Bacitracin 500 μg/g or (2nd choice) erythromycin 0.5% ophthalmic ointment:
  - Apply with a cotton-tipped applicator.
  - The frequency and duration of treatment are guided by the severity (2)[C].
- Topical corticosteroids (short term) may be useful for eyelid or ocular surface inflammation. The minimum effective dose should be used; long-term use should be avoided if possible (2,3)[C].
- For patients with meibomian gland dysfunction inadequately controlled with eyelid hygiene, consider doxycycline 100 mg/d or tetracycline 1,000 mg/d in divided doses, tapered after clinical improvement (2–4 weeks) to doxycycline 50 mg/d or tetracycline 250–500 mg/d (2)[C].
- Since aqueous tear deficiency is common in blepharitis, use twice-daily artificial tears in addition to eyelid hygiene and medications.

- Contraindications: Allergy to medication; tetracyclines are not for use in pregnancy, nursing women, or children <8 years of age.
- Precautions: Tetracyclines may cause photosensitivity; sunscreen is recommended. Corticosteroids may increase intraocular pressure and risk of cataract.

Second Line
- Topical fluoroquinolones (e.g., gatifloxacin 0.3%, levofloxacin 0.5%, or moxifloxacin 0.5%) may be helpful for persistent or recurrent staphylococcal blepharitis or for those patients who prefer a solution.
- Seborrheic blepharitis may respond to antifungal agents such as a short course of itraconazole (4)[C].

ADDITIONAL TREATMENT
General Measures
- Promote proper eyelid hygiene (2)[C]:
  - Apply warm compresses for several minutes once daily to soften adherent encrustations.
  - The eyelid margins then are scrubbed gently with eyelid cleanser or diluted baby shampoo twice a day to remove adherent material and clean the meibomian gland orifices (5)[C].
- Brief, gentle massage of the eyelids can help to express meibomian secretions in patients with meibomian gland dysfunction (2)[C].
- Discontinue soft contact lenses use during an acute case of blepharitis.

Issues for Referral
Chronic recurrent blepharitis requires referral to an ophthalmologist for evaluation as to whether patient should continue soft lens use.

 ## ONGOING CARE

FOLLOW-UP RECOMMENDATIONS
Patient Monitoring
- Patients should schedule a return visit if their condition worsens despite treatment.
- Return visit intervals for patients with severe disease vary.
- If corticosteroid is prescribed, reevaluate within a few weeks to measure intraocular pressure and determine response to therapy.

PATIENT EDUCATION
- "Blepharitis Fact Sheet" from the American Academy of Ophthalmology
- Advise patient that blepharitis is a chronic condition, prone to recurrence if eyelid hygiene is not maintained after antibiotic treatment is discontinued.

PROGNOSIS
- Symptoms frequently can be improved but rarely are eliminated.
- Long-term eyelid hygiene is required for control.

COMPLICATIONS
- Stye and chalazion
- Scarring of eyelid margin
- Corneal infection

REFERENCES

1. Tsai T, O'Brien JM. Masquerade syndromes: malignancies mimicking inflammation in the eye. Int Ophthalmol Clin. 2002;41:115–31.
2. American Academy of Ophthalmology Cornea/External Disease Panel, Preferred Practice Patterns Committee. Preferred Practice Pattern: Blepharitis. San Francisco: AAO. 2003.
3. Abelson MB, et al. Blepharitis Hiding in plain sight. Rev Ophthalmol. May 15, 2004.
4. Ninomiya J, Nakabayashi A, Higuchi R, et al. A case of seborrheic blepharitis; treatment with itraconazole. Nippon Ishinkin Gakkai Zasshi. 2002;43:189–91.
5. McCulley JP, Shine WE. Changing concepts in the diagnosis and management of blepharitis. Cornea. 2000;19:650–8.

ADDITIONAL READING
- Lemp MA. Contact lenses and associated anterior segment disorders: dry eye, blepharitis, and allergy. Ophthalmol Clin North Am. 2003;16:463–9.
- McCulley JP, Shine WE. Eyelid disorders: the meibomian gland, blepharitis, and contact lenses. Eye Contact Lens. 2003;29:S93–5; discussion S115–8, S192–4.

See Also (Topic, Algorithm, Electronic Media Element)
Conjunctivitis, Acute; Dry Eye Syndrome (Keratoconjunctivitis Sicca)

 ## CODES

ICD9
373.00 Blepharitis, unspecified

CLINICAL PEARLS
- Blepharitis is often a chronic condition; symptoms frequently can be improved but rarely are eliminated.
- Promote proper eyelid hygiene.
- Bacitracin ophthalmic ointment is the 1st-line treatment if Staphylococcus is suspected.

BODY DYSMORPHIC DISORDER

Dawn S. Tasillo, MD

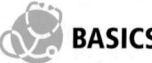 **BASICS**

DESCRIPTION

Body dysmorphic disorder (BDD) is a dysmorphic disorder in which patients have a pervasive subjective feeling of ugliness of some aspect of their appearance despite a normal or near-normal appearance:

- Diagnostic criteria according to the *DSM-IV*:
  – Preoccupation with an imagined defect in appearance. If there is a minor physical anomaly, the concern is excessive.
  – The preoccupation causes clinically significant distress or impairment in social, occupational, or other important areas of function.
  – The preoccupation is not accounted for by another mental disorder.

EPIDEMIOLOGY

- High comorbidity with depressive disorders
- Usually begins during adolescence, with a common average age of onset between 15 and 30 years
- Women are affected somewhat more often than men.
- Affected patients are likely to be unmarried.
- Different cultural beliefs may influence or amplify preoccupations:
  – Adolescents usually present similar to adults.
  – Can present in childhood, often with refusing to attend school or planning suicide
- Onset can be gradual or abrupt.
- Often a delay in diagnosis until 10–15 years after the onset

Prevalence

- <1% in general population
- More common in women than men
- 5–40% in individuals with anxiety or depressive disorders
- 6–15% in cosmetic surgery patients and in dermatologic clinics

RISK FACTORS

- Genetic predisposition
- Shyness, perfectionism, or anxious temperament
- Childhood adversity:
  – Teasing or bullying
  – Poor peer relationships
  – Social isolation
  – Lack of support of family
  – Sexual abuse
- History of dermatologic or other physical stigmata
- Being more aesthetically sensitive than average
- Low self-esteem

PATHOPHYSIOLOGY

- Not well understood
- A cognitive behavioral model has been described in which an external representation of the person's appearance (i.e., a photograph or mirror reflection) creates a distorted mental image. Through selective attention, awareness of the image and its specific features is increased. The affected individual becomes preoccupied by the distorted image; this is maintained by various safety and submissive behaviors meant to decrease scrutiny by others, but which may increase the individual's abnormal self-image and thus reinforces the behavior.
- Magnetic resonance imaging studies note left cerebral hemisphere hyperactivity, which may imply abnormal visual information processing, leading to selective recall of details and perception of distortions that do not exist (1).

ETIOLOGY

Not known, but likely multifactorial involving genetic, biological, and environmental factors

COMMONLY ASSOCIATED CONDITIONS

- Depression
- Social phobia
- Bipolar disorder
- Eating disorders
- Obsessive-compulsive disorder
- Suicide (up to 25%)
- Delusional disorder (27–39%)

 DIAGNOSIS

HISTORY

- Determine and validate the patient's concern.
- Determine the severity of the disorder.
- Quantify the amount of time spent worrying about the "distorted" appearance.
- Determine what is done to hide or eliminate the problem.
- Determine the degree to which the defect affects school, job, or social life.
- Rule out other psychiatric disorders.
- Signs and symptoms may include:
  – Preoccupation that ≥1 features are unattractive, ugly, or deformed
  – Can involve any part of the body, but usually involves the skin, hair, or facial features:
    ○ Women are more likely to be preoccupied with their weight, hips, legs, and breasts.
    ○ Men are more likely to be preoccupied with their height, body hair, body build, and genitals.
- Nature of the preoccupation can change with time
- Have little insight
- Tend to display delusions of reference

- Large amounts of time are consumed by behaviors to examine the perceived defect repeatedly, disguise it, or improve it:
  – Mirror gazing
  – Excessive grooming
  – Camouflaging the "defect"
  – Skin picking
  – Reassurance seeking
  – Dieting
  – Pursuing dermatologic treatment or cosmetic surgery
- Tend to avoid social interactions
- Trouble staying in school, maintaining a job, or maintaining significant relationships:
  – Tend to be unhappy with results of dermatologic and cosmetic procedures

PHYSICAL EXAM

- Important to do a mental status examination:
  – Look for:
    ○ Depression
    ○ Suicidal ideation
    ○ Anxiety
  – Rule out organic factors by reviewing:
    ○ Orientation
    ○ Memory
    ○ Ability to concentrate
- Rule out actual physical pathology.

DIAGNOSTIC TESTS & INTERPRETATION

- Several modules have been developed to assist with the diagnosis and severity rating of BDD (1).
- Administered by a trained clinician, these include:
  – The BDD Examination
  – Yale Brown Obsessive–Compulsive Scale modified for BDD

DIFFERENTIAL DIAGNOSIS

- Normal concerns about appearance
- Eating disorders: BDD differs from an eating disorder in that an eating disorder involves a preoccupation with overall body shape and weight, and with BDD the preoccupation is with only a specific body part.
- Obsessive–compulsive disorder (OCD): While BDD may be a version of OCD, the diagnosis differs in that in OCD, the obsessions and compulsions are not just restricted to appearance, as they are in BDD.
- Gender identity disorder
- Major depressive episode
- Narcissistic personality disorder
- Avoidant personality disorder
- Social phobia
- Schizophrenia
- Trichotillomania
- Hypochondriasis
- Delusional disorder, somatic type
- Koro: A culture-related syndrome seen in Southeast Asia that involves a preoccupation that the genitals (penis, labia, nipples, or breast) are shrinking and disappearing into the abdomen

TREATMENT

- In any patient with a coexisting mental disorder, such as a depressive or anxiety disorder, the coexisting disorder should be treated with the appropriate psychotherapy or pharmacotherapy.
- Cognitive behavior therapy has been shown to be very effective (2,3)[A]:
  - Behavioral experiments
  - Graded exposure tasks
  - Imagery rescripting
  - Cognitive restructuring
  - Reverse role-playing
  - Relaxation
- Support groups
- Psychotherapy may be effective.
- Therapy with and for family members, spouses, or significant others

MEDICATION

- Results from the small number of available randomized controlled trials suggest that selective serotonin reuptake inhibitors (SSRIs) may be useful in treating patients with BDD (2)[A].
- SSRIs are currently considered the medication of choice for BDD (4).

First Line
SSRI:

- Not an approved use by the FDA
- Patients with and without a delusional disorder did equally well with an SSRI.
- Maximum tolerated dose should be taken for at least 12–16 weeks
- Dosages may need to be higher than typically recommended for an eating disorder.

Second Line
Add a low-dose antipsychotic drug to an SSRI if there is failure to respond to ≥2 SSRIs.

ADDITIONAL TREATMENT
Issues for Referral
- Referral to a psychiatrist for diagnosis and therapy can be helpful and necessary for difficult cases.
- Regular counseling

SURGERY/OTHER PROCEDURES
- Studies investigating the rate of BDD among persons who seek appearance-enhancing treatments suggest that approximately 5–15% of individuals who seek these treatments suffer from BDD (5).
- Retrospective reports suggest that persons with BDD rarely experience improvement in their symptoms following these treatments, leading some to suggest that BDD is a contraindication to cosmetic surgery and other treatments.

 ONGOING CARE

FOLLOW-UP RECOMMENDATIONS
Patient Monitoring
Many patients have substantial improvement in core BDD symptoms, psychosocial functioning, quality of life, suicidality, and other aspects of BDD when treated with appropriate pharmacotherapy that targets BDD symptoms (4).

PATIENT EDUCATION
- Phillips KA. *The Broken Mirror: Understanding and Treating Body Dysmorphic Disorder*. Revised and expanded. New York: Oxford University Press, 2005.
- Butler Hospital's Body Dysmorphic Disorder and Body Image Program at http://www.butler.org/body.cfm?id=123

PROGNOSIS
- Continuous course with periods of waxing and waning in the intensity of symptoms
- The longer the duration and the more severe the symptoms, the less the chance of partial or full remission.

COMPLICATIONS
- Repeated surgical or dermatologic procedures
- Inability or limited ability to function in society
- Comorbid conditions
- Poor social relations
- Poor self-esteem
- Suicide

REFERENCES

1. Feusner et al. Abnormalities of visual processing and frontostriatal systems in body dysmorphic disorder. *Arch Gen Psychiatry*. 2010;67(2): 197–205.
2. Ipser JC, Sander C, Stein DJ. Pharmacotherapy and psychotherapy for body dysmorphic disorder. *Cochrane Database Syst Rev*. 2009;CD005332.
3. Buhlmann U, Reese HE, Renaud S, et al. Clinical considerations for the treatment of body dysmorphic disorder with cognitive-behavioral therapy. *Body Image*. 2008.
4. Phillips KA, Hollander E. Treating body dysmorphic disorder with medication: evidence, misconceptions, and a suggested approach. *Body Image*. 2008.
5. Sarwer DB, Crerand CE. Body dysmorphic disorder and appearance enhancing medical treatments. *Body Image*. 2008.
6. Albertini RS, Philips KA. Thirty-three cases of body dysmorphic disorder in children and adolescents. *J Am Acad Child Psy*. 1999;38:453–9.

ADDITIONAL READING

- *American Psychiatric Association: Diagnostic and Statistical Manual of Mental Disorders*, Fourth Edition, *Text Revision*. Washington, DC: American Psychiatric Association. 2000:507–10.
- Philips KA, et al. Predictors of remission from body dysmorphic disorder: a prospective study. *J Ner Ment Dis*. 2005;193:564–7.
- Phillips KA. *The Broken Mirror: Understanding and Treating Body Dysmorphic Disorder. Revised and expanded*. New York: Oxford University Press, 2005.
- Phillips KA. The presentation of body dysmorphic disorder in medical settings. *Prim Psychiatry*. 2006;13:51–9.
- Rief W, Buhlmann U, Wilhelm S, et al. The prevalence of body dysmorphic disorder: a population-based survey. *Psychol Med*. 2006;36:877–85.
- Sadock BJ, Sadock VA. *Kaplan & Sadock's Synopsis of Psychiatry*, 9th ed. Philadelphia: Lippincott Williams & Wilkins. 2003:653–5.
- Slaughter JR, Sun AM. In pursuit of perfection: a primary care physician's guide to body dysmorphic disorder. *Am Fam Physician*. 1999;60:1738–42.

 CODES

ICD9
300.7 Hypochondriasis

CLINICAL PEARLS

- An eating disorder involves a preoccupation with overall body shape and weight, while in body dysmorphic disorder, the preoccupation is with only a specific body part (6).
- In obsessive-compulsive disorder, the obsessions and compulsions are not just restricted to appearance, as in body dysmorphic disorder.
- If the patient insists she has a physical defect and wants it surgically corrected but you don't appreciate a physical defect, after validating the patient's concerns, refer to a psychiatrist for further evaluation before performing the procedure. Most patients with body dysmorphic disorder are not content after the procedure, and their concerns persist.

BONE TUMOR, PRIMARY MALIGNANT

Nathan P. Falk, MD
Ashley Falk, MD

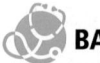

BASICS

DESCRIPTION
- Primary malignant bone tumors are rare.
- Osteogenic sarcomas arise from mesenchymal cells capable of differentiating into bone, cartilage, or fibrous tissue. Three histologic types:
  - Osteosarcoma: Characterized by the production of osteoid or immature bone by the malignant cells; has multiple subtypes
  - Chondrosarcoma: Cellular cartilaginous tumor with abundant binucleate cells, myxoid areas, pushing borders; lacks osteoid
  - Fibrosarcoma: Spindle cells and collagen; no osteoid
- Ewing sarcoma: Small, round blue-cell neoplasm
- Malignant fibrous histiocytoma (MFH): Pleomorphic sarcoma of storiform (starlike) pattern without differentiation; 10-year survival 20% for high grade, 90% for low grade
- Giant cell tumor of bone: Has both benign (90%) and malignant forms; often recurs
- Chordoma: Develops from remnants of primitive notochord at base of skull or sacrum; rare; slowly progressive; recurrent; cure possible

EPIDEMIOLOGY
Incidence
- Rare: 2,380 primary bone tumors diagnosed per year in US; 1,470 deaths (1)
- Osteosarcoma most common; chondrosarcoma, 2nd; Ewing sarcoma, 3rd
- Predominant age:
  - Bone tumors account for 6% of childhood malignancies.
  - Osteosarcoma: Bimodal: Ages 13–16 and >65 years
  - Chondrosarcoma: 3rd–7th decades
  - Fibrosarcoma: 2nd–6th decades
  - Ewing sarcoma: Children and teenagers usually 10–15 years old (70% of Ewing patients <20 years of age)
  - MFH: Adults and elderly
  - Chordoma: >30 years of age
- Predominant gender:
  - For most, Male = Female.
  - Osteosarcoma, Male > Female (1.5:1), and chondrosarcoma, Male > Female (2:1).
- Race:
  - Ewing sarcoma is significantly more common in Caucasian than in African-American children (2).
  - Osteosarcoma is slightly more common in African-American than in Caucasian children.

RISK FACTORS
- Previous irradiation is a risk factor for osteosarcoma and MFH.
- Rapid bone growth, teenage growth spurt
- Fibrous dysplasia

Genetics
- Genetic risk factors include
  - Bone dysplasias:
    - Paget disease risk factor for osteosarcoma
    - Multiple hereditary exostosis: Chondrosarcoma
    - Multiple enchondromatosis (Ollier disease): Chondrosarcoma
    - Enchondromatosis and hemangiomatosis (Maffucci syndrome)
  - Germ-line retinoblastoma, especially after radiation: Osteosarcoma
  - Li-Fraumeni syndrome (germ-line *p53* mutation)
  - Rothmund-Thomson syndrome (autosomal recessive association of congenital bone defects, hair and skin dysplasias, hypogonadism, and cataracts)
- Tumor genetics:
  - Ewing sarcoma has chromosomal translocation t(11;22)(q24;q12) in 90% of tumors and resulting EW5-FLI1 fusion protein.
  - Ewing sarcoma breakpoint region *EWSR1* gene encodes a putative ribonucleic acid (RNA)–binding protein.
  - Ewing sarcoma caveolin-1 overexpression is necessary for malignant tumor growth (3).
  - Osteosarcoma shows loss of retinoblastoma and *p53* suppressor genes and amplification of the genes *C-myc, mdm-2, SAS*, and *cyclin-dependent kinase.*

GENERAL PREVENTION
Irradiation is the only known environmental risk factor.

ETIOLOGY
- Generally unknown
- Malignant fibrous histiocytoma often follows irradiation or arises in old bone infarct.
- Osteosarcoma has association with loss of suppressor retinoblastoma and *p53* genes.
- Chondrosarcoma may arise in preexisting enchondroma or exostosis.

COMMONLY ASSOCIATED CONDITIONS
- Genetic conditions listed previously
- Patients with enchondromatosis more often die of gastrointestinal (GI) malignancies than of metastatic chondrosarcoma.

DIAGNOSIS

HISTORY
- Pain with weight bearing, at rest, and at night; often dull or aching
- Swelling
- Tenderness
- Fracture with minor trauma (pathologic fracture present in 10–15% of cases)
- Minor injury may bring attention to lesion.

PHYSICAL EXAM
- Bone tenderness
- Palpable bony or soft tissue mass
- Rectal exam, if risk for prostate cancer, should be done to exclude prostate nodules.

DIAGNOSTIC TESTS & INTERPRETATION
Lab
Initial lab tests
- Calcium, phosphate, alkaline phosphatase, lactate dehydrogenase (LDH)
- 50% of osteosarcomas have an elevated alkaline phosphatase.
- Ewing sarcoma may be associated with an elevated erythrocyte sedimentation rate (ESR) and LDH.
- Prostate-specific antigen to exclude prostatic carcinoma
- Thyroid function tests to exclude thyroid carcinoma
- Elevated ESR and white blood cells (WBCs) in osteomyelitis
- Serum protein electrophoresis and urine electrophoresis to exclude myeloma

Imaging
Initial approach
- Plain films provide important information regarding the nature of the lesion and guide further testing.
- Classic plain-film findings include "onion skin" for Ewing sarcoma and Codman triangle formation and soft tissue "sunburst" for osteosarcoma.
- Bone scan is done prior to biopsy to look for other lesions.
- CT scan for cortical destruction and internal calcification or ossification
- MRI determines the extent of marrow involvement and associated soft tissue mass.
- Osteosarcoma: Location of lesion important: Surface osteosarcomas often may be cured by surgery alone.
- Chest radiograph and CT scan for metastatic disease
- Abdominal CT scan, MRI, or renal ultrasound
- Mammogram to exclude breast carcinoma

Diagnostic Procedures/Surgery
- Open biopsy or needle biopsy: Needle biopsies may not provide enough tissue.
  - Frozen section problematic if calcified
  - Touch prep
  - Permanent section
  - Snap freezing
  - Electron microscopy
  - Cytogenetic and molecular studies
  - DNA indices
  - Immunoperoxidase staining
  - Immunophenotyping to rule out lymphoma
- Biopsy tract should be excised in continuity with the tumor at the time of resection (4).
- Biopsy of associated soft tissue mass may lessen the risk of pathologic fracture.

Pathological Findings
- Histology and special studies in combination with radiographic findings confirm the diagnosis.
- 90% of osteosarcomas are high-grade intramedullary tumors.
- Conventional osteosarcomas have histologic subtypes: Osteoblastic, chondroblastic, or fibroblastic depending on the predominant cellular component, but all are managed similarly.

- Osteosarcoma may express *Her-2/neu*, indicating, if present, a more aggressive tumor, but one that may respond more favorably to trastuzumab (Herceptin).
- Ewing sarcoma expresses MIC-2 protein (CD99).
- Electron microscopy: Glycogen granules in Ewing sarcoma

DIFFERENTIAL DIAGNOSIS

- Metastatic cancer: Breast, prostate, thyroid, lung, kidney
- Hematologic malignancy:
  – Myeloma, especially in patients >40 years of age
  – Lymphoma at any age
- Benign bone tumors: Endochondroma, osteochondroma, nonossifying fibroma, chondroblastoma, osteoid osteoma, osteoblastoma, periosteal chondroma, (benign) giant cell tumor, chondromyxoid fibroma
- Other space-occupying lesions: Aneurysmal bone cyst, unicameral bone cyst, fibrous dysplasia, eosinophilic granuloma
- Infection (osteomyelitis)
- Metabolic bone disease (osteopenia, Paget, hyperparathyroidism)
- Synovial diseases (pigmented villonodular synovitis, synovial chondromatosis, degenerative or inflammatory synovitis)
- Myositis ossificans and repair reaction to trauma
- Avascular necrosis

TREATMENT

MEDICATION

- Neoadjuvant chemotherapy treats micrometastatic disease, allows time for ordering replacement prosthesis and bone graft, and allows in vivo assessment of response to chemotherapy (5,6)[C].
- Osteosarcoma:
  – Standard agents: Doxorubicin, cisplatin, ifosfamide, and methotrexate (MTX)
  – Recurrent disease: High-dose (HD) MTX, doxorubicin, and cisplatin
- Chondrosarcoma is not likely to respond to chemotherapy.
- MFH: Less histologic response to chemotherapy than conventional osteosarcoma; survival similar
- Ewing sarcoma response to induction chemotherapy important prognostic factor:
  – A dramatic decrease in size of Ewing sarcoma usually occurs after initial chemotherapy.
  – Adjuvant chemotherapy improves cure rate dramatically; cure rate is 10–20% with surgery or radiation alone.
  – Standard agents: Vincristine, doxorubicin, and cyclophosphamide, alternating with ifosfamide, etoposide
- Precautions:
  – Left ventricular dysfunction with doxorubicin; cumulative dose >450 mg/m^2 increases risk.
  – With HD MTX, hydration, alkalinization of the urine, and close monitoring of plasma levels are needed.
- Significant adverse effects:
  – Myelosuppression
  – Renal tubular dysfunction with ifosfamide
  – Renal and hepatic dysfunction and GI mucositis with MTX
  – Nephrotoxicity and ototoxicity with cisplatin

SURGERY/OTHER PROCEDURES

- Complete surgical resection with adequate margins is crucial (7)[C].
- Chondrosarcoma in the extremities should be treated exclusively by surgery, unless it is of the mesenchymal or dedifferentiated high-grade variety.
- Ewing sarcoma is radiosensitive; however, surgery with limb salvage is increasingly accepted.
  – Surgery is preferred if lesion is resectable.
  – Despite irradiation, local recurrence is common in up to 25% with pelvic lesions.
  – After neoadjuvant chemotherapy, reassess resectability of lesion; either surgery or irradiation.
  – Nonresectable tumors may be irradiated.
  – Adjuvant radiotherapy is used for Ewing sarcoma only in some circumstances.
- Limb salvage is employed whenever a safe margin can be obtained.
  – Primary goal is eradication of disease.
  – Secondary goal is preservation of function.
- In selected patients, limb salvage does not increase risk of death.
- Limb-sparing surgery may require endoprosthesis or bone graft (allograft or homograft).
- Rotation-plasty is a procedure used when tumor dictates resection of the distal femur.
  – Lower leg is spared and rotated 180 degrees; tibia is fused to femur.
  – Reattached, reversed ankle serves as knee joint. Prosthesis is fitted to (reversed) foot.

ONGOING CARE

FOLLOW-UP RECOMMENDATIONS
Patient Monitoring

- Blood counts for myelosuppression
- Serial electrocardiograms (ECGs) when Adriamycin is being used; granulocyte colony-stimulating factor (G-CSF) is often used to minimize neutropenia.
- Chest radiographs should be obtained every 2 months for the 1st year, every 3 months for the 2nd year, and every 4 months for the 3rd year.
- CT scans of the lungs are repeated every 6 months during the 1st 2 years.
- Ewing sarcoma may recur >5 years after diagnosis.

PATIENT EDUCATION

Refer to local branch of American Cancer Society for information and support groups.

PROGNOSIS

- With amputation alone, 80% of patients with osteosarcoma had pulmonary metastatic disease by 2 years. With chemotherapy, the 5-year disease-free survival rate is 50–85% (8)[C].
- Favorable prognostic factors for MFH and osteosarcoma include responsiveness to chemotherapy, distal portions of the extremities, small size, and age >10 years.
- Most chondrosarcomas are of lower grade and have a low risk of metastatic spread and low incidence of local recurrence after adequate surgery.
- MFH, osteosarcoma, and Ewing sarcoma have an overall 50% survival with combined treatment modalities.

COMPLICATIONS

- For limb salvage with any primary malignant bone tumor, potential complications include leg-length discrepancy, infection, wound dehiscence, skin-coverage problems, and artery and nerve injury.
- Nonunion of bone grafts and mechanical loosening of prosthetic implants
- Local recurrence risk for osteosarcoma with limb salvage is <10%.
- Micrometastatic disease may have occurred by the time of presentation and can appear at any time during the course of treatment or follow-up.
- Thoracotomy and continued chemotherapy are often recommended for metastatic disease to the lung.
- Ewing sarcoma metastatic to the lung is often diffuse and not amenable to resection.

REFERENCES

1. Jemal A, Siegel R, Ward E, et al. Cancer statistics, 2008. *CA Cancer J Clin*. 2008;58:71–96.
2. Heare T, Hensley MA, Dell'Orfano S. Bone tumors: osteosaroma and Ewing's sarcoma. *Current Opinion in Pediatrics*. 2009;21:365–372.
3. Lewis VO. What's new in musculoskeletal oncology. *J Bone Joint Surg Am*. 2007;89:1399–407.
4. Schajowicz F, McGuire MH. Diagnostic difficulties in skeletal pathology. *Clin Orthop Rel Res*. 1991;240:281–310.
5. Longhi A, Pasini E, Bertoni F, et al. Twenty-year follow-up of osteosarcoma of the extremity treated with adjuvant chemotherapy. *J Chemother*. 2004;16:582–8.
6. Mendelsohn J. Jeremiah Metzger Lecture. Targeted cancer therapy. *Trans Amer Clin Climatol Assoc*. 2000;111:95–110.
7. Siegel HJ, Pressey JG. Current concepts on the surgical and medical management of osteosarcoma. *Expert Rev Anticancer Ther*. 2008;8:1257–69.
8. Bruland OS, Høifødt H, Saeter G, et al. Hematogenous micrometastases in osteosarcoma patients. *Clin Cancer Res*. 2005;11:4666–73.

 CODES

ICD9

- 170.0 Malignant neoplasm of bones of skull and face, except mandible
- 170.1 Malignant neoplasm of mandible
- 170.9 Malignant neoplasm of bone and articular cartilage, site unspecified

CLINICAL PEARLS

- Osteosarcoma variants, such as parosteal, periosteal, and intraosseous osteosarcoma, are lower-grade lesions with a more favorable prognosis; they often do not require chemotherapy.
- Other variants and postirradiation and post-Paget osteosarcoma metastasize early.

BORDERLINE PERSONALITY DISORDER

Heath A. Grames, PhD
W. Jeff Hinton, PhD

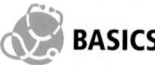 **BASICS**

DESCRIPTION
Beginning no later than adolescence or early adulthood, borderline personality disorder (BPD) is a consistent and pervasive pattern of an unstable affect and sense of self, impulsivity, and volatile interpersonal relationships (1):
- Common behaviors and variations:
  – Self-mutilation (pinching, scratching, cutting)
  – Suicide (ideation, history of attempts, plans)
  – Splitting (idealizing then devaluing people and relationships)
  – Presentation of helplessness or victimization
  – Emotional pain (may look for physical diagnoses)
  – May be high utilizer of medical services
  – High rate of associated mental disorders (see Associated Conditions)
- Patients with this disorder typically display little insight into their behavior.

Geriatric Considerations
Illness (both acute and chronic) may exacerbate BPD behaviors and may lead to intense feelings of fear and helplessness. Manifestations may decrease with age.

Pediatric Considerations
Diagnosis is rarely made in children. Must first rule out Axis I disorders and behavior related to a general medical condition or to the developmental cycle of the child.

Pregnancy Considerations
Physical and social changes may induce stress or increased fears, resulting in possible escalation of borderline behaviors.

EPIDEMIOLOGY
- Predominant age: Onset no later than adolescence or early adulthood (may go undiagnosed for years)
- Predominant sex: Female > Male

Prevalence
- General population: 2%
- Estimated lifetime prevalence: 10–13%
- 20–30% of patients in primary care outpatient settings have a personality disorder.
- 20% of patients in psychiatry inpatient settings have BPD.

RISK FACTORS
- Biological relatives with the disorder
- Childhood sexual and/or physical abuse and neglect
- Physical illness and external social factors may exacerbate borderline personality behaviors.

Genetics
1st-degree relatives are at greater risk for this disorder (undetermined whether due to genetic or psychosocial factors).

GENERAL PREVENTION
- Tends to be a multigenerational problem
- Children, caregivers, and significant others should have some time and activities away from the borderline individual, which may protect them.

ETIOLOGY
Undetermined, but generally accepted that PDs are due to a combination of the following:
- Hereditary temperamental traits
- Environment (i.e., history of childhood sexual and/or physical abuse, history of childhood neglect, ongoing conflict in home)
- Developmental traits

COMMONLY ASSOCIATED CONDITIONS
Other psychiatric disorders, including:
- Co-occurring PDs, frequent
- Mood disorders, common
- Anxiety disorders, common
- Substance-related disorders, common
- Eating disorders, common
- Post-traumatic stress disorder, common

 DIAGNOSIS

- The comprehensive evaluation should focus on (2):
  – Comorbid conditions
  – Functional impairments
  – Needs/goals
  – Adaptive/maladaptive coping styles
  – Psychosocial stressors
  – Patient strengths
- Initial assessment should focus on determining treatment setting (2):
  – Establish treatment agreement with patient and outline treatment goals.
  – Assess suicide ideation and self-harm behavior.
  – Assess for psychosis.
  – Hospitalization is necessary if patient presents a threat of harm to self or others.

HISTORY
- Clinic visits for problems that do not have biological findings
- Problems with medical staff members
- Idealizing or unexplained anger at physician
- History of unrealistic expectations of physician (e.g., "I know you can take care of me." "You're the best, unlike my last provider.")
- Obtain collateral information (i.e., from family, partner) about patient behaviors.

PHYSICAL EXAM
Possible scarring from self-mutilation (look on arms and legs where hidden by clothing, but can occur on other parts of the body)

DIAGNOSTIC TESTS & INTERPRETATION
- Consider age of onset. To meet criteria for BPD, borderline pattern will be present from adolescence or early adulthood.
- Formal psychological testing
- Rule out personality change due to a general medical condition (GMC) (1):
  – Traits may emerge due to the effect of a GMC on the central nervous system.
- Rule out symptoms related to chronic substance use.
- If symptoms begin later than early adulthood or are related to trauma (e.g., after a head injury), a GMC, or substance use, then consider other diagnoses.
- Increased diagnostic accuracy may be facilitated by utilizing the Structured Clinical Interview for DSM-IV Axis II disorders (SCID-II) (3).

Diagnostic Procedures/Surgery
Patient must meet at least 5 of the following criteria (1):
- Attempt to avoid abandonment
- Volatile interpersonal relationships
- Identity disturbance
- Impulsive behavior:
  – In ≥2 areas
  – Impulsive behavior is self-damaging.
- Suicidal or self-mutilating behavior
- Mood instability
- Feeling empty
- Is unable to control anger, or finds it difficult
- Paranoid or dissociative when under stress

DIFFERENTIAL DIAGNOSIS
- Mood disorders:
  – Look at baseline behaviors when considering BPD vs mood disorder.
  – BPD symptoms increase the likelihood of misdiagnosing bipolar disorder (4).
- Psychotic disorder:
  – With BPD, only occurs under intense stress and is not characteristic of disorder
- Other PD:
  – Consider patient's thoughts, feelings, and behavior to differentiate borderline from other PDs.
  – High co-occurrence of borderline and other PDs
- General medical condition (GMC):
  – Traits may emerge due to the effect of a GMC on the central nervous system.
- Chronic substance abuse

 TREATMENT

- Patient may need to be placed on suicide watch.
- Inpatient hospitalization is ineffective in changing Axis II disorder behaviors.
- Inpatient hospital services for conditions related to Axis II disorder should be limited and of short duration to decrease dependence. Hospitalization should be considered for:
  – Adjusting medications
  – Implementing psychotherapy for crisis intervention
  – Stabilizing patient (psychosocial stressors)
- Extended inpatient hospitalization should be considered for the following reasons (2)[C]:
  – Persistent/severe suicidal ideation or risk to others
  – Nonadherence to outpatient or partial hospitalization treatments
  – Comorbid Axis I disorders that may increase threat to life for the patient (i.e., eating disorders, mood disorders)
  – Comorbid substance abuse or dependence that is unresponsive to outpatient or partial hospitalization treatments

MEDICATION
- While there are no specific medications approved by the U.S. Food and Drug Administration (FDA) to treat BPD, American Psychiatric Association (APA) guidelines recommend pharmacotherapy to manage symptoms (2)[B].
- Treat symptoms (5)[C].

- Treat Axis I disorders (2)[B].
- Consider high rate of self-harm and suicidal behavior in patients with BPD when prescribing (6)[C].
- Depression/anxiety (7)[A]:
  – SSRIs
- Impulsive, aggressive, or history of bipolar disorder (5)[C]:
  – Mood stabilizer
- Psychosis, paranoid or hostile behavior, debilitating anxiety (5)[C]:
  – Atypical antipsychotic
- APA guideline recommendations (2)[B]:
  – Affective dysregulation: SSRI and monoamine oxidase inhibitors (MAOIs)
  – Impulsive-behavioral control: SSRIs and mood stabilizers
  – Cognitive-perceptual symptoms: Antipsychotics

ADDITIONAL TREATMENT
General Measures
- Focus on patient management rather than on "fixing" behaviors.
- Schedule consistent appointment follow-ups to relieve patient anxiety.
- Meet with and rely on treatment team to avoid splitting of team by patient and to provide opportunity for team to discuss issues with patient.
- Psychotherapy (referral to mental health therapist) is considered treatment of choice (2,8,9)[A].

Issues for Referral
- If hospitalized, probably for suicide risk, mood or anxiety disorders, or substance-related disorders
- Urgency for scheduled follow-up depends on community resources (i.e., Do outpatient day programs for suicidal patients exist? What substance abuse programs are available?):
  – With increased risk for self-harm or self-defeating behaviors and low community resources, the patient can/will use increased need for frequent visits.
- Treatment of Axis II disorder should include psychotherapy and/or psychiatry (2)[B].

Additional Therapies
Consider referring patient for specialty mental health behavioral services, including (2,10):
- Dialectic behavioral therapy (DBT)
- Psychoanalytic-oriented day hospital therapy
- Transference-focused psychotherapy

IN-PATIENT CONSIDERATIONS
Hospitalization is necessary if patient presents a threat of harm to self or others.

Initial Stabilization
- Assess suicidal ideation.
- Consider inpatient treatment if crisis intervention is warranted.
- If psychotic, consider antipsychotic medications (5).

Admission Criteria
Refer to inpatient or outpatient psychiatry services if harm to self or others is expressed:
- Call police or admit for inpatient services immediately if patient is psychotic and/or presents risk of harm to self or others.

Nursing
Nurses can be helpful in managing patient and calling the patient as needed (contact with the patient helps relieve patient stress).

Discharge Criteria
- Patient should not present risk of harm to self or others.
- Patient should have safety plan.
- Routine follow-up should be scheduled with psychiatrist, mental health therapist, or primary care provider.

 ## ONGOING CARE
FOLLOW-UP RECOMMENDATIONS
- Schedule routine follow-up with patient (relieves patient anxiety about medical care relationship with physician).
- Focus primarily on medical conditions and comorbid Axis I disorders.
- Exercise to decrease stress
- Find time to relax: Remove self from daily problems (teaches self-management).

Patient Monitoring
Monitor for suicidal or other self-harm behaviors.

PATIENT EDUCATION
As appropriate, provide patient education about the disorder, treatment, and self-care (2).

PROGNOSIS
- Borderline behaviors may decrease with age (1) and over time (9).
- Treatment is complex and takes time.
- Medical focus is on patient management and caring for medical and Axis I disorders (11).

REFERENCES

1. American Psychiatric Association. *Diagnostic and Statistical Manual of Mental Disorders*. 4th ed. Washington, DC: American Psychiatric Association; 1994.
2. American Psychiatric Association: *Practice guideline for the treatment of patients with borderline personality disorder*. Arlington, VA: American Psychiatric Association, 2001.
3. First MB, Gibbon M, Spitzer RL, Williams JBW, Benjamin LS. *Structured Clinical Interview for DSM-IV Axis II Personality Disorders, (SCID-II)*. Washington, D.C.: American Psychiatric Press, Inc., 1997.
4. Ruggero CJ, Zimmerman M, Chelminski I, Young D. Borderline personality disorder and the misdiagnosis of bipolar disorder. *Journal of Psychiatric Research*. 2010;44:405–408.
5. Ward RK. Assessment and management of personality disorders. *Am Fam Phys*. 2004;70:1505–12.
6. Makela EH, Moeller KE, Fullen JE, et al. Medication utilization patterns and methods of suicidality in borderline personality disorder. *Ann Pharmacother*. 2006;40:49–52.
7. Binks CA, Fenton M, McCarthy L, et al. Pharmacological interventions for people with borderline personality disorder. *Cochrane Database Syst Rev*. 2006;1. Art. No.: CD005653. DOI:10.1002/14651858.CD005653.
8. Kraus G, Reynolds DJ. The "A-B-C's" of the cluster B's: identifying, understanding, and treating cluster B personality disorders. *Clin Psychol Rev*. 2001;21:345–73.
9. Oldham JA. *Guideline watch: practice guideline for the treatment of patients with borderline personality disorder*. Arlington, VA: American Psychiatric Association, 2005.
10. Binks CA, Fenton M, McCarthy L, et al. Psychological therapies for people with borderline personality disorder. *Cochrane Database Syst Rev*. 2006;1. Art. No.: CD005652. DOI:10.1002/14651858.CD005652.
11. Koenigsberg HW, Woo-Ming AM, Siever LJ. Pharmacological treatments of personality disorders. In: Nathan PE, Gorman JM, eds. *A Guide to Treatments that Work*. 2nd ed. New York: Oxford University Press, 2002:625–41.

ADDITIONAL READING

- Battle CL, Shea MT, Johnson DM, et al. Childhood maltreatment associated with adult personality disorders: findings from the Collaborative Longitudinal Personality Disorders Study. *J Personal Disord*. 2004;18:193–211.
- Bellino S, Paradiso E, Bogetto F. Efficacy and tolerability of pharmacotherapies for borderline personality disorder. *CNS Drugs*. 2008;22:671–92.

 ## CODES

ICD9
301.83 Borderline personality disorder

CLINICAL PEARLS
- Borderline PD should be viewed as a chronic condition.
- Borderline PD patients are at increased risk for suicide attempts.
- If there are problems with the patient disrespecting the physician or support staff, clear guidelines should be established with the treatment team and then with the patient.
- If you are considering terminating your relationship with the patient, the patient may improve if he or she is warmly confronted about certain behaviors and is given clear guidelines on how to behave in the clinic. As it is the patient's job to follow the guidelines, it is you and your team's job to enforce the guidelines. Finally, designate a case management nurse or well-trained support staff person who can be the primary contact person for the patient.
- Have an agenda when you visit with PD patients. Be cordial—they deserve the same professionalism any patient gets. Help your patient understand that she can have 1 to 2 issues discussed per clinic visit. Frequently scheduled visits can help with this.
- Patients will benefit from regularly scheduled psychotherapy treatment in conjunction with or in addition to regularly scheduled office visits. Psychotherapy can help maximize physician performance by becoming the "home" for mental health treatment, leaving the physician to focus on the patient's immediate physical/medical issues.

BOTULISM

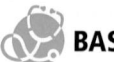

Payal S. Patel, DO

BASICS

DESCRIPTION
- Botulism is a muscle-paralyzing illness caused by a neurotoxin made by the bacterium *Clostridium botulinum*.
- Characterized by acute onset of bilateral cranial nerve involvement (diplopia, difficulty swallowing or speaking) associated with symmetric descending weakness, intact mental state, no fever, and no sensory dysfunction
- 7 types of *C. botulinum* (A–G) are distinguished by their antigenic characteristics. Types A, B, E, and, in rare cases, F, cause disease in humans.
- Forms include:
  - Foodborne: Caused by ingestion of preform toxin
  - Infant botulism: Caused by ingestion of *C. botulinum* that produce toxin in the gastrointestinal (GI) tract
  - Wound: Caused by wound infection with *C. botulinum* that secretes the toxin
  - Aerosolized/inhalational botulinum: Bioterrorism attack potential because of high toxicity; <1 μg is lethal human dose
  - Injection related: Rare
  - Adult colonization botulism: Rare
- System(s) affected: Neuromuscular; Respiratory; GI
- Diagnosis is made through history and clinical exam.
- Laboratory confirmation demonstrates presence of toxin in serum, stool, or wound; or culturing *C. botulinum* from stool, wound, or food
- Treatment should not wait for laboratory confirmation.
- Synonym(s): Sausage poisoning; Kerner disease
- A purified and diluted form of Type A neurotoxin is used to produce Botox injections.

EPIDEMIOLOGY
Incidence
- Average of 110 cases of botulism reported annually in US
- ~20% of cases are foodborne; 30–40% wound-related; 65% infant botulism
- Wound botulism incidence increasing due to IV heroin use and cocaine abuse
- Hidden or intestinal: More common in disorders of the GI tract, such as prior surgery, Crohn disease, or recent antibiotic use
- Inhalation: Only a single incident involving 3 laboratory workers has been described.

Prevalence
- Predominant age:
  - Foodborne: Mean age is 46 years; range of 3–78 years
  - Infantile: Mean age of onset 13 weeks, with range of 1–63 weeks
  - Wound: Median age is 41 years with a range of 23–58 years
- Predominant gender:
  - Foodborne and infantile: Male = Female
  - Wound: Female > Male

RISK FACTORS
- Foodborne: Ingestion of home-canned or prepared contaminated foods
- Infantile: From ingestion of honey or corn syrup; breastfeeding (controversial)
- Wound: IV drug use (black tar heroin; IM/SC) or "skin popping"

GENERAL PREVENTION
- Foodborne: Proper handling, processing, preparation (heating), and storage of food; avoid eating food from bulging cans and food that smells/looks spoiled.
- Infant: Avoid honey before 1 year of age.
- Wound: Proper wound care
- Health care providers: Standard precautions
- If meningitis is suspected in patients with flaccid paralysis, medical personnel should use droplet precautions.
- Heat potentially contaminated food or drink to an internal temperature of 85°C for at least 5 minutes.
- After exposure to *C. botulinum* toxin, clothing and skin should be cleaned with soap and water.
- Contaminated objects or surfaces should be cleaned with 0.1% bleach solution. All food suspected of contamination should be promptly removed from potential consumers.

PATHOPHYSIOLOGY
- Disease results from hematogenous spread of toxin from mucosal surface (stomach, small intestine) or from an infected wound.
- The toxin prevents acetylcholine release at presynaptic membranes, blocking neuromuscular transmission in cholinergic nerve fibers.

ETIOLOGY
- Toxin produced by *C. botulinum*, an encapsulated, anaerobe, gram-positive, spore-forming, rod-shaped bacillus
- Ingestion of *C. botulinum* neurotoxins (A, B, and E most common)
- Foodborne, usually from home-canned vegetables, prepared foods, or foods incubated in anaerobic conditions
- Infantile from ingestion of spores in environment or occasionally in honey
- Wound due to contamination with toxin-producing *C. botulinum*
- Inadvertent: IM injections of botulinum toxin

DIAGNOSIS

HISTORY
- Foodborne:
  - Incubation: Typically 12–36 hours after toxin ingestion. Rare case as late as 10 days after ingestion.
  - Wound and infant botulism: Incubation time cannot be ascertained.
  - Inhalational: Same as foodborne botulism
- Adults: Acute onset of symmetric neuropathies. Difficulty in swallowing or speaking, dry mouth. Diplopia, blurred vision, dilated or nonrelated ptosis (drooping eyelids).
- Symmetric descending, flaccid paralysis in oriented, afebrile patient
- Respiratory dysfunction

- Infant botulism: Disease presentation and severity variable:
  - Constipation, shortly followed by weakness, feeding difficulties, descending or global hypotonia, drooling, anorexia, irritability, and weak cry
- Ask about diet, travel, drug use, and other persons with same symptoms.

PHYSICAL EXAM
- General appearance: Oriented, flaccid, may complain of malaise, dizziness, nausea, vomiting
- Vital signs, afebrile (fever may occur in wound botulism due to secondary infection), normal blood pressure
- Head, eyes, ears, nose, throat: Dry mouth
- Chest/lungs: Respiratory muscle weakness, respiratory dysfunction, paralysis
- Heart: Normal or slow rate
- Abdomen: Distention, constipation (early sign in infant form); may be absent in wound form
- Genitourinary: Urinary retention
- Neurologic:
  - Symmetrical descending weakness beginning with the cranial nerves
  - Ptosis; extraocular muscle paresis; fixed, dilated pupils; dysphagia
  - Infant botulism: Poor muscle tone (loss of head control and facial expression), poor feeding (loss of suck), drooling, feeding difficulties, weak cry
  - Diminished or absent deep tendon reflexes

DIAGNOSTIC TESTS & INTERPRETATION
Lab
Initial lab tests
- Laboratory confirmation is done by demonstrating the presence of toxin in serum or stool, or by culturing *C. botulinum* from stool, wounds, or food.
- Mouse neutralization assay confirmation:
  - Standard method of diagnosis (1)[B]
  - Available from Centers for Disease Control and some state laboratories; takes ~4 days for results
- Routine tests (complete blood count, electrolytes, liver function tests, urinalysis) generally not helpful/show no characteristic abnormalities
- Cerebrospinal fluid testing: Normal helps differentiate from Guillain-Barré syndrome. Occasionally a borderline elevation in protein is seen.
- Toxin detected in gastric contents, serum, stool, and suspected food and containers:
  - PCR tests are also available for rapid detection of clostridia in food samples (2)[B].
- A normal Tensilon test helps to differentiate botulism from myasthenia gravis; borderline can occur in botulism

Imaging
CT or MRI to rule out neurologic pathology

Diagnostic Procedures/Surgery
Electrophysiology testing:
- Presumptive evidence in patients with negative bioassay studies (3)[C]
- Brief, small-amplitude motor potential with incremental response on repetitive nerve stimulation

DIFFERENTIAL DIAGNOSIS
- Adult botulisms:
  - Guillain-Barré syndrome
  - Encephalitis, meningitis
  - Tick paralysis
  - Myasthenia gravis
  - Eaton Lambert myasthenic syndrome
  - Cerebrovascular accident: Basilar artery stroke
  - Congenital neuropathy or myopathy
  - Sepsis
  - Hypokalemic periodic paralysis
  - Poliomyelitis
  - Other poisonings (organophosphate, shellfish, *Amanita* mushrooms, atropine, and aminoglycosides)
  - Miller-Fisher variant of Guillain-Barré syndrome
  - Diphtheritic neuropathy
  - Carbon monoxide intoxication
  - Hypermagnesemia
- Infant botulism:
  - Sepsis
  - Meningitis
  - Electrolyte–mineral imbalance
  - Reye syndrome
  - Congenital myopathy
  - Leigh disease
  - Werdnig-Hoffman disease

 TREATMENT

MEDICATION
First Line
- Antitoxin therapy with trivalent A-B-E antitoxin:
  - Call CDC Assistance (770) 488-7100
  - Initiating botulinum antitoxin therapy is primarily based on symptoms and physical examination findings that are consistent with botulism (4)[B].
  - Early administration is important (4)[B].
  - Horse serum derived: Up to 20% reaction incidence. Consider skin testing or pretreatment with steroids or antihistamines.
- Infantile:
  - Treatment with human botulism immune globulin (BIG-IV or Baby BIG) for botulism types A and B (5)[B]
  - Available only through the California State Health Department (510) 540-2646 or (510) 231-7600
- Wound:
  - Antitoxin therapy with trivalent A-B-E antitoxin, 1 vial IV and 1 vial IM, repeat in 2–4 hours if persistent symptoms
  - Antibiotics unproven by clinical trial, but widely used and recommended:
    o Penicillin G (3 million units IV q4h in adults)
    o Metronidazole (500 mg IV q8h) for penicillin-allergic patients
  - Vaccine: Pentavalent vaccine available:
    o Efficiency in terrorist attack is unknown
    o Newer vaccines being developed

Second Line
Supportive care, including mechanical ventilation (6)[C]

Pregnancy Considerations
Safety of botulism antitoxin during pregnancy and breastfeeding unknown or controversial (6)

ADDITIONAL TREATMENT
Issues for Referral
- Nutrition: For hyperalimentation and later, tube feeding
- Physical/occupational therapy: Including swallow evaluation

Additional Therapies
- Stress ulcer and deep vein thrombosis prophylaxis
- Pulmonary and physical rehabilitation

SURGERY/OTHER PROCEDURES
Wound excision/debridement

IN-PATIENT CONSIDERATIONS
Initial Stabilization
Hospital admission with meticulous airway management

Admission Criteria
All suspected cases must be admitted.

IV Fluids
Keep patient well hydrated.

Nursing
- Prevent decubitus ulcer, IV line infections, other nosocomial infections
- Before administration of antitoxin, skin testing should be performed for sensitivity.

 ONGOING CARE

FOLLOW-UP RECOMMENDATIONS
Outpatient follow-up with physical/occupational therapy, nutrition specialist, and psychiatry as needed

Patient Monitoring
- Pulmonary function testing
- Cardiorespiratory monitoring

DIET
Nasogastric feedings, if needed

PATIENT EDUCATION
- Spores destroyed by pressure cooking at 250°F (120°C) for 30 minutes
- Toxin destroyed by boiling for 10 minutes or cooking at 175°F (80°C) for 30 minutes
- Avoid honey in 1st year of life.
- Avoid IV drug use.
- Do not eat/sample foods that look and smell rotten or come from bulging cans.

PROGNOSIS
- Delay in administering antitoxin: Most important factor affecting clinical course and outcome (4)[B]
- Mortality: Overall 7–10%; <5% if infection is treated, but approaches 60% if untreated (6)
- Mortality for patients >60 years is twice that of younger patients
- Full recovery may take months.
- Significant health, functional, and social limitations several years after infection (7)[C]:
  - Recovery follows the regeneration of new neuromuscular connections.
  - 2–8 weeks of ventilator support may be required in more severe cases.
- Dyspnea with severe ptosis and pupil abnormality has been shown to correlate with severe illness and respiratory failure (8)[C].
- Increased incubation time has been shown to correlate with better outcomes (8)[C].

COMPLICATIONS
- Nosocomial infections, including aspiration pneumonia and ventilator-associated pneumonia
- Hypoxic tissue damage
- Death

REFERENCES
1. Lindström M, Korkeala H. Laboratory diagnostics of botulism. *Clin Microbiol Rev*. 2006;19:298–314.
2. Fach P, Micheau P, Mazuet C, et al. Development of real-time PCR tests for detecting botulinum neurotoxins A, B, E, F producing Clostridium botulinum, Clostridium baratii and Clostridium butyricum. *J Appl Microbiol*. 2009;107:465–73.
3. Bayrak A, et al. Electrophysiologic findings in a case of severe botulism. *J Neurol Sci*. 2006;23:49–53.
4. Dembek ZF, Smith LA, Rusnak JM. Botulism: cause, effects, diagnosis, clinical and laboratory identification, and treatment modalities. *Disaster Med Public Health Prep*. 2007;1:122–34.
5. Arnon SS, Schechter R, Maslanka SE, et al. Human botulism immune globulin for the treatment of infant botulism. *N Engl J Med*. 2006;354:462–71.
6. O'Brien KK, Higdon ML, Halverson JJ. Recognition and management of bioterrorism infections. *Am Fam Physician*. 2003;67:1927–34.
7. Gottlieb SL, Kretsinger K, Tarkhashvili N, et al. Long-term outcomes of 217 botulism cases in the Republic of Georgia. *Clin Infect Dis*. 2007;45:174–80.
8. Witoonpanich R, Vichayanrat E, Tantisiriwit K, et al. Survival analysis for respiratory failure in patients with food-borne botulism. *Clin Toxicol (Phila)*. 2010;48:177–83.
9. Botulism Facts for Healthcare Providers. Accessed 5/30/2010 at http://emergency.cdc.gov/agent/botulism/hcpfacts.asp.

See Also (Topic, Algorithm, Electronic Media Element)
Food Poisoning, Bacterial

 CODES

ICD9
- 005.1 Botulism food poisoning
- 040.42 Wound botulism

CLINICAL PEARLS
- Botulinum antitoxin should be administered as soon as possible; don't wait for lab results.
- Medical care providers who suspect botulism in a patient should immediately call their state health department's emergency 24-hour telephone number.
- A helpful mnemonic to recall progression of symptoms is the "dozen D's": Dry mouth, diplopia, dilated pupils, droopy eyes, droopy face, diminished gag reflex, dysphagia, dysarthria, dysphonia, difficulty lifting head, descending paralysis, and diaphragmatic paralysis (9)

BRAIN ABSCESS

Nathan Weldon, MD

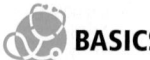

BASICS

DESCRIPTION
- Single or multiple abscesses within the brain, usually occurring secondary to a focus of infection outside the central nervous system
- May mimic brain tumor, but generally evolves more rapidly (over days to weeks)
- Starts as a cerebritis, becomes necrotic, and subsequently becomes encapsulated
- Synonym(s): Cerebral abscess

Geriatric Considerations
Age does not affect outcome as much as the abscess size and state of neurologic dysfunction at presentation.

Pediatric Considerations
- About 1/3 of the cases in pediatric age group
- Rarely found in infants <1 year of age
- Cyanotic congenital heart disease frequently associated

EPIDEMIOLOGY
- Predominant age: Median age 30–40 years, although brain abscess occurs at all ages
- Predominant sex: Male > Female (2:1)

Incidence
Infrequent, but increasing due to increase in immune-suppressed individuals, opportunistic pathogens, and resistance to antibiotics (1)

RISK FACTORS
- HIV/AIDS
- Immunocompromised state
- IV drug abuse

Genetics
No known genetic pattern

GENERAL PREVENTION
- Adequate treatment of otitis media, mastoiditis, sinusitis, dental abscess, other ear/nose/throat (ENT) infections
- Prophylactic antibiotics after compound skull fracture or penetrating head wound

ETIOLOGY
- Hematogenous source is most common overall for single or multiple cerebral abscesses.
- Direct extension from otitis, mastoiditis, sinusitis, or dental infection
- Cranial osteomyelitis
- Penetrating skull trauma
- Prior craniotomy
- Bacteremia from lung abscess, pneumonia
- Bacterial endocarditis
- Fungal infection of the nasopharynx
- *Toxoplasma gondii* (in AIDS patients)
- Cyanotic congenital heart disease
- IV drug use
- No source found in 20%.

- Most common infective organisms: Streptococci, staphylococci (especially after neurosurgery), enteric gram-negative bacilli and anaerobes (usually same as source of infection), *Nocardia*
- Brain abscess associated with HIV infection is assumed to be due to *T. gondii*.
- The frontal lobe of the brain is the most common site for an abscess.

COMMONLY ASSOCIATED CONDITIONS
- AIDS
- Congenital heart disease

DIAGNOSIS

HISTORY
- Recent onset of headache becoming severe
- New focal neurological deficit
- Altered mental status progressing to stupor and coma
- Nausea and vomiting
- Seizures

PHYSICAL EXAM
- Afebrile or low-grade fever
- Papilledema
- Neck stiffness
- Focal neurologic signs depending on location

DIAGNOSTIC TESTS & INTERPRETATION
Abscess culture: Predominant organisms include *Toxoplasma* (AIDS), *Staphylococcus* (trauma), aerobic or anaerobic bacteria, fungi (rare).

ALERT
- Lumbar puncture often contraindicated
- Prior administration of antibiotics may alter lab results.

Lab
Initial lab tests
- White blood cell (WBC) count may be normal or mildly elevated.
- Blood studies: Mild PMN leukocytosis; elevated erythrocyte sedimentation rate (ESR)
- Culture and susceptibilities of the abscess material

Imaging
- Search for primary source of infection, depending on suspected source.
- Solitary intracerebral abscess suggests a direct contiguous source such as sinus or ear infection.
- Multiple cerebral abscesses suggest hematological spread.
- Head computed tomography (CT) and magnetic resonance imaging (MRI) are the diagnostic methods of choice. Specific findings are dependent on stages of the abscess (2)[B].
- CT provides sufficient diagnostic information in most cases (3)[B], including skull fracture, sinus infection, or otic source.
- Consider cardiac echo, chest x-ray, and chest CT if cardiac or pulmonary source suspected
- Radionuclide [117]In-labeled leukocytes may distinguish abscess from neoplasm.

Diagnostic Procedures/Surgery
- Lumbar puncture often contraindicated
- Surgical burr hole with aspiration to make a specific bacteriologic diagnosis

Pathological Findings
- Suppuration, liquefaction, or encapsulation, depending on stage of evolution
- Fibrosis

DIFFERENTIAL DIAGNOSIS
- Brain tumors
- Cysticercosis
- Stroke
- Resolving intracranial hemorrhage
- Subdural empyema
- Extradural abscess
- Encephalitis

TREATMENT

Immediate neurosurgical consult is indicated for suspected CNS abscess.

MEDICATION
- Antibiotics according to organism and sensitivities, if known
- Initial empiric treatment according to suspected source
- Hematogenous sources should cover MRSA initially, and should include vancomycin, and may be broadened to include metronidazole and a 3rd-generation cephalosporin.
- For dental source, penicillin G and metronidazole are reasonable initial choices.
- For otogenic or sinus source, coverage should include metronidazole and either ceftriaxone or cefotaxime.
- For gastrointestinal or genitourinary source, consider a 3rd-generation cephalosporin such as cefotaxime to cover gram negatives.
- For traumatic source, consider vancomycin plus either ceftriaxone or cefotaxime.
- Hospital-acquired sources, including postsurgical abscess, consider vancomycin and cefepime or ceftazidime
- If MSSA is isolated, change vancomycin to oxacillin or nafcillin.
- Use vancomycin in penicillin-sensitive patients.
- Generally a 6–8-week course of parenteral antibiotics is required.
- If brain abscess associated with HIV/AIDS:
  – Daily doses of sulfadiazine and pyrimethamine
  – Lifelong therapy in AIDS patients
- Anticonvulsants:
  – Phenytoin until abscess resolves or perhaps longer
  – Monitor anticonvulsant levels.
- Following a neurosurgical procedure, use corticosteroids such as dexamethasone to reduce edema. Taper rapidly. Use is usually limited to 1 week.
- Contraindications: Sensitivity or allergy to any prescribed medications

- Precautions:
  - Sulfadiazine is poorly water-soluble. Patients must maintain adequate hydration or risk developing crystalluria.
  - Decrease dosage of penicillin in patients with renal dysfunction.
  - Monitor serum levels of anticonvulsants.
  - A dose of pyrimethamine is required for the treatment of toxoplasmosis, which may approach toxic levels. The patient should be observed for folic acid deficiency and treated with folinic acid (leucovorin) 5–15 mg (p.o., IM, IV) if necessary.
- Significant possible interactions: Refer to the manufacturer's literature.

ADDITIONAL TREATMENT
General Measures
- Palliative and supportive
- Treatment of brain abscess requires a combination of antimicrobial agents, surgical intervention, and eradication of the primary foci of infection (4)[A].
- Initial medical therapy includes broad-spectrum antibiotics pending determination of the causative organism.
- Determination of point of entry and source of infection is critical to effective treatment (5).
- Medical therapy only may be indicated:
  - For surgically inaccessible lesions or multiple abscesses
  - For abscesses in early cerebritis stage
  - For small (<2.5 cm) abscesses
- Antibiotic therapy may be directed toward most likely organism if no specific organism is identified.
- Monitor clinical response to antibiotic therapy.

Issues for Referral
Neurosurgery for all patients. Consider infectious disease and neurology consultations if available.

SURGERY/OTHER PROCEDURES
- Mandatory when neurologic deficits are severe or progressive
- Often used when the abscess is in the posterior fossa or is the result of trauma
- Type of surgical treatment used depends on the patient's clinical status, the neuroradiographic characteristics of the abscess, and the experience of the surgeon(s) carrying out the procedure (4).
- Abscess drainage via a needle under stereotactic CT guidance through a burr hole under local anesthesia is the most rapid and effective surgical method of treatment and may be repeated if needed.
- Craniotomy: If abscess is large or multilocular
- In general, similar outcomes for stereotactic-guided drainage or craniotomy (6)

IN-PATIENT CONSIDERATIONS
Initial Stabilization
Inpatient care for close observation, diagnostic evaluation, and specialty consultation (neurology, neurosurgery, or infectious disease)

Admission Criteria
Upon diagnosis for close monitoring, IV antibiotics, and possible surgery. A brain abscess often requires admission to an intensive care unit (ICU), and may be the complication of ICU patients with neurologic injury, contributing significantly to morbidity and mortality (7)[B].

IV Fluids
IV fluids if nausea and vomiting present

Discharge Criteria
When patient is asymptomatic, afebrile, and responding to therapy as determined by serial imaging studies

ONGOING CARE
FOLLOW-UP RECOMMENDATIONS
- Bed rest until infection controlled and abscess evacuated or resolving, then as tolerated
- May need long-term rehabilitative care

Patient Monitoring
- Postsurgical monitoring as needed
- Serial CT or MRI for at least 3 months to evaluate the therapeutic response, confirm progressive resolution, detect new lesions, and manage complications.

DIET
IV fluids if significant nausea and vomiting

PATIENT EDUCATION
- Brain Research Foundation, 208 S. LaSalle Street, Suite 1426, Chicago, IL 60604; (312) 782-4311.
- Pri-Med Patient Education Center: Brain Abscess at http://www.patienteducationcenter.org/aspx/HealthELibrary/HealthETopic.aspx?cid=210320

PROGNOSIS
- The route of spread, the type and virulence of the organism, thickness of the capsule, location and number of abscesses in the brain, and immune status of the host are important determinants of outcome (1).
- Survival: >80% with early diagnosis and treatment
- In 1 retrospective analysis, 80% of patients recovered fully or had minimal incapacity and 10% died (3)[B].
- Patients with underlying cranial neoplasms or medical conditions have worse outcomes than those with a contiguous focus of infection or posttraumatic abscess (3)[B].

COMPLICATIONS
- Permanent neurologic deficits
- Surgical complications
- ICU-related complications
- Recurrent abscess
- Seizures
- Death

REFERENCES
1. Sundaram C, Lakshmi V. Pathogenesis and pathology of brain abscess. *Indian J Pathol Microbiol.* 2006;49:317–26.
2. Foerster BR, Thurnher MM, Malani PN, et al. Intracranial infections: clinical and imaging characteristics. *Acta Radiol.* 2007;48:875–93.
3. Carpenter J, Stapleton S, Holliman R. Retrospective analysis of 49 cases of brain abscess and review of the literature. *Eur J Clin Microbiol Infect Dis.* 2007;26:1–11.
4. Lu CH, et al. Strategies for the management of bacterial brain abscess. *J Clin Neurosci.* 2006;13(10):979–85. Epub 2006 Oct 23.
5. Bernardini GL. Diagnosis and management of brain abscess and subdural empyema. *Curr Neurol Neurosci Rep.* 2004;4:448–56.
6. Smith SJ, Ughratdar I, MacArthur DC et al. Never go to sleep on undrained pus: a retrospective review of surgery for intraparenchymal cerebral abscess. *Br J Neurosurg.* 2009;23:412–7.
7. Ziai WC, Lewin JJ. Update in the diagnosis and management of central nervous system infections. *Neurol Clin.* 2008;26:427–68, viii.

ADDITIONAL READING
- Alangaden G, Chandrasekar PH et al. Case 10-2010: a woman with weakness and a mass in the brain. *N Engl J Med.* 2010;363:395; author reply 395–6.
- Chang YT, Lu CH, Chuang MJ, Huang CR, Chuang YC, Tsai NW, Chen SF, Chang CC, Chang WN et al. Supratentorial deep-seated bacterial brain abscess in adults: clinical characteristics and therapeutic outcomes. *Acta Neurol Taiwan.* 2010;19:174–9.
- Mace SE et al. Central nervous system infections as a cause of an altered mental status? What is the pathogen growing in your central nervous system? *Emerg Med Clin North Am.* 2010;28:535–70.
- Patron V, Orsel S, Caire F, Aubry K, Jégoux F et al. Transethmoidal Drainage of Frontal Brain Abscesses. *Surgical innovation.* 2010;
- Shachor-Meyouhas Y, Bar-Joseph G, Guilburd JN, Lorber A, Hadash A, Kassis I et al. Brain abscess in children—epidemiology, predisposing factors and management in the modern medicine era. *Acta Paediatr.* 2010;99:1163–7.

CODES
ICD9
324.0 Intracranial abscess

CLINICAL PEARLS
- Headache and altered mental status are common presenting symptoms of a brain abscess.
- Determination of point of entry and source of infection is essential for adequate treatment.
- Treatment of brain abscess may require a combination of antimicrobial agents for 6–8 weeks, surgical intervention, and eradication of the primary foci of infection.
- Serial head CTs for at least 3 months can help to evaluate a patient's response to therapies.

BRAIN INJURY, TRAUMATIC

Dana M. Collaguazo, MD

BASICS

DESCRIPTION
- A dynamic process with initial bleeding followed by secondary injury due to cerebral edema, continued bleeding
- Frequently related to rapid deceleration, as in motor vehicle or diving accidents, or blunt trauma
- System(s) affected: Cardiovascular; Endocrine/Metabolic; Nervous
- Synonym(s): Head injury

EPIDEMIOLOGY
Incidence
- 1.7 million per year
- 1,365,000 emergency department visits per year
- 275,000 hospitalizations per year
- 52,000 deaths per year

Prevalence
- Predominant age: 0–4, 15–19, and over 65 years
- Predominant gender: Male > Female

RISK FACTORS
Alcohol, prior head injury, contact sports; "heading" soccer balls may cause long-term cognitive loss.

Geriatric Considerations
Subdural hematomas are common after fall or blow; symptoms may be subtle.

GENERAL PREVENTION
- Safety education
- Seat belts, bicycle and motorcycle helmets
- Protective headgear for contact sports

PATHOPHYSIOLOGY
Initial intracranial bleeding followed by secondary injury due to cerebral edema, continued bleeding, etc.

ETIOLOGY
- Motor vehicle accident (17%)
- Falls (35%)
- Assault
- Child abuse:
  - Consider if dropped or fell <4 feet (e.g., off bed, couch) and significant injury present or any retinal hemorrhages

COMMONLY ASSOCIATED CONDITIONS
Alcohol and drug abuse

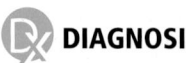

DIAGNOSIS

HISTORY
- Loss of consciousness (LOC)
- Headache
- Vomiting
- Amnesia
- Epidural hemorrhage from blunt trauma is generally acute, 30% with a "lucid interval" (initial LOC followed by recovery of consciousness, then LOC recurs and persists)
- Subdural hemorrhage usually has a slower onset and may present weeks after the initial injury, especially in the elderly.

PHYSICAL EXAM
- Focal neurologic signs and symptoms
- Evidence of increased intracranial pressure (ICP) (elevated BP, decreased pulse rate, or slow or irregular breathing [Cushing triad]—only 30% have all 3)
- Decorticate or decerebrate posturing (bad prognostic signs)
- Seizures
- Signs of basilar skull fracture: Raccoon eyes, battle sign, hemotympanum, CSF rhinorrhea or otorrhea (see Diagnostic Procedures)
- Unilateral dilated pupil in an alert patient is not consistent with impending herniation, as such patients are always unconscious.

DIAGNOSTIC TESTS & INTERPRETATION
Lab
Initial lab tests
- Evaluate for coagulopathy.
- Type and screen for possible surgical intervention.
- Perform drug and alcohol screening.

Imaging
Initial approach
CT, noncontrast, is study of choice to review bone windows, tissue windows, and subdural space:
- NEXUS II study (1)[B] demonstrated 8 clinical criteria that indicate a low likelihood of significant TBI when absent:
  - Evidence of significant skull fracture (depressed, basilar, or diastatic)
  - Altered level of alertness
  - Neurologic deficit
  - Persistent vomiting
  - Presence of scalp hematoma
  - Abnormal behavior
  - Coagulopathy
  - Age >65

Follow-Up & Special Considerations
Skull radiographs are not helpful in most cases, but can be done to document child abuse.

Diagnostic Procedures/Surgery
- CSF rhinorrhea:
  - Contains glucose; nasal mucus does not
  - Check for the double-halo sign: If nasal discharge contains CSF and blood, 2 rings appear when placed on filter paper—a central ring followed by a paler ring.
- Placement of ICP monitor when indicated
- Serial neurologic exams
- Neuropsychometric testing when able

Pathological Findings
- Epidural, subdural, or intraparenchymal hemorrhage
- Coup or contrecoup injury
- Evolving, diffuse axonal injury is a principal cause of neurologic sequelae with mild head trauma.

DIFFERENTIAL DIAGNOSIS
Other causes of altered mental status (e.g., toxicologic, infectious, metabolic, vascular causes)

TREATMENT

MEDICATION
First Line
- Pain: Morphine 1–2 mg IV p.r.n. with caution as can depress mental status further and alter serial neurologic evaluations
- Increased ICP:
  - Mannitol: 0.25–2 g/kg (0.25–1 g/kg in children) given over 30–60 minutes in patients with adequate renal function; should not be used unless there is evidence of increased ICP; prophylactic use is associated with worse outcomes
  - Lasix: 20–40 mg IV to promote diuresis:
    - Neither furosemide nor mannitol should be given to a hypotensive patient.
  - Hypertonic saline: 2 mL/kg IV decreases ICP without adverse hemodynamic status and may have beneficial effects on immune system and excitatory neurotransmitters (2)[B].
- Sedation:
  - Propofol: Preferred due to short duration of action, which allows serial neurologic exams
- Seizures:
  - Phenytoin (Dilantin): 15 mg/kg IV (1 mg/kg/min IV, not to exceed 50 mg/min). Stop infusion if QT interval increases by >50%.
  - Lorazepam (Ativan): 1–2 mg (0.1 mg/kg in children) IV
  - Phosphenytoin (Cerebyx): 15 mg/kg IV, not to exceed 150 mg/min. May give IM.
  - Levetiracetam (Keppra): May be desirable; lower complication rates, but prospective studies are needed. Use at neurosurgeon's instruction (3)[C].
- Contraindications: Allergy

Second Line
- Diuretics and IV β-blockers (e.g., esmolol or labetalol) can be used to maintain mean arterial pressure between 130 and 70 mm Hg.
- Nitrates may be helpful; however, may increase ICP
- Antibiotics (e.g., cefazolin): Given if penetrating trauma is present; prophylactic antibiotics are not useful in basilar skull fractures.

ADDITIONAL TREATMENT
General Measures
- Acute management depends on severity of injury. Most patients need no interventions.
- Immediate goal: Determine who needs further therapy, imaging studies (CT), and hospitalization to prevent further injury.
- For the severely injured patient:
  - Avoid hypotension or hypoxia. Head injury causes increased ICP secondary to edema, and perfusion pressure must be maintained.
  - Hyperventilation is controversial. Prophylactic hyperventilation for those without signs or symptoms of increased ICP is contraindicated and may cause additional injury secondary to vasoconstriction (4)[B].

– Hypothermia: Although no difference is seen in mortality, may have marginal benefit, especially in patients with elevated ICP refractory to other methods (5)[B].

– Seizure prophylaxis does not change outcomes (such as death rates) but may prevent seizures. Consider phenytoin or levetiracetam for 1 week postinjury.

- Manage breakthrough seizures with lorazepam.
- Brain tissue oxygen probes can measure brain tissue hypoxia (<10 mm Hg is associated with worse outcomes) and may help define treatment parameters in acute traumatic brain injuries (6)[A].

Issues for Referral
Consult neurosurgery for:

- All penetrating head trauma
- All abnormal head CTs

SURGERY/OTHER PROCEDURES
Depends on neurosurgical consult

IN-PATIENT CONSIDERATIONS
Initial Stabilization
- ABCs take priority over head injury.
- C-spine immobilization should be considered in all head trauma.

Admission Criteria
- Abnormal CT
- Abnormal Glasgow coma scale
- Clinical evidence of basilar skull fracture
- Persistent neurologic deficits (e.g., confusion, somnolence)
- Patient with no competent adult at home for observation
- Possibly admit: LOC, amnesia, etc.

IV Fluids
Use normal saline for resuscitation fluid.

Discharge Criteria
Normal CT with return to normal mental status and responsible adult to observe patient at home (see Patient Monitoring)

 ## ONGOING CARE

FOLLOW-UP RECOMMENDATIONS
- Schedule regular follow-up within a week to determine return to activities.
- Rehabilitation indicated following a significant acute injury. Set realistic goals.

Patient Monitoring
Any patient discharged should have "head injury instructions" to watch for symptoms indicating need for further intervention (e.g., changing mental status, worsening headache, focal findings). Give to a competent adult who will observe the patient. A patient who deteriorates is not likely to remember or act on any instructions.

DIET
As tolerated

PATIENT EDUCATION
Proper counseling, symptomatic management, and gradual return to normal activities are essential to prevent a posttraumatic neurosis that can become refractory to treatment.

PROGNOSIS
- Gradual improvement for many
- 30–50% of severe head injuries may be fatal.
- Prolonged coma may be followed by satisfactory outcome.
- Predicting outcome is difficult, and patients may improve for years.

Geriatric Considerations
- Poorer prognosis with increasing age. Patients 75 and older have the highest rate of TBI hospitalizations and death.

Pediatric Considerations
- Outcome is more positive, except in severe TBI.

COMPLICATIONS
- Delayed hematomas
- Chronic subdural hematoma, which may follow even "mild" head injury, especially in the elderly. Often presents with headache and decreased mentation.
- Delayed hydrocephalus
- Emotional disturbances and psychiatric disorders resulting from head injury may be refractory to treatment.
- Seizure disorders: In 50% of penetrating head injuries, in 20% of severe closed head injuries, and in <5% of head injuries overall. Hematomas significantly increase risk of epilepsy.
- The postconcussion syndrome can follow mild head injury without LOC and includes headaches, dizziness, fatigue, and subtle cognitive or affective changes.
- 2nd-impact syndrome occurs when the CNS loses autoregulation. An individual with a minor head injury is returned to a contact sport and, following even minor trauma (e.g., whiplash), the patient will lose consciousness and herniate within 1–2 minutes, with a 50% mortality. A similar syndrome of "malignant edema" can occur in children with even a single injury.
- Increased risk for Alzheimer disease, Parkinson disease, and other brain disorders whose prevalence increases with age

REFERENCES

1. Mower WR, Hoffman JR, Herbert M, et al. Developing a decision instrument to guide computed tomographic imaging of blunt head injury patients. *J Trauma*. 2005;59:954–9.
2. Vincent JL, Berré J. Primer on medical management of severe brain injury. *Crit Care Med*. 2005;33: 1392–9.
3. Szaflarski JP, Meckler JM, Szaflarski M, et al. Levetiracetam use in critically ill patients. *Neurocrit Care*. 2007;7:140–7.
4. Stocchetti N, Maas AI, Chieregato A, et al. Hyperventilation in head injury: a review. *Chest*. 2005;127:1812–27.
5. Henderson WR, Dhingra VK, Chittock DR, et al. Hypothermia in the management of traumatic brain injury. A systematic review and meta-analysis. *Intensive Care Med*. 2003;29:1637–44.
6. Maloney-Wilensky E, Gracias V, Itkin A, et al. Links brain tissue oxygen and outcome after severe traumatic brain injury: A systematic review. *Crit Care Med*. 2009 Apr 20. [Epub ahead of print].

ADDITIONAL READING

- Faul M, Xu L, Wald MM, Coronado VG. *Traumatic brain injury in the United States: emergency department visits, hospitalizations, and deaths*. Atlanta GA: Centers for Disease Control and Prevention, National Center for Injury Prevention and Control, 2010.
- Meloney-Wilensky E, Gracias V, Itkin A et al. Brain tissue oxygen and outcome after severe traumatic brain injury: a systematic review. *Crit Care Med*. 2009;37(6):2057–63.

See Also (Topic, Algorithm, Electronic Media Element)
Brain Injury–Post Acute Care Issues; Postconcussive Syndrome; Seizure Disorders

 ## CODES

ICD9
- 852.00 Subarachnoid hemorrhage following injury, without mention of open intracranial wound, with state of consciousness unspecified
- 853.00 Other and unspecified intracranial hemorrhage following injury, without mention of open intracranial wound, with state of consciousness unspecified
- 854.00 Intracranial injury of other and unspecified nature, without mention of open intracranial wound, with state of consciousness unspecified

CLINICAL PEARLS

- Head injury is a dynamic process: Initial bleeding followed by secondary injury due to cerebral edema, continued bleeding, etc.
- Patients with history of head injury should have imaging if any of the following are present: Evidence of skull fracture, altered consciousness, neurologic deficit, persistent vomiting, scalp hematoma, abnormal behavior, coagulopathy, age >65
- Patient with normal head CT who has returned to normal mental status may be discharged to home with a competent adult observer for 24 hours.
- Strict criteria exist for patients to return to normal sport activity following head injury to avoid the 2nd-impact syndrome, which has 50% mortality.
- Predicting outcome is difficult, and patients may improve for years.

BRAIN INJURY–POST ACUTE CARE ISSUES

Maria I. Aguilar, MD

 BASICS

DESCRIPTION

Traumatic brain injury (TBI) is a brain injury due to externally inflicted trauma; may result in significant impairment of an individual's physical, cognitive, and psychosocial functioning. TBI: leading mortality cause in North America for ages 1–45.

EPIDEMIOLOGY

- Predominant age: Highest incidence in the very young (ages 0–4), in persons 15–24 years of age and those >75 years old
- Predominant sex: Male > Female (2:1)

Incidence

- 1.2–1.7 million Americans sustain TBI per year.
- 50,000 deaths per year
- 80,000–90,000 sustain long-term disabilities

Prevalence

5.3 million Americans are living with TBI-related disabilities for which they require long-term assistance with activities of daily living.

RISK FACTORS

- High risk: Male, age 15–34
- Moderate risk <5 years and >60 years
- Lower socioeconomic status (head injury)

GENERAL PREVENTION

Improved safety standards and programs designed to minimize injury from vehicular-related events (motor vehicle, motorcycle, bicycle, pedestrian), falls, violence, sports, and recreation provide best prevention against TBI (1)[C].

PATHOPHYSIOLOGY

- Cortical contusions due to coup–contrecoup injuries. While axonal rupture from shear and tensile forces can occur at the time of severe head injury, milder degrees of axonal damage may play a role in mild TBI.
- Disruption of axonal neurofilament organization impairs axonal transport, leading to axonal swelling, Wallerian degeneration, and transection.
- Release of excitatory neurotransmitters acetylcholine, glutamate, and aspartate, and generation of free radicals may contribute to secondary injury.

ETIOLOGY

- Leading causes of TBI: falls and motor vehicle accidents (MVA). Violence-related TBI has increased during the past decade and accounts for about 10% of all cases. Sports and recreation injuries are also an important cause of TBI, especially in teenagers and young adults.
- As the conflict in the Middle East continues, the number of soldiers returning to the US with diagnosed and undiagnosed blast-related TBI will continue to increase.

COMMONLY ASSOCIATED CONDITIONS

- Psychosis
- Suicide attempts
- Substance abuse
- Attention deficit disorder

 DIAGNOSIS

HISTORY

- Non-neurologic complications: Pulmonary, metabolic and endocrinologic, nutritional, GI, musculoskeletal, genitourinary, dermatologic, chronic pain
- Most neurologic complications are apparent within the 1st days following injury. Long-term sequelae include seizures, headache, hydrocephalus, visual defects, neuroendocrine abnormalities, and movement and sleep disorders.
- Cognitive consequences: Memory impairment, difficulties in attention and concentration, language deficits, visual perception problems, and poor problem-solving, reasoning, insight, judgment, and information processing
- Behavioral problems: Decreased ability to initiate responses, verbal and physical aggression, agitation, learning difficulties, shallow self-awareness, altered sexual functioning, impulsivity, social disinhibition
- Psychological consequences: Mood disorders, personality changes, altered emotional control, depression, anxiety
- Social consequences: Risk of suicide, divorce, unemployment, economic strain, alcohol/substance abuse.

Pediatric Considerations

Interactions of physical, cognitive, and behavioral sequelae interfere with new learning. Effects of early TBI may not become apparent until later in the child's development.

PHYSICAL EXAM

- TBI's severity is classified based on the Glasgow Coma Scale (GCS) as follows: Mild injury GCS 13–15; moderate injury GCS 9–12; severe injury GCS 8 or less.
- Glasgow Coma Scale (GCS). For all 3 categories, score best response:

Verbal response	Score
Oriented	5
Confused	4
Inappropriate words	3
Incomprehensible speech	2
No response	1
Eye opening	
Spontaneous	4
To speech	3
To pain	2
No response	1
Motor response	
Obeys commands	6
Localizes pain	5
Withdraws from pain	4
Abnormal flexion to pain	3
Abnormal extension to pain	2
No response	1

DIAGNOSTIC TESTS & INTERPRETATION

- Evoked potentials (auditory, visual, somatosensory)
- Behavioral assessment, neuropsychological testing, vocational assessment
- Cognitive test for orientation and arousal; use Western Neuro Sensory Stimulation Profile or Galveston Orientation Amnesia Test
- Electroencephalograph (EEG)

Lab
Initial lab tests
As needed for suspected metabolic complications

Imaging
Initial approach
- Bone scan: Heterotopic ossification
- CT: Hydrocephalus, atrophy, hematoma
- Video fluoroscopic swallowing study
- MRI to evaluate diffuse axonal injury
- EEG: To evaluate subclinical seizure activity. Limited predictive value in the setting of acute TBI.

Pathological Findings
- Evidence of microscopic axonal injury, axon retraction bulbs, and microglial clusters
- Hydrocephalus with periventricular edema
- Joint contractures result in collagen cross-linking: Decreased range of motion
- Heterotopic ossification: Disorganized osteoid calcification in soft tissue

DIFFERENTIAL DIAGNOSIS

- The diagnosis of pain following TBI can be difficult in light of limitations imposed by cognitive, language, and behavioral deficits.
  - Dysautonomia: Tachypnea, hypertension, painful posturing/contractions, diaphoresis
  - Neuropathic pain: Burning, shocklike, or pins and needles; allodynia/hyperpathia. 3 most common: Complex regional pain syndrome, central pain syndrome, and peripheral neuropathy.
  - Spasticity or spastic dystonia
  - Headache: Posttraumatic headache, hydrocephalus, increased intracranial pressure
  - Myofascial pain syndrome
  - Neurogenic heterotopic ossification: Bone formation in soft tissue
  - Deep vein thrombosis
  - Constipation and urinary retention
  - Trauma: Fractures, musculoskeletal injuries
  - Shoulder: Subluxation, acromioclavicular separation, rotator cuff tendonitis/tear
- Chronic infection, depression, hypothyroidism, hydrocephalus, intracerebral hemorrhage, seizures, fractures, tracheal stricture, pain, alcohol, drugs, polypharmacy, and/or central nervous system depressant

TREATMENT

MEDICATION

- Psychostimulants may affect speed of cognitive processing, mood, and behavior:
  - Methylphenidate 20–40 mg/d in 2 divided doses; dextroamphetamine [B]
  - Also likely to improve memory, attention, concentration, and mental processing in children/adults (2)[A]

- Agitation:
  - Treat epilepsy or depression 1st.
  - Minimize the use of antipsychotics and benzodiazepines, as they worsen cognition.
  - β-Blockers have best evidence for efficacy in agitation/aggression (3)[A].
  - Antidepressants (SSRIs) and AEDs in the context of an affective disorder or epilepsy, respectively, may help agitation/aggression (4)[B].
  - If necessary, use antipsychotics of the atypical class (clozapine, olanzapine, quetiapine, risperidone, and ziprasidone) (5)[B].
- Abulia (lack of initiative): Amantadine (Symmetrel), bromocriptine, methylphenidate, levodopa (5)[C].
- Epilepsy: American Academy of Physical Medicine and Rehabilitation does not recommend AEDs for preventing late (>7 days post TBI) posttraumatic seizures (6)[B]. If epilepsy occurs, avoid phenobarbital; too sedating (6).
- Spasticity caution: Be aware of potential negative consequences of all agents:
  - Use dantrolene sodium 25–200 mg/d divided t.i.d.; baclofen; intrathecal baclofen; diazepam, clonidine, tizanidine, and gabapentin; botulinum toxin injections for focal spasticity (7)[B].
- Neurogenic bladder: Oxybutynin 2.5 mg t.i.d.– 10 mg q.i.d. if bladder pressures low and/or postvoid residuals low (1)[B]
- Bowel routine: Stool softener such as docusate sodium (daily) combined with laxative (night before suppository), high-fiber diet, and suppository (every other day) (1)[C]
- Heterotopic ossification: Indomethacin 25–50 mg t.i.d. If severe, progressive, or history of GI ulceration, then etidronate (Didronel) 20 mg/kg for 6 months or alendronate 20 mg/d (1)[C].
- Neurobehavioral problems: Weak evidence supports psychostimulants as effective in treatment of inattention, apathy, and slowness; high-dose β-blockers in treatment of agitation and aggression; and anticonvulsants and antidepressants in treatment of agitation and aggression with an affective disorder (4)[B].
- Precautions: Medications may have significant adverse effects in persons with TBI and can impede rehabilitation progress.

ADDITIONAL TREATMENT
General Measures
- Diminished level of arousal: Identify best modality for communication, assess functional skills (proper seating, hand function) with behaviorist/neuropsychologist.
- Social work (family education and long-term planning) and nursing
- Reduce sedatives
- Neurogenic bladder—treat urinary tract infection:
  - If postvoid residual <50 mL, then try regular voiding routine q2h
  - If still incontinent, add oxybutynin
  - If still incontinent, try condom catheter during the day; incontinence pads at night.
  - If high postvoid residuals or high pressure bladder or dyssynergic bladder on urodynamics: Intermittent catheter q4–6h
- Neurogenic bowel: Regular bowel routine
- Contractures and spasticity; stretching:
  - If no progress after 4 weeks, consider serial casting or custom-made orthotic
  - Contractures >45°: Consider tendon release.

- Heterotopic ossification: Stretch soft tissue to decrease maturation of osteoid, consider orthotics/splinting, bone scan at baseline
- Skin: Turn patient q2h; avoid sitting such as in bed at 45°, observe for erythema around tube sites, and rule out latex allergy.
- Respiratory: Night humidification for tracheotomy
- Endocrine: Monitor fluid balance
- Dental: Assessment and radiographs
- Rehabilitative practices: Rehabilitative programs should be interdisciplinary, comprehensive, and include cognitive and behavioral assessment and intervention (1)[C]

Issues for Referral
- Refer to multidisciplinary rehabilitation programs.
- Suicide attempts and ideation (SI) are more prevalent in people with TBI, even after controlling for psychiatric disorders (8)[C]. Assess hopelessness and SI proactively.

COMPLEMENTARY AND ALTERNATIVE MEDICINE
- Cognitive exercises (including computer-assisted strategies), compensatory devices (memory books, paging systems), psychotherapy, behavior modification, vocational rehabilitation, school rehabilitation, nutritional support, music and art therapy, therapeutic recreation
- Hyperbaric oxygen therapy (HBOT) cannot be routinely recommended for patients with TBI because of few trials, methodologic shortcomings, and poor reporting (9)[A].

 ## ONGOING CARE

FOLLOW-UP RECOMMENDATIONS
Patient Monitoring
Patients make slow, steady gains; review medical status monthly.

DIET
- Ensure adequate hydration; 2–2.5 L of water/d.
- Bolus feeds preferred if fed by gastrostomy.
- Upright and quiet for 1/2 hour following feeds, as aspiration can occur even with a g-tube
- Early feeding is associated with trend toward better survival and disability outcomes (10)[A].

PATIENT EDUCATION
- For information and family support groups:
  - Brain Injury Information Network www.tbinet.org/
  - Brain Injury Association of America www.biausa.org/
- Families need support, advocacy, education, information (verbally and written), opportunity to have input regarding priorities and treatment plans, and to discuss limits of treatment for patient (advance directive).

PROGNOSIS
- Most rapid return of function is during 1st 2 years, but some improve slowly for 5–10 years
- Highly variable (80% of individuals with severe injuries become independent in dressing and self-care at 1 year)
- Negative prognostic factors:
  - Age >40 years old
  - Abnormal pupillary responses or extraocular eye movements
  - Prolonged coma
- Abnormal evoked potentials

- Accurate prediction of return to work is not feasible, with rates in the 12–70% range.

COMPLICATIONS
Major affective disorder (depression, psychosis) in up to 50% of patients, family and caregiver burnout, substance abuse, social isolation, dental caries, osteoporosis, aspiration pneumonia, pressure ulcers, dysphagia, esophagitis, bladder incontinence, contractures/spasticity

REFERENCES

1. Consensus conference. Rehabilitation of persons with traumatic brain injury. NIH Consensus Development Panel on Rehabilitation of Persons With Traumatic Brain Injury. JAMA. 1999;282: 974–83.
2. Siddall OM. Use of methylphenidate in traumatic brain injury. Ann Pharmacother. 2005;39: 1309–13.
3. Fleminger S, et al. Pharmacological management for agitation and aggression in people with acquired brain injury. Cochrane Database Syst Rev. 2003/2006;(1):CD003299.
4. Deb S, Crownshaw T. The role of pharmacotherapy in the management of behaviour disorders in traumatic brain injury patients. Brain Inj. 2004;18:1–31.
5. Elovic EP, et al. The use of atypical antipsychotics in traumatic brain injury. J Head Trauma Rehab. 2003;18(2):177–95.
6. Bushnik T, et al. Medical and social issues related to posttraumatic seizures in persons with traumatic brain injury. J Head Trauma Rehab. 2004;19(4):296–304.
7. Zafonte R, et al. Acute care management of post-TBI spasticity. J Head Trauma Rehab. 2004;19(2):89–100.
8. Simpson G, Tate R, et al. Suicidality in people surviving a traumatic brain injury: prevalence, risk factors and implications for clinical management. Brain Inj. 2007;21:1335–51.
9. Bennett M, Heard R. Hyperbaric oxygen therapy for multiple sclerosis. Cochrane Database Syst Rev. 2004:CD003057.
10. Perel P, Yanagawa T, Bunn F, et al. Nutritional support for head-injured patients. Cochrane Database Syst Rev. 2006:CD001530.

CODES

ICD9
- 339.20 Post-traumatic headache, unspecified
- 854.00 Intracranial injury of other and unspecified nature, without mention of open intracranial wound, with state of consciousness unspecified
- 907.0 Late effect of intracranial injury without mention of skull fracture

CLINICAL PEARLS

- TBI can cause both neurologic and non-neurologic manifestations.
- Best approach to treatment includes multi- and interdisciplinary team member participation.
- TBI can lead to devastating sequelae; prevention is key.

BRANCHIAL CLEFT FISTULA

Timothy L. Black, MD

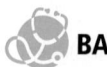 **BASICS**

DESCRIPTION

- A congenital, abnormal tract connecting the skin of the neck with an internal structure, resulting from failure of closure of 1 of the 4 branchial clefts
- May involve branchial clefts I–IV, which develop in the 4th gestational week
- System(s) affected: Skin/Exocrine

Pediatric Considerations
Almost all occur in the pediatric age group.

EPIDEMIOLOGY

- Predominant age: By definition, all are present at birth, although they may remain unnoticed for some time. (Branchial cleft cysts may not present until later childhood.) (1)[C]
- Predominant sex: Unknown

Incidence
Unknown

Prevalence
Unknown

RISK FACTORS
Positive family history

Genetics
10% have family history.

PATHOPHYSIOLOGY

- Both respiratory and squamous epithelium alone or in combination may line branchial anomalies (2)[C].
- Squamous epithelium is found more commonly in cysts.
- Ciliated, columnar epithelium is found more commonly in sinuses and fistulae.

ETIOLOGY

- The 1st branchial cleft contributes to the tympanic cavity and eustachian tube. Related fistulae are very rare and tend to be infra- or retroauricular. (Preauricular cysts and sinuses are not thought to be of branchial cleft origin.) The first branchial cleft anomalies enter the external auditory canal and/or the middle ear
- The 2nd branchial cleft forms the hyoid bone and tonsillar fossa. Related fistulae (most common variant) course between the internal and external carotid arteries. Internal opening usually at level of tonsillar fossa. External opening along anterior border of sternocleidomastoid muscle (1)[C]. 2nd branchial cleft lesions represent 90% or more of all branchial cleft lesions.
- 3rd and 4th branchial clefts form parathyroid glands, thymus, and portions of thyroid (parafollicular cells). Fistulae are rare; those from third cleft course posterior to carotid artery; both should have external ostia on lower anterior neck. Sinus tracts (also called pyriform sinuses) originate in the pyriform sinus and course adjacent to the thyroid cartilage (3)[C]. 3rd branchial cleft anomalies represent 2–8% of all branchial anomalies.

COMMONLY ASSOCIATED CONDITIONS
Microtia and aural atresia occur with failure of development of 1st branchial cleft.

 DIAGNOSIS

HISTORY

- History of drainage from cervical area
- Neck abscess or suppurative thyroiditis

PHYSICAL EXAM

- Presence of tiny external opening usually on mid-to-lower neck along anterior border of sternocleidomastoid muscle
- Spontaneous mucoid drainage
- External openings may also be marked by a skin tag or cartilage.
- Infection may rarely be the presenting sign, with erythema, swelling, pain, or fever.
- 10% are bilateral.
- Small orifices located in the mid-neck, most commonly along the anterior border of the sternocleidomastoid muscle (less commonly in the lower neck or postauricular)
- Third branchial cleft anomalies are predominantly left-sided (89%) (4)[B].

DIAGNOSTIC TESTS & INTERPRETATION
Lab
Culture if signs of infection

Imaging
- Computed tomography (CT) of neck with IV contrast occasionally beneficial in 3rd and 4th branchial cleft fistulas/sinus (3)[C].
- CT may demonstrate fistula tract in up to 64% of cases (2)[C].
- Magnetic resonance imaging and ultrasound may occasionally be useful.
- Barium esophagogram may demonstrate the fistula (may have a sensitivity rate of 50–80% when used to evaluate 3rd and 4th branchial anomalies (2)[C].

Diagnostic Procedures/Surgery
- Sinogram or fistulogram may be done, but is of little value.
- Pharyngoscopy may occasionally be useful.

Pathological Findings
- Lined by stratified squamous epithelium; may contain hair follicles, sweat glands, sebaceous glands, or cartilage
- Some are lined by ciliated columnar epithelium.

DIFFERENTIAL DIAGNOSIS
- External sinuses
- Cystic hygroma
- Dermoid cysts
- Lymphadenopathy

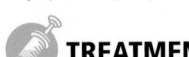 TREATMENT
- Surgical excision
- Outpatient status usually appropriate

SURGERY/OTHER PROCEDURES
- Small transverse incision at external ostium with careful dissection of fistula (1)[C]
- Stepladder incisions may be needed.
- End of fistula ligated flush with pharyngeal mucosa. 1st branchial cleft lesions may require larger incision (1)[C].
- Methylene blue injection into fistula may be useful.
- Drains are not used.
- Antibiotics only for infection
- Patients with abscess related to 3rd branchial cleft anomalies frequently require initial incision and drainage (4)[B]:
  - Incision and drainage failure rate of 94% at 1st attempt
  - Virtually all require resection.
  - Those with acute suppurative thyroiditis may require partial thyroidectomy with resection.
- Endoscopic cauterization of the internal orifice has been successfully used in some cases.

ONGOING CARE

FOLLOW-UP RECOMMENDATIONS
Patient Monitoring
- Follow at weekly intervals if infected until resolution, then excision
- Postoperative visit at 2 weeks

PROGNOSIS
Good

COMPLICATIONS
- Facial nerve injury
- Hypoglossal nerve injury
- Spinal accessory nerve injury
- Vagus nerve injury
- Infection
- Carotid artery injury
- Possible recurrence if any epithelium remains
- Neoplastic degeneration of branchial remnants (about 250 reported cases) if not resected

REFERENCES

1. Roback SA, Telander RL. Thyroglossal duct cysts and branchial cleft anomalies. *Sem Ped Surg.* 1994;3:142–46.
2. Waldhausen JH et al. Branchial cleft and arch anomalies in children. *Semin Pediatr Surg.* 2006;15:64–9.
3. Liberman M, Kay S, Emil S, et al. Ten years of experience with third and fourth branchial remnants. *J Ped Surg.* 2002;37:685–90.
4. Nicoucar K, Giger R, Jaecklin T, Pope HG, Dulguerov P et al. Management of congenital third branchial arch anomalies: a systematic review. *Otolaryngol Head Neck Surg.* 2010;142:21–28.e2.

CODES

ICD9
744.41 Branchial cleft sinus or fistula

CLINICAL PEARLS
- Most common: 2nd branchial cleft; results in an opening in the mid-neck at the anterior border of the sternocleidomastoid muscle, together with a history of an occasional droplet of fluid, is diagnostic. Radiographic confirmation is not needed; surgical excision as an outpatient is both diagnostic and therapeutic.
- Branchial cleft remnants, sinuses, and cysts are the result of failure of branchial cleft to complete its normal development.

BREAST ABSCESS
Anya S. Koutras, MD

 BASICS

DESCRIPTION
- Collection of pus, usually localized
- Can be associated with lactation or fistulous tracts secondary to squamous epithelial neoplasm or duct occlusion
- System(s) affected: Skin/Exocrine
- Synonym(s): Mammary abscess; peripheral breast abscess; subareolar abscess; puerperal abscess

Pregnancy Considerations
Most commonly associated with postpartum lactation

EPIDEMIOLOGY
Predominant age:
- Puerperal abscess: Premenopausal
- Subareolar abscess: Postmenopausal
- Predominant sex: Female

Incidence
- 0.1–0.5% of breast-feeding women
- Puerperal abscess rare after 1st 6 weeks of lactation

RISK FACTORS
- Puerperal mastitis: 5–11% go on to abscess (most often due to inadequate therapy). Risk factors for mastitis are those that result in milk stasis (infrequent feeds, missing feeds).
- Poor latch, damaged nipple, illness in mother or baby, rapid weaning, breast pressure, blocked nipple pore or duct, maternal stress or fatigue, maternal malnutrition
- General factors: Diabetes, rheumatoid arthritis
- Steroids, silicone/paraffin implants, lumpectomy with radiation, heavy cigarette smoking
- Nipple retraction

GENERAL PREVENTION
- Prevention of mastitis
- Early treatment of mastitis with milk expression and cold compresses
- Early treatment with antibiotics

ETIOLOGY
- Delayed treatment of mastitis
- Puerperal abscesses: Blocked lactiferous duct
- Subareolar abscess: Squamous epithelial neoplasm with keratin plugs or ductal extension with associated inflammation
- Peripheral abscess: Stasis of the duct

 DIAGNOSIS

- Tender breast lump, fluctuant, usually unilateral
- Systemic malaise (though usually less malaise than with mastitis)
- Fever

HISTORY
Tender breast lump, usually unilateral

PHYSICAL EXAM
- Erythema
- Draining pus
- Local edema
- Nipple and skin retraction
- Proximal lymphadenopathy

DIAGNOSTIC TESTS & INTERPRETATION
Lab
- Leukocytosis
- Elevated sedimentation rate
- Culture and sensitivity of drainage to identify pathogen, usually *Staphylococci* or *Streptococci*. *E. coli* is 3rd most common. Nonlactational abscess associated with anaerobic bacteria.

Imaging
- Ultrasound
- Mammogram

Diagnostic Procedures/Surgery
- Aspiration for culture
- Fine-needle aspiration not accurate to exclude carcinoma

Pathological Findings
- Squamous metaplasia of the ducts
- Intraductal hyperplasia
- Epithelial overgrowth
- Fat necrosis
- Duct ectasia

DIFFERENTIAL DIAGNOSIS
- Carcinoma (inflammatory or primary squamous cell)
- Tuberculosis (may be associated with HIV infection)
- Actinomycosis
- Typhoid
- Sarcoid
- Granulomatous disease
- Syphilis
- Foreign body reactions (e.g., to silicone and paraffin)
- Mammary duct ectasia
- Hydatid cyst
- Sebaceous cyst

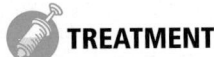 **TREATMENT**

MEDICATION

- Combine antibiotics with drainage for cure
- Culture midstream sample of milk for mastitis, abscess fluid for breast abscess
- NSAIDs
- Dicloxacillin 500 mg q.i.d. for 10–14 days
- If no response in 24–48 hours, switch to cephalexin 500 mg q.i.d. for 10–14 days:
  – Or amoxicillin-clavulanate (Augmentin) 250 mg t.i.d.
- Clindamycin 300 mg t.i.d. if anaerobes suspected
- Contraindications: Allergy to the antibiotic
- Precautions: Refer to manufacturer's profile for each drug
- New techniques include percutaneous intracavitary urokinase irrigation for large abscesses in nonlactating women (1)[C]

ADDITIONAL TREATMENT
General Measures
- Cold compresses for pain control
- Important to continue to breast-feed or express milk

COMPLEMENTARY AND ALTERNATIVE MEDICINE
Lecithin supplementation

SURGERY/OTHER PROCEDURES
- Aspiration under ultrasound (1,2)[B],(3)[C]
- Needle aspiration alone (without antibiotics) may be effective for small breast abscesses (4)[A].

- If aspiration and antibiotics fail, incision and drainage with removal of loculations
- Biopsy of all nonpuerperal abscesses to rule out carcinoma
- Open all fistulous tracts, especially in nonlactating abscesses

IN-PATIENT CONSIDERATIONS
Initial Stabilization
Outpatient, unless systemically immunocompromised or septic

 ONGOING CARE

FOLLOW-UP RECOMMENDATIONS
Patient Monitoring
Ensure resolution to exclude carcinoma.

PATIENT EDUCATION
- Care of wound
- Breast-feeding precautions

PROGNOSIS
- Complete healing expected in 8–10 days
- Subareolar abscesses frequently recur, even after I&D and antibiotics; may require surgical removal of ducts.

COMPLICATIONS
Fistula

REFERENCES

1. Schwarz RJ, Shrestha R. Needle aspiration of breast abscesses. *Am J Surgery*. 2001;182:117.
2. Dener C, Inan A. Breast abscesses in lactating women. *World J Surgery*. 2003;27:130.
3. Christensen AF, Al-Suliman N, Nielsen KR, et al. Ultrasound-guided drainage of breast abscesses: results in 151 patients. *Br J Radiol*. 2005;78:186–8.
4. Thirumalaikumar S, Kommu S et al. Best evidence topic reports. Aspiration of breast abscesses. *Emerg Med J*. 2004;21:333–4.

ADDITIONAL READING
- Berná-Serna JD, Berná-Mestre JD, Galindo PJ, et al. Use of urokinase in percutaneous drainage of large breast abscesses. *J Ultrasound Med*. 2009;28: 449–54.
- Dabbas N, Chand M, Pallett A, Royle GT, Sainsbury R et al. Have the organisms that cause breast abscess changed with time?–implications for appropriate antibiotic usage in primary and secondary care. *Breast J*. 2010;16:412–5.
- Jahanfar S, Ng CJ, Teng CL et al. Antibiotics for mastitis in breastfeeding women. *Cochrane Database Syst Rev*. 2009;CD005458.

 CODES

ICD9
- 611.0 Inflammatory disease of breast
- 675.14 Postpartum abscess of breast

CLINICAL PEARLS
- 5–11% of cases of puerperal mastitis go on to abscess (most often due to inadequate therapy for mastitis). Risk factors for mastitis are those that result in milk stasis (infrequent feeds, missing feeds).
- Abscess not associated with lactation should prompt coverage with antibiotics that cover anaerobic bacteria.
- Treatment is antibiotic and aspiration, with I&D, with breakup of loculations reserved for those failing more conservative management.

BREAST CANCER

Susan E. Donohue, MD
David S. Shepro, MD

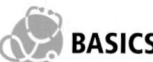 **BASICS**

DESCRIPTION
Common malignant tumor that originates from epithelial cells of breast tissue

EPIDEMIOLOGY
Incidence
- 123 cases per 100,000 women per year in 2006 (1)
- Invasive cancer new cases in 2009: Women: 194,280
- In situ cancer new cases in 2009: 62,280 (85% ductal carcinoma in situ)
- Breast cancer (BC) deaths: 40,480
- Lifetime risk BC: 1 in 8 (12%)
- Lifetime risk BC death: 1 in 35
- Most common malignancy in women in US, second only to lung cancer as cause of cancer death (2)

Prevalence
2.5 million women in the US

RISK FACTORS
- Female, family history, nulliparity and/or older age at first live birth, early menarche, delayed menopause, increasing patient age, personal history of BC
- Prior chest radiation (lymphoma), DES
- Prolonged hormone replacement therapy (HRT), high ethyl alcohol (ETOH) use, high body mass index (BMI), physical inactivity

Genetics
- BRCA1 and BRCA2
- Other genes: ATM, CHEK2, p53
- Cowden syndrome (PTEN): Hamartomas skin, mucosa, bones, central nervous system (CNS), thyroid (benign and malignant)
- Li-Fraumeni syndrome (TP53): Autosomal dominance, Ca in CNS, leukemia, sarcoma, adrenal cortex
- Criteria for additional risk evaluation/gene testing:
  – BC at age ≤50 years
  – 2 breast primaries of breast/ovary cancer in single patient or ≥2 breast primary cancers or breast + ovary cancer same side of family
  – Clustering of BC with thyroid Ca, sarcoma, adrenal cortex, endometrial, pancreas, CNS, leukemia/lymphoma same side of family
  – FH BC susceptibility gene
  – Ashkenazi Jewish with breast/ovary cancer at any age
  – Any male breast cancer
  – Ovarian cancer in family

GENERAL PREVENTION
- Avoid risk factors when possible.
- Selective estrogen receptor modulators
- For hereditary breast and/or ovarian cancer (3):
  – Begin at age 18–25: BSE (beginning at 18 years), clinical breast exam, yearly mammogram and breast magnetic resonance imaging (MRI) (at 25)
  – Discuss risk-reducing mastectomy. Counsel, suggest risk-reducing salpingo-oophorectomy ideally between 35 and 40 or after completion of child-bearing.

PATHOPHYSIOLOGY
- Estrogen/progesterone induce cyclin D1 and c-myc expression
- Bcl-2 commonly overexpressed
- Estrogen receptor (ER) not expressed in 1/3 BC:
  – Mutations of cell adhesion molecules
  – Epidermal growth factors (EGF, c-erb-B2 [HER2])
  – IGF family
  – TGF-β family
  – BRCA1 and BRCA2 may function in cell cycle progression and in DNA repair.

 DIAGNOSIS

HISTORY
- Mass, pain, redness, nipple retraction, nipple discharge
- Symptoms of metastatic disease
- Family history

PHYSICAL EXAM
- Careful clinician breast exam:
  – Evidence suggests that clinical exam of breast produces a reduction in breast cancer mortality.
- Regional lymph node exam
- Evaluate possible metastatic disease.
- Psychosocial evaluation

DIAGNOSTIC TESTS & INTERPRETATION
Lab
Initial lab tests
New BC:
- Complete blood count, liver function tests/alkaline phosphatase
- Chest imaging
- Optional bone scan, computed tomography (CT) abdomen/pelvis
- Tumor markers usually not indicated for early BC

Imaging
Initial approach
- Screening for BC:
  – X-ray mammography decreases BC mortality
  – Digital mammography may benefit. Computer-aided detection (CAD) increases sensitivity and decreases specificity.
  – MRI: BRCA1 or 2, lifetime breast cancer risk of ≥20%, prior chest radiation, other factors increasing risk
  – Ultrasound: Limited data in women with dense breasts
- Diagnosis of BC:
  – X-ray, ultrasound-guided biopsy/aspirate
  – MRI commonly used to define disease in breast and presence of multifocal/multicentric ipsilateral disease

Follow-Up & Special Considerations
Staging of BC:
- CT, bone scan (back pain)
- MRI especially if CNS/spinal cord symptoms

Diagnostic Procedures/Surgery
- Primary tumor: Fine-needle aspiration, biopsy
- Genomic assay on formalin-fixed tissue for select ER-positive/node-negative (Oncotype DX)

Pathological Findings
- Histology:
  – Ductal/lobular/other
  – Benign/malignant
  – Tumor size
  – Inflammatory component
  – Invasive/noninvasive
  – Margins
  – Nodal involvement
  – Nodal micrometastases: Increased risk of disease recurrence
- Estrogen receptor
- Progesterone receptor
- HER-2 assay

DIFFERENTIAL DIAGNOSIS
- Benign breast disease
- Infection

TREATMENT

MEDICATION

- Prevention:
  - Risk assessment tool at http://www.cancer.gov/bcrisktool/
  - Assertive screening/surveillance
  - Risk-reducing mastectomy
  - Risk-reducing bilateral salpingo-oophorectomy for breast and ovary cancer
  - Surgery
  - Chemoprevention/hormone therapy:
    - Risk reduction for ER-positive tumors
    - No demonstration of increased survival
- Hormone therapy for ER-positive tumors:
  - Tamoxifen
  - Ovarian ablation
  - Aromatase inhibitors
- Adjuvant:
  - Hormone therapy for ER-positive tumors:
    - Tamoxifen
    - Ovarian ablation with surgery or gonadotropin-releasing hormone agonists/antagonism
    - Aromatase inhibitors
  - Cytotoxic therapy:
    - Anthracyclines, alkylating agents, taxanes, antimetabolites
    - Pre-op (neoadjuvant) vs post-op (adjuvant)
    - Combinations of above
    - Dose-dense versus non–dose-dense
  - Anti-HER2/neu antibody in select HER2/neu-positive patients:
    - Monitor cardiac toxicity, especially with anthracycline.
- Advanced disease:
  - Hormone therapy
  - Cytotoxic therapy
  - Bisphosphonates to decrease skeletal complications
  - Antivascular endothelial growth factor (VEGF) antibody
  - Anti-HER2/neu antibody in select HER2/neu-positive patients

ADDITIONAL TREATMENT
Additional Therapies
Prevention therapy discussed in Treatment section

COMPLEMENTARY AND ALTERNATIVE MEDICINE
Research before prescribing

SURGERY/OTHER PROCEDURES
- Breast-conserving partial mastectomy/lumpectomy therapy if possible:
  - Negative margins
  - Tumor usually <5 cm
  - No prior breast radiation
- Mastectomy:
  - Large tumors
  - Young women with known BRCA
  - Consider immediate or delayed reconstruction.
- Radiation therapy should be initiated without delay:
  - After breast-conserving therapy
  - Postmastectomy in select high-risk patients
  - Palliation of metastatic disease

 ONGOING CARE

FOLLOW-UP RECOMMENDATIONS
- Interval history/physical every 4–6 months for 1st year and while receiving adjuvant therapy, then yearly (4):
  - Recognize increased risk of ovarian cancer
  - Rare: AML (therapy-induced), angiosarcoma (radiation), endometrial cancer (tamoxifen/postmenopause)
- Other signs/symptoms to monitor/manage related to chemo, hormone, radiation:
  - Hot flashes
  - Sexual dysfunction
  - Arthralgias (aromatase)
  - Cognitive dysfunction
  - Depression
  - Fatigue
  - BMI
  - Osteopenia or osteoporosis
  - Cardiovascular disease, congestive heart failure
  - Deep vein thrombosis
  - No evidence to support the use of "tumor markers" for BC/routine bone scan, CT scans, MRI, positron emission tomography (PET), ultrasound in the symptomatic patient
- Mammogram/imaging every 12 months (and 6–12 months postradiation therapy if breast conserved)
- Assess bone health.
- Gynecologic exam for women on tamoxifen every 12 months

Patient Monitoring
- Continue screening mammograms.
- Bone density
- Annual gynecologic exam if uterus present and on tamoxifen

DIET
- Evidence that certain lifestyle characteristics are risk factors for BC (obesity, increased alcohol consumption)
- No evidence that lifestyle modification changes BC risk

PROGNOSIS
- Influenced by age, menopausal status, stage of disease, ER and PR status, many other characteristics
- Risk of BC recurrences are maintained for life and are not limited by number of years postdiagnosis/therapy.
- Some patients with limited metastatic disease have a better prognosis.

COMPLICATIONS
- Spinal cord compression
- Hypercalcemia
- Visceral metastatic disease
- Emotional issues, especially depression and body-image alteration
- Postoperative lymphedema
- Therapy-induced toxicity

REFERENCES
1. National Cancer Institute, US National institutes of Health. 2009/2010 Update http://progressreport. cancer.gov/doc_detail.asp?pid=1&did=2009&chid =93&coid=920&mid=.
2. The NCCN Practice Guidelines in Oncology (Version 1. 2009) © 2009 Breast Cancer National Comprehensive Cancer Network, Inc. Accessed 6/14/2009 at http://www.nccn.org.
3. Robson M, Offit K. Clinical practice. Management of an inherited predisposition to breast cancer. *N Engl J Med.* 2007;357:154–62.
4. Hayes DF. Clinical practice. Follow-up of patients with early breast cancer. *N Engl J Med.* 2007;356: 2505–13.

ADDITIONAL READING

Pruthi S, Brandt KR, Degnim AC, et al. A multidisciplinary approach to the management of breast cancer, part 1: prevention and diagnosis. *Mayo Clin Proc.* 2007;82:999–1012.

CODES

ICD9
- 174.0 Malignant neoplasm of nipple and areola of female breast
- 174.1 Malignant neoplasm of central portion of female breast
- 174.9 Malignant neoplasm of breast (female), unspecified site

CLINICAL PEARLS
- Pursue/refer all abnormal breast PE/imaging findings.
- Normal mammography does not exclude possibility of cancer with a palpable mass.

BREAST-FEEDING

Julie Scott Taylor, MD, MSc
Kathy Mariani, MD

BASICS

- Breast-feeding is the natural process of feeding an infant human milk directly from the breast.
- Breast milk feeding is the process of feeding a child human milk that has been expressed either by hand or by pump.
- The American Academy of Pediatrics (AAP), the American Academy of Family Physicians, and other medical organizations recommend exclusive breast-feeding for approximately the 1st 6 months of life and support for breast-feeding for the 1st year and beyond as long as mutually desired by mother and child (1).

DESCRIPTION

- Maternal benefits (as compared to mothers who do not breast-feed) include: (2)
  - Decreased postpartum bleeding (due to oxytocin release)
  - Decreased risk of postpartum depression
  - Easier postpartum weight loss
  - Delayed postpartum fertility
  - Decreased risk of breast and ovarian cancer
  - Decreased risk of type 2 diabetes
  - Increased sense of well-being (endorphin response)
  - Increased bonding
  - Convenience
  - Cost
- Infant benefits (as compared with children who are formula-fed) include: (2)
  - Ideal food: Easily digestible, nutrients well absorbed, less constipation
  - Lower rates of virtually all infections via maternal antibody protection
    ○ Fewer respiratory and gastrointestinal infections
    ○ Decreased incidence of otitis media
    ○ Decreased severe lower respiratory infection
  - Decreased incidence of obesity
  - Decreased incidence of allergies and atopic dermatitis in childhood
  - Decreased incidence of type I and 2 diabetes
  - Decreased risk of childhood leukemia
  - Decreased risk of sudden infant death syndrome
  - Decreased mortality
  - Increased attachment between mother and baby

EPIDEMIOLOGY

Incidence
According to the most recent National Immunization Survey, for births in the US in 2007(3):

- Any breast-feeding: 75.0%
- Breastfeeding at 6 months: 43.0%
- Breastfeeding at 12 months: 22.4%
- Exclusive breast-feeding at 3 months: 33.0%
- Exclusive breast-feeding at 6 months: 13.3%

RISK FACTORS
Breast surgery, especially reduction surgery, prior to pregnancy may disrupt breast milk production in the future.

GENERAL PREVENTION
Maternal avoidance diets during lactation not recommended to prevent allergic disease (4)[B]

PATHOPHYSIOLOGY
The overarching mechanism of milk production is based on supply and demand.

- Stimulation of areola causes secretion of oxytocin.
- Oxytocin is responsible for let-down reflex when milk is ejected from cells into milk ducts.
- Sucking stimulates secretion of prolactin, which triggers milk production. Thus, milk is made in response to nursing and increases supply.
  - Endocrine/Metabolic: Thyroid dysfunction may cause delayed lactation or decreased milk production.

COMMONLY ASSOCIATED CONDITIONS
- Breast milk jaundice should be considered if jaundice persists for greater than 1 week in an otherwise healthy, well-hydrated newborn. It peaks at 10–14 days.
- Other causes, such as hypothyroidism and infection, should be considered.

DIAGNOSIS

PHYSICAL EXAM
- Examine breasts, ideally during pregnancy, looking for scars or inverted nipples.
- Breast cancer incidence low but possible in premenopausal women.
  - A breast lump should be followed to complete resolution or worked up if present and not just attributed to changes from lactation.

TREATMENT

ADDITIONAL TREATMENT
General Measures
- Flat or inverted nipples:
  - When stimulated, inverted nipples will retract inward, flat nipples remain flat; check for this on initial prenatal physical.
  - Nipple shells, a doughnut-shaped insert, can be worn inside the bra during the last month of pregnancy to gently force the nipple through the center opening of the shell.
  - Babies can nurse successfully even if the shell does not correct the problem before birth.
- Contraindications to breast-feeding are few:
  - Maternal HIV infection
  - Active tuberculosis
  - Substances of abuse and some medications that will pass into human milk (5)[B]
  - Infants with galactosemia should not be fed with breast milk.
  - Maternal hepatitis is not a contraindication to breast-feeding.

Issues for Referral
- Refer to trained physician, nurse, or lactation consultant for inpatient and/or outpatient teaching.
- Frequent follow-up if having problems with latching, sore nipples, or inadequate milk production.

COMPLEMENTARY AND ALTERNATIVE MEDICINE
Fenugreek may increase breast milk production. Suggested dose: 3 tablets t.i.d. Safety is not established.

IN-PATIENT CONSIDERATIONS
Initial Stabilization
- Initiate breast-feeding immediately after birth, ideally placing the infant at the mother's breast in the delivery room.
- Get mother in a comfortable position, usually sitting or reclining with the baby's head in crook of her arm.
  - Side-lying position often useful following cesarean-section delivery.
- Bring baby to mother to decrease stress on mother's back.
- Baby's belly and mother's belly should face each other or touch ("belly to belly"). Initiate the rooting reflex by tickling baby's lips with nipple or finger. As baby's mouth opens wide, mother guides her nipple to back of her baby's mouth while pulling the baby closer. This will ensure that the baby's gums are sucking on the areola, not the nipple (6)[C].
- Feed every 2–4 hours, 20 minutes per side.
- Rooming-in to encourage on-demand feeding (6)
- Observation of a nursing session by an experienced physician, nurse, or lactation consultant
- Avoid supplementation with formula or water.
- Review expectations, techniques, and feeding cues.
- Be very encouraging.

ONGOING CARE

FOLLOW-UP RECOMMENDATIONS
- See mother and baby within a few days of hospital discharge.
- Primary care-initiated interventions to promote breast-feeding have been shown to be successful with respect to child and maternal health outcomes.

Patient Monitoring
- Monitor infant's weight and output closely.
- Supplementation with infant formula recommended only if infant has lost 7% or more of birth weight, shows signs of dehydration such as decreased urine output, or has less than 3 small stools a day.
- Given that the mechanism of milk production is supply and demand, supplementation without persistent and regular breast stimulation with frequent feedings or breast pump use will decrease milk production and decrease breast-feeding success.

DIET
- For mothers:
  - Continue prenatal vitamins.
  - Drink plenty of fluids: 12.5 cups or 3.0 L of fluids per day.
  - Breast-feeding mothers require 1,800–2,300 calories per day; ~500 more than pre-pregnancy needs.
  - Gassy foods such as cabbage may cause baby to have colic.
  - American Academy of Pediatrics (AAP) suggests limiting maternal caffeine to 300 mg/day.
  - Alcohol should be avoided. 1–2 drinks/week of alcohol may be okay, but mothers should avoid nursing 2–3 hours after a drink. Only <2% of alcohol is passed to baby via breast milk.

- For infants:
  – In 2008, the AAP increased its recommended daily intake of vitamin D in infants to 400 IU. For exclusively breast-fed babies, this will require taking a vitamin supplement such as Poly-Vi-Sol or Vi-Daylin vitamin drops, 0.5 cc/day, beginning at 2 months of age.
  – In 2010, the AAP recommended adding supplementation for breast-fed infants with oral iron 1 mg/kg per day beginning at age 4 months (7).
    ○ Preterm infants fed human milk should receive an iron supplement of 2 mg/kg per day by 1 month of age, and this should be continued until the infant is weaned to iron-fortified formula or begins eating complementary foods that supply the 2 mg/kg of iron.
  – Fluoride supplement unnecessary until 6 months of age.

PATIENT EDUCATION
- The US Preventive Services Task Force (USPSTF) recommends structured breast-feeding education and behavioral counseling programs to promote breast-feeding.
- Regular promotion of advantages of breast-feeding (8)[C]
- Emphasize importance of exclusive breast-feeding for 1st 4 weeks of life to allow adequate buildup of sufficient milk supply.
- Discuss woman's postpartum plans (i.e., if going to work). Emphasize possibility of nursing part-time after returning to work or nursing until weaning the week before returning to work.
- Immediate breast-feeding after the birth.
- Milk will not come in before 3rd day postpartum.
- Frequent nursing (8–12 feedings per 24 hours) will lead to milk coming in sooner and in greater quantities.
- Baby should have 5–8 wet diapers per day and 2–5 bowel movements per day.
- After day 4 of life, should gain 4–7 oz per week
- See in office within a few days of discharge, especially if 1st time breastfeeding
- Signs of adequate nursing:
  – Breasts become hard before and soft after feeding.
  – 6 or more wet diapers in 24 hours
  – Baby satisfied; appropriate weight gain (average 1 oz/day in 1st few months)
- Growth spurts: Anticipate these ~10 days, 6 weeks, 3 months, and 4–6 months. Baby will nurse more often at these times for several days. This will increase milk production to allow for further adequate growth.
- The AAP recommends supplementation with vitamin D starting at age 2 months and iron starting at age 4 months (7,9).
- Weaning:
  – Exclusive breast milk is optimal food for 1st 6 months.
  – Solid food may be introduced at 6 months.
  – For mothers going to work, start switching the baby to breast milk feeding or formula feeding during the hours mother will be gone about a week ahead of time. Do this by dropping a feeding every few days and substituting pumped breast milk or formula, preferably given by another caregiver.

- Family planning:
  – Lactational amenorrhea method (LAM): Breast-feeding may be used as effective birth control option if (1) infant is less than 6 months old, (2) infant is exclusively breast-feeding, and (3) mother is amenorrheic (10).
  – Other options include barrier methods, implants, Depo-Provera, oral contraception, and intrauterine devices.
  – Most providers use progesterone-only birth control pills in the early postpartum period.
- The Academy of Breastfeeding Medicine (ABM), a worldwide organization of physicians dedicated to the promotion, protection and support of breastfeeding and human lactation. www.bfmed.org
- La Leche League at www.llli.org
- Protecting, Promoting and Supporting Breastfeeding: The Special Role of Maternity Services, a joint WHO/UNICEF statement published by the World Health Organization. http://www.unicef.org/newsline/tenstps.htm
- Thomas Hale's Medications and Mother's Milk: A Manual of Lactational Pharmacology.

COMPLICATIONS
- Plugged duct:
  – Mother is well except for sore lump in 1 or both breasts without fever
  – Use moist, hot packs on lump prior to and during nursing.
  – More frequent nursing on affected side; ensure good technique
- Mastitis (see topic Mastitis):
  – Sore lump in 1 or both breasts plus fever and/or redness on skin overlying lump
  – Use moist, hot packs on lump prior to and during nursing; more frequent nursing on affected side.
  – Antibiotics covering for *Staphylococcus aureus* (the most common organism) for at least 7 days (11)
  – Other possible sources of fever should be ruled out, endometritis, pyelonephritis in particular.
  – Mother should get increased rest; use acetaminophen (Tylenol) as necessary.
  – Fever should resolve within 48 hours or consider changing antibiotics. Lump should also resolve. If it continues, an abscess may be present, requiring surgical drainage.
- Milk supply inadequate:
  – Check infant weight gain.
  – Review signs of adequate supply; technique, frequency, and duration of nursing.
  – Check to see if mother has been supplementing, thereby decreasing her own milk production.
- Sore nipples:
  – Check technique.
  – Baby should be taken off the breast by breaking the suction with a finger in the mouth.
  – Air-dry nipples after each nursing and/or coat with expressed breast milk.
  – Do not wash nipples with soap and water.
  – Check for signs of thrush in baby and on mother's nipple. If affected, treat both.
- Engorgement:
  – Usually develops after milk 1st comes in (day 3 or 4)
  – Signs are warm, hard, sore breasts.
  – To resolve, offer baby more frequent nursing
    ○ May have to hand express a little milk to soften areola enough to let baby latch on.
    ○ Breast-feed long enough to empty breasts.
  – Generally resolves within a day or 2.

REFERENCES
1. http://www.aap.org/advocacy/releases/feb05breastfeeding.htm
2. *Breastfeeding and Maternal and Infant Health Outcomes in Developed Countries [Structured Abstract]*. Rockville, MD: Agency for Healthcare Research and Quality, 2007. Available at: http://www.ahrq.gov/clinic/tp/brfouttp.htm.
3. http://www.cdc.gov/breastfeeding/pdf/BreastfeedingReportCard2010.pdf
4. U.S. Department of Health and Human Services. *Healthy People 2010*, Conference ed. Vols I and II. Washington, DC: U.S. Department of Health and Human Services, Public Health Service, Office of the Assistant Secretary for Health, January 2000.
5. Berlin CM, Briggs GG. Drugs and chemicals in human milk. *Semin Fetal Neonatal Med*. 2005;10:149–59.
6. Sinusas K, Gagliardi A. Initial management of breast-feeding. *Am Fam Phys*. 2001;15;64:981–8.
7. http://www.aap.org/pressroom/Ironfinal.pdf
8. Chung M, Raman G, Trikalinos T, Lau J, Ip S et al. Interventions in primary care to promote breastfeeding: an evidence review for the U.S. Preventive Services Task Force. *Ann. Intern. Med*. 2008;149:565–82.
9. Casey CF, Slawson DC, Neal LR et al. Vitamin D supplementation in infants, children, and adolescents. *Am Fam Physician*. 2010;81:745–8.
10. http://www.llli.org/ba/Aug93.html
11. Jahanfar S, Ng CJ, Teng CL et al. Antibiotics for mastitis in breastfeeding women. *Cochrane Database Syst Rev*. 2009;CD005458.

ADDITIONAL READING
- Cramton R, Zain-Ul-Abideen M, Whalen B et al. Optimizing successful breastfeeding in the newborn. *Curr Opin Pediatr*. 2009;21:386–96.
- Grummer-Strawn LM, Shealy KR et al. Progress in protecting, promoting, and supporting breastfeeding: 1984–2009. *Breastfeeding medicine: the official journal of the Academy of Breastfeeding Medicine*. 2009;4 (Suppl 1):S31–9.

 ## CODES

ICD9
V24.1 Postpartum care and examination of lactating mother

CLINICAL PEARLS
- Breast milk is the optimal food for infants with myriad health benefits for mothers and children.
- USPSTF recommends structured education to promote breast-feeding.
- Vitamin D and iron supplementation should begin at 2 and 4 months of age, respectively, for exclusively breast-fed infants.

BREECH BIRTH

Kimberle Vore, MD

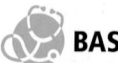 **BASICS**

DESCRIPTION

At the time of delivery, the fetal buttocks or lower limbs are the presenting part in the maternal pelvis:

- Frank breech: Fetal hips flexed and knees extended with feet near the shoulders (45–60% of breech presentations at term)
- Footling or incomplete breech: Foot or knee presenting (25–35% of breech presentations)
- Complete breech: Hips and knees flexed (as if squatting) (5–15% of breech presentations)

EPIDEMIOLOGY

Prevalence

- 3–4% of singleton term deliveries and up to 15–30% of low-birth-weight infants (<2,500 g)
- Breech presentation is common in early pregnancy. At 25–26 weeks, ~20–30% of singleton fetuses are in breech position, but this decreases near term.

RISK FACTORS

- Previous history of breech birth
- Fetal anomalies; see Genetics.
- Low-birth-weight or premature infant
- Oligohydramnios
- Uterine anomalies, including bicornate uterus
- Uterine relaxation associated with great parity
- Uterine overdistention as in polyhydramnios or multiple gestation
- Placenta previa
- Placental implantation in cornual-fundal region
- Pelvic contractures or irregularly shaped pelvis, such as android or platypelloid pelvis
- Pelvic tumors

Genetics

Fetal anomalies, including anencephaly, hydrocephalus, trisomy 21 and 18, Potter syndrome, and myotonic dystrophy, have higher incidences of breech birth.

GENERAL PREVENTION

- Antenatal folate therapy to decrease risk of neural tube defects
- Prevention of fetal anomalies by tight glucose control in diabetics

COMMONLY ASSOCIATED CONDITIONS

- See Risk Factors.
- Congenital hip dislocation has higher incidence in infants with breech presentation at term.

 DIAGNOSIS

HISTORY

Mother reports kicking in lower abdomen

PHYSICAL EXAM

- Anus palpable on digital vaginal exam
- Leopold maneuver reveals ballottable head in fundal region.
- Presenting part not palpable in pelvis near term

DIAGNOSTIC TESTS & INTERPRETATION

Imaging

Initial approach

Ultrasound confirms presenting part

Diagnostic Procedures/Surgery

- Near-term women should be examined to determine presenting part.
- If breech is suspected, an ultrasound should be done to confirm presenting part.
- When breech presentation is confirmed, the options of external version or elective cesarean section should be discussed with the patient.

Pathological Findings

Congenital malformation among term breech infants: Overall incidence 6–9%

DIFFERENTIAL DIAGNOSIS

- Face vs. breech presentation on vaginal exam
- In breech presentation, greater trochanter and anus form a straight line. In face presentation, mouth and malar bones form a triangle.

 TREATMENT

ADDITIONAL TREATMENT

General Measures

- Continuous electronic fetal monitoring during labor
- Breech presentation may be converted to vertex by external version.
- American College of Obstetricians and Gynecologists (ACOG) recommends external version at term. Decision for mode of delivery should depend on the experience of the health provider, with planned cesarean delivery for persistent breech presentation likely to be preferred.
- In 2000, the Term Breech Trial showed decreased perinatal and neonatal morbidity and mortality in planned breech cesarean delivery (1) [NNT 30] vs. planned breech vaginal delivery. There was no difference in maternal morbidity or mortality (1)[B].
- In 2005, a large observational prospective study showed no difference in neonatal outcomes when vaginal breech candidates were carefully selected and followed strict protocols (2).

Additional Therapies

External cephalic version:

- Conversion of breech to vertex can be attempted after 36 weeks of gestation and, if successful, allows for vaginal vertex delivery. Success rates 48–78%, with reversion rates back to breech of 2% (3)[B].
- External cephalic version associated with risk (1–2%) of umbilical cord entanglement, abruptio placenta, preterm labor, premature rupture of membranes, fetal brachycardia, fetal–maternal hemorrhage, and severe maternal discomfort.
- Prior to procedure, tocolytics are usually administered and RhoGAM is given to Rh-negative mothers (3)[B].
- External cephalic version should be attempted only with continuous fetal heart monitoring in the delivery suite, where immediate cesarean delivery can be done (3)[C].
- Contraindications to external cephalic version include multiple pregnancy, nonreassuring fetal monitoring, placenta previa, premature rupture of membranes, placental abruption, uterine malformation, oligohydramnios, or major fetal anomalies.
- Predictors of successful external cephalic version include multiparity, relaxed abdominal wall, adequate amniotic fluid, nonfrank breech, floating presenting part, posterior placenta, and average maternal body weight.

SURGERY/OTHER PROCEDURES

- Breech delivery is accomplished either vaginally or by cesarean section (4).
- Most physicians and patients opt for elective cesarean delivery for breech presentation near term, which is usually planned for the 39th week of pregnancy.
- When a patient presents in labor with the fetus in breech position, a decision about a trial of labor or immediate cesarean section must be made. Ideally, this decision is made prior to onset of labor.
- Obtain ultrasound to document fetal presentation, check for fetal abnormalities, and estimate fetal weight in deciding candidacy for vaginal delivery.
- Vaginal breech delivery may be appropriate in the following situations:
  - Breech presentation in advanced labor
  - Delivery of a 2nd twin in nonvertex presentation
  - Fetus too immature to survive
  - Fetus with congenital defects incompatible with life
  - Multiparous mother, estimated fetal weight not greater than that of siblings delivered by uncomplicated SVD

- Cesarean section procedure:
  – Prepare for cesarean section by starting IV fluids and obtaining blood type and screen, in all patients, in case needed for emergency.
  – A low transverse cesarean section may need to be extended vertically if there is difficulty with head entrapment (this extension produces a weak scar).
  – General anesthesia with isoflurane can rapidly relax the uterus and allow delivery of an entrapped after-coming head.
  – Delivery is usually accomplished with spinal anesthesia.
  – Cord blood gases should be obtained following delivery.
- Vaginal delivery procedures:
  – The candidate for vaginal delivery needs to be attended by a birth attendant skilled in breech delivery, a scrubbed assistant, an anesthesiologist capable of rapid induction of general anesthesia, and an individual skilled in neonatal resuscitation.
  – Epidural is preferred anesthesia.
  – Leave membranes intact as long as possible to prevent possible cord prolapse.
  – The patient should not push until fully dilated due to risk of partial delivery through a cervix that is not fully dilated, which can lead to head entrapment.
  – Consider cutting a large episiotomy to allow sufficient room for delivery.
  – Use abdominal guidance of fetal head to keep it flexed as it descends into the pelvis.
  – The infant should not be touched before the umbilicus crosses the maternal perineum. Traction prior to this point constitutes a complete breech extraction and is associated with higher risk of perinatal morbidity and mortality.
  – With the fetal back anterior, maintain downward traction while grasping the fetal hips until the scapula becomes visible.
  – Check for nuchal arm.
  – As 1 axilla becomes visible, rotate the infant until the shoulders are oriented anteriorly and posteriorly, allowing their delivery.
  – The fetal head is delivered in a face-down position with either piper forceps or manual flexion of the head.
  – Cord blood gases should be obtained following delivery.

IN-PATIENT CONSIDERATIONS
Admission Criteria
- For planned C-section
- For labor and delivery

IV Fluids
Maintain IV access and hydration status with lactated Ringer's or saline solution.

Discharge Criteria
- After delivery once stable
- 1–4 days after delivery depending on vaginal vs. breech delivery

 ONGOING CARE

FOLLOW-UP RECOMMENDATIONS
Routine postpartum care

Patient Monitoring
Continuous electronic fetal monitoring during labor

DIET
NPO

PATIENT EDUCATION
Educate patient about increased risk of fetal distress and fetal trauma in both cesarean and vaginal breech delivery compared to vaginal vertex delivery.

PROGNOSIS
- Perinatal morbidity and mortality are much higher in breech births. A large proportion of the deaths are related to congenital abnormalities.
- Successful external cephalic version at term significantly lowers cesarean rate (15)[A].
- For infants 750–1,500 g or <32 weeks gestational age, a much higher rate of cerebral hemorrhage and perinatal death is associated with vaginal compared to cesarean delivery.

COMPLICATIONS
- Trauma to the head, soft tissue, brachial plexus, and spinal cord; not always prevented by cesarean
- Entrapment of fetal head
- Asphyxia secondary to cord compression or prolapse
- Congenital hip dislocation

REFERENCES
1. Hannah ME, Hannah WJ, Hewson SA et al. Planned caesarean section versus planned vaginal birth for breech presentation at term: a randomised multicentre trial. Term Breech Trial Collaborative Group. *Lancet.* 2000;356:1375–83.
2. Goffinet F, Carayol M, Foidart J et al. Is planned vaginal delivery for breech presentation at term still an option? Results of an observational prospective survey in France and Belgium. *Am J Obstet Gynecol.* 2006;194:1002–11.
3. American College of Obstetricians and Gynecologists. External cephalic version. Practice Bulletin No. 13. February, 2000.
4. American College of Obstetricians and Gynecologists, Committee on Obstetric Practice. ACOG committee opinion. Mode of term singleton breech delivery. Practice Bulletin No. 340. July, 2006. American College of Obstetricians and Gynecologists.
5. Tan JM, Macario A, Carvalho B et al. Cost-effectiveness of external cephalic version for term breech presentation. *BMC Pregnancy Childbirth.* 2010;10:3.

ADDITIONAL READING
Kotaska A, Menticoglou S, Gagnon R et al. Vaginal delivery of breech presentation. *J Obstet Gynaecol Can.* 2009;31.

See Also (Topic, Algorithm, Electronic Media Element)
Placenta Previa; Preterm Labor

 CODES

ICD9
- 652.10 Breech or other malpresentation successfully converted to cephalic presentation, unspecified as to episode of care
- 652.20 Breech presentation without mention of version, unspecified as to episode of care
- 652.80 Other specified malposition or malpresentation, unspecified as to episode of care

CLINICAL PEARLS
- Vaginal breech delivery is associated with increased risk of prolapsed cord and/or cord compression; fetal hypoxia; nuchal arm, with attendant risk of trauma, including humerus fracture, clavicle fracture, and nerve palsies; and entrapment of fetal head.
- External version after 36 weeks gestation may allow for vaginal vertex delivery with decreased risk of infant and maternal morbidity.
- If a patient goes into labor prior to a planned elective cesarean breech delivery, which is usually scheduled at 39–40 weeks gestation, she should go immediately to the hospital.
- Risks of cesarean delivery include infection, bleeding, and possible damage to maternal bladder or bowel; there is a slightly increased risk of maternal mortality compared with vaginal vertex delivery. Maternal recovery time is almost always longer with cesarean delivery.

BRONCHIECTASIS

Dylan C. Kwait, MD

 BASICS

DESCRIPTION
- Bronchiectasis is an irreversible dilation of 1 or more airways accompanied by recurrent transmural bronchial infection/inflammation and chronic mucopurulent sputum production.
- Generally classified into cystic fibrosis (CF) and noncystic fibrosis (non-CF) bronchiectasis.

EPIDEMIOLOGY
- Predominant age: Most commonly presents in 6th decade of life (1)
- Predominant sex: Female > Male (1)

Incidence
Incidence has decreased in the US for 2 reasons:
- Widespread childhood vaccination against pertussis (2)
- Effective treatment of childhood respiratory infections with antibiotics (1)

Prevalence
- Prevalence in adult US population estimated to be >110,000 affected individuals (1)
- Internationally, prevalence increases with age from 4.2 per 100,000 persons aged 18–34 years to 271.8 per 100,000 among those aged 75 years or older (3).

RISK FACTORS
- Nontuberculous mycobacterial infection is both a cause and a complication of non-CF bronchiectasis (4).
- Severe respiratory infection in childhood (measles, adenovirus, influenza, pertussis, or bronchiolitis)
- Systemic diseases (e.g., rheumatoid arthritis and connective tissue disorders)
- Chronic rhinosinusitis
- Recurrent pneumonia
- Aspirated foreign body
- Immunodeficiency

GENERAL PREVENTION
- Routine immunizations against pertussis, measles, Haemophilus influenza type B, influenza, and pneumococcal pneumonia
- Genetic counseling where congenital condition may increase likelihood of bronchiectasis
- Smoking cessation counseling

PATHOPHYSIOLOGY
Vicious circle hypothesis: Transmural infection, generally by bacterial organisms, causes inflammation and obstruction of airways. Damaged airways and dysfunctional cilia foster bacterial colonization, which leads to further inflammation and obstruction (2)[A].

ETIOLOGY
- CF bronchiectasis: Bronchiectasis due to cystic fibrosis
- Non-CF bronchiectasis:
  - Most cases are idiopathic.
  - Most commonly associated with non-CF bronchiectasis is childhood infection (2).

COMMONLY ASSOCIATED CONDITIONS
- Mucociliary clearance defects:
  - Primary ciliary dyskinesia
  - Young syndrome (secondary ciliary dyskinesia)
  - Kartagener syndrome
- Other congenital conditions:
  - α1-Antitrypsin deficiency
  - Marfan syndrome
  - Cartilage deficiency (Williams-Campbell syndrome)
- Chronic obstructive pulmonary disease
- Postinfectious conditions:
  - Bacteria (H. influenzae and P. aeruginosa)
  - Mycobacterial infections (TB and MAC)
  - Whooping cough
  - Aspergillus species
  - Viral (HIV, adenovirus, measles, influenza virus)
- Immunodeficient conditions:
  - Primary: Hypogammaglobulinemia
  - Secondary: Allergic bronchopulmonary aspergillosis, post-transplantation
- Sequelae of toxic inhalation or aspiration (e.g., chlorine, luminal foreign body)
- Rheumatic/chronic inflammatory conditions:
  - Rheumatoid arthritis
  - Sjögren syndrome
  - Systemic lupus erythematosus
  - Inflammatory bowel disease
- Miscellaneous:
  - Yellow nail syndrome

 DIAGNOSIS

- Typical symptoms include chronic productive cough, wheezing, and dyspnea.
- Symptoms are often accompanied by repeated respiratory infections (5).
- Once diagnosed, investigation of possible causes and associated conditions is essential.

HISTORY
- Time course of illness
- Any predisposing factors (congenital, infectious, and/or exposure-related)
- Immunization history

PHYSICAL EXAM
Symptoms are commonly present for many years and include (1,2):
- Chronic cough (90%)
- Sputum may be copious and purulent (90%).
- Rhinosinusitis (60–70%)
- Fatigue may be a dominant symptom (70%).
- Dyspnea (75%)
- Chest pain may be pleuritic (20–30%).
- Hemoptysis (20–30%)
- Wheezing (20%)
- Bibasilar crackles (60%)
- Rhonchi (44%)
- Digital clubbing (3%)

DIAGNOSTIC TESTS & INTERPRETATION
- Spirometry:
  - Limited use in diagnosis
  - Characterized by moderate airflow obstruction and hyperresponsive airways (1)
  - FEV1 <80% predicted and FEV1/FVC <0.7 (6)
- Special tests:
  - Ciliary biopsy by electron microscopy

Lab
- Sputum culture (1):
  - H. influenzae, nontypeable form (42%)
  - P. aeruginosa (18%)
  - Cultures may also be positive for S. pneumoniae, M. catarrhalis, MAC, and Aspergillus.
  - 30–40% of all isolates will show no growth.
- Special tests:
  - Sweat test for CF
  - PPD test for TB
  - Skin test for Aspergillus
  - HIV
  - Serum immunoglobulins to test for humoral immunodeficiency

Imaging
- Chest radiograph:
  - Nonspecific findings; sensitivity and specificity are too low to confirm the diagnosis (6).
  - Increased lung markings (1)
  - May appear normal
- Chest CT:
  - Noncontrast high-resolution chest CT is most important diagnostic tool (2).
  - Bronchi are dilated and do not taper.
  - Varicose constrictions and balloon cysts may also be appreciated (2).

Diagnostic Procedures/Surgery
Interventional bronchoscopy may be used to obtain cultures and evacuate sputum.

Pathological Findings
Bronchoscopy findings include (2):
- Dilation of airways
- Thickened bronchial walls with necrosis of bronchial mucosa
- Peribronchial scarring

DIFFERENTIAL DIAGNOSIS
- CF
- Chronic obstructive pulmonary disease
- Asthma
- Chronic bronchitis
- Pulmonary TB
- Allergic bronchopulmonary aspergillosis

 TREATMENT

- Non-CF bronchiectasis: Determining cause of exacerbations, promoting good bronchopulmonary hygiene via daily airway clearance, and surgical resection of damaged lung if necessary
- Medical management: Reduce morbidity by controlling symptoms and preventing disease progression.
- Patients with non-CF bronchiectasis may not respond to CF treatment regimens in the same way as patients with CF (4)[A].

MEDICATION
- Treat acute exacerbations with short courses of antibiotics.
- Frequent exacerbations may be treated with prolonged and aerosolized antibiotics (5)[A].
- The role of mucolytics, anti-inflammatory agents, and bronchodilators is still unclear (5)[A].

First Line
- Antibiotics:
  - Useful in acute exacerbations
  - Chronic therapy decreases sputum volume and purulence, but does not diminish the frequency of exacerbations (7)[A].
  - Patients may require twice usual dose and longer treatment (7–14 days) (6)[B].
  - Sputum culture and sensitivity should direct therapy; antibiotic selection complicated by wide range of pathogens and resistant organisms.
  - Should be administered IV in cases of severe infection:
    - Augmentin (6)[B]: 500 mg p.o. every 8–12 hours for 7–10 days. Pediatric: Base dosing on amoxicillin content.
    - Trimethoprim/sulfamethoxazole (6)[B]: 160 mg TMP/800 mg SMX p.o. every 12 hours for 10–14 days. Pediatric: ≥2 months, 8 mg/kg TMP and 40 mg/kg SMX p.o. per 24 hours, administered in 2 divided doses every 12 hours for 10 days
    - Doxycycline and cefaclor given orally are also effective (6)[B].
    - Nebulized aminoglycosides (tobramycin): 300 mg by aerosol b.i.d. (8)[B]
    - Macrolides: Appear to have immunomodulatory benefits (1)[A]
- Bronchodilators:
  - Chronic use of β_2–agonists (e.g., albuterol) reverses airflow obstruction (1)[A].
- Inhaled corticosteroids:
  - There is insufficient evidence to recommend use of inhaled steroids in adults with stable-state bronchiectasis (9)[A].
  - A therapeutic trial of inhaled steroids may be justified in adults with difficult-to-control symptoms and in certain subgroups (9)[A].
  - Decrease sputum and tend to improve lung function (6)[B]:
    - Fluticasone: 110–220 μg inhaled b.i.d.

Second Line
Other broad-spectrum antimicrobials, including antipseudomonals

ADDITIONAL TREATMENT
General Measures
- Dry powder mannitol improves tracheobronchial clearance (1)[A].
- Maintain hydration (nebulized saline may be used) (2)[A].
- Noninvasive positive-pressure ventilation (2)[A]

Issues for Referral
May require pulmonologist for bronchoscopy and/or long-term management

Additional Therapies
Sputum clearance techniques, including physiotherapy (percussion and postural drainage) and pulmonary rehabilitation (improves exercise tolerance) (1)[A]

SURGERY/OTHER PROCEDURES
- Surgery if area of bronchiectasis is localized and symptoms remain intolerable despite medical therapy or if disease is life-threatening (5)[A]
- Surgery effectively improves symptoms in 80% of these cases (1)[A].

IN-PATIENT CONSIDERATIONS
For non-CF bronchiectasis, determine cause of exacerbations, promoting good bronchopulmonary hygiene via daily airway clearance, and surgical resection when necessary.

Initial Stabilization
Hemoptysis, although rare, may occur and can be life-threatening.

 ## ONGOING CARE

Long-term outpatient treatment recommendations for bronchiectasis in children (10)[B]:
- Children with CF- and non–CF-related bronchiectasis should be treated by comprehensive interdisciplinary chronic disease management programs.
- Pathogen-directed aerosolized tobramycin treatment should be used long term on a regular basis to improve the course of CF-related bronchiectasis.
- Oral macrolide antibiotic use short term (up to 6 months) improves lung function among children with CF-related bronchiectasis.
- Long-term antibiotic use (oral or aerosolized) in children with non–CF-related bronchiectasis has not been studied enough to warrant routine use.
- Hypertonic saline administered by inhalation used long term (48 weeks) improves lung function and is safer when used with pretreatment bronchodilator therapy among children who have CF.
- Nebulized dornase improves multiple pulmonary outcomes of children who have CF and is indicated for long-term use.
- The risks for long-term oral corticosteroid use outweigh pulmonary benefits in the treatment of CF-related bronchiectasis.
- High-dose ibuprofen therapy reduces the rate of decline among children with mild CF-related bronchiectasis and is indicated for long-term use.
- Mucolytic agents, airway hydrating treatments, anti-inflammatory therapy, CPT, and bronchodilator therapy have not been studied sufficiently long term in children with non–CF-related bronchiectasis to merit their routine use.

FOLLOW-UP RECOMMENDATIONS
Regular exercise is recommended.

Patient Monitoring
- Serial spirometry, every 2–5 years, to monitor the course of the disease (1)[A]
- Routine microbiological sputum analysis (1)[A]

PATIENT EDUCATION
American Lung Association, 1740 Broadway, New York, NY 10019; (212) 315-8700, http://www.lungusa.org

PROGNOSIS
- Mortality rate (death due directly to bronchiectasis) is 13% (1).
- *Pseudomonas* infection is associated with poorer prognosis (1).

COMPLICATIONS
- Hemoptysis
- Recurrent pulmonary infections
- Pulmonary hypertension
- Cor pulmonale
- Lung abscess

REFERENCES

1. King P, Holdsworth S, Freezer N, et al. Bronchiectasis. *Intern Med J*. 2006;36:729–37.
2. Barker AF. Bronchiectasis. *N Engl J Med*. 2002;346:1383–93.
3. Pappalettera M, Aliberti S, Castellotti P, et al. Bronchiectasis: an update. *Clin Respir J*. 2009;3: 126–34.
4. Bilton D. Update on non-cystic fibrosis bronchiectasis. *Curr Opin Pulm Med*. 2008; 14:595–9.
5. ten Hacken NH, Wijkstra PJ, Kerstjens HA. Treatment of bronchiectasis in adults. *BMJ*. 2007;335:1089–93.
6. Bradley J, Lavery K, Rendall J, et al. Managing bronchiectasis. *Practitioner*. 2006;250:194, 197, 199–200 passim.
7. Evans DJ, Bara AI, Greenstone M. Prolonged antibiotics for purulent bronchiectasis. *Cochrane Database Syst Rev*. 2006;4:CD00284.
8. Lobue PA. Inhaled tobramycin: not just for cystic fibrosis anymore? *Chest*. 2005;127:1098–101.
9. Kapur N, Bell S, Kolbe J, et al. Inhaled steroids for bronchiectasis. *Cochrane Database Syst Rev*. 2009:CD000996.
10. Redding GJ. Bronchiectasis in children. *Pediatr Clin North Am*. 2009;56:157–71,xi.

ADDITIONAL READING
Pasteur MC, Bilton D, Hill AT, British Thoracic Society Bronchiectasis non-CF Guideline Group, et al. British Thoracic Society guideline for non-CF bronchiectasis. *Thorax*. 2010;65(Suppl 1):i1–58.

See Also (Topic, Algorithm, Electronic Media Element)
Cystic Fibrosis; Chronic Obstructive Pulmonary Disease; Asthma; Pulmonary Tuberculosis; Aspergillosis; Kartagener Syndrome

 ## CODES

ICD9
- 494.0 Bronchiectasis without acute exacerbation
- 494.1 Bronchiectasis with acute exacerbation

CLINICAL PEARLS
- Symptoms of bronchiectasis include chronic productive cough, wheezing, and dyspnea, often accompanied by repeated respiratory infections.
- CXR has poor sensitivity and specificity for the diagnosis; noncontrast high-resolution chest CT is the most important diagnostic tool.
- Treat acute exacerbations with short courses of antibiotics; frequent exacerbations may be treated with prolonged and aerosolized antibiotics.

BRONCHIOLITIS
Dennis E. Hughes, DO

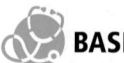

BASICS

DESCRIPTION
- Inflammation and obstruction of small airways and reactive airways generally affecting infants and young children
- May be seasonal (winter and spring) and often occurs in epidemics
- Usual course: Insidious, acute, progressive
- Leading cause of hospitalizations in infants and children
- Predominant age: Newborn–2 years (peak age <6 months). Neonates are not protected despite transfer of maternal antibody.
- Predominant sex: Male > Female

EPIDEMIOLOGY
Incidence
- 21% in North America
- 18.8% (90,000 annually) of all pediatric hospitalizations (excluding live births) in children <2 years of age
- Incidence increasing since 1980

RISK FACTORS
- Smoking exposure
- Low birth weight
- Immunodeficiency
- Formula feeding (not breastfed)
- Contact with infected person (primary mode of spread)
- Children in daycare environment
- Heart-lung transplantation patient
- Adults: Exposure to toxic fumes, connective tissue disease

GENERAL PREVENTION
- Handwashing
- Contact isolation of infected babies
- Persons with colds should keep contacts with infants to a minimum
- Palivizumab (Synagis), a monoclonal product, administered monthly, October–May, 15 mg/kg IM; used for respiratory syncytial virus prevention in high-risk patients (1):
  – 32–35-week gestation and <3 months old at the start of RSV season with at least 1 risk factor: Either attending daycare or with a sibling <5 years old at home
  – 28–32-week gestation and <6 months old
  – <28 weeks gestation and <12 months old
  – Moderately severe bronchopulmonary dysplasia and up to 2 years old
  – Hemodynamically significant congenital heart disease (until age 6 months)
  – Once begun, continue through end of season regardless of age attained
- Respiratory syncytial virus immune globulin, a human blood product, can also be used in at-risk patients. Monthly infusions of 750 mg/kg, October–May.

PATHOPHYSIOLOGY
- Infection results in necrosis and lysis of epithelial cells and subsequent release of inflammatory mediators.
- Edema and mucus secretion that, combined with accumulating necrotic debris and loss of cilia clearance, results in luminal obstruction.
- Ventilation-perfusion mismatching resulting in hypoxia
- Air trapping is due to dynamic airways narrowing during expiration, which increases work of breathing.

ETIOLOGY
Respiratory syncytial virus accounts for 70–85% of all cases, but parainfluenza virus, adenovirus, rhinovirus, influenza virus, *Mycoplasma pneumoniae*, and *Chlamydia pneumoniae* have all been implicated.

Pediatric Considerations
Prior infection does not seem to confer subsequent immunity.

COMMONLY ASSOCIATED CONDITIONS
- Upper respiratory congestion
- Conjunctivitis
- Pharyngitis
- Otitis media
- Diarrhea

DIAGNOSIS

Consensus is that history and physical examination should be the basis for the diagnosis of bronchiolitis (2).

HISTORY
- Irritability
- Anorexia
- Fever
- Noisy breathing (due to rhinorrhea)
- Cough
- Grunting
- Cyanosis
- Apnea
- Vomiting

PHYSICAL EXAM
- Tachypnea
- Retractions
- Rhinorrhea
- Wheezing
- Upper respiratory findings: Pharyngitis, conjunctivitis, otitis

DIAGNOSTIC TESTS & INTERPRETATION
Routine laboratory and other ancillary testing not warranted

Lab
Initial lab tests
- Arterial oxygen saturation by pulse oximetry (<94% significant)
- Rapid respiratory viral antigen testing (not usually necessary during respiratory syncytial virus [RSV] season because the disease is managed symptomatically, but may be useful for epidemiologic, hospital cohorting purposes, or in the very young to reduce unnecessary other workup):
  – Sensitivity 87–91%; specificity 96–100% (2)

Imaging
Initial approach
Chest x-ray (CXR):
- Increased anteroposterior diameter
- Flattened diaphragm
- Air trapping
- Patchy infiltrates
- Focal atelectasis: Right upper lobe common
- Peribronchial cuffing

Pathological Findings
- Abundant mucous exudate
- Mucosal: Hyperemia, edema
- Submucosal lymphocytic infiltrate, monocytic infiltrate, plasmacytic infiltrate
- Small airway debris, fibrin, inflammatory exudate, fibrosis
- Peribronchiolar mononuclear infiltrate

DIFFERENTIAL DIAGNOSIS
- Other pulmonary infections such as pertussis, croup, or bacterial pneumonia
- Aspiration
- Vascular ring
- Foreign body
- Asthma
- Heart failure
- Gastroesophageal reflux
- Cystic fibrosis

TREATMENT

Mainstay of therapy is supportive to prevent hypoxia and dehydration.

MEDICATION
First Line
- Oxygen
- Nebulized albuterol (0.15 mg/kg) is often tried for acute symptoms; a trial of therapy may be reasonable in the presence of a bronchospastic component, but no benefit noted in several high-quality studies (3)[B].
- Epinephrine aerosols (0.5 mL of 2.25% solution in 3 mL NS) also may be tried. Benefit remains unproved, but some studies support short-term improvement in outpatient settings (4,5)[B].
- Corticosteroids:
  - Oral dexamethasone (1 mg/kg loading dose, then 0.6 mg/kg b.i.d. for 5 days) reduced subsequent hospitalization. A recent multiple-center trial found no difference in admission rates or respiratory assessment scores in children treated with 1 mg/kg dexamethasone (6)[B].
  - Nebulized dexamethasone (2–4 mg in 3 mL NS) may have anecdotal benefit; studies show mixed results.

Second Line
- Antibiotics only if secondary bacterial infection present (rare) (7)[B]
- Heliox therapy (70% helium–30% oxygen) may be of benefit early in moderate-to-severe bronchiolitis to reduce amount of respiratory distress (8).
- Ribavirin (palivizumab):
  - Updated AAP guidelines for use (for prevention in high-risk children)
  - Inhaled antiviral agent active against RSV
  - Nebulize via small-particle aerosol generator.
  - Pregnant women should not be exposed.

ADDITIONAL TREATMENT
- Nebulized hypertonic (3%) saline has recently been studied and may decease LOS in hospitalized patients (5).
- Positive pressure ventilation (PPV) in the form of CPAP can be used in cases of respiratory failure. There is limited clinical evidence other than observational studies (5).
- Leukotriene receptor antagonists currently show no sustained benefit (5).

IN-PATIENT CONSIDERATIONS
Bronchiolitis can be associated with apnea.

Initial Stabilization
Supplemental oxygen for pulse oximetry <94% on room air

Admission Criteria
- Respiratory rate >45/min with respiratory distress or apnea
- Hypoxia is common; evidence-based cutoff requiring admission is not available (only "D" level-expert opinion), so clinical criteria are more helpful.
- Ill or toxic appearance
- Underlying heart, respiratory condition, or immune suppression
- High risk for apnea (<30 days of age, preterm birth [<37 weeks]) (7)[B]
- Dehydrated or unable to feed
- Uncertain home care
- Use of Respiratory Distress Assessment Instrument can aid in determining admission vs discharge. Scoring based on quantification and quality of wheezes, retractions, and respiratory rate (6).

IV Fluids
Indicated only if tachypnea precludes oral feeding. Weight-based maintenance rate plus insensible losses

Discharge Criteria
Normal respiratory rate and no oxygen requirement (recent small studies suggest that after a period of observation, children can be safely discharged on home oxygen)

 ONGOING CARE

FOLLOW-UP RECOMMENDATIONS
Patient Monitoring
- Hospitalization is usually only required if oxygen is a requirement or unable to feed/drink.
- For a hospitalized patient, monitor as needed depending on the severity of the infection.
- If the patient is receiving home care, follow daily by telephone for 2–4 days; the patient may need frequent office visits.

PATIENT EDUCATION
- American Academy of Pediatrics: http://www.aap.org
- American Academy of Family Physicians: http://www.familydoctor.org

PROGNOSIS
- In most cases, recovery is complete within 7–14 days.
- Mortality statistics differ, but probably <1%.
- High-risk infants (bronchopulmonary dysplasia, congenital heart disease) may have a prolonged course.

COMPLICATIONS
- Bacterial superinfection
- Bronchiolitis obliterans
- Apnea
- Respiratory failure
- Death
- Increased incidence of development of reactive airway disease (asthma)

REFERENCES

1. *REDBOOK: Report of the Committee on Infectious Disease*. American Academy of Pediatrics. 2009
2. Cincinnati Children's Hospital Medical Center. Evidence-based clinical practice guideline for medical management of bronchiolitis in children less than 1 year of age presenting with a first time episode. Cincinnati (OH): Cincinnati Children's Hospital Medical Center; 2006. May. 13p (85 references)
3. Patel H, et al. A randomized, controlled trial of the effectiveness of nebulized therapy with epinephrine compared with albuterol and saline in infants hospitalized for acute viral bronchiolitis. *J Ped*. 2002;141(6):818–24.
4. Mull CC, Scarfone RJ, Ferri LR, et al. A randomized trial of nebulized epinephrine vs albuterol in the emergency department treatment of bronchiolitis. *Arch Pediatr Adolesc Med*. 2004;158:113–8.
5. Petruzella FD, Gorelick MH et al. Current therapies in bronchiolitis. *Pediatr Emerg Care*. 2010;26: 302–7.
6. Corneli HM, Zorc JJ, Majahan P, et al. A multicenter, randomized, controlled trial of dexamethasone for bronchiolitis. *N Engl J Med*. 2007;357:331–9.
7. Spurling GKP, et al. Antibiotics for bronchiolitis in children. *Cochrane Database Syst Rev*. 2007;1: CD005189. DOI:10.1002/14651859, CD005189.pub2.
8. Liet JM, Ducruet T, Gupta V, Cambonie G et al. Heliox inhalation therapy for bronchiolitis in infants. *Cochrane Database Syst Rev*. 2010;4:CD006915.

ADDITIONAL READING
- Bush A, Thomson AH. Acute bronchitis. *BMJ*. 2007;335:1037–41.
- Everard ML. Acute bronchiolitis and croup. *Pediatr Clin North Am*. 2009;56:119–33, x–xi.
- Worrall G. Bronchiolitis. *Can Fam Physician*. 2008;54:742–3.
- Yanney M, Vyas H. The treatment of bronchiolitis. *Arch Dis Child*. 2008;93:793–8.

 CODES

ICD9
466.19 Acute bronchiolitis due to other infectious organisms

CLINICAL PEARLS
- Bronchiolitis is the leading cause of hospitalizations in infants and children.
- Treatment is primarily supportive.
- Antibiotics not helpful in the majority of cases
- Parental education of expected course of illness important
- Be aware of new Synagis treatment guidelines for premature infants.

BRONCHITIS, ACUTE
Alan J. Cropp, MD

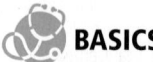 **BASICS**

DESCRIPTION
- Inflammation of trachea, bronchi, and bronchioles resulting from a respiratory tract infection or chemical irritant (1,2)
- Cough is the predominant symptom (3).
- Generally self-limited, with complete healing and full return of function
- Most infections are viral if no underlying cardiopulmonary disease is present.
- Synonym(s): Tracheobronchitis, chest cold

Geriatric Considerations
Can be serious, particularly if part of influenza, with underlying chronic obstructive pulmonary disease (COPD) or congestive heart failure (CHF) (3)

Pediatric Considerations
- Usually occurs in association with other conditions of upper and lower respiratory tract (trachea usually involved) (4)
- If repeated attacks occur, child should be evaluated for anomalies of the respiratory tract, including immune deficiencies or for chronic asthma.
- When acute bronchitis is caused by respiratory syncytial virus (RSV), it may be fatal.

EPIDEMIOLOGY
- Predominant age: All ages
- Predominant gender: Male = Female.

Incidence
- ~5% of adults per year (3)
- A common cause of infection in children (4)

Prevalence
Results in 10–12 million office visits per year (3)

RISK FACTORS
- Infants
- Elderly
- Air pollutants
- Smoking
- Secondhand smoke
- Environmental changes
- Chronic bronchopulmonary diseases
- Chronic sinusitis
- Tracheostomy
- Bronchopulmonary allergy
- Hypertrophied tonsils and adenoids in children
- Immunosuppression:
  - Immunoglobulin deficiency
  - HIV infection
  - Alcoholism
- Gastroesophageal reflux disease (GERD)

Genetics
No known genetic pattern

GENERAL PREVENTION
- Avoid smoking.
- Control underlying risk factors (i.e., asthma, sinusitis, and reflux).
- Avoid exposure, especially day care.
- Pneumovax, influenza immunization

PATHOPHYSIOLOGY
Acute bronchitis causes an injury to the epithelial surfaces, resulting in an increase in mucous production (2) and thickening of the bronchiole wall (1).

ETIOLOGY
- Viral infections, such as adenovirus, influenza A and B, parainfluenza virus, coxsackievirus, RSV, rhinovirus, coronavirus (types 1–3), herpes simplex virus
- Bacterial infections, such as *Chlamydia pneumoniae* [Taiwan acute respiratory (TWAR) agent], *Mycoplasma, Bordetella pertussis, Haemophilus influenzae, Streptococcus pneumoniae, Moraxella catarrhalis*, and *Mycobacterium tuberculosis*
- Secondary bacterial infection as part of an acute upper respiratory infection
- Possibly fungal infections
- Chemical irritants

COMMONLY ASSOCIATED CONDITIONS
- Allergic rhinitis
- Sinusitis
- Pharyngitis
- Epiglottitis (rare but can be rapidly fatal)
- Coryza
- Croup
- Influenza
- Pneumonia
- Asthma
- COPD/emphysema
- GERD

 DIAGNOSIS

HISTORY
- Sudden onset of cough and no evidence of pneumonia, asthma, exacerbation of COPD, or the common cold (3)
- Cough is initially dry and unproductive, then productive; later, mucopurulent sputum, which may indicate secondary infection
- Dyspnea, wheeze, fever, and fatigue may occur.
- Possible contact with others who have respiratory infections (1)

PHYSICAL EXAM
- Fever
- Tachypnea
- Pharynx injected
- Rales, rhonchi, wheezing
- No evidence of pulmonary consolidation

DIAGNOSTIC TESTS & INTERPRETATION
Lab
Initial lab tests
- Sputum culture/sensitivity if purulent
- Influenza titers (if appropriate for time of year)
- White blood cell (WBC)

Follow-Up & Special Considerations
- Arterial blood gases: Hypoxemia (rarely)
- Pulmonary function tests (seldom needed during acute stages): Increased residual volume, decreased maximal expiratory rate (2)

Imaging
Initial approach
Chest radiograph:
- Lungs normal if uncomplicated
- Helps to rule out other diseases (pneumonia) or complications

DIFFERENTIAL DIAGNOSIS
- Common cold
- Acute sinusitis
- Bronchopneumonia
- Influenza
- Bacterial tracheitis
- Bronchiectasis
- Asthma
- Reactive airways dysfunction syndrome (RADS)
- Allergy
- Eosinophilic pneumonitis
- Aspiration
- Retained foreign body
- Inhalation injury
- Cystic fibrosis
- Bronchogenic carcinoma
- Heart failure
- GERD

 TREATMENT

MEDICATION

> **ALERT**
> Antibiotics are usually not recommended (1,3,5)[A] unless a treatable pathogen has been identified or significant comorbidities are present.

First Line
- Amantadine or rimantadine therapy if influenza A is suspected; most effective if started within 24–48 h of development of symptoms [also consider oseltamivir (Tamiflu) or zanamivir (Relenza)]
- Decongestants if accompanied by sinus condition (1)
- Antipyretic analgesic, such as aspirin, acetaminophen, or ibuprofen
- Antibiotics if a treatable cause (i.e., pertussis) is identified (5)[A]:

- Amoxicillin 500 mg q8h or trimethoprim-sulfamethoxazole DS q12h for routine infection
  - Penicillins and trimethoprim-based regimens seem to be equivalent in terms of effectiveness and toxicity for acute bacterial exacerbations of chronic bronchitis (ABECB) (6)[B].
  - Clarithromycin (Biaxin) 500 mg q12h or azithromycin (Zithromax) Z-pack for penicillin allergy or *Mycoplasma* infection: In patients with acute bronchitis of a suspected bacterial cause, azithromycin tends to be more effective in terms of lower incidence of treatment failure and adverse events than amoxicillin or amoxycillin-clavulanicacid (7)[B].
  - Doxycycline 100 mg/d × 10 days if *Moraxella*, *Chlamydia*, or *Mycoplasma* suspected
  - Quinolone for more serious infections or other antibiotic failure or in elderly or patients with multiple comorbidities
  - Macrolide for pertussis (1)[A]
- Cough suppressant for troublesome cough (not with COPD); guaifenesin with codeine or dextromethorphan (3)[A]
- Inhaled beta agonist (e.g., albuterol) or in combination with steroids for cough with bronchospasm (2,3)[B]
- Consider steroids for bronchospasm
- Contraindication(s): Doxycycline should not be used during pregnancy or in children.
- Precautions:
  - Watch for theophylline toxicity with macrolides and quinolones.
  - Multiple antibiotics have the potential to interfere with the effectiveness of oral contraceptives.

Second Line
- Other antibiotics if indicated by sputum culture (*Moraxella* needs a different set of antibiotics)
- Antivirals
- Other macrolides or quinolones based on pathogen and sensitivity

ADDITIONAL TREATMENT
General Measures
- Rest
- Stop smoking/avoid smoke.
- Steam inhalations
- Vaporizers
- Adequate hydration
- Antitussives
- Antibiotics are usually not recommended (1,3,5)[A].
- Treat associated illnesses (e.g., GERD).

Issues for Referral
- Complications, such as pneumonia or respiratory failure
- Comorbidities, such as COPD
- Cough lasting longer than 3 months

Additional Therapies
Antipyretic for fever (e.g., acetaminophen, aspirin, or ibuprofen)

COMPLEMENTARY AND ALTERNATIVE MEDICINE
Throat lozenges for pharyngitis

IN-PATIENT CONSIDERATIONS
Initial Stabilization
- Outpatient, unless elderly or complicated by severe underlying disease
- May require supplemental oxygen in selected patients
- Bronchodilators if patient is bronchospastic

Admission Criteria
- Hypoxia
- Severe bronchospasm
- Exacerbation of underlying disease

IV Fluids
May be helpful if patient is dehydrated

Nursing
- Ensure patient comfort and monitor for signs of deterioration, especially if underlying lung disease exists.
- May need to follow oxygen saturation in patients with underlying lung disease

Discharge Criteria
Improvement in symptoms and comorbidities

 ## ONGOING CARE

FOLLOW-UP RECOMMENDATIONS
- Usually a self-limited disease not requiring follow-up
- Cough may linger for several weeks.
- In children, if recurrent, need to consider other diagnoses, such as asthma (4)

Patient Monitoring
- Oximetry until no longer hypoxemic
- Recheck for chronicity.

DIET
Increased fluids (3–4 L/d) while febrile

PATIENT EDUCATION
- For patient education materials favorably reviewed on this topic, contact the American Lung Association, 1740 Broadway, New York, NY 10019, (212) 315-8700; www.lungusa.org.
- American Academy of Family Physicians: www.familydoctor.org

PROGNOSIS
- Usual: Complete resolution
- Can be serious in the elderly or debilitated
- Cough may persist for several weeks after an initial improvement (1,2).
- Postbronchitic reactive airways disease (rare)
- Bronchiolitis obliterans and organizing pneumonia (rare)

COMPLICATIONS
- Superinfection such as bronchopneumonia
- Bronchiectasis
- Hemoptysis
- Acute respiratory failure
- Chronic cough

REFERENCES
1. Wenzel RP, Fowler AA. Clinical practice. Acute bronchitis. *N Engl J Med*. 2006;355:2125–30.
2. Knutson D, Braun C. Diagnosis and management of acute bronchitis. *Am Fam Physician*. 2002;65: 2039–44.
3. Braman SS. Chronic cough due to acute bronchitis: ACCP evidence-based clinical practice guidelines. *Chest*. 2006;129:95S–103S.
4. Fleming DM, Elliot AJ. The management of acute bronchitis in children. *Expert Opin Pharmacother*. 2007;8:415–26.
5. Fahey T, et al. Antibiotics for acute bronchitis. *Cochrane Database Syst Rev*. 2004;4:CD000245. DOI:10.1002/14651858.CD000245.pub2.
6. Korbila IP, Manta KG, Siempos II, et al. Penicillins vs trimethoprim-based regimens for acute bacterial exacerbations of chronic bronchitis: Meta-analysis of randomized controlled trials. *Can Fam Physician*. 2009;55:60–7.
7. Panpanich R, Lerttrakarnnon P, Laopaiboon M. Azithromycin for acute lower respiratory tract infections. *Cochrane Database Syst Rev*. 2008; CD001954.

See Also (Topic, Algorithm, Electronic Media Element)
Asthma; Chronic Obstructive Pulmonary Disease and Emphysema
Algorithm: Cough

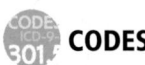 ## CODES

ICD9
466.0 Acute bronchitis

CLINICAL PEARLS
- Acute bronchitis is a common and generally self-limited disease.
- Usually does not require treatment with antibiotics
- Cough may linger for several weeks.
- Recurrent or seasonal episodes may suggest another disease process, such as asthma.

BRUCELLOSIS

Nancy J. Snapp, MD, MPH

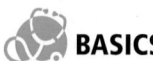 **BASICS**

DESCRIPTION
- Systemic bacterial infection caused by *Brucella sp.* in infected animal products or vaccine
- Incubation period usually 5–60 days, but highly variable and may be several months
- Characterized by intermittent or irregular fevers, with symptoms ranging from subclinical disease to infection of almost any organ system
- Bone and joint involvement common
- May be chronic or recurrent
- System(s) affected: Cardiovascular; Endocrine/Metabolic; GI; Musculoskeletal; Nervous; Pulmonary; Renal/Urologic; Skin/Exocrine
- Synonym(s): Undulant fever; Malta fever

Pediatric Considerations
May be mild, subclinical

Pregnancy Considerations
High rates of miscarriage or abortion (can occur in subclinical cases). Early antibiotic treatment is preventive.

EPIDEMIOLOGY
- Predominant age: All ages, but especially 20–60 years (occupational exposure), sometimes children (milk-related outbreaks)
- Predominant gender:
  - Male > Female (occupational exposure)
  - Female ≥ Male (milk exposure)

Incidence
~100 per year (0.34/100,000), but probably underreported (1,2)

Prevalence
- Common in developing countries; consider in immigrants
- Highest rates in Hispanic population along US–Mexico border
- Considered a potential biologic terror agent in aerosolized form
- Reportable in all states except Nevada

RISK FACTORS
- In US, from occupational exposure to infected animals (especially cattle, sheep): Veterinarians, meat processors, farm workers who may experience accidental exposure to vaccine
- Consumer exposure to unpasteurized milk products, cheese, especially Hispanics along US–Mexico border
- Exposure while traveling in countries where endemic (Mediterranean, Middle East, North and East Africa, central Asia, India, Mexico, Central and South America)
- Worse in chronically ill, immunosuppressed, and malnourished
- Iron deficiency increases susceptibility.

Genetics
- Some evidence for intrauterine transmission
- Some complications may have genetic predisposition (2).

GENERAL PREVENTION
- Avoid infected dairy products.
- For occupational exposure, use caution, animal vaccination, protective goggles, protective gloves. Possibility exists for future human vaccine.
- Postexposure prophylaxis same as treatment in large-scale exposure such as bioterrorism
- Susceptible to heat, disinfectant, but can survive in dust, soil, or water for weeks

ETIOLOGY
- *Brucella* ingestion from tissue or milk
- Worst disease: *B. melitensis*, *B. suis*; also *B. canis*, *B. abortus*; enters through mucous membrane or broken skin; occasionally inhaled
- Facultative intracellular parasite
- Person-to-person transmission rare; sexual, vertical, and possibly breast milk; case report of neonatal brucellosis from a blood transfusion
- Potential airborne biologic weapon

 DIAGNOSIS

PHYSICAL EXAM
- Fever (may be undulant, increased in afternoon and evening, maximum 101–104°F daily), weakness, headache, sweating, chills, generalized aching, arthralgia (90%) (2)[A]
- Also common: Weight loss, depression, irritability, hepatosplenomegaly (20–30%)
- Hepatic dysfunction (abnormal liver function test): 30–60%
- GI symptoms (unusual)
- Lymphadenopathy, especially cervical, inguinal (12–21%)
- Orchitis, epididymitis (normal urinalysis) (2–40%)
- Nephritis, prostatitis (rare)
- Cystitis
- Pulmonary: Cough or other pulmonary symptoms; radiograph may be normal (15–25%)
- Cutaneous: Many transient, nonspecific rashes have been described; also, purpura from thrombopenia (5%)
- Visual disturbances, eye pain
- Chronic fatigue syndrome and various neuropsychiatric symptoms described. Relationship is unclear.
- Also localized suppurative infections (see Complications)
- Malodorous perspiration (2)
- Noncaseating granulomas (1); possibly some

DIAGNOSTIC TESTS & INTERPRETATION
Lab
Initial lab tests
- Isolation of organism from blood, discharge, bone, or other tissue: Bone marrow is gold standard (3)[A]:
  - Fastidious and slow growing
  - Watch for 3–4 weeks, with periodic subcultures

- Automated systems shorten time, but not all recognize brucellosis.
  - Polymerase chain reaction (PCR) accurate, including nonblood samples, but not available in most clinical labs (3)[A]
  - Skin tests not standardized; not recommended for diagnosis
- Acute illness: Blood culture positive 70%, bone marrow 90%
- May have thrombocytopenia, disseminated intravascular coagulation, granulopenia, lymphopenia, lymphocytosis
- 30–60% with abnormal liver function test
- Up to 70% may have normal labs.
- Serology: Use at least 2 tests to confirm (4)[A]:
  - *Brucella* standard tube agglutination paired sera, >1:160 or 4× rise (cheapest)
  - Easy, accurate, and rapid dipstick for IgM now exists for developing countries.
- More effective enzyme linked immunosorbent assay (ELISA), indirect fluorescent antibody test, Coombs tests, immunocapture-agglutination (*Brucella* apt). With ELISA, IgM, IgG, or IgA may be present at low levels >1 year even if treated.
- IgM increases initially for several weeks, declines by 3 months
- IgG begins to rise in 2 weeks, may stay up (low levels) for >1 year if treated or not treated (although IgM increase may be lower or gone by 6 months if treated; can also persist >1 year at low levels). IgG titer rises again with reinfection or reactivation. IgG and IgA titer >1:160 at 1 year implies ongoing disease (4)[A].
- New research: Gene cloning and amplification for discriminatory markers detection and strain differences; PCR-ELISA
- Drugs that may alter lab results: None
- Disorders that may alter lab results:
  - Serologic cross-reaction with *F. tularensis*, *Yersinia enterocolitica*, *V. cholerae*, or vaccinated patients
  - Has been misdiagnosed in culture as *Moraxella phenylpyruvica*

Imaging
- Bone scan, computed tomography, depending on location
- Chest x-ray: Pleural effusion, lung cavitation
- Joint radiographs frequently normal, requiring scan or magnetic resonance imaging

Diagnostic Procedures/Surgery
Bone marrow biopsy, biopsy of affected area

Pathological Findings
- Facultative intracellular gram-negative coccobacillus; can survive inside phagocytic cells, circulation lymph nodes, and into circulation
- Immune reaction in arthritis, including elevated C3, C4; antinuclear antibody, and rheumatoid factor
- Variable tissue reaction depending on site, organisms; causes local microabscesses

DIFFERENTIAL DIAGNOSIS

- Many nonspecific systemic febrile illnesses; a great mimic
- Tularemia
- Psittacosis
- Rickettsial disease
- Tuberculosis
- Visceral leishmaniasis
- Other disease of infected organs
- HIV infection

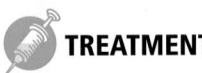

TREATMENT

MEDICATION

First Line

- Optimal therapy includes 2 drugs, at least 1 with good intracellular penetration. In some cases, 3 drugs may give a better long-term cure.
- Longer courses (months) may improve relapse rate in complicated disease.
- Rifampin 600–1,200 mg and doxycycline 200 mg given together every day for at least 6 weeks (possibly for several months with severe complications):
  - 5–10% relapse rate, not related to drug resistance; use same drugs for relapse
  - Usual cause is localized sequestration of organisms or noncompliance with medication (5)[A]
- Steroids in Herxheimer reaction, severe illness, and pancytopenia
- Contraindications:
  - Avoid doxycycline in children and pregnant women (affects bone).
- Precautions:
  - May get Herxheimer reaction when therapy initiated
- Significant possible interactions:
  - Rifampin is a potent inducer for the hepatic P450 enzyme system, and may increase metabolism of many drugs metabolized by the liver.
  - Doxycycline: Antacids, anticoagulants, barbiturates, carbamazepine, hydantoins, cimetidine, digoxin, insulin, iron salts, lithium, methoxyflurane, oral contraceptives, penicillins, sodium bicarbonate

Second Line

- Doxycycline orally b.i.d. and streptomycin by injection is very effective (streptomycin currently not available in the US except by special request from Centers for Disease Control); slightly more effective than doxycycline/rifampin, especially with spondylitis, but more toxic and less convenient (5).
- In children and pregnant women, rifampin 15 mg/kg for 4–5 weeks plus cotrimoxazole for 6 weeks or gentamicin for 7 days or netilmicin 5–6 mg/kg IM. Significant cotrimoxazole resistance in some countries (1)[A].
- Ofloxacin or ciprofloxacin plus rifampin effective in a recent study, but not as effective as 1st-line treatment (6)[A],(7)[B].
- Sensitivities don't reflect in vivo action (2)[A].

ADDITIONAL TREATMENT

General Measures

- Supportive care
- In milk-related or occupational outbreak, look for other cases.
- Bed rest during febrile periods and restricted activity in acute cases

Issues for Referral

Need for procedures

SURGERY/OTHER PROCEDURES

Specific complications may require surgical drainage or valve replacement (endocarditis).

IN-PATIENT CONSIDERATIONS

Admission Criteria

- Outpatient in mild cases, hospitalization in severe illness
- Cardiac care unit for patients with complicating cardiac disease

ONGOING CARE

FOLLOW-UP RECOMMENDATIONS

Patient Monitoring

- Check serology at 6 months and 1 year for chronic disease (difficult to evaluate if continuing exposure).
- Investigate any suspicion of recurrence.
- PCR recently shown to be sensitive and specific for monitoring treatment relapse

DIET

- No special diet
- May need to provide supplemental foods, such as milkshakes, to counter weight loss

PATIENT EDUCATION

- Food Safety and Inspection Service, Office of Public Awareness, Department of Agriculture, Room 1165-S, Washington, DC 20205; (202)720-9904; http://www.fsis.usda.gov/
- Education about exposure

PROGNOSIS

- Untreated case fatality <2%
- Most cases resolve with treatment in 2–3 weeks in acute uncomplicated cases, but at least 6 weeks treatment recommended

COMPLICATIONS

- Relapse rate overall: 5–10%
- Complications present: 10–15% (4)[A]
- Localized suppurative infections: Osteoarticular (20–85%). Includes arthritis (possibly also immune effect), bursitis, tenosynovitis, osteomyelitis, sacroiliitis, vertebral or paraspinous abscess
- Endocarditis: Rare, but main cause of death in brucellosis
- Thrombophlebitis
- Neurobrucellosis: Most are meningeal. Also peripheral neuritis (usually single; bilateral is possible), encephalitis, myelitis, radiculopathy. Possibly neuropsychiatric symptoms.
- Intrinsic ocular lesions: Uveitis, retinal thrombophlebitis, nummular keratitis
- Pneumonitis with pleural effusion
- Hepatitis
- Cholecystitis
- Chronic infection: Persistent (>1 year) signs of infection, elevated titers, occasional bacteria in blood or tissue. Chronic fatigue syndrome with everything negative is controversial.

REFERENCES

1. Sauret JM, Vilissova N. Human brucellosis. *J Am Board Fam Pract*. 2002;15:401–6.
2. Pappas G, et al. Brucellosis. *N Eng J Med*. 2005; 352(22):2325–36.
3. Al Dahouk S, Tomaso H, Nöckler K, et al. Laboratory-based diagnosis of brucellosis–a review of the literature. Part I: Techniques for direct detection and identification of Brucella spp. *Clin Lab*. 2003;49:487–505.
4. Al Dahouk S, Tomaso H, Nöckler K, et al. Laboratory-based diagnosis of brucellosis–a review of the literature. Part II: serological tests for brucellosis. *Clin Lab*. 2003;49:577–89.
5. Pappas G, et al. New approaches to the antibiotic treatment of brucellosis. *Intl J Antimicrob Ag*. 2005;26(2):101–5.
6. Skalsky K, Yahav D, Bishara J, et al. Treatment of human brucellosis: systematic review and meta-analysis of randomised controlled trials. *BMJ*. 2008;336:701–4.
7. Keramat F, Ranjbar M, Mamani M, Hashemi SH, Zeraati F, et al. A comparative trial of three therapeutic regimens: ciprofloxacin-rifampin, ciprofloxacin-doxycycline and doxycycline-rifampin in the treatment of brucellosis. *Trop Doct*. 2009;39:207–10.

CODES

ICD9

023.9 Brucellosis, unspecified

CLINICAL PEARLS

- Infection is caused by infected animal products or animal vaccine. More common outside US. In US, most cases result from occupational exposure to infected animals (especially cattle, sheep): Veterinarians, meat processors, and farm workers who may experience accidental exposure to vaccine and ingestion of raw milk.
- Characterized by intermittent or irregular fevers, with symptoms ranging from subclinical disease to infection of almost any organ system
- Concern that this may become a weaponized bioterrorism agent

BULIMIA NERVOSA

Jeffrey L. Goodie, PhD
Pamela M. Williams, MD, Lt Col, USAF, MC

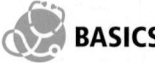

BASICS

DESCRIPTION
- A pattern of discrete periods of uncontrolled eating, followed by compensatory behaviors
- System(s) affected: Oropharyngeal; Endocrine/Metabolic; Gastrointestinal; Dermatologic; Cardiovascular; Nervous

EPIDEMIOLOGY
- Predominant age: Adolescents and young adults
- Mean age of onset: 18–21 years
- Predominant sex: Female > Male (10–20:1)

Incidence
28.8 women, 0.8 men per 100,000 per year

Prevalence
- 1–3% in women 16–35 years old
- 0.5% in young men (higher among gay and bisexual men)

RISK FACTORS
- Female gender
- History of obesity and dieting
- Body dissatisfaction
- Critical comments by family or others about weight, body shape, or eating
- Severe life stressor
- Low self-esteem
- Perceived pressure to be thin
- Perfectionist or obsessive thinking
- Poor impulse control, alcohol misuse
- History of anorexia nervosa (AN)
- Environment stressing high achievement, competition, thinness, or physical fitness (e.g., armed forces, ballet, cheerleaders, gymnastics, or models)
- Family history of substance abuse, affective disorders, eating disorder, or obesity
- Early feeding problems
- Low birth weight for gestational age
- Hyporeactivity at birth
- Type I diabetes
- Sexual abuse is not causally related to bulimia.

GENERAL PREVENTION
- Prevention programs can reduce risk factors and future onset of eating disorders (1)[C].
- Target adolescents and young women 15 years or older.
- Encourage realistic and healthy weight management strategies and attitudes.
- Decrease body dissatisfaction.
- Promote self-esteem.
- Reduce focus on thin as ideal.
- Moderate overly high self-expectations.
- Decrease anxiety/depressive symptoms.
- Improve stress management.

ETIOLOGY
Combination of biological, psychological, environmental, and social factors. Unique contribution of any specific factor remains unclear.

COMMONLY ASSOCIATED CONDITIONS
- Major depression and dysthymia
- Anxiety disorders
- Substance abuse/dependence
- Bipolar disorder
- Obsessive-compulsive disorder
- Borderline personality disorder
- Schizophrenic disorder

DIAGNOSIS

DSM-IV-TR criteria:
- Recurrent episodes of binge eating (2 times per week for 3 months):
  – Eating in a discrete period more than most people would eat during that time
  – Perceived lack of control during binges
- Recurrent inappropriate compensatory behavior (2 times per week for 3 months)
- Purging and nonpurging subtypes:
  – Purging: Often by self-induced vomiting, laxatives, diuretics
  – Nonpurging: Binges followed by sharply restricted diet and/or vigorous exercise
- Body shape and weight significantly affect self-evaluation.
- Does not occur during AN episodes
- Psychological self-report screening tests:
  – Eating Attitudes Test
  – Eating Disorder Inventory
  – Eating Disorder Screen for Primary Care
  – Bulimia Test (revised)
  – Bulimia Investigatory Test Edinburgh
  – SCOFF (sick, control, one, fat, food)

HISTORY
- Patients unlikely to self-identify binge eating or purging behaviors; corroborate with parent/relative
- Unhappiness and/or preoccupation with weight and diet attempts
- Pattern of restricting diet, binge eating, and purging behaviors:
  – Binge is context-specific; amount can vary
  – Vomiting (often with little effort)
  – Vigorous aerobic exercise
  – Distress/shame related to loss of control
- Depressed mood and self-depreciation following the binges
- Relief and increased ability to concentrate following the purges
- Other possible signs and symptoms:
  – Requesting weight loss help and mildly underweight to overweight
  – Diet pill, diuretic, laxative, ipecac, and thyroid medication use/abuse
  – Menstrual disturbance
  – Fatigue and lethargy
  – Abdominal pain, bloating, constipation, diarrhea, rectal prolapse
  – Sore throat
  – Frequent fluctuations in weight
  – Omission/underdosing insulin in diabetes patients

PHYSICAL EXAM
- Often normal
- Bradycardia
- Eroded tooth enamel
- Asymptomatic, noninflammatory parotid gland enlargement
- Epigastric tenderness to palpation
- Calluses, abrasions, bruising on hand, thumb
- Peripheral edema

DIAGNOSTIC TESTS & INTERPRETATION
All lab results may be within normal limits and are not necessary for diagnosis.

Lab
- Blood work:
  – Hypokalemia, hypochloremia
  – Hypomagnesemia, hyponatremia, hypocalcemia, hypophosphatasemia
  – Alkalosis
  – Elevated blood urea nitrogen
  – Hypoglycemia
- Urinalysis:
  – Increased urine-specific gravity

Diagnostic Procedures/Surgery
Electrocardiogram
- Bradycardia or arrhythmias
- Conduction defects
- Depressed ST segment due to hypokalemia

Pathological Findings
- Esophagitis
- Acute pancreatitis
- Cardiomyopathy and muscle weakness due to ipecac abuse
- Delayed or arrested skeletal growth
- Stress fracture
- Irreversible dental erosions
- Osteopenia/osteoporosis

DIFFERENTIAL DIAGNOSIS
- Anorexia, binge eating/purging type
- Major depressive disorder
- Anxiety disorders
- Psychogenic vomiting
- Malabsorption
- Addison disease
- Celiac disease
- Diabetes mellitus
- Hyperthyroidism; hypothyroidism
- Hyperpituitarism
- Hypothalamic brain tumor
- Kleine-Levin syndrome
- Body dysmorphic disorder
- Borderline personality disorder

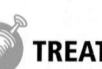

TREATMENT

- Cognitive behavioral therapy (CBT) should be considered as 1st-line treatment (2,3,4)[A].
- Guided self-help therapies may be effective (3,4)[B].

MEDICATION
First Line

- Selective serotonin reuptake inhibitors (SSRIs), particularly fluoxetine (Prozac) at 60 mg, are effective in reducing symptoms with relatively few side effects. Higher doses than standard doses for depression are often needed (3,5,6)[B]:

– Combination of medication and CBT has been shown to have added benefit over medication or therapy alone (6).

- To prevent relapse, maintain antidepressant at full therapeutic dose for at least 1 year.
- Bupropion not recommended due to its association with seizures in patients who purge.
- Misrepresentation and nonadherence may be more likely in this population.
- Precautions:
  – Serious toxicity following overdose is common.
  – Patients may vomit medications.

Second Line
- Ondansetron (Zofran) 4–8 mg t.i.d. between meals can help prevent vomiting.
- Psyllium (Metamucil) preparations, 1 tbs q.h.s. with glass of water, can prevent constipation during laxative withdrawal.

ADDITIONAL TREATMENT
Most patients can be treated as outpatients.

General Measures
- Psychotherapies should be employed as 1st-line treatments.
- Multidisciplinary team:
  – Primary care physician, behavioral health provider, nutritionist
- Build trust; increase motivation for change.
- Assess psychological and nutritional status.
- Consider evidence-based self-help program.
- Cognitive behavioral therapy for bulimia nervosa (2,3,4,5)[A]:
  – 16–20 50-minute appointments
  – Involve patient in establishing goals.
  – Self-monitoring of food intake, frequency of binges/purges, related antecedents, consequences, thoughts, and emotions
  – Self-monitoring of weight once per week
  – Educate about ineffectiveness of purging for weight control and adverse outcomes.
  – Establish prescribed eating plan to develop regular eating habits; realistic weight goal.
  – Gradually introduce feared foods into diet.
  – Problem-solve how to cope with triggers.
  – Decrease ruminations about calories, weight, and purging.
  – Challenge fear of loss of control.
  – Establish relapse prevention plan.
  – Gradual laxative withdrawal
- Interpersonal therapy (2,3)[B]:
  – May act more slowly than CBT
- Transdiagnostic cognitive-behavioral therapy
- Dialectical behavior therapy
- Family therapy for adolescents
- Nutritional education, relaxation techniques
- Educate patient to brush teeth and use baking soda to rinse mouth after vomiting.

Issues for Referral
Patients with bulimia require a multidisciplinary team, including a primary care physician, behavioral health provider, and a nutritionist.

COMPLEMENTARY AND ALTERNATIVE MEDICINE
Bright light therapy may help (3).

IN-PATIENT CONSIDERATIONS
- If possible, admit to a specialized eating disorders unit.
- Supervised meals and bathroom privileges

- Monitor weight and physical activity.
- Monitor electrolytes.
- Gradually shift control to patients as they demonstrate responsibility.

Admission Criteria
Hospitalize if severe malnutrition, dehydration, electrolyte disturbances, cardiac dysrhythmia, uncontrolled binging and purging, psychiatric emergency, or if outpatient treatment failed

 ## ONGOING CARE

FOLLOW-UP RECOMMENDATIONS
Patient Monitoring
- Binge-purge activity, including antecedents and consequences
- Level of exercise activity
- Self-esteem, comfort with body and self
- Ruminations and depressive symptoms
- Repeat any abnormal lab values weekly or monthly until stable.

DIET
- Balanced diet, normal eating pattern
- Reintroduce feared foods.

PATIENT EDUCATION
The following books may be useful for guided self-help treatment programs:
- Fairburn CG. *Overcoming Binge Eating.* New York, NY: Guilford Press; 1995.
- McCabe RE, McFarlane TL, Olmstead MP. *Overcoming Bulimia: Your Comprehensive, Step-by-Step Guide to Recovery.* Oakland, CA: New Harbinger; 2003.

PROGNOSIS
- After effective cognitive behavioral treatment:
  – In the short-term, 50% of treated individuals do not meet criteria for diagnosis.
  – In the long-term (2–10 years), 70% may be asymptomatic.
  – Symptomatic individuals may demonstrate remissions, relapses, subclinical, or other eating-related behaviors.
- Untreated:
  – Likely to remain chronic/relapsing problem
- Greater weight fluctuations, other impulsive behaviors, and personality disorder diagnoses may predict poor prognosis.

COMPLICATIONS
- Drug and alcohol abuse
- Osteopenia/osteoporosis
- Stress fracture
- Gastric dilatation
- Mallory-Weiss tears
- Spontaneous pneumomediastinum
- Potassium depletion; cardiac arrhythmia; cardiac arrest
- Suicide

Pregnancy Considerations
Maternal and fetal problems if pregnant:
- Binging/purging behaviors may persist, increase, or decrease with pregnancy.
- Increased risk for preterm delivery, operative delivery, and infants with low birth weight, smaller head circumference, and/or microcephaly; should be managed as high risk

REFERENCES
1. Stice E, Shaw H, Marti CN. A meta-analytic review of eating disorder prevention programs: encouraging findings. *Annu Rev Clin Psychol.* 2007;3:207–31.
2. Hay PP, Bacaltchuk J, Stefano S, Kashyap P et al. Psychological treatments for bulimia nervosa and binging. *Cochrane Database Syst Rev.* 2009; CD000562.
3. Shapiro JR, Berkman ND, Brownley KA, et al. Bulimia nervosa treatment: a systematic review of randomized controlled trials. *Int J Eat Disord.* 2007;40:321–36.
4. NICE. *Eating disorders–core interventions in the treatment of anorexia nervosa, bulimia nervosa, and related eating disorders.* NICE Clinical Guideline no 9. London: NICE, 2004: Available at: http://www.nice.org.uk. Accessed July 17, 2008.
5. *Practice guideline for the treatment of patients with eating disorders,* 3rd edition. American Psychiatric Association. Available at http://www.psych.org. Accessed February 22, 2007.
6. Bacaltchuk J, Hay P, Trefiglio R. Antidepressants versus psychological treatments and their combination for bulimia nervosa. *Cochrane Database Sys Rev.* 2001(4):CD003385.

ADDITIONAL READING
- McElroy SL, Guerdjikova AI, Martens B, et al. Role of antiepileptic drugs in the management of eating disorders. *CNS Drugs.* 2009;23:139–56.
- Powers PS, Bruty H. Pharmacotherapy for eating disorders and obesity. *Child Adolesc Psychiatr Clin N Am.* 2009;18:175–87.

See Also (Topic, Algorithm, Electronic Media Element)
Anorexia Nervosa; Hyperkalemia; Laxative Abuse; Salivary Gland Tumors
Algorithm: Weight Loss

 ## CODES

ICD9
307.51 Bulimia nervosa

CLINICAL PEARLS
- Particularly among young women with a risk factor, asking "Are you satisfied with your eating patterns?" and/or "Do you worry that you have lost control over how much you eat?" may help to screen for those with an eating problem. A brief, standardized screening measure (e.g., SCOFF, ESP, EAT) will help to identify those who may need a broader assessment.
- Binging and purging behaviors can be seen in anorexia nervosa as well.
- Consider using a stepped-care approach. Start with a guided self-help program using instructional aids, next begin cognitive behavioral therapy (e.g., 16–20 sessions over 4–5 months).
- SSRIs, particularly fluoxetine (60 mg daily), may be helpful as a 1st step or as an adjunctive treatment.

BUNION

Linda Sinclair, MD
Jason Kittler, MD, PhD, JD

BASICS

DESCRIPTION
- Commonly known as a bunion, a hallux valgus deformity consists of a lateral deviation of the great toe (hallux) with medial deviation of the first metatarsal. There is often lateral rotation of the toe such that the nail faces medially (eversion) (1).
- Pressure at the head of the first metatarsal forces it to move medially. The hallux is forced laterally and a misalignment between the first metatarsal and the hallux develops. This results in a medial prominence of the first metatarsophalangeal (MTP) joint and a potentially painful and/or debilitating deformity.
- Strain on the medial collateral ligament along the MTP joint leads to loss of tensile strength, and eventually rupture, which decreases the medial stabilization of the joint (2).
- Changes in muscle positioning and tightening of the lateral collateral ligament can allow for the adductor hallucis muscle to pull unopposed, which can lead to hallux rotation (1).
- System(s) affected: Musculoskeletal/Skin

EPIDEMIOLOGY
- Predominant age: More common in adults
- Predominant sex: Female > Male
- Prevalence increases with age.

RISK FACTORS
- Familial predisposition
- Abnormal anatomy/mechanics
- Joint hypermobility or laxity
- Pronation of hindfoot
- Achilles tendon contracture
- Pes planus (fallen arches)
- Metatarsus primus varus
- Amputation of 2nd toe
- Inflammatory joint disease
- Neuromuscular disorders
- Exacerbated by improper footwear, especially tight-fitting or pointed shoes (3)

GENERAL PREVENTION
No known effective prevention exists, given that the etiology is poorly understood.

ETIOLOGY
The exact etiology of hallux valgus is unknown, but the disease is thought to be multifactorial. The risk factors listed above may all contribute to the development of the disease.

COMMONLY ASSOCIATED CONDITIONS
- Medial bursitis of the 1st MTP joint (most common)
- Hammertoe deformity of the second phalanx
- Plantar callus
- Central metatarsalgia
- Metatarsalgia of MTP joint
- Degeneration of 1st metatarsal head cartilage
- Pronated feet
- Ankle equinus
- Ingrown toenail
- Entrapment of the medial dorsal cutaneous nerve
- Synovitis of the MTP joint (1,3)

DIAGNOSIS

- Most often made on clinical exam
- Radiography for staging purposes

PHYSICAL EXAM
- Pain or deformity at the 1st digit (great toe)
- Increased valgus angle at the 1st MTP joint
- Medial eminence of 1st metatarsal
- Bursal inflammation/ulceration over medial surface
- Painful callus development on 2nd toe
- Displacement of the 1st digit above/below 2nd digit
- Lateral deviation of other digits
- Impaired gait
- To perform a complete exam, the physician should:
  - Observe the patient in sitting and standing positions, as weight bearing often accentuates the deformity.
  - Assess the magnitude of hallux valgus deformity, including any rotation of the 1st digit.
  - Measure the active/passive range of motion of the 1st MTP joint.
  - Assess the congruency of the 1st MTP joint by passive correction of the deformity.
  - Assess for pain and/or crepitus with movement of 1st MTP joint (may indicate degenerative osteoarthritis and change management).
  - Assess the neurovasculature of the foot.
  - Assess the gait of the patient (3)[C].

DIAGNOSTIC TESTS & INTERPRETATION
Imaging
Weight-bearing anteroposterior, lateral, and oblique radiographs may be obtained. The radiographs are used to make the following measurements:
- Hallux abductus (HA) angle: Created by the bisection of the longitudinal axis of the hallux and the longitudinal axis of the first metatarsal.
  - A normal angle is <20° (1).
  - Deformity is considered severe when HA angle is >40° (2).

- Intermetatarsal (IM) angle: Created by the bisection of the longitudinal axes of the first and second metatarsals.
  - A normal angle is <9° (1).
  - Deformity is considered severe when IM angle is >16° (2).
- Medial prominence of the 1st metatarsal head: Note erosions or squaring.
- MTP joint congruency: A congruent joint displays no lateral subluxation of the proximal phalanx on the metatarsal head.

DIFFERENTIAL DIAGNOSIS
- Trauma:
  - Turf toe
  - Sesamoiditis
  - Stress fracture
- Infection:
  - Osteomyelitis
  - Septic arthritis
- Joint disorder:
  - Osteoarthritis
  - Rheumatoid arthritis
  - Gout
- Tendon disorder:
  - Tendinosis
  - Tenosynovitis
  - Tendon rupture
- Other:
  - Bursitis
  - Ganglia
  - Foreign-body granuloma

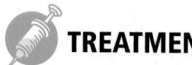

TREATMENT

Hallux valgus deformity will not resolve without treatment. Surgical treatment is more effective in improving patient outcomes than conservative therapy, although evidence is limited (4)[A].

MEDICATION
While no medication is available to treat the underlying cause of hallux valgus, nonsteroidal anti-inflammatory agents can be used for relief of pain and swelling (5)[C]. As with the use of any medication, patients should be evaluated for contraindications and monitored for adverse reactions.

B

ADDITIONAL TREATMENT

Conservative treatments (e.g., orthoses and night splints) did not appear to be any more beneficial in improving outcomes and preventing progression than no treatment (4). Evidence suggests that custom-made orthoses are a safe intervention that may slightly decrease pain at 6 and 12 months (but no continued decrease in pain after 12 months) compared to no treatment; however, this improvement is less than that seen with surgical interventions (see below) (6).

General Measures

Despite the lack of strong evidence supporting the clinical efficacy of conservative therapy, a number of nonoperative modalities have been recommended to attempt to alleviate symptoms and decrease the rates of progression of hallux valgus deformity before surgical referral (5)[C]:

- Shoe modification: Low-heeled, wide shoes to alleviate pressure on MTP joint
- Orthoses: Shoe inserts may alter abnormal foot rotation
- Night splinting: May help balance supporting ligaments
- Stretching to improve intrinsic foot muscle strength
- Bunion pads: To decrease friction on the MTP joint
- Ice: To reduce inflammation

COMPLEMENTARY AND ALTERNATIVE MEDICINE

Marigold ointment may reduce pain and soft tissue swelling over an 8-week period (7)[C].

SURGERY/OTHER PROCEDURES

Surgery is indicated if patient has severe pain, dysfunction, or symptoms that do not improve with conservative therapy. Surgery is shown to be more beneficial than conservative therapy, and patient should be referred to a podiatric foot and ankle surgeon (5)[A]. More than 150 different surgical techniques have been performed, but evidence is too limited to show which form of surgery is more effective (4)[A]. It is important that patients have realistic expectations about surgical outcomes. Patients may not be able to fit into smaller shoes after surgery, and the great toe may not appear straight. Choice of surgical technique will depend on severity of disease. Examples include:

- Arthrodesis: Fusion of the 1st MTP joint
- Arthroplasty: Removing the joint or replacing it with a prosthesis
- Exostectomy/bunionectomy: Removing the medial bony prominence of the MTP joint
- Lapidus procedure: Fusion at the 1st metatarsocuneiform joint
- Soft-tissue procedure: To alter the function of surrounding ligaments and tendons
- Osteotomy and realignment
- Keller's arthroplasty: Removal of the medial eminence on the metatarsal head and removal of part of the proximal phalanx, leaving a flexible joint

 ONGOING CARE

FOLLOW-UP RECOMMENDATIONS

Activity after surgery is indicated to decrease joint stiffness. Post-operative treatment may include physical therapy, physiotherapy, use of supportive shoe, continuous passive motion or manual manipulation. Although there is little evidence to support clinical efficacy, physical therapy and gait training after surgery may improve ability to weight bear and ambulate after surgery (8) and passive motion may improve time to recovery and range of motion of MTP (4). Early weight bearing has not been found to be detrimental to final outcome (4). Refer to specific recommendation made by patient's surgeon.

PROGNOSIS

Patient outcome varies depending on individual factors, severity, and treatment modality used. The radiological HA angle is a predictor of surgical correction; patients with a HA angle <37° have a higher chance of having the deformity corrected with surgery compared to patients with a HA angle >37° (9).

COMPLICATIONS

All surgery carries the risk of wound infection or poor wound healing. Additional complications may include:

- Early swelling
- Hallux varus
- Recurrence of bunion
- Decreased sensation over the 1st metatarsal or phalanx (5)

REFERENCES

1. Ferrari J, et al. Hallux valgus deformity (bunion). *Article from UpToDate*. Lasted updated 2/22/2010.
2. Glasoe WM, Nuckley DJ, Ludewig PM et al. Hallux valgus and the first metatarsal arch segment: a theoretical biomechanical perspective. *Phys Ther*. 2010;90:110–20.
3. Coughlin MJ. Hallux valgus. *J Bone Joint Surg Am*. 1996;78:932–66.
4. Ferrari J, et al. Interventions for treating hallux valgus (abductovalgus) and bunions. *Cochrane Database of Systematic Reviews*. 1, 2009.
5. Vanore JV, Christensen JC, Kravitz SR et al. Diagnosis and treatment of first metatarsophalangeal joint disorders. Section 1: Hallux valgus. *J Foot Ankle Surg*. 2003;42:112–23.
6. Hawke F, et al. Custom-made foot orthoses for the treatment of foot pain. *Cochrane Database of Systematic Reviews*. 1, 2009.
7. Khan MT. The podiatric treatment of hallux abducto valgus and its associated condition, bunion, with Tagetes patula. *J Pharm Pharmacol*. 1996;48: 768–70.
8. Schuh R, Hofstaetter SG, Adams SB et al. Rehabilitation after hallux valgus surgery: importance of physical therapy to restore weight bearing of the first ray during the stance phase. *Phys Ther*. 2009;89:934–45.
9. Deenik AR, de Visser E, Louwerens JW et al. Hallux valgus angle as main predictor for correction of hallux valgus. *BMC Musculoskelet Disord*. 2008;9:70.

ADDITIONAL READING

- Ashman CJ, Klecker RJ, Yu JS. Forefoot pain involving the metatarsal region: differential diagnosis with MR imaging. *Radiographics*. 2001;21:1425–40.
- Klosok JK, Pring DJ, Jessop JH, et al. Chevron or Wilson metatarsal osteotomy for hallux valgus. A prospective randomised trial. *J Bone Joint Surg Br*. 1993;75:825–9.

 CODES

ICD9

727.1 Bunion

CLINICAL PEARLS

- When bunions occur in children or adolescents, the condition may be termed juvenile or adolescent hallux valgus, respectively, and is thought to have an etiology different from that in the adult population.
- Also known as a bunionette, a tailor's bunion is a lateral prominence of the 5th metatarsal head.
- Patients should avoid any footwear with high heels, pointed toe boxes, or inadequate space for the toes to reduce the risk of bunions. Women's high-heeled shoes and cowboy boots often fall into this category.

BURNS

Timothy L. Black, MD
James P. Miller, MD

 BASICS

DESCRIPTION
- Tissue injuries caused by application of heat, chemicals, electricity, or irradiation to the tissue
- Extent of injury (depth of burn) is result of intensity of heat (or other exposure) and duration of exposure.
  - 1st degree involves superficial layers of epidermis.
  - 2nd degree involves varying degrees of epidermis (with blister formation) and part of the dermis.
  - 3rd degree involves destruction of all skin elements (full thickness) with coagulation of subdermal plexus.
- System(s) affected: Endocrine/Metabolic; Skin/Exocrine

Geriatric Considerations
- Prognosis is poorer for severe burns.
- Patients >60 years of age account for 11% of burns.

Pediatric Considerations
Consider child abuse or neglect when dealing with hot-water burns in children.

EPIDEMIOLOGY
- Predominant age: 30 years; 13% infants; 11% >60 years of age
- Predominant gender: Males account for 70%

Incidence
Per year in US:
- 1.2–2 million burns, 700,000 emergency room visits, 45,000–50,000 hospitalizations, 3,900 deaths owing to burn-related complications
- In children: 250,000 burns, 15,000 hospitalizations, 1,100 deaths
- Estimated total cost of $2 billion annually for burn care
- 75% of deaths owing to house fires

RISK FACTORS
- Water heaters set too high
- Workplace exposure to chemicals, electricity, or irradiation
- Young children and older adults with thin skin are more susceptible to injury.
- Carelessness with burning cigarettes: Related to 18% of fatal fires in 2006
- Inadequate or faulty electrical wiring
- Lack of smoke detectors: Lacking or nonfunctioning smoke alarms are implicated in 63% of residential fires.
- Arson: Cause of 27% of fires that resulted in fatalities in 2006

GENERAL PREVENTION
- Home safety education should be a key mechanism for injury prevention.
  - Home education families were more likely to have safe hot-water temperatures.
  - Home education results in more families having functioning smoke alarms and increased use of fire guards.

- There is no evidence that home education results in increasing the chance of possessing a fire extinguisher.
- Home education did not improve the odds of keeping hot drinks or food out of reach of children and did not increase the safe storage of matches.
- There is a lack of evidence that home safety education with or without the provision of safety equipment results in a reduction of thermal injuries.
- Skin grafts or newly epithelialized skin is highly sensitive to sun exposure and thermal extremes.

ETIOLOGY
- Open flame and hot liquid are most common (heat usually ≥45°C): Flame burns more common in adults; scald burns more common in children.
- Caustic chemicals or acids (may show little signs or symptoms for the 1st few days)
- Electricity (may have significant injury with very little damage to overlying skin)
- Excess sun exposure

COMMONLY ASSOCIATED CONDITIONS
Smoke inhalation syndrome:
- May involve thermal burn to respiratory mucosa (e.g., trachea, bronchi) as well as carbon monoxide inhalation
- Occurs within 72 h of burn
- Should be suspected in all burns occurring in an enclosed space

 DIAGNOSIS

HISTORY
- History of source of burn
- In children, check for consistency between the history and the burn's physical characteristics.

PHYSICAL EXAM
- 1st degree:
  - Erythema of involved tissue
  - Skin blanches with pressure.
  - Skin may be tender.
- 2nd degree:
  - Skin is red and blistered.
  - Skin is very tender.
- 3rd degree:
  - Burned skin is tough and leathery.
  - Skin is not tender.
- Rule of nines (1)[C]:
  - Each upper extremity: Adult and child 9%
  - Each lower extremity: Adult 18%; child 14%
  - Anterior trunk: Adult and child 18%
  - Posterior trunk: Adult and child 18%
  - Head and neck: Adult 10%; child 18%
- Careful documentation of extent of burn and the estimated depth of burn
- Check for any signs suggestive of potential airway involvement: Singed nasal hair, facial burns, carbonaceous sputum, progressive hoarseness, or tachypnea.

DIAGNOSTIC TESTS & INTERPRETATION
- Children: Glucose (hypoglycemia may occur in children because of limited glycogen storage)
- Smoke inhalation: Arterial blood gas, carboxyhemoglobin
- Electrical burns: Electrocardiogram (ECG), urine myoglobin, creatine kinase isoenzymes

Lab
- Hematocrit
- Type and cross
- Electrolytes, including blood urea nitrogen (BUN) and creatinine
- Urinalysis

Imaging
- Chest radiograph
- Xenon scan useful in suspected smoke inhalation

Diagnostic Procedures/Surgery
Bronchoscopy may be necessary in smoke inhalation to evaluate lower respiratory tract.

 TREATMENT

- Prehospital care (1)[C]:
  - Remove patient from source of burn.
  - Extinguish and remove all burning clothing.
  - Remove all rings, watches, and jewelry.
  - Room-temperature water may be poured onto burn, but only in the 1st 15 minutes following burn exposure.
  - Wrap patient to prevent hypothermia.
  - All patients to receive 100% O$_2$ via face mask
- Hospitalization for all serious burns:
  - 2nd-degree burns >10% of body surface area (BSA)
  - Any 3rd-degree burn
  - Burns of hands, feet, face, or perineum
  - Electrical/lightning burns
  - Inhalation injury
  - Chemical burns
  - Circumferential burn
- Transfer to burn center for (1)[C]
  - 2nd- and 3rd-degree burns >10% of BSA in patients <10 years and >50 years of age
  - 2nd-degree burns >20% of BSA and full-thickness burns >5% BSA in any age range
  - Burns of hands, feet, face, or perineum
  - Electrical or lightning burns
  - Inhalation injury
  - Chemical burns
  - Circumferential burn

MEDICATION
First Line
- Morphine: Small, frequent IV doses (0.1 mg/kg per dose in children; 2.5–20 mg q2–6h in adults)
- Silver sulfadiazine (Silvadene): Apply topically to burn site (can cause leukopenia).
- Neosporin or bacitracin ointment: Apply to facial burns.
- Mupirocin: Has potent inhibitory activity against methicillin-resistant *Staphylococcus aureus* (MRSA) (2)[B]
- Acticote A.B. (a dressing consisting of two sheets of high-density polyethylene mesh coated with nanocrystalline silver) has a more controlled, prolonged release of silver, allowing less frequent dressing changes (2)[B].

- Electrical burn with myoglobinuria will require alkalinization of urine and mannitol.
- No indication for prophylactic antibiotics.
- Consider H_2 blockers or proton-pump inhibitors (e.g., cimetidine, ranitidine, famotidine, lansoprazole, or nizatidine) for stress ulcer prophylaxis in severely burned patients.
- Tetanus toxoid/tetanus immunoglobulin
- There is no clear indication for prophylactic systemic antibiotics (2)[B].
- Use of VAC system may result in a low-protease environment with higher levels of angiogenic factor [vascular endothelial growth factor (VEGF)] during wound healing, leading to more chaotic, hyperkeratinized, thickened epidermis when compared with a standard hydrocolloid dressing (3)[C].

Second Line
- Mafenide (Sulfamylon) for full-thickness burn (*Caution:* Metabolic acidosis)
- Silver nitrate 0.5% (messy, leaches electrolytes from burn, causes water toxicity)
- Povidone–iodine (Betadine) may result in iodine absorption from burn and "tan eschar." Makes débridement more difficult.
- Travase (enzymatic débridement)

ADDITIONAL TREATMENT
General Measures
- Based on depth of burns and accurate estimate of total BSA involved (rule of nines)
- Quick estimate (for smaller burns): The surface area of the patient's hand is ~1% of the BSA.
- Tetanus prophylaxis (if not current)
- Remove all rings, watches, and other items from injured extremities to avoid tourniquet effect.
- Remove clothing, and cover all burned areas with dry sheets.
- Flush area of chemical burn (for ~2 h).
- 100% oxygen administration for all major burns; consider early intubation.
- Do not apply ice to burn site.
- Nasogastric tube (high risk of paralytic ileus)
- Foley catheter
- Pain relief:
  – IV meperidine (Demerol), morphine, or methadone for severe pain
  – Oral analgesics, such as acetaminophen (Tylenol) with codeine, acetaminophen with oxycodone (Percocet), or acetaminophen with hydrocodone (Lortab) for moderate pain
- ECG monitoring in 1st 24 h following electrical burn
- Whirlpool hydrotherapy followed by silver sulfadiazine (Silvadene) occlusive dressings in severe burns
- Daily or b.i.d. cleansing with dressing changes
- Epilock or Elasto-Gel may be used as dressing in selected patients (especially useful for outpatient treatment of minor burns).

- Burn fluid resuscitation (1)[C]:
  – Calculate fluid resuscitation from time of burn, not from time treatment begins.
  – 2–4 mL Ringer's lactate × body weight (kg) × % BSA burn (1/2 given in 1st 8 hours, in 2nd 8 hours, and in 3rd 8 hours); in children, this is given in addition to maintenance fluids and is adjusted according to urine output and vital signs.
  – Colloid solutions are not recommended during the 1st 12–24 h of resuscitation (1)[C],(4)[A].
- Other: Use of biologic membranes or skin substitutes may be indicated for burn coverage.
- Inhalation injury:
  – Intubation, ventilation with positive end-expiratory pressure assistance
  – Hyperbaric oxygen treatment may be useful in patients with carbon monoxide levels >25%, patients with coma, focal neurologic deficit, ischemic ECG changes, and pregnant patients (1)[C].

SURGERY/OTHER PROCEDURES
- Escharotomy may be necessary in constricting circumferential burns of extremities or chest.
- Tangential excision with split-thickness skin grafts
- Early excision of burns results in a significant reduction in mortality (excluding patients with inhalational injury) and a significant decrease in hospital length of stay (5)[B].

 ## ONGOING CARE

FOLLOW-UP RECOMMENDATIONS
Early mobilization is the goal.

DIET
- High-protein, high-calorie diet when bowel function resumes
- Nasogastric tube feedings may be required in early postburn period.
- Total parenteral nutrition if n.p.o. expected for >5 days

PATIENT EDUCATION
- Use of sunscreen
- Access to electrical cords/outlets
- Isolate household chemicals
- Use low-temperature setting for water heater (below 54°C)
- Household smoke detectors with special emphasis on maintenance
- Family/household evacuation plan
- Proper storage and use of flammable substances
- Burn management: www.aafp.org/afp/20001101/2029ph.html
- Burn prevention: www.aafp.org/afp/20001101/2032ph.html

PROGNOSIS
- 1st-degree burn: Complete resolution
- 2nd-degree burn: Epithelialization in 10–14 days (deep 2nd-degree burns probably will require skin graft)
- 3rd-degree burn: No potential for reepithelialization; skin graft required
- Length of hospital stay and need for ICU care depend on extent of burn, smoke inhalation, and age.

- A 50% survival rate can be expected with a 62% burn in patients aged 0–14 years, 63% burn in patients aged 15–40 years, 38% burn in patients aged 40–65 years, and 25% burn in patients >65 years of age (1)[C].
- 90% of survivors can be expected to return to an occupation as remunerative as their preburn employment.

COMPLICATIONS
- Gastroduodenal ulceration (curling ulcer)
- Marjolin ulcer: Squamous cell carcinoma developing in old burn site
- Burn wound sepsis: most commonly *S. aureus* (including MRSA), vancomycin-resistant enterococci, and gram-negative organisms (2)[B]
- Pneumonia
- Decreased mobility with possibility of future flexion contractures
- Hypertrophic scarring common with burns

REFERENCES
1. Teague H, Sweneki SA, Tang A. The burned patient: assessment, diagnosis, and management in the ED. *Trauma Reports.* 2005;6:1–12.
2. Church D, Elsayed S, Reid O, Winston B, Lindsay R, et al. Burn wound infections. *Clin Microbiol Rev.* 2006;19:403–34.
3. Caulfield RH, Tyler MP, Austyn JM, et al. The relationship between protease/anti-protease profile, angiogenesis and re-epithelialisation in acute burn wounds. *Burns.* 2008;34:474–86.
4. Roberts I, Alderson P, Bunn F, et al. Colloids versus crystalloids for fluid resuscitation in critically ill patients (Review). *Cochrane Database Sys Rev.* 2006; Vol 1.
5. Ong YS, Samuel M, Song C. Meta-analysis of early excision of burns. *Burns.* 2006;32:145–50.

 ## CODES

ICD9
949.0 Burn of unspecified site, unspecified degree

CLINICAL PEARLS
- 1st degree:
  – Erythema of involved tissue
  – Skin blanches with pressure.
  – Skin may be tender.
- 2nd degree:
  – Skin is red and blistered.
  – Skin is very tender.
- 3rd degree:
  – Burned skin is tough and leathery.
  – Skin is not tender.

BURSITIS

J. Herbert Stevenson, MD

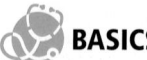 **BASICS**

DESCRIPTION

A *bursa* is a sac that is formed or found in areas subject to friction, such as locations where tendons pass over bony landmarks. Most common sites are subdeltoid, olecranon, prepatellar, trochanteric, and radiohumeral. Bursae essentially lubricate the region with synovial fluid:

- Large bursae usually communicate with joints and are responsible for retaining the synovial fluid in place.
- Bursae are fluid-filled sacs that serve as a cushion between tendons and bones.
- E.G. Bywaters, an English rheumatologist, found at least 78 bursae symmetrically placed on each side of the body.
- System(s) affected: Musculoskeletal

Pediatric Considerations
- Bursitis is less common in the pediatric population.

EPIDEMIOLOGY
Predominant age:
- 15–50 years (most common in skeletally mature)
- Traumatic bursitis more likely in patients < 35 years of age

Incidence
- Common
- Trochanteric pain: 1.8/1,000 per year (1)[B]

RISK FACTORS
Individuals who engage in repetitive and vigorous training or others who suddenly increase their level of activity (e.g., "weekend warriors")

GENERAL PREVENTION
- Appropriate warm-up and cool-down maneuvers, avoidance of overuse, or inadequate rest between workouts
- Range-of-motion exercises
- Maintain high level of fitness and general good health

ETIOLOGY
- Bursitis may be acute or chronic
- Many types of bursitis, including infectious, traumatic, inflammatory, and gouty
- Less often rheumatoid disease or tuberculosis as well as gout and pseudogout

COMMONLY ASSOCIATED CONDITIONS
- Tendinitis
- Sprains, strains
- Associated stress fractures

 DIAGNOSIS

PHYSICAL EXAM
- Pain/tenderness
- Decreased range of motion of affected region (rare except at shoulder)
- Erythema if infection present
- Swelling
- Crepitus sometimes found

DIAGNOSTIC TESTS & INTERPRETATION
Consider ECG (if left shoulder pain mimics cardiac pain)

Lab
- The following may help in differentiating soft tissue disease from rheumatic and connective tissue disease:
  - CBC
  - ESR
  - Serum protein electrophoresis
  - Rheumatoid factor
  - Serum uric acid
  - Phosphorus
  - Alkaline phosphatase
  - Blood testing for syphilis
  - Joint fluid analysis and culture (when indicated)
- Drugs that may alter lab results:
  - ESR rate may be increased with coexistent use of methyldopa, methysergide, penicillamine, theophylline, vitamin A.
  - ESR may be decreased with coexistent use of quinine, salicylates, and drugs that cause a high glucose level.

Imaging
- MRI may prove beneficial if diagnosis is unclear.
- Calcific deposits may be seen on plain radiograph.
- Ultrasound (2)[B]

Diagnostic Procedures/Surgery
- Aspiration of swollen bursa and evaluation of synovial fluid; the clinician must differentiate infected from inflammatory bursitis:
  - Fluid WBC 2–5,000/uL imply inflammatory, whereas >5,000 imply infectious cause.
  - Fluid analysis, Gram-stain, culture, and crystal analysis required to make the diagnosis.
- If the Gram-stain and culture yield an infective cause, treat with appropriate antibiotics. If the etiology is inflammatory, give local care.

Pathological Findings
- Acute with early inflammation: Bursa is distended with watery or mucoid fluid.
- Infection: Purulent fluid on aspiration
- Chronic:
  - Bursal wall is thickened, and inner surface is shaggy and trabeculated.
  - The space is filled with granular, brown, inspissated blood admixed with gritty, calcific precipitations.
  - Upper extremity tendinitis and bursitis are usually the result of repetitive microtrauma, probably resulting in disruption of fibers, leading to pain, spasm, and disability.

DIFFERENTIAL DIAGNOSIS
- Septic arthritis
- Gout, pseudogout
- Rheumatic disorders
- Osteoarthritis
- Tendinitis, strains, and sprains
- Lyme arthritis

TREATMENT

Outpatient; refer only difficult cases

MEDICATION

First Line
- NSAIDs or aspirin (3,4)[C]
- Antibiotic therapy if infection present; cover for staph and strep species (most common) (5)[B]
- Contraindications: Refer to manufacturer's profile of each drug.
- Precautions: Refer to manufacturer's profile of each drug.
- Significant possible interactions: Refer to manufacturer's profile of each drug.

Second Line
- Injectable corticosteroids once infectious etiology ruled out (3)[C],(4)[B],(6)[C],(7)[B]
- Systemic steroids provide limited short-term benefit (8)[B]

ADDITIONAL TREATMENT

General Measures
- Conservative therapy consists of rest, ice, and local care; elevation, gentle compression (often referred to as RICE therapy [rest-ice-compression-elevation])
- Compression with Ace wrap or neoprene sleeve
- Bursa aspiration
- Corticosteroid injection if infectious etiology ruled out
- Treatment of any underlying infection

SURGERY/OTHER PROCEDURES

Surgical excision in severe cases unresponsive to conservative treatments (5)[B]

 ONGOING CARE

FOLLOW-UP RECOMMENDATIONS
Rest and elevation of affected extremity

Patient Monitoring
- Discontinue NSAIDs as soon as possible to avoid side effects.
- Some patients may require repeated injections (usually no more than 3) of a corticosteroid and lidocaine (3,6)[C].

DIET
Consider changes if bursitis is directly related to obesity/crystalline deposition.

PROGNOSIS
- Most bouts of bursitis heal without sequelae.
- Repetitive acute bouts may lead to chronic bursitis, necessitating repeated joint/bursal aspirations or, eventually, surgical excision of involved bursa.

COMPLICATIONS
- Septic bursitis may extend to the nearby joint.
- Acute bursitis may progress to chronic.
- Severe long-range limitation of motion

REFERENCES

1. Lievense A, Bierma-Zeinstra S, Schouten B, et al. Prognosis of trochanteric pain in primary care. *Br J Gen Pract*. 2005;55:199–204.
2. Finlay K, Friedman L. Ultrasonography of the lower extremity. *Orthop Clin North Am*. 2006;37: 245–75, v.
3. Talia AH, Cardone D. Diagnostic and therapeutic injection of the shoulder region. *Am Fam Phys*. 2003;67(6):1271–8.
4. McFarland EG, Gill HS, Laporte DM, et al. Miscellaneous conditions about the elbow in athletes. *Clin Sports Med*. 2004;23:743–63, xi–xii.
5. Small LN, Ross JJ. Suppurative tenosynovitis and septic bursitis. *Infect Dis Clin North Am*. 2005;19: 991–1005, xi.
6. Cardone D, Tallia AH. Diagnostic and therapeutic injection of the hip and knee. *Am Fam Phys*. 2003;67(10):2147–53.
7. Buchbinder R, et al. Corticosteroid injection for shoulder pain. *Cochrane Database Sys Rev*. 2003; Issue Jan. 1.
8. Buchbinder R, Hoving JL, Green S, et al. Short course prednisolone for adhesive capsulitis (frozen shoulder or stiff painful shoulder): a randomised, double blind, placebo controlled trial. *Ann Rheum Dis*. 2004;63:1460–9.

ADDITIONAL READING

Cardone D, Tallia AH. Diagnostic and therapeutic injection of the elbow. *Am Fam Phys*. 2002;66(11): 2097–3100.

See Also (Topic, Algorithm, Electronic Media Element)
Tendinitis
Video: Olecranon Bursitis Aspiration

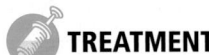 CODES

ICD9
727.3 Other bursitis disorders

CLINICAL PEARLS

Remember RICE acronym for conservative therapy:
- Rest affected area
- Ice inflammed bursa
- Compression (with Ace wrap or neoprene sleeve)
- Elevate joint

CANDIDIASIS

Brock D. Lutz, MD
Ronald A. Greenfield, MD

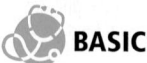

BASICS

DESCRIPTION
Candida albicans and related species cause a variety of infections:

- Cutaneous syndromes include erosio interdigitalis blastomycetica, folliculitis, balanitis, intertrigo, paronychia, onychomycosis, diaper rash, perianal candidiasis, and the syndromes of chronic mucocutaneous candidiasis.
- Mucous membrane infections include oral candidiasis (thrush), esophagitis, and vaginitis.
- The most serious manifestations of candidiasis are candidemia and hematogenously disseminated invasive candidiasis. This article discusses candidemia and hematogenously disseminated candidiasis.

EPIDEMIOLOGY
- Predominant age: All ages are susceptible to hematogenously disseminated candidiasis; premature neonates are at particularly high risk.
- Predominant sex: Male = Female (hematogenously disseminated candidiasis)

Incidence
≥20/100,000 persons per year

Prevalence
Data not available

RISK FACTORS
- Neutropenia
- Corticosteroid treatment
- HIV infection
- Diabetes mellitus
- Mucocutaneous colonization/infection
- Broad-spectrum antibacterial chemotherapy
- Recent chemotherapy or radiation
- Indwelling intravascular access devices
- Cardiothoracic or abdominal surgery
- Parenteral nutrition
- Prolonged hospital stay
- Intensive care unit (ICU) stay
- Burns
- End-stage renal disease
- Bone marrow or solid organ transplant recipient
- Cancer
- Premature birth

GENERAL PREVENTION
- Polyenes, azoles, and echinocandins reduce the incidence of candidiasis in patients undergoing induction therapy for acute leukemia or bone marrow or stem cell transplantation (1)[A].
- Fluconazole prophylaxis in high-risk ICU patients reduces the incidence of invasive candidiasis (2)[A]. See Medications.

PATHOPHYSIOLOGY
An acute suppurative infection in which polymorphonuclear host defense is the critical element

ETIOLOGY
- *Candida albicans* is the most frequent pathogen. Other important human pathogens include *C. tropicalis, C. krusei, C. stellatoidea, C. pseudotropicalis, C. guilliermondi, C. parapsilosis, C. lusitaniae, C. rugosa, C. lambica,* and *C. glabrata*.
- *Candida* species colonize human mucocutaneous surfaces; most infections are endogenously acquired from this reservoir.
- Human-to-human transmission of *Candida* occurs in some settings.

COMMONLY ASSOCIATED CONDITIONS
See Risk Factors.

DIAGNOSIS

HISTORY
- Several days of fever that is unresponsive to broad-spectrum antibiotics
- Prolonged intravenous catheterization
- A history of several key risk factors
- Be alert to organ system dysfunction.

PHYSICAL EXAM
- Fever
- Malaise
- Tachycardia
- Hypotension
- Altered mental status
- Hepatosplenomegaly
- Maculopapular or nodular skin rash

Pediatric Considerations
- For an infant with thrush, be sure to also check for candidal diaper dermatitis. Also, there is often a concomitant infection.
- Fever
- Macronodular skin lesions (10%)
- Candidal endophthalmitis (10–28%)
- Generally patients are ill and may manifest septic shock.

DIAGNOSTIC TESTS & INTERPRETATION
- The diagnosis is established by isolating the causative organism from blood cultures or other normally sterile body sites or by demonstration of organisms in histopathologic specimens of normally sterile tissues.
- Isolation of *Candida* from multiple sites should raise the diagnostic suspicion of hematogenously disseminated invasive candidiasis.
- *Candida* species isolated from a normally sterile site should be identified to the species level (1)[A].
- Because fluconazole-resistant *C. albicans* and particularly nonalbicans species are reported with increasing frequency, fluconazole susceptibility testing should be performed before treatment with fluconazole (1)[B].

Imaging
- Generally not specifically useful in diagnosis of hematogenously invasive disseminated candidiasis. However, multisite metastasis of infection is common.
- In the syndrome of hepatosplenic candidiasis (chronic systemic candidiasis), imaging of the liver and spleen by liver scan, ultrasound, computed tomography (CT), or magnetic resonance imaging (MRI) may suggest this syndrome as the cause of persistent fever and liver dysfunction in patients who have recently recovered from neutropenia.

Diagnostic Procedures/Surgery
- If blood cultures remain consistently negative, aspiration or excisional biopsy of sites of focal infection may be useful in diagnosis.
- Aspiration and biopsy of skin lesions occasionally seen with hematogenously disseminated candidiasis are also useful.

Pathological Findings
Characteristic histopathology of lesions of *Candida* invasion of visceral organs is microabscess formation.

DIFFERENTIAL DIAGNOSIS
Includes a variety of cryptic bacterial infections and, in the neutropenic host, multiple opportunistic infections

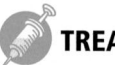

TREATMENT

Inpatient for hematogenously disseminated invasive candidiasis

MEDICATION
- Echinocandins (3)[A]:
  - An initial therapy of choice for any patient with candidemia (1)[A]
  - Patients with initial echinocandin therapy may have a survival advantage.
  - Caspofungin: Administer 70 mg IV dose on day 1 followed by 50 mg/d IV for 2 weeks after last positive sterile site culture if no evident metastatic infection.
  - Modify dose for severe hepatic insufficiency.
  - *C. parapsilosis* has reduced sensitivity to echinocandins.
  - The echinocandins anidulafungin and micafungin have similar efficacy.
- Fluconazole:
  - An initial therapy of choice for some patients (1)[A]
  - Because it is fungistatic rather than fungicidal, it should not be used for treatment of patients with severe neutropenia or severe immunosuppression.
  - It should only be used after confirmation of in vitro susceptibility in patients with azole therapy in prior 3 months.
  - Should be used empirically only in institutions with a very low prevalence of resistance
  - Useful for switch therapy after demonstration of in vitro susceptibility after initial therapy with an echinocandin or amphotericin

- For 1st week, administer 400–800 mg/d IV, followed by additional IV or oral therapy at the same dose for ≥2 weeks after the last positive blood culture or last evidence of infection. Higher doses of fluconazole may be required if non-*Albicans* species are known or suspected, because they carry a higher likelihood of drug resistance.
  - *C. krusei* and many *C. glabrata* are resistant to fluconazole.
- Liposomal amphotericin B:
  - Can be used as an initial therapy for any patient with candidemia (1)[A]. Cautious use is indicated given relative risks of toxicity compared to alternative therapies.
  - Usual dosage is 3 mg/kg/d IV.
  - *C. lusitaniae* may be resistant.
  - Consider higher doses for *C. krusei* or *C. glabrata* (5–10 mg/kg/d).
- Other azole antifungals, depending on activity and safety (itraconazole and voriconazole)
- Contraindications:
  - The safety of amphotericin B therapy in pregnant patients has not been established.
  - Echinocandins are pregnancy Category C.
- Precautions:
  - Liposomal amphotericin B:
    - The toxicity is less common than with conventional amphotericin B, but may still be formidable. Acute reactions (fever, rigors, and hypotension) may occur during the initiation of therapy. Ameliorate or eliminate by premedication with acetaminophen or ibuprofen. Use meperidine if needed to abort rigors.
    - Azotemia may occur. Maintenance of optimal fluid status and prevention of dehydration help minimize the risk of azotemia. "Sodium loading" with 1 L half-normal saline daily may decrease renal toxicity.
    - Significant hypokalemia and renal tubular acidosis may develop. Significant hypomagnesemia may worsen hypokalemia.
    - Anemia commonly develops in patients on protracted therapy, but is almost always reversible.
    - Headache and phlebitis are common. Use central venous access for administration.
    - Leukopenia, thrombocytopenia, and liver function abnormalities are rare.
- Itraconazole, voriconazole, caspofungin, anidulafungin, and micafungin do not enter the urinary stream in sufficient concentrations to treat urinary tract infections (UTIs).
- Significant possible drug-drug interactions:
  - Echinocandins:
    - Potentially important interactions with carbamazepine, phenytoin, cyclosporine, tacrolimus, sirolimus, non-nucleoside reverse transcriptase inhibitors, and rifampin.
  - Liposomal amphotericin B:
    - Concomitant therapy with cyclosporine or other nephrotoxic agents, such as aminoglycosides or vancomycin, may increase the risk of amphotericin-induced nephrotoxicity.
  - Fluconazole and other azoles:
    - Potentially important drug-drug interactions may occur in patients receiving oral hypoglycemics, coumarin-type anticoagulants, phenytoin, cyclosporine, rifampin, theophylline, or terfenadine or astemizole.

- These drug-drug interactions are more likely with itraconazole and voriconazole than with fluconazole.

ADDITIONAL TREATMENT
General Measures
- Fluid and electrolyte therapy are often required.
- Hemodynamic and respiratory support may be required in seriously ill patients.
- The removal of potentially infected intravascular access devices is imperative.

Issues for Referral
Invasive *Candida* infections should be managed with the assistance of an infectious disease specialist.

SURGERY/OTHER PROCEDURES
Drainage of abscess (by any means clinically feasible) is necessary for resolution. Removal of any indwelling contaminated device or catheter is necessary.

IN-PATIENT CONSIDERATIONS
IV Fluids
Generally necessary in critically ill patients

 ## ONGOING CARE

FOLLOW-UP RECOMMENDATIONS
Patients should receive follow-up visit ~6 weeks after end of therapy and be screened for metastatic infection complications by history and physical exam.

Patient Monitoring
- Evaluate complete blood count (CBC), serum electrolytes, and serum creatinine at least twice weekly in patients on liposomal amphotericin B therapy.
- If blood cultures are positive, they should be repeated until negative. Therapy must be extended in this case.

DIET
Popular literature has reports of diet being linked to yeast overgrowth and subsequent chronic fatigue; randomized controlled trials suggest following a low-sugar, low-yeast diet has no benefit over general healthy eating for symptoms of fatigue (4)[B].

PATIENT EDUCATION
Advise patients of the nature of the infection and the toxicities associated with therapy.

PROGNOSIS
Overall mortality for patients with hematogenously disseminated candidiasis is 40–75%, with mortality attributable to candidemia being 15–37%.

COMPLICATIONS
- Systemic inflammatory response syndrome
- Pyelonephritis
- Endophthalmitis
- Endocarditis, myocarditis, pericarditis
- Arthritis, chondritis, osteomyelitis
- Pneumonitis
- Central nervous system infection

REFERENCES
1. Spellberg BJ, Filler SG, Edwards JE. Current treatment strategies for disseminated candidiasis. *Clin Infect Dis*. 2006;42:244–51.
2. Vardakas KZ, Samonis G, Michalopoulos A, et al. Antifungal prophylaxis with azoles in high-risk, surgical intensive care unit patients: a metaanalysis of randomized, placebo-controlled trials. *Crit Care Med*. 2006;34:1216–24.
3. Sucher AJ, Chahine EB, Balcer HE. Echinocandins: The Newest Class of Antifungals (October) (CE). *Ann Pharmacother*. 2009.
4. Hobday RA, Thomas S, O'Donovan A, et al. Dietary intervention in chronic fatigue syndrome. *J Hum Nutr Diet*. 2008;21:141–9.

ADDITIONAL READING
- Benjamin DK, Stoll BJ, Fanaroff AA, et al. Neonatal candidiasis among extremely low birth weight infants: risk factors, mortality rates, and neurodevelopmental outcomes at 18 to 22 months. *Pediatrics*. 2006;117:84–92.
- Golan Y, Wolf MP, Pauker SG, et al. Empirical anti-Candida therapy among selected patients in the intensive care unit: a cost-effectiveness analysis. *Ann Intern Med*. 2005;143:857–69.
- Ha JF, Italiano CM, Heath CH, et al. Candidemia and invasive candidiasis: a review of the literature for the burns surgeon. *Burns: Journal of the International Society for Burn Injuries*. 2010.
- Ostrosky-Zeichner L, Pappas PG. Invasive candidiasis in the intensive care unit. *Crit Care Med*. 2006;34:857–63.
- Worthington HV, Clarkson JE, Khalid T, et al. Interventions for treating oral candidiasis for patients with cancer receiving treatment. *Cochrane Database Syst Rev*. 2010;7:CD001972.

See Also (Topic, Algorithm, Electronic Media Element)
Vulvovaginitis, Candidal

 ## CODES

ICD9
- 112.0 Candidiasis of mouth
- 112.1 Candidiasis of vulva and vagina
- 112.2 Candidiasis of other urogenital sites

CLINICAL PEARLS
- Fluconazole prophylaxis in high-risk ICU patients reduces the incidence of invasive candidiasis.
- Caspofungin or another of the echinocandins is initial therapy of choice for any patient with candidemia (1)[A].

CANDIDIASIS, MUCOCUTANEOUS

Sheila O. Stille, DMD, MAGD
Hugh J. Silk, MD

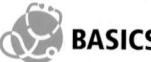 **BASICS**

DESCRIPTION
- A mucocutaneous disorder caused by infection with various *Candida* sp.
- Areas include:
  - GI
    - Oropharyngeal candidiasis: Mouth, pharynx
    - Angular cheilitis: Fissures at mouth corners
    - Candida esophagitis: Esophagus
    - GI candidiasis: Gastritis, +/− ulcers, associated with thrush; in tract or perianal
  - Non-Gastrointestinal
    - Candida vulvovaginitis: Vaginal mucosa and/or cutaneous aspects of the vulva
    - Candidal balanitis: Glans penis
    - Candidal paronychia: Nail bed of a digit
    - Folliculitis: Hair follicles
    - Interdigital candidiasis: Webs of the digits
- System(s) affected: Oropharynx; GI; Skin/Exocrine; Genitourinary
- Synonym(s): Monilia; thrush; yeast

ALERT
Vaginal antifungal creams and suppositories can weaken condoms and diaphragms.

Pregnancy Considerations
No known fetal complications of maternal *Candida*

EPIDEMIOLOGY
- Common in the US, very common with immunodeficiency and/or uncontrolled diabetes
- Predominant age: None:
  - Infants and seniors: Thrush and cutaneous infections (infant diaper rash)
  - Women of childbearing age: Vaginitis
  - Prepubertal or postmenopausal: Yeast vaginitis uncommon
  - Predominant sex: Female > Male (because of vaginitis)

Incidence
Not well studied, but some estimate 50/100,000

Prevalence
Candida colonization: >50% of US population

RISK FACTORS
- Immunosuppression
- Hormonal fluctuations in females
- Antibacterial therapy, especially broad-spectrum antibiotics
- Douches, chemical irritants, and other vaginitides can predispose to yeast vaginitis
- Dentures
- Birth control pills
- Hyperglycemia

Genetics
Chronic mucocutaneous candidiasis is a heterogeneous, genetic syndrome; usually presents in childhood, but mode of inheritance has not been clarified.

GENERAL PREVENTION
- Minimize antibiotic use
- Minimize inhaled and systemic steroid use; rinse mouth after inhaled steroid use
- Avoid douching, chemicals (i.e., spermicides)
- Treat other vaginitides
- Minimize moist environments (e.g., wear cotton underwear)
- Clean dentures appropriately; have new, well-fitting dentures fabricated
- Control diabetes (if present)

ETIOLOGY
C. albicans predominant (responsible for 80–92% vulvovaginal candidiasis and 70–80% oral isolates)

COMMONLY ASSOCIATED CONDITIONS
- HIV and other leukopenias
- Diabetes mellitus
- Cancer and other immunosuppressive disorders
- Disorders requiring corticosteroids (1) or other immunosuppressive chemotherapy

 DIAGNOSIS

- NOTE: *Candida* is normal flora, in very small amounts, in oral cavity, GI tract, and female genital tract.
- In children:
  - Oral: White, raised, painless, distinct patches within the mouth; can be wiped off to reveal red base, sometimes with pinpoint bleeding
  - Perineal: Erythematous maculopapular rash with satellite pustules or papules
  - Angular cheilitis: Painful fissures in mouth corners, often cracked and bleeding
- In adults:
  - Vulvovaginal lesions; thin to thick whitish cottage cheese-like discharge; red patches in vagina or perineum; symptoms range from none to intense pruritus/burning
- In immunocompromised hosts:
  - Oral: White, raised, painless, distinct patches; red, slightly raised patches; thick, dark-brownish coating; deep fissures
  - Esophagitis: Dysphagia, odynophagia, retrosternal pain; usually with thrush
  - GI symptoms: Ulcerations, pain
  - Balanitis: Erythema, linear erosions, scaling; possible dysuria
  - Angular cheilitis (see In children)
  - Folliculitis: Follicular pustules
  - Interdigital: Redness, itchiness at base of fingers and/or toes susceptible to maceration

DIAGNOSTIC TESTS & INTERPRETATION
Imaging
Barium swallow: Esophageal candidiasis may reveal a cobblestone appearance, fistulas, or esophageal dilatation (from denervation)

Diagnostic Procedures/Surgery
- KOH prep: A sample of the discharge or coating of the infected area or ulcer is needed.
- Esophagitis may require biopsy.
- Oral hyperplastic candidiasis should be biopsied to rule out carcinoma.
- HIV seropositivity plus thrush with dysphagia relieved by antifungal treatment are acceptable criteria for diagnosis of *Candida* esophagitis.

Pathological Findings
- Slide preparation: Mycelia (hyphae) or pseudomycelia (pseudohyphae) yeast forms; *Candida* does not induce an increased PMN leukocyte response.
- Biopsy: Epithelial parakeratosis with PMNs in superficial layers; PAS staining reveals presence of candidal hyphae.

DIFFERENTIAL DIAGNOSIS
- For oral candidiasis:
  - Leukoplakia
  - Lichen planus
  - Geographic tongue
  - Herpes simplex
  - Erythema multiforme
  - Pemphigus
- Baby formula or breast milk can mimic thrush
- Hairy leukoplakia: Does not rub off to erythematous base; usually on lateral tongue
- Angular cheilitis from vitamin B or iron deficiency, staph infection, or edentulous over closure
- *Bacterial vaginosis* and *Trichomonas vaginalis* tend to have more odor, itch, and have a different discharge, but symptoms that are similar to those of *Candida vaginalis* include:
  - Marked vulvar irritation
  - Labial erythema
  - External dysuria
  - Vaginal tenderness

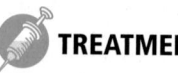 **TREATMENT**

MEDICATION
First Line
- Vaginal (choose 1):
  - Miconazole (Monistat) 2% cream: 1 applicator or 1 100–200-mg suppository, intravaginally q.h.s. for 7 days
  - Clotrimazole (Gyne-Lotrimin, Mycelex): Intravaginal tablets (100 mg q.h.s. for 6–7 days, 200 mg q.h.s. for 3 days; 500 mg daily for 1 day), or 1% cream (1 applicator q.h.s. for 6–7 days)
  - Fluconazole 150 mg PO in 1 dose.
  - Nystatin (Mycostatin, Nilstat): 100,000 U/g cream (1 applicator) or 100,000 U tablets (1 tablet) intravaginally 1 × day for 7–14 days
- Oropharyngeal:
  - Mild disease:
    - Clotrimazole (Mycelex): 10 mg troche, suck on over 20 minutes 5 times a day for 7–14 days, or
    - Nystatin suspension: 100,000 U/ml given 4–6 times daily, or
    - Nystatin pastilles: 200,000 U each, administered 4 times daily for 7–14 days (2)[B]
    - Denture wearers:
      - Nystatin ointment: 100,000 U/g on fitting surfaces of denture and corners of mouth for 3 weeks
      - Remove dentures at night; clean twice weekly with diluted (1:20) bleach
  - Moderate to severe disease:
    - Fluconazole : 100–200 mg (3 mg/kg) daily for 7–14 days

- Esophagitis:
  – Fluconazole: 100 mg/d for 14–21 days, load with 200 mg
  – Itraconazole (Sporanox):
    ○ Solution: 1–200 mg daily for 7–14 days
    ○ Capsules: 200 mg/d (take with food) for 2–3 weeks
- GI: Therapy not well defined
- Any site during pregnancy

Pregnancy Considerations
Miconazole is usually the drug of choice.

Second Line
- Vaginal:
  – Terconazole (Terazol): Recurrent cases: 0.4% cream (1 applicator q.h.s. for 10–14 days of induction therapy); 0.8% cream/80-mg suppositories (1 applicator or 1 suppository q.h.s. for 3 days)
  – Prophylaxis: fluconazole, 150 mg once per week for 6 months to prevent recurrent infections
- Oropharyngeal:
  – Clotrimazole troches at a dosage of 10 mg 5 times daily
  – Nystatin oral suspension (100,000 U/mL):
    ○ Children: 5–10 mL 4 times daily for 10 days directly to oral lesions
    ○ Infants: 0.5 mL in each cheek 4 times daily for 10 days
    ○ Adults: Swish for as long as reasonable and swallow 5–10 mL 4 times daily for 14 days; prophylaxis is achieved with above dosages 2–5 times a day.
  – Fluconazole: 100 mg/d for 7–14 days (load immunocompromised patient with 200 mg)
  – Itraconazole (Sporanox) suspension: 200 mg (20 mL) daily; swish and swallow for 7–14 days; capsules: 200 mg/d (take with food) for 2–4 weeks
  – Miconazole oral gel (20 mg/mL): q.i.d., swish for as long as reasonable and swallow
  – Amphotericin B (Fungizone) oral suspension (100 mg/mL): 1 mL 4 times daily, swish for as long as reasonable and swallow; use between meals
  – Ketoconazole: 200–400 mg PO daily for 14–21 days
- Esophagitis:
  – Oral fluconazole at a dosage of 200–400 mg (3–6 mg/kg) daily for 14–21 days
  – Amphotericin B (variable dosing) i.v. dose of 0.3–0.7 mg/kg daily, or an echinocandin should be used for patients who cannot tolerate oral therapy
- Continue all treatments until 2 days after disappearance of infection:
  – Contraindications:
    ○ Ketoconazole, itraconazole, or nystatin (if swallowed): Severe hepatotoxicity
    ○ Amphotericin B: Renal failure
  – Precautions:
    ○ Miconazole: Can potentiate the effect of warfarin, but drug of choice in pregnancy
    ○ Fluconazole: Renal excretion; rare hepatotoxicity; resistance frequent
    ○ Itraconazole: Doubling the dosage results in ~3-fold increase in itraconazole plasma concentrations

- Possible interactions (rarely seen with creams, lotions, or suppositories):
  – Fluconazole:
    ○ Rifampin: Decreased fluconazole concentrations
    ○ Tolbutamide: Decreased tolbutamide concentrations
    ○ Warfarin, phenytoin, cyclosporine: Altered metabolism; check levels
  – Itraconazole: Potent CYP 3A4 inhibitor. Carefully assess all coadministered medications.

ADDITIONAL TREATMENT
General Measures
Screen severely immunodeficient patients at routine visits.

Issues for Referral
- Patients without obvious reasons for recurrent superficial candidal infections
- GI candidiasis

Additional Therapies
- For infants with thrush: Boil pacifiers and bottle nipples; assess mom's breasts/nipples for candida infections as well
- For denture-related candidiasis, disinfection of the denture, in addition to antifungal therapy

COMPLEMENTARY AND ALTERNATIVE MEDICINE
Probiotics: *Lactobacillus* and *Bifidobacterium* may inhibit *Candida sp* (3).

IN-PATIENT CONSIDERATIONS
Nursing
Staff for the elderly patients should be properly trained in oral hygiene. Protocols for brushing, proper denture care, and moistening the oral cavity can reduce candidal infections in the elderly.

ONGOING CARE

FOLLOW-UP RECOMMENDATIONS
Patient Monitoring
Immunocompromised persons may benefit from regular symptom evaluation plus routine KOH preps during vaginal and oral exams.

DIET
Active-culture yogurt or other live lactobacillus may decrease colonization; indeterminate evidence

PATIENT EDUCATION
- Advise patients at risk for recurrence about antibacterial therapy overgrowth (1)[B]
- "zole-type" medications are Category C

PROGNOSIS
- For immunocompetent individuals: Benign course, excellent prognosis
- For immunosuppressed persons: *Candida* may become an AIDS-defining illness, and chronicity may cause much morbidity

COMPLICATIONS
In immunosuppressed persons, complications depend on the severity of the immune status. In HIV infection, moderate immunosuppression (e.g., CD4 200–500 cells/mm^3) may be associated with chronic candidiasis. In severe immunosuppression (e.g., CD4 <100 cells/mm^3), thrush may lead to esophagitis, then a full-systemic infection involving every organ system, particularly renal.

REFERENCES

1. Kyrmizakis DE, Papadakis CE, Lohuis PJ, et al. Acute candidiasis of the oro- and hypopharynx as the result of topical intranasal steroids administration. *Rhinology*. 2000;38:87–9.
2. Pappas PG, Kauffman CA, Andes D, et al. Clinical practice guidelines for the management of candidiasis: 2009 update by the Infectious Diseases Society of America. *Clin Infect Dis*. 2009;48: 503–35.
3. Strus M, Kucharska A, Kukla G, et al. The in vitro activity of vaginal Lactobacillus with probiotic properties against Candida. *Infect Dis Obstet Gynecol*. 2005;13:69–75.

ADDITIONAL READING

- Achkar JM, Fries BC, et al. Candida infections of the genitourinary tract. *Clin Microbiol Rev*. 2010;23: 253–73.
- Pappas PG, Kauffman CA, Andes D, et al. Clinical practice guidelines for the management of candidiasis: 2009 update by the Infectious Diseases Society of America. *Clin Infect Dis* 2009;48(5): 503–35. PubMed.
- Terai H, Shimahara M. Tongue pain: burning mouth syndrome vs Candida-associated lesion. *Oral Dis*. 2007;13:440–2.

See Also (Topic, Algorithm, Electronic Media Element)
Candidiasis; HIV Infection and AIDS

 CODES

ICD9
- 112.0 Candidiasis of mouth
- 112.1 Candidiasis of vulva and vagina
- 112.2 Candidiasis of other urogenital sites

CLINICAL PEARLS

- The diagnosis of candidiasis is generally made clinically, but may include KOH. Rarely, a culture of skin scrapings or even a biopsy is needed for resistant strains or to explore the differential.
- Transmission from person to person is rare. Rarely, *Candida* vaginitis may be sexually transmitted.
- If tongue pain continues after treatment, consider burning mouth syndrome.
- Topical antifungals rarely cause problems, but oral medications may have hepatic side effects.
- Amphotericin B can cause nephrotoxicity.

CARBON MONOXIDE POISONING

Robert De Marco, MD

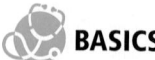 **BASICS**

DESCRIPTION

Carbon monoxide (CO) is the leading cause of poisoning death in the US. CO is an odorless, tasteless, colorless gas produced by combustion of carbon-containing compounds:

- CO inhalation leads to displacement of oxygen from binding sites on hemoglobin.
- Detrimental effects are related to tissue hypoxia from decreased oxygen content and a shift of the oxyhemoglobin dissociation curve to the left.
- CO binds to cytochrome oxidase, impairing mitochondrial function, and to cytochrome oxidase, affecting muscle function.
- CO binding to myoglobin affects muscle activity.
- System(s) affected: Cardiovascular; Musculoskeletal; Nervous

Pregnancy Considerations

Tissue hypoxia includes the fetus. CO poisoning may cause significant fetal abnormalities, depending on the developmental stage. Also, adult hemoglobin holds oxygen less tightly than does fetal hemoglobin. Therefore, a pregnant mother potentially may be unaffected while the fetus is affected.

EPIDEMIOLOGY

Incidence

- 40,000 emergency department visits annually
- 5,000–6,000 deaths annually in the US
- Inadvertent CO poisoning likely causes 500 deaths annually.
- Intentional CO poisoning is approximately 10 times higher.
- Unintended poisoning is most common during winter months in cold climates.
- 10,000 individuals miss 1 or more days of work due to CO poisoning.

RISK FACTORS

- Smoke inhalation
- Being in a closed space with a faulty furnace or stove or running engine
- Cigarette smoking
- Employment in a coal mine, as an auto mechanic, paint stripper, or in the solvent industry
- Improperly vented fuel-burning devices:
  – Kerosene heaters, charcoal grills, camping stoves, gasoline-powered generators, wood stoves
  – Open-air exposure to motorboat exhaust
- Underground utility electrical cable fires produce large amounts of CO, which can seep into adjacent buildings and homes.

GENERAL PREVENTION

- Appropriate ventilation, especially where there are fuel-burning devices
- Use of CO monitors
- Public education
- Determining the mechanism of exposure is critical in cases of accidental poisoning in order to limit future risk

PATHOPHYSIOLOGY

- CO is rapidly absorbed in lungs.
- CO has ~250 times the affinity for hemoglobin that oxygen has.
- CO binds to hemoglobin to form carboxyhemoglobin (COHb), resulting in impaired oxygen-carrying capacity, utilization, and delivery:
  – Leftward shift of the oxyhemoglobin dissociation curve occurs.
  – CO interferes with peripheral oxygen utilization by inactivating cytochrome oxidase.
- Delayed neurologic sequelae, probably due to lipid peroxidation by toxic oxygen species generated by xanthine oxidase.
- The half-life of CO while the patient is breathing room air is ~300 minutes, while breathing high-flow oxygen via a nonrebreathing face mask is ~90 minutes, and with 100% hyperbaric oxygen is ~30 minutes.

ETIOLOGY

- CO inhalation
- Inhaled or ingested methylene chloride (from paint remover [dichloromethane]) is metabolized to CO by the liver, causing CO toxicity in the absence of ambient CO.

COMMONLY ASSOCIATED CONDITIONS

CO and cyanide poisoning can occur simultaneously following smoke inhalation (synergistic effect).

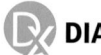 **DIAGNOSIS**

- Acute CO poisoning is suggested by history, physical examination, and an elevated COHb.
- Chronic CO intoxication is difficult to diagnose.
- Pulse oximetry cannot screen for CO exposure because it does not differentiate carboxyhemoglobin from oxyhemoglobin.

HISTORY

- Tinnitus
- Headaches
- Dizziness, nausea, vomiting, or diarrhea
- Weakness or fatigue
- Flushing
- Syncope
- Angina

PHYSICAL EXAM

- "Cherry red" appearance of the lips and skin
- In absence of trauma or burns, look for altered mental status.
- Impaired judgment, respiratory depression, arrhythmias, hypotension
- Cyanosis or tachypnea
- A careful neurologic examination is crucial.
- Visual-field defects, blindness, papilledema, or nystagmus
- Central nervous system depression
- Ataxia
- Seizures
- Coma
- Angina
- Tachycardia or cardiac dysrhythmias
- Cardiopulmonary arrest

DIAGNOSTIC TESTS & INTERPRETATION

Lab

Initial lab tests

- Measurement of COHb
- Check CO level via co-oximetry of arterial or venous blood (some authors question their accuracy).
- Check acid-base status on blood gas.
- Electrocardiogram (EKG) in all patients
- Cardiac enzymes in:
  – ≥65 years
  – Patient with cardiac risk factors

Follow-Up & Special Considerations

Think of CO poisoning in younger patients with chest pain or symptoms suggestive of ischemia.

Imaging

Head computed tomography scan is helpful to rule out other causes of neurologic decompensation.

DIFFERENTIAL DIAGNOSIS

- Cyanide toxicity
- Acute viral syndrome
- Other causes of mental status changes: Metabolic, drugs, infectious, trauma

 TREATMENT

MEDICATION

- Prompt removal from the source of CO
- Institution of 100% oxygen by high-flow mask or endotracheal tube
- 100% normobaric oxygen for all suspected victims of CO poisoning, regardless of pulse oximetry or arterial PO_2(1)[B]

ADDITIONAL TREATMENT
General Measures
- Removal from source
- Rapid reduction in tissue hypoxia with 100% oxygen to reduce the half-time of elimination of CO to 90 minutes
- Supportive care as necessary
- Intubation and mechanical ventilation may be necessary for severe intoxication. All patients who are comatose or have severely impaired mental status should be intubated and mechanically ventilated without delay (1)[B].
- Volume resuscitation

Additional Therapies
- 100% oxygen by tight-fitting nonrebreathing mask
- Hyperbaric oxygen for severe poisoning or in the following conditions (2)[B]:
  – CO level >20% in a pregnant patient
  – Loss of consciousness
  – Severe metabolic acidosis (pH <7.1)
  – Possible end-organ ischemia (EKG changes, chest pain, altered mental status)
- For mild poisoning (carboxyhemoglobin levels <30%); no signs or symptoms of cardiovascular or neurologic dysfunction:
  – Treatment: Admission if carboxyhemoglobin >25%
  – Symptomatic medication for headache
  – 100% oxygen by nonrebreathing mask until carboxyhemoglobin <5%
  – Patients with underlying heart disease should be admitted, regardless of level of carboxyhemoglobin
- For moderate poisoning (carboxyhemoglobin 30–40%); no signs or symptoms of cardiovascular or neurologic dysfunction:
  – Treatment: Admission
  – Cardiovascular status should be followed closely, even in the absence of clear cardiac effects
  – Determination of acid–base status: Corrected by oxygen
  – 100% oxygen by nonrebreathing mask until carboxyhemoglobin <5%
- For severe poisoning (carboxyhemoglobin >40%); cardiovascular or neurologic functional impairment at any carboxyhemoglobin level:
  – Treatment: Admission
  – Cardiovascular function monitoring
  – Acid–base status monitoring
  – 100% oxygen by nonrebreathing mask until carboxyhemoglobin <5%
  – Hyperbaric oxygen immediately if available; if unavailable, treat as in moderate poisoning
- If no improvement occurs in cardiovascular or neurologic function within 4 hours, transport the patient to the nearest facility with hyperbaric oxygen, regardless of distance.

IN-PATIENT CONSIDERATIONS
Patients often present in clusters, with similar symptoms and a common environment.

Initial Stabilization
- Emergency department (ED) for mild poisoning
- Inpatient treatment for moderate or severe poisoning

Admission Criteria
Patients whose symptoms do not resolve, who demonstrate EKG or laboratory evidence of severe poisoning, or who have other medical or social cause of concern should be hospitalized.

Discharge Criteria
Patients with mild symptoms from accidental poisoning can be managed in the ED and safely discharged.

 ONGOING CARE

FOLLOW-UP RECOMMENDATIONS
Rest until carboxyhemoglobin reduced and symptoms abate

Patient Monitoring
- Measurement of carboxyhemoglobin levels
- Arterial blood gases
- Psychiatric evaluation and follow-up for intentional exposure

PATIENT EDUCATION
- Professional installation and maintenance of combustion devices: 1-800-638-2772; Consumer Products Safety Commission hotline
- CO detector installation in homes, especially near bedrooms and potential sources

PROGNOSIS
Most survivors recover completely, with only a minority developing chronic neuropsychiatric impairment.

COMPLICATIONS
- Myocardial infarction
- Pulmonary edema (congestive heart failure)
- Pneumonia (aspiration)
- Anoxic encephalopathy
- Long-term neuropsychiatric complications:
  – Intellectual deterioration
  – Memory impairment
- Dysrhythmia
- Shock
- Rhabdomyolysis, personality changes:
  – Irritability
  – Aggressiveness
  – Violence
- Moodiness

Geriatric Considerations
- Higher incidence of cardiovascular and neurologic disease, increasing complications
- Atherosclerosis with chronic exposure

REFERENCES
1. Hampson NB, Scott KL, Zmaeff JL. Carboxyhemoglobin measurement by hospitals: implications for the diagnosis of carbon monoxide poisoning. *J Emerg Med*. 2006;31:13–6.
2. Kao LW, Nañagas KA. Carbon monoxide poisoning. *Emerg Med Clin North Am*. 2004;22:985–1018.

ADDITIONAL READING
- Insufficient evidence to establish usefulness of hyperbaric oxygen for carbon monoxide poisoning. *Cochrane Library*. 2005;1:CD002041.
- Internet resources available at: http://www.cpsc.gov.
- Juurlink DN, Buckley NA, Stanbrook MB, et al. Hyperbaric oxygen for carbon monoxide poisoning. *Cochrane Database Syst Rev*. 2005:CD002041.
- Satran D, Henry CR, Adkinson C, et al. Cardiovascular manifestations of moderate to severe carbon monoxide poisoning. *J Am Coll Cardiol*. 2005;45:1513–6.
- World Health Organization's List of International Poison Control Centers www.who.int/ipcs/poisons/centre/directory/en.

 CODES

ICD9
986 Toxic effect of carbon monoxide

CLINICAL PEARLS
- The most appropriate intervention in the management of a CO-poisoned patient is a prompt removal from the source of CO and institution of 100% oxygen by high-flow face mask or endotracheal tube.
- Consider CO poisoning in younger patients with chest pain or ischemia.

CARDIAC ARREST

Aman D. Sabharwal, MD
Marc Grossman, MD

 BASICS

DESCRIPTION
- The absence of effective mechanical cardiac activity
- This section is not a substitute for an AHA-approved Advanced Cardiac Life Support (ACLS) course and is intended only as a quick reference.
- Synonym(s): Code blue in many institutions

Geriatric Considerations
Low rate of survival and poor long-term outcome. Be aware of Do Not Resuscitate orders on patients at risk.

Pediatric Considerations
Bradycardia is linked to hypoxia. Bradycardia is the most common initial form of cardiac arrest and is often the response to hypoxia. Adequate oxygenation and ventilation are critical.

Pregnancy Considerations
- Displace the uterus to the left either manually or by placing a rolled towel under the right hip. If the patient cannot be resuscitated within 5–15 minutes, consider emergency C-section to relieve uterine obstruction and increase blood return to the heart. This may also be done to save the fetus if fetus has reached gestational age of viability.
- Consider amniotic fluid embolism or eclampsia-related seizures as precipitating factors.

EPIDEMIOLOGY
- Predominant age: Risk increases with age
- Predominant sex: Male > Female

Incidence
0.5–1.5/1,000 persons per year

RISK FACTORS
- Male gender
- Advanced age
- Hypercholesterolemia
- HTN
- Cigarette smoking
- Family history of atherosclerosis
- Diabetes
- Cardiomyopathy
- Prolonged QT

ETIOLOGY
- Asystole (confirm in 2 leads)
- Ventricular fibrillation (VF)
- Pulseless ventricular tachycardia (VT)
- Pulseless electrical activity (PEA, previously known as electrical mechanical dissociation [EMD])
- Consider possible reversible causes (5 Hs and 4 Ts):
  – Hypoxia, severe hypovolemia, hyper- and hypokalemia [H+] (acidosis), hypothermia
  – Cardiac tamponade, tension pneumothorax, thrombosis (pulmonary embolism, myocardial infarction), tablets (medications and overdoses)

COMMONLY ASSOCIATED CONDITIONS
- Coronary artery disease/ACS (cardiac arrest may be presenting symptom)
- Valvular heart disease
- HTN

 DIAGNOSIS

- Loss of consciousness secondary to CNS hypoperfusion
- Absence of pulses in large arteries
- Apnea or agonal breathing
- Cyanosis or pallor

HISTORY
- Witnessed or unwitnessed
- Seizure activity
- History or risk factors
- Associated trauma

PHYSICAL EXAM
- Check pupils: May indicate drug overdose. Cannot interpret if patient has received atropine.
- Check pulse.
- Check lungs (i.e., did patient have respiratory decline prior to cardiac decline?).
- Check for dialysis shunt: Patients on dialysis are at increased risk for electrolyte imbalance causing arrest (especially hyperkalemia).

DIAGNOSTIC TESTS & INTERPRETATION
Lab
- Fingerstick glucose
- ABG
- Cardiac enzymes (troponin, CK, CK-MB); consider serial enzymes
- Chemistry and/or electrolyte panel
- CBC with platelets
- Drug levels (toxicology screen, acetaminophen/aspirin levels, history of specific medication (e.g., digoxin, antiepileptics)
- Blood type and cross, if indicated

Imaging
- CXR for endotracheal tube (ET) placement, pneumothorax; consider emergency echocardiogram for pericardial effusion and assessment of cardiac motion.
- Once stabilized, consider CT scan of brain.

Diagnostic Procedures/Surgery
- ECG
- 2-dimensional echocardiogram
- Airway management/intubation
- Peripheral IV access as close to central circulation as possible; intraosseous if no venous access. Avoid placement of central line during CPR. If must place during CPR, use femoral approach. Many medications may be administered by endotracheal tube if access otherwise unobtainable (double dose and flush with saline).
- Pericardiocentesis for cardiac tamponade
- Needle decompression/chest tube for pneumothorax

TREATMENT

- Prompt initiation of CPR, particularly chest compressions (push hard, push fast, and don't interrupt!), and immediate defibrillation (in witnessed VF and pulseless VT but not in PEA) are 1st priority (1)[A]:
  – In unwitnessed arrest, complete 1–2 minutes of CPR before attempting defibrillation (2)[A].
- Establishing IV access, intubation, and medications are 2nd priority.
- Continue CPR for 1–2 minutes following return of a potentially perfusing rhythm before stopping for pulse check, except for witnessed arrest with prompt return of rhythm following defibrillation.

MEDICATION
First Line
- Vascular access for medications: IV or intraosseous
- Consider medications after initiation of CPR and defibrillation attempt. Medications should be administered during CPR as soon as possible following a rhythm check.
- Epinephrine: 1 mg IV q3–5 min (1)[B] *OR* vasopressin 40 U IV single dose (1)[B] can be used once in lieu of the 1st or 2nd dose of epinephrine in VT or VF, but not in PEA:
  – Vasopressin is not recommended in children.
  – Pediatric dose of epinephrine: 0.01 mg/kg
- Atropine for asystole; consider in PEA with absolute bradycardia: 1 mg q3–5 min IV push to total dose of 3 mg (1)[C]:
  – Pediatric dose: 0.02 mg/kg
  – Minimum dose: 0.1 mg; maximum single dose is 0.5 mg in child, 1.0 mg in adolescent
- Magnesium sulfate: 1–2 g diluted in 10 mL D_5W IV push in suspected torsades de pointes (1)[B]:
  – Magnesium is relatively contraindicated in renal failure, but given the consequences of not correcting this rhythm, contraindication is only relative in this setting.
- Antiarrhythmics:
  – Consider if VT/VF unresponsive to 2–3 shocks and 1st dose of vasopressor
  – Amiodarone is drug preferred by AHA. Dosing: 300 mg IV push followed by 2nd dose of 150 mg IV (1)[B]
  – Amiodarone for perfusing tachyarrhythmias: Loading dose of 5 mg/kg IV or IO over 20–60 minutes, maximum dose 15 mg/kg/d
  – Lidocaine: Initial dose, 1–1.5 mg/kg IV; repeat loading dose of 1–1.5 mg/kg can be given at 5–10-minute intervals if VT/VF persist to maximum dose of 3 mg/kg (1)[C], then followed by drip if perfusing rhythm recovered

- Endotracheal medications (NAVEL): Narcan, atropine, vasopressin (and Valium), epinephrine, or lidocaine. Each may be placed in 5–10 mL of normal saline or sterile water and given by ET followed by bagging. Dosage should be 2–2.5 times recommended IV dose. IV or IO is preferred.

Second Line
- Procainamide: 30 mg/min IV in refractory VF/VT (maximum dose: 17 mg/kg) is permissible. However, because the time to a useful level by infusion is so long, it is unlikely to be of benefit in cardiac arrest, but may be useful in perfusing tachycardias (1)[C].
- Calcium: May be useful in hyperkalemia, ionized hypokalemia secondary multiple transfusions, and Ca+ channel blocker toxicity; otherwise, no clear benefit is shown
- High-dose epinephrine: No survival benefit is seen with high dose (0.1 mg/kg), but may be considered in exceptional situations, such as β-blocker or calcium channel blocker overdose.
- Bicarbonate: 1 mEq/kg IV only in known preexisting bicarbonate-responsive acidosis, hyperkalemia, or to alkalinize the urine in known responsive overdoses (i.e., tricyclics, aspirin). Also may be considered in patients with prolonged or unknown down-time (1)[C].

ADDITIONAL TREATMENT
General Measures
- Perform CPR: Fast (100/min) and hard, with minimal interruptions (1)[B]
- 80–100 bpm without interruption of CPR
- Sequence should be:
  – CPR
  – Rhythm check
  – Resume CPR
  – Shock/meds (charge defibrillator and administer drugs during CPR)
  – Continue CPR (after shocking) for 5 cycles before rechecking rhythm (repeat as needed) (1)[B]
- In VF/pulseless VT, 1 shock should be delivered, and continue sequence above (1)[B]:
  – Monophasic automatic external defibrillators (AEDs) initial and subsequent shocks at 360 J
  – Biphasic AEDs:
    ○ 150–200 J for biphasic truncated exponential waveform
    ○ 120 J for rectilinear biphasic waveform
    ○ If not specified on the biphasic defibrillator, use default of 200 J
  – Subsequent shocks should be same or higher energy
  – Pediatric manual defibrillation energy should be 2 J/kg for 1st attempt and 4 J/kg for following attempts.
- Consider possible causes of VT/VF, including hypoxia, hyperkalemia, hypokalemia, preexisting acidosis, drug overdose, and hypothermia.
- Administer 100% oxygen by bag-valve-mask or ET.

- IV and IO are preferred methods of medication administration, followed by ET tube.
- Start IV lines as close to the heart as possible. Large-bore peripheral lines can deliver fluid more quickly than a triple-lumen catheter (avoid central line placement during CPR).
- Use an end-tidal CO_2 monitor to assess gas exchange, if available. Esophageal intubation will produce a very low end-tidal CO_2 and requires proper reintubation (1). Use of sodium bicarbonate will increase ET-CO_2 levels.
- Consider termination of efforts if no reversible underlying cause is found.

Issues for Referral
- Consider communication with medical examiner's office.
- Consider communication with organ/tissue bank.

Additional Therapies
Consider mild therapeutic hypothermia after resuscitation (to 32–34°C for 12–24 hours if initial rhythm was VF). Most benefit is seen in VF as initial rhythm and short down-time (less than 25 minutes) but may be considered with any patient with return of spontaneous circulation (ROSC) and coma state.

IN-PATIENT CONSIDERATIONS
Initial Stabilization

- Decreasing the EMS response interval increases survival (1)[A].
- Home use of automatic external defibrillators does not improve survival (3).

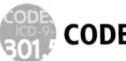 **ONGOING CARE**

FOLLOW-UP RECOMMENDATIONS
Patient Monitoring
Admit to ICU or CCU on continuous monitoring

PROGNOSIS
- Outcome is related to underlying disease, age, duration of arrest, and other factors.
- Outcome is poor if:
  – >4 minutes to CPR or >8 minutes to ACLS
  – Arrest occurs out of hospital
  – Resuscitation effort >30 minutes
- ~17% survive in-hospital arrest.
- ~1-10% survive to leave the hospital in out-of-hospital arrest, varying by geographic region.
- ~10-15% of those with VF survive.
- If arrest is out-of-hospital without return of vital signs from ALS prehospital care, patient is unlikely to respond to ED resuscitation efforts.
- If ROSC with coma, strongly consider induced hypothermia to improve neurologic outcome (number needed to treat in VF = 6).

COMPLICATIONS
- Significant neurologic, hepatic, renal, or cardiac ischemic injury
- Rib fractures, hemopneumothorax, abdominal organ injury from CPR

REFERENCES
1. Hypothermia after Cardiac Arrest Study Group. Mild therapeutic hypothermia to improve the neurologic outcome after cardiac arrest. *N Engl J Med*. 2002;346:549–56.
2. Wik L, Hansen TB, Fylling F, et al. Delaying defibrillation to give basic cardiopulmonary resuscitation to patients with out-of-hospital ventricular fibrillation: a randomized trial. *JAMA*. 2003;289:1389–95.
3. Bardy GH, Lee KL, Mark DB, et al. Home use of automated external defibrillators for sudden cardiac arrest. *N Engl J Med*. 2008;358:1793–804.

ADDITIONAL READING
2005 American Heart Association Guidelines for Cardiopulmonary Resuscitation and Emergency Cardiovascular Care. *Circulation*. 2005;112(Suppl I): IV-1–IV-203.

See Also (Topic, Algorithm, Electronic Media Element)
Algorithm: Coronary Syndrome, Acute

CODES

ICD9
427.5 Cardiac arrest

CLINICAL PEARLS
- Prompt initiation of CPR, particularly chest compressions (*push hard, push fast, and don't interrupt!*), and immediate defibrillation (in witnessed VF and pulseless VT but not in PEA) are 1st priority.
- In unwitnessed arrest, complete 1–2 minutes of CPR before attempting defibrillation.
- Get ECG following return of circulation to evaluate for acute coronary syndrome.
- Epinephrine is the first drug to give in any case requiring CPR:
  – Avoid use of central lines during CPR; intraosseous and endotracheal routes are preferred if peripheral access is not attainable.

C

CARDIAC TAMPONADE

Parag Goyal, MD
Rishi Vohora, DO

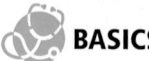 **BASICS**

DESCRIPTION

- A rapid or slow accumulation of fluid within the pericardium that causes compression of the chambers of the heart, impairing diastolic filling and ultimately leading to cardiovascular collapse.
- Tamponade can be acute or subacute, depending on the etiology:
  - Acute: Rapid accumulation (usually blood) within a stiff, noncompliant pericardium
  - Subacute: Gradual increase of a preexisting effusion, with limited accommodative pericardial stretch
- Variants include low-pressure and regional tamponade:
  - Low-pressure: Occurs when left- and right-sided pressures equalize at lower pressures; occurs when a decrease in intravascular volume makes an unchanged preexisting effusion hemodynamically significant (1)
  - Regional: Occurs when a loculation or hematoma limits diastolic filling

EPIDEMIOLOGY

Incidence
Difficult to assess due to absence of population-based studies

Prevalence
Difficult to assess due to absence of population-based studies

PATHOPHYSIOLOGY

- As a pericardial effusion accumulates, it overcomes the pericardium's intrinsic compliance yielding increased intrapericardial pressure. This pressure eventually exceeds intracardiac diastolic pressures, compresses the chambers of the heart, and limits diastolic filling with subsequent reduction of cardiac output.
- Diastolic filling is decreased first in the more compliant right-sided chambers (RA, then RV), followed by decrease of the left side. Tamponade is defined as the critical point at which diastolic equalization of the left and right ventricles occurs, total venous return drops, and cardiac output falls.
- The hemodynamic significance of the effusion depends on:
  - Rate of accumulation
  - Compliance of the pericardium to accommodate the enlarging effusion

ETIOLOGY

- Acute tamponade (most commonly from a rapidly accumulating hemopericardium, with sometimes as little as 50–100 mL of fluid):
  - Penetrating or blunt trauma
  - Iatrogenic instrumentation (cardiac surgery, central lines, pacer wire migration, peripherally inserted central catheter lines)
  - Aortic dissection
  - Rupture of cardiac free wall, ventricular aneurysm, or coronary artery. These most commonly occur during the postmyocardial infarction (MI) period.

- Subacute tamponade (any condition that causes a pericardial effusion) (2):
  - Idiopathic pericarditis (20%)
  - Iatrogenic effusions (16%) (see above)
  - Malignancy (13%): Breast, lung, lymphoma, leukemia, or radiation pericarditis
  - Idiopathic effusion (9%)
  - Acute MI (8%): Can complicate 15% of MIs and <1% of MIs treated with thrombolysis (2)
  - End-stage renal disease (ESRD) (6%): Usually blood urea nitrogen >60 mg/dL, but hemodialysis is an independent risk factor
  - Congestive heart failure (CHF) (5%): Effusions seen in 14% of CHF
  - Collagen vascular disease (5%): Systemic lupus erythematosus, rheumatoid arthritis (RA)
  - Infection (4%):
    ○ HIV
    ○ Bacterial infection: *Staphylococcus aureus*, *Mycobacterium tuberculosis*, *Streptococcus pneumoniae* (rare)
    ○ Fungal infection: *Histoplasmosis capsulatum*
    ○ Viral infection: Coxsackie group B, influenza, enteric cytopathogenic human orphan, herpes
  - Hypothyroidism with myxedema
  - Massive fluid resuscitation
  - Coagulopathies
- Low-pressure tamponade:
  - Patients with preexisting effusions who receive hemodialysis or diuretics thus reducing intravascular volume
- Regional tamponade:
  - Localized hematomas after cardiac surgery or post-MI

 DIAGNOSIS

HISTORY

- Dyspnea: Most sensitive symptom (88%) (2)
- Vague chest pain or an overall subjective sense of discomfort
- Syncope or presyncopal symptoms
- Altered mentation from poor perfusion
- Nausea or abdominal pain from hepatic venous engorgement
- In acute presentations, look for history of recent trauma, surgery, vascular instrumentation
- In subacute presentations, patients may have histories of known preexisting effusions with new or worsening exertional dyspnea.

PHYSICAL EXAM

- Only sign may be pulseless electrical activity
- Beck triad: Distant heart sounds, hypotension, distended neck veins:
  - Pertains specifically to acute tamponade
  - Subacute tamponade: Beck triad is often absent, and blood pressure (BP) may be normal or elevated (2).
- Most sensitive physical findings on exam (2):
  - Pulsus paradoxus (82%).
  - Tachypnea (80%)
  - Tachycardia (77%)
  - Jugular venous distention (76%)
- Pulsus paradoxus: Defined as an exaggerated drop in systolic blood pressure (SBP) (usually >10 mm Hg) during inspiration:

- This is due to the fact that the normal transmission of pressure from the intrapleural to intrapericardial cavity does not occur. Therefore, with inspiration, there is a relative decrease in the pressures across the pulmonary vascular bed with a relatively fixed left atrial pressure. This leads to decreased pulmonary venous drainage into the left atrium and therefore a decrease in left-sided stroke volume with inspiration (3).
  - Likelihood ratio (LR) for >12 mm Hg: 5.9; likelihood ratio (LR) for >10 mm Hg: 3.3
  - Can be absent in the settings of hypovolemia, severe AI, severe LV dysfunction, ASD, or in patients with positive-pressure ventilation (4)
  - Can also be seen in the setting of acute pulmonary embolus, RV infarction, and COPD
  - Can be false positive in severe lung disease
  - Performed best via sphygmomanometer by the following steps:
    ○ Insufflate cuff >20 mm Hg beyond systolic pressure.
    ○ Slowly deflate cuff and record pressure at which Korotkoff sounds are slightly audible at expiration only.
    ○ Further deflate cuff and record pressure at which Korotkoff sounds are equally audible at inspiration and expiration.
    ○ If these 2 pressures differ by >10 mm Hg, pulsus paradoxus is present.
- Respiratory distress, but with surprisingly little or no pulmonary edema
- Jugular venous distention with a rapid systolic (X) descent and absent diastolic (Y) descent
- Narrow pulse pressure (due to limited stroke volume and increased peripheral vascular resistance)
- Signs of cardiogenic shock: Low BP with poor mentation and cool, poorly perfused extremities
- Kussmaul sign (elevation of jugular venous distention with inspiration caused by increased right-sided pressure)
- Increased peripheral (right-sided) edema due to impaired venous return
- Right upper quadrant tenderness due to hepatic engorgement
- Increased area of cardiac dullness outside the apical point of maximum impulse

DIAGNOSTIC TESTS & INTERPRETATION

Electrocardiogram (ECG):

- Sinus tachycardia
- Low-voltage QRS, defined as <5 mm in limb leads and <10 mm in precordial leads; sensitivity of 42%
- Signs of pericarditis (except in uremic pericarditis): Initially diffuse ST segment elevation and PR segment depression of pericarditis; later stages exhibit T-wave inversions that may be transient or permanent
- Electrical alternans (QRS and/or P-wave beat-to-beat variation in axis and/or amplitude) is only seen in 10–20% of cases of tamponade. However, it is the most specific ECG finding for tamponade (4).

Lab
Initial lab tests
- Acute tamponade (trauma and preoperative labs):
  - Complete blood count (CBC), serum chemistries, coagulation panel, ethanol, drugs of abuse, UA

- Subacute tamponade (evaluate cause of the effusion):
  – CBC, serum chemistries, erythrocyte sedimentation rate, cardiac enzymes, antinuclear antibodies, rheumatoid factor
  – Fluid analysis of glucose, protein, cell count, lactate dehydrogenase, amylase, cholesterol, cytology, complement levels, Gram stain, and cultures (including bacterial, viral, acid-fast bacilli, and fungal cultures)

Imaging
Initial approach
- Chest radiograph:
  – May show enlargement of cardiac shadow (if >200 mL fluid present)
  – Cardiomegaly is 89% sensitive.
- Echocardiography (5):
  – Diastolic chamber collapse: RA collapse in late diastole (more sensitive 55–60%, less specific 50–68%) and RV collapse in early diastole (less sensitive 38–48%, more specific 84–100%) (3)
  – Doppler flow: An exaggerated increase through tricuspid valve (>40% variation) and exaggerated decrease (>25% variation) through mitral valve. High sensitivity (75%) and specificity (91%).
  – Inferior vena cava (IVC) distention with <50% collapse during inspiration (3)
  – Compression of pulmonary trunk
  – Paradoxical motion of interventricular septum
  – Swinging heart
- CT: Helpful in evaluating cause (i.e., aortic dissection) and characterizing the effusion (i.e., blood, pus, serous). A pericardial effusion with any of the following is suggestive of tamponade (3):
  – IVC diameter 2 × aorta
  – Reflux of contrast into IVC and/or azygous vein
  – Compression of coronary sinus
  – Flattening of anterior surface of heart and concave chamber deformity
  – Bowing of the IV septum into the LV
- MRI (3):
  – Can detect fluid collection as small as 30 mL
  – Highly effective in evaluating the composition of pericardial effusion
  – Use is limited due to emergent nature of tamponade.

Diagnostic Procedures/Surgery
Right heart catheterization:
- Diastolic pressures of RA and RV are increased and eventually equalize with the left-sided chambers and the intrapericardial pressure (usually at 15–20 mm Hg) (4).
- The dip and plateau pattern of constriction or restriction pericardial disease is absent.

DIFFERENTIAL DIAGNOSIS
- Any condition causing obstructive or cardiogenic shock, such as massive pulmonary embolism, tension pneumothorax, anterior wall MI, MI with valve rupture or dysfunction, or constrictive/restrictive pericarditis
- Of note, effusive-constrictive pericarditis can be especially difficult to distinguish from tamponade because it involves an effusion that is present with chamber collapse but is not the reason for the collapse. Differentiation can be made on echo by close examination of the diastolic filling patterns:
  – In tamponade, chamber filling is decreased but continuous throughout diastole.
  – In constrictive pericarditis, there is a surge of filling at the beginning of diastole, but is minimal during the rest of the diastolic cycle.

TREATMENT
MEDICATION
First Line
Fluid resuscitation:
- Fluid bolus is temporizing in acute setting.
- In subacute tamponade, most agree that while all patients do not universally benefit from fluid, those with hypotension do (6)[B].

Second Line
- Vasopressors if necessary: Dobutamine thought to maintain better cardiac output and delivery of oxygen than does norepinephrine.
- Benefit of inotropes is unclear.
- High-dose anti-inflammatory medications for pericarditis

ADDITIONAL TREATMENT
General Measures
- Maintain hemodynamic stability until definitive drainage.
- ICU monitoring
- Consider Swan-Ganz catheter if time allows.

Additional Therapies
- Hemodialysis for ESRD if patient is not in extremis (volume overload can be a cause for increasing pericardial effusions in ESRD)
- Minimize positive end expiratory pressure and pressure support if mechanically ventilated to preserve cardiac filling (4)[A].

SURGERY/OTHER PROCEDURES
Drainage is the definitive treatment (7)[A]. For acute traumatic tamponade: Prepare operating room for definitive cardiac repair via subxiphoid pericardotomy or full surgical thoracotomy. Pericardiocentesis is NOT the definitive treatment, as coagulated blood within the pericardium makes aspiration limited and hemorrhage from the cardiac injury usually refills the sac immediately. However, if there is hypotension despite fluid, a pericardiocentesis can be attempted in the emergency room (ER). For subacute tamponade: Pericardiocentesis may be guided by CT (98% success rate), fluoroscopy (93%), or ultrasound (93% for effusions >10 mm; only 58% in smaller effusions). Blind approach may be necessary in sudden cardiovascular collapse (73% success rate). An 18-G spinal needle is used, and, with the aid of a guide wire, a pigtail catheter can be introduced into the pericardium to prevent reaccumulation (7)[A]. The catheter can usually be pulled once it is draining <50 mL/d (4)[A]. If pericardiocentesis is unsuccessful in the setting of cardiovascular collapse, an immediate thoracotomy in ER is indicated (8)[B].

IN-PATIENT CONSIDERATIONS
Admission Criteria
Requires ICU-level monitoring

ONGOING CARE
FOLLOW-UP RECOMMENDATIONS
Follow-up echocardiogram may be used to evaluate for recurrence of effusions (7)[A].

PROGNOSIS
Acute traumatic tamponade: 70–80% survival rate quoted for level-1 trauma centers (8).

COMPLICATIONS
- Chamber lacerations
- Pneumothorax
- Ventricular tachycardia

REFERENCES
1. Sagristà-Sauleda J, Angel J, Sambola A, et al. Low-pressure cardiac tamponade: clinical and hemodynamic profile. *Circulation.* 2006;114: 945–52.
2. Roy CL, Minor MA, Brookhart MA, et al. Does this patient with a pericardial effusion have cardiac tamponade? *JAMA.* 2007;297:1810–8.
3. Restrepo CS, Lemos DF, Lemos JA, et al. Imaging findings in cardiac tamponade with emphasis on CT. *Radiographics.* 2007;27:1595–610.
4. Spodick DH. Acute cardiac tamponade. *N Engl J Med.* 2003;349:684–90.
5. Wann S, Passen E et al. Echocardiography in pericardial disease. *J Am Soc Echocardiogr.* 2008;21:7–13.
6. Sagristà-Sauleda J, Angel J, Sambola A, et al. Hemodynamic effects of volume expansion in patients with cardiac tamponade. *Circulation.* 2008;117:1545–9.
7. Cheitlin MD, Armstrong WF, Aurigemma GP, et al. ACC/AHA/ASE 2003 guideline update for the clinical application of echocardiography: summary article: a report of the American College of Cardiology/American Heart Association Task Force on Practice Guidelines (ACC/AHA/ASE Committee to Update the 1997 Guidelines for the Clinical Application of Echocardiography). *Circulation.* 2003;108:1146–62.
8. Fitzgerald M, et al. Definitive management of acute cardiac tamponade secondary to blunt trauma. *Emerg Med Australasia.* 2005;17:494–9.

ADDITIONAL READING
Hoit BD et al. Pericardial disease and pericardial tamponade. *Crit Care Med.* 2007;35:S355–64.

CODES
ICD9
423.3 Cardiac tamponade

CLINICAL PEARLS
- Pericardial tamponade is a potentially reversible cause of pulseless electrical activity: Perform emergent pericardiocentesis as diagnostic and therapeutic maneuver.
- Checking for pulsus parodoxicus may be a useful bedside maneuver with reasonable sensitivity in most cases, although nonspecific.
- Acute tamponade from trauma or intrapericardial rupture presents with much more rapid clinical deterioration than does subacute tamponade due to sudden rises in pericardial pressure and inability of the pericardium to stretch to accommodate the effusion.

C

CARDIOMYOPATHY, END STAGE

Timothy P. Fitzgibbons, MD

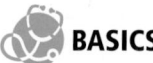 **BASICS**

DESCRIPTION

In 1995, the World Health Organization (WHO) defined cardiomyopathy as a "disease of the myocardium associated with cardiac dysfunction." The WHO proposed a classification system based on pathophysiology. Each class may be caused by many disorders, and some disorders may overlap classes:

- Classification of cardiomyopathy:
  – Dilated (systolic):
    ○ Characterized by dilation and reduced systolic function of 1 or both ventricles
  – Hypertrophic (diastolic):
    ○ Left and/or right ventricular hypertrophy with normal to reduced end diastolic volumes
    ○ May include asymmetric septal hypertrophy
    ○ Cause of sudden cardiac death in young athletes
  – Restrictive (diastolic):
    ○ Restrictive filling and reduced diastolic volume of either or both ventricles
    ○ Systolic function may be near normal.
    ○ Etiology: Idiopathic, amyloidosis, etc.
  – Arrhythmogenic right ventricular (RV) dysplasia:
    ○ Fibrofatty replacement of the RV
    ○ May present with arrhythmia or sudden cardiac death in the young
  – Unclassified:
    ○ Cases that do not fit easily into 1 group (i.e., noncompacted myocardium)
  – Specific: Includes patients with cardiomyopathy in association with a known systemic disorder:
    ○ Ischemic
    ○ Valvular
    ○ Hypertensive
    ○ Inflammatory
    ○ Metabolic
    ○ Peripartum
- End-stage cardiomyopathy patients have stage D heart failure or severe symptoms at rest refractory to standard medical therapy.
- System(s) affected: Cardiovascular; Renal

Pediatric Considerations
Etiology: Idiopathic, viral, congenital heart disease, and familial

Pregnancy Considerations
May occur in women postpartum

EPIDEMIOLOGY
Predominant age: Ischemic cardiomyopathy is the most common etiology; predominantly patients >50 years. Consider uncommon causes in young.

Incidence
- 60,000 patients <65 die each year from end-stage heart disease.
- 35,000–70,000 people might benefit from cardiac transplant or chronic support.

Prevalence
Most rapidly growing form of heart disease

RISK FACTORS
- Hypertension
- Hyperlipidemia
- Obesity
- Diabetes mellitus
- Smoking
- Physical inactivity
- Excessive alcohol intake
- Dietary sodium
- Obstructive sleep apnea
- Chemotherapy

Genetics
Hypertrophic, dilated cardiomyopathy, and arrhythmogenic RV dysplasia may present as familial syndromes with autosomal-dominant inheritance.

GENERAL PREVENTION
Reduce salt and water intake; home blood pressure (BP) and daily weight measurement

ETIOLOGY
The most frequent causes are in bold:
- **Ischemic heart disease: Most common etiology; up to 66% of patients**
- **Hypertension**
- **Familial cardiomyopathies**
- Congenital heart disease
- Peripartum/postpartum
- Toxic/metabolic causes:
  – **Alcoholism**
  – Radiation
  – Beriberi
  – Cobalt
  – Selenium deficiency
  – Thyrotoxicosis
- Infectious causes:
  – **Viral** (e.g., HIV, Coxsackie virus)
  – Diphtheria
  – Toxoplasmosis
  – Trichinosis
  – Trypanosomiasis
  – Acute rheumatic fever
- Inherited disorders of metabolism:
  – Glycogen storage disease
  – Pompe disease
  – Hurler syndrome
  – Hunter syndrome
  – Fabry disease
- Inherited neuromuscular disorders:
  – Duchenne muscular dystrophy
  – Friedreich ataxia
- Drugs:
  – Chemotherapy: Anthracyclines, cyclophosphamide, Herceptin

- Inflammatory/infiltrative causes:
  – Giant cell myocarditis
  – Loeffler eosinophilia
  – Sarcoidosis
  – Amyloidosis
  – Hemochromatosis
- Idiopathic
- Other causes:
  – **Tachycardia-mediated cardiomyopathy**
  – Valvular heart disease
  – Endomyocardial fibrosis

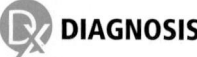 **DIAGNOSIS**

HISTORY
- Dyspnea at rest or with exertion
- Paroxysmal nocturnal dyspnea
- Orthopnea
- Postprandial dyspnea
- Right upper quadrant pain or bloating
- Fatigue
- Syncope
- Edema

PHYSICAL EXAM
- Tachypnea
- Low pulse pressure
- Cool extremities
- Jugular venous distention
- Bibasilar rales
- Tachycardia
- Displaced point of maximal impulse (PMI)
- S3 gallop
- Blowing systolic murmur
- Hepatosplenomegaly
- Ascites
- Edema

DIAGNOSTIC TESTS & INTERPRETATION
- Electrocardiogram: Left ventricular (LV) hypertrophy, interventricular conduction delay, atrial fibrillation, evidence of prior Q-wave infarction
- Cardiopulmonary exercise testing: Maximal oxygen consumption <10 mL/kg/mm correlates with 50% 1-year mortality, and >18 mL/kg/mm correlates with >90% 1-year survival. Used in stable outpatients to estimate prognosis and prior to cardiac transplant referral.

Lab
- Hyponatremia
- Prerenal azotemia
- Anemia
- Mild elevation in troponin
- Elevated B-type natriuretic peptide (BNP) or pro-BNP
- Mild hyperbilirubinemia
- Elevated liver function tests
- Elevated uric acid

Imaging
- Chest radiograph:
  - Cardiomegaly
  - Increased vascular markings to the upper lobes
  - Pleural effusions may or may not be present.
- Echocardiography:
  - In dilated cardiomyopathy, 4-chamber enlargement and global hypokinesis are present.
  - In hypertrophic cardiomyopathy, severe left ventricular (LV) hypertrophy is present.
  - Segmental contraction abnormalities of the LV are indicative of previous localized myocardial infarction.
- Cardiac magnetic resonance imaging:
  - May be useful to characterize certain nonischemic cardiomyopathies

Diagnostic Procedures/Surgery
Cardiac catheterization:
- Helpful to rule out ischemic heart disease
- Characterize hemodynamic severity
- Pulmonary artery catheters may be reasonable in patients with refractory heart failure (HF) to help guide management (1)[C].

DIFFERENTIAL DIAGNOSIS
- Severe pulmonary disease
- Primary pulmonary hypertension
- Recurrent pulmonary embolism
- Constrictive pericarditis
- Hypothyroidism
- Some advanced forms of malignancy
- Anemia
- Chronic illness

TREATMENT

See "Congestive Heart Failure" for detailed treatment protocols.

MEDICATION
First Line
- Systolic failure syndromes:
  - Angiotensin-converting enzyme (ACE) inhibitors:
    - Lisinopril, 5–40 mg/d or captopril, 6.25–50 mg t.i.d. (1)[A]
  - Loop diuretics:
    - May need to be given IV initially and then orally as patient stabilizes
    - Furosemide 40–120 mg/d or t.i.d. (1)[A]
  - β-blockers:
    - Use with caution in acutely decompensated or low cardiac output states.
    - Metoprolol succinate, 12.5–200 mg/d; carvedilol, 3.125–25 mg b.i.d.; or bisoprolol, 1.25–10 mg/d (1)[A]
  - Aldosterone antagonists:
    - Patients with New York Heart Association (NYHA) III-IV congestive heart failure (CHF), ejection fraction (EF) <35%, on standard therapy; spironolactone, 12.5–25 mg/d (2)[A]
  - Digoxin, 0.125–0.250 mg/d for symptomatic patients on standard therapy (1)[A]

- Diastolic failure:
  - Few evidence-based therapies for diastolic heart failure. Empiric management goals include:
    - Management of hypertension
    - Reduction of congestive states (i.e., diuretics)
    - Prevention of progression of left ventricular hypertrophy (i.e., renin-angiotensin-aldosterone system blockade)
    - Maintenance of sinus rhythm
- Contraindications:
  - β-blockers: Low cardiac output, 1st- or 2nd-degree heart block
  - Ca-blockers (non-dihydropyridine): Low cardiac output, heart block
  - Aldosterone antagonists: Oliguria, anuria, renal dysfunction
  - Loop diuretics: Hypokalemia, hypomagnesemia
  - ACE inhibitors: Pregnancy, angioedema
- Precautions:
  - In patients with chronic kidney disease, digoxin dosage should be 0.125 mg/d or less, and drug levels followed carefully to avoid toxicity.
  - Closely monitor electrolytes.
  - ACE inhibitors: Initiate with care if BP is low. Begin with low-dose captopril, such as 6.25 mg t.i.d.
  - β-blockers: Avoid in patients with evidence of poor tissue perfusion; they may further depress systolic function.
  - Milrinone, amrinone: Contraindicated for long-term use due to increased mortality

Second Line
- Combination hydralazine/isosorbide dinitrate is recommended in addition to standard treatment in African American patients with class III–IV symptoms (1)[A], and for all patients with reduced EF and symptoms incompletely responsive to ACE inhibitor and beta blocker (3).
- Angiotensin receptor blockers as an alternative to, or in addition to, ACE inhibitors
- Inotropic therapy (e.g., dobutamine or milrinone) for support prior to surgery or cardiac transplantation

ADDITIONAL TREATMENT
General Measures
- Reduction of filling pressures
- Treatment of electrolyte disturbances

Issues for Referral
Management by a heart failure team improves outcomes and facilitates early transplant referral.

Additional Therapies
- Prophylactic implantable cardioverter defibrillator (ICD) should be considered for patients with an LVEF <30% (1)[A].
- Biventricular pacing should be considered for patients with QRS interval >120 ms, LVEF <35%, and class III CHF despite medical therapy (1)[A]. MADIT-CRT data suggests patients with class II and possibly class I may also benefit (4)[A].
- Patients with severe, refractory HF with no reasonable expectation of improvement should not be considered for an ICD (1)[C].
- Consideration of an LV assist device as "permanent" or destination therapy is reasonable in selected stage D patients.

ONGOING CARE

DIET
Low fat, low salt, fluid restriction

PROGNOSIS
20–40% of patients in NYHA functional class IV die within 1 year. With a transplant, a 1-year survival is as high as 94%.

COMPLICATIONS
Worsening CHF, syncope, renal failure, arrhythmias, or sudden death

REFERENCES
1. Richardson P, McKenna W, Bristow M, et al. Report of the 1995 World Health Organization/International Society and Federation of Cardiology Task Force on the Definition and Classification of cardiomyopathies. *Circulation*. 1996;93:841–2.
2. Nohria A, Lewis E, Stevenson LW. Medical management of advanced heart failure. *JAMA*. 2002;287:628–40.
3. 2009 Focused update: ACCF/AHA guidelines for the diagnosis and management of heart failure in adults: a report of the American College of Cardiology Foundation/American Heart Association Task Force on Practice Guidelines. *Circulation*. 2009;119:1977–2016.
4. Moss AJ, Hall WJ, Cannom DS, et al. Cardiac-Resynchronization Therapy for the Prevention of Heart-Failure Events. *N Engl J Med*. 2009.

ADDITIONAL READING
Hunt SA, et al. ACC/AHA 2005 guideline update for the diagnosis and management of chronic heart failure in adults. *J Am Coll Cardiol*. 2005;46:1116–43.

See Also (Topic, Algorithm, Electronic Media Element)
Alcohol Withdrawal; Alcohol Abuse and Dependence; Amyloidosis; Congestive Heart Failure; Diabetes Mellitus, Type 1; Diabetes Mellitus, Type 2; Hypertension; Hypothyroidism, Adult; Idiopathic Hypertrophic Subaortic Stenosis; Malnutrition, Protein-Calorie; Rheumatic Fever; Sarcoidosis

CODES

ICD9
- 425.4 Other primary cardiomyopathies
- 425.5 Alcoholic cardiomyopathy
- 425.8 Cardiomyopathy in other diseases classified elsewhere

C

CAROTID SINUS SYNDROME

George E. Kikano, MD

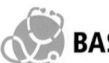 **BASICS**

DESCRIPTION

- Baroreceptors in the carotid sinus and aortic arch normally influence blood pressure (BP) and heart rate. An endogenous increase in BP or external pressure on the carotid sinus increases the baroreceptor firing rate and activates vagal efferents, resulting in a bradycardia and/or drop in BP.
- In carotid sinus syndrome, stimulation of 1 or both hypersensitive carotid sinuses may produce brief episodes of faintness or loss of consciousness.
- Carotid sinus syndrome is defined as an asystole of ≥ 3 seconds and/or a drop in systolic BP of ≥ 50 mm Hg elicited by cardiac sinus pressure.
- 4 types are described:
  - Cardioinhibitory: Vagally mediated, causing bradycardia, sinus arrest, or atrioventricular block for >3 seconds
  - Vasodepressor: A sudden drop of peripheral vascular resistance leads to a >50 mm Hg decrease in systolic BP without change in heart rate, or to a >30 mm Hg symptomatic drop in systolic BP.
  - Mixed: Combined cardioinhibitory and vasodepressor changes
  - Cerebral: Extremely rare; carotid sinus hypersensitivity occurs without bradycardia or hypotension.
- System(s) affected: Cardiovascular; Nervous
- Synonym(s): Carotid sinus syncope; Carotid sinus hypersensitivity

EPIDEMIOLOGY
- Predominant age: Elderly
- Predominant sex: Male > Female (2:1)

Geriatric Considerations
- More likely to occur in elderly
- Can be a cause of unexplained frequent falls

Incidence
- 35 million cases are reported every year.
- Incidence increases with age

Prevalence
- In 2 large studies of patients with syncope, 6–14% had carotid sinus hypersensitivity.
- In patients >80 years of age with unexplained syncope, prevalence of carotid sinus syndrome may be as high as 40%.

RISK FACTORS
- Diffuse atherosclerosis
- Age

ETIOLOGY
- Idiopathic
- Carotid body tumors
- Inflammatory and malignant lymph nodes in the neck
- Metastatic cancer

COMMONLY ASSOCIATED CONDITIONS
- Sick sinus syndrome
- Atrioventricular block
- Coronary artery disease

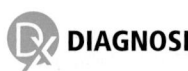 **DIAGNOSIS**

HISTORY
- Syncope
- Unexplained falls
- Abnormal gait and balance
- Absence of postictal symptoms

PHYSICAL EXAM
- Bradycardia
- Hypotension
- Pallor
- Abnormal visual acuity
- Diaphoresis
- Orthostatic vital signs (exclude orthostatic hypotension)

DIAGNOSTIC TESTS & INTERPRETATION
Electrocardiogram (ECG)

Imaging
Carotid duplex scan

Diagnostic Procedures/Surgery
- Special test: Unilateral carotid sinus pressure "massage" for 5–10 seconds:
  - With the patient in the supine position and while the BP and ECG are monitored, manual pressure on the carotid sinus causes asystole or reproduces the symptoms (commonly but somewhat erroneously termed "massage")
  - Diagnostic yield may be increased by combining with tilt-table testing.
  - Contraindications to this test include:
    ○ Carotid bruit
    ○ History of stroke or transient ischemic attack
    ○ Recent myocardial infarction
    ○ History of ventricular tachycardia or fibrillation
- The test can be falsely positive in elderly patients.

Pathological Findings
Pressure on the carotid sinus causes asystole of >3 seconds (cardioinhibitory) and/or a drop in systolic BP ≥ 50 mm Hg.

DIFFERENTIAL DIAGNOSIS
- Neurocardiogenic syncope
- Postural hypotension
- Primary autonomic insufficiency
- Hypovolemia
- Dysrhythmias
- Sick sinus syndrome
- Cerebrovascular insufficiency
- Other causes of syncope

TREATMENT

MEDICATION

First Line

- Anticholinergics: Atropine (acutely) for cardioinhibitory type
- α-Sympathomimetics: Ephedrine, midodrine
- Precautions: Concomitant usage of digitalis, β-blockers, clonidine, and α-methyldopa may accentuate response to carotid sinus massage.

Second Line

Fludrocortisone can be used to improve orthostatic symptoms in patients with vasodepressor response.

ADDITIONAL TREATMENT

General Measures

- No treatment is required for asymptomatic individuals.
- Support hose may help with vasodepressor symptoms.
- Dietary high-salt intake may be helpful.

Issues for Referral

Symptomatic patients need to be referred for further evaluation.

SURGERY/OTHER PROCEDURES

- Carotid sinus denervation by surgery or radiation therapy for selected patients
- Adventitial stripping is a surgical technique that is effective and relatively safe in many patients.
- Permanent pacing may help prevent recurrent symptoms in patients with cardioinhibitory component.
- Carotid endarterectomy for patients with atheroma

 ONGOING CARE

PATIENT EDUCATION

- Avoid pressure on the neck, tight collars, and neckties.
- Restrictions on driving or other potentially hazardous activities until cleared by the physician
- Take medications as prescribed.
- Avoid medications that might cause hypotension.

PROGNOSIS

- May be serious if syncope is associated with atheromatous narrowing of sinus artery or basilar artery
- Recurrence rate is difficult to quantify.

COMPLICATIONS

- Frequent falls, leading to injuries and fractures
- Rarely, sudden death from asystole

ADDITIONAL READING

- ACC/AHA/NASPE 2002 Guideline update for implantation of cardiac pacemakers and antiarrhythmia devices: Summary article. A report of the American College of Cardiology/American Heart Association task force on practice guidelines (ACC/AHA/NASPE committee to update the 1998 pacemaker guidelines).
- Alboni P, Brignole M, Menozzi C, et al. Diagnostic value of history in patients with syncope with or without heart disease. *J Am Coll Cardiol*. 2001;37:1921–8.
- Bartoletti A, Fabiani P, Bagnoli L, et al. Physical injuries caused by a transient loss of consciousness: main clinical characteristics of patients and diagnostic contribution of carotid sinus massage. *Eur Heart J*. 2008;29:618–24.

- Davies AJ, Kenny RA. Frequency of neurologic complications following carotid sinus massage. *Am J Cardiol*. 1998;81:1256–7.
- Humm AM, Mathias CJ. Unexplained syncope–is screening for carotid sinus hypersensitivity indicated in all patients aged >40 years? *J Neurol Neurosurg Psychiatry*. 2006;77:1267–70.
- Kenny RA, Richardson DA, Steen N, et al. Carotid sinus syndrome: a modifiable risk factor for nonaccidental falls in older adults (SAFE PACE). *J Am Coll Cardiol*. 2001;38:1491–6.
- Kerr SR, Pearce MS, Brayne C, et al. Carotid sinus hypersensitivity in asymptomatic older persons: implications for diagnosis of syncope and falls. *Arch Intern Med*. 2006;166:515–20.
- Mathias CJ, Deguchi K, Schatz I. Observations on recurrent syncope and presyncope in 641 patients. *Lancet*. 2001;357:348–53.

See Also (Topic, Algorithm, Electronic Media Element)

Syncope

 CODES

ICD9
337.01 Carotid sinus syndrome

CLINICAL PEARLS

- Pressure on the carotid sinus causes asystole of >3 seconds (cardioinhibitory) and/or a drop in systolic BP ≥50 mm Hg, reproducing symptoms.
- It is clinically important to distinguish carotid sinus syndrome from sick sinus syndrome.
- The finding of carotid sinus hypersensitivity does not exclude other causes of syncope.

CAROTID STENOSIS

Charles Strom, MD
Jeremy Golding, MD

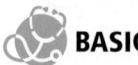 **BASICS**

DESCRIPTION
- Narrowing of carotid artery lumen, typically due to atherosclerotic changes in the vessel wall. Atherosclerotic plaques are responsible for 90% of extracranial carotid lesions and up to 30% of all ischemic strokes.
- Carotid lesions classified by:
  - Symptom status
    - Asymptomatic: Tend to be homogenous and stable
    - Symptomatic (stroke, transient cerebral ischemic event): Tend to be heterogeneous and unstable
  - Degree of stenosis
    - High grade: 80–99% stenosis
    - Moderate grade: 50–79% stenosis
    - Low grade: <50% stenosis

EPIDEMIOLOGY
More common in men and with increasing age (see Risk Factors)

Incidence
Unclear (asymptomatic patients often go undiagnosed)

Prevalence
- Of patients aged >50 years, 4.8% of men and 2.2% of women have moderate (≥50%) stenosis (1).
- Of patients aged >70 years, moderate stenosis affects 12.5% of men and 6.9% of women (1).

RISK FACTORS
- Nonmodifiable factors: Advanced age, hypercoagulable states, male sex, family history, carotid bruit, cardiac disease, race (African American, Latino)
- Modifiable factors: Smoking, hyperlipidemia, sedentary lifestyle, elevated body mass index, use of oral contraceptive pills, hypertension (HTN), diabetes mellitus, history of transient ischemic attack (TIA) or stroke, EtOH/drug abuse, low serum folate levels, elevated anticardiolipin antibodies, fibrinogen, or homocysteine levels

Genetics
Increased incidence among family members:
- Direct genetic factors (increased carotid artery stenosis/plaque formation seen in homozygotes):
  - apoE lipoprotein [varepsilon]4 polymorphism
  - TT Leu554Phe E-selectin variant
  - Apolipoprotein 5 (APOA5) 56C >G variant
- Genetically linked factors:
  - Hypercoagulability, diabetes mellitus, race, HTN, family history, obesity

GENERAL PREVENTION
- Antihypertensive therapy
- Statin therapy in appropriate candidates

PATHOPHYSIOLOGY
Atherosclerosis formation begins during adolescence, consistently at carotid bifurcation. The carotid bulb has unique blood-flow dynamics. Hemodynamic disturbances cause endothelial injury and dysfunction. Plaque formation in vessel wall results, and stenosis then ensues.

ETIOLOGY
Initial cause not well understood, but certain risk factors are frequently present (see Risk Factors). Tensile stress on the vessel wall, turbulence, and arterial wall shear stress seem to be involved.

COMMONLY ASSOCIATED CONDITIONS
- TIA/stroke
- Coronary artery disease (CAD)/myocardial infarction (MI)
- Peripheral vascular disease (PVD)
- HTN
- Diabetes mellitus
- Hyperlipidemia
- Hypercoagulable states

 DIAGNOSIS

Screening for carotid stenosis is not recommended. However, in the setting of symptoms suggestive of stroke or TIA, workup for this condition may be indicated.

HISTORY
- Identification of modifiable and nonmodifiable comorbidities (see Risk Factors)
- History of cerebral ischemic event
- Stroke, TIA, amaurosis fugax (monocular blindness), aphasia
- CAD/MI
- PVD
- Full review of systems, with focus on risk factors for:
  - Cardiovascular disease
  - Stroke (HTN and arrhythmia)

PHYSICAL EXAM
- Lateralizing neurologic deficits:
  - Contralateral motor and/or sensory deficit
- Monocular blindness (amaurosis fugax):
  - Hollenhorst plaques on retinal examination
- Cerebellar abnormalities:
  - Binocular vision loss, falls without syncope, vertigo, loss of coordination
- Carotid bruit (low sensitivity and specificity)

DIAGNOSTIC TESTS & INTERPRETATION
Lab
Initial lab tests
- Complete blood count with differential
- Basic metabolic panel
- ESR (if temporal arteritis a consideration)
- Glucose/HbA1c
- Fasting lipid profile
- Hypercoagulable workup if (+) risk factors

Follow-Up & Special Considerations
Proceed to imaging if suggestion of stenosis from history or physical examination.

Imaging
Initial approach
Duplex ultrasound identifies ≥50% stenosis with 98% sensitivity and 88% specificity (2)[A]. Doppler ultrasound determines degree of stenosis by assessing velocity of blood flow through stenotic vessel. Although findings should be confirmed by angiogram (magnetic resonance [MR], computed tomography [CT], or contrast), ultrasound is increasingly used to screen prior to surgical assessment.

Follow-Up & Special Considerations
Other noninvasive imaging techniques can add detail to duplex results:
- CT angiography:
  - 88% sensitivity and 100% specificity
  - Requires contrast load with risk for subsequent renal morbidity
- MR angiography:
  - 95% sensitivity and 90% specificity (3)[A]
  - Evaluates cerebral circulation (extracranial and intracranial) as well as aortic arch and common carotid artery
  - Tends to overestimate degree of stenosis

Diagnostic Procedures/Surgery
Contrast angiography is the traditional gold standard for diagnosis:
- Delineates anatomy pertaining to aortic arch and proximal vessels
- However, procedure is invasive and has multiple risks:
  - Dye allergy and renal toxicity
  - Stroke
  - Should be used only when other tests are not conclusive

Pathological Findings
- Stenosis consistently occurs at carotid bifurcation, with plaque formation most often at proximal internal carotid artery:
  - Plaque thickest at carotid bifurcation
  - Plaque occupies intima and inner media, avoids outer media and adventitia

- Plaque histology:
  - Homogenous (stable) plaques, seldom hemorrhage or ulcerate:
    o Fatty streak and fibrous tissue deposition
    o Diffuse intimal thickening
  - Heterogenous (unstable) plaques, may hemorrhage or ulcerate:
    o Presence of lipid-laden macrophages, necrotic debris, cholesterol crystals
    o Ulcerated plaques
  - Soft and gelatinous clots with platelets, fibrin, and red and white blood cells

DIFFERENTIAL DIAGNOSIS
- Aortic valve stenosis
- Aortic arch atherosclerosis
- Arrhythmia with cardiogenic embolization
- Migraine
- Brain tumor
- Metabolic disturbances
- Functional/psychologic deficit
- Seizure

TREATMENT

Smoking cessation, good control of blood pressure, and use of antiplatelet medication and statin medication is the primary treatment for both asymptomatic and symptomatic carotid stenosis (4).

MEDICATION
- Antihypertensives:
  - Thiazide diuretic ± angiotensin-converting enzyme inhibitor (5)[A]
- Statins (5)[A]
- Antiplatelet (5)[A] agents:
  - Aspirin 81–325 mg daily
  - Clopidogrel 75 mg daily
  - Aspirin/dipyridamole

ADDITIONAL TREATMENT
General Measures
- Lifestyle modifications
- Control of HTN, generally with target <140/90
- Avoidance of cigarettes
- Dietary control and weight loss

Issues for Referral
- For acute symptomatic stroke, order imaging and contact neurology.
- For known carotid stenosis, some suggest duplex imaging every 6 months if stenosis is >50% and patient is a surgical candidate.

SURGERY/OTHER PROCEDURES
Goal: Prevention of stroke:
- Carotid endarterectomy (CEA) may be indicated in:
  - Asymptomatic patients with >60–70% stenosis, but the absolute reduction in stroke risk is small, and long-term benefit is critically dependent upon low perioperative stroke rate (≤3% morbidity and mortality). CEA for asymptomatic carotid disease remains controversial.
  - Symptomatic patients: Number needed to treat (NNT) to prevent 1 disabling stroke or death over 2–6 years is 15 for patients with severe stenosis (stenosis >70–80%) and 21 for patients with less severe stenosis (50–70%). Good outcomes depend upon surgeons and centers with <6% perioperative stroke risk.

- Regional anesthesia may be preferable to general (fewer strokes, arrhythmias, and MIs).
- Carotid angioplasty with stent placement is an alternative option in symptomatic high-risk patients with >80% stenosis.

IN-PATIENT CONSIDERATIONS
Initial Stabilization
Rapid evaluation for symptoms compatible with TIA should be obtained in the emergency department or inpatient setting.

Admission Criteria
Any patient with presentation of acute symptomatic carotid stenosis should be hospitalized for further diagnostic workup and appropriate therapy.

IV Fluids
Not necessary

Discharge Criteria
24–48 hours post-CEA, if ambulating, taking adequate p.o. intake, and neurologically intact

ONGOING CARE

FOLLOW-UP RECOMMENDATIONS
Patient Monitoring
After CEA, overnight in postanesthesia care unit or step-down:
- Duplex at 2–6 weeks postop
- Duplex every 6–12 months

DIET
- NPO postop (in case return to operating room)
- Low fat, low cholesterol, low salt at discharge

PATIENT EDUCATION
- Signs and symptoms of TIA/stroke:
  - Lateralizing neurologic deficits, monocular blindness, aphasia
- Diet and lifestyle modification

PROGNOSIS
Risk proportional to degree of stenosis

COMPLICATIONS
- Untreated:
  - TIA/stroke
- Postoperative (s/p CEA):
  - Perioperative (within 30 days):
    o Stroke/death, cranial nerve injury, hemorrhage, hemodynamic instability, MI (because of comorbid CAD)
  - Late (>30 days postop):
    o Recurrent stenosis, false aneurysm at surgical site

REFERENCES

1. de Weerd M, Greving JP, de Jong AW, et al. Prevalence of Asymptomatic Carotid Artery Stenosis According to Age and Sex. Systematic Review and Metaregression Analysis. *Stroke*. 2009.
2. Jahromi AS, Cinà CS, Liu Y, et al. Sensitivity and specificity of color duplex ultrasound measurement in the estimation of internal carotid artery stenosis: a systematic review and meta-analysis. *J Vasc Surg*. 2005;41:962–72.
3. Nederkoorn PJ, van der Graaf Y, Hunink MG. Duplex ultrasound and magnetic resonance angiography compared with digital subtraction angiography in carotid artery stenosis: a systematic review. *Stroke*. 2003;34:1324–32.
4. *Cochrane Database Syst Rev*. 2010;(2):CD005953.
5. Sacco RL, Adams R, Albers G, et al. Guidelines for prevention of stroke in patients with ischemic stroke or transient ischemic attack: a statement for healthcare professionals from the American Heart Association/American Stroke Association Council on Stroke: co-sponsored by the Council on Cardiovascular Radiology and Intervention: the American Academy of Neurology affirms the value of this guideline. *Stroke*. 2006;37:577–617.

ADDITIONAL READING

Barnett HJ, Taylor DW, Eliasziw M, et al. Benefit of carotid endarterectomy in patients with symptomatic moderate or severe stenosis. North American Symptomatic Carotid Endarterectomy Trial Collaborators. *N Engl J Med*. 1998;339:1415–25.

See Also (Topic, Algorithm, Electronic Media Element)
Algorithms: Transient Ischemic Attack; Stroke; Hypercholesterolemia

CODES

ICD9
433.10 Occlusion and stenosis of carotid artery without mention of cerebral infarction

CLINICAL PEARLS
- Atherosclerosis is responsible for 90% of all cases of carotid artery stenosis.
- The greater the degree of stenosis, the greater the risk of embolism and stroke.
- Amaurosis fugax (monocular blindness) is often described as "curtain pulled over eye" and is concerning for further ischemic events.
- Duplex is the best initial imaging modality.
- Medical management is the cornerstone of treatment, with surgical management in carefully selected cases and situations

CARPAL TUNNEL SYNDROME

Jay U. Howington, MD

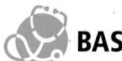 **BASICS**

DESCRIPTION

- Carpal tunnel syndrome is the most common cause of peripheral nerve compression.
- The median nerve is compressed as it traverses the carpal tunnel in the wrist and hand.
- The tunnel is composed of the carpal bones dorsally and the transverse carpal ligament ventrally. It contains flexor tendons and the median nerve.
- Symptoms tend to affect the dominant hand, but >50% of patients experience bilateral symptoms.
- System(s) affected: Musculoskeletal; Nervous

Pregnancy Considerations
Not uncommon during pregnancy

EPIDEMIOLOGY

- Predominant age: 40–60
- Predominant sex: Female > Male (3:1–10:1) (1)

Incidence
- Two peaks: Late 50s in women and late 70s when the sex ratio is more equal
- Older patients tend to have more severe carpal tunnel syndrome (59% >65 have thenar atrophy) (2).

Prevalence
Most common entrapment neuropathy. Most recent estimates of prevalence indicate that the disorder occurs in 346/100,000 population.

RISK FACTORS

- No clear evidence that repetitive flexion and extension of the wrist may influence the development of carpal tunnel syndrome.
- Occupation as a seamstress or computer operator may exacerbate carpal tunnel syndrome. There is, however, no universal agreement that carpal tunnel syndrome is job-related.
- Obesity is a risk factor in younger patients.

Genetics
Unknown; however, a familial type has been reported.

GENERAL PREVENTION
Take a break once an hour when doing repetitive work involving hands.

ETIOLOGY

- Disorders affecting the musculoskeletal system in the region of the wrist, including:
  - Trauma or Colles fracture
  - Degenerative joint disease
  - Rheumatoid arthritis
  - Ganglion cyst
  - Scleroderma
- Hypothyroidism and diabetes are frequently associated with this condition, which also occurs with increased frequency during pregnancy.

- Other miscellaneous causes include:
  - Acromegaly
  - Lupus erythematosus
  - Leukemia
  - Pyogenic infections
  - Sarcoidosis
  - Primary amyloidosis
  - Paget disease
- Hyperparathyroidism, hypocalcemia

COMMONLY ASSOCIATED CONDITIONS
- Diabetes
- Obesity
- Pregnancy

 DIAGNOSIS

HISTORY
- Burning pain and/or tingling in the fingers, particularly at night (acroparesthesias):
  - The altered sensation (tingling or prickling) is characteristically confined to the thumb and the index and middle fingers, but many patients do not distinguish this localization and feel the entire hand is affected.
- Arm pain
- Symptoms characteristically are relieved by shaking or rubbing the hands.
- During waking hours, symptoms occur when driving the car, reading the newspaper, and occasionally when using the hands for repetitive maneuvers.

PHYSICAL EXAM

- Positive Tinel sign: Tapping of the wrist proximal to the carpal tunnel may produce electric sensation perceived by the patient, a sign of nerve compression (50% sensitivity and 77% specificity) (3)[A].
- Positive Phalen sign: Holding the wrist flexed for 60 seconds may precipitate the paresthesias experienced by the patient (68% sensitivity and 73% specificity) (3)[A].
- Finger sensory loss
- Wasting of the thenar and hypothenar muscles is a late sign.
- Weakness of the hand, however, for such tasks as opening jars is often noted by the patient early in the disorder.

DIAGNOSTIC TESTS & INTERPRETATION
Lab
- No laboratory test is diagnostic.
- Normal serum TSH and normal serum glucose may be helpful in excluding conditions associated with carpal tunnel syndrome.

Initial lab tests
- Special tests:
  - Electromyography:
    - Will be abnormal in >85% of cases
    - Prolonged distal latency of the median motor nerves may be seen.
    - The most sensitive indicator is the median sensory distal latency, which is prolonged. Further, the sensory nerve action potential may be reduced or unobtainable.
    - Not required as a diagnostic test where clinical symptoms are well defined or to predict surgical outcome (3)[A]
- Stimulation of the ulnar nerve should be done as well to exclude generalized polyneuropathy.

Imaging
Initial approach
- Special radiographic views of the carpal tunnel may be obtained. These are of limited usefulness unless heterotopic calcification can be identified.
- Magnetic resonance neurography may be used to confirm compression of the median nerve in the carpal tunnel and to assess the success of surgical decompression.

Diagnostic Procedures/Surgery
A BP tourniquet to cut off circulation to the arm may precipitate symptoms promptly.

DIFFERENTIAL DIAGNOSIS
- Cervical spondylosis
- Generalized peripheral neuropathy
- Brachial plexus lesion
- Pronator syndrome
- Anterior interosseous syndrome

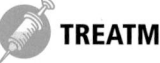 **TREATMENT**

MEDICATION
First Line
NSAIDs such as ibuprofen, 800 mg b.i.d. or t.i.d., or naproxen sodium, 500 mg b.i.d., may provide significant relief of symptoms in many patients:
- Contraindications: GI intolerance
- Precautions: GI side effects of NSAIDs may preclude their use in selected patients.

Second Line
Oral steroid

ADDITIONAL TREATMENT
General Measures
- Splinting of the wrist in extension while sleeping may provide significant relief of symptoms. Prolonged use of splinting, if possible, may allow some symptoms to resolve.
- Injection of the carpal tunnel with steroid may provide significant temporary relief. This is particularly useful during pregnancy. Can be expected to provide relief for up to 1 month or longer.
- The combination of splinting and steroid injections provides long-term relief in only 10% of cases and is not better than either treatment in isolation (4,5)[A].

COMPLEMENTARY AND ALTERNATIVE MEDICINE
Despite studies, no data exists to support use of vitamin B_6 in the prevention or treatment of carpal tunnel syndrome.

SURGERY/OTHER PROCEDURES
- Surgical decompression of the carpal tunnel by dividing the transverse carpal ligament completely provides almost total relief of symptoms in >95% of patients.
- Surgical decompression is usually done as an outpatient procedure under local anesthesia.
- Healing of the incision generally takes 2 weeks; an additional 2 weeks of recuperation may be required before the hand can be fully used for tasks requiring strength.
- Recent randomized, controlled studies indicate that surgery is more effective than splinting at 18 months (6,7)[A].
- Open vs endoscopic procedures produce similar outcomes at 1 year and approach should be driven based upon surgeon and patient preference (8)[A].

IN-PATIENT CONSIDERATIONS
Initial Stabilization
- Outpatient
- Outpatient surgery

 ONGOING CARE

FOLLOW-UP RECOMMENDATIONS
Patient Monitoring
- Patients treated with wrist splints or other palliative measures such as cortisone injections will require follow-up in the ensuing 4–12 weeks to assess the success of treatment modalities.
- Patients treated surgically rarely experience recurrence of the disorder. Routine follow-up once healing of the incision has occurred is not necessary.

PATIENT EDUCATION
Carpal Tunnel Syndrome Foundation. For patient education materials favorably reviewed on this topic, contact: American Academy of Family Physicians Foundation, P.O. Box 8418, Kansas City, MO 64114, (800) 274-2237, Ext. 4400.

PROGNOSIS
Untreated, more severe cases of the condition can be expected to lead to numbness and weakness in the hand, with atrophy of hand muscles and permanent loss of function of the extremity.

COMPLICATIONS
- Postoperative infection (rare)
- Injury to recurrent branch of the nerve

REFERENCES

1. Nordstrom DL, DeStefano F, Vierkant RA, et al. Incidence of diagnosed carpal tunnel syndrome in a general population. *Epidemiology.* 1998;9:342–5.
2. Blumenthal S, Herskovitz S, Verghese J. Carpal tunnel syndrome in older adults. *Muscle Nerve.* 2006;34:78–83.
3. Jordan R, Carter T, Cummins C. A systematic review of the utility of electrodiagnostic testing in carpal tunnel syndrome. *Br J Gen Pract.* 2002;52:670–3.
4. Graham RG, et al. A prospective study to assess the outcome of steroid injections and wrist splinting for the treatment of carpal tunnel syndrome. *Plas Reconst Surg.* 2004;113:550–6.
5. Marshall S, Tardif G, Ashworth N et al. Local corticosteroid injection for carpal tunnel syndrome. *Cochrane Database Syst Rev.* 2007;CD001554.
6. Verdugo RJ, Salinas RA, Castillo JL, et al. Surgical versus non-surgical treatment for carpal tunnel syndrome. *Cochrane Database Syst Rev.* 2008:CD001552.
7. Gerritsen AA, de Vet HC, Scholten RJ, et al. Splinting vs surgery in the treatment of carpal tunnel syndrome: a randomized controlled trial. *JAMA.* 2002;288:1245–51.
8. Scholten RJ, Mink van der Molen A, Uitdehaag BM, Bouter LM, de Vet HC et al. Surgical treatment options for carpal tunnel syndrome. *Cochrane Database Syst Rev.* 2007;CD003905.

ADDITIONAL READING
Cudlip SA, Howe FA, Clifton A, et al. Magnetic resonance neurography studies of the median nerve before and after carpal tunnel decompression. *J Neurosurg.* 2002;96:1046–51.

See Also (Topic, Algorithm, Electronic Media Element)
Arthritis, Rheumatoid; Hypoparathyroidism; Scleroderma; Systemic Lupus Erythematosus (SLE) Algorithms: Carpal Tunnel Syndrome; Pain in Upper Extremity

 CODES

ICD9
354.0 Carpal tunnel syndrome

CLINICAL PEARLS
- The altered sensation (tingling or prickling) in carpal tunnel syndrome is characteristically confined to the thumb and the index and middle fingers, but many patients do not distinguish this localization and feel the entire hand is affected.
- Tinel and Phalen signs have poor sensitivity and specificity.
- Normal serum TSH and normal serum glucose may be helpful in excluding conditions associated with carpal tunnel syndrome.
- Strongly consider surgical treatment for moderate and severe cases. Atrophy is a late finding indicating severe disease.

C

CATARACT

Christopher Gudas, MD
John W. Gittinger, Jr., MD

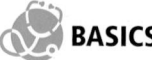 **BASICS**

DESCRIPTION

A *cataract* is any opacity or discoloration of the lens, localized or generalized; the term is usually reserved for changes that affect visual acuity:

- Etymology: From Latin *catarractes*, for "waterfall"; named after foamy appearance of opacity
- Leading cause of blindness worldwide, an estimated 20 million people
- Types include:
  - Age-related ("senile"): 90% of total
  - Congenital (1/250 newborns; 10–38% of childhood blindness)
  - Systemic disease associated (myotonic dystrophy, atopic dermatitis)
  - Metabolic (diabetes via accelerated sorbitol pathway, hypocalcemia, Wilson disease)
  - Secondary to associated eye disease, so-called complicated (e.g., uveitis associated with juvenile rheumatoid arthritis or sarcoid, tumor such as melanoma or retinoblastoma)
  - Traumatic (e.g., heat, electric shock, radiation, concussion, perforating eye injuries, intraocular foreign body)
  - Toxic/nutritional (e.g., corticosteroids, medications)
- Morphologic classification:
  - Nuclear: Exaggeration of normal aging changes of *central* lens nucleus, often associated with myopia due to increased refractive index of lens (some elderly patients consequently may be able to read again *without spectacles,* so-called second sight of the aged)
  - Cortical: Outer portion of lens; may involve anterior, posterior, or equatorial cortex; radial, spokelike opacities
  - Subcapsular: Posterior subcapsular cataract has more profound effect on vision than nuclear or cortical cataract; patients particularly troubled under conditions of miosis; near vision frequently impaired more than distance vision
- System(s) affected: Nervous

Geriatric Considerations
Some degree of cataract formation is expected in all people >70 years of age.

Pediatric Considerations
See Congenital Cataracts; may present as leukocoria.

Pregnancy Considerations
See Congenital Cataracts (i.e., medications, metabolic dysfunction, intrauterine infection, and malnutrition).

EPIDEMIOLOGY

Incidence
- Nearly 48% of the 37 million cases of blindness worldwide result from cataracts.
- Leading cause of treatable blindness and vision loss in developing countries
- Predominant age: Depends on type of cataract
- Predominant sex: Male Female (perhaps *slight* female predominance of cortical cataract)

Prevalence
- Cataract type and prevalence highly variable based on population demographic
- It is estimated that 50% of people 65–74 years of age and 70% of people >75 years of age have age-related cataract change.

RISK FACTORS
- Aging
- Cigarette smoking
- Ultraviolet B (UVB) sunlight exposure
- Diabetes
- Prolonged high-dose steroids
- Positive family history (see Genetics)
- Alcohol

Genetics
- Congenital sometimes associated (e.g., heredofamilial systemic disorders [Laurence-Moon-Biedl syndrome], chromosomal disorders [Down syndrome]) (1)[A]
- Genetics of age-related cataract not yet established, but likely multifactorial contribution (2)

GENERAL PREVENTION
- Use of UVB protective glasses (2,3)[A]
- Avoidance of tobacco products (2,3)[A]
- Effective control of diabetes (2,3)[A]
- Care with high-dose, long-term steroid use (systemic therapy > inhaled treatment) (2)[B]
- Protective methods using pharmaceutical intervention (e.g., antioxidants, ASA, hormone replacement therapy [HRT]) show no proven benefit to date (2,3)[C].

ETIOLOGY
- Age-related cataract:
  - Continual addition of layers of lens fibers throughout life creates hard, dehydrated lens nucleus that impairs vision (nuclear cataract).
  - Aging alters biochemical and osmotic balance required for lens clarity; outer lens layers hydrate and become opaque, adversely affecting vision.
- Congenital:
  - Usually obscure cause
  - Drugs (corticosteroids in 1st trimester, sulfonamides)
  - Metabolic diabetes in mother, galactosemia in fetus
  - Intrauterine infection during 1st trimester (e.g., rubella, herpes, mumps)
  - Maternal malnutrition
- Other cataract types:
  - Common feature is a biochemical/osmotic imbalance that disrupts lens clarity
  - Local changes in lens protein distribution lead to light scattering (lens opacity).

COMMONLY ASSOCIATED CONDITIONS
- Diabetes (especially with poor control)
- Myotonic dystrophy (90% of patients develop visually innocuous change in 3rd decade; becomes disabling in 5th decade)
- Atopic dermatitis: 10% of patients with severe AD develop cataracts in 2nd–4th decades, often bilateral.
- Neurofibromatosis type 2
- Associated ocular disease or "secondary cataract" (e.g., chronic anterior uveitis, acute [or repetitive] angle-closure glaucoma or high myopia)
- Drug-induced (e.g., steroids, chlorpromazine)
- Trauma

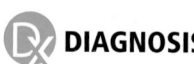 **DIAGNOSIS**

HISTORY
- Age-related cataract:
  - Blurred vision, distortion, or "ghosting" of images
  - Problems with visual acuity in bright light or night driving (glare)
  - Falls or accidents; injuries (e.g., hip fracture)
- Congenital: Often asymptomatic, or parents notice child's visual inattention or strabismus
- Other types of cataract:
  - May present with decreased visual acuity
  - Appropriate history or signs to help in diagnosis

PHYSICAL EXAM
- Age-related cataract: Lens opacity on eye examination
- Congenital:
  - Lens opacity present at birth or within 3 months of birth
  - Leukocoria (white pupil), strabismus, nystagmus, signs of associated syndrome (as with Down or rubella syndrome)
  - *Note:* Always must rule out ocular tumor; early diagnosis and treatment of retinoblastoma may be lifesaving.
- Other types of cataract: May present with decreased visual acuity

DIAGNOSTIC TESTS & INTERPRETATION
- Visual quality assessment: Glare testing, contrast sensitivity sometimes indicated
- Retinal/macular function assessment: Potential acuity meter testing

Lab
Diabetic control: HbA1c; hyperglycemic state creates an osmotic change within the lens and may alter visual acuity and refractive measurement.

Pathological Findings
Consistent with lens changes found in the type of cataract; however, diagnosis is made by clinical examination.

DIFFERENTIAL DIAGNOSIS
An opaque-appearing eye may be due to opacities of the cornea (e.g., scarring, edema, calcification), lens opacities, tumor, or retinal detachment. Biomicroscopic examination (slit lamp) or careful ophthalmoscopic exam should provide diagnosis:
- In the elderly, visual impairment is often due to multiple factors, such as cataract and macular degeneration, both contributing to visual loss.
- Age-related cataract is significant if symptoms and ophthalmic exam support cataract as a major cause of vision impairment.
- Congenital lens opacity in the absence of other ocular pathology may cause severe amblyopia.
- *Note:* Cataract *does not* produce a relative afferent pupillary reaction defect. Abnormal pupillary reactions mandate further evaluation for other pathology.

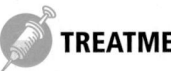 **TREATMENT**

- Outpatient (usually) or inpatient surgery
- ~1.64 million cataract extractions in US yearly

MEDICATION
There is currently no medication to prevent or slow the progression of cataracts.

ADDITIONAL TREATMENT
Issues for Referral
If patient has cataract and symptoms do not seem to support recommended surgery, a 2nd opinion by another ophthalmologist may be indicated.

SURGERY/OTHER PROCEDURES
- Age-related cataract:
  - Surgical removal is indicated if visual impairment–producing symptoms are distressing to the patient, interfering with lifestyle or occupation, or posing a risk for fall or injury.
  - Because significant cataract may develop gradually, the patient may not be aware of how it has changed his or her lifestyle. Physician may note a significant cataract, and patient reports "no problems." Thus, evaluation requires effective physician–patient exchange of information.
  - Surgical technique: Cataract extraction via small incisions, followed by implantation of a prosthetic intraocular lens; lenses have power calculated based on size of the eye and curvature of cornea usually to correct for distance vision; surgery performed on 1 (worse) eye, with contralateral surgery only after recovery and if deemed necessary; generally takes less than an hour depending on surgical technique
  - Anesthesia: Usually local with sedation and monitoring of vital signs
  - Preoperative evaluation: By the primary-care physician; patients on anticoagulants may need to be temporarily discontinued 1–2 weeks before surgery if possible (but not always necessary; thus, need to discuss with ophthalmologist); patients who have ever taken an α-blocker should alert their ophthalmologist (risk of intraoperative floppy iris syndrome)
  - Postoperative care: Usually protective eye shield as directed, topical antibiotic, and steroid ophthalmic medications; avoid lifting or bending over for a few weeks.
- Congenital cataract:
  - Treatment is surgical removal of cataract. Newborn may require surgery within days to reduce risk of severe amblyopia. Use of lens implants is controversial.
  - Postoperative care: Long-term patching program for good eye to combat amblyopia; refractive correction of operative eye, with multiple repeat examinations; challenging for physician and parents

 ONGOING CARE

FOLLOW-UP RECOMMENDATIONS
Patient Monitoring
- As cataract progresses, an ophthalmologist may change spectacle correction to maintain vision. When this is no longer successful and *interferes with patient's activities of daily living* (ADLs), surgery is indicated.
- Following surgery, spectacle correction may be required to maximize near and/or far visual acuity. Refraction is usually prescribed several weeks after surgery.

PATIENT EDUCATION
See Surgery.
PROGNOSIS
- Ocular prognosis good after cataract removal if no prior ocular disease: 95% of otherwise healthy eyes achieve best corrected visual acuity of 20/40 or better (90% when all eyes are considered, including comorbidity such as diabetes and glaucoma).
- In congenital cataracts, prognosis often is poorer because of the high risk of amblyopia.
COMPLICATIONS
- Vary widely from delay in visual recovery or protracted visual discomfort to blindness and loss of eye
- Nearly all reported complications occur rarely (<2% of eyes) except for posterior capsule opacification (~25% of eyes, usually treated with Nd-YAG laser capsulotomy in office).

REFERENCES

1. Tasman W, ed. *Duane's Ophthalmology.* Philadelphia: JB Lippincott Co, 2002.
2. Abraham AG, Condon NG, West Gower E. The new epidemiology of cataract. *Ophthalmol Clin North Am.* 2006;19:415–25.
3. Asbell PA, Dualan I, Mindel J, et al. Age-related cataract. *Lancet.* 2005;365:599–609.

ADDITIONAL READING

Bradford CA, ed. *Basic Ophthalmology.* 8th ed. San Francisco: American Academy of Ophthalmology; 2004.

See Also (Topic, Algorithm, Electronic Media Element)
Algorithm: Cataracts

CODES

ICD9
- 366.9 Unspecified cataract
- 366.10 Senile cataract, unspecified
- 743.30 Congenital cataract, unspecified

CELIAC DISEASE

Brandi Kelly, PharmD
Gary Mark McWilliams, MD

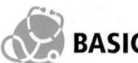 **BASICS**

DESCRIPTION
- Classically, a chronic diarrheal disease characterized by intestinal malabsorption of virtually all nutrients and precipitated by eating gluten-containing foods. Multiple forms exist.
- Nondiarrheal form may actually be more common (intestinal villous atrophy produces vitamin and mineral malabsorption)
- System(s) affected: Gastrointestinal
- Synonym(s): Sprue; Gluten enteropathy; Celiac sprue

EPIDEMIOLOGY
Incidence
- Disease primarily of individuals of Northern European ancestry
- Predominant sex: Female > Male (3:2)

Prevalence
~1 in 133 persons in US

RISK FACTORS
- 1st-degree relatives: 10% incidence
- 71% in monozygotic twins

Genetics
HLA-DQ2 and/or DQ8 closely associated (testing may be indicated if indeterminate small bowel pathology)

GENERAL PREVENTION
Avoid all gluten-containing products (wheat, barley, rye, and possibly oat products).

ETIOLOGY
Sensitivity to gluten, specifically gliadin fraction

COMMONLY ASSOCIATED CONDITIONS
- May have secondary lactase deficiency
- Extraintestinal manifestation may include marked decrease in bone density
- Dermatitis herpetiformis common
- Autoimmune thyroiditis
- Diabetes, type 1 (prevalence of celiac disease in type 1 diabetes is 3–8%)
- Elevated AST and ALT
- Recurrent fetal loss or infertility
- IBS (irritable bowel syndrome) (1)[A]
- Restless legs syndrome (2)

Pregnancy Considerations
- Celiac disease may be an underappreciated cause of male and female infertility. Consider celiac disease in pregnant women with severe anemia.

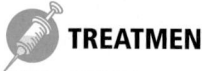 **DIAGNOSIS**

HISTORY
- Diarrhea
- Steatorrhea
- Muscle cramps
- Iron-deficiency anemia
- Nervousness
- Weight loss
- Failure to thrive (slowing velocity of weight gain)
- Weakness
- Lassitude
- Fatigue
- Large appetite
- Explosive flatulence
- Abdominal pain, nausea, vomiting rare
- Recurrent aphthous stomatitis
- Abdominal distention

Pediatric Considerations
- Failure to thrive and delayed growth with short stature may be early manifestations. A few children may outgrow intolerance to wheat after prolonged gluten-free diets, but should be cautioned to watch for signs of recurrence in middle age.

DIAGNOSTIC TESTS & INTERPRETATION
Lab
Initial lab tests
Positive IgA antiendomysial antibodies and IgA tissue transglutaminase (sensitivity 90–98%, specificity 98%) when on normal (nongluten-free) diet

Follow-Up & Special Considerations
- IgA-deficient patients have false-negative IgA antiendomysial and IgA antitransglutaminase antibodies
- tTG (the tissue transglutaminase antibody test) is the preferred test (over the deamidated gliadin peptide [DGP] antibody) (3,4)[A].
- 72-hour fecal fat showing >7% fat malabsorption
- Elevated liver function tests
- d-Xylose test showing malabsorption
- Decreased calcium
- Increased prothrombin time (PT)
- Decreased neutral fats
- Decreased cholesterol
- Decreased vitamin A
- Decreased vitamin B_{12} (rare)
- Decreased vitamin D
- Decreased vitamin C
- Decreased folic acid
- Decreased iron (common)
- Decreased total protein
- Decreased hemoglobin (common)

Imaging
Initial approach
Upper GI series showing flocculation of barium, edema, and flattening of mucosal folds

Follow-Up & Special Considerations
Evaluate for osteoporosis

Diagnostic Procedures/Surgery
- Endoscopy with diagnostic biopsy of the duodenal mucosa with repeat endoscopy and normal biopsy on a gluten-free diet is necessary before a firm diagnosis can be made.
- In general, diagnosis should not be made based on serology alone.

Pathological Findings
Small bowel biopsy:
- Flattened villi, hyperplasia and lengthening of crypts, infiltration of plasma cells, and lymphocytes in lamina propria

DIFFERENTIAL DIAGNOSIS
- Short bowel syndrome
- Pancreatic insufficiency
- Crohn disease
- Whipple disease
- Hypogammaglobulinemia
- Tropical sprue
- Lymphoma
- AIDS
- Acute enteritis
- Giardiasis
- Eosinophilic gastroenteritis
- Pancreatic disease

 TREATMENT

MEDICATION
First Line
Usually none: Gluten-free diet is treatment

Second Line
- In refractory disease, consider:
  - Steroids (prednisone, 40–60 mg/d p.o. in cases of refractory sprue)
  - Azathioprine (immunosuppressants should be used with caution; use may lead to lymphoma in celiac disease)
  - Cyclosporine
  - Infliximab
  - Cladribine
- Patients may require supplemental calcium, calcium carbonate, 500 mg p.o. b.i.d., and vitamin D (ergocalciferol) 10–100 g/d; in severe malabsorption, up to 2.5 mg/d may be required.

ADDITIONAL TREATMENT

General Measures
- Removal of gluten from the diet. Rice, corn, and soybean flour are safe, palatable substitutes.
- Levels of IgA antigliadin normalize with gluten abstinence.

Issues for Referral
- Additional nutritional support
- Refractory disease

 ONGOING CARE

FOLLOW-UP RECOMMENDATIONS
- Consultation with dietitian
- Screening for osteoporosis

Patient Monitoring
- Repeat endoscopy after 6–8 weeks on a gluten-free diet (in selected cases).
- IgA antigliadin assay may be used to monitor response to gluten-free diet.

DIET
Removal of gluten: Wheat, rye, barley, and those with gluten additives. This can be a challenging diet (especially learning sources of "hidden" gluten) and should be coordinated with a skilled dietitian.

PATIENT EDUCATION
- Discuss importance of recognizing gluten in various products.
- Highlight potential complications and outcomes of failing to follow a gluten-free diet.

PROGNOSIS
- Good with correct diagnosis and adherence to gluten-free diet
- Patient should feel better in 7 days.
- All symptoms usually disappear in 4–6 weeks.
- It is unknown whether strict dietary adherence decreases cancer risk.

COMPLICATIONS
- Malignancy: <10% of patients (50% of whom have small bowel lymphoma)
- Refractory sprue:
  - May respond to prednisone 40–60 mg/d p.o.
  - Refractory sprue unresponsive to corticosteroid therapy raises the specter of adult-onset autoimmune enteropathy or cryptic T-cell lymphoma. In this circumstance, screening for antienterocyte autoantibodies and careful scrutiny of the small intestine, including retroperitoneal lymph node biopsy with full-thickness small bowel biopsy, may be needed.
- Chronic ulcerative jejunoileitis:
  - Associated with multiple ulcers, intestinal bleeding, strictures, perforation, obstruction, and peritonitis
  - 7% mortality
- Osteoporosis secondary to decreased vitamin D and calcium absorption
- Dehydration
- Electrolyte depletion
- Refractory cases may need total parenteral nutrition.

REFERENCES

1. Ford AC, Chey WD, Talley NJ, et al. Yield of diagnostic tests for celiac disease in individuals with symptoms suggestive of irritable bowel syndrome: systematic review and meta-analysis. *Arch Intern Med*. 2009;169:651–8.
2. Weinstock L, Walters A, Mullin G, et al. Celiac disease is associated with restless legs syndrome. *Dig Dis Sci*. 2010;55:1667–73.
3. Lewis NR, Scott BB et al. Meta-analysis: deamidated gliadin peptide antibody and tissue transglutaminase antibody compared as screening tests for coeliac disease. *Aliment Pharmacol Ther*. 2010;31:73–81.
4. van der Windt DA, Jellema P, Mulder CJ, Kneepkens CM, van der Horst HE et al. Diagnostic testing for celiac disease among patients with abdominal symptoms: a systematic review. *JAMA*. 2010;303:1738–46.

ADDITIONAL READING

- AGA Institute. AGA Institute Medical Position Statement on the Diagnosis and Management of Celiac Disease. *Gastroenterology*. 2006;131: 1977–80.
- Celiac Disease: A Hidden Epidemic by Peter Green.
- Celiac Sprue Association (CSA) http://www.csaceliacs.org.
- *Guidelines for a Gluten-free Lifestyle*, 3rd. ed. Celiac Disease Foundation. http://www.celiac.org.
- Quick Start Diet Guide: Celiac Disease Foundation (CDF) & Gluten Intolerance Group (GIG). http://www.celiac.org,http://www.gluten.net.

See Also (Topic, Algorithm, Electronic Media Element)
Algorithms: Diarrhea, Chronic; Malabsorption Syndrome

 CODES

ICD9
579.0 Celiac disease

CLINICAL PEARLS
- Common condition (1 in 133)
- Characterized by mucosal inflammation and villous atrophy
- Associated with malabsorption of nutrients
- Treatment is gluten-free diet.
- Test for celiac disease in patients with IBS.

C

CELLULITIS

Laura Sullivan Eurich, MD
Frank J. Domino, MD

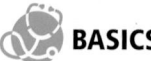 **BASICS**

DESCRIPTION
- A diffuse and nonpurulent infection of the skin and subcutaneous tissue. It initially affects the epidermis and dermis layers of the skin, and may subsequently spread within the superficial fascia.
- Several entities are recognized:
  - Cellulitis of the extremities
  - Recurrent cellulitis of the leg after saphenous vein removal
  - Dissecting cellulitis of the scalp
  - Facial cellulitis
  - Perianal cellulitis
  - *Pseudomonas* cellulitis
- System(s) affected: Skin/Exocrine

EPIDEMIOLOGY
- Cellulitis can affect any part of body, but commonly affects the extremities or head.
- Predominant age:
  - Perianal cellulitis: Principally in children
  - Facial cellulitis: In adults, usually <45 years; in children, <3 years
- Predominant sex: Male = Female (perianal cellulitis more common in boys)

Incidence
24.6 cases per 1,000 person-years

Prevalence
Unknown

RISK FACTORS
- Previous trauma (e.g., laceration, puncture, human or animal bite)
- Surgical procedures (saphenous vein removal, breast cancer axillary node dissection, or lymph node dissection for pelvic malignancy)
- Lower extremity lymphedema secondary to radical pelvic surgery, radiation therapy, chronic venous insufficiency
- Preexisting skin infections: Impetigo, ulceration, intertrigo, tinea pedis
- Immunocompromised patients, diabetics, IV drug users, cirrhotics, chronic renal disease, neutropenics

Geriatric Considerations
In cellulitis of lower extremities, older patients are more prone to develop thrombophlebitis.

GENERAL PREVENTION
- Avoid trauma, swimming with skin abrasions, and human or animal bites.
- Wear support stockings to decrease peripheral edema.
- Maintain good skin hygiene, especially with minor cuts.
- Maintain tight glycemic control and proper foot care for diabetics.

PATHOPHYSIOLOGY
Cellulitis is caused by bacterial penetration through a break in the skin integrity. Hyaluronidase mediates subcutaneous spread.

ETIOLOGY
- According to site (*S. aureus* most common overall):

  - Cellulitis of the extremities: Group A streptococcus, *Staphylococcus aureus*

- Recurrent cellulitis of the leg: Non–group A β-hemolytic streptococci (groups C, G, and B)
- Dissecting cellulitis of the scalp: *S. aureus*
- Facial cellulitis in adults: *Haemophilus influenzae* type B
- Facial cellulitis in children: *H. influenzae* type B, patients >3 years with portal of entry: Staphylococcal and streptococcal
- Synergystic necrotizing cellulitis: Mixed aerobic-anaerobic flora
- Intravenous drug use: MRSA, streptococci, Enterobacteriaceae, *Pseudomonas*, fungi
- Specific diseases:
  - Diabetes mellitus: *S. aureus*, streptococci, gram-negative bacilli, anaerobes
  - Human bites: *Eikenella corrodens*
  - Animal bites (e.g., cat, dog): *Pasteurella multocida*, *Capnocytophaga canimorsus*
- Patient groups:
  - Neonates: Group B streptococcus
  - Immunocompromised:
    - Bacteria (e.g., *Serratia*, *Proteus*, and other Enterobacteriaceae)
    - Fungi (e.g., *Cryptococcus neoformans*)
    - Atypical mycobacterium
  - Cirrhotics:
    - *Campylobacter fetus*, *Coliforms*, *Vibrio vulnificus*
  - Environmental and occupational exposures:
    - *Erysipelothrix rhusiopathiae* in patients handling fish, shellfish, meat, and poultry
    - *Vibrio* sp: Saltwater exposure
    - *Aeromonas hydrophila*: Freshwater exposure
    - *Pseudomonas aeruginosa:* Hot-tub exposure

COMMONLY ASSOCIATED CONDITIONS
- Facial cellulitis in children:
  - Upper respiratory tract infection
  - Unilateral or bilateral otitis media
  - Meningitis
- Perianal cellulitis:
  - Pharyngitis may precede infection.

 DIAGNOSIS

HISTORY
- Previous trauma, surgery, or animal/human bites
- High-risk comorbidities, trauma, surgery, bites

PHYSICAL EXAM
- Localized pain and tenderness (1)[A]
- Erythema
- Fever
- Chills
- Malaise
- Regional lymphadenopathy: Face, periorbital region, neck, or extremities
- Decreased visual activity and compromised extraocular movements
- Purulent drainage from burrowing interconnecting abscesses
- Itching
- Burning
- Irritability
- Intense perianal erythema or itching
- Pain on defecation
- Blood-streaked stools

- Area of local inflammation with redness, warmth, edema, tenderness, itchiness, poorly demarcated margins, regional lymphadenopathy.

DIAGNOSTIC TESTS & INTERPRETATION
Diagnosis based primarily on skin appearance and clinical setting, but laboratory, pathology, and imaging modalities can confirm diagnosis.

Lab
Initial lab tests
- Aspirates from point of maximum inflammation yield a 45% positive culture rate compared with a 5% rate from leading-edge culture; recommended in patients with systemic toxicity, immunocompromised, recurrent cellulitis, comorbidities, or special exposures (1)[B].
- Blood cultures: Potential pathogens isolated in <5% of patients. Better yield in patients with systemic symptoms (i.e., fever, tachycardia, hypotension, etc.). Blood cultures in children are more likely to show a contaminant than a true positive (2)[C].
- Mild leukocytosis with a left shift (1)[C]
- Mildly elevated erythrocyte sedimentation rate or C-reactive protein

Imaging
Initial approach
- Plain radiographs or computed tomography useful if a subjacent osteomyelitis, fracture, or early necrotizing fasciitis is suspected.
- Magnetic resonance imaging is helpful in differentiating cellulitis from necrotizing fasciitis.
- Ultrasonography is helpful in detecting subcutaneous accumulation of pus, and aids in guiding aspiration.
- Gallium[67] scintillography is helpful for detecting cellulitis superimposed on recently increasing chronic lymphedema of a limb.

Diagnostic Procedures/Surgery
- Skin biopsy is not indicated in immunocompetent mild cellulitis.
- Lumbar puncture should be considered for all children with *H. influenzae* type B cellulitis or patients with meningeal signs associated with facial cellulitis.
- Gram stain of cellulitis aspirate may be useful for making preliminary microbial diagnosis to direct specific antibiotic therapy.

Pathological Findings
Biopsy of skin shows marked infiltration of the dermis with eosinophils and inflammatory changes.

DIFFERENTIAL DIAGNOSIS
- Toxic shock syndrome
- Bursitis
- Acute dermatitis
- Herpes zoster
- Deep vein thrombosis
- Insect stings
- Acute gout, pseudogout
- Necrotizing fasciitis or myositis
- Gas gangrene
- Deep venous thrombophlebitis
- Herpetic whitlow
- Osteomyelitis
- Cutaneous diphtheria
- Erythema chronicum migrans

TREATMENT

MEDICATION
First Line
Treat 5–15 days or longer, depending on clinical response, and guided by culture results whenever possible. Use IV therapy for rapidly spreading infection or significant comorbidities:

- Empiric therapy or mild cellulitis infection (activity against β-hemolytic streptococci and methicillin-susceptible *S. aureus*): Oral dicloxacillin, cephalexin, clindamycin, or IV cefazolin, oxacillin, or nafcillin
- Parenteral therapy if severely ill or unable to tolerate oral therapy: Include penicillinase-resistant penicillins, a 1st-generation cephalosporin; if penicillin-allergic, use clindamycin or vancomycin
- Necrotizing fasciitis and gas gangrene: Use parenteral clindamycin and penicillin
- Recurrent infection underlying predisposing conditions, previous episode of proven methicillin-resistant *Staphylococcus aureus* (MRSA) infection, or systemic toxicity:
  – Use agents with activity against MRSA: Parenteral vancomycin or oral trimethoprim-sulfamethoxazole (TMP/SMX), doxycycline or minocycline, or clindamycin
- Mild early-suspected streptococcal etiology: Aqueous penicillin G, 600,000 U, then IM procaine penicillin at 600,000 U q8h–q12h.
- Freshwater exposure: Penicillinase-resistant: Penicillin plus gentamicin or fluoroquinolone
- Saltwater exposure: Doxycycline 200 mg IV in divided doses
- Human or animal bites: Oral amoxicillin-clavulanate or IV ampicillin-sulbactam or ertapenem in patients. If mildly allergic to penicillin, use cefoxitin or carbapenems. For severe penicillin reactions, use doxycycline, TMP/SMX, or a fluoroquinolone plus clindamycin.
- Facial cellulitis in adults and children (*H. influenza* B): Cefotaxime IV (1)[B]
- Diabetic foot infection: Ampicillin/sulbactam 3 g IV q6h or imipenem/cilastatin, or meropenem. Alternative: Combinations targeting anaerobes as well as gram-positive and gram-negative aerobes
- Severe infection, toxicity, immunocompromised patients, or worsening infection despite empirical therapy: Consider agents effective against MRSA (i.e., vancomycin, linezolid, tigecycline, quinupristin/dalfopristin, or daptomycin). Switch to oral dicloxacillin, cephradine, cephalexin, or cefadroxil when symptoms begin to resolve (3)[A].
- Recurrent streptococcal cellulitis: Penicillin IV 250 mg b.i.d., or if penicillin-allergic, use erythromycin 250 mg once or twice daily

ALERT
If community-acquired MRSA is a concern, treatment options (7–14 days) include:

- Trimethoprim/sulfamethoxazole: DS (160 mg TMP and 800 mg of SMX) 1–2 PO b.i.d. daily; doxycycline: 100 mg PO b.i.d., *or*
- Clindamycin: 300–600 mg PO t.i.d.

Pediatric Considerations
- Review contraindications, including patient allergies to antibiotics as well as organ failure.

- Avoid doxycycline in children ≤8 years old and during pregnancy.
- Now that children are HIB-vaccinated, the most common predisposing conditions are conjunctivitis or an infected wound near the eye, rather than bacteremia (4)[A].

Second Line
Mild infection:

- Penicillin allergy: Erythromycin 500 mg PO q6h
- Cephalexin remains a cost-effective therapy for outpatient management of cellulitis at current estimated MRSA levels.

ADDITIONAL TREATMENT
General Measures
- Immobilization and elevation of the involved limb to reduce swelling
- Sterile saline dressings to decrease local pain
- Cool aluminum acetate compresses for pain relief
- Edema: Compression stocking, pneumatic pumps, and diuretic therapy
- Adjuvant corticosteroids (prednisone 0.5 mg/kg/d for 5–8 days) if partial response to parenteral antibiotics and hemorrhagic or bullous cellulitis
- Treat intertrigo with topical antifungals (miconazole, clotrimazole, or terbinafine).

Issues for Referral
Consider consulting Infectious Disease if patient is immunocompromised, not responding to treatment, or infection is severe.

SURGERY/OTHER PROCEDURES
- Debridement for gas and purulent matter collections
- Intubation or tracheotomy may be needed for cellulitis of the head or neck.

IN-PATIENT CONSIDERATIONS
Admission Criteria
- Severe infection, suspicion of deeper or rapidly spreading infection, tissue necrosis, or severe pain
- Marked systemic toxicity or worsening symptoms that do not resolve after 24–48 hours of therapy
- Patients with underlying risk factors or severe comorbidities

Nursing
- Ambulate patient in mild infection
- Bed rest in severe infection
- Elevate extremity to reduce swelling

ONGOING CARE

FOLLOW-UP RECOMMENDATIONS
Patient Monitoring
- Repeat needle aspirate culture.
- Repeat blood count if patient was toxic.
- Repeat lumbar puncture in case of meningitis.
- Consider prophylaxis of deep vein thrombosis.
- Symptomatic improvement usually occurs within 24–48 hours of therapy; however, visible improvement may take up to 72 hours.
- Cutaneous inflammation may worsen in first 24 hours due to inflammatory response from release of bacterial antigens.

PATIENT EDUCATION
- Practice good skin hygiene, especially with minor cuts.
- Report early skin changes to physician.

PROGNOSIS
With adequate antibiotic treatment, outlook is good.

COMPLICATIONS
- Bacteremia
- Local abscesses
- Superinfection with gram-negative organisms
- Lymphangitis, especially in recurrent cellulitis
- Thrombophlebitis or venous thrombosis of lower extremities in older patients
- Bacterial meningitis
- Gangrenous disorder

REFERENCES

1. Swartz MN. Clinical practice. Cellulitis. *N Engl J Med*. 2004;350:904–12.
2. Sadow KB, Chamberlain JM. Blood Cultures in the Evaluation of Children with Cellulitis. *Pediatrics*. 1998;101;e4.
3. Daum RS. Clinical practice. Skin and soft-tissue infections caused by methicillin-resistant Staphylococcus aureus. *N Engl J Med*. 2007;357: 380–90.
4. Rimon A, Hoffer V, Prais D, et al. Periorbital cellulitis in the era of Haemophilus influenzae type B vaccine: predisposing factors and etiologic agents in hospitalized children. *J Pediatr Ophthalmol Strabismus*. 2008;45:300–4.

ADDITIONAL READING

- Chira S, Miller LG et al. Staphylococcus aureus is the most common identified cause of cellulitis: a systematic review. *Epidemiol Infect*. 2010;138: 313–7.
- Wells RD, Mason P, Roarty J, et al. Comparison of initial antibiotic choice and treatment of cellulitis in the pre- and post-community-acquired methicillin-resistant Staphylococcus aureus eras. *Am J Emerg Med*. 2009;27:436–9.

CODES

ICD9
- 682.0 Cellulitis and abscess of face
- 682.1 Cellulitis and abscess of neck
- 682.9 Cellulitis and abscess of unspecified sites

CLINICAL PEARLS
- Most common overall causes of cellulitis are *Staphylococcus aureus* and group A Streptococcus.
- Consider MRSA if cellulitis is not responding to antibiotics in the 1st 48 hours.
- Rapid expansion of infected area with red/purple discoloration and severe pain may suggest necrotizing fasciitis requiring urgent surgical evaluation.

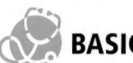

BASICS

DESCRIPTION
- Acute, spreading infection involving the fat and/or muscle within the bony orbit posterior to the orbital septum
- Synonym(s): Postseptal cellulitis

ALERT
Prompt diagnosis and intervention are critical, since delayed treatment can result in sustained or permanent vision loss, intracranial complications, and even death.

EPIDEMIOLOGY
- Occurs more commonly in the winter because of increased incidence of sinusitis (12)[C]
- No racial predilection or difference in frequency between the sexes in adults
- More common in children. Male > Female (2:1).
- The median age of children hospitalized with orbital cellulitis is 7–12 years.

RISK FACTORS
- Continuous sinusitis is the most common risk factor, accounting for up to 80–90% of cases (1,3)[C].
- Orbital trauma
- Dental or intracranial infection
- Retained orbital foreign body
- Preorbital or facial cellulitis
- Facial skin infection (i.e., impetigo, infected insect bite, acne, eczema)
- Acute dacryocystitis
- Acute dacryoadenitis
- Orbital mucopyocele
- Ophthalmologic surgery (for strabismus or detached retina, blepharoplasty, radial keratotomy, peribulbar anesthesia)

Genetics
No known genetic predisposition

GENERAL PREVENTION
- Appropriate treatment of bacterial sinusitis
- Proper postoperative wound care

PATHOPHYSIOLOGY
Orbital cellulitis often develops as a complication of acute sinusitis, as the sinuses are major components of the walls of the orbit.

ETIOLOGY
- Most common organisms (2,3)[C]:
  - *Staphylococcus aureus*
  - *Streptococcus pneumoniae*
- Less common organisms:
  - *Moraxella catarrhalis*
  - *Haemophilus influenza*
  - Nonspore–forming anaerobes
  - Group A β-hemolytic streptococcus
  - *Pseudomonas aeruginosa*
  - Fungal pathogens
  - *Mycobacterium tuberculosis*
  - *Mycobacterium avium* complex
- Since the introduction of routine vaccination in 1990, *Haemophilus influenzae* B is no longer a leading cause of orbital cellulitis (2,3)[B].

COMMONLY ASSOCIATED CONDITIONS
- More than 80% of orbital cellulitis cases result from contiguous sinusitis.
- Some cases are related to trauma, dental diseases, or hematogenous infection dissemination.

DIAGNOSIS

Chandler staging of orbital cellulitis is still widely used today (1,3)[C]:

- Stage I: Preorbital cellulitis (considered a different entity) (1,3)[B]
- Stage II: Edema of orbital lining, chemosis, proptosis, limitation of extraocular movement, fever
- Stage III: Include stage II with a subperiosteal abscess. Occasional vision loss.
- Stage IV: Orbital abscess. Ophthalmoplegia with visual loss.
- Stage V: Extension of the infection to the cavernous sinus, subdural space, meninges, or brain

HISTORY
- Malaise and fever
- Most patients with history of sinusitis, dental infection, or history of eye surgery or trauma
- Diffuse unilateral periorbital edema and erythema
- Chemosis (conjunctival swelling)
- Pain with eye movement
- Restricted extraocular mobility
- Diplopia
- Proptosis and globe displacement
- Blurred vision or loss of vision

ALERT
Ophthalmoplegia, mental status changes, contralateral cranial nerve palsy, or bilateral orbital cellulitis may herald intracranial involvement.

PHYSICAL EXAM
- Thorough inspection of the eye and surrounding structures
- Inspection of nasal vaults and sinus palpation for evidence of acute sinusitis
- Ocular motility testing
- Visual acuity testing

DIAGNOSTIC TESTS & INTERPRETATION
Lab
- Complete blood count with differential, C-reactive protein, and erythrocyte sedimentation rate
- Cultures can be obtained from sinus aspirates and abscesses.
- Cultures of eye secretions or nasopharyngeal aspirates are likely to be contaminated by normal flora, but may be helpful in identifying antibiotic-resistant organisms.
- Cultures from orbital and sinus abscesses are more likely to yield positive results, although these should be limited to cases where invasive procedures are clinically indicated.
- Blood cultures should be obtained prior to initiation of antibiotic therapy (more likely to be positive in children <5 years old) (3)[C].

Follow-Up & Special Considerations
A full septic evaluation, including lumbar puncture, should be considered before antibiotic administration in any toxic-appearing patient, or in the presence of any signs or symptoms suggestive of meningitis (3)[C].

Imaging
- Stage I: Preorbital cellulitis. Computed tomography (CT) scan normal.
- Stage II: CT scan shows no subperiosteal abscess. Might see mucosal edema or swelling.
- Stage III: CT scan shows subperiosteal abscess, globe displacement, and intraconal involvement of extraocular muscles.
- Stage IV: CT scan shows proptosis, abscess formation involving the extraocular muscles and orbital fat, and periosteal rupture (2,3,4)[C].

Initial approach
- Contrast CT is the most widely used modality for evaluating orbital cellulitis (5)[B]:
  - Consider CT imaging if concern for stage III or IV disease (5)[C]
  - Thin sections (2 mm) CT, coronal and axial views with bone windows
  - Differentiate preorbital from orbital cellulitis.
  - Confirm extension of inflammation into orbit, detect coexisting sinus disease, and identify orbital or subperiosteal abscesses.
  - Deviation of medial rectus on the affected side indicates intraorbital involvement.
- Magnetic resonance imaging offers superior resolution of soft tissue infections and is the modality of choice for identification of cavernous sinus thrombosis.
- Ultrasonography can be useful in ruling out orbital myositis, locating foreign bodies or abscesses, and following the progression of a drained abscess.

DIFFERENTIAL DIAGNOSIS
- Periorbital cellulitis:
  - Stage I orbital cellulitis in Chandler classification. Now it is mostly considered to be a different entity (1)[B].
  - Induration, erythema, warmth, and tenderness of the periorbital soft tissues
  - Extraocular motion is not affected and should be full.
  - Mostly caused by trauma (1)[C]
  - The inflammation does not extend into the bony orbit (1)[B].
- Idiopathic orbital inflammatory disease (3)[C]:
  - Usually no prodromal symptoms such as fever or malaise
- Atopic dermatitis
- Contact dermatitis
- Rosacea
- Trauma, including insect bites
- Conjunctivitis
- Blepharitis
- Hordeolum
- Herpes or varicella lesions
- Rapidly progressive tumors:
  - Rhabdomyosarcoma
  - Lymphoma
  - Leukemia
- Ruptured dermoid cyst

TREATMENT

- Once diagnosed with orbital cellulitis, the patient should be admitted to a hospital for treatment and careful monitoring of ocular status.
- Stage II: Intravenous antibiotics
- Stage III: Intravenous antibiotics first; surgical intervention if no improvement within 24–48 hours of medical treatment or worsening signs discovered (impaired vision, complete ophthalmoplegia, or well-defined periosteal abscess.
- Stage IV: Intravenous antibiotics and surgical drainage (2,4)[C]

MEDICATION

- Empiric antibiotic therapy at all ages should provide coverage for pathogens associated with acute sinusitis (*S. pneumoniae*, *H. influenzae*, *M. catarrhalis*, *S. pyogenes*), as well as for *S. aureus* and anaerobes.
- IV antibiotic treatment should be modified accordingly when microbiological sensitivities return. Duration of IV therapy is usually a week, based on clinical picture.
- Oral antibiotic therapy should continue for 2–3 weeks. Longer duration (3–6 weeks) is recommended for patients with severe sinusitis and bony destruction.

First Line
- Mainstay of therapy is broad-spectrum IV antibiotics: Ampicillin/sulbactam (Unasyn) or cefuroxime plus metronidazole or clindamycin if concurrent anaerobic infection is suspected (2)[C]:
  – Ampicillin/sulbactam 1.5 to 3 g IV q6h for adult; 200-300 mg/kg/d divided q6h for children
  – Cefuroxime 150 mg/kg/d divided q8h
  – Clindamycin, 600–900 mg IV q8h for adults; 25–40 mg/kg/d IV q6–8h for children
  – Metronidazole 30–35 mg/kg/d divided q8h
- In severe, culture-proven methicillin-resistant *Staphylococcus aureus* infection, vancomycin remains parenteral drug of choice (2)[C]:
  – Vancomycin 1g IV q12h for adults; 40 mg/kg/d IV divided q8–12h, max daily dose 2 g for children
- Nafcillin or oxacillin plus cefotaxime or ceftriaxone can also be considered as initial IV treatment:
  – Nafcillin or oxacillin 2 g IV q4h for adults; 200 mg/kg/d divided q6–8h for children, max daily dose 12 g

Second Line
If the patient is penicillin-allergic, clindamycin with a fluoroquinolone (ciprofloxacin or levofloxacin) (>18 years only) may be used; or vancomycin and a fluoroquinolone can be used. In children, consider clindamycin with cefazolin or clindamycin with vancomycin:
- Ceftriaxone 2 g IV q12h for adults; 80–100 mg/kg/g divided q12h for children, max daily dose 4 g
- Cefotaxime 2 g IV q4h for adults; 150–200 mg/kg/d divided q6–8h, max daily dose 12 g for children
- Ciprofloxacin or levofloxacin 500 mg q12h (>18 years only)

ADDITIONAL TREATMENT
Steroid use is still controversial. Short-term systemic steroid may be recommended for use in orbital cellulitis secondary to sinusitis (3)[C].

Issues for Referral
- Ophthalmology and otolaryngology should be consulted early when orbital cellulitis is suspected.
- Infectious disease consultation should be considered if available.
- Neurology or neurosurgery should be consulted if intracranial spread is suspected (3,4)[B].

SURGERY/OTHER PROCEDURES
- IV antibiotic therapy is still the best initial therapy. Surgical intervention is warranted when a patient has visual impairment, complete ophthalmoplegia, or well-defined large abscess (>10 mm) on presentation or no clinical improvement after 24 hours of antibiotic therapy.
- Treatment of choice for brain abscess is surgical excision or drainage with 4–8 weeks of antibiotics.
- Surgical interventions include external ethmoidectomy, endoscopic ethmoidectomy, uncinectomy, antrostomy, and subperiosteal drainage (1)[C].

IN-PATIENT CONSIDERATIONS
Patients with orbital cellulitis should be admitted for IV antibiotics and repeated eye examination to evaluate progression of infection or involvement of optic nerve (1,2,3)[A].

ONGOING CARE

FOLLOW-UP RECOMMENDATIONS
Patient Monitoring
- Visual acuity testing at least daily
- Pupillary light reflex monitored at least daily

ALERT
Close monitoring is indicated, as complications can develop rapidly.

PATIENT EDUCATION
- Maintain good skin hygiene.
- Avoid skin trauma.
- Promptly report periorbital swelling and/or erythema to health care professional.

COMPLICATIONS
- Complications can develop rapidly and include permanent vision loss, central nervous system involvement, and even death.
- Permanent vision loss:
  – Corneal opacification
  – Endophthalmitis
  – Septic uveitis or retinitis
  – Exudative retinal detachment
  – Globe rupture due to significantly increased intraocular pressure
  – Orbital compartment syndrome, compression of orbital soft tissues and optic nerve
  – Optic neuritis
  – Thrombophlebitis of ocular veins
  – Central retinal artery occlusion
  – Acute infarction of retina and choroids
- Central nervous system complications:
  – Intracranial abscess
  – Meningitis
  – Cavernous sinus thrombosis (2,3,4)[B]

REFERENCES

1. Botting AM, McIntosh D, Mahadevan M. Paediatric pre- and post-septal peri-orbital infections are different diseases A retrospective review of 262 cases. *Int J Pediatr Otorhinolaryngol*. 2008.
2. Hauser A, Fogarasi S et al. Periorbital and orbital cellulitis. *Pediatr Rev*. 2010;31:242–9.
3. Kloek CE, Rubin PA. Role of inflammation in orbital cellulitis. *Int Ophthalmol Clin*. 2006;46:57–68.
4. Brook I et al. Microbiology and antimicrobial treatment of orbital and intracranial complications of sinusitis in children and their management. *Int J Pediatr Otorhinolaryngol*. 2009;73:1183–6.
5. Rudloe TF, Harper MB, Prabhu SP, Rahbar R, Vanderveen D, Kimia AA et al. Acute periorbital infections: who needs emergent imaging? *Pediatrics*. 2010;125:e719–26.

ADDITIONAL READING

- Cannon PS, Mc Keag D, Radford R, Ataullah S, Leatherbarrow B et al. Our experience using primary oral antibiotics in the management of orbital cellulitis in a tertiary referral centre. *Eye (Lond)*. 2009;23:612–5.
- Ryan JT, Preciado DA, Bauman N, et al. Management of pediatric orbital cellulitis in patients with radiographic findings of subperiosteal abscess. *Otolaryngol Head Neck Surg*. 2009;140:907–11.
- Yang M, Quah BL, Seah LL, Looi A et al. Orbital cellulitis in children-medical treatment versus surgical management. *Orbit*. 2009;28:124–36.

CODES

ICD9
376.01 Orbital cellulitis

CLINICAL PEARLS

- Most of orbital cellulitis cases result from contiguous sinusitis.
- Patients should be admitted to the hospital for monitoring and IV antibiotic treatment if orbital cellulitis is diagnosed.
- Ophthalmoplegia, mental status changes, contralateral cranial nerve palsy, or bilateral orbital cellulitis may herald intracranial involvement.
- Ophthalmology and otolaryngology should be consulted early when orbital cellulitis is suspected.

Fozia A. Ali, MD

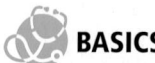 BASICS

DESCRIPTION
- An acute, spreading infection of the skin and subcutaneous tissue of the area surrounding the eye, usually secondary to external inoculation, but the inflammation does not extend into the bony orbit
- Synonym(s): Preseptal cellulitis

ALERT
It is important to distinguish periorbital cellulitis from orbital cellulitis (restricted extraocular mobility, diplopia, proptosis, and globe displacement vision loss), which is a potentially life-threatening condition.

EPIDEMIOLOGY
Occurs more commonly in children, with mean age 21 months

Incidence
Increased incidence in the winter months (due to increased number of cases of sinusitis)

RISK FACTORS
- Contiguous spread from upper respiratory infection
- Sinusitis
- Local skin trauma
- Insect bite
- Puncture wound
- Bacteremia

Genetics
No known genetic predisposition

GENERAL PREVENTION
- Avoid dermatologic trauma.
- Avoid swimming in fresh or salt water with skin abrasion.

PATHOPHYSIOLOGY
- An understanding of the anatomy of the eyelid is important in distinguishing preseptal from orbital cellulitis. The orbital septum is a sheet of connective tissue that extends from the orbital bones to the margins of the upper and lower eyelids, and it acts as a barrier to infection deep in the orbital structures. Infection of the tissues superficial to the orbital septum is called preseptal cellulitis, whereas infection deep in the orbital septum is termed orbital cellulitis.

- Periorbital cellulitis classically arises from a contiguous infection of soft tissues of the face, secondary to:
  – Sinusitis (via lamina papyracea)
  – Local trauma
  – Insect or animal bites
  – Foreign bodies

ETIOLOGY
- Common organisms:
  – *Streptococcus pneumoniae*
  – *Staphylococcus aureus*
  – *Streptococcus pyogenes*
- Atypical organisms:
  – *Acinetobacter sp.*
  – *Nocardia brasiliensis*
  – *Bacillus anthracis*
  – *Pseudomonas aeruginosa*
  – *Neisseria gonorrhoeae*
  – *Proteus sp.*
  – *Pasteurella multocida*
  – *Mycobacterium tuberculosis*
  – *Trichophyton sp.* (ringworm)
- Since the introduction of routine vaccination in 1990, *Haemophilus influenzae* B is no longer a leading cause of orbital cellulitis.

DIAGNOSIS

HISTORY
- Induration, erythema, warmth, and/or tenderness of periorbital soft tissues
- Chemosis (conjunctival swelling), proptosis, pain with extraocular eye movements
- Fever (although not necessary for diagnosis)

ALERT
Pain with eye movement and conjunctival swelling can occur, although both should raise the suspicion for orbital cellulitis.

PHYSICAL EXAM
- Thorough inspection of the eye and surrounding structures is key part in physical exam.
- Erythema, swelling, and tenderness of lids without orbital congestion. Violaceous discoloration of eyelid is more commonly associated with *Haemophilus influenza*.

- Also look for any break in skin if history of trauma causing periorbital cellulitis. Look for vesicle to rule out herpetic infection.
- Inspection of nasal vaults and sinus palpation for signs of acute sinusitis
- Ocular motility and visual acuity testing to rule out orbital cellulitis

DIAGNOSTIC TESTS & INTERPRETATION
Lab
- Complete blood count with differential
- Blood cultures

Follow-Up & Special Considerations
Children with periorbital or orbital cellulitis often have underlying sinusitis. If the child is febrile and appears toxic, blood cultures should be performed and lumbar puncture considered.

Imaging
If suspicious for orbital involvement, computed tomography (CT) scan can be used to evaluate the extent of infection and detect orbital inflammation or abscess (1)[B]. The classic sign of orbital cellulitis on CT scan is bulging of the medial rectus. CT should be performed with contrast, thin sections (2 mm), coronal and axial views with bone windows.

DIFFERENTIAL DIAGNOSIS
- Orbital cellulitis: Orbital cellulitis may have the same signs and symptoms in the periorbital tissue, but also results in proptosis, edema of the conjunctiva, ophthalmoplegia, or decreased visual acuity.
- Abscess
- Dacryocystitis
- Hordeolum
- Allergic inflammation
- Orbital or periorbital trauma
- Idiopathic orbital inflammatory syndrome
- Rapidly progressive tumors:
  – Rhabdomyosarcoma
  – Retinoblastoma
  – Lymphoma
- Leukemia

TREATMENT

MEDICATION

- Empiric antibiotic treatment regimens are based on coverage of the most likely organisms, paying attention to local resistance patterns and the pathogens usually associated with sinusitis.
- Uncomplicated post-traumatic:
  – Usually due to skin flora, including *Staphylococcus* and *Streptococcus*
  – Cephalexin, dicloxacillin, clindamycin
- Extension from sinusitis:
  – Amoxicillin, clavulanate, 3rd-generation cephalosporin
- Bacteremic cellulitis:
  – May be associated with meningitis
  – Ceftriaxone plus vancomycin to cover methicillin-resistant *Staphylococcus aureus*
- Duration of therapy should be 7–10 days:
  – If symptoms do not improve within 24 hours, IV antibiotic therapy is indicated (2)[B].

ADDITIONAL TREATMENT
Issues for Referral
Although treatment may consist of intravenous antibiotics alone, management should be in consultation with otolaryngologists and ophthalmologists, especially when there is concern of orbital cellulitis.

SURGERY/OTHER PROCEDURES
Orbital surgery is indicated if the patient:

- Fails to respond
- No improvement by 24–48 hours
- Visual impairment
- Complete ophthalmoplegia
- Well-defined periosteal abscess (1,2)
- Deteriorates clinically despite treatment
- Has worsening visual acuity or pupillary changes
- Develops an abscess, except in selected pediatric cases of medial subperiosteal abscess, which may be successfully treated medically. Abscess formation necessitates incision and drainage.
- Endoscopic and transcaruncular surgery has been successfully employed to treat subperiosteal and intraorbital abscesses.

IN-PATIENT CONSIDERATIONS
- Mild cases in adults and children >1 year can be managed on an outpatient basis, provided the patient is stable and without systemic signs of toxicity.
- Preseptal cellulitis in children <4 years may warrant hospitalization and the use of intravenous antibiotics.

Admission Criteria
Consider hospitalization and IV antibiotics:

- For children <1 year
- Patients who have not been immunized for *S. pneumoniae* or *H. influenza*
- If no signs of clinical improvement are apparent after 24 hours of oral antibiotics

Discharge Criteria
- There are no strict guidelines to indicate when to switch therapy from parenteral to oral agents.
- Generally, we switch to oral therapy after the patient is afebrile and the skin findings have begun to resolve, which usually takes 3–5 days. Once we switch to oral therapy, it should be continued for 2–3 weeks. The longer duration is recommended for those patients with severe ethmoid sinusitis associated with bony destruction.

ONGOING CARE

FOLLOW-UP RECOMMENDATIONS
Patient Monitoring
The patient should be monitored for signs of orbital involvement, including decreased visual acuity or painful/limited ocular motility.

PATIENT EDUCATION
- Maintain good skin hygiene.
- Avoid skin trauma.
- Report early skin changes to health care professional.

PROGNOSIS
With adequate antibiotic treatment, outlook is good. Response to antibiotics in children with periorbital cellulitis usually is rapid, and a 10-day course of treatment generally is sufficient.

COMPLICATIONS
- Orbital cellulitis
- Abscess formation
- Scarring
- Delay in diagnosis and adequate treatment may result in serious complications, including blindness.

REFERENCES

1. Beech T, Robinson A, McDermott AL, et al. Paediatric periorbital cellulitis and its management. *Rhinology*. 2007;45:47–9.
2. Hennemann S, et al. Clinical inquiries. What is the best initial treatment for orbital cellulitis in children? *J Fam Prac*. 2007;56(8):662–4.
3. Georgakopoulos CD, Eliopoulou MI, Stasinos S, Exarchou A, Pharmakakis N, Varvarigou A et al. Periorbital and orbital cellulitis: a 10-year review of hospitalized children. *European journal of ophthalmology*. 2010.

ADDITIONAL READING

- *Br J Ophthalmol*. 2008;92:1337–41 doi:10.1136/bjo.2007.128975.
- Goldstein SM, Shelsta HN. Community-acquired Methicillin-resistant Staphylococcus aureus Periorbital Cellulitis: A Problem Here to Stay. *Ophthal Plast Reconstr Surg*. 2009;25:77.
- http://emedicine.medscape.com/article/798397-overview.

CODES

ICD9
682.0 Cellulitis and abscess of face

CLINICAL PEARLS

- Preseptal and orbital cellulitis occur most commonly in children.
- A multidisciplinary approach is needed in managing children with this condition, and CT scan of the patient's sinuses is essential to differentiate from orbital cellulitis.
- Early detection of periorbital cellulitis is important to prevent complications.
- The 2 most important factors for periorbital cellulitis are upper respiratory infection and eyelid trauma; sinusitis is more associated with orbital cellulitis (3)[C].

C

CEREBRAL PALSY

Jessica Hahn, MD
Beverly L. Nazarian, MD

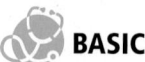 **BASICS**

DESCRIPTION

Cerebral palsy (CP): A group of chronic disorders of movement and posture caused by *nonprogressive* lesions in the developing brain. Some *activity limitation* must result from the motor impairment, and this motor dysfunction may be accompanied by impairment in other areas.

EPIDEMIOLOGY

Incidence

- Overall, 1.5–2.5 per 1,000 live births
- Incidence increases as gestational age (GA) at birth decreases (1):
  – 146/1,000 for GA of 22–27 weeks
  – 62/1,000 for GA of 28–31 weeks
  – 7/1,000 for GA of 32–36 weeks
  – 1/1,000 for GA of 37+ weeks

Prevalence

3–4/1,000 of the population

RISK FACTORS

- Prenatal:
  – Congenital anomalies
  – Multiple gestation
  – In utero stroke
  – Intrauterine infection (chorioamnionitis, TORCH)
  – Antepartum bleeding
  – Maternal factors (cognitive impairment, seizure disorders, hyperthyroidism)
  – Abnormal fetal position (e.g., breech)
- Perinatal:
  – Preterm birth
  – Low birth weight
  – Periventricular leukomalacia
  – Perinatal hypoxia/asphyxia
  – Intracranial hemorrhage/intraventricular hemorrhage
  – Neonatal seizure or stroke
  – Hyperbilirubinemia
- Postnatal:
  – Traumatic brain injury or stroke
  – Sepsis, meningitis, encephalitis
  – Asphyxia

Genetics

There are emerging reports of associations between cerebral palsy and candidate genes:

- Thrombophilic, cytokines, and apolipoprotein E

GENERAL PREVENTION

- Magnesium sulfate administration to mothers at risk for preterm delivery has a neuroprotective effect and reduces CP risk (2).
- Improved management of hyperbilirubinemia with decrease in kernicterus has greatly reduced dyskinetic CP.
- Prevention or reduction of chorioamnionitis and premature births (3)

PATHOPHYSIOLOGY

- Multifactorial; CP results from static injury or lesions in the developing brain, occurring prenatally, perinatally, or postnatally.
- Cytokines and free radicals and inflammatory response are likely contributing factors.

ETIOLOGY

- 50% of cases: Etiology is not established; most likely multifactorial.
- Spastic CP is most common, usually related to premature birth, with either periventricular leukomalacia or germinal matrix hemorrhage.
- Dyskinetic CP, often resulting from kernicterus, is now rare due to improved management of hyperbilirubinemia.

COMMONLY ASSOCIATED CONDITIONS

- Seizure disorder (22–40%)
- Cognitive impairment (23–44%)
- Behavior difficulties
- Speech and language disorders (42–81%)
- Sensory impairments:
  – Hearing deficits
  – Visual (62–71%):
    ○ Poor visual acuity, strabismus (50%), or hemianopsia
- Feeding impairment, swallowing dysfunction, and aspiration
- Poor dentition, excessive drooling
- Gastrointestinal conditions:
  – Constipation (59%), vomiting (22%), or gastroesophageal reflux
- Decreased linear growth or osteopenia
- Weight abnormalities (under- and overweight)
- Bowel and bladder incontinence
- Orthopedic: Contractures, hip subluxation/dislocation, or scoliosis

 DIAGNOSIS

- A clinical diagnosis including:
  – Delayed motor milestones
  – Abnormal tone
  – Abnormal neurological exam suggesting a cerebral etiology
  – Absence of regression
  – Absence of underlying syndromes or alternative explanation for etiology
- Although the pathological lesion is static, clinical presentation may change as the infant grows and matures.
- Accurate early diagnosis remains difficult. Neurologic abnormalities observed in the first 1–2 years of life may resolve. Caution against diagnosis of CP before age 2.

HISTORY

- Presentation: Parental concerns over movements or motor development
- Ask about:
  – Prenatal, perinatal, and postnatal risk factors
  – Neurobehavioral signs:
    ○ Poor feeding/frequent vomiting
    ○ Irritability
  – Timing of motor milestones:
    ○ Delay in milestones is not sensitive or specific until after 6 months of age.
  – Abnormal spontaneous general movements
  – Asymmetry of movements, such as early hand preference
  – Symptoms of other conditions
- Regression of motor skills *does not* occur with cerebral palsy.

PHYSICAL EXAM

- Assess for 1 or more type of neurological impairment:
  – Spasticity: Increased tone/reflexes/clonus
  – Dyskinesia: Abnormal movements
  – Hypotonia: Decreased tone
  – Ataxia: Abnormal balance/coordination
- Areas of exam:
  – Tone: May be increased or decreased.
  – Trunk and head control: Often poor, but may be advanced due to high tone
  – Persistence of primitive reflexes
  – Asymmetry of movement or reflexes
  – Brisk DTRs
  – Clonus
  – Delayed motor milestones:
    ○ Serial exams most effective
  – Gait and stance:
    ○ Scissoring gait
    ○ Toe-walking
- Specific subtypes best diagnosed after 5 years of age:
  – Spastic hemiplegic CP:
    ○ Unilateral spasticity
  – Spastic diplegic CP:
    ○ Bilateral spasticity with leg > arm involvement
  – Spastic quadriplegic CP:
    ○ Bilateral spasticity with arm > or = leg involvement
  – Dyskinetic CP:
    ○ Dystonia-hypertonia and reduced movement
    ○ Choreoathetosis: Irregular spasmodic involuntary movements of the limbs or facial muscles
  – Ataxic CP:
    ○ Loss of orderly muscular coordination
  – Mixed

DIAGNOSTIC TESTS & INTERPRETATION

Cerebral palsy is a clinical diagnosis based on history, physical, and risk factors. Diagnostic tests rule out other conditions.

Lab

- Laboratory testing is not needed to make diagnosis, but can sometimes help to exclude other etiologies.
- Testing for metabolic and genetic syndromes (4):
  – Not routinely obtained in the evaluation for CP
  – If no specific etiology is identified by neuroimaging, or if there are atypical features in clinical presentation, genetic or metabolic testing may be useful.
  – Detection of certain brain malformations may warrant genetic or metabolic testing to identify syndromes.
- Screening for coagulopathies:
  – Diagnostic testing for coagulopathies should be considered in children with hemiplegic CP with cerebral infarction identified on neuroimaging (4)[C].

Imaging

- Neuroimaging is not essential, but recommended in children with CP for whom the etiology has not been established (4)[C].

- Magnetic resonance imaging (MRI) is preferred to computed tomography (CT) scanning (4)[C].
- Abnormalities in 80–90% of patients (5)[A]:
  - Brain malformation, cerebral infarction, intraventricular or other intracranial hemorrhage, periventricular leukomalacia, ventricular enlargement, or other cerebrospinal fluid (CSF) space abnormalities

Diagnostic Procedures/Surgery

- Assessing the functional impact of cerebral palsy can help to determine appropriate services and prognosis:
  - The Gross Motor Function Classification System is commonly used
  - A score of II or higher is considered significant. A score of IV or V indicates more severe involvement.
- Screening for comorbid conditions: Developmental delay/cognitive impairment, basion/hearing impairments, speech and language disorders, or feeding/swallowing dysfunction

Pathological Findings

Perinatal brain injury may include:

- White matter damage:
  - Most common in premature infants
  - Periventricular leukomalacia:
    - Gliosis with or without focal necrosis with resulting cysts and scarring
    - May be multiple lesions of various ages
    - Necrosis can lead to cysts/scarring.
  - Germinal matrix hemorrhage:
    - May lead to intraventricular hemorrhage
- Grey matter damage:
  - More common in term infants
  - Cortical infarcts, focal neuronal damage, myelination abnormalities

DIFFERENTIAL DIAGNOSIS

Benign congenital hypotonia, Brachial plexus injury, Familial spastic paraplegia, Dopa-responsive dystonia, Transient toe-walking, Muscular dystrophy, Metabolic disorders (e.g., glutaric aciduria type 1), Mitochondrial disorders, Genetic disorders (e.g., Rett syndrome)

 TREATMENT

Focuses on control of symptoms: Spasticity, management of comorbid conditions, improvement in functioning, and quality of life

MEDICATION

First Line

- Baclofen (6)[C]:
  - γ-aminobutyric acid B (GABA$_B$) agonist, facilitates presynaptic inhibition of mono- and polysynaptic reflexes
  - Adults: Initial dose is 5 mg t.i.d. and increase dosage every 3 days to an average maintenance dose of 20 mg t.i.d. 80 mg/24-hr maximum
  - Pediatric dose (>2 y/o): Initial 10–15 mg/24 hrs. Titrate to effective dose. <8 y/o = 40 mg/24 hrs. maximum. >8 y/o 60 mg/24 hrs. maximum
- Intrathecal Baclofen (Baclofen Pump):
  - Continuous intrathecal route allows greater maximal response with smaller dosage
  - Significantly reduces spasticity in children with cerebral palsy
  - Multiple adverse effects due to catheter placement and medication side effects
- Diazepam (6)[C]:
  - A GABA$_A$ agonist, facilitating CNS inhibition at spinal and supraspinal levels to reduce spasticity

---

- Adult dose: 2–12 mg/dose p.o. q6–12 hrs.
- Pediatric dose (<12 yrs): 0.12–0.8 mg/kg/24 h. p.o., divided q6–8h.
- Botulinum toxin type A:
  - Injected directly into muscles of interest
  - Acts at neuromuscular junction to inhibit the release of acetylcholine
  - Chemically denervates muscles, reducing tone
  - Lasts for 12–16 weeks following injection

Second Line

The following medications are used far less frequently:

- Dantrolene:
  - Limits calcium release from muscles, reducing spasticity
  - Adult dosing: 25 mg p.o. daily titrated to effective dose, maximum 100 mg p.o. q.i.d.
  - Pediatric dosing: 0.5 mg/kg p.o. daily titrated to effective dose, maximum 12 mg/kg/24 hrs.
- Tizanidine and other α-adrenergic agents:
  - α-adrenergic agonist, presynaptically inhibits motor activation, reducing spasticity
  - Adult dosing: 4 mg/day p.o., titrate to effective dose, up to 8 mg p.o. q4–6h, 36 mg/24 hrs. maximum
- Gabapentin:
  - Anticonvulsant structurally similar to GABA, increases levels of GABA in brain and reduces spasticity
  - Adult dosing: Titrate to starting dose 100 mg t.i.d. starting dosage, maximum dose 3600 mg/day in divided dosing

ADDITIONAL TREATMENT

- Care needs to be multidisciplinary, usually including specialists from orthopedics, neurology, ophthalmology, and physiatry, as well as physical, occupational, and speech therapists.
- "Medical home" with PCP (7) which requires:
  - Identification of patient's and family's needs for support, respite, and community resources
  - Care coordination among medical providers and with community agencies
  - Collaboration with schools and transition to adult care

General Measures

- Referral to early intervention for children ages 0–3 is essential.
- Various therapy modalities enhance functioning:
  - Physical therapy: Posture stability and gait, motor strength and control, contracture prevention
  - Occupational therapy: Functional activities of daily living and other fine motor skills
  - Speech therapy: Verbal and nonverbal speech and aid in feeding
- Equipment optimizes participation in activities:
  - Orthotic splinting: Maintains functional positioning and prevents contractures
    - AFOs (ankle-foot orthosis)
    - DAFOs (dynamic ankle-foot orthosis)
  - Spinal bracing (body jacket) may slow scoliosis.
  - Augmentative communication: Pictures, switches, or computer systems for nonverbal individuals
  - Electrical stimulation: Therapeutic and functional
  - Use of adaptive equipment such as standers to allow weight bearing
  - Mobility: Crutches, walkers, wheelchairs

COMPLEMENTARY AND ALTERNATIVE MEDICINE

- Hyperbaric oxygen: Conflicting results
- Hippotherapy: Therapeutic horse riding
- Aquatic therapy

SURGERY/OTHER PROCEDURES

- Dorsal root rhizotomy: Selectively cutting dorsal rootlets from L1–S2:
  - Best for patients with normal intelligence with spastic diplegia
  - Minimizes spasticity in lower limbs, but associated with adverse effects
- Surgical treatment of joint dislocations/subluxation, scoliosis management, tendon lengthening, etc.

 ONGOING CARE

PROGNOSIS

Reduced lifespan only in most severely affected.

REFERENCES

1. Himpens E, Van den Broeck C, Oostra A et al. Prevalence, type, distribution, and severity of cerebral palsy in relation to gestational age: a meta-analytic review. Dev Med Child Neurol. 2008;50:334–40.
2. Doyle LW, Crowther CA, Middleton P, et al. Magnesium sulphate for women at risk of preterm birth for neuroprotection of the fetus. Cochrane Database Syst Rev. 2009:CD004661.
3. Shatrov JG, Birch SC, Lam LT et al. Chorioamnionitis and cerebral palsy: a meta-analysis. Obstet Gynecol. 2010;116:387–92.
4. Ashwal S, Russman BS, Blasco PA et al., Practice parameter: diagnostic assessment of the child with cerebral palsy: report of the Quality Standards Subcommittee of the American Academy of Neurology and the Practice Committee of the Child Neurology Society. Neurology. 2004; 62:851–63.
5. Korzeniewski SJ, Birbeck G, Delano MC et al., A systematic review of neuroimaging for cerebral palsy. J Child Neurol. 2008;23:216–27.
6. Montané E, Vallano A, Laporte JR. Oral antispastic drugs in nonprogressive neurologic diseases: a systematic review. Neurology. 2004;63:1357–63.
7. Cooley WC, American Academy of Pediatrics Committee on Children With Disabilities. Providing a primary care medical home for children and youth with cerebral palsy. Pediatrics. 2004;114:1106–13.

 CODES

ICD9

- 343.0 Congenital diplegia
- 343.1 Congenital hemiplegia
- 343.2 Congenital quadriplegia

CLINICAL PEARLS

- Management should focus on maximizing functioning and quality of life with multidisciplinary team approach.
- Regression of motor skills does not occur with cerebral palsy.

C

CERVICAL HYPEREXTENSION INJURIES

Francesca L. Beaudoin, MS, MD
Stephanie Carreiro, MD

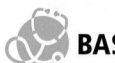

BASICS

DESCRIPTION
- Group of injuries involving the neck that result from a rapid, forceful, backwards motion
- May involve:
  - Injury to vertebral and paravertebral structures: Fractures, dislocations, ligamentous tears, and disc disruption/subluxation
  - Spinal cord injury: Traumatic central cord syndrome (CCS) secondary to cord compression or vascular insult
  - Vascular injury: Vertebral artery or carotid artery dissection
  - Soft tissue injury around cervical spine: Cervical strain/sprain
- System(s) affected: Musculoskeletal; Nervous; Vascular
- Synonym(s): Cervical acceleration-deceleration injury

EPIDEMIOLOGY
- Predominant age: Trauma and sports injuries more common in young adults (average age 29.4 years); however, CCS mostly seen in older population (average age 53 years)
- Predominant sex: Male > Female
- 25% spinal injuries caused by hyperextension

Incidence
In the US:
- Cervical fractures: 2–5/100 blunt trauma patients
- Central cord syndrome: 3.6/100,000 people/year
- Cervical artery dissection: 3 /100,000 people/year
- Cervical strain: 3 /1,000 people/year

RISK FACTORS
- Pre-existing spinal stenosis is present in >50% of cases of CCS, which may be:
  - Acquired: Prior trauma, spondylosis
  - Congenital: Klippel-Feil syndrome (congenital fusion of any 2 cervical vertebra) with cervical stenosis
- Conditions predisposing to spinal rigidity, such as ankylosing spondylitis, increase risk of vertebral fractures.

GENERAL PREVENTION
Wear seat belts and use proper safety equipment in sports activities.

ETIOLOGY
Trauma due to motor vehicle accidents, sports injuries, falls, and assaults.

COMMONLY ASSOCIATED CONDITIONS
Closed head injuries (concussion, cerebral contusions, intracranial bleeding), facial fractures, thoracic/lumbar spinal injury

DIAGNOSIS

HISTORY
Usually acute presentation with mechanism of cervical hyperextension (see Etiology) and complaints of neck pain, stiffness or headaches, +/− neurologic symptoms

PHYSICAL EXAM
- External signs of trauma on the head and neck such as abrasions, lacerations, hematomas, or contusions
- Presence, severity, and location of neck tenderness:
  - Posterior midline, bony point tenderness concerning for bony injury
  - Paraspinal or lateral soft tissue tenderness suggestive of muscular/ligamentous injury.
  - Anterior tenderness concerning for carotid injury
- Range-of-motion (ROM) limitation
- Neurologic exam: Paresthesias/numbness, weakness
- CCS:
  - Typical symptom distribution: Distal > proximal, upper extremity > lower extremity
  - Extremity weakness/paralysis
  - Variable sensory changes below level of lesion (including paresthesias and dysesthesia)
  - Bladder/bowel dysfunction

DIAGNOSTIC TESTS & INTERPRETATION
Imaging
Initial approach
- Low-risk patients can be cleared clinically (without radiographic evaluation) using either the Canadian C-Spine Rule (CCR) or the National Emergency X-ray Utilization Study (NEXUS) Criteria:
  - CCR: Clinically clear a stable, adult patient with no history of cervical spine disease/surgery if all of the following conditions are met:
    - GCS = 15
    - Nonintoxicated patients without a distracting injury
    - No dangerous mechanism or extremity paresthesias
    - At least 1 "low-risk factor" (i.e., simple rear-end MVA, ambulation at the accident scene, no midline cervical tenderness, delayed onset of neck pain or sitting position at the time of exam)
  - NEXUS: Clinically clear if all of the following are met:
    - No alteration of mental status or intoxication
    - No focal neurodeficits
    - No distracting injury
    - No posterior, midline c-spine tenderness
  - Reported sensitivity/specificity: CCR (99.4%/45.1%), NEXUS (90.7%/36.8%) (1)[A]
- If imaging is required, choose from the following options based on the suspected injury and level of clinical suspicion:
  - Plain radiographs: Recommended by some in patients who cannot be cleared clinically but still are in low-suspicion category: Sensitivity for c-spine injury as low as 52% (2)[B]:
    - Static: Lateral, anterior-posterior (A-P) and odontoid views; in addition to bony abnormalities, may show prevertebral soft tissue swelling
    - Dynamic: Flexion/extension, only if asymptomatic and no neurologic deficits or mental impairment. Evaluates spine stability and union by amount of movement in fractures during or after treatment. Of limited utility in the acute setting given that technically adequate films are difficult to obtain in patients with restricted ROM (3)[C].
  - CT: Axial CT from occiput to T1 with coronal and sagittal reconstructions: Rapidly replacing plain radiography as the test of choice for cases with moderate to high clinical suspicion of c-spine injury given high sensitivity (95–99%) (2,4)[B]

  - MRI: Diagnostic test of choice in CCS with direct visualization of traumatic cord lesions (edema or hematomyelia), soft tissue compressing cord, and/or stenosis of canal. Also detects ligamentous injury and abnormalities of intervertebral discs and soft tissues, but modality is poor with fractures and is prone to false-positive results due to nonspecific findings.
  - CTA/MRA: Visualization of cervical and cerebral vascular structures to detect carotid or vertebral artery dissections

Follow-Up & Special Considerations
Cervical strain: May repeat flexion/extension lateral cervical spine views to confirm stability once muscular spasms have resolved

Pathological Findings
- Vertebral fractures: See General Measures.
- CCS: Currently thought to be due to axonal disruption within the white matter of the lateral column, particularly the corticospinal tracts
- Vascular dissection: Intimal disruption, leading to thrombosis and embolization
- Models of acute cervical strain/sprain based on animal, cadaver, and postmortem studies show myofascial tearing, edema, and inflammation; facet joint capsular pain may also play a role.
- Stretching or rupture of spinal ligaments
- Injuries to intervertebral discs

DIFFERENTIAL DIAGNOSIS
- Acute or chronic disc pathology (including herniation or internal disruption)
- Osteoarthritis
- Cervical radiculopathy
- For CCS:
  - Bell cruciate palsy
  - Bilateral brachial plexus injuries
  - Carotid or vertebral artery dissection

Geriatric Considerations
- Degenerative disease of c-spine may be confused with acute traumatic change on imaging; CT imaging more helpful to distinguish the 2
- Osteoporosis increases risk of fracture.

Pediatric Considerations
Consider SCI without radiographic abnormality, which has a high incidence at <9 years and accounts for up to 50% of all pediatric cervical spine injuries. MRI may help detect the injury.

TREATMENT

MEDICATION
- CCS: Methylprednisolone IV 30 mg/kg over 15 minutes, then 45 minutes later; start continuous infusion by IV 5.4 mg/kg/h for 24 hours. Further improvement in motor function recovery may be seen if infusion is given for 48 hours, especially if bolus dose is given 3–8 hours after injury (5)[A].
- Carotid/vertebral dissection: Anticoagulation with IV heparin, followed by warfarin therapy for 3–6 months, then long term antiplatelet therapy is currently recommended. However, an antiplatelet agent is recommended as the sole initial therapy in patients with contraindications to anticoagulation.

- Cervical strain: Muscle relaxants, acetaminophen/nonsteroidal anti-inflammatory agents +/- opiate analgesics are commonly used

ADDITIONAL TREATMENT
General Measures
- Fractures:
  - Stability determined by imaging; decompression and stabilization are indicated in:
    ○ Incomplete SCIs with spinal canal compromise
    ○ Clinical deterioration or failure to improve despite conservative management
  - Hangman fracture: Traumatic spondylolisthesis of C2 (the "axis") with bilateral fractures through C2 pedicles, often with anterior subluxation of C2 over C3: Can be unstable:
    ○ Managed with halo vest immobilization for 12 weeks until repeated flexion/extension films normalize
    ○ Unstable if C2 subluxation over C3; >50% of vertebral body of C3 in anteroposterior diameter, or if excessive angulation of C2 over C3
  - Odontoid fracture: Treated according to type:
    ○ I: Through apex; usually stable; external immobilization with a cervical collar or halo vest for up to 12 weeks
    ○ II: Most common, at base of dens, usually unstable; nonunion rates of up to 67% with halo immobilization alone, especially with dens displacement >6 mm or age >50 years
    ○ III: Through C2 body, usually stable; initially immobilized in halo or cervical collar for 12–20 weeks (6)[B]
  - Hyperextension teardrop fractures:
    ○ If stable, rigid collar or cervicothoracic brace for 8–14 weeks
    ○ If unstable, halo brace for up to 3 months
- CCS: Neck immobilization with cervical collar, PT/OT
- Cervical strain: Treatment depends on severity:
  - No evidence that immobilization is beneficial; may use soft cervical collar for up to 10 days for symptomatic relief; otherwise, early mobilization and activity as tolerated

Issues for Referral
- When cervical spine injury is suspected, the patient should be immobilized and sent to the emergency department for evaluation.
- Emergent consultation from a spinal surgeon (neurosurgery and/or orthopedics) is indicated if there is any concern for unstable fracture or spinal cord injury.

COMPLEMENTARY AND ALTERNATIVE MEDICINE
Acupuncture for chronic neck pain resulting from cervical strain

SURGERY/OTHER PROCEDURES
- Hangman's fracture: Consider surgical fixation in cases of excessive angulation or subluxation, disruption of intervertebral disc space or failure to obtain alignment with external orthosis (6)[B].
- Odontoid fractures:
  - Type II: Early surgical stabilization recommended in setting of age >50 years old, dens displacement >5 mm and in certain fracture patterns
  - Type III: Surgical intervention often reserved for cases of nonunion/malunion after trial of external immobilization

- Hyperextension teardrop fractures: Consider surgical repair if unstable with neurologic deficit
- CCS:
  - If occurs in setting of unstable injury and/or herniated disc, surgical decompression/fixation is indicated
  - Otherwise, surgery considered when neurologic function plateaus or deteriorates (7)[B]

IN-PATIENT CONSIDERATIONS
Initial Stabilization
Advanced Trauma Life Support (ATLS) protocol with backboard and collar

Admission Criteria
Varies by injury; clinical judgment, radiographic findings, and need for operative intervention influence decision

 ## ONGOING CARE

FOLLOW-UP RECOMMENDATIONS
Follow-up depends on the severity of injury, but all patients with hyperextension injuries should receive follow-up care.

Patient Monitoring
Patients with known injuries will often be followed with serial radiographs under the care of a specialist.

PATIENT EDUCATION
For patient instruction on prevention: THINK FIRST Foundation at: http://www.thinkfirst.org.

PROGNOSIS
- Overall, the most important prognostic factor is the initial neurologic status.
- Fracture dislocation:
  - Hangman fracture: 93–100% fusion rate after 8–14 weeks external immobilization
  - Odontoid fracture, fusion rate by type: Type I approximately 100% with external immobilization alone; Type III, 85% with external immobilization, 100% with surgical fixation (6)
- CCS:
  - Spontaneous recovery of motor function in >50% of cases over several weeks
  - Younger patients (<50 years old) are more likely to regain function.
  - Leg, bowel, and bladder functions return first; upper extremities follow, but recovery is often incomplete, especially manual dexterity (7)
- Cervical strain: 50% of patients continue to have neck pain at 1 year:
  - Greater initial disability, symptom severity, and psychological factors also predict slower recovery.
  - Prognostic factors for development of late whiplash syndrome (>6 months of symptoms affecting normal activity) include increased initial pain intensity, pain-related disability, and cold hyperalgesia.

COMPLICATIONS
- Nonunion/malunion of fractures
- Persistent instability requiring 2nd procedure
- Reactions and infection related to orthosis
- Embolic ischemic events and pseudoaneurysm formation after vascular dissection
- Persistent symptoms and pain/late whiplash syndrome

REFERENCES
1. Stiell IG, Clement CM, McKnight RD, Brison R, Schull MJ, Rowe BH, Worthington JR, Eisenhauer MA, Cass D, Greenberg G, MacPhail I, Dreyer J, Lee JS, Bandiera G, Reardon M, Holroyd B, Lesiuk H, Wells GA et al. The Canadian C-spine rule versus the NEXUS low-risk criteria in patients with trauma. *N Engl J Med.* 2003;349:2510–8.
2. Holmes JF, Akkinepalli R et al. Computed tomography versus plain radiography to screen for cervical spine injury: a meta-analysis. *J Trauma.* 2005;58:902–5.
3. Insko EK, Gracias VH, Gupta R, Goettler CE, Gaieski DF, Dalinka MK et al. Utility of flexion and extension radiographs of the cervical spine in the acute evaluation of blunt trauma. *J Trauma.* 2002;53:426–9.
4. Como JJ, Diaz JJ, Dunham CM, Chiu WC, Duane TM, Capella JM, Holevar MR, Khwaja KA, Mayglothling JA, Shapiro MB, Winston ES et al. Practice management guidelines for identification of cervical spine injuries following trauma: update from the eastern association for the surgery of trauma practice management guidelines committee. *J Trauma.* 2009;67:651–9.
5. Bracken MB. Steroids for acute spinal cord injury. Cochrane injuries group. *Cochrane Database Syst Rev.* 2008;3.
6. Pryputniewicz DM, Hadley MN et al. Axis fractures. *Neurosurgery.* 2010;66:68–82.
7. Aarabi B, Koltz M, Ibrahimi D et al. Hyperextension cervical spine injuries and traumatic central cord syndrome. *Neurosurg Focus.* 2008;25:E9.

See Also (Topic, Algorithm, Electronic Media Element)
Cervical Spinal Injury

 ## CODES

ICD9
- 847.0 Neck sprain
- 952.00 C1-c4 level spinal cord injury, unspecified
- 952.03 C1-c4 level with central cord syndrome

CLINICAL PEARLS
- Suspect SCI until exam and imaging suggest otherwise.
- Follow NEXUS or Canadian Cervical Spine rules on every patient with potential neck injury to determine imaging needs, but use clinical judgement!
- Inquire about preexisting cervical spine injuries or conditions, especially in the elderly, as they may increase risk of injury or alter radiographic interpretation.
- Consider vascular dissection when neurologic deficits are inconsistent with level of known injury.

CERVICAL MALIGNANCY

Amos O. Adelowo, MD, MPH
Antonella M. Leary, MD

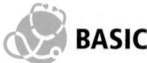 BASICS

DESCRIPTION
- Invasive cancer of the uterine cervix
- Commonly involves the vagina, parametria, and pelvic side walls
- Invasion of bladder, rectum, and other pelvic sites in advanced disease
- Disease prognosis differs with tumor stage.

EPIDEMIOLOGY
Incidence
- Worldwide, cervical cancer ranks 2nd among all malignancies for women (1).
- Higher incidence of cervical cancer in developing countries, contributing up to 83% of reported cases annually
- In the US, it is the 3rd most common gynecologic cancer and the 6th most common solid malignant neoplasm among women.
- Median age at diagnosis is bimodal: 35–50 years and >65 years

Prevalence
- In 2007, the American Cancer Society (ACS) estimated 11,150 new cases with 3,670 deaths from the malignancy.
- In 2008, the number of new cases decreased to 11,070 and the number of deaths increased to 3,870.
- African Americans and women in lower socioeconomic groups have the highest age-standardized cervical cancer death rates.
- Hispanic and Latino women have the highest incidence rate of the malignancy.

RISK FACTORS
- Strong association with sexually transmitted HPV infection
- Other risk factors include:
  - Early coitarche
  - Multiple sexual partners
  - Unprotected sex
  - A history of STDs
  - Nonbarrier methods of birth control
  - Low socioeconomic status
  - High parity
  - Cigarette smoking
  - Immunosuppression
  - DES exposure in utero
  - Lack of regular Pap smears

Genetics
Not an inherited disease

GENERAL PREVENTION
- Patient education regarding safer sex, condom use, decreasing number of sexual partners (2)[A]
- Smoking cessation
- Gardasil vaccine (3): Quadrivalent vaccine containing proteins from HPV strains 6, 11, 16, and 18. Recommended age of vaccination is 11–12 years, but can be given from age 9–26:
  - Vaccine is a series of 3 IM injections, with the 2nd and 3rd following 3 and 6 months after the 1st (4)[B].
- Regular screening: Pap smears and pelvic exams at appropriate intervals according to American College of Obstetricians and Gynecologists and the American Cancer Society
- Despite HPV vaccination, cervical cancer screening will remain the main preventive measure for both vaccinated and nonvaccinated women, but the nature of screening and management of women with cervical disease is being adapted to the new technologies (5).

PATHOPHYSIOLOGY
- Arise from preexisting dysplastic lesions usually following HPV infection
- Pattern of local growth may be exophytic or endophytic.
- Lymphatic spread typically through cervical lymphatic drainage
- Local tumor extension involving the bladder, ureters, rectum, and distant metastasis from hematogenous spread

ETIOLOGY
- Epidemiologic and experimental evidence supports oncogenic strains of HPV 16 and 18 as etiologic agents in cervical carcinogenesis.
- Association with the E6 and E7 oncogenic proteins responsible for malignant cell transformation by inactivation of the p53 and Rb tumor suppressor genes
- Slow progression from dysplasia to invasive cancer

COMMONLY ASSOCIATED CONDITIONS
- Condyloma acuminata
- Preinvasive/invasive lesions of the vulva and vagina

 DIAGNOSIS

HISTORY
- May be asymptomatic
- Most common symptom is vaginal bleeding, often postcoital.
- Other gynecological symptoms include intermenstrual or postmenopausal bleeding and vaginal discharge.
- Other less common symptoms include low back pain with radiation down posterior leg, lower extremity edema, vesicovaginal and rectovaginal fistula, and urinary symptoms.

PHYSICAL EXAM
- Most patients have a normal physical exam.
- Thorough external genitalia and internal vaginal exam is needed to look for lesions:
  - Cervix may appear grossly normal with microinvasive disease.
  - Lesions may be exophytic, endophytic, polypoid, papillary, ulcerative, or necrotic.
  - Watery, purulent, or bloody discharge.
- Bimanual and rectovaginal examination for uterine size, vaginal wall, rectovaginal septum, parametrial, uterosacral, and pelvic sidewall involvement.
- Enlarged supraclavicular or inguinal lymphadenopathy, lower extremity edema, ascites, or decreased breath sounds with lung auscultation may indicate metastases.
- Examination under anesthesia for extent of pelvic tumor spread

DIAGNOSTIC TESTS & INTERPRETATION
Lab
Initial lab tests
- Pap smear
- CBC may show anemia.
- LFTs
- BUN and creatinine
- Urinalysis may show hematuria.

Follow-Up & Special Considerations
Prompt follow-up for test results and treatment plans

Imaging
Initial approach
CXR, IV pyelogram (IVP), CT scan of abdomen and pelvis, MRI, and PET scan:
- Evaluation of lung, lymph node, and distal organ metastasis; hydronephrosis; local extracervical invasion

Follow-Up & Special Considerations
Prompt multidisciplinary plan of care

Diagnostic Procedures/Surgery
- Biopsy of gross lesion
- Colposcopy with biopsy of abnormal blood vessels, irregular surface contour with loss of surface epithelium as indicated
- Endocervical curettage and cervical conization as indicated to determine depth of invasion and presence of lymphovascular involvement
- Cystoscopy to evaluate bladder invasion
- Proctoscopy for invasion into rectum

Pathological Findings
- Majority of cases (80%) are invasive squamous cell types usually arising from the ectocervix.
- Adenocarcinoma comprise 10–15% of cervical cancer arising from endocervical mucus-producing glandular cells.
- Other cell types that may be present include:
  - Rare mixed cell types
  - Neuroendocrine tumors
  - Sarcomas, lymphomas, melanomas

DIFFERENTIAL DIAGNOSIS
- Marked cervicitis and erosion
- Glandular hyperplasia
- STD
- Herpetic ulcer or chancre
- Cervical condyloma
- Cervical leiomyoma
- Cervical polyps
- Metastasis from endometrial carcinoma or gestational trophoblastic disease

 TREATMENT

MEDICATION
- Cisplatin, hydroxyurea, and fluorouracil have been used as adjuvant sensitizer to radiation therapy, but standard of care remains cisplatin as a radiosensitizer.
- Cisplatin/carboplatin, etoposide (VP-16), ifosfamide, and bleomycin have been used as adjuvant therapy for recurrent, metastatic disease.

ADDITIONAL TREATMENT
General Measures
Improve nutritional state, correct any anemia, and treat any vaginal and/or pelvic infections.

Issues for Referral
Multidisciplinary management of patients as needed and in a timely fashion

Additional Therapies
- Radiation therapy forms the cornerstone of advanced-stage cervical cancer.
- Combination of external beam pelvic radiation and brachytherapy is usually employed.
- If para-aortic nodal metastases are evident, then extended-field radiation can be added to treat affected lymph nodes.
- Chemoradiation with cisplatin-containing regimen has been associated with superior survival rates compared with pelvic and extended-field radiation alone.

SURGERY/OTHER PROCEDURES
- Removal of precursor lesions (CIN) by LEEP, cold knife conization, laser ablation, or cryotherapy (6)[A]
- Stage IA1 (lesions with <3 mm invasion from basement membrane): Cervical conization with total hysterectomy later when child-bearing is completed; otherwise, total hysterectomy
- Stage IA2 (lesions with >3 mm but <5 mm invasion from the basement membrane) and stages IB1, IB2, IIA: Option of radical hysterectomy, bilateral pelvic lymphadenectomy, and para-aortic node sampling or primary radiation with brachytherapy and teletherapy
- Stage IVA (lesions limited to central metastasis to the bladder and/or rectum): Pelvic exenteration may be feasible.
- Radiotherapy:
  - For stage IB2 or higher:
    - Brachytherapy with intracavitary radium or cesium or interstitial cesium needles to treat the central tumor sites
    - Teletherapy with external radiation to treat tumor metastasis in the pelvic walls
  - For localized persistent or recurrent disease, radiation therapy or pelvic exenteration as appropriate
- Stage IVB disease has poor prognosis and is treated with goal of palliation.

IN-PATIENT CONSIDERATIONS
Initial Stabilization
- Active vaginal bleeding can be controlled with timely vaginal packing and radiation therapy.
- Recognition of ureteral blockage, hydronephrosis, urosepsis, and timely intervention

Admission Criteria
- Signs of active bleeding
- Urinary symptoms
- Dehydration
- Complications from surgery, chemotherapy, or radiation

IV Fluids
Adequate hydration and electrolyte repletion as needed

Nursing
Routine perioperative and postoperative care; pre- and postchemoradiation care

Discharge Criteria
Discharge criteria based on multidisciplinary assessment, including physicians, physical therapists, long- or short-term rehabilitation, home nursing care, or hospice.

Pregnancy Considerations
- Generally, the choice of treatment depends on the severity of the abnormal Pap smear, the length of gestation, the patient's wish to continue pregnancy to attainment of fetal lung maturity, and the treating physician's comfort level in delaying definitive therapy.
- Clinical stage at diagnosis is the single most important prognostic factor during pregnancy.
- If treatment is delayed, the patient must receive close follow-up care, with its frequency dependent on the severity of the disease.

 ONGOING CARE

FOLLOW-UP RECOMMENDATIONS
Patient Monitoring
- With completion of definitive therapy, each patient is evaluated with physical/pelvic examinations and Pap smears:
  - Every 3 months for 1–2 years
  - Every 6 months until the 5th year
  - Yearly thereafter
- Signs of cancer recurrence are unexplained weight loss, leg edema, and pelvic or thigh pain.

DIET
As appropriate

PATIENT EDUCATION
Patient education material available through the American Cancer Society at www.cancer.org

PROGNOSIS
After commonly accepted surgical and radiation treatments, 5-year survival:

Stage	5-yr Survival (%)
1	80
2	65
3	30
4	15

COMPLICATIONS
- Loss of ovarian function from radiotherapy or indication for bilateral oophorectomy
- Hemorrhage
- Pelvic infection
- Genitourinary fistula
- Bladder dysfunction
- Ureteral obstruction with renal failure
- Bowel obstruction
- Pulmonary embolism

REFERENCES
1. Scarinci IC, Garcia FA, Kobetz E, Partridge EE, Brandt HM, Bell MC, Dignan M, Ma GX, Daye JL, Castle PE et al. Cervical cancer prevention: new tools and old barriers. *Cancer*. 2010;116:2531–42.
2. Martin-Hirsch PL, et al. Surgery for cervical intraepithelial neoplasia. Cochrane Gynaecological Cancer Group. *Cochrane Database of Syst Rev.* 2007:3.
3. Kinney W, Stoler MH, Castle PE et al. Special commentary: patient safety and the next generation of HPV DNA tests. *Am J Clin Pathol*. 2010;134:193–9.
4. Markowitz LE, Dunne EF, Saraiya M, et al. Quadrivalent Human Papillomavirus Vaccine: Recommendations of the Advisory Committee on Immunization Practices (ACIP). *MMWR Recomm Rep.* 2007;56:1–24.
5. Grce M, Matovina M, Milutin-Gasperov N, Sabol I et al. Advances in cervical cancer control and future perspectives. *Coll Antropol*. 2010;34:731–6.
6. http://www.cancer.gov.

ADDITIONAL READING
- American Cancer Society: Cancer Facts and Figures 2007. Atlanta: American Cancer Society, 2007.
- Herrero R, Hildesheim A, Bratti C, et al. Population-based study of human papillomavirus infection and cervical neoplasia in rural Costa Rica. *J Natl Cancer Inst*. 2000;92:464–74.
- Jemal A, Siegel R, Ward E, et al. Cancer statistics, 2008. *CA Cancer J Clin*. 2008;58:71–96.
- Morris M, Eifel PJ, Lu J, et al. Pelvic radiation with concurrent chemotherapy compared with pelvic and para-aortic radiation for high-risk cervical cancer. *N Engl J Med*. 1999;340:1137–43.

See Also (Topic, Algorithm, Electronic Media Element)
Abnormal Pap and Cervical Dysplasia

 CODES

ICD9
- 180.0 Malignant neoplasm of endocervix
- 180.1 Malignant neoplasm of exocervix
- 180.8 Malignant neoplasm of other specified sites of cervix

CLINICAL PEARLS
- Worldwide, cervical cancer ranks 2nd among all malignancies for women.
- Women with cervical cancer may be asymptomatic and have a normal physical exam.
- Cervical carcinoma is clinically staged.
- Radiation therapy forms the cornerstone of advanced-stage cervical cancer.

CERVICAL POLYPS

Nicole D. Pilevsky, MD

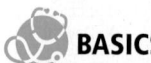 **BASICS**

DESCRIPTION
- Pedunculated masses, usually single, that vary in size from a few millimeters to 3 cm, that protrude from the cervix and may bleed
- System(s) affected: Reproductive

Geriatric Considerations
Rare

Pediatric Considerations
Rare

Pregnancy Considerations
Delay removal of polyps until postpartum unless bleeding or cervical dilation is found.

EPIDEMIOLOGY
- Predominant age: 40–60 years
- Predominant sex: Female only

Incidence
Common

RISK FACTORS
None

GENERAL PREVENTION
None known

PATHOPHYSIOLOGY
Hyperplastic proliferation of cervical or endometrial cells

ETIOLOGY
- Unknown for most cases
- Secondary reaction to cervical inflammatory or hormonal stimulation
- Extremely rare incidence of dysplasia or malignancy

COMMONLY ASSOCIATED CONDITIONS
There is some possibility of coexisting endometrial polyps.

 DIAGNOSIS

Cervical polyps are typically painless.

HISTORY
- The majority of cervical polyps are asymptomatic.
- Some cause abnormal vaginal bleeding or discharge:
  – Intermenstrual bleeding
  – Postcoital or postmenopausal bleeding
  – Leukorrhea

PHYSICAL EXAM
- Polyp may be an incidental finding on routine speculum exam.
- Document its location and size.

DIAGNOSTIC TESTS & INTERPRETATION
Lab
Send polyp for pathologic analysis.

Imaging
Sonohysterography may be helpful if there is suspicion of multiple polyps or to determine if polyp is originating from the endometrium.

Diagnostic Procedures/Surgery
Perform Pap smear before treatment if the patient is due for screening.

Pathological Findings
- Benign hyperplastic endocervical epithelium, often with a large number of blood vessels involved
- Extremely rare incidence of dysplasia or malignancy:
  – Most atypia is found in the teens and 20s.
  – Most cancers are found in women >48 years.
- Case reports of lymphoma and sarcoma botryoides

DIFFERENTIAL DIAGNOSIS
- Prolapsed submucous myoma or endometrial polyp
- Other causes of intermenstrual bleeding
- Decidualized endometrium

TREATMENT

- There is no absolute need to remove a polyp unless there is a suspicion of malignancy, but removal may stop bleeding.
- Smaller polyps may be removed in the office as long as hemostatic agents are available. The polyp is grasped with a ring forceps and twisted on its stalk until it detaches. Local anesthetic is not generally necessary. Silver nitrate or Monsel solution may be applied if cautery is needed. Sessile polyps may be removed using an electrosurgical loop (with local anesthetic).
- Larger polyps may require removal in an operating room.

SURGERY/OTHER PROCEDURES
Outpatient management usually. If polyps are treated in the operating room, hysteroscopy may be a useful adjunct (1).

IN-PATIENT CONSIDERATIONS
Admission Criteria
Uncontrolled hemorrhage

 ONGOING CARE

FOLLOW-UP RECOMMENDATIONS
Following removal, avoid sexual intercourse, tampons, and douching for 2 weeks.

Patient Monitoring
Recheck at routine appointments or as needed.

PATIENT EDUCATION
Given the possibility of incomplete excision, patients should be educated about symptoms.

PROGNOSIS
Recurrence not likely with complete excision

COMPLICATIONS
Bleeding and mild pain with removal

REFERENCE
1. Stamatellos I, Stamatopoulos P, Bontis J. The role of hysteroscopy in the current management of the cervical polyps. *Arch Gynecol Obstet*. 2007.

ADDITIONAL READING
Schnatz PF, Ricci S, O'Sullivan DM. Cervical polyps in postmenopausal women: is there a difference in risk? *Menopause*. 2009.

 CODES

ICD9
622.7 Mucous polyp of cervix

CLINICAL PEARLS
- There is no absolute need to remove a polyp unless there is a suspicion of malignancy, but removal may stop bleeding.
- Cervical polyps are extremely rarely cancerous.
- Smaller polyps may be removed in the office as long as hemostatic agents are available. Larger polyps may be removed in the operating room.

C

CERVICAL SPINE INJURY

Caroline Tschibelu, MD
Otis Warren, MD

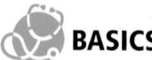 **BASICS**

DESCRIPTION
- Cervical spine injuries can result in vertebral fracture, ligamentous injury, or spinal cord injury.
- Vertebral and ligamentous injuries can cause cervical spine instability leading to cord injury.

EPIDEMIOLOGY
Incidence
- There are an estimated 12,000 new cases of spinal cord injury per year in the United States, with over half involving the cervical spine.
- Primarily affects young adults with active lifestyles, but the elderly are also affected due to prevalence of degenerative joint disease and increased risk of falls.
- Average age at time of injury: 39.5
- Male-to-female ratio: 4:1

RISK FACTORS
Anatomic irregularities:
- Degenerative joint disease (particularly the elderly)
- Osteoporosis
- Spinal canal stenosis
- Spina bifida

Genetics
Inherited connective tissue disorders (e.g., familial cervical spondylosis, a spondylitis)

GENERAL PREVENTION
- Use seat belts and child safety seats.
- Avoidance of high-risk activities such as driving while intoxicated
- Treatment of osteoporosis (e.g., calcium and vitamin D supplement, HRT, bisphosphonates)
- Fall prevention for the elderly

PATHOPHYSIOLOGY
4 major vertebral and ligamentous injuries are classified by mechanism:
- Flexion:
  - Simple wedge compression fracture:
    - Anterior compression fracture of vertebrae
    - Nuchal ligament stretch but not disruption
    - Diminished vertebral body height on x-ray
    - Stable fracture
  - Flexion teardrop fracture:
    - Anteroinferior vertebral body fracture
    - Displaced anterior fragment ("teardrop")
    - Posterior and anterior ligamentous disruption
    - Extremely unstable, high risk of cord injury
  - Anterior subluxation:
    - Posterior ligament rupture without fracture
    - Rarely associated with neurologic deficit
    - Seen on flexion-extension views
    - Treated as unstable due to risk while in flexion, but not unstable by definition
  - Bilateral facet dislocation:
    - More severe anterior subluxation
    - Includes disruption of annulus, anterior, and posterior ligaments
    - Inferior facets move superior and anterior to the superior facets, causing displacement.
    - Neurologic injury related to disk herniation
  - Clay shoveler fracture:
    - Oblique fracture at base of spinous process
    - Occurs with abrupt flexion with simultaneous contraction of lower neck and upper body

  - Also occurs with blunt trauma
  - Avulsed fragment seen on lateral views
  - Stable fracture, low risk for neurologic deficit
- Flexion–rotation:
  - Unilateral facet dislocation:
    - Less anterior displacement than bilateral
  - Rotary atlantoaxial dislocation (C1–C2):
    - Specific type of unilateral facet dislocation
    - Asymmetry of the lateral masses of C1 seen
    - Considered unstable due to location
- Extension:
  - Hangman fracture:
    - Traumatic spondylolisthesis of C2
    - Bilateral fractures through C2 pedicles
    - Unstable fracture, but cord injury rare
  - Extension teardrop fracture:
    - Avulsion fracture from stretch on anterior longitudinal ligament, causing anteroinferior bony fragment
    - Commonly found at lower cervical levels
    - Cord injury possible due to ligamenta flava encroaching into spinal canal
    - Unstable fracture in extension
  - Fracture of C1 posterior arch:
    - Stable fracture
  - Posterior atlantoaxial dislocation (C1–C2):
    - Cord injury possible
- Vertical compression (from axial load):
  - Jefferson fracture:
    - Burst fracture of C1 ring
    - Instability determined by severity of transverse ligamentous disruption
    - Unstable if more than 25% loss of height
  - Occipital condyle fracture:
    - Can be avulsion or compression fracture
    - Associated with cranial nerve deficits
- Unclear mechanisms:
  - Odontoid (dens) fracture, part of C2 (axis):
    - Type I: Involving tip of dens
    - Type II: Involving base of dens
    - Type III: Extends into body of axis
    - Types II and III can become unstable.
  - Atlanto-occipital dislocation:
    - Brainstem stretch may cause immediate respiratory arrest and death.
- Spinal cord injury (SCI):
  - Complete cord injury: Characterized by complete loss of sensory and motor functions below injury through S4–S5. Can also present with priapism, urinary retention, and bladder distention.
  - Incomplete deficits: Sensory and motor functions partially preserved below injury. Sensory preserved to a greater degree because sensory tracts peripherally located. Incidence of incomplete cord injury has increased compared to complete injury with implementation of ATLS protocols for all trauma patients (1). Most SCI are mixed injuries but there are some specific syndromes:
    - Central cord syndrome: Most common incomplete injury; motor deficits greater in upper than lower extremities. Sensory loss in the distribution of a "cape" and due to watershed injury affecting long fiber tracts; may be due to hyperextension.
    - Anterior cord syndrome: Posterior columns spared; affects spinothalamic, corticospinal, anterior, and lateral columns; loss of pain, temperature, motor with preserved vibration and position sense below the lesion

    - Posterior cord syndrome: Sensory deficits more pronounced than motor, due to contusion of posterior columns
    - Brown-Sequard syndrome: Ipsilateral motor loss and vibration sensation deficits with contralateral loss of pain and temperature sensation; hemisection of cord most often due to penetrating trauma

ETIOLOGY
Traumatic injury to the head or neck from:
- Motor vehicle accidents or falls
- Violence, commonly gunshot wounds
- High-risk or high-impact sports

COMMONLY ASSOCIATED CONDITIONS
- Intracranial hemorrhage
- Skull and facial fractures
- Thoracolumbar spine injury
- Other: Visceral/extremities injuries in polytrauma

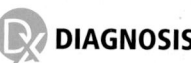 **DIAGNOSIS**

HISTORY
- History of traumatic injury to head or neck
- Neck pain or neurologic symptoms
- Past medical history, including medications
- Substance abuse or intoxication

PHYSICAL EXAM
- Midline cervical tenderness on palpation
- Limited or painful cervical range of motion
- Weakness, paresthesias, or numbness on complete neurological exam
- Abnormal rectal tone

DIAGNOSTIC TESTS & INTERPRETATION
Lab
Initial lab tests
- Complete blood count, basic metabolic panel
- Urine toxicology, blood alcohol level

Imaging
Initial approach
- Standard trauma series includes 5 x-ray views. However, if high suspicion for c-spine injury, consider CT as 1st-line imaging.
- Use Canadian C-spine Rules (CCR) or NEXUS Low-Risk Criteria (LRC) to decide when not to radiograph:
  - CCR, no imaging needed if (2)[A]:
    - Patient is alert (GCS = 15) and stable
    - No high-risk factors, no dangerous mechanism, no paresthesias, age <65
    - A low-risk factor (simple rear-end MVA, ambulatory, delayed pain, absence of midline tenderness) in a patient who can rotate neck 45 degrees left and right
  - NEXUS LRC, no imaging needed if (3)[A]:
    - No posterior midline cervical tenderness
    - Alert, without evidence of intoxication
    - No focal neurologic deficit
    - No painful distracting injury
- 2003 prospective cohort of 8,283 patients found CCR superior to NEXUS LRC.
- CT is superior to radiography in higher risk patients with decreased mentation.
- If C7–T1 cannot be visualized, consider CT.

Geriatric Considerations
In the geriatric population, avoid sedating medications. Strongly consider CT of cervical spine due to degenerative disease.

Pediatric Considerations
- Subluxation more likely than fracture
- Larger head size increases risk of cord injury
- C1–C3 more likely affected in children under 8
- Some sources support CT scan as 1st-line in children under 14, but risk of radiation outweighs the benefits in asymptomatic children (4)[B].
- Spinal Cord Injury Without Radiographic Abnormality (SCIWORA): Neurologic deficits without signs of bony or ligamentous injury on adequate radiographs or CT. SCIWORA primarily seen in children due to ligamentous laxity and incomplete ossification of the spine. Consider MRI to better visualize ligamentous injury in this population.

Follow-Up & Special Considerations
- If negative cervical spine CT with persistent midline tenderness, consider MRI in 72 hours.
- Flexion–extension radiographs were considered if the patient was alert and cooperative with persistent concern for ligamentous cervical spine injury not seen on standard x-rays. They are falling out of favor due to MRI ability to detect those injuries and because they may worsen spinal injury.
- MRI has NPV of 100% for noninjury, including injuries not seen on x-rays or CT (5)[A].

Diagnostic Procedures/Surgery
CT angiography of carotid or vertebral arteries if concerned for associated vascular injury

Pathological Findings
- Vertebral fractures on x-rays or CT
- Ligamentous tear or soft tissue edema on MRI
- Spinal cord entrapment on MRI

 ## TREATMENT

MEDICATION
- Pain control
- Steroid treatment controversial for cord injury because effectiveness uncertain:
  - Methylprednisolone: Bolus: 30 mg/kg, then 5.4 mg/kg/h for the next 23 hours if within 3 hours of injury; if within 3–8 hours of injury, treat for total of 48 hours (6)[A]
- Increased risk of infection, GI bleeding, and steroid myopathy with steroid use (7)[C]

ADDITIONAL TREATMENT
General Measures
Long-term cervical collar or halo-style orthosis if evidence of vertebral, ligamentous, or cord injury

Issues for Referral
Orthopedics and/or neurosurgery

COMPLEMENTARY AND ALTERNATIVE MEDICINE
Massage therapy for residual muscular pain or spasm

SURGERY/OTHER PROCEDURES
Surgical stabilization used for a minority of cases

IN-PATIENT CONSIDERATIONS
Initial Stabilization
Follow the Advanced Trauma Life Support (ATLS) algorithm.

ALERT
- Immediately place patient in cervical collar if:
  - High-impact accident
  - Facial trauma, head injury, or direct cervical injury
  - Altered consciousness
- Presents from home after recent injury, despite functional status or time elapsed
- If transporting, use a backboard with stabilizing blocks to maintain neutral position.
- Keep oxygen saturation normal to prevent further cord injury from hypoxia.

Admission Criteria
- Respiratory: Oxygen requirements
- Cardiovascular: Hemodynamic instability
- Neurologic: Focal neurological findings, limited independent function, or concern for delayed intracranial bleed
- Surgical: Awaiting surgical stabilization

IV Fluids
Volume resuscitation or pressors as needed

Nursing
Frequent neurologic checks and use of appropriate, well-fitted collar

Discharge Criteria
Patient can be discharged if:
- Cleared according to NEXUS or CCR criteria or after neurology/orthopedic consults
- Ligamentous injury is present or suspected and sent home in cervical orthosis
- Stable vertebral fracture present and sent home in a cervical orthosis
- In permanent halo device and placed in a rehabilitation facility

 ## ONGOING CARE

FOLLOW-UP RECOMMENDATIONS
Follow-up required if discharged with a collar

Patient Monitoring
If spinal cord injury, high cervical fracture, respiratory failure, or hemodynamic instability, critical care monitoring required

DIET
- n.p.o. until alert and protecting airway
- Early nutrition due to hypermetabolic state related to trauma and injury

PATIENT EDUCATION
- The national spinal cord injury association: http://www.spinalcord.org 1-800-962-9629
- NINDS spinal cord injury information page: http://www.ninds.nih.gov/disorders/sci/sci.htm

PROGNOSIS
Function after 1 year postinjury indicates long-term function.

COMPLICATIONS
- Common complications of cervical trauma:
  - Chronic musculoskeletal pain
  - Herniated discs
  - Chronic radiculopathy
- Common complications of spinal cord injury:
  - Pneumonia
  - Deep vein thrombosis
  - Pulmonary embolus
  - Pressure ulcers
  - Wound infections
  - Urinary tract infections
  - Chronic pain
  - Depression
  - Renal failure
- Death in cord injury patients usually related to pneumonia, pulmonary embolus, or sepsis.

REFERENCES
1. O'Dowd JK et al. Basic principles of management for cervical spine trauma. *Eur Spine J.* 2010;19 Suppl 1:S18–22.
2. Stiell IG, Wells GA, Vandemheen KL, et al. The Canadian C-spine rule for radiography in alert and stable trauma patients. *JAMA.* 2001;286:1841–8.
3. Hoffman JR, Mower WR, Wolfson AB, et al. Validity of a set of clinical criteria to rule out injury to the cervical spine in patients with blunt trauma. National Emergency X-Radiography Utilization Study Group. *N Engl J Med.* 2000;343(2):94–9.
4. Jimenez RR, DeGuzman MA, Shiran S, et al. CT versus plain radiographs for evaluation of c-spine injury in young children: do benefits outweigh risks? *Pediatr Radiol.* 2008;38:635–44.
5. Muchow RD, Resnick DK, Abdel MP. Magnetic resonance imaging (MRI) in the clearance of the cervical spine in blunt trauma: a meta-analysis. *J Trauma.* 2008;64(1):179–89.
6. Bracken MB. Steroids for acute spinal cord injury. *Cochrane Database Syst Rev.* 2002:CD001046.
7. Wuermser L, Ho CH, Chiodo AE, et al. Spinal Cord Injury Medicine: Acute Care Management of Traumatic and Nontraumatic Injury. *Arch Phys Med Rehabil.* 2007;88(1):S55–S61.

 ## CODES

ICD9
- 805.00 Closed fracture of cervical vertebra, unspecified level
- 952.00 C1-c4 level spinal cord injury, unspecified
- 952.05 C5-c7 level spinal cord injury, unspecified

CLINICAL PEARLS
- Suspect cervical injury in any patient with facial or head trauma, especially if obtunded or intoxicated.
- Perform a comprehensive neurologic exam.
- Follow clear imaging guidelines, such as the Canadian C-spine Rules.
- Although controversial, consider early steroids if spinal cord injury suspected.

CERVICAL SPONDYLOSIS

Eric J. Kujawski, DO
Kenneth M. Bielak, MD
Brian K. Linn, MD

 BASICS

DESCRIPTION

Considered the most common progressive disorder of the cervical spine due to the process of noninflammatory degeneration of the facet joints and intervertebral discs and osteophyte formation:

- Seen as a natural process of aging, most people remain asymptomatic.
- Symptomatic patients fall into three groups: Axial neck pain, cervical radiculopathy, and cervical myelopathy.
- System(s) affected: Musculoskeletal; Neurological
- Synonym(s): Cervical arthritis; Cervical myelopathy; Cervical osteophyte; Cervicalgia

Geriatric Considerations

- Patients <55 usually present due to a herniated disc.
- Patients >55 usually have osteophyte formation with canal or foraminal stenosis.
- Rule out myelopathy before considering conservative treatment.

Pediatric Considerations

Symptoms are less common, but radiographic changes can be seen as early as skeletal maturity.

EPIDEMIOLOGY

Incidence

Predominant sex: Male > Female (3:2)

Prevalence

- 10% by age 25
- 95% by age 65

RISK FACTORS

- Aging
- Smoking
- Laborers
- Congenital spinal canal narrowing

PATHOPHYSIOLOGY

- Loss of disc height:
  - Desiccation leads the nucleus pulposus to lose elasticity and become smaller and more fibrous.
  - The annulus fibrosus takes on more weight and can bulge into the spinal canal.
  - Loss of height begins ventrally, leading to loss of cervical lordosis and a resulting focal kyphosis.

- Osteophyte formation:
  - Bare edges of the vertebral bodies
  - Uncovertebral joints
  - Facet joints (C5–C7 most common)
- Thickened laminae
- Thickened or ossified posterior longitudinal ligament
- Thickened or buckling ligamentum flavum
- Vertebral artery involvement

COMMONLY ASSOCIATED CONDITIONS

See Etiology

 DIAGNOSIS

HISTORY

- Gradual chronic onset is more common than acute presentation. Radiculopathy can be acute, subacute, or chronic.
- Generally worse with movement. Common complaint of neck being "stiff."
- Pain in the posterior neck and trapezius muscle associated at times with radiation into the arms
- Scapular pain
- Arm pain usually on the outer aspect of the arm at least to the elbow (coronary heart pain is almost always on the inner aspect of the arm)
- Radicular pain may be present without neck pain.
- Loss of neck extension
- Lateral flexion is limited while erect but improves while lying down.
- Tenderness of biceps and pectoralis major in C5–C6 segment disease
- Tenderness of triceps in C6–C7 disease
- Long tract signs and positive Babinski may develop in severe cases with myelopathy.

PHYSICAL EXAM

- Tenderness over the affected segments
- Palpation occasionally reproduces radicular pain.
- Coughing, sneezing, Valsalva, and certain cervical movements can increase radicular pain.
- The "shoulder abduction sign" relieves pain in some patients. The patient holds the arm over their head and rests the wrist or forearm on top of the head.

DIAGNOSTIC TESTS & INTERPRETATION

Lab

Initial lab tests

Only if diagnosis is in question:

- Erythrocyte sedimentation rate
- Rheumatoid factor
- Complete blood count with differential

Imaging

Initial approach

X-rays of cervical spine, anteroposterior (AP), lateral, open-mouth odontoid, and obliques. Osteophytes and/or joint space narrowing will be evident (1)[C].

Follow-Up & Special Considerations

- CT or MRI scans are valuable in cases where surgery is contemplated or the diagnosis is in doubt.
- Degenerative changes and disc herniations are commonly seen in asymptomatic patients, so correlation with neurological exam is needed.
- MRI better depicts cord changes, enlargement, compression, or atrophy.
- CT shows bony changes better, especially foraminal stenosis (2)[B].
- CT myelography in place of MRI in patients with metal hardware or pacemaker (3)[C]

Diagnostic Procedures/Surgery

Electromyogram (EMG) and nerve conduction studies may be needed to rule out other neurological causes. These studies are usually not needed in most patients with well-defined radiculopathy and correlating radiology findings.

DIFFERENTIAL DIAGNOSIS

- Cervical strain
- Rheumatoid arthritis
- Polymyalgia rheumatica
- Bone metastases
- Thoracic outlet syndrome
- With radiculopathy or myelopathy symptoms:
  - Multiple sclerosis
  - Syringomyelia
  - Tumor
  - Epidural abscess
  - Amyotrophic lateral sclerosis
  - Cervical herniated disc
  - Herpes zoster
  - Lyme radiculopathy
  - Diabetic polyradiculopathy

TREATMENT

MEDICATION

First Line

- NSAIDs (ibuprofen 800 mg t.i.d. 7–14 days or naproxen 500 b.i.d. 7–14 days) (4)[C]:
  - Contraindications: Gastrointestinal bleeding or ulcer
  - Precautions in patients with renal disease, hepatic disease, or coagulation disorders
- Acetaminophen 650 mg/dose 5 × per 24 hours or maximum of 3250 mg/day
- Muscle relaxants (up to 2 weeks) (4)[C]
- Topical pain relief cream (ketoprofen 20%, cyclobenzaprine 2%, lidocaine 10%; apply sparingly 2–3 × daily)
- Lidocaine or diclofenac patches
- Anticonvulsants for radiculopathy (gabapentin, pregabalin, tiagabine, or oxcarbazepine) (4)[C]

Second Line

- Short course of oral corticosteroids may benefit patients with acute radicular pain
- Facet joint steroid injections (3)[B]
- Opioids in patients who do not improve with other conservative treatments and are not surgical candidates.

ADDITIONAL TREATMENT

General Measures

- Avoidance of any provocative activities
- Physical therapy with exercise and gradual mobilization (5)[C]
- Return to normal activities as soon as possible.
- Conservative treatment for patients with only axial pain:
  - Oral analgesics (NSAIDS)
  - A short course of oral corticosteroids
  - Referral to physical therapy
  - Use of a cervical pillow
  - Soft cervical collar (up to 2 weeks)
  - Isometric exercises
- Patients with radicular pain with only paresthesia or numbness and no specific weakness:
  - Conservative treatment for 6–12 weeks
  - Facet joint injections if continued symptoms after conservative treatment
  - Epidural steroid injections (4)[C]
- Patients with myelopathy:
  - Surgical decompression is indicated (6)[B].

Issues for Referral

Immediate referral to an orthopedic surgeon for symptoms of myelopathy (gait disturbances, frequent falls, bowel or bladder dysfunction, loss of dexterity, Babinski sign, clonus, hyperreflexia)

Additional Therapies

- Cervical traction unit: 8–12 lbs at 24 degree angle of flexion for 15–20 minute intervals (3)[C]
- Avoid high-velocity manual manipulative therapy.

SURGERY/OTHER PROCEDURES

Surgical decompression for myelopathy can be beneficial in early cases. (5,6)[B]

ONGOING CARE

FOLLOW-UP RECOMMENDATIONS

Referral indicated for continued severe pain with conservative treatment, significant or progression of neurological deficits, or any sign/symptoms of myelopathy

Patient Monitoring

Follow-up visit in 3–4 weeks for evaluation of neurologic status. If no change, follow at intervals of 3–6 months, depending on severity of symptoms.

PATIENT EDUCATION

Patients should immediately report any weakness, eye symptoms, bladder or bowel incontinence, gait disturbance, loss of dexterity, or fine motor control.

PROGNOSIS

75% of patients have complete or significant relief of symptoms with nonoperative approach (4)[B].

REFERENCES

1. Pateder DB, Berg JH, Thal R et al. Neck and shoulder pain: differentiating cervical spine pathology from shoulder pathology. *J Surg Orthop Adv*. 2009;18:170–4.
2. Binder AI. Cervical spondylosis and neck pain. *BMJ*. 2007;334:527–31.
3. Eubanks JD. Cervical Radiculopathy: Nonoperative Management of Neck Pain and Radicular Symptoms. *American Family Physician*. 2010;81(1):33–40.
4. Mazanec D, Reddy A. Medical management of cervical spondylosis. *Neurosurgery*. 2007;60:S43–50.
5. Rao RD, Currier BL, Albert TJ., et al. Degenerative cervical spondylosis: clinical syndromes, pathogenesis, and management. *J Bone Joint Surg Am*. 2007;89:1360–78.
6. Hsu W, Dorsi MJ, Witham TF et al. Surgical Management of Cervical Spondylotic Myelopathy. *Neurosurgery quarterly*. 2009;19:302–307.

ADDITIONAL READING

- Robinson J, Kothari M. Treatment of Cervical Radiculopathy. Retrieved July 6, 2008, from http://www.utdol.com.
- Shedid D, Benzel EC. Cervical spondylosis anatomy: pathophysiology and biomechanics. *Neurosurgery*. 2007;60(1 Supp1 1):S7–13.

- Woiciechowsky C, et al. Degenerative spondylolisthesis of the cervical spine. *European Spine Journal*. 2004;13:680–4.
- Young WF. Cervical spondylotic myelopathy: a common cause of spinal cord dysfunction in older persons. *Am Fam Physician*. 2000;62:1064–70, 1073.

See Also (Topic, Algorithm, Electronic Media Element)

See videos: Neck Stretch with a Towel; Neck Extension in Prone; Neck Stretches - Chin Tucks; Neck Trigger Point Massage - Trapezius

CODES

ICD9

- 721.0 Cervical spondylosis without myelopathy
- 721.1 Cervical spondylosis with myelopathy

CLINICAL PEARLS

- Noninflammatory degeneration of the facet joints and intervertebral discs
- Considered a natural process of aging, most people remain asymptomatic:
  - Symptomatic patients fall into three groups: Axial neck pain, cervical radiculopathy, and cervical myelopathy.
- Patients <55 usually present due to herniated disc.
- Patients >55 usually present due to radicular symptoms related to osteophyte formation or foraminal stenosis.
- Diagnosis via X-rays of cervical spine, AP, lateral, open-mouth odontoid, and obliques
- Referral indicated for continued severe pain with conservative treatment, significant or progression of neurological deficits, or any sign/symptoms of myelopathy
- 75% of patients have complete or significant relief of symptoms with nonoperative approach.

CERVICITIS, ECTROPION AND TRUE EROSION

Jeremy Golding, MD
Barbara A. Majeroni, MD

 BASICS

DESCRIPTION
Cervicitis refers to inflammatory changes of the cervix.
- Ectropion: Presence of cervical columnar cells on the vaginal portion of the cervix (portio); often seen during adolescence and during pregnancy
- True erosion: Loss of overlying cervical epithelium owing to trauma (e.g., forceful insertion of vaginal speculum in patient with atrophic mucosa)
- System(s) affected: Reproductive

Geriatric Considerations
- Chronic cervicitis in postmenopausal women may be related to lack of estrogen.
- The possibility of infectious cervicitis should not be overlooked in geriatric patients because many remain sexually active.

Pregnancy Considerations
- Doxycycline should not be used during pregnancy.
- Screen all pregnant women for infectious cervicitis because of the risk of transmission to the fetus.

Pediatric Considerations
Infectious cervicitis in children should lead to an investigation for possible sexual abuse.

EPIDEMIOLOGY
Incidence
- Cervicitis: Cervicitis-specific data are not available. Based on CDC 2006 data:
  - Chlamydia incidence: Total actual cases reported to CDC were >1 million. CDC estimates 3 million new cases of chlamydia infection in both genders yearly.
  - Gonorrhea: Total actual cases reported to CDC approximately 358,000 both genders. CDC estimates actual incidence 700,000 new cases in both genders yearly.
  - Trichomoniasis: CDC estimates 7.4 million new cases in women and men yearly.
- Ectropion: Common with oral contraceptive use; very common in pregnant women
- True erosion: Occasionally seen in postmenopausal women
- Predominant age: 15–19 years
- Predominant sex: Women, especially sexually active women

RISK FACTORS
- Cervicitis:
  - Multiple sexual partners
  - Adolescence and young adulthood
  - Unprotected sex
  - History of STD
  - Smoking
  - Other reproductive tract infections: Vaginitis, PID
  - Foreign objects: Pessary, diaphragm, cervical cap, etc.
- Ectropion: Adolescence, pregnancy
- True erosion: Estrogen deficiency, trauma

GENERAL PREVENTION
- Sexually transmitted infection (gonorrhea, chlamydia, trichomoniasis):
  - Follow CDC-recommended screening measures: The US Preventive Services Task Force recommends screening for chlamydial infection in all sexually active nonpregnant young women ≤24 years and for older nonpregnant women who are at increased risk, but no routine screening for women >24 years not at increased risk (1)[C].
  - Treat sexual partners of infected women.
  - Advise use of condom during coitus.
- Estrogen deficiency: Estrogen replacement therapy

ETIOLOGY
- Cervicitis: C. trachomatis, N. gonorrhoeae, T. vaginalis, herpes simplex virus (HSV), mycoplasmas (e.g., M. genitalium), Ureaplasma, cytomegalovirus
- Non-sexually transmitted infectious cervicitis can be caused by β-hemolytic streptococcus or E. coli.
- Noninfectious causes include chemical irritation (e.g., from douching or latex exposure) and local trauma from vaginal foreign bodies such as diaphragms or cervical caps.
- Often no specific etiology is identified.
- Ectropion:
  - Hormonal changes with oral contraceptive use (especially with progesterone) or pregnancy
  - Resulting from cervical laceration during childbirth
- True erosion: Injury to atrophic epithelium owing to estrogen deficiency in menopause

 DIAGNOSIS

HISTORY
Patient may complain of vaginal discharge, dyspareunia, or bleeding/spotting following intercourse or may be asymptomatic.

PHYSICAL EXAM
- Cervicitis: Purulent vaginal discharge, cervical friability, erythema, ulceration (HSV); punctate hemorrhage causes "strawberry" cervix appearance in trichomoniasis.
- Ectropion: Cervix appears red, owing to the color of the columnar epithelium.
- True erosion: Vaginal bleeding, sharply defined ulcers of cervix
- Cervical motion tenderness may be appreciated on bimanual pelvic exam (suggests PID).

DIAGNOSTIC TESTS & INTERPRETATION
Lab
- Saline and KOH preparation of cervical and vaginal smears (endocervical sample with >10 WBC/hpf suggests cervicitis)
- Nucleic acid amplification tests: More sensitive and also may be used on urine, self-obtained vaginal swabs, and endocervical specimens (2)[A]. (Sensitivity and specificity between 95% and 99% for both gonorrhea and chlamydia.)
- Vaginal wet mount for T. vaginalis
- If ulcerations are present, culture for HSV.
- Pap smear of cervix

Diagnostic Procedures/Surgery
Colposcopy may be helpful in cases of chronic inflammation with a biopsy of suspicious areas.

Pathological Findings
- Cervicitis: Acute and chronic inflammatory changes, presence of infective organisms
- Ectropion: None/squamous metaplasia
- True erosion: Sharply defined ulcer borders, loss of epithelium

DIFFERENTIAL DIAGNOSIS
- Cervical dysplasia
- Carcinoma of the cervix
- Bacterial vaginosis (discharge is noninflammatory)

 TREATMENT

Cervicitis increases HIV viral RNA present in vaginal secretions, so treatment of cervicitis therefore may reduce risk of HIV transmission in those with HIV and cervicitis (2).

MEDICATION
First Line
- If infectious cervicitis suspected, treat without awaiting culture results: Ceftriaxone (Rocephin) 125 mg single dose IM, followed by either doxycycline (Vibramycin) 100 mg PO b.i.d. × 7 days or azithromycin (Zithromax) 1 g single dose (3)[A]. Option of Rocephin and azithromycin removes patient-compliance factor because they are 1-time doses.
- Trichomoniasis: Metronidazole 2 g once or 500 mg b.i.d. × 7 days or 1 g b.i.d. × 2 doses
- Known or suspected chlamydial infection: For nonpregnant women, azithromycin 1 g PO once or doxycycline 100 mg b.i.d. PO × 7 days; for pregnant women, azithromycin 1 g once or erythromycin base 500 mg q.i.d. PO × 7 days or erythromycin ethylsuccinate 800 mg q.i.d. × 7 days

- Ectropion: None, unless patient is extremely symptomatic with copious discharge. In that case, acid-buffered vaginal jelly can be used to decrease discharge. Cautery can be used but generally is considered overly invasive.
- True erosion: Estrogen, conjugated vaginal cream daily for 1–2 weeks, followed by maintenance cream twice weekly or oral HRT
- Contraindications:
  - Metronidazole: Older references state that metronidazole is relatively contraindicated during 1st trimester of pregnancy. More recent meta-analyses suggest absence of teratogenicity. Treatment of trichomoniasis may be deferred until 2nd trimester if clinician remains concerned by product labeling.
  - Doxycycline: Pregnancy or lactation
  - Estrogen: See extended list of contraindications to estrogen use in standard texts.
- Precautions:
  - Metronidazole: See above; disulfiram reaction with ethanol ingestion
  - Doxycycline: Possible fetal harm if used during pregnancy; staining of the infant's teeth if used during breast-feeding; allergy; photosensitization
  - Erythromycin: Nausea or vomiting
  - Estrogens: History of estrogen-dependent neoplasms; history of thromboembolic diseases. See extended list of contraindications to estrogen therapy in standard texts.
- Significant possible interactions:
  - Metronidazole: Ethanol
  - Doxycycline: Dairy products, iron preparations, warfarin, and oral contraceptives (advise use of alternative contraceptive method)
  - Erythromycin: Theophylline (elevated theophylline level)
  - Estrogen: N/A

Second Line
- Cefixime 400 mg PO single dose is an acceptable alternative to ceftriaxone.
- The rise of quinolone-resistant *N. gonorrhoea* has prompted a change in CDC recommendations concerning management of gonococcal disease (3)[A]. Quinolones are no longer recommended for primary management. The exception to this recommendation occurs only if the patient is penicillin-allergic and the organism is known to be sensitive to quinolones. The lack of availability of spectinomycin in the US creates a problem for patients with gonorrhea and true penicillin allergy. It seems reasonable to treat with a quinolone as below, with follow-up testing to ensure eradication in this case. Quinolones are contraindicated in pregnancy:
  - Ofloxacin (Floxin) 400 mg PO single dose
  - Ciprofloxacin (Cipro) 500 mg PO single dose
  - Levofloxacin (Levaquin) 250 mg PO single dose

- Alternative to metronidazole for trichomoniasis: Tinidazole 2 g PO × 1 dose
- Estrogen deficiency: A number of estrogen vaginal preparations are available commercially.

SURGERY/OTHER PROCEDURES
Chronic cervicitis with negative cultures that does not respond to empirical medical treatment may be treated with cryosurgery, electrocautery, or loop excision.

- Adverse effects of cautery or cryosurgery can include cervical stenosis, which may affect fertility.

 ## ONGOING CARE

FOLLOW-UP RECOMMENDATIONS
Patient Monitoring
- Follow-up assay is recommended in pregnant patients to document infection eradication.
- Estrogen deficiency: Re-examine in 1 month to confirm healing.

ALERT
Follow-up nucleic acid amplification tests should not be done <3 weeks after treatment because of false-positive results owing to dead organisms.

PATIENT EDUCATION
If the etiology of a patient's cervicitis is confirmed to be a sexually transmittable infection, educate patient on the necessity of treating her sexual partners to avoid reinfection.

PROGNOSIS
- Cervicitis: Excellent healing after infection is eradicated
- Ectropion: Spontaneous regression postpartum and with cessation of use of oral contraceptives
- True erosion: Spontaneous healing

COMPLICATIONS
Cervicitis owing to *C. trachomatis* or *N. gonorrhoeae* is associated with an 8–10% risk of developing subsequent PID. Adolescents are a high-risk group for reinfection with sexually transmitted organisms, and screening frequency should be once/twice yearly in this population.

REFERENCES

1. US Preventive Services Task Force. Screening for chlamydial infection: U.S. Preventive Services Task Force recommendation statement. *Ann Intern Med*. 2007;147:128–34.
2. Cook RL, Hutchison SL, Østergaard L, et al. Systematic review: noninvasive testing for Chlamydia trachomatis and Neisseria gonorrhoeae. *Ann Intern Med*. 2005;142:914–25.
3. Centers for Disease Control and Prevention. *Sexually transmitted diseases: Treatment guidelines 2006. MMWR*.

ADDITIONAL READING

- Arráiz R N, Colina Ch S, Marcucci J R, et al. Mycoplasma genitalium detection and correlation with clinical manifestations in population of the Zulia State, Venezuela. *Rev Chilena Infectol*. 2008;25:256–61.
- Brocklehurst P. Antibiotics for gonorrhea in pregnancy. *Cochrane Database Syst Rev*. 2006: 1. Accessed February 20, 2006.
- Johnson LF, Lewis DA. The Effect of Genital Tract Infections on HIV-1 Shedding in the Genital Tract: A Systematic Review and Meta-Analysis. *Sex Transm Dis*. 2008.
- Simpson T, Oh MK. Urethritis and cervicitis in adolescents. *Adolescent Med Clin*. 2004;15: 153–271.
- Wilson JF et al. In the clinic. Vaginitis and cervicitis. *Ann Intern Med*. 2009;151.

 ## CODES

ICD9
- 616.0 Cervicitis and endocervicitis
- 622.0 Erosion and ectropion of cervix

CLINICAL PEARLS

- If infectious cervicitis is suspected, treatment of choice is ceftriaxone 125 mg IM plus azithromycin 1 g PO × 1 dose. Do not wait for test results.
- Encourage patient to have sexual partner(s) treated.
- Quinolones are no longer recommended to treat gonorrhea.
- Lubricants (e.g., KY Jelly) do not alter Pap smear results, so small quantities may be used when performing Pap smears.
- Positive results for *N. gonorrhoeae* or chlamydia should be reported to local or state health department.

CHANCROID

Jeffery T. Kirchner, DO

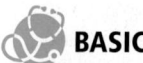 **BASICS**

DESCRIPTION
A sexually transmitted disease characterized by painful genital ulcerations and inflammatory inguinal adenopathy. Although uncommon in the US, it is found worldwide. Chancroid is endemic in developing countries, especially sub-Saharan Africa, and is a co-factor for HIV transmission.

EPIDEMIOLOGY
Incidence
- <50 cases reported to Centers for Disease Control (CDC) in 2004–2007 (from only 8 states)
- Actual numbers are considered higher due to lack of testing and thus underreporting.

Prevalence
- Endemic in developing countries, but actual prevalence is unknown due to lack of testing
- Thought to be extremely common in sub-Saharan Africa, southeast Asia, Latin America

RISK FACTORS
- Multiple sexual partners
- Uncircumcised men
- Prostitutes may be carriers.
- Patients presenting with other genital ulcerative diseases

GENERAL PREVENTION
Condom use

PATHOPHYSIOLOGY
Involves attachment of the bacteria to susceptible cells. Cytotoxin is secreted, which may play a role in epithelial injury and ulcer formation. Dendritic cells and natural killer cells respond to *H. ducreyi*, and this innate host response determines bacterial clearance versus disease progression.

ETIOLOGY
Haemophilus ducreyi (gram-negative rod)

COMMONLY ASSOCIATED CONDITIONS
- Syphilis: Concurrent in 10% of patients
- Herpes simplex virus or HIV infection

 DIAGNOSIS

HISTORY
- Exposure to infected individual, but often not helpful or obtained
- Incubation period typically lasts 4–10 days.

PHYSICAL EXAM
- Tender erythematous genital papule that progresses into a pustule that erodes into an ulcer. Infected persons commonly have >1 ulcer.
- Typical ulcer is 1–2 cm, but size is variable.
- Ulcers are painful, with erythematous base and clearly demarcated borders, which are sometimes undermined.
- Common sites for ulcers in men include the penile shaft, glans, and meatus.
- Common sites for ulcers in women include labia, introitus, and perianal areas.

- Inguinal lymphadenitis with abscess (bubo) formation occurs in ~50% of men but less common in women.
- Buboes arise 1–2 weeks after ulceration, are typically painful
- Buboes may spontaneously rupture if the primary disease is untreated.
- Atypical presentations include folliculitis and foreskin abscess.

DIAGNOSTIC TESTS & INTERPRETATION
Lab
CDC criteria for presumptive diagnosis:
- Definite: Isolation of *H. ducreyi* from a lesion
- Probable: Clinical findings *plus* negative darkfield exam, negative serologic test for syphilis, negative cultures for herpes simplex virus (HSV), or a clinical presentation not typical for HSV.

Initial lab tests
- "School of fish" pattern on Gram stain with organisms clumped in long parallel strands
- Serologic testing for antibody to *H. ducreyi* with enzyme linked immunosorbent assay
- Culture of the organism on Mueller-Hinton agar with incorporated vancomycin but sensitivity is <80%.
- Multiplex polymerase chain reaction (PCR) has sensitivity of 95–98%, but no Food and Drug Administration-approved tests in the US; available from some commercial labs

Follow-Up & Special Considerations
All patients should also be tested for syphilis and HSV.

Diagnostic Procedures/Surgery
Gram stain and culture of exudate (1):
- Aspiration of inguinal bubo (lymph node)
- PCR testing of ulcer exudate for *H. ducreyi* DNA
- Darkfield examination of exudate to rule out *Treponema pallidum* infection
- Culture or PCR testing for HSV

DIFFERENTIAL DIAGNOSIS
- Syphilis (*Treponema pallidum*)
- Genital herpes (HSV-1 and -2)
- Lymphogranuloma venereum (*Chlamydia trachomatis*)
- Granuloma inguinale (donovanosis)
- Drug eruption; Behçet disease

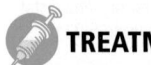

TREATMENT

MEDICATION
First Line
Azithromycin: 1 g p.o. single dose (2,3)[A]:
- Ceftriaxone 250 mg IM single dose

Second Line
- Ciprofloxacin 500 mg p.o. b.i.d. for 3 days (2,3)[A]
- Erythromycin base 500 mg q.i.d. for 7 days (2,3)[A]
- Contraindications:
  - Allergy to the medication
  - Ciprofloxacin during pregnancy and lactation and in patients <18 years

ADDITIONAL TREATMENT
General Measures
- Outpatient treatment
- Saline or Burrow's solution to soak ulcers
- Aspiration of buboes if >5 cm; approached through adjacent skin. Also consider incision and drainage for larger lesions.

ALERT
HIV disease may affect treatment response.

ONGOING CARE

FOLLOW-UP RECOMMENDATIONS
Patient Monitoring
- Avoid sexual activity until ulcers are resolved.
- Clinical improvement usually occurs within 48 hours.
- Patients should be reexamined 3–7 days after initiation of therapy and followed closely until all clinical signs of infection are resolved.
- Baseline syphilis serology and at 3 months
- Baseline HIV testing and at 3 months post-treatment

PATIENT EDUCATION
- Sexual counseling
- Use of condoms
- Local wound care
- Treatment of all sexual partners with same regimen as index
- HIV testing

PROGNOSIS
- Full clinical resolution with appropriate treatment
- Failure to respond may be due to incorrect diagnosis, coinfection with syphilis or HIV, medication nonadherence, or resistant *H. ducreyi*.
- 5% relapse after treatment.

COMPLICATIONS
- Phimosis
- Balanoposthitis
- Rupture of buboes with fistula formation and scarring

REFERENCES

1. Alfa M et al. The laboratory diagnosis of Haemophilus ducreyi. *Can J Infect Dis Med Microbiol*. 2005;16:31–4.
2. Lewis DA. Chancroid: Clinical manifestations, diagnosis, and management. *Sex Transm Inf*. 2003;79:68–71.
3. Centers for Disease Control and Prevention. Sexually transmitted diseases treatment guidelines—2006. *MMWR*. 2006;55:17–18.

ADDITIONAL READING

- Centers for Disease Control and Prevention. STD Surveillance. Division of STD Prevention—January 13, 2009.
- Janowicz DM, Li W, Bauer ME et al. Host-pathogen interplay of Haemophilus ducreyi. *Curr Opin Infect Dis*. 2010;23:64–9.
- Janowicz DM, Ofner S, Katz BP, et al. Experimental infection of human volunteers with Haemophilus ducreyi: fifteen years of clinical data and experience. *J Infect Dis*. 2009;199:1671–9.
- Montero JA. Chancroid: An update. *Infect Med*. 2002;191:174–8.
- Rosen T, Vandergriff T, Harting M. Antibiotic use in sexually transmissible diseases. *Dermatol Clin*. 2009;27:49–61.

 ## CODES

ICD9
099.0 Chancroid

CLINICAL PEARLS
- Chancroid is a rare disorder in the US but more common elsewhere.
- Characterized by genital papules that progress to pustules that open, producing painful ulcers
- Treatment of choice is azithromycin 1 gm once.
- Treat sexual partners even in the absence of signs or symptoms of disease.

CHARCOT JOINT

Patrick W. Joyner, MD
Kristyn Fagerberg, MD

 BASICS

In 1868, a French neurologist, Jean Martin Charcot, first described rapid joint deterioration in patients with tabes dorsalis. However, in 1703, Dr. William Musgrave first reported swollen, inflamed joints in a paralyzed patient. In 1936, Dr. William Jordan first described an association of diabetes mellitus with neuropathic changes in the foot and ankle.

DESCRIPTION
- A progressive destructive arthritis secondary to peripheral neuropathy and loss of pain sensation. The affected joints are subjected to repeated stress that is unrecognized by the patient, therefore causing continuous damage to the underlying bone and cartilage.
- Most often seen in tarsal and tarsometatarsal joints, less in metatarsophalangeal and talotibial joints. May also be seen in knee, hip, spine.
- Upper extremity joints rarely are involved.
- Diabetes mellitus (DM) is the most common cause in the US.
- 3 stages are identified:
  – Fragmentation/destruction
  – Coalescence
  – Consolidation/resolution
- Patients suspected to have a Charcot neuropathy should be referred to an orthopedic foot and ankle surgeon or podiatrist for follow-up and treatment.
- System(s) affected: Musculoskeletal; Endocrine; Neurologic
- Synonym(s): Neuropathic joint disease; Neuropathic arthropathy

EPIDEMIOLOGY
- Primarily seen in 5th and 6th decades
- Male = Female
- Bilateral involvement in 9–35% of cases

Incidence
- 0.1–0.4% in patients with DM
- 5–9% of patients with peripheral neuropathy

Prevalence
0.1% in all patients, up to 13% in high-risk diabetes foot clinics

RISK FACTORS
- >15-year history of diabetes
- Poor blood sugar control
- Poor foot hygiene; poor-fitting shoes, socks
- Diabetes mellitus is the most common cause in the United States.
- Globally, other medical conditions, such as syphilis and leprosy, are also risk factors.

Genetics
Family history of DM

GENERAL PREVENTION
- Excellent control of blood sugar
- Diabetic foot care
- Well-fitting footwear with adequate support
- Frequent exam of feet for signs of pressure sores or ulcerations
- Good foot hygiene

PATHOPHYSIOLOGY
Exact cause unknown, 3 major theories:
- Autonomic neuropathy: Autonomic neuropathy leads to local increase in blood flow, which leads to osteopenia secondary to increased osteoclastic activity.
- Neurotraumatic: Repetitive microtrauma not sensed by the patient leads to osseous destruction and progressive damage to ligaments, articular surfaces, and may lead to fractures and subluxation.
- Neurovascular: Underlying medical disorder creates hypervascularity; this in conjunction with increased osteoclastic resorption and osteoporosis. Both mechanisms in the setting of microfractures and subchondral collapse will lead to joint destruction.

ETIOLOGY
Many causes of peripheral neuropathy:
- Diabetes mellitus
- Multiple sclerosis
- Raynaud disease
- Any connective tissue disease (i.e., scleroderma, rheumatoid arthritis)
- Syphilis/tabes dorsalis
- Syringomyelia, upper extremity disease
- Meningomyelocele
- Frequent intra-articular steroid injections
- Alcoholism
- Pernicious anemia
- Charcot-Marie-Tooth disease
- Leprosy (Hansen disease)
- Renal dialysis
- Amyloidosis

 DIAGNOSIS

- Findings frequently confused with cellulitis
- Symptoms usually unilateral
- Significant swelling:
  – Early: Large effusion
  – Late: Swelling usually resolved
- Local increased warmth: 3–7°C higher than unaffected extremity
- Skin erythema:
  – Classically will resolve with elevation; helps to differentiate from infection (erythema from infection would not be affected by elevation)
- Effusion in joint
- Loss of distal sensation
- Skin intact
- Decreased pain, proprioception in affected limb
- Laxity/instability of joint:
  – May lead to calluses and/or ulcerations

HISTORY
- Long-standing diabetes
- May recall predisposing trauma, such as ankle twist/sprain, object dropped on foot
- May present with pain; however, proportionally less pain than expected by appearance
- Limited motion

- Diffuse swelling
- Erythema
- Can affect any number of joints. Charcot joint has been reported in the following anatomic locations: Spine, shoulder, elbow, wrist, hand, hip, knee, ankle, and foot

PHYSICAL EXAM
- Localized warmth, swelling, erythema
- Brodsky test: Elevating the foot should resolve swelling.
- Neurologic exam:
  – Findings normally symmetric, sensory, and distal
  – Absent sensation on 4/10 sites using 5.07 g monofilament
  – Decreased or absent reflexes
  – Loss of pain, proprioception, and vibratory sensation
- Foot deformities:
  – Corns/calluses
  – Collapse of arch
  – Collapse of tarsal bones causing rocker-bottom foot
  – Protruding osteophytes
  – Plantar ulcer
- Peripheral circulation often normal

DIAGNOSTIC TESTS & INTERPRETATION
Resolution of erythema with elevation of affected extremity

Lab
- Blood sugar, hemoglobin A1c
- White blood cells may be elevated in osteomyelitis.
- Erythrocyte sedimentation rate: Elevated in osteomyelitis
- Basic metabolic panel: Blood urea nitrogen, creatinine to rule out renal disease
- B_{12}/folate, hematocrit, mean corpuscular volume
- Rapid plasma reagin, FTA-ABS to rule out syphilis
- Elevated alkaline phosphatase, calcium, parathyroid hormone, and low phosphate to rule out metabolic bone disease

Imaging
- Radiographs:
  – Early changes:
    ○ Slight fracture with joint subluxation
    ○ Joint effusion
    ○ Joint space narrowing
    ○ Sclerosis of subchondral bone
    ○ Bone fragmentation
  – Late changes:
    ○ Marked articular destruction
    ○ Fractures
    ○ Hypertrophic changes: Periarticular new bone, osteophytes, osseous debris, may look like severe arthritis
    ○ Bone resorption
    ○ Subluxation
    ○ Intra-articular loose bodies
    ○ Osteolysis
    ○ Large osteophytes
    ○ Atrophic changes: Massive bone resorption, joint disintegration, may look like chronic infection
- May be difficult to differentiate radiograph findings from those of osteomyelitis

- Magnetic resonance imaging (MRI): Assists in ruling out osteomyelitis, but can be difficult because joint will most likely have increased signal secondary to edema.
- Bone scan in conjunction with a tagged WBC scan: Assists in ruling out osteomyelitis:
  - Indium[111] more specific than technetium[99]

Initial approach
Rule out underlying neurologic disorder.

Diagnostic Procedures/Surgery
Arthrocentesis:

- Fluid for culture and sensitivity if osteomyelitis suspected
- Presence of WBC, calcium pyrophosphate dihydrate (CPPD) crystals
- Rule out malignancy of any cause for concern

DIFFERENTIAL DIAGNOSIS
- Cellulitis
- Osteomyelitis
- Osteonecrosis
- Advanced osteoarthritis
- Calcium pyrophosphate dihydrate crystal deposition disease
- Neoplasm

 ## TREATMENT

- Early recognition of diabetic foot pathology
- No weight-bearing on affected extremity
- Total contact cast (gold standard)
- Reconstruction of foot to help prevent ulceration if conservative management fails. However, cannot be performed until erythema has resolved (i.e., late phase).

MEDICATION
Because pathophysiology is thought to involve increased osteoclastic activity, bisphosphonates have been used to halt progression of disease:

- Pamidronate, alendronate shown to give clinical improvement (1)[A]
- Bisphosphonates

ADDITIONAL TREATMENT
General Measures
- Goal of treatment is to restore joint stability and limit progression of disease.
- After casting, various braces are used to protect affected extremity:
  - Ankle-foot orthotic, rocker-bottom shoes, Charcot restraint orthotic walker, prefabricated pneumatic walking brace, custom prescription footwear
- Strict blood sugar control to limit progression of peripheral neuropathy

Additional Therapies
- Protective treatment with bracing, orthotics
- Radiotherapy does not appear to benefit healing of acute Charcot feet in people with diabetes (2)[B].

SURGERY/OTHER PROCEDURES
- Surgical treatment is reserved for severe cases and/or failure of conservative treatment.
- Surgery is indicated when a risk of skin ulceration, unstable fracture, or dislocation is present, or failure of medical therapy.

- Procedures performed vary, depending on joints involved and surgeon experience:
  - Exostosectomy of bony projections
  - Open reduction internal fixation
  - Osteotomy
  - Arthrodesis, with or without tendon lengthening
  - Amputation
  - Use of external fixation if poor skin quality or increase risk of postoperative healing complications
- Any surgical treatment should be delayed until after early fragmentation and inflammatory stages.
- Patients treated surgically often have long healing times.

IN-PATIENT CONSIDERATIONS
Initial Stabilization
- Immobilization of joint is initial treatment:
  - Casting:
    - Provides full immobilization
    - Casts must be checked weekly for correct fit, especially if underlying ulceration of skin.
    - Casts should be changed every 1–2 weeks.
    - Time in cast determined by clinical and radiographic measures
    - Total-contact cast better disperses pressure. Ensure pressure points are well padded, as these patients frequently have severely limited to no sensation and will likely not be aware of the development of pressure ulcer.
  - Brace/orthotic:
    - Alternative to casting
    - Removable
    - Patients may be noncompliant, and may not be able to sense a poor-fitting brace.
- Immobilization needed for minimum of 6 months; possibly 1 year or longer
- Also necessary to reduce stress on affected joint by limiting pressure:
  - Non-weight-bearing preferred, partial weight-bearing at minimum

Admission Criteria
Foot ulceration, suspicion of associated osteomyelitis, fractures

 ## ONGOING CARE

FOLLOW-UP RECOMMENDATIONS
- Activity: Non- or partial weight-bearing initially
- Regular follow-up with podiatrist to maintain strict foot care

Patient Monitoring
- Regular monitoring of blood sugar, HbA1C
- After initial radiographs, repeat films should be obtained in 4–6 weeks.

Geriatric Considerations
Because most cases occur in patients >50, diabetic patients in this age group should be counseled about the symptoms and signs of neuropathic joint disease. The benefits of good blood sugar control should be discussed.

PATIENT EDUCATION
Multidisciplinary team approach

PROGNOSIS
- Patients often are immobilized for several months.
- Usually non-weight-bearing of extremity for an average of 6 months if surgery is required
- Total healing may take years to achieve.

- Patients must be vigilant about preventing further injury, receiving regular footcare, examining feet daily, and noting swelling and/or temperature of joints.
- Maintain strict diabetic control:
  - Especially critical if patient to undergo surgery. Increased likelihood of non-union, wound healing complications, and postoperative infection if diabetes not well controlled.

COMPLICATIONS
- Unidentified fractures can lead to debilitating joint deformities and skin ulcerations, increasing risk of infection.
- Collapse and inversion of arch into clubfoot or rocker-bottom foot
- Amputation

REFERENCES
1. Anderson JJ, et al. Bisphosphonates for the treatment of Charcot neuroarthropathy. *J Foot Ankle Surg*. 2004;43(5):285–9.
2. Chantelau E, et al. Palliative radiotherapy for acute osteoarthropathy of diabetic feet: A preliminary study. *Pract Diabetes Int*. 1997;14(6):154–6.

ADDITIONAL READING
Jude EB, et al. Medical treatment of Charcot's arthropathy. *J Am Podiatric Med Assoc*. 2002;92(7): 381–3.

 ## CODES

ICD9
- Neuropathic joint disease (Charcot's joints):
  - 094.0 Tabes dorsalis
  - 250.60 Diabetes mellitus with neurological manifestations, Type II or unspecified type, not stated as uncontrolled
- 713.5 Arthropathy associated with neurological disorders

CLINICAL PEARLS
- The most common presenting symptoms of Charcot joint are significant unilateral swelling, warmth, and erythema, usually in the feet. Patients may or may not recall minor preceding trauma.
- The goal of early prolonged immobilization is to prevent repetitive trauma and progression of arthropathy. Significant complications, such as severe foot deformities, ulcerations leading to infections, and amputation, can result if treatment is delayed.

CHICKENPOX (VARICELLA ZOSTER)
Kay A. Bauman, MD, MPH

 BASICS

DESCRIPTION
- Common, highly contagious generalized exanthem characterized by the development of crops of pruritic vesicles on the skin and mucous membranes.
- Fever in up to 70% of persons.
- Virus is spread by respiratory (airborne) droplets, direct contact with varicella vesicles, or rarely zoster lesions.
- Virus establishes latency in the dorsal root ganglia; reactivation results in herpes zoster or "shingles."
- Outbreaks tend to occur late winter to early spring in temperate climates.
- The usual incubation period is 14–16 days (range, 10–21). Patients are infectious from ~48 hours before appearance of the rash until the final lesions have crusted. Historically, most people acquire chickenpox during childhood and develop lifelong immunity. (1) Now it is an immunizable disease.
- System(s) affected: Nervous; Skin/Exocrine
- Synonym(s): Varicella

EPIDEMIOLOGY
- Predominant age: Peak incidence preschoolers to 9 years, but may occur at any age
- Predominant gender: Male = Female

Incidence
- Decreasing incidence since vaccine available: Estimated at 3.5 million cases annually prior to vaccine introduction with an incidence rate of 8–9% in children 1–9 years of age. Reported US varicella cases 1991: 147,076; reported for 2007: 40,146; reported for 2008: 30,386 (2,3).
- Prior to vaccine availability, ~100 deaths in the US/year were reported; for 2008, only 2 deaths were reported. (3,4,5)

RISK FACTORS
- No prior history of varicella infection
- Immunosuppressed patients (especially children with leukemia/lymphoma in remission or receiving high-dose corticosteroids)

Geriatric Considerations
- Infection more severe in adults than in children
- Latent varicella infection may reactivate and cause the exanthem known as shingles or zoster.
- Herpes zoster vaccine, a live attenuated vaccine licensed in 2006, is now recommended for persons ≥60 to prevent zoster (shingles):
  – 1-time dose. Recommended for those previously infected with varicella (chickenpox); those never infected should receive regular varicella vaccine (6). Dose: 0.65ml SQ, available as single dose vial.
- Most common cause of death: Primary viral pneumonia

Pediatric Considerations
- Neonates born to mothers who develop chickenpox from 5 days before to 2 days after delivery are at risk for serious disease. Must give varicella-zoster immune globulin
- Varicella bullosa seen mainly in children <2 years. Lesions appear as bullae instead of vesicles. The clinical course does not change.
- Most common cause of death: Septic complications and encephalitis
- Avoid aspirin/acetylsalicylic acid in children because of link to Reye syndrome.

Pregnancy Considerations
- Risk of transplacental infection after maternal infection is 25%.
- Congenital malformations are seen in 2% (1) of patients when the fetus is infected during the 1st or 2nd trimesters, characterized by limb atrophy and scarring of the skin of the extremities and occasional CNS and eye manifestations.
- Morbidity is increased in women infected during pregnancy (e.g., pneumonia).

GENERAL PREVENTION
- Exposed, susceptible people should be considered at risk and potentially infectious for 21 days.
- Isolate hospitalized patients.
- Passive immunization with IM varicella-zoster immune globulin given within 96 hours (preferably within 72 hours) of exposure to ensure efficacy (1):
  – Recommended for people exposed to chickenpox or shingles within 96 hours who are immunocompromised, ≥15 years old without prior history of chickenpox, newborns of mothers with onset of chickenpox <5 days before delivery or <2 days after delivery. Exposure criteria: Continued household contact, prolonged face-to-face contact (same room), or indoor playmate >1 hour
- Active immunization after exposure: Shown to prevent or reduce significantly the severity of varicella if given within 72 hours postexposure.
- Active immunization: Varicella virus vaccine (Varivax): Live attenuated vaccine approved by FDA in 1995 for pediatrics immunization and recommended by Advisory Committee on Immunization Practices for immunization of healthy patients ≥12 months who have not had chickenpox
- 12 months–12 years old: Initial dose 0.5 mL SC at age 12–15 months; 2nd dose age 4–6 years. Prelicensure studies showed efficacy rates: 70–90% against any disease and 95% against severe disease 7–10 years after vaccination. Other studies showed 100% efficacy at 1 year and 98% at 2 years after vaccination. More recent studies show rates of 85–94% effectiveness, the higher end for the prevention of severe disease. The 2-dose regimen is even more effective, with rates of 96–98% effectiveness. Breakthrough disease generally has <50 lesions, shorter duration of illness, and lower incidence of fever (7)[A].
- ≥13 years: 2 0.5 mL SC doses 4–8 weeks apart, seroconversion rates 78–82% after 1 dose, 99% after 2 doses (1). Adults have efficacy rates in the lower end of this range.

- Vaccine side effects are pain and redness at vaccine site.
- The newly approved MMRV vaccine which combines the measles, mumps, and rubella vaccine with varicella is equally effective. There are rare reports of an increased risk of febrile seizures 5–12 days after vaccination in 1/2300-2600 patients (8)[A].
- May be considered for a subset of HIV-positive children in CDC class I with CD4 >25% (1):
  – Vaccine recipients should avoid contact with immunocompromised people and pregnant women who have never had chickenpox and their newborns, for up to 6 weeks after vaccination.
  – Children needing catch-up vaccination need at least 3 months between doses 1 and 2.

PATHOPHYSIOLOGY
- Skin lesions identical histologically to those of herpes simplex virus.
- In fatal cases, intranuclear inclusions can be found in the endothelium of blood vessels and most organs.

ETIOLOGY
- Varicella-zoster virus is a member of the α-Herpesviridae subfamily; a double-stranded DNA virus.
- Reservoir is humans

 DIAGNOSIS

HISTORY
- Prodromal symptoms: Fever, malaise, anorexia, mild headache
- Malaise, muscle aches, arthralgias, and headache more common in adults (2)
- Subclinical in ~4% of cases

PHYSICAL EXAM
- Characteristic rash: Crops of "teardrop" vesicles on erythematous bases
- Lesions erupt in successive crops
- Progress from macule to papule to vesicle, then begin to crust
- Pruritic rash is present in various stages of development
- Lesions may be present on mucous membranes, both oral and vaginal

DIAGNOSTIC TESTS & INTERPRETATION
Generally used for complicated cases and epidemiologic studies

Lab
Initial lab tests
- Leukocyte count may be normal, low, or mildly increased.
- Marked leukocytosis suggests secondary infection.
- Multinucleated giant cells visible on Tzanck smear from scrapings of vesicles
- Isolated virus from human tissue culture

Follow-Up & Special Considerations
- Visualization of the virus by electron microscopy, tissue culture (costly), and various methods of acute and convalescent sera collection: Latex agglutination (most available), enzyme immunoassay, indirect immunofluorescence antibody, fluorescent antibody to membrane assay, or PCR assay, which can detect wild from vaccine viral strains (1)
- Vaccine-modified cases can be more difficult to diagnose; consider PCR testing of skin lesions (9)[B].

DIFFERENTIAL DIAGNOSIS
- Herpes simplex virus infection
- Herpes zoster
- Impetigo
- Coxsackievirus infection
- Scabies
- Dermatitis herpetiformis
- Drug rash
- Rickettsial pox infection

TREATMENT

Outpatient except for complicating emergencies

MEDICATION
First Line
- Supportive: Antipyretics for fever; avoid aspirin in children
- Local and/or systemic antipruritic agents for itching
- In immunocompromised patients: Varicella-zoster immune globulin available for passive immunization. Varicella-zoster immune globulin must be given within 96 hours after exposure to be beneficial. After 4th day postexposure, wait for rash to develop, then give acyclovir 500 mg/m^2/d q8 h for 7 days.
- Acyclovir: Decreases duration of fever and shortens time of viral shedding. Recommended for adolescents, adults, and high-risk patients. Most beneficial if initiated early in the disease ($\leq$24 h).
  - 2–16-year-old patients: 20 mg/kg/dose (max. 800 mg/dose), q.i.d. for 5 days
  - Adults: 800 mg, 5 times daily.
- Contraindications:
  - Hypersensitivity to the drug
- Precautions
  - Possible renal insufficiency with acyclovir
  - Significant possible interactions
  - Concurrent administration of probenecid increases half-life; increased effects with zidovudine (e.g., drowsiness, lethargy)

Second Line
- Famciclovir: 500 mg t.i.d. for 7–10 days (adults)
- Valacyclovir: 1 g t.i.d. for 7–10 days (adults)

ADDITIONAL TREATMENT
General Measures
- Supportive/symptomatic treatment
- Antihistamines and/or Aveeno or oatmeal baths as needed for itch
- Acetaminophen and/or ibuprofen as needed
- Nail clipping in children to prevent scarring or secondary infection from itching

ONGOING CARE

FOLLOW-UP RECOMMENDATIONS
Patient Monitoring
- Usually none needed in mild cases. If complications occur, intensive supportive care may be required.
- Activity as tolerated. Children may return to school when lesions have scabbed.

DIET
No special diet

PATIENT EDUCATION
- In the healthy child, chickenpox is rarely serious and recovery is complete
- Confers lifelong immunity
- 2nd attack rare, but subclinical infection can occur; happens occasionally after vaccination in children
- Infection latent and may recur years later as herpes zoster in adults (and sometimes in children)
- Fatalities rarely occur from complications

COMPLICATIONS
- Although only 2% of cases are reported after 2nd decade, 35% of deaths occur in this age group (2)
- Secondary bacterial infection: Cellulitis, abscess, erysipelas, sepsis, septic arthritis/osteomyelitis, or staphylococcal pyomyositis
- Pneumonia: 20–30% of adults with chickenpox have lung involvement, 1/400 are hospitalized (2)
- Encephalitis (the most common CNS complication)
- Meningitis
- Reye syndrome
- Purpura
- Thrombocytopenia
- Glomerulonephritis
- Arthritis
- Hepatitis

REFERENCES

1. American Academy of Pediatrics. *Report of the Committee on Infectious Diseases (Red Book)*. Elk Grove Village, IL: American Academy of Pediatrics, 2003.
2. Goldman L, Bennett JC, ed. *Cecil Textbook of Medicine*, 21st ed. Philadelphia: WB Saunders, 2000.
3. Centers for Disease Control and Prevention. *MMWR* 2010;58:869.
4. Centers for Disease Control and Prevention. Summary of Notifiable Diseases, US, 1991. *MMWR.* 1992;40(No. 53).
5. Centers for Disease Control and Prevention (CDC). Varicella-related deaths–United States, January 2003-June 2004. *MMWR Morb Mortal Wkly Rep.* 2005;54:272–4.
6. *The Medical Letter.* 2006;48:73–4.
7. Marin M, Güris D, Chaves SS, Schmid S, Seward JF, Advisory Committee on Immunization Practices, Centers for Disease Control and Prevention (CDC) et al. Prevention of varicella: recommendations of the Advisory Committee on Immunization Practices (ACIP). *MMWR Recomm Rep.* 2007;56:1–40.
8. Marin M, Broder KR, Temte JL, Snider DE, Seward JF, Centers for Disease Control and Prevention (CDC) et al. Use of combination measles, mumps, rubella, and varicella vaccine: recommendations of the Advisory Committee on Immunization Practices (ACIP). *MMWR Recomm Rep.* 2010;59:1–12.
9. Leung J, Harpaz R, Baughman AL, Heath K, Loparev V, Vázquez M, Watson BM, Schmid DS et al. Evaluation of laboratory methods for diagnosis of varicella. *Clin Infect Dis.* 2010;51:23–32.

ADDITIONAL READING
- Campos-Outcalt D. Varicella vaccination: 2 doses now the standard. *J Fam Pract.* 2008;57:38–40.
- Galea SA, Sweet A, Beninger P, Steinberg SP, Larussa PS, Gershon AA, Sharrar RG et al. The safety profile of varicella vaccine: a 10-year review. *J Infect Dis.* 2008;197 (Suppl 2):S165–9.

See Also (Topic, Algorithm, Electronic Media Element)
Herpes Zoster

CODES

ICD9
052.9 Varicella without mention of complication

CLINICAL PEARLS
- Infection is more likely to produce serious illness in adults than in children.
- All people being immunized should receive two doses of vaccine, preferably at least 3 months but no fewer than 28 days apart.
- Herpes zoster vaccine (Zostavax) recommended for persons $\geq$60 years of age to prevent shingles (zoster).

CHILD ABUSE

Karen A. Hulbert, MD

 BASICS

DESCRIPTION
- Types of abuse: Neglect (most common and highest mortality), physical abuse, emotional/psychological abuse, sexual abuse—often in combination
- Child Abuse Hotline by state: http://www.childwelfare.gov/responding/reporting.cfm or call 800-4-A-Child (800-422-4453)
- System(s) affected: Gastrointestinal (GI); Endocrine/Metabolic; Musculoskeletal; Nervous; Renal; Reproductive; Skin/Exocrine; Psychiatric
- Synonym(s): Suspected nonaccidental trauma, child maltreatment, child neglect

EPIDEMIOLOGY
Prevalence
- An estimated 905,000 children in the US were victims of child abuse or neglect in 2006 out of approximately 3.6 million who received investigation (1).
- It is estimated that the actual number of victims is 3× greater than number reported
- Remains the 4th leading cause of childhood death in the US (2)

RISK FACTORS
- All ages; Male = Female:
  - Risk of physical abuse increases with age
  - Risk of fatal abuse more common <age 2
  - Physical abuse 2.1× higher among children with disabilities (3)
- Poverty, drug abuse, lower educational status, parental history of abuse, mentally ill parent/maternal depression, poor support network, and domestic violence:
  - Child abuse may be 4.9× more likely in family with spouse abuse (3)
  - Children in households with unrelated adults 50× more likely to die of inflicted injuries (3)
  - Adults who were abused as children are at much higher risk of becoming abusers than those not raised with abuse

GENERAL PREVENTION
- Know your patients and document their family situations; have increased suspicion to screen for risk factors at prenatal, postnatal, pediatric visit.
- Physicians can educate parents on range of normal behaviors to expect in infants and children:
  - Anticipatory guidance on ways to handle crying infants; methods of discipline for toddlers
- Train first responders—teachers, childcare workers—to look for signs of abuse
- Early childhood home visitation programs recommended to reduce maltreatment in high-risk families (4)[A]
- More research urgently needed to assess effectiveness of interventions such as parenting programs on ability to reduce abuse and neglect

COMMONLY ASSOCIATED CONDITIONS
- Failure to thrive
- Prematurity
- Developmental deficits
- Poor school performance
- Poor social skills
- Low self-esteem, depression

 DIAGNOSIS

Documentation:
- Information in the medical record is an important piece of evidence for investigation and litigation (5)[C]
- Critical elements include (5)[C]:
  - Brief statement of child's disclosure or caregiver's explanation, including any alternate explanations offered
  - Time the incident occurred and date/time of disclosure
  - Whether witnesses were present
  - Developmental abilities of child
  - Objective medical findings
  - Interpretation of the findings
- DO NOT use terms such as "rule out," "R/O," and "alleged." They may cause ambiguity; clearly state physician opinion (5)[C].
- Documentation should include disposition of patient and record any report made to child protective services (5)[C].

HISTORY
- Use nonjudgmental, open-ended questions (ask: who, what, when, and where; NEVER why)
- Use quotes whenever possible
- Document past medical and developmental history, child's temperament, interactions among family members.
- Suggestive of intentional trauma:
  - No explanation or vague explanation (3)
  - Important detail of explanation changes dramatically (3)
  - Explanation is inconsistent with pattern, age, or severity (3)
  - Explanation is inconsistent with child's physical or developmental abilities (3)
  - Different witnesses provide markedly different history (3)
  - Considerable delay in seeking treatment
- Nonspecific symptoms of abuse:
  - Behavior changes; self-destructive behavior
  - Anxiety and/or depression
  - Sleep disturbances, night terrors
  - School problems

PHYSICAL EXAM
- General assessment for signs of physical abuse, neglect, self-injurious behaviors (6)[C]
- Thorough physical exam:
  - Skin, head, eyes, ears, nose, and mouth
  - Chest/abdomen
  - Genital (consider exam under sedation) or refer to ED
  - Extremities with focus on inner arms and legs
  - Growth data
- Maintain high index of suspicion for occult head, chest, and abdominal trauma
- Physical abuse:
  - Skin markings (e.g., lacerations, burns, ecchymoses, linear/shaped contusions, bites)
  - Immersion injuries with clearly distinguished outlines (e.g., from boiling water)
  - Oral trauma (e.g., torn frenulum, loose teeth)
  - Ear trauma (e.g., signs of ear pulling)
  - Eye trauma (e.g., hyphema, hemorrhage)
  - Head/abdominal blunt trauma
  - Fractures

- Sexual abuse:
  - Unexplained penile, vaginal, hymenal, perianal, or anal injuries/bleeding/discharge
  - Pregnancy or sexually transmitted infections (STIs)
  - Sperm is a definitive finding of child abuse
- Neglect:
  - Child may be undersized or unkempt
  - Rashes
  - Fearful or too trusting
  - Clinging to or avoiding caregiver
  - Flat or balding occiput
  - Abnormal development or growth parameters
- Measurements, photographs, careful descriptions are critical for accurate diagnosis
- Collaboration with specialist and child abuse assessment team (3)[C]

DIAGNOSTIC TESTS & INTERPRETATION
Lab
Initial lab tests
- Lab testing should be directed by history and physical exam:
  - Urinalysis (e.g., abdominal/flank/back/genital trauma)
  - Complete blood chemistry. Consideration of coagulation studies and platelet count (e.g., rule out bleeding disorder, abdominal trauma) as appropriate.
  - Electrolytes, creatinine, blood urea nitrogen, glucose
  - Liver and pancreatic function tests (e.g., abdominal trauma)
  - Guaiac stool (abdominal trauma)
- In cases of suspected neglect:
  - Stool exam, calorie count, purified protein derivative and anergy panel, sweat test, lead and zinc levels
- In cases of suspected sexual abuse:
  - STI testing: Gonorrhea, chlamydia, trichomonas; also consider HIV, HSV, hepatitis panel, syphilis (6)[C]
  - Serum pregnancy test (6)[C]

Follow-Up & Special Considerations
Bruising is a common presenting feature:
- Bruising in babies that are not independently mobile is very uncommon (<1%) (7)[A]
- Patterns suggestive of abuse (7)[A]:
  - Bruises seen away from bony prominences
  - Bruises to face, back, abdomen, arms, buttocks, ears, hands
  - Multiple bruises in clusters
  - Multiple bruises of uniform shape
  - Bruises that carry imprint of an implement

Imaging
Initial approach
Imaging should be directed by history and injury/condition:
- All children with fractures and children with suspicious injuries under age 2:
  - Skeletal survey (3)[B]: X-rays include 2 views of each extremity, skull: (AP) and lateral, spine: AP and lateral, chest x-ray, and/or rib (posterior), abdomen, pelvis, hands, and feet
  - Consider bone scan for acute rib fractures and subtle long bone fractures (3)[B]

- Intracranial and extracranial injury:
  – CT scan of head (3)[B]
  – Consider MRI of head/neck for better dating of injuries, looking at subtle findings, intercerebral edema, or hemorrhage (3)[B]
- Intra-abdominal injuries:
  – CT scan of abdomen

Diagnostic Procedures/Surgery
Sexual abuse:
- Consider photocolposcopy
- <72 hours from time of abuse: Collect samples for the forensic laboratory (contact authorities for appropriate protocol) (6)[C]

Pathological Findings
- Spiral fractures in nonambulatory patients (children that are not walking or cruising should not have bruising or fractures from "falls")
- Chip or bucket-handle fractures
- Epiphysial/metaphysial rib fractures in infants
- Rupture of liver/spleen in abdominal blunt trauma
- Retinal hemorrhages in shaken baby syndrome

DIFFERENTIAL DIAGNOSIS
- Physical trauma (including but not limited to):
  – Accidental injury; toxic ingestion
  – Bleeding disorders (e.g., classic hemophilia)
  – Metabolic diseases; congenital conditions
  – Conditions with skin manifestations (e.g., mongolian spots, Henoch-Schönlein purpura, meningococcemia, erythema multiforme, hypersensitivity, car seat burns, staphylococcal scalded skin syndrome, chickenpox, impetigo)
  – Cultural practices (e.g., cupping, coining)
- Neglect (including but not limited to):
  – Endocrinopathies (e.g., diabetes mellitus)
  – Constitutional
  – GI (clefts, malabsorption, irritable bowel)
  – Seizure disorder
  – Sudden infant death syndrome (SIDS)
- Skeletal trauma (including but not limited to):
  – Obstetrical trauma
  – Nutritional (scurvy, rickets)
  – Infection (congenital syphilis, osteomyelitis)
  – Osteogenesis imperfecta
- Neoplasm

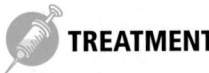 TREATMENT

MEDICATION
First Line
Antibiotics as indicated for treatment of documented STIs or infection

Second Line
Consider antidepressants if needed.

ALERT
Emergency contraception reduces rate of pregnancy after sexual assault if given within 5 days
- Levonorgestrel 1.5 mg as a single dose as effective as 2 split doses (0.75 mg each) 12 hours apart (8)[A]

ADDITIONAL TREATMENT
General Measures
- Always explain what the physical exam will involve and why certain procedures are necessary.
- Examine child in a comfortable setting.
- Allow child to choose who will be in the room.
- Use appropriate positions to examine the anal and genital areas of young children (6)[C].
- Test for STIs before treatment (6)[C].

Issues for Referral
- Consider managing in ER to collect forensic specimens and maintain chain of evidence.
- Mandatory reporting to child protective authorities

SURGERY/OTHER PROCEDURES
As clinically indicated

IN-PATIENT CONSIDERATIONS
Initial Stabilization
As clinically indicated

Admission Criteria
- Moderate-to-severe injuries or unstable
- Acute psychological trauma
- If safety of child outside the hospital cannot be guaranteed

IV Fluids
As clinically indicated

Nursing
As clinically indicated

Discharge Criteria
- Child should be sent to another relative or into foster care if the suspected abuser lives with the child.
- Counseling for individual and family
- After initial evaluation, consider referral to sexual assault center.

 ONGOING CARE

FOLLOW-UP RECOMMENDATIONS
As clinically indicated

Patient Monitoring
- Refer to the state protective services
- Monitor injury healing over time
- Follow-up assessment for STIs that may not present acutely (e.g., HPV, herpes) (6)[C]

DIET
Routine

PATIENT EDUCATION
As clinically indicated

PROGNOSIS
Without intervention, child abuse is often a chronic and escalating phenomenon.

COMPLICATIONS
- Long-term physical and psychological damage
- Death

REFERENCES

1. Department of Health and Human Services, Administration on Children, Youth, and Families (ACF). Child Maltreatment 2006.
2. Deaths: Leading Causes for 2006. *Natl Vital Stat Rep*. 2010;58;14:1–100.
3. Kellogg ND, American Academy of Pediatrics Committee on Child Abuse and Neglect. Evaluation of suspected child physical abuse. *Pediatrics*. 2007; 119(6):1232–41.
4. Hahn RA, Bilukha OO, Crosby A et al. First reports evaluating the effectiveness of strategies for preventing violence: early childhood home visitation. Findings from the Task Force on Community Preventive Services. *MMWR Recomm Rep*. 2003;52(RR-14):1–9.
5. Jackson A, et al: Let the Record Speak: Medicolegal Documentation in Cases of Child Maltreatment. *Clin Ped Emerg Med*. 2006;7:181–5.
6. Nancy Kellogg and the Committee on Child Abuse and Neglect. The evaluation of sexual abuse in children. *Pediatrics*. 2005;116:506–12.
7. Maguire S, Mann MK, Sibert J, et al. Are there patterns of bruising in childhood which are diagnostic or suggestive of abuse? A systematic review. *Arch Dis Child*. 2005;90:182–6.
8. Cheng L, Gülmezoglu AM, Van Oel CJ, et al. Interventions for emergency contraception. *The Cochrane Database of Systematic Reviews*. 2004, Issue 3.

ADDITIONAL READING
Child Abuse Evaluation & Treatment for medical providers (http://www.ChildAbuseMD.com).

 CODES

ICD9
- 995.50 Unspecified child abuse
- 995.51 Child emotional/psychological abuse
- 995.52 Child neglect (nutritional)

CLINICAL PEARLS
- High index of suspicion important for both prevention (knowing risk factors, ways to intervene) and recognition of abuse.
- Neglect is the most common and lethal form of abuse and should be aggressively reported.
- Detailed exam with documentation is key.
- Mandated reporting is required for suspected child abuse and neglect (reasonable suspicion); the physician does not have to prove abuse before reporting.
- Child Abuse Hotline by state: http://www.childwelfare.gov/responding/reporting.cfm or call 800-4-A-Child (800-422-4453).

CHLAMYDIA PNEUMONIAE

Lawrence M. Hwang, MD
Daniel T. Lee, MD

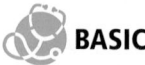 **BASICS**

DESCRIPTION

- *Chlamydia pneumoniae*, an obligate intracellular, gram-negative bacterium, has been established as an important cause of adult and pediatric respiratory disease and is capable of causing persistent latent infection.
- Humans are the only known reservoir.
- 1st recognized as a respiratory pathogen in 1989
- System(s) affected: Respiratory; Cardiovascular; Neurologic
- Synonym(s): Taiwan acute respiratory agent; *Chlamydophila pneumoniae*

EPIDEMIOLOGY

- Incubation period is approximately 30 days.
- Predominant age: More common in elderly; less common in children 2 months–5 years
- Serologic evidence of acute and chronic infection found in 1/3 of patients with acute chronic obstructive pulmonary disease (COPD) exacerbation, often together with other concurrent bacterial infection

Incidence

- Overall incidence rate of *C. pneumoniae* is unknown
- No particular seasonal variation
- Outbreaks have occurred among military recruits, university students, and nursing home residents.

Prevalence

- Accounts for 5–20% of community-acquired pneumonia in adults and children. Greatly varied rates exist between study locations.
- Most cases occur sporadically, although intrafamilial spread also occurs.

Pediatric Considerations

Uncommon in children 2 months–5 years of age

GENERAL PREVENTION

- As transmission is via contact with respiratory secretions, advise hand-washing and avoid exposure to infected persons.
- Flu and pneumococcal vaccines for high-risk groups

PATHOPHYSIOLOGY

Infection with *C. pneumoniae* and resultant host responses may lead to mucus production in the nasal passages, sinuses, bronchial tree, and alveoli, along with nasopharyngeal and airway inflammation and bronchospasm.

COMMONLY ASSOCIATED CONDITIONS

- COPD
- Asthma
- HIV infection
- Cystic fibrosis
- Diabetes mellitus
- Atherosclerosis
- Multiple sclerosis
- Alzheimer disease

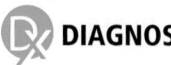 **DIAGNOSIS**

Geriatric Considerations

- Usually more severe disease in older adults, and more common in the elderly who also have concomitant medical problems.
- Elderly patients less likely to exhibit respiratory symptoms with pneumonia and may present with altered mental status or history of falls.

HISTORY

- Spectrum of illness may vary from mild and self-limited to severe pneumonia.
- Onset often gradual with delayed presentation
- Sore throat and hoarseness may precede cough by a week or more, giving biphasic appearance to illness (uncommon in *Legionella*, less common in *Mycoplasma*, *Streptococcus pneumoniae*, and *Haemophilus influenzae*).
- Dry cough
- Low grade fever (usually early in illness)
- Chills
- Rhinitis
- Headache
- Malaise
- Myalgias
- Sinus congestion
- Nausea
- Altered mental status

PHYSICAL EXAM

- General appearance usually nontoxic, unless extremely ill
- Fever
- Tachypnea
- Tachycardia
- Diminished breath sounds
- Crackles or wheezing
- Bronchial breath sounds
- Percussion dullness and egophony less sensitive but more specific for pneumonia
- Pharyngeal erythema (without exudates)
- Retropharyngeal lymphoid granulation

DIAGNOSTIC TESTS & INTERPRETATION
Lab
Initial lab tests

- Multiple unreliable laboratory methods for diagnosis including culture, antigen detection, serology, PCR.
- Leukocyte count usually normal or low, but may be mildly elevated
- Blood cultures recommended if toxic and requiring ICU admission; otherwise not likely to be helpful
- Culture has traditionally been the gold standard diagnostic method (1)[A]:
  – Many limitations include technical complexity, limited availability, and variable yield (1)[A]
  – Most easily cultured in HL or HEp2 cells (culture is 10–80% sensitive and >95% specific) (2)[A]
- Testing with microimmunofluorescence (MIF) is recommended by CDC, as enzyme immunoassay testing is less specific. However, MIF testing is not standardized for *C. pneumoniae* and may also lack specificity and sensitivity (2)[A].
  – 4-fold increase in IgG titer diagnostic of acute infection (10–100% sensitivity) (2)[A]
  – Presence of IgM antibody ($\geq$1:16) (1)[A]
  – Single IgG titers are discouraged (1)[A]
- Complement fixation for *Chlamydia* is widely available but cannot distinguish *C. pneumonia* from *Chlamydophila psittaci*.
- PCR from pharyngeal swab or bronchioalveolar lavage specimen (30–95% sensitivity, >95% specificity) (2)[A]

Imaging
Initial approach

- Patients with suspected community-acquired pneumonia who are more than mildly ill should be evaluated with a chest x-ray (CXR) (2)[A].
  – CXR may be abnormal even in clinically mild disease.
- Variable radiographic abnormalities include unilateral and bilateral infiltrates and pleural effusions. Single, subsegmental funnel-shaped or circumscribed infiltrate is common.

Diagnostic Procedures/Surgery

Although serology is 95% specific, definitive diagnosis requires a positive culture or PCR testing (2)[A].

DIFFERENTIAL DIAGNOSIS
- Other causes of atypical pneumonia, including *M. pneumoniae* and *L. pneumophila*
- Other bacterial causes of pneumonia, including *S. pneumoniae*. *H. influenzae*, *Moraxella catarrhalis*, and *Staphylococcus aureus*
- Respiratory viruses: Adenovirus, influenza A, influenza B, parainfluenza virus, and respiratory syncytial virus
- Endemic fungal pathogens: Blastomycosis, coccidioidomycosis, histoplasmosis
- Bioterrorism agents: Anthrax, plague, tularemia
- Conditions that mimic community-acquired pneumonia: Acute respiratory disease syndrome, atelectasis, idiopathic pulmonary fibrosis, neoplasm, pulmonary embolus, sarcoidosis, congestive heart failure

 TREATMENT

MEDICATION
- β-Lactam antibiotics and sulfasoxazole not effective for *C. pneumoniae*.
- An advantage in clinical efficacy or mortality by empiric coverage of atypical pathogens in patients with community-acquired pneumonia has not been shown (3)[A].
- The treatment course may be extended by several weeks in certain patients whose symptoms have not resolved.

First Line
- Azithromycin: 500 mg on day 1, then 250 mg on days 2–5 *OR*
- Clarithromycin: 500 mg q12h for 10–14 days *OR*
- Doxycycline, 100 mg q12h for at least 14 days (4)[C]:
  - Tetracycline not for use during pregnancy or in children <8 years
  - Tetracycline may cause photosensitivity; sunscreen is recommended.
    - Tetracyclines may increase the anticoagulant effect of warfarin.

Second Line
- Alternative drugs: Erythromycin base, 250–500 mg q.i.d. for 14–21 days
- Levofloxacin, 250–500 mg/d (PO or IV) or other respiratory fluoroquinolones have good bioavailability and the convenience of once-daily dosing, but are recommended for use only when patients have failed treatment with a 1st-line drug, or have had recent antibiotics, significant comorbidities, or allergies to alternatives.

Pregnancy Considerations
Tetracyclines and fluoroquinolones are contraindicated.

COMPLEMENTARY AND ALTERNATIVE MEDICINE
In small studies, manipulative treatment was shown to reduce duration of intravenous antibiotic treatment and days in the hospital for hospitalized elderly patients with pneumonia (5)[C].

IN-PATIENT CONSIDERATIONS
- Usually outpatient care for most. Those with severe pneumonia or coexisting illness may require hospitalization.
- Pneumonia severity index or other validated prediction rule can assist in predicting those patients with community-acquired pneumonia with higher morbidity and those requiring hospitalization (6)[A].

Initial Stabilization
Infection in debilitated or hospitalized patients can be severe. Stabilize respiratory distress as per advanced cardiac life support protocol.

IV Fluids
Increased fluids generally recommended

Discharge Criteria
Reversal of any respiratory distress, with the patient tolerating oral medications, otherwise stable medically, and stable for discharge per the clinical judgment of the physician

 ONGOING CARE

FOLLOW-UP RECOMMENDATIONS
Patient Monitoring
- Weekly patient monitoring until well
- Follow-up chest x-ray for resolution
- Reinfection is possible
- Some reports of individuals who are persistently culture-positive despite antibiotic treatment

PROGNOSIS
- Pneumonia is especially life-threatening in older adults and patients with other illnesses that affect the lungs (e.g., asthma, COPD) or the immune system (e.g., diabetes), with an overall 0.5–29% mortality rate.
- Estimated mortality rate from *C. pneumoniae* is 9%, but this may be an overestimate due to the number of subclinical cases.
- Death usually from secondary infection or underlying comorbidity

COMPLICATIONS
- Reactive airway disease
- Erythema nodosum
- Otitis media
- Endocarditis
- Pericarditis or myocarditis
- Meningoencephalitis
- Associated with atherosclerotic disease: *C. pneumoniae* has been cultured from atherosclerotic plaque in patients with coronary artery disease, but treatment has not been shown to affect mortality.

REFERENCES
1. Kumar S, Hammerschlag MR. Acute respiratory infection due to Chlamydia pneumoniae: current status of diagnostic methods. *Clin Infect Dis.* 2007;44:568–76.
2. Lutfiyya MN, et al. Diagnosis and treatment of community-acquired pneumonia. *AFP.* 2006;73:3:442–50.
3. Shefet D, et al. Empiric antibiotic coverage of atypical pathogens for community acquired pneumonia in hospitalized adults. *Cochrane Database Syst Rev.* 2006;1:CD004418.
4. Kauppinen M, Saikku P. Pneumonia due to Chlamydia pneumoniae: prevalence, clinical features, diagnosis, and treatment. *Clin Infect Dis.* 1995;21(Suppl 3):S244–52.
5. Noll DR, Shores JH, Gamber RG, et al. Benefits of osteopathic manipulative treatment for hospitalized elderly patients with pneumonia. *J Am Osteopath Assoc.* 2000;100:776–82.
6. Fine MJ, Auble TE, Yealy DM, et al. A prediction rule to identify low-risk patients with community-acquired pneumonia. *N Engl J Med.* 1997;336:243–50.

ADDITIONAL READING
- Blasi F, Tarsia P, Aliberti S. Chlamydophila pneumoniae. *Clin Microbiol Infect.* 2009;15:29–35.
- Miyashita N, et al. Clinical presentation of community-acquired *Chlamydia pneumonia* in adults. *Chest.* 2002;121:1176–81.
- Thibodeau KP, et al. Atypical pathogens and challenges in community-acquired pneumonia. *AFP.* 2004;69:7:1701–6.

See Also (Topic, Algorithm, Electronic Media Element)
Algorithm: Cough, Chronic

 CODES

ICD9
483.1 Pneumonia due to chlamydia

CLINICAL PEARLS
- *C. pneumoniae* is a significant cause of adult and pediatric pneumonias.
- Formal and accurate diagnosis of *C. pneumoniae* is difficult due to lack of standardized diagnostic tests. Culture remains the gold standard.
- Initial treatment should include tetracyclines, macrolides, and quinolones.

CHLAMYDIAL SEXUALLY TRANSMITTED DISEASES

Autumn Davidson, MD
Jeremy Golding, MD

 BASICS

DESCRIPTION

- An obligate intracellular membrane-bound prokaryotic organism, *C. trachomatis* is the most common bacterial sexually transmitted infection in the US.
- Transmitted through vaginal, anal, or oral sex. May also occur vertically from mother to infant during vaginal birth.
- Screening has increased over the last 20 years, but remains suboptimal with annual screening rates of only 42% among sexually active females ages 16–25 in 2007.
- Majority of cases are asymptomatic (75–90% females, 50–75% males)
- If untreated, may lead to pelvic inflammatory disease, ectopic pregnancies, and infertility.
- System(s) affected: Reproductive

Pregnancy Considerations
Perinatal acquisition may result in neonatal pneumonia and/or conjunctivitis.

EPIDEMIOLOGY
Incidence
- Mandatory reporting started in 1985 with national data showing steady increase in incidence since.
- 1.2 million *reported* cases in 2008, with >3 million estimated cases yearly in the US. Increasing incidence reflects greater screening and improved testing modalities.

Prevalence
- 401.3 per 100,000 people in the US in 2008. This was a 9.2% increase from 2007.
- Populations most affected: Young females, particularly those of ethnic minority groups
- Peak incidence: Late teens, early 20s
- Predominant sex: Females have higher reported incidence and prevalence than males, but this likely reflects increased testing in females.
- Minorities bear the highest burden, with infection rates among blacks in 2008, 8× that of whites. Rates among American Indian/Alaska natives and Hispanics were 4.9 and 2.9 times higher than whites, respectively. Rates higher in US southern states as compared with the Northeast.

RISK FACTORS
Risk correlates with:
- Number of lifetime sexual partners
- Number of concurrent sexual partners
- Use of oral contraceptives (due to resulting cervical ectopy)
- Younger age (highest in females 15–19 years, males 20–24 years)
- Black/Hispanic/American Indian and Alaskan native ethnicity (1)

GENERAL PREVENTION
- Populations with prevalence >5% should be screened at least annually (2). Screen if: New or >1 sex partner in past 6 months, attending an adolescent or family-planning clinic or an STD or abortion clinic, attending a jail or other detention-center clinic, rectal pain, discharge or tenesmus, testicular pain, testing of any individual with urethral or cervical discharge.
- All sexually active women <25 years of age should be screened at least yearly, and repeat testing in approximately 3 months is recommended for those who screen positive, not as test of cure but because reinfection rate is high regardless of whether the sexual partner is treated (2)[A].
- Screening sexually active men <25 years is controversial but should be strongly considered in high-risk populations (3,4)[A].

ETIOLOGY
C. trachomatis serotypes D–K

COMMONLY ASSOCIATED CONDITIONS
- Females:
  - PID: As many as 40% of untreated women will develop PID
  - Infertility
  - Ectopic pregnancies
  - Chronic pelvic pain
  - Mucopurulent cervicitis with cervical edema and propensity to bleed during speculum
  - Urethral syndrome (common in women with dysuria, frequency and pyuria in the absence of infection with uropathogen)
- Males:
  - Epididymitis
  - Nongonococcal urethritis
  - Reiter's syndrome (HLA-B27)
  - Proctitis (Men who have sex with men)
- Neonates:
  - Inclusion conjunctivitis
  - Otitis media
  - Pneumonia
- Diseases caused by other chlamydial species:
  - Lymphogranuloma venereum: *C. trachomatis* serotypes L1–L3
  - Trachoma: *C. trachomatis* serotypes A–C

DIAGNOSIS

- Majority of patients are asymptomatic. Of those with symptoms, the most common are as follows:
  - In females: Mucopurulent vaginal discharge, dysuria (urethral syndrome), bartholinitis, abdominopelvic pain (endometritis, salpingitis/PID), right upper quadrant pain (Fitz-Hugh-Curtis perihepatitis syndrome)
  - In males: Dysuria, urethral discharge (urethritis), scrotal pain (epididymitis), rectal pain or discharge (proctitis), acute arthritis (Reiter syndrome)
  - In infants: Conjunctivitis, pneumonitis, carriage in pharynx/gastrointestinal tract

- Lymphogranuloma venereum (LVG) (*C. trachomatis* serovars L1, L2, or L3): Primary lesion is a small genital or rectal papule that may ulcerate at the site of transmission after an incubation period of 3–30 days. Most common manifestation in heterosexuals is unilateral tender lymphadenopathy. With rectal transmission, LGV causes an invasive proctocolitis, which may be scarring and cause strictures.

HISTORY
- Complete sexual history, including number of sex partners lifetime and past year, prior history of sexually transmitted infections, use of barrier protection, exchange of money or drugs for sex, oral or anal receptive intercourse
- Symptom history, with onset date for each symptom

PHYSICAL EXAM
- Men and women:
  - External genitalia (rash? lesions?)
  - Urethra (discharge?)
  - Inguinal lymph nodes
  - Pharynx and perianal area, if history indicates
- In addition, for women:
  - Cervix (discharge? motion tenderness?)
  - Uterus, ovaries, adnexae

DIAGNOSTIC TESTS & INTERPRETATION
Lab
- Test of choice: Nucleic acid amplification tests (NAAT)
  - Amplified molecular testing (e.g., PCR, ligase chain reaction, specific dynamic action, human chorionic somatotropin, thyroid microsomal antigen): Sensitivity >95%; specificity >99%. Urine equally as sensitive as cervical swab. Patient self-collected vaginal swabs have also been shown to be effective. Lab tests may remain positive for as long as 3 weeks after successful treatment
- Chlamydial cell culture: Sensitivity 50–90%; specificity >99%
- Enzyme immunoassay: Sensitivity 40-60%; specificity >99%
- Direct fluorescent antibody detection: Sensitivity 50–70%; specificity >99%
- Specimens should contain cell scrapings rather than inflammatory discharge because the organism lives only inside the epithelial cells.

Imaging
Imaging not indicated for initial screening; consider pelvic ultrasound/CT if high clinical suspicion for PID or tubo-ovarian abscess.

Initial approach
Offer testing for other STDs including gonorrhea, HIV, syphilis, and for HPV

Follow-Up & Special Considerations
Test of cure not routinely recommended with exceptions for the following patients: Those in whom symptoms persist, those in whom adherence to medication regimens may not be complete, and pregnant females.

DIFFERENTIAL DIAGNOSIS
- *N. gonorrhoeae:* Urethritis, proctitis, epididymitis, cervicitis, PID, Bartholin abscess, perihepatitis
- *Mycoplasma* or *U. urealyticum:* Urethritis, epididymitis, Reiter disease, PID
- *C. trachomatis* (serotypes L1–L3): LGV, Proctitis

TREATMENT

MEDICATION

First Line
Treatment of chlamydial urethritis, cervicitis (including sexual partners of infected persons):
- Azithromycin 1 g PO single dose, or
- Doxycycline: 100 mg PO b.i.d. × 7 days

Pregnancy Considerations
- In pregnant women: Tetracycline and ofloxacin are contraindicated during pregnancy; consider azithromycin or amoxicillin
  - Azithromycin as above, or
  - Amoxicillin 500 mg PO t.i.d. × 7 days
- 1st-line PID treatment (outpatient):
  - Ceftriaxone 250 mg IM × 1 PLUS Doxycycline 100 mg PO × 14 days with or without Metronidazole 500 mg PO b.i.d. × 14 days, or
  - Cefoxitin 2g IM × 1 with Probenecid 1 g PO × 1 PLUS doxycycline 100 mg PO × 14 days with or without Metronidazole 500 mg PO b.i.d. × 14 days
- 1st-line PID treatment parenteral therapy: See "Pelvic Inflammatory Disease"
- 1st-line treatment of LGV: Doxycycline 100 mg b.i.d. × 21 days or erythromycin base 500 mg orally q.i.d. × 21 days
- Tetracyclines may cause photosensitivity; sunscreen is recommended. Avoid concurrent administration of tetracyclines with antacids, dairy products, or iron.
- Practitioners may elect to give azithromycin and ceftriaxone together to the patient in the office to reduce patient noncompliance.

Pregnancy Considerations
Tetracyclines (e.g., doxycycline) and quinolones (e.g., ofloxacin, levofloxacin) are contraindicated in pregnant women.

Pediatric Considerations
Tetracyclines and quinolones are contraindicated in children.

Second Line
- 2nd-line therapy for chlamydial urethritis/cervicitis
- Erythromycin base: 500 mg PO q.i.d. × 7 days
- Erythromycin ethylsuccinate: 800 mg PO q.i.d. × 7 days
- Ofloxacin: 300 mg PO b.i.d. × 7 days
- Levofloxacin: 500 mg PO daily × 7 days

ADDITIONAL TREATMENT
Expedited partner therapy (EPT) is the practice of physicians delivering medications or prescriptions to sexual partners of persons infected with STIs without clinical assessment of the partners.

- Treatment of sexual partners is a key component to STI control. EPT has been shown to be more effective than traditional partner referral in reducing recurrence rates.
- EPT is currently legal is 23 states, "potentially allowable" in 19 states, and illegal in 8. The logistics of this practice differ from state to state and continue to evolve.
- For an updated review on the legal status of EPT, please refer to the CDC website on this subject: http://www.cdc.gov/std/ept/legal/default.htm.

General Measures
- All patients with known or suspected chlamydia should be tested for gonorrhea, syphilis, and HIV (the latter requires individual counseling and consent) (2)[C].
- Ensure females are up to date with pap smears.
- Some experts recommend that all patients treated for chlamydia should be treated empirically for gonorrhea simultaneously, unless they are known to be negative for gonorrhea by sensitive lab testing.
- All partners of patients treated for chlamydia should be tested, if possible. They should be treated empirically rather than waiting for test results. They should also be treated empirically even if they were not tested.

IN-PATIENT CONSIDERATIONS
Treatment of PID: Trend toward outpatient treatment. However, decision to hospitalize made on case-by-case basis. Those falling into the following categories recommended for inpatient treatment: Pregnancy, lack of response or intolerance to oral meds, suspicion of poor compliance/nonadherence to therapy, severe clinical illness (fevers, severe vomiting, or abdominal pain), pelvic abscess, possible need for surgical intervention.

Initial Stabilization
Outpatient treatment, unless patient is moderately or severely ill with PID or other complications

Admission Criteria
As outlined above

ONGOING CARE

FOLLOW-UP RECOMMENDATIONS
Abstinence from sexual contact until diagnosis and treatment complete for patient and all partners

Patient Monitoring
- It is not routine to test the patient to see if a cure has been obtained, except in pregnancy. However, retesting of infected women at 3 months is indicated because of high risk of reinfection (2,5)[A].
- Sexual partners must be evaluated and treated empirically, if necessary, to prevent passing the disease back and forth between partners. Partnerships with local public health departments should be fostered to assist with partner tracing.
- Lack of resolution or recurrence of symptoms must be reported immediately to the physician, and severe cases of urethritis/cervicitis, as well as the chlamydial syndromes, should be seen in follow-up after completion of therapy.
- Up to 25% of asymptomatic patients screened for chlamydia may not return for treatment after chlamydia culture results. Strategies must be developed to ensure treatment can be instituted.

PATIENT EDUCATION
- Suggest risk-reduction counseling and encourage delay of initiation of sexual activity, especially in younger adolescents.
- Encourage safe-sex practices, such as barrier protection (condoms particularly).
- Inform about serious sequelae of chlamydial disease, such as tubal infertility or chronic pelvic pain.
- Stress the need to finish entire course of antibiotics.

PROGNOSIS
Prognosis is good with early and compliant therapy; however, because of the asymptomatic nature of the early disease and the population affected, symptomatic PID still accounts annually for 2.5 million outpatient visits and >250,000 hospitalizations.

COMPLICATIONS
- Both sexes: Enhancement of transmission of and susceptibility to HIV
- Males: Transient oligospermia and postepididymitis urethral stricture (rare)
- Females: Tubal infertility (most common cause of acquired infertility), tubal (ectopic) pregnancy, chronic pelvic pain

REFERENCES
1. http://www.cdc.gov/std/chlamydia/default.htm#stat.
2. Centers for Disease Control and Prevention. Sexually transmitted disease treatment guidelines 2006. MMWR. 2006;55:No. RR-11.
3. Turner CF, Rogers SM, Miller HG, et al. Untreated gonococcal and chlamydial infection in a probability sample of adults. JAMA. 2002;287:726–33.
4. http://www.cdc.gov/std/chlamydia/ChlamydiaScreening-males.pdf.
5. Hosenfeld CB, Workowski KA, Berman S, Zaidi A, Dyson J, Mosure D, Bolan G, Bauer HM et al. Repeat infection with Chlamydia and gonorrhea among females: a systematic review of the literature. Sex Transm Dis. 2009;36:478–89.

See Also (Topic, Algorithm, Electronic Media Element)
Cervicitis; Epididymitis' Gonococcal Infections; HIV Infection and AIDS; Pelvic Inflammatory Disease; Syphilis; Urethritis

CODES

ICD9
- 099.55 Other venereal diseases due to chlamydia trachomatis, unspecified genitourinary site
- 616.11 Vaginitis and vulvovaginitis in diseases classified elsewhere

CLINICAL PEARLS
- C. trachomatis infection is common (but usually asymptomatic) in sexually active teens and young adults.
- Chlamydia infection is the most common cause of acquired infertility in the US.
- To prevent recurrence, treat patients and their partners concurrently.
- ACOG estimates that 40% of untreated chlamydial infections progress to PID, and 1 in 5 cases of PID lead to infertility.
- 2006 was the 1st year that new reported chlamydial cases in the US exceeded 1 million, and this is with only half the eligible sexually active women being screened.
- If all eligible women were screened, we would annually prevent an estimated 60,000 cases of PID, 8,000 cases of chronic pelvic pain, and over 7,000 cases of infertility.

CHOLANGITIS, ACUTE

Mallika Mundkur, MD
John M. Levey, MD

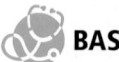 **BASICS**

DESCRIPTION

- An ascending bacterial infection of the bile duct system occurring in the context of a partial or complete obstruction of the biliary tree, most commonly caused by gallstones.
- Classically, presents with the clinical triad of fever, jaundice, and right upper quadrant (RUQ) pain (Charcot triad) or the pentad of fever, jaundice, RUQ pain, mental status changes and hypotension (Reynold pentad)
- Severity of the syndrome may range from mild to life-threatening
- Management includes medical and/or surgical interventions.
- System(s) affected: GI; Hepatobiliary

EPIDEMIOLOGY

- Predominant age: 55–70 years; rare in children, more common in adults
- The data on gender distribution is inconsistent; some studies note that though gallstones are more frequent in females than males, the frequency of cholangitis is equivalent between sexes.

RISK FACTORS

- As cholangitis often occurs secondary to gallstone obstruction, many of the risk factors for developing cholangitis are the same as those for developing gallstones: Populations such as Native Americans and African Americans with sickle cell disease
- Any condition that predisposes to bile stasis increases risk for cholangitis, including biliary strictures, biliary malignancies causing narrowing of the duct, or pancreatic tumors compressing the ductal system extrinsically.
- Endoscopic or surgical manipulation
- Parasitic infections of the Hepatobiliary system (*Ascaris lumbricoides, Clonorchis sinensis, Opisthorchis viverrini*)
- Biliary stents

GENERAL PREVENTION

Ensure surgical clearance of retained choledocholithiasis (CBD) stones at time of cholecystectomy with endoscopic or radiographic cholangiography or provide adequate drainage of the biliary tree

PATHOPHYSIOLOGY

- The composition of bile includes antibacterial components, such as immunoglobulins.
- The flow of bile from the liver to the GI tract via the ampulla enhances the maintenance of the bile as a sterile fluid.
- Obstruction to the flow of bile predisposes the system to an infection that festers in the biliary system and may ascend higher in the biliary tree.
- If the infection ascends unopposed to penetrate the hepatic circulation, the patient may present with generalized infection, severe sepsis, and a poor outcome.

ETIOLOGY

- *Escherichia coli, Klebsiella pneumoniae,* and *Streptococcus faecalis* are the most commonly cultured organisms from the bile of patients with cholangitis.
- *Bacteroides fragilis, Enterococcus, Enterobacter,* and *Pseudomonas* are also reported to have been frequently isolated from the bile of affected patients.

COMMONLY ASSOCIATED CONDITIONS

- Choledocholithiasis
- Malignant tumors
- Benign strictures
- Biliary-enteric anastomosis
- Invasive procedures
- Foreign bodies
- Parasites
- Secondary sclerosing cholangitis
- Immunosuppression

 DIAGNOSIS

HISTORY

- Although the classic presentation, as per Charcot triad, includes fever, jaundice, and RUQ abdominal pain, the full triad is present in only approximately 2/3 of patients.
- More atypical presentations often occur in the elderly, who may present later in the evolution of the disease with sudden decompensation from sepsis.
- Reynold pentad includes the 3 symptoms of Charcot triad (fever, jaundice, RUQ abdominal pain) as well as the additional features of disorientation and hypotension. The presence of the pentad suggests a much more severe manifestation of the disease.

PHYSICAL EXAM

Patient may have only 1 or 2 of the following symptoms, and the abdominal exam may be unrevealing:

- RUQ pain, not severe; abdominal exam may be similar or identical to that with acute cholecystitis
- Jaundice
- Chills and fever
- Shock
- CNS depression

DIAGNOSTIC TESTS & INTERPRETATION
Lab

- Complete blood count: Elevated white blood cell count (WBC), neutrophil predominant
- Liver function tests: Elevated bilirubin, GGT, alkaline phosphatase, transaminases
- Serum amylase and lipase (stone impacted at level of the ampulla)
- Blood cultures: Occasionally positive for growth, depending on severity of infection
- WBC $\geq$20,000, and *T. Bili* $\geq$10 mg/dl are selective predictors of adverse outcomes (1)[B].

Imaging
- See Diagnostic Procedures.
- CT may be helpful to distinguish suppurative from nonsuppurative cholangitis (2)[C].

Diagnostic Procedures/Surgery
- Ultrasound (US) will rapidly diagnose gallstones and CBD dilatation
  - However, cholangiography is the definitive diagnostic test.
- Percutaneous transhepatic cholangiography or endoscopic retrograde cholangiopancreatography (ERCP) allow for both diagnostic confirmation and therapeutic intervention.
- ERCP allows for procedures such as stone extraction, stent-placement and sphincterotomy.
- MRCP is a newer noninvasive method of imaging the bile duct using magnetic resonance technology; may be useful in confirming biliary pathology prior to ERCP, and has high sensitivity and specificity for primary sclerosing cholangitis (3)[A].

DIFFERENTIAL DIAGNOSIS
- Acute cholecystitis
- Mirizzi syndrome
- Biliary leaks
- Oriental cholangiohepatitis
- Pyogenic liver abscess
- Hepatitis
- Infected choledochal cysts
- Acute pancreatitis
- Perforated duodenal ulcer
- Pelvic inflammatory disease with peritonitis
- Kidney stones
- Pancreatitis
- Right lower-lobe pneumonia

 TREATMENT

- Monitor airway, breathing, and circulation, resuscitate as needed; intravenous crystalloid
- Make patient NPO, and if vomiting, place nasogastric tube

MEDICATION
Management consists of intravenous antibiotics, fluid resuscitation, and biliary drainage.
- The initial empiric antibiotic therapy should be broad-spectrum until results of blood cultures are obtained, at which time the regimen should be modified according to the organism isolated

- Little data is available on the best initial antibiotic regimen, but sample initial broad-spectrum regimens are listed below in no particular order:
  - Monotherapy with a beta-lactam/beta-lactamase inhibitor, such as ampicillin-sulbactam (3 g every 6 hours) OR piperacillin/tazobactam (4.5 g every 6 hours) OR ticarcillin-clavulanate (3.1 g every 4 hours)
  - Metronidazole (500 mg IV every eight hours) PLUS a 3rd-generation cephalosporin, such as ceftriaxone (1 g IV every 24 hours)
  - Metronidazole (500 mg IV every eight hours) PLUS a fluoroquinolone (ciprofloxacin 400 mg IV every 12 hours or levofloxacin 500 mg IV daily)
  - Monotherapy with a carbapenem, such as imipenem (500 mg every six hours) OR meropenem (1 g every 8 hours) OR ertapenem (1 g daily)

ADDITIONAL TREATMENT
- The majority of patients will respond to antibiotics and conservative management and will be able to undergo elective biliary drainage.
- Approximately 1/5 of patients will require urgent biliary decompression, requiring invasive procedures that include ERCP with sphincterotomy, percutaneous transhepatic decompression, open surgical decompression, or T-tube placement
- Indications for urgent decompression include: Prolonged persistence of abdominal pain, mental status changes, fever >39C (102 F), hypotension not adequately responsive to fluid resuscitation

SURGERY/OTHER PROCEDURES
- Patients who do not respond to antibiotics and supportive care require emergency decompression of the biliary duct system. This may be accomplished by surgery, endoscopy, or transhepatic cholangiography.
- In case of obstruction secondary to stones, endoscopic papillotomy and stone extraction will drain the duct, may be definitive treatment of the underlying cause, and are shown to reduce mortality.

IN-PATIENT CONSIDERATIONS
See Treatment.

 ONGOING CARE

FOLLOW-UP RECOMMENDATIONS
Some patients with recurrent symptoms of cholangitis may require maintenance antibiotics and imaging to exclude liver abscess.

DIET
NPO until acute phase is terminated.

PATIENT EDUCATION
For patient education materials favorably reviewed on this topic, contact National Digestive Diseases Information Clearinghouse, Box NDDIC, Bethesda, MD 20892, (301) 468-6344.

PROGNOSIS
- Historically the mortality rate was 100%.
- With current medical and surgical interventions, mortality from acute cholangitis has now decreased to approximately 5%.
- Coexistent cardiac or kidney impairment, malignancies, and hepatic abscesses worsen the prognosis of affected individuals.

COMPLICATIONS
- Hepatic abscess
- Sepsis
- Hepatic dysfunction
- Acute renal failure

REFERENCES

1. Rosing DK, De Virgilio C, Nguyen AT, et al. Cholangitis: analysis of admission prognostic indicators and outcomes. *Am Surg.* 2007;73: 949–54.
2. Lee NK, Kim S, Lee JW, et al. Discrimination of suppurative cholangitis from nonsuppurative cholangitis with computed tomography (CT). *Eur J Radiol.* 2008.
3. Dave M, Elmunzer BJ, Dwamena BA et al. Primary sclerosing cholangitis: meta-analysis of diagnostic performance of MR cholangiopancreatography. *Radiology.* 2010;256:387–96.

ADDITIONAL READING

Magnuson TH, Bender JS, Duncan MD., et al. Utility of magnetic resonance cholangiography in the evaluation of biliary obstruction. *J Am Coll Surg.* 1999;189: 63–71; discussion 71–2.

See Also (Topic, Algorithm, Electronic Media Element)
Cholelithiasis

 CODES

ICD9
576.1 Cholangitis

CLINICAL PEARLS
- The complete Charcot triad is present in only 2/3 of patients.
- Ultrasound helps with diagnosis, but ERCP is both diagnostic and therapeutic.

CHOLEDOCHOLITHIASIS

David Carne, MD

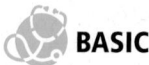

BASICS

DESCRIPTION
- Stones in common bile duct (CBD)
- 3 types: Cholesterol (majority), calcium bilirubinate or pigment, and mixed stones
- Pigment stones may form de novo in the CBD.
- System(s) affected: Gastrointestinal; Hepatobiliary
- Synonym(s): CBD stones; CBD calculi

EPIDEMIOLOGY
Incidence
- 700,000 cholecystectomies performed annually in US:
  - 4.6–20% of patients with gallstones have choledocholithiasis discovered at time of cholecystectomy, depending on whether routine cholangiography is used.
- Increases with age (30–50% of patients >60 years old with gallstones have CBD stones):
  - On average, present 10 years older than cholelithiasis patients
- Incidence of gallstones in US is 10–20%: Individuals >60 years old is up to 40%
- Internationally, incidence is increased due to parasitic infections such as *Ascaris lumbricoides*.
- Choledocholithiasis found with intraoperative cholangiography may be a false positive and may pass spontaneously without intervention.

Prevalence
Predominant sex: Female > Male

RISK FACTORS
- Cholelithiasis (most CBD stones migrate from the gallbladder [GB] into CBD)
- Pancreatitis (30%)
- Obesity
- Higher consumption of long-chain saturated fatty acids (1)[A]
- Chronic hemolysis
- Estrogen exposure
- Weight loss >25% of original weight after bariatric surgery (2)[A]
- Prior cholecystectomy:
  - <2 years prior: Considered a "retained" stone
  - >2 years prior: Considered "recurrent" stone

Genetics
- MDR3 defects may predispose to bile sludge formation, cholelithiasis, cholestasis of pregnancy, and subsequent choledocholithiasis.
- Increased prevalence in Hispanic population

GENERAL PREVENTION
- Maintain a normal weight.
- Avoid rapid weight loss.
- Regular exercise

PATHOPHYSIOLOGY
CBD stones may be primary or secondary:
- Primary stones form within the biliary tract: Caused by any condition leading to bile stasis or chronic bactibilia
- Secondary stones form within the gallbladder

ETIOLOGY
- Cholelithiasis: Majority of stones
- Chronic hemolytic states
- Formation of de novo pigment stones:
  - Dilated, sclerosed, or strictured ducts (e.g., from recurrent cholangitis)

- Hepatobiliary parasitism (*Ascaris lumbricoides* or *Clonorchis sinensis*)

COMMONLY ASSOCIATED CONDITIONS
- Cholelithiasis, cholecystitis, cholangitis
- Gallstone pancreatitis

- Colorectal adenomas: Strong association between cholelithiasis and multiple (>/= 3) lesions [adjusted OR 2.39, 95% CI 1.21–4.72] and left-sided colorectal adenomas [adjusted OR 1.82, 95% CI 1.28–2.59] (3)[A]
- Cholangiocarcinoma [OR = 23.97, 95% CI 2.9–198.9] (4)[A]; cholecystectomy does not change risk.

DIAGNOSIS

HISTORY
- Asymptomatic (30–50%)
- Right upper quadrant pain. Moderate/intense spasmodic pain, often intermittent, transient, recurrent:
  - May radiate to right shoulder/back
  - Worse after eating fatty or greasy foods
  - Occurs within minutes following meals
  - Pain not relieved by antacids
- Secondary effects of obstruction:
  - Clay-colored stool
  - Tea-colored urine
  - Jaundice
  - Nausea/vomiting
  - Pruritus
  - Pancreatitis (epigastric pain radiating to back, etc.)
  - Hepatomegaly
- Infection that may progress to cholangitis and septic shock:
  - Fever, chills
  - Hypotension, flushing
- History of CBD strictures, recurrent sclerosing cholangitis, sphincter of Oddi dysfunction, cystic dilation
- Weight loss

PHYSICAL EXAM
- Moderate right upper quadrant tenderness on palpation
- Jaundice
- Fever
- Anorexia
- Fever, RUQ pain, and jaundice (Charcot triad) strongly indicative of cholangitis:
  - With severe cholangitis: Shock and mental status changes possible (Reynolds pentad)
- Palpable gallbladder (less common)
- Rebound tenderness or guarding absent

DIAGNOSTIC TESTS & INTERPRETATION
Lab
Initial lab tests
- Lab tests may be entirely normal.
- Direct hyperbilirubinemia (with total serum bilirubin >3 mg/dL) indicates obstruction
- Leukocytosis
- Blood cultures positive in 30–60% of patients with cholangitis
- Alkaline phosphatase and gamma-glutamyl-transpeptidase elevated with CBD obstruction
- Combination of a dilated common bile duct, elevated alkaline phosphatase, and ALT has modest

sensitivity and high specificity for patients with cholelithiasis and choledocholithiasis
- Possible elevation of pancreatic enzymes
- Increased liver transaminases

Imaging
Initial approach
- Imaging is the most effective method of confirming suspected choledocholithiasis.
- Transabdominal ultrasound:
  - Fastest modality
  - Poorly confirms/excludes CBD stones (sensitivity 15–50%, specificity 75%)
  - Can detect dilation of CBD, but difficult to identify stones
  - A dilated CBD is found in only half of those with choledocholithiasis.
- Endoscopic ultrasound:
  - Sensitivity 88–97% and specificity 96–100% improved over transabdominal U/S
  - More invasive and increased cost
- Magnetic resonance cholangiopancreatography (MRCP):
  - Sensitivity 92%, specificity 97%
  - Most accurate noninvasive test; no contrast required (5)[A]
  - Preferred by patients over endoscopic retrograde cholangiopancreatography (ERCP), no associated morbidity, and may be less costly than diagnostic ERCP (6)[A]
  - May miss calculi smaller than 5 mm
- Abdominal CT:
  - Less sensitive than MRCP, but faster
  - Good at detecting CBD dilation, complications, and delineating surrounding structures (e.g., pancreas)
- Cholescintigraphy (HIDA/DISIDA scan): CBD radionuclide imaging. Isotope derivatives taken up by hepatocytes and excreted into biliary tree. Can be used to assess for bile duct obstruction, cystic duct obstruction, or bile leakage:
  - May be combined with CCK to observe GB function and estimate GB "ejection fraction"

Diagnostic Procedures/Surgery
- Cholangiography is the gold standard for determining the presence of CBD stones:
  - ERCP (sensitivity 90–95%, specificity 95%): Most common diagnostic modality. Allows for papillotomy/stone extraction at time of diagnosis.
  - Percutaneous transhepatic cholangiography (PTC): Puncture of hepatic duct by needle, injection of radiopaque dye, and subsequent radiograph imaging of abdomen. Used in place of ERCP in patients with extensive bile duct stone disease or in whom ERCP would be difficult.
  - Intraoperative cholangiography (IOC): Contrast inserted via opening in cystic duct during cholecystectomy. Ongoing debate if IOC should be routinely performed during cholecystectomy.
- Endoscopic ultrasound: More likely to detect stones than transabdominal route (sensitivity 85–97%, specificity 96–100%)
- Intraoperative intraluminal ultrasonography:
  - Can be performed during laparoscopic or open procedures
  - May be indicated in patients with contrast dye allergy
- Postoperative studies:
  - MRI (MRCP) can be commonly used postoperatively to diagnose CBD stone.

– T-tube cholangiography
- Choledochoscopy can be used to extract stones intraoperatively or via t-tube tract.

DIFFERENTIAL DIAGNOSIS
- Biliary stricture
- Narrowed biliary–enteric anastomosis
- Cholangitis (acute or primary sclerosing)
- Cholangiocarcinoma
- Sphincter of Oddi dysfunction
- Biliary parasites
- Papillary stenosis
- Blood clots

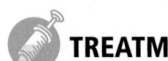

TREATMENT
MEDICATION
- The obstruction needs to be removed. If not symptomatic and small, stones may pass spontaneously.
- Antibiotics are used if infection is suspected (cholangitis) and need to cover enteric flora.
- Broad-coverage antibiotics (substitute fluoroquinolones for penicillin-allergic patients). Routinely prescribed for prophylaxis, although a 2003 study suggests prophylactic antibiotics did not prevent cholangitis in those with choledocholithiasis:
  – Piperacillin-tazobactam (Zosyn) 3.375 g IV q6h
  – Ampicillin-sulbactam (Unasyn) 1.5–3.0 g (1–2 g ampicillin + 0.5–1 g sulbactam) IV/IM q6–8h; not to exceed 8 g/d ampicillin or 4 g/d sulbactam
- Fluoroquinolones have good biliary penetration:
  – Levofloxacin 250–500 mg IV or p.o. once daily
  – Ciprofloxacin 200 mg IV/p.o. b.i.d.
- Duration of therapy depends on rapidity of response, subsequent surgery, and presence of bacteremia, as well as correction of biliary obstruction.
- Addition of metronidazole for anaerobic coverage in sepsis/infection, elderly patients, and patients with previous biliary manipulation (not necessary with newer broad-spectrum penicillins):
  – Metronidazole 500 mg IV q8h
- Consider stress ulcer prophylaxis.
- DVT prophylaxis

SURGERY/OTHER PROCEDURES
- Endoscopic CBD stone removal: Often performed following endoscopic cholangiography or following stone identification by other modalities:
  – Relatively low complication rate (mortality 0.5%, pancreatitis 1–8%, perforation 0.4%, bleeding from sphincterotomy 1–2%, cholangitis 1%)
  – Up to 90% success rate
- Surgical CBD stone removal: High success rate (75–95%) and few complications:
  – Laparoscopic: Often performed at the time of cholecystectomy. May be preferable to pre-/postoperative ERCP once laparoscopy has been initiated (7)[A],(8)[B].
  – 1-stage management of symptomatic CBD stones with laparoscopic cholecystectomy + laparoscopic common bile duct exploration is associated with less morbidity and mortality (7% and 0.19%, respectively) than 2-stage management utilizing ERCP/ES (endoscopic sphincterotomy) followed by laparoscopic cholecystectomy (13.5% and 0.5%) (9)[A].
  – Using a CBD lumen catheter may be considered if laparoscopic common bile duct exploration is not feasible and the chance of a CBD stone is less than 65% (9)[A].

– Open choledochotomy: Rarely used. Only for complex cases where laparoscopic and endoscopic techniques fail unless patient already undergoing an open procedure.
- Lithotripsy through a cholangioscope passed via duodenoscope to crush stones with a basket or fracture them with a laser or electrohydraulic method
- Surgical drainage via external catheter or by papillotomy through ampulla of Vater
- Indications for drainage: Sphincter of Oddi sclerosis or dysfunction, multiple or primary CBD stones, or previous stone
- Laparoscopic cholecystectomy with IOC is definitive treatment, unless patient unable to tolerate surgery
- New emerging techniques such as single port cholecystectomy and natural orifice transluminal endoscopic surgery (NOTES) cholecystectomy may offer advantages: Reduced abdominal pain, lower rates of wound infections, and reduced incidence of hernia formation (10)[B]

IN-PATIENT CONSIDERATIONS
Initial Stabilization
n.p.o. and antibiotics if infection suspected or with biliary manipulation

Admission Criteria
To control serious infection and urgently decompress common bile duct

Nursing
Early ambulation

Discharge Criteria
When stable

 # ONGOING CARE
FOLLOW-UP RECOMMENDATIONS
Retained stone extraction 6 weeks after placement of biliary drain

Patient Monitoring
- Liver function tests and bilirubin levels
- WBC and pancreatic enzymes
- Patients with weight loss >25% from original weight after bariatric surgery may benefit from U/S surveillance and subsequent cholecystectomy if gallstones are identified (2)[A].

PROGNOSIS
- With endoscopic or surgical treatment, prognosis is good.
- Untreated, 55% of patients experience complications.
- Filling defects found on intraoperative cholangiograms: 25% are false positives; 25% will pass spontaneously by 6 wks

COMPLICATIONS
- Cholangitis: Most frequent (60%)
- Retained CBD stones (2–10%)
- Pancreatitis
- Biliary enteric fistula
- Hemobilia
- Liver dysfunction/failure
- Bile duct injury

REFERENCES
1. Tsai CJ, Leitzmann MF, Willett WC, et al. Long-chain saturated fatty acids consumption and risk of gallstone disease among men. *Ann Surg.* 2008;247:95–103.
2. Li VK, Pulido N, Fajnwaks P, et al. Predictors of gallstone formation after bariatric surgery: a multivariate analysis of risk factors comparing gastric bypass, gastric banding, and sleeve gastrectomy. *Surg Endosc.* 2009.
3. Yamaji Y, Okamoto M, Yoshida H, et al. Cholelithiasis Is a Risk Factor for Colorectal Adenoma. *Am J Gastroenterol.* 2008.
4. Welzel TM, Mellemkjaer L, Gloria G, et al. Risk factors for intrahepatic cholangiocarcinoma in a low-risk population: A nationwide case-control study. *Int J Cancer.* 2006.
5. Romagnuolo J, Bardou M, Rahme E, et al. Magnetic resonance cholangiopancreatography: a meta-analysis of test performance in suspected biliary disease. *Ann Intern Med.* 2003;139: 547–57.
6. Kaltenthaler E, Vergel YB, et al. A systematic review and economic evaluation of magnetic resonance cholangiopancreatography compared with diagnostic endoscopic retrograde cholangiopancreatography. *Health Technol Assess.* 2004;8(10):iii, 1–89.
7. Tranter SE, Thompson MH. Comparison of endoscopic sphincterotomy and laparoscopic exploration of the common bile duct. *Br J Surg.* 2002;89:1495–504.
8. Nathanson LK, O'Rourke NA, Martin IJ, et al. Postoperative ERCP versus laparoscopic choledochotomy for clearance of selected bile duct calculi: a randomized trial. *Ann Surg.* 2005;242:188–92.
9. Kharbutli B, Velanovich V. Management of Preoperatively Suspected Choledocholithiasis: A Decision Analysis. *J Gastrointest Surg.* 2008.
10. Auyang ED, Hungness ES, Vaziri K, et al. Natural orifice translumenal endoscopic surgery (NOTES): dissection for the critical view of safety during transcolonic cholecystectomy. *Surg Endosc.* 2009.

ADDITIONAL READING
Padda MS, Singh S, Tang SJ, et al. Liver test patterns in patients with acute calculous cholecystitis and/or choledocholithiasis. *Aliment Pharmacol Ther.* 2009.

See Also (Topic, Algorithm, Electronic Media Element)
Cholangitis (acute); Cholecystitis; Cholelithiasis; Jaundice

 # CODES
ICD9
- 574.30 Calculus of bile duct with acute cholecystitis without mention of obstruction
- 574.40 Calculus of bile duct with other cholecystitis, without mention of obstruction
- 574.50 Calculus of bile duct without mention of cholecystitis, without mention of obstruction

CLINICAL PEARLS
- Stones in the common bile duct may originate there (primary) or in the gallbladder (secondary) and then migrate to CBD.
- Cholangiography is "gold standard" for diagnosis.
- ERCP offers both diagnostic and therapeutic options.
- Cholangitis is most frequent complication.

C

CHOLELITHIASIS

Hongyi Cui, MD, PhD
John J. Kelly, MD

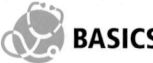 **BASICS**

DESCRIPTION
Cholelithiasis manifests in cholesterol, pigment, or mixed stones formed and contained in the gallbladder:
- Synonym(s): Gallstones

Pediatric Considerations
- Uncommon at <10 years of age
- Associated with blood dyscrasia
- Most gallstones in pediatric population are pigment stones.

EPIDEMIOLOGY
Incidence
- Increased in Native Americans and Hispanics
- Increases with age by 1–3% per year; peaks at 7th decade
- 2% of the US population develops gallstones annually.

Prevalence
- Population: 8–10% of US
- Predominant sex: Female > Male (2–3:1)

RISK FACTORS
- Age (peak in 60–70s)
- Female gender
- Caucasian, Hispanic, or Native American descent
- Hereditary (such as patients carrying the p.D19H variant for the hepatocanalicular cholesterol transporter ABCG5/ABG8 have an increased risk for gallstones)
- Metabolic syndrome (i.e., obesity, dyslipidemia, hypertension, and type 2 diabetes)
- Pregnancy and multiparity
- Cholestasis in association with prolonged fasting and long-term total parenteral nutrition
- Rapid weight loss following bariatric surgery
- Metabolic changes in association with short gut syndrome, terminal ileal resection, and inflammatory bowel disease
- Hemolytic disorders (e.g., hereditary spherocytosis and sickle cell anemia) and cirrhosis (for black or pigment stones)
- Medications (such as early use of birth control pills; estrogen replacement therapy at high doses)
- Biliary tract infection (such as liver flukes) and stricture (for intraductal formation of brown pigment stones)

Genetics
Animal studies indicate that gallstone formation is a dominant trait determined by at least 2 genes; susceptible strains fail to downregulate cholesterol synthesis during cholesterol feeding.

GENERAL PREVENTION
- Ursodiol (Actigall) taken during rapid weight loss prevents gallstone formation (1)[A]
- Regular exercise and dietary modification may reduce the incidence of gallstone formation.

PATHOPHYSIOLOGY
Gallstone formation is a complex process mediated by genetic, metabolic, immune, and environmental factors.

ETIOLOGY
- Production of bile supersaturated with cholesterol (cholesterol stones)
- Decrease in bile content of either phospholipid (lecithin) or bile salts
- Biliary stasis or impaired gallbladder motility
- Generation of excess unconjugated bilirubin in patients with hemolytic diseases; passage of excess bile salt into the colon with subsequent absorption of excess unconjugated bilirubin in patients with inflammatory bowel disease or after distal ileal resection (black or pigment stones)
- Hydrolysis of conjugated bilirubin or phospholipid by bacteria in patients with biliary tract infection or stricture (brown stones or primary bile duct stones; rare in the Western world and common in Asia)

COMMONLY ASSOCIATED CONDITIONS
90% of people with gallbladder carcinoma have gallstones.

 DIAGNOSIS

HISTORY
- Mostly asymptomatic (80%):
  - 5–10% become symptomatic each year.
  - Over their lifetime, <1/2 of the patients with gallstones develop symptoms.
- Episodic right upper quadrant or epigastric pain lasting longer than 15 minutes and sometimes radiating to the back (biliary colic), usually postprandially; the majority of patients will develop recurrent symptoms after the 1st episode.
- Nausea
- Vomiting
- Fatty food intolerance (not proven)
- Indigestion or bloating sensation

PHYSICAL EXAM
- Physical exam is usually normal in patients with cholelithiasis.
- Epigastric and/or right upper quadrant tenderness (Murphy's sign) when in association with cholecystitis
- Fever and jaundice in patients with choledocholithiasis and cholangitis; jaundice can also be caused by extrinsic compression of the bile duct by a stone in the gallbladder or cystic duct (Mirizzi syndrome)
- Flank and periumbilical ecchymoses (Cullen sign and Grey-Turner sign) in patients with acute hemorrhagic pancreatitis
- In patients with concomitant acute calculus cholecystitis and gallbladder cancer, a mass in the right upper quadrant may be palpated.

DIAGNOSTIC TESTS & INTERPRETATION
Lab
- No lab study is specific for cholelithiasis.
- Leukocytosis and elevated C-reactive protein level are associated with acute calculus cholecystitis.

Imaging
- Ultrasound (best technique to diagnose gallstones and differentiate from cholecystitis). Ultrasound can detect gallstones in 97–98% of patients. Thickening of the gallbladder wall (5 mm or greater), pericholecystic fluid, and direct tenderness when the probe is pushed against the gallbladder

(sonographic Murphy sign) are all radiographic signs of acute calculus cholecystitis.
- Computed tomography scan (no advantage over ultrasound except in detecting distal common bile duct stones)
- Magnetic resonance cholangiopancreatography is reserved for cases of suspected common bile duct stones due to high cost.
- Endoscopic ultrasound has been shown to be as sensitive as endoscopic retrograde cholangiopancreatography (ERCP) for detection of common bile duct stones in patients with gallstone pancreatitis.
- Hepatobiliary iminodiacetic acid (HIDA) scan is useful in differentiating acalculous cholecystitis from other causes of abdominal pain. False-positive results can arise from fasting status or insufficient resistance of the sphincter of Oddi. CCK-HIDA is specifically used to diagnose gallbladder dysmotility disorder (i.e., biliary dyskinesia).
- 10–30% of gallstones are radiopaque calcium or pigment-containing gallstones and are more likely to be visible on plain x-ray. A "porcelain gallbladder" is a calcified gallbladder, visible by x-ray; associated with gallbladder cancer (25%).

Pathological Findings
- Pure cholesterol stones have a white or slightly yellow color.
- Pigment stones may be black or brown. Black stones contain polymerized calcium bilirubinate, most often secondary to cirrhosis or hemolysis, and almost always form in the gallbladder. Brown stones are associated with biliary tract infection, caused by bile stasis, and as such may form either in the bile ducts or gallbladder.

DIFFERENTIAL DIAGNOSIS
- Peptic ulcer diseases
- Gastritis
- Hepatitis
- Pancreatitis
- Cholangitis
- Gallbladder cancer
- Gallbladder polyps
- Acalculous cholecystitis
- Biliary dyskinesia
- Biliary tree stricture
- Choledocholithiasis
- Choledochocyst
- Coronary artery disease
- Esophageal motility disorders
- Appendicitis
- Pneumonia
- Renal stones

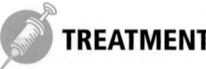 **TREATMENT**

Geriatric Considerations
Age alone should not alter the therapy plan.

MEDICATION
First Line
- Analgesics for pain relief
- Oral dissolution therapy is rarely used today.
- Antibiotics are indicated in patients with signs of acute cholecystitis.

- Prophylactic antibiotics in low-risk patients do not prevent infections for laparoscopic cholecystectomies (2)[A].

Second Line
Nonsteroidal anti-inflammatory drugs (NSAIDs) may have a role in pain relief, given that prostaglandins are important in the development of pain.

ADDITIONAL TREATMENT
General Measures
- Treat only symptomatic gallstones and observe asymptomatic stones.
- Attempt conservative therapy during pregnancy. If necessary, perform surgery preferentially in the 2nd trimester.
- Prophylactic cholecystectomy for patients with calcified (porcelain) gallbladder (risk for gallbladder cancer), and patients with recurrent pancreatitis due to microlithiasis
- In morbidly obese patients, simultaneous cholecystectomy may be performed in combination with bariatric procedures in an effort to reduce later stone-related complications.

Issues for Referral
Patients with retained or recurrent bile duct stones following cholecystectomy should be referred to gastroenterology for ERCP.

SURGERY/OTHER PROCEDURES
- Surgical intervention should be considered for patients who have symptomatic cholelithiasis or gallstone-related complications such as cholecystitis (3)[B].
- Laparoscopic cholecystectomy is currently the standard of care for most cases (4)[B]. In well-selected patients, single incision/port laparoscopic cholecystectomy is a novel method for the treatment of symptomatic cholelithiasis. Natural orifice transluminal endoscopic surgery (NOTES) is still at an experimental stage, and NOTES cholecystectomy is only available in a limited number of specialized centers:
  - Surgery-related complications include common bile duct injury (0.5%), right hepatic duct/artery injury, retained stones, cystic duct or duct of Luschka leak, biloma formation, or bile duct stricture in the long term.
  - Conversion to open procedure based on the judgment of the operating surgeon
  - Intraoperative cholangiogram (IOC) may help delineate bile duct anatomy when dissection proves difficult. Selective or routine use of IOC is a topic of debate, but may be associated with earlier recognition and decreased incidence of bile duct injury (5)[B].
- Open cholecystectomy is indicated for gallbladder cancer diagnosed preoperatively.
- Percutaneous cholecystostomy (PC) in high-risk patients with cholecystitis or gallbladder empyema. PC may also be used in patients with symptoms of cholecystitis for >72 hrs in which altered anatomy might significantly increase the surgical risk. Interval cholecystectomy is usually advisable after the resolution of cholecystitis and optimization of associated medical conditions to prevent recurrent cholecystitis.

IN-PATIENT CONSIDERATIONS
For patients with symptomatic cholelithiasis, laparoscopic cholecystectomy has become an outpatient procedure; for patients who developed gallstone-related complications (i.e., cholecystitis,

cholangitis, and pancreatitis), inpatient care is necessary.

Initial Stabilization
- Patients are treated during the acute phase with nothing by mouth (n.p.o.), intravenous fluids, and antibiotics.
- Adequate pain control with narcotics and/or NSAIDs is also needed.

 ONGOING CARE

FOLLOW-UP RECOMMENDATIONS
Patient Monitoring
- Medical attention if asymptomatic stones become symptomatic
- Patients on oral dissolution agents should be followed up with liver enzyme, serum cholesterol, and imaging studies.

DIET
A low-fat diet may be helpful.

PATIENT EDUCATION
- Change in lifestyle (e.g., regular exercise) and dietary modification (low-fat diet and reduction of total calorie intake) may reduce gallstone-related hospitalizations.
- Patients with asymptomatic gallstones should be educated about the typical symptoms of biliary colic and gallstone-related complications.

PROGNOSIS
- <1/2 of patients with gallstones become symptomatic.
- Cholecystectomy: Mortality <0.5% elective, 3–5% emergency; morbidity <10% elective, 30–40% emergency
- ~10–15% of the patients will have associated choledocholithiasis.
- After cholecystectomy, stones may recur in the bile duct.

COMPLICATIONS
- Acute cholecystitis (90–95% secondary to gallstones)
- Gallbladder empyema
- Gallstone pancreatitis
- Acute cholangitis
- Common bile duct stones with obstructive jaundice
- Biliary-enteric fistula
- Gallstone ileus
- Gallbladder perforation
- Peritonitis and sepsis
- Liver abscess
- Gallbladder cancer
- Mirizzi syndrome (bile duct obstruction caused by gallstones lodged in gallbladder or cystic duct)

REFERENCES
1. Uy MC, Talingdan-Te MC, Espinosa WZ, et al. Ursodeoxycholic Acid in the Prevention of Gallstone Formation after Bariatric Surgery: A Meta-analysis. *Obes Surg.* 2008.
2. Zhou H, Zhang J, Wang Q, et al. Meta-analysis: Antibiotic prophylaxis in elective laparoscopic cholecystectomy. *Aliment Pharmacol Ther.* 2009; 29:1086–95.
3. Bellows CF, Berger DH, Crass RA. Management of gallstones. *Am Fam Phys.* 2005;72:637–42.
4. Shamiyeh A, Wayand W. Current status of laparoscopic therapy of cholecystolithiasis and common bile duct stones. *Dig Dis.* 2005;23: 119–26.
5. Connor S, Garden OJ. Bile duct injury in the era of laparoscopic cholecystectomy. *Br J Surg.* 2006;93: 158–68.

ADDITIONAL READING
- Bogue CO, Murphy AJ, Gerstle JT, et al. Risk factors, complications, and outcomes of gallstones in children: a single-center review. *J Pediatr Gastroenterol Nutr.* 2010;50:303–8.
- Gurusamy KS, Samraj K, et al. Cholecystectomy versus no cholecystectomy in patients with silent gallstones. *Cochrane Database Syst Rev.* 2007; CD006230.
- Keus F, Gooszen HG, van Laarhoven CJ, et al. Open, small-incision, or laparoscopic cholecystectomy for patients with symptomatic cholecystolithiasis. An overview of Cochrane Hepato-Biliary Group reviews. *Cochrane Database Syst Rev.* 2010;:CD008318.
- Lammert F, Miquel JF. Gallstone disease: From genes to evidence-based therapy. *J Hepatol.* 2008.
- Sakorafas GH, Milingos D, Peros G, et al. Asymptomatic cholelithiasis: is cholecystectomy really needed? A critical reappraisal 15 years after the introduction of laparoscopic cholecystectomy. *Dig Dis Sci.* 2007;52:1313–25.

See Also (Topic, Algorithm, Electronic Media Element)
Cholangitis (acute); Cholecystitis; Choledocholithiasis

 CODES

ICD9
- 574.00 Calculus of gallbladder with acute cholecystitis, without mention of obstruction
- 574.10 Calculus of gallbladder with other cholecystitis, without mention of obstruction
- 574.20 Calculus of gallbladder without mention of cholecystitis, without mention of obstruction

CLINICAL PEARLS
- Laparoscopic cholecystectomy has become the most frequently used procedure; lithotripsy and oral dissolution therapy may be considered in rare circumstances.
- Acute acalculous cholecystitis is associated with bile stasis and gallbladder ischemia.
- Prophylactic cholecystectomy is not indicated in patients with diabetes and asymptomatic gallstones. There is no evidence that asymptomatic diabetics are at increased risk of developing complications of gallstone disease.
- The best imaging modality for the diagnosis of gallstones is transabdominal ultrasound (sensitivity of 97% and specificity of 95%); not sensitive for occult gallstones or microlithiasis (stones smaller than 5 mm).
- Think of gallstones in the post-bariatric surgery patient complaining of "gas pains" as they are adjusting to their new diet.

CHOLERA

Abdulrazak Abyad, MD, PhD, MBA, MPH, AGSF, AFCHSE

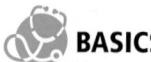 **BASICS**

DESCRIPTION
An acute infectious disease caused by *Vibrio cholerae* (El Tor type is responsible for the most recent epidemic; the other type, classic, is found only in Bangladesh). Characteristics include severe diarrhea with extreme fluid and electrolyte depletion, vomiting, muscle cramps, and prostration. (New serotype now in Bangladesh, India [0139]. Important because of lack of efficacy of standard vaccine.):
- Usual course: Acute, chronic, and relapsing
- Clinical course is 3–5 days; in the early stages, a severely affected patient can lose 1 L/h.
- Endemic areas: India, Southeast Asia, Africa, Middle East, southern Europe, Oceania, South and Central America
- System(s) affected: Gastrointestinal
- Synonym(s): Asiatic cholera; Epidemic cholera; Rice-water diarrhea; Cholera gravis

Pediatric Considerations
- Breastfeeding protects against cholera.
- Vaccine not recommended for children <6 months

EPIDEMIOLOGY
- Predominant age: All ages
- Predominant sex: Male = Female

Incidence
Since 1817, 7 cholera epidemics have occurred.

Prevalence
About 0.01 cases/100,000. The few cases in the US have been found in returning travelers or are associated with food brought into this country illegally.

RISK FACTORS
- Traveling or living in epidemic/endemic areas
- Exposure to contaminated food or water
- Person-to-person transmission (rare)
- In endemic areas, children <5 years
- Attack more severe in patients with blood group O compared with AB
- People with low gastric acid secretion
- Gastrectomy
- Patients on acid-suppressing medications

GENERAL PREVENTION
- Water purification
- Careful food selection (e.g., no unpeeled raw fruits or vegetables, no raw or undercooked seafood)
- Enteric precautions
- Tetracycline for social contacts of an index case
- Natural infection confers long-lasting immunity.

- Prophylactic vaccine:
  - 50% effective for 3–6 months
  - Not recommended unless required by destination country and, if so, a single dose is sufficient.
  - Concomitant administration with yellow fever vaccine may result in reduced vaccine response to yellow fever.
  - Invariably associated with local side effects
  - Systemic side effects of fever and malaise
  - Newer oral killed-whole-cell vaccines provide longer immunity in adults, often up to 2 years from a single dose, and up to 3 or 4 years with annual boosters (1)[A].

  - There are a number of vaccines being developed, including:
    ○ Wyeth-Ayerst parenteral whole vaccine directed at *V. cholerae* O1 not effective
    ○ CVD 103-HgR highly protective against moderate and severe cholera
    ○ The WC/rBS stimulate both antibacterial and antitoxic antibodies.

ETIOLOGY
- Enterotoxin elaborated by gram-negative bacteria
- *Cholerae* (O-group 1)
- Human host
- Contaminated food
- Contaminated water
- Contaminated shellfish

COMMONLY ASSOCIATED CONDITIONS
Increased risk of disease with gastric achlorhydria

 DIAGNOSIS

PHYSICAL EXAM
- Abdominal discomfort
- Anorexia
- Anuria
- Apathy
- Cyanosis
- Decreased skin turgor
- Dehydration
- Diarrhea, painless
- Distant heart sounds
- Diuresis, sudden
- Dysrhythmias
- Fever
- Hypotension
- Hypothermia
- Hypovolemic shock
- Increased or decreased bowel sounds
- Lethargy
- Listlessness
- Malaise

- Oliguria
- Rice-water diarrhea
- Seizures
- Sunken eyes
- Tachycardia
- Thirst
- Vomiting
- Washerwoman's fingers
- Weak peripheral pulses
- Weakness

DIAGNOSTIC TESTS & INTERPRETATION
Lab
- Stool culture: On selective media (thiosulfate citrate bile salts sucrose [TCBS])
- Typed antisera-specific agglutination
- Dark-field microscopy: Characteristic vibrio motility in stool
- Increased vibriocidal antibodies in nonimmunized patient
- Laboratory abnormalities of severe dehydration:
  - Acidemia
  - Acidosis
  - Hypokalemia
  - Hyponatremia
  - Hypochloremia
  - Hypoglycemia
  - Increased specific gravity
  - Polycythemia
  - Mild neutrophilic leukocytosis

Imaging
- Abdominal film: Ileus
- Chest radiograph: Microcardia

Diagnostic Procedures/Surgery
Physical examination and medical history that includes recent travel

Pathological Findings
- Electron microscopy: Organism adheres to mucosa.
- Intact mucosa
- Increased cellularity of lamina propria
- Increased cellularity of mucosa
- Vascular congestion
- Lymphoid hyperplasia of Peyer patches
- Lymphoid hyperplasia of mesenteric lymph nodes
- Lymphoid hyperplasia of spleen
- Cerebral edema
- Acute tubular necrosis
- Vacuolar hypokalemic nephropathy
- Pulmonary edema
- Hyaline membranes
- Bronchopneumonia
- Focal myocardial damage
- Lipid-depleted adrenals
- Tubularization of zona fasciculata

DIFFERENTIAL DIAGNOSIS
Other causes of severe diarrhea and dehydration (e.g., infection with Shigella, *Escherichia coli*, venous viruses)

TREATMENT

- Primary goal is to replenish fluid losses
- Rehydration in 2 phases: Rehydration and maintenance
- Practical guidelines for the treatment of cholera are as follows:
  - Evaluate the degree of dehydration upon arrival.
  - Rehydrate the patient in 2 phases. These include rehydration (for 2–4 h) and maintenance (until diarrhea abates).
  - Register output and intake volumes on predesigned charts, and periodically review these data.
  - Only use the intravenous route:
    ○ During the rehydration phase for severely dehydrated patients for whom an infusion rate of 50–100 mL/kg/h is advised
    ○ For moderately dehydrated patients who do not tolerate the oral route
    ○ During the maintenance phase in patients considered high stool purgers (i.e., >10 mL/kg/h)
  - During the maintenance phase, use ORS at a rate of 800–1000 mL/h. Match ongoing losses with ORS administration.
  - Reduced osmolarity ORS may cause low blood sodium levels with cholera (2)[A].
  - Discharge patients to the treatment center if oral tolerance is greater than or equal to 1,000 mL/h, urine volume is greater than or equal to 40 mL/h, and stool volume is less than or equal to 400 mL/h.

MEDICATION
First Line
- Oral rehydration therapy for mild disease:
  - Oral rehydration solution (ORS) commercial brands available (Pedialyte, Rehydralyte, Resol, Rice-Lyte) or
  - Oral rehydration solution formula from World Health Organization, per liter:
    ○ Sodium chloride 3.5 g
    ○ Potassium chloride 1.5 g
    ○ Glucose 20 g
    ○ Trisodium citrate 2.9 g
    ○ Parenteral rehydration
- Rehydration for severely dehydrated patients:
  - IV rehydration (Ringer lactate) is followed by oral or nasogastric administration of glucose or sucrose-electrolyte solution.
  - Antibiotics:
    ○ For older children and adults: Doxycycline (Vibramycin): 300 mg once or 100 mg b.i.d. for 3 days or tetracycline 50 mg/kg/d for 3 days
    ○ For young children: Trimethoprim-sulfamethoxazole (SMX-TMP, Bactrim, Septra) 8 mg/kg trimethoprim plus 40 mg/kg sulfamethoxazole per day, divided q.12 h. This dosage is equivalent to 1 mL/kg of trimethoprim-sulfamethoxazole suspension.
    ○ In pregnant patients: Furazolidone 100 mg q.i.d. for 7–10 days

- Contraindications:
  ○ Tetracycline: Not for use in pregnant patients or children <8 years old
  ○ Furazolidone and alcohol in combination may cause disulfiram-like reaction
- Precautions:
  ○ Tetracycline: May cause photosensitivity; sunscreen recommended
- Significant possible interactions:
  ○ Tetracycline: Avoid concurrent administration with antacids, dairy products, or iron.

Second Line
In young children: Furazolidone (Furoxone) 5–10 mg/kg/d divided q.6 h for 3 days

ADDITIONAL TREATMENT
General Measures
- Determination of the amount of fluid loss (may compare patient's previous with current weight)
- Rehydration therapy: Oral for mild-to-moderate cases. Patients with severe dehydration may require IV fluid replacement.

IN-PATIENT CONSIDERATIONS
Initial Stabilization
Outpatient for mild cases, inpatient for moderate-to-severe cases

ONGOING CARE

FOLLOW-UP RECOMMENDATIONS
Bed rest until symptoms resolve and strength returns

Patient Monitoring
Observe patient until symptoms are resolved.

DIET
Small, frequent meals when vomiting stops and appetite returns

PATIENT EDUCATION
- Centers for Disease Control and Prevention. Traveler's Information Hotline: (404) 332-4559 (available 24 hours via a touch-tone telephone)
- International Association for Medical Assistance to Travelers, 417 Center St., Lewiston, NY 14092; (716) 754-4883
- U.S. Centers for Disease Control and Prevention does not expect a major outbreak of cholera in the US, but has issued a "Cholera Preparedness Plan" outlining steps for proper surveillance, treatment, laboratory diagnosis, investigation of outbreaks, and public education.

PROGNOSIS
- Prompt p.o. or IV treatment can save lives.
- Appropriate disposal of human waste
- Antibiotic treatment reduces duration and infectivity of disease.
- Mortality <1% with appropriate supportive care
- Mortality higher with untreated hypovolemic shock

COMPLICATIONS
- Hypovolemic shock
- Chronic biliary infection
- Up to 50% mortality with untreated shock
- Intermittent stool shedding

REFERENCES
1. Shears P. Recent developments in cholera. *Curr Opin Infect Dis*. 2001;14:553–8.
2. Graves PM, Deeks JJ, Demicheli V et al. Vaccines for preventing cholera. *Cochrane Infectious Diseases Group Cochrane Database of Systematic Reviews*. 1, 2009.

ADDITIONAL READING
- Murphy C, Hahn S, Volmink J. Reduced osmolarity oral rehydration solution for treating cholera. *Cochrane Database of Systematic Reviews*. 2004, Issue 4. Art. No.: CD003754. DOI:10.1002/14651858.CD003754.pub2.
- Olsson L, Parment PA. Present and future cholera vaccines. *Expert Rev Vaccines*. 2006;5:751–2.

See Also (Topic, Algorithm, Electronic Media Element)
Diarrhea, Acute; Oral Rehydration

 CODES

ICD9
001.9 Cholera, unspecified

CLINICAL PEARLS
- To avoid cholera while traveling, pay scrupulous attention to drinking only safe water and monitor personal hygiene.
- Currently available vaccine is of limited efficacy and should not be relied upon to prevent disease.
- During acute infection, patients may lose as much as 1 liter per hour in diarrhea and must be hydrated vigorously, then maintained on maintenance fluids until diarrhea abates.

CHRONIC COUGH

Jacqueline L. Olin, MS, PharmD, BCPS, CPP
Susan Ziglar, MD

BASICS

DESCRIPTION
- Chronic cough persists >8 weeks in adults.
- Subacute cough describes cough lasting 3–8 weeks.
- In children, chronic cough is defined as cough for >4 weeks in duration.
- Patients present because of fear of the causative illness (e.g., cancer), as well as annoyance, self-consciousness, and hoarseness.
- Patients with stress urinary incontinence may find cough particularly troubling.
- At the primary care level, COPD and smoking-related cough are most common causes.
- System(s) affected: Gastrointestinal; Pulmonary

EPIDEMIOLOGY
- Predominant age: All age groups
- Predominant sex: Male = Female

Incidence
Recurrent cough has been reported at 3–40% by various population estimates.

Prevalence
Chronic cough is one of the most common reasons for primary care visits.

RISK FACTORS
Although various conditions may contribute to chronic cough, the main causes include smoking and pulmonary diseases.

PATHOPHYSIOLOGY
Varies with findings and disorders implicated

ETIOLOGY
- Often multiple etiologies, but most are related to bronchial irritation. Most frequent etiologies (account for >90% of cases) in nonsmokers include:
  - Upper airway cough syndrome (UACS) (postnasal drip syndrome)
  - Asthma
  - Nonasthmatic eosinophilic bronchitis (NAEB)
  - GERD
- Other causes:
  - Chronic smoking or exposure to smoke or pollutants
  - Aspiration
  - Bronchiectasis
  - ACE inhibitor therapy
  - Pertussis
  - Tuberculosis
  - Cystic fibrosis
  - Chronic interstitial lung disease
  - Restrictive lung disease
  - Neoplasms: lung or laryngeal cancer, other
  - Psychogenic (habit cough)

COMMONLY ASSOCIATED CONDITIONS
Patients with UACS, asthma, and GERD may present with chronic cough as the only symptom and not the usual symptoms associated with the diagnoses.

DIAGNOSIS

HISTORY
- The age of the patient, presence of associated signs/symptoms, medical history, medication history (ACE inhibitor), environmental exposures, potential for aspiration, and smoking history may make some causes more likely.
- The character of cough or description of sputum quality is rarely helpful in predicting the underlying cause.
- Cough diaries have not correlated well with objective measures.
- Various ambulatory systems for recording cough are under development.

PHYSICAL EXAM
- Signs and symptoms are variable and related to the underlying cause; usually a nonproductive cough with no other signs or symptoms.
- Possible signs and symptoms of UACS, sinusitis, GERD, congestive heart failure
- Absence of additional signs/symptoms of a particular condition not necessarily helpful (75% of GERD patients have no other signs or symptoms)

DIAGNOSTIC TESTS & INTERPRETATION
Extensive testing only if indicated by the history and physical. Simple testing (CXR, sinus CT) is followed by empiric therapy directed at likely underlying etiology.

Pediatric Considerations
Children with chronic cough should undergo, at a minimum, spirometry and chest radiograph (if age-appropriate).

Lab
Initial lab tests
As indicated by history and physical
Follow-Up & Special Considerations
If clinically indicated:
- Sweat chloride testing
- Sputum for eosinophils and cytology

Imaging
Initial approach
If clinically indicated: CXR
Follow-Up & Special Considerations
If clinically indicated:
- Chest CT
- Endoscopy

Diagnostic Procedures/Surgery
If diagnosis suspected and inadequate response to initial measures, procedures can be considered:
- Pulmonary function testing
- Purified protein derivative (PPD) skin testing
- 24-hour esophageal pH monitor
- Bronchoscopy if necessary
- Endoscopic or video fluoroscopic swallow evaluation or barium esophagram
- Sinus CT
- Ambulatory cough monitoring and cough challenge with citric acid or capsaicin (at specialized cough clinic)
- Echocardiogram

Pathological Findings
Specific to underlying cause

TREATMENT

- With chronic cough, empiric treatment should be directed at the most common causes (UACS, asthma, GERD, NAEB) (1)[C].
- Oral antihistamine/decongestant therapy with a 1st-generation antihistamine should be initial empiric treatment (1)[C].
- In patients with cough associated with the common cold, nonsedating antihistamines were not found to be effective in reducing cough (1)[C].
- In stable patients with chronic bronchitis, therapy with ipratropium bromide may reduce chronic cough (2)[C].
- Centrally-acting antitussive drugs (codeine, dextromethorphan) are recommended for short-term symptomatic relief of coughing in patients with chronic bronchitis (2)[C]:
  - These agents have limited efficacy in cough due to upper respiratory infections (2)[C].
- For cough associated with lung cancer, the use of narcotic cough suppressants is recommended (2)[C].

C

Pediatric Considerations

- In 2008, the FDA issued a public health advisory stating that OTC cough and cold medicines, including antitussives, expectorants, nasal decongestants, antihistamines, or combinations should not be given to children <2 years.
- The American Academy of Pediatrics does not recommend central cough suppressants for treating any kind of cough (1)[B].
- In children <14 years old, when pediatric recommendations are not available, adult recommendations should be used with caution (1)[C].
- Some children with recurrent cough and no evidence of airway obstruction may benefit from an inhaled β-agonist (3)[C].

MEDICATION

Treatments (antacids, bronchodilators, inhaled corticosteroids, proton pump inhibitors, antibiotics) should be directed at the specific cause of cough.

First Line

- In adults, oral antihistamine/decongestant therapy should be empiric treatment. Multiple formulations are available OTC in combination with other ingredients. Advise patients to review labels carefully or consult pharmacist.
  - Chlorpheniramine 2 mg/phenylephrine 5 mg/ Acetaminophen 325 mg (Tylenol Allergy Multi-Symptom) 2 caplets or gelcaps PO q12h (Maximum 12 caplets or gelcaps in 24 hours: Age >12 years.
- Central cough suppressants for short-term symptomatic relief of nonproductive cough:
  - Dextromethorphan 10–20 mg PO q4h: Age >12 years. Use 5–10 mg PO q4h for age 6–12 years.
  - Narcotics: Codeine 15–30 mg PO q6h; hydrocodone (Vicodin) 5 mg PO q6h; hydrocodone (Tussionex Pennkinetic) 10 mg (5 mL) PO q12h for age 12 or over

Second Line

- A peripherally acting antitussive agent has been used.
  - Benzonatate (Tessalon Perles) 100–200 mg PO three times daily as needed (Maximum 600 mg daily): Age >10
- Results from a small randomized placebo-controlled trial (n = 27) demonstrated subjective cough score improvement in patients using slow-release morphine sulfate. Patients had failed with other antitussive therapies. Side effects included constipation and drowsiness and there were no discontinuations due to adverse events (4)[C].
  - Morphine was administered 5–10 mg PO twice daily.
- For patients with cystic fibrosis, amiloride may increase cough clearance.

ADDITIONAL TREATMENT
General Measures

- In patients with chronic cough, considerations for potential etiology should include asthma (1)[B] or UACS (1)[C].
- With concomitant complaints of heartburn and regurgitation, GERD should be considered as a potential etiology (1)[C].
- 90% of patients will have resolution of cough after smoking cessation (1)[A].
- When indicated, ACE inhibitor therapy should be switched in patients in whom intolerable cough occurs (1)[A].
- Empiric treatment of postnasal drip and GERD.
- Consider nonpharmacological options such as warm fluids, hard candy, or nasal drops. In infants and children, can try clearing secretions with a bulb syringe.
- Attempt maximal therapy for single most likely cause for several weeks, then search for coexistent etiologies.

Issues for Referral

Refer based on specific diagnosis for cough.

SURGERY/OTHER PROCEDURES

Fundoplication may be effective for cough secondary to refractory GERD.

 ONGOING CARE

FOLLOW-UP RECOMMENDATIONS

Consider stepwise withdrawal of medications after resolution of cough.

Patient Monitoring

Frequent follow-up is necessary to assess the effectiveness of the treatment and the addition of other medications as needed.

DIET

Patients with GERD may benefit by avoiding ethanol, caffeine, nicotine, citrus, tomatoes, chocolate, and fatty foods.

PATIENT EDUCATION

- Reassure patient that most cases do not have life-threatening causes and that the condition can usually be managed effectively.
- Counsel that several weeks to a month may be needed for significant reduction or total elimination of cough.
- Prepare the patient for the possibility of multiple diagnostic tests and therapeutic regimens, because the treatment is very often empiric.

PROGNOSIS

- >80% of patients can be effectively diagnosed and treated using a systematic approach.
- Cough from any cause may take weeks to months until resolution, and resolution depends greatly on efficacy of treatment directed at underlying etiology.

COMPLICATIONS

- Cardiovascular: Arrhythmias, syncope
- Stress urinary incontinence
- Abdominal and intercostal muscle strain
- GI: Emesis, hemorrhage, herniation
- Neurologic: Dizziness, headache, seizures
- Respiratory: Pneumothorax, laryngeal, or tracheobronchial trauma
- Skin: Petechiae, purpura, disruption of surgical wounds
- Medication side effects
- Other: Negative impact on quality of life

REFERENCES

1. Irwin RS, Baumann MH, Bolser DC, et al. Diagnosis and management of cough executive summary: ACCP evidence-based clinical practice guidelines. *Chest*. 2006;129:1S–23S.
2. Bolser DC. Cough suppressant and pharmacologic protussive therapy: ACCP evidence-based clinical practice guidelines. *Chest*. 2006;129:238S–249S.
3. Gupta A, et al. Management of chronic non-specific cough in childhood: An evidence-based review. *Arch Dis Child Educ Pract Ed*. 2007; 92:ep33–ep39.
4. Morice AH, Menon MS, Mulrennan SA et al. Opiate therapy in chronic cough. *Am J Respir Crit Care Med*. 2007;175:312–5.

ADDITIONAL READING

Pavord ID, Chung KF. Management of chronic cough. *Lancet*. 2008;371:1375–84.

See Also (Topic, Algorithm, Electronic Media Element)

Asthma; Bronchiectasis; Congestive Heart Failure; Eosinophilic Pneumonias; Gastroesophageal Reflux Disease (GERD); Laryngeal Cancer; Lung, Primary Malignancies; Pertussis; Pulmonary Edema; Rhinitis, Allergic; Sinusitis; Tuberculosis
Algorithm: Cough, Chronic

CODES

ICD9
786.2 Cough

CLINICAL PEARLS

- Chronic cough is defined as a cough that persists for >8 weeks in adults.
- In patients with chronic cough, most frequent etiologies include a history of smoking, asthma, UACS, and GERD.
- In 2008, the FDA issued a public health advisory stating that OTC cough and cold medicines should not be given to children <2 years.
- Consumer Healthcare Products Association (CHPA) members are voluntarily changing OTC product labels to state "do not use" in children <4 years old. New child-resistant packaging and measuring devices are being developed.

CHRONIC FATIGUE SYNDROME

Joan M. Stachnik, PharmD, BCPS
Anthony Valdini, MD

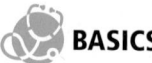 **BASICS**

DESCRIPTION

- A condition characterized by profound mental and physical exhaustion, with at least 6 months presence of multiple systemic and neuropsychiatric symptoms. At least 4 of 8 associated conditions are required per Centers for Disease Control and Prevention (CDC) definition:
  - Impaired memory
  - Sore throat
  - Tender lymph nodes
  - Persistent muscle or joint pain
  - New headaches
  - Unrefreshing sleep
  - Postexertion malaise
- Must have a new or definite onset (not lifelong). Fatigue is not relieved by rest and results in >50% reduction in previous activities (occupational, educational, social, and personal). Other potential medical causes must be ruled out.

EPIDEMIOLOGY

- Predominant age: 20–50 years
- Predominant sex: Male < Female
- All socioeconomic groups
- Because of cultural differences in presentation, doctors in less developed countries may not recognize the syndrome, making an accurate prevalence difficult to determine (1).
- Various associations between ethnicity and incidence have been reported. Higher rates found in ethnic minorities (Native Americans, Latinos, and African Americans) compared to white populations, based on population studies. Service-based studies (tertiary care) have reported higher rates among whites, or no association between incidence and ethnicity (2).

Incidence
Available studies have focused on prevalence of the disorder.

Prevalence
Estimates vary widely and depend upon case definition and population studied, but a reasonable estimate using a strict case definition is 100 cases per 100,000 population. Community-based studies have reported prevalence rates of 0.23% and 0.42%.

RISK FACTORS
Possible predisposing factors include (3,4):
- Personality characteristics (neuroticism and introversion)
- Lifestyle:
  - Childhood inactivity or overactivity
  - Inactivity in adulthood after infectious mononucleosis
  - Familial predisposition
  - Comorbid mood disorders of depression and anxiety
- Long-standing medical conditions in childhood
- Childhood trauma (emotional, physical, sexual abuse)

Genetics
- Higher concordance has been reported among monozygotic twins compared with dizygotic twins.
- Gender may be a significant predictor

ETIOLOGY
- Unknown and likely multifactorial:
  - Possible interaction between genetic predisposition, environmental factors, an initiating stressor, and perpetuating factors
- Physiologic or environmental stressor could be precipitant.
- Many patients with chronic fatigue recall significant stressors (e.g., major medical procedure, loss of a loved one, loss of employment) in months before symptoms began.
- Systems hypothesized to contribute to physiology include:
  - Neuroendocrine (e.g., diminished cortisol response to increased corticotropin concentrations)
  - Immune (e.g., increased C-reactive protein and beta-2 microglobulin) (5)
  - Neuromuscular (e.g., dysfunction of oxidative metabolism) (5)
- Serotonergic (e.g., hyperserotonergic mechanisms or upregulation of serotonin receptors).

COMMONLY ASSOCIATED CONDITIONS
- Common comorbidities include:
  - Fibromyalgia
  - Irritable bowel syndrome
  - Temporomandibular joint disorder
  - Anxiety disorders
  - Major depression
  - Post-traumatic stress disorder (including physical and/or sexual past abuse)
  - Domestic violence
- Exclusions:
  - Patients are excluded from chronic fatigue syndrome (CFS) definition until 2 years after resolution of substance/alcohol abuse and 5 years after resolution of anorexia nervosa or bulimia.

 DIAGNOSIS

HISTORY
See "Description" for CFS historical features.

PHYSICAL EXAM
Complete physical examination to rule out other medical causes for symptoms. Note: Tender adenopathy is one of the defining criteria.

DIAGNOSTIC TESTS & INTERPRETATION
No single diagnostic test available

Lab
Standard laboratory tests are recommended to rule out other causes for symptoms (6):
- Chemistry panel
- Complete blood count (CBC)
- Urinalysis
- Thyroid-stimulating hormone (TSH)
- Erythrocyte sedimentation rate (ESR) or C-reactive protein
- Liver function

- Screen for drugs of abuse
- Age-/gender-appropriate cancer screening
- Additional studies, if clinical findings are suggestive (6):
  - Antinuclear antibodies (if +ESR)
  - Rheumatoid factor (if +ESR)
  - Creatine kinase
  - Tuberculin skin test
  - Serum cortisol
  - Human immunodeficiency virus (HIV)
  - Lyme serology
  - Gluten sensitivity (IgA tissue transglutaminase)

Follow-Up & Special Considerations
- Assessment for comorbid psychiatric disorders.
- Assessment for personality and psychosocial factors and maladaptive coping styles.
- In patients with sleep disturbance, polysomnography may reveal a treatable comorbid disease.

Imaging
No applicable imaging tests available

DIFFERENTIAL DIAGNOSIS
- Insomnia: Primary (no clear etiology) vs. secondary (due to anxiety, depression, environmental factors, poor sleep hygiene, etc.)
- Idiopathic chronic fatigue (i.e., fatigue of unknown cause for >6 months without meeting criteria for CFS)
- Morbid obesity, body mass index (BMI) >40
- Malignancy
- Autoimmune disease
- Localized infection (e.g., occult abscess)
- Chronic or subacute bacterial disease (e.g., endocarditis)
- Lyme disease
- Fungal disease (e.g., histoplasmosis, coccidioidomycosis)
- Parasitic disease (e.g., amebiasis, giardiasis, helminth infestation)
- HIV-related disease
- Psychiatric disorders:
  - Major depression
  - Somatization disorder
- Chronic inflammatory disease (sarcoidosis, Wegener granulomatosis)
- Known chronic viral disease (HIV)
- Neuromuscular disease (multiple sclerosis, myasthenia gravis)
- Endocrine disorder (hypothyroidism, Addison disease, Cushing's syndrome, diabetes mellitus)
- Iatrogenic (e.g., medication side effects)
- Toxic agent exposure
- Other known or defined systemic disease (chronic pulmonary, cardiac, hepatic, renal, or hematologic disease)
- Pregnancy until 3 months post-partum
- Physiologic fatigue (inadequate or disrupted sleep, menopause)
- *Weakness* and *sleepiness* can indicate a different etiology.

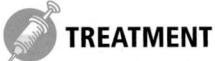 TREATMENT

MEDICATION

- No established pharmacologic treatment recommendations
- Studies have been conducted with antidepressants, immunoglobulins, hydrocortisone, and modafinil. None have shown clear benefit (6).
- If insomnia present, use of non-addicting sleep aids (hydroxyzine, trazodone, doxepin, etc.) may improve outcomes.

ADDITIONAL TREATMENT

General Measures

- Two treatments have been shown effective, often used in combination (7,8,9):
  - Individual cognitive behavioral therapy (CBT): Challenge fatigue-related cognition. Plan social and occupational rehabilitation.
  - Graded exercise therapy (GET): Track amount of exercise patient can do without exacerbating symptoms and gradually increase the intensity and duration. Both involve a carefully planned balance between activity and rest.
- Patients learn how to gradually increase activity in a way that will not exacerbate their illness. Vigorous exercise can trigger relapse, perhaps related to immune dysregulation; therefore, activity plan must be carefully monitored (8).
- Improves functional capacity and diminishes sense of fatigue (9).
- GET is more effective when delivered with educational interventions, explaining symptoms, and encouragement with telephone reminders (9).
- The duration of illness does not predict treatment outcome, so this approach can be applied to patients with chronic symptoms.

Issues for Referral

- Psychiatrist to assess for comorbid disorders if screening indicates need
- Rehabilitative medicine

COMPLEMENTARY AND ALTERNATIVE MEDICINE

- Although complementary and alternative medicines have been suggested, data are insufficient to recommend their use.
- Social support groups have not proven to be effective.

 ONGOING CARE

FOLLOW-UP RECOMMENDATIONS

- Gradual increase in physical exercise with scheduled rest periods.
- Avoid extended periods of rest.

Patient Monitoring

Although no consensus exists, periodic re-evaluation is appropriate for support, relief of symptoms, and assessment for other possible causes of symptoms.

DIET

- No diet has been shown to be effective for treatment of CFS.
- A BMI of 40 has been associated with fatigue in general. Whether weight loss improves symptoms in such patients has yet to be tested.

PATIENT EDUCATION

- Patient education is an important part of treatment of CFS, such as education on the benefits of cognitive therapies, lifestyle changes, and pharmacologic therapy directed at specific associated symptoms.
- Chronic Fatigue and Immune Dysfunction Syndrome Association of America: www.cfids.org
- CDC Chronic Fatigue Syndrome: www.cdc.gov

PROGNOSIS

- Fluctuating course
- Generally, improvement is slow, with a course of months to years.
- An estimated 5% fully recover.

COMPLICATIONS

- Depression
- Unemployment. Although studies document improvement with treatment, fewer than 1/3 of patients in trials return to work (10).
- Polypharmacy

REFERENCES

1. Cho HJ, Menezes PR, Hotopf M et al. Comparative epidemiology of chronic fatigue syndrome in Brazilian and British primary care: prevalence and recognition. *Br J Psychiatry*. 2009;194:117–22.
2. Dinos S, Khoshaba B, Ashby D et al. A systematic review of chronic fatigue, its syndromes and ethnicity: prevalence, severity, co-morbidity and coping. *Int J Epidemiol*. 2009;38:1554–70.
3. Viner R, Hotopf M. Childhood predictors of self reported chronic fatigue syndrome/myalgic encephalomyelitis in adults: national birth cohort study. *BMJ*. 2004;329:941.
4. Heim C, Wagner D, Maloney E, et al. Early adverse experience and risk for chronic fatigue syndrome: results from a population-based study. *Arch Gen Psychiatry*. 2006;63:1258–66.
5. Fulle S, Pietrangelo T, Mancinelli R et al. Specific correlations between muscle oxidative stress and chronic fatigue syndrome: a working hypothesis. *J Muscle Res Cell Motil*. 2007;28:355–62.
6. Baker R, Shaw EJ. Diagnosis and management of chronic fatigue syndrome or myalgic encephalomyelitis (or encephalopathy): summary of NICE guidance. *BMJ*. 2007;335:446–8.
7. Margo KL, Margo GM. Two therapies lift mood in chronic fatigue syndrome. *Current Psychiatry*. 2006;5:91–100.
8. Nijs J, Paul L, Wallman K. Chronic fatigue syndrome: an approach combining self-management with graded exercise to avoid exacerbations. *J Rehabil Med*. 2008;40:241–7.
9. Price JR, Mitchell E, Tidy E, et al. Cognitive behaviour therapy for chronic fatigue syndrome in adults. *Cochrane Database Syst Rev*. 2008:CD001027.
10. Cairns R, Hotopf M. A systematic review describing the prognosis of chronic fatigue syndrome. *Occup Med-Oxford*. 2005;55:20–31.

ADDITIONAL READING

- Adams D, Wu T, Yang X et al. Traditional Chinese medicinal herbs for the treatment of idiopathic chronic fatigue and chronic fatigue syndrome. *Cochrane Database Syst Rev*. 2009;CD006348.
- Baker R, Shaw EJ et al. Diagnosis and management of chronic fatigue syndrome or myalgic encephalomyelitis (or encephalopathy): summary of NICE guidance. *BMJ*. 2007;335:446–8.
- Prins JB, van der Meer JW, Bleijenberg G et al. Chronic fatigue syndrome. *Lancet*. 2006;367: 346–55.
- Rimes KA, Chalder T et al. Treatments for chronic fatigue syndrome. *Occup Med (Lond)*. 2005;55: 32–9.

See Also (Topic, Algorithm, Electronic Media Element)

Algorithm: Fatigue

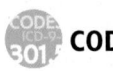 CODES

ICD9
780.71 Chronic fatigue syndrome

CLINICAL PEARLS

- CFS and depression can be comorbid. However, to differentiate between the two, sore throat, tender lymph nodes, and post-exercise fatigue are much more characteristic of CFS.
- Although a number randomized controlled trials on various pharmacologic agents (e.g., antidepressants, immune modulators) have been conducted, no single agent has been shown to be consistently effective.
- About 70% of patients show improvement with cognitive behavioral therapy, compared to 55% with graded exercise therapy; in many cases, these two treatments can be undertaken in combination.
- There are many more patients with idiopathic chronic fatigue than true CFS. To diagnose CFS, CDC criteria need to be met; standardized instruments (SF-36, Symptom Index) have been shown to be of use in the empirical diagnosis of CFS.

C

CHRONIC KIDNEY DISEASE

Lisa Pelunis-Messier, PharmD
Mhd Basheer Rahmoun, MD

 BASICS

Chronic kidney disease (CKD) is defined as:
- Kidney damage for ≥3 months, defined by structural or functional abnormalities of the kidney, with or without decrease in glomerular filtration rate (GFR), by either pathologic abnormalities or markers of damage, including abnormalities in blood or urine tests or imaging studies, *or*
- GFR <60 mL/min/1.73 m^2 for ≥3 months, with or without kidney damage (1)

DESCRIPTION
- CKD is classified into 5 stages by GFR estimated by Modification of Diet in Renal Disease (MDRD) equation:
  - Stage 1: Kidney damage with GFR >90 mL/min/ 1.73 m^2
  - Stage 2: Kidney damage with mild ↓ GFR 60–89 mL/min/1.73 m^2
  - Stage 3: Moderate ↓ GFR 30–59 mL/min/1.73 m^2
  - Stage 4: Severe ↓ GFR 15–29 mL/min/1.73 m^2
  - Stage 5: Kidney failure: GFR <15 mL/min/1.73 m^2 or dialysis
- System(s) affected: Renal/Urinary; Cardiovascular; Skeletal; Endocrine; Metabolic; Hematologic; Lymphatic; Immune; Neurologic
- Synonym(s): Chronic renal failure; Chronic renal insufficiency

Geriatric Considerations
GFR normally decreases with age, despite normal creatinine (Cr).

ALERT
- Adjust renally cleared drugs for GFR in elderly.
- Use nephrotoxic agents with caution in elderly.

Pediatric Considerations
- CKD definition is not applicable for children <6 years; lower GFR even when corrected for body surface area.
- Estimated GFR based on serum Cr can be compared with normative age-appropriate values to detect renal impairment.

Pregnancy Considerations
- Renal function in CKD may deteriorate during pregnancy.
- Cr >1.5 and hypertension are major risk factors for worsening renal function.
- Increased risk of premature labor, preeclampsia, and/or fetal loss
- Angiotensin-converting enzyme (ACE) inhibitors and angiotensin receptor blockers (ARBs) are contraindicated due to teratogenicity.
- Use diuretics with caution.

EPIDEMIOLOGY
- Majority of people with CKD in stages 1–3
- African Americans are 4 times more likely to develop chronic kidney failure than Caucasians.
- Predominant sex: For the CKD stages, was similar in both sexes; however, incidence rate of end-stage renal disease (ESRD) is males 409/million > females 276/million (USRDS 2004).

Incidence
- An estimated annual incidence of CKD was 1700/million population.
- Estimated ESRD patients by 2010: 129,200 ± 7742 new patients; 651,330 ± 15,874 long-term ESRD; 520,240 ± 25,609 dialysis; 178,806 ± 4349 with functioning transplants; and 95,550 ± 5478 patients on waiting lists

Prevalence
The unadjusted prevalence and incidence rates of ESRD (stage 5) are 1585 and 350.7/million, respectively. These numbers do not reflect the burden of earlier stages of CKD (1–40, which are estimated to affect 13.2% of population nationwide, or 26.3 million Americans (2).

RISK FACTORS
- Type 1 or 2 diabetes mellitus (most common)
- Age >60 years
- Cardiovascular disease (e.g., hypertension [HTN] [common])
- Acute kidney injury
- Urinary tract obstruction (e.g., benign prostatic hyperplasia)
- Autoimmune disease/vasculitis/connective tissue disorder
- Family history of CKD
- Nephrotoxic drugs (lithium, salicylate, high doses NSAIDs)
- Congenital anomalies; obstructive uropathy; renal aplasia/hypoplasia/dysplasia; reflux nephropathy
- Hyperlipidemia
- Low income/education/ethnic minority status
- Obesity/smoking
- Neoplasia

Genetics
- Alport syndrome, Fabry disease, sickle cell anemia, systemic lupus erythematosus (SLE), and autosomal-dominant polycystic kidney disease can lead to CKD
- Polymorphisms in gene that encodes for podocyte mom muscle myosin IIA are more common in African Americans than Caucasians and appear to increase risk for nondiabetic ESRD (3)

GENERAL PREVENTION
- Treat reversible causes: Hypovolemia, infections, diuretics, drugs (NSAIDS, aminoglycosides, IV contrast).
- Treat risk factors: diabetes mellitus, HTN, hyperlipidemia, smoking, and obesity.
- Adjust medication doses to prevent renal toxicity.

PATHOPHYSIOLOGY
Progressive destruction of kidney nephrons; GFR will drop gradually, and plasma Cr values will approximately double with 50% reduction in GFR and 75% loss of functioning nephrons mass.

ETIOLOGY
- Renal parenchymal/glomerular:
  - Nephritic: hematuria, red blood cell (RBC) casts, HTN, variable proteinuria:
    - Focal proliferative: IgA nephropathy, SLE, Henoch-Schoenlein purpura, Alport syndrome; proliferative glomerulonephritis; crescentic glomerulonephritis

  - Diffuse proliferative: Membranoproliferative glomerulonephritis, SLE, cryoglobulinemia, rapidly progressive glomerulonephritis (RPGN), Goodpasture syndrome.
  - Nephrotic: proteinuria (>3.5 g/day), hypoalbuminemia, hyperlipidemia and edema:
    - Minimal change disease, membranous nephropathy, focal segmental glomerulosclerosis
    - Amyloidosis, diabetic nephropathy
- Vascular: HTN, thrombotic microangiopathies, vasculitis (Wegener), scleroderma
- Interstitial-tubular: Infections, obstruction, toxins, allergic interstitial nephritis, multiple myeloma, connective tissue disease, cystic disease
- Postrenal: Obstruction (benign prostatic hyperplasia), neoplasm, neurogenic bladder

COMMONLY ASSOCIATED CONDITIONS
- HTN, Diabetes mellitus, Cardiovascular disease

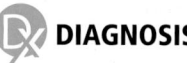 **DIAGNOSIS**

HISTORY
- Oliguria, nocturia, polyuria, hematouria, change in urinary frequency
- Bone disease
- Fatigue, depression, weakness
- Pruritus
- Metallic taste in mouth, anorexia, nausea, vomiting
- Dyspnea
- Hypertension
- Poorly controlled diabetes with retinopathy, neuropathy
- Hyperlipidemia
- Claudication, restless legs

PHYSICAL EXAM
- Volume status (pallor, blood pressure/orthostatics; edema; jugular venous distention; weight)
- Skin: Sallow complexion, uremic frost
- Ammonialike odor (uremic fetor)
- Cardiovascular: Assess for murmurs, bruits, pericarditis
- Chest: Pleural effusion
- Rectal: Enlarged prostate
- Central nervous system: (Asterixis, confusion, seizures, coma), peripheral neuropathy

DIAGNOSTIC TESTS & INTERPRETATION
Lab
Initial lab tests
- GFR can be estimated by MDRD equation:
  - GFR(mL/min/1.73 m^2) = 186 × {[serum Cr μmol/1/88.4] − 1.154} × {age (years) − 0.203} × 0.742 for females, or 1.21 for males
- Cr clearance (CrCl) can be calculated using Cockroft-Gault formula:
  - CrCl (male) = ([140-age] × weight(kg)/(serum Cr X72)
  - CrCl (female) = CrCl (male) × 0.82
- Urine analysis:
  - Urine microscopy: White blood cell/RBC casts, dysmorphic RBCs
  - Urine electrolytes: Sodium, Cr, urea (if on loop diuretics)

- Proteinuria/albuminuria
  - 24-hour urine collection: >20–200 μg/min
  - Spot urine sample: >30–300mg/L
  - Albumin/Cr ratio (ACR): $\geq$3.5 mg/mmol (Females); 2.5 mg/mmol (males)
- Hematology:
  - Normochromic, normocytic anemia, increased bleeding time
- Chemistry:
  - Elevated BUN, Cr, Hyperkalemia
  - Increased parathyroid hormone, decreased 25-(OH) Vitamin D
  - Hypocalcemia, Hyperphosphatemia
  - Hyperlipidemia
  - Metabolic acidosis
  - Decreased albumin

ALERT
Drugs that may alter lab result:
- Cimetidine: Inhibits Cr secretion
- Trimethoprim: Inhibits Cr secretion
- Cefoxitin and flucytosine: Increases serum Cr
- Diltiazem and verapamil: Have significant antiproteinuric effects in patients with >300 mg/day of proteinuria

Follow-Up & Special Considerations
- Serology: ANA; antineutrophil cyplasmic antibody; complements (C3, C4, CH50); anti-GBM antibodies; hepatitis B, C; and HIV screening
- If proteinuria in patient >45 years, serum and urine immunoelectrophoresis

Imaging
- Ultrasound: Small, echogenic kidneys; may see obstruction (e.g., hydronephrosis); cysts; kidneys may be enlarged with HIV and diabetic nephropathy.
- Doppler ultrasound to assess for renovascular disease, thrombosis
- Noncontrast CAT scan: Obstruction; calculi; cysts; neoplasm; renal artery stenosis
- MRI/MRA; avoid gadolinium because of the risk of nephrogenic systemic fibrosis.
- Renal arteriogram for renal artery stenosis can be therapeutic (angioplasty or stenting).
- Renal scan to screen for differential function between kidneys

Diagnostic Procedures/Surgery
Biopsy: Hematuria, proteinuria, acute/progressive renal failure, nephritic or nephrotic syndrome

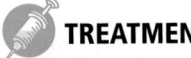 ## TREATMENT

MEDICATION
- Hypertension: Goal is blood pressure <130/80:
  - ACE inhibitors or ARBs for blood pressure control and antiproteinuric effect
    - Potential for hyperkalemia
    - Can tolerate up to 30% rise in serum Cr unless hyperkalemia develops
    - If goal not reached, add diuretic (thiazides, then loop diuretic), followed by diltiazem or verapamil or a β-blocker
    - Aldosterone antagonists for antiproteinuric effect; hyperkalemia potential.
- Secondary hyperparathyroidism:
  - Cinacalcet, paricalcitol (decrease PTH levels)
  - Recommended serum phosphate maintenance Levels for CKD patients (4)

Stage	mg/dL	mmol/L
Normal Range *may vary by institution*	2.5–4.5	0.81–1.45
Stage 3 and 4 CKD (not on dialysis)	2.7–4.6	0.87–1.49
Stage 5 and ALL stages on dialysis	3.0–5.0	1.13–1.78

- Stages 3–5 CKD (not on dialysis): Restrict dietary phosphate to 900 mg/day
  - Calcium-containing phosphate binders (with meals): Calcium carbonate, calcium acetate—risk of hypercalcemia
  - Non-calcium phosphate binders (to be taken with meals): sevelamer, lanthanum
  - Vitamin D: Inactive vitamin D 25 (ergocalciferol or cholecalciferol), calcitriol (active vitamin D 1,25 [OH])
    - Vitamin D may increase absorption of phosphate by intestines and should not be started until serum phosphate concentration is controlled
- Anemia: Ferrous sulfate, erythropoietin:
  - Indication: Start when Hgb <10 g/dL; goal range 11–12 g/dL—not to exceed 13 g/dL
- Hyperlipidemia: Statins
- Glycemic control: Goal HbA1c <7; avoid metformin owing to the risk of metabolic acidosis.
- Metabolic acidosis: Start treatment when bicarb <20 mEq/L; goal >23 mEq/L.
  - Sodium bicarbonate: Daily dose of 0.5 to 1 mEq/kg per day
  - Sodium citrate: Should be avoided in patients taking aluminum-containing antacid

ADDITIONAL TREATMENT
General Measures
- Minimize radiocontrast exposure; prehydrate; N-acetylcysteine use is controversial.
- Renal replacement: Prepare for dialysis or transplant when GFR <30 mL/min/1.73 m².
- Vaccines: Pneumococcal; influenza
- Encourage smoking cessation.

Issues for Referral
- Nephrology consultation early to slow progression
- If GFR <15 immediate referral; 15<GFR<29 urgent referral; 30<GFR<59 routine referral in presence of risk factors; 60<GFR<89 no referral required unless other problem present

SURGERY/OTHER PROCEDURES
Placement of dialysis access or transplantation for ESRD

IN-PATIENT CONSIDERATIONS
Admission Criteria
Uremia: nausea/vomiting, fluid overload, pericarditis, uremic encephalopathy, resistant hypertension, hyperkalemia, metabolic acidosis, hyperphosphatemia (consider dialysis)

 ## ONGOING CARE

DIET
Nutrition consult for CKD diet:
- For GFR <60 mL/min/1.73 m², assess protein and energy intake; important to maintain adequate nutrition.
- Restricted intake of phosphates
- Sodium restriction
- Potassium restriction if hyperkalemic

PATIENT EDUCATION
National Kidney Federation patient Web site at: http://www.kidney.org/patients

PROGNOSIS
Patients with CKD gradually progress to ESRD

COMPLICATIONS
HTN, anemia, 2° hyperparathyroidism, renal osteodystrophy, sleep disturbances, infections, malnutrition, increased magnesium, platelet dysfunction/bleeding, pseudogout, gout, metabolic calcification, sexual dysfunction

REFERENCES
1. K/DOQI clinical practice guidelines for chronic kidney disease: evaluation, classification, and stratification. *Am J Kidney Dis*. 2002;39(2 Suppl 1):S1–266.
2. Coresh J, Selvin E, Stevens LA, Manzi J, Kusek JW, Eggers P, Van Lente F, Levey AS et al. Prevalence of chronic kidney disease in the United States. *JAMA*. 2007;298:2038–47.
3. MYH9 is associated with nondiabetic end-stage renal disease in African Americans. *Nat Genet*. 2008;40(10):1185–92. Epub 2008 Sep 14
4. KDIGO Clinical Practice guidelines for the diagnosis, evaluation, and treatment of chronic kidney disease-mineral and bone disorder (CKD-MBD). *Kidney Int* 2009;76(Suppl 113):S1.

See Also (Topic, Algorithm, Electronic Media Element)
Proteinuria; Hydronephrosis; Nephrotic Syndrome; Polycystic Kidney Disease
Algorithm: Anuria or Oliguria

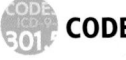 ## CODES

ICD9
- 585.1 Chronic kidney disease, stage i
- 585.2 Chronic kidney disease, stage ii (mild)
- 585.3 Chronic kidney disease, stage iii (moderate)

CLINICAL PEARLS
- Patient education is important in slowing the progression of CKD.
- Maintaining blood pressure <130/80 is crucial.
- Prevent and treat reversible causes of renal dysfunction.

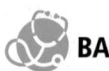

BASICS

DESCRIPTION
- Chronic obstructive pulmonary disease (COPD) encompasses several diffuse pulmonary diseases, including chronic bronchitis, asthma, cystic fibrosis, bronchiectasis, and emphysema:
  - The term usually describes a mixture of chronic bronchitis and emphysema.
  - Characterized by airflow limitation that is not fully reversible, is progressive, and inflammation is present (1,2,3)
- Chronic bronchitis is defined clinically by increased mucus production and recurrent cough present on most days for at least 3 months during at least 2 consecutive years.
- Emphysema is the destruction of interalveolar septa; it occurs in the distal or terminal airways and involves both airways and lung parenchyma.

EPIDEMIOLOGY
Incidence
Affects ~10–20% of adults; >100,000 deaths/year in US

Prevalence
- 14 million people have chronic bronchitis; 2 million people have emphysema.
- 4th leading cause of death in US

RISK FACTORS
- Smoking
- Passive smoking, especially adults whose parents smoked
- Severe viral pneumonia early in life
- Aging
- Alcohol consumption
- Airway hyperactivity

Genetics
- Chronic bronchitis is not a genetic disorder.
- Antiprotease deficiency (due to α_1 antitrypsin deficiency) is an inherited, rare disorder due to 2 autosomal-codominant alleles.

GENERAL PREVENTION
- Avoidance of smoking is the most important preventive measure.
- Passive smoke also has been shown to be harmful.
- Early detection through pulmonary function tests (PFTs) in high-risk patients may be useful in preserving remaining lung function.

PATHOPHYSIOLOGY
- Impaired gas (CO_2 and O_2) exchange
- Airway obstruction by mucus in chronic bronchitis (1)
- Destruction of lung parenchyma in emphysema

ETIOLOGY
Cigarette smoking, air pollution, antiprotease deficiency (α_1 antitrypsin), occupational exposure (firefighters), infection possibly (viral), occupational pollutants (cadmium, silica)

COMMONLY ASSOCIATED CONDITIONS
- Lung cancer
- Coronary artery disease
- Chronic sinusitis
- Malnutrition
- Laryngeal carcinoma
- Acute bronchitis
- Sleep apnea
- Chronic respiratory failure
- Osteoporosis

DIAGNOSIS

HISTORY
- Patient's habits with regard to tobacco should be discussed. Also review possible causes of exacerbation (e.g., recent infection) and history of cough, sputum, and dyspnea (1).
- Chronic bronchitis: Cough, sputum production, frequent infections, intermittent dyspnea, wheeze, hemoptysis, morning headache, pedal edema
- Emphysema: Minimal cough, scant sputum, dyspnea, weight loss, occasional infections

PHYSICAL EXAM
- Rarely diagnostic for COPD (3)
- Chronic bronchitis: Cyanosis, wheezing, weight gain, diminished breath sounds, distant heart sounds
- Emphysema: Barrel chest, minimal wheezing, accessory muscles used, pursed lip breathing, cyanosis slight or absent, breath sounds diminished

DIAGNOSTIC TESTS & INTERPRETATION
Lab
Initial lab tests
- Chronic bronchitis:
  - Arterial blood gases (ABGs) may show hypercapnia and hypoxia.
  - Hemoglobin may be increased.
- Emphysema:
  - Normal serum hemoglobin or polycythemia
  - Normal $PaCO_2$ on ABGs unless forced expiratory volume in 1 second (FEV1) <1 L, in which case it can be elevated.
  - Mild hypoxia

Follow-Up & Special Considerations
- Consider checking continuous overnight oximetry in selected patients.
- α_1-antitrypsin screening for those with COPD <45 years old or a blood relative with this disease

Imaging
Initial approach
- Chronic bronchitis chest x-ray (CXR): Increased bronchovascular markings and cardiomegaly
- Emphysema CXR: Small heart, hyperinflation, flat diaphragms, and possibly bullous changes

Follow-Up & Special Considerations
Chest computed tomography may show diffuse bullous changes or upper lobe predominance.

Diagnostic Procedures/Surgery
- PFTs:
  - Not indicated during acute exacerbation
  - Decreased FEV_1 and resulting reduction in FEV_1/FVC (forced vital capacity) ratio
  - Poor or absent reversibility to bronchodilator
  - Normal or reduced FVC
  - Normal or increased total lung capacity
  - Increased residual volume and functional residual capacity
  - Diffusing capacity is normal or reduced.
- Nocturnal oximetry

Pathological Findings
- Chronic bronchitis:
  - Bronchial mucous gland enlargement
  - Increased number of secretory cells in surface epithelium
  - Thickened small airways from edema and inflammation
  - Smooth muscle hyperplasia
  - Mucus plugging
  - Bacterial colonization of airways
- Emphysema:
  - Entire lung affected
  - Bronchi usually clear of secretions
  - Anthracotic pigment
  - Alveoli enlarged with loss of septa
  - Cartilage atrophy
  - Bullae

DIFFERENTIAL DIAGNOSIS
- Asthma
- Bronchiectasis
- Lung cancer
- Acute viral infection
- Normal aging of lungs
- Occupational asthma
- Chronic pulmonary embolism
- Sleep apnea
- Primary alveolar hypoventilation
- Chronic sinusitis
- Reactive airways dysfunction syndrome
- Congestive heart failure (CHF)
- Bronchiolitis obliterans
- Gastroesophageal reflux disease

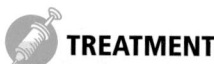

TREATMENT

MEDICATION
Medications help to reduce symptoms and exacerbations (3) and may prevent progression of disease (4,5)[A].

First Line
- Anticholinergics (2)[A]:
  - Ipratropium (Atrovent), tiotropium (Spiriva): 1 inhalation daily (6)[A]
  - AND/OR
- Long-acting β-agonists:
  - Salmeterol (Serevent), formoterol (Foradil) 1 inhalation q12h or arformoterol (Brovana), formoterol (Perforomist) nebulized q12h (6)[A]

Second Line
- Trial of inhaled corticosteroids for moderate or severe disease (4)[A]. 10–20% of patients may have salutary response. Discontinue if no benefit in symptoms or objective measures in 6–8 weeks:
  - May initiate earlier if suggestion of asthmatic component to disease
  - Systemic corticosteroids; prednisone (Deltasone) can be given orally 7.5–15 mg/d
  - Consider pulse dosing (40 mg/d) with taper depending on length of therapy. Most useful in bronchitis with some reversibility (1)[A].
  - Among patients with COPD, inhaled corticosteroid use for at least 24 weeks is associated with a significantly increased risk of serious pneumonia, without a significantly increased risk of death (7)[A].
- Theophylline (1)[A]: 400 mg/d; increase by 100–200 mg in 1–2 weeks, if necessary:

- Reduce dosage in patients with impaired renal or liver function, age >55, or CHF.
- Monitor serum level. Therapeutic range is 8–13 μg/mL (1)[A].
- Combination of inhaled corticosteroid, long-acting β-agonist, and anticholinergic indicated for severe disease (6)[A]
- Mucolytic agents may improve secretions but do not improve outcomes.
- Low-dose macrolides (clarithromycin or erythromycin) to decrease inflammation (8)[A]
- α1-antitrypsin, if deficient: 60 mg/kg weekly to maintain level exceeding 80 mg/dL
- Low-dose macrolides (clarithromycin, zithromycin, or erythromycin) to decrease inflammation
- Precautions:
  - Sympathomimetics: Excessive use may be dangerous. May need to reduce dosage or use levalbuterol (Xopenex) in patients with cardiovascular disease, hypertension (HTN), hyperthyroidism, diabetes, or convulsive disorders.
  - Anticholinergics: Narrow-angle glaucoma, benign prostatic hyperplasia, bladder-neck obstruction
  - Corticosteroids may mask infection or predispose to infection, especially fungal; subcapsular cataracts; glaucoma; adrenocortical insufficiency; psychic derangements; gastrointestinal bleeding; diabetes mellitus, reactivation of tuberculosis
- Sympathomimetics may be aerosolized.
- Anticholinergics: Ipratropium (Atrovent) may be aerosolized or combined with albuterol (Combivent).

ADDITIONAL TREATMENT
General Measures
- Smoking cessation: This is the most important intervention to decrease risk (3).
- Mucolytic agents
- Aggressive treatment of infections (3)[A]
- Treat any reversible bronchospasm.
- Home oxygen: May improve survival in hypoxemia and cor pulmonale, and should be initiated early in these conditions if oxygen <89% (8)[A]
- Influenza and pneumococcal immunizations

Issues for Referral
Severe exacerbation, frequent hospitalizations, age <40, rapid progression, weight loss, severe disease, or surgical evaluation

Additional Therapies
- Adequate hydration and pulmonary hygiene
- Consider postural drainage, flutter valve, or other devices to assist mucus clearance.
- Pulmonary rehabilitation may be of benefit (9).
- Occasionally, intermittent noninvasive ventilation may be of benefit with severe chronic respiratory failure (4)[A].

SURGERY/OTHER PROCEDURES
- Lung reduction surgery (selected cases)
- Lung transplantation (selected cases)

IN-PATIENT CONSIDERATIONS
Initial Stabilization
- Outpatient treatment is usually adequate.
- Supplemental oxygen and short-acting bronchodilators should be given in the emergency room (3)[A].
- Acute respiratory failure may require intensive care unit and mechanical ventilation.

Admission Criteria
- Exacerbation with acute decompensation (hypoxemia, hypercarbia) due to infection
- Need for mechanical ventilation
- Serious comorbidities, such as decompensated congestive heart failure (CHF)

Nursing
- Teach proper inhaler use.
- Monitor fluid balance.

Discharge Criteria
- Not waking at night due to dyspnea (3)
- Ability to ambulate
- Patient should have adequate gas exchange.
- Hypoxia can be treated with home O_2 (may only be temporary) (2)[A].
- Inhaled β-agonist therapy no more frequently than q4h (3).

 ## ONGOING CARE

FOLLOW-UP RECOMMENDATIONS
- May taper oral steroids as outpatient
- If pneumonia caused exacerbation, need to follow CXR until clear.

Patient Monitoring
- Severe or unstable patients should be seen monthly. When stable, see every 6 months.
- Check theophylline level with dose adjustment, then check every 6–12 months.
- With home O_2, check ABGs yearly or with change in condition. Monitor O_2 saturation (pulse oximetry) more frequently.
- Some patients only desaturate at night, thus only need nocturnal O_2.
- Avoid travel at high altitude.
- Discuss advance directive and health care proxy.
- Yearly PFTs

DIET
A high-protein diet is suggested. Decreased carbohydrates may benefit those with hypercarbia.

PATIENT EDUCATION
Printed material available from National Jewish Hospital in Denver, CO. Local branch of American Lung Association also has informational material.

PROGNOSIS
- Patient's age and postbronchodilator FEV_1 are the most important predictors of prognosis. Young age and FEV_1 >50% predicted to have a good prognosis. Older patients do worse.
- Supplemental O_2, when indicated, is shown to increase survival (may only need at night).
- Smoking cessation improves prognosis.
- Malnutrition, cor pulmonale, hypercapnia, and pulse >100 indicate a poor prognosis.

COMPLICATIONS
- Infections
- Cor pulmonale
- Secondary polycythemia
- Bullous lung disease
- Acute or chronic respiratory failure
- Pulmonary HTN
- Malnutrition
- Pneumothorax
- Poor sleep quality
- Arrhythmias

REFERENCES
1. Braman SS. Chronic cough due to chronic bronchitis: ACCP evidence-based clinical practice guidelines. *Chest.* 2006;129:104S–115S.
2. Celli BR. Update on the management of COPD. *Chest.* 2008;133:1451–62.
3. Wilt TJ, Niewoehner D, MacDonald R, et al. Management of stable chronic obstructive pulmonary disease: a systematic review for a clinical practice guideline. *Ann Intern Med.* 2007;147:639–53.
4. Maclay JD, Rabinovich RA, MacNee W. Update in chronic obstructive pulmonary disease 2008. *Am J Respir Crit Care Med.* 2009;179:533–41.
5. Rubins JB, Raci E, Kunisaki KM. Managing stable COPD in 2009: incorporating results from recent clinical studies into a goal-directed approach for clinicians. *Postgrad Med.* 2009;121:104–12.
6. Rabe KF, Hurd S, Anzueto A, et al. Global strategy for the diagnosis, management, and prevention of chronic obstructive pulmonary disease: GOLD executive summary. *Am J Respir Crit Care Med.* 2007;176:532–55.
7. Singh S, Amin AV, Loke YK. Long-term use of inhaled corticosteroids and the risk of pneumonia in chronic obstructive pulmonary disease: a meta-analysis. *Arch Intern Med.* 2009;169:219–29.
8. Cosio BG, Agustí A et al. Update in chronic obstructive pulmonary disease 2009. *Am J Respir Crit Care Med.* 2010;181:655–60.
9. Casaburi R, ZuWallack R. Pulmonary rehabilitation for management of chronic obstructive pulmonary disease. *N Engl J Med.* 2009;360:1329–35.

See Also (Topic, Algorithm, Electronic Media Element)
Bronchitis, Acute
Algorithms: Clubbing; Cyanosis

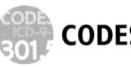 ## CODES

ICD9
- 492.8 Other emphysema
- 493.20 Chronic obstructive asthma, unspecified
- 496 Chronic airway obstruction, not elsewhere classified

CLINICAL PEARLS
- Screening PFTs should be done on all high-risk patients.
- Check overnight oximetry when daytime saturation is borderline.
- Influenza and pneumococcal vaccines should be kept up to date.
- Smoking cessation counseling, if applicable, is a critical component of care.

Pink puffer
Blue

CHRONIC PAIN MANAGEMENT: AN EVIDENCE BASED APPROACH

Irene C. Coletsos, MD
Gail Gazelle, MD

 BASICS

- Defined as pain that extends beyond time of tissue healing or pain that cannot be explained by levels of pathology observed
- Because of changes in CNS, chronic pain becomes a disease state itself, continuing well beyond the initial event.
- Patients who experience chronic pain fall into three categories:
  - Those with known physical illnesses or traumas as the etiology of the chronic pain.
  - No identified physical etiology known to cause chronic pain, >50% of patients.
  - Those with psychiatric comorbidities.

EPIDEMIOLOGY
In the US, an estimated 35.5% of the residents suffer from chronic pain, the majority of which manage without use of chronic narcotics.

Prevalence
In the US, pain is the most common reason patients seek medical care. An estimated 50 million Americans suffer from chronic pain, and it is the major cause of adult disability.

RISK FACTORS
- Traumatic: Amputations, falls, motor vehicle accidents, repetitive motion injuries, sports injuries, work related injuries
- Postsurgical: e.g., failed back surgery, incisional pain, phantom limb pain, postthoracotomy syndrome.
- Medical conditions: Arthritis, back disease, cancer, fibromyalgia; neuropathies (diabetes, HIV, multiple sclerosis, shingles, past chemotherapy), radiculopathies; poststroke syndrome, spinal cord injuries
- Cancer
- Psychiatric comorbidities: Anxiety, borderline personality disorders, depression, dysthymia, post-traumatic stress disorder (PTSD), schizoaffective disorders, somatic disorders, the sequela of childhood sexual abuse
- Aging: Increased incidence with age, but should not be considered a "normal" part of aging
- Idiopathic: No pathological cause found despite repeated testing
- Secondary gain: Factitious disorder, malingering, Münchhausen's

GENERAL PREVENTION
- Avoidance of work-related injuries through the use of ergonomically correct workplace design
- Exercise and physical therapy to help prevent work-related low back pain
- Varicella vaccine and rapid treatment of shingles to lower risk of postherpetic neuralgia
- Tight glycemic control for diabetic patients, alcohol cessation for alcoholics, smoking cessation to avoid neuropathies

PATHOPHYSIOLOGY
With intense, repeated, or prolonged stimulation of damaged or inflamed tissues, the threshold for activating primary afferent pain fibers is lowered, the frequency of firing is higher, and there is increased response to noxious stimuli. The amygdala is thought to help modulate the relationship between pain and the emotions that may accompany it, such as anxiety and depression.

 DIAGNOSIS

Chronic pain can be divided into 3 general categories:
- Nociceptive pain (2 types):
  - Somatic: Incisional, bone, soft-tissue disease. Well localized, dull, aching, throbbing, or gnawing
  - Visceral: Affecting viscera; poorly localized; described as deep, dull, and aching; may refer to sites remote from lesion
- Neuropathic pain: See "Neuropathic Pain."
- Sympathetically maintained pain: Peripheral nerve injury can cause severe burning pain associated with swelling of the affected limb, focal change in sweat production, and skin texture. Example: Complex regional pain syndrome.

HISTORY
- Use standardized tools to document baseline experience: Pain—Brief Pain Inventory (short form); Mood—Patient Health Questionnaire-9 (PHQ-9); Alcohol use—Alcohol Use Disorders Identification Test (AUDIT).
- Issues with substance abuse ("How many times in the last 12 months did you use an illegal drug or a prescription drug for nonmedical reasons?"); personal trauma; how patients have treated their pain in the past; and their current goals for pain relief (1)
  - Pain initiation, character and intensity (scale of 0–10, 10 being the worst)
  - Modifying factors (what lessens it and what makes it worse)
  - Questions about functioning—how the pain affects the patient's ability to carry on his/her life and job
  - Mood and sensory experience accompanying the pain
  - Past medical history, including arthritis, neoplasm, surgery, trauma, childhood or current abuse, psychiatric illness, substance abuse

PHYSICAL EXAM
- Physical exam begins in the waiting room. Note movement from chair to standing, ambulation. Does the patient change gait, grimace, express pain?
- Muscle wasting, localized tenderness, swelling, erythema, or increased warmth, muscle weakness. For joint pain, check passive and active range of motion.
- Neurological exam: Motor strength, reflexes, and sensation to light touch, noxious touch, and vibration; deep palpation of trigger points
- In chronic regional pain syndrome: Pain, swelling, limited range of motion, vasomotor instability, and skin changes (cyanosis, mottling, increased sweating, abnormal hair growth) in the affected area. Relief of the pain with a sympathetic block is diagnostic.

DIAGNOSTIC TESTS & INTERPRETATION
Lab
Testing should be directed at the differential diagnosis regarding the area/body system involved.
Initial lab tests
- Complete blood count, erythrocyte sedimentation rate
- Urine drug screen (Urine Qualitative analysis for drugs of abuse and quantitative analysis of medication patient is reported to be using) and serum toxicology
- If abdominal: Liver function tests, amylase, lipase
- If pelvic: Ultrasound and possibly further imaging studies to rule out ovarian cancer
- If joint pain: RF, ANA, studies for Lyme disease, gonorrhea, septic arthritis

Follow-Up & Special Considerations
- Complex regional pain syndrome is possible, a ganglion block or sympathetic block can be diagnostic and possibly prevent the development of a chronic pain syndrome.
- If using opioids, order random urine drug screens: Qualitative analysis for drugs of abuse, quantitative analysis of the drug you are prescribing and urinalysis to confirm the specimen is in fact urine.

Diagnostic Procedures/Surgery
Consider referral to a pain center for interventional diagnostics such as facet joint blocks (to help diagnose facet joint disease); a nerve root block (to evaluate level of radicular pain); sacroiliac joint injection (to evaluate sacroiliac joint pain) (2).

DIFFERENTIAL DIAGNOSIS
- Abdominal adhesions, migraines, arthritis, bipolar disorder/depression, bursitis, chronic fatigue, drug abuse, endometriosis, fibromyalgia, lumbar degenerative disc disease, malignancy, neuromas, tendinitis
- Domestic abuse and violence, malingering, somatic disorders; Münchhausen syndrome and Münchhausen by proxy (in older children who are protecting the care provider who has been abusing the child)
- Diversion: Unintended use of a prescription medication for a nonmedical reason; for narcotics, it would include drug seeking to resell

 TREATMENT

- Trust between health care provider and patient
- Maintain clear boundaries: call frequency, amount of phone time, behavior toward staff
- Team approach: Involve family members, primary care doctor, substance abuse specialist, counselor, physical and occupational therapist, psychiatrist; relaxation training, spiritual counseling, complementary medicine. Patients cared for by multidisciplinary teams report a reduction in the intensity of their pain a year after these interventions (2).

MEDICATION

Sequential time-limited trials of medications, starting at low doses and gradually increasing until either effect or dose-limiting side effects are reached.

- For mild to moderate chronic pain:
  - Acetaminophen: Daily dose not to exceed total 4 grams in healthy adults and 2 grams in the elderly or those with hepatic disease or active or past history of alcohol use.
  - Nonsteroidal anti-inflammatory drugs (NSAIDS): Patients taking aspirin for cardiovascular protection should avoid the added gastrointestinal toxicity of NSAIDs. Cox-2 selective inhibitors should be used with caution because of cardiac risks.
  - "Weak" opioids, including codeine, hydrocodone, and tramadol. Avoid tramadol in elderly or patients at risk for seizures.
- For neuropathic pain (chronic low back pain, fibromyalgia, etc:
  - See "Neuropathic Pain" topic.
  - Classes of medications for neuropathic pain: (1) tricyclic, selective serotonin reuptake inhibitor (SSRIs), and selective serotonin-norepinephrine reuptake inhibitor (SSNRI) antidepressants; (2) anticonvulsants; (3) antiarrhythmics; (4) opioids, particularly methadone.
  - Example: Combination of amitriptyline or duloxetine + gabapentin.
- For moderate-to-severe nonneuropathic chronic pain:
  - Strong opioids: Bind to central nervous system opioid receptors. Includes morphine, oxycodone, oral hydromorphone, oral morphine, Fentanyl. Check coanalgesic tables for differential dosing. Note no evidence supports any of these strong opioids as superior or having improved side-effect profile. Morphine should be avoided in patients with significant renal insufficiency. Methadone: Only opioid that acts as N-methyl-D-aspartate receptor antagonist; is uniquely effective in neuropathic pain. Methadone has many drug interactions, and is easy to cause overdose. Methadone can contribute to potentially fatal cardiac arrhythmias.
  - Buprenorphine: A mixed opioid agonist and antagonist
  - Once stable dose of opioids is established, change to sustained-release formulations. Short-acting formulations only for break-through pain.
  - Common side effects: Constipation: senna and bisacodyl should be prescribed at time opioids are started. Also: nausea, sedation, mental status changes, pruritus.
  - Miscellaneous agents:
    ○ Capsaicin, found in hot chili peppers, depletes substance P in nociceptors.
    ○ Topical NSAIDS
    ○ Cannabinoids where legal

ALERT

All patients on chronic opioids should be managed with a "pain contract," random urine drug screening, and a "zero tolerance" approach when diversion is suspected.

ADDITIONAL TREATMENT

General Measures

Keep a "pain diary" to record pain, better or worse, and how much medication is taken.

COMPLEMENTARY AND ALTERNATIVE MEDICINE

- Acupuncture: Efficacy in chronic neck, back pain, and fibromyalgia
- Exercise: Efficacy in low back pain and fibromyalgia
- Improved mood and coping skills with behavioral and cognitive behavioral therapies (CBT). CBT may also decrease disability from chronic pain.
- Mind-body interventions: Yoga, tai chi, hypnosis, progressive muscle relaxation
- Children with chronic headaches, abdominal pain, etc: biofeedback, cognitive behavioral therapy, hypnosis, and relaxation exercises.

IN-PATIENT CONSIDERATIONS

Discharge Criteria

Discharge should include planning for:

- Chronic medication management (adding a stool regimen for opioids, adding liver and kidney function tests for chronic acetaminophen and NSAID use).
- Education and prescriptions for "rescue" medication doses for breakthrough pain.
- PT/OT, psychiatry, acupuncture, group/individual counseling, addiction counseling, stress-reduction techniques.

 ONGOING CARE

FOLLOW-UP RECOMMENDATIONS

Patient Monitoring

- Contract between care provider and patient for all patients taking opioids. It should include:
  - 1 prescribing clinician (or designee)
  - No after-hours prescriptions or early refills
  - Mandatory police reports for medication thefts
  - Pain contracts (e.g., http://www.ohsu.edu/ahec/pain/med_contractlf.pdf)
- Random urine drug tests to reduce diversion and confirm no other illicit substances
- Taper and discontinue medications if patient does not benefit or side effects outweigh benefits, or if medications are abused or suspect diversion (1).
- Scheduled follow-up where patient's pain, function, and engagement in treatment (ex. physical therapy, occupational therapy, psychology therapies) (1)
- Scheduled follow-up appointments in which patient's mood is evaluated. Poorly controlled chronic pain is a risk factor for suicidality.

PATIENT EDUCATION

American Chronic Pain Association: http://www.theacpa.org

COMPLICATIONS

Substance abuse:

- Addiction: Includes 1 or more of following: Impaired control over drug use, compulsive use, and continued use despite harm. Taking drug for non-prescribed reasons.
- Physical dependence: Withdrawal syndrome produced by abrupt cessation or rapid dose reduction. Is a physiologic phenomenon
- Tolerance: A state of adaptation in which exposure to a drug induces changes that result in a diminution of 1 or more of the drug's effects over time.
- Addiction is common, but "problematic drug seeking behavior," due to other difficulties, including homelessness (loss of medications, improper dosing), genetic predispositions, and use of pain medications to self-treat anxiety or depressive disorder.

- Diversion: Selling drugs or giving them to persons other than for whom they are prescribed.

ALERT

Death: The rate of unintentional death due to opioid toxicity doubled between 1999 and 2005, accounting for more than 10,000 deaths. Narcotic overdose is the leading cause of accidental death of adults 25–55 (surpassing motor vehicle accidents) CDC/HVSS.

REFERENCES

1. Chou R, Fanciullo GJ, Fine PG, Adler JA, Ballantyne JC, Davies P, Donovan MI, Fishbain DA, Foley KM, Fudin J, Gilson AM, Kelter A, Mauskop A, O'Connor PG, Passik SD, Pasternak GW, Portenoy RK, Rich BA, Roberts RG, Todd KH, Miaskowski C, American Pain Society-American Academy of Pain Medicine Opioids Guidelines Panel et al. Clinical guidelines for the use of chronic opioid therapy in chronic noncancer pain. *J Pain*. 2009;10:113–30.
2. American Society of Anesthesiologists Task Force on Chronic Pain Management, American Society of Regional Anesthesia and Pain Medicine et al. Practice guidelines for chronic pain management: an updated report by the American Society of Anesthesiologists Task Force on Chronic Pain Management and the American Society of Regional Anesthesia and Pain Medicine. *Anesthesiology*. 2010;112:810–33.

See Also (Topic, Algorithm, Electronic Media Element)

Federation of State Medical Boards of the United States, Inc. Model Policy for the Use of Controlled Substances for the Treatment of Pain: www.painpolicy.wisc.edu/domestic/model04.pdf

 CODES

ICD9

- 338.4 Chronic pain syndrome
- 338.21 Chronic pain due to trauma
- 338.22 Chronic post-thoracotomy pain

CLINICAL PEARLS

- Start with the presumption the patient's pain is *real*, even if pathophysiological evidence for it cannot be found.
- In taking the history, keep in mind that past/active sexual/domestic abuse can present as chronic physical pain.
- Have the patient keep a "pain diary."
- Emphasize that being pain free may not be possible, but that better function and quality-of-life can be shared goals.
- Written contracts and random urine testing for patients prescribed chronic opioids

CIRRHOSIS OF THE LIVER

Anne M. Walsh, PA-C, MMSc
Jill A. Grimes, MD

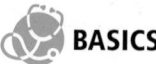 **BASICS**

DESCRIPTION
A chronic disease in which liver cell injury causes inflammation, necrosis, and stellate cell activation. Fibrosis replaces normal liver tissue and destroys the liver's vascular and lobular architecture, progressively diminishing blood flow and decreasing function. End result is liver failure and/or cancer.

Geriatric Considerations
- Jaundice and encephalopathy more common

Pediatric Considerations
- Inborn errors of metabolism (e.g., tyrosinemia), congenital anomalies (e.g., biliary atresia)

EPIDEMIOLOGY
- Predominant age: 40–50 years old
- Predominant sex: Male > female; but more females get cirrhosis from alcohol abuse.
- 12th leading cause of death in all US adults

RISK FACTORS
- Alcohol abuse
- IV drug abuse
- Obesity

Genetics
Hemochromatosis, Wilson disease, and Alpha-1-antitrypsin deficiency in adults

GENERAL PREVENTION
- Counsel patients to prevent risk factors for chronic liver disease (e.g., alcohol abuse); over 80% of chronic liver disease is preventable.
- Limit alcohol consumption to <2 drinks/day and advise weight loss for obesity
  - Raised BMI and alcohol consumption are both linked to liver disease, with evidence of a supra-additive interaction between the two. (1)[A]

ETIOLOGY
- Alcohol abuse (~60%)
- Chronic hepatitis B and/or C (~10%)
- Nonalcoholic steatohepatitis/obesity (~10%)
- Biliary obstruction (~10%)
- Hemochromatosis (~5%)
- Rare metabolic, genetic, toxic, infectious disorders (~5%)

COMMONLY ASSOCIATED CONDITIONS
- Diabetes
- Alcoholism
- Drug abuse
- Depression
- Obesity

 DIAGNOSIS

HISTORY
- Review risk factors (alcohol abuse, viral hepatitis; family history of primary liver cancer, other liver disease, or autoimmune disease)
- Symptoms:
  - Fatigue, malaise, weakness
  - Anorexia, weight loss (gain if ascites/edema)
  - Right upper abdominal pain
  - Absent/irregular menses
  - Diminished libido, erectile dysfunction
  - Tea-colored urine, clay-colored stools
  - Edema, abdominal swelling/bloating
  - Bruising, bleeding, hematemesis, hematochezia, melena
  - Pruritus
  - Night blindness

PHYSICAL EXAM
Physical exam may be normal until end-stage disease develops.
- Skin changes:
  - Spider angiomata
  - Palmar erythema
  - Jaundice, scleral icterus
  - Ecchymoses
  - Caput medusa
  - Hyperpigmentation
- Hepatomegaly (small liver in end-stage disease)
- Splenomegaly if portal hypertension
- Central obesity
- Abdominal fluid wave, shifting dullness if ascites present
- Gynecomastia
- Dupuytren contractures
- Pretibial, presacral pitting edema
- Asterixis
- Mental status changes
- Muscle wasting, weakness

DIAGNOSTIC TESTS & INTERPRETATION
Lab
- ALT and AST mildly elevated; typically AST > ALT. Enzymes normalize as cirrhosis progresses.
- Elevated alkaline phosphatase (ALP), gamma-glutamyl transpeptidase (GGT), and total/direct bilirubin, indicates cholestasis
- Decreased platelet count from portal hypertension with splenomegaly
- Impaired synthetic liver function:
  - Low albumin and cholesterol
  - Prolonged prothrombin (PT), international normalized ratio (INR), partial thromboplastin time (PTT)
- Progressive cirrhosis:
  - Elevated ammonia level; decreased blood urea nitrogen (BUN), sodium, and potassium
- Alpha-fetoprotein level at diagnosis to screen for hepatocellular carcinoma (HCC)

Follow-Up & Special Considerations
To determine specific etiology consider:
- Hepatitis B surface antigen (HBsAg), core antibody (HBcAb), and surface antibody (HBsAb)
- Hepatitis C antibody
- Serum ethanol and GGT if suspected ongoing alcohol abuse
- Antimitochondrial antibody to screen for primary biliary cirrhosis
- Anti–smooth muscle and antinuclear antibodies to screen for chronic active (autoimmune) hepatitis
- Iron saturation (>50%) and ferritin (markedly increased) to screen for hemochromatosis; if abnormal, check hemochromatosis (HFE) genetics/mutation analysis
- Alpha-1-antitrypsin phenotype to screen for deficiency
- Ceruloplasmin level to screen for Wilson disease; if low, check copper excretion (serum copper plus 24-hour urine copper)

Imaging
- Abdominal ultrasound (US) every 6–12 months to screen for hepatocellular carcinoma
- Doppler US of hepatic/portal veins
- MRI to clarify patency of blood vessels and collaterals; best follow-up test for HCC if alpha-fetoprotein elevated and/or liver mass found on US

Diagnostic Procedures/Surgery
- Liver biopsy: percutaneous if INR <1.5 and no ascites; otherwise, transjugular biopsy
- Liver-spleen scan to diagnose portal hypertension if patient cannot be biopsied
- Endoscopy if portal hypertension, R/O esophageal varices/portal hypertensive gastropathy (2)[C]

Pathological Findings
- Fibrosis and regenerative nodules are general features of cirrhosis on biopsy
- Other histologic findings vary with etiology:
  - Alcoholic liver disease: Steatosis, polymorphonuclear leukocyte (PMN) infiltrate, ballooning degeneration of hepatocytes, Mallory bodies, giant mitochondria
  - Chronic hepatitis B and C: Periportal lymphocytic inflammation
  - Nonalcoholic steatohepatitis: Identical to alcoholic liver disease, confirmed by history. Steatosis may be absent in advanced disease ("burned-out NASH")
  - Biliary cirrhosis: PMN infiltrate in wall of bile ducts, inflammation increased in portal spaces, progressive loss of bile ducts in portal spaces
  - Hemochromatosis: Intrahepatic iron stores increased (iron stain or weighted biopsy tissue)
  - Alpha-1-antitrypsin deficiency: Positive Periodic Acid-Schiff (PAS) bodies in hepatocytes

DIFFERENTIAL DIAGNOSIS
- Diffuse hepatic parenchymal disease (e.g., fatty liver)
- Other causes of portal hypertension (e.g., portal vein thrombosis, lymphoma)
- Metastatic or multifocal cancer in the liver
- Vascular congestion (e.g., cardiac cirrhosis)
- Reversible (e.g., acute alcoholic hepatitis)

TREATMENT

Outpatient care except for major gastrointestinal bleeding, altered mental status, sepsis/infection, rapidly progressing hepatic decompensation, renal failure

MEDICATION
As indicated to treat the underlying cause (*Note prescribing precautions in decompensated cirrhosis*):
- Hepatitis C: Combination therapy with pegylated-interferon alpha 2a or 2b SC once weekly plus ribavirin 200 mg 2–3 pills PO b.i.d. for 6–12+ months eradicates virus permanently ("sustained viral response" or SVR) in ~50% of patients overall and in 80–90% of genotypes 2/3
- Hepatitis B: lamivudine 100 mg PO daily; adefovir, 10 mg PO daily; entecavir, 0.5–1 mg PO daily; or telbivudine, 600 mg PO daily until resistance develops; alternatively peginterferon alpha 2a SC weekly for 48 weeks. Due to high rates of resistance, combination recommended (3)[C].

- Biliary cirrhosis: ursodeoxycholic acid (Ursodiol) 10–15 mg/kg PO daily, indefinitely (2)[A]
- Wilson disease: penicillamine 1–3 g/d or tetrathiomolybdate, 100–400 mg/d. After 1 year, zinc acetate 250 mg b.i.d. for maintenance
- Autoimmune (chronic active) hepatitis: prednisone 5–20 mg/d with or without azathioprine (Imuran) 0.5–1 mg/kg; adjust to keep transaminase levels normal.
- Esophageal varices: propranolol 40–160 mg, or nadolol 10 mg daily, to lower portal pressure by 20 mm Hg, systolic pressure to 90–100 mm Hg, and pulse rate by 25% (2)[A]
- Ascites/edema: Low-sodium (<2 g/day) diet and spironolactone, 100–400 mg daily with or without furosemide, 40–160 mg PO daily; torsemide may substitute for furosemide.
- Encephalopathy: lactulose 15 mL b.i.d., titrate to induce 3 loose bowel movements daily. Neomycin or rifaximin may be combined with lactulose (4).
- Pruritus: Ursodiol and antihistamines (e.g., hydroxyzine).
- Renal insufficiency: Stop diuretics, nephrotoxic drugs; normalize electrolytes; hospitalize for plasma expansion or dialysis.
- Prophylactic antibiotics for invasive procedures, GI bleeding, or history of spontaneous bacterial peritonitis (2)[A]
- Proton pump inhibitor for esophageal varices requiring banding or portal hypertensive gastropathy (5)[C]
- Recombinant factor VIIa to correct bleeding shows no survival benefit (4).

ADDITIONAL TREATMENT
General Measures
- Patients *must* abstain from alcohol, drugs, liver toxic medications, and herbs.
- Immunize for pneumococcal disease, hepatitis A and B, influenza.
- Nonalcoholic steatohepatitis (NASH): Weight reduction, exercise, optimal control of lipids/glucose.

Issues for Referral
Liver transplant evaluation at first onset complications (ascites, variceal bleed, encephalopathy), jaundice, or liver lesion suggestive of hepatocellular carcinoma, and/or when evidence of hepatic dysfunction develops (Child-Turcotte-Pugh >7 and MELD >10) (6)[C].

COMPLEMENTARY AND ALTERNATIVE MEDICINE
- Milk thistle (silymarin) may lower transaminases and improve symptoms; likely safe but offers no effect on overall mortality (7)[C]. *Caution*: Some preparations may contain hepatoxins and may interfere with INR and transaminase monitoring.
- Many herbal medications are liver toxic.

SURGERY/OTHER PROCEDURES
- Varices: Endoscopic ligation; 4–6 treatments typical (if acute bleed, use pre-esophagogastroduodenoscopy [EGD] octreotide as vasoconstrictor); transjugular intrahepatic shunt (TIPS) second-line or salvage therapy for acute bleed (8)
- Ascites: If tense, therapeutic paracentesis every 2 weeks PRN; caution if pedal edema absent.
- Fulminant hepatic failure: Liver transplantation
- Hepatocellular carcinoma: Curable if small with radiofrequency ablation or resection and transplant

IN-PATIENT CONSIDERATIONS
Admission Criteria
Major gastrointestinal (GI) bleeding, altered mental status, sepsis/infection, rapidly progressing hepatic decompensation, renal failure

 ## ONGOING CARE

FOLLOW-UP RECOMMENDATIONS
Regular conditioning may help fatigue.

Patient Monitoring
- Once stable, monitor liver enzymes, platelets, and PT every 6–12 months.
- Patients >55 years old, with chronic hepatitis B or C, elevated INR, or low platelets are highest risk for HCC. Check alpha-fetoprotein and liver ultrasound every 6–12 months for screening in cirrhotics (4)[A].
- Endoscopy at diagnosis and every 2 years to screen for varices.

DIET
Protein 1–1.5 g/kg of body weight, high fiber, daily multivitamin (without iron), and <2 g/d sodium (essential if ascites/edema). A high-protein diet may precipitate encephalopathy, but protein restriction is no longer recommended (4). Coffee consumption has a graded and inverse association with liver cancer (9)[B].

PATIENT EDUCATION
- Educate caregivers on when to seek emergency care (e.g., hematemesis, altered mental status).
- Maintain sobriety/recovery/smoking cessation (includes no cannabis).
- Hepatitis A/B immunization and hepatitis C transmission precautions

PROGNOSIS
- At diagnosis of cirrhosis, expect 5–20 years of asymptomatic disease.
- At onset of complications, expect death within 5 years without transplant:
  – 5% per year develop HCC
  – 50% of cirrhotics develop ascites over 10 years; 50% 5-year survival if ascites develop
  – Acute variceal bleed most common fatal complication; carries 30% mortality
  – Median survival at onset decompensation (ascites, variceal bleed, encephalopathy) is 1.5 years (4).
  – With transplant, 85% survive 1 year; posttransplant deaths ~5% per year
- Fewer than 25% of eligible patients are transplanted due to donor organ shortage.

COMPLICATIONS
- Ascites
- Edema
- Infections
- Encephalopathy
- GI bleed: Esophageal varices, gastropathy, colopathy
- Hepatorenal syndrome
- Hepatopulmonary syndrome
- Hepatocellular carcinoma
- Fulminant hepatic failure
- Complications posttransplant (e.g., surgical, rejection, infections)

REFERENCES
1. Hart CL, Morrison DS, Batty GD, Mitchell RJ, Davey Smith G. Effect of body mass index and alcohol consumption on liver disease: analysis of data from two prospective cohort studies. *BMJ*. 2010;340:c1240.
2. Talwalkar JA, Kamath PS. Influence of recent advances in medical management on clinical outcomes of cirrhosis. *Mayo Clin Proc*. 2005;80:1501–8.
3. Lok AS, McMahon BJ. Chronic hepatitis B. *Hepatology*. 2007;45:507–39.
4. Garcia-Tsao G. Managing the Complications of Cirrhosis, Hepatitis Annual Update 2008, Clinical Care Options Hepatitis, http://clinicaloptions.com/Hepatitis/Annual%20Updates/2008%20Annual%20Update.aspx
5. Nietsch HH. Management of portal hypertension. *J Clin Gastroenterol*. 2005;39:232–6.
6. Murray KF, Carithers RL, AASLD. AASLD practice guidelines: Evaluation of the patient for liver transplantation. *Hepatology*. 2005;41:1407–32.
7. Rambaldi A, Jacobs BP, Iaquinto G, et al. Milk thistle for alcoholic and/or hepatitis B or C virus liver diseases. Cochrane Hepato-Biliary Group *Cochrane Database Syst Rev*. 2006;Issue 4.
8. Garcia-Tsao G, Sanyal AJ, Grace ND. et al. Prevention and management of gastroesophageal varices and variceal hemorrhage in cirrhosis. *Hepatology*. 2007;46:922–38.
9. Hu G, Tuomilehto J, Pukkala E. et al. Joint effects of coffee consumption and serum gamma-glutamyltransferase on the risk of liver cancer. *Hepatology*. 2008.

ADDITIONAL READING
- Lebrec D, Thabut D, Oberti F et al. Pentoxifylline does not decrease short-term mortality but does reduce complications in patients with advanced cirrhosis. *Gastroenterology*. 2010;138:1755–62.
- Singal A, Volk ML, Waljee A, et al. Meta Analysis: Surveillance with Ultrasound for Early Stage Hepatocellular Carcinoma in Patients with Cirrhosis. *Aliment Pharmacol Ther*. 2009.

See Also (Topic, Algorithm, Electronic Media Element)
Algorithm: Cirrhosis

 ## CODES

ICD9
- 571.2 Alcoholic cirrhosis of liver
- 571.5 Cirrhosis of liver without mention of alcohol

CLINICAL PEARLS
- 80% of chronic liver disease that leads to cirrhosis is preventable (primarily alcoholic).
- Check immunity to hepatitis A and B and vaccinate if not immune
- Check abdominal ultrasounds every 6 months for early detection of hepatocellular carcinoma

C

CLAUDICATION

William J. Knaus, II, MD
Arabinda Chatterjee, MD, FRCS, MS, D. Urology

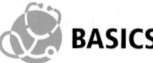 BASICS

DESCRIPTION
- Reproducible, exercise-induced muscle pain in the extremities associated with peripheral arterial disease:
  - Generally occurs in the lower extremities
- Intermittent claudication is the most common symptom of patients with peripheral arterial disease:
  - <20% of patients with peripheral arterial disease report typical symptoms.

EPIDEMIOLOGY
- 2/3 of patients with peripheral arterial disease are asymptomatic.
- Predominant sex: Male > Female (<2:1 ratio).

Incidence
- Incidence is related to age: 0.07% of men 35–44 years old and 1.4% of men > 65 years old develop the disease per year.
- Diabetic patients have an incidence 4–6 times greater than nondiabetic patients.

Prevalence
2–3% of men >60 years of age have symptomatic peripheral arterial disease compared to 1–2% of same-aged women.

RISK FACTORS
- Cigarette smoking:
  - 90% of all patients with claudication
- Diabetes mellitus
- Hypertension
- Hypercholesterolemia
- Family history
- Obesity
- Preexisting heart disease (15% of CHD patients have vascular disease in other beds)
- Advanced age

GENERAL PREVENTION
- Frequent walking exercises
- Smoking cessation
- Diet, lipid, and glucose control

PATHOPHYSIOLOGY
Atherosclerotic stenosis or occlusion of arterial flow diminishes blood pressure to the muscles of an extremity. Symptoms are generally exacerbated by exercise when blood-flow demand exceeds supply distal to the area of stenosis or occlusion and reduces tissue perfusion.

ETIOLOGY
- Sites affected depend upon the area of arterial supply involved.
- Symptoms occur distal to the area of arterial stenosis or occlusion.
- Superficial-femoral disease: Most common area associated with claudication. Pain may extend to the calf.
- Aortoiliac disease: Pain may extend from buttock to thigh.
- Femoropopliteal disease: Pain may extend from calf to foot.
- Subclavian, axillary, and brachial disease: Pain may extend to the upper extremity.

COMMONLY ASSOCIATED CONDITIONS
- Other manifestations of atherosclerosis:
  - Myocardial infarction
  - Carotid artery occlusive disease
  - Renovascular occlusive disease
  - Hypertension
- Of all patients with peripheral artery disease, 25–68% have concurrent coronary artery disease and 34–50% have a concomitant cerebrovascular disease (1)[B].

 DIAGNOSIS

- Patients will limit their walking based on their symptoms:
  - Symptom continuum ranges from calf muscle fatigue to severe cramps and pain.
  - Pain occurring at rest is an ominous presentation.
- Cold feet are an early warning symptom.
- Paresthesias or numbness are later symptoms:
  - Diabetics less likely to report pain
- Rubor in dependent limb
- Leg color may darken to a dusky crimson when in lowered position.
- Lower extremities are hairless.
- Nonhealing ulcer is associated with poor circulation.
- Can lead to marked limitation of daily activities (1)

HISTORY
- Reproducible pain associated with restricted walking distance and relieved by rest.
- The Edinburgh is a questionnaire with the following criteria required for PVD diagnosis (sensitivity: 99%, specificity: 91%) (2):
  - Leg pain occurs with walking.
  - Pain does not have onset while standing or sitting.
  - Pain occurs while walking fast or uphill.
  - Pain resolves within 10 minutes of standing still.
- Modifiers:
  - Pain occurring even at normal pace on level ground suggests severe claudication.
  - Classic pain location is in the calf; thigh or buttock pain without calf pain is atypical.

PHYSICAL EXAM
- Signs of peripheral vascular disease: Abnormal skin coloration (pallor, rubor), cool feet, atrophy of nails, delayed capillary refill, loss of hair
- Diminished or absent femoral, popliteal, posterior tibial, or dorsalis pedis pulses (3)[B].

DIAGNOSTIC TESTS & INTERPRETATION
Lab
Initial lab tests
- Fasting lipid panel, fasting glucose
- Blood pressure readings in both arms
- ABI (arterial brachial index)
- Measuring fibrinogen and homocysteine and manipulation if elevated have not led to improved outcomes, so is not recommended.

Imaging
- Digital-subtraction angiography: The gold standard
- Contrast-enhanced magnetic resonance angiography: Highly accurate and reliable in identifying >50% stenosis (sensitivity 95%, specificity 97%)
- CT angiography (sensitivity 91%, specificity 91%)
- Duplex ultrasound (sensitivity 88%, specificity 96%) (4)

Diagnostic Procedures/Surgery
- The ankle–brachial index (ABI) is the systolic BP taken by a Doppler at the dorsalis pedis divided by the systolic pressure taken in the brachial artery. Sensitivity 95%, specificity 90%.
- Normal value is minimally ≥1. ABI <0.9 correlates with at ≥50% stenosis of at least 1 vessel (5)[B]:
  - ABI between 0.4 and 0.9 suggests stenosis and correlates with clinical claudication.
  - ABI <0.5 suggests multisegmental arterial stenoses.
  - ABI of <0.3 correlates with probable tissue death and/or rest pain.
- Photoplethysmography is another diagnostic option to evaluate blood pressure in the lower extremities.

DIFFERENTIAL DIAGNOSIS
- Osteoarthritis: Weight-bearing worsens pain.
- Pseudoclaudication: Attributed to spinal cord impingement or spinal stenosis. Relieved by sitting or squatting:
  - Neither pseudoclaudication nor osteoarthritis affects the arterial-brachial index.
- Thromboarterial occlusive disease (Buerger)
- Cystic adventitial disease
- Extraluminal compression (e.g., popliteal artery entrapment syndrome)
- Leriche syndrome: Lower extremity claudication, absence of femoral pulse, impotence, buttock muscle wasting
- Compartment syndrome
- Venous congestion

TREATMENT

- Smoking cessation
- Frequent exercise regimens are a mainstay of therapy:
  – Supervised routines are more effective (6).
  – Consider referral to physical therapy or supervised exercise program to develop structure to patient's exercise pattern
- Recommended exercise regimen:
  – Improve walking distance by 150% over 3–12 months.
  – Recommend treadmill walking until pain elicited (7).
  – Then, briefly rest until symptoms subside, then resume.
  – Goal is 30–60 minutes per day, minimally 3 days per week for 3 months.

MEDICATION
First Line
- Antiplatelet therapy is recommended lifelong in patients with symptomatic disease (8):
  – Aspirin should be considered for all patients. It has no proven benefit for decreasing lower extremity claudication, but may be beneficial in reducing sequelae due to atherosclerotic disease:
    ○ Dose: Aspirin 80–325 mg PO/day
  – Clopidogrel (Plavix) can be used if aspirin is not tolerated. There is no evidence supporting dual antiplatelet therapy (8).
  – Ticlopidine (Ticlid) is effective in reducing mortality, but due to its side effect profile, is not preferred.
- Cilostazol (Pletal) improves maximal and pain-free walking distance (9).
- Recommended for moderate to severe disabling intermittent claudication that is unresponsive to exercise regimens in patients who are not candidates for surgical or percutaneous intervention (8):
  – Dose: 100 mg PO b.i.d.
  – Precautions: Headache occurs in >30% of patients taking cilostazol.
  – Contraindication: Patients with symptoms of congestive heart failure.
  – Significant possible drug-drug interactions: Use caution when combining with drugs metabolized by the cytochrome-P450 3A4 isoenzyme.
- HMG-CoA reductase inhibitor with a low-density lipoprotein goal of ≤100 mg/dL (≤70 for high-risk patients) (7)
- Pentoxifylline 400 mg t.i.d. with meals; reduces symptoms by 25% but no more effectively than placebo, so is only used if exercise and other measures have failed.

Second Line
- Pentoxifylline (Trental): There is conflicting evidence regarding its efficacy in improving walking distance. 400mg PO t.i.d. (8)
- Arginine: 3g PO t.i.d.
- Propionyl levocarnitine: 1–2 g PO b.i.d.
- Ginkgo biloba: 120–160 mg PO b.i.d.
- Vitamin E: 50 mg PO per day (10)
- Naftidrofuryl (11)
- Prostaglandin analogues and stimulants continue to be investigated (12).

ADDITIONAL TREATMENT
General Measures
- Eliminate risk factors whenever possible.
- Smoking cessation is critical to success and is the single most important intervention.
- Optimize diet with low-fat and low-cholesterol regimen.
- Exercise is essential to management, significantly improving maximal walking time, distance to claudication, and calf blood flow.

COMPLEMENTARY AND ALTERNATIVE MEDICINE
Naftidrofuryl (unavailable in US; Cochrane review found clinical benefit to its use)

SURGERY/OTHER PROCEDURES
- Revascularization is reserved for a minority of patients:
  – Indications:
    ○ Severe claudication in which symptoms limit lifestyle or job performance
    ○ Unresponsive to exercise and medical management
- Angioplasty is preferred for patients with favorable anatomic features and younger patients (≤50 years old).
- Arterial-bypass surgery is recommended for older patients (≥50 years old) or with less certain anatomical features.
- Stenting modalities continue to be investigated (7).

 ONGOING CARE

FOLLOW-UP RECOMMENDATIONS
- Recommend continued, frequent exercise.
- Consider referral to vascular surgeon or cardiologist for follow-up of unresponsive or advanced cases.
- Peripheral noninvasive vascular studies every 6 months.
- If findings suggest condition of patient is worsening, this would be indication for surgery.

DIET
Cardiovascular diet (low-fat, low-cholesterol) is recommended.

PATIENT EDUCATION
- Encourage an exercise program, smoking cessation, healthy dietary choices, management of blood glucose levels in diabetic patients, and blood-pressure control.
- Reassurance that most patients improve walking distance over time and symptoms generally improve

PROGNOSIS
- Patients should experience gradual improvement with an intense walking program, appropriate medical therapy, as well as modification of risk factors.
- Disease progression may include rest pain, tissue loss, and gangrene.
- Select patients may require revascularization.

COMPLICATIONS
- Severe cases can result in tissue loss and gangrene, possibly requiring amputation of affected area.
- Largely affects patients with advanced, uncontrolled diabetes mellitus.
- Risk of venous thrombosis is increased due to the low-flow state indicated by claudication.

REFERENCES
1. Hiatt WR. The U.S. experience with cilostazol in treating intermittent claudication. *Atherosclerosis Suppl*. 2006;6:21–31.
2. Leng GC, Fowkes FG. The Edinburgh Claudication Questionnaire: an improved version of the WHO/Rose Questionnaire for use in epidemiological surveys. *J Clin Epidemiol*. 1992;45:1101–9.
3. Khan NA, Rahim SA, Anand SS et al. Does the clinical examination predict lower extremity peripheral arterial disease? *JAMA*. 2006;295:536–46.
4. Collins R, Burch J, Cranny G et al. Duplex ultrasonography, magnetic resonance angiography, and computed tomography angiography for diagnosis and assessment of symptomatic, lower limb peripheral arterial disease: systematic review. *BMJ*. 2007;334:1257.
5. Feringa HHH et al. The long-term prognostic value of the resting and postexercise ankle brachial index. *Arch Int Med*. 2006;166:529–35.
6. Watson L, Ellis B, Leng GC. Exercise for intermittent claudication. *Cochrane Database Syst Rev*. 2008:CD000990.
7. White C. Clinical practice. Intermittent claudication. *N Engl J Med*. 2007;356:1241–50.
8. Sobel M, Verhaeghe R. Antithrombotic therapy for peripheral artery occlusive disease: American College of Chest Physicians Evidence-Based Clinical Practice Guidelines (8th Edition). *Chest*. 2008;133:815S–843S.
9. Robless P, Mikhailidis DP, Stansby GP. Cilostazol for peripheral arterial disease. *Cochrane Database Syst Rev*. 2008:CD003748.
10. Kleijnen J, Mackerras D. Vitamin E for intermittent claudication. *Cochrane Database Syst Rev*. 2000: CD000987.
11. De Backer T, Vander Stichele R, Lehert P et al. Naftidrofuryl for intermittent claudication: meta-analysis based on individual patient data. *BMJ*. 2009;338:b603.
12. Reiter M, Bucek RA, Stümpflen A, et al. Prostanoids for intermittent claudication. *Cochrane Database Syst Rev*. 2004:CD000986.

 CODES

ICD9
- 440.21 Atherosclerosis of native arteries of the extremities with intermittent claudication
- 443.9 Peripheral vascular disease, unspecified

CLINICAL PEARLS
- Mainstay of treatment involves gradual increase in exercise in supervised setting and maximizing reduction of CHD risk factors: Smoking cessation, LDL reduction, glucose control in diabetes, etc.
- Available revascularization techniques include catheter-based balloon dilation with or without luminal stenting, endarterectomy, arterial reconstruction with an anatomically placed bypass graft, or with an extra-anatomically placed bypass prosthesis. Selection is based on patient risk, surgeon experience, and pattern of occlusions.
- Indications for revascularization are critical limb ischemia, patients with repeated atheroembolism, or severe lifestyle-limiting symptoms.

C

CLOSTRIDIUM DIFFICILE INFECTION

Aman D. Sabharwal, MD
Nathan T. Connell, MD

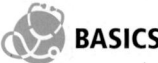 **BASICS**

DESCRIPTION
- *Clostridium difficile* is a gram-positive, spore-forming anaerobic bacillus.
- Infection caused by *C. difficile* is usually linked to broad-spectrum antibiotic use.
- Severity of infection can range from diarrhea to colitis to perforation to death.
- System(s) affected: GI
- Synonyms(s): *C. difficile*–associated disease or diarrhea (CDAD); antibiotic-associated diarrhea; *C. diff*

EPIDEMIOLOGY
Incidence
- Most cases of *C. difficile* infection occur in hospitals or long-term care facilities at a rate of 25–80 per 100,000 occupied bed-days (1).
- For outpatient setting, the rate is ~7.7 cases per 100,000 person-years.

Prevalence
- *C. difficile* causes ~25% of all cases of antibiotic-associated diarrhea.
- C. *difficile* infections account for ~25% of all nosocomial antibiotic associated infections (1).

RISK FACTORS
- Exposure to all antimicrobial agents (except aminoglycosides) is associated with *C. difficile* infection.
- Patients in health care settings have a higher risk of developing *C. difficile* infection.
- Age >65 years
- Duration of stay in the hospital
- Nasogastric intubation
- Previous *C. difficile* infection
- Severe primary illness
- Controversial: Use of anti-ulcer medications
- Chemotherapy
- Perioperative antibiotic prophylaxis:
  – Even if patients receive no other antibiotics other than perioperative prophylaxis, they are still at risk for developing *C. difficile* infection (2).

Geriatric Considerations
C. difficile is the most common cause of acute diarrheal illness in long-term care facilities. These patients are older and receive more antibiotics and antacids than the general public; thus, it is difficult to determine which factors contribute most to this increased risk.

Pediatric Considerations
Neonates have a higher rate of *C. difficile* colonization (25–80%), yet they are much less likely to be symptomatic than adults, possibly due to immature toxin receptors.

Genetics
No known genetic factors

GENERAL PREVENTION
- Implementation of a comprehensive infection-control program has resulted in a decrease in the incidence of *C. difficile* infection
- Disinfection with hypochlorite solution
- Handwashing with soap and water:
  – Alcohol-based hand gels do not kill spores.
- Reduction in the use of rectal thermometers
- Reduction of unnecessary broad-spectrum antibiotic use
- Isolation of infected patients and use of contact precautions
- Education of hospital personnel

PATHOPHYSIOLOGY
- *C. difficile* can thrive in the colon and cause infection if disruption of the normal flora and ingestion of *C. difficile* occur.
- *C. difficile* spores can survive for months.
- Host factors such as the presence of antibodies to *C. difficile* toxins can reduce the severity and prevent recurrences of infection.
- *C. difficile* produces toxins that are essential for disease to occur:
  – Toxins A (enterotoxin) and B (cytotoxin) attract neutrophils and monocytes, and degrade colonic epithelial cells, causing colitis, pseudomembrane colitis, and watery diarrhea.
  – BI/NAP1 strain of *C. difficile* has been shown to produce more virulent characteristics (3).
  – Binary toxin produces a virulent form of disease (different from toxin A or B); this may result in increased rates of colectomies and mortality.
  – Binary toxin has been identified in ~6% of clinical *C. difficile* isolates obtained in the US and Europe.

ETIOLOGY
- Altered colonic mucosa
- *C. difficile* spore ingestion
- Active toxin release

 DIAGNOSIS

HISTORY
- Recent antibiotic use (especially broad-spectrum fluoroquinolones and cephalosporins)
- Diarrhea that is watery, foul-smelling
- Fever (typically <10%)
- Recent hospitalizations or stay at nursing facility

PHYSICAL EXAM
- Mild disease:
  – Mild lower abdominal cramping pain
- Moderate disease:
  – Fever
  – Nausea and vomiting
- Severe disease:
  – Peritonitis
  – Ileus
  – Hypovolemia
- Mild abdominal tenderness to peritonitis, depending on severity
- Hypovolemia

DIAGNOSTIC TESTS & INTERPRETATION
Markers of severe or fulminant infection include hypotension, sepsis, markedly elevated white blood cell count, and bandemia. Other signs include obstruction, perforation, toxic megacolon, colonic-wall thickening, or ascites.

Lab
- ELISA for toxins:
  – Available within several hours
  – Sensitivity 63–99%
  – Specificity 75–100%
  – Some labs only test for toxin A, others test for A and B.
- Tissue culture cytotoxicity assay:
  – Takes 24–48 hours for results; labor-intensive
  – Sensitivity 67–100%
  – Specificity 85–100%
- Microbiology culture:
  – Nontoxin-producing strains also detected
  – Mostly used to evaluate epidemiology studies
- PCR-based testing is currently research-based.
- Repeat testing during the same episode of diarrhea is discouraged (3).

Imaging
- Plain films may show thumbprinting and colonic distension.
- CT radiography may show mucosal wall thickening, thickened colonic wall, and pericolonic inflammation.

Diagnostic Procedures/Surgery
- Endoscopy can be used to evaluate for pseudomembranes and exclude other conditions.
- Flexible sigmoidoscopy may miss 15–20% of pseudomembranes that may be more proximal in the colon.
- Colonoscopy evaluates the entire colon: Used when diagnosis is in doubt or severity demands rapid diagnosis

Pathological Findings
Pseudomembranes consist of inflammatory and cellular debris that forms visible exudates that can obscure the underlying mucosa. These exudates have a yellow to grayish color.

DIFFERENTIAL DIAGNOSIS
- Food poisoning
- Enteric infections
- Antibiotic-associated diarrhea

 TREATMENT

MEDICATION
If clinically indicated (moderate-to-severe diarrhea, fever, significant leukocytosis, abdominal pain, etc.), consider antimicrobial against *C. difficile* (4)[A].

First Line
- Metronidazole is the drug of choice for mild-to-moderate *C. difficile* infection due to low cost and prevention of the emergence of vancomycin-resistant organisms (3)[A]:
  – 500 mg p.o. 3 times a day for 10–14 days
  – If patient is unable to take oral medications, then IV metronidazole or intraluminal vancomycin can be used.

- Vancomycin is first-line therapy in patients with severe or fulminant *C. difficile* infection. Vancomycin is also first-line therapy for the 3rd and subsequent relapse in fewer than 6 months (3):
  - 125 mg p.o. 4 times a day for 10–14 days
  - Vancomycin retention enema if unable to take p.o. or there is evidence of poor GI motility.
- For the first recurrence of *C. difficile* infection, the treatment is the same as the initial treatment, although current severity of illness should be taken into account. For subsequent relapses, use oral vancomycin as treatment in a pulse-taper format. Consultation with an infectious diseases specialist is recommended.

ALERT
When using vancomycin for treatment of *C. difficile* infection, oral or rectal formulations must be used since IV formulations are not excreted into the colonic lumen.

Second Line
- Vancomycin (4,5)[A]:
  - 125 mg p.o. 4 times a day for 10–14 days
  - Indicated for patients who cannot tolerate or have failed metronidazole therapy, and for those who are pregnant
- Immunoglobulin IV (IVIG) has been used in special cases.

ADDITIONAL TREATMENT
General Measures
- Avoid antimotility agents and opiates (4,6)[A].
- Avoid use of proton pump inhibitors (PPIs) unless absolutely necessary, as they have been associated with a 42% increased risk of recurrence if used concurrently with treatment for *C. difficile* colitis (7).

COMPLEMENTARY AND ALTERNATIVE MEDICINE
- Probiotics (*Lactobacilli* and *Saccharomyces)* have shown conflicting data, and have been associated with increased bacteremia (3):
  - Use oral *Lactobacilli* with caution if also using vancomycin, since the latter antibiotic is active against *Lactobacilli*.
- Fecal transplant in severe or relapsing disease

SURGERY/OTHER PROCEDURES
If *C. difficile* infection progresses to toxic megacolon, peritonitis, or sepsis after initiation of treatment, other therapeutic options should be explored, including a surgical consult (4,5)[A].

IN-PATIENT CONSIDERATIONS
Initial Stabilization
- Current nonessential antibiotic therapy should be discontinued if possible (3,4)[A].
- Institute supportive therapy with fluids and electrolytes if needed (3,4)[A].

Admission Criteria
- Hypovolemia
- Comorbid conditions
- Inability to keep up with enteric losses
- Hematochezia
- Electrolyte disturbances

IV Fluids
- Infuse to keep patient euvolemic
- Once over acute phase, patient can be weaned off IV fluids.

Nursing
See General Prevention.

Discharge Criteria
- Improved diarrhea severity and frequency
- Tolerating both medications and p.o.
- Afebrile

ONGOING CARE

FOLLOW-UP RECOMMENDATIONS
- Many patients can be treated as outpatients.
- Bed rest during acute phase

Patient Monitoring
- Relapses of colitis will occur in 15–30%.
- Relapses typically occur 2–10 days after discontinuation of antibiotics.
- Repeat treatment with 14-day course of antibiotics will result in 40% cure rate.
- The management of the first relapse following therapy for *C. difficile* diarrhea and colitis does not differ substantially from treatment of the initial episode.
- Administration of vancomycin or metronidazole every other day or every 3rd day allows spores to germinate on the off days and then be killed when the antibiotics are taken again.
- For multiple relapses, some success has been reported with the following oral vancomycin taper regimen:
  - Week 1: 125 mg q.i.d.
  - Week 2: 125 mg b.i.d.
  - Week 3: 125 mg daily
  - Week 4: 125 mg every other day
  - Weeks 5 and 6: 125 mg every 3 days
- If continued infection, consider pulse therapy with vancomycin in consultation with an infectious disease specialist.

DIET
No restrictions; as tolerated

PATIENT EDUCATION
Patients should be kept informed of the progress of disease and taught to practice good hygiene (i.e., handwashing).

PROGNOSIS
- Majority of patients will improve with conservative management and antibiotics
- 1–3% of patients will develop severe colitis requiring emergency colectomy.

REFERENCES
1. McDonald LC, Owings M, Jernigan DB. Clostridium difficile infection in patients discharged from US short-stay hospitals, 1996–2003. *Emerg Infect Dis*. 2006;12:409–15.
2. Carignan A, Allard C, Pépin J, et al. Risk of Clostridium difficile infection after perioperative antibacterial prophylaxis before and during an outbreak of infection due to a hypervirulent strain. *Clin Infect Dis*. 2008;46:1838–43.
3. Cohen SH, Gerding DN, Johnson S, Kelly CP, Loo VG, McDonald LC, Pepin J, Wilcox MH et al. Clinical practice guidelines for Clostridium difficile infection in adults: 2010 update by the society for healthcare epidemiology of America (SHEA) and the infectious diseases society of America (IDSA). *Infect Control Hosp Epidemiol*. 2010;31:431–55.
4. Bartlett JG. Narrative review: the new epidemic of Clostridium difficile-associated enteric disease. *Ann Intern Med*. 2006;145:758–64.
5. McFarland LV. Alternative treatments for *Clostridium difficile* disease: What really works? *J Med Micro*. 2005;54:101–11.
6. Koo HL, Koo DC, Musher DM, et al. Antimotility agents for the treatment of Clostridium difficile diarrhea and colitis. *Clin Infect Dis*. 2009;48: 598–605.
7. Linsky A, Gupta K, Lawler EV, Fonda JR, Hermos JA et al. Proton pump inhibitors and risk for recurrent Clostridium difficile infection. *Arch Intern Med*. 2010;170:772–8.

ADDITIONAL READING

McFarland LV. Meta-analysis of probiotics for the prevention of antibiotic associated diarrhea and the treatment of Clostridium difficile disease. *Am J Gastroenterol*. 2006;101:812–22.

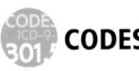

CODES

ICD9
008.45 Intestinal infection due to clostridium difficile

CLINICAL PEARLS

- Treatment of asymptomatic patients is not recommended.
- Therapeutic response should be based on clinical signs and symptoms. Patients may shed organism or toxin for weeks after treatment.

COLIC, INFANTILE

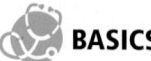

Daniel T. Lee, MD
Leanne Zakrzewski, MD

BASICS

DESCRIPTION
- Colic is defined as excessive crying in an otherwise healthy baby.
- A commonly used criteria is the Wessel criteria, or the "rule of 3": Crying lasts for >3 hours a day, >3 days a week, and persists >3 weeks.
- Many clinicians no longer use the criterion of persistence for >3 weeks because few parents or clinicians will wait that long before evaluation or intervention.
- Some clinicians feel that colic represents the extreme end of the spectrum of normal crying, whereas most feel that colic is a distinct clinical entity.

EPIDEMIOLOGY
Incidence
- Predominant age: Between 2 weeks and 4 months of age
- Predominant sex: Male = Female.

Prevalence
- Probably between 10% and 25% of infants
- Range is somewhere between 8% and 40% of infants

Pediatric Considerations
This is a problem during infancy.

RISK FACTORS
Physiologic predisposition in infant, but no definitive risk factors have been established.

GENERAL PREVENTION
Colic is generally not preventable.

ETIOLOGY
The cause is unknown. Factors that may play a role include
- Infant gastroesophageal reflux disease
- Allergy to cow's milk, soy milk, or breast milk protein
- Fruit juice intolerance
- Swallowing air during the process of crying, feeding, or sucking
- Overfeeding or feeding too quickly; underfeeding also has been proposed.
- Inadequate burping after feeding
- Family tension
- Parental anxiety, depression, and/or fatigue
- Parent-infant interaction mismatch
- Baby's inability to console itself when dealing with stimuli
- Increased gut hormone motilin, causing hyperperistalsis
- Tobacco smoke exposure
- Disorder of impaired synchronization between infant arousal and environment (1)[C]

DIAGNOSIS

HISTORY
- Evaluation for Wessel criteria: Crying lasts for >3 hours per day, >3 days per week, and persists >3 weeks
- The colicky episodes may have a clear beginning and end.
- The crying is generally spontaneous, without preceding events triggering the episodes.
- The crying is typically different from normal crying. Colicky crying may be louder, more turbulent, variable in pitch, and appear more like screaming.
- The infant may be difficult to soothe or console regardless of how the parents try to help.
- The infant acts normally when not colicky.
- Assess the support system of caregivers and families, including coping skills.

PHYSICAL EXAM
- A comprehensive physical exam is normal.
- Since excessive crying may be a risk factor for shaken baby syndrome or other forms of child abuse (2)[B], be sure to examine the child carefully for signs of shaken baby syndrome or other forms of child abuse.

DIAGNOSTIC TESTS & INTERPRETATION
Diagnostic Procedures/Surgery
A thorough history and physical examination should be performed to rule out other causes. Otherwise, no diagnostic procedures or surgery is indicated.

DIFFERENTIAL DIAGNOSIS
Any organic cause for excessive or qualitatively different crying in infants such as
- Infections such as meningitis, sepsis, otitis media, or urinary tract infection
- GI issues such as gastroesophageal reflux, intussusception, lactose intolerance, constipation, anal fissure, or strangulated hernia
- Trauma such as foreign bodies, corneal abrasion, occult fracture, digit or penile hair tourniquet, or child abuse

TREATMENT

MEDICATION
- Dicyclomine (Bentyl) has been proven beneficial, but the potential serious adverse effects such as apnea, seizures, and syncope have precluded its use. Further, the manufacturer has made the medication contraindicated for infants <6 months of age (3,4)[B].
- Simethicone has not been shown to be beneficial (3,4)[B].

ADDITIONAL TREATMENT
General Measures
- Soothe by holding and rocking the baby (3)[C].
- Use pacifier (3)[C].
- Use of gentle rhythmic motion (e.g., strollers, infant swings, car rides) (3)[C].
- Place near "white noise" (e.g., vacuum cleaner, clothes dryer, white noise machine) (3)[C].
- Crib vibrators or car-ride simulators have not proven to be helpful (3,5)[B].
- Increased carrying or use of infant carrier did not improve colic (3,5)[B].
- Employ the "5 S's" (need to be done concurrently):
  - Swaddling: Tight wrapping with blanket; may be especially beneficial in infants <8 weeks of age (6)[B]
  - Side/stomach: Laying baby on side or stomach
  - Shushing: Loud white noise
  - Swinging: Rhythmic, jiggly motion
  - Sucking: Sucking on anything (e.g., nipple, finger, pacifier) (3)[C]

Issues for Referral

Excessive vomiting, poor weight gain, recurrent respiratory diseases, or bloody stools should prompt referral to a specialist.

COMPLEMENTARY AND ALTERNATIVE MEDICINE

- Herbal teas and supplements may help but are not recommended because of limited, inconclusive evidence. For example,
  - One study concluded that herbal teas containing mixtures of chamomile, vervain, licorice, fennel, and balm-mint used up to t.i.d. may be beneficial (4)[B]. However, the study used dosages of up to 150 cc t.i.d., raising clinical concerns that this dosage may impair needed milk consumption in infants and may be impractical to administer. Additionally, preparations used in the study may not be commercially available in the US.
  - A second double-blind, randomized trial of 0.1% fennel seed oil emulsion versus placebo demonstrated a decrease in colic symptoms according to the Wessel criteria. However, this preparation of fennel seed oil is not commercially available in the US, and the long-term health effects are unknown (7).
- A home-based intervention focusing on reducing infant stimulation and synchronizing infant sleep-wake cycles with the environment, as well as parental support, was effective (1)[B].
- Use of music may help (8,9)[C].
- Chiropractic treatment has shown no benefit over placebo (3)[C].
- Infant massage has not been shown to be helpful (3)[B].

 ONGOING CARE

FOLLOW-UP RECOMMENDATIONS

Frequent outpatient visits as needed for parental reassurance, education, and monitoring and to ensure the health of the infant and parents

Patient Monitoring

Follow for proper feeding, growth, and development.

DIET

- If breast-feeding:
  - Continue breast-feeding. Switching to formula probably will not help (3)[C].
  - Possible therapeutic benefit from eliminating milk products, eggs, wheat, and nuts from the diet of breast-feeding mothers (3,5)[B].
  - Along with eliminating the preceding foods from the maternal diet, removing soy, nuts, and fish may be beneficial (10)[C].
  - Probiotics (Lactobacillus reuteri) have been shown to be beneficial in a small study of breast-fed infants (11).

- If formula feeding:
  - Feeding the infant in a vertical position using a curved bottle or bottle with collapsible bag may help to reduce air swallowing.
  - Consider a 1-week trial of hypoallergenic formulas, such as whey hydrolysate (e.g., Good Start) or casein hydrolysate (e.g., Alimentum, Nutramigen, Pregestimil) (4,5)[B].
  - American Academy of Pediatrics concluded that there is no proven role for soy formula in the treatment of colic (12)[C].
  - Adding fiber to formula has not been shown to be helpful (5,8)[B].
- Supplementing with sucrose solution may be helpful, but the effect may be short-lived (<1 h) (4,5)[B].
- Use of lactase enzymes in formula or breast milk or given directly to the infant has no therapeutic benefit (5)[B].

PATIENT EDUCATION

- Reassure parents that colic is not the result of bad parenting, and advise parents about having proper rest breaks, adequate sleep, and help in caring for the infant.
- Explain spectrum of crying behavior.
- Avoid overfeeding or underfeeding.
- Instruct in better feeding techniques such as improved bottles (low air, curved) and sufficient burping after feeding.
- Colic: What You Should Know at www.aafp.org/afp/2004/0815/p741.html

PROGNOSIS

- Usually subsides by 3–6 months of age
- Despite apparent abdominal pain, colicky infants eat well and gain weight normally.
- A handful of studies indicate that temper tantrums may be more common among formerly colicky infants, as studied in toddlers up to 4 years of age (13,14).
- Colic has no bearing on the baby's intelligence or future development.

COMPLICATIONS

Colic is self-limiting and does not result in lasting effects to infant or maternal mental health (15)[C].

REFERENCES

1. Keefe MR, Lobo ML, Froese-Fretz A, et al. Effectiveness of an intervention for colic. Clin Pediatr (Phila). 2006;45:123–33.
2. Reijneveld SA, van der Wal MF, Brugman E, et al. Infant crying and abuse. Lancet. 2004;364: 1340–2.
3. Roberts DM, Ostapchuk M, O'Brien JG. Infantile colic. Am Fam Physician. 2004;70:735–40.
4. Wade S, Kilgour T. Extracts from "clinical evidence": Infantile colic. BMJ. 2001;323: 437–40.
5. Garrison MM, Christakis DA. A systematic review of treatments for infant colic. Pediatrics. 2000; 106:184–90.
6. van Sleuwen BE, L'hoir MP, Engelberts AC, et al. Comparison of behavior modification with and without swaddling as interventions for excessive crying. J Pediatr. 2006;149:512–7.
7. Alexandrovich I, Rakovitskaya O, Kolmo E, Sidorova T, Shushunov S et al. The effect of fennel (Foeniculum Vulgare) seed oil emulsion in infantile colic: a randomized, placebo-controlled study. Altern Ther Health Med. 58–61.
8. Clemons RM. Issues in newborn care. Prim Care. 2000;27:251–67.
9. McCollough M, Sharieff GQ. Common complaints in the first 30 days of life. Emerg Med Clin North Am. 2002;20:27–48, v.
10. Hill DJ, Roy N, Heine RG, et al. Effect of a low-allergen maternal diet on colic among breastfed infants: a randomized, controlled trial. Pediatrics. 2005;116:e709–15.
11. Savino F, Pelle E, Palumeri E, et al. Lactobacillus reuteri (American Type Culture Collection Strain 55730) versus simethicone in the treatment of infantile colic: a prospective randomized study. Pediatrics. 2007;119:e124–30.
12. O'Connor NR. Infant formula. Am Fam Physician. 2009;79:565–70.
13. Canivet C, Jakobsson I, Hagander B et al. Infantile colic. Follow-up at four years of age: still more "emotional". Acta Paediatr. 2000;89:13–7.
14. Rautava P, Lehtonen L, Helenius H, Sillanpää M et al. Infantile colic: child and family three years later. Pediatrics. 1995;96:43–7.
15. Clifford TJ, Campbell MK, Speechley KN, et al. Sequelae of infant colic: evidence of transient infant distress and absence of lasting effects on maternal mental health. Arch Pediatr Adolesc Med. 2002;156:1183–8.

 CODES

ICD9
789.7 Colic

CLINICAL PEARLS

- Colic is defined as excessive crying in an otherwise healthy baby.
- Excessive crying may be a risk factor for shaken baby syndrome or other forms of child abuse.
- Provide advice, support, and reassurance to parents (3)[B].
- Prevent caregiver burnout by advising parents to get proper rest breaks, sleep, and help in caring for the infant.

COLONIC POLYPS

Macario C. Corpuz, Jr., MD
Pamela Lynn Grimaldi, DO

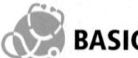 **BASICS**

DESCRIPTION

- A colonic polyp is an intraluminal outgrowth arising from the large intestinal epithelial lining, which is usually benign. The potential for malignant transformation necessitates close evaluation and monitoring. (See Colorectal Malignancy.)
- 3 types:
  – Adenomatous: May become malignant:
    ○ Villous: Polyps tend to be larger, most likely to become malignant (10%)
    ○ Tubular (75%)
    ○ Tubulovillous (15%)
  – Hyperplastic: Rarely become malignant
  – Inflammatory: No malignant potential

EPIDEMIOLOGY

- Varies considerably worldwide. Industrialized countries are generally at greater risk compared to the rest of the world.
- Age is an important determinant in the US and other high-risk countries.
- Adenomas more common in men than women

Incidence

- Estimated 5% of the US population
- ~20% of middle-aged and older adults
- 50% seen in ≥50 years

Prevalence

Average prevalence of 25% before age 40 to as high as 55% at age 80

RISK FACTORS

- Advancing age
- Male
- Obesity

- Family history of polyposis, polyps, or colorectal cancer (CRC)
- Inflammatory bowel disease
- Current cigarette smoking
- Excessive alcohol intake: >8 drinks of beer or spirits a week (1)
- Sedentary lifestyle

Genetics

May occur in the setting of genetic syndromes that are associated with gene mutations

GENERAL PREVENTION

- Diet: High-fiber diet has been a controversial risk. Two recent studies stressed that doubling fiber intake can significantly reduce colorectal cancer risk (2,3).
- Avoid smoking.
- Limit alcohol intake.
- Calcium supplement: Shown reduction of colorectal adenoma recurrence (4)
- Vitamin D, folic acid, vitamin B6
- Aspirin. Three randomized controlled trials (RCT) revealed that ASA caused significant reduction in the recurrence of sporadic adenomatous polyps after 1 to 3 years while short-term studies support regression of colorectal adenomas in FAP (5).

PATHOPHYSIOLOGY

- Adenomatous polyps: Formed from abnormal proliferation and from dysplasia
- Nonadenomatous polyps: Result from abnormal mucosal maturation, inflammation, or architecture

ETIOLOGY

Unknown. May be related to environmental and genetic factors.

COMMONLY ASSOCIATED CONDITIONS

Associated with several hereditary disorders:

- Familial adenomatous polyposis (FAP)
- Peutz-Jeghers syndrome
- Gardner syndrome
- Hereditary nonpolyposis colon cancer (HNPCC)

 DIAGNOSIS

HISTORY

- Asymptomatic
- Hematochezia
- Melena
- Diarrhea or constipation
- Anemia
- Fatigue
- Abdominal pain

PHYSICAL EXAM

- Usually normal
- Rectal lesions may be felt by digital examination.

DIAGNOSTIC TESTS & INTERPRETATION

Lab

Initial lab tests

- Complete blood count (CBC): Anemia
- Electrolyte abnormalities: In villous adenoma

Diagnostic Procedures/Surgery

- Colonoscopy (6): Standard of goal. Most sensitive test available but its sensitivity is a concern. Chromoscopy enhances the detection of neoplastic lesions in the colon and the rectum (7).
- Chromoscopy: Studies are examining narrow-band imaging for histologic differentiation between adenomatous and hyperplastic polyps (7,8).
- CT colonography (formerly known "Virtual colonoscopy")
- Sigmoidoscopy
- Air-contrast barium enema: Misses small lesions
- Fecal occult blood test (FOBT): Many false positive results
- Fecal DNA testing
- Some polyps are more likely to become malignant, hence, they require histopathologic evaluation.

Pathological Findings

- Villous adenoma:
  - Gross: Velvety, multiple-frond projections
  - Micro: Glands proliferate in fingerlike projections, malignant degenerations
- Tubular adenoma:
  - Gross: Smooth, firm, pink surface; microlobulated; fissures; pedunculated
  - Glands proliferate in tubular fashion, nuclei elongated, hyperchromatic

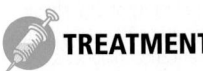 ## TREATMENT

SURGERY/OTHER PROCEDURES

- Endoscopic polypectomy: Major risks include perforation and bleeding
- Colonic resection: For multiple intestinal polyps associated with FAP

 ## ONGOING CARE

FOLLOW-UP RECOMMENDATIONS

Benign polyps should have follow-up colonoscopy every 3–5 years.

Patient Monitoring

Offer CRC screening for average risk patients beginning at age 50, earlier for at-risk patients. Most guidelines recommend to stop screening if life expectancy is less than 10 years.

DIET

Calcium supplementation might contribute a moderate degree to the prevention of colorectal adenomatous polyps (4).

PROGNOSIS

- Curable with polypectomy
- Projection estimates suggested that 50% of postpolypectomy patients will have a recurrence within 7.6 years; hence, need follow-up (9).

- Adenomatous polyps may undergo malignant transformation if not removed.
- Multiple polyps are particularly at increased risk of developing colorectal cancer.

COMPLICATIONS

Perforation with colonoscopy is rare.

REFERENCES

1. Anderson JC, Alpern Z, Sethi G, et al. Prevalence and risk of colorectal neoplasia in consumers of alcohol in a screening population. *Am J Gastroenterol.* 2005;100:2049–55.
2. Asano TK, McLeod RS. Dietary fibre for the prevention of colorectal adenomas and carcinomas. *Cochrane Database of Systematic Reviews.* 2002, Issue 1. Art. No.: CD003430. DOI:10.1002/14651858.CD003430.
3. Peters, Ulrike, et al. "Dietary fibre and colorectal adenoma in a colorectal cancer early detection programme." *Lancet.* 361.9368 (2003):1491–5.
4. Weingarten MA, Zalmanovici A, Yaphe J. Dietary calcium supplementation for preventing colorectal cancer and adenomatous polyps. *Cochrane Database Syst Rev.* 2008:CD003548.
5. Asano T, McLeod R. Non steroidal anti-inflammatory drugs (NSAID) and aspirin for preventing colorectal adenomas and carcinomas *Cochrane Database of Systematic Reviews.* 2010;2:CD004079.
6. Kim DH, Pickhardt PJ, Taylor AJ, et al. CT colonography versus colonoscopy for the detection of advanced neoplasia. *N Engl J Med.* 2007;357:1403–12.
7. Brown SR, et al. Chromoscopy versus conventional endoscopy for the detection of polyps in the colon and rectum. *Cochrane Database Syst Rev.* 2007;4:CD006439. DOI:10.1002/14651858.CD006439.pub2.
8. Rastogi, Amit, et al. "Recognition of surface mucosal and vascular patterns of colon polyps by using narrow-band imaging: interobserver and intraobserver agreement and prediction of polyp histology." *Gastrointestinal endoscopy.* 2009;69(Suppl 3):716–22.
9. Yood, Marianne Ulcickas, et al. "Colon polyp recurrence in a managed care population." *Archives of internal medicine.* 163.4 (2003):422–6.

ADDITIONAL READING

- Elwood PC, Gallagher AM, Duthie GG, et al. Aspirin, salicylates, and cancer. *Lancet.* 2009;373:1301–9.
- Kumar D, et al. *Pathologic Basis of Disease,* 7th ed. 2005;856–870.
- Larsen IK, Grotmol T, Almendingen K, et al. Lifestyle as a predictor for colonic neoplasia in asymptomatic individuals. *BMC Gastroenterol.* 2006;6:5.
- Seong-Eun K, et al. An association between obesity and the prevalence of colonic adenoma according to age and gender. *J Gastroenterol.* 2007;42(8).

See Also (Topic, Algorithm, Electronic Media Element)

Algorithm: Bleeding, GI

 ## CODES

ICD9
211.3 Benign neoplasm of colon

CLINICAL PEARLS

- Villous adenomatous polyps are the "villains" (most likely to become malignant).
- Hyperplastic polyps rarely become cancer.
- Up to 50% of patients who have polyps removed have recurrent polyps.

COLORECTAL CANCER

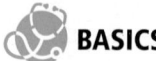

Stephen M. Scott, MD, MPH

BASICS

DESCRIPTION
- Colorectal cancer (CRC) denotes a neoplasm that develops in the colon or rectum.
- CRC is the 3rd leading cause of cancer-related death in the US when men and women are considered separately; however, it is the 2nd leading cause when both sexes are combined.

EPIDEMIOLOGY
Incidence
In 2008, an estimated ~148,810 new cases of CRC were diagnosed, and 49,960 deaths occurred from CRC.

Prevalence
- The overall lifetime risk for developing CRC in the US is about 1 in 19 (5.4%).
- Death rates have been declining due to improved screening, prevention, and treatment.

RISK FACTORS
- Age: > 90% of people diagnosed with CRC are >50.
- Personal history of colorectal polyps:
  – Risks increase with multiple polyps, villous polyps, and larger polyps.
- Personal history of cancer:
  – Rectal cancer has a higher incidence of local recurrence than proximal cancers (20–30% vs. 2–4%)
- History of inflammatory bowel disease:
  – The prevalence of CRC in ulcerative colitis and Crohn disease is about 3%, with a cumulative risk of CRC of 2% at 10 years, 8% at 20 years, and 18% at 30 years (1,2).
- Family history of CRC (although most CRCs occur in people without a family history):
  – The risk doubles in those who have a single 1st-degree relative with a history of CRC.
  – The risk is > double for those who have a history of CRC or polyps in:
    ○ Any 1st-degree relative <60 years old
    ○ ≥2 1st-degree relatives, regardless of age
- Inherited syndromes:
  – Familial adenomatous polyposis (FAP):
    ○ Affected individuals develop hundreds to thousands of polyps in colon and rectum.
    ○ CRC usually present by age 40
    ○ Accounts for about 1% of CRCs
  – Hereditary nonpolyposis colon cancer (HNPCC, also called Lynch syndrome):
    ○ Often develops at a relatively young age
    ○ Lifetime risk of CRC 70–80%
    ○ Accounts for about 3–4% of all CRCs
  – Peutz-Jeghers syndrome:
    ○ Individuals may have freckles (mouth, hands, feet) and large polyps in gastrointestinal (GI) tract.
    ○ Greatly increased risk for CRC and cancers
- Race and ethnicity:
  – African Americans have highest CRC incidence and mortality rates in US.
  – Several different gene mutations have been identified among Ashkenazi Jews.

- Miscellaneous:
  – *Streptococcus bovis* bacteremia is associated with CRC.
  – Patients with acromegaly are at increased risk.

Genetics
- Most result from acquired DNA mutation
- There does not seem to be a single genetic pathway to CRC, although mutations are frequently seen in APC, K-Ras, p53, and SMAD4.
- A small percentage of colon cancers are known to be caused by inherited gene mutations:
  – APC, a tumor suppressor gene, is altered in FAP.
  – Genes encoding DNA repair enzymes implicated in HNPCC: MLH1, MSH2, MSH6, PMS1, PMS2, and others
  – STK11, a tumor suppressor gene, is altered in Peutz-Jeghers syndrome.

GENERAL PREVENTION
- Diets high in fruits and vegetables have been linked with decreased risk; those high in red and processed meats may increase CRC risk.
- People who are physically inactive are at higher risk for CRC.
- Long-term smokers are more likely than nonsmokers to develop and die from CRC.
- CRC has been linked to heavy alcohol consumption; may be related to low folic acid.
- Some studies suggest that vitamin D, calcium, and folate may lower CRC risk.
- NSAIDs may reduce risk in some groups; however, experts do not recommend NSAID use as a cancer prevention strategy in people at average risk for CRC.
- Colon cancer screening is one of the most powerful tools in preventing colon cancer:
  – The United States Preventive Services Task Force (USPSTF) strongly recommends that clinicians screen men and women between the ages of 50 and 75 for CRC (3)[A].
  – Current screening recommendations from the American Cancer Society include completing 1 of the following tests (1)[C]:
    ○ Fecal occult blood testing (FOBT) annually
    ○ Fecal immunochemical test (FIT) annually
    ○ Stool DNA test (sDNA), interval uncertain
    ○ Flexible sigmoidoscopy every 5 years
    ○ Double-contrast barium enema every 5 years
    ○ Colonoscopy every 10 years
    ○ Computed tomography (CT) colonography every 5 years (colonoscopy completed if positive)
  – The USPSTF does not recommend barium enema as a screening test and concludes that the evidence is insufficient to assess the benefits and harms of CT colonography and stool DNA testing as screening modalities for CRC (2)[A].
  – Digital rectal exam (DRE), alone or in combination with a 1-sample FOBT or FIT test, is not an acceptable method for CRC screening.

- Screening in high-risk groups:
  – People with a personal history of polyps need more frequent colonoscopy screening, depending on risk (i.e., 1 or 2 <1 cm polyps with low-grade dysplasia is deemed low-risk and may warrant repeat colonoscopy in 5–10 years; decision is influenced by family history, age, quality of initial colonoscopy, and patient comorbidities).
  – People who have a family history of CRC should begin colonoscopy at age 40 or 10 years younger than the age of relative at cancer diagnosis, whichever is earlier.
  – People with a family history of polyps should begin colonoscopy screening at age 40.
  – People with inflammatory bowel disease (IBD) should have regular surveillance colonoscopy with biopsies to detect dysplasia; guidelines for timing and location vary by professional society, but generally indicate starting surveillance by about 8 years of onset of disease followed by surveillance every 1–2 years.
  – Genetic testing may be appropriate for individuals with a strong family history of CRC or polyps:
    ○ Family members of a person affected by HNPCCC should start colonoscopy screening during their early 20s.
    ○ Individuals who test positive for the gene linked to FAP should start colonoscopy screening in their teens.

PATHOPHYSIOLOGY
The progression from the 1st abnormal cells to the appearance of CRC usually occurs over 10–15 years, a disease characteristic that contributes to the effectiveness of prevention.

ETIOLOGY
Multiple genetic and environmental factors have been linked to the development of CRC.

DIAGNOSIS

HISTORY
- Many patients with CRC are asymptomatic.
- Common presenting symptoms and signs in symptomatic patients include:
  – Abdominal pain or cramping
  – Change in bowel habits (constipation, diarrhea, narrowing of stool)
  – Rectal bleeding, dark stools, or blood in stool
  – Weakness or fatigue
  – Weight loss
  – Anemia
- Other presentations may include symptoms due to the presence of metastatic lesions (lymph nodes, liver, lung, peritoneum), fever of unknown origin, and *S. bovis* or *Clostridium septicum* sepsis.

PHYSICAL EXAM
- Weight loss
- Palpable abdominal mass
- Signs of anemia (i.e., conjunctival pallor)

DIAGNOSTIC TESTS & INTERPRETATION
Lab
Initial lab tests
- Complete blood count (CBC) (to evaluate anemia)
- Liver function (CRC may spread to the liver)

Imaging
Initial approach
- CT scanning to evaluate the presence of metastatic disease
- Chest X-ray (CXR) may be used to evaluate the presence of chest metastases.
- Endoscopic ultrasound (EUS) may be used to evaluate the extent of rectal cancers; endorectal magnetic resonance imaging (MRI) may also provide further detail.
- Intraoperative ultrasound may be used to evaluate solid organs (such as the liver) after tumor resection.

Follow-Up & Special Considerations
- X-ray, CT, and/or MRI examinations may be used to monitor the presence or absence of CRC.
- Positron emission tomography (PET) may be used in some cases to detect metastatic disease.

Diagnostic Procedures/Surgery
- Biopsy is usually performed (most often during colonoscopy) if CRC is suspected.
- CT needle-guided biopsy may be needed to evaluate a suspected tumor or metastasis.

Pathological Findings
- The American Joint Committee on Cancer (AJCC) TNM criteria and Duke's criteria are most often used for staging. TNM staging for CRC is:
  – Stage 0: Limited to the mucosa (*carcinoma in situ* or *intramucosal carcinoma*, Tis, N0, M0)
  – Stage I: Through the muscularis mucosa into the submucosa or muscularis propria; no invasion of lymph nodes or distant sites (T1, N0, M0 or T2, N0, M0)
  – Stage IIA: Invades serosa; no lymph nodes or distant sites (T3, N0, M0)
  – Stage IIB: Through the wall of the colon or rectum and into adjacent tissues or organs; no lymph nodes or distant sites (T4, N0, M0)
  – Stage IIIA: Through mucosa into submucosa or muscularis propria with spread to 1–3 lymph nodes; no distant sites (T1, N1, M0 or T2, N1, M0)
  – Stage IIIB: Through colon or rectum with or without invasion of adjacent tissues or organs plus spread to 1–3 lymph nodes; no distant sites (T3, N1, M0, or T4, N1, M0)
  – Stage IIIC: Through colon or rectum and spread to 4 or more nearby lymph nodes; no distant sites (any T, N2, M0)
  – Stage IV: Any level of invasion with spread to distant site (any T, any N, M1)
- CRCs are graded on a 4-point scale from G1–G4. G1–G2 may be called low-grade and G3–G4 high-grade.

DIFFERENTIAL DIAGNOSIS
- >95% of CRCs are adenocarcinomas.
- Other colonic tumors include carcinoid tumors, lymphomas, and Kaposi's sarcoma in HIV.
- Many conditions can mimic CRC, including other cancers, hemorrhoids, inflammatory bowel disease, infection, and extrinsic masses (i.e., cysts, abscesses).

TREATMENT
MEDICATION
Surgical resection is the primary treatment for colorectal cancer. Chemotherapeutic regimens for metastatic disease may extend overall survival from 6 months to approximately 2 years. Adjuvant chemotherapy is most clearly beneficial for stage III (node-positive) disease, in which reductions of approximately 30% may be achieved in both disease recurrence and overall survival, compared with nontreated controls.

First Line
Chemotherapeutic agents include fluorouracil (5-FU), capecitabine (Xeloda, which is available in oral tablet form and is converted by body to 5-FU), irinotecan (Camptosar), and oxaliplatin (Eloxatin).

Geriatric Considerations
Elderly tend to tolerate CRC chemotherapy fairly well and should be considered when appropriate.

Second Line
Targeted therapies may be used alongside 1st-line agents or by themselves if 1st-line agents are ineffective:
- Bevacizumab (Avastin) is a monoclonal antibody that targets vascular endothelial growth factor (VEGF); inhibits angiogenesis.
- Cetuximab (Erbitux) and panitumumab (Vectibix) are monoclonal antibodies that target epidermal growth factor receptor (EGFR).

COMPLEMENTARY AND ALTERNATIVE MEDICINE
- May serve as an adjunct to treatment for CRC
- 70–75% of cancer survivors report using at least 1 type of complementary and alternative medicine (CAM), and almost all report that the alternative therapy improved their well-being.

SURGERY/OTHER PROCEDURES
- Surgery is the primary treatment for CRC:
  – May involve segmental resection, hemicolectomy, or colectomy, as well as resection of nodes, depending on size and invasion
  – Laparoscopic-assisted colectomy is an emerging option for earlier-stage tumors.
  – Surgery for rectal cancer may include local transanal, low anterior, or abdominoperineal resection, or pelvic exenteration.
- Radiation therapy is most often used for peritoneal or rectal cancers; it is rarely used for metastatic disease due to side effects.

ONGOING CARE
FOLLOW-UP RECOMMENDATIONS
Patient Monitoring
- People with a personal history of proximal cancer (nonrectal) should have follow-up colonoscopy in 1 year, and if normal, in 3 and 5 years subsequently.
- Carcinoembryonic antigen (CEA) and/or CA 19-9 are used to detect recurrence in people treated for CRC. (Note: CEA levels may be elevated in ulcerative colitis, nonmalignant GI tumors, liver disease, lung disease, and in smokers.)

PATIENT EDUCATION
- NCI: What You Need to Know About Cancer of the Colon and Rectum: http://www.cancer.gov/cancertopics/wyntk/colon-and-rectal

- AAFP: Colorectal Cancer Screening (includes Spanish): http://familydoctor.org/online/famdocen/home/common/cancer/risk/556.html

PROGNOSIS
5-year relative survival rate is determined by stage (adjusted for patients dying of other diseases): Stage I: 92%; Stage II: 73%; Stage III: 56%; Stage IV: 8% (2)[A]

COMPLICATIONS
- Colorectal surgery: Pain, deep vein thrombosis (DVT), anastomotic leaks, infection, scarring, bowel obstruction
- Chemotherapy: Hair loss, nausea, vomiting, bruising, fatigue, increased risk for infections
- Radiation therapy: Skin irritation, nausea, rectal pain, incontinence, bladder irritation, fatigue, and sexual problems

REFERENCES
1. American cancer society guidelines for the early detection of cancer. Available at: http://www.cancer.org/docroot/PED/content/PED_2_3X_ACS_Cancer_Detection_Guidelines_36.asp?sitearea=PED. Accessed 9/30/2008.
2. O'Connell JB, Maggard MA, Ko CY. Colon cancer survival rates with the new American Joint Committee on Cancer sixth edition staging. *J Natl Cancer Inst.* 2004;96:1420–5.
3. Screening: Colorectal cancer. Available at: http://www.ahrq.gov/clinic/uspstf/uspscolo.htm. Accessed 9/30/2008.

ADDITIONAL READING
- Konda A, Duffy MC. Surveillance of patients at increased risk of colon cancer: inflammatory bowel disease and other conditions. *Gastroenterol Clin North Am.* 2008;37:191–213, viii.
- National Cancer Institute. At: http://www.cancer.gov/cancertopics/types/colon-and-rectal.
- National Colorectal Cancer Roundtable. At: http://www.nccrt.org.

CODES
ICD9
- 153.9 Malignant neoplasm of colon, unspecified site
- 154.0 Malignant neoplasm of rectosigmoid junction
- 154.1 Malignant neoplasm of rectum

CLINICAL PEARLS
- The USPSTF recommends screening beginning at age 50, and notes that evidence supports several different screening regimens.
- 10% of cases of CRC occur in people younger than age 50. People who have a family history of CRC should begin colonoscopy at age 40, or 10 years younger than the age of relative at cancer diagnosis, whichever is earlier.
- Iron deficiency anemia in the elderly should prompt a search for CRC, and should not be attributed to normal aging.

COMPLEMENTARY AND ALTERNATIVE MEDICINE

Jennifer A. Caragol, MD
Anna Svircev, DO, MPH
Andrew Bentley, MS

BASICS

Complementary and alternative medicine (CAM) are medical and health care systems, practices, and products that are not presently considered part of conventional medicine. The National Center for Health Statistics (NCHS) 2007 survey reports that 38% of adult Americans and 12% of children use some form of CAM, and this percentage is increasing as CAM healing practices and products become better known and more accessible. Medical professionals who incorporate CAM into their medical practice will often refer to their health care model as "integrative medicine."

DESCRIPTION
- Definitions and additional terms:
  - Complementary medicine is used with conventional medicine to address a health concern. For example, massage plus physical therapy to address low back pain, or medication plus osteopathic manipulation to address recurrent headaches.
  - Alternative medicine is used in place of conventional medicine to promote healing of conditions that cannot be explained by the conventional biomedical model or for which the effectiveness of therapy is not yet established by clinical research.
  - Integrative medicine is the combination of allopathic medicine with CAM, and may be provided to the patient by a single licensed medical professional versed in CAM or by a group of diverse health care providers. For example, a nurse on the oncology unit who integrates healing touch into the care of the patient.
  - Holistic is a descriptive term for a practitioner's approach to patient care. A holistic practitioner assesses the emotional, spiritual, mental, and physical state of wellness of the client and then works to provide comprehensive care. A holistic practice may include practitioners of different disciplines to best address all aspects of wellness or illness.
- Biologically based therapies: Diets, herbals, vitamins, supplements, flower essences
- Manipulative and body-based methods:
  - Massage therapy is the manipulation of the soft tissues of the body whereby the licensed practitioner uses knowledge of anatomy and physiology to restore function, promote relaxation, and relieve pain. There are several different types of massage.
  - Osteopathic manipulative medicine focuses on the musculoskeletal system. It includes indirect techniques, e.g., muscle energy, myofascial release, osteopathy in the cranial field, and strain-counterstrain approach, as well as direct action techniques (high-velocity thrusts).
  - Craniosacral therapy is a gentle manual treatment focusing on the release of bony and fascial restrictions in the craniosacral system, which includes the cranium, sacrum, spinal cord, meninges, and cerebrospinal fluid. Cranial osteopathy was developed in the early 1900s by American osteopath Dr. William Sutherland, who researched the subtle movements of the cranial

bones and developed techniques to help release restrictions between sutures.
  - Chiropractic therapy is a discipline that focuses on the musculoskeletal and nervous systems and how imbalances in these systems can affect general health. It is most often used to treat back pain, neck pain, and joint pain. Doctors of chiropractic (DCs) complete 4–5 years of intensive training in anatomy, physiology, and manipulation.
- Mind-body medicine:
  - Meditation, traditionally a form of spiritual practice, is a practice of detachment in which a person sits quietly, generally focusing on the breath while releasing all thoughts from the mind with the intention to center the self, restore balance, and enhance well-being.
  - Spiritual practices/prayer
  - Yoga is an exercise of mindfulness, meditation, strength, and balance with the goal of achieving enlightenment. It is comprised of asanas (postures) and pranayamas (focused breathing). The discipline of yoga originated in India and has been practiced for thousands of years. Variations of yoga including Hatha, Raja, Jnana, Bhaki, and Tantra.
  - Aromatherapy utilizes highly concentrated plant extracts to stimulate physical, emotional, and energetic healing processes. These aromatic oils are rubbed on the skin, aerosolized, or used in compresses.
  - Tai chi and qigong are Chinese exercise systems that combine meditation, regulated breathing, and flowing dancelike movements to enhance and balance chi (qi), or life force energy.
- Alternative medical systems:
  - Traditional Chinese medicine incorporates Chinese herbs and acupuncture. Acupuncture is the practice of regulating chi by inserting hair-thin needles at specific points along meridian pathways of the body. Chi movement is responsible for animating and protecting the body; relieving pain; and regulating blood, oxygen, and nourishment to every cell.
  - Ayurvedic medicine originated in India and is one of the world's oldest medical systems. It utilizes healing modalities and herbs to integrate and balance the body, mind, and spirit.
  - Homeopathy is a system of therapy based on the concept that very dilute quantities of an offending agent can stimulate the body's own immune system to produce a reaction against this offense, thereby healing itself. In general, homeopathic remedies are considered safe and unlikely to cause serious adverse reactions.
  - Naturopathy is based on providing natural and minimally invasive options for prevention and treatment of disease. Treatment regimens can include herbs, vitamins, supplements, dietary counseling, homeopathic remedies, manipulative therapies, acupuncture, and hydrotherapy. 4-year doctoral training programs are available; however, because only 16 states have licensing laws for naturopathic physicians, patients are encouraged to research their prospective naturopath's credentials.

- Energy therapies:
  - Reiki, which means source energy, from Japan. Laying hands lightly on the patient or holding the hands just above the body, the Reiki practitioner facilitates spiritual and physical healing by replenishing and strengthening the patient's life force energy.
  - Healing touch designed by a registered nurse. Practitioners use their hands to clear, energize, and balance a patient's energy field to enhance well-being.
- Common reasons patients choose CAM:
  - Conventional medicine has been unsuccessful in fully addressing ailment.
  - Preventative health care
  - Desire for a holistic and natural approach to well-being
  - Preference for noninvasive treatment options
  - Concern about side effects of prescription medication
  - Desire for spiritual support to be incorporated into healing practice
  - Cultural or familial belief system may be more aligned with "natural" solutions not provided for or supported by the standard allopathic model of health care.

EPIDEMIOLOGY
- All ages use CAM, but is most prevalent among adults aged 30–69 years
- Gender ratio: Female predominance
- College graduates and residents from Western states are more likely to use CAM.
- 10 most utilized CAM therapies based on the NCHS 2007 survey; prayer is also reported. These 10 CAM therapies were used by the indicated percentage of survey participants:
  - Prayer/self (43%)
  - Prayer/others (24.4%)
  - Natural products (17.7%)
  - Deep breathing (12.7%)
  - Prayer group (9.6%)
  - Meditation (9.4%)
  - Chiropractic and osteopathic (8.6%)
  - Massage (8.3%)
  - Yoga (6.1%)
  - Diet-based therapies (3.6%)
  - Progressive relaxation (2.9%)
  - Guided imagery (2.2%)
  - Homeopathic treatment (1.8%)

TREATMENT

- Evidence supports both safety and efficacy:
  - Meditation for lowering blood pressure (1)
  - Acupuncture for chronic low back pain (2)
  - Spinal manipulative therapy for prophylactic treatment of headaches
  - Manipulation, massage, and mobilization for acute low back and posterior neck pain
  - Massage therapy to promote weight gain in preterm infants
  - Acupuncture for nausea and vomiting
  - Tai chi for improving balance and decreasing the risk of and fear of falling in elderly (3)
  - Aromatherapy massage for temporary relief of anxiety or depression in cancer patients (4)

C

- Mind-body techniques for migraines, chronic pain, and insomnia
- Homeopathic remedy for the treatment of chemotherapy-induced stomatitis in children (5)
- Riboflavin for migraine prophylaxis (6)
- Horse chestnut seed extract to improve lower leg venous tone, pain, and edema
- Glucosamine and chondroitin sulfate for osteoarthritis and knee pain
- Yoga and meditation appear to improve endothelial function in patients with CAD.
- Yoga can have a potential beneficial effect on depressive disorders.
• Evidence supports safety, but evidence regarding efficacy is inconclusive:
- Saw palmetto for benign prostatic hyperplasia
- Acupuncture for recurrent headache
- Homeopathy for induction and augmentation of labor
- Dietary fat reduction for certain types of cancer
- Mind-body techniques for metastatic cancer
- Copper and magnetic bracelets for pain
• Evidence supports efficacy, but evidence regarding safety is inconclusive:
- St. John's wort extract for depression
- Ginkgo biloba for cognitive function in dementia
• Evidence indicates serious risk:
- Delay in seeking medical care or replacement of curative conventional treatments
- Injections of unapproved substances
- Use of toxic herbs or substances
- Known herb-drug interactions

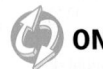 ONGOING CARE

PATIENT EDUCATION
• National Library of Medicine: Alternative medicine (www.nlm.nih.gov)
• The National Center for Complementary and Alternative Medicine (nccam.nih.gov)

COMPLICATIONS
• Potentially toxic herbs:
- Serious adverse events from herbal remedies remain extremely rare.
- Some ethnic medicines, as those prescribed by practitioners of Ayurveda or traditional Chinese medicine, may intentionally contain heavy metals or other toxic substances. These are usually listed by their pharmacopial names, e.g., *qian dan* = lead oxide.
- Bitter orange (*Citrus sinensis*): Sympathomimetic; increases heart rate (HR), blood pressure (BP)
- California poppy (*Eschscholzia californica*): May cause respiratory depression, drowsiness; contains opioids
- Cascara sagrada (*Frangula purshiana*): Depletes serum potassium
- Chaparral (*Larrea tridentata*): Hepatotoxic
- Ephedra (*Ephedra* species): Sympathomimetic; increases HR, BP; insomnia, gastric distress
- Ginkgo (*Ginkgo biloba*): Extravasation, increased bleeding time
- Guarana (*Paullinia cupana*): Tachycardia, hypertension; contains caffeine
- Kava (*Piper methysticum*): Decreases utilization of niacin; possibly hepatotoxic
- Licorice (*Glycyrrhiza* species): Long-term use depletes serum potassium
- Lily of the valley (*Convallaria majalis*): Contains cardiac glycosides

- Poke root (*Phytolacca* species): Strong gastric irritant, may cause sedation
- Senna (*Cassia senna*): Depletes serum potassium
- Snakeroot (*Aristolochia* species): Nephrotoxic
- Wormwood (*Artemisia absinthum*): Elevates serotonin level, may raise BP
- Yohimbe (*Pausinystalia yohimbe*): Elevates BP
• Important herbal–medication interactions:
- Ginkgo and St. John's wort account for most herb–drug interactions described in the medical literature.
- Angelica, dong quai (*Angelica* species): Additive effect with calcium channel blockers
- Bitter melon (*Momordicacharantia*): Additive effect with other hypoglycemic agents
- Cascara sagrada (*Frangula purshiana*): Shortens transit time of intestinally absorbed drugs; Potential for causing hypokalemia may potentiate digoxin toxicity
- Chamomile (*Anthemis, Matricaria* species): Antagonistic interaction with benzodiazepines
- Echinacea (*Echinacea* species): May counteract immunosuppressants
- Garlic (*Allium sativum*): Modest anticoagulant effect; decreases levels of saquinavir
- Guarana (*Paullina cupana*): Contains caffeine; may inhibit platelet aggregation
- Ginkgo (*G. biloba*): Dangerous synergistic effect with anticoagulants (1)
- Ginseng (*Panax* species): Potentiates dopaminergic drugs; counteracts phenothiazines
- Kava (*Piper methysticum*): Additive effect with sedatives
- Kelp (*Laminaria* species): May interfere with thyroxine and liothyronine
- Lemon Balm (*Melissa officinalis*): Additive effect with sedatives; binds TSH and may interfere with thyroid testing and function
- Licorice (*Glycyrrhiza* species): Increases potential for digoxin toxicity; depletes potassium
- Lobelia (*Lobelia* species): Potentially counteracts β_2 adrenergic bronchodilators
- Meadowsweet (*Filipendula ulmaria*): Increased anticoagulant effect; contains salicylates
- Motherwort (*Leonurus cardiaca*): Can potentiate digoxin; contains cardiac glycosides
- Milk thistle (*Silybum marianum*): Might accelerate clearance of liver-metabolized drugs
- Pumpkin seed (*Cucurbita pepo*): Elevates levels of androgenic drugs
- Red clover (*Trifolium pratense*): Partial agonistic/antagonistic interaction with estrogens
- Saw palmetto (*Serenoa repens*): May potentiate or antagonize androgenic drugs
- Soy isoflavones (*Glycine max*): Partial agonistic/antagonistic interaction with estrogens
- St. John's wort (*Hypericum perforatum*): Induces CYP450 pathways, reducing levels of many drugs (2)
- Tobacco (*Nicotiana tabacum*): May counteract β-blockers
- Uva ursi (*Arctostaphylos uva-ursi*): Interferes with action of other diuretics; may cause faster clearance of kidney-metabolized drugs
- Valerian (*Valeriana officinalis*): Potential for interference with valproic acid derivatives
- Willow bark (*Salix alba*): Additive effect with anticoagulants; contains salicylates

• Vitamins and minerals with potential toxicity:
- Iron is a leading cause of accidental poisoning in children under 6. Minerala (i.e., potassium, calcium, magnesium, zinc, copper, and selenium) may cause toxicity
- Fat-soluble vitamins have the potential to cause hypervitaminosis
  ○ Vitamin A is most common cause of hypervitaminosis
  ○ β-carotene may have a limited potential for overdose.
- Vitamin A: Pseudotumor cerebri, hepatic damage, loss of appetite, osteomalacia
- Vitamin D: Constipation, hypercalcemia
- Vitamin E: Coagulopathy, fatigue, pain in extremities

REFERENCES
1. Anderson JW, Liu C, Kryscio RJ. Blood pressure response to transcendental meditation: a meta-analysis. *Am J Hypertens*. 2008;21:310–6.
2. Manheimer E, White A, Berman B, et al. Meta-analysis: acupuncture for low back pain. *Ann Intern Med*. 2005;142:651–63.
3. Sattin RW, Easley KA, Wolf SL, et al. Reduction in fear of falling through intense tai chi exercise training in older, transitionally frail adults. *J Am Geriatr Soc*. 2005;53:1168–78.
4. Wilkinson SM, Love SB, Westcombe AM, et al. Effectiveness of aromatherapy massage in the management of anxiety and depression in patients with cancer: a multicenter randomized controlled trial. *J Clin Oncol*. 2007;25:532–9.
5. Oberbaum M, Yaniv I, Ben-Gal Y, et al. A randomized, controlled clinical trial of the homeopathic medication TRAUMEEL S in the treatment of chemotherapy-induced stomatitis in children undergoing stem cell transplantation. *Cancer*. 2001;92:684–90.
6. Schoenen J, Jacquy J, Lenaerts M. Effectiveness of high-dose riboflavin in migraine prophylaxis. A randomized controlled trial. *Neurology*. 1998;50: 466–70.

ADDITIONAL READING
• Bent S et al. Herbal medicine in the United States: review of efficacy, safety, and regulation: grand rounds at University of California, San Francisco Medical Center. *J Gen Intern Med*. 2008;23:854–9.
• Rakel D, Faas N. *Complementary Medicine in Clinical Practice*. Boston: Jones and Bartlett, 2006.

CLINICAL PEARLS
1/3 of adults and >10% of children use CAM; best evidence examples include:
• Meditation for lowering blood pressure (1)
• Acupuncture for chronic low back pain (2)
• Spinal manipulative therapy for prophylactic treatment of headaches

COMPLEX REGIONAL PAIN SYNDROME

Dennis E. Hughes, DO

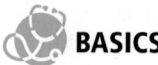 **BASICS**

Multidisciplinary approach with physical, occupational, and recreational therapy involvement

DESCRIPTION
- Pain syndrome after injury to bone and soft tissue; pathogenesis is obscure. Evidence suggests that these syndromes involve areas of the brain and nervous system.
  - Type I: No nerve injury [reflex sympathetic dystrophy (RSD)]
  - Type II: Associated with a demonstrable nerve injury (causalgia)
- System(s) affected: Nervous
- Synonym(s): Traumatic erythromelalgia, Weir Mitchell causalgia, causalgia, reflex sympathetic dystrophy, posttraumatic neuralgia, sympathetically maintained pain

EPIDEMIOLOGY
- Predominant age: Mean age 36–46 years (1)
- Predominant gender: Female > Male (3:1, 60–81%) (1)
- Extremely rare in children

Incidence
26.2/100,000 person-years, but may be higher owing to misdiagnosis initially

Prevalence
~6 million in the US

RISK FACTORS
- Minor or severe trauma (upper extremity fracture noted in 44%)
- Surgery
- Lacerations
- Burns
- Frostbite
- Casting
- Penetrating injury

Genetics
No known genetic pattern

GENERAL PREVENTION
- Early mobilization after fracture, stroke, and myocardial infarction has proven benefit in reducing incidence of complex regional pain syndrome (CRPS).
- 1 study of wrist fractures found that addition of 500 mg/d of vitamin C lowered rates of CRPS (2).

PATHOPHYSIOLOGY
Poorly understood activation of abnormal sympathetic reflex that lowers pain threshold

ETIOLOGY
Other than known nerve injury (type II or causalgia), no known definitive pathogenesis

COMMONLY ASSOCIATED CONDITIONS
- Serious injury to bone and soft tissue
- Herpes zoster
- Postherpetic neuralgia results from partial or complete damage to afferent nerve pathways.
- Pain occurs in dermatomes as a sequela of herpes zoster.

 DIAGNOSIS

Unprovoked pain is the hallmark of the condition.

HISTORY
- Inciting injury ranges from minor sprains to major trauma
- Hyperhydrosis
- Thermal hypersensitivity
- Hair loss
- Burning paroxysms of pain
- Increased symptoms during emotional stress
- Muscle spasms
- Hypersensitivity to light touch
- Mottled skin
- Partial motor paralysis

PHYSICAL EXAM
- Smooth, glossy skin
- Guarding of extremity
- Diminished hair

DIAGNOSTIC TESTS & INTERPRETATION
Lab
Initial lab tests
- Complete blood count (CBC) (3)
- Erythrocyte sedimentation rate (ESR) (3)

Imaging
Initial approach
- Plain radiographs may show patchy demineralization within 3–6 weeks of onset of CRPS and more pronounced than one would see from disuse alone (3).
- 3-phase bone scanning has varying sensitivity but is most accurate for support of the diagnosis when there is diffuse activity (especially on phase 3) (1,3).
- Bone densometry (3)

Diagnostic Procedures/Surgery
- Electromyelography (EMG) shows nerve injury with type II CRPS (3).
- Sudomotor function testing (resting sweat testing, resting skin temperature, quantitative sudomotor axon reflex testing—all related to increased autonomic activity of the affected limb) (1)

Pathological Findings
- Partial or complete damage to afferent nerve pathways and probably reorganized central pain pathways
- Nerves most commonly involved are median and sciatic.
- Atrophy in affected muscles
- Incomplete nerve plexus lesion

DIFFERENTIAL DIAGNOSIS
- Infection
- Hypertrophic scar
- Bone fragments
- Neuroma
- CNS tumor or syrinx

 TREATMENT

MEDICATION
First Line
- No single drug or combination of drugs has produced consistent results; early therapy is beneficial.
- α-Adrenergic blockers: Phenoxybenzamine: 40–120 mg/d PO in divided doses; the initial dose should not exceed 10 mg.
- Miscellaneous: Prednisone: 30 mg/d PO × 2–3 weeks, then tapered over 2–4 weeks (4)[B]
- Tricyclic antidepressants (response to each may be variable; therefore, several should be considered) (3,4)[C]:
  - Amitriptyline (Elavil): 25–100 mg/d at bedtime
  - Nortriptyline (Pamelor): 25–100 mg/d
- Anticonvulsants (serum drug level monitoring may be needed, except for clonazepam; individualize doses):
  - Carbamazepine (Tegretol): 200–1,000 mg/d PO
  - Phenytoin (Dilantin): 100–300 mg/d PO
  - Clonazepam (Klonopin): 1–10 mg/d PO
  - Valproic acid (Depakene): 750–2,250 mg/d PO, maximum of 60 mg/kg
  - Gabapentin: 100 mg/d at bedtime up to 600–1,200 mg t.i.d. (3,4)[B]

- Skeletal muscle relaxant: Baclofen: 10–40 mg/d PO; may act synergistically with carbamazepine and phenytoin (3)
- Contraindications: Refer to manufacturer's literature.
- Precautions: Refer to manufacturer's literature.
- Significant possible interactions: Many exist within this group of drugs. Refer to the manufacturer's literature for each drug.

Second Line
Bisphosphonates have the potential to reduce pain associated with bone loss in patients with CRPS (5)[B].

ADDITIONAL TREATMENT
General Measures
Discourage maladaptive behaviors.

Issues for Referral
- After 2 months of the illness, psychological evaluation generally is indicated to identify and treat any comorbid conditions (1)[C].
- Refer the patient to a specialty pain clinic in difficult cases (many advocate early referral to an expert in the management to reduce duration of symptoms).

Additional Therapies
- Available information about treatment is based on small studies or treatment reports; therefore, therapy remains largely empirical.
- Treatment response can be predicted by diagnosis (type I versus type II).
- Type I:
  – Physical therapy
  – Transcutaneous nerve stimulation
  – Psychotherapy

COMPLEMENTARY AND ALTERNATIVE MEDICINE
- Vitamin C (500 mg/d) may help to prevent CRPS in those with wrist fracture (2).
- Briskly rub the affected part several times per day.
- Acupuncture
- Hypnosis can be suggested.
- Relaxation training (alternate muscle relaxing and contracting)
- Biofeedback
- Mirror therapy (6)[A]

SURGERY/OTHER PROCEDURES
- Type II responds more favorably to nerve-directed treatment.
  – Sympathetic blocks
  – Sympathectomy (4)[C]
- Anesthetic blockade (chemical or surgical) of sympathetic nerve function:
  – Transient relief suggests that chemical or surgical sympathectomy will be helpful (1)[C].
  – Little in the way of quality clinical trials exist to support local sympathetic blockage as the "gold standard" of therapy (7).
- IV regional sympathetic block with guanethidine or reserpine by pain specialist or anesthetist
- Transcutaneous electric nerve stimulation (controversial)
- Inject myofascial painful trigger points
- Spinal cord stimulation (3)[C]
- Intrathecal analgesia (3)[C]

IN-PATIENT CONSIDERATIONS
Admission Criteria
Only for proposed surgical therapy

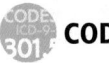 **ONGOING CARE**

FOLLOW-UP RECOMMENDATIONS
Weekly to monitor progress and initiate additional modalities as needed

PATIENT EDUCATION
- Stress need to remain active physically.
- Instruct carefully about any prescribed medications.
- Reflex Sympathetic Dystrophy Syndrome Association, www.rsds.org, (203) 877-3790 or American RSD Hope Group, www.rsdhope.org, (207) 583-4589

PROGNOSIS
Most improve with early treatment (1)

COMPLICATIONS
- Depression
- Disability
- Opioid dependence

REFERENCES
1. Rho RH, Brewer RP, Lamer TJ, et al. Complex regional pain syndrome. *Mayo Clin Proc.* 2002;77: 174–80.
2. Ghai B, Dureja GP. Complex regional pain syndrome: a review. *J Postgrad Med.* 2004;50: 300–7.
3. Cepeda MS, Carr DB, Lau J. Local anesthetic sympathetic blockade for complex regional pain syndrome. *Cochrane Database Syst Rev.* 2005:CD004598.
4. Malis A. Sympathetectomy for neuropathic pain. *The Cochrane Collaboration,* 2007.
5. Brunner F, Schmid A, Kissling R, et al. Biphosphonates for the therapy of complex regional pain syndrome I—Systematic review. *Eur J Pain.* 2008.
6. Ezendam D, Bongers RM, Jannink MJ et al. Systematic review of the effectiveness of mirror therapy in upper extremity function. *Disabil Rehabil.* 2009;31:2135–49.
7. Harden RN. Pharmacotherapy of complex regional pain syndrome. *Am J Phys Med Rehab.* 2005;84: s17–s28.

ADDITIONAL READING
Lang L, et al. *Living with RSDS. Your Guide to Coping with Reflex Sympathetic Dystrophy Syndrome.* Oakland CA: New Harbinger, 2003.

See Also (Topic, Algorithm, Electronic Media Element)
Algorithm: Pain in Upper Extremity

 CODES

ICD9
- 337.20 Reflex sympathetic dystrophy, unspecified
- 337.21 Reflex sympathetic dystrophy of the upper limb
- 337.22 Reflex sympathetic dystrophy of the lower limb

CLINICAL PEARLS
- Pain control and early mobility are key to recovery.
- Regional sympathetic blocks may be useful.
- Use multidisciplinary approach.

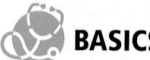

CONCUSSION

J. Herbert Stevenson, MD

BASICS

DESCRIPTION
- A complex pathophysiologic process affecting brain function, induced by traumatic biomechanical forces that generally resolves over 7–10 days.
- Concussion severity can only be determined in retrospect.
- System(s) affected: Cardiovascular; Endocrine/Metabolic; Nervous; Psychiatric
- Synonym(s): Mild traumatic brain injury (TBI)

Pediatric Considerations
Children (ages 5–18) should not be allowed to return to training or play that same day and not until completely symptom-free. Resolution of symptoms and clinical findings often take longer in the pediatric athlete.

EPIDEMIOLOGY
- Predominant age: 12–24 years
- Predominant sex: Male > Female
- Usually related to accidents, sometimes sports related

Incidence
- 0.14–3.66 injuries/100 players each season at high school level
- 0.5–3.0 injuries/1,000 athlete exposures at college level (1)
- Average annual incidence 503:100,000.
- ~1.5 million cases of TBI in US annually, 85% of which are considered mild TBI.
- ~10% of TBIs are related to sports or cycling injuries.
- Among the 5–14 age group, 26.4% of mild TBI is related to sports or cycling (2).

RISK FACTORS
Contact sports, particularly football, and history of recent concussion.

GENERAL PREVENTION
- Educate athletes, coaches, parents, and officials on signs and symptoms of concussions.
- Rule enforcement in sports (e.g., penalties for spearing or head-to-head contact)
- Consideration of rule changes in sports to decrease dangerous plays
- Current protective headgear for contact sports decreases facial injuries, but has not been shown to decrease the overall concussion risk.
- Useful web site: www.thinkfirst.ca/default.asp

PATHOPHYSIOLOGY
Concussion represents a functional brain injury rather than a structural brain injury. The neurobiologic cascade has been shown to include excitatory amino acid release, ionic flux, hyperglycolysis, and reduced cerebral blood flow.

ETIOLOGY
- Falls
- Sports related
- Motor vehicle accidents

 ## DIAGNOSIS

HISTORY
- Cognitive symptoms:
  - Confusion
  - Post-traumatic amnesia (PTA)
  - Retrograde amnesia (RGA)
  - Loss of consciousness (LOC)
  - Disorientation
  - Feeling "in a fog," "zoned out"
  - Inability to focus
  - Delayed verbal and motor responses
  - Slurred/incoherent speech
  - Excessive drowsiness
- Somatic:
  - Headache
  - Fatigue
  - Disequilibrium, dizziness
  - Visual disturbances
  - Phonophobia
- Affective:
  - Emotional lability
  - Irritability
- Sleep Disturbance

PHYSICAL EXAM
Variable and dependent on degree of injury:
- ABCs if seen acutely
- External evidence of major trauma
- Focal neurologic signs and symptoms
- Musculoskeletal: Evaluate for possible C-spine injury and stability.
- Detailed neurologic exam including:
  - State of alertness
  - Orientation
  - 3- or 5-word recall at 5 minutes
  - Concentration/attention (serial 3s or 7s)
  - Cerebellar function and postural stability assessment

DIAGNOSTIC TESTS & INTERPRETATION
- The sideline assessment of concussion (SAC) scale has been validated to drop from baseline after a concussion and return to baseline once symptoms clear.
- Serial cognitive evaluations should be done by an experienced health care provider using the neurologic exam listed above or by using other assessment tools such as the sport concussion assessment tool (SCAT) (3)[C].
- Computerized neurocognitive testing to date lacks sufficient evidence on validity, cost effectiveness, and improved management to warrant global usage (4)[B].
- Current gold standard is evaluation and treatment by a trained physician. Until improved outcomes, validity, and cost-effectiveness of computerized testing are established, use should be limited to experimental situations or possibly in management of complex concussions.

Lab
Generally not necessary.

Imaging
- Structural neuroimaging is usually normal in the setting of concussion.
- Consider MRI or CT with prolonged LOC, focal neurologic deficit, or overall worsening symptoms.
- Role of functional MRI is largely experimental and unvalidated at this time.
- Consider C-spine films.

Diagnostic Procedures/Surgery
Serial neurologic exams at least every 10–15 minutes until symptoms are clearing and patient is stabilizing or patient has been transported to hospital for further evaluation.

DIFFERENTIAL DIAGNOSIS
- Concussion
- Subdural hematoma
- Epidural hematoma
- Cerebral contusion
- Facial or skull fracture

 ## TREATMENT

MEDICATION
- Ibuprofen or acetaminophen may be used as adjunct pain management for headache once structural brain injury ruled out.
- Prolonged symptoms such as sleep disturbance or anxiety, may benefit from appropriate pharmacologic treatment for symptom relief.

ADDITIONAL TREATMENT
General Measures
- Acute management depends on severity of injury. Most patients need only physical and cognitive rest, serial clinical evaluations to include neurologic checks, and a plan for follow-up evaluation (1)[C].
- Prolonged LOC, abnormal neurologic exam, or deteriorating symptoms necessitate urgent or emergent referral to the hospital for further evaluation (1)[C].

Issues for Referral
- Most concussions can be managed by primary care physicians using the standard guidelines for return to play; generally, referral to a specialist is not needed.
- Patients with a complex or atypical concussion, or who have suffered recurrent concussions should be referred to a sports medicine physician or neurologist for management and clearance prior to returning to sports activities.

SURGERY/OTHER PROCEDURES
Generally not indicated, unless signs of more severe TBI present, with increased intracranial pressure or large bleed.

IN-PATIENT CONSIDERATIONS
Initial Stabilization
- ABCs take priority over head injury and concussion.
- C-spine immobilization should be considered in all head trauma.

Admission Criteria
- Progressive neurologic symptoms, including deterioration of mental status, seizures, and focal neurologic signs
- No competent adult at home

Discharge Criteria
- Improving mental status at or near baseline
- Competent adult at home for patient observation (see Patient Monitoring)

ONGOING CARE

FOLLOW-UP RECOMMENDATIONS
- Any athlete with a suspected concussion should be withheld that day from sports participation and not returned till a concussion has been ruled out or a diagnosed concussion has been appropriately treated as noted below (3).
- Current recommendation on treatment involves an asymptomatic graduated return to play as follows (3)[C]:
  - Complete rest until symptom-free, including cognitive rest (e.g., video games, and potentially scholastic activities)
  - May then begin gradual reintroduction of activity as long as symptom free. Each step should be generally done 24 hours apart.
    ○ Light aerobic exercise
    ○ Sport-specific exercise
    ○ Noncontact training drills
    ○ Full contact training
    ○ Game play
- If postconcussive symptoms occur (exertional headache, visual disturbance, or disequilibrium), decrease level of activity until again asymptomatic, and progress again in 24 hours.

- High-risk athletes for more prolonged recovery include pediatric athletes, athletes with mood disorders, athletes with learning disabilities, and athletes with migraine headaches. These athletes should have a slower return to play progression and may require more intensive evaluation (formal neuropsychologic, balance, symptom testing).
- Athletes with multiple concussions should have slower return to play and may benefit from sports medicine consultation or neurology referral.

Patient Monitoring
- Written instructions regarding postconcussion management should be given to a competent adult describing signs to watch for and when to bring the patient back for further evaluation.
- Have a follow-up plan prior to discharge to home, ideally to be seen within a few days.
- Instruct patients and families regarding postconcussive symptoms, including the cognitive, somatic, and affective symptoms listed earlier.
- Ensure adequate rest and symptom-free return to both school and sports-related activities.

DIET
As tolerated.

COMPLICATIONS
- Delayed hematomas, including subdural hematomas, can present minutes to hours after initial injury, necessitating serial neurologic checks and close observation.
- Postconcussion syndrome occurs when symptoms of concussion, such as headache, fatigue, memory changes, or emotional lability, are persistent and last >1–3 months.
- Recurrent concussions can lead to second-impact syndrome or can occur with less and less impact force. Symptoms can persist longer than a 1st concussion, and progression to chronic cognitive and psychiatric symptoms is possible.
- Second-impact syndrome describes an additional insult or injury to the brain after a concussion and before the brain has had adequate time to completely recover. A rare, but life-threatening, cerebral edema after repeated head injury can occur. The etiology is thought to be due to loss of regulation of either cerebral circulation or glucose metabolism in the concussed brain.
- Chronic traumatic brain injury with chronic cognitive, mood, and potential Parkinson-type symptoms (5).

REFERENCES

1. Concussion (mild traumatic brain injury) and the team physician: a consensus statement. *Med Sci Sports Exerc*. 2006;38:395–9.
2. Bazarian JJ, McClung J, Shah MN et al. Mild traumatic brain injury in the United States, 1998–2000. *Brain Inj*. 2005;19:85–91.
3. McCrory P, Meeuwisse W, Johnston K, et al. Consensus Statement on Concussion in Sport: the 3rd International Conference on Concussion in Sport held in Zurich, November 2008. *Br J Sports Med* 2009;42(Suppl 1):i76–90.
4. Randolph C, McCrea M, Barr W. Is neuropsychological testing useful in the management of sport-related concussion? *J Athletic Train*. 2005;40(3):136–51.
5. Guskiewicz KM, Marshall SW, Bailes J et al. Association between recurrent concussion and late-life cognitive impairment in retired professional football players. *Neurosurgery*. 2005;57:.

ADDITIONAL READING

- Halstead ME, Walter KD. Council on Sports Medicine and Fitness et al. American Academy of Pediatrics. Clinical report–sport-related concussion in children and adolescents. *Pediatrics*. 2010;126:597–615.
- Mayers L. Return-to-play criteria after athletic concussion: a need for revision. *Arch Neurol*. 2008;65:1158–61.

See Also (Topic, Algorithm, Electronic Media Element)
Brain Injury, Traumatic; Brain Injury, Post Acute Care Issues; Postconcussive Syndrome; Seizure Disorders

CODES

ICD9
- 310.2 Postconcussion syndrome
- 850.9 Concussion, unspecified

CLINICAL PEARLS
- Most symptoms resolve completely within 7–10 days, but each person recovers at a different rate, and some symptoms may continue for weeks to months.
- Some athletes notice worsening symptoms, such as headache or nausea, while concentrating. If symptoms worsen while in class, they should stay home from school until their symptoms clear.
- Generally, patients who have been observed for at least 1–2 hours and are stable or improving do not need to be roused from sleep.
- When symptom-free at rest, the athlete may begin a gradual ramp-up of activity over 3–5 days, as listed above. If symptoms recur during any level of play, the athlete should postpone further activity for at least another 24 hours.

CONDYLOMATA ACUMINATA

Timothy R. McCurry, MD
Sujata Sharma, MD

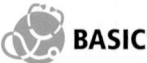 **BASICS**

DESCRIPTION
Condylomata acuminata are soft, skin-colored, fleshy warts that are caused by human papillomavirus (HPV):

- HPV types 6, 11, 16, 18, 31, 33, and 35 associated with condylomata acuminata
- Highly contagious; incubation period may be from 1–6 months.
- Warts appear singly or in groups, small or large; on the vagina, cervix, around the external genitalia and rectum, and in the urethra and anus. Reports of conjunctival, nasal, oral, and laryngeal warts and occasionally the throat.
- System(s) affected: Skin/Exocrine; Reproductive

Pediatric Considerations
Consider sexual abuse if seen in children, although they can be infected by other means (e.g., transfer from wart on another child's hand).

Pregnancy Considerations
- Warts often grow larger during pregnancy and regress spontaneously after delivery. Use cryotherapy.
- Virus does not cross the placenta. Treatment during pregnancy is somewhat controversial. Cesarean section is not absolutely indicated.
- Few documented cases of HPV transmission to infant at time of delivery have resulted in laryngeal papillomas, a rare and life-threatening condition.
- HPV vaccination is contraindicated in pregnancy.

EPIDEMIOLOGY
- Most common viral sexually transmitted infection (STI) in the US
- Predominant age: 15–30 years old
- Predominant sex: Male = Female

Incidence
- Venereal warts are increasing in an ever-younger population. A recent study of 487 college women showed an infection rate of 48%.
- Increased size and number in immunocompromised patients

Prevalence
- Peak prevalence in ages 17–33
- Minimum of 10–20% of sexually active women may be infected with HPV. Studies in men suggest a similar prevalence.
- Pregnancy and immunosuppression favor recurrence and increasing growth of lesions.

RISK FACTORS
- Young adults and adolescents
- Multiple sexual partners
- Not using condoms
- Possibly subclinical infection
- Young age of commencing sexual activity
- Cigarette smoking: Tobacco smoke has been shown to reduce cellular protection by decreasing cervical keratinocyte production.
- Poor hygiene
- History of genital warts

GENERAL PREVENTION
- Use of condoms (preventive effects not adequately evaluated; 40% of infected men have scrotal warts)
- Abstinence until treatment completed
- Circumcision may prevent recurrence in some men.
- Quadrivalent HPV vaccine available against genital warts and cervical cancer. This vaccination is targeted to adolescents before the period of their greatest risk for exposure to HPV. The vaccine does not treat previous infections:
  - Immunity has been documented to last at least 5 years after HPV vaccination.
  - The use of 4 HPV-specific virion protein capsids address the 2 most common HPV serotypes to be contracted in 6 and 11, and the 2 most cancer-promoting types in 16 and 18 (Gardasil) (1,2).
  - HPV quadrivalent vaccine protects against some types of condyloma-producing virus.
  - Quadrivalent vaccine, females and males (1) ages 9–26: Vaccine is administered IM; 3 doses to achieve optimal seroconversion.
  - Vaccination regimen: 0.5 mL IM injection first dose, and at months 2 and 6 after first dose to complete vaccination.
  - Observe recipients of vaccine for syncopal response.
- Bivalent HPV vaccine is available but does not cover the common viruses that cause condyloma lesions (Cervarix) (2).

ETIOLOGY
HPV is a circular double-stranded DNA molecule. There are >70 HPV subtypes. Types 6 and 11 cause common venereal warts. Cervical dysplasia and carcinoma in situ associates with types 16, 18, 31, 33, and 35.

COMMONLY ASSOCIATED CONDITIONS
- >90% of cervical cancer associated with HPV
- STIs (i.e., gonorrhea, syphilis, chlamydia); AIDS

 DIAGNOSIS

HISTORY
Explore sexual history, contraception use, and other lifestyle issues.

- Pruritus
- Vaginal discharge
- Irritation (burning and redness)

PHYSICAL EXAM
- Multiple fingerlike projections; soft, sessile; smooth or rough
- Perianal condylomata acuminata usually rough and cauliflower-like
- Male sites include frenulum, corona, glans, prepuce, meatus, shaft, and scrotum.
  - Penile lesions often smooth and papular; occur in groups of 3 or 4
- Female sites include labia, clitoris, periurethral area, perineum, vagina, and cervix (flat lesions).
- Bleeding (result of trauma)
- Perianal area (both sexes)

DIAGNOSTIC TESTS & INTERPRETATION
Acetowhitening test: Subclinical lesions can be visualized by wrapping the penis with gauze soaked with 5% acetic acid for 5 minutes. Using a 10× hand lens or colposcope, warts appear as tiny white papules. A shiny white appearance of the skin represents foci of epithelial hyperplasia (subclinical infection); not highly specific, low positive predictive value.

Lab
- Serologic tests for syphilis negative
- Pap smear

Diagnostic Procedures/Surgery
Biopsy with highly specialized identification techniques rarely useful. HPV DNA detected through polymerase chain reaction

- Colposcopy
- Antroscopy, anoscopy, urethroscopy may be required

Pathological Findings
- Possible cervical dysplasia
- Sometimes difficult to differentiate from squamous cell carcinoma

DIFFERENTIAL DIAGNOSIS
- Condylomata lata (flat warts of syphilis)
- Lichen planus
- Normal sebaceous glands
- Seborrheic keratosis
- Molluscum contagiosum
- Keratomas, micropapillomatosis
- Scabies
- Crohn disease
- Skin tags
- Melanocytic nevi
- Vulvar intraepithelial neoplasia
- Buschke-Lowenstein tumor

TREATMENT

MEDICATION
First Line
- Imiquimod (Aldara): self-treatment with a 5% cream applied overnight 3 times weekly until warts resolve for up to 16 weeks. The skin is then washed with soap and water 6 to 10 hours after application (3,4)
  - Precautions: Imiquimod has been noted to weaken condoms and diaphragms; therefore, patients should refrain from sexual contact while the cream is on the skin (3).
- Cryotherapy: Liquid nitrogen is applied to warts for 2 5- to 10-second bursts; usually requires 2–3 weekly sessions (3,5).
- Podophyllin in tincture of benzoin. Apply directly to warts. Leave on for 1–4 hours, then wash off. Repeat treatment every 7 days until gone (in-office procedure) or (3,6)
- Podofilox (Condylox): Apply to external warts (affected area) every 12 hours (allowing to dry) for 3 consecutive days. May repeat after 4 days (home application) (3,6).
- Trichloroacetic acid: 25–85%. Apply only to warts. Use powder/talc to remove unreacted acid. Repeat in office at weekly intervals.
- Trichloroacetic acid is ideal for isolated lesions in pregnant women.

- Intralesion interferon has been shown to be effective in refractory cases and should be reserved for such cases (7,8).
- Oral:
  – Oral cimetidine: 30–40 mg/kg divided t.i.d. for 3 months in children with genital and perigenital condyloma. It is used as a primary and adjunctive therapy (9).
- Contraindications:
  – Podophyllin: Do not use in pregnant patients or on oral, cervical, urethral, or perianal warts. Can use on limited number of vaginal warts with careful drying after application. It is recommended that no more than 0.5 mL should be used.
  – Cryotherapy: Cryoglobulinemia
- Precautions:
  – Podophyllin: To minimize local and systemic reactions, wash treated areas 1–4 hours after application and use ointments to protect surrounding skin from contact with podophyllin.
  – Cryotherapy: None
  – Electrocautery: Do not use in patients with pacemaker.

Second Line
- External (penile and perianal):
  – Podophyllin (3)
  – Podofilox (Condylox) self-treatment (3)
  – Intralesional interferon
  – Small study of topical use of Calmette-Guérin bacillus for penile lesions (10)
  – Cidovir 1% topical applied once daily for 5 contiguous days per week for 6 cycles (11)
- Urethral meatus:
  – Podophyllin (3)
  – Cryrotherapy (3,5)
  – Topical fluorouracil is no longer recommended due to severe side effects and teratogenicity. However, for refractory cases intralesional injection with fluorouracil/epinephrine/bovine collagen gel has been proven effective in phase clinical trials (12).
- Anal:
  – Trichloroacetic acid: Apply weekly (13).
  – Topical fluorouracil is no longer recommended.
- Uterine/cervix
  – Trichloroacetic acid and Cryrotherapy are treatment options (3).
  – Oral isotretinoins can be used for the treatment of recalcitrant condyloma acuminata of the cervix (note special prescription monitoring for this class of medications) (14).

ADDITIONAL TREATMENT
Pregnancy Considerations
- Podophyllin, podofilox, and fluorouracil should not be used in pregnancy due to the concern of possible teratogenicity (3).
- Surgical excision, trichloroacetic acid, Cryotherapy, and electrocautery are treatment options during pregnancy to minimize neonatal exposure to the virus (3).

General Measures
- May resolve spontaneously
- Change therapy if no improvement after 3 treatments, no complete clearance after 6 treatments, or therapy's duration or dosage exceeds manufacturer's recommendations.
- Appropriate screening/counseling of partners

SURGERY/OTHER PROCEDURES
- Larger warts require laser treatment or electrocoagulation including infrared therapy (15)
  – Precaution: Laser treatment may create smoke plumes that may contain HPV; therefore, it is recommended that physicians performing this procedure should wear appropriate masks.
- Surgical excision for large warts
- Intraurethral, external (penile and perianal), anal, and oral lesions can be treated with fulgurating CO_2 laser. Oral or external penile/perianal lesions can also be treated with electrocautery or surgery (3).

 ## ONGOING CARE

FOLLOW-UP RECOMMENDATIONS
No restrictions, except for sexual contact
Patient Monitoring
- Patients seen every 2 weeks until lesions resolve and have annual Pap test
- Patients should also follow up 3 months after completion of treatment
- Persistent warts require biopsy.
- Sexual partners require monitoring.
- Treatment does not decrease transmissible infectivity.

PATIENT EDUCATION
- Provide pamphlets on HPV, STI prevention, and condom use.
- Emphasize the need for women to get regular Pap smears.

PROGNOSIS
- Warts will clear with treatment or resolve spontaneously, but recurrences are frequent and may necessitate repeated treatment.
- Some studies identified 3 independent risk factors for condylomatous relapse: Positive HIV status, male gender, and Langerhans cell level: Cell level per millimeter of anal tissue (15 vs. 30)
- Without treatment, may remain stable, worsen, or resolve completely
- Asymptomatic infection persists indefinitely.

COMPLICATIONS
- Cervical dysplasia
- Malignant change: Progression to cancer rarely, if ever, occurs.
- Male urethral obstruction
- The prevalence of high-grade dysplasia and cancer in anal canal is higher in HIV-positive than in HIV-negative patients, probably because of HPV activity.

REFERENCES
1. Centers for Disease Control and Prevention (CDC) et al. FDA licensure of quadrivalent human papillomavirus vaccine (HPV4, Gardasil) for use in males and guidance from the Advisory Committee on Immunization Practices (ACIP). MMWR Morb Mortal Wkly Rep. 2010;59:630–2.
2. Markowitz LE, Dunne EF, Saraiya M, et al. Quadrivalent human papillomavirus vaccine: Recommendations of the Advisory Committee on Immunization Practices (ACIP). MMWR Recomm Rep. 2007;56(RR-2):1–24.
3. Charles M, Kodner MD, Soraya Nasraty MD. University of Louisville School of Medicine, Louisville, Kentucky. Am Fam Physician. 2004; 70(12):2335–2342.
4. Edwards L. Imiquimod in clinical practice. Aust J Dermatol. 1998;39(Suppl 1):S14–S16.
5. Maw RD et al. Treatment of anogenital warts. Dermatol Clin. 1998;16:829–34, xv
6. Lacey CJ, et al. Randomised controlled trial and economic evaluation of podophyllotoxin solution, podophyllotoxin cream, and podophyllin in the treatment of genital warts. Sex Transm Infect 2003;79:270.
7. Welander CE, Homesley HD, Smiles KA, Peets EA et al. Intralesional interferon alfa-2b for the treatment of genital warts. Am. J. Obstet. Gynecol. 1990;162:348–54.
8. Klutke JJ, Bergman A. Interferon as an adjuvant treatment for genital condyloma acuminatum. Int J Gynaecol Obstet. 1995;49:171.
9. Franco I. Oral cimetidine for the management of genital and perigenital warts in children. J Urol. 2000;164:1074–5.
10. Böhle A, Büttner H, Jocham D. Primary treatment of condylomata acuminata with viable bacillus Calmette-Guerin. J Urol. 2001;165:834–6.
11. Snoeck R, Bossens M, Parent D, Delaere B, Degreef H, Van Ranst M, Noël JC, Wulfsohn MS, Rooney JF, Jaffe HS, De Clercq E et al. Phase II double-blind, placebo-controlled study of the safety and efficacy of cidofovir topical gel for the treatment of patients with human papillomavirus infection. Clin Infect Dis. 2001;33:597–602.
12. Swinehart JM, Sperling M, Phillips S, Kraus S, Gordon S, McCarty JM, Webster GF, Skinner R, Korey A, Orenberg EK. Intralesional fluorouracil/ epinephrine injectable gel for treatment of condylomata acuminata. A phase 3 clinical study. Arch Dermatol. 1997;133(1):67–73.
13. Sobhani I, Vuagnat A, Walker F, et al. Prevalence of high-grade dysplasia and cancer in the anal canal in human papillomavirus-infected individuals. Gastroenterology. 2001;120:857–66.
14. Georgala S, Katoulis AC, Georgala C, Bozi E, Mortakis A et al. Oral isotretinoin in the treatment of recalcitrant condylomata acuminata of the cervix: a randomised placebo controlled trial. Sex Transm Infect. 2004;80:216–8.
15. Bekassy Z, Weström L et al. Infrared coagulation in the treatment of condyloma acuminata in the female genital tract. Sex Transm Dis. 1987;14: 209–12.

ADDITIONAL READING
- Beutner KR, Spruance SL, Hougham AJ, et al. Treatment of genital warts. J Am Acad Dermatol 1998;38:230.
- Workowski KA, Berman SM. Sexually transmitted diseases treatment guidelines, 2006. MMWR Recomm Rep. 2006;55:1–94.

 ## CODES

ICD9
078.11 Condyloma acuminatum

C

CONGESTIVE HEART FAILURE

Jeremy Golding, MD

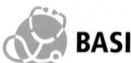 **BASICS**

DESCRIPTION

Congestive heart failure (CHF) (better term: heart failure [HF], because not all heart failure is *congestive*) affects both the cardiovascular and pulmonary systems. It is the principal complication of heart disease. The heart is unable to fill and/or pump blood sufficiently to meet tissue metabolic needs. Heart failure may involve the left heart, the right heart, or be biventricular. New York Heart Association (NYHA) Classification is a fundamental descriptive system used for classifying patients with HF: NYHA I—Asymptomatic; NYHA II—Symptomatic with moderate exertion; NYHA III—Symptomatic with mild exertion and may limit activities of daily living; NYHA IV—Symptomatic at rest.

EPIDEMIOLOGY

Medicare spends more to diagnose and treat heart failure than any other medical condition.

Incidence
- 500,000 new cases annually
- In 2002, the direct cost exceeded $15 billion.

Prevalence
- About 5 million people in the US have heart failure.
- <1% in those <50, increasing to 10% of those older than age 80
- Primarily a disease of the elderly; 75% of hospital admissions for HF are in persons >65.

RISK FACTORS
- For development of heart failure: Coronary artery disease (CAD) and myocardial infarction (MI), hypertension (HTN) (80% of cases of HF in the US caused by either CAD or HTN), valvular heart disease, diabetes mellitus, cardiotoxic medications
- For heart failure exacerbation: Sodium intake and/or fluid excess, nonadherence to medication regimen, arrhythmia (e.g., atrial fibrillation), ischemic ventricular dysfunction, negative inotropic drugs (e.g., calcium blocker, introduction of beta-blocker), excessive physical, emotional, or environmental stress, thyrotoxicosis, pregnancy, or increased metabolic demand

Genetics
Familial cardiomyopathy predisposes to development of heart failure (rare).

GENERAL PREVENTION
Control blood pressure (BP) and other risk factors. Thiazide diuretics and angiotensin-converting enzyme (ACE) inhibitors are superior to other agents in preventing development of heart failure.

PATHOPHYSIOLOGY
2 physiologic components explain most of the clinical findings of congestive heart failure:
- Systolic dysfunction: An *inotropic* abnormality, often due to MI or dilated or ischemic cardiomyopathy, resulting in diminished systolic emptying (ejection fraction <45%)
- Diastolic dysfunction: A *compliance* abnormality, often due to hypertensive cardiomyopathy, in which the ventricular relaxation is impaired (ejection fraction >45%)
- Patients with systolic dysfunction may also have diastolic dysfunction.

ETIOLOGY
- Coronary artery disease and ischemia, myocardial infarction
- Myocarditis and cardiomyopathy: Alcoholic, viral, longstanding HTN, drugs (e.g., chemotherapeutic agents), muscular dystrophy, amyloidosis (infiltrative), sarcoidosis (infiltrative), postpartum state, infectious (e.g., Chagas disease), HIV
- Valvular and vascular abnormalities: Aortic stenosis or regurgitation, rheumatic heart disease (mitral and aortic valvular disease). Renal artery stenosis, usually bilateral, may cause recurrent "flash" pulmonary edema, especially in setting of severe chronic hypertension.
- Chronic lung disease and pulmonary hypertension (right heart failure)
- Volume overload (requires extreme overload in patients with normal hearts and kidneys)
- Arrhythmias (atrial fibrillation and other tachyarrhythmias, high-grade heart block)
- Misc: High-output states: Hyperthyroidism, anemia, cardiac depressants (beta blocker overdose)

COMMONLY ASSOCIATED CONDITIONS
Dysrhythmia, followed by pump failure, are the leading causes of death in this condition.

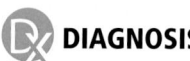 **DIAGNOSIS**

HISTORY
- Dyspnea on exertion: Cardinal sign of left heart failure. Deteriorating exercise capacity: Easy fatigue, generalized weakness.
- Nocturnal nonproductive cough, orthopnea, and paroxysmal nocturnal dyspnea; sometimes frothy or pink sputum
- Wheezing, especially nocturnal in absence of history of asthma or infection (cardiac asthma). Cheyne-Stokes breathing
- Anorexia/cachexia and/or fullness or dull pain in right upper quadrant (hepatic distension in right heart failure)
- Edema often with cool extremities due to peripheral vasoconstriction. Abdominal bloating (ascites) or anasarca. Cyanosis.

PHYSICAL EXAM
Rales (crackles) and sometimes wheezing, peripheral edema, S3 gallop, hepatomegaly, hepatojugular reflux, ascites, hypotension

DIAGNOSTIC TESTS & INTERPRETATION
Diagnosis of heart failure in patients with known heart failure and heart failure exacerbation should be primarily clinical, with laboratory data as adjunctive and indicative of complications.

Lab
Initial lab tests
- β-type natriuretic peptide (BNP) and N-type pro-BNP may be helpful in:
  - Emergency department (ED) setting to help differentiate the cause of dyspnea (BNP <100 essentially rules out HF as cause of dyspnea with NPV of ~99%. Most dyspneic patients with HF have BNP>400.)
  - Titrating treatment, because its value changes rapidly with LV functional status (unclear, however, that BNP-guided therapy improves outcomes) (1)

- BNP values of 100–400 are most problematic, as they may indicate heart failure or may be due to conditions like pulmonary embolism, renal failure, acute coronary syndromes, and pulmonary hypertension.
  - Patients may have BNP elevation due to heart failure, but acute dyspnea may be from another cause (like pneumonia or pulmonary embolism).
- Lab findings in early and mild-to-moderately severe CHF include respiratory alkalosis, mild azotemia, decreased erythrocyte sedimentation rate (ESR), proteinuria (usually <1 g/24 h), elevated creatinine, dilutional hyponatremia (poor prognosis), and rarely hyperbilirubinemia.

Imaging
Initial approach
Chest x-ray (CXR) (changes lag clinical symptoms by up to 6 hours): Increased heart size, vascular redistribution/cephalization with "butterfly" pattern of pulmonary edema, interstitial and alveolar edema, Kerley B lines, pleural effusions

Diagnostic Procedures/Surgery
Determination of ejection fraction is critical to proper diagnosis and management of heart failure:
- Echocardiographic study is most useful single test to determine ejection fraction and valvular abnormalities. May be repeated if change suspected in underlying cardiac status.
- Nuclear imaging to estimate left and right ventricular size, perfusion and systolic function.

Pathological Findings
- Cardiac pathology depends upon underlying process (etiology) of heart failure.
- Noncardiac findings: Liver is engorged, firm, and fluid-filled. Microscopic analysis reveals dilated central hepatic veins and sinusoids. Late/chronic findings include hemosiderin deposits in lungs and "nutmeg" liver with centrilobular necrosis.

DIFFERENTIAL DIAGNOSIS
Simple dependent edema, pulmonary embolism, exertional asthma, cardiac ischemia with angina, chronic obstructive pulmonary disease (COPD), constrictive pericarditis, nephrotic syndrome, cirrhosis, venous occlusive disease with subsequent peripheral edema, High-output states: Anemia, sepsis, hyperthyroidism

 TREATMENT

MEDICATION
Diuretics are used initially in fluid-overload acute heart failure, with nitrates added if needed. Nitrates are primary therapy in ischemic acute heart failure (flash pulmonary edema), with diuretics secondary. Once acute HF is stabilized, an ACE inhibitor or beta-blocker should be started. Instruct patients not to use nonsteroidal anti-inflammatory drugs (NSAIDs), which markedly worsen HF. Avoid use of diltiazem and verapamil in patients with systolic dysfunction.

First Line
- ACE inhibitors:
  - Used to decrease afterload: Shown to increase survival, improve general symptomatology and overall exercise capacity in patients in all NYHA classifications; benefit greatest for patients with systolic dysfunction and post-MI. NNT approx 25/year for mortality (2).

- Angiotensin receptor blockers (ARBs) have fewer side effects than ACE inhibitors, but are less effective than ACE inhibitors and are therefore not 1st-line treatment.
- β-blockers used in systolic or diastolic HF (Note: Initiate in hospital or outpatient setting in hemodynamically stable patients at low dose and titrate upward slowly); NNT = 25 for mortality. Evidence mounting for titration to heart rate rather than specific dose:
  - Carvedilol: 3.125 mg b.i.d. to a maintenance of 25 mg b.i.d.; Metoprolol succinate extended release: 12.5 mg/d to a maximum of 200 mg/d (Note: Metoprolol tartrate may be equivalent but is taken b.i.d.) or bisoprolol 1.25–10 mg once daily
- Digoxin reduces symptoms, but has not shown any effect on mortality (2):
  - In patients with preserved renal function (creatinine clearance >50 mL/min), the recommended dose is 0.125 mg/d.
  - Levels lower than used for atrial fibrillation are effective and safer
- Diuretics helpful to manage volume overload:
  - Furosemide (Lasix): 20–320 mg IV/IM/p.o.
  - Metolazone (Zaroxolyn): 2.5–20 mg/d p.o.
  - Spironolactone (only diuretic to reduce mortality when added to standard therapy in NYHA Class III and IV, and probably Class II): 12.5–25 mg/d p.o.; maximum 50 mg/d p.o. Caution regarding hyperkalemia (2).
- Vasodilators:
  - IV nitroglycerin may be of short-term benefit to decrease preload, afterload, and systemic resistance, especially in acute heart failure.
  - The combination of hydralazine (75 mg/d divided b.i.d. or t.i.d.) and isosorbide dinitrate (40 mg q.i.d.) is effective for African Americans (2) or if unable to take ACE inhibitors or an ARB.
- Fish oil/omega-3 fatty acids: 1 gm daily of n-3 PUFA reduced mortality and time to hospitalization (NNT approx 170/year) (3)

Second Line
- Dobutamine in outpatient basis with intermittent infusions. Despite improving quality of life, it reduces short-term survival.
- Nesiritide is approved for short-term use in decompensated heart failure. It is a recombinant form of human brain-type natriuretic peptide. Should not be used in ED. No better than nitroglycerine for most, and may increase mortality.

ADDITIONAL TREATMENT
Device therapy for heart failure increasingly successful, especially biventricular pacing for ventricular dyssynchrony and implantable cardiac defibrillators (AICDs):

- Biventricular pacing indicated for NYHA II, III (especially) or IV with low EF who are on optimal management for at least 6 months (2), with QRS >0.120 msec and who remain significantly symptomatic. Improves symptoms and may improve survival.
- AICD: Improve survival in dilated cardiomyopathy (4) and are recommended for: Primary prevention in patients with ischemic heart disease (HD) who are post-MI, LVEF<30%, Class 2 or 3 HF on optimal medical therapy, and >1 year estimated survival (2)[A], as well as for nonischemic HF EF<30%. Not indicated in Stage D (end-stage) HF.
- Treat anemia. Target minimum Hct at least 30 and possibly somewhat higher. Improves quality of life and may reduce mortality (5).

Additional Therapies
Home oxygen for pulse oximetry <89% (resting or with activity)

SURGERY/OTHER PROCEDURES
- Heart valve surgery if defective heart valve is responsible; mitral valve repair especially helpful if mitral regurgitation is aggravating condition.
- Cardiac transplantation to be considered in patients <55 and without other disqualifying medical problems who are developing CHF unresponsive to other therapeutic maneuvers, and who are considered to have a life expectancy of >1 year.

IN-PATIENT CONSIDERATIONS
Initial Stabilization
Sublingual nitroglycerin is rapid-onset and reduces both pre- and afterload. Bilevel positive airway pressure (BiPap) may help delay or avoid intubation, and often gives rapid symptomatic relief. Morphine titrated to reduce anxiety/air hunger.

Admission Criteria
Acute change in heart failure, with pulmonary edema accompanied by decreased oxygenation, change in mental status, with acute renal insufficiency, or significant hyponatremia

IV Fluids
Limit. Avoid sodium-containing fluids unless necessary to urgently correct hyponatremia. Fluid restriction is best for nonurgent correction of hyponatremia.

Discharge Criteria
Subjective improvement, resting heart rate (HR) <100, systolic BP >80 mm Hg, heart failure outpatient education performed

 ## ONGOING CARE

FOLLOW-UP RECOMMENDATIONS
Critical patient education performed at all outpatient and inpatient physician visits "MAWDS":
- **M**edications: Take every day; don't skip.
- **A**ctivity: A little every day, don't overdo
- **W**eight: Daily. If gain >2 lb in a day or 5 lb above ideal, CALL!
- **D**iet: Eat less than 2,000 mg Na+ daily.
- **S**ymptoms: Know the signs of worsening HF (cough, weight gain, worsening or rest dyspnea, swelling) and call the doctor early! Quit smoking, if a smoker!

Patient Monitoring
Rapid office follow-up after hospitalization and home health monitoring by specially trained nurses have both been shown to decrease frequency of hospitalizations.

DIET
Reduce sodium load (2 g).

PATIENT EDUCATION
- American Heart Association, 7320 Greenville Avenue, Dallas, TX 75231, (214) 373-6300
- American College of Cardiology, 911 Old Georgetown Road, Bethesda, MD 20814, (301) 897-5400

PROGNOSIS
After symptoms develop, 1-year mortality approximately 25% and 5-year mortality ~50%

COMPLICATIONS
- Sudden death (arrhythmic)
- Acute pulmonary edema and death

REFERENCES
1. Porapakkham P, Porapakkham P, Zimmet H, Billah B, Krum H et al. B-type natriuretic peptide-guided heart failure therapy: A meta-analysis. *Arch Intern Med*. 2010;170:507–14.
2. Hunt SA, Abraham WT, Chin MH, et al. 2009 Focused update incorporated into the ACC/AHA 2005 Guidelines for the Diagnosis and Management of Heart Failure in Adults A Report of the American College of Cardiology Foundation/American Heart Association Task Force on Practice Guidelines. *J Am Coll Cardiol*. 2009; 53:e1–e90.
3. Gissi-Hf Investigators. Effect of n-3 polyunsaturated fatty acids in patients with chronic heart failure (the GISSI-HF trial): a randomised, double-blind, placebo-controlled trial. *Lancet*. 2008.
4. Moss AJ, Hall WJ, Cannom DS, et al. Cardiac-Resynchronization Therapy for the Prevention of Heart-Failure Events. *N Engl J Med*. 2009.
5. Ngo K, Kotecha D, Walters JAE, Manzano L, Palazzuoli A, van Veldhuisen DJ, Flather M. Erythropoiesis-stimulating agents for anaemia in chronic heart failure patients. *Cochrane Database of Systematic Reviews* 2010, Issue 1. Art. No.: CD007613. DOI:10.1002/14651858. CD007613.pub2

ADDITIONAL READING
Hernandez AF, et al. Relationship between early physician follow-up and 30-day readmission among Medicare beneficiaries hospitalized for heart failure. *JAMA*. 2010;303:1716.

See Also (Topic, Algorithm, Electronic Media Element)
Algorithms: Congestive Heart Failure; Congestive Heart Failure, Treatment

 ## CODES

ICD9
428.0 Congestive heart failure, unspecified

CLINICAL PEARLS
- Have patients weigh themselves daily and report weight gains of greater than 2 pounds in a day or 5 pounds above dry weight.
- An echocardiogram is the key test in initial workup of heart failure.
- Beta-blockers and ACE inhibitors are the core medications for management of this condition.
- Consider referral for biventricular pacing in patients with bundle branch block, and AICD in those with low EF.

C

CONJUNCTIVITIS, ACUTE

Frances Y. Wu, MD

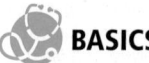 **BASICS**

DESCRIPTION
- Inflammation of the bulbar and/or palpebral conjunctiva <4 weeks duration
- System(s) affected: Nervous; Skin/Exocrine
- Synonym(s): Pink eye

Geriatric Considerations
Suspect autoimmune, systemic, or irritative conditions

Pediatric Considerations
- Neonatal conjunctivitis may be gonococcal, chlamydial, irritative, or related to dacryocystitis.
- Pediatric emergency room study; 78% positive bacterial cult, mostly *H. influenzae*; 13% no growth; other studies showed greater than 50% adenovirus
- Daycare regulations sometimes require any child with presumed conjunctivitis to be treated with a topical antibiotic despite the lack of evidence.

EPIDEMIOLOGY
- Predominant age:
  - Pediatric: Viral, bacterial
  - Adult: Viral, bacterial, allergic
- Predominant sex: Male = Female

Incidence
In the US: Variable, but accounts for 1–2% of all ambulatory office visits

RISK FACTORS
- History of contact with infected persons
- Sexually transmitted disease (STD) contact: Gonococcal, chlamydial, syphilis, or herpes
- Contact lenses: Pseudomonal or acanthamoeba keratitis
- Epidemic bacterial (streptococcal) conjunctivitis reported in school settings

GENERAL PREVENTION
- Wash hands frequently.
- Demonstrate eye dropper technique: Eye is closed and head back, several drops at nasal margin; open eyes to allow liquid to enter. Never touch tip of dropper to skin or eye.

ETIOLOGY
- Viral:
  - Adenovirus (common cold) or Coxsackie
  - Enterovirus (acute hemorrhagic conjunctivitis)
  - Herpes simplex
  - Herpes zoster or varicella
  - Measles, mumps, or influenza
- Bacterial:
  - *Staphylococcus aureus* or *epidermidis*
  - *Streptococcus pneumoniae*
  - *Haemophilus influenzae* (children)
  - *Pseudomonas* species or anaerobes (in contact lens users)
  - Acanthamoeba from contaminated contact lens solution may cause keratitis.
  - *Neisseria gonorrhoeae* and *meningitidis*
  - *Chlamydia trachomatis*: Gradual onset >4 weeks
- Allergic:
  - Hay fever, seasonal allergies, atopy

- Nonspecific:
  - Irritative: Topical medications, wind, dry eye, ultraviolet light exposure, smoke
  - Autoimmune: Sjögren, pemphigoid, Wegener granulomatosis
  - Rare: Rickettsial, fungal, parasitic, tuberculosis, syphilis, Kawasaki, chikungunya, Graves, gout, carcinoid, sarcoid, psoriasis, Stevens-Johnson, Reiter syndrome

COMMONLY ASSOCIATED CONDITIONS
- Viral infection (e.g., common cold)
- STD

 DIAGNOSIS

HISTORY
- RED FLAG: Any decrease in visual acuity is not consistent with conjunctivitis alone; must document normal vision for diagnosis of isolated conjunctivitis.
- Viral: Contact or travel:
  - May start with 1 eye, then both
  - If herpetic, recurrences or vesicles on skin
- Bacterial: Difficult to distinguish from viral, unless contact lens user. Assume bacterial in contact lens wearer unless cultures negative. If recent STD, suspect chlamydia or GC
- Allergic: Itching, atopy, seasonal, dander
- Irritative: Feels dry, exposure to wind, tear film deficit may persist 30 days after acute conjunctivitis, chemicals, or drug: Atropine, aminoglycosides, iodide, phenylephrine, antivirals, bisphosphonates, retinoids, topiramate, chamomile, COX-2 inhibitors
- Foreign body: Redness may persist 24 hours after removal.

PHYSICAL EXAM
- General: Common to all types of conjunctivitis:
  - Red eye, conjunctival injection
  - Foreign body sensation
  - Eyelid sticking or crusting, discharge
  - Normal visual acuity and pupillary reactivity
- Viral:
  - Palpable preauricular lymphadenopathy may be present.
  - Severe viral: Herpes simplex or zoster:
    ○ Burning sensation, rarely itching
    ○ Unilateral, herpetic skin vesicles in herpes zoster
    ○ Palpable preauricular node
- Bacterial (non-STD): May be epidemic:
  - Mild pruritus, discharge mild to heavy
  - Conjunctival chemosis/edema
  - If contact lens user, must rule out pseudomonal (or other bacterial) keratitis
- Bacterial: Gonococcal (or meningococcal) hyperacute infection:
  - Rapid onset 12–24 hours
  - Severe purulent discharge
  - Chemosis/conjunctival/lid edema
  - Rapid growth of superior corneal ulceration
  - Preauricular adenopathy
  - Signs of STDs (chlamydia, GC, HIV, etc.)
- Allergic:
  - Itching predominant
  - Seasonal or dander allergies
  - Chemosis/conjunctival/eyelid edema

- Nonspecific irritative:
  - Dry eyes, intermittent redness, chemical/drug exposure
  - Foreign body: May have redness and discharge 24 hours after removal
- Must document normal visual acuity
- Cornea should be clear and without fluorescein uptake. If cloudy or signs of keratitis, consult ophthalmologist.
- Recommend fluorescein exam:
  - Evert lid to inspect for foreign bodies.
- Skin: Look for herpetic vesicles, nits on lashes (lice), scaliness (seborrhea), or styes
- Limbal flush at corneal margin if uveitis
- If pupil is irregular (i.e., penetrating foreign body), emergent referral
- Discharge but no conjunctival injection: Blepharitis

DIAGNOSTIC TESTS & INTERPRETATION
Lab
- Usually not needed initially for the most common causes
- Culture swab if STD suspected, very severe symptoms, or patient is a contact lens user

Diagnostic Procedures/Surgery
- Fluorescein exam for ulcer or abrasion on cornea
- Small superficial foreign bodies may be removed with irrigation or moistened swab.

DIFFERENTIAL DIAGNOSIS
- Uveitis (iritis, iridocyclitis, choroiditis): Limbal flush (red band at corneal margin), hazy anterior chamber, and decreased visual acuity
- Penetrating ocular trauma: Emergently hospitalize
- Acute glaucoma (emergency): Headache, corneal clouding, poor visual acuity
- Corneal ulcer(s) or foreign body: Lesions on fluorescein exam
- Dacryocystitis: Tenderness and swelling over tear sac (below medial canthus)
- Scleritis and episcleritis: Red injected vessels radially oriented, sectoral (pie wedge), nodularity of sclera
- Ophthalmia neonatorum: Neonates in 1st 2 days of life (gonococcal; 5–12 days of life): Chlamydial, HSV, very rare Neisseria meningitidis. Consider specialty consultation for required systemic therapy.
- Blepharitis: Lid margins inflamed and producing itching, scale, or discharge, but no conjunctival injection.

 TREATMENT

MEDICATION
First Line
- Viral (nonherpetic):
  - Artificial tears for symptomatic relief
  - Vasoconstrictor/antihistamine (e.g., naphazoline/pheniramine) q.i.d. for severe itching
  - May consider topical antibiotic (see bacterial below) if return to daycare requires treatment (1)[C]
- Viral (herpetic) (by ophthalmologist):
  - Trifluridine: 1% drops 1 q2h (2)[C]
  - Acyclovir oral: 400 mg 5 × day for herpes simplex virus (HSV) (use 800 mg for zoster) × 7 days

- Bacterial (non-STD) self-limited 5–7 days, so treatment is optional (and should take cost and bacterial resistance-production factors into consideration), although it may shorten the symptoms by half a day (3)[A]. Alternative strategy: Delay treatment until 3rd day (using simple warm moist towel cleansing of closed eye), same duration of symptoms (4)[B]. Contact lens wearers should be referred for evaluation of possible keratitis:
  – Trimethoprim/polymyxin ophthalmic: 1 drop q4h (while awake) for 5 days or
  – Erythromycin ophthalmic ointment: 1/2 inch b.i.d.–q.i.d. for 5 days or
  – Sodium sulfacetamide (10% solution:) 2 drops q4h (while awake) for 5 days or
  – Tobramycin 0.3% ophthalmic drops/ointment q4h (drops) to q8h (ointment)
- Bacterial (gonococcal) hospitalize for IV ceftriaxone:
  – If no corneal lesions, ceftriaxone 1 g IM as single dose and topical bacitracin ophthalmic ointment 1/2 inch q.i.d. Chlamydial in neonates requires oral erythromycin ethylsuccinate 30 mg/kg daily q6h p.o. × 14 d, max 3 g/d.
- Allergic and atopic (by increasing approximate cost: All are efficacious, but evidence favoring one over another is inconclusive):
  – Ketotifen 0.25% 1 drop b.i.d. (5)[A]
  – Cromolyn (Opticrom) 4%, q.i.d. (4)[A]
  – Epinastine (Elestat) 0.05% b.i.d. (5)[A]
  – Ketorolac 0.1% 1 drop q.i.d. (5)[A]
  – Emedastine 0.05% 1 drop q.i.d. (5)[A]
  – Azelastine 0.05% 1 drop b.i.d. (4)[A]
  – Olopatadine 0.1% 1 drop b.i.d. or 0.2% 1 drop daily (5)[A]

  – Oral nonsedating antihistamines (Zyrtec [cetirizine] 10 mg/d, Allegra [fexofenadine] 60 mg b.i.d.), etc., to treat nasal and urticarial symptoms
  – Oral antihistamine (e.g., diphenhydramine 25 mg t.i.d.) in severe cases
- Contraindications: Avoid topical steroids unless able to monitor intraocular pressure. Also case report of HSV keratitis presenting without distinguishing findings from viral conjunctivitis would discourage initial use of steroids.
- Precautions:
  – Do not allow dropper to touch eye
  – Vasoconstrictor/antihistamine: Rebound vasodilation after prolonged use

Second Line
- Viral and allergic: Numerous over-the-counter products
- Bacterial: Polymyxin-gramicidin, ciprofloxacin

ADDITIONAL TREATMENT
General Measures
- Appropriate health care: Outpatient
- Eyelid cleansing with wet cloth up to q.i.d.
- Stop use of contact lenses while red
- Patching of eye not beneficial
- Avoid irritants such as smoke, wind, and sun

Issues for Referral
Any significantly decreased visual acuity, herpetic keratitis, or contact lens-related bacterial conjunctivitis: Ophthalmologic consultation

COMPLEMENTARY AND ALTERNATIVE MEDICINE
As it is usually benign and self-limited, saline flushes and other placebos would be expected to work.

SURGERY/OTHER PROCEDURES
No surgery for this condition. Other eye surgeries may be delayed until resolution of this condition.

IN-PATIENT CONSIDERATIONS
Acute gonococcal conjunctivitis (or very rare case of meningococcal conjunctivitis) would require inpatient treatment with ceftriaxone 50 mg/kg IV every day (pediatric), 1 gm IM x 1 (adult) along with ophthalmologic consultation.

Admission Criteria
Penetrating ocular trauma, GC

 ## ONGOING CARE
FOLLOW-UP RECOMMENDATIONS
- If not resolved within 5–7 days, alternate diagnoses should be considered or consultation obtained.
- Children may be excluded from school until eye is no longer red if viral or bacterial, depending on school policy. Allergic conjunctivitis should be able to return to school with doctor's note.

Patient Monitoring
Referral if worse in 24 hours

PATIENT EDUCATION
- Patients should not wear contacts until their eyes are fully healed (typically 1 week).
- Patients should throw away current pair of contacts.
- Patients should throw away any eye makeup that they have been using, especially mascara.
- Cool, moist compresses can ease irritation and itch.

PROGNOSIS
- Viral: 5–10 days for pharyngitis with conjunctivitis, 2 weeks with adenovirus
- Herpes simplex: 2–3 weeks
- Bacterial: Self-limited; treated, 2–5 days; untreated, 5–7 days

COMPLICATIONS
- Corneal scars with herpes simplex
- Lid scars or entropion with varicella zoster
- Corneal ulcers or perforation, very rapid with gonococcal
- Hypopyon: Pus in anterior chamber
- Chlamydial neonatal ophthalmia: Could have concomitant pneumonia
- Otitis media may follow *H. influenzae* conjunctivitis.
- The very rare Neisseria meningitidis conjunctivitis may be followed by meningitis.

REFERENCES
1. David SP. Should we prescribe antibiotics for acute conjunctivitis? *Am Fam Physician.* 2002;66: 1649–50.
2. Greenberg MF, Pollard ZF. The red eye in childhood. *Pediatr Clin North Am.* 2003;50:105–24.
3. Sheikh A, Hurwitz B. Antibiotics vs. placebo for acute bacterial conjunctivitis. *Cochrane database of Systematic Reviews.* 2006, Issue 2. Art.No. CD001211.
4. Bielory L, Lien KW, Bigelsen S. Efficacy and tolerability of newer antihistamines in the treatment of allergic conjunctivitis. *Drugs.* 2005;65:215–28.
5. Chigbu DI et al. The management of allergic eye diseases in primary eye care. *Cont Lens Anterior Eye.* 2009;32:260–72.

ADDITIONAL READING
- Everitt HA, Little PS, Smith PW. A randomised controlled trial of management strategies for acute infective conjunctivitis in general practice. *BMJ.* 2006;333:321.
- Gupta R, Levent F, Healy CM, et al. Unusual soft tissue manifestations of Neisseria meningitidis infections. *Clin Pediatr (Phila).* 2008;47:400–3.
- Hamerlynck JV, Rietveld RP, Hooft L. [From the Cochrane Library: Marginally higher chance of cure by antibiotic treatment in acute bacterial conjunctivitis] *Ned Tijdschr Geneeskd.* 2007;151: 594–6.
- Huang T, Wang Y, Liu Z, et al. Investigation of tear film change after recovery from acute conjunctivitis. *Cornea.* 2007;26:778–81.
- Rose PW, Harnden A, Brueggemann AB, et al. Chloramphenicol treatment for acute infective conjunctivitis in children in primary care: a randomised double-blind placebo-controlled trial. *Lancet.* 2005;366:37–43.

See Also (Topic, Algorithm, Electronic Media Element)
Rhinitis, Allergic
Algorithm: Eye Pain

 ## CODES
ICD9
- 077.99 Unspecified diseases of conjunctiva due to viruses
- 372.00 Acute conjunctivitis, unspecified
- 771.6 Neonatal conjunctivitis and dacryocystitis

CLINICAL PEARLS
- Conjunctivitis does not alter visual acuity; decreased acuity or photophobia should prompt consideration of more serious ophthalmic disorders.
- Culture discharge in all contact lens wearers, consider referral and remind patient to throw away current contacts and avoid contacts until eyes fully healed.
- Antibiotic therapy is of no value in viral conjunctivitis (most cases of infectious conjunctivitis), and does not significantly alter the course of most types of bacterial conjunctivitis (so is optional in these cases).

C

CONSTIPATION

Robert A. Baldor, MD
Abdulrazak Abyad, MD, PhD, MBA, MPH, AGSF, AFCHSE

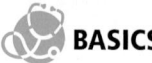

BASICS

A group of syndromes with similar findings that include unsatisfactory defecation characterized by infrequent stools, difficult stool passage, or both. Characteristics include fewer than 3 bowel movements a week, hard stools, excessive straining, prolonged time spent on the toilet, a sense of incomplete evacuation, and abdominal discomfort/bloating.

DESCRIPTION
- System(s) affected: Gastrointestinal (GI)
- Synonym(s): Obstipation

Geriatric Considerations
Increased incidence of colorectal neoplasms with age may be associated with constipation; thus, new onset of constipation after 50 years of age is considered a "red flag."

Pediatric Considerations
Consider Hirschsprung disease (absence of colonic ganglion cells): 25% of all newborn intestinal obstructions, milder cases diagnosed in older children with chronic constipation, abdominal distension, decreased growth. 5:1 male:female ratio. Associated with inherited conditions such as Down syndrome.

EPIDEMIOLOGY
- Predominant age: May affect all ages, but more pronounced in children and elderly
- Predominant sex: Female > Male (2:1)
- Non-whites > whites

Incidence
- 5 million office visits annually
- 100,000 hospitalizations

Prevalence
~15% of population effected

RISK FACTORS
- Extremes of life (very young and very old)
- Polypharmacy
- Sedentary lifestyle or condition
- Improper diet and inadequate fluid intake

Genetics
Unknown, but condition may be familial

GENERAL PREVENTION
High-fiber diet, adequate fluids, exercise, and bowel training to "obey the urge" to defecate are useful preventive strategies.

PATHOPHYSIOLOGY
- As food leaves the stomach, the ileocecal valve relaxes (gastroileal reflex) and chyme enters the colon (1–2 L/day). Peristaltic contractions move the chyme through the colon into the rectum. In the colon, sodium is actively absorbed in exchange for potassium and bicarb—water follows because of the generated osmotic gradient. The chyme is converted into feces (200–250 mL).
- Normal transit time for a meal to reach the cecum is 4 hours, and to the pelvic colon 8 hours later. Transit then slows to the anus. Rectal distention initiates the defecation reflex.

- Defecation follows as a reflex that can be inhibited by voluntarily contracting the external sphincter or facilitated by straining to contract the abdominal muscles while voluntarily relaxing the anal sphincter. The *urge to defecate* occurs as rectal pressures increase. Distention of the stomach by food also initiates rectal contractions and a desire to defecate.

ETIOLOGY
- Primary constipation:
  – Slow colonic transit time (13%)
  – Pelvic floor/anal sphincter dysfunction (25%)
  – Functional—normal transit time and sphincter function, yet problems (bloating, abdominal discomfort, perceived difficulty going, presence of hard stools) (69%)
- Secondary constipation:
  – Irritable bowel syndrome (IBS)
  – Endocrine dysfunction (diabetes mellitus, hypothyroid)
  – Metabolic disorder (increased calcium, decreased potassium)
  – Mechanical (obstruction, rectocele)
  – Pregnancy
  – Neurologic disorders (Hirschsprung, multiple sclerosis, spinal cord injuries)
- Medication effect:
  – Anticholinergic effects (antidepressants, narcotics, antipsychotics)
  – Antacids (calcium, aluminum)
  – Calcium channel blockers

COMMONLY ASSOCIATED CONDITIONS
- Debility, either general as in the aged or that imposed by specific underlying illness
- Dehydration
- Hypothyroidism
- Hypokalemia
- Hypercalcemia

DIAGNOSIS

A group of syndromes with similar findings that include unsatisfactory defecation characterized by infrequent stools, difficult stool passage, or both.

ALERT
Red flags:
- New onset after age of 50
- Hematochezia/melena
- Unintentional weight loss
- Anemia
- Neurological defects

HISTORY
Ask about the Rome III criteria (1):
- At least 2 of the following, for 12 weeks, in the previous 6 months:
  – Fewer than 3 stools/week
  – Straining at least 1/4 of the time
  – Hard stools at least 1/4 of the time
  – Need for manual assist at least 1/4 of the time
  – Sense of incomplete evacuation at least 1/4 of the time
  – Sense of anorectal blockade at least 1/4 of the time
- Loose stools rarely seen without use of laxatives

PHYSICAL EXAM
- Digital rectal exam (masses, pain, stool, fissures, hemorrhoids, anal tone)
- Abdominal/gynecological exam (masses, pain)
- Neurological exam

DIAGNOSTIC TESTS & INTERPRETATION
For the most part, this is a clinical diagnosis, as evidence to support the use of routine labs/x-rays/scoping is lacking in the workup of constipation (2).

Lab
Initial lab tests
However, the American Gastroenterological Association guidelines suggest complete blood count, BS, TSH, calcium, and creatinine routinely and sigmoid/colonoscopy if red flags are present (3).

Imaging
Initial approach
If condition is refractory to empiric approach, pursue further testing:
- Colonoscopy
- Barium enema to look for obstruction and/or megarectum, megacolon, or Hirschsprung disease

Follow-Up & Special Considerations
Measure colonic transit time by ingesting radiopaque (Sitz-Mark) markers:
- Plain abdominal film obtained 5 days later (120 hours): Retention >20% markers indicates slow transit
- Markers seen exclusively in distal colon/rectum suggests defecatory disorder.

Diagnostic Procedures/Surgery
Consider referral to evaluate defecation:
- Balloon expulsion
- Defecography using a barium paste
- Anorectal manometry with a rectal catheter

Pathological Findings
- None in common, functional constipation
- Paucity or absence of intramural enteric ganglia in certain cases of congenital or acquired megacolon
- Neuromuscular abnormalities in certain cases of pseudo-obstruction

DIFFERENTIAL DIAGNOSIS
- Congenital:
  – Hirschsprung disease/syndrome
  – Hypoganglionosis
  – Congenital dilation of the colon
  – Small left colon syndrome
- Meconium ileus
- Other causes of abdominal pain

TREATMENT

Address immediate concerns:
- Bloating/discomfort/straining: Osmotic agents
- Post-op, childbirth, hemorrhoids, fissures: Stool softener to make defecation easier
- Stimulants and suppositories
- Manual disimpaction as needed, then approach the chronic condition

MEDICATION

- In patients with no known secondary causes of constipation, conservative nonpharmacologic treatment measures generally are recommended, including:
  - Regular exercise
  - Increased fluid intake
  - Bowel habit training
- Other nonpharmacologic therapies include:
  - Biofeedback therapy
  - Behavior therapy
  - Electric stimulation

First Line

Bulking agents (need to be accompanied by adequate amounts of liquid to be useful):

- Hydrophilic colloids (bulk-forming agents):
  - Psyllium (Konsyl, Metamucil, Perdiem Fiber): 1 rounded tsp in liquid p.o. daily up to t.i.d.
  - Bran methylcellulose (Citrucel): 1 rounded tsp in 8 oz cold water p.o. daily up to t.i.d.
  - Polycarbophil (Mitrolan, FiberCon): 1 g p.o. q.i.d.
- Stool softeners:
  - Docusate sodium (Colace): 100 mg b.i.d.
- Osmotic laxatives:
  - Polyethylene glycol (MiraLax) (0.8 mg/kg/d) 17 g daily (current evidence shows PEG to be superior to lactulose) (4)[A]
  - Saccharines Lactulose (Chronulac) 15–60 ml q.h.s. (flatulence, bloating, cramping side effects)
  - Sorbitol 15–60 ml q.h.s. (as effective as lactulose)
  - Magnesium salts (Milk of Magnesia) avoid in renal insufficiency

Second Line

Stimulants (irritate bowel causing muscle contraction; usually combined with a softener; work in 8–12 hours)

- Senna/docusate (Senokot-S, ex-lax) 1–2 capsules or 15–30 mL at bedtime
- Bisacodyl/docusate (Dulcolax, Correctol) 2–3 tablets daily
- Casanthranol/docusate (Peri-Colace) lubricants (contain mineral oil, coating the stool)

ALERT

- Short-term use only. Can bind fat-soluble vitamins with the potential for deficiencies. May similarly decrease absorption of some drugs.
- Avoid in those at risk for aspiration (lipid pneumonia).
- Suppositories:
  - Osmotic: Sodium phosphate
  - Lubricant: Glycerin
  - Stimulatory: Bisacodyl
- Enemas:
  - Sodium phosphate (Fleet enema)
  - Lubiprostone (Amitiza): A selective chloride channel activator; 24 mcg b.i.d.

Pregnancy Considerations

- Avoid in pregnancy and breastfeeding
- Prokinetic agents (partial 5-HT4 agonists): Have been withdrawn due to cardiac side effects (tegaserod [Zelnorm], cisapride [Propulsid])
- Other agents not approved by the Food and Drug Administration:
  - Misoprostol (Cytotec) : A prostaglandin that increases colonic motility (5)
  - Colchicine: Neurogenic stimulation to increase colonic motility (6)

ADDITIONAL TREATMENT

General Measures

- Attempt to eliminate medications that may cause or worsen constipation
- Increase fluid intake
- Increase fiber in diet
- Enemas if other methods fail

Additional Therapies

Biofeedback with artificial silicon stool

SURGERY/OTHER PROCEDURES

Surgery rarely indicated

IN-PATIENT CONSIDERATIONS

Nursing

Manual disimpaction occasionally required in difficult chronic situations

 ONGOING CARE

FOLLOW-UP RECOMMENDATIONS

Encourage exercise and physical activity.

Patient Monitoring

If what seems to be simple, functional constipation persists, further investigate for a possible organic cause.

DIET

Increase fiber, but bloating and gas can be problematic:

- Gradually increase intake to 25 grams/day over a 6-week period.
- Insoluble, less fermentable fiber, like wheat bran, tends to be better tolerated.
- Bran (hard outer layer of cereal grains)
- Vegetables and fruits
- Whole grain foods
- Encourage liberal intake of fluids.

PATIENT EDUCATION

- Occasional mild constipation is normal.
- Instruction in consistent bowel training; the best time to move bowels is in the morning, after eating breakfast, when the normal bowel transit and defecation reflexes are typically functioning to move the bowels.

PROGNOSIS

- Constipation that is only occasional, brief, and responsive to simple measures is harmless.
- That which is habitual can be a lifelong nuisance.
- Those with neurologic compromise can suffer from ill effects such as obstipation and impaction to toxic megacolon.
- No evidence for dependence
- No evidence for harm from stimulant use; melanosis coli may develop, but it is a benign condition (7)

COMPLICATIONS

- Volvulus
- Toxic megacolon
- Acquired megacolon: In severe, long-standing cases
- Fluid and electrolyte depletion: Laxative abuse
- Rectal ulceration (stercoral ulcer) related to recurrent fecal impaction
- Anal fissures

REFERENCES

1. Longstreth GF, Thompson WG, Chey WD, et al. Functional bowel disorders. *Gastroenterology*. 2006;130:1480–91.
2. American College of Gastroenterology Chronic Constipation Task Force. An evidence-based approach to the management of chronic constipation in North America. *Am J Gastroenterol*. 2005;100 (Suppl 1):S1–4.
3. Locke GR, Pemberton JH, Phillips SF. American Gastroenterological Association Medical Position Statement: guidelines on constipation. *Gastroenterology*. 2000;119:1761–6.
4. Lee-Robichaud H, Thomas K, Morgan J et al. Lactulose versus Polyethylene Glycol for Chronic Constipation. *Cochrane Database Syst Rev*. 2010;7:CD007570–
5. Roarty TP, Weber F, Soykan I, et al. Misoprostol in the treatment of chronic refractory constipation: results of a long-term open label trial. *Aliment Pharmacol Ther*. 1997;11:1059–66.
6. Verne GN, Davis RH, Robinson ME, et al. Treatment of chronic constipation with colchicine: randomized, double-blind, placebo-controlled, crossover trial. *Am J Gastroenterol*. 2003;98: 1112–6.
7. Müller-Lissner SA, Kamm MA et al. Myths and misconceptions about chronic constipation. *Am J Gastroenterol*. 2005;100:232–42.

ADDITIONAL READING

- Spinzi G, Amato A, Imperiali G et al. Constipation in the elderly: management strategies. *Drugs Aging*. 2009;26:469–74.
- van Dijk M, Benninga MA, Grootenhuis MA, et al. Chronic childhood constipation: A review of the literature and the introduction of a protocolized behavioral intervention program. *Patient Educ Couns*. 2007.

 CODES

ICD9
564.00 Constipation, unspecified

CLINICAL PEARLS

- Constipation can be characterized as unsatisfactory defecation, with infrequent stools, difficult stool passage, or both, for 3 months.
- Functional constipation (normal transit time and sphincter function) seen most often
- Workup is necessary in the presence of red flags: Onset >50 yrs, hematochezia/melena, unintentional weight loss, anemia, neurological defects
- Best evidence for effectiveness is for osmotic agents (polyethylene glycol [PEG]).

CONTRACEPTION

Kristen Kelly, MD
Jeremy Golding, MD

 BASICS

DESCRIPTION
- Methods to prevent pregnancy
- Mechanisms include prevention/delay of ovulation, inhibition of sperm entry into the uterus, or interference with implantation of fertilized ovum.
- Natural family planning limits coitus to presumably nonfertile portions of the menstrual cycle.
- The most effective method of contraception is permanent sterilization. Reversal of sterilization may be difficult if not impossible.

Pediatric Considerations
Use of estrogen prior to pubertal growth spurt may reduce ultimate height due to epiphysial closure.

EPIDEMIOLOGY
Incidence
- ~98% of women of reproductive age have used some form of contraception, but 1/3–1/2 of pregnancies are unplanned or unwanted (1).
- OCs are leading method (31% of women) in the US, followed by tubal sterilization (1).
- Factors in choice of contraceptive method include efficacy, convenience, adverse effects, and affordability.

RISK FACTORS
Unintended pregnancy:
- Young adolescents
- Lower socioeconomic population
- Those with limited knowledge and access to reproductive service

 DIAGNOSIS

DIAGNOSTIC TESTS & INTERPRETATION
Lab
- No routine testing is needed prior to initiating contraception except reassurance that the patient is not pregnant (by history or laboratory).
- If family history of thrombophilia, consider testing for the specific defect (if known) or common disorders (factor V Leiden, prothrombin gene G20210A mutation) prior to initiation of hormonal contraception.

 TREATMENT

CDC issued comprehensive guidelines in 2010 for use of contraceptive methods in patients with medical conditions (2).

MEDICATION
- Spermicides:
  - All contain nonoxynol-9; may alter vaginal flora and mucosal barrier
- Sponge:
  - 2-inch circular disk that contains nonoxynol-9. Moisten with water before insertion in vagina; effective for 24 hours.

- OCs:
  - Side effects minimized with pills having <50 μg estrogen. OCs with 35 μg of ethinyl estradiol provide the same blood hormone levels as 50 μg of mestranol.
  - Progestational agents vary. Newer progestogens are less androgenic and have less effect on lipoproteins (clinical significance unknown). Possible increased risk of thrombosis with desogestrel (3)[C].
  - Continuous pill (e.g., Seasonale with 84 active days and 7 inactive) used for endometriosis and premenstrual dysphoric disorder. Any monophasic may be used for continuous cycling: Skip the last 7 pills and begin new pack (off-label indication).
  - If adverse effects occur, pill may be changed based on nature of adverse reaction.
  - Progestin-only is the preferred OC for breast-feeding mothers, especially in the first few months of nursing because combined estrogen-progestin can suppress milk production.
- Weekly hormonal patch (Ortho-Evra):
  - Patch must be changed weekly; contains 20 μg ethinyl estradiol and 150 μg norelgestromin
  - Produces higher serum estrogen levels than oral 20 μg pill
  - Patch may cause local skin irritation.
  - Not as reliable in women >90 kg
- Vaginal contraceptive ring (NuvaRing):
  - Flexible polymer ring containing 15 μg ethinyl estradiol and 120 μg etonogestrel; inserted into vagina for 3 weeks per cycle (also may be used for continuous cycling for 4 weeks [off label])
- Medroxyprogesterone (Depo-Provera), also known as depot-medroxyprogesterone acetate (DMPA):
  - 150 mg IM or 104 mg/0.65 mL SC, both are given every 3 months
  - Contraceptive levels of hormone persist for up to 4 months (2–4-week margin of safety).
  - Potential for decreased bone mineral density if used for >2 years:
    - Recommend that women take 1300 mg of calcium and 400 IU of vitamin D when using DMPA (4).
- IUD:
  - ParaGard (Copper T): Interferes with sperm transport and ova fertilization; approved for up to 10 years, but likely remains effective for longer. May increase menstrual blood loss. Also effective as postcoital contraceptive up to 5 days from intercourse.
  - Mirena (Levonorgestrel intrauterine system):
    - T-shaped IUD that releases 20 μg of levonorgestrel per day (very low serum levels)
    - Approved for use up to 5 years; has been used off label for up to 7
    - Expect irregular menstrual spotting initially and then possibly amenorrhea after 6–9 months of use.
    - Ideally, insert during menses (ensures patient is not pregnant).
  - The literature on IUD use among adolescents is scant and obsolete. Nevertheless, published reports are generally reassuring (5), and both types of IUD are now commonly used in adolescents and other nulliparous women.

- Etonogestrel implant (Implanon):
  - Small, single, plastic rod that is implanted into the superficial subcutaneous tissue of the upper arm and provides continuous contraception via progestin hormone. This prevents ovulation and thickens cervical mucus to halt fertilization. Effective for up to 3 years.
  - The device may be inserted only by trained and certified providers, as improper placement may result in unintended pregnancy, pain, infection, and difficult removal.
  - Menstrual irregularities are common the 1st 6–12 months (and beyond); some will not have menses after 1 year, although others may have continuing irregular spotting for years.
- Emergency contraception: Start within 72 hours for maximum effectiveness, but evidence supports up to 120 hours:
  - Levonorgestrel: 1.5 mg taken as 2 0.75 mg tablets (Plan B), or 1 1.5 mg tablet (Plan B 1-Step). Less nausea and slightly more effective than the "Yuzpe regimen" (see below) (6):
    - Available over the counter, but may be less expensive for many women if prescribed
    - Prescription is needed for women under age 17.
  - Estradiol/levonorgestrel (Preven, Ovral, Ogestrel): "Yuzpe regimen" 50 μg/0.25 mg, 2 tablets q12h (4 tablets total). Other OCs may be used as long as dose of estrogen component ≥100 μg/dose. *Note*: Antinausea medication (e.g., Phenergan) given 1–2 hours before the doses
  - Copper-bearing IUD (Paragard): Insert up to 5 days after intercourse; over 99% effective in preventing pregnancy and continues to provide contraception for up to 10 years.
  - Ulipristal acetate (Ella) 30 mg approved by FDA in 2010. Selective progesterone modulator, approved for use up to 5 days following unprotected intercourse
- Contraindications: Hormonal contraceptives, especially those containing estrogen (WHO Medical Eligibility Criteria for Contraceptive Use): History of coronary artery disease (CAD) or multiple risk factors (age >55, smoking, high blood pressure, diabetes mellitus); history of deep vein thrombosis (DVT)/pulmonary embolism (PE); history of cerebrovascular accident (CVA); history of migraines at age >35 or migraine at any age with aura; current or past breast cancer; active liver disease or hepatic tumor; pregnancy; unexplained abnormal uterine bleeding without further investigation. Relative contraindication: Smokers >35. Healthy nonsmokers may use oral contraceptives until menopause.

ALERT
Significant possible interactions due to increased metabolism of hormones (use higher estrogen dose and/or add barrier method):

ADDITIONAL TREATMENT
General Measures
Nondrug methods:
- Latex condom
- Diaphragm: Needs fitting
- IUD: Contraindications include pregnancy, undiagnosed genital bleeding, uterine anomalies, and large fibroids (3)[C].

- Periodic abstinence:
  - Calendar method: Track length of last 6 cycles; fertility period is calculated by subtracting 18 from the number of days of shortest cycle and 11 from number of days in longest cycle. Example: If shortest cycle is 28 days and longest cycle is 31 days, fertile period is from day 10–20.
  - Symptothermal method: Calculate the 1st day of abstinence by subtracting 21 from the length of the shortest menstrual cycle in the previous 6 months, or the 1st day cervical mucus is detected, whichever comes first. End calculated as 3 days after body temperature rises 1°C.
  - Withdrawal method: Male partner withdraws from vagina before ejaculation. Failure occurs if withdrawal is not timed accurately or if the pre-ejaculatory fluid contains sperm.
- Lactation delays resumption of ovulation postpartum due to prolactin-induced inhibition of gonadotropin-releasing hormone (GNRH) release. Breast-feeding is effective contraception only if (1) the infant is <6 months old, (2) the infant is exclusively breast-feeding, and (3) the mother has not resumed her regular menses (lactational amenorrhea method or LAM) (7).

SURGERY/OTHER PROCEDURES
Permanent sterilization:

- Tubal sterilization in the female
- Hysteroscopic sterilization via polyester fibers (Essure): Polyester fibers with a coiled spring are introduced into each fallopian tube by transcervical route. Requires another contraceptive to be used for 3 months after procedure (3)[C].
- Vasectomy in the male

 ## ONGOING CARE

FOLLOW-UP RECOMMENDATIONS
Patient Monitoring
- Pelvic exam and Pap smear per guidelines
- Sexually transmitted disease (STD) testing per guidelines
- Check for IUD 1 month after insertion. Spontaneous expulsion rate highest in first month. Pt should monitor presence of string monthly following menses.
- OC users: Monitor BP 3 months after starting, then annual follow up

DIET
Vitamin C and some herbals such as St. John's wort may alter estrogen levels, reducing efficacy or causing breakthrough bleeding.

PATIENT EDUCATION
- Condoms: Water-based lubricants (inside and outside) reduce the risk of breakage. Withdraw penis before it becomes flaccid.
- IUD: Check string periodically.
- Diaphragm:
  - Refit after childbirth or if weight changes by more than 10%.
  - Before inserting, 1 Tbs of water-soluble spermicidal jelly or cream should be placed in the dome.
  - Leave in at least 6 hours after coitus. If coitus is repeated before 6 hours, insert another teaspoon of spermicidal jelly into the vagina without removing the diaphragm.

- Female condom:
  - New condom required for each sex act
- OC:
  - Pill should be taken same time each day.
  - If a pill is missed, take 2 the following day, but use a barrier method until next period.
- Emergency contraception prevents pregnancy via several proposed mechanisms, including inhibition of sperm motility, alterations in tubal transport, unfavorable uterine receptivity, and/or fertilization inhibition. Emergency contraception does not affect an established pregnancy: 1-888-NOT-2-LATE or http://www.planbonestep.com/

COMPLICATIONS
- Hormonal contraceptives, serious:
  - Thromboembolism
  - Hypertension
  - Myocardial infarction, stroke
- OCs, minor:
  - Nausea and vomiting: Take after eating.
  - Breakthrough bleeding: Usually self-limiting after 3 months; if persists, change pill
  - Amenorrhea: Pregnancy must be ruled out.
  - Cyclic weight gain: Use smallest dose of estrogen available.
  - Breast tenderness: Rare with low-dose pill
  - Depression: Rare with low-dose pill
  - Chloasma: Stop pill or cover with makeup
  - Acne or hirsutism: Change to a less androgenic progesterone
  - Cholestatic jaundice: Stop pill; do not restart
  - Weight gain throughout cycle: Use triphasic pill to minimize dose of progesterone or use newer progesterone.
- Injectable contraceptive (Depo-Provera):
  - Irregular bleeding: No treatment needed; nonsteroidal anti-inflammatory drug (NSAID) may help
  - Weight gain
  - Amenorrhea: Common after 1 year of use
  - Possible ↑ bone resorption and ↓ bone mineral density (BMD), but rapid recovery following discontinuation. Food and Drug Administration (FDA) recommends BMD for use >2 years and to consider periodic estrogen.
- Sponge and diaphragm:
  - Associated with toxic shock syndrome
- IUD:
  - Pelvic inflammatory disease (PID) or salpingitis: Device removal is not necessary for mild PID treated as outpatient. For infections requiring hospitalization, most recommend that device be removed.
  - Heavy bleeding and cramps: Remove device.
  - Although absolute risk is no higher than without IUD, pregnancy, when it occurs, is more likely to be ectopic.

REFERENCES

1. CDC National Center for Health Statistics. *Use of Contraception and Use of Family Planning Services*: United States: 1992–2002. Hyattsville, MD; 2004.
2. Division of Reproductive Health, National Center for Chronic Disease Prevention and Health Promotion, Centers for Disease Control and Prevention (CDC), Farr S, Folger SG, Paulen M, Tepper N, Whiteman M, Zapata L, Culwell K, Kapp N, Cansino C et al. U.S. Medical Eligibility Criteria for Contraceptive Use, 2010: adapted from the World Health Organization Medical Eligibility Criteria for Contraceptive Use, 4th edition. *MMWR Recomm Rep*. 2010;59:1–86.
3. Hatcher RA, Zietman M, Cwiak C, et al. *A Pocket Guide to Managing Contraception*. 8th ed. Tiger, GA: Bridging the Gap Foundation; 2005.
4. Schrager SB. DMPA's effect on bone mineral density: A particular concern for adolescents. *J Fam Pract*. 2009;58:E1–8.
5. Deans EI, Grimes DA. Intrauterine devices for adolescents: a systematic review. *Contraception*. 2009;79:418–23.
6. Cheng L, Gülmezoglu AM, Piaggio G, et al. Interventions for emergency contraception. *Cochrane Database Syst Rev*. 2008;CD001324.
7. Academy of Breastfeeding Medicine Clinical Protocol #13: Contraception during breastfeeding. 2005. Available at http://www.bfmed.org/Resources/Protocols.aspx

ADDITIONAL READING

- Hughes H. Postpartum contraception. *J Fam Health Care*. 2009;19:9–10, 12.
- Mestad RE, Kenerson J, Peipert JF. Reversible contraception update: the importance of long-acting reversible contraception. *Postgrad Med*. 2009; 121:18–25.
- Naz RK, Rowan S. Update on male contraception. *Curr Opin Obstet Gynecol*. 2009;21:265–9.

See Also (Topic, Algorithm, Electronic Media Element)
Thrombophilia, Factor V Leiden, Prothrombin Gene Mutation

 ## CODES

ICD9
- V25.01 General counseling on prescription of oral contraceptives
- V25.02 General counseling on initiation of other contraceptive measures
- V25.03 Encounter for emergency contraceptive counseling and prescription

CLINICAL PEARLS

- Hormonal and IUD contraceptives may be initiated immediately ("Quick-Start") as long as likelihood of established pregnancy is low.
- Quick-start may reduce risk of pregnancy occurring before next last menstrual period (LMP), and may improve long-term adherence.
- Clearly established benefits of OCs include reduction in ovarian cancer, endometrial cancer, ectopic pregnancies, and PID; less dysmenorrhea and anemia; reduced number of functional ovarian cysts, a regular menstrual cycle; improvement in acne.
- Barrier contraceptives lower the risk of STDs.

COR PULMONALE

Parag Goyal, MD
Oscar Starobin, MD

 BASICS

DESCRIPTION
- Enlargement and subsequent dysfunction and failure of the right ventricle (RV) in the presence of pulmonary arterial hypertension secondary to abnormalities of the lungs, thorax, pulmonary ventilation or circulation
- May occur in acute or chronic setting:
  - Acute: Rapid increase of pulmonary arterial pressure causing RV overload and resulting dysfunction/failure
  - Chronic: Progressive hypertrophy and dilation of RV over months to years, with eventual dysfunction/failure

EPIDEMIOLOGY
- Approximately, 6–7% of all types of adult heart disease in US
- Between 10% and 30% of heart failure admissions in the US are the result of cor pulmonale (1).

Incidence
Difficult to assess. Best estimate is 1/10,000–3/10,000 per year (2).

Prevalence
Difficult to assess. Best estimate is 2/1,000–6/1,000 (2).

RISK FACTORS
- Acute cor pulmonale is most commonly caused by massive pulmonary embolism (PE):
  - Risk factors associated with PE include:
    - Vessel injury
    - Stasis
    - Hypercoagulable states
- Chronic cor pulmonale is most commonly caused by COPD and/or pulmonary arterial hypertension (PAH).
  - Risk factors associated with COPD and/or PAH include:
    - Tobacco use
    - Living at high altitudes
    - Industrial exposures such as asbestos
    - Alpha-1-antitrypsin deficiency
    - Connective tissue disease

GENERAL PREVENTION
- Prevention of pulmonary embolism via deep venous thrombosis prophylaxis when necessary
- Early detection and timely management of COPD to delay its progression
- Management of underlying disease, including aggressive correction of hypoxia and acidosis, that may contribute to worsening pulmonary hypertension

PATHOPHYSIOLOGY
- Acute: A sudden event, such as large pulmonary embolism, increases resistance to blood flow in the pulmonary vasculature, causing a quick and significant increase of pressure proximally. The RV is unable to overcome this pressure, leading to low cardiac output and RV failure.
- Chronic: PAH develops from many possible etiologies, although predominantly from alveolar hypoxia. The RV is initially able to compensate for this increased pressure through concentric hypertrophy. However, worsening pulmonary hypertension eventually overcomes the RV's

accommodative abilities, leading to dilation of the RV. This results in both systolic and diastolic dysfunction, causing reduced cardiac output and right-sided heart failure.

ETIOLOGY
- Lung disease: COPD including emphysema and chronic bronchitis (80–90%) (3), cystic fibrosis, restrictive and interstitial lung disease, including scleroderma and sarcoidosis, pulmonary thromboembolism, tumor emboli, idiopathic pulmonary arterial hypertension
- Hematological abnormalities: Sickle cell anemia, polycythemia vera
- Neuromuscular disease: Amyotrophic lateral sclerosis, myasthenia gravis, Guillain-Barré syndrome, polio, spinal cord injuries
- Disorders of ventilator control: Primary central hypoventilation, sleep apnea syndromes
- Thoracic cage deformities: Kyphoscoliosis
- Collagen vascular disease
- Left ventricular failure is NOT considered a cause of cor pulmonale.

COMMONLY ASSOCIATED CONDITIONS
Pulmonary arterial hypertension (PAH): Classically defined as the presence of a resting mean pulmonary artery pressure (PAP) >20 mm Hg, though some sources define as >25 mm Hg at rest and >30 mm Hg with exercise

 DIAGNOSIS

HISTORY
- Dyspnea, orthopnea
- Fatigue, lethargy, syncope
- Cyanosis, pallor, diaphoresis
- Pleuritic chest pain, cough, hemoptysis
- Exertional angina
- Hoarseness secondary to compression of the left recurrent laryngeal nerve by enlarged pulmonary vessels
- Anorexia and/or right upper quadrant discomfort from hepatic congestion
- Cardiovascular collapse, shock, and/or cardiac arrest may occur in acute setting or advanced chronic setting.

PHYSICAL EXAM
- Peripheral edema is the most common sign of right heart failure (RHF), though it is nonspecific.
- Tachypnea, wheeze
- Increased intensity of pulmonic component of 2nd heart sound (P2)
- Splitting of S2 over the cardiac apex with inspiration
- Audible S3 or S4
- Pansystolic murmur heard best at right midsternal border increasing with inspiration, consistent with tricuspid regurgitation (typically a late sign).
- Early diastolic murmur heard best at left upper sternal border, consistent with pulmonary regurgitation.
- Right ventricular heave
- Jugular venous distension with inspiration (Kussmaul sign)
- Prominent a and v waves on jugular venous pulse tracing
- Hepatomegaly

- Signs of DVT, such as tenderness or unilateral swelling, may or may not be present.

DIAGNOSTIC TESTS & INTERPRETATION
ECG (poor sensitivity; up to 67% patients will have normal findings) (1):
- Rightward P-wave axis deviation
- Peaked P waves anteriorly and in inferior leads (i.e., "P pulmonale")
- $S_1S_2S_3$ pattern, or $S_1Q_3T_3$, inverted pattern (McGinn-White pattern)
- RV hypertrophy (high specificity, low sensitivity)
- Right bundle-branch block
- Low-voltage QRS

Lab
Initial lab tests
- CBC and serum chemistries may be obtained to rule out other conditions:
  - Lab findings such as polycythemia and hypercapnia may be present due to COPD.
  - LFTs may be elevated due to hepatic congestion secondary to RV failure.
- Pulmonary function testing may show airflow obstruction with reduced PO_2, or other findings associated with COPD.
- Arterial blood gas, indicated for acute respiratory distress, may show hypercapnic acidosis and hypoxemia.
- BNP and cardiac troponins may be elevated secondary to RV stretch.

Imaging
- Chest x-ray:
  - Cardiomegaly
  - Increased width of right descending pulmonary artery
  - Left main pulmonary artery prominence below the aortic knob
- 2-dimensional echocardiogram:
  - RV mid-wall hypokinesis/akinesis plus normokinesis/hyperkinesis of RV apex (McConnell sign) are associated with acute cor pulmonale caused by acute pulmonary embolism.
  - RV dilatation and/or hypertrophy may be indicative of chronic cor pulmonale.
  - Doppler echocardiography with saline contrast to estimate tricuspid regurgitation is the most reliable noninvasive estimation of pulmonary artery pressure (PAP).
- Spiral CT scan of chest:
  - Most accurate modality for diagnosing emphysema and interstitial lung disease
  - Test of choice for assessment of acute pulmonary embolism
- V/Q scan may be used to assess for pulmonary embolism in acute cor pulmonale.
- MRI commonly used, as it can characterize right ventricular size, mass morphology, and gross function

Diagnostic Procedures/Surgery
- Right heart catheterization is the gold standard for quantitation of ventricular and pulmonary pressures, and exclusion of congenital heart disease as etiology. Right heart catheterization is also recommended to assess vasoreactivity prior to implementing calcium channel blocker therapy.

- Pulmonary function tests should be performed in patients with a suggestive history of underlying lung disease and in those with normal cardiac function.

DIFFERENTIAL DIAGNOSIS
- Right-sided heart failure secondary to left-sided heart failure
- Right-sided cardiomyopathy, ischemic or nonischemic
- Tricuspid valvulopathy
- Severe congenital pulmonary hypertension secondary to congenital heart disease with left-to-right shunting, most frequently from unrepaired nonrestrictive ventricular septal defect (VSD)

 TREATMENT

Reduce disease burden via oxygenation, preservation of cardiac function, and attenuation of PAH (4).

MEDICATION
- Oxygenation:
  - Oxygen:
    - Long-term continuous oxygen therapy improves the survival of hypoxemic patients with COPD and cor pulmonale.
    - All patients with pulmonary hypertension whose PaO_2 is consistently <55 mm Hg or saturation ≤88% at rest, during sleep, or with ambulation should be prescribed oxygen to keep O_2 >90 mm Hg (5)[A].
- Preservation of cardiac function:
  - Diuretics: Decrease RV filling pressures; also improves peripheral edema secondary to right heart failure:
    - Furosemide: Starting at 20–80 mg p.o./IV, titrate and increase dose per diuresis.
    - Excessive volume depletion should be avoided.
    - Monitor closely for metabolic alkalosis, as this may suppress ventilatory drive and contribute to hypoxia.
  - Cardiac glycosides:
    - Impact of digoxin on cor pulmonale alone is unclear
    - Digoxin may be appropriate in the presence of co-existent left ventricular systolic failure.
    - Digoxin may also be appropriate in the presence of atrial fibrillation as adjunct for rate control.
- Amelioration of PAH:
  - Calcium channel blockers (CCB) (4):
    - May be used as adjunctive therapy in those with low-to-moderate disease
    - Vasodilator therapy to reduce pulmonary vascular resistance has been shown to be effective in a small subset of patients (10%).
    - Vasoreactivity trial should be attempted with short-acting vasodilator at cardiac catheterization to determine likelihood of response. Reduction of >20% PAP without reduction of cardiac output should prompt adding CCB such as nifedipine, diltiazem, amlodipine to treatment regimen.
    - Repeat vasoreactivity trial via cardiac catheterization is recommended at 3-6 months following initiation of CCB therapy to assess sustained response. For nonsustained response, discontinue CCB and pursue alternative medications (6).

- For nonresponse or unsustained response to CCB, treatment with phosphodiesterase inhibitors, endothelin receptor antagonists, and/or prostanoids may be appropriate based on World Health Organization (WHO) classification (6):
  - WHO Class I: Supportive therapy.
  - WHO Class II: Monotherapy is recommended with either phosphodiesterase inhibitor or endothelin receptor antagonist.
  - WHO Class III: Combination therapy may be used with phosphodiesterase inhibitor, endothelin receptor antagonist, or prostanoids. There is currently little randomized data on which combination is most efficacious (7).
  - WHO Class IV: Epoprostenol IV is 1st-line therapy in critically ill patients; other classes of drugs may also be added for combination therapy.
  - Phosphodiesterase inhibitors: Vasodilates by increasing cAMP and therefore increasing nitric oxide, an endogenous vasodilator. Sildenafil, tadalafil; Endothelin receptor antagonists: Vasodilates by blocking the function of endothelin, a potent vasoconstrictor. Bosentan, Ambrisentan, Sitaxsentan.
  - Prostanoids: Vasodilates by mimicking endogenous vasodilators. Iloprost Inhaled. IV may also be used; evidence to date limited to expert opinion. Treprostinil SC. IV may also be used; evidence to date limited to expert opinion. Beraprost PO Epoprostenol IV: Currently recommended for WHO Class IV only.
- Anticoagulation:
  - Recommended for patients with underlying thromboembolic disease
  - Recommended for patients with cor pulmonale in association with idiopathic pulmonary arterial hypertension (5)[B]
  - Use in secondary causes of PAH is widely accepted, though little supportive evidence to date (8)
  - In general, warfarin is recommended unless contraindications. Target international normalized ratio (INR) for prophylaxis is 2–3.

ADDITIONAL TREATMENT
General Measures
- Treat underlying disease.
- Supportive therapy as necessary:
  - Continuous positive airway pressure or bilevel positive airway pressure may be used for hypoxia/sleep disorders.
  - Ventilation using positive-pressure masks, negative-pressure body suits, or mechanical ventilation is suggested for patients with neuromuscular disease.
  - Phlebotomy may be indicated for severe polycythemia (hematocrit >55%).

Issues for Referral
Patients with cor pulmonale should be referred to a cardiologist or pulmonologist for expert consultation.

SURGERY/OTHER PROCEDURES
Moderate-to-severe disease refractory to medication may require atrioseptostomy and/or lung transplantation.

 ONGOING CARE

Referral of patients with PAH to a specialized center with close follow-up is strongly recommended.

DIET
Salt and fluid restriction

PATIENT EDUCATION
- Smoking cessation and avoidance of exposure to secondary smoke is strongly recommended.
- Exertional activity should be limited.
- Pregnancy should be avoided in PAH.

PROGNOSIS
- Patients with cor pulmonale resulting from COPD have a greater likelihood of dying than do similar patients with COPD alone.
- The pulmonary artery pressure (PAP) is a reliable indicator of prognosis; higher pressure is associated with worse prognosis.
- In patients with COPD and mild disease (PAP 20–35 mm Hg), 5-year survival is 50%.

REFERENCES
1. Han MK, McLaughlin VV, Criner GJ, Martinez FJ et al. Pulmonary diseases and the heart. *Circulation.* 2007;116:2992–3005.
2. Naeije R et al. Pulmonary hypertension and right heart failure in chronic obstructive pulmonary disease. *Proc Am Thorac Soc.* 2005;2:20–2.
3. Weitzenblum E, Chaouat A et al. Cor pulmonale. *Chron Respir Dis.* 2009;6:177–85.
4. Hoeper MM et al. Drug treatment of pulmonary arterial hypertension: current and future agents. *Drugs.* 2005;65:1337–54.
5. Badesch DB, Abman SH, Simonneau G, et al. Medical therapy for pulmonary arterial hypertension: updated ACCP evidence-based clinical practice guidelines. *Chest.* 2007;131: 1917–28.
6. Barst RJ, Gibbs JS, Ghofrani HA, Hoeper MM, McLaughlin VV, Rubin LJ, Sitbon O, Tapson VF, Galiè N et al. Updated evidence-based treatment algorithm in pulmonary arterial hypertension. *J Am Coll Cardiol.* 2009;54:S78–84.
7. Benedict N, Seybert A, Mathier MA et al. Evidence-based pharmacologic management of pulmonary arterial hypertension. *Clin Ther.* 2007;29:2134–53.
8. Alam S, Palevsky HI. Standard therapies for pulmonary arterial hypertension. *Clin Chest Med.* 2007;28:91–115, viii.

See Also (Topic, Algorithm, Electronic Media Element)
Pulmonary Embolism; Chronic Obstructive Pulmonary Disease and Emphysema; Pulmonary Arterial Hypertension, Idiopathic; Congestive Heart Failure

 CODES

ICD9
- 415.0 Acute cor pulmonale
- 416.9 Chronic pulmonary heart disease, unspecified

CLINICAL PEARLS
- Continuous, long-term oxygen therapy improves life expectancy and quality of life in cor pulmonale.
- Referral of patients with PAH to a specialized center is strongly recommended.

CORNEAL ABRASION AND ULCERATION

Ken S. Ota, DO

 BASICS

DESCRIPTION
- Corneal abrasions result from scratching, denuding, abrading, or cutting of the outermost layer of the eye. They are usually due to trauma, but can occur spontaneously as well.
- Corneal ulcers usually represent an infection of the cornea by bacteria, viruses, or fungi as a result of breakdown in the protective epithelial barrier:
  - Both corneal abrasions and ulcerations can result in scarring, which may impair vision.
  - Both lesions can occur centrally or marginally.

EPIDEMIOLOGY
Incidence
- Corneal abrasion is the most common ophthalmologic visit to the emergency department and is commonly seen in urgent care as well.
- Ulceration is also common in the US.

RISK FACTORS
- Any abrasive injury
- Contact lenses (especially soft lenses)
- Blepharitis
- Dry eye syndrome
- Entropion (with lashes scratching cornea)
- Chronic topical steroid use
- Abuse of topical anesthetics
- Autoimmune disorders
- Vitamin A deficiency
- Chronic corneal exposure (Bell palsy, exophthalmos, etc.)
- Recent eye surgery
- Optic neuropathy

GENERAL PREVENTION
- Eye protection to avoid injury during work, crafts, and sport
- Proper contact lens handling
- Artificial tears for those with inability to blink or known dry eyes

ETIOLOGY
- Corneal abrasions typically result from accidental trauma (i.e., fingernail scratch).
- Corneal ulcers result from presence of an entryway to the external eye through dry eye, burns, abrasion, contact lenses, inappropriate use of topical anesthetics, antibiotics, or antiviral drops, immunosuppressant drugs, diabetes, or immunodeficiency.
- Causative agents of ulceration:
  - Gram-positive organisms (staphylococci, streptococci, and bacilli)
  - Anaerobes (cocci, bacilli)
  - Gram-negative organisms (*Pseudomonas*, diplococci, and rods)
  - Viruses, such as herpes
  - Fungal organisms (*Candida, Aspergillus, Fusarium, Acanthamoeba*) in agricultural workers or associated with ocular corticosteroid use
  - Peripheral ulcerative keratitis usually caused by autoimmune disorders such as rheumatoid arthritis (RA), systemic lupus erythematosus (SLE), scleroderma, etc.
  - Vitamin A deficiency may cause corneal necrosis or keratomalacia.

COMMONLY ASSOCIATED CONDITIONS
- Chronic ulcerations may be associated with neurotrophic keratitis due to lack of 5th nerve innervation of the cornea. Individuals with thyroid disease, diabetes, or immunosuppressive conditions are particularly at risk.
- Any cause of fat malabsorption may be associated with vitamin A deficiency.

 DIAGNOSIS

HISTORY
- History remarkable for contact lens use, dry eyes, rubbing eye, history of trauma from foreign body or chemical burn, or history of connective tissue disorder
- Signs and symptoms of abrasion or ulceration include sudden onset of eye pain, photophobia, tearing, foreign-body sensation, blurring of vision, and/or conjunctival injection.
- Abrasions and ulcerations are usually unilateral.

PHYSICAL EXAM
- Visual acuity may be decreased if abrasion of ulcer is centrally located.
- Conjunctival injection
- Increased lacrimation on affected side
- Photophobia
- Lesion seen on slit lamp exam and area of damage shows fluorescein uptake; staining seen using Wood lamp or cobalt blue slit lamp

DIAGNOSTIC TESTS & INTERPRETATION
Lab
Initial lab tests
- Culture ulcer and contact lens if applicable.
- *Note:* Pretreatment with topical antibiotics may alter culture results.

Diagnostic Procedures/Surgery
Scrapings of the corneal ulcer for culture and sensitivities ideally should be done before beginning local antibiotics. The sample should be plated directly onto the culture medium.

Pathological Findings
Scrapings for Gram and Giemsa stain may demonstrate bacteria, yeast, or intranuclear inclusions that may aid in the diagnosis.

DIFFERENTIAL DIAGNOSIS
- Foreign bodies
- Keratitis
- Herpes simplex or zoster
- Bilateral or true idiopathic lesions may suggest basement membrane dystrophy.

 TREATMENT

MEDICATION
First Line
- Pain reduction can be achieved with ophthalmic NSAIDs (1)[A].
- Some ophthalmic NSAIDs include ketorolac 0.5% [Acular], diclofenac 0.1% [Voltaren], and bromfenac 0.09% [Xibrom].
- Ophthalmic antibiotics may help prevent further infection and ulceration of corneal abrasions (2)[C].
- Some ophthalmic antibiotics include chloramphenicol 1% [Chloroptic], ciprofloxacin 0.3% [Ciloxan], ofloxacin 0.3% [Ocuflox], gentamicin 0.3%, and erythromycin 0.5%. Note: ointment preparations may be more soothing to the eye than solutions.

- Eye patching is not helpful and may be harmful; thus, it is not recommended (3)[A].
- Consultation with an ophthalmologist is recommended for all ulcers to help determine appropriate therapy (4)[C].
- Topical gentamicin and tobramycin are effective against *Pseudomonas, Enterobacter, Klebsiella*, and aerobic gram-negative organisms; cephalosporins (e.g., cefazolin 50 mg/mL) also may be used.
- Fungal keratitis is treated with a protracted course of topical antifungal agents.
- Herpetic keratitis should be treated initially with trifluridine. Vidarabine and acyclovir are alternatives (5)[A].

Second Line
- Supplemental topical cycloplegia (i.e., homatropine 5% and cyclopentolate 1%) has not been found to be beneficial (6)[B].
- Oral analgesic medication if topical analgesia not adequate

ADDITIONAL TREATMENT
General Measures
- Corneal abrasions can be managed by primary care physicians (7)[C]. See indications for referral below.
- All patients with corneal ulceration should be referred immediately to an ophthalmologist.
- For corneal ulcerations, appropriate antimicrobial therapy should be instituted after cultures have been obtained.
- Eye patching is not recommended (3)[A].
- Corneal abrasions should be evaluated regularly to determine if ophthalmology referral is necessary.

Issues for Referral
Refer to ophthalmologist if there is a history of significant ocular trauma, if corneal infection is suspected, or if a recurrent or nonhealing abrasion is encountered despite standard treatment (7)[C].

 ## ONGOING CARE
FOLLOW-UP RECOMMENDATIONS
Patient Monitoring
The patient should be monitored every 1–3 days, depending on the depth/severity of the abrasion, until healed.

PATIENT EDUCATION
Prevention of abrasions and proper handling of contact lenses can prevent recurrence of corneal ulcers.

PROGNOSIS
Corneal abrasions and ulcerations should improve daily and heal with appropriate therapy. If healing does not occur or the lesion extends, obtain an ophthalmology consultation.

COMPLICATIONS
Recurrence, scarring of the cornea, loss of vision, and corneal perforation

REFERENCES

1. Weaver CS, Terrell KM et al. Evidence-based emergency medicine. Update: do ophthalmic nonsteroidal anti-inflammatory drugs reduce the pain associated with simple corneal abrasion without delaying healing? *Ann Emerg Med*. 2003;41:134–40.
2. Upadhyay MP, Karmacharya PC, Koirala S, Shah DN, Shakya S, Shrestha JK, Bajracharya H, Gurung CK, Whitcher JP et al. The Bhaktapur eye study: ocular trauma and antibiotic prophylaxis for the prevention of corneal ulceration in Nepal. *Br J Ophthalmol*. 2001;85:388–92.
3. Turner A, Rabiu M et al. Patching for corneal abrasion. *Cochrane Database Syst Rev*. 2006; CD004764.
4. Wirbelauer C. Management of the red eye for the primary care physician. *Am J Med*. 2006;119: 302–6.
5. Wilhelmus KR. Therapeutic interventions for herpes simplex virus epithelial keratitis. *Cochrane Database Syst Rev*. 2007;CD002898.
6. Carley F, Carley S et al. Towards evidence based emergency medicine: best BETs from the Manchester Royal Infirmary. Mydriatics in corneal abrasion. *Emerg Med J*. 2001;18:273.
7. Fraser S et al. Corneal abrasion. *Clin Ophthalmol*. 2010;4:387–90.

ADDITIONAL READING

- Ehler JP, Shah CP, Fenton GL. The Wills Eye Manual: Office and Emergency Room Diagnosis and Treatment of Eye Disease. Baltimore: Lippincott, Williams and Wilkins; 2008.
- Morden NE, Berke EM. Topical fluoroquinolones for eye and ear. *Am Fam Physician*. 2000;62:1870–6.
- Watson SL, Barker NH. Interventions for recurrent corneal erosions. *Cochrane Database Syst Rev*. 2007;CD001861.

 ## CODES

ICD9
- 370.00 Corneal ulcer, unspecified
- 918.1 Superficial injury of cornea

CLINICAL PEARLS

- Contact lens use should be discontinued while corneal abrasion or ulcer is healing.
- Eye patching is not recommended.
- Prescribe topical and/or oral analgesic medication for symptom relief and consider ophthalmic antibiotics.
- Prompt referral to an ophthalmologist should be made for suspicion of an ulcer, recurrence of abrasion, retained foreign body, or lack of improvement despite therapy.
- Appropriate antimicrobial therapy should be instituted immediately when corneal infection is suspected.

C

CORNS AND CALLUSES

Neil J. Feldman, DPM

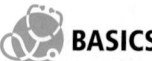 **BASICS**

DESCRIPTION
- A callus (tyloma) is a diffuse area of hyperkeratosis, usually without a distinct border.
- Typically the result of exposure to repetitive forces, including friction and mechanical pressure. Tend to occur on the palms of hands and soles of feet.
- A corn (heloma) is a circumscribed hyperkeratotic lesion with a central conical core of keratin that causes pain and inflammation. The conical core in a corn is a thickening of the stratum corneum.
- Hard corn or heloma durum (more common): More often on toe surfaces, especially 5th toe (PIP) joint
- Soft corn (heloma molle): Commonly in the interdigital space
- Digital corns are also known as clavi.
- Intractable plantar keratosis are usually located under a metatarsal head (1st and 5th most common), are typically more difficult to resolve, and resistant to usual conservative treatments.

EPIDEMIOLOGY
Corns and calluses have the largest prevalence of all foot disorders.

Incidence
Incidence of corns and calluses increases with age. Less common in pediatric patients. Women affected more often than men. Blacks report corns and calluses 30% more often than whites.

Prevalence
- 9.2 million Americans
- Nearly 38/1,000 people affected

RISK FACTORS
- Extrinsic factors producing pressure, friction, and local stress:
  - Ill-fitting shoes
  - Not using socks, gloves
  - Manual labor
  - Walking barefoot
  - Activities that increase stress applied to skin of hands or feet (running, walking, sports)
- Intrinsic factors:
  - Bony prominences: Bunions
- Enlarged bursa or abnormal foot function/structure: Hammertoe, claw toe, or mallet toe deformity

Genetics
No true genetic basis identified, since most corns and calluses are due to mechanical stressors on the foot/hands.

GENERAL PREVENTION
External irritation is by far the most common cause of calluses and corns. General measures to reduce friction on the skin are recommended to reduce incidence of callus formation. Examples include wearing shoes that fit well and using socks and gloves.

Geriatric Considerations
- In elderly patients, especially those with neurologic or vascular compromise, skin breakdown from calluses/corns may lead to increased risk of infection/ulceration. 30% of foot ulcers in the elderly arise from eroded hyperkeratosis. Regular foot exams are emphasized for these patients, as well as diabetic patients.

PATHOPHYSIOLOGY
Increased activity of keratinocytes in superficial layer of skin leading to hyperkeratosis. This is a normal response to excess friction, pressure, or stress.

ETIOLOGY
- Calluses typically arise from repetitive friction, motion, or pressure to skin.
- Soft corns arise from increased moisture from perspiration leading to maceration of the skin along with mechanical irritation, especially between toes.
- Hard corns are an extreme form of callus with a keratin-based core. Often found on the digital surfaces and commonly linked to bony protrusions causing skin to rub against shoe surfaces.

COMMONLY ASSOCIATED CONDITIONS
- Foot ulcers, especially in diabetic patients or patients with neuropathy or vascular compromise
- Infection; look for warning signs of:
  - Spreading or redness around sore
  - Pus-like drainage
  - Increased pain/swelling
  - Fever
  - Change in color of fingers or toes
- Signs of gangrene

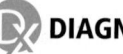 **DIAGNOSIS**

- Most commonly a clinical diagnosis based on visualization of the lesion.
- Examination of footwear may also provide clues

HISTORY
- Careful history can usually pinpoint cause.
- Ask about neurologic and vascular history and diabetes. These may be risk factors for progression of corns/calluses to frank ulcerations and infection.

PHYSICAL EXAM
- Calluses:
  - Thickening of skin without distinct borders
  - Often on feet, hands; especially over palms of hands, soles of feet
  - Colors from white to gray-yellow, brown, red
  - May be painless or tender
  - May throb or burn
- Corns:
  - Hard corns: Commonly on dorsum of toes or dorsum of 5th PIP joint:
    - Varied texture: Dry, waxy, transparent, to a hornlike mass
    - Distinct borders
    - More common to feet
    - Often painful
  - Soft corns:
    - Often between toes, especially between 4th and 5th digits at the base of the webspace
    - Often yellowed, macerated appearance
    - Often extremely painful

DIAGNOSTIC TESTS & INTERPRETATION
Imaging
Initial approach
- Radiographs may be warranted if no external cause found. Look for abnormalities in foot structure, bone spurs.
- Use of metallic radiographic marker and weight-bearing films often highlights the relationship between the callus and bony prominence.

Diagnostic Procedures/Surgery
Biopsy with microscopic evaluation in rare cases

Pathological Findings
Abnormal accumulation of keratin in epidermis, stratum corneum

DIFFERENTIAL DIAGNOSIS
- Plantar warts (typically a loss of skin lines within the wart)
- Porokeratoses (blocked sweat gland)

 ## TREATMENT

MEDICATION
- Most therapy for corns and calluses can be done as self-care in the home.
- Use bandages, soft foam padding, or silicone sleeve over the affected area to decrease friction on the skin and promote healing with digital clavi.
- Use socks or gloves regularly.
- Use lotion/moisturizers for dry calluses and corns.
- Keratolytic agents such as urea or ammonium lactate can be applied safely.
- Use sandpaper discs or pumice stones over hard, thickened areas of skin.

Geriatric Considerations
- Use of salicylic acid corn plasters can cause skin breakdown and ulceration in patients with thin, atrophic skin; diabetes; and those with vascular compromise. The skin surrounding the callus will often turn white and can become quite painful.

ADDITIONAL TREATMENT
General Measures
- Debridement of affected tissue and use of protective padding
- Low-heeled shoes, soft upper with deep and wide toebox
- Extra-width shoes for 5th toe corns
- Avoidance of activities that contribute to painful lesions
- Prefabricated or custom orthotics

Issues for Referral
- May benefit from referral to podiatrist if use of topical agents and shoe changes are ineffective.
- Abnormalities in foot structure may require surgical treatment.
- Diabetic, vascular, and neuropathic patients may benefit from referral to podiatrist for regular foot exams to prevent infection, ulceration.

COMPLEMENTARY AND ALTERNATIVE MEDICINE
- Many OTC topical ointments and lotions available for calluses (Keralac, Callex, urea, Lac-Hydrin). Do not use on broken skin.
- Epsom salt soaks for 5–10 minutes at a time

SURGERY/OTHER PROCEDURES
- Surgical treatment of areas of protruding bone where corns and calluses form
- Rebalancing of foot pressure through functional foot orthotics
- Shaving or cutting off hardened area of skin using a chisel or 15-blade scalpel. For corns, remove keratin core and place pad over area during healing.

IN-PATIENT CONSIDERATIONS
Admission Criteria
- Admission usually not necessary, unless progression to ulcerated lesion with signs of severe infection, gangrene
- May require aggressive debridement in operating room should an abscess or deep-space infection be suspected.

Nursing
Wound care, dressing changes for infected lesions

 ## ONGOING CARE

PATIENT EDUCATION
- General information available at: http://www.mayoclinic.com/health/corns-and-calluses/DS00033/DSECTION=9
- American Podiatric Medical Association. Available at: http://www.apma.org

PROGNOSIS
Complete cure is possible once factors causing injury are eliminated.

COMPLICATIONS
Ulceration, infection

ADDITIONAL READING
- Freeman DB. Corns and calluses resulting from mechanical hyperkeratosis. *Am Fam Physician*. 2002;65:2277–80.
- Pinzur MS, Slovenkai MP, Trepman E, et al. Guidelines for diabetic foot care: recommendations endorsed by the Diabetes Committee of the American Orthopaedic Foot and Ankle Society. *Foot Ankle Int*. 2005;26:113–9.
- Theodosat A. Skin diseases of the lower extremities in the elderly. *Dermatol Clin*. 2004;22:13–21.

 ## CODES

ICD9
700 Corns and callosities

CLINICAL PEARLS
Most therapy for corns and calluses can be done as self-care in the home using padding over the affected area to decrease friction.

COSTOCHONDRITIS

Scott A. Fields, MD

 BASICS

DESCRIPTION
- Anterior chest wall pain associated with pain and tenderness of the costochondral and costosternal regions
- System(s) affected: Musculoskeletal
- Synonym(s): Costosternal syndrome; Parasternal chondrodynia; Anterior chest wall syndrome; Tietze disease and syndrome; Chondrocostal junction syndrome

Pediatric Considerations
Pay special attention to psychogenic chest pain in children who perceive family discord.

EPIDEMIOLOGY
- Predominant age: 20–40 years
- Predominant gender: Female

Incidence
~10% of chest pain complaints; 15–20% of teenagers with chest pain may have costochondritis.

RISK FACTORS
- Unusual physical activity or overuse
- Recent trauma (including motor vehicle accident, domestic violence, etc.) or new activity
- Recent upper respiratory infection (URI)

ETIOLOGY
- Not fully understood
- Trauma
- Overuse

COMMONLY ASSOCIATED CONDITIONS
URI

DIAGNOSIS

- Insidious onset
- Pain, usually sharp, sometimes pleuritic
- Pain involves multiple locations, the 2nd–5th costal cartilages are most often involved.
- Pain worsens with movement and breathing.
- Heat often relieves pain.
- Chest tightness is often associated with the pain.
- Pain sometimes radiates into arm.
- Nonsuppurative edema and tenderness at rib articulations
- Redness and warmth at sites of tenderness

HISTORY
A complete and thorough history is mandatory for the diagnosis, with special emphasis on cardiac risk factor evaluation.

PHYSICAL EXAM
A physical exam to exclude more serious conditions that may present with chest pain is necessary for the diagnosis. Tenderness elicited over the costochondral junctions is necessary to establish the diagnosis, but does not completely exclude other causes of chest pain.

Geriatric Considerations
- Often presents with multiple problems capable of causing chest pain, making a thorough history and physical exam imperative.

DIAGNOSTIC TESTS & INTERPRETATION
Lab
- The diagnosis of costochondritis is primarily based on a thorough history and physical exam.
- Laboratory exams should be used only if concern exists regarding other elements of the differential diagnosis.
- Erythrocyte sedimentation rate is inconsistently elevated.

Imaging
No imaging is indicated for the diagnosis of costochondritis; chest x-ray normal.

Diagnostic Procedures/Surgery
None indicated for the diagnosis of costochondritis

Pathological Findings
Costochondral joint inflammation

DIFFERENTIAL DIAGNOSIS
- Cardiac:
  - Coronary artery disease
  - Aortic aneurysm
  - Mitral valve prolapse
  - Pericarditis
  - Myocarditis
- Gastrointestinal:
  - Gastroesophageal reflux
  - Peptic esophagitis
  - Esophageal spasm
  - Gastritis
- Musculoskeletal:
  - Fibromyalgia
  - Slipping rib syndrome involves the lower ribs
  - Costovertebral arthritis
  - Painful xiphoid syndrome
  - Rib trauma with swelling
  - Thoracic disc compression
  - Ankylosing spondylitis
  - Epidemic myalgia
  - Precordial catch syndrome
- Psychogenic:
  - Anxiety disorder
  - Panic attacks
  - Hyperventilation
- Respiratory:
  - Asthma
  - Pulmonary embolism
  - Pneumonia
  - Chronic cough
  - Pneumothorax
- Other:
  - Domestic violence and abuse
  - Herpes zoster
  - Spinal tumor
  - Metastatic cancer
  - Substance abuse (cocaine)

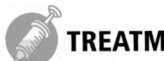 TREATMENT

Reassurance of benign nature of condition

MEDICATION
First Line
Nonsteroidal anti-inflammatory drugs (aspirin, ibuprofen, naproxen, or diclofenac). Narcotics rarely indicated (1,2)[C].

Second Line
Acetaminophen (1,2)[C]

ADDITIONAL TREATMENT
General Measures
- Patient reassurance, rest, and heat (or ice massage)
- Stretching exercises

COMPLEMENTARY AND ALTERNATIVE MEDICINE
Limited data on use of manipulation or ice massage, but may be safely tried if patient interested

IN-PATIENT CONSIDERATIONS
Admission Criteria
Only indicated if differential diagnosis is unclear and cardiac or other more serious etiology of chest pain is being considered (3)[C]

Discharge Criteria
When diagnosis is established

 ONGOING CARE

FOLLOW-UP RECOMMENDATIONS
Follow-up within 1 week if diagnosis is unclear

DIET
Normal

PATIENT EDUCATION
Educate the patient in regard to the self-limited (although potentially recurrent) nature of the illness. Instruct patient on proper physical activity regimens to avoid overuse syndromes. Also stress importance of avoiding sudden, significant changes in activity.

PROGNOSIS
- Self-limited illness, although sometimes chronic
- Often recurs

COMPLICATIONS
Incomplete attention to differential diagnosis or inappropriate interventions in a desire to ensure that a more life-threatening diagnosis is not missed

REFERENCES

1. Freeston J, Karim Z, Lindsay K, et al. Can early diagnosis and management of costochondritis reduce acute chest pain admissions? *J Rheumatol*. 2004;31:2269–71.
2. Jensen S. Musculoskeletal causes of chest pain. *Aust Fam Physician*. 2001;30:834–9.
3. Mukamel M, Kornreich L, Horev G, et al. Tietze's syndrome in children and infants. *J Pediatr*. 1997;131:774–5.

ADDITIONAL READING

- Disla E, Rhim HR, Reddy A, et al. Costochondritis. A prospective analysis in an emergency department setting. *Arch Intern Med*. 1994;154:2466–9.
- Gregory PL, Biswas AC, Batt ME. Musculoskeletal problems of the chest wall in athletes. *Sports Med*. 2002;32:235–50.
- Rovetta G, Sessarego P, Monteforte P et al. Stretching exercises for costochondritis pain. *G Ital Med Lav Ergon*. 169–71.

See Also (Topic, Algorithm, Electronic Media Element)
Algorithm: Chest Pain

 CODES

ICD9
733.6 Tietze's disease

CLINICAL PEARLS
- A very common disorder, accounting for perhaps 10% of all cases of chest pain, and a greater percentage in teenagers and young adults
- Educate the patient in regard to the self-limited (although potentially recurrent) nature of the illness. Instruct patient on proper physical activity regimens to avoid overuse syndromes. Also stress importance of avoiding sudden, significant changes in activity.
- Consider an anxiety disorder as a contributor to all cases of persistent chest pain, whether musculoskeletal or cardiac.

COUNSELING TYPES

William T. Garrison, PhD

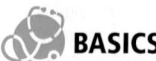 **BASICS**

DESCRIPTION

- Psychotherapeutic and counseling interventions play an important role in the management of chronic- and acute-onset diseases and disorders. They are typically the primary initial mode of evaluation and/or treatment for most mild-to-moderate psychiatric disorders that reach criteria using the DSM or ICD diagnostic classification systems. Treatment and successful control of either medical or psychological conditions require some form of professional counseling experience. Best outcomes occur when they are employed by a skilled practitioner. However, psychotherapy differs from generic counseling, which can take many forms and is delivered commonly in nonmedical settings with mixed results.
- Counseling approaches are usually tailored to the specific presenting problem or issue, and serve educational and emotional support functions. Typically, such counseling in medical settings will be time-limited and problem-focused, and is often not intended to lead to major medical symptom relief or major behavioral changes.
- The goals of psychotherapy range from increasing individual psychological insight and motivation for change, reduction of interpersonal conflict in the marriage or family, reduction of chronic or acute emotional suffering, and reversal of dysfunctional or habitual behaviors. There are several general types of psychotherapy, starting with individual, marital, or family approaches. In addition, a number of psychological theories guide various methods and treatment philosophies. The following is a brief overview of commonly used psychotherapeutic and counseling methods.
- Psychodynamic therapy: Unconscious conflict manifests as patient's symptoms/problem behaviors:
  - Short-term (4–6 mo) and long-term (1 yr+)
  - Focus is on increasing insight of underlying conflict to initiate symptomatic change.
  - Therapist actively helps patient identify patterns of behavior stemming from existence of an unconscious conflict.
- Cognitive behavioral therapy (CBT): Patterns of thoughts and behaviors can lead to development and/or maintenance of symptoms. Thought patterns may not accurately reflect reality and may lead to psychological distress:
  - Therapy aims at modifying thought patterns by increasing cognitive flexibility and changing dysfunctional behavioral patterns.
  - Encourages patient self-monitoring
  - Uses therapist-assisted challenges to patient's basic beliefs/assumptions
  - May utilize *exposure*, a procedure derived from basic learning theories
  - Can be offered in group or individual formats
  - Therapist role is suggestive and supportive.

- Dialectical behavior therapy (DBT): Techniques such as social skills training, mindfulness, and problem solving are used to modulate impulse control and affect management:
  - Derivative of CBT
  - Originally used in treatment of patients with self-destructive behaviors (e.g., cutting, suicide attempts)
  - Seeks to change rigid patterns of cognitions and behaviors that have been maladaptive
  - Utilizes both individual and group treatment modalities
  - Therapist takes an active role in interpretation and support.
- Interpersonal psychotherapy: Interpersonal relationships in a patient's life are linked to symptoms. Therapy seeks to alleviate symptoms and improve social adjustment through exploration of patients' relationships and experiences. Focus is on 1 of 4 potential problem areas:
  - Grief
  - Interpersonal role disputes
  - Role transitions
  - Interpersonal deficits: Therapist works with the patient in resolving the problematic interpersonal issues to facilitate change in symptoms
- Family therapy: Focuses on the family as a unit of intervention:
  - Uses psychoeducation to increase patient's and family's insight
  - Trains in communication and problem-solving skills
- Motivational interviewing: Focuses on motivation as a key to successful change process:
  - Short term
  - Focuses on identifying discrepancies between goals and behavior
  - "5 A's" model is a brief counseling framework developed specifically for physicians to effect behavioral change in patients:
    ○ Assess for a problem.
    ○ Advise making a change.
    ○ Agree on action to be taken.
    ○ Assist with self-care support to make the change.
    ○ Arrange follow-up to support the change.
- Counseling (heterogeneous treatment):
  - Often focuses on situational factors maintaining symptoms
  - Often encourages utilization of community resources
- Behavioral therapy: Relatively nontheoretical approach to behavioral change or symptom reduction/eradication through application of principles of stimulus and response

Pediatric Considerations

- Important distinctions are made between psychotherapy and counseling for children/teens compared to adults/couples.
- The focus of evaluation must include attention to parent and family processes and factors. Interventions typically include interactions and sessions with parents, as well as collateral work with teachers and other school personnel.
- Younger children will often be evaluated and diagnosed through behavioral descriptions provided by parents and other adults who know them well, as well as through direct observation and/or play techniques. Children of all ages should be screened using behavioral checklists that are norm-referenced for age.
- Any child or teenager who requests counseling should be interviewed initially by the primary care provider and referred appropriately. Most referrals will be in response to parental request, however.
- Psychotherapeutic interventions with the strongest empirical basis with children include behavior therapy/modification, CBT, and family/parenting therapy. Play therapy has the least empirical support, and insight-oriented therapies appear to be more effective with older children (>11 years).
- There is controversy regarding the efficacy of psychopharmacologic treatment in preadolescents, although clear benefits have been demonstrated in some studies. Treatment guidelines for mild-to-moderate depressed mood and/or anxiety disorders typically recommend pediatric CBT initially, and studies have supported this approach.

EPIDEMIOLOGY

- ~18.8 million adults suffer from clinical depression, and 20 million suffer from a diagnosable anxiety disorder.
- 1 in 4 Americans report seeking some form of mental health treatment in their adult life. This includes generic counseling in nonmedical settings such as work, clergy, or school settings, but also includes visits to primary care providers. It is estimated that between 3.5% and 5% of adults in the US actually participate in formal mental health psychotherapy annually.
- Public health experts report that the majority of those adults with diagnosable psychiatric disorders, however, do not receive professional mental health services. This is due to multiple factors, including failure to identify, noncompliance with psychiatric referral, regional shortages of providers, economic barriers, and excessive time duration from referral to available service.

- A large study conducted between 1987 and 1997 concluded that the percentage of adults in psychotherapy remained relatively stable over that decade, the use of psychopharmacology doubled, and older adults (ages 55–64) increasingly sought psychotherapy services. In that same study, it was found that psychotherapy duration (number of sessions) decreased substantially and about 1/3 of psychotherapy patients only attended 1 or 2 sessions.

RISK FACTORS
The need for psychotherapy or counseling services is directly and indirectly associated with a host of socioeconomic and biogenetic factors, including the general effects of poverty, family or marital dysfunction, life stressors, medical diseases or conditions, and individual biologic predisposition to mental health disorders.

GENERAL PREVENTION
It is generally assumed that early identification and intervention of child and adolescent psychopathology increases the likelihood of reducing the risk for adult psychopathology, but this has not been sufficiently validated in all categories of psychological disorders. Data support such claims in disorders such as childhood attention deficit hyperactivity disorder, anxiety disorders, and habit disorders of childhood, however.

 ## TREATMENT

MEDICATION

- Psychotherapy is most likely to be accompanied by use of pharmaceutical adjuncts in moderate-to-severe cases of psychological dysfunction that do not respond to other therapies, or in cases of extremely poor quality of life or high risk. The most common examples are in cases of clinical depression or anxiety that clearly incapacitates the patient or significantly reduces their quality of life. Patients at risk for suicide or who represent a danger to others are also candidates for acute psychopharmacotherapy. Studies suggest that verbal and behaviorally oriented therapies can add efficacy to medication treatment in both depression and anxiety.
- There is controversy in the research field regarding the efficacy of medication alone vs psychotherapy alone vs combined treatments. The most recent consensus has been that combined treatments in moderate-to-severe psychological dysfunction are most likely to render positive short-term results and increase the likelihood such effects can be sustained over time.

ADDITIONAL TREATMENT
General Measures
There is evidence of a "dose effect" in psychotherapy outcomes research, with some investigators suggesting that 6–8 sessions are necessary to yield positive initial effects, and upwards of 15–20 sessions for longer-term, sustainable therapeutic effects. This dose effect may not be applicable to counseling services with primarily informational or emotional/supportive functions.

Additional Therapies
- Anxiety disorders:
  – Panic disorder with and without agoraphobia (1)[A]: CBT, psychodynamic therapy
  – Generalized anxiety disorder: CBT (2)[A]
  – Obsessive-compulsive disorder: CBT (3)[A]
  – Post-traumatic stress disorder: CBT
  – Specific phobia: CBT
  – Social phobia: CBT (4)[A]
- Mood disorders:
  – Unipolar depression: CBT, interpersonal therapy, psychodynamic therapy (5)[A]
  – Bipolar disorder: Family therapy, interpersonal therapy, CBT
  – Schizophrenia: Psychodynamic therapy, family therapy, CBT
- Eating disorders:
  – Binge eating disorder: CBT, interpersonal therapy
  – Bulimia nervosa: CBT, interpersonal therapy
- Personality disorders:
  – Borderline: DBT, CBT
- Substance-use disorders:
  – Alcohol: Counseling, CBT, motivational interviewing
  – Cocaine: CBT, counseling
  – Heroin: CBT, counseling
  – Smoking: 5 A's
- Somatoform disorders:
  – Hypochondriasis: CBT
  – Body dysmorphic disorder: CBT

COMPLEMENTARY AND ALTERNATIVE MEDICINE
A host of nonempirically based psychological and nutritional therapies can be found outside of mainstream medicine and psychological science. Very little or no evidence exists to support such experimental therapies, but all have the considerable power of the placebo effect fueling their anecdotal supports or claims. Placebo effects are also thought to be further enhanced by the use of ingested or applied substances that create perceived or real physiologic changes in the patient.

REFERENCES

1. Furukawa TA, et al. Combined psychotherapy plus antidepressants for panic disorder with or without agoraphobia. *Cochrane Database Sys Rev.* 2007;2: CD004364.
2. Hunot V, et al. Psychological therapies for generalized anxiety disorder. *Cochrane Database Sys Rev.* 2007;2.
3. Eddy KT, Dutra L, Bradley R, et al. A multidimensional meta-analysis of psychotherapy and pharmacotherapy for obsessive-compulsive disorder. *Clin Psychol Rev.* 2004;24:1011–30.
4. Rodebaugh TL, Holaway RM, Heimberg RG. The treatment of social anxiety disorder. *Clin Psychol Rev.* 2004;24:883–908.
5. Bortolotti B, Menchetti M, Bellini F, et al. Psychological interventions for major depression in primary care: a meta-analytic review of randomized controlled trials. *Gen Hosp Psychiatry.* 2008;30: 293–302.

 ## CODES

ICD9
- V65.49 Other specified counseling
- V65.8 Other reasons for seeking consultation

CLINICAL PEARLS

- Combined medication and psychotherapeutic treatments in moderate-to-severe psychological dysfunction are most likely to render positive short-term results and increase the likelihood such effects can be sustained over time. Relapse is common over time and/or as treatments are discontinued.
- There is evidence of a "dose effect" in psychotherapy outcomes research, with some investigators suggesting that 6–8 sessions are necessary to yield positive initial effects, and upwards of 15–20 sessions for longer-term, sustainable therapeutic effects. This dose effect may not be applicable to counseling services with primarily informational or emotional/supportive functions. Since many patients cease attendance to psychotherapy sessions after one or a few sessions, most interventions of this type cannot be accurately evaluated by the referring provider.

CROHN DISEASE

Gary I. Levine, MD

 BASICS

DESCRIPTION

Idiopathic inflammatory disease of the alimentary tract that may present anywhere in the GI tract; most commonly found in the terminal ileum (60%), but may be limited to the colon in 15–20%, proximal small bowel 10%:

- Transmural disease
- May involve multiple regions of the intestine in between normal sections (skip lesions)

EPIDEMIOLOGY

Incidence

- Annual incidence of 3–7 cases per 100,000
- In US, more common in whites
- Predominant age: 15–25 years; 2nd, smaller peak in ages 55–65 years
- Female > Male
- 2–4 × increased risk in Ashkenazi Jewish ethnicity

Prevalence

20–100 per 100,000

RISK FACTORS

Cigarette smoking (2 × higher risk in smokers)

Genetics

- 15% of patients have 1st-degree relatives with inflammatory bowel disease, and develop the disease with similar patterns and age of onset.
- Chances of having a child with Crohn disease = 5% if mother has CD, 36% if both parents have CD

PATHOPHYSIOLOGY

- Segmental disease with patchy distribution and variable severity
- Strictures common; may prevent passage of the endoscope
- Aphthous ulcers found on mucosal surfaces
- Histologic features: Transmural inflammation, crypt abscesses, noncaseating granulomas

ETIOLOGY

- Combination of genetic factors, environmental factors, and immunologic abnormalities:
  - IBD locus on chromosome 16 - CARD15/NOD2; also on chromosomes 5q, 6p, and 19
- Idiopathic, immune-mediated Th-1 cells organize cell-mediated response, which involves tumor necrosis factor, interferon, and interleukin 12

COMMONLY ASSOCIATED CONDITIONS

- Arthritis, skin lesions, erythema nodosum, nonspecific rashes, pyoderma gangrenosum; gallstones; sclerosing cholangitis in ~10%
- Increased risk of both colorectal cancer and small bowel cancer: RR = 5–20 (1)

 DIAGNOSIS

PHYSICAL EXAM

- Vary with area of intestinal involvement:
  - Diarrhea occurs in most patients.
  - Abdominal pain in 2/3; occasional mass
  - Weight loss, malaise
  - Growth failure in children
  - Low-grade fever
  - Fistula: Perirectal, bladder, skin, vagina
  - Extraluminal disease (25–35%): Skin, iritis, arthritis, sclerosing cholangitis, multifocal osteomyelitis
- Small-bowel disease only (15–30%):
  - Diarrhea prominent, including nocturnal
  - Vague abdominal pain frequent
  - Intestinal obstruction (1/3): Cramping abdominal pain precedes for months.
  - Bleeding in 20%, rarely massive
  - Perianal disease, including fistulae
- Colon disease only (25–30%):
  - Diarrhea prominent, including nocturnal
  - Hematochezia
  - Abdominal pain in 50%, relieved by stooling
  - Perianal disease in 40%, fistulae
  - Weight loss prominent
  - Megacolon in 10%
  - Intestinal obstruction occasional
- Colon and small-bowel disease (40–60%):
  - Intestinal obstruction much more common than in other types

DIAGNOSTIC TESTS & INTERPRETATION

Constellation of barium-identified distribution of lesions, endoscopic findings, and biopsies usually establish the diagnosis.

Lab

- Anemia (microcytic) is common.
- Albumin level decreased in severe cases
- Serum electrolytes imbalance
- Steatorrhea
- Elevated sedimentation rate, C-reactive protein
- Vitamin levels to evaluate specific nutrient deficiency (vitamin B_{12}, fat-soluble vitamins)
- Serologic biomarkers:
  - Used as adjuncts to other diagnostic modalities and clinical judgement
  - May predict disease behavior, but do not correlate with disease activity
  - ASCAs (anti-saccharomyces cerevisiae antibodies)
    - Elevated in Crohn disease (50–60% of patients) and ulcerative colitis (10–15%)
  - Atypical pANCA (perinuclear antineutrophil cytoplasmic antibody) titer:
    - Elevated in ulcerative colitis (40–80%) and Crohn disease (5–25%)
  - Antiglycan antibody titer
    - Highly specific, poor sensitivity for CD Dx
    - ALCA, ACCA, AMCA:
  - Anti-OmpC antibody
    - 55% CD, 10% UC
  - Anti-I2 IgA
    - 30–50% CD, 10% UC
  - Anti-pancreatic antibodies
    - 30% CD, 2–6% UC
  - Anti-CBir1 antibodies
    - 50% CD, 6% UC

Imaging

- Barium radiographs: Enema and small bowel:
  - Loss of smooth mucosa, undermined ulcers, narrowed lumen (string sign), fistulae, skip areas
- CT scans:
  - Thickening of bowel wall, strictures, and dilatation; abscess and fistulae; perirectal disease
  - CT enterography (CTE): Superior to plain CT
    - IV contrast and low-density oral contrast
- MR enteroscopy (MRE): Superior to CTE for pelvic soft tissue and perianal fistulae
  - Safer in pregnancy and renal insufficiency
- Ultrasound:
  - May identify bowel wall thickening, distinguish fibrosis from edema

Diagnostic Procedures/Surgery

- Colonoscopy; EGD; small bowel capsule endoscopy: 40–70% diagnostic yield in CD (contraindicated if strictures)
- Double balloon endoscopy: Use when capsule endoscopy contraindicated or obstructive symptoms
- Biopsy of mucosa helpful but not diagnostic: Helps rule out other causes

Pathological Findings

- All layers of intestinal wall, with inflammation in at least focal areas in >95% of cases
- Skip areas; granuloma in up to 50% of resected specimen; fat hypertrophy

DIFFERENTIAL DIAGNOSIS

- Appendicitis; ulcerative, collagenous, lymphocytic, ischemic or drug-induced colitis; radiation enteritis
- PID, endometriosis, IBS, diverticulitis, infection, malignancy, or small bowel disease

TREATMENT

General treatment goals include the reduction of abdominal pain, diarrhea, fatigue, anemia, nutritional deficiencies, extraintestinal manifestations, hospitalizations, surgeries, abcesses, fistulas, infections, and malignancies.

MEDICATION

First Line

- Traditional "step up" therapy. 5-ASA derivatives and adrenocorticosteroids are used to induce remission, and azathioprine and 6-MP are used to maintain remission. Treatment also includes appropriate symptomatic measures and supportive care (e.g., antispasmodic and antidiarrheals).
- "Top down" therapy. Anti-TNF alpha agents and immunomodulators as initial treatment if high risk of rapidly progressive disease.
- To induce remission in naive patient, relapse, or severe sx:
  - Sulfasalazine or mesalamine: 2–4 g/d
    - Useful in mild disease
    - Sulfasalazine more effective in CD colitis
    - Add folic acid 1–2 mg/day
  - Prednisone: 40–60 mg/d O:
    - For moderate disease, small bowel CD
    - 50% become steroid-dependent or resistant within 1 year
    - Not effective for maintaining remission

- Budesonide: 9 mg/day can be administered topically or orally; synthetic glucocorticoid with reduced bioavailability:
  - Alternative to prednisone in patients requiring long-term steroid use
  - Partially avoids steroid complications
- Antibiotics:
  - Ciprofloxacin 1 g/day
  - Rifaximin 800 mg b.i.d.: 50% achieve remission in 6–12 weeks
- Enteral nutritional therapy:
  - 60% remission rate, requires feeding tube
- To achieve remission in patients who relapse with prednisone tapering or fail to respond, or to maintain remission:
  - Add azathioprine (Imuran) 2–3 mg/kg/d or mercaptopurine (6-MP) 1–1.5 mg/kg/d. If good response, taper steroid, effective in maintaining remission:
    - Check TPMT levels prior to beginning therapy—predictive of development of leukopenia. Full level: Use normal dose; intermediate level: Use 1/2 normal dose; zero–low level: Do not use azathioprine or 6-MP
  - Methotrexate 25 mg IM weekly to achieve remission, then 15 mg/week to maintain remission as an alternative to 6-MP or azathioprine
    - Add folic acid 1–2 mg/day, monitor LFTs.
- If inadequate response to achieve or maintain remission or for Rx of symptomatic nonresponsive fistulas or extraintestinal manifestations, maintain patient on immunosuppressant and start a course of anti-TNF monoclonal antibody:
  - Infliximab (Remicade)
    - Chimeric (75% human and 25% murine) IgG-1 monoclonal antibody vs TNF
    - 5 mg/kg infusion, repeat at 2 wks, 6 wks, then every 8 wks; can increase to 10 mg/kg if needed
    - Used with azathioprine, 6-MP, or methotrexate to reduce infliximab antibody formation
    - Increases risk of TB 7 ×, need to screen for latent TB prior to starting this medication
    - Active intra-abdominal abscess is a contraindication to use.
  - Adalimumab (Humira):
    - Recombinant human IgG-1 monoclonal antibody vs TNF
    - Given by subcutaneous injection
    - Used with infliximab failure or intolerance
  - Certolizumab pegol (Cimzia):
    - Pegylated 95% humanized Fab fragment of anti-TNF monoclonal antibody
    - Given by subcutaneous injection
    - Used with infliximab failure or intolerance
  - Natalizumab (Tysabri):
    - Humanized IgG4 monoclonal antibody vs alpha 4 integrin-mediated leukocyte migration
    - Used in CD patients with active inflammation not responsive to or unable to tolerate anti TNF alpha Rx
    - Increased risk of JC virus progressive multifocal leukoencephalopathy
- If tenesmus or bleeding prominent:
  - Mesalamine enema or hydrocortisone enema maintenance therapy
- Predominantly perirectal disease with fistulae:
  - Metronidazole (Flagyl) 250 mg t.i.d. for maximum of 8 weeks
- Patients with joint, eye, and skin extraintestinal manifestations:
  - Unresponsive to mesalamine, occasionally responsive to prednisone
  - Usually responsive to infliximab

- For all well-controlled patients:
  - Loperamide (Imodium) 2 mg to control diarrhea to avoid interference with daily life

Second Line
- Cyclosporine: Has assisted in closing fistulae when other measures fail; otherwise, not useful
- Tacrolimus: Reserved for nonresponders

ADDITIONAL TREATMENT
General Measures
- Attention to maintaining weight and nutrition
- Physical rest and relief of emotional stress
- Perirectal disease: Sitz baths, soap and water after stooling, surgical drainage of perirectal abscesses, surgical treatment of recurrent fistulae if medical management fails
- Folate supplementation may potentially decrease risk for malignancy (2)[B].

Additional Therapies
Vaccinations:
- Hepatitis B, HPV, pneumococcus, influenza, varicella; give at disease ONSET

COMPLEMENTARY AND ALTERNATIVE MEDICINE
Trichuris suis (porcine whipworm) ova administration has been effective in clinical trials in inducing and maintaining remission without significant side effects.

SURGERY/OTHER PROCEDURES
- Palliative, not curative: Laparoscopic or open
- Relapse rates after intestinal resection:
  - 5 years: 30–35%; 10 years: 50–55%; 15 years: 60–75%; 25 years: 95%
- Indications:
  - Failure of medical management
  - Total or recurrent intestinal obstruction or abscess
  - Perforation, hemorrhage, fistula, failure to thrive
  - Toxic megacolon, extensive disease, or cancer
  - Failure of ostomy to function after ≥1 year

 ONGOING CARE

FOLLOW-UP RECOMMENDATIONS
Patient Monitoring
- Regular assessment (every 3–6 months if patient is stable), particularly status of weight, pain, diarrhea, hemoglobin, and sed rate
- Crohn Disease Activity Index (CDAI) score is an objective measure for recording disease activity that can be used to assess response to therapy:
  - <150 = remission, 150–220 = mild disease, 221–400 = moderate disease, >400 = severe disease
- Surveillance colonoscopy beginning 8 years after Crohn colitis diagnosis and every 1–3 years thereafter (1)[B]:
  - Biopsy any abnormal mucosa or stricture
  - 4-quadrant biopsy of normal mucosa every 10 cm
- Check liver tests yearly.
- Check vitamin B_{12} level in those with ileal disease or ileal resection.
- Check folate level in all on 5-aminosalicylate; use supplements in all.
- Follow CBC, LFTs, and consider monitoring 6-MMP and 6-TG levels in patients on AZA or 6-MP.
- Follow LFTs in patients on methotrexate.

DIET
- If fat malabsorption, diminish fat in diet.
- If strictures or recurrent obstruction, avoid highly fibrous substances.

- If diarrhea prominent, increase dietary fiber (sometimes recommended), decrease fat.
- Enteral nutrition preferred over parenteral

PATIENT EDUCATION
Crohn and Colitis Foundation of America, Inc., 11th floor, Park Ave. South, NY 10016, Phone (800) 343–3637.

PROGNOSIS
- Chronic condition with variable but nearly certain progression
- Average patient has surgery every 7 years: Short-bowel syndrome common after >4 surgeries:
  - 50–75% require surgery after 5 years, 70–90% after 10 years
- Most are able to maintain normal life.
- Fertility rate is the same as population at large.
- Pregnancy
  - Increased risk of spontaneous abortion/stillbirth; preterm birth and low birth weight infant; labor and delivery complications
  - No increased risk of congenital malformations
  - Risk of disease flare is same if pregnant or not pregnant.

COMPLICATIONS
- Fistulae (15%): Perirectal, cutaneous, enterovaginal, and enterovesicular
- Extraluminal disease (25%): Skin, uveal tract, joint, bone, and biliary tract
- Colon perforation, toxic megacolon, sepsis, hemorrhage, ischemia, gallstones in >25%, osteoporosis
- Depression and anxiety in 15%, 3 × normal population
- Colon cancer:
  - Extensive colon disease associated with 6 × increased risk of adenocarcinoma (3)

REFERENCES
1. Rubin DT, Kavitt RT. Surveillance for cancer and dysplasia in inflammatory bowel disease. *Gastroenterol Clin North Am*. 2006;35:581–604.
2. Chan EP, Lichtenstein GR. Chemoprevention: risk reduction with medical therapy of inflammatory bowel disease. *Gastroenterol Clin North Am*. 2006;35:675–712.
3. Jess T, Gamborg M, Matzen P, et al. Increased risk of intestinal cancer in Crohn's disease: a meta-analysis of population-based cohort studies. *Am J Gastroenterol*. 2005;100:2724–9.

 CODES

ICD9
- 555.0 Regional enteritis of small intestine
- 555.1 Regional enteritis of large intestine
- 555.2 Regional enteritis of small intestine with large intestine

CLINICAL PEARLS
- Crohn disease involves skip areas; ulcerative colitis extends continuously from rectum.
- Surgery is not curative; it is palliative. Recurrence is common after surgery.
- Cancer risk is greatest with Crohn colitis, and surveillance colonoscopy is strongly recommended.

CROUP (LARYNGOTRACHEOBRONCHITIS)

Garreth C. Biegun, MD

 BASICS

DESCRIPTION
- Croup is a subacute viral illness characterized by upper-airway symptoms such as barking cough, stridor, and fever. "Croup" is used to refer to viral laryngotracheitis or laryngotracheobronchitis (LTB), though it is sometimes used for LTB with pneumonitis, bacterial tracheitis, or spasmodic croup.
- Most common cause of upper-airway obstruction or stridor in children
- System(s) affected: Pulmonary; Respiratory
- Synonym(s): Croup; Infectious croup; Viral croup; LTB
- Spasmodic croup: Noninfectious form with sudden resolution:
  - No fever or radiographic changes
  - Initially treated as croup
  - Usually self-limited and resolves with mist therapy at home
  - Often recurs on same night or in 2–3 nights

EPIDEMIOLOGY
- Predominant age (1):
  - Common, 7 months to 3 years
  - Most common in 2nd year of life
  - Rare >6 years
- Predominant sex: Male > Female (1.5:1) (1)
- Timing:
  - Any time of year possible, but most common in fall and winter (with parainfluenza 1 and respiratory syncytial virus [RSV])

Incidence
- 6 cases of croup per year per 100 children <6 years old
- 1.5–6% of cases require hospitalization.
- 2–6% of those require intubation.
- Decreasing incidence in the US and Canada

RISK FACTORS
- Past history of croup
- Recurrent upper respiratory infections
- Atopic disease increases risk of spasmodic croup.

PATHOPHYSIOLOGY
- Subglottic region/larynx is entirely encircled by the cricoid cartilage.
- Inflammatory edema and subglottic mucus production decrease airway radius.
- Small children have small airways with more compliant walls.
- Negative-pressure inspiration pulls airway walls closer together.
- Small decrease in airway radius causes significant increase in resistance (Poiseuille law: Resistance proportional to $1/radius^4$).

ETIOLOGY
- Usually viruses that initially infect oropharyngeal mucosa and then migrate inferiorly
- Parainfluenza virus:
  - Most common pathogen: 75% of cases
  - Type 1 is most common, causing 18% of all cases of croup.
  - Types 2, 3, and 4 are also common.
  - Type 3 may cause a particularly severe illness.

- Other viruses:
  - RSV
  - Paramyxovirus
  - Influenza virus type A or B
  - Adenovirus
  - Rhinovirus
  - Enteroviruses (Coxsackie and Echo)
  - Reovirus
  - Measles virus where vaccination not common
- *Haemophilus influenzae* type B now rare with routine immunization (2)
- May have bacterial cause: *Mycoplasma pneumoniae* has been reported.

COMMONLY ASSOCIATED CONDITIONS
If recurrent (>2 episodes in a year) or in 1st 90 days of life, consider host factors:
- Underlying anatomic abnormality (e.g., subglottic stenosis)
- Paradoxical vocal cord dysfunction
- Gastroesophageal reflux disease
- Prolonged neonatal intubation

 DIAGNOSIS

- Most children who present with acute onset of barky cough, stridor, and chest-wall indrawing have croup.
- Croup is a clinical diagnosis; labs and imaging serve only ancillary purposes (3).
- Classic "seal-like" barking, spasmodic cough
- May have biphasic stridor
- Low-grade to moderate fever
- Upper-respiratory infection prodrome lasting 1–7 days
- Severity usually determined by clinical observation for signs of respiratory effort: Nasal flaring, retractions, tripoding, sniffing position, abdominal breathing, tachypnea. Late: Hypoxia/cyanosis or fatigue.
- Westley Croup Scale (≤2 mild; 3–7 moderate; ≥8 severe):
  - Level of consciousness: Normal, including sleep = 0; disoriented = 5
  - Cyanosis: None = 0; with agitation = 4; at rest = 5
  - Stridor: None = 0; with agitation = 1; at rest = 2
  - Air entry: Normal = 0; decreased = 1; markedly decreased = 2
  - Retractions: None = 0; mild = 1; moderate = 2; severe = 3
- Nontoxic-appearing child: Normal voice, no drooling
- No change in stridor with positioning
- Nontender larynx
- Inflamed subglottic region with normal-appearing supraglottic region

HISTORY
- 2–3 days nonspecific prodromal syndrome with low-grade fever, coryza, rhinorrhea
- Onset and recurrence at night when child is sleeping
- Symptoms often resolve en route to hospital as child is exposed to cool night air.
- Lack of prodrome indicates spasmodic croup.

PHYSICAL EXAM
- Pulse oximetry often is normal because there is no disturbance of alveolar gas exchange.
- Overall appearance: Child comfortable or struggling?
- Work of breathing: Labored or comfortable?
- Sound of breathing and voice: Hoarse, stridor, inspiratory wheezing, short sentences?
- Observed/subjective tidal volume: Sufficient for child size?

DIAGNOSTIC TESTS & INTERPRETATION
Lab
- No laboratory abnormality is diagnostic.
- White blood cells may be low, normal, or elevated.
- Lymphocytosis expected but not required
- Rapid antigen or viral culture tests are available in some centers:
  - Guide isolation precautions not management

Imaging
- Posteroanterior and lateral neck films show funnel-shaped subglottic region with normal epiglottis: "Steeple," "hour glass," or "pencil point" sign (present in 40–60% of children with laryngotracheobronchitis).
- CT may be more sensitive for defining etiology of obstruction in a confusing clinical picture.
- Patient should be monitored during imaging; progression of airway obstruction may be rapid.

Pathological Findings
- Inflammatory reaction of respiratory mucosa
- Loss of epithelial cells
- Thick mucoid secretions

DIFFERENTIAL DIAGNOSIS
- Epiglottitis: Currently rare
- Foreign-body aspiration
- Subglottic stenosis (congenital or acquired)
- Bacterial tracheitis
- Simple upper-respiratory infection
- Retropharyngeal or peritonsillar abscess
- Trauma
- Allergic reaction (acute angioneurotic edema)
- Airway anomalies (e.g., tracheo/laryngomalacia)
- Subglottic hemangioma

 TREATMENT

MEDICATION
First Line

- Well established in literature; cornerstones of treatment are immediate nebulized epinephrine and dexamethasone (4)[A].
- Racemic or L-epinephrine (equal efficacy and side-effect profiles; L-epinephrine is used for most other hospital purposes and is less expensive):
  - Racemic epinephrine: 0.05 mL/kg/dose (max, 0.5 mL) of 2.25% solution nebulized in normal saline total volume 3 mL (5)[A](6)[B]
  - L-epinephrine: 0.5 mL/kg per dose (max of 5 mL) of a 1:1000 dilution
  - Onset in 1–5 minutes, duration 2 hours
  - Repeat as necessary if side effects tolerated
  - Must observe child for 3–4 hours

- Corticosteroids: (7)[A]:
  – Dexamethasone (cheapest, most literature, easiest), 0.15–0.6 mg/kg; higher doses have been traditional care, but studies have proven 0.15 mg/kg has equal efficacy (8). Single dose, IV/IM/PO have proven equal efficacy (9)[A]
  – Nebulized budesonide also proven effective (10)[B]
  – Onset by 6 hours
- Heli-Ox: A helium-oxygen mixture:
  – Smaller, lower-mass helium molecule (compared to nitrogen) theoretically maintains laminar flow in narrower airways, serves as bridge therapy to steroids.
  – Minimum 60% helium must be used; 70% preferable; 79% if patient has no O_2 requirement
  – There is limited data. Anecdotal reports and 1 case series support its use, but 2 prospective studies showed no benefit (11,12). Also, a Cochrane review found insufficient evidence to support the use of Heliox in croup (13).
- Antibiotics not indicated in this viral illness:
  – Antecedent or subsequent bacterial infection is possible but uncommon.
- Oxygen as needed
- Contraindications, precautions, and significant possible interactions: Refer to the manufacturer's literature.

Second Line
Amantadine for influenza A: 100 mg PO b.i.d. for 3–5 days

ADDITIONAL TREATMENT
General Measures
- Minimize labs, imaging, and other procedures that upset the child; agitation that worsens tachypnea is more detrimental than accepting a clinical diagnosis.
- Electrocardiogram monitoring and pulse oximetry:
  – Frequent checks are more sensitive to worsening disease than is pulse-oximetry.

COMPLEMENTARY AND ALTERNATIVE MEDICINE
- Mist therapy often helps with symptoms. Do not use high-temperature misters (e.g., tea kettles) due to risk of burns. Sitting with child in bathroom with hot shower running is a good steam generator.
- Some children respond well to cold, dry air.

SURGERY/OTHER PROCEDURES
- Intubation rarely required; tube 0.5–1 mm smaller than normal:
  – After trial of medical management, intubation is for fatigue due to work of breathing or beginning total obstruction; not secondary to low oxygen saturation.
  – Extubate in 3–5 days when there is an appropriate air-leak around the endotracheal tube.
- Tracheotomy: Rarely, maintenance 3–7 days

IN-PATIENT CONSIDERATIONS
Initial Stabilization
- Outpatient care in mild cases
- Admission for patients who do not respond to therapy, or who have O_2 requirement, pneumonia, or congestive heart failure
- In most cases, emergency department observation after medical management is sufficient.

Admission Criteria
Minor cases need no visit to hospital or primary care physician (PCP):
- No stridor at rest, no difficulty breathing
- Child able to tolerate PO liquids
- No underlying medical condition
- Caretakers able to assess changes to clinical picture and reassess medical care

Discharge Criteria
Patients who maintain a good response to medical therapy for 3–4 hours (after epinephrine dose) may be safely discharged as long as they have reliable caretakers and good access to medical services if symptoms return (14)[C].

 ## ONGOING CARE

FOLLOW-UP RECOMMENDATIONS
Patient Monitoring
Most patients will be seen in ED or PCP office setting. Some will be overnight by telephone.

DIET
- NPO and IV fluids for severe cases
- Frequent small feedings with increased fluids for mild cases

PATIENT EDUCATION
- Must keep patient quiet; crying may exacerbate symptoms.
- Educate parents about when to seek emergency care if mild cases progress.
- Emotional support and reassurance for the patient

PROGNOSIS
- Up to 1/3 of patients will have recurrence.
- Recovery is usually full and without lasting effects.

COMPLICATIONS
- Rare
- Subglottic stenosis in intubated patients
- Bacterial tracheitis
- Cardiopulmonary arrest
- Pneumonia

REFERENCES
1. Cherry JD. Clinical practice. Croup. N Engl J Med. 2008;358:384–91.
2. Sobol SE, Zapata S. Epiglottitis and croup. Otolaryngol Clin North Am. 2008;41:551–66, ix.
3. Everard ML. Acute bronchiolitis and croup. Pediatr Clin North Am. 2009;56:119–33, x–xi.
4. Johnson DW, Jacobson S, Edney PC, et al. A comparison of nebulized budesonide, and intramuscular dexamethasone, and placebo for moderately severe croup. N Engl J Med. 1998; 339:498–503.
5. Westley CR, Cotton EK, Brooks JG. Nebulized racemic epinephrine by IPPB for the treatment of croup: a double-blind study. Am J Dis Child. 1978;132:484–7.
6. Waisman Y, Klein BL, Boenning DA, et al. Prospective randomized double-blind study comparing L-epinephrine and racemic epinephrine aerosols in the treatment of laryngotracheitis (croup). Pediatrics. 1992;89:302–6.
7. Russell K, Wiebe N, Saenz A, et al. Glucocorticoids for croup. Cochrane Database Syst Rev. 2004;CD001955.
8. Dobrovoljac M, Geelhoed GC et al. 27 years of croup: an update highlighting the effectiveness of 0.15 mg/kg of dexamethasone. Emerg Med Australas. 2009;21:309–14.
9. Geelhoed GC, Turner J, MacDonald WB. Efficacy of a small single dose of oral dexamethasone for outpatient croup: A double-blind placebo controlled clinical trial. Br Med J. 1996; 313(7050):140–2.
10. Cetinkaya F, Tüfekçi BS, Kutluk G. A comparison of nebulized budesonide, and intramuscular, and oral dexamethasone for treatment of croup. Int J Pediatr Otorhinolaryngol. 2004;68:453–6.
11. Vorwerk C, Coats TJ. Use of helium-oxygen mixtures in the treatment of croup: a systematic review. Emerg Med J. 2008;25:547–50.
12. Gupta VK, Cheifetz IM. Heliox administration in the pediatric intensive care unit: an evidence-based review. Pediatr Crit Care Med. 2005;6:204–11.
13. Vorwerk C, Coats T et al. Heliox for croup in children. Cochrane Database Syst Rev. 2010; 2:CD006822-.
14. Klassen TP. Croup. A current perspective. Pediatr Clin North Am. 1999;46:1167–78.

ADDITIONAL READING
Bjornson CL, Johnson DW. Croup. Lancet. 2008;371: 329–39.

See Also (Topic, Algorithm, Electronic Media Element)
Bronchiolitis; Epiglottitis; Tracheitis, Bacterial

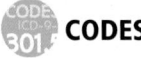 ## CODES

ICD9
464.4 Croup

CLINICAL PEARLS
- Parainfluenza virus is the most common pathogen.
- Also caused by RSV, paramyxovirus, influenza virus type A or B, adenovirus, rhinovirus, enteroviruses (Coxsackie and Echo)
- Established efficacy of inhaled epinephrine and corticosteroids
- Lateral neck films show funnel-shaped subglottic region with normal epiglottis: "Steeple," "hour glass," or "pencil point" sign (present in 40–60% of children with laryngotracheobronchitis).

CRYOGLOBULINEMIA

Luke Godwin, MD
Fred Schiffman, MD

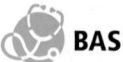 **BASICS**

DESCRIPTION

- Cryoglobulinemia is a state characterized by the presence of cryoglobulins in a patient's serum.
- Cryoglobulins are circulating immunoglobulins that precipitate at cold temperatures (below 37°C) and dissolve on rewarming.
- Clinical symptoms are often secondary to either small vessel occlusion and a hyperviscosity syndrome in Type I cryoglobulins, or the formation of cryoglobulin-containing immune complexes leading to vasculitis in Type II and Type III cryoglobulins (i.e., "mixed cryoglobulinemia"):
  - Type I
    - Monoclonal immunoglobulin (Ig); IgM is most common
    - 10–15% of all cryoglobulinemia
    - Less frequently IgG, IgA, free Ig light chains
  - Type II
    - Monoclonal IgM with rheumatoid factor activity (anti-IgG), which forms an immune complex with polyclonal IgG
    - 50–60% of all cryoglobulinemia
    - Monoclonal fraction rarely IgG or IgA
  - Type III:
    - Polyclonal IgM with rheumatoid factor activity (anti-IgG), which forms an immune complex with polyclonal IgG
    - 25–30% of cryoglobulinemia

EPIDEMIOLOGY

- No adequate epidemiological studies regarding overall prevalence
- Healthy patients may have low concentrations of cryoglobulins present in the serum (<0.06 g/L)
- Clinically relevant cryoglobulinemia is far more common in patients with chronic infections and/or inflammation

RISK FACTORS

- Type I: Associated with lymphoproliferative disorders:
  - Multiple myeloma
  - Waldenström's macroglobulinemia
  - Chronic lymphocytic leukemia (CLL)
  - Monoclonal gammopathy of unknown significance (MGUS)
  - B-cell lymphoma
- Type II (mixed cryoglobulinemia):
  - Main association with hepatitis C
  - 40–90% of patients with mixed cryoglobulinemia are hepatitis C positive
  - Higher association with hepatitis C compared to type III cryoglobulinemia
  - Also associated with Sjögren's syndrome, HIV, and other autoimmune/connective tissue disease

- Type III (mixed cryoglobulinemia):
  - Like Type II, also associated with chronic infection and inflammatory states:
    - Autoimmune disease: SLE, RA, IBD
    - Infection: EBV, CMV, TB, HIV, subacute endocarditis
  - Significant hepatitis C virus association, just less than type II

PATHOPHYSIOLOGY

- Exact mechanism of cold insolubility in these cryoproteins is unknown. Hypotheses include reduced concentrations of sialic acid and galactose in the Fc region of Ig, as well as steric conformation changes due to temperature variation.
- Type I:
  - An underlying lymphoproliferative disorder causes monoclonal B cell proliferation.
  - B cells produce cryoglobulin, which precipitates, causing hyperviscosity and vessel damage.
- Types II and III:
  - B cell hyperactivation (from hepatitis C virus or another chronic inflammatory state) produces immunoglobulin with rheumatoid factor activity, which leads to immune complex formation.
  - Immune complex deposition and subsequent complement activation causes small-vessel damage.

ETIOLOGY

Hepatitis C correlation:

- Hepatitis C virus displays lymphotropism. The E2 capsid protein of HCV binds site to CD81, a site present on hepatocytes, T lymphocytes, and B lymphocytes.
- Patients infected with HCV who have mixed cryoglobulinemia (MC) have been found to have higher viral loads than patients with HCV and no MC.

COMMONLY ASSOCIATED CONDITIONS

- NOTE: See above for specific association by cryoglobulinemia type classification
- Infections:
  - Viral: Hepatitis C, hepatitis B, hepatitis A, HIV, Epstein-Barr virus, VZV, cytomegalovirus, HTLV-1, adenovirus, influenza virus, parvovirus B19, rubella virus
  - Bacterial: Lyme disease, syphilis, Q fever, poststreptococcal nephritis, subacute bacterial endocarditis, leprosy, TB, brucella
  - Fungal: Coccidiomycosis
  - Parasitic: Kala-azar toxoplasmosis, echinococcosis, malaria, schistosomiasis, trypanosomiasis

- Hematologic disease:
  - Non-Hodgkin lymphoma
  - Chronic lymphocytic leukemia
  - Multiple myeloma
  - Waldenström's macroglobulinemia
  - Hodgkin lymphoma
  - Chronic myeloid leukemia
  - Castleman disease
  - Thrombocytopenic thrombotic purpura
  - Cold agglutinin disease
- Autoimmune diseases:
  - Sjögren syndrome
  - Systemic lupus erythematosus
  - Polyarteritis nodosa
  - Systemic sclerosis
  - Rheumatoid arthritis
  - Autoimmune thyroiditis
  - Temporal arteritis
  - Dermatomyositis/polymyositis
  - Henoch-Schönlein disease
  - Sarcoidosis
  - Inflammatory bowel disease
  - Pemphigus vulgaris

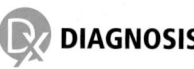 **DIAGNOSIS**

- Type I:
  - Commonly asymptomatic
  - More frequent association with signs of peripheral vessel occlusion, less with signs of vasculitis. Think of Raynaud's phenomenon, acrocyanosis, livedo reticularis, purpura, ulcers, gangrene.
- Types II and III: Mixed cryoglobulinemia syndrome
  - Caused by immune complex-mediated vasculitis
  - Characterized by Meltzer's triad:
    - Purpura
    - Weakness
    - Arthralgias
  - Multiple organ involvement is common:
    - Cutaneous vasculitis, purpura
    - Membranoproliferative glomerulonephritis (nephropathy)
    - Peripheral neuropathy

HISTORY

- Constitutional/nonspecific: Fever, myalgias, arthralgia, malaise, generalized weakness, sensory changes
- Hyperviscosity: Blurring of vision, headache, vertigo, dizziness, diplopia, ataxia, confusion, dementia, stroke
- Past medical history: Risk factors for hepatitis C, lymphoproliferative disorders

PHYSICAL EXAM
- Skin: Purpura (intermittent, palpable, beginning in legs), ulcers, Raynaud phenomenon, livedo reticularis, acrocyanosis
- Gastrointestinal: Hepatomegaly, splenomegaly
- Endocrine: Lymphadenopathy
- Extremities: Synovitis, signs of peripheral vascular occlusion
- Neurological: Peripheral neuropathy

DIAGNOSTIC TESTS & INTERPRETATION
Important to rule out other small-vessel vasculitis (see section Differential Diagnosis) (1)

Lab
Initial lab tests
- General:
  - Complete blood count (CBC), with peripheral smear
  - Electrolytes
  - Liver function tests (LFTs)
  - Blood urea nitrogen (BUN), creatinine
  - Urinalysis
  - Rheumatoid factor
- Specific:
  - Serological test for cryoglobulins (blood collection and initial storage needs to be at 37°C); following detection of cryoglobulins, further testing including electrophoresis and immunofixation should be completed.
  - Serum complement levels (low C4, normal or slightly decreased C3)
  - Serologic tests for hepatitis B and C
  - Rheumatologic (e.g., antinuclear antibody, ANCA)

Diagnostic Procedures/Surgery
Check main organ systems involved:
- Kidneys: Proteinuria, microscopic hematuria, arterial hypertension common at diagnosis
- Nervous system: Peripheral neuropathy in types II and III cryoglobulinemia
- Liver: Normal or increased liver enzymes, steatosis, chronic hepatitis, cirrhosis

Pathological Findings
- Renal biopsy: Most common type of nephropathy is membranoproliferative glomerulonephritis
- Bone marrow: May be indicated for type I cryoglobulinemia; examination often reveals underlying hematological condition
- Liver biopsy: Inflammation is graded; fibrosis is staged

DIFFERENTIAL DIAGNOSIS
- Possible causes of small-vessel vasculitis: Henoch-Schönlein purpura, lupus vasculitis, rheumatoid vasculitis, Sjögren syndrome vasculitis, hypocomplementemic urticarial vasculitis, Behçet syndrome, Goodpasture syndrome, serum sickness vasculitis, drug-induced immune complex vasculitis, infection-induced immune complex vasculitis, ANCA-associated vasculitis, paraneoplastic syndrome-associated vasculitis, inflammatory bowel disease-associated vasculitis
- Possible causes of hyperviscosity: Waldenstrom macroglobulinemia, polycythemia, sickle cell anemia, malaria, babesiosis

 TREATMENT
- Most important to treat underlying disease
- Treat according to individual patient and severity of symptoms
- Mild disease treated with cold avoidance, analgesics, nonsteroidal anti-inflammatory drugs
- Intensive therapy with steroids, plasmapheresis, or cytotoxic agents only for organ-threatening or recalcitrant disease
- Type I:
  - Cytotoxic treatment of lymphoproliferative disease as appropriate
- Types II and III:
  - Antiviral hepatitis C treatment as appropriate

MEDICATION
- Hepatitis C-associated:
  - Antiviral therapy: Combination therapy of pegylated interferon (PEG-INF)α and ribavirin
- Non-hepatitis C-associated:
  - Immunosuppression, low-dose corticosteroids
- Rituximab: this chimeric monoclonal antibody directed against CD20 has shown some efficacy in treating both type I and mixed cryoglobulinemias, and should be considered in severely symptomatic patients.

ADDITIONAL TREATMENT
Plasmapheresis:
- For severe clinical manifestations of disease
- Used alongside immunosuppressive treatment to avoid rebound phenomena

 ONGOING CARE

DIET
At least one small study has suggested that a low antigen content (LAC) diet can be helpful in improving the symptoms of cryoglobulinemia. The hypothesized mechanism is a reduction in antigen input load for the reticuloendothelial system that allows that system to more efficiently process circulating immune complexes.

PATIENT EDUCATION
http://www.vasculitisfoundation.org/

PROGNOSIS
There seems to be no increased morbidity or mortality risk with cryoglobulinemia over the associated underlying conditions.

REFERENCES
1. Sargur R, White P, Egner W et al. Cryoglobulin evaluation: best practice? *Ann. Clin. Biochem.* 2010;47:8–16.

ADDITIONAL READING
- Alpers CE, Smith KD et al. Cryoglobulinemia and renal disease. *Curr Opin Nephrol Hypertens.* 2008;17:243–9.
- Dammacco F, Sansonno D, Piccoli C. , et al. The cryoglobulins: an overview. *Eur J Clin Invest.* 2001;31:628–38.
- Dispenzieri A et al. Symptomatic cryoglobulinemia. *Curr Treat Options Oncol.* 2000;1:105–18.
- Ferri C, Antonelli A, Mascia MT et al. B-cells and mixed cryoglobulinemia. *Autoimmun Rev.* 2007;7:114–20.
- Sansonno D, Carbone A, De Re V et al. Hepatitis C virus infection, cryoglobulinaemia, and beyond. *Rheumatology (Oxford).* 2007.
- Tedeschi A, Baratè C, Minola E, et al. Cryoglobulinemia. *Blood Rev.* 2007.

 CODES

ICD9
- 273.1 Monoclonal paraproteinemia
- 273.2 Other paraproteinemias

CLINICAL PEARLS
- Cryoglobulins are circulating immunoglobulins that precipitate at cold temperatures (below 37°F) and dissolve on rewarming.
- Type I: Associated with lymphoproliferative disorders (e.g., multiple myeloma, Waldenstrom macroglobulinemia, MGUS, CLL)
- Type II (mixed cryoglobulinemia): Main association with hepatitis C (40–90% are hepatitis C positive)
- Type III (mixed cryoglobulinemia): High association with chronic infection and inflammatory states
- Initial laboratory evaluation: CBC with peripheral smear, electrolytes, LFTs, BUN, creatinine, urinalysis, rheumatoid factor
- Specific:
  - Serological test for cryoglobulins (blood collection and initial storage needs to be at 37°C); electrophoresis and immunofixation if cryoglobulins present
  - Serum complement levels (low C4, normal or slightly decreased C3)
  - Serologic tests for hepatitis B and C
  - Rheumatologic (ANA, ANCA)

C

CRYPTORCHIDISM
Pamela I. Ellsworth, MD

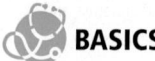 **BASICS**

DESCRIPTION
- Incomplete or improper descent of 1 or both testicles; normally, descent is in the 7th–8th month of gestation. The cryptorchid testis may be palpable or nonpalpable.
- Types of cryptorchidism:
  - Abdominal: Located inside the internal ring
  - Canalicular: Located between the internal and external rings
  - Ectopic: Located outside the normal path of testicular descent from abdominal cavity to scrotum; may be ectopic to perineum, femoral canal, superficial inguinal pouch (most common), suprapubic area, or opposite hemiscrotum
  - Retractile: Fully descended testis that moves freely between the scrotum and the groin
  - Iatrogenic: Previously descended testis becomes undescended secondary to scar tissue after inguinal surgery, such as an inguinal hernia repair or hydrocelectomy.
  - Also may be referred to as *palpable* versus *nonpalpable*
- System(s) affected: Reproductive
- Synonym(s): Undescended testes (UDT)

Pediatric Considerations
- This problem is usually detectable at birth or soon thereafter.
- If surgery is to be the treatment, it should be performed during the 1st 6–9 months of life (1).
- Puberty: If unilateral cryptorchidism is discovered at or after puberty, the usual treatment is orchiectomy.

EPIDEMIOLOGY
Incidence
- Predominant age: Premature newborns
- Predominant sex: Male only

Prevalence
- In the US, cryptorchidism occurs in 3% of full-term and 33% of premature newborn males.
- Spontaneous testicular descent occurs by age 1–3 months in 50–70% of full-term males with cryptorchidism.
- Descent at 6–9 months of age is rare.

RISK FACTORS
- Family history of cryptorchidism: Boys with UDTs: 4% of their fathers and 6.2–9.8% of their brothers have UDTs (23,).
- Low birth weight, prematurity, and small for gestational age are associated with a substantial increase in incidence of cryptorchidism, which may reach 20–25% in infants with birth weight less than 2.5 kg (4).

Genetics
Occurrence of UDT in siblings as well as fathers suggests a genetic etiology.

ETIOLOGY
- Not fully known
- May involve alterations in
  - Mechanical factors (gubernaculum, length of vas deferens and testicular vessels, groin anatomy, epididymis, cremasteric muscles, and abdominal pressure), hormonal factors (gonadotropin, testosterone, dihydrotestosterone, and müllerian inhibiting substance) and neural factors (ilioinguinal nerve and genitofemoral nerve)
  - Major regulators of testicular descent from intraabdominal location into the bottom of the scrotum are the Leydig cell–derived hormones testosterone and insulin-like growth factor 3 (IGF-3).
  - Mutations in the gene for IGF-3 and in the androgen receptor gene have been recognized as causes of cryptorchidism as well as chromosomal alterations.
  - Environmental factors acting as endocrine disruptors of testicular descent also may contribute to the etiology of cryptorchidism (5).

COMMONLY ASSOCIATED CONDITIONS
- Inguinal hernia/hydrocele
- Abnormalities of vas deferens and epididymis
- Intersex abnormalities
- Hypogonadotropic hypogonadism
- Germinal cell aplasia
- Prune-belly syndrome
- Meningomyelocele
- Hypospadias
- Wilms tumor
- Prader-Willi syndrome
- Kallman syndrome
- Cystic fibrosis

℞ DIAGNOSIS

HISTORY
≥1 testicles in a site other than the scrotum; may be an isolated defect or associated with other congenital anomalies

PHYSICAL EXAM
- Performed with warm hands, with child in sitting, standing, and squatting position
- A Valsalva maneuver and applied pressure to lower abdomen may help to identify the testes, especially a gliding testis.
- Failure to palpate a testis after repeated exams suggests an intraabdominal or atrophic testis.
- An enlarged contralateral testis in the presence of a nonpalpable testis suggests testicular atrophy/absence.

DIAGNOSTIC TESTS & INTERPRETATION
Lab
Initial lab tests
- In boys ≤3 months of age with bilateral nonpalpable UDTs, luteinizing hormone, follicle-stimulating hormone, and testosterone levels are helpful to determine whether the testes are present.
- >3 months of age, a human chorionic gonadotropin (hCG) stimulation test to determine presence/absence of testicular tissue (hCG 2,000 IU/d × 3 days, and check testosterone before and after stimulation)

Follow-Up & Special Considerations
In newborns and children <6–12 months of age, periodic examination to determine if testis is palpable and descended prior to considering further intervention

Imaging
Initial approach
- Ultrasonography has a sensitivity of 76%, a specificity of 100%, and an accuracy of 84% in the diagnosis on nonpalpable UDT, whereas MRI has a sensitivity of 86%, a specificity of 79%, and an accuracy of 85% (6)[C].
- CT scan findings in children are inconsistent.

Diagnostic Procedures/Surgery
Laparoscopy is useful in a child with nonpalpable cryptorchidism to accurately confirm testicular absence or presence and to determine the feasibility of performing a standard orchiopexy (7)[C].

Pathological Findings
- Higher incidence of carcinoma in UDT and alterations in spermatogenesis
- Histologic changes occur by 1.5 years of age and include smaller seminiferous tubules, fewer spermatogonia, and more peritubular tissue.

DIFFERENTIAL DIAGNOSIS
- Retractile testis (hypermobile testis): A normally descended testis that ascends into the inguinal canal because of an active cremasteric reflex (more common in males 4–6 years of age)
- Atrophic testis: May occur as a result of neonatal torsion
- Vanished testis may be the result of a lack of development or in utero torsion.

TREATMENT

MEDICATION

- The International Health Foundation recommends biweekly hCG injections for 5 weeks: 250 (IU) for infants, 500 IU for children ≤6 years of age, and 1,000 IU for children ≥6 years of age.
- Success rates for descent into the scrotum range from 0–55% (8)[B].
  - The more distal the testis, the more likely the descent.
  - A systematic review with a meta-analysis of randomized clinical trials concluded that the evidence for the use of hCG versus gonadotropin-releasing hormone (GnRH) shows advantages for hCG but noted that the evidence was based on few trials (9)[B].
- Contraindications: hCG therapy is contraindicated in patients with a clinically apparent inguinal hernia, those with a history of previous ipsilateral groin surgery, or those with ectopic testicles. Also refer to manufacturer's literature.
- Precautions: (1) May induce precocious puberty; discontinue drug; effects should reverse in 4 weeks; (2) premature epiphyseal closure
- Significant possible interactions: Refer to manufacturer's literature.
- GnRH is approved for use in Europe, and neoadjuvant GnRH therapy may improve fertility index in UDT (10)[C].

ADDITIONAL TREATMENT

General Measures
- Rule out retractile testis.
- Appropriate health care: Outpatient until surgery performed
- Administration of chorionic gonadotropin may cause testicular descent in some boys. Reports of efficacy are inconsistent.

Issues for Referral
- Bilateral nonpalpable UDTs
- ≥1 testes not descended by 6 months to 1 year of age

SURGERY/OTHER PROCEDURES
- Reasons to consider: Avoids torsion, averts trauma, decreases but does not eliminate risk of malignancy, and prevents further alterations in spermatogenesis
- Orchiopexy should be performed by age 1. Alterations in germ cell count in the cryptorchid testis have been identified by age 2.
- Laparoscopy is performed first if testis is nonpalpable.
- If palpable, an inguinal approach is usually performed. Prepubertal approach is considered in select situations, but may increase the risk of hernia (11)[C].

ONGOING CARE

FOLLOW-UP RECOMMENDATIONS
Initial follow-up within 1 month of surgery and periodically thereafter to assess testicular size/growth

Patient Monitoring
- Patients should be followed after surgery to evaluate testicular growth.
- Testicular tumors occur mainly during or after puberty; thus these children should be taught self-examination when they are older.

DIET
No restrictions

PATIENT EDUCATION
Discuss with parents about causes, available treatments, and possible effects on patient's reproductive potential; also increased risk for testicular cancer and need for regular self-examination.

PROGNOSIS
- Disorder is usually corrected with medical or surgical therapy; however, possible lifelong consequences.
- If testicle is absent or orchiectomy is required, may consider placement of testicular prosthesis.
- Early orchidopexy may decrease risk of testicular damage and risk of malignancy.

COMPLICATIONS
- Progressive failure of spermatogenesis, if left untreated; even with orchiopexy, the fertility rate is still reduced, especially with bilateral UDTs.
- Spermatogenesis is related to the duration of cryptorchidism and the location of the testis.
- Formerly bilaterally cryptorchid men have a greater decrease in fertility compared with unilateral cryptorchid male and the general male population.
- Abnormalities also have been identified in the contralateral descended testis, although less severe.

ALERT
- There is a 4–7× higher risk of developing testicular cancer in a male with a history of UDT (2)[C], but early orchidopexy appears to decrease the risk of cancer.
- Hernia development (25%)

REFERENCES

1. Lee PA. Fertility after cryptorchidism: epidemiology and other outcome studies. *Urology*. 2005;66: 427–31.
2. Cortes D. Cryptorchidism: Aspects of pathogenesis, histology and treatment. *Scan J Nephrol*. 1998;9:54.
3. Scorer CG, Farrington HG. *Congenital Deformities of the Testes and Epididymis*. London: Butterworths, 1971.
4. Cryptorchidism: a prospective study of 7500 consecutive male births, 1984–8. John Radcliffe Hospital Cryptorchidism Study Group. *Arch Dis Child*. 1992;67(7):892–9.
5. Foresta C, Zuccarello D, Garolla A, Ferlin A et al. Role of hormones, genes, and environment in human cryptorchidism. *Endocr Rev*. 2008;29: 560–80.
6. Kanemoto K, Hayashi Y, Kojima Y, et al. Accuracy of ultrasonography and magnetic resonance imaging in the diagnosis of non-palpable testis. *Int J Urol*. 2005;12:668–72.
7. Patil KK, et al. Laparoscopy for impalpable testis. *Br J Urol*. 2005;95:704–8.
8. Henna MR, Del Nero RG, Sampaio CZ, et al. Hormonal cryptorchidism therapy: systematic review with metanalysis of randomized clinical trials. *Pediatr Surg Int*. 2004;20:357–9.
9. Henna MR, Del Nero RG, Sampaio CZ, Atallah AN, Schettini ST, Castro AA, Soares BG et al. Hormonal cryptorchidism therapy: systematic review with metanalysis of randomized clinical trials. *Pediatr Surg Int*. 2004;20:357–9.
10. Schwentner C, Oswald J, Kreczy A, et al. Neoadjuvant gonadotropin-releasing hormone therapy before surgery may improve the fertility index in undescended testes: a prospective randomized trial. *J Urol*. 2005;173:974–7.
11. Al-Mandil M, Khoury AE, El-Hout Y, Kogon M, Dave S, Farhat WA et al. Potential complications with the prescrotal approach for the palpable undescended testis? A comparison of single prescrotal incision to the traditional inguinal approach. *J Urol*. 2008;180:686–9.

ADDITIONAL READING

Berkowitz GS, Lapinski RH, Dolgin SE, et al. Prevalence and natural history of cryptorchidism. *Pediatrics*. 1993;92:44–9.

CODES

ICD9
752.51 Undescended testis

CLINICAL PEARLS

- If testicular descent does not occur by 6–9 months of age, it is unlikely to occur. Therefore, refer patients to a urologist if a testes has not descended by 6 months to 1 year of age.
- Children with bilateral nonpalpable UDTs require laboratory evaluation to determine if viable testicular tissue is present.
- The risk of infertility is increased with bilateral UDTs.

CUBITAL TUNNEL SYNDROME

Joseph Blazuk, MD
Mark Kaplan, MD

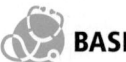 BASICS

DESCRIPTION
- Compression of the ulnar nerve on the medial aspect of the elbow where it enters the cubital tunnel. Often resulting in elbow pain and paresthesias of the forearm, wrist, 4th and 5th fingers.
- Synonym(s): Ulnar neuropathy

EPIDEMIOLOGY
- Predominant sex: Male > Female (3–8 times more common)
- Elbow is most common site of compression of ulnar nerve. Less common sites of entrapment include the arcade of Struthers, the medial intermuscular septum, the medial epicondyle, and the deep flexor pronator aponeurosis.
- 2nd most common nerve compression of upper extremity (behind median nerve compression in carpal tunnel) (1)

RISK FACTORS
- Patients who sleep or position themselves with their elbows bent, their arms overhead, or both
- Athletes in throwing sports, racquet sports, weightlifting, and skiing
- Preexisting polyneuropathy
- Patients with end-stage renal disease on hemodialysis
- Patients placed in dependent positioning (surgery, ICU)

GENERAL PREVENTION
- Avoid long periods with elbows bent or pressure on elbows.
- Sleep with elbows straight and avoid sleeping with arms overhead.
- Keep proper posture when working at a desk.

PATHOPHYSIOLOGY
- The ulnar nerve is the terminal branch of the medial cord of the brachial plexus and is composed from the C8 and T1 nerve roots.
- The ulnar nerve becomes more superficial as it enters the ulnar sulcus ~3.5 cm proximal to the medial epicondyle. The nerve courses posterior to the medial epicondyle and medial to the olecranon, then enters the cubital tunnel (2).
- The cubital tunnel is a fibro-osseous canal. The roof is defined by the arcuate ligament of Osbourne. The floor consists of the medial collateral ligament of the elbow, the joint capsule, and the olecranon.
- Elbow flexion increases distance from medial epicondyle to olecranon 5 mm for every 45°.
- Elbow flexion places stress on medial collateral ligament, overlying retinaculum, and ulnar nerve.
- Shape of cubital tunnel changes from a circle to an oval, with a 2.5-mm loss of height with elbow flexion.

- Loss of height of cubital tunnel with elbow flexion decreases tunnel volume by 55%, which doubles intraneural pressure on the ulnar nerve from 7–14 mm Hg.
- Maximal pressure on the ulnar nerve in cubital tunnel is created by shoulder abduction, elbow flexion, and wrist extension.

ETIOLOGY
- Elbow flexion decreases volume of cubital tunnel, causing compression of ulnar nerve.
- Compression of ulnar nerve causes pain at medial aspect of elbow and symptoms at forearm and hand.
- Caused by constricting fascial bands, subluxation of ulnar nerve over medial epicondyle, cubitus valgus, bony spurs, hypertrophied synovium, tumors, ganglia, or direct compression of ulnar nerve as it crosses cubital tunnel

COMMONLY ASSOCIATED CONDITIONS
- Ulnar nerve subluxation
- Osteoarthritis of elbow joint

 DIAGNOSIS

HISTORY
- Nocturnal elbow pain
- Medial elbow pain
- Paresthesias along lateral forearm, wrist, and 4th and 5th digits
- Paresthesias may be intermittent at first and then become more constant.
- History of trauma over the area
- Repetitive elbow flexion and extension activities (such as in hammering)
- Overhead throwing athlete with repetitive elbow motion
- Chronic symptoms: Loss of grip strength and loss of fine motor skills in hand

PHYSICAL EXAM
- Inspect carrying angle of both elbows.
- Palpate medial epicondyle and cubital tunnel for areas of tenderness or ulnar nerve subluxation.
- Check elbow range of motion.
- Positive Hoffman-Tinel test (tapping over ulnar nerve) (3)
- Pain on palpating over ulnar nerve
- Atrophy of intrinsic muscles
- Loss of sensation at ulnar side of 5th digit
- Wasting of hypothenar muscles and flexion contracture of 4th and 5th digits (ulnar claw)
- Wartenberg sign is clawing or abduction of the 5th digit with extension.
- Assess ability to cross 2nd and 3rd digits.

- Evaluate grip and pinch strength for weakness.
- Check vibration and light touch sensation.
- Recently, the "scratch-collapse test" has been described. The patient faces the examiner with arms adducted, elbows flexed, hands outstretched, and wrists at neutral. The patient resists bilateral shoulder adduction and internal rotation as examiner applies these forces to the forearm. The examiner "scratches" or swipes fingertips over course of compressed ulnar nerve. The force is then reapplied to the forearm. A positive result occurs when the patient has a temporary loss of external rotation resistance tone.
- Sensitivity for the scratch collapse was 69% compared with 54% and 46% for Tinel test and elbow flexion-compression test, respectively. Tinel test, however, had the highest negative predictive value (98%) of all tests for cubital tunnel (4).

DIAGNOSTIC TESTS & INTERPRETATION
McGowan grades quantify the degree of physical exam findings and are specific for cubital tunnel syndrome:
- McGowan Grade I: No wasting or weakness of intrinsic muscles, feeling of clumsiness in affected hand, mild paresthesias in ulnar nerve distribution
- McGowan Grade II: Intermediate lesions with weak interossei and muscle wasting
- McGowan Grade III: Severe lesions with paralysis of interossei and a marked weakness of the hand

Imaging
Initial approach
- X-rays may reveal osteophytes impinging on the area. Include anterior posterior (AP) lateral, and cubital tunnel views (3). Radiographs may also show signs of instability, deformity from old trauma, or presence of a supracondylar process (which can cause median nerve compression).
- Cubital tunnel view: Elbow is maximally flexed and x-ray beam is shot as an AP view of the distal humerus.

Follow-Up & Special Considerations
- Chest x-ray if patient has history of smoking and ulnar nerve symptoms (to exclude Pancoast tumor in apical lung)
- Magnetic resonance imaging shows inflammation and irritation of ulnar nerve.
- High-resolution ultrasound

Diagnostic Procedures/Surgery
- Corticosteroid injection into ulnar groove
- Electromyogram (EMG) is not essential when diagnosis is obvious on clinical exam. Use to determine the efficacy of conservative treatment or when the diagnosis is unclear.
- EMG is considered positive if motor conduction delay across the elbow is <50 m/s or difference between motor velocity across elbow and below the elbow is >10 m/s.
- Nerve conduction studies

Pathological Findings

Inflammation and swelling of ulnar nerve

DIFFERENTIAL DIAGNOSIS

- Cervical disc lesion
- Thoracic outlet syndrome
- Carpal tunnel syndrome
- Medial epicondylitis
- Thoracic outlet syndrome
- Pancoast syndrome
- Metabolic disorders creating peripheral neuropathies
- Multiple sclerosis and other myelopathies

 TREATMENT

Mild cubital tunnel syndrome can often be treated without surgery. If provocative causes can be identified and avoided, there is tendency for spontaneous recovery. Patients with constant symptoms and/or muscle atrophy typically require surgical intervention.

MEDICATION

First Line

Nonsteroidal anti-inflammatory drugs or other analgesic

Second Line

Corticosteroid (injection)

ADDITIONAL TREATMENT

General Measures

- Rest
- Avoidance of aggravating activities
- Conservative treatment is initial approach if no motor weakness.
- Instruct patient to avoid periods of prolonged elbow flexion.
- Instruct patient to avoid long periods of pressure and compression on ulnar nerve at elbow.
- Ice/heat for symptom relief
- Splint or brace while sleeping to keep affected elbow in extension and take pressure off cubital tunnel (e.g., wrap towel around elbow and hold in place with tape; use a small size soft knee splint but wear it on the elbow, tie a scarf around waist then around wrist)
- Physical therapy (nerve mobilization techniques)
- Workplace modifications (e.g., correct posture, avoid long periods with elbows bent)
- Avoid any activities that bring about symptoms.
- Otherwise activity as tolerated

Issues for Referral

Failure of conservative treatment, loss of grip strength, flexion contracture of 4th and 5th digits, positive EMG for motor conduction delay

Additional Therapies

- Corticosteroid injection into ulnar groove
- Use 1 mL lidocaine and 20–40 mg methylprednisolone injected into ulnar groove, parallel to ulnar nerve (3).
- Hand therapy and custom splint prescription

COMPLEMENTARY AND ALTERNATIVE MEDICINE

Vitamin B$_6$ (100 mg/d) not found to be effective in randomized trials

SURGERY/OTHER PROCEDURES

- Goal of surgery is to create more space for ulnar nerve (5).
- Many surgical treatments exist for the treatment of cubital tunnel syndrome. *In situ* decompression, transposition of the ulnar nerve into the subcutaneous, intramuscular, or submuscular plane, or medial epicondylectomy have all been shown to be effective in the treatment of this disease process. Comparative studies have shown some short–term advantages to one or another technique, but overall results between the treatments have essentially been equivocal. The choice of surgical treatment is based on multiple factors, and a single surgical approach cannot be applied to all clinical situations (2).

 ONGOING CARE

FOLLOW-UP RECOMMENDATIONS

Patient Monitoring

- In severe cases, the nerve damage may be permanent and the patient may not recover.
- The longer the nerve has been irritated, the more difficult it is to recover fully.

DIET

No restrictions

PATIENT EDUCATION

- Use correct posture; avoid putting pressure on your elbows, and place padding under your elbows.
- Inability to straighten fingers is often a sign of severe ulnar nerve damage. Patients with this level of irritation usually do not recover, even with surgery.

PROGNOSIS

- Both conservative and surgical methods result in 85–90% good-to-excellent results.
- For McGowan Grade III: Anterior intramuscular transposition has best outcome (6)[C].

COMPLICATIONS

Anterior transposition may have recurrent subluxation of the ulnar nerve.

REFERENCES

1. Fernandez E, Pallini R, Lauretti L, et al. Neurosurgery of the peripheral nervous system: cubital tunnel syndrome. *Surg Neurol*. 1998;50: 83–5.
2. Palmer BA, Hughes TB et al. Cubital tunnel syndrome. *J Hand Surg Am*. 2010;35:153–63.
3. Chumbley EM, O'Connor FG, Nirschl RP. Evaluation of overuse elbow injuries. *Am Fam Physician*. 2000; 61:691–700.
4. Cheng CJ, Mackinnon-Patterson B, Beck JL, Mackinnon SE et al. Scratch collapse test for evaluation of carpal and cubital tunnel syndrome. *J Hand Surg Am*. 2008;33:1518–24.
5. Mowlavi A, Andrews K, Lille S, et al. The management of cubital tunnel syndrome: a meta-analysis of clinical studies. *Plast Reconstr Surg*. 2000;106:327–34.
6. Bartels RH, Menovsky T, Van Overbeeke JJ, et al. Surgical management of ulnar nerve compression at the elbow: an analysis of the literature. *J Neurosurg*. 1998;89:722–7.

ADDITIONAL READING

Cutts S. Cubital tunnel syndrome. *Postgrad Med J*. 2007;83:28–31.

See Also (Topic, Algorithm, Electronic Media Element)

Ulnar Collateral Ligament Injury; Medial Epicondylitis; Lateral Epicondylitis

 CODES

ICD9

354.2 Lesion of ulnar nerve

CLINICAL PEARLS

- Elbow flexion decreases depth of cubital tunnel, thus putting pressure on ulnar nerve.
- Sleeping with elbow bent and arm overhead can cause symptoms.
- Improper posture when working at a desk can cause symptoms.
- Conservative treatment consists of ice, rest, hand therapy, splint fabrication, and activity modifications.
- Both conservative and surgical methods result in good-to-excellent results 85–90% of the time.

CUSHING DISEASE AND CUSHING SYNDROME

David M. Barclay, III, MD, MPH, FAAFP
Colleen Veloski, MD

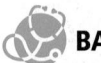 **BASICS**

DESCRIPTION
- Clinical abnormalities associated with chronic exposure to excessive amounts of cortisol (the major adrenocorticoid)
- Cushing disease is defined as glucocorticoid excess due to excessive adrenocorticotropic hormone (ACTH) secretion from a pituitary tumor. This is the most common cause of primary Cushing syndrome.
- Cushing syndrome is defined as excessive corticosteroid exposure from exogenous sources (medications) or endogenous sources (pituitary, adrenal, pulmonary, etc., or tumor)
- System(s) affected: Endocrine/Metabolic; Musculoskeletal; Skin/Exocrine; Cardiovascular; Neuropsychiatric

Pediatric Considerations
- Rare in infancy and childhood
- Most cases in children <8 years are a result of malignant adrenal tumors.

Pregnancy Considerations
Pregnancy may exacerbate disease.

EPIDEMIOLOGY
Incidence
Uncommon: 0.7–2.4 per million per year

Prevalence
In difficult-to-control diabetic patients with obesity and hypertension, prevalence has been reported at 2–5%.

RISK FACTORS
- Predominant sex: Female > Male (slightly). Cushing syndrome is equally prevalent in both sexes.
- Pituitary tumor
- Adrenal mass
- Neuroendocrine tumor (e.g., bronchial carcinoid)
- Prolonged use of corticosteroids

Genetics
- Multiple endocrine neoplasia type I
- Carney complex (an inherited multiple neoplasia syndrome)
- McCune-Albright syndrome (mutation of GNAS1 gene)

GENERAL PREVENTION
Avoid corticosteroid exposure when possible.

PATHOPHYSIOLOGY
- Disease: Pituitary tumor causing excess ACTH (corticotropin)
- Syndrome: Excessive corticosteroid exposure from exogenous sources (medications) or endogenous sources (pituitary, adrenal, pulmonary, etc., or tumor)

ETIOLOGY
- Exogenous glucocorticoids or ACTH
- Endogenous ACTH-dependent hypercortisolism (80–85%):
  – ACTH-secreting pituitary tumor: 70%
  – Ectopic ACTH production (e.g., small-cell carcinoma of lung, bronchial carcinoid): 20%
- Endogenous ACTH-independent hypercortisolism: 15–20%:
  – Adrenal adenoma
  – Adrenal carcinoma
  – Macronodular or micronodular hyperplasia

 DIAGNOSIS

HISTORY
- Weight gain: 95% (1)[B]
- Decreased libido: 90%
- Menstrual irregularity: 80%
- Hirsutism: 75%
- Depression/emotional lability: 50–80%
- Easy bruising: 65%
- Proximal muscle weakness: 60%
- Diabetes or glucose intolerance: 60%

PHYSICAL EXAM
- Obesity: 95%
- Facial plethora: 90%
- Moon face (facial adiposity): 90%
- Thin skin: 85%
- Hypertension: 75%
- Skeletal growth retardation in children (epiphyseal plates remain open): 70–80%
- Purple striae on the skin
- Increased adipose tissue in neck and trunk
- Acne

DIAGNOSTIC TESTS & INTERPRETATION
Lab
Initial lab tests
- For initial evaluation, order either late-night salivary cortisol or 24-hour urinary-free cortisol. In normal circadian rhythm, cortisol secretion is highest in the morning and lowest between 11 PM and midnight. The nadir of serum cortisol is maintained in pseudo-Cushing (e.g., obesity, alcoholism, depression), but not in Cushing syndrome.
- Elevated late-night salivary cortisol provides sensitivity and specificity >90–95% (2,3)[B]. (Contact local lab for instructions to obtain this test.)
- 24-hour urinary-free cortisol level: Obtain ≥3 samples to rule out intermittent hypercortisolism if results are normal and suspicion is high. Also measure 24-hour urinary creatinine excretion to verify adequacy of collection. Results may be falsely low if glomerular filtration rate <30 mL/min. Overall sensitivity and specificity varies, but has been reported to be 90–97% and 85–96%, respectively (2)[B].
- Midnight plasma cortisol: Try to obtain samples on 3 consecutive nights. A late evening serum cortisol >7.5 μg/dL has a sensitivity of 96% and a specificity of 100% (4)[B].

- Persistently elevated serum cortisol implies Cushing syndrome; nadir of serum cortisol is maintained in obese patients, but not in those with Cushing.
- Low-dose dexamethasone suppression testing is no longer used as 1st-line testing. Dexamethasone 1 mg is given between 11 PM and midnight, and fasting plasma cortisol is measured between 8 and 9 AM the following morning. A serum cortisol level below 1.8 μg/dL excludes Cushing syndrome, but specificity is limited. The presence of pseudo-Cushing states (depression, obesity, etc.), hepatic or renal disease, or any drug that induces cytochrome P-450 enzymes may cause a false result.
- High-dose dexamethasone suppression testing: This test is used to distinguish between an ACTH-secreting pituitary tumor and an ectopic ACTH-secreting tumor. 0.5 mg dexamethasone is given q.6h for 8 doses, with serum cortisol measured at 2 and 6 hours after last dose. Sensitivity 79%, specificity 74%.

ALERT
- Antiepileptic drugs, progesterone, oral contraceptives, rifampin, and spironolactone may cause a false-positive dexamethasone suppression test.
- Corticotropin-releasing hormone (CRH) after dexamethasone: This test is used to distinguish Cushing syndrome from pseudo-Cushing syndrome. Dexamethasone 0.5 mg is given q.6h for 48 hours starting at noon. CRH (1 μg/Kg) is given 2 hours after the last dose of dexamethasone. Plasma cortisol is >1.4 μg/dL 15 minutes after CRH in patients with Cushing syndrome but not in those with pseudo-Cushing (5)[B].

Imaging
Initial approach
- Chest radiograph
- Lumbar spine radiograph:
  – Osteoporosis is common
- Pituitary MRI scan if pituitary tumor suspected
- Abdominal CT scan if adrenal disease suspected
- Chest CT scan if ectopic ACTH secretion is suspected and inferior petrosal sinus sampling rules out pituitary source (6)[C]
- Octreotide scintigraphy to look for occult ACTH-secreting tumor

Diagnostic Procedures/Surgery
- Diagnostic procedure depends on circumstances and clinical judgment
- Inferior petrosal sinus sampling with CRH stimulation if ACTH-dependent tumor suspected (6)[C]

Pathological Findings
- Thyroid function suppressed
- Hypertension
- Dyslipidemia
- Polycystic ovarian syndrome/hyperandrogenism
- Oligomenorrhea/hypogonadism
- Myopathy/cutaneous wasting
- Neuropsychiatric problems
- Nodular adrenal disease
- Hypercoagulable state
- Osteoporosis
- Nephrolithiasis
- Growth hormone reduced

DIFFERENTIAL DIAGNOSIS
- Obesity
- Diabetes mellitus
- Hypertension
- Metabolic syndrome X
- Polycystic ovarian disease
- Hypercortisolism secondary to alcoholism (pseudo-Cushing)

TREATMENT

MEDICATION
- Drugs are not usually effective as the primary long-term treatment, and are used primarily either in preparation for surgery or as adjunctive treatment after surgery, pituitary radiotherapy, or both.
- Metyrapone, ketoconazole, and mitotane can all be used to lower cortisol by directly inhibiting synthesis and secretion in the adrenal gland. As initial treatment, remission rates up to 85% (6,7)[C].

SURGERY/OTHER PROCEDURES
- Tumor-specific surgery:
  - Trans-sphenoidal surgery for Cushing disease offers selective microadenectomy of the ACTH-producing adenoma, leaving the remaining pituitary intact (remission rate 60–80%).
  - For Cushing syndrome, resection of the ACTH-producing tumor is optimal treatment.
- Adrenal surgery:
  - For unilateral adrenal adenomas, laparoscopic surgery is treatment of choice.
  - For patients with Cushing disease, bilateral laparoscopic adrenalectomy is used more often, especially when the disease is severe or because of patient preference.
  - Pituitary radiotherapy can be used to treat persistent hypercortisolism after trans-sphenoidal surgery.

ONGOING CARE

PATIENT EDUCATION
- Comprehensive teaching to help patient cope with lifelong treatment may be needed, including:
  - Diet and monitoring weight daily
  - Early treatment of infections
  - Emotional lability prevention
- Refer to National Adrenal Disease Foundation: NADF 505 Northern Blvd. Great Neck, NY 11021; (516) 407-4992

PROGNOSIS
- Generally chronic course with cyclic exacerbations and rare remissions
- Guardedly favorable prognosis with surgery
- 20% long-term recurrence rate after surgery; more frequent following surgery for benign adrenal tumors:
  - Poor with small cell carcinoma of the lung producing ectopic hormone; neuroendocrine tumors (bronchial carcinoid) have much better prognosis (4)[C]

COMPLICATIONS
- Osteoporosis
- Increased susceptibility to infections
- Metastases of malignant tumors
- Increased cardiovascular risk even after treatment
- Lifelong glucocorticoid dependence following treatment with bilateral adrenalectomy
- Nelson syndrome (pituitary tumor) after treatment with bilateral adrenalectomy

REFERENCES

1. Newell-Price J, Bertagna X, Grossman AB, et al. Cushing's syndrome. *Lancet*. 2006;367:1605–17.
2. Putignano P, et al. Midnight salivary cortisol versus urinary free and midnight serum cortisol as screening tests for Cushing's syndrome. *J Clin Endocrinol Metabol*. 88(9):4153–7.
3. Yaneva M, Mosnier-Pudar H, Dugué MA et al. Midnight salivary cortisol for the initial diagnosis of Cushing's syndrome of various causes. *J Clin Endocrinol Metab*. 2004;89:3345–51.
4. Isidori AM, et al. The ectopic adrenocorticotropin syndrome: Clinical features, diagnosis, management and long term follow up. *J Clin Endocrinol Metabol*. 2006;91(2):371–7.
5. Yanovski JA, Cutler GB, Chrousos GP et al. Corticotropin-releasing hormone stimulation following low-dose dexamethasone administration. A new test to distinguish Cushing's syndrome from pseudo-Cushing's states. *JAMA*. 1993; 269:2232–8.
6. Findling JF, et al. Cushing's syndrome: Important issues in diagnosis and management. *J Clin Endocrinol Metabol*. 2006;10:3746–53.
7. Nieman LK, Ilias I. Evaluation and treatment of Cushing's syndrome. *Am J Med*. 2005;118: 1340–6.

See Also (Topic, Algorithm, Electronic Media Element)
Algorithm: Cushing Syndrome

CODES

ICD9
255.0 Cushing's syndrome

CLINICAL PEARLS

- Cushing disease is due to excessive ACTH secretion from a pituitary tumor, resulting in corticosteroid excess.
- Cushing syndrome is due to excessive corticosteroid exposure from exogenous sources (medications) or endogenous sources (pituitary, adrenal, pulmonary, etc. or tumor).

CUTANEOUS DRUG REACTIONS

Nikki D.Y. Tang, MD
Nathaniel J. Jellinek, MD

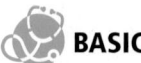

BASICS

DESCRIPTION
- An adverse cutaneous reaction in response to administration of a drug
- Cutaneous eruptions are the most common negative reactions to medications.
- Reactions are divided into immunologic and nonimmunologic reaction types.
- Morbilliform and urticarial eruptions are most common, but multiple morphologic types may occur.
- System(s) affected: Skin/Mucosa/Exocrine; Hematologic/Lymphatic/Immunologic
- Synonym(s): Drug eruptions; Drug rash; Dermatologic drug reactions' Dermatitis medicamentosa; Fixed drug eruption

Geriatric Considerations
- Possibly more likely in this age group due to greater number of medications
- Severe systemic reactions with greater morbidity

Pediatric Considerations
May occur in this age group

EPIDEMIOLOGY
- Predominant age: Geriatric, but all ages affected
- Predominant sex: Female > Male

Incidence
- In the US: 2–5% of inpatients, 0–8% overall, highest for antibiotic use (1–8%)
- Most are mild and resolve after removal of the offending agent, but severe and potentially fatal reactions may affect 1 in 1,000 inpatients.
- Likelihood of developing a cutaneous reaction is 10-fold greater in immunocompromised state

RISK FACTORS
Concurrent infections, immunocompromise (e.g., HIV, cancer, chemotherapy), metabolic disorders, large number of medications

GENERAL PREVENTION
- Always question patients about prior adverse drug events.
- Be aware of any potential cross-reactions.

PATHOPHYSIOLOGY
- Most drug reactions are nonimmunologic. Mechanisms include drug accumulation, idiosyncratic reactions (e.g., amoxicillin in infectious mononucleosis), direct release of mast-cell mediators (NSAID shift in leukotriene production causing histamine release), Jarisch-Herxheimer phenomenon, overdosage, phototoxic dermatitis, intolerance, or adverse effects.
- Reactions may be immunologically mediated, IgE-dependent, immune complex–dependent, cytotoxic, or most commonly delayed-type (type 4 hypersensitivity).

ETIOLOGY
- More than 700 drugs are known to cause a dermatologic reaction. Temporal relationship and type of reaction may elucidate the causative agent:
  - Acneform: OCPs, corticosteroids, iodinated compounds, hydantoins, lithium
  - Erythema multiforme: Sulfonamides, penicillins, barbiturates, hydantoins, NSAIDs, tetracycline, Cefaclor, Terbinafine
  - Erythema nodosum: OCPs, sulfonamides, penicillins
  - Fixed drug eruptions: OCPs, barbiturates, salicylates, tetracycline, sulfonamides
  - Lichenoid: Sildenafil, gold, antimalarials, thiazides, captopril
  - Photosensitivity: Doxycycline, thiazides, sulfonylureas, quinolones
  - Vasculitis: Thiazides, gold, sulfonamides, NSAIDs, tetracycline
  - Bullous: NSAIDs, thiazides, barbiturates, captopril
  - Skin necrosis: Warfarin, heparin
- Particularly common offenders: Antibiotics, NSAIDs, phenytoin, allopurinol, warfarin, gold, lithium

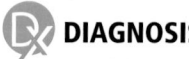

DIAGNOSIS

HISTORY
- Medications within past month: All oral, parenteral, and topical agents; all OTC drugs; vitamins, homeopathic, and herbal remedies
- Inquire about previous adverse reactions to medications.
- Ask about multiple courses of therapy or long-term use of a drug that can induce allergic sensitization.
- Consider other etiologies, including bacterial infections and viral exanthems.

PHYSICAL EXAM
May present as a number of different eruption types, including but not limited to:
- Morbilliform eruptions (exanthems):
  - Most frequent cutaneous reaction (28–95%) (1)[A]
  - May be indistinguishable from viral exanthem
  - Erythematous macules and papules; confluent, symmetric, and pruritic
  - Most common on trunk and in dependent areas
  - Onset 7–21 days after initiation
- Urticaria:
  - Also very common reaction
  - Pruritic erythematous wheals distributed anywhere on the body, including mucous membranes
  - 40% progress to angioedema, appearing as nonpitting edema without erythema or margins (2)[C]
  - May be annular in pediatric patient
  - Individual lesions fade within 24 hours, but new urticaria may develop.
- Fixed drug eruptions:
  - Single or multiple, round, sharply defined, dark violaceous plaques with gray center that leave residual macular hyperpigmentation
  - Appear shortly after drug exposure and reappear in the same location after drug ingestion; lesions can occur anywhere: Favored sites include mouth, genitalia, and acral areas
  - Onset usually 2 hours after ingestion of drug
  - Some patients have a refractory period during which the drug fails to activate lesions.
- Eczematous reactions:
  - Pruritic scalelike erythematous lesions typically on flexor surfaces of arms or legs
- Erythema multiforme (EM):
  - EM minor:
    - Target and bullous lesions predominantly on the extremities

- Association with herpes simplex virus much more commonly than any drug
- EM major:
  - Stevens-Johnson syndrome (SJS): Widespread skin and mucous membrane involvement with large atypical targetoid lesions with <10% skin sloughing; 5%-15% mortality (3)[C]
  - Toxic epidermal necrolysis (TEN): More extensive lesions with sloughing >30% of body surface, often with confluent areas of necrosis; 30% mortality (4)[C] with secondary infection and sepsis major concerns
  - Typical onset 1–3 weeks after starting offending agent
- Exfoliative erythroderma/dermatitis:
  - Erythema or eczema and scaling of over 50% of body surface
  - Lymphadenopathy, hepatosplenomegaly, leukocytosis, eosinophilia, or anemia may be present.
  - Potentially life-threatening
  - Difficult to distinguish between drug etiology, inflammatory etiology, cutaneous lymphoma etiology
- Acral erythema (erythrodysesthesia):
  - Common reaction to chemotherapeutic agents
  - Erythema, edema, and tenderness of palms and soles
  - Resolves in 2–4 weeks
- Lichen planuslike eruptions:
  - Violaceous, pruritic papules on extensor surfaces
  - Reticular pattern, buccal mucosa
- Photosensitivity reaction:
  - Phototoxic reactions within 24 hours of light exposure with exaggerated sun burn reaction
  - Photoallergic reactions; less common, more pruritic than painful, caused by UVA exposure
- Acneform eruptions:
  - Pustular lesions, but unlike true acne (no comedones)
- Vasculitis:
  - Petechiae or purpura concentrated on lower legs
  - Fever, myalgias, arthritis, and abdominal pain may also be present.
- Hypersensitivity syndrome (e.g., drug rash with eosinophilia and systemic symptoms—DRESS):
  - Related to anticonvulsants, sulfonamides, dapsone, minocycline, allopurinol
  - Classic triad of fever, exanthem, and internal organ involvement. May also present with pharyngitis and lymphadenopathy.
  - Internal organ involvement: 80% hepatic, 40% renal, 33% pulmonary (5)[C]
  - Atypical lymphocytosis with prominent eosinophilia (6)[C]
  - Onset 2–8 weeks, but may develop 3 months or later into therapy
- Acute generalized exanthematous pustulosis (AGEP):
  - Fever with multiple small, sterile, nonfollicular pustules on erythematous background with desquamation after 7–10 days
  - Appears similar to pustular psoriasis, but AGEP has more marked leukocytosis with neutrophilia and eosinophilia
  - Short time to onset (24 h to 2 weeks)

- Serum sicknesslike reaction:
  - Fever, nonspecific cutaneous eruption, arthralgias
  - Onset 7–14 days
  - Related to antibiotics, minocycline (6)[C]:
    ○ Detailed observation and morphologic description of all lesions facilitates diagnosis.
    ○ Nikolsky sign (epidermis sloughs with lateral pressure; may constitute medical emergency)
- Sweet syndrome (acute febrile neutrophilic dermatosis):
  - Fever, neutrophilia, tender reddish-blue or violet papules, plaques, or nodules, with or without pustules or vesicles that spontaneously resolve
  - May have oral ulcers or ocular manifestations such as conjunctivitis
  - Classically seen in young women after a mild respiratory illness, but 7–56% associated with malignancy (7)[C]
  - Also associated with G-CSF, GM-CSF administration
- Dermatomyositislike:
  - Similar cutaneous findings (e.g., Gottron papules), but lack muscle involvement and antinuclear antibodies

DIAGNOSTIC TESTS & INTERPRETATION
Lab
Initial lab tests
- Routine laboratory tests generally are nonspecific and not helpful.
- Significant eosinophilia may be related to more severe disease in allergic reactions (4)[C].
- Special tests dependent on suspected mechanism (8)[C]:
  - Type I: Skin testing, RAST, serum tryptase
  - Type II: Direct or indirect Coombs test
  - Type III: ESR, C-reactive protein, ANA, antihistone antibody, tissue biopsy for immunofluorescence studies
  - Type IV: Patch testing, lymphocyte proliferation assay (investigational)
- Cultures may be useful to exclude infectious causes.

Imaging
For vasculitic eruptions, chest radiography and urinalysis

Diagnostic Procedures/Surgery
- Withdrawal of suspected offending agent and observation for resolution
- Punch biopsy sometimes helpful for fixed drug eruptions

Pathological Findings
Nonspecific histologic findings are superficial infiltrates composed variably of lymphocytes, neutrophils, and eosinophils (9).

DIFFERENTIAL DIAGNOSIS
- Viral exanthem: Presence of fever, lymphocytosis, and other systemic findings may help differentiate
- Primary dermatosis: Correlation of drug withdrawal to rash resolution may clarify diagnosis; skin biopsy may be helpful.

 TREATMENT

MEDICATION
- Depends on the type of eruption; symptomatic treatment may be useful; most require no specific therapy except withdrawal of offending drug.
- Anaphylaxis or widespread urticaria: Epinephrine 1:1,000, 0.01 mL/kg (0.3 mL maximum) SC
- Acute urticaria (<6 weeks): First- or second-generation H1 antihistamines are mainstay of therapy (2)[A].
- Chronic urticaria (>6 weeks): Antihistamines, doxepin in increasing doses and antileukotriene medications are options (2)[A]. H4 receptor antagonists may be more beneficial than H1 receptor antagonists (8)[C].
- Anaphylaxis, severe urticaria, or erythema multiforme: Corticosteroids parenterally as indicated by condition; or prednisone p.o. 1 mg/kg in tapering doses (2)[A]
- Chronic erythema multiforme associated with herpes simplex: Prophylactic acyclovir (10)[A]
- Topical lubricants, emollients for eczematous reactions
- Topical corticosteroids (Groups I–III) for limited eczematous-type eruptions or lichenoid eruptions
- Contraindications, precautions, and significant possible interactions: Refer to manufacturer's information.

ADDITIONAL TREATMENT
General Measures
- Appropriate health care, monitor for signs of impending cardiovascular collapse:
  - Urticaria or bullous lesions, angioedema, and generalized erythroderma are all potentially more serious than other types of reactions; therefore, possible offending medications should be discontinued immediately, medical evaluation as soon as possible
  - Anaphylactic reactions, Stevens-Johnson syndrome, extensive bullous reactions, or TEN: Consider inpatient treatment.
- In patients on multiple medications, the decision to discontinue each medication should be based on the likelihood of each individual medication causing the reaction (e.g., 7% for penicillins, sulfonamides) and the risk/benefit ratio of continuing each medication.
- Do not rechallenge with drugs causing urticaria, bullae, angioedema, anaphylaxis, or erythema multiforme.
- Consider continuation of medications through morbilliform eruptions unless severe.

 ONGOING CARE

FOLLOW-UP RECOMMENDATIONS
Patient Monitoring
- For urticarial, bullous, or erythema multiformelike lesions, close patient follow-up needed
- Patients with serious reactions (anaphylaxis, angioedema) should be given EpiPen for secondary prevention
- Label the patient's chart with the suspected agent and type of reaction.

PATIENT EDUCATION
American Academy of Dermatology, (708) 330-0230

PROGNOSIS
- Eruptions generally fade within days after removing offending agent
- Anaphylaxis, angioedema, and bullous reactions are potentially fatal.

COMPLICATIONS
- Anaphylaxis
- Bone marrow suppression
- Hepatitis (dapsone, hydantoin)
- Cross-reaction to chemically similar agents in future

REFERENCES
1. Bigby M. Rates of cutaneous reactions to drugs. *Arch Dermatol*. 2001;137:765–70.
2. Amar SM & Dreskin SC. Urticaria. *Prim Care Clin Office Pract*. 2008;(35):141–57.
3. Hazin R, Ibrahimi OA, Hazin MI, Kimyai-Asadi A et al. Stevens-Johnson syndrome: pathogenesis, diagnosis, and management. *Ann. Med*. 2008;40:129–38.
4. Granowitz EV & Brown RB. Antibiotic adverse reactions and drug interactions. *Crti Care Clin*. 2008:412–42.
5. Chen YC, Chiu HC, Chu CY et al. Drug Reaction With Eosinophilia and Systemic Symptoms: A Retrospective Study of 60 Cases. *Archives of dermatology*. 2010;
6. Knowles SR & Shear NH. Recognition and management of severe cutaneous drug reactions. *Dermatol Clin*. 2007;25:245–53.
7. Cohen PR, Kurzrock R et al. Sweet's syndrome: a neutrophilic dermatosis classically associated with acute onset and fever. *Clin. Dermatol*. 2000;18: 265–82.
8. Sicherer SH, et al. Advances in allergic skin disease, anaphylaxis and hypersensitivity reactions to foods, drugs and insects in 2007. *J All Clin Immunol*. 2008:1351–7.
9. Gerson D et al. Cutaneous drug eruptions: A 5-year experience. *J Am Acad Dermatol*. 2008;59;6:995–9.
10. Tatnall FM, Schofield JK, Leigh IM et al. A double-blind, placebo-controlled trial of continuous acyclovir therapy in recurrent erythema multiforme. *Br J Dermatol*. 1995;132:267–70.

 CODES

ICD9
- 693.0 Dermatitis due to drugs and medicines taken internally
- 708.0 Allergic urticaria

CLINICAL PEARLS
- Virtually any drug can cause any rash; antibiotics are the most common culprits causing cutaneous drug reactions.
- Focus on drug history with new suspicious skin eruptions.
- Morbilliform rashes are the most frequent.
- Usually self-limited after withdrawal of offending agent.
- Symptoms such as tongue swelling/angioedema, skin necrosis, blisters, high fever, dyspnea, and mucous membrane erosions signify more severe drug reactions.

CUTANEOUS SQUAMOUS CELL CARCINOMA

Herbert P. Goodheart, MD

 BASICS

- Squamous cell carcinoma (SCC) is a malignant epithelial tumor arising from keratinocytes of the epidermis. Cutaneous (nonmucous membrane) SCC is the second most common form of skin cancer. Lesions most frequently occur on sun-exposed sites of elderly, fair-skinned individuals. The majority of SCCs arise in solar keratoses *(actinic keratoses)*. Such actinically derived SCCs that develop from solar keratoses are slow-growing, minimally invasive, unaggressive; and the prognosis is usually excellent because distant metastases that arise from these lesions are extremely rare. An SCC may appear de novo without a preceding solar keratosis. SCCs may also develop from causes other than sun exposure. For example, an SCC may arise in an old burn scar or from sites previously exposed to ionizing radiation. An SCC may also emerge from preexisting human papilloma virus infection *(verrucous carcinoma)*. An SCC is capable of locally infiltrative growth, spread to regional lymph nodes, and distant metastasis, most often to the lungs. When metastases from SCC do occur, they are more likely to result from lesions that appear on the ears or on the vermilion border of the lips or from tumors >2 cm in diameter. Other risks for metastasis include lesions that arise on mucous membranes, from sites that received ionizing radiation, on the skin of organ transplant recipients, in chronic inflammatory lesions (e.g., discoid lupus erythematosus), or in long-standing scars or cutaneous ulcers (e.g., venous stasis ulcers) or other nonhealing wounds.
- System(s) affected: Skin/Exocrine
- Synonym(s): Squamous cell carcinoma of the skin; Epidermoid carcinoma; Prickle cell carcinoma

EPIDEMIOLOGY
- Predominant age: Elderly population
- Predominant sex: Males > Females
- More common in geographic areas that have a high frequency of sun exposure

Incidence
- The dramatic escalating incidence in the US due to an increase in sun exposure in the general population, aging of the population, earlier and more frequent diagnosis of SCC, and a rising number of immunosuppressed patients
- The incidence is highest in Australia and in the Sun Belt of the US.

ALERT
Bowen disease and frank squamous cell carcinoma are 2 of the few skin cancers that should be considered in blacks. These non–sun–related skin cancers tend to arise on the extremities de novo or in an old scar or in a lesion of discoid lupus erythematosus.

RISK FACTORS
- Older age
- Male sex: However, incidence is increasing in females due to lifestyle changes (e.g., suntan parlors, shorter dresses, etc.)
- Chronic sun exposure: SCC is noted more frequently in those with a greater degree of outdoor activity (e.g., farmers, sailors, gardeners).
- Patients with multiple solar keratoses are at increased risk.
- Personal or family history of skin cancer

- Northern European descent
- Fair complexion, fair hair, light eyes
- Poor tanning ability, with tendency to burn
- Organ transplant recipients, chronic immunosuppression
- Exposure to chemical carcinogens (e.g., arsenic, tar) or ionizing radiation
- Therapeutic UV and ionizing radiation exposure
- Defects in cell-mediated immunity related to lymphoproliferative disorders (CLL, lymphoma)
- Human papillomavirus (HPV) infection (certain subtypes)
- Chronic scarring and inflammatory conditions
- Specific genodermatoses (e.g., xeroderma pigmentosum)

Genetics
- Persons of Irish or Scottish ancestry have the highest prevalence of SCC.
- SCC is relatively rare in people of African and Asian descent, although it is the most common form of skin cancer in these populations.
- Patients with oculocutaneous albinism are at greater risk.

GENERAL PREVENTION
Sun-avoidance measures: Sunscreens, hats, etc. Sunglasses with UV protection. Tinted windshields and side windows in cars. Sun-protective garments.

ETIOLOGY
- Exact mechanisms are not established; however, it is well known that ultraviolet radiation damages skin cell nucleic acids (DNA) resulting in a mutant clone of the gene p53. This leads to uncontrolled growth of skin cells. Ultraviolet radiation also suppresses the immune response preventing recovery from this damage.
- Epidemiologic and experimental evidence suggests the following as causative agents: Sunlight (solar radiation), radiation exposure, tanning parlors, PUVA phototherapy exposure, inorganic arsenic exposure, coal tar and other oil derivatives
- Immunosuppression by medications or disease such as HIV

COMMONLY ASSOCIATED CONDITIONS
- Solar keratosis (some investigators consider a solar keratosis to be an early squamous cell carcinoma, although relatively few ultimately are found to develop into an SCC)
- Keratoacanthoma
- Cutaneous horn
- Actinic cheilitis (solar keratoses of the mucous membranes of the lips) and leukoplakia of lip
- Xeroderma pigmentosum, albinism, and vitiligo
- Immunosuppression
- Chronic skin ulcers and chronic thermal burns

DIAGNOSIS

HISTORY
Often a family or personal history of skin cancer

PHYSICAL EXAM
- Lesions occur chiefly on chronically sun-exposed areas:
  - The face and the backs of the forearms and hands
  - Bald areas of the scalp and top of ears in men
  - The sun-exposed "V" of the neck, as well as the posterior neck below the occipital hairline

  - In elderly females, lesions tend to occur on the legs and other sun-exposed locations.
  - In blacks: Equal frequency in sun-exposed and unexposed areas
- Clinical appearance:
  - Generally slow-growing, firm, hyperkeratotic papules, nodules, or plaques
  - Most SCCs are asymptomatic, although bleeding, pain, and tenderness (all of which are unusual) may be noted.
  - Lesions may have a smooth, verrucous, or papillomatous surface.
  - Varying degrees of ulceration, erosion, crust, or scale
  - Color is often red to brown, tan, or pearly, and may be indistinguishable from basal cell carcinoma

DIAGNOSTIC TESTS & INTERPRETATION
Diagnostic Procedures/Surgery
- Surgical biopsy to ensure diagnosis: Shave biopsy, punch biopsy, excisional biopsy, incisional biopsy
- Sentinel lymph node biopsy has been used to identify micrometastases in a small number of patients with high-risk SCC and clinically negative nodes. Complete lymphadenectomy of the draining nodal basin has also been suggested for high-risk tumors.

Pathological Findings
- Noninvasive SCC is characterized by an intraepidermal proliferation of atypical keratinocytes. Hyperkeratosis, acanthosis, and confluent parakeratosis are seen within the epidermis. Cellular atypia, including pleomorphism, hyperchromatic nuclei, and mitoses, are prominent. Atypical keratinocytes may be found in the basal layer and often extend deeply down hair follicles, but they do not invade the dermis.
- In the in situ type of SCC (*Bowen disease*), only the full thickness of the epidermis is involved. The basement membrane remains intact.
- An invasive squamous cell carcinoma penetrates through the basement membrane into the dermis. It has various levels of anaplasia and may manifest relatively few to multiple mitoses and display varying degrees of differentiation, such as keratinization.
- Poorly differentiated tumors are clinically more aggressive. SCCs proliferate 1st by local invasion. Metastases, when they do occur, spread via local lymph ducts to local lymph nodes.

DIFFERENTIAL DIAGNOSIS
- Solar keratosis (*actinic keratosis*). Early SCC lesions may be clinically difficult, if not impossible, to distinguish from a precursor solar keratosis.
- Basal cell carcinoma may be also indistinguishable from an SCC, particularly if the lesion is ulcerated.
- Verruca vulgaris

ALERT
- The appearance of common warts is often similar to that of SCC lesions.
- A subungual SCC can easily be mistaken for a verruca.
- Seborrheic keratosis: "Stuck on" appearance
- Keratoacanthoma: This lesion also may be clinically impossible to differentiate from an SCC:
  - Occurs in the elderly >60 years
  - Fast growing
  - A nodular lesion that usually has a characteristic central crater

– If ignored, lesions may involute spontaneously.
– Resembles an SCC histologically and is considered by some dermatologists and dermatopathologists to be a low-grade variant of an SCC. (Some investigators feel that it should be treated as an SCC.)

- Melanoma:
  – Amelanotic melanoma and ulcerated melanoma may also be impossible to distinguish from an SCC.
- Clinical variants of SCC:
  – Bowen disease (*squamous cell carcinoma in situ*): This is a solitary lesion that resembles a scaly psoriatic or eczematous plaque. By definition, the atypia of SCC in situ involves the full thickness of the epidermis without invasion into the dermis.
  – Cutaneous horn: SCC with an overlying cutaneous horn. A cutaneous horn represents a fingernail platelike keratinization produced by the SCC. Bowen disease may also produce a cutaneous horn on its surface.
  – HPV-associated SCC: Virally induced SCC most commonly manifests as a new or enlarging warty growth on the penis, vulva, perianal area, or periungual region.
  – Erythroplasia of Queyrat refers to Bowen disease of the glans penis, which manifests as 1 or more velvety red plaques.
  – Subungual SCC: Such lesions typically mimic a wart and are misdiagnosed prior to biopsy.
  – Anogenital SCC: SCC in the anogenital region may manifest as a moist, red plaque on the glans penis or perianal area; indurated or ulcerated lesions may be seen on the vulva, external anus, or scrotum.
  – Verrucous carcinoma, a subtype of SCC, can be locally destructive but rarely metastasizes. Lesions are "cauliflowerlike" verrucous nodules or plaques.

TREATMENT

MEDICATION
First Line
- Immunotherapy:
  – Imiquimod (Aldara) (1,2) 5% cream is approved for the treatment of solar keratoses, genital warts, and for superficial basal cell carcinomas. It is now being used "off-label" for SCC in situ (Bowen disease), and may have some utility in treating selected patients who have highly differentiated SCCs.
- In patients with multiple or recurrent SCCs, chemoprevention with systemic retinoids (3,4) such as acetrecin may be effective for reducing the number of new SCCs; shown to be beneficial in treating existing SCCs or at reducing the risk of recurrence after treatment.

Second Line
- Photodynamic therapy (PDT): Treatment with PDT involves the application of a photosensitizer (given topically or systemically) followed by exposure to a light source. PDT is used primarily to treat large numbers of solar keratoses and is not recommended for treatment of invasive SCC.
- Radiotherapy is a primary treatment option that is generally restricted to older patients who are physically debilitated or are unable to undergo, or refuse to undergo, excisional surgery.
- Topical chemotherapy: Topical formulations of 5-fluorouracil (5-FU) are available for the treatment of Bowen disease and solar keratoses.
- Intralesional 5-FU has also been used to successfully treat keratoacanthomas.

SURGERY/OTHER PROCEDURES
- Electrocautery (electrodesiccation) and curettage (ED&C):
  – For small lesions (generally <1 cm) on flat surfaces (e.g., forehead, cheek) and SCC in situ (Bowen disease). ED&C may be used to treat superficially invasive SCCs without high-risk characteristics, but it is not appropriate for certain high-risk anatomic locations (see below).
  – Cryosurgery with LN$_2$ in selected lesions, such as Bowen disease
- Total excision, which is the preferred method of therapy for SCC, permitting histologic diagnosis of the tumor margins
- Micrographic (Mohs) surgery is a microscopically controlled method of removing skin cancers that allows for controlled excision and maximum preservation of normal tissue. It has the highest cure rate of all surgical treatments. Mohs surgery may be indicated for:
  – Large or invasive carcinomas
  – Recurrent SCCs
  – Lesions with a poorly delineated clinical border
  – An SCC within an orifice (e.g., ear canals or nostrils)
  – Locations where preservation of normal tissue is extremely important (e.g., tip of the nose, eyelids, ala nasi, ears, lips, and glans penis)
  – Bone or cartilage invasion
  – A lesion in an area of late radiation change
  – Micrographic (Mohs) surgery provides the best available cure rates (94–99%) for SCC.
- Metastatic disease requires aggressive management by a multidisciplinary team involving plastic, ENT/maxillofacial, a general surgeon, or a surgical oncologist.

ONGOING CARE

FOLLOW-UP RECOMMENDATIONS
Patient Monitoring
After therapy, periodic skin exam every month for 3 months, 6 months after treatment, and then yearly

ALERT
- SCCs that arise in areas of non-sun–exposed skin or those that originate de novo on areas of sun-exposed skin have a greater tendency to metastasize.
- An SCC arising on a mucous membrane, one arising from a chronic ulcer, or one arising in an immunocompromised patient should be regarded as potentially metastatic.

PATIENT EDUCATION
Skin self-exam, encourage sun avoidance techniques, sunscreens, etc. Artificial tanning devices should be avoided.

PROGNOSIS
- 90–95% cure rate with appropriate treatment
- Head and neck lesions have better prognosis (5).
- The ability to produce scale (*keratinization*) indicates a tendency for a lesion to be more differentiated and less likely to metastasize.
- Softer, nonkeratinizing lesions are not as well differentiated and thus are more likely to spread.
- Lesions ≥2 cm more prone to recur
- SCCs that are deeply invasive in subcutaneous fat or deeper, or those that have perineural involvement, are more likely to metastasize.
- When SCC does metastasize, it usually occurs within several years from the time of diagnosis and involves draining lymph nodes.
- Once nodal metastasis of cutaneous SCC has occurred, the overall 5-year survival rate has historically been in the range of 25–35%.

ALERT
An SCC that is histopathologically described as being "poorly differentiated" should be treated more aggressively.

COMPLICATIONS
Untreated, SCC becomes indurated, with a tendency to ooze, ulcerate, or bleed. Local recurrence. Metastatic disease.

REFERENCES
1. Patel GK, Goodwin R. Imiquimod 5% cream monotherapy for cutaneous *squamous cell carcinoma in situ* (Bowen's disease): A randomized, double-blind, placebo-controlled trial. *J Am Acad Dermatol*. 2006;54(1):25–32.
2. Hengge UR, Schaller J. Successful treatment of invasive squamous cell carcinoma using topical imiquimod. *Arch Dermatol*. 2004;140:404–6.
3. Harwood CA, Leedham-Green M, Leigh IM, et al. Low-dose retinoids in the prevention of cutaneous squamous cell carcinomas in organ transplant recipients: a 16-year retrospective study. *Arch Dermatol*. 2005;141:456–64.
4. Chen K, Craig JC, Shumack S. Oral retinoids for the prevention of skin cancers in solid organ transplant recipients: a systematic review of randomized controlled trials. *Br J Dermatol*. 2005;152:518–23.
5. Clayman GL, Lee JJ, Holsinger FC, et al. Mortality risk from squamous cell skin cancer. *J Clin Oncol*. 2005;23:759–65.

ADDITIONAL READING
Schmults CD. High-risk cutaneous squamous cell carcinoma: identification and management. *Adv Dermatol*. 2005;21:133–52.

CODES

ICD9
- 173.0 Other malignant neoplasm of skin of lip
- 173.1 Other malignant neoplasm of skin of eyelid, including canthus
- 173.2 Other malignant neoplasm of skin of ear and external auditory canal

CLINICAL PEARLS
- An early lesion of SCC is difficult to distinguish from a solar keratosis.
- SCCs that develop from solar keratoses are generally unaggressive.
- An SCC arising on a mucous membrane such as the glans penis, lip, or from a chronic ulcer, or one arising in an immunocompromised patient, is potentially metastatic.

CUTANEOUS T-CELL LYMPHOMA

Sandra Cuellar, PharmD, BCOP
Paul G. Rubinstein, MD

BASICS

Cutaneous T-cell lymphomas are a rare group of mature T-cell lymphomas presenting primarily in the skin. These diseases involve overlap of the disciplines of dermatology, medical oncology, and radiation oncology. Other than allogeneic stem cell transplant, there are no curative therapies for this disease (1,2,3,4).

DESCRIPTION
- A heterogeneous group of relatively uncommon extranodal non-Hodgkin lymphomas
- This section focuses on mycosis fungoides (MF), the most common type of cutaneous lymphoma. For other subtypes, please consult the reference section.

EPIDEMIOLOGY
- Median age at diagnosis is 55–60; however, it can occur in children and young adults (2).
- Male:Female = 2:1 (2)
- African American incidence greater compared to whites (2)

Incidence
0.4 cases per 100,000 per year

RISK FACTORS
No compelling evidence that mycosis fungoides is caused by viral infection or chemical exposure

Genetics
- Clonal T-cell receptor gene rearrangements are detected in most cases (4).
- No recurrent, mycosis fungoides-specific chromosomal translocations have been identified (2).
- Loss at chromosome 10q and abnormalities in the tumor suppressor genes p15, p16, and p53 are common (2,4).

PATHOPHYSIOLOGY
- Malignancy of CD4$^+$ helper T cells
- Malignant cells have a high affinity to the epidermis.
- Malignant T cells are also activated T cells (CD45RO$^+$) and produce cytokines, such as IL-4 and IL-5, which can lead to eosinophilia and atopylike symptoms.

ETIOLOGY
Unknown

DIAGNOSIS

- Diagnostic algorithm for MF is a point-based system. Points are scored for clinical, histopathologic, molecular biological, and immunopathological categories. A diagnosis of MF is made when a total of 4 points or more are determined (5).
- Clinical criteria: Patient has persistent and/or progressive patches and plaques plus lesions in a non-sun-exposed location, size/shape variation of lesions, poikiloderma (5)
- Histopathologic criteria: Superficial lymphoid infiltrate present plus epidermotropism without spongiosis, lymphoid atypia (5)
- Molecular biological criteria: Clonal TCR gene rearrangement is present (5).
- Immunopathologic criteria: <50% of T cells express CD2, CD3, CD5; <10% of T cells express CD 7; there is discordance of the epidermal and dermal cells with regard to expression of CD2, CD3, CD5, or CD7 (5)

PHYSICAL EXAM
- Examination of the entire skin, with assessment of percent of involved body surface area (%BSA), and lesions found, is critical.
- Pink scaly patches and plaques, typically in sun-protected areas such as the buttocks, thighs, and breasts
- Cutaneous tumors and ulcerations
- Exfoliative erythroderma
- Palmoplantar keratoderma (thickened scaly skin on palms and soles)
- Lymphadenopathy can be present in later stages.
- Hepatosplenomegaly can be present at late stages.

DIAGNOSTIC TESTS & INTERPRETATION
Lab
- Complete blood count (CBC) with differential and platelets and Sézary screen
- Polymerase chain reaction (PCR) of peripheral blood to detect clonal rearrangement of the T-cell receptor
- Flow cytometric studies to establish the presence of Sézary cells. Markers for CD3,4,7,8,26 need to be analyzed.
- If the CD4:CD8 ratio of >10, a circulating clonal T-cell population is identified, a positive Sézary cell count of over 1000 cells/mm^3 is found, this is consistent with Sézary syndrome; see below.
- Comprehensive metabolic profile
- LDH

Imaging
- Computed tomography (CT) of the neck, chest, abdomen for T2 disease or greater (see staging system described below)
- Chest x-ray should be used in limited disease without any palpable lymphadenopathy.

Diagnostic Procedures/Surgery
- Skin biopsy: Diagnostic procedure of choice
- Lymph node biopsy if there is clinical adenopathy or advanced disease
- Bone marrow biopsy for unexplained hematologic abnormality: Not normally done

Pathological Findings
- Skin biopsy shows superficial bandlike infiltrate, epidermotropism of lymphocytes, Pautrier microabscesses, and dermal infiltrates of atypical cells in tumors (5).
- Cells are usually CD3+, CD4+, CD45RO+, CD8−.
- Loss of T-cell antigens such as CD2, CD3, CD5, and CD7 is often seen.
- Sézary syndrome is diagnosed when Sézary cells are found in the peripheral circulation. Sézary cells are defined as atypical lymphocytes with cerebriform nuclei. Generalized erythroderma and lymphadenopathy usually accompanies this blood finding to complete the syndrome (2):
  – Sézary syndrome (leukemic phase of cutaneous T-cell lymphoma) is defined by the following: If the CD4:CD8 ratio >10, a circulating clonal T-cell population is identified, a positive Sézary cell count of over 1,000 cells/mm^3, a CD4/CD26- greater than or equal to 30% of all of the lymphocytes in the presence of a clonal T-cell population (2)
- Large cell transformation of cutaneous T-cell lymphoma is a rare and lethal event. If 25% of large cells are found on a biopsy taken from an MF lesion, this represents a transformation from an indolent lymphoma, MF, to a very aggressive form of cutaneous T-cell lymphoma. It is refractory to most chemotherapies, and overall survival is limited to just months (1,3,6).
- The treatment of the disease and prognosis (see prognosis section below) is determined by the stage (6):
  – Staging is done based on physical exam and pathology. Bone marrow biopsy is not needed for staging of the disease. The TNMB staging system ([T]umor, [N]ode, [M]Visceral, and [B]lood involvement with Sézary cells):
    ○ T1: Patches or plaques involving <10% of total body surface area
    ○ T2: Patches, papules, and/or plaques involving ≥10% of total body surface area
    ○ T3: 1 or more cutaneous tumors (≥1 cm in diameter)
    ○ T4: Erythroderma (>80% of total body surface area)

- ○ N0: Lymph nodes clinically uninvolved
- ○ N1: Lymph nodes clinically enlarged but not histologically involved
- ○ N2: Lymph nodes clinically normal but histologically involved
- ○ N3: Lymph nodes clinically enlarged and histologically involved
- ○ M0: No visceral organ involvement
- ○ M1: Visceral involvement with pathological confirmation
- ○ B0: Absence of significant blood involvement (<5% of peripheral blood lymphocytes are Sézary cells)
- ○ B1: Low blood tumor burden (>5% of the peripheral blood lymphocytes are Sézary cells)
- ○ B2: High blood tumor burden: >1000/microliter Sézary cells
- Stage groups:
  - IA: T1N0M0B0-1
  - IB: T2N0M0B0-1
  - II: T1-2N1-2M0B0-1
  - IIB: T3N0-2M0B0-1
  - III: T4N0-2M0B0-1
  - IIIA: T4N0-2M0B0
  - IIIB: T4N0-2M0B1
  - IVA1: T1-4N0-2M0B2
  - IVA2: T1-4N3M0B0-2
  - IVB: T1-4N0-3M1B0-2

DIFFERENTIAL DIAGNOSIS

- Patches and plaques seen in MF resemble lesions of:
  - Eczema
  - Parapsoriasis
  - Atopic dermatitis
  - Photodermatitis
  - Drug eruptions
  - Psoriasis
  - Contact dermatitis
- Cutaneous tumors:
  - Similar to other cutaneous lymphomas
- Erythroderma, though rare, can present like:
  - Atopic dermatitis
  - Contact dermatitis
  - Drug eruptions
  - Erythrodermic psoriasis

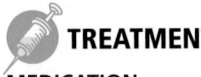

TREATMENT

MEDICATION

- Therapy must be individualized. No universally accepted standard approach exists to treat this disease. The stage of disease dictates the aggressiveness and type of therapy (13):
- T1 and T2 disease:
  - Topical potent corticosteroids
  - Topical mechlorethamine (nitrogen mustard)
  - Topical bis-chlor-nitrosourea
  - Topical bexarotene
  - Phototherapy: Psoralen and ultraviolet A light (PUVA) or narrow-band UVB
  - Oral retinoids (bexarotene)
  - Oral methotrexate
  - Radiation therapy (See Issues for Referral section below)

- T3 disease:
  - Oral retinoids (bexarotene)
  - Interferon α-2b
  - Denileukin diftitox
  - Chemotherapy: If the disease progresses on the above therapies, gemcitabine or pegylated doxorubicin is usually used first-line. If the disease continues to progress, low-dose methotrexate, bortezomib, cyclophosphamide, and fludarabine are used as second-line therapy. Stem cell transplantation can also be used in certain cases; see below.
- T4 disease and Sézary syndrome:
  - Oral retinoids (bexarotene)
  - Interferon α-2b
  - Denileukin diftitox
  - Phototherapy
  - Vorinostat (an oral deacetylase inhibitor)
  - Romidepsin (an injectable deacetylase inhibitor)
  - Extracorporeal photopheresis
  - Chemotherapy: If the disease progresses on the above therapies, gemcitabine or pegylated doxorubicin is usually used first-line. If the disease continues to progress, low-dose methotrexate, bortezomib, cyclophosphamide, and fludarabine are used as second-line therapy. Stem cell transplantation can also be used in certain cases; see below.
  - Stem cell transplantation (reserved for extensive and/or refractory disease)

ADDITIONAL TREATMENT
General Measures

- Most patients are managed on an outpatient basis.
- Treatment should be individualized for each patient, based on their extent of disease and side effects of possible therapies (1,3).
- Skin lesions commonly become infected, and treatment with antibiotic may be necessary.

Issues for Referral

- Dermatology manages early disease.
- Hematology-oncology is involved for later-stage diseases.
- Radiation oncology can be referred for limited disease or to treat extensive or painful skin lesions when refractory to chemotherapy.

Additional Therapies

Localized or total skin electron-beam therapy can be used in most stages of disease, either as monotherapy or in combination with other agents.

ONGOING CARE

FOLLOW-UP RECOMMENDATIONS
Patient Monitoring
Must be individualized

PATIENT EDUCATION
Patient information can be found at:

- American Academy of Dermatology Web site: http://www.aad.org
- Cutaneous Lymphoma Foundation Web site: http://www.clfoundation.org

PROGNOSIS

- MF is a chronic disease, though early-stage disease is curable.
- Survival by stage:
  - Stage 1A: Survival similar to age-/sex-matched individuals without disease
  - Stage IB and IIA: 11 years
  - Stage IIB: 3.2 years
  - Stage III: 4.6 years
  - Stage IVA or B: 13 months

COMPLICATIONS

- Immunosuppression from the disease and treatments can lead to infections.
- Skin lesions commonly become infected and can lead to sepsis.

REFERENCES

1. Horwitz SM, Olsen EA, Duvic M, et al. Review of the treatment of mycosis fungoides and Sézary syndrome: a stage-based approach. *J Natl Compr Canc Netw.* 2008;6:436–42.
2. Hwang ST, Janik JE, Jaffe ES, et al. Mycosis fungoides and Sézary syndrome. *Lancet.* 2008;371: 945–57.
3. Prince HM, Whittaker S, Hoppe RT et al. How I treat mycosis fungoides and Sézary syndrome. *Blood.* 2009;114:4337–53.
4. Girardi M, Heald PW, Wilson LD. The pathogenesis of mycosis fungoides. *N Engl J Med.* 2004;350: 1978–88.
5. Pimpinelli N, Olsen EA, Santucci M, et al. Defining early mycosis fungoides *J Am Acad Dermatol.* 2005;53(6):1053–63.
6. Willemze R, Jaffe ES, Burg G, et al. WHO-EORTC classification for cutaneous lymphomas. *Blood.* 2005;105:3768–85.

 # CODES

ICD9
202.10 Mycosis fungoides, unspecified site

CYCLIC VOMITING SYNDROME

Salwa Khan, MD, MHS

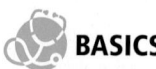 **BASICS**

DESCRIPTION
An idiopathic chronic functional GI disorder characterized by discrete, recurrent, stereotypical episodes of high-intensity nausea and vomiting lasting hours to days, separated by symptom-free intervals
Cyclic vomiting syndrome (CVS) has a phasic pattern with four distinct phases.

- Interepisodic: Symptom-free period
- Prodromal: Often marked by nausea $\pm$ abdominal pain; able to take oral medications
- Vomiting: Nausea, vomiting, and retching
- Recovery: Nausea remits and patient has recovered appetite, strength, and energy.

EPIDEMIOLOGY
Incidence
Unknown
Prevalence
- 0.04–1.9%
- Whites more affected than other races
- Predominant sex: Female > Male (55:45).

RISK FACTORS
- Family history of migraine headaches
- Depression
- Anxiety
- Chronic cannabis use
Genetics
- Possible matrilineal inheritance
- A3243G mitochondrial DNA mutation
- Ion-channel mutations

GENERAL PREVENTION
- Handwashing to prevent upper respiratory infection (URI)
- Adequate sleep
- Avoiding triggers
- Psychological testing and stress-reduction techniques

PATHOPHYSIOLOGY
- Unknown
- Strong link between CVS and migraine, with similar symptoms, common coexistence in patients, and effectiveness of antimigraine therapy
- Proposed mechanism:
  - Heightened neuronal excitability owing to enhanced ion permeability, mitochondrial deficits, or hormonal state → increased susceptibility to physical or psychological trigger → release of corticotropin-releasing-factor (CRF) → vomiting
  - Vomiting perpetuated by altered brain stem regulation → sustained vomiting

ETIOLOGY
- Unknown
- Possible maternal inheritence
- Multiple theories:
  - GI motility dysfunction
  - Autonomic dysfunction
  - Mitochondrial enzymopathies
  - Food allergy or intolerance

COMMONLY ASSOCIATED CONDITIONS
- Irritable bowel syndrome (67%)
- Headaches (52%)
- Motion sickness (46%)
- Migraines (11–40%)
- Seizure disorder (5.6%)

 DIAGNOSIS

HISTORY
- Children with CVS often present with bilious emesis (83%), severe abdominal pain (80%) and/or hematemesis.
- The North American Society for Pediatric Gastroenterology, Hepatology, and Nutrition consensus statement recommends the following criteria to be fulfilled to diagnose CVS:
  - At least 5 attacks in any interval or a minimum of 3 attacks during a 6-month period
  - Episodic attacks of intense nausea and vomiting lasting 1 h to 10 days and occurring at least 1 week apart
  - Stereotypical pattern and symptoms in the individual patient
  - Vomiting during attacks occurs at least 4 times/h for at least 1 h
  - Return to baseline health between episodes
  - Not attributed to another disorder

PHYSICAL EXAM
Dehydration evaluation (seen in 30%):
- Orthostatic hypotension
- Tachycardia
- Skin turgor, decreased
- Mucous membranes, dry

DIAGNOSTIC TESTS & INTERPRETATION
Lab
There are no specific laboratory findings to diagnose CVS. Initial tests are mainly for screening purposes and to exclude other diagnoses.

Initial lab tests
- Electrolytes: Hypokalemia (Addison disease would show hyponatremia and hypoglycemia.)
- Complete blood count (CBC): Hemoconcentration and leukocytosis
- Amylase and lipase to check for pancreatitis
- Erythrocyte sedimentation rate (ESR)
- Hepatic transaminases: To exclude hepatitis or gallbladder disease
- Urinalysis: Granular casts, ketosis
- Urine pregnancy test
- Lactate, ammonia, amino acids, urine organic acids during an acute episode for young children to exclude metabolic diseases

Follow-Up & Special Considerations
Counseling:
- Anxiety and depression management
- Cannabis cessation (if applicable)

Imaging
Initial approach
- Upper GI series to exclude malrotation
- Small bowel follow-through
- Abdominal ultrasound to exclude transient hydronephrosis, gallstones, and ureteropelvic junction obstruction

Follow-Up & Special Considerations
CT scan of head, abdomen, and pelvis to evaluate biliary and urinary tracts and exclude structural reason

Diagnostic Procedures/Surgery
- Esophagogastroduodenoscopy (EGD): To evaluate for clinical suspicion of peptic ulcer disease or sign of hematemesis
- Electroencephalogram (EEG): Seizure disorder evaluation
- Gastric emptying studies
- Autonomic testing
- Neuropsychiatric testing

DIFFERENTIAL DIAGNOSIS
- Evaluate for causes of vomiting:
  - GI: Surgical and nonsurgical
  - Urologic
  - Renal
  - Gynecologic
  - Neurologic
  - Endocrinologic
  - Ear/nose/throat (ENT)
  - Psychiatric, including Münchausen by proxy
  - Metabolic
- Any child with suspected CVS should be evaluated for a possible metabolic or neurologic etiology of their symptoms if:
  - Child is <2 years of age.
  - Vomiting episodes are associated with other concurrent illnesses, prior fasting, or increased protein uptake.
  - Any focal findings on neurologic exam
  - Hypoglycemia, anion-gap metabolic acidosis, hyperammonia, or other findings suggestive of metabolic disorders

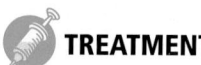 **TREATMENT**

MEDICATION
First Line
Lifestyle changes including avoidance of sleep deprivation, triggering foods, and motion sickness may reduce episode frequency. Prophylactic pharmacotherapy can be considered if the child is having repeated episodes requiring frequent hospitalization and school absences.

- Prophylactic: Decreases frequency or severity by >50%:
  - Amitriptyline (67–73%): Children >5 years: 0.3–0.5 mg/kg/d; adults: 50–75 mg/kg/d (1,2,3)[C]
  - Propranolol (57%): Children: 0.5 mg/kg/d divided b.i.d.–t.i.d.; adults: 10–20 mg/d b.i.d.–t.i.d. (4)[C]
  - Cyproheptadine (39–66%): Children <5 years: 0.3 mg/kg/d divided b.i.d.–t.i.d.; appetite stimulant (1)[C]

- Abortive:
  – Ondansetron: Children: 0.3–0.4 mg/kg/dose q6h; adults: 4 mg IV/PO q6–8h (5)[C]
  – Lorazepam: Children: 0.05–0.1 mg/kg/dose IV (not to exceed 4 mg/dose); adults: 1–2 mg IM/IV q4–6h p.r.n.) (5)[C]
  – Sumatriptan: >40 kg/20 mg intranasal p.r.n. (5)[C]

Second Line
- Prophylactic: Decreases frequency or severity by >50%:
  – Phenobarbital (79%): 2–3 mg/kg/d (4)[C]
  – Erythromycin (75%): 20 mg/kg/d divided b.i.d.–t.i.d. (4)[C]
- Abortive:
  – Hydromorphone: Children: 0.015 mg/kg/dose IV for 1 dose; adults: 3 mg p.r.n. or 0.5–2 mg IM/SC × 1 dose (4,5)[C]
  – Diphenhydramine: Children: 1.25 mg/kg/dose q6h, not to exceed 300 mg/d; adults: 25–50 mg q4–6h p.r.n. (4,5)[C]

ADDITIONAL TREATMENT
General Measures
- Patient reassurance
- Nonstimulating environment
- Relaxation techniques
- Avoid recreational drugs

Issues for Referral
Mental health, weekly appointments

Additional Therapies
Relaxation techniques:
- Deep breathing
- Biofeedback
- Guided imagery

COMPLEMENTARY AND ALTERNATIVE MEDICINE
Coenzyme Q may play a role in helping CVS (6)[A].

IN-PATIENT CONSIDERATIONS
Initial Stabilization
- IV fluids
- IV ondansetron and lorazepam
- Analgesia for pain

Admission Criteria
- Dehydration requiring >2 L of IV fluids
- Failure of outpatient management
- Increased anion gap that reflects severe dehydration or metabolic decompensation

IV Fluids
Replacement of ongoing losses; may consider 10% dextrose-containing fluids to attenuate any metabolic crisis

Nursing
- Decrease stimulation; avoid noise and bright light.
- Supportive care
- Encourage relaxation techniques
- Avoid unnecessary interruptions during sleep

Discharge Criteria
- Resolution of vomiting phase
- Pain managed with oral analgesia
- Euvolemia
- Appropriate oral intake

 ## ONGOING CARE

FOLLOW-UP RECOMMENDATIONS
Patient Monitoring
- Weekly appointments for severe cases
- Monitoring of emesis-associated laboratory values: Hypokalemia, acid–base disturbances, ketosis
- Regular outpatient visits for support

DIET
- Foods rich in carbohydrates, proteins, vitamins, and minerals
- Limit fats and spicy foods.
- Avoid trigger foods: Chocolate, cheese, and monosodium glutamate (MSG).
- Regular meal schedules
- Maintenance of good hydration

PATIENT EDUCATION
- Information and explanation about CVS may greatly alleviate the burden of illness among older patients.
- Maintain vomiting diary to note patterns, which helps to identify potentially avoidable triggers in 75% of children.
- Stress management techniques
- Good sleep hygiene
- Regular, moderate exercise
- Online resources such as the Cyclic Vomiting Syndrome Association Web site at www. cvsaonline.org

PROGNOSIS
- Usually lasts 2.5–5.5 years
- Vomiting resolves in 60% of children with CVS.
- However, many children will continue to have somatic symptoms, including headache and abdominal pain.
- 37% develop recurrent/migraine headaches.
- 50–75% with prophylactic treatment are asymptomatic at 1 year.

COMPLICATIONS
Occur during vomiting phase:
- Dehydration
- Electrolyte derangement, including the syndrome of inappropriate antidiuretic hormone (SIADH)
- Hematemesis
- Peptic esophagitis
- Mallory-Weiss tear
- Weight loss
- Hypovolemic shock

REFERENCES
1. Andersen JM, Sugerman KS, Lockhart JR, et al. Effective prophylactic therapy for cyclic vomiting syndrome in children using amitriptyline or cyproheptadine. *Pediatrics*. 1997;100:977–81.
2. Prakash C, Clouse RE. Cyclic vomiting syndrome in adults: clinical features and response to tricyclic antidepressants. *Am J Gastroenterol*. 1999;94: 2855–60.
3. Hejazi RA, Reddymasu SC, Namin F, Lavenbarg T, Foran P, McCallum RW et al. Efficacy of tricyclic antidepressant therapy in adults with cyclic vomiting syndrome: a two-year follow-up study. *J Clin Gastroenterol*. 2010;44:18–21.
4. Pareek N, et al. Cyclic vomiting syndrome: What a gastroenterologist needs to know. *Am J Gastroenterology*. 2007;102(12):2832–40.
5. Li BU. Cyclic Vomiting Syndrome. *Curr Treat Options Gastroenterol*. 2000;3:395–402.
6. Boles RG, Lovett-Barr MR, Preston A, Li BU, Adams K et al. Treatment of cyclic vomiting syndrome with co-enzyme Q10 and amitriptyline, a retrospective study. *BMC Neurol*. 2010;10:10.

ADDITIONAL READING
- Cyclic Vomiting Syndrome Association: Website: http://www.cvsaonline.org/
- Fitzpatrick E, Bourke B, Drumm B, Rowland M et al. Outcome for children with cyclical vomiting syndrome. *Arch. Dis. Child*. 2007;92:1001–4.
- Fleisher DR. Empiric guidelines for the management of cyclic vomiting syndrome. Available at: http://www.ch.missouri.edu/fleisher.
- Li BU, Balint JP. Cyclic vomiting syndrome: evolution in our understanding of a brain-gut disorder. *Adv Pediatr*. 2000;47:117–60.
- Li BU, Lefevre F, Chelimsky GG, et al. North American Society for Pediatric Gastroenterology, Hepatology, and Nutrition consensus statement on the diagnosis and management of cyclic vomiting syndrome. *J Pediatr Gastroenterol Nutr*. 2008;47:379–93.
- National digestive diseases information clearinghouse: http://www.digestive.niddk.nih.gov.

 ## CODES

ICD9
536.2 Persistent vomiting

CLINICAL PEARLS
- Identify patterns and triggers for cycles.
- Encourage sleep hygiene, stress management, and appropriate diet.
- Treatment in the vomiting phase requires pharmacologic and psychosocial interventions.
- Educating families about CVS can help to reduce the burden of illness among patients.

C

CYSTIC FIBROSIS

Michael S. Stalvey, MD
Christian Müller, PhD
Terence R. Flotte, MD

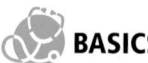 **BASICS**

DESCRIPTION
- Cystic fibrosis (CF) is an autosomal-recessive genetic condition that most prominently affects the lungs and pancreas.
- The intestinal tract, liver, endocrine system, reproductive organs, and skin can all be involved.
- Initially a pediatric disease, CF has become a chronic pediatric and adult medical condition as improvements in medical care have led to a dramatic increase in long-term survival.

EPIDEMIOLOGY
CF is the most common lethal inherited disease in Caucasians and is found in every racial group.

Incidence
- Prevalence varies according to country and ethnic background.
- Number of infants born with CF in relation to the total number of live births in the US:
  - 1 in 2,270 Ashkenazi Jewish Caucasian
  - 1 in 3,000 Caucasians
  - 1 in 10,000 Hispanics
  - 1 in 15,000 African Americans
  - 1 in 35,000 Asian Americans (reported frequency in Japan of 1 in 35,000) (1,2)[A]

Prevalence
- As per the 2008 CF Foundation Patient Registry, there are 30,000 patients with CF living in the US (3).
- ~1,000 new diagnoses are made annually (3).

RISK FACTORS
CF is a single-gene disorder. The severity of the phenotype can be affected by the specific CFTR mutation (most predictive of pancreatic disease), other modifier genes (CFTM1 for meconium ileus), and environmental factors, such as environmental tobacco smoke exposure, gastroesophageal reflux, and severe respiratory virus infections.

Genetics
CFTR gene (cystic fibrosis transmembrane conductance regulator). More than 1,500 mutations exist that can cause phenotypic CF, all of which are recessively inherited. Most common is loss of the phenylalanine residue at 508th position (deltaF508), which accounts for ~2/3 of affected alleles in the CF population in the US (2)[A].

GENERAL PREVENTION
- ACOG recommends genetic analysis for all North American couples planning a pregnancy, with appropriate counseling to identified carriers. Genetic analysis of siblings of known CF patients is highly recommended.
- Newborn screening for CF is offered throughout the United States. Identification of an affected newborn in a family has resulted in a reduction in the incidence of new cases, allowing genetic counseling prior to the birth of subsequent siblings.
- Prevention or amelioration of complications of CF can be accomplished through early diagnosis (by newborn screening or otherwise) followed by referral to an accredited regional CF center.

PATHOPHYSIOLOGY
- Abnormal CFTR function leads to abnormally viscous secretions that alter organ function.
- The lungs; obstruction, infection, and inflammation negatively affect lung growth, structure, and function:
  - Decreased mucociliary clearance
  - Infection is accompanied by an intense neutrophilic response.
  - Degradation of supporting tissues causes bronchiectasis and eventual failure.

COMMONLY ASSOCIATED CONDITIONS
- The GI tract:
  - Pancreatic exocrine insufficiency (85–90%):
    - Malabsorption of fat, protein, and fat-soluble vitamins (A, D, E, and K)
  - Hepatobiliary disease (11%) (3)[A]:
    - Focal biliary cirrhosis
    - Cholelithiasis
  - Meconium ileus at birth (10–15%)
  - Distal intestinal obstruction syndrome (DIOS): Intestinal blockage that typically occurs in older children and adults
- Endocrine:
  - CF-related diabetes (CFRD) (3)[A]:
    - May present as steady decline in weight, lung function, or increased frequency of exacerbation
    - Leading comorbid complication (21.5%)
    - Result of progressive insulin deficiency
    - Early screening and treatment may improve reduced survival found in CFRD (4).
  - Bone mineral disease (11.1%) (3)[A]
  - Hypogonadism:
    - Frequent low testosterone levels in men
    - Menstrual irregularities are common.
- Reproductive organs:
  - Congenital absence of the vas deferens: Obstructive azoospermia in 98% of males

Pregnancy Considerations
- Originally considered too dangerous for women with CF, successful pregnancies are occurring more frequently (3)[A].
- Pulmonary disease may worsen during pregnancy.

DIAGNOSIS

- General (any age):
  - Family history
  - Chronic/recurrent respiratory symptoms, including airway obstruction and infections
  - Persistent infiltrates on chest x-rays
  - Hypochloremic metabolic acidosis
- Neonatal:
  - Meconium ileus
  - Prolonged jaundice
- Infancy:
  - Failure to thrive
  - Chronic diarrhea
  - Anasarca/hypoproteinemia
  - Pseudotumor cerebri (vitamin A deficiency)
  - Hemolytic anemia (vitamin E deficiency)

- Childhood:
  - Recurrent endobronchial infection
  - Bronchiectasis
  - Recurrent sinusitis
  - Steatorrhea
  - Rectal prolapse
  - DIOS (distal intestinal obstruction syndrome)
  - Poor growth
  - Allergic bronchopulmonary aspergillosis
- Adolescence and adulthood:
  - Recurrent endobronchial infection
  - Bronchiectasis
  - Allergic bronchopulmonary aspergillosis
  - Chronic sinusitis
  - Hemoptysis
  - Pancreatitis
  - Portal hypertension
  - Azoospermia
  - Delayed puberty

HISTORY
Suspected in any child with failure to thrive, steatorrhea, and recurrent respiratory problems

PHYSICAL EXAM
- Respiratory:
  - Rhonchi and/or crackles
  - Hyper-resonance on percussion
  - Nasal polyps
- Gastrointestinal: Hepatosplenomegaly when cirrhosis present
- Other: Digital clubbing, growth retardation, and pubertal delay

DIAGNOSTIC TESTS & INTERPRETATION
Lab
Initial lab tests
- Newborn screening (42.8% of new cases) (3)[A]
- Sweat test (gold standard):
  - Sweat chloride:
    - >60 mmol/L is positive for CF.
    - <40 mmol/L is normal.
- CFTR mutation analysis:
  - Limited panel testing: Allele-specific PCR identifies >90% of mutations; finite chance of false-negative. Full sequence testing more costly and time-consuming. Greater sensitivity than PCR in patients of non-European descent.

Follow-Up & Special Considerations
- Sputum culture (common CF organisms)
- Pulmonary function tests (PFTs)
- 72-hour fecal fat
- Stool elastase
- Oral glucose tolerance test (OGTT)

Imaging
Initial approach
Chest x-ray:
- Hyperinflation early in disease
- Bronchial thickening and plugging
- Nodular densities, patchy atelectasis, and confluent infiltrates
- Bronchiectasis

Follow-Up & Special Considerations
- Head CT: Abnormal sinus CT findings are nearly universal in CF and may include mucosal thickening, intraluminal sinus polyps, and sinus effusions. Many children with CF never develop aerated frontal sinuses.
- Chest CT (not routine): Useful when unusual findings noted on CXR

Diagnostic Procedures/Surgery
- Flexible bronchoscopy
- Bronchoalveolar lavage

DIFFERENTIAL DIAGNOSIS
- Pulmonary:
  - Difficult-to-manage asthma
  - Chronic bronchitis
  - Recurrent pneumonia
  - Chronic/recurrent sinusitis
- GI:
  - Celiac disease
  - Protein-losing enteropathy
  - Pancreatitis of unknown etiology
  - Shwachman-Diamond syndrome

 # TREATMENT

MEDICATION
- Pulmonary:
  - Antibiotics, oral:
    - *S. aureus*: Bactrim or cephalexin
    - *P. aeruginosa*: Fluoroquinolones
    - Azithromycin (anti-inflammatory properties) (5)[A]
  - Antibiotics, inhaled:
    - TOBI (tobramycin 300 mg/dose via nebulizer)
    - Colistin (more commonly used in Europe)
    - Cayston (aerosolized aztreonam) 75 mg t.i.d. following bronchodilator use for 28 days (6)
  - Antibiotics, IV:
    - *S. aureus*: Zosyn or nafcillin
    - MRSA: Vancomycin or linezolid
    - *P. aeruginosa*: Zosyn or ceftazidime plus aminoglycoside (tobramycin)
    - *B. cepacia*: ≥3 drugs based on synergy studies
  - Inhalation therapy:
    - β-agonist in conjunction with chest physiotherapy
    - Recombinant human DNAse (7)[A]
    - Hypertonic saline (8)[A]
  - Anti-inflammatory agents:
    - Oral steroids (useful in setting of ABPA)
    - Ibuprofen (high dose)
- GI:
  - Pancreatic enzymes:
    - Use in pancreatic-insufficient patients.
  - Vitamin supplementation:
    - Fat-soluble vitamins (A, D, E, and K)
  - Liver disease (cholestasis):
    - Ursodeoxycholic acid

ADDITIONAL TREATMENT
General Measures
- Yearly influenza vaccination for all CF patients >6 months of age (3)
- Avoidance of smoke

Issues for Referral
All patients should be followed in a CF center (accredited sites are listed at www.cff.org).

Additional Therapies
- Airway clearance techniques (9)[A]
- Routine chest physiotherapy with postural drainage is critical in prevention of pulmonary exacerbations:
  - VEST (airway clearance system)
  - Flutter valve or acapella
- Endocrine:
  - CFRD: Dietary restrictions should be avoided.
  - CF-related bone disease: Consider bisphosphonate therapy.

SURGERY/OTHER PROCEDURES
- Lung transplantation reserved for patients with limited life expectancy (FEV$_1$ <30% predicted):
  - 158 patients with CF underwent lung transplantation during 2008 (3)[A].
  - 5-year post-transplant survival is 32.9–62% (10,11)[A].
- Liver transplantation is reserved for progressive liver failure and/or portal hypertension with GI bleeding.

IN-PATIENT CONSIDERATIONS
Initial Stabilization
Nasal cannula oxygen when the patient is hypoxic (SaO$_2$ <90%)

Admission Criteria
- Pulmonary exacerbation (most common reason for admission):
  - Increased cough, sputum production, and decreased pulmonary function
  - Change in lung examination (rales, retractions, tachypnea)
  - New abnormalities on CXR
  - Decreased energy level, appetite, and weight loss
  - Fever, leukocytosis, elevation of acute-phase reactants
- Bowel obstruction (due to distal intestinal obstruction syndrome, or DIOS, previously known as meconium ileus equivalent or MIE)
- Pancreatitis (in pancreatic-sufficient patients)

IV Fluids
- Increased salt loss increases risk of hyponatremic hypochloremic dehydration.
- Cautious use of IV fluids with worsening lung disease

Nursing
Nursing assignments should involve only one CF patient per nurse for isolation purposes.

 # ONGOING CARE

FOLLOW-UP RECOMMENDATIONS
- Upon discharge for a pulmonary exacerbation, follow up with their CF provider within 2–4 weeks
- Routine clinic visits every 3 months, with airway cultures and pulmonary function testing
- Annual comprehensive nutritional evaluation with morphometric analysis
- Yearly OGTT after 10 years of age (3)
- Bone densitometry every 1–4 years after age 18

DIET
High-calorie, high-fat diet with added salt

PATIENT EDUCATION
Cystic Fibrosis Foundation: www.cff.org

PROGNOSIS
- Most recent median survival is 37.4 years, as of 2008 CF Foundation Patient Registry (3)[A]
- Progression of lung disease usually determines length of survival.

REFERENCES
1. Palomaki GE, FitzSimmons SC, Haddow JE. Clinical sensitivity of prenatal screening for cystic fibrosis via CFTR carrier testing in a United States panethnic population. *Genet Med*. 2004;6: 405–14.
2. O'Sullivan BP, Freedman SD et al. Cystic fibrosis. *Lancet*. 2009;373:1891–904.
3. Cystic Fibrosis Foundation Patient Registry, 2008 Annual Data Report. Bethesda, Maryland, 2009.
4. Moran A, Dunitz J, Nathan B, Saeed A, Holme B, Thomas W et al. Cystic fibrosis-related diabetes: current trends in prevalence, incidence, and mortality. *Diabetes Care*. 2009;32:1626–31.
5. Saiman L, Marshall BC, Mayer-Hamblett N, et al. Azithromycin in patients with cystic fibrosis chronically infected with Pseudomonas aeruginosa: a randomized controlled trial. *JAMA*. 2003;290:1749–56.
6. O'Sullivan BP, Yasothan U, Kirkpatrick P, et al. Inhaled aztreonam. *Nat Rev Drug Discov*. 2010;9: 357–8.
7. Jones AP et al. Recombinant human deoxyribonuclease for cystic fibrosis. *Cochrane Database Sys Rev*. 2003;(3):CD001127.
8. Donaldson SH, Bennett WD, Zeman KL, et al. Mucus clearance and lung function in cystic fibrosis with hypertonic saline. *N Engl J Med*. 2006;354:241–50.
9. Main E et al. Conventional chest physiotherapy compared to other airway clearance techniques for cystic fibrosis. *Cochrane Database Sys Rev*. 2005;(1):CD002011.
10. Allen J, Visner G. Lung transplantation in cystic fibrosis—primum non nocere? *N Engl J Med*. 2007;357:2186–8.
11. Meachery G, De Soyza A, Nicholson A, et al. Outcomes of Lung transplantation for Cystic Fibrosis in a large United Kingdom cohort. *Thorax*. 2008.

 ## CODES

ICD9
- 277.00 Cystic fibrosis without mention of meconium ileus
- 277.01 Cystic fibrosis with meconium ileus
- 277.02 Cystic fibrosis with pulmonary manifestations

CLINICAL PEARLS
- CF must be considered in ANY child with chronic diarrhea, especially if associated with poor growth or failure to thrive.
- All children with nasal polyps should be evaluated.
- Children with CF may present with generalized edema due to protein/calorie malnutrition.
- The presence of digital clubbing or bronchiectasis should always trigger consideration of CF.
- A rapid decline in pulmonary function suggests the acquisition of resistant organisms (such as *B. cepacia*), CF-related diabetes, ABPA, or GE reflux disease.

CYTOMEGALOVIRUS INCLUSION DISEASE

Bonnie W. Lau, MD, PhD
Penelope Dennehy, MD

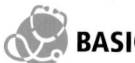 **BASICS**

Cytomegalovirus (CMV) infection is highly prevalent as illustrated by seroprevalence in 40–100% of the population (1). Serious disease can result in the perinatal period and in immunocompromised patients. Immunocompetent patients may become symptomatic with reinfection with different CMV strains. Prompt treatment and prophylaxis are the current mainstays of infection control.

DESCRIPTION
- β-infection from cytomegalovirus (CMV), a DNA virus in the *Herpesvirus* family
- Primary infection: Often asymptomatic; may remain latent throughout a person's life if no immunocompromise
- Severe disease can result from primary infection of newborns or reactivation in setting of immunocompromise or organ transplantation.
- Name derives from the infected cells, which are large and contain intranuclear inclusions, described as "owl's eye" inclusions
- Not highly contagious:
  - Spread via close contact with persons shedding virus from saliva, urine, blood, breast milk, or semen.
  - Also acquired via infected transplant organs.
  - Any organ can be affected.
- Categories of CMV infections:
  - Congenital: Vary greatly from mild viremia in a normal infant to the cause of abortion, stillbirth, postnatal morbidity and death from hemorrhage, anemia, or liver or central nervous system damage (including hearing loss, developmental delay and mental retardation) (2)
  - Acute infection in a normal host: Symptomatic infection commonly presents with acute mononucleosis syndrome (3).
  - Latent infection: Higher IgG titers may contribute to development of atherosclerotic disease (4).
  - Infection in bone marrow and solid organ transplant patients:
    - Bone marrow transplant: Usually interstitial pneumonia
    - Liver transplant: Hepatitis
    - Kidney transplant: CMV syndrome
  - Infection in patients with AIDS: Most commonly retinitis, 2nd most common is colitis, followed by esophagitis and neurologic disease (5)
  - Infections in other immunocompromised patients: Pulmonary, gastrointestinal (GI), or renal disease
- System(s) affected: Ophthalmic; Pulmonary; GI; Neurologic; Renal; Skin/Exocrine
- Synonym(s): Giant cell inclusion disease; CID CMV

Pregnancy Considerations
- CMV infection during pregnancy can be hazardous to the fetus.
- May lead to stillbirth, brain damage, birth defects, or to severe neonatal illness.

Pediatric Considerations
- May occur congenitally or postnatally.
- Breastfeeding can transmit virus to high-risk preterm infants. However there is low risk of symptomatic disease and no evidence of long-term sequelae from transmission from breastfeeding. Currently there are no recommendations for avoidance or treated breast milk (6).

EPIDEMIOLOGY
Incidence
- Common, but frequently asymptomatic
- <2–3 cases of end-organ disease per 100 person-years in HIV patients
- CMV infection is even more prevalent in populations at higher risk for HIV infection (IV drug users 75%, homosexual males 90%).
- Predominant age: All ages, peaks at <3 months, 16–40 years, and 40–75 years
- Predominant sex: Male > Female

Prevalence
- Occurs worldwide
- 40–100% of the general US population is seropositive from prior exposure during childhood or early adulthood (1).
- 20% of children in the US are seropositive before reaching puberty (1).
- Most common perinatally transmitted infection: 0.2–2.2% of births in the US (7)

RISK FACTORS
- HIV infection with specific risks, including:
  - CD4 count <50 cells/μL (5)[B]
  - Absence of treatment with or failure to respond to ART (5)[B]
  - Previous opportunistic infections (5)[B]
  - HIV viral load >100,000 (5)[B]
- Organ transplantation
- Blood transfusion
- Immunocompromise
- Living in closed population
- Corticosteroid therapy
- Day care environment, infant or geriatric (8)[B]
- For congenital infection, maternal infection during pregnancy
- Low socioeconomic status (7)[C]
- Critically ill immunocompetent adults in intensive care unit settings (up to 1/3 develop CMV, primarily between days 4–12 after admission) (9)[A]

GENERAL PREVENTION
- Handwashing/basic hygiene (8)[A]
- Avoid immunosuppression
- Highly active antiretroviral therapy (HAART) is the best method for high-risk HIV patients (1)[A].
- Chronic maintenance therapy for life in HIV patients with CMV end-organ disease unless successfully treated with ART (3)[A]
- Options include:
  - Parenteral or oral ganciclovir (3)[A]
  - Parenteral foscarnet (3)[A]
  - Combined parenteral ganciclovir and foscarnet (3)[A]
  - Parenteral cidofovir (3)[A]
  - Ganciclovir administration via intraocular implant or repetitive intravitreous injection of fomivirsen (3)[A]
- CMV antibody+, HIV+ children who are severely immunosuppressed require oral ganciclovir 30 mg/kg t.i.d. (8)[C]
- Antiviral suppression of CMV reactivation in CMV+ transplant recipients or recipients of CMV+ organs:
  - Solid organ transplant: Prophylactic or preemptive treatment with oral ganciclovir, valganciclovir (10)[A]
  - Bone marrow transplant: IV ganciclovir
- CMV immunoglobulins decrease rate of severe disease after liver transplant (11)[A] and decrease incidence of disease after renal transplant.

ETIOLOGY
- Primary infection
- Reinfection with different CMV strains
- Reactivation of latent virus in patients who are immunosuppressed

COMMONLY ASSOCIATED CONDITIONS
- AIDS
- Corticosteroid therapy
- Leukemia
- Lymphoma

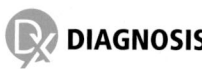 **DIAGNOSIS**

- Congenital:
  - Asymptomatic cytomegaloviremia
  - Symptomatic: Small for gestational age, purpura/petechiae, jaundice, hepatosplenomegaly, chorioretinitis, microcephaly, intracranial calcifications, hearing impairment
  - 90% have late complications: Sensorineural hearing loss occurs in 14%; 3–5% moderate to severe (11)[A]
  - Mental retardation, chorioretinitis, optic atrophy, seizures, learning disabilities (7)
- Acquired: Acute infection in a normal host:
  - Usually asymptomatic
  - Mononucleosis syndrome: Fever, malaise, sore throat, headache, antibiotic rash (3)
  - Less common: Exudative pharyngitis, splenomegaly, cervical adenopathy, rash (3)
- Infections in AIDS patients:
  - Retinitis: Usually unilateral, floaters, scotomata, peripheral field defects. Diagnosis made when characteristic retinal changes noted by ophthalmologist on funduscopic exam (5)
  - Colitis: Fever, weight loss, anorexia, abdominal pain, diarrhea, malaise; hemorrhage or perforation rare but serious (5)
  - Esophagitis: Fever, odynophagia, nausea, abdominal discomfort (5)
  - Pneumonitis: Dyspnea with or without exertion, nonproductive cough, hypoxemia (5)
  - Neurologic disease: Dementia, lethargy, confusion, fever, focal neurologic signs (5)
- Infections in transplant recipients:
  - Persistent fever (most common) (8)
  - Bone marrow transplant: Interstitial pneumonia (10)
  - Liver transplant: Hepatitis (10)
  - Kidney transplant: CMV syndrome (fever, leucopenia, atypical lymphocytes, hepatomegaly, myalgia, arthralgia) (10)

DIAGNOSTIC TESTS & INTERPRETATION

Lab

- Acute infection in a normal host:
  - Elevated liver transaminases in 92%, although transaminases rarely increase to >5 times normal ranges (3)
  - Anemia (3)
  - Thrombocytopenia (3)
  - Positive cold agglutinins (3)
  - Lymphocytosis with >10% atypical (3)
  - Negative heterophil antibody test (rules out Epstein Barr virus mononucleosis) (3)
  - Positive CMV IgM antibodies; may not peak until 4–7 weeks after acute infection (3)
  - CMV IgG should increase 4–fold during acute infection (3)
- Congenital/infant:
  - <12 months: Positive CMV antibody indicates maternal infection, but not necessarily child infection (8)
  - >12 months: Positive CMV antibody assay or culture indicates previous infection, but not necessarily active disease (8)
  - Recovery of virus from tissue in symptomatic patient (GI or pulmonary tissue) indicates infection, although 1–6 weeks are required for distinctive cytopathic events to occur (8)
  - Quantitative DNA polymerase chain reaction (PCR) evidences disease and can be used to monitor therapy (8)
  - Direct hyperbilirubinemia >3 mg/dL (8)
  - Thrombocytopenia (<75,000/mL) (7)
  - Elevated liver transaminases (7)
- Immunocompromised:
  - Viremia: PCR, antigen assays (pp65 lower-matrix protein in leukocytes), blood culture, although viremia can be present without CMV disease (5)[A]
  - Serum CMV antibodies not useful; can be falsely negative due to immunosuppression (5)[C]
  - Neurologic disease: CMV detected in cerebrospinal fluid or brain tissue clinches diagnosis. Enhanced by PCR analysis (5)[A].

Imaging

- Head computed tomography or magnetic resonance imaging: Periventricular enhancement (CMV neurologic disease)
- Chest X-ray: Interstitial infiltrates (CMV pneumonitis)

Diagnostic Procedures/Surgery

- Bronchoscopy: Identification of CMV inclusion bodies in lung tissue in context of pulmonary infiltrates (pneumonitis)
- Endoscopic exam of GI tract: Mucosal ulcerations and colonoscopic, rectal, or esophageal biopsy (colitis, esophagitis) (5)[B]

Pathological Findings

Giant cells with basophilic inclusion bodies (owl's eye)

DIFFERENTIAL DIAGNOSIS

- Congenital: Toxoplasmosis, rubella, herpes, syphilis
- Acquired in immunocompetent: Epstein-Barr virus (EBV) mononucleosis, viral hepatitis
- Acquired immunocompromised: Other viral, bacterial, fungal opportunistic infections

 TREATMENT

MEDICATION

First Line

- Congenital disease: Ganciclovir 12 mg/kg IV q12h for 6 weeks (7)[B]
- Pediatric disseminated disease: IV ganciclovir (3)[A]
- CMV mononucleosis/asymptomatic viremia: No treatment (5)
- Retinitis: Effective treatments include the following and should be chosen in consultation with a specialist:
  - Oral valganciclovir (for peripheral lesions) (5)[A]
  - IV ganciclovir followed by oral valganciclovir (5)[A]
  - IV foscarnet (5)[A]
  - IV cidofovir (5)[A]
  - Ganciclovir intraocular implant with oral or IV valganciclovir (5)[A]
  - Treat until CD4 >100 for 3–6 months (5)[A]
- Colitis or esophagitis: IV ganciclovir or foscarnet for 21–28 days or until symptom resolution (5)[B]
- Neurologic disease: Prompt treatment with ganciclovir and foscarnet (5)[B]
- CMV disease in transplant patients: IV ganciclovir for 2–4 weeks (10)[B]

Second Line

- Adult CMV retinitis: Fomivirsen (7)[A]
- Pediatric disseminated disease: Foscarnet 60 mg/kg q8h for 14–21 days (7)[A], combination ganciclovir and foscarnet (7)[B]
- CMV disease in transplant patients: Valganciclovir (10)[C]
- CMV in bone marrow transplant patients:
  - Prophylaxis: Valacyclovir (10)[B]
  - Preemptive: Foscarnet (10)[B]

 ONGOING CARE

FOLLOW-UP RECOMMENDATIONS

Bed rest

Patient Monitoring

- CMV urine culture at birth for all HIV-infected or -exposed (8)[C] and annual testing for CMV seronegative/HIV+ children (8)[C]
- Patients with CD4 counts <50 should have ophthalmologic screening every 3–6 months (8)[C].
- Patients on therapy should be followed for neutropenia, anemia, and thrombocytopenia.

DIET

Normal

PROGNOSIS

Severe disease with primary infection in newborns and reactivation in immunocompromised

COMPLICATIONS

- Congenital: Hearing loss, mental retardation, optic atrophy, seizures, learning disabilities
- Colitis: Hemorrhage and perforation

REFERENCES

1. Salzberger B, Hartmann P, Hanses F, et al. Incidence and prognosis of CMV disease in HIV-infected patients before and after introduction of combination antiretroviral therapy. *Infection.* 2005;33:345–9.
2. Yinon Y, Farine D, Yudin MH et al. Cytomegalovirus infection in pregnancy. *J Obstet Gynaecol Can.* 2010;32:348–54.
3. Taylor GH. Cytomegalovirus. *Am Fam Phys.* 2003;67(3):519–24.
4. Crumpacker CS. Invited commentary: human cytomegalovirus, inflammation, cardiovascular disease, and mortality. *Am J Epidemiol.* 2010;172(4):372–4.
5. Benson CA, Kaplan JE, Masur H, et al. Treating opportunistic infections among HIV-infected adults and adolescents: recommendations from CDC, the National Institutes of Health, and the HIV Medicine Association/Infectious Diseases Society of America. *MMWR Recomm Rep.* 2004;53:1–112.
6. Kurath S, Halwachs-Baumann G, Müller W et al. Transmission of cytomegalovirus via breast milk to the prematurely born infant: a systematic review. *Clin Microbiol Infect.* 2010;16:1172–8.
7. Mofenson LM, Oleske J, Serchuck L et al. Treating opportunistic infections among HIV-exposed and infected children: recommendations from CDC, the National Institutes of Health, and the Infectious Diseases Society of America. *MMWR Recomm Rep.* 2004;53:1–92.
8. Cohen J, et al. *Infectious diseases*, 2nd ed. New York: Elsevier, 2004.
9. Osawa R, Singh N. Cytomegalovirus infection in critically ill patients: a systematic review. *Crit Care.* 2009;13:R68.
10. Razonable RR, Emery VC, 11th Annual Meeting of the IHMF (International Herpes Management Forum). Management of CMV infection and disease in transplant patients. 27–29 February 2004. *Herpes.* 2004;11:77–86.
11. Grosse SD, Ross DS, Dollard SC. Congenital cytomegalovirus (CMV) infection as a cause of permanent bilateral hearing loss: a quantitative assessment. *J Clin Virol.* 2008;41:57–62.

ADDITIONAL READING

- Patel R, Paya CV. Infections in solid-organ transplant recipients. *Clin Microbiol Rev.* 1997;10:86–124.
- Sun HY, Wagener MM, Singh N. Prevention of posttransplant cytomegalovirus disease and related outcomes with valganciclovir: a systematic review. *Am J Transplant.* 2008;8:2111–8.

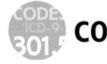 CODES

ICD9

- 078.5 Cytomegaloviral disease
- 771.1 Congenital cytomegalovirus infection

CLINICAL PEARLS

- CMV mono has much less cervical adenopathy and/or splenomegaly than EBV mono in adults.
- CMV is a major cause of sensorineural hearing loss in young children.

DE QUERVAIN TENOSYNOVITIS

J. Herbert Stevenson, MD

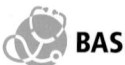 **BASICS**

DESCRIPTION

De Quervain tenosynovitis is a stenosis of the 1st dorsal compartment of the wrist including the extensor pollicis brevis (EPB) and abductor pollicis longus (APL). It is an inflammation or thickening of the tendon sheath that surrounds EPB and the APL, which leads to pain with certain movements of the thumb.

EPIDEMIOLOGY

- Predominant age: 30–50 years old
- Predominant sex: Female < Male (women 6–10× more likely than men)

Incidence

Common condition

RISK FACTORS

- Women age 30–50
- Pregnancy (primarily 3rd trimester and postpartum)
- Individuals participating in golf, fly fishing, and racquet sports
- Repetitive motions with the hand/thumb requiring forceful grasping or wrist ulna/radial deviation; often seen in carpenters and machine operators

GENERAL PREVENTION

Avoidance of repetitive actions of the thumb associated with forceful grasping or repetitive wrist ulna/radial deviation (e.g., hammering)

PATHOPHYSIOLOGY

Repetitive actions of the wrist and the thumb results in microtrauma and thickening of the surrounding tendon and tendon sheath (EPB, APL). This thickening causes inflammation and pain with movements of the thumb and wrist and may elicit pain over the radial styloid as they rub over the prominence.

ETIOLOGY

- Repetitive movements of the wrist and thumb and activities that require forceful grasping
- Trauma
- Systemic diseases (e.g., rheumatoid arthritis)

 DIAGNOSIS

HISTORY

- Patients may complain of gradual worsening pain along their thumb and radial aspect of their wrist with certain movements, including ulnar deviation of the wrist.
- Usually insidious in onset
- Usually no associated trauma

PHYSICAL EXAM

- Pain and swelling is present over the radial styloid, which may be exacerbated when patients move their thumb or make a fist.
- Crepitus with movement of the thumb may be felt or heard.
- Occasionally, slight swelling at the base of the thumb and wrist is noted.
- Decreased range of motion of the thumb
- Swelling and tenderness may be appreciated over the distal radius.
- Pain over the 1st extensor compartment on resisted thumb abduction or extension
- Crepitus may be associated with movement of the thumb.

DIAGNOSTIC TESTS & INTERPRETATION

Finkelstein test is pathognomonic for De Quervain tenosynovitis. This test involves patient flexing thumb in palm, while the examiner ulnar deviates the wrist. The test is positive if patient's symptoms are reproduced.

Lab

No labs are indicated.

Imaging

This disease is primarily a clinical diagnosis, but if the diagnosis is questionable, then radiographs of the wrist may be indicated to rule out other pathology. Radiographs may rule out CMC arthritis, which can be misdiagnosed as De Quervain. MRI is the test of choice to rule out coexisting soft tissue injury or wrist joint pathology.

Pathological Findings

Inflamed and thickened retinacular sheath of the tendon

DIFFERENTIAL DIAGNOSIS

- Fracture of the scaphoid
- Dorsal wrist ganglion
- Osteoarthritis of the 1st carpometacarpal joint
- Flexor carpi radialis tendonitis
- Infectious tenosynovitis
- Tendonitis of the wrist extensors
- Intersection syndrome
- Trigger thumb

 TREATMENT

- Rest and immobilization may be helpful early in the disease process. This is achieved with the use of a thumb spica splint.
- NSAIDs may help along with the splint to decrease the inflammation.

MEDICATION

First Line

Immobilization and NSAIDs

Second Line

Corticosteroid injection of the tendon sheath has shown significant cure rates. An 83% success rate after single injection has been reported (1)[B]. Additional injections are sometimes required.

ADDITIONAL TREATMENT

General Measures

- If full relief is not being achieved, a corticosteroid injection of the tendon sheath has been shown to result in 83% cure rate (1)[B].
- Anatomic variants may complicate treatment, including 2 tendon sheaths in the 1st compartment or the EPB tendon may travel in a separate compartment.
- Surgery is indicated for cases not responding to 3–6 months of conservative treatment. Surgery has been found to result in 91% cure rate (2)[B].

Issues for Referral

Referral to a hand surgeon is indicated if no improvement is noted after conservative treatments.

Additional Therapies

- Hand therapy along with iontophoresis/phonophoresis may help improve outcomes for moderate cases.
- Patients may incorporate thumb-stretching exercises into their rehabilitation.

SURGERY/OTHER PROCEDURES

Only indicated for patients who have failed conservative treatment. Surgical release has shown cure rates of up to 91% (2)[B].

IN-PATIENT CONSIDERATIONS

Initial Stabilization

- Splinting of the thumb (thumb spica splint or dorsal hood splint)
- Rest
- Ice (15–20 minutes 5–6× a day)
- Anti-inflammatory medications

ONGOING CARE

FOLLOW-UP RECOMMENDATIONS

- Additional corticosteroid injection may be performed at 4–6 weeks if symptoms are not significantly reduced.
- Avoid repetitive activities and motions that aggravate the pain.

DIET

As tolerated

PATIENT EDUCATION

Modification of activities eliciting pain, such as repetitive movement of the wrist and thumb, and forceful grasping.

PROGNOSIS

Prognosis is extremely good with conservative treatments. 95% success rates have been shown with conservative therapy over 1 year, although up to 1/3 of patients will have recurrence (3)[A]. Surgery has shown success in 91% of patients who did not improve with conservative therapy.

COMPLICATIONS

- Most complications are secondary to the treatment modalities. This includes gastrointestinal, renal, and hepatic injury secondary to NSAIDs.
- Nerve damage may occur during surgery.
- Hypopigmentation, fat atrophy, bleeding, and infection are potential adverse events from corticosteroid injections.
- If not treated correctly, loss of flexibility of the thumb due to fibrosis may occur.

REFERENCES

1. Richie CA, Briner WW. Corticosteroid injection for treatment of de Quervain's tenosynovitis: a pooled quantitative literature evaluation. *J Am Board Fam Pract*. 2003;16:102–6.
2. Ta KT, Eidelman D, Thomson JG. Patient satisfaction and outcomes of surgery for de Quervain's tenosynovitis. *J Hand Surg [Am]*. 1999;24:1071–7.
3. Jirarattanaphochai K, Saengnipanthkul S, Vipulakorn K, et al. Treatment of de Quervain disease with triamcinolone injection with or without nimesulide. A randomized, double-blind, placebo-controlled trial. *J Bone Joint Surg Am*. 2004;86-A:2700–6.

ADDITIONAL READING

- Rettig AC. Athletic injuries of the wrist and hand. Part II overuse injuries of the wrist and traumatic injuries of the hand. *Am J Sport Med*. 2004;32: 262–73.
- Rossi R, et al. De Quervain Disease in volleyball players. *Am J Sport Med*. 2005;33:424–7.
- Tallia AF, Cardone DA. Diagnostic and therapeutic injection of the wrist and hand region. *Am Fam Physician*. 2003;67:745–50.

See Also (Topic, Algorithm, Electronic Media Element)

Algorithm: Pain in upper extremity

 CODES

ICD9
727.04 Radial styloid tenosynovitis

CLINICAL PEARLS

- Repetitive movements of the wrist and thumb and activities that require forceful grasping are the most common causes of De Quervain tenosynovitis.
- De Quervain tenosynovitis is a stenosis of the 1st dorsal compartment of the wrist including the EPB and APL. It is an inflammation or thickening of the tendon sheath that surrounds EPB and the APL, which leads to pain with certain movements of the thumb.
- It is diagnosed via the Finkelstein test, which is pathognomonic for De Quervain tenosynovitis. This test involves patient flexing thumb in palm, while the examiner ulnar deviates the wrist. The test is positive if patient's symptoms are reproduced.
- Activity can be as-tolerated, using pain as a threshold; however, most people require modification of their activities to assist with rehabilitation and improvement.

D

DECOMPRESSION SICKNESS

Elise R. Bender, MD

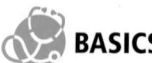

BASICS

DESCRIPTION
- Also known as "caisson disease" or "the bends"
- Occurs most often in SCUBA diving, free diving, high altitude flying, and aerospace events
- Rapid decrease in environmental pressure causing inert gases (usually nitrogen) to form bubbles in tissues or to obstruct small blood vessels, causing symptoms
- Type I (mild):
  – Musculoskeletal (70–85%): Mild joint pain that increases with time; most commonly shoulder or elbow pain
  – Cutaneous (10–15%): Rash, pruritus, edema
- Type II (serious):
  – Neurologic (10–15%): Headache, visual disturbance, paresthesias, paresis, paralysis, bladder or bowel incontinence, vertigo, memory loss, ataxia, seizures
  – Pulmonary (2–5%): Nonproductive cough, wheezing, pharyngeal irritation, chest discomfort on inspiration, respiratory distress
  – Death

Pregnancy Considerations
- A pregnant patient with decompression sickness is a priority, because the fetus may be affected and at greater risk for arterial gas emboli.
- No contraindication to recompression therapy during pregnancy

EPIDEMIOLOGY
- Predominant age: 20–29 years (although there is a trend toward increased susceptibility with increase in age, especially over age 42)
- Predominant sex: Male (although no evidence suggests increased male susceptibility)

Incidence
3.1/10,000 dives

Prevalence
<1% even in high-density diving areas and areas of caisson work

RISK FACTORS
- Large pressure reduction (i.e., flying after diving)
- Multiple repetitive SCUBA dives or ascents to altitudes above 18,000 feet
- High rate of ascent or decompression
- Previous decompression injury
- Obesity
- Cold-water diving
- Poor physical conditioning
- Vigorous physical activity
- Dehydration
- Local injury
- Patent foramen ovale or any intracardiac right-to-left shunt (increased risk of neurologic symptoms)

Genetics
No known genetic predisposition

GENERAL PREVENTION
- Travel by air after SCUBA diving should be restricted for 12 hours (after 1 dive per day) or 48 hours (after multiple dives or decompression).
- Chronic obstructive lung disease, cystic fibrosis, bronchiectasis, interstitial lung disease, or a history of thoracic surgery or prior pneumothorax should be absolute contraindications to diving.
- Intracardiac right-to-left shunts (e.g., patent foramen ovale, atrial septal defect, ventricular septal defect, patent ductus arteriosus, etc.) may be contraindications to diving.
- Follow decompression tables (Navy, National Association for Underwater Instructors [NAUI], Professional Association for Diving Instructors [PADI]) for diving to depth (>33 feet).
- Use dive computers that calculate nitrogen content of various tissues to estimate decompression limit.
- Breathing pure oxygen before exposure to a low barometric pressure environment (prebreathing) may decrease the risk of developing altitude decompression syndrome (1).
- Pre-dive oral hydration may also reduce bubble formation (2).
- Repeated dives and physical activity may have a protective effect (3).

PATHOPHYSIOLOGY
- As divers descend to increased pressures, the solubility of nitrogen in tissues increases.
- As the diver ascends, this dissolved gas may come out of solution and form bubbles, which can cause symptoms by blocking vessels, compressing tissue, or activating inflammatory cascades.
- Excess gas can be eliminated via respiration, so allowing for adequate breathing time is essential in disease prevention.

ETIOLOGY
- Rapid ascent from diving (depth >33 feet)
- Rapid ascent/decompression in an airplane
- Tunnel work (caisson disease)
- Inadequate pressurization/denitrogenation when flying
- Flying to high altitude too soon after diving

COMMONLY ASSOCIATED CONDITIONS
- Pulmonary barotrauma (pulmonary edema and hemorrhage; pneumomediastinum; pneumothorax; arterial gas embolism)
- Ear, sinus, or dental barotraumas
- Nitrogen narcosis
- Dysbaric osteonecrosis

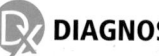

DIAGNOSIS

HISTORY
- Recent history of diving or high-altitude flying, or occupational exposures to pressurized environments (e.g., miners, construction workers, divers, pilots)
- 75% present within 1 hour; 90% present within 12 hours; but can present >24 hours after diving
- Localized joint pain (e.g., elbow, shoulder, knee, hip, wrist, ankle) ranges from dull ache to severe.
- Localized pruritus, which usually resolves without treatment, but may be painful (cutis marmorata)
- Painful lymphedema
- Headache, visual field deficits
- Confusion, memory loss, unexplained fatigue
- Seizures, dizziness/vertigo, nausea/vomiting
- Urinary and rectal incontinence
- Rapidly ascending paraplegia
- Substernal chest pain
- Coughing paroxysms (Behnken sign)
- Hemoptysis
- Coma, death

PHYSICAL EXAM
- Complete neurological exam required to rule out serious disease
- May see increased joint pain with active and passive motion
- Cutaneous and lymphatic signs:
  – Localized edema (mainly on chest and torso), lymphadenopathy
  – Localized erythema
  – Sharply defined area of pallor on tongue (Liebermeister sign)
  – Skin lesions:
    ○ Painful, pruritic, blotchy, red rash on torso
    ○ Burning blebs on skin
  – Joints:
    ○ Erythema and edema on periarticular surfaces
- Ataxia, nystagmus
- Arrhythmia, bradycardia, or tachycardia
- Hypotension
- Tachypnea

DIAGNOSTIC TESTS & INTERPRETATION
Lab
Initial lab tests
- Arterial blood gases:
  – May show decreased Po_2, decreased Pco_2, and metabolic acidosis
- Electrolytes, creatinine, BUN
- CBC:
  – Thrombocytopenia, increased hematocrit in severe cases due to dehydration
- Coagulation tests:
  – May see increased fibrin split products, increased prothrombin time
- Carboxyhemoglobin
- EEG:
  – Irregular slowing with cerebral bends

Imaging
Initial approach
- Chest X-ray:
  – Pneumothorax, mediastinal emphysema, right-sided heart enlargement
- Plain radiograph or ultrasound:
  – Gas bubbles in joints, tendons, bursae, muscles
- CT scan all patients with history of trauma or neurologic signs.
- MRI not very helpful in initial DCS:
  – Consider in spinal cord evaluation for continued symptoms

Diagnostic Procedures/Surgery
Test of pressure to ascertain response:
- Trial of recompression to 2.8 atmosphere absolute (ata)/100% oxygen for 10 minutes

DIFFERENTIAL DIAGNOSIS
- Arterial gas embolism
- Traumatic injury to extremity
- Cerebrovascular accident
- Musculoskeletal strains
- Urticaria
- Malingering
- Carbon monoxide poisoning

 TREATMENT

MEDICATION
First Line
- 100% oxygen via tight nonrebreathing mask
- Isotonic fluid resuscitation:
  – Avoid D5W, hypotonic solutions in cord injury
  – No experimental or clinical studies support use of volume expanders (dextran, albumin).
- Steroids:
  – Advocated by some for the assumed vasogenic edema seen in decompression sickness
  – Controversial and not proven in controlled clinical trials
  – If prescribed, do not use for >4 days
- Diazepam: 5–15 mg IV (IM absorption unpredictable) for inner ear decompression sickness:
  – Relieves vertigo, nausea, and vomiting
  – Contraindications: Hypersensitivity to benzodiazepines, acute narrow-angle glaucoma
  – Precautions:
    ○ Monitor respiratory status, BP, and heart rate.
    ○ Reduce dose in elderly and patients with hepatic dysfunction.
  – Significant possible interactions: Benzodiazepines potentiate the effects of other CNS depressants.

Second Line
Adjunctive therapy:
- NSAIDs (tenoxicam) or use of heliox may reduce the number of recompressions required (although neither improves the odds of recovery).
- Digitalization for CHF/tachycardia
- Aminophylline *not* useful for decompression sickness
- Roles of steroids and heparin not determined

ADDITIONAL TREATMENT
General Measures
- Rapid referral to hyperbaric chamber facility
- Position in left lateral decubitus position (Durant maneuver)
- Trendelenburg is no longer recommended

Issues for Referral
- Prehospital: Referral through Divers' Alert Network (DAN; 919-684-8111) to nearest hyperbaric facility for recompression test
- Although recompression therapy is best administered as early as possible, some patients may still benefit even 6–9 days after the incident.

Additional Therapies
- Hyperbaric decompression (hyperbaric therapy for at least 4 hours)
- Transport via ground, low-altitude airplane, or aircraft pressurized to sea level

IN-PATIENT CONSIDERATIONS
IV Fluids
Isotonic fluid resuscitation

Nursing
Bed rest when neurologic involvement present

Discharge Criteria
Patients may be sent home when only cutaneous symptoms are present or if the appropriate response to therapy is observed in the emergency department.

 ONGOING CARE

FOLLOW-UP RECOMMENDATIONS
Patient Monitoring
Symptomatic assessment

DIET
Normal

PATIENT EDUCATION
- SCUBA divers should be certified by an appropriate diving agency: NAUI, PADI, SSI, or YMCA.
- Sport divers who have not been diving for >6 months should review diving principles/skills via a refresher course.

PROGNOSIS
- Excellent for early symptomatic presentation, referral, and treatment
- Related to duration and severity of symptoms prior to treatment
- 16% of patients have residual symptoms for up to 3 months.

COMPLICATIONS
- Oxygen toxicity with seizures (infrequent and unpredictable)
- Neurologic sequelae for nonresponders
- Long-term risk of aseptic necrosis

REFERENCES
1. Castagna O, Gempp E, Blatteau JE. Pre-dive normobaric oxygen reduces bubble formation in scuba divers. *Eur J Appl Physiol*. 2009.
2. Gempp E, Blatteau JE, Pontier JM, et al. Preventive Effect Of Pre-Dive Hydration On Bubble Formation In Divers. *Br J Sports Med*. 2008.
3. Pontier JM, Guerrero F, Castagna O. Bubble formation and endothelial function before and after 3 months of dive training. *Aviat Space Environ Med*. 2009;80:15–9.

ADDITIONAL READING
- Barratt DM, Harch PG, Van Meter K. Decompression illness in divers: a review of the literature. *Neurologist*. 2002;8:186–202.
- Bennett MH, Lehm JP, Mitchell SJ, et al. Recompression and adjunctive therapy for decompression illness. *Cochrane Database Syst Rev*. 2007;CD005277.
- British Thoracic Society Fitness to Dive Group, Subgroup of the British Thoracic Society Standards of Care Committee. British Thoracic Society guidelines on respiratory aspects of fitness for diving. *Thorax*. 2003;58:3–13.
- DAN Annual Diving Report: 2007 Edition.
- DAN Scuba Diving Medical Services: http://www.diversalertnetwork.org/medical.
- Information from your family doctor: Medical problems of recreational scuba diving. *Am Fam Physician*. 2001;63(11):2225–6.
- Newton, HB. Neurologic complications of scuba diving. *Am Fam Physician*. 2001;63(11):2211–8.
- Sheffield PJ. Flying after diving guidelines: a review. *Aviat Space Environ Med*. 1990;61:1130–8.
- Sulaiman ZM, Pilmanis AA, O'Connor RB. Relationship between age and susceptibility to altitude decompression sickness. *Aviat Space Environ Med*. 1997;68(8):695–8.
- Tetzlaff K, Shank ES, Muth CM. Evaluation and management of decompression illness—an intensivist's perspective. *Intensive Care Med*. 2003;29:2128–36.

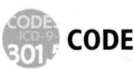 CODES

ICD9
993.3 Caisson disease

CLINICAL PEARLS
- If the patient only has musculoskeletal and skin complaints, you should still worry about neurologic or pulmonary issues as well. 71% of nervous system decompression sickness presents with skin/limb bends.
- 75% of patients present within 1 hour; 90% present within 12 hours; but some patients may still present >24 hours after diving.
- If recompression therapy is delayed several days, you should still proceed. Early administration is best, but patients may benefit even 6–9 days after the incident.
- Travel by air after SCUBA diving should be restricted for 12 hours (after 1 dive per day) or 48 hours (after multiple dives or decompression).

DEEP VEIN THROMBOPHLEBITIS (DVT)

Alfonso J. Tafur, MD
Denisse Tafur Chang, MD

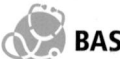

BASICS

DESCRIPTION
- Development of blood clot within the deep veins, usually accompanied by inflammation of the vessel wall.
- The major clinical consequences are embolization, usually to the lung, and postphlebitic syndrome.
- System(s) affected: Cardiovascular

EPIDEMIOLOGY
- The age- and gender-adjusted incidence of VTE is 100 times higher in the hospital than in the community (1).
- 1/3 of VTE cases die within 30 days, 1/5 will have sudden death due to PE. The 28-day DVT fatality rate is 9%.

Incidence
- In the US, VTE occurs for the 1st time in 100 persons per 100,000 per year.
- Approximately 2/3 of the new VTE cases are DVT alone.
- Higher incidence among Caucasians and African Americans relative to Hispanics and Asians
- Complicates approximately 1 in 1,000 pregnancies.

Prevalence
Variable; dependent on medical condition or procedure:
- 22–52% of the patients with PE have DVT.
- 25% of patients with superficial venous thrombosis (2)
- Present in 11% of patients with acquired brain injury entering to neurorehabilitation

RISK FACTORS
- Acquired: Age, previous thrombosis, immobilization, major surgery, orthopedic surgery, malignancy, oral contraceptives, hormonal replacement therapy, antiphospholipid syndrome, polycythemia vera, paroxysmal nocturnal hemoglobinuria, prolonged travel, pregnancy/puerperium
- Inherited: Antithrombin deficiency, protein C deficiency, protein S deficiency, factor V Leiden R506Q, prothrombin G20210A, dysfibrinogenemia
- Mixed/unknown: Hyperhomocysteinemia, high levels of factor VIII, activated protein C resistance not factor V Leiden, high levels of factor IX, high levels of thrombin activatable fibrinolysis inhibitor (TAFI), high levels of factor XI

Genetics
- Factor V Leiden is found in 5% of the population and in 20% of all VTE events. It is the most common thrombophilia. Homozygosity is found in 1 per 5,000 persons. It increases the risk of VTE 3- to 8-fold in heterozygous carriers and 50- to 80-fold in homozygous.
- PT20210A is found in 3% of Caucasians. Increases the risk of thrombosis about 3-fold.

GENERAL PREVENTION
- Mechanical thromboprophylaxis is recommended in patients with high bleeding risk and as an adjunct to anticoagulant based thromboprophylaxis. Mechanical measures include early ambulation, graduated compression stockings, venous foot pump, intermittent pneumatic compression.
- Level of risk
  - With minor surgery in mobile patient or fully mobile medical patients, risk of VTE <10%; early ambulation recommended
  - With medical patients on bed rest, general, and gynecologic or urologic surgeries, risk of VTE 10-40%; prophylactic LMWH, low-dose UFH or Fondaparinux recommended
- Hip or knee arthroplasty, major trauma, spinal cord injury, or hip fracture surgery, risk of VTE is 40–80%; LMWH, Fondaparinux, or oral vitamin K antagonist [INR 2-3] recommended

ETIOLOGY
Factors involved may include venous stasis, endothelial injury, and abnormalities of coagulation.

DIAGNOSIS

Wells criteria
- Active cancer within 6 months +1
- Paralysis or immobilization of lower extremity +1; Recent bedridden >3 days or major surgery within 4 weeks +1
- Tenderness/cord along vein +1
- Entire leg swollen +1
- Calf circumference >3 cm vs other leg +1
- Alternative diagnosis likely −2
- Interpretation
  - High probability +3
  - Moderate probability +3
  - Low probability 0

HISTORY
- Establish pretest probability based on Wells criteria.
- Classify as "Provoked" or "Idiopathic." Determine the presence of risk factors including family history.
- Clinical assessment of bleeding risk: bleeding with previous history of anticoagulation, history of liver disease, recent interventions, history of gastrointestinal bleed.

PHYSICAL EXAM
Physical exam is only 30% accurate for DVT. Resistance to dorsiflexion of the foot (Homan sign) is unreliable. Palpable tender cords are helpful if present but are often not present. Erythema over area of thrombosis (often not present). Fever is occasionally present. Swelling of collateral veins. Massive edema with cyanosis is a medical emergency (phlegmasia cerulea dolens, rare). Pain on medial tibia percussion (Lisker sign). Pain on compression of calf against tibia in the anteroposterior plane (Bancroft or Moses sign).Thoracic outlet maneuvers in Upper extremity DVT. Attention to signs of possible malignancy.

DIAGNOSTIC TESTS & INTERPRETATION
Lab
- D-dimer (sensitive but not specific; has a high NPV); most protocols are used to rule out DVT in low pretest probability cases: If D-dimer negative, DVT is ruled out with low pretest probability cases. Do not order D-dimer if pretest probability is moderate or high.
- CBC, platelet count, activated partial thromboplastin time (aPTT), prothrombin time (PT)/international normalized ratio (INR)

- In young patients with idiopathic or recurrent VTE consider:
  - Factor V Leiden, G20210A prothrombin, serum homocysteine, factor VIII level, and lupus anticoagulant
  - Protein C and S levels, antithrombin activity, anticardiolipin antibodies.
- Testing for genetic polymorphisms CYP2C9 and VK0RC1 (www.warfarindosing.org for current recommendations)
- Thrombosis lowers antithrombin III; workup for deficiency performed after therapy completed. Secondary antithrombin deficiency is more common than primary.

Imaging
- Compression ultrasound (US): Noninvasive; sensitive and specific for popliteal, femoral thrombi, but has poor ability to detect calf vein thrombi
- Contrast venography: Gold standard, is technically difficult, risk of morbidity
- Impedance plethysmography: As accurate as duplex ultrasound, less operator dependency, but poor at detecting calf vein thrombi; not widely available
- Magnetic resonance venography: As accurate as contrast venography; may be useful for patients with contraindications to IV contrast
- ^{125}I-fibrinogen scan: Detects only active clot formation; very good at detecting ongoing calf thrombi; takes 4 hours for results

DIFFERENTIAL DIAGNOSIS
Cellulitis, fracture, ruptured synovial cyst (Baker cyst), lymphedema, muscle strain/tear, extrinsic compression of vein (for example, by tumor or enlarged lymph nodes), compartment syndrome, localized allergic reaction, filariasis (in developing countries)

TREATMENT

MEDICATION
- All DVTs should receive treatment. Consider starting therapy even before confirmation in patients with high pre-test probability.
- 2008 American College of Chest Physicians Guidelines recommend low molecular weight heparin [LMWH], unfractionated heparin [UFH] (either IV, or fixed-dose or adjusted-dose subcutaneous heparin), or fondaparinux and warfarin for at least 5 days until the INR is 2–3 for 24 hours (3)[A].

First Line
- Unfractionated heparin (UFH):
  - IV drip: Initial dose of 80 units/kg or 5,000 Units followed by continuous infusion of 18 units/kg/ hour. Target an APTT ratio >1.5. The APTT prolongation shall correspond to a 0.3 to 0.7 anti Xa level.
  - SC UFH: Monitored: 17,500 units or 250 units/kg b.i.d. with APTT adjustment to an equivalent to 0.3–0.7 anti Xa. Alternatively, fixed dose: 333 units/kg followed by b.i.d. dose 250 units/kg.
- Enoxaparin (Lovenox): 1 mg/kg/dose subcutaneously every 12 hours or 1.5 mg/kg/dose per day
- Dalteparin (Fragmin): 200 IU/kg subcutaneously every 24 hours

- Fondaparinux (Arixtra): 5 mg (body weight <50 kg), 7.5 mg (body weight = 50–100 kg), or 10 mg (body weight >100 kg) subcutaneously once daily.
- Maintenance therapy:
  – Warfarin (Coumadin): 5 mg/d for 3 days, then adjust to a target INR of 2–3.
- Adverse effects:
  – Heparin or LMWH: Bleeding, edema, injection site irritation, skin eruptions, hematoma, thrombocytopenia
  – Fondaparinux: Bleeding, injection site irritation, rash, fever, anemia
  – Warfarin: Bleeding, skin necrosis, teratogenicity
- Contraindications:
  – Heparin or LMWH: Bleeding, heparin hypersensitivity, heparin-induced thrombocytopenia (HIT), ITP, infants/neonates
  – Fondaparinux: Bleeding, endocarditis, renal failure, thrombocytopenia
  – Warfarin: Current bleeding, alcoholism, preeclampsia, pregnancy, surgery, high fall risk

Second Line
If warfarin is contraindicated, heparin can be given by intermittent subcutaneous self-injection.

Pregnancy Considerations
- Warfarin (Coumadin) is a teratogen; treat with full-dose heparin initially, followed by subcutaneous heparin starting at 15,000 units every 12 hours.
- Warfarin is safe with breast-feeding.
- LMWH, dalteparin, and fondaparinux are pregnancy category B.

ADDITIONAL TREATMENT
Additional Therapies
- Discharge with compression stockings 30–40 mm Hg. Stress use to prevent post-phlebitic syndrome. Continue compression therapy for 2 years.
- Intermittent pneumatic compression may be tried in patients with significant edema.

SURGERY/OTHER PROCEDURES
- In selected patients with proximal DVT (Iliofemoral DVT, <2 weeks of symptoms, good functional status, >1 year of life expectancy), catheter directed thrombolysis or open thrombectomy may be considered.
- When anticoagulants have failed or are contraindicated, filtering devices are recommended.

IN-PATIENT CONSIDERATIONS
Admission Criteria
Admission for: Respiratory distress, proximal VTE, candidates for thrombolysis, active bleeding, renal failure, phlegmasia cerulea dolens, history of heparin-induced thrombocytopenia

Nursing
Limb elevation

Discharge Criteria
Medically stable and properly anticoagulated; overlap of anticoagulation and warfarin monitoring may be done as an outpatient

 ## ONGOING CARE

FOLLOW-UP RECOMMENDATIONS
- Gradual resumption of normal activity, with avoidance of prolonged immobility.
- Duration of warfarin treatment after DVT:
  – 3 months for treatment of a DVT secondary to a reversible risk factor
  – Patients with unprovoked DVT shall be considered for prolonged secondary prophylaxis:
    ○ In patients who have completed 3 months of anticoagulation after an unprovoked VTE, a positive D Dimer 1 month after discontinuation of therapy correlates with the risk of VTE recurrence (4).
    ○ Tailoring the anticoagulation duration base on recanalization ultrasound evidence, may reduce the rate of recurrent VTE (5).
  – Consider prolonged secondary prophylaxis (1 year or indefinitely): Recurrent DVT; PE; active cancer (LMWH preferred over warfarin); life-threatening event (large pulmonary embolism, limb-threatening DVT); cerebral or visceral vein thrombosis; antithrombin deficiency with event; homozygous for factor V Leiden; combined clotting disorders (e.g., combined heterozygous factor V Leiden and PT20210A); antiphospholipid syndrome

Patient Monitoring
- Monitor platelet count while on heparin.
- Monitoring with LMWH and fondaparinux: Periodic platelet count. An anti-factor Xa activity level may help guide titration of therapy.
- Investigate significant bleeding (e.g., hematuria or GI hemorrhage) because anticoagulant therapy may unmask a preexisting lesion (e.g., cancer, peptic ulcer disease, or arteriovenous malformation).

DIET
Patients taking warfarin must be aware that foods high in vitamin K can affect INR.

PATIENT EDUCATION
- Patients should wear compression stockings post-DVT; these can be cumbersome and uncomfortable; however, they can reduce the risk of DVT recurrence and post-phlebitic syndrome.
- Dietary habits should be discussed when warfarin is initiated to ensure that intake of vitamin K-rich foods are identified.

PROGNOSIS
- 20% of untreated proximal (e.g., above the calf) DVTs progress to pulmonary emboli, and 10–20% of those are fatal; with anticoagulant therapy, mortality is decreased 5–10-fold.
- DVT confined to the infrapopliteal veins has a small risk of embolization, but can propagate into the proximal system. Best treatment uncertain, but most recommend 6–12 weeks of anticoagulation.

COMPLICATIONS
- Pulmonary embolism (fatal in 10–20%)
- Arterial embolism (paradoxical embolization) with AV shunting
- Chronic venous insufficiency
- Postphlebitic syndrome (pain and swelling in affected limb without new clot formation)
- Treatment-induced hemorrhage
- Soft tissue ischemia associated with massive clot and high venous pressures: phlegmasia cerulea dolens (rare, but a surgical emergency)

REFERENCES

1. Heit JA, Melton LJ, Lohse CM, et al. Incidence of venous thromboembolism in hospitalized patients vs community residents. *Mayo Clin. Proc.* 2001;76:1102–10.
2. Decousus H, Quéré I, Presles E, et al. Superficial venous thrombosis and venous thromboembolism: a large, prospective epidemiologic study. *Ann Intern Med.* 2010;152:218–24.
3. Kearon C, Kahn SR, Agnelli G, et al. Antithrombotic therapy for venous thromboembolic disease: American College of Chest Physicians Evidence-Based Clinical Practice Guidelines (8th Edition). *Chest.* 2008;133:454S–545S.
4. Palareti G, Cosmi B, Legnani C, et al. D-dimer testing to determine the duration of anticoagulation therapy. *N Engl J Med.* 2006; 355:1780–9.
5. Prandoni P, Prins MH, Lensing AW, et al. Residual thrombosis on ultrasonography to guide the duration of anticoagulation in patients with deep venous thrombosis: a randomized trial. *Ann Intern Med.* 2009;150:577–85.

See Also (Topic, Algorithm, Electronic Media Element)
Antithrombin Deficiency; Factor V Leiden; Protein C Deficiency; Protein S Deficiency; Prothrombin 20210 (Mutation); Pulmonary Embolism

 ## CODES

ICD9
- 453.40 Acute venous embolism and thrombosis of unspecified deep vessels of lower extremity
- 453.41 Acute venous embolism and thrombosis of deep vessels of proximal lower extremity
- 453.42 Acute venous embolism and thrombosis of deep vessels of distal lower extremity

CLINICAL PEARLS

- Many cases are asymptomatic and are diagnosed after embolization.
- 25% of the patients with superficial thrombophlebitis will have DVT at presentation.
- Heparin and warfarin should overlap for a minimum of 5 days or longer to achieve target INR.
- Consider thoracic outlet syndrome in upper extremity DVT .
- Do a cancer-oriented review of systems and age- and gender-appropriate cancer screening in: Recurrent VTE, Not catheter associated Upper extremity DVT, bilateral lower extremity DVT, intra-abdominal DVT.

D

DEHYDRATION

Nitin Aggarwal, MD
Julie Scott Taylor, MD, MSc

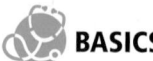

BASICS

DESCRIPTION
- Dehydration is a state of negative fluid balance.
- There are 2 types of dehydration:
  – Water loss dehydration (hyperosmolar, associated with either increased sodium or glucose)
  – Salt and water loss dehydration (hyponatremia)

EPIDEMIOLOGY
- Dehydration is the cause of 10% of all pediatric hospitalizations in the US.
- Gastroenteritis, one of the leading causes of dehydration, leads to hospital admission in 13 out of 1,000 children <5 years each year in the US (1).

Incidence
- There are more than a half million hospital admissions annually in the US for dehydration (2).
- 7.8% of hospitalized older persons have the diagnosis of dehydration (3).
- Worldwide, ~3–5 billion cases of acute gastroenteritis occur each year in children <5 years, resulting in nearly 2 million deaths (1).

RISK FACTORS
- Children <5 years old at highest risk
- Elderly
- Decreased cognition

Genetics
Some underlying causes of dehydration have a genetic component (diabetes), while others do not (gastroenteritis).

PATHOPHYSIOLOGY
- Negative fluid balance occurs when ongoing fluid losses exceed fluid intake.
- Fluid losses can be insensible (sweat, respiration), obligate (urine, stool), or abnormal (diarrhea, vomiting, osmotic diuresis in diabetic ketoacidosis).
- Negative fluid balance can ultimately lead to severe intravascular volume depletion and ultimately end-organ damage from inadequate perfusion.
- The elderly are at increased risk as kidney function, urine concentration, thirst sensation, aldosterone secretion, release of vasopressin, and renin activity are all significantly lowered with age. (4)

ETIOLOGY
- Decreased intake
- Increased output: Vomiting, diarrheal illnesses, sweating, frequent urination
- 3rd-spacing of fluids: Effusions, ascites, capillary leaks from burns or sepsis

COMMONLY ASSOCIATED CONDITIONS
- Hypo-/hypernatremia
- Hyperkalemia
- Hyperglycemia
- Hypovolemic shock
- Renal failure

DIAGNOSIS

Calculate % dehydration = (preillness weight – illness weight)/preillness weight × 100:

PHYSICAL EXAM
- Vitals: Pulse, BP, temperature
- Weight loss: <5%, 10%, or >15%
- Mental status
- Head: Sunken anterior fontanelle (for infants)
- Eyes: Sunken, +/– tear production
- Mucous membranes: Tacky, dry, or parched
- Capillary refill: Ranges from brisk to >3 sec

DIAGNOSTIC TESTS & INTERPRETATION
Lab
- For mild dehydration: Generally not necessary
- For moderate to severe dehydration:
  – Blood work including electrolytes, blood urea nitrogen (BUN), creatinine, and glucose
  – Urinalysis (specific gravity, hematuria, glucosuria)

Pediatric Considerations
Infants and the elderly may not concentrate urine maximally, so a nonelevated specific gravity should not be reassuring.

Imaging
Imaging does not play a role in diagnosis of dehydration, unless diagnosis of the specific medical condition causing the dehydration requires imaging.

DIFFERENTIAL DIAGNOSIS
- Decreased intake:
  – Ineffective breast-feeding
  – Inadequate thirst response
  – Anorexia
  – Malabsorption
  – Metabolic disorder
  – Obtunded state
- Excessive losses:
  – Gastroenteritis
  – Diarrhea
  – Febrile Illness
  – Diabetes/diabetic ketoacidosis (DKA)/hyperosmolar hyperglycemic state (HHS)
  – Diabetes insipidus
  – Intestinal obstruction
  – Inadequate intravascular volume
  – Sepsis

TREATMENT

MEDICATION
First Line
- If the patient is experiencing excessive vomiting, consider using an antiemetic.
- Antiemetic medications that are currently available include ondansetron, granisetron, tropisetron, dolasetron, ramosetron, promethazine, dimenhydrinate, metoclopramide, domperidone, droperidol, prochlorperazine, and trimethobenzamide.
- One randomized controlled trial (RCT) showed that a single oral dose of ondansetron reduced gastroenteritis-related vomiting and facilitated oral rehydration therapy (ORT) without significant adverse events (6)[B].

Clinical Finding (5)	Mild Dehydration	Moderate Dehydration	Severe Dehydration
% Dehydration: Children	5–10%	10–15%	>15%
% Dehydration: Adults	3–5%	5–10%	>10%
General Condition: Infants	Thirsty, alert, restless	Lethargic or drowsy	Limp, cold, cyanotic extremities, may be comatose
General Condition: Older Children	Thirsty, alert, restless	Alert, postural dizziness	Apprehensive, cold, cyanotic extremities, muscle cramps
Quality of radial pulse	Normal	Thready or weak	Feeble or impalpable
Quality of respiration	Normal	Deep	Deep and rapid/tachypnea
Blood Pressure	Normal	Normal to Low	Low (shock)
Skin Turgor	Normal skin turgor	Reduced skin turgor, cool skin	Skin tenting, cool, mottled, acrocyanotic skin
Eyes	Normal	Sunken	Very sunken
Tears	Present	Absent	Absent
Mucous Membranes	Moist	Dry	Very dry
Urine Output	Normal	Reduced	None passed in many hours
Anterior Fontanelle	Normal	Sunken	Markedly sunken

GENERAL PREVENTION
- Patient/parent education on the early signs of dehydration
- Regular hand washing decreases the spread of contagious viral gastroenteritis.

Geriatric Considerations
A systematic approach in assessing risk factors is necessary for early prevention and management of dehydration in the elderly, especially those in long-term care facilities.

HISTORY
- Fever
- Intake (including description and amount)
- Diarrhea (including duration, frequency, consistency, +/– mucus or blood)
- Vomiting (including duration, frequency, consistency, +/– bilious/nonbilious)
- Urination pattern
- Sick contacts
- Medication history (e.g., diuretics, laxatives)

Second Line

- 2 RCTs found that in children with mild to moderate dehydration, loperamide reduced the duration of diarrhea compared with placebo. Another RCT found no significant difference. There is insufficient evidence to assess the risk of adverse effects (6)[B].
- In children ages 3–12 with mild diarrhea and minimal dehydration, loperamide improves diarrhea duration and frequency when used with oral rehydration (7)[A].

Pediatric Considerations

Given a higher risk for serious adverse events, loperamide is not indicated for children <3 years old with acute diarrhea (7)[A].

ADDITIONAL TREATMENT

Issues for Referral

- If dehydration is severe, or depending on underlying etiology, critical care referral and intensive care unit (ICU)-level care may be warranted.
- Consider surgical consultation for acute abdominal issues.

SURGERY/OTHER PROCEDURES

For specific underlying causes of dehydration, such as intestinal obstruction or appendicitis

IN-PATIENT CONSIDERATIONS

Initial Stabilization

- Stabilize ABCs.
- If mild dehydration, try oral rehydration therapy (ORT): See Oral Rehydration.
- If excessive vomiting or severe dehydration with shock, start IV access and IV fluids immediately.

Admission Criteria

- Intractable vomiting or diarrhea
- Electrolyte abnormalities
- Hemodynamic instability
- Inability to tolerate ORT

IV Fluids

- Stage I:
  - For moderate to severe dehydration in children: Isotonic saline or Ringer's lactate solution bolus of 10–20 mL/kg. May repeat up to 60 mL/kg; if still hemodynamically unstable, consider colloid replacement (blood, albumin, fresh frozen plasma) and address other causes for shock.
  - For moderate to severe dehydration in adults: Isotonic saline or Ringer's lactate 20 mL/kg/hour until normal state of consciousness returns or vital signs stabilize. Also consider colloid replacement if continued fluids required beyond 3L.
- Stage II: Replace fluid deficit along with maintenance over 48 hours. Fluid deficit = preillness weight – illness weight.
- An alternative IVF treatment option for moderate (10%) dehydration in children: (8)
  - Bolus with NS/LR at 20 mL/kg for 1 hour
  - Replete fluid deficit with D5 1/2NS + 20 mEq KCl/L at 10 mL/kg for 8 hours (hours 2–9)
  - Replete 1.5× maintenance fluids with D5 1/4NS + 20 mEq/L of KCl for 16 hours (hours 10–24)
- An alternative to IV fluids is hypodermoclysis, the subcutaneous infusion of fluids into the body.
  - Hypodermoclysis is indicated for the hydration of patients with mild to moderate dehydration who do not tolerate oral intake because of cognitive impairment, severe dysphagia, advanced terminal illness or intractable vomiting. It is also indicated

to prevent dehydration, especially in frail elderly residents living in long-term care settings who reject the oral route for any reason.
  - It can also be a useful technique in rehydration for patients in whom IV access is difficult to obtain.
  - Hypodermoclysis is not indicated in patients with severe dehydration or shock, patients with coagulopathy or receiving full anticoagulation, patients with severe generalized edema (anasarca) or congestive heart failure, and those with fluid overload (9).

Nursing

- Strict I & Os.
- Document all oral and IV intake carefully.
- Document output of urine and stool, which may include weighing wet diapers.

Discharge Criteria

- Intake > output
- Underlying etiology treated and improving

ONGOING CARE

FOLLOW-UP RECOMMENDATIONS

Activity as tolerated

- If mild to moderate dehydration, the patient may be mobile without restrictions, although watch for orthostasis/falls.
- If moderate to severe dehydration, bed rest.

Patient Monitoring

Ongoing surveillance for recurrence

DIET

- Bland food such as a BRAT diet (bananas, rice, apples, toast)
- If diarrhea, avoid dairy for 48 hours after symptoms resolve. 1 systematic review of weak RCTs and 3 of 5 subsequent RCTs found that lactose-free feeds reduced the duration of diarrhea in children with mild to severe dehydration, compared with lactose-containing feeds. However, 2 subsequent RCTs found no difference between lactose-free and lactose-containing feeds in duration of diarrhea. (1)[A]
- Small frequent sips of room-temperature liquids
- For children, Pedialyte (liquid or Popsicles)
- Continue breast-feeding ad lib.

PATIENT EDUCATION

- Patients should go to the nearest emergency facility or call 911 if they or their child feels faint or dizzy when rising from a sitting or lying position, becomes lethargic and/or confused, or complains of a rapid heart rate.
- Patients should call their physician if they are unable to keep down any fluids, vomiting has been going on >24 hours in an adult or >12 hours in a child, diarrhea has lasted >2 days in an adult or child, an infant or child is much less active than usual or is very irritable, or if adult or child has excessive urination, especially if there is a history or family history of diabetes or diuretics administration.
- Patient information on dehydration at: http://www.mayoclinic.com/health/dehydration/DS00561
- Additional patient information at: http://familydoctor.org/online/famdocen/home/children/parents/common/stomach/196.html
- Treating gastroenteritis and dehydration in children at: http://www.aafp.org/afp/991201ap/991201a.html

PROGNOSIS

Self-limited if treated early. Potentially fatal.

COMPLICATIONS

- Seizures
- Renal failure
- Cardiovascular arrest

REFERENCES

1. Dalby-Payne J, et al. Clinical evidence concise: Gastroenteritis in children. Am Fam Physician. 2008;77(3):353. Available at: http://www.aafp.org/afp/20080201/bmj.html.
2. Xiao H, Barber J, Campbell ES et al. Economic burden of dehydration among hospitalized elderly patients. Am J Health Syst Pharm. 2004;61:2534–40.
3. Thomas DR, Cote TR, Lawhorne L, Levenson SA, Rubenstein LZ, Smith DA, Stefanacci RG, Tangalos EG, Morley JE, Dehydration Council et al. Understanding clinical dehydration and its treatment. J Am Med Dir Assoc. 2008;9:292–301.
4. Wotton K, Crannitch K, Munt R et al. Prevalence, risk factors and strategies to prevent dehydration in older adults. Contemp Nurse. 2008;31:44–56.
5. Gorelick MH, Shaw KN, Murphy KO et al. Validity and reliability of clinical signs in the diagnosis of dehydration in children. Pediatrics. 1997;99:E6-
6. Leung AK, Robson WL. Acute gastroenteritis in children: role of anti-emetic medication for gastroenteritis-related vomiting. Paediatr Drugs. 2007;9:175–84.
7. Barclay L, et al. Adjunctive loperamide therapy reduces acute diarrhea in children. Available at: http://www.medscape.com/viewarticle/554475.
8. Holliday MA, Ray PE, Friedman AL. Fluid therapy for children: facts, fashions and questions. Arch Dis Child. 2007;92:546–50.
9. Lopez JH, Reyes-Ortiz CA. Subcutaneous hydration by hypodermoclysis. Reviews in Clinical Gerontology. 2010;20(02):105–113.

See Also (Topic, Algorithm, Electronic Media Element)

Oral Rehydration

CODES

ICD9

- 276.1 Hyposmolality and/or hyponatremia
- 276.51 Dehydration

CLINICAL PEARLS

- Dehydration is the result of a negative fluid balance, when ongoing fluid losses exceed fluid intake for a variety of reasons.
- Dehydration is a common cause of hospitalization in both children and the elderly.
- Begin by assessing level of dehydration and determining the underlying cause.
- Treatment is directed at restoring fluid balance via oral rehydration therapy or IV fluids and treating underlying causes.

DELIRIUM

Jonathan M. Flacker, MD

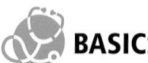 **BASICS**

DESCRIPTION
- A neurologic complication of illness and/or medication(s) especially common in older patients
- A medical emergency requiring immediate evaluation to decrease morbidity and mortality
- System(s) affected: Nervous
- Synonym(s): Acute confusional state; Altered mental status; Organic brain syndrome; Acute mental status change

EPIDEMIOLOGY
- Predominant age: Older persons
- Predominant sex: Male = Female

Incidence
>50% in high-risk older patients

Prevalence
- 10% in older emergency room patients
- 10–40% in hospitalized older patients
- 25% in older post–acute care patients
- Highest rates (>50%) in intensive care unit (ICU), post-hip fracture repair, post-cardiothoracic surgery

RISK FACTORS
- Predisposing risk factors:
  - Advanced age
  - Prior cognitive impairment
  - Functional impairment
  - High blood urea nitrogen: Creatinine ratio
  - Dehydration
  - Malnutrition
  - Hearing or vision impairment
  - Frailty
- Precipitating risk factors:
  - Severe illness in any organ system(s)
  - Need for a urinary catheter
  - >3 medications
  - Specific medications, especially long-acting sedative hypnotics (e.g., diazepam and flurazepam), narcotics (especially meperidine), and anticholinergics (especially diphenhydramine)
  - Pain
  - Any adverse iatrogenic event

GENERAL PREVENTION
Follow treatment approach.

PATHOPHYSIOLOGY
- Neuropathophysiology is not clearly defined; cholinergic deficiency is a leading hypothesis.
- Multicomponent approach addressing contributing factors can reduce incidence and complications.

ETIOLOGY
- Usually multifactorial
- Often interaction between predisposing and precipitating risk factors
- With more predisposing factors (i.e., frail patients), fewer precipitating factors needed to produce delirium
- If few predisposing factors (e.g., very robust patients), more precipitating factors needed to manifest delirium

COMMONLY ASSOCIATED CONDITIONS
Multiple, but most common are:
- New medicine or medicine changes
- Infections (especially lung and urine, but meningitis needs consideration as well)

- Toxic-metabolic (especially low sodium, elevated calcium, renal failure, and hepatic failure)
- Heart attack
- Stroke
- Alcohol or drug withdrawal
- Preexisting cognitive impairment increases risk.

 DIAGNOSIS

- The Confusion Assessment Method (CAM) may be used either pre- or post-hospital, or in hospital, and has been adapted for ICU setting (CAM-ICU).

ALERT
- Key diagnostic features of the CAM (1):
  - Acute change in mental status that fluctuates
  - Abnormal attention and **either** disorganized thinking **or** altered level of consciousness
- Any of the following nondiagnostic symptoms may be present:
  - Short- and long-term memory problems
  - Sleep-wake cycle disturbances
  - Hallucinations and/or delusions
  - Emotional lability
  - Tremors and asterixis
- Subtypes based on level of consciousness:
  - Hyperactive delirium (15%): Patients are loud, rambunctious, and disruptive.
  - Hypoactive delirium (20%): Quietly confused; may sit and not eat, drink, or move
  - Mixed delirium (50%): Features of both hyperactive and hypoactive delirium
  - Normal consciousness delirium (15%): Still display disorganized thinking, along with acute onset, inattention, and fluctuation

HISTORY
- Time course of mental status changes
- Recent medication changes
- Symptoms of infection
- New neurologic signs

PHYSICAL EXAM
- Comprehensive cardiorespiratory exam is essential.
- Focal neurologic signs usually absent
- Formal mini mental state exam is not diagnostic, but is helpful as structured interview and followed serially over time.

DIAGNOSTIC TESTS & INTERPRETATION
Electrocardiogram as necessary

Lab
Guided by history and physical exam

Initial lab tests
- Complete blood count
- Electrolytes, blood urea nitrogen, and creatinine
- Urinalysis, urine culture
- Medication levels (digoxin, theophylline where applicable)

Follow-Up & Special Considerations
If the above does not indicate a precipitator of delirium, consider:
- Arterial blood gases
- Troponin
- Toxicology screen
- Liver panel
- Thyroid-stimulating hormone

Imaging
Guided by history and physical exam

Initial approach
- Chest radiograph for most
- Other if indicated by history and exam

Follow-Up & Special Considerations
Non-contrast-enhanced head computed tomography scan if:
- Unclear diagnosis
- Recent fall
- Receiving anticoagulants
- New focal neurologic signs
- Need to rule out increased intracranial pressure before lumbar puncture

Diagnostic Procedures/Surgery
- Lumbar puncture:
  - Rarely necessary
  - Perform if clinical suspicion of a central nervous system (CNS) bleed or infection is high
- Electroencephalogram:
  - Rarely necessary; consider after above evaluation if:
    - Diagnosis remains unclear
    - Suspicion of seizure activity

DIFFERENTIAL DIAGNOSIS
- Depression (slow onset, disturbance of mood, normal level of consciousness, and fluctuates over weeks to months)
- Dementia (insidious onset, memory problems, normal level of consciousness, and fluctuates over days to weeks)
- Psychosis (rarely sudden onset in older adults)

 TREATMENT

- Stabilize vitals if needed.
- Ensure immediate evaluation. Addressing 6 risk factors (i.e., cognitive impairment, sleep deprivation, dehydration, immobility, vision impairment, and hearing impairment) in at-risk hospitalized patients can reduce the incidence of delirium by 33%.

MEDICATION
- Nonpharmacologic approaches are preferred for initial treatment.
- Medications often treat only the symptoms and do not address the underlying cause.

First Line
- Neuroleptics:
  - Haloperidol (Haldol): Initially, 0.25–0.5 mg p.o./IM/IV unless urgent sedation needed; reevaluate and potentially redose hourly
  - Quetiapine (Seroquel): 25 mg/d to b.i.d.
  - Risperidone (Risperdal): 0.25–0.5 mg/d p.o.
- Short-acting benzodiazepines if neuroleptics do not work or should be avoided:
  - Lorazepam (Ativan): Initially, 0.25–0.5 mg p.o./IM/IV q6–8h; may need to adjust to effect (caution in patients with impaired liver function)
- Contraindications: Avoid neuroleptics in patients with parkinsonism or Parkinson disease
- Precautions: Neuroleptics may cause extrapyramidal effects, and benzodiazepines may lead to sedation. Both increase the risk of falls.

Second Line
- Olanzapine (Zyprexa): 2.5–5.0 mg/d p.o.
- Despite multiple trials there is no evidence to support the use of cholinesterase inhibitors in the prevention or treatment of delirium,

ADDITIONAL TREATMENT
General Measures
- Postoperative patients should be monitored and treated for the following:
  – Myocardial infarction/ischemia
  – Pulmonary complications/pneumonia
  – Pulmonary embolism
  – Urinary or stool retention (attempt catheter removal by postoperative day 2)
- Anesthesia route (general epidural) does not affect the risk of delirium.
- Multifactorial treatment: Identify contributing factors and provide preemptive care to avoid iatrogenic problems (1,2)[A] with special attention to:
  – CNS oxygen delivery (attempt to attain the following):
    ○ SaO_2 >90% with goal of SaO_2 >95%
    ○ Systolic blood pressure <2/3 of baseline or >90 mm Hg
    ○ Hematocrit >30%
- Fluid/electrolyte balance:
  – Sodium, potassium, and glucose normal (glucose <300 mg/dL in diabetics)
  – Treat fluid overload or dehydration.
- Treat pain:
  – Schedule acetaminophen (1 g q.i.d.) if daily pain
  – Morphine or oxycodone for breakthrough pain if acetaminophen ineffective

ALERT
- Avoid meperidine (Demerol) (2)[A].
- Eliminate unnecessary medications:
  – Investigate new symptoms as potential medication side effects.
- Regulate bowel/bladder function:
  – Bowel movement at least every 48 hours
  – Screen for urinary retention or incontinence, especially after catheter removal.
- Prevent major hospital-acquired problems:
  – 6-inch-thick foam mattress overlay or a pressure-reducing mattress
  – Avoid urinary catheter.
  – Incentive spirometry, if bed-bound
  – SC heparin 5,000 U b.i.d., if bed-fast
  – Environmental stimulation:
    ○ Glasses and hearing aids
    ○ Clock and calendar
    ○ Soft lighting
    ○ Radio, tapes, and television, if desired
  – Sleep:
    ○ Quiet environment
    ○ Soft music
    ○ Therapeutic massage
- Restraints do not reduce risk of falls/injury:
  – Use only in the most difficult-to-manage patients, as briefly as possible

Issues for Referral
Psychiatric and/or neurologic assessment helpful if delirium not easily explainable after full evaluation

Additional Therapies
Early mobilization critical:
- Out of bed on hospital day 2 (or postoperative day 1) if no contraindications
- Out of bed several hours daily if able
- Daily therapy if not ambulating independently
- Daily therapy if not functionally independent

IN-PATIENT CONSIDERATIONS
General measures described above are also applicable to delirium prevention.

Admission Criteria
New delirium is a medical emergency and requires admission, except in the setting of palliative home care.

IV Fluids
As needed for dehydration

Nursing
- Institute skin care program for patients with established incontinence.
- Turning regimen if at risk of pressure ulcers
- Soft restraints are acceptable for a short time only if needed for protection of patient and others.

Discharge Criteria
- Resolution of precipitating factor(s)
- Safe discharge site if still delirious

 ## ONGOING CARE

FOLLOW-UP RECOMMENDATIONS
- If delirium at discharge, will usually be followed in post-acute facility
- If no delirium at discharge, follow up with primary care physician in 1–2 weeks.
- As tolerated
- Early physical therapy consultation to prevent deconditioning

Patient Monitoring
- Evaluate and assess mental status daily.
- Depends on specific conditions present

DIET
- Dentures used properly
- Proper positioning for meals
- Assistance with meals when necessary
- Nutritional supplements (1–3 cans daily) if intake is poor
- Temporary nasogastric tube if unable to eat and bowels working

PROGNOSIS
- Usually improves with treatment of underlying condition, but may become chronic
- Delirium complicating medical illness significantly increases a person's chance of dying from that illness

COMPLICATIONS
- Falls
- Pressure ulcers
- Malnutrition
- Functional decline
- Oversedation
- Polypharmacy

REFERENCES

1. Fong TG, Tulebave SR, Inouye SK. Delirium in elderly adults: Diagnosis, prevention, and treatment. Nature Reviews Neurology 2009;5: 210–220.
2. Hopkins RO, Jackson JC. Assessing neurocognitive outcomes after critical illness: are delirium and long-term cognitive impairments related? *Curr Opin Crit Care*. 2006;12:388–94.

ADDITIONAL READING

- Hshieh TT, Fong TG, Marcantonio ER, Inouye SK et al. Cholinergic deficiency hypothesis in delirium: a synthesis of current evidence. *J Gerontol A Biol Sci Med Sci*. 2008;63:764–72.
- van Eijk MM, van Marum RJ, Klijn IA, de Wit N, Kesecioglu J, Slooter AJ et al. Comparison of delirium assessment tools in a mixed intensive care unit. *Crit Care Med*. 2009;37:1881–5.
- Yang FM, Marcantonio ER, Inouye SK, Kiely DK, Rudolph JL, Fearing MA, Jones RN et al. Phenomenological subtypes of delirium in older persons: patterns, prevalence, and prognosis. *Psychosomatics*. 2009;50:248–54.

See Also (Topic, Algorithm, Electronic Media Element)
Substance Use Disorders; Dementia; Depression
Algorithm: Delirium

 ## CODES

ICD9
- 293.0 Delirium due to conditions classified elsewhere
- 293.1 Subacute delirium
- 293.9 Unspecified transient mental disorder in conditions classified elsewhere

CLINICAL PEARLS

- The Confusion Assessment Method (CAM) criteria for delirium are acute onset of fluctuating mental status, inattention, disorganized thinking, AND EITHER disorganized thinking or altered level of consciousness.
- In the absence of active monitoring, the hypoactive subtype of delirium can easily be missed.
- Addressing 6 risk factors (i.e., cognitive impairment, sleep deprivation, dehydration, immobility, vision impairment, and hearing impairment) in at-risk hospitalized patients can reduce the incidence of delirium by 33%.
- Delirium may not resolve as soon as the treatable contributors are fixed; resolution may take weeks or months. Rarely will become chronic.
- Avoid diphenhydramine in older patients. Nonpharmacologic measures are preferable as a sleep aid, but if needed, zolpidem (5 mg hs) or trazodone (25 mg hs) are reasonable alternatives.

DEMENTIA

Alicia R. Desilets, PharmD
Karen Bryant, MD

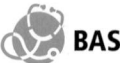 BASICS

DESCRIPTION
Dementia is a decline in cognitive function potentially caused by a number of disorders:
- Alzheimer dementia (AD):
  - Progressive deterioration of higher cortical functioning
- Vascular dementia (VaD):
  - Usually correlated with a cerebrovascular event and/or cerebrovascular disease
  - Stepwise deterioration with periods of clinical plateaus
- Lewy body dementia:
  - Fluctuating cognition associated with parkinsonism, hallucinations and delusions, gait difficulties, and falls
- Frontotemporal dementia:
  - Language difficulties, personality changes, and behavioral disturbances

EPIDEMIOLOGY
Prevalence
- In patients ≥71 years old:
  - AD: 70%
  - VaD: 17%
  - Other: 13%
- AD 60–64 years: <1%, approximately doubles every 5 years after age 60
- Estimated 5.2 million Americans had AD in 2008:
  - 5 million >65 years old; 200,000 <65 years

RISK FACTORS
- Increasing age
- Women > Men
- Lower educational status
- Genetic predisposition
- Head injury early in life
- Sedentary lifestyle
- Hypertension: AD; VaD
- Hypercholesterolemia: AD; VaD
- Diabetes: VaD
- Cigarette smoking: VaD

Genetics
- Heterogenous: Sporadic AD, ApoE4 allele on chromosome 19
- Familial: <0.1% AD, autosomal dominant

GENERAL PREVENTION
Data supporting specific preventative measures are limited and not conclusive:
- Smoking cessation
- Physical and mental activity
- Treatment of hypertension, hypercholesterolemia, and diabetes

ETIOLOGY
- AD:
  - Several mechanisms have been investigated.
  - Neurofibrillary tangles: Unable to support microtubules
  - Neuritic plaques (amyloid β-peptide):
    - Accumulation may lead to impaired cognitive function.
  - Other: Inflammatory mechanisms, oxidative:
    - Stress, mitochondrial dysfunction, apoptosis

- VaD:
  - Cerebral atherosclerosis or emboli with clinical or subclinical infarcts

COMMONLY ASSOCIATED CONDITIONS
- Anxiety and depression
- Delirium
- Behavioral disturbances (agitation, aggression)
- Sleep disturbances
- Caregiver stress

DIAGNOSIS

HISTORY
Probable diagnosis AD (1)[A]:
- Age between 40 and 90 (usually >65)
- Progressive cognitive decline of insidious onset
- No disturbances of consciousness
- Deficits in >2 areas of cognition
- No other explainable cause of symptoms
- Specifically, rule out thyroid disease, vitamin deficiency (B$_{12}$), grief reaction
- Supportive factors: Family history

PHYSICAL EXAM
- No disturbances of consciousness
- Cognitive decline demonstrated by standardized instruments, including:
  - Mini-Mental Status Exam
  - ADAS-Cog
  - Clock draw test
  - Change test
- Deficits in >2 areas of cognition

DIAGNOSTIC TESTS & INTERPRETATION
Lab
Initial lab tests

- Used to rule out other causes (1)[A]:
  - Comprehensive metabolic profile
  - Complete blood count
  - Thyroid stimulating hormone
  - Vitamin B$_{12}$ level
  - Neuroimaging (preferably magnetic resonance imaging [MRI] of brain)
- Select patients:
  - HIV
  - Rapid plasma reagin
  - Erythrocyte sedimentation rate
  - Folate
  - Heavy metal screen
  - Toxicology screen

Imaging
Tests that support the diagnosis:
- Cerebral atrophy on neuroimaging
- Normal lumbar puncture

Initial approach

- Early age of onset (<65 years old), rapid progression, focal neurologic deficits, cerebrovascular disease risk, or atypical symptoms: Neuroimaging (MRI or computed tomography) to rule out other causes (1)[A]
- Important findings:
  - AD: Diffuse cerebral atrophy starting in association areas, hippocampus, amygdala
  - VaD: Old infarcts, including lacunes

Diagnostic Procedures/Surgery
Positron emission tomography scan not routinely recommended; has been approved to differentiate between Alzheimer disease and frontotemporal dementia (2)[A]

Pathological Findings
AD:
- Neurofibrillary tangles: Abnormally phosphorylated tau protein
- Senile plaques: Amyloid precursor protein derivatives
- Microvascular amyloid

DIFFERENTIAL DIAGNOSIS
- Mild cognitive impairment
- Major depression
- Medication side effect
- Chronic alcohol use
- Delirium
- Subdural hematoma
- Normal pressure hydrocephalus
- Brain tumor
- Thyroid disease
- Parkinson disease
- Vitamin B$_{12}$ deficiency
- Toxins (aromatic hydrocarbons, solvents, heavy metals, marijuana, opiates, sedative-hypnotics)

TREATMENT

MEDICATION
First Line

- Cognitive dysfunction, mild (2)[A]:
  - Cholinesterase inhibitors: Donepezil (Aricept), 5–10 mg/d; rivastigmine (Exelon), 1.5–6 mg b.i.d., transdermal system 4.6 mg/24 hours and 9.5 mg/24 hours; galantamine (Razadyne), 4–12 mg b.i.d., extended release 8–24 mg/d:
    - Adverse events: Nausea, vomiting, diarrhea, anorexia, nightmares
    - Galantamine warning: Associated with mortality in patients with mild cognitive impairment in clinical trial
- Cognitive dysfunction, moderate to severe (2)[A]:
  - Cholinesterase inhibitors OR
  - Memantine (Namenda) 5–20 mg/d:
    - Adverse events: Dizziness, confusion, headache, constipation
  - OR combination cholinesterase inhibitor and memantine
- Commonly associated conditions:
  - Psychosis and agitation/aggressive behavior:
    - Antipsychotics: Initiate low doses, haloperidol 0.25–0.5 mg/d; risperidone 0.25–1 mg/d; clozapine 12.5 mg/d; olanzapine 1.25–5 mg/d; quetiapine 12.5–50 mg/d; aripiprazole 5 mg/d; ziprasidone 20 mg/d (2)[A]
    - Atypical antipsychotics associated with a better side effect profile; quetiapine and aripiprazole often 1st-line due to decreased extrapyramidal side effects

ALERT

- Black box warning on atypical antipsychotics due to increased mortality found when used in elderly patients with dementia
- Depression:
  - Selective serotonin reuptake inhibitors (SSRIs): Initiate low doses, citalopram (Celexa) 10 mg/d; escitalopram (Lexapro) 5 mg/d; sertraline (Zoloft) 25 mg/d (2)[A]
  - Adverse events: Nausea, vomiting, agitation, parkinsonian effects, sexual dysfunction, hyponatremia
  - Fluoxetine (Prozac) and paroxetine (Paxil) should be avoided in elderly patients.
- Sleep disturbances:
  - Mirtazapine (7.5–60 mg) or trazodone (25–100 mg) at bedtime if also has depression (2)[A]
  - Atypical antipsychotics if psychotic symptoms present (2)[A]
  - Zolpidem (5–10 mg); zaleplon (5–10 mg) (2)[A]
  - Benzodiazepines only for short term if anxiety or as needed: Lorazepam 0.5–1.0 mg; oxazepam 7.5–15 mg (2)[A]

Second Line

Associated conditions:

- Depression: Venlafaxine, mirtazapine and bupropion (2)[A]
- Psychosis and agitation/aggressive behavior:
  - Some data for SSRIs (2)[A]
  - Benzodiazepines if agitation with anxiety; in elderly, use as needed (2)[A]

Geriatric Considerations

- Initiate pharmacotherapy at low doses and titrate slowly up if necessary.
- If benzodiazepines indicated for anxiety, choose drug with short half-life
- Watch decreased renal function and hepatic metabolism.

ADDITIONAL TREATMENT

Behavioral modification:

- Socialization such as adult day care to prevent isolation and depression
- Sleep hygiene program as alternative to pharmaceuticals for sleep disturbance
- Scheduled toileting to prevent incontinence

General Measures

- Daily schedules and written directions
- Emphasis on nutrition, personal hygiene, accident-proofing the home, safety issues, sleep hygiene and supervision
- Socialization (adult day care)
- Sensory stimulation (display of clocks and calendars) in the early to mid stages
- Discussion with the family concerning support and advance directives

Issues for Referral

- Neuropsychiatric evaluation particularly helpful in early stages or mild cognitive impairment
- Assessment and management of:
  - Cognitive problems
  - Mood disorders (e.g., depression, anxiety)
  - Psychosis
  - Behavioral problems (e.g., agitation, aggression)

COMPLEMENTARY AND ALTERNATIVE MEDICINE

- Vitamin E is no longer recommended due to lack of evidence and possible association with an increase in mortality (2)[A].
- Ginkgo biloba should not be recommended due to lack of evidence (2)[A].
- Huperzine-A appears to have potential in small trials; however, until clinical evidence can firmly establish its role, it should not be recommended.
- Use of nonsteroidal anti-inflammatory drugs, selegiline, and estrogen should not be recommended due to lack of efficacy and safety data (2)[A].

IN-PATIENT CONSIDERATIONS

Admission Criteria

- Patients who cannot be treated in an outpatient setting
- Patients who may require geripsychiatric admission for aggressive behaviors

 ONGOING CARE

FOLLOW-UP RECOMMENDATIONS

Patient Monitoring

- Progression of cognitive impairment by use of standardized tool (e.g., MMSE, ADAS-Cog)
- Development of behavioral problems
- Adverse events of pharmacotherapy
- Nutritional status
- Caregiver evaluation of stress
- Evaluate issues that may affect quality of life.

PATIENT EDUCATION

- Safety concerns
- Long-term issues: Management of finances, medical decision making, possible placement when appropriate
- Advance directives

PROGNOSIS

- AD: Progressive disease (variable rates) leading to profound cognitive impairment:
  - Without treatment average decline on MMSE of 2 points per year
- VaD: Less likely to be progressive, but cognitive improvement is unlikely
- Secondary dementias: Treatment of the underlying condition may lead to improvement.

COMPLICATIONS

- Wandering
- Falls with injury:
  - Hip fracture
  - Head trauma
  - Subdural hematoma
- Aspiration pneumonia in end stage
- Caregiver burnout

REFERENCES

1. Blass DM, Rabins PV. In the clinic. Dementia. *Ann Intern Med*. 2008;148:ITC4–1-ITC4-16.
2. APA Work Group on Alzheimer's Disease and other Dementias, Rabins PV, Blacker D, et al. American Psychiatric Association practice guideline for the treatment of patients with Alzheimer's disease and other dementias. Second edition. *Am J Psychiatry*. 2007;164:5–56.

ADDITIONAL READING

- Birks J. Cholinesterase inhibitors for Alzheimer's disease. *Cochrane Database Syst Rev*. 2006; CD005593.
- Blennow K, de Leon MJ, Zetterberg H. Alzheimer's disease. *Lancet*. 2006;368:387–403.
- Burns A, Iliffe S. Alzheimer's disease. *BMJ*. 2009;338:b158.
- Lleó A, Greenberg SM, Growdon JH. Current pharmacotherapy for Alzheimer's disease. *Annu Rev Med*. 2006;57:513–33.
- Lyketsos CG, Colenda CC, Beck C, et al. Position statement of the American Association for Geriatric Psychiatry regarding principles of care for patients with dementia resulting from Alzheimer disease. *Am J Geriatr Psychiatry*. 2006;14:561–72.

See Also (Topic, Algorithm, Electronic Media Element)

Algorithm: Dementia

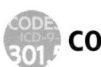 CODES

ICD9

- 290.0 Senile dementia, uncomplicated
- 290.40 Vascular dementia, uncomplicated
- 331.0 Alzheimer's disease
- 331.82 Dementia with Lewy bodies

CLINICAL PEARLS

- Dementia is loss of cognitive function in multiple areas.
- Time is diagnostic; AD is a progressive disease that will manifest with continual decline over time.
- Medications for AD show a small, statistically significant improvement in some cognitive measures, but it remains unclear if the improvement is clinically significant.

DENTAL INFECTION

Sheila O. Stille, DMD, MAGD
John J. Gentile, DMD

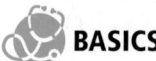 **BASICS**

DESCRIPTION
- Very painful area ± swelling in the head and neck region arising from the teeth and supporting structures. If left untreated, can lead to serious and potentially life-threatening illnesses.
- Assume any head and neck infection or swelling to be odontogenic in origin until proven otherwise.

EPIDEMIOLOGY
Incidence
- Caries is a contagious bacterial infection that is transmitted vertically from caregivers.
- The introduction of fluoride has dramatically decreased dental caries.

Prevalence
25% of children between ages of 5 and 17 years account for 80% of caries in the US (1).

RISK FACTORS
- Low socioeconomic status
- Poor access to care
- Fear of dentist
- Poor oral hygiene
- Poor nutrition
- Prior trauma to the teeth or jaws
- Heavily restored dentition
- Inadequate fluoride
- Gingival recession (increased risk of root caries)
- Physical and mental disabilities
- Decreased salivary flow
- Use of anticholinergic medications

GENERAL PREVENTION
- Preventable, contagious bacterial infection (*S. mutans*)
- Majority of dental problems can be avoided through flossing, brushing with fluoride toothpaste, and biannual cleaning (2)[B]
- Avoid smoking; linked to severe periodontal disease
- Good control of systemic diseases, i.e., diabetes

PATHOPHYSIOLOGY
Caries or trauma can lead to pulpal death, which in turn, leads to infection of pulp and/or abscess of adjacent tissues via direct or hematogenous bacterial colonization.

ETIOLOGY
- *Streptococcus mutans* vertically transmitted to newly dentate infants from caregivers
- Acidic secretions from *Streptococcus mutans* are implicated in early caries.
- Often polymicrobial
- Anaerobes, including *Pepto streptococci, Bacteroides, Prevotella,* and *Fusobacterium,* have been implicated. *Lactobacilli* may subsequently be involved.

COMMONLY ASSOCIATED CONDITIONS
- Rampant caries throughout dentition; multiple missing teeth
- Periodontal abscess
- Soft tissue cellulitis
- Pericoronitis
- Periodontitis

 DIAGNOSIS

HISTORY
- Pain at infected site or referred to ears, jaw, cheek, or sinuses
- Sensitivity to hot or cold stimuli
- Unprovoked, intermittent, or constant throb along nerve pathway
- Pain on biting
- Bleeding or purulent drainage from gingival tissues
- When severe infection (systemic):
  – Fever
  – Difficulty breathing or swallowing
  – Death
- Children <4 years with stiff neck, sore throat, and dysphagia should be worked up for retropharyngeal abscess secondary to molar infection.

PHYSICAL EXAM
- Gingival edema and erythema
- Cheek or intraoral swelling
- Presence of fluctuant mass
- Suppuration of gingival margin or tooth
- Lymphadenopathy
- Severe infection may present with dysphagia, fever, and signs of airway compromise.

DIAGNOSTIC TESTS & INTERPRETATION
Lab
Initial lab tests
- No initial labs needed, unless patient looks acutely ill
- If acutely ill:
  – Consider complete blood count with differential.
  – Culture and sensitivity; if abscess present, aspirate pus. Test for aerobes and anaerobes.
  – Note: Multiple organisms involved; most likely anaerobic gram-negative rods and anaerobic gram-positive cocci (2).

Imaging
Initial approach
- Individual dental films of suspected teeth
- Panoramic film of the teeth and jaw for evaluation of the extent of infection

Follow-Up & Special Considerations
Computed tomography scan can be used to determine the extent and density of the swelling, locating the abscess within the soft tissue and bone. This aids in determining treatment course.

DIFFERENTIAL DIAGNOSIS
- Bacterial or viral throat infection
- Otitis media
- Sinusitis
- Viral or aphthous stomatitis
- Temporomandibular joint (TMJ) dysfunction (myofascial pain)
- Parotitis
- Cyst
- Jaw pain can be anginal equivalent, especially in women, and especially lower-left portion of the jaw.

 TREATMENT

- Place patient on appropriate antibiotic, if indicated.
- Tend to appropriate pain control: Anti-inflammatory agents
- Refer to dentist as soon as possible for definitive treatment: Root canal or extraction
- If infection is severe, consider hospitalization with IV antibiotics until stabilized. Patient may need incision and drainage of abscess.

MEDICATION

First Line
- Penicillin VK loading dose of 1,000 mg, followed by 500 mg q.i.d. for 7–10 days. In children, 40–60 mg/kg/d divided q.i.d.
- Amoxicillin loading dose of 1,000 mg, followed by 500 mg t.i.d. for 7–10 days. In children, 40–60 mg/kg/d divided t.i.d.
- If penicillin-allergic, use clindamycin

Second Line
If long-standing infection or previously treated infection that does not respond to 1st-line treatment:
- Oral clindamycin 300 mg t.i.d. for 7–10 days
- If severe infection, load with clindamycin 600 mg, 900 mg IV, then 300 mg q6h; consider double coverage with metronidazole

ADDITIONAL TREATMENT

General Measures
- Ibuprofen 600–800 mg (or 10 mg/kg) q6h, or acetaminophen 650–1,000 mg (10–15 mg/kg) q4–6h
- For more severe pain, consider acetaminophen or ibuprofen + opioids.
- Can consider local anesthetic nerve block with long-acting anesthetic (bupivacaine) as adjunct; avoid penetrating infection with needle to avoid tracking infection

Issues for Referral
A dentist should be consulted and follow-up definitive care appointment should be secured prior to discharge from medical office, emergency room, or hospital unit.

SURGERY/OTHER PROCEDURES
- Incision and drainage of abscess should be performed if abscess is large and fluctuant.
- Root canal or extraction should be performed as definitive treatment.

IN-PATIENT CONSIDERATIONS

Initial Stabilization
- Secure airway, if compromised, with either endotracheal intubation or tracheotomy.
- IV fluid resuscitation with normal saline may be indicated in acutely ill patients.

Admission Criteria
Criteria for hospital admission include swelling involving deep spaces of the neck, unstable vital signs, fever, chills, confusion or delirium, or evidence of invasive infection.

Nursing
- Ensure good oral hygiene.
- Rinse mouth with chlorhexidine gluconate 2 times per day.
- Use warm salt water rinses several times per day to encourage drainage, especially after incision and drainage.

Discharge Criteria
Discharge patient if:
- Airway not compromised
- Abscess and sepsis eliminated
- Able to take p.o. intake and ambulate

 ONGOING CARE

Educate patient in need for proper oral hygiene, need for follow-up dental care, need for routine dental care, and stress medical complications that can and have occurred due to lack of dental care.

FOLLOW-UP RECOMMENDATIONS
- Follow-up with dentist within 24 hours.
- Ensure adequate p.o. intake, including protein.

DIET
- Maintain a healthy diet. Bacteria thrive on refined sugar and starch.
- Avoid sugary foods that stick between the teeth.

Pediatric Considerations
In children, limit the frequency of sugary drinks, and advise against sleeping with a bottle to decrease the chance of dental caries.

PATIENT EDUCATION
- Biannual dental visits
- Nutritional education
- Limit the frequency of sugar/carbonated drinks and sugary or sticky foods.
- In young children, avoid sleeping with a bottle to decrease the chance of dental caries.
- Brush and floss daily.
- Caretakers should tend to their personal oral hygiene, +/− chlorhexidine rinses in 1st 3 years of the child's life to decrease the risk of transmission of the caries causing microorganisms.

PROGNOSIS
Prognosis is excellent with proper treatment.

COMPLICATIONS
- Ludwig angina
- Retropharyngeal and mediastinal infection
- Osteomyelitis
- Endocarditis
- Submental infection
- Submandibular infection
- Can cause unstable diabetes in diabetics/worsen preexisting heart disease
- Possible link to preterm labor
- Brain abscess/death

REFERENCES

1. Kaste LM, Selwitz RH, Oldakowski RJ, et al. Coronal caries in the primary and permanent dentition of children and adolescents 1-17 years of age: United States, 1988–1991. *J Dent Res.* 1996;75 Spec No:631–41.
2. Lockhart PB, ed. *Dental Care of the Medically Complex Patient*, 5th ed. New York: Elsevier, 2004.

ADDITIONAL READING

- Cliff K, et al. An evidence-based update of the use of analgesics in dentistry. *Periodontology.* 2008; 46(1):143–164.
- Marinho VCC, et al. Topical fluoride (toothpastes, mouthrinses, gels or varnishes) for preventing dental caries in children and adolescents. Cochrane Oral Health Group. *Cochrane Database Syst Rev.* 2007;(4):CD002781.
- Matijevi S, Lazi Z, Kulji-Kapulica N, et al. Empirical antimicrobial therapy of acute dentoalveolar abscess. *Vojnosanit Pregl.* 2009;66:544–50.
- Stefanopoulos PK, Kolokotronis AE. Controversies in antibiotic choices for odontogenic infections. *Oral Surg Oral Med Oral Pathol Oral Radiol Endod.* 2006;101:697–8.
- Stefanopoulos PK, Kolokotronis AE. The clinical significance of anaerobic bacteria in acute orofacial odontogenic infections. *Oral Surg Oral Med Oral Pathol Oral Radiol Endod.* 2004;98:398–408.
- Vargas CM, Crall JJ, Schneider DA. Sociodemographic distribution of pediatric dental caries: NHANES III, 1988–1994. *J Am Dent Assoc.* 1998;129:1229–38.
- Vellappally S, Fiala Z, Smejkalová J, et al. Smoking related systemic and oral diseases. *Acta Medica (Hradec Kralove).* 2007;50:161–6.

 CODES

ICD9
- 521.00 Dental caries, unspecified
- 522.5 Periapical abscess without sinus
- 528.3 Cellulitis and abscess of oral soft tissues

CLINICAL PEARLS
- Do not ignore toothache pain.
- Treat patients with facial swelling aggressively, as infections can spread quickly.

DENTAL TRAUMA

Sheila O. Stille, DMD, MAGD
John J. Gentile, DMD

BASICS

DESCRIPTION
Loss or fracture of a tooth and/or supporting bone due to trauma. Trauma can result in shifting of remaining teeth, loss of teeth, loss of alveolar bone, displaced or nonunion of maxilla and/or mandible, resulting in functional and aesthetic deformities that may become difficult to correct.

EPIDEMIOLOGY
- Dental injuries of the teeth, supporting bone, and surrounding soft tissue constitute 7% of all physical injuries.
- Causes: Falls/sports, 63%; assault, 17%; auto or motorcycle accidents, 2%
- Male > Female (2–3:1)

Prevalence
- Prevalence: 5% of all school-age children; 7–13% in primary dentition, 1–16% in permanent dentition
- Affects 13% of population <12 years

RISK FACTORS
- Physical and mental disabilities
- Contact sports without wearing proper protective equipment, i.e., helmets, mouth guards
- Age: Youth <12 years
- Tongue rings
- Prior dental trauma
- Male gender

GENERAL PREVENTION
- Mouth guards and helmets may prevent traumatic dental injuries during sport exercises like football, soccer, baseball, hockey, bicycling, or skateboarding.
- Avoid tongue piercings.
- Wear seat belts while in the car.
- Monitor home for slippery areas.
- Childproof house gates and pad sharp table edges.

PATHOPHYSIOLOGY
Direct force sufficient to overcome the bond between the tooth and periodontal ligament within the alveolar socket or disruption of enamel and dentin. Force against maxilla or mandibular arch great enough to cause fracture.

COMMONLY ASSOCIATED CONDITIONS
- Tooth loss can cause loss of space in dental arch.
- Malocclusion causing functional problems
- Trauma to dentition resulting in pulpitis, which causes necrosis of the pulp
- Child abuse: Be alert for history inconsistent with injuries.

DIAGNOSIS

HISTORY
- Assess ABCs.
- Determine nature, time of injury; associated injuries
- Dental fractures:
  - Ask patient if they have possession of missing tooth pieces or swallowed/aspirated teeth.
  - Assess extent of fracture: Enamel only; enamel and dentin; enamel, dentin, and pulp; root fracture
- Concussion of teeth; subluxed; intruded; extruded
- Tooth avulsion:
  - Time out of socket (critical to management and prognosis)
  - Location of tooth when recovered
  - Type of tooth transfer media (milk, water, towel, etc.)
- Maxilla or mandibular fracture
- Consider child abuse in patients with dental fractures.

PHYSICAL EXAM
- Inspect the surrounding tissue for laceration, ecchymosis, embedded tooth fragments, or foreign bodies.
- Classify fracture by Ellis classification:
  - Ellis I fracture involves only the enamel.
  - Ellis II fracture includes enamel and dentin (pale yellow material underlying the enamel).
  - Ellis III fracture involves enamel, dentin, and pulp (red material under dentin).
- Check for sensitivity to hot/cold/percussion.
- Check if the tooth is mobile: Palpate tooth and surrounding bone.
- Check for mandibular fracture: Percuss/twist with tongue blade to evaluate.
- Bimanual palpation for maxilla fracture/alveolar fracture
- If tooth missing, investigate for intrusion of tooth or root fragment in socket.

DIAGNOSTIC TESTS & INTERPRETATION
Lab
Initial lab tests
No initial labs needed, unless patient appears acutely ill.

Imaging
Initial approach
Panoramic radiograph of the teeth and jaw for evaluation of the extent of injury; computed tomography (CT) scan only needed if other associated head trauma.

Follow-Up & Special Considerations
Chest x-ray may be needed for lost avulsed teeth: May be in trachea, lungs, esophagus, or stomach

DIFFERENTIAL DIAGNOSIS
- Crown fracture
- Root fracture
- Subluxation of tooth
- Extrusion/intrusion of tooth
- Trismus

TREATMENT

Assess ABCs for other problems associated with the traumatic injury.

MEDICATION
First Line
- Pain management:
  - Ibuprofen 600–800 mg (or 10 mg/kg) q6h, or acetaminophen 650–1,000 mg (10–15 mg/kg) q4–6h
  - For more severe pain, consider acetaminophen or ibuprofen + opioids.
  - Can consider local anesthetic nerve block with long-acting anesthetic (bupivacaine) as adjunct
- Antibiotics for fractures or avulsions to prevent complications:
  - Penicillin VK 500 mg q.i.d. for 7 days in adults. For children, 10 mg/kg/dose q.i.d.
  - Clindamycin 150–300 mg t.i.d. (or 5–7.5 mg/kg/dose) in penicillin-allergic patients

Second Line
- Phenoxymethyl penicillin 200–500 mg p.o. q6h for children <12 years
- Clindamycin 150–300 mg t.i.d. (or 5–7.5 mg/kg/dose) in penicillin-allergic patients

ADDITIONAL TREATMENT
General Measures
- Fractured teeth:
  - Ellis I: Smooth edges with emery board or dental drill; cosmetic repair can be done by dentist in follow-up.
  - Ellis II and III: Cover exposed area with calcium hydroxide paste (Dycal). Tooth must be dry before adding Dycal. If not available, Coe-Pak (zinc oxide preparation) can be used. Wrap preparation around fractured tooth edge. Follow up with dentist within 24 hours, if other injuries permit.
- Primary goal of reimplantation/repositioning is to protect periodontal ligament; tooth pulp may die, but tooth can be saved by root canal.
- Subluxation (abnormal mobility) of teeth:
  - Patient should be referred to dentist as soon as possible to evaluate for possible repositioning and splinting.
  - Nonrigid splint should be placed ASAP.
- Intrusion (apical displacement of tooth into the alveolar bone):
  - Primary teeth should be left alone to allow for spontaneous eruption after dental follow-up.
  - For permanent teeth, do not reposition; refer to oral surgeon ASAP. Attempts to reposition may cause compromise of blood supply to supporting bone and nerve. Alveolar bone may have necrosis, causing bony defect. Tooth usually needs to be extracted when bone heals.

- Avulsed teeth: Dental emergency:
  - Time is of the essence when reimplanting teeth.
  - If primary tooth: Do not reimplant. If unsure, consult dentist.
  - If permanent tooth: Avoid touching tooth root, handle only by the crown; rinse with normal saline. Minimize trauma to socket. If dirt or large clot in socket, perform gentle irrigation of the socket with normal saline and light aspiration of blood clot before implantation.
  - If tooth is outside of socket <20 minutes, attempt implantation of tooth and stabilize with resin/metal splint, or, if not available, zinc oxide (Coe-Pak) splint.
  - If tooth is outside of socket 20–60 minutes, soak tooth in Hanks solution for 30 minutes to preserve pH. If Hanks is not available, use saline. Attempt implantation and stabilization.
  - If tooth is outside of socket >60 minutes, soak tooth in citric acid and fluoride for 30 minutes; attempt reimplantation and stabilization. If citric acid/fluoride not available, use Hanks or saline.
  - Consult dentist for follow-up and for any questions.
- Soft foods only for 10–14 days, depending on injury.
- Jaw fracture:
  - Assess for displacement.
  - If nerve impingement, immediate surgery needed. Contact oral surgeon ASAP.
  - If not displaced or no indication of nerve impingement, have patient see oral surgeon within 24 hours for fixation.

Issues for Referral
- All patients should be referred to a dentist for follow-up.
- Splints are typically maintained in place for 7–10 days for subluxed teeth and 2–8 weeks for avulsed teeth. Alveolar fractures should be splinted for 4–6 weeks and can take up to 6 months to heal.
- Avulsed teeth continue to deteriorate up to 36 months after injury and typically require root canal therapy.
- Oral surgeon should follow jaw fractures in consultation with general dentist.

Additional Therapies
Tetanus booster should be considered if tetanus coverage is uncertain or if tooth has been in contact with soil or deep lacerations present.

COMPLEMENTARY AND ALTERNATIVE MEDICINE
- Acupuncture (1)[C]
- Clove oils (2)[C]

SURGERY/OTHER PROCEDURES
Oral surgeon referral within 1 hour if patient has alveolar bone fracture or jaw fracture. Reduction is easier before swelling.

IN-PATIENT CONSIDERATIONS
Initial Stabilization
Secure airway if compromised with either endotracheal intubation or tracheotomy.

Admission Criteria
Criteria for hospital admission include swelling compromising airway, mental status change due to concussion or hypoxia, after aspiration of teeth, or unstable vital signs.

IV Fluids
IV fluid resuscitation with normal saline may be indicated in septic patients.

Nursing
Ensure excellent oral hygiene. Rinse mouth with chlorhexidine gluconate to minimize bacterial load in oral cavity.

Discharge Criteria
Discharge patient when:
- Abscess and sepsis have been eliminated
- Patient able to take in adequate p.o. and ambulation
- Cleared from concussion

 ## ONGOING CARE

FOLLOW-UP RECOMMENDATIONS
Follow-up with dentist or oral surgeon within 24 hours after any dental trauma:
- Restrict use of pacifiers if dental injuries are involved.
- Ellis III fractures in children <12 years are likely to get infected; clinicians should consider antibiotic coverage.

Patient Monitoring
Biannual cleaning and follow-up. First 36 months most critical to long-term prognosis.

DIET
Avoid any solid food before following up with dentist, and maintain diet as directed by dentist.

PATIENT EDUCATION
- Use a soft toothbrush and soft diet for 10–14 days after dental trauma. Rinse with chlorhexidine 0.1% twice a day for 1 week to prevent plaque and debris accumulation (3)[A].
- If tooth avulsion occurs, handle tooth only by the crown.
- Cold milk is the best transportation medium before coming to the emergency room, as it maintains the periodontal ligament for about 3 hours and has pH and osmolarity to maintain vitality of the cells. Saline or saliva is a good substitute. Water is the least desirable transport medium because it is a hypotonic solution that can lyse the cells.

PROGNOSIS
- <20 minutes of tooth separation from socket: Good prognosis
- >60 minutes of tooth separation: Poor prognosis for tooth reattachment
- Alveolar fracture: Poor prognosis for teeth involved
- Jaw fracture: Good prognosis with proper reduction/fixation

COMPLICATIONS
- Tooth loss
- Infection
- Cosmetic and/or functional deformity
- Anesthesia/paraesthesia of nerve entrapment with fractured jaw, especially mandibular fracture

REFERENCES
1. NIH Consensus Conference. Acupuncture. *JAMA*. 1998;280:1518–24.
2. Alan S. Marathon Man lessons for dental pain. *Emerg Med News*. 2005;27(9):20–21.
3. Flores MT, Andersson L, Andreasen JO, et al. Guidelines for the management of traumatic dental injuries. II. Avulsion of permanent teeth. *Dent Traumatol*. 2007;23:130–6.

ADDITIONAL READING
- Andreasen JO, Lauridsen E, Christensen SS. Development of an interactive dental trauma guide. *Pediatr Dent*. 2009;31:133–6.
- Celenk S, Sezgin B, Ayna B, et al. Causes of dental fractures in the early permanent dentition: a retrospective study. *J Endod*. 2002;28:208–10.
- Evidence-based review of clinical studies on trauma. *J Endod*. 2009;35:1160–2.
- Flores MT, Andersson L, Andreasen JO, et al. Guidelines for the management of traumatic dental injuries. I. Fractures and luxations of permanent teeth. *Dent Traumatol*. 2007;23:66–71.
- Flores MT, Andreasen JO, Bakland LK, et al. Guidelines for the evaluation and management of traumatic dental injuries. *Dent Traumatol*. 2001;17:193–8.
- Ong CKS, et al. An evidence-based update of the use of analgesics in dentistry. *Periodontology*. 2008;46(1):143–164.
- Vellappally S, Fiala Z, Smejkalová J, et al. Smoking related systemic and oral diseases. *Acta Medica (Hradec Kralove)*. 2007;50:161–6.
- Wilson S, et al. Epidemiology of dental trauma treated in an urban pediatric emergency department. *Pediatr Emerg Care*. l997;13:12–15.

 ## CODES

ICD9
- 802.20 Closed fracture of unspecified site of mandible
- 873.63 Open wound of internal structures of mouth, tooth (broken) (fractured) (due to trauma), uncomplicated
- 873.73 Open wound of internal structures of mouth, tooth (broken) (fractured) (due to trauma), complicated

CLINICAL PEARLS
- Do not reimplant primary teeth. Reimplant permanent teeth ASAP.
- Milk is the best transportation medium before coming to emergency room (ER), as it maintains the periodontal ligament for about 3 hours and has protective pH and osmolarity. Saline or saliva is a good substitute. Water is the least desirable transport medium because it is a hypotonic solution.
- Consider child abuse in younger patients.
- Young children are more likely to get infection after Ellis fractures; consider antibiotic coverage.
- Ensure tetanus vaccination is updated.

DEPENDENT PERSONALITY DISORDER

Heath A. Grames, PhD
W. Jeff Hinton, PhD

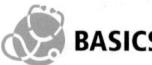 **BASICS**

DESCRIPTION
Beginning no later than adolescence or early adulthood, a consistent and pervasive pattern of dependency on others to make even the most trivial decisions, feelings of incompetence, and an excessive need for care by others (1):
- Common behaviors and variations:
  – Can be very clingy to caregivers
  – May isolate contact they have with other people to interactions with caregivers
  – May be very agreeable or submissive with others (even when they don't agree) out of fear of losing support/approval
  – May experience large amounts of distress when faced with decisions
  – May experience fear when alone
  – Lack of independence/fear of independence
  – Above behaviors are in excess of cultural norms
- Patients with this disorder typically display little insight into their behavior.

Geriatric Considerations
Illness (acute and chronic) may exacerbate dependent personality disorder (DPD) behaviors and may lead to intense feelings of fear and helplessness.

Pediatric Considerations
Diagnosis is rarely made for children/adolescents (may not be appropriate due to dependency needs of children/adolescents). Axis I disorders must be ruled out, as well as behavior related to a general medical condition or to the developmental cycle of the child. For diagnosis, baseline behaviors must be representative of DPD for a duration of at least 1 year.

Pregnancy Considerations
Physical and social changes may induce stress or increase fears, which may result in increased dependent behaviors. Distinguish this disorder from increased dependency due to pregnancy (i.e., when there is no, or poor, support system).

EPIDEMIOLOGY
- Predominant age: Onset no later than adolescence or early adulthood (may go undiagnosed for years)
- Predominant sex: Female > Male

Prevalence
- DPD accounts for 20–30% of all personality disorders in primary care outpatient settings (2).
- DPD is among the most common personality disorder in mental health clinics.

RISK FACTORS
- Chronic or severe illness or disability in children
- Childhood/adolescent separation anxiety
- Parenting style that does not encourage age-appropriate independence

GENERAL PREVENTION
Children with chronic illness or handicap may be more susceptible to DPD. When possible, foster appropriate independence in the face of disability.

ETIOLOGY
Undetermined; however, generally accepted that it is due to a combination of the following:
- Hereditary temperamental traits
- Environment (e.g., not allowed independence; age-appropriate)
- Developmental traits

COMMONLY ASSOCIATED CONDITIONS
- Co-occurring personality disorders: Frequent
- Increased risk with mood anxiety and adjustment disorders

 DIAGNOSIS

Due to high co-occurrence with other Axis II disorders, assess suicide ideation and self-harm behavior.

HISTORY
- Difficulty making decisions (even trivial decisions) without a great deal of reassurance and coaxing (1)
- Dramatic/urgent demands for medical attention (even when symptoms are not painful or life-threatening)
- May actively attempt to prolong illness or seek unnecessary medical procedures (3)
- Perception that he or she needs to be taken care of
- Clingy/demanding
- Seeks primary care provider and other caregivers to make decisions
- Once physician is in role of caregiver, may become submissive, agreeable (fear of losing relationship)
- Important to obtain collateral information (i.e., from family, partner) about patient behaviors
- Ask about substance abuse.

DIAGNOSTIC TESTS & INTERPRETATION
- Consider age of onset. To meet criteria for DPD, dependent pattern will be present from early adulthood.
- If symptoms begin later than early adulthood or are related to trauma (e.g., after a head injury), a general medical condition (GMC), or substance, consider other diagnoses.
- Rule out personality change due to a GMC:
  – Traits may emerge due to the effect of a GMC on the central nervous system (1).
- Rule out symptoms related to chronic substance abuse.
- Consider referring patient for formal psychological testing.
- Diagnostic accuracy may be improved through the utilization of the Structured Clinical Interview for DSM-IV Axis II Disorders (SCID-II) (4).

Diagnostic Procedures/Surgery
Must meet at least 5 of the following criteria for diagnosis (1):
- Indecisive: Needs support/reassurance from others to make decisions
- Defers personal responsibility (decision making, life choices) to others
- Does not voice disagreement with others without difficulty out of fear of losing relationship
- Not including realistic fears of abuse/retribution
- Difficulty starting/doing projects independently
- Seeks nurturance/support from others, even at great personal costs
- Experiences discomfort with solitude; fears having to care for self

DIFFERENTIAL DIAGNOSIS
Other psychiatric conditions, such as:
- Mood disorders:
  – Consider baseline behaviors when considering DPD vs mood disorder.
- Anxiety disorders:
  – With DPD, chronic baseline behaviors will suggest personality disorder (does not only occur at moments of stress or with Axis I disorders).

- Adjustment disorder:
  – Differentiate in that dependence from stressor is not chronic and is related to stressor
- Other personality disorder:
  – Consider patient's thoughts, feelings, and behavior to differentiate dependence from other personality disorders.
  – High co-occurrence of DPD and other personality disorders, especially borderline, histrionic, and avoidant
- General medical condition:
  – Traits may emerge due to the effect of a GMC on the central nervous system.
- Chronic substance abuse

TREATMENT

- Inpatient hospitalization is relatively ineffective in changing Axis II disorder behaviors.
- Inpatient hospital services for conditions related to dependent personality disorder should be limited and of short duration to decrease dependence (decreasing likelihood of behavior change).
- Hospitalization should be considered for the following:
  – Adjust medications.
  – Implement psychotherapy for crisis intervention.
  – Stabilize patient (psychosocial stressors).
- If suicidal, may need suicide watch and receive appropriate psychiatric care.

MEDICATION

- No medications treat DPD.
- Treat symptoms and Axis I disorders (2)[C].
- Depression/anxiety (2)[C]:
  – Serotonin reuptake inhibitors
  – Benzodiazepines (short-term) if needed for anxiety symptom relief

ADDITIONAL TREATMENT
General Measures

- Focus on patient management rather than fixing or curing behaviors (2)[C].
- Schedule follow-up to relieve patient stress.
- Meet with and rely on treatment team to avoid burnout and to provide opportunity for team to discuss issues with patient.
- As necessary, refer patient to mental health therapist.

Issues for Referral
Treatment for Axis II disorder should include psychotherapy and/or psychiatry.

Additional Therapies
- Consider referring patient for specialty mental health services.
- Cognitive behavioral therapy has demonstrated some success with Axis II disorders in general.

IN-PATIENT CONSIDERATIONS
Admission Criteria
Refer to inpatient or outpatient psychiatry services if harm to self or others is expressed by the patient and/or suspected by the primary care provider.

ONGOING CARE

FOLLOW-UP RECOMMENDATIONS
- Schedule routine follow-up with patient (relieves patient anxiety about medical care relationship with physician).
- Nurses can be helpful in managing the patient and calling the patient as needed (contact with the patient helps relieve patient stress).
- Focus should be on medical conditions and comorbid Axis I disorders.

PROGNOSIS
- Medical focus is on patient management and caring for medical and Axis I disorders (3).
- With appropriate treatment, including mental health services, patient is viewed as treatment-responsive (5).

REFERENCES

1. American Psychiatric Association. *Diagnostic and Statistical Manual of Mental Disorders*. 4th ed., text revision. Washington, DC: American Psychiatric Association; 2000.
2. Ward RK. Assessment and management of personality disorders. *Am Fam Physician*. 2004;70:1505–12.
3. Feder A, Robbins SW, Ostermeyer B. Personality disorders. In: Feldman, Christensen JF, eds. *Behavioral Medicine in Primary Care: A Practical Guide*. 2nd ed. New York: McGraw-Hill, 2003;231–52.
4. First MB, Gibbon M, Spitzer RL, Williams JBW, Benjamin LS. *Structured clinical interview for DSM-IV Axis II personality disorders, (SCID-II)*. Washington, DC: American Psychiatric Press, Inc., 1997.
5. Eskedal GA, Demetri JM. Etiology and treatment of cluster C personality disorders. *J Mental Health Counsel*. 2006;28:1–17.

CODES

ICD9
301.6 Dependent personality disorder

CLINICAL PEARLS

- To determine whether a patient has a DPD vs dependent behavior from an Axis I or substance-related disorder or from a general medical condition, note that personality disorders are chronic, so look at baseline behavior. Patients with DPD must have developed the personality disorder traits during adolescence or early adulthood rather than after a medical or Axis I change.
- In the outpatient setting, frequent, short visits help patients with DPD to calm their fears of losing support and help providers with time management. When possible, always have an appointment scheduled so patients can look forward to their next visit.
- To feel less overwhelmed when you are seeing a DPD patient, have an agenda ready for the visit. Be cordial—they deserve the same professionalism any patient gets. Address 1–2 issues per clinic visit.
- Many patients will benefit from additional psychotherapy treatments that target thoughts and behaviors associated with clients' underlying dependency needs.

DEPRESSION

Deborah S. Clements, MD

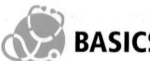 **BASICS**

DESCRIPTION

Depression is a primary mood disorder characterized by a depressed mood and/or decreased interest in things that used to give pleasure (anhedonia) during the same 2-week period, and representing a change from previous functioning:

- Synonym(s): Unipolar affective disorder
- System(s) affected: Nervous

EPIDEMIOLOGY

Incidence
Affects >78 million in the US

Prevalence
- 15% lifetime risk of having major depressive disorder (MDD)
- 4th most common reason to visit a physician

RISK FACTORS
- Female > Male (2:1)
- Predominant age: 1st onset usually in late 20s (earlier in women than men)
- Elderly (≥65)
- History of behavioral disorders
- Presence of chronic disease(s)
- Recent myocardial infarction/stroke
- Peptic ulcer disease
- Strong family history (depression, bipolar, suicide, alcoholism, other substance abuse)
- Domestic abuse or violence
- Substance abuse and dependence
- Losses and stressors
- Single, divorced, or unhappily married

Genetics
Multiple gene loci place a person at increased risk when faced with environmental stressors.

PATHOPHYSIOLOGY
- Changes in receptor–neurotransmitter relationship in the limbic system:
  - Serotonin and norepinephrine are the primary neurotransmitters involved; dopamine, acetylcholine, and γ-aminobutyric acid have also been involved.
- As action potential is passed on, the neurotransmitter is:
  - Reabsorbed into the neuron, where it is either destroyed by an enzyme or actively removed by a reuptake pump and stored until needed or
  - Destroyed by monoamine oxidase in the mitochondria
- Symptoms related to decreased levels of norepinephrine (dullness and lethargy) and serotonin (irritability, hostility, and suicidal ideation)

ETIOLOGY
- Impaired synthesis of neurotransmitters
- Increased metabolism of neurotransmitters
- Environmental factors and learned behavior may affect neurotransmitters and/or have an independent influence on depression.

COMMONLY ASSOCIATED CONDITIONS
- Manic depression (bipolar disorder)
- Cyclothymic and grief reactions
- Anxiety disorders
- Schizophrenia/schizoaffective disorders
- Psychophysiologic disorders
- Physical disorders
- Substance abuse

 DIAGNOSIS

HISTORY
- Depressed mood most of the day, nearly every day
- Anhedonia
- Depression is probable when at least 4 of the following exist in addition to depressed mood or anhedonia:
  - Appetite: Significant weight gain or loss when not dieting (change of >5% of body weight in 1 month)
  - Sleep disturbance: Insomnia or hypersomnia nearly every day
  - Fatigue: Out of proportion to the amount of energy expended
  - Psychomotor retardation or agitation: Restlessness, irritability, or withdrawal
  - Poor self-image: Worthlessness, excessive or inappropriate guilt
  - Concentration: Diminished thinking or concentration, poor memory, indecisiveness
  - Suicidal ideation: Recurrent thoughts of death; sometimes, as patients begin to recover, they gain enough energy to think about and sometimes attempt suicide.

Geriatric Considerations
- Can present with pseudodementia
- More common in elderly and difficult to precisely diagnose due to medical comorbidities (highest rates of depression are associated with stroke, coronary artery disease, cancer, Parkinson disease, and Alzheimer disease)

Pediatric Considerations
Depression occurs in children and can present with somatic complaints, irritability (versus depressed mood), and social withdrawal.

PHYSICAL EXAM
Vital signs and complete physical exam with special attention paid to:
- Thyroid
- Cardiac exam, listening for arrhythmias
- Mental status, including affect

DIAGNOSTIC TESTS & INTERPRETATION
Lab
Initial lab tests
Labs may not be necessary, but are sometimes used to rule out other diagnoses:
- Thyroid-stimulating hormone
- Complete blood count
- Chem 7, including blood sugar
- Calcium
- Liver function tests

Follow-Up & Special Considerations
Electrocardiogram to rule out arrhythmia

Imaging
Initial approach
Electroencephalogram, computed tomography, or magnetic resonance imaging of brain to rule out organic brain disease if suspected

Diagnostic Procedures/Surgery
- Depression is primarily a clinical diagnosis made by eliciting personal, family, social, and psychosocial factors.
- Validated standard rating scales can assist:
  - Clinical Global Impressions Scale
  - Montgomery-Asberg Depression Rating Scale
  - Hamilton Rating Scale for Depression
  - Beck Depression Inventory

DIFFERENTIAL DIAGNOSIS
- Dysthymic disorder
- Bipolar disorder
- Organic brain diseases
- Endocrine/thyroid disorders, diabetes
- Metabolic abnormalities (hypercalcemia)
- Adrenal disease (Cushing)
- Liver/renal failure
- Malignancy
- Chronic fatigue syndrome
- Lupus
- Nutritional: Pernicious anemia, pellagra
- Medications: Abuse, side effects, overdose
- Substances: Abuse, dependence, withdrawal

 TREATMENT

MEDICATION
First Line
- Selective serotonin reuptake inhibitors (SSRIs):
  - Fluoxetine (Prozac): 20–80 mg/d
  - Sertraline (Zoloft): 50–200 mg/d
  - Paroxetine (Paxil): 10–50 mg/d
  - Paroxetine CR (Paxil CR): 12.5–62.5 mg/d
  - Citalopram (Celexa): 20–60 mg/d
  - Escitalopram (Lexapro): 10–20 mg/d
- Others:
  - Venlafaxine (Effexor): 75–375 mg/d (divided doses)
  - Venlafaxine XR (Effexor XR): 75–225 mg/d
  - Bupropion (Wellbutrin): 100–450 mg/d (divided doses, t.i.d.)
  - Bupropion SR (Wellbutrin SR): 100–450 mg/d (divided doses, b.i.d.)
  - Bupropion XL (Wellbutrin XL): 150–300 mg/d
  - Duloxetine (Cymbalta): 30–60 mg/d

Second Line

- Tricyclic antidepressants (TCAs) with sedating properties *condensed list*:
  – Amitriptyline (Elavil): 50–150 mg/QHS, max 300
  – Nortriptyline (Pamelor): 75–150 mg QHS
  – Doxepin (Prudoxin, Zonalon): 75–150 mg QHS
- TCAs with activating properties *condensed list*:
  – Imipramine (Tofranil, Tofranil-PM): 150–200 mg QHS
  – Desipramine (Norpramin): 150–300 mg/d
- α_2-antagonists (sedating):
  – Mirtazapine (Remeron): 15–45 mg QHS
- SSRI/antagonists:
  – Trazodone: 150 mg/d (divided doses), maximum 600 mg/d (divided doses)
- Precautions:
  – Bupropion: Increased risk of seizures
  – TCAs: Advanced age, glaucoma, benign prostate hypertrophy, hyperthyroidism, cardiovascular disease, liver disease, urinary retention, MAOI treatment, potential for fatal overdose
  – SSRIs: Abrupt discontinuation may result in withdrawal symptoms (i.e., dizziness), may raise serum levels of other drugs
- Significant potential interactions:
  – TCAs: Amphetamines, barbiturates, clonidine, epinephrine, ethanol, norepinephrine, MAOIs: Allow 14-day washout period before starting MAOIs, propoxyphene
  – SSRIs and MAOIs: 14-day washout before instituting therapy
  – Venlafaxine may cause fatal serotonin syndrome
  – MAOIs: Significant drug and food interactions limit use, but can be useful in refractory cases.

ALERT

Black-box warning: Increased risk of suicidality in children, adolescents, and young adults up to age 25 treated with SSRI antidepressant medications. Although this has not been extended to adults, suicide risk assessments are warranted for all patients.

Geriatric Considerations

Reduce dosage of medications (1/2 usual starting dose); may need to treat longer than younger adults.

Pediatric Considerations

Reduce dosage of medications in adolescents; also see Alert.

Pregnancy Considerations

SSRIs: If possible, taper and discontinue. (Paroxetine is Category D; the rest of SSRIs are Category C.)

ADDITIONAL TREATMENT

General Measures

Psychotherapeutic interventions act synergistically with pharmacologic therapy.

Additional Therapies

Electroconvulsive therapy for refractory cases

COMPLEMENTARY AND ALTERNATIVE MEDICINE

Use in mild depression; evidence is inconsistent:

- Hypericum perforatum (St. John's wort) (1)[A]: Be aware of multiple drug interactions.
- SAM-e (S-adenosyl methionine): 400–1,600 mg/d (2)[A]

IN-PATIENT CONSIDERATIONS

Admission Criteria

Inpatient care is indicated for severely depressed, psychotic, or suicidal patients.

Discharge Criteria

Depressive symptoms improving, no longer suicidal

ONGOING CARE

FOLLOW-UP RECOMMENDATIONS

Patient Monitoring

- See within 2 weeks after starting medication.
- During follow-up, evaluate the side effects, dosage, and effectiveness of the medication.
- Follow up every 2 weeks until improvement.
- Follow up every 3 months thereafter.
- Explain treatment must continue for at least 6 months to 2 years; longer with family history, severe depression, and in the very young.

PATIENT EDUCATION

- Depression is a medical illness, not a character defect.
- Stress need for long-term treatment and follow-up, which includes lifestyle changes.
- 30 minutes of moderate-intensity exercise, 3–5 days per week for healthy adults (3)[A]

PROGNOSIS

- 70% significant improvement
- It has been shown that of patients with a single depressive episode, 50% develop a recurrent episode.

COMPLICATIONS

- Suicide
- Lower quality-of-life

REFERENCES

1. Keller MB. Issues in treatment-resistant depression. *J Clin Psychiatry*. 2005;66(Suppl 8):5–12.
2. Institute for Clinical Systems Improvement. *Major Depression in Adults in Primary Care*. Bloomington, MN: Institute for Clinical Systems Improvement; 2006.
3. American Psychiatric Association. *Diagnostic and Statistical Manual of Mental Disorders DSM-IV-TR*. 4th ed. [text revision]. Washington, DC: American Psychiatric Publishing, 2000.

ADDITIONAL READING

- Adams SM, Miller KE, Zylstra RG. Pharmacologic management of adult depression. *Am Fam Physician*. 2008;77:785–92.
- Fochtmann LJ, et al. *Guideline Watch: Practice Guideline for the Treatment of Patients with Major Depressive Disorder*, 2nd ed. Accessed June 1, 2008 at: http://www.psych.org/psych_pract/treatg/pg/prac_guide.cfm.
- Halfin A. Depression: the benefits of early and appropriate treatment. *Am J Manag Care*. 2007; 13:S92–7.

- Kessler RC, Berglund P, Demler O, et al. The epidemiology of major depressive disorder: results from the National Comorbidity Survey Replication (NCS-R). *JAMA*. 2003;289:3095–105.
- Kocsis JH, et al. Prevention of recurrent episodes of depression with venlafaxine ER in a 1-year maintenance phase from the PREVENT Study. *J Clin Psychiatry*. 2007;68:1012–23.
- Kornstein SG, Bose A, Li D, et al. Escitalopram maintenance treatment for prevention of recurrent depression: a randomized, placebo-controlled trial. *J Clin Psychiatry*. 2006;67:1767–75.
- Maurer D, Colt R. An evidence-based approach to the management of depression. *Prim Care*. 2006; 33:923–41.
- Roose SP, Sackeim HA, Krishnan KR, et al. Antidepressant pharmacotherapy in the treatment of depression in the very old: a randomized, placebo-controlled trial. *Am J Psychiatry*. 2004;161: 2050–9.
- Skultety KM, Rodriguez RL. Treating geriatric depression in primary care. *Curr Psychiatry Rep*. 2008;10:44–50.
- Thase ME. Treatment of severe depression. *J Clin Psychiatry*. 2000;61(Suppl 1):17–25.

See Also (Topic, Algorithm, Electronic Media Element)

Algorithms: Depressive Episode, Major; Depressed Mood Resulting from Medical Illness

CODES

ICD9

- 296.20 Major depressive affective disorder, single episode, unspecified degree
- 296.30 Major depressive affective disorder, recurrent episode, unspecified degree
- 311 Depressive disorder, not elsewhere classified

CLINICAL PEARLS

- The relationship (therapeutic alliance) between the patient and health care provider is important to the success of treatment.
- Depression management has 2 main goals:
  – Remission: Absence of depressive symptoms with return to full functioning
  – Recovery: No longer meets MDD criteria for at least 8 weeks
- Given the high recurrence rates, long-term treatment is often necessary.

DEPRESSION, ADOLESCENT

Alyssa H. Tran, DO

 BASICS

DESCRIPTION
- Primary mood disorder characterized by sadness or irritability and a loss of self-worth and interest in typically pleasurable activities
- Depression in adolescents is undertreated, as an estimated 70–80% of these patients do not receive appropriate care.
- Dysthymic disorder is differentiated from major depression by less intense symptoms that are more persistent, lasting at least 1 year.
- Depressive disorder NOS is diagnosed when an adolescent presents with depressive symptoms but does not meet the criteria for other diagnoses.
- Treatment-resistant depression is a failure of treatment with 2 antidepressants administered in adequate dosage for at least 6 weeks.
- Depression is more likely to present as irritability or somatic complaints in adolescents (vs acutely depressed mood in adults). Adolescents may present with symptoms primarily when alone or with family, often "fine with friends." Symptoms may include declining grades, change in friends, or experimentation with drugs.

EPIDEMIOLOGY
Incidence
15–20% during adolescence

Prevalence
0.4–8.3% of adolescents. At least twice as common in females.

RISK FACTORS
- Female gender
- Prior depressive episodes
- History of anxiety disorders, ADHD, and/or learning disabilities
- Chronic illness
- Hormonal changes during puberty
- Use of certain medications (e.g., isotretinoin [Accutane]) (1)
- Family history: Risk is increased 3–6 times if 1st-degree relative has a major affective disorder.
- General stressors, such as socioeconomic deprivations, adverse life events/experiences, difficulties with peers, loss of a loved one, academic difficulties
- Childhood neglect or abuse
- Cigarette smoking
- Presence of specific serotonin-transporter gene variants (2)

Genetics
Studies have shown a 76% concordance rate in monozygotic twins reared together and a 67% concordance rate among those reared apart, along with a 19% concordance rate in dizygotic twins reared together.

GENERAL PREVENTION
Insufficient evidence supports the universal implementation of depression prevention programs (psychological and social) (3)[B]. May be a small benefit to regular exercise in preventing episodes of depression (4)[B]

PATHOPHYSIOLOGY
Still fairly unclear, but low functional levels of neurotransmitters may produce symptoms. Decreased norepinephrine may cause dullness and lethargy. Decreased serotonin may cause irritability, hostility, and suicidal ideation.

ETIOLOGY
External factors may affect neurotransmitters or independently affect depression

COMMONLY ASSOCIATED CONDITIONS
- Eating disorders (especially bulimia)
- Substance abuse
- Anxiety disorders
- Behavioral disorders (i.e., ADHD, oppositional defiant disorder, conduct disorder)
- Learning disorders
- Somatization disorders
- Depression in the adolescent population typically emerges after the comorbid disorder (except for substance abuse and conduct disorders).

 DIAGNOSIS

HISTORY
- According to the DSM-IV, adolescents must display EITHER (3) depressed or irritable mood OR (4) loss of interest or pleasure (anhedonia) for most of the day, nearly every day, for at least 2 weeks, causing significant distress or functional impairment.
- In addition, 4 or more of the following symptoms must be present during the same 2-week period:
  – Change in appetite with weight loss or gain (change of >5% of body weight in 1 month)
  – Insomnia or hypersomnia nearly every day
  – Psychomotor agitation or retardation:
    ○ Adolescents will commonly talk or move more slowly and produce less speech with longer response latencies, and may display a flat affect.
    ○ Conversely, they may present with restlessness, excessive movements, and verbal outbursts.
  – Fatigue or loss of energy
  – Feelings of excessive guilt or worthlessness: Adolescents may be extremely self-critical, unable to identify positive self-attributes, or feel they deserve to be punished for things that are not their fault.
  – Indecisiveness or impaired thinking or concentration: School performance may decline significantly.
  – Recurring thoughts of death or suicide or actual attempts at suicide
- Symptoms must not: Meet the criteria for a mixed manic episode (suggestive of bipolar disorder); be due to the effects of a drug or other condition; be secondary to bereavement

PHYSICAL EXAM
Psychomotor retardation or agitation may be present.

ALERT
Clinicians should carefully assess patients for signs of self-injury (wrist lacerations) or abuse.

DIAGNOSTIC TESTS & INTERPRETATION
Lab
Initial lab tests
May be used to rule out other diagnoses (i.e., CBC, TSH, glucose, mono spot)

Imaging
Initial approach
CT or MRI of brain only if brain disease is suspected

Diagnostic Procedures/Surgery
- Depression is primarily diagnosed after conducting a formal clinical interview with the adolescent, combined with supporting information obtained from caregivers and teachers.
- The following standardized tests can be useful as screening tools and to monitor response to treatment, but should not be used as the sole basis for diagnosis:
  – Beck Depression Inventory (BDI): All ages
  – Child Depression Inventory (CDI): Ages 7–17
  – Reynolds Adolescent Depression Scale (RADS): Teenagers in grades 7–12
  – Guidelines for Adolescent Preventive Services (GAPS): To be delivered to parents, younger and older adolescents during their 11–17-year-old annual health visits
- Suicide risk assessment should be performed.
- Office-based screening/case finding questionnaires have minimal impact on the detection, management, or outcome of depression by clinicians (5)[A].

DIFFERENTIAL DIAGNOSIS
- Normal bereavement
- Substance-induced mood disorder
- Bipolar disorder
- Mood disorder secondary to a medical condition
- Endocrine diseases (hypo- or hyperthyroidism)
- Organic CNS diseases
- Malignancy
- Infectious mononucleosis
- Anemia
- Medication side effects (isotretinoin)
- Chronic diseases (diabetes)

 TREATMENT

Pediatric depression is often managed by primary care providers rather than psychiatrists (6).

MEDICATION
First Line
- Fluoxetine (Prozac): Starting dose 10 mg/day. Effective dose 20–60 mg/day: Fluoxetine is the only SSRI approved by the FDA for the treatment of depression in adolescence (7)[B].
- Careful monitoring of the patient for suicidal thoughts and behavior is required, given the possible increased risk while taking any antidepressant. However, completed suicide rates are higher in areas where SSRIs are not prescribed to adolescents (7)[C].

Second Line
- The following SSRIs are NOT approved by the FDA for treatment of adolescent depression, but may be tried as 2nd-line agents at the clinician's discretion (7)[B]:
  – Citalopram (Celexa): Starting dose 10 mg/day. Effective dose 20–60 mg/day.
  – Escitalopram (Lexapro): Starting dose 5 mg/day. Effective dose 10–20 mg/day.

– Fluvoxamine (Luvox): Starting dose 50 mg/day. Effective dose 150–300 mg/day.
– Paroxetine (Paxil) : Starting dose 10 mg/day. Effective dose 20–60 mg/day.
– Sertraline (Zoloft): Starting dose 25 mg/day. Effective dose 50–200 mg/day.

- Venlafaxine (Effexor), nefazodone, mirtazapine, and bupropion may be tried in adolescents who have failed SSRIs, but no evidence supports the use of these atypical antidepressants in this population.
- Tricyclic antidepressants have not been proven to be effective in adolescents and should NOT be used (7,8)[A].

ADDITIONAL TREATMENT

General Measures

- Cognitive behavioral therapy (CBT) is effective in the treatment of mild-to-moderate adolescent depression (7)[A]:
  – Goal is to alter a patient's negative thoughts and behaviors to improve his or her mood by encouraging pleasurable activities (behavioral activation), reducing negative thoughts (cognitive restructuring), and improving assertiveness and problem-solving skills to reduce feelings of hopelessness.
  – Interpersonal psychotherapy (IPT) and family therapy may also be helpful: Treatment targets a patient's interpersonal problems to improve both interpersonal functioning and his or her mood.
- Regular exercise may help reduce depressive symptoms (4)[B].

Issues for Referral

Referral to a child psychiatrist is recommended for adolescents with severe, recurrent, or treatment-resistant depression. Referrals are also recommended if the patient has comorbidities or if the clinician is uncomfortable prescribing complex therapies.

COMPLEMENTARY AND ALTERNATIVE MEDICINE

No evidence supports the use of St. John's wort or acupuncture.

IN-PATIENT CONSIDERATIONS

Admission Criteria

Indicated if an adolescent is severely depressed, psychotic, suicidal, or homicidal

Nursing

Patient may need one-on-one supervision or routine checks for safety if suicidal ideation is present.

 ONGOING CARE

Treatment for at least 6 months reduced the likelihood of suicide attempts compared with treatment for less than 8 weeks (9).

FOLLOW-UP RECOMMENDATIONS

- Systematic and regular tracking of goals and outcomes from treatment should be performed, including assessment of depressive symptoms and functioning in home, school, and peer settings (9).
- Recommendations from National Guideline Clearinghouse: Treatment (9):
  – After initial diagnosis of mild depression, clinicians should consider a period of active support and monitoring before starting other evidence-based treatment.

– If a primary care provider (PCP) identifies an adolescent with moderate or severe depression or complicating factors/conditions such as coexisting substance abuse or psychosis, consultation with a mental health specialist should be considered. Appropriate roles and responsibilities for ongoing management by the PCP and mental health clinicians should be communicated and agreed upon. The patient and family should be consulted and approve the roles of the PC and mental health professionals.
– PCPs should recommend scientifically tested and proven treatments (i.e., psychotherapies such as cognitive behavioral therapy [CBT] or interpersonal therapy [IPT] and/or antidepressant treatment such as selective serotonin reuptake inhibitors [SSRIs]) whenever possible and appropriate to achieve the goals of the treatment plan.
– PCPs should monitor for the emergence of adverse events during antidepressant treatment.

- Recommendations from National Guideline Clearinghouse: Outgoing management (9):
  – Systematic and regular tracking of goals and outcomes from treatment should be performed, including assessment of depressive symptoms and functioning in several key domains: home, school, and peer settings.
  – Diagnosis and initial treatment should be reassessed if no improvement is noted after 6–8 weeks of treatment. Mental health consultation should be considered.
  – For patients who achieve only partial improvement after diagnostic and therapeutic approaches have been exhausted (including exploration of poor adherence, comorbid disorders, and ongoing conflicts or abuse), a mental health consultation should be considered.
  – PCPs should actively support depressed adolescents who are referred to mental health to ensure adequate management. PCPs may also consider sharing care with mental health agencies/professionals when possible. Appropriate roles and responsibilities regarding the provision and coordination of care should be communicated and agreed upon by the PCP and the mental health specialist.

Patient Monitoring

- Once started on antidepressants, patients should be seen weekly for the 1st month, biweekly for the 2nd month, and at least monthly thereafter: Careful monitoring for suicidal thoughts or behavior is required, particularly in the 1st 2 months after initiation or dose increase.
- Length of medication treatment:
  – First episode: Minimum 6 months followed by a slow taper over 6–8 weeks
  – Second episode: At least 1 year
  – Third episode: 1–3 years
  – >3 episodes: Lifelong
- Adverse effects (i.e., nausea, headaches, behavioral activation, etc.) occur in up to 93% of patients treated with SSRIs. Therefore, routine monitoring and discussion of possible medication side effects is critical for depressed youth who are treated with antidepressants.

PATIENT EDUCATION

Educate patients and parents about mental health and the fact that depression is a medical illness, not a character defect.

PROGNOSIS

- If left untreated, major depressive episode in adolescents typically lasts 7–9 months, with 90% resolving within 2 years.
- CBT alone is effective treatment in 40–50%.
- Combination therapy of CBT with fluoxetine results in improvement in 71% of patients.
- Recurrence is 40% by 2 years and 70% by 5 years.

COMPLICATIONS

- Lack of improvement in symptoms
- School failure or refusal
- Suicide

REFERENCES

1. Wysowski DK, Pitts M, Beitz J. An analysis of reports of depression and suicide in patients treated with isotretinoin. *J Am Acad Dermatol*. 2001;45:515–9.
2. Hariri AR, Mattay VS, Tessitore A, Kolachana B, Fera F, Goldman D, et al. Serotonin transporter genetic variation and the response of the human amygdala. *Science*. 2002;297:400–3.
3. Merry S, et al. Psychological and/or educational interventions for the prevention of depression in children and adolescents. Cochrane Depression, Anxiety and Neurosis Group. *Cochrane Database Syst Rev*. 2007:4.
4. Larun L, et al. Exercise in prevention and treatment of anxiety and depression among children and young people. Cochrane Depression, Anxiety and Neurosis Group. *Cochrane Database Syst Rev*. 2007:4.
5. Gilbody S, et al. Screening and case finding instruments for depression. Cochrane Depression, Anxiety and Neurosis Group. *Cochrane Database Syst Rev*. 2007:4.
6. Cheung AH, Dewa CS, Levitt AJ, et al. Pediatric depressive disorders: management priorities in primary care. *Curr Opin Pediatr*. 2008;20:551–9.
7. Bhatia SK, Bhatia SC. Childhood and adolescent depression. *Am Fam Physician*. 2007;75:73–80.
8. Hazell P, et al. Tricyclic drugs for depression in children and adolescents. Cochrane Depression, Anxiety and Neurosis Group. *Cochrane Database Syst Rev*. 2007:4.
9. Cheung AH, Zuckerbrot RA, Jensen PS, et al. Guidelines for Adolescent Depression in Primary Care (GLAD-PC): II. Treatment and ongoing management. *Pediatrics*. 2007;120:e1313–26.

 CODES

ICD9

- 296.20 Major depressive affective disorder, single episode, unspecified degree
- 296.30 Major depressive affective disorder, recurrent episode, unspecified degree
- 311 Depressive disorder, not elsewhere classified

CLINICAL PEARLS

- Adolescent depression is underdiagnosed and often presents with irritability and anhedonia.
- CBT combined with fluoxetine is most efficacious for adolescents with major depression.
- Referral to a child psychiatrist is appropriate for complex cases.

DEPRESSION, GERIATRIC

Anna Mirk, MD
Frederick Wu, MD

BASICS

DESCRIPTION
Depression is a primary mood disorder characterized by a depressed mood and/or a markedly decreased interest or pleasure in normally enjoyable activities for at least 2 weeks and causing significant distress or impairment in daily functioning.

EPIDEMIOLOGY
Prevalence rates among the elderly vary, largely depending on the specific diagnostic instruments used and their current health and/or home environment:
- 1–3% of community-dwelling elderly
- 7.5% seen in primary care clinics
- 10–21% of hospitalized elderly patients
- 12–27% of nursing home residents

RISK FACTORS
- General:
  - Chronic physical health condition(s)
  - History of mental health problems
  - Death of a loved one
  - Caregiving
  - Social isolation
  - Lack or loss of social support
  - Significant loss of independence
  - Uncontrolled pain
  - Insomnia/sleep disturbance
- Prevalence of depression in medical illness:
  - Stroke (22–50%)
  - Cancer (18–50%)
  - Myocardial infarction (15–45%)
  - Parkinson disease (10–39%)
  - Rheumatoid arthritis (13%)
  - Diabetes mellitus (5–11%)
  - Alzheimer's dementia (5-15%)
- Suicide:
  - Suicide is the 11th leading cause of death in the US for all ages.
  - Suicide rates are higher for Americans age >65 compared to the general population (approximately 15 per 100,000 people).
  - Suicide rates are highest for males aged >75 (rate 38.5 per 100,000).

PATHOPHYSIOLOGY
- There are still significant gaps in the understanding of the underlying pathophysiology.
- Ongoing research has identified several possible mechanisms, including:
  - Monoamine transmission and associated transcriptional and translational activity
  - Epigenetic mechanisms and resilience factors
  - Neurotrophins, neurogenesis, neuroimmune systems, and neuroendocrine systems

ETIOLOGY
Depression appears to be a complex interaction between heritable and environmental factors.

DIAGNOSIS

HISTORY
- Depressed mood most of the day, nearly every day, and/or loss of interest or pleasure in life
- Other common symptoms include:
  - Feeling hopeless, helpless, or worthless
  - Insomnia and loss of appetite/weight (alternatively, hypersomnia with increased appetite/weight in atypical depression)
  - Fatigue and loss of energy
  - Somatic symptoms (headaches, chronic pain)
  - Neglect of personal responsibility or care
  - Psychomotor retardation or agitation
  - Diminished concentration, indecisiveness
  - Thoughts of death or suicide

Screening with **SIGECAPS**:
- **S**LEEP: Changes in sleep habits from baseline, including excessive sleep, early waking, or inability to fall asleep
- **I**NTEREST: Loss of interest in previously enjoyable activities
- **G**UILT: Guilt that may or may not focus on a specific problem or circumstance
- **E**NERGY: Perceived lack of energy
- **C**ONCENTRATION: Inability to concentrate on specific tasks
- **A**PPETITE: Increase or decrease in appetite
- **P**SYCHOMOTOR: Restlessness and agitation, or the perception that everyday activities are too strenuous to manage
- **S**UICIDALITY: Desire to end life or hurt oneself, harmful thoughts directed internally, or thoughts of homicidality

DIAGNOSTIC TESTS & INTERPRETATION
Lab
Initial laboratory evaluation is done primarily to rule out potential medical factors that could be causing symptoms.

Initial lab tests
- Thyroid-stimulating hormone (TSH)
- Complete blood count with differential
- Comprehensive metabolic panel, including liver function
- Urine drug screen
- Vitamin B_{12}

Follow-Up & Special Considerations
Additional testing for possible confounding medical and cognitive disorders as warranted

Diagnostic Procedures/Surgery
Validated screening tools and rating scales:
- Geriatric Depression Scale: 15- or 30-point scales
- Patient Health Questionnaire (PHQ-2 or PHQ-9)
- The Hamilton Depression Rating Scale
- The Beck Depression Inventory

DIFFERENTIAL DIAGNOSIS
Concurrent medical conditions, cognitive disorders, and medications may produce neurovegetative symptoms that may mimic depression:
- Medical conditions: e.g., hypothyroidism, B_{12} deficiency, liver or renal failure, cancers, stroke
- Medication induced: e.g., interferon-α, β-blockers, isotretinoin
- Dementia and neurodegenerative disorders
- Delirium
- Psychiatric disorders: e.g., bipolar disorder, dysthymic disorder, anxiety disorders, substance abuse-related mood disorders, psychotic disorders

TREATMENT

Although response alone, usually interpreted as a 50% reduction in symptoms, can be clinically meaningful, the goal is to treat patients to the point of remission (i.e., essentially the absence of depressive symptoms).

MEDICATION
- Typically more conservative initial dosing and titration of antidepressants in the elderly, starting with 1/2 of the usual initiation dose and increasing within a couple of weeks if tolerated
- Continue titrating dose every 3–4 weeks as appropriate. It is important to reach an adequate treatment dose.

First Line
- Selective serotonin reuptake inhibitors (SSRIs) have been found to be effective in treating depression in the elderly (1,2)[A].
- No single SSRI clearly outperforms others in the class; choice of medication often reflects side effect profile or practitioner familiarity:
  - Citalopram: Start at 10 mg/day. Treatment range 20–60 mg/day.
  - Sertraline: Start at 25 mg/day. Treatment range 50–200 mg/day.
  - Escitalopram: Start at 5–10 mg/day. Treatment range 10-20 mg/day.
  - Fluoxetine: Start at 10 mg/day. Treatment range 20–60 mg/day.
  - Paroxetine: Start at 10 mg/day. Treatment range 20–60 mg/day.
- SSRIs should not be used concomitantly with monoamine oxidase inhibitors (MAOIs).

Second Line
- Atypical antidepressants: More effective than placebo in treatment of depression in the elderly, although additional studies are needed to better delineate patient factors that determine response (3)[A]:
  - Bupropion (immediate, sustained/twice a day, and extended/once daily available): Start at 100 mg/day. Increase dose in 3 days. Treatment range 200-300 mg/day. Avoid in patients with elevated seizure risk.
  - Venlafaxine (immediate and sustained release available): Start at 37.5 mg and titrate weekly. Treatment range 75–300 mg/day. May be associated with elevated blood pressure at higher doses.

– Duloxetine: Start at 30 mg/day. Treatment range 30–60 mg/day. Also may be associated with elevated blood pressure.
– Mirtazapine: Start at 7.5–15 mg/nightly. Treatment range 15–45 mg/day. Can produce problems with weight gain, sedation, and cognitive dysfunction.

- For patients who have not responded to initial SSRI trial:
  – Switch to a different SSRI medication, switch to an atypical antidepressant, or augment initial antidepressant with bupropion (4,5,6)[B].

ADDITIONAL TREATMENT

- Tricyclic antidepressants (TCAs) have been shown to be effective in treating depression in the elderly (1,2)[A]. However, they are difficult for elderly patients to tolerate due to side effect profile and are potentially lethal in overdose, limiting their use as initial treatment agents.
- Although not FDA approved, buspirone, lithium, or triiodothyronine are sometimes used off-label to augment a primary antidepressant (6)[B].
- Monoamine oxidase inhibitors (MAOIs) also appear more effective than placebo in the treatment of depression in the elderly (1)[A]. They are not used frequently in clinical practice due to potential side effects and necessary dietary restrictions.

General Measures
Psychotherapy: Studies do show some benefit in depressed elderly patients (7)[B]:
- Cognitive behavioral therapy
- Problem-solving therapy
- Interpersonal therapy
- Psychodynamic psychotherapy

Issues for Referral
Depression with suicidal ideation, psychotic depression, bipolar disorder, co-morbid substance abuse issues, severe or refractory illness

Additional Therapies
- Electroconvulsive therapy (ECT): Has been shown to produce remission of depressive symptoms in the elderly (8)[B]. It should be considered as initial option for patients with severe or psychotic depression.
- Exercise: May be beneficial for depression in the elderly population (9,10)[B].

COMPLEMENTARY AND ALTERNATIVE MEDICINE

- St. John's wort may have minimal benefit (11)[A].
- Tryptophan and hydroxytryptophan: 150–300 mg/d; possible efficacy, additional investigation required (12)[B],(13)

IN-PATIENT CONSIDERATIONS
Inpatient care indicated for imminent safety risk (e.g., acutely suicidal patients) or for those patients unable to care adequately for themselves due to depression.

 ## ONGOING CARE

FOLLOW-UP RECOMMENDATIONS
Due to the delay of benefit following initiation of antidepressant therapy (2–4 weeks), it is necessary to ensure open communication with the patient to prevent premature discontinuation of therapy. An adequate explanation of potential side effects with instructions to call the office before discontinuing therapy is imperative.

Patient Monitoring
- A patient with severe depression who exhibits suicidality may require admission to an appropriate facility.
- Monitor for worsening anxiety symptoms or increase in suicidality.

DIET
No dietary restrictions are necessary, except for patients taking MAOIs, which necessitate dietary restriction of foods high in tyramine.

PATIENT EDUCATION
- Depression is a treatable illness.
- Medications may need to be taken for at least 2–4 weeks before any beneficial effect is noted.
- Depression is often a recurring illness.
- National Suicide Prevention Lifeline at 1-800-273-TALK (8255) is a free, 24-hour hotline available to anyone in suicidal crisis or emotional distress. Calls will be routed to the nearest crisis center.

PROGNOSIS
- Treatment outcomes in the elderly may be worse than in the general population, possibly mediated by physical comorbidities and other factors.
- Depending on the population studied and specific clinical measures used, estimates vary for initial clinical response and remission (between 30% and 70%).

COMPLICATIONS
- Impairment in social, occupational, or interpersonal functioning
- Difficulty performing activities of daily living (ADLs) and self-care
- Increase in medical services utilization and increased costs of care
- Suicide

REFERENCES

1. Wilson K, Mottram PG, Sivananthan A, et al. Antidepressants versus placebo for the depressed elderly. *Cochrane Database of Systematic Reviews* 2001, Issue 1. Edited (no change to conclusions), published in Issue 1, 2009.
2. Mottram PG, Wilson K, Strobl JJ. Antidepressants for depressed elderly. *Cochrane Database of Systematic Reviews* 2006, Issue 1. Edited (no change to conclusions), published in Issue 1, 2009.
3. Nelson JC, Delucchi K, Schneider LS, et al. Efficacy of second generation antidepressants in late-life depression: a meta-analysis of the evidence. *Am J Geriatr Psychiatry.* 2008;16:558–67.
4. Ruhe HG, Huyser J, et al. Switching antidepressants after a first selective serotonin reuptake inhibitor in major depressive disorder: a systematic review. *J Clin Psychiatry* 2006;67(12):1836–1855.
5. Rush AJ, Trivedi MH, et al. Bupropion-SR, sertraline, or venlafaxine-XR after failure of SSRIs for depression. *N Engl J Med.* 2006;354(12):1231–1242.
6. Trivedi MH, Fava M, et al. Medication Augmentation after the Failure of SSRIs for Depression. *New England Journal of Medicine.* 2006;354(12):1243–1252.
7. Wilson KC, Mottram PG, Vassilas CA, et al. Psychotherapeutic treatments for older depressed people. *Cochrane Database Syst Rev.* 2008; CD004853.
8. Van der Wurff FB, et al. Electroconvulsive therapy for the depressed elderly. *Cochrane Database Sys Rev.* 2003;CD003593. DOI:10.1002/14651858. CD003593.
9. Blake H, Mo P, Malik S, et al. How effective are physical activity interventions for alleviating depressive symptoms in older people? A systematic review. *Clin Rehabil.* 2009.
10. Sjösten N, Kivelä SL et al. The effects of physical exercise on depressive symptoms among the aged: a systematic review. *Int J Geriatr Psychiatry.* 2006;21:410–8.
11. Linde K, et al. St. John's wort for depression. *Cochrane Database Sys Rev.* 2005;CD000448. DOI:10.1002/14651858.CD000448.pub2.
12. Shaw K, Turner J, DelMar C. Tryptophan and 5-hydroxytryptophan for depression. *Cochrane Database Sys Rev.* 2002;CD003198. DOI:10.1002/14651858.CD003198.
13. Sarris J, Schoendorfer N, Kavanagh DJ. Major depressive disorder and nutritional medicine: a review of monotherapies and adjuvant treatments. *Nutr Rev.* 2009;67:125–31.

See Also (Topic, Algorithm, Electronic Media Element)
Algorithms: Depressive Episode, Major; Depressed Mood Resulting from Medical Illness

 ## CODES

ICD9
- 290.21 Senile dementia with depressive features
- 311 Depressive disorder, not elsewhere classified

CLINICAL PEARLS

- Depression is not a normal part of aging.
- Depression in the elderly may be difficult to precisely diagnose due to medical and cognitive comorbidities.
- Depression may present primarily with cognitive dysfunction. Cognitive function may improve with treatment of the depression.
- A multidisciplinary approach to the treatment of depression is often most efficacious.
- SSRIs are considered first-line therapy for safety and tolerability. A full remission may take upwards of 12 weeks of treatment. Long-term treatment may be needed to prevent recurrence.

DEPRESSION, POSTPARTUM
Karla M. Rodriguez, MD
Nancy Byatt, DO, MBA

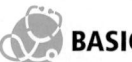 **BASICS**

DESCRIPTION
Major depressive disorder (MDD) that recurs or has its onset in the postpartum period. May also occur in mothers adopting a baby or in fathers (1).

EPIDEMIOLOGY
Incidence
10–15% of mothers within 1st year of giving birth (2)

Prevalence
- Controversial; assessments range from 10–20% during the early postpartum weeks
- Investigators have reported elevated depressive symptoms in 30–50% of women during the early postpartum period with continued symptoms throughout the 1st postpartum year (3).

RISK FACTORS
- Previous episodes of postpartum depression
- History of MDD
- MDD during pregnancy
- Anxiety during pregnancy (4)
- History of premenstrual dysphoria
- Family history of depression (5)
- Unwanted pregnancy
- Socioeconomic stress
- Low self-esteem
- Young maternal age
- Alcohol abuse
- Marital conflict
- Multiple births (6)
- Lack of social and family support system (7)
- Postpartum pain, sleep disturbance, and fatigue
- Assisted reproductive technology pregnancy (8)
- Recent immigrant status
- Increased stressful life events
- History of childhood sexual abuse
- Decision to decrease antidepressants during pregnancy

GENERAL PREVENTION
- Universal screening during the 3rd trimester to diagnose depression and risk factors for depression and to allow initiation of treatment before or immediately after delivery (9)[A]
- Postpartum screening using Edinburgh Postnatal Depression Scale within 4-6 weeks post-delivery (9)[A]
- Continuation of antidepressants in high-risk women during pregnancy may prevent postnatal depression.
- Provide postnatal visits and psychotherapy and/or education for high-risk women.
- Use of depression care manager who provides education, routine telephone contact, and follow-up in order to engage women in treatment

PATHOPHYSIOLOGY
May be related to sensitivity in hormonal fluctuations, including estrogen, progesterone, and other gonadal hormones, as well as neuroactive steroids; cytokines; HPA axis hormones; and altered fatty acid, oxytocin, and arginine vasopressin levels (4)

ETIOLOGY
Multifactorial, including biologic–genetic predisposition in terms of neurobiologic deficit, destabilizing effects of hormone withdrawal at birth, inflammation, and psychosocial stressors (2)

COMMONLY ASSOCIATED CONDITIONS
- Bipolar mood disorder
- Depressive disorder not otherwise specified
- Dysthymic disorder
- Cyclothymic disorder
- Major depressive disorder (10)

 DIAGNOSIS

HISTORY
- Increased/decreased sleep
- Decreased interest in formerly compelling or pleasurable activities
- Guilt, low self-esteem
- Decreased energy
- Decreased concentration
- Increased/decreased appetite
- Psychomotor agitation or retardation
- Suicidal ideation

DIAGNOSTIC TESTS & INTERPRETATION
Lab
Initial lab tests
Thyroid-stimulating hormone (TSH) (11)[A]

Diagnostic Procedures/Surgery
- Edinburgh Postnatal Depression Scale is the primary screening tool.
- Beck, Hamilton, and Zung depression inventories may provide information about the severity of the depression and suicidal risks.
- Edinburgh Postnatal Depression Scale (Partner Version). To be completed by mother's partner to obtain his/her view of mother's depression.

DIFFERENTIAL DIAGNOSIS
- Baby blues: Not a psychiatric disorder, mood lability, resolves within days
- Postpartum psychosis: A psychiatric emergency
- Postpartum anxiety/panic disorder
- Postpartum obsessive-compulsive disorder
- Hypothyroidism
- Postpartum thyroiditis: Can occur in up to 7.5% of patients and can present as depression (12)[A]
- Sleep apnea

 TREATMENT

MEDICATION
First Line
- Selective serotonin reuptake inhibitors (SSRIs) are generally effective and safe:
  – Fluoxetine (Prozac): 20–80 mg/d p.o. (most activating of all SSRIs); less expensive
  – Sertraline (Zoloft): 50–200 mg/d p.o. (sedating)
  – Paroxetine (Paxil): 20–60 mg/d p.o. (sedating)
  – Citalopram (Celexa): 20–60 mg/d p.o.

- Tricyclic antidepressants (TCAs) effective and less expensive, yet are lethal in overdose and have unfavorable side effects:
  – Avoid TCAs in mothers with a history of suicide attempts.
- Bupropion (Wellbutrin): 150–450 mg/d p.o. in patients with depression plus psychomotor retardation, hypersomnia, and with weight gain. Bupropion is less likely to cause weight gain or sexual dysfunction and is highly activating.
- Mirtazapine (Remeron): 15–45 mg/d p.o. q.h.s. May assist with sleep restoration and weight gain; no sexual dysfunction
- Venlafaxine (Effexor XR): A dual-action antidepressant that blocks the reuptake of serotonin in doses of up to 150 mg/d and then blocks the reuptake of norepinephrine in doses of 150–450 mg/d p.o.
- Bipolar disorder requires treatment with mood stabilizer.
- Among breastfeeding mothers:
  – Weigh potential efficacy of treatment with antidepressant, risks of exposure to infant, and known negative effects of not treating on child development.
  – All antidepressants are excreted in breast milk, but are generally compatible with lactation.
  – Paroxetine and sertraline offer best safety profile during lactation.
  – Start with low doses and increase slowly. Monitor infant for adverse side effects.
  – Minimize infant exposure to medication by avoiding breastfeeding at time of peak concentration.
  – Consider continuing medication that is efficacious while monitoring infant carefully, rather than switching antidepressants (4,13)[B].
  – For further information: *Medications and Mother's Milk* by Thomas Hale, PhD

Second Line
Electroconvulsive therapy (ECT): May be indicated in patients who cannot tolerate antidepressant medication, are actively engaged in suicidal self-destructive behaviors, or have a previous history of response to ECT (14)[C]

ADDITIONAL TREATMENT
General Measures
- Most patients respond to outpatient individual psychotherapy in combination with pharmacotherapy.
- Support/therapy groups may be helpful.
- Assess suicidal ideation.
- Assess homicidal ideation and thoughts of harming baby. Thoughts of harming baby require immediate hospitalization.
- Visiting nurse services can provide direct observations of the mother about safety issues and mother–child bonding (10)[A].

Issues for Referral
- Obtain psychiatric consultation for patients with psychotic symptoms.
- Immediate hospitalization is mandatory if delusions or hallucinations are present.
- Hospitalization is indicated if mother's ability to care for self and/or infant is significantly compromised.

Additional Therapies

- Psychoeducation, including providing reading material for the patient and family (10)[C]
- Psychotherapy: Interpersonal psychotherapy, cognitive behavioral therapy, and psychodynamic psychotherapy shown to be effective (4)[C]

COMPLEMENTARY AND ALTERNATIVE MEDICINE

- Breastfeeding is effective in reducing stress and protecting maternal mood (11)[A].
- Infant massage, infant sleep intervention, exercise, and bright light therapy may be beneficial (4)[B],(15)[A].

IN-PATIENT CONSIDERATIONS

ALERT

Obtain psychiatric consultation for patients with psychotic symptoms. If delusions or hallucinations are present, immediate hospitalization is mandatory. The psychotic mother should *not* be left alone with the baby.

Admission Criteria

Presence of suicidal or homicidal ideation and/or psychotic symptoms and/or thoughts of harming baby and/or inability to care for self or infant, severe weight loss

Discharge Criteria

- Absence of suicidal or homicidal ideation and/or psychotic symptoms and/or thoughts of harming baby
- Mother must be able to care for self and infant.

 ONGOING CARE

FOLLOW-UP RECOMMENDATIONS

Patient Monitoring

- Collaborative care approach, including primary care visits and case manager follow-ups
- Consultation with the infant's doctor, particularly if mother is breastfeeding while taking psychotropic medications

DIET

- Good nutrition and hydration, especially when breastfeeding
- The addition of a multivitamin with minerals and Ω-3 fatty acids may be helpful.

PATIENT EDUCATION

- *This Isn't What I Expected: Overcoming Postpartum Depression*, by Karen R. Kleinman and Valerie Davis Radkin
- *Down Came the Rain: My Journey Through Postpartum Depression*, by Brooke Shields, 2005
- *Behind the Smile: My Journey Out of Postpartum Depression*, by Marie Osmond, Marcie Wilkie, and Judith Morre, 2001
- *A Medication Guide for Breastfeeding Moms*, by Thomas Hale and Ghia Mcafee, 2008
- Web resources:
  - Postpartum support international: http://www.postpartum.net
  - http://www.4women.gov
  - La Leche League: http://www.lalecheleague.org
  - http://toxnet.nlm.nih.gov
  - www.mededppd.org
  - www.womensmentalhealth.org
  - www.motherrisk.org

PROGNOSIS

- Treatment of maternal depression to remission has been shown to have a positive impact on children's mental health (13)[B].
- Some patients, particularly those with undertreated or undiagnosed depression, may develop chronic depression requiring long-term treatment (16)[A].
- Untreated maternal depression is linked to impaired child development, including poor cognitive functioning and emotional maladjustment in infants and children (4,13)[B].
- Postpartum psychosis associated with tragic outcomes, such as maternal suicide and infanticide (2,16)[C]

COMPLICATIONS

- Suicide
- Self-injurious behavior
- Psychosis
- Neglect of baby
- Harm to the baby (12)[A]

REFERENCES

1. Paulson JF, Dauber S, Leiferman JA. Individual and combined effects of postpartum depression in mothers and fathers on parenting behavior. *Pediatrics*. 2006;118:659–68.
2. Brett K, et al. Prevalence of self-reported postpartum depressive symptoms: 17 Sate, 2004–2005. *MMWR Weekly*. 2008;361–6.
3. Mayberry J, et al. Depression symptom prevalence and demographic risk factors among U.S. women during the 1st 2 years postpartum. *J Obstet Gynecol Neo Nurs*. 2007;542–9.
4. Pearlstein T, Howard M, Salisbury A, et al. Postpartum depression. *Am J Obstet Gynecol*. 2009;200:357–64.
5. Davey HL, Tough SC, Adair CE, et al. Risk Factors for Sub-Clinical and Major Postpartum Depression Among a Community Cohort of Canadian Women. *Matern Child Health J*. 2008.
6. Choi Y, Bishai D, Minkovitz CS. Multiple births are a risk factor for postpartum maternal depressive symptoms. *Pediatrics*. 2009;123:1147–54.
7. Lee AM, et al. Prevalence, course, risk factors for antenatal anxiety and depression. *Obstet Gyn*. 2007;5:1102–12.
8. Monti F, et al. Depressive symptoms during late pregnancy and early adulthood following assisted reproductive technology. *Fertility Sterility*. 2008;1–7.
9. Jomeen J, et al. Replicability and stability of the multidimensional model of the Edinburgh Postnatal Depression Scale I late pregnancy. *J Psychiatr Mental Health Nurs*. 2007;14:319–24.
10. Howard LM, et al. Antidepressant prevention of postnatal depression. *PLoS Medicine*. 2006;3:1741–2.
11. Kendall-Tackett K. A new paradigm for depression in new mothers: The central role of inflammation and how breastfeeding and anti-inflammatory treatments protect maternal health. *Intl Breastfeeding J*. 2007;2:6.
12. Harrington AR, Greene-Harrington CC. Healthy Start screens for depression among urban pregnant, postpartum and interconceptional women. *J Natl Med Assoc*. 2007;99:226–31.
13. Freeman MP. Breastfeeding and antidepressants: clinical dilemmas and expert perspectives. *J Clin Psychiatry*. 2009;70:291–2.
14. Forray A, Ostroff RB. The use of electroconvulsive therapy in postpartum affective disorders. *J ECT*. 2007;23:188–93.
15. Daley AJ, Macarthur C, Winter H. The role of exercise in treating postpartum depression: a review of the literature. *J Midwifery Womens Health*. 2007;52:56–62.
16. Tammentie T, Tarkka MT, Astedt-Kurki P, et al. Family dynamics and postnatal depression. *J Psychiatr Ment Health Nurs*. 2004;11:141–9.
17. Musters C, McDonald E, Jones I. Management of postnatal depression. *BMJ*. 2008;337:a736.

ADDITIONAL READING

- Gjerdingen D, et al. Stepped care treatment of postpartum depression. *Women's Health Issues*. 2007;18:44–52.
- Sit DK, Wisner KL et al. Identification of postpartum depression. *Clin Obstet Gynecol*. 2009;52:456–68.

 CODES

ICD9

- 296.20 Major depressive affective disorder, single episode, unspecified degree
- 296.30 Major depressive affective disorder, recurrent episode, unspecified degree
- 648.44 Postpartum mental disorders of mother

CLINICAL PEARLS

- PPD is a common, debilitating medical condition that impairs a mother's ability to function and interact with her infant and family.
- Universal screening for PPD is recommended during the 3rd trimester and at regular intervals during the postpartum period.
- Early diagnosis and treatment are vital, as untreated PPD can lead to developmental difficulties for the infant and prolonged disability and suffering for the mother (4,17)[B].
- Breastfeeding is recommended for maternal and child health. There are several medication options for treating depression in mothers that are safe for breastfeeding infants.

DERMATITIS, ATOPIC

Dennis E. Hughes, DO

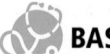 **BASICS**

DESCRIPTION
- Chronic, relapsing, pruritic eczematous condition affecting characteristic sites
- System(s) affected: Skin/Exocrine
- Synonym(s): Eczema; Atopic eczema; Atopic neurodermatitis; Constitutional dermatitis; Besnier prurigo

EPIDEMIOLOGY
Environmentally triggered in susceptible individuals

Incidence
- 45% of all cases begin in the 1st 6 months of life.
- 70% of affected children will have a spontaneous remission before adolescence.

Prevalence
- Mainly childhood disease; affects 10% of all children
- Also may have late-onset dermatitis in adults
- Visits for the condition have been rising over the last 10 years.
- Asians and blacks affected more often than whites
- 60% for one affected parent; rises to 80% if both parents affected

RISK FACTORS
- "Itch-scratch cycle"
- Skin infections
- Emotional stress
- Irritating clothes and chemicals
- Excessively hot or cold climate
- Food allergy in children (in some cases)
- Exposure to tobacco smoke
- Family history of atopy:
  - Asthma
  - Allergic rhinitis

Genetics
- Arises from gene-gene and gene-environment interactions
- Both epidermal and immune coding likely involved

PATHOPHYSIOLOGY
- Alteration in stratum corneum results in transepidermal water loss.
- Epidermal adhesion is reduced either as a result of genetic mutation or as a result of inflammatory response.
- Interleukin 31 (IL-31) upregulation is thought to be a major factor in pruritus rather than histamine excess.

COMMONLY ASSOCIATED CONDITIONS
- Food sensitivity/allergy in many cases
- Asthma
- Allergic rhinitis
- Hyper-IgE syndrome (Job syndrome):
  - Atopic dermatitis
  - Elevated IgE
  - Recurrent pyodermas
  - Decreased chemotaxis of mononuclear cells

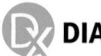 **DIAGNOSIS**

HISTORY
Pruritus is the most common symptom.

PHYSICAL EXAM
- Distribution of lesions:
  - Infants: Trunk, face, and flexural surfaces; diaper-sparing
  - Children: Antecubital and popliteal fossae
  - Adults: Hands, feet, face, neck, upper chest, and genital areas
- Morphology of lesions:
  - Infants: Erythema and papules; may develop oozing, crusting vesicles
  - Children and adults: Lichenification and scaling are typical with chronic eczema as a result of persistent scratching and rubbing (lichenification rare in infants).
- Associated signs:
  - Facial erythema, mild to moderate
  - Perioral pallor
  - Infraorbital fold (Dennie sign/Morgan line)
  - Dry skin
  - Increased palmar linear markings
  - Pityriasis alba (hypopigmented asymptomatic areas on face and shoulders)
  - Keratosis pilaris

DIAGNOSTIC TESTS & INTERPRETATION
Lab
Initial lab tests
- No test is diagnostic.
- Serum IgE levels are elevated in as many as 80% of affected individuals.
- Eosinophilia tends to correlate with disease severity.

Pathological Findings
- Epidermis thickened and hyperkeratotic
- Perivascular inflammation of dermis

DIFFERENTIAL DIAGNOSIS
- Photosensitivity rashes
- Contact dermatitis (especially if only the face is involved)
- Scabies
- Seborrheic dermatitis (especially in infants)
- Psoriasis or lichen simplex chronicus if only localized disease is present in adults
- Rare conditions of infancy:
  - Histiocytosis X
  - Wiskott-Aldrich syndrome
  - Ataxia-telangiectasia syndrome
- Ichthyosis vulgaris

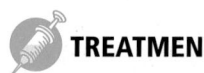 **TREATMENT**

Pediatric Considerations
Chronic potent fluorinated corticosteroid use may cause striae, hypopigmentation, or atrophy, especially in children.

MEDICATION
First Line
- Frequent systemic lubrication with thick emollient creams (e.g., Eucerin, Vaseline) over moist skin is the mainstay of treatment before any other intervention is considered.
- Infants and children: 0.5–1% topical hydrocortisone creams or ointments (1)[C]
- Adults: Higher-potency topical corticosteroids in areas other than face and skin folds
- Short-course higher-potency corticosteroids for flares; then return to the lowest potency (creams preferred) that will control dermatitis (2)[C]. Hypopigmentation can occur even with short-term use.
- Antihistamines for pruritus (e.g., Hydroxyzine 10–25 mg at bedtime and as needed)

Second Line

- Topical immunomodulators (tacrolimus or pimecrolimus) for episodic use for children >2 years of age. There is a black box warning from the Food and Drug Administration regarding potential cancer risk (3).
- Plastic occlusion in combination with topical medication to promote absorption
- For severe atopic dermatitis, consider systemic steroids × 1–2 weeks [e.g., Prednisone 2 mg/kg/d PO (maximum 80 mg/d) initially, tapered over 7–14 days].
- Topical tricyclic doxepin as a 5% cream may decrease pruritus.
- Modified Goeckerman regimen (tar and ultraviolet light)
- Immune modifiers (methotrexate, azathioprine, cyclosporine)

ADDITIONAL TREATMENT

General Measures

- Decrease stress if possible.
- Avoid agents that may cause irritation (e.g., wool, perfumes).
- Minimize sweating.
- Lukewarm (not hot) baths
- Minimize use of soap (superfatted soaps best).
- Frequent systemic lubrication with thick emollient creams (e.g., Eucerin) over moist skin
- Sun exposure may be helpful.
- Humidify the house.
- Avoid excessive contact with water.
- Avoid lotions that contain alcohol.
- If very resistant to treatment, search for a coexisting contact dermatitis.

Issues for Referral

- Ophthalmology evaluation for persistent vernal conjunctivitis
- If using topical steroids around eyes for extended periods, ophthalmology follow-up for cataract evaluation

Additional Therapies

- Methods to reduce house mite allergens (micropore filters on heating, ventilation, and air-conditioning systems, impermeable mattress covers) (4)[C]
- Behavioral relaxation therapy to reduce scratching (4)[B]

COMPLEMENTARY AND ALTERNATIVE MEDICINE

- Evening primrose oil (includes high content of fatty acids):
  - May decrease prostaglandin synthesis
  - May promote conversion of linoleic acid to omega-6 fatty acid
- Probiotics may reduce the severity of the condition, reducing medication use (4)[C].

 ## ONGOING CARE

FOLLOW-UP RECOMMENDATIONS

Patient Monitoring

Evaluate to ensure that secondary bacterial or fungal infection does not develop as a result of disruption of the skin barrier.

DIET

- Trials of elimination may find certain "triggers" in some patients.
- Breast-feeding in conjunction with maternal hypoallergenic diets may decrease the severity in some infants.

PATIENT EDUCATION

- http://www.add.org/public/publications/pamplets/eczemaatopicdermatitis.htm
- National Eczema Association: www.nationaleczema.org

PROGNOSIS

- Chronic disease
- Declines with increasing age
- 90% of patients have spontaneous resolution by puberty.
- Localized eczema (e.g., chronic hand or foot dermatitis, eyelid dermatitis, or lichen simplex chronicus) may continue in some adults.

COMPLICATIONS

- Cataracts are more common in patients with atopic dermatitis.
- Skin infections (usually *Staphylococcus aureus*); sometimes subclinical
- Eczema herpeticum:
  - Generalized vesiculopustular eruption caused by infection with herpes simplex or vaccinia virus
  - Causes acute illness requiring hospitalization
- Atrophy and/or striae if fluorinated corticosteroids are used on face or skin folds
- Systemic absorption may occur if large areas of skin are treated, particularly if high-potency medications and occlusion are combined.

REFERENCES

1. Bieber T. Atopic dermatitis. *N Engl J Med*. 2008;358:1483–94.
2. Williams HC. Clinical practice. Atopic dermatitis. *N Engl J Med*. 2005;352:2314–24.
3. Trammell S, Shakil A, Wilder L, et al. Clinical inquiries. What is the role of tacrolimus and pimecrolimus in atopic dermatitis? *J Fam Pract*. 2005;54:714–6.
4. Weston S, et al. Effects of probiotics on atopic dermatitis: A randomized controlled trial. *Arch Disease Child*. 2005;90:892–897.

ADDITIONAL READING

Hill DJ, Hosking CS, Food Allergy and Atopic Dermatitis in Infancy: An Epidemiological Study. *Padiatr Allergy Immunol*. 2004;15(5):421–7.

See Also (Topic, Algorithm, Electronic Media Element)

Algorithm: Rash, focal

CODES

ICD9

691.8 Other atopic dermatitis and related conditions

CLINICAL PEARLS

- Institute early and proactive treatment to reduce inflammation.
- Monitor for secondary bacterial infection.
- Frequent systemic lubrication with thick emollient creams (e.g., Eucerin, Vaseline) over moist skin is the mainstay of treatment before any other intervention is considered.
- Use the lowest-potency topical steroid that controls symptoms.

DERMATITIS, CONTACT

Aamir Siddiqi, MD

 BASICS

DESCRIPTION
- The cutaneous reaction to an external substance
- Primary irritant dermatitis is due to direct injury of the skin. It affects individuals exposed to specific irritants and generally produces discomfort immediately after exposure.
- Allergic contact dermatitis (ACD) affects only individuals previously sensitized to the substance. It represents a delayed hypersensitivity reaction, requiring several hours for the cascade of cellular immunity to be completed to manifest itself.
- System(s) affected: Skin/Exocrine
- Synonym(s): Dermatitis venenata

EPIDEMIOLOGY
Common

Incidence
Occupational contact dermatitis: 20.5/100,000 workers

Prevalence
- Contact dermatitis represents >90% of all occupational skin disorders.
- Predominant sex: Male = Female:
  - Variations due to differences in exposure to offending agents as well as normal cutaneous variations between male and female (eccrine and sebaceous gland function and hair distribution)

Geriatric Considerations
Increased incidence of irritant dermatitis secondary to skin dryness

Pediatric Considerations
Increased incidence of positive patch testing due to better delayed hypersensitivity reactions

RISK FACTORS
- Occupation
- Hobbies
- Travel
- Cosmetics
- Jewelry

Genetics
Increased frequency of ACD in families with allergies

GENERAL PREVENTION
- Avoid causative agents.
- Use of protective gloves (with cotton lining) may be helpful (1)[A].

PATHOPHYSIOLOGY
Hypersensitivity reaction to a substance generating cellular immunity response

ETIOLOGY
- Plants:
  - Rhus-urushiol: Poison ivy, oak, sumac
  - Primary contact: Plant (roots/stems/leaves)
  - Secondary contact: Clothes/fingernails (not blister fluid)
- Chemicals:
  - Nickel: Jewelry, zippers, hooks, and watches
  - Potassium dichromate: Tanning agent in leather
  - Paraphenylenediamine: Hair dyes, fur dyes, and industrial chemicals
  - Turpentine: Cleaning agents, polishes, and waxes
  - Soaps and detergents
- Topical medicines:
  - Neomycin: Topical antibiotics
  - Thimerosal (Merthiolate): Preservative in topical medications
  - Anesthetics: Benzocaine
  - Parabens: Preservative in topical medications
  - Formalin: Cosmetics, shampoos, and nail enamel

 DIAGNOSIS

HISTORY
- Itchy rash
- Assess for prior exposure to irritating substance

PHYSICAL EXAM
- Acute:
  - Papules, vesicles, bullae with surrounding erythema
  - Crusting and oozing
  - Pruritus
- Chronic:
  - Erythematous base
  - Thickening with lichenification
  - Scaling
  - Fissuring
- Distribution:
  - Where epidermis is thinner (eyelids, genitalia)
  - Areas of contact with offending agent (e.g., nail polish)
  - Palms and soles more resistant
  - Deeper skin folds spared
  - Linear arrays of lesions
  - Lesions with sharp borders and sharp angles are pathognomonic.
- Well-demarcated area with a papulovesicular rash

DIAGNOSTIC TESTS & INTERPRETATION
Diagnostic Procedures/Surgery
Consider patch tests for suspected allergic trigger (systemic corticosteroids or recent, aggressive use of topical steroids may alter results) (2)[B]

Pathological Findings
- Intercellular edema
- Bullae

DIFFERENTIAL DIAGNOSIS
- Based on clinical impression:
  - Appearance, periodicity, and localization
- Groups of vesicles:
  - Herpes simplex
- Diffuse bullous or vesicular lesions:
  - Bullous pemphigoid
- Photodistribution:
  - Phototoxic/allergic reaction to systemic allergen
- Eyelids:
  - Seborrheic dermatitis
- Scaly eczematous lesions:
  - Atopic dermatitis
  - Nummular eczema
  - Lichen simplex chronicus
  - Stasis dermatitis
  - Xerosis

TREATMENT

MEDICATION

First Line
- Topical medications:
  – Lotion of zinc oxide, talc, menthol 0.25%, phenol 0.5% (Gold Bond, others)
  – Corticosteroids for allergic contact dermatitis as well as irritant dermatitis (1)[A]:
    o High-potency steroids: Fluocinonide (Lidex) 0.05% ointment t.i.d.–q.i.d.
    o Use high-potency steroids only for a short time and then switch to low- or medium-potency steroid cream or ointment.
    o Caution regarding face/skin folds: Use lower-potency steroids and avoid prolonged usage. Switch to lower-potency topical steroid once the acute phase is resolved.
- Calamine lotion for symptomatic relief
- Topical antibiotics for secondary infection (bacitracin, erythromycin)
- Systemic:
  – Antihistamine:
    o Hydroxyzine: 25–50 mg p.o. q.i.d., especially useful for itching
    o Diphenhydramine: 25–50 mg p.o. q.i.d.
  – Corticosteroids:
    o Prednisone: Taper starting at 60–80 mg/d p.o., over 10–14 days
    o Used for moderate-to-severe cases
    o May use burst dose of steroids for up to 5 days
  – Antibiotics for secondary skin infections:
    o Dicloxacillin: 250 mg p.o. q.i.d. for 7–10 days
    o Amoxicillin-clavulanate (Augmentin): 500 mg p.o. b.i.d. for 7–10 days
    o Erythromycin: 250 mg p.o. q.i.d. in penicillin-allergic patients
- Precautions:
  – Antihistamines may cause drowsiness.
  – Prolonged use of potent topical steroids may cause local skin effects (atrophy, stria, telangiectasia).
  – Use tapering dose of oral steroids if using more than 5 days.

Second Line
Other topical or systemic antibiotics, depending on organisms and sensitivity

Pregnancy Considerations
Usual cautions with medications

ADDITIONAL TREATMENT

General Measures
- Removal of offending agent:
  – Avoidance
  – Work modification
  – Protective clothing
  – Barrier creams, especially high-lipid content moisturizing creams (e.g., Keri lotion, petrolatum, coconut oil) (3)[A]
- Topical soaks with cool tap water, Burow solution (1:40 dilution), saline (1 tsp/pint water), or silver nitrate solution (25.5%)
- Lukewarm water baths
- Aveeno oatmeal baths
- Emollients (white petrolatum, Eucerin)

Issues for Referral
May need referral to a dermatologist or allergist if refractory to conventional treatment

COMPLEMENTARY AND ALTERNATIVE MEDICINE
The use of complementary and alternative treatment is a supplement and not an alternative to conventional treatment (4).

IN-PATIENT CONSIDERATIONS

Admission Criteria
Rarely will need hospital admission

 # ONGOING CARE

FOLLOW-UP RECOMMENDATIONS
Stay active, but avoid overheating.

Patient Monitoring
- As necessary for recurrence
- Patch testing for etiology after resolved

DIET
No special diet

PATIENT EDUCATION
- Avoidance of irritating substance
- Cleaning of secondary sources (nails, clothes)
- Fallacy of blister fluid spreading disease

PROGNOSIS
- Self-limited
- Benign

COMPLICATIONS
- Generalized eruption secondary to autosensitization
- Secondary bacterial infection

REFERENCES

1. Saary J, Qureshi R, Palda V, et al. A systematic review of contact dermatitis treatment and prevention. *J Am Acad Dermatol*. 2005;53:845.
2. Saripalli YV, Achen F, Belsito DV. The detection of clinically relevant contact allergens using a standard screening tray of twenty-three allergens. *J Am Acad Dermatol*. 2003;49:65–9.
3. Hachem JP, De Paepe K, Vanpée E, et al. Efficacy of topical corticosteroids in nickel-induced contact allergy. *Clin Exp Dermatol*. 2002;27:47–50.
4. Noiesen E, Munk MD, Larsen K, et al. Use of complementary and alternative treatment for allergic contact dermatitis. *Br J Dermatol*. 2007.

See Also (Topic, Algorithm, Electronic Media Element)
Algorithm: Rash, Focal

 ## CODES

ICD9
- 692.0 Contact dermatitis and other eczema due to detergents
- 692.3 Contact dermatitis and other eczema due to drugs and medicines in contact with skin
- 692.4 Contact dermatitis and other eczema due to other chemical products

CLINICAL PEARLS
- Anyone exposed to irritants or allergic substances is predisposed to contact dermatitis, especially in occupations that have high exposure to chemicals.
- The most common allergens causing contact dermatitis are plants of the *Toxicodendron* genus (poison ivy, poison oak, poison sumac).
- The usual treatment for contact dermatitis is avoidance of the allergen or irritating substance and temporary use of topical steroids.
- A contact dermatitis rash presents in a nondermatomal geographic fashion, due to the skin being in contact with an external source.

D

DERMATITIS, DIAPER

Dennis E. Hughes, DO

 BASICS

DESCRIPTION
- Diaper dermatitis is a rash occurring under the covered area of a diaper. The rash may be a direct result of wearing the diaper, aggravated by the diaper, or coincidental with a rash that appears elsewhere on the body.
- System(s) affected: Skin/Exocrine
- Synonym(s): Diaper rash

Geriatric Considerations
Incontinence is a significant cofactor.

EPIDEMIOLOGY
Incidence
- The most common dermatitis found in infancy
- Peak incidence: 7–12 months of age, then decreases

Prevalence
Prevalence has been variably reported from 4–35% in the 1st 2 years of life.

RISK FACTORS
- Infrequent diaper changes
- Waterproof diapers
- Improper laundering
- Family history of dermatitis
- Hot, humid weather
- Recent treatment with oral antibiotics
- Diarrhea (>3 stools per day increases risk)
- Dye allergy
- Prior history of eczema may increase risk.

GENERAL PREVENTION
Attention to hygiene during bouts of diarrhea

PATHOPHYSIOLOGY
- Fecal proteases and lipases are irritants.
- Superhydrase urease enzyme found in the stratum cornium liberates ammonia from cutaneous bacteria.
- Fecal lipase and protease activity is increased by acceleration of GI transit; thus a higher incidence of irritant diaper dermatitis is observed in babies who have had diarrhea in the previous 48 h.

- Once the skin is compromised, secondary infection by *Candida albicans* is common. 40–75% of diaper rashes that last >3 days are colonized with *C. albicans*.
- Bacteria may play a role in diaper dermatitis through reduction of fecal pH and resulting activation of enzymes.
- Allergy is exceedingly rare as a cause in infants.

ETIOLOGY
- Wet skin from prolonged contact with urine or feces resulting in susceptibility to chemical, enzymatic, and physical injury; wet skin is also penetrated more easily.
- Some have raised the possibility of contact allergy from the dye in disposable diapers.

COMMONLY ASSOCIATED CONDITIONS
- Contact (allergic or irritant) dermatitis
- Seborrheic dermatitis
- Psoriasis
- Candidiasis
- Atopic dermatitis

 DIAGNOSIS

HISTORY
- Onset, duration, and change in the nature of the rash
- Presence of rashes outside the diaper area
- Associated scratching or crying
- Contact with infants with a similar rash
- Recent illness, diarrhea, or antibiotic use
- Fever
- Pustular drainage
- Lymphangitis

PHYSICAL EXAM
- Mild forms consist of shiny erythema ± scale.
- Margins are not always evident.
- Moderate cases have areas of papules, vesicles, and small superficial erosions.
- It can progress to well-demarcated ulcerated nodules that measure 1 cm or more in diameter.
- It is found on the prominent parts of the buttocks, medial thighs, mons pubis, and scrotum.
- Skin folds are spared or involved last.
- *Tidemark dermatitis* refers to the bandlike form of erythema of irritated diaper margins.
- Diaper dermatitis can cause an id (autoeczematous) reaction outside the diaper area.

DIAGNOSTIC TESTS & INTERPRETATION
Lab
Initial lab tests
- Rarely needed
- Consider a culture of lesions or a KOH preparation.

Follow-Up & Special Considerations
- The finding of anemia in association with hepatosplenomegaly and the appropriate rash may suggest a diagnosis of Langerhans cell histiocytosis or congenital syphilis.
- Finding mites, ova, or feces on a mineral oil preparation of a burrow scraping can confirm the diagnosis of scabies.

Pathological Findings
- Biopsy is rare.
- Histology may reveal acute, subacute, or chronic spongiotic dermatitis.

DIFFERENTIAL DIAGNOSIS
- Contact dermatitis
- Seborrheic dermatitis
- Candidiasis
- Atopic dermatitis
- Scabies
- Acrodermatitis enteropathica
- Letterer-Siwe disease
- Congenital syphilis
- Child abuse
- Streptococcal infection
- Kawasaki disease
- Biotin deficiency
- Psoriasis
- HIV infection

TREATMENT

See "General-Measures" for 1st-line approach.

MEDICATION
First Line
- For a pure contact dermatitis, a low-potency topical steroid (hydrocortisone 0.5–1% t.i.d.) and removal of the offending agent should suffice.
- If candidiasis is suspected or diaper rash persists, use an antifungal such as miconazole nitrate 2% cream, miconazole powder, econazole (Spectazole), clotrimazole (Lotrimin), or ketoconazole (Nizoral) cream at each diaper change (1)[B].
- If inflammation is prominent, consider a very low-potency steroid cream such as hydrocortisone 0.5–1% t.i.d. along with an antifungal cream ± a combination product such as clioquinol-hydrocortisone (Vioform–hydrocortisone) cream (1)[B].
- If a secondary bacterial infection is suspected, use an antistaphylococcal oral antibiotic or mupirocin (Bactroban) ointment topically.
- Precautions: Avoid high- or moderate-potency steroids often found in combination steroid antifungal mixtures (1)[B].

Second Line
Sucralfate paste for resistant cases

ADDITIONAL TREATMENT
General Measures
- Expose the buttocks to air as much as possible (1).
- Avoid waterproof pants during treatment (day or night); they keep the skin wet and subject to rash or infection.
- Change diapers frequently, even at night, if the rash is extensive (2).
- Superabsorbable diapers are beneficial (1,2)[B].
- Discontinue using baby lotion, powder, ointment, or baby oil (except zinc oxide).
- Disposable baby wipes contain substances that induce contact or irritant dermatitis, such as fragrance, benzalkonium chloride, and isothiazolinone or alcohol.
- Apply zinc oxide ointment or other barrier cream to the rash at the earliest sign and b.i.d. or t.i.d. (e.g., Desitin or Balmex). Thereafter, apply to clean, thoroughly dry skin (1).
- Use mild soap, and pat dry.
- Cornstarch can reduce friction. Talc powders that do not enhance the growth of yeast can provide protection against frictional injury in diaper dermatitis but do not form a continuous lipid barrier layer over the skin and obstruct the skin pores. These treatments are not recommended.

Issues for Referral
Consider if a systemic disease such as Langerhans cell histiocytosis, acrodermatitis enteropathica, or HIV infection is suspected.

IN-PATIENT CONSIDERATIONS
Admission Criteria
- Febrile neonates
- Recalcitrant rash suggestive of immunodeficiency
- Toxic-appearing infants

Nursing
Assist 1st-time parents with hygiene education.

 ONGOING CARE

FOLLOW-UP RECOMMENDATIONS
Patient Monitoring
Recheck weekly until clear; then at times of recurrence.

PATIENT EDUCATION
Patient education is vital to the treatment and prevention of recurrent cases.

PROGNOSIS
- Quick, complete clearing with appropriate treatment
- Secondary candidal infections may last a few weeks after treatment is begun.

COMPLICATIONS
- Secondary bacterial infection [consider community-acquired methicillin-resistant *Staphylococcus aureus* (MRSA) in pustular dermatitis that does not respond to normal therapy]
- Rare complication is inoculation with group A β-hemolytic *Streptococcus* resulting in necrotizing fascitis.
- Secondary yeast infection

REFERENCES
1. Scheinfeld N. Diaper dermatitis: A review and brief survey of eruptions of the diaper area. *Am J Clin Derm*. 2005;6:273–81.
2. Janniger CK, Thomas I. Diaper dermatitis: an approach to prevention employing effective diaper care. *Cutis*. 1993;52:153–5.

ADDITIONAL READING
- Alberta L, et al. Diaper dye dermatitis. *Pediatrics*. 2005;116(3):450–2.
- Kazaks EL, et al. Diaper dermatitis. *Pediatr Clin North Am*. 2000;47(4):909–19.

See Also (Topic, Algorithm, Electronic Media Element)
Algorithm: Rash, Focal

 CODES

ICD9
- 112.3 Candidiasis of skin and nails
- 691.0 Diaper or napkin rash

CLINICAL PEARLS
- Hygiene is the main preventative measure.
- Look for secondary infection in persistent cases.

D

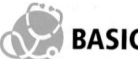

BASICS

DESCRIPTION
- Exfoliative dermatitis (ED), or *erythroderma*, is a rare disorder characterized by a generalized (often >90% of body) scaling eruption of most, if not all, of the skin.
- It may appear suddenly or gradually, occasionally accompanied by fever, chills, and lymphadenopathy.
- It arises idiopathically or secondary to an underlying cutaneous or systemic disease or as a reaction to medications.
- Cutaneous involvement consists of redness and/or scaling of most of the skin.
- When fulminant, this reaction is potentially life-threatening.
- System(s) affected: Skin/Exocrine
- Synonym(s): Erythroderma; Exfoliative erythroderm; Red man syndrome (*homme rouge*); Pityriasis rubra

EPIDEMIOLOGY
The vast majority of patients are older than 40 years of age and are mostly males.

Incidence
- In the US: Rare; estimated 1% of hospitalizations for skin disease
- Predominant age: >40 years, except when it results from atopic dermatitis, seborrheic dermatitis, staphylococcal scalded-skin syndrome, or hereditary ichthyosis, all of which are most common in the pediatric age group.
- Predominant sex: Male > Female (2–4:1)

RISK FACTORS
- Underlying diseases as noted below
- Male sex
- Age >40 years

PATHOPHYSIOLOGY
Arises idiopathically or secondary to an underlying cutaneous or systemic disease, or as a reaction to medications

COMMONLY ASSOCIATED CONDITIONS
- The most common associated conditions or diseases that have been reported to present with or develop into exfoliative dermatitis include:
  - In adults, psoriasis most frequently
  - In children, most often secondary to severe atopic dermatitis
  - Drug reactions
  - Idiopathic in up to 20–30% of cases

- Less commonly, ED has been noted as a finding in the following skin disorders:
  - Allergic contact dermatitis
  - Stasis dermatitis with secondary autoeczematization
  - Pityriasis rubra pilaris (a rare disorder of keratinization)
  - Graft-versus-host disease
  - Seborrheic dermatitis (Leiner disease) in infants
  - Ichthyosiform dermatoses
  - Pemphigus foliaceus
  - Papulosquamous dermatitis of AIDS
  - Fungal disease with id reaction
- Other rare reported associations include:
  - Reiter syndrome
  - SLE
  - Hailey-Hailey disease
  - Norwegian scabies
  - Sarcoidosis
  - Lichen planus
  - Dermatomyositis
- Medications: May occur as a reaction to the following drugs: Allopurinol, antimalarials, aspirin, barbiturates, captopril, codeine, cefoxitin, cimetidine, dapsone, gold salts, hydantoin, isoniazid, lithium, NSAIDs, omeprazole, para-aminosalicylic acid, penicillin, phenylbutazone, phenothiazine, St. John's wort, sulfonamide, sulfonylurea, thalidomide, and vancomycin
- May occur as a complication or presenting symptom of the following malignancies:
  - Mycosis fungoides (cutaneous T-cell lymphoma)
  - Sézary syndrome (leukemic variant of mycosis fungoides)
  - Hodgkin disease
  - Non-Hodgkin lymphoma and leukemia

DIAGNOSIS

- Diagnosis is made on a clinical basis.
- Determination of the cause is often elusive, but history is the most important aid in finding the underlying etiology of ED.

PHYSICAL EXAM
- Nail dystrophy in 40%
- Fever in 40–50%
- Chills
- Malaise/weakness
- Eosinophilia (30%)
- Hepatomegaly (20%)
- Splenomegaly when underlying lymphoma/leukemia is present
- Alopecia
- Hypoproteinemia

- Dehydration
- High-output cardiac failure
- Tachycardia (40%)
- In time, lichenification may occur.
- Postinflammatory dyspigmentation (hyper- or hypopigmented areas of the skin)
- Eliciting a history of drug ingestion or a preexisting dermatosis or disease may be valuable.
- Infrequently, the characteristic lichenification of atopic dermatitis or the nail pitting that suggests psoriasis or islands of sparing in pityriasis rubra pilaris may be found.
- There is marked generalized erythema followed by scaling.
- Pruritus may be severe.
- Edema and increased warmth of the skin
- Pedal or pretibial edema
- Lymphadenopathy, usually a reactive type (*dermatopathic lymphadenopathy*) is often present.
- Most often, primary lesions that might offer clues to making an etiologic diagnosis are obscured or lacking.

DIAGNOSTIC TESTS & INTERPRETATION
Lab
None are diagnostic; however, may have elevated WBC count with eosinophilia, anemia, elevated ESR, decreased albumin, and electrolyte abnormalities

Imaging
CXR and other imaging procedures as indicated to investigate any underlying disease process

Diagnostic Procedures/Surgery
- Laboratory testing can provide serologic evidence of Sézary syndrome or leukemia.
- Patch testing during a period of remission may uncover a contact allergen.
- Skin biopsy (lymph node or bone marrow) as indicated to investigate an underlying disease process
- Further tests are performed if suggested by the review of systems and physical examination.

Pathological Findings
- May have characteristics of an underlying cutaneous disease; however, findings are most often nonspecific and consist of hyperkeratosis, parakeratosis, and acanthosis in the epidermis and edema, vasodilation, and perivascular infiltrates with lymphocytes, histiocytes, and eosinophils in the dermis
- Repeated or multiple biopsies are sometimes helpful in finding an underlying cause.

DIFFERENTIAL DIAGNOSIS

- Extensive acute eczematous dermatoses, such as contact dermatitis and drug eruptions
- Toxic epidermal necrolysis
- Staphylococcal scalded-skin syndrome
- Erythema multiforme major

 TREATMENT

- Cool tap water dressings
- Application of intermediate-strength topical steroids (e.g., triamcinolone cream 0.025–0.1%) beneath wet dressings
- Cool colloid baths with oatmeal (e.g., Aveeno)
- Local bland moisturizing ointments/lotions
- Systemic antibiotics if signs of secondary infection are observed
- Antihistamines act primarily as sedatives.

ALERT
Systemic steroids may be helpful in some cases, but should be avoided in suspected cases of psoriasis.

MEDICATION
First Line
- Midpotency topical steroids
- In addition, treatment specific to any underlying infection or disease should be provided.
- Systemic steroids: Initial dosage equivalent to prednisone 40 mg/d with increases in dosage by 20 mg/d if there is no response after 3–4 days. Subsequently, dosage should be tapered as symptoms are controlled.
- Oral retinoids: If psoriasis is determined to be the underlying cause of the ED, an oral retinoid such as isotretinoin probably is a better choice than systemic steroids, which may exacerbate psoriasis.

Second Line
- When psoriasis is the underlying cause, cyclosporine, methotrexate, etretinate, phototherapy, photopheresis, photochemotherapy, as well as monoclonal antibodies such as infliximab and alemtuzumab may be effective.
- Photochemotherapy also may be useful therapy for treating ED associated with mycosis fungoides.
- Oral acitretin and isotretinoin have been used when pityriasis rubra pilaris is the underlying cause.
- Antimetabolites/cytotoxic drugs
- Bexarotene
- Infliximab (1)
- Etanercept (2)

ADDITIONAL TREATMENT
General Measures
- Outpatient care except in patients with complications of secondary infection, dehydration, or heart failure
- Withdrawal of any implicated medications or treatment of any identified underlying infection/disease
- Protection from development of hypothermia
- When ED evolves rapidly, the patient frequently requires hospitalization, where measures such as fluid replacement, temperature control, and expert topical skin care are available.

IN-PATIENT CONSIDERATIONS
Admission Criteria
- Impending or actual heart failure
- Inability to control ED on an outpatient basis

Nursing
Bed rest, cool compresses, lubrication with emollients, antipruritic therapy with oral antihistamines, and low- to intermediate-strength topical steroids

 ONGOING CARE

DIET
- Increased fluid intake
- Ensure adequate nutrition with emphasis on sufficient protein intake.

PROGNOSIS
- The prognosis of ED depends largely on underlying etiology.
- In patients with an identified underlying cause, the course and prognosis generally will parallel those of the primary disease. For example, in patients who have underlying psoriasis or atopic dermatitis, the progression of disease generally is gradual.
- ED due to a drug eruption usually clears after the drug is discontinued.
- A study of erythrodermic pediatric patients indicated that age <3 years, fever, ill appearance, hypotension, and elevated creatinine levels are poor prognostic signs, and the possibility of toxic shock syndrome should be considered.
- Acute, severe episodes, particularly in elderly persons or in persons with preexisting heart disease, also have a more guarded prognosis.
- In patients with idiopathic ED, the prognosis is poor, and recurrences are not uncommon.

COMPLICATIONS
- Secondary infection, sepsis
- A marked loss of exfoliated scales (uncontrolled mitosis and desquamation) and an increase in cutaneous blood perfusion may contribute to:
  – Dehydration/electrolyte disturbances
  – Hypoalbuminemia
  – Edema
  – Heat loss and hypothermia
  – Possible high-output cardiac failure and death
- Depending on the underlying cause and possible complications, the overall mortality ranges from 20–40%.

REFERENCES

1. Rongioletti F, Borenstein M, Kirsner R, et al. Erythrodermic, recalcitrant psoriasis: clinical resolution with infliximab. *J Dermatolog Treat.* 2003;14:222–5.
2. Querfeld C, Guitart J, et al. Successful treatment of recalcitrant, erythroderma-associated pruritus with etanercept. *Arch Dermatol.* 2004;140(12):1539–40.

ADDITIONAL READING

- Byer RL, Bachur RG. Clinical deterioration among patients with fever and erythroderma. *Pediatrics.* 2006;118:2450–60.
- Heald P. The treatment of cutaneous T-cell lymphoma with a novel retinoid. *Clin Lymphoma.* 2000:1S45–1S49.
- Okoduwa C, Lambert WC, Schwartz RA, et al. Erythroderma: review of a potentially life-threatening dermatosis. *Indian J Dermatol.* 2009;54(1):1–6.
- Ott H, Hütten M, Baron JM, et al. Neonatal and infantile erythrodermas. *J Dtsch Dermatol Ges.* 2008;6:1070–85; quiz 1086.
- Pruszkowski A, Bodemer C, Fraitag S, et al. Neonatal and infantile erythrodermas: a retrospective study of 51 patients. *Arch Dermatol.* 2000;136:875–80.
- Tomi NS, Kränke B, Aberer E. Staphylococcal toxins in patients with psoriasis, atopic dermatitis, and erythroderma, and in healthy control subjects. *J Am Acad Dermatol.* 2005;53:67–72.

See Also (Topic, Algorithm, Electronic Media Element)
Algorithm: Rash, Focal

 CODES

ICD9
695.89 Other specified erythematous conditions

CLINICAL PEARLS

- In its more severe manifestations, ED is a medical and dermatologic emergency.
- In many cases, the underlying cause is never established.

DERMATITIS HERPETIFORMIS

Anne M. Mahoney, MD
Amit Garg, MD

BASICS

DESCRIPTION
- Dermatitis herpetiformis (DH) is a chronic, intensely pruritic papulovesicular eruption involving primarily extensor skin surfaces (elbows, knees, buttocks, back) and the scalp.
- DH is distinguished from other bullous diseases by characteristic histologic and immunologic findings, as well as associated gluten-sensitive enteropathy (1).
- Within the spectrum of gluten-sensitive disorders, which include celiac disease (CD), some forms of IgA nephropathy, and gluten-sensitive ataxia (2)
- System(s) affected: Skin
- Synonym(s): Duhring disease

EPIDEMIOLOGY
- Occurs most frequently in those of Northern European origin
- Rare in persons of Asian or African-American origin
- Predominant age: Most common between the ages of 30 and 40 years but may occur in children
- Predominant sex: Male > Female (1.4:1 in the US, 2:1 worldwide)

Incidence
0.98/100,000 persons per year in US

Prevalence
11/100,000 persons in US population; as high as 39/100,000 persons worldwide

RISK FACTORS
- Gluten-sensitive enteropathy (GSE): >90% of those with DH will have GSE, which may be asymptomatic.
- Family history of DH or CD

Genetics
- High incidence of human leukocyte antigen A1, B8, DR3, and DQ2 (1)
- Strong association with combination of alleles DQA1*0501 and DQB1*02 OR DQA1*03 and DQB1*0302 (3)

GENERAL PREVENTION
Gluten-free diet (GFD) results in improvement of DH and reduces dependence on medical therapy. GFD also may prevent complications associated with DH.

PATHOPHYSIOLOGY
- Evidence suggests that epidermal transglutaminase (eTG) 3, a keratinocyte enzyme involved in cell envelope formation, is the autoantigen in DH (4).
- eTG is highly homologous with tissue transglutaminase (tTG), which is the antigenic target in celiac disease (3).
- The initiating event for DH is presumed to be the interaction of wheat peptides with TTGs, which results in activation of T cells and the humoral immune system.
- IgA antibodies against tTGs cross-react with eTG and result in IgA-eTG immune complexes that are deposited in the papillary dermis. Subsequent activation of complement and recruitment of neutrophils to the area result in inflammation and blistering.
- Skin eruption may be delayed 5–6 weeks after exposure to gluten.

- Gluten applied directly to the skin does not result in the eruption, whereas gluten taken by mouth or rectum does. This implies necessary processing by the GI system (2).

ETIOLOGY
Thought to be autoimmune or immune complex–mediated (3)

COMMONLY ASSOCIATED CONDITIONS
- Gluten-sensitive enteropathy
- Gastric atrophy, hypochlorhydria, pernicious anemia
- Gastrointestinal lymphoma, non-Hodgkin lymphoma
- Hyperthyroidism, hypothyroidism, thyroid nodules, thyroid cancer
- Down syndrome
- Glomerulopathy
- Autoimmune disorders, including systemic lupus erythematosus, dermatomyositis, Sjögren syndrome, rheumatoid arthritis, Raynaud phenomenon, insulin-dependent diabetes mellitus, myasthenia gravis, Addison disease, vitiligo, alopecia, and psoriasis

DIAGNOSIS

Diagnosis of DH involves a clinicopathologic correlation among clinical presentation, histologic and direct immunofluorescence evaluation, serology, and response to therapy or diet restriction.

HISTORY
- Waxing and waning, intensely pruritic eruption with papules and tiny vesicles
- Eruption may worsen with gluten intake.
- GI symptoms may be absent or may not be reported until prompted.

PHYSICAL EXAM
- Symmetric, grouped, erythematous papules and vesicles
- Only erosions, excoriations, and hyperpigmentation secondary to scratching may be apparent on presentation (5).
- Areas involved include extensor surfaces of elbows (90%), knees (30%), shoulders, buttocks, and sacrum. The scalp is also frequently affected. Oral lesions are rare. Palms and soles are spared (5).
- The eruption in children is similar to that in adults (2).
- Adults with associated enteropathy are most often asymptomatic, with <10% complaining of bloating, diarrhea, or steatorrhea.
- Children with associated enteropathy may present with abdominal pain, diarrhea, iron deficiency, and reduced growth rate (5).

DIAGNOSTIC TESTS & INTERPRETATION
The "gold standard" for diagnosing DH is direct immunofluorescence on skin, which demonstrates that granular IgA is deposited in the dermal papillae (5)[A].

Lab
Initial lab tests
- IgA TTG antibodies: Detection of tTG antibodies was noted to be 94.4% sensitive and 92.3% specific for DH in patients on unrestricted diets (6).

- IgA eTG antibodies: Antibodies to eTG, the primary autoantigen in DH, were shown to be more sensitive than antibodies to tTG in the diagnosis of patients with DH on unrestricted diets (95% vs 79%) (7).
- IgA endomysial antibodies: Have a sensitivity between 50% and 100% and a specificity close to 100% in patients on unrestricted diets (5)

Follow-Up & Special Considerations
Serologic assessment of anti-tTG and anti-endomysial antibodies (EMA) may be useful in monitoring major deviations from GFD (5).

Diagnostic Procedures/Surgery
Skin biopsy for hematoxylin and eosin stain and for direct immunofluorescence on skin

Pathological Findings
- Direct immunofluorescence of skin reveals a granular pattern of IgA deposition in the dermal papillae (5).
- Histopathology with routine staining reveals neutrophilic microabscesses in dermal papillae and also may show subepidermal blistering (2).

DIFFERENTIAL DIAGNOSIS
- In adults (5):
  - Bullous pemphigoid: Linear deposition of C3 and IgG at the basement membrane zone
  - Linear IgA disease: Homogeneous and linear deposition of IgA at the basement membrane zone, absence of GSE
  - Transient acantholytic dermatosis
  - Urticaria: Wheals, angioedema, dermal edema
  - Erythema multiforme
- In children (5):
  - Atopic dermatitis: Face and flexural areas
  - Scabies: Interdigital areas, axillae, genital region
  - Papular urticaria: Dermal edema
  - Impetigo

TREATMENT

MEDICATION
- Disease control is achieved with dietary modification, medication, or both.
- Medication is useful for immediate symptom management.
- A GFD is necessary for long-term management of underlying gluten sensitivity.
- Interdisciplinary treatment involves outpatient care with a dermatologist as well as consultations with a gastroenterologist and a registered dietician.

First Line
- Dapsone is the most widely used medication for DH (2)[A].
- It is the only medication approved by the Food and Drug Administration for use in this disease. Adult doses range from 25–400 mg/d, which result in improvement of symptoms within 24–48 h. Use of a minimum effective dose is recommended. Average maintenance dose is 1 mg/kg/d. Minor outbreaks on the face and scalp are common even with treatment.
- Dapsone works by inhibiting neutrophil recruitment, inhibiting the respiratory burst of neutrophils, and protecting cells from neutrophil-mediated injury, thereby suppressing the skin reaction. It has no role in preventing IgA deposition or mitigating the immune reaction in the gut (2).

- Precautions:
  - Common side effects include nausea, vomiting, headache, dizziness, and weakness
  - A drop in hemoglobin of 1–2 g is characteristic with dapsone 100 mg/d.
  - G6PD deficiency increases severity of hemolytic stress. Dapsone should be avoided if possible in those who are G6PD-deficient.
  - Dose-related methemoglobinemia may occur, typically with doses >100 mg/d.
  - Other adverse events include toxic hepatitis, cholestatic jaundice, hypoalbuminemia, sensory and motor neuropathy, psychosis, infectious mononucleosis syndrome with fever and lymphadenopathy, agranulocytosis, aplastic anemia, leukopenia, exfoliative dermatitis, erythema multiforme, erythema nodosum, and urticaria.
  - The drug is secreted in breast milk and will produce hemolytic anemia in infants.

ALERT
- Monitor for potentially fatal sulfone syndrome: Fever, jaundice and hepatic necrosis, exfoliative dermatitis, lymphadenopathy, methemoglobinemia, and hemolytic anemia.
- Can occur 48 h or 6 months after treatment, most often 5 weeks after initiation

Pediatric Considerations
- <2 years: Dosing not established
- >2 years: 0.5–1.0 mg/kg/d

Pregnancy Considerations
- Category C: Safety during pregnancy is not established.
- Adherence to a strict GFD 6–12 months before conception should be considered with the hope of eliminating need for dapsone during pregnancy.

Second Line
Sulfasalazine (1–2 g/d), sulphamethoxypyridazine (0.25–1.5 g/d): Side effects include nausea, vomiting, anorexia, hypersensitivity reactions, hemolytic anemia, proteinuria, and crystalluria (5).

ALERT
- Prior to treatment, monthly for the first 3 months of treatment and biannually thereafter, complete blood count (CBC) with differential and urinalysis with urine microscopy should be done (5).
- Colchicine, prednisone, tetracycline plus nicotinamide, minocycline, cyclosporine, and topical steroids are 3rd-line medications.

ADDITIONAL TREATMENT
GFD:
- Average of 2 years is often necessary for diet to completely eliminate skin eruptions, and lesions usually recur within 12 weeks of gluten reintroduction (5).
- Fundamentals of the GFD (8):
  - Grains that should be avoided:
    - Wheat (includes spelt, kamut, semolina, and triticale)
    - Rye
    - Barley (including malt)
  - Safe grains (gluten-free):
    - Rice
    - Amaranth
    - Buckwheat
    - Corn
    - Millet
    - Quinoa
    - Sorghum
    - Teff (an Ethiopian cereal grain)
    - Oats
  - Sources of gluten-free starches that can be used as flour alternatives:
    - Cereal grains: Amaranth, buckwheat, corn, millet, quinoa, sorghum, teff, rice (white, brown, wild, basmati, jasmine), and montina
    - Tubers: Arrowroot, jicama, taro, potato, and tapioca
    - Legumes: Chickpeas, lentils, kidney beans, navy beans, pea beans, peanuts, and soybeans
    - Nuts: Almonds, walnuts, chestnuts, hazelnuts, and cashews
    - Seeds: Sunflower, flax, and pumpkin

 ## ONGOING CARE

FOLLOW-UP RECOMMENDATIONS
Patient Monitoring
If treating with dapsone:
- Obtain baseline CBC and liver function tests.
- Quantify G6PD prior to initiating treatment in Asians, African Americans, and those of southern Mediterranean origin.
- Check CBC weekly for 1st month, monthly for the next 5 months, and semiannually thereafter.
- Check chemistry profile every 6 months.
- Patient should be made aware of potential hemolytic anemia and the signs associated with methemoglobinemia.

DIET
- 87% of patients showed complete remission of skin manifestations after 18 months of a GFD (9)[C].
- Improvement in cutaneous disease and normalization of small bowel mucosa result from strict compliance with a GFD in most patients (5)[C].

PATIENT EDUCATION
- American Academy of Dermatology, 930 N. Meacham Road., P.O. Box 4014, Schaumburg, IL 60168-4014; (708) 330-0230
- Gluten Intolerance Group of North America, 31214–124 Ave. SE, Auburn, WA 98092; phone (206) 246-6652; fax (206) 246-6531; www.gluten.net
- The Celiac Disease Foundation, 13251 Ventura Blvd., #1, Studio City, CA 9160; phone (818) 990-2354; fax (818) 990-2379

PROGNOSIS
- Lifelong disease
- Remission in 10–20%
- Skin disease responds readily to dapsone.
- Strict adherence to a GFD improves clinical symptoms and decreases dapsone requirement. GFD is the only sustainable method of eliminating cutaneous and GI disease. Dapsone does not alter GI mucosal pathology.
- Occasional new lesions (2–3 per week) are to be expected and are not an indication for altering daily dosage.
- Risk of lymphoma may be decreased in those who maintain a GFD.

COMPLICATIONS
- Malnutrition, weight loss
- Abdominal pain, dyspepsia
- Nutritional deficiencies (folate, B_{12}, iron)
- Osteoporosis
- Chronic fatigue
- Autoimmune diseases
- Lymphomas

REFERENCES
1. Patrício P, Ferreira C, Gomes MM, Filipe P et al. Autoimmune bullous dermatoses: a review. *Ann N Y Acad Sci*. 2009;1173:203–10.
2. Nicolas ME, Krause PK, Gibson LE, et al. Dermatitis herpetiformis. *Int J Dermatol*. 2003;42:588–600.
3. Kárpáti S et al. Dermatitis herpetiformis: close to unravelling a disease. *J Dermatol Sci*. 2004;34:83–90.
4. Sárdy M, Kárpáti S, Merkl B, et al. Epidermal transglutaminase (TGase 3) is the autoantigen of dermatitis herpetiformis. *J Exp Med*. 2002;195:747–57.
5. Caproni M, Antiga E, Melani L, et al. Guidelines for the diagnosis and treatment of dermatitis herpetiformis. *J Eur Acad Dermatol Venereol*. 2009.
6. Caproni M, Cardinali C, Renzi D, et al. Tissue transglutaminase antibody assessment in dermatitis herpetiformis. *Br J Dermatol*. 2001;144:196–7.
7. Rose C, Armbruster FP, Ruppert J, Igl BW, Zillikens D, Shimanovich I et al. Autoantibodies against epidermal transglutaminase are a sensitive diagnostic marker in patients with dermatitis herpetiformis on a normal or gluten-free diet. *J Am Acad Dermatol*. 2009;61:39–43.
8. Green PH, Cellier C. Celiac disease. *N Engl J Med*. 2007;357:1731–43.
9. Nino M, Ciacci C, Delfino M. A long-term gluten-free diet as an alternative treatment in severe forms of dermatitis herpetiformis. *J Dermatolog Treat*. 2007;18:10–2.

ADDITIONAL READING
Desai AM, Krishnan RS, Hsu S. Medical pearl: Using tissue transglutaminase antibodies to diagnose dermatitis herpetiformis. *J Am Acad Dermatol*. 2005;53:867–8.

See Also (Topic, Algorithm, Electronic Media Element)
Celiac Disease
Algorithm: Rash, Focal

 ## CODES

ICD9
694.0 Dermatitis herpetiformis

CLINICAL PEARLS
- DH is a chronic, intensely pruritic papulovesicular eruption involving primarily extensor skin surfaces symmetrically as well as the scalp.
- Strong association with gluten-sensitive enteropathy
- Diagnosed by skin biopsy with direct immunofluorescence
- 1st-line treatment: Dapsone

DERMATITIS, SEBORRHEIC

Juan Qiu, MD, PhD

 BASICS

DESCRIPTION
Chronic, superficial, recurrent inflammatory rash affecting sebum-rich, hairy regions of the body, especially scalp, eyebrows, and face

EPIDEMIOLOGY
Incidence
- Predominant age: Infancy, adolescence, and adulthood
- Predominant sex: Male > Female

Prevalence
Seborrheic dermatitis: 3–5%

RISK FACTORS
- Parkinson disease
- AIDS (disease severity correlated with progression of immune deficiency)
- Emotional stress
- Medications may flare or induce seborrheic dermatitis: Auranofin, aurothioglucose, buspirone, chlorpromazine, cimetidine, ethionamide, gold, griseofulvin, haloperidol, interferon alfa, lithium, methoxsalen, methyldopa, phenothiazine, psoralen, stanozolol, thiothixene, trioxsalen

Genetics
Positive family history; no genetic marker identified to date

GENERAL PREVENTION
Seborrheic skin should be washed more often than usual.

PATHOPHYSIOLOGY
Helper T cells, phytohemagglutinin and concanavalin stimulation, and antibody titers are depressed compared with those of control subjects.

ETIOLOGY
- Skin surface yeasts *Malassezia* (formerly *P. ovale*) may be a contributing factor (1).
- *Malassezia* spp. may have a role in T-cell suppression and complement activation.
- The mite *D. folliculorum* may have a direct or indirect role.
- Genetic and environmental factors: Flares are common with stress or illness.
- Parallels increased sebaceous gland activity in infancy and adolescence or as a result of some acnegenic drugs

COMMONLY ASSOCIATED CONDITIONS
- Parkinson disease
- AIDS

 DIAGNOSIS

The diagnosis of seborrheic dermatitis usually can be made by history and physical examination.

HISTORY
- Intermittent active phases manifest with burning, scaling, and itching alternating with inactive periods; activity is increased in winter and early spring, with remissions commonly occurring in summer.
- Infants:
  - Cradle cap: Greasy scaling of scalp, sometimes with associated mild erythema
  - Diaper and/or axillary rash
  - Age at onset typically ~1 month
  - Usually resolves by 8–12 months
- Adults:
  - Red, greasy, scaling rash in most locations consisting of patches and plaques with indistinct margins
  - Red, smooth, glazed appearance in skin folds
  - Minimal pruritus
  - Chronic waxing and waning course
  - Bilateral and symmetric
  - Most commonly located in hairy skin areas: Scalp and scalp margins, eyebrows and eyelid margins, nasolabial folds, ears and retroauricular folds, presternal area, and middle to upper back, buttock crease, inguinal area, genitals, and armpits

PHYSICAL EXAM
- Scalp appearance varies from mild, patchy scaling to widespread, thick, adherent crusts. Plaques are rare.
- Seborrheic dermatitis can spread onto the forehead, the posterior part of the neck, and the postauricular skin, as in psoriasis.
- Skin lesions manifest as branny or greasy scaling over red, inflamed skin.
- Hypopigmentation is seen in blacks.
- Infectious eczematoid dermatitis, with oozing and crusting, suggests secondary infection.
- Seborrheic blepharitis may occur independently.

DIAGNOSTIC TESTS & INTERPRETATION
Diagnostic Procedures/Surgery
Consider biopsy if:
- Usual therapies fail
- Petechiae noted
- Histiocytosis X suspected
- Fungal cultures in refractory cases or when pustules and alopecia are present

Pathological Findings
Nonspecific changes:
- Hyperkeratosis, acanthosis, accentuated rete ridges, focal spongiosis, and parakeratosis are characteristic.
- Parakeratotic scale around hair follicles and mild superficial inflammatory lymphocytic infiltrate

DIFFERENTIAL DIAGNOSIS
- Atopic dermatitis: Distinction may be difficult in infants.
- Psoriasis:
  - Usually knees, elbows, and nails are involved.
  - Scalp psoriasis will be more sharply demarcated than seborrhea, with crusted, infiltrated plaques rather than mild scaling and erythema.
- *Candida*
- Tinea cruris or capitis: Suspect these when usual medications fail or if hair loss occurs.
- Eczema of auricle or otitis externa
- Rosacea
- Discoid lupus erythematosus: Skin biopsy will be beneficial.
- Histiocytosis X: May appear as seborrheic-type eruption
- Dandruff: Scalp only, noninflammatory

TREATMENT

MEDICATION
First Line
- Cradle cap: Use a coal tar shampoo or ketoconazole (Nizoral) shampoo if the nonmedicated shampoo is ineffective (2).
- Adults:
  - Topical antifungal agents:
    - Ketoconazole 2% foam or shampoo twice a week for clearance, then once a week or every other week for maintenance
    - Ketoconazole (Nizoral) cream may be used to clear scales in other areas.
    - Ciclopirox 1% shampoo twice weekly (1)[B]
  - Topical corticosteroids:
    - Begin with 1% hydrocortisone, and advance to more potent (fluorinated) steroid preparations as needed.

- Avoid continuous use of the more potent steroids to reduce the risk of skin atrophy, hypopigmentation, or systemic absorption (especially in infants and children).
  - Precautions: Fluorinated corticosteroids and higher concentrations of hydrocortisone (e.g., 2.5%) may cause atrophy or striae if used on the face or on skin folds.
  - Other topical agents:
    - Coal tar1% shampoo twice a week
    - Selenium sulfide 2.5% shampoo twice a week
    - Zinc pyrithione shampoo twice a week
    - Lithium succinate ointment twice a week
- Once controlled, washing with zinc soaps or selenium lotion with periodic use of steroid cream may help to maintain remission.

Second Line
- Calcineurin inhibitors:
  - Pimecrolimus 1% cream twice daily
  - Tacrolimus 0.1% ointment twice daily
- Systemic antifungal therapy:
  - Data are limited.
  - For moderate to severe seborrheic dermatitis:
    - Ketoconazole 200 mg/d
    - Itraconazole 200 mg/d
    - Daily regimen for 1–2 months followed by twice-weekly dosing for chronic treatment
    - Monitor potential hepatotoxic effects.

ADDITIONAL TREATMENT
General Measures
- Increase frequency of shampooing.
- Sunlight in moderate doses may be helpful.
- Cradle cap:
  - Frequent shampooing with a mild, nonmedicated shampoo
  - Remove thick scale by applying warm mineral oil, and then wash off an hour later with a mild soap and a soft-bristle toothbrush or terrycloth washcloth (2).
- Adults: Wash all affected areas with antiseborrheic shampoos. Start with over-the-counter brands (Tegrin, Selsun Blue), and increase to more potent preparations (containing coal tar, sulfur, selenium, or salicylic acid) if no improvement is noted (2).
- For dense scalp scaling, 10% liquor carbonic detergens in Nivea oil may be used at bedtime, covering the head with a shower cap. This should be done nightly for 1–3 weeks.

Issues for Referral
No response to 1st-line therapy and concerns regarding systemic illness (HIV, etc.)

 ONGOING CARE

FOLLOW-UP RECOMMENDATIONS
Patient Monitoring
Every 2–12 weeks as necessary depending on disease severity and degree of patient sophistication

PATIENT EDUCATION
http://familydoctor.org/online/famdocen/home/common/skin/disorders/157.html

PROGNOSIS
- In infants, seborrheic dermatitis usually remits after 6–8 months.
- In adults, seborrheic dermatitis is usually chronic and unpredictable, with exacerbations and remissions. Disease is usually easily controlled with shampoos and topical steroids.

COMPLICATIONS
- Skin atrophy or striae are possible from fluorinated corticosteroids, especially if used on the face.
- Glaucoma can result from use of fluorinated steroids around the eyes.
- Photosensitivity is caused occasionally by tars.
- Herpes keratitis is a rare complication of herpes simplex: Instruct patient to stop eyelid steroids if herpes simplex develops.

REFERENCES
1. Shuster S, Meynadier J, Kerl H, et al. Treatment and prophylaxis of seborrheic dermatitis of the scalp with antipityrosporal 1% ciclopirox shampoo. *Arch Dermatol*. 2005;141:47–52.
2. Johnson BA, Nunley JR. Treatment of seborrheic dermatitis. *Am Fam Physician*. 2000;61:2703–10, 2713–4.

ADDITIONAL READING
- Darabi K, Hostetler SG, Bechtel MA, et al. The role of Malassezia in atopic dermatitis affecting the head and neck of adults. *J Am Acad Dermatol*. 2008.
- Karincaoglu Y, Tepe B, Kalayci B, et al. Is Demodex folliculorum an aetiological factor in seborrhoeic dermatitis? *Clin Exp Dermatol*. 2009.

- Naldi L, Rebora A. Clinical practice. Seborrheic dermatitis. *N Engl J Med*. 2009;360:387–96.
- Shemer A, Kaplan B, Nathansohn N, et al. Treatment of moderate to severe facial seborrheic dermatitis with itraconazole: an open non-comparative study. *Isr Med Assoc J*. 2008;10:417–8.
- Shin H, Kwon OS, Won CH, et al. Clinical efficacies of topical agents for the treatment of seborrheic dermatitis of the scalp: A comparative study. *J Dermatol*. 2009;36:131–7.

See Also (Topic, Algorithm, Electronic Media Element)
Algorithm: Rash, Focal

 CODES

ICD9
- 690.10 Seborrheic dermatitis, unspecified
- 690.11 Seborrhea capitis
- 690.12 Seborrheic infantile dermatitis

CLINICAL PEARLS
Search for an underlying systemic disease in a patient who is unresponsive to usual therapy.

D

DERMATITIS, STASIS
Joseph A. Florence, MD

 BASICS

DESCRIPTION
- Chronic, eczematous, erythremic, scaling, and noninflammatory edema of the lower extremities accompanied by cycle of scratching, excoriations, weeping, crusting, and inflammation in patients with chronic venous insufficiency, due to impaired circulation and other factors (nutritional edema)
- Clinical skin manifestation of chronic venous insufficiency usually appears late in the disease
- May present as a solitary lesion
- System(s) affected: Skin/Exocrine
- Synonym(s): Gravitational eczema; Varicose eczema; Venous dermatitis

EPIDEMIOLOGY
Incidence
- In the US: Common in patients >50 (6–7%)
- Predominant age: Adult, geriatric
- Predominant sex: Female > Male

Geriatric Considerations
- Common in this age group
- Estimated to affect 15–20 million patients >50 years in the US

RISK FACTORS
- Atopy
- Superimposition of itch–scratch cycle
- Trauma
- Previous deep vein thrombosis (DVT)
- Previous pregnancy
- Prolonged medical illness
- Obesity
- Secondary infection
- Low-protein diet
- Old age
- Deposition of fibrin around capillaries
- Microvascular abnormalities
- Ischemia
- Genetic propensity
- Edema
- Tight garments that constrict the thigh
- Vein stripping
- Vein harvesting for coronary artery bypass graft surgery
- Previous cellulitis

Genetics
Familial link probable

GENERAL PREVENTION
- Use compression stockings to avoid recurrence of edema and to mobilize the interstitial lymphatic fluid from the region of stasis dermatitis.
- Topical lubricants twice a day to prevent fissuring and itching

ETIOLOGY
- Incompetence of perforating veins causing blood to backflow to the superficial venous system leading to venous hypertension (HTN) and cutaneous inflammation
- Continuous presence of edema in ankles, usually present because of venous valve incompetency (varicose veins)
- Weakness of venous walls in lower extremities
- Trauma to edematous, eczematized skin
- Itch may be caused by inflammatory mediators (from mast cells, monocytes, macrophages, or neutrophils) liberated in the microcirculation and endothelium
- Abnormal leukocyte-endothelium interaction is proposed to be a major factor.
- A cascade of biochemical events leads to ulceration.
- Is associated with amlodipine therapy
- Elevated homocysteine has been noted in patients with stasis dermatitis.

COMMONLY ASSOCIATED CONDITIONS
- Varicose veins
- Venous insufficiency
- Other eczematous disease

 DIAGNOSIS

HISTORY
- Erythema, scaling, edema of lower extremities
- Pruritus
- Excoriations
- Weeping, crusting, inflammation of the skin
- Noninflammatory edema precedes the skin eruption and ulceration.
- Edema initially develops around the ankle.
- Itching, pain, and burning may precede skin signs, which are aggravated during evening hours (1)[B].
- Insidious onset
- Usually bilateral
- Description may include aching/heavy legs

PHYSICAL EXAM
- Evaluation of the lower extremities characteristically reveals:
  - Bilateral scaly, eczematous patches, papules, and/or plaques
  - Violaceous (sometimes brown), erythematous-colored lesions due to deoxygenation of venous blood (postinflammatory hyperpigmentation and hemosiderin deposition within the cutaneous tissue)
- Distribution: Medial aspect of ankle with frequent extension onto the foot and lower leg
- Brawny induration
- Stasis ulcers (frequently accompany stasis dermatitis) secondary to cuts, bruises, and excoriations to the weakened skin around the ankle

- Mild pruritus, pain (if ulcer present)
- Varicosities are often associated with ulcers.
- Clinical inspection reveals erythematous color with increased pigmentation, swelling, and warmth.
- Skin changes are more common in the lower 3rd of the extremity and medially.
- Early signs include prominent superficial veins and pitting ankle edema.
- May present as a solitary lesion (2)[C]

DIAGNOSTIC TESTS & INTERPRETATION
Lab
Initial lab tests
Culture stasis ulcers if bacterial infection is suspected.

Imaging
Initial approach
Duplex ultrasound imaging is helpful in diagnosis (3)[C].

Diagnostic Procedures/Surgery
Rule out arterial insufficiency (check peripheral pulses, leg blood pressures).

Pathological Findings
Chronic inflammation, characterized histologically by proliferation of small blood vessels in the papillary dermis

DIFFERENTIAL DIAGNOSIS
- Other eczematous diseases:
  - Atopic dermatitis
  - Uremic dermatitis
  - Contact dermatitis (due to topical agents used to self-treat)
  - Neurodermatitis
  - Arterial insufficiency
  - Sickle cell disease causing skin ulceration
  - Cellulitis
  - Erysipelas
- Tinea dermatophyte infection
- Pretibial myxedema
- Nummular eczema
- Lichen simplex chronicus
- Xerosis
- Asteatotic eczema
- Amyopathic dermatomyositis

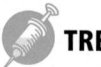 **TREATMENT**

MEDICATION
First Line
- Use of antibiotics topically or systemically is controversial, as stasis ulcer may not be infected.
- Antibiotics are indicated if bacterial infection is present, or may be used empirically if bacterial infection is suspected.
- If ulcer is present, local povidone-iodine treatment is as effective as systemic antibiotics (4)[B].
- If secondary infection, treat with oral antibiotics for *Staphylococcus* or *Streptococcus* organisms (e.g., dicloxacillin 250 mg q.i.d., cephalexin 250 mg q.i.d. or 500 mg b.i.d., or levofloxacin 250 mg q.i.d.).

- Gram-negative colonization: Treat with topical antimicrobial agents (e.g., benzoyl peroxide, acetic acid, silver nitrate, or Hibiclens) or broad-spectrum topical antibiotics (e.g., neomycin or bacitracin-polymyxin B [Polysporin]).
- 5% Aluminum acetate (Burow solution) wet dressings and cooling pastes
- Topical triamcinolone 0.1% (Kenalog, Aristocort) cream/ointment t.i.d. or topical betamethasone
- Betamethasone valerate (Valisone) 0.1% cream/ointment/solution t.i.d. (5)[A]
- Topical antipruritic: Pramoxine, camphor, menthol, and doxepin
- Systemic steroids for severe cases
- Calcium dobesilate has been shown to be an effective adjuvant therapy (6)[B].
- Vitamin supplementation in patients with hyperhomocysteinemia (7)[C]
- Evidenced-based treatment options for associated venous ulcers include aspirin and pentoxifylline (8)[B].

Second Line
- Consider antibiotics on basis of culture results of exudate from ulcer craters.
- Lubricants when dermatitis is quiescent
- Chronic stasis dermatitis can be treated with topical emollients (e.g., white petroleum, lanolin, Eucerin).
- Antipruritic medications (e.g., diphenhydramine, cetirizine hydrochloride, desloratadine)

ADDITIONAL TREATMENT
If the patient is on amlodipine therapy consider discontinuing amlodipine (9)[B].

General Measures
Primary role of treatment is to reverse effects of venous HTN. Appropriate health care:
- Outpatient:
  - Reduce edema (8)[B]:
    - Leg elevation: Heels higher than knees, knees higher than hips
    - Compression therapy: Elastic bandage wraps: Ace bandages or Unna paste boot (zinc gelatin) if lesions are dry or compression stockings (Jobst or nonfitted type) (10,11)[A]
    - Pneumatic compression devices
    - Diuretic therapy
  - Treat infection:
    - Débride the ulcer base of necrotic tissue.
    - Improvement of lipodermatosclerosis
  - Activity:
    - Avoid standing still.
    - Stay active and exercise regularly.
    - Elevate foot of bed unless contraindicated.
- Inpatient for vein stripping, sclerotherapy, or skin grafts:
  - Venous ulcer treatment includes autolytic, biologic, chemical, mechanical, and surgical:
    - Autolytic: Hydrogels, alginates, hydrocolloids, foams, and films
    - Biologic: Topical application of granulocyte macrophage colony-stimulating factor promotes healing of ulcers.

- Chemical: Enzyme débriding agents
- Mechanical: Wet to dry dressings, hydrotherapy, and irrigation
- Surgical modifying cause of venous HTN, treat ulcer by graft

SURGERY/OTHER PROCEDURES
Sclerotherapy and surgery may be required.

 ONGOING CARE

FOLLOW-UP RECOMMENDATIONS
Patient Monitoring
If Unna boot compression is used: Cut off and reapply boot once a week (restricts edema and prevents scratching).

DIET
- No special diet
- Lose weight, if overweight

PATIENT EDUCATION
- Stress staying active to keep circulation and leg muscles in good condition. Walking is ideal.
- Keep legs elevated while sitting or lying.
- Don't wear girdles, garters, or pantyhose with tight elastic tops.
- Don't scratch.
- Elevate foot of bed with 2–4-inch blocks.

PROGNOSIS
- Chronic course with intermittent exacerbations and remissions
- The healing process for ulceration is often prolonged and may take months.

COMPLICATIONS
- Sensations of itching, pain, and burning have negative impact on the quality of life
- Secondary bacterial infection
- DVT
- Bleeding at dermatitis sites
- Squamous cell carcinoma in edges of long-standing stasis ulcers
- Scarring, which in turn leads to further compromise to blood flow and increased likelihood of minor trauma

REFERENCES

1. Duque MI, Yosipovitch G, Chan YH, et al. Itch, pain, and burning sensation are common symptoms in mild to moderate chronic venous insufficiency with an impact on quality of life. *J Am Acad Dermatol*. 2005;53:504–8.
2. Weaver J, Billings SD et al. Initial presentation of stasis dermatitis mimicking solitary lesions: a previously unrecognized clinical scenario. *J Am Acad Dermatol*. 2009;61:1028–32.
3. Coleridge-Smith P, Labropoulos N, Partsch H, et al. Duplex ultrasound investigation of the veins in chronic venous disease of the lower limbs–UIP consensus document. Part I. Basic principles. *Eur J Vasc Endovasc Surg*. 2006;31:83–92.
4. Daróczy J. Quality control in chronic wound management: the role of local povidone-iodine (Betadine) therapy. *Dermatology*. 2006;212 (Suppl 1):82–7.
5. Weiss SC, Nguyen J, Chon S, et al. A randomized controlled clinical trial assessing the effect of betamethasone valerate 0.12% foam on the short-term treatment of stasis dermatitis. *J Drugs Dermatol*. 2005;4:339–45.
6. Kaur C, Sarkar R, Kanwar AJ, et al. An open trial of calcium dobesilate in patients with venous ulcers and stasis dermatitis. *Int J Dermatol*. 2003;42: 147–52.
7. Kartal Durmazlar SP, Akgul A, Eskioglu F et al. Hyperhomocysteinemia in patients with stasis dermatitis and ulcer: A novel finding with important therapeutic implications. *J Dermatolog Treat*. 2009;1–4.
8. Collins L, Seraj S et al. Diagnosis and treatment of venous ulcers. *Am Fam Physician*. 2010;81: 989–96.
9. Gosnell AL, Nedorost ST et al. Stasis dermatitis as a complication of amlodipine therapy. *J Drugs Dermatol*. 2009;8:135–7.
10. Partsch H, Flour M, Coleridge Smith P. Indications for compression therapy in venous and lymphatic disease Consensus based on experimental data and scientific evidence. Under the auspices of the IUP. *Int Angiol*. 2008;27:193–219.
11. Coleridge-Smith PD. Leg ulcer treatment. *J Vasc Surg*. 2009;49:804–8.

ADDITIONAL READING

- Antignani PL. Classification of chronic venous insufficiency: a review. *Angiology*. 2001; 52 (Suppl 1):S17–26.
- Durmazlar SPK, Akgul A, Eskioglu F. Hyperhomocysteinemia in patients with stasis dermatitis and ulcer: A novel finding with important therapeutic implications. *J Dermatolog Treat*. 2009;20:3;1–4.

See Also (Topic, Algorithm, Electronic Media Element)
Varicose Veins
Algorithm: Rash, focal

 CODES

ICD9
- 454.1 Varicose veins of lower extremities with inflammation
- 459.81 Venous (peripheral) insufficiency, unspecified

CLINICAL PEARLS

Treatment of edema associated with stasis dermatitis via elevation and/or compression stockings is essential for optimal results.

DIABETES INSIPIDUS

Kristine Willett, PharmD
Susan White, MD

BASICS

DESCRIPTION
- A condition of intense thirst (polydipsia) and excessive urination (polyuria) owing to the kidneys' inability to conserve water as they filter blood.
- Most commonly, this results from decreased pituitary secretion of vasopressin [central diabetes insipidus (DI)] or failure of response to vasopressin (nephrogenic DI).
- Rarely, DI can be induced by pregnancy (gestational DI)
- System(s) affected: Endocrine/Metabolic

EPIDEMIOLOGY
Incidence
- 1/25,000 persons
- May occur in 18.3% following transsphenoidal microsurgery
- Causes of DI:
  - 30% idiopathic
  - 25% brain tumors (malignant or benign)
  - 16% head trauma
  - 20% after cranial surgery

Prevalence
- Vasopressin deficiency may occur at any age.
- Nephrogenic DI is usually manifest in infancy.
- Nephrogenic DI is encountered in males more commonly, reflecting its X-linked mode of inheritance.

RISK FACTORS
- Intracranial neoplasm
- Infection
- Following surgery
- Drug-induced (amphotericin B, colchicine, demeclocycline, foscarnet, gentamicin, lithium, loop diuretics, methoxyflurane)
- Head trauma
- Genetic predisposition

Genetics
- Central DI: Familial cases of vasopressin deficiency have been reported (commonly autosomal dominant; >20 mutations have been identified), but the disease usually is isolated and often secondary to other disorders.
- Nephrogenic DI:
  - Most common is an X-linked defect in the V_2 receptor that binds antidiuretic hormone (ADH).
  - Autosomal dominant or recessive defects in the aquaporin-2 gene that encodes an ADH-responsive water channel

PATHOPHYSIOLOGY
- Central DI:
  - Inadequate secretion of vasopressin may be due to loss or malfunction of the neurosecretory neurons that make up the neurohypophysis (posterior pituitary) and the pituitary stalk.
  - Posterior pituitary lesions rarely cause DI because ADH is produced in the hypothalamus and therefore still would be secreted.
- Nephrogenic DI:
  - Inadequate response of kidney to vasopressin
  - A disorder of renal tubular function resulting in inability to respond to vasopressin in absorption of water

ETIOLOGY
- Central DI (inadequate secretion of vasopressin; may be idiopathic or familial):
  - Idiopathic
  - Trauma/head injury: A study of 89 patients with traumatic brain injury found that primary hormonal dysfunction (including DI) occurred in 21% of patients and tended to occur in patients with the lowest Glasgow Outcome Scale scores (1).
  - Neurosurgery
  - Tumors (e.g., craniopharyngioma, lymphoma, metastasis)
  - Infections (e.g., meningitis, encephalitis)
  - Granulomas (e.g., sarcoid, histiocytosis)
  - Hypoxic encephopathy
  - Vascular disorders
  - Inheritable defects (rare, occurs in 1–2%)
- Nephrogenic DI (inadequate response of kidneys to vasopressin):
  - Familial genetic defect in resorption of water in renal collecting ducts, including X-linked V_2 receptor mutation and autosomal recessive aquaporin-2 mutation
  - Drug induced (amphotericin B, colchicine, demeclocycline, foscarnet, gentamicin, lithium, loop diuretics, methoxyflurane)

COMMONLY ASSOCIATED CONDITIONS
- Potassium depletion
- Chronic hypercalcemia
- Tumors
- Infection:
  - Encephalitis
  - Tuberculosis
  - Syphilis
- Xanthomatosis
- Pyelonephritis
- Renal amyloidosis
- Sjögren syndrome
- Sickle-cell anemia
- Multiple myeloma
- Wolfram syndrome (DIDMOAD: *DI, diabetes mellitus, optic atrophy, deafness*)

DIAGNOSIS

The diagnosis of DI may be difficult to make because the clinical presentation depends on the cause, severity, and other medical conditions that may or may not be present. The course of DI not associated with brain injury tends to be indolent and, as long as water is available, may be hard to detect. Polyuria is highly variable, as is tolerance for dehydration.

HISTORY
- Thirst/polydipsia (with a particular preference for cold or iced drinks)
- Polyuria (3–20 L/d)
- Nocturia, bed wetting
- Dehydration
- Headache
- Visual disturbances
- Rate of onset of polydipsia is more rapid in central DI than in nephrogenic DI.
- Family history of polyuria
- In children, enuresis, anorexia, linear growth defects, and frequent fatigue may be found.
- In infants, crying, irritability, poor growth, hyperthermia, and weight loss are often found.

PHYSICAL EXAM
Signs of dehydration and an enlarged bladder may be present, but otherwise the exam is usually unremarkable.

DIAGNOSTIC TESTS & INTERPRETATION
Lab
- Low urine specific gravity and osmolality are indicative of DI.
- Urine/plasma osmolality ratio and plasma vasopressin concentration results may be difficult to interpret; low ratios may be found in patients with primary polydipsia.
- Water deprivation test (Miller-Moses test) to evaluate the ability to concentrate urine; aids in determining etiology.
  - Water is withheld, and urine and plasma osmolality are measured at hourly intervals.
  - A rise in urine osmolality indicates an intact ADH response.
  - A rise in plasma osmolality or stable urine osmolality indicates poor ADH response.
  - Perform the test during the day, not overnight, to avoid serious volume depletion or hypernatremia.
  - If the results support the diagnosis, desmopressin should be administered to test renal concentrating ability.

Initial lab tests
- Serum electrolyte levels
- Serum glucose to rule out diabetes mellitus
- Urine osmolality
- Urine specific gravity
- Urine electrolytes; hypokalemia and hypercalcemia alter the ability to concentrate urine.

- Plasma vasopressin or urinary vasopressin following osmotic stimulus, such as fluid restriction or administration of hypertonic saline
- Drugs that may alter lab results: Lithium, demeclocycline, and methoxyflurane may induce vasopressin insensitivity.

Imaging
Head MRI

Initial approach
If the diagnosis of DI is made, appropriate studies for cause, including MRI of the brain, must be performed.

Pathological Findings
Degeneration of neurosecretory neurons in the neurohypophysis

DIFFERENTIAL DIAGNOSIS
- Diabetes mellitus and other causes of polydipsia and polyuria
- Increased solute load for excretion, as occurs with high salt intake; osmotic diuresis
- Psychogenic polydipsia (ultimately impairs vasopressin secretion)

 TREATMENT

MEDICATION
- Therapy depends on type of DI.
- Central DI (23):
  – Desmopressin (DDAVP), a derivative of vasopressin, may be given orally, parenterally (IV, IM, SQ), or intranasally.
    ○ Intranasally (100 μg/mL solution), recommended initial dose is 10 μg at bedtime to relieve nocturia; may dose twice daily if symptoms persist in daytime.
    ○ Orally available as 0.1- to 0.2-mg tablets; recommended initial dose in children >4 years of age is 0.05 mg twice daily.
  – Thiazide diuretic dosed once or twice daily
- Nephrogenic DI (23):
  – Does not respond to desmopressin (DDAVP)
  – Remove offending agent(s).
  – Correct electrolyte imbalances (i.e., hypokalemia, hypocalcemia).
  – Pitressin has vasopressor and ADH activity, increasing water resorption at collecting ducts.
    ○ Adults: 5–10 units SC q3–6h; children: 2.5–10 units SC b.i.d. to q.i.d.
    ○ Major side effect is coronary artery constriction.
    ○ Contraindicated in patients with hypertension, angina, coronary heart disease
    ○ Pregnancy category B
  – Chlorpropamide (Diabinese) promotes renal response to ADH.
    ○ Adult 125–250 mg PO b.i.d.; not recommended for pediatric patients
    ○ Contraindicated in type I diabetes mellitus, severe renal or hepatic impairment, thyroid dysfunction
    ○ Pregnancy category C
    ○ Hypoglycemia may occur.

- Contraindications: Use desmopressin with caution in the immediate postoperative period for intracranial lesions because of possible cerebral edema.
- Precautions: An overdose of desmopressin may produce water intoxication and hyponatremia in patients with excessive water intake.

First Line
- Desmopressin is the treatment of choice in patients with central DI or gestational DI (pregnancy category B).

ADDITIONAL TREATMENT
General Measures
- Control fluid balance, and prevent dehydration.
- Careful follow-up and management of electrolytes
- Check weight daily.
- Provide good skin and mouth care.
- Nephrogenic DI: Correct hypercalcemia and hypokalemia, and discontinue causative medications (2)[A].

Issues for Referral
- Dilatation of urinary tract (may be secondary to large urine volumes)
- Complications of primary disease (tumor, histiocytosis, etc.)
- In congenital nephrogenic DI, an associated retardation of mental development may occur in some patients.
- Subnormal growth rate

 ONGOING CARE

FOLLOW-UP RECOMMENDATIONS
Continuing care is provided on an outpatient basis with self-medication.

Patient Monitoring
- Regular follow-up at 2- to 3-week intervals initially and 3–4 months later
- Adjust treatment on the basis of urine and electrolyte concentrations.
- Following moderate to severe traumatic brain injury, testing should done 6 and 12 months after injury.

DIET
- Normal, with free access to fluids
- Young infants with nephrogenic DI may benefit from low-solute formula.
- A low-sodium, low-protein diet may reduce urine output in nephrogenic DI.

PATIENT EDUCATION
- Reassurance of good prognosis
- Monitor medications/urinary pattern.
- Special precautions during travel, hot weather, exertion, and times of vomiting or diarrhea to avoid dehydration

PROGNOSIS
- Most reversible cases of nephrogenic DI are caused by medications, and patient symptoms improve with removal of the offending agent (4)[A]. Lithium may cause irreversible DI (4)[A].
- Generally good prognosis depending on underlying disorder

COMPLICATIONS
- Dilatation of the urinary tract has been observed (probably secondary to large volume of urine).
- Complications of the primary disease (tumor histiocytosis, etc.) should be anticipated. In congenital nephrogenic DI, an associated retardation of mental development may occur in some patients (cause undetermined).
- Without treatment, dehydration can lead to confusion, stupor, and coma.
- Subnormal growth rate

REFERENCES
1. Karhulik D, Zapletalova J, Frysak Z, et al. Dysfunction of hypothalamic-hypophysial axis after traumatic brain injury in adcults. *J Neurosurg.* 2009;0:1–4. Posted online November 20, 2009.
2. Makaryus AN, McFarlane SI. Diabetes insipidus: diagnosis and treatment of a complex disease. *Cleve Clin J Med.* 2006;73:65–71.
3. www.diabetesinsipidus.org
4. Garofeanu CG, Weir M, Rosas-Arellano MP, et al. Causes of reversible nephrogenic diabetes insipidus: a systematic review. *Am J Kidney Dis.* 2005;45:626–37.

ADDITIONAL READING
- Fukuda I, Hizuka N, Takano K. Oral DDAVP is a good alternative therapy for patients with central diabetes insipidus: experience of five-year treatment. *Endocr J.* 2003;50:437–43.
- Nemergut EC, Zuo Z, Jane JA, et al. Predictors of diabetes insipidus after transsphenoidal surgery: a review of 881 patients. *J Neurosurg.* 2005;103: 448–54.

 CODES

ICD9
253.5 Diabetes insipidus

CLINICAL PEARLS
- To distinguish primary polydipsia from DI in a patient with polyuria, a patient with primary polydipsia will have a normal response to a water restriction test and normal levels of plasma ADH.
- Vasopressin (IM) had been used previously but has been replaced by desmopressin, which provides the antidiuretic but not the vasoconstrictive activity of vasopressin for the treatment of central DI.
- The goal in adult patients with congenital nephrogenic DI is to prevent dehydration by ensuring proper fluid intake. Genetic testing should be recommended for access to genetic counseling and to facilitate newborn screening.

DIABETES MELLITUS, TYPE 1

Alfred Chege Gitu, MD

BASICS

DESCRIPTION
- Chronic disease caused by pancreatic insufficiency (deficiency) of insulin production
- Results in hyperglycemia and end-organ complications (e.g., accelerated atherosclerosis, neuropathy, nephropathy, and retinopathy)
- Features include:
  – Patients are insulinopenic and require insulin.
  – Ketosis
  – Usually rapid onset
  – Nutritional status: Normal or thin physique
- System(s) affected: Endocrine/Metabolic

Pregnancy Considerations
- During embryogenesis, hyperglycemia increases the incidence of congenital malformations. Tight control of blood sugar prior to conception is important.
- Women with microalbuminuria during the 1st trimester are at increased risk for preeclampsia and preterm delivery.
- A safe pregnancy is possible with vaginal delivery of a term baby. Close monitoring of blood sugar during labor is important.

EPIDEMIOLOGY
- Mean age of onset 8–12 years, peaking in adolescence
- Onset 1.5 years earlier in girls than boys
- Rapid decline in incidence after adolescence
- Overall incidence increasing worldwide
- Age of presentation has a bimodal distribution, being highest at ages 4–6 and 10–14 yrs.

Incidence
- 15/100,000 per year
- Racial predilection for whites
- African Americans have lowest overall incidence.

Pediatric Considerations
- Although onset is usually before the age of 19 yrs, true type 1 diabetes can occur for the first time in patients who are well into their 30s.
- Young children are more likely to present in diabetic ketoacidosis (DKA) due to atypical presentation, and because they may not express thirst or obtain fluids as readily as older children or adults.

RISK FACTORS
- Certain human leukocyte antigen (HLA) types
- Presence of a specific 64,000 mw protein may be responsible for antibody formation.
- Family history: Insulin-dependent or noninsulin-dependent diabetes in any 1st-degree relatives
- Dietary factors: Breastfeeding may provide a degree of protection against the disease, whereas exposure to cow's milk at an early age is associated with an increased risk of the disease.
- Maternal age at birth may play a role (1).
- Slightly greater risk for a child if the father has type 1 diabetes

Genetics
- Mode of genetic expression not clear
- Genes located on major histocompatibility complex on chromosome 6

- HLA DR3 and DR4 are individually associated with an increased risk; if a person is carrying both susceptibility genes, the relative risk is increased.
- HLA B8 and B15 associated with increased risk

PATHOPHYSIOLOGY
- Alteration in immunologic integrity, placing the β cell at special risk for inflammatory damage, accounts for most cases
- Autoantibodies to islet cells, glutamic acid decarboxylase (GAD), tyrosine phosphatase antibodies, and insulin identified in certain cases (type 1A diabetes)
- Some idiopathic cases (type 1B) have no evidence of autoimmune or other reason for beta cell damage.

ETIOLOGY
- Inherited defect
- Associated environmental triggers: None have been verified:
  – Viruses (such as mumps, coxsackie, cytomegalovirus, and hepatitis viruses)
  – Diet high in nitrosamines
  – Environmental toxins
- Emotional and physical stress

COMMONLY ASSOCIATED CONDITIONS
- Autoimmune diseases, such as hypothyroidism and Addison disease:
  – Screening regularly for hypothyroidism is particularly important in females.
- Diabetes mellitus can also be seen as part of multiple endocrine adenomatosis.

DIAGNOSIS

DIAGNOSTIC TESTS & INTERPRETATION
Lab
- Criteria for the diagnosis of diabetes:
  – Fasting glucose >126 mg/dL (7.0 mmol/L) OR
  – Random of >200 mg/dL (11.1 mmol/L) in a patient with classic symptoms of hyperglycemia OR
  – Oral glucose tolerance test; plasma glucose ≥200 mg/dL 2 hours after a glucose load of 1.75 g/kg (max. dose 75g) OR
  – Glycated hemoglobin (HbA1c) level ≥6.5% (2)[C]
- Other tests to consider:
  – Serum electrolytes, especially in sicker patients who may have ketoacidosis
  – Urinalysis for glucose and ketones and microalbuminuria
  – Pancreatic autoantibodies (to diagnose type 1A diabetes):
    ○ Islet cells, insulin, GAD, tyrosine phosphatase antibodies
  – Complete blood count (white blood cell count and hemoglobin may be elevated)
- C-peptide insulin level if needed to differentiate from type 2 diabetes

Pathological Findings
Inflammatory changes, lymphocytic infiltration around the islets of Langerhans, or islet cell loss

HISTORY
- Polyuria and polydipsia:
  – Polyuria may present as nocturia, bedwetting, or incontinence in a previously continent child.
  – Polyuria may be difficult to appreciate in diaper-clad children.

- Weight loss 10–30%:
  – Often almost devoid of body fat at diagnosis
  – Due to hypovolemia and increased catabolism
- Prolonged or recurrent candidal infection, usually in the diaper area
- Increased fatigue, lethargy, muscle cramps
- Irritability and emotional lability, headaches, abdominal discomfort, nausea
- Vision changes, such as blurriness
- Altered school or work performance
- Anxiety attacks

DIFFERENTIAL DIAGNOSIS
- Benign renal glycosuria
- Glucose intolerance
- Type 2 noninsulin-dependent diabetes:
  – Obese children might have maturity-onset diabetes of the young (MODY)
- Secondary diabetes:
  – Pancreatic disease (chronic pancreatitis, cystic fibrosis, hereditary hemochromatosis)
  – Hormonal disorders (pheochromocytoma, multiple endocrine adenomatosis)
  – Inborn errors of metabolism (glycogen storage disease, type 1)
  – Hereditary neuromuscular disease
  – Progeroid syndromes
  – Obesity (Prader-Willi syndrome)
  – Cytogenetic syndromes (trisomy 21, Klinefelter, and Turner syndromes)
  – Drug- or chemical-induced glucose intolerance: Glucocorticosteroids, HIV protease inhibitors, atypical antipsychotics, tacrolimus, cyclosporine
- Acute poisonings (salicylate poisoning can cause hyperglycemia and glycosuria, and may mimic diabetic ketoacidosis)

TREATMENT

MEDICATION
- All type 1 diabetes patients will require some form of insulin supplementation.
- Types of insulin:
  – Long-acting insulin analogues (insulin glargine [Lantus] and insulin detemir [Levemir]). These should not be mixed with other insulins in the same syringe.
  – Intermediate-acting insulin (NPH)—Humulin N or Novolin N—can be mixed with other insulins.
  – Short-acting (regular) insulin: Novolin R or Humulin R
  – Very rapid-acting insulin analogues (insulin lispro [Humalog], insulin aspart [Novolog], and insulin glulisine [Apidra])

First Line
- Flexible intensive insulin therapy is the gold standard.
- Frequent daily injections (FDI) or continuous subcutaneous insulin infusion (CSII) have equal efficacy.
- Total initial dose is 0.2–0.4 units per gg/day for insulin-naive patients.
- 40–60% of total dose given as basal insulin, and the rest as bolus insulin

- FDI regime:
  – Basal, long-acting insulin once or twice a day
  – Prandial, short-acting insulin based on number of carbohydrate portions (e.g., 1:10, meaning 1 unit of insulin for every 10 g of carbohydrate to be eaten)
  – Correctional short-acting mealtime insulin based on premeal blood glucose level (e.g., BS-100/50, meaning if the blood glucose is >150, subtract 100 from the BG level, and divide that number by 50)
  – Administration of the mealtime insulin before a meal may be more efficacious than during or after the meal.
- CSII regime:
  – May use regular insulin or rapid-acting insulin analogues
  – Basal insulin is infused continuously at a preset rate, and bolus doses are given with meals as above.

Second Line
- Conventional insulin therapy
- Once to twice daily injections with NPH mixed with regular or rapid-acting insulin in the same syringe
- Not physiologic, but lower cost and fewer injections may improve compliance in the less motivated patient.
- Premixed insulin available as NPH/regular (Novolin or Humulin 70/30) or NPH/rapid-acting insulin (e.g., Novolog 75/25 Mix or Humulin 75/25 Mix)
- Pancreatic transplantation is usually reserved for patients with end-stage renal failure, who may receive kidney-pancreatic transplants at the same time.
- Oral hypoglycemics not indicated in type 1 diabetes (except in obese patients, who may have MODY; or a combination of type 1 and type 2): Metformin (Glucophage)

ADDITIONAL TREATMENT
General Measures
- Overall control of carbohydrate metabolism for the very young child:
  – Normoglycemia (adjusted for age): Strive for blood glucose levels in range of 80–150 mg/dL (4.4–8.3 mmol/L) all the time (80–120 in older patients)
  – Very tight control might be dangerous in young children due to risk of repeated hypoglycemia.
  – Hemoglobin A1c target levels:
    ○ Children <6 years: 7.5–8.5%
    ○ Children 6–12 years: <8.0%
    ○ Adolescents 13–19: <7.5% (<7.0% if achieved without excessive hypoglycemia)
    ○ Nonpediatric patients: <6.0%
- Normal growth and development, and overall good health (asymptomatic):
  – Reach optimal height for genetic potential
  – Appropriate and timely pubertal maturation
  – Coping psychosocial development: Normal school or work attendance and performance; normal goals/career plans. Screen adolescents annually for depression.
- Prevent acute complications, including:
  – Hypoglycemic insulin reactions
  – Ketoacidosis
- Delay or prevent chronic complications.

IN-PATIENT CONSIDERATIONS
Newly diagnosed type 1 diabetics may require hospitalization during initiation of insulin therapy.

 ONGOING CARE

FOLLOW-UP RECOMMENDATIONS
- Normal; full participation in sports activities
- Regular aerobic exercise is recommended.

Patient Monitoring
- Blood pressure (BP) monitoring at every office visit (3)[C]
- Monitor height, weight, and sexual maturation (in children).
- Daily home blood glucose monitoring with home blood glucose meter: Blood tests should be done at least 4–6 times daily (more frequently in pump patients) for optimal monitoring.
- Quarterly measurement of hemoglobin A1c
- Annual screenings after 5 years of diabetes, sooner if glycemic control is suboptimal:
  – Microalbuminuria for earliest signs of possible nephropathy
  – If elevated, depending on level, even if BP is normal, consider an angiotensin-converting enzyme inhibitor (such as Vasotec [enalapril])
  – Ophthalmology exam (after 3–5 years of diabetes, also depending on glycemic control); regularly thereafter
  – Yearly lipid profile, thyroid levels, blood chemistries, complete blood count
  – Annual influenza vaccine

DIET
- American Diabetic Association diet:http://www.diabetes.org/food-and-fitness/food/
- Carbohydrate counting using insulin-to-carbohydrate ratio with all meals and snacks. Allows patient flexibility of eating and ability to eat almost anything.

PROGNOSIS
- Initial remission or honeymoon phase with decreased insulin needs and easier control, usually 3–6 months and rarely beyond a year
- Progression to total diabetes when endogenous insulin is insignificant; usually is gradual, but stress or illness initiate it suddenly
- Current prognosis:
  – Increasing longevity and quality of life with careful blood glucose monitoring and improvement in insulin delivery regimens
- At this time, reduced life expectancy, but has improved greatly over the past 20 years

COMPLICATIONS
- Microvascular disease (retinopathy, nephropathy, neuropathy)
- Hyperlipidemia
- Macrovascular disease (coronary and cerebral artery disease)
- Chronic foot ulcers/amputations
- Hypoglycemia
- Diabetic ketoacidosis
- Excessive weight gain
- Increased risk for preeclampsia and preterm delivery (4)
- Driving mishaps (5)
- Psychologic problems of chronic disease

REFERENCES

1. Cardwell CR, Stene LC, Joner G, Bulsara MK, Cinek O, Rosenbauer J, Ludvigsson J, Jané M, Svensson J, Goldacre MJ, Waldhoer T, Jarosz-Chobot P, Gimeno SG, Chuang LM, Parslow RC, Wadsworth EJ, Chetwynd A, Pozzilli P, Brigis G, Urbonaite B, Sipetic S, Schober E, Devoti G, Ionescu-Tirgoviste C, de Beaufort CE, Stoyanov D, Buschard K, Patterson CC et al. Maternal age at birth and childhood type 1 diabetes: a pooled analysis of 30 observational studies. *Diabetes*. 2010;59:486–94.
2. THE INTERNATIONAL EXPERT COMMITTEE. International Expert Committee Report on the Role of the A1C Assay in the Diagnosis of Diabetes. *Diabetes Care*. 2009.
3. American Diabetes Association (ADA). Standards of medical care in diabetes. V. Diabetes care. *Diabetes Care*. 2006;29(Suppl 1):S8–17.
4. Jensen DM, Damm P, Ovesen P, Mølsted-Pedersen L, Beck-Nielsen H, Westergaard JG, Moeller M, Mathiesen ER et al. Microalbuminuria, preeclampsia, and preterm delivery in pregnant women with type 1 diabetes: results from a nationwide Danish study. *Diabetes Care*. 2010;33:90–4.
5. Cox DJ, Ford D, Gonder-Frederick L, Clarke W, Mazze R, Weinger K, Ritterband L et al. Driving mishaps among individuals with type 1 diabetes: a prospective study. *Diabetes Care*. 2009;32: 2177–80.

ADDITIONAL READING

Silverstein J, Klingensmith G, Copeland K, et al. Care of children and adolescents with type 1 diabetes: a statement of the American Diabetes Association. *Diabetes Care*. 2005;28:186–212.

See Also (Topic, Algorithm, Electronic Media Element)
Diabetes Mellitus, Type 2; Diabetic Ketoacidosis (DKA)

 CODES

ICD9
- 250.01 Diabetes mellitus without mention of complication, type I (juvenile type), not stated as uncontrolled
- 250.03 Diabetes mellitus without mention of complication, type I (juvenile type), uncontrolled

CLINICAL PEARLS

- Polyuria may present as nocturia, bedwetting, or incontinence in a previously continent child.
- Young children are more likely to present in DKA because they may not express thirst or obtain fluids as readily as older children or adults.
- Onset usually before the age of 19 yrs, but type 1 diabetes can present in patients who are well into their 30s.
- Obese children might have MODY.

DIABETES MELLITUS, TYPE 2
Ramothea L. Webster, MD, PhD

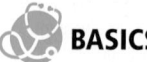

BASICS

DESCRIPTION
- Diabetes mellitus (DM) type 2 manifests in nonketotic hyperglycemia, insulin resistance, and relative impairment in insulin secretion.
- System(s) affected: Endocrine/Metabolic; Nervous; Renal/Urologic; Cardiovascular

Geriatric Considerations
- Significant contributing factor to blindness, renal failure, and lower limb amputations
- Dietary restrictions for elderly patients with DM in long-term facilities is not warranted; give regular diet.

Pediatric Considerations
Incidence is increasing dramatically, possibly related to increases in childhood obesity.

Pregnancy Considerations
First-line drug is insulin (class B), but may consider glyburide (class B) only after the 1st trimester or metformin (class B)

EPIDEMIOLOGY
Incidence
300/100,000; Male, 230/100,000; Female, 340/100,000

Prevalence
- 5,000/100,000; within race: 7.2% whites, 9% Hispanics, 11.2% blacks, and 35% Pima Indians
- If diagnosed <40, average reduction in life-years is 12 Yr (male) and 19 Yr (female).
- Lifetime risk of developing diabetes if born in 2000 is 33% (male) and 39% (female)

RISK FACTORS
- Family history: 1st-degree relative
- Gestational diabetes (GDM)
- Obesity: Induces resistance to insulin-mediated peripheral glucose uptake
- Ethnicity: African American, Latino, Native American, Asian American, and Pacific Islander
- Impaired fasting glucose (IFG) or impaired glucose tolerance (IGT)

Genetics
- Strong polygenic familial susceptibility
- Concordance nearly complete in identical twins

GENERAL PREVENTION
- Lose 5–10% body weight, exercise 150 min/week, and decrease fat and caloric intake
- Protein increases insulin response, but not to exceed 15% of caloric intake

PATHOPHYSIOLOGY
- Decrease in peripheral insulin effects ("insulin resistance") and resultant progressive loss of β-cell function and mass
- Cellular damage due to inability of cells to regulate uptake of glucose during hyperglycemic events via mitochondrial superoxide production to capillary endothelial cells in retina, mesangial cells in renal glomerulus, and to neurons and Schwann cells in peripheral nerves (1)[A].

ETIOLOGY
- Genetic factors (β-cell dysfunction, defects in insulin action, diseases of the exocrine pancreas, i.e., cystic fibrosis)
- Obesity, immune-mediated, infection, hemochromatosis
- Drug- or chemical-induced (e.g., medications used for psychosis, HIV, or transplant recipients)

COMMONLY ASSOCIATED CONDITIONS
- Hypertension
- Hyperlipidemia
- Impotence
- Stroke
- Peripheral neuropathy
- Syndrome X/metabolic syndrome
- Renal insufficiency/failure
- Cardiovascular disease
- Retinopathy
- Infertility
- Pancreatic cancer
- Polycystic ovary syndrome
- Acanthosis nigricans

DIAGNOSIS

HISTORY
Polyuria, polydipsia, polyphagia, weight loss, weakness, fatigue, and frequent infections

PHYSICAL EXAM
Complications of hyperglycemia: Retinopathy, neuropathy, and poor wound healing

DIAGNOSTIC TESTS & INTERPRETATION
- According to the ADA, IFG 100–125mg/dL, and IGT 140–199 mg/dL 2 hours after ingestion of 75g of glucose are prediabetes categories (1)[A].
- Glucose tolerance test (GTT) is usually not necessary, except when diagnosing gestational diabetes.
- HbA_{1c} has advantages over fasting plasma glucose (FPG) for diagnosis and analysis (2)[A].
- HbA_{1c} approximately ≤8.5% is mostly due to postprandial hyperglycemia and less fasting hyperglycemia, whereas HbA_{1c} ≥8.5% is mostly due to fasting hyperglycemia and less by postprandial hyperglycemia (1)[A].

Lab
- Criteria for diagnosis:
  - HbA_{1c} ≥6.5% on 2 or more occasions is diagnostic; HbA_{1c} between 5.7–6.4% is prediabetes (2)[A].
  - Symptoms of diabetes plus random plasma glucose ≥200 mg/dL (11.1 mmol/L), or
  - FPG ≥126 mg/dL (7.0 mmol/L) on 2 occasions, or
  - 2-hour plasma glucose ≥200 mg/dL (11.1 mmol/L) during oral GTT with 75-g glucose load (3)[A]
- Drugs that may alter lab results: Atypical antipsychotics, pentamidine, nicotinic acid, glucocorticoids, thyroid hormone, diazoxide, beta-adrenergic agonists, thiazides, Dilantin, alpha-interferon, and some fluoroquinolones

DIFFERENTIAL DIAGNOSIS
- Type 1 DM
- GDM

TREATMENT

- Goal FPG <110 mg/dL (5.5 mmol/L)
- Use drugs from different classes to achieve adequate control.
- Insulin might be the next best addition if uncontrolled by oral agents
- Goals remain unclear; some data suggest best A1C ~ 7.5%; ADA endorses <7.5%
- If HbA_{1c} >8%, consider starting 2 oral agents (3)[B].

MEDICATION
First Line
- Metformin: Preferred 1st medication because of its effects on weight loss and insulin resistance
- The following classes of agents may be used alone or in combination:
  - Biguanides
    - Metformin (Glucophage, Fortamet, Riomet, Glumetza): 500–1000 mg b.i.d.–t.i.d. or ER 1000–2000 mg qpm, max 2550 mg/d, except Glumetza, 2000 mg/d
    - Avoid situations that increase risk for lactic acidosis: Renal insufficiency, radiocontrast agents, surgery, or acute illnesses i.e., liver disease, cardiogenic shock, pancreatitis, or hypoxia
    - Caution with congestive heart failure (CHF), alcohol abuse, elderly, or with tetracycline
  - Sulfonylureas
    - Glipizide (Glucotrol): 2.5–40 mg/d; dosage >10 mg/d given b.i.d., take 30 minutes before meals
    - Glipizide extended-release: 5–20 mg/d
    - Glyburide (DiaBeta, Glynase, Micronase): 1.25–20 mg/d, Glynase 0.75–12 mg/d
    - Glimepiride (Amaryl): 1–8 mg/d
    - Caution with renal, liver, or thyroid disease, sulfa allergy, Cr CL <50, late pregnancy
    - Chlorpropamide (Diabinese): 100–500mg/d, max 750 mg/d
  - Thiazolidinediones
    - Pioglitazone (Actos): 15–45 mg/d
    - Monitor serum transaminase q2mo for the 1st year, contraindicated for liver disease and symptomatic heart failure patients; may cause or exacerbate CHF and myocardial infarction.
  - Alpha-glucosidase inhibitors
    - Acarbose (Precose): 25–100 mg t.i.d.
    - Miglitol (Glyset): 25–100 mg t.i.d.
    - Take at beginning of meals to decrease postprandial glucose peaks.
    - Poor patient compliance due to gastrointestinal symptoms
    - Avoid in renal insufficiency, inflammatory bowel disease, colonic ulceration, or partial bowel obstruction.
  - Dipeptidyl peptidase-4 inhibitor:
    - Sitagliptin (Januvia): 100 mg/d
    - Vildagliptin (Galvus): Awaiting FDA approval
    - Renally excreted; therefore, adjust dosage for renal patients.
- Precautions: Warn patients of signs of hypo- and hyperglycemia:
  - Combination of metformin and sulfonylurea can increase patient's relative risk of cardiovascular hospitalization or mortality

- Significant possible interactions:
  - Drugs that may potentiate sulfonylureas: Salicylates, clofibrate, warfarin (Coumadin), ethanol, and ACE inhibitors
  - Thiazides can cause IGT.
  - Gatifloxacin can cause either severe hypo- or hyperglycemia.
  - TZD pioglitazone may decrease effectiveness of oral contraceptives.
  - Drug binders, such as cholestyramine resin, should be taken at least 2 hours apart from alpha-glucosidase inhibitors

ALERT
Avandia: Associated with an increased risk of heart attack, stroke, and CHF. As of fall 2010, Avandia has been suspended in Europe; in U.S., is restricted to only when other diabetes medicine have failed and patients are aware of the drug's cardiovascular risks.

Second Line
- Insulin: Rapid (Aspart, Lispro, Glulisine), short (regular insulin), intermediate (NPH), and long/peakless (Glargine) or long/peak (Detemir):
  - Can be given up to t.i.d.
  - May be used in combination with oral agents, or with an insulin of a different half-life
  - Most often required in late stages of type 2 DM, when oral agents fail to control glucose levels
  - Insulindetemir (Levemir) or insulin glargine (Lantus): 0.5–1 U/kg/d, onset 1 hour, no true peak, duration 6–23 hours, given QHS or b.i.d.; start with 10 U SC QHS, then increase by 1 Unit daily until FPG <100.
  - Long-acting insulins have a lower risk of hypoglycemia and lower variability than other insulins
- Amylinomimetic:
  - Pramlintide (Symlin): 60–120 μg SC qAC:
  - When used with insulin, may cause severe hypoglycemia
  - Preprandial insulins, short-acting or rapid-acting, should be reduced by 50% at initiation of drug.
  - Contraindicated in patients with gastroparesis
  - Drug interactions: Anticholinergic drugs or agents that slow intestinal absorption of nutrients
- GLP-1 (glucagonlike peptide-1) receptor agonist
  - Exenatide (Byetta): 5–10 μg SC b.i.d. within 60 minutes before meals and at least 6 hours apart
  - Liraglutide (Victoza): 0.6 mg SQ per day for 1 week, then increase to 1.2; max 1.8 mg/day; less expensive and better tolerated than exenatide; should not be used in patients with history or family history of medullary thyroid cancer or MEN type II (black box warning) (4)[A]
- Promotes weight loss, increases high-density lipoprotein cholesterol, and decreases diastolic blood pressure (BP)
- Sulfonylureas should be decreased to reduce the chance of hypoglycemia. Patients should be advised to take other oral medications 1 hour before injecting Exenatide.
- Meglitinides:
  - Repaglinide (Prandin): 0.5–4 mg before meals; may be useful in patients with sulfa allergy or renal impairment
  - Nateglinide (Starlix): 60–120 mg before meals t.i.d.

ADDITIONAL TREATMENT
General Measures
- Foot exam every visit for neuropathy (monofilament), arterial insufficiency, and ulcers

- Nephropathy: Urine analysis to check microalbumin yearly
- Retinopathy: Yearly eye exams
- NCEP guidelines recommend a low-density lipoprotein cholesterol goal of <70 mg/dL in patients with existing cardiovascular disease (CVD) or risk factors for CVD.
- Strict control of hypertension (goal BP <130/80 mm Hg)
- Low-dose aspirin is recommended for all adults with diabetes, unless there is a contraindication.
- ACEI/ARB 1st-line hypertension drug (3)[A]; if contraindicated, consider a calcium channel blocker

COMPLEMENTARY AND ALTERNATIVE MEDICINE
- Cinnamon has no statistical significance with improving HbA$_{1c}$ or lipid parameters, but has shown improvements with FBG in patients with DM types 1 or 2. Its role in preventing DM is unknown.
- Chromium studies have shown reduction in HbA$_{1c}$ and FBG in patients with diabetes, although further studies are needed to fully understand its role in diabetes treatment and prevention.

 ## ONGOING CARE

FOLLOW-UP RECOMMENDATIONS
Regular aerobic exercise about 150 min/week can improve glucose tolerance and decrease medication requirements (3)[A]. Lifestyle modifications with pharmacotherapy can delay progression from prediabetes to diabetes (1)[A].

Patient Monitoring
- Office visits every 2–4 months
- Monitor glucose, HbA$_{1c}$, lipids, BP, body weight, and renal function.
- HbA$_{1c}$ twice a year for glycemic-controlled patients and quarterly for uncontrolled or change-in-therapy patients (3)[A]

DIET
ADA suggests mild caloric restriction to achieve mild to moderate weight loss. Carbohydrates should consist of <45%–65% of caloric consumption/day; fat <30%; protein <15%; and fiber 50 g/day (3)[A].

PATIENT EDUCATION
ADA patient education materials

PROGNOSIS
In susceptible individuals, complications begin to appear 10–15 years after onset, but can be present at time of diagnosis since disease may go undetected for years.

COMPLICATIONS
- Damage of macro- and microvascular arterial cell walls
- Peripheral neuropathy
- Proliferative retinopathy
- Nephropathy and chronic renal failure
- Atherosclerotic CVD and peripheral vascular disease
- Hyperosmolar coma

- Gangrene of extremities
- Blindness
- Glaucoma
- Cataracts
- Skin ulceration
- Charcot joints

REFERENCES
1. Blonde L et al. Current antihyperglycemic treatment guidelines and algorithms for patients with type 2 diabetes mellitus. *Am J Med*. 2010;123:S12–8.
2. The International Expert Committee. International Expert Committee Report on the Role of the A1C Assay in the Diagnosis of Diabetes. *Diabetes Care*. 2009.
3. American Diabetes Association. Standards of medical care in diabetes-2010. *Diabetes Care*. 2010;33(suppl 1)S11–S61.
4. Fakhoury WK, Lereun C, Wright D et al. A meta-analysis of placebo-controlled clinical trials assessing the efficacy and safety of incretin-based medications in patients with type 2 diabetes. *Pharmacology*. 2010;86:44–57.

See Also (Topic, Algorithm, Electronic Media Element)
Diabetes Mellitus, Type 1; Diabetic Ketoacidosis (DKA); Hypertension, Essential
Algorithm: Diabetes Mellitus, Type 2

 ## CODES

ICD9
- 250.00 Diabetes mellitus without mention of complication, type ii or unspecified type, not stated as uncontrolled
- 250.02 Diabetes mellitus without mention of complication, type ii or unspecified type, uncontrolled

CLINICAL PEARLS
- Screening: ≥45 years with a body mass index (BMI) ≥25 kg/m^2 or <45 years, overweight (BMI >25 kg/m^2), and other risk factors. Repeat every 3 years; if IFG or IGT, check every 1–2 years
- Criteria for testing children for DM II is: Overweight (BMI >85th percentile; weight for height >85th percentile or weight >120% of ideal height). Plus any 2 risk factors below:
  - Family history with 1st- or 2nd-degree relatives
  - Race/ethnicity
  - Signs of insulin resistance or conditions associated with insulin resistance (AN, hypertension, hyperlipidemia, or PCOS)
  - Maternal history of DM or GDM
  - Start at age 10 or at onset of puberty, whichever comes first
  - Frequency: every 2 years

DIABETIC KETOACIDOSIS (DKA)

Francesca L. Beaudoin, MS, MD
Nadine T. Himelfarb, MD

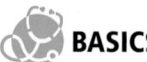 **BASICS**

DESCRIPTION
- A true medical emergency secondary to severe insulin deficiency and characterized by hyperglycemia, ketosis, and metabolic acidosis
- System(s) affected: Endocrine/Metabolic

EPIDEMIOLOGY
Incidence
- In US: 46 episodes/10,000 diabetic patients; 2/100 patient-years of type 1 diabetes mellitus (DM)
- Predominant age: 0–19 years
- Predominant sex: Male = Female.

RISK FACTORS
- Type 1 > type 2 DM
- Younger patients at higher risk

GENERAL PREVENTION
- Close monitoring of glucose during periods of stress, infection, and trauma
- Careful insulin control and monitoring of the blood glucose level
- "Sick day" management instructions

PATHOPHYSIOLOGY
A relative or absolute deficiency of insulin, exacerbated by an increase in counterregulatory hormones (e.g., catecholamines, cortisol, glucagon, and growth hormone) leading to a hyperglycemic crisis

ETIOLOGY
- Noncompliance/insufficient insulin: 25%
- Infection: 30–40%
- 1st presentation of DM: 10–20%
- Myocardial infarction (MI): 5–7%
- No cause identified: 10–30%
- Cerebrovascular accident (CVA)
- Medications (corticosteroids, thiazides)
- Drugs (cocaine)
- Trauma
- Surgery
- Emotional stress
- Pregnancy

COMMONLY ASSOCIATED CONDITIONS
Complications of chronic DM such as nephropathy, neuropathy, and retinopathy

 DIAGNOSIS

HISTORY
- Recent illness
- Changes in diet or medications
- Missed insulin doses
- Polyuria, nocturia
- Polydipsia
- Generalized weakness
- Malaise, lethargy
- Anorexia or increased appetite
- Nausea, vomiting
- Abdominal pain
- Decreased perspiration
- Fever
- Confusion
- Coma

PHYSICAL EXAM
- Hypotension
- Tachycardia
- Hypothermia or fever
- Tachypnea, Kussmaul respirations
- Fruity odor to breath (acetone smell)
- Decreased reflexes
- Abdominal tenderness
- Decreased bowel sounds
- Dry mucus membranes, poor skin turgor
- Decreased perspiration
- Confusion
- Coma
- Attempt to find precipitating cause (i.e., source of infection).

DIAGNOSTIC TESTS & INTERPRETATION
- Electrocardiogram (ECG):
  – Usually shows sinus tachycardia
  – Look for changes consistent with electrolyte abnormalities and ischemia/MI
- Urine and blood cultures
- Consider lumbar puncture (meningitis)

Lab

ALERT
- Hyponatremia: Hyperglycemia or hypertriglyceridemia may cause an artificially low or very low sodium concentration. The measured sodium is suppressed by 1.6 mg/dL for every 100 mg/dL of glucose over normal.
- Hyperglycemia (usually 250–800 mg/dL)
- Serum ketosis: Check β-hydroxybutyrate (β-HB) instead of ketones to evaluate ketosis (1)[B]. With concomitant lactic acidosis, acetoacetate production may be inhibited in the presence of high levels of β-HB. Nitroprusside reaction, which measures only acetoacetate, may not be strongly positive.
- Urine ketosis (may be falsely negative initially; urinalysis (UA) may only identify acetoacetate and not β-HB)
- Glycosuria
- Hyperamylasemia, hyperlipasemia
- Hypertriglyceridemia/hypercholesterolemia
- Increased creatinine and blood urea nitrogen (BUN): Markedly increased serum ketones may cross-react and cause a falsely high serum creatinine
- HCO_3 (usually $\leq$15 mEq/L)
- Decreased calculated total-body K^+: Severe acidosis gives an artificially high K^+ level.
- Metabolic acidosis on arterial blood gases
- Increased serum osmolality
- Increased anion gap
- Elevated base deficit

Initial lab tests
- Complete blood count, electrolytes, BUN, creatinine
- Serum β-HB or ketones
- Arterial blood gases; venous blood gases (VBGs) also may be used (VBG pH 0.03 lower)

Imaging
- Chest X-ray to rule out pulmonary infection
- Head CT scan if suspected CVA or cerebral edema

Diagnostic Procedures/Surgery
Only if surgical problem is the underlying precipitant (e.g., appendicitis)

DIFFERENTIAL DIAGNOSIS
- Hyperosmolar nonketotic coma
- Alcoholic ketoacidosis
- Starvation ketosis
- Toxic ingestions (e.g., salicylates)
- Lactic acidosis
- Acute hypoglycemic coma
- Uremia/chronic renal failure

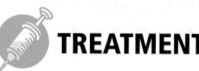 **TREATMENT**

- Oxygen and airway management as needed
- Establish IV access
- Cardiac monitoring
- Start isotonic crystalloid solution (0.9% saline)
- Fingerstick glucose testing
- Empirical naloxone if altered mental status

MEDICATION
First Line

- Insulin: IV infusion of regular insulin at 0.1 unit/kg/h; may use IM or SC route, but IV is recommended for moderate to severe DKA (1,2)[B].
- Potassium: Falsely elevated owing to acidosis; start replacement when K^+ $\leq$5.0 mg/dL and urine output is adequate. Start 30–40 mEq/L IV fluids. Increase rate (up to 60 mEq/L) if K^+ $\leq$3.5 mg/dL (2,1)[A].
  – Hold insulin if K^+ $\leq$2.5 mg/dL; give IV potassium 1 mEq/kg over 1 h.
  – For each 0.1 unit of pH, serum K^+ will change by $\sim$0.6 mEq in opposite direction.
- Phosphorus: Routine replacement may lead to hypocalcemia; if very low (<1.0), give 1/3 of K^+ replacement as KPhos.
- Sodium bicarbonate: No demonstrable benefit with a pH >7.0 (1,2)[B]; rehydration usually leads to resolution of acidosis. Consider its use in patients with arterial pH <6.9 or patients with life-threatening hyperkalemia.
- Magnesium: If Mg $\leq$1.8 mg/dL and the patient is symptomatic, consider replacement.
- Precautions:
  – If the patient is on an insulin pump, it should be stopped.
  – Double insulin if no response in serum glucose over 1st 2 h.
  – If blood glucose does not fall by $\sim$75 mg every 2 h, increase insulin rate.
  – If using bicarbonate, add 50–100 mEq NaHCO$_3$ to 1 L 0.45% saline or 150 mEq NaHCO$_3$ to 1 L D$_5$W and give over 1 h. Once a pH of 7.1 has been reached, infusion should be stopped.

Second Line
Insulin, SC or IM: Load with 0.3 unit/kg SC, followed by 0.1 unit/kg/h. Space dosing to q2h once glucose <250 mg/dL.

ADDITIONAL TREATMENT
General Measures
- All but mild cases require inpatient management; severe DKA requires an ICU setting.
- Goals:
  - Fluid resuscitation
  - Insulin therapy
  - Resolution of anion-gap acidosis
  - Correction of electrolytes
- Laboratory testing during management:
  - Serum glucose every 1–2 h until stable
  - Electrolytes, phosphorous, and venous pH every 2–6 h as needed

Pediatric Considerations
- Children with moderate to severe DKA should be transferred to the nearest pediatric critical-care hospital.
- In 0.3–1% of children/adolescents, fluid resuscitation and treatment may result in marked mental deterioration, including development of coma 4–6 h after therapy has begun; death is 21–24%.
  - Think of cerebral edema secondary to rapid IV hydration.
  - Diagnose by CT scan.
  - Treat with IV bolus of mannitol 1 g/kg in 20% solution.
  - If no response, hyperventilation to a pCO$_2$ of 28 mm Hg.

Geriatric Considerations
Must be careful with impaired renal function or congestive heart failure when correcting fluid and electrolyte abnormalities.

Pregnancy Considerations
- Pregnancy itself is diabetogenic. It also results in a compensated respiratory alkalosis (HCO$_3$ 19–20 mEq/L) with theoretically reduced buffering capacity. Therefore, pregnant patients are more susceptible to DKA.
- Euglycemic DKA
- Increased risk of preeclampsia and fetal death
- β-Tocolytics and corticosteroids can trigger DKA.
- Perinatal death: 9–35%

IN-PATIENT CONSIDERATIONS
Admission Criteria
ADA admission guidelines: Blood glucose >250 mg/dL; pH <7.3; HCO$_3$ ≤15 mEq/L; ketones in urine; ICU setting for severe DKA (3)

IV Fluids
- 10–20 mL/kg over the 1st h, then 500 mL/h (~0.7 mL/kg/h) for 4 h or until hemodynamics improve; then 250 mL/h (3.5 mL/kg/h) until tolerating PO
- Switch to 5% dextrose in 0.45% saline at maintenance rate when serum glucose <250 mg/dL. Maintain blood glucose between 150 and 250 mg/dL. Too rapid correction of fluid balance may precipitate cerebral edema (1)[C]. If the blood glucose level is falling too rapidly, consider using a 10% dextrose solution instead.

Pediatric Considerations
Bolus 10–20 mL/kg initially; 4-h fluid total should be <50 mL/kg to reduce chance of cerebral edema.

Discharge Criteria
Discharge when DKA has resolved: glucose <200 mg/dL; pH >7.3; bicarbonate >18 mEq/L; additionally, patients must be tolerating PO intake and able to resume home medication regimen, and the underlying precipitant (e.g., infection) must be identified and treated.

ONGOING CARE

FOLLOW-UP RECOMMENDATIONS
Bed rest

Patient Monitoring
- Monitor mental status, vital signs, and urine output q30–60min until improved, then q2–4h every 24 h.
- Monitor blood sugar q1h until <300 mg/dL, then q2–6h.
- Monitor electrolytes (Na, K, HCO$_3$) q2h.
- Monitor phosphate, calcium, and magnesium q4–6h.

DIET
- NPO initially
- Advance to preketotic diet when nausea and vomiting are controlled.
- Avoid foods with high glycemic index (e.g., soft drinks, white bread, etc.).

PROGNOSIS
- 16% of all diabetes-related fatalities
- Death 1–2%
- In children <10 years of age, DKA causes 70% of diabetes-related fatalities.

COMPLICATIONS
- Cerebral edema
- Pulmonary edema
- Vascular thrombosis
- Hypokalemia
- Cardica dysrhythmia

- MI
- Acute gastric dilatation
- Late hypoglycemia
- Erosive gastritis
- Infection, mucormycosis
- Respiratory distress

REFERENCES
1. Agus MS, Wolfsdorf JI. Diabetic ketoacidosis in children. *Pediatr Clin North Am.* 2005;52: 1147–63, ix.
2. Kitabchi AE, Umpierrez GE, Murphy MB, et al. Hyperglycemic crises in diabetes. *Diabetes Care.* 2004;27 (Suppl 1):S94–102.
3. American Diabetes Association. Hospital admission guidelines for diabetes. *Diabetes Care.* 2004;27 (Suppl 1):S103.

ADDITIONAL READING
- Carroll MA, Yeomans ER. Diabetic ketoacidosis in pregnancy. *Crit Care Med.* 2005;33:S347–53.
- Trachtenbarg DE. Diabetic ketoacidosis. *Am Fam Physician.* 2005;71:1705–14.

See Also (Topic, Algorithm, Electronic Media Element)
Diabetes Mellitus, Type 1

CODES

ICD9
- 250.12 Diabetes mellitus with ketoacidosis, type ii or unspecified type, uncontrolled
- 250.13 Diabetes mellitus with ketoacidosis, type I (juvenile type), uncontrolled

CLINICAL PEARLS
- Admit if blood glucose >250 mg/dL, pH <7.3, HCO$_3$ ≤15 mEq/L, and ketones in urine.
- Potassium is falsely elevated owing to acidosis; start replacement when K$^+$ ≤5.0 mg/dL and urine output is adequate.

DIABETIC POLYNEUROPATHY

Samir Malkani, MD

 BASICS

DESCRIPTION
Peripheral nerve dysfunction seen in diabetes; several patterns described:
- Symmetric polyneuropathy:
  - Distal sensory or sensorimotor
  - Proximal lower extremity polyneuropathy
- Focal and multifocal neuropathy:
  - Cranial neuropathy
  - Focal limb neuropathy
  - Diabetic amyotrophy
  - Truncal neuropathy
- Autonomic neuropathies
- Chronic inflammatory demyelinating polyneuropathy (CIDP)

EPIDEMIOLOGY
Prevalence
- Prevalence increases with diabetes duration
- Generalized polyneuropathy:
  - 10% at diabetes diagnosis
  - 50% at 25 years
  - Cross-sectional prevalence: 15% by symptoms; 50% by nerve conduction
- Autonomic neuropathy: 16.7% in a UK study

RISK FACTORS
- Poor glycemic control
- Duration of diabetes
- Older age
- Presence of retinopathy

GENERAL PREVENTION
Maintenance of normal blood sugar

PATHOPHYSIOLOGY
- >1 pathogenetic factor may operate
- Metabolic derangement due to hyperglycemia:
  - Aldose reductase converts excess glucose to sorbitol, which causes nerve damage
  - Nonenzymatic glycation of neural proteins and lipids forms damaging advanced glycosylation end products
  - Protein kinase C activation causes vascular endothelial changes
  - Oxidative stress from excessive production of reactive oxygen species
- Vasculopathy causing nerve ischemia: Likely in mononeuropathies

ETIOLOGY
Diabetes mellitus (type 1 and 2)

DIAGNOSIS

HISTORY
- Most common form: Symmetric distal sensory or sensorimotor polyneuropathy:
  - Distressing numbness, tingling, pain of legs/feet, usually worse at night; allodynia; hyperalgesia
  - Sometimes silent and unnoticed by patient
  - Ataxia due to proprioceptive loss
  - Neuropathic foot ulcers due to analgesia and repetitive injury
  - Neuropathic degeneration of foot joints
  - Hands involved late
  - Distal muscle involvement, usually mild
- Symmetric proximal polyneuropathy:
  - Proximal leg weakness and wasting
  - Muscles of shoulder girdle rarely involved
  - Pain and sensory changes less prominent
- Focal cranial or limb mononeuropathy:
  - May involve 3rd, 4th, 6th, or 7th cranial nerve
  - Femoral, sciatic, or peroneal neuropathy: Weakness or pain in nerve distribution
  - Any major peripheral nerve can be involved
- Truncal neuropathies: Painful radiculopathy over dermatomes
- Diabetic amyotrophy (this term is used for a lumbar radiculoplexopathy):
  - Unilateral hip, thigh pain
  - Pelvic girdle, thigh weakness, atrophy
  - Recovery over months
- Diabetic autonomic neuropathy:
  - Gastrointestinal: Nocturnal diarrhea, sometimes alternating with constipation; gastroparesis with postprandial fullness; nausea and vomiting
  - Cardiovascular: Postural dizziness; increased risk for coronary event; exercise intolerance
  - Urogenital: Urinary hesitancy, overflow incontinence; erectile dysfunction; vaginal dryness; sexual dysfunction
  - Sudomotor: Anhidrosis or hyperhydrosis; gustatory sweating of head and upper body
- CIDP: Progressive, severe motor loss
- Diabetic cachexia: Weight loss and depression with polyneuropathy

PHYSICAL EXAM
- Symmetric distal polyneuropathy:
  - "Stocking-and-glove" distal sensory loss
  - Large-fiber neuropathy: Loss of vibratory perception and light touch (10-G monofilament)
  - Small-fiber involvement: Loss of temperature and pinprick
  - Absent ankle reflexes
  - Wasting, weakness of small muscles in foot; changes to arch of foot or clawing of toes
  - With small-fiber involvement, there may be lack of objective sensory deficit despite pain
- Symmetric proximal polyneuropathy:
  - Proximal leg, arm wasting and weakness
  - Loss of patellar reflexes

- Focal cranial or limb mononeuropathy:
  - 3rd cranial nerve palsy: Painful ophthalmoplegia and ptosis; preserved pupillary reflexes (in contrast to compressive palsies)
  - 6th cranial nerve: Lateral gaze palsy
  - Femoral neuropathy: Weakness of lower leg extension; hip flexion; quadriceps wasting; absent patellar reflex; sensory loss in anterior thigh
  - Sciatic neuropathy: Pain or sensory loss in back of thigh and leg; weakness of hamstrings, lower leg muscles
  - Peroneal neuropathy: Foot drop
- Truncal neuropathies: Sensory loss along dermatome
- Lumbar radiculoplexopathy (amyotrophy):
  - Weakness and wasting pelvic girdle and thigh
  - Sensory loss in L2–L3
  - Absent patellar reflex
- Autonomic neuropathy:
  - Cardiovascular: Resting tachycardia; orthostatic hypotension
  - Gastroparesis: Postprandial distension; gastric splash
- CIDP: Motor weakness

DIAGNOSTIC TESTS & INTERPRETATION
Lab
Initial lab tests
- Fasting plasma glucose, 2-hr glucose tolerance test or hemoglobin A1c for diagnosis and to assess glycemic control
- Serum B_{12} levels
- Thyroid function
- Creatinine and blood urea nitrogen
- Syphilis testing
- Serum protein electrophoresis
- In mononeuropathy/mononeuritis multiplex, test for vasculitis, paraproteinemia, and sarcoid.

Imaging
Initial approach
In radiculopathy or mononeuropathy, imaging studies to exclude compressive lesions

Diagnostic Procedures/Surgery
- Quantitative sensory testing for vibratory and thermal thresholds:
  - Standardized measures for assessing severity and risk of foot ulceration
- Electromyogram nerve conduction velocity (1):
  - Useful to confirm mononeuropathy and entrapment syndromes
  - Sensitive but nonspecific index of presence and severity of diabetic polyneuropathy
  - In small unmyelinated fiber painful neuropathy, test may be normal
- Lumbar puncture:
  - In CIDP, elevation of spinal fluid protein
- Skin biopsy (1):
  - Enables direct study of small nerve fibers that are difficult to assess electrophysiologically
- Corneal confocal microscopy (2):
  - Noninvasive approach based on examination of corneal innervation

Pathological Findings
- In peripheral nerve, Wallerian degeneration, focal axonal swellings containing neurofilaments, axonal atrophy, and demyelination are seen.
- Thick neural capillary basement membrane
- Obliterative microvascular lesions and perivascular inflammation

DIFFERENTIAL DIAGNOSIS
- Uremic polyneuropathy
- Drug-induced:
  – Antineoplastic drugs: Cisplatin, vincristine
  – Isoniazid
  – Amiodarone
- Toxic:
  – Chronic arsenic poisoning
  – n-Hexane, methyl-n-butyl ketone
- Nutritional deficiency:
  – Usually associated with alcoholism
- Paraneoplastic polyneuropathy
- Hypothyroidism

 ## TREATMENT

MEDICATION
First Line
- Management of pain and sensory neuropathy:
  – Tricyclic antidepressants (TCAs) (1,3,4)[A]:
    ○ Analgesia may be related to effects on sodium channels
    ○ Amitriptyline 25–150 mg at bedtime
    ○ Nortriptyline (25–150 mg); desipramine (25–200 mg) less sedating than amitriptyline
    ○ Anticholinergic side effects may occur.
  – Calcium channel modulators: Gabapentin (1,34)[A]:
    ○ Fewer side effects than TCAs
    ○ Act on subunits of voltage-gated calcium channels (same site as pregabalin)
    ○ Dose titration is from 300–1,200 mg t.i.d.
    ○ Reduce dose in renal insufficiency
    ○ Adverse effects: Dizziness, fatigue, edema
  – Calcium channel modulators: Pregabalin (34)[A]
    ○ Binds Ca^{2+} channel-associated protein $\alpha_2\text{-}\delta$, inhibits neurotransmitter release
    ○ Usual dose 150–600 mg
    ○ Adverse effects are dizziness and edema.
  – Duloxetine (3 ,4)[A]:
    ○ Selective serotonin and norepinephrine uptake inhibitor
    ○ Usual dose is 60–120 mg/d
    ○ Adverse effects are nausea and dizziness.
- Management of autonomic neuropathy (3):
  – Orthostatic hypotension:
    ○ Fludrocortisone
    ○ Midodrine
  – Gastroparesis:
    ○ Metoclopramide or domperidone
    ○ Erythromycin
  – Diabetic diarrhea:
    ○ Loperamide
    ○ Clonidine
    ○ Octreotide
    ○ Antibiotics for bacterial overgrowth
  – Erectile dysfunction:
    ○ Phosphodiesterase-5 inhibitors
    ○ Prostaglandin E_1 injection
    ○ Mechanical devices
  – Hyperhidrosis:
    ○ Propantheline

Geriatric Considerations
- Anticholinergic effects of TCAs may cause urinary retention, arrhythmias

Second Line
- Antidepressants:
  – Venlafaxine (75–225 mg daily) (4)[B]:
    ○ Serotonin norepinephrine reuptake inhibitor
  – Selective serotonin reuptake inhibitors (4)[B]:
    ○ Paroxetine and citalopram demonstrate some efficacy.
- Anticonvulsants:
  – Carbamazepine (1,3)[B]:
    ○ Alleviates pain by blocking sodium channels
    ○ Dose 400–1,200 mg/d
  – Lamotrigine/topiramate 200–600 mg (1,3)[B]
- Topical therapies:
  – Capsaicin 0.075% cream applied t.i.d. 3[B]:
    ○ Depletes C fibers in skin of substance P
  – Lidocaine 5% (700 mg) patches applied daily to feet (3)[B]:
    ○ Causes sodium channel blockade
- Opiate analgesia:
  – Tramadol 100–400 mg daily (1,3):
    ○ Nonnarcotic medication; binds opiate receptors; fewer opiate side effects
  – Oxycodone (1,3)[A]:
    ○ Controversial due to dependence potential
- α-Lipoic Acid (4)[B]:
  – Antioxidant properties may limit free radical-mediated damage
  – 600 mg oral daily dose; showed benefit in small studies

ADDITIONAL TREATMENT
General Measures
- Maintain blood glucose close to normal.
- Provide appropriate footwear to prevent pressure damage to insensate feet.

Issues for Referral
If CIDP suspected, refer to neurologist for investigation and treatment

Additional Therapies
- Transcutaneous electrical nerve stimulation
- Percutaneous nerve stimulation
- Electrical spinal cord stimulation

COMPLEMENTARY AND ALTERNATIVE MEDICINE
Acupuncture (1)[C]: Placebo response possible, as trials were unblinded

SURGERY/OTHER PROCEDURES
Electrical spinal cord stimulation (1)

 ## ONGOING CARE

PROGNOSIS
- Generalized symmetric polyneuropathies:
  – Usually slow chronic progression
  – Insensitive but painless foot as pain lessens
- Focal neuropathies:
  – Recovery over months to years

COMPLICATIONS
- Claw foot deformity
- Neurotropic ulceration:
  – Painless ulcers on weightbearing area
  – Callus formation precursor to ulceration
- Neuropathic arthropathy:
  – Results in complete disorganization of joint structure in foot, Charcot joint

REFERENCES
1. Boulton AJ, Malik RA, Arezzo JC, et al. Diabetic somatic neuropathies. *Diabetes Care*. 2004;27: 1458–86.
2. Zochodne DW. Diabetic polyneuropathy: an update. *Curr Opin Neurol*. 2008;21:527–33.
3. Unger J, et al. Recognition and management of diabetic neuropathy. *Primary Care: Clin Office Pract*. 2007;34:887–913.
4. Ziegler D et al. Painful diabetic neuropathy: advantage of novel drugs over old drugs? *Diabetes Care*. 2009;32 (Suppl 2):S414–9.

ADDITIONAL READING
- Boulton AJ, Vinik AI, Arezzo JC, et al. Diabetic neuropathies: a statement by the American Diabetes Association. *Diabetes Care*. 2005;28:956–62.
- Casellini CM, Vinik AI et al. Clinical manifestations and current treatment options for diabetic neuropathies. *Endocr Pract*. 2007;13:550–66.
- Wong MC, Chung JW, Wong TK. Effects of treatments for symptoms of painful diabetic neuropathy: systematic review. *BMJ*. 2007;335:87.

See Also (Topic, Algorithm, Electronic Media Element)
Diabetes Mellitus, Type 1; Diabetes Mellitus, Type 2

CODES

ICD9
- 250.60 Diabetes mellitus with neurological manifestations, type ii or unspecified type, not stated as uncontrolled
- 250.61 Diabetes mellitus with neurological manifestations, type I (juvenile type) not stated as uncontrolled
- 250.62 Diabetes mellitus with neurological manifestations, type ii or unspecified type, uncontrolled

CLINICAL PEARLS
- Occasionally, when glycemic control improves dramatically, as can occur when treatment for diabetes is initiated, there may be a worsening of neuropathy symptoms. Symptoms usually stabilize and gradually improve as glycemic control is maintained.
- It is common to combine agents with different mechanisms of action in the management of neuropathic pain. Topical therapies can also be combined with systemic therapies.

DIARRHEA, ACUTE

Cheryl Abel, PharmD
Jill A. Grimes, MD

 BASICS

DESCRIPTION
- Abnormal increase in stool frequency or liquidity in an otherwise healthy individual
- Often self-limiting; <14 days duration
- Acute viral diarrhea (50–70%):
  – Most common form; usually occurs for 1–3 days; self-limited
  – Causes changes in small intestinal cell morphology, such as villous shortening and an increase in the number of crypt cells
- Bacterial diarrhea (15–20%):
  – Develop 6–24 hours after infected food ingested
  – Suspect if simultaneous illness is present in others who have shared contaminated food
- Protozoal infections (10–15%):
  – Cause prolonged, watery diarrhea (travelers from areas with contaminated water supply)
- Traveler's diarrhea typically begins 3–7 days after arrival in foreign location; often quite acute.
- System(s) affected: Endocrine/Metabolic; Gastrointestinal

EPIDEMIOLOGY
Predominant age: All ages

Prevalence
- 11% of the general population
- Highest in children <5 years old

RISK FACTORS
- Individual from an industrialized country visiting a developing country
- Immunocompromised host
- Antibiotic use
- Day care attendance; nursing home residency

GENERAL PREVENTION
- Frequent handwashing; proper hygiene
- Rotavirus vaccine
- Strict food handling
- Care during foreign travel to avoid brushing teeth with contaminated water, ingesting ice cubes, or eating cold salads or meats
- Probiotics may be used to help prevent traveler's diarrhea (1)[A].

ETIOLOGY
- Bacterial:
  – *Escherichia coli*
  – *Salmonella*
  – *Shigella*
  – *Campylobacter jejuni*
  – *Vibrio parahaemolyticus*
  – *Vibrio cholerae*
  – *Yersinia enterocolitica*
  – *Clostridium difficile*
  – *Staphylococcus aureus*
  – *Bacillus cereus*
- Viral:
  – Rotavirus
  – Norwalklike virus (Norovirus)

- Protozoal:
  – *Giardia lamblia*
  – *Cryptosporidium*
  – *Entamoeba histolytica*
  – *Isospora belli*

Pediatric Considerations
- Rotavirus is a common cause of viral diarrhea in the winter months and is accompanied by vomiting.
- Other etiologies include overfeeding, medications, cystic fibrosis, and malabsorption.

COMMONLY ASSOCIATED CONDITIONS
- Diabetes mellitus
- Ileal resection
- Gastrectomy
- Hyperthyroidism

 DIAGNOSIS

HISTORY
- Anorexia ± vomiting
- Malaise
- Headache
- Myalgia
- Assess stool characteristics: Frequency and quantity, presence of mucous or blood, consistency (2)[A]
- Travel history, day care attendance, ingestion of raw or undercooked meat, raw seafood, unpasteurized milk, sick contacts (2)[A]
- With *Giardia*: Cramping; pale, greasy stools; fatigue; weight loss; chronicity

PHYSICAL EXAM
- Loose liquid stools ± blood or mucus
- Fever
- Abdominal pain and distension
- Determine hydration status; look for decreased skin turgor, dry mucous membranes, hypotension, or decreased urination:
  – In children: Absence of tears, depressed fontanelles, dry diapers
- Abdominal exam to rule out potential surgical causes of diarrhea such as appendicitis or pelvic abscess

Geriatric Considerations
Watery diarrhea with chronic constipation may be caused by fecal impaction or obstructing neoplasm.

Pregnancy Considerations
Dehydration may lead to preterm labor.

DIAGNOSTIC TESTS & INTERPRETATION
Lab
Initial lab tests
- Consider testing if diarrhea is prolonged
- Complete blood count:
  – Increased white blood cells with a left shift may indicate an infectious process.
  – A decreased hemoglobin/hematocrit may indicate anemia from blood loss.
- Serum electrolytes:
  – Increased sodium from dehydration
  – Decreased potassium from diarrhea

- Blood urea nitrogen, creatinine: Elevated in dehydration
- pH: Hyperchloremic acidosis
- Stool sample:
  – Occult blood present in inflammatory bowel disease, bowel ischemia, bacterial infections
  – Fecal leukocytes present in diarrhea caused by *Salmonella, Campylobacter, Yersinia*
  – For community-acquired or traveler's diarrhea >1 day or accompanied by fever or bloody stools: Culture or test for *Salmonella, Shigella, Campylobacter, E. coli* O157:H7. If antibiotics or chemotherapy in recent weeks, *C. difficile* toxin A and B (2)[B].
  – For nosocomial diarrhea (onset ≥3 days in hospital): Test for *C. difficile* toxins A and B. Also consider bacterial cultures listed above in patients with bloody stools or infants (2)[B].
  – For diarrhea >7 days: Stool ova and parasites (O & P) plus bacterial cultures if immunocompromised (2)[B]
  – *Giardia* enzyme linked immunosorbent assay: >90% sensitive in at-risk population, consider prior to O & P

Imaging
Abdominal radiographs (flat plate and upright) indicated with abdominal pain or evidence of obstruction to rule out toxic megacolon and bowel ischemia

Diagnostic Procedures/Surgery
Sigmoidoscopy indicated with bloody diarrhea or suspected pseudomembranous or ulcerative colitis

Pathological Findings
- Viral diarrhea: Changes in small intestine cell morphology that include villous shortening, increased number of crypt cells, and increased cellularity of the lamina propria
- Bacterial diarrhea: Bacterial invasion of colonic wall leads to mucosal hyperemia, edema, and leukocytic infiltration.

DIFFERENTIAL DIAGNOSIS
- Inflammatory bowel disease
- Drugs (cholinergic agents, magnesium-containing antacids)
- Pseudomembranous colitis secondary to antibiotic use
- Diverticulitis
- Spastic (irritable) colon
- Fecal impaction
- Malabsorption
- Zollinger-Ellison syndrome
- Ischemic bowel
- Gastrinoma

TREATMENT

MEDICATION

First Line

- Loperamide: 4 mg followed by 2-mg capsule after each unformed stool (see precautions below)
- Bismuth subsalicylate: 30 mL every 1/2 hour until 8 doses; may be helpful in mild diarrhea
- If diarrhea persists and a bacterial or parasitic organism is identified, antibiotic therapy should be started:
  – Giardia: Metronidazole 250 mg t.i.d. for 5 days
  – E. histolytica: Metronidazole 750 mg t.i.d. for 10 days
  – Shigella: Trimethoprim-sulfamethoxazole (Bactrim DS) 160 mg/800 mg b.i.d. for 5 days, or ciprofloxacin 500 mg b.i.d. for 3 days
  – Campylobacter: Erythromycin 500 mg q.i.d. for 5 days or ciprofloxacin 500 mg b.i.d. for 3 days
  – C. difficile: Discontinue antibiotics if possible. Consider metronidazole 500 mg t.i.d. for 10–14 days if diarrhea persists or worsens.
  – Traveler's diarrhea: Ciprofloxacin 750 mg 1 dose or, if severe, 500 mg divided p.o. twice a day for 3 days or TMP/SMX (Bactrim DS) 1 tab twice a day for 3 days
- Contraindications:
  – Antibiotics are contraindicated in Salmonella infections unless caused by S. typhosa or the patient is severely ill.
  – Avoid alcoholic beverages with metronidazole due to the possibility of a disulfiram reaction.
  – Antibiotics are not indicated in foodborne toxigenic diarrhea.
- Precautions:
  – Antiperistaltic agents (e.g., loperamide) should be used with caution in patients suspected of having infectious diarrhea (especially if E. coli 0157:H7 suspected) or antibiotic-associated colitis.
  – Antiperistaltic agents may speed recovery from traveler's diarrhea when used in combination with antibiotics (3)[A].
  – Doxycycline, sulfamethoxazole-trimethoprim, and ciprofloxacin may cause photosensitivity; use sunscreen.
- Significant possible interactions:
  – Salicylate absorption from bismuth subsalicylate can cause toxicity in patients already taking aspirin-containing compounds and may alter anticoagulation control in patients taking Coumadin.
  – Ciprofloxacin and erythromycin increase theophylline levels.

Second Line

- Doxycycline: 100 mg b.i.d. for 3 days
- Diphenoxylate-atropine in nonpregnant adults
- Tinidazole or selnidazole for E. histolytica
- Oral vancomycin for C. difficile infections

ADDITIONAL TREATMENT

General Measures

Replace lost fluid and electrolytes (2)[A]:

- Clear liquids at room temperature, such as tea, broth, carbonated beverages (without caffeine), and rehydration fluids (e.g., Gatorade) to replace lost fluid.
- Packets of rehydration salts (1 packet to be diluted in 1 quart of water); drink until thirst is quenched (helps replace electrolytes); treatment of choice for pediatric patients
- ORS (oral rehydration solutions): Polymer-based ORS may be superior to glucose-based ORS in watery diarrhea (4)[A].
- IV fluids if patient cannot tolerate oral rehydration

COMPLEMENTARY AND ALTERNATIVE MEDICINE

- In children with acute infectious diarrhea, treatment with probiotics appears to be safe and effective for reducing the duration and frequency of diarrhea (5)[B].
- In patients being treated with antibiotics, administration of a probiotic at levels above 10^{10}/g may prevent diarrhea (6)[A].
- Zinc supplementation can decrease diarrhea-related morbidity and mortality (7)[A].

IN-PATIENT CONSIDERATIONS

Initial Stabilization

Outpatient health care except for complicating emergencies (dehydration)

ONGOING CARE

DIET

- Early refeeding is encouraged.
- During periods of active diarrhea, avoid coffee, alcohol, dairy products, most fruits, vegetables, red meats, and heavily seasoned foods.
- Begin by eating clear soup with rice, salted crackers, dry toast or bread, and sherbet.
- As stooling rate decreases, slowly add to diet baked potato and chicken soup with noodles.
- As stool begins to retain shape, add to diet baked fish, poultry, applesauce, and bananas.
- The traditional bananas, rice, applesauce, toast diet has little evidence-based support despite heavy clinical use.

PATIENT EDUCATION

See guidelines in Prevention section.

PROGNOSIS

This common problem is rarely life-threatening if adequate hydration is maintained.

COMPLICATIONS

- Dehydration
- Sepsis
- Shock
- Anemia

REFERENCES

1. McFarland LV et al. Meta-analysis of probiotics for the prevention of traveler's diarrhea. Travel Med Infect Dis. 2007;5:97–105.
2. Guerrant RL, Van Gilder T, Steiner TS, et al. Practice guidelines for the management of infectious diarrhea. Clin Infect Dis. 2001;32:331–51.
3. Riddle MS, Arnold S, Tribble DR et al. Effect of adjunctive loperamide in combination with antibiotics on treatment outcomes in traveler's diarrhea: a systematic review and meta-analysis. Clin Infect Dis. 2008;47:1007–14.
4. Gregorio GV, Gonzales ML, Dans LF, et al. Polymer-based oral rehydration solution for treating acute watery diarrhoea. Cochrane Database Syst Rev. 2009;CD006519.
5. Chen CC, Kong MS, Lai MW, Chao HC, Chang KW, Chen SY, Huang YC, Chiu CH, Li WC, Lin PY, Chen CJ, Li TY et al. Probiotics have clinical, microbiologic, and immunologic efficacy in acute infectious diarrhea. Pediatr Infect Dis J. 2010;29:135–8.
6. McFarland LV et al. Evidence-based review of probiotics for antibiotic-associated diarrhea and Clostridium difficile infections. Anaerobe. 2009;15:274–80.
7. Walker CL, Black RE et al. Zinc for the treatment of diarrhoea: effect on diarrhoea morbidity, mortality and incidence of future episodes. Int J Epidemiol. 2010;39 (Suppl 1):i63–9.

ADDITIONAL READING

- Dupont HL. Systematic review: the epidemiology and clinical features of travellers' diarrhoea. Aliment Pharmacol Ther. 2009.
- Marcos LA, DuPont HL. Advances in defining etiology and new therapeutic approaches in acute diarrhea. J Infect. 2007;55:385–93.

See Also (Topic, Algorithm, Electronic Media Element)

Botulism; Cholera; Food Poisoning, Bacterial

CODES

ICD9
- 005.9 Food poisoning, unspecified
- 008.5 Bacterial enteritis, unspecified
- 009.2 Infectious diarrhea

CLINICAL PEARLS

- Viruses, especially norovirus, are the most common causes of acute diarrheal illness in the US:
  – Antibiotics are not generally needed for routine bacterial causes of gastroenteritis.
- Early refeeding and use of probiotics is encouraged.
- Loperamide and bismuth are useful antidiarrheal medications.
- Bismuth can cause transient black tongues and stools.

DIARRHEA, CHRONIC

Cheryl Abel, PharmD
Jill A. Grimes, MD

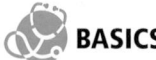 **BASICS**

DESCRIPTION
Chronic diarrhea refers to an increase in frequency or decrease in fecal consistency (typically >3 loose stools per day) for >4 weeks:
- Causes include inflammatory diarrhea, osmotic diarrhea (malabsorption), secretory diarrhea, and intestinal dysmotility.
- System(s) affected: Gastrointestinal

Geriatric Considerations
Patients with lifelong diarrhea may suffer increasing difficulty with advanced age.

EPIDEMIOLOGY
Prevalence
Depends on criterion used, but approximately 5% of US population is affected.

RISK FACTORS
- Female > Male
- Inflammatory:
  - AIDS
  - Infections
  - Radiation
  - Family history
- Osmotic:
  - Infectious
  - Abdominal surgery: Cholecystectomy, resection, vagotomy
  - Chronic alcohol abuse
  - Sorbitol, fructose, lactose, gluten
- Secretory: Distal ileal surgery
- Altered intestinal motility:
  - Diabetes
  - Fecal impaction
  - Neurologic diseases
- Factitious: Laxative use

Genetics
- Celiac sprue and inflammatory bowel disease may be familial.
- Lactose intolerance: Increased incidence in certain geographic regions

GENERAL PREVENTION
Refrain from dietary or pharmacologic agents that may precipitate a diarrhea event.

PATHOPHYSIOLOGY
Incomplete absorption of water from intestinal lumen

ETIOLOGY
- Inflammatory diarrhea:
  - Inflammatory bowel disease
  - Radiation enterocolitis
  - Eosinophilic gastroenteritis
  - Hypersensitivity (e.g., food allergy)
  - AIDS

- Infectious diarrhea:
  - Parasites (e.g., *Giardia lamblia, Isospora*)
  - Helminths (e.g., Strongyloides)
  - Bacterial (e.g., *Mycobacterium avium intracellulare, Clostridium difficile*)
- Osmotic diarrhea:
  - Celiac disease
  - Lactase deficiency
  - Pancreatic insufficiency
  - Bacterial overgrowth
  - Thyrotoxicosis
  - Whipple disease
  - Abetalipoproteinemia
  - Postsurgical (short gut, peptic ulcer disease [PUD] surgery)
  - Drugs: Osmotically active agents, antibiotics, nonsteroidal anti-inflammatory drugs (NSAIDs), prostaglandins, colchicine, metformin, digoxin, selective serotonin reuptake inhibitors (SSRIs), antineoplastic agents
  - Herbal products: St. John's wort, echinacea, feverfew, garlic, saw palmetto, ginseng, cranberry extract, pokeroot tea, aloe vera
- Secretory diarrhea:
  - Carcinoid syndrome
  - Zollinger-Ellison syndrome
  - Vasoactive intestinal peptide-secreting pancreatic adenomas
  - Medullary carcinoma of thyroid
  - Villous adenoma of rectum
  - Microscopic colitis (collagenous, lymphocytic)
  - Choleraic diarrhea: Excessive secretion of electrolytes
  - Diabetes mellitus
  - Laxatives (phenolphthalein, cascara, senna, aloe)
  - Toxins (arsenic, mushrooms, insecticides, alcohol)
- Altered intestinal motility (most common in clinical practice)
- Irritable bowel syndrome (most common in young females)
- Fecal impaction
- Neurologic diseases
- Diabetes: Increased transit and possible bacterial overgrowth
- In children: Secondary to dietary products (e.g., fructose and apple juice)

COMMONLY ASSOCIATED CONDITIONS
- Immune-complex-mediated extraintestinal complications of inflammatory bowel disease (IBD)
- Arthritis, uveitis, pyoderma gangrenosum, nephritis

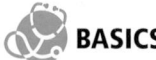 **DIAGNOSIS**

HISTORY
- Review the onset, pattern, duration, frequency of loose stools, and stool characteristics.
- Asses for fecal incontinence, aggravating factors (diet, stress), mitigating factors (diet, drugs), travel, or other exposures.
- Check for weight loss.
- Review previous evaluation.
- Appropriate review of systems for underlying causes; hyperthyroidism, diabetes mellitus, collagen vascular diseases, tumor syndromes, AIDS, Ig deficiencies (review the Rome Criteria for IBS) (1)[C]:
  - ≥3 months of abdominal discomfort, relieved with defecation and associated with a change in frequency and consistency of stool
  - >2 of the following altered stools, at least 25% of the time:
    ○ Frequency
    ○ Form (e.g., loose or hard stools)
    ○ Stool passage (sensation of incomplete evacuation after bowel movements, straining, or urging)
    ○ Passing mucus

PHYSICAL EXAM
- General: Fluid balance, nutrition
- Skin: Flushing, rashes, dermatographism
- Thyroid: Mass
- Chest: Wheezing
- Heart: Murmur
- Abdomen: Hepatomegaly, mass, ascites, tenderness
- Anorectal: Sphincter competence, fecal occult blood test
- Extremities: Edema

DIAGNOSTIC TESTS & INTERPRETATION
Lab
Initial lab tests
- Complete blood count (CBC) with differential, electrolytes, total protein, albumin, thyroid-stimulating hormone (TSH), amylase/lipase (if weight loss)
- If celiac disease suspected: Antiendomysial antibody (AEA), transglutimase antibody (TGA), Ig A
- Initial stool analysis: WBCs, electrolytes, pH, fecal occult blood, fat output (Sudan stain), laxative screen
- Stool ova and parasites
- *C. difficile* toxin (if history of antibiotic use)
- Modified Ziehl-Neelson stain if immunocompromised (*Cryptosporidium*)

Follow-Up & Special Considerations
- When tumor syndrome suspected: Gastrin, calcitonin, vasoactive intestinal peptide, somatostatin, urine excretion of 5-hydroxy acetic acid, metanephrine, histamine
- 24-hour stool collection: Weight (g/24 hours), pH, electrolytes, osmolality

Imaging
Initial approach
- Plain film abdomen
- Flexible sigmoidoscopy with (if >45 years old) or without (if <45) barium enema (2)[B]
- Computed tomography (CT) to rule out pancreatic cancer/chronic pancreatitis if abnormal pancreatic enzymes or evidence of malabsorption

Diagnostic Procedures/Surgery
- Colonoscopy/sigmoidoscopy for inflammatory lesions; if occult blood in stool ± iron deficiency
- Barium enema with small bowel follow-through can help evaluate the small bowel.
- If barium enema is negative and diarrhea persists, biopsies are indicated.
- Esophagogastroduodenoscopy (EGD) with small bowel biopsies if malabsorption disorder suspected

Pathological Findings
- When present, the findings are those of the associated or underlying disease.
- None seen in functional disorder
- Melanosis coli suggests cathartic abuse.

DIFFERENTIAL DIAGNOSIS
- Functional disorder
- Inflammatory bowel disease: Look for systemic illness or extraintestinal manifestations (arthritis, pyoderma gangrenosum, erythema nodosum, uveitis, or vasculitis).
- Factitious: Psychiatric disease or past history
- Irritable bowel syndrome (IBS): Alternating diarrhea and constipation
- Tropical sprue
- Tuberculosis enteritis
- Chronic radiation enterocolitis
- Colonic neoplasm
- Diverticular disease
- Lactose intolerance (uncommon)

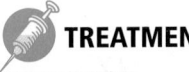 TREATMENT

MEDICATION
First Line
Opioid agonists are considered 1st-line symptomatic treatment relief of diarrhea:
- Diphenoxylate-atropine (Lomotil): 5–20 mg/d or loperamide (Imodium) 4–16 mg/d, doses calculated and timed according to patient's weight and individual needs
- Contraindicated in infectious diarrhea and ulcerative colitis toxic megacolon

Second Line
- Cholestyramine (Questran) for bile salt malabsorption, certain postsurgical patients (3)[C]:
  – 4–8 g t.i.d.
  – May interfere with absorption of fat-soluble vitamins and other medications

- Lactase (Lactaid, Lactrase) for lactose intolerance: Chew/swallow 3 original-strength tablets or 1 fast-acting tablet with 1st bite of food containing dairy products.
- Budesonide exhibits high clinical and histological response rates in collagenous colitis (pooled OR for clinical response 12.32 (95% CI 5.53-27.46) with NNT of 2 patients (4)[A]:
  – 9 mg p.o. daily for 6–8 weeks
- Steroids and sulfasalazine derivatives in inflammatory bowel disease
- Octreotide (Sandostatin): In carcinoid and other peptide-secreting tumors, dumping syndrome, chemotherapy-induced diarrhea:
  – 200–300 SC μg/d in 2–4 divided doses
  – Can be switched to IM depot form (Sandostatin LAR) 20 mg intragluteally q4wk. Reevaluate after 2 months.

ADDITIONAL TREATMENT
There is little evidence to support treating children with antimicrobials for persistent diarrhea (5)[A].

General Measures
- Unless the patient is hypotensive or an electrolyte abnormality or deconditioning is present, outpatient therapy is adequate.
- Fluids with electrolyte supplementation

SURGERY/OTHER PROCEDURES
For villous adenomas, hormone-producing tumors, and refractory ulcerative colitis

 ONGOING CARE

DIET
- Abstain from gluten products, sorbitol, lactose-containing products, and food allergens.
- In irritable bowel syndrome, add dietary fiber (e.g., 20–30 g/d supplemental fiber).

PATIENT EDUCATION
- Reassure that normal frequency varies widely.
- Restrict colon stimulants.
- Dietary consult when appropriate

PROGNOSIS
Variable, from a short (factitious and altered intestinal motility) and treatable course, to a chronic illness (e.g., Crohn disease, ulcerative colitis)

COMPLICATIONS
- Fluid and electrolyte abnormalities
- Malnutrition
- Anemia

REFERENCES
1. Longstreth GF, Thompson WG, Chey WD, et al. Functional bowel disorders. *Gastroenterology*. 2006;130:1480–91.
2. Thomas PD, Forbes A, Green J, et al. Guidelines for the investigation of chronic diarrhoea, 2nd edition. *Gut*. 2003;52 (Suppl 5):v1–15.
3. Ung KA, Gillberg R, Kilander A, et al. Role of bile acids and bile acid binding agents in patients with collagenous colitis. *Gut*. 2000;46:170–5.
4. Chande N, McDonald JWD, MacDonald JK. Interventions for treating collagenous colitis. *Cochrane Database of Systematic Reviews*. 2008, Issue 2. Art. No.: CD003575. DOI:10.1002/14651858.CD003575.pub5.
5. Abba K, Sinfield R, Hart CA, Garner P, et al. Antimicrobial drugs for persistent diarrhoea of unknown or non-specific cause in children under six in low and middle income countries: systematic review of randomized controlled trials. *BMC Infect. Dis.* 2009;9:24.

ADDITIONAL READING
- Baber KF, Anderson J, Puzanovova M, Walker LS, et al. Rome II versus Rome III classification of functional gastrointestinal disorders in pediatric chronic abdominal pain. *J. Pediatr. Gastroenterol. Nutr.* 2008;47:299–302.
- Fan X, Sellin JH. Review article: Small intestinal bacterial overgrowth, bile acid malabsorption and gluten intolerance as possible causes of chronic watery diarrhea. *Aliment Pharmacol Ther*. 2009.
- Nwachukwu CE, Okebe JU, et al. Antimotility agents for chronic diarrhoea in people with HIV/AIDS. *Cochrane Database Syst Rev*. 2008;CD005644.
- Saxena S, Mitton SG, Pollok R et al. Chronic diarrhoea in a teenager. *BMJ*. 2008;337:a430.

See Also (Topic, Algorithm, Electronic Media Element)
Algorithm: Diarrhea, Chronic

 CODES

ICD9
787.91 Diarrhea

CLINICAL PEARLS
- The most common causes are functional disorders such as IBS, IBD, malabsorptive syndromes, chronic infections, and idiopathic secretory diarrhea.
- Opioids and opioid agonists (loperamide, diphenoxylate-atropine) should be considered as 1st-line for symptomatic relief of chronic, noninfectious diarrhea.
- The evaluation and treatment of diarrheal syndromes is often a multistep process that requires ruling out a wide variety of entities. However, most cases can be diagnosed through careful history and physical examination and select laboratory studies.

DIFFUSE INTERSTITIAL LUNG DISEASE

Jacqueline L. Olin, MS, PharmD, BCPS, CPP
Julie Scott Taylor, MD, MSc

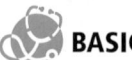 **BASICS**

DESCRIPTION
- Interstitial lung diseases (ILDs) represent a diverse group of chronic progressive lung diseases associated with alveolar inflammation and/or potentially irreversible pulmonary fibrosis.
- >200 individual diseases may present with similar characteristics, making ILD difficult to classify.
- A classification scheme proposed by the American Thoracic Society and European Respiratory Society includes these subtypes:
  - Known causes (environmental, occupational, or drug-associated disease)
  - Systemic disorders (sarcoidosis, Wegener granulomatosis, collagen vascular disease, etc.)
  - Rare lung diseases (pulmonary histiocytosis, lymphangioleiomyomatosis, etc.)
  - Idiopathic interstitial pneumonias (IIPs)
- Based on clinical, radiologic, and histologic features, IIPs are further subclassified into the following diagnoses:
  - Idiopathic pulmonary fibrosis (IPF), characterized by progressive dyspnea, cough, restrictive lung disease, and a specific histopathologic pattern
  - IIPs other than IPF (including nonspecific interstitial pneumonia [NSIP], respiratory bronchiolitis-associated ILD [RBILD], acute interstitial pneumonia [AIP], bronchiolitis obliterans with organizing pneumonia [BOOP], etc.)
- The classification of IIPs and relationships between the subtypes continues to be an area of controversy.

Pediatric Considerations
Interstitial lung disease (ILD) in infants and children represents a heterogeneous group of respiratory disorders that are mostly chronic and associated with high morbidity and mortality. In children, ILD is difficult to diagnose, as no classification scheme is entirely satisfactory (1). Classification can center around whether disease is primarily a pulmonary process or if symptoms occur as a result of a systemic disorder.

EPIDEMIOLOGY
Incidence
- Due to lack of consistency in disease presentation and definition, epidemiologic data are not well defined. Exact incidence has been difficult to determine because of differences in case definitions and procedures used in diagnosis.
- Ranges cited for incidence of IPF: 6.8–16.3 per 100,000 (2)
- According to the National Heart, Lung, and Blood Institute, about 50,000 new cases of IPF are diagnosed each year in the US.

Prevalence
- Exact prevalence has been difficult to determine because of differences in case definitions and procedures used in diagnosis.
- Ranges cited for prevalence of IPF: 14–42.7 per 100,000 (2) and above 175 per 100,000 in the older population (3)

RISK FACTORS
- Environmental or occupational exposure to inorganic or organic dusts
- 66–75% of patients with ILD have a history of smoking.
- Due to diversity of diseases, age is not a reliable predictor of pathology:
  - Most patients with connective tissue disease-related pathology and inherited subtypes present between ages 20 and 40.
  - Patients with IPF are typically age 50 or older.

Genetics
Some studies suggest that some subtypes of ILD may be associated with specific predisposing genes and environmental exposures; however, the role of genetic factors is unknown at this time; ~10% of IPF cases are inherited.

GENERAL PREVENTION
Avoiding environmental/occupational exposure to organic or inorganic dust and smoking cessation may reduce incidence or improve clinical course in patients with established ILD.

PATHOPHYSIOLOGY
- Alveolar inflammation may progress into irreversible fibrosis.
- Varying degrees of ventilatory dysfunction occur among the ILD subtypes.
- ILD associated with collagen vascular disease and systemic connective disorders can manifest involvement of skin, joints, muscular, and ocular systems.

ETIOLOGY
Some types of ILD are associated with specific exposures:
- Medications (amiodarone, antibiotics [especially nitrofurantoin], chemotherapy agents, gold, illicit drugs)
- Inorganic dusts (silicates, asbestos, talc, mica, coal dust, graphite)
- Organic dusts (moldy hay, inhalation of fungi, bacteria, animal proteins)
- Metals (tin, aluminum, cobalt, iron, barium)
- Gases, fumes, vapors, aerosols

COMMONLY ASSOCIATED CONDITIONS
- Many systemic disorders and primary diseases are associated with ILD.
- A partial list includes:
  - Collagen vascular disease
  - Sarcoidosis
  - Amyloidosis
  - Goodpasture syndrome
  - Churg-Strauss syndrome
  - Wegener granulomatosis

DIAGNOSIS
- Diagnosis should be based on clinical, radiologic, and histologic data.
- A multidisciplinary consensus is recommended for diagnosis since even among experts, diagnostic criteria are subject to interpretation.

HISTORY
- Symptoms may include progressive exertional dyspnea and nonproductive cough.
- Patients may also present with hemoptysis (due to idiopathic alveolar hemosiderosis) or fatigue.
- Obtaining a history of illness duration (acute vs chronic), potential environmental/occupational exposures, travel, and medical conditions (including systemic diseases) is important in assessing the cause of the ILD.
- Some cases of lung disease may occur weeks to years after discontinuation of an offending agent.

PHYSICAL EXAM
Physical findings are usually nonspecific. Some common features include:
- Rales
- Inspiratory "squeaks"
- Clubbing of the digits
- Cyanosis in advanced disease

DIAGNOSTIC TESTS & INTERPRETATION
Lab
Initial lab tests
- Arterial blood gas (ABG)
- If a systemic disorder is suspected, consider obtaining an antinuclear antibody (ANA), rheumatoid factor (RF), erythrocyte sedimentation rate (ESR), and antineutrophil cytoplasmic antibodies (ANCA).

Follow-Up & Special Considerations
If indicated, hypersensitivity pneumonitis panel, plasma angiotensin-converting enzyme (ACE) concentration (sarcoidosis)

Imaging
Patients may also present initially with an abnormal chest x-ray (CXR) as compared with previous imaging.

Initial approach
CXR

Follow-Up & Special Considerations
High-resolution computed tomography (HRCT) of the chest is the most useful tool for distinguishing among ILD subclasses, especially in those patients with normal CXRs.

Diagnostic Procedures/Surgery
- Pulmonary function testing (PFT; spirometry, lung volumes, carbon monoxide diffusing capacity):
  - Commonly demonstrates a restrictive defect (decreased vital capacity and total lung capacity)
- Bronchoscopy:
  - Bronchoalveolar lavage (BAL) cellular analysis studies may be useful in distinguishing some subtypes (including sarcoidosis, hypersensitivity pneumonitis, cancer), but its role in diagnosis, prognostication, and assessment of disease progression is not clear (4).
  - Bronchoscopic transbronchial lung biopsy may help diagnose sarcoidosis and, on occasion, is sufficiently supportive of other ILD diagnoses.
- Thoracoscopic surgery for lung biopsy has the greatest diagnostic specificity for ILDs, but is less frequently used given improved specificity of HRCT. It may be indicated if a specific diagnosis cannot be determined from transbronchial biopsy, HRCT, etc., or if deemed necessary prior to further treatment.

Pathological Findings

- The diagnostic classifications of IIPs are based on histopathologic patterns seen on lung biopsy.
- The major histologies include an inflammation and fibrotic and granulomatous patterns.
- Characteristic changes on HRCT may help to distinguish between subtypes:
  – Reticulonodular, ground-glass opacities, and, in later stages, honeycombing may be seen.
  – Associated hilar and mediastinal adenopathy are characteristic of stage I and II sarcoidosis.
- No specific test is the "gold standard," which emphasizes the importance of a multidisciplinary consensus for diagnosis with clinical, radiological, and pathological findings.

DIFFERENTIAL DIAGNOSIS

- Acute pulmonary edema
- Diffuse hemorrhage
- Atypical pneumonia
- Diffuse bronchoalveolar cell carcinoma or lymphatic spread of tumor

TREATMENT

- Evidence does not support the routine use of any specific therapy for ILD in general, and especially IPF.
- A single randomized-controlled trial did not demonstrate survival benefit of home oxygen use in ILD (5).
- There is no evidence that any pharmacologic therapies improve survival or quality of life (6)[B].
- Corticosteroids have a role in some ILD subtypes. (7)[A]
- Current evidence does not clearly support routine use of noncorticosteroid anti-inflammatory agents for IPF, including cyclosporine, azathioprine, colchicines, cyclophosphamide, cytokines, methotrexate, or interferon (8).
- Phase II studies of bosentan and etanercept had demonstrated trends towards improvement in some quality-of-life measures. A recent study showed limited effect of bosentan on health-related quality-of-life measures in a subset of patients who underwent lung biopsy (9).

MEDICATION

First Line

- In general, corticosteroids are most effective for certain ILDs, especially exacerbations of sarcoidosis, NSIP, BOOP, and hypersensitivity pneumonitis. However, response rates have been variable across and within subtypes. The optimal dose and duration of therapy is unknown.
- Common starting dose of prednisone is 0.5–1 mg/kg/d for 4–12 weeks, with potential up-titration to 0.5 mg/kg based on patient response.

Second Line

- 2nd-line agents have been used for IPF alone or in combination with steroids, with limited success rates:
  – Azathioprine was studied at 2–3 mg/kg/d (not to exceed 200 mg/d; adjusted to the nearest 25-mg dose increment) in combination with prednisone and ultimately as a steroid-sparing agent.
  – Cyclosporine has been studied in a limited number of patients.
  – The addition of acetylcysteine (1,800 mg/d for 12 months) to therapy with azathioprine and prednisone in IPF was studied in a double-blind, placebo-controlled trial. Improvements in vital

capacity and carbon monoxide diffusing capacity were noted in the acetylcysteine-treated patients.
  – Pirfenidone, an orally active antifibroblast agent, currently submitted for Food and Drug Administration (FDA) approval, demonstrated potentially promising treatment effects in phase III trials of patients with IPF.
- Several 2nd-line agents have been used in Wegener granulomatosis:
  – Cyclophosphamide is commonly used in treatment of Wegener granulomatosis. It is given 1.5–2 mg/kg/d p.o. for 3–6 months.
  – Methotrexate has been used in treatment of mild Wegener granulomatosis in combination with corticosteroids. A studied dosing regimen consisted of an initial methotrexate dose of 0.3 mg/kg (maximum dose of 15 mg) once weekly, with 2.5 mg titration each week (maximum dose of 25 mg/wk).
  – Other 2nd-line agents that have been studied include mycophenolate mofetil and rituximab.

ADDITIONAL TREATMENT

General Measures

- Avoid/minimize offending environmental/occupational exposures.
- Smoking cessation
- Discontinue culprit medications.
- Supplemental oxygen, if indicated

Issues for Referral

Patients benefit from ongoing care by a pulmonary specialist.

SURGERY/OTHER PROCEDURES

Single- or double-lung transplantation may be a treatment of last resort in some patients. However, some ILDs associated with systemic disease may recur in the recipient lung.

ONGOING CARE

FOLLOW-UP RECOMMENDATIONS

Follow-up testing should include PFTs, cardiopulmonary stress test, pulse oximetry, and CXR.

Patient Monitoring

Patients must be carefully monitored for objective response to treatments and adverse effects.

PATIENT EDUCATION

- Wide degree of prognostic variation occurs among ILD subtypes.
- National Heart, Lung, and Blood Institute at http://www.nhlbi.nih.gov/health/dci/Diseases/ipf/ipf_whatis.html

PROGNOSIS

Overall prognosis is varied among subtypes. IPF confers the worst prognosis (50–80% mortality in 5 years). Some entities, including hypersensitivity pneumonitis, nonspecific interstitial pneumonia, and cryptogenic organizing pneumonia, have a good prognosis.

COMPLICATIONS

- Cor pulmonale
- Pneumothorax
- Progressive respiratory failure

REFERENCES

1. Clement A, Eber E. Interstitial lung diseases in infants and children. *Eur Respir J.* 2008;31:658–66.
2. Raghu G, Weycker D, Edelsberg J, et al. Incidence and prevalence of idiopathic pulmonary fibrosis. *Am J Respir Crit Care Med.* 2006;174:810–6.
3. Rogliani P, Mura M, Assunta Porretta M, et al. New perspectives in the treatment of idiopathic pulmonary fibrosis. *Ther Adv Respir Dis.* 2008;2:75–93.
4. Reynolds HY et al. Present status of bronchoalveolar lavage in interstitial lung disease. *Curr Opin Pulm Med.* 2009;15:479–85.
5. Crockett AJ, Cranston JM, Antic N et al. Domiciliary oxygen for interstitial lung disease. *Cochrane Database Syst Rev.* 2001;CD002883.
6. King TE. Clinical advances in the diagnosis and therapy of the interstitial lung diseases. *Am J Respir Crit Care Med.* 2005;172:268–79.
7. Richeldi L, Davies HR, Ferrara G et al. Corticosteroids for idiopathic pulmonary fibrosis. *Cochrane Database Syst Rev.* 2003;CD002880.
8. Davies HR, et al. Immunomodulatory agents for idiopathic pulmonary fibrosis. *Cochrane Database Syst Rev.* 2006;(3).
9. Raghu G, King TE, Behr J et al. Quality of life and dyspnoea in patients treated with bosentan for idiopathic pulmonary fibrosis (BUILD-1). *Eur Respir J.* 2010;35:118–23.

ADDITIONAL READING

- Behr J, Thannickal VJ. Update in diffuse parenchymal lung disease 2008. *Am J Respir Crit Care Med.* 2009;179:439–44.
- Demedts M, Behr J, Buhl R, et al. High-dose acetylcysteine in idiopathic pulmonary fibrosis. *N Engl J Med.* 2005;353:2229–42.
- Dinwiddie R. Treatment of interstitial lung disease in children. *Paediatr Respir Rev.* 2004;5:108–15.
- King TE Jr, Behr J, Brown K et al. BUILD-1: a randomized placebo-controlled trial of bosentan in idiopathic pulmonary fibrosis. *Am J Respir Crit Care Med.* 2008;177:75–81.

CODES

ICD9

515 Postinflammatory pulmonary fibrosis

CLINICAL PEARLS

- ILD differs from COPD; anatomically, ILD involves the lung parenchyma (i.e., alveoli) and COPD involves both airways and alveoli.
- In some cases, for ILD due to organic or inorganic dust or drug-related ILD, avoiding or minimizing offending environmental/occupational exposures, medications, and smoking may alter the severity of disease, but other general preventative measures are not known at this time.
- A wide degree of prognostic variation occurs among different subtypes of ILD. For example, death is rare with cryptogenic organizing pneumonia, but acute interstitial pneumonia has 60% mortality in <6 months. Refer the patient to a pulmonologist for a thorough evaluation.

DIGITALIS TOXICITY

Katherine Boyle, MD
Kathryn W. Weibrecht, MD

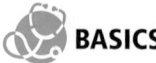 **BASICS**

DESCRIPTION
- A life-threatening condition resulting from intoxication by digitalis (digoxin) when used for chronic therapy, from accidental or intentional overdose, or from ingestion of naturally occurring compounds containing cardiac glycosides (e.g., foxglove, oleander)
- Can be acute or chronic
- System(s) affected: Cardiovascular; Gastrointestinal; Ocular; Central Nervous System

EPIDEMIOLOGY
Incidence
About 1.1% of outpatients on digitalis glycosides per year develop toxicity, with as many as 10–20% of nursing home residents annually experiencing some degree of digoxin-related toxicity.

Prevalence
In 2007, the American Association of Poison Control Centers' National Poison Data System reported more than 2,500 cases of cardiac glycoside overdose.

RISK FACTORS
- Advanced age
- Renal failure
- Hypoxemia
- Electrolyte disturbances:
  - Hypokalemia
  - Hypomagnesemia
  - Hypernatremia
  - Hypercalcemia
- Acid–base disturbances
- Decompensating congestive heart failure
- Myocardial infarction
- Myocarditis
- Recent cardiac surgery
- Hypothyroidism
- Cor pulmonale

GENERAL PREVENTION
- Use caution when prescribing digitalis if the patient is taking medications that interfere with digoxin metabolism or clearance.
- Adjust dosing when there are circumstances that increase total body levels of the drug (e.g., acute or chronic renal failure), increase cardiac sensitivity (e.g., ischemia, myocarditis), or increase bioavailability by altering gut flora (e.g., macrolides).
- Prescribe lower doses of digoxin (0.125 mg/day instead of 0.25 mg/day) (1). Digoxin is effective in heart failure at much lower levels than necessary for rate control in atrial fibrillation.

PATHOPHYSIOLOGY
- Digitalis inhibits Na^+-K^+-ATPase in myocytes, resulting in an increase in intracellular sodium and a decrease in the transmembrane sodium gradient.
- The loss of the sodium gradient decreases the drive of the Na^+-Ca^{2+} transporter, leading to increased intracellular calcium and thus increased inotropy.

- At high/toxic digoxin concentrations, elevated intracellular calcium generates small depolarizations, and the additive effects of these depolarizations produce dysrhythmias.
- Digitalis also acts on the parasympathetic system resulting in increased vagal tone and slowing AV node conduction.
- The combination of these effects can cause tachyarrhythmias and conduction block, which can present simultaneously.

ETIOLOGY
- Chronic therapy
- Intentional overdose (suicide attempt)
- Accidental overdose (children)
- Prescription/administration error
- Electrolyte disturbances
- Renal failure or any condition that decreases clearance of the drug
- Poisoning with plants containing cardiac glycosides (e.g., oleander, foxglove, lily of the valley)
- Concurrent use of medications:
  - Antibiotics: Rifampin, tetracycline, macrolides
  - Selective serotonin reuptake inhibitors (SSRIs)
  - Calcium channel blockers: Diltiazem, verapamil
  - Antiarrhythmics: Quinidine, amiodarone
  - Diuretics: Spironolactone
  - β-blockers

COMMONLY ASSOCIATED CONDITIONS
- Renal failure
- Congestive heart failure
- Dehydration
- Syncope

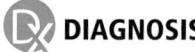 **DIAGNOSIS**

HISTORY
- For patients at risk for toxicity from chronic use, ask about new medications or new or worsened cardiac or renal disease.
- For suspected accidental overdose in children, a careful history of childproofing and available medications should be obtained.
- As with all suspected or confirmed intentional ingestions, ask about timing of ingestions and coingestions.
- Signs and symptoms generally nonspecific:
  - Anorexia
  - Nausea
  - Vomiting
  - Diarrhea
  - Visual disturbances (e.g., yellow halos)
  - Mydriasis
  - Confusion
  - Fatigue
  - Restlessness
  - Weakness
  - Headache
  - Depression
  - Hallucinations
  - Neuralgias
  - Vertigo

DIAGNOSTIC TESTS & INTERPRETATION
Lab
Initial lab tests
- Na^+, K^+, Cl^-, $HCO3^-$, Mg^+, Ca^+, blood urea nitrogen (BUN), Cr, and cardiac enzyme biomarkers
- Serum digoxin level: Total:
  - The accepted therapeutic range in serum is 0.8–2.0 ng/mL (for rate control in atrial fibrillation), with toxicity more common above 2.5 ng/mL (1)[B].
  - Toxicity may occur with plasma digoxin levels within therapeutic range, especially in chronic overdose (2)[C].
  - Digoxin level may be falsely high if measured <6 hours after acute ingestion or last dose (1)[C].
  - Non-digoxin cardiac glycoside (e.g., foxglove, oleander) may cross-react and generate a positive/elevated level; a negative level does not rule out exposure.
- Free serum digoxin level:
  - Free levels are useful for monitoring response to therapy after digoxin-specific Fab antibody fragments are given (Fab bound to digoxin increases the total digoxin level).
- Potassium:
  - In acute toxicity, hyperkalemia can be common, life-threatening, and predictive of lethality (1)[B].
  - Hypokalemia potentiates digoxin toxicity.

Diagnostic Procedures/Surgery
- Electrocardiogram (EKG):
  - Digoxin has been reported to cause a wide variety of rhythm disturbances, so consider the diagnosis with any sudden change in cardiac rhythm. Look for rhythms that suggest increased automaticity and/or delayed conduction (2)[C].
  - Characteristic EKG changes ("digitalis effect") can occur at therapeutic levels:
    - Prolonged PR segment
    - T-wave changes, prolonged QT interval, scooping of ST segment
  - EKG changes relatively specific for digitalis toxicity:
    - Accelerated junctional rhythm
    - Bidirectional ventricular tachycardia
    - New-onset Mobitz type I AV block
    - Nonparoxysmal atrial tachycardia with AV block
  - Other associated rhythms:
    - Ventricular ectopy, premature ventricular contractions
    - High-degree heart block
    - Sinus bradycardia
    - Sinus bradycardia with junctional tachycardia
    - Ventricular fibrillation or tachycardia
    - Atrial flutter
  - Digoxin toxicity is less likely to cause supraventricular tachycardia, rapid atrial fibrillation, or Mobitz Type II AV block.
- For suspected intoxication with naturally occurring cardiac glycosides, consider early consultation with a medical toxicologist or poison control center for help in identifying the toxic source and to guide treatment decisions.

DIFFERENTIAL DIAGNOSIS
- Conduction abnormalities:
  - Sick sinus syndrome
  - AV nodal dysfunction
- Medication effect
- Electrolyte disturbances
- Other causes of life-threatening arrhythmia

 TREATMENT

MEDICATION
First Line
- Digoxin-specific Fab antibody fragments (Digibind)
- Indications:
  - Treatment of severe, life-threatening arrhythmias due to digitalis toxicity (3)[A]:
    - Sustained ventricular arrhythmias
    - Advanced AV block
    - Asystole
  - Hemodynamic instability
  - Plasma potassium concentration >5 mEq/L in the setting of acute overdose
  - Plasma digoxin concentration above 10 ng/mL (at steady state)
  - Acute ingestion of >10 mg digoxin in adults or >4 mg in children
- Dosage of Digibind:
  - If possible, obtain a total digoxin level before administration.
  - Use free levels to monitor treatment response.
  - To calculate Digibind dosage (1)[A]:
    - Number of vials = Ingested amount (mg) × 0.8/0.5
    - Number of vials = Digoxin level (ng/mL) × weight (kg)/100
  - Unknown acute ingestion or drug level:
    - Empiric dose is 10 vials (4)[C].
  - Dosing for children is the same as for adults.
  - Slow administration increases the efficiency and elimination of digoxin (5)[C].
  - Onset of action for reversal of digoxin toxicity is rapid (minutes) (1)[C].
- Adverse reactions:
  - Hypokalemia: Monitor potassium carefully, since rapid development of hypokalemia can occur after Digibind therapy (1)[A].
  - Exacerbation of heart failure, increased ventricular response in atrial fibrillation, and hypersensitivity reactions can occur (1)[A].

Second Line
- Activated charcoal (1)[C]:
  - Consider in acute or overdose settings
  - Increases GI elimination and systemic clearance
- Magnesium: 2 g IV initially, consider maintenance infusion (3)[C]
- Temporary pacing if no Digibind available (3)[C]
- Hemodialysis can be used to treat hyperkalemia, but is not effective for reversal of toxicity because of the extensive tissue distribution of digoxin (1)[C].

ADDITIONAL TREATMENT
General Measures
- Discontinue digoxin and other medications that interact with digoxin or exacerbate dysrhythmias.
- Correct electrolyte abnormalities and monitor potassium levels:
  - Maintain potassium in high–normal range.
  - Treat hyperkalemia with sodium bicarbonate, insulin, glucose, and Kayexalate.
  - Treat hypokalemia cautiously.
  - Do not use calcium salts, which can worsen ventricular arrhythmias by further increasing intracellular calcium (2)[C].
- For chronic toxicity, treat the underlying cause.

IN-PATIENT CONSIDERATIONS
Initial Stabilization
- Manage airway
- IV access/fluid resuscitation
- Supplemental oxygen
- Atropine for symptomatic bradycardia (1)[C]
- Temporary cutaneous pacing (1)[C]
- Hemodynamically unstable patients should receive Digibind as soon as possible (3)[A].

Admission Criteria
All patients with suspected digoxin toxicity who have cardiac dysrhythmias, toxic digoxin levels, or hyperkalemia should be admitted for continuous cardiac monitoring.

IV Fluids
Administration of appropriate IV fluids depends on underlying etiology for toxicity (e.g., decompensated congestive heart failure vs acute renal failure secondary to dehydration).

Discharge Criteria
Patients should remain in the hospital until the signs and symptoms have resolved and the serum digoxin level ≤2 ng/mL.

 ONGOING CARE

FOLLOW-UP RECOMMENDATIONS
- Psychiatric referral is indicated for all intentional overdoses.
- In chronic toxicity, close follow-up by a primary care physician or cardiologist is recommended if digoxin therapy is continued after discharge.

Patient Monitoring
- Digoxin levels should be monitored in acute toxicity. However, Digibind administration can interfere with the assay and give unreliable results.
- Electrolytes, especially potassium, should be carefully monitored.
- Medications that may have precipitated or contributed to digoxin intoxication should be discontinued and restarted when clinical symptoms have resolved.
- EKG and cardiac monitoring should continue until resolution of dysrhythmias.

PROGNOSIS
Moderate/major morbidity or death has been reported from 20–25% of exposures treated in hospitals (6).

REFERENCES
1. Bauman JL, Didomenico RJ, Galanter WL. Mechanisms, manifestations, and management of digoxin toxicity in the modern era. *Am J Cardiovasc Drugs*. 2006;6:77–86.
2. Hauptman PJ, Kelly RA. Digitalis. *Circulation*. 1999;99:1265–70.
3. ACC/AHA/ESC 2006 guidelines for management of patients with ventricular arrhythmias and the prevention of sudden cardiac death-executive summary: A report of the American College of Cardiology/American Heart Association Task Force and the European Society of Cardiology Committee for Practice Guidelines. *Circulation*. 2006;114: 1088–1132.
4. Brubacher JR, Heller MB, Ravikumar PR, et al. Treatment of Toad Venom Poisoning with Digoxin-Specific Fab Fragments. *Chest*. 1996;110:1282–1288.
5. Lapostolle F, Borron S, Verdier C, et al. Digoxin-specific Fab fragments as single first-line therapy in digitalis poisoning. *Crit Care Med*. 2008;36(11):3014–3018.
6. Lapostolle F, Borron SW, Verdier C, et al. Assessment of digoxin antibody use in patients with elevated serum digoxin following chronic or acute exposure. *Intensive Care Med*. 2008;34: 1448–1453.

ADDITIONAL READING
- Rajapakse S. Management of yellow oleander poisoning. *Clinical Toxicology*. 2009;47(3): 206–212.
- Roberts DM, Buckley N. Antidotes for acute cardenolide (cardiac glycoside) poisoning (Review). *Cochrane Database of Systematic Reviews*. 2006; Issue 4.

 CODES

ICD9
972.1 Poisoning by cardiotonic glycosides and drugs of similar action

CLINICAL PEARLS
- The onset of vague symptoms accompanied by dysrhythmia should raise suspicion of toxicity by digitalis or other cardiac glycosides (e.g. foxglove, oleander).
- Toxicity may develop even when digoxin serum levels are within normal therapeutic range.
- Digoxin-specific Fab antibody fragments are the treatment of choice for severe, life-threatening arrhythmias due to digitalis toxicity.

DIPHTHERIA

Richard Kent Zimmerman, MD, MPH
Gregory A. Poland, MD

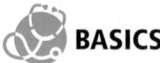 **BASICS**

DESCRIPTION

- Acute respiratory tract infection caused by *Corynebacterium diphtheriae*, usually producing a membranous pharyngitis
- Incubation period 2–5 days typically (range 1–10)
- Infection usually occurs during fall and winter in temperate regions. In the tropics, seasonal trends are less distinct.
- Transmission by respiratory route from infected person or carrier. Humans are the only reservoir.
- Several forms occur:
  – Membranous pharyngotonsillar diphtheria: The membrane is gray, adheres to the pharynx, and is surrounded by erythema. The underlying mucosa bleeds when the membrane is removed.
  – Nasal diphtheria: Unilateral discharge
  – Obstructive laryngotracheitis: Complication when membrane descends into larynx or bronchial tree. When it breaks up in young children, total obstruction of the airway may occur.
  – Cutaneous diphtheria: Punched-out ulcer covered by gray membrane (particularly in tropics and among homeless). Peaks August–October in southern US.
- System(s) affected: Cardiovascular; Nervous; Skin/Exocrine; Respiratory

EPIDEMIOLOGY

- Predominant age: Children <15 years old and poorly immunized adults
- Predominant sex: Male = Female

Incidence

In the US: For noncutaneous form, 1.6 in 100 million. Diphtheria is a rare condition in the US today. Fairly recent outbreaks have occurred in the independent states of the former Soviet Union.

RISK FACTORS

- Crowded living conditions
- Inadequate immunization
- Lower socioeconomic status
- Native Americans
- Alcoholism
- Travelers: Outbreaks have occurred in various countries; see CDC's travel Web site.

GENERAL PREVENTION

Prevention is by immunization:

- Children age 6 weeks up to 7 years of age should receive doses at 2, 4, 6, and 15–18 months and 4–6 years of age with 0.5 mL of DTaP vaccine IM. If the pertussis component is contraindicated, then pediatric diphtheria tetanus (DT) should be used. A booster dose of adult Tdap should be given at age 11–12 years.
- Unimmunized persons ≥7 years should receive 2 doses of adult Td 4–8 weeks apart with a 3rd dose 6–12 months later. 0.5 mL of Td should be given. Subsequently, booster doses with Td should be given every 10 years to all individuals without a contraindication. CDC currently recommends that Tdap substitute for 1 of the recommended decennial Td boosters.
- Immunized individuals may develop diphtheria, but their course is milder; immunization protects against the toxin, not infection or microbial carriage in the nose, pharynx, or skin. Disinfect all articles in contact with patient.
- Close contacts should be cultured and given antibiotic prophylaxis, regardless of immunization status.
- Contacts should receive an age-appropriate diphtheria toxoid-containing vaccine unless given a booster within the past 5 years.
- Contacts should receive a diphtheria toxoid-containing vaccine unless vaccinated within the past 5 years.

PATHOPHYSIOLOGY

Toxigenic strains produce an exotoxin that inhibits protein synthesis in all cell types.

ETIOLOGY

C. diphtheriae infection

 DIAGNOSIS

- Membranous pharyngotonsillar diphtheria:
  – Initially, white-to-yellow membrane, which is easily removed
  – Adherent, whitish-gray, leathery membrane on tonsils or pharynx
  – Removing membrane causes bleeding of mucosa.
  – Injected pharynx
  – Membrane may become black due to hemorrhage.
  – Sore throat
  – Cervical adenopathy with swelling
  – Malaise and prostration
  – Enlarged, tender cervical and submandibular lymph nodes
  – May progress to edematous, swollen neck (bull neck)
  – Paralysis of soft palate
  – Low-grade fever of 37.8–38.8°C (100–100.9°F)
  – Thrombocytopenia and purpura
- Nasal diphtheria:
  – Serosanguineous or seropurulent discharge and excoriations
  – Often, discharge is unilateral.
  – Often chronic, mild course
- Obstructive laryngotracheitis:
  – Hoarseness
  – Croupy cough
  – Progresses to dyspnea and stridor
  – Labored breathing
  – Thick speech
- Cutaneous diphtheria:
  – On skin, conjunctiva, vulva, vagina, and penis
  – Primary cutaneous diphtheria: Starts as tender pustule on lower extremity and becomes deep, round, punched-out ulcer covered by grayish membrane
  – Secondary infection of preexisting wound, purulent exudate, partial membrane

DIAGNOSTIC TESTS & INTERPRETATION

Lab

- Gram-positive rods in the pathognomonic Chinese character configuration
- Moderate leukocytosis
- Thrombocytopenia
- Transient albuminuria
- In experienced hands, methylene-blue stains can assist in a presumptive diagnosis.
- Culture from nose and throat beneath membrane and plate on special media; inform lab that diphtheria is suspected.
- Should test for toxigenicity of strain
- Serial ECGs and cardiac enzymes to detect myocarditis
- Delayed peripheral nerve conduction velocities
- Culture on special media (cystine-tellurite blood agar or modified Tinsdale agar) is positive in 8–12 hours if not previously treated with an antibiotic. Laboratory must be alerted to use special media.
- Toxin production confirmed by modified Elek test.
- Polymerase chain reaction
- Drugs that may alter lab results:
  – If an antibiotic was used, then ≥5 days may be required for the culture to grow on medium.

Pathological Findings

- Pleomorphic gram-positive rods
- Necrotic epithelium
- Hyaline degeneration

DIFFERENTIAL DIAGNOSIS

- Bacterial pharyngitis including group A Streptococcus
- Viral pharyngitis
- Mononucleosis
- Oral syphilis
- Candidiasis
- Vincent angina
- Acute epiglottitis

TREATMENT

MEDICATION

First Line
- Both antitoxins and antibiotics are needed for noncutaneous diphtheria.
- Diphtheria antitoxin, equine: Use 20,000–40,000 U of antitoxin for laryngeal or pharyngeal disease of <48 hours' duration; 40,000–60,000 U for nasopharyngeal lesions; 80,000–120,000 U for extensive disease ≥3 days or swelling of the neck (bull neck) (1)[B].
- Some experts recommend treating cutaneous disease with 20,000–40,000 U of antitoxin, while others doubt its value when there are no signs of systemic disease.
- Antitoxin is obtained from the CDC under Investigation New Drug protocol at 770-488-7100.
- Erythromycin parenterally or p.o., 40–50 mg/kg/d; maximum of 2 g/d for 14 days (2)[B], or penicillin G IM or IV for 14 days, or penicillin G procaine IM for 14 days. For cutaneous diphtheria, 10 days of one of these antibiotics.
- Precautions:
  – Equine antitoxin: 7% of patients are sensitive to equine antitoxin and need desensitization. Always test for hypersensitivity to antitoxin prior to its administration:
    ○ 1st, a drop of 1:100 dilution of antitoxin is placed on a scratch on the forearm, read at 15–20 minutes. If negative, an intradermal skin test is done with 1:1,000 dilution (0.02 mL). A positive reaction is the development of urticaria within 20 minutes of injection.
    ○ If no reaction to 1st intradermal, then repeat test with a 1:100 dilution
    ○ If the person has a negative history for animal allergy, has not previously received animal serum, and had a negative scratch test, then 1:100 dilution may be used initially.

Second Line
DL-carnitine 100 mg/kg/d b.i.d. p.o. in children for 4 days in myocarditis is experimental

ADDITIONAL TREATMENT
Antibiotics recommended for close contacts (oral erythromycin for 10 days or single IM penicillin G benzathine). Contacts should receive an age-appropriate diphtheria toxoid-containing vaccine unless given a booster within the past 5 years. Contacts who are children <7 years and who lack their 4th dose of DTaP should be vaccinated. Antibiotics recommended for carriers.

General Measures
- Appropriate health care:
  – Inpatient, initially hospitalized in unit that can monitor cardiac and respiratory status (must act on presumptive diagnosis because therapy cannot wait for culture confirmation)
  – Droplet isolation for pharyngeal diphtheria until cultures on 2 consecutive days are negative. The 1st culture must be taken at least 24 hours after the cessation of antibiotic therapy.
  – Contact precautions for cutaneous diphtheria.

- Have intubation or tracheostomy readily available. For laryngeal disease, laryngoscopy is desirable. Intubation or tracheostomy should be considered early for laryngeal disease.
- Avoid hypnotics and sedatives while monitoring respiratory status.

Additional Therapies
Physical therapy in convalescence for range of motion exercises to prevent contractions

 ONGOING CARE

FOLLOW-UP RECOMMENDATIONS
Rest for at least 3 weeks until risk of developing myocarditis has passed.

Patient Monitoring
- ECG, cardiac enzymes, and respiratory status. Serial ECG 2–3 times per week for 4–6 weeks to detect myocarditis
- Elimination of the organism should be documented by 2 negative cultures 24 hours apart. The 1st culture should 24 hours after the completion of antimicrobial therapy.
- During convalescence, patients should be immunized against diphtheria, because infection does not necessarily confer immunity.

DIET
Liquid to soft as tolerated

PATIENT EDUCATION
Explain aspects of illness and complications.

PROGNOSIS
- <5% mortality rate unless respiratory form for which case-fatality rate is 5–10%
- Prognosis guarded until recovery
- In convalescing patients, 5–10% persistence in nasopharynx
- Worse prognosis if myocarditis

COMPLICATIONS
- Myocarditis (10–25%) may occur early.
- Cranial and peripheral neuropathy (2–6 weeks after onset)
- ECG abnormalities in 2/3 of patients, including bundle branch block, tachycardia, atrial or ventricular fibrillation, and extrasystoles
- Right-sided heart failure
- Local paralysis of soft palate and posterior pharynx demonstrated by regurgitation of fluids through the nares
- Peripheral and cranial neuropathy affecting primarily motor nerve functions. Motor dysfunction starts proximally and extends distally. It usually resolves slowly.
- Syndrome resembling Guillain-Barré

REFERENCES
1. Hrobjartsson A, et al. The controlled clinical trial turns 100 years: Fibiger's trial of serum treatment of diphtheria. *Br Med J*. 1998;317:1243–5.
2. Kneen R, Pham NG, Solomon T, et al. Penicillin vs. erythromycin in the treatment of diphtheria. *Clin Infect Dis*. 1998;27:845–50.

ADDITIONAL READING
- American Academy of Pediatrics. Diphtheria. In Pickering LK: *Red Book: 2009 Report of the Committee on Infectious Diseases*. 28th Edition. Elk Grove Village, IL: American Academy of Pediatrics, 2009:280–3.
- Karam AG, Cherry JD. Hypotonic and Hyporesponsive Episodes After Diptheria-Tetanus-Acellular Pertussis Vaccination. *Pediatr Infect Dis J*. 2007;26:966–7.
- The original streptomycin trial paper: Fibiger J. Om Serumbehandling af Difteri. *Hospitalstidende*. 1898;6:309–25, 337–50

See Also (Topic, Algorithm, Electronic Media Element)
http://www.cdc.gov/vaccines/vpd-vac/diphtheria
http://wwwnc.cdc.gov/travel/yellowbook/2010/chapter-2/diphtheria.aspx

CODES

ICD9
- 032.0 Faucial diphtheria
- 032.2 Anterior nasal diphtheria
- 032.3 Laryngeal diphtheria

CLINICAL PEARLS
- Close contacts should be cultured, checked for immunization status, and considered for antimicrobial prophylaxis (penicillin or erythromycin).
- Past infection does not necessarily confer immunity.
- Alert lab if sending a culture because *C. diphtheriae* requires a special media to grow.

D

DISSEMINATED INTRAVASCULAR COAGULATION (DIC)

Jan Cerny, MD, PhD
Eva Medvedova, MD

BASICS

DESCRIPTION
- Acquired syndrome characterized by diffuse activation of intravascular coagulation arising from different causes. It can originate from and cause damage to the microvasculature, which, if sufficiently severe, can produce organ dysfunction.
- Occurring in complications of obstetrics (eg, abruptio placentae, fetus retention, amniotic fluid embolism), infection (especially gram-negative), malignancy (uncontrolled, metastatic tumor or leukemia), trauma, and other severe illnesses
- System(s) affected: Hematologic/Lymphatic/Immunologic
- Synonym(s): Consumptive coagulopathy; DIC

EPIDEMIOLOGY
Incidence
Unknown

Prevalence
- Predominant age: None
- Predominant sex: Male = Female

RISK FACTORS
See Etiology

GENERAL PREVENTION
Aggressive interventions aimed at early treatment of the underlying clinical conditions

PATHOPHYSIOLOGY
- Systemic formation of fibrin is the result of the simultaneous coexistence of:
  - Increased thrombin generation via tissue factor/factor VII mediated pathway
  - Suppression of the physiologic anticoagulant pathways:
    - Antithrombin due to consumption, degradation, and impaired synthesis
    - Proteins C and S due to decreased levels of thrombomodulin
  - Impaired fibrinolysis (early on):
    - Sustained increase in plasminogen activator inhibitor, type 1
- Increased fibrinolysis (late during the process) leads to bleeding.

ETIOLOGY
Causes can be classified as acute or chronic, systemic or localized:
- Sepsis/severe infection (any microorganism)
- Trauma (polytrauma, neurotrauma)
- Obstetric complications (amniotic fluid embolism, abruptio placentae)
- Solid tumors and leukemias (especially acute promyelocytic leukemia)
- Vascular disorders, such as Kasabach-Merritt syndrome, large vascular aneurysms, and thrombosis
- Organ destruction (severe pancreatitis, severe liver failure)
- Severe toxic or immunologic reactions:
  - Snake bite
  - Recreational drugs
  - Transfusion reactions
  - Transplant rejection
  - Thermal injury
- Infant and adult respiratory distress syndrome
- Neonatal purpura fulminans

COMMONLY ASSOCIATED CONDITIONS
Thromboembolic phenomena are associated with venous thrombosis, thrombotic vegetations on the aortic heart valve, arterial emboli, and neonatal purpura fulminans (homozygous protein C or protein S deficiency).

Pediatric Considerations
Neonatal purpura fulminans is associated with DIC and protein C or protein S deficiency (homozygous).

DIAGNOSIS

Symptoms and signs are related to the underlying disease process and disseminated intravascular coagulation.

HISTORY
Symptoms of microvascular thrombosis (e.g., renal failure), as well as diffuse bleeding

PHYSICAL EXAM
- Bleeding manifestations:
  - Skin (petechiae, purpura, ecchymosis, generalized oozing from venipuncture sites and wounds)
  - Renal (hematuria)
  - Gastrointestinal (mucous membranes and intestinal bleeding)
  - Neurologic (hemorrhagic infarction, massive intracerebral bleeding)
  - Respiratory (epistaxis, pulmonary hemorrhage)
- Microvascular thrombosis:
  - Skin (skin infarction, digital gangrene)
  - Gastrointestinal (mucosal ulcerations, bowel infarction)
  - Renal (oliguria, anuria, uremia)
  - Pulmonary (hypoxemia, acute respiratory distress syndrome)
  - Neurologic (convulsions, delirium, coma, multifocal cortical infarction)

DIAGNOSTIC TESTS & INTERPRETATION
No single laboratory test is sensitive and specific enough to allow a definitive diagnosis of DIC.

Lab
- Thrombocytopenia
- Increased partial thromboplastin time (PTT)
- Increased prothrombin test (PT)
- Decreased fibrinogen (serial levels)
- Increased fibrin degradation product (FDP)
- Positive D-dimer
- Decreased antithrombin III, decreased protein C
- Microangiopathic hemolytic anemia (schistocytes, increased lactate dehydrogenase levels, low hemoglobin)
- Decreased factor VIII (can help differentiate DIC vs liver failure—normal in liver failure)

Initial lab tests
Diagnostic algorithm for overt DIC (International Society on Thrombosis and Haemostasis)
- Assess if underlying disease is known to be associated with DIC:
  - YES: Proceed with this algorithm.
  - NO: Do not use this algorithm.
- Order global coagulation tests (PT, PTT, fibrinogen, soluble fibrin monomers, or FDPs)
- Score global coagulation test results:
  - Platelet count (>100 = 0, <100 = 1, <50 = 2)
  - Elevated fibrin-related markers (no increase = 0, moderate increase = 1, strong increase = 3)
  - Prolonged PT (<3 seconds = 0, >3 but <6 seconds = 1, >6 seconds = 2)
  - Fibrinogen level (>1 g/l = 0, <1 g/l =1)
- Calculate score:
  - If ≥5: Compatible with DIC, repeat scoring daily. If <5: Suggestive (not affirmative for nonovert DIC: Repeat in 1–2 days).

Follow-Up & Special Considerations
Frequent follow-up of initially abnormal laboratory tests to see effect of therapeutic interventions

DIFFERENTIAL DIAGNOSIS

- Fulminant liver failure or massive hepatic necrosis
- Vitamin K deficiency
- Thrombotic thrombocytopenic purpura
- Hemolytic–uremic syndrome
- Heparin-induced thrombocytopenia
- Primary fibrinolysis
- HELLP syndrome in pregnancy (hemolysis, elevated liver function, and low platelets)

 TREATMENT

Heterogeneity of the underlying disorders and the clinical presentations makes the therapeutic approach to DIC difficult:

- Appropriate health care: Inpatient and often intensive care unit (depending on underlying condition)
- Treat underlying condition (e.g., evacuation of uterus in abruptio placentae; broad-spectrum antibiotics for gram-negative sepsis)
- Supportive care with transfusions in patients who are bleeding, going for surgery, or at high risk of bleeding. Do not treat abnormal laboratory parameters:
  – Fresh frozen plasma
  – Platelet concentrates
  – Cryoprecipitate or fibrinogen concentrates
- Anticoagulants remain very controversial. Deep venous thrombosis prophylaxis is recommended in patients who are not bleeding.
- Restoration of anticoagulant pathways:
  – Recombinant human-activated protein C (benefit only in carefully selected patients at high risk of death from sepsis. The drug should only be administered in an Intensive Care Unit (ICU) when patient is monitored by trained personnel) (1)[A].
  – Activated factor VII use remains controversial.

MEDICATION

- Broad-spectrum antibiotics for sepsis
- Recombinant human-activated protein C in severe sepsis (1)

SURGERY/OTHER PROCEDURES

Surgical treatment or procedures should be considered, especially if they are treating the underlying condition (e.g., evacuation of uterus in abruptio placentae; some trauma or bleeding situations).

IN-PATIENT CONSIDERATIONS

Initial Stabilization

- Treat underlying disorder.
- Frequent monitoring of clinical and laboratory response

Admission Criteria

Usually dictated by severity of underlying condition. Some cases can be managed on a standard ward, but ICU care is typical.

Discharge Criteria

Once clinical and laboratory criteria are significantly improved and underlying reason for DIC is under control

 ONGOING CARE

FOLLOW-UP RECOMMENDATIONS

Patient Monitoring

- Monitor closely until much improved
- Serial platelet count, coagulation tests, and fibrinogen levels to see effect of therapeutic interventions

PROGNOSIS

- Related to the severity of cause
- Decreased antithrombin level is a poor prognostic factor in DIC.

COMPLICATIONS

- Acute renal failure
- Shock
- Cardiac tamponade
- Hemothorax
- Intracerebral hematoma
- Various thrombotic complications, including myocardial infarction, stroke, gangrene, and loss of digits

REFERENCE

1. Vincent JL, Bernard GR, Beale R, et al. Drotrecogin alfa (activated) treatment in severe sepsis from the global open-label trial ENHANCE: further evidence for survival and safety and implications for early treatment. *Crit Care Med.* 2005;33:2266–77.

ADDITIONAL READING

- Franchini M, Lippi G, Manzato F. Recent acquisitions in the pathophysiology, diagnosis and treatment of disseminated intravascular coagulation. *Thromb J.* 2006;4:4.
- Levi M. Disseminated intravascular coagulation. *Crit Care Med.* 2007;35:2191–5.
- Levi M, Toh CH, Thachil J, Watson HG et al. Guidelines for the diagnosis and management of disseminated intravascular coagulation. British Committee for Standards in Haematology. *Br J Haematol.* 2009;145:24–33.
- Taylor FB, Toh CH, Hoots WK, et al. Towards definition, clinical and laboratory criteria, and a scoring system for disseminated intravascular coagulation. *Thromb Haemost.* 2001;86:1327–30.

 CODES

ICD9

286.6 Defibrination syndrome

CLINICAL PEARLS

Treat underlying condition(s); transfusions represent supportive measures.

Transfusions are not indicated in patients with abnormal laboratory parameters without clinical bleeding.

DISSOCIATIVE DISORDERS

Moshe S. Torem, MD, DLFAPA

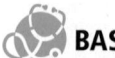 **BASICS**

DESCRIPTION
- Dissociative disorders bring about a sudden change in state of consciousness, identity, motor behavior, thoughts, feelings, and perception of reality so that these functions do not operate congruently.
- Numerous pathologic symptoms can be experienced, but all patients experience dysphoria, suffering, and maladaptive functioning.
- Disorders include dissociative amnesia, dissociative fugue, dissociative identity disorder, depersonalization disorder, and dissociative disorder not otherwise specified. Some authors may include somnambulism (sleepwalking disorder), conversion reactions, pseudo-epilepsy, and (in some cultures) a variety of possession syndromes.
- System(s) affected: Nervous
- Synonym(s): Hysterical neurosis, dissociative type; Ganser syndrome (1)

Geriatric Considerations
Decrease in frequency and intensity of dissociative symptoms; medication side effects are more likely

Pediatric Considerations
Suspect abuse or neglect.

EPIDEMIOLOGY
Incidence
- Predominant age: Adolescents and young to middle-age adults; rare as a new illness in the elderly. If untreated, it may linger from childhood into adulthood and old age.
- Predominant sex: Female > Male (2:1)

Prevalence
- Transient symptoms of depersonalization or derealization in the general population are common.
- Lifetime prevalence rate is 26–74%.
- 31–66% occurring at the time of a traumatic event
- Up to 70% of young adults report short periods of dissociative experiences that are self-limiting and resolve spontaneously without any treatment.
- Dissociative amnesia occurs in 2–7% of the general population.

RISK FACTORS
- Exposure to neglect, abuse, and trauma in childhood (2)
- Physical, emotional, verbal, or sexual abuse in childhood
- Sudden and severe trauma or threat to psychologic or physical integrity
- Sudden and unexpected exposure to watching others being killed or severely injured (as in an industrial or car accident)
- Tendency to cope with life's stresses by excessively using an escape mechanism of daydreaming and/or dissociation
- A preponderance of coping with trauma and internal or interpersonal conflicts by the use of dissociation
- Psychologic/social support to cope with the trauma/abuse was unavailable.
- Family history of dissociative disorders or posttraumatic stress disorder (PTSD)

GENERAL PREVENTION
- Child abuse prevention via parent education and community agency intervention
- Crisis intervention following individual trauma or disasters may prevent dissociative disorders.

PATHOPHYSIOLOGY
- All disorders share symptoms that:
  - Cause significant distress or impairment in social, occupational, or other important areas of functioning
  - Are not due to the direct physiologic effects of a substance (e.g., drug of abuse, a medication) or a general medical condition (e.g., temporal lobe epilepsy)
- Dissociative amnesia:
  - ≥1 episodes of inability to recall important personal information too extensive to be explained by ordinary forgetfulness
  - Not occurring during another psychiatric illness and not due to effects of chemical substance (e.g., drug abuse or medication)
  - Not due to a neurologic or other medical condition (e.g., epilepsy, head trauma)
- Dissociative fugue:
  - Sudden unexpected travel away from home or customary place of work with an inability to recall one's past
  - Confusion about personal identity or assumption of a new identity
  - Above symptoms do not occur during course of dissociative identity disorder.
  - Symptoms cause significant distress or impairment in social, occupational, or other activities of daily living (ADLs).
- Dissociative identity disorder:
  - Presence of ≥2 distinct identities or personality states (each with its own relatively enduring pattern of perceiving, relating to, and thinking about the environment and self)
  - At least 2 of these identities or personality states recurrently take control of the person's behavior.
  - Inability to recall important personal information that cannot be explained by ordinary forgetfulness
  - Reports of lost time, distortion, and lapses
  - Experiencing voices from inside one's head
  - Chronic headaches not due to other diagnoses
  - History of severe emotional or physical abuse as a child
  - Referring to self as he/she, we, they, us
  - Abnormal eating behaviors
  - Flashbacks
  - Feelings of derealization
  - Feelings of depersonalization
  - Amnesia about important childhood events
  - Personal objects and belongings that cannot be accounted for
  - Disowning unrecalled behaviors
  - Different handwriting styles
  - Different signatures and names
  - Sudden mood changes
  - Sudden behavioral changes (e.g., from adult to young child)
  - Episodes of déjà vu and déjà entendu
  - Feeling controlled by another person from within
  - Self-inflicted violence such as wrist cutting

- Depersonalization disorder:
  - Persistent or recurrent experiences of feeling detached from, and as if an outside observer of, mental processes or body (e.g., feeling like as if in a dream)
  - During the depersonalization experience, reality testing remains intact.
  - The depersonalization causes clinically significant distress or impairment in social, occupational, or other important areas of functioning.
  - The depersonalization experience does not occur exclusively during the course of another mental disorder, such as schizophrenia, panic disorder, acute stress disorder, or another dissociative disorder, and is not due to the direct physiological effects of a substance (e.g., a drug of abuse, a medication) or a general medical condition (e.g., temporal lobe epilepsy).
- Dissociative disorder not otherwise specified: Predominant feature is a dissociative symptom (e.g., a disruption in the usually integrated functions of consciousness, memory, identity, or perception of the environment) that does not meet the criteria for any other specific dissociative disorder. Examples:
  - Clinical presentations similar to dissociative identity disorder (DID) that fail to meet the full diagnostic criteria for DID
  - Derealization unaccompanied by depersonalization in adults
  - States of dissociation that occur in individuals who have been subjected to periods of prolonged and intense coercive persuasion (e.g., brainwashing, thought reform, or indoctrination while captive)
  - Dissociative trance disorder: Single or episodic disturbances in the state of consciousness, identity, or memory that are indigenous to particular locations and cultures. Dissociative trance involves narrowing of awareness, of immediate surroundings, or stereotyped behaviors or movements that are experienced as being beyond one's control.
  - Possession trance: Involves replacement of the customary sense of personal identity, attributed to the influence of a spirit, power, deity, or other person, and is associated with stereotyped involuntary movements or amnesia. This may be the most common dissociative disorder in Asia. Examples: *amok*, *bebainan* (Indonesia), *latah* (Malaysia), *pibloktoq* (Arctic). The dissociative or trance disorder is not a normal part of a broadly accepted collective cultural or religious practice.
  - Loss of consciousness, stupor, or coma not attributed to a general medical condition
- Ganser syndrome: Rare dissociative disorder characterized by nonsensical or wrong answers to questions or doing things incorrectly (e.g., $2 + 2 = 5$) when not associated with dissociative amnesia or dissociative fugue

ETIOLOGY
Common link to a history of trauma

COMMONLY ASSOCIATED CONDITIONS
See Risk Factors.

DIAGNOSIS

HISTORY
Patient's personal history should be complemented with history obtained from a family member.

DIAGNOSTIC TESTS & INTERPRETATION
Lab
Initial lab tests
- Electroencephalogram to rule out epilepsy
- Polysomnogram to rule out sleep disorders

Follow-Up & Special Considerations
- Toxicology screening may be helpful.
- Computed tomography scan and magnetic resonance imaging of the head to rule out organic brain disorders

Imaging
Follow-Up & Special Considerations
- Avoid sleep deprivation.
- Avoid substance abuse.

Diagnostic Procedures/Surgery
- Neuropsychologic testing to rule out learning disabilities and cognitive deficits due to early dementia or borderline mental retardation
- Psychologic testing to identify specific disorders, personality structure, and dynamics
- Dissociation scales help assess the tendency to dissociate in daily living activities
- Amobarbital (Amytal) interviews (narcoanalysis) and interviews under hypnosis may be useful in selected cases.

DIFFERENTIAL DIAGNOSIS
- Other mental/central nervous system disorder: Schizophrenia, depression, anxiety disorder, bipolar, PTSD, obsessive-compulsive disorder, identity disorder, phobic disorders, and eating disorders
- Other: Extreme sensory deprivation, epilepsy, dementia, encephalitis, head trauma, migraine, cerebral vascular disease, brain tumors
- Endocrinopathy: Hypoglycemia, hypothyroidism, hyperthyroidism
- Miscellaneous: Huntington disease, carbon monoxide poisoning, mescaline intoxication, botulism, hyperventilation

 TREATMENT

MEDICATION
First Line
- No medications are specifically curative. The following have been helpful:
  – Antidepressants for depression
  – Benzodiazepines for anxiety
  – Propranolol (80–400 mg/d) for flashbacks and other dissociative symptoms (off label)
  – Neuroleptics (low doses) for psychotic symptoms
  – Mood swings in dissociative disorders do not respond to the use of mood stabilizers.
- Precautions:
  – Potential abuse with short-acting benzodiazepines
  – Overdose/suicide potential with tricyclic antidepressants (TCAs)
  – Very low doses of neuroleptics can be used without producing tardive dyskinesia.
  – Atypical neuroleptics may be associated with hyperglycemia.
- Significant possible interactions:
  – Avoid monoamine oxidase inhibitors with TCAs or selective serotonin reuptake inhibitors.

Second Line
- Anxiety symptoms:
  – Buspirone (BuSpar), 30–80 mg/d for anxiety
- Obsessive-compulsive and/or depressive symptoms: Consider psychotropic medications.
- Atypical neuroleptics have recently been found useful for the control of self-inflicted violence or psychotic symptoms. Consider medications with the lowest effective dose.

ADDITIONAL TREATMENT
General Measures
- Individual psychotherapy plus behavior modification and in selective cases hypnotherapy (3)
- Adjuncts: Group therapy, expressive art therapy, occupational and recreational therapy when not associated with dissociative amnesia or dissociative fugue

Issues for Referral
Dissociative disorders are best treated by a well-trained mental health professional.

IN-PATIENT CONSIDERATIONS
Initial Stabilization
- Outpatient, individual psychotherapy
- At times of crisis: Intensive hospital-based treatment (as a protection for patients with suicidal or homicidal impulses)
- Use inpatient care to verify diagnosis with special tests and begin a treatment program.
- Note: Treatment emphasis should be on progress in the adaptive functions with daily living activities, symptom alleviation, ego strengthening, and preventing regressions.

 ONGOING CARE

PATIENT EDUCATION
- Self-hypnosis, relaxation exercises, guided imagery, mindfulness meditation
- Encourage patients to get educated about their condition and be inspired by those who got better and recovered:
  – Benson, H. The Relaxation Response. New York: HarperCollins, 2000.
  – Kabat-Zinn J. Coming to Our Senses. New York: Hyperion, 2005.
  – Rossman, ML. Guided Imagery for Self-Healing. Novato, CA: New World Library, 2000.
  – Sizemore C. A Mind of My Own. New York: W. Morrow, 1989.
  – Tart TC. Living the Mindful Life. Boston: Shambhala Publications, 1994.
  – Steinberg, M & Schnall, M. The Stranger in the Mirror. New York: HarperCollins, 2001.

PROGNOSIS
- Ranges from spontaneous improvement in cases of dissociative amnesia, dissociative fugue, and depersonalization disorder to acute and chronic morbidity in others
- Without treatment, a dissociative identity disorder patient may have a healthy functioning facade, with episodes of depression, confusion, mood swings, etc. With age, the intensity and frequency of dissociative experiences may decrease and crystallize around 1–2 major personality states.
- Effective treatment produces partial or full recovery for many patients.

COMPLICATIONS
Self-inflicted violence, suicide attempts, substance abuse, chemical dependency

REFERENCES
1. American Psychiatric Association. Diagnostic and Statistical Manual of Mental Disorders. 4th ed. Washington, DC: American Psychiatric Association; 1994:477–91.
2. Savitz JB, van der Merwe L, Newman TK, et al. The relationship between childhood abuse and dissociation. Is it influenced by catechol-O-methyltransferase (COMT) activity? Int J Neuropsychopharmacol. 2008;11:149–61.
3. Maldonado JR, et al. Treatment for dissociative disorders. In: Natham P, Gorman JM, eds. A guide to treatments that work, 2nd ed. England: Oxford University; 2002:463–96.

ADDITIONAL READING
- Alvi T & Minhas FA. Type of Presentation of Dissociative Disorder and Frequency of Co-morbid Depressive Disorder. J Coll Physicians Surg Pak. 2009;19:113–16.
- Espirito-Santo H, Pio-Abreu JL. Psychiatric symptoms and dissociation in conversion, somatization and dissociative disorders. Aust N Z J Psychiatry. 2009;43:270–6.
- Foote B, Smolin Y, Neft DI, et al. Dissociative disorders and suicidality in psychiatric outpatients. J Nerv Ment Dis. 2008;196:29–36.
- Maaranen P, Tanskanen A, Hintikka J, et al. The course of dissociation in the general population: a 3-year follow-up study. Compr Psychiatry. 2008; 49:269–74.
- Ozturk E, Sar V. Somatization as a predictor of suicidal ideation in dissociative disorders. Psychiatry Clin Neurosci. 2008;62:662–8.
- Phillips KA, et al. Special DSM-V issues on anxiety, obsessive-compulsive spectrum, posttraumatic, and dissociative disorders. Depress Anxiety. 2010; 27:91–92.
- Ross CA. Borderline personality disorder and dissociation. J Trauma Dissoc. 2007;8:71–80.
- Simeon D, et al. Temporal disintegration in depersonalization disorder. J Trauma Dissoc. 2007;8:11–24.

 CODES

ICD9
- 300.12 Dissociative amnesia
- 300.13 Dissociative fugue
- 300.14 Dissociative identity disorder

CLINICAL PEARLS
- Focus on improving and maintaining adaptive functioning with ADLs.
- Symptom stabilization and ego-strengthening come before exploration of past trauma.
- Regularly assess and reassess levels of functioning. Prevent unnecessary regressions.

DIVERTICULAR DISEASE

David M. Navel, MD
Justin M. Bailey, MD

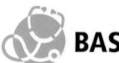 **BASICS**

DESCRIPTION
- Diverticular disease includes asymptomatic diverticula, symptomatic uncomplicated diverticular disease (recurrent pain, distention), diverticulitis, and diverticular hemorrhage
- Diverticula: Saclike protrusion of the mucosal and submucosal wall
  - Diverticulosis develops more commonly in countries where people eat a low-fiber diet.
  - In Western societies, 90–95% are found in the sigmoid colon, whereas Asian populations have more right-sided disease.
  - Diverticula number increase with age.
- Diverticular hemorrhage: Occurs in 3–5% of patients with diverticular disease:
  - Accounts for >40% of lower GI bleeds and 17–40% of cases of hematochezia in general
  - Bleeding is more common from right-sided diverticula.
- Diverticulitis: The most usual clinical complication, affects 10–25% of patients
- Complicated diverticulitis includes associated abscess, perforation, fistula, or stricture.
- System(s) affected: GI

EPIDEMIOLOGY
Incidence
- Diverticula in up to 20% general population, but increases progressively with age reaching up to 2/3 of people by the 8th decade
- Diverticulitis: 2,400–3,800/100,000
- Yearly mortality rate: 2.5/100,000

Prevalence
- Predominant age: <10% of people <40 years old, 2/3 of people in their 80s have diverticula
- Predominant sex: Male = Female overall, but more male <65 and female >65 years old

RISK FACTORS
- Age >40
- Low-fiber diet
- Sedentary lifestyle, obesity
- Previous diverticulitis and number of diverticula
- NSAID use may increase the risk of perforation.

Genetics
- No known genetic pattern
- Asian populations have a higher predominance of right-sided disease.

GENERAL PREVENTION
High-fiber diet; best with >30 g/day of fiber

ETIOLOGY
- Increased intraluminal pressure from dense, fiber-depleted stools and abnormal colonic motility
- Occur at areas of weakness from junctures of penetrating arteries in the muscular wall
- Bleeding is caused by medial thinning of the vasa recta and weakening of the artery.
- Diverticulitis occurs when increased pressures and fecal particles cause local inflammation and necrosis.

COMMONLY ASSOCIATED CONDITIONS
Connective tissue diseases, colon cancer, and inflammatory bowel disease

DIAGNOSIS

HISTORY
- Diverticulosis:
  - 80–85% of patients remain asymptomatic. Of the 15–20% with symptoms, 1–2% will need hospitalization and 0.5% will need surgery.
  - Pain: Dull, colicky, mostly in left lower quadrant, can be worse after eating, some relief following bowel movement or passage of flatus
  - Diarrhea or constipation
- Diverticulitis: Uncomplicated (75%) and complicated (25%):
  - Pain: Acute onset, mostly localized in left lower quadrant; prominently associated with tenderness in same region
  - Fever with chills as severity increases
  - Anorexia, nausea (20–62%), or vomiting
  - Constipation (50%) or diarrhea (25–35%)
  - Dysuria, frequency if bladder involved
  - Pneumaturia, fecaluria if colovesical fistula develops
- Diverticular hemorrhage:
  - Melena, hematochezia,
  - Painless rectal bleeding

PHYSICAL EXAM
- Diverticulosis:
  - Abdomen normal or distended and tympanitic
  - Absent signs of peritoneal inflammation
- Diverticulitis:
  - Rebound tenderness, involuntary guarding, or boardlike rigidity
  - Palpable mass (20%) that is tender, firm, or fixed
  - Abdomen distended and tympanitic
  - Bowel sounds depressed or could be exaggerated if obstruction ensues
  - Rectal exam may reveal tenderness, induration, or mass in the cul-de-sac.
  - Enterocutaneous, enterovaginal, and perirectal fistulae may be the initial manifestation.

DIAGNOSTIC TESTS & INTERPRETATION
Lab
Initial lab tests
- White blood cell count normal in diverticulosis; usually elevated with immature polymorphs in diverticulitis (normal in up to 45% of diverticulitis patients)
- Hemoglobin low, if bleeding present
- Erythrocyte sedimentation rate elevated in diverticulitis
- Urine analysis may be abnormal with microscopic pyuria, hematuria, pneumaturia, or fecaluria possibly suggesting fistula formation.
- Urine culture: Persistent infection in colovesical fistula
- Blood culture: Positive in diverticulitis with generalized peritonitis
- Drugs that may alter lab results:
  - Steroids
  - Other immunosuppressive drugs
- Disorders that may alter lab results:
  - Severe malnutrition

Imaging
Initial approach
- Diverticulosis:
  - Symptomatic uncomplicated disease: Consider a colonoscopy or a barium enema to rule out malignancy or colitis.
  - Recurrent uncomplicated diverticular disease: Evaluate by either a CT scan or a barium enema.
- Diverticulitis:
  - Plain film abdomen supine and upright; useful in peritonitis and perforation
  - Patients with suspected diverticulitis should have a CT scan with intravenous, oral, and rectal contrast to rule out complicated disease (1)[A].
  - CT may help in determining degree of acute perforation when present and assist in surgical planning.
  - Ultrasound has been shown to be effective in identifying diverticulitis in the acute setting (2)[B].
  - Avoid endoscopy or barium enemas due to risk of extravasation into the peritoneum.
- Diverticular hemorrhage/hematochezia:
  - Endoscopy is generally considered the test of choice for the evaluation of lower GI bleeding (3).
  - Angiography is used if massive bleeding obscures endoscopy or when endoscopy cannot visualize a source (3). It may also be used in some institutions as a primary evaluation tool for patients with acute lower GI bleeding.

Follow-Up & Special Considerations
- After resolution of an initial episode of acute diverticulitis, the colon should be evaluated with endoscopy to exclude any associated malignancies, strictures, or inflammatory bowel disease (1).
- After an episode of lower GI bleeding, colonoscopy should be performed to exclude neoplasia (2).

Diagnostic Procedures/Surgery
- For evaluation of hematochezia in suspected diverticular hemorrhage:
  - A nasogastric tube should be placed to exclude upper GI sources of bleeding (3).
  - 99mTc-pertechnetate–labeled red blood cell scans can be used before angiography to evaluate if angiography can be effective or not in revealing a source; however, this has not been studied in a comparison trial (3).
- For diverticulitis, gallium- or indium-labeled leukocytes to localize abscess (rarely used)

Pathological Findings
- Right-sided diverticula are true diverticula (all layers of the colonic wall).
- Left-sided diverticula are actually pseudodiverticula (outpouchings of the mucosa and submucosa).
- Surgical and autopsy studies show mycosia, a constellation of thickened circular muscle (pseudohypertrophy due to increased elastin in the taeniae), short taeniae, and luminal narrowing.
- Diverticulitis: Inflammation with lymphocytic infiltrate, ulceration, mucin depletion necrosis, Paneth cell metaplasia, and cryptitis.

DIFFERENTIAL DIAGNOSIS

Irritable bowel syndrome, lactose intolerance, carcinoma, inflammatory bowel disease, fecal impaction, incarcerated hernia, gallbladder disease, angiodysplasia, colitis, acute appendicitis, ectopic pregnancy

Pregnancy Considerations
- Rule out ectopic pregnancy.
- Carefully select antibiotic use in pregnant women due to teratogenicity of some medications.

 TREATMENT

MEDICATION
First Line
- Diverticulosis:
  - High fiber intake is recommended (preferably above 20–30 g/day).
- Symptomatic uncomplicated diverticular disease in the absence of a history of complicated disease can be treated with cyclical rifaximin or mesalamine continuously.
- Diverticulitis:
  - Oral antibiotics for outpatient treatment of mild disease: Cover for anaerobes and gram-negative rods with:
    ○ A quinolone (ciprofloxacin or levofloxacin) plus metronidazole (Flagyl) *OR*
    ○ Bactrim plus metronidazole
  - More severe cases in hospitals use intravenous antibiotics:
    ○ Mild/moderate disease: Zosyn or Unasyn or Ertapenem
    ○ Severe disease: Imipenem or Meropenem
  - Recurrences of acute diverticulitis may be decreased by using mesalamine ± rifaximin (4)[A] or probiotics
- Diverticular bleeding:
  - Consider Vasopressin 0.2–0.3 units/min through selective intra-arterial catheter
- Precautions:
  - Avoid morphine and other opiates that may increase intraluminal pressure or promote ileus.
  - Increased fiber intake is not recommended in the acute management of diverticulitis.

Second Line
- For outpatient therapy, Augmentin or Moxifloxacin
- For mild/moderate inpatient therapy:
  - Intravenous quinolone (ciprofloxacin or levofloxacin) + metronidazole or tigecycline
- For severely ill patients:
  - Ampicillin + metronidazole + a quinolone *OR*
  - Ampicillin + metronidazole + an aminoglycoside (if renal function allows)

ADDITIONAL TREATMENT
General Measures
- Diverticulosis: Outpatient with fiber supplements to soften stools
- Outpatient diverticulitis: Pain, tenderness, leukocytosis, but no toxicity or peritoneal signs; treat with oral antibiotics. 1–2% of subjects require hospitalization for toxicity, septicemia, peritonitis, or failure of symptoms to be resolved in a few days. Up to 30% of patients may require surgery at 1st episode of diverticulitis. Up to 50% of all patients with diverticulitis eventually may come to surgery.
- Toxic patients require hospitalization, bowel rest with clear liquids or nothing by mouth, and intravenous antibiotics at least until there is a positive response.

- Symptomatic improvement is expected within 2–3 days of initiating antibiotics, and antibiotics continued for 7–10 days (2).
- 80% of diverticular hemorrhages will resolve spontaneously (3).

Issues for Referral
Acutely suspected perforation, peritoneal signs, persistent lower GI bleeding requiring multiple transfusions

COMPLEMENTARY AND ALTERNATIVE MEDICINE
Probiotics may have benefit in symptomatic uncomplicated diverticular disease.

SURGERY/OTHER PROCEDURES
- Indication for emergent surgery: Peritonitis, uncontrolled sepsis, visceral perforation, colonic obstruction, or acute deterioration
- Surgery for nonemergent state controversial, sometimes even in complicated cases of diverticulitis (5)
- Elective surgery after acute diverticulitis: Decision for elective resection should be made on a case-by-case basis (1)[B].
  - After 1st episode, there is a 33% chance of a recurrence; if it does recur, there is a 66% chance of a 3rd bout.
  - Most complicated cases occur on the 1st presentation with subsequent presentations being uncomplicated (5).
  - Emergent surgery carries a 9-fold increase in mortality when compared to elective resection (6).
  - Elective resection is typically advised after recovery from a complicated diverticulitis treated nonoperatively (1)[B].
  - Age: Younger patients more likely to have recurrence; but should not determine the need for surgery.
  - Immunocompromised patients: More likely to present with acute complicated diverticulitis, fail medical management and have complications from elective surgery.
- Large abscesses (>4 cm) are usually drained radiologically and many of these patients can be acutely managed nonoperatively. As stated above, the ASCRS generally recommends elective resection after resolution of such a case (1)[B].
- In diverticular hemorrhage, patients requiring more than 4 units of red blood cells transfused have a 60% chance of requiring surgical intervention to stop bleeding. Patients requiring <4 units typically do not need surgery (3).

IN-PATIENT CONSIDERATIONS
Initial Stabilization
Intravenous fluids, analgesics, antibiotics, nasogastric suction

Admission Criteria
~1–2% of subjects require hospitalization for toxicity, septicemia, peritonitis

 ONGOING CARE

DIET
- NPO during acute diverticulitis; progress to fluids, then high-fiber as bowel function returns
- Patients with known diverticulosis should eat a high-fiber diet (>30 g/day) to prevent recurrence.
- Nuts, corn, and popcorn do not increase risk for diverticulosis or diverticular complications (7).

PROGNOSIS
- Good with early detection and treatment of complications.
- Recurrence risk increases with each bout.
- If diverticular bleeding, rebleeding occurs in up to 6%.

COMPLICATIONS
Hemorrhage, perforation, peritonitis, obstruction, abscess, or fistula

REFERENCES
1. Standards Committee of The American Society of Colon and Rectal Surgeons, Rafferty J, Shellito P, et al. Practice Parameters for Sigmoid Diverticulitis. *Dis Colon Rectum*. 2006.
2. Stollman NH, Raskin JB. Diagnosis and management of diverticular disease of the colon in adults. Ad Hoc Practice Parameters Committee of the American College of Gastroenterology. *Am J Gastroenterol*. 1999;94:3110–21.
3. Zuccaro G. Management of the adult patient with acute lower gastrointestinal bleeding. American College of Gastroenterology. Practice Parameters Committee. *Am J Gastroenterol*. 1998;93:1202–8.
4. Gatta L, Vakil N, Vaira D, Pilotto A, Curlo M, Comparato G, Leandro G, Ferro U, Lera M, Milletti S, Di Mario F et al. Efficacy of 5-ASA in the treatment of colonic diverticular disease. *J Clin Gastroenterol*. 2010;44:113–9.
5. Nelson RS, Ewing BM, Wengert TJ, et al. Clinical outcomes of complicated diverticulitis managed nonoperatively. *Am J Surg*. 2008;196:969–72; discussion 973–4.
6. Novitsky YW, Sechrist C, Payton BL, et al. Do the risks of emergent colectomy justify nonoperative management strategies for recurrent diverticulitis? *Am J Surg*. 2008.
7. Strate LL, Liu YL, Syngal S, et al. Nut, corn, and popcorn consumption and the incidence of diverticular disease. *JAMA*. 2008;300:907–14.

 CODES

ICD9
- 562.00 Diverticulosis of small intestine (without mention of hemorrhage)
- 562.01 Diverticulitis of small intestine (without mention of hemorrhage)
- 562.02 Diverticulosis of small intestine with hemorrhage

CLINICAL PEARLS
- Diverticula occur in up to 20% of general population, but increases progressively with age, reaching up to 2/3 of people by the 8th decade.
- Patients with known diverticulosis should eat a high-fiber diet to prevent recurrence, and nuts, corn, and popcorn do not increase risk for diverticular complications.
- WBC are not elevated in up to 45% of cases of diverticulitis

DOMESTIC VIOLENCE

Rhonda A. Faulkner, PhD
Meg Lekander, MD

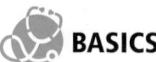 **BASICS**

DESCRIPTION
- Domestic violence (DV) is behavior in any relationship that is used to gain or maintain power and control over an intimate partner.
- May include physical, sexual, and/or emotional abuse, economical or psychological actions, or threats of actions that influence another person.
- Although women are at greater risk of experiencing DV, it occurs among patients of any race, age, sexual orientation, religion, gender, socioeconomic background, and education level.
- Synonym(s): Intimate partner violence (IPV); Spousal abuse; Family violence

EPIDEMIOLOGY
Incidence
Approximately 8%; women were more likely to report partner violence than men (1)[B]

Prevalence
- Domestic violence occurs in 1 in 4 American families. In the US, 2–4 million women are abused by an intimate partner each year. Nearly 5.3 million incidents of DV occur each year among US women ≥18 years, and 3.2 million incidents among men.
- DV results in nearly 2 million injuries and 2,000–4,000 deaths nationwide each year.
- Reportedly, 30% of women and 22% of men have experienced physical, sexual, or psychological IPV during their lifetime in the U.S.
- DV is estimated to affect at least 1/3 of patients cared for by primary care physicians, with 5% of women patients in current abusive relationship.

Geriatric Considerations
- ~4–6% of elderly are abused, with ~1–2 million elderly persons experiencing abuse and/or neglect each year. In 90% of cases, the perpetrator is a family member.
- Elder abuse is any form of mistreatment that results in harm or loss to an older person; may include physical, sexual, emotional, financial abuse, and/or neglect.

Pediatric Considerations
- >3 million children aged 3–17 years are at risk of witnessing acts of DV.
- Approximately 1 million abused children are identified in the US each year.
- Children living in violent homes are at increased risk of physical, sexual, and/or emotional abuse; anxiety and depression; decreased self-esteem; emotional, behavioral, social, and physical disturbances.

Pregnancy Considerations
DV occurs during 7–20% of pregnancies. Women with unintended pregnancy are at 3 times greater risk of DV compared with those whose pregnancy was planned. 25% of abused women report exacerbation of abuse during pregnancy.

RISK FACTORS
Patient/victim risk factors:
- Substance abuse
- Poverty/financial stressors/unemployment
- Recent loss of social support
- Family disruption and life cycle changes
- History of abusive relationships or witness to abuse as child
- Mental or physical disability in family
- Social isolation
- Pregnancy

Abuser risk factors:
- Substance abuse (e.g., heavy drinking)
- Young age
- Unemployment
- Low academic achievement
- Witnessing or experiencing violence as child
- Depression
- Personality disorders

Relational risk factors:
- Marital conflict
- Marital instability
- Economic stress
- Traditional gender role norms
- Poor family functioning

Geriatric Considerations
Factors associated with the abuse of older adults include increasing age, nonwhite race, low income status, functional impairment, cognitive disability, substance use, poor emotional state, low self-esteem, cohabitation, and lack of social support.

Pediatric Considerations
Factors associated with child abuse or neglect include low-income status, low maternal education, nonwhite race, large family size, young maternal age, single-parent household, parental psychiatric disturbances, and presence of a stepfather.

 DIAGNOSIS

- DV is often underdiagnosed, with only 10–12% of physicians conducting routine screening.
- Although prevalence of DV in primary care settings is 7–50%, <15% are screened.
- Pregnancy increases risk.
- 15–20% of women in US emergency departments are there related to DV.
- Barriers to screening: Time constraints, discomfort with the subject, fear of offending the patient, and lack of perceived skills and resources to manage DV.
- Abused patients may refuse to disclose abuse for many reasons:
  - Not feeling emotionally ready to admit the reality of the situation
  - Shame and self-blame
  - Feelings of failure if abuse is admitted
  - Fear of rejection by the physician
  - Fear of retribution from abuser
  - Belief that abuse will not happen again
  - Believe that no alternatives or available resources exist

- Physicians should introduce the subject of DV in a general way (i.e., "I routinely ask all patients about domestic violence. Have you ever been in a relationship where you were afraid?").
- How to screen:
  - Screen patient alone, without partner or others present
  - Ask screening questions in patient's primary language; do not use children or other family members as interpreters
- Partner violence screening:
  - "Have you ever been hit, kicked, punched, or otherwise hurt by someone?"
  - "Have you ever been verbally threatened or abused by someone?
  - "Do you feel safe in your current relationship?"
  - "Is there a partner from a previous relationship who is making you feel unsafe now?"
  - "Has your child(ren) ever witnessed anything violent or frightening in your home, neighborhood, or school?"
- CDC-recommended RADAR system:
  - R: Routinely screen every patient; make screening a part of everyday practice in prenatal, postnatal, routine gynecologic visits, and annual health screenings.
  - A: Ask questions directly, kindly, and be nonjudgmental.
  - D: Document findings in the patient's chart using the patient's own words, with details. Use body maps and photographs as necessary.
  - A: Assess the patient's safety and see if the patient has a safety plan.
  - R: Review options for dealing with domestic violence with the patient and provide referrals.
- Additional DV screening tools:
  - SAFE Questions:
    - Stress/Safety: "Do you feel safe in your relationship?"
    - Afraid/Abused: "Have you ever been in a relationship where you were threatened, hurt, or afraid?"
    - Friends/Family: "Are your friends or family aware that you have been hurt? Could you tell them, and would they be able to give you support?"
    - Emergency Plan: "Do you have a safe place to go and the resources you need in an emergency?"
  - HITS screening tool (1-never, 2-rarely, 3-sometimes, 4-often, 5- frequently; Score >9 is considered abuse):
    - How often does your partner: Hurt you (physically)?; Insult you?; Threaten you with harm?; Scream or curse at you?

HISTORY
- Pregnancy difficulties such as poor/late prenatal care, low-birth-weight babies. and perinatal deaths
- Pelvic and abdominal pain, chronic without demonstrable pathology
- Headaches
- Back pain
- Gynecologic disorders
- Sexually transmitted infections including HIV/AIDS
- Central nervous system disorders
- Gastrointestinal disorders

- Depression
- Suicidal ideation
- Anxiety
- Fatigue
- Substance abuse
- Eating disorders
- Overuse of health services/frequent emergency room visits
- Noncompliance

PHYSICAL EXAM
- Psychological signs and symptoms:
  - Signs of Battered Woman Syndrome &/or PTSD (flat affect/avoidance of eye contact; evasiveness; heightened startle response; sleep disturbance; traumatic flashbacks)
  - Depression, anxiety, chronic fatigue, substance abuse
  - Suspicious partner accompaniment at appointment; overly solicitous partner and/or refusal to leave exam room
- Physical signs and symptoms:
  - Tympanic membrane rupture
  - Rectal or genital injury (centrally located injuries with bathing-suit pattern of distribution—concealable by clothing)
  - Head and neck injuries (site of 50% of abusive injuries)
  - Facial scrapes, loose or broken tooth, bruises, cuts, or fractures to face or body
  - Knife wounds, cigarette burns, bite marks, welts w/outline of weapon (such as belt buckle)
  - Broken bones
  - Defensive posture injuries
  - Injuries inconsistent with the explanation given
  - Injuries in various stages of healing

DIAGNOSTIC TESTS & INTERPRETATION
- The US Preventive Services Task Force (USPSTF) found insufficient evidence to recommend for/against routine screening of parents or guardians for the physical abuse or neglect of children, of women for intimate partner violence, or of older adults or their caregivers for elder abuse.
- Other recommendations:
  - American College of Physicians recommends routine screening for DV in primary care settings and when women present for emergency care with traumatic injuries.
  - US Surgeon General and American Association of Family Practitioners recommend that physicians consider the possibility of DV as a cause of illness and injury.

Pediatric Considerations
American Academy of Pediatrics (AAP) and American Medical Association (AMA) recommend that physicians remain alert for signs and symptoms of child physical and sexual abuse in the routine exam.

Pregnancy Considerations
ACOG and AMA guidelines on DV recommend that physicians should routinely assess all pregnant women for DV.

Lab
Initial lab tests
LFTs, amylase, lipase if abdominal trauma is suspected

TREATMENT
- Treatment includes: Initial diagnosis; ongoing medical care; emotional support, counseling, and patient education regarding the DV cycle; referrals to community and supportive services as needed.
- Upon diagnosis, offer validation and emotionally supportive statements:
  - "You are not to blame. I am sorry this is happening to you. There is no excuse for DV."
  - Remind patient of your commitment to confidential communication.
- Listen and respond to safety issues for the patient:
  - "Are you afraid to go home?"
  - "Are there guns in the home?"
- Provide information about DV and help where needed:
  - "DV is a health issue for you (and your children)."
- Make referrals to local resources:
  - "Do you need or want to access a safety shelter or DV service agency?"
  - "Do you want police intervention and if so, would you like me to call the police so they can make a report with you?"
  - Offer numbers to local resources and National DV Hotline: 1.800.799.SAFE (open 24/7; can provide physicians in every state with information on local resources).
- Document findings:
  - Use patient's own words regarding injury and abuse.
  - Legibly document injuries: Use a body map.
  - If possible, take instant photographs of patient's injuries if given patient consent.
- Make patient safety plan.
- If patient is planning to leave:
  - Is there a friend or supportive family member nearby with whom the patient can stay?
  - Does patient want to go to a DV shelter or contact police; obtain an order of protection?
- If patient is not planning to leave:
  - Can she or he anticipate the escalation of violence and take precautions?
  - Are there weapons in the home?
- Preparing patient to get away in an emergency:
  - Encourage patient to keep the following items in a safe place: Keys (house and car); important papers (Social Security card, birth certificates, photo ID/driver's license, passport, green card); cash, food stamps, credit cards; medication for self and children; children's immunization records; important phone numbers/addresses (friends, family, local shelters); personal care items, extra glasses, etc.
  - Encourage patient to arrange a signal with someone to let that person know when she or he needs help.

ADDITIONAL TREATMENT
- National DV Hotline: 1.800.799.SAFE (7233)
- Post in all exam rooms posters in both English and Spanish; available at http://www.thehotline.org/resources/resource-download-center/

General Measures
- Reporting child and elder abuse to protective services is mandatory in most states. Several states have laws requiring mandatory reporting of IPV.
- Contact the local DV program to find out about laws and community resources before they are needed.
- Display resource materials (National DV Hotline: 1.800.799.SAFE) in the office, all exam rooms, and restrooms.

ONGOING CARE
FOLLOW-UP RECOMMENDATIONS
- Schedule prompt follow-up appointment.
- Inquire about what has happened since last visit.
- Review medical records and ask about past episodes to convey concern for the patient and a willingness to address this health issue openly.
- DV often requires multiple interventions over time before it is resolved.

PATIENT EDUCATION
- Counsel patients about nonviolent ways to resolve conflict.
- Educate patients about the cycle of violence.
- Counsel parents about developmentally appropriate ways to discipline their children.
- Educate parents about the negative consequences of arguments on children and each other.
- National Coalition Against Domestic Violence: www.ncadv.org
- CDC: www.cdc.gov/violenceprevention

PROGNOSIS
Most DV perpetrators do not voluntarily seek therapy unless pressured by partners or upon legal mandate. Current evidence is insufficient on effectiveness of therapy for perpetrators.

REFERENCE
1. Walton MA, Murray R, Cunningham RM, Chermack ST, Barry KL, Booth BM, Ilgen MA, Wojnar M, Blow FC et al. Correlates of intimate partner violence among men and women in an inner city emergency department. *J Addict Dis.* 2009;28:366–81.

ADDITIONAL READING
MacMillan HL, Wathen CN, Jamieson E, et al. Screening for intimate partner violence in health care settings: A randomized trial. *JAMA.* 2009;302:493–501.

CODES
ICD9
- 995.50 Unspecified child abuse
- 995.51 Child emotional/psychological abuse
- 995.52 Child neglect (nutritional)

CLINICAL PEARLS
- Display resource materials in the office (e.g., posting Abuse Awareness posters/National DV Hotline, 1.800.799.SAFE, in both English and Spanish, in all exam rooms and restrooms).
- Despite lack of data, screen all women: "Have you ever been threatened, hit, kicked, or are you afraid of your partner?"
- For those who screen positive, offer resources, reassure confidentiality, and provide close follow-up.

DOWN SYNDROME

Michele Roberts, MD, PhD

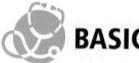 **BASICS**

DESCRIPTION
- Congenital condition associated with mental retardation and an increased risk of multisystem medical problems
- One of the most common identifiable causes of mental retardation
- System(s) affected: Neurologic (100%); Cardiac (40–50%); Gastrointestinal (GI) (8–12%)
- Etiology: The presence of all or part of an extra chromosome 21
- Synonym(s): Trisomy 21; DS

Pediatric Considerations
- Congenital heart disease is major cause of morbidity/mortality. Murmur may not be present at birth. Delay in recognition may lead to irreversible pulmonary hypertension.
- Early treatment of subclinical thyroid disease may improve growth and development (1)[B].

Geriatric Considerations
- Life expectancy has increased to 56 years in 2008 (2).
- Age-related health issues occur at earlier age than in general population.
- Communication difficulties may interfere with prompt recognition of:
  - Alzheimer disease, which is more prevalent and may occur at a younger age, and other psychiatric illness
  - Thyroid/autoimmune disorders
  - Cataracts/hearing loss

Pregnancy Considerations
- Most DS males are infertile:
- Females are subfertile but can conceive:
  - 36% of reported offspring have DS
  - Assess mental and physical fitness to carry pregnancy/care for child

EPIDEMIOLOGY
Incidence
In the US, 1 in 700 live births
Prevalence
350,000 persons in the US

RISK FACTORS
- DS occurs in all races with equal frequency.
- Risk increases dramatically with mother's age:
  - Age 20, 1 in 1,445
  - Age 35, 1 in 270
  - Age 37, 1 in 100
  - Age 45, 1 in 25
- With prenatal screening of older mothers, relatively more DS infants are born to younger mothers.

Genetics
- Online Mendelian Inheritance in Man (OMIM) #190685
- Inheritance: Most commonly sporadic nondisjunction resulting in trisomy 21

- Chance of having another child with DS is:
  - 1% (or age risk, whichever is greater) after conceiving a pregnancy with nondisjunction trisomy 21
  - 10–15% for mothers and 3–5% for fathers who carry a balanced translocation
  - 100% if the parental translocation is 21:21(45,t [21:21])
- Unclear after child with mosaic DS, but ~1%
- Chromosome 21 has been sequenced; it is the smallest human chromosome.
- The majority of identifiable phenotypic characteristics associated with DS map to a 37–44 Mb region of distal 21q. Broad susceptibility regions for 25 phenotypes have been identified, arguing against a single Down syndrome critical region (DSCR) (3).

GENERAL PREVENTION
- No prevention for nondisjunction
- The American College of Medical Genetics and the American College of Obstetrics and Gynecology recommend that all pregnant women be offered prenatal screening for DS.
- Preimplantation diagnosis with in vitro fertilization (IVF) or prenatal diagnosis and termination are current options.
- Maternal prenatal screening includes:
  - Pregnancy-associated plasma protein A (PAPP-A): 1st trimester
  - Quadruple test: 2nd trimester
  - Sequential/integrated screen combines both
  - Ultrasound (nuchal translucency or NT)
- Chorionic villi sampling or amniocentesis: if high a priori risk or positive screen

ETIOLOGY
- Trisomy 21: In 95% of patients, an extra chromosome 21 is found in all cells due to nondisjunction usually in maternal meiosis.
- Translocation DS: In 3% of patients, extra chromosome 21q material is translocated to another chromosome (usually 13, 14, or 21). For translocation trisomy 21, 2/3 are new, 1/3 have a parental carrier:
  - Translocation DS more likely if mother <30 years of age
- Mosaic trisomy 21: Found in 2% of patients with DS. Manifestations may be milder.

COMMONLY ASSOCIATED CONDITIONS
- Cardiac:
  - Congenital heart defects (40–50%):
  - Mostly endocardial cushion or ventricular septal defect (VSD)
- GI/growth:
  - Structural defects (12%):
    - Duodenal or anal atresia/stenosis
    - Hirschsprung disease, annular pancreas
  - Gastroesophageal reflux
  - Constipation
  - Celiac disease
- Pulmonary:
  - Tracheal stenosis/tracheoesophageal fistula
  - Pulmonary hypertension
  - Obstructive apnea
- Genitourinary:
  - Cryptorchidism, hypospadias
  - Renal anomaly

- Hematologic/neoplastic:
  - Macrocytosis (66%)
  - Transient leukemoid reaction (10%):
    - Generally resolves spontaneously, but can be preleukemic (AMKL) in 20–30%
  - Leukemia (0.5–1%):
  - Acute lymphoblastic leukemia (ALL) risk: 10–20 × that of ALL in non-DS
  - Decreased risk of most solid tumors; increased risk of germ cell tumors
- Endocrine:
  - Hypothyroidism: Congenital or acquired (20–40%)
  - Diabetes
  - Hypogonadism
- Skeletal:
  - Altered growth pattern
  - Atlantoaxial instability (15%); 2% symptomatic
  - Ligamentous laxity
  - Scoliosis (some cases have adult onset)
  - Hip problems (8%)
- Immune/rheumatologic:
  - Abnormal immune function with increased rate of and mortality from infection, especially respiratory
  - Increased risk of autoimmune disorders including thyroid, celiac disease, lupus
- Neurologic:
  - Mental retardation ranging from near-normal to severe. Average is moderate retardation.
  - Seizures:
    - Infantile spasms (5–10%)
    - Increased risk child-/adult-onset seizures
  - Alzheimer disease: 100% develop neuropathologic changes, though not all develop symptoms
- Psychiatric:
  - Emotional/conduct disorders (25–33%)
  - Depression: Up to 10% of adults
- Sensory:
  - Hearing loss (60–90%):
    - Mostly conductive due to high frequency of asymptomatic middle ear effusion
  - Visual impairment (60–70%): Mostly strabismus, nystagmus, cataracts
- Dermatologic, worsens with increasing age:
  - Palmoplantar hyperkeratosis (>75%), atopic or seborrheic dermatitis (50%), onychomycosis (50%), syringomas (30%), furunculosis/folliculitis (15%)

 DIAGNOSIS

- The mother should be informed of the diagnosis promptly by a physician (preferably the obstetrician and pediatrician, or family physician), on the basis of clinical observations and before the karyotype is available, but with consideration of extenuating circumstances (e.g., mother's medical condition).
- The spouse/partner and infant should be present unless this would cause undue delay. The meeting should be private.
- Refer to the baby by name.
- The physician should be knowledgeable on the subject of DS, and should conduct a discussion with content that is current, respectful, balanced, informative, and realistic but not overly pessimistic, concentrating on what is relevant to the first year of life.

HISTORY
85% of mothers of infants with DS learn of the diagnosis postnatally

PHYSICAL EXAM
- DS-specific growth curves should be used.
- Infants and children:
  - Brachycephaly (100%)
  - Hypotonia (80%)
  - Small ears, often low set and simplified
  - Upslanting palpebral fissure (90%)
  - Epicanthic folds (90%)
  - Brushfield spots
  - Depressed nasal bridge
  - Short neck, often with increased nuchal folds
  - Abnormal dermatoglyphics, including single palmar crease, single flexion crease on 5th finger
  - Increased space between toes 1–2; 5th finger clinodactyly; brachydactyly
- Adults: Features may become less obvious.

DIAGNOSTIC TESTS & INTERPRETATION
Lab
Initial lab tests
- A chromosome test is definitive and should always be done at the time of clinical suspicion.
- Parental chromosome study indicated only if translocation DS found in child.

Imaging
Initial approach
- Echocardiogram at the time of diagnosis. A ventricular septal defect (VSD)/endocardial cushion defect may not be apparent at birth.
- Radiographs of neck currently recommended for all children once between ages 3 and 5 years.

Follow-Up & Special Considerations
- Repeat neck films for minor trauma, neck pain, long-tract symptoms, or breathing problems.
- Cardiac follow-up as indicated

Pathological Findings
Upslanting palpebral fissures, epicanthic folds, 5th-finger clinodactyly, and single palmar crease individually may be a benign familial trait. Unilateral single palmar crease seen in 4% of general population; bilateral in 1%.

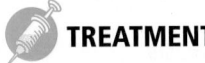 **TREATMENT**

ADDITIONAL TREATMENT
General Measures
Genetic evaluation and counseling

Issues for Referral
- Infant stimulation programs
- Physical/occupational/speech therapy
- Special needs educational support
  - Inclusion programs generally work well.

COMPLEMENTARY AND ALTERNATIVE MEDICINE
- Antioxidant therapy has theoretical basis for future benefits, although a 2008 randomized controlled trial provided no evidence to support the use of antioxidant or folinic acid supplements in children with Down syndrome (4).
- Vitamin E, selenium, and zinc may be beneficial (5)[C].
- Many unproven and dangerous procedures and therapies are offered to vulnerable parents:
  - Craniosacral manipulation is dangerous due to potential atlantoaxial instability.

- Sicca is illegal in US, potentially dangerous, and without any evidence of benefit.
- Piracetam is much publicized, without scientific evidence of benefit.

SURGERY/OTHER PROCEDURES
Repair of congenital anomalies is appropriate. Plastic surgery for facial features generally not recommended.

IN-PATIENT CONSIDERATIONS
Discharge Criteria
If the social situation indicates adoption, there are families specifically seeking to adopt DS children.

 ONGOING CARE

FOLLOW-UP RECOMMENDATIONS
Patient Monitoring
Surveillance recommendations (6,7,8)[C] (repeat additionally for clinical suspicion):
- Vision: Assess for strabismus, cataracts, and nystagmus at birth and on each routine visit:
  - Should be seen by ophthalmologist by 6 months and every 2 years in early childhood, annually in later childhood and adulthood
- Hearing: Neonatal screen with ABR or OAE, then audiogram every 6 months until age 3 years, then annual hearing assessment
- Thyroid: Initial newborn screen. Repeat thyroid-stimulating hormone (TSH) at 6 months, 12 months, and then annually.
- Screening for celiac disease is controversial, but does not appear to be cost effective.
- C-spine flexion/extension films once at 3–5 years of age and as indicated clinically.
- Echocardiogram for all newborns, regardless of murmur. Monitor clinically for later cardiac complications throughout life.

DIET
- No special diet, but caloric needs are lower in adolescents/adults with DS than in their peers
- Obesity is prevalent at all ages.
- No scientific evidence to support megavitamin therapy and dietary supplements that are widely discussed in the lay press

PATIENT EDUCATION
- National Down Syndrome Congress (800) 232-NDSC http://www.ndsccenter.org
- National Down Syndrome Society (800) 221-4602 http://www.ndss.org
- Dr. Len Leshin, a pediatrician whose son has Down syndrome, has written an extensive collection of accurate and accessible articles about Down syndrome: http://www.ds-health.com/
- The Down Syndrome Research Foundation provides information on the latest research and educational programs for people with Down syndrome: http://dsrf.org/index.cfm?fuseaction=publications.dsq

PROGNOSIS
- Associated congenital anomalies are the immediate concern during the newborn period.
- Adults can often work in protected situations; a few are largely independent.
- Earlier onset of age-related health issues, shortened life expectancy.
- Clinical Alzheimer disease in at least 1/3 of patients after age 35 years

REFERENCES
1. van Trotsenburg AS, Vulsma T, van Rozenburg-Marres SL, et al. The effect of thyroxine treatment started in the neonatal period on development and growth of two-year-old Down syndrome children: a randomized clinical trial. *J Clin Endocrinol Metab*. 2005;90:3304–11.
2. http://www.ndss.org.
3. Lyle R, Béna F, Gagos S et al. Genotype-phenotype correlations in Down syndrome identified by array CGH in 30 cases of partial trisomy and partial monosomy chromosome 21. *Eur J Hum Genet*. 2009;17:454–66.
4. Ellis JM, Tan HK, Gilbert RE, et al. Supplementation with antioxidants and folinic acid for children with Down's syndrome: randomised controlled trial. *BMJ*. 2008;336:594–7.
5. Roizen NJ. Complementary and alternative therapies for Down syndrome. *MRDD Res Rev*. 2005;11:149–55.
6. American Academy of Pediatrics: Health supervision for children with Down syndrome *Pediatrics*. 2001;107:442–9.
7. Cohen WI. Current dilemmas in Down syndrome clinical care. *Am J Med Genet*. 2006;142C:141–8.
8. Smith DS. Health care management of adults with Down syndrome. *Am Fam Physician*. 2001;64: 1031–8.

ADDITIONAL READING
- Mégarbané A, Ravel A, Mircher C et al. The 50th anniversary of the discovery of trisomy 21: the past, present, and future of research and treatment of Down syndrome. *Genet Med*. 2009;11:611–6.
- Ranweiler R. Assessment and care of the newborn with down syndrome. *Adv Neonatal Care*. 2009;9:17–24.
- Reynolds T, Vranken G, Van Nueten J, et al. Down's syndrome screening: population statistic dependency of screening performance. *Clin Chem Lab Med*. 2008;46:639–47.
- Roizen NJ, Patterson D. Down's syndrome. *Lancet*. 2003;361:1281–9.
- Skotko BG, Capone GT, Kishnani PS, et al. Postnatal diagnosis of Down syndrome: synthesis of the evidence on how best to deliver the news. *Pediatrics*. 2009;124:e751–8.

See Also (Topic, Algorithm, Electronic Media Element)
Algorithm: Mental Retardation

 CODES

ICD9
758.0 Down's syndrome

CLINICAL PEARLS
- DS can affect all systems, including neurologic, cardiac, gastrointestinal, and endocrine.
- As life expectancy increases, regular health monitoring can improve outcomes.

DUMPING SYNDROME

Hongyi Cui, MD, PhD
John J. Kelly, MD

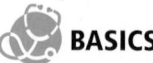 **BASICS**

DESCRIPTION
Gastrointestinal and vasomotor symptoms resulting from rapid gastric emptying and delivery of large amounts of hyperosmolar content into the small intestine. Usually occurs following gastric and esophageal surgery (gastrectomy, vagotomy, pyloroplasty, esophagectomy, Nissen fundoplication, or gastric bypass procedures).

EPIDEMIOLOGY
- Overall, about 10% of patients following gastric surgery and up to 50% of patients who undergo esophagectomy develop dumping symptoms.
- Predominant age: Middle age to elderly
- Predominant sex: Female > Male

Incidence
- In the US, 0.9% of proximal gastric vagotomy without any drainage procedure; 10–22% truncal vagotomy and drainage. After partial gastrectomy, 14–20% of patients develop symptoms of dumping.
- It is a prominent feature after bariatric surgery. Over 70% of patients that have undergone gastric bypass procedure experience varying degree of dumping symptoms. It is regarded as a beneficial feature of gastric bypass surgery since patients learn to avoid calorie-rich foods and eat small meals.

RISK FACTORS
Accelerated gastric emptying resulting from gastric surgery is a main risk factor for dumping syndrome. In fact, the severity of dumping syndrome is proportional to the rate of gastric emptying. The common gastric surgical procedures associated with dumping syndrome are:
- Bariatric surgery (i.e., Roux-en-Y gastric bypass)
- Gastric drainage procedures (e.g., pyloroplasty)
- Partial gastrectomy
- Total gastrectomy. Those with pouch formation have significantly less dumping and heartburn (1)[A].
- Esophagectomy
- Antiulcer surgery (e.g., vagotomy)
- Antireflux surgery (e.g., Nissen fundoplication, especially in pediatric patients)

GENERAL PREVENTION
- Dietary modifications (i.e., eating frequent, small, dry meals that contain limited amount of refined carbohydrates; restrict fluids to between meals; avoid milk products and increase protein/fat intake and supplement dietary fibers, etc.)
- Postural changes (i.e., lying supine for 30 minutes after meals)

ETIOLOGY
The pathogenesis of dumping syndrome is multifactorial. It includes at least the following interplaying factors:
- Alterations in the storage function of the stomach and/or the pyloric emptying mechanism, leading to rapid delivery of hyperosmolar material into the intestine. This results in fluid shifts from the intravascular compartment into the bowel lumen, leading to rapid small-bowel distention and an increase in the frequency of bowel contractions (early dumping).
- Supraphysiologic release of various GI peptides/vasoactive mediators, leading to paradoxical vasodilation in a relatively volume-contracted state.
- Reactive hypoglycemia secondary to hyperinsulinemia caused by high concentration of carbohydrates in the proximal small intestine and rapid absorption of glucose (late dumping).
- Pancreatic islet cell hyperplasia, rather than late dumping, is thought to be the underlying mechanism for hyperinsulinemic hypoglycemia with nesidioblastosis after gastric bypass.

COMMONLY ASSOCIATED CONDITIONS
- Peptic ulcer disease
- Reactive hypoglycemia
- Gastrectomy/vagotomy/pyloroplasty
- Esophagectomy
- After Nissen fundoplication for reflux disease in pediatric population
- After gastric bypass procedure for morbid obesity

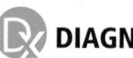 **DIAGNOSIS**

A suggestive symptom profile in a patient who has undergone gastric (including bariatric) or esophageal surgery warrants the investigation for dumping syndrome.

HISTORY
- History of gastric procedures
- GI symptoms (in early dumping):
  - Cramping abdominal pain
  - Diarrhea (postprandial)
  - Borborygmi
  - Bloating or epigastric fullness
  - Nausea/vomiting
- Systemic/vasomotor symptoms (both early and late dumping):
  - Palpitations
  - Diaphoresis
  - Faintness, fatigue, and headache
  - Flushing
  - Light-headedness and desire to lie down
  - Confusion and syncope
  - Malnutrition and weight loss

- Early dumping symptoms include gastrointestinal (abdominal pain, nausea, bloating, borborygmi and diarrhea, etc.) and vasomotor (perspiration and facial flushing, a desire to lie down, palpitations, weakness and syncope, etc.) symptoms; late dumping symptoms include perspiration, palpitations, hunger, weakness, confusion and syncope, etc.

PHYSICAL EXAM
- Diagnosis is mainly based on typical symptoms in patients with history of gastric procedures. A diagnostic scoring system has been developed by Sigstad based on various weighting factors allocated to the symptoms of dumping. A score index >7 is suggestive of dumping syndrome. The score index is very helpful in assessing a response to therapy.
- No physical signs are specific for dumping syndrome.

DIAGNOSTIC TESTS & INTERPRETATION
Lab
- Postprandial hypoglycemia
- Anemia
- Hypoalbuminemia
- Drugs that may alter lab results: Insulin
- Disorders that may alter lab results: Diabetes mellitus

Imaging
- Upper gastrointestinal series: Barium rapidly emptying from stomach
- Nuclear medicine gastric emptying study
- Endoscopy (to define anatomy and exclude mechanical obstruction)

Diagnostic Procedures/Surgery
- Dumping syndrome is a clinical diagnosis based on typical symptoms in patients who have undergone gastric surgery.
- Oral glucose challenge test (i.e., oral intake of 50 grams of glucose following 10-hour fasting) can elicit typical signs and symptoms in patients with dumping syndrome. A rise in heart rate by 10 beats per minute or more in the first hour is diagnostic.
- Hydrogen breath test after oral ingestion of glucose is also a sensitive test.

DIFFERENTIAL DIAGNOSIS
- Mechanical obstruction
- Gastroenteric fistula
- Celiac sprue
- Crohn disease
- Pancreatic exocrine insufficiency
- Neuroendocrine tumors (e.g., carcinoid)
- Irritable bowel syndrome
- Lactose intolerance

TREATMENT

Dietary modifications are the mainstay of treatment in patients with dumping syndrome. Medical therapy is effective in patients with incapacitating symptoms who fail dietary modifications. Remedial surgery is only considered in patients refractory to medical management.

MEDICATION
First Line
- Octreotide (Sandostatin) 100–500 μg SC b.i.d. Can be very expensive (2)[B]. Patients may have increased steatorrhea during octreotide treatment, and pancreatic enzyme supplement is effective in relieving this symptom.
- Late dumping symptoms can be ameliorated by the α-glucosidase inhibitor acarbose (100–200 mg, PO t.i.d.), which lowers blood glucose by delaying GI absorption of carbohydrates.
- Pectin/guar gum are effective by delaying glucose absorption and prolonging small bowel transit time.

Second Line
Anticholinergics: Results generally are disappointing.

ADDITIONAL TREATMENT
General Measures
Most patients can be managed conservatively with dietary modification and medical treatment. Only a small percentage of patients ultimately require surgical intervention.

Additional Therapies
Continuous trophic enteral feeding via a jejunostomy has been reported to be an effective approach in patients refractory to all other treatment measures.

SURGERY/OTHER PROCEDURES
- Remedial surgery only if dietary and medical management unsuccessful and symptoms debilitating; the results are variable and unpredictable. A proper selection of the surgical intervention is very important. Most patients with dumping syndrome as a result of gastric bypass will find that the effects ameliorate with time (>2 years).
- Options of surgery include Roux-en-Y conversion (from Billroth I and II), pyloric reconstruction (for patients who have severe dumping following pyloroplasty), reversed jejunal segment (for patients who failed Roux-en-Y reconstruction), and conversion of Billroth II to Billroth I anastomosis.

- Patients with refractory dumping symptoms after loop gastrojejunostomy may benefit from simple takedown of the anastomosis; conversion to Roux-en-Y gastrojejunostomy is a reasonable option for patients with disabling dumping after distal gastrectomy. Other procedures have been attempted with limited success.
- The syndrome of hyperinsulinemic hypoglycemia with nesidioblastosis (a hyperplasia of islet cells) after Roux-en-Y gastric bypass (>1–2 year post-op) can usually be managed with low-carbohydrate diet and alpha-glucosidase inhibitors. Subtotal or total pancreatectomy (as has been suggested in the literature) is usually unnecessary.

 ONGOING CARE

FOLLOW-UP RECOMMENDATIONS
Lying supine for 30 minutes after eating or when symptoms occur may reduce the chance of syncope.

Patient Monitoring
Follow to be sure of adequate nutrition.

DIET
- Low-carbohydrate, high-protein diet
- Add dietary fiber.
- Milk or milk products should be avoided.
- Frequent small meals with minimal liquid
- Avoid hyperosmolar liquids.

PATIENT EDUCATION
National Digestive Diseases Information Clearinghouse, Box NDDIC, Bethesda, MD 20892, (301) 468-6344, digestive.niddk.nih.gov

PROGNOSIS
Favorable

COMPLICATIONS
- Hypoglycemia
- Malnutrition and weight loss
- Electrolyte disturbances, including hypokalemia

REFERENCES
1. Gertler R, Rosenberg R, Feith M, Schuster T, Friess H et al. Pouch vs. no pouch following total gastrectomy: meta-analysis and systematic review. *Am J Gastroenterol*. 2009;104:2838–51.
2. Ukleja A. Dumping syndrome: pathophysiology and treatment. *Nutr Clin Pract*. 2005;20:517–25.

3. Gonzalez-Sánchez JA, Corujo-Vázquez O, Sahai-Hernández M. Bariatric surgery patients: reasons to visit emergency department after surgery. *Bol Asoc Med P R*. 2007;99:279–83.
4. Penning C, Vecht J, Masclee AA. Efficacy of depot long-acting release octreotide therapy in severe dumping syndrome. *Aliment Pharmacol Ther*. 2005;22:963–9.
5. Bouras EP, Scolapio JS. Gastric motility disorders: management that optimizes nutritional status. *J Clin Gastroenterol*. 2004;38:549–57.

ADDITIONAL READING

Tack J, Arts J, Caenepeel P et al. Pathophysiology, diagnosis and management of postoperative dumping syndrome. *Nat Rev Gastroenterol Hepatol*. 2009;6: 583–90.

See Also (Topic, Algorithm, Electronic Media Element)
Diarrhea, Chronic; Hypoglycemia, Non-diabetic; Peptic Ulcer Disease
Algorithm: Diarrhea, Chronic

 CODES

ICD9
564.2 Postgastric surgery syndromes

CLINICAL PEARLS

- Vagotomy affects gastric emptying through increased gastric tone and decreased receptive relaxation.
- Dumping syndrome is the most common cause for ER presentation after bariatric surgery (3)[B].
- An increase in heart rate of 10 BPM is noted after glucose challenge (50 g oral glucose) in patients with dumping syndrome.
- Depot octreotide has shown some promise as an alternative to standard SC octreotide (4)[B].
- Some side effects of octreotide are gallstones, steatorrhea, and diarrhea (5)[B].

DUPUYTREN CONTRACTURE

Jeffrey F. Minteer, MD

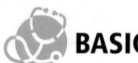

BASICS

DESCRIPTION
- Palmar fibromatosis; due to progressive fibrous proliferation and tightening of the fascia inside the palms, resulting in flexion deformities and loss of function
- Not the same as "trigger finger," which is caused by thickening of the distal flexor tendon
- Similar change may rarely occur in plantar fascia; it usually appears simultaneously.
- System(s) affected: Musculoskeletal

EPIDEMIOLOGY
Prevalence
- Unknown in United States
- Norway: 9% males and 3% females

RISK FACTORS
- Smoking (mean 16 pack-years, odds ratio 2.8)
- Increasing age
- Male/Caucasian
- Workers exposed to vibration
- Diabetes mellitus (1/3 affected, increases with time, usually mild; middle and ring finger involved)
- Epilepsy
- Chronic illness (e.g., pulmonary tuberculosis, liver disease, HIV)
- Hypercholesterolemia
- Alcohol consumption

Genetics
- Autosomal-dominant with variable penetrance
- 68% of male relatives of affected patients develop disease at some time

GENERAL PREVENTION
Avoid risk factors, especially with a strong family history.

ETIOLOGY
Unknown; possibly a T-cell–mediated autoimmune disorder

COMMONLY ASSOCIATED CONDITIONS
- Alcoholism
- Epilepsy
- Diabetes mellitus
- Chronic lung disease
- Occupational hand trauma (vibration white finger)
- Shoulder–hand syndrome
- Status postmyocardial infarction
- Hypercholesterolemia
- Carpal tunnel syndrome

DIAGNOSIS

HISTORY
- Caucasian male aged 50–60 years
- Family history
- Mild pain early
- Unilateral or bilateral (50%)
- Right hand more frequent
- Ring finger more frequent
- Ulnar digits more affected than radial digits

PHYSICAL EXAM
- Painless plaques or nodules in palmar fascia
- Extends into a cordlike band in the palmar fascia
- Skin adheres to fascia and becomes puckered.
- Nodules can be palpated under the skin.
- Digital fascia becomes involved as disease progresses
- Reduced flexibility of metacarpophalangeal (MCP) and proximal interphalangeal (PIP) joints
- No sign of inflammation
- Web space contractures
- Dupuytren diathesis can involve plantar (Ledderhose—10%) and penile (Peyronie—2%) fascia
- Knuckle pads over PIP
- Disease stages:
  – Early: Skin pits (can also be seen in nevoid basal cell cancer and palmar keratosis)
  – Intermediate: Nodules and cords
  – Late: Contractures

DIAGNOSTIC TESTS & INTERPRETATION
Diagnostic Procedures/Surgery
Magnetic resonance imaging (MRI) can assess cellularity of lesions that correlate with higher recurrence after surgery.

Pathological Findings
- Myofibroblasts
- 1st stage (proliferative): Increased myofibroblasts
- 2nd stage (residual): Dense fibroblast network
- 3rd stage (involutional): Myofibroblasts disappear

DIFFERENTIAL DIAGNOSIS
- Early for callosity
- Tendon abnormalities
- Camptodactyly: Early teens; tight fascial bands on ulnar side of small finger
- Diabetic cheiroarthropathy: All 4 fingers
- Volkmann ischemic contracture

TREATMENT

MEDICATION
First Line
- Steroid injection for an acute tender nodule, painful knuckle pad
- Clostridial collagenase injections (FDA approved 2010):
  – Degrades collagen to allow manual rupture of diseased cord
  – Best for isolated cord of MCP joint
  – Recurrence rate at 8 years 67% in MCP joints but less severe than initial contracture (1)[B]

Second Line
- Topical high-potency steroids: Case report of improvement with clobetasol 0.1% b.i.d. and at bedtime for 2–4 weeks
- Surgery for contracture >30%

ADDITIONAL TREATMENT

General Measures
- Physiotherapy alone is ineffective:
  - Intermittent splinting unlikely to be effective
  - Continuous splinting may be helpful in pre- and postoperative
- Isolated involvement of palmar fascia can be followed.
- MCP joint involvement can be followed if flexion contracture is <30°.

Issues for Referral
- Any involvement of PIP joints
- MCP joints contracted >30°
- Positive Hueston test

Additional Therapies
- Continuous elongation technique is useful to prepare a severely contracted PIP joint for surgery. The digit can frequently be completely extended; however, it will relapse if surgery is not performed.
- Prophylactic external beam radiation: 87% either no progression or improvement at 12 months; concern about local effects in a benign disease
- Intraoperative 5-fluorouracil ineffective
- Percutaneous and needle fasciotomy:
  - Best for MCP joint
  - Recurrence common
  - Not indicated in severe or recurrent disease

SURGERY/OTHER PROCEDURES
- Selective fascial ray release/partial fasciectomy (2)[B]
- Indications:
  - Any involvement of the PIP joints
  - MCP joints are contracted at least 30°.
  - Positive Hueston tabletop test: When the palm is placed on a flat surface, the digits cannot be simultaneously placed fully on the same surface as the palm because of flexion contractures.

- May require skin grafts for wound closure with severe cutaneous shrinkage. Reports of clinical regression with continuous passive skeletal traction in extension and under a skin graft.
- 80% have full range of movement if operated on early.
- Amputation of little finger if severe and deforming
- MCP joints respond better than PIP joints, especially if contracted >45°.

 ## ONGOING CARE

FOLLOW-UP RECOMMENDATIONS
Patient Monitoring
Regular follow-up by physician every 6 months–1 year

PATIENT EDUCATION
- Avoid risk factors, especially with a strong family history.
- Mild disease: Passively stretch digits twice a day and avoid recurrent gripping of tools.

PROGNOSIS
- Unpredictable, but usually slowly progressive
- 10% may regress spontaneously.
- Patients likely to have aggressive disease if 1 or more of the following are present: Age <40 years at onset, knuckle pads, positive family history, bilateral disease involving radial side of hand
- Recurrence rate after surgery is high; more with aggressive features
- Prognosis better for MCP joint vs PIP joint after surgery and collagenase injection

COMPLICATIONS
- Postsurgery development of reflex sympathetic dystrophy
- Postoperative recurrence or extension in 46–80%
- Postoperative hand edema and skin necrosis
- Digital infarction

REFERENCES
1. Watt AJ, Curtin CM, Hentz VR et al. Collagenase injection as nonsurgical treatment of dupuytren's disease: 8-year follow-up. *J Hand Surg Am*. 2010;35:534–9, 539.e1.
2. van Rijssen AL, Werker PM et al. [Treatment of Dupuytren's contracture; an overview of options] *Ned Tijdschr Geneeskd*. 2009;153:A129.
3. Rayan GM. Clinical presentation and types of Dupuytren's disease. *Hand Clin*. 1999;15:87–96, vii.

ADDITIONAL READING
- Hunt TR. What is the appropriate treatment for Dupuytren contracture? *Cleve Clin J Med*. 2003;70:96–7.
- Hurst LC, Badalamente MA, Hentz VR, Hotchkiss RN, Kaplan FT, Meals RA, Smith TM, Rodzvilla J, CORD I Study Group et al. Injectable collagenase clostridium histolyticum for Dupuytren's contracture. *N Engl J Med*. 2009;361:968–79.
- Rayan GM. Duypuytren Disease: Anatomy, Pathology, Presentation, and Treatment. *J of Bone & Joint Surgery*. 2007;89(1):189–98.

 ## CODES

ICD9
- 728.6 Contracture of palmar fascia
- 728.71 Plantar fascial fibromatosis

CLINICAL PEARLS
- 90% of cases are progressive.
- Refer those with any involvement of the PIP joints or MCP involvement >30°.
- Neither surgical nor enzymatic fasciotomy offers a cure with high rate of recurrence (3)

DYSFUNCTIONAL UTERINE BLEEDING

Meaghan Delaney, MD
Debra Papa, MD
Ginger Allister, MD

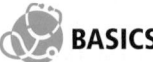

BASICS

DESCRIPTION
- Dysfunctional uterine bleeding (DUB) is irregular (usually heavy, prolonged, or frequent) bleeding that occurs in the absence of anatomic pathology
- Associated with anovulatory menstrual cycles
- Typically a diagnosis of exclusion: Need to exclude anatomic pathology and medical illnesses
- Systems affected: Endocrine/Metabolic, Reproductive

EPIDEMIOLOGY
- Predominant age: 12–50 years
- Predominant gender: Female only
- Adolescents and perimenopausal women are most often affected

Incidence
Accounts for 5–10% of outpatient gynecologic visits

Prevalence
Abnormal uterine bleeding occurs in:
- ~ 1 in 3 women of reproductive age
- ~1 in 10 post-menopausal women

RISK FACTORS
Risk factors for endometrial cancer (which can cause DUB):
- Age >40
- Obesity
- Diabetes Mellitus
- Nulliparity
- Early menarche or late menopause (>55 years)
- Hypertension
- Chronic anovulation or infertility
- Unopposed estrogen therapy
- History of breast cancer or endometrial hyperplasia
- Tamoxifen use
- Family history: Gynecologic, breast, or colon cancer

Genetics
Unclear

PATHOPHYSIOLOGY
- Disruption of normal hormonal sequence of ovulatory menstrual cycle
- Anovulation accounts for 90% of DUB:
  - Loss of cyclic endometrial stimulation
  - Elevated estrogen levels stimulate endometrial growth
  - Endometrium does not shed and eventually outgrows blood supply
  - Tissue breaks down and sloughs from uterus

ETIOLOGY
The diagnosis of DUB is made when pathologic causes of abnormal bleeding have been ruled out:
- Pregnancy
  - Ectopic pregnancy, threatened or incomplete abortion, or hydatidiform mole
- Reproductive pathology & structural disorders
  - Uterus: leiomyomas, endometritis, hyperplasia, polyps, trauma
  - Adnexa: Salpingitis, functional ovarian cysts
  - Cervix: Cervicitis, polyps, sexually transmitted diseases (STDs), trauma
  - Vagina: Trauma, foreign body
  - Vulva: Lichen sclerosis, STDs

- Malignancy of the vagina, cervix, uterus, & ovaries
- Systemic diseases
  - Inflammatory bowel disease
  - Hematologic disorders (Von Willebrand's disease, thrombocytopenia, etc.)
  - Advanced or fulminant liver disease
  - Chronic renal disease
- Diseases causing anovulation
  - Hyper/hypothyroidism
  - Adrenal disorders
  - Pituitary disease (prolactinoma)
  - Polycystic ovarian syndrome (PCOS)
  - Eating disorders
- Medications (iatrogenic causes)
  - Anticoagulants
  - Steroids
  - Tamoxifen
  - Hormonal medications: Intrauterine devices (IUDs)
  - Selective-serotonin reuptake inhibitors
  - Antipsychotic medications
- Other causes of abnormal uterine bleeding:
  - Excessive weight gain
  - Increased exercise
  - Stress

DIAGNOSIS

A thorough medical, surgical, social, and family history should be obtained.

HISTORY
- History of bleeding:
  - Onset, severity (quantified in pad/tampon use, presence & size of clots)
  - Association with other factors (i.e. coitus, contraception, weight loss/gain)
- Menstrual history:
  - Unpredictable or episodic, heavy or light bleeding
  - Menstrual symptoms do not typically precede bleeding
- Review of symptoms (exclude symptoms of pregnancy, symptoms of bleeding disorders, bleeding from other orifices, stress, exercise, recent weight change, visual changes, headaches, galactorrhea)
- Medication history (evaluate for use of aspirin, anticoagulants, hormones, herbal supplements)

ALERT
Postmenopausal bleeding is any bleeding that occurs >1 year after the last menstrual period; cancer must always be ruled out

PHYSICAL EXAM
Discover anatomic or organic causes of DUB:
- Assess hemodynamic stability
- Evaluate for:
  - Obesity (BMI)
  - Pallor
  - Visual field defects (pituitary lesion)
  - Hirsutism or acne (hyperandrogenism)
  - Goiter
  - Galactorrhea (hyperprolactinemia)
  - Purpura, ecchymosis (bleeding disorders)
- Pelvic exam:
  - Evaluate for uterine irregularities
  - Check for foreign bodies
  - Rule out rectal or urinary tract bleeding

- Include Pap smear and tests for STDs

Pediatric Considerations
Premenarchal children with vaginal bleeding should be evaluated for foreign bodies, physical/sexual abuse, possible infections, and signs of precocious puberty.

DIAGNOSTIC TESTS & INTERPRETATION
Lab
Not always necessary

Initial lab tests
- Urine human chorionic gonadotropin (rule out pregnancy and/or hydatiform mole)
- Complete blood count (CBC)
- Thyroid-stimulating hormone (TSH) (1)[B]
- Prolactin level
- Consider other tests based on differential diagnosis:
  - Follicle-stimulating hormone (FSH) to evaluate for hypo/hypergonadotropism
  - Coagulation studies & factors (2)[A]
  - Liver function tests
  - 17-hydroxyprogestrone
  - Androgenic hormones
  - *Neisseria gonorrhea, Chlamydia trachomatis* tests

Imaging
Initial approach
- Transvaginal ultrasound (TVUS):
  - Indications: postmenopausal patients, suspicion of pregnancy or anatomic abnormalities, PCOS
  - High sensitivity for endometrial carcinoma in postmenopausal women (3)[A]. If ≤4 mm, endometrial cancer unlikely
  - If endometrial thickness >5 mm, proceed to endometrial biopsy (EMB)
- Saline infusion sonohistogram: Often superior to TVUS in screening for anatomic abnormalities (4). Can perform if TVUS suspicious for lesion.

Diagnostic Procedures/Surgery
- Pap smear to exclude cervical cancer
- Endometrial biopsy (EMB) should be performed in women:
  - Women >35 years of age with DUB to rule out cancer or premalignancy
  - Women with endometrial thickness >5 mm
  - Women aged 18–35 with DUB and risk factors for endometrial cancer (see Risk Factors)
  - Perform ≥day 18 of cycle if known; secretory endometrium confirms ovulation occurred
  - Does not diagnose leiomyosarcoma or fibroids because lesions are deep to endometrial lining
- Dilation & curettage:
  - Performed if bleeding is heavy, uncontrolled, and/or failed emergent medical management
  - If unable to perform EMB in office
- Hysteroscopy if lesion suspected (diagnostic and therapeutic)

Pathological Findings
Pap smear could reveal carcinoma or inflammation indicative of cervicitis. Most EMBs show proliferative or dyssynchronous endometrium (suggesting anovulation)

DIFFERENTIAL DIAGNOSIS
See Etiology

TREATMENT

Attempt to diagnose other causes of bleeding prior to instituting therapy.

MEDICATION

First Line

- Acute, emergent, nonovulatory bleeding: (5)
  - Conjugated equine estrogen (Premarin): 25 mg IV Q4H (maximum of 6 doses) or 2.5 mg PO Q6H should control bleeding in 12–24 hours (6)[A]
  - Then change to OCP or progestin for cycle regulation
- Acute, nonemergent, nonovulatory:
  - Combination OCP with ≥30 mcg estrogen given as a taper. An example of a tapered dose: 4 pills/d until bleeding stopped for 24 hours; 3 pills/d for 3 days; 2 pills/d for 3 days.
  - Then begin once-a-day regimen (7)[B]
- Nonacute, nonovulatory:
  - OCPs: 20–35 mcg estrogen plus progesterone (mono- or triphasic)
  - Progestins: Medroxyprogesterone acetate (Provera) 10 mg/d for 5–10 days each month. Daily progesterone for 21 days per cycle results in significantly less blood loss (8)[A].
  - Levonorgestrel intrauterine devices (Mirena) are most effective (9)[A].
- Do not use estrogen if contraindications are present
- Precautions:
  - Exclude endometrial hyperplasia & carcinoma before administering estrogen
  - Consider deep vein thrombosis prophylaxis when treating with high-dose estrogens
  - Failed medical treatment requires further workup
  - Smokers >35 years of age should be counselled on the risk of thromboembolic disease when using OCPs

Second Line

- Gonadotropin-releasing hormone (GnRH) agonists create a hypogonadotropic state, usually used as a bridge to definitive therapy.
- Danazol (Danocrine 200–400 mg/d) is more effective than nonsteroidal anti-inflammatory drugs (NSAIDs), but is limited by androgenic side effects & cost (10)[A]. It has been essentially replaced by GnRH agonists.
- Antifibrinolytics like tranexamic acid (Lysteda, 650mg, 2 tabs three times daily (max of 5 days during menstruation) (11)[A].

ADDITIONAL TREATMENT

General Measures

NSAIDs (naproxen sodium 500 mg BID, mefenamic acid 500 mg TID, ibuprofen 600–1,200 mg/d):

- Decreases amount of blood loss compared to placebo (10)[A]
- Diminishes pain

Issues for Referral

- If an obvious cause for vaginal bleeding is not found in a pediatric patient, refer to a pediatric endocrinologist.
- Patients with persistent bleeding despite medical treatment require reevaluation and referral to a gynecologist.

Additional Therapies

- Antiemetics if treating with high-dose estrogen
- Iron supplementation if anemia (usually iron deficiency) is identified

SURGERY/OTHER PROCEDURES

- Hysterectomy if endometrial cancer, if medical therapy fails, or uterine pathology
- Endometrial ablation is less expensive than hysterectomy with high satisfaction; medical treatment does not have to fail first (12)[A]

IN-PATIENT CONSIDERATIONS

Initial Stabilization

With acute bleeding, replace volume with crystalloid and blood as necessary

Admission Criteria

Significant hemorrhage causing acute anemia with signs of hemodynamic instability

Nursing

Pad counts and clot size can be helpful to determine and monitor amount of bleeding

Discharge Criteria

- Hemodynamic stability
- Control of vaginal bleeding

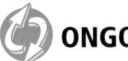 **ONGOING CARE**

FOLLOW-UP RECOMMENDATIONS

Routine follow-up with a primary care or ob/gyn provider

Patient Monitoring

Women treated with estrogen or OCPs should keep a menstrual diary to document bleeding patterns & their relation to therapy.

DIET

No restrictions

PATIENT EDUCATION

- Explain possible/likely etiologies
- Answer all questions, especially those related to cancer and fertility
- http://www.acog.org

PROGNOSIS

- Varies with pathophysiologic process
- Most anovulatory cycles can be treated with medical therapy and do not require surgical intervention.

COMPLICATIONS

- Iron-deficiency anemia
- Uterine cancer in cases of prolonged unopposed estrogen stimulation

REFERENCES

1. Albers J, et al. Abnormal uterine bleeding. *Am Fam Physician*. 2004;69:8.
2. Kouides PA, et al. Hemostasis and menstruation: Appropriate investigation for underlying disorders of hemostasis in women with extensive menstrual bleeding. *Fertil Steril*. 2005;84(5):1345–51.
3. Dijkhuizen FP, et al. The accuracy of transvaginal ultrasonography in the diagnosis of endometrial abnormalities. *Obstet Gynecol*. 1996;87(3):345–9.
4. Maness DL, Reddy A, Harraway-Smith CL, Mitchell G, Givens V et al. How best to manage dysfunctional uterine bleeding. *J Fam Pract*. 2010;59:449–58.
5. Casablanca Y. Management of dysfunctional uterine bleeding. *Obstet Gynecol Clin North Am*. 2008;35:219–34.
6. DeVore GR, et al. Use of intravenous Premarin in the treatment of dysfunctional uterine bleeding: A double-blind randomized control study. *Obstet Gynecol*. 1982;59(3):285–91.
7. Rimsza ME. Dysfunctional uterine bleeding. *Pediatr Rev*. 2002;23(7):227–33.
8. Lethaby A, et al. Cyclical progestogens for heavy menstrual bleeding. *Cochrane Database Syst Rev*. 2004.
9. Lethaby A, et al. Progesterone or progesterone-releasing intrauterine systems for heavy menstrual bleeding. *Cochrane Database Syst Rev*. 2005.
10. Lethaby A, et al. Nonsteroidal anti-inflammatory drugs for heavy menstrual bleeding. *Cochrane Database Syst Rev*. 2004.
11. Lethaby A, et al. Antifibrinolytics for heavy menstrual bleeding. *Cochrane Database Syst Rev*. 2004.
12. Lethaby A, et al. Endometrial resection and ablation versus hysterectomy for heavy menstrual bleeding. *Cochrane Database Syst Rev*. 2004.

ADDITIONAL READING

- Chen EC, Danis PG, Tweed E et al. Clinical inquiries. Menstrual disturbances in perimenopausal women: what's best? *J Fam Pract*. 2009;58:E3.
- LaCour DE, Long DN, Perlman SE et al. Dysfunctional uterine bleeding in adolescent females associated with endocrine causes and medical conditions. *J Pediatr Adolesc Gynecol*. 2010;23:62–70.

See Also (Topic, Algorithm, Electronic Media Element)

Menorrhagia; Dysmenorrhea
Algorithm: Menorrhagia

 CODES

ICD9

626.8 Other disorders of menstruation and other abnormal bleeding from female genital tract

CLINICAL PEARLS

- Uterine bleeding in premenarchal & postmenopausal women is always abnormal and should prompt immediate evaluation.
- Dysfunctional uterine bleeding is irregular bleeding occurring in the absence of pathology, making it a diagnosis of exclusion.
- Anovulation accounts for 90% of DUB.
- An endometrial biopsy should be performed in all women >35 years of age with DUB to rule out cancer or premalignancy, and considered in women aged 18–35 with DUB and risk factors for endometrial cancer.

DYSHIDROSIS

Katherine A. Mansalis, MD
Rebecca A. Frye, DO

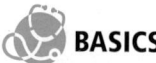 BASICS

DESCRIPTION
- A skin rash (dermatitis) of which there are several different classes within the family "dyshidrosis" and strict definitions are disputed.
- Dyshidrotic eczema:
  – Common, chronic, or recurrent, nonerythematous, vesicular eruption primarily of the palms, soles, and interdigital areas
  – Associated with burning, itching, and pain
- Pompholyx (from Greek, "bubble"):
  – Rare condition characterized by abrupt onset of large bullae, primarily on hands
  – Sometimes used interchangeably with dyshidrosis, although many believe them to be discrete entities
- Lamellar dyshidrosis:
  – Fine, spreading exfoliation of the superficial epidermis in the same distribution as described above
- System(s) affected: Dermatologic; Exocrine; Immunologic
- Synonym(s): Pompholyx; Cheiropompholyx; Keratolysis exfoliativa; Dyshidrotic eczema; Vesicular palmoplantar eczema; Desquamation of interdigital spaces; Palmar pompholyx reaction

EPIDEMIOLOGY
Incidence
- Incidence is 0.5%.
- Mean age of onset is <40 years.
- Male = Female
- Comprises 5–20% of hand eczema cases

Prevalence
20 cases per 100,000

RISK FACTORS
- Many risk factors are disputed in the literature, with none being consistently associated
- Atopy
- Other dermatologic conditions:
  – Atopic dermatitis (early in life)
  – Contact dermatitis (later in life)
  – Dermatophytosis
- Sensitivity to
  – Foods
  – Drugs: neomycin, quinolones, acetaminophen, and oral contraceptives
  – Nickel (seen in patients treated with disulfiram, which causes a high serum level of nickel)
  – Smoking in males

Genetics
- Atopy: 50% of patients with dyshidrotic eczema have atopic dermatitis.
- Rare autosomal dominant form of pompholyx found in Chinese population maps to chromosome 18q22.1–18q22.3

GENERAL PREVENTION
- Control emotional stress.
- Avoid excessive sweating.
- Avoid exposure to irritants.
- Avoid diet high in metal salts (chromium, cobalt, nickel).

PATHOPHYSIOLOGY
- Exact mechanism unknown; thought to be multifactorial
- On dermatopathology, vesicles are found in spongiotic dermatitis
- Thick stratum corneum of palmar and plantar skin keeps the vesicles intact

ETIOLOGY
- Exact cause not known
- Aggravating factors (debated):
  – Hyperhidrosis (in 40% of patients with the condition)
  – Climate: Hot or cold weather; humidity
  – Nickel sensitivity
  – Irritating compounds and solutions
  – Stress
  – Dermatophyte infection
  – Prolonged wear of occlusive gloves
  – Intravenous immunoglobulin therapy
  – Smoking

COMMONLY ASSOCIATED CONDITIONS
- Atopic dermatitis
- Allergic contact dermatitis
- Parkinson disease

℞ DIAGNOSIS

HISTORY
- Episodes of pruritic rash alternating with periods that are symptom free
- Recent emotional stress
- Familial or personal history of atopy
- Exposure to allergens or irritants (1):
  – Occupational, dietary, or household
  – Cosmetic and personal hygiene products
- Costume jewelry use
- IV immunoglobulin therapy
- HIV
- Smoking

PHYSICAL EXAM
- Symmetric distribution on the palms and soles; also may affect the dorsal aspects of hands and feet
- Early findings:
  – 1–2 mm, clear nonerythematous deep-seated vesicles
- Late findings:
  – Unroofed vesicles with inflamed bases
  – Desquamation
  – Peeling, rings of scale, or lichenification common

DIAGNOSTIC TESTS & INTERPRETATION
Lab
Initial lab tests
Skin culture in suspected secondary infection (most commonly *staph aureus*) (2)

Follow-Up & Special Considerations
Consider antibiotics based on culture results and severity of symptoms.

Diagnostic Procedures/Surgery
- Diagnosis is based on clinical exam
- Patch test (to elicit allergic cause)
- KOH wet mount (if concerned about dermatophyte infection)

Pathological Findings
- Fine 1–2-mm spongiotic vesicles intraepidermally with little to no inflammatory changes
- No eccrine glandular involvement

DIFFERENTIAL DIAGNOSIS
- Vesicular tinea pedis/manus
- Vesicular id reaction
- Contact dermatitis (allergic or irritant)
- Chronic vesicular hand dermatitis
- Drug reaction
- Dermatophytid
- Bullous disorders: Dyshidrosiform bullous pemphigoid, pemphigous, bullous impetigo, epidermolysis bullosa
- Pustular psoriasis
- Acrodermatitis continua
- Erythema multiforme
- Herpes infection
- Pityriasis rubra pilaris
- Vesicular mycosis fungoides

TREATMENT

Identification and avoidance of aggravating factors.

MEDICATION

First Line

- Mild cases: Topical steroids (high potency) (2)[B]
- Moderate to severe cases:
  - Ultrahigh-potency topical steroids with occlusion over treated area (3)[B]
  - Psoralens plus UV therapy (PUVA), either oral *or* immersion in psoralens (4)[B]:
    - Oral 8-methoxypsoralen (8-MOP) dose: 0.6 mg/kg taken 1 h prior to UVA irradiation
    - Immersion in 8-MOP: Solution of 5 mg/L of water × 15 minutes immediately preceding UVA irradiation
- Recurrent cases (3)[C]:
  - Systemic steroids at onset of itching prodrome
  - Single morning dose of 60 mg × 3–4 days every 2–4 months

Second Line

- Topical calcineurin inhibitors (mitigate the long term risks of topical steroid use):
  - Topical tacrolimus (5)[A]
  - Topical pimecrolimus (5)[A]
- Oral cyclosporine (2)[A]
- Injections of botulinum toxin type A (BTXA) (5)[A]
  - Newer topical forms of BTXA currently being developed and show promise
- Systemic alitretinoin (5)[A]
- Topical bexarotene (a retinoid X receptor agonist approved for use in cutaneous T-cell lymphoma) (5)[B]
- Methotrexate (5)[C]

ADDITIONAL TREATMENT

- Radiation therapy (6)[C]
- UV-free phototherapy (5)[C]

General Measures

- Avoid possible causative factors: Stress, chemical irritants, nickel, occlusive gloves, smoking, sweating
- Moisturizers/emollients for symptomatic relief
- Foot care:
  - Wear shoes with leather rather than rubber soles (e.g., sneakers).
  - Wear socks made of cotton instead of synthetic materials.
  - Remove shoes and socks whenever possible to allow sweat evaporation and to apply lubricants.

Issues for Referral

- Allergist (if allergen testing required)
- Psychologist (if stress modification needed)

COMPLEMENTARY AND ALTERNATIVE MEDICINE

- Topical treatments to minimize pruritus (not curative) (2)[C]: Burrow solution (aluminum acetate) or vinegar compress
- Exposure to sunlight as maintenance therapy (7)[C]
- Dandelion juice (avoid in atopic patients) (5)[C]

ONGOING CARE

FOLLOW-UP RECOMMENDATIONS

Patient Monitoring

- Dyshidrotic Eczema Area and Severity Index (DASI)
- Parameters used in the DASI score:
  - Number of vesicles per square centimeter
  - Erythema
  - Desquamation
  - Severity of itching
  - Surface area affected
- Grading: Mild (0–15), moderate (16–30), severe (31–60)
- Monitor BP and glucose in patients receiving systemic corticosteroids.
- Monitor for adverse effects of medications.

DIET

- Consider diet low in metal salts if there is history of nickel sensitivity (2)[A].
- Updated recommendations for low-cobalt diet are available (8).

PATIENT EDUCATION

- Instructions on self-care, complications, and avoidance of triggers/aggravating factors
- Suggested web site for patients: www.nlm.nih.gov

PROGNOSIS

- Condition is benign.
- Usually heals without scarring
- Lesions often resolve spontaneously but resolve more quickly with appropriate treatment (9).
- Recurrence is common.

COMPLICATIONS

- Secondary bacterial infections (*staphylococcus aureus* most common)
- Dystrophic nail changes
- Fissures
- Skin tightening/discomfort
- Psychological distress

REFERENCES

1. Guillet MH, Wierzbicka E, Guillet S, et al. A 3-year causative study of pompholyx in 120 patients. *Arch Dermatol*. 2007;143:1504–8.
2. Lofgren SM. Dyshidrosis: Epidemiology, clinical characteristics, and therapy. *Dermatitis*. 2006;17:165–81.
3. Chen J, et al. The gene for a rare autosomal dominant form of pompholyx maps to chromosome 18q22.1–18q22.3. *J Invest Dermatol*. 2006;126: 300–4.
4. Tzaneva S, Kittler H, Thallinger C, et al. Oral vs. bath PUVA using 8-methoxypsoralen for chronic palmoplantar eczema. *Photodermatol Photoimmunol Photomed*. 2009;25:101–5.
5. Wollina U. Pompholyx: what's new? *Expert Opinion in Investigational Drugs*. 2008;17:897–904.
6. Sumila M, Notter M, Itin P, et al. Long-term Results of Radiotherapy in Patients with Chronic Palmo-plantar Eczema or Psoriasis. *Strahlentherapie und Onkologie*. 2008;184:218–223.
7. Leti M. Exposure to sunlight as adjuvant therapy for dyshidrotic eczema. *Med Hypotheses*. 2009.
8. Stuckert J, Nedorost S. Low-cobalt diet for dyshidrotic eczema patients. *Contact Dermatitis*. 2008;59:361–5.
9. Rashid RD, Salah W, Keuer EJ. Vexing Vesicles. *Journal of Medicine*. 2007;120:589–590.

ADDITIONAL READING

- Thiers BH. What's new in dermatologic therapy. *Dermatol Ther*. 2008 Mar–Apr;21:142–9.
- Veien NK. Acute and Recurrent Vesicular Hand Dermatitis. *Dermatologic Clinics*. 2009;27:337–353.

See Also (Topic, Algorithm, Electronic Media Element)

Algorithm: Rash, Focal

CODES

ICD9
705.81 Dyshidrosis

CLINICAL PEARLS

- Dyshidrosis is a transient, recurrent vesicular eruption most commonly of the palms, soles, and interdigital areas.
- The etiology and pathophysiology are unknown but are most likely related to a combination of genetic and environmental factors.
- The best prevention is limiting exposure to irritating agents.
- Treatments are based on severity of disease and include topical steroids, UV therapy, botulinum toxin A, and various immunosuppressants.
- The condition is benign and usually heals spontaneously and without scarring. Medical treatment decreases healing time and risk for progression to secondary bacterial infection.

DYSMENORRHEA

Janice E. Daugherty, MD

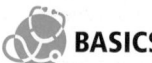

BASICS

DESCRIPTION
- Pelvic pain occurring at or around the time of menses; a leading cause of absenteeism for women <30 years
- Primary dysmenorrhea: Without pathologic physical findings
- Secondary dysmenorrhea: Often more severe than primary, having a secondary pathologic (structural) cause
- Classified by severity:
  - Mild: Pelvic discomfort, cramping, or heaviness on 1st day of bleeding with no associated symptoms
  - Moderate: Discomfort occurring on 1st 2–3 days of menses and accompanied by mild malaise, diarrhea, and headache
  - Severe: Intense, cramp-like pain lasting 2–7 days, often with nausea, diarrhea, back pain, thigh pain, and headache
- System(s) affected: Reproductive
- Synonym(s): Menstrual cramps

EPIDEMIOLOGY
- Predominant age:
  - Primary: Teens to early 20s
  - Secondary: 20s–30s
- Predominant sex: Female only

Prevalence
- >50% of adult females have menstrual pain.
- 10% are incapacitated for 1–3 days each cycle.

RISK FACTORS
- Primary:
  - Nulliparity
  - Obesity
  - Cigarette smoking
  - Positive family history
- Secondary:
  - Pelvic infection
  - Sexual transmitted diseases (STDs)
  - Endometriosis

Genetics
Not well studied

GENERAL PREVENTION
- Primary: Choose a diet low in animal fats, dairy products, and eggs. Increase vegetables, raw seeds, and nuts to increase production of beneficial prostaglandins. Consider supplementation with zinc 30 mg, taken 1–3 times daily for 1–4 days prior to the expected onset of menses [C].
- Secondary: Reduce risk of STDs

PATHOPHYSIOLOGY
See Etiology.

ETIOLOGY
- Primary: Elevated production (2–7 times normal) of prostaglandins and other mediators in the uterus that produce uterine ischemia through:
  - Platelet aggregation
  - Vasoconstriction
  - Uterine contractions generating pressures higher than the systemic blood pressure (BP)
- Secondary:
  - Congenital abnormalities of uterine or vaginal anatomy
  - Cervical stenosis
  - Pelvic infection
  - Adenomyosis

- Endometriosis
- Pelvic tumors, especially leiomyomata (fibroids)
- Uterine polyps
- Copper-containing intrauterine device (IUD)

Pediatric Considerations
Onset with first menses raises probability of genital tract anatomic abnormality, such as transverse vaginal septum, minimally perforate hymen, and uterine anomalies.

COMMONLY ASSOCIATED CONDITIONS
- Obesity
- Hyperestrogenic states
- Longer menstrual cycle length

DIAGNOSIS

- Primary: History is characteristic.
- Based on characteristic history of cramping pain felt in suprapubic or low back
- Patients may have associated diarrhea, headache, or pain radiating into inner thighs.

HISTORY
- Onset of symptoms
- Recurrence at or just before the onset of the menstrual flow:
  - Pelvic pain occurring between menstrual periods is not likely to be dysmenorrhea.
- Relief associated with:
  - Continued bleeding for the usual duration
  - Use of analgesics, especially nonsteroidal anti-inflammatory drugs (NSAIDs)
  - Orgasm
  - Local heat application
- Response to dietary supplements or NSAIDs helps confirm diagnosis.

PHYSICAL EXAM
- Primary: Physical exam is typically normal.
- Secondary: Exam may show evidence of uterine enlargement, tenderness, irregularity, or fixation.

DIAGNOSTIC TESTS & INTERPRETATION
Lab
- Pregnancy test to rule out ectopic pregnancy
- Cervical cultures to rule out infection
- Drugs that may alter lab results:
  - Antibiotics

Follow-Up & Special Considerations
Counsel regarding appropriate preventive measures for sexually transmitted infection and pregnancy.

Imaging
Initial approach
- Primary: Consider pelvic ultrasound to rule out secondary abnormalities if history is not characteristic.
- Secondary: Ultrasound or laparoscopy to define anatomy

Diagnostic Procedures/Surgery
Laparoscopy is rarely needed.

Pathological Findings
- Primary:
  - None
- Secondary:
  - Uterine enlargement
  - Leiomyomata
  - Ligamentous thickening
  - Fixation of pelvic structures

- Endometritis
- Salpingitis
- Adenomyosis

DIFFERENTIAL DIAGNOSIS
- Primary:
  - History is characteristic
- Secondary:
  - Pelvic or genital infection
  - Complication of pregnancy
  - Missed or incomplete abortion
  - Ectopic pregnancy
  - Uterine or ovarian neoplasm
  - Endometriosis
  - Urinary tract infection (UTI)
  - Complication of intrauterine device

Pregnancy Considerations
Consider ectopic pregnancy in differential diagnosis of pelvic pain with vaginal bleeding.

TREATMENT

- Reassure patient that treatment success is very likely with adherence to recommendations.
- Relief may require the use of several treatment modalities at the same time.

MEDICATION
First Line
- NSAIDs (1): All NSAIDs studied have been found equally effective in the relief of dysmenorrhea. As NSAIDs work by inhibiting prostaglandin synthesis, taking them at the very onset of menses (or whenever the cramping starts) provides the most relief.
  - Ibuprofen 400–600 mg q6h
  - Naproxen sodium 550 mg q12h
- Combination oral contraceptives in monthly and especially in 3–5-month cycles may improve or eliminate dysmenorrhea, although they may be associated with increased breakthrough menstrual spotting (2)[B]:
  - Combination oral contraceptives containing 20 mcg or less of ethinyl estradiol have not been found effective in reducing menstrual pain.
- Potential contraindications to NSAIDs and combination oral contraceptive (OC) methods:
  - Platelet disorders
  - Gastric ulceration or gastritis
  - Thromboembolic disorders
  - Vascular disease
  - Other contraindications to oral contraceptives
- Precautions:
  - Gastrointestinal irritation
  - Lactation
  - Coagulation disorders
  - Impaired renal function
  - Congestive heart failure (CHF)
  - Liver dysfunction
- Significant possible interactions:
  - Coumadin-type anticoagulants
  - Aspirin with other NSAIDs
  - Methotrexate
  - Furosemide
  - Lithium

Second Line

- Mefenamic acid 500 mg at once, then 250 mg q6h may be tried if other NSAIDs are ineffective, as it blocks production of prostaglandins as well as already-formed prostaglandins (1)[A].
- Progestin-containing IUD (Mirena) in suitable candidates

ADDITIONAL TREATMENT
General Measures

- General physical conditioning, exercise to raise endorphins
- Transcutaneous electrical nerve stimulation (3)[B]
- Secondary dysmenorrhea: Treatment of infections; suppression of endometrium if endometriosis is suspected

COMPLEMENTARY AND ALTERNATIVE MEDICINE

- Because of low methodologic quality and small sample size in 30 different randomized controlled trials (RCTs), there is no convincing evidence for acupuncture in the treatment of primary dysmenorrhea (4)[A].
- However, in individual studies, acupuncture has been shown to be effective for both treatment and prevention. The lack of significant adverse effects of acupuncture, compared with common effects of NSAIDs including GI bleeding, blood pressure elevation, and potential renal impairment make acupuncture a choice to be considered early in the treatment plan (5,6,7).
  - Acupressure at Sanyinjiao (SP6) is quickly effective and can be taught to women for self-treatment.
  - Acupuncture at SP6, with or without 60 HZ, 2–3 mV electrical stimulation, was significantly more effective than ibuprofen.
  - Acupuncture at Hegu (LI4) and Taichong (LR3) was effective in decreasing menstrual pain.
  - Ear acupressure at appropriate points with vaccaria seeds was significantly more effective than indomethacin.
  - For endometriosis, acupuncture was more effective than oral danazol to decrease pain, irregular menstruation, back pain, and perineal swelling.
- Aromatherapy with lavender, clary sage, rose oils, and abdominal massage decreases intensity of pain (8)[B].
- Osteopathic manipulation, including pressure over the sacrum, can decrease the intensity of menstrual pain (9)[B].

SURGERY/OTHER PROCEDURES

- Adenomyosis may require hysterectomy.
- Uterine artery embolization may be an alternative to hysterectomy for patients with leiomyomata (fibroid tumors) (10).

IN-PATIENT CONSIDERATIONS

Both primary and secondary dysmenorrhea are usually managed in the outpatient setting.

Initial Stabilization

- Primary: Outpatient care
- Secondary: Usually outpatient care

 ONGOING CARE

FOLLOW-UP RECOMMENDATIONS
Normal

DIET

- Several dietary supplements have been found to be effective at treating dysmenorrhea:
  - Vitamin B1 100 mg daily
  - Fish oil 3,000–5,000 mg + vitamin E 1.5 mg daily (vitamin E is preservative)
  - Diosmin 450 mg + hesperidin 50 mg t.i.d. with onset of menses
  - Magnesium 400 mg daily (11)
- Several dietary supplements are possibly effective, although have not studied in large trials:
  - Vitamin E 200 mg b.i.d. beginning 2 days before expected menses and continuing for the 1st 3 days of bleeding (12)[B]
  - Vitamin B1 (thiamine) 100 mg/d p.o. for at least 90 days (13)[C]
  - Fish oil capsule 1,000 mg daily for 2 months (14)[B]
  - Zinc 30 mg 1–3 times daily for 1–4 days preceding expected menses has been found effective for prevention (15)[C].
- Low-fat vegetarian diet significantly decreases pain.

PATIENT EDUCATION

Reassure patient that primary dysmenorrhea is treatable with use of dietary supplements and/or NSAIDs prior to menses and/or oral contraceptives, and that it will usually abate with age and parity.

PROGNOSIS

- Primary: Improves with age and parity
- Secondary: Likely to require therapy based on underlying cause

COMPLICATIONS

- Primary: Anxiety and/or depression
- Secondary: Infertility from underlying pathology

REFERENCES

1. Marjoribanks J, Proctor ML, Farquhar Cl. Nonsteroidal anti-inflammatory drugs for primary dysmenorrhoea (Cochrane Review). *The Cochrane Library*. 2003;4.
2. Proctor ML, Roberts H, Farquhar CM. Combined oral contraceptive pill (OCP) as treatment for primary dysmenorrhoea (Cochrane Review). In: *The Cochrane Library*. 2003;4.
3. Milsom I, Hedner N, Mannheimer C. A comparative study of the effect of high-intensity transcutaneous nerve stimulation and oral naproxen on intrauterine pressure and menstrual pain in patients with primary dysmenorrhea. *Am J Obstet Gynecol*. 1994;170:123–9.
4. Yang H, Liu CZ, Chen X, et al. Systematic review of clinical trials of acupuncture-related therapies for primary dysmenorrhea. *Acta Obstet Gynecol Scand*. 2008:1–9.
5. Proctor ML, Smith CA, Farquhar CM, et al. Transcutaneous electrical nerve stimulation and acupuncture for primary dysmenorrhoea (Cochrane Review). 2003;4.
6. Zhao L, Li P. A survey of acupuncture treatment for primary dysmenorrhea. *J Tradit Chin Med*. 2009;29:71–6.

7. Ziaei S, Zakeri M, Kazemnejad A, et al. A randomised controlled trial of vitamin E in the treatment of primary dysmenorrhoea. *BJOG*. 2005;112:466–9.
8. Han SH, Hur MH, Buckle J, Choi J, Lee MS, et al. Effect of aromatherapy on symptoms of dysmenorrhea in college students: A randomized placebo-controlled clinical trial. *J Altern Complement Med*. 2006;12:535–41.
9. Chadwick K and Morgan A. The efficacy of osteopathic treatment for primary dysmenorrhea in young women. *The AAO Journal: A Publication of the American Academy of Osteopathy*. 1996 Fall;6(3):15–17, 29–31.
10. Bradley LD et al. Uterine fibroid embolization: a viable alternative to hysterectomy. *Am J Obstet Gynecol*. 2009;201:127–35.
11. Guerrera MP, Volpe SL, Mao JJ et al. Therapeutic uses of magnesium. *Am Fam Physician*. 2009;80:157–62.
12. Transdermal nitroglycerine in the management of pain associated with primary dysmenorrhoea: a multinational pilot study. The Transdermal Nitroglycerine/Dysmenorrhoea Study Group. *J Int Med Res*. 1997;25:41–4.
13. French L. Dysmenorrhea. *Am Fam Physician*. 2005;71:285–91.
14. Harel Z, Biro FM, Kottenhahn RK et al. Supplementation with omega-3 polyunsaturated fatty acids in the management of dysmenorrhea in adolescents. *Am J Ob Gyn*. 1996;174:1335–8.
15. Eby G. Zinc treatment prevents dysmenorrhea. *Med Hypoth*. 2007;69.2:297–301.

ADDITIONAL READING

- Cho SH, Hwang EW et al. Acupuncture for primary dysmenorrhoea: a systematic review. *BJOG*. 2010;117:509–21.
- Giudice LC et al. Clinical practice. Endometriosis. *N Engl J Med*. 2010;362:2389–98.
- Sanfilippo J, Erb T. Evaluation and management of dysmenorrhea in adolescents. *Clin Obstet Gynecol*. 2008;51:257–67.
- Stones RW, Mountfield J. Interventions for treating chronic pelvic pain in women (Cochrane Review). *The Cochrane Library*. 2003;4.
- White AR. A review of controlled trials of acupuncture for women's reproductive health care. *J Fam Plan Reprod Health Care*. 2003;29:233–6.

See Also (Topic, Algorithm, Electronic Media Element)
Endometriosis
Algorithm: Pelvic Girdle Pain

 CODES

ICD9
625.3 Dysmenorrhea

CLINICAL PEARLS

- Dysmenorrhea is a leading cause of absenteeism for women <30 years old.
- Lifestyle and dietary supplement therapies are preferable for long-term treatment, as they have equal or greater efficacy and pose fewer health risks than NSAIDs or hormonal contraceptives.
- All NSAIDs studied have been found equally effective in the relief of dysmenorrhea.

DYSPAREUNIA

Scott T. Henderson, MD

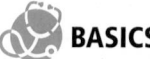 **BASICS**

DESCRIPTION
- Recurrent and persistent genital pain associated with sexual activity that is not exclusively due to lack of lubrication or vaginismus
- May be the result of organic, emotional, or psychogenic causes:
  - Primary: Present throughout one's sexual history
  - Secondary: Arising from some specific event or condition (e.g., menopause, drugs)
  - Superficial: Pain at or near the introitus or vaginal barrel associated with penetration
  - Deep: Pain after penetration located at the cervix or lower abdominal area
  - Complete: Present under all circumstances
  - Situational: Occurring selectively with specific situations
- System(s) affected: Reproductive

EPIDEMIOLOGY
- Predominant age: All ages
- Predominant sex: Female > Male.

Incidence
More than 50% of all sexually active women will report dyspareunia at some time.

Geriatric Considerations
Incidence increases dramatically in postmenopausal women primarily because of vaginal atrophy.

Prevalence
- Most sexually active women will experience dyspareunia at some time in their lives.
  - ~15% (4–40%) of adult women will have dyspareunia on a few occasions during a year.
  - ~1–2% of women will have painful intercourse on a more-than-occasional basis.
- Male prevalence is ~1%.

RISK FACTORS
- Fatigue
- Stress
- Diabetes
- Estrogen deficiency:
  - Menopause
  - Lactation
- Vaginal surgery
- Alcohol/marijuana consumption
- Medication side effects (antihistamines, tamoxifen, bromocriptine, low-estrogen oral contraceptives, depo-medroxyprogesterone, desipramine)

Pregnancy Considerations
Pregnancy is a potent influence on sexuality; dyspareunia is common.

PATHOPHYSIOLOGY
See Etiology section.

ETIOLOGY
- Disorders of vaginal outlet:
  - Adhesions
  - Clitoral irritation
  - Decreased lubrication
  - Episiotomy scars
  - Fissures
  - Hymenal ring abnormalities
  - Infections
  - Lichen planus
  - Lichen sclerosus
  - Postmenopausal atrophy
  - Trauma
  - Vulvar papillomatosis
  - Vulvar vestibulitis/vulvodynia
- Disorders of vagina:
  - Abnormality of vault owing to surgery or radiation
  - Congenital malformations
  - Decreased lubrication
  - Infections
  - Inflammatory or allergic response to foreign substance
  - Masses or tumors
  - Pelvic relaxation resulting in rectocele, uterine prolapse, or cystocele
- Disorders of pelvic structures:
  - Endometriosis
  - Levator ani myalgia
  - Malignant or benign tumors of the uterus
  - Ovarian pathology
  - Pelvic adhesions
  - Pelvic inflammatory disease
  - Pelvic venous congestion
  - Prior pelvic fracture
- Disorders of the GI tract:
  - Constipation
  - Crohn disease
  - Diverticular disease
  - Fistulas
  - Hemorrhoids
  - Inflammatory bowel disease
- Disorders of the urinary tract:
  - Interstitial cystitis
  - Ureteral or vesical lesions
- Male:
  - Cancer of penis
  - Genital muscle spasm
  - Infection or irritation of penile skin
  - Infection of seminal vesicles
  - Lichen sclerosus
  - Musculoskeletal disorders of pelvis and lower back
  - Penile anatomy disorders
  - Phimosis
  - Prostate infections and enlargement
  - Testicular disease
  - Torsion of spermatic cord
  - Urethritis

- Psychological disorders:
  - Anxiety
  - Conversion reactions
  - Depression
  - Fear
  - Hostility toward partner
  - Phobic reactions
  - Psychological trauma

COMMONLY ASSOCIATED CONDITIONS
Vaginismus

Pregnancy Considerations
- Episiotomies do not have a protective effect (1)[A].
- Mediolateral episiotomy increases the risk of dyspareunia compared with no episiotomy (2)[B].

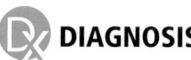 **DIAGNOSIS**

HISTORY
- Include menstrual, obstetric, reproductive, and sexual histories.
- Identify pain characteristics.
  - Onset and duration
  - Location
  - Intensity/quality: Varying degrees of pelvic/genital pressure, aching, tearing, and/or burning
  - Pattern (precipitating or aggravating factors): When pain occurs (at entry, during or after intercourse)
  - Relief measures (avoid intercourse, change positions, have intercourse only at certain times of the month)
- Question for history of domestic violence or history of rape.

PHYSICAL EXAM
- A complete exam, including a focused pelvic exam, to identify pathology and provide patient education
- Since exam often reproduces the pain, it must include inspection and palpation of vaginal area and urethral structures as well as palpation of the uterus.

DIAGNOSTIC TESTS & INTERPRETATION
Lab
Initial lab tests
Based on history and exam findings:
- Wet mount
- Gonorrhea culture
- Chlamydia culture
- Herpes culture
- Urine analysis
- Urine culture
- Pap smear

Imaging
Initial approach
Limited and based on history and exam findings
Follow-Up & Special Considerations
- Voiding cystourethrogram if urinary tract involvement
- GI contrast studies if GI symptoms
- Ultrasound and CT scan are of limited value; perform if clinically indicated.

Diagnostic Procedures/Surgery
Based on history and exam findings:
- Colposcopy and biopsy if vaginal/vulvar lesions
- Laparoscopy if complex deep-penetration pain
- Cystoscopy if urinary tract involvement
- Endoscopy if GI involvement

Pathological Findings
Depend on etiology

DIFFERENTIAL DIAGNOSIS
Vaginismus

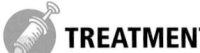 **TREATMENT**

- Primary dyspareunia might be related to vaginismus, low libido, and/or arousal disorders.
- Endocrine factors, such as primary amenorrhea, might reduce the biologic basis of sexual response.
- If pain prevents penetration, severe vaginismus may be present.

MEDICATION
First Line
Depends on the etiology:
- Antibiotics, antifungals, or antivirals as indicated for infection
- Estrogen for vaginal and vulvar atrophy
- Analgesics and topical anesthetics for pain
- Lubricants for dryness
- Vulvar vestibulitis/vulvodynia may respond to tricyclic antidepressants or gabapentin.

ADDITIONAL TREATMENT
General Measures
- Educate the patient and partner as to the nature of the problem. Reassure them that the problem can be solved.
- If an organic cause is identified during the initial evaluation, initiate specific treatment.
- Once organic causes are ruled out, treatment is a multidimensional and multidisciplinary approach (2)[C].
  – Individual behavioral therapy: Indicated to help the patient deal with intrapersonal issues and assess the role of the partner
  – Couple behavioral therapy:
    ○ Indicated to help resolve interpersonal problems
    ○ May involve short-term structured intervention or sexual counseling
    ○ Designed to systemically desensitize uncomfortable sexual responses and intercourse through a series of interventions over a period of weeks
    ○ Interventions range from muscle relaxation and mutual body massage to sexual fantasies and erotic massage.

Issues for Referral
Referral for long-term therapy may be necessary.

Additional Therapies
No benefit of therapeutic ultrasound (3)[A]

COMPLEMENTARY AND ALTERNATIVE MEDICINE
- Sitz baths may relieve painful inflammation.
- Perineal massage

SURGERY/OTHER PROCEDURES
- Laparoscopic excision of endometriotic lesions has shown benefit (4)[B].
- Surgical vestibulectomy can be considered if conservative measures fail with vulvar vestibulitis.

 ONGOING CARE

FOLLOW-UP RECOMMENDATIONS
Patient Monitoring
- Outpatient follow-up depends on therapy.
- Every 6–12 months once resolved

DIET
A high-fiber diet may help if constipation is a contributing cause.

PATIENT EDUCATION
- Boston Women's Health Book Collective. *Our Bodies, Ourselves: A New Edition for a New Era.* New York: Simon & Schuster, 2005
- Kegel exercise information
- Provide couples with information about sexual arousal techniques.

PROGNOSIS
Most patients will respond to treatment.

REFERENCES
1. Carroli G, Mignini L. Episiotomy for vaginal birth. *Cochrane Database Syst Rev.* 2009;CD000081.
2. Crowley T, Richardson D, Goldmeier D, et al. Recommendations for the management of vaginismus: BASHH Special Interest Group for Sexual Dysfunction. *Int J STD AIDS.* 2006;17:14–8.
3. Sartore A, De Seta F, Maso G, et al. The effects of mediolateral episiotomy on pelvic floor function after vaginal delivery. *Obstet Gynecol.* 2004;103: 669–73.
4. Ferrero S, Abbamonte LH, Giordano M, et al. Deep dyspareunia and sex life after laparoscopic excision of endometriosis. *Hum Reprod.* 2006.

ADDITIONAL READING
- Boardman LA, Stockdale CK et al. Sexual pain. *Clin Obstet Gynecol.* 2009;52:682–90.
- Frank JE, Mistretta P, Will J. Diagnosis and treatment of female sexual dysfunction. *Am Fam Physician.* 2008;77:635–42.
- Steege JF, Zolnoun DA. Evaluation and treatment of dyspareunia. *Obstet Gynecol.* 2009;113:1124–36.

See Also (Topic, Algorithm, Electronic Media Element)
Balanitis; Endometriosis; Pelvic Inflammatory Disease (PID); Sexual Dysfunction in Women; Vaginismus; Vulvovaginitis, Prepubescent; Vulvovaginitis, Estrogen Deficient
Algorithms: Dyspareunia; Discharge, Vaginal

 CODES

ICD9
- 302.76 Dyspareunia, psychogenic
- 625.0 Dyspareunia

CLINICAL PEARLS
- Determine whether patient feels pain before, during, or after intercourse to help identify cause.
  – Pain before intercourse suggests a phobic attitude toward penetration and/or the presence of vestibulitis.
  – Pain during intercourse combined with the location of the pain is most predictive of the causes of pain.
  – Introital pain after intercourse suggests vestibulitis in women of childbearing age, hypertonic pelvic floor, or vulvovaginal dystrophia.
- Primary dyspareunia might be related to vaginismus, low libido, and/or arousal disorders.
- Episiotomy does not offer any benefit in the prevention of dyspareunia; a mediolateral episiotomy in fact may cause more future discomfort.

DYSPEPSIA, FUNCTIONAL

Anthony M. Zizza, III, MD
Randall S. Pellish, MD

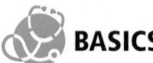 BASICS

DESCRIPTION

- A condition characterized by the presence of chronic intermittent symptoms for at least 3 months of epigastric pain, postprandial fullness, early satiety, or epigastric burning without mucosal lesions or other structural abnormalities of the gastrointestinal (GI) tract (1)[A]
- Analogous to irritable bowel syndrome (IBS) of the upper GI tract
- System(s) affected: GI
- Synonym(s): Nonulcer dyspepsia; Moynihan dyspepsia; Pseudo-ulcer dyspepsia; Phantom ulcer; Nonorganic dyspepsia; Nervous dyspepsia

EPIDEMIOLOGY

Incidence
- Common in US
- Affecting 15–20% of patients referred to gastroenterologists
- Accounts for 60% of patients with dyspepsia

Prevalence
- Predominant age: Adults, but can be seen in children
- Predominant gender: Females > Males

RISK FACTORS
- Other functional disorders
- Anxiety
- Depression

Genetics
Possible link to G-protein β-3 subunit 825 CC genotype and serotonin transport genes

GENERAL PREVENTION
Avoid foods and habits known to exacerbate symptoms (see Diet).

PATHOPHYSIOLOGY
- Not well understood
- Motility disorder
- Possible visceral hypersensitivity to gastric distention
- Psychosocial factors

ETIOLOGY
- Often unknown; may be of several different etiologies
- Evanescent ulcers (20–30% go on to develop ulcers)
- Gastric motility disorder (delayed or accelerated)
- Visceral hypersensitivity
- Impaired gastric accommodation

- Controversial relationship to *Helicobacter pylori*
- Adverse drug effects
- Carbohydrate malabsorption
- Food intolerance
- Psychosocial factors

COMMONLY ASSOCIATED CONDITIONS
Other functional bowel disorders

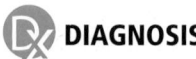 DIAGNOSIS

HISTORY
- Belching
- Aerophagia, gaseousness, abdominal distension
- Borborygmus
- Epigastric pain, gnawing or burning; eating may improve or worsen symptoms
- Substernal pain, gnawing, or burning
- Early satiety
- Anorexia, nausea, or vomiting
- Change in bowel habits
- Abdominal tenderness
- Stress, anxiety, depression
- Exclude (2)[A]:
  – IBS
  – Peptic ulcer disease
  – Malignancy
  – Biliary tract disease
  – Gastroesophageal reflux disease (GERD)
  – Medication-induced dyspepsia

Pediatric Considerations
Look for family system dysfunction.

Pregnancy Considerations
Pregnancy may exacerbate condition.

Geriatric Considerations
Cancer risk is higher.

PHYSICAL EXAM
To rule out other disorders

DIAGNOSTIC TESTS & INTERPRETATION
Lab
Initial lab tests
- Complete blood count
- Chemistry panel
- *H. pylori* serology
- Stool for occult blood

Imaging
Initial approach
- Extensive workup only in patients with *alarm symptoms*:
  – Onset of symptoms >45–55 years (3)[B]
  – Unexplained weight loss
  – Change in stool caliber
  – With symptoms and signs suggesting more serious disease
  – Who need added reassurance
  – Who are younger and do not respond rapidly to empiric treatment
- Usual:
  – Endoscopy (2)[A],(4)
  – Upper GI series
  – Test and treat for *H. pylori* (in areas of high prevalence) (3)[B]
- Sometimes:
  – Barium enema
  – Gallbladder studies for right upper quadrant pain (e.g., ultrasound or gallbladder cholecystokinin function testing)
  – Nuclear medicine gastric emptying study (in selected cases)

Diagnostic Procedures/Surgery
- Esophageal manometry (rarely needed)
- 24-hour intraesophageal pH monitoring (rarely needed unless dysphagia is present)

Pathological Findings
None (by definition)

DIFFERENTIAL DIAGNOSIS
- GERD
- Cholecystitis
- Peptic ulcer disease
- Gastric cancer
- Esophageal spasm
- Malabsorption syndromes
- Pancreatic disease
- IBS
- Aerophagia
- Ischemic heart disease
- Diabetes mellitus
- Thyroid disease
- Connective tissue disorders
- Conversion disorder

TREATMENT

MEDICATION

First Line
- 40% of patients improve with placebo.
- Acid reduction drugs:
  - H₂ antagonists: Ranitidine, others
  - Over-the-counter omeprazole (5)[A]
  - *H. pylori* eradication (often does not relieve symptoms, but may be worth trying)
- Contraindications:
  - Avoid magnesium-containing antacids in patients with significant renal dysfunction.
- Precautions:
  - Monitor H₂ antagonist dosages in patients with renal disease.
  - Calcium-containing antacids may precipitate the formation of kidney stones.
- Significant possible interactions:
  - H₂ blockers interact with drugs metabolized by and affecting the liver.

Second Line
- Gastric motility drugs (2)[A]:
  - Metoclopramide (Reglan); although neurologic side effects are significant
  - Erythromycin
- Amitriptyline: 50 mg q.h.s.
- Selective serotonin reuptake inhibitors
- Itopride (6)[C]:
  - Placebo-controlled trial showed symptom improvement.
  - Mechanism unknown, requires more studies

ADDITIONAL TREATMENT

General Measures
- Appropriate health care: Outpatient
- Supportive measures:
  - Reassurance
  - Do not investigate excessively.
  - Dietary changes (see Diet)
  - Elevate head of bed (where applicable).
  - Maintain ideal body weight.
  - Explore psychological issues.

Additional Therapies
- Stress reduction:
  - Relaxation techniques
  - Physical exercise
  - Reflux precautions where applicable
- Psychological therapy (1)[B]:
  - Cognitive behavioral therapy
  - Hypnotherapy
  - Psychotherapy

COMPLEMENTARY AND ALTERNATIVE MEDICINE
In combination with caraway oil, peppermint oil can be used for reducing symptoms of nonulcer dyspepsia (7).

 ONGOING CARE

FOLLOW-UP RECOMMENDATIONS

Patient Monitoring
- Usual duration of medication is 4 weeks, then 2 weeks intermittently for exacerbations. If chronic medication use is needed, endoscopy evaluation is indicated.
- Continue observation to provide support and reassurance.
- Minimize diagnostic studies unless disabling symptoms persist or new problems arise.

DIET
- Symptoms are frequently triggered or exacerbated by fatty foods (8).
- Eat frequent small meals.
- AVOID:
  - Foods known to exacerbate symptoms
  - Regular and decaffeinated coffee
  - Tea, cocoa, and chocolate
  - Heavy alcohol use
  - Cigarette smoking
  - Aspirin-containing compounds and NSAIDs

PATIENT EDUCATION
Prevention: Continue healthy habits listed under Treatment and Diet (i.e., avoid activities known to exacerbate problems, maintain healthy lifestyle, continue stress-reduction techniques).

PROGNOSIS
Long-term or chronic symptoms with symptom-free periods

COMPLICATIONS
Iatrogenic, from evaluation to rule out serious pathology

REFERENCES

1. Drossman DA. The functional gastrointestinal disorders and the Rome III process. *Gastroenterol*. 2006;130:1377–90.
2. Dickerson LM, et al. Evaluation and management of nonulcer dyspepsia. *Am Fam Phys*. 2004;70: 107–14.
3. Kandulski A, Venerito M, Malfertheiner P, et al. Therapeutic strategies for the treatment of dyspepsia. *Expert Opin Pharmacother*. 2010;11: 2517–25.
4. Delaney B, Ford AC, Forman D, et al. Initial management strategies for dyspepsia. *Cochrane Database Syst Rev*. 2005:CD001961.
5. Moayyedi P, et al. The efficacy of proton pump inhibitors in nonulcer dyspepsia: A systematic review and economic analysis. *Gastroenterol*. 2004;127:1329–37.
6. Holtmann G, Talley NJ, Liebregts T, et al. A placebo-controlled trial of itopride in functional dyspepsia. *N Engl J Med*. 2006;354:832–40.
7. Madisch A, Holtmann G, Mayr G, et al. Treatment of functional dyspepsia with a herbal preparation. A double-blind, randomized, placebo-controlled, multicenter trial. *Digestion*. 2004;69:45–52.
8. Pilichiewicz AN, Feltrin KL, Horowitz M, et al. Functional Dyspepsia Is Associated With a Greater Symptomatic Response to Fat But Not Carbohydrate, Increased Fasting and Postprandial CCK, and Diminished PYY. *Am J Gastroenterol*. 2008.

ADDITIONAL READING

- Choung RS, et al. Novel mechanisms in functional dyspepsia. *W J Gastroenterol*. 2006;12:673–7.
- Faure C, Patey N, Gauthier C, Brooks EM, Mawe GM et al. Serotonin signaling is altered in irritable bowel syndrome with diarrhea but not in functional dyspepsia in pediatric age patients. *Gastroenterology*. 2010;139:249–58.
- Keohane J, et al. Functional dyspepsia and nonerosive reflux disease: Clinical interactions and their implications. *Med Gen Med*. 2007;9:31.

See Also (Topic, Algorithm, Electronic Media Element)
Dyspepsia, Endoscopic-Negative Reflux Disease, Gastritis; Irritable Bowel Syndrome
Algorithms: Dyspepsia; Epigastric Pain; Esophageal Regurgitation

 CODES

ICD9
536.8 Dyspepsia and other specified disorders of function of stomach

CLINICAL PEARLS
- When no organic cause for dyspepsia is found, it is considered functional or idiopathic.
- Extensive diagnostic testing is not recommended unless the patient presents with alarm symptoms (vomiting, early satiety, weight loss, or anemia).
- Consider empiric treatment with acid suppressants or *H. pylori* eradication if serology is positive.

DYSPHAGIA

Archit Sharma, MD
Mark D. Goodman, MD

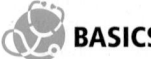 **BASICS**

Difficulty or discomfort during the progression of the alimentary bolus from the mouth to the stomach

DESCRIPTION
- Difficulty in swallowing
- A disorder of transferring the food bolus from oropharynx to esophagus or of impairment in transport of the bolus through the esophagus
- Commonly divided based on:
  - Anatomical standpoint: Oropharyngeal or esophageal dysfunction
  - Pathophysiological standpoint: Structure-related or functional causes
- Associated symptoms: *Odynophagia* (painful swallowing); *globus* (lump in throat)
- System(s) affected: GI; Nervous

EPIDEMIOLOGY
Incidence
- In US: 7% incidence lifetime
- Predominant age: All ages; increasing prevalence with age
- Predominant sex: Male = Female

Prevalence
- 16–22% of people >50 years
- Up to 60% of nursing home residents
- 25% of hospitalized patients

RISK FACTORS
- Children: Hereditary and/or congenital malformations
- Adults: Age >50 years (esophageal cancer, neurologic disorders) more likely
- Smoking, excess alcohol, obesity
- Long history of GERD
- Medications (quinine, potassium chloride, vitamin C, tetracycline, Bactrim, clindamycin, NSAIDs, and others)
- Neurologic events or diseases (CVA, neuromuscular disease, multiple sclerosis, Parkinson disease, ALS)
- Trauma or irradiation of head, neck, and chest

GENERAL PREVENTION
- Observe feeding of infants closely for aspiration; have suction available.
- Correct poorly fitting dentures in older patients.
- Avoid drinking alcohol with meals.
- Give consideration to positioning during meals, texture of foods being eaten
- In infants/children: Discuss underlying problem and therapy for recurrent aspiration.
- Positioning and texture in older adults, dentures, supervision to prevent aspiration

ETIOLOGY
- In children:
  - Malformations: Congenital (esophageal atresia, cleft palate, choanal atresia, TE fistula, Zenkers diverticulum)
  - Malformations: Acquired (corrosive or herpetic esophagitis)
  - Neuromuscular/neurologic: Delayed maturation, CP, MD, poliomyelitis
  - GERD

- In adults (esophageal):
  - Structural: Tumors (cancer or benign), strictures (peptic, chemical, trauma, radiation), lower esophageal rings (Schatzki rings), esophageal webs
  - Mechanical: Extrinsic compression from enlarged left atrium, aortic aneurysm, aberrant subclavian artery (termed dysphagia lusoria), substernal thyroid, cervical bony exostosis, and thoracic tumor
  - GERD
  - Neuromuscular: Achalasia, diffuse esophageal spasm, hypertensive lower esophageal sphincter, scleroderma, myasthenia gravis, nutcracker esophagus
- In adults (oropharyngeal):
  - CVA
  - Parkinson disease
  - Neurodegenerative diseases (MS, ALS, Huntington disease, pseudobulbar palsy)
  - Zenker diverticulum
  - Myasthenia gravis
  - Polio
  - Cricopharyngeal achalasia
  - Cervical spondylosis (cervical osteophytes)
  - Obstructive lesions (tumors, inflammatory masses)

Pediatric Considerations
- Congenital malformations
- Tonsillar hypertrophy, large tongue, dental problems (overbite)

Geriatric Considerations
- Poor dentition and/or dentures
- Drug-induced

COMMONLY ASSOCIATED CONDITIONS
- Esophageal carcinoma
- GERD-induced peptic stricture
- Dysphagia lusoria (extrinsic compression)
- Achalasia
- Symptomatic diffuse esophageal spasm
- Eosinophilic esophagitis
- Foreign body
- Scleroderma
- Myasthenia gravis
- CVA

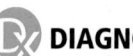 **DIAGNOSIS**

ALERT
Rapidly progressive symptoms and/or profound weight loss is indicative of malignant process; requires immediate attention; should undergo endoscopy with/without biopsy

HISTORY
- Is the dysphagia for solids, liquids, or both? Which started first?
- Does the food bolus feel stuck? If so, where?
- Are there symptoms of oropharyngeal dysfunction?
- Do you have any cough while swallowing? Is it early in swallowing or late?
- Is the dysphagia intermittent or progressive?
- Have you ever brought food back up or vomited?
- Is there a history of chronic heartburn?
- How much alcohol and/or tobacco do you use?
- Are there associated symptoms such as weight loss or chest pain?

- What medications are being taken?
- Is there odynophagia? (Does it hurt with just solid food or both solid and liquids?)
- Is there any halitosis?

PHYSICAL EXAM
- Oropharyngeal type:
  - Choking with swallowing
  - Coughing with swallowing
  - Nasal speech (wet voice)
  - Hoarseness of voice
  - Sialorrhea (drooling of saliva)
  - Frequent respiratory infections
  - Weight loss
  - Dysarthria
  - Nasopharyngeal regurgitation with swallowing
- Esophageal type:
  - Pressure sensation in midchest (localizing below suprasternal notch highly likely to be esophageal disorder); narrow the diagnostic possibilities by asking if this occurs for solids, liquids, or both.
  - Oral or pharyngeal regurgitation
  - Recurrent aspiration pneumonia
  - Weight loss
  - Symptoms of GERD
- Neck and oral cavity for lesions, masses, goiter
- Signs of collagen: Vascular disease
- Detailed neurologic exam, especially cranial nerves with gag reflex testing (CVA, neuromuscular disease, Parkinson)
- In infants:
  - Breastfeeding problems
  - Vomiting or spitting up during feeds
  - Lengthy feeding or eating times (>30 min)

DIAGNOSTIC TESTS & INTERPRETATION
- In infants/children:
  - Observe sucking/eating.
  - Attempt to pass NG tube to assess esophageal patency.
  - Radiography of neck and chest
  - Contrast radiography
  - Endoscopy
- In adults:
  - Barium swallow
  - Fiberoptic endoscopic examination of swallowing (FEES)
  - Gastroesophageal endoscopy
  - Barium cine/video esophagogram
  - Ambulatory 24-h pH testing
  - Esophageal manometry
  - Videofluoroscopic swallowing study (VFSS)

Lab
As suggested by specific differential diagnosis under consideration

Initial lab tests
- CBC to screen for infectious and inflammatory condition
- Serum protein and albumin levels for nutritional assessment
- Thyroid function studies to detect dysphagia associated with hypothyroidism or hyperthyroidism

Imaging
- Barium swallow
- CT scan of chest
- MRI of brain and cervical spine
- Videofluoroscopic swallowing study (VFSS)

Diagnostic Procedures/Surgery
- Endoscopy with biopsy
- Esophageal manometry
- Esophageal pH monitoring

Pathological Findings
- Squamous cell or adenocarcinoma
- Barrett metaplasia
- Fibrous tissue of a ring, web, or stricture
- Loss of smooth muscle (scleroderma)
- Acute or chronic inflammatory changes
- Oropharyngeal lesions

DIFFERENTIAL DIAGNOSIS
- Cardiac chest pain
- Globus hystericus
- Functional heartburn or dysphagia

 TREATMENT

MEDICATION
- For spasms: Calcium channel blockers: Nifedipine (Procardia) 10–30 mg t.i.d.; amitriptyline 0.5–2 mg/kg q.h.s.; dicyclomine (Bentyl) 20 mg q.i.d.
- For esophagitis:
  – Antacids: Tums, Mylanta, Maalox
  – H$_2$ blockers: Cimetidine (Tagamet), ranitidine (Zantac), nizatidine (Axid), famotidine (Pepcid)
  – Proton pump inhibitors: Omeprazole (Prilosec), lansoprazole (Prevacid), rabeprazole (AcipHex), esomeprazole (Nexium), pantoprazole (Protonix)
  – Prokinetic agents: Metoclopramide (Reglan), erythromycin (Ery-Tab)
- Contraindications:
  – Anticholinergics: Obstructive uropathy, glaucoma, myasthenia gravis, achalasia, dementia/delirium, advanced age
  – Nitrates: Early MI, severe anemia, increased ICP, HTN
- Investigational: Cilostazol for dysphagia in poststroke patients is under investigation; may improve swallowing and reduce risk of aspiration pneumonia; mechanism is not completely understood
- Precautions: May need to use liquid forms of medications, as patients might have difficulty swallowing pills

ADDITIONAL TREATMENT
General Measures
- Exclude cardiac disease.
- Ensure airway and pulmonary function.
- Assess nutritional status.
- Speech therapy evaluation is helpful.

Issues for Referral
- Need for endoscopy, refractory: Gastroenterology
- Failure of dilation or medications: Surgery for esophageal myotomy

Additional Therapies
Speech therapy for swallowing assessment, dietary and positioning recommendations, and muscle-strengthening exercise; no eating at bedtime; remaining upright after eating

SURGERY/OTHER PROCEDURES
- Esophageal dilatation (pneumatic or bougie)
- Esophageal stent; laser for cancer palliation
- Treatment for underlying problem (e.g., thyroid goiter, vascular ring, esophageal atresia)
- Nd: YAG laser incision of lower esophageal rings refractory to dilation

- Photodynamic therapy (cancer)
- Cricopharyngeal myotomy for oropharyngeal dysphagia
- Surgery for Zenker diverticulum, refractory strictures, or myotomy for achalasia
- Nissens fundoplication to prevent reflux

IN-PATIENT CONSIDERATIONS
Initial Stabilization
- Outpatient for conditions where patient is able to maintain nutrition and has little risk of complications
- Hospitalization may be required for either infants or adults when dysphagia is associated with total or near-total obstruction of esophageal lumen.
- Endoscopy and/or esophageal dilation may be needed for stenoses and strictures (often recur).
- Surgery may be required in either benign or malignant processes.

Admission Criteria
- Complete or partial esophageal obstruction with malnutrition or hypovolemia/dehydration
- Comorbid conditions complicating etiology of dysphagia
- Enteral feeding might be required in patients with:
  – Impaired level of consciousness
  – Massive aspiration or recurrent respiratory infections
  – Esophageal obstruction

IV Fluids
For dehydrated, hypovolemic patients and patients with impaired consciousness

Nursing
- Monitor for aspiration.
- Ensure correct posture of patient while feeding.
- Consider bedside screening tests using water swallowing and pulse oximetry to screen neurologic patients for dysphagia (1)[A].

Discharge Criteria
- Correction of dysphagia
- Tolerating adequate diet without nausea/pain
- Adequate nutritional intake
- Control of pain syndrome

 ONGOING CARE

FOLLOW-UP RECOMMENDATIONS
- No restrictions
- Sit upright for meals, stay upright afterward; appropriately fitting dentures
- Follow speech therapy/swallow therapy recommendations.
- Strengthening exercises and rehab for post-CVA

Patient Monitoring
Related to specific etiology of the dysphagia

DIET
Depends on etiology and severity:
- Counsel the patient on avoiding irritating drugs.
- Counsel the patient on the importance of chewing food well.
- Speech therapy texture recommendations like mechanical soft diet or pureed diet

PATIENT EDUCATION
Dietary modification, no eating at bedtime, remaining upright after eating, pharmacologic therapy, smoking cessation

PROGNOSIS
Course and prognosis vary with specific diagnosis (cancer, poor; esophageal peptic stricture, good).

COMPLICATIONS
- Aspiration/aspiration pneumonia
- Esophageal "asthma"
- Upper respiratory tract infections
- Malnutrition
- Esophagitis: Reflux based or pill induced
- Death

REFERENCE
1. Bours GJ, Speyer R, Lemmens J, et al. Bedside screening tests vs. videofluoroscopy or fibreoptic endoscopic evaluation of swallowing to detect dysphagia in patients with neurological disorders: systematic review. *J Adv Nurs.* 2009;65:477–93.

ADDITIONAL READING
- Rofes L, Arreola V, Almirall J, Cabré M, Campins L, García-Peris P, Speyer R, Clavé P et al. Diagnosis and Management of Oropharyngeal Dysphagia and Its Nutritional and Respiratory Complications in the Elderly. *Gastroenterology research and practice.* 2011;2011.
- Speyer R, Baijens L, Heijnen M, Zwijnenberg I et al. Effects of therapy in oropharyngeal dysphagia by speech and language therapists: a systematic review. *Dysphagia.* 2010;25:40–65.
- White GN, O'Rourke F, Ong BS, Cordato DJ, Chan DK et al. Dysphagia: causes, assessment, treatment, and management. *Geriatrics.* 2008;63:15–20.

See Also (Topic, Algorithm, Electronic Media Element)
Esophageal Tumors; Gastroesophageal Reflux Disease

 CODES

ICD9
- 530.3 Stricture and stenosis of esophagus
- 750.3 Congenital tracheoesophageal fistula, esophageal atresia and stenosis
- 787.20 Dysphagia, unspecified

CLINICAL PEARLS
- Careful history taking of types of food involved, progression, and associated symptoms will help to determine where the problem is.
- The alarm symptoms to look for are weight loss, chest pain, rapid progression, and risk factors such as chronic GERD and alcohol or tobacco use.
- A barium study (esophagram) is the first step in evaluating patients with dysphagia if you suspect obstruction or achalasia, and then endoscopy; or directly to endoscopy if achalasia is less likely.
- An EGD with esophageal biopsies should be considered in patients with intermittent solid-food dysphagia to rule out eosinophilic esophagitis even if they have normal endoscopic findings.

ECTOPIC PREGNANCY

Janelle M. Evans, MD
Shaila V. Chauhan, MD

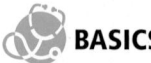 **BASICS**

DESCRIPTION
- Ectopic: Pregnancy occurs outside the confines of the uterine cavity
- Tubal: Pregnancy implanted in any portion of the fallopian tube
- Abdominal: Pregnancy implanted intra-abdominally, most commonly in the posterior cul-de-sac
- Heterotopic: Pregnancy implanted intrauterine and a separate pregnancy implanted outside uterine cavity
- Ovarian: Implantation of pregnancy in ovarian tissue
- Cervical: Implantation in cervix (associated with large blood loss)
- Intraligamentary: Implantation of pregnancy within the broad ligament

EPIDEMIOLOGY
Incidence
- 108,800 cases in 1992 in the US according to Centers for Disease Control census (most recent data available)
- 15.8 per 1,000 total reported pregnancies, or 9.5 per 10,000 women
- 28,000 hospitalizations reported in 2006 in the US for ectopic pregnancy
- Heterotopic pregnancy, although rare (1:30,000), occurs with greater frequency in women undergoing in vitro fertilization (IVF) (1–2/1,000)
- Leading cause of 1st-trimester maternal death and accounts for 9% of national pregnancy deaths

Prevalence
- Predominant age: >40% occur in women between ages 20 and 29
- 12–15% recurrence rate if prior ectopic pregnancy

RISK FACTORS
- History of tubal surgery (7:1,000 for tubal ligation)
- Previous ectopic pregnancy
- History of pelvic inflammatory disease (PID), endometritis, or current gonorrhea/chlamydia infection
- Pelvic adhesive disease (infection, prior surgery)
- Use of an intrauterine device: Reduction of the absolute risk of ectopic pregnancy overall, but increased likelihood of pregnancy being ectopic if pregnancy occurs
- Use of assisted reproductive technologies in up to 4% (e.g., IVF, embryo transfer)
- Diethylstilbestrol exposure in utero
- Cigarette smoking
- Some evidence that vaginal douching is a modifiable risk factor
- Patients with disorders that affect ciliary motility may be at increased risk.

GENERAL PREVENTION
- Reliable contraception or abstinence
- Screening and treatment of sexually transmitted diseases (gonorrhea, chlamydia) that can cause PID and tubal scarring

PATHOPHYSIOLOGY
- 98% of ectopic pregnancies occur in the fallopian tube, 70% in the ampullary portion of the tube, 12% in the isthmus, 11% in the fimbria, and 2% in the cornua.
- Abdominal pregnancies account for 1.3% of all ectopics; ovarian and cervical sites account for 0.2% each.

ETIOLOGY
- For a tubal pregnancy:
  – Damage or compromise to the integrity of the fallopian tubes leads to dysfunction of the tubal cilia, which are required for proper movement of the fertilized ovum to the uterine cavity.
  – Scarring or narrowing of the tube damages tubal integrity.
- Other locations are rare and may occur from reimplantation of an aborted tubal pregnancy or uterine structural abnormalities (mainly cervical pregnancy).

 DIAGNOSIS

HISTORY
- In more than half of presenting cases, patients have sudden-onset abdominal pain coupled with cessation of menses or irregular menses.
- Nausea and/or vomiting
- Abdominal pain or mass
- Referred shoulder pain (secondary to hemoperitoneum)

PHYSICAL EXAM
- Abdominal tenderness
- Vaginal bleeding
- Palpable mass on pelvic exam
- Cervical motion tenderness may also be appreciated.
- In cervical cases, an hourglass-shaped cervix might be noted.
- In cases of rupture and intraperitoneal bleeding, signs of shock such as pallor, tachycardia, and hypotension may be present.

DIAGNOSTIC TESTS & INTERPRETATION
Lab
Initial lab tests
- Human chorionic gonadotropin (HCG): Serial quantitative serum levels normally increase by ~66% every 48 hours:
  – Abnormal rise should prompt workup for gestational abnormalities.
- Serial hematocrit and abdominal exams to quantify blood loss only if not immediately going to the operating room
- Serum progesterone level (>20 mg/mL associated with lower risk of ectopic pregnancy)

Imaging
Initial approach
- Transvaginal ultrasound (TVUS) is the gold standard for diagnosis (1)[A]:
  – Doppler flowmetry is usually coupled with ultrasound for more accurate diagnosis.
- Magnetic resonance imaging is also useful, but costly, and rarely used if ultrasound is available.

Follow-Up & Special Considerations
Consider TVUS in the 1st trimester of future pregnancies.

Pathological Findings
- Tubal pregnancy: Chorionic villi within the tubal wall
- Ovarian pregnancy (Spiegelberg criteria):
  – Pregnancy found displacing or replacing the ovarian tissue
  – Possible utero-ovarian ligament attachment
  – Ovarian tissue identified as part of gestational sac
- Abdominal pregnancy—primary form:
  – Both ovaries and tubes appear normal.
  – No uteroperitoneal fistula is present.
  – Limited to peritoneal attachment of conceptus
- Cervical pregnancy: Villi seen in the cervical canal
- Intraligamentary pregnancy: The products of conception (POCs) are within the confines of the broad ligament.

DIFFERENTIAL DIAGNOSIS
- Missed or threatened abortion
- Appendicitis
- Salpingitis, PID
- Ruptured corpus luteum or hemorrhagic cyst
- Ovarian tumor, benign or malignant
- Ovarian torsion
- Endometrioma
- Cervical cancer
- Cervical phase of uterine abortion

 TREATMENT

MEDICATION
- Methotrexate: Primary treatment for unruptured tubal pregnancy or for remaining POCs after laparoscopic salpingotomy. It inhibits DNA synthesis via folic acid antagonism.
- Most effective when pregnancy is <3 cm diameter, HCG <5,000 mIU/mL, and no fetal heart rate is seen. Success rate is 85–90% with proper selection.
- Dosage:
  – Single: IM methotrexate: 50 mg/m^2 of body surface area; may repeat once (preferred method) if <15% decline in HCG by day 7
  – Multidose: Methotrexate 1 mg/kg IM/IV every other day, with leucovorin 0.1 mg/kg IM in between. Maximum 4 doses; course may be repeated 7 days after last dose if necessary.

- Contraindications:
  – Hemodynamic instability or any evidence of rupture
  – Fetal heart rate seen
  – Large gestational sac (>3 cm)
  – Noncompliance or limited access to hospital or transportation
- Precautions:
  – Immunologic, hematologic, renal, gastrointestinal, hepatic, and pulmonary disease, or interacting medications
- Pretreatment testing: serum HCG, complete blood count, liver and renal function tests, type and screen
- Patient counseling: During therapy, refrain from use of alcohol, aspirin, nonsteroidal anti-inflammatory drugs, or folate supplements (decreases efficacy of MTX), avoid excessive sun exposure

ADDITIONAL TREATMENT
- After evidence of repeat medical failure or rupture, surgery is necessary.
- Follow all patients treated medically to an HCG of 0 to prevent surgical intervention.
- Expectant management in asymptomatic patients with no evidence of rupture or hemodynamic instability coupled with an appropriately low BHCG, no evidence of fetal cardiac activity

Issues for Referral
- Co-manage with or refer to a gynecologist for medical treatment.
- Consult a gynecologist for surgical care.

COMPLEMENTARY AND ALTERNATIVE MEDICINE
Watchful waiting: If no clear adnexal mass and low HCG (usually 1,000–2,000), may follow with HCG/ultrasound. Rare cases of rupture have been described with low quants.

SURGERY/OTHER PROCEDURES
- Indications include ruptured ectopic, inability to comply with medical follow-up, previous tubal ligation, known tubal disease or current heterotopic pregnancy, desire for permanent sterilization at time of diagnosis
- Laparoscopy is 1st-line surgical management.
- Salpingostomy preferred in patients who wish to maintain fertility:
  – Slightly higher recurrence rate than with salpingectomy
  – Slightly higher rate of persistent trophoblastic tissue with laparoscopy vs open laparotomy (8% vs 3.4%)
- Salpingectomy indicated for uncontrolled bleeding, recurrent ectopic pregnancy, severely damaged tube, gestational sac >4 cm, or patient desire for sterilization

IN-PATIENT CONSIDERATIONS
Initial Stabilization
Surgical emergency:
- 2 IV access lines should be placed immediately if suspicion of rupture; aggressive resuscitation as needed
- Blood product transfusion and fluids if necessary en route to operating room
- In cases of shock, pressors and cardiac support may be necessary.

Admission Criteria
Fails criteria for methotrexate management, suspicion of rupture, orthostatic, shock, and severe abdominal pain requiring IV narcotics

Nursing
Strict input/output, hourly vitals, orthostatics if mobile, frequent abdominal exams, serial hematocrit, pad counts if heavy vaginal bleeding

Discharge Criteria
Afebrile; abdominal pain resolving or resolved

ONGOING CARE

FOLLOW-UP RECOMMENDATIONS
Patient Monitoring
- Serial serum quantitative HCG until level drops to negative
- Pelvic ultrasound for persistent or recurrent masses
- Pain control: Brief course of narcotics usually necessary
- Liver and renal function tests following methotrexate administration
- Delay of subsequent pregnancy for at least 3 months after treatment with methotrexate due to teratogenicity

DIET
- Avoid foods and vitamins high in folate due to interaction with methotrexate efficacy.
- Maintain excellent hydration.

PROGNOSIS
- Recurrence rate 12–15% for ectopic pregnancy
- Future fertility depends on fertility prior to ectopic, history of tubal compromise
- Referral to reproductive endocrinology appropriate if infertility persists beyond 12–18 months

COMPLICATIONS
- Hemorrhage and hypovolemic shock
- Persistent trophoblastic tissue after medical or surgical management
- Infection
- Infertility (more commonly with salpingectomy)
- Blood transfusions with associated infections/transfusion reaction
- Disseminated intravascular coagulation

REFERENCE

1. *Ann Emerg Med*. 2010;56(6):674–683.

ADDITIONAL READING

- ACOG practice bulletin. Medical management of tubal pregnancy. Number 3, December 1998. Clinical management guidelines for obstetrician-gynecologists. American College of Obstetricians and Gynecologists. *Int J Gynaecol Obstet*. 1999;65: 97–103.
- Bisharah M, Tulandi T. Laparoscopic surgery in pregnancy. *Clin Obstet Gynecol*. 2003;46:92–7.
- Braude P, Rowell P. Assisted conception. III–problems with assisted conception. *BMJ*. 2003;327:920–3.
- Centers for Disease Control and Prevention. Sexually Transmitted Disease Surveillance 2007. Atlanta, GA: U.S. Department of Health and Human Services; December 2008.
- Centers for Disease Control and Prevention. Sexually Transmitted Disease Surveillance 2007. Atlanta, GA: U.S. Department of Health and Human Services; December 2008.
- Elson J, et al. Expectant management of tubal ectopic pregnancy: Prediction of successful outcome using decision tree analysis. *Ultrasound Obstet Gynecol*. 2004;23:552–6.
- Hajenius PJ, Mol F, Mol BW, et al. Interventions for tubal ectopic pregnancy. *Cochrane Database Syst Rev*. 2007;CD000324.
- Lipscomb GH. Medical therapy for ectopic pregnancy. *Semin Reprod Med*. 2007;25:93–8.
- Mol F, Mol BW, Ankum WM, et al. Current evidence on surgery, systemic methotrexate and expectant management in the treatment of tubal ectopic pregnancy: a systematic review and meta-analysis. *Hum Reprod Update*. 2008.
- Murray H, et al. Diagnosis and treatment of ectopic pregnancy. *Can Med Assoc J*. 2005;173(8): 905–912.
- Nama V, Manyonda I. Tubal ectopic pregnancy: diagnosis and management. *Arch Gynecol Obstet*. 2008.
- Ramakrishnan K, Scheid DC. Ectopic pregnancy: expectant management of immediate surgery? *J Fam Pract*. 2006;55:517–22.
- Tay JI, Moore J, Walker JJ. Ectopic pregnancy. *BMJ*. 2000;320:916–9.

 # CODES

ICD9
- 633.00 Abdominal pregnancy without intrauterine pregnancy
- 633.10 Tubal pregnancy without intrauterine pregnancy
- 633.20 Ovarian pregnancy without intrauterine pregnancy

CLINICAL PEARLS

- Ectopic pregnancy is the leading cause of 1st-trimester maternal death and accounts for 9% of national pregnancy deaths.
- 98% of ectopic pregnancies occur in the fallopian tube.
- TVUS is the gold standard for diagnosis.
- When an ectopic pregnancy is <3 cm diameter, HCG <5,000 mIU/mL, and no fetal heart rate is seen, a single dose of methotrexate is the preferred medical treatment, with a success rate of 85–90%.
- Indications for surgery include ruptured ectopic, inability to comply with medical follow-up, previous tubal ligation, known tubal disease or current heterotopic pregnancy, or desire for permanent sterilization at time of diagnosis.

EJACULATORY DISORDERS

Andrew Leone, MD
Kyle D. Wood, MD

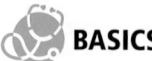

BASICS

DESCRIPTION
- Premature/rapid ejaculation: Inability to control the ejaculatory reflex is the most common type of sexual dysfunction affecting all age groups:
  - American Urological Association (AUA) 2003 Guidelines definition: "Ejaculation that occurs sooner than desired, either before or shortly after penetration, causing distress to either one or both partners." (1)
  - Natural biologic response is to ejaculate within 2–5 minutes after vaginal penetration.
  - Ejaculatory control is an acquired behavior that increases with experience.
- Delayed (retarded) ejaculation: Prolonged time to ejaculate despite desire, stimulation, and erection.
- Aspermia (lack of sperm in the ejaculate):
  - Anejaculation: Lack of emission or contractions of bulbospongiosus muscle
  - Retrograde ejaculation: Partial or complete ejaculation of semen into the bladder
  - Obstruction: Ejaculatory duct obstruction or urethral obstruction
- Painful ejaculation: Genital or perineal pain during or after ejaculation
- Ejaculatory anhedonia: Normal ejaculation lacking orgasm or pleasure
- Hematospermia: Presence of blood in the ejaculate
- Ejaculatory duct obstruction
- System(s) affected: Nervous; Reproductive
- Synonym(s): Premature ejaculation; rapid ejaculation; retarded ejaculation; retrograde ejaculation; anejaculation; inhibited orgasm in males; ejaculatory dysfunction

EPIDEMIOLOGY
- Premature ejaculation is common. Reported prevalence in US males ages 18–59: 21%
- Retarded ejaculation is reported in ~5–8% of men between 18 and 59, but <3% experience the problem for >6 months.
- Predominant age: All sexually mature age groups
- Predominant sex: Male only

Prevalence
20% of men affected

RISK FACTORS
See Etiology

PATHOPHYSIOLOGY
Male sexual response:
- Erection mediated by parasympathetic nervous system
- Ejaculation consists of 2 phases:
  - Emission phase: Semen is deposited into urethra by contraction of prostate, seminal vesicles, and vas deferens. Under autonomic sympathetic control.
  - Ejaculation phase: Semen is forcibly propelled out of urethra by rhythmic contractions of the bulbospongiosus and ischiocavernosus muscles. This is mediated by the somatic nervous system on the motor branches of the pudendal nerve.
- Bladder neck contracture occurs during the above process and is induced by alpha-adrenergic receptors to ensure anterograde ejaculation.

- Orgasm: The pleasurable sensation associated with ejaculation (cerebral cortex) (2)

ETIOLOGY
- Untreated erectile dysfunction is the most common treatable cause.
- Premature ejaculation (many potential causes but all without evidence base):
  - Penile hypersensitivity
  - 5-hydroxytryptamine (5-HT)-receptor sensitivity
  - Sexual inexperience
  - High level of sexual arousal and/or long interval since last ejaculation
  - Fear of sexual transmitted diseases (STDs)
  - Anxiety
  - Guilty feelings about sex
  - Lack of privacy
  - Interpersonal maladaptation (e.g., marital problems, unresponsiveness of partner)
- Retarded ejaculation:
  - Rarely may be caused by an underlying painful disorder (e.g., prostatitis, seminal vesiculitis)
  - May be psychogenic as part of erectile dysfunction
  - Sexual performance anxiety and other psychosocial factors
  - Some drugs may impair ejaculation (e.g., certain monoamine oxidase inhibitors [MAOIs], selective serotonin reuptake inhibitors [SSRIs], α- and β-blockers, thiazides, antipsychotics, tricyclic and quadricyclic antidepressants, nonsteroidal anti-inflammatory drugs [NSAIDs], opiates, or alcohol).
- Never any ejaculate:
  - Congenital structural disorder (Müllerian duct cyst, Wolffian abnormality)
  - Acquired (radical prostatectomy, postinfectious, post-traumatic, T10–12 neuropathy)
- Anejaculation:
  - Medications (α- and β-blockers, benzodiazepines, SSRIs, MAOIs, TCAs, antipsychotics, aminocaproic acid)
  - Diabetes mellitus (DM) (neuropathy)
  - Retroperitoneal lymph node dissection
  - Sympathetic nerve injury (spinal cord injury, intraoperative injury)
  - Radical prostatectomy
- Retrograde ejaculation:
  - Transurethral resection of the prostate (25%) or other prostate resection procedures
  - Surgery on the neck of the bladder
  - Extensive pelvic surgery
  - Retroperitoneal lymph node dissection for testicular cancer (also may produce failure of emission)
  - Neurologic disorders (multiple sclerosis, DM)
  - Medications (alpha-blockers, in particular tamsulosin, ganglion blockers, antipsychotics)
  - Urethral stricture
  - Trauma
- Painful ejaculation:
  - Infection or inflammation (orchitis, epididymitis, prostatitis, urethritis)
  - Ejaculatory duct obstruction
  - Seminal vesicle calculi
  - Obstruction of the vas deferens
  - Psychological

- Ejaculatory anhedonia:
  - Medications
  - Psychological
  - Hormonal imbalances
  - Decreased libido
- Hematospermia:
  - Inflammation/infection
  - Calculi: Bladder, seminal vesicle, prostate, urethra
  - Trauma to genital area, i.e., cycling or constipation
  - Obstruction
  - Cyst
  - Tumor (prostate cancer [1–3% present with hematospermia])
  - Arteriovenous malformations
  - Iatrogenic
  - Hypertension
- Endocrinopathies can result in ejaculatory dysfunction

COMMONLY ASSOCIATED CONDITIONS
- Neurologic disorders (e.g., multiple sclerosis)
- Diabetes mellitus
- Prostatitis
- Ejaculatory duct obstruction
- Urethral stricture
- Psychologic disorders
- Endocrinopathies
- Relationship/interpersonal difficulties

DIAGNOSIS

- Ejaculation occurs before individual wishes.
- Ejaculation does not occur following normal stimulation (including masturbation).

HISTORY
- Detailed sexual history, including:
  - Time frame of the problem
  - Evaluation of the quality of patient's sexual response
  - Sense of ejaculatory control and sexual distress
  - Overall assessment of the relationship
- Detailed history of recent and current medications
- History of past trauma or recent infections
- Past surgical history with particular attention to genitourinary surgeries
- Inquire about home remedies attempted.
- Many men do not distinguish initially between problems related to erection and ejaculation.
- Some men have unrealistic expectations of ejaculatory response and frequency.
- Include the sexual partner in the interview, especially if the patient expresses a belief that he is not meeting his partner's needs.
- In review of systems, elicit any evidence of testosterone deficiency or prolactin excess for diagnosis of anhedonia.

PHYSICAL EXAM
- Look for multiple sclerosis, spinal cord injury, and emotional disorders
- Thorough genitourinary (GU) exam, including (3):
  - Size and texture of testes and epididymis
  - Verification of the presence of the vas deferens
  - Location and patency of urethral meatus
  - Digital rectal examination to evaluate prostate consistency and size and possible midline lesions

DIAGNOSTIC TESTS & INTERPRETATION
Lab
- Laboratory test results may be normal.
- Fasting blood sugar to rule out diabetes
- Postorgasmic urinalysis will confirm retrograde ejaculation. Sperm, fructose level, and viscosity can be measured.
- Anejaculation will have fructose negative, sperm negative, nonviscous postorgasmic urinalysis.
- In painful ejaculation, urinalysis and urine culture
- If prostate cancer is considered, check prostate-specific antigen (PSA).
- In anhedonia, consider checking testosterone, prolactin, and thyroid levels.

Imaging
- In hematospermia, painful ejaculation, or if ejaculatory duct obstruction is considered, transrectal ultrasound (TRUS) may be helpful.
- TRUS-guided seminal vesicle aspiration; if ejaculatory duct obstruction is present, then the aspirate will contain sperm.
- If suspicious of anatomic abnormality, can use ultrasound and/or MRI

 ## TREATMENT
MEDICATION
- Premature ejaculation:
  – Treating underlying erectile dysfunction (if identified) may allow for a decrease in the rapidity.
  – Behavioral/sex therapy is important when appropriate.
  – Topical anesthetic gel applied (2.5% prilocaine + 2.5 % lidocaine (EMLA)) 2.5 g under a condom for 30 minutes prior to intercourse
  – Experimental PSD502 topical aerosol preparation of lidocaine/prilocaine effective in phase III trials (4)
  – Clomipramine 20–50 mg/d or sertraline 25–200 mg/d, fluoxetine 5–20 mg/d, or paroxetine 10–40 mg/d have been shown to delay ejaculation.
  – Clomipramine shown to be the most effective, but has higher rate of side effects
  – On-demand use of clomipramine 20–40 mg 4–24 hours before intercourse or sertraline 50 mg 4–8 hours before intercourse or paroxetine 20 mg 3–4 hours before intercourse
  – Switching antidepressants to bupropion, nefazodone, mirtazapine, or possibly trazodone may eliminate drug-induced ejaculatory disturbance.
- Delayed (retarded) ejaculation:
  – Retarded orgasm and ejaculation in patients who must continue SSRIs may respond to bupropion, buspirone, cyproheptadine, or yohimbine supplementation before intercourse.
  – Some evidence that cyproheptadine and amantadine may be helpful (5)
- Anejaculation/retrograde ejaculation:
  – Alpha-agonists and antihistamines can be helpful but are not approved by Food and Drug Administration (FDA):
    ○ Pseudoephedrine 60 mg p.o. every day to q.i.d.
    ○ Imipramine 25 mg p.o. b.i.d.
    ○ Ephedrine sulfate 50 mg p.o. q.i.d.
- Painful ejaculation:
  – Treat underlying infection/inflammatory process
  – Alpha-blockers may have some benefit

ADDITIONAL TREATMENT
General Measures
- Identifying any medical cause (even if not reversible) helps patient accept condition.
- Improve partner communication.
- Psychological counseling may be beneficial for some patients.
- Reduce performance pressure through reassurance.
- Use of a variety of resources may be necessary (e.g., psychiatrist, psychologist, sex therapist, vascular surgeon, urologist, endocrinologist, neurologist).
- Premature ejaculation
  – Use sensate focus therapy (gradual progression of nonsexual contact to sexual contact)
  – Quiet vagina: Female partner stops moving just prior to ejaculation
  – Techniques to learn ejaculatory control (e.g., coronal squeeze technique [squeezing the glans penis until ejaculatory urge ceases] or start-and-stop technique [cessation of penile stimulation when ejaculation approaches and resumption of stimulation when ejaculatory feeling ends])
- Delayed ejaculation:
  – Change medications to an antidepressant that is less likely to cause delayed ejaculation (citalopram, fluvoxamine, nefazodone).
  – If patient has diabetes, better control of diabetes may improve ejaculation.
  – Penile vibratory stimulation (not frequently used)
- Anejaculation/retrograde ejaculation:
  – Discontinue offending medication(s).
  – Diabetic control
  – If urethral obstruction present, referral to urology for management
  – Retrograde ejaculation may be helped if intercourse occurs when bladder is full.
  – Consider penile vibratory stimulation (effective in spinal cord injuries greater than T10) or electroejaculation (place on monitor if lesions above T6 since autonomic dysreflexia may result) to collect sperm in anejaculation cases.
- Painful ejaculation:
  – Counseling may be beneficial.
  – If seminal vesicle stones possible, refer to urology.
- Hematospermia:
  – If persistent or high degree of suspicion for abnormality, refer to urologist for proper evaluation.

Issues for Referral
The following conditions, when suspected, should be referred to a urologist:
- Ejaculatory duct obstruction
- Seminal vesicle or prostatic stones
- Urethral obstruction
- Vas deferens obstruction
- Calculi
- Persistent or severe hematospermia

SURGERY/OTHER PROCEDURES
Surgical treatment of ejaculatory duct obstruction:
- Transurethral resection of the ejaculatory ducts

 ## ONGOING CARE
PATIENT EDUCATION
See General Measures

PROGNOSIS
Often improves with therapy and counseling

COMPLICATIONS
Psychologic impact on some males: Signs of severe inadequacy, self-doubt, additional anxiety, and guilt

REFERENCES
1. Montague DK, Jarow J, Broderick GA, et al. AUA guideline on the pharmacologic management of premature ejaculation. *J Urol*. 2004;172:290–4.
2. Master VA, Turek PJ. Ejaculatory physiology and dysfunction. *Urol Clin North Am*. 2001;28: 363–75, x.
3. Schuster TG, Ohl DA. Diagnosis and treatment of ejaculatory dysfunction. *Urol Clin North Am*. 2002;29:939–48.
4. Dinsmore WW, Wyllie MG. PSD502 improves ejaculatory latency, control and sexual satisfaction when applied topically 5 min before intercourse in men with premature ejaculation: results of a phase III, multicentre, double-blind, placebo-controlled study. *BJU Int*. 2009.
5. McMahon CG, Abdo C, Incrocci L, et al. Disorders of orgasm and ejaculation in men. *J Sex Med*. 2004;1:58–65.

ADDITIONAL READING
- Mercer CH, et al. Sexual function problems and health seeking behaviour in Britain: Probability sample survey. *Br Med J*. 2003;327:426–7.
- Richardson D, Goldmeier D, BASHH Special Interest Group for Sexual Dysfunction. Recommendations for the management of retarded ejaculation: BASHH Special Interest Group for Sexual Dysfunction. *Int J STD AIDS*. 2006;17:7–13.
- Waldinger MD. Premature ejaculation: definition and drug treatment. *Drugs*. 2007;67:547–68.

CODES

ICD9
- 302.75 Premature ejaculation
- 608.87 Retrograde ejaculation

CLINICAL PEARLS
- If erectile dysfunction is contributing to ejaculatory difficulty, management of erectile dysfunction should precede attempted management of ejaculatory disorders.
- Medications should always be thoroughly reviewed, as they may be the primary cause of ejaculatory disorders.
- A multidisciplinary approach, including the primary care physician, urologists, psychologists, and other appropriate health care professionals, is essential to the proper treatment of ejaculatory disorders.

ELDER ABUSE
Thomas Price, MD

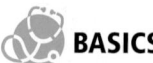

BASICS

DESCRIPTION
Elder abuse, or elder mistreatment, is a condition where the physical, psychological, or financial well-being of an older adult is infringed upon through intentional acts or lack of action, even if harm is not intended. 3 basic entities comprise this problem:
- Abuse: Includes physical, sexual, or psychological harm
- Neglect: Withholding of necessary treatments or services
- Exploitation: Use of an older adult's property counter to their needs or benefit

EPIDEMIOLOGY
Incidence
2–10% of persons worldwide over the age of 65 suffer abuse on an annual basis, as many as 1 new case every 8 hours (1)

Prevalence
1–2 million seniors affected in the US as of 2003 data (1)

RISK FACTORS
- 5 major risk factors (2):
  - Shared living situation (abuser/victim)
  - Dementia or other cognitive impairment
  - Social isolation (abuser or victim)
  - Mental illness/alcohol abuse (abuser)
  - Financial/material dependence (abuser) on the victim
- The presence of all of these risk factors does not convey increased diagnostic accuracy; likewise, the absence of all risk factors does not preclude abuse.

GENERAL PREVENTION
- Improve patient social contact and support.
- Monitor patients for self-neglect and functional decline.
- Recognition of caregiver stressors and burden
- Assist management of behavioral and functional changes that occur in dementia
- While several screening tools exist, screening questionnaires are not helpful in patients with cognitive impairment (3). Common screening questions include:
  - "Have you felt unsafe at home?"
  - "Has anyone hurt you, called you names, or taken things from you?"
  - " What happens when you disagree with [caregiver]?"

ETIOLOGY
The most common scenario of abuse is a caregiver with poor family/social support who is providing care for an older person with a degree of disability. These caregivers are often relatives of the possible victim. Abuse can occur in any setting (home, assisted living, nursing home), and any older person with an impaired ability to defend or care for themself can be at risk.

COMMONLY ASSOCIATED CONDITIONS
- Nearly 2/3 of patients diagnosed as suffering from elder abuse had dementia in an international study (4)[B].
- Older patients that are admitted with a geriatric syndrome of "failure to thrive" may be victims and should be screened for abuse.

DIAGNOSIS

As neglect and exploitation are more common forms of elder mistreatment than abuse, the history is extremely important and will allow the practitioner to develop their own suspicion threshold for an individual case.

HISTORY
- Interviewing the patient separate from the suspected abuser is helpful. The patient may give vague explanations of the causes of injury, or may refuse to answer questions.
- A history of dementia or functional decline can be associated with increased risk, as is an increase in physical and psychological aggression as is often seen in dementia.
- Observe interaction between patient and caregiver: Suspicion is raised if there is withdrawal of patient from caregiver, or caregiver interrupting the patient and providing answers for them. Caregivers with anxiety, depression, and reduced social support are more likely to mistreat their care recipients (3)[C].

PHYSICAL EXAM
- Documentation of abnormal findings on physical exam may be used as evidence in court cases and should not include subjective or editorial comments or conclusions.

- Context of the physical condition of the patient is important. If they are examined in their own bed, look for bedding or mattress soiled by bodily fluids. If found in sheets, copious flakes of skin or shedded hair can point to restricted mobility and care:
  - Appearance of poor personal hygiene
  - Bruises and soft tissue injury:
    - Common areas include surfaces of the upper back, upper arms, and lower legs
    - Lesions with shapes (such as buckles, snaps, or buttons) suggest prolonged immobility or blunt trauma
  - Pressure ulcers can indicate neglect but are equivocal outside of context.
  - Poor dentition or evidence of oral sores, candidiasis, etc.
  - Findings of lice, scabies, or saprophytes
- Fearful or withdrawn affect
- A genital exam is indicated if sexual abuse is suspected, but should be performed with a documented chaperone of the patient's gender. The use of a rape kit if trained personnel is available may be appropriate.

DIAGNOSTIC TESTS & INTERPRETATION
Lab
The following workup is recommended:
- Urine and blood screen for narcotics, intoxicants, and other psychoactive agents (extended panels may be necessary depending on your laboratory)
- Nutritional assessment, including appropriate serology (albumin, prealbumin, iron), blood count, and extended blood chemistry
- Additional labs to consider in patients with cognitive impairment: Thyroid stimulating hormone, syphilis serology, vitamin B_{12} level
- Assessment of infection (may include urinalysis and culture, chest radiograph, blood count, and cultures)
- If sexual abuse suspected, culture and microscopy of any present exudate or residue and viral serology (rape kit lab package)

Imaging
- Radiographic imaging of areas below soft tissue injury is indicated if there is evidence of infection (osteomyelitis) at a pressure ulcer site or bruising of a limb (fracture).
- If physical abuse is suspected and cognitive impairment present, then cranial imaging looking for hemorrhage (subdural, etc.) is indicated.

Diagnostic Procedures/Surgery
- Pulse test: Check blood pressure and pulse in presence and absence of suspected abuser. Elevation of either in the presence of the suspected abuser should raise suspicion. Useful in patients with dementia or other condition that makes history taking difficult.
- Documentation: Practitioners may make statements of "suspected mistreatment" but should avoid making definitive diagnosis of abuse in their initial assessment.

DIFFERENTIAL DIAGNOSIS
- Self-neglect is a condition where a patient fails to provide adequate self-care. It can occur in patients with cognitive impairment and may be a sign of early-stage dementia. It is also seen in patients with psychiatric disorders such as schizophrenia and depression. Many consider this a condition related to elder abuse and place it in the category of elder mistreatment.
- Alzheimer's disease alone can manifest with poor nutrition, withdrawal from society, and feelings of persecution.
- Delusions due to dementia, such as the Alzheimer's type, may manifest early with accusations of theft and deception.
- Parkinson's disease patients often fall and may exhibit fractures and bruises on a frequent basis that may mimic recurrent physical abuse.
- Coagulopathy such as due to use of antiplatelet or warfarin therapy can cause easy bruising of the forearms, but usually spares the upper arm.
- Adenocarcinoma of the lung, prostate, and colon can present with weight loss, apathy, and pressure ulcers.
- Pancreatic adenocarcinoma may present with severe weight loss, depression, and a failure-to-thrive picture.
- Hypothyroidism can present with apathy, weight loss, and confusion that may be confused for neglect.
- Chronic lung disease can present as weight loss, reduced functional reserve, and withdrawal.
- Acute psychosis can be due to infection, medications, or metabolic disturbances and may result in delusional accusations of harm and neglect.
- Impaired financial status often leads to a lack of access to appropriate food, clothing, shelter, and medical care.

 ## TREATMENT

In most states, the physician or allied health care worker is a mandated reporter of suspicion of elder abuse. This does not put a burden of charge on the physician.

IN-PATIENT CONSIDERATIONS
Initial Stabilization
Patient's living situation must be explored and determination of a safe alternative environment made. This is usually in conjunction with a social worker.

Admission Criteria
- Victims of elder abuse should be admitted to the hospital (observation status) if there are no safe discharge alternatives.
- Often, these victims will have acute or chronic medical illness that requires medical attention and possible conversion from observation to inpatient status.
- Cases of suspected abuse *must be reported* to the state's Adult Protective Services agency or a designated alternative (e.g., if patient resides in nursing home, then report to that state's regulatory entity). Social services may help. If physical harm has occurred, consider reporting to local law enforcement for investigation.
- Hospital security may need to be notified if restricted visitor access to a patient is required and the patient's name may be hidden from the public hospital census.

Discharge Criteria
Victims should not be discharged back to a potentially abusive environment without active investigation or protection (e.g., court order). Alternatives to discharge to the unsafe environment may include:
- Another friend or family member
- Nursing home
- Personal care home
- Assisted living facility
- Local victims rescue or sheltering program if available

 ## ONGOING CARE

FOLLOW-UP RECOMMENDATIONS
Victims of abuse should not be discharged without adequate follow-up, including:
- Primary care physician visit in 1 week
- Follow up with Adult Protective Services or other agency
- Home Health Agency for assessment of safety (physical therapy)
- Follow up with appropriate psychiatric or psychological care.

Patient Monitoring
Frequent follow-up with appropriate state agency as discussed above

PATIENT EDUCATION
To locate Elder Abuse Hotline in your state, go to: http://www.nccafv.org/state_elder_abuse_hotlines.htm

PROGNOSIS
Patients with corroborated elder abuse have a 3-fold increase in mortality over 10 years when compared to controls (5)[B].

COMPLICATIONS
Victims of elder abuse who are seen by an Adult Protective Services caseworkers are 4 times more likely to be admitted to a nursing home (6)[B].

REFERENCES

1. National Center on Elder Abuse. *Elder Abuse Prevalence and Incidence*. Washinton, DC: American Public Human Services Association: 2005.
2. Lachs MS, Pillemer K et al. Elder abuse. *Lancet*. 2004;364:1263–72.
3. Wiglesworth A, Mosqueda L, Mulnard R, Liao S, Gibbs L, Fitzgerald W et al. Screening for abuse and neglect of people with dementia. *J Am Geriatr Soc*. 2010;58:493–500.
4. Cooper C, Katona C, Finne-Soveri H, Topinková E, Carpenter GI, Livingston G et al. Indicators of elder abuse: a crossnational comparison of psychiatric morbidity and other determinants in the Ad-HOC study. *Am J Geriatr Psychiatry*. 2006;14:489–97.
5. Lachs MS, Williams CS, O'Brien S, Pillemer KA, Charlson ME et al. The mortality of elder mistreatment. *JAMA*. 1998;280:428–32.
6. Lachs MS, Williams CS, O'Brien S, Pillemer KA, et al. Adult protective service use and nursing home placement. *Gerontologist*. 2002;42:734–9.

 ## CODES

ICD9
- 995.80 Unspecified adult maltreatment
- 995.82 Adult emotional/psychological abuse
- 995.83 Adult sexual abuse

CLINICAL PEARLS

Patients with dementia or other psychiatric illness may accuse caregivers of physical harm or theft due to disease-induced elusions. Corroborating evidence may be needed to support suspicion of abuse, but these claims should not be summarily dismissed.

E

ENCEPHALITIS, VIRAL

Mary Cataletto, MD
Paul J. Lee, MD
Margaret McCormick, MS, RN

 BASICS

DESCRIPTION
- Inflammatory process of the brain associated with clinical evidence of neurologic dysfunction
- System(s) affected: Nervous
- Synonym(s): Meningoencephalitis

EPIDEMIOLOGY
Incidence
3.5–7.4/100,000 persons/year

Prevalence
- Seasonal variation: (e.g., arboviruses, enteroviruses, mumps, varicella)
- Nonseasonal: Most others (e.g., herpes simplex virus [HSV])

RISK FACTORS
- Age: Increased incidence in infants and elderly
- Contact with animals or insect vectors
- Impaired immune status
- Ingestions (e.g., raw meat)
- Occupation (e.g., lab or animal-care workers)
- Recreational activities (e.g., camping, hunting)
- Transfusion and transplantation
- Travel to endemic areas
- Recent vaccinations or unvaccinated status

GENERAL PREVENTION
- Appropriate clothing to protect against mosquitos
- Use of mosquito repellants (DEET, Picaridin)
- Avoidance and removal of ticks
- Elimination of mosquito breeding sources
- Vaccines, when available

PATHOPHYSIOLOGY
- Most common entry site is through the blood.
- Specific cell lines may be infected and are associated with specific symptom complexes:
  - Neurons: Associated with seizures
  - Oligodendroglia: May cause demyelination alone, cortical infection, or reactive parenchymal swelling; changes in state of consciousness
  - Brainstem neurons: Coma, respiratory failure
  - Microglia, macrophages: Neurologic dysfunction
- Pathologic changes seen with postinfectious and postvaccinal encephalomyelitis include perivascular infiltration of mononuclear inflammatory cells.

ETIOLOGY
- Vaccines have changed epidemiology in US.
- Despite extensive evaluations, the etiologic agent is frequently not identified (32–75%).
- Most commonly identified etiologies in US: HSV, West Nile, enteroviruses

COMMONLY ASSOCIATED CONDITIONS
- Seizures
- Hyperthermia
- Increased intracranial pressure (ICP)
- Inappropriate ADH

DIAGNOSIS

- Seek epidemiologic clues and assess risk factors in all patients with encephalitis (1)[A].
- Consider acute disseminated encephalomyelitis (ADEM) with history of recent infectious illness or vaccination associated with clinical presentation of encephalitis (2)[B].
- Specific diagnostic studies should be done in the majority of patients (see testing section) (2)[A].

HISTORY
General and specific neurological findings may include headache, fever, nausea/vomiting, altered consciousness

PHYSICAL EXAM
- General signs:
  - Rash
  - Mucus membrane lesions
  - Concurrent or prodromal upper respiratory findings
  - Parotitis
  - Erythema nodosum
- Neurologic findings:
  - Altered level of consciousness
  - Acute cognitive dysfunction
  - Behavioral changes
  - Neck stiffness
  - Focal neurologic signs
  - Motor weakness
- Other:
  - Loss of temperature or vasomotor control
  - Diabetes insipidus
  - Syndrome of inappropriate secretion of antidiuretic hormone

DIAGNOSTIC TESTS & INTERPRETATION
Lab
- Recommended general diagnostic studies for all suspected encephalitis patients (diagnostic studies outside of the CNS):
  - Blood cultures (2)[B]
  - Serum samples: Should be obtained at time of initial presentation and stored for future studies
- Additional studies based on risk factors and clinical findings may include:
  - Cultures of stool, nasopharynx, sputum (2)[B]
  - Skin scrapings of active vesicles (DFA testing to identify viral antigen)
  - Biopsy of specific tissues with culture, antigen detection, nucleic acid amplification testing and histology (2)[A]
  - Serologic testing: IgM antibodies (2)[A], IgM and IgG capture ELISAs
  - Plaque reduction neutralization
  - Acute and convalescent-phase serum to show seroconversion: Not helpful to initiate therapy but may be helpful for the retrospective diagnosis of a specific pathogen (2)[B]
  - Serum IgG antibodies should be considered in patients where the encephalitis may be the result of reactivation of a previously acquired infection.
  - Nucleic acid amplification tests (such as PCR) (2)[B]

Initial lab tests
- Lumbar puncture is essential (unless specific contraindication) (2)[A]:
  - CSF shows pleocytosis (10–2,000 cells/mm³). Mononuclear cells usually predominate. Finding of CSF eosinophils may suggest certain pathogens (e.g., highest with helminths but can also be seen with other pathogens).
  - CSF glucose normal or mildly depressed
  - CSF protein usually mild or moderately increased
  - Direct examination of CSF fluid with Gram stain for bacteria, acid fast stain for *Mycobacteria*, by India ink for *Cryptococcus*, wet preparation for free living amoeba, Giemsa stain for trypanosomes
  - CSF culture for bacteria, mycobacteria, fungi, amoeba, and viruses
  - CSF culture for viruses has limited value; not routinely recommended
  - CSF nucleic acid amplification tests (e.g., PCR) (2)[A]; herpes simplex PCR should be performed on all specimens (2)[A]; if negative, consider repeat in 3–7 days in those with compatible clinical syndrome or temporal lobe localization on neuroimaging (2)[B]
  - Viral-specific IgM (2)[A]
- In up to 10% of cases with viral encephalitis, CSF findings are normal.

Follow-Up & Special Considerations
- PCR may be negative early on; repeat in 48–72 hours; may be useful in detecting herpesvirus, enterovirus, seasonal and 2009 H1N1 influenza virus, and polyomavirus.
- Rapid Influenza Diagnostic Tests (RIDTs) may be helpful in diagnosing seasonal and 2009 H1N1 in a clinically useful time frame. However, their sensitivity ranges from 10–70% and the currently available RIDTs cannot distinguish between the different influenza A subtypes (seasonal H1N1 vs. 2009 H1N1 vs H3N2).

Imaging
Initial approach
- MRI: Most sensitive and most specific; however, in some cases it may be normal either initially or during clinical course (3)[A].
- Diffusion-weighted imaging is superior to conventional MRI in encephalitis caused by herpes simplex, enterovirus, and West Nile virus.
- FLAIR (fluid attenuated inversion recovery) imaging may be helpful with enterovirus 71 encephalitis, flaviviruses, and Eastern equine encephalitis.
- CT, with and without contrast enhancement, if MRI not an option (2)[B]
- FDG-PET not routinely recommended, but may be helpful as an adjunct diagnostic tool

Follow-Up & Special Considerations
Imaging studies (e.g., CT, MRI, brain scan) may be normal early; later, nonspecific abnormalities may be seen (exception: herpes simplex encephalitis).

Diagnostic Procedures/Surgery
- CXR may be helpful
- EEG is nondiagnostic but may be useful in early herpes simplex encephalitis and less commonly in other herpes viruses (VAV, EBV, HHV6). It is recommended for all patients with encephalitis (2)[A].
- Serologic testing
- Brain biopsy: Rarely used and not routinely recommended. Consider in patients with encephalitis of unknown etiology whose condition is deteriorating despite treatment with acyclovir (2)[B].

Pathological Findings
- Prominent inflammatory reaction in meninges and in a perivascular distribution
- Swelling and degenerative changes of neural elements

DIFFERENTIAL DIAGNOSIS
- Vasculitis
- Paraneoplastic syndromes
- Postinfectious encephalitis
- Postimmunization encephalitis
- ADEM
- Secondary encephalopathy

TREATMENT
- Most will require intensive care.
- Initial empiric therapy includes prompt administration of intravenous acyclovir (unless there is a contraindication).
- When appropriate, combine with appropriate therapy for bacterial, rickettsial, or ehrlichial infection.
- Once an etiologic agent has been identified, therapeutic intervention should be reevaluated, focusing on pathogen-specific therapy and discontinuing therapy if there is no available therapy against the specific etiologic agent.

MEDICATION
- No specific drug therapy is available for most types of viral encephalitis.
- Antiviral agents are available for encephalitides caused by herpes viruses, especially HSV, and for both seasonal and 2009 H1N1 influenza viruses.
- Acyclovir is recommended as initial treatment for all patients with suspected encephalitis as soon as possible, pending results of diagnostic studies (2)[A].
- Appropriate antiviral therapy (i.e., Oseltamivir or Zanamivir) should be started as soon as possible for hospitalized patients with neurologic symptoms and suspected seasonal or 2009 H1N1 influenza infection (4)[C].
- Empiric antimicrobial therapy should be initiated if indicated by the clinical history or specific epidemiologic factors (2)[A].
- Doxycycline should be added to empiric regimen when clinical clues suggest rickettsial or ehrlichial infection (2)[A].
- Once etiology is determined, treat specifically.

ADDITIONAL TREATMENT
General Measures
- Supportive therapy
- Monitoring for drug-related toxicities

Issues for Referral
- Monitoring and management of ICP
- Evaluation and treatment of seizures
- Multidisciplinary teams often provide care.

Additional Therapies
Adjunctive agents: Limited data; consider risks and benefits; infectious disease consultation should be considered.
- IFN alpha: Tried with West Nile virus encephalitis; results inconclusive
- IFN alpha 2b (limited series): Reduce severity and duration of complications of St. Louis *encephalitis virus meningoencephalitis* (further studies are necessary).
- Intravenous immunoglobulin containing high anti–West Nile virus antibody titers in patients with West Nile virus nueroinvasive disease (in trial)

SURGERY/OTHER PROCEDURES
The following procedures may be required during stabilization and care:
- Intracranial pressure monitor
- Intubation
- Mechanical ventilation
- Central line for hemodynamic monitoring
- Arterial line
- Central line for total parenteral nutrition
- Nasogastric tube placement
- Foley catheter placement

IN-PATIENT CONSIDERATIONS
- Admit suspected cases of encephalitis to hospital for evaluation, supportive care, and treatment. Most will require intensive care services.
- Although standard isolation precautions are appropriate for most viral encephalitides, droplet precautions are necessary for patients with confirmed or suspected seasonal or 2009 H1N1 influenza infection.

Initial Stabilization
- Protect airway when appropriate.
- When indicated:
  – Supplemental oxygen
  – Intubation and mechanical ventilatory support
- Assessment and management of circulatory status, fluids, glucose, and electrolytes
- Precautions for seizure and altered mental status
- Consider isolation for immunosuppressed patients and those with exanthems.

Admission Criteria
- Suspicion of encephalitis
- Altered level of consciousness
- Need for intensive monitoring
- Need for airway protection, cardiopulmonary support

IV Fluids
- Monitor glucose, chemistries, and fluid balance
- Monitor for SIADH
- Monitor for drug-specific toxicities

Nursing
- Isolation should be considered for immunosuppressed patients and those with exanthems.
- Precautions for seizure and altered mental status
- Comfort measures to reduce headache
- Injury prevention and safety
- Monitor level of consciousness, neurologic signs, cardiorespiratory parameters, and fluid balance.
- Establish and maintain open lines of communication with patient and family.

- Educate families about the importance of vaccines when available and postexposure prophylaxis for seasonal or 2009 H1N1 influenza virus.
- Skin care to prevent decubitus ulcers

Discharge Criteria
Resolution of acute symptoms:
- No longer need hospital-level care
- Outpatient services in place if needed

 ONGOING CARE

Patients with suspected or proven encephalitis are best cared for, at least initially, in an intensive care unit.

FOLLOW-UP RECOMMENDATIONS
- Postencephalitis sequelae are primarily neurologic, and follow-up should be guided by patient's condition (e.g., anticonvulsants for seizures).
- Physical therapy may be necessary.

Patient Monitoring
Postencephalitis patients should be followed carefully after discharge. Specialty services and follow-up may be required.

DIET
Guided by clinical condition

PATIENT EDUCATION
- DEET-containing mosquito repellants
- Avoidance of outdoor activities during periods of peak mosquito activity
- Use of protective clothing
- Adequate vector control and environmental sanitation
- Vaccines when available
- http://www.mayoclinic.com/health/encephalitis/DS00226

PROGNOSIS
Often difficult to predict; prognosis related to etiologic agent, age, and clinical course

COMPLICATIONS
Vary with age, etiologic agent, and clinical course

REFERENCES
1. Hinson VK, Tyor WR. Update on viral encephalitis. *Curr Opin Neurol*. 2001;14:369–74.
2. Mandell G, et al. *Principles & Practice of Infectious Diseases*, 6th ed. New York: Elsevier, 2005: 1143–7.
3. Chaudhuri A, Kennedy PG. Diagnosis and treatment of viral encephalitis. *Postgrad Med J*. 2002;78:575–83.
4. CDC. Neurologic Complications Associated with Novel Influenza A (H1N1) Virus Infection in Children — Dallas, Texas, May 2009. *MMWR* 2009;58:773–8.

 CODES

ICD9
049.9 Unspecified non-arthropod-borne viral diseases of central nervous system

CLINICAL PEARLS
- Neurologic signs are unlikely to distinguish etiologies, but location and type of skin lesions may be helpful.
- Think of ADEM if there is a history of recent mild viral illness.

E

ENCOPRESIS

Jay Gar-Yee Fong, MD
William T. Garrison, PhD

 BASICS

DESCRIPTION
- The involuntary or intentional passage of feces into clothing or other inappropriate places by a child 4–18 years of age:
  - Age may be chronologic or developmental.
  - Absence of underlying organic process explaining these symptoms
  - At least 1 event per month for 3 months
  - Classified into functional constipation (retentive encopresis) and functional nonretentive fecal incontinence (FNRFI): Both cause fecal incontinence, but no constipation in FNRFI. Functional constipation more common.
- System(s) affected: GI; Psychological
- Synonym(s): Fecal incontinence

EPIDEMIOLOGY
Incidence
Predominant sex: Male > Female (3:1). Constipation accounts for 3% of general pediatric referrals; up to 84% of constipated children have fecal incontinence at some point.

Prevalence
1–3% of children >4 years of age

RISK FACTORS
- Male gender
- Constipation
- Very low birth weight
- Painful defecation
- Difficulty with bowel training, including pressure related to early daycare placement
- Organic/anatomic causes
- Anxiety and depression

Genetics
None known, although incidence may be higher in children with family history of constipation

GENERAL PREVENTION
Family education regarding constipation, avoid toilet training prior to readiness, optimal feeding, early detection of problems. Look for signs of relapse: Large-caliber stools, decrease in stool frequency, and soiling.

PATHOPHYSIOLOGY
- In 90% of cases, encopresis develops as a consequence of chronic constipation with resulting overflow incontinence, which typically is termed *retentive encopresis*. The other 10% are caused by specific organic etiologies.
- Chronic constipation due to irregular and incomplete evacuation results in progressive rectal distension and stretching of both the internal and external anal sphincters.
- As the child habituates to chronic rectal distension, he or she may no longer sense the normal urge to defecate. Eventually, soft or liquid stool begins to leak around the retained fecal mass, resulting in fecal soiling.
- Many children voluntarily withhold stool in response to the urge to defecate for fear of pain.

ETIOLOGY
- Psychological:
  - Stool withholding, fear, anxiety
  - Difficulty with toilet training, including unusual anxiety or conflict with parent
  - Resistance to using public toilet facilities, such as school bathrooms or outdoor toilets
  - Known association with sexual abuse in boys; likely similar association in girls as well
  - Developmental delay
- Anatomic:
  - Rectal distension and desensitization
  - Anal fissure or painful defecation
  - Muscle hypotonia
  - Slow intestinal motility
  - Hirschsprung disease
  - Cystic fibrosis
  - Spinal cord defects, e.g., spina bifida
  - Congenital anorectal malformations
  - Anal stenosis
  - Anterior displacement of the anus
  - Postoperative stricture of anus or rectum
  - Pelvic mass
  - Neurofibromatosis
- Dietary or metabolic:
  - Lack of fiber
  - Excessive protein or milk intake
  - Inadequate water intake
  - Hypothyroidism
  - Hypercalcemia
  - Hypokalemia
  - DI or DM
  - Food allergy
  - Gluten enteropathy
- Medication side effects

COMMONLY ASSOCIATED CONDITIONS
- Constipation (common)
- Developmental and behavioral diagnoses
- Cerebral palsy (intermediate)
- Cystic fibrosis (intermediate)
- Hirschsprung disease (common)
- Urinary incontinence

 DIAGNOSIS

HISTORY
- Look for signs/symptoms of constipation:
  - Hard, large-caliber stools
  - <3 defecations/week
  - Pain or discomfort with stool passage, withholding of stool
  - Blood on stools
  - Decreased appetite
  - Abdominal pain improving with stool passage
  - Hiding while defecating before child is toilet trained; avoiding use of the toilet
  - Diet low in fiber or fluids, high in dairy
  - Passed stool within 1st 48 h of life
  - Pasty stool found on underclothes
  - Recurrent UTIs
- Abrupt onset after age 5 years more likely to be associated with psychological trauma
- Overlap with ADD common in children >5 years of age
- Medications such as opiates, phenobarbital, and TCAs
- Family history of constipation

PHYSICAL EXAM
- Detailed history and physical exam usually make the diagnosis without need for lab testing.
- Neurologic exam of lower extremities and perineal area with attention to S1–S4 distribution, perineal sensation, cremasteric reflex, and anal sphincter tone
- Genital area
- Digital rectal exam: Assess for anal fissures, sphincter tone, rectal distension/impaction, presence of occult or visible blood
- Abdominal exam: Mild abdominal distension; palpable stool in left lower quadrant.

DIAGNOSTIC TESTS & INTERPRETATION
Lab
Most cases of fecal incontinence do not require extensive lab work.

Initial lab tests
Done to rule out organic causes when conventional treatment fails: UA/urine culture: UTI/glucosuria; Thyroid function tests: Hypothyroidism; electrolyte panel including calcium may show hypokalemia, hypercalcemia, or hyperglycemia

Follow-Up & Special Considerations
Failure to pass meconium within 48 h of birth, failure to thrive, bloody diarrhea, or bilious vomiting in neonate is almost always associated with aganglionic megacolon, and that history would warrant a barium enema and/or rectal biopsy. Constipation and diarrhea, rash, failure to thrive, or recurrent pneumonia should prompt evaluation for cystic fibrosis. Celiac disease should also be a consideration. Patients with abdominal distension or ileus should be evaluated for possible obstruction.

Imaging
Abdominal plain films may be useful if an impaction is suspected but not detected by abdominal or rectal exam.

Initial approach
Comprehensive history and physical exam. Management includes education, disimpaction if necessary, prevention, and follow-up.

Diagnostic Procedures/Surgery
Manometric studies may be useful in patients who have constipation that does not respond to treatment.

 TREATMENT

A treatment approach that integrates both laxative treatment and behavioral therapy improves continence in children with fecal incontinence over laxative treatment alone (1).

MEDICATION
- Remove stool impaction, then start maintenance treatment program.
- No randomized, controlled studies have compared methods of disimpaction: Can use oral agents, enemas, and rectal suppositories; oral agents least traumatic. Glycerin suppositories best option for infants.

First Line
- Disimpaction with PEG has been shown to be more effective than lactulose in 1 study (2)[B]:

– Give 17 g (240 mL) water or juice: 1–1.5 g/kg/d × 3 days for disimpaction
– 0.26–0.084 g/kg/d for maintenance

- Disimpaction with mineral oil for child >1 year also effective; give 15–30 mL/year of age to maximum of 240 mL:
  – Maintenance: 1–3 mL/kg/d or divided b.i.d.
  – May mix with orange juice to make palatable; *avoid in infants to avoid aspiration and lipoid pneumonia*
- Other maintenance regimens include:
  – Milk of magnesia (MOM) 400 mg (5 mL): 103 mL/kg/d b.i.d. (3)[A]
  – Lactulose 10 g (15 mL) 1–3 mL/kg/d b.i.d.
  – Senna syrup 8.8 g sennoside (5 mL): Age 2–6 years: 2.5–7.5 mL/d b.i.d.; age 6–12 years: 5–15 mL/d b.i.d.
  – Bisacodyl suppository 10 mg: 0.5–1 suppository once or twice per day

Second Line
Another disimpaction protocol is as follows:
- Give 1 oz (28.4 g) of mineral oil the 1st day.
- On the next day, give 1–3 enemas until clear; this may be repeated over the next 1–2 days.
- Give an oil-retention enema.
- Follow the oil-retention enema with hypophosphate enemas (e.g., sodium phosphate [Fleet] 1 oz [28.4 g] per 20 lb [9.1 kg]) of body weight *or*
- Normal saline enemas: 2 tsp table salt/qt (946 mL) of warm water, and give 2 oz (60 mL)/year of age to a maximum of 16 oz (480 mL)

ADDITIONAL TREATMENT
General Measures
- Anticipatory guidance relative to toilet training beginning at 18 months, with special attention to when children should reduce reliance on diapers or pull-ups during the daytime hours
- Eliminate impaction prior to maintenance Rx.
- Avoid frequent and repeated rectal exams, enemas, and suppositories, especially in infants.
- Once stools seem regular in frequency, child should sit on toilet b.i.d. at the same time each day for 10–15 minutes and for 10–15 minutes after meals. Incorporate positive reinforcement for successfully produced bowel movements.

Issues for Referral
If symptoms do not improve after 6 months of good compliance with a multifactorial treatment model, refer to pediatric GI for further evaluation.

Additional Therapies
Behavioral treatment and counseling

COMPLEMENTARY AND ALTERNATIVE MEDICINE
- Behavioral treatment is recommended as an adjunct to medical therapy in children with functional constipation (4)[A].
- Children who receive behavioral treatment in addition to medications are more likely to have resolution of encopresis at 3 and 6 months than children who get medication alone.
- Biofeedback is not recommended because it does not improve outcomes when it is combined with medical therapy for functional constipation in children (1)[B].

SURGERY/OTHER PROCEDURES
Some children who have ongoing constipation that is refractory to a combination of medical and behavioral therapy should be considered for evaluation with anorectal manometry to evaluate for internal anal sphincter achalasia (or ultrashort-segment Hirschsprung's disease). If present, this condition can be treated successfully in the majority of patients with an internal sphincter myectomy.

IN-PATIENT CONSIDERATIONS
Initial Stabilization
Hospital admission and abdominal films may be necessary to ensure complete removal of impaction. This may include gastric administration of balanced electrolyte–polyethylene glycol solutions if the patient cannot tolerate the medication by mouth. Serial abdominal films as well as careful observation of the rectal effluent can help to determine when the patient is adequately treated.

Admission Criteria
Admission criteria should include:
- Continued soiling and recurrent impaction on outpatient medical therapy, whether from lack of medication efficacy or patient medication nonadherence
- Decreased p.o. intake for fluid and food
- Vomiting or obstructive-type symptoms

IV Fluids
IV fluids should be considered when the pediatric patient is heading toward dehydration while undergoing bowel cleanout.

Nursing
Nursing is essential to observing and documenting the stool consistency and clarity.

Discharge Criteria
Stools that are becoming more loose in consistency and clear in appearance would signify a successful inpatient endpoint for discharge consideration. In addition, an abdominal radiograph that shows much less fecal loading as compared with a pretreatment radiograph in combination with serial abdominal exams can provide additional evidence that the patient is ready for discharge.

ONGOING CARE
FOLLOW-UP RECOMMENDATIONS
Patient Monitoring
- Continue the maintenance treatment program for at least 6 months, possibly 1–2 years.
- Visits every 4–10 weeks for support and to ensure compliance; more often with oppositional or anxious children.
- Telephone availability to adjust doses and to provide continued encouragement to caregivers
- Treat redevelopment of impaction promptly.
- Chief target behaviors in a behavior plan for such children include compliance with medication, compliance with sits, and self-initiation of bathroom visits.
- Children who do not progress with a well-designed behavior plan should be referred for more in-depth mental health evaluation and counseling.

DIET
Hydration, high fiber, decrease or avoid cow's milk products if a trial shows this to be helpful. Avoid excessive bananas, rice, apples, and gelatin.

PATIENT EDUCATION
- Education and demystifying of the process
- Careful and full explanation of the treatment plan and dietary changes
- Avoid punishment for soiling.

- In children >4 years of age, explain to parents how overreliance on diapers and pull-ups, while convenient, can prolong the problem.
- Always attempt to use positive reinforcement 1st for successful toilet sits and medication compliance.
- If positive approach is unsuccessful, consider removing daily desired privileges (e.g., TV, video games, time with friends, etc.) for noncompliance with behavioral plan. Some children respond better to use of a token economy (chips or tickets to earn privileges the child desires).

PROGNOSIS
- Initial good response with a high relapse rate due to noncompliance by parents and/or child
- Depending on the study, anywhere from 30–50% of children still may have encopresis after 5 years of treatment.
- Children with psychosocial or emotional problems that preceded the encopresis are more recalcitrant to treatment.

COMPLICATIONS
- Colitis due to excessive enema/suppository
- Perianal dermatitis
- Anal fissure

REFERENCES
1. Brazzelli M, et al. Behavioural and cognitive interventions with or without other treatments for the management of faecal incontinence in children. *Cochrane Database Syst Rev.* 2008;3:CD002240.
2. Loening-Baucke V, Pashankar DS. A randomized, prospective, comparison study of polyethylene glycol 3350 without electrolytes and milk of magnesia for children with constipation and fecal incontinence. *Pediatrics.* 2006;118:528–35.
3. Baker S, et al. Evaluation and the treatment of constipation in infants and children: Recommendation of the north American Society for Pediatric Gastroenterology, Hepatology, and Nutrition. *J Pediatr Gastroenterol Nutr.* 2006; 43e1–13.
4. Borowitz SM, et al. Treatment of childhood encopresis: A randomized trial comparing 3 treatment protocols. *J Ped Gastroenterol Nutr.* 2002;34:378–84.

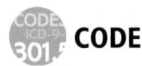 ## CODES

ICD9
- 307.7 Encopresis
- 787.60 Full incontinence of feces
- 787.62 Fecal smearing

CLINICAL PEARLS

Most children (84%) with constipation have some fecal incontinence, but diagnosis of encopresis requires at least 1 event per month for 3 months. 90% of encopresis results from chronic constipation. Address toddler constipation early (decrease excessive milk intake, increase fruits/vegetables) to avoid future issues.

E

ENDOCARDITIS, INFECTIVE

William L. Marshall, MD

 BASICS

DESCRIPTION
- An infection primarily of the valvular endocardium; and occasionally, the mural endocardium
- System(s) affected: Cardiovascular; Endocrine/Metabolic; Hematologic/Lymphatic; Immunologic; Pulmonary; Renal/Urologic; Skin/Exocrine; Neurologic
- Synonym(s): Bacterial endocarditis; Subacute bacterial endocarditis; Acute bacterial endocarditis

EPIDEMIOLOGY
Incidence
In the US: 1.5–6.2/100,000

Geriatric Considerations
- Incidence increased in the elderly
- Cumulative rate of endocarditis at 1 year after prosthetic valve replacement: 1.5–3.0%
- At 5 years: 3–6%
- Highest risk during 6-month period following valve replacement

RISK FACTORS
- Injection drug use
- IV catheterization
- Certain malignancies (colon cancer)
- High-risk cardiac conditions:
  - Prosthetic cardiac valve
  - Previous infective endocarditis (IE)
  - Congenital heart disease (CHD):
    - Unrepaired cyanotic CHD, including palliative shunts and conduits
    - Repaired CHD with prosthetic device during the prior 6 months
    - Repaired CHD with residual defects at or near the site of prosthetic material
    - Cardiac transplantation recipients who develop valvulopathy (1)[B]

GENERAL PREVENTION
- Maintain good oral hygiene.
- Antibiotic prophylaxis is now only recommended for people with cardiac conditions predicting the highest risk of adverse outcome from IE (1).
- Procedures requiring prophylaxis:
  - Oral/upper respiratory tract: Manipulation of gingival tissue or periapical region of teeth or perforation of the oral mucosa (1)[C], invasive respiratory procedures involving incision, or biopsy of the respiratory mucosa:
    - Prophylaxis for dental/oral procedures (1)[C]
  - Amoxicillin: 2 g PO (if penicillin-allergic, clindamycin 600 mg PO) 30–60 min before procedure
  - Alternative: Ampicillin 2 g IV/IM (penicillin-allergic patients, clindamycin 600 mg IV), or
  - Cephalexin 2 g PO, or
  - Azithromycin/clarithromycin 500 mg PO, or
  - Cefazolin/ceftriaxone 1 g IV/IM 30 minutes before procedure
  - Pediatric doses: Amoxicillin 50 mg/kg PO; cephalexin 50 mg/kg PO; clindamycin 20 mg/kg PO; and ampicillin or ceftriaxone 50 mg/kg IM/IV
  - GI/GU: Only consider coverage for enterococcus (with penicillin, ampicillin, piperacillin, or vancomycin) for patients with an established infection undergoing procedures (1)[B].

- Cardiac valvular surgery or placement of prosthetic intracardiac/intravascular materials (1)[B], perioperative prophylaxis with cefazolin 1–2 g IV 30 min preop, or vancomycin 15 mg/kg 60 min preop in the penicillin-allergic patient
- Skin: Incision and drainage of infected tissue; patients should receive treatment with agents active against skin pathogens, e.g., cefazolin 1–2 g IV q8h or vancomycin 15 mg/kg q12h in the penicillin-allergic patient or where MRSA is suspected.

ETIOLOGY
- Acute endocarditis:
  - Gram-positive: *Staphylococcus aureus*; *Streptococcus* groups A, B, C, G; *Streptococcus pneumoniae*; *Staphylococcus lugdunensis*; *Enterococcus* spp.
  - Gram-negative: *Haemophilus influenzae* or *parainfluenzae*; *Neisseria gonorrhoeae*
- Subacute endocarditis:
  - Gram-positive: α-Hemolytic streptococci (Viridans group strep), *Streptococcus bovis*, *Enterococcus* spp., *S. aureus*, *Staphylococcus epidermidis*
  - HACEK organisms: **H**aemophilus aphrophilus or paraprophilus, **A**ctinobacillus actinomycetemcomitans, **C**ardiobacterium hominis, **E**ikenella corrodens, **K**ingella kingae
- Endocarditis in IV drug abusers (tricuspid valve):
  - Gram-positive: *S. aureus*, *Enterococcus* spp.
  - Gram-negative: *Pseudomonas aeruginosa*, *Burkholderia cepacia*, other bacilli
  - *Candida* spp.
- Early prosthetic-valve endocarditis (<60 days after valve implantation):
  - Gram-positive: *S. aureus*, *Staphylococcus epidermidis*
  - Gram-negative bacilli
  - Fungi: *Candida* spp., *Aspergillus* spp.
- Late prosthetic-valve endocarditis (>60 days after valve implantation):
  - Gram-positive: α-Hemolytic streptococci, *Enterococcus* spp., *S. epidermidis*
  - Fungi: *Candida* spp., *Aspergillus* spp.
- Culture-negative endocarditis:
  - *Bartonella quintana* (homeless people)
  - *Bartonella henselae* (cat owners)
  - Fastidious organism: *Brucella* spp., fungi, *Coxiella burnetii* (Q fever), *Chlamydia trachomatis*, *Chlamydia psittaci*, HACEK organisms
  - Use of antibiotics prior to blood cultures
  - *Abiotrophia* (formerly B6 deficient streptococci)

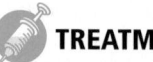 **DIAGNOSIS**

- Modified Duke Criteria for Diagnosis of IE (2)[B] (definite: 2 major criteria, or 1 major and 3 minor criteria, or 5 minor criteria; possible: 1 major and 1 minor criteria, or 3 minor criteria)

- Major clinical criteria:
  - Positive blood culture:
    - Typical microorganism for infective endocarditis (viridans strep., *S. aureus*, or community-acquired *Enterococcus*) from 2 separate blood cultures, or
    - Persistently positive blood culture
  - Single positive blood culture for *C. burnetii* or anti–phase-1 IgG antibody titer >1:800

- Positive transesophageal echocardiogram recommended with prosthetic valves and "possible IE," or with complicated IE):
  - Oscillating mass on valve or supporting structures, in the path of regurgitant jets, on implanted material, or
  - Periannular abscess, or
  - New partial dehiscence of prosthetic valve
  - New valvular regurgitation (change in preexisting murmur not sufficient)
- Minor criteria:
  - Predisposing heart condition or IV-drug use
  - Fever ≥38.0°C (100.4°F)
  - Vascular phenomena: Major arterial emboli, septic pulmonary infarcts, mycotic aneurysm, intracranial hemorrhage, conjunctival hemorrhage, Janeway lesions
  - Immunologic phenomena: Glomerulonephritis, Osler nodes, Roth spots, rheumatoid factor
  - Microbiologic evidence: Positive blood culture, but not of major criterion (excluding single positive cultures for coagulase-negative staphylococci and organisms that do not cause endocarditis) or serologic evidence of infection with an organism likely to cause infective endocarditis

DIAGNOSTIC TESTS & INTERPRETATION
Lab
- Positive blood cultures drawn >2 hours apart
- Leukocytosis in acute endocarditis
- Anemia in subacute endocarditis
- Elevated ESR, CRP
- Decreased C3, C4, CH50 in subacute endocarditis
- Hematuria, microscopic or macroscopic
- Rheumatoid factor in subacute endocarditis
- Consider serologies for *Chlamydia*, Q fever, and *Bartonella* in "culture-negative" endocarditis.

Imaging
- Transthoracic or transesophageal echocardiogram
- CT scan may be useful in locating abscesses (e.g., splenic abscess).

Pathological Findings
- Vegetations are composed of platelets, fibrin, and colonies of microorganisms. Destruction of valvular endocardium, perforation of valve leaflets, rupture of chordae tendineae, abscesses of myocardium, rupture of sinus of Valsalva, and pericarditis may occur.
- Emboli, infarction, abscesses, and/or infarction may be found in any organ.
- Immune-complex glomerulonephritis

DIFFERENTIAL DIAGNOSIS
- Marantic endocarditis; Connective tissue diseases; Fever of unknown origin
- Intra-abdominal infections; Rheumatic fever; Salmonellosis
- Malignancy; Tuberculosis; Atrial myxoma; Septic thrombophlebitis; Infected central venous catheter

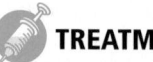 **TREATMENT**

MEDICATION
First Line
- PCN-susceptible Viridans group streptococci or *S. bovis*, native valve:
  - Pen G 12–18 million U/d IV either continuously or in 4–6 equally divided doses *or* ceftriaxone 2 g/d IV/IM in 1 dose, both for 4 weeks (3)[A]

- For prosthetic valve infection, Pen G 24 million units/d IV either continuously or 4–6 equally divided doses for 6 weeks or ceftriaxone 2 g/d IV/IM in 1 dose ± gentamicin 3 mg/kg IV/IM q24h for 2 weeks (peak gentamicin level 3 mcg/ml and trough <1 mcg/ml)
- PCN-resistant Viridans group streptococci or *S. bovis,* native valve:
  - Pen G 24 million U/d IV either continuously or in 6 equally divided doses or ceftriaxone 2 g/d IV/IM in 1 dose for 4 weeks plus gentamicin 3 mg/kg IV/IM q24h for 2 weeks (peak gentamicin level 3 mcg/ml and trough <1 mcg/ml) (3)[B]
  - Regimen for prosthetic valve infection is equivalent, but length of therapy is 6 weeks for all antibiotics.
- *Staphylococcus* on native valve:
  - Oxacillin-sensitive: Oxacillin or nafcillin 2 g IV q4h for 4–6 weeks. Use of gentamicin 1 mg/kg q8h IV/IM for the 1st 3–5 days does not improve survival and increases the chance of nephrotoxicity (4).
  - Oxacillin-resistant: Vancomycin 15 mg/kg/d IV q12h for 6 weeks for goal trough of 15–20 mcg/ml (3)[B]
- Daptomycin may also be considered for continued outpatient therapy (5).
- *Staphylococcus* of prosthetic valve:
  - Oxacillin-sensitive: Oxacillin or nafcillin 12 g/d IV in 6 equally divided doses plus rifampin 300 mg IV/PO q8h, for 6 weeks, plus gentamicin 1 mg/kg q8h IV/IM for the 1st 2 weeks (peak gentamicin level 3 mcg/ml and trough <1 mcg/ml) (3)[B]
  - Oxacillin-resistant: Vancomycin 15 mg/kg IV q12h, plus rifampin 300 mg IV/PO q8h, both for 6 weeks, plus gentamicin 3 mg/kg/d IV/IM in 2–3 doses for the 1st 2 weeks (peak gentamicin level 3 mcg/ml and trough <1 mcg/ml) (3)[B]
- Pan-sensitive *Enterococcus,* native or prosthetic valve: Ampicillin 2g IV q4h OR Pen G 18–30 million units/d IV either continuously or in 6 equally divided doses, plus gentamicin 1 mg/kg IV q8h for 4–6 weeks (peak gentamicin level 3 mcg/ml and trough <1 mcg/ml) (3)[A] Consider expert consultation for resistant enterococci.
- HACEK organisms: Ceftriaxone 2 g IM or IV q24h for 4 weeks (3)[B] OR ampicillin-sulbactam 2g IV q6h for 4 weeks (3)[B] OR Ciprofloxacin 1 g/d PO or 800 mg/d IV in 2 equally divided doses for 4 weeks (3)[C]
- Precautions:
  - In patients with renal impairment, dosage adjustment should be made for penicillin G, gentamicin, cefazolin, ampicillin, ampicillin/sulbactam, ciprofloxacin, and vancomycin.
  - Rapid infusion of vancomycin <1 hour may cause "red-man syndrome; due to histamine release, not an allergic reaction; will disappear when rate of infusion is reduced.
- Significant possible interactions:
  - Vancomycin plus gentamicin increases renal toxicity.
  - Rifampin increases the requirement for Coumadin and oral hypoglycemic agents.

Second Line
For patients allergic to penicillin:

- Penicillin-susceptible or resistant Viridans group streptococci or *S. bovis:* Vancomycin 30 mg/kg (not to exceed 2 g/d) IV for 4 weeks (6 weeks for prosthetic valve endocarditis) for goal trough of 10–15 mcg/ml (3)[B]

- *Enterococcus,* native or prosthetic valve: Desensitization to penicillin should be considered. Vancomycin 15 mg/kg (usual dose, 1 g) IV q12h, plus gentamicin or streptomycin (peak gentamicin level 3 mcg/ml and trough <1 mcg/ml) for 4–6 weeks (6 weeks for prosthetic valve endocarditis) (3)[B].
- *Staphylococcus* of native valve: Cefazolin 2 g IV q8h (not to be used in patients with immediate-type hypersensitivity to penicillin) for 4–6 weeks (3)[B] OR vancomycin 30 mg/kg (usual dose, 1 g) IV q12h for a goal trough of 15–20 mcg/ml, for 6 weeks (3)[B]

SURGERY/OTHER PROCEDURES
Surgical therapy (i.e., valve replacement) should be considered for:

- CHF due to valve incompetence (3)[B]
- Embolic event in 1st 2 weeks of antibiotic therapy (3)[B] and stroke if hemorrhage has been excluded (6)[B]
- Persistent bacteremia after 1 week of antibiotic therapy or infection caused by resistant organisms (e.g., fungus, *Pseudomonasaeruginosa,* S. marcescens) (3)[B], *S. aureus* on a prosthetic valve, or most cases of relapsing IE (6)[B]
- Valve dehiscence, perforation, rupture or fistula, heart block, or large perivalvular abscess (3,7)[B]. Anterior mitral valve leaflet vegetation >10 mm in size, persistent vegetation after systemic embolization (3)[B], or increase in vegetation size despite antibiotic therapy (3,7)[C]
- Early prosthetic valve IE (6)[B]

ONGOING CARE

FOLLOW-UP RECOMMENDATIONS
Patient Monitoring
- Check gentamicin peak (~3 μg/mL) and trough (<1 μg/mL) levels if used for >5 days, and with renal dysfunction.
- Check vancomycin trough (15–20 μg/mL) levels in all patients (8)[B].
- Perform twice-weekly BUN and serum creatinine while on gentamicin.
- Consider audiometry baseline and follow-up during long-term aminoglycoside therapy.
- Baseline EKG, and monitor EKG for conduction disturbances/MI in initial weeks.
- TTE at the end of therapy
- Blood cultures q48h until negative

PROGNOSIS
Regardless of the mode of treatment, the mortality for IE remains high.

COMPLICATIONS
- Arterial emboli and infarcts (e.g., myocardial infarction, mesenteric, splenic, cerebral infarct)
- Infectious emboli (e.g., abscesses of heart, lung, brain, meninges, bone, pericardium)
- Inflammatory/immune disorders (e.g., arthritis, myositis, glomerulonephritis)
- Miscellaneous complications (e.g., CHF, ruptured valve cusp, sinus of Valsalva aneurysm, cardiac arrhythmia, intra- and extracranial mycotic aneurysms)

REFERENCES
1. Wilson W, et al. Prevention of infective endocarditis. Guidelines from the American Heart Association. A Guideline from the American Heart Association Rheumatic Fever, Endocarditis, and Kawasaki Disease Committee, Council on Cardiovascular Disease in the Young, and the Council on Cardiology, Council on Cardiovascular Surgery and Anesthesia, and the Quality of Care and Outcomes Research Interdisciplinary Working Group. *Circulation.* 2007; epub 19 Apr. 2007.
2. Li JS, Sexton DJ, Mick N, et al. Proposed modifications to the Duke criteria for the diagnosis of infective endocarditis. *Clin Infect Dis.* 2000;30:633–8.
3. Baddour LM, Wilson WR, Bayer AS, et al. Infective endocarditis: diagnosis, antimicrobial therapy, and management of complications: a statement for healthcare professionals from the Committee on Rheumatic Fever, Endocarditis, and Kawasaki Disease, Council on Cardiovascular Disease in the Young, and the Councils on Clinical Cardiology, Stroke, and Cardiovascular Surgery and Anesthesia, American Heart Association: endorsed by the Infectious Diseases Society of America. *Circulation.* 2005;111:e394–434.
4. Cosgrove SE, Vigliani GA, Campion M, et al. Initial Low-Dose Gentamicin for Staphylococcus aureus Bacteremia and Endocarditis Is Nephrotoxic. *Clin Infect Dis.* 2009.
5. Rehm S, Campion M, Katz DE, et al. Community-based outpatient parenteral antimicrobial therapy (CoPAT) for Staphylococcus aureus bacteraemia with or without infective endocarditis: analysis of the randomized trial comparing daptomycin with standard therapy. *J Antimicrob Chemother.* 2009.
6. Prendergast BD, Tornos P et al. Surgery for infective endocarditis: who and when? *Circulation.* 2010; 121:1141–52.
7. Paterick TE, Paterick TJ, Nishimura RA, et al. Complexity and subtlety of infective endocarditis. *Mayo Clin Proc.* 2007;82:615–21.
8. Rybak M, Lomaestro B, Rotschafer JC, et al. Therapeutic monitoring of vancomycin in adult patients: a consensus review of the American Society of Health-System Pharmacists, the Infectious Diseases Society of America, and the Society of Infectious Diseases Pharmacists. *Am J Health Syst Pharm.* 2009;66:82–98.

CODES

ICD9
421.0 Acute and subacute bacterial endocarditis

CLINICAL PEARLS
- Antibiotic prophylaxis is now only recommended for people with artificial heart valves, past history of IE, certain congenital heart diseases, and cardiac transplants with a heart-valve problem.
- Mitral valve prolapse by itself is no longer an indication for antibiotic prophylaxis.

E

ENDOMETRIAL CANCER AND UTERINE SARCOMA

Michael P. Hopkins, MD, MEd
Jonna M. Quinn, DO

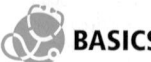 **BASICS**

DESCRIPTION
- Endometrial cancer: Malignancy of the endometrial lining of the uterus
  - Two types
    - I: estrogen dependent, lower grade, better prognosis
    - II: estrogen independent, higher grade, more aggressive
- Cell types: Adenocarcinoma, adenosquamous (malignant squamous elements), clear cell, and papillary serous
- Sarcomas: Malignancy of the uterine mesenchyme and mixed tumors:
  - Mixed müllerian sarcoma (carcinosarcoma): Heterologous sarcoma elements are not native to the müllerian system (e.g., cartilage or bone); homologous sarcoma elements are native to the müllerian system.
  - Endometrial stromal sarcoma develops from the stromal component of the endometrium.
  - Leiomyosarcoma develops in the myometrium or rarely in a myoma (fibroid).
  - Poorer prognosis
- Predominant age:
  - Endometrial cancer: The majority are postmenopausal
    - Median age: 66 years old
  - Sarcomas: Age 40–69 years old
- System(s): Reproductive
- Synonym(s): Uterine cancer; Endometrial cancer; Corpus cancer

Pregnancy Considerations
This malignancy is not associated with pregnancy.

EPIDEMIOLOGY
Incidence
- Most common gynecologic malignancy, 4th most common cancer in women, 8th leading cause of cancer-related death in women
- ~40,000 new cases per year and 7,000 deaths per year

Prevalence
500,000 women in the US

RISK FACTORS
- Early menarche/late menopause
- Nulliparity
- Personal or family history of colon or reproductive system cancer
- Obesity
- Diabetes mellitus
- Hypertension
- Polycystic ovarian syndrome
- Menstrual irregularities
- Endometrial hyperplasia
- Unopposed estrogens
- Tamoxifen
- Age
- Prior pelvic irradiation (sarcoma)

Genetics
- Endometrial: Lynch syndrome (hereditary nonpolyposis colorectal cancer)
- Sarcoma: African American

GENERAL PREVENTION
- In young women who are obese or anovulatory, the risk of endometrial cancer can be reduced by taking oral contraceptive pills, permanently losing weight, or taking cyclic progesterone to prevent unopposed estrogens effects on the uterus.
- Estrogen replacement therapy should always include progesterone unless the woman has undergone a hysterectomy.
- Cigarette smoking has been associated with a lower risk of endometrial cancer; however, it is not recommended secondary to its many health risks.

PATHOPHYSIOLOGY
Continuous estrogen stimulation unopposed by progesterone

ETIOLOGY
- Endometrial: Unopposed estrogen:
  - Estrogen replacement therapy without concomitant progesterone increases the risk. Addition of progesterone decreases risk to that of general population
- Sarcomas: Etiology unknown

COMMONLY ASSOCIATED CONDITIONS
- Endometrial Hyperplasia: 1–25% will progress to endometria adenocarcinoma
  - Simple without Atypia
  - Complex without Atypia
  - Simple with Atypia
  - Complex with Atypia
    - 43% with Complex Hyperplasia with Atypia have concurrent endometrial cancer
- Endometrial cancer patients should be screened regularly for breast and colon cancer because of an increased risk of these cancers.
- Patients who have breast or colon cancer are at increased risk for endometrial cancer.
- Granulosa cell tumors of the ovary produce estrogen; these patients will have an increased risk of endometrial cancer.

DIAGNOSIS

HISTORY
- Endometrial cancer:
  - Postmenopausal bleeding is the most frequent sign. Any spotting or abnormal discharge mandates evaluation.
- Sarcoma:
  - Mixed müllerian sarcoma: Bleeding and prolapsing tissue, pain
  - Leiomyosarcoma: Increasing size of presumed uterine myomas, pain

PHYSICAL EXAM
Pelvic exam: Enlarged uterus

DIAGNOSTIC TESTS & INTERPRETATION
Lab
Initial lab tests
- Liver and renal function tests
- Levels of cancer antigen 125 (CA-125) may be elevated when intra-abdominal disease is present.

Follow-Up & Special Considerations
- A biopsy of a pregnant uterus can produce tissue that looks hyperplastic or premalignant.
- Pap smear is rarely positive.

Imaging
Initial approach
- Transvaginal ultrasound usually shows increased endometrial thickness.
- CXR: Most common site of metastases is the lungs.
- Mammogram and colonoscopy: Endometrial cancer is associated with breast and colon cancer.

Follow-Up & Special Considerations
- CT scan, bone scan, liver spleen scan: Not part of the routine evaluation, but may be needed if suspected metastasis
- MRI has been reported to show the depth of myometrial penetration accurately but is not always cost effective.

Diagnostic Procedures/Surgery
- Office endometrial biopsy (90% accurate). If this is negative with high suspicion for cancer, a dilation and curettage is necessary. Endometrial stromal sarcoma and leiomyosarcoma are rarely diagnosed preoperatively.
- Fractional dilation and curettage is 99% accurate except in cases of sarcoma.
- Hysteroscopy may be associated with higher risk of positive washings/cytology – controversial

Pathological Findings
- Stage I (confined to corpus uteri):
  - A. No or less than half myometrial invasion
  - B. Invision equal to or more than half the myometrium
- Stage II: Tumor invades cervical stroma, but does not extend beyond the uterus
- Stage III: Local and/or regional spread
  - A. Uterine serosal and or adnexal invasion
  - B. Vaginal and/or parametrial involvement
  - C. Metastases to pelvic and/or para-aortic lymph nodes
    - IIIC1: +pelvic nodes
    - IIIC2: +para-aortic LN +/– positive pelvic lymph nodes
  - Stage IV: Tumor invades bladder and/or bowel mucosa, and or distant metastases
    - A. Tumor invades bladder and/or bowel mucosa,
    - B. Distant metastases, including intra-abdominal metastases and/or inguinal lymph nodes
- FIGO Staging System: revised 2009 (1)

DIFFERENTIAL DIAGNOSIS
- Atypical complex hyperplasia: A premalignant lesion of the endometrium
- Cervical cancer
- Ovarian cancer invading the uterus
- Endometriosis
- Adenomyosis

TREATMENT

MEDICATION

First Line

- Endometrial:
  - Chemotherapy for advanced or recurrent disease incurable with surgery and radiation (2,3)[A]:
    - Doxorubicin + Cisplatin + Paclitaxel
    - Paclitaxel + Carboplatin
  - Hormonal therapy:
    - Medroxyprogesterone acetate: For recurrence or metastases (2)[A]
    - Megestrol (Megace) 160 mg/d for 3 months for women with premalignant lesions, atypical complex hyperplasia, or well-differentiated endometrial cancer patients desiring fertility. Follow with dilation and curettage to determine cancer resolution.
    - Levonorgestrel containing IUD: As above for patients desiring future fertility
- Sarcoma:
  - Chemotherapy:
    - Doxorubicin as single-agent or in combination (4)[A]
  - Hormonal:
    - Tamoxifen or aromatase inhibitors- not fully studied
    - Progesterones

Second Line

Ondansetron (Zofran), dronabinol (Marinol), metoclopramide (Reglan), and others to control nausea from chemotherapy

ADDITIONAL TREATMENT

General Measures

- Main treatment for uterine cancer is surgery
- Radiation is used to prevent tumor recurrence at the vaginal cuff.

Issues for Referral

Patients should be referred to gynecologic oncologist, radiation oncologist, and medical oncologist as indicated.

Additional Therapies

Radiation therapy:

- Nonoperative candidates: Radiation therapy alone (5)[A]
- Low-risk: No adjuvant radiation therapy (5)[A]
- Intermediate-risk: Consider adjuvant vaginal brachytherapy. Reduces local recurrences but has no effect on overall survival (5)[A].
- High-risk: Chemotherapy and radiation therapy in some cases.

SURGERY/OTHER PROCEDURES

Surgical staging:

- Extrafascial hysterectomy and bilateral salpingo-oophorectomy
- Cytologic washings
- Pelvic and para-aortic lymph node dissection
- Omental sampling as indicated
- Optimal tumor debulking

Geriatric Considerations

Older (especially obese) patients may be at high risk for surgery. Alternative radiation therapy can be considered.

IN-PATIENT CONSIDERATIONS

Admission Criteria

- Excessive vaginal bleeding
- Preoperative stabilization

Nursing

Routine; ensure postoperative pain is controlled.

Discharge Criteria

Postsurgical criteria: Pain controlled, tolerating diet, ambulating, and voiding

ONGOING CARE

FOLLOW-UP RECOMMENDATIONS

Speculum and rectovaginal exam every 3–4 months for 2–3 years then every 6 months for 3 years then annually for life

Patient Monitoring

CXR annually

DIET

As tolerated and according to comorbidities

PATIENT EDUCATION

Following surgery:

- No intercourse for ~6 weeks
- No lifting >10–15 lbs
- No driving until pain free
- Do not expect resumption of full activity for 6 weeks.

PROGNOSIS

5-year survival rates:

- Uterine Adenocarcinoma

Stage	Survival (%)
IA	88
IB	75
II	69
IIIA	58
IIIB	50
IIIC	47
IVA	17
IVB	15

- Uterine Sarcoma

Stage	Survival (%)
I	70
II	45
III	30
IV	15

COMPLICATIONS

- Surgical: Excessive bleeding, wound infection, lymphedema, DVT, and damage to the urinary or intestinal systems
- Radiation: Diarrhea, ileus, bowel obstruction or fistula, radiation cystitis, proctitis, vaginal stenosis, DVT
- Chemotherapy: Per the drug given

REFERENCES

1. Creasman W. Revised FIGO staging for carcinoma of the endometrium. *Int J Gynaecol Obstet*. 2009; 105(2):109. Epub 2009 Apr 3. PubMed PMID: 19345353.
2. Polyzos NP, Pavlidis N, Paraskevaidis E, et al. Randomized evidence on chemotherapy and hormonal therapy regimens for advanced endometrial cancer: an overview of survival data. *Eur J Cancer*. 2006;42:319–26.
3. Fleming GF, Brunetto VL, Cella D, et al. Phase III trial of doxorubicin plus cisplatin with or without paclitaxel plus filgrastim in advanced endometrial carcinoma: a Gynecologic Oncology Group Study. *J Clin Oncol*. 2004;22:2159–66.
4. Bramwell VH, Anderson D, Charette ML, et al. Doxorubicin-based chemotherapy for the palliative treatment of adult patients with locally advanced or metastatic soft tissue sarcoma. *Cochrane Database Syst Rev*. 2003:CD003293.
5. Einhorn N, Tropé C, Ridderheim M., et al. A systematic overview of radiation therapy effects in uterine cancer (corpus uteri). *Acta Oncol*. 2003;42: 557–61.

ADDITIONAL READING

- American Cancer Society, 2010 http://www.cancer.org.
- American College of Obstetricians & Gynecologists (ACOG), http://www.acog.com.
- American College of Obstetricians and Gynecologists. ACOG practice bulletin, clinical management guidelines for obstetrician-gynecologists, number 65, August 2005: management of endometrial cancer. *Obstet Gynecol*. 2005;106:413–25.
- Gadducci A, Cosio S, Romanini A, et al. et al. The management of patients with uterine sarcoma: A debated clinical challenge. *Crit Rev Oncol Hematol*. 2007.
- Humber C, et al. Chemotherapy for advanced, recurrent or metastatic endometrial carcinoma. *Cochrane Database Syst Rev*. 2005;(4):CD003915.

See Also (Topic, Algorithm, Electronic Media Element)

Cervical Malignancy
Algorithm: Pelvic Pain

 CODES

ICD9

182.0 Malignant neoplasm of corpus uteri, except isthmus

CLINICAL PEARLS

- Most common presenting symptom is abnormal uterine bleeding.
- Primary cause is unopposed estrogen.
- Endometrial thickness on transvaginal ultrasound of less than 5 mm makes endometrial cancer very unlikely.
- Primary treatment is with surgery with possible chemotherapy ± radiation.

ENDOMETRIOSIS

Ginger Allister, MD
Julie Scott Taylor, MD, MSc

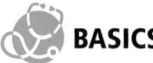

BASICS

DESCRIPTION
- Endometriosis is a common, recurring disease in females of reproductive age that may even persist into early menopause (1).
- Heterotopic islands of endometrial glands and stroma found outside the uterus:
  - Pelvic sites: Peritoneal surfaces (bladder, cul-de-sac, pelvic walls, ligaments, and fallopian tubes), vagina, cervix, lymph nodes, ovaries, bowel
  - Distant sites: Abdominal wall, spleen, gallbladder, stomach, nasal mucosa, spinal canal, lungs, breasts, diaphragm, pleura, pericardium
- Classified as peritoneal, ovarian, or deep endometriosis
- Staged according to the American Society for Reproductive Medicine surgical scoring system:
  - Based on disease severity: Extent and characteristics of endometrial implants and adhesions
  - Stage I (minimal) to IV (severe)
- System affected: Reproductive
- Synonym: Endometriosis externa

ALERT
Staging is useful in therapeutic planning but does not correlate with severity of pain or predict response to treatment for symptoms or infertility.

EPIDEMIOLOGY
Incidence
- Affects 0.5–5% of fertile women
- Found in 30-50% of infertile women (2)
- Found in 50-60% of women and adolescent females with pelvic pain (3)

Pediatric Considerations
Endometriosis may begin with puberty, causing debilitating pelvic pain and severe dysmenorrhea associated with missed school, social, and family activities.

Pregnancy Considerations
Pelvic endometriosis is generally ameliorated with pregnancy, but infertility is significantly associated with the disease itself.

Geriatric Considerations
Although menopause often results in resolution of symptoms, pelvic endometriosis may extend into menopause and is exacerbated by hormone replacement therapy (HRT).

Prevalence
- Predominant sex: Female only
- Affects 6-10% of reproductive-age women

RISK FACTORS
- Diethylstilbestrol (DES) exposure in utero
- Low birth weight
- Obstruction of menstrual flow (Müllerian anomalies)
- Prolonged exposure to endogenous estrogen
  - Early menarche
  - Short menstrual cycles
  - Late menopause
  - Delayed childbearing
  - Obesity
- Hereditary/genetic predisposition

- Exposure to endocrine-disrupting chemicals
- Increased dietary intake of red meat and trans fats

Genetics
Genetic predisposition is common.

GENERAL PREVENTION
- Prevention is not possible, but some factors are considered protective:
  - Fruits, green vegetables, n-3 long-chain fatty acids
  - Multiple pregnancies
  - Prolonged lactation
- Early diagnosis and treatment might help prevent the possible sequelae.

PATHOPHYSIOLOGY
- Not fully understood; tendency for abnormal endometrial tissue to implant and proliferate, causing chronic peritoneal inflammation
- Endometrial-associated infertility is multifactorial:
  - Pelvic inflammation
  - Anatomic disruption of pelvic structures (involvement of the fallopian tube may cause isthmic tubal obstruction)
  - Proliferation and activation of peritoneal macrophages (may predispose to gamete phagocytosis)
  - Alteration in eutopic endometrium

ETIOLOGY
Not fully understood. Theories:
- Sampson theory: Retrograde menstruation results in peritoneal implantation and disease
  - Affected women have an immune dysfunction that prevents clearing of implants
- Halban theory: Distant disease probably caused by hematogenous/lymphatic dissemination or metaplastic transformation
- Coelomic metaplasia: Coelomic epithelium undergoes metaplasia, forming functioning endometrium

COMMONLY ASSOCIATED CONDITIONS
Associated with increased risk of other autoimmune diseases (3). Increased risk of ovarian, endometrioid, and clear-cell cancers as well as other cancers (non-Hodgkin's lymphoma)

DIAGNOSIS

- Diagnosis can be challenging because symptoms overlap with many other gynecological and nongynecological conditions.
- A complete medical, surgical, social, and family history should be collected from patients.
- A complete physical exam, including a pelvic exam, should be performed.

HISTORY
- Dysmenorrhea (50–90% of cases)
- Dyspareunia
- Chronic pelvic pain (≥6 months) that worsens with time and activity
  - Intermittent or continuous
  - Dull, throbbing, or sharp
- Premenstrual spotting
- Dyschezia
- Cyclic nausea, abdominal distention, and early satiety

- Painful defecation
- Hematochezia
- Hematuria
- Infertility
- Spontaneous abortion (theoretical)
- History of pelvic pain, infertility, and hysterectomy in 1st- or 2nd-degree relative

PHYSICAL EXAM
- Focal pain/tenderness on pelvic exam (associated with endometriosis in 66% of patients) (3)
- Pelvic mass
- Immobile pelvic organs (frozen pelvis)
- Rectovaginal exam revealing uterosacral nodules, beading, or tenderness

DIAGNOSTIC TESTS & INTERPRETATION
Lab

Initial lab tests
No special labs; CA-125 levels are not recommended (poor sensitivity and specificity) and may be falsely elevated due to peritoneal irritation.

Imaging
Initial approach
- Routine imaging is not recommended.
- If history and physical exam reveal adnexal pain or tenderness with/without fullness on pelvic exam:
  - Transvaginal ultrasound (US) and MRI are equally effective in detecting ovarian endometriomas. Sensitivity 80–90% and specificity 60-98% for both (3)
  - US is preferred (less costly).
  - Both modalities are poor in detecting peritoneal implants and adhesions.

Diagnostic Procedures/Surgery
- Definitive diagnosis is made via visualization of lesions during surgery (laparoscopy or laparotomy).
- Hysterosalpingography for tubal occlusion (proximal or distal) and periadnexal adhesions

Pathological Findings
- Red and blue-black lesions, adhesions, and "chocolate cysts"
- Endometrial glands and stroma on histologic analysis of biopsied lesions

DIFFERENTIAL DIAGNOSIS
Differential diagnosis of pelvic pain includes all causes of acute abdomen, and:
- Complications of intrauterine or ectopic pregnancy
- Pelvic adhesions
- Acute salpingitis/Pelvic inflammatory disease
- Ruptured ovarian cyst
- Uterine leiomyomas
- Adenomyosis
- Irritable bowel syndrome
- Inflammatory bowel disease
- Intussusception
- Urinary tract infection (UTI)/Cystitis
- Interstitial cystitis
- Malignancies
- Depression
- History of sexual abuse
- Myofascial pain

TREATMENT

MEDICATION
Medications may be helpful in treatment symptoms of pain and dysmenorrhea, but symptoms frequently recur.

First Line
Empirical medical treatment is indicated for symptom management, but has not been shown to improve fertility (4):
- Nonsteroidal anti-inflammatory drugs (NSAIDs) initiated at the beginning or just before menses
- Cyclic combined oral contraceptive pills (OCPs)

Second Line
- Continuous combined OCPs. Switch from cyclic to continuous OCPs for 3–6 months if symptoms persist or in chronic, noncyclic pelvic pain
- Progestogens
  - Levonorgestrel IUD (Mirena), especially for symptomatic rectovaginal endometriosis (although not FDA approved) or instead of continuous OCPs in pain that persists despite 1st-line treatment
  - Medroxyprogesterone acetate 150 mg IM or 104 mg SC every 3 months
- GnRH agonists inhibit pituitary gonadotropin synthesis and induce a hypoestrogenic state (3)[A]:
  - Leuprolide acetate (Depo-Lupron) 3.75 mg IM each month or 11.25 mg IM every 3 months (gluteal)
  - Nafarelin (Synarel) intranasal spray 400 μg/day divided into 2 inhalations per day, 1 in each nostril (start between days 2–4 of menstrual cycle)
  - Goserelin (Zoladex) implant 3.6 mg SC in upper abdominal wall every 28 days for 6 months
- GnRH agonists should be given with estrogen-progestogen add-back therapy to minimize effects of hypoestrogenism (most importantly reduced bone mineral density) (3)[A]:
  - Norethindrone acetate 5 mg p.o. once daily
  - Conjugated equine estrogen 0.635 mg p.o. once daily
- Danazol was an early treatment (now 2nd-3rd line). Use limited by androgenic side effects.

ADDITIONAL TREATMENT
General Measures
Calcium / vitamin D supplementation (1,000–1,500 mg/day) is recommended when using GnRH agonists to prevent calcium loss.

Issues for Referral
- Early referral to a board-certified reproductive endocrinologist or gynecologist with expertise in infertility if the patient has difficulty conceiving
- Other indications for referral to a gynecologist include:
  - Need for definitive diagnosis (failure to respond to a conservative 1st-line therapy)
  - Chronic pelvic pain
  - Adolescent with severe dysmenorrhea/dyspareunia

Additional Therapies
Regular exercise and counseling for pain-management strategies (avoidance of narcotics is ideal)

COMPLEMENTARY AND ALTERNATIVE MEDICINE
- Physical therapy (3)[C]
- Acupuncture (3)[C]

SURGERY/OTHER PROCEDURES
Surgery (laparoscopy or laparotomy) is both diagnostic and therapeutic (1st line or when conservative measures fail):
- Peritoneal endometriosis: Laser ablation, excision, or fulguration,
- Ovarian endometriosis (endometriomas) >3 cm: Ablation, excision, drainage

ALERT
- Surgery for endometriomas may decrease ovarian reserve in advanced disease.
- Lysis of adhesions (LOA)
- Hysterectomy with bilateral salpingo-oophorectomy for debilitating symptoms refractory to other medical or surgical treatments (3)[C]
  - Relieves pain in 80–90% but pain recurs in 10% within 1–2 years after surgery
  - Postoperative hormone replacement should include estrogen and progestogen (3)[C]
- Interruption of nerve pathways:
  - Laparoscopic ablations and presacral neurectomy improve dysmenorrhea (3)[A].

  Fertility procedures:
- Ablation of lesions with LOA is recommended to treat infertility in Stage I–II disease (3)[A]
  - Spontaneous conception should be attempted for 1 year prior to assisted reproduction techniques
- GnRH agonists 3–6 months before in vitro fertilization (IVF) significantly increases live birth rates (3)[A].
  - Disease does not endanger IVF pregnancies.

 ONGOING CARE

FOLLOW-UP RECOMMENDATIONS
Routine gynecological care with Pap smears, mammograms, etc.

Patient Monitoring
- Symptomatic and asymptomatic pelvic masses <5 cm may be followed with serial US
- Patients on GnRH agonist therapy should have serum estradiol levels monitored to assess degree of hypoestrogenemia & efficacy of add-back therapy: Maintaining estradiol between 30–45 pg/mL (109–164 pmol/L) prevents bone loss without stimulating disease
- Endometriosis is likely an independent risk factor for the development of epithelial ovarian cancer.

DIET
No restrictions.

PATIENT EDUCATION
- American Congress of Obstetrics and Gynecology at www.acog.org
- American Academy of Family Physicians at www.familydoctor.org

PROGNOSIS
- Excellent, especially if diagnosis and treatment plans are initiated early in disease course
- Poor for recovery of fertility if the disease has progressed to stage III or IV

COMPLICATIONS
Possible sequelae include chronic pelvic pain, repetitive surgical intervention, costs, infertility, and the psychological manifestations thereof.

REFERENCES
1. Ozkan S, Murk W, Arici A. Endometriosis and infertility: epidemiology and evidence-based treatments. *Ann N Y Acad Sci.* 2008;1127:92–100.
2. Härkki P, Tiitinen A, Ylikorkala O et al. Endometriosis and assisted reproduction techniques. *Ann N Y Acad Sci.* 2010;1205: 207–13.
3. Giudice LC et al. Clinical practice. Endometriosis. *N Engl J Med.* 2010;362:2389–98.
4. Rodgers AK, et al. Treatment strategies for endometriosis. *Exp Opin Pharmacother.* 2008;9(2): 243–55.

ADDITIONAL READING
- Davis L, Kennedy SS, Moore J, et al. Modern combined oral contraceptives for pain associated with endometriosis. *Cochrane Database Syst Rev.* 2007:CD001019.
- de Ziegler D, Borghese B, Chapron C et al. Endometriosis and infertility: pathophysiology and management. *Lancet.* 2010;376:730–8.
- Ferrero S, Remorgida V, Venturini PL et al. Current pharmacotherapy for endometriosis. *Expert Opin Pharmacother.* 2010;11:1123–34.
- Harada T, Taniguchi F et al. Dienogest: a new therapeutic agent for the treatment of endometriosis. *Womens Health (Lond Engl).* 2010;6:27–35.
- Hughes E, Brown J, Collins JJ, et al. Ovulation suppression for endometriosis. *Cochrane Database Syst Rev.* 2007:CD000155.
- Jacobson TZ, Duffy JM, Barlow D, Koninckx PR, Garry R et al. Laparoscopic surgery for pelvic pain associated with endometriosis. *Cochrane Database Syst Rev.* 2009:CD001300.
- Nothnick WB et al. Endometriosis: in search of optimal treatment. *Minerva Ginecol.* 2010;62: 17–31.
- Vercellini P, Somigliana E, Viganò P, et al. Endometriosis: current and future medical therapies. *Best Pract Res Clin Obstet Gynaecol.* 2008;22: 275–306.

See Also (Topic, Algorithm, Electronic Media Element)
Algorithm: Pelvic Pain

 CODES

ICD9
- 617.0 Endometriosis of uterus
- 617.1 Endometriosis of ovary
- 617.2 Endometriosis of fallopian tube

CLINICAL PEARLS
- Severe dysmenorrhea and dyspareunia are never normal. Failure to respond to NSAIDs and/or OCPs warrants further investigation.
- In patients suspected of having endometriosis, always perform a rectovaginal exam looking for uterosacral tenderness, nodules, and beading.

E

ENDOMETRITIS AND OTHER POST-PARTUM INFECTIONS

Justin P. Lavin, Jr., MD
Allison Kreiner, MD

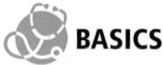 **BASICS**

DESCRIPTION
- Bacterial infection of the genital tract, usually within the 1st week after delivery, but can occur 1–6 weeks postpartum
- Endometritis (infection of the endometrium) is the most common postpartum infection.
- Less common are postpartum infections of the myometrium and parametrial tissues, vaginal and cervical infections, perineal cellulitis, pelvic cellulitis, septic pelvic vein thrombophlebitis, and parametrial phlegmon.
- System: Reproductive
- Synonym(s): Postpartum infection; endometritis; endoparametritis; endomyometritis; myometritis; endomyoparametritis; metritis; metritis with pelvic cellulitis

EPIDEMIOLOGY
Incidence
- Predominant age: Women of childbearing years
- Predominant sex: Female only

Prevalence
- Occurs in 1–3% of all births
- 10 times more likely with cesarean section:
  - 2–15% prior to labor
  - 30–35% after labor without prophylaxis
  - 2–15% after labor with prophylaxis
  - Accounts for 7% of maternal deaths
  - 4th leading cause of maternal mortality

RISK FACTORS
- Cesarean delivery is the most important risk factor
- Chorioamnionitis
- Bacterial vaginosis
- Group B streptococcal colonization of genital tract
- HIV infection
- Prolonged labor
- Prolonged rupture of membranes
- Multiple vaginal examinations
- Internal fetal monitoring during labor
- Operative vaginal delivery
- Manual extraction of the placenta
- Low socioeconomic status

GENERAL PREVENTION
- Avoid unnecessary vaginal examinations.
- Treat chorioamnionitis during labor.
- Spontaneous placental extraction
- Avoid retained placental fragments or membranes.
- Antibiotic prophylaxis for 3rd- and 4th-degree laceration (1)[B]
- Use of aseptic technique during operative vaginal delivery
- No data to support antibiotic prophylaxis for operative vaginal delivery (2)[A]
- Administering prophylactic antibiotics prior to skin incision in cesarean delivery (as opposed to the prior practice of waiting to cord clamping) is considered the standard of care. Antibiotics should be administered within 1 hour of the surgery start time. There is a 40% reduction in postpartum maternal infections without any increase in neonatal infectious outcomes or difficulty in evaluating the neonate (3)[B].
- Extending the spectrum of coverage to include not only a cephalosporin but also azithromycin decreases the incidence of infections (4)[A],(5)[B].

ETIOLOGY
- Endometritis commonly follows chorioamnionitis.
- Other infections follow trauma to the perineum, vagina, cervix, and uterus.
- Infection is nearly always polymicrobial and involves organisms that have ascended from the lower genital tract:
  - Aerobic isolates in 70%: *Streptococcus faecalis, S. agalactiae, S. viridans, Staphylococcus aureus, Escherichia coli*
  - Anaerobic isolates in 80%: *Peptococcus* sp., *Peptostreptococcus* sp., *Clostridium* sp., *Bacteroides bivius, B. fragilis, Fusobacterium* sp.
- Other genital mycoplasmata; role in endometritis unclear
- *Chlamydia trachomatis* responsible for some late (2–10 days) postpartum endometritis (see Medication, Second Line)
- Range of number of isolates is 1–8

COMMONLY ASSOCIATED CONDITIONS
- Chorioamnionitis
- Wound infection

DIAGNOSIS

HISTORY
- Fever, chills, malaise, headache, anorexia
- Abdominal pain

PHYSICAL EXAM
- Oral temperature >38.7°C (101.6°F) in 1st 24 hours postpartum or >38°C (100.4°F) in 2 of 1st 10 days postpartum (excluding 1st 24 hours)
- Tachycardia
- Uterine tenderness on exam
- Other localized tenderness on exam
- Purulent or malodorous lochia
- Heavy vaginal bleeding
- Ileus
- Group A or B streptococcal bacteremia may have no localizing signs.

DIAGNOSTIC TESTS & INTERPRETATION
Lab
Initial lab tests
- Complete blood count (CBC): Interpret with care, because *physiologic leukocytosis may be as high as 20,000 white blood cells (WBCs)*
- 2 sets of blood cultures (especially if sepsis is suspected)
- Note: Diagnosis is usually made clinically, but consider additional testing, including:
  - Genital tract cultures and rapid test for group B streptococci, which may be done while patient is in labor
  - Amniotic fluid Gram stain: Usually polymicrobial
  - Uterine tissue cultures: Prep the cervix with Betadine and use a shielded specimen collector or Pipelle. Difficult to obtain without contamination.

Imaging
Initial approach
If patient is not responsive to antibiotics in 24–48 hours:
- Ultrasound (US) for retained products of conception, pelvic abscess, or mass
- Computed tomography (CT) or magnetic resonance imaging (MRI) looking for pelvic vein thrombophlebitis, abscess, or deep-seated wound infection

Diagnostic Procedures/Surgery
Paracentesis or culdocentesis with culture rarely is necessary.

Pathological Findings
- Superficial layer of infected necrotic tissue in microscopic sections of uterine lining
- >5 neutrophils per HPF in superficial endometrium; ≥1 plasma cell in endometrial stroma
- Thrombosis of any of the pelvic veins, including the vena cava
- Phlegmon on leaves of the broad ligament
- Abscess

DIFFERENTIAL DIAGNOSIS
- Urinary tract infection
- Viral syndrome
- Dehydration
- Pneumonia
- Wound infection
- Thrombophlebitis
- Thyroid storm
- Mastitis

TREATMENT

MEDICATION

First Line

- Clindamycin 900 mg IV every 8 hours plus gentamicin 5 mg/kg IV every 24 hours (6)[A]
- Potential side effects include nephrotoxicity, ototoxicity, pseudomembranous colitis, or diarrhea (in up to 6%).

Second Line

- Clindamycin 900 mg IV every 8 hours plus aztreonam 1–2 g every 8 hours (6)[A].
- Metronidazole 500 mg every 12 hours plus penicillin 5 million units every 6 hours. *OR*
- Ampicillin 2 g every 6 hours plus gentamicin 5 mg/kg every 24 hours (6)[A].
- Cefoxitin 2 g IV every 6 hours. Add ampicillin 2 g IV every 6 hours, if clinical failure after 48 hours (6)[A]
- Cefotetan 2 g IV every 12 hours. Add ampicillin 2 g IV every 6 hours, if clinical failure after 48 hours (6)[A].
- Note: Base therapy on cultures, sensitivities, and clinical response
- Contraindications:
  - Drug allergy
  - Renal failure (aminoglycosides)
  - Avoid sulfa, tetracyclines, and fluoroquinolones before delivery and if breastfeeding. Metronidazole is relatively contraindicated if breastfeeding; however, clinical scenario should be considered.
- Precautions:
  - Clindamycin and other antibiotics occasionally cause pseudomembranous colitis.
- Significant possible interactions: Refer to the manufacturer's literature for each drug.
- Note: Consider adding a macrolide antibiotic (for chlamydia coverage) for infections occurring after 48 hours.
- Note: Heparin may be indicated for septic pelvic vein thrombophlebitis; requires 10 days of full anticoagulation.

SURGERY/OTHER PROCEDURES

- Curettage of retained products of conception
- Surgery to drain an abscess
- Surgery to decompress the bowel
- Surgical drainage of a phlegmon is not advised unless it is suppurative.

IN-PATIENT CONSIDERATIONS

Initial Stabilization

- Inpatient care for severe infection
- Low-grade endometritis may respond to outpatient treatment with oral antibiotics (see "Medication, Second Line").
- Most infections (94%) occur after hospital discharge.
- IV antibiotics and close observation for severe infections

- Open and drain infected wounds.
- Normalize fluid status.
- Note: Amnioinfusion during labor may decrease infections when membranes have been ruptured for >6 hours (7)[B].

ONGOING CARE

FOLLOW-UP RECOMMENDATIONS

Patient Monitoring

- Individualize according to severity
- IV antibiotics can be stopped when the patient is afebrile for 24–48 hours.
- Oral antibiotics on discharge are not necessary, except in cases of bacteremia; then continue oral antibiotics to complete a 7-day course.

DIET

As tolerated, although may be limited by ileus

PATIENT EDUCATION

- Advise patient to call her doctor if she has fever >38°C (100.4°F) postpartum, heavy vaginal bleeding, foul-smelling lochia, or other symptoms of infection.
- Information available at: http://www.healthline.com/yodocontent/pregnancy/infections-postpartum-endometritis.html

PROGNOSIS

- With supportive therapy and appropriate antibiotics, most patients improve within a few days.
- If no improvement occurs on antibiotics, consider retained placental fragments or membranes, abscess, wound infection, hematoma, cellulitis, phlegmon, or septic pelvic vein thrombosis.

COMPLICATIONS

- Resistant organisms
- Peritonitis
- Pelvic abscess
- Septic pelvic thrombophlebitis
- Ovarian vein thrombosis
- Sepsis
- Death

REFERENCES

1. Duggal N, Mercado C, Daniels K, et al. Antibiotic prophylaxis for prevention of postpartum perineal wound complications: a randomized controlled trial. *Obstet Gynecol.* 2008;111:1268–73.
2. Liabsuetrakul T, et al. Antibiotic prophylaxis for operative vaginal delivery. *Cochrane Databse Sys Rev.* 2009;1:CD004455.
3. Owens SM, Brozanski BS, Meyn LA, Wiesenfeld HC et al. Antimicrobial prophylaxis for cesarean delivery before skin incision. *Obstet Gynecol.* 2009;114:573–9.
4. Costantine MM, Rahman M, Ghulmiyah L, et al. Timing of perioperative antibiotics for cesarean delivery: a metaanalysis. *Am J Obstet Gynecol.* 2008;199:301.e1–6.

5. Tita AT, Owen J, Stamm AM, et al. Impact of extended-spectrum antibiotic prophylaxis on incidence of postcesarean surgical wound infection. *Am J Obstet Gynecol.* 2008;199:303.e1–3.
6. French LM, Smaill F. Antibiotic regimens for endometritis after delivery. *Cochrane Database Sys Rev.* 2009;1:CD001067.
7. Parilla BV, McDermott TM. Prophylactic amnioinfusion in preganancies complicated by chorioamnionitis: a prospective randomized trial. *Am J Perinatol.* 1998;15:649–52.

ADDITIONAL READING

- Belfort MA, Clark SL, Saade GR, Kleja K, Dildy GA, Van Veen TR, Akhigbe E, Frye DR, Meyers JA, Kofford S et al. Hospital readmission after delivery: evidence for an increased incidence of nonurogenital infection in the immediate postpartum period. *Am J Obstet Gynecol.* 2010;202:35.e1–7.
- Maharaj D. Puerperal pyrexia: a review. Part I. *Obstet Gynecol Surv.* 2007;62:393–9.
- Maharaj D. Puerperal pyrexia: a review. Part II. *Obstet Gynecol Surv.* 2007;62:400–6.

See Also (Topic, Algorithm, Electronic Media Element)

Algorithm: Pelvic Pain

CODES

ICD9

- 615.9 Unspecified inflammatory disease of uterus
- 670.04 Major puerperal infection unspecified, postpartum

CLINICAL PEARLS

- Endometritis is a postpartum complication causing fever and uterine tenderness that occurs in 1–3% of all births.
- Infection is nearly always polymicrobial and involves organisms that have ascended from the lower genital tract.
- Evidence supports antibiotic prophylaxis prior to skin incision for all cesarean deliveries, but not for operative vaginal deliveries.
- Recommended treatment of endometritis is clindamycin 900 mg IV evert 8 hours and gentamicin 5 mg/kg every 24 hours until the patient is afebrile for 24–48 hours.
- Antibiotics can be stopped completely when the patient has been afebrile for 24–48 hours, except in cases of documented bacteremia, which require a 7-day course of therapy.

E

ENURESIS

Melanie J.S. Malec, MD

 BASICS

DESCRIPTION
- Nocturnal enuresis (NE): Repeated spontaneous voiding of discrete amounts of urine during sleep after the anticipated age of bladder control (age 5)
- Daytime incontinence: Uncontrollable leakage of urine while awake
- Classification:
  - Primary NE: 1% of adult population; 80% of all cases; child/adult who has never established urinary continence on consecutive nights for a period of 6 months or more
  - Secondary NE: 20% of cases; resumption of enuresis after at least 6 months of urinary continence
- Also categorized as:
  - Monosymptomatic NE (uncomplicated): Bed wetting without lower urinary tract symptoms other than nocturia and no history of bladder dysfunction
  - Nonmonosymptomatic NE: Bed wetting with lower urinary tract symptoms such as frequency, urgency, daytime wetting, hesitancy, straining, weak or intermittent stream, posturination dribbling, lower abdominal or genital discomfort, sensation of incomplete emptying
- Adult-onset NE with absent daytime incontinence is a serious symptom; complete urologic evaluation and therapy are warranted; usually associated with diurnal symptoms, voiding dysfunction, and urinary incontinence (UI).
- System(s) affected: Nervous; Renal/Urologic
- Synonym(s): Bed wetting; Sleep enuresis; Nocturnal incontinence; Primary nocturnal enuresis

EPIDEMIOLOGY
Incidence
- Dependent upon family history
- Spontaneous resolution: 15% per year, 99% children are dry by age 15

Prevalence
- Very common. Affects 5–7 million children in the US
- 40% of 3 year olds; 10% of 6 year olds; 3% of 12 year olds; 1% of adults
- Predominant sex: Male > Female (3:1)
- Predominant timing: Nocturnal > Day (3:1)

Geriatric Considerations
Infrequent; often associated with daytime incontinence (formerly referred to as diurnal enuresis)

RISK FACTORS
- Family history
- Stressors (emotional, environmental) common in secondary enuresis (e.g., divorce, death)
- Constipation and encopresis
- Organic disease: 1% of monosymptomatic NE (e.g., urologic and nonurologic causes)
- Psychological disorders:
  - Comorbid disorders are highest with secondary NE: Depression, anxiety, social phobias, conduct disorder, hyperkinetic syndrome, internalizing disorders
  - Association with attention deficit hyperactivity disorder (ADHD; more pronounced in older children ages 9–12 years); 30% greater chance of enuretic events

- Abuse; victims may present with NE; 11% sexually abused girls
- Altered mental status or impaired mobility

Genetics
Most commonly, NE is an autosomal dominant inheritance pattern with high penetrance (90%); more heritable in boys than in girls:
- 1/3 of all cases are sporadic.
- 4 loci associated with NE identified (chromosomes 8, 12, 13, and 22)
- Higher rates in monozygotic versus dizygotic twins (68% vs. 36%)
- 75% of children with enuresis have a 1st-degree relative with the condition.
- If both parents had NE, risk in child is 77%; 44% if 1 parent affected. Parental age of resolution often predicts when child's enuresis should resolve.

GENERAL PREVENTION
No known measures

PATHOPHYSIOLOGY
A disorder of sleep arousal, a low nocturnal bladder capacity, and nocturnal polyuria are the three factors that interrelate to cause nocturnal enuresis (1).

ETIOLOGY
- Both functional and organic causes; many theories, none absolutely confirmed
- Primary NE owing to disparity between bladder capacity, nocturnal urine production, and the child's failure to awaken in response to a full bladder
- Detrusor instability
- Deficiency of arginine vasopressin (AVP); owing to decreased inherent nocturnal AVP or decreased AVP stimulation secondary to an empty bladder (bladder distension stimulates AVP)
- Maturational delay of CNS
- Severe NE with some evidence of interaction between bladder overactivity and brain arousability: Association between children with severe NE and frequent cortical arousals in sleep
- Organic urologic causes in 1–4% of enuresis in children: Urinary tract infection (UTI), occult spina bifida, ectopic ureter, lazy bladder syndrome, irritable bladder with wide bladder neck, posterior urethral valves
- Organic nonurologic causes: Epilepsy, diabetes mellitus, food allergies, obstructive sleep apnea, chronic renal failure, hyperthyroidism, pinworm infection, sickle-cell disease
- No evidence of sleep disorder/altered sleep pattern; NE occurs in all stages of sleep.

COMMONLY ASSOCIATED CONDITIONS
- Obstructive sleep apnea syndrome; ↑ atrial natriuretic factor → inhibits renin-angiotensin-aldosterone pathway → ↑ diuresis
- Constipation (1/3 of NE patients)
- Behavioral problems

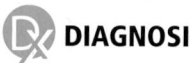 **DIAGNOSIS**

HISTORY
- Age of onset, duration, severity
- Lower urinary tract symptoms
- Constipation and encopresis (15% with comorbid encopresis)
- Daily intake patterns
- Voiding and elimination patterns
- Psychosocial history
- Family history of enuresis
- Investigation and previous treatment history

PHYSICAL EXAM
- ENT: Evaluation for adenotonsillar hypertrophy
- Abdomen: Enlarged bladder, kidneys, or fecal masses or impaction
- Look for dimpling or tufts of hair on sacrum
- Genital urinary exam:
  - Males: Meatal stenosis, hypospadias, epispadias, phimosis
  - Females: Vulvitis, vaginitis, labial adhesions, ureterocele at introitus; wide vaginal orifice with scar or healed laceration may be evidence of abuse.
- Rectal exam: Tone and constipation
- Neurologic exam

DIAGNOSTIC TESTS & INTERPRETATION
Lab
Initial lab tests
- Only obligatory test in children is urinalysis.
- Urinalysis and culture: UTI, pyuria, hematuria, proteinuria, glycosuria, and poor concentrating ability (low specific gravity) may suggest organic etiology, especially in adults.

Follow-Up & Special Considerations
Select tests for diagnosing causes of secondary enuresis: Serum glucose, blood urea nitrogen (BUN), creatinine, thyroid-stimulating hormone (TSH).

Imaging
Initial approach
- Urinary tract imaging is usually not necessary.
- If abnormal clinical findings or adult onset: Renal ultrasound (US) and bladder US IV pyelogram, voiding cystourethrogram, or retrograde pyelogram as indicated
- Spine radiographs for spina bifida occulta

Follow-Up & Special Considerations
In children, imaging and urodynamic studies are helpful for significant daytime symptoms, history of UTIs, suspected structural abnormalities, and refractory cases.

Diagnostic Procedures/Surgery
Urodynamic studies may be beneficial in adults and nonmonosymptomatic NE.

Pathological Findings
- Dysfunctional voiding
- Detrusor instability and/or reduced bladder capacity most common findings

DIFFERENTIAL DIAGNOSIS
- Primary NE:
  - Delayed physiologic urinary control
  - UTI (both)
  - Spina bifida occulta
  - Obstructive sleep apnea (both)
  - Idiopathic detrusor instability

- Previously unrecognized myelopathy or neuropathy (e.g., multiple sclerosis, tethered cord, epilepsy)
- Anatomic urinary tract abnormally (e.g., ectopic ureter)
• Secondary NE:
  - Bladder outlet obstruction
  - Neurologic disease, neurogenic bladder (e.g., spinal cord injury)

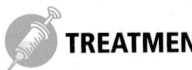 TREATMENT

Combined therapy (e.g., enuresis alarm, bladder training, motivational therapy, and pelvic floor muscle training) is more effective than each component alone or than pharmacotherapy (2)[A].

MEDICATION
First Line

• Desmopressin (DDAVP): Synthetic analogue of vasopressin that decreases nocturnal urine output (3)[A]:
  - Adults only: 20 μg intranasally at bedtime
  - As of 2007, USFDA recommends against use in children due to reports of severe hyponatremia resulting in seizures and deaths in children using intranasal formulations of desmopressin (45)[A].
  - Oral DDAVP: dose dependent: begin at 0.2 mg tablet taken at bedtime on empty stomach; may titrate to 0.6 mg
    ○ Maximally effective in 1 h; cleared within 9 h
    ○ Trial nightly for 6 months then stop for 2 weeks for test of dryness
    ○ Suspend dose in children who experience acute condition affecting fluid/electrolyte balances (fever, vomiting, diarrhea, vigorous exercise)
  - 10–60% success; safe even when used for >12 months; high relapse rate after discontinuation without a structured withdrawal program
• Anticholinergics:
  - Oxybutynin (Ditropan, Ditropan XL, Oxytrol patch): Anticholinergic; smooth muscle relaxant, antispasmodic; may increase functional bladder capacity and aids in timed voiding
    ○ Ditropan: Adults and children >5 years of age: 5 mg PO t.i.d.–q.i.d.; children 1–5 years of age: 0.02 mg/kg/dose b.i.d.–q.i.d. (syrup 5 mg/5 mL)
    ○ Ditropan XL: Adults: 5 mg/d PO; increase to 30 mg/d PO (5-, 10-mg tabs)
    ○ Oxytrol patch: 1 patch every 3–4 days (3.9 mg/patch) (periodic trials off the medication, i.e., weekends or weeks at a time, will help determine efficacy and resolution of primary disturbance)
    ○ Ditropan 5–10 mg at night; 30–50% success; 50% relapse after stopped
  - Tolterodine (Detrol, Detrol LA): Anticholinergic; fewer side effects than Ditropan:
    ○ Detrol: 1–2 mg PO b.i.d.
    ○ Detrol LA: 2–4 mg/d

Pediatric Considerations

USFDA recommends against using intranasal formulations of desmopressin in children due to reports of severe hyponatremia resulting in seizures and deaths (45)[A].

Second Line

• Imipramine (Tofranil): Tricyclic antidepressant, anticholinergic effects; increases bladder capacity, antispasmodic properties
  - Primarily in adults; use in children reserved for resistant cases
  - Dose: Adults, 25–75 mg and children >6 years, 10–25 mg PO at bedtime; increase by 10–25 mg at 1- to 2-week intervals; treat for 2–3 months; then taper;
  - 25–30% success when used >3 months
  - Pretreatment ECG recommended to identify underlying rhythm disorders
• Precautions:
  - Oxybutynin: Glaucoma, myasthenia gravis, GI or genitourinary obstruction, ulcerative colitis, megacolon; use a decreased dose in the elderly.
  - Tolterodine: Urinary retention, gastric retention, or uncontrolled narrow-angle glaucoma; significant drug interactions with CYP2D6, CYP3A3/4 substrates
  - DDAVP: Avoid in patients at risk for electrolyte changes or fluid retention (congestive heart failure [CHF], renal insufficiency).
  - Imipramine: Do not use with monoamine oxidase inhibitors (MAOIs), hypotension, and arrhythmias; low toxic therapeutic ratio.
• Combination therapy with DDAVP and oxybutynin has better results than individual use.
• Prostaglandin inhibitors (e.g., indomethacin) have been studied; may increase bladder capacity.

ADDITIONAL TREATMENT
General Measures

• Use non-pharmacologic approaches as 1st line before prescribing medications (6)[A].
• Simple behavioral interventions (e.g., scheduled wakening, positive reinforcement, bladder training, minimizing fluid/caffeine 2 hours prior to sleep, limiting dairy consumption to 4 hours prior to bedtime)
• Motivational therapy
• Enuresis alarms (bells or buzzers)
  - 66–70% success rate; must be used nightly for 3–4 months; offers cure; significant parental involvement; disruption of sleep for entire family

Issues for Referral

• Primary NE: Persistent enuresis despite nonpharmacologic and pharmacologic therapies
• Diurnal incontinence or nonmonosymptomatic enuresis with voiding dysfunction or underlying medical condition

Additional Therapies

Individual psychotherapy, crisis intervention, and family therapy

COMPLEMENTARY AND ALTERNATIVE MEDICINE

Acupuncture and hypnosis are other treatments offered; few data support their use (7,8)[B]

SURGERY/OTHER PROCEDURES

Only for surgically correctable causes (e.g., tethered cord, ectopic ureter, benign prostatitic hypertrophy, obstructive sleep apnea)

 ONGOING CARE

FOLLOW-UP RECOMMENDATIONS
Patient Monitoring

Follow patient until condition resolved. Monitor therapy.

DIET

Limit fluid and caffeine intake prior 2 hours to bedtime. Limit dairy products 4 hours prior to bedtime (decrease osmotic diuresis).

PATIENT EDUCATION

Web resources for alarms and supplies:
• http://www.bedwettingstore.com/index.htm
• http://www.pottypager.com/

PROGNOSIS

In children, NE usually self-limiting; 1% will persist as adult; evaluate for organic causes.

COMPLICATIONS

UTI, perineal excoriation, psychological disturbance (especially in children)

REFERENCES

1. Robson WL. Current management of nocturnal enuresis. *Curr Opin Urol.* 2008;18:425–30.
2. Zaffanello M, Giacomello L, Brugnara M, et al. Therapeutic options in childhood nocturnal enuresis. *Minerva Urol Nefrol.* 2007;59:199–205.
3. Vande Walle J, Stockner M, Raes A, et al. Desmopressin 30 years in clinical use: a safety review. *Curr Drug Saf.* 2007;2:232–8.
4. Graham KM, Levy JB et al. Enuresis. *Pediatr Rev.* 2009;30:165–72; quiz 173.
5. http://www.fda.gov/Drugs/DrugSafety/PostmarketDrugSafetyInformationforPatientsandProviders/ucm107924.htm
6. Robson WL et al. Clinical practice. Evaluation and management of enuresis. *N Engl J Med.* 2009; 360:1429–36.
7. Neveus T, Eggert P, Evans J et al. Evaluation of and treatment for monosymptomatic enuresis: a standardization document from the International Children's Continence Society. *J Urol.* 2010;183: 441–7.
8. Libonate J, Evans S, Tsao JC et al. Efficacy of acupuncture for health conditions in children: a review. *Scientific World Journal.* 2008;8:670–82.

See Also (Topic, Algorithm, Electronic Media Element)

Incontinence, Urinary Adult Female; Incontinence, Urinary Adult Male
Algorithm: Enuresis

 CODES

ICD9
• 307.6 Enuresis
• 788.30 Urinary incontinence, unspecified
• 788.36 Nocturnal enuresis

CLINICAL PEARLS

• Diagnosis is usually made based on history, physical examination, and urinalysis.
• If the condition is not distressing to child and caretakers, treatment is unnecessary.
• Dryness is possible for most children.

EPICONDYLITIS

Shawn M. Ferullo, MD

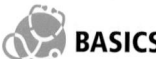 **BASICS**

DESCRIPTION
- Tendon injury characterized by pain and tenderness at the tendinous origins of the wrist flexors/extensors on the epicondyles of the humerus
- May be acute (traumatic) or chronic (overuse)
- 2 types:
  - Medial epicondylitis or "golfer's elbow":
    - Involvement of the wrist flexors and pronators on the medial epicondyle
  - Lateral epicondylitis or "tennis elbow":
    - Involvement of the wrist extensors and supinators on the lateral epicondyle
- May be caused by many different athletic or occupational activities
- Common in carpenters, plumbers, gardeners, and politicians
- Usually occurs unilaterally on the epicondyles of the dominant arm
- Lateral epicondyle involvement is more common than medial.

EPIDEMIOLOGY
- Predominant age: >40
- Predominant sex: Male = Female

Incidence
- Very common site of overuse injury
- Lateral > Medial

RISK FACTORS
Repetitive wrist motions:
- Flexion/pronation → medial
- Extension/supination → lateral

GENERAL PREVENTION
- Limit overuse of the wrist flexors, extensors, pronators, and supinators.
- Use proper techniques when working.
- Use lighter tools that have smaller grips.

PATHOPHYSIOLOGY
- Acute (tendonitis):
  - Inflammatory response to injury
- Chronic (tendonosis):
  - Overuse injury
  - Tendon degeneration, fibroblast proliferation, microvascular proliferation, lack of inflammatory response

ETIOLOGY
- Repetitive wrist motions
- Tool/racquet gripping
- Shaking hands
- Sudden maximal muscle contraction
- Direct blow

 DIAGNOSIS

HISTORY
- Occupational activities
- Sport participation
- Direct trauma
- Duration of symptoms
- Treatments or medication use
- Pain with gripping
- Sensation of mild forearm weakness

PHYSICAL EXAM
- Localized pain just proximal to the affected epicondyle
- Increased pain with wrist flexion/pronation (medial)
- Increased pain with wrist extension/supination (lateral)
- Medial epicondylitis:
  - Tenderness at origin of wrist flexor tendons
  - Increased pain with resisted wrist flexion and pronation
  - Normal elbow range of motion
  - Increased pain with gripping
- Lateral epicondylitis:
  - Tenderness at origin of wrist extensors
  - Increased pain with resisted wrist extension/supination
  - Normal elbow range of motion
  - Increased pain with gripping

DIAGNOSTIC TESTS & INTERPRETATION
Imaging
- None required
- Anterior-posterior/lateral radiograph if decreased range of motion or trauma
- Magnetic resonance imaging for recalcitrant cases

Diagnostic Procedures/Surgery
Local injection of anesthetic to document resolution of symptoms

DIFFERENTIAL DIAGNOSIS
- Elbow osteoarthritis
- Fractures of the epicondyles
- Posterior interosseous nerve entrapment (lateral)
- Ulnar neuropathy (medial)
- Synovitis
- Medial collateral ligament injury
- Referred pain from shoulder or neck

 TREATMENT

- May take weeks to months to resolve
- Majority of patients will improve with conservative treatment
- Relative rest with reduction of aggravating activities
- Changing technique of activities
- Ice to area for 10 minutes b.i.d.
- Elbow straps during activity (counterforce bracing) (1)[B]

MEDICATION
First Line
Nonsteroidal anti-inflammatory drugs (NSAIDs): Good for short-term relief. There are no data to support long-term usefulness (2)[B].

Second Line
Corticosteroid injections (3)[B] help relieve pain in acute setting; no effect in long-term outcome.

ADDITIONAL TREATMENT

Physical therapy:

- Begin once acute pain resolved
- Focus on eccentric strength training.
- Grip exercises
- Ultrasound (4)[B]
- Corticosteroid iontophoresis

General Measures

Relative rest

Issues for Referral

Failure of conservative therapy

Additional Therapies

- Botulinum toxin injections (5)[B]
- Platelet-rich plasma injections (6)[C]:
  - Involves the injection of a concentrated portion of the patient's plasma. Specifically, the platelet-rich portion of plasma is used. The localized injection of the concentrate leads to a local inflammatory response causing the platelets to degranulate, releasing growth factors, which then stimulate the physiologic healing cascade.
- Prolotherapy:
  - Involves the injection of a dextrose solution into and around the tendon attachment. This stimulates a localized inflammatory response, leading to increased blood supply to the area, which increases the flow of nutrients and healing mediators to stimulate tendon healing.
  - Research is currently being performed to look at efficacy of use in epicondylitis.

COMPLEMENTARY AND ALTERNATIVE MEDICINE

Acupuncture (7)[A]

SURGERY/OTHER PROCEDURES

- May be indicated in refractory cases
- Involves debridement and release of the involved tendons
- Can be performed open or arthroscopically (1)[B]

 ONGOING CARE

PROGNOSIS

Good: Majority resolve with conservative care

REFERENCES

1. Dunkow PD, Jatti M, Muddu BN. A comparison of open and percutaneous techniques in the surgical treatment of tennis elbow. *J Bone Joint Surg.* 2004;86-B:701.
2. Green S, et al. Non-steroidal anti-inflamatory drugs for treating lateral elbow pain in adults. *Cochrane Database Syst Rev.* 2001;(4):CD002267.
3. Assendelft W, Green S, Buchbinder R, et al. Tennis elbow (lateral epicondylitis). *Clin Evid.* 2002: 1290–300.
4. Smidt N, van der Windt DA, Assendelft WJ, et al. Corticosteroid injections, physiotherapy, or a wait-and-see policy for lateral epicondylitis: a randomised controlled trial. *Lancet.* 2002;359: 657–62.
5. Wong SM, Hui AC, Tong PY, et al. Treatment of lateral epicondylitis with botulinum toxin: a randomized, double-blind, placebo-controlled trial. *Ann Intern Med.* 2005;143:793–7.
6. Mishra A, Pavelko T. Treatment of chronic elbow tendinosis with buffered platelet-rich plasma. *Am J Sports Med.* 2006;34:1774–8.
7. Trinh KV, Phillips SD, Ho E, et al. Acupuncture for the alleviation of lateral epicondyle pain: a systematic review. *Rheumatology (Oxford).* 2004;43:1085–90.

ADDITIONAL READING

Wilson JJ, Best TM. Common overuse tendon problems: A review and recommendations for treatment. *Am Fam Physician.* 2005;72:811–8.

See Also (Topic, Algorithm, Electronic Media Element)

Algorithm: Pain in Upper Extremity

 CODES

ICD9

- 726.31 Medial epicondylitis
- 726.32 Lateral epicondylitis

CLINICAL PEARLS

- Tendon injury characterized by pain and tenderness at the tendinous origins of the wrist flexors/extensors on the epicondyles of the humerus
- 2 types:
  - Medial epicondylitis or "golfer's elbow":
    ○ Involvement of the wrist flexors and pronators on the medial epicondyle
  - Lateral epicondylitis or "tennis elbow":
    ○ Involvement of the wrist extensors and supinators on the lateral epicondyle
- May take weeks to months to resolve
- Majority of patients will improve with conservative treatment.
- NSAIDs 1st line; steroid injection 2nd line
- Ice to area for 10 minutes b.i.d.
- Elbow straps during activity (counterforce bracing)
- Physical therapy as symptoms improve

E

EPIDIDYMITIS

Andrew Leone, MD
Kyle D. Wood, MD

BASICS

- Acute epididymitis: Pain for <6 weeks
- Chronic epididymitis: Pain for >3 months

DESCRIPTION

Inflammation (infectious or noninfectious) of epididymis resulting in scrotal pain and swelling, induration of the posterior epididymis, and eventual scrotal wall edema, involvement of the adjacent testicle, and hydrocele formation:

- System(s) affected: Reproductive
- Synonym(s): Epididymo-orchitis
- Classification: Infectious (bacterial, viral, fungal, parasitic) versus sterile (chemical, traumatic, autoimmune, idiopathic, industrial, noninfectious, vasoepididymal reflux syndrome, vasal reflux syndrome); chronic versus acute

EPIDEMIOLOGY

- Predominant age: Usually younger, sexually active men or older men with urinary tract infections; in older men usually secondary to bladder outlet obstruction
- Predominant sex: Male only

Pediatric Considerations

Occurs in prepubertal boys: Epididymitis is found to be the most common cause of acute scrotum, more common than testicular torsion.

Incidence

- Common (600,000 cases annually in United States)
- 1 in 1,000 males per year

Prevalence

Common

RISK FACTORS

- Urinary tract infection (UTI), prostatitis
- Indwelling urethral catheter
- Urethral instrumentation or transurethral surgery
- Urethral or meatal stricture
- Transrectal prostate biopsy
- Prostate brachytherapy (seeds) for prostate cancer
- Anal intercourse
- High-risk sexual activity
- Strenuous physical activity
- Prolonged sedentary periods
- Bladder obstruction (benign prostatic hyperplasia, prostate cancer)
- HIV-immunosuppressed patient
- Severe Behçet disease
- Presence of foreskin (1)
- Constipation
- Sterile epididymitis:
  - Increased intra-abdominal pressure (occupation requiring frequent physical strain):
    - ○ Military recruits, especially who begin their physically unprepared
    - ○ Laborers; Restaurant kitchen workers
    - ○ Full bladder during intense physical exertion

GENERAL PREVENTION

- Vasectomy or vasoligation during transurethral surgery
- Safer sexual practices
- Mumps vaccination
- Antibiotic prophylaxis for urethral manipulation

- Early treatment of prostatitis/benign prostatic hyperplasia
- Avoid vigorous rectal exam with acute prostatitis.
- Sterile epididymitis:
  - Emptying the bladder prior to physical exertion
  - Physically conditioning the body prior to engaging in regular intense physical exertion (2)
  - Treating constipation

PATHOPHYSIOLOGY

- Infectious epididymitis:
  - Retrograde spread of urine or urinary bacteria from the prostate or urethra via the ejaculatory ducts and the vas deferens into the epididymis; rarely, hematogenous spread
  - Causative organism is identified in 80% of patients, and varies according to patient age.
- Sterile epididymitis:
  - Urine in full bladder when exposed to increased intra-abdominal pressure is pushed through internal urethral sphincter (located at proximal end of prostatic urethra).
  - Reflux of urine through orifice of ejaculatory ducts at verumontanum may occur with history of urethritis/prostatitis, as inflammation may produce rigidity in musculature surrounding orifice to ejaculatory ducts, holding them open.
  - Exposure of epididymis to foreign fluid may produce inflammatory reaction within 24 hours

ETIOLOGY

- <35 years and sexually active:
  - Usually *Chlamydia trachomatis* or *Neisseria gonorrhoeae*
  - Look for serous urethral discharge (chlamydia) or purulent discharge (gonorrhea).
  - With anal intercourse, likely *Escherichia coli* or *Haemophilus influenzae*
- >35 years:
  - Coliform bacteria usually, but sometimes *Staphylococcus aureus* or *S. epidermidis*
  - In elderly men, often with distal urinary tract obstruction, BPH, UTI, or catheterization
  - Tuberculosis, if sterile pyuria and nodularity of vas deferens (hematogenous spread)
  - Sterile urine reflux after transurethral prostatectomy
  - Granulomatous reaction following BCG intravesical therapy for bladder cancer
- Prepubertal boys:
  - Usually coliform bacteria
  - Evaluate for underlying congenital abnormalities, such as vesicoureteral reflux, ectopic ureter, or anorectal malformation (rectourethral fistula).
- Amiodarone may cause noninfectious epididymitis; resolves with decreasing drug dosage.
- Syphilis, blastomycosis, coccidioidomycosis, and cryptococcosis are rare causes, but brucellosis can be a common cause in endemic areas (3).

COMMONLY ASSOCIATED CONDITIONS

- Prostatitis/Urethritis/Orchitis
- Hemospermia
- Constipation
- Urinary Tract Infection

DIAGNOSIS

- Scrotal pain, sometimes radiating to the groin region, may begin acutely over several hours.
- Urethral discharge or symptoms of UTI, such as frequency of urination, dysuria, cloudy urine, or hematuria (4)
- Initially, only the posterior-lying epididymis, usually the lowermost tail section, is very tender and indurated; will eventually progress to involvement of body and head of epididymis.
- Elevation of the testes/epididymis improves the discomfort (Prehn sign).
- Entire hemiscrotum becomes swollen and red, the testis becomes indistinguishable from the epididymis, the scrotal wall becomes thick and indurated, and reactive hydrocele may occur.
- Sterile epididymitis:
  - Unilateral scrotal pain and swelling preceded by intense physical exertion by several hours. Patient may recall full bladder prior to exertion.
  - No symptoms of infection

Pediatric Considerations

- In prepubertal patients, may be postinfectious inflammatory condition; treat with anti-inflammatories, analgesics, and usually no antibiotics (5)
- Bacteremia from *Haemophilus influenzae* infection may produce acute epididymitis.
- In adolescent males, particularly >13 years old, must rule out testicular torsion.
- History not helpful in distinguishing epididymitis from testicular torsion.

Geriatric Considerations

- Diabetics with sensory neuropathy may have pain despite severe infection/abscess.

PHYSICAL EXAM

- The tail of the epididymis is larger in comparison to the contralateral side.
- Epididymis is markedly tender to palpation.
- Cremasteric reflex should be present in epididymitis; if absent, suspect testicular torsion.

DIAGNOSTIC TESTS & INTERPRETATION

Lab

Initial lab tests

- Urinalysis (pyuria and bacteriuria suggestive of infectious origin)
- Urine culture (negative does not rule out)
- GC/chlamydia testing (urethral swab or urine testing)
- Gram stain urethral discharge
- White blood cell count may be elevated.
- Urinalysis clear and culture-negative suggest sterile epididymitis

Imaging

- If testicular torsion cannot be excluded (especially in pediatrics), Doppler ultrasound test of choice (6)
- In adult men, Doppler ultrasound: Sensitivity and specificity of 100% in evaluation of acute scrotum, but usually not needed (7)

Follow-Up & Special Considerations

Pediatric Considerations

Further radiographic imaging in children should be done to rule out anatomic abnormalities:

Diagnostic Procedures/Surgery
This is a clinical diagnosis.

Pathological Findings
- Epididymis:
  - Surrounding tissue fibrosis and scarring
  - Interstitial nonspecific acute infiltration, edema, congestion, PMNs, and lymphocytes
  - Fine inflammatory adhesions
  - Can progress to abscess or necrosis (2)
- Vas deferens:
  - Possible fibrosis of this structure

DIFFERENTIAL DIAGNOSIS
- Epididymal congestion following vasectomy
- Testicular torsion
- Torsion of testicular appendages
- Orchitis
- Testicular malignancy
- Testicular trauma
- Epididymal cyst
- Inguinal hernia
- Urethritis
- Spermatocele
- Hydrocele
- Hematocele
- Varicocele
- Epididymal adenomatoid tumor
- Epididymal rhabdomyosarcoma
- Vasculitis (Henoch-Schönlein purpura)

 ## TREATMENT

- Bed rest or restriction on activity
- Athletic scrotal supporter
- Scrotal elevation
- Ice pack/warm compress
- If chemical epididymitis:
  - Cessation of strenuous physical activity for several weeks
  - Empty bladder prior to strenuous exercises.

MEDICATION
First Line
- <35 years, for chlamydia: Doxycycline 100 mg PO bid for 10 PO ceftriaxone 250 mg IM × 1. Treat sexual partner(s) (8).
- If penicillin-allergic or participates in insertive anal intercourse: Ciprofloxacin (Cipro) 500 mg PO bid or ofloxacin (Floxin) 200 mg PO bid for 10 days
- Older men with bacteriuria:
  - Levofloxacin (Levaquin) 500 mg PO every day for 7–10 days (8)
  - Ofloxacin 300 mg orally bid for 10 days (8)
  - Ciprofloxacin (Cipro) 500 mg PO bid or ciprofloxacin (Cipro XL) 1000 mg/day for 10–14 days
- Analgesia (infectious and chemical epididymitis):
  - Nonsteroidal anti-inflammatory drugs (NSAIDs) (e.g., naproxen or ibuprofen) for mild to moderate pain
  - Consider corticosteroid if patient cannot tolerate NSAID.
  - Acetaminophen-codeine or acetaminophen-oxycodone for moderate-to-severe pain
- Septic or toxic patient:
  - 3rd-generation cephalosporin or aminoglycoside
- For Beçhet, sarcoid, Henoch Schönlein purpura:
  - Corticosteroids such as methylprednisolone 40 mg/day recommended

Second Line
- Trimethoprim-sulfamethoxazole (Bactrim, Septra) double-strength PO bid for 10–14 days; increasing bacterial resistance may limit effectiveness.
- Add rifampin (rifampicin) or vancomycin as required.

ADDITIONAL TREATMENT
General Measures
Spermatic cord block with local anesthesia in severe cases

Issues for Referral
- If suspicion is high for testicular torsion or cancer, consult urologist.
- If failed medical management, should be referred to urologist to rule out anatomic abnormality or to diagnosis chemical epididymitis.

SURGERY/OTHER PROCEDURES
- Vasostomy to drain infected material if severe or refractory case
- Scrotal exploration if unable to clinically distinguish between epididymitis or testicular torsion
- Drainage of abscesses, epididymectomy (acute suppurative), or epididymo-orchiectomy in severe cases refractory to antibiotics
- Surgery to correct underlying anatomic abnormality or obstruction

IN-PATIENT CONSIDERATIONS
Initial Stabilization
- The majority of cases can be managed with outpatient care.
- Inpatient care needed if septic or if surgery is scheduled

Admission Criteria
- Intractable pain
- Sepsis
- Abscess
- Persistent vomiting
- Purulent drainage

 ## ONGOING CARE

FOLLOW-UP RECOMMENDATIONS
Patient Monitoring
- Office visits until all signs of infection have cleared
- In chemical epididymitis, follow-up in 4 weeks to assess efficacy of NSAIDs and lifestyle changes

DIET
If constipation is contributing to chemical epididymitis, consider a high-fiber diet.

PATIENT EDUCATION
- Stress completing course of antibiotics, even when asymptomatic.
- Early recognition and treatment of UTI or prostatitis
- Safer sexual practices
- If chemical epididymitis, then educate on noninfectious etiology and proper lifestyle changes

PROGNOSIS
- Pain improves within 1–3 days, but induration may take several weeks/months to completely resolve.
- If bilateral involvement, sterility may result.
- In chemical epididymitis, symptoms resolve in usually <1 week

COMPLICATIONS
- Recurrent epididymitis
- Infertility
- Oligospermia
- Testicular necrosis or atrophy
- Secondary abscess formation
- Fournier gangrene (necrotizing synergistic infection)

REFERENCES
1. Bennett RT, Gill B, Kogan SJ. Epididymitis in children: the circumcision factor? *J Urol*. 1998;160:1842–4.
2. Wolin LH. On the etiology of epididymitis. *J Urol*. 1971;105:531–3.
3. Akinci E, Bodur H, Cevik MA, et al. A complication of brucellosis: epididymoorchitis. *Int J Infect Dis*. 2006;10:171–7.
4. Tracy CR, Steers WD, Costabile R. Diagnosis and management of epididymitis. *Urol Clin North Am*. 2008;35:101–8; vii.
5. Somekh E, Gorenstein A, Serour F. Acute epididymitis in boys: evidence of a post-infectious etiology. *J Urol*. 2004;171:391–4; discussion 394.
6. Trojian TH, Lishnak TS, Heiman D. Epididymitis and orchitis: an overview. *Am Fam Physician*. 2009;79:583–7.
7. Süzer O, Ozcan H, Küpeli S, et al. Color Doppler imaging in the diagnosis of the acute scrotum. *Eur Urol*. 1997;32:457–61.
8. Drugs for sexually transmitted infections. *Treat Guidel Med Lett*. 2007;5:81–8.

 ## CODES

ICD9
- 604.90 Orchitis and epididymitis, unspecified
- 604.91 Orchitis and epididymitis in diseases classified elsewhere
- 604.99 Other orchitis, epididymitis, and epididymo-orchitis, without mention of abscess

CLINICAL PEARLS
- With epididymitis, the pain is more gradual in onset, and the tenderness is mostly posterior to the testis. With testicular torsion, the symptoms are quite rapid in onset, the testis will be higher in the scrotum and may have a transverse lie, and the cremasteric reflex will be absent. The absence of leukocytes on urine analysis and decreased blood flow on scrotal ultrasound with Doppler will suggest torsion.
- Prostatic massage is contraindicated in epididymitis because the risk for worsening local infection and potential for sepsis is increased with acute prostatitis.
- Chemical epididymitis is a clinical diagnosis of exclusion, and infectious causes are much more common, but certain occupations, such as soldiers and laborers, must be considered.

EPIGLOTTITIS

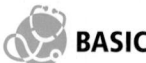

Vassiliki P. Syriopoulou, MD

 BASICS

DESCRIPTION
- An illness with acute onset characterized by inflammation and edema of the supraglottic structures, epiglottis, vallecula, arytenoepiglottic folds, and arytenoids
- System(s) affected: Pulmonary
- Synonym(s): Supraglottitis

EPIDEMIOLOGY
Incidence
- Has decreased dramatically since the introduction of the *Haemophilus influenzae* type b (Hib) vaccine in the mid-1980s (1,2)
- In adults: 1–3 per 100,000 per year
- In the pre-vaccine era, the most commonly affected group was children 2–4 years old.
- With use of Hib vaccine, the predominant age is shifting to older children (median age, 7 years) and adults (1,2).
- Predominant sex: Male > Female (1.8:1)

Prevalence
More prevalent in countries without universal immunization

RISK FACTORS
- Absence of immunization against Hib
- Immunocompromise

GENERAL PREVENTION
- *H. influenzae* type B vaccine is effective, although not 100% protective.
- Rifampin prophylaxis (20 mg/kg/d for 4 days, maximum daily dose 600 mg) for all household and daycare contacts of invasive Hib. Family and close contacts may be asymptomatic carriers of Hib.

Pediatric Considerations
Rare since introduction of Hib vaccine

Geriatric Considerations
Rare

PATHOPHYSIOLOGY
- In epiglottitis, usually a local invasion of the epiglottis occurs, followed by bacteremia.
- The epiglottis, aryepiglottic folds, false vocal cords, and supraglottic structures become inflamed and edematous, leading to narrowed airway and respiratory compromise.
- Inspiratory airway occlusion often occurs prior to total occlusion from supraglottic edema.

ETIOLOGY
- Bacterial:
  - Hib
  - *Streptococcus pyogenes*
  - *Streptococcus pneumoniae*
  - *Staphylococcus aureus*
  - Other bacteria
- Fungal
- Viral
- Traumatic: Caustic ingestion
- Allergic reactions

 DIAGNOSIS

HISTORY
- Sudden onset of severe symptoms and a fulminant course over a period of hours, unless airway control and medical management are initiated promptly.
- Fever is the 1st symptom, followed by stridor and labored breathing.
- Dysphagia, refusal to eat, drooling, and sore throat are common.
- Muffled voice/cry (vs hoarseness in croup)
- Minimal cough (vs barking cough in croup)
- Usually no history of prodromal upper respiratory infection (vs positive history in croup)
- In adults, presentation is more indolent (sore throat and odynophagia are the predominant symptoms).

PHYSICAL EXAM
- Toxic appearance/shock (occasionally, due to associated septicemia)
- Marked restlessness, irritability, and anxiety are common.
- Airway obstruction resulting in respiratory distress
- Tripod position (sitting propped up on hands with head forward and tongue out)
- Stridor softer and less prominent than in croup
- Anterior neck exam may reveal tender adenopathy.
- Definitive diagnosis is established by visualizing a swollen and erythematous epiglottis during careful exam of the oropharynx, although this should not normally be attempted without specific training and equipment available to manage an obstructed airway, such as in an operating room.
- Cyanosis indicates a poor prognosis.

DIAGNOSTIC TESTS & INTERPRETATION
Lab
Initial lab tests
- Blood culture (positive in >75–90% of children with Hib-acute epiglottitis). *Do not* visualize/swab epiglottis except in controlled environment (e.g., operating room). Blood tests are also contraindicated until airway is secured.
- Epiglottic swab culture (positive in 70%)
- Complete blood count: Leukocytosis with left shift
- Hib antigen test in serum/urine useful in children with previous antibiotic treatment
- Hypoxia usually not present until airway obstructed

Imaging
Initial approach
- Lateral neck radiographs typically show an enlarged edematous epiglottis (the thumbprint sign) (1,3); however, radiographs are contraindicated because of danger of sudden complete airway obstruction with delay of important airway intervention.
- If radiographs are obtained, ensure adequate staff in case complete airway obstruction occurs.
- Chest x-rays after intubation to check position of endotracheal tube and to rule out pneumonia, which may occur as a complication.

Diagnostic Procedures/Surgery
- Visualization of epiglottis with tongue depressor is contraindicated because of danger of sudden complete airway obstruction.
- Controlled visualization of epiglottis at intubation in operating room is diagnostic (cherry red, edematous epiglottis).
- Lumbar puncture is indicated if there is clinical suspicion of meningitis.
- In an adult, indirect laryngoscopy is generally safe.

DIFFERENTIAL DIAGNOSIS
- Viral croup (laryngotracheobronchitis)
- Acute angioneurotic edema (no fever)
- Aspirated foreign body (history, no fever)
- Bacterial tracheitis (pseudomembranous croup)
- Retropharyngeal or peritonsillar abscess
- Diphtheria in an unimmunized patient (often an adult)
- Sepsis from other cause

TREATMENT

There are 2 key aspects to the treatment of acute epiglottitis:
- Maintenance of an adequate airway should be the primary concern (1,2,3)[C].
- Administration of antimicrobial agents

MEDICATION
First Line
- Begin empiric antibiotic promptly after blood and epiglottic cultures are obtained. Use antibiotics guided by cultures thereafter. Duration of antimicrobial: 7–10 days (1,3)[C]
- Cefotaxime (Claforan) 100–200 mg/kg/d q8h IV (1,3)[C]
- Ceftriaxone (Rocephin) 50–100 mg/kg/d q12h IV (1,3)[C]

Second Line
- Other 3d- or 4th-generation cephalosporins IV or only ampicillin if Hib is sensitive (3)[C]
- Ampicillin-sulbactam (Unasyn) 150 mg/kg/d q6h, IV
- The role of steroids and racemic epinephrine remains controversial (1,3)[C].
- Antipyretics if necessary

ADDITIONAL TREATMENT
General Measures
- Each institution should have an emergency protocol involving a team of emergency room physicians, pediatricians, anesthesiologists, surgeons, pediatric intensivists, and pediatric intensive care unit (ICU) nurses (principles are similar for pediatric and adult patients).
- Call anesthesiologist to bedside.
- Have equipment for intubation and needle cricothyrotomy or percutaneous tracheostomy at bedside.
- Notify operating room (OR).
- Notify pediatric surgeon or ear/nose/throat (ENT) specialist for standby in OR in case tracheostomy becomes necessary.
- Keep patient quiet, calm, sitting up (in parent's arms).
- Avoid venipuncture, blood gases, oxygen masks, IV lines, injections, monitors, and radiographs.
- Judicious use of sedation that does not depress respirations may be appropriate.
- Racemic epinephrine is without benefit.
- Avoid examining the pharynx.
- Transport patient and parent together to OR in a wheelchair.

- Intubate all patients, preferably in OR under controlled circumstances by experienced anesthesiologist, with surgeon or ENT specialist on standby for emergency tracheostomy.
- Tracheostomy is not indicated unless intubation is unsuccessful (1,2,3)[C].
- Tape airway securely in place, and use a bite block if indicated.
- Splint elbows and restrain arms to avoid self-extubation.
- Use humidity and avoid T-piece (traction increases risk of accidental extubation).
- Continuous positive airway pressure, mechanical ventilation, and sedation are usually unnecessary.
- Pay attention to supervision and pulmonary suctioning to minimize risk of endotracheal tube plugs.

SURGERY/OTHER PROCEDURES
Emergency tracheotomy may be necessary (1,2,3)[C].

IN-PATIENT CONSIDERATIONS
Initial Stabilization
Acute epiglottitis is a medical emergency. During acute illness, hospitalize patient in ICU (1,2,3)[C].

Admission Criteria
Whenever the diagnosis of epiglottitis is suspected, immediate hospitalization is required.

IV Fluids
Initially, while intubated

Nursing
Expert respiratory nursing care is essential.

Discharge Criteria
Extubated patients afebrile in good clinical condition

 ONGOING CARE

FOLLOW-UP RECOMMENDATIONS
Immunization

Patient Monitoring
- Rule out secondary foci of infection.
- Observe swallowing ability and presence of an air leak around endotracheal/nasotracheal tube.
- Follow-up with laryngoscopy prior to extubation (advocated by some).
- Observe in ICU for 24 hours following extubation.

DIET
IV fluid initially, then nasogastric feedings while intubated

PATIENT EDUCATION
Reassurance about treatment and outcome

PROGNOSIS
- Most patients can be extubated after 24–48 hours.
- Morbidity and mortality are low with appropriate intervention.

COMPLICATIONS
- Pneumonia, meningitis, septic arthritis, cervical adenitis, and cellulitis (rare)
- Progression of infection to deep neck tissue
- Epiglottic abscess
- Septic shock (~1%)
- Pneumothorax (rare)
- Death from asphyxia

REFERENCES

1. Mayo-Smith MF, Spinale JW, Donskey CJ, et al. Acute epiglottitis. An 18-year experience in Rhode Island. *Chest*. 1995;108:1640–7.
2. Guldfred LA, Lyhne D, Becker BC. Acute epiglottitis: epidemiology, clinical presentation, management and outcome. *J Laryngol Otol*. 2008;122:818–23.
3. Glynn F, Fenton JE. Diagnosis and management of supraglottitis (epiglottitis). *Curr Infect Dis Rep*. 2008;10:200–4.

ADDITIONAL READING

- Cheung CS, Man SY, Graham CA, Mak PS, Cheung PS, Chan BC, Rainer TH et al. Adult epiglottitis: 6 years experience in a university teaching hospital in Hong Kong. *Eur J Emerg Med*. 2009;16:221–6.
- Sobol SE, Zapata S et al. Epiglottitis and croup. *Otolaryngol Clin North Am*. 2008;41:551–66, ix

 CODES

ICD9
- 464.30 Acute epiglottitis without mention of obstruction
- 464.31 Acute epiglottitis with obstruction
- 487.1 Influenza with other respiratory manifestations

CLINICAL PEARLS
- Acute epiglottitis is a medical emergency and requires immediate hospitalization. The airway must be secured before transport of all patients with suspected epiglottitis. Transport must be done by an experienced team.
- Evident respiratory distress, stridor, drooling, and shorter duration of symptoms are clinical features associated with a higher likelihood of airway obstruction in children with epiglottitis.
- Security of the airway is always of primary concern in acute epiglottitis; failure to intervene prior to loss of the airway associated with an increase in mortality. Avoid interventions that may upset the child, and proceed directly to operating room in parent's lap
- Avoid use of tongue blade, which may worsen obstruction. Direct laryngoscopy should be done in OR.

E

EPISTAXIS

Julie Yeh, MD, MPH

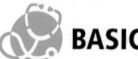 **BASICS**

DESCRIPTION
- Hemorrhage from the nose involving either the anterior or posterior mucosal surfaces
- Synonym(s): Nosebleed

EPIDEMIOLOGY
Incidence
- In the US: Common
- Estimated lifetime incidence approximately 60%
- Bimodal, with peaks in children up to 15 and in adults >50
- Rare in children under age 2

RISK FACTORS
- Local irritation from multiple causes (see Etiology)
- Medications/supplements, including aspirin and clopidogrel

GENERAL PREVENTION
- Humidification at night
- Cut fingernails to minimize picking.

PATHOPHYSIOLOGY
- Local vs systemic disease. Large majority are due to local causes.
- Anterior: 90–95% of all cases (Kiesselbach plexus)
- Posterior: Usually branches of sphenopalatine arteries: May be asymptomatic or may present with other symptoms

ETIOLOGY
- Idiopathic
- Local inflammation/irritation:
  – Infection
  – Irritant inhalation
  – Topical steroid use
  – Septal deviation (more air movement on 1 side)
  – Low humidity
- Trauma:
  – Epistaxis digitorum (nose picking)
  – Foreign bodies
  – Septal perforation
  – Sinus fracture

COMMONLY ASSOCIATED CONDITIONS
- Vascular malformation/telangiectasia
- Neoplasm (rare, but consider in persistent unilateral cases)
- Systemic:
  – Coagulopathy, primary or iatrogenic
  – Thrombocytopenia
  – Cirrhosis
  – Renal failure
  – Alcoholism
- No proven association with HTN, but may make control of bleeding more difficult.

 DIAGNOSIS

HISTORY
- Initial presentation, including detail on where bleeding started (which side?)
- Trauma, including nose picking
- Previous episodes
- Comorbid conditions
- Current medications, including over-the-counter and supplements

PHYSICAL EXAM
- Blood loss through 1 or both nostrils in the majority of cases is due to anterior nasal septal bleeding and can often be directly visualized.
- Examiner should wear protective gear, including gown, gloves, and goggles.
- Patient seated, head forward, to avoid blood going down the posterior pharynx.

DIAGNOSTIC TESTS & INTERPRETATION
Indicated only in complicated cases
Lab
Lab testing is not indicated in the majority of uncomplicated cases in which bleeding is reasonably easily controlled and is not truly hemorrhagic.

Initial lab tests
- For recurrent or intractable cases
- CBC, platelet count, prothrombin time
- Cross-match when appropriate
- Toxicology screen when nasal use of illicit drugs is suspected

Imaging
For most cases, imaging not indicated

Diagnostic Procedures/Surgery
Nasal endoscopy

DIFFERENTIAL DIAGNOSIS
- Diagnosis usually apparent; the differential for the etiology is key
- Posterior bleeding must be included in the differential for any chronic blood loss.

Pediatric Considerations
More likely anterior, idiopathic, and recurrent

Geriatric Considerations
More likely to be posterior bleed

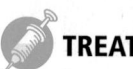 **TREATMENT**

- Most cases managed as outpatient
- Patient applies direct pressure by pinching the lower part of the nose for 5–20 minutes without a break. This will stop active bleeding in the majority of patients.
- An ice pack placed over the dorsum of the nose may help with hemostasis.
- Inspect the nasal septum for the bleeding site.

MEDICATION
First Line
If general measures fail, affected naris may be sprayed with topical vasoconstrictor such as phenylephrine or oxymetazoline.

Second Line
NosebleedQR: A nonprescription powder of hydrophilic polymer with potassium salt; induces formation of scab

ADDITIONAL TREATMENT

- Nasal packing: Either with ribbon gauze or preformed nasal tampons
- FloSeal: A biodegradable hemostatic sealant (a thrombin-type gel) in 1 study more effective and better tolerated than packing (1)[B]
- If an actively bleeding anterior septal site is visualized, this may be treated with gentle and specific silver nitrate cautery for ~10 seconds for definitive treatment.
- Limit to 1 side of septum, or wait 4–6 weeks in between treatments to reduce risk of perforation (2).
- Posterior: Posterior packing or tamponade with balloon devices (Foley catheter has been used)
- Recurrent epistaxis: Cochrane Review of issue in children shows no difference in effectiveness between antiseptic nasal cream, petroleum jelly, silver nitrate cautery, or no treatment (3)[A]:
  – Silver nitrate cautery followed by 4 weeks of antiseptic cream may be better than antiseptic cream alone (4)[B].

General Measures
Resuscitation as indicated. Use universal "ABC" approach.

Issues for Referral
- Posterior bleeding, frequently requires an otolaryngology consultation
- Intractable bleeding. May require more specialized measures:
  – Endoscopic laser or electrocauterization
  – Angiography with arteriolar embolization

SURGERY/OTHER PROCEDURES
- Packing:
  – Layering of Vaseline ribbon gauze:
    ○ For gauze packing, be certain both ends of the ribbon gauze protrude from the nostril.
    ○ The packing is layered from the floor upward.
    ○ Secure packing with gauze across the outside of the nostril
  – Nasal tampon may be used after lubricating the tip with KY Jelly or antibiotic cream or ointment.
  – Additional saline may be needed to expand the tampon if the bleeding has slowed.
  – Merocel and Rapid Rhino packs are easier to use than gauze packing and are usually well tolerated.

- Posterior bleed:
  – In the emergent setting, this may be attempted utilizing a Foley catheter or a specific posterior packing balloon.
  – With both methods, the tubing is introduced through the nose similar to the passage of a nasogastric tube. Once it reaches the posterior oral pharynx, the balloon is inflated and the tubing is pulled back outward to tamponade the posterior bleeding source:
    ○ If using a Foley catheter (10–14 French), the balloon can be inflated with 10 mL of saline.
    ○ Traction is maintained with an umbilical cord clamp with adequate padding between the clip and the nose to avoid injury.

IN-PATIENT CONSIDERATIONS
Consider for elderly or for patients with posterior bleeding or coagulopathy. May also consider if significant comorbidities.

Initial Stabilization
Universal "Airway/Breathing/Circulation" (ABC) approach. Stop blood loss.

Admission Criteria
- Posterior bleed
- Hemodynamic changes
- Clotting dysfunction

 ONGOING CARE

FOLLOW-UP RECOMMENDATIONS
Patient Monitoring
- When significant blood loss, hemodynamic monitoring
- With packing, 24-hour minimum; some authors recommend 3–5 days. The latter recommendation carries the risk of mucosal injury and toxic shock syndrome. The former has the risk of rebleed, which usually occurs between 24 and 48 hours.

PATIENT EDUCATION
- Demonstrate proper pinching pressure techniques.
- Avoidance of trauma or irritants is key.
- Management of systemic illness and proper use of medication

PROGNOSIS
- Most are self-limited.
- Good results with proper treatment

COMPLICATIONS
- Septal perforation
- Pressure-induced tissue necrosis of the nasal mucosa
- Toxic shock syndrome with packing
- Arrhythmias triggered by packing

REFERENCES

1. Mathiasen RA, Cruz RM. Prospective, randomized, controlled clinical trial of a novel matrix hemostatic sealant in patients with acute anterior epistaxis. *Laryngoscope.* 2005;115:899–902.
2. Hanif J, Tasca RA, Frosh A, et al. Silver nitrate: histological effects of cautery on epithelial surfaces with varying contact times. *Clin Otolaryngol Allied Sci.* 2003;28:368–70.
3. Burton MJ, Dorée CJ. Interventions for recurrent idiopathic epistaxis (nosebleeds) in children. *Cochrane Database Syst Rev.* 2004:CD004461.
4. Calder N, Kang S, Fraser L, Kunanandam T, Montgomery J, Kubba H et al. A double-blind randomized controlled trial of management of recurrent nosebleeds in children. *Otolaryngol Head Neck Surg.* 2009;140:670–4.

ADDITIONAL READING

- Douglas R, Wormald PJ. Update on epistaxis. *Curr Opin Otolaryngol Head Neck Surg.* 2007;15:180–3.
- Gifford TO, Orlandi RR. Epistaxis. *Otolaryngol Clin North Am.* 2008;41:525–36, viii.
- Kucik CJ, et al. Management of epistaxis. *Am Fam Physician.* 2005;7(2).
- Robertson S, Kubba H. Long-term effectiveness of antiseptic cream for recurrent epistaxis in childhood: five-year follow up of a randomised, controlled trial. *J Laryngol Otol.* 2008:1–4.
- Viehweg TL, Roberson JB, Hudson JW. Epistaxis: diagnosis and treatment. *J Oral Maxillofac Surg.* 2006;64:511–8.

 CODES

ICD9
784.7 Epistaxis

CLINICAL PEARLS
- Most episodes are anterior in etiology and respond to timed pressure over the anterior nares for 5–20 minutes.
- Most are idiopathic or as a result of nose picking.
- Posterior nosebleeds can be asymptomatic or present with nausea, hematemesis, or heme-positive stool.

EPSTEIN-BARR VIRUS INFECTIONS

Dennis E. Hughes, DO

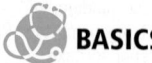 **BASICS**

DESCRIPTION
- Epstein-Barr virus (EBV) is the cause of heterophile-positive infectious mononucleosis.
- All seropositive persons actively shed the virus in the saliva.
- System(s) affected: Hemic/Lymphatic/Immunologic

EPIDEMIOLOGY
Incidence
Worldwide, infects >90% of people (antibody-positive) (1)

Prevalence
- Military and college student groups have the most active infection rate (0.1–0.48%) (2).
- Predominant age: 10–19 years (2)
- By young adult life, 60–90% of persons are antibody-positive to EBV; antibodies persist for lifetime (1).
- Predominant gender: Male = Female

RISK FACTORS
- Age
- Sociohygienic level
- Geographic location
- Close, intimate contact
- EBV may play a cofactor role in chronic inflammatory and autoimmune diseases such as multiple sclerosis (MS) (3)[C].

GENERAL PREVENTION
- Avoiding close physical contact with persons known to be currently symptomatic
- Good handwashing and hygiene
- EBV vaccine currently under development

PATHOPHYSIOLOGY
- A polyclonal B-cell proliferative response is characteristic of infectious mononucleosis. Relatively few circulating lymphocytes are infected by EBV and represent <0.1% of circulating mononuclear cells in the acute illness.
- EBV is tropic for B-lymphocytes, which are infected in the oropharynx through salivary exchange; infected B cells then circulate in the blood and are distributed to the bone marrow and lymphoreticular system.
- EBV can also be found in infected epithelial cells of the buccal mucosa, salivary glands, tongue, and endocervix; this suggests that chronic epithelial replication brings about continuous reinfection of B lymphoid cells.
- Immune T-cell responses to latently infected B cells account for the clinical findings.

ETIOLOGY
EBV, a member of the herpesvirus (DNA virus) group

COMMONLY ASSOCIATED CONDITIONS
- Infectious mononucleosis: The symptomatic primary EBV infection seen in otherwise healthy older children, adolescents, and young adults:
  - Clinical features vary in severity and duration: In children, generally mild; in adults, more severe and protracted.
  - Incubation period is 30–50 days.
- X-linked lymphoproliferative syndrome (Duncan disease)
- Lymphoproliferative syndromes due to EBV infections in transplant patients
- Lymphomas (B-cell lymphoblastic, T cell)
- Lymphocytic interstitial pneumonitis
- Hairy leukoplakia of the tongue and central nervous system (CNS) lymphomas in AIDS patients
- Burkitt lymphoma
- Nasopharyngeal carcinoma
- Parotid carcinoma
- Hodgkin lymphoma

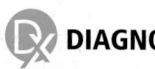 **DIAGNOSIS**

HISTORY
- May begin abruptly or insidiously
- Syndrome of fatigue, malaise, and sore throat
- In adults, temperature may rise to 103°F (39.4°C) and gradually fall over a variable period of 7–10 days; in severe cases, temperature elevations of 104–105°F (40.0–40.6°C) may persist for 2 weeks.
- Children usually have a low-grade fever or may be afebrile.
- Diffuse hyperemia and hyperplasia of oropharyngeal lymphoid tissue
- Gelatinous, grayish-white exudative tonsillitis persists for 7–10 days in 50%.
- Petechiae develop at border of hard and soft palates in 60%.
- Axillary, epitrochlear, popliteal, inguinal, mediastinal, and mesenteric nodes may also be affected (95% of patients) (2).
- Lymph node enlargement subsides over days or weeks.
- Chest pain (myocarditis and pericarditis)

PHYSICAL EXAM
- Fever, lymphadenopathy, pharyngitis in >50%, with palatal petechiae and hepatosplenomegaly ~10% (1,4)
- Tender lymphadenopathy (cervical nodes are most commonly enlarged)
- Splenomegaly in 50%
- Skin manifestations (3–16%):
  - Erythematous macular or maculopapular rash
  - Petechial and purpuric exanthems have been reported.
  - Rash location: Trunk and upper arms; occasionally the face and forearms involved

DIAGNOSTIC TESTS & INTERPRETATION
Lab
Initial lab tests
- Complete blood count (CBC) with differential
- Lymphocytes and atypical lymphocytes:
  - Increased numbers of lymphocytes (especially atypical lymphocytes; may be up to 70% of leukocytes) in peripheral blood
  - In 1st week after onset, white blood cell (WBC) count is normal or moderately decreased. By the 2nd week, lymphocytosis develops with >10% atypical lymphocytes (4).
  - During early illness, atypical lymphocytes are B cells transformed by the EBV; later, atypical cells are primarily T cells having an immunoregulatory function.
- Antibodies:
  - Heterophile antibodies in 80–90% of adults
  - Heterophile antibody is an IgM response, which appears during the 1st or 2nd week of illness and persists for 3–6 months.
  - In general, agglutinin titer is higher in infectious mononucleosis than in other disorders; an unabsorbed heterophile titer >1:128 and 1:40 or higher after absorption is significant.
- Specific antibodies to EBV-associated antigens:
  - Develop regularly in infectious mononucleosis
  - Viral capsid-specific IgM and IgG are present early in illness; viral capsid-IgM responses disappear after several months, whereas viral capsid-IgG antibodies persist for life.
- Liver function studies; AST and ALT elevations and hyperbilirubinemia are common; frank jaundice is rare.
- Disorders that may alter lab results: Atypical lymphocytes are not specific for EBV infections and may be present in other clinical conditions, including rubella, infectious hepatitis, allergic rhinitis, asthma, and primary atypical pneumonia:
  - In infectious mononucleosis, increased numbers of atypical forms are present in peripheral blood; in other disorders, quantitative percentage is usually less.

Follow-Up & Special Considerations
Abnormal hepatic enzymes in 80% of patients for several weeks after onset; hepatomegaly in 15–20%

Imaging
Initial approach
- Abdominal ultrasound to monitor for splenic enlargement is not supported routinely (2).
- Consider for those wishing to return to strenuous activity or contact sports at day 21 of illness to evaluate for resolution of splenomegaly.

Diagnostic Procedures/Surgery
Chest x-ray (CXR):
- Hilar adenopathy may be observed in infectious mononucleosis cases with extensive lymphoid hyperplasia.

Pathological Findings
- Mononuclear infiltrations involve lymph nodes, tonsils, spleen, lungs, liver, heart, kidneys, adrenal glands, skin, and CNS.
- Bone marrow hyperplasia develops regularly, and small granulomas may be present; these are nonspecific and have no prognostic significance.

DIFFERENTIAL DIAGNOSIS
- Streptococcal pharyngitis and tonsillitis
- Diphtheria
- Blood dyscrasias
- Rubella
- Measles
- Viral hepatitis
- Cytomegalovirus
- Toxoplasmosis

 TREATMENT

MEDICATION
- Antimicrobial agents (usually a penicillin) if throat culture is positive for group A, beta-hemolytic streptococci (5)
- Warm saline gargles for the pain of pharyngeal involvement and enlarged lymph nodes
- Corticosteroids:
  - Support unclear; may provide some symptomatic relief, but no improvement in resolution of illness
  - Consider in severe pharyngotonsillitis with oropharyngeal edema and airway encroachment. Dexamethasone (0.3 mg/kg/day) may be used for 1–3 days (2,5,6)[B].
  - Also for patients with marked toxicity or major complications (e.g., hemolytic anemia, thrombocytopenic purpura, neurologic sequelae, myocarditis, pericarditis) (1)
- Precautions: Refer to the manufacturer's literature.

ADDITIONAL TREATMENT
General Measures
- The treatment is chiefly supportive.
- Nonsteroidal anti-inflammatory drugs
- During acute stage, limit activity for 4 weeks to reduce potential complications (splenic rupture, etc.) and aid in recovery.

SURGERY/OTHER PROCEDURES
With profound thrombocytopenia, refractory to corticosteroid therapy, splenectomy may be necessary.

IN-PATIENT CONSIDERATIONS
Admission Criteria
- Inability to eat food or drink fluids
- Splenic rupture

 ONGOING CARE

FOLLOW-UP RECOMMENDATIONS

> **ALERT**
> Rupture of the spleen may be fatal if not recognized, and requires blood transfusions, treatment for shock, and splenectomy. Occurrence is estimated at 0.1% (2).

Patient Monitoring
- Avoid contact sports, heavy lifting, and excess exertion until spleen and liver have returned to normal size.
- Eliminate alcohol or exposure to other hepatotoxic drugs until liver function tests return to normal.
- Monitor patients closely during the 1st 2–3 weeks after the onset of symptoms. Thereafter, follow patients until their symptoms subside.
- Rarely, laboratory results resolve more slowly, and symptoms (malaise, fatigue, intermittent sore throat, lymphadenopathy) may persist for several months (4).

DIET
No restrictions. Hydration during acute phase is very important.

PATIENT EDUCATION
Mononucleosis on Familydoctor.org

PROGNOSIS
- Vast majority will be recovered by 4 weeks.
- Fatigue symptoms may persist for months (2).

COMPLICATIONS
- Neurologic (rare):
  - Aseptic meningitis
  - Bell palsy
  - Meningoencephalitis
  - Guillain-Barré syndrome
  - Transverse myelitis
  - Cerebellar ataxia
  - Acute psychosis
- Hematologic (rare):
  - Thrombocytopenia, slight to moderate, early in illness
  - Hemolytic anemia with marked neutropenia during early weeks
  - Aplastic anemia
  - Agammaglobulinemia
- Pneumonitis
- Splenic rupture:
  - Rare, but most often occurs in 1st 21 days of illness

REFERENCES
1. Cohen JI. Epstein-Barr virus infection. *N Engl J Med*. 2000;343:481–92.
2. Ebell MH. Epstein-Barr virus infectious mononucleosis. *Am Fam Physician*. 2006;70(7): 1279–88.
3. Pohl D. Epstein-Barr virus and multiple sclerosis. *J Neurol Sci*. 2009.
4. Rea TD, Russo JE, Katon W, et al. Prospective study of the natural history of infectious mononucleosis caused by Epstein-Barr virus. *J Am Board Fam Pract*. 2001;14:234–42.
5. Halstead ME, Bernhardt DT. Common infections in the young athlete. *Pediatr Ann*. 2002;31:42–8.
6. Thompson SK, Doerr TD, Hengerer AS. Infectious mononucleosis and corticosteroids: management practices and outcomes. *Arch Otolaryngol Head Neck Surg*. 2005;131:900–4.

ADDITIONAL READING
Roy M, Bailey B, Amre DK, et al. Dexamethasone for the treatment of sore throat in children with suspected infectious mononucleosis: a randomized, double-blind, placebo-controlled, clinical trial. *Arch Pediatr Adolesc Med*. 2004;158:250–4.

CODES

ICD9
075 Infectious mononucleosis

CLINICAL PEARLS
- False-negative monosport (heterophile antibody) in the 1st 10–14 days of illness
- 98% have fever, sore throat, cervical node enlargement, and tonsillar hypertrophy.
- Although splenic rupture is extremely rare, athletic activity should be curtailed for 3–4 weeks.
- Lab shows a lymphocytosis, not a monocytosis.

E

ERECTILE DYSFUNCTION

Michael C. Barros, PharmD, BCPS
Erica Tavares, PharmD, RPh
Frank J. Domino, MD

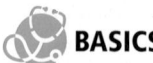 **BASICS**

DESCRIPTION

- Inability to achieve or maintain an erection sufficient for satisfactory sexual performance (1)[C]
- Erectile dysfunction is sometimes assumed to be a symptom of the aging process in men, but it can likely result from concurrent medical conditions of the patient or from medications that patients may be taking to treat those conditions.
- Normal penile erection requires full functioning of the vascular, nervous, and hormonal systems.
- System(s) affected: Cardiovascular; Nervous; Urologic; Reproductive
- Synonym: Impotence

EPIDEMIOLOGY

Prevalence

- Overall prevalence for erectile dysfunction per the Massachusetts Male Aging Study (2):
  - 52% in men age 40–70 years
  - Age-related increase ranging from 12.4% in men age 40–49 years up to 46.6% in men age 50–69 years
- A study of US health professionals found prevalence of sexual dysfunction 12% in men <59 years old, 22% age 60–69 years, and 30% >69 years old (3).

RISK FACTORS

- Age
- Cardiovascular disease
- Diabetes
- Metabolic syndrome
- Lower urinary tract systems of benign prostatic hyperplasia
- Medications that induce erectile dysfunction
- Urologic surgery or trauma/injury to pelvic area or spinal cord
- Central neurologic and endocrinologic conditions
- Substance abuse
- Psychological conditions: stress, anxiety, or depression
- Smoking

Genetics

Rarely related to chromosomal disorders

ETIOLOGY

- Erectile dysfunction may result from problems with systems required for normal penile erection:
  - Vascular: Diseases that compromise blood flow:
    ○ Peripheral vascular disease, arteriosclerosis, essential hypertension
  - Neurologic: Diseases that impair nerve conduction to brain or penile vasculature:
    ○ Spinal cord injury, trauma (bicycling accident), stroke, diabetes
  - Endocrine: Diseases associated with changes in testosterone, luteinizing hormone, prolactin levels
  - Psychological: Patients suffering from malaise, depression, performance anxiety, or Alzheimer's disease

- Social habits such as smoking or excessive alcohol intake
- Medications may cause erectile dysfunction.
- Structural injury or trauma

Geriatric Considerations

Aging alone is not a cause.

COMMONLY ASSOCIATED CONDITIONS

- Cardiovascular disease
  - Men with erectile dysfunction have a greater likelihood of having angina, myocardial infarction, stroke, transient ischemic attack, congestive heart failure, or cardiac arrhythmia compared to men without erectile dysfunction (3).
- Diabetes
- Psychiatric disorders

 DIAGNOSIS

- Inability to maintain erection satisfactory for intercourse
- Inability to achieve erection
- Reduced body hair
- Thyromegaly
- Gynecomastia
- Testicular atrophy or absence
- Deformed penis
- Peripheral vascular disease
- Neuropathy

HISTORY

- Identify concurrent medical illnesses or surgical procedures
- Social history: Smoking, ethanol intake, recreational drug use
- List of prescription and nonprescription medications

PHYSICAL EXAM

- Assess vital signs (blood pressure and heart rate)
- Signs and symptoms of hypogonadism: Gynecomastia, small testicles, decreased body hair
- Abnormal penile curvature (Peyronie's disease)
- Assess for central obesity, thyroid goiter
- Detailed examination of the cardiovascular, neurologic, and genitourinary systems
  - Check femoral and lower extremity pulses to assess vascular supply to genitals
  - Check anal sphincter tone and genital reflexes for adequate nerve supply
  - Digital rectal exam for patients age >50 years to rule out benign prostatic hyperplasia (BPH)
- Screen for cardiovascular risk factors

DIAGNOSTIC TESTS & INTERPRETATION

- Nocturnal penile tumescence and rigidity assessment
- Consider the following only in rare circumstances, when indicated:
  - 24-hour urine zinc
  - Dorsal nerve somatosensory-evoked potentials
  - Sacral evoked response

- Penile–brachial blood pressure (BP)
- Aortogram
- Selective pudendal angiogram
- Dynamic cavernosography
- Penile BP
- Optional diagnostic tests: psychological or psychiatric evaluation

Lab

Initial lab tests

- Fasting serum glucose
- Lipid profile
- Serum testosterone levels drawn in the morning (2 serial levels are needed to confirm hypogonadism)
- Thyroid-stimulating hormone
- Prolactin

Imaging

Doppler, angiogram, cavernosogram

Diagnostic Procedures/Surgery

International Index of Erectile Function (IIEF) Survey may be used to assess the severity of a patient's erectile dysfunction. The survey is also available in an abbreviated form (IIEF-5).

DIFFERENTIAL DIAGNOSIS

- Endocrine:
  - Thyroid dysfunction
  - Low testosterone
  - High prolactin
  - Diabetes
  - High estrogen effect
  - Renal failure
  - Zinc deficiency
- Neurologic: Central, Spinal, Peripheral
- Vascular: Arterial insufficiency, Cavernosal insufficiency, Venous insufficiency
- Medication: β-blockers, thiazides, antidepressants
- Psychological: Depression, Schizophrenia, Relationship disorders, Personality disorders, Anxiety
- Structural:
  - Microphallus, Chordee and Peyronie's disease, Cavernosal scarring
  - Phimosis, Hypospadias
- Postsurgical sequelae

 TREATMENT

Use least invasive therapy first; reserve more invasive therapies for nonresponders.

MEDICATION

First Line

Phosphodiesterase type 5 (PDE-5) inhibitors are effective in the treatment of erectile dysfunction associated with diabetes mellitus and spinal cord injury, and sexual dysfunction associated with antidepressants (3).

- Sildenafil (Viagra): Usual daily dose: 25–100 mg within 30–60 min of sexual intercourse on an empty stomach, at least 2 hours before meals. Duration up to 4 hours.

- Vardenafil (Levitra): Usual daily dose 5–20 mg within 30–60 minutes of sexual intercourse on an empty stomach, at least 2 hours before meals. Duration up to 4 hours.
- Tadalafil (Cialis): Usual daily dose 5–20 mg, 2 hours before intercourse. May take without regard to meals. Duration up to 36 hours.

Geriatric Considerations
- Use doses at the lower end of the dosing range for elderly patients:
  – Sildenafil 25 mg daily
  – Vardenafil 5 mg daily
- Adverse effects of PDE-5 inhibitors: Headache, facial flushing, dyspepsia, nasal congestion, dizziness, hypotension, increased sensitivity to light (sildenafil and vardenafil), vision changes, lower back pain (tadalafil), and priapism (with excessive doses)

Second Line
- Penile injectables:
  – Alprostadil, also known as prostaglandin E_1, causes smooth muscle relaxation of the arterial blood vessels and sinusoidal tissues in the corpora. Available in 2 formulations:
    ○ Alprostadil (Caverject): Usual dose: 10–20 mcg, with max dose of 60 mcg. Injection should be made at right angles into one of the lateral surfaces of the proximal third of the penis using a 0.5-inch 27- or 30-gauge needle. Do not use >3 times a week or > once in 24 hours. Patient to notify physician if erection lasts >4 hours for immediate attention. Apply manual pressure at site of injection to prevent hematoma formation. Use with caution in patients with sickle cell disease: Initial trial dose should be administered under supervision of a physician
    ○ Alprostadil may also be combined with papaverine (Bimix) plus phentolamine(Tri-Mix).
    ○ Alprostadil (Muse) urethral suppository: 125-, 250-, 500-, and 1,000-mcg pellets. Administer 5–50 minutes before intercourse. No more than 2 doses in 24 hours are recommended.
- Miscellaneous:
  – Testosterone replacement regimens for patients with primary or secondary hypogonadism as confirmed by decreased libido and low testosterone concentrations.
    ○ Testosterone patch (Testoderm) 4 mg/patch, 6 mg/patch: Apply 4–6 mg/day to scrotum
    ○ Testosterone patch (Testoderm TTS) 4 mg/patch, 6 mg/patch: Apply 4–6 mg/day to arm, buttock, back
    ○ Testosterone patch (Androderm) 2.5 mg/patch: Apply 2.5–5 mg/day to arm, back, abdomen, thigh
    ○ Testosterone gel (AndroGel 1%) 5 g/packet, 10 g/packet: Apply 5–10 g/day to shoulders, upper arms, abdomen
    ○ Testosterone cypionate (Depo-Testosterone) 100 mg/mL, 200 mg/mL
    ○ Testosterone enanthate (Delatestryl) 100 mg/mL, 200 mg/mL: Inject 200–400 mg intramuscularly every 2-4 weeks
  – Contraindications:
    ○ Avoid injections in patients with bleeding disorders, sickle cell disease or trait, and penile deformities.
    ○ Avoid use in patients with known allergies to constituents.
    ○ Nitroglycerin (or other nitrates) and phosphodiesterase inhibitors: Potential for severe, potentially fatal hypotension

– Precautions:
  ○ Testosterone: Urinary retention, acne, sodium retention, and gynecomastia
  ○ Injection therapy: Priapism, fibrosis, hypotension, and nausea
  ○ Urethral suppositories: Penile pain and irritation, as well as testicular pain
  ○ Sildenafil: Hypotension (caution for patients on nitrates)
  ○ PDE-5 inhibitors: Use caution with congenital prolonged QT syndrome, class Ia or II antiarrhythmics, nitroglycerin, α-blockers (e.g., terazosin, tamsulosin), retinal disease, unstable cardiac disease, liver and renal failure
– Significant possible interactions:
  ○ PDE-5 inhibitor concentration is affected by CYP3A4 inhibitors (e.g., erythromycin, indinavir, ketoconazole, ritonavir, amiodarone, cimetidine, clarithromycin, delavirdine, diltiazem, fluoxetine, fluvoxamine, grapefruit juice, itraconazole, nefazodone, nevirapine, ritonavir, saquinavir, and verapamil). Serum concentrations and/or toxicity may be increased. Lower starting doses should be used in these patients.
  ○ PDE-5 inhibitor concentration may be reduced by rifampin and phenytoin.

ADDITIONAL TREATMENT
General Measures
- Penile prosthesis should be reserved for patients who have failed 1st- or 2nd-line therapies.
- Psychotherapy alone or in combination with psychoactive drugs may be helpful in men whose erectile dysfunction is caused by depression or anxiety.
- Weight loss and increased physical activity for obese men with erectile dysfunction.
- Improve partner communication.
- Reduce performance pressure.
- Try vacuum erectile device or oral therapy (can be used in conjunction with intracavernous injections). Do not use vacuum devices in men with sickle cell anemia or blood dyscrasias, or those on anticoagulants.
- Use of psychiatrists, psychologists, sex therapists, vascular surgeons, urologists, endocrinologists, neurologists, or plastic surgeons is often necessary for refractory cases.

COMPLEMENTARY AND ALTERNATIVE MEDICINE
Yohimbine and herbal therapies are not recommended for the treatment of erectile dysfunction (1).

SURGERY/OTHER PROCEDURES
Penile prosthesis is the most invasive treatment of erectile dysfunction and is reserved for patients who do not respond or are not candidates for oral or injectable therapies. Penile arterial reconstructive surgery is controversial.

 ONGOING CARE

FOLLOW-UP RECOMMENDATIONS
Patient Monitoring
Treatment should be assessed at baseline and after the patient has completed at least 1–3 weeks of a specific treatment: Monitor the quality and quantity of penile erections and Monitor the level of satisfaction patient achieves.

DIET
Diet and exercise recommended to achieve a normal body mass index; limit alcohol

PROGNOSIS
- All commercially available PDE-5 inhibitors are equally effective. In the presence of sexual stimulation, sildenafil produces satisfactory erections in 56–82% of patients. Similar results are seen in 65–80% of patients taking vardenafil and 62–77% in patients taking tadalafil:
  – Lower success rates with diabetes mellitus or who have postoperative nerve damage.
- Overall effectiveness is 70–90% for intracavernosal alprostadil and 43–60% for intraurethral alprostadil (4,5).
- Penile prostheses are associated with a 90% patient satisfaction rate, and the surgical success rate after insertion is 82–98% (4).

REFERENCES
1. Montague DK, Jarrow JP, Broderick GA, Dmochowski RR, Heaton JP, Lue TF, et al. *The Management of Erectile Dysfunction: An Update.* Linthicum, MD: American Urological Association, 2006.
2. Johannes CB, Aranjo AB, Feldman HA, et al. Incidence of erectile dysfunction in men 40-69 years old: Longitudinal results from the Massachusetts Male Aging Study. *J Urol.* 2000;163:460–3.
3. Heidelbaugh JJ et al. Management of erectile dysfunction. *Am Fam Physician.* 2010;81:305–12.
4. Lue TF. Erectile dysfunction. *N Engl J Med.* 2000;342:1802–13.
5. McVary KT. Clinical practice. Erectile dysfunction. *N Engl J Med.* 2007;357:2472–81.

CODES

ICD9
- 302.72 Psychosexual dysfunction with inhibited sexual excitement
- 607.84 Impotence of organic origin

CLINICAL PEARLS
- Nitrates should be withheld for 24 hours after sildenafil or vardenafil administration and for 48 hours after use of tadalafil.
- Reserve surgical treatment for patients who do not respond to drug treatment.
- The use of PDE-5 inhibitors with alpha-adrenergic antagonists may increase the risk of hypotension. Tamsulosin is the least likely to cause orthostatic hypotension.
- Consult a cardiologist for use of PDE-5 inhibitors in patients with left ventricular dysfunction or NYHA class II. Do not use in patients with NYHA class III or IV.

ERYSIPELAS

James G. Anderson, MD
Richard A. Moriarty, MD

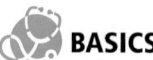

BASICS

DESCRIPTION
- Distinct form of cellulitis notable for acute, well-demarcated, superficial bacterial skin infection with lymphatic involvement almost always caused by *Streptococcus pyogenes*. Usually acute, but a chronic recurrent form also exists (1).
- System(s) affected: Skin/Exocrine
- Synonym(s): Saint Anthony's fire

EPIDEMIOLOGY
- Predominant age: Infants, children, and adults >40 years. Greatest in elderly (>75 years).
- Predominant sex: Male = Female
- Affects all races

Incidence
- Erysipelas occurs in about 1 person/1,000/year (2)
- Incidence on the rise since the 1980s (3)

Prevalence
Unknown

RISK FACTORS
- Toe-web intertrigo and lymphedema (2)
- Skin barrier disruption (surgical incisions, insect bites, eczematous lesions, local trauma, abrasions, dermatophytic infections)
- Fissured skin (especially at the nose and ears)
- Leg ulcers/stasis dermatitis
- Venous or lymphatic insufficiency (saphenectomy, varicose veins of leg, phlebitis, radiotherapy, mastectomy, lymphadenectomy)
- Chronic diseases (diabetes, malnutrition, nephrotic syndrome, heart failure)
- Immunocompromised (HIV) or debilitated
- Alcohol abuse
- Morbid obesity
- Recent streptococcal pharyngitis

GENERAL PREVENTION
- Good skin hygiene.
- Appropriate management of underlying medical condition that might predispose to the condition: Tinea pedis, stasis dermatitis, etc.
- Men who shave within 5 days of facial erysipelas are more likely to have a recurrence.
- With recurrences, search for other possible source of streptococcal infection (e.g., tonsils, sinuses).
- Compression stockings should be encouraged for patients with lower extremity edema.
- Consider suppressive prophylactic antibiotic therapy in patients with ≥2 episodes in a 12-month period.

PATHOPHYSIOLOGY
- Group A streptococci induce inflammation and activation of the contact system, releasing proteinases and pro-inflammatory cytokines.
- The generation of antibacterial peptides and the release of bradykinin, a proinflammatory peptide, increase vascular permeability and induce fever and pain.
- The M proteins from the group A streptococcal cell wall interact with neutrophils, leading to the secretion of heparin-binding protein, an inflammatory mediator that also induces vascular leakage.

- These cascades of reactions lead to the symptoms seen in erysipelas: Fever, pain, erythema, and edema

ETIOLOGY
- Group A β-hemolytic streptococci primarily; occasionally other streptococcus groups C or G
- Rarely, group B streptococci or *Staphylococcus aureus* may be involved.

Pediatric Considerations
- Group B streptococcus may be a cause in neonates/infants.

DIAGNOSIS

- Prodromal symptoms may include chills, malaise, moderate- to high-grade fever, headache, vomiting, and anorexia, usually in the 1st 48 hours.
- Arthralgias

ALERT
Important to differentiate erysipelas from MRSA infection, which usually has an indurated center, significant pain, and later evidence of abscess formation

PHYSICAL EXAM
- Vital signs: Moderate- to high-grade fever with resultant tachycardia. Hypotension may occur.
- Fever may be a differentiating factor among other skin infections.
- Headache and vomiting may be prominent.
- Acute onset of erythematous patch
- Sharply demarcated, raised border, fiery-red plaque that spreads circumferentially over hours/days
- Lesion characteristically hot, indurated, tender with marked swelling
- Peau d'orange appearance
- Vesicles and bullae may form, but are not uniformly present.
- Desquamation may occur later.
- Location:
  - Lower extremity 70–80% of cases
  - Face involvement is less common (5–20%), especially nose and ears
  - Chronic form usually recurs at site of the previous infection, and may recur years after initial episode.
- Patients on systemic steroids may be more difficult to diagnose because signs and symptoms of the infection may be masked by anti-inflammatory action of the steroids.
- Systemic toxicity resolves rapidly with treatment; skin lesions desquamate on days 5–10, but usually heal without scarring.

Pediatric Considerations
- Abdominal involvement more common in infants, especially around umbilical stump
- Face, scalp, and leg common in older children

Geriatric Considerations
- Fever may not be as prominent.
- More prone to complications

- High-output cardiac failure may occur in debilitated patients with underlying cardiac disease.
- Face and lower extremity are most common areas
- Integument: Hot, tender, erythematous, superficial plaque with sharply demarcated borders. Facial involvement presents in a butterfly pattern. Pustules characteristically absent.
- Lymphatics: Regional lymphadenopathy, lymphangitic streaking

DIAGNOSTIC TESTS & INTERPRETATION
Lab
- Classic erysipelas can be diagnosed and treated without laboratory workup. Reserve diagnostic for severely ill, toxic patients or those who are immunosuppressed.
- Leukocytosis
- Blood culture (<5% positive)
- Elevated erythrocyte sedimentation rate (ESR) and C-reactive protein (CRP)
- Streptococci may be cultured from exudate or noninvolved sites.
- Antistreptolysin, streptozyme, anti-DNase, and antihyaluronidase titers may not be helpful acutely.

Imaging
Usually not indicated

Pathological Findings
- Dermal and epidermal edema, extending into the subcutaneous tissues
- Peau d'orange appearance caused by edema in the superficial tissue surrounding the hair follicles
- Vasodilation and enlarged lymphatics
- Mixed interstitial infiltrate mainly consisting of neutrophils and mononuclear cells
- Endothelial cell swelling
- Gram-positive cocci in lymphatics and tissue with rare invasion of local blood vessels
- Fibrotic thickening of lymphatic vessel walls with possible luminal occlusion may be seen in recurrent erysipelas.

DIFFERENTIAL DIAGNOSIS
- Cellulitis (margins are less clear)
- Necrotizing fasciitis (systemic illness and more pain)
- Dermatophytes
- Impetigo (blistered or crusted appearance; superficial)
- Ecthyma (ulcerative impetigo)
- Herpes zoster (dermatomal distribution)
- Erythema annulare centrifugum (raised pink-red ring or bulls-eye marks)
- Contact dermatitis (no fever, pruritic)
- Giant cell urticaria (transient, wheal-appearance, severe itching)
- Angioneurotic edema (no fever)
- Scarlet fever (widespread rash with indistinct borders and without edema; rash is most common early in skin folds; develops generalized "sandpaper" feeling as it progresses)
- Toxic shock syndrome (diffuse erythema with evidence of multiorgan involvement)
- Lupus (of the face; less fever, positive antinuclear antibodies)
- Polychondritis (common site is the ear)

- Tuberculoid leprosy
- Inflammatory breast carcinoma
- Other bacterial infections to consider:
  - Meat, shellfish, fish, and poultry workers: *Erysipelothrix rhusiopathiae* (known as erysipeloid)
  - Human bite: *Eikenella corrodens*
  - Cat or dog bite: *Pasteurella multocida* or *Capnocytophaga canimorsus*
  - Salt water exposure: *Vibrio vulnificus*
  - Fresh or brackish water exposure: *Aeromonas hydrophilia*

 TREATMENT

Infectious Diseases Society of America guidelines for the diagnosis and management of skin and soft tissue infections recommends penicillin, either p.o. or parenterally, depending on clinical severity, as the treatment of choice for erysipelas (4).

MEDICATION
First Line
- Adults:
  - Mild: Penicillin VK 500 mg p.o. q6h for 10–14 days (improvement in 24–48 hours) or penicillin G procaine 0.6–1.2 million U IM b.i.d. for 10 days (4)[A]
  - Moderate-severe: Cefazolin 1–2 grams q8h IM/IV or ceftriaxone 1 gram q24h IM/IV
- Children:
  - Penicillin VK:
    - <12 years: 25–50 mg/kg/d p.o. div. q6–8h with max: 3 g/d
    - >12 years: Adult dose
  - Penicillin G procaine:
    - <30 kg: 300,000 U/d IM
    - >30 kg: Adult dose
- Nafcillin or oxacillin 2.0 g IV q4h or penicillin G parenterally is recommended for severe or complicated cases (1 million–2 million units q4–6h).
- No reported group A streptococci resistance to beta-lactam antibiotics
- In chronic recurrent infections, prophylactic treatment after the acute infection resolves:
  - Penicillin G benzathine 1.2 million U IM q month, or Penicillin VK 250 mg p.o. b.i.d.
- If staphylococcal infection is suspected or patient is acutely ill, a beta-lactamase-stable antibiotic should be considered.
- Consider community-acquired methicillin-resistant *Staphylococcus aureas* (MRSA) and, depending on regional sensitivity, may treat MRSA with trimethoprim-sulfamethoxazole, clindamycin, or tetracycline. If resistance is a concern or patient is clinically unstable, treat with vancomycin, daptomycin, or linezolid.

Second Line
- Cephalosporins:
  - Cephalexin:
    - Children: 25 mg/kg/d p.o. divided q6h
    - Adults: 500 mg p.o. q6h
  - Cefazolin:
    - Children: 50 mg/kg/d IV divided q8h
    - Adults: 1 g IV q8h
  - Contraindications: Allergy
  - Pregnancy Category B
- Clindamycin for penicillin-allergic patients in regions with high macrolide resistance:
  - Children: 10-25 mg/kg/d p.o. divided q6–8h or alternatively: 15–25 mg/kg/d IV/IM divided q6–8h

- Adults: 150–450 mg p.o. q6h or alternatively: 600–2,700 mg/d IV/IM divided q6–12h
  - Use IV for severe infections.
- Macrolides in penicillin-allergic patients:
  - Azithromycin 500 mg on day 1, then 250 mg/d for 4 days or clarithromycin 500 mg b.i.d. for 10 days
  - Macrolide resistance among group A streptococci has increased regionally in the US, but there has never been penicillin or cephalosporin resistance reported.
- Recurrent erysipelas in adults:
  - Pen V 250 mg p.o. b.i.d.
  - Azithromycin 500 mg/d p.o.
  - Clarithromycin 500 mg/d p.o.

ADDITIONAL TREATMENT
Consider prednisolone 30 mg daily with taper over 8 days as optional adjunct for treatment of uncomplicated erysipelas in adults (5)[B].

General Measures
- Symptomatic treatment of myalgias and fever
- Adequate fluid intake
- Local treatment with cold compresses
- Elevation of affected extremity
- Appropriate therapy for any underlying predisposing condition

Issues for Referral
Recurrent infection, treatment failure

IN-PATIENT CONSIDERATIONS
Initial Stabilization
Outpatient care

Admission Criteria
- Patient with systemic toxicity
- Patient with high-risk factors (elderly, lymphedema, postsplenectomy, diabetes, etc.)

IV Fluids
IV therapy if systemic toxicity or unable to tolerate p.o.

Discharge Criteria
No evidence of systemic toxicity with improvement of erythema and swelling

 ONGOING CARE

FOLLOW-UP RECOMMENDATIONS
Bed rest with elevation of extremity during acute infection, then activity as tolerated

Patient Monitoring
Patients should be treated until all symptoms and skin manifestations have resolved.

DIET
No special diet

PATIENT EDUCATION
Stress importance of completing medication regimen prescribed

PROGNOSIS
- Patients should recover fully if adequately treated.
- Mortality less than 1% in patients receiving appropriate treatment.
- Bullae formation suggests longer disease course, and often indicates a concomitant *Staphylococcus aureus* infection that may require antibiotic coverage for MRSA.
- Chronic edema/scarring may result from chronic recurrent cases.
- Rarely, obstructive lymphadenitis may result from chronic recurrent cases.

COMPLICATIONS
- Recurrent infection
- Abscess (suggests staphylococcal infection)
- Necrotizing fasciitis
- Lymphedema
- Bacteremia (which may lead to sepsis or involvement of other organ systems)
- Sepsis
- Pneumonia (due to sepsis or toxin-producing organism)
- Meningitis (due to sepsis or toxin-producing organism)
- Embolism
- Gangrene
- Bursitis
- Septic arthritis, tendinitis, or osteitis

REFERENCES
1. Gabillot-Carré M, Roujeau JC. Acute bacterial skin infections and cellulitis. *Curr Opin Infect Dis*. 2007;20:118–23.
2. Bernard P. Management of common bacterial infections of the skin. *Curr Opin Infect Dis*. 2008;21:122–8.
3. Celestin R, Brown J, Kihiczak G, et al. Erysipelas: a common potentially dangerous infection. *Acta Dermatovenerol Alp Panonica Adriat*. 2007;16:123–7.
4. Stevens DL, et al. Practice guidelines for the diagnosis and management of skin and soft tissue infections. *Clin Infect Dis*. 2005;41:1973.
5. Bergkvist PI, Sjöbeck K et al. Antibiotic and prednisolone therapy of erysipelas: a randomized, double blind, placebo-controlled study. *Scand J Infect Dis*. 1997;29:377–82.

ADDITIONAL READING
Breen JO et al. Skin and soft tissue infections in immunocompetent patients. *Am Fam Physician*. 2010;81:893–9.

 CODES

ICD9
035 Erysipelas

CLINICAL PEARLS
- Athlete's foot is the most common portal of entry for this superficial bacterial skin infection caused by *Streptococcus pyogenes*.
- Erysipelas is distinguished from cellulitis by its sharp, shiny, fiery-red, raised border.
- In recurrent cases, search for other possible source of streptococcal infection (e.g., tonsils, sinuses, intertrigo).
- Most erysipelas infections now occur on the legs, rather than the face.

ERYTHEMA MULTIFORME

Congjun Yao, MD

BASICS

- Erythema multiforme (EM) is an acute, self-limited hypersensitivity reaction:
  - Mostly triggered by infectious agents (more than 50% by herpes simplex virus [HSV]-1 or -2) or drugs (1,2)[B]
  - Involving the skin and sometimes the mucous membrane, most commonly the mouth
  - Skin lesions include typical target or "iris" lesions, flat or raised atypical lesions, macules with or without blisters.
- Currently, there are no universal diagnostic criteria for EM. It was previously considered to be a spectrum of disease, consisting of EM, EM major, Stevens-Johnson syndrome (SJS), and toxic epidermal necrolysis (TEN). However, it appears to be a growing consensus that EM is a distinct condition from SJS and TEN due to the differences in clinical presentation, histopathology manifestation, patient demographics, possible etiology and pathogenesis, and treatment plan (1,2,3,4)[C].

DESCRIPTION
- Two subtypes, erythema multiforme minor (EMm) and erythema multiforme major (EMM), with the former involving none or 1 mucous membrane, and the latter involving at least 2 mucous sites (1)[C]
- Recurrent EM has a mean number of 6 attacks (range 2–24) per year and a mean duration of 9.5 years (range 2–36) (1)[B].
- System(s) affected: Skin/Exocrine
- Synonym(s): Erythema polymorphe

EPIDEMIOLOGY
Incidence
The annual incidence in the US has been estimated at between 0.01 and 1% (4)[C].

Prevalence
- Predominant age: Peak incidence in 20s and 40s; rare <age 3 and >age 50
- Predominant sex: Male > Female (3:2 to 2:1) (1,2)[C]

RISK FACTORS
Previous history of erythema multiforme

Genetics
Strong association with HLA-DQ3 in herpes-related cases. Possible association in recurrent cases with HLA-B15, -B35, -A33, -DR53, DQB1*0301, and DQW3 (1)[C]

GENERAL PREVENTION
- Known or suspected etiologic agents should be avoided.
- Acyclovir may help prevent herpes-related erythema multiforme (1,2)[B].

PATHOPHYSIOLOGY
- The exact pathophysiology of EM is unknown.
- Possible immunologically mediated lymphocytic reaction to an infectious agent or a drug at the dermal-epithelial junction
- HSV-triggered EM seems to involve CD4+ T-cell infiltration and associated IFN-γ activation.
- Drug-triggered EM involves CD8+ T-cells and associated TNF-α activation (4)[C].

ETIOLOGY
- Most cases appear to be due to a preceding infection.
- Viral infections, particularly herpes simplex (accounting for more than 50% of cases); also Epstein-Barr, coxsackie, echovirus, varicella, mumps, poliovirus, hepatitis C, cytomegalovirus, HIV, molluscum contagiosum virus
- Bacterial infections, particularly *Mycoplasma pneumoniae;* other occasional reported bacterial infections include *Treponema Pallidum* and *Gardnerella vaginalis*
- Fungal infection, including *Histoplasma capsulatum* and *Coccidioides immitis*
- Medications, including sulfonamides, penicillins, barbiturates, hydantoins, nonsteroidal anti-inflammatory drugs (NSAIDs), phenothiazines. Other sparsely reported medications include candesartan, cilexetil, rofecoxib, metformin, bupropion, ciprofloxacin, sorafenib, gemfibrozil, risperidone, paclitaxel, metoprolol, adalimumab, etanercept, and infliximab.
- Vaccines: Tetanus/diphtheria, bacillus Calmette-Guérin, oral polio, hepatitis B, human papillomavirus
- Protozoan infections
- Radiation therapy
- Premenstrual hormone changes
- Sarcoidosis

COMMONLY ASSOCIATED CONDITIONS
Any of the infections or diseases listed under Etiology

DIAGNOSIS

Diagnose clinically by careful review of the history and detailed physical examination. No specific labs are required for the diagnosis.

HISTORY
- Absent or mild prodromal symptoms.
- Preceding HSV infection (over 50% of cases) 10–15 days before the skin eruptions (1,2)[B]
- Rash involving the skin and sometimes the mucous membrane, most commonly the mouth

PHYSICAL EXAM
- Skin pleomorphic eruption with a mixture of macules, papules of various sizes, and target lesions:
  - Typical target lesions: Raised and cyanotic center, edematous light intermediate ring and bright erythematous border (three zones)
  - Flat or raised atypical target lesions: 2 zones only (center and intermediate ring) with poorly defined border

  - Symmetrically distributed rash, mainly on the palms, soles, dorsum of the hands, and extensor surface of the extremities and the face
  - Lesions may coalesce and become generalized.
  - Body surface area with epidermal detachment <10% (1,2,3,4)[B]
- Mucosal involvement:
  - Minimal involvement in EM minor; if present, most commonly involves the mouth
  - At least 2 mucosal sites involved in EM major, including eyes (conjunctivitis, keratitis), mouth (stomatitis, cheilitis), and probable trachea, bronchi, gastrointestinal tract, or genital tract (balanitis and valvulitis)
  - Multiple papules and vesicles, superficial irregular erosions, shallow painful ulcers with erythematous margin (1)[C]

DIAGNOSTIC TESTS & INTERPRETATION
Lab
- No specific lab test is indicated to make the diagnosis of EM (1,2,3,4)[B].
- Skin biopsy of lesional and perilesional tissue in equivocal conditions (1,2,3,4)[C]
- Direct and indirect immunofluorescence to differentiate EM from other vesiculobullous diseases (1)[C]. Indirect immunofluorescence is detected on a biopsy of perilesional skin, and direct immunofluorescence is detected from a blood sample.
- HSV tests in recurrent EM (serologic tests, swab culture, or tests using skin biopsy sample to check HSV antigens or DNA in keratinocytes by immunofluorescence or polymerase chain reaction (PCR)) (4)[C]
- Antibody staining to IFN-γ and TNF-α to differentiate HSV-associated EM and drug-associated EM (4)[C]
- Elevated *M. pneumonia* antibody titer in *M. pneumonia* infection–associated EM (1)[C]

Imaging
Initial approach
No specific imaging studies are indicated in most cases.

Follow-Up & Special Considerations
Chest x-ray may be necessary if an underlying pulmonary infection (*M. pneumonia* infection) is suspected.

Pathological Findings
- A predominantly perivascular inflammatory infiltrate with CD4+ T lymphocytes and histocytes in papillary dermis and the epidermal-dermal junction
- Focal necrotic keratinocytes mainly in the basal layer
- Dermal edema (1,2,4)[C]

DIFFERENTIAL DIAGNOSIS
- Stevens-Johnson syndrome (3)[C]:
  - Different pattern and location of the skin lesions. No typical target lesion. Atypical flat target lesions or macules, generalized or mainly in the trunk
  - Blisters and skin detachment less than 10% of the total body surface area
  - Usually with systemic complications (i.e., Central Nervous System, lung, gastrointestinal system, kidney)
  - 1–5% mortality rate

- Toxic epidermal necrolysis (1,3)[C]:
  – Blisters and skin detachment more than 30% of the total body surface area
  – 10–30% mortality rate
- Urticaria
- Necrotizing vasculitis
- Drug eruptions
- Contact dermatitis
- Pityriasis rosea
- Herpes simplex
- Secondary syphilis
- Ringworm
- Pemphigus vulgaris
- Pemphigoid
- Dermatitis herpetiformis
- Herpes gestationis
- Septicemia
- Serum sickness
- Viral exanthems
- Rocky Mountain spotted fever
- Collagen vascular diseases
- Mucocutaneous lymph node syndrome
- Meningococcemia
- Lichen planus
- Behçet syndrome
- Recurrent aphthous ulcers
- Herpetic gingivostomatitis
- Granuloma annulare

 TREATMENT

MEDICATION
First Line

- Treatment of any underlying or causative disease (1,2)[B]
- Withdrawal of any drugs that might be the cause (1,2)[B]
- Symptomatic treatment with oral antihistamines and topical corticosteroids for mild cases (1,2)[B]
- Early treatment with acyclovir may lessen the number and duration of cutaneous lesions for patients with coexisting or recent HSV infection (2)[B]:
  – Acyclovir for adults: 200 mg, 5 times a day for 7–10 days in the onset of EM
  – For pediatric patients: 10 mg/kg or 500 mg/s^2, 3 times a day for 7–10 days
- Recurrent EM may be treated with oral acyclovir (400 mg 2 times per day) , even if HSV infection has not been confirmed (2)[B].
- Valacyclovir (Valtrex, 500–1,000 mg per day) and famciclovir (Famvir, 125–250 mg per day) may be tried in patients who are resistant to acyclovir (2)[C]:
  – Reduce the dosage once the patient is recurrence-free for 4 months, and eventually discontinue the drug.

Second Line
- Recurrent EM cases nonresponsive to antiviral therapy could also try dapsone (100–150 mg per day), azathioprine (Imuran, 100–150 mg per day), thalidomide (100–200 mg per day), mycophenolate mofetil (CellCept <2 g daily), hydroxychloroquine (<400 mg daily), colchicine (<1.2 mg daily) (25)[C].

- Cyclosporine given intermittently (4 mg/kg per day for a week) may also be used for recurrent EM (2)[C].
- Systemic steroid use is controversial, because it may decrease the patient's resistance to HSV and increase recurrent HSV infection (1,2)[C].
- Precautions: Refer to the manufacturer's profile of each drug.
- Significant possible interactions: Refer to the manufacturer's profile of each drug.

ADDITIONAL TREATMENT
General Measures
- Meticulous wound care and Burow's solution or Domeboro solution dressings for severe cases with epidermal detachment
- Mouth washes with warm saline or a solution of diphenhydramine, lidocaine (Xylocaine), and Kaopectate for oral lesions to provide symptomatic relief and oral hygiene, and to facilitate oral intake

IN-PATIENT CONSIDERATIONS
Admission Criteria
- Care at home
- Hospitalization needed for fluid, electrolyte management if patient with severe mucous membrane involvement, impaired oral intake and dehydration.
- IV antibiotics if secondary infection develops

 ONGOING CARE

FOLLOW-UP RECOMMENDATIONS
Patient Monitoring
- The disease is self-limiting.
- Complications are rare, with no mortality.

DIET
As tolerated with increased fluid intake

PATIENT EDUCATION
- The disease is self-limiting. However, the recurrence risk may be 30%.
- Antiviral therapy with acyclovir may reduce the duration and frequency of outbreaks.
- Avoid any identified etiological agents.

PROGNOSIS
- Rash evolves over 1–2 weeks and subsequently resolves within 2–6 weeks, generally without scarring or sequelae.
- Following resolution, there may be some postinflammatory hyper- or hypopigmentation.

COMPLICATIONS
Secondary infection

REFERENCES

1. Al-Johani KA, Fedele S, Porter SR. Erythema multiforme and related disorders. *Oral Surg Oral Med Oral Pathol Oral Radiol Endod*. 2007.
2. Lamoreux MR, Sternbach MR, Hsu WT. Erythema multiforme. *Am Fam Physician*. 2006;74:1883–8.
3. Auquier-Dunant A, Mockenhaupt M, Naldi L, et al. Correlations between clinical patterns and causes of erythema multiforme majus, Stevens-Johnson syndrome, and toxic epidermal necrolysis: results of an international prospective study. *Arch Dermatol*. 2002;138:1019–24.
4. Aurelian L, Ono F, Burnett J. Herpes simplex virus (HSV)-associated erythema multiforme (HAEM): a viral disease with an autoimmune component. *Dermatol Online J*. 2003;9:1.
5. Wetter DA, Davis MD et al. Recurrent erythema multiforme: clinical characteristics, etiologic associations, and treatment in a series of 48 patients at Mayo Clinic, 2000 to 2007. *J Am Acad Dermatol*. 2010;62:45–53.

ADDITIONAL READING

- Chen M, Doherty SD, Hsu S et al. Innovative uses of thalidomide. *Dermatol Clin*. 2010;28:577–86.
- Nikkels AF, Pièrard GE. Treatment of mucocutaneous presentations of herpes simplex virus infections. *Am J Clin Dermatol*. 2002;3:475–87.
- Williams PM, Conklin RJ. Erythema multiforme: a review and contrast from Stevens-Johnson syndrome/toxic epidermal necrolysis. *Dent Clin North Am*. 2005;49:67–76, viii.

See Also (Topic, Algorithm, Electronic Media Element)
Cutaneous Drug Reactions; Dermatitis Herpetiformis; Herpes Gestationalis; Urticaria; Stevens-Johnson Syndrome; Toxic Epidermic Necrotisis

 CODES

ICD9
695.10 Erythema multiforme, unspecified

CLINICAL PEARLS

- EM is diagnosed clinically by careful review of the history, through detailed physical examination, and by excluding other similar disorders. No lab tests are required for the diagnosis.
- Typical lesions are pleomorphic macules, papules, and characteristic target or "iris" lesions
- Lesions are symmetrically distributed on palms, soles, dorsum of the hands, and extensor surfaces of extremities and face. Mucosal involvement is minimal.
- Management of EM involves determining the etiology when possible. The first step is to treat the suspected infection or discontinue the causative drug.
- Complications are rare. Most cases are self-limited. However, the recurrence risk may be as high as 30%.
- Recurrent cases often are secondary to herpes simplex infection. Antiviral therapy may be beneficial.

E

ERYTHEMA NODOSUM

Sophia L. Delano, MD
Nikki Levin, MD, PhD

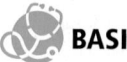 BASICS

DESCRIPTION
- A delayed-type hypersensitivity reaction to infectious agents, medications, or malignancies, or in the setting of autoimmune disorders, presenting as a subcutaneous panniculitis
- Clinical pattern of multiple, bilateral, erythematous, tender subcutaneous nodules that undergo a characteristic pattern of color changes, similar to that seen in bruises. Unlike erythema induratum, the lesions of erythema nodosum do not typically ulcerate.
- Occurs most commonly on the shins, less commonly on the thighs and forearms
- May be accompanied by fever and arthralgias
- Often idiopathic but may be associated with a number of clinical entities
- Usually remits spontaneously in weeks to months without scarring or atrophy
- Synonym(s): Dermatitis contusiformis

Pregnancy Considerations
May have repeat outbreaks during pregnancy

EPIDEMIOLOGY
Incidence
- 1-5/100,000
- Predominant age: 20–30 years
- Predominant sex: Female > Male (3:1).

Prevalence
Varies geographically depending on the prevalence of disorders associated with erythema nodosum

RISK FACTORS
See "Etiology."

ETIOLOGY
- Idiopathic: 37–60%
- Bacterial: Streptococcal infections (most common cause in children), tuberculosis, leprosy, tularemia, gonorrhea, *Yersinia enterocolitica*, *Campylobacter*, *Salmonella*, *Shigella*
- Sarcoid

- Drugs: Sulfonamides, amoxicillin, oral contraceptives, bromides
- Pregnancy
- Fungal: Dermatophytes, coccidioidomycosis, histoplasmosis, blastomycosis
- Viral/chlamydial: Infectious mononucleosis, lymphogranuloma venereum, paravaccinia
- Enteropathies: Ulcerative colitis, Crohn disease, Behçet disease (1), celiac disease (2)
- Malignancies: Lymphoma/leukemia, sarcoma, after radiation therapy

COMMONLY ASSOCIATED CONDITIONS
See "Etiology."

DIAGNOSIS

HISTORY
- Increasingly tender and aching nodules on the legs, usually over the shins.
- Fever, malaise, chills, fatigue
- Eruptions often preceded by symptoms of pharyngitis or upper respiratory infection
- Headache
- Arthralgias

PHYSICAL EXAM
- Initially warm, tender, brightly erythematous nodules, which may be raised, on anterior shins; lesions become bluish and fluctuant, gradually fading to yellowish, resembling a bruise.
- May occur on any area with subcutaneous fat
- Diameter usually 2–6 cm, but may rarely be larger

DIAGNOSTIC TESTS & INTERPRETATION
Diagnosis is usually clinical.
Lab
- Erythrocyte sedimentation rate (ESR). May be elevated or normal.
- Complete blood count (CBC): Mild leukocytosis
- Antistreptolysin titers may be elevated.
- Throat culture (usually negative because the infection typically resolves before lesions appear)
- Stool culture and leukocytes, if indicated
- Skin testing for mycobacteria, if indicated
- Drugs that may alter lab results: Antecedent antibiotics may affect cultures.

Imaging
CXR for hilar adenopathy or infiltrates related to sarcoidosis or tuberculosis

Diagnostic Procedures/Surgery
Deep incisional skin biopsy including subcutaneous fat; rarely necessary except in atypical cases with ulceration, duration greater than 12 weeks or a presentation that does not include skin lesions.

Pathological Findings
- Septal panniculitis without vasculitis.
- Neutrophilic infiltrate in septa of fat tissue early in course.
- Actinic radial (Miescher's) granulomas, consisting of collections of histocytes around a central stellate cleft, may be seen (3).
- Fibrosis, paraseptal granulation tissue, lymphocytes, and multinucleated giant cells predominate late in course.

DIFFERENTIAL DIAGNOSIS
- Nodular vasculitis or erythema induratum (warm ulcerating calf nodules)
- Superficial thrombophlebitis
- Cellulitis
- Septic emboli
- Weber-Christian disease (violaceous, scarring nodules)
- Lupus panniculitis
- Cutaneous polyarteritis nodosa
- Sarcoidal granulomas
- Cutaneous T-cell lymphoma
- Erythema nodosum leprosum (clinically similar to EN but shows vasculitis on histopathology)
- Vasculitis

TREATMENT

All medications listed as treatment for erythema nodosum are off-label uses of the medications. There are no FDA-approved medications for erythema nodosum.

MEDICATION
First Line
- Medication usually more effective in acute than in chronic disease
- Condition often self-limited
- Nonsteroidal anti-inflammatory drugs (NSAIDs):
  – Ibuprofen: 400 mg po q4–6 hours (not to exceed 3200 mg per day)
  – Indomethacin: 25–50 mg po t.i.d.
  – Naproxen (Naprosyn): 250–500 mg po b.i.d.

- Aspirin: 325 mg 1–2 tablets po q4–6 hours (not to exceed 12 tablets a day); use enteric-coated tablets to decrease GI upset.
- Contraindications:
  – Active or recent peptic ulcer disease
  – History of hypersensitivity to NSAIDs
- Precautions:
  – GI upset/bleeding
  – Fluid retention
  – Dose reduction in elderly, especially those with renal disease, diabetes, or heart failure
  – May mask fever
  – NSAIDs may elevate liver function tests.
- Significant possible interactions:
  – May blunt antihypertensive effects of diuretics and β-blockers
  – NSAIDs can elevate plasma lithium levels.
  – Caution is advised with naproxen or any highly protein-bound drug because it may compete for albumin binding and elevate levels.
- NSAIDs can cause significant elevation and prolongation of methotrexate levels.

Second Line
- Potassium iodide 400–900 mg/d divided 2–3×/day × 3–4 weeks (for persistent lesions). Need to monitor for hypothyroidism with prolonged use. Pregnancy Class D.
- Corticosteroids for severe, refractory cases in which an infectious workup is negative. Prednisone 1mg/kg/d for 1–2 weeks often helps resolve the lesions (4). Potential side effects include hyperglycemia, hypertension, weight gain, mood changes, bone loss, osteonecrosis, myopathy.
- Recent reports of improvement with colchicine 0.6–1.2 mg b.i.d.
- Hydroxychloroquine, thalidomide and cyclosporine may also be used.

ADDITIONAL TREATMENT
General Measures
- Mild compression bandages and leg elevation may reduce pain. (Wet dressings, hot soaks, and topical medications are not useful.)
- Discontinue potentially causative drugs.
- Treat underlying disease.

COMPLEMENTARY AND ALTERNATIVE MEDICINE
Vitamin B12 replacement. A single case report of resolution of lesions with B12 replacement in a patient who had B12 deficiency and erythema nodosum (5).

IN-PATIENT CONSIDERATIONS
Admission Criteria
Occasionally, admission may be needed for the antecedent illness (e.g., tuberculosis).

 ## ONGOING CARE

FOLLOW-UP RECOMMENDATIONS
- Keep legs elevated.
- Elastic wraps or support stockings may be helpful when patients are ambulating.

Patient Monitoring
Monthly follow-up or as dictated by underlying disorder

DIET
No restrictions

PATIENT EDUCATION
- Lesions will resolve over a few weeks to months.
- No scarring is anticipated.
- Joint aches and pains may persist.
- <20% recur.

PROGNOSIS
- Individual lesions resolve generally within 2 weeks.
- Total time course of 6–12 weeks but may vary with underlying disease.
- Joint aches and pains may persist for years.
- Lesions do not scar.
- Recurrences in 12–14% of patients: Occurs over variable periods, averaging several years; seen most often in sarcoid, streptococcal infection, pregnancy, and oral contraceptive use

COMPLICATIONS
- Vary according to underlying disease
- None expected from lesions of erythema nodosum

REFERENCES

1. Psychos DN, Voulgari PV, Skopouli FN, et al. Erythema nodosum: the underlying conditions. *Clin Rheumatol*. 2000;19:212–6.
2. Bartyik K, Várkonyi A, Kirschner A, et al. Erythema nodosum in association with celiac disease. *Pediatr Dermatol*. 2004;21:227–30.
3. Schwartz RA, Nervi SJ et al. Erythema nodosum: a sign of systemic disease. *Am Fam Physician*. 2007;75:695–700.
4. Requena L, Yus ES et al. Erythema nodosum. *Dermatol Clin*. 2008;26:425–38, v
5. Volkov I, et al. Successful treatment of chronic erythema nodosum with vitamin B12. *J Am Board Fam Pract*. 2005;18:6.

ADDITIONAL READING

- González-Gay MA, García-Porra C, Pujol RM, et al. Erythema nodosum: a clinical approach. *Clin Exp Rheumatol*. 2001;19:365–8.
- Habif T. *Clinical Dermatology*, 4th ed. St. Louis, MO: CV Mosby, 2004.
- Requena L, et al. Erythema nodosum. *Dermatol Online J*. 2002;8:4.
- Wolff K, et al., eds. *Fitzpatrick's Dermatology in General Medicine*, 7th ed. New York: McGraw-Hill Professional, 2007.

 ## CODES

ICD9
695.2 Erythema nodosum

CLINICAL PEARLS
- Lesions of erythema nodosum appear to be erythematous patches, but when palpated, their underlying nodularity is appreciated.
- Erythema nodosum in the setting of hilar adenopathy may be seen with multiple etiologies and does not exclusively indicate sarcoidosis.
- In patients with a history of Hodgkin lymphoma, erythema nodosum may be a warning of impending recurrence.

E

ERYTHROBLASTOSIS FETALIS

Donald A.F. Nelson, MD

 BASICS

DESCRIPTION
- Hemolytic anemia of the fetus or newborn caused by transplacental transmission of maternal antibody
- When severe, the anemia may result in extramedullary hematopoiesis, secondary organ dysfunction, heart failure, hydrops, and death.
- The term *erythroblastosis* refers to the presence of immature erythrocytes in the peripheral blood from accelerated hematopoiesis.
- System(s) affected: Cardiovascular; Hemic/Lymphatic/Immunologic; Nervous
- Synonym(s): Erythroblastosis neonatorum; Hemolytic disease of the fetus and newborn (HDFN); Congenital anemia of the newborn; Immune hydrops fetalis; Icterus gravis neonatorum

EPIDEMIOLOGY
- Predominant age: Affects fetus and newborn
- Predominant sex: Male = Female

Incidence
Universal screening for Rh sensitization and widespread use of RhIG in 3rd trimester and/or at birth have made this disease relatively rare.

RISK FACTORS
Prior transfusion with incompatible blood:

Pregnancy Considerations
- Any Rh-positive pregnancy in an Rh-negative woman (~9% of pregnancies have an Rh-negative mother with an Rh-positive fetus)
- Without prophylactic immunotherapy (RhIG), risk of Rh sensitization is up to 16% during or after term pregnancy, ~3% for spontaneous abortion, and 5–6% for surgical abortion.
- Sensitization by exposure to fetal blood may also occur with ectopic pregnancy, amniocentesis, chorionic villus sampling, placental trauma or manipulation, and placental abruption.
- Prophylaxis with Rho(D) immune globulin (RhIG) reduces risk of sensitization to <1% of susceptible pregnancies (1).
- Universal screening for Rh sensitization and widespread use of RhIG in 3rd trimester and/or at birth have made this disease relatively rare.

Genetics
- May occur when the fetus inherits a paternal blood group antigen lacking in the mother
- The Rh D antigen is most frequently implicated (for more on inheritance of Rh antigens, see Rh Incompatibility).
- In cases of a heterozygous paternal genotype, new DNA techniques now make it possible to diagnose the fetal blood type through free fetal DNA in maternal plasma (2).

GENERAL PREVENTION
- RhIG (RhoGAM, Rhophylac, HyperRHO) given prophylactically to unsensitized, Rh-negative pregnant women at risk. Usually at 28–32 weeks' gestation and at birth if infant is Rh-positive (see Rh Incompatibility).
- Artificial insemination with sperm from antigen-negative donor for isoimmunized woman whose partner is antigen-positive

ETIOLOGY
- Maternal isoimmunization to Rh antigen by transfusion of Rh-positive blood
- Maternal isoimmunization from exposure to fetal Rh antigens in prior or current pregnancy
- Maternal isoimmunization to other blood group antigens (e.g., Kell, Duffy, Kidd, M, Diego, S) is unusual, but may cause serious disease (3).

 DIAGNOSIS

PHYSICAL EXAM
- Pallor
- Respiratory distress
- Jaundice
- Hepatomegaly
- Splenomegaly
- Ascites
- Purpura/bleeding problems
- Edema
- Anasarca (extreme generalized edema)
- Hydrops (fluid accumulation in ≥2 or more fetal compartments, including ascites, pericardial effusion, pleural effusion, and skin edema)
- Hypotension/shock
- Fetal death in utero

DIAGNOSTIC TESTS & INTERPRETATION
Lab
Initial lab tests
- Complete blood count:
  - Anemia
  - Thrombocytopenia
  - Nucleated red blood cells on differential count
- Reticulocytosis
- Hyperbilirubinemia (indirect bilirubin)
- Elevated amniotic fluid bilirubin (δ OD 450)
- Positive indirect Coombs test (antibody screen) during pregnancy
- Positive direct Coombs test
- If paternity is certain, paternal blood typing may exclude pregnancy from being at risk.

Follow-Up & Special Considerations
- Maternal antibody titer measured by 20 weeks and q.4wk. during pregnancy. A titer of 1:16 or greater, particularly if rising, indicates need for further testing (3)[C].
- Formerly, periodic amniocentesis for photometric determination of amniotic fluid bilirubin levels was the preferred method of monitoring in pregnancies with elevated antibody titers. Results estimated the extent of fetal hemolysis. High fluid bilirubin levels indicated the need for percutaneous umbilical blood sampling (cordocentesis) to determine the degree of fetal anemia (3)[C].
- Improvements in fetal ultrasonography now permit assessment of fetal anemia by Doppler measurement of flow velocity in the fetal middle cerebral artery. This noninvasive procedure is gradually replacing invasive methods for monitoring affected pregnancies (3)[C].
- Fetal heart rate testing/ultrasonography to assess fetal status (3)[C]
- Amniocentesis for fetal lung maturity at the point of pregnancy when early delivery is a management option, especially after 34 weeks (3)[C]
- Prior administration of Rho(D)IG during pregnancy may lead to weakly (false) positive indirect Coombs test in mother and direct Coombs test in infant.

Imaging
Initial approach
- Serial peak middle cerebral artery velocities by Doppler ultrasonography to detect/assess fetal anemia (2).
- Ultrasound may demonstrate hepatomegaly, abdominal enlargement, ascites, or signs of hydrops.
- When there is a history of an affected fetus or infant, maternal titers are no longer predictive of risk in subsequent pregnancies (2).

Follow-Up & Special Considerations
Fetus may be severely affected without hydrops; the presence or absence of hydrops on ultrasonography is poor at predicting the need for intervention.

Diagnostic Procedures/Surgery
- Amniocentesis
- Umbilical cord blood sampling

Pathological Findings
- Erythroid hyperplasia of bone marrow
- Extramedullary hematopoiesis
- Hepatomegaly
- Splenomegaly
- Cardiac enlargement
- Pulmonary hemorrhages
- Enlargement, edema of placenta

DIFFERENTIAL DIAGNOSIS

- Fetal blood loss anemia
- Twin-to-twin transfusion
- Arteriovenous or cardiac malformations
- Hereditary hemolytic anemias
- Drug-induced hemolytic anemia
- Nonimmune fetal hydrops
- Hemolysis from intrauterine infection (syphilis, toxoplasmosis, cytomegalovirus, others)

 TREATMENT

MEDICATION

First Line

- IG infusion has been used antenatally in combination with intrauterine transfusion to reduce the number of transfusions needed (4)B].
- IG infusion in the newborn can reduce the number of exchange transfusions or the duration of phototherapy required for treatment (4)B].

Second Line

- Maternal plasmapheresis combined with IG infusion has been used successfully in some severe cases (5)C].
- Diuretics or inotropic agents may be used in addition to transfusion to manage heart failure in the newborn.

ADDITIONAL TREATMENT

General Measures

Depending on severity of involvement, treatment of infant may include:

- Intrauterine transfusion: Intravascular approach via the umbilical vein is becoming preferred over the intraperitoneal approach and appears to be more effective.
- Early delivery
- Phototherapy
- Transfusion after delivery
- Exchange transfusion
- Diuretics and digoxin for hydrops

Issues for Referral

- Affected pregnancies are usually managed at the tertiary care level by perinatologists because of the specialized, somewhat hazardous, treatment measures involved.
- Delivery should occur in an institution capable of performing exchange transfusion, even if only mild involvement of the infant is expected.
- Infants with moderate or severe disease require neonatal intensive care.

 ONGOING CARE

PROGNOSIS

- 50% of affected infants have mild disease and require no treatment (or treatment of anemia and jaundice only after delivery) and can be delivered at or near term.
- 30% have moderate disease with anemia and hepatomegaly. They require close follow-up of the pregnancy for signs of deterioration, which may require early delivery after 32–34 weeks or intrauterine transfusion prior to that age. After delivery, exchange transfusion is usually needed to treat anemia and hyperbilirubinemia.
- 20% have fetal hydrops, require intrauterine transfusion, and delivery as early as 32–34 weeks.
- Disease severity tends to worsen in successive affected pregnancies.
- Hydrops is associated with a poorer prognosis.
- Without treatment, overall perinatal mortality is ~50%.
- With appropriate monitoring and treatment, most infants do well, even those requiring intrauterine transfusion, and perinatal mortality has been reduced to 2–3% (1).
- Long-term studies have revealed normal neurologic outcomes in more than 90% of cases (2).

COMPLICATIONS

- Fetal distress requiring emergent delivery
- Fetal death in utero
- DIC
- Pregnancy loss from umbilical blood sampling
- Pregnancy loss from intrauterine transfusion
- Asphyxia
- Neonatal hemolytic anemia, mild to severe
- Neonatal anemia from hematopoietic suppression after intrauterine transfusion
- Pulmonary edema
- Congestive heart failure
- Shock
- Neonatal jaundice, mild to severe
- Kernicterus

REFERENCES

1. Bowman J. Thirty-five years of Rh prophylaxis. *Transfusion*. 2003;43:1661–6.
2. Moise KJ. Management of rhesus alloimmunization in pregnancy. *Obstet Gynecol*. 2008;112:164–76.
3. Management of alloimmunization during pregnancy. *ACOG Practice Bulletin 75*. Aug 2006.
4. Alcock GS, et al. Immunoglobulin infusion for isoimmune haemolytic jaundice in neonates. *Cochrane Database Sys Rev*. 2006;1.
5. Ruma MS, et al. Combined plasmapheresis and IV immune globulin for the treatment of severe maternal red cell alloimmunization. *Am J Obstet Gynecol*. 2007;196:138.e1–138.e6.

 CODES

ICD9

- 773.0 Hemolytic disease of fetus or newborn due to Rh isoimmunization
- 773.1 Hemolytic disease of fetus or newborn due to abo isoimmunization
- 773.2 Hemolytic disease of fetus or newborn due to other and unspecified isoimmunization

CLINICAL PEARLS

- Prior administration of Rho(D)IG during pregnancy may lead to weakly (false) positive indirect Coombs test in mother and direct Coombs test in infant.
- Ultrasound is poor at predicting need for intervention.
- As for prognosis, 50% of affected infants have mild disease and require minimal treatment, 30% have moderate disease with anemia and hepatomegaly, and 20% have fetal hydrops.
- With appropriate monitoring and treatment, most infants do well, even those requiring intrauterine transfusion.
- Perinatal mortality has been reduced to 2–3% for this rare condition.

E

ESOPHAGEAL VARICES

James G. Nee, MD

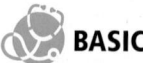

BASICS

DESCRIPTION
- Dilated collateral veins in the lamina propria of the distal esophagus connecting the portal and systemic circulations
- Results from chronic hypertension in the portal circulation due to increased resistance to blood flow.
- Increased pressure and turbulent flow within these vessels as well as their superficial location in the distal esophagus make them prone to rupture with significant morbidity and mortality.

EPIDEMIOLOGY
- Esophageal varices occur in ~50% of patients with cirrhosis.
- 50% of patients with esophageal varices bleed during their lifetime.
- Bleeding from esophageal varices is associated with 15–20% mortality.
- Predominant sex: Male > Female

RISK FACTORS
Cirrhosis of the liver

Genetics
No known pattern

GENERAL PREVENTION
- Endoscope esophagus annually in patients with cirrhosis
- Consider use of nonselective beta-blockers or obliteration of varices with esophageal banding for those intolerant of medication to prevent bleeding.

PATHOPHYSIOLOGY
Portal hypertension is caused by elevated portal pressure due to splanchnic arteriolar vasodilatation and increased resistance through dilated hepatic sinusoids.

ETIOLOGY
- Portal hypertension is defined as a pressure gradient >10 mm Hg.
- Cirrhosis accounts for >90% of cases. Alcohol and hepatitis C are the most common etiologies.
- Hemochromatosis, hepatitis B, nonalcoholic fatty liver disease, biliary cirrhosis, and autoimmune cirrhosis account for remainder. Extrahepatic portal vein thrombosis from umbilical vein infection, trauma, chronic pancreatitis, thrombotic conditions, and polycythemia.
- Malignant invasion of liver sinusoids or portal vein; seen in lymphoma, leukemia, hepatocellular carcinoma, and pancreatic carcinoma.
- Metabolic diseases altering liver sinusoids—amyloid, Gaucher disease, fatty liver
- Budd-Chiari syndrome
- Veno-occlusive disease

COMMONLY ASSOCIATED CONDITIONS
- Portal hypertensive gastropathy
- Hemorrhoids

DIAGNOSIS

- GI bleeding:
  - 75% of time, painless hematemesis and/or melena
  - Occult bleeding with anemia 25%
- Signs of cirrhosis

HISTORY
- Generally a history of cirrhosis or liver disease
- Painless hematemesis or melena

PHYSICAL EXAM
- Possible hypotension/tachycardia
- Small, hard liver
- Splenomegaly
- Ascites
- Visible abdominal periumbilical collateral circulation (Caput medusae)
- Spider angiomata on upper chest/back
- Palmar erythema

DIAGNOSTIC TESTS & INTERPRETATION
Lab
Initial lab tests
- Anemia related to blood loss
- Possibly abnormal liver function tests, thrombocytopenia, prolonged prothrombin time or low albumin-reflecting cirrhosis

Imaging
Initial approach
- Barium swallow:
  - Adequate for advanced varices, but is insensitive to small ones
  - Precludes possible urgent endoscopy
- Doppler sonography: Demonstrates patency, diameter, and flow in portal vein, and splenic vein, and large collaterals intra-abdominally.
- MRI:
  - Demonstrates large vascular channels intra-abdominally, and in the mediastinum.
  - Can demonstrate patency of the intrahepatic portal vein and splenic vein
- Venous phase celiac arteriography: Demonstrates portal vein and its collaterals, also can diagnose hepatic vein occlusion.

Diagnostic Procedures/Surgery
- Esophagoscopy as part of esophagogastroduodenoscopy:
  - Can identify and treat varices that appear as protruding submucosal veins in the distal 3rd of the esophagus.
  - Can identify actively bleeding varices as well as those with stigmata of recent hemorrhage.
  - Can treat actively bleeding vessels with sclerotherapy or esophageal band ligation or can obliterate vessels to prevent rebleeding. Can also identify associated conditions, including gastric varices and portal hypertensive gastropathy.
- Capsule endoscopy has acceptable sensitivity and specificity for detecting varices, and may be an alternative for those unwilling to undergo an EGD (1)[A].

- Endoscopic ultrasound is particularly sensitive to gastric varices.
- Portal pressure measurement:
  - Radiologist introduces a catheter retrograde into the hepatic vein in a wedged position to occlude flow.
  - The catheter is withdrawn to a free position and pressure again measured. The difference between wedged and free is the portal pressure. If <12 mm Hg, bleeding is less likely. Progressive increases above 12 correlate with the likelihood of hemorrhage
  - This is sometimes used to monitor successful treatment with beta-adrenergic blocking agent though it is not widely available.

Pathological Findings
- Extensive collateral circulation in the mediastinum and in the abdomen in addition to large vessels in the submucosa of the esophagus
- When bleeding occurs, these large veins explode into the submucosa of esophagus and rupture into the lumen.

DIFFERENTIAL DIAGNOSIS
- Upper GI bleeding:
  - Pulmonary bleeding; hemoptysis
  - Peptic ulcer disease
  - Gastric or esophageal malignancy
  - Arteriovenous malformation (AVM)
  - Nosebleed
- Lower GI bleeding:
  - Hemorrhoids
  - Colonic neoplasia
  - Diverticulosis
  - AVMs

TREATMENT
MEDICATION
- For varices
  - β-Blockers: Decrease risk of first bleed by 45–50% in primary prophylaxis of variceal hemorrhage (2)[A]
  - Propranolol: 40 mg b.i.d. increase until heart rate decreased by 25% from baseline
  - Nadolol 80 mg daily, increase as above
  - Isosorbide mononitrate further reduces portal pressure. Begin at 20 mg b.i.d. No significant benefit in preventing first bleeds when given in combination with β-blockers. Should not be given as monotherapy (3)[B].
  - During banding or sclerotherapy: Proton pump inhibitor, such as lansoprazole 30 mg/d until varices obliterated
- During bleeding, consider antibiotic prophylaxis for spontaneous peritonitis and other infections with ciprofloxacin for 7–10 days.
- Contraindications: Severe asthma with β-blockers
- Precautions: Symptomatic hypotension

First Line
β-Blockers, proton pump inhibitors, antibiotics

Second Line
Isosorbide mononitrate

ADDITIONAL TREATMENT

General Measures

- Treat co-morbidities, generally related to cirrhosis.
- Hospital management of bleeding varices:
  - Appropriate resuscitation and maintenance of blood volume
  - Treat coagulopathy, if necessary.
  - IV somatostatin to lower portal venous pressure usually used as adjuvant to endoscopic management. Begin with IV bolus of 50 mg followed by drip of 50 mg/h (4)[A].
  - Urgent upper endoscopy for diagnosis and treatment. Variceal band ligation or sclerotherapy for bleeding varices or those not bleeding, which are medium to large in size, to decrease risk of bleeding. Variceal band ligation is preferred due to better bleeding cessation with fewer complications (5)[A].
  - Vasoactive drugs may be safe and effective whenever endoscopic therapy is not promptly available and seems to be associated with less adverse events than emergency sclerotherapy (6,7)[A].
  - Pharmacotherapy may be as effective as endoscopic therapy in reducing rebleeding rates and all-cause mortality (8)[A].
  - Pharmacotherapy plus endoscopic intervention is more effective than endoscopic intervention alone (8)[A].
  - Repeat ligation or sclerosant injection if bleeding recurs.
  - If endoscopic treatment fails to stop bleeding or cannot be accomplished, may need to use Sengstaken Blakemore or Minnesota tube to stabilize patient for a transjugular intrahepatic portosystemic shunt.
- Management of nonbleeding varices:
  - If ligation started, usually in medium to large varices (grade 2–4), repeat banding at 1- to 3-week intervals. 4–6 treatments are usually required to obliterate varices.
  - For those not treated endoscopically, begin nonselective β-blockers such as propranolol or nadolol. Increase dose for goal of heart rate reduction of 25% of baseline (SBP >90, HR >50). For those who do not tolerate the side effects of this regimen, proceed with endoscopic variceal band ligation as primary prophylaxis (9)[A].
  - If bleeding recurs, or portal pressure measurement shows portal pressure still >12 mm Hg, isosorbide mononitrate may be added, though endoscopic band ligation preferred if possible (10)[B].
  - Refractory bleeding may require use of transjugular intrahepatic portasystemic shunt (TIPS) or portocaval shunt (11)[B]
  - Refer for liver transplantation where appropriate.

Issues for Referral

Primarily those associated with liver transplantation

SURGERY/OTHER PROCEDURES

- Endoscopic variceal ligation: Preferred approach to those who cannot tolerate β-blockers.
- Endoscopic sclerotherapy
- Transjugular intrahepatic portasystemic shunt (TIPS)
- Portacaval shunt
- Esophageal transection

- Liver transplantation
- In patients with current or prior bleeding from esophageal varices, endoscopic variceal ligation is superior to endoscopic sclerotherapy (12)[A].

IN-PATIENT CONSIDERATIONS

Admission Criteria

Inpatient for acute bleeding

Discharge Criteria

Cessation of bleeding, stability of other comorbidities

 ONGOING CARE

FOLLOW-UP RECOMMENDATIONS

Patient Monitoring

- Close monitoring of vital signs if actively bleeding
- Endoscopic variceal ligation, repeated every 1–4 weeks until varices eradicated
- All patients with cirrhosis should undergo endoscopy to document the presence of varices and risk of hemorrhage (2)[B].
- If TIPS or other portacaval shunt, repeat endoscopy only if clinically bleeding
- If TIPS present, follow-up as recommended by radiologist; usually Doppler sonogram every 6 months

PATIENT EDUCATION

- Appropriate to cirrhosis
- National Digestive Information Clearinghouse, 2 Information Way, Bethesda, MD 20892 (digestive.niddk.nih.gov/) or American Liver Foundation, 1425 Pompton Way, Cedar Grove, NJ 07009 (www.liverfoundation.org)

PROGNOSIS

- Depends heavily on ability to treat or reverse underlying condition
- In those with cirrhosis, 1 year survival for those who are alive 2 weeks after variceal bleed is ~50%.

COMPLICATIONS

- Bleeding
- Gastric or other uncommon varices may occur following successful eradication of esophageal varices.
- Esophageal varices can recur after obliteration.

REFERENCES

1. Lu Y, Gao R, Liao Z, et al. Meta-analysis of capsule endoscopy in patients diagnosed or suspected with esophageal varices. *World J Gastroenterol*. 2009;15:1254–8.
2. Groszmann RJ, Garcia-Tsao G, Bosch J, et al. Beta-blockers to prevent gastroesophageal varices in patients with cirrhosis. *N Engl J Med*. 2005;353: 2254–61.
3. D'Amico , et al. Pharmacological treatment of portal hypertension: an evidence based approach. *Semin Lever Dis*. 1999;19:475.
4. Zhou Y, Qiao L, Wu J, et al. Comparison of the efficacy of octreotide, vasopressin, and omeprazole in the control of acute bleeding in patients with portal hypertensive gastropathy: a controlled study. *J Gastroenterol Hepatol*. 2002;17:973–9.
5. Laine L, el-Newihi HM, Migikovsky B, et al. Endoscopic ligation compared with sclerotherapy for the treatment of bleeding esophageal varices. *Ann Intern Med*. 1993;119:1–7.
6. D'Amico G, Pagliaro L, Pietrosi G, Tarantino I et al. Emergency sclerotherapy versus vasoactive drugs for bleeding oesophageal varices in cirrhotic patients. *Cochrane Database Syst Rev*. 2010;3:CD002233.
7. Lo GH et al. Management of acute esophageal variceal hemorrhage. *Kaohsiung J Med Sci*. 2010;26:55–67.
8. Ravipati M, Katragadda S, Swaminathan PD et al. Pharmacotherapy plus endoscopic intervention is more effective than pharmacotherapy or endoscopy alone in the secondary prevention of esophageal variceal bleeding: a meta-analysis of randomized, controlled trials. *Gastrointest Endosc*. 2009;70:658–664.e5.
9. Boyer TD. Primary prophylaxis for variceal bleeding: are we there yet? *Gastroenterology*. 2005;128:1120–2.
10. Merkel C., et al. Randomised trial of nadolol alone or with isosorbide mononitrate for primary prophylaxis of variceal bleeding in cirrhosis. *Lanc*. 1996;348:1677.
11. Sanyal AJ, Freedman AM, Luketic VA, et al. Transjugular intrahepatic portosystemic shunts for patients with active variceal hemorrhage unresponsive to sclerotherapy. *Gastroenterology*. 1996;111:138–46.
12. Qureshi W, Adler DG, Davila R, et al. ASGE Guideline: the role of endoscopy in the management of variceal hemorrhage, updated July 2005. *Gastrointest Endosc*. 2005;62:651–5.

ADDITIONAL READING

Cheung J, Zeman M, van Zanten SV., et al. Systematic review: secondary prevention with band ligation, pharmacotherapy or combination therapy after bleeding from esophageal varices. *Aliment Pharmacol Ther*. 2009.

See Also (Topic, Algorithm, Electronic Media Element)

Cirrhosis of the Liver; Hemorrhoids; Portal Hypertension

 CODES

ICD9

- 456.0 Esophageal varices with bleeding
- 456.1 Esophageal varices without mention of bleeding
- 456.20 Esophageal varices in diseases classified elsewhere, with bleeding

CLINICAL PEARLS

- Esophageal varices occur in ~50% of patients with cirrhosis.
- 50% of patients with esophageal varices bleed during their lifetime.
- Bleeding from esophageal varices is associated with 15–20% mortality.
- Endoscopy can identify and treat actively bleeding varices.

Jonathon M. Firnhaber, MD

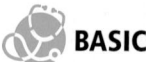 **BASICS**

DESCRIPTION
- A postural (occurring with voluntary maintenance of a position against gravity) or kinetic (occurring during voluntary movement) flexion–extension tremor that is slow and rhythmic and primarily affects the hands and forearms, head, and voice with a frequency of 4–12 Hz.
- Older patients tend to have lower frequency tremors, while younger patients exhibit frequencies in the higher range.
- May be familial, sporadic, or associated with other movement disorders
- Can begin at any age, but the incidence and prevalence increase with age
- The tremor can be exacerbated by emotional or physical stresses, fatigue, and caffeine.

EPIDEMIOLOGY
Essential tremor is the most common pathological tremor in humans.

Incidence
- Can occur at any age, but bimodal peaks exist in the 2nd and 6th decades
- Incidence rises significantly after age 49.
- System(s) affected: Neurologic; Musculoskeletal; ENT (voice)

Prevalence
0.4–5% of the general population

RISK FACTORS
Genetics
- Positive family history in 50–70% of patients; autosomal dominant inheritance is demonstrated in many families, but twin studies suggest that environmental factors are also involved.
- There is a link to genetic loci on chromosomes 2p22–25, 3q13, and 6p23. In addition, a Ser9Gly variant in the dopamine D_3 receptor gene on 3q13 has been suggested as a risk factor.

PATHOPHYSIOLOGY
Suspected to originate from an abnormal oscillation within thalamocortical and cerebello-olivary loops, as lesions in these areas tend to reduce essential tremor. Essential tremor is not a homogenous disorder; many patients have other motor manifestations and nonmotor features, including cognitive and psychiatric symptoms.

COMMONLY ASSOCIATED CONDITIONS
Can be present in 10% of patients with Parkinson disease (PD); characteristics of PD that distinguish it from essential tremor include 3- to 5-Hz resting tremor; accompanying rigidity, bradykinesia, or postural instability; and no change from alcohol consumption.

 DIAGNOSIS

HISTORY
- Core criteria for diagnosis:
  - Bilateral action (postural or kinetic) tremor of the hands and forearms (but not rest tremor)
  - Absence of other neurologic signs, with the exception of cogwheel phenomenon
  - May have isolated head tremor with no signs of dystonia
- Secondary criteria include long duration (>3 years), positive family history, and beneficial response to alcohol (1)[C].

PHYSICAL EXAM
- Tremor can affect upper limbs (~95% of patients).
- Less commonly, the tremor affects head (~34%), lower limbs (~30%), voice (~12%), tongue (~7%), face (~5%), and trunk (~5%).

DIAGNOSTIC TESTS & INTERPRETATION
Lab
Initial lab tests
- Ceruloplasmin and serum copper to rule out Wilson disease
- Thyroid-stimulating hormone to rule out thyroid dysfunction
- Serum electrolytes, blood urea nitrogen, creatinine

Imaging
Initial approach
Brain magnetic resonance imaging (MRI) usually is not necessary or indicated unless Wilson disease is found or exam implies central lesion.

Diagnostic Procedures/Surgery
Electromyogram usually is not necessary.

Pathological Findings
Posture-related tremor

DIFFERENTIAL DIAGNOSIS
- Wilson disease
- Hyperthyroidism
- Multiple sclerosis
- Dystonic tremor
- Cerebellar tremor
- Asterixis
- Psychogenic tremor
- Drug-induced tremor [valproic acid, selection serotonin reuptake inhibitors, steroids, lithium, cyclosporine, β-adrenergic agonists, ephedrine, theophylline, tricyclic antidepressants (TCAs), antipsychotics]
- PD is manifested by a tremor at rest.

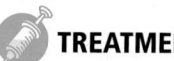 **TREATMENT**

MEDICATION
Pharmacologic treatment should be considered when tremor interferes with activities of daily living or causes psychological distress.

First Line
- Propranolol 60–320 mg/d in divided doses or in long-acting formulation reduces limb-tremor magnitude by ~50%, and almost 70% of patients experience improvement in clinical rating scales. There is insufficient evidence to recommend propranolol for vocal tremor. Single doses of propranolol, taken before social situations that are likely to exacerbate tremor, are useful for some patients.

- Primidone 25 mg q.h.s., gradually titrated to 150–300 mg q.h.s., improves tremor amplitude by 40–50%. Maximum dose is 750 mg/d, with doses greater than 250 mg/d typically divided to b.i.d. or t.i.d. Low-dose therapy (<250 mg/d) is just as effective as high-dose (750 mg/d) therapy.
- Propranolol and primidone have similar efficacy when used as initial therapy for limb tremor; both carry a level A recommendation.

Second Line

- Topiramate at a mean dose of 292 mg/d demonstrated significantly greater reduction in tremor rating scale (TRS) compared with placebo (7.7 vs 0.08; $p <.005$; baseline TRS = 37.0) in a small study combining results of 3 double-blind randomized controlled trials following a common protocol (2)[B]. Use is limited by dropout rates as high as 40% due to appetite suppression, weight loss, paresthesias, and concentration difficulties.
- Gabapentin up to 400 mg t.i.d.
- Sotalol, nadolol, and atenolol are alternative β-blockers; each has less evidence than propranolol to support use.
- Clonazepam and alprazolam should be used with caution because of abuse potential.
- Clozapine has shown efficacy at doses of 6–75 mg/d but is recommended only for refractory cases of limb tremor because of a 1% risk of agranulocytosis.
- Other medications that have been used to treat essential tremor include acetazolamide, flunarizine, levetiracetam, methazolamide, olanzapine, pregabalin, sodium oxybate, and zonisamide.
- Botulinum toxin A injections should be offered as a treatment option for cervical dystonia (Level A recommendation from American Association of Neurology), and may be offered for blepharospasm, focal upper extremity dystonia, adductor laryngeal dystonia and upper extremity essential tremor (3)[B]. Limited data support its use for head and voice tremor (4).

ADDITIONAL TREATMENT
Issues for Referral
Referral to a neurologist can help to differentiate those with dystonia, neuropathic tremor, PD, or drug-induced tremor.

SURGERY/OTHER PROCEDURES
- Deep brain stimulation may be used to treat medically refractory limb tremor and has fewer adverse effects than thalamotomy.
- Bilateral thalamic stimulation is effective in reducing tremor and functional disability; however, dysarthria is a possible complication.
- Unilateral thalamotomy may be used to treat limb tremor that is refractory to medical management.
- Bilateral thalamotomy is not recommended because of adverse side effects.

 ## ONGOING CARE

DIET
Avoid caffeine.

PROGNOSIS
Tremor tends to worsen with age, increasing in amplitude.

REFERENCES

1. Bain P, Brin M, Deuschl G, et al. Criteria for the diagnosis of essential tremor. *Neurology*. 2000;54:S7.
2. Connor GS, Edwards K, Tarsy D. Topiramate in essential tremor: findings from double-blind, placebo-controlled, crossover trials. *Clin Neuropharmacol*. 2008;31:97–103.
3. Simpson DM, et al. Therapeutics and Technology Assessment Subcommittee of the American Academy of Neurology. Assessment: Botulinum neurotoxin for the treatment of movement disorders (an evidence-based review): report of the Therapeutics and Technology Assessment Subcommittee of the American Academy of Neurology. *Neurology*. 20086;70(19):1699–1706.
4. Zesiewicz TA, et al. Practice parameter: Therapies for essential tremor: Report of the Quality Standards Subcommittee of the American Academy of Neurology. 2005;28;64(12):2008–20.

ADDITIONAL READING

Sullivan KL, Hauser RA, Zesiewicz TA. Essential tremor. Epidemiology, diagnosis, and treatment. *Neurologist*. 2004;10:250–8.

 ## CODES

ICD9
333.1 Essential and other specified forms of tremor

CLINICAL PEARLS

- Core criteria for diagnosis of essential tremor include bilateral action (intention) tremor of the hands, forearm, and/or head without resting component.
- Beneficial response to alcohol and positive family history help to differentiate essential tremor from PD; PD is characterized by tremor at rest.
- 10% of patients with PD will have both resting tremors of PD and essential (intention) tremors.
- Wilson disease, thyroid disease, and medication effect should be ruled out.
- Brain MRI is usually not necessary or indicated.
- 1st-line treatments include propranolol and primidone.

E

EUSTACHIAN TUBE DYSFUNCTION

Teresa V. Chan, MD

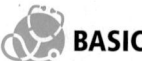 **BASICS**

DESCRIPTION
- Eustachian tube dysfunction (ETD) is classically described as a functional or structural obstruction of the eustachian tube. The eustachian tube does not open or close properly in response to pressure changes within the middle ear or outside the ear.
- Acute ETD may occur in the setting of pressure changes (e.g., plane travel) or acute upper airway inflammation (e.g., URI, sinusitis).
- Chronic ETD may lead to negative middle ear pressure, retracted tympanic membrane, serous effusions, otitis media, adhesive otitis media, or cholesteatoma.
- Patulous eustachian tube (PET), a distinct entity, is failure of the eustachian tube to close. It is often manifested as autophony, when an individual's own breathing and voice sounds excessively loud.
- System(s) affected: Auditory
- Synonym(s): Auditory tube dysfunction; Eustachian tube disorder; Blocked eustachian tube; Patulous eustachian tube

ALERT
- Sudden single-sided deafness (SSNHL) can be misdiagnosed as ETD.
- A simple 512-Hz tuning fork test lateralizes to the opposite ear in sudden sensorineural hearing loss and to the affected ear in ETD with conductive hearing loss.
- Any sudden sensorineural hearing loss is a medical emergency and should be referred to an otolaryngologist immediately.
- Treatment of SSNHL with high-dose steroids should begin ASAP, ideally within 14 days of onset.

EPIDEMIOLOGY
- Most common in children <5 years of age (1)
- Usually decreases with age but may persist into adulthood in some patients

Pediatric Considerations
Refer to an otolaryngologist if hearing loss or recurrent or chronic middle ear infections.

RISK FACTORS
- Adult and pediatric:
  - Tobacco and pollutant exposure, GERD, allergy, chronic sinusitis, sleep apnea with continuous positive airway pressure use, adenoid hypertrophy or nasopharyngeal mass, neuromuscular disease, altered immunity
  - Native American, Inuit, Australian Aborigine
- Pediatric:
  - 2nd-hand smoke, prematurity and low birth weight, young age, daycare, exposure to many other children, crowded living conditions, low socioeconomic status, prone sleeping position, prolonged bottle use
  - Craniofacial abnormalities (e.g., cleft palate, Down syndrome)

Pregnancy Considerations
- ETD may be exacerbated by rhinitis of pregnancy.
- Symptoms typically resolve postpartum.

Genetics
Twin studies show a genetic component (1). Specific genetic cause is still undefined.

GENERAL PREVENTION
- Control sources of upper airway inflammation: Allergens, GERD, URIs
- Autoinsufflation of middle ear (i.e., blow gently against pinched nostril and closed mouth)
- Avoid exposure to pressure changes (e.g., plane flight, scuba diving) in the setting of URI.
- Avoid exposure to environmental irritants: Smoking and 2nd-hand smoke

PATHOPHYSIOLOGY
- ETD is failure of the system at the proximal end (ET, palate, nasal cavities, and nasopharynx) to regulate the middle ear and mastoid gas cell system at its distal end.
- Eustachian tube functions:
  - Ventilation/regulation of middle ear pressure
  - Protection from nasopharyngeal secretions
  - Drainage of middle ear fluid
  - ET is closed at rest and opens with yawning, swallowing, and sneezing.
- Cycle of dysfunction: Structural or functional obstruction of the ET compromises 3 functions of this system:
  - Negative pressure develops in middle ear.
  - Serous exudate is drawn from the middle ear mucosa by negative pressure or refluxed into the middle ear if the ET opens momentarily.
  - Infection of static fluid causes edema and release of inflammatory mediators, which exacerbates cycle of inflammation and obstruction.
- Pathologic constriction of the ET in adults and children with chronic otitis media (COM) or in monkeys with a chemically or mechanically damaged tensor veli palatini (1)

ETIOLOGY
- In children, a horizontal ET predisposes to difficulties with ventilation and drainage (1).
- Shorter ET predisposes to reflux (1).
- Adenoid hypertrophy can block the torus tubarius (proximal opening of the ET) (1).
- In adults, paradoxical closing with swallowing has been noted in a majority of patients (1).

COMMONLY ASSOCIATED CONDITIONS
- Hearing loss
- Middle ear effusion
- Cholesteatoma
- Allergic rhinitis
- Chronic sinusitis
- URI
- Adenoid hypertrophy
- GERD
- Cleft palate
- Down syndrome
- Obesity
- Nasopharyngeal carcinoma or other tumor

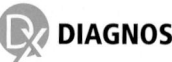 **DIAGNOSIS**

HISTORY
- Fullness, pressure, clogged feeling in the ear
- Otalgia or ear discomfort
- Relieved by "popping ears" (i.e., yawn or swallow tenses the tensor veli palatini, causing the ET to dilate)
- Hearing loss
- Symptoms: Unilateral or bilateral

- Tinnitus (usually popping, fluttering, clicking instead of high-pitched ringing)
- Dizziness or lightheadedness
- Recent onset vs chronic lifelong problem
- History of previous ear infections
- Previous ear surgeries, including tubes
- Constant vs waxing and waning symptoms
- Smoking history
- Antecedent URI
- Difficulty breathing through nose
- Allergic symptoms
- Trauma
- Voice change (hypo- or hypernasal voice, consider NP mass or palatal dysfunction)
- Recent flying or diving

ALERT
Unilateral symptoms and/or recent onset of symptoms in the absence of identifiable cause for ETD warrants workup for nasopharyngeal process such as tumor (1)[A].

PHYSICAL EXAM
- Pneumatic otoscopy: Retracted tympanic membrane, decreased movement, effusion
- Toynbee maneuver: View changes of the drum while patient autoinsufflates against closed lips and pinched nostrils. May show various degrees of retraction:
  - Entire drum may be retracted and "lateralize" with insufflation.
  - Posterosuperior quadrant (pars flaccida) may form a retraction pocket. Early on, this can be "lateralized" with autoinsufflation. If long-standing or severe, this pocket is well established and even may be scarred down to the middle ear mucosa or filled with cholesteatoma.
- Nasopharyngoscopy: Adenoid hypertrophy or nasopharyngeal mass
- Anterior rhinoscopy: Nasal obstruction, turbinate hypertrophy
- Tuning fork test: 512-Hz fork lateralizes to affected ear in setting of conductive hearing loss.

DIAGNOSTIC TESTS & INTERPRETATION
Imaging
- Radiologic studies are not performed routinely if clinical signs/symptoms suggest ETD.
- CT scan may show middle ear/mastoid opacification or other sequelae of chronic ETD and OM.
- Lateral neck film may help to confirm diagnosis of adenoid hypertrophy in an uncooperative pediatric patient.

Diagnostic Procedures/Surgery
- Tympanometry: Type B or C tympanograms indicate fluid or retraction, respectively. Negative middle ear peak pressures seen even with normal (type A) tympanograms.
- Audiogram may show conductive hearing loss.

Pathological Findings
- Blockage of the ET orifice by mucopurulent nasal discharge or edema
- Compression of the orifice by adenoid tissue
- Hypertrophy of the peritubal tonsil
- Paradoxical ET closure when swallowing
- Atrophy of the orifice
- In over 1/3 of patients, endoscopic findings were normal (2).

DIFFERENTIAL DIAGNOSIS

- SSNHL (a medical emergency)
- Tympanic membrane perforation
- Barotrauma
- TMJ disorder
- Ménière disease
- Superior semicircular canal dehiscence
- Skull base tumor

 ## TREATMENT

- Reduce cycle of infection/inflammation.
- Tympanostomy tubes ± adenoidectomy when indicated for recurrent ear infections or severe progressive retractions

MEDICATION

- Few data exist demonstrating efficacy for ETD.
- Initiate treatment based on individual patient's symptoms and possible cause.
- Decongestants (1)[C]: There are common ingredients in many OTC brands; encourage patients to read labels. In general, avoid prolonged use of intranasal decongestants >3 days; use with caution in patients with hypertension or cardiac risk factors:
  - Phenylephrine (Neo-synephrine Nasal Spray, Sudafed PE oral) Adults: 1 (10 mg) tablet or 1 spray each nostril every 4 hours p.r.n., children (<4y) 1 tsp (2.5 mg) q4h p.r.n.
  - Pseudoephedrine (Sudafed), Adults: 2 (30 mg) tablets every 4–6 hours p.r.n., children <12 y: 1 tablet every 4–6 hours p.r.n.
  - Oxymetazoline (Afrin Nasal Spray), Adults: 1–2 sprays each nostril every 12 hours p.r.n.
  - Xylometazoline (Otrivin Nasal Spray), Adults 2 sprays of 0.1% solution each nostril every 8 hours p.r.n., children (2–12 y): 2 sprays of 0.05% solution each nostril every 8 hours p.r.n.
- Nasal steroids (may be beneficial for those with allergic rhinitis) (1)[B]:
  - Beclomethasone (Beconase, Vancenase), Adults and children >12 y: 1–2 sprays each nostril b.i.d., children 6-12 y, 1 spray each nostril b.i.d. Not recommended for children <6 y.
  - Budesonide (Rhinocort): Adults and children >6 y, 1 spray each nostril daily
  - Ciclesonide (Omnaris) (a prodrug that is activated on nasal mucosa): Adults and children >6 y: 2 sprays each nostril daily
  - Flunisolide (Nasarel, Nasalide): Adults and children >6 y: 2 sprays each nostril b.i.d.
  - Fluticasone furoate (Veramyst): Adults and children >12 y: 2 sprays each nostril daily; children 2–11 y: 1 spray each nostril daily
  - Fluticasonepropionate (Flonase): Adults 1–2 sprays each nostril daily; children >4 y: 1 spray each nostril daily
  - Triamcinolone (Nasacort): Adults and children >6 y: 1–2 sprays each nostril daily, children 2–5 y; 1 spray each nostril daily
- 2nd-generation H$_1$ antihistamines (may be beneficial for those with allergic rhinitis) (1)[B]:
  - Loratadine (Claritin) (tablets, redi-tabs and liquid available): Adults and children >6 y: 10 mg orally daily, children 2–6 y: 5 mg orally daily
  - Desloratadine (Clarinex) (tablets, redi-tabs and liquid available): Adults and children >12 y: 5 mg orally daily, children 6-11 y: 2.5 mg orally daily, children 12 m-5 y: 1.25 mg orally daily, children 6–11 m: 1 mg orally daily

- Fexofenadine (Allegra) (tablets, redi-tabs and liquid available): Adults and children >12 y: 60 mg orally b.i.d. or 180 mg orally daily, children 6–11 y: 30 mg orally b.i.d.
  - Cetirizine (Zyrtec) (tablets, chewable tablets or liquid available): Adults and children >6 y: 5–10 mg orally daily, children 6 months-5 y: 2.5–5 mg orally daily or divided b.i.d.
  - Levocetirizine (Xyzal) (tablets and liquid available): Adults and children >12 y: 2.5–5 mg orally q.p.m., children 6–11 y: 2.5 mg orally q.p.m., children 6 m–5 y: 1.25 mg orally q.p.m.
- Antihistamine nasal sprays:
  - Olopatadine (Patanase) (antihistamine): Adults and Children >12y: 2 sprays each nostril BID, Children 6–11y: 1 spray each nostril BID
  - Azelastine (Astepro or Astelin) (antihistamine), Adults and children >12 y: 1–2 sprays each nostril b.i.d., children 6–11 y: 1 spray each nostril b.i.d.
- Antibiotics (not routinely used unless ETD is associated with acute OM):
  - Amoxicillin, 1st-line (1)[A]: Adults and children >3 months: 25 mg/kg/day in divided doses every 12 hours or 20 mg/kg/day in divided doses every 8 hours, children <12 weeks: 30 mg/kg/day divided q12h
  - Treatment for 10 days is most effective (1)[B].
- If ETD leads to OM associated with tympanic membrane perforation or if ventilation tube present, topical antibiotic drops are more efficacious than oral antibiotics (1)[A]:
  - Ciprofloxacin-dexamethasone (Ciprodex): 4–5 drops b.i.d. × 7 days
  - Ciprofloxacin–hydrocortisone suspension (Cipro HC) 3–5 drops b.i.d. × 7 days
  - Neomycin–polymyxin–hydrocortisone suspension (Cortisporin) 3–4 drops q.i.d. × 10 days
  - Ofloxacin (Floxin): 5 drops b.i.d. × 10 days
- Pain control, anti-inflammatory: Acetaminophen, NSAIDs

ADDITIONAL TREATMENT
General Measures
- Reduce cycle of inflammation with decongestants, antihistamines, topical steroids, antireflux medications, and antibiotics when indicated.
- Culture-directed antibiotics are 90% effective in treating sequela of ETD (chronic suppurative otitis media [CSOM] and mastoiditis) (1)[B].

Issues for Referral
Refer to an otolaryngologist if conservative 1st-line medications have provided no relief of symptoms or for surgical consideration.

SURGERY/OTHER PROCEDURES
- Myringotomy and pressure equalization tube placement to ventilate middle ear, relieve pressure, and prevent sequelae of chronically retracted drum (1)[A]
- Adenoidectomy if tissue is present:
  - In children, 1st set of tubes alone, then adenoidectomy in conjunction with second set of tubes if problems recur (1)[A]
  - Some advocate adenoidectomy even in absence of excess tissue; reduces frequency and number of subsequent tubes (3)[A].
- Direct nasopharyngoscopy and biopsy if mass
- Mastoidectomy for associated sequelae (e.g., chronic otomastoiditis, cholesteatoma)

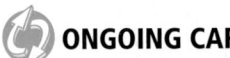 ## ONGOING CARE

FOLLOW-UP RECOMMENDATIONS
- Monitor pressure equalization tubes every 6–8 months in children and every 6–12 months in adults.
- Monitor tympanic membrane retraction pocket for progression every 6–12 months to allow for early intervention for erosion or cholesteatoma.
- Avoid pressure changes (e.g., scuba diving, plane flights) with URI (1)[C].

DIET
- Generally no restrictions; avoid foods that would exacerbate reflux symptoms.
- In newborns, breastfeeding has been associated with a lower incidence of ETD and OM (1)[A].

PROGNOSIS
- May resolve with age in pediatric patients
- For some, it is a chronic disorder; current treatments provide symptomatic relief; usually require prolonged use.

COMPLICATIONS
Morbidity related to hearing compromise or associated chronic ear infections

REFERENCES

1. Bluestone CD. Studies in otitis media: Children's Hospital of Pittsburgh-University of Pittsburgh progress report–2004. *Laryngoscope.* 2004;114:1–26.
2. Butler CC, Van Der Voort JH. Oral or topical nasal steroids for hearing loss associated with otitis media with effusion in children. *Cochrane Database Syst Rev.* 2002:CD001935.
3. Bluestone CD, Hebda PA, Alper CM, et al. Recent advances in otitis media. 2. Eustachian tube, middle ear, and mastoid anatomy; physiology, pathophysiology, and pathogenesis. *Ann Otol Rhinol Laryngol Suppl.* 2005;194:16–30.

See Also (Topic, Algorithm, Electronic Media Element)
Algorithm: Ear Pain

 ## CODES

ICD9
381.81 Dysfunction of eustachian tube

CLINICAL PEARLS

- SSNHL can be missed diagnosed as ETD, and the optimal window to commence high-dose steroids is lost.
- A simple 512-Hz tuning fork test lateralizes to the opposite ear in sudden sensorineural hearing loss and to the affected ear in ETD with conductive hearing loss.
- Any sudden sensorineural hearing loss is a medical emergency and should be referred to an otolaryngologist immediately.
- Treatment of SSNHL with high-dose steroids should begin ASAP, ideally within 14 days of onset.

E

FACTITIOUS DISORDER/MÜNCHAUSEN SYNDROME

Irene C. Coletsos, MD
William G. Elder, Jr., PhD
Harold J. Bursztajn, MD

 BASICS

DESCRIPTION
- Patients appear ill because they are feigning, exaggerating, or inducing symptoms.
- A mental disorder because the patient has an abnormal need for a sick role. Patients are aware of but will deny their deceit.
- Becomes apparent when there is a disease history stated in absence of symptoms, when symptom patterns are puzzling, or when there are nonhealing or unremitting symptoms despite adequate and correct treatment
- In factitious disorder by proxy, or Munchausen by proxy, an individual falsifies or induces illness in another person to vicariously accrue emotional payoffs, including sympathy, admiration, and/or feelings of power over care providers. Children are the usual victims and the mother is the usual perpetrator. The updated term for this activity is medical child abuse.
- Types of factitious disorder:
  – Factitious disorder with predominantly physical signs and symptoms:
    ○ Typically simulates 1 physical disease
  – Factitious disorder with predominantly psychological signs and symptoms:
    ○ These patients mimic the behavior of people with mental illnesses, claiming they are hearing voices or having visual hallucinations. In Ganser syndrome, patients may also give wrong answers to simple questions.
  – Münchausen syndrome is an extreme form usually with predominantly physical symptoms. Patients spend much of their lives seeking medical care from different providers and hospitals (changing hospitals when treatment is refused) and are willing to undergo painful procedures and surgeries to maintain their sick role. Named after an 18th-century nobleman who told tall tales.

EPIDEMIOLOGY
Incidence
Estimates vary on the incidence of medical child abuse. In the US, an estimated 200 new cases of serious abuse are expected to be uncovered yearly.

Prevalence
Factitious disorder with predominantly physical signs and symptoms: ∼1–5% of people presenting with medical illness, according to some studies, but hard to estimate due to the secretive nature of the disorder. Identified as the probable cause of 3–9% of fevers of unknown origin in prospective studies.

RISK FACTORS
- Abuse/deprivation in childhood
- Childhood traumas, including hospitalizations
- Growing up with ill or emotionally unavailable caretakers
- Experience as health care professional
- Female gender 2:1 in factitious disorder
- Male gender 2:1 Münchausen syndrome
- Most by-proxy presentations involve a mother inducing symptoms in a child. Siblings of children known to have suffered this abuse are at grave risk.

ETIOLOGY
- The psychological basis is thought to be an unresolved sense of deprivation from childhood that, in a time of stress in adulthood, leads to a false claim of medical illness in order to get care. In Münchausen, this behavior is chronic.
- Personality predisposition and shaping may be factors, evident in the high degree of deceitfulness, lack of remorse, disregard for safety, inability to manage work and interpersonal situations, and failure to conform to social norms.

COMMONLY ASSOCIATED CONDITIONS
- History of many medical procedures
- Substance abuse
- Suicide attempts
- Psychiatric comorbidities, including adjustment disorder, borderline personality disorder, depression, somatoform disorder, eating disorders
- In medical child abuse, the siblings of the currently affected child may have been improperly diagnosed with a rare, intractable condition or may even have died.
- Delusional disorder

 DIAGNOSIS

HISTORY
- A patient will relate a history of disease symptoms, often with "classic" textbook details, but has no signs of disease on examination. Or, if signs are noted, there may be evidence they were self-inflicted or are not medically caused.
- Careful elicitation of the developmental history may reveal early abuse or deprivations (1)[C].

PHYSICAL EXAM
- Normal, or evidence of self-inflicted wounds, such as scars
- Old wound with fresh bleeding (1)[C]
- Abscesses and rashes
- Tenderness on palpation with no tenderness noted by patient when the same areas are auscultated with pressure applied

DIAGNOSTIC TESTS & INTERPRETATION
Lab
- Abnormal urine studies not reproducible if the patient is directly observed. (Patients may surreptitiously heat their thermometers or contaminate urine specimens.)
- Skin infection (abscesses, IV sites, Foley sites): Culture may show infection via *E. coli*, presumably a patient's own fecal material.
- Repeated blood cultures showing uncommon pathogens in a patient who is immunocompetent and has no history of IV drug use (2)[C]
- Lab results fail to show the expected disease markers suggested by the reported symptoms.
- Agents taken to mimic disease states (insulin, to produce hypoglycemia; thyroxine or Cytomel to produce hyperthyroidism; laxative or diuretics, to produce hypokalemia; self-injection of epinephrine or isoproterenol hydrochloride, to mimic Cushing disease; warfarin, to produce bleeding; quinidine, to produce purpura; alkylating agents, to produce pancytopenia)

Diagnostic Procedures/Surgery
- Patients often undergo many diagnostic or surgery procedures before the psychological nature of their illness is discovered. Procedures are often welcomed by the patient and, in the cases of medical child abuse, by the patient's caregiver. Avoid if possible.
- Psychological testing (3)[B]:
  – The Minnesota Multiphasic Personality Inventory, neuropsychological tests, and forensic tests are sensitive to faking and identify unusual profiles associated with factitious disorders.
- Cameras and other means of surveillance have frequently been used accidentally or purposely to detect patients or parents feigning or inflicting illness. Check with hospital attorney.

DIFFERENTIAL DIAGNOSIS
- Factious disorders are mental disorders where the patient has an abnormal need to maintain a sick role. Factitious disorders may be contrasted with other mental disorders where symptoms are beyond the patient's control, such as delusional disorders with bizarre somatic beliefs, and somatoform disorders such as hypochondriasis, conversion, and somatization disorders where the patient has and experiences symptoms for psychological reasons:
  – In hypochondriasis the person believes or fears that they have a disorder. Anxiety is marked.
  – Somatization disorder involves recurrent physical symptoms, such as gastrointestinal (GI), sexual, pain, and neurologic symptoms where these symptoms cannot be explained fully by physical disorder. Worsens in times of stress and begins in late adolescence.
  – Conversion disorder manifests in pseudoneurological symptoms classically originating from an unconscious psychological conflict.
- Factitious disorders may be contrasted with malingering where secondary gain is sought such as financial goal or avoiding responsibility and as a result of a conscious decision.
- Cultural differences in expressing pain and experiencing illness
- Occult medical illness (early stages of disease when blood tests may still show negative results)
- Unusual presentations of disease
- False-negative lab results
- For factitious disorder with predominantly psychological signs and symptoms, in addition to psychiatric illnesses that can have true psychotic symptoms, consider other medical etiologies:
  – Drugs, ingested as prescribed or abused (i.e., benzodiazepines, cocaine, PCP, steroids)
  – Poisoning (alcohol, lead, mercury)
  – Stroke or traumatic brain injury
  – Also consider:
    ○ Infection (especially sepsis)
    ○ Postsurgical anesthesia
    ○ Pneumonia (especially in older patients)
    ○ Urinary tract infection (especially in older patients)
    ○ Thiamine deficiency/Wernicke encephalopathy

ALERT

- Factitious disorder (or Münchausen syndrome) by proxy is a form of abuse.
- Parent may injure their child and then bring the child to care with a false history.
- Parents may appear overly involved and comfortable in the hospital setting, and not saddened or frightened by the child's illnesses.
- A child in this situation may become quite ill, can have frequent hospitalizations, and may die from injuries.
- Older children who are victims of Münchausen by proxy may collude with the care provider who is victimizing them in order to maintain their relationship with the care provider (4)[C].
- Take steps to protect the child and siblings. Medical providers are legally required to report this and other types of abuse. Most experts recommend a multisystem approach that includes separating children from the abuser; therapy for the abuser, the abuser's significant other, and children; court monitoring to determine when/if the abuser can be reunited with children; medical monitoring to make sure future medical care for the child is warranted (and not part of an on-going abuse). Visits between the abuser and child can be therapeutic, but all must be carefully monitored to prevent the abuser from giving the child any food/drinks or medicine (5).

TREATMENT

ADDITIONAL TREATMENT
General Measures

- When possible, review medical and mental health records and mental health history. Mental disorders may be initially denied (3)[B].
- In cases of known or suspected factitious disorder, emergency department providers protect the patients (and protect themselves legally) by proceeding with the necessary treatment (e.g., if the patient has swallowed a foreign object, consult GI), putting the patient under observation during the hospital stay (to avoid having the patient inflict further self-injury), and consulting psychiatry as part of the treatment plan (6)[C].
- Management may be limited to clinician recognition of the disorder and making sure patients are not offered unnecessary drugs, risky procedures, or surgeries (7).
- Directly confronting patients ("You did this to yourself!") is usually met with angry denial. The patients often leave and try to get the treatment they had wanted from other providers and hospitals. Face-saving techniques that allow patients to give up their symptoms without being humiliated are thought to be more effective (8)[C].
- For example:
  - Patients with factitious disorder may accept a frank but empathetic assessment that their actions themselves constitute the disorder (6).
  - The Inexact Interpretation method may eventually help the patient begin to understand that the self-harm is part of a pattern of trying to cope with (usually) unresolved childhood stresses, without directly accusing them of the self-harm. For example, if a patient with a history of

childhood abuse at the hands of a parent is believed to be creating/reinfecting a skin wound, a provider can say: "I think your anger at your parent is making it more difficult for you to heal. It could also make it more difficult for you to work with your doctors." This type of interaction has been found to advance the therapy and can help lessen the inclination to self-harm (8)[C].
  - A double-blind diagnostic explanation may assist remission (8)[C]. The clinician should perform a thorough physical examination and go through a rapport-building interview. The diagnosis is then delivered in 2 parts:
    ○ Part 1: "Sometimes people do things to make themselves ill. We call doing that factitious disorder."
    ○ Part 2: "Your problem is unusual and I believe it will respond to 1 more attempt to treat it. If that doesn't improve it, it is likely that you have a factitious disorder." The medical therapy should be a benign one, such as biofeedback, self-hypnosis, or, in the case of a "nonhealing" skin wound (due to a patient's persistent reinfecting of it), a skin graft and antibiotics.
- In treating perpetrators of by proxy/medical child abuse: They must be able to admit what they have done, have an appropriate emotional response, have strategies in place to treat their own emotional issues without abusing those they care for, and can demonstrate, over time (6 months to a year), that they have put those strategies in place. One mode of therapy is "story construction," in which abusers can be helped to construct life narratives that explain why they were abusive, but then create alternative narratives that would prevent them from abusing in the future. The clinician advising the court on possible reunification of the abuser and child(ren) should be different from the one offering therapy. Despite therapy and intervention, relapse risk is high (9).
- In all clinical settings, be aware of the possibility of countertransference. Remain aware of personal responses and feelings toward these patients. Anger at these patients hinders the therapeutic alliance, and could lead to missed diagnoses. On the other hand, overidentification with these patients (who are often health care providers themselves) interferes with the timely identification of this syndrome and treatment (6)[C]. In all cases, consider consulting with a psychiatrist or psychologist (7)[B].

IN-PATIENT CONSIDERATIONS
Initial Stabilization

- Form an alliance with the patient, identifying their suffering.
- Seek a detailed history of childhood events. Health history of parents and siblings may reveal early traumas to the patient (3)[B].

Admission Criteria

- Patients whose behavior threatens their own lives should be considered for an emergency inpatient psychiatric commitment and evaluation (10)[C].
- In by proxy/medical child abuse cases, children may have to be hospitalized for monitored detoxification from the unneeded medications they had been given.

Nursing

IV and other in-room equipment should be monitored for tampering.

ONGOING CARE

PROGNOSIS

- Fair to poor especially if etiology underlying the disorder cannot be addressed
- The long-term outcomes of patients with untreated factitious disorder has been judged to be worse than those with other severe mental disorders such as schizophrenic, bipolar, and delusional disorders.

COMPLICATIONS

Patient illness or death from self-harm and unnecessary medical interventions

REFERENCES

1. Peebles R, Sabella C, Franco K, et al. Factitious disorder and malingering in adolescent girls: Case series and literature review. Clin Pediatr. 2005;44(3):237–43.
2. Galanos J, Perera S, Smith H, et al. Bacteremia due to three Bacillus species in a case of Munchausen's syndrome. J Clin Microbiol. 2003;41:2247–8.
3. Binder LM, Campbell KA. Medically unexplained symptoms and neuropsychological assessment. J Clin Experiment Neuropsychol. 2004;26(3): 369–92.
4. Awadallah N, Vaughan A, Franco K, et al. Munchausen by proxy: a case, chart series, and literature review of older victims. Child Abuse Negl. 2005;29:931–41.
5. Schreier H et al. On the importance of motivation in Munchausen by Proxy: the case of Kathy Bush. Child Abuse Negl. 2002;26:537–49.
6. Jagoda P. Factitious disorder in the emergency department. Primary Psychiatry. 2009;16(1): 61–66.
7. Krahn LE, Li H, O'Connor MK. Patients who strive to be ill: factitious disorder with physical symptoms. Am J Psychiatry. 2003;160(6):1163–8.
8. Eisendrath SJ. Factitious physical disorders. West J Med. 1994;160:177–9.
9. Sanders MJ, Bursch B et al. Forensic assessment of illness falsification, Munchausen by proxy, and factitious disorder, NOS. Child Maltreat. 2002;7:112–24.
10. Johnson BR, Harrison JA. Suspected Munchausen's syndrome and civil commitment. J Am Acad Psychiatry Law. 2000;28:74–6.

CODES

ICD9

- 300.16 Factitious disorder with predominantly psychological signs and symptoms
- 300.19 Other and unspecified factitious illness
- 301.51 Chronic factitious illness with physical symptoms

CLINICAL PEARLS

- Atypical emotional responses to illness are telling.
- Respond as you would to someone who cannot control self-harm rather than someone who wants to deceive you.
- In cases of by proxy disorders/medical child abuse, watch for children growing more ill after parental visits.

FACTOR V LEIDEN

Marc Jeffrey Kahn, MD
Rebecca Kruse-Jarres, MD, MPH

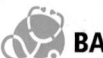 **BASICS**

DESCRIPTION
- Factor V Leiden is a genetic disease that is the most common hereditary cause of venous thrombosis. It leads to resistance to activated protein C.
- System(s) affected: Cardiovascular; Gastrointestinal; Hemic/Lymphatic/Immunologic; Nervous; Pulmonary; Reproductive
- Synonym(s): Factor V Leiden thrombophilia; factor V Leiden mutation

Pediatric Considerations
Increased thrombosis risk in patients with factor V Leiden

Pregnancy Considerations
Heterozygous patients are not at increased risk for thromboembolism or fetal loss.

EPIDEMIOLOGY
- Predominant age: Thrombosis typically occurs after the 2nd decade.
- Predominant sex: Male = Female

Prevalence
- ~3–12% of Caucasians are affected:
  − The mutation is rare in other ethnic groups.
- ~15–20% of patients who present with thrombosis have factor V Leiden.

RISK FACTORS
- Risk for venous embolism is 2.7-fold in heterozygous and 18-fold in homozygous factor V Leiden individuals, compared with individuals without the mutation.
- Oral contraceptives increase the risk of thrombosis:
  − In homozygotes, the risk increases 100-fold; in heterozygotes, 35-fold.
  − The increased risk is halved when the patient uses desogestrel-containing oral contraceptives.
- Hormone replacement therapy (HRT) and selective estrogen receptor modulators (SERMs) both increase the risk of thrombosis, and in patients with factor V Leiden, that risk is increased substantially.
- Pregnancy and homozygous factor V Leiden increase the risk of thrombosis 7–16-fold during pregnancy and the puerperium. Other complications of pregnancy may be increased in patients with factor V Leiden.
- Recurrence risk after an initial thrombosis is not increased in individuals who are heterozygous for factor V Leiden mutation. Data is conflicting in individuals who are homozygous, but it may not be increased (1).

Genetics
- Deep and superficial thrombosis of the venous system occurs with an odds ratio of 50–100 times greater for homozygotes.
- The odds ratio is closer to 2.5 times greater for heterozygotes.

GENERAL PREVENTION
Patients with factor V Leiden without thrombosis do not require prophylactic anticoagulation.

PATHOPHYSIOLOGY
- Point mutation causing substitution of arginine for glycine in residue 506 of factor V gene, rendering it less susceptible to inactivation by activated protein C
- Activated protein C is generated when protein C binds to its endothelial receptor, thrombomodulin.
- Activated protein C and its cofactor, protein S, lead to inactivation of factors V and VIII.
- Factor V Leiden is the most common cause of resistance to activated protein C.

ETIOLOGY
Genetic defect

COMMONLY ASSOCIATED CONDITIONS
Venous thrombosis

 DIAGNOSIS

HISTORY
- Previous thrombosis
- Family history of thrombosis
- Family history of factor V Leiden mutation

PHYSICAL EXAM
- Arterial thrombosis is rare in adults with factor V Leiden.
- Thrombosis in unusual locations, such as the sagittal sinus, mesentery, and portal systems, is less common in patients with factor V Leiden than in patients with deficiency of protein C or S.
- Obstetric complications and venous thrombosis are increased in patients with factor V Leiden, and especially in those taking oral contraceptives.

DIAGNOSTIC TESTS & INTERPRETATION
Lab
Initial lab tests
- Genetic test: DNA-based test for factor V mutation; is reliable while on anticoagulation
- Functional test: Plasma-based coagulation assay using factor V–deficient plasma to which patient plasma is added along with purified activated protein C. The relative prolongation of the activated partial thromboplastin time (aPTT) is used to assay for the defect. May be unreliable while taking heparin products (2).

Imaging
Initial approach
- Extremity ultrasound for deep vein thrombosis (DVT)
- V/Q scan of spiral CT for pulmonary embolism (PE)

Follow-Up & Special Considerations
- Ultrasound may not show DVT acutely; repeat in 1–2 days if strong suspicion.
- V/Q scan may be difficult to interpret in patients with other lung disease.

Diagnostic Procedures/Surgery
Magnetic resonance angiography (MRA), venography, or arteriography to detect thrombosis

Pathological Findings
Venous thrombus

DIFFERENTIAL DIAGNOSIS
- Protein C deficiency
- Protein S deficiency
- Antithrombin deficiency
- Other causes of activated protein C resistance (e.g., antiphospholipid antibodies)
- Dysfibrinogenemia
- Dysplasminogenemia
- Homocystinemia
- Prothrombin 20210 mutation
- Elevated factor VIII levels

 TREATMENT

Indicated for thrombosis

MEDICATION
First Line
- Low-molecular-weight heparin (LMWH) (2)[A]:
  − Enoxaparin (Lovenox): 1 mg/kg SC b.i.d., start warfarin simultaneously, continue Lovenox for at least 5 days and until international normalized ratio (INR) is >2.0, at which time it can be stopped
  − Fondaparinux (Arixtra): 7.5 mg SC daily
  − Tinzaparin (Innohep): 175 anti-Xa IU/kg SC daily for 6 days and patient is adequately anticoagulated with warfarin (INR of at least 2 for 2 consecutive days)
  − Dalteparin (Fragmin): 200 IU/kg SC daily
- Oral anticoagulant:
  − Warfarin (Coumadin) 5 mg daily p.o. initially and adjusted to an INR of 2–3
- Contraindications:
  − Active bleeding precludes anticoagulation (2)[A].
  − Risk of bleeding is a relative contraindication to long-term anticoagulation (2)[A].
  − Warfarin is contraindicated in patients with history of warfarin skin necrosis (2)[A].
  − Warfarin is contraindicated in pregnancy.
- Precautions:
  − Observe patient for signs of embolization, further thrombosis, or bleeding.
  − Avoid IM injections. Periodically check stool and urine for occult blood; monitor complete blood counts (CBCs), including platelets.
  − Heparin: Thrombocytopenia and/or paradoxic thrombosis with thrombocytopenia
  − Warfarin: Necrotic skin lesions (typically breasts, thighs, or buttocks)
  − LMWH: Adjust dosage in renal insufficiency. May also need dose adjustment in pregnancy (check anti-Xa level)

- Significant possible interactions:
  - Agents that intensify the response to oral anticoagulants: Alcohol, allopurinol, amiodarone, anabolic steroids, androgens, many antimicrobials, cimetidine, chloral hydrate, disulfiram, all nonsteroidal anti-inflammatory drugs (NSAIDs), sulfinpyrazone, tamoxifen, thyroid hormone, vitamin E, ranitidine, salicylates, acetaminophen
  - Agents that diminish the response to anticoagulants: Aminoglutethimide, antacids, barbiturates, carbamazepine, cholestyramine, diuretics, griseofulvin, rifampin, oral contraceptives

Second Line
- Heparin 80 mg/kg IV bolus followed by 18 g/kg/hour continuous infusion
- Adjust dose depending on aPTT.
- In patients requiring large daily doses of heparin, measure an anti-Xa level for dose guidance.
- Alternatively, unfractionated heparin can be given at 35,000 U per 24 hours SQ, with subsequent dosing to maintain a therapeutic aPTT (3)[C].

ADDITIONAL TREATMENT
General Measures
- Patients with factor V Leiden and a 1st thrombosis should be anticoagulated initially with heparin or LMWH (4)[A].
- Treatment with LMWH is recommended over unfractionated heparin, unless the patient has severe renal failure (3)[B].
- Treat as outpatient, if possible (3)[B].
- Initiate warfarin with heparin on the 1st treatment day, and discontinue heparin after 5 days and when INR >2.0 (3)[A].
- Patients should be maintained on warfarin with an INR of 2–3 for at least 6 months (3)[A].
- Recurrent thrombosis requires indefinite anticoagulation (4)[B].
- Compression stockings for prevention

Issues for Referral
- Recurrent thrombosis on anticoagulation
- Difficulty anticoagulating
- Genetic counseling

SURGERY/OTHER PROCEDURES
- Anticoagulation must be held for surgical interventions.
- For most patients with deep vein thrombosis (DVT), recommendations are against routine use of vena cava filter in addition to anticoagulation (3)[A].
- Thrombectomy may be necessary in some cases.

IN-PATIENT CONSIDERATIONS
Initial Stabilization
Heparin

Admission Criteria
Complicated thrombosis, such as pulmonary embolus

Nursing
- Teach LMWH and warfarin use.
- See above for drug interactions.

Discharge Criteria
Stable on anticoagulation

 ## ONGOING CARE

FOLLOW-UP RECOMMENDATIONS
Patient Monitoring
Warfarin use requires periodic (~monthly after initial stabilization) INR measurements, with a goal of 2–3 (2)[A].

DIET
- No restrictions
- Foods rich in vitamin K may interfere with anticoagulation with warfarin.

PATIENT EDUCATION
- Patients should be educated about:
  - Use of oral anticoagulant therapy
  - Avoidance of NSAIDs while on warfarin
- The role of family screening is unclear, as most patients with this mutation do not have thrombosis. In a patient with a family history of factor V Leiden, consider screening during pregnancy or if considering oral contraceptive use.

PROGNOSIS
- Most patients heterozygous for factor V Leiden do not have thrombosis.
- Homozygotes have about a 50% lifetime incidence of thrombosis.
- Recurrence rates after a 1st thrombosis are not clear, with some investigators finding rates as high as 5% and others finding rates similar to the general population.
- Despite the increased risk for thrombosis, factor V Leiden does not increase overall mortality.

COMPLICATIONS
- Recurrent thrombosis
- Bleeding on anticoagulation

REFERENCES
1. Lijfering WM, Middeldorp S, Veeger NJ, Hamulyák K, Prins MH, Büller HR, van der Meer J et al. Risk of recurrent venous thrombosis in homozygous carriers and double heterozygous carriers of factor V Leiden and prothrombin G20210A. *Circulation*. 2010;121:1706–12.
2. Moll S. Thrombophilias–practical implications and testing caveats. *J Thromb Thrombolysis*. 2006; 21:7–15.
3. Büller HR, Agnelli G, Hull RD, et al. Antithrombotic therapy for venous thromboembolic disease: the Seventh ACCP Conference on Antithrombotic and Thrombolytic Therapy. *Chest*. 2004;126: 401S–428S.
4. Kim RJ, Becker RC. Association between factor V Leiden, prothrombin G20210A, and methylenetetrahydrofolate reductase C677T mutations and events of the arterial circulatory system: a meta-analysis of published studies. *Am Heart J*. 2003;146:948–57.

ADDITIONAL READING
Seligsohn U, Lubetsky A. Genetic susceptibility to venous thrombosis. *N Engl J Med*. 2001;344: 1222–31.

See Also (Topic, Algorithm, Electronic Media Element)
Thrombosis; Deep Vein Thrombophlebitis (DVT)

 ## CODES

ICD9
289.81 Primary hypercoagulable state

CLINICAL PEARLS
- Extremely rare in Asian and African populations
- Asymptomatic patients with factor V Leiden do not need anticoagulation.

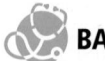

FAILURE TO THRIVE (FTT)

Jessica Davidson, MD

BASICS

DESCRIPTION
- Failure to thrive (FTT) is a general sign characterized by failure of physical growth, malnutrition, and potential retardation of development in children. The term is usually based on weight. In severe cases, it may lead to decreased length and/or head circumference.
- FTT describes a child with any of the following growth abnormalities:
  - Weight for age <5th percentile on >1 occasion
  - Weight that drops 2 or more major percentile lines on the standard growth charts
  - Weight <80% ideal body weight (IBW) based on National Center for Health Statistics' growth charts
  - Weight for height <10th percentile
  - Height for age <10th percentile
- Note that children with Down syndrome, intrauterine growth restriction (IUGR), premature infants, and infants with other syndromes follow different growth patterns.

EPIDEMIOLOGY
Incidence
- Predominant age: 6–12 months; most <3 years but can occur in older age groups
- Predominant sex: Male = Female

Prevalence
- Difficult to ascertain, as many studies do not exclude low birth weight (LBW) infants.
- As many as 10% of children seen in primary care have signs of growth failure.
- 1–5% of pediatric inpatient admissions are for evaluation of FTT.

RISK FACTORS
- Psychosocial risks:
  - Poverty is the leading risk factor.
  - Other risk factors include parent(s) with mental health disorder or limiting cognitive impairment, parent(s) with poor parenting skills or hypervigilant parents, families with unique health/nutritional beliefs, history of physical or emotional abuse, substance abuse, and social isolation
- Medical risks:
  - Intrauterine exposures, history of IUGR (symmetric or asymmetric), congenital abnormalities, premature or sick newborn, infant with physical deformity, acute or chronic medical conditions, developmental delay

Pregnancy Considerations
FTT is linked to intrauterine exposures, IUGR, and prematurity.

Genetics
No consistent genetic pattern but genetic disorders and inborn errors of metabolism can lead to FTT.

GENERAL PREVENTION
- Adequate parenting/caregiving skills
- Stable home life

PATHOPHYSIOLOGY
- Inadequate caloric intake (most frequent)
- Inadequate caloric absorption
- Excessive caloric expenditure
- Defective utilization

ETIOLOGY
- Traditional classifications of FTT have been listed as organic and nonorganic but most cases are a combination of these factors.
- Many cases of FTT begin with organic etiology. However, as the problem progresses, the caregivers and child begin to have interaction difficulties that also need to be addressed.
- Causes of FTT can be grouped by pathophysiology (including examples):
  - Inadequate intake: Breastfeeding difficulty, incorrect formula preparation, poor transition to food (6–12 months), poor feeding habits (e.g., excessive juice, avoidance of high calorie foods), mechanical problems (e.g., oropharyngeal dysfunction, congenital anomalies, GERD, CNS or PNS anomalies), poverty, neglect, poor parent-child interaction
  - Inadequate absorption: Necrotizing enterocolitis, short gut syndrome, biliary atresia, liver disease, cystic fibrosis, celiac disease, milk protein allergy, vitamin/mineral deficiency
  - Increased expenditure: Hyperthyroidism, congenital heart disease, chronic lung disease, HIV, congenital immunodeficiencies, malignancy, renal disease
  - Defective utilization: Metabolic disorders, congenital infections
- NOTE: Approximately 25% of children will decrease their weight or height by more than 25 percentile points in the first . years of life. These children are falling to their genetic potential or demonstrating constitutional growth delay (slow growth with a bone age less than chronologic age). After shifting down, these infants grow at a normal rate along their new percentile and do not have FTT.

DIAGNOSIS

HISTORY
- Prenatal history
- Developmental history
- Past medical history: Any acute or chronic disease that would affect caloric intake, digestion/absorption, cause increased energy need, or defective utilization
- Medication history, including complementary and alternative medications
- Family history: Stature of parents and growth trajectories of siblings; chronic diseases; genetic disorders; developmental delay
- Diet history from birth: Breast or formula feeding; timing and introduction of solids; who feeds the child, when, and how often; placement of child during feeds; amounts consumed; beverages consumed; snacking; vomiting or stooling associated with feeds
- Social history: Family composition, socioeconomic status, child-rearing beliefs, stressors, parental depression, parental substance abuse, caretaker personal history of abuse/neglect
- Review of systems: Anorexia, activity level, mental status, fevers, dysphagia, vomiting, gastro-esophageal reflux (GER), stooling pattern/consistency; dysuria; urinary frequency

PHYSICAL EXAM
- Accurate measurement of height, weight, and head circumference on National Center for Health Statistics (NCHS) growth charts

(www.cdc.gov/growthcharts). Be sure that parameters are correctly plotted.
- Observe for signs of dehydration or severe malnutrition
  - Severity of malnutrition assessed via Gomez classification: Compare current weight for age with expected weight for age (50th percentile): Severe: <60% of expected; Moderate: 61–75%; Mild: 76–90%
- Medical disease that may be contributing to malnutrition
- Dysmorphic features
- Mental status (alert, responsive to stimuli)
- Any signs of physical abuse and/or neglect
- Observe interaction with caregivers and feeding techniques, specifically bonding and social/psychological cues

DIAGNOSTIC TESTS & INTERPRETATION
- Routine newborn screen in infants.
- Labs useful only in approximately 1.4% of cases.
- A period of re-nutrition is preferable prior to extensive lab workup.

Lab
Labs should be ordered based on history and physical exam findings and the age of the patient.

Initial lab tests
- CBC
- Electrolytes, serum BUN and creatinine
- Urinalysis and urine culture
- Erythrocyte sedimentation rate (ESR)
- Lead level
- If severe malnutrition is evident also include: Albumin, alkaline phosphatase, calcium, and phosphorus
- Other tests as dictated by the history and exam:
  - Thyroid-stimulating hormone (TSH), amylase and lipase, serum zinc level, iron studies, karyotype, genetic testing, sweat chloride test, stool for ova and parasite, guaiac, alpha-1-antitrypsin and elastase, RAST testing for IgE food allergies, tissue transglutaminase and total IgA (celiac sprue), P-ANCA and ASCA (anti-Saccharomyces cerevisiae antibodies for IBD), TB test, HIV ELISA, hepatitis A, B, other infections

Follow-Up & Special Considerations
- Evaluation by a multidisciplinary team including primary care physicians (PCPs), dietitians, occupational, physical and speech therapists, social workers, developmental specialists, psychiatrists, psychologists, visiting nurses, and/or child protection services.
- Evaluation should include a home visit by the child's PCP or visiting nurse for observation of infant, interaction with caretakers, and home environment
- Prospective food diary over 3–5 day
- Individual or family counseling for caregivers, parenting classes

Imaging
Not routine. Performed only as indicated by specific history or physical exam findings.

Initial approach
- Skeletal survey if suspicion or evidence of physical abuse
- Radiographs for bone age (wrist film)
- Swallowing studies, small bowel follow through
- Brain imaging if microcephalic and/or neurologic findings on examination.

DIFFERENTIAL DIAGNOSIS
- Consider by system and disease process. Also consider psychosocial factors and abuse.
- Differentiate based on growth patterns:
- If low weight for age, normal linear growth, normocephalic OR low weight for age, followed by decreased linear growth OR low weight for age, leading to decreased linear growth and decreased head circumference (w/o neurological signs) = INADEQUATE NUTRITION (most common)
  - Consider the following:
    - Inadequate food offered
    - Poor appetite
    - Oral aversion or food aversion
    - Oromotor dysfunction
    - Maldigestion/malabsorption
    - Hypermetabolic state
- If low linear growth with normal weight for length OR low linear growth and proportionately low weight and decreased head circumference = short stature
  - Consider the following:
    - Genetic potential
    - Genetic syndromes
    - Teratogens
    - Endocrine disorder
- If microcephaly with prominent neurologic signs with poor growth secondary to presumed neurologic disorder
  - Consider the following:
    - TORCHES
    - Genetic syndromes
    - Teratogens
    - Brain injury (i.e., hypoxic/ischemic)

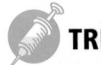

TREATMENT

MEDICATION
- Increase (and document) caloric intake.
- Consider multivitamin supplementation.

ADDITIONAL TREATMENT
General Measures
- Treatment is to improve nutrition to allow catch-up growth (weight gain 2–3 times greater than average for age).
- May use either of the following to calculate energy needs:
  - Increase intake 50% greater than the dietary reference intake (DRI) for age:
    - 0–6 months: 108 kcal/kg per day
    - 6–12 months: 98 kcal/kg per day
    - 1–3 years: 102 kcal/kg per day (1)[B]
  - General guideline for caloric requirements for infants with poor growth (for catch-up growth):
    - kcal/kg/d required = [RDA for age (kcal/kg) × Ideal wt. for ht.] / Actual wt., where ideal wt. for ht. is the median wt. for the patient's ht. (from NCHS curves)
- Rapid high-calorie intake can cause diarrhea, malabsorption, hypokalemia, hypophosphatemia. Therefore, increasing formulas above 24 kcal/oz is not recommended.
- The target energy intake should be slowly increased to goal over 5–7 days.
- Catch-up growth should be seen in 2–7 days.
- Accelerated growth should be continued for 4–9 months to restore weight and height:
  - Manage organic causes.
  - Establish appropriate nutritional intake.

- Assist with social and family problems (WIC Program, food stamps, and other transitional assistance).

Issues for Referral
Multidisciplinary care is key. Referrals are dictated by the known or suspected cause of FTT.

Additional Therapies
- In severe cases, nasogastric (NG) tube feedings can be used to supplement oral feedings.
- Gastrostomy may also be considered.

IN-PATIENT CONSIDERATIONS
Most cases of FTT can be managed as outpatients.

Initial Stabilization
- During catch-up growth, some children will develop nutritional recovery syndrome.
  - Symptoms include sweating, increased body temperature, hepatomegaly (increase glycogen deposits), widening of cranial sutures (brain growth > bone growth), increased periods of sleep, fidgetiness and mild hyperactivity.
- There may also be an initial period of malabsorption with resultant diarrhea.

Admission Criteria
Consider hospitalization if outpatient management fails, severe malnutrition or dehydration exists, and/or psychosocial situation presents harm to child.

Discharge Criteria
Catch-up growth should be seen in 2–7 days. If this is not seen, reevaluation of causes is needed.

 ONGOING CARE

FOLLOW-UP RECOMMENDATIONS
- When the etiology is organic, follow-up depends on the particular disease involved.
- Close long-term follow-up with frequent visits is important to create and maintain a healthy, supportive environment.
- If the family fails to comply, child protection authorities must be notified.

DIET
- Consider the presence of vegetarian or all-soy diets that may contribute to FTT. Safe vegetarian diets for children do exist, but must be chosen carefully.
- Nutritional requirements for a "normal" child:
  - Infant:
    - 110 kcal/kg, decreased to 100 kcal/kg at 6 months; if breastfed, ensure feeding occurs 8 times/day (minimum) w/ 5 minutes at each breast
    - Between 6 and 12 months, milk provides most of calories, but pureed foods should be consumed several times a day during this period
  - Toddler:
    - Minimum 5.5 oz/kg (110 kcal/kg) of formula; ensure proper formula mixing; if breastfed, ensure adequate supplemental foods
    - By middle of 2nd postnatal year, non-milk foods should provide at least 50% of caloric intake: 3 meals plus 2 nutritional snacks, 16–32 oz. milk/day, avoid juice and soda, and feed in a social environment
  - Rate of weight gain expected for age:
    - 0–3 months: 26–31 g/d
    - 3–6 months: 17–18 g/d
    - 6–9 months: 12–13 g/d
    - 9–12 months: 9 g/d
    - 1–3 years: 7–9 g/d

PATIENT EDUCATION
- Educate parents regarding infant social and physiological cues, formula/food preparation, proper feeding techniques, and importance of relaxed mealtimes
- When environmental deprivation is established, attempting to educate in a nonpunitive way is essential.
- Assist family with financial and nutritional assistance programs.
- Failure to Thrive: Why Is My Child Underweight? Available at http://www.aafp.org/afp/20030901/886ph.html
- The Women, Infants, and Children Program (WIC) provides Federal grants to states for supplemental foods, health care referrals, and nutrition education for low-income pregnant, breastfeeding, and non-breastfeeding postpartum women, and to infants and children up to age five who are found to be at nutritional risk. http://www.fns.usda.gov/wic/

PROGNOSIS
- Many children with FTT show adequate improvement in dietary intake with intervention.
- A significant proportion (1/3–1/2) will have long-term cognitive or behavioral abnormalities, the etiology of which is unclear.
- FTT may stunt neurologic development especially if head circumference is affected.
- Children with FTT are at increased risk for future undernutrition, overnutrition, and eating disorders.

REFERENCE
1. Krugman SD, Dubowitz H. Failure to thrive. *Am Fam Physician.* 2003;68:879–84.

See Also (Topic, Algorithm, Electronic Media Element)
Down Syndrome; Turner Syndrome; Irritable Bowel Syndrome
Algorithm: Failure to Thrive

 CODES

ICD9
783.41 Failure to thrive

CLINICAL PEARLS
- FTT is usually multifactorial. A multidisciplinary team approach to diagnosis and treatment is critical to help children with FTT and their families.
- Accurate weight and length and head circumference should be followed regularly.

F

FATTY LIVER SYNDROME

Dhvani Shah, MD
Edward Feller, MD

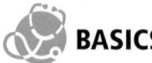

BASICS

Nonalcoholic fatty liver disease (NAFLD) describes a spectrum of fatty changes in the liver ranging from asymptomatic hepatic steatosis (fatty liver) to nonalcoholic steatohepatitis (NASH) and cirrhosis. NAFLD may be implicated to up to 90% of patients with asymptomatic, mild aminotransferase elevation not caused by alcohol, viral hepatitis, or medications.

DESCRIPTION
- Fatty liver:
  - Reversible condition where large vacuoles of triglyceride fat accumulate in hepatocytes; liver biopsy diagnosis usually shows fatty deposits in >30% of liver cells; No necrosis, no fibrosis
  - ALT and AST enzymes usually normal but may be elevated, rarely >3–4× the upper limit of normal
- NAFLD:
  - Fatty liver not due to excess alcohol consumption
  - Risk factors include associated obesity, metabolic syndrome, dyslipidemia, insulin resistance, and type 2 diabetes.
- NASH:
  - Progressive form of NAFLD; liver biopsy diagnosis of fatty deposits in >50% of liver cells associated with acute and chronic inflammation and fibrosis
  - Asymptomatic; ALT and AST elevated, generally <3–4× the upper limit of normal
  - Disease may progress to cirrhosis and/or hepatocellular cancer; incomplete data exists to assess natural history, although some evidence indicates that 30% with NASH have progression of fibrosis over 5 years.
- Both diseases usually identified in the 4th and 5th decade but may occur at any age,
- Synonym(s): Steatosis; Steatonecrosis; Nonalcoholic fatty liver disease (NAFLD); Steatohepatitis; Nonalcoholic steatohepatitis (NASH)

Pregnancy Considerations
- A severe complication of 3rd trimester is acute fatty liver of pregnancy. May be associated with signs of preeclampsia.
- Abrupt onset of confusion and restlessness with possible jaundice and right upper quadrant pain
- ALT and AST always elevated, usually <1000 IU/liter
- Emergency liver biopsy confirms diagnosis.
- Prompt delivery corrects the liver disease.
- Recurrence rare in subsequent pregnancies.

EPIDEMIOLOGY
NAFLD is the most common chronic liver disease globally, usually as benign, asymptomatic fatty liver (steatosis). NASH may be symptomatic with potential for progressive inflammation and fibrosis.

Incidence
- Present in up to 2/3 of obese (BMI >30) and in 90% of morbidly obese (BMI >39)
- Present in 5–10% type 2 DM patients
- Predominant age: 40s–50s; does occur in children
- Predominant sex: Male = Female

Prevalence
US prevalence is estimated at 6–24%

RISK FACTORS
- Obesity: BMI >30; DM; Hypertension; Hyperlipidemia (Metabolic syndrome)
- Protein–calorie malnutrition

- TPN >6 weeks
- Severe acute weight loss, including starvation and bariatric surgery
- Organic solvent (e.g., chlorinated hydrocarbons, toluene) exposure; vinyl chloride; hypoglycin A
- Gene for hemochromatosis or other conditions with increased iron stores
- Drugs: Tetracycline, glucocorticoids, tamoxifen, methotrexate, valproic acid, fialuridine, most chemotherapy regimes, and nucleoside analogues

Pediatric Considerations
- Reye syndrome: Fatty liver with encephalopathy characterized by
  - Vomiting with dehydration; usually postviral URI
  - Progressive CNS damage
  - Signs of hepatic injury: Liver morphologically shows extensive fatty vacuolization.
  - Hypoglycemia
- Etiology unknown; viral agents and drugs, especially salicylates, are implicated.
- Mortality rate 50%
- Tx: Mannitol, IV glucose, and FFP

Genetics
Largely unknown; carriers of hemochromatosis gene are more likely to be affected; possible genetic variants in the apolipoprotein C3 gene may play a role in fatty liver disease, insulin resistance, and hypertriglyceremia.

GENERAL PREVENTION
- Avoid excessive alcohol intake: >30 g/d for men, >20 g/d for women.
- Maintain or attain appropriate BMI.
- Avoid hepatotoxic medications
- Obtain HAV and HBV vaccination if not immune
- Obtain Pneumovax and yearly influenza vaccination.

PATHOPHYSIOLOGY
Primary pathophysiological derangement is *insulin resistance*, which leads to increased lipolysis, triglyceride synthesis, and increased hepatic uptake of fatty acids.

ETIOLOGY
- NAFLD: Most commonly an impaired ability of the liver to remove fatty acids
- NASH: "Two-hit" hypothesis involving macrovascular steatosis due to increased hepatic lipid synthesis, reduced transfer of lipids from the liver, and increasing insulin resistance with increased hepatic oxidative stress (1). Mitochondrial damage leading to impaired restoration of ADT stores, lipid peroxidation, and increased iron stores each have been found in 25–40% of the NASH patients.

COMMONLY ASSOCIATED CONDITIONS
Preeclampsia in pregnancy-related disease, central obesity, type 2 diabetes, insulin resistance, hyperlipidemia, hypertension

DIAGNOSIS

- Consider hepatic steatosis in any patient with asymptomatic aminotransferase elevation
- NAFLD can be present with normal or fluctuating AST and ALT.
- NASH has no distinguishing historical or laboratory features from other chronic liver disorders.

- Index of suspicion is higher in patients with associated risk factors such as metabolic syndrome, insulin resistance, or obesity.
- Noninvasive biomarkers of steatosis or fibrosis are not sufficiently reliable for diagnosis. Liver biopsy is the definitive diagnostic test. Biopsy should be considered when the results are likely to change management decisions.

HISTORY
Typically asymptomatic but some may experience fatigue and/or abdominal fullness

PHYSICAL EXAM
Hepatomegaly: Incidentally observed enlarged liver or spleen on physical exam or imaging.
Most common signs (each is infrequent):
- Liver pain or tenderness
- Mild to marked hepatomegaly
- Splenomegaly
- Limited to advanced cases: cutaneous stigmata of chronic liver disease or portal hypertension, variceal hemorrhage, ascites, hepatic encephalopathy, edema

DIAGNOSTIC TESTS & INTERPRETATION
Lab
- Liver function tests: Both ALT and AST may be elevated
  - Nonalcoholic, usually ALT:AST >1
  - If alcohol-induced, usually AST:ALT ≥2; serum alkaline phosphatase and direct bilirubin may be mildly elevated.
  - If advanced cirrhosis is present, marked, nonspecific enzyme abnormalities may exist.
- Level of enzyme elevation does not correlate with degree of fibrosis (2)[C].
- Severity in acute liver disease is marked by defects in ability to produce plasma proteins (serum albumin, prothrombin time), which are also clues to chronic hepatic disorders. Thrombocytopenia may be indicative of chronic liver disease and portal hypertension.
- Lipids almost always abnormal with elevated cholesterol, LDL, triglyceride, and decreased HDL
- Biomarkers of inflammation, increased oxidative stress or hepatocyte apoptosis such as ROS, leptin, adiponectin, CRP, serum caspase, and cytokeratin 18 remain investigational but may help differentiate NASH from NAFLD.

Initial lab tests
Serologic studies for viral hepatitis are vital: Serum ALT and AST, alkaline phosphatase, direct and total bilirubin, albumin and globulin, CBC, serum electrolytes, BUN, and creatinine

Follow-Up & Special Considerations
Patients with NAFLD have a 13% increase in carotid intima–media thickness; consider carotid ultrasound to assess (3)[A].

Imaging
- Fatty liver can be identified on ultrasound as hyperechoic liver and remains the 1st-line imaging modality for assessment of liver function test abnormalities; other imaging modalities such as MRI or CT may also be used; imaging modalities such as Fibroscan and magnetic resonance spectroscopy are currently being evaluated (4)[B].

- No imaging modality can distinguish between simple steatosis from NASH.

Diagnostic Procedures/Surgery
- Liver biopsy is the only reliable diagnostic method; however it is not without risk, cost, and sampling error.
- Predictors associated with increased risk of fibrosis on biopsy are BMI >30, age >50, insulin resistance or diabetes mellitus, and elevated serum aminotransferases.

Pathological Findings
- Anatomic pathology liver biopsy is the gold standard to differentiate fatty liver with good prognosis from NASH (2)[B].
- In NASH, steatosis, ballooning, and lobular inflammation are considered common set of minimal criteria for diagnosis; other findings that are common but not necessary include mild-moderate portal inflammation, acidophil bodies, perisinusoidal zone 3 fibrosis, megamitochondria, and Mallory hyaline in hepatocytes (5)[B].
- Staging is based largely on the extent of fibrosis.

DIFFERENTIAL DIAGNOSIS
- Viral hepatitis
- Alcoholic fatty liver (history of alcoholism may be difficult to document or exclude)
- Drug- or toxin-induced hepatitis
- Occupational exposure
- Metabolic liver disease
- Autoimmune hepatitis
- Celiac disease
- Muscle disease if nonhepatic cause of elevated ALT and ALT are possible

 ## TREATMENT

Lifestyle modification through diet and exercise is the primary recommendation for patients with NAFLD and especially those with NASH. There have been a number of studies looking at the use of insulin-sensitizing and hepatoprotective agents; however currently there is no proven medication treatment regimen besides interventions that produce sustained weight loss, regular exercise, and diet composition modification.

MEDICATION
No specific therapy currently exists, but several promising agents are under investigation.
- There have been several studies that show drugs improving insulin resistance for patients with NAFLD may have a favorable role, but they are not definitive. These include metformin and pioglitazone (6)[A].
- Vitamins E and C have been shown to show mild improvement in hepatic steatosis and some improvement in inflammation (7)[B].
- Several other drugs have been studied in small pilot trials and animal studies. These include fibrates, gemfibrozil, statins, betaine, angiotensin-receptor blockers, and ursodeoxycholic acid. However, validation in larger randomized controlled studies have yet to be undertaken (7)[B].

ADDITIONAL TREATMENT
General Measures
- Aerobic exercise should occur 3× weekly for 20–45 minutes at the least.
- DM should be tightly regulated.
- Other components of metabolic syndrome such as hypertension, dyslipidemia, and obesity should be treated.
- All alcohol use should be discontinued permanently (2)[C].
- Avoid hepatotoxic medications.

Issues for Referral
Individuals with persistent elevation of liver enzymes 2–3 times above the upper limit of normal or with fibrosis on liver biopsy benefit from regular hepatologist follow-up.

COMPLEMENTARY AND ALTERNATIVE MEDICINE
Be wary of potential hepatotoxicity of complementary medications, which may also contain impurities.

SURGERY/OTHER PROCEDURES
Newer bariatric procedures have been found to have a positive impact on NASH (2)[B]. However careful case selection assessing risk-benefit ratio is vital since natural history is generally uncomplicated.

 ## ONGOING CARE

FOLLOW-UP RECOMMENDATIONS
Patient Monitoring
- Repeat liver function tests yearly.
- Perform yearly US or CT scan to document diminution in fat.
- Changes toward normal provide major motivation to continue lifestyle changes.
- Routine repeat liver biopsy is not recommended (2)[C].

DIET
Diet low in fat; low in simple carbohydrates; low in high fructose corn syrup; devoid of industrial trans fats; and replete with vitamins, minerals, and natural antioxidants; avoidance of alcohol

PATIENT EDUCATION
Planning for lifelong change in eating, exercise, and alcohol use is required.

PROGNOSIS
Within the spectrum of NALFD, only NASH has been convincingly shown to have a progressive course, potentionally leading to cirrhosis, hepatocellular carcinoma, or liver failure.
- Cirrhosis develops in 25% of patients >20–30 years of age, with liver failure from cirrhosis occurring in 1–5%.
- Transplantation is effective, but NASH may recur after transplantation (2)[C].

COMPLICATIONS
Progressive disease may be complicated by features of decompensated cirrhosis and portal hypertension, such as ascites, encephalopathy, bleeding varices, hepato-renal or hepatopulmonary syndromes.

REFERENCES
1. Edmison J, McCullough AJ et al. Pathogenesis of non-alcoholic steatohepatitis: human data. *Clin Liver Dis*. 2007;11:75–104, ix
2. Ghali P, et al. The spectrum of nonalcoholic fatty liver disease. *J Clin Outcomes Managem*. 2005;12:585–93.
3. Sookoian S, Pirola CJ. Non-alcoholic fatty liver disease is strongly associated with carotid atherosclerosis: A systematic review. *J Hepatol*. 2008.
4. Rafiq N, Younossi ZM et al. Nonalcoholic fatty liver disease: a practical approach to evaluation and management. *Clin Liver Dis*. 2009;13:249–66.
5. Brunt EM et al. Nonalcoholic steatohepatitis. *Semin. Liver Dis*. 2004;24:3–20.
6. Angelico F, Burattin M, Alessandri C, Del Ben M, Lirussi F. Drugs improving insulin resistance for non-alcoholic fatty liver disease and/or non-alcoholic steatohepatitis. *Cochrane Database of Systematic Reviews*. 2007, Issue 1. Art. No.: CD005166. DOI:10.1002/14651858. CD005166.pub2.
7. Torres D, Harrison S. Diagnosis and Therapy of Nonalcoholic Steatohepatitis. *Gastroenterology*. 2008;134:1682–1698.
8. Schwimmer JB, Pardee PE, Lavine JE, et al. Cardiovascular risk factors and the metabolic syndrome in pediatric nonalcoholic fatty liver disease. *Circulation*. 2008;118:277–83.

See Also (Topic, Algorithm, Electronic Media Element)
Alcohol Abuse and Dependence; Cirrhosis of the Liver; Diabetes Mellitus, Type 2; Metabolic Syndrome

 ## CODES

ICD9
- 571.0 Alcoholic fatty liver
- 571.8 Other chronic nonalcoholic liver disease

CLINICAL PEARLS
- NAFLD: Spectrum of liver damage ranging from simple steatosis to NASH, advanced fibrosis, and, rarely, progression to cirrhosis. Once thought to be benign, it is increasingly recognized as a major cause of liver-related morbidity and mortality.
- NAFLD: Most common cause of liver disease in children. Overweight children with NAFLD are more likely to have metabolic syndrome and central obesity; elevated levels of total cholesterol, LDL cholesterol and triglyceride; low HDL cholesterol levels; elevated blood pressure, and impaired fasting glucose (8)[B].
- NAFLD: A major cause of asymptomatic mild serum aminotransferase elevation.
- Benefit of statins in hypercholesterolemic patients generally outweighs risk of hepatotoxicity. Continue statins and monitor hepatic enzymes.

F

FECAL IMPACTION

Benjamin Hilliker, MD
Eric Schmidt, MD

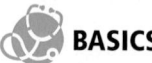 **BASICS**

DESCRIPTION
- Incomplete evacuation of feces, leading to formation of a large, firm, immovable mass of stool in the rectum (70%), sigmoid flexure (20%), or proximal colon (10%)
- System(s) affected: GI
- Synonym(s): Terminal reservoir syndrome

EPIDEMIOLOGY
Incidence
- General population: 1% (1,000/100,000)
- Children: 1.5%
- Nursing home residents: 30%
- Constipation more common in women, nonwhites, low income, <12 years of education (1)[C]
- Predominant age: >60 years
  Predominant sex:
- No sex preponderance in adults
- Among children, 75% are boys.

Geriatric Considerations
- Much more likely to occur in patients >80 years of age
- Megarectum may be present in physically and mentally impaired elderly.
- Constipation appears to correlate with decreased caloric intake in the elderly.

RISK FACTORS
- Institutionalization
- Psychogenic illness
- Immobility, inactivity
- Pica
- Excessive seed consumption (common in Middle East cultures), leading to rectal seed bezoars
- Chronic renal failure; renal transplant recipients
- Urinary incontinence
- Cognitive decline
- Constipation
- Heavy metal ingestion
- Poor toileting routines

Pediatric Considerations
- Habitual neglect of defecation urge, because of interference with play, may promote impaction.
- Fecal impaction has been reported to occur in >50% of all children with chronic constipation.

Genetics
Fecal impaction of the cecum may be seen in cystic fibrosis.

GENERAL PREVENTION
- Establish regular, consistent toilet time using gastrocolic reflex (2)[C]
- Maintain adequate hydration
- Maintain high-fiber diet (2)[C]
- Regular exercise (2)[B]

- Install user-friendly commodes.
- Psyllium 7–24 g PO daily (1)[B]
- Use periodic enemas, if indicated
- Periodic polyethylene glycol powder (MiraLax): 1 heaping tsp in 8 oz (240 mL) water daily × 2 weeks (1)[A]
- Lactulose 30–60 mL/d (1)[A]

PATHOPHYSIOLOGY
- The rectosigmoid colon dilates to accommodate mass, which, in turn, is not pliable enough to pass through the disproportionately small anal canal as a result of the patient's weak defecation effort.
- Impacted stool may exist as a single mass (stercolith) or as a composite of small, rounded fecal particles (scybalum).

ETIOLOGY
- Diet lacking in fiber
- Drug side effects (2)[C]:
  – Stimulant laxatives
  – Opiates
  – Benzodiazepines
  – Tricyclic antidepressants
  – Phenothiazines
  – Antihypertensives (calcium channel blockers)
  – Aluminum (sucralfate, antacids)
  – Iron
  – Antispasmodics
  – Vinca alkaloids
  – 5HT3 antagonist
- Painful rectal conditions inhibiting voluntary defecation (e.g., anal fissure, hemorrhoids, fistulas)
- Neoplastic or inflammatory obstructing lesions (e.g., rectal bezoars)
- Neurogenic disorders:
  – Hirschsprung disease
  – Chagas disease
  – DM
  – Autonomic neuropathy
  – Multiple sclerosis
  – Spinal cord injury
  – Cauda equine
  – Parkinson disease
- Nonneurogenic:
  – Hypothyroidism
  – Hypokalemia
  – Hypercalcemia
  – Anorexia nervosa
  – Systemic sclerosis
  – Myotonic dystrophy
- Excess of GI inhibitory hormones (e.g., prolactin, endorphins, glucagon, secretin)
- Severe idiopathic chronic constipation
- Irritable bowel syndrome
- Pelvic floor dysfunction
- Pelvic floor dyssynergia
- Encopresis

COMMONLY ASSOCIATED CONDITIONS
- Pulmonary aspiration
- Urinary tract obstruction
- Recurrent UTIs
- Intestinal obstruction
- Spontaneous perforation of colon

- Stercoral ulceration
- Hernia
- Volvulus
- Megacolon or megarectum
- Rectal prolapse
- Pneumothorax
- Hypoxia
- Hypovolemic shock
- Iliac occlusion

Pregnancy Considerations
Impaction can produce dysfunctional labor, dystocia.

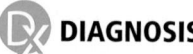 **DIAGNOSIS**

HISTORY
- Fecal incontinence, interpreted as diarrhea
- Postprandial abdominal pain
- Tenesmus
- Colic
- Nausea
- Vomiting
- Anorexia
- Weight loss
- Headache
- General malaise
- Agitation; confusion
- Urinary frequency
- Urinary incontinence

PHYSICAL EXAM
The general physical exam is not helpful in most patients.
- Weight loss
- Dehydration
- Agitation; confusion
- Fever to 39.4°C (103°F)
- Tachycardia
- Tachypnea
- Digital rectal exam:
  – Identify fissures or hemorrhoids.
  – Loss of sphincter tone: Neurologic disorders
- Large mass of stool palpable in lower left quadrant and rectal vault

DIAGNOSTIC TESTS & INTERPRETATION
Lab
Often normal
- Leukocytosis to 15,000 WBCs/mm^3
- Hyponatremia
- Hypokalemia
- Hypercalcemia
- TSH
- Stool may be positive for occult blood.
- Anemia, owing to chronic blood loss
- Pediatrics:
  – Antigliadin and antiendomysium antibodies
  – Lead

Geriatric Considerations
- Measure TSH, electrolyte activity, and BUN in elderly patients presenting with impaction.

Imaging

- Plain abdominal radiography may reveal stool or signs of obstruction if digital exam unrevealing.
- Stool retention is associated with megacolon.
- Barium enema can differentiate feces from tumor.

Diagnostic Procedures/Surgery

Sigmoidoscopy may be used to clarify the nature of a rectosigmoid mass.

DIFFERENTIAL DIAGNOSIS

- Irritable bowel syndrome
- Gastroenteritis, colitis
- Diverticulitis
- Appendicitis
- Carcinoma of the colon

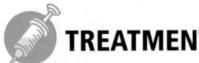 **TREATMENT**

MEDICATION

- A daily 1-L bolus of polyethylene glycol–electrolyte (GoLYTELY) solution given over 4–6 hours up to 3 days (2)[B]
- Polyethylene glycol-electrolyte (GoLYTELY) is better than lactulose in outcomes of frequency per week, form of stool, relief of abdominal pain, and the need for additional products (3)[A].
- Disimpaction in children; Consider combination:
  – Day 1: 1–2 phospho-soda enemas, 1 oz/10 kg; 4.5 oz maximum
  – Day 2: Bisacodyl suppository per rectum daily or b.i.d.
  – Day 3: Bisacodyl tablet PO every day or b.i.d.
  – Repeat 3-day cycle if needed once or twice.
- High-dose mineral oil: 15–30 mL PO per year of age per day to 8 oz maximum daily; b.i.d. for 3 days. Avoid if aspiration risk.
- Enemas: 1–2 oz/10 kg to 4.5 oz maximum, daily; b.i.d. for 1–2 days
- Children with constipation or fecal impaction who are treated with polyethylene glycol–electrolyte (GoLYTELY) have demonstrated consistently good outcomes. Dosages range from 0.3–0.7 g/kg/day (4)[A].
- Enemas and polyethylene glycol-electrolyte (GoLYTELY) were equally effective in treating fecal impaction in children. Polyethylene glycol-electrolyte (GoLYTELY) caused more fecal incontinence with comparable behavior scores (5)[B].
- Methylnaltrexone (Relistor) is approved for opioid-induced constipation by the FDA and can be considered in patients who do not have a reasonable response to a laxative regimen. Its use may be limited by cost (6)[B].
- Precautions:
  – Use magnesium citrate with caution in patients with renal insufficiency.
  – Be careful with lactulose; colonic distension can result from its bacterial fermentation.

ADDITIONAL TREATMENT

General Measures

- Manual fragmentation and extraction of fecal mass (after lubrication with lidocaine jelly) may be attempted.
- Larger masses can be disimpacted with water jet directed through fiberoptic sigmoidoscope.
- Enemas containing 20% water-soluble contrast material (Hypaque) may help.

- If incomplete fragmentation: Suppositories or enemas with mineral oil, tap water, or sodium phosphate
- Ensure minimum fluid intake of 1.5–2.0 L/d.

Issues for Referral

In the pediatric population, consultation with a pediatric gastroenterologist should be considered in children in whom oral or rectal medication is ineffective for disimpaction and in whom dietary changes and laxative therapy are ineffective.

COMPLEMENTARY AND ALTERNATIVE MEDICINE

Biofeedback improves constipation in patients with dyssynergic bowel function (7)[B].

SURGERY/OTHER PROCEDURES

- Laparotomy necessary only in extreme cases (2)[B]
- Electrohydraulic lithotripsy has been used to safely remove large, calcified fecaliths.

IN-PATIENT CONSIDERATIONS

Admission Criteria

- Disimpaction usually is performed in outpatient setting.
- Hospitalization is necessary if several attempts at outpatient management have failed.
- Presence of complications

 ONGOING CARE

FOLLOW-UP RECOMMENDATIONS

Increased activity is important.

Patient Monitoring

<1 bowel movement every other day may lead to impaction.

DIET

- High fiber
- Home remedy: Mix 2 cups bran, 2 cups applesauce, and 1 cup unsweetened prune juice; refrigerate; take 2–3 tbs b.i.d.

PATIENT EDUCATION

- Avoid catharsis.
- Comprehensive program, including use of laxative, behavior changes, dietary changes
- Effective education of the parents and child with regard to constipation is crucial in changing chronic behavior patterns.
- No hot water, soap, or hydrogen peroxide enemas. They may burn or irritate rectal mucosa, causing bleeding.

PROGNOSIS

- Reimpaction is likely if program is not followed.
- Prognosis is poor for perforation with peritonitis.
- Mortality with impaction and obstruction is highest in the very young and the very old (up to 16%).

COMPLICATIONS

- Sepsis
- Hypotension
- Instrumental perforation
- Bleeding
- Postoperative obstruction

REFERENCES

1. Brandt LJ, Prather CM, Quigley EM, et al. Systematic review on the management of chronic constipation in North America. *Am J Gastroenterol.* 2005;100 (Suppl 1):S5–S21.
2. Hsieh C. Treatment of constipation in older adults. *Am Fam Physician.* 2005;72:2277–84.
3. Lee-Robichaud H, Thomas K, Morgan J, Nelson RL et al. Lactulose versus Polyethylene Glycol for Chronic Constipation. *Cochrane Database Syst Rev.* 2010;7:CD007570.
4. Candy D, Belsey J. Macrogol (polyethylene glycol) laxatives in children with functional constipation and faecal impaction: a systematic review. *Arch Dis Child.* 2009;94:156–60.
5. Bekkali N, van den Berg M, Dijkgraaf M, van wijk P, Bongers EJ, Liem O, Benninga M. Rectal Fecal Impaction Treatment in Childhood Constipation: Enemas versus High Doses Oral PEG. *Pediatrics* 2009;124;e1108–e1115.
6. Enck R. An Overview of Constipation and Newer Therapies. *American Journal of Hospice & Palliative Medicine.* 2009;26(3):157–158.
7. Rao SS, Seaton K, Miller M, et al. Randomized controlled trial of biofeedback, sham feedback, and standard therapy for dyssynergic defecation. *Clin Gastroenterol Hepatol.* 2007;5:331–8.

ADDITIONAL READING

- Constipation Guideline Committee of the North American Society for Pediatric Gastroenterology, Hepatology and Nutrition. Evaluation and treatment of constipation in infants and children: recommendations of the North American Society for Pediatric Gastroenterology, Hepatology and Nutrition. *J Pediatr Gastroenterol Nutr.* 2006;43: e1–13.
- Tariq SH. Geriatric fecal incontinence. *Clin Geriatr Med.* 2004;20:571–87, ix.

See Also (Topic, Algorithm, Electronic Media Element)

Constipation; Diarrhea, Chronic; Encopresis

CODES

ICD9
560.32 Fecal impaction

CLINICAL PEARLS

- Any elderly person with a fever of uncertain cause should be considered to have a fecal impaction until you can disprove it with a DRE.
- When treating chronic pain patients with opioid preparations, be sure to supplement with stool softeners or osmotic laxatives. Hydrophilic colloid (fiber) is not that helpful in frail, end-of-life, or nonmobile patients.

F

FEMALE ATHLETE TRIAD

Rahul Kapur, MD, CAQSM
Natasha Harrison, MD
Kristyn Newhall, MD

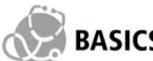

BASICS

Consisting of three interrelated spectrums of:
- Low energy availability
- Menstrual dysfunction
- Decreased bone health

DESCRIPTION
- First recognized in 1992.
- 2007 American College of Sports Medicine (ACSM) criteria recommends to consider each component of the triad as a continuous spectrum. The criterion of disordered eating has been replaced by "low energy availability with or without an eating disorder." Amenorrhea is considered within a spectrum from "eumenorrhea" to "functional hypothalamic amenorrhea." The endpoint diagnosis of osteoporosis has been replaced by a spectrum from "optimal bone health" to "osteoporosis." The ACSM 2007 revision underscores the importance of energy availability as the 1st step in the propagation of the triad, emphasizing that without correction of this triad component, full recovery is not possible (1).
- Energy availability: The dietary energy intake minus exercise energy expenditure, which represents the amount of dietary energy remaining for body functions after exercise training. When energy availability is low, the body compensates to restore energy balance by reducing mechanisms of cellular maintenance, thermoregulation, growth and reproduction. Athletes with low energy availability may develop an imbalance by increasing training disproportionately to energy intake, while others may reduce energy intake by restricting, fasting, bingeing and purging, or by using diet pills, laxatives, diuretics, or enemas. Only some of these athletes will meet the (DSM-IV) criteria for eating disorders including anorexia nervosa and bulimia nervosa.
- Menstrual dysfunction: A spectrum ranging from eumenorrhea to amenorrhea, allowing for the inclusion of athletes who have low estrogen levels but may still experience menstruation:
  – This spectrum includes luteal suppression (shortened luteal phase, prolonged follicular phase and decreased estradiol level), anovulation, oligomenorrhea (menstrual cycle greater than 35 days) and primary and secondary hypothalamic amenorrhea. Primary amenorrhea, though less common, can occur in young athletes. Secondary amenorrhea is defined as the absence of menstrual cycles for greater than three months after menarche has occurred.
  – Hypothalamic suppression is the most common cause of secondary amenorrhea in these athletes, although other causes must be ruled out prior to attributing the problem to low energy availability.
- Bone health: Bone health exists on a spectrum from optimal bone health to osteoporosis, a skeletal disorder characterized by compromised bone strength predisposing a person to an increased fracture risk. Bone health refers to bone strength, or bone mineral density (BMD), as well as bone quality. Current technology allows for the measurement of bone density but not quality, which helps to explain why 2 athletes with the same BMD may have very different bone fracture histories:
  – Athletes with a BMD Z-score that is 2 standard deviations (SD) below the mean are termed low bone density below the expected range for age for premenopausal women and low bone density for chronologic age for children.
  – Because most athletes have a higher BMD than nonathletes, the ACSM recommends physicians consider further workup for any athlete with a Z-score <−1.0, even in the absence of fracture (2).

EPIDEMIOLOGY
Unknown as often hidden by patients

Prevalence
- Prevalence unclear; data suggests between 3.4–4.3%. The 2 other triad studies, found all 3 components of triad in 2.7% of collegiate and 1.2% of high school athletes (1,3).
- Disordered eating: Prevalence of clinically diagnosed (DSM-IV) eating disorders in elite athletes 25–31% vs 5.5-9% in the general population.
- Menstrual dysfunction: Prevalence of secondary amenorrhea found to be as high as 69% in dancers and 65% in long-distance runners compared to 2–5% in the general population. Majority exhibit a luteal deficiency or anovulatory cycle in 1 in 3 menstrual cycles.
- Bone health: A systematic review of past studies using the World Health Organization (WHO) criteria for low BMD revealed prevalence of osteopenia (T-score between −1.0 and −2.5) from 22–50% in female athletes, compared to 12% in the normal population and of osteoporosis (T-score ≤ −2.5) as high as 13%, compared to 2.3% in the normal population.

RISK FACTORS
- Sports with an aesthetic component, e.g., ballet, figure skating, gymnastics, distance running, diving and swimming, or sports with weight classifications, e.g., martial arts and wrestling. Frequent weigh-ins, consequences for weight gain, domineering coaches or parents, and a win-at-all-cost attitude increase risk of developing the triad.
- A lack of family or social support, either secondary to intense training hours causing social isolation or entering a new environment (boarding school or college)
- Athlete with comorbid psychological conditions, e.g., anxiety, depression, and/or obsessive-compulsive disorder is more likely to develop the triad (3).

GENERAL PREVENTION
- Education of athletes, coaches, trainers, parents, and physicians about the triad is crucial. Young athletes are extremely impressionable and may turn negative comments and unhealthy advice from adults into maladaptive eating and exercising habits.
- Primary care physicians should screen all adolescents for disordered eating, menstrual dysfunction, and injury history.
- Athletes presenting with "red flag" conditions such as fractures, weight changes, fatigue, amenorrhea, bradycardia, orthostatic hypotension, syncope, arrhythmia, electrolyte abnormalities, or depression should also be screened for the triad.

PATHOPHYSIOLOGY
- Current theory is based on a baseline caloric deficit or low energy availability causing a disruption in the hypothalamic-pituitary-ovarian axis, decreasing the pulsatile release of gonadotropin-releasing hormone (GnRH).
- Low energy availability alters the levels of various metabolic hormones including insulin, cortisol, growth hormone, insulin-like growth factor-1 (ILGF-1), 3.3.5-triiodothyronine (T3) and leptin, some of which are thought to play a role in the regulation of GnRH secretion. Low GnRH levels subsequently decrease luteinizing hormone (LH) and follicle-stimulating hormone (FSH) levels causing a decrease in estrogen production, resulting in varying degrees of menstrual dysfunction.
- Estrogen deficiency also negatively affects bone density and a chronic state of malnutrition reduces the rate of bone formation and increases the rate of bone resorption. This change in increased bone resorption and declined rate of bone formation began within 5 days of energy availability reduction (1,4).

COMMONLY ASSOCIATED CONDITIONS
- Anorexia nervosa or bulimia nervosa
- Psychological disorders including low self-esteem, depression, and anxiety. In one study, 5.4% of athletes with eating disorders reported suicide attempts (5).
- Low BMD predisposes athletes to stress fractures and may not be fully reversible. This may lead to an even higher rate of fractures as these athletes reach postmenopausal status.

DIAGNOSIS

- The female athlete triad is a clinical diagnosis based mainly on patient history.
- Screening for the female athlete triad should occur at annual sports physicals, routine exams, and acute visits for any concerning complaints or components of the triad (1)[C].

HISTORY
- A 24-hour food recall diary may be helpful in this process. Athletes should be assessed for menstrual history (including oral contraceptive use), fracture history, and symptoms of depression (5)[C].
- Special dietary practices, eating behaviors, and weight changes should also be collected.
- Body image, fear of weight gain, fluctuations in weight, history of disordered eating, and use of laxatives, diet pills, or enemas are crucial to understanding the extent of the disease.

PHYSICAL EXAM
- Height, weight, and vital signs
- Common findings in patients with disordered eating include bradycardia, orthostatic hypotension, hypothermia, cold or cyanotic extremities, lanugo, hypercarotenemia, parotid gland enlargement or tenderness, epigastric tenderness, eroded tooth enamel, and knuckle or hand calluses (Russell sign) (5)[C].
- Patients with primary amenorrhea should undergo a pelvic exam to determine the presence of a uterus. A pelvic exam in patients with secondary amenorrhea

is warranted to rule out anomalies. Vaginal atrophy may be present in the hypoestrogen state (1)[C].

DIAGNOSTIC TESTS & INTERPRETATION
Lab
- Electrolytes and kidney function, complete blood count with differential, erythrocyte sedimentation rate, thyroid stimulating hormone (TSH), 25 vitamin D, and urinalysis.
- Primary evaluation for secondary amenorrhea includes a urine pregnancy test, follicle stimulating hormone, luteinizing hormone, prolactin and thyroid stimulating hormone (1)[B].

Imaging
- Electrocardiogram (EKG) to rule out a prolonged QT interval. The QT interval may be prolonged even in the absence of electrolyte abnormalities (5)[C].
- Evidence for bone mineral density testing by dual-energy x-ray absorptiometry (DXA) is controversial. Current guidelines recommend DXA studies for patients with disordered eating, eating disorders, amenorrhea, or oligomenorrhea for at least 6 months and/or patients with a history of stress fractures or fractures from minimal trauma. In patients with persistent components of the triad, reevaluation by the same DXA machine is recommended in 12 months from initial scan (1)[C].

DIFFERENTIAL DIAGNOSIS
The diagnosis of each component of the female athlete triad must be one of exclusion. Patients must be screened for anorexia nervosa and bulimia nervosa using the DSM-IV criteria. Similarly, before presuming a diagnosis of hypothalamic amenorrhea secondary to energy deficit, the following groups of diagnoses must be ruled out:
- Pregnancy
- Hypothalamic dysfunction: Psychological stress induced amenorrhea, medication induced amenorrhea, Kallmann syndrome
- Pituitary dysfunction: Prolactinoma or other pituitary neoplasm, Sheehan syndrome, sarcoidosis, empty-sella syndrome
- Ovarian dysfunction: Polycystic ovarian syndrome, premature ovarian failure, menopause, gonadal dysgenesis, Turner syndrome, ovarian neoplasm, autoimmune disease
- Uterine dysfunction: Asherman syndrome, absence of uterus
- Endocrine abnormalities: Thyroid dysfunction, Cushing syndrome (3)[B]

 TREATMENT

- The treatment goal is to optimize nutritional status by establishing healthy eating behaviors and treating any associated maladaptive thought processes or psychological disorders.
- A multidisciplinary team including a physician (or other health care provider), registered dietitian and a mental health provider is crucial for treatment (1)[C]. Diet and exercise behaviors must be modified by a combination of increasing dietary intake and reducing energy expenditure. Nutritional counseling by a registered dietitian is necessary for energy availability estimates as well as modification of eating behaviors. Individual, group and family psychotherapy may also be needed for the full treatment of the triad (5)[B]. Communication with team coaches, trainers, and family is also a critical intervention.

- Studies have shown a positive energy availability of more than 30 kcal/kg of fat-free muscle mass/day is sufficient to restore menstrual cycling, while an energy availability of more than 45 kcal/kg of fat-free muscle mass/day is likely needed for BMD improvement. Increases in body weight have been accompanied by improved BMD by up to 5% per year in previously amenorrheic athletes (1).

MEDICATION
The use of oral contraceptive pills (OCPs), hormone replacement therapy (HRT), and/or bisphosphonates has not been clearly shown to increase BMD or aid in the restoration of normal menstrual cycling. OCPs can be considered to minimize further bone loss in patients over age 16, who, despite adequate nutrition and body weight gain, continue to have decreasing BMD and functional hypothalamic amenorrhea (1)[C].

ADDITIONAL TREATMENT
Issues for Referral
Referrals to registered dietitians, mental health professionals who specialize in disordered eating behaviors, and sports medicine specialists for treatment of fractures often are needed (1)[C].

IN-PATIENT CONSIDERATIONS
Patients with disordered eating or clinically diagnosable eating disorders must be evaluated for potentially life-threatening conditions requiring hospital admission including bradycardia, severe orthostatic hypotension, significant electrolyte imbalances, hypothermia, arrhythmias, or prolonged QT interval on EKG (3,5)[C].

 ONGOING CARE

- Patients with components of the triad should undergo frequent monitoring by all members of the multidisciplinary treatment team. In order to continue training and competing, athletes with disordered eating or clinically diagnosable eating disorders must agree to the following criteria:
  - To comply with all treatment strategies; to be closely monitored by heath care providers; to place treatment goals over training goals; and to modify the type, duration, and intensity of training or competition if necessary.
- Athletes with disordered eating behaviors who do not comply with this agreement may need to be restricted from training (1)[C].

PATIENT EDUCATION
All young female patients should be counseled on the importance of proper nutrition, calcium, and vitamin D intake and the benefits of regular weight-bearing exercise. Patients presenting with one or more components of the triad should be educated about the short-term and long-term effects of low BMD (6).

PROGNOSIS
- The short- and long-term prognosis for patients with female athlete triad is dependent on time to diagnosis and treatment. Assuming early intervention with a multidisciplinary team, prognosis is very good. With adequate treatment and an increase in energy availability, patients will regain normal menstrual cycling and fertility and begin to increase BMD.

- Because the triad often occurs within the age window of optimal bone strengthening, patients with a prolonged disease course may suffer from complications of decreased bone mineral density throughout their adolescent and adult life. In addition, patients with disordered eating behaviors may require long-term ongoing therapy to manage their disease (3).

REFERENCES

1. Otis CL, Drinkwater B, Johnson M, et al. American College of Sports Medicine position stand. The Female Athlete Triad. *Med Sci Sports Exerc.* 1997;29:i–ix.
2. International Society for Clinical Densitometry Writing Group for the ISCD Position Development Conference. Diagnosis of osteoporosis in men, women, and children. *J Clin Densitom.* 2004;7: 17–26.
3. Hobart JA, Smucker DR. The female athlete triad. *Am Fam Physician.* 2000;61:3357–64, 3367.
4. The female athlete triad. *Med Sci Sports Exerc.* 2007;39:1867–82.
5. American Psychiatric Association Working Group on Eating Disorders. Treatment of patients with eating disorders, third edition. *Am J Psychiatry.* 2006;163:4–54.
6. American Academy of Pediatrics. Committee on Sports Medicine and Fitness. Medical concerns in the female athlete. *Pediatrics.* 2000;106:610–3.

See Also (Topic, Algorithm, Electronic Media Element)
Algorithms: Amenorrhea, Secondary; Amenorrhea, Primary; Weight Loss

 CODES

ICD9
- 307.50 Eating disorder, unspecified
- 626.0 Absence of menstruation
- 733.00 Osteoporosis, unspecified

CLINICAL PEARLS
- The female athlete triad consists of three related spectrums of energy availability, menstrual function, and BMD. Athletes may exhibit varying degrees of dysfunction along each of the 3 spectra.
- Regular screening of adolescent and adult females at all routine and relevant acute visits is critical to early diagnosis and intervention.
- Immediate intervention by a multidisciplinary team including physicians, registered dietitians, mental heath professionals, coaches, trainers, and parents is crucial to minimize further bone loss, recover bone mineral density, and regain menstrual cycling.

FEVER OF UNKNOWN ORIGIN (FUO)

Scott T. Henderson, MD

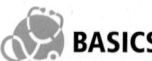

BASICS

DESCRIPTION
- Classic definition by Petersdorf and Beeson:
  - Fever over 38.3°C on several occasions
  - Fever duration at least 3 weeks
  - Uncertain diagnosis after 1 week of study in the hospital
- Modifications to the definition have been proposed, including eliminating the in-hospital evaluation and shortening the exam time.
- Some have suggested expansion of the definition to include nosocomial, neutropenic, and HIV-associated fevers that may not be prolonged.

EPIDEMIOLOGY
Incidence
No data on actual incidence

RISK FACTORS
- Recent travel
- Exposure to biologic or chemical agents
- HIV-infected patients with advanced disease
- Persons in AIDS risk group
- Elderly
- Drug abuse
- Immigrants
- Young female health care workers; consider factitious fever

ETIOLOGY
- >200 causes; each with prevalence 5% or less
- Infection:
  - Abdominal abscesses
  - Amebic hepatitis
  - Catheter infections
  - Cytomegalovirus
  - Endocarditis/pericarditis
  - HIV (late stage)
  - Mycobacterial infection (often with advanced HIV)
  - Osteomyelitis
  - Renal
  - Sinusitis
  - Wound infections
  - Other miscellaneous infections
- Neoplasms:
  - Atrial myxoma
  - Colon cancer
  - Hepatoma
  - Lymphoma
  - Leukemia
  - Solid tumors (hypernephroma)
- Collagen vascular disease:
  - Giant cell arteritis
  - Polyarteritis nodosa
  - Polymyalgia rheumatica
  - Systemic lupus erythematosus
  - Rheumatic fever
  - Rheumatoid arthritis

- Other causes:
  - Alcoholic hepatitis
  - Cerebrovascular accident
  - Cirrhosis
  - Drug fever/medication induced:
    - Allopurinol, captopril, carbamazepine, cephalosporins, cimetidine, clofibrate, erythromycin, heparin, hydralazine, hydrochlorothiazide, isoniazid, meperidine, methyldopa, nifedipine, nitrofurantoin, penicillin, phenytoin, procainamide, quinidine, sulfonamides
  - Endocrinologic diseases
  - Factitious/fraudulent fever
  - Granulomatous diseases
  - Occupational causes
  - Periodic fever
  - Pulmonary emboli/deep vein thrombosis
  - Thermoregulatory disorders
- In up to 20% of cases, the cause of the fever will not be identified despite thorough workup.

Geriatric Considerations
- Most common causes are acute leukemia, Hodgkin lymphoma, intra-abdominal infections, TB, and temporal arteritis

Pediatric Considerations
- Infections and collagen-vascular diseases are the most likely etiology.
- Inflammatory bowel disease is the common etiology in older children and adolescents.

DIAGNOSIS

HISTORY
- History should focus on relevant symptoms:
  - Constitutional symptoms almost always accompany a fever:
    - Chills, night sweats, myalgias, weight loss with an intact appetite (infectious)
    - Arthralgias, myalgias, fatigue (inflammatory)
    - Fatigue, night sweats, weight loss with loss of appetite (neoplasms)
- Past medical history should include information about previously treated chronic infections and any prior diagnosis of cancer.
- Past surgical history should include specific information about type of surgery performed, postoperative complications, and any indwelling foreign materials.
- Obtain a comprehensive list of all medications, including over-the-counter and herbal remedies.
- Family history to identify prior illnesses in family members that may have a genetic link, such as periodic fever syndromes, and recent illnesses in family members to which the patient may have been exposed

ALERT
Special attention should be paid to travel, occupational, sexual, and drug exposure.

Geriatric Considerations
- Signs and symptoms in the elderly are much more nonspecific.
- Coexisting diseases and numerous medications may cloud features.

PHYSICAL EXAM
- Physical exam should focus on areas that have high diagnostic yield:
  - Fundoscopic exam for choroid tubercles or Roth spots; temporal artery palpation; gums and oral cavity; auscultation for bruits and murmurs; abdominal palpation for organomegaly; rectal examination; testicular examination; palpate for adenopathy; skin and nail bed exam for clubbing, nodules, lesions, and rashes; focal neurologic signs; bony tenderness; and joint effusion
- Repeated exams are essential to determine cause.

DIAGNOSTIC TESTS & INTERPRETATION
Lab
Initial lab tests
- Complete blood count
- Peripheral blood smear
- Liver function tests
- C-reactive protein
- Erythrocyte sedimentation rate
- HIV antibody test
- Blood cultures (not to exceed 6 sets)
- Urinalysis and urine culture

Geriatric Considerations
- Residents of long-term care facilities have unique guidelines; review advanced directives first to determine if any testing should be done.
- Blood cultures are shown to have lower yield (1)[A].

Follow-Up & Special Considerations
- Rheumatoid factor and antinuclear antibody test
- Serologic tests: Epstein-Barr, hepatitis, syphilis, Lyme disease, Q fever, cytomegalovirus, amebiasis, coccidioidomycosis
- Serum ferritin
- Serum protein electrophoresis
- Sputum and urine cultures for TB
- Thyroid function tests
- Tuberculin skin test:
  - May not be helpful if anergic or acute infection
  - If test negative, repeat in 2 weeks

Imaging
Initial approach
- CXR
- CT scan or MRI of abdomen and pelvis (plus directed biopsy, if indicated) (2)[C]

Follow-Up & Special Considerations
- Technetium-based scan if infectious process or tumor suspected (2)[B]
- PET scan using the radiolabeled glucose analogue ^{18}F-fluorodeoxyglucose if infectious process, inflammatory process, or tumor suspected; PET scans have a high negative predictive value (3)[B]

- Ultrasound of abdomen and pelvis (plus directed biopsy, if indicated) if mass lesions, renal obstruction, or gallbladder/biliary tree pathology suspected
- ECG if cardiac valve lesions (endocarditis), atrial myxomas, or pericardial effusion suspected (transthoracic vs transesophageal)
- Leg Doppler if deep vein thrombosis/pulmonary embolism suspected
- CT scan of chest if pulmonary emboli suspected
- Indium-labeled leukocyte scanning if inflammatory process suspected
- Bone scan if osteomyelitis or metastatic disease suspected

Diagnostic Procedures/Surgery
- Liver biopsy if granulomatous disease suspected (2)[C]
- Temporal artery biopsy, particularly in the elderly (2)[B]
- Lymph node, muscle or skin biopsy if clinically indicated
- Bone marrow biopsy if clinically indicated
- Spinal tap if clinically indicated

Pathological Findings
Depends on etiology

DIFFERENTIAL DIAGNOSIS
See Etiology.

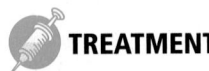

TREATMENT

MEDICATION
First Line
- 1st-line drugs are dependent on the diagnosis.
- Evidence does not support treatment of fever (4)[C].

Pediatric Considerations
- Aspirin should be avoided in children because of the risk of Reye syndrome.

Second Line
If the patient has symptoms with the fever or continues to decline, a therapeutic trial may be indicated:
- Antibiotic trial based on patient's history
- Antituberculous therapy if there is a high risk for granulomatous disease pending culture results
- Steroid trial based on patient's history (once occult malignancy is ruled out)

ALERT
If a steroid trial is initiated, patient may have a relapse after treatment or if certain conditions (such as TB) have been undiagnosed.

ADDITIONAL TREATMENT
General Measures
- Attempt to determine the etiology before initiating the therapy.
- Avoid therapeutic trials unless as a last resort and only if therapy is reasonably specific.
- "Shotgun" approaches are condemned, as they obscure the clinical picture, have untoward effects, and do not solve the problem (2)[C].

Additional Therapies
With temperature elevations, patients will have increased caloric and fluid demands.

SURGERY/OTHER PROCEDURES
Need for exploratory laparotomy has been largely eliminated with the advent of more sophisticated tests and imaging modalities.

IN-PATIENT CONSIDERATIONS
Admission Criteria
- Reserved for the ill and debilitated
- Consider if factitious fever has been ruled out or an invasive procedure is indicated

 ## ONGOING CARE

FOLLOW-UP RECOMMENDATIONS
Patient Monitoring
If the etiology of the fever remains unknown, repeat the history and physical exam along with screening lab studies.

DIET
With temperature elevations, patients will have increased caloric and fluid demands.

PATIENT EDUCATION
Maintain an open line of communication between physician and patient/family as the workup progresses:
- The extended time required in establishing a diagnosis can be frustrating.

PROGNOSIS
- Depends on etiology and age:
  – Patients with HIV have the highest mortality.
- 1-year survival rates reflecting deaths due to all causes

Age	Survival
<35	91%
35–64	82%
>64	67%

COMPLICATIONS
Dependent on etiology

Pregnancy Considerations
Fever is known to increase the risk of neural tube defects and trigger preterm labor.

REFERENCES

1. High KP, Bradley SF, Gravenstein S, et al. Clinical practice guideline for the evaluation of fever and infection in older adult residents of long-term care facilities: 2008 update by the Infectious Diseases Society of America. *J Am Geriatr Soc*. 2009;57: 375–94.
2. Mourad O, Palda V, Detsky AS. A comprehensive evidence-based approach to fever of unknown origin. *Arch Intern Med*. 2003;163:545–51.
3. Keidar Z, Gurman-Balbir A, Gaitini D, Israel O et al. Fever of unknown origin: the role of 18F-FDG PET/CT. *J Nucl Med*. 2008;49:1980–5.
4. Plaisance KI, Mackowiak PA. Antipyretic therapy: physiologic rationale, diagnostic implications, and clinical consequences. *Arch Intern Med*. 2000;160: 449–56.

ADDITIONAL READING

- Cunha BA. Fever of unknown origin: Clinical overview of classic and current concepts. *Infect Dis Clin N Am*. 2007;21:867–915.
- Cunha BA. Fever of unknown origin: Focused diagnostic approach based on clinical clues from the history, physical examination, and laboratory tests. *Infect Dis Clin N Am*. 2007;21:1137–87.
- Williams J, Bellamy R et al. Fever of unknown origin. *Clin Med*. 2008;8:526–30.

See Also (Topic, Algorithm, Electronic Media Element)
Arthritis, Juvenile Idiopathic; Colorectal Cancer; Cytomegalovirus Inclusion Disease; Endocarditis, Infective; Giant Cell Arteritis; Hepatoma; HIV Infection and AIDS; Leukemia; Osteomyelitis; Polyarteritis Nodosa; Polymyalgia Rheumatica; Pulmonary Embolism; Rheumatic Fever; Sinusitis; Stroke (Brain Attack); Lupus Erythematosus, Discoid; Algorithms: Fever, Acute; Fever of Unknown Origin; Fever in the First 3 Months of Life

 ## CODES

ICD9
780.60 Fever, unspecified

CLINICAL PEARLS

- The history, exam, and test should focus on the relevant causes of FUO:
  – A sequential approach leads to a rational sequentially diagnosis or rules out causes of FUO.
- A "shotgun" approach to treatment should be avoided; empiric therapy should be used only in carefully defined circumstances.
- FUO cases that defy precise diagnosis after intensive investigation and prolonged observation generally carry a favorable prognosis.
- In many cases, FUO in older persons may represent atypical, nonclassic presentations of common infectious and noninfectious diseases.

F

FIBROCYSTIC CHANGES OF THE BREAST

Katherine M. Callaghan, MD
Dawn S. Tasillo, MD

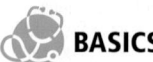 **BASICS**

DESCRIPTION
- Fibrocystic changes of the breast (FCC) is a generalized term for a heterogeneous group of changes affecting the stromal and glandular tissues of the breast.
- The most common of all benign breast conditions
- Commonly presents as mastalgia, engorgement, increased breast nodularity, and/or cysts:
  - Mastalgia (breast pain) is usually in upper outer quadrants of breast, bilateral, and may radiate to shoulders or upper arms.
  - Localized pain may occur with a rapidly enlarging cyst.
  - Nodules are usually small (2–10 mm), diffuse, and bilateral, with a rubbery consistency.
  - Cysts are more common in women in their 40s.
  - Larger cysts may have consistency of a water-filled balloon.
- Symptoms are most prominent in premenstrual (luteal) phase.
- System(s) affected: Endocrine/Metabolic; Reproductive
- Synonym(s): Fibrocystic breast disease; Mammary dysplasia; Chronic cystic mastitis

EPIDEMIOLOGY
Most common in women of reproductive years; occasionally seen after menopause with hormone replacement

Incidence
Unknown but very frequent

Prevalence
Present in up to 90% of women during their lifetime

RISK FACTORS
- The effect of consumption of methylxanthine-containing substances (e.g., coffee, tea, cola, and chocolate) has not been found to be a contributing factor (1)[A].
- Diet high in fruits and vegetables and high parity independently decrease risk of FCC (2)
- Diet high in saturated fats may increase risk of FCC

PATHOPHYSIOLOGY
May be the result of an exaggerated response of breast tissue to cycling hormones or a subtle imbalance in the ratio of estrogen to progesterone

ETIOLOGY
Estrogen likely a causative factor for many (3)[B]

 DIAGNOSIS

HISTORY
- May present in 3 overlapping, indistinct stages:
  - Mastoplagia and mastalgia, which may subside after menses; common in women in their 20s
  - Adenosis: Appearance of multiple small breast nodules; common in women in their 30s
  - Cystic phase: Tender cysts, usually small but up to 5 cm in diameter; common in women in their 40s
- Family history of breast disease (benign or malignant)

PHYSICAL EXAM
- With patient in supine position and rotated on contralateral hip, evaluate all breast tissue from sternum to midaxillary line, from clavicle to mammary ridge.
- Using fingertip, proceed in a linear fashion from top of sternum past breast tissue using 3 different depths of pressure at each palpation. Continue superiorly again to clavicle in a "lawnmower" fashion.
- Quantitate size, consistency, mobility, location, and skin changes.
- Findings in FCC may include:
  - Smooth, tense, or fluctuant masses
  - Bilateral masses
  - Breast thickening
  - Nipple discharge
- Palpate for axillary lymph nodes.

DIAGNOSTIC TESTS & INTERPRETATION
Evaluation should focus on excluding breast cancer. Testing may be conducted based on level of clinical suspicion.

Imaging
Initial approach
- Ultrasound (US): Signs of malignancy include irregular mass, clustered masses, calcifications, architectural distortion, dilated duct; US is useful for differentiating cystic from solid lesions.
- Mammography may reveal mass or dense tissue ± calcifications.

Follow-Up & Special Considerations
- Mammogram may be normal in presence of malignancy and difficult to interpret in women <35 years of age due to dense breast tissue; US may be helpful.
- Magnetic resonance imaging is indicated in patients with *BRCA1* or *BRCA2* mutation or in any woman with 25% or greater lifetime risk for breast cancer (4).

Diagnostic Procedures/Surgery
- Fine-needle aspiration (FNA) and biopsy:
  - Allows differentiation of cystic and solid lesions
  - Aspirate may be straw-colored, dark brown, or green.
  - Cells sent for cytology can reveal cancer with high accuracy.
  - Low morbidity
- If mass disappears, no further evaluation is necessary (including cytologic evaluation of aspirated fluid).

Pathological Findings
- Atypia: Relative risk of 4.24 for eventual breast cancer
- Proliferative changes without atypia: Relative risk of 1.88 for eventual breast cancer
- Nonproliferative changes: Relative risk of 1.27 for eventual breast cancer (5)

DIFFERENTIAL DIAGNOSIS

- Pain: Mastitis, costochondritis, pectoralis muscle strain, neuralgia, breast cancer, angina pectoris, gastroesophageal reflux, superficial phlebitis of the thoracoepigastric vein (Mondor disease)
- Masses: Breast cancer, sebaceous cyst, fibroadenoma, lipoma, fat necrosis
- Skin changes: Breast cancer (peau d'orange: Thickened skin similar to peel of an orange), eczema

TREATMENT

- After ruling out malignancy by means of imaging and diagnostic procedures, FCC may not require treatment and often resolves with time.
- Cool compresses and a well-fitting, supportive bra (worn day and night) may be useful for symptom relief.

MEDICATION

First Line

For cyclic pain and swelling: Nonsteroidal anti-inflammatory drugs:

- Ibuprofen 400 mg q.i.d./p.r.n.
- Naproxen 500 mg b.i.d./p.r.n.

Second Line

- Oral contraceptives may be useful in modulating symptoms or in preventing the development of new changes.
- For severe pain, consider (6):
  - Danazol (Danocrine) 100–400 mg/d divided in 2 doses × 4–6 months
  - Bromocriptine 2.5 mg b.i.d. × 3 months
  - Tamoxifen 10 mg/d × 3–6 months

ADDITIONAL TREATMENT

Issues for Referral

- If discrete lesion in a woman ≤35 years, US then refer to a surgeon
- If discrete lesion in a woman >35 years, diagnostic mammography ± US then refer to surgeon

COMPLEMENTARY AND ALTERNATIVE MEDICINE

Evidence supporting evening primrose oil, vitamin E, or pyridoxine as treatment for the discomforts of FCC is insufficient to draw conclusions about effectiveness (1).

SURGERY/OTHER PROCEDURES

Breast cyst aspiration can be both diagnostic and therapeutic.

ONGOING CARE

FOLLOW-UP RECOMMENDATIONS

Condition is benign, chronic, and recurrent.

Patient Monitoring

- Patient needs to be assessed with clinical examination, radiologic studies, and sometimes biopsy to be certain a lump is not malignant.
- Follow-up times are variable depending on the clinical situation.
- US is useful to differentiate cysts from solid lesions and in evaluating women <35 years of age for FCC but is not useful for screening.
- Screening mammograms should be obtained yearly after age 40.
- Aspiration cytology is useful for diagnosis of cysts and solid lesions. The false-positive rate ranges from 0–5.8%. The false-negative rate ranges from 1.7–22%.
- When physical examination, mammography, and FNA are used in combination, detection rates for breast cancer range from 93–100%.

PATIENT EDUCATION

- Patient info on fibrocystic breasts from the Mayo Foundation for Medical Education and Research: http://www.mayoclinic.com/health/fibrocystic-breasts/DS01070
- Info on breast cancer prevention from the National Cancer Institute: http://www.cancer.gov or 1-800-4-CANCER

REFERENCES

1. Horner NK, Lampe JW. Potential mechanisms of diet therapy for fibrocystic breast conditions show inadequate evidence of effectiveness. *J Am Diet Assoc.* 2000;100:1368–80.
2. Wu C, Ray RM, Lin MG, et al. A case-control study of risk factors for fibrocystic breast conditions: Shanghai Nutrition and Breast Disease Study, China, 1995-2000. *Am J Epidemiol.* 2004;160: 945–60.
3. Meisner AL, Fekrazad MH, Royce ME. Breast disease: benign and malignant. *Med Clin North Am.* 2008;92:1115–41, x.
4. Morris E. Diagnostic breast MR imaging: Current status and future directions. *Radio Clin N Am.* 2007;45(5).
5. Hartmann LC, Sellers TA, Frost MH, et al. Benign breast disease and the risk of breast cancer. *N Engl J Med.* 2005;353:229–37.
6. Srivastava A, Mansel RE, Arvind N, Prasad K, Dhar A, Chabra A et al. Evidence-based management of Mastalgia: a meta-analysis of randomised trials. *Breast.* 2007;16:503–12.

ADDITIONAL READING

- Kutson D, et al. Screening for breast cancer: current recommendations and future directions. *Am Fam Phys.* 2007;7(11):1660–6.
- Santen RJ, Mansel R. Benign breast disorders. *N Engl J Med.* 2005;353:275–85.
- Saslow D, et al. American Cancer Society guidelines for breast screening with MRI as an adjunct to mammography. *CA J Clin.* 2007;57(2):75–89.

CODES

ICD9

- 610.0 Solitary cyst of breast
- 610.1 Diffuse cystic mastopathy
- 610.2 Fibroadenosis of breast

CLINICAL PEARLS

- Immediate office aspiration of breast cysts is a relatively easy procedure and often provides pain relief.
- If a mass is still present after cyst aspiration, patient may need surgery.

F

FIBROMYALGIA

Jhilam Biswas, MD
Robert E. Berry, Jr., MD

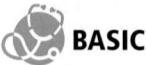 **BASICS**

DESCRIPTION
- Noninflammatory soft tissue pain disorder diagnosed by:
  - ≥3 months' duration
  - Widespread musculoskeletal pain
  - Excess tenderness in at least 11 of 18 defined anatomic sites
- Synonym(s): Fibrositis

EPIDEMIOLOGY
Incidence
- Predominant sex: Female > Male (6× more common in females)
- Predominant age: 30–60 years

Prevalence
- 2% of adult U.S. population
- Uncommon juvenile form with 1% prevalence
- Up to 8% of population >70 years of age may meet diagnostic criteria

RISK FACTORS
- Female gender
- Lower socioeconomic status
- Poor functional status
- Negative/stressful life events

Genetics
- Odds ratio may be as high as 8.5 for 1st-degree relatives, but shared environmental factors may play a role.
- Co-aggregates with mood disorders in families

GENERAL PREVENTION
No specific prevention known

ETIOLOGY
- Combination of:
  - Abnormal responsiveness or dysfunction of nervous system
  - Genetic/familial/environmental factors
  - Mood or anxiety disorder
- In 50% of patients, starts after a negative event or flulike illness

COMMONLY ASSOCIATED CONDITIONS
- Chronic fatigue syndrome
- Irritable bowel syndrome
- Headaches
- Mood disorders
- Anxiety disorders
- Unexplained pelvic pain
- Bladder dysfunction syndromes
- Multiple chemical sensitivities
- Temporomandibular joint (TMJ) syndrome

 DIAGNOSIS

- Signs and symptoms are chronic in nature.
- Nonrestorative sleep with early morning awakening in an unrefreshed state
- Pain is increased with anxiety and/or stress.
- Pain improved by mild physical activity or vacations (stress-relieving situations)
- Generalized fatigue or tiredness
- Anxiety
- Chronic headache
- Alternating diarrhea, constipation, and tenesmus
- Subjective complaints of swelling or numbness
- Dizziness
- Depression
- Reduced physical endurance
- Decreased social interaction

HISTORY
- >3 months of symptoms of widespread musculoskeletal pain unexplained by other diagnoses (diagnosis of exclusion)
- Fatigue
- Sleep disturbances
- Female usually of age 20–65 years
- Impaired social/occupational functioning
- Depressed/anxiety symptoms
- Absence of identifiable contributing disease
- Adverse effect of medication excluded (eg, statins)

PHYSICAL EXAM
- Multiple painful sites may be present; patient may have general hyperalgesia. There will be an absence of features in the joints or skin of any inflammatory musculoskeletal disease.
- Neurological exam may show some abnormalities in hoarseness and gait.
  - 4 kg of pressure (whitens examiner's nail bed) manually applied to specific sites, referred to as *trigger points*, causes significant pain.
    - Insertion of suboccipital muscle
    - Middle upper trapezius muscle
    - Under the lower sternocleidomastoid muscle
    - Near the 2nd costochondral junction
    - Origin of the supraspinatus muscle
    - 2 cm distal to lateral epicondyle
    - Upper outer quadrant of the buttocks
    - At the prominence of the greater trochanter
    - At the medial fat pad of the knee

DIAGNOSTIC TESTS & INTERPRETATION
Lab
Initial lab tests
Testing done to exclude other diseases:
- Normal Westergren erythrocyte sedimentation rate and/or C-reactive protein
- Normal muscle enzymes (creatine kinase and aldolase)
- Normal thyroid-stimulating hormone

- Normal complete blood count with differential
- Normal renal and liver function
- 25 OH vitamin D
- Antinuclear antibodies not helpful if preceding tests are normal

Imaging
Not indicated except to exclude other diagnoses

Diagnostic Procedures/Surgery
- Sleep studies if indicated to rule out obstructive sleep apnea or narcolepsy as cause of fatigue
- Neuropsychiatric testing for vegetative symptoms (SIGECAPS, HAM-D)
  - Depression
  - Anxiety
  - Cognitive disturbance
  - Memory

DIFFERENTIAL DIAGNOSIS
- Overlap syndromes:
  - Chronic fatigue syndrome
  - Myofascial pain (more localized than fibromyalgia)
- Common coexisting disorders:
  - Connective tissue diseases
  - Psychiatric illness
  - Sleep disorders
  - TMJ syndrome

TREATMENT

- Multicomponent nonpharmacologic treatment along with medication shown to be effective in the short term in reducing key symptoms

- Essential nonpharmacologic elements include engaging in exercise, education on condition, and psychotherapy. Some weak data exists that short-term benefit may result from hydrotherapy (1,2)[A].

- Mainstay of therapy includes tricyclic antidepressants or cyclobenzaprine, daily aerobic exercise, sleep hygiene, and careful attention to mental status plus psychotherapy (cognitive behavioral therapy, etc.)

- Medications have shown to decrease pain, fatigue, depressed mood, sleep disturbance, and health-related quality of life.

MEDICATION
Nonsteroidal anti-inflammatory drugs are less likely to help because there is no identified inflammation, except as an additional pain measure.

ALERT
Avoid narcotics.

First Line
- Amitriptyline 25–50 mg p.o. at bedtime (1,2,3)[A]: Alternative: Desipramine (less sedating)
- Cyclobenzaprine 10–30 mg p.o. at bedtime (3)[A]
- Acetaminophen 325–1000 mg p.o. q.i.d. p.r.n.
- Tramadol 200–300 mg/d p.o. divided doses (3)[A]
- Combinations of acetaminophen and tramadol effective for pain control
- Gabapentin 1200–2400 mg/d p.o. b.i.d.–t.i.d.; start with lower doses (3)[A]. May be considered 1st line if exercise and TCAs are not sufficient at controlling pain scores.

Second Line

- Pregabalin 300–600 mg/day p.o. b.i.d.–t.i.d.; start with 150 mg/day and then advance as needed. Most improvement shown at 450 mg/day p.o. (4).
- Duloxetine 60 mg p.o. b.i.d.
- Milnacipran 100 mg/day or 200 mg/day p.o. (became available in 2009)
- Fluoxetine 20–80 mg/d p.o. (higher doses may be needed) (3)[A]
- Clonazepam 0.5 mg p.o. at bedtime may help sleep.
- Combinations of medicines such as amitriptyline and fluoxetine may be tried.

ADDITIONAL TREATMENT

General Measures

- Patient understanding of the illness and goals of therapy are key.
- Low-impact cardiovascular exercise is useful as long as the exercise program continues. Strength training has also shown improvement (4)[A].
- Cognitive behavioral therapy (3)[A]
- Stress management
- Patient education; consider group format (3)[A]
- Sleep hygiene
- Psychosocial support
- Consider job/workplace modifications.

Issues for Referral

Referrals for nonresponders may go to rheumatology, psychiatry, and pain management centers.

COMPLEMENTARY AND ALTERNATIVE MEDICINE

- Physical therapy may be helpful as part of conditioning program/fitness.
- Moderate efficacy shown in some studies for:
  – Hydrotherapy (5)[A]
  – Hypnotherapy
  – Biofeedback
- Weak evidence for efficacy:
  – Chiropractic
  – Acupuncture
  – Massage therapy
  – Electrotherapy
  – Ultrasonography

Pregnancy Considerations

May require therapy modification

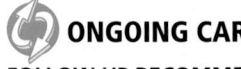 ## ONGOING CARE

FOLLOW-UP RECOMMENDATIONS

Encourage full activity as able, especially with fitness exercises.

Patient Monitoring

- For efficacy of therapy at 2–4 weeks
- For medication side effects every 3–6 months

DIET

No restrictions; no proven efficacy of any specific diet

PATIENT EDUCATION

It is very important that the patient understand the diagnosis and participate in developing and continuing a treatment program.

PROGNOSIS

- 50% with partial remission after 2–3 years of therapy
- Typically has fluctuating, chronic course
- Poorer outcome with:
  – Longer illness duration
  – More severe symptoms
  – Depression
  – Advanced age
  – Lack of social support

COMPLICATIONS

Chronic pain, chronic loss of work

REFERENCES

1. Hauser W, Bernhard M, Schiltenwolf M. Efficacy of multicomponent treatment in fibromyalgia syndrome: A meta-analysis of randomized controlled clinical trials. *Arth and Rheum*. 2009; 61(2):216–224.
2. Hauser W, Bernandy K, Uceyler N, Sommer C. Treatment of fibromyalgia syndrome with antidepressants: A meta-analysis. *JAMA*. 2009;301(2):198–209.
3. Goldenberg DL, Burckhardt C, Crofford L. Management of fibromyalgia syndrome. *JAMA*. 2004;292:2388–95.
4. Busch AJ, et al. Exercise for treating fibromyalgia. *Cochrane Database Syst Rev*. 2007:4CD003786.
5. McVeigh JG, McGaughey H, Hall M, Kane P. The effectiveness of hydrotherapy in the management of fibromyalgia syndrome: a systematic review. *Rheumatology International*. 2008;29(2):119–30.

ADDITIONAL READING

- Aaron LA, Burke MM, Buchwald D. Overlapping conditions among patients with chronic fatigue syndrome, fibromyalgia, and temporomandibular disorder. *Arch Intern Med*. 2000;160:221–7.
- Abeles AM, Pillinger MH, Solitar BM, et al. Narrative review: the pathophysiology of fibromyalgia. *Ann Intern Med*. 2007;146:726–34.

- American College of Rheumatology. Practice guidelines, patient education. At http://www.rheumatology.org.
- Arnold LM. Biology and therapy of fibromyalgia. New therapies in fibromyalgia. *Arthritis Res Ther*. 2006;8:212.
- Carville SF, Arendt-Nielsen S, Bliddal H, et al. EULAR evidence-based recommendations for the management of fibromyalgia syndrome. *Ann Rheum Dis*. 2008;67:536–41.
- National Fibromyalgia Association. At http://www.fmaware.org.
- Moore RA, Straube S, Wiffen PJ, Derry S, McQuay H. Pregabalin for acute and chronic pain in adults. *Chchrane Database of Syst Rev*. 2009;(3): CD007076.

See Also (Topic, Algorithm, Electronic Media Element)

Algorithm: Fatigue

 ## CODES

ICD9

729.1 Myalgia and myositis, unspecified

CLINICAL PEARLS

- Coexisting severe complaints of chronic pain, fatigue, multiple symptoms in the *absence* of laboratory or physical exam findings
- Biologic basis is still unclear, but the disease is considered a disorder of pain regulation termed *central sensitization*.
- Overlap with stress, depression, and anxiety must be recognized in treatment plan.
- Best outcomes occur in patients who understand their illness and are willing to engage in multimodal treatment, including medications, exercise, psychotherapy, and changing lifestyle habits.

FOLLICULITIS

Lewis C. Rose, MD

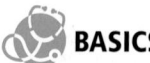 **BASICS**

DESCRIPTION
- Inflammation of hair follicle caused by infection, chemical irritation, or physical injury
- Divided into superficial and deep folliculitis
- Eosinophilic pustular folliculitis (EPF), also known as Ofuji disease, is a distinct entity with sterile papules or pustules.
- Folliculitis decalvans is a rare inflammatory scalp disorder of middle-aged adults, with diagnostic overlap with perifolliculitis capitis abscedens et suffodiens.
- System(s) affected: Skin/Exocrine

EPIDEMIOLOGY
Incidence
- Predominant age: All ages
- Predominant sex: Male > Female

Pregnancy Considerations
Pruritic folliculitis of pregnancy is a rare disorder that resolves spontaneously after delivery.

RISK FACTORS
- Frequent shaving
- Pre-existing dermatoses
- Occlusive dressing
- Occlusive clothing
- Obesity
- Immunosuppression
- Long-term antibiotic use
- Use of hot tubs or saunas
- Diabetes mellitus
- Close contacts with individuals with methicillin-resistant *Staphylococcus aureus* (MRSA) infections
- As an occasional complication of therapeutic epilation with intense pulsed light

GENERAL PREVENTION
- Practice good personal hygiene; avoid reinfection from contaminated clothing and washcloths.
- Minimize friction from clothing.
- Avoid shaving.

PATHOPHYSIOLOGY
Predisposing factors to folliculitis:
- Nasal carriage of *Staphylococcus aureus*
- Exposure to pools and hot tubs contaminated with *Pseudomonas aeruginosa* (may be due to inadequate chlorination)
- Candida folliculitis related to recent antibiotic or corticosteroid use

ETIOLOGY
- Staphylococcal infection
- Pityrosporum folliculitis may mimic acne.
- *Demodex* mite infection on the face and scalp
- *Malassezia* may cause folliculitis of the scalp.
- Herpes simplex is an uncommon cause.
- Herpes zoster may cause an area of folliculitis in an unusual location.
- As a reaction to cutaneous larva migrans infestation
- Pseudofolliculitis barbae may mimic true folliculitis.
- MRSA due to increasing incidence of community-acquired infections
- Pseudomonal folliculitis commonly erupts quickly after soaking in an infected spa or hot tub.
- Transplant patients taking sirolimus are at risk for scalp folliculitis.
- Eosinophilic folliculitis is uncommon in completely healthy adults, being more common in immunosuppressed patients, but in Japan it occurs as Ofuji disease.

COMMONLY ASSOCIATED CONDITIONS
- Conjunctivitis
- External otitis

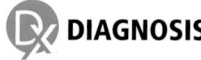 **DIAGNOSIS**

HISTORY
- Pustular rash occurring on hair-bearing skin, especially the face (beard), proximal limbs, and scalp
- Pseudomonal folliculitis appears as a widespread rash mainly on the trunk and limbs when the growing hair curls around and penetrates the skin, provoking a foreign-body reaction.
- Gram-negative folliculitis occurs from long-term antibiotic therapy.
- Pityrosporum folliculitis occurs more often in warm, humid climates and more frequently in immunocompromised patients.
- Herpes folliculitis occurs from infection with herpes 1 and 2.

PHYSICAL EXAM
- Characteristic lesions are multiple small papules and pustules, usually measuring ≤5 mm in diameter with erythematous base pierced by a central hair.
- In pseudofolliculitis barbae, curled beard hairs with chisel-like tip may turn around and penetrate into the skin.

DIAGNOSTIC TESTS & INTERPRETATION
Lab
Initial lab tests
- Gram stain
- Potassium hydroxide preparation to look for budding yeast or hyphae
- Culture
- Biopsy
- Fasting blood sugar
- HIV status

Diagnostic Procedures/Surgery
Incision and drainage is rarely used because the scar formation may be ugly; disorder may return.

Pathological Findings
- Superficial/deep: Moderately intense infiltrate of inflammatory cells
- Pseudofolliculitis: Perifollicular inflammatory infiltrate
- Eosinophilic folliculitis: Collection of eosinophils within superficial follicle

DIFFERENTIAL DIAGNOSIS
- Acne vulgaris
- Acneiform eruptions
- Cutaneous candidiasis
- Contact dermatitis
- Milia:
  - Miliaria
- Papular urticaria
- Insect bite

TREATMENT
MEDICATION
- Systemic antibiotics do not appear to be helpful.
- Staphylococcal folliculitis:
  - Mupirocin applied 2–5 times per day is drug of choice; oral agents are reserved for widespread disease.
  - Dicloxacillin: 250 mg q.i.d. p.o. for 14 days
  - Cephalosporin (Cephalexin): 250 mg q.i.d. or 1,000 mg b.i.d. for 10 days
- For MRSA:
  - Clindamycin 150–450 mg p.o. q6–8h for 10 days
  - Bactrim DS 1 b.i.d. for 10 days
  - Minocycline or doxycycline 100 mg p.o. b.i.d. for 10 days
- Pseudomonal folliculitis:
  - Usually self-limited; no antibiotic indicated
  - If severe or persistent, adults can use ciprofloxacin 500 mg or ofloxacin 400 mg b.i.d. p.o. for 10 days
- EPF:
  - Topical corticosteroids
  - Itraconazole or fluconazole
  - Topical tacrolimus ointment
  - Indomethacin
  - UVB light

- Herpetic folliculitis:
  - Valacyclovir 500 b.i.d. for 5 days
  - Famciclovir 125 mg b.i.d. for 5 days
  - Acyclovir 800 b.i.d. for 5 days
- Recurrent disease:
  - Vitamin C (1 g/d × 4–6 weeks)
  - Mupirocin nasal ointment (5 days)
  - Low-dose clindamycin (150 mg/d × 3 months)

ADDITIONAL TREATMENT
General Measures
- Antibacterial soaps (Dial, Chlorhexidine)
- Good handwashing techniques
- Warm compresses
- Clean shaving instruments each day.
- Change towels/washcloths and sheets daily.
- Avoid nose picking.
- For obese individuals, weight reduction may be helpful.

Issues for Referral
Persistent cases

SURGERY/OTHER PROCEDURES
Incision and drainage is rarely used because the scar formation may be ugly, and disorder may return.

ONGOING CARE
FOLLOW-UP RECOMMENDATIONS
Patient Monitoring
- Resistant cases should be followed every 2 weeks until cleared.
- 1 return visit in 2 weeks if symptoms abate

DIET
For obese individuals, weight reduction may be helpful.

PATIENT EDUCATION
Avoid shaving in involved areas.

PROGNOSIS
- Usually resolves with treatment
- May recur in *Staphylococcus* carriers
- Mupirocin may be required on nares of patient to treat carrier state.
- Family carriers may also require treatment.
- Resistant or severe cases may warrant testing for diabetes mellitus or immunodeficiency.

COMPLICATIONS
- Primary complication of concern is recurrent folliculitis
- May progress to become furuncles or abscesses

ADDITIONAL READING
- Böer A, Herder N, Winter K, et al. Herpes folliculitis: clinical, histopathological, and molecular pathologic observations. *Br J Dermatol*. 2006;154:743–6.
- Ellis E, et al. Eosinophilic pustular folliculitis: a comprehensive review of treatment options. *Am J Dermatol*. 2004;5(93):189–97.
- Sladden MJ, et al. More common skin infections in children. *Br Med J*. 2005;330(7501):1194–8.

See Also (Topic, Algorithm, Electronic Media Element)
Algorithm: Rash, Focal

 ## CODES

ICD9
704.8 Other specified diseases of hair and hair follicles

CLINICAL PEARLS
- Folliculitis is a pyoderma localized to hair follicles.
- The lesions of folliculitis measure ≤5 mm in size, are erythematous, pruritic, and usually cluster in groups.
- Systemic antibiotics do not appear to be helpful in treating folliculitis.
- Consider MRSA in difficult-to-treat cases.

F

FOOD ALLERGY

Stanley Fineman, MD

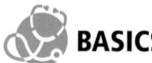 **BASICS**

DESCRIPTION
- Hypersensitivity reaction caused by certain foods
- System(s) affected: GI; Hemic/Lymphatic/Immunologic; Pulmonary; Skin/Exocrine
- Synonym(s): Allergic bowel disease; dietary protein-sensitivity syndrome

EPIDEMIOLOGY
- Predominant age: All ages, but more common in infants and children
- Predominant sex: Male > female (2:1)

Incidence
Prospective studies indicate that ~2.5% of infants experience hypersensitivity reactions to cow's milk in their 1st year of life (1)[B].

Prevalence
- The prevalence of IgE-mediated food allergy is likely between 1–2% in the US. (2,3)[A]
- In young children, the most common food allergies are cow's milk (2.5%), egg (1/3%), peanut (0.8%), and wheat (0.4%).
- Adults tend to have allergies to shellfish (2%), peanut (0.6%), tree nuts (0.5%), and fish (0.4%). (3)[B]
- In general, only 3–4% of children >4 years have persisting food allergy; therefore, it is frequently a transient phenomenon.
- 20% of children with peanut protein allergy outgrow their sensitivity by school age (4,3)[B].

RISK FACTORS
- Persons with allergic or atopic predisposition have increased risk of hypersensitivity reaction to food.
- Family history of food hypersensitivity

Genetics
In family members with a history of food hypersensitivity, the probability of food allergy in subsequent siblings may be as high as 50%.

GENERAL PREVENTION
Avoidance of offending food

PATHOPHYSIOLOGY
Allergic response owing to immunologic mechanisms, such as the classic IgE allergic response or nonimmunologic-mediated mechanisms

ETIOLOGY
- Any food or ingested substance can cause allergic reactions:
  - Most commonly implicated foods include cow's milk, egg whites, wheat, soy, peanuts, fish, tree nuts (walnut and pecan), shellfish, melons, sesame seeds, and sunflower seeds.
- Several food dyes and additives can elicit allergic-like reactions.

 DIAGNOSIS

PHYSICAL EXAM
- GI (system usually affected):
  - More common: Nausea, vomiting, diarrhea, abdominal pain, occult bleeding, flatulence, and bloating
  - Less common: Malabsorption, protein-losing enteropathy, eosinophilic-enteritis, colitis
- Dermatologic:
  - More common: Urticaria/angioedema, atopic dermatitis, pallor, or flushing
  - Less common: Contact rashes
- Respiratory:
  - More common: Allergic rhinitis, asthma and bronchospasm, cough, serous otitis media
  - Less common: Pulmonary infiltrates (Heiner syndrome), pulmonary hemosiderosis
- Neurologic:
  - Less common: Migraine headaches
- Other symptoms:
  - Systemic anaphylaxis, vasculitis

DIAGNOSTIC TESTS & INTERPRETATION
Lab
- Eosinophilia in blood or tissue suggests atopy
- Epicutaneous (prick or puncture) allergy skin tests are used for documenting IgE-mediated immunologic hypersensitivity.
- Skin testing using the suspect food may be helpful. When fresh food skin testing is negative, an oral challenge may be completed to accurately determine the clinical hypersensitivity. The overall agreement between allergy skin testing and oral food challenge is 60% (i.e., a positive skin test showing a positive challenge reaction to a particular food) (5)[A].
- Food-specific IgE assays can also detect specific IgE antibodies to offending foods:
  - In certain laboratories, the ImmunoCap food-specific IgE was almost as accurate as a skin test in predicting positive oral challenges (6)[B].
- Periodic monitoring of the peanut-specific IgE levels every 2 years may be helpful. If the level of peanut-specific IgE falls below 0.5 kU/L, then a cautious oral challenge under the supervision of an allergist may be considered. A fresh food skin test with peanut protein should be considered prior to the oral challenge.
- Patch tests for foods are reported to be useful for determining delayed-sensitivity immunologic reactions, which are reported in patients with eosinophilic esophagitis and atopic dermatitis, although the addition of these is considered of marginal benefit (7)[B].

- Leukocyte histamine release and assays for circulating immune complexes are predominantly research procedures and are of limited use in clinical practices:
  - Assays for IgG and IgG 4 subclass antibodies are commercially available.
  - No convincing data suggest that these tests are reliable for the diagnosis of food allergy.
- The provocative injection and sublingual provocative tests are both highly controversial and have been proven to be useless for the diagnosis of food allergy.
- The leukocytotoxic assay is an unproven diagnostic procedure and is not useful for the diagnosis of allergy (8)[A]

Diagnostic Procedures/Surgery
Elimination and challenge test is the best procedure for confirming food allergy:
- The suspected food is eliminated from the diet for 1–2 weeks.
- The patient's symptoms are monitored. If the patient's symptoms disappear or substantially improve, an oral challenge with the suspected food should be performed under medical supervision.
- Optimally, this challenge should be performed in a double-blind, placebo-controlled manner.
- Patients with a history of anaphylaxis should not have an oral challenge unless lack of significant IgE sensitivity can be documented.
- Most allergic reactions will occur within 30 minutes–2 hours after the challenge, although late reactions have also been described, which may occur from 12–24 hours.

Pathological Findings
Pathologic findings are not common in food allergies; however, inflammatory changes can sometimes be seen in the GI tract.

DIFFERENTIAL DIAGNOSIS
- A careful history is necessary to document a temporal relationship with the manifestations of suspected food hypersensitivity.
- The GI, dermatologic, respiratory, neurologic, or other systemic manifestations may mimic a variety of clinical entities.

TREATMENT

MEDICATION

- Patients with significant type 1, IgE-mediated hypersensitivity should have epinephrine for auto-injection available in case of accidental ingestion and resulting severe anaphylactic reaction.
- Symptomatic treatment for milder reactions (e.g., antihistamine)
- The use of cromolyn has been suggested but is not practical for use in most patients with food allergy.

ADDITIONAL TREATMENT

General Measures

- Avoidance of the offending food is the most effective mode of treatment for patients with food allergies.
- Those patients with exquisite and severe allergy hypersensitivity to a food should be more cautious in their avoidance of that food. They should carry epinephrine for self-administration in the event that the offending food is ingested unknowingly and a subsequent immediate reaction develops.
- Immunotherapy or hyposensitization with food extracts by various routes, including subcutaneous immunotherapy or sublingual neutralization, are not recommended. Research studies are in progress, but immunotherapy with foods is considered experimental at this time.

COMPLEMENTARY AND ALTERNATIVE MEDICINE

There are reports of benefit using various Chinese herbal medicines in laboratory animals with induced food allergy. Benefits have not been reported in humans at this time.

ONGOING CARE

FOLLOW-UP RECOMMENDATIONS

Patient Monitoring

As needed

DIET

- As determined by tests and clinical evaluation
- Strict avoidance of offending food

PATIENT EDUCATION

- Patients should be counseled by a dietitian to be sure that they maintain a nutritionally sound diet despite avoiding those foods to which the patient is sensitive.
- Patient support: Food Allergy and Anaphylaxis Network: 4744 Holly Ave., Fairfax, VA 22030-5647; 703-691-3179; Web site http://www.foodallergy.org
- Other information available at http://www.acaai.org and http://www.aaaai.org

PROGNOSIS

- Most infants will outgrow their food hypersensitivity by 2–4 years.
  - It may be possible to reintroduce the offending food cautiously into the diet (particularly helpful when the food is one that is difficult to avoid). It is critical that a specific IgE to the offending food is checked, optimally by fresh food allergy skin test, and is negative prior to an oral challenge.
  - 20% of young children with peanut allergy experience resolution by age of 5 years (4)[B].
- Adults with food hypersensitivity (particularly to milk, fish, shellfish, or nuts) tend to maintain their allergy for many years.

COMPLICATIONS

- Anaphylaxis
- Angioedema
- Bronchial asthma
- Enterocolitis
- Eosinophilic esophagitis
- Eczematoid lesions

REFERENCES

1. Høst A, Halken S. A prospective study of cow milk allergy in Danish infants during the first 3 years of life. Clinical course in relation to clinical and immunological type of hypersensitivity reaction. *Allergy.* 1990;45:587–96.
2. Chafen JJ, Newberry SJ, Riedl MA, Bravata DM, Maglione M, Suttorp MJ, Sundaram V, Paige NM, Towfigh A, Hulley BJ, Shekelle PG et al. Diagnosing and managing common food allergies: a systematic review. *JAMA.* 2010;303:1848–56.
3. Sicherer SH, Sampson HA et al. Food allergy. *J Allergy Clin Immunol.* 2010;125:S116–25.
4. Sicherer SH, Sampson HA et al. Peanut allergy: emerging concepts and approaches for an apparent epidemic. *J Allergy Clin. Immunol.* 2007;120.
5. Sampson HA. Utility of food-specific IgE concentrations in predicting symptomatic food allergy. *J Allergy Clin Immunol.* 2001;107:891–6.
6. Maloney JM, Rudengren M, Ahlstedt S, et al. The use of serum specific IgE measurements for the diagnosis of peanut, tree nut, and seed allergy. *J Allergy Clin Immunol.* 2008.
7. Spergel JM, Brown-Whitehorn T, Beausoleil JL, Shuker M, Liacouras CA et al. Predictive values for skin prick test and atopy patch test for eosinophilic esophagitis. *J Allergy Clin Immunol.* 2007;119:509–11.
8. Bernstein IL, Li JT, Bernstein DI, et al. Allergy diagnostic testing: an updated practice parameter. *Ann Allergy Asthma Immunol.* 2008;100:S1–148.
9. Chapman JA, Bernstein IL. Food Allergy: a practice parameter. *Ann Allergy Asthma Immunol.* 2006;96:S1–S68.
10. Greer FR, Sicherer SH, Burks AW, et al. Effects of early nutritional interventions on the development of atopic disease in infants and children: the role of maternal dietary restriction, breastfeeding, timing of introduction of complementary foods, and hydrolyzed formulas. *Pediatrics.* 2008;121: 183–91.

See Also (Topic, Algorithm, Electronic Media Element)

Celiac Disease; Irritable Bowel Syndrome; Anaphylaxis

CODES

ICD9

- 708.0 Allergic urticaria
- 995.60 Anaphylactic shock due to unspecified food
- 995.7 Other adverse food reactions, not elsewhere classified

CLINICAL PEARLS

- Recent studies suggest that up to 20% of children with peanut allergy may outgrow their sensitivity.
  - Periodic monitoring of the peanut-specific IgE levels every 2 years may be helpful. If the level of peanut-specific IgE falls below 0.5 kU/L, then a cautious oral challenge under the supervision of an allergist may be considered. A fresh food skin test with peanut protein should be considered prior to the oral challenge.
- Oral itching following ingestion of fresh fruit may be a warning of risk for anaphylaxis, but may only represent oral allergy syndrome.
  - This syndrome is the result of cross-reacting proteins in pollens (example: Patients sensitive to birch tree pollen frequently have this cross-reactivity to fresh apples and pears. Cooked fruits are usually tolerated) (9)[B].
- Current evidence does not support a major role for maternal dietary restrictions during pregnancy or lactation in the prevention of atopic disease in infants. It is generally recommended to exclusively breast-feed for the first 6 months of life, particularly when there is a family history of atopy and food allergy. Although solid foods should not be introduced before 4–6 months of age, there is no convincing evidence that delaying their introduction beyond this period has a significant protective effect on the development of allergies (10)[B].

F

FOOD POISONING, BACTERIAL

Thomas J. Hansen, MD

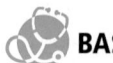 **BASICS**

DESCRIPTION
- Food poisoning, also called foodborne infection, is an illness resulting from the consumption of contaminated food.
- The illness may be produced by bacterial infection or by toxins produced by the bacteria.
- The most commonly recognized foodborne infections are those caused by the bacteria *Campylobacter*, *Salmonella*, and *E. coli* 0157:H7 (1).

EPIDEMIOLOGY
Incidence
In the US, it is estimated that there are more than 76 million cases of foodborne poisoning annually, resulting in 325,000 hospitalizations and 5,000 deaths (1).

RISK FACTORS
- Travel to developing countries
- Improper food storage or handling
- Cross-contamination during preparation of food
- Weakened immune system, pregnancy, very young age
- Underlying gastrointestinal disorders
- Patients taking antacids, H-2 blockers, and proton pump inhibitors (2)

GENERAL PREVENTION
- When preparing food at home (3):
  - Clean
    - Wash hands, cutting boards and surfaces before food preparation and after preparing each food item.
    - Wash fresh produce thoroughly before eating.
  - Separate
    - Keep raw meat, poultry, fish, and their juices away from other food.
  - Cook: Thoroughly cook meat to the following temperature:
    - Fresh beef, veal, and lamb: 145° F
    - Fresh pork: 160°F
    - Ground beef, pork, veal, lamb, egg dishes: 160°F
    - Poultry: 165° F. Cook chicken eggs thoroughly until the yolk is firm.
  - Chill
    - Refrigerate leftovers within 2 hours in clean, shallow, covered containers. If the temperature is above 90°F, refrigerate within 1 hour.
- When traveling to underdeveloped countries (4):
  - Eat only foods that are freshly prepared.
  - Avoid beverages diluted with nonpotable water, such as ice and milk.
  - Avoid food washed in nonpotable water, such as salads.
  - Other risky foods include raw or undercooked meat and seafood, unpeeled raw fruits and vegetables.
  - Bottled, carbonated, and boiled beverages are generally safe to drink.

- Bismuth subsalicylate (Pepto-Bismol), two 262-mg tablets four times daily has been shown to protect travelers to developing countries approximately 60% of the time. However, it is not recommended for persons taking anticoagulants or other salicylates (5).

ETIOLOGY
- Short incubation period (1–6 hours)
  - *Bacillus cereus* (preformed enterotoxin)
    - Food sources: Improperly cooked rice/fried rice and red meats.
    - Causes sudden onset of severe nausea and vomiting. Diarrhea may be present.
  - *Staphylococcus aureus*
    - Food sources: Unrefrigerated or improperly refrigerated meats, potato and egg salads.
    - Causes sudden onset of severe nausea and vomiting. Abdominal cramps and fever may be present.
- Medium incubation period (8–16 hours)
  - *Bacillus cereus* (toxin)
    - Food sources: Meat, stew gravy, vanilla sauce.
    - Causes watery diarrhea, abdominal cramps, nausea.
  - *Clostridium perfringens*
    - Food sources: Dry or precooked meats and poultry
    - Causes watery diarrhea, nausea, abdominal cramps.
- Long incubation period (> 16 hours)
  - Toxin-producing organisms
    - *Clostridium botulinum*: Food source is home-canned or improperly canned commercial foods. Causes vomiting, diarrhea, blurred vision, diplopia, dysphagia, and descending muscle weakness.
    - *Enterohemorrhagic E. coli*: Food sources are undercooked beef, especially hamburger, unpasteurized milk, raw fruits and vegetables, and contaminated water. Causes severe diarrhea that is often bloody, abdominal pain, vomiting. More common in children <4 years of age.
    - *Enterotoxigenic E. coli*: Food sources are foods or water contaminated by human feces. Causes watery diarrhea, abdominal cramps, and vomiting.
    - *Vibrio cholerae*: Food sources are contaminated water, fish, and shellfish, especially food sold by street vendors. Causes profuse watery diarrhea and vomiting which can lead to severe dehydration and death within hours.
  - Invasive organisms
    - *Campylobacter jejuni*: Food sources are raw and undercooked poultry, unpasteurized milk, contaminated meats. Causes diarrhea (may be bloody), cramps, vomiting, and fever.
    - *Salmonella*: Food sources are contaminated eggs, poultry, unpasteurized milk or juice, cheese, contaminated raw fruits and vegetables. Causes diarrhea, fever, abdominal cramps, vomiting.

- *Shigella*: Food sources are food or water contaminated by human fecal material. Causes abdominal cramps, fever, diarrhea.
- *Vibrio parahaemolyticus*: Food source is raw shellfish. Causes nausea vomiting, diarrhea, and abdominal pain.
- *Vibrio vulnificus:* Food source is undercooked and raw seafood; wounds exposed to sea water. Causes vomiting, diarrhea, abdominal pain, bacteremia, wound infections. Can be fatal in patients with liver disease or who are immunocompromised.
- *Y. pentoerocolitica* and *Y. pseudotuberculosis*: Food sources are undercooked pork, unpasteurized milk, tofu, contaminated water. Causes appendicitis-like symptoms: abdominal pain, fever, diarrhea, and vomiting; occurs primarily in older children and younger adults (6).

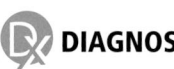 **DIAGNOSIS**

HISTORY
- Food poisoning most often presents as gastroenteritis (5).
- Most cases of gastroenteritis have a viral etiology. Suspect bacterial food poisoning when multiple persons become ill after eating the same meal, possibly with high fever and blood or mucus in stool.
- Suspect bacterial gastroenteritis if traveling in or recent travel to an underdeveloped country (5,7).
- Timing and presentation can aid in establishing an etiology (6).

PHYSICAL EXAM
- The physical exam should focus on signs of dehydration, including evaluating skin turgor and mucous membranes, and observing for hypotension or orthostatic changes.
- The abdominal exam should focus on abdominal distension with tenderness, suggestive of bowel obstruction. Auscultation may demonstrate increased bowel sound in obstruction or decreased bowel sounds with an ileus (7).

DIAGNOSTIC TESTS & INTERPRETATION
Lab
Initial lab tests
- Culture of stool and sensitivity, fecal leukocytes, and Hemoccult testing; consider ova and parasites if history of foreign travel or symptoms lasting longer than 2 weeks.
- BMP and white blood cell count if diarrhea is severe, temperature >101.5°F (38.5°C), persistently bloody stools, severe abdominal pain, or if patient is immunocompromised, elderly, or very young

Follow-Up & Special Considerations
Epidemiologic investigation may be warranted.

DIFFERENTIAL DIAGNOSIS
- Infectious gastroenteritis of any kind
- *C. difficile* colitis
- Inflammatory bowel disease
- Appendicitis and other acute abdominal surgical processes

 TREATMENT

- Most cases of food poisoning are self-limiting and do not require medication.
- A health care provider should be consulted for food poisoning if the following are present: High fever (≥101.5° F); blood in the stools; prolonged vomiting; signs of dehydration (decrease in urination, a dry mouth and throat, and feeling dizzy when standing up); diarrheal illness that lasts more than 3 days (4)[C].

First Line
Children, the elderly and pregnant patients with sign of mild diarrhea should be started on oral rehydration solution to prevent dehydration (2)[B].

Second Line
- For severe cases of food poisoning, the following medications are recommended:
- *Bacillus cereus:*
  – Supportive care only.
- *Campylobacter jejuni:*
  – Supportive care only.
- *Clostridium botulinum:*
  – Supportive care. Antitoxin can be helpful if administered early in the course of the illness.
- *Clostridium perfringens:*
  – Supportive care only.
- *Enterohemorrhagic E. coli:*
  – Supportive care only. Closely monitor renal function, hemoglobin and platelets. Infection associated with hemolytic uremic syndrome (HUS).
- *Enterotoxigenic E. coli* (common cause of traveler's diarrhea):
  – Generally self-limited. Antibiotics shorten course of illness.
  – Children: Azithromycin 10 mg/kg/day for 3 days or Ceftriaxone 50 mg/kg/day for 3 days
  – Adults: Ciprofloxacin 500 mg once a day for 3 days or SMX/TMP one DS tab twice daily for 3 days.
- *Salmonella:*
  – Children: Ceftriaxone: 100 mg/kg/day divided into two doses for 7–10 days or Azithromycin 20 mg/kg/day for 7 days.
  – Adults: Levofloxacin 500 mg a day for 7–10 days or azithromycin 500 mg daily for 7 days. Either can be given for 14 days for immunosuppressed patients.

- *Shigella:*
  – Children: Azithromycin 10 mg/kg/day for 3 days or Ceftriaxone 50 mg/kg/day for 3 days.
  – Adults: Metronidazole 500 mg three times a day for 10–14 days or Vancomycin 125 mg four times a day for 10–14 days or Rifaximin 400 mg four times a day for 10–14 days.
- *Staph. aureus:*
  – Supportive care only.
- *Vibrio cholerae:*
  – Children: Erythromycin 30 mg/kg/day given three times a day for 3 days or Azithromycin 10 mg/kg/day for three days.
  – Adults: Doxycycline 300 mg one time dose or Tetracycline 500 mg four times a day for 3 days or Erythromycin 250 mg three times a day for 3 days or Azithromycin 500 mg a day for three days.
- *Vibrio parahaemolyticus:*
  – Supportive care only.
- *Vibrio vulnificus:*
  – Adults: Minocycline or Doxycycline 100 mg twice daily plus either Cefotaxime 2 gm IV every eight hours or Ceftriaxone 1 g IV daily with doses appropriately adjusted for underlying renal or hepatic disease.
- *Yersinia:*
  – Supportive care only (6)[C]

ADDITIONAL TREATMENT
Loperamide 4 mg initially, then 2 mg after each loose stool to a maximum of 16 mg in a 24-hour period may be used unless high fever, bloody diarrhea, and/or severe abdominal pain are present (signs of enteroinvasion).

 ONGOING CARE

DIET
- Avoid food while nausea is present but drink plenty of fluids.
- As the nausea subsides, drink adequate fluids, eat small, low-fat meals, and rest.
- Nursing infants should continue to be breastfed on demand, and infants and older children should be offered their usual food (5).

PROGNOSIS
Most infections are self-limited and will resolve over the course of 4–5 days.

COMPLICATIONS
- Dehydration
- Hemolytic uremic syndrome
- Guillain-Barré syndrome after Campylobacter enteritis
- Reiter syndrome
- *Clostridium difficile* colitis after antibiotic use
- Postinfectious irritable bowel (5)

REFERENCES

1. U.S. Food and Drug Administration, Foodborne Illness-Causing Organisms in the U.S.-What You Need to Know. October 2008, http://www.fda.gov/Food/ResourcesForYou/Consumers/ucm103263.htm
2. Ang JY, Mathur A. Traveler's Diarrhea: Updates for Pediatricians. *Pediatric Annals* 2008;37:814–820.
3. http://www.fsis.usda.gov/PDF/Kitchen_Companion.pdf
4. http://www.cdc.gov/ncidod/dbmd/diseaseinfo/foodborneinfections_g.htm#howtreated
5. Yates J. Traveler's diarrhea. *Am Fam Physician*. 2005;71:2095–100.
6. American Medical Association, Diagnosis and Management of Foodborne Illnesses: A Primer for Physicians and Other Health Care Professionals, February 2004, http://www.ama-assn.org/ama1/pub/upload/mm/36/2004_food_table_bact.pdf
7. Scorza K, Williams A, Phillips JD, Shaw J. Evaluation of Nausea and Vomiting. *Am Fam Physician*. 2007;76:76–84.

ADDITIONAL READING

- Diagnosis and management of foodborne illnesses: A primer for physicians. *MMWR Recomm Rep.* 2004;53(RR04):1–33.
- Reduced osmolarity oral rehydration solution. *Cochrane Database Syst Rev.* 2007, Issue 3.
- The Community Summary Report on Trends and Sources of Zoonoses and Zoonotic Agents in the European Union in 2007. *The European Food Safety Authority Journal.* 2009;223.

See Also (Topic, Algorithm, Electronic Media Element)
Appendicitis, Acute; Botulism; Brucellosis; Dehydration; Diarrhea, Acute; Guillain-Barré Syndrome; Hypokalemia; Intestinal Parasites; Salmonella Infection; Typhoid Fever

 CODES

ICD9
- 003.9 Salmonella infection, unspecified
- 005.89 Other bacterial food poisoning
- 008.00 Intestinal infection due to e. coli, unspecified

CLINICAL PEARLS

- Consider bacterial food poisoning when multiple people present with symptoms after ingesting the same food and show fevers and blood or mucus in stool, or have recently returned from a developing nation.
- Consider antibiotics in a prolonged febrile state with blood/mucus in stool, septicemic states, and traveler's diarrhea.
- Reintroduce food as soon as tolerated; limit high-fat foods and foods high in simple sugars. Lactose limitation is controversial.

F

FRAGILE X SYNDROME

Thomas J. Hansen, MD

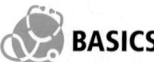 **BASICS**

DESCRIPTION
- Fragile X syndrome is the most common inherited form of mental retardation (also referred to as mental impairment).
- Among the genetic causes of mental impairment, FXS is the second most common cause following Down syndrome.
- In addition to mental impairment, FXS is characterized by a group of symptoms that may include specific physical features, distinctive behavior patterns, defective speech and language, and cognitive deficits (1).
- Synonyms: Marker X syndrome; Martin-Bell syndrome; Escalante's syndrome

EPIDEMIOLOGY
- Although this condition is seen in both sexes, males are usually more severely affected than females.
- Affected males almost always have mental impairment, mostly of moderate severity.
- Only 1/3–1/2 of the affected females have mental impairment, usually in the mild-to-moderate range (1).

Prevalence
- FXS with full mutation is seen in 1:4,000 males and 1:8,000 females (2).
- FXS with premutation is seen in 1:800 males and 1:200 females (1).

RISK FACTORS
Genetics
- This is an X-linked dominant disorder with variable penetrance.
- The syndrome is caused by an abnormal expansion of CGG (cytosine-guanine-guanine) on the fragile X mental retardation 1 (FMR1) gene. FMR1 normally synthesizes the fragile X protein (FMRP), but mutations in FMR1 lead to a lack of FMRP synthesis, which is important for normal brain development (3).
- The number of CGG repeats in the FMR1 gene are classified as:
  – Full mutation (>200 CGG repeats)
  – Premutation (approximately 6–200 CGG repeats)
- Most males with full mutation have mental impairment in addition to some form of the physical and behavioral features.
- Males with premutation have normal intelligence but have an increased risk for tremor-ataxia syndrome between the ages of 50 and 60.
- Females with full mutation have an approximate 50% chance of having mental impairment in addition to some form of physical and behavioral features.

- Females with premutation have normal intelligence but have a 20% risk for premature ovarian failure.
- Since a male has only one X chromosome, it is never passed on to his son. He will pass the affected chromosome to all of his daughters.
- An affected female has a 50% chance of passing her affected chromosome to all of her offspring.

COMMONLY ASSOCIATED CONDITIONS
- Autistic spectrum disorder (2)
- Connective tissue manifestations, including flat feet and inguinal hernias (2)
- Mitral valve prolapse (develops during adolescence and adulthood) (2)
- Recurrent otitis media and sinusitis in childhood (2)
- Seizure disorder (15–20% for boys and 5% for girls) (3)
- Social phobias and other anxiety disorders (3)

 DIAGNOSIS

HISTORY
- Family history of mental impairment, particularly with multiple male relatives
- Family history of premature ovarian failure (POF) or fragile X-related tremor ataxia syndrome
- Delay of 1 or more developmental milestones, especially when there is mental impairment in the family (1)
- After the 1st year of life, delay in speech and language along with impaired fine motor skills

Pediatric Considerations
Average age at the time of diagnosis is 8 years, reflecting the subtlety of features in young children (1).

PHYSICAL EXAM
- Physical characteristics, which become more prominent with advancing age, include (2):
  – Large anterior fontanelle and macrosomia at birth
  – Macrocephaly
  – Prominent forehead
  – Pale blue iris
  – Long and thin face with a prominent jaw
  – Large ears
  – Midface hypoplasia
  – High arched palate
  – Dental overcrowding
  – Inability to touch the lips with the tongue
  – Soft stretchy skin
  – Plantar and hallucal crease
  – Single palmar crease
  – Double-jointed thumb
  – Hyperextensible metacarpophalangeal joints
  – Mitral valve prolapse
  – Pectus excavatum
  – Scoliosis
  – Pes planus
  – Macro-orchidism (usually seen after puberty)

- Cognitive deficits: Delayed language, math skills, problem-solving, abstract thinking, visuospatial abilities, short-term memory, adaptive behavior, and social skills (2)
- Behavioral characteristics include poor eye contact, tactile defensiveness, hand flapping, hand biting, perseverative speech (2), inattention, hypersensitivity to stimuli, overarousability, hyperactivity, and (mostly in men) explosive and aggressive behavior to others or self (3).

DIAGNOSTIC TESTS & INTERPRETATION
Diagnosis of FXS is made by DNA-based molecular tests, such as Southern blot test and PCR, to isolate the FMR1 gene mutation. Indications for testing include:
- Patients with a family history of mental impairment or FXS
- Any child with developmental delay of uncertain etiology or autism
- Individual with mental impairment of unknown etiology
- Women with premature ovarian failure of unknown cause
- Individuals with late-onset intentional tremor or ataxia, especially with a family history of movement disorders, FXS, or undiagnosed mental impairment
- Prenatal testing is offered only if maternal premutation or full mutation is present:
  – Chorionic villus sampling or amniocentesis is used for prenatal diagnosis.
  – Preimplantation genetic diagnosis may be another option for women with a premutation FXS; however, there are several limitations to this approach.

Imaging
Initial approach

Newborn screening for FXS is not routine at the present time (4)[B].

DIFFERENTIAL DIAGNOSIS
- Pervasive developmental disorder
- Learning disability
- Autism
- ADHD
- Other causes of mental impairment

TREATMENT

Treatment is usually supportive.

MEDICATION

Depending on the clinical presentation, pharmacotherapy may include (5)[B]:
- Atypical antipsychotics
- Selective serotonin reuptake inhibitors (SSRIs)
- Antiepileptics
- Methylphenidates
- Dextroamphetamines
- Clonidine
- Guanfacine

ADDITIONAL TREATMENT

Nonpharmacologic therapies are of tremendous value (6)[B] and include:
- Behavior therapy
- Speech and language therapy
- Psychotherapy and counseling
- Occupational and physical therapy
- Social skill training, support group
- Special education and preschool intervention programs (6)

Issues for Referral
- The proband and his or her family should be referred for genetic counseling and tested for the FMR1 gene.
- Also see Additional Treatment section.

ONGOING CARE

PATIENT EDUCATION
- In young females with FXS who are planning for future pregnancies, one should review the reproductive options, such as egg donation, prenatal diagnosis, adoption, and preimplantation genetic diagnosis.
- Useful Web sites:
  - The National Fragile X Foundation (http://www.fragilex.org)
  - FRAXA Research Foundation (http://www.fraxa.org)
  - Gene Tests (www.genetests.org, www.geneclinics.org)
  - American College of Medical Genetics (www.acmg.net/resources/policies/pol014.asp)
  - Dolan DNA Learning Center: Your Gene, Your Health (www.ygyh.org)
  - National Institute of Child Health and Human Development (www.nichd.nih.gov)

PROGNOSIS
- Patients with FXS have a normal lifespan.
- About 20–33% of women carrying a premutation for FXS are at increased risk for premature ovarian failure.
- 1/3 of males and, to a lesser extent, the females carrying the premutation are at increased risk for late-onset (>50 years of age) progressive neurodegenerative disorder. It is characterized by intentional tremor and ataxia, called fragile X-associated tremor/ataxia syndrome (FXTAS). Other associated findings include parkinsonism, autonomic dysfunction, peripheral neuropathy, and dementia.

REFERENCES

1. Wattendorf DJ, Muenke M. Diagnosis and management of fragile X syndrome. *Am Fam Physician*. 2005;72:111–3.
2. Visootsak J, Warren ST, Anido A, et al. Fragile X syndrome: an update and review for the primary pediatrician. *Clin Pediatr (Phila)*. 2005;44:371–81.
3. Tsiouris JA, Brown WT. Neuropsychiatric symptoms of fragile X syndrome: pathophysiology and pharmacotherapy. *CNS Drugs*. 2004;18:687–703.
4. Bailey DB, Skinner D, Davis AM, et al. Ethical, legal, and social concerns about expanded newborn screening: fragile X syndrome as a prototype for emerging issues. *Pediatrics*. 2008;121:e693–704.
5. Hagerman RJ, Berry-Kravis E, Kaufmann WE, et al. Advances in the treatment of fragile X syndrome. *Pediatrics*. 2009;123:378–90.
6. Solomon M, Hessl D, Chiu S, et al. A genetic etiology of pervasive developmental disorder guides treatment. *Am J Psychiatry*. 2007;164:575–80.

ADDITIONAL READING

- American College of Obstetricians and Gynecologists Committee on Genetics. ACOG committee opinion. No. 338: Screening for fragile X syndrome. *Obstet Gynecol*. 2006;107:1483–5.
- Garber KB, Visootsak J, Warren ST. Fragile X syndrome. *Eur J Hum Genet*. 2008.
- Huber K. Fragile X syndrome: molecular mechanisms of cognitive dysfunction. *Am J Psychiatry*. 2007;164: 556.

- McConkie-Rosell A, Finucane B, Cronister A, et al. Genetic counseling for fragile x syndrome: updated recommendations of the national society of genetic counselors. *J Genet Couns*. 2005;14:249–70.
- Orr HT, Zoghbi HY. Trinucleotide repeat disorders. *Annu Rev Neurosci*. 2007;30:575–621.
- Penagarikano O, Mulle JG, Warren ST. The pathophysiology of fragile x syndrome. *Annu Rev Genomics Hum Genet*. 2007;8:109–29.
- Wiesner GL, Cassidy SB, Grimes SJ, et al. Clinical consult: developmental delay/fragile X syndrome. *Prim Care*. 2004;31:621–5, x.

See Also (Topic, Algorithm, Electronic Media Element)
Algorithm: Mental Retardation

CODES

ICD9
759.83 Fragile x syndrome

CLINICAL PEARLS
- FXS is the most common inherited form of mental retardation.
- FXS is an X-linked dominant disorder with variable penetrance. Therefore, although this condition is seen in both sexes, males are usually more severely affected than females.
- Newborn screening for FXS is not routine.
- The average age at the time of diagnosis is 8 years old.

F

FROSTBITE

Alan M. Ehrlich, MD

 BASICS

DESCRIPTION
- A localized complication of exposure to cold, causing tissue to freeze, resulting in diminished blood flow to the affected part (especially hands, face, or feet)
- System(s) affected: Endocrine/Metabolic; Skin/Exocrine
- Synonym(s): Dermatitis congelationis; Frostnip; Environmental injuries

EPIDEMIOLOGY
- Predominant age: All ages
- Predominant sex: Male = Female

RISK FACTORS
- Previous cold-related injury
- Decreased caloric intake (<1,500 calories/day)
- Dehydration or hypovolemia
- Impaired cerebral function
- Under the effects of alcohol or drug abuse
- Underlying psychiatric disturbance
- Ambient temperature ≤−17.8°C (0°F)
- Smoker
- Elderly
- Lean body mass
- Low level of fitness
- Lack of proper clothing or shelter
- Raynaud phenomenon
- Constriction from excessively tight clothing (including too many layers of socks)
- Vehicular failure leading to prolonged cold exposure

GENERAL PREVENTION
- Dress in layers with appropriate cold-weather gear.
- Avoid clothing that is too constricting.
- Cover exposed areas and extremities appropriately.
- Prepare properly for trips to cold climates.
- Avoid alcohol.

PATHOPHYSIOLOGY
- Ice crystals form intracellularly.
- Dehydration, enzymatic destruction, and ultimately cell death occur.
- In severe cases, deep-tissue freezing may occur with damage to underlying blood vessels, muscles, and nerve tissue.

ETIOLOGY
- Prolonged exposure to cold
- Refreezing thawed extremities

COMMONLY ASSOCIATED CONDITIONS
Alcohol and/or drug abuse

 DIAGNOSIS

HISTORY
- Throbbing pain
- Paresthesia
- Excessive sweating
- Joint pain

PHYSICAL EXAM
- Feet, hands, and face most commonly affected
- Injured area appears cold, hard, and white and is anesthetic to touch. It progresses to blotchy-red, swollen, and painful regions after rewarming.
- 1st degree: Redness and edema without blister formation
- 2nd degree: Redness, edema, and blister formation
- 3rd degree: Same as above with addition of hemorrhagic vesicles
- 4th degree: Necrosis and gangrene
- Pallor
- Loss of cutaneous sensation
- Numbness
- Limited movement of affected joints
- Subcutaneous edema
- Hyperemia
- Blistering
- Blue discoloration
- Skin necrosis
- Gangrene

DIAGNOSTIC TESTS & INTERPRETATION
ECG in hypothermia may show bradycardia, atrial fibrillation, atrial flutter, ventricular fibrillation, diffuse T-wave inversion, Osborn waves (upward-going "hump" following S wave in the RS–T segment)

Lab
- May show signs of hemoconcentration such as elevated hemoglobin or high BUN/creatinine ratio
- Liver function tests for decreased hepatic function

Imaging
- Triple-phase bone scan can identify tissue viability at early stage and facilitate early debridement.
- Other imaging techniques sometimes used include MRI/MRA, infrared thermography, angiography, digital plethysmography, and laser Doppler studies.

Pathological Findings
- Ice crystallization in the intravascular extracellular space
- Atrophy
- Fibroblastic proliferation
- Skin necrosis

DIFFERENTIAL DIAGNOSIS
- Frostnip, a superficial cold injury that does not cause permanent damage
- Chilblains (pernio), an inflammatory reaction to short-term cold, wet exposure without tissue freezing
- Immersion syndrome (trench foot), inflammatory reaction to prolonged cold, wet exposure, typically socks or footwear

TREATMENT

Geriatric Considerations
- Associated disease states increase mortality
- Periarticular osteoporosis complicates
- More prone to hypothermia

Pediatric Considerations
Loss of epithelial growth centers

> **ALERT**
> Acidosis

MEDICATION
First Line
- tPA administered within 24 hours of injury may prevent damage from thrombosis and may reduce amputation rate (1,2)[C].
- Tetanus toxoid
- Penicillin G 500,000 units every 6 hours for 48–72 hours prophylactically (3)[B]
- Ibuprofen 400 mg every 12 hours to inhibit prostaglandins (3)[C]
- NSAIDs for mild-moderate pain. For severe pain, narcotic analgesia.
- Precautions: tPA should not be used with history of recent bleeding, stroke, ulcer, etc.

Second Line
Vasodilators such as iloprost and pentoxifylline have been tried with some success (3)[C].

ADDITIONAL TREATMENT
General Measures
- If transport time will be short (1–2 hours at most), the risks posed by improper rewarming or refreezing outweigh the risks of delaying treatment for deep frostbite (4)[C].

- If transport will be prolonged (more than 1–2 hours), frostbite will often thaw spontaneously. It is more important to prevent hypothermia than to rewarm frostbite rapidly in warm water. This does not mean that a frostbitten extremity should be kept in the cold to prevent spontaneous rewarming. Anticipate that frostbitten areas will rewarm as a consequence of keeping the patient warm and protect them from refreezing at all costs (4)[C].
- Rapid rewarming (3)[B]:
  – Immerse frozen body part in warm water (37–39°C [99–102°F]) for 15–30 minutes or until thawing is complete.
  – Continue rewarming until a red/purple color appears and the affected part becomes pliable.
  – It is critical not to allow refreezing after thawing has occurred.
- After rewarming, injured parts should be covered with nonadhesive dressings, splinted, and elevated.
- Remove jewelry and clothing, if present, from the affected area.
- Application of aloe vera every 6 hours
- Sterile cotton between fingers or toes, if applicable, to prevent maceration
- Keep the patient dry.
- If conscious, give the patient warm fluids with high sugar content.
- Prevent infection once treatment begins.
- Institute ongoing whirlpool therapy for cleansing and debridement.
- Prevent damage to other body parts.
- Prohibit use of nicotine-containing products (including cigarettes) or other vasoconstrictive agents.
- Maintenance: Gastric lavage, peritoneal dialysis, hemodialysis, and mediastinal lavage if needed (using warmed fluids)

Additional Therapies
- Heated oxygen
- Warm intravenous fluids via central venous pressure line

SURGERY/OTHER PROCEDURES
- Urgent surgery rarely needed except fasciotomy for compartment syndrome (suspect if tissue swollen and compartment pressures greater than 37–40 mm Hg)
- Surgical debridement as needed to remove necrotic tissue
- Amputation should not be considered until it is definite that tissues are dead: May take ~3 weeks to know whether the tissue is permanently injured

IN-PATIENT CONSIDERATIONS
Initial Stabilization
- Institute emergency measures for hypothermic patient without pulse or respiration. Such measures may include CPR and internal warming with warm intravenous fluids and warm oxygen (see topic Hypothermia).
- Prevent refreezing.

- It may be necessary to keep the frostbitten part frozen until the patient can be transported to a care facility. Prolonged freezing is preferable to warming and refreezing (5)[C].
- Remove nonadherent wet clothing.
- Treat for hypothermia.
- Treat for pain:
  – NSAIDs and/or narcotics if needed
- Do not rub areas to warm them; increased tissue damage may occur (1)[C].
- Do not allow patient with frostbitten feet to walk except when the life of the patient or rescuer is in danger (4)[C].

Admission Criteria
Hospitalization generally recommended (2)

 ONGOING CARE

FOLLOW-UP RECOMMENDATIONS
Outpatient or inpatient, depending on severity:
- As tolerated; protect injured body parts
- Initiate physical therapy once healing progresses sufficiently.

Patient Monitoring
- Preferably electronic probe for temperature monitoring (rectal or vascular)
- Follow-up for physical therapy progress, infection, other complications

DIET
- As tolerated
- Warm oral fluids

PATIENT EDUCATION
- Refer to local library for information.
- Provide education on:
  – Exposure protection
  – Early signs and symptoms of frostbite

PROGNOSIS
- Anesthesia and bullae may occur.
- The affected areas will heal or mummify without surgery; the process may take 6–12 months for healing.
- Patient may be sensitive to cold and experience burning and tingling.
- Cyanotic nonblanching skin and blisters with dark fluid suggest worse prognosis (5)[C].

COMPLICATIONS
- Hyperglycemia
- Acidosis
- Refractory arrhythmias
- Tissue loss: Distal parts of an extremity may undergo spontaneous amputation
- Gangrene
- Death

REFERENCES
1. Bruen KJ, Ballard JR, Morris SE, et al. Reduction of the incidence of amputation in frostbite injury with thrombolytic therapy. *Arch Surg.* 2007;142: 546–51; discussion 551–3.
2. Jurkovich GJ. Environmental cold-induced injury. *Surg Clin North Am.* 2007;87:247–67, viii.
3. Imray C, Grieve A, Dhillon S, Caudwell Xtreme Everest Research Group et al. Cold damage to the extremities: frostbite and non-freezing cold injuries. *Postgrad Med J.* 2009;85:481–8.
4. State of Alaska Cold Injury Guideline: Alaska Multi-level 2003 Version. http://www.chems. alaska.gov/EMS/documents/AKColdInj2005.pdf.
5. Biem J, Koehncke N, Classen D, et al. Out of the cold: management of hypothermia and frostbite. *CMAJ.* 2003;168:305–11.

ADDITIONAL READING
- Cappaert TA, Stone JA, Castellani JW, et al. National Athletic Trainers' Association position statement: environmental cold injuries. *J Athl Train.* 2008;43: 640–58.
- Murphy JV, Banwell PE, Roberts AH, et al. Frostbite: pathogenesis and treatment. *J Trauma.* 2000;48: 171–8.
- Reamy BV. Frostbite: review and current concepts. *J Am Board Fam Pract.* 1998;11:34–40.
- Twomey JA, Peltier GL, Zera RT. An open-label study to evaluate the safety and efficacy of tissue plasminogen activator in treatment of severe frostbite. *J Trauma.* 2005;59:1350–4; discussion 1354–5.

See Also (Topic, Algorithm, Electronic Media Element)
Hypothermia
Algorithm: Hypothermia

 CODES

ICD9
- 991.0 Frostbite of face
- 991.1 Frostbite of hand
- 991.2 Frostbite of foot

CLINICAL PEARLS
- Frostbite is considered a tetanus-prone injury. Treat as any injury involving tissue destruction.
- Avoid rewarming en route to the hospital if there is a chance of refreezing. Avoid burns to affected areas, which may be numb and insensitive to heat.

F

FROZEN SHOULDER

J. Herbert Stevenson, MD
Jeffrey Manning, MD

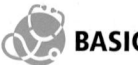

BASICS

DESCRIPTION
- Syndrome of painful restriction of active and passive range of motion (ROM) in 1 or both shoulders. Idiopathic adhesive capsulitis has 3 stages: Painful, adhesive, and recovery.
- System(s) affected: Musculoskeletal
- Synonym(s): Pericapsulitis; adherent bursitis; obliterative bursitis; adhesive capsulitis

EPIDEMIOLOGY
- Predominant age: 40–70 years
- Predominant sex: Female > Male

Geriatric Considerations
Common

Pediatric Considerations
Rare, but reported

Pregnancy Considerations
Primary (idiopathic): 2–3%

Prevalence
- General population is reported to be 2%.
- 11% in unselected individuals with diabetes

RISK FACTORS
- Systemic diseases (See Etiology. Diseases and conditions associated with secondary adhesive capsulitis) (1)[A]
- Prolonged immobilization
- Age (more common in elderly)
- Diabetes
- Thyroid disease

Genetics
Frequent trisomy 7 and trisomy 8 identified in fibroblasts

GENERAL PREVENTION
- Early ROM exercises after injury
- Stretching, frequent physical activity
- Avoid extended periods of immobilization.

PATHOPHYSIOLOGY
A chronic inflammatory response with fibroblastic proliferation, which may be immunomodulated (2)[B]

ETIOLOGY
Idiopathic (primary)

COMMONLY ASSOCIATED CONDITIONS
- Trauma
- Diabetes (most common)
- Postinflammatory
- After cerebrovascular accident or myocardial infarction (MI)
- After mastectomy (immobilization is the speculated cause)
- Hypothyroidism/hyperthyroidism
- Avascular necrosis
- Tuberculosis
- Scleroderma; rheumatoid arthritis
- Lung cancer or chronic lung disease

DIAGNOSIS

HISTORY
- Subacute onset of shoulder pain and decreased ROM without trauma
- Night pain often interrupting sleep
- Pain aggravated with movement and alleviated with rest
- Pain and tenderness to palpation:
  - May interrupt sleep
- Preceding injury, illness, or immobilization (secondary adhesive capsulitis)
- Loss of active and passive ROM in all planes
- Loss of natural arm swing with gait
- Because of compensatory scapular elevation (to lift the arm), muscles may be painful and spastic.
- Muscle atrophy and weakness with time
- Inability to reach into a back pocket or fasten the back of a garment
- Stages of adhesive capsulitis:
  - Painful stage (weeks to months):
    - Pain with movement
    - Generalized shoulder ache that is difficult to pinpoint
    - Muscle spasm
    - Increasing pain at night and at rest
  - Adhesive stage (up to 1 year):
    - Less pain
    - Increasing stiffness and restriction of movement
    - Decreasing pain at night and at rest
    - Discomfort felt at extreme ranges of movement
  - Recovery stage (weeks to months):
    - Decreased pain
    - Marked restriction with slow, gradual increase in range of motion
    - Recovery is spontaneous, frequently incomplete.

PHYSICAL EXAM
- Possible diffuse shoulder tenderness, but discrete point tenderness makes the diagnosis less likely.
- Marked limitation of passive and active shoulder abduction, flexion, internal and external rotation
- Normal 5/5 strength in all planes
- Hawkins, Neer, Yergason, and Speed testing can be positive.
- No neurovascular deficits

DIAGNOSTIC TESTS & INTERPRETATION
Lab

Initial lab tests
No lab is diagnostic for frozen shoulder, but may be required to rule out other disorders if suspected, such as systemic autoimmune disease.

Imaging
Initial approach
- Plain radiograph [anteroposterior (AP), axillary, supraspinatus outlet views] to rule out osteoarthritis, calcific tendinitis, avascular necrosis, osteomyelitis, fracture, dislocation, and tumor:
  - AP: Check osteopenia, fractures, dislocations, and superior migration of humeral head.
  - Axillary: Check subluxation or articular head damage (Bankart or Hills-Sachs lesions).
  - Supraspinatus outlet views: Check supraspinatus outlet narrowing to rule out acromial impingement.
- Arthrography:
  - Joint volume is reduced to 5–10 mL (normal, 20–30 mL).
  - Since this is invasive, arthrography is reserved for patients with uncertain diagnosis.
- Consider magnetic resonance imaging (MRI) to evaluate rotator cuff, evaluating for thickening of the shoulder capsule and to rule out other shoulder disorders.

Diagnostic Procedures/Surgery
- Joint aspiration if septic joint is suspected (rarely necessary)
- Arthroscopy to visualize fibrous bands in the joint space (rarely necessary)

Pathological Findings
- Active process of hyperplastic fibroplasia and excessive type III collagen secretion that lead to soft tissue contractures
- Fibrous bands traversing the glenohumeral joint space (occasional)
- Surgical findings of adherence of capsule to humeral head

DIFFERENTIAL DIAGNOSIS
- Rotator cuff strain/tear/impingement syndrome
- Bicipital/rotator/calcific tendinitis
- Septic arthritis
- Bursitis
- Polymyalgia rheumatica
- Glenohumeral or acromioclavicular joint osteoarthritis
- Cervical osteoarthritis/strain/disc disease
- Rheumatoid arthritis
- Bony neoplasm/metastases
- Dislocation
- Fracture (distal clavicle, proximal humerus)
- Avascular necrosis
- Fibromyalgia
- Myofascial pain syndrome
- Myelomeningocele
- Thoracic outlet syndrome
- Parkinson disease

TREATMENT

Make patient aware of a 6–18-month recovery.

MEDICATION

First Line
- Nonsteroidal anti-inflammatory drugs (NSAIDs) during painful stage
- Acetaminophen if NSAIDs contraindicated
- Opioid analgesics (with physical therapy) if NSAIDs contraindicated and not responding
- Oral corticosteroids: 3–4-week taper (40 mg, 30 mg, 20 mg, 10 mg, then discontinue) (3)[A]
- Contraindications:
  – NSAIDs: Gastrointestinal (GI) ulcer disease/bleeding
  – Renal disease: See the manufacturer's literature.

Second Line
- Low-dose tricyclic antidepressants (e.g., amitriptyline) may help with pain and sleep.
- Subacromial bursa corticosteroid injection (4,5)[A]:
  – Increased ROM and decreased pain temporarily

ADDITIONAL TREATMENT
- Glenohumeral corticosteroid injection (e.g., triamcinolone, betamethasone) (4,5)[A]:
  – Does not shorten recovery, but may aid in decreasing discomfort with mobility exercises (controversial)
- Glenohumeral distention arthrography (controversial)
- Iontophoresis (electromotive drug administration) is generally not recommended in this condition.

General Measures
- Control of pain and preservation of mobility
- Avoid prolonged immobilization.
- Heat and/or ice
- Address underlying causes of secondary adhesive capsulitis (see Differential Diagnosis).
- Physical therapy

Issues for Referral
Not responding to conservative treatment within 3 months, but usually self-limiting

Additional Therapies
- Low-power laser therapy (6)[C]
- Physical therapy:
  – Avoid in the painful stage, as it will aggravate symptoms.
  – Focus on passive and active ROM exercises in the adhesive and recovery stages.

COMPLEMENTARY AND ALTERNATIVE MEDICINE
- Osteopathic manipulative technique may help decrease pain and increase shoulder ROM.
- Electroacupuncture or interferential electrotherapy may be of benefit (7)[C].

SURGERY/OTHER PROCEDURES
- Arthroscopic lysis of adhesions and manipulation under anesthesia are reserved for refractory cases.
- Arthroscopic capsular release with manipulation can offer good results to refractory cases (8,9,10)[A].

IN-PATIENT CONSIDERATIONS
Initial Stabilization
Outpatient care

ONGOING CARE

FOLLOW-UP RECOMMENDATIONS
Monthly follow-up to determine ongoing treatment plan

Patient Monitoring
Close monitoring and frequent encouragement are usually needed for successful recovery.

DIET
No restrictions

PATIENT EDUCATION
- Long-term course of treatment until resolution of symptoms
- Stretching exercises daily or b.i.d. during and after improvement
- Codman exercises: Sit sideways in a straight chair; rest armpit on the back of the chair; swing the arm slowly in circles. Start with smaller circles and then bigger circles (clockwise and counterclockwise).
- Climbing the wall: Put the hand flat on a wall in front of you; use the fingers to "climb" the wall; pause 30 seconds every few inches.
- Reaching: Put everyday objects on a high shelf so that reaching is done more often.

PROGNOSIS
- Disorder is considered self-limiting (11)[A]
- Adhesive capsulitis may last from 6–9 months to as long as 1–3 years:
  – Painful stage: 2–6 months
  – Adhesive stage: 4–6 months
  – Recovery stage: 1–3 months

COMPLICATIONS
- Long-term loss of some mobility (7–30%) or function (rare)
- Residual pain and stiffness
- Long-term disability

REFERENCES

1. Milgrom C, Novack V, Weil Y, Jaber S, Radeva-Petrova DR, Finestone A. Risk factors for idiopathic frozenshoulder. *Israel Medical Association Journal: Imaj*. 2008;10(5):361–4.
2. Hand GC, Athanasou NA, Matthews T, Carr AJ. The pathology of frozenshoulder. *Journal of Bone & Joint Surgery - British Volume*. 2007;89(7):928–32.
3. Buchbinder R, Green S, Youd JM, Johnston RV. Oral steroids for adhesive capsulitis. *Cochrane Database of Systematic Reviews*. 2006.
4. Arroll B, Goodyear-Smith F. Corticosteroid injections for painful shoulder: a meta-analysis. *Br J Gen Pract*. 2005;55(512):224–8. Review.
5. Arslon S, et al. Comparison of the efficacy of local corticosteroid injection and physical therapy for the treatment of adhesive capsulitis. *Rheumatol Int*. 2001;21:20–3.
6. Stergioulas A. Low-power laser treatment in patients with frozenshoulder: preliminary results. *Photomedicine and Laser Surgery*. 2008;26(2):99–105.
7. Cheing GL, So EM, Chao CY. Effectiveness of electroacupuncture and interferential electrotherapy in the management of frozenshoulder. *Journal of Rehabilitation Medicine*. 2008;40(3):166–70.
8. Liem D, Meier F, Thorwesten L, Marquardt B, Steinbeck J, Poetzl W. The influence of arthroscopic subscapularis tendon and capsule release on internal rotation strength in treatment of frozenshoulder. *American Journal of Sports Medicine*. 2008;36(5):921–6.
9. Ozbaydar MU, Tonbul M, Altun M, et al. [Arthroscopic selective capsular release in the treatment of frozen shoulder] *Acta Orthop Traumatol Turc*. 2005;39:104–13.
10. Pearsall AW, Osbahr DC, Speer KP. An arthroscopic technique for treating patients with frozen shoulder. *Arthroscopy*. 1999;15:2–11.
11. Hand C, Clipsham K, Rees JL, Carr AJ. Long-term outcome of frozenshoulder. *Journal of Shoulder & Elbow Surgery*. 2008;17(2):231–6.

ADDITIONAL READING
- Daigneault J, et al. Shoulder pain in older people. *J Am Geriatr Soc*. 1998;46:1145–51.
- Siegel LB, et al. Adhesive capsulitis: A sticky issue. *Am Fam Physician*. 1999;59:1843–51.
- Woodward T, et al. The painful shoulder. II: Acute and chronic disorders. *Am Fam Physician*. 2000;61:3291–3300.

CODES

ICD9
726.0 Adhesive capsulitis of shoulder

CLINICAL PEARLS
- Syndrome of painful restriction of active and passive ROM commonly occurring in elderly
- Consider in symptomatic diabetic patients
- Primary cause is idiopathic.
- Treatment mainly consists of conservative measures: NSAIDs, corticosteroid injection, physical therapy.
- Prognosis is generally good, with self-limiting course over months to years.

F

FURUNCULOSIS

Zoltan Trizna, MD, PhD

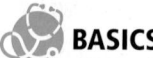

BASICS

DESCRIPTION
Acute bacterial abscess of a hair follicle (often *Staphylococcus aureus*):
- System(s) affected: Skin/Exocrine
- Synonym(s): Boils

EPIDEMIOLOGY
Incidence
- Predominant age:
  – Adolescents and young adults
  – Clusters have been reported in teenagers living in crowded quarters, within families, or in high school athletes.
- Predominant sex: Male = Female

Prevalence
Exact data are not available.

RISK FACTORS
- Carriage of pathogenic strain of *Staphylococcus* sp. in nares, skin, axilla, and perineum
- Rarely, polymorphonuclear leukocyte defect or hyperimmunoglobulin E–*Staphylococcus* sp. abscess syndrome
- Diabetes mellitus, malnutrition, alcoholism, obesity, atopic dermatitis
- Primary immunodeficiency disease and AIDS (common variable immunodeficiency, chronic granulomatous disease, Chediak-Higashi syndrome, C3 deficiency, C3 hypercatabolism, transient hypogammaglobulinemia of infancy, immunodeficiency with thymoma, Wiskott-Aldrich syndrome)
- Secondary immunodeficiency (e.g., leukemia, leukopenia, neutropenia, therapeutic immunosuppression)
- Medication impairing neutrophil function (e.g., omeprazole)

Genetics
Unknown

GENERAL PREVENTION
Patient education regarding self-care (see General Measures); treatment and prevention are interrelated.

PATHOPHYSIOLOGY
Infection spreads away from hair follicle into surrounding dermis.

ETIOLOGY
Pathogenic strain of *S. aureus* (usually); increasing incidence of community-acquired methicillin-resistant *S. aureus* (CA-MRSA)

COMMONLY ASSOCIATED CONDITIONS
- Usually normal immune system
- Diabetes mellitus
- Polymorphonuclear leukocyte defect (rare)
- Hyperimmunoglobulin E–*Staphylococcus* sp. abscess syndrome (rare)
- See Risk Factors.

DIAGNOSIS

HISTORY
- Located on hair-bearing sites, especially areas prone to friction or repeated minor traumas (e.g., underneath belt, anterior aspects of thighs, nape, buttocks)
- No initial fever or systemic symptoms
- The folliculocentric nodule may enlarge, become painful, and develop into an abscess (frequently with spontaneous drainage).

PHYSICAL EXAM
- Painful erythematous papules/nodules (1–5 cm) with central pustules
- Tender, red, perifollicular swelling, terminating in discharge of pus and necrotic plug
- The lesions may be solitary or clustered.

DIAGNOSTIC TESTS & INTERPRETATION
Lab
Initial lab tests
Culture of the purulent contents
Follow-Up & Special Considerations
- Immunoglobulin levels in rare (e.g., recurrent or otherwise inexplicable) cases
- If culture grows gram-negative bacteria or fungus, consider polymorphonuclear neutrophil leukocyte functional defect

Pathological Findings
Histopathology (though a biopsy is rarely needed):
- Perifollicular necrosis containing fibrinoid material and neutrophils
- At deep end of necrotic plug, in subcutaneous tissue, is a large abscess with a Gram stain positive for small collections of *S. aureus*.

DIFFERENTIAL DIAGNOSIS
- Folliculitis
- Pseudofolliculitis
- Carbuncles
- Ruptured epidermal cyst
- Myiasis (larva of botfly/tumbafly)
- Hidradenitis suppurativa
- Atypical bacterial or fungal infections

TREATMENT

MEDICATION
First Line
- If suspect CA-MRSA, see Second Line.
- If abscesses multiple, if lesions have marked surrounding inflammation, cellulitis, systemic symptoms such as fever, or if immunocompromised:
  – Obtain culture, and place on antibiotics directed at *S. aureus* × 10–14 days.
  – Dicloxacillin (Dynapen, Pathocil) 500 mg p.o. q.i.d. *or*
  – Cephalexin 250 mg p.o. q.i.d. *or*
  – Clindamycin 150 mg q.i.d. if penicillin-allergic
- Suppression of pathogenic strain (if topical treatment fails):
  – Dicloxacillin/cloxacillin 500 mg b.i.d. × 10–14 days
  – Cephalexin or clindamycin (if penicillin-allergic)
  – If preceding fails, dicloxacillin/cloxacillin 500 mg plus rifampin 600 mg p.o. daily × 7–10 days *or* clindamycin 150 mg/d × 3 months (1)[C]
- Contraindications: Allergy to the particular drug selected
- Precautions: Cloxacillin and dicloxacillin: Anaphylactic reaction

Second Line
- Resistant strains of *S. aureus* (MRSA): Clindamycin 300 mg q6h or doxycycline 100 mg q12h or TMP-SMX DS 1 tab q8h or minocycline 100 mg q12h (2)[C]
- If known or suspected impaired neutrophil function (e.g., impaired chemotaxis, phagocytosis, superoxide generation), add vitamin C 1,000 mg/d × 4–6 weeks (prevents oxidation of neutrophils)
- If fail with antibiotic regimens:
  - May try oral pentoxifylline 400 mg t.i.d. × 2–6 months (3)[C]
  - Contraindications: Recent cerebral and/or retinal hemorrhage; intolerance to methylxanthines (e.g., caffeine, theophylline); allergy to the particular drug selected
  - Precautions: Prolonged prothrombin time (PT) and/or bleeding; if on warfarin, frequent monitoring of PT

ADDITIONAL TREATMENT
General Measures
- Moist, warm compresses (provide comfort, encourage localization/pointing/drainage) 30 minutes q.i.d.
- If pointing or large, incise and drain
- Consider packing.
- Routine culture not necessary for localized abscess in nondiabetic patients with normal immune system
- Systemic antibiotics usually unnecessary, unless extensive surrounding cellulitis or fever
- If recurrent, usually related to chronic skin carriage of *Staphylococci* (nares or on skin). Treatment goals are to decrease or eliminate pathogenic strain *or* suppress pathogenic strain:
  - Culture nares, skin, axilla, and perineum (culture nares of family members).
  - Apply mupirocin ointment to anterior nares b.i.d. × 5 days (patient and family members/carriers).
  - Culture anterior nares every 3 months. If failure, retreat with mupirocin or consider oral antibiotics (4)[C].
  - See Medications, First Line, Suppression of Pathogenic Strain.

- Especially in recurrent cases, wash entire body and fingernails (with nailbrush) daily for 1–3 weeks with povidone–iodine (Betadine), hexachlorophene (Hibiclens), or pHisoHex soap (all can cause dry skin)
- Sanitary practices: Change towels, washcloths, and sheets daily; clean shaving instruments; avoid nose picking; change wound dressings frequently; do not share items of personal hygiene.

 ## ONGOING CARE

FOLLOW-UP RECOMMENDATIONS
Patient Monitoring
Instruct patient to see physician if compresses unsuccessful

DIET
Unrestricted

PROGNOSIS
- Self-limited: Usually drains pus spontaneously and will heal with or without scarring within several days
- Recurrent/chronic: May last for months or years

COMPLICATIONS
- Scarring
- Bacteremia
- Seeding (e.g., septal/valve defect, arthritic joint)

REFERENCES

1. Klempner MS, Styrt B. Prevention of recurrent staphylococcal skin infections with low-dose oral clindamycin therapy. *JAMA*. 1988;260:2682–5.
2. *Up To Date 2007*. Impetigo, Folliculitis, Furunculosis, and Carbuncles.
3. Wahba-Yahav AV. Intractable chronic furunculosis: prevention of recurrences with pentoxifylline. *Acta Derm Venereol*. 1992;72:461–2.
4. Doebbeling BN, et al. Long Term Efficacy of Intranasal Mupirocin, A Prospective Cohort Study of Staphylococcal Aureus. *Arch Int Med*. 1994;154:1505.
5. Winthropp KL, et al. An outbreak of mycobacterium furunculosis associated with footbaths at a nail salon. *N Engl J Med*. 2002;346(18):1366–71.

ADDITIONAL READING

Frazee BW, Lynn J, Charlebois ED, Lambert L, Lowery D, Perdreau-Remington F et al. High prevalence of methicillin-resistant Staphylococcus aureus in emergency department skin and soft tissue infections. *Ann Emerg Med*. 2005;45:311–20.

See Also (Topic, Algorithm, Electronic Media Element)
Folliculitis; Hidradenitis Suppurativa

 ## CODES

ICD9
680.9 Carbuncle and furuncle of unspecified site

CLINICAL PEARLS
- The pathogens may be different in different localities. Keep up-to-date with the locality-specific epidemiology.
- If few, furuncles/furunculosis do not always need antibiotic treatment. If systemic symptoms (e.g., fever), cellulitis, or multiple lesions occur, oral antibiotic therapy is needed.
- Other treatments for MRSA include linezolid p.o. or IV and IV vancomycin.
- Folliculitis, furunculosis, and carbuncles are parts of a spectrum of pyodermas.
- Other causative organisms include anaerobic (e.g., *Escherichia coli, Pseudomonas aeruginosa,* and *Streptococcus faecalis*), anaerobic (e.g., *Bacteroides, Lactobacillus, Peptobacillius*), and *Peptostreptococcus*), and *Mycobacteria* (5).

F

GALACTORRHEA

Katherine M. Callaghan, MD
Dawn S. Tasillo, MD

 BASICS

DESCRIPTION
- Milky nipple discharge not associated with gestation. Galactorrhea does not include serous, purulent, or bloody nipple discharge.
- System(s) affected. Endocrine/Metabolic; Nervous; Reproductive
- Synonym(s): Disordered lactation; Nipple discharge

Pregnancy Considerations
- Most cases of galactorrhea during pregnancy are physiologic.
- Adenomas can grow rapidly during pregnancy.

EPIDEMIOLOGY
- Predominant age: 15–50 years
- Predominant sex: Female > Male (rare, 20% of patients with *MEN1* have prolactinomas)

Prevalence
1–50% of nonpregnant reproductive-age women

GENERAL PREVENTION
Keep medication causes in mind.

PATHOPHYSIOLOGY
Disorders of lactation are associated with hyperprolactinemia from overproduction or loss of inhibitory regulation by dopamine.

ETIOLOGY
- Nipple stimulation
- Pituitary gland overproduction:
  – Prolactinoma, acromegaly, empty sella, lymphocytic hypophysitis
- Hypothalamic region dysregulation:
  – Craniopharyngiomas, meningiomas, dysgerminomas, tumors, sarcoid, irradiation, vascular insult, stalk disruption, or dissection
- Medications that suppress dopamine:
  – Phenothiazines, atypical antipsychotics, selective serotonin reuptake inhibitors, tricyclic antidepressants, butyrophenones, cimetidine, ranitidine, reserpine, alpha methyl-dopa, verapamil, estrogens, isoniazid, opioids, stimulants, neuroleptics, metoclopramide, domperidone, protease inhibitors (1)
- Chest wall conditions:
  – Zoster, fibrocystic breast disease, or surgical or other trauma
- Postoperative condition, especially oophorectomy

- Other causes:
  – Primary hypothyroidism, cirrhosis, Cushing disease, ectopic prolactin secretion, renal failure, sarcoid, lupus, multiple sclerosis, polycystic ovary syndrome
- Physiologic with pregnancy or up to 6 months after stopping lactation
- Chiari-Frommel:
  – Galactorrhea >6 months postpartum
- Idiopathic:
  – Normal prolactin levels

COMMONLY ASSOCIATED CONDITIONS
See Etiology.

 DIAGNOSIS

- Findings vary with causes
- Signs/symptoms of associated conditions:
  – Adrenal insufficiency, acromegaly, hypothyroidism, chest wall conditions

HISTORY
- Usually bilateral milky nipple discharge
- Hypogonadism from hyperprolactinemia:
  – Oligomenorrhea, amenorrhea
  – Inadequate luteal phase, anovulation, infertility
  – Decreased libido (especially in affected males)
- Mass effects from pituitary enlargement:
  – Headache, cranial neuropathies
  – Bitemporal hemianopsia, amaurosis, scotomata

PHYSICAL EXAM
Breast examination should be performed with attention to the presence of spontaneous or induced nipple discharge.

DIAGNOSTIC TESTS & INTERPRETATION
Formal visual field testing if pituitary adenoma suspected

Lab
- Check prolactin level and thyroid-stimulating hormone.
- Check pregnancy test, liver, and renal functions.
- Consider follicle-stimulating hormone and luteinizing hormone if amenorrheic.
- Consider growth hormone levels if acromegaly suspected.
- Check adrenal steroids if signs of Cushing disease.
- Drugs that may alter lab results:
  – See medications that can cause hyperprolactinemia.

- Situations that may alter lab results:
  – See Etiology.
  – Lab evaluation of prolactin may be falsely elevated by a recent breast examination, vigorous exercise, sexual activity, or high-carbohydrate diet. Consider repeating the test under different circumstances if the value is borderline (30–40) elevated.

Follow-Up & Special Considerations
- Prolactin levels may fluctuate. Elevated prolactin levels should be confirmed with at least 1 additional level drawn in a fasting, nonexercised state, with no breast stimulation (2).
- Prolactin levels above 200 ng/mL are highly suggestive of a pituitary adenoma (2).

Imaging
Pituitary magnetic resonance imaging (MRI) with gadolinium enhancement if the serum prolactin level is significantly elevated (>200 ng/mL) or if a pituitary tumor is otherwise suspected

Diagnostic Procedures/Surgery
Confirm that microscopic evaluation of secretions is lipoid.

Pathological Findings
None unless pituitary resection required

DIFFERENTIAL DIAGNOSIS
- Primary hypothyroidism
- Nonmilky nipple discharge:
  – Intraductal papilloma
  – Fibrocystic disease
- Purulent breast discharge:
  – Mastitis
  – Breast abscess
  – Impetigo
  – Eczema
- Bloody breast discharge:
  – Consider malignancy

 TREATMENT

- Treat underlying cause if possible.
- Idiopathic galactorrhea (normal prolactin levels) does not require treatment.
- Treat to manage symptoms, reduce patient anxiety, and restore fertility.
- Reduce tumor size or prevent progression to prevent neurologic sequelae.
- If microadenoma, watchful waiting can be appropriate, as 95% do not enlarge.
- Treat asymptomatic tumors if >10 mm.
- Discontinue offending medications.

MEDICATION

- The dopamine agonists work to reduce prolactin levels and shrink tumor size. Therapy is suppressive, not curative.
- Treatment is discontinued when tumor size has reduced or regressed completely or after pregnancy has been achieved.
- Contraindications are similar for all and include:
  - Uncontrolled hypertension
  - Sensitivity to ergot alkaloids
  - Preeclampsia
- Precautions:
  - Nausea, vomiting, and drowsiness are common.
  - Orthostasis, lightheadedness, or syncope
  - Hypertension, seizures, acute psychosis, and digital vasospasm are rare.
- Significant possible interactions:
  - Phenothiazines, butyrophenones, other drugs listed under "Etiology"
- Bromocriptine:
  - Start at 1.25 mg/d p.o. with food and increase weekly by 1.25 mg/d until therapeutic response achieved. (Usually 2.5–15 mg/d, divided once daily/3 times daily.)
  - More expensive and more frequent dosing; however, most providers have experience with this effective drug.
  - Long-term treatment can cause woody fibrosis of the pituitary gland.
- Cabergoline (Dostinex):
  - Start at 0.25 mg p.o. weekly and increase by 0.25 mg monthly until prolactin levels normalize. Usual dose ranges from 0.25 mg–1 mg p.o. once or twice weekly.
  - More effective and better tolerated than bromocriptine
  - Convenient dosing
  - Although cabergoline has been associated with valvular heart disease in patients treated for Parkinson disease, the lower doses used in treatment of prolactinomas have not been adequately studied (3).

SURGERY/OTHER PROCEDURES

- Surgery:
  - Macroadenomas need surgery if medical management does not halt growth, if neurologic symptoms persist, if size >10 mm, or if patient cannot tolerate medications. Also considered in young patients with microadenomas in order to avoid long-term medical therapy (4).
  - Trans-sphenoidal pituitary resection
  - 50% recurrence after surgery

- Radiotherapy:
  - Radiation is an alternate tumor therapy for macroprolactinomas not responsive to other modes of treatment:
    - 20–30% success rate
    - 50% risk of panhypopituitarism after radiation
    - Risk of optic nerve damage (5)
- Gamma knife is effective with high-volume surgeons (1)[B].

 ## ONGOING CARE

FOLLOW-UP RECOMMENDATIONS

- Outpatient care unless pituitary resection required
- Bromocriptine patients need adequate hydration.

Patient Monitoring

- Varies with cause; check prolactin levels every 6 weeks until normalized, then every 6–12 months
- Monitor visual fields and/or MRI at least yearly until stable.

DIET

No restrictions

PATIENT EDUCATION

- Warn about symptoms of mass enlargement in pituitary.
- Discuss treatment rationale and risks of treating or not.
- Patient education material available from American Family Physician: http://www.aafp.org/afp/20040801/553ph.html

PROGNOSIS

- Depends on underlying cause
- Symptoms can recur after discontinuation of medication.
- Surgery can have 50% recurrence (6).
- Prolactinomas <10 mm can resolve spontaneously.

COMPLICATIONS

- Depends on underlying cause
- If enlarging pituitary adenoma, risk of permanent visual field loss
- Panhypopituitarism can complicate radiation or surgical therapy.
- Osteoporosis if amenorrhea persists without estrogen replacement

REFERENCES

1. Molitch M. Medication-induced hyperprolactinemia. *Mayo Clin Proc Rochester*. 2005;80(8):1050–8.
2. Leung AK, Pacaud D. Diagnosis and management of galactorrhea. *Am Fam Physician*. 2004;70:543–50.
3. Kars M, Pereira A, Bax J, et al. Cabergoline and cardiac valve disease in prolactinoma patients:Additional studies during long-term treatment are required. *Eur J Endocrinol*. 2008.
4. Mancini T, Casanueva FF, Giustina A. Hyperprolactinemia and prolactinomas. *Endocrinol Metab Clin North Am*. 2008;37:67–99.
5. Prabhakar VK, Davis JR. Hyperprolactinaemia. *Best Pract Res Clin Obstet Gynaecol*. 2007.
6. Schlechte JA. Long-term management of prolactinomas. *J Clin Endocrinol Metab*. 2007;92:2861–5.

See Also (Topic, Algorithm, Electronic Media Element)

Hyperprolactinemia

 ## CODES

ICD9

- 611.6 Galactorrhea not associated with childbirth
- 676.60 Galactorrhea associated with childbirth, unspecified as to episode of care

CLINICAL PEARLS

- Galactorrhea is a common disorder, affecting between 1% and 50% of reproductive-age, nonlactating women.
- Lab evaluation of prolactin may be falsely elevated due to recent sexual activity, breast examination, exercise, or high-carbohydrate diet. Repeat any borderline elevation before continuing evaluation or initiating treatment.
- Most cases may be adequately evaluated by thyroid-stimulating hormone, prolactin, and human chorionic gonadotropin measurement, with additional testing as suggested by the presence of other symptoms or signs.
- Evaluate prolactin >200 ng/mL (or suspicion of pituitary macroadenoma) with a gadolinium-enhanced MRI.

G

GAMBLING ADDICTION

Amy Shah, MD
Christopher C. White, MD, JD

 BASICS

DESCRIPTION
Gambling is the act of placing something of value at risk in the hopes of gaining something of greater value. Gambling addiction is an impulse-control disorder ranging in severity from problem gambling to the more severe pathologic gambling (PG). Disordered gambling is a dynamic behavior, and patients frequently move in both directions along the continuum of normal and PG behavior over relatively short time periods. Gambling addiction is further categorized into levels:
- Level 0: Nongamblers
- Level 1: Gambled without adverse consequences
- Level 2: Experienced negative consequences from gambling behavior but do not meet criteria for PG
- Level 3: Gambling meets *Diagnostic and Statistical Manual of Psychological Disorders*, Fourth Edition (DSM-IV), criteria for PG: Persistent and recurrent maladaptive gambling behavior indicated by ≥5 DSM-IV criteria.
- Level 4: Seeking help for gambling addiction regardless of degree of gambling addiction

EPIDEMIOLOGY
- Predominant sex: Male > Female
- The younger the person starts gambling, the more likely he or she is to become a pathologic gambler.
- A higher likelihood exists if parents have PG.
- Family history of substance abuse and mental disorders

Incidence
There are limited incidence studies, but some research states that the number of people affected by gambling addiction remains stable over time.

Prevalence
- According to the National Gambling Impact Study Commission, prevalence of problem and pathologic gambling was 1.7–7.3% of adults in the 17 states where surveys were done.
- 0.2–2.1% of the world's population meets diagnostic criteria for level 3 pathologic gamblers, with prevalence changing little over time.

GENERAL PREVENTION
Focus on treatment, patient education, and awareness of risk factors, associated conditions, and warning signs of pathologic or problematic gambling behaviors.

RISK FACTORS
- Some types of gambling present a greater risk to cause PG than other types: pull tabs, casino gambling, and bingo and cards outside a casino.
- Being involved with several gaming modalities is related to PG and suggests that the gambler is very captivated with risking money for excitement as opposed to risking money for social pleasure or for an interest in sports.
- Alcohol abuse and dependence are correlated with problem gambling.
- Lower socioeconomic status positively correlates with increased gambling pathology because these persons have few financial resources and cannot recover as easily from losses. Persons even may believe that gambling is a way to ease their financial burden.

Genetics
SLC6A4 serotonin transporter gene has been associated with PG in males but not females.

PATHOPHYSIOLOGY
- The brains of pathologic gamblers may have some predisposition to illness. Functional MRI studies indicate that the ventromedial prefrontal cortex is less activated when gambling stimuli are presented to pathologic gamblers.
- Abnormalities in the neurotransmitters serotonin, norepinephrine, dopamine, and glutamate may be implicated in PG.
  - Norepinephrine: Still unclear but plays a part in arousal or excitement
  - Serotonin: Involved in impulse control
  - Dopamine: May induce reversible PG in Parkinson patients who take dopamine agonists

COMMONLY ASSOCIATED CONDITIONS
- Poor nutrition
- Stress-related medical conditions (e.g., PUD, hypertension, migraine)
- Suicidal ideation and attempts
- Substance abuse disorder
- Attention deficit–hyperactivity disorder (ADHD)
- Bipolar disorder and other mood disorders
- Impulse-control disorders
- Personality disorders
- Incarceration
- Financial problems

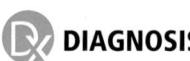 **DIAGNOSIS**

DSM-IV criteria for PG:
- Persistent and recurrent maladaptive gambling behavior, as indicated by five or more of the following:
  - Preoccupation with gambling
  - Need to gamble with increasing amounts of money to achieve the desired excitement
  - Repeated unsuccessful efforts to control, cut back, or stop gambling
  - Restless or irritable when attempting to cut down or stop gambling
  - Gambles as a way of escaping from problems or of relieving a dysphoric mood
  - After losing money gambling, often returns another day to get even
  - Lies to family members, therapist, or others to conceal the extent of involvement with gambling
  - Has committed illegal acts such as forgery, fraud, theft, or embezzlement to finance gambling
  - Has jeopardized or lost a significant relationship, job, or educational or career opportunity because of gambling
  - Relies on others to provide money to relieve a desperate financial situation caused by gambling
- The gambling behavior is not better accounted for by a manic episode.

HISTORY
- Preoccupation with gambling
- Preoccupation with money
- Unexplained new financial problems
- New participation in illegal or dishonest money-making endeavors or activities
- Disruptions in personal life or career
- Patient may ask his or her family and friends to pay off his or her debts ("bailing them out").

DIAGNOSTIC TESTS & INTERPRETATION
- Lie/bet method: Have you ever had to lie to people important to you about how much you gambled? Have you ever felt a need to bet more money?
  - A patient who answers at least one question with a "Yes" screens positively for PG.
  - This test has been shown to have >85% specificity and >95% sensitivity (1).
- South Oaks Gambling Screen (SOGS):
  - 20-question screen for PG
  - Score of 3–4 suggests problem gambling.
  - Score of 5 or more indicates probable PG.
  - Criticized as overestimating the number of pathologic gamblers and being too lengthy to administer (2)[B].
- Gamblers Anonymous 20 questions:
  - Easily obtainable from Gamblers Anonymous Web site
  - Scores of >7 are indicative of problem/PG.

Imaging
- Neuroimaging research indicates that the neural structures of the mesolimbic pathway are involved in PG, including the orbitofrontal cortex, amygdala, and ventral striatum/nucleus accumbens.
- There are some data to suggest the idea that because there is lower activity in the ventral striatum when receiving a reward in PG, these patients have decreased sensitivity to reward.

DIFFERENTIAL DIAGNOSIS
- Social gambling
- Professional gambling
- Bipolar disorder, manic episode
- Substance use disorder
- Personality disorder

 TREATMENT

In order to treat PG, treat the comorbidities first. The usual comorbid disorders are substance abuse, bipolar disorder, ADHD, and other impulse-control disorders. There is no Food and Drug Administration (FDA)–approved therapy for PG. Nonpharmacologic therapies are more effective than pharmacologic therapies. There are some data suggesting that gambling abstinence is not necessary for treatment; patients still can exhibit controlled gambling.

MEDICATION
- Selective serotonin reuptake inhibitors (SSRIs):
  - Beneficial for treating comorbid impulse-control disorders
  - Used to treat gambling addiction because of link with serotonergic dysfunction: Some studies show that low levels of serotonin cause a suppression of inhibitory responses.
  - Citalopram (Celexa) has shown significant improvement on all gambling measures, including number of days gambled, urge to gamble, and preoccupation with gambling. Celexa is also a low-cost medication with few drug interactions.
  - Fluvoxamine (Luvox) has been shown to be effective in a short-term acute trial as well.
  - Use of paroxetine (Paxil) in PG needs further studies.
- Modafinil helps pathologic gamblers with high impulsivity but increases gambling behavior in low-impulsivity pathologic gamblers. Modafinil shows decreases in motivation to gamble, risky decision making, and impulsivity in high-impulsivity pathologic gamblers (3)[B].
- Valproate and carbamazepine, as well as lithium carbonate, are effective treatments (3)[A].
- Opiate antagonists have the ability to decrease dopamine release in the dopamine reward pathway. Naltrexone and nalmefene are efficacious for PG and reduce urges to gamble. Positive family history of alcoholism predicted a positive response to opiate antagonist treatment (3).
- Selected antipsychotics have been shown to be ineffective in PG (i.e., olanzapine is not efficacious for the treatment of PG, and haloperidol may increase the desire to gamble in pathological gamblers) (3)[B].
- N-acetylcysteine (NAC), a glutamate-modulating agent, causes significant improvements in gambling thoughts and behaviors.

ADDITIONAL TREATMENT
- Patients are often forced to come in for treatment after an ultimatum, such as threat of divorce or prosecution.
- Patients' personal characteristics (i.e., pride, denial, or impatience) can hinder therapy.
- Additionally, pathologic gamblers may leave when therapy does not work fast enough.
- Mental health workers must avoid negative transference.
- Because of increased suicide rates, patients may need to be hospitalized acutely for safety and to prevent gambling.
- Since patients are at increased risk from mental and physical illness, they benefit from relaxation exercises to reduce stress, identify triggers, substitute gambling with other activities, and a complete physical and lab work with nutrition evaluation.

General Measures
- Get a sense of the patient's readiness for change.
- Provide intervention/patient education. While there are no FDA-approved drug treatments for PG, make clinically based medication recommendations.
- Screen for and treat comorbid conditions.

- Provide referrals:
  - Addiction psychiatrist/counselor
  - Gamblers Anonymous
  - Consumer credit organizations
  - Bankruptcy lawyers
  - Gam-Anon for family members

Additional Therapies
- Cognitive-behavioral therapy (CBT):
  - The main effective interventions for CBT are psychoeducation, cognitive restructuring, problem solving, social skills training, and relapse prevention. Studies indicated that CBT resulted in significant improvement for short-term therapy (4)[A].
  - CBT may be done in several formats: Individual, group, brief group, and dual diagnosis. All these formats have been shown to be effective. Group therapy is favored because patients are often extroverted. Couple or family therapy also may be used.
- Gamblers Anonymous:
  - A 12-step program similar to Alcoholics Anonymous for a person suffering from a gambling addiction
  - Dropout rate is high if this is the only means of therapy (1)[B].
  - Patients may deny need to attend in the 1st place, and for that reason, Gamblers Anonymous may not be appropriate for patients who are in the precontemplation stage.
- Motivational enhancement therapy (MET):
  - Provides nonargumentative exploration of patient's stage of change
  - Patient receives positive reinforcement from clinician.
  - Motivational enhancement strategies support self-efficacy.
  - Improves patient rapport; aids in removing barriers to treatment
  - In one study, MET alone did not show any improvement, but MET and CBT together improved outcome measures (3)[B].

 ONGOING CARE

FOLLOW-UP RECOMMENDATIONS
Patients seeking treatment for gambling addiction should be followed routinely by physicians and counselors to monitor the response to treatment, tolerance to medications, and possibility of relapse.

PATIENT EDUCATION
- Gamblers Anonymous:
  - http://www.gamblersanonymous.org
  - National hotline 1-888-GA-HELPS (888-424-3577)
- Gam-Anon: Support group for spouses, family, or close friends of compulsive gamblers: http://www/gam-anon.org
- Responsible Gambling Council: http://www.responsiblegambling.org
- Humphrey H. This Must Be Hell: A Look at Pathological Gambling. IUniverse, 2000.
- Lee B. Born to Lose: Memoirs of a Compulsive Gambler. Hazelden, 2005.

PROGNOSIS
- Patients with gambling addiction can be treated, but many relapse.
- 36–39% of patients did not experience any gambling-related problems according to one study, and only 7–12% sought formal treatment or Gamblers Anonymous meetings.
- Roughly 1/3 of patients who have a gambling addiction recover without any intervention.

REFERENCES

1. Potenza MN, Fiellin DA, Heninger GR, et al. Gambling: an addictive behavior with health and primary care implications. *J Gen Intern Med*. 2002;17:721–32.
2. Rossow I and Molde H. Chasing the criteria: comparing SOGS-RA and the Lie/Bet screen to assess prevalence of problem gambling and "at-risk" gambling among adolescents. *Journal of Gambling Issues*. 2006;(18):57–71.
3. Leung KS, Cottler LB. Treatment of pathological gambling. *Curr Opin Psychiatry*. 2009;22:69–74.
4. Hodgins DC, Peden N. Cognitive-behavioral treatment for impulse control disorders. *Rev Bras Psiquiatr*. 2007.

ADDITIONAL READING
- Brewer JA, Potenza MN. The neurobiology and genetics of impulse control disorders: Relationships to drug addictions. *Biochem Pharmacol*. 2007.
- Potenza MN. Review. The neurobiology of pathological gambling and drug addiction: an overview and new findings. *Philos Trans R Soc Lond B Biol Sci*. 2008.

CODES

ICD9
- 312.31 Pathological gambling
- V69.3 Gambling and betting

CLINICAL PEARLS
- There are several brief screening strategies that can be used to identify PG, including the lie/bet method, the SOGS, and the Gamblers Anonymous 20 questions.
- To treat PG, 1st treat comorbidities such as substance abuse, bipolar disorder, ADHD, and other impulse-control disorders.
- Nonpharmacologic therapies are more effective than pharmacologic therapies. There is no FDA-approved therapy for PG.
- Patients seeking treatment for gambling addiction should be followed routinely by physicians and counselors to monitor the response to treatment, tolerance to medications, and possibility of relapse.

GANGLION CYST

Christopher Garofalo, MD

BASICS

- Ganglions are common benign tumors.
- Can be located throughout the body and usually located adjacent to joints and tendons, mostly on wrist, foot, ankle
- Average size is 3 cm.
- Most are not symptomatic except for changing size.

EPIDEMIOLOGY
- Can affect all age groups but unusual in children
- Most common in young adults
- Mucous cysts are usually seen in older patients.
- Hand and wrist ganglions are commonly seen in dorsal wrist, radial wrist, and dorsum of the DIP joint (which is referred to as a mucous cyst).
- 60–70% of hand and wrist ganglions are in dorsal wrist, 15–20% are at the volar wrist.

Prevalence
- Prevalence of wrist ganglia in patients presenting with wrist pain has been reported as 19%.
- Prevalence of ganglia in patients with a palpable mass in the wrist has been reported as 27%.

RISK FACTORS
- No specific risk factors
- No known occupational risk factors

PATHOPHYSIOLOGY
Pathogenesis is unclear. Several theories:
- Herniation of synovial lining creating a one-way valve; this is supported by dye studies that show communication of fluid from the wrist joint into the cyst but not from the cyst to the joint.
- Ganglions are benign tumors of synovium. However, pathologic analysis of surgical specimens from ganglion excision do not show a synovial lining, which brings these theories into question.
- A rent in the joint capsule or tendon sheath allows synovial fluid to leak, irritating surrounding tissue, which creates a pseudocapsule and ganglion and would explain why no lining is seen on pathology.
- Mucoid degeneration of collagen fibers in the joint with the collagen products forming a pool of hyaluronic acid and then a cyst
- Recurrent stress and microtrauma at the synovial-capsular interface may stimulate mucin production by mesenchymal cells or fibroblasts.

ETIOLOGY
- Etiology is unknown.
- May be associated with trauma but majority of patients cannot recall specific trauma

COMMONLY ASSOCIATED CONDITIONS
Mucous cysts are usually associated with some level of osteoarthritis of DIP joint.

DIAGNOSIS

- Usually made on basis of history and physical examination
- Patients usually present when there is pain, increased size, interference with activities, or weakness.

HISTORY
- Patients usually present with asymptomatic mass present for months or years, decreasing and increasing in size.
- Mostly asymptomatic but can be associated with pain, limitations in activity.
- 1/3 of patients presenting with ganglion cyst elected for surgical intervention (1).

PHYSICAL EXAM
- Mass is compressible, subcutaneous, transilluminating, slightly mobile; no overlying skin changes.
- Extension of wrist often elicits pain at the site.
- Small ganglions may only be palpable in full wrist flexion.
- Occult ganglions are not palpable but can be quite painful.

DIAGNOSTIC TESTS & INTERPRETATION
Most ganglions do not require imaging to confirm diagnosis unless unclear wrist pain presents.

Imaging
- Several options:
  – Ultrasound
  – MRI
  – Bone scintigraphy, arthroscopy
- Ultrasound and MRI have similar rates of sensitivity and specificity.
- Scintigraphy is less specific.
- Ultrasound is less expensive than MRI but more operator-dependent.
- Arthroscopy is both diagnostic and therapeutic but should be considered when initial workup is nondiagnostic and conservative treatment effective.

Initial approach
Most are apparent clinically and do not need imaging

Pathological Findings
- Gross pathologic evaluation shows that cysts are often multilobulated.
- Microscopic exam reveals outer wall w/several layers of randomly oriented collagen fibers, relatively acellular with a few fibroblasts and mesenchymal cells in the collagen fibers.
- As pathology does not show an epithelial lining it is therefore not a true cyst.
- Fluid contains glucosamine, albumin, globulin, hyaluronic acid.
- Ganglions are histopathologically identical regardless of anatomic location.

DIFFERENTIAL DIAGNOSIS
- A mobile mass of extensor tendons of wrist may be a ganglion or tendon sheath, giant cell tumor, tenosynovitis from infection or inflammation.
- Other tumors include lipoma, sarcoma, hamartoma, interosseous neuroma.
- Firm mass may represent osteophyte.

TREATMENT

3 primary treatment options (2):
- Reassurance that ganglia is not likely to be malignant or to cause damage, and observation; 33% dorsal ganglions and 45% volar ganglions resolve spontaneously by 6 years, up to 80% of ganglion in children resolve.
- Closed rupture, historically by hitting cyst with a book; results in initial decreased clinical symptoms by 22–66% but often leads to recurrence
- Aspiration can be done in an office under local anesthesia with 18-gauge or larger needle.
- Studies demonstrate mixed results on aspirations of a ganglion; evidence supporting injecting steroids is weak, and splinting after the procedure may help cure rate but recurrence may be as high as 80% after single aspiration. This can be reduced to 20% with multiple aspirations.
- Volar ganglion are not aspirated due to risk of neurovascular structures:
  – Mucous cysts can be aspirated but recurrence is over 50% and pain may not resolve if it is due to underlying osteoarthritis.
- Surgical excision

- 6-year study comparing aspiration to surgery to watchful waiting found:
  - Recurrence rates: 58% after aspiration, 39% after surgery, and 58% in untreated patients;
  - Satisfaction: 81% aspiration, 83% surgery, and 53% who were reassured, a significant difference
  - Persistent pain: 23% of patients who were satisfied vs 45% who were unsatisfied
  - No significant difference seen in pain, weakness, or stiffness between groups
  - Significant improvement in pain was seen in all groups.
  - Authors conclude that neither aspiration nor surgical excision provides a clear long-term benefit over the natural history of wrist ganglion, and the only benefit of surgery is early resolution of the appearance of the ganglia (3)[C].
- Bottom line:
  - Surgical excision yields less risk of recurrence but similar rates of pain, weakness, stiffness as aspiration or reassurance.
  - Patient satisfaction is higher with excision or aspiration; however, longer time out of work is seen with excision compared with aspiration and reassurance.

SURGERY/OTHER PROCEDURES

- Risks of surgery include:
  - Cosmesis, functioning
  - Sensory and motor dysfunction
  - Infection
  - Joint instability
- 2 methods:
  - Arthroscopic compared to open excision: After 1 year, approximately 10% had recurrence; no significant difference in surgical approaches (4)[C].

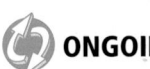 ## ONGOING CARE

May require supervised hand therapy after surgical repair to aid in pain reduction, improve stiffness and function

FOLLOW-UP RECOMMENDATIONS

- Hand therapy may be helpful if ganglion symptoms persist despite rest.
- Improved resolution rates with multiple aspirations
- Splinting is often used after surgical repair and follow-up with orthopedics occurs for several weeks; hand therapy may be indicated for residual symptoms.

PROGNOSIS

- Very good
- Up to 50% will resolve with watchful waiting.
- Higher rate of resolution in children

COMPLICATIONS

- Risk of recurrence is present regardless of treatment; no specific recommendations to minimize this risk.
- Risks of surgical excision include:
  - Residual pain
  - Poor cosmesis
  - Neuropathy
  - Stiffness and instability of the wrist, especially scapholunate ligament instability; also may require open excision if arthroscopic fails to resolve symptoms

REFERENCES

1. Wong AS, Jebson PJ, Murray PM, et al. The Use of Routine Wrist Radiography is Not Useful in the Evaluation of Patients with a Ganglion Cyst of the Wrist. *Hand*. 2007;2:117–9.
2. Thommasen HV. Management of the occassional wrist ganglion. *Can J Rural Med*. 2006;11:51–53.
3. Dias JJ, Dhukaram V, Kumar P. The natural history of untreated dorsal wrist ganglia and patient reported outcome 6 years after intervention. *J Hand Surg Eur*. 2007;32:502–8.
4. Kang L, Akelman E, Weiss AP. Arthroscopic versus open dorsal ganglion excision: a prospective, randomized comparison of rates of recurrence and of residual pain. *J Hand Surg [Am]*. 2008;33:471–5.

ADDITIONAL READING

- Dias J, Buch K. Palmar wrist ganglion: does intervention improve outcome? A prospective study of the natural history and patient-reported treatment outcomes. *J Hand Surg [Br]*. 2003;28:172–6.
- Goldsmith S, Yang SS. Magnetic resonance imaging in the diagnosis of occult dorsal wrist ganglions. *J Hand Surg Eur Vol*. 2008;33:595–9.
- Lowden CM, Attiah M, Garvin G, et al. The prevalence of wrist ganglia in an asymptomatic population: magnetic resonance evaluation. *J Hand Surg [Br]*. 2005;30:302–6.

- Lowden CM et al. The prevalence of wrist ganglia in an asymptomatic population: Magnetic resonance evaluation. *Journal of Hand Surgery*. 2005;30B:3: 302–6.
- Rizzo M, Berger RA, Steinmann SP, et al. Arthroscopic resection in the management of dorsal wrist ganglions: results with a minimum 2-year follow-up period. *J Hand Surg [Am]*. 2004;29:59–62.
- Thornburg LE. Ganglions of the hand and wrist. *J Am Acad Orthop Surg*. 1999;7:231–8.

See Also (Topic, Algorithm, Electronic Media Element)

Algorithm: Pain in Upper Extremity

 ## CODES

ICD9

- 727.41 Ganglion of joint
- 727.42 Ganglion of tendon sheath
- 727.43 Ganglion, unspecified

CLINICAL PEARLS

- Ganglia are the most common masses in the wrist and are not true cysts.
- Typical history and examination will make the diagnosis in most cases; plain films are expensive and not indicated.
- Can consider MRI or ultrasound if occult ganglion is suspected
- Available treatment options have similar rates of recurrence and symptoms over 6 years, so watchful waiting is indicated initially. Refer to orthopedics when ganglion causes symptoms, limits function.
- Bottom line:
  - Surgical excision yields less risk of recurrence but similar rates of pain, weakness, stiffness as aspiration or reassurance.
  - Patient satisfaction is higher with excision or aspiration; however, longer time out of work is seen with excision compared with aspiration and reassurance.

G

GASTRIC MALIGNANCY

Scott T. Henderson, MD

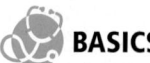 **BASICS**

DESCRIPTION
- May occur anywhere in the stomach
- Infiltration to lymph nodes, omentum, lungs, and liver is rapid.
- Uncommon in US natives
- Synonym(s): Linitis plastica

Pediatric Considerations
Rare

Pregnancy Considerations
- Rarely diagnosed during pregnancy
- Prognosis is poor if diagnosed.

EPIDEMIOLOGY
- Predominant age: >55 (2/3 >65)
- Predominant gender: Male > Female (1.7:1)
- Incidence is decreasing globally, but it remains the 2nd leading cause of cancer death.

Incidence
- 5.9/100,000 males (North America)
- 2.5/100,000 females (North America)
- 21,130 new cases per year (US)

RISK FACTORS
- *Helicobacter pylori* infection
- Achlorhydria
- Atrophic gastritis/intestinal metaplasia
- Pernicious anemia
- Prior gastric resection
- Polyps or dysplasia anywhere in alimentary canal
- Familial polyposis
- Barrett esophagus
- Smoking/tobacco abuse
- Patients in lower socioeconomic classes are at greater risk of developing gastric tumors.
- Diet rich in additives (e.g., smoked, pickled, or salted foods; highly spiced Asian foods)
- Low consumption of fruits and vegetables
- Overweight and obesity; strength of association increases with increasing BMI (1)[A]
- Ethnic background: Hispanic, Japanese, Chilean, Costa Rican:
  - Migrants from high-incidence areas (e.g., Iceland, Chile, or Japan) to low-incidence areas maintain an increased risk, whereas their offspring have an occurrence rate that corresponds to that of the new location.

Genetics
- More common in people with blood group A
- 2–4 times more common in 1st-degree relatives
- 1–3% of gastric cancers are associated with inherited gastric cancer predisposition syndromes, known as hereditary diffuse gastric cancer.

GENERAL PREVENTION
- A healthy lifestyle (not smoking, not consuming excess alcohol, avoiding obesity, and maintaining a good diet) is associated with reduced risk of gastric cancer:
  - Diets including 5–20 servings of both fruits and vegetables each week reduce the risk of gastric malignancy by ~1/2.
- Insufficient data to establish that screening would decrease mortality in US population
- Screening may be of benefit in high-prevalence areas.

ETIOLOGY
Unknown

COMMONLY ASSOCIATED CONDITIONS
- Giant hypertrophic gastritis (Ménétrier disease)
- Intestinal metaplasia of the stomach
- Atrophic gastritis
- *H. pylori* infection

 DIAGNOSIS

HISTORY

> **ALERT**
> - Symptoms present late in the course.
> - Anorexia/weight loss (70–80%)
> - Cachexia
> - Early satiety
> - Nausea and vomiting
> - Change in bowel habits
> - Chronic noncolicky abdominal pain (especially in epigastrium):
>   - Ranges from postprandial fullness to severe steady pain (70%)
>   - Unrelieved by antacids
>   - Exacerbated by food
>   - Relieved by fasting
> - Gross GI bleeding (10%)
> - Dysphagia (rare)

PHYSICAL EXAM
- Abdominal palpation for masses and/or ascites
- Palpation for lymph nodes:
  - Left supraclavicular node (Virchow)
  - Sister Mary Joseph nodule at umbilicus
- Assess for jaundice

DIAGNOSTIC TESTS & INTERPRETATION
Lab
Initial lab tests
- CBC and platelet count:
  - Hemoglobin <12 g/dL (1.86 mmol/L)
  - Hematocrit <35 (0.35)
- Serum chemistry analysis:
  - Albumin 3.0 g/dL
- Coagulation studies
- *H. pylori* testing
- Stool guaiac

Follow-Up & Special Considerations
Pentagastrin test (stomach pH <6):
- Pernicious anemia may cause a false-positive pentagastrin test.

Imaging
Initial approach
CT scan of chest and abdomen with intravenous contrast and gastric distension with oral contrast or water should be performed routinely (2)[B].

Follow-Up & Special Considerations
In females, consider pelvic ultrasound or CT scan.

Diagnostic Procedures/Surgery
- Upper endoscopy for direct visualization, cytology, and biopsy
- Endoscopic ultrasound is most accurate preoperative staging tool.
- Laparoscopy may be useful in select patients for staging (3)[C].

Pathological Findings
- Adenocarcinomas: 90% (Types: Intestinal and diffuse [linitis plastica])
- Gastric lymphomas, sarcomas, and other rare types: 10%

DIFFERENTIAL DIAGNOSIS
- Angiodysplasia of the colon
- Carcinoma of body or tail of the pancreas
- Carcinoma of the colon
- Crohn disease
- Eosinophilic gastroenteritis
- Functional dyspepsia
- Gastric lymphoma
- Giant hypertrophic gastritis
- GI sarcoidosis
- Peptic ulcer with or without hemorrhage
- Small intestinal lymphoma

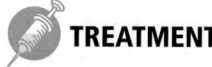 **TREATMENT**

MEDICATION
First Line
Combination chemotherapy improves survival compared to single-agent 5-FU (4)[A]:
- Among the combination chemotherapy regimens studied, best survival results are achieved with regimens containing 5-FU, anthracyclines, and cisplatin.
- In this category, epirubicin, cisplatin, and continuous-infusion 5-FU are tolerated best.

Second Line
- Ondansetron (Zofran), dronabinol (Marinol), metoclopramide (Reglan), and others for nausea control
- Pain control with opioids

ADDITIONAL TREATMENT
General Measures
- Multidisciplinary treatment is mandatory.
- Surgical excision of the tumor is only potentially curative option:
  – Extent of lymph nodes resection is controversial (5)[B].
  – Endoscopic mucosal resection for early gastric cancer and high-grade dysplasia may be curative.
  – Even patients with incurable lesions should be offered an attempt at surgical reduction of the tumor:
    ○ Surgical reduction offers the best form of palliation and improves the likelihood of benefit if chemotherapy and/or radiation therapy is administered.
- Adjuvant chemotherapy may provide benefit compared to surgery alone (4)[A].
- Compared to best supportive care, chemotherapy significantly improves survival.
- Radiation therapy:
  – Used in combination with surgery and/or chemotherapy
  – Little benefit when used alone because of the radiation resistance of gastric tumors
  – Does have use in the palliation of pain, bleeding, and obstruction

Issues for Referral
Referral to a high-volume surgery center is usually indicated.

Additional Therapies
- The neoadjuvant use of radiotherapy is not recommended outside clinical trials.
- Role of treatment with anti-HER2 monoclonal antibodies being studied based on the evidence of HER2 overexpression in gastric cancer

COMPLEMENTARY AND ALTERNATIVE MEDICINE
Commonly used but with little supportive evidence

SURGERY/OTHER PROCEDURES
- Radical subtotal gastrectomy with gastrojejunostomy or gastroduodenostomy is the usual treatment of choice:
  – Large part of the stomach along with the greater and lesser omentum is removed en bloc.
  – Splenectomy or distal pancreatectomy is also sometimes performed.
  – Direct extensions also excised
- Total gastrectomy indicated only if necessary to remove the local lesion
- Local excision, endoscopic laser therapy, or electrocautery for palliation of incurable lesion by resection of bleeding area or area of obstruction

IN-PATIENT CONSIDERATIONS
Admission Criteria
- Inpatient care common, but depends on stage at time of diagnosis
- Most of the follow-up treatment is outpatient.

 ONGOING CARE

FOLLOW-UP RECOMMENDATIONS
Routine, frequent follow-up to monitor disease state, assess treatments, monitor for recurrence/metastasis, and assess nutritional status

Patient Monitoring
Monitor vitamin B_{12} and iron levels following surgical resection; supplement if indicated.

DIET
- Patients at high nutritional risk should be considered for preoperative nutritional support.
- All patients undergoing surgery should be considered for early postoperative nutritional support:
  – Enteral route preferred
  – Consider placement of jejunostomy feeding tube.

PATIENT EDUCATION
- Contact local the American Cancer Society.
- Cancer Research Institute Helpbook: What to Do If Cancer Strikes. FDR Station, Box 5199, New York, NY 10150–5199.

PROGNOSIS
- Because most lesions do not produce symptoms until late in course, gastric carcinomas are usually advanced at the time of diagnosis.
- Overall 5-year relative survival rate is 24% (if local disease 61%, regional spread 24%, distant spread 3%).
- Early gastric cancers are usually detected as incidental findings or when screening endoscopy is performed in endemic areas.
- Primary gastric lymphoma is more treatable than gastric adenocarcinoma:
  – 5-year survival rate is 40–60% with subtotal gastrectomy followed by combination chemotherapy.

COMPLICATIONS
- Early lymphatic spread
- Aggressive metastatic disease (especially hepatic, cerebral, peritoneum, and pulmonary)
- Anemia (especially pernicious)
- Pyloric stenosis
- Dumping syndrome may occur following gastric surgery.

REFERENCES

1. Yang P, Zhou Y, Chen B, et al. Overweight, obesity and gastric cancer risk: Results from a meta-analysis of cohort studies. *Eur J Cancer.* 2009.
2. Scottish Intercollegiate Guidelines Network (SIGN). Management of oesophageal and gastric cancer. A national clinical guideline. Edinburgh (Scotland): Scottish Intercollegiate Guidelines Network (SIGN); 2006 Jun.
3. Sarela AI, Lefkowitz R, Brennan MF, et al. Selection of patients with gastric adenocarcinoma for laparoscopic staging. *Am J Surg.* 2006;191:134–8.
4. Wagner AD, Unverzagt S, Grothe W, Kleber G, Grothey A, Haerting J, Fleig WE et al. Chemotherapy for advanced gastric cancer. *Cochrane Database Syst Rev.* 2010;3:CD004064.
5. McCulloch P, et al. Extended versus limited lymph nodes dissection technique for adenocarcinoma of the stomach (Cochrane Review). In: *The Cochrane Library*, Issue 4. Chichester, UK: John Wiley and Sons, 2005.

ADDITIONAL READING

- Clark CJ, Thirlby RC, Picozzi V, et al. Current problems in surgery: gastric cancer. *Curr Probl Surg.* 2006;43:566–670.
- Khushalani N. Cancer of the esophagus and stomach. *Mayo Clin Proc.* 2008;83:712–22.
- Maconi G, Manes G, Porro GB. Role of symptoms in diagnosis and outcome of gastric cancer. *World J Gastroenterol.* 2008;14:1149–55.
- Wagner AD, et al. Chemotherapy for advanced gastric cancer (Cochrane Review). In: *The Cochrane Library*, Issue 4. Chichester, UK, 2005.
- Wagner AD, Moehler M. Gastric cancer: development of targeted therapies in advanced disease. *Curr Opin Oncol.* 2009.
- Wang YP, et al. Endoscopic mucosal resection for early gastric cancer. In: *The Cochrane Library*, Issue 1. Chichester, UK: John Wiley and Sons, 2006.

See Also (Topic, Algorithm, Electronic Media Element)
Multiple Endocrine Neoplasia (MEN)

 CODES

ICD9
- 151.0 Malignant neoplasm of cardia
- 151.1 Malignant neoplasm of pylorus
- 151.9 Malignant neoplasm of stomach, unspecified site

CLINICAL PEARLS
- Accurate preoperative staging is necessary to enhance survival.
- Endoscopic ultrasound is the most accurate preoperative staging tool.
- To enhance survival therapy with surgery, combination chemotherapy and radiation is necessary.

G

GASTRITIS

Michelle Whitehurst-Cook, MD

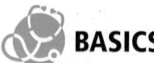 **BASICS**

DESCRIPTION

Inflammatory reaction in the stomach. Typically involves the mucosa; seldom the full thickness of the stomach wall:

- Patchy erythema of gastric mucosa: A common endoscopic finding; usually insignificant
- Erosive gastritis: A reaction to mucosal injury by a noxious chemical agent (e.g., drugs [especially NSAIDs] or alcohol)
- Reflux gastritis:
  - A reaction to protracted reflux exposure to bile and pancreatic juice, usually associated with a defective pylorus
  - Typically limited to the prepyloric antrum
- Hemorrhagic gastritis (stress ulceration):
  - A reaction to hemodynamic disorder (e.g., hypovolemia or hypoxia [as in shock])
  - Also common in ICUs
  - Seen after severe burns
  - Seen after significant physical trauma
- Infectious gastritis:
  - Commonly associated with *Helicobacter pylori* (possibly causative, maybe opportunistic)
  - Viral infection, usually as a component of systemic infection, is common.
  - Significant infection by other specific microbes is rare.
- Gastric mucosal atrophy, sometimes called atrophic gastritis:
  - Frequent, in varying degrees, in the elderly
  - Invariable in primary (pernicious) anemia
  - Autoimmune disease
- Synonym(s): Erosive gastritis; Reflux gastritis; Hemorrhagic gastritis; Acute gastritis
- Neutrophil cellular infiltration in acute gastritis
- Patches of lymphoid follicles noted in chronic gastritis, along with plasma cells and macrophages; antibodies to parietal cells and intrinsic factor
- More than 50% of humans are colonized with *H. pylori*.

Geriatric Considerations
Persons >60 often harbor *H. pylori* infection.

Pediatric Considerations
Gastritis rarely occurs in infants or children.

EPIDEMIOLOGY

- Predominant age: All ages
- Predominant sex: Male = Female

RISK FACTORS

- Age >60
- Exposure to potentially noxious drugs or chemical agents, including alcohol or NSAIDS
- Hypovolemia, hypoxia (shock)
- Autoimmune diseases (thyroid and diabetes mellitus I)
- Family history of *H. pylori* and/or gastric cancer

Genetics
Unknown

GENERAL PREVENTION

- Patients should be warned of known or potentially injurious drugs or chemical agents.
- Patients liable to hypovolemia or hypoxia (especially patients confined to an intensive care ward) should receive prophylactic therapy with antacids.
- H_2 receptor antagonists, prostaglandins, or sucralfate used frequently in the ICU, burn and trauma victims
- Consider testing for *H. pylori* (and eradicating if present) in patients facing long-term NSAID therapy (1)[A].

ETIOLOGY

- Bacterial infection (e.g., *H. pylori*) most common cause
- Alcohol
- Aspirin and other NSAIDs
- Bile reflux
- Pancreatic enzyme reflux
- Stress (hypovolemia or hypoxia)
- Radiation
- *Staphylococcus aureus* exotoxins
- Viral infection
- Pernicious anemia
- Gastric mucosal atrophy
- Portal HTN gastropathy
- Emotional stress

COMMONLY ASSOCIATED CONDITIONS

- Gastric or duodenal peptic ulcer
- Primary (pernicious) anemia
- Portal HTN
- Development of gastric lymphoma linked to the lymphoid follicles

 DIAGNOSIS

HISTORY

- Nondescript epigastric distress, often aggravated by eating, often severe, burning
- Anorexia
- Nausea, with or without vomiting
- Significant bleeding is unusual except in hemorrhagic gastritis.
- Hiccups
- Bloating or abdominal fullness

PHYSICAL EXAM

- Mild epigastric tenderness
- May have heme-positive stool
- Stool may be black in color.

DIAGNOSTIC TESTS & INTERPRETATION

- Special tests:
- ^{13}C-urea breath test for *H. pylori* (not widely available)
- Serologic test available for *H. pylori,* serum IgG (office and clinical laboratory); inexpensive
- Gastric acid analysis may be abnormal, but is not a reliable indicator of gastritis.

Lab
- Usually unremarkable, except when blood loss results in anemia
- Drugs that may alter lab results: Antibiotics or omeprazole may affect urea breath test for *H. pylori*.

Imaging
Nuclear scintigraphy is not done clinically.

Diagnostic Procedures/Surgery
Gastroscopy, usually with biopsy, is essential for a precise diagnosis. (Recommended if there is a poor response to the initial treatment.)

Pathological Findings
Acute or chronic inflammatory infiltrate in gastric mucosa, often with distortion or erosion of adjacent epithelium. Presence of *H. pylori* may be confirmed.

DIFFERENTIAL DIAGNOSIS

- Functional gastrointestinal disorder
- Peptic ulcer disease
- Linitis plastica
- Viral gastroenteritis
- Pancreatic disease
- Gastric cancer (elderly)
- Cholecystitis
- Pancreatic disease (inflammation vs tumor)

TREATMENT

MEDICATION

- Antacids: Best given in liquid form, 30 mL 1 hour after meals and at bedtime; useful mainly as an emollient
- H_2 receptor antagonists (e.g., cimetidine [Tagamet]): Oral cimetidine 300 mg q6h (or ranitidine [Zantac] or famotidine [Pepcid] or nizatidine [Axid]). Not shown to be clearly superior to antacids (2)[C]:
  – For severely ill patients: "Priming" dose of 300 mg IV, then a steady infusion of 37.5–75 mg per hour, dissolved in the running fluid
- Sucralfate (Carafate): 1 g q4–6h on an empty stomach; rationale uncertain, but empirically helpful
- Prostaglandins (e.g., misoprostol [Cytotec]): Can help allay gastric mucosal injury, suggested dosage of 100–200 mcg q.i.d.
- PPIs may be used if there is no response to antacids or H_2 receptor blockers
- To eradicate *H. pylori*:
  – "Quadruple therapy" is advised: PPI plus bismuth (Pepto-Bismol) 30 mL liquid or 2 tablets q.i.d. for 4 weeks plus metronidazole 250 mg q.i.d. for the 1st week, plus tetracycline 250 mg q.i.d. or amoxicillin 250 mg t.i.d. for 2–4 weeks has equal efficacy of "triple therapy" with PPI plus clarithromycin 500 mg b.i.d. for 2 weeks plus amoxicillin 250 mg t.i.d. for 2 weeks:
    ○ "Quadruple therapy" yields similar eradication rates to "triple therapy" (3)[A].
  – "Dual therapy" with omeprazole 20 mg b.i.d. plus amoxicillin 500 mg q.i.d. for 2 weeks
  – A short-course therapy with 1 week of metronidazole, omeprazole, and clarithromycin b.i.d. is 90% effective
- Contraindications: Hypersensitivity to the drug(s)
- Precautions:
  – If bismuth is prescribed, warn the patient about the side effect of stool becoming black.
  – Refer to the manufacturer's profile of each drug.
- Significant possible interactions: Refer to the manufacturer's profile of each drug.

ADDITIONAL TREATMENT
General Measures
- Treatment of *H. pylori* is required to relieve symptoms, no specific therapy for the "gastritis" (4)[C]
- Parenteral fluid and electrolyte supplements required if vomiting prevents food intake

- Consider discontinuing NSAIDs or adding misoprostol.
- Encourage alcohol and smoking cessation.
- Endoscopy indicated for patients not responsive to treatment (4)[C]

IN-PATIENT CONSIDERATIONS
Gastritis may occur in ICU patients.

Initial Stabilization
Outpatient, except for severe hemorrhagic gastritis

 ONGOING CARE

FOLLOW-UP RECOMMENDATIONS
Usually no restrictions

Patient Monitoring
- Gastroscopy should be repeated after 6 weeks if gastritis has been severe or if symptomatic response to treatment has not been achieved.
- Patients with chronic gastritis are at increased risk for gastric carcinoma (lymphoma or adenocarcinoma).

DIET
Restrictions, if any, depend on the severity of the symptoms (e.g., bland, light, soft foods); it is wise to avoid caffeine and spicy foods, as well as alcohol.

PATIENT EDUCATION
- Explanation, reassurance
- Smoking cessation
- Dietary changes
- Relaxation therapy

PROGNOSIS
- Most cases clear spontaneously when the cause has been identified and treated.
- Recurrence of *H. pylori* infection may require a repeated course of treatment.

COMPLICATIONS
Bleeding from extensive mucosal erosion or ulceration

REFERENCES

1. Lanza FL, Chan FK, Quigley EM, Practice Parameters Committee of the American College of Gastroenterology et al. Guidelines for prevention of NSAID-related ulcer complications. *Am J Gastroenterol*. 2009;104:728–38.
2. Nazareno J, Driman DK, Adams P. Is Helicobacter pylori being treated appropriately? A study of inpatients and outpatients in a tertiary care centre. *Can J Gastroenterol*. 2007;21:285–8.
3. Luther J, Higgins PD, Schoenfeld PS, Moayyedi P, Vakil N, Chey WD et al. Empiric quadruple vs. triple therapy for primary treatment of Helicobacter pylori infection: Systematic review and meta-analysis of efficacy and tolerability. *Am. J. Gastroenterol*. 2010;105:65–73.
4. Wu JC, Sung JJ. Ulcer and gastritis. *Endoscopy*. 2002;34:104–10.
5. Lee JH, Kim N, Chung JI, et al. Long-term follow up of Helicobacter pylori IgG serology after eradication and reinfection rate of H. pylori in South Korea. *Helicobacter*. 2008;13:288–94.

ADDITIONAL READING

- de Bortoli N, Leonardi G, Ciancia E, et al. Helicobacter pylori eradication: a randomized prospective study of triple therapy versus triple therapy plus lactoferrin and probiotics. *Am J Gastroenterol*. 2007;102:951–6.
- Lahner E, Annibale B, Delle Gave G. Systemic Review: Heliocobacter pylori infection and impaired drug absorption. *Alimentary Pharmacology & Therapeutics*. 2009;(294):379–86.

CODES

ICD9
- 535.40 Other specified gastritis (without mention of hemorrhage)
- 535.50 Unspecified gastritis and gastroduodenitis (without mention of hemorrhage)
- 535.51 Unspecified gastritis and gastroduodenitis with hemorrhage

CLINICAL PEARLS

- Over half the population is colonized with *H. pylori*.
- *H. pylori* is the most common cause of gastritis.
- *H. pylori* antibodies decline in the year after treatment, but cannot be used to determine eradication (5)[B].
- *H. pylori* antibody titers rise significantly with reinfection.

G

GASTROESOPHAGEAL REFLUX DISEASE

Ruben Peralta, MD

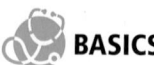 **BASICS**

DESCRIPTION
Reflux of gastroduodenal contents into the esophagus, larynx, or lungs, with or without resultant esophageal inflammation

Pediatric Considerations
Symptoms (vomiting, weight loss, failure to thrive) usually resolve by 18 months.

EPIDEMIOLOGY
Incidence
Pediatric Considerations
Children affected: 1/300–1,000

Prevalence
- Prevalence of gastroesophageal reflux disease (GERD): 10–20% in the US
- Prevalence of Barrett esophagus: 1.5%
- 65% adults have had heartburn; 15% have weekly symptoms
- In an European population-based study, reflux symptoms were found only in 40% of subjects with Barrett esophagus, and in one-third of patients with documented esophagitis (1)

RISK FACTORS
- Obesity
- Alcohol use
- Smoking (2)
- Caffeine use
- Position of the *acid pocket* above the diaphragm in patients with hiatal hernia (see below) (3,4)

Genetics
Gene polymorphism identified

GENERAL PREVENTION
Pediatric Considerations
- Positional treatment: Use infant seat for 2–3 hours after meals; thickened feedings
- Avoid alcohol, nicotine, and caffeine.
- Avoid lying down immediately after a meal.
- Elevate head of bed.

ETIOLOGY
- Occurs with loss of the normal pressure gradient between the lower esophageal sphincter (LES) and the stomach
- Most commonly due to inappropriate relaxation of LES:
  - Foods (high fat, spicy, citrus, chocolate, peppermint, onions)
  - Medications (anticholinergic, smooth muscle relaxants, i.e., calcium channel blockers, nitrates)
- Other contributing factors include:
  - Pregnancy (progestational hormones decrease LES pressure)
  - Ineffective peristalsis
  - Scleroderma
  - Delayed gastric emptying
  - Positional: Recumbency, bending
- Obesity

COMMONLY ASSOCIATED CONDITIONS
- Reflux esophagitis: Due to exposure to acid, pepsin; classified as erosive (mucosal damage apparent, ulcers, friability) or nonerosive

- Extraesophageal reflux:
  - Aspiration
  - Chronic cough
  - Laryngitis, vocal cord granuloma
  - Sinusitis
  - Otitis media
- Halitosis
- Hiatal hernia: The position of the *acid pocket* (the zone of high acidity detected in the proximal stomach after a meal) above the diaphragm in patients with hiatal hernia is a major risk factor (3,4).
- Peptic stricture: In 10% with GERD
- Barrett esophagus
- Esophageal adenocarcinoma

 DIAGNOSIS

- Heartburn (70–85%)
- Regurgitation of digested food (60%)
- Anginalike chest pain (33%)
- Abdominal pain (29%)
- Hoarseness (21%)
- Dysphagia (for solids; if solids and liquids, consider another cause) (20%)
- Bronchospasm (asthma) (15–20%)
- Aspiration (14%)
- Chronic cough
- Loss of dental enamel

HISTORY
- Heartburn: Retrosternal burning
- Regurgitation; sour or acid taste in mouth
- Symptoms with bending or recumbency
- Extraesophageal symptoms (e.g., cough)
- Diet, alcohol, smoking, and caffeine
- Diagnosis often made based on history alone, followed by a 1-week empiric trial with an antacid regimen

DIAGNOSTIC TESTS & INTERPRETATION
- Treated empirically if no red flags (dysphagia odynophagia, weight loss, early satiety, anemia, new onset, male >45 years) suggesting need to screen for more serious disease
- 24-hour pH monitoring: Gold standard for diagnosis; records number of reflux episodes and number that occur supine or upright; can be correlated with symptom diary
- Esophageal manometry records pressure of LES and effectiveness of peristalsis.

Lab
Check for anemia due to bleeding esophageal erosions or due to poor B_{12} absorption on proton pump inhibitor (PPI).

Imaging
Barium swallow:
- Presence of a sliding hiatal hernia appears to be a predictor of reflux esophagitis.
- Mucosal irregularity due to inflammation and edema

Diagnostic Procedures/Surgery
- Endoscopy:
  - Not part of initial workup, unless anemia, unintentional weight loss, progressive dysphagia, gastrointestinal bleeding, persistent vomiting, palpable epigastric mass, suspicion based on imaging study

  - Recommended for patients >55 who continue with symptoms after 4 weeks of treatment
  - Confirm mucosal injury; look for Barrett esophagus; biopsy for adenocarcinoma
  - ~50–70% of patients with heartburn have negative findings on endoscopy (nonerosive or endoscopy-negative reflux disease).
- Savary-Miller classification:
  - For grading esophagitis based on endoscopic findings:
    - Grade I: ≥1 nonconfluent reddish spots, with or without exudate
    - Grade II: Erosive and exudative lesions in the distal esophagus; may be confluent, but not circumferential
    - Grade III: Circumferential erosions in the distal esophagus
    - Grade IV: Chronic complications such as deep ulcers, stenosis, or scarring with Barrett metaplasia

Pathological Findings
- Acute inflammation (especially eosinophils)
- Hyperplasia of the basal zone of the epithelium seen in 85%
- Barrett epithelial change: Gastric columnar epithelium replaces squamous epithelium in distal esophagus

DIFFERENTIAL DIAGNOSIS
- Infectious esophagitis (*Candida*, herpes, HIV, cytomegalovirus)
- Chemical esophagitis (lye ingestion)
- Pill-induced esophagitis
- Radiation injury
- Crohn disease
- Angina
- Stricture
- Esophageal carcinoma
- Achalasia
- Scleroderma
- Peptic ulcer disease.

 TREATMENT

MEDICATION
First Line
- Stepped therapy (5):
  - Phase I: Lifestyle and diet modifications, antacids plus H_2 blockers or PPIs
  - Phase II: Symptoms persist, consider endoscopic evaluation
  - Phase III: Surgery
- H_2 blockers in equipotent oral doses (e.g., cimetidine 800 mg b.i.d. or 400 mg q.i.d., or ranitidine 150 mg b.i.d., or famotidine 20 mg b.i.d., or nizatidine 150 mg b.i.d.)
- PPIs: Irreversibly bind proton pump, onset of effect 4 days. Include omeprazole 20 mg/d, lansoprazole 30 mg/d, pantoprazole 40 mg/d, rabeprazole 20 mg/d, esomeprazole 40 mg/d
- Erosive esophagitis: PPI given for 8 weeks will be effective for healing in 90%. PPI more effective than H_2 blocker for healing erosive esophagitis.

Pediatric Considerations
Antacids or liquid histamine type 2 blockers, omeprazole, metoclopramide

Second Line
- Antacids and agents like Sucralfate may relieve breakthrough symptoms.
- Metoclopramide: 5–10 mg before meals
- Precautions:
  – Blood dyscrasias with PPIs and H_2 blockers
  – H_2 blockers must be renally dosed.
  – Metoclopramide is a dopamine blocker; risk of dystonia and tardive dyskinesia
  – On PPI, monitor B_{12}; B_{12} and iron absorption and calcium absorption compromised on PPI
- Significant possible interactions:
  – PPIs and H_2 blockers: Multiple cytochrome P450 drug interactions; examples include warfarin, phenytoin, antifungals

ADDITIONAL TREATMENT
General Measures
Lifestyle changes are 1st intervention:
- Elevate head of bed and avoid lying down soon after meals.
- Avoid stooping, bending, tight-fitting garments.
- Avoid medications that relax the LES (anticholinergic, calcium channel blockers).
- Lose weight.
- Stop smoking.
- Avoid alcohol.

SURGERY/OTHER PROCEDURES
Open or laparoscopic Nissen fundoplication to increase pressure gradient between stomach and esophagus by wrapping gastric fundus around distal esophagus, often circumferential (360-degree fundoplication) (6):
- Indications: Evidence of severe esophageal injury, incomplete response to medical treatment, medication treatment that has been or is expected to be prolonged
- Rule out esophageal dysmotility prior to surgery. If motility problems, consider a partial (270-degree, Toupet) wrap.
- Open and laparoscopic procedures both produce >90% response, equally effective for symptom reduction, quality of life, and decreased need for medications (6)[B],(7)[A].
- Cost analysis has indicated that if patient requires >10 years of PPI treatment, surgery may be more cost-effective.

Pediatric Considerations
- Surgery for severe symptoms (apnea, choking, persistent vomiting)

 ONGOING CARE

FOLLOW-UP RECOMMENDATIONS
Patient Monitoring
- Follow symptomatically.
- Repeat endoscopy at 4–8 weeks for poor symptomatic response to medical therapy, especially in older patients.
- Current guideline is endoscopic surveillance every 2–5 years in patients with Barrett esophagus, assuming treatment if cancer is detected.

DIET
Avoid foods that make symptoms worse.

PATIENT EDUCATION
- Chocolate, peppermint, citrus, onions, spicy foods, and foods high in fat can make GERD symptoms worse.

- Eat small meals.
- Avoid lying down soon after meals.
- Elevate head of bed.
- Lifestyle changes, such as losing weight and smoking cessation, avoiding alcohol and caffeine helps.

PROGNOSIS
- Symptoms and esophageal inflammation often return promptly when treatment is withdrawn; to prevent relapse of symptoms, patients should be treated with continued antisecretory therapy:
  – PPI maintenance therapy may improve quality of life better than H_2 blocker maintenance.
  – Full-dose PPIs more effective than 1/2 dose for maintenance (7)[A]
  – In erosive esophagitis, daily maintenance therapy with a PPI has been proven to prevent relapse; intermittent PPI therapy has not been proven effective (8)[A].
- In terms of symptom reduction, medical and surgical therapy is equally effective (7)[A].
- Antireflux surgery:
  – 90–94% symptom response
  – 5% continued symptoms, should have anatomy evaluated by esophagram
  – Long-term follow-up shows some surgically treated patients may eventually require medical therapy.
- Regression of Barrett epithelium does not routinely occur, despite aggressive medical or surgical therapy (9).

COMPLICATIONS
- Peptic stricture: 10–15%
- Barrett esophagus: 10%:
  – Adenocarcinoma from Barrett epithelium (rate of cancer development 0.5% annually)
- Extraesophageal symptoms: 5–10%, including hoarseness, aspiration, including aspiration pneumonia
- Bleeding due to mucosal injury
- Noncardiac chest pain

Geriatric Considerations
Complications more likely (e.g., aspiration pneumonia)

REFERENCES
1. Ronkainen J, Aro P, Storskrubb T, Johansson SE, Lind T, Bolling-Sternevald E, Vieth M, Stolte M, Talley NJ, Agréus L et al. Prevalence of Barrett's esophagus in the general population: an endoscopic study. *Gastroenterology*. 2005;129: 1825–31.
2. Dent J, El-Serag HB, Wallander MA, et al. Epidemiology of gastro-oesophageal reflux disease: a systematic review. *Gut*. 2005;54: 710–7.
3. Beaumont H, Bennink RJ, de Jong J, Boeckxstaens GE et al. The position of the acid pocket as a major risk factor for acidic reflux in healthy subjects and patients with GORD. *Gut*. 2010;59:441–51.
4. McColl KE, Clarke A, Seenan J et al. Acid pocket, hiatus hernia and acid reflux. *Gut*. 2010;59: 430–1.
5. Mine S, Iida T, Tabata T, et al. Management of symptoms in step-down therapy of gastroesophageal reflux disease. *J Gastroenterol Hepatol*. 2005;20:1365–70.

6. Bais JE, Bartelsman JF, Bonjer HJ, et al. Laparoscopic or conventional Nissen fundoplication for gastro-oesophageal reflux disease: randomised clinical trial. The Netherlands Antireflux Surgery Study Group. *Lancet*. 2000;355:170–4.
7. Agency for Healthcare Research and Quality. Comparing effectiveness of management strategies for gastroesophageal reflux disease. An update to the 2005 report. Available at: http://effectivehealthcare.ahrq.gov. Accessed July 7, 2010.
8. Zacny J, Zamakhshary M, Sketris I, et al. Systematic review: the efficacy of intermittent and on-demand therapy with histamine H2-receptor antagonists or proton pump inhibitors for gastro-oesophageal reflux disease patients. *Aliment Pharmacol Ther*. 2005;21:1299–312.
9. Spechler SJ, Lee E, Ahnen D, Goyal RK, Hirano I, Ramirez F, Raufman JP, Sampliner R, Schnell T, Sontag S, Vlahcevic ZR, Young R, Williford W et al. Long-term outcome of medical and surgical therapies for gastroesophageal reflux disease: follow-up of a randomized controlled trial. *JAMA*. 2001;285:2331–8.
10. Chang AB, Lasserson TJ, Kiljander TO, Connor FL, Gaffney JT, Garske LA et al. Systematic review and meta-analysis of randomised controlled trials of gastro-oesophageal reflux interventions for chronic cough associated with gastro-oesophageal reflux. *BMJ*. 2006;332:11–7.

ADDITIONAL READING
- Fuccio L, Zagari RM, Eusebi LH, Laterza L, Cennamo V, Ceroni L, Grilli D, Bazzoli F et al. Meta-analysis: can Helicobacter pylori eradication treatment reduce the risk for gastric cancer? *Ann Intern Med*. 2009;151:121–8.
- Reid BJ, Li X, Galipeau PC, Vaughan TL et al. Barrett's oesophagus and oesophageal adenocarcinoma: time for a new synthesis. *Nat Rev Cancer*. 2010;10:87–101.

See Also (Topic, Algorithm, Electronic Media Element)
Algorithms: Dyspepsia; Epigastric Pain; Esophageal Regurgitation

 CODES

ICD9
- 530.11 Reflux esophagitis
- 530.81 Esophageal reflux

CLINICAL PEARLS
- There is no evidence to support that treatment with PPI causes regression of Barrett esophagus or inhibits progression of esophageal dysplasia beyond benefits of symptomatic relief.
- GERD treatments are used to treat chronic cough. Meta-analysis of randomized clinical trials suggest PPIs help with cough resolution in some adults (10)[A].
- The role of *H. pylori* as an etiologic agent in GERD remains controversial.

GENERALIZED ANXIETY DISORDER

Michelle A. Tinitigan, MD

 BASICS

DESCRIPTION
- Anxiety disorders are characterized by excessive worry that is difficult to control with at least 3 of the following symptoms: Restlessness, irritability, difficulty concentrating, muscle tension, sleep disturbances, and being easily fatigued. Symptoms must be distressing or impairing and not adequately explained by another related disorder (1).
- Occurs gradually, is recurrent and remains chronic if not treated (1).

ALERT
Individuals with an anxiety disorder have a 15–20% lifetime risk of committing suicide.

Pediatric Considerations
Children and adolescents often present with worries concerning performance or competence.

EPIDEMIOLOGY
Prevalence
- Lifetime prevalence: 5–6% using the *Diagnostic and Statistical Manual of Mental Disorders, Fourth Edition* (DSM-IV) criteria; however, the European Study of the Epidemiology of Mental Disorders gives a lower estimate of 2.8% (1).
- Primary-care setting prevalence: 5–8%
- Twice as common in women and commonly seen in middle age, with prevalence rates rising after age 35 in women and after age 45 in men (1)

RISK FACTORS
- Risk factors during childhood: Maternal internalizing symptoms (i.e., the mother's symptoms of anxiety and depression manifesting as insomnia, hopelessness, tension, somatic complaints), maltreatment, internalizing, conduct problems, and negative emotionality
- Family history
- History of other anxiety or mood disorders
- More common in ethnic minorities and in low socioeconomic status; some controversy over whether this results from more realistic worry about life situation

Genetics
Genetic factors play only a modest role in etiology of GAD. Heritability of female twin pairs was 30%.

PATHOPHYSIOLOGY
- Maladaptive response to stressful stimuli involving norepinephrine, serotonin, and γ-amino butyric acid
- Possible relationship between hypothalamic-pituitary-adrenal axis abnormalities and potential role of cholecystokinin

ETIOLOGY
GAD is likely a combination of genetic, developmental, and neurobiologic factors.

COMMONLY ASSOCIATED CONDITIONS
High rate of psychiatric comorbidity in patients with GAD, with 61% having multiple anxiety disorders, and 79% with more than 1 Axis I disorder (1); 35–50% of patients with major depression meet criteria for GAD.

 DIAGNOSIS

- A 7-item anxiety questionnaire, GAD-7, has been developed in a primary care setting .
- Self-assessment screening tool; positive screen (score $\geq$8) should be followed by a clinician interview to establish a diagnosis.
- The first 2 items of GAD-7 (referred to as GAD-2), with a cutoff score of $\geq$3 warranting further evaluation; may be equally sensitive to GAD-7.

HISTORY
- Initial interview: Unhurried and open-ended; when appropriate, family members should be involved.
- Medical history: Focused on contributing factors (e.g., medication side effects, substance abuse, or current medical condition)
- Psychosocial history: Screen for comorbid psychiatric disorders (major depression or agoraphobia), life stressors, family history, current social history, substance abuse history (including caffeine, nicotine, and alcohol), past sexual history, physical and emotional abuse, or emotional neglect.
- Diagnostic criteria from *DSM-IV* for GAD:
  - Excessive anxiety and worry about a number of events or activities, occurring more days than not for at least 6 months, that is out of proportion to the likelihood or impact of feared events, causing clinically significant social distress or functional impairment in social, occupational, or other important areas of functioning (2)
  - Anxiety is associated with at least 3 of the following somatic complaints: Restlessness, irritability, impaired concentration, muscle tension, fatigue, insomnia.
  - Affected patients have little insight into the connection between reported worries, current life stress, and their physical symptoms.
- Explore for causes of anxiety that may lead to other anxiety disorders.
  - Embarrassment in public (social phobia)
  - Having a panic attack (panic disorder)
  - Obsessions and rituals (OCD)
  - Separation from relatives (separation anxiety disorder)
  - Body image (anorexia nervosa)
  - Assess for suicidality.
- Anxiety disorders have been shown to independently increase the risk of suicidality (panic disorder and social phobia more than GAD and OCD).

PHYSICAL EXAM
- Signs of common somatic symptoms include trembling, muscle tension, or muscle aches
- Examine thyroid for signs of hyperthyroidism.
- Cardiac exam for tachycardia or atrial fibrillation

DIAGNOSTIC TESTS & INTERPRETATION
Lab
Initial lab tests
- Complete blood count, comprehensive metabolic panel, thyroid-stimulating hormone, urinalysis
- ECG (in patients >40 years of age with chest pain or palpitations)
- Serum or urine toxicology screen or drug levels if substance-induced anxiety suspected

DIFFERENTIAL DIAGNOSIS
- Other anxiety disorders: OCD, separation anxiety disorder, social phobia, posttraumatic stress disorder (PTSD,) adjustment disorder with anxious mood, panic disorder, anorexia nervosa, hypochondriasis, somatization disorder
- Anxiety disorder owing to a general medical condition: Pheochromocytoma, hyperthyroidism, atrial fibrillation, stroke, parathyroid illness, vestibular nerve disease, mitral valve prolapse
- Anxiety associated with psychotic disorder or mood disorder; substance-induced anxiety disorder
- Dementia
- Medication-induced anxiety (e.g., steroids, thyroxine, theophylline, neuroleptics, selective serotonin reuptake inhibitors [SSRIs], tricyclic antidepressants, antihistamines, idiosyncratic reactions to other medications)

 TREATMENT

MEDICATION
First Line
- SSRIs:
  - Paroxetine: 20 mg daily (number needed to treat [NNT] = 6.7)
    - May start at lower doses of 5–10 mg/d × 1 week to minimize adverse effect of restlessness and insomnia [C]. Geriatric: 10 mg every morning; increase by 10 mg weekly to a maximum dose of 40 mg daily.
  - Escitalopram: Maintenance: 10–20 mg daily; geriatric: 10 mg daily; citalopram has shown efficacy in older patients ($\geq$60 years old).
  - Sertraline: 25 mg daily; maintenance: 50–200 mg daily; may start at lower doses of 12.5–25 mg daily × 1 week to minimize adverse effects (e.g., agitation, headache, diarrhea, nausea, insomnia)
  - In children: sertraline, fluoxetine, and fluvoxamine are effective in treating the symptoms of GAD in children and adolescents; should be reserved for individuals who have not responded to psychological therapies because of the risk of possible suicidal thoughts or behaviors.
- Serotonin norepinephrine reuptake inhibitors (SNRIs):
  - Venlafaxine: Initial: 37.5–75 mg daily; increase by 37.5-mg increments every 1–2 weeks until a dose of 150–300 mg is attained (NNT = 5.06).
  - Duloxetine: Initial: 30 mg PO daily × 1 week; then 60 mg PO daily

Second Line
- If monotherapy fails, try augmentation with a drug from another class, switch to drug with a different mechanism, or addition of psychotherapy. Second line drugs include:
- Azapirones:
  - Buspirone (NNT = 4.4)
    - 15–30 mg b.i.d.; 30–60 mg/d given in 2 or 3 divided doses
    - Slow onset of action: Several weeks; variable intolerability
    - Appears to be useful in the treatment of GAD, especially for benzodiazepine-naive patients, because it may be less addictive than benzodiazepines.
    - May alleviate decreased libido, diminished sexual arousal, or impaired orgasm associated with the use of antidepressants

- Tricyclic antidepressants (TCAs):
  - Imipramine 75 mg PO daily; increase to maximum of 200 mg/d (NNT = 4.07). May start at 10–20 mg at night, and titrate up to 75–300 mg at night. Usual maintenance: 50–150 mg/d. Geriatric: 25–75 mg at night; maximum of 200 mg/d
- Benzodiazepines (should be tapered as the antidepressant dose is titrated to therapeutic levels after 6–8 weeks):
  - Clonazepam: 0.25–0.5 mg PO b.i.d., titrated up to 1 mg b.i.d. or t.i.d.
  - Lorazepam: 0.5–1.0 mg PO t.i.d., titrated up to 1 mg PO t.i.d. or q.i.d.
  - Diazepam: 2–10 mg PO 2–4 times daily as needed; geriatric: 2–2.5 mg PO once or twice daily; increase gradually
    - Have a rapid onset of action and are effective in GAD
    - Often recommended as adjunctive therapy to help patients in acute crisis or while waiting for a SSRI/SNRI to take effect.
    - Not recommended as monotherapy for depression, dysthymia, obsessive-compulsive disorder, and PTSD, which commonly occur with GAD.
    - Use for short-term treatment duration (up to 4 weeks) to avoid the risk of physical dependence and withdrawal (rebound anxiety).
    - Tapering usually takes months, with about 10% reduction per week.
    - If symptoms recur, it may be difficult to differentiate between benzodiazepine withdrawal or recurrence of GAD symptoms; symptoms that worsen within 2 weeks are most likely due to benzodiazepine withdrawal and suggest that the taper rate be decreased slightly.
    - Avoid in patients with polydrug or alcohol use, chronic pain disorders, and severe personality disorders owing to high risk of dependence.
- Antihistamines
  - Hydroxyzine: Should not be used as 1st therapy because of associated side effects (in particular, sedation and anticholinergic effects), slow onset of action, and lack of efficacy for comorbid disorders (3).
- Pregabalin
  - Approved in Europe for treatment of GAD
  - Improves both psychic and somatic symptoms in adults with GAD, including the elderly (4)
  - Discontinuation symptoms if abruptly stopped.
- Atypical antipsychotic
  - Quetiapine 50–150 mg daily
    - Could be considered after other classes of drugs have proved ineffective or when certain types of symptoms are present (5)
    - Most trials used this for augmentation; however, more trials are needed to validate the efficacy of this class of drug

Pregnancy Considerations
- Paroxetine (Paxil): Association with congenital heart (septal) defects in 1st-trimester exposure and with persistent pulmonary hypertension in 3rd-trimester exposure; Category D; fetal echocardiography should be considered for women who are exposed in early pregnancy.
- Venlafaxine (Effexor): Association with congenital heart defects in 1st-trimester exposure
- Benzodiazepines: 1st-trimester exposure is associated with craniofacial deformities. Maternal benzodiazepine use shortly before delivery is associated with floppy infant syndrome.

ADDITIONAL TREATMENT
Propranolol is not recommended for the treatment of GAD (no significant efficacy over placebo after 3 weeks in one randomized, controlled trial).

General Measures
Both psychological and medication therapies are effective and work well when used together.

Issues for Referral
Refer to a psychiatrist for comorbid depression, for prolonged use of benzodiazepines, and for patients with suicidal ideation.

Additional Therapies
- Patient surveys have shown a preference for psychological therapy to medications (6).
- Cognitive-behavioral therapy is frequently recommended as the 1st-line psychological treatment for GAD and has been shown to be superior to placebo in alleviating the symptoms of GAD.

COMPLEMENTARY AND ALTERNATIVE MEDICINE
- Kava is not recommended for the treatment of anxiety. Associated with fatal hepatotoxicity, and the FDA has issued a safety alert.
- Valerian is marketed principally for insomnia but also has been used as a mild sedative for anxiety disorders.
  - Clinical studies are inconclusive about effectiveness for treatment of insomnia; mild sedative effects in animals; no human studies available
  - Few adverse effects reported, but no data about long-term safety

IN-PATIENT CONSIDERATIONS
Initial Stabilization
Evaluate for suicidality, and begin pharmacologic treatment as soon as possible. Faster-acting medications (e.g., benzodiazepines) may be required for initial stabilization.

Admission Criteria
Inpatient admission is generally not necessary unless the patient expresses suicidal ideation.

Discharge Criteria
When suicidal ideation is no longer present and treatment has been started

 ## ONGOING CARE

FOLLOW-UP RECOMMENDATIONS
- Efficacy, medication tolerance, symptoms, and side effects should be assessed within 2 weeks of starting any new treatment.
- Once the patient has begun to experience relief from symptoms, follow-up should be every 4 weeks.

DIET
Patients should discontinue or limit consumption of caffeine and other stimulant-type food/beverages.

PATIENT EDUCATION
- Patients should be presented with both medication and psychological treatment options.
- Patients treated with benzodiazepines should be made aware of the potential for dependence and the resulting short-term nature of this type of treatment.

PROGNOSIS
- GAD is a chronic disorder that rarely goes into remission, with long-term recovery achieved in only 1/3 of patients.

- Many patients will need chronic treatment with medication to prevent relapse; other patients may be treated with intermittent courses of acute treatment.
- Patients experience fluctuating levels of symptoms provoked by stressful life events. Augment treatment as needed.

REFERENCES
1. Davidson J, Feltner D, Dugar A. Management of Generalized Anxiety Disorder in Primary Care: Identifying the Challenges and Unmet Needs. *Prim Care Companion J Clin Psychiatry* 2010;12(2): e1–e13.
2. American Psychiatric Association. *Diagnostic and Statistical Manual of Mental Disorders*, 4th ed, Primary Care Version (DSM-IV-PC). American Psychiatric Association, Washington, DC, 1995.
3. Bandelow B, Zohar J, Hollander E, et al. World Federation of Societies of Biological Psychiatry (WFSBP) guidelines for the pharmacological treatment of anxiety, obsessive-compulsive and post-traumatic stress disorders-first revision. *World J Biol Psychiatry.* 2008;9:248–312.
4. Montgomery S, Chatamra K, Pauer L, Whalen E, Baldinetti F et al. Efficacy and safety of pregabalin in elderly people with generalised anxiety disorder. *Br J Psychiatry.* 2008;193:389–94.
5. Bandelow B, Chouinard G, Bobes J, Ahokas A, Eggens I, Liu S, Eriksson H et al. Extended-release quetiapine fumarate (quetiapine XR): a once-daily monotherapy effective in generalized anxiety disorder. Data from a randomized, double-blind, placebo- and active-controlled study. *Int J Neuropsychopharmacol.* 2010;13:305–20.
6. Hunot V, Churchill R, Teixeira V, et al. Psychological therapies for generalized anxiety disorder. *Cochrane Database of Systematic Reviews.* 2007, Issue 1. Art. No.: CD001848. DOI:10.1002/14651858.CD001848.pub4.

See Also (Topic, Algorithm, Electronic Media Element)
Depression

 ## CODES

ICD9
300.02 Generalized anxiety disorder

CLINICAL PEARLS
- GAD is defined as excessive anxiety and worry more days than not for a period of 6 months or more, which the patient has a difficult time controlling and which causes significant impairment and distress.
- Patients should be evaluated for medical conditions that can cause hyperarousal and other anxiety disorders.

G

GIARDIASIS

Jill A. Grimes, MD

BASICS

DESCRIPTION
- Intestinal infection caused by the protozoan parasite *Giardia lamblia* (1)
  - *G. lamblia* is also called *G. duodenalis* and *G. intestinalis*.
- Infection results from ingestion of the cysts, which excyst into trophozoites. These colonize the small intestine and cause symptoms.
- Cycle is continued when the trophozoites encyst in the small intestine and water, food, or hands are contaminated by feces of the infected person.
- Most infections result from fecal–oral transmission or ingestion of contaminated water (such as while swimming) and are less commonly the result of contaminated food.

EPIDEMIOLOGY
- Predominant age: All ages, but most common in early childhood ages 1–9 and adults 35–44 (2)[A]
- Predominant gender: Male > Female (slightly)

Pediatric Considerations
Common in early childhood

Prevalence
- 5% of patients with stools submitted for ova and parasite exams
- >19,000 cases/year in the United States (although it is not reportable in Indiana, Kentucky, Mississippi, North Carolina, and Texas)

RISK FACTORS
- Daycare centers
- Anal intercourse
- Wilderness camping
- Travel to developing countries
- Children adopted from developing countries
- Public swimming pools

Genetics
No known genetic risk factors

GENERAL PREVENTION
- Good hand-washing when caring for diapered children
- Water purification when camping and when traveling to developing countries
- Cooking all foods

PATHOPHYSIOLOGY
Giardia trophozoites colonize the surface of the proximal small intestine. The mechanism by which they cause diarrhea is unknown.

ETIOLOGY
Protozoan parasite (*G. lamblia*) infection acquired through fecal–oral transmission or ingestion of contaminated water, less commonly from contaminated food

COMMONLY ASSOCIATED CONDITIONS
Hypogammaglobulinemia and possibly IgA deficiency; diarrhea more severe and prolonged in these patients

DIAGNOSIS

HISTORY
- ~25–50% of infected persons are symptomatic.
- Chronic diarrhea (lasting >5–7 days and frequently weeks)
- Abdominal bloating
- Flatulence
- Loose, greasy, foul-smelling stools
- Weight loss
- Nausea
- Lactose intolerance

PHYSICAL EXAM
Nonspecific; abdominal bloating and afebrile

DIAGNOSTIC TESTS & INTERPRETATION
Lab
Initial lab tests
- Stool for ova and parasites:
  - Repeated 3 times if necessary
  - Cysts are seen in fixed or fresh stools and, occasionally, trophozoites are found in fresh diarrheal stools.

- Fluorescent antibody (FA) and ELISA tests of fecal specimens are available. *A single FA or ELISA is at least as sensitive as 3 stools for ova and parasites.*
- Polymerase chain reaction (PCR) techniques have been found to be more sensitive than microscopy, but have not been widely adopted secondary to cost (3).

Follow-Up & Special Considerations
String test (Enterotest): A gelatin capsule on a string is swallowed and left in the duodenum for several hours or overnight. The end of the string is then visualized microscopically.

Diagnostic Procedures/Surgery
Esophagogastroduodenoscopy with biopsy and sample of small intestinal fluid

Pathological Findings
Intestinal biopsy shows flattened, mild lymphocytic infiltration and trophozoites on the surface.

DIFFERENTIAL DIAGNOSIS
- Includes other etiologies of small intestinal diarrhea
- Infectious causes include cryptosporidiosis, isosporiasis, and cyclosporiasis.
- Other causes of malabsorption include celiac sprue, tropical sprue, bacterial overgrowth syndromes, and Crohn ileitis.
- Irritable bowel is suspected when diarrhea is not accompanied by weight loss.

TREATMENT

Outpatient for mild cases, inpatient if symptoms are severe enough to cause dehydration

MEDICATION
First Line
- Metronidazole (Flagyl): 250 mg t.i.d. for 5–7 days (4)[B]
- Tinidazole 2 g single dose (50 mg/kg up to 2 g for children) (4)[B]
- Albendazole 400 mg once daily for 5 days:
  - Albendazole has comparable effectiveness to metronidazole with fewer side effects and low cost (5)[A].

- Precautions:
  - Theoretical risk of carcinogenesis with metronidazole
- Significant possible interactions: Occasional disulfiram reaction with metronidazole or tinidazole

Pregnancy Considerations
- Concern for potential teratogenicity of medications; consult infectious disease specialist or gastroenterologist for symptomatic disease
- Contraindications: Relatively contraindicated in pregnancy, especially 1st trimester

Second Line
- Furazolidone: 8 mg/kg/d t.i.d. for 10 days (slightly less effective, but commonly used in pediatrics because it is well tolerated)
- Paromomycin (Humatin): A nonabsorbable aminoglycoside that is probably less effective but commonly recommended in pregnancy because of theoretical risk of teratogenicity of other agents
- Quinacrine: 100 mg t.i.d. for 5–7 days; was the treatment of choice for giardiasis, but is withdrawn from the market in US
- Nitazoxanide suspension was approved by the FDA in 2003 for treatment of giardiasis in children ages 1–11. Children ages 1–4 receive 100 mg b.i.d. and ages 5–11 receive 200 mg b.i.d. for 3 days (1)[B].

ADDITIONAL TREATMENT
Lactose intolerance may follow Giardia infection and be a cause of persistent diarrhea post treatment.

General Measures
- Medical therapy for all infected individuals
- Fluid replacement if dehydrated

ONGOING CARE

FOLLOW-UP RECOMMENDATIONS
Patient Monitoring
Symptoms, weight, stool exams

DIET
Good nutrition, low lactose, low fat, monitor for dehydration

PATIENT EDUCATION
Hand washing may be more important than water purification to prevent transmission in outdoor recreationalists (6)[A].

PROGNOSIS
- Untreated giardiasis lasts for weeks.
- Patients usually (90%) respond to treatment within a few days:
  - Most nonresponders or relapses respond to a 2nd course with the same or a different agent.

COMPLICATIONS
Malabsorption and weight loss

REFERENCES

1. Yoder JS, Beach MJ, Centers for Disease Control and Prevention (CDC). Giardiasis surveillance–United States, 2003–2005. *MMWR Surveill Summ*. 2007;56:11–8.
2. Yoder JS, Harral C, Beach MJ, Centers for Disease Control and Prevention (CDC) et al. Giardiasis surveillance - United States, 2006-2008. *MMWR Surveill Summ*. 2010;59:15–25.
3. Haque R, Roy S, Siddique A, et al. Multiplex real-time PCR assay for detection of Entamoeba histolytica, Giardia intestinalis, and Cryptosporidium spp. *Am J Trop Med Hyg*. 2007;76:713–7.
4. Fallah M, Rabiee S, Moshtaghi AA. Comparison between efficacy of a single dose of tinidazole with a 7-day standard dose course of metronidazole in giardiasis. *Pakistan Journal of Medical Sciences*. 2007;23(1):43–6.
5. Solaymani-Mohammadi S, Genkinger JM, Loffredo CA, Singer SM et al. A meta-analysis of the effectiveness of albendazole compared with metronidazole as treatments for infections with Giardia duodenalis. *PLoS Negl Trop Dis*. 2010;4:e682.
6. Welch TP et al. Risk of giardiasis from consumption of wilderness water in North America: a systematic review of epidemiologic data. *Int J Infect Dis*. 2000;4:100–3.

ADDITIONAL READING
- Pawlowski SW, Warren CA, Guerrant R: Diagnosis and treatment of acute or persistent diarrhea. *Gastroenterology*. 2009;136(6):1874–86.
- Shields JM, Gleim ER, Beach MJ. Prevalence of Cryptosporidium spp. and Giardia intestinalis in Swimming Pools, Atlanta, Georgia. *Emerg Infect Dis*. 2008;14:948–50.

See Also (Topic, Algorithm, Electronic Media Element)
Algorithm: Diarrhea, Chronic

CODES

ICD9
007.1 Giardiasis

CLINICAL PEARLS
- Daycare facilities and public swimming pools are common sources of *Giardia* (don't assume camping or travel is required).
- Treatment with metronidazole is often poorly tolerated, but has higher cure rates.
- Most treatment failures respond to a second course of antibiotics (whether or not you switch drugs).

G

GILBERT DISEASE

Robert A. Marlow, MD, MA

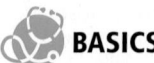 **BASICS**

DESCRIPTION
Mild chronic or intermittent unconjugated hyperbilirubinemia (not due to hemolysis) with otherwise normal liver function (1)

Pediatric Considerations
Rare for the disorder to be diagnosed before puberty

Pregnancy Considerations
The relative fasting that may occur with morning sickness can elevate the bilirubin level.

EPIDEMIOLOGY
- Predominant age: Present from birth, but most often presents in the 2nd or 3rd decade of life; heterozygous for single abnormal gene
- Predominant sex: Male > Female (2–7:1)

Prevalence
Prevalence in the US: ~7% of the population (2)

RISK FACTORS
Male gender

Genetics
A gene defect resulting in reduced bilirubin uridine diphosphate–glucuronosyltransferase-1 appears to be necessary but not sufficient for Gilbert syndrome (3).

ETIOLOGY
The hyperbilirubinemia results from impaired hepatic bilirubin clearance (~30% of normal). Hepatic bilirubin conjugation (glucuronidation) is reduced, although this is likely not the only defect.

COMMONLY ASSOCIATED CONDITIONS
Gilbert disease may be part of a spectrum of hereditary disorders that includes types I and II Crigler-Najjar syndrome.

 DIAGNOSIS

HISTORY
No significant symptoms, although a variety of nonspecific symptoms have been described.

PHYSICAL EXAM
No abnormal physical findings other than occasional mild jaundice

DIAGNOSTIC TESTS & INTERPRETATION
Lab
- Bilirubin: Elevated but <6 mg/dL (103 μmol/L) and usually <3 mg/dL (51 μmol/L), virtually all unconjugated (indirect)
- Complete blood count (CBC) with peripheral smear is normal.
- Reticulocyte count is normal.
- Liver function tests (aspartate aminotransferase [AST], alanine transaminase [ALT], alkaline phosphatase, and glutamyl transpeptidase [GGT] are normal.
- Fasting and postprandial serum bile acids are normal.
- Up to 60% of patients have clinically insignificant mild hemolysis that frequently can only be detected with sophisticated red cell survival studies.
- Drugs that may alter lab results: Bilirubin level may be raised by nicotinic acid and lowered by phenobarbital.
- Disorders that may alter lab results: Bilirubin levels increase during fasting and may increase during a febrile illness.

Diagnostic Procedures/Surgery
- A liver biopsy is not usually needed to exclude other diagnoses (2).
- Some clinicians recommend confirming the diagnosis by reducing daily caloric intake to 400 kcal for 48 hours, which results in a 2- to 3-fold increase in unconjugated bilirubin.
- After 12 hours of fasting, an increase of total bilirubin to >1.9 mg/dL 2 hours after an oral dose of rifampin 900 mg distinguishes patients with Gilbert disease with a sensitivity of 100% and a specificity of 100% (4).

DIFFERENTIAL DIAGNOSIS
- Hemolysis
- Ineffective erythropoiesis (megaloblastic anemias, certain porphyrias, thalassemia major, sideroblastic anemia, severe lead poisoning, congenital dyserythropoietic anemias)
- Cirrhosis
- Chronic persistent hepatitis
- Pancreatitis
- Biliary tract disease

TREATMENT

Outpatient. The most important treatment is to make a positive diagnosis of Gilbert disease to reassure the patient and prevent further unnecessary procedures.

 ## ONGOING CARE

FOLLOW-UP RECOMMENDATIONS

Patient Monitoring

If history, physical exam, and laboratory tests are normal, see the patient on 2–3 further occasions during the ensuing 12–18 months. If the patient develops no symptoms, reticulocytosis, or new liver function abnormalities, make the diagnosis of Gilbert disease.

PATIENT EDUCATION

Reassure the patient that the condition is benign with no known sequelae.

PROGNOSIS

The disorder is benign with an excellent prognosis. There is some preliminary evidence that patients with Gilbert disease may have a lower incidence of cardiovascular disease (56). Elevated levels of bilirubin may exert an antioxidation effect (6).

COMPLICATIONS

No known complications

REFERENCES

1. Bosma PJ. Inherited disorders of bilirubin metabolism. *J Hepatol*. 2003;38:107–17.
2. Radu P, Atsmon J. Gilbert's syndrome–clinical and pharmacological implications. *Isr Med Assoc J*. 2001;3:593–8.
3. Bosma PJ, Chowdhury JR, Bakker C, et al. The genetic basis of the reduced expression of bilirubin UDP-glucuronosyltransferase 1 in Gilbert's syndrome. *N Engl J Med*. 1995;333:1171–5.
4. Murthy GD, Byron D, Shoemaker D, et al. The utility of rifampin in diagnosing Gilbert's syndrome. *Am J Gastroenterol*. 2001;96:1150–4.
5. Inoguchi T, Sasaki S, Kobayashi K, Takayanagi R, Yamada T et al. Relationship between Gilbert syndrome and prevalence of vascular complications in patients with diabetes. *JAMA*. 2007;298: 1398–400.
6. Bulmer AC, Blanchfield JT, Toth I, Fassett RG, Coombes JS et al. Improved resistance to serum oxidation in Gilbert's syndrome: a mechanism for cardiovascular protection. *Atherosclerosis*. 2008;199:390–6.

ADDITIONAL READING

Strassburg CP et al. Pharmacogenetics of Gilbert's syndrome. *Pharmacogenomics*. 2008;9:703–15.

 ## CODES

ICD9

277.4 Disorders of bilirubin excretion

CLINICAL PEARLS

- The most important reason to make the diagnosis of Gilbert disease is to reassure the patient that this is a benign condition with no known sequelae and to prevent unnecessary procedures.
- A liver biopsy is not usually needed to rule out other liver diseases. The diagnosis can be confirmed by otherwise normal liver function tests, no evidence of hemolysis, and the response to fasting or a dose of rifampin.
- The etiology of Gilbert disease can result when the patient has a gene defect resulting in reduced conjugation of bilirubin. The gene defect is necessary, but not sufficient to produce Gilbert disease.

G

GINGIVITIS

Hugh J. Silk, MD
Sheila O. Stille, DMD, MAGD
Liang Zhao, MD

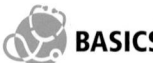 **BASICS**

DESCRIPTION
Gingivitis is a reversible form of inflammation of the gingiva. It is a mild form of periodontal disease. Classification includes:

- Plaque-induced
- Not plaque-induced (acute necrotizing gingivitis, Vincent disease, denture-related)
- Modified by systemic factors (e.g., pregnancy, HIV, diabetes, leukemia)
- Modified by medications (antihypertensives, antipsychotics, antiepileptics, hormones)
- Modified by malnutrition (vitamin deficiencies)
- System(s) affected: Gastrointestinal
- Synonym(s): Mild periodontal disease; Gum disease

Geriatric Considerations
More frequent in this age group (owing more to lifelong accumulation than to increased susceptibility)

Pediatric Considerations
Mild cases common in children (most common form of pediatric periodontal disease) and usually require no specific interventions

Pregnancy Considerations
- Very common in pregnant women; hormonal effect
- Hyperplasia
- Common; self-limited

EPIDEMIOLOGY
- Predominant age: >35 years old (but as young as 5)
- Predominant sex: Male = Female

Prevalence
- ~50% of children
- ~90% of adolescents and adult population
- ~30–75% of pregnant women

RISK FACTORS
- Poor dental hygiene/plaque formation
- Pregnancy
- Diabetes mellitus
- Malocclusion or dental crowding
- Smoking
- Mouth breathing
- Faulty dental restoration
- HIV-positive; AIDS
- Stress
- Vitamin C deficiency; coenzyme Q10 deficiency
- Dental appliances (dentures, braces)
- Eruption of primary or secondary teeth

- Necrotizing ulcerative gingivitis:
  – Stress
  – Lack of sleep
  – Malnutrition
  – Viral illness
  – Typically younger patients
- Bronchial asthma (1)
- Rheumatoid arthritis (2)

Genetics
Possible genetic link (up to 30% of population). Rare condition called hereditary gingival fibromatosis associated with hirsutism

GENERAL PREVENTION
- Good oral hygiene:
  – Adults
    ○ Regular twice daily brushing with fluoride toothpaste and increased benefit of using circular oscillating electric brush rather than regular brush (3)
    ○ Daily flossing
  – Pediatrics
    ○ Regular twice daily brushing with fluoride toothpaste with parental supervision until full manual dexterity (~age 8)
    ○ Regular flossing if no spaces between teeth
- Cleaning by a dentist or hygienist every 6 months or more frequently if indicated

PATHOPHYSIOLOGY
Inflammation of gingiva that may progress to deeper inflammation (see "Periodontitis")

ETIOLOGY
- Noncontagious
- Inadequate plaque removal
- Blood dyscrasias (pregnancy)
- Oral contraceptives
- Allergic reactions
- Nutritional deficiencies
- Vasoconstriction (nicotine)
- Endocrine/hormonal variations:
  – Pregnancy
  – Menses
  – Menarche
- Chronic debilitating disease
- Vincent disease:
  – Synergistic infection with fusiform bacillus (*Fusobacterium* spp.) and spirochete (*Borrelia vincentii*)

COMMONLY ASSOCIATED CONDITIONS
- Periodontitis
- Glossitis
- Pedunculated growths (pyogenic granulomata)

 DIAGNOSIS

HISTORY
- Gum swelling and edema (usually painless)
- Gum erythema
- Bleeding of gums when brushing, flossing, or eating
- Inquire about HIV risk, pregnancy, nutritional deficiencies, diabetes, and other risk factors as indicated (See "Risk Factors").
- Smoking history
- Oral hygiene, dental visit history

PHYSICAL EXAM
- Normal gums should appear pink, firm, and shiny
- Gum swelling and edema (usually painless)
- Erythema
- Bleeding with manipulation of gums
- Change of normal gum contours
- Plaque and calculus (not easily removed)
- Edema of interdental papillae
- HIV gingivitis:
  – Also called linear gingival erythema
  – Narrow band of bright red inflamed gum surrounding neck of tooth
  – Painful
  – Bleeds easily
  – Rapid destruction of tissue
- Vincent disease:
  – Ulcers
  – Fever
  – Malaise
  – Regional lymphadenopathy
  – Pain
  – Mouth odor

DIAGNOSTIC TESTS & INTERPRETATION
Lab
Initial lab tests
- Possible smear or culture to identify causative agent (HIV gingivitis includes gram-negative anaerobes, enteric strains, and candida)
- Labs for contributing conditions (HIV, pregnancy, diabetes, nutritional deficiencies)

Imaging
Initial approach
No tests usually needed

Pathological Findings
- Acute or chronic inflammation
- Hyperemic capillaries
- Polymorphonuclear infiltration
- Papillary projections in subepithelial tissue
- Fibroblasts

DIFFERENTIAL DIAGNOSIS
- Periodontitis (deeper inflammation to connective tissue, ligaments, and alveolar bone)
- Glossitis
- Desquamative gingivitis (painful, persistent, usually middle-aged women)
- Pericoronitis (gum flap traps food and plaque over partially erupted molar), common in adolescence
- Gingival ulcers (aphthous, herpetic, malignancy, TB, syphilis)
- Specific forms of gingivitis: See "Description" including acute necrotizing ulcerative gingivitis (Vincent disease) and HIV gingivitis (linear gingival erythema)

 ## TREATMENT

MEDICATION
First Line
- Chlorhexidine rinses or varnishes may be used (4)
- Antibiotics indicated only for acute necrotizing ulcerative gingivitis (Vincent disease)
- Antibiotics:
  – Penicillin V: Pediatric dose, 25–50 mg/kg/d divided q6h; adult dose, 250–500 mg q6h, OR
  – Erythromycin: Pediatric dose 30–40 mg/kg/d divided q6h; adult dose, 250 mg q6h
- Topical corticosteroids:
  – Triamcinolone (0.147 mg/g) in Orabase (spray), applied locally t.i.d., q.i.d.
- Contraindications:
  – Allergy to specific medication
- Precautions:
  – Erythromycin frequently causes significant gastrointestinal issues.

Second Line
- Acetaminophen or ibuprofen for any pain (rare)
- Other antibiotics or antifungal rinses or systemics according to culture or smear
- Decapinol oral rinse (surfactant that acts as a physical barrier, making it harder for bacteria to stick to tooth surfaces) to reduce bacteria (not recommended for pregnant women or children under 12). Should be used in conjunction with other oral hygiene practices when those practices alone are not enough.

ADDITIONAL TREATMENT
General Measures
- Stop any contributing medications
- Remove irritating factors (plaque, calculus, faulty dentures)
- Good oral hygiene (see "General Prevention")
- Regular dental checkups (for scaling and polishing if plaque and/or tartar are present)
- No smoking
- Warm saline rinses b.i.d.

Issues for Referral
- Dental referral for cleanings and further treatment as needed
- If gingivitis becomes periodontitis, deep root scaling and planing may be indicated.

COMPLEMENTARY AND ALTERNATIVE MEDICINE
- Bilberry: Potentially helpful in reducing inflammation and stabilizing collagen tissue
- Coenzyme Q10: Topically, to restore coenzyme Q10 deficiency
- Replace any other deficiencies (e.g., vitamin C).

SURGERY/OTHER PROCEDURES
- Debridement for acute necrotizing gingivitis
- Minor surgery may be necessary to correct tissue overgrowth for gingivitis caused by medicines.

 ## ONGOING CARE

FOLLOW-UP RECOMMENDATIONS
- Outpatient
- No restrictions

Patient Monitoring
Until clear; dental follow-up for continued cleanings and secondary prevention

DIET
- Well-balanced diet that includes fruits, vegetables, vitamin C; avoid sugary snacks and drinks, which contribute to plaque formation.
- Soft foods during flare if significant inflammation/bleeding for a few days

PATIENT EDUCATION
- Good oral hygiene including twice daily brushing with fluoridated toothpaste and daily flossing; regular dental visits
- Printable and viewable patient information available under "periodontal diseases" from the American Dental Association at http://www.ada.org; and the American Academy of Periodontology at http://www.perio.org

PROGNOSIS
- Usual course: Acute, relapsing, intermittent, chronic
- Prognosis: Generally favorable, responds well to appropriate treatment
- Left untreated may progress to periodontitis (controversial), which is a major cause of tooth loss

COMPLICATIONS
Severe periodontal disease (which is associated with heart disease, diabetes, and preterm birth)

REFERENCES

1. Mehta A, Sequeira PS, Sahoo RC, et al. Is bronchial asthma a risk factor for gingival diseases? A control study. *N Y State Dent J*. 2009;75:44–6.
2. Nilsson M, Kopp S. Gingivitis and periodontitis are related to repeated high levels of circulating tumor necrosis factor-alpha in patients with rheumatoid arthritis. *J Periodontol*. 2008;79:1689–96.
3. Deery C, Heanue M, Deacon S, et al. The effectiveness of manual versus powered toothbrushes for dental health: a systematic review. *J Dent*. 2004;32:197–211.
4. Puig-Silla M, Montiel-Company JM, Almerich-Silla JM. Use of chlorhexidine varnishes in preventing and treating periodontal disease. A review of the literature. *Med Oral Patol Oral Cir Bucal*. 2008;13:E257–60.

ADDITIONAL READING

- Armitage GC. Development of a classification system for periodontal diseases and conditions. *Ann Periodont*. 1999;4:1.
- Coventry J, Griffiths G, Scully C et al. Periodontal disease: ABC of oral health. *Br Med J*. 2000;321:36–9.
- Genco RJ. Current view of risk factors for periodontal diseases. *J Periodontol*. 1996;67: 1041–9.
- Loesche WJ, Grossman NS. Periodontal disease as a specific, albeit chronic, infection: diagnosis and treatment. *Clin Microbiol Rev*. 2001;14:727–52.
- New Oral Rinse Helps Treat Gingivitis. FDA Consumer [serial on the Internet]. (2005, July), [cited July 22, 2008]; 39(4):5–6. Available from: Alt HealthWatch.
- Oliver RC, Brown LJ, Loer H. Peridontal disease in the United States population. *J Peridontol*. 1998; 69(2):269–78.

See Also (Topic, Algorithm, Electronic Media Element)
Glossitis, Dental Infection
Algorithm: Bleeding Gums

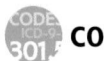 ## CODES

ICD9
- 523.00 Acute gingivitis, plaque induced
- 523.01 Acute gingivitis, non-plaque induced
- 523.10 Chronic gingivitis, plaque induced

CLINICAL PEARLS
- Gingivitis may be treated with regular dental cleanings, good oral hygiene, and use of chlorhexidine rinses.
- Untreated, gingivitis may progress to periodontitis, a possible contributor to systemic inflammation and its consequences (such as coronary artery disease and preterm labor).
- New onset or difficult to treat gingivitis, consider differential of etiology - pregnancy, HIV, diabetes, medications, vitamin deficiencies .

G

GLAUCOMA, PRIMARY CLOSED-ANGLE

Samantha R. Llanos, PharmD, RPh
Mark Iverson, MD

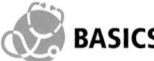 **BASICS**

DESCRIPTION
- Acute-angle closure (the term *glaucoma* is added when glaucomatous optic neuropathy is present):
  - At least 2 of the following symptoms: Ocular pain; N/V; intermittent blurred vision with halos, *plus*
  - At least 3 of the following signs: Intraocular pressure (IOP) >21 mm Hg; conjunctival injection; corneal epithelial edema; mid-dilated nonreactive pupil; shallower chamber in the presence of occlusion
- Primary-angle closure (the term *glaucoma* is added when glaucomatous optic neuropathy is present):
  - Occludable drainage angle *plus* signs that the peripheral iris has obstructed the trabecular meshwork (e.g., elevated IOP, lens opacities)
- Chronic angle-closure glaucoma: Refers to an eye with permanent closure of areas of the anterior chamber angle by peripheral anterior synechiae

Geriatric Considerations
Increased risk with age and prior history of cataract, hyperopia, and/or uveitis

Pediatric Considerations
Rare

Pregnancy Considerations
Medications used may cross the placenta and be excreted into breast milk.

EPIDEMIOLOGY
- 6th and 7th decades of life
- Female > Male
- Inuit and Asian > African and European
- Most common form of glaucoma worldwide, but only 10% of glaucoma in the US

Prevalence
Acute-angle closure glaucoma occurs in 1 in 1,000 Caucasians; 1 in 100 Asians; 2–4 in 100 Eskimos (lifetime)

RISK FACTORS
- Hyperopia
- Age >40–50 years old
- Shallow anterior chamber
- Female gender
- Family history of angle closure
- Asian or Inuit descent
- Pseudoexfoliation
- Medications that may induce angle-closure glaucoma:
  - Angiotensin-converting enzyme inhibitors (rare)
  - Adrenergic agonists (albuterol)
  - Anticholinergics
  - Antihistamines
  - Antidepressants: Selective serotonin reuptake inhibitors, TCAs
  - Cholinergic agents (pilocarpine)
  - Noncatecholamine adrenergic agonists
  - Sulfa-based drugs
  - Topiramate
  - Warfarin (rare)

Genetics
Polygenic inheritance: 1st-degree relatives have a 2–5% lifetime risk.

GENERAL PREVENTION
- Routine eye exam with gonioscopy for high-risk populations
- United States Preventive Services Task Force: Insufficient evidence to recommend for or against screening adults for glaucoma

PATHOPHYSIOLOGY
- Peripheral iris apposition to the trabecular meshwork obstructs the outflow of aqueous humor through the trabecular meshwork, which causes elevation in IOP.
- The underlying mechanism is anterior lens displacement or other anatomic abnormality, leading to pupillary block in which aqueous humor egress through the pupil is limited. This causes pressure to build posterior to the iris, leading to anterior iris displacement.

ETIOLOGY
Predisposing ocular anatomy

COMMONLY ASSOCIATED CONDITIONS
- Cataract
- Hyperopia
- Microphthalmos
- Systemic hypertension

 DIAGNOSIS

HISTORY
- Patient's previous medical and ophthalmologic history
- Family history of glaucoma
- Obtain history of prescription and over-the-counter medications
- Precipitating factors (dim light, meds)
- Review of symptoms
- Acute:
  - Severe unilateral ocular pain
  - Blurred vision
  - Lacrimation
  - Photophobia
  - Halos around lights/objects
  - Frontal, ipsilateral, headache
  - Nausea and vomiting
- Chronic:
  - May have subacute symptoms (intermittent subacute attacks)
  - Compromised peripheral, then central vision
  - May be asymptomatic

PHYSICAL EXAM
- Includes, but is not limited to, the following in the undilated eye (1)[C]:
  - Visual acuity
  - Visual field testing and ocular motility
  - Pupil size and reactivity (mid-dilated, minimally reactive)
  - External examination
  - Undilated fundus exam (congestion, cupping, atrophy of optic nerve)
  - Slit-lamp biomicroscopy (anterior segments)
  - Tonometry (determination of IOP)
  - Gonioscopy (visualization of the angle)

- Acute:
  - Elevated intraocular pressure (usually 40–80 mm Hg)
  - Corneal microcystic edema (haze)
  - Lid edema, conjunctival hyperemia, and circumcorneal injection (ciliary flush)
  - Fixed mid-dilated pupil (often oval) and firm globe
  - Shallow anterior chamber, often with inflammatory reaction (cell and flare)
  - Blepharospasm (severe cases)
  - Pain with eye movement
  - Closed angle by gonioscopy
- Chronic:
  - Multiple peripheral anterior synechiae
  - Normal or elevated intraocular pressure
  - Increased cup-to-disc ratio or excavation of disc
  - Glaucoma flecks (lens) and iris atrophy (previous acute attacks)

DIAGNOSTIC TESTS & INTERPRETATION
Imaging
Ultrasound biomicroscopy

Diagnostic Procedures/Surgery
Careful ophthalmic examination, including gonioscopy and tonometry (1,2,3)[C]

Pathological Findings
- Corneal stromal and epithelial edema
- Endothelial cell loss (guttata)
- Iris stromal necrosis
- Anterior subcapsular cataract (*glaukomflecken*)
- Optic disc congestion, cupping, excavation
- Optic nerve atrophy

DIFFERENTIAL DIAGNOSIS
- Acute orbital compartment syndrome
- Traumatic hyphema
- Conjunctivitis, episcleritis
- Corneal abrasion
- Glaucoma, malignant or neovascular
- Herpes zoster ophthalmicus
- Iritis and uveitis
- Orbital/periorbital infection
- Plateau iris syndrome
- Vitreous or subconjunctival hemorrhage
- Tight necktie, causing increased IOP

 TREATMENT

Goals of Treatment
- Reduce acutely increased IOP.
- Remove anything causing pupillary block .
- Treat residual increased IOP caused by permanent trabecular meshwork dysfunction.

MEDICATION
- Practically speaking, acute angle glaucoma is managed with oral mannitol **or** glycerin for a rapid decrease in IOP, and then, once the cornea clears, a peripheral iridotomy is done.

- Initiate medical therapy first, using some or all of the following (1)[C],(4)[B]:

– Topical/systemic carbonic anhydrase inhibitor
  ○ Acetazolamide (Diamox) 500 mg IV *plus/or* 500 mg PO; dorzolamide 2% eyedrops or brinzolamide (Azopt) 1% suspension; 1 drop in affected eye q8h.
  ○ Contraindications/precautions: Sulfa-allergy (risk of cross-sensitivity), bitter taste, eyelid reactions
– β-Blockers:
  ○ Timolol (Timoptic) 0.5% solution, levobunolol (Betagan) 0.5% solution *or* betaxolol (Betoptic) 0.5% solution; also carteolol (generic) 1% solution or metipranolol (OptiPranolol) 0.3% solution, 1 drop in affected eye q12h.
  ○ Contraindications/precautions: Decompensated heart failure, sinus bradycardia ≥2nd-degree heart block, severe COPD/asthma; increased risk of bradycardia or heart block with digoxin, verapamil, diltiazem, or clonidine; effect on IOP may be lessened in patients taking oral β-blockers
– α-Agonists:
  ○ Apraclonidine (Iopidine) 0.5–1% solution, 1 drop in affected eye q8h; brimonidine 1 drop 2–3 times daily
  ○ Prostaglandin analogs: latanoprost (Xalatan), travoprost (Travatan), bimatoprost (Lumigan) 1 drop daily. Precautions: Irreversible changes to iris, eyelid and eyelash pigmentation, eyelash growth, itching, redness, edema
– Topical steroid: (Prednisolone 1% solution) 1–2 drops 2–4+ times daily
– Miotics:
  ○ Pilocarpine (2–4% solution, 1 drop in affected eye q6–8h); do not use unless directed by ophthalmologist .
  ○ Carbachol 3% solution, 1 drop 4 times daily or echothiophate iodide (phospholine iodide) 0.125% solution, 1 drop twice daily
  ○ Precautions: May worsen the condition due to anterior rotation of the lens-iris diaphragm, impaired night vision,
– Hyperosmotic agents:
  ○ Glycerin, 1–2 g/kg PO, repeat q5h p.r.n.; isosorbide, 1.5 g/kg PO; mannitol 20% solution, 1.5–2 g/kg over 30 minutes
  ○ Precautions: Glycerin-caution in patients with congestive heart failure or diabetes; mannitol-caution in patients with congestive heart failure or renal failure

ADDITIONAL TREATMENT
General Measures
- For acute form:
  – Manage extraocular symptoms, such as nausea and pain.
  – Obtain immediate ophthalmology consult.
- Ocular goals of therapy through medical and surgical treatment:
  – Reduce IOP to <35 mm Hg or by >25% of presenting IOP (4)[B].
  – Prevent damage to the optic nerve.
  – Prevent central retinal artery occlusion.
  – Prevent or reverse angle closure.

Additional Therapies
- Initiate immediate emergency ophthalmologic treatment.
- Keep patient supine.

SURGERY/OTHER PROCEDURES
- Acute (1,5)[B]:
  – Laser peripheral iridotomy per ophthalmology (1,5)[B]
  – Perform surgical iridectomy if laser is not possible.
- Chronic:
  – Goniosynechialysis
  – Phacoemulsification

IN-PATIENT CONSIDERATIONS
Admission Criteria
- Patient requires metabolic ± electrolyte and volume status monitoring (with osmotic agents)
- Maintain ophthalmology follow-up.

IV Fluids
IV access

Nursing
Implement emergency ophthalmic plan of care.

Discharge Criteria
Patient is stable for outpatient follow-up.

 # ONGOING CARE

FOLLOW-UP RECOMMENDATIONS
- Schedule immediate ophthalmologic follow-up.
- Hospital admission if clinically warranted

Patient Monitoring
- Postsurgical follow-up
- Fellow eye evaluation
- Chronic monitoring post acute attack per ophthalmology

DIET
Regular as tolerated

PATIENT EDUCATION
- Advise patient to seek emergency medical attention if experiencing a change in visual acuity, blurred vision, eye pain, or headache.
- New medication counseling
- If narrow angles but no peripheral iridotomy performed: Avoid decongestants, motion sickness medications, adrenergic agents, antipsychotics, antidepressants, and anticholinergic agents.
- Proper eyedrop administration technique
- Patients with significant visual impairment should be referred to vision rehab and social services
- Patient education materials:
  – Glaucoma Research Foundation at: http://www.glaucoma.org
  – National Eye Institute at: http://www.nei.nih.gov
  – Glaucoma handout from American Academy of Family Physicians
  – Handout on using glaucoma eyedrops in Am Fam Physician 1999;59(7):1882

PROGNOSIS
- With timely treatment, most patients do not have permanent vision loss.
- Depends on:
  – Time to treatment
  – Underlying eye disease
  – Ethnicity

COMPLICATIONS
- Chronic corneal edema
- Corneal fibrosis and vascularization
- Iris atrophy
- Cataract
- Optic atrophy
- Malignant glaucoma
- Central retinal artery/vein occlusion
- Permanent decrease in visual acuity
- Repeat episode
- Fellow eye attack

REFERENCES
1. American Academy of Ophthalmology. *Primary angle closure preferred practice pattern*. San Francisco: American Academy of Ophthalmology, 2005. Available at: http://www.aao.org.
2. Asrani S, Sarunic M, Santiago C, et al. Detailed visualization of the anterior segment using fourier-domain optical coherence tomography. *Arch Ophthalmol*. 2008;126:765–71.
3. Barkana Y, Dorairaj SK, Gerber Y, et al. Agreement between gonioscopy and ultrasound biomicroscopy in detecting iridotrabecular apposition. *Arch Ophthalmol*. 2007;125:1331–5.
4. Choong YF, Irfan S, Menage MJ. Acute angle closure glaucoma: an evaluation of a protocol for acute treatment. *Eye*. 1999;13(Pt 5):613–6.
5. Saw SM, Gazzard G, Friedman DS. Interventions for angle-closure glaucoma: an evidence-based update. *Ophthalmology*. 2003;110:1869–78; quiz 1878-9, 1930.

ADDITIONAL READING
Tripathi RC, Tripathi BJ, Haggerty C. Drug-induced glaucomas: mechanism and management. *Drug Saf*. 2003;26:749–67.

See Also (Topic, Algorithm, Electronic Media Element)
Glaucoma, Primary Open-Angle

 ## CODES

ICD9
- 365.20 Primary angle-closure glaucoma, unspecified
- 365.22 Acute angle-closure glaucoma
- 365.23 Chronic angle-closure glaucoma

CLINICAL PEARLS
- Examiner can determine if patient is hyperopic by observing the *magnification* of the patient's face through their glasses (myopic lenses minify).
- A careful history may reveal similar episodes of angle closure that resolved spontaneously.
- Miotics are ineffective in the setting of high IOP (due to iris sphincter ischemia) and can potentially worsen angle closure by causing anterior rotation of the lens–iris diaphragm.

GLAUCOMA, PRIMARY OPEN-ANGLE

Richard W. Allinson, MD

 BASICS

DESCRIPTION
- Primary open-angle glaucoma (POAG) is an optic neuropathy resulting in visual field loss frequently associated with increased intraocular pressure (IOP).
- Normal IOP is 10–22 mm Hg. However, glaucomatous optic nerve damage also can occur with normal IOP and as a secondary manifestation of other disorders, such as corticosteroid-induced glaucoma.
- System(s) affected: Nervous
- Synonym(s): Chronic open-angle glaucoma

Pregnancy Considerations
Prostaglandins should be avoided during pregnancy in the treatment of POAG.

EPIDEMIOLOGY
Incidence
- Predominant age: Usually >40 years
- Increases with age
- Predominant gender: Male = Female

Prevalence
Prevalence of POAG in persons >40 years of age is ~1.8%.

Geriatric Considerations
Increasing prevalence with increasing age

RISK FACTORS
- Increased IOP
- Myopia
- DM
- African American
- Elderly
- Positive family history
- Central corneal thickness <550 μm
- Larger vertical cup-to-disc ratio
- Larger horizontal cup-to-disc ratio
- Disc hemorrhage
- Prolonged use of topical, periocular, inhaled, or systemic corticosteroids

Genetics
A family history of glaucoma increases the risk for developing glaucoma.

GENERAL PREVENTION
- Genetic testing may help to screen for POAG.
- Possible reduced risk of open-angle glaucoma with long-term use of oral statins

PATHOPHYSIOLOGY
- Abnormal aqueous outflow resulting in increased IOP
- Normally, aqueous is produced by the ciliary epithelium of the ciliary body and is secreted into the posterior chamber of the eye.
- Aqueous then flows through the pupil and enters the anterior chamber to be drained by the trabecular meshwork in the iridocorneal angle of the eye into the Schlemm canal and into the venous system of the episclera.
- 5–10% of the total aqueous outflow leaves via the uveoscleral pathway.

ETIOLOGY
- Impaired aqueous outflow through the trabecular meshwork
- Increased resistance within the aqueous drainage system

COMMONLY ASSOCIATED CONDITIONS
DM

 DIAGNOSIS

HISTORY
Painless, slowly progressive visual loss; patients are generally unaware of the visual loss until late in the disease. Central visual acuity remains unaffected until late in the disease.

PHYSICAL EXAM
- Increased IOP
- Cup-to-disc ratio (C:D) >0.5: Normal eyes show a characteristic configuration for disc rim thickness of inferior ≥ superior ≥ nasal ≥ temporal (ISNT rule).
- Earliest visual field defects are paracentral scotomas and peripheral nasal steps.

DIAGNOSTIC TESTS & INTERPRETATION
Imaging
Initial approach
- Optical coherence tomography can be useful in the detection of glaucoma by measuring the thickness of the retinal nerve fiber layer (RNFL).
- RNFL is thinner in patients with glaucoma.
- RNFL thickness is affected by age, ethnicity, axial length, and optic disc area. RNFL tends to be thinner with older age, Caucasians, greater axial length, and smaller optic disc area.
- Factors associated with variability in RNFL thickness measurements include signal-strength variability, low analysis confidence, and low RNFL thickness.

Diagnostic Procedures/Surgery
- Visual field testing: Perimetry
- Tonometry to measure IOP
- Ophthalmoscopy to assess optic nerve for glaucomatous damage

Pathological Findings
- Atrophy and cupping of optic nerve
- Loss of retinal ganglion cells and their axons produces defects in the retinal nerve fiber layer.

DIFFERENTIAL DIAGNOSIS
- Normal-tension glaucoma
- Optic nerve pits
- Anterior ischemic optic neuropathy
- Compressive lesions of the optic nerve or chiasm
- Posthemorrhagic (shock optic neuropathy)

 TREATMENT

MEDICATION
- >1 medication, with different mechanisms of action, may be needed.
- When ≥3 medications are required, compliance is difficult, and surgery may be needed. Ocular hypotensive agent categories:
  - β-Adrenergic antagonists (nonselective and selective): Decrease aqueous formation: Timolol 0.5% 1 drop in affected eye q12h
  - Parasympathomimetics (miotic), including cholinergic (direct-acting) and anticholinesterase agents (indirect-acting parasympathomimetic): Increase aqueous outflow:
    - Pilocarpine 1–4% 1 drop in affected eye b.i.d.–q.i.d. (cholinergic)
    - Demecarium bromide 0.125% 1 drop in affected eye b.i.d. (anticholinesterase)
- Carbonic anhydrase inhibitors (oral, topical): Decrease aqueous formation:
  - Acetazolamide 250 mg p.o. q.i.d.
  - Dorzolamide 2% 1 drop t.i.d.
- Adrenergic agonists (nonselective and selective α_2-adrenergic agonists):
  - Epinephrine 0.5–2% 1 drop b.i.d. and dipivefrin 0.1% 1 drop b.i.d. (nonselective agents) increase aqueous outflow through the trabecular meshwork and increase uveoscleral outflow.
  - Brimonidine tartrate 0.1% 1 drop t.i.d. (α_2-adrenergic agonist) decreases aqueous formation and increases uveoscleral outflow.
- Prostaglandin analogues: Enhance uveoscleral outflow: Latanoprost 0.005% 1 drop at bedtime
- Hyperosmotic agents: Increase blood osmolality, drawing water from the vitreous cavity:
  - Mannitol 20% solution administered IV at 2 g/kg of body weight
  - Glycerin 50% solution administered orally; dosage is usually 4–7 oz
- Contraindications:
  - Nonselective β-adrenergic antagonists: Avoid in asthma, COPD, 2nd- and 3rd-degree A-V block, and decompensated heart failure. Betaxolol is a selective β-adrenergic antagonist and is safer in pulmonary disease.
  - Parasympathomimetics (miotic): Indirect-acting parasympathomimetic agents increase risk of ocular and systemic side effects and are used rarely.
  - Carbonic anhydrase inhibitors:
    - Do not use with sulfa drug allergies.
    - Do not use with cirrhosis because of the risk of hepatic encephalopathy.
  - Adrenergic agonists: Caution recommended when using brimonidine and MAO inhibitor or TCA and in patients with vascular insufficiency. Brimonidine can cause excessive sleepiness and lethargy in children.
  - Prostaglandin analogues: Caution with uveitis and avoided during pregnancy.
  - Hyperosmotic agents:
    - Glycerin can produce hyperglycemia or ketoacidosis in diabetic patients.
    - Can cause congestive heart failure
    - Do not use in patients with anuria.

- Precautions:
  - β-Adrenergic antagonists: Caution with obstructive pulmonary disease, heart failure, and DM
  - Parasympathomimetics (miotic): Cause pupillary constriction and may cause decreased vision in patients with a cataract, and may cause an eye ache or myopia due to increased accommodation. All miotics break down the blood–aqueous barrier and may induce chronic iridocyclitis.
  - Adrenergic agonists (e.g., brimonidine): Caution with vascular insufficiency
  - Prostaglandin analogues may cause increased pigmentation of the iris and periorbital tissue (eyelid):
    - ○ Increased pigmentation and growth of eyelashes
    - ○ Should be used with caution in active intraocular inflammation (iritis/uveitis)
    - ○ Caution is also advised in eyes with risk factors for herpes simplex, iritis, and cystoid macular edema.
    - ○ Macular edema may be a complication associated with treatment.
  - Hyperosmotic agents: Caution in diabetics, dehydrated patients, and those with cardiac, renal, and hepatic disease
- Significant possible interactions: β-Adrenergic antagonists: Caution in patients taking calcium antagonists because of possible A-V conduction disturbances, left ventricular failure, or hypotension
- Parasympathomimetics (miotic): Indirect-acting parasympathomimetic agents, anticholinesterase eye drops, can reduce serum pseudocholinesterase levels. If succinylcholine is used for induction of general anesthesia, prolonged apnea may result.

ADDITIONAL TREATMENT
General Measures
- Early Manifest Glaucoma Trial:
  - Early treatment delays progression.
  - The magnitude of initial IOP reduction influences disease progression (1)[A].
- Ocular Hypertension Treatment Study:
  - Patients who only had increased IOP in the range of 24–32 mm Hg were treated with topical ocular hypotensive medication.
  - Treatment produced ~20% reduction in IOP.
  - At 5 years, treatment reduced the incidence of POAG by >50%: 9.5% in the observation group vs 4.4% in the medication-treated group (2)[A]
- The Collaborative Normal-Tension Glaucoma Study Group:
  - Therapeutic intervention that resulted in a 30% decrease in IOP and helped to prevent progression of visual field loss (3)[A]
- The Advanced Glaucoma Intervention Study:
  - Eyes were randomized to laser trabeculoplasty or filtering surgery when medical therapy failed.
  - In follow-up, if the IOP was always <18 mm Hg, the visual fields tended to stabilize. When IOP was >17 mm Hg more than 1/2 of the time, patients tended to have worsening of their visual fields (4)[A].
  - Whites did better with trabeculectomy first, whereas African Americans did better with argon laser trabeculoplasty as the initial procedure.

- Collaborative Initial Glaucoma Treatment Study:
  - Both initial medical and surgical treatment achieved significant IOP reduction, and both had little visual field loss over time (5)[A].

SURGERY/OTHER PROCEDURES
- Argon laser trabeculoplasty (ALT):
  - Applied to 180 degrees of the trabecular meshwork
  - Improves aqueous outflow
  - The Glaucoma Laser Trial Research Group showed in newly diagnosed, previously untreated patients with POAG that ALT was as effective as topical glaucoma medication within the 1st 2 years of follow-up.
  - Usually reserved for patients needing better IOP control while taking topical glaucoma drops
- Trabeculectomy (glaucoma filtering surgery):
  - Usually reserved for patients needing better IOP control after maximal medical therapy and who may have previously undergone an ALT
  - Mitomycin C can be applied at the time of surgery to increase the chances of a surgical success.
  - Subconjunctival bevacizumab may be a beneficial adjunctive therapy for reducing late surgical failure after trabeculectomy.
- Shunt (tube) surgery:
  - For example, Molteno and Ahmed devices
  - Generally reserved for difficult glaucoma cases in which conventional filtering surgery has failed or is likely to fail
- Tube Versus Trabeculectomy (TVT) Study:
  - After 3 years of follow-up, both procedures were associated with similar intraocular pressure reduction and the number of glaucoma medications needed (6)[A].
- Ciliary body ablation: Indicated to lower IOP in patients with poor visual potential or those who are poor candidates for filtering or shunt procedures

 ONGOING CARE

FOLLOW-UP RECOMMENDATIONS
Patient Monitoring
- Monitor vision and IOP every 3–6 months.
- Visual field testing every 6–18 months
- Optic nerve evaluation every 3–18 months depending on POAG control
- A worsening of the mean deviation by 2 dB on the Humphrey field analyzer and confirmed by a single test after 6 months had a 72% probability of progression.
- The IOP response to ocular hypotensive agents tends to be reduced in persons with thicker corneas.

PATIENT EDUCATION
POAG is a silent robber of vision, and patients may not appreciate the significance of their disease until much of their visual field is lost.

PROGNOSIS
- With standard glaucoma therapy, the rate of visual field loss in POAG is slow.
- Patients still may lose vision and develop blindness, even when treated appropriately.
- The rate of legal blindness from POAG over a follow-up of 22 years is 19%.

COMPLICATIONS
Blindness

REFERENCES
1. Heijl A, Leske MC, Bengtsson B, et al. Reduction of intraocular pressure and glaucoma progression: results from the Early Manifest Glaucoma Trial. *Arch Ophthalmol*. 2002;120:1268–79.
2. Kass MA, Heuer DK, Higginbotham EJ, et al. The Ocular Hypertension Treatment Study: a randomized trial determines that topical ocular hypotensive medication delays or prevents the onset of primary open-angle glaucoma. *Arch Ophthalmol*. 2002;120:701–13; discussion 829–30.
3. Comparison of glaucomatous progression between untreated patients with normal-tension glaucoma and patients with therapeutically reduced intraocular pressures. Collaborative Normal-Tension Glaucoma Study Group. *Am J Ophthalmol*. 1998;126:487–97.
4. The Advanced Glaucoma Intervention Study (AGIS): 7. The relationship between control of intraocular pressure and visual field deterioration. The AGIS Investigators. *Am J Ophthalmol*. 2000;130: 429–40.
5. Lichter PR, et al. CIGTS Study Group. Interim clinical outcomes in the Collaborative Initial Glaucoma Treatment Study comparing initial treatment randomized to medications or surgery. *Ophthalmol*. 2001;108:1943–53.
6. Gedde SJ, Schiffman JC, et al. Three-Year Follow-up of the Tube Versus Trabeculectomy Study. *Am J Ophthalmol*. 2009;148:670–684.

CODES

ICD9
365.11 Primary open angle glaucoma

CLINICAL PEARLS
- Topical or systemic steroids can cause the IOP to increase.
- Pain is not a frequent symptom of POAG.
- Painless, slowly progressive visual loss; patients generally are unaware of the visual loss until late in the disease. Central visual acuity remains unaffected until late in the disease.
- Patients still may lose vision and develop blindness, even when treated appropriately.

G

GLOMERULONEPHRITIS, ACUTE

Carla M. Nester, MD

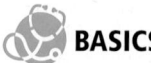 **BASICS**

DESCRIPTION

- Acute glomerulonephritis (GN) is an inflammatory process involving the glomerulus of the kidney, resulting in a clinical syndrome consisting of hematuria, proteinuria, hypertension, and renal insufficiency.
- Acute glomerulonephritis may be one of many primary diseases, or it may present as part of a systemic disease:
  – Postinfectious GN
  – IgA nephropathy–Henoch Schönlein purpura
  – Antiglomerular basement membrane disease (anti-GBM disease)
  – Antineutrophil cytoplasmic antibody (ANCA)-associated GN
  – Membranoproliferative GN (MPGN)
  – Lupus nephritis
  – Cryoglobulin-associated GN
- Clinical severity ranges from asymptomatic microscopic or gross hematuria to a rapid loss of kidney function (rapidly progressive glomerulonephritis: RPGN).

ALERT
Urgent investigation and treatment are required to avoid irreversible loss of kidney function.

EPIDEMIOLOGY
- Postinfectious GN:
  – Most commonly follows group A beta-hemolytic *Streptococcus* infection, but can occur as a result of other infections.
  – Onset occurs 1–3 weeks after an infectious process (throat or skin).
  – Accounts for 80% of acute GN in children
- IgA nephropathy:
  – Most common form of primary acute GN
  – Occurs mainly in the 2nd and 3rd decades
  – Male:Female: 3:1
  – Incidence differs geographically: Asia > US
- Anti-GBM disease:
  – Also known as Goodpasture disease
  – A noted cause of the pulmonary–renal syndrome
  – Occurs most commonly in the 2nd or 3rd decade
  – Male:Female: 6:1
- ANCA-associated GN:
  – Uncommon: Often has a relapsing and remitting course
  – 3 disease presentations:
    ○ Wegener granulomatosis
    ○ Churg-Strauss disease
    ○ Microscopic polyangiitis
  – Older patients are more commonly affected, though this GN can affect any age group.
- MPGN:
  – May be primary or secondary
  – May present in the setting of a systemic viral or rheumatic illness
- Lupus nephritis:
  – 30–70% of systemic lupus patients will have renal involvement.
- Cryoglobulin-associated vasculitis:
  – 80% of cases are associated with hepatitis C infection.

RISK FACTORS
- Epidemics of nephritogenic strains of streptococci are triggers for postinfectious GN.
- Hepatic cirrhosis and celiac disease place patients at risk for IgA nephropathy.
- Anti-GBM disease has been associated with influenza A infection and inhaled hydrocarbon solvent exposure.
- ANCA-associated GN is increased in settings where there is increased silica exposure (i.e., earthquakes and farming).
- Complement factor abnormalities and infection with hepatitis B and/or C are known to be associated with MPGN.
- Infection with hepatitis C is a risk factor for developing cryoglobulinemic GN.
- Mutations in alternate complement pathway genes are associated with membranoproliferative glomerulonephritis.

Genetics
There are likely to be genetic factors that play a role in susceptibility to many of the acute GNs, though these have not been sufficiently defined to be useful clinically.

GENERAL PREVENTION
Early detection is paramount.

ETIOLOGY
- In general, an immunologic mechanism triggers inflammation and proliferation of glomerular tissue.
- Postinfectious GN:
  – Host immune reaction to nephritogenic strains of streptococci are triggers.
- IgA nephropathy:
  – Relates to an abnormal glycosylation of IgA
- Anti-GBM disease:
  – Caused by autoantibodies that target type IV collagen of basement membranes
- ANCA-associated GN:
  – Autoantibodies against neutrophil granules are involved in the pathogenesis.
- MPGN:
  – An immune or genetic etiology is presumed, which triggers renal deposits and inflammation.
- Lupus nephritis:
  – An immune complex-mediated glomerular disease
- Cryoglobulin-associated GN:
  – An immune etiology is presumed, but not clearly defined.

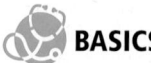 **DIAGNOSIS**

HISTORY
- Patients may complain of cola- or tea-colored urine and decreased urine volume.
- Edema occurs in many patients, typically face and lower extremities
- Shortness of breath may occur with significant fluid overload.
- Generalized malaise

- Patients may also present with complaints more specific to the associated disease:
  – Joint pain or rash in lupus nephritis
  – Hemoptysis in anti-GBM disease
  – Sinusitis and pulmonary infiltrates in ANCA-associated GN
  – Abdominal pain and purpura in IgA-Henoch Schönlein purpura
  – Purpura and skin vasculitis in cryoglobulinemia-associated GN

PHYSICAL EXAM
- A complete physical exam may discover clues to systemic disease as a potential cause.
- Sinus disease: ANCA-associated GN
- Pharyngitis or impetigo: Postinfectious GN
- Pulmonary abnormality: Anti-GBM disease or lupus nephritis
- Hepatomegaly or liver tenderness could point to cryoglobulinemia-associated GN or IgA nephropathy.
- Purpura may point to ANCA-associated GN or Henoch Schönlein purpura GN.

DIAGNOSTIC TESTS & INTERPRETATION
Lab
- Urinalysis with examination of sediment:
  – Dysmorphic red blood cells (RBCs) or RBC casts on urine microscopy indicate glomerular hematuria and suggest the diagnosis of an acute glomerulonephritis.
- Electrolytes, blood urea nitrogen, creatinine, complete blood count
- Antistreptolysin O titer
- Streptozyme
- Complement levels (C3 and C4):
  – C3 complement levels are abnormal in postinfectious GN; C3 and C4 are abnormal in lupus nephritis and MPGN; C4 can be low in cryoglobulinemia.
- Proteinuria:
  – 24-hour collection or random urine protein/creatinine ratio
- Antinuclear antibody to rule out lupus nephritis
- ANCA antibody screen:
  – MPO and PR3 antibodies
- Anti-GBM antibody
- Hepatitis B antigen
- Hepatitis C antibody

Imaging
A chest x-ray may be useful to define the significance of hemoptysis or a suspected infiltrate on exam.

Pathological Findings
Renal biopsy:
- If clinical picture is consistent with postinfectious GN in a child, a biopsy may not be needed.
- If there is clinical suspicion for other causes of acute GN, renal biopsy should be done.
- Light microscopy:
  – Diffuse hypercellularity suggests a proliferative disease such as IgA nephropathy, lupus nephritis, or postinfectious GN.

- Immunofluorescence:
  - IgA staining is pathognomonic for IgA nephropathy, with the absence of staining suggesting ANCA-associated GN.
- Electron microscopy:
  - The location of immunoglobulin deposits is useful in pointing to a particular diagnosis.

DIFFERENTIAL DIAGNOSIS

- The differential for hematuria (without clear indication that it is from a glomerular origin) should include trauma, prostate diseases, urologic cancer, or renal stone disease.
- If the urine blood is felt to be of glomerular origin, the differential should include each of the glomerular diseases that can present as an acute glomerulonephritis.

 ## TREATMENT

Supportive in post infectious

MEDICATION

First Line
- Hypertension:
  - Diuretics are useful, given that salt retention and edema are often present.
  - Calcium channel blockers
  - Avoid angiotensin-converting enzyme inhibitors if significant renal dysfunction is present.
- Peripheral edema:
  - Loop diuretics are often required due to the degree of edema.
- Pulmonary edema:
  - Oxygen and diuretic
- Hyperkalemia:
  - Sodium polystyrene sulfonate (Kayexalate) resin: 15 g p.o. every day to q.i.d. in 10% sorbitol
- Acidosis: Sodium bicarbonate 1–2 mEq/kg per dose (1–2 mmol/kg per dose) IV or p.o.

Second Line
- Each of the glomerular diseases often requires a specific treatment plan based on renal biopsy results; therefore, a nephrologist is often guiding care at this point.
- Pulse methylprednisolone has been reported to be useful in rapidly progressive forms of glomerulonephritis (1,2)[A].
- Crescents noted on renal biopsy are treated with the alkylating agent known as cyclophosphamide (1,2)[A].
- ANCA-associated renal disease, anti-GBM disease, and proliferative forms of lupus are treated with steroids plus either cyclophosphamide or mycophenolate (1,2,3,4,5)[A].
- Plasmapheresis has been shown to be effective in cases of pulmonary hemorrhage and in some patients who present in renal failure (2)[A].
- Dialysis may be needed for uremia, hyperkalemia refractory to medical management, intractable acidosis, and diuretic-resistant pulmonary edema.

ADDITIONAL TREATMENT

Issues for Referral
Consultation with a nephrologist is often required in order to assist with renal biopsy to confirm diagnosis and to assist with management.

IN-PATIENT CONSIDERATIONS

Admission Criteria
Consider admission for patients with no urine output, significant hypertension, and suspicion of pulmonary hemorrhage or fluid overload that is compromising heart or respiratory function.

Discharge Criteria
Hemodynamically stable patients without complications may be managed as outpatients.

 ## ONGOING CARE

FOLLOW-UP RECOMMENDATIONS

Patient Monitoring
Depends on type of glomerulonephritis:

- Regular blood pressure checks and urinalysis to detect recurrence; assessment of renal function to detect acute or follow chronic renal disease as a result of the primary event; and regular clinical assessment to detect suspicious symptoms that may herald a recurrence (i.e., rash, joint complaint, hemoptysis)
- Periodic reassessment of serology tests to detect asymptomatic individuals

DIET
- No-added-salt diet and fluid restriction until edema and hypertension clear
- Avoid high-potassium foods if significant renal dysfunction is present.

PATIENT EDUCATION
- National Kidney Foundation, 30 E. 33rd Street, Suite 1100, New York, NY 10016; (212) 889-2210
- Web site: http://vsearch.nlm.nih.gov/vivisimo/cgi-bin/query-meta?v%3Aproject=medlineplus&query=glomerulonephritis&x=48&y=10 - then search under the individual disease

PROGNOSIS
- In general, the prognosis depends on the cause of the glomerulonephritis.
- The GN may be self-limited (i.e., postinfectious GN) or part of a chronic disease that makes the possibility of recurrence likely.

COMPLICATIONS
- Hypertensive retinopathy and encephalopathy
- Rapidly progressive glomerulonephritis
- Microscopic hematuria may persist for years.
- Chronic kidney disease
- Nephrotic syndrome ($\sim$10%)

REFERENCES

1. Flanc RS, Roberts MA, Strippoli GF, et al. Treatment for lupus nephritis. *Cochrane Database Syst Rev.* 2004;CD002922.
2. Walters G, Willis NS, Craig JC. Interventions for renal vasculitis in adults. *Cochrane Database Syst Rev.* 2008;CD003232.
3. Hu W, Liu C, Xie H, et al. Mycophenolate Mofetil Versus Cyclophosphamide for Inducing Remission of ANCA Vasculitis with Moderate Renal Involvement. *Nephrol Dial Transplant.* 2007.
4. Walsh M, James M, Jayne D, et al. Mycophenolate Mofetil for Induction Therapy of Lupus Nephritis: A Systematic Review and Meta-Analysis. *Clin J Am Soc Nephrol.* 2007.
5. Isenberg D, Appel GB, Contreras G, Dooley MA, Ginzler EM, Jayne D, Sánchez-Guerrero J, Wofsy D, Yu X, Solomons N et al. Influence of race/ethnicity on response to lupus nephritis treatment: the ALMS study. *Rheumatology (Oxford).* 2010;49:128–40.

ADDITIONAL READING

Kaplan AA et al. The use of apheresis in immune renal disorders. *Ther Apher Dial.* 2003;7:165–72.

See Also (Topic, Algorithm, Electronic Media Element)
Hyperkalemia; Hypertensive Emergencies; Renal Failure, Acute
Algorithm: Hematuria

 ## CODES

ICD9
580.9 Acute glomerulonephritis with unspecified pathological lesion in kidney

CLINICAL PEARLS
- Dysmorphic RBCs and RBC casts are a key component of the urinalysis in glomerulonephritis.
- Postinfectious GN in children is typically a self-limited disease.
- Searching for other organ involvement is useful in establishing a definitive diagnosis.
- With discovery of a GN, monitor the initial renal function labs frequently to identify a rapidly progressive GN.

G

GLOSSITIS

Karyn M. Sullivan, PharmD, MPH
George Abraham, MD, MPH

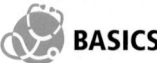 **BASICS**

DESCRIPTION
- An acute or chronic inflammation of the tongue, either as primary disease or a symptom of systemic disease
- System(s) affected: Gastrointestinal
- Common forms:
  – Atrophic glossitis (AG) or smooth tongue
  – Benign migratory glossitis (BMG) or geographic tongue or erythema migrans
  – Median rhomboid glossitis (MRG)
  – Herpetic geometric glossitis (HGG)

EPIDEMIOLOGY
- Predominant age: All ages
- Predominant gender:
  – Male > Female (3:1, MRG)
  – Female > Male (BMG)

Geriatric Considerations
Many patients with glossitis due to nutrition deficiencies are postmenopausal or elderly.

Prevalence
Varies; usual reported range: 1–14%

RISK FACTORS
- Poor nutrition
- Dentures
- Piercings
- Allergic background (e.g., asthma, eczema, hay fever)
- Smoking, smokeless tobacco
- Alcoholism
- Anxiety, stress
- Depression
- Hormonal disturbances
- Oral contraceptives
- Advancing age
- Immunocompromised state

Genetics
Familial history may be present with BMG.

GENERAL PREVENTION
- Evaluation of nutritional status, including B-vitamin deficiencies, anemias
- Cessation of tobacco use (including smokeless)
- Assess for irritation from teeth, dentures, or piercings.

PATHOPHYSIOLOGY
Tongue:
- AG: Atrophy of filiform papillae
- BMG: Erythematous, yellow-white lesions (dorsum)
- MRG: Atrophic filiform, plaque-like lesions (midline)
- HGG: Linear fissures (dorsum)

ETIOLOGY
- Systemic:
  – Nutritional deficiencies (e.g., B_{12}, folic acid)
  – Anemia (pernicious, iron deficiency)
  – HIV (opportunistic infections such as candidiasis, herpes simplex virus [HSV]; or HIV-associated changes such as loss of papillae)
  – Broad-spectrum antibiotics
  – Topical or inhaled corticosteroids
  – Various other medications (e.g., captopril, clarithromycin, enalapril, lansoprazole, lithium, metronidazole, nonsteroidal anti-inflammatory drugs)
- Local:
  – Infections (e.g., HSV, Epstein-Barr virus, candidiasis)
  – Trauma (ill-fitting dentures, piercings, burns, convulsive seizures)
  – Primary irritants (alcohol, tobacco, hot foods, spices, excessive peppermint, citrus)
  – Sensitization with chemical irritants (e.g., dyes, mouthwash, toothpaste, systemic drugs)
  – Malignancy (95% are squamous cell)

COMMONLY ASSOCIATED CONDITIONS
- Fissured tongue (BMG)
- HIV infection (rare)
- Reiter syndrome (rare)
- Down syndrome (rare)
- Crohn disease (rare)
- Celiac disease (possible correlation)

 DIAGNOSIS

Some symptoms of glossitis have no organic cause. Treat symptoms and reevaluate if no improvement.

HISTORY
- Many cases are asymptomatic.
- Oral discomfort
- Burning sensation on tongue (often associated with nutritional deficiency)
- Sensitivity to hot or spicy foods
- Sensation of foreign body in the mouth
- Paroxysmal ear pain
- Swollen or painful submandibular lymph nodes
- Symptoms tend to wax and wane (BMG).

PHYSICAL EXAM
- AG: Smooth, glossy, red or pink tongue (1,2)[B]
- BMG: Erythematous and white patches on the dorsum of tongue; lesions may lack papillae; irregular (maplike) and migratory lesions (3)[B]
- MRG: Erythematous, shiny, rhomboid-shaped plaque in middle of tongue; hypertrophic or atrophic surface changes (3,2)[B]
- HGG: Linear fissures on dorsal tongue; geometric pattern is common; herpetic lesions usually are absent on other mucosal surfaces (3)[B]

DIAGNOSTIC TESTS & INTERPRETATION
Lab
Serum B_{12}, folic acid, complete blood count (CBC) with differential, ferritin, RPR, TSH

Initial lab tests
- AG: Test for B_{12}, folic acid, iron deficiency (1)[B]
- BMG: None (3,4)[B]
- MRG: Viral culture, fungal smear (3)[B]
- HGG: Viral culture, Tzanck smear (3)[B]

Diagnostic Procedures/Surgery
- Biopsy solitary lesions that do not respond to treatment (3,4)[B].
- 10% potassium hydroxide scrapings for suspected candidiasis (1)[B]

Pathological Findings
Vary according to underlying causes

DIFFERENTIAL DIAGNOSIS
- Irritation fibroma
- Mucocele
- Granular cell tumor
- Tertiary syphilis
- Drug reaction
- Lichen planus
- Squamous cell carcinoma (rarely) (5)[C]

Pediatric Considerations
Differential diagnosis includes local trauma and severe neutropenia (4)[B].

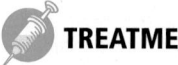 **TREATMENT**

MEDICATION
- AG:
  – Vitamin B_{12}, folic acid, iron (if deficient)
  – For candidiasis: Nystatin oral suspension 100,000 units/mL swish and spit 5 mL q.i.d. *OR* clotrimazole 1–2 troches 4–5 times a day (3)[B]
- BMG:
  – Usually no treatment
  – The following agents may be used to reduce tongue sensitivity or if lesions recur: Antihistamines, such as diphenhydramine liquid: Rinse with 5–10 mL, holding it over the tongue for a few minutes and then swallowing, 3–4 times a day (may also dilute in a 1:4 ratio with water) (2,6)[B] *OR* Miracle Mouthwash: Swish and spit 5 mL, 3–4 times a day *OR* topical steroid gels, such as 0.1% triamcinolone oral dental paste (Oralone) (2)[B]

- MRG:
  - Usually no treatment
  - Topical antifungals (nystatin oral suspension or clotrimazole troches) may provide temporary improvement (3)[B].
- HGG:
  - Oral antivirals such as acyclovir 200 mg 5 times daily (3)[B],(7)[C]

    Contraindications:
- Nystatin oral suspension: Hypersensitivity to nystatin products
- Clotrimazole troche: Hypersensitivity to clotrimazole
- Diphenhydramine:
  - Hypersensitivity to diphenhydramine
  - Newborns or premature infants
  - Nursing mothers
- Acyclovir (oral): Hypersensitivity to acyclovir or valacyclovir
- Triamcinolone (oral paste): corticosteroid hypersensitivity
- Precautions:
  - Clotrimazole troche: Hepatic impairment
  - Diphenhydramine:
    - May cause excitation in young children
    - Concurrent monoamine oxidase inhibitor (MAOI) therapy
    - Concurrent use of central nervous system (CNS) depressants
    - Decreases mental alertness and psychomotor performance
    - Older adults are more susceptible to side effects.
    - Bladder neck obstruction
    - Symptomatic prostatic hypertrophy
    - Narrow-angle glaucoma
    - History of bronchial asthma, increased intraocular pressure, hyperthyroidism, cardiovascular disease, or hypertension
  - Acyclovir (oral):
    - Maintain adequate hydration.
    - Geriatric patients (due to age-related decline in renal function)
    - Renal impairment
  - Triamcinolone (oral paste): Infections or sores in the mouth
- Significant possible interactions:
  - Diphenhydramine: Alcohol (increased sedation)
  - Acyclovir (oral): Meperidine (increased risk of CNS stimulation and seizures)
- Adverse effects:
  - Clotrimazole troche:
    - Nausea, vomiting, or diarrhea
    - Mild elevations in serum glutamic-oxaloacetic transaminase (SGOT) levels
  - Diphenhydramine:
    - Sedation
    - Dizziness
    - Urinary retention
  - Acyclovir (oral):
    - Nausea, vomiting, and diarrhea
    - Myalgia
    - Transient renal impairment
  - Triamcinolone (oral paste):
    - Burning
    - Itching
    - Irritation

Pediatric Considerations
- Diphenhydramine liquid: Rinse with 5–10 mL (depending on age and weight), holding it over the tongue for a few minutes and then swallowing, 3–4 times a day (6)[B].
- Topical antifungal/steroid agent: Triamcinolone acetonide 0.1% in nystatin suspension (8)[B]
- Alkaline saline mouth rinse (8)[B]
- Topical anesthetics/coating agents: 1:1 mixture of diphenhydramine liquid and Maalox (8)[B]

ADDITIONAL TREATMENT
General Measures
- Usually outpatient
- Avoid any possible sensitizing irritants or agents (such as acidic or spicy foods and drinks).
- Analgesics when needed
- Request dental evaluation.
- Scrupulous oral hygiene

IN-PATIENT CONSIDERATIONS
Initial Stabilization
If glossitis is secondary to a severe primary condition, attend to any acute needs of the primary problem.

 ## ONGOING CARE

FOLLOW-UP RECOMMENDATIONS
If lesions do not heal, biopsy is indicated.

Patient Monitoring
Revisit periodically when needed until healing occurs.

DIET
Bland or liquid diet

PATIENT EDUCATION
- Proper diet and nutrition
- Avoid irritants such as cigarette smoking and acidic or spicy foods.
- Maintain good oral hygiene.

PROGNOSIS
Prompt improvement when cause can be identified and treated

COMPLICATIONS
- Recurrence: Evaluate for systemic etiology.
- Chronicity: If not healing, biopsy is indicated

REFERENCES

1. Terai H, Shimahara M. Atrophic tongue associated with Candida. *J Oral Pathol Med*. 2005;34:397–400.
2. Reamy BV, Derby R, Bunt CW. Common tongue conditions in primary care. *Am Fam Phys*. 2010;81:627–34.
3. Byrd JA, Bruce AJ, Rogers RS. Glossitis and other tongue disorders. *Dermatol Clin*. 2003;21:123–34.
4. Assimakopoulos D, Patrikakos G, Fotika C, et al. Benign migratory glossitis or geographic tongue: an enigmatic oral lesion. *Am J Med*. 2002;113:751–5.
5. Nelson BL, Thompson L. Median rhomboid glossitis. *Ear Nose Throat J*. 2007;86:600–1.
6. Sigal MJ, Mock D. Symptomatic benign migratory glossitis: report of two cases and literature review. *Pediatr Dent*. 1992;14:392–6.
7. Grossman ME, Stevens AW, Cohen PR. Brief report: herpetic geometric glossitis. *N Engl J Med*. 1993;329:1859–60.
8. Oh TJ, Eber R, Wang HL. Periodontal diseases in the child and adolescent. *J Clin Periodontol*. 2002;29:400–10.

See Also (Topic, Algorithm, Electronic Media Element)
Candidiasis; HIV Infection and AIDS; Vitamin Deficiency

 ## CODES

ICD9
529.0 Glossitis

CLINICAL PEARLS
- An acute or chronic inflammation of the tongue, either as primary disease or a symptom of systemic disease
- Common forms:
  - Atrophic glossitis (AG): Smooth, glossy, red or pink tongue
  - Benign migratory glossitis (BMG) or geographic tongue or erythema migrans: Erythematous and white patches on the dorsum of tongue; lesions may lack papillae; irregular (maplike) and migratory lesions
  - Median rhomboid glossitis (MRG): Erythematous, shiny, rhomboid-shaped plaque in middle of tongue; hypertrophic or atrophic surface changes
  - Herpetic geometric glossitis (HGG): Linear fissures on dorsal tongue; geometric pattern is common; herpetic lesions usually are absent on other mucosal surfaces.
- Testing: Serum B_{12}, folic acid, CBC with differential, ferritin, RPR, TSH

GLUCOSE INTOLERANCE

Dylan C. Kwait, MD
Robert A. Baldor, MD

BASICS

DESCRIPTION
- Glucose intolerance is characterized by hyperglycemia resulting from defects in glucose and fat metabolism. Overt diabetes is classified as type 1 (T1DM), type 2 (T2DM), and gestational (GDM). Hyperglycemia not sufficient to meet the diagnostic criteria for diabetes is termed prediabetes and is categorized as either impaired fasting glucose (IFG) or impaired glucose tolerance (IGT).
- IFG and IGT are risk factors for developing diabetes and moderately increase the risk of cardiovascular disease (1)[A].

EPIDEMIOLOGY
- Diabetes affects almost 6% of the world's population.
- ~97% of diabetic patients have T2DM.
- ~41 million people in the US aged 40–74 have prediabetes.

Incidence
- Incidence of both T1DM and T2DM is increasing worldwide.
- Incidence of T1DM ranges from 7.61–25.7/100,000/year in North America.

Prevalence
Prevalence of T2DM ranges from 6.69–28.2% in North America.

RISK FACTORS
- Type 1 diabetes:
  - 1st-degree relative with T1DM
- Prediabetes and type 2 diabetes:
  - BMI ≥25 kg/m
  - Physical inactivity:
    ○ Obesity increases the risk of developing T2DM 10-fold in women and 11.2-fold in men.
  - 1st- or 2nd-degree relative with T2DM
  - Race/ethnicity: African American, Latino, Native American, Asian American, Pacific Islander
  - Many patients with T2DM also have the metabolic syndrome, which is characterized by central adiposity, insulin resistance, dyslipidemia, and hypertension.
- Gestational diabetes:
  - Delivery of a baby weighing >9 lbs
  - Marked obesity

Genetics
- Type 1 diabetes:
  - Multiple genetic predispositions and poorly defined environmental factors contribute to T1DM:
    ○ HLA-DR3 and HLA-DR4 associations exist with linkage to the DQA and DQB genes
- Type 2 diabetes:
  - A stronger genetic predisposition than T1DM, but the genetics are complex and ill defined

GENERAL PREVENTION
- A decrease in excess body fat provides the greatest risk reduction (2)[B].
- Screening for prediabetes and diabetes should be performed at 3-year intervals beginning at age 45 (3)[B]:
  - Screen at younger ages or with increased frequency in those with additional risk factors or a BMI ≥25 kg/m (3)[B].
- Patients with either IFG or IGT benefit from moderate weight loss (5–10%) and aerobic physical activity (150 min/week) (1)[A]:
  - Metformin, acarbose, and orlistat effectively decrease the rate of progression to diabetes (4)[B].
- Patients with IFG or IGT should be monitored for diabetes every 1–2 years (3)[B].
- Patients with other cardiovascular risk factors (e.g., dyslipidemia, HTN, tobacco use) should receive appropriate counseling to modify diet and exercise.

Pregnancy Considerations
- Screening for diabetes in pregnancy is based on risk factor analysis.
- Women with gestational diabetes should be screened for diabetes 6–12 weeks postpartum (3)[B].

ETIOLOGY
- Type 1 diabetes:
  - Cellular-mediated autoimmune pathologic process leading to destruction of pancreatic islet β-cells and ultimately absolute insulin deficiency
- Type 2 diabetes:
  - A multiorgan disease characterized by chronic and progressive insulin resistance and relative insulin deficiency:
    ○ Insulin resistance initially leads to an increase in functional β-cell mass, but this compensatory measure is often insufficient and relative insulin deficiency, glucose intolerance, and hyperglycemia result.
  - Autoimmune destruction of β-cells does not occur.
  - Arises in part due to genetic susceptibility, but the current epidemic is more likely due to a trend toward increased energy intake and decreased physical activity

COMMONLY ASSOCIATED CONDITIONS
- Hypertension
- Dyslipidemia
- Acanthosis nigricans
- Polycystic ovary syndrome
- Patients with T1DM are prone to other auto-immune disorders including celiac sprue, Grave disease, Hashimoto thyroiditis, Addison disease, vitiligo, myasthenia gravis, and pernicious anemia (3)[A].

DIAGNOSIS

HISTORY
- Characteristics of the onset of disease (e.g., DKA, routine lab evaluation)
- Diet and exercise history
- History of diabetes-related complications:
  - Microvascular: Eye, kidney, nerve
  - Macrovascular: Cardiac, cardiovascular disease, peripheral artery disease
  - Other: Sexual dysfunction, gastroparesis
- Tobacco and alcohol use
- Polyuria
- Polydipsia
- Unexplained weight loss (sometimes accompanied by polyphagia)
- Blurred vision

PHYSICAL EXAM
- Blood pressure, including orthostatics
- Dorsalis pedis and posterior tibialis pulses
- Funduscopic exam
- Thyroid palpation
- Skin exam (for acanthosis nigricans and insulin injection sites), trophic changes on toes
- Neurological exam:
  - Patellar and Achilles reflexes
  - Proprioception, vibration, and monofilament sensation tests

DIAGNOSTIC TESTS & INTERPRETATION
- Prediabetes (3)[B]:
  - Categorized as IFG when diagnosed using Hb1ic or a fasting plasma glucose (FPG); IGT when diagnosed using the oral glucose tolerance test (OGTT):
    ○ IFG:
      ▪ HbA1c between 5.7 and 6.4% (5)[A]
      ▪ FPG ≥100 mg/dL and <126 mg/dL
    ○ IGT: A 2-hour plasma glucose between 140 mg/dL and 199 mg/dL following ingestion of a 75-g glucose load
  - Glucose tolerance test (GTT) is usually not necessary, except when diagnosing gestational diabetes.
  - HbA1c has advantages over fasting plasma glucose (FPG) for diagnosis.
- Diabetes (3)[B]:
  - Diagnosed using any 1 of the following (on 2 or more occasions):
    ○ HbA1c ≥6.5% is diagnostic (5)[A].
    ○ Symptoms of diabetes plus:
      ▪ Random plasma glucose (measured at any time of day, regardless of time since last meal) ≥200 mg/dL; or
      ▪ FPG ≥126 mg/dL; or
      ▪ A 2-hour plasma glucose ≥200 mg/dL following ingestion of a 75-g glucose load is diagnostic.

Lab
- Hemoglobin A1C
- Fasting lipid profile
- Liver function tests
- Test for microalbuminemia
- Serum creatinine and calculated GFR
- Thyroid-stimulating hormone

DIFFERENTIAL DIAGNOSIS
Diabetes insipidus

 TREATMENT

Glycemic control and the preservation of beta cell function are central to the treatment of T1DM and T2DM.

MEDICATION
Noninsulin glucose-lowering agents:
- Sulfonylureas and meglitinides
- Metformin and acarbose: Reduce rates of glucose appearance in the circulation
- Thiazolidinediones: Modify fat-induced insulin resistance (3)[B]
- Incretins (exenatide and sitagliptin) do not cause the weight gain associated with other noninsulin glucose-lowering agents, and may actually cause significant weight loss (6)[B].

First Line
- Type 1 diabetes:
  – Insulin: Combination of intermediate- or long-acting basal insulin with premeal rapid- or short-acting insulin (3)[B]
- Type 2 diabetes:
  – Metformin combined with intensive, multidisciplinary lifestyle modification (7)[A]

Second Line
Type 2 diabetes:
- Any of the following oral agents may be used in combination with metformin. Up to 3 oral agents may be used concurrently, but initiation of insulin therapy is preferred if treatment goals cannot be met using 2 oral agents (7)[A]:
  – Sulfonylurea
  – Glitazones
  – Acarbose

ALERT
- Metformin can cause lactic acidosis, a potentially fatal complication, in geriatric patients and patients with renal dysfunction and congestive heart failure (3)[B].
- Thiazolidinediones, including Avandia, Avandamet, and Avandaryl, may cause or exacerbate congestive heart failure in some patients. Initiation of these drugs in patients with established NYHA class III or IV heart failure is contraindicated. After initiation of Avandia, Avandamet, or Avandaryl, and after dose increases, observe patients carefully for signs and symptoms of heart failure (including excessive, rapid weight gain, dyspnea, and/or edema) (8)[B].

ADDITIONAL TREATMENT
Weight loss of 5–10% improves glycemic control, increases insulin sensitivity, improves lipids, and lowers blood pressure (6)[B].

Issues for Referral
- Eye exam at time of initial diagnosis and annually thereafter
- Diabetes educator/registered dietician
- Exercise physiologist

IN-PATIENT CONSIDERATIONS
Initial Stabilization
- Monitor blood glucose levels, which should be considered an additional "vital sign."

- Critically ill and postsurgical diabetic patients usually require intravenous infusion of regular insulin:
  – Sliding-scale insulin regimens are ineffective and are not recommended (3)[B].
  – Prandial insulin doses should be given in relation to meals after correcting for pre-meal hyperglycemia.
- Monitor hospitalized patients closely for hypoglycemia.

Admission Criteria
- Diabetic ketoacidosis
- Nonketotic hyperosmolar syndrome

Discharge Criteria
Patient is no longer acidotic and has been transitioned from intravenous insulin to either subcutaneous insulin delivery or oral agents with appropriate glycemic control.

 ONGOING CARE

FOLLOW-UP RECOMMENDATIONS
- At least 150 min/week of moderate-intensity aerobic exercise and/or at least 90 min/week of vigorous aerobic exercise (3)[B]
- Resistance exercise improves insulin sensitivity to the same extent as aerobic exercise; resistance training 3 times/week is recommended for those with T2DM (3)[B]

Patient Monitoring
- Self-monitoring of blood glucose
- The A1C should be measured at least twice a year in patients meeting treatment goals, and quarterly in those whose therapy has changed or who are not meeting glycemic goals (3)[B]:
  – Therapeutic goal is to achieve an A1C (<7%) as close to normal as possible in the absence of hypoglycemia (3)[B].
- Blood pressure should be routinely measured.
- Annual testing for lipid abnormalities and microalbuminuria
- Annual dilated fundal exam
- Annual foot exam including monofilament testing for distal polyneuropathy

DIET
- Monitor carbohydrate intake: Match doses of insulin and insulin secretagogues to the carbohydrate content of meals (9)[B].
- Low-fat (<25%) intake (9)[B]:
  – Saturated fat intake should be <7% of total calories.
  – Minimize *trans* fat intake.
- Low-sodium intake (9)[B]
- High fiber (~50 g fiber/d, 14 g fiber/1,000 kcal) and whole-grain intake (9)[B]
- Maximize low-glycemic index foods.
- Moderate alcohol intake

PROGNOSIS
- When appropriately treated, diabetes is not in itself a terminal disease.
- Most negative sequelae can be averted with consistent, longitudinal glycemic control.

COMPLICATIONS
- Cardiovascular disease
- Sexual dysfunction
- Gastroparesis
- Nephropathy and potential for renal failure
- Retinopathy and potential for loss of vision
- Peripheral and autonomic neuropathy

REFERENCES

1. Ford ES, Zhao G, Li C et al. Pre-diabetes and the risk for cardiovascular disease: a systematic review of the evidence. *J Am Coll Cardiol*. 2010;55: 1310–7.
2. Biuso TJ, Butterworth S, Linden A. A conceptual framework for targeting prediabetes with lifestyle, clinical, and behavioral management interventions. *Dis Manag*. 2007;10:6–15.
3. American Diabetes Association. Standards of medical care in diabetes-2010. *Diabetes Care*. 2010;33(Suppl. 1):11–61.
4. Swanson A, Watrin K, Wilder L et al. Clinical Inquiries: How can we keep impaired glucose tolerance and impaired fasting glucose from progressing to diabetes? *J Fam Pract*. 2010;59: 532–3.
5. The International Expert Committee. International Expert Committee Report on the Role of the A1C Assay in the Diagnosis of Diabetes. *Diabetes Care*. 2009.
6. Pi-Sunyer X. The metabolic syndrome: how to approach differing definitions. *Med Clin North Am*. 2007;91:1025–40, vii.
7. Saenz A, et al. Metformin monotherapy for type 2 diabetes mellitus. *Cochrane Database Sys Rev*. 2005;CD002966.
8. http://www.fda.gov/cder/drug/InfoSheets/HCP/rosiglitazone200707HCP.htm#2007_7
9. American Diabetes Association, Bantle JP, Wylie-Rosett J, Albright AL, Apovian CM, Clark NG, Franz MJ, Hoogwerf BJ, Lichtenstein AH, Mayer-Davis E, Mooradian AD, Wheeler ML et al. Nutrition recommendations and interventions for diabetes: a position statement of the American Diabetes Association. *Diabetes Care*. 2008; 31(Suppl 1):S61–78.

ADDITIONAL READING

Adeghate E, Schattner P, Dunn E. An update on the etiology and epidemiology of diabetes mellitus. *Ann N Y Acad Sci*. 2006;1084:1–29.

See Also (Topic, Algorithm, Electronic Media Element)
Algorithm: Hypoglycemia

 CODES

ICD9
- 790.21 Impaired fasting glucose
- 790.22 Impaired glucose tolerance test (oral)
- 790.29 Other abnormal glucose

CLINICAL PEARLS

- HbA1c ≥6.5% is diagnostic for diabetes and has advantages over fasting plasma glucose (FPG).
- Glucose tolerance test (GTT) is usually not necessary, except when diagnosing gestational diabetes.

G

GONOCOCCAL INFECTIONS

Paul E. Lyons, MD

BASICS

DESCRIPTION
Gonorrhea is a sexually or vertically transmitted bacterial infection that has a predilection for epithelial cells.

- Caused by the gram-negative intracellular diplococci, *Neisseria gonorrhoeae*; virtually any mucosal membrane can be infected.
- Infection commonly manifests itself as urethritis, salpingitis, cervicitis, pelvic inflammatory disease (PID), epididymitis, or proctitis.
- Hematogenous dissemination may also occur and lead to fever, skin lesions, arthralgias, purulent arthritis, tenosynovitis, endocarditis or, rarely, meningitis.
- Asymptomatic carrier state can occur in both sexes.
- In newborns, gonococcal ophthalmia neonatorum, a purulent conjunctivitis, may occur after vaginal delivery by an infected mother and may lead to blindness if not treated promptly.
- System(s) affected: Cardiovascular; Musculoskeletal; Nervous; Reproductive; Skin/Exocrine
- Synonym(s): GC; Clap

EPIDEMIOLOGY
- Predominant age: 15–24 years
- Predominant sex: Prior to 1996, rates of gonorrhea among men were higher than rates among women. However, gonorrhea rates in women are now slightly higher than in men.

Incidence
- In 2008, 336,742 cases were reported to the Centers for Disease Control (CDC), resulting in rate of 111.6/100,000 US population.
- Highest rates are among black women aged 15–19 (2,934.6 /100,000)
- Blacks (625/100,000) have 20.2 times greater rate than whites (31/100,000)

Prevalence
As a treatable disease, incidence and prevalence of diagnosed disease are approximately equal. The asymptomatic nature of the disease (especially among women) would suggest that the prevalence is higher than the reported incidence.

RISK FACTORS
- History of previous gonorrhea infection
- Sexual exposure to an infected individual without barrier protection (condom)
- Other sexually transmitted infections
- New or multiple sexual partners
- Inconsistent condom use
- Sex work
- Drug use
- Infants: Passage through infected birth canal of mother
- Children: Sexual abuse by infected individual
- Autoinoculation (finger to eye)
- For PID: Use of intrauterine devices

Genetics
Individuals with congenital deficiency of late components of complement cascade (C7,8,9) are prone to develop dissemination of local gonococcal infections.

GENERAL PREVENTION
- Condoms offer partial protection, but must be used for oral, anal, and vaginal intercourse to be effective.
- Sexual contacts should be treated.

PATHOPHYSIOLOGY
Infection requires 4 steps:
- Mucosal attachment
- Local penetration/invasion
- Local proliferation
- Inflammatory response or dissemination

ETIOLOGY
N. gonorrhoeae (gonococcus)

COMMONLY ASSOCIATED CONDITIONS
Other sexually transmitted infections:
- Chlamydia
- Syphilis
- HIV
- Hepatitis B
- Herpes

DIAGNOSIS

HISTORY
- For all patients: Sexual history including number of partners and age of onset of sexual activity, new/recent change in sexual partner, contact with sex workers, condom use, history of STIs, menses, and possibility of pregnancy
- Patients should be screened for additional STIs, including HIV
- For patients with symptoms: Onset, context, duration, timing, severity, associated symptoms, and modifying factors of symptoms
- Remember 10% males and 20–40% of women are asymptomatic.
- Patients with symptoms should also be asked about symptomatic partner(s).
- Signs and symptoms may include:
  – General: Urinary symptoms: Urinary frequency, urgency, dysuria
  – Urethral symptoms: Copious urethral discharge, meatus and anterior urethral inflammation
  – Ocular symptoms: Purulent discharge, conjunctivitis, chemosis, eyelid edema, corneal ulceration
  – Pharyngeal symptoms:
    ○ Pharyngeal infection: Asymptomatic infection (98%), sore throat, exudative pharyngitis (<1%)
  – GI symptoms: Acute diarrhea
  – Males: Scant to copious purulent urethral discharge (82%); dysuria (53%); testicular pain (1%); asymptomatic infection (10%), proctitis
  – Females: Asymptomatic cervical infection (20%), endocervical discharge (96%), vaginal discharge, Bartholin gland abscess, dysmenorrhea, menometrorrhagia, abdominal pain/tenderness, cervical motion tenderness, rebound, infertility, chronic pelvic pain
  – Either sex, for receptive anal intercourse: Rectal discharge, tenesmus, rectal burning, asymptomatic
  – Disseminated syndromes:
    ○ Fever, chills, malaise, tenosynovitis, dermatitis, polyarthralgia, purulent arthritis

  ○ Endocarditis: Rapid cardiac valve destruction, high fevers
  ○ Meningitis: Meningeal signs, headache, skin lesions, fever, altered mental status

PHYSICAL EXAM
A full physical exam with an emphasis on vital signs, throat, abdomen, pelvic/rectal, genital, skin, and joints

DIAGNOSTIC TESTS & INTERPRETATION
Lab
Initial lab tests
CDC recommends nucleic acid amplification as the most sensitive and specific test for *N. gonorrhoeae*. Other options include:
- Genital culture
- Consider adding pharyngeal culture in adolescents (1)[A]
- Gram stain (recommended for urethritis)
- Urethral smear, sensitivity in symptomatic male: ≥95%. Sensitivity of endocervical smear in infected woman: 40–60%. Specificity: 100%
- DNA probes and PCR sensitivity: 92–99% dependent on population. Specificity: >97%; can replace culture
- Sensitivity of blood culture in disseminated disease: 50%. Sensitivity of joint fluid culture in septic arthritis: 50%
- If a clinical consideration, order with chlamydia, rapid plasma reagin (RPR), and HIV testing

Follow-Up & Special Considerations
- Test-of-cure testing is not generally recommended.
- Follow-up testing may be considered in cases of recurrent infection and/or in areas where significant antibiotic resistance exists.

Imaging
Initial approach
Imaging is not generally recommended for initial evaluation of uncomplicated gonococcal urethritis or clinically apparent PID.

Follow-Up & Special Considerations
Pelvic ultrasound or CT scan may demonstrate thick, dilated fallopian tubes or abscess formation.

Diagnostic Procedures/Surgery
Culdocentesis may demonstrate free purulent exudate and provide material for gram staining and culture. Gram staining material from unroofed skin lesions may show typical organisms.

Pathological Findings
- Exudate of polymorphonuclear leukocytes is typical.
- Gram-negative intracellular *diplococci*
- Nonpathologic gram-negative *diplococci* may be found in extragenital locations. For this reason, gram stain of pharyngeal or rectal swabs is not recommended.

DIFFERENTIAL DIAGNOSIS
- *Chlamydia trachomatis*
- Urinary tract infections
- Nongonococcal vaginitis
- Nongonococcal urethritis

TREATMENT

MEDICATION

Because of the public health importance of untreated gonococcal infection, only antibiotics with a demonstrated success rate of 95% or higher should be used.

First Line
- Uncomplicated gonorrheal infection of the cervix, urethra, or rectum:
  - Ceftriaxone, 125 mg IM in a single dose or Cefixime, 400 mg PO in a single dose plus treatment for chlamydia
  - Note: During pregnancy, ceftriaxone is treatment of choice.
  - Pharyngitis: Ceftriaxone, 125 mg IM once
  - Conjunctivitis: Ceftriaxone, 1 g IM
  - PID: Outpatient regimens (for inpatient regimens, see citations):
    ○ Ceftriaxone, 250 mg IM once *plus* Doxycycline, 100 mg PO b.i.d. for 14 days *with or without* Metronidazole, 500 mg PO b.i.d. for 14 days
- Disseminated infection in adults:
  - Ceftriaxone, 1 g IM or IV q24h for 24–48 hours, also treat for chlamydial infection. Then for 1 week:
    ○ Cefixime, 400 mg PO b.i.d.
- Meningitis and endocarditis:
  - Ceftriaxone, 1–2 g IV q12h 10–14 days for meningitis; 4 weeks for endocarditis
- Treatment of infants and children: <45 kg (patients >45 kg should receive full adult dose)
- Uncomplicated genital, pharyngeal, rectal, or conjunctival infection, and infants born to mothers with untreated gonorrhea:
  - Ceftriaxone, 125 mg IM in single dose
  - Disseminated infections: Ceftriaxone, 25–50 mg/kg IV or IM daily, or cefotaxime, 25 mg/kg IV or IM q12h; bacteremia: 7 days; meningitis: 10–14 days; endocarditis: 4 weeks
- Ophthalmic neonatorum prophylaxis: Single application of:
  - Erythromycin (0.5%) ophthalmic ointment *or* tetracycline ophthalmic ointment (1%)
- Contraindications: Tetracyclines such as doxycycline are contraindicated in pregnancy and young children.
- Precautions: Refer to the manufacturer's profile of each drug.
- Significant possible interactions: Refer to the manufacturer's profile of each drug.
- Note: All medication recommendations from source

Second Line
- No 2nd-line agent available in the US for gonococcal infections:
  - Recent gonococcal isolates within the US have demonstrated significant rates of resistance to both azithromycin and quinolones. Neither is currently recommended for treatment.
  - Progressive resistance to sulfonamides, penicillins, tetracyclines, fluoroquinolones and now developing resistance in Asia, Australia, and elsewhere to 3rd-generation cephalosporins makes prevention critically important (2)[B].
- PID can be treated with clindamycin and gentamicin.
- For treatment options other than those listed in previous section, please see CDC report on sexually transmitted diseases treatment guidelines at: http://www.cdc.gov/std/treatment/2006/updated regimens.htm

ADDITIONAL TREATMENT

General Measures
Counseling concerning risk reduction and condom use

IN-PATIENT CONSIDERATIONS

Initial Stabilization
In rare cases, individual may be hemodynamically unstable from sepsis; stabilize with IV fluids if necessary.

Admission Criteria
- Hematogenously disseminated infection
- Pneumonia or eye infection in infants
- PID: If unable to take oral medications, significant tubo-ovarian abscess, or patient is pregnant

IV Fluids
Indicated for patients whose presenting complaints include significant nausea/vomiting with clinical evidence of dehydration

ONGOING CARE

FOLLOW-UP RECOMMENDATIONS

Patient Monitoring
US Preventive Services Task Force (USPSTF) recommends:
- Screen all sexually active women if they are at increased risk of infection (which includes having a new partner).
- Insufficient evidence to recommend screening men at increased risk of infection
- No screening for men or women not at increased risk of infection
- Strongly recommend prophylactic ocular topical medication for all newborns (3)[C].

PATIENT EDUCATION
- Counseling concerning risk reduction and condom use
- Counseling concerning future fertility
- Encourage patient and partner HIV testing.
- This is a reportable disease:
  - Reportable diseases are diseases considered to be of great public health importance. Local, state, and national agencies require that such diseases be reported when they are diagnosed. All states have a reportable diseases list. Most of these lists are similar. Gonorrhea is generally a mandatory written-report disease. A provider must contact both the state health department and the CDC.

PROGNOSIS
With adequate, early therapy, complete cure with return to normal function is the rule.

COMPLICATIONS
- Infertility
- Urethral stricture
- Corneal scarring
- Destruction of joint articular surfaces
- Cardiac valves

Pediatric Considerations
Vertical transmission to newborn infants is a significant risk among patients with gonococcal infection at the time of delivery.

Pregnancy Considerations
USPSTF found insufficient evidence to recommend for or against routine screening for gonorrheal infection in pregnant women who are not at increased risk for infection (3)[C].

REFERENCES

1. Giannini CM, Kim HK, Mortensen J, Mortensen J, Marsolo K, Huppert J et al. Culture of non-genital sites increases the detection of gonorrhea in women. *J Pediatr Adolesc Gynecol*. 2010;23: 246–52.
2. Barry PM, Klausner JD. The use of cephalosporins for gonorrhea: the impending problem of resistance. *Expert Opin Pharmacother*. 2009; 10:555–77.
3. US Preventive Services Task Force. Screening for Gonorrhea: Recommendation Statement. AHRQ Publication No. 05-0579-A. Rockville MD: Agency for Healthcare Research and Quality, May 2005. Available at: http://www.ahrq.gov/clinic/uspstf05/gonorrhea/gonrs.htm.

ADDITIONAL READING

- Centers for Disease Control and Prevention (CDC). Increases in fluoroquinolone-resistant Neisseria gonorrhoeae among men who have sex with men—United States, 2003, and revised recommendations for gonorrhea treatment, 2004. *MMWR Morb Mortal Wkly Rep*. 2004;53:335–8.
- *MMWR Morb Mortal Wkly Rep*. Update to CDC's sexually transmitted diseases treatment guidelines, 2006: fluoroquinolones no longer recommended for treatment of gonococcal infections. 2007;56(14): 332–6.

See Also (Topic, Algorithm, Electronic Media Element)
Chlamydial Sexually Transmitted Diseases; Pelvic Inflammatory Disease (PID); Syphilis; HIV Infection and AIDS

CODES

ICD9
- 098.0 Gonococcal infection (acute) of lower genitourinary tract
- 098.10 Gonococcal infection (acute) of upper genitourinary tract, site unspecified
- 098.11 Gonococcal cystitis (acute)

CLINICAL PEARLS

- The USPSTF recommends screening sexually active women at high risk of infection. High risk of infection is defined as <35 years of age, history of previous gonorrhea infection or other STD, NEW or multiple sexual partners, inconsistent condom use, sex work, and drug use.
- The USPSTF does not recommend routine screening of men at high risk or anyone at low risk.
- Patients testing positive for gonorrhea should also be considered for additional STI testing including chlamydia, syphilis, HIV, and hepatitis.
- Treat also for chlamydia, unless chlamydia infection ruled out.

G

GOUT

Janice A. Litza, MD
Jacob L. Bidwell, MD

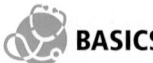

BASICS

DESCRIPTION
- Gout refers to a group of disorders related to hyperuricemia. Although hyperuricemia is necessary for the development of gout, it is not the only determining factor.
- Characterized by deposition of monosodium urate (MSU) crystals in tissue, resulting in acute and chronic arthritis, soft tissue masses called tophi, urate nephropathy, and uric acid nephrolithiasis
- Natural history involves 4 stages:
  – Asymptomatic hyperuricemia
  – Acute arthritis
  – Intercritical gout
  – Chronic tophaceous gout
- Acute gouty arthritis can affect ≥1 joints. The 1st metatarsophalangeal joint is most commonly involved at presentation (podagra).
- Other common sites include midtarsal, ankle, and knee joints.
- After an initial attack, patients can be attack-free for months or even years. Some patients will develop more frequent attacks or go on to develop chronic tophaceous gout.
- Management involves treating acute attacks and preventing recurrent disease by long-term reduction of serum uric acid levels through pharmacology and lifestyle adjustments.

Geriatric Considerations
- Presentation may lack acute pain, swelling, and inflammation
- More common in women >80
- Can present with tophi and finger joint pain
- Commonly triggered by diuretic use, especially in women

Pediatric Considerations
Often due to an inborn error of metabolism or other disease

EPIDEMIOLOGY
Incidence
Increases with age, especially in women

Prevalence
6 per 1,000 population for men; 1 per 1,000 population for women

RISK FACTORS
- Hyperuricemia
- Male gender (age <65)
- Increasing age
- Ethanol ingestion (beer and liquor > wine)
- Obesity (50%)
- Hypertension (50%)
- Diabetes
- Medications: Diuretics induce 20% of secondary gout
- Diet: High-purine animal-origin foods (e.g., meats and seafood)
- Family history
- Keto- and lactic acidosis
- Surgery or trauma
- Renal impairment
- Hypothyroidism

- Parathyroid disease
- Hyperlipidemia types II, IV, V
- Paget disease
- Hyperproliferative skin disorders (psoriasis)
- Lymphoproliferative disorders, hemolytic anemia, hemoglobinopathies, pernicious anemia
- Glycogen storage diseases

Genetics
- Primary gout runs in families and follows multifactorial inheritance.
- Phosphoribosyl pyrophosphate (PRPP) deficiency and hypoxanthine-guanine-phosphoribosyltransferase (HGPRT) deficiency are inherited enzyme defects associated with a primary overproduction of uric acid.
- URAT1 (urate transporter) deficiency is also a hereditary enzyme defect resulting in primary underexcretion of uric acid.

GENERAL PREVENTION
- Treat underlying cardiovascular risk factors.
- Maintain weight at optimal BMI of <26.
- Regular exercise
- Diet modification
- Reduce alcohol consumption (beer and liquor).
- Maintain fluid intake and avoid dehydration.

PATHOPHYSIOLOGY
- Humans have a narrow window for urate to remain soluble before crystal precipitation due to lack of uricase enzyme.
- Precipitation of MSU crystals can occur in the synovium, joint cartilage, kidneys, and soft tissue.
- MSU crystals can initiate and sustain an inflammatory response, leading to an acute gout attack.
- Chronic and untreated hyperuricemia lead to tophi formation in and around the joint space.
- Tophi contribute to chronic synovitis, often resulting in joint damage.

ETIOLOGY
- Increased uric acid production
- Impaired renal excretion of uric acid
- Enzyme defects
- Increased purine turnover
- Dehydration or starvation

COMMONLY ASSOCIATED CONDITIONS
- Metabolic syndrome (obesity, hyperglycemia, hyperlipidemia, hypertension [HTN])
- Myeloproliferative disorders
- Lymphoproliferative disorders
- Alcoholism
- Endocrinopathies
- Lesch-Nyhan syndrome

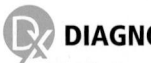

DIAGNOSIS

HISTORY
- Rapid onset of severe pain, usually beginning in early morning with 1 or 2 joints (75% are monoarticular) +/− fever
- Soft tissue redness, swelling, warmth
- Exquisite tenderness

- 1st metatarsophalangeal joint in 50% of initial attacks
- Acute untreated attacks last 2–21 days.
- Recurrent attacks last longer and occur more frequently with each recurrence.
- Between attacks, absence of inflammation (until the chronic or tophaceous phase occurs)
- Rarely polyarticular
- Migratory polyarthritis is a rare presentation.
- 50% untreated develop chronic arthritis
- Subcutaneous or intraosseous nodules (20%), referred to as tophi, may affect ears (antihelix), extensor aspects of peripheral joints (e.g., olecranon), cornea, aorta, spine, even intracranial space (1).
- Pain with urination secondary to uric acid renal stones

PHYSICAL EXAM
- Examine suspected joint(s) for tenderness, swelling, and range of motion (ROM).
- Assess for presence of firm nodules known as tophi.

DIAGNOSTIC TESTS & INTERPRETATION
Lab
Initial lab tests
- Synovial fluid analysis: Urate crystals, (negatively birefringent under polarizing microscopy), cell count (white blood count [WBC] usually 5,000–50,000/mm^3; predominantly neutrophils); culture to rule out infection
- Blood studies: Elevated serum uric acid level, complete blood count (can show elevated WBC during acute attack)
- Urine studies: Urine analysis, 24-hour urine testing for uric acid and creatinine (urate excretion will likely not be accurate during an acute attack)

Imaging
Initial approach
- Radiograph is usually normal early in disease.
- Radiograph in chronic gout reveals "punched-out" erosions (lytic areas), often with periosteum overgrowing the erosion ("overhanging edge").
- Urate kidney stones are radiolucent, and thus invisible on radiograph.

Diagnostic Procedures/Surgery
- Arthrocentesis with polarizing optical examination
- Biopsy of synovial membrane or SC nodule, processing the specimen anhydrously (urate is water-soluble)

Pathological Findings
- Acute arthritis: Neutrophilic infiltrate throughout synovium
- Chronic arthritis: Intra-articular and periarticular tophi
- Tophi: Macrophages surround MSU crystals, forming a granuloma.
- Gouty nephropathy: MSU crystals deposited in medullary interstitium

DIFFERENTIAL DIAGNOSIS
- Septic arthritis
- Pseudogout (calcium pyrophosphate deposition disease)
- Cellulitis
- Reactive arthritis

- Amyloidosis
- Osteoarthritis
- Hyperparathyroidism
- Spondyloarthropathy
- Rheumatoid arthritis (rarely)

 TREATMENT

- Key component is lifestyle adjustment to avoid triggers and reduce risk
- Chronic treatment indicated if >2 attacks per year, tophi present, radiographic evidence of joint damage (2)[C]
- Goal for chronic treatment is serum uric acid less than 6 mg/dL (2)[B]

MEDICATION
First Line
- Acute attack:
  – Nonsteroidal anti-inflammatory drugs (NSAIDs) (e.g., naproxen and indomethacin) at full dosage:
    ○ Taper a few days after symptoms resolve.
    ○ Use limited by GI side effects, including GI bleeding (1)[A]
- Chronic treatment:
  – Urate-lowering agents should not be prescribed until 2–3 weeks after acute attack has resolved, but should be continued if patient is taking them prior to attack.
- Xanthine oxidase inhibitors:
  – Allopurinol start at 100 mg daily and adjusted every 2–4 weeks until goal of serum uric acid is <6mg/dL for 3–6 months (2)[B]:
    ○ Monitor for hypersensitivity reactions: Rash, hepatitis, interstitial nephritis, and toxic epidermal necrolysis.
    ○ Coprescribe with colchicine 0.5–1 mg/d OR low-dose NSAIDs daily upon initiation of treatment to prevent rebound acute gout attacks (2)[B].
  – Febuxostat:
    ○ Approved by Food and Drug Administration (FDA) 2/2009 for gout
    ○ Benefits include more selective xanthine oxidase inhibitor and no renal dose adjustment
    ○ Starting dose 40 mg daily, titrate to 80 mg daily to goal serum uric acid of <6 mg/dL (3,4)[B]

Second Line
- Acute attack:
  – Colchicine: Should be used within 12–24 hours of attack onset. 1 mg followed by 0.5 mg q2h until absence of symptoms or GI side effects occur (nausea, vomiting, diarrhea) (1)[A].
  – Systemic corticosteroids (5)[B]
  – Intra-articular long-acting corticosteroid is useful if 1 or a few joints involved (2)[B]
  – Adrenocorticotropic hormone (ACTH) 25 USP units SC for acute small-joint monoarticular gout. 40 USP units IM or IV for larger joints or polyarticular gout (2)[B].
- Chronic treatment:
  – Uricosuric agents
  – Use in patients refractory to allopurinol or in whom allopurinol is contraindicated. Ideal for patients <60 years with CrCl >80 mL/min, 24-hour urinary uric acid excretion ≤700 mg on normal diet, and without history of renal calculi:

○ Probenecid: Start at 250 mg p.o. b.i.d. and gradually increase to 500–2,000 mg p.o. (in 2 doses) until desired SUA in those with normal renal function (2)[B].
○ Sulfinpyrazone: Start at 50 mg p.o. b.i.d. and gradually increase to 100–400 mg (in 2 doses) daily until desired SUA in those with normal renal function (2)[B].
○ Initially coprescribe all uricosurics with either colchicine 0.5–1 mg/d for up to 6 months OR low-dose NSAIDs for up to 6 weeks.
– Fenofibrate and losartan or amlodipine: Consider as alternative therapy for hyperlipidemia and HTN, respectively. Modest uricosuric effect (2,6)[B].
– Ongoing studies: Puricase (PEG-uricase) for refractory chronic gout (7)[B]

ADDITIONAL TREATMENT
General Measures
Apply ice packs and rest affected joint.

SURGERY/OTHER PROCEDURES
Large tophi that are infected or interfering with joint motion may need to be surgically removed.

 ONGOING CARE

FOLLOW-UP RECOMMENDATIONS
Patient Monitoring
Related to medicinal control of the acute attack and suppressing attacks:
- CBC, renal, liver function tests (LFTs), and urinalysis at 1 week, 6 weeks, and every 3 months

DIET
- Reduce ingestion of purine-rich foods of animal origin (meat and shellfish).
- Avoid alcoholic beverages, specifically beer and liquor.
- Increase low-fat dairy foods.
- Maintain adequate hydration.
- Consider additional vitamin C 500 mg daily (8).

PATIENT EDUCATION
Gout and Uric Acid Education Society: http://www.gouteducation.org

PROGNOSIS
- Gout can usually be successfully managed with proper treatment.
- Recurrent attacks may require long-term uric acid-lowering therapy.
- During the 1st 6–12 months of uricosuric or allopurinol therapy, acute gout attacks may occur.

COMPLICATIONS
- Increased susceptibility to infection
- Urate nephropathy
- Renal stones
- Nerve/spinal cord impingement

REFERENCES
1. Schlesinger N, Schumacher R, Catton M, et al. Colchicine for acute gout. *Cochrane Database Syst Rev.* 2006;CD006190.
2. Zhang W, Doherty M, Bardin T, et al. EULAR evidence based recommendations for gout. Part II: Management. Report of a task force of the EULAR Standing Committee for International Clinical Studies Including Therapeutics (ESCISIT). *Ann Rheum Dis.* 2006;65:1312–24.
3. Bruce SP. Febuxostat: a selective xanthine oxidase inhibitor for the treatment of hyperuricemia and gout. *Ann Pharmacother.* 2006;40:2187–94.
4. Schumacher HR, Becker MA, Wortmann RL, et al. Effects of febuxostat versus allopurinol and placebo in reducing serum urate in subjects with hyperuricemia and gout: A 28-week, phase III, randomized, double-blind, parallel-group trial. *Arthritis Rheum.* 2008;59:1540–8.
5. Janssens H, et al. Systemic corticosteroids for acute gout. *Cochrane Database Syst Rev.* 2008;16(2):CD005521.
6. Høieggen A, Alderman MH, Kjeldsen SE, et al. The impact of serum uric acid on cardiovascular outcomes in the LIFE study. *Kidney Int.* 2004;65:1041–9.
7. Sundy JS, Ganson NJ, Kelly SJ, et al. Pharmacokinetics and pharmacodynamics of intravenous PEGylated recombinant mammalian urate oxidase in patients with refractory gout. *Arthritis Rheum.* 2007;56:1021–8.
8. Huang HY, Appel LJ, Choi MJ, et al. The effects of vitamin C supplementation on serum concentrations of uric acid: results of a randomized controlled trial. *Arthritis Rheum.* 2005;52:1843–7.

ADDITIONAL READING
- Eggebeen AT. Gout: an update. *Am Fam Physician.* 2007;76:801–8.
- Keith MP, Gilliland WR. Updates in the management of gout. *Am J Med.* 2007;120:221–4.
- Liote F, et al. Gout: Update on some pathogenic and clinical aspects. *Rheum Dis Clin N Am.* 2006;32:295–311.
- Rott KT, Agudelo CA. Gout. *JAMA.* 2003;289:2857–60.
- Terkeltaub RA. Clinical practice. Gout. *N Engl J Med.* 2003;349:1647–55.

See Also (Topic, Algorithm, Electronic Media Element)
Alcohol Abuse and Dependence; Anemia, Sickle Cell

CODES
ICD9
- 274.00 Gouty arthropathy, unspecified
- 274.9 Gout, unspecified
- 274.10 Gouty nephropathy, unspecified

CLINICAL PEARLS
- MSU crystals found in synovial fluid aspirate are pathognomonic for gout.
- Acute gout and sepsis can coexist.
- Asymptomatic hyperuricemia does not require treatment.
- Presentation may vary by age and gender.

GRANULOMA ANNULARE

Ronald Adler, MD

 BASICS

DESCRIPTION
A benign skin condition characterized by grouped papules, which typically occur in an annular pattern. 4 variants have been described, the most common of which is localized granuloma annulare (GA). The other types are generalized (or disseminated), subcutaneous, and perforating.

EPIDEMIOLOGY
Incidence
GA is not common, though its occurrence in the general population is unknown. It is seen more often in women, with a ratio of 2:1 over men. The age distribution varies by type, as follows:
- Localized: Children and adults <30 years old
- Generalized: Bimodal: Children <10 and adults 30–60 years old
- Subcutaneous: Children 2–10 years old
- Perforating: Typically children, but also young adults

Prevalence
Among cases of GA, the approximate distribution is as follows:
- Localized: 75%
- Generalized: 10–15%
- Subcutaneous: <5%
- Perforating: <5% (perhaps higher in Hawaii)

RISK FACTORS
No definite risk factors have been identified. There is weak evidence for possible associations with diabetes mellitus, TB, HIV, EBV and other viral infections, trauma, insect bites, and malignancies.

Genetics
There is some evidence for a possible hereditary component.

GENERAL PREVENTION
There are no established strategies for preventing GA.

ETIOLOGY
The cause of GA remains unknown, though it is probably immunologic.

COMMONLY ASSOCIATED CONDITIONS
See Risk Factors. These noted associations are not common.

 DIAGNOSIS

HISTORY
Cutaneous lesions of GA are generally asymptomatic. They may persist for months or years; longer duration is more often seen in the generalized subtype. They typically resolve spontaneously and they may recur.

PHYSICAL EXAM
- Localized: Small (1–2 mm) papules arranged in a ring, which may enlarge from 5 mm–5 cm. Color may range from flesh tones to red. The most common locations are the dorsal aspects of the distal extremities.
- Generalized: Similar to localized, but a higher number of lesions, which are more widespread, often larger, and typically persist longer.
- Subcutaneous: Firm, nontender, subcutaneous nodule, which tends to grow rapidly. Usually solitary, but may occur in groups. Most common location is lower extremities, especially pretibial; other sites include upper extremities, scalp, buttocks.
- Perforating: Papules may be up to 4 mm and display umbilication, crusting, or scale. Lesions are often generalized and may occur anywhere.

DIAGNOSTIC TESTS & INTERPRETATION
Lab
Initial lab tests
Diagnosis is typically established by the history and physical, so lab investigations are rarely needed. Skin scraping/KOH test may be useful for excluding a fungal process.

Imaging
Initial approach
Rarely indicated, but may occasionally be useful in the workup of suspected subcutaneous subtype

Diagnostic Procedures/Surgery
Occasionally, biopsy is required to confirm the diagnosis. This is most commonly the case for subcutaneous subtype.

DIFFERENTIAL DIAGNOSIS
- Localized: Tinea corporis, annular lichen planus, necrobiosis lipoidica, pityriasis rosea, erythema migrans of Lyme disease, leprosy
- Generalized: Sarcoidosis, lichen planus, cutaneous metastases
- Subcutaneous: Rheumatoid nodule
- Perforating: Molluscum contagiosum

TREATMENT

MEDICATION

- There is no strong evidence supporting any treatment intervention for GA. Multiple therapies have been tried (particularly in generalized cases), and the following medications may be of some use:
  - Corticosteroids, either by intralesional injection or topical application (with or without occlusion)
  - Tacrolimus
  - Pimecrolimus
  - Imiquimod
  - Isotretinoin
  - Dapsone
  - Hydroxychloroquine
  - Cyclosporine
  - Niacinamide
  - Infliximab
  - Doxycycline
  - Allopurinol
- Other therapies:
  - Psoralen ultraviolet A (PUVA)
  - Cryotherapy

ADDITIONAL TREATMENT
General Measures
Given that GA is an asymptomatic condition that is likely to resolve spontaneously, the clinician's primary role after diagnosis is to educate the patient regarding the anticipated natural history and to provide reassurance.

 ONGOING CARE

FOLLOW-UP RECOMMENDATIONS
Routine follow-up is not required. However, if treatment is initiated, follow-up may be important to monitor for possible adverse effects associated with treatment.

PATIENT EDUCATION
The patient should be informed that GA is a benign, self-limited condition that may persist a long time, resolve, and recur.

PROGNOSIS
Many cases resolve spontaneously, though recurrence—typically at the original site—is common.

COMPLICATIONS
Complications of treatment are much more likely than complications from GA.

ADDITIONAL READING

- Cyr PR. Diagnosis and Management of Granuloma Annulare. *Amer FP*. 2006;74(10):1729–34.
- Duarte AF, Mota A, et al. Generalized granuloma annulare - response to doxycycline. *J Eur Acad Dermat and Vener*. 2009;23:84–5.
- Mazzatenta C, Ghilardi A, Grazzini M. Treatment of disseminated granuloma annulare with allopurinol: case report. *Dermatologic Therapy*. 2010;23:S24–7.

 CODES

ICD9
695.89 Other specified erythematous conditions

CLINICAL PEARLS

This condition is benign. Most proposed treatments are not. *Primum non nocere*.

G

GRANULOMA INGUINALE

Omar A. Khan, MD, MHS

 BASICS

DESCRIPTION
Granuloma inguinale is a primarily sexually transmitted, chronic bacterial infection caused by *Calymmatobacterium granulomatis* (which some authorities classify as *Klebsiella granulomatis*), formerly known as *Donovania granulomatis*, an intracellular gram-negative bacillus.
- Also known as *donovanosis*
- Causative organism similar to *Klebsiella* spp., leading to discussions on nomenclature
- Usually manifests as genital or anal lesions
- Sexual/anal intercourse is the main source.
- Also can be acquired via fecal route, passage through an infected birth canal, or contact with laps of infected individuals (children)
- Granuloma inguinale is a risk factor for acquiring HIV infection.
- Four varieties of skin lesions exist: ulcerovegetative, cicatricial, nodular, and verrucous.

EPIDEMIOLOGY
- <100 cases annually in the US (mostly foreign travel)
- Endemic: Tropical and subtropical regions (e.g., New Guinea, Caribbean, West Indies, southern India, sub-Saharan Africa, Southeast Asia, Australia, Brazil)
- Incidence higher in blacks in US
- Predominant sex: Males slightly more susceptible
- Predominant age: 20–40 years; rarely seen in children or elderly; no congenital cases reported

RISK FACTORS
- Residing or traveling in underdeveloped parts of tropical/subtropical countries
- Sexual contact with travelers to endemic area
- Males having unprotected sex with males
- Anal intercourse
- Low socioeconomic background
- HIV positivity

GENERAL PREVENTION
- Safe sex practices
- If infection likely, avoid sexual contact; notify partners.
- Examples of prevention include barrier methods of contraception, avoidance of high-risk sexual activity, and appropriate gynecologic screening (including during the course of pregnancy).
- Sexual contacts within 60 days prior to symptom onset should be evaluated and offered treatment.
- Remaining up to date on HIV care

PATHOPHYSIOLOGY
- Repeated is exposure necessary for clinical infection to occur.
- Communicable as long as the infected person remains untreated and bacteria are present

ETIOLOGY
Bacterial infection caused by caused by the bacillus *Klebsiella/Calymmatobacterium granulomatosis* (previously known as *Donovania granulomatis*)

COMMONLY ASSOCIATED CONDITIONS
Can be associated with other sexually transmitted infections (STIs), including HIV infection

 DIAGNOSIS

HISTORY
- Sexual contact ± genital lesions
- Recent travel
- History of HIV infection or other STIs
- Subcutaneous nodules or superficial blisters in the genital area that develop into open sores, usually painless

PHYSICAL EXAM
- Incubation period varies: 1–15 weeks.
- Begins with subcutaneous nodules or superficial blisters in the genital area; may spread to inguinal folds and lead to surrounding depigmentation
- Blister becomes a slowly enlarging open sore; usually painless; may emit a foul odor
- Four types, commonly classified as
  - Ulcerovegetative: This is the most common. The ulcers are fairly large, with raised margins and a prominently erythematous appearance. The base is friable and thus bleeds easily.
  - Cicatricial: This consists of dry ulcers that may coalesce into a plaque.
  - Nodular: Isolated pruritic red nodules are the prominent feature; may develop into the ulcerative type. Owing to their resemblance, these lesions should be distinguished from the buboes of other conditions.
  - Verrucous or hypertrophic: Rare; proliferative reaction; forms large vegetative masses resembling warts
- Genital involvement in 90%, inguinal in 10%
- Males: Lesions usually occur on the genitalia, including the penis and scrotum.
- Association with uncircumcised men if occurring in low-hygiene situations
- Females: Lesions usually occur on the genitalia; about 10% of lesions may be cervical.
- 10–50% infected men and women have lesions in the anal area.

- Extragenital involvement (6%):
  - The most common extragenital sites of infection are the GI tract (including the oral cavity and anus), lymph nodes (may present as pseudobuboes), and hematogenous spread to intraabdominal organs and, rarely, bony structures.

DIAGNOSTIC TESTS & INTERPRETATION
- Mostly a clinical diagnosis; most labs do not have a culture available.
- Consider testing for mimics and common coinfections.
- Staining and biopsy are also appropriate, but results are difficult to assess and not always accurate.

Lab
- Most effective diagnostic method is direct visualization of the organisms within the macrophages, seen as safety pin–shaped intracytoplasmic inclusions (Donovan bodies).
- Tissue crush preparations from ulcer edge may be performed via punch biopsy, curettage, or a thin wedge of skin. Use of Wright-Giemsa or Warthin-Starry stain can help in the visualization of Donovan bodies.
- Polymerase chain reaction (PCR) used for research; may be available clinically in some settings
- Indirect immunofluorescence technique is not accurate for confirming the diagnosis.
- Pap smears may identify Donovan bodies on routine cervical screening.
- Test for other STIs and HIV infection because multiple infections frequently coexist.

Imaging
Consider radiographs if bony involvement is suspected.

DIFFERENTIAL DIAGNOSIS
- Lymphogranuloma venereum
- Condyloma lata of syphilis
- Chancroid
- HIV-associated herpetic ulcers
- Carcinoma of the penis, vulva, or cervix
- Tuberculosis of the cervix

TREATMENT

Usually can be treated in an outpatient setting with appropriate antibiotics and clinical monitoring

MEDICATION

First Line
- All regimens should be administered for 3 weeks or until ulcer resolution.
- Azithromycin: 1 g/d PO 1st day, 500 mg/d after that
- Trimethoprim-sulfamethoxazole DS (Bactrim) PO b.i.d. (avoid in pregnancy)
- Doxycycline: 100 mg PO b.i.d. (avoid in pregnancy)
- HIV-associated granuloma inguinale may take longer to heal; the addition of an aminoglycoside is highly recommended.

Second Line
- Ciprofloxacin: 750 mg PO b.i.d. × 3 weeks (avoid in pediatric and pregnant patients)
- Erythromycin base: 500 mg PO q.i.d. for 3 weeks (use as 1st line in pregnancy)
- Gentamicin: 1 mg/kg IM/IV t.i.d. in pregnancy or if other regimens are ineffective in 1st few days of treatment
- Single-dose regimens of ciprofloxacin, azithromycin, and ceftriaxone have been reported anecdotally.

Pediatric Considerations
Children born to mothers with untreated genital lesions of donovanosis are at risk of infection, and a course of prophylactic antibiotics should be considered.

Pregnancy Considerations
- Use erythromycin, 500 mg PO q.i.d. ± aminoglycoside.
- Doxycycline and ciprofloxacin are contraindicated in pregnancy.
- Sulfonamides are relatively contraindicated.

ADDITIONAL TREATMENT

General Measures
- Empirical treatment should be comprehensive and cover all likely pathogens.
- Antimicrobials given for at least 3 weeks and continued until reepithelialization of the ulcer
- If the ulcer does not respond within the 1st few days of treatment, add an IV aminoglycoside.
- Relapse may occur up to 18 months after treatment.
- Tetracycline is no longer recommended owing to bacterial resistance.
- Care must be taken with pregnant and pediatric patients when choosing antimicrobials.

Issues for Referral
- Surgical referral (e.g., urologic, gynecologic, colorectal), based on complications
- Infectious disease consultation may be helpful if coexisting HIV infection or other STIs are present or suspected.

SURGERY/OTHER PROCEDURES
May need surgical correction for disfiguring genital lesions, abscess drainage, or correction of urethral/lymphatic obstruction

IN-PATIENT CONSIDERATIONS

Initial Stabilization
Usually not a concern unless patient presents with a surgical complication such as lymphatic or urethral obstruction

Admission Criteria
- Extensive, chronic, or necrotizing lesions
- Hematogenous dissemination
- Patient compliance with outpatient regimen a concern

Nursing
- Wound care as needed
- Monitoring for evidence of secondary bacterial infection (i.e., careful review of vital signs)

Discharge Criteria
- Surgical clearance if surgical complications were part of the reason for admission
- Ability to access and tolerate oral antimicrobials if needed
- Clinical improvement

ONGOING CARE

FOLLOW-UP RECOMMENDATIONS
If treated in a timely manner, lesions usually resolve.

Patient Monitoring
- Monitor for hyperkalemia with extended TMP-SMX treatment.
- Other monitoring varies per treatment regimen.
- Monitor patient until resolution of symptoms.

PATIENT EDUCATION
- Patient rapport is critical because many patients may present late secondary to low self-esteem.
- Counseling on safe sex practices should be provided.

PROGNOSIS
- Goal of treatment is to reduce morbidity and prevent complications.
- Relapse may occur up to 18 months after treatment.
- If untreated, lesions may expand for years.

COMPLICATIONS
- Carcinoma (in 0.25%): Squamous cell carcinoma of the penis, vulva, or cervix
- After ulcer healing, fibrosis, stricture formation, phimosis, and scarring can occur, leading to deformity and functional disability.
- Balanitis and secondary infection of ulcers
- Elephantiasis of the genitals may occur secondary to lymphatic obstruction.
- Extragenital involvement with potential fatal spread to the viscera
- Recurrent disease even months to years after treatment (usually associated with HIV infection)

ADDITIONAL READING
- CDC. Sexually transmitted diseases treatment guidelines 2006. *MMWR*. 2006;55:1–118.
- Richens J. Donovanosis (granuloma inguinale). *Sex Transm Inf*. 2006;82(Suppl 4):21–2.
- Velho PE, de Souza EM, Belds Jr. W. Donovanosis. *The Brazilian Journal of Infectious Diseases* 2008;12(6):521–525.

CODES

ICD9
099.2 Granuloma inguinale

CLINICAL PEARLS
- The disease is transmitted usually through sexual activity, including vaginal and anal sex. It can, however, be transmitted through breaks in the skin, such as contact with ulcers of an infected person.
- Antibiotic treatment is available and must be tailored to the patient (e.g., pediatric, pregnant, coexisting conditions).
- It can be transmitted through an infected birth canal from a pregnant woman to her fetus.

G

GRANULOMA, PYOGENIC

Augustine J. Sohn, MD, MPH

 BASICS

DESCRIPTION
- Benign, acquired, solitary vascular proliferation that involves exposed areas such as distal extremities (especially the hands) and face as well as oral cavity (most frequently the gingiva)
- System(s) affected: Gastrointestinal (e.g., colon, small intestine); Skin/Exocrine; External ear canal, eye (e.g., eyelid, lacrimal sac)
- Synonym(s): Pregnancy tumor; Granuloma gravidum; Granuloma telangiectaticum; Lobular capillary hemangioma

EPIDEMIOLOGY
Mean age of patients with pyogenic granuloma is 40.5 years.

Incidence
- In children, accounts for <1% of all skin nodules
- 5% of pregnant women are affected in the US.

Prevalence
Unknown

RISK FACTORS
- Pregnancy
- Trauma
- Intraoral trauma or surgery

GENERAL PREVENTION
Good oral hygiene

ETIOLOGY
- Thought to be an aberrant healing response to minor trauma in many cases
- May be related to hormonal changes in pregnancy
- Not caused by bacterial infection, but associated with capillary proliferation
- Not considered a hemangioma or neoplasm

 DIAGNOSIS

HISTORY
- Solitary lesion that develops rapidly from days to weeks after minor trauma and bleeds easily
- Grows early in pregnancy and partially regresses postpartum

PHYSICAL EXAM
- Most commonly located at head and neck lesion and upper extremities (1)[C]
- Among oral lesions, gingiva is the most common location (2)[C]
- Bright red, purple, yellow, or brown with moist and sometimes scaly appearing surface
- Ranges from a few millimeters to 2–3 cm in diameter (usually <1 cm); giant lesions may rarely occur on areas such as the foot
- Soft; sessile or pedunculated
- Granular, smooth, or slightly nodular

DIAGNOSTIC TESTS & INTERPRETATION
Diagnostic Procedures/Surgery
Excisional biopsy

Pathological Findings
Micro:
- Small, endothelial-lined vascular spaces
- Loose or dense connective tissue stroma
- Acute and chronic inflammatory cells
- No true granuloma formation
- Abundant mitotic activity

DIFFERENTIAL DIAGNOSIS
- Peripheral ossifying granuloma
- Giant cell granuloma
- Odontogenic fibroma
- Kaposi sarcoma
- Malignant melanoma
- Angiolymphoid hyperplasia with eosinophilia
- Metastatic carcinoma
- Pilomatricoma
- In AIDS patients: Bacillary angiomatosis, deep mycoses

TREATMENT

SURGERY/OTHER PROCEDURES
- Surgical excision with simple closure gives the best result with least recurrence (3)[C].
- Shave excision with cautery may be optimal treatment for a lesion on fingertips (1)[C].
- Topical imiquimod may be useful for children (4)[C].
- Electrosurgery (electrodesiccation and curettage)
- Topical phenol may be used for periungual lesion (5)[C]
- CO_2-laser destruction
- Excision must be adequate to avoid recurrence. Even a small fragment of tissue left behind may lead to recurrence.
- Excisional biopsy should be tried in all situations if possible to ensure a proper diagnosis (i.e., not missing malignancies like amelanotic melanoma or basal cell carcinoma) (1)

ONGOING CARE

PATIENT EDUCATION
Patient should avoid trauma to area following excision.

PROGNOSIS
- Some lesions spontaneously resolve on their own (usually within 6 months).
- Complete resolution is expected with adequate excision.

COMPLICATIONS
Recurrence: After removal or destruction of solitary lesion, multiple satellite lesions can form around original treatment site.

REFERENCES

1. Giblin AV, Clover AJ, Athanassopoulos A, Budny PG et al. Pyogenic granuloma - the quest for optimum treatment: audit of treatment of 408 cases. *Journal of plastic, reconstructive & aesthetic surgery : JPRAS.* 2007;60:1030–5.
2. Gordón-Nñez MA, Carvalho MD, Benevenuto TG, Lopes MF, Silva LM, Galvão HC et al. Oral Pyogenic Granuloma: A Retrospective Analysis of 293 Cases in a Brazilian Population. *Journal of oral and maxillofacial surgery : official journal of the American Association of Oral and Maxillofacial Surgeons.* 2010;
3. Gilmore A, Kelsberg G, Safranek S et al. Clinical inquiries. What's the best treatment for pyogenic granuloma? *J Fam Pract.* 2010;59:40–2.
4. Tritton SM, Smith S, Wong LC, Zagarella S, Fischer G et al. Pyogenic granuloma in ten children treated with topical imiquimod. *Pediatr Dermatol.* 269–72.
5. Iglesias ME, DE Bengoa Vallejo RB et al. Topical Phenol as a Conservative Treatment for Periungual Pyogenic Granuloma. *Dermatologic surgery : official publication for American Society for Dermatologic Surgery [et al.].* 2010;

CODES

ICD9
686.1 Pyogenic granuloma of skin and subcutaneous tissue

CLINICAL PEARLS

- Benign, acquired, solitary vascular proliferation that involves exposed areas such as distal extremities and face as well as oral cavity
- Due mainly to aberrant healing response to minor trauma in many cases
- Excision must be adequate to avoid recurrence.
- Excisional biopsy recommended to ensure proper diagnosis (and to not miss a malignant lesion)
- Excision with primary closure or excision with cautery should be the first choice for treatment in most of the lesions.

G

GRAVES DISEASE

Katharine Barnard, MD

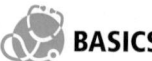 **BASICS**

DESCRIPTION
Graves disease is an autoimmune disease in which thyroid-stimulating antibodies cause increased thyroid function. In addition to hyperthyroidism, classic findings are goiter and ophthalmopathy.

EPIDEMIOLOGY
Prevalence
- Overall prevalence of hyperthyroidism is estimated to be 2% for women and 0.2% for men.
- Graves disease accounts for 60–80% of all cases of hyperthyroidism.
- Predominant age: 30–40 years

RISK FACTORS
- Female sex (due to sex steroids)
- Postpartum period
- Stressful life events (1)
- Medications: Iodine, amiodarone, lithium, HAART, rarely immune-modulating medications (i.e., interferon)
- Smoking (higher risk of developing ophthalmopathy)

Genetics
Higher risk with personal or family history of any autoimmune disease, especially Hashimoto's thyroiditis

GENERAL PREVENTION
Screening TSH in asymptomatic patients is not recommended. No data conclusively show that treatment of subclinical thyroid dysfunction improves quality of life or clinical outcome measures (2).

PATHOPHYSIOLOGY
- Excessive production of TSH receptor antibodies from B cells primarily within the thyroid, likely due to genetic clonal lack of suppressor T cells
- Binding of these antibodies to TSH receptors in the thyroid causes increased production of thyroid hormone.
- Binding to similar antigen in retro-orbital connective tissue causes ocular symptoms.

COMMONLY ASSOCIATED CONDITIONS
- Mitral valve prolapse
- Hypokalemic periodic paralysis

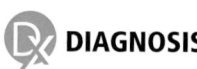 **DIAGNOSIS**

Thyroid hormone controls metabolic rate and affects many organ systems. Hyperthyroid patients appear hypermetabolic, with increased adrenergic tone.

HISTORY
- Tachycardia, palpitations
- Tremor, restlessness
- Anxiety, emotional lability, insomnia
- Sweating, heat intolerance
- Pruritus, skin changes
- Weight loss
- Fatigue, shortness of breath (due to muscle weakness)
- Oligo-/amenorrhea (women), erectile dysfunction (men), gynecomastia
- Loose, frequent stools

- Blurred vision or diplopia, lacrimation, photophobia, gritty sensation in eyes (ocular dryness), retro-orbital discomfort, painful eye movement, loss of color vision or visual acuity
- Worsening of chronic medical conditions (anxiety or Bipolar disorder, glucose intolerance, heart failure or angina)

Geriatric Considerations
Elderly patients may not display classic symptoms; may present with atrial fibrillation or weight loss

PHYSICAL EXAM
- Thyroid: Enlarged, nontender, and without nodules; possible bruit (increased blood flow)
- Integumentary: Fine hair, warm skin, onycholysis of nails, palmar erythema, possible pretibial myxedema, possible hyperpigmented plaques (dermopathy)
- Cardiac: Resting tachycardia, hyperdynamic circulation, possible atrial fibrillation
- Ophthalmologic (present in 50% of cases): Lid lag, lid retraction, proptosis, corneal irritation, ophthalmoplegia; papilledema and loss of color vision may signify optic neuropathy
- Extremities: Tremor, hyper-reflexia, proximal myopathy; rarely, soft tissue edema of extremities and clubbing of digits (acropachy)

DIAGNOSTIC TESTS & INTERPRETATION
Lab
Initial lab tests
- TSH is initial test. Very low or undetectable TSH confirms hyperthyroidism.
- Next, check T_4 level. T_4 will be high in Graves.

Pregnancy Considerations
Thyroid-stimulating hormone (TSH) level at 36 weeks gestation is most predictive of neonatal hyperthyroidism. This should be checked even in post-treatment pregnant patients taking thyroid hormone replacement.

Imaging
Initial approach
After confirming suppressed TSH and high T_4, next step is radioactive iodine uptake (RAIU) and scan. Graves patients will have diffuse, elevated RAIU (vs focal/nodular elevated uptake in adenoma and multinodular goiter, and decreased uptake in thyroiditis).

DIFFERENTIAL DIAGNOSIS
- Toxic multinodular goiter (multiple hormone-producing nodules)
- Toxic adenoma (single hormone-producing nodule)
- Thyroiditis (hormone leakage):
  - Subacute, usually postviral (thyroid will be tender)
  - Lymphocytic, including postpartum
  - Hashimoto's thyroiditis (anti-TPO antibodies may stimulate TSH receptors)
- Iatrogenic (treatment-induced):
  - Iodine-induced (dietary, radiographic contrast, or medications)
  - Amiodarone
  - Thyroid hormone over-replacement (accidental or intentional)
- Tumor:
  - Pituitary adenoma producing TSH
  - HCG-producing tumors (stimulate TSH receptors)
  - Extraglandular thyroid hormone production (i.e., struma ovarii or metastatic thyroid cancer)

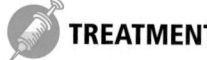 **TREATMENT**

MEDICATION
Goal of therapy is to correct the hypermetabolic state with the fewest side effects and lowest incidence of post-treatment hypothyroidism.

Pediatric Considerations
- Pediatric cases need treatment, as spontaneous remission occurs in only 30% of cases or less.
- Radioactive iodine is treatment of choice: Fewer side effects, higher cure rate, and no observed increase in future cancer risk or genetic damage. Higher dose radioactive iodine seems to confer even less risk of thyroid cancer than low dose, and so is preferable (3).

First Line
Radioactive iodine:
- Concentrates in the thyroid gland and destroys thyroid tissue
- Treatment of choice in the US for Graves disease
- High cure rate with single treatment, especially with high-dose regimen
- Risks: Side effects (neck soreness, flushing, decreased taste); worsening ophthalmopathy (15% incidence, higher in smokers) (4); post-treatment hypothyroidism (80% incidence, not dosage-dependent); radiation thyroiditis (1% incidence); need to adhere to safety precautions until radiation is eliminated from the body
- Pretreatment with antithyroid medication should be considered in patients with severe disease as symptom control and to reduce risk of post-treatment radiation thyroiditis. Pretreatment may, however, reduce cure rate with radioactive iodine so is not uniformly recommended.
- May be repeated in as soon as 4 months if needed

Pregnancy Considerations
- Radioactive iodine is contraindicated in pregnancy and lactation. There is no effect on future fertility, but it is recommended to avoid pregnancy for 4 months after receiving radioactive iodine.
- Antithyroid drugs: Methimazole (MMI) and propothiouracil (PTU):
  - Compete with the thyroid for iodine, thereby decreasing the synthesis of thyroid hormone; PTU also blocks peripheral conversion of T_4 to T_3
  - Treatment of choice for children and for adults who refuse radioactive iodine
  - May use as pretreatment (symptom control) for older or cardiac patients before radioactive iodine or surgery
  - MMI is usually first choice due to lower cost and once-daily dosing
  - No improvement in remission rates noted with higher-dose MMI; therefore, lowest effective dose should be used (5)
  - Minor side effects (<5% incidence), which may be controlled by switching from one agent to another: Rash, fever, arthralgias, GI side effects
  - Major side effects, which necessitate a change in treatment:
    - Polyarthritis (1–2%)
    - Agranulocytosis (<0.5%)
    - Elevated liver enzymes (30% with PTU) or hepatitis (rare)
    - Cholestasis and jaundice (occurs rarely with MMI)

- Discontinue treatment after 1 year if patient is euthyroid and thyroid-stimulating antibody level is undetectable.
- 60% remission rate with 2 years of treatment (standard regimen); newer studies suggest no increased benefit to treatment beyond 18 months (6)
- Relapse rate of up to 50% in patients who respond initially; higher relapse rate if smoker, large goiter, or positive thyroid-stimulating antibodies at the end of treatment

Pregnancy Considerations
PTU is preferred in pregnancy, as MMI crosses the placenta and may have risks of congenital malformation and for congenital hypothyroidism. Either is safe in breastfeeding (7).

Second Line
Plasmapheresis is under investigation as a treatment option (8).

ADDITIONAL TREATMENT
Issues for Referral
- Endocrinologist:
  - Radioactive iodine therapy
  - Pregnant or breastfeeding patient
  - Graves ophthalmopathy (also should see ophthalmologist)
- Surgeon:
  - Failed drug therapy, or refusing RAI
  - Obstruction
  - Cosmesis

Additional Therapies
- Beta-blockers provide prompt control of adrenergic symptoms. Can be started while workup is in progress. Long-acting propranolol is used most commonly, and titrated to symptom control (40–320 mg daily). Calcium channel blockers are an alternative for heart rate control in patients who cannot take beta-blockers (8).
- Symptom control may be achieved with iodides, which block conversion of T_4 to T_3, and inhibit TSH release. Use for pregnant patients who do not tolerate antithyroid medication, or in conjunction with antithyroid medications. Should not be used long-term (may cause paradoxical increase in TSH release) or in combination with radioactive iodine.
- For corneal protection: Tinted glasses when outdoors, artificial tears, patching or taping the lids at night
- For proptosis: Oral steroid (prednisone 60–80 mg daily for 2–4 weeks, then tapered off)
- For dermopathy, if local discomfort at site of plaques: Topical corticosteroid

SURGERY/OTHER PROCEDURES
- Surgery may be indicated if medication fails, if patient refuses RAI, or in the case of severe disease in second trimester of pregnancy.
- Subtotal thyroidectomy preserves some thyroid function and only holds 25% post-op incidence of hypothyroidism, but has less predictable outcome; therefore, total thyroidectomy is now standard of care. Studies show no increased risk of permanent complications (hypoparathyroidism or laryngeal nerve damage) with total thyroidectomy (9).

IN-PATIENT CONSIDERATIONS
Indications for hospital admission:
- Thyroid storm (rare but life-threatening complication of Graves, with exaggerated symptoms: Tachycardia, hyperpyrexia, neurologic compromise, and GI/liver dysfunction; may be precipitated by trauma, infection, iodine load, or surgery). Admit to ICU for symptom control and antithyroid medications.
- Ophthalmopathy with visual impairment. Admit with ophthalmology consult.
- Severe cardiac symptoms (CHF, rapid atrial fibrillation, angina). Admit for rate control and cardiology consult.

 ## ONGOING CARE

FOLLOW-UP RECOMMENDATIONS
Patient Monitoring
- Monitoring is for resolution of hyperthyroidism and for development of hypothyroidism.
- Check TSH and T_4 levels every 1–2 months for first 6 months after treatment, then every 3 months for a year, then every 6–12 months thereafter. For patients on treatment with PTU and MMI, check anti-TSH receptor antibodies at 12 months of treatment to determine possibility of discontinuing medication.

Pregnancy Considerations
Postpartum exacerbation of hyperthyroidism is common for women not currently under treatment, so TSH and symptoms should be monitored.

DIET
Nutritional supplementation with L-carnitine may diminish hyperthyroid symptoms and may decrease bone demineralization (10).

PATIENT EDUCATION
Adherence to follow-up (surveillance) recommendations and medication regimens are the most important ways to achieve a good outcome and promote lifelong health.

PROGNOSIS
- Generally good with treatment
- May have irreversible ocular, cardiac, and psychiatric consequences
- Increased morbidity and mortality due to osteoporosis, atherosclerotic disease, insulin resistance and obesity, and endothelial cell dysfunction (thromboembolic risk) (8,11)

COMPLICATIONS
Hypothyroidism is most common consequence of treatment (25-80% depending on treatment modality). Patients should be monitored annually, even if asymptomatic.

REFERENCES
1. Matos-Santos A. Relationship between number of and impact of stressful life events and the onset of Graves Disease and toxic multinodular goitre. *Clin Endocrinol*. 2007;55(1).
2. Helfand M, U.S. Preventive Services Task Force. Screening for subclinical thyroid dysfunction in nonpregnant adults: a summary of the evidence for the U.S. Preventive Services Task Force. *Ann Intern Med*. 2004;140:128–41.
3. Rivkees SA, Dinauer C. An optimal treatment for pediatric graves' disease is radioiodine. *J Clin Endocrinol Metab*. 2007;92:797–800.
4. Woeber KA. The year in review: the thyroid. *Ann Intern Med*. 1999;131:959–62.
5. Benker G, Reinwein D. Is there a methimazole dose effect on remission rate in Graves Disease? Results from a longterm prospective study. *Clin Endocrinol*. 2004;49(4).
6. Maugendre D, Gatel A. Antithyroid drugs and Graves Disease - prospective randomized assessment of longterm treatment. *Clin Endocrinol*. 2004;50(1).
7. Streetman DD, Khanderia U. Diagnosis and treatment of Graves disease. *Ann Pharmacother*. 2003;37:1100–9.
8. Reid JR, Wheeler SF. Hyperthyroidism: diagnosis and treatment. *Am Fam Physician*. 2005;72: 623–30.
9. Barakate MS, Agarwal G. Total thyroidectomy is now the preferred option for the surgical management of Graves Disease. *ANZ Journal of Surgery*. 2002;72(5).
10. Benvenga S, Ruggeri RM, Russo A, et al. Usefulness of L-carnitine, a naturally occurring peripheral antagonist of thyroid hormone action, in iatrogenic hyperthyroidism: a randomized, double-blind, placebo-controlled clinical trial. *J Clin Endocrinol Metab*. 2001;86:3579–94.
11. Burggraaf J, Lalezari S, Emeis JJ, et al. Endothelial function in patients with hyperthyroidism before and after treatment with propranolol and thiamazol. *Thyroid*. 2001;11:153–60.

ADDITIONAL READING
AACE Thyroid Task Force. American Association of Clinical Endocrinologists medical guidelines for clinical practice for the evaluation and treatment of hyperthyroidism and hypothyroidism. *Endocr Pract*. 2002;8(6).

See Also (Topic, Algorithm, Electronic Media Element)
Algorithms: Weight Loss; Cardiac Arrhythmias; Anxiety

 ## CODES

ICD9
- 242.00 Toxic diffuse goiter without mention of thyrotoxic crisis or storm
- 242.01 Toxic diffuse goiter with mention of thyrotoxic crisis or storm

CLINICAL PEARLS
Thyroid hormone controls metabolic rate and affects many organ systems. Hyperthyroid patients appear hypermetabolic, with symptoms and signs of increased adrenergic tone.

G

GROWTH HORMONE DEFICIENCY
Lee A. Mancini, MD, CSCS, CSN

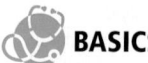 **BASICS**

DESCRIPTION
- Inadequate production of growth hormone (GH, also called *somatotropin*) in either adults or children
- GH is a polypeptide hormone that stimulates growth and cell reproduction.
- *Hypopituitarism* is often used to describe growth hormone deficiency (GHD). However, hypopituitarism is actually defined as GHD plus a deficiency in at least 1 other anterior pituitary hormone.
- *Panhypopituitarism* is defined as a deficiency in all the hormones produced in the pituitary gland.
- System(s) affected: Endocrine; Musculoskeletal
- Synonym(s): Hypopituitarism

EPIDEMIOLOGY
Incidence
- Most common cause of GHD in children is idiopathic.
- Most common cause of GHD in adults is a pituitary adenoma or treatment of the adenoma with surgery or radiotherapy:
  - 76% of patients with GHD had a pituitary tumor.
  - 13% had an extrapituitary tumor.
  - 8% the cause was unknown
  - 1% had sarcoidosis.
  - 0.5% had Sheehan syndrome.

Prevalence
- In children, isolated GHD has been reported to affect 1 in 4,000.
- Adult-onset idiopathic GHD is extremely rare.

RISK FACTORS
Genetics
A variety of congenital genetic causes of GHD:
- Transcription factor defects (PIT-1, PROP-1, LHX3/4, HESX-1, and PITX-2)
- GHRH receptor gene defects
- GH secretagogue receptor gene defects
- GH gene defects
- GH receptor/postreceptor defects
- Prader-Willi syndrome

PATHOPHYSIOLOGY
- GHD is caused by a complete lack of GH production or a decline in GH production. There are multiple causes.
- Hypothalamus secretes GH-releasing hormone (GHRH), which stimulates the pituitary to secrete GH. Somatostatin is secreted by the hypothalamus to inhibit GH secretion. When GH pulses are secreted into the blood, then insulinlike growth factor (IGF)-1 is released. GHD may result from disruption of the GH axis at numerous places—in the higher brain, the hypothalamus, or the pituitary gland.

ETIOLOGY
- Congenital:
  - Genetic (see Genetics)
  - Structural brain defects:
    - Agenesis of corpus callosum
    - Septo-optic dysplasia
    - Empty sella syndrome
    - Encephalocele
    - Hydrocephalus
    - Arachnoid cyst
  - Associated midline facial defects:
    - Single central incisor
    - Cleft lip/palate
- Acquired:
  - Trauma:
    - Perinatal
    - Postnatal
  - Central nervous system (CNS) infection
  - Tumors of hypothalamus or pituitary:
    - Pituitary adenoma
    - Craniopharyngioma
    - Rathke cleft cyst
    - Glioma/astrocytoma
    - Germinoma
    - Metastatic
  - Cranial irradiation
  - Surgery

COMMONLY ASSOCIATED CONDITIONS
- Macroadenoma
- Sarcoidosis
- Sheehan syndrome

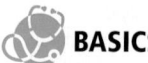 **DIAGNOSIS**

HISTORY
- Adults:
  - Fatigue
  - Muscle weakness
  - Depression
  - Social withdrawal
  - Poor memory
  - Loss of strength
  - Loss of stamina
- Children:
  - Slower muscular development and delayed gross motor milestones such as standing, walking, and jumping
  - Important questions to ask:
    - Birth weight and length
    - Height of parents
    - Timing of puberty in parents
    - Previous growth points
    - Nutritional history
    - General health of child

PHYSICAL EXAM
- Children with GHD:
  - Most common presentation is short stature
  - Newborns may present with hypoglycemia, jaundice, or micropenis.
  - Severe GHD children have maxillary hypoplasia and forehead prominence; kewpie doll appearance.
  - Accurately measure height and weight.
  - Assess pubertal status using Tanner staging system.
- Adults:
  - Decreased lean body mass
  - Poor bone density

DIAGNOSTIC TESTS & INTERPRETATION
Lab
Initial lab tests
- IGF-1, IGFBP-3
- Multiple GH levels
- Thyroid-stimulating hormone (TSH) (hypothyroidism should be excluded as a cause)
- Serum electrolytes (low bicarbonate levels may indicate renal tubular acidosis)
- Complete blood count (CBC) and erythrocyte sedimentation rate (ESR)
- Karyotype

Follow-Up & Special Considerations
- Testing for GHD by random measurement of GH in a single blood sample is not beneficial, as GH is nearly undetectable for most of the day.
- In children, evaluate those who have significant discrepancy between growth curve.
- Low levels of IGF-1 and IGF binding protein (IGFBP)-3
- Multiple blood-sample testing for GH levels

Imaging
Initial approach
Radiograph of left hand and wrist to determine skeletal age in children

Follow-Up & Special Considerations
Brain magnetic resonance imaging (MRI) to evaluate for a tumor may be ordered.

Diagnostic Procedures/Surgery
Provocative tests:
- Give a dose of an agent that in a normal person causes a surge in the release of GH: Common agents used include argine, clonidine, glucagons, insulin, levodopa, and propranolol (1)[C]
- After agent is given, GH serum levels are drawn every 15 minutes.
- GH levels are checked for over 60 minutes.

DIFFERENTIAL DIAGNOSIS
- Turner syndrome
- Renal failure
- Small size for gestational age in newborns
- Prader-Willi syndrome
- Idiopathic short stature
- Noonan syndrome
- Russell-Silver syndrome
- Down syndrome

 ## TREATMENT

MEDICATION
- GHD is treated with GH replacement.
- In 1985, GH was synthetically produced from recombinant DNA.
- Several medications are approved for GHD treatment in children:
  - Liquid solutions for SC injection: These are available in multidose pen devices. Daily therapy is more effective than 3-times-a-week therapy. The recommended dose is 0.04 mg/kg/d for children (2)[C].

- Encapsulated GH in glycolide microspheres for deep SC administration. Either 1.5 mg/kg body weight once a month or 0.75 mg/kg twice a month.
- Geref (sermorelin) has been removed from the market. It is a synthetic growth hormone-releasing hormone.
- Several growth hormone-releasing peptides (GHRPs) or nonpeptide analogs are to be evaluated in children and adults. It is too early to evaluate their long-term safety and efficacy.

ADDITIONAL TREATMENT
Issues for Referral
Patients with GHD would benefit from a referral to an endocrinologist.

 ## ONGOING CARE

FOLLOW-UP RECOMMENDATIONS
- Children: Regular follow-up with a pediatric endocrinologist
- Adults: Follow-up with an endocrinologist is recommended.

DIET
No restrictions

PROGNOSIS
- In children, the prognosis for GHD is good. GH therapy is effective.
- 5 independent predictors of pubertal growth:
  - Gender
  - Age at onset of puberty
  - Age at end of growth
  - Dose of growth hormone at onset of puberty
  - Deviation of target height from height at onset of puberty

COMPLICATIONS
- In children:
  - Slipped capital femoral epiphysis
  - Scoliosis
- In adults and children:
  - Unmet expectations
  - Metabolic effects
  - Antibodies to growth hormone
  - Cancer: Lymphoma, tumor recurrence
  - Fluid retention: Pseudotumor cerebri, carpal tunnel syndrome, pancreatitis, and edema

REFERENCES
1. Molich ME, et al. Clinical practice guideline: Evaluation and treatment of adult growth hormone deficiency. An endocrine society clinical practice guideline. *J Clin Endocrinol Metabol*. 2006;91: 1621–34.
2. deMuink Keizer-Schrama SM, et al. Dose-response study of biosynthetic human growth hormone in GH-deficient children: Effects on axiological and biochemical parameters. *J Clin Endocrinol Metabol*. 1992;74:898.

ADDITIONAL READING
- Hoffman AR, et al. Efficacy and tolerability of an individualized dosing regimen for adult growth hormone replacement therapy in comparison with fixed body weight-based dosing. *J Clin Endocrinol Metabol*. 2004;87:1974–9.
- Rosenfield RG, et al. Diagnostic controversy: the diagnosis of childhood growth hormone deficiency revisited. *J Clin Endocrinol Metabol*. 1995;80:1532.

See Also (Topic, Algorithm, Electronic Media Element)
Pituitary Tumors

 ## CODES

ICD9
- 253.2 Panhypopituitarism
- 253.3 Pituitary dwarfism

CLINICAL PEARLS
- Most common cause of GHD in children is idiopathic.
- Most common cause of GHD in adults is pituitary adenoma.
- Treatment of pituitary adenoma is either surgery or radiotherapy.
- All patients taking replacement GH therapy need to have their IGF-1 level monitored.

G

GUILLAIN-BARRÉ SYNDROME

Sheela Swaminatha, MD

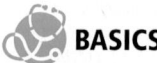 **BASICS**

DESCRIPTION
- A group of autoimmune diseases targeted at the peripheral nerves and causing acute progressive weakness, usually an ascending paralysis
- Divided into 2 forms:
  - Demyelinating: Acute inflammatory demyelinating polyradiculoneuropathy (AIDP): >90% of cases in Western countries
  - Axonal injury: Uncommon; poor prognosis:
    - Acute motor axonal neuropathy (AMAN): 5% of cases; predominant motor involvement; acute flaccid paralysis with rapid recovery; >50% in northern China; recent *Campylobacter jejuni* gastroenteritis; often summer epidemics in children and adults
    - Acute motor-sensory axonal neuropathy (AMSAN): Hyperacute course: Leads to profound weakness with muscle wasting; poor prognosis
- Occurs mostly in adults
- Synonym(s): Acute inflammatory demyelinating polyradiculopathy; Landry-Guillain-Barré-Strohl syndrome; Acute inflammatory neuropathy; Acute idiopathic polyneuritis; Acute immune-mediated polyneuritis; Landry ascending paralysis

ALERT
30% of the patients have respiratory paralysis requiring mechanical ventilation, but complete or substantial recovery is the natural disease course.

Geriatric Considerations
Worse prognosis >60 years of age

Pediatric Considerations
Disease tends to be milder in children.

Pregnancy Considerations
Uncommon in pregnancy

EPIDEMIOLOGY
Incidence
In the US: 1.8/100,000 (0.8/100,000 in children <18 years of age; 3.2/100,000 in adults >60 years of age)

Prevalence
- In the US: 3–10/100,000
- Predominant age: All ages
- Predominant sex: Male > Female (1.5:1)
- Nonseasonal, nonepidemic

RISK FACTORS
Diabetes mellitus (DM), recent surgery, organ transplantation (i.e., immunosuppression)

PATHOPHYSIOLOGY
Autoimmune disorder targeted against myelin and/or axons of peripheral nerves causing destruction of peripheral nerves in susceptible individuals

ETIOLOGY
Unclear; may be related to viral or bacterial infection

COMMONLY ASSOCIATED CONDITIONS
- Vaccinations: Swine flu (but not other influenza vaccine) and rabies
- Inactivated flu vaccines cause an estimated 1.6 additional cases of Guillain-Barré syndrome per million vaccinations (1)[A].

- 2009 data reveal no increased incidence of Guillain-Barré syndrome (GBS) with the Gardasil vaccine for human papillomavirus (HPV) compared with age-matched controls; incidence was 0.2/100,000 doses (2)[A],(3).
- Malignancies, Hodgkin lymphoma

 DIAGNOSIS

HISTORY
- Upper respiratory or diarrheal disease within previous 1–3 weeks in 50–70%: *C. jejuni* (~40%), cytomegalovirus (13%), Epstein-Barr virus (10%), *Mycoplasma pneumoniae* (5%), or HIV
- Dysesthesias, paresthesias of feet and hands are usually the earliest symptoms.
- Pain common, especially back pain; can radiate to the legs; no myalgias
- Gait disorder common in all age groups; most common presentation in children
- Neck muscle weakness, dysphagia, and dysarthria are predictors of respiratory failure.
- Most patients reach the plateau phase within 3 weeks of admission, and muscle strength is expected to improve.

PHYSICAL EXAM
- Acute, symmetric, and usually ascending weakness of limbs within days of dysesthesias (4)[A]
- Areflexia or hyporeflexia and muscle weakness, decreased position and vibratory sensation
- Respiratory muscle paralysis 30% if untreated
- Cranial nerve involvement <50%; usually facial weakness, 10–20% ophthalmoparesis
- Dysautonomia (50%): Labile blood pressure, arrhythmias, ileus, urinary retention; more common when seen with severe quadriparesis and respiratory failure
- Miller-Fisher variant: Ophthalmoplegia, ataxia, areflexia

DIAGNOSTIC TESTS & INTERPRETATION
Lab
Initial lab tests
- CSF: Elevated protein and normal white blood cells (WBCs; albuminocytologic dissociation) are characteristic, except that in patients with HIV aseptic meningitis, cell counts may be high. There is a normal opening pressure.
- Blood: Complete blood count (CBC), renal and hepatic function; when appropriate, rheumatoid factor, antineutrophil cytoplasmic antibodies, Sjögren syndrome A&B antibody, angiotensin-converting enzyme (ACE) level, cryoglobulinemia, D-aminolevulinic acid, and Lyme titer
- Urine: 24-hour urine for light chains
- Optional: Drug/toxin, heavy metal screen, HIV; in children, may check arylsulfatase A activity

Follow-Up & Special Considerations
- Special test: Serum anti-GM1 antibody titer in axonal variant (2)[B]; 30% of patients have elevated anti-GM1 antibodies.
- Anti-GQ1$_b$ in ophthalmoplegia form of GBS (Miller-Fisher variant) (5)

- Disorders that may alter lab results: Demyelinating neuropathy of DM may have CSF similar to that of GBS; however, GBS usually has higher CSF protein (>0.4 g/dL).
- Protein normal in 50% patients in 1st week of illness

Imaging
Initial approach
CXR

Follow-Up & Special Considerations
MRI of spinal cord if myelopathy or cord lesion suspected. Diffuse dorsal root enhancement seen on MRI with gadolinium supports GBS.

Diagnostic Procedures/Surgery
- Lumbar puncture for CSF analysis
- Nerve conduction studies (most sensitive test):
  - Initially, may show prolonged F-wave latency
  - Conduction block is common in GBS and characteristic of acquired demyelinating neuropathy.
  - Prolonged distal latency and slowing of conduction velocity in 2 nerves each in arms or legs
  - Formal pulmonary function test (includes negative inspiratory force [NIF] and forced vital capacity [FVC])
  - 12-lead ECG

Pathological Findings
Sural nerve biopsy not indicated unless necessary to rule out vasculitis or amyloidosis: Multifocal inflammatory cell infiltration with segmental demyelination and relative axonal sparing in GBS; axonal degeneration in axonal form of GBS; sensory neuronopathy in so-called Miller-Fisher syndrome

DIFFERENTIAL DIAGNOSIS
- Brain:
  - Acute cerebrovascular strokes (e.g., basilar artery thrombosis)
  - Encephalitis
- Spinal cord syndromes:
  - Transverse myelitis: Can have identical initial presentation
  - Cord compression
  - Carcinomatous meningoradiculitis
- Motor neuron disorder: Poliomyelitis
- Peripheral neuropathy associated with:
  - Vasculitis (e.g., polyarteritis nodosa, Wegner, Churg-Strauss, nonsystemic vasculitis limited to peripheral nerve)
  - Disimmune process (e.g., paraneoplastic syndrome, sensory gangliopathy, angiofollicular lymphoma)
  - Acute ICU neuromyopathy, critical illness neuropathy, ICU myopathy
  - Toxin (e.g., arsenic or thallium poisoning, vitamin B$_6$ overdose, glue sniffing, chemotherapeutics, organophosphates, neurotoxic fish)
  - Infectious (e.g., tick paralysis, diphtheria, Lyme)
  - Flaring of hereditary/congenital neuropathy (e.g., porphyria, Fabry, mitochondria cytopathy)
- Neuromuscular junction:
  - Myasthenia gravis
  - Eaton-Lambert
  - Botulism
  - Hypermagnesemia
- Muscle:
  - Polymyositis
  - Periodic paralysis (hypokalemia)
  - Toxic myopathy
- Psychiatric: Hysteria

TREATMENT

MEDICATION

- Immune globulin IV 2 g/kg over 5 days:
  - In severe disease, intravenous immunoglobulin started within 2 weeks from onset hastens recovery as much as plasma exchange (6)[A] *or*
- Plasmapheresis on 5 alternate days for a total of 250 mL/kg (7):
  - Requires vascular access
  - May be difficult in hemodynamically unstable patient given fluid shifts during plasma exchange
- Corticosteroids given alone do not significantly hasten recovery from GBS or affect the long-term outcome (8)[A].

ADDITIONAL TREATMENT

General Measures

- Tachyarrhythmias: May not require treatment
- Bradyarrhythmias: If symptomatic, atropine
- Sinus arrest and complete heart block: Temporary pacemaker
- Constipation/ileus from autonomic neuropathy: Laxatives, enemas
- Sucralfate 1 g b.i.d. in mechanically ventilated or nonsteroidal anti-inflammatory drug (NSAID) users
- Urinary retention from autonomic neuropathy: Catheterization
- Depression: Frequent reminders that recovery is the rule; avoid antidepressants.

Additional Therapies

There is no role for high-dose corticosteroids (7).

COMPLEMENTARY AND ALTERNATIVE MEDICINE

Lipoic acid for neuropathic pain control

IN-PATIENT CONSIDERATIONS

Initial Stabilization

- Admitted to ICU; 50% of those need mechanical ventilation; 10–20% of patients have mild disease without need of immune globulin IV or plasmapheresis (9)[A].
- Serial FVC, NIF, and oximetry; intubation for respiratory distress or FVC <20 mL/kg (<1 L in adults), NIF >−20, or difficulty swallowing/aspiration from bulbar palsy; use caution—unfavorable NIF and FVC may precede dyspnea or appreciable rise in pCO_2 on arterial blood gases (ABGs).
- Hypertension (HTN):
  - Often does not need treatment
  - In severe HTN, use morphine bolus to prevent congestive heart failure (CHF).
- Hypotension: Trendelenburg position and volume expansion; pressors if needed
- Pain: Common; can be severe and recalcitrant; analgesics including opioids; carbamazepine; transcutaneous electrical nerve stimulation (TENS)
- Aspiration precautions

Admission Criteria

Any patients suspected of GBS

Nursing

- Prevent complications of immobilization with physical therapy, pneumatic compressor, or subcutaneous heparin.
- Respiratory care and frequent turning; aspiration precaution
- Monitor bowel and bladder function for retention/ileus.

Discharge Criteria

Transfer to rehabilitation facility if patient is able to walk in the plateau phase. Discharge if in the recovery phase.

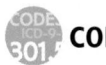

ONGOING CARE

FOLLOW-UP RECOMMENDATIONS

FVC is the best measurement, as opposed to oximetry/ABGs, which are normal until respiratory failure has occurred.

Patient Monitoring

- Accessory muscle for respiration and spirometry/vital capacity 4×/day at bedside
- Bulbar weakness and airway secretions
- Mechanical ventilation for airway protection or vital capacity <15 mL/kg of body weight or maximum inspiratory pressure ≤25 cm H_2O
- Telemetry monitoring for cardiac condition

DIET

No special diet; enteral feedings if intubated

PATIENT EDUCATION

Important to emphasize expectation of full/significant recovery, regardless of treatment

PROGNOSIS

- If untreated, 3 phases of illness:
  - Initial progression phase 24 hours–3 weeks; >50% reach nadir before 14 days; highest risk of death and complications during this phase (10)[A].
  - Plateau phase same duration as initial phase
  - Recovery phase 1–6 months; in adults, no discernible improvement after 2 years
- Mortality (most often from dysautonomia or complications): 2–5%
- Complete recovery: 50%
- Some residual disability: 45%
- Severe permanent disability: 5%
- Miller-Fisher variant often has more benign prognosis with mean recovery in ~10 weeks.
- Relapses may occur both before and after recovery; acute inflammatory demyelinating polyradiculoneuropathy is the initial presentation of 2% of chronic inflammatory demyelinating polyradiculoneuropathy patients.
- Poor prognostic signs:
  - Rapid progression to severe disease (<7 days)
  - Mechanical ventilation
  - Nerve conduction studies: Compound muscle action potential <10% or mean distal motor amplitude <20%
  - Acute motor axonal neuropathy (see Differential Diagnosis)
  - Preceding *C. jejuni* infection
  - Age >60 years

COMPLICATIONS

- Paralysis, permanent residual weakness
- Respiratory failure, mechanical ventilation
- Hypotension, HTN, labile blood pressure
- Cardiac arrhythmias
- Ileus
- Urinary retention
- Aspiration, pneumonia, sepsis
- Deep vein thrombosis, pulmonary embolism
- Psychiatric problems, including depression

REFERENCES

1. Jefferson T, Di Pietrantonj C, Rivetti A, Bawazeer GA, Al-Ansary LA, Ferroni E et al. Vaccines for preventing influenza in healthy adults. *Cochrane Database Syst Rev.* 2010;7:CD001269.
2. Hiraga A, Mori M, Ogawara K, et al. Recovery patterns and long term prognosis for axonal Guillain-Barré syndrome. *J Neurol Neurosurg Psychiatry.* 2005;76:719–22.
3. Slade BA, Leidel L, Vellozzi C, et al. Postlicensure safety surveillance for quadrivalent human papillomavirus recombinant vaccine. *JAMA.* 2009;302:750–7.
4. Ruts L, van Koningsveld R, van Doorn PA. Distinguishing acute-onset CIDP from Guillain-Barré syndrome with treatment related fluctuations. *Neurology.* 2005;65:138–40.
5. Chiba A, Kusunoki S, Obata H, et al. Serum anti-GQ1b IgG antibody is associated with ophthalmoplegia in Miller Fisher syndrome and Guillain-Barré syndrome: clinical and immunohistochemical studies. *Neurology.* 1993;43:1911–7.
6. Hughes RA, Swan AV, van Doorn PA et al. Intravenous immunoglobulin for Guillain-Barré syndrome. *Cochrane Database Syst Rev.* 2010;6:CD002063.
7. Hughes RA, Wijdicks EF, Barohn R, et al. Practice parameter: immunotherapy for Guillain-Barré syndrome: report of the Quality Standards Subcommittee of the American Academy of Neurology. *Neurology.* 2003;61:736–40.
8. Hughes RA, Swan AV, van Doorn PA et al. Corticosteroids for Guillain-Barré syndrome. *Cochrane Database Syst Rev.* 2010;2:CD001446.
9. Moussouttas M, Chandy D, Dyro F. Fulminant acute inflammatory demyelinating polyradiculoneuropathy: case report and literature review. *Neurocrit Care.* 2004;1:469–73.
10. Green DM, Ropper AH. Mild Guillain-Barré syndrome. *Arch Neurol.* 2001;58:1098–101.

CODES

ICD9
357.0 Acute infective polyneuritis

CLINICAL PEARLS

- GBS is treatable, and if recognized and addressed early, few patients die from this condition.
- The natural history of GBS is to resolve, and treatment with IVIG or plasmapheresis may speed rate of recovery.
- The most useful diagnostic tests are lumbar puncture and a nerve conduction study.
- If GBS is suspected, initial evaluation must include an FVC and NIF to assess for respiratory compromise.

G

GYNECOMASTIA

Timothy L. Black, MD

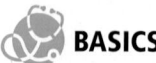 **BASICS**

DESCRIPTION
- Benign glandular enlargement of male breast that is generally bilateral (may be asymmetric or unilateral):
  - Type 1: Benign adolescent hypertrophy; physiologic discoid subacute mass
  - Type 2: Physiologic gynecomastia; generalized enlargement to greater degree
  - Type 3: Simulated by obesity
  - Type 4: Pectoral muscle hypertrophy
- System(s) affected: Endocrine/Metabolic; Skin/Exocrine
- Synonym(s): Male breast hypertrophy

EPIDEMIOLOGY
- Predominant age: Puberty; >65 years of age (especially with weight gain)
- Predominant sex: Male only

Pediatric Considerations
Transient gynecomastia is seen in neonatal boys.

Geriatric Considerations
Drug-induced form is more common in geriatric patients.

Prevalence
- 38–64% of pubertal males may have mild form. Usual onset is 11–12 years of age, with resolution by age 16–17 years.
- Nonpubertal forms are rare except when drug-induced.

RISK FACTORS
- Obesity
- Liver disease
- Renal disease
- Recovery from prolonged severe illness associated with malnutrition and weight loss (refeeding gynecomastia)
- Multiple therapeutic as well as nontherapeutic drugs (e.g., spironolactone, cimetidine, ranitidine, omeprazole, isoniazid, ketoconazole, amlodipine, captopril, diltiazem, enalapril, nifedipine, verapamil, diazepam, haloperidol, digitalis, statin drugs, anabolic steroids, androgens, estrogens, growth hormone, amphetamines, heroin, methadone, marijuana, and ethanol, among others) (1)
- Family history

Genetics
Some instances of familial gynecomastia may be inherited as male-limited autosomal trait.

GENERAL PREVENTION
In men taking estrogen for prostate cancer: Low-dose radiation prior to institution of diethylstilbestrol

PATHOPHYSIOLOGY
The cause of pubertal gynecomastia is not clear (2)[C].
- May be related to transient imbalance of androgens and estrogens
- May be related to higher leptin levels (may result in altered local estrogen levels)

ETIOLOGY
- Physiologic: Transient in neonatal boys and at puberty:
  - 60–90% of newborn males develop transient breast enlargement related to transplacental estrogen.
  - In pubertal boys, may require 1–3 years to regress or may not regress at all
  - Men age 60–90 years may develop gynecomastia related to declining levels of testosterone.
- Exposure to a high level of estrogen compared with testosterone concentration
- Identifiable syndrome/cause found in 12% of pubertal boys (3)[C]
- Tumors: Estrogen-secreting, gonadotropin-secreting, prolactin-secreting pituitary adenomas, hepatic fibrolamellar carcinoma
- Drugs (10–25% of gynecomastia) (1): Hormones, marijuana, digitalis, spironolactone, cimetidine, ketoconazole, phenytoin, furosemide, verapamil, cytotoxic drugs, antihypertensives, sedatives, antidepressants, amphetamines, heroin, methadone, anabolic steroids (2)[C]
- Systemic disorders: Cirrhosis, thyrotoxicosis, renal failure
- Androgen production deficiency
- Androgen-insensitivity syndromes
- Idiopathic (25% of gynecomastia)

COMMONLY ASSOCIATED CONDITIONS
- Peutz-Jeghers syndrome
- Male pseudohermaphroditism
- Hyperthyroidism
- Hypothyroidism
- Hepatic disease
- Prostate carcinoma
- Adrenal neoplasms (adenoma or carcinoma)
- Renal disease or dialysis
- True hermaphrodism
- Klinefelter syndrome
- Testicular failure (enzymatic defects of testosterone production, androgen insensitivity)
- Testicular neoplasms (germ cell, Leydig cell, Sertoli cell tumors)

 DIAGNOSIS

HISTORY
- Determine onset and duration of symptoms.
- Investigate concurrent drug treatments.

PHYSICAL EXAM
- Careful breast exam to evaluate characteristics of breast:
  - May involve 1 or both breasts
  - Usually asymptomatic but may be tender if it has developed rapidly
  - Usually located concentrically beneath the nipple and areola
- Abdominal exam
- Testicular exam
- Rectal exam

DIAGNOSTIC TESTS & INTERPRETATION
- Most cases in teenage boys are self-limiting and require reassurance alone.
- Full endocrine investigations may be indicated if symptoms of other disease states are indicated.
  - Thyroid function studies, testosterone, estradiol, beta human chorionic gonadotropin, luteinizing hormone (LH), liver functions tests, GGT, prolactin, α-fetoprotein

Lab
Laboratory evaluation rarely indicated in teenage boys

Initial lab tests
If worsening symptoms or clinical suspicion of secondary cause, consider
- Human chorionic gonadotropin (hGC) levels: High levels may indicate choriocarcinoma or other hCG-secreting tumor.
- Plasma testosterone and LH measurements: Help diagnose hypogonadism
- Serum estradiol (E_2)

- Serum prolactin
- Prostate-specific antigen (PSA)
- Liver function tests (LFTs)
- Others if clinically indicated (e.g., thyroid function, chromosomal analysis)

Follow-Up & Special Considerations
Disorders that may alter lab results:

- Cirrhosis
- Thyrotoxicosis
- Renal failure

Imaging

- CT scan of chest and abdomen if adrenal or extragonadal germ cell tumor is suspected
- Testicular ultrasound if there is a palpable mass or abnormality of one or both testicles (rarely indicated)
- MRI of pituitary fossa if prolactin levels are elevated (to exclude a prolactinoma)

Diagnostic Procedures/Surgery
Biopsy, if suspicious

Pathological Findings

- Dense, periductal, hyaline, collagenous connective tissue
- Hyperplastic ductal lining
- Plasma cell infiltrate

DIFFERENTIAL DIAGNOSIS

- Obesity with increase in adipose tissue
- Carcinoma of male breast
- Lipomas
- Neurofibromas
- Cystic hygroma

 TREATMENT

- In teenage males, only reassurance and follow-up are usually indicated.
  - Spontaneous resolution in majority with the first 1–2 years
  - Persistent idiopathic gynecomastia in 7–8% of teenage boys at 3 years following diagnosis (2)[C]
- There is little evidence to recommend medical treatment of idiopathic gynecomastia in pediatric patients at this time (4).
- Consider medication or illicit drug use in adult males before initiating treatment.

MEDICATION

- Danazol (100 mg b.i.d. × 1 week followed by 100 mg t.i.d. × 2–6 weeks) (5)[B]:
  - Effective in 80% of patients
  - Especially effective in reducing tenderness
  - Dose can be repeated for responders.
  - Drug is licensed for treatment of gynecomastia in the UK.
- Tamoxifen (20–40 mg/d) has been used (5)[B]:
  - May be effective in 78–83% of men with gynecomastia
  - Less effective in breasts with a large amount of fatty tissue
  - May have high relapse rate
  - Short-term tamoxifen treatment also has been used successfully in the treatment of pubertal gynecomastia (6)[C].

- Anastrazole has been studied in pediatric patients with idiopathic gynecomastia and is not effective (4).
- Timing of treatment with medications may influence patient response.
  - Treatment early in the course of developing gynecomastia may be more beneficial (2)[C].
- Testosterone may be of some benefit but has not been well studied and is used infrequently.
- Clomiphene has been used infrequently.

ADDITIONAL TREATMENT
General Measures

- Correct underlying disorder.
- Withdraw causative drug (if feasible).
- Observe with reassurance that the problem is transient.

Issues for Referral
Refer to endocrinologist if abnormally elevated hormone levels are confirmed.

SURGERY/OTHER PROCEDURES

- Biopsy if suspicious for cancer:
  - Needle biopsy or excisional biopsy
  - Gynecomastia is felt to be a risk factor for the development of male breast cancer (7).
- Subcutaneous mastectomy for severe, painful, or persistent cases or for patients with psychologic concerns (8)[C]:
  - Usually performed as outpatient surgery
  - General anesthesia required
  - Liposuction of the subcutaneous tissue may be required as well as skin removal if the breast is pendulous (9).

 ONGOING CARE

FOLLOW-UP RECOMMENDATIONS
No restrictions

Patient Monitoring

- Every 3–6 months for physiologic gynecomastia
- Until well for nonphysiologic gynecomastia

DIET

- No special diet
- If obesity a problem, weight-loss diet

PATIENT EDUCATION
Surgical procedures for gynecomastia in pubertal boys are rarely covered by insurance because most insurance companies consider these procedures to be cosmetic.

PROGNOSIS

- Type 1: Resolves spontaneously
- Type 2: Clears without treatment (may take up to 2 years)
- Type 3: Little change without substantial weight loss
- Drug-induced: Drug withdrawal should result in resolution of gynecomastia in most cases.
- Other causes: Outcome depends on etiology.
- Good results with subcutaneous mastectomy

COMPLICATIONS

- Nipple inversion may occur following SC mastectomy.
- Asymmetry of breasts
- Postoperative fluid collection
- Withdrawal behavior related to drugs
- Depression
- Weight gain may be associated with danazol treatment.

REFERENCES

1. Eckman A, Dobs A. Drug-induced gynecomastia. *Expert Opin Drug Saf*. 2008;7:691–702.
2. Nordt CA, Divasta AD. Gynecomastia in adolescents. *Curr Opin Pediatr*. 2008;20:375–82.
3. Sher ES, et al. Evaluation of boys with marked breast development at puberty. *Clin Ped*. 1998;37:367–72.
4. Ma NS, Geffner ME. Gynecomastia in prepubertal and pubertal men. *Curr Opin Pediatr*. 2008;20:465–70.
5. Devalia HL, Layer GT et al. Current concepts in gynaecomastia. *Surgeon*. 2009;7:114–9.
6. Derman O, Kanbur NO, Kutluk T. Tamoxifen treatment for pubertal gynecomastia. *Int J Adolesc Med Health*. 2003;15:359–63.
7. Brinton LA, Carreon JD, et al. Etiologic factors for male breast cancer in the U.S. Veterans Affairs medical care system database. *Breast Cancer Res Treat*, epub ahead of print, 2009.
8. Gabra H, et al. Gynaecomastia in the adolescent: A surgically relevant condition. *Eur J Ped Surg*. 2004;14:3–6.
9. Cordova A, Moschella F. Algorithm for clinical evaluation and surgical treatment of gynaecomastia. *J Plast Reconstr Aesthet Surg*. 2007.

See Also (Topic, Algorithm, Electronic Media Element)
Algorithm: Gynecomastia

 CODES

ICD9
611.1 Hypertrophy of breast

CLINICAL PEARLS

- The initial workup of gynecomastia is history, physical exam, and fasting labs including serum hCG, testosterone, LH, E_2, prolactin, PSA, and LFTs.
- Lab tests do not need to be done in boys with suspected pubertal gynecomastia, but they should be considered if the gynecomastia persists for >1 year.

G

HAMMER TOES

Bryan Beutel, MD
Martin Kerzer, MD

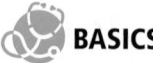 **BASICS**

Hammer toes are classified as a form of lesser toe (digits 2–5) deformities.

DESCRIPTION
- Plantar flexion deformity of the proximal interphalangeal joint (PIPJ) with varying degrees of hyperextension of the metatarsophalangeal (MTP) and distal interphalangeal (DIP) joints (1). Occurs primarily in sagittal plane.
- Can be flexible, semirigid, or fixed:
  – Flexible: Passively correctable to neutral position
  – Semirigid: Partially correctable to neutral position
  – Fixed: Not passively correctable to neutral position

EPIDEMIOLOGY
Most common deformity of lesser toes, typically affecting only one or two digits; 2nd toe most commonly involved

Incidence
- Undefined with limited data
- Can range from 1–20%
- Increases with age, duration of deformity (from flexible to rigid)

Prevalence
- More common in women than men (2):
  – Female predominance from 2.5:1 to 9:1, depending on age group
- Blacks more affected than whites (2)

RISK FACTORS
- Pes cavus and planus
- Hallux valgus
- Metatarsus adductus
- Ankle equinus
- Neuromuscular disease (rare)
- Trauma
- Improperly fitted shoes (e.g., with narrow toe box) and/or hosiery
- Abnormal metatarsal and/or digit length
- Inflammatory joint disease (e.g., rheumatoid arthritis)
- Connective tissue disease
- Diabetes mellitus

Genetics
- Specific genetic markers not identified
- Seen more frequently in families

GENERAL PREVENTION
- No documented means of prevention
- Modification of shoewear using pressure dispersive devices improves pain (1).
- Foot orthoses modulate biomechanical dysfunction and muscular imbalance, thereby preventing progression (2)
- Control of predisposing factors (e.g., inflammatory joint disease) may slow progression

PATHOPHYSIOLOGY
- Any biomechanical dysfunction that results in loss of function of extensor digitorum longus (EDL) tendon at PIPJ and the flexor digitorum longus (FDL) tendon at the MTP joint. The intrinsic muscles sublux dorsally as the MTP hyperextends. This results in plantar flexion of the PIPJ and hyperextension of the MTP joint (2).
- Specific pathomechanics vary by etiology
  – Toe length discrepancy or narrow toe box induces PIPJ flexion by forcing digit to accommodate shoewear. May also lead to MTP joint synovitis secondary to overuse, with elongation of plantar plate and MTP joint hyperextension.
  – Rheumatoid arthritis causes MTP joint destruction and resultant subluxation

ETIOLOGY
- Congenital
- Acquired:
  – Any condition that compromises intra-articular and periarticular tissues, such as 2nd ray longer than 1st, inflammatory joint disease, improper fitting shoes, and trauma (1)
    ○ Damage to joint capsule, collateral ligaments, or synovia leads to unstable PIPJ or MTP joint.

COMMONLY ASSOCIATED CONDITIONS
- Hallux valgus
- Cavus foot
- Metatarsus adductus
- Dorsal callus

 DIAGNOSIS

History and physical exam often sufficient for diagnosis of hammer toes. Additional testing available to exclude other conditions

HISTORY
- Location, duration, severity, and rate of progression of foot deformity (3)[C]
- Type, location, duration of pain
  – Patients often relate sensation of lump on plantar aspect of MTP joint.
- Degree of functional impairment
- Factors that improve and exacerbate the condition
- Type of footwear and hosiery worn
- Peripheral neurological symptoms
- Any prior treatment rendered

PHYSICAL EXAM
- Note MTP joint hyperextension, PIPJ flexion, and DIPJ extension.
- Observe any adjacent toe deformities (e.g., hallux valgus, flexion contractures).
- Assess degree of flexibility and reducibility of deformity in both weightbearing and nonweightbearing positions (2)[C].
- Note any hyperkeratosis over the joint, ulcers, clavi (dorsal PIPJ, metatarsal head), adventitious bursa, erythema, or skin breakdown (2).
- Palpate for pain over dorsal aspect of PIPJ or MTP joint.
- Drawer test of MTP joint
- Palpate webspaces to exclude interdigital neuroma.
- Neurovascular evaluation (e.g., pulses, sensation, muscle bulk)

DIAGNOSTIC TESTS & INTERPRETATION
Lab
Initial lab tests
- Not required unless clinically indicated to rule out suspected metabolic or inflammatory arthropathies (2)[C]
  – Rheumatoid factor, ANA, HLA-B27 serologies for inflammatory disease

Imaging
Initial approach
Weightbearing x-rays of affected foot in anterior-posterior (AP), lateral, and oblique views (2)[C]
- AP view superior for assessing MTP subluxation or dislocation
- Lateral view best for evaluation of gross hammer toe deformity

Follow-Up & Special Considerations
MRI or bone scan if suspect osteomyelitis

Diagnostic Procedures/Surgery
- Nerve conduction studies or EMG if suspect neurologic disorder
- Doppler or plethysmography if impaired circulation and surgery is considered
- Computerized weightbearing pressure testing indicated only in setting of neuromuscular deficiencies of toes

Pathological Findings
Histologic evaluation typically not necessary before treatment

DIFFERENTIAL DIAGNOSIS
Hammer toe: Hyperextension of the MTP and DIP joints and plantar flexion of the PIP joint
- Claw toe: Dorsiflexion of MTP joint and plantar flexion of the DIP joint
- Mallet toe: Fixed or flexible deformity of the distal interphalangeal (DIP) joint of the toe
- Overlapping 5th toe
- Interdigital neuroma
- Plantar plate rupture
- Nonspecific synovitis of MTP joint
- Exostosis
- Arthritis (e.g., rheumatoid, psoriatic)
- Fracture

TREATMENT

Goal of treatment is to reduce or relieve symptoms so that patients may return to their normal activity level. Management includes surgical and nonsurgical interventions. Mild cases, however, may not require treatment.

MEDICATION
Indicated if adequate pain relief achievable nonsurgically or patient is poor surgical candidate

First Line
- Nonsteroidal anti-inflammatory drugs (NSAIDs) may be helpful in managing symptoms of pain, as well as soft tissue and joint inflammation.
- Contraindications: Gastrointestinal bleeding or active intracranial bleed; thrombocytopenia; coagulation defects; necrotizing enterocolitis; significant renal dysfunction

Second Line
Anti-inflammatory (cortisone) injectables if local inflammation or bursitis exists (1)[C]

ADDITIONAL TREATMENT
General Measures
Nonsurgical (conservative) treatment includes:
- Shoe modifications, such as wider and/or deeper toe box, may be used to accommodate the deformity and decrease the pressure over osseous prominences. Avoid high-heeled shoes (2)[C].
- Toe sleeve or orthodigital padding of the hammer toe prominence (4)[C]
- Hammer toe straightening orthotics or taping to reduce flexible deformities
- Debridement of hyperkeratotic lesions is effective in reducing symptoms. Topical keratolytics may be helpful (2)[C].
- Shoe orthotics may be used to control abnormal biomechanical influences.
- Physical therapy for stretching and strengthening of the toes may help to preserve flexibility.

Issues for Referral
If nonsurgical (conservative) treatment is unsuccessful and/or impractical or patient has combined deformity of MTP joint, PIPJ, and/or DIPJ, then patient may be referred to an orthopedic surgeon or surgical podiatrist for surgical interventions.

SURGERY/OTHER PROCEDURES
- Surgical procedures for the correction of hammer toes rely on the degree and flexibility of the contracture(s) and the related abnormalities that exist.
- Surgical interventions for <u>flexible</u> hammer toes include (1,4)[C]:
  - PIPJ arthroplasty (most common)
  - Flexor tendon lengthening/flexor tenotomy
  - Extensor tendon lengthening/tenotomy/MTP joint capsulotomy
  - Exostosectomy
  - Implant arthroplasty
- Surgical interventions for semirigid/rigid hammer toes include (1,4)[C]:
  - PIPJ resection arthroplasty or arthrodesis
  - Girdlestone-Taylor flexor-to-extensor transfer
  - Metatarsal shortening (Weil osteotomy)
  - Exostosectomy
  - Diaphysectomy of the proximal phalanx (less common)
  - Middle phalangectomy (less common)
  - Soft tissue releases/lengthening
- Procedures may be performed as isolated operations or in conjunction with other procedures
- Contraindications for surgery: Active infection, inadequate vascular supply, and desire for cosmesis alone

ONGOING CARE

FOLLOW-UP RECOMMENDATIONS
- Radiographs should be taken immediately following surgery or at the first postoperative visit. Subsequent x-rays may be taken as needed.
- Full weightbearing in a postoperative (surgical) shoe or other device is indicated based on the procedure(s) performed and on the individual patient.
- Elevate the foot above nose to minimize swelling, which can lead to pain and delay wound healing.
- Return to regular shoewear depends on the postoperative course.
- Role and efficacy of postoperative physical therapy (3 times per week for 2–3 weeks) unclear

Patient Monitoring
In the absence of complications, the patient should be seen initially within the 1st week following the procedure(s). Frequency of subsequent visits is determined based on the procedure(s) performed and the postoperative course.

PATIENT EDUCATION
- Patients should be aware of mild to moderate swelling and plantar foot discomfort that may persist for many (1–6) months after surgery and may limit footwear options until resolved.
- MTP joint and PIPJ may remain stiff for extended period of time.
- "Molding" of the operative toe (assumes shape of adjacent toes)
- Encourage patients to wear shoes of adequate size with rounded or squared toe box in future.

PROGNOSIS
- Nonoperative (conservative) treatment usually alleviates pain; however, the deformity may progress despite diligent care.
- Surgical treatment of flexible hammer toe deformity reliably corrects the deformity and alleviates pain. Recurrence and progression are common, especially if the patient resumes wearing improperly fitted shoes.
- Surgical treatment of fixed hammer toe deformity provides reliable deformity correction and pain relief. Recurrence is uncommon.

COMPLICATIONS
- Common complications specific to digital surgery include, but are not limited to, the following:
  - Persistent edema
  - Recurrence of deformity
  - Residual pain
  - Excessive stiffness
  - Metatarsalgia
- Less common complications include the following:
  - Numbness (e.g., digital nerve palsy)
  - Flail toe
  - Symptomatic osseous regrowth
  - Malposition of toe
  - Malunion/nonunion
  - Infection
  - Vascular impairment (e.g., toe ischemia, gangrene)

REFERENCES

1. Academy of Ambulatory Foot and Ankle Surgery: Hammertoe Syndrome. National Guideline Clearinghouse. 2003.
2. Clinical Practice Guideline Forefoot Disorders Panel of the American College of Foot and Ankle Surgeons: Diagnosis and Treatment of Forefoot Disorders. Section 1: Digital Deformities. *The Journal of Foot & Ankle Surgery.* 2009;48(2): 230–8.
3. Schrier JC, Verheyen CC, Louwerens JW. Definitions of hammer toe and claw toe: an evaluation of the literature. *J Am Podiatr Med Assoc.* 2009;99: 194–7.
4. Smith BW, Coughlin MJ et al. Disorders of the lesser toes. *Sports Med Arthrosc.* 2009;17:167–74.

ADDITIONAL READING

- Miller JM, Blacklidge DK, Ferdowsian V, Collman DR et al. Chevron arthrodesis of the interphalangeal joint for hammertoe correction. *J Foot Ankle Surg.* 2010;49:194–6.
- O'Kane C, Kilmartin T. Review of proximal interphalangeal joint excisional arthroplasty for the correction of second hammer toe deformity in 100 cases. *Foot Ankle Int.* 2005;26:320–5.
- Pietrzak WS, Lessek TP, Perns SV. A bioabsorbable fixation implant for use in proximal interphalangeal joint (hammer toe) arthrodesis: biomechanical testing in a synthetic bone substrate. *J Foot Ankle Surg.* 2006;45:288–94.

See Also (Topic, Algorithm, Electronic Media Element)
Algorithm: Foot Pain

CODES

ICD9
- 735.4 Other hammer toe (acquired)
- 755.66 Other congenital anomalies of toes

CLINICAL PEARLS
- Hammer toe is plantar flexion deformity of PIPJ.
- Patients may complain of pain at the PIPJ or MTP joint.
- Perform a careful inspection and examination of foot, especially PIPJ and MTP joint.
- Initial management of hammer toe deformity consists of conservative therapy; however, if unsuccessful, surgical interventions are indicated.
- Well-fitting shoewear is vital to minimizing recurrence after treatment.

H

HEADACHE, CLUSTER

David Cachia, MD
Ann Mitchell, MD

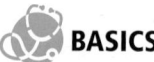

BASICS

DESCRIPTION
- Primary headache disease
- Multiple attacks of short-lived, excruciating, unilateral, sharp, searing, or piercing pain, typically localized in the periorbital area and temple accompanied by signs of ipsilateral autonomic dysfunction. *Severe* pain syndrome.
- Underdiagnosed and suboptimally treated
- Autonomic symptoms: Parasympathetic hyperactivity signs (ipsilateral lacrimation, eye redness, and nasal congestion) and sympathetic hypoactivity (ipsilateral ptosis and miosis)
- Attacks are without prodrome, rapidly escalating in intensity usually within 15 minutes, frequently have a circadian rhythmicity, and often wake patients 60–90 minutes after falling asleep. In contrast to other headache syndromes, the severe pain may cause patients to pace restlessly and occasionally exhibit agitated behavior.
- Individual attacks last 15–180 minutes if untreated and occur from once every other day to 8 times per day. 2 forms exist (ICHD-2 criteria):
  - Episodic: At least 2 cluster periods lasting 7 days–1 year, separated by a pain-free interval of >1 month (80–90% of cases)
  - Chronic: Cluster-free interval of <1 month in a 12-month period or greater

EPIDEMIOLOGY
Incidence
1 year incidence of 53 per 100,000

Prevalence
- Lifetime prevalence 124 per 100,000
- Predominant sex: Male > Female (4.3:1)
- Mean age of onset: Between 29.6 and 35.7 years
- Episodic cluster headaches (CH) > chronic CH

RISK FACTORS
- Male gender
- Age >30 years
- Cigarette smoking
- Family history of CH
- Alcohol induces attacks during a cluster, but not during remission.
- Small amounts of vasodilators (e.g., alcohol, nitroglycerin)
- Strong odors

Genetics
- Usually sporadic inheritance
- Autosomal-dominant inheritance in about 5% of cases, autosomal recessive or multifactorial pattern in other families
- Exact transmission pattern still debated
- 1st-degree relatives carry 5–18-fold; 2nd-degree 1–3-fold increased relative risk of disease.

PATHOPHYSIOLOGY
- Unknown
- Unlikely to arise from a single trigger zone
- Proposed mechanisms include:
  - Pain: Activation of trigeminal nerve
  - Autonomic symptoms: Activation of craniofacial parasympathetic nerve fibers secondary to pathological activation of trigemino-autonomic brainstem reflex. Trigger of trigeminofacial reflex

might be in hypothalamus also explaining cyclical nature of cluster headache.

ETIOLOGY
Unknown

COMMONLY ASSOCIATED CONDITIONS
- Increased risk of suicide secondary to the extreme nature of the pain
- Medication-overuse headache
- History of migraine, frequently in female patients
- Sleep apnea
- Increased prevalence of cardiac right-to-left shunt and patent foramen ovale

DIAGNOSIS

- Diagnosis is clinical.
- *International Classification of Headache Disorders* (2nd edition) criteria:
  - At least 5 attacks of severe or very severe unilateral orbital, supraorbital, or temporal pain lasting 15–180 minutes if untreated
- At least 1 of the following:
  - Ipsilateral
    - ○ Conjunctival injection or lacrimation
    - ○ Nasal congestion and/or rhinorrhea
    - ○ Eyelid edema
    - ○ Forehead and facial sweating
    - ○ Miosis and/or ptosis
  - Sense of restlessness or agitation
- Attack frequency: 1 every other day to 8 per day
- Not attributed to another disorder
- Episodic CH: At least 2 cluster periods lasting 7 days–1 year, separated by a pain-free interval of >1 month (80–90% of cases)
- Chronic CH: Cluster-free interval of <1 month in ao12-month period or greater

PHYSICAL EXAM
- Acute distress, crying, screaming, restless, and/or agitated during attacks.
- Ipsilateral lacrimation, injected conjunctivea, ptosis, and miosis
- Nasal stuffiness or rhinorrhea
- Bradycardia or tachycardia
- Nausea

DIAGNOSTIC TESTS & INTERPRETATION
- Diagnosis is primarily clinical; lab tests are not generally indicated.
- Consider neuroimaging (MRI/CT head and vascular imaging of brain):
  - Atypical CH presentation
  - Abnormal neurological exam
  - Suspect secondary CH (see differential diagnosis)

DIFFERENTIAL DIAGNOSIS
- Other trigeminal autonomic cephalgias: Paroxysmal hemicrania, short-lasting unilateral neuralgiform headache attacks with conjunctival injection and tearing (SUNCT)
- Hemicrania continua, hypnic headaches, trigeminal and other facial neuralgias, migraine, temporal arteritis, herpes zoster
- Secondary cluster headache:
  - Vertebral or carotid artery dissection
  - Brain arteriovenous malformations
  - Intracranial artery aneurysms
  - Pituitary adenomas

- Nasopharyngeal carcinoma
- Maxillary sinus foreign body/sinusitis
- Cavernous hemangioma
- Meningiomas/carcinomas/metastases

TREATMENT

Many of the medications discussed below are used off-label in the treatment of cluster headache.

MEDICATION
- Avoid pain therapy, especially narcotic analgesics, for acute attacks.
- Goal is abortion of acute attack and prophylaxis for expected duration of the cluster.
- Assess cardiovascular risk before instituting a vasoactive drug such as ergotamine or sumatriptan.

First Line
- For acute attacks:
  - Oxygen: 100% at least 6–12 L/min for 15 minutes via nonrebreathing mask. Relief within 15 minutes. Avoid in severe COPD as might affect hypoxic respiratory drive (1)[A].
  - Sumatriptan (Imitrex): 6 mg SC, maximum 12 mg/24 hours with at least 1 hour between injections (2)[A]. Relief in 10 minutes. Adverse effects: Nonischemic chest pain, distal paresthesias, injection site reactions, nausea and vomiting, fatigue. Triptans contraindicated in ischemic cardiac disease, stroke, uncontrolled hypertension, Prinzmetal angina, basilar migraine, hemiplegic migraine, ischemic bowel disease, and peripheral vascular disease.
  - Sumatriptan nasal spray: 20 mg effective within 30 minutes. Common adverse effect: Bitter taste (3)[B]
  - Zolmitriptan nasal spray: 5 mg and 10 mg dosage both effective to relieve headaches at 30 minutes (4)[A].
  - Zolmitriptan tablet:5 mg and 10 mg tablets shown to be superior to placebo at 30 minutes with episodic CH, but not chronic CH (5)[B]

- Prophylaxis to shorten cluster period and severity and to prevent expected attacks.
  - Verapamil*: Starting dose should be 240 mg to 360 mg daily. (120 mg t.i.d. or in SR formulation). Increase by 80 mg every 2 weeks with ECG control, until 720 mg dose is reached. Recommended clinical dose is 480 mg daily (6). If exceeded, informed consent has to be obtained. Doses up to 1200 mg daily may be required. Has many drug-drug interactions, as it is a CYP3A4 inhibitor. Adverse effects include hypotension, arrhythmias, AV block, bradycardia, pr-prolongation, syncope, gum and ankle swelling, constipation, CHF.
  - Lithium*: One study compared lithium 800 mg daily to placebo in episodic CH. No difference in percentage of patients having cessation of attacks, although those on lithium felt subjectively better. Another study compared verapamil 360 mg daily to lithium 900 mg daily. 50% of verapamil group and 37% in lithium group improved (7)[C]. Seems more effective in chronic CH. Side effects: Confusion, dizziness, diabetes insipidus, polyuria, hypothyroidism, tremor, bradycardia, muscle hyperexcitability, headaches. Monitor levels, liver, renal, and thyroid function. Caution with nephrotoxic drugs, diuretics.

– *Though both verapamil and lithium are given a class C rating based on the trials done, extensive clinical experience as prophylaxis for cluster headaches is available. Verapamil is hence considered 1st-line prophylactic treatment.

Second Line
- Acute attack:
  – Lidocaine/Cocaine: 10% (1 ml) of lidocaine or 40–50 mg of 10% cocaine intranasal. Most common side effects are nasal congestion, unpleasant lidocaine taste.
  – Octreotide: SC 100 μg. Can be considered in patients when triptans are contraindicated. Main side effect is gastrointestinal upset.
- Prophylaxis:
  – Civamide: 100 μL of 0.025% into each nostril daily. Only studied in episodic CH. Most common SE were nasal burning, lacrimation, pharyngitis, rhinorrhea.
  – Melatonin: 10 mg showed reduction in daily headache frequency vs placebo. No SE were reported.
  – Sodium valproate: Did not show any benefit vs placebo. Not advised as preventive treatment.
  – Methylsergide: No studies available to confirm efficacy. Has serious adverse effects including pulmonary and retroperitoneal fibrosis. Cannot be given with triptans and ergots. Avoid use.

ADDITIONAL TREATMENT
Transitional preventive treatment:
- Used until longer-term preventive treatment becomes effective. Longer-term maintenance agents are started concurrently.
  – Steroids: Only 1 study using oral prednisone and it had serious limitations (8). In practice, a commonly used regime is prednisone 60 mg daily for 3 days, then decreased by 10 mg every 3 days for a total of 18 days of treatment. Adverse effects for short-term use: Insomnia, psychosis, hyponatremia, edema, hyperglycemia, peptic ulcer.
  – Suboccipital steroid injection: One class I RCT showed benefit after 72 hours. 12.46 mg betamethasone dipropionate, 5.26 mg betamethasone disodium phosphate, and 0.5 ml 2% Xylocaine used.
  – Dihydroergotamine: 1 mg SC/im b.i.d. for several days
  – Ergotamine tartrate: 1 mg/2 mg daily or in divided doses. Contraindicated with triptans.
- Dihydroergotamine and ergotamine (no trials to prove efficacy)
- See "Acute and preventive pharmacologic treatment of cluster headache" by Francis et al. under Additional Reading

General Measures
- Avoid major changes in sleep habits.
- Stop smoking.
- Avoid use of alcohol during cluster period.
- Avoid prolonged physical exertion.
- Avoid extreme changes in altitude due to changes in oxygen levels.
- Avoid exposure to chemical agents/solvents.

Pregnancy Considerations
Collaboration between headache specialist, obstetrician, and pediatrician strongly encouraged. For abortive treatment, oxygen is most appropriate 1st-line therapy with nasal formulation of sumatriptan (pregnancy category B) or nasal lidocaine (pregnancy category B) as appropriate second line therapies. As preventive therapy, verapamil (pregnancy category C)

and steroids (pregnancy category C) remain the preferred options.

Issues for Referral
Consider a neurology or headache center referral for refractory or complicated patients.

SURGERY/OTHER PROCEDURES
- Surgery may be considered for patients who are refractory to or have contraindications to medical therapy.
- The costs and potential benefits of surgery must be carefully weighed. There is a paucity of long-term outcomes data, and available efficacy data are often conflicting.
- Various techniques focused on ablation of segments of trigeminal nerve root and sphenopalatine ganglion
- Occipital nerve:
  – 2 reports of occipital nerve stimulation found that approximately 60% of patients responded to treatment as defined by >50% reduction in headache severity or frequency.
- Deep brain stimulation (DBS):
  – Of the posterior inferior hypothalamus
  – Latest data showing that therapeutic effect of DBS might be related not to direct stimulation of hypothalamus but might modulate a local cluster headache generator in hypothalamus or mesencephalic gray matter or through non-specific anti-nociceptive mechanisms (9).

IN-PATIENT CONSIDERATIONS
Admission Criteria
Suicidal ideation, unwilling to contract for safety

ONGOING CARE
FOLLOW-UP RECOMMENDATIONS
Patient Monitoring
- Anticipate cluster bouts and initiate early prophylaxis.
- Watch for adverse medication response and side effects.
- Watch for unmasking of underlying cardiovascular disorder.
- Educate patient and family.

PROGNOSIS
- Unpredictable course
- With aging attack frequency often decreases
- Poor prognosis associated with older age of onset, male gender, disease duration of >20 years for episodic form.
- Possibility of transformation of episodic cluster to chronic cluster and occasionally chronic cluster to episodic cluster

COMPLICATIONS
- Side effects of medication, including unmasking of coronary heart disease
- Potential for drug abuse
- Problems with high-flow oxygen in patients with COPD or in those who smoke

REFERENCES
1. Cohen AS, Burns B, Goadsby PJ et al. High-flow oxygen for treatment of cluster headache: a randomized trial. *JAMA*. 2009;302:2451–7.
2. Ekbom K, Monstad I, Prusinski A, et al. Subcutaneous sumatriptan in the acute treatment of cluster headache: a dose comparison study. The Sumatriptan Cluster Headache Study Group. *Acta Neurol Scand*. 1993;88:63–9.
3. van Vliet JA, Bahra A, Martin V, Ramadan N, Aurora SK, Mathew NT, Ferrari MD, Goadsby PJ et al. Intranasal sumatriptan in cluster headache: randomized placebo-controlled double-blind study. *Neurology*. 2003;60:630–3.
4. Rapoport AM, Mathew NT, Silberstein SD, Dodick D, Tepper SJ, Sheftell FD, Bigal ME et al. Zolmitriptan nasal spray in the acute treatment of cluster headache: a double-blind study. *Neurology*. 2007;69:821–6.
5. Bahra A, Gawel MJ, Hardebo JE, Millson D, Breen SA, Goadsby PJ et al. Oral zolmitriptan is effective in the acute treatment of cluster headache. *Neurology*. 2000;54:1832–9.
6. Tfelt-Hansen P, Tfelt-Hansen J et al. Verapamil for cluster headache. Clinical pharmacology and possible mode of action. *Headache*. 2009;49:117–25.
7. Bussone G, Leone M, Peccarisi C, Micieli G, Granella F, Magri M, Manzoni GC, Nappi G et al. Double blind comparison of lithium and verapamil in cluster headache prophylaxis. *Headache*. 1990;30:411–7.
8. Jammes JL et al. The treatment of cluster headaches with prednisone. *Dis Nerv Syst*. 1975;36:375–6.
9. Fontaine D, Lanteri-Minet M, Ouchchane L, Lazorthes Y, Mertens P, Blond S, Geraud G, Fabre N, Navez M, Lucas C, Dubois F, Sol JC, Paquis P, Lemaire JJ et al. Anatomical location of effective deep brain stimulation electrodes in chronic cluster headache. *Brain*. 2010;133:1214–23.

ADDITIONAL READING
Francis GJ, Becker WJ, Pringsheim TM et al. Acute and preventive pharmacologic treatment of cluster headache. *Neurology*. 2010;75:463–73.

See Also (Topic, Algorithm, Electronic Media Element)
Algorithm: Headache, Chronic

CODES

ICD9
- 339.00 Cluster headache syndrome, unspecified
- 339.01 Episodic cluster headache
- 339.02 Chronic cluster headache

ICD10
G44.0 Cluster headache syndrome

CLINICAL PEARLS
- Patients are often agitated during the headache (vs the quiet and withdrawn appearance of a migraine).
- Alcohol is only a trigger during clusters (not during remission).
- Oxygen and triptans are 1st-line therapy, not narcotics.
- Patients on verapamil should have EKG monitoring, those on lithium should have lithium levels checked.

HEADACHE, TENSION

Kaelen C. Dunican, PharmD, RPh
Jill A. Grimes, MD

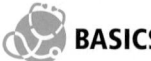 **BASICS**

DESCRIPTION
- Headache typically characterized by bilateral mild to moderate pain and pressure. May be associated with pericranial tenderness at the base of the occiput.
- 2 types:
  - Episodic tension-type headache (ETTH) divided into:
    ○ Infrequent: <1 day per month
    ○ Frequent: ≥1 but <15 days per month
  - Chronic tension-type headache (CTTH): ≥15 days per month for >3 months
- Synonym(s): Muscle contraction headache; Stress headache

EPIDEMIOLOGY
Most common type of primary headache

Prevalence
- Lifetime prevalence is 79%.
- More prevalent in female gender
- Prevalence of CTTH is 3%.
- Prevalence of ETTH decreases with age, whereas the prevalence of CTTH increases with age.

RISK FACTORS
Associated with triggers/precipitating factors:
- Stress
- Change in sleep regimen
- Skipping meals
- Certain foods (caffeine, alcohol, chocolate)
- Physical exertion
- Environmental factors (sun glare, odors, smoke, noise, lighting)
- Poor or sustained posture
- Female hormonal changes
- Medications (e.g., nitrates, selective serotonin reuptake inhibitors [SSRIs], antihypertensives)
- Overuse of abortive headache medication

Genetics
An increased genetic risk has been suggested by studies, particularly for CTTH.

GENERAL PREVENTION
- Identification and avoidance of triggers/precipitating factors
- Minimize emotional stress.
- Encourage relaxation techniques:
  - Biofeedback, relaxation therapy, and physical therapy
  - Consider counseling/psychotherapy.

PATHOPHYSIOLOGY
- Debatable: Peripheral and/or central mechanisms
- Activation of peripheral nociceptors leads to muscle tenderness in ETTH.
- Central sensitization is associated with CTTH:
  - Nitric oxide may play an important role in central sensitization.
  - Debatable: Low platelet serotonin
- Peripheral: May provoke the central mechanism leading from ETTH to CTTH

ETIOLOGY
Stress is the most frequently reported precipitating factor.

COMMONLY ASSOCIATED CONDITIONS
- 83% of patients with migraine headaches also suffer from tension-type headaches.
- Debatable: Increased prevalence of comorbid anxiety and depression

 DIAGNOSIS

Diagnosis is based on clinical symptoms:
- Diagnostic criteria provided by the International Headache Society (1):
  - Headache lasting 30 minutes–7 days
  - At least 2 of the following:
    ○ Bilateral location
    ○ Pressing/tightening (nonpulsating) quality
    ○ Mild or moderate intensity
    ○ Not aggravated by routine physical activity
  - Not associated with nausea or vomiting (chronic type may be associated with nausea)
  - No more than 1 of the following:
    ○ Photophobia or phonophobia
- Headache not due to another disorder
- Fronto-occipital or generalized pain (dull, pressing, or bandlike)
- Associated symptoms:
  - Fatigue
  - Irritability
  - Difficulty concentrating
  - Muscular tightness, tenderness, or stiffness in neck, occipital, and frontal regions

HISTORY
Obtain a thorough headache history to rule out other headache disorders, including severity, symptoms, onset, location and radiation of pain; quality of pain; concurrent medical conditions and medications; recent trauma or other procedures.

PHYSICAL EXAM
- General physical exam: Vital signs, funduscopic and cardiovascular assessment, and palpation of the head and neck
- Neurologic exam: Mental status, pupillary responses, motor-strength testing, deep tendon reflexes, sensation, cerebellar function, gait testing, and signs of meningeal irritation

Geriatric Considerations
- Onset of new headache in patients >40 years is cause for careful study, including imaging.

DIAGNOSTIC TESTS & INTERPRETATION
Labs and neuroimaging (computed tomography [CT] or magnetic resonance imaging [MRI]) are only necessary when a secondary cause is suspected:
- Atypical pattern of headache (doesn't fit specific category such as migraine, cluster, or tension) (2)[A]
- Focal neurologic findings
- New onset after age 40 years
- Sudden onset or worsening with exertion or Valsalva (2)[A]

Imaging
- CT scan, with and without contrast, is as sensitive as MRI and is the test of choice.
- MRI when lesions of the posterior fossa or aneurysm is the concern

DIFFERENTIAL DIAGNOSIS
- Migraine headache
- Cluster headache
- Head trauma
- Subarachnoid hemorrhage
- Subdural hematoma
- Unruptured vascular malformation
- Ischemic cerebrovascular disease
- Temporal arteritis
- Arterial hypertension (HTN)
- Cerebral venous thrombosis
- Benign intracranial HTN
- Intracranial neoplasm, infection, or meningitis
- Low cerebrospinal fluid pressure
- Medication (nonprescription analgesic dependency, nitrates)
- Caffeine dependency
- Metabolic disorders (hypoxia, hypercapnia, hypoglycemia)
- Toxic effects from drugs or fumes
- Temporomandibular joint syndrome
- Eyes: Glaucoma, refractive errors
- Sinusitis or middle-ear infection
- Cervical spondylosis
- Severe anemia or polycythemia
- Uremia and hepatic disorders
- Paget disease of bone

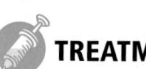 **TREATMENT**

- Nonsteroidal anti-inflammatory drugs (NSAIDs), acetaminophen (APAP), and aspirin (ASA) are effective for short-term pain relief of ETTH (3)[A].
- NSAIDs are most effective and should be considered 1st line for acute ETTH (3)[A].
- Tricyclic antidepressants (TCAs) are effective prophylaxis of CTTH (3)[A],(4).

MEDICATION
Choice of simple analgesic is based on patient-specific parameters:
- NSAIDs should be considered 1st line in most patients:
  - Ibuprofen and naproxen may be preferred due to better gastrointestinal (GI) tolerability
- APAP should be considered for patients taking warfarin, unable to tolerate NSAIDs, or allergic to ASA or NSAIDs

First Line
- For acute attack (ETTH): NSAIDs, APAP, or ASA:
- NSAIDs:
  - Ibuprofen (Motrin, Advil) 400–800 mg; may repeat q8h PRN (maximum 3.2 g/d)
  - Naproxen (Naprosyn) 375–500 mg or naproxen sodium (Aleve, Anaprox) 440–550 mg; may repeat q8–12h PRN (maximum 1,250 mg naproxen base/d)
  - Ketoprofen (Orudis) 12.5–50 mg; may repeat q6–8h PRN (maximum 300 mg/d)
  - Diclofenac (Voltaren, Cataflam) 50–100 mg; may repeat q8h PRN (maximum 150 mg/d)
- Contraindications:
  - ASA or NSAID allergy or bronchospasm, renal disease, bleeding disorders, increased risk of cardiovascular events (myocardial infarction [MI], stroke, new onset, or worsening of HTN)

- Drug interactions: Antihypertensives, anticoagulants, antiplatelet drugs, ASA, lithium, methotrexate
- Adverse effects:
  – Epigastric distress, peptic ulcer
- APAP (Tylenol) 1,000 mg; may repeat q6h PRN (maximum 4 g/d):
  – Adverse effects (rare): Rash, pancytopenia, liver damage
  – Precaution: Hepatic impairment, consumption of ≥3 alcoholic beverages per day
- Aspirin 500–1,000 mg; may repeat q6h PRN (maximum 4 g/d):
  – Contraindication: ASA or NSAID allergy or bronchospasm, bleeding disorders
  – Drug interactions: Anticoagulants, antiplatelet drugs, angiotensin-converting enzyme inhibitors, β-blockers, corticosteroids, NSAIDs, sulfonylureas
  – Adverse effects: GI irritation/bleeding, thrombocytopenia
- Caffeine combinations: 130 mg caffeine with 500 mg APAP and/or 500 mg ASA q6h PRN
- Isometheptene/dichloralprnhenazone/APAP (Midrin, Duradrin): 1–2 caps q4h PRN (max 8/d)
- Prophylaxis for CTTH: TCAs (amitriptyline, [Elavil]): 10–75 mg/d:
  – Contraindications: Acute recovery phase of MI, use of monamine oxidase inhibitors (MAOIs) within 14 days
  – Drug interactions: Clonidine, MAOIs, quinolone antibiotics, SSRIs, sympathomimetics, azole antifungals, valproic acid
  – Adverse effects: Drowsiness, dry mouth, tachycardia, heart block, blurred vision, urinary retention, seizure

Second Line
- For acute attack (ETTH):
  – Caffeine combinations: 130 mg caffeine with 500 mg APAP and/or 500 mg ASA q6h PRN
  – Isometheptene/dichloralprnhenazone/APAP (Midrin, Duradrin): 1–2 caps q4h PRN (max 8/d)
  – Narcotic analgesics (rarely indicated; consider secondary causes of headache or secondary gain, such as drug-seeking behavior for personal use or diversion/sale)
  – Ketorolac: 60 mg IM single dose
- For CTTH prophylaxis: (although limited evidence of benefit, all are widely used for prophylaxis) (5)
  – Alternative TCAs:
    ○ Desipramine (Norpramin) 50–100 mg/d
    ○ Imipramine (Tofranil) 50–100 mg/d
    ○ Nortriptyline (Pamelor) 25–50 mg/d
    ○ Protriptyline (Vivactil) 25 mg/d
  – Tizanidine 2 mg/d increase up to 8 mg t.i.d.

ALERT
Use of abortive agents >2 days per week may lead to *medication-overuse headaches*; must withdraw acute treatment to diagnose

Pediatric Considerations
ASA and antidepressants are contraindicated.

ADDITIONAL TREATMENT
The combination of stress management therapy and a TCA (amitriptyline) may be most effective for CTTH.

General Measures
Relief measures: Relaxation routines; rest in quiet, dark room; hot bath or shower; massage of back of neck and temples

Additional Therapies
- Cognitive behavioral interventions such as stress management programs may be helpful.
- Physical therapy, including positioning, ergonomic instruction, massage, transcutaneous electrical nerve simulation, application of heat or cold, and spinal manipulation, may provide limited value.
- Evidence regarding the usefulness of relaxation, biofeedback, and cognitive behavioral therapies is conflicting.

COMPLEMENTARY AND ALTERNATIVE MEDICINE
- Drugs with limited clinical evidence for prevention CTTH:
  – Mirtazapine 15–30 mg/d
  – Topiramate 100 mg/d
  – Venlafaxine XR (Effexor XR): 37.5–300 mg/d
- Drugs with conflicting clinical evidence for CTTH:
  – Tizanidine 2–6 mg t.i.d.
  – Botulinum toxin type A 2–12 U injected into tender cranial muscles
  – Memantine 20–40 mg/day
- Alternative agents:
  – Tiger Balm or peppermint oil applied topically to the forehead may be effective for ETTH.
  – Limited evidence supports use of acupuncture (6)[A].

IN-PATIENT CONSIDERATIONS
Initial Stabilization
Outpatient treatment

ONGOING CARE

FOLLOW-UP RECOMMENDATIONS
- Regulate sleep schedule.
- Regular exercise

DIET
- Identification and avoidance of dietary triggers
- Regulate meal schedule.

PATIENT EDUCATION
For additional information, contact:
- National Headache Foundation (888-643-5552, http://www.headaches.org)
- American Council for Headache Education (800-255-ACHE, http://www.achenet.org)

PROGNOSIS
- Usually follows a chronic course when life stressors are not changed
- Most cases are intermittent.

COMPLICATIONS
- Lost days of work and productivity (>CTTH)
- Cost to health system
- Dependence/addiction to narcotic analgesics
- GI bleeding from NSAID use

REFERENCES

1. Headache Classification Subcommittee of the International Headache Society. The international classification of headache disorders: 2nd edition. *Cephalalgia*. 2004;24:1–151.
2. Detsky ME, McDonald DR, Baerlocher MO, Tomlinson GA, McCrory DC, Booth CM et al. Does this patient with headache have a migraine or need neuroimaging? *JAMA*. 2006;296:1274–83.
3. Lenaerts ME. Pharmacotherapy of tension-type headache (TTH). *Expert Opin Pharmacother*. 2009;10:1261–71.
4. Moja PL, Cusi C, Sterzi RR, et al. Selective serotonin re-uptake inhibitors (SSRIs) for preventing migraine and tension-type headaches. *Cochrane Database Syst Rev*. 2005:CD002919.
5. Verhagen AP, Damen L, Berger MY, Passchier J, Koes BW et al. Lack of benefit for prophylactic drugs of tension-type headache in adults: a systematic review. *Fam Pract*. 2010;27:151–65.
6. Linde K, Allais G, Brinkhaus B, Manheimer E, Vickers A, White AR et al. Acupuncture for tension-type headache. *Cochrane Database Syst Rev*. 2009;CD007587.

See Also (Topic, Algorithm, Electronic Media Element)
Algorithm: Headache, Chronic
Videos: Neck Stretch with Towel; Neck Extension in Prone; Neck Stretches - Chin Tucks; Neck Trigger Point Massage—Trapezius

CODES

ICD9
307.81 Tension headache

CLINICAL PEARLS

- Tension-type headache may be difficult to distinguish from migraine without aura. A tension-type headache is typically described as bilateral, mild to moderate, dull pain, whereas a migraine is typically pulsating; unilateral; and associated with nausea, vomiting, and photophobia or phonophobia.
- Evidence suggests that NSAIDs may be more effective than APAP for episodic tension-type headache. Consider APAP for patients who cannot tolerate or have a contraindication to NSAIDS. APAP 500 mg may not be as effective as 1,000 mg.
- CTTH is difficult to treat, and these patients are more likely to develop medication-overuse headache. Clinical evidence supports the use of amitriptyline plus stress-management therapy for CTTH.
- Medication-overuse headaches must be avoided by limiting use of abortive agents to no more than 2 days per week.

H

HEARING LOSS

Teresa V. Chan, MD

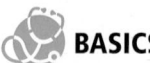 **BASICS**

DESCRIPTION

- Reduction in hearing manifested as decreased ability to detect or comprehend sound or speech
- May be conductive hearing loss (CHL or air-bone gap), sensorineural hearing loss (SNHL), or both
- System(s) affected: Auditory; External and middle ear (CHL), or inner ear (SNHL)

ALERT

- Any sudden SNHL (usually unilateral) is a medical emergency and should be referred to an otolaryngologist immediately.
- Treatment with high-dose steroids (1 mg/kg/d prednisone for 14 days, followed by taper) should begin ASAP, ideally within 1–2 weeks of onset.
- A simple 512-Hz tuning fork test lateralizes to unaffected ear in sudden SNHL (emergency) and lateralizes to the affected ear in CHL (not an emergency).

EPIDEMIOLOGY

- Predominant age: All ages affected; common in children (CHL) and elderly (SNHL)
- Predominant sex: Male = Female

Incidence

Hearing loss by age group:

- 3 in 10 people >60 years old
- 1 in 6 people ages 41–59 years old
- 1 in 14 people ages 29–40 years old
- At least 1.4 million children (18 or younger)

Prevalence

Hearing loss has doubled in the US during the past 30 years: 13.2 1971 to 28.2 million in 2000

Geriatric Considerations

- Age-related hearing loss is the most common cause in the US.
- ~50% of people >85 years have hearing loss.
- Hearing aids are underutilized.
- Loss of communication is a source of emotional stress and a physical risk for elderly.

Pediatric Considerations

Congenital hearing loss:

- 1–3/1,000 infants have hearing loss.
- Mandatory newborn screening (OAE and ABR testing is ideal)
- NICU screening before discharge
- Audiologic testing after major intracranial infection (meningitis)

Pregnancy Considerations

Otosclerosis (a CHL) can worsen during pregnancy.

RISK FACTORS

- Conductive:
  - Allergy
  - Chronic sinusitis
  - Cigarette smoking, 2nd-hand smoke
  - Sleep apnea with CPAP use
  - Adenoid hypertrophy
  - Nasopharyngeal mass
  - Eustachian tube dysfunction
  - Head trauma
  - Neuromuscular disease

  - Family history/heredity
  - Altered immunity
  - Prematurity and low birth weight
  - Young age
  - Craniofacial abnormalities (e.g., cleft palate, Down syndrome)
  - 3rd mobile window (superior canal dehiscence or large vestibular aqueduct)
- Sensorineural:
  - Aging/older age
  - Loud noise/acoustic trauma
  - Dizziness/vertigo: Especially Ménière disease or history of labyrinthitis
  - Medications (aminoglycosides, loop diuretics, quinine, aspirin, chemotherapeutic agents)
  - Bacterial meningitis
  - Head trauma
  - Atherosclerosis
  - Vestibular schwannoma/skull base neoplasm
  - Previous ear surgery
- Sensorineural, pediatric-specific:
  - Postnatal asphyxia
  - NICU hospitalization
  - Mechanical ventilation lasting ≥5 days
  - In utero infections (TORCH)
  - Toxemia of pregnancy
  - Maternal diabetes
  - Rh incompatibility
  - Prematurity or birth weight <1,500 g
  - Hyperbilirubinemia; exchange transfusions
  - Anomalous temporal bone (Mondini or large vestibular aqueduct)
  - Infectious diseases: Chickenpox, measles, encephalitis, influenza, mumps

Genetics

- Connexin 26 (13q11–12): Most common cause of nonsyndromic genetic hearing loss
- Mitochondrial mutations or disorders:
  - May predispose to aminoglycoside ototoxicity
- Otosclerosis: Familial; no clear genetic cause
- Most common congenital syndromes:
  - Hemifacial microsomia
  - Stickler syndrome
  - Congenital cytomegalovirus
  - Usher syndrome
  - Branchio-oto-renal syndrome
  - Pendred syndrome
  - CHARGE association
  - Neurofibromatosis type II
  - Waardenburg syndrome

GENERAL PREVENTION

- Limit noise exposure; use hearing protection when exposure cannot be avoided.
- Avoid ear canal instrumentation (Q-tips, etc.).
- Limit ototoxic medications.

PATHOPHYSIOLOGY

- CHL:
  - Hearing loss can result from middle ear effusion, obstruction of canal (cerumen/foreign body, osteomas/exostoses, cholesteatoma, tumor), loss of continuity (ossicular discontinuity), stiffening of the components (myringosclerosis, tympanosclerosis, and otosclerosis), and loss of the pressure differential across the TM (perforation).

- SNHL:
  - Damage along the pathway from oval window, cochlea, auditory nerve, and brainstem. Examples include vascular/metabolic insult, mass effect, infection and inflammation, acoustic trauma (see below).
  - Noise-induced hearing loss is caused by acoustic insult that affects outer hair cells in organ of Corti causing them to be less stiff. Over time, severe damage occurs with fusion and loss of stereocilia. Eventually may progress to inner hair cells and auditory nerve as well.
- Large vestibular aqueduct or superior canal dehiscence: 3rd mobile window shunts acoustic energy away from cochlea.

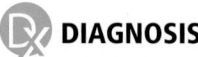 **DIAGNOSIS**

HISTORY

- Difficulty hearing:
  - Rapid vs gradual decline: Rapid (<2 weeks' duration) is a medical emergency. If suspect sudden SNHL, refer to ENT ASAP.
  - Difficulty with discrimination
  - Difficulty hearing in crowds
  - Frequently having to ask speakers to repeat
  - Friends/family complain of hearing loss
  - TV, phone volume increasing
- Tinnitus, bilateral or unilateral
- Otalgia
- Otorrhea, clear or purulent
- Dizziness or vertigo
- Ear fullness
- Autophony (hearing own voice louder or echoing)
- Facial nerve twitching or asymmetry
- Depression
- Anxiety
- History of ear infections or ear surgeries
- History of trauma or noise exposure
- Family history of hearing loss
- History of recent viral infection
- Nasal obstruction
- Frequent epistaxis

PHYSICAL EXAM

- 512-Hz tuning fork tests:
  - Sensorineural loss:
    - Placed on the forehead: Lateralizes to nonaffected ear (Weber test)
    - Placed on the mastoid and then next to ear; heard louder next to ear (Rinne test)
  - Conductive loss:
    - Placed on the forehead or teeth lateralizes to affected or symptomatic ear
    - Placed on the mastoid and then next to ear; heard louder behind the ear on the side of conductive deficit
- Otoscopy: Assess for deformity, canal patency, and otorrhea, TM integrity/retraction/mobility with insufflation, canal, or middle ear mass.
- Facial symmetry
- Cranial nerve exam
- Nasopharyngoscopy: Adenoid hypertrophy or nasopharyngeal mass (mandatory in adult patient with new unilateral serous effusion)
- Pediatric: Survey for syndromic anomalies

DIAGNOSTIC TESTS & INTERPRETATION
Lab
Often labs are not needed. If indicated:
- Pendred syndrome (goiter, mental retardation + SNHL): Perchlorate test, thyroid function tests
- Alport syndrome (nephritis + SNHL): Urinalysis, renal function tests
- Jervell and Lange-Nielsen syndrome (syncope, family history of sudden death + SNHL): EKG
- Any pediatric patient with SNHL: Genetic testing for connexin 26, mitochondrial studies
- TORCH screening test
- RPR confirmed with FTA-ABS
- Lyme titer in endemic areas
- Antinuclear antibodies and sedimentation rate as a screen for autoimmune disease

Imaging
Often imaging is not required; if indicated:
- Fine-cut CT temporal bones without contrast
- MRI of brain and brainstem with gadolinium

Diagnostic Procedures/Surgery
- Audiometry: Pure tone (air and bone), speech testing, and impedance (middle ear pressure) testing
- Tympanometry: Type B or C tympanograms indicate fluid or retraction, respectively. Negative middle ear peak pressures seen even with normal (Type A) tympanograms.
- Other tests:
  - Auditory brainstem response
  - Otoacoustic emissions: Echo of the cochlea
  - Behavioral (visual reinforcement) audiometry; used in children 6 months–5 years
- Myringotomy for aspiration of middle ear fluid is both diagnostic and therapeutic.

Pathological Findings
Varies depending on etiology

DIFFERENTIAL DIAGNOSIS
- Conductive:
  - Cerumen impaction/foreign body
  - Perforation of tympanic membrane
  - Middle ear fluid (serous otitis media)
  - Acute otitis media
  - Adhesive otitis media
  - Cholesteatoma
  - Ossicular erosion (infection, cholesteatoma)
  - Myringosclerosis/tympanosclerosis
  - Temporal bone fracture
  - Otosclerosis
  - Congenital malleus fixation
  - Glomus tumor
  - Congenital aural atresia
  - Osteogenesis imperfecta
  - Superior canal dehiscence
- Sensorineural:
  - Presbycusis (hearing loss related to aging)
- Noise-induced (recreational, occupational)
  - Ménière disease
  - Ototoxicity (aspirin, quinine, aminoglycosides)
  - Viral labyrinthitis
  - Cerebellopontine angle tumor
  - Large vestibular aqueduct syndrome
  - Syndromic hearing loss
  - Congenital cochlear malformation
  - Labyrinthine artery infarct
  - Idiopathic
  - Syphilis
  - CMV
  - Rubella

- Temporal bone fracture
- Metabolic (hyper/hypothyroid)
- Paget disease
- Perilymphatic (inner ear) fistula
- Autoimmune disease

TREATMENT
- Early detection: If sudden single-sided deafness, refer ASAP to otolaryngologist for hearing testing and prompt steroid therapy.
- Hearing rehabilitation: Hearing aids, cochlear implants for patients with bilateral severe to profound hearing loss

MEDICATION
- Depends on cause. Hearing loss is a broad topic with many possible etiologies.
- Sudden SNHL: High-dose oral steroids: 1 mg/kg or 60–100 mg/d prednisone or 12–16 mg/d dexamethasone for 14 days, followed by a taper:
  - Some recent papers suggest simultaneous use of oral and intratympanic steroid use results in better outcomes. There is an ongoing multi-center trial comparing the efficacy of oral steroids and intratympanic steroids (1)[A],(2).
  - Evidence is conflicting regarding use of systemic steroids in sudden SNHL (2)[A].
- Vasodilators and vasoactive substances are being used to treat idiopathic SNHL, but evidence is conflicting (3)[A].

ADDITIONAL TREATMENT
Issues for Referral
- Audiology: If hearing loss is suspected, referral to audiology is warranted. Audiologists also provide hearing aid options and maintenance.
- Genetics: If congenital syndrome or familial hearing loss is suspected
- Speech therapist: If speech delay or speech impediment is present
- Endocrinology: Pendred syndrome, other associated endocrine disorder (hypo-/hyperthyroidism)
- Cardiology: Jervell and Lange-Nielsen syndrome
- Ophthalmology: Usher syndrome
- Neurosurgery: CPA lesion, intracranial complication of middle ear disease

SURGERY/OTHER PROCEDURES
- CHL often has surgical options for repair:
  - Tympanostomy and tube placement
  - Tympanoplasty
  - Mastoidectomy
  - Ossicular chain reconstruction
  - Stapedectomy/stapedotomy
  - Canaloplasty
- Those with profound bilateral SNHL may qualify for cochlear implantation.

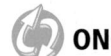

ONGOING CARE
FOLLOW-UP RECOMMENDATIONS
Patient Monitoring
Audiogram and clinical exam are primary means of monitoring patient.

DIET
Salt restriction to 2 g/d is helpful for Ménière disease patients.

PROGNOSIS
SNHL is usually permanent and progressive.

COMPLICATIONS
Acute middle ear problems may become chronic (perforations, cholesteatoma).

REFERENCES
1. Plontke SK, Löwenheim H, Mertens J, et al. Randomized, double blind, placebo controlled trial on the safety and efficacy of continuous intratympanic dexamethasone delivered via a round window catheter for severe to profound sudden idiopathic sensorineural hearing loss after failure of systemic therapy. Laryngoscope. 2009;119: 359–69.
2. Wei BP, Mubiru S, O'Leary S et al. Steroids for idiopathic sudden sensorineural hearing loss. Cochrane Database Syst Rev. 2006;CD003998.
3. Agarwal L, Pothier DD et al. Vasodilators and vasoactive substances for idiopathic sudden sensorineural hearing loss. Cochrane Database Syst Rev. 2009;CD003422.

ADDITIONAL READING
- Chau JK, Lin JR, Atashband S, Irvine RA, Westerberg BD et al. Systematic review of the evidence for the etiology of adult sudden sensorineural hearing loss. Laryngoscope. 2010;120:1011–21.
- For information on NIH-funded study. Available at: http://www.suddendeafness.org
- National Institute on Deafness and Other Communication Disorders. At: http://www.nidcd. nih.gov/health/hearing/.
- Ragab A, Shreef E, Behiry E, et al. Randomised, double-blinded, placebo-controlled, clinical trial of ozone therapy as treatment of sudden sensorineural hearing loss. J Laryngol Otol. 2008:1–7.

CODES
ICD9
- 389.00 Conductive hearing loss, unspecified
- 389.10 Sensorineural hearing loss, unspecified
- 389.20 Mixed hearing loss, unspecified

CLINICAL PEARLS
- In sudden hearing loss, if a 512-Hz tuning fork test (Weber test) lateralizes to the *unaffected ear*, suspect sensorineural causes (emergent evaluation needed), but if it lateralizes to the *affected* ear, the diagnosis is conductive hearing loss (not an emergency).
- ~50% of people >85 years have hearing loss, so encourage screening and treatment, especially in patients with early dementia (to maximize sensory input and sort out confusion vs lack of hearing).

H

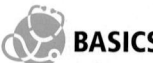

BASICS

DESCRIPTION
- A continuum of increasingly severe heat illnesses caused by dehydration, electrolyte losses, and failure of the body's thermoregulatory mechanisms
  - Heat exhaustion is an acute heat injury with hyperthermia owing to dehydration.
  - Heat stroke is extreme hyperthermia with thermoregulatory failure and profound CNS dysfunction.
- System(s) affected: Endocrine/Metabolic; Nervous
- Synonym(s): Heat illness; Heat injury; Hyperthermia; Heat collapse; Heat prostration

Geriatric Considerations
Elderly persons are more susceptible.

Pediatric Considerations
Children are more susceptible.

Pregnancy Considerations
Pregnant women may be more prone to volume depletion with heat stress.

EPIDEMIOLOGY
- Predominant age: More likely in children or elderly
- Predominant sex: Male = Female

Incidence
Depends on intensity of heat; estimate of 20/100,000 persons per season

Prevalence
- Depends on predisposing conditions in combination with environmental factors
- Roughly 240 deaths per year in the US

RISK FACTORS
- Poor acclimatization to heat or poor physical conditioning
- Salt or water depletion
- Obesity
- Acute febrile or GI illnesses
- Chronic illnesses: Uncontrolled diabetes mellitus or hypertension, cardiac disease
- Alcohol and other substance abuse
- High heat and humidity, poor air circulation in environment
- Heavy, restrictive clothing
- Nutritional supplementation that includes ephedra

GENERAL PREVENTION
- Most important factor in preventing heat stress is adequate fluid replacement.
- Allow acclimatization to hot weather through proper conditioning and activity modification.
- Dress appropriately with loose-fitting, open-weave, light-colored clothing.

PATHOPHYSIOLOGY
Only those associated with major organ system failure

ETIOLOGY
Failure of heat-dissipating mechanisms or an overwhelming heat stress leading to a rise in core temperature, dehydration, and salt depletion

DIAGNOSIS

- Heat exhaustion: Symptoms are milder than in heat stroke, with no severe CNS derangements.
  - Fatigue and lethargy
  - Weakness
  - Dizziness
  - Nausea, vomiting
  - Myalgias
  - Headache
  - Profuse sweating
  - Tachycardia
  - Hypotension
  - Lack of coordination
  - Agitation
  - Intense thirst
  - Hyperventilation
  - Paresthesias
  - Core temperature elevated but <103°F (<39.4°C)

- Heat stroke: Divided into two categories: Classic and exertional
  - Classic: Caused by environmental exposure, primarily in elderly or chronically ill patients, and may develop gradually over days
  - Exertional: Typically younger, very active patients; rapid onset
    - Exhaustion
    - Confusion, disorientation
    - Delirium
    - Coma
    - Hot, flushed, and dry skin (sweating may continue in exertional heat stroke)
    - Core temperature >105°F (>40.5°C)

DIAGNOSTIC TESTS & INTERPRETATION
Lab
- Used primarily to detect end-organ damage
- Electrolytes, urinalysis
- Creatinine, blood urea nitrogen
- Liver enzymes, muscle enzymes (creatine phosphokinase)
- Complete blood count
- Increased urine specific gravity
- Results of these studies may indicate hypernatremia, hyperchloremia, and hemoconcentration.
- Drugs that may alter lab results: Diuretics

Diagnostic Procedures/Surgery
Rectal temperature monitoring

DIFFERENTIAL DIAGNOSIS
- Other causes of elevated temperature, dehydration, or circulatory collapse
- Febrile illnesses, sepsis
- Drug-induced fluid loss
- Cardiac arrhythmia or infarction
- Acute cocaine intoxication
- Neuroleptic malignant syndrome
- Malignant hyperthermia (an autosomally inherited disorder of skeletal and cardiac muscle in which patients have abnormal muscle metabolism on exposure to halothane or skeletal muscle reactants)

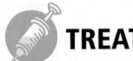

TREATMENT

MEDICATION

First Line
No medications are required in the initial management. Use isotonic saline solution to rehydrate (1,2)[C].

Second Line
- Consider immunomodulators such as corticosteroids (2)[C].
- Iced gastric, bladder, or peritoneal lavage (1,2)[C]
- Dantrolene 2–4 mg/kg for chemically assisted cooling (2)[C]
- In disseminated intravascular coagulopathy (DIC), consider appropriate replacement therapy.

ADDITIONAL TREATMENT

General Measures
- Fluid and electrolyte replacement with hypotonic oral fluids or IV 0.5–1.0 L normal saline
- Consider central venous pressure (CVP) monitoring.
- Body immersion in ice water (1,2)[C]
- Evaporative cooling: Spraying water over the patient and facilitating evaporation and convection with the use of fans (1,2)[C]
- Immersing the hands and forearms in cold water (1,2)[C]
- Use of ice or cold packs in the neck, groin, and axillae (3)

IN-PATIENT CONSIDERATIONS

Initial Stabilization
- Emergency treatment; best in a hospital setting
- Rapid cooling; remove clothing, wet patient down, apply ice packs.

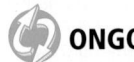

ONGOING CARE

FOLLOW-UP RECOMMENDATIONS
Rest with legs elevated (1,2)[C]

Patient Monitoring
- Rectal temperature monitoring: Cooling may be discontinued when the core temperature drops to 102°F (38.9°C) and stabilizes.
- Heat stroke patients may require airway management, hemodynamic monitoring, and careful fluid and electrolyte administration and monitoring.
- Consider CVP monitoring.

DIET
- Cool or cold clear liquids only (noncarbonated)
- Avoid caffeine.
- Unrestricted sodium

PATIENT EDUCATION
- The key to prevention is proper hydration.
- Stress the importance of proper conditioning and acclimatization.
- Instruct patients to recognize heat stress signs and symptoms.
- Maintain as much skin exposure as possible in hot, humid conditions while using proper sun block protection.
- Avoid dehydration with proper fluids during activity or exercise: 8 oz fluid intake for every 15 minutes of moderate exercise.
- Never leave children unattended in cars during hot weather.
- Try to gain access to air-conditioned environment during hot weather.

PROGNOSIS
- Good when mental function is not altered and when serum enzymes are not elevated; recovery is within 24–48 h in most cases.
- The mortality rate for heat stroke (10–80%) is directly related to the duration and intensity of hyperthermia, as well as to the speed and effectiveness of diagnosis and treatment.

COMPLICATIONS
- May involve failure of any major organ system
- Cardiac arrhythmias or infarction
- Pulmonary edema, acute respiratory distress syndrome
- Coma, seizures
- Acute renal failure
- Rhabdomyolysis
- DIC
- Hepatocellular necrosis

REFERENCES

1. Cleary M. Predisposing risk factors on susceptibility to exertional heat illness: clinical decision-making considerations. *J Sport Rehabilitation*. 2007;16(3): 204–14.
2. Muldoon S, et al. Identification of risk factors for exertional heat illness: A brief commentary on genetic testing. *J Sport Rehabilitation*. 2007; 16(3):222–26.
3. Gaffin SL, Gardner JW, Flinn SD. Cooling methods for heatstroke victims. *Ann Intern Med*. 2000;132: 678.

ADDITIONAL READING

- American College of Sports Medicine, Armstrong LE, Casa DJ, Millard-Stafford M, Moran DS, Pyne SW, Roberts WO et al. American College of Sports Medicine position stand. Exertional heat illness during training and competition. *Med Sci Sports Exerc*. 2007;39:556–72.
- Bouchama A, Knochel JP. Heat stroke. *N Engl J Med*. 2002;346:1978–88.
- Charaton F. Ephedra supplement may have contributed to sportsman's death. *Br Med J*. 2003;326:464.
- Glazer JL. Management of heatstroke and heat exhaustion. *Am Fam Physician*. 2005;71(11): 2133–40.
- Smith JE. Cooling methods used in the treatment of exertional heat illness. *Br J Sports Med*. 2005;39: 503–7; discussion 507.
- Yeo TP. Heat stroke: a comprehensive review. *AACN Clin Issues*. 2004;15:280–93.

CODES

ICD9
- 992.0 Heat stroke and sunstroke
- 992.5 Heat exhaustion, unspecified

CLINICAL PEARLS
- The diagnosis of heat stroke relies on both hyperthermia and CNS dysfunction (e.g., irritability, ataxia, confusion, seizures, or coma).
- Start the cooling process immediately when heat exhaustion or heat stroke is recognized, beginning with wetting the skin with a cool mist and giving oral rehydration solutions containing saline, if alert and oriented.

H

HEMATURIA

Tracy O. Middleton, DO

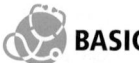 **BASICS**

DESCRIPTION
- Blood or red blood cells (RBCs) in the urine
- May be:
  – Gross (visible) or microscopic (nonvisible)
  – Symptomatic or asymptomatic

EPIDEMIOLOGY
Prevalence
- Microscopic hematuria in school-aged children: 0.5–2% (1)
- Microscopic hematuria in asymptomatic adults varies from 0.19–21%, depending on population studied (2,3).

RISK FACTORS
- Smoking
- Occupational exposures (dyes, rubber or tire manufacturing) (urothelial cancer)
- Analgesic abuse (e.g., phenacetin)
- Medications (e.g., cyclophosphamide)
- Pelvic irradiation
- Chronic infection, especially with calculi
- Recent upper respiratory tract infection
- Positive family history of renal diseases (stones, glomerulonephritis)
- Underlying primary renal disorder

ETIOLOGY
- Trauma:
  – Exercise-induced (resolves with rest)
  – Abdominal trauma and/or pelvic fracture with renal, bladder, or ureteral injury
  – Iatrogenic from abdominal or pelvic surgery; chronic indwelling catheters
  – Foreign body, physical/sexual abuse
- Neoplasms:
  – Malignancies: 30% of adult patients with gross hematuria and ~10% with microscopic hematuria have a malignancy (2). Urothelial carcinoma of the bladder and renal tumors are of greatest concern in adults.
  – Benign tumors
  – Endometriosis of the urinary tract (suspect in females with cyclic hematuria)
- Inflammatory causes:
  – Urinary tract infection (UTI): The most common cause of hematuria in adults
  – Renal diseases: Radiation nephritis, radiation cystitis, acute and chronic tubulointerstitial nephritis (due to drugs, infections, systemic disease)
  – Glomerular disease:
    ○ Goodpasture syndrome (antiglomerular basement membrane disease; autoimmune; associated pulmonary hemorrhage)
    ○ IGA nephropathy
    ○ Lupus nephritis
    ○ Henoch-Schönlein purpura
    ○ Membranoproliferative glomerulonephritis
    ○ Post-streptococcal glomerulonephritis
    ○ Rapidly progressive glomerulonephritis
    ○ Wegener granulomatosis
  – Endocarditis/visceral abscesses
  – Other infections: Schistosomiasis, TB, syphilis

- Metabolic causes:
  – Calculus disease (85% of patients have hematuria):
    ○ Hypercalciuria: A common cause of both gross and microscopic hematuria in children (1)
    ○ Hyperuricosuria
- Congenital/familial causes:
  – Cystic disease: Polycystic kidney disease, solitary renal cyst
  – Benign familial hematuria or thin basement membrane nephropathy (autosomal dominant)
  – Alport syndrome (X-linked in 85%; hematuria, proteinuria, hearing loss, corneal abnormalities) (4)
  – Fabry disease (X-linked recessive inborn error of metabolism; vascular kidney disease)
  – Nail-patella syndrome (autosomal dominant; nail and patella hypoplasia; hematuria in 33%)
  – Renal tubular acidosis type 1 (autosomal dominant or autoimmune)
- Hematologic causes:
  – Bleeding dyscrasias (e.g., hemophilia)
  – Sickle cell anemia/trait (renal papillary necrosis)
- Vascular causes:
  – Hemangioma
  – Arteriovenous malformations (rare)
  – Nutcracker syndrome: Compression of left renal vein and subsequent renal parenchymal congestion
  – Renal artery/vein thrombosis
  – Arterial emboli to kidney
- Chemical causes:
  – Nephrotoxins: Aminoglycosides, cyclosporine
  – Other drugs: Analgesics, oral contraceptives, Chinese herbs
- Obstruction:
  – Strictures or posterior urethral valves
  – Hydronephrosis, from any cause
  – Benign prostatic hyperplasia: Rule out other causes of hematuria.
- Other causes: Loin pain hematuria (most often in young women on oral contraceptives)

 DIAGNOSIS

HISTORY
Considerations:
- Burning, urgency, frequency: UTI
- Dark cola-colored urine: Glomerular origin
- Arthritis/arthralgias/rash: Lupus, vasculitis, Henoch-Schönlein purpura
- Flank pain: Stones, infarction, pyelonephritis
- Recent upper respiratory infection (URI): PSGN, MPGN; concurrent URI: IgA nephropathy
- Excessive vitamin use: Stones
- Marathon runner: Traumatic, rhabdomyolysis
- Travel: Schistosomiasis, tuberculosis
- Painless hematuria and/or weight loss: Malignancy
- Family history: Alport disease (hereditary nephritis), sickle cell, polycystic, IgA nephropathy, thin basement membrane disease

PHYSICAL EXAM
Considerations:
- Elevated BP, edema, and weight gain: Glomerular disease
- Fever: Infection
- Palpable kidney: Neoplasm, polycystic
- Genitalia: Look for meatal erosion, lesions

DIAGNOSTIC TESTS & INTERPRETATION
Pediatric Considerations
- Consider glomerulonephritis, Wilms tumor, child abuse
- Isolated asymptomatic microscopic hematuria may not need full workup, and in fact, these pediatric patients rarely need cystoscopy, but they must be observed for development of HTN, gross hematuria, or proteinuria (1,4)[B].
- Gross, or symptomatic, hematuria needs a full workup.
- If eumorphic RBCs, consider ultrasound (rule out stones, congenital abnormalities) and urinary Ca:Cr ratio (hypercalcemia) (4).
- If dysmorphic RBCs, consider renal consult.
- Renal ultrasound identifies most congenital and malignant conditions; CT reserved for cases of suspected trauma or stones (4)

Geriatric Considerations
- Suspect UTI, sometimes occult
- More likely to have malignant etiology
- Workup includes imaging, cytology, and cystoscopy.

Lab
Initial lab tests
- Urine dipstick:
  – False-negatives are rare, but can be caused by high-dose vitamin C.
  – False-positives: Oxidizers (povidone, bacterial peroxidases, bleach), myoglobin, alkaline urine (>9), semen, food coloring, food (beets, blackberries, rhubarb, paprika) (5)
  – Phenazopyridine may discolor the dipstick, making interpretation difficult.
  – Proteinuria (large) suggests glomerular disease.
- Microscopic urinalysis should always be done to confirm dipstick findings and quantify RBCs (6):
  – American Urological Association (AUA) defines clinically significant microscopic hematuria as ≥3 RBCs/hpf on microscopic evaluation of sediment from 2 of 3 properly collected specimens (2,5)[C]:
    ○ Criterion is based on a midstream, fresh, clean-catch voided urine sample (7)[C].
  – Exclude factitious or nonurinary causes, such as menstruation, mild trauma, exercise, poor collection technique, chemical/drug causes, through cessation of activity/cause and a repeat urinalysis in 48 hours (1,2)[C].
- Differentiate intrinsic renal disease from other causes. Indicators of renal disease are significant (>500 mg/day) proteinuria, red cell casts (pathognomonic of glomerular disease), dysmorphic RBCs, and increased creatinine (7)[C].
- Urine culture if suspected infection/pyuria (4)
- In patients at high risk for urothelial cancer (e.g., former smokers, age >40, occupational exposures, etc.):
  – Urine cytology; preferably 1st void of morning on 3 consecutive days (AUA recommendation) (2)[C]:
    ○ Patients with symptoms of bladder cancer should be evaluated with cystoscopy and bladder wash cytology.

- If persistent microscopic hematuria:
  – Renal function tests: BUN and creatinine
  – PT/INR for patients on warfarin or suspected of abusing warfarin
  – CBC:
    ○ Elevated white blood cells with deeper infections
    ○ Anemia is unlikely from hematuria, although gross hematuria may produce significant blood loss.
  – Urine Ca:Cr ratio >0.2 mg/mg is suggestive of hypercalcuria in children >6 years (4).

Follow-Up & Special Considerations
Other tests depend on suspected etiology: STD testing, ANCA, C3, C4, ASO titer, hemoglobin electrophoresis (4)

Imaging
Initial approach
- Multidetector CT urography (MDCTU):
  – An exam of the urinary tract by MDCT in the excretory phase, following IV contrast
  – Should be considered as the initial imaging of choice in nonpregnant adults with unexplained hematuria, especially if risk factors are present (5,8)[B]
  – Highly specific (>95%) and relatively sensitive for the diagnosis of urinary tract neoplasms, especially when >1 cm (8)[B]
  – Higher radiation dose; weigh risk of disease vs risk of radiation exposure (9)[B]
  – Does not obviate the need for cystoscopy, particularly in high-risk patients (8)[B]
  – Visualization of ureters is discontinuous.
  – Less cost-efficient
- CT:
  – Perform unenhanced helical CT as 1st test for suspected stone disease (2)[B].
- Intravenous urography (IVU):
  – Limited sensitivity for small renal masses and for differentiating cystic from solid masses (7)[C]
  – Addition of ultrasound or CT often necessary to evaluate renal parenchyma (7)[C]
  – Potential reactions to IV iodine contrast media
- Renal US:
  – Best for differentiating cystic from solid masses
  – Sensitive for hydronephrosis
  – No radiation or iodinated contrast exposure
  – Cost-efficient
  – Poor sensitivity for small renal masses (<3 cm) (7)[C]
  – Main disadvantage is inability to thoroughly evaluate the urothelium for transitional cell cancer
- MRI:
  – Similar to CT in sensitivity for renal masses
  – No radiation exposure
  – Least cost-efficient
  – Limited ability to reliably detect urinary tract calcifications (9)[B]

Pregnancy Considerations
Renal ultrasound is initial imaging choice for pregnant or pediatric patients (5)[C].

Follow-Up & Special Considerations
In the case of glomerulonephritis, consider CXR to rule out cardiac enlargement, effusions, or pulmonary bleeding (5)[C].

Diagnostic Procedures/Surgery
- Renal biopsy:
  – May be necessary to diagnose glomerulonephritis or in the face of increasing renal insufficiency

- Retrograde pyelogram:
  – Used to further evaluate filling defects detected on other modalities (9)[B]
  – Reserved for patients in which findings on MDCTU are equivocal or increased radiation is not justifiable (9)[B]
  – Sensitive for small lesions of supravesicular collecting system
  – Requires cystoscopy
- Cystoscopy:
  – Best for evaluation of bladder pathology, especially small urothelial carcinomas (2)[B]
  – Fluorescence can be used to enhance detection of flat lesions (10)[C].
  – AUA recommends all patients with hematuria who are >40, younger with risk factors for bladder cancer, and/or those with abnormal cytology receive cystoscopy (2,7)[C].
- Ureteroscopy/pyeloscopy:
  – For visualization of suspected supravesical collecting system lesions
  – Biopsy, excision, fulguration, or extraction of lesions/stones possible
  – Requires anesthesia
  – Requires cystoscopy
  – Risk of injury to collecting system

Pathological Findings
Glomerulonephritis

 TREATMENT

MEDICATION
None indicated for undiagnosed hematuria

ADDITIONAL TREATMENT
Issues for Referral
Prompt nephrology referral for proteinuria, red cell casts, and elevated serum creatinine (2,7)[C]

SURGERY/OTHER PROCEDURES
Gross hematuria: Clots may require continuous bladder irrigation with a large-bore Foley catheter (2- or 3-way catheter may be helpful) to prevent clot retention.

 ONGOING CARE

FOLLOW-UP RECOMMENDATIONS
After initial workup, 35% of patients remain without a diagnosis.

Patient Monitoring
Although some experts still recommend periodic urinalysis and cytology, more recent literature suggests after thorough initial negative investigations (imaging, cystoscopy, cytology) no follow-up is indicated unless new symptoms or frank hematuria develops (3)[B].

DIET
Not restricted, except in certain conditions (e.g., increased fluids for stones or clots; restricted animal proteins in stone disease)

PROGNOSIS
- Generally excellent for common causes of hematuria
- Poorer for malignant tumors and certain types of nephritis

REFERENCES

1. Bergstein J, Leiser J, Andreoli S. The clinical significance of asymptomatic gross and microscopic hematuria in children. *Arch Pediatr Adolesc Med*. 2005;159:353–5.
2. McDonald MM, Swagerty D, Wetzel L. Assessment of microscopic hematuria in adults. *Am Fam Physician*. 2006;73:1748–54.
3. Mishriki SF, Nabi G, Cohen NP. Diagnosis of urologic malignancies in patients with asymptomatic dipstick hematuria: prospective study with 13 years' follow-up. *Urology*. 2008;71:13–6.
4. Massengill SF. Hematuria. *Pediatr Rev*. 2008;29:342–8.
5. Choyke PL. Radiologic evaluation of hematuria: guidelines from the American College of Radiology's appropriateness criteria. *Am Fam Physician*. 2008;78:347–52.
6. Rao PK, Gao T, Pohl M, Jones JS et al. Dipstick pseudohematuria: unnecessary consultation and evaluation. *J Urol*. 2010;183:560–4.
7. Grossfeld GD, Wolf JS, Litwan MS, et al. Asymptomatic microscopic hematuria in adults: summary of the AUA best practice policy recommendations. *Am Fam Physician*. 2001;63:1145–54.
8. Sudakoff GS, Dunn DP, Guralnick ML, et al. Multidetector computerized tomography urography as the primary imaging modality for detecting urinary tract neoplasms in patients with asymptomatic hematuria. *J Urol*. 2008;179:862–7; discussion 867.
9. O'Connor OJ, McSweeney SE, Maher MM. Imaging of hematuria. *Radiol Clin North Am*. 2008;46:113–32, vii.
10. Sharma S, Ksheersagar P, Sharma P et al. Diagnosis and treatment of bladder cancer. *Am Fam Physician*. 2009;80:717–23.

See Also (Topic, Algorithm, Electronic Media Element)
Algorithm: Hematuria

 CODES

ICD9
- 599.70 Hematuria, unspecified
- 599.71 Gross hematuria
- 599.72 Microscopic hematuria

CLINICAL PEARLS

- Screening asymptomatic patients for microscopic hematuria is not recommended (2,4,10)[A].
- Asymptomatic hematuria and hematuria persisting after treatment of UTIs must be evaluated (2)[B].
- After initial workup, 35% of patients remain without a diagnosis.
- Routine use of anticoagulants should not cause hematuria unless there is an underlying urologic abnormality (2)[B].

H

HEMOCHROMATOSIS

Robert A. Marlow, MD, MA

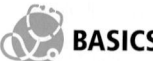 **BASICS**

DESCRIPTION
Hemochromatosis is a hereditary disorder in which the small intestine absorbs excessive iron (1,2):

- Early clinical features include arthralgia, fatigue, and decreased libido.
- Late effects include cirrhosis of the liver, diabetes, hypermelanotic pigmentation of the skin, and heart failure.
- Because there is no mechanism to excrete excess iron, the excess is stored in muscle and in organs, including the liver, pancreas, and heart, eventually resulting in severe damage to the affected organs.
- Liver damage ultimately may result in hepatocellular carcinoma.
- System(s) affected: Endocrine/Metabolic
- Synonym(s): Bronze diabetes; Troisier-Hanot-Chauffard syndrome

EPIDEMIOLOGY
Incidence
- Predominant age: Metabolic abnormality is congenital, but symptoms usually present in the 5th and 6th decades.
- Predominant sex: Gene frequency: Male = Female, although clinical signs are more frequent in men (8:1 male:female ratio) (3)

Prevalence
3/1,000 people (heterozygote frequency, 1/10) (4): The most common genetic abnormality in the US

Pediatric Considerations
Rarely, iron overload may occur as early as 2 years of age. The disorder can be diagnosed before iron overload is clinically apparent.

RISK FACTORS
- The disease is a genetic disorder.
- Affected individuals should not ingest iron supplements, eat raw shellfish, or eat large quantities of iron-rich food such as red meat.
- Alcohol increases the absorption of iron. (As many as 41% of patients with symptomatic disease are alcoholic.)
- Loss of blood, such as that which occurs during menstruation and pregnancy, delays the onset of symptoms.

Genetics
- Genetically heterogeneous disorder of iron overload; types 1, 2, and 3 are autosomal recessive; type 4 is autosomal dominant. Neonatal hemochromatosis is rare.
- Penetrance is incomplete; expressivity is variable.
- Factors contributing to variable expressivity include different mutations in the same gene, mitigating or exacerbating genes, and environmental factors.

GENERAL PREVENTION
- Family members of affected individuals should be screened.
- Screening of population is *not* recommended because the vast majority of those with homozygous hematomachrosis will remain asymptomatic and have a normal life span.
- Pregnant women with the disorder should avoid iron supplements.

ETIOLOGY
- Type 1 hemochromatosis is caused by mutations in the *HFE* gene; type 2 by mutations in either the *HFE2* gene or *HAMP* gene; type 3 by mutations in the *TFR2* gene; and type 4 by mutations in the *SLC40A1* gene. The cause of neonatal hemochromatosis is unknown.
- The mechanism for increased iron absorption in the face of excessive iron stores is not clear. Iron metabolism appears normal in this disease except for a higher level of circulating iron.
- Iron overload may be caused by thalassemia, sideroblastic anemia, liver disease, excess iron intake, or chronic transfusion.

COMMONLY ASSOCIATED CONDITIONS
See Complications.

 DIAGNOSIS

HISTORY
- Weakness (83%)
- Abdominal pain (58%)
- Arthralgia (43%)
- Loss of libido or potency (38%)
- Amenorrhea (22%)
- Dyspnea on exertion (15%)
- Neurologic symptoms (6%)
- Symptoms of diabetes

PHYSICAL EXAM
- Hepatomegaly (83%)
- Increased skin pigmentation (75%)
- Loss of body hair (20%)
- Splenomegaly (13%)
- Peripheral edema (12%)
- Jaundice (10%)
- Gynecomastia (8%)
- Ascites (6%)
- Testicular atrophy
- Hepatic tenderness

DIAGNOSTIC TESTS & INTERPRETATION
After the diagnosis is established, consider having the patient take an oral glucose tolerance test to rule out diabetes and undergo an echocardiogram to rule out cardiomyopathy.

Lab
- Transferrin saturation (serum iron concentration ÷ total iron-binding capacity × 100): >70% is virtually diagnostic of iron overload; 45% or higher warrants further evaluation. Iron supplements and transfusions may elevate serum iron.
- Serum ferritin: >300 μg/L for men and postmenopausal women and 200 μg/L for premenopausal women (5); may be elevated by inflammatory reactions, other forms of liver disease, certain tumors (e.g., acute granulocytic leukemia), and rheumatoid arthritis
- Urinary iron
- Increased urine hemosiderin
- Hyperglycemia
- Decreased FSH
- Decreased LH
- Decreased testosterone
- Increased serum glutamic-oxaloacetic transaminase
- Hypoalbuminemia

Imaging
Not indicated unless used to evaluate suspected liver disease

Diagnostic Procedures/Surgery
- Liver biopsy for stainable iron is the standard for diagnosis. Presence or absence of cirrhosis also can be ascertained. However, with the availability of genetic testing, liver biopsy is not frequently necessary to confirm the diagnosis (5)[C].
- DNA PCR testing for *HFE* gene mutations C282Y and H63D: Present in 85–90% of patients
- Homozygosity for the C282Y mutation with biochemical evidence for iron overload can confirm the diagnosis.

Pathological Findings
- Increased hepatic parenchymal iron stores
- Hepatic fibrosis and cirrhosis with hepatomegaly
- Pancreatic enlargement
- Excess hemosiderin in liver, pancreas, myocardium, thyroid, parathyroid, joints, skin
- Cardiomegaly
- Joint deposition of iron

DIFFERENTIAL DIAGNOSIS
- Repeated transfusions
- Hereditary anemias with ineffective erythropoiesis
- Alcoholic cirrhosis
- Porphyria cutanea tarda
- Atransferrinemia
- Excessive ingestion of iron (rare)

TREATMENT

MEDICATION

- None. Only when phlebotomy is not feasible or in the presence of severe heart disease should the iron-chelating agent deferoxamine (Desferal) be considered.
- Hepatitis A and hepatitis B immunizations should be done if there is no evidence of previous exposure (6).

ADDITIONAL TREATMENT

General Measures

- Remove excess iron by repeated phlebotomy once or twice weekly to establish and maintain a mild anemia (hematocrit of 35–39%) (5)[C].
- When the patient finally becomes iron deficient, a lifelong maintenance program of 2–6 phlebotomies a year to keep storage iron normal; maintain serum ferritin ≤50 μg/L

IN-PATIENT CONSIDERATIONS

Initial Stabilization

Outpatient treatment

ONGOING CARE

FOLLOW-UP RECOMMENDATIONS

Full activity unless there is significant heart disease

Patient Monitoring

- Measure hematocrit before each phlebotomy; skip phlebotomy if hematocrit <36%.
- Schedule an additional phlebotomy when hematocrit >40%.
- When anemia becomes refractory, repeat transferrin saturation and serum ferritin to confirm depletion of iron stores.
- When iron stores are depleted, 2–6 phlebotomies a year should keep iron stores normal; maintain serum ferritin ≤50 μg/L.
- During maintenance therapy, measure transferrin saturation and serum ferritin yearly.

DIET

- An iron-poor diet is not of significant benefit.
- Avoid alcohol, iron-fortified foods, iron-containing supplements, and uncooked shellfish (increased susceptibility to *Vibrio* sp).
- Restrict vitamin C to small doses between meals.
- Tea chelates iron and may be drunk with meals.

PATIENT EDUCATION

- Iron Overload Diseases Association, Inc., 525 Mayflower Rd, West Palm Beach, FL 33405.
- American Hemochromatosis Society, Inc., 4044 W. Lake Mary Blvd., Unit 104, Lake Mary, FL 32746-2012.

PROGNOSIS

- Patients diagnosed before cirrhosis develops and treated with phlebotomy have a normal life expectancy.
- Life expectancy is reduced in patients with cirrhosis and DM and those who require >18 months of phlebotomy therapy to return iron stores to normal.
- Patients with ferritin levels <1,000 μg/L are unlikely to have cirrhosis (3,4).

COMPLICATIONS

- Cirrhosis
- Hepatoma (only in patients with cirrhosis)
- Diabetes mellitus
- Cardiomyopathy
- Arthritis
- Hypogonadism

REFERENCES

1. Pietrangelo A. Hereditary hemochromatosis–a new look at an old disease. *N Engl J Med*. 2004;350: 2383–97.
2. Janssen MC, Swinkels DW et al. Hereditary haemochromatosis. *Best Pract Res Clin Gastroenterol*. 2009;23:171–83.
3. Allen KJ, Gurrin LC, Constantine CC, Osborne NJ, Delatycki MB, Nicoll AJ, McLaren CE, Bahlo M, Nisselle AE, Vulpe CD, Anderson GJ, Southey MC, Giles GG, English DR, Hopper JL, Olynyk JK, Powell LW, Gertig DM et al. Iron-overload-related disease in HFE hereditary hemochromatosis. *N Engl J Med*. 2008;358:221–30.
4. Brandhagen DJ, Fairbanks VF, Baldus W. Recognition and management of hereditary hemochromatosis. *Am Fam Phys*. 2002;65:853–60.
5. Qaseem A, Aronson M, Fitterman N, et al. Screening for hereditary hemochromatosis: a clinical practice guideline from the American College of Physicians. *Ann Intern Med*. 2005;143:517–21.
6. Alexander J, Kowdley KV. Hereditary hemochromatosis: genetics, pathogenesis, and clinical management. *Ann Hepatol*. 2005;4: 240–7.

ADDITIONAL READING

- Adams PC, Barton JC et al. Haemochromatosis. *Lancet*. 2007;370:1855–60.
- Phatak PD, Bonkovsky HL, Kowdley KV et al. Hereditary hemochromatosis: time for targeted screening. *Ann Intern Med*. 2008;149:270–2.
- U.S. Preventive Services Task Force. Screening for hemochromatosis: recommendation statement. *Ann Intern Med*. 2006;145:204–8.

CODES

ICD9

- 275.01 Hereditary hemochromatosis
- 275.03 Other hemochromatosis

CLINICAL PEARLS

- The best laboratory tests available to screen a patient initially for hemochromatosis are serum ferritin and transferrin saturation. An elevated transferrin saturation is the earliest abnormality in hemochromatosis. Ferritin is a sensitive measure of iron overload but can be elevated in a variety of infectious and inflammatory conditions without iron overload being present.
- Liver biopsy need not be done to confirm the diagnosis or to check for cirrhosis if the patient is homozygous for C282Y or is heterozygous for C282Y/H63D. If the patient's serum ferritin is <1,000 μg/L, LFTs are normal, and hepatomegaly is not present, cirrhosis is very unlikely, so liver biopsy is not needed.
- Initially, a patient with hemochromatosis should have a phlebotomy weekly until the serum ferritin is <50 μg/L and the transferrin saturation falls to <30%. Then lifelong maintenance therapy of 2–6 phlebotomies a year is mandatory to keep the ferritin <50 μg/L and the transferrin saturation <50%.
- Most patients with hemochromatosis go undiagnosed. Because treatment with phlebotomy will prevent all complications when begun early, physicians should consider the diagnosis of hemochromatosis much more frequently. However, the US Preventive Services Task Force recommends against routine screening of asymptomatic average-risk populations.

H

HEMOPHILIA

Robyn D. Wing, MD
Patricia McQuilkin, MD

BASICS

DESCRIPTION
- Inherited bleeding disorders caused by a deficiency of coagulant factor VIII (hemophilia A) or factor IX (hemophilia B, also called Christmas Disease). They are clinically indistinguishable but can be differentiated by assays that detect levels of factors VIII and IX.
- Disease severity is determined by the levels of the coagulant factor present:
  - Severe: <1%
  - Moderate: 1–5%
  - Mild: >5%
- Patients with >25% factor activity rarely bleed; however, bleeding after major surgery may occur in patients or carriers with factor VIII levels in the range of 25–35%.
- Synonym(s): Christmas Disease (hemophilia B)

EPIDEMIOLOGY
- Congenital conditions: X-linked–recessive, therefore, they affect males almost exclusively.
- Females are generally asymptomatic carriers unless their factor level is <40%.

Incidence
Incidence of hemophilia A is 1:5,000 live male births; hemophilia B, 1:30,000 live male births.

Prevalence
Affect 500,000 worldwide; 2/3 undiagnosed

RISK FACTORS
Genetics
- Both hemophilia A and B are X-linked–recessive.
- 30% of cases are due to spontaneous mutation.

GENERAL PREVENTION
Consider testing family members for carrier status. 1/3 will have factor levels low enough to cause clinically significant bleeding. Some may wish to use this information in reproductive decision making.

PATHOPHYSIOLOGY
- When blood vessel walls are damaged, exposure of subendothelial tissue initiates the primary hemostatic response, with plasma proteins and platelets interacting with this tissue to generate the platelet plug. Vascular injury also activates the coagulation pathway, which generates thrombin, an element essential to the creation of the fibrin net that stabilizes the platelet plug.
- Deficiencies in factor VIII or factor IX impair the coagulation pathway such that the platelet plug is inadequately stabilized, leading to excessive bleeding.

DIAGNOSIS

- Initial presentation:
  - May be known due to family history. All male infants born to known carriers should have factor level testing.
  - Intracranial bleeding, bleeding with circumcision, dental work, surgery, or injury
  - Excessive bruising, hematomas, hemarthroses
- Bleeding:
  - Depends on disease severity:
    - Severe: Spontaneous bleeding

- Moderate: Bleeding with mild to moderate trauma
    - Mild: Bleeding with major trauma or surgery
  - Joints: Most common sites are ankle (children) and elbows, knees, and ankles (adolescents and adults). May present as irritability or decreased use of limb in an infant. In adults, prodromal stiffness and acute pain and swelling of joint:
    - Progressive arthropathy: Repeated bleeding into a joint damages cartilage and subchondral bone, causing fixed joints and resultant muscle wasting, which may significantly impair mobility.
  - Muscles: Hematoma formation most common in quadriceps, iliopsoas, and forearm
  - Gastrointestinal (GI) tract: Hematomas of bowel wall can cause obstruction or intussuception, as well as pain mimicking appendicitis.
  - Central nervous system (CNS): Intracranial hemorrhage
  - Genitourinary (GU) tract: Hematuria
  - Post-traumatic: Delayed bleeding after injury or surgical procedures
- Compartment syndrome and ischemic nerve damage from large hematomas may occur, for example, femoral nerve neuropathy due to undetected retroperitoneal hemorrhage.
- Pseudotumor syndrome: Untreated hemorrhage causing a hematoma, which calcifies (named because it can be mistaken for cancer)

DIAGNOSTIC TESTS & INTERPRETATION
Lab
Initial lab tests
- Hemophilia A: Diagnostic test is low factor VIII
- Hemophilia B: Diagnostic test is low factor IX
- Activated partial thromboplastin time (PTT): Prolonged
  - Corrected when mixed with normal plasma in absence of inhibitors
- Prothrombin time (PT): Normal
- Platelet count: Normal
- Bleeding time: Prolonged in 15–20% of patients with hemophilia A:
  - Recent aspirin use will increase bleeding time and can lead to confusion with Von Willebrand disease.

Follow-Up & Special Considerations
Inhibitors to factor VIII and IX (see Complications):
- Should be periodically measured with the Bethesda inhibitor assay, which quantifies the antibody titer
- Screen before invasive procedures and at regular intervals.

Diagnostic Procedures/Surgery
Prenatal diagnosis: Genetic testing of a sample of chorionic villus or fluid obtained at amniocentesis

Pathological Findings
In affected joints: Synovial hemosiderosis, articular cartilage degeneration, thickening of periarticular tissues, bony hypertrophy

DIFFERENTIAL DIAGNOSIS
- Von Willebrand disease
- Vitamin K deficiency (factor IX is vitamin K–dependent)
- Other factor deficiencies, afibrinogenemia, dysfibrinogenemia, fibrinolytic defects, platelet disorders
- Child abuse

TREATMENT

MEDICATION
First Line
- Primary prophylaxis:
  - Standard of care for patients with severe hemophilia
  - Regular and long-term treatment with deficient factor
  - Goal is to maintain the factor level above 1%, converting patient to moderate or mild hemophilia.

  - 3 times a week factor infusion for hemophilia A and twice weekly infusions for hemophilia B have been demonstrated to reduce bleeding into joints, better prevent joint damage, and decrease frequency of hemorrhages when compared with patients treated on demand (1)[B].
  - Optimal age to start treatment has not been established. Consensus is that it should be initiated before joint bleeds begin in order to most reduce the risk of subsequent arthropathy (usually within the first 2 years of life) (2)[B].
  - Questions remain about what dose of factor should be provided, when to escalate therapy, and how long prophylaxis should be given (1)[B].

  - Barriers include cost and the need for frequent venous access. Stable venous access can be attained by CVLs or AV fistulae.
- On-demand therapy:
  - Hemophilia A:
    - Desmopressin (DDAVP): For mild hemophilia. Raises factor VIII levels by stimulating release of factor VIII from endothelial storage sites.
      - IV or SubQ: 0.3 mcg/kg infused 30 minutes prior to procedure; may repeat if needed
      - Intranasal: >50 kg = 150 mcg to each nostril (total = 300 mcg). <50 kg = 150 mcg to 1 nostril.
      - Adverse effect: Hyponatremic seizures, especially in children. Need to restrict fluids and watch sodium levels and urine output
      - Children may have a lower therapeutic response, which may increase with age (3)[B].
    - Purified factor VIII: Plasma-derived factor replacement is treated to inactivate viruses, an important innovation, because pooled plasma used previously carried high risk of HIV, hepatitis B, and hepatitis C transmission.
    - Recombinant factor VIII: Treatment of choice. Dosing: 1 U of factor VIII (the amount in 1 mL of plasma)/kg body weight will raise the plasma level of the recipient by 2%. Half-life of factor VIII is 8–12 hours. Therefore, b.i.d. or t.i.d. dosing is required with frequent factor-level checks.
  - Hemophilia B:
    - Purified factor IX
    - Recombinant factor IX: Treatment of choice. Dosing: 1 U/kg will raise levels 1%. Half-life of factor IX is 16–17 hours.
  - Amount and duration of factor replacement depends on location and severity of the bleed:
    - A target factor level of >30% is generally sufficient for mild bleeding episodes.
    - Major hemorrhages and large muscle bleeds require correction to levels between 50% and 100%.

○ Life-threatening bleeds require levels between 80–100%, which should be sustained with bolus dosing or continuous infusion.
– Both hemophilia A and B:
○ Antifibrinolytic agents: Enhance clot stabilization by inhibiting plasminogen activation. Effective in controlling mucosal bleeding, such as bleeding in oral cavity, epistaxis, and menorrhagia. Can also be used prophylactically, for example, prior to tooth extractions. Tranexamic acid (25 mg/kg p.o. every 6–8 hours or 10 mg/kg IV every 6–8 hours) and aminocaproic acid (Amicar) are also used (4)[B].

Second Line
Patients with inhibitors:
- Low-titer (<5 BU/mL): Transient antibodies, which can be overcome with high amounts or longer duration of factor concentrate
- High-titer: Cannot be treated with deficient factor concentrates; must bypass the deficient factor in the clotting cascade
  – Prothrombin complex concentrates and activated prothrombin complex concentrates (aPCC) may be used (both contain factors II, VII, IX, and X).
    ○ Risk of thrombus formation and disseminated intravascular coagulation (DIC) when used repeatedly or in higher doses.
    ○ FEIBA VH dose: 50–100 U/kg every 8–12 hours, but not to exceed 200 U/kg/day (5)[C].
  – Recombinant activated factor VII (rFVIIa): Avoids the risk associated with pooled donor plasma and does not cause a rise in antibody titer. However, it promotes coagulation only at the local level because it requires tissue factor to be active.
    ○ rFVIIa dose: 90–120 mcg/kg every 2 to 3 hours or single dose of 270 mcg/kg for target joint bleeds (5)[B]
- Immune tolerance induction: Protocols to eliminate inhibitors. Regimens include frequent exposure to high-dose factor VIII therapy over 12–18 months, with or without immunosuppressive therapy (corticosteroids, cyclophosphamide, Rituximab), until tolerance develops. Success rate shown to be 60–80% (6)[B].

ADDITIONAL TREATMENT
General Measures
- Avoid aspirin or other nonsteroidal anti-inflammatory drugs.
- Treat early; symptoms may occur before bleeding is clinically apparent.
- For surgical prophylaxis:
  – If major surgery is undertaken, factor levels should be maintained at >50% for at least 2–3 weeks after the procedure.
  – Dental extractions: Antifibrinolytics (Amicar, tranexamic acid) may be used.
  – Small procedures: may use DDAVP
- Hepatitis A and B vaccinations are recommended.
- Encourage physical activity. Patients should avoid high-impact contact sports.
- Female carriers: Majority of females are asymptomatic carriers, although an occasional carrier will bleed at time of surgery.

COMPLEMENTARY AND ALTERNATIVE MEDICINE
Gene therapy:
- Replacement of defective factor gene sequence with a corrected version, which would allow for increased factor production
- Animal studies have demonstrated safe, long-term expression of clotting factors using multiple gene-transfer strategies, but these findings have not been successful in patients (7)[B].
- Dramatic improvements could be seen with even minimal increases in factor levels. For example, a patient may improve from a severe to a mild phenotype by increasing factor from <1% to >5%.

SURGERY/OTHER PROCEDURES
In patients with hemophilic arthropathy from recurrent hemarthrosis:
- Surgical or radionuclide synovectomy
- Total joint replacement

 ONGOING CARE

FOLLOW-UP RECOMMENDATIONS
Restrict activities in proportion to the degree of factor deficiency, with efforts to maintain a normal life and adequate physical condition.

Patient Monitoring
Regular evaluations every 6–12 months, including a musculoskeletal evaluation, an inhibitor screen, liver tests, and tests for antibodies to hepatitis viruses and HIV

PATIENT EDUCATION
- National Hemophilia Foundation at: http://www.hemophilia.org
- World Federation of Hemophilia at: http://www.wfh.org

PROGNOSIS
- Survival is normal for those with mild disease; mortality is increased 2–6-fold in those with moderate to severe disease.
- At one time, AIDS surpassed intracranial hemorrhage as the leading cause of death in hemophilia. Risk for HIV infection has declined significantly due to development of recombinant and virus-inactivated factor-replacement products.
- Hemophilic arthropathy is the main cause of morbidity in patients with severe hemophilia, as repeated hemarthroses result in eventual deformity and progressive disability.

COMPLICATIONS
- Hemophilic arthropathy: Symptoms include pain, limitation of motion, and contractures.
- Transmission of bloodborne infections, such as hepatitis A, B, C, D, and HIV. This risk has now been greatly reduced.
  – Hepatitis B and C increases risk for cirrhosis and hepatocellular cancer.
- Development of inhibitor autoantibodies: IgG antibodies that neutralize the deficient factor
  – More common in those with hemophilia A (20–30% of patients compared to 5% in hemophilia B) (6)[B]
  – More common in patients with severe disease requiring multiple transfusions
  – Risk factors for inhibitor development include:
    ○ Specific genetic defect (family history); null mutations have higher inhibitor incidence

○ Very low or no circulating factor, therefore requiring multiple transfusions
○ Age of 1st exogenous factor exposure; previous studies report a higher incidence of developing antibodies in those exposed to exogenous factor at <6 months of age, but new studies show this may be due to severity of disease (8)[B].
○ Concurrent inflammation/infection when administering factor (5)[B] (e.g., surgical prophylaxis).
○ Duration of factor exposure (5)[B]
– No increased risk of bleeding, but when bleeding occurs, it is more difficult to achieve hemostasis due to decreased response to factor replacement

REFERENCES

1. Manco-Johnson MJ, Abshire TC, Shapiro AD, et al. Prophylaxis versus episodic treatment to prevent joint disease in boys with severe hemophilia. *N Engl J Med.* 2007;357:535–44.
2. Carcao M, Chambost H, Ljung R et al. Devising a best practice approach to prophylaxis in boys with severe haemophilia: evaluation of current treatment strategies. *Haemophilia.* 2010;16(Suppl 2):4–9.
3. Castaman G et al. Desmopressin for the treatment of haemophilia. *Haemophilia.* 2008;14(Suppl 1):15–20.
4. Price VE, Hawes SA, Chan AK. A practical approach to hemophilia care in children. *Paediatr Child Health.* 2007;12:381–3.
5. Kempton CL, White GC et al. How we treat a hemophilia A patient with a factor VIII inhibitor. *Blood.* 2009;113:11–7.
6. Carcao M, Lambert T et al. Prophylaxis in haemophilia with inhibitors: update from international experience. *Haemophilia.* 2010;16(Suppl 2):16–23.
7. Murphy SL, High KA. Gene therapy for haemophilia. *Br J Haematol.* 2008;140:479–87.
8. Gouw SC, van der Bom JG, Marijke van den Berg H et al. Treatment-related risk factors of inhibitor development in previously untreated patients with hemophilia A: the CANAL cohort study. *Blood.* 2007;109:4648–54.

 CODES

ICD9
- 286.0 Congenital factor viii disorder
- 286.1 Congenital factor ix disorder
- 286.2 Congenital factor xi deficiency

CLINICAL PEARLS
- Hemophilia A and B are X-linked recessive conditions, affecting males almost exclusively.
- The severity of disease varies based on amount of factor present.
- Standard of care for treatment now includes primary prophylaxis with recombinant factor, as well as on-demand factor replacement with recombinant factor.
- Inhibitor formation should be suspected when treatment with deficient factor fails to correct coagulopathy.

HEMORRHOIDS

Juan Qiu, MD, PhD

 BASICS

DESCRIPTION
- Varicosities of the hemorrhoidal venous plexus
- External hemorrhoids are located below the dentate line and covered by squamous epithelium.
- Internal hemorrhoids are located above the dentate line.
- Both types of hemorrhoids often coexist.
- Classification of internal hemorrhoids:
  – 1st degree: Hemorrhoids do not prolapse.
  – 2nd degree: Prolapse through the anus on straining but reduce spontaneously
  – 3rd degree: Protrude and require digital reduction
  – 4th degree: Cannot be reduced
- Hemorrhoids often progress from itching, bleeding stage to protrusion with easy reduction, then difficult reduction, and finally rectal prolapse. Thrombosis may occur at any protrusion stage.

Geriatric Considerations
Common in elderly along with rectal prolapse

Pediatric Considerations
- Uncommon in infants and children. Look for underlying cause (e.g., venacaval or mesenteric obstruction, cirrhosis, portal HTN).
- Occasionally, as in adults, hemorrhoids may result from chronic constipation, fecal impaction, and straining at stool. Surgery is rarely required in children.

Pregnancy Considerations
- Common in pregnancy
- Usually resolves after pregnancy
- No treatment required, unless extremely painful

EPIDEMIOLOGY
- Predominant age: Adults; peak between 45 and 65 years old
- Predominant sex: Male = Female

Incidence
Common

Prevalence
About 4–5% in general population in US

RISK FACTORS
- Pregnancy
- Pelvic space-occupying lesions
- Liver disease
- Portal HTN
- Constipation
- Occupations that require prolonged sitting
- Loss of muscle tone in old age, rectal surgery, episiotomy, anal intercourse
- Obesity
- Chronic diarrhea

Genetics
No known genetic pattern

GENERAL PREVENTION
- Avoid constipation with high-fiber diet and hydration.
- Lose weight, if overweight.
- Avoid prolonged sitting on the toilet.

ETIOLOGY
- Dilated veins of hemorrhoidal plexus
- Tight internal anal sphincter
- Abnormal distention of the arteriovenous anastomosis
- Prolapse of the cushions and the surrounding connective tissues

COMMONLY ASSOCIATED CONDITIONS
- Liver disease
- Pregnancy
- Portal HTN
- Constipation

 DIAGNOSIS

Diagnosis is usually made by history and inspection of the perineum, rectal exam, and anoscopy.

HISTORY
- All cases:
  – Classically, bright red blood per rectum; may be scant blood on toilet paper, or copious in the toilet bowl
  – Constipation or diarrhea
  – Straining with defecation
- Small or minimal external hemorrhoids: Episodic bleeding on stool or toilet paper, pruritus
- More extensive internal hemorrhoids: Feeling of incomplete evacuation

PHYSICAL EXAM
- Anorectal exam including anoscopy
- Inspection following straining at stool
- For protruding hemorrhoids: Mass, more prominent bleeding
- If not reducible, increased risk of strangulation and/or thrombosis with acute pain
- External hemorrhoids cause pain; internal hemorrhoids generally do not.
- Thrombosed hemorrhoids present as acute discomfort and the presence of a painful mass.

DIAGNOSTIC TESTS & INTERPRETATION
Diagnostic Procedures/Surgery
Sigmoidoscopy or colonoscopy depending on coexistent risk factors for malignancy in patients who present with bleeding.

DIFFERENTIAL DIAGNOSIS
- Rectal or anal neoplasia
- Condyloma
- Skin tag
- Inflammatory bowel disease (1)[B]
- Anal fistula, fissure, or abscess (2)[B]

 TREATMENT

All these treatments, except surgical, are outpatient with quick recovery time, usually <48 hours.

MEDICATION
- Prevention:
  – Fiber supplements
  – Stool softeners
- Pain:
  – Hydrocortisone ointment (0.5–1.0%)
  – Analgesic sprays or ointments—benzocaine, dibucaine (Nupercainal). Use sprays with caution as they may contain alcohol that can cause burning sensation when applied.
- Pruritus: Hydrocortisone (Anusol-HC, Cortifoam) ointment
- Bleeding:
  – Astringent suppositories (Preparation H)
  – Hydrocortisone (Anusol; Cortifoam) ointment
- Treatment for special cases:
  – Thrombosed external hemorrhoids: Fairly common complication of hemorrhoidal disease. With conservative treatment, the thrombus will be absorbed over the course of weeks and pain improves within 2–3 days (1)[B].
  – With severe acute pain, prompt excision should be performed under local anesthetic and the wound left open without packing. Sitz baths, topical anesthetics, and mild pain relievers for 1st 7–10 days after excision (1)[B].
  – Strangulated hemorrhoid: From irreducible 3rd- or 4th-degree hemorrhoid. If untreated, can progress to ulceration and thrombosis. Treatment requires urgent or emergent hemorrhoidectomy.
  – Acute hemorrhoidal bleeding associated with portal HTN: Bleeding can be life-threatening. Treatment should be suture of the bleeding site with incorporation of the mucosa, submucosa, and internal sphincter. Coagulopathy should be corrected.

ADDITIONAL TREATMENT

General Measures

- Hemorrhoids are a recurrent disease, even after surgical excision; measures for prevention should be taken.
- For mild symptoms or prevention:
  - Avoid prolonged sitting at stool.
  - Avoid straining.
  - Avoid constipation by eating a high-fiber diet or by taking fiber supplements; if necessary, take regular stool softeners.
  - Regular exercise
- For pain, sitz baths warm water or hypertonic Epsom salts (1 cup per 2 quarts of water)
- Mild and minimal hemorrhoids respond to changed diet, relief of constipation, and brief stooling.
- Pruritus or mild discomfort after stooling responds to hydrocortisone ointment, anesthetic ointments or sprays, and warm sitz bath.
- Constipation relief, anal hygiene, local ointments, and sitz baths are effective through the stage of easy reduction, but the more severe stages require rubber band ligation or rectal surgery.

SURGERY/OTHER PROCEDURES

- Indications: Failure of medical and nonoperative therapy, symptomatic 3rd- or 4th-degree (3) symptoms (3) in presence of a concomitant anorectal condition requiring surgery, or patient preference (2)[B],(3)
- Incision of thrombosed hemorrhoid: For severe pain
- Severe protruding hemorrhoids:
  - Rubber band ligation (internal hemorrhoids only)
  - Sclerotherapy: For symptomatic prolapsed stage I or II hemorrhoids; care must be (4) taken injecting near periprostatic parasympathetic nerves. Not for advanced disease or if evidence of infection, inflammation, ulceration is present (1)[B]:
    - Cryotherapy is no longer recommended due to high rate of complications (2)[B].
  - Prolapsed rectum:
    - Requires surgical correction
  - Surgical resection:
    - Gold standard: Conventional hemorrhoidectomy should be considered for grade III hemorrhoids not responding to banding, mixed internal and external, grade IV hemorrhoids, or when complicated by fissures, fistula, or extensive skin tags.

- Newer technique:
  - Stapled hemorrhoidopexy; less painful than traditional surgery, but higher incidence of recurrences (5)[B]
  - Ligasure hemorrhoidectomy; reduces operating time, is superior in patient tolerance, and is equally effective as conventional hemorrhoidectomy in long-term symptom control

ONGOING CARE

FOLLOW-UP RECOMMENDATIONS

- Encourage physical fitness.
- Avoid prolonged sitting and straining on the toilet.

Patient Monitoring

As needed, depending on treatment

DIET

High-fiber, adequate fluids

PROGNOSIS

- Spontaneous resolution
- Recurrence

COMPLICATIONS

- Thrombosis
- Ulceration
- Anemia (rare)
- Incontinence
- Pelvic sepsis following hemorrhoidectomy (5)[B]

REFERENCES

1. Kaidar-Person O, Person B, Wexner SD. Hemorrhoidal disease: A comprehensive review. *J Am Coll Surg.* 2007;204:102–17.
2. Clinical Practice Committee, American Gastroenterological Association. American Gastroenterological Association medical position statement: Diagnosis and treatment of hemorrhoids. *Gastroenterology.* 2004;126:1461–2.
3. Castellvi J, Sueira A, Espinosa J, Vallet J, Gil V, Pi F. Ligasure versus diathermy hemorrhoidectomy under spinal anesthesia or pudendal block with ropivacaine: a randomized prospective clinical study with 1-year follow-up. *Int J Colorectal Dis.* Published online: 25 April 2009.
4. Nienhuiji S, de Hingh I. Conventional versus LigaSure hemorrhoidectomy for patients with symptomatic hemorrhoids (Review). *The cochrane Library* 2009, Issue 2.
5. Nisar PJ, Acheson AG, Neal KR, et al. Stapled hemorrhoidopexy compared with conventional hemorrhoidectomy: systematic review of randomized, controlled trials. *Dis Colon Rectum.* 2004;47:1837–45.

ADDITIONAL READING

- Giordano P, Gravante G, Sorge R, Ovens L, Nastro P. Long-term Outcomes of stapled hemorrhoidopexy vs conventional hemorrhoidectomy. *Arch Surg.* 2009;144(3):266–72.
- Reese GE, von Roon AC, Tekkis PP et al. Haemorrhoids. *Clin Evid (Online).* 2009.

See Also (Topic, Algorithm, Electronic Media Element)

Colorectal Malignancy; Portal Hypertension

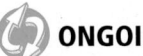 CODES

ICD9

- 455.0 Internal hemorrhoids without mention of complication
- 455.1 Internal thrombosed hemorrhoids
- 455.2 Internal hemorrhoids with other complication

CLINICAL PEARLS

- Hemorrhoids are uncommon in inflammatory bowel disease, and pain is most related to perianal inflammation, irritation, and swelling. Anal hygiene and symptomatic pain relief are the treatments of choice.
- No pain is associated with internal hemorrhoids. Pain occurs with external hemorrhoids only.

H

HENOCH-SCHÖNLEIN PURPURA

Kimberly A. Pesaturo, PharmD
Evan R. Horton, PharmD
Amy Pelletier, DO

 BASICS

DESCRIPTION
- Henoch-Schönlein purpura (HSP) is an immunologically mediated, nonthrombocytopenic, purpuric, systemic vasculitis involving small blood vessels (1).
- HSP is often self-limiting but can result in long-term renal damage (1).

EPIDEMIOLOGY
Incidence
- Up to 20.4/100,000 children <17 years of age per year, but incidence is variable (2)
- Predominant age: Highest incidence between 4 and 6 years of age (2)
- Most common in Caucasians, Japanese, and Native Americans (2)
- Low incidence in Africans and African Americans (2)
- Predominant sex: Male > Female (approximately 1.2:1) (2)

Prevalence
- Year-round occurrence
- More common in late fall to early spring (3)

RISK FACTORS
Genetics
Possible genetic predisposition (1)

PATHOPHYSIOLOGY
- Immune-mediated disorder involving IgA complexes (specifically IgA1) that form and deposit in affected areas, triggering localized inflammation (1)
- Results in leukocytoclastic vasculitis and small blood vessel necrosis
- Proliferative glomerulonephritis with IgA deposit may be seen (4).

ETIOLOGY
- No single etiologic agent has been identified.
- Many cases are associated with preceding infections, usually involving group A β-hemolytic streptococci (3).
- Also reported following infections with (but not limited to): parvovirus B19, adenovirus, hepatitis A and B viruses, Coxsackie virus, Epstein-Barr virus, varicella virus, *B. henselae*, *H. pylori*, and *M. pneumoniae* (3).
- Rare reports after drug ingestion, insect bites, and some vaccines

DIAGNOSIS

Palpable purpura with lower limb predominance with one or more of the following (4):
- Abdominal pain
- Biopsy with predominant IgA
- Arthralgia or arthritis
- Renal involvement (hematuria or proteinuria)

HISTORY
- Previous disease: Infections such as streptococcal infections, upper respiratory infections, and hepatitis (3)
- Rash: Initially may resemble urticaria prior to developing into palpable purpura (1)
- Headache
- Cough
- Vomiting
- Abdominal pain is the most common gastrointestinal symptom (1).
- Transient arthritis of joints, most frequent in lower-limbs (knees and ankles) (1)
- Edema of the periorbital region or ankles
- Hematuria
- Testicular pain or scrotal swelling (1)

PHYSICAL EXAM
- Hypertension may be present.
- Rash is the hallmark of HSP (1). Rash may be petechial or purpuric in a pressure-dependent, symmetric distribution, usually predominating on lower limbs.
  - Rash may be briefly preceded by joint involvement or abdominal pain.
  - Skin lesions may spread to face and trunk; bullous lesions can develop.
- Abdomen often tender to palpation. Some form of bleeding may occur.
  - Abdominal symptoms may precede the rash by up to 2 weeks.
  - Intussusception is a possible complication.
- Orchitis (less common) may occur and can mimic testicular torsion.
  - Swelling and bruising may be noted on the scrotum.
  - Testicular torsion also has been reported.
- Joints (mainly lower limb) should be examined for swelling and limited range of motion.
- CNS involvement may present with headaches, seizures, or behavioral changes (less common).
- Rare pulmonary involvement may be noted.

DIAGNOSTIC TESTS & INTERPRETATION
No definitive tests confirm the diagnosis of HSP.

Lab
The following labs may be useful in diagnosing HSP (1,3):
- CBC:
  - Normal platelet count differentiates from thrombocytopenic purpura.
  - Hemoglobin is usually normal; leukocytosis, eosinophilia especially, may be present.
  - Can detect anemia if there is GI blood loss.
- ESR:
  - Normal or elevated
- Prothrombin (PT) and partial thromboplastin time (PTT):
  - Normal
- IgA:
  - Often elevated in the acute phase of illness, with normal or increased IgG and IgM
- C3/C4:
  - Normal; sometimes decreased
- Antinuclear antibody:
  - Negative
- Throat culture for group A β-hemolytic streptococci:
  - Positive in up to 75% of patients
- Anti-streptolysin O titer:
  - Determines preceding streptococcal infection
- Serum basic/comprehensive chemistries:
  - Elevated BUN and creatinine levels and decreased protein and albumin are seen with renal involvement.
- Urinalysis:
  - Gross hematuria and proteinuria are present in many patients. Microscopic blood, RBCs, WBCs, and casts suggest glomerulonephritis.
- Blood culture:
  - Evaluate for sepsis or bacteremia
- Stool guaiac

Imaging
The following imaging tests may be useful (1):
- Abdominal ultrasound for thickened bowel wall intussusception
- Abdominal radiograph
- Renal tract ultrasound
- CXR

Diagnostic Procedures/Surgery
- Renal biopsy: Severe renal failure
  - Epithelial crescent formation on renal biopsy suggests significant renal damage and inflammation.
- Skin biopsy of purpura: IgA deposition

DIFFERENTIAL DIAGNOSIS
- Petechial and purpuric rashes seen in thrombocytopenia from:
  - Idiopathic thrombocytopenic purpura
  - Sepsis/infection: meningococcemia, Rocky Mountain spotted fever
  - Leukemia
  - Hemolytic-uremic syndrome
  - Coagulopathies
- Vasculitic rashes may result from primary and secondary vasculitides.
  - Polyarteritis nodosa
  - Wegener granulomatosis
  - Infection related
  - Connective tissue diseases (e.g., systemic lupus erythematosus) or Berger disease
  - Infantile acute hemorrhagic edema
  - Rheumatoid arthritis
  - Rheumatic fever
  - Kawasaki disease
- Other: Acute abdomen, bacterial endocarditis, abuse (3)

TREATMENT

MEDICATION
- HSP without nephritis usually resolves spontaneously without specific therapy.
- Early oral prednisone (1–2 mg/kg/day of prednisone for two weeks) may reduce intensity of joint and abdominal pain (5)[B].
- Patients with severe renal damage should be considered for aggressive therapy with high-dose steroids and/or immunosuppressants or plasmapheresis; evidence is inconclusive (3)[C].
- Dapsone 1–2 mg/kg/d may be considered for skin rash (6)[C].
- Analgesics and NSAIDs may be used for analgesia, but salicylates and other agents that affect platelet function should be avoided if GI tract bleeding is present.
  - NSAIDs should be avoided in patients with renal disease (3).

ADDITIONAL TREATMENT
General Measures
- Treatment of hypertension may delay or prevent progression of renal disease in patients with glomerulonephritis.
- Rest and elevation of affected areas may limit purpura (3).

Issues for Referral
Pediatric nephrology and/or dermatology

IN-PATIENT CONSIDERATIONS
Hospitalization is often unnecessary. Severe complications may require admission.

Admission Criteria
- Gastrointestinal hemorrhage
- Protein-losing enteropathy requiring total parenteral nutrition
- Renal disease
- Hypertension
- Pulmonary hemorrhage

IV Fluids
Hydration should be maintained.

ONGOING CARE

FOLLOW-UP RECOMMENDATIONS
Patient Monitoring
- Patients should be seen weekly during the acute illness. Visits should include history and physical exam, along with BP measurement and urinalysis.
- All patients, even those who did not present with renal involvement, should have urine checked for blood weekly for 6 months and then monthly for 3 years because deterioration of renal function has been observed years after presentation in some patients.
- Women with a history of HSP should be monitored for proteinuria and HTN during pregnancy.

PATIENT EDUCATION
American Family Physician handout on HSP at www.aafp.org/afp/980800ap/980800b.html

PROGNOSIS
- Generally excellent: Most patients are improved within 4 weeks of HSP onset.
- Younger age is associated with better prognosis.
- Recurrence within 1st 6 months in up to 33% (3)
- Extent of renal disease often dictates long-term prognosis (3).

COMPLICATIONS
- Hypertension
- End-stage renal disease
- Intussusception (most common GI tract complication, affecting 1–5% of patients)
- Protein-losing enteropathy
- Hemorrhagic pancreatitis
- Hydrops of the gallbladder
- Intestinal strictures
- Bowel perforations, ischemia, and infarctions, obstructions
- GI hemorrhage
- Pseudomembranous colitis
- Appendicitis
- Skin necrosis
- Subarachnoid, subdural, and cortical hemorrhage and infarction
- Peripheral mononeuropathies and polyneuropathies (Guillain-Barré syndrome)
- Pulmonary hemorrhage (uncommon but may result in death)
- Torsion of the testis and appendix testes and priapism
- Scrotal swelling and pain
- CNS complications
- Myocarditis

REFERENCES
1. McCarthy HJ, Tizard EJ. Diagnosis and management of Henoch-Schönlein purpura. Eur J Pediatr. 2010;169:643–650.
2. Gardner-Medwin JM, Dolezalova P, Cummins C, et al. Incidence of Henoch-Schönlein purpura, Kawasaki disease, and rare vasculitides in children of different ethnic origins. Lancet. 2002;360:1197–202.
3. Reamy BV, Williams PM, Lindsay TJ. Henoch-Schönlein purpura. Am Fam Physician. 2009;80(7):697–704.
4. Ozen S, Pistorio A, Iusan SM, et al. EULAR/PRINTO/PRES criteria for Henoch-Schönlein purpura, childhood polyarteritis nodosa, childhood Wegener granulomatosis and childhood Takayasu arteritis: Ankara 2008. Part II: final classification criteria. Ann Rheum Dis. 2010;69:798–806.
5. Weiss PF, Feinstein JA, Luan X, et al. Effects of corticosteroid on Henoch-Schönlein purpura: a systematic review. Pediatrics. 2007;120:1079–87.
6. Iqbal H, Evans A. Dapsone therapy for Henoch-Schönlein purpura: a case series. Arch Dis Child. 2005;90:985–6.

ADDITIONAL READING
- González LM, Janniger CK, Schwartz RA. Pediatric Henoch-Schönlein purpura. Int J Dermatol. 2009;48:1157–1165.
- Roberts PF, Waller TA, Brinker TM, et al. Henoch-Schönlein purpura: a review article. South Med J. 2007;100:821–4.

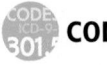 CODES

ICD9
287.0 Allergic purpura

CLINICAL PEARLS
- Rash is the hallmark of HSP.
- HSP without renal involvement is often self-limiting.
- All patients, even those who did not present with renal involvement, should have urine checked for blood weekly for 6 months and then monthly for 3 years because deterioration of renal function has been observed years after presentation in some patients.

H

HEPARIN-INDUCED THROMBOCYTOPENIA

Adam B. Pesaturo, PharmD, BCPS
Patrick Mailloux, DO

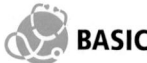 **BASICS**

DESCRIPTION
- Unexplained decrease in platelet count in a patient treated with heparin:
  - Minimum platelet count fall between 30% and 50% from baseline
- Antibody-mediated prothrombotic disorder initiated by heparin administration
- Idiosyncratic reaction
- 2 types: Nonimmune heparin-associated thrombocytopenia (previously called HIT type I) and HIT (previously called HIT type II):
  - Nonimmune heparin-associated thrombocytopenia: More common, onset 1–4 days after starting heparin, mild thrombocytopenia (>100,000), few complications
  - HIT: Less common, onset 5–14 days after primary exposure to heparin, thrombocytopenia often <100,000 but usually >20,000, high risk of thrombosis:
    - Presentation of thrombocytopenia can be immediate if recent heparin exposure within past 100 days

EPIDEMIOLOGY
Incidence
- 10–15% of heparin-treated patients will experience decrease in platelet count.
- 0.3–3% will develop HIT.

RISK FACTORS
- Postsurgical > medical > obstetric:
  - Postcardiopulmonary bypass being the most significant risk factor
- Bovine unfractionated heparin (UFH) > porcine UFH > low-molecular-weight heparin (LMWH)
- Female > Male
- Heparin duration >4 days

GENERAL PREVENTION
- Inquire about recent heparin exposure and any prior history of HIT
- Proper documentation of past HIT reactions in patient's medical record
- No form of heparin should ever be administered once the diagnosis of HIT is confirmed.

PATHOPHYSIOLOGY
- Nonimmune heparin-associated thrombocytopenia: Potentially a result from direct platelet membrane binding with heparin
- HIT: Heparin can cause an increase in the blood concentration of platelet factor 4 (PF4), a chemokine. PF4 will form a complex with heparin. This heparin/PF4 complex can, in turn, stimulate the production of specific antiheparin/PF4 complex antibodies. These antibodies cause platelet activation and a prothrombotic state. Ultimately, this hypercoagulable state leads to thromboembolic complications in many patients.

COMMONLY ASSOCIATED CONDITIONS
- Venous thrombosis: Deep venous thrombosis (DVT), pulmonary embolism (PE), adrenal vein thrombosis with hemorrhagic infarction
- Arterial thrombosis
- Skin lesions
- Acute systemic reactions

 DIAGNOSIS

- Nonimmune heparin-associated thrombocytopenia: Asymptomatic drop in platelet count
- HIT: Thrombocytopenia or thrombosis with the presence of heparin-dependent antibodies:
  - A clinicopathologic syndrome, meaning the foundation for diagnosis is based on both clinical and serologic findings

HISTORY
- Duration of current heparin therapy
- Previous exposure to heparin, including heparin flushes and heparin-coated catheters
- In patients being treated with heparin for thrombosis in which thrombosis recurs during therapy, consider HIT as a potential cause.
- Pretest probability for HIT can be calculated using the "4T's" methodology (1).

PHYSICAL EXAM
- Signs of venous or arterial thrombosis
- Skin necrosis (begins with erythema, progressing to ecchymosis and necrosis)
- Ischemic changes (signs of limb, renal, splenic, mesenteric ischemia)
- Bleeding (less common)

DIAGNOSTIC TESTS & INTERPRETATION
Lab
- Serial platelet counts in patients receiving heparin: Check platelets at baseline, 24 hours, and then every other day for first 14 days (2)[B].
- Confirmatory lab tests needed for a clinical diagnosis can use 1 of 3 serologic assays:
  - Enzyme-linked immunosorbent assay (ELISA) (antigenic assay): Up to 99% sensitive, poor specificity; thus, has an excellent negative predictive value for HIT
  - Heparin-induced platelet activation (platelet activation test): High specificity and low sensitivity
  - Serotonin release assay (platelet activation test): High specificity and moderate sensitivity
- Either a platelet activation assay or an antigenic assay alone may not be adequate for clinical diagnosis; their use in combination is usually recommended.
- The diagnostic interpretation of these laboratory tests must be made in the context of the clinical estimation of the pretest probability of HIT since HIT is a clinicopathologic syndrome. Patients may form heparin-dependent antibodies and still not develop HIT (3).

DIFFERENTIAL DIAGNOSIS
Other potential causes of thrombocytopenia include (list is not all-inclusive):
- Sepsis and other infections
- Drug reactions
- Autoimmune
- Transfusion reactions
- Physical destruction (i.e., during cardiopulmonary bypass)

 TREATMENT

Treatment is by prompt withdrawal of heparin and replacement with a suitable alternative anticoagulant.

MEDICATION
- Most patients will require anticoagulation either because of:
  - Preexisting thrombosis OR
  - Risk of thrombosis during 30 days after HIT diagnosis; consider anticoagulation for 30 days (4)[B]
- Dosing of anticoagulant will depend on indication (prophylaxis vs treatment):
  - In cases where there is clinically a low suspicion/pretest probability of HIT and laboratory confirmation is pending, it may be appropriate to continue antithrombotic prophylaxis using nonheparin anticoagulants.
  - In cases with high suspicion/pretest probability of HIT and laboratory confirmation is pending, it is appropriate to begin anticoagulation treatment with a nonheparin product.
- Direct thrombin inhibitors (DTI) (lepirudin, argatroban, and bivalirudin):
  - They reduce relative risk of thrombosis by 30%, on average (2)[B].
  - DTIs can produce misleading elevation in international normalized ratio (INR) (most likely an in vitro reaction) (5):
    - Argatroban > bivalirudin > lepirudin
  - Lepirudin:
    - Initial dose 0.1 mg/kg/hr, decrease dose with reduced renal function
    - Dose adjustments based on active partial thromboplastin time (aPTT) (goal: 1.5–2 times patient baseline); check aPTT every 4 hours until steady state within goal aPTT range is achieved
  - Argatroban:
    - Initial dose is 2 mcg/kg/min, decrease dose with reduced hepatic function or with critical illness
    - Dose adjustments based on aPTT similar to lepirudin, except aPTT is initially checked every 2 hours
  - Bivalirudin:
    - Favorable pharmacologic profile; however, evidence for use is insufficient compared to lepirudin and argatroban
    - Initial dose is a 0.1 mg/kg bolus, followed by a continuous infusion rate of 0.2 mg/kg/hr, reduced dose with renal insufficiency (CrCl <30 mL/min)
    - Dose adjustments based on aPTT

- Factor Xa inhibitor (fondaparinux):
  - Reports of its use theorized to be useful; however, there is minimal data supporting its efficacy for HIT, and an ideal dose has yet to be determined.
  - Association with the development of HIT has been reported (6)[C]
  - Optional agent for thromboembolic prophylaxis when practitioner wants to avoid heparin
  - Avoid in patients with renal dysfunction (CrCl <30 mL/min).
- Warfarin:
  - Must anticoagulate with an immediate-acting agent before starting warfarin
  - Use of warfarin without other anticoagulants should be avoided, as it can cause thrombosis (2)[A].
  - Begin warfarin after platelet count >150,000 (2)[B]
  - Discontinue other anticoagulant and continue only warfarin after INR is therapeutic (2–3) for at least 5 days (2)[A]. This management differs from the normal heparin-to-warfarin transition in other conditions requiring anticoagulation.
- Low-molecular-weight heparin (LMWH):
  - Although LMWH has a lower risk of initiating a HIT reaction, it should NOT be used when antibodies are already present. These antibodies can cross-react with LMWH and induce thrombosis and thrombocytopenia (2)[A].

ADDITIONAL TREATMENT
General Measures
- Discontinue all heparin products, including flushes and heparin-coated catheters.
- Nonimmune heparin-associated thrombocytopenia generally resolves when heparin is stopped:
  - Consider a nonheparin alternative like fondaparinux if pharmacologic DVT prophylaxis is warranted.
- Avoid platelet transfusions (2)[C].
- Adverse reaction to heparin should be clearly documented in medical record with instruction to avoid all heparin products in the future.
- For patients with a documented history of HIT, under special circumstances only (such as the need for cardiopulmonary bypass), the use of heparin for a short duration may be acceptable if the absence of heparin/PF4 complex antibodies can be documented (7)[C].

IN-PATIENT CONSIDERATIONS
Nursing
- Avoid heparin flushes.
- Avoid platelet transfusion.
- Clearly document reaction in all medical records to avoid the future use of heparin.

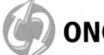

ONGOING CARE
FOLLOW-UP RECOMMENDATIONS
- The transition period of anticoagulation with a DTI and warfarin in patients with HIT can be problematic.
- The INR while administering both a DTI and warfarin should be therapeutic (2–3) for at least 5 days before discontinuing the DTI.
- Warfarin therapy should not be commenced until the platelet count has stabilized within a normal range.
- DTIs can prolong INR; therefore, if INR is >4 while on both warfarin and a DTI, temporarily hold the DTI for 4–6 hours and recheck INR; this second INR will represent only the anticoagulant effect of warfarin.

Patient Monitoring
- Serial platelet counts
- Monitor PTT or INR as determined by the anticoagulation agent

PATIENT EDUCATION
- Patient should inform all health care providers of any previous adverse reaction to heparin.
- HIT information available at: http://medlibrary.org/medwiki/Heparin-induced_thrombocytopenia

PROGNOSIS
- Thrombosis in HIT has 20–30% mortality, with additional morbidity from stroke and limb ischemia
- Platelet counts normalize within weeks after stopping heparin.
- Risk of delayed thrombosis, especially in the first 30 days

REFERENCES
1. Lo GK, Juhl D, Warkentin TE, Sigouin CS, Eichler P, Greinacher A et al. Evaluation of pretest clinical score (4 T's) for the diagnosis of heparin-induced thrombocytopenia in two clinical settings. *J Thromb Haemost*. 2006;4:759–65.
2. Warkentin TE, Greinacher A, Koster A, et al. Treatment and prevention of heparin-induced thrombocytopenia: American College of Chest Physicians Evidence-Based Clinical Practice Guidelines (8th Edition). *Chest*. 2008;133: 340S–380S.
3. Shantsila E, Lip GY, Chong BH. Heparin-induced thrombocytopenia: a contemporary clinical approach to diagnosis and management. *Chest*. 2009;135:1651–64.
4. Dager WE, Dougherty JA, Nguyen PH, et al. Heparin-Induced Thrombocytopenia: Treatment Options and Special Considerations. *Pharmacotherapy*. 2007;27:564–87.
5. Warkentin TE, Greinacher A, Craven S, et al. Differences in the clinically effective molar concentrations of four direct thrombin inhibitors explain their variable prothrombin time prolongation. *Thromb Haemost*. 2005;94:958–64.
6. Warkentin TE, Maurer BT, Aster RH. Heparin-induced thrombocytopenia associated with fondaparinux. *N Engl J Med*. 2007;356:2653–5; discussion 2653–5.
7. Warkentin TE, Kelton JG et al. Temporal aspects of heparin-induced thrombocytopenia. *N Engl J Med*. 2001;344:1286–92.

ADDITIONAL READING
- HIT information. Available at: http://www.heparininducedthrombocytopenia.com/.
- Martel N, Lee J, Wells PS. Risk for heparin-induced thrombocytopenia with unfractionated and low-molecular-weight heparin thromboprophylaxis: a meta-analysis. *Blood*. 2005;106:2710–5.
- Smythe MA, Koerber JM, Mattson JC. The Incidence of Recognized Heparin-Induced Thrombocytopenia in a Large Tertiary Care, Teaching Hospital. *Chest*. 2007.

 CODES

ICD9
289.84 Heparin-induced thrombocytopenia (HIT)

CLINICAL PEARLS
- Heparin exposure through virtually any preparation (including LMWH), any dose, or any route can cause HIT.
- LMWH is contraindicated in HIT; although LMWH is less likely to cause HIT, once HIT is present, the antibodies will cross-react and continue to cause a HIT reaction.
- If a patient is suspected of HIT (with or without confirmatory testing), immediately discontinue of all forms of heparin.
- Patients will require anticoagulation either because of preexisting thrombosis or the risk of thrombosis in first 30 days after HIT.
- A DTI should be used until a patient's INR is therapeutic (2–3) on warfarin for at least 5 days.
- The key to avoiding sequelae from HIT is awareness, vigilance, and a high degree of suspicion.

H

HEPATIC ENCEPHALOPATHY

Walter M. Kim, MD, PhD
Jyoti Ramakrishna, MD

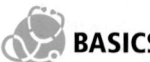

BASICS

DESCRIPTION
- Reversible altered mental and neuromotor functioning associated with acute or chronic liver disease and/or portal systemic shunting of blood
- The prominent features are confusion, impaired arousability, and a "flapping tremor" (asterixis).
- System(s) affected: Gastrointestinal (GI); Nervous
- Synonym(s): HE; Hepatic coma; Liver coma; Portosystemic encephalopathy

EPIDEMIOLOGY
Predominant sex: Male = Female (reflecting underlying liver disease)

Prevalence
- Occurs in 1/3 of cirrhosis cases
- Occurs in all cases of fulminant hepatic failure
- Present in nearly 1/2 of patients who require transplantation
- Parallels the age predominance of fulminant liver disease: Peaks in the 40s; cirrhosis peaks in the late 50s; may occur at any age

RISK FACTORS
In patients with underlying liver disease, precipitating factors include:
- Infection (overt or occult, including spontaneous bacterial peritonitis)
- GI hemorrhage
- Use of sedative or opiate drugs
- Electrolyte disturbance (K^+, Mg^{2+}, or other electrolyte depletion)
- Transjugular intrahepatic portosystemic shunt (TIPS)

Genetics
- Unknown
- Conditions such as cystic fibrosis, α-1-antitrypsin deficiency, and Wilson disease can contribute to HE.

GENERAL PREVENTION
- Recognition of early signs and seeking of prompt treatment
- Avoidance of nonessential medications, particularly opiates and sedatives

PATHOPHYSIOLOGY
- Failure of liver to detoxify agents noxious to the central nervous system (e.g., ammonia, mercaptans, fatty acids)
- Increased aromatic and reduced branched chain amino acids in blood
- These act as false neurotransmitters, possibly interacting with the gamma-aminobutyric acid receptor.

ETIOLOGY
- Shunting of intestinal blood through the severely diseased liver without the intervention of viable liver cells
- Most common in long-standing cirrhosis of the liver with spontaneous shunting of intestinal blood through collaterals
- Shunting of such blood through collateral circulation or surgically constructed portacaval shunts
- TIPS, a widely used radiologically inserted shunt to lower portal pressure, produces HE.
- Acute onset of HE: Search for risk factors.

COMMONLY ASSOCIATED CONDITIONS
- Occurs rarely with portacaval shunt with normal liver function
- May occur as a complication of acute fatty liver of pregnancy

DIAGNOSIS

HISTORY
Preexisting liver disease

PHYSICAL EXAM
- Ages 10–60 years:
  - Prominent signs of underlying liver disease (50%); jaundice most common, ascites 2nd most common
  - GI hemorrhage with hematemesis or melena: 20%
  - Systemic infection, urinary tract or pulmonary: 20%
  - 4 stages of confusion and degree of obtundation described:
    - Stage 1: Forgetfulness, disturbance in nocturnal sleep, daytime drowsiness
    - Stage 2: Mild confusion, drowsy but arousable
    - Stage 3: Patient arousable, markedly confused, with limited orientation and inability to follow commands
    - Stage 4: Patient is unable to be aroused and exhibits extensive posturing.
  - Handwriting and hand coordination deteriorate in stages 1 and 2
  - Asterixis prominent in stage 2
  - Reflexes symmetrically hyperactive in stage 3
  - Psychotic thoughts infrequent
  - Mental and neurologic signs change rapidly (over 6–12 hours)
- Age >60:
  - Signs of underlying liver disease diminish (25%)
  - Confusion more prominent
  - Precipitating GI hemorrhage or infection less often identified
  - Remains in stage 1 or 2 for many days
  - Progression slower
- Age <10:
  - Signs of underlying liver disease prominent; usually fulminant hepatic failure or extremely advanced cirrhosis
  - Progression through the stages very rapid, often 6–12 hours
  - Wilson disease can imitate HE.
- Vital signs:
  - Bradycardia
  - Increased blood pressure suggestive of increased intracranial pressure
- Jaundice, ascites, and other correlates of liver disease
- Central nervous system exam pertaining to stage of HE: Assess short-term memory and presence of asterixis.

DIAGNOSTIC TESTS & INTERPRETATION
- The clinical setting and findings are adequate to establish diagnosis in 80% of the cases.
- The treatment response often confirms the diagnosis.
- Electroencephalogram: Shows symmetric slowing of basic (α) rhythm common with other forms of metabolic encephalopathy (1)[A]; useful to a limited extent
- Visual evoked potential: Specific in stages 2, 3, and 4
- Number connection test, line drawing test, clicker flicker frequency test, and other psychometric tests may be used to assess for minimal HE (2)[A].

Lab
- Liver tests, including aspartate aminotransferase, alanine aminotransferase, and serum albumin to evaluate severity of underlying liver disease
- Prothrombin time elevated in liver failure
- Elevated ammonia often present (3)[A]; levels affected by infusion of amino acid solutions, opiate administration producing severe constipation, uremia, and rapid and severe tissue breakdown, massive burns, trauma, or infection
- Hematology to identify anemia and signs of infection
- Standard biochemistry profile to identify hypokalemia, bilirubinemia, altered calcium status, hypomagnesemia, and hypoglycemia
- Blood urea nitrogen:creatinine ratio >20 suggestive of GI bleeding or dehydration
- Blood, urine, and ascitic fluid cultures to identify infection, if clinically indicated
- Consider arterial blood gases.
- Toxicology screen for illicit drugs

Imaging
- Useful only to rule out other diagnoses
- Computed tomography scan of the head may be most useful (4)[A].
- Magnetic resonance imaging may demonstrate increased T1 signal in globus pallidus.

Diagnostic Procedures/Surgery
Electroencephalogram has typical rhythm (see above).

Pathological Findings
- Brain edema in 100% of fatal cases
- Glial hypertrophy in chronic encephalopathy

DIFFERENTIAL DIAGNOSIS
- Metabolic encephalopathy related to anoxia, hypoglycemia, hypokalemia, hypo- or hypercalcemia, or uremia
- Head trauma, concussion, subdural hematoma
- Transient ischemic attack, ischemic stroke
- Alcohol withdrawal syndrome
- Alcohol intoxication
- Toxic confusion due to medication or drugs
- Meningitis
- Wilson disease
- Reye syndrome

TREATMENT

MEDICATION
First Line
- Lactulose syrup (laxative action decreases colonic transit time, and bacterial digestion acidifies colon promoting excretion of ammonia): 30–60 mL of 50% solution 4 times daily. Diminish to 15–30 mL twice daily when ≥3 bowel movements occur daily.
- Lactulose enema (for patients who cannot tolerate oral lactulose or have suspected ileus): 300 mL plus 700 mL tap water

- If worsening occurs or no improvement in 2 days, add antibiotics:
  – Rifaximin: 400 mg 3 times a day (nonabsorbable antibiotic) (5)[A]
  – Neomycin: 1–2 g per day divided q6–8h, if renal status is good
  – Metronidazole and vancomycin are alternative antibiotics.
- Antacids as needed
- Contraindications:
  – Total ileus
  – Hypersensitivity reaction
- Precautions:
  – Hypokalemia
  – Electrolyte imbalance
  – Renal failure
- For significant possible interactions, refer to manufacturer's profile of each drug.

Second Line
Flumazenil

ADDITIONAL TREATMENT
General Measures
- Identify and vigorously treat precipitating causes: GI bleeding, infection, sedative drugs, and electrolyte imbalance are most common.
- Stage 2 or higher: Ensure adequate fluid intake and at least 1000 kcal (4.19 megajoules) daily; avoid hypoglycemia.
- Give initial enema to all patients without diarrhea.
- If clumsiness and poor judgment are prominent, be sure the patient has the care needed to avoid falls, cuts on broken glass, smoking burns, and machinery/auto accidents.
- Avoid sedative or opiate medications. Benzodiazepine sedatives and opiate derivatives, such as diphenoxylate/atropine, have caused liver coma.
- Stage 4: Protect the airway, as aspiration is common (tracheal intubation is often used); feed intravenously or with jejunal feeding tube.

Issues for Referral
Refer early to a transplant center.

COMPLEMENTARY AND ALTERNATIVE MEDICINE
Probiotics and prebiotics have been associated with improvement of HE through modulation of gut flora (6)[C].

SURGERY/OTHER PROCEDURES
- Artificial liver perfusion devices have proven useful in fulminant hepatic failure to bridge the patient until a donor liver is available for transplantation.
- Stage 3 and 4 patients should be considered for liver transplantation.

IN-PATIENT CONSIDERATIONS
Initial Stabilization
- Monitor closely in stages 1 and 2 when diagnosis is clear and watch for progression.
- Inpatient management for stages 3 and 4
- Stage 3 or 4 in fulminant hepatic failure is a strong indication for evaluation for liver transplantation; transfer to a transplant center should be considered.

 ONGOING CARE

FOLLOW-UP RECOMMENDATIONS
- Activity as tolerated
- Avoid driving or operating machinery.

Patient Monitoring
- To optimize treatment, a trail-making test should be followed (a pencil/paper connect-the-dots according to numbers). Apply to stage 1 and 2 patients to determine how much maintenance treatment is needed and what diet is appropriate. The test should be run daily at first and then at each visit when changes in drugs and diet are made.
- Patients with changed findings should be seen twice weekly.
- Stable patients should be seen monthly.
- Number connection test or line drawing test at each office visit
- In cirrhosis, evaluate for transplantation; death likely in 24 months

DIET
- Integrate with needs of underlying liver disease.
- Lower total protein (0.8–1.2 g/kg/day); vegetable protein diets are better tolerated than animal protein diets; special IV/enteral formulations with increased branched chain amino acids are available.
- Stage 3 and 4 patients need parenteral nutrition or jejunal feeds.
- As coma improves, increase dietary protein as tolerated.
- Have dietitian instruct patient in eating lower-protein diet.

PATIENT EDUCATION
Pamphlets suitable for patient and family are available from the American Association for the Study of Liver Diseases, 1729 King Street, Suite 200, Alexandria, Virginia 22314; (703) 299–9766; www.aasld.org.

PROGNOSIS
- Acute or fulminant disease: With adequate aggressive treatment, disappears without residue or recurrence
- Chronic disease:
  – Coma returns
  – With each recurrence, becomes more and more difficult to treat
  – Plateau of maximum improvement shows a decrement over several years such that the degree of improvement with treatment is less and less; the mortality rate is 80%

COMPLICATIONS
- Recurrence
- With many recurrences, permanent basal ganglion injury (non-Wilsonian hepatolenticular degeneration)
- Hepatorenal syndrome

REFERENCES

1. Saxena N, Bhatia M, Joshi YK, et al. Electrophysiological and neuropsychological tests for the diagnosis of subclinical hepatic encephalopathy and prediction of overt encephalopathy. *Liver*. 2002;22:190–7.
2. Weissenborn K, Ennen JC, Schomerus H, et al. Neuropsychological characterization of hepatic encephalopathy. *J Hepatol*. 2001;34:768–73.
3. Ong JP, Aggarwal A, Krieger D, et al. Correlation between ammonia levels and the severity of hepatic encephalopathy. *Am J Med*. 2003;114:188–93.
4. Quero Guillén JC, Herrerías Gutiérrez JM. Diagnostic methods in hepatic encephalopathy. *Clin Chim Acta*. 2006;365:1–8.
5. Bass NM, Mullen KD, Sanyal A, Poordad F, Neff G, Leevy CB, Sigal S, Sheikh MY, Beavers K, Frederick T, Teperman L, Hillebrand D, Huang S, Merchant K, Shaw A, Bortey E, Forbes WP et al. Rifaximin treatment in hepatic encephalopathy. *N Engl J Med*. 2010;362:1071–81.
6. Liu Q, Duan ZP, Ha DK, et al. Synbiotic modulation of gut flora: effect on minimal hepatic encephalopathy in patients with cirrhosis. *Hepatology*. 2004;39:1441–9.
7. Als-Nielsen B, et al. Non-absorbable disaccharides for hepatic encephalopathy: Systematic review of randomised trials. *Br Med J*. 2004;328:1046–1511.

ADDITIONAL READING

- Blei AT, Córdoba J, Practice Parameters Committee of the American College of Gastroenterology. Hepatic Encephalopathy. *Am J Gastroenterol*. 2001;96:1968–76.
- Ferenci P, Lockwood A, Mullen K, et al. Hepatic encephalopathy—definition, nomenclature, diagnosis, and quantification: final report of the working party at the 11th World Congresses of Gastroenterology, Vienna, 1998. *Hepatology*. 2002;35:716–21.
- Kircheis G, Fleig WE, Görtelmeyer R, et al. Assessment of low-grade hepatic encephalopathy: A critical analysis. *J Hepatol*. 2007.
- Mas A et al. Hepatic encephalopathy: from pathophysiology to treatment. *Digestion*. 2006; 73(Suppl 1):86–93.

See Also (Topic, Algorithm, Electronic Media Element)
Algorithm: Delirium

 CODES

ICD9
572.2 Hepatic encephalopathy

CLINICAL PEARLS
- Closely monitor the mental status of your patient for confusion/drowsiness and through psychometric testing to determine if your patient with liver disease is developing HE.
- Although questions regarding the superiority of lactulose over antibiotics have been raised (7), at present, there is not sufficient evidence to change our current treatment recommendations.
- It is recommended that all patients with HE receive a liver transplantation evaluation.

H

HEPATITIS A

J. Scott Gaertner, MD

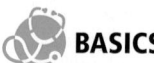 **BASICS**

DESCRIPTION
Infection with the hepatitis A virus (HAV) primarily involving the liver

EPIDEMIOLOGY
Pediatric Considerations
- Disease is often milder or asymptomatic in pediatric population.
- 70% of infections are asymptomatic in children <6 years of age.
- Hepatitis A infection severity increases with age.

Incidence
- In 2007 there were 2,979 HAV infections reported in the US.
- Prior to release of HAV vaccine, there were 22,000–36,000 cases reported per year in the US (1)[B].
- Estimated cases: 25,000 HAV infections in 2007 (lowest ever recorded in US)
- 1.1/100,000 incidence in US
- Predominant sex: Male = Female

Prevalence
Antibodies in 33% of US population

RISK FACTORS
- Foreign travel to developing countries accounts for over 50% of cases in North America and Europe.
- Employment in health care
- Household exposure
- Intimate exposure, especially men who have sex with men
- Institutionalized individuals
- Clotting factor disorders such as hemophilia
- Blood exposure/transfusion rare

Genetics
Autoimmune hepatitis is associated with human leukocyte antigen class II; DR3 and DR4 after active infection with HAV, although rare

GENERAL PREVENTION
- HAV vaccines: Havrix and Vaqta:
  - 0.5 mL IM for children >1 year. 1 mL IM for adults. 2nd dose at 6–12 months.
  - Separate syringe site from immunoglobulin
  - Used for travelers, day care staff/children, custodial facility employees, sewage workers, military, homosexual men, and food handlers. American Academy of Pediatrics recommends routine administration of HAV vaccine to all children 12–23 months of age in all states, according to the Centers for Disease Control-approved immunization schedule.
  - In 2007, self-reporting studies estimated vaccination coverage among adults aged 18–49 years at 12.1% (1)[B].
  - 98% seroprotection at 10 years after primary hepatitis A vaccine
  - HIV infected adults should receive 3 doses at weeks 0, 4, and 24.
  - HAV and hepatitis B virus: Twinrix
- Passive immunization: Immunoglobulin:
  - 0.02–0.06 mL/kg IM given within 2 weeks after exposure prevents illness 80–90%
  - HAV vaccine has similar efficacy to immunoglobulin in postexposure prophylaxis if given within 2 weeks
  - Use immunoglobulin in cases where travelers need immediate protection.
  - Use 0.06 mL/kg q.5 months for long-term travelers if unable to receive vaccine.
  - Do not give immunoglobulin with measles, mumps, rubella, or varicella vaccine.
- Good sanitation
- Good hygiene, including hand washing, especially food handlers, health care, and day care workers
- HAV is NOT killed by freezing.
- HAV is killed by:
  - Heating to 185°F for 60 seconds
  - Chlorine
  - Iodine

Pediatric Considerations
Children <1 year of age

Pregnancy Considerations
Pregnant females who will be traveling

PATHOPHYSIOLOGY
- Hepatitis A vaccine is a single-stranded linear RNA enterovirus and a member of the *Picornaviridae* family.
- Humans are the only natural host.

ETIOLOGY
- Incubation 2–6 weeks (mean of 4 weeks)
- Greatest infectivity is during the 2 weeks before the onset of clinical illness.
- Infection occurs after eating or drinking food or water contaminated with HAV or direct contact with infected person who has poor personal hygiene.
- Food can become contaminated if handled by an infected individual with poor personal hygiene.
- Shellfish, such as clams and oysters, may be contaminated if harvested from waters contaminated with HAV.
- Bloodborne transmission occurs but is rare.
- No chronicity in HAV

COMMONLY ASSOCIATED CONDITIONS
- Arthritis
- Urticaria
- Anemia
- Immune complex nephritis

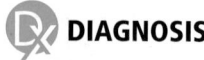 **DIAGNOSIS**

HISTORY
- Fever: 60%
- Malaise: 67%
- Nausea and vomiting
- Anorexia: 54%
- Dark urine: 84%
- Transient pale stools
- Right upper abdominal pain
- Fatigue
- Myalgias
- Symptom severity has direct correlation to age.
- Pediatric cases frequently asymptomatic

PHYSICAL EXAM
- Hepatomegaly
- Fever
- Jaundice
- Icterus
- Right upper abdominal tenderness

DIAGNOSTIC TESTS & INTERPRETATION
Lab
Initial lab tests
- Aspartate aminotransferase (AST) and alanine aminotransferase (ALT) elevated. May exceed 10,000. ALT usually >AST.
- Anti-HAV immunoglobulin M: Positive at time of onset of symptoms
- Anti-HAV immunoglobulin G: Appears soon after IgM and generally persists for years
- Alkaline phosphatase: Mildly elevated
- Bilirubin: Conjugated and unconjugated fractions usually increased. Usually follows rises in ALT and AST.

- Prothrombin time and partial thromboplastin time: Usually remains normal or near normal range:
  – Significant rises should raise concern
- Complete blood count: Mild leukocytosis. Aplasia and pancytopenia are rare:
  – Initial thrombocytopenia may predict illness severity.
- Albumin, electrolytes, and glucose
- Urinalysis: Bilirubinuria

Follow-Up & Special Considerations
Illness usually resolves within 4 weeks from onset of symptoms.

Imaging
- Usually not needed
- Consider ultrasound to rule out differential diagnosis

Initial approach
Bed rest and appropriate nutrition/hydration

Follow-Up & Special Considerations
Usually can be managed outpatient

Diagnostic Procedures/Surgery
Liver biopsy usually not necessary

Pathological Findings
- Pronounced portal inflammation
- Immunofluorescent stains for HAV-antigen positive
- Positive serum markers in hepatitis A:
  – Acute disease: Anti-HAV IgM and IgG positive
  – Recent disease: Anti-HAV IgM and IgG positive
  – Previous disease: Anti-HAV IgM negative and IgG positive

DIFFERENTIAL DIAGNOSIS
- Other hepatitis virus infections B, C, D, E
- Infectious mononucleosis
- Primary or secondary hepatic malignancy
- Ischemic hepatitis
- Drug-induced hepatitis
- Alcoholic hepatitis
- Autoimmune hepatitis
- Wilson disease

 # TREATMENT

MEDICATION
Postexposure prophylaxis to persons within 2 weeks of exposure to hepatitis A virus:
- Administer hepatitis A vaccine to persons between the ages of 1 and 40.
- Administer immunoglobulin to persons <1 and >40 years of age.

First Line
- No antiviral medications indicated, as spontaneous resolution occurs in almost all patients.
- Steroids not indicated unless patient with autoimmune hepatitis

Second Line
- Antiemetics: Metoclopramide 5–20 mg IV/IM t.i.d.
- IV fluids

ADDITIONAL TREATMENT
General Measures
- Monitor coagulation defects, fluid and electrolytes, acid-base imbalance, hypoglycemia, and impairment of renal function.
- Report acute cases to local public health department.

Issues for Referral
- Dictated by severity of illness
- Hepatic failure

COMPLEMENTARY AND ALTERNATIVE MEDICINE
Avoid botanicals with hepatotoxicity potential, including:
- Barberry
- Comfrey
- Golden ragwort
- Groundsel
- Huang qin
- Kava kava
- Pennyroyal
- Sassafras
- Senna
- Valerian
- Wall germander
- Wood sage

SURGERY/OTHER PROCEDURES
Liver transplant in fulminant hepatic failure

IN-PATIENT CONSIDERATIONS
Initial Stabilization
Treatment is usually outpatient

Admission Criteria
Dictated by severity of illness

IV Fluids
Treat dehydration and electrolyte imbalances.

Nursing
Routine

 # ONGOING CARE

FOLLOW-UP RECOMMENDATIONS
Return to work/school 10–14 days after onset of symptoms with diligence to hygiene

Patient Monitoring
- Monitor coagulation defects, fluid and electrolytes, acid-base imbalance, hypoglycemia, and impairment of renal function.
- Report acute cases to local public health department.
- Usually infectious 4 weeks from initial symptoms

DIET
- Adequate balanced nutrition
- Avoid alcohol.
- Avoid medications that may accumulate in the liver.

PATIENT EDUCATION
- Segregation of food handlers with HAV
- HAV immunity after infection

PROGNOSIS
- Excellent
- Mortality 0.2%

COMPLICATIONS
- Coagulopathy, encephalopathy, and renal failure
- Relapsing HAV: Usually milder than the initial case. Positive anti-HAV IgM. Total duration usually less than 9 months.
- Prolonged cholestasis: Characterized by protracted periods of jaundice and pruritus (>3 mo). Resolves without intervention.
- Autoimmune hepatitis: Good response to steroids
- Hepatic failure: Rare (1–2%)

REFERENCE

1. *Vaccine*. 2009 Feb 25;27(9):1301–5. Epub 2009 Jan 20. Hepatitis A vaccination coverage among adults aged 18–49 years in the United States. Lu PJ, Euler GL, Hennessey KA, Weinbaum CM.

ADDITIONAL READING

- Abreu C. *Acta Med Port*. 2007;20(6):557–66. Epub 2008 Feb 13.
- Bianco E, De Masi S, Mele A, Jefferson T. *Digest Liver Disease*. 2004;36(12):834–42.
- Garner-Spitzer E, Kundi M, Rendi-Wagner P, et al. Correlation between humoral and cellular immune responses and the expression of the hepatitis A receptor HAVcr-1 on T cells after hepatitis A re-vaccination in high and low-responder vaccinees. *Vaccine*. 2008.
- Gilroy, Richard K. eMedicine from WebMD. AAFP. *Hepatitis A*. May 30, 2006.
- Launay O, Grabar S, Gordien E, et al. Immunological efficacy of a three-dose schedule of hepatitis A vaccine in HIV-infected adults: HEPAVAC study. *J Acquir Immune Defic Syndr*. 2008;49:272–5.
- Weiland O. Lakartidningen, 2008;105(19): 1371–2.

See Also (Topic, Algorithm, Electronic Media Element)
Hepatitis B; Hepatitis C
Algorithm: Hyperbilirubinemia

 # CODES

ICD9
070.1 Viral hepatitis a without mention of hepatic coma

CLINICAL PEARLS

- Hepatitis A vaccine 2 doses 6–12 months apart
- Indicated for travelers, day care staff/children, custodial facility employees, sewage workers, military, homosexual men, and food handlers
- HAV disease severity directly correlates with age; children are often asymptomatic.

H

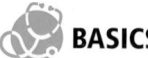

HEPATITIS B

Anne M. Walsh, PA-C, MMSc
Jill A. Grimes, MD

BASICS

DESCRIPTION
Systemic viral infection that may cause acute and chronic liver disease and hepatocellular carcinoma (HCC)

EPIDEMIOLOGY
Incidence
- Predominant age: All ages
- Predominant sex: Fulminant hepatitis B virus (HBV): Male > Female (2:1)
- 60,000 new infections in US in 2008, 70% due to IV drug use

Prevalence
- 2 million people in US with chronic HBV:
  – 5,000 deaths per year
- 350–400 million persons with chronic HBV worldwide:
  – 1,000,000 deaths/year:
    ○ 10th leading cause of death
    ○ 2nd most important carcinogen (behind tobacco)
    ○ 25% of chronic carriers die of cirrhosis or HCC.
    ○ 75% of chronic carriers are Asian.

RISK FACTORS
- Screen high-risk groups with HBsAg/sAb (1)[A]:
  – Persons born in endemic areas (45% of world)
  – Hemodialysis patients
  – IV drug users (IVDU), past or present
  – Men who have sex with men (MSM)
  – HIV- and HCV-positive patients
  – Household members of HBsAg carriers
  – Sexual contacts of HBsAg carriers
  – Inmates of correctional facilities
  – All patients with chronically elevated aminotransferases (ALT/AST)
- Vaccinate all above groups if negative.
- Additional risk factors:
  – Needle stick/occupational exposure
  – Recipients of blood/products
  – Transplanted organ recipient
  – Intranasal drug users
  – Body piercing/tattoos

Genetics
Family history of HBV and/or HCC to determine exposure and future HCC risk

Pediatric Considerations
- Shorter acute course; fewer complications
- 90% of vertical/perinatal infections become chronic.

Marker	Acute Infection	Chronic Infection	Inactive Carrier	Resolved Infection
HBsAg	+	+	+	–
HBsAb	–	–	–	+
HBcAb	+ IgM	– IgM; + total/IgG	+	+
HBeAg	+	±	–	–
HBeAb	–	–/+	+	±
HBV DNA	Present	Present	Low–negative	
	Negative ALT	Marked elevation	Transient mild elevation	Normal

Pregnancy Considerations
- Screen all pregnant women for HBsAg (1)[A].
- High viral load at 28 weeks treated with oral meds from 32 weeks on reduces perinatal transmission (2)[B].

- Infant of HBV-infected mother needs HBIg (0.5 mL) plus HBV vaccine within 12 hours of birth and HBV series at 1 and 6 months (1)[A].
- Breastfeeding safe if HBIg and HBV vaccine administered and nipples without fissures
- HIV coinfection significantly increases risk of vertical transmission.
- Continue medications if pregnancy occurs while on oral antiviral therapy to prevent acute flare.

GENERAL PREVENTION
- Most effective: HBV vaccination series (3 doses):
- Vaccinate:
  – All infants at birth
  – All at-risk patients (see Risk Factors)
  – Health care and public safety workers at high risk
  – Sexual contacts of HBsAg carriers
  – Household contacts of HBsAg carriers
- Proper hygiene/sanitation by health care workers, IVDU, tattoo/piercing artists
  – Barrier precautions, safe handling of needles, proper sterilization of equipment
- Do not share personal items exposed to blood (e.g., nail clipper, razor, toothbrush).
- Advocate safe sexual practices, including use of condoms.
- HBsAg carriers cannot donate blood, tissue, or organs.
- Postexposure (e.g., needlestick): HB immune globulin (HBIg) 0.06 mL/kg in <24 hours

ETIOLOGY
HBV is a DNA virus of the family *Hepadnaviridae*.

COMMONLY ASSOCIATED CONDITIONS
Arthritis, polyarteritis nodosa, membranous glomerulopathy, anemia (including aplastic anemia), dermatitis, cardiomyopathy, hepatitis D virus infection, metabolic syndrome

DIAGNOSIS

HISTORY
- Exposure: Detailed family and social history
- Acute HBV:
  – Fever
  – Malaise/fatigue/arthralgias/myalgias
  – Anorexia/nausea/vomiting
  – Jaundice/scleral icterus
  – Dark urine/pale stools
  – Right upper quadrant abdominal pain
  – Headache/meningismus (occasional)
- Chronic HBV: Typically asymptomatic

PHYSICAL EXAM
- Acute: Ill-appearing; jaundice/scleral icterus; right upper quadrant tenderness, hepatomegaly
- Typically normal in noncirrhotic chronic HBV

DIAGNOSTIC TESTS & INTERPRETATION
Lab
Initial lab tests
- AST/ALT: Marked elevation in acute HBV, particularly of ALT, 400 to several thousand IU/mL (may be normal or mildly elevated in chronic HBV)
  – Elevate before bilirubin elevates
- Bilirubin: Normal to markedly elevated in acute HBV, conjugated/unconjugated
  – Last test to normalize as acute infection resolves
- Alkaline phosphatase: Mild elevation
- HBcAb IgM may be the only early finding ("window period," when HBsAg/sAb–).
- For acute hepatitis
  – Monitor PT, albumin, electrolytes, glucose, CBC
  – If severe acute HBV, check for superinfection with hepatitis D (HDV).
  – Hepatitis B serologic markers
- Hepatitis B e antigen (HBeAg+) indicates high replication/infectivity; confirmed with high HBV DNA ($\geq 10^5$ copies/mL); these patients benefit from medical therapy.
- HBV precore mutants have undetectable HBeAg despite active viral replication (confirm with HBV DNA level) as well as antibody to e antigen (HBeAb+).
- Screen for HIV, HCV, and immunity to HAV (HAV Ab total/IgG).

Follow-Up & Special Considerations
HBsAg+ persistence >6 months = chronic HBV
- Measure HBV DNA level and ALT every 3–6 months.
- Measure baseline α-fetoprotein (AFP).
- Follow HBeAg for loss (every 6–12 months).
- Lifetime monitoring for progression, need for treatment, and screening for HCC

Imaging
- Ultrasound to demonstrate ascites, exclude obstruction, screen for HCC
- Contrast CT or MRI if abnormal ultrasound or elevated AFP

Diagnostic Procedures/Surgery
Liver biopsy determines extent of injury, excludes other liver disease, guides therapy.

Pathological Findings
Liver biopsy in chronic HBV may show interface hepatitis and variable inflammation, necrosis, cholestasis, fibrosis, cirrhosis, or chronic active hepatitis.

DIFFERENTIAL DIAGNOSIS
- EBV; CMV; hepatitis A,C, or E
- Drug-induced, alcoholic, or autoimmune hepatitis
- Wilson disease or rheumatologic/immunologic disorders

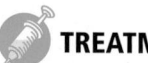

TREATMENT

MEDICATION
First Line
- Acute HBV:
  – Supportive care; antiviral therapy not indicated; spontaneously resolves in 95% of immunocompetent adults

- Chronic HBV: Treatment based on HBeAg status:
  - FDA-approved drugs: Lamivudine 100 mg, adefovir 10 mg, entecavir 0.5–1 mg, telbivudine 600 mg, or tenofovir 300 mg, all given PO every day; pegylated interferon (peg-IFN) α2a SC weekly (1)[A]

Table 2 Chronic Hepatitis B Therapy (1)

HBeAg	HBV DNA Viral Load	ALT*	Recommendation
(+)	≥20,000 IU/mL	Elevated	Treat w/mono or combination therapy
(−)	≥2,000 IU/mL	Elevated	(see above)
(+)	≤20,000 IU/mL	Any	Monitor q6–12mo
(−)	≥2,000 IU/mL	Normal	Biopsy; treat if disease
(+)	≥20,000 IU/mL	Normal	(see above)
(−)	≤2,000 IU/mL	Any	Monitor q6–12mo
Cirrhosis	Any	Any	Treat with combination tx (3)
Decomp	Any	Any	Treat + transplant

*ALT elevated if >2 × ULN; ULN for male = 30 IU/mL and for female = 19 IU/mL

- Lamivudine no longer recommended 1st-line due to high rates of resistance
- Entecavir, tenofovir, peg-IFN are preferred 1st-line agents (1,4)[A]
- Oral agents given for extended period:
  - If HBeAg+, treat 6–12 months post loss of eAg/gain of eAb (1)[A]
  - If HBeAg−, treat indefinitely or until HBsAg clearance (1)[A]
- Change/add drug based on development of resistance:
  - Confirm patient compliance with medications before assuming resistance.
  - Combination therapy lowers rate of resistance.
- Dose adjustment made for elevated creatinine
- Standard IFN (Intron A) no longer used in favor of peg-IFN:
  - Peg-IFN (Pegasys) injections given weekly for 48 weeks
  - Best efficacy in genotype A
  - Contraindicated if decompensated cirrhosis
- Goals of therapy: Undetectable HBV DNA, normalization of ALT, loss of HBeAg and appearance of HBeAb; loss of HBsAg (occurs only with IFN therapy)
- Precautions:
  - Oral drugs: Renal insufficiency, acute flare if discontinued, resistance/mutation development
  - Peg-IFN: Coagulopathy, myelosuppression, depression/suicidal ideation
- Interactions: Refer to manufacturer's profile.

Second Line
Emtricitabine effective; pending FDA approval

ADDITIONAL TREATMENT
General Measures
- Monitor coagulation, electrolytes, glucose, renal function, acid/base
- Report all HBsAg+ to public health department
- Providers must be familiar with medication risks/benefits/side effects, monitoring for development of resistance, and HCC screening guidelines.

Issues for Referral
- Refer all HBsAg+ patients to experienced gastroenterologist/hepatologist for consideration of antiviral therapy.

- Refer to liver transplant program ASAP if fulminant acute hepatitis, end-stage liver disease, or HCC. Resection/ablation of early or noncirrhotic HCC yields excellent outcomes posttransplant.

COMPLEMENTARY AND ALTERNATIVE MEDICINE
No evidence to support alternative treatments

SURGERY/OTHER PROCEDURES
Liver transplantation, operative resection, radiofrequency ablation

IN-PATIENT CONSIDERATIONS
Outpatient treatment usually successful in acute HBV

Admission Criteria
- Worsening course (marked increase in bilirubin, transaminases, or symptoms)
- Hepatic failure (high PT, low albumin)

 ## ONGOING CARE

FOLLOW-UP RECOMMENDATIONS
Activity as tolerated; bed rest during acute symptoms (abdominal pain, N/V, jaundice)

Patient Monitoring
- Vaccinate for HAV if seronegative (1)[B].
- Monitor serial ALT and HBV DNA:
  - High ALT + low HBV DNA associated with favorable response to therapy
- Serologic markers: Useful for evaluation of recovery or progression to chronicity (see chart)
- Metabolic complications and renal function
- WBC/platelets with IFN therapy
- Monitor HBV DNA q3–6 months during therapy:
  - Undetectable DNA at week 24 of oral drug therapy associated with low resistance at year 2.
- Monitor for complications (ascites, encephalopathy, variceal bleed) in cirrhosis.

DIET
Adequate calories, balanced nutrition

PATIENT EDUCATION
- Acute HBV:
  - Review transmission precautions (1)[C] and vaccinate seronegative family members and sexual partners (1)[A].
  - Symptoms, especially fatigue, may take several months to resolve.
- Chronic HBV:
  - Alcohol/smoking increase progression of liver disease and should be avoided.
  - If treated, strict compliance with oral medication is critical to prevent flare.

- Patient education materials in English and Spanish available at http://www.cdc.gov/hepatitis/B/PatientEduB.htm.

PROGNOSIS
- 95% of adults recover from acute infection.
- Severity of encephalopathy predicts survival in fulminant hepatic failure.
- Acute HBV: Mortality 1%
- Acute HBV + HDV: Mortality 2–20%
- Chronic HBV:
  - 0.5% per year spontaneously resolve
  - 25% suffer premature death from cirrhosis or HCC.
  - Baseline DNA predictive: Risk of HCC rises with rate of viral replication, even if no cirrhosis
  - US and AFP q 6–12 months for screening (patient-specific guidelines) (1,3)[B]

COMPLICATIONS
- Acute or subacute hepatic necrosis; cirrhosis; hepatic failure
- Hepatocelluar carcinoma (all chronic HBV patients are at risk)
- Severe flare of chronic HBV with corticosteroids:
  - Avoid if able; taper very slowly if used.
- Reactivation of resolved infection if immunosuppressed (e.g., chemotherapy): Prophylactic premedication recommended if HBsAg+ (1,3).

REFERENCES
1. Lok AS, McMahon BJ. Chronic hepatitis B. *Hepatology.* 2007;45:507–39.
2. Tran T, et al. Management of the pregnant hepatitis B patient. *Curr Hep Rep.* 2008;7:12–7.
3. Weinmaum C, et al. Recommendations for identification and public health management of persons with chronic hepatitis B infection. *MMWR.* 2008;57:1–20.
4. Woo G, Tomlinson G, Nishikawa Y, Kowgier M, Sherman M, Wong DK, Pham B, Ungar WJ, Einarson TR, Heathcote EJ, Krahn M et al. Tenofovir and Entecavir are Most Effective Antiviral Agents for Chronic Hepatitis B; A Systematic Review and Bayesian Meta-Analyses. *Gastroenterology.* 2010;

See Also (Topic, Algorithm, Electronic Media Element)
Hepatitis A; Hepatitis C; Cirrhosis of the Liver
Algorithm: Hyperbilirubinemia

 ## CODES

ICD9
- 070.30 Viral hepatitis b without mention of hepatic coma, acute or unspecified, without mention of hepatitis delta
- 070.32 Chronic viral hepatitis b without mention of hepatic coma without mention of hepatitis delta

CLINICAL PEARLS
- All patients born in endemic countries should be screened with HBsAg.
- Patients with chronic HBV need lifetime monitoring for progressive disease and HCC.

H

HEPATITIS C

Anne M. Walsh, PA-C, MMSc
Frank J. Domino, MD

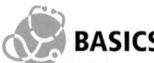 **BASICS**

DESCRIPTION
Systemic viral infection primarily involving liver; can result in acute and chronic disease

EPIDEMIOLOGY
- Predominant age: All ages; most new diagnoses 40–60 years old
- Predominant sex: Both sexes; Male = Female

Geriatric Considerations
Age >60 less likely to respond; treat earlier if able

Pediatric Considerations
- Prevalence: 0.3%
- Fewer symptoms or abnormal liver tests; more likely to clear spontaneously; slower rate of progression

Pregnancy Considerations
- Vertical transmission 1–5% if HIV negative
- Breastfeeding safe if no fissures (1)
- Ribavirin is teratogenic; contraindicated in pregnancy and in male partners of pregnant or impregnable women without contraception

Incidence
- 40,000 new cases of *chronic* hepatitis C virus (HCV) per year in US:
  – Reports of *acute* infections rare (asymptomatic)
  – 2/3 of people with chronic HCV are undiagnosed.
- Rate of new infections reduced since 1992 when effective donor blood screening began

Prevalence
- ~4 million in US (1.8%) ever infected (HCV Ab+)
- ~3 million have chronic HCV (HCV RNA+)
- ~10,000 deaths annually
- Most common cause of chronic liver disease & liver transplant
- Genotype 1 predominant (75% of cases)

RISK FACTORS
- Screen all patients with persistently elevated alanine aminotransferase (ALT) and all patients with known risk factors (1)[B]:
  – Hemodialysis
  – Blood +/– product transfusion before 1992
  – Hemophilia treatment before 1987
  – IV drug use:
    ○ 60–70% of new infections
    ○ *High transmission first use; "once" is high risk*
  – Sexually active homosexual male
  – HIV or hepatitis B infection
  – Household exposure to infected body fluids
  – Organ transplant recipients before 1992
  – Children of HCV+ mothers (test >18 months age)
  – Current sexual partners of HCV+ persons
- Possible risk factors:
  – Inhaled cocaine use; shared works
  – Body piercing and tattoos
  – Unsterile medical equipment
  – Health care worker/occupational risks low unless needlestick
- Universal screening is not recommended.

GENERAL PREVENTION
- No vaccine or postexposure prophylaxis available
- HCV Ab+ does not confer immunity to reinfection.
- Do not share razors/toothbrushes/nail clippers.

- Use and dispose of needles and soiled items properly.
- Sexual transmission rare in long-term partners (1.5%) if monogamous (1)[C].

ETIOLOGY
Single-stranded RNA virus of family *Flaviviridae*

COMMONLY ASSOCIATED CONDITIONS
- Diabetes, metabolic syndrome, iron overload, depression, substance abuse/recovery, autoimmune and hematologic disease
- HIV and hepatitis B coinfections

 DIAGNOSIS

HISTORY
- Determine exposure: *complete* social history
- Chronic HCV: Vast majority mildly symptomatic (nonspecific fatigue) or asymptomatic elevated ALT/aspartate aminotransferase (AST)
- Acute HCV: *If* symptoms develop (rare):
  – Onset 2+ weeks postexposure
  – Persist 2–12 weeks
  – Spontaneous clearance more likely:
    ○ Fever
    ○ Malaise/fatigue, arthralgias/myalgias
    ○ Nausea/vomiting/anorexia
    ○ Jaundice/icterus/pruritis
    ○ Dark urine/ Pale stools
    ○ Right upper quadrant (RUQ) pain

PHYSICAL EXAM
- Typically normal unless advanced fibrosis/cirrhosis
- May have RUQ tenderness/hepatomegaly

DIAGNOSTIC TESTS & INTERPRETATION
Lab
Initial lab tests
- AST/ALT:
  – Normal or transiently elevated in chronic HCV
  – ALT usually 1–2 × ULN; AST may be normal or elevated but < ALT
  – AST/ALT ratio ≥1 associated with cirrhosis; if ratio >2, rule out alcohol abuse
  – Marked elevation only in acute hepatitis (400 to several thousand U/L)
  – If acute, serial PT to monitor for liver failure
- Alkaline phosphatase and GGT: Usually normal; more likely abnormal if cirrhosis, alcohol/fatty liver, or biliary obstruction
- Bilirubin: Normal in chronic HCV unless end-stage disease; markedly elevated in acute HCV (both direct/indirect); occurs after ALT/AST increase, ≥6 weeks post-exposure
- Albumin and PT normal until liver failure
- Anti-HCV negative until 8–9 weeks postexposure
- HCV RNA is positive 1–3 weeks postexposure
- Persistent HCV RNA >6 months = chronic HCV
- False(+) antibody: Autoimmune disease; false (–): immunosuppressed
- Screen for other liver disease (see Differential Diagnosis):
  – Ferritin (moderately high levels typical in HCV), Ceruloplasmin, ANA, α1-Antitrypsin phenotype, Fasting glucose/lipid panel
- If chronic, baseline α-fetoprotein (AFP) serum markers in Hepatitis C diagnosis

Follow-Up & Special Considerations
Vaccinate if seronegative for hepatitis A/B (1)[C].

Imaging
- US: Hepatomegaly, fatty liver, R/O mass
- MRI with contrast if US or AFP abnormal; Early cirrhosis not detectable by imaging

Diagnostic Procedures/Surgery
Liver biopsy recommended in chronic HCV to determine extent of injury, exclude other disease, guide treatment, and determine prognosis (2)[C]

Pathological Findings
- Periportal lymphocytic inflammation with or without necrosis, steatosis, cholestasis, fibrosis, iron
- Inflammation: Grade 0–4; Fibrosis: Stage 0–4

DIFFERENTIAL DIAGNOSIS
- Hepatitis A or B; EBV, CMV
- Acute/chronic alcoholic hepatitis
- Nonalcoholic steatohepatitis (NASH)
- Hemochromatosis, Wilson disease, α1–Antitrypsin deficiency
- Ischemic, drug induced, or autoimmune hepatitis

Serum Markers in Hepatitis C Diagnosis

Result	Marker (Lab Test)
(+)	Anti-HCV (antibody): • ELISA III • RIBA (distinguishes false-positive HCV Ab from spontaneous clearance)
(+)	HCV RNA (viral load); • Qualitative (TMA) • Quantitative, confirms (+) qualitative (PCR or bDNA)
1, 2, 3, 4, or 6 (rare) (also >50 subtypes)	Genotype: (1)[A] • Indeterminate if RNA too low, spontaneous clearance, or false positive anti-HCV • Best response to therapy: 2a, 2b, 3a • Least responsive: 1a, 1b

 TREATMENT

MEDICATION

- Acute HCV: Antiviral therapy highly effective if given within 12 wks of infection (2)[B]:
  – Pegylated interferon (IFN) alone or in combination with low-dose ribavirin, for 12–24 weeks
- Chronic HCV: Antiviral therapy variably effective
  – Peg-IFN/ribavirin combined therapy (1,3)[A]:
    ○ Peg-IFN α2b 1.5 μg/kg SC weekly *OR*
    ○ Peg-IFN α2a 180 mcg SC weekly *WITH*
    ○ Ribavirin 800–1,400 mg p.o., divided, b.i.d. (weight-based)

  – Duration of therapy: 24–72 weeks based on genotype, presence of cirrhosis, HIV coinfection, and rate/degree viral response (check DNA at 4, 12, 24 wks)

- 32–36 weeks of HCV RNA undetectability optimal duration for genotype 1 (4)
- 24 weeks sufficient for genotype 2/3 if early viral response (EVR):
  - Cirrhosis lowers sustained viral response (SVR) by 50% in all genotypes.
  - Dose-reduced ribavirin/therapy interruption, especially before RNA negative, reduces SVR (5)[B]
- Contraindications:
  - Mouse IG, egg, or neomycin allergy
  - Pregnancy/breastfeeding
  - Decompensated liver disease or renal failure
  - Untreated psychiatric disease
  - Corticosteroid use or uncontrolled autoimmune disease
  - DDI in HIV patients (substitute comparable agent)
- Precautions:
  - Disorders of coagulation, anemia or myelosuppression
  - Seizures
  - Depression/suicidal ideation; psychiatric clearance and monitoring recommended
  - Retinopathy (diabetic/hypertensive) needs ophthalmology clearance/monitoring

ADDITIONAL TREATMENT
General Measures
- Report acute cases to health department
- Pretreatment patient counseling is critical.
- Control all other conditions prior to treatment (lipids, glucose, gout, mood, etc.).
- Side effects of IFN/ribavirin:
  - Fatigue, weight loss, insomnia, headache, depression/irritability, cognitive changes, nausea, rash, cough, thyroiditis, alopecia (temporary)
  - Premedicate injections with acetaminophen or NSAIDs if not contraindicated; early and prophylactic treatment of somatic and psychiatric side effects is key to adherence (4).
- Growth factors help maintain dose and tolerability (erythropoietin for ribavirin-induced anemia, G-CSF for IFN-induced neutropenia); however, not associated w/ improved SVR (5)[C]
- Team (PCP, GI, counselor, help line/support group, insurance disease management program, family, 12-step sponsor) improves outcomes (4).

Issues for Referral
- Refer all patients to a gastroenterologist or hepatologist experienced with HCV therapy (2)[C]; clinical trial if patient is uninsured.
- Refer to liver transplant program if fulminant acute hepatitis, at 1st complication of end-stage disease, or at diagnosis HCC (2)[A].

Additional Therapies
- Interferon-alfacon-1 (consensus IFN, Infergen) up to 37% cure rate in nonresponders/relapsers (6)[C].
- Addition of third drug (telaprivir, boceprevir) offers improved SVR but increased adverse effects; FDA approval is pending.

COMPLEMENTARY AND ALTERNATIVE MEDICINE
- No medical evidence exists for using herbal or alternative therapy in HCV/cirrhosis/HCC (1)[C].
- Milk thistle (silymarin) generally safe and may reduce ALT but does not eradicate virus nor improve outcomes; avoid while on IFN.
- Rate of HCC tripled in patients on herbal therapy compared to IFN therapy (3).

 ## ONGOING CARE
FOLLOW-UP RECOMMENDATIONS
- If treatment is deferred, annual liver function tests; monitor for complications/associated conditions; and maintain sobriety/recovery.
- No need to monitor serial viral load unless on antiviral therapy; unrelated to disease severity or prognosis, and individual lab assays not well standardized.
- In cirrhosis, lifetime risk HCC 20%; screen with US/AFP every 6–12 months (2)[C].

Patient Monitoring
- Serial ALT/AST; serial fasting glucose
- Serial Hgb/Hct, white blood cells, absolute neutrophil count, platelets
- Follow electrolytes, TSH, renal function, PT
- HCV qualitative RNA negativity at week 4 is rapid viral response (RVR); confers ~90% chance of SVR in all genotypes (1)
- HCV quantitative RNA negativity (or drop of ≥2 log) at week 12 is EVR; confers good chance SVR
- SVR also more likely in patients with (4):
  - Age ≤40; Female gender; Caucasian race
  - Absence of bridging fibrosis/cirrhosis
  - HCV RNA <800,000 IU/mL
  - Genotypes 2 and 3
  - BMI <30 kg/m^2
  - Absence of insulin resistance and steatosis
  - Absence of HIV
  - Recent infection (e.g., needle stick)
- HCV RNA level without 2 log drop at week 24 indicates nonresponse; consider switching to interferon alfacon-1 (Infergen, daily injections) and continue combination therapy ≥6 months.
- HCV RNA positive but ≥2 log drop indicates extending current therapy may be beneficial; continue up to 72 weeks if tolerated (4)[C] or switch to Infergen.
- Monitor for decompensation (low albumin, ascites, encephalopathy, GI bleed) in cirrhotics.
- Goal of therapy is SVR: Eradication of HCV by negative qualitative RNA (TMA) 6 months post-treatment (relapse extremely rare after 6 months)

DIET
- Healthy diet (low-fat, high-fiber) and exercise to prevent/treat obesity/fatty liver
- Extra protein and fluids while on IFN therapy

PATIENT EDUCATION
- Educate patients to avoid alcohol, tobacco, and drugs (including marijuana) at diagnosis; refer to rehab/12-step program and monitor for relapse.
- Caution patients against Internet/alternative medicine claims of false cures.
- Recommend avoidance of herbs (may contain hepatotoxins and contaminants) as well as hepatotoxic medications and vitamins/supplements.

PROGNOSIS
- 70–80% of acute infections become chronic.
- 30% of chronic infections will progress to cirrhosis at a rate of 1–3%/year over 10–30 years.
- 30% of cirrhosis progresses to liver failure and/or cancer (HCC); more rapid if:
  - Older age when infected; Male gender; Alcohol/substance abuse
  - HIV or HBV coinfection; Insulin resistance/diabetes (7)

- IFN therapy, regardless of viral response, slows/improves progressive fibrosis and reduces risk HCC.
- Chronic HCV is *curable* in ~50% of cases; in noncirrhotic genotype 2 or 3, cure rate ~90%

COMPLICATIONS
- Acute/subacute hepatic necrosis, liver failure, transplant and complications, death
- HCC: Risk factors include cirrhosis, age >55, male, obesity/diabetes/fatty liver, and ongoing alcohol/tobacco/marijuana/drug use.

REFERENCES
1. Ghany M, Strader D et al. AASLD Practice Guidelines: Diagnosis, Management, and Treatment of Hepatitis C: An Update. *Hepatology*. 2009;49:1335–74.
2. Chronic Hepatitis C: Current Disease Management, NIH Pub. no. 07-4230 Nov. 2006. Available at: http://digestive.niddk.nih.gov/ddiseases/pubs/chronichepc/ Accessed 5/15/10.
3. Plequezuelo M, et al. Does HCV antiviral therapy decrease the risk of hepatocellular carcinoma? *Curr Hepatitis Rep*. 2008;7:72–9.
4. Agudelo E, et al. Optimizing therapy in treatment-naïve genotype 1 patients. *Curr Hepatitis Rep*. 2008;7:64–71.
5. Shiffman ML. Optimizing the current therapy for chronic hepatitis C virus: peginterferon and ribavirin dosing and the utility of growth factors. *Clin Liver Dis*. 2008;12:487–505, vii.
6. Leevy CB. Consensus interferon and ribavirin in patients with chronic hepatitis C who were nonresponders to pegylated interferon alfa-2b and ribavirin. *Dig Dis Sci*. 2008;53:1961–6.
7. Zein N. Steatosis and metabolic syndrome: An emerging enigma in the natural history of chronic hepatitis C. *Curr Hepatitis Rep*. 2008;7:61–3.

See Also (Topic, Algorithm, Electronic Media Element)
Hepatitis A; Hepatitis B; Cirrhosis of the Liver
Algorithm: Hyperbilirubinemia

CODES
ICD9
- 070.54 Chronic hepatitis c without mention of hepatic coma
- 070.70 Unspecified viral hepatitis c without hepatic coma

CLINICAL PEARLS
- Hepatitis A&B vaccines if seronegative.
- 1 in 10 patients with hepatitis C have no identifiable risk factors.
- 15–25% of infected persons spontaneously clear their infection without treatment.

H

HEPATITIS, AUTOIMMUNE

Vilas Patwardhan, MD
Rashmi V. Patwardhan, MD

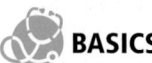 **BASICS**

DESCRIPTION
- Autoimmune hepatitis (AIH) is a chronic inflammatory disorder of the liver, of unknown etiology, characterized by interface hepatitis, hypergammaglobulinemia, and autoantibodies.
- Type I (classic, most common):
  – Affects all age groups
- Type II (ALKM-1):
  – Primarily affects young females and children
- Type III (SLA/LP) is clinically identical to type I, but with different antibody profile:
  – Least well-established type

EPIDEMIOLOGY
Incidence
1.9 per 100,000 per year
Prevalence
16.9 per 100,000

RISK FACTORS
- Female sex
- Bimodal age distribution: Adolescents and adults in the 4th–6th decades are most at risk.
- Associated autoimmune conditions (see Associated Conditions)

Genetics
- Associated with HLA B8, DR3, and DR4
- Recent data show associations between microsatellite markers on chromosomes 11 and 18 (D11S902 and D18S464) and type I AIH (1).

PATHOPHYSIOLOGY
Chronic inflammation of the liver leads to fibrosis and eventually cirrhosis in advanced cases. Acute fulminant inflammation can lead to acute liver failure in the absence of cirrhosis.

ETIOLOGY
Unknown

COMMONLY ASSOCIATED CONDITIONS
- Type I diabetes mellitus
- Thyroiditis
- Immune-mediated hemolytic anemia
- Idiopathic thrombocytopenic purpura
- Celiac sprue
- Ulcerative colitis
- Vitiligo
- Rheumatoid arthritis
- Primary biliary cirrhosis and primary sclerosing cholangitis occasionally overlap with AIH (1).

DIAGNOSIS

HISTORY
- Symptoms range from asymptomatic to vague nonspecific symptoms to acute fulminant hepatic failure.
- 40% of cases are abrupt in onset.
- Course is often fluctuating.
- Right upper quadrant (RUQ) pain, nausea, jaundice, pruritus
- Fatigue, anorexia, arthralgias (usually of the small joints)
- Often history of other autoimmune disorders, especially in type II AIH

PHYSICAL EXAM
Physical exam may be normal at the time of presentation:
- Hepatomegaly, splenomegaly, jaundice
- Stigmata of chronic liver disease

DIAGNOSTIC TESTS & INTERPRETATION
Simplified criteria for the diagnosis of AIH by the International Autoimmune Hepatitis Group, 2008 (1)[C] based on:
- IgG:
  – 1 point for IgG >16 g/L and 2 points for IgG >18 g/L
  – 1 point for antinuclear antibodies (ANA) or antismooth muscle antibodies (ASMA >1:40)
  – 2 points for ANA, ASMA >1:80
- Autoantibodies:
  – 2 points for positive soluble liver antigen (SLA)
- Histology:
  – 2 points for histology typical for AIH
- Exclusion of viral hepatitis:
  – 2 points for negative viral hepatitis markers
- Diagnosis:
  – 6 points or greater made diagnosis of AIH very likely
  – 8 points confirmed definite AIH

Lab
Initial lab tests
- AST, ALT, alkaline phosphatase:
  – AST and ALT >2–10 times normal (2,3)[C]
  – Alk phos:AST (or ALT) ratio of <1.5 suggests AIH (2)[C]
- IgG >1.5–2.0 times normal suggests AIH (2,3)[C]

- Autoantibodies with titers >1:40–80 suggests AIH, including (2,3)[C]:
  – Antinuclear antibodies (ANA)
  – Antismooth muscle antibodies (ASMA)
  – Antibodies to liver/kidney microsomes (ALKM-1) (suggests type II AIH)
  – Antiliver cytosol 1 antibodies (LC-1) (suggests type II AIH) (2,3)[C]
  – Antisoluble liver antigen/liver-pancreas antibodies (SLA/LP) in type III (4)[C]:
    ○ Presence of antimitochondrial antibodies makes AIH less likely.
- Autoantibodies are suggestive but are not diagnostic by themselves.
- If patient negative for conventional autoantibodies but AIH is suspected, other serological markers, including at least anti-SLA and atypical pANCA, should be tested (5)[B]

Imaging
RUQ ultrasound and cholangiography can help distinguish obstructive from nonobstructive liver injury.

Diagnostic Procedures/Surgery
Liver biopsy

Pathological Findings
- Interface hepatitis; plasma cell infiltrate and rosettes also common (1)[C]
- Portal mononuclear cell infiltrate (3)[C]
- Eosinophils frequently present (3)[C]
- Biliary tree generally spared (3)[C]
- Fibrosis usually present with bridging in advanced cases (3)[C]

DIFFERENTIAL DIAGNOSIS
- AIH is a diagnosis of exclusion; hereditary, viral, and drug-induced causes must be ruled out.
- Primary biliary cirrhosis
- Primary sclerosing cholangitis
- Acute or chronic viral hepatitis
- Steatohepatitis (alcoholic or nonalcoholic)
- Systemic lupus erythematosus
- Wilson disease
- Hemochromatosis
- α1-Antitrypsin deficiency
- Drug-induced hepatitis (e.g., minocycline, isoniazid, methyldopa, nitrofurantoin, atorvastatin) (2,3)

TREATMENT

MEDICATION
- Treatment generally indicated in the following conditions (4,6)[C]:
  - AST >10 times normal
  - AST >5 times normal with serum gamma globulin >2 times normal
  - Histological features of bridging necrosis or multiacinar necrosis
- Treatment generally indicated in pediatric patients
- Treatment may be deferred in the following situations (4)[C]:
  - Asymptomatic interface hepatitis without necrosis
  - AST <5 times normal
  - Inactive cirrhosis
  - Decompensated inactive cirrhosis

First Line
- Prednisone (10–30 mg) with azathioprine (50–100 mg) (2,3,4)[B]:
  - Preferred therapy
- Prednisone (20–60 mg) alone (2,3,4)[B]
- Combination therapy preferred for the following conditions (3,4,6)[C]:
  - Osteoporosis
  - Postmenopause
  - Diabetes
  - HTN
  - Obesity
  - Acne
  - Depression
- Prednisone alone preferred for the following conditions (3,4,6)[C]:
  - TPMT deficiency
  - Cytopenias
  - Pregnancy

Second Line
- 6-Mercaptopurine may be substituted for azathioprine (2,4)[C].
- Cyclosporine may be used in children who do not tolerate prednisone or who are steroid-resistant (1,2,4)[C].
- Cyclophosphamide, mycophenate mofetil, deflazacort, and tacrolimus have shown some benefit in small trials (1,2)[C].

ADDITIONAL TREATMENT
General Measures
Keep patient comfortable, with analgesics and antiemetics as necessary.

Geriatric Considerations
Use corticosteroids with caution in the elderly.

Pediatric Considerations
AIH is often more advanced in children, and treatment is generally advised.

Pregnancy Considerations
- AIH is associated with increased risk of low birth weight, prematurity, and fetal demise.
- Pregnancy is not a contraindication to treatment.
- Patients may require less immunosuppression during pregnancy.
- β-Blockers and short 2nd stage of labor recommended if varices are present in 2nd trimester.

SURGERY/OTHER PROCEDURES
Liver transplant for liver failure

IN-PATIENT CONSIDERATIONS
Admission Criteria
- No strict criteria; clinical judgment based on patient symptoms
- Severe cases should be admitted for monitoring of and to prevent fulminant hepatic failure.

IV Fluids
If significant nausea or vomiting occurs, replace fluid losses.

ONGOING CARE

FOLLOW-UP RECOMMENDATIONS
Follow AST, ALT, autoantibodies, IgG, and histology.

Patient Monitoring
- Although clinical and laboratory findings can resolve within 2 weeks, treatment should be continued for at least 3–6 months after this because histologic improvement lags behind clinical improvement (3,4)[C].
- Liver biopsy should be obtained before discontinuing or reducing the maintenance immunosuppressive dose (4)[C].
- Liver biopsy may also be helpful for monitoring. Biopsy is suggested 1 year after normalization of laboratory values and/or 2 years after initial presentation (3)[C].
- Monitor AST, ALT, and autoantibodies regularly after discontinuing therapy. May decrease frequency of monitoring if no relapse occurs:
  - Treatment of relapse is the same as initial presentation of AIH.
- Long-term maintenance therapy is indicated for multiple relapses.
- Consider screening for hepatocellular carcinoma in patients with cirrhosis every 6–12 months with ultrasound and α-fetoprotein measurements or yearly liver MRI.

DIET
As tolerated

PATIENT EDUCATION
- Diet to control weight and lipids is advised.
- Avoid hepatotoxic drugs such as alcohol and acetaminophen.

PROGNOSIS
- Untreated 5- and 10-year survival rates are 50% and 10%, respectively (1,2)[C].
- With treatment, survival >80% at 20 years (no statistical difference from general population) (3,4)[C]

- 80–90% will relapse following discontinuation of therapy (6)[C].
- 10% of patients will fail immunosuppressive therapy. These patients will ultimately need liver transplant (6)[C].
- Survival after liver transplant is 80–90% at 5 years and 75% at 10 years with recurrence of AIH up to 42% (3,6)[C].

COMPLICATIONS
- Fulminant hepatic failure requiring liver transplant
- Cirrhosis
- Hepatocellular carcinoma in patients who develop cirrhosis

REFERENCES

1. Teufel A, Galle PR, Kanzler S. Update on autoimmune hepatitis. *World J Gastroenterol.* 2009;15:1035–41.
2. Manns MP, Vogel A. Autoimmune hepatitis, from mechanisms to therapy. *Hepatology.* 2006;43: S132–44.
3. Krawitt EL. Autoimmune hepatitis. *N Engl J Med.* 2006;354:54–66.
4. Al-Khalidi JA, Czaja AJ. Current concepts in the diagnosis, pathogenesis, and treatment of autoimmune hepatitis. *Mayo Clin Proc.* 2001;76:1237–52.
5. Manns MP, Czaja AJ, Gorham JD, Krawitt EL, Mieli-Vergani G, Vergani D, Vierling JM, American Association for the Study of Liver Diseases et al. Diagnosis and management of autoimmune hepatitis. *Hepatology.* 2010;51:2193–213.
6. Heathcote J. Treatment Strategies for Autoimmune Hepatitis. *Am J Gastroenterol.* 2006;101: S630–S632.

See Also (Topic, Algorithm, Electronic Media Element)
Algorithm: Hyperbilirubinemia

CODES

ICD9
571.42 Autoimmune hepatitis

CLINICAL PEARLS
- Treatment must continue for 3–6 months despite clinical and lab findings returning to normal within weeks.
- Alk phos: AST (or ALT) ratio of <1.5 suggests AIH.
- Children generally require treatment, but adults may not progress enough to require medications.

H

HEPATOMA

Michael Engels, MD
Nadeem Anwar, MD

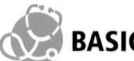 **BASICS**

DESCRIPTION
Primary malignant tumor of the liver arising from hepatic parenchymal cells (hepatocytes), blood vessels, or cholangioles within the liver, excluding gallbladder and biliary passages; with the exception of the rare fibrolamellar type, 85% are associated with an underlying liver disease, usually cirrhosis.

EPIDEMIOLOGY
Incidence
- 5th most common malignancy worldwide
- 3–4 new cases/100,000 of the US population per year
- Among known cirrhotics, 2–5 cases/100 cirrhotics/year

Prevalence
- Asians > whites > blacks > Hispanics > Native Americans
- Predominant age: Mean age 55–62 years in West, 2–3 decades earlier in Asia and Africa
- Predominant sex: Male > Female (3–4:1)

RISK FACTORS
- For hepatocellular carcinoma (HCC):
  - 80–90% HCC occurs in context of cirrhosis (1)[B]
  - HCC can occur with cirrhosis from any cause: Hepatitis B and C, alcoholism, hemochromatosis, nonalcoholic steatohepatitis, α_1–antitrypsin deficiency, biliary cirrhosis, autoimmune hepatitis, Wilson's disease
  - Fungal aflatoxins (contaminants of grain in Africa and Asia) have a synergistic effect with other causes of liver disease.
  - Choledochal cysts
  - Clonorchiasis
  - Tyrosinemia
  - Nonalcoholic fatty liver disease/nonalcoholic steatohepatitis (2)[C]
- For fibrolamellar type: Risk factors unknown
- For angiosarcoma: Vinyl polymer

Genetics
No known genetic pattern

GENERAL PREVENTION
- The major risk factor for HCC is cirrhosis from any cause. Prevention of cirrhosis and monitoring for tumors in patients with or at risk for cirrhosis are keys to prevention.
- Prevent hepatitis B virus (HBV) and hepatitis C virus (HCV) infection/cirrhosis. Safe sexual practices; avoid shared drug paraphernalia; HBV vaccination in high-risk individuals and all children
- Treat chronic HBV and HCV with lamivudine, adefovir, entecavir, tenofovir, or ribavirin/pegylated interferon according to guidelines to avoid cirrhosis.
- Avoid excessive alcohol use.
- Screening for cancer in at-risk individuals by ultrasonography every 6–12 months

- High risk:
  - HBV
  - HCV
  - Alcoholic cirrhosis
  - Genetic hemochromatosis
  - Primary biliary cirrhosis
  - HCC progresses gradually from dysplastic nodules through eventual vascular invasion (usually occurs after tumor reaches 2 cm diameter). For patients at risk, liver imaging should be done every 6 months (3)[B].
- Patients exposed to 10 years or more of vinyl chloride should have sonography every 6 months. New nodules should be biopsied promptly.

ETIOLOGY
- Cirrhosis accounts for 80–90% HCC. Alcoholic cirrhosis is most important in Western world. Reported risk of hepatoma in alcoholic cirrhosis is 3–10% with micronodular pattern.
- HBV and HCV independent and synergistic risk factors for HCC:
  - Associated with >70% of cases worldwide
  - Most important factor in Africa and Asia
- Chronic alcohol use
- Chronic smoking
- Mycotoxins (aflatoxins): Metabolite of the fungus *Aspergillus flavus* that contaminates foods
- Vinyl polymer, but not the finished product, produces angiosarcoma.

COMMONLY ASSOCIATED CONDITIONS
See Risk Factors.

 DIAGNOSIS

- In children:
  - Feminization, precocious puberty
  - Palpable nodule on liver
  - In children aged 2–6 years, abdominal mass in liver, abdominal pain, irregular hepatomegaly
- In adults:
  - Known cirrhosis or prominent clinical signs of cirrhosis: 80%
  - Abdominal pain: 80%; right upper quadrant, dull ache to severe
  - Hepatomegaly: 80–90%; irregular, nodular, firm to hard, tender
  - Weight loss: 30%
  - Hepatic arterial bruit: 20%
  - Friction rub: Rare; more common in metastatic liver disease
  - Nausea, vomiting
  - Paraneoplastic syndrome: Hypertrophic osteoarthropathy, carcinoid syndrome, feminization, polycythemia
  - Hemoperitoneum: Most common tumor cause
  - Unexplained deterioration of stable cirrhosis
  - Budd-Chiari syndrome

DIAGNOSTIC TESTS & INTERPRETATION
Lab
- Liver function test abnormalities
- Rare paraneoplastic syndrome: Erythrocytosis, elevated calcium, low glucose
- Tumor markers:
  - α-Fetoprotein (AFP): Single most important lab test for diagnosis of HCC
  - AFP has low sensitivity for detecting early HCC (25–60% sensitivity, 80% specificity), and it is not recommended as a screening test unless ultrasound (US) is not available (1)[B].
  - Level >400 ng/mL (>400 μg/L) is diagnostic. Level >200 ng/mL highly suspicious for HCC; level does not correlate with prognosis; useful in monitoring for recurrence
  - Fibrolamellar carcinoma usually does not produce AFP.
- Disorders that may alter lab results (all cause a slight elevation in AFP):
  - Acute or chronic hepatitis
  - Germ cell tumors
  - Pregnancy

Imaging
- US (3)[B]:
  - Capable of detecting tumor >1 cm, performance dependent on examiner, technology, cirrhosis (cirrhosis decreases sensitivity)
  - May be positive when AFP is normal
  - Has been useful in serially following cases of cirrhosis to identify hepatocellular cancer when <2 cm and curable
  - If US positive, computed tomography (CT) scan or magnetic resonance imaging (MRI) to confirm (3)[B]
  - Also may be used to guide percutaneous liver biopsy and to guide other percutaneous guided therapy (injection or ablation)
- CT scan:
  - Can detect tumors at 1 cm
  - Valuable in determining extrahepatic spread of the disease
- Positron emission tomography (PET)/PET-CT improves CT detection rates.
- MRI: More sensitive than helical CT scan for early detection of HCC; may help to differentiate benign from malignant tumors; helpful in delineating the details of tumor and invasion of vessels
- Imaging of focal hepatic mass >2 cm with certain characteristic contrast enhancement features can be sufficient for diagnosis (3)[B].
- Hepatic arteriography: Less commonly used as MRI technology improves; used to define vascular anatomy for resection or embolization

Diagnostic Procedures/Surgery
- Tissue diagnosis must be made for mass seen on imaging with atypical findings for HCC or in a noncirrhotic liver. Tissue confirmation is also useful to rule out metastases from other primary sites (3)[B].
- Liver biopsy: Usually US- or CT-guided when nodules are not palpable
- Laparoscopy: Occasionally used to evaluate extent in cirrhosis

Pathological Findings

- Nodular: 75%; usually in cirrhotic liver
- Massive: Common in children and noncirrhotic livers; more prone to rupture
- Diffuse: Rare; a large part of liver is involved
- Hepatocellular origin: Most commonly multicentric, well differentiated; usually superimposed on underlying cirrhosis

DIFFERENTIAL DIAGNOSIS

- Early asymptomatic tumor; underlying liver conditions:
  - Cirrhosis
  - Chronic hepatitis
  - Benign liver nodules
  - Hamartoma
  - Hemangioma
  - Metastatic adenocarcinoma
  - Gallstones
  - Gallbladder polyp
- Late symptomatic tumor with hepatomegaly:
  - Hepatic cyst
  - Adenoma
  - Hemangioma
  - Abscess
  - Metastatic malignancy of liver
  - Cirrhosis
  - Thrombosis of hepatic veins, portal vein, or inferior vena cava
  - Active viral hepatitis or alcoholic hepatitis
- Ruptured tumor: All causes of acute abdomen
- Traumatic hemoperitoneum

TREATMENT

MEDICATION

- Chemotherapy offers no survival benefit.
- Treatment of hepatoma in patients with HCV with pegylated interferon-α and ribavirin prolongs survival and improves quality of life.

SURGERY/OTHER PROCEDURES

- Surgical resection and liver transplantation offer highest cure rate in HCC (1)[B]:
  - Resection should be considered in children and may include up to 1 lobe of the liver.
  - In noncirrhotic patients with HCC, if preserved liver function, no portal hypertension, resection is preferred treatment. Transplantation is preferred treatment for all others who meet transplantation criteria (1)[B].
  - Advanced liver disease, medical comorbidities, extrahepatic metastases are common and result in only 15–30% of HCC patients being eligible for resection (1)[B].
  - High cure rate for both surgical options when ≤3 or fewer nodules, each <5 cm
- Percutaneous treatments best for unresectable disease, as bridge to surgical resection/transplantation, and for early-stage tumors not eligible for surgery
  - Radiofrequency ablation (RFA) considered superior to alcohol injection for localized therapy (4)[B]
  - Recent trials showed similar survival rates for RFA vs surgical resection in small HCCs, but insufficient evidence to change recommendations favoring surgery at this time (5)[B].

- Embolization of the tumor-supplying artery with chemotherapy, under radiographic guidance, is effective palliation and may make surgery possible (6)[B].
- For patients not appropriate for surgery, 2 approaches:
  - Regional transarterial therapy (which delivers chemotherapy directly to the tumor via its immediate blood supply) for intermediate-stage tumors
  - Local chemical and thermal ablative therapies (which cause tumor necrosis by injecting the agent into the tumor itself) for early-stage tumors
  - The 2 approaches can be used together and may yield a better outcome than either treatment alone (6)[B].
- Fibrolamellar variant should be treated by surgical resection, which yields excellent survival.

 ## ONGOING CARE

FOLLOW-UP RECOMMENDATIONS
Patient Monitoring
- After successful resection, a high risk for recurrence
- Check AFP every 3 months.
- Ultrasound every 4–6 months

DIET
Attention to nutrition: High-calorie diet

PATIENT EDUCATION
Emphasize preventive measures and HBV vaccine.

PROGNOSIS
- Unresectable symptomatic tumors: Grave; patients seldom live >6 months.
- Resectable asymptomatic tumors:
  - Surgery is curative in >70% of children, 40% of adults
  - Surgery is curative in >80% of tumors <3 cm in cirrhotics.
- Transplantation: Same survival as that for tumor-free patients when hepatoma is incidentally discovered or is <2 cm in diameter; 5-year survival rate of >70% with 1 lesion <5 cm or maximum of 3 lesions <3 cm (UNOS criteria) (3)[B]

COMPLICATIONS
- Rupture
- Hemoperitoneum
- Liver failure
- Cachexia
- Metastases to other organs
- Thrombosis of portal, hepatic, renal veins

REFERENCES

1. Cha CH, Saif MW, Yamane BH, Weber SM et al. Hepatocellular carcinoma: current management. *Curr Probl Surg*. 2010;47:10–67.
2. Siegel AB, Zhu AX et al. Metabolic syndrome and hepatocellular carcinoma: two growing epidemics with a potential link. *Cancer*. 2009;115:5651–61.
3. El-Serag HB, Marrero JA, Rudolph L, Reddy KR et al. Diagnosis and treatment of hepatocellular carcinoma. *Gastroenterology*. 2008;134:1752–63.
4. Cho YK, Kim JK, Kim MY, Rhim H, Han JK et al. Systematic review of randomized trials for hepatocellular carcinoma treated with percutaneous ablation therapies. *Hepatology*. 2009;49:453–9.
5. Delis S, Bakoyiannis A, Papailiou J, Tassopoulos N, Dervenis C et al. Liver resection vs radio-frequency ablation in the treatment of small hepatocellular carcinoma. *Surg Oncol*. 2009;
6. Garrean S, Hering J, Helton WS, et al. A primer on transarterial, chemical, and thermal ablative therapies for hepatic tumors. *Am J Surg*. 2007;194:79–88.

ADDITIONAL READING

- Colli A, Fraquelli M, Casazza G, et al. Accuracy of ultrasonography, spiral CT, magnetic resonance, and alpha-fetoprotein in diagnosing hepatocellular carcinoma: a systematic review. *Am J Gastroenterol*. 2006;101:513–23.
- Stipa F, Yoon SS, Liau KH, et al. Outcome of patients with fibrolamellar hepatocellular carcinoma. *Cancer*. 2006;106:1331–8.

 ## CODES

ICD9
155.0 Malignant neoplasm of liver, primary

CLINICAL PEARLS

- With benign liver tumors, most patients will have normal liver function tests; 97% with HCC will have at least 1 abnormal test.
- Fibrolamellar carcinoma, which occurs at younger age (mean 25 years), is more likely to present with resectable lesions and higher cure rate after resection (6)[B].
- In Africa and Asia, there is a younger onset (3rd and 4th decades); Male:Female ratio is 6–7:1; aflatoxin and HBV are the major factors; more progressive and fulminant; more likely to be unresectable at presentation.

H

HEPATORENAL SYNDROME

Saira Khan, MD

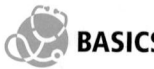

BASICS

- Hepatorenal syndrome (HRS): development of renal failure in patients with end-stage liver disease (ESLD) who have portal hypertension (HTN) and ascites with poor prognosis
- Histological appearance of the kidneys is normal; they may resume normal function following liver transplantation.

DESCRIPTION
- HRS is a diagnosis of exclusion.
- Spontaneous bacterial peritonitis (SBP) frequently precipitates HRS (approximately 1/3 of patients with SBP will develop HRS) and should be ruled out in all ESLD patients. Prompt therapy with IV antibiotics and albumin decreases the risk of developing HRS.
- HRS is a functional disorder (reversal of renal dysfunction by liver transplantation restores renal function).
- HRS classification:
  – Type 1: Rapidly progressive decline in serum creatinine >2.5 or a >50% drop in GFR in 2 weeks
  – Type 2: Slowly progressive (>2 weeks), less severe, usually associated with ascites resistant to diuretics
- System(s) affected: Endocrine/Metabolic; Gastrointestinal (GI); Hemic/Lymphatic/Immunologic; Nervous; Renal/Urologic
- Synonym(s): Renal failure of cirrhosis; functional renal failure of cirrhosis; hepatic nephropathy; Heyde syndrome; oliguric renal failure of cirrhosis; hemodynamic renal failure of cirrhosis

EPIDEMIOLOGY
- Up to 40% of patients with cirrhosis and ascites will develop HRS during the natural history of the disease.
- Predominant age: Usually after 4th decade (increased incidence of alcoholic cirrhosis)
- Predominant gender: Male > Female

Incidence
Unclear; explicit differentiation between HRS and acute tubular necrosis (ATN) or prenal state not always made:
- In a prospective study of 229 the incidence of HRS in nonazotemic cirrhotic patients with ascites was reported as 18% at 1 year and 39% at 5 years. For acute fulminant liver disease: the incidence of HRS is 20–30% at 1 year.
- Estimate: 32–41/100 admitted to the hospital for cirrhosis with ascites develop HRS by 2 and 5 years

RISK FACTORS
- Any reduction of effective blood volume in cirrhosis, including:
  – Volume depletion (excessive diuretics, large-volume paracentesis, etc.)
  – Excessive diarrhea (lactulose-induced) or vomiting
- Infections: Spontaneous bacterial peritonitis (SBP), bacteremia
- Reduction in venous return with tense ascites
- GI bleeding (e.g., variceal bleeding)
- Protein-calorie malnutrition, especially with alcoholic cirrhosis
- Alcohol abuse

Genetics
Only as risk for liver disease (e.g., infantile or autosomal-recessive polycystic kidney disease or a1-antitrypsin deficiency)

GENERAL PREVENTION
- Avoid volume depletion in cirrhotic patients.
- Early diagnosis and aggressive treatment of infections in cirrhotic patients is essential.
- Careful management of patients with cirrhosis to prevent common precipitants (listed above)
- Encourage alcohol cessation in patients who abuse alcohol.

PATHOPHYSIOLOGY
- Severe renal vasoconstriction from generalized vasodilation (especially in splanchnic circulation). Pooling of blood occurs in areas of vasodilation, causing reduction of effective arterial volume (EAV). Splanchnic vasodilation is mediated by vasodilator substances from high endothelial sheer stress from portal hypertension.
- Increased cardiac output initially maintains renal blood flow; later decreased EAV activates other compensatory mechanisms: renin-angiotensin, sympathetic nervous system, and ADH, causing vasoconstriction. HRS develops when increased cardiac output and renal intrinsic vasodilators can no longer counteract decreased EAV and renal vasoconstriction. AKI then develops from decreased renal blood flow.
- Renal vasoconstriction results in retention of sodium and water aggravating ascites and edema. ADH release secondary to decreased EAV also results in water retention, which explains the Hyponatremia in HRS.
- SBP and other infections are a common precipitating factors of HRS in which vasoactive cytokines such as nitric oxide are produced, mediating splanchnic vasodilation. Reduction in EAV from hemorrhage, diarrhea, or vomiting large volume paracentesis may also precipitate HRS. NSAIDs also cause HRS by inhibiting renal prostaglandin synthesis.

ETIOLOGY
- HRS may develop in patients with:
  – ESLD or acute fulminant hepatitis from:
    ○ Alcohol, medications, viral hepatitis, or malignancy
- Any other injury that leads to cirrhosis (e.g., *Schistosoma*)

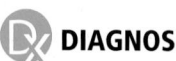

DIAGNOSIS

Other causes of AKI must be excluded before diagnosing HRS. If no ascites, oligoria, and hyponatremia, then HRS is *unlikely*.

HISTORY
- AKI progresses more rapidly in HRS type I, and patients are more severely ill as compared to patients with HRS type 2.
- Uremic encephalopathy on hepatic encephalopathy may cause severe deterioration of mental status.
- Patient with advanced or severe acute liver failure presenting with declining renal function
- May have history of infection, bleeding, overdiuresis, alcohol binge

PHYSICAL EXAM
- Oliguria (urine output <500 mL/d) in the setting of cirrhosis
- Jaundice
- Signs of portal hypertension: Ascites, encephalopathy, splenomegaly
- GI bleeding
- Poor nutritional status
- Spider angioma
- Peripheral vasodilation
- Tachycardia and bounding pulse

DIAGNOSTIC TESTS & INTERPRETATION
- Key aspect of diagnosis: Lack of improvement in renal function following diuretic withdrawal and expansion of plasma with intravenous albumin for at least 48 hours to rule out prerenal azotemia.
- The presence of proteinuria, hematuria, and sediment abnormalities in ESLD patient is diagnosis other that HRS.
- Heavy proteinuria and RBC casts suggest glomerular disease.

Lab
Initial lab tests
- Azotemia in the setting of cirrhosis with appropriate spot urine values (consistent with normal tubular function):
  – Urine sodium <10 mEq/L (10 mmol/L)
  – Fractional excretion of sodium <1%
  – No significant proteinuria
  – Urine/plasma creatinine >30:1
  – Osmolality: Mild to moderate reduction in concentrating ability (400–600 mOsm/kg/water)
  – All reversible causes should be ruled out (e.g., prerenal azotemia, obstruction).
- Urinalysis: Absence of ATN casts; <500 mg/dL protein, high specific gravity
- Minor criteria:
  – Urine volume <500 mL/d
  – Urine red blood cells <50/high-power field
  – Serum sodium <130 mEq/L
- Other:
  – Prolonged prothrombin time
  – Decreased serum albumin concentration
  – Elevated bilirubin

Imaging
Renal ultrasound should be performed to rule out hydronephrosis or obstruction as the cause of AKI.
Initial approach
- Renal ultrasound shows normal kidneys without obstruction.
- Although experimental presently, renal Doppler ultrasonography appears to have predictive value in separating cirrhotics who will develop HRS from those who will not based on resistive index.

Diagnostic Procedures/Surgery
Early nephrology consultation should be considered, and renal biopsy may be required if there is unclear cause of AKI.

Pathological Findings
- Liver: Cirrhosis or acute fulminant failure
- Kidneys: Would function if transplanted into hosts without liver disease; a functional renal derangement only

DIFFERENTIAL DIAGNOSIS

For abrupt onset of oliguria in cirrhosis:

- Intravascular volume depletion
- GI fluid loss
- Cardiac failure (possibly alcoholic cardiomyopathy)
- Postrenal; obstruction
- Interstitial nephritis (drug-induced)
- Intrinsic renal disease
- Renal artery or renal vein occlusion by thrombosis (1)

 TREATMENT

- Definitive treatment is liver transplant.
- Goals: Decreasing the incidence of HRS, hemodynamic stabilization, and possible improvement in renal function
- Prevention of SBP by long-term treatment with quinolone in selected patients with ascites. Treatment in SBP with 2 doses of IV albumin 1.5 mg/kg upon diagnosis and 1.0 mg/kg 48 hours later has shown to significantly reduce the incidence of HRS by 10% compared with 33% in patients who were not given the treatment with albumin.
- Supportive therapy (dialysis) to prolong survival for possible liver transplant
- Initial therapy includes administration of plasma volume expanders, such as albumin or fresh frozen plasma (FFP).

MEDICATION

In several trials reversal of HRS has been reported in 25–83% of patients treated with pressor agents plus albumin compared to 8.7–12.5% of patients treated with albumin alone.

First Line

- Combination therapy with midodrine (selective a-1 agonist) and octreotide (somatostatin analog) plus albumin infusion found to improve renal function and improve mortality rates compared to administration of dopamine. Doses used in 1 study were midodrine 7.5–12.5 mg t.i.d. and octreotide 100–200 mg SC t.i.d. titrated to an increase in mean arterial pressure of at least 15 mm Hg (1)[B].
- Judicious use of loop diuretics

Second Line

- Low-dose dopamine once thought to be beneficial; however, not proven in clinical studies (2)
- Vasopressin analogs (terlipressin and ornipressin) combined with plasma volume expanders such as albumin and FFP demonstrate some effect on short-term improvement in renal function and reduction in mortality:
  - May act as a bridge to liver transplantation
  - Additional evidence needed (3)[B]
- Terlipressin is unavailable in US at this time, but works in reversal of renal function (4)[A].
- Recent studies suggest potential benefit of noradrenaline combined with albumin, comparable to terlipressin. More research needed (5)[B].
- Ornipressin may be associated with ischemic complications (6).
- Under investigation: N-acetylcysteine, extracorporeal albumin dialysis

ADDITIONAL TREATMENT
General Measures

- Supportive:
  - Avoid iatrogenic events that precipitate HRS, including excessive volume contraction in cirrhotic inpatients.

- Avoid nonsteroidal anti-inflammatory drugs (NSAIDs), demeclocycline, aminoglycosides, or other nephrotoxins.
- Diagnose and treat correctable causes of azotemia in cirrhosis:
  - ○ Try volume expanders (100 g of albumin in 500 mL of normal saline).
  - ○ Maximize left ventricular function, if possible.
  - ○ Relieve urinary obstruction when present.
- Other:
  - HRS in the setting of acute liver failure may reverse if the liver regenerates or patient gets a liver transplant.

Additional Therapies

- Dialysis: Indicated only as ancillary support for patients awaiting liver transplant or in patients with acute, potentially reversible liver failure
- Continuous venovenous hemofiltration may also be beneficial for patients awaiting transplant, particularly in the setting of hemodynamic instability (7).

SURGERY/OTHER PROCEDURES

- Liver transplantation, when feasible, is the only curative treatment.
- In some studies, transjugular intrahepatic portosystemic shunt (TIPS) has been shown to improve renal function; use is limited by high MELD scores in patients with HRS and high incidence of encephalopathy post-TIPS (2).

IN-PATIENT CONSIDERATIONS
Initial Stabilization

- Maintenance of volume status in cirrhosis
- Type 1 HRS will likely require hospitalization, whereas type 2 HRS may be managed in outpatient setting.

 ONGOING CARE

FOLLOW-UP RECOMMENDATIONS
Patient Monitoring

- Close follow-up with liver disease specialist as an outpatient
- Monitor urine output, renal and hepatic function, and serum electrolytes, particularly potassium.

DIET

- Salt restriction to ≤88 mmol per day (≤2,000 mg) to slow ascites accumulation
- Inpatient: Free water restriction in patients prone to hyponatremia

PATIENT EDUCATION

- In alcoholic cirrhosis, abstention from alcohol is essential and may prevent further deterioration of cirrhosis.
- Discuss importance of adherence to low-sodium diet.

PROGNOSIS

- Grave without liver transplant in cirrhosis or without regeneration of the liver in acute fulminant failure
- The patient may be supported with hemodialysis, continuous arteriovenous hemofiltration, or continuous arteriovenous hemodialysis and transjugular portosystemic stent-shunt prior to organ availability for transplantation.
- The time and degree of renal recovery after liver transplantation is variable, depending on the pretransplant renal function, but a substantial number of patients do show significant renal improvement.

COMPLICATIONS

- Death: 30-day mortality is extremely high in type 1 HRS.
- Dialysis dependency/end-stage renal disease in type 2 HRS
- Bleeding
- Damage to, and failure of, many organ systems
- End-stage kidney disease
- Fluid overload with congestive heart failure or pulmonary edema
- Hepatic coma
- Secondary infections

REFERENCES

1. Angeli P, Volpin R, Gerunda G, et al. Reversal of type 1 hepatorenal syndrome with the administration of midodrine and octreotide. *Hepatology.* 1999;29:1690–7.
2. Wadei HM, Mai ML, Ahsan N, et al. Hepatorenal syndrome: pathophysiology and management. *Clin J Am Soc Nephrol.* 2006;1:1066–79.
3. Gluud LL, et al. Terlipressin for hepatorenal syndrome. *Cochrane Database Syst Rev.* 2006:4.
4. Fabrizi F, Dixit V, Messa P, et al. Terlipressin for hepatorenal syndrome: A meta-analysis of randomized trials. *Int J Artif Organs.* 2009;32:133–40.
5. Alessandria C, Ottobrelli A, Debernardi-Venon W, et al. Noradrenalin vs terlipressin in patients with hepatorenal syndrome: a prospective, randomized, unblinded, pilot study. *J Hepatol.* 2007;47:499–505.
6. Guevara M, et al. Hepatorenal syndrome. *Dig Dis.* 2005;23:45–47.
7. Arroyo V, Guevara M, Ginès P. Hepatorenal syndrome in cirrhosis: pathogenesis and treatment. *Gastroenterology.* 2002;122:1658–76.

ADDITIONAL READING

Venkat, Deepak and K.K. Hepatorenal Syndrome. *Southern Medical Journal.* 2010;103:654–59.

See Also (Topic, Algorithm, Electronic Media Element)

Acetaminophen Poisoning; Cirrhosis of the Liver; Hepatitis A; Hepatitis B; Hepatitis C; Renal Failure, Acute; Schistosomiasis of the Liver, Chronic

 CODES

ICD9
572.4 Hepatorenal syndrome

CLINICAL PEARLS

- HRS is a diagnosis of exclusion. Other causes of acute renal failure must be ruled out.
- HRS stems from hemodynamic changes associated with advanced liver disease, without intrinsic renal abnormalities.
- Treat correctable causes of azotemia. Initial therapy includes volume expansion, with albumin if possible.
- Liver transplantation is the treatment of choice.

H

HERNIA
Leah A. Burnett, MD

 BASICS

DESCRIPTION
This topic pertains to external hernias of the groin and abdominal wall. These are an abnormal protrusion of the contents of the abdominal cavity through a fascial defect in the abdominal wall:

- Definitions:
  - Reducible: Extruded sac and its contents can be returned to its original intra-abdominal position, either spontaneously or with gentle manual manipulation.
  - Irreducible/incarcerated: Extruded sac and its contents cannot be returned to its original intra-abdominal position.
  - Strangulated: Compromise of blood supply to hernia sac contents
  - Richter: Partial circumference of bowel is incarcerated or strangulated. Partial wall damage may occur, increasing potential for bowel rupture and peritonitis.
  - Sliding (wall of a viscus forms part of the wall of the inguinal hernia sac)R-cecum, L-sigmoid colon
- Types:
  - Groin: Inguinal and femoral
  - Inguinal:
    o Direct inguinal: Acquired; herniation through defect in transversalis fascia of abdominal wall medial to inferior epigastric vessels; increased frequency with age as fascia weakens
    o Indirect inguinal: Congenital; herniation lateral to the inferior epigastric vessels, through internal inguinal ring into inguinal canal. A "complete hernia" is one that descends into the scrotum, while an "incomplete hernia" remains within the inguinal canal.
  - Pantaloon: Combination of direct and indirect inguinal hernia with protrusion of abdominal wall on both sides of the epigastric vessels
  - Femoral: Descends through the femoral canal deep to the inguinal ligament. Because of the narrow neck of a femoral hernia, this type of hernia is especially prone to incarceration and strangulation.
  - Other: Obturator, sciatic, perineal
  - Incisional or ventral: Iatrogenic, herniation through a defect in the anterior abdominal wall at the site of a prior surgical incision
  - Umbilical: Defect occurs at umbilical ring tissue
  - Epigastric: Protrudes through the linea alba above the level of the umbilicus. These may develop at exit points of small paramidline nerves and vessels, or through an area of congenital weakness in the linea alba.
- Other:
  - Interparietal (e.g., Spigelian hernia): Hernia sac insinuates itself between layers of the abdominal wall; strangulation common, often mistaken for tumor or abscess

Geriatric Considerations
Abdominal wall hernias increase with advancing age, with significant increase in risk during surgical repair.

Pregnancy Considerations
- Increased intra-abdominal pressure and hormone imbalances may contribute to increased risk of abdominal wall hernias.
- Umbilical hernias associated with multiple, prolonged deliveries

EPIDEMIOLOGY
Incidence
- 75–80% groin hernias, including inguinal and femoral
- 2–20% incisional/ventral, depending on whether surgery was associated with infection or contamination
- 3–10% umbilical, considered congenital
- 1–3% other
- Groin:
  - 6–27% lifetime risk in adult men
  - Approximately 50% of children under 2 will have a patent processus vaginalis, decreasing to 40% after age 2. Only between 25% and 50% will become clinically significant.
  - Inguinal hernia found in less than 5% of newborns, but M:F ratio is 10:1
  - Increased incidence in premature infants (1)[B]
  - Increased incidence in patients with abdominal aortic aneurysms
- Incisional/ventral: ~10–23% of abdominal surgeries complicated by an incisional hernia.
- Umbilical: 10–20% of newborns (2)

Prevalence
- Inguinal hernias more prevalent in men; femoral and umbilical hernias are more prevalent in women.
- Incisional/ventral hernias are more prevalent in obese or overweight men, as well as more prevalent among smokers. The opposite may be true for inguinal hernias (3)[C].

RISK FACTORS
Increased abdominal pressure, coughing, heavy lifting, constipation or straining with stool, pregnancy, ascites, prostatism, obesity, advancing age and loss of tissue turgor, smoking, steroid use, low birth weight, prematurity

Genetics
No known genetic pattern

PATHOPHYSIOLOGY
Loss of tissue strength and elasticity, especially with aging or congenital defect in abdominal fascia

ETIOLOGY
In general, a defect in the fascia of the abdominal wall. Most pediatric hernias are congenital defects (e.g., patent processus vaginalis), while most adult hernias are a result of acquired weakness in the tissues of the anterior abdominal wall.

COMMONLY ASSOCIATED CONDITIONS
Obesity, chronic obstructive pulmonary disease, multiple abdominal surgeries, pregnancy, advanced age, Ehlers-Danlos, Marfan, Hurler-Hunter, PKD, osteogenesis imperfecta, Beckwith-Wiedemann syndrome, Down syndrome, abdominal aortic aneurysm

 DIAGNOSIS

HISTORY
- While many hernias are asymptomatic, symptoms may include pain, nausea, vomiting, bloating, and relief with reclining.
- Hernia may be directly observed as protrusion through abdominal wall during maneuvers that increase intra-abdominal pressure.

PHYSICAL EXAM
- Examination should initially occur with patient standing and examiner placing finger in inguinal canal via the scrotum. Exam should also be performed with patient in supine position and with cough.
- Inguinal (superior to inguinal ligament):
  - Direct inguinal hernia: Finger in inguinal canal finds defect of the transversalis fascia as a deep (posterior to anterior) bulge palpated by pad of finger with increased intra-abdominal pressure.
  - Indirect inguinal hernia: Finger in inguinal canal finds a persistent process vaginalis as a bulge (lateral to medial) palpated by fingertip, and may extend down into scrotum.
- Femoral (inferior to inguinal ligament): Bulge in upper middle thigh; neck of the sac will protrude lateral to and below a finger placed on the pubic tubercle
- Umbilical: Palpable protrusion at umbilius
- Incisional/ventral: Palpable protrusion at site of prior abdominal incision
- Epigastric: Majority occur just off midline, above umbilicus.

DIAGNOSTIC TESTS & INTERPRETATION
Imaging
Initial approach
Hernia evaluation rarely require imaging; reserve for suspected abdominal hernia or unclear diagnosis. Plain radiographs are often used to look for evidence of obstructive signs including dilated proximal bowel and bowel stacking.
- Ultrasonography can be used to assess inguinal hernias.
- CT or tangential radiography may also be used; best for incisional and abdominal wall hernias.
- Herniography is no longer recommended but may be useful in interpreting obscure hernia symptoms in an atypical presentation (4)[A].
- CT Imaging is frequently used to evaluate post-surgical patients with complaints of abdominal pain and is considered the gold standard there.

Pediatric Considerations
- There is insufficient evidence for contralateral exploration in pediatric patients, except using ultrasonography.

Follow-Up & Special Considerations
For occult hernias not be well appreciated on exam or with imaging, diagnostic laparoscopy may be beneficial.

DIFFERENTIAL DIAGNOSIS
Lymphadenopathy, hydrocele, lipoma, varices, cryptorchidism, abscess, tumor, sports hernia (athletic pubalgia), pelvic fractures, adductor tears, omphalomesenteric duct, urachal cyst.

TREATMENT

Acute setting:

- Pain medication recommended for symptomatic hernias.
- Strangulated hernias should be surgically repaired as early as possible to prevent complications such as necrosis and viscus perforation.
- Manual reduction of incarcerated hernia improves outcomes by allowing for elective repair after improvement of acute swelling and inflammation (5).
- Complication rate is near 20 times greater in emergent repair of pediatric inguinal hernias than elective procedures (6)[A].

MEDICATION

- Antibiotics: Antibiotic prophylaxis did not reduce wound infections after groin hernia repairs.
- Pain: Local anesthetic during surgical repair results in significant in reduction of postoperative pain (6)[A]. Tension-free procedures such as Lichtenstein may be performed under local anesthesia.

ADDITIONAL TREATMENT
Geriatric Considerations
Use of a truss (external supportive device) for direct inguinal hernias common; no data exists on their long-term efficacy, and are often considered a temporizing measure

Issues for Referral
Warn patients of symptoms or signs of incarceration or strangulation (acute abdominal pain, fever, bloody bowel movements) mandate immediate self-referral to emergency room.

SURGERY/OTHER PROCEDURES

All inguinal hernias should be surgically repaired, but watchful waiting in the asymptomatic patient is a safe option if significant comorbidities may compromise emergent repair (6)[A]:

- Incarceration and strangulation are absolute indications for hernia repair.
- Contraindications: Patients who are not surgical candidates based on cardiovascular risk factors:
  – Elective repair should be avoided in pregnant patients or those with active infections.
- Special considerations:
  – Umbilical hernias < 0.5 cm usually obliterate and can be managed by observation (2).
  – Umbilical hernias in children age 2–4 years may be observed as there is a high rate of spontaneous closure.
  – Semielective surgical repair can be safe during pregnancy if delayed until after 2nd trimester.
  – Women had lower recurrence rates with laparoscopic methods than with Lichtenstein open method.
  – Ascites is not a strict contraindication for surgical repair. There is a greater risk of strangulation and complication without repair than the increased risks associated with repair in the presence of ascites.
  – The more emergent hernia operations can be performed using the same methods for nonacute situations. However, incarceration with strangulation my require laparotomy with partial bowel resection.

- Gold standard:
  – Inguinal hernia:
    ○ Open: Lichtenstein with mesh (37%) or mesh plug (34%): Decreased recurrence rates (6)[A]
    ○ Laparoscopic (14%) with mesh: Decreased hospital stay and postoperative pain (6)[A]
      ■ Requires general anesthesia.
      ■ Transabdominal preperitoneal (TAPP) versus total extraperitoneal (TEP)
    ○ Pediatric: Recovery and outcome similar after open and laparoscopic repair. Laparoscopic hernia repair associated with increased operation/anesthesia time and postoperative pain.
  – Incisional/ventral:
    ○ Laparoscopic repair with mesh for simple, noncomplex hernias
    ○ Open repair with mesh for complex or recurrent hernias
  – Umbilical:
    ○ Pediatric: Open excision and closure with suture
    ○ Adult: Open repair with mesh or plug may reduce hernia recurrence.
- Newer techniques:
  – Prolene hernia system
  – Biologic wound closure system: Reduced recurrence in contaminated procedures
- Complications:
  – Recurrence
  – Postoperative pain, temporary or chronic: Improved in laparoscopic approach versus open
  – Wound infection
  – Injury to cord structures in inguinal herniorrhaphy

ONGOING CARE

PATIENT EDUCATION
Cleveland Clinic: http://my.clevelandclinic.org/disorders/hernia/hic_hernia.aspx
- Groin hernias: University of Chicago Children's Hospital: http://www.uchicagokidshospital.org/specialties/general-surgery/patient-guides/inguinal-hernia.html
- Incisional/ventral: Society of American Gastrointestinal and Endoscopic Surgeons: http://sages.org/sagespublication.php?doc=PI10
- Umbilical hernias: Boston Children's Hospital: http://www.childrenshospital.org/az/Site1018/mainpageS1018P0.html

PROGNOSIS
- Groin (pediatric): Low recurrence rates (<3%) with surgical treatment; may spontaneously resolve in infants.
- Groin (adult): ≥1%/year risk of bowel strangulation without surgical treatment; 0–10% postoperative recurrence rates, depending on surgeon experience level and method
- Incisional/ventral: 3–5% postoperative occurrence: 2–17% post repair recurrence, increased to 20–46% in larger hernias
- Umbilical (pediatric):
  – High rate of spontaneous resolution
  – Hernia less likely to close further in older children and in children with larger defects
- Umbilical (adult): Up to 11% postoperative recurrence rate
- Epigastric: Most will ultimately become incarcerated and/or strangulated without surgical treatment. Recurrence is high due to frequency of missed defects during repair.

REFERENCES

1. Brandt ML. Pediatric hernias. *Surg Clin North Am.* 2008;88:27–43, vii-viii.
2. Snyder CL. Current management of umbilical abnormalities and related anomalies. *Semin Pediatr Surg.* 2007;16:41–9.
3. Rosemar A, Angerås U, Rosengren A. Body mass index and groin hernia: a 34-year follow-up study in Swedish men. *Ann Surg.* 2008;247:1064–8.
4. Ng TT, Hamlin JA, Kahn AM. Herniography: analysis of its role and limitations. *Hernia.* 2008.
5. Lau ST, Lee YH, Caty MG. Current management of hernias and hydroceles. *Semin Pediatr Surg.* 2007;16:50–7.
6. Matthews RD, Neumayer L. Inguinal hernia in the 21st century: an evidence-based review. *Curr Probl Surg.* 2008;45:261–312.

See Also (Topic, Algorithm, Electronic Media Element)
Algorithms: Lower Abdominal Pain (R, Lt.); Intestinal Obstruction; Pelvic Pain

CODES

ICD9
- 550.10 Unilateral or unspecified inguinal hernia, with obstruction, without mention of gangrene
- 550.90 Unilateral or unspecified inguinal hernia, without mention of obstruction or gangrene
- 552.00 Unilateral or unspecified femoral hernia with obstruction

CLINICAL PEARLS

- Groin: Inguinal and femoral:
- Inguinal:
  – Direct inguinal: Acquired; herniation through defect in transversalis fascia of abdominal wall medial to inferior epigastric vessels; increased frequency with age as fascia weakens
  – Indirect inguinal: Congenital; herniation lateral to the inferior epigastric vessels through internal inguinal ring into inguinal canal. A "complete hernia" is one that descends into the scrotum, while an "incomplete hernia" remains within the inguinal canal.
  – Pantaloon: Combination of direct and indirect inguinal hernia with protrusion of abdominal wall on both sides of the epigastric vessels
  – Femoral: Descends through the femoral canal deep to the inguinal ligament. Because of the narrow neck of a femoral hernia, this type of hernia is especially prone to incarceration and strangulation.
  – Other: Obturator, sciatic, perineal
- Incisional or ventral: Iatrogenic; herniation through a defect in the anterior abdominal wall at the site of a prior surgical incision
- Umbilical: Defect occurs at umbilical ring tissue.
- Epigastric: Protrudes through the linea alba above the level of the umbilicus. These may develop at exit points of small paramidline nerves and vessels, or through an area of congenital weakness in the linea alba.

H

HERPANGINA

Aamir Siddiqi, MD

 BASICS

DESCRIPTION
- Infectious disease caused by coxsackievirus group A
- Characteristics:
  - Fever of short duration
  - Typical vesicular or ulcerated lesions in the posterior pharynx or on the soft palate
  - Incubation period is 4 days.
- Usual course: Acute and self-limited
- System(s) affected: Endocrine/Metabolic; GI

EPIDEMIOLOGY
Incidence
- Year round in tropical climate; summer and fall in temperate climate (1)[B]
- Predominant age: 3 months–16 years
- Predominant sex: Male = Female.

RISK FACTORS
Contact with infected person

GENERAL PREVENTION
- Avoid contact with infected individual.
- The mode of transfer is fecal-oral, so general hygiene (hand-washing) is suggested.

ETIOLOGY
- Common: Coxsackievirus A, types 1–10, 16, and 22 (2)[B]
- Infrequent:
  - Coxsackievirus B, types 1–5
  - Echovirus, types 6, 9, 11, 17, 22, and 25
  - Other enterovirus (3)[B]

 DIAGNOSIS

HISTORY
The patient may have low- or high-grade fever, general malaise, sore throat, and characteristic oropharyngeal lesions.

PHYSICAL EXAM
- Bilateral discrete vesicles, gray base
- Erythematous patches
- Vesicles may rupture to form ulcers.
- Posterior pharynx location: Pharynx, tonsils, soft palate, little involvement of anterior 2/3 of mouth
- Oropharyngeal lesions in the form of vesicles with erythematous edges
- Anorexia
- Drooling
- Sore throat
- Fever
- Malaise
- Irritability
- Listlessness
- Local pain
- Emesis
- Backache
- Headache
- Coryza
- Diarrhea

DIAGNOSTIC TESTS & INTERPRETATION
- This is a clinical diagnosis, so tests are usually not necessary.
- Complement fixation
- Hemagglutinin inhibition tests
- Serum antibodies to coxsackievirus: Titers should show a 4-fold rise in serial samples.

Lab
- Generally no lab work is necessary.
- Slight leukocytosis
- Positive viral culture—mouth washings, stool

DIFFERENTIAL DIAGNOSIS
- Herpes simplex:
  - Multiple ulcers on lips and anterior mouth
  - Diagnose with herpes culture.
- Drug reactions: Cutaneous lesions often present (urticaria, erythema multiforme)
- Recurrent aphthous stomatitis:
  - Buccal, labial, alveolar, mucosal ulcers
  - Recurrent crops
  - Few systemic symptoms
- Lichen planus: Painful ulcer, white lacy pattern on mucosa or may have cutaneous lesions that are purple and pruritic
- Hand, foot, and mouth disease: Classic distribution of vesicular rash on hands, buttocks, feet, and mouth

TREATMENT

Benign and self-limited course of the disease should be explained to the patient.

MEDICATION

- Analgesics: Acetaminophen, nonsteroidal anti-inflammatory drugs (NSAIDs; ibuprofen or naproxen)
- Topical anesthetics: Viscous lidocaine2% solution
- Mouthwash: Aqueous solution of 1% dyclonine and 1% diphenhydramine (Benadryl) in 50% attapulgite (Kaopectate)

ADDITIONAL TREATMENT

General Measures
- Self-limited
- Palliative and supportive
- Hydration

COMPLEMENTARY AND ALTERNATIVE MEDICINE

Myrrh, an herbal antimicrobial, can improve the blister healing process and provide an analgesic effect, reducing the discomfort of topical ulcerations.

IN-PATIENT CONSIDERATIONS

Initial Stabilization
Outpatient

 ONGOING CARE

FOLLOW-UP RECOMMENDATIONS
- No restrictions
- As tolerated, with no limitations

Patient Monitoring
Hydration

DIET
- Clear liquids
- Nonirritating foods such as milk products will be more palatable.

PROGNOSIS
Complete recovery

COMPLICATIONS
Complications are rare.
- Exanthem
- Aseptic meningitis
- Myocarditis
- Encephalitis

REFERENCES

1. Chen KT, Chang HL, Wang ST, et al. Epidemiologic features of hand-foot-mouth disease and herpangina caused by enterovirus 71 in Taiwan, 1998–2005. *Pediatrics*. 2007;120:e244–52.
2. Melnick JL. Enteroviruses: Polioviruses, coxsackieviruses, echoviruses, and newer enteroviruses. In: *Field's Virology*. 1990:549–98.
3. Chang LY, Tsao KC, Hsia SH, et al. Transmission and clinical features of enterovirus 71 infections in household contacts in Taiwan. *JAMA*. 2004;291:222–7.
4. Frydenberg A, Starr M. Hand, foot and mouth disease. *Aust Fam Physician*. 2003;32:594–5.

See Also (Topic, Algorithm, Electronic Media Element)
Herpes Simplex

CODES

ICD9
074.0 Herpangina

CLINICAL PEARLS

- Herpangina occurs commonly during the summer season.
- It is not practical to keep children out of school or child care because virus may be shed in feces for weeks (4)[B].
- Herpangina is caused most commonly by coxsackievirus A but less commonly also may be caused by coxsackievirus B, enterovirus, and echovirus.
- Herpangina predominantly affects newborns and younger children.
- Herpangina is a clinical diagnosis; lab tests are not needed.

H

HERPES EYE INFECTIONS

Matthew J. Dykhuizen, MD
Frank J. McCabe, MD

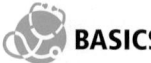 **BASICS**

DESCRIPTION
- Eye infection (blepharitis, conjunctivitis, keratitis, uveitis, retinitis, glaucoma, or optic neuritis) caused by herpes simplex virus (HSV) types 1 and 2 or varicella-zoster virus (VZV)
- Categories: Neonatal, primary, and recurrent:
  - Classically causes a dendritic keratitis best seen with fluorescein staining
  - Reactivation of latent infection is most common.
  - Primary HSV keratitis is more common in children.
- System(s) affected: Eye; Skin; Central Nervous System (CNS) (neonatal)
- Synonyms: HSV keratitis; herpes zoster ophthalmicus (HZO)

EPIDEMIOLOGY
- Predominant age: HSV, any age; zoster, usually older people
- Predominant sex: Male = Female

Incidence
- HSV (in US): 20,000 new ocular cases/year; 28,000 reactivations/year; 1/10,000 infants with neonatal HSV
- Zoster: 0.5–3.4 total HZ cases/1,000 individuals per year; lifetime risk of HZ is 10–20%
  - HZO represents 10–25% of all cases of HZ.
  - 90% of adults are serologically positive.

Prevalence
149 per 100,000 person-years

RISK FACTORS
- Increased age (>50)
- HSV history or close contact with HSV-infected person
- History of varicella infection
- Reactivating factors:
  - UV light, illness, stress, menstruation, local trauma, primary/secondary immunosuppression

ALERT
Consider primary/secondary immunodeficiency disorders in all zoster patients <40 (e.g., AIDS, malignancy)

GENERAL PREVENTION
- Contact precautions with active lesions
- VZV can be spread to those who have not had chickenpox or are not immunized.
- Antiviral prophylaxis while on topical steroids

- Varicella vaccination (Zostavax): Single 0.65 mL SQ dose. No booster. No need to inquire about history of varicella or to perform testing for antibody. Can be given to those with prior zoster episode. Not used in treatment of acute zoster or postherpetic neuralgia (PHN).
- Acyclovir 400 mg p.o. b.i.d.: Reduces recurrence by 50% (1,2)[A]; may not be cost-effective (3)

ALERT
Zoster vaccination contraindicated if HIV-positive, other immunocompromised state, or active untreated tuberculosis (TB) (4)

Pregnancy Considerations
- Pregnant women without history of chickenpox should avoid contact with persons with active zoster.
- Pregnancy increases risk of recurrence.
- Vaccine is contraindicated, as it is a live vaccine.

PATHOPHYSIOLOGY
- HSV and VZV are members of the *Herpesviridae* group (DNA viruses).
- Primary infection from contact with infected person leads to a latent state within trigeminal ganglia (HZO).
- Reactivation of virus affecting the ophthalmic branch is common and can lead to direct ocular involvement.

ETIOLOGY
- Primary infections:
  - Neonatal usually HSV-2
  - Primary ocular HSV usually HSV-1
- Recurrent infections:
  - Reactivation from trigeminal ganglion
  - HSV-1, HSV-2, or VZV

COMMONLY ASSOCIATED CONDITIONS
Primary and secondary immunocompromised states

 DIAGNOSIS

HISTORY
- Varies according to the virus and the ocular structures involved
- History of varicella or herpes simplex infection
- Eye pain, headache, photophobia, tearing, ocular redness, discharge
- Decreased or blurry vision

PHYSICAL EXAM
- Varies according to the virus and the ocular structures involved (HSV most commonly affects the corneal epithelium; VZV most commonly affects corneal stroma and uvea)
- Fever, malaise
- Decreased visual acuity
- Conjunctival infection
- Decreased corneal sensation
- Corneal scar
- Slit lamp exam:
  - Fluorescein and rose bengal stain: Dendritic corneal epithelial staining pattern
  - Anterior chamber cells if uveitis present

ALERT
Unilateral dermatomal vesicular rash most commonly in ophthalmic branch (V_1) of trigeminal nerve (VZV):
- Hutchinson sign: Vesicular lesion on nose from VZV indicates an increased risk of HZO due to involvement of nasociliary branch of trigeminal nerve, which also innervates the eye.

DIAGNOSTIC TESTS & INTERPRETATION
Lab
Initial lab tests
- Typically none needed, as diagnosis is primarily based on history and physical exam
- Other:
  - Corneal swab for HSV DNA by polymerase chain reaction (PCR) (PPV = 96%)
  - If vesicle present, can perform a Tzanck smear for VZV or HSV (multinucleated giant cells)
  - Antibody titers to asses exposure only; DFA (direct fluorescent antibody); tissue culture

ALERT
- Urgent ophthalmology referral for slit lamp exam, dilated fundus exam, and intraocular pressure measurement
- Evaluate zoster patients <40 for possible immunodeficiency.

DIFFERENTIAL DIAGNOSIS
- Any other cause of red, painful eye:
  - Bacterial, fungal, allergic, or other viral conjunctivitis
  - Acute angle closure glaucoma
  - Iritis or scleritis
- Corneal abrasion, recurrent corneal erosion, toxic conjunctivitis

TREATMENT

MEDICATION
First Line
- Skin and eyelid lesions:
  - Bacitracin or erythromycin b.i.d.
  - Eyelid margin involvement:
    - Trifluorothymidine (Viroptic) 1% drops or vidarabine 3% ointment 5 times per day
  - Zoster: Acyclovir 800 mg p.o. 5 times per day for 10 days or famciclovir 500 mg p.o. t.i.d. for 7 days if started within 3 days of onset and active lesions are present
  - Severe or persistent zoster: Acyclovir 5–10 mg/kg IV q8h for 5–10 days; hospitalize if indicated for systemic disease or if immunocompromised
  - Options for postherpetic neuralgia (PHN):
    - Prednisone 60 mg p.o. for 3–7 days and taper over 1–2 weeks (H$_2$-blocker such as cimetidine while on prednisone)
    - Amitriptyline 25 mg p.o. t.i.d.
    - Capsaicin cream (not near the eye), lidocaine cream/patch, gabapentin
- HSV corneal epithelial disease:
  - Trifluorothymidine 1% drops q2h (agent of choice) or vidarabine 3% ointment 5 times per day or 0.15% ganciclovir or 3% acyclovir; taper over 10–21 days based on response (1,5)[A]
  - If severe HSV infection: Acyclovir 400 mg p.o. 5 times per day; if immunocompromised, 800 mg p.o. 5 times per day
  - Epithelial debridement: Removes virus quickly
  - Avoid topical steroids
- HSV stromal keratitis or uveitis (without epithelial disease):
  - Cycloplegia with scopolamine 0.25% or cyclopentolate 1% drops t.i.d.
  - Prednisolone acetate 1% drops q.i.d. with slow taper (5)[A]
  - Consider systemic steroids in severe uveitis.
  - Trifluorothymidine 1% drops q.i.d. for prophylaxis while on topical steroids
- Herpes zoster ophthalmicus:
  - Acyclovir 800 mg p.o. 5 times per day for 10–14 days or valacyclovir 1 g p.o. t.i.d. for 7–10 days or famciclovir 500 mg p.o. t.i.d. for 7–10 days (start antiviral within 72 hours of rash onset)
  - If immunocompromised: Acyclovir 30 mg/kg/d in 3 divided doses for 7 days
  - Prednisolone acetate 1% drops q.i.d. with slow taper
  - Cycloplegic agent if anterior uveitis present

ALERT
- Topical steroids:
  - Should only be prescribed by an ophthalmologist
  - Contraindicated with active corneal epithelial disease, which is best monitored with a slit lamp
  - Can increase intraocular pressure, cause corneal thinning, and, with long-term use, cause cataracts
- Topical antiviral agents:
  - Toxic to corneal epithelium
- Acyclovir:
  - Reduce dosage in renal insufficiency
- Prednisone:
  - Contraindicated in immunocompromised patients

Pregnancy Considerations
Systemic steroids and acyclovir should not be used in pregnancy.

Second Line
- Idoxuridine 0.5% ointment or 0.1% drops 5 times per day (1)[A]
- Nonsteroidal anti-inflammatory drugs (NSAIDs) p.o. for scleritis associated with zoster. Acyclovir 2 g/day p.o. in divided doses over 10 days in patients intolerant of topical antivirals (1,3)[A].

ADDITIONAL TREATMENT
General Measures
- Cool compresses
- Artificial tears
- P.o. pain medications
- Avoid contact with nonimmune people.

Issues for Referral
Emergent or urgent ophthalmology referral, depending on severity of disease

Additional Therapies
Recurrent HSV requires suppressive therapy:
- Acyclovir 800 mg p.o. daily or valacyclovir 500 mg p.o. daily

SURGERY/OTHER PROCEDURES
Corneal transplantation for severe scarring or perforation

IN-PATIENT CONSIDERATIONS
Admission Criteria
- Severe systemic VZV disease
- Systemic HSV in children

Discharge Criteria
Resolution of systemic disease

ONGOING CARE

FOLLOW-UP RECOMMENDATIONS
Patient Monitoring
- Monitor with slit lamp exam every 1–2 days until improvement, then every 3–4 days until epithelial defect resolves.
- Weekly after epithelial disease resolves until off topical antivirals

PATIENT EDUCATION
Educate patient about importance of early recognition of recurrent symptoms and need for prompt evaluation and treatment.

PROGNOSIS
- Many cases are self-limited but, depending on the ocular structure involved, can lead to permanent blindness, especially in the setting of recurrent disease.
- Recurrent ocular HSV:
  - HSV epithelial disease without treatment, 40% resolve without sequelae; with treatment, 90–95% resolve without complication

Pediatric Considerations
- Neonatal primary HSV often disseminated with high mortality rate; 37% have vision worse than 20/200
- Pediatric cases more likely to be bilateral (26%); recurrent (48% in 15 months) and may cause amblyopia

COMPLICATIONS
- Recurrence
- Corneal neovascularization and scarring resulting in poor vision
- Neurotrophic ulcer with perforation
- Secondary bacterial or fungal infection
- Secondary glaucoma in 10%
- PHN in 20–40% with VZV, typically longer-lasting in older patients
- Vision loss from optic neuritis or chorioretinitis

REFERENCES
1. Wilhelmus KR. Interventions for herpes simplex virus epithelial keratitis. *Cochrane Database Sys Rev.* 2008;3:CD002898.
2. Uchoa UB, Rezende RA, Carrasco MA, et al. Long-term acyclovir use to prevent recurrent ocular herpes simplex virus infection. *Arch Ophthalmol.* 2003;121:1702–4.
3. Lee P, Zhang P. Economic analysis in eye disease. *Arch Ophthalmol.* 2003;121:115–6.
4. Oxman MN, Levin MJ, Johnson GR, et al. A vaccine to prevent herpes zoster and postherpetic neuralgia in older adults. *N Engl J Med.* 2005;352:2271–84.
5. Tullo A. Pathogenesis and management of herpes simplex virus keratitis. *Eye.* 2003;17:919–22.

See Also (Topic, Algorithm, Electronic Media Element)
Algorithm: Eye Pain

CODES

ICD9
- 053.20 Herpes zoster dermatitis of eyelid
- 053.21 Herpes zoster keratoconjunctivitis
- 053.22 Herpes zoster iridocyclitis

CLINICAL PEARLS
- HSV and VZV can lead to a wide array of ocular manifestations, ranging from self-limited disease to potentially vision-threatening disease and complications.
- An ophthalmologist should be consulted before prescribing topical steroids.
- Hutchinson sign (vesicular lesion on nose from VZV) is a strong indicator of HZO.
- Zostavax is effective at preventing zoster and decreasing the duration of PHN.

H

HERPES SIMPLEX
Michelle Whitehurst-Cook, MD

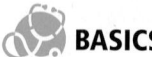 **BASICS**

DESCRIPTION
- Viral disease with many manifestations
- Usually seen as painful vesicles that often occur in clusters on skin, cornea, or mucous membranes
- May occur as encephalitis, pneumonia, or disseminated infection, and/or skin lesions including but not limited to oral and genital sites

EPIDEMIOLOGY
- Predominant age: Affects all ages
- Predominant sex: Male = Female

Incidence
29.2/100,000 office visits per year

Prevalence
- Widespread; 0.65–25% of adults may be excreting herpes simplex virus type 1 or 2 (HSV-1, HSV-2) at any given time.
- Prevalence of antibodies varies from 30% in higher socioeconomic strata to 100% in lower socioeconomic strata; 20,000–70,000/100,000

RISK FACTORS
- Immune compromise (brief, as with occurrence of other illness or stress; or more chronic, as with chemotherapy, malignancy, or AIDS). Children with eczema are at higher risk.
- Newborns: If exposed to actively infected mother via birth canal, or if exposed to case in nursery (insufficient maternal passive antibody transfer); risk greatest for neonate of mother with active primary herpes simplex infection. Those with active disease should avoid exposing newborns.
- Prior HSV infection
- Sexual intercourse with infected person (condoms may help prevent HSV, but location of lesions may limit effectiveness)
- Occupational exposure (medical/dental risk more for HSV-1 whitlow and general community for HSV-2 whitlow)

Pregnancy Considerations
- Caesarean section and/or acyclovir indicated if any active genital lesions (or prodrome) present at the time of delivery; consider if primary genital herpes occurred within 4 weeks of expected delivery (1,2)[C]
- Avoid fetal scalp electrodes if mother has history of genital HSV.
- Risk of viral shedding at delivery from asymptomatic recurrent genital HSV is low (~1.6%); not predicted by monitoring cultures

Geriatric Considerations
Decreased immunologic competence of old age may increase risk.

GENERAL PREVENTION
- Avoid contact with immunocompromised people.
- Wash hands often.
- Kissing, sharing beverages from the same container, sharing food utensils or toothbrushes can transmit HSV

- Genital herpes: Avoid sexual contact while disease is active (recognizing herpes simplex is transmitted even when disease appears to be inactive); discuss condom benefits and limits, and reinforce benefits of mutually monogamous sexual relations.

ETIOLOGY
HSV, a DNA virus of 2 major types: HSV-1 and HSV-2. Most often, HSV-1 is associated with oral lesions and HSV-2 with genital lesions, but reverse also occurs.

COMMONLY ASSOCIATED CONDITIONS
Erythema multiforme: 50% of associated cases are caused by HSV I or II (3).

 DIAGNOSIS

PHYSICAL EXAM
- Vesicles: Usually cluster and open as painful ulcerated lesions, often with erythematous base
- Herpetic whitlow: Localized primary infection on a finger with intense itching and pain, followed by vesicles that may coalesce with swelling and erythema, and may mimic pyogenic paronychia; neuralgia, and axillary adenopathy sometimes occur; heals over 2–3 weeks without incision. Primary inoculation of other abraded skin may occur (e.g., herpes gladiatorum in wrestlers).
- Primary herpetic gingivostomatitis and pharyngitis: 1st infection with HSV-1 usually in early childhood; incubation from 2–12 days, then fever, sore throat, pharyngeal edema, and erythema; small vesicles develop on pharyngeal and oral mucosa, rapidly ulcerate, and increase in number to involve soft palate, buccal mucosa, tongue, floor of mouth, and often lips and cheeks; tender gums may bleed; fetid breath, cervical adenopathy; fever, general toxicity, poor oral intake, and drooling contribute to dehydration; autoinoculation of other sites may occur; resolves in 10–14 days.
- Primary genital herpes: See Herpes, Genital.
- Primary herpes keratoconjunctivitis: By HSV-1 usually; may present as unilateral conjunctivitis with regional adenopathy, as blepharitis with vesicles on lid margin, as keratitis with dendritic lesions, or with punctate opacities; lasts 2–3 weeks; systemic involvement prolongs process
- Eczema herpeticum: Diffuse pox-like eruption complicating atopic dermatitis; 1 cause of Kaposi varicelliform eruption; sudden appearance of lesions in typical atopic areas (upper trunk, neck, head); high fever, local edema, adenopathy
- Umbilicated vesicles develop hemorrhagic crust or become pustular; vesicles appear in crops for up to a week; significant fluid or blood loss and secondary bacterial infections may cause fatality; may occur in severe burn patients and go unrecognized under the eschar
- Neonatal herpes simplex: Perinatal primary infection is life-threatening and usually acquired by vaginal birth of infected mother; fetal risk and neonatal risk are greater in mothers with primary genital herpes infection because shedding is more prolonged and the inoculum is greater; incubation from 5–7 days usually (rarely 4 weeks); cutaneous, mucous membrane, or ocular signs in only 70%:
  – Congenital infection via prenatal transplacental virus transfer may present with jaundice, hepatosplenomegaly, disseminated intravascular coagulation, encephalitis, seizures, temperature instability, chorioretinitis, and/or conjunctivitis

with or without skin vesicles; neurologic morbidity worse with HSV-2 than with HSV-1 in neonates; fatal hepatic or adrenal necrosis may occur.
- Recurrent diseases from endogenous reactivation include:
  – Herpes labialis: Recurrent lesions on lips with HSV-1; usually <1 recurrence per 6 months, but 5–25% may have >1 attack per month; precipitating events may be sunlight, fever, trauma, menses, stress; prodrome of pain, burning, itching may last 6–48 hours before vesicles appear, often at vermilion border, with increased pain; vesicles ulcerate and crust within 48 hours; heals within 8–10 days generally; may have local adenopathy
  – Ocular herpes: May recur as keratitis, blepharitis, or keratoconjunctivitis; patients may have dendritic ulcers, decreased corneal sensation, less visual acuity; uveitis may cause permanent visual loss
  – Recurrent genital herpes (herpes progenitalis): See Herpes, Genital.

DIAGNOSTIC TESTS & INTERPRETATION
Screen for other STIs with primary genital herpes.

Lab
- Tzanck smear shows multinucleated giant cells with 12–15 nuclei, often with eosinophilic intranuclear inclusions (scrape material from lesion onto slide, fix with ethanol or methanol, stain with Giemsa or Wright preparation; alternatively, spray slide with cytologic fixative and stain as for Pap smear); varicella (herpes zoster) has identical findings.
- HSV culture: Only 1/2 of true positives available in 2 days; rest may take 6 days or longer to be positive; not reliable near delivery
- Newer type-specific antibody tests can reliably distinguish between HSV-1 and HSV-2.
- Primary infection is ruled out with initially high titers or <4-fold rise of titers between acute and convalescent sera.
- Immunoglobulin M HSV antibodies may appear in 1st 4 weeks of life in infected infants.

Diagnostic Procedures/Surgery
Occasionally a biopsy is needed.

Pathological Findings
- See Tzanck prep above.
- Intraepithelial edema (ballooning degeneration) and intracellular edema
- A brain biopsy (in encephalitis) has hemorrhagic necrosis of gray and white matter with acute and chronic inflammation, thrombosis and fibrinoid necrosis of parenchymal vessels, and intranuclear inclusions in astrocytes, oligodendroglia, and neurons.

DIFFERENTIAL DIAGNOSIS
- Impetigo: Straw-colored vesicles that crust
- Aphthous stomatitis: Grayish, shallow erosions with ring of hyperemia, usually only anterior in mouth and lips
- Herpes zoster: Unilateral dermatome distribution
- Syphilitic chancre: Usually painless ulcer
- Herpangina: Vesicles predominate on anterior tonsillar pillars, soft palate, uvula, and oropharynx but not more anteriorly on lips or gums (usually caused by group A coxsackievirus)
- Stevens-Johnson syndrome
- Other causes of Kaposi varicelliform eruption are varicella and coxsackievirus A16.

TREATMENT

Pediatric Considerations
Neonates with possible exposure to HSV at birth or later with signs of infection (lethargy, poor feeding, fever, lesions): Culture urine, stool, cerebrospinal fluid, eyes, throat; treat immediately with IV acyclovir if HSV illness suspected (1)[C].

MEDICATION
First Line
- Acyclovir:
  – Short half-life and poor bioavailability require a frequent dosing schedule
  – Primary herpes labialis: 15 mg/kg (up to 200 mg) p.o. for 5 doses daily for 7–10 days significantly decreases disease duration and infectivity (4)[B]:
    ○ Early treatment is more effective but does not decrease recurrent outbreaks.
  – Recurrent herpes labialis: Treatment speeds healing time of discomfort and lesions compared to placebo (4)[A]:
    ○ Acyclovir 400 mg p.o. 5 times per day for 5 days
  – Primary genital herpes: 400 mg p.o. t.i.d. or 200 mg p.o. for 5 doses daily for 7–10 days
  – Recurrent genital herpes: 800 mg p.o. b.i.d. or 200 mg p.o. for 5 doses daily for 7–10 days; for chronic suppression in persons with frequent recurrences, 400 mg b.i.d.
  – Neonatal herpes simplex or encephalitis: 20 mg/kg IV over 1 hour q8h for 14–21 days
  – Primary herpes gingivostomatitis, recurrent herpes labialis, and other HSV skin infections: 200 mg p.o. q4h for 5 doses daily for 10 days
  – In pregnancy: May give orally for 1st episode of genital herpes or severe recurrent herpes. Give IV for severe or complicated disease.
- Penciclovir (Denavir): Oroherpes recurrence: 1% cream q2h while awake for 4 days
- Valacyclovir (Valtrex):
  – Better bioavailability orally than acyclovir; is converted to acyclovir
  – Recurrent herpes labialis:
    ○ Valacyclovir 2g po BID for a single day (4)[A]
  – Primary genital herpes: 1 g p.o. b.i.d. for 10 days
  – Recurrent genital herpes: 500 mg p.o. b.i.d. for 3 days; chronic suppression, 1 g p.o. daily (10 or more recurrences per year) or 500 mg p.o. daily (9 or fewer recurrences per year)
- Famciclovir (Famvir):
  – Converted to penciclovir, with longer intracellular half-life and higher levels than those of acyclovir
  – Primary genital herpes: 250 mg p.o. t.i.d. for 7–10 days
  – Recurrent genital herpes: 125 mg p.o. b.i.d. for 5 days OR now single-day dosing of 1000 mg p.o. b.i.d.
  – Chronic suppression, 250 mg p.o. b.i.d.
- Contraindications for acyclovir, valacyclovir, and famciclovir: Hypersensitivity or intolerance
- Precautions:
  – Reduce dosage in renal insufficiency for acyclovir, valacyclovir, and famciclovir.
  – Acyclovir may produce encephalopathic reactions, particularly in the elderly.
  – Valacyclovir: Thrombotic thrombocytopenia purpura/hemolytic uremic syndrome reported in some immunocompromised persons in trials on high doses (8 g daily) for cytomegalovirus suppression

- Significant possible interactions: Probenecid with IV acyclovir and possibly probenecid with valacyclovir may reduce renal clearance and elevate antiviral drug levels.

Second Line
- Foscarnet:
  – Drug of choice for acyclovir resistance in immunocompromised persons with systemic HSV
  – 40 mg/kg IV q8h (assume valacyclovir and famciclovir resistance also if acyclovir resistance occurs)
- Other topicals: Ophthalmic preparations for herpes keratoconjunctivitis; acyclovir, vidarabine (Vira-A), idoxuridine, and trifluorothymidine; refer to ophthalmologist

- Topical acyclovir and penciclovir improve healing times for recurrent herpes labialis by approximately 10% (5)[A].

ADDITIONAL TREATMENT
General Measures
- Limited skin lesions (as in recurrent herpes labialis) may benefit from early unroofing of vesicles and application of Campho-Phenique.
- Intermittent, cool, moist dressings with Domeboro or Burrow solution
- Inability to void due to painful lesions is helped by pouring a cup of warm water over genitals while urinating or by sitting in a warm bath while urinating.
- Children with gingivostomatitis or extensive skin disease (eczema herpeticum) may require intravenous hydration and volume replacement.
- In pregnant women: Caesarean section and/or acyclovir indicated if any active genital lesions (or prodrome) present at time of delivery; consider if primary genital herpes occurred within 4 weeks of expected delivery (1,2)[C].

IN-PATIENT CONSIDERATIONS
Initial Stabilization
Outpatient treatment

 ONGOING CARE

FOLLOW-UP RECOMMENDATIONS
No restrictions

Patient Monitoring
Observe for disappearance of lesions and resolution of systemic manifestations.

DIET
Avoid acidic foods with gingivostomatitis.

PATIENT EDUCATION
Reassure to reduce stigma

PROGNOSIS
- The usual course of the primary disease is 2 weeks; expect frequent recurrences.
- Recurrences respond well to treatment.
- The duration of the recurrence varies.
- Viral shedding in recurrence is briefer than with the primary disease.
- Newborns or immunocompromised individuals are at risk for major morbidity or mortality.

COMPLICATIONS
- Herpes encephalitis: A brain biopsy may be needed for diagnosis.
- Herpes pneumonia
- Aseptic meningitis
- Herpes viremia

REFERENCES
1. Rudnick CM, Hoekzema GS. Neonatal herpes simplex virus infections. *Am Fam Physician*. 2002;65:1138–42.
2. Beauman JG. Genital herpes: A review. *Am Fam Physician*. 2005;72:1527–34, 1541–42.
3. Lamoreux MR, Sternbach MR, Hsu WT. Erythema multiforme. *Am Fam Physician*. 2006;74:1883–8.
4. Cernik C, Gallina K, Brodell RT et al. The treatment of herpes simplex infections: an evidence-based review. *Arch Intern Med*. 2008;168:1137–44.
5. Harmenberg J, Oberg B, Spruance S et al. Prevention of ulcerative lesions by episodic treatment of recurrent herpes labialis: A literature review. *Acta Derm Venereol*. 2010;90:122–30.

ADDITIONAL READING
- Chayavichitsilp P, Buckwalter JV, krakowski AC, Friedlander SF. Herpes Simplex, *Pediatr Rev*. 2009;30(4):119–29.
- Crosby RA, Head S, DiClemente RJ, et al. Do protective behaviors follow the experience of testing positive for herpes simplex type 2? *Sex Transm Dis*. 2008;35:787–90.

See Also (Topic, Algorithm, Electronic Media Element)
Herpes, Genital
Algorithm: Genital Ulcers

CODES

ICD9
- 054.3 Herpetic meningoencephalitis
- 054.6 Herpetic whitlow
- 054.9 Herpes simplex without mention of complication

CLINICAL PEARLS
- 25–30% of the US population has genital herpes, and more than 80% of the US population is seropositive for herpesvirus infection.
- Prevalence varies significantly by race and socioeconomic group.
- Most individuals are unaware that they have been infected.
- Chronic suppression for those with frequent recurrences remains effective even after several years of treatment; recurrences naturally become less frequent over time, however.

H

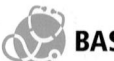 *Robert J. Hyde, MD*

BASICS

DESCRIPTION
- Usually presents as a painful unilateral vesicular eruption within a dermatome
- Results from reactivation of varicella-zoster virus (human herpesvirus type 3)
- Postherpetic neuralgia (PHN) is usually defined as pain persisting at least 1 month after rash has healed. Because of variable definitions of PHN used in research, the term *zoster-associated pain* may be more clinically useful.
  - System(s) affected: Nervous; Integumentary; Exocrine
  - Synonym(s): Shingles

EPIDEMIOLOGY
Predominant sex: Male = Female.

Incidence
- 215/100,000/year; incidence is increasing as population ages.
- Active herpes zoster: 23.9/100,000
- PHN: 86/100,000
- Increases with age: 80% of cases occur in persons >20 years of age (2.2–3.4 per 1,000 aged 20–50 years; 10 per 1,000 aged >80 years)
- PHN increases dramatically with age (4% aged 30–50 years; 50% aged >80 years).

Prevalence
Occurs in 10–20% of the population at some time

Pregnancy Considerations
May occur during pregnancy.

Geriatric Considerations
- Increased incidence of zoster outbreaks
- Increased incidence of PHN

Pediatric Considerations
- Occurs less frequently in children.
- Has been reported in newborns primarily infected in utero.

RISK FACTORS
- The vast majority of persons affected have no underlying illness.
- Increasing age
- Reduced immunity associated with some malignancies (e.g., lymphoma, etc.)
- Treatment of malignancy (chemotherapy or radiotherapy)
- HIV infection
- Use of immunosuppressant drugs after organ transplant surgery or for disease management
- Spinal surgery

GENERAL PREVENTION
- Herpes zoster vaccination is available and recommended for patients ≥60 years of age.
- Zoster patients may transmit virus-causing varicella (chickenpox) to susceptible persons.

ETIOLOGY
Reactivation of varicella zoster virus (human herpesvirus type 3) from dorsal root or cranial nerve ganglia

COMMONLY ASSOCIATED CONDITIONS
Immunocompromised individuals, including HIV infection, posttransplantation, immunosuppressive drugs, and malignancy

 ## DIAGNOSIS

PHYSICAL EXAM
- Prodromal phase (sensations over involved dermatome prior to rash):
  - Tingling
  - Itching
  - Boring or knifelike pain
- Acute phase:
  - Constitutional symptoms variable (e.g., fatigue, malaise, headache, low-grade fever)
  - Dermatomal rash
  - Weakness (1% may have weakness in distribution of rash)
  - Initially erythematous and maculopapular; evolves rapidly to grouped vesicles
  - Vesicles become pustular and/or hemorrhagic in 3–4 days.
  - Resolution of rash, with crusts separating by 14–21 days
- Possible sine herpete (zoster without rash) and other chronic disorders associated with varicella-zoster virus without the typical rash
- Chronic phase:
  - PHN (15% overall; increases with age)
  - A small percentage (1–5%) may affect the motor nerves, causing weakness (called *zoster motorius*), facial nerve (e.g., Ramsay Hunt syndrome), spinal motor radiculopathies

DIAGNOSTIC TESTS & INTERPRETATION
Lab
- Rarely necessary because clinical appearance is usually sufficiently distinctive
- Viral culture
- Tzanck smear (does not distinguish from herpes simplex, and false-negative results occur)
- Polymerase chain reaction analysis
- Immunofluorescent antigen staining
- Varicella-zoster-specific immunoglobulin M

Pathological Findings
- Multinucleated giant cells with intralesional inclusion
- Lymphatic infiltration of sensory ganglia with focal hemorrhage and nerve cell destruction

DIFFERENTIAL DIAGNOSIS
- Rash:
  - Herpes simplex virus
  - Coxsackievirus
  - Contact dermatitis
  - Superficial pyoderma
- Pain:
  - Cholecystitis
  - Appendicitis
  - Nephrolithiasis
  - Pleuritis
  - Myocardial infarction
  - Diabetic neuropathy

 ## TREATMENT

MEDICATION
First Line
- Acute treatment:
  - Antiviral agents initiated within 72 h of rash may relieve symptoms, speed resolution of rash, and prevent and/or ameliorate PHN (1)[A].
  - Valacyclovir: 1,000 mg t.i.d. × 7 days
  - Famciclovir: 500 mg t.i.d. × 7 days
  - Acyclovir: 800 mg q4h (5 doses daily) × 7 days
- Analgesics (acetaminophen, nonsteroidal anti-inflammatory drugs, opioids)
- Corticosteroids to prevent postherpetic neuralgia remain unproven; may help acute pain symptoms but theoretically may increase risk of dissemination. If used, should be in combination with antiviral therapy (2).
- Treatment of complications:
  - Secondary bacterial skin infections: Silver sulfadiazine topically and/or systemic antibiotics
- PHN and zoster-associated pain (1):
  - Tricyclic antidepressants (TCAs; amitriptyline 25 mg at bedtime and other low-dose TCAs) relieve pain acutely and may reduce pain duration.
  - Lidocaine patch 5% (Lidoderm) applied after skin rash closure over painful areas (limit 3 patches simultaneously or trim a single patch) for up to 12 h has been reported to be effective in 1 limited trial.
  - Gabapentin: 100–600 mg t.i.d. for pain and other quality-of-life indicators; limited by adverse effects
  - Opioids, capsaicin cream, and other analgesics may be useful adjuncts.
  - Pregabalin: 50–100 mg t.i.d. reduces pain, but usefulness is limited by side effects.

- Prevention of PHN and zoster-associated pain: No treatment has been shown to prevent PHN completely, but treatment may shorten duration and/or reduce severity of symptoms (3).
  - Antiviral therapy with valacyclovir, famciclovir, or acyclovir given during acute skin eruption may be effective in limiting the duration of pain.
  - Low-dose amitriptyline in the same dosage as for treatment of PHN but started within 72 h of rash onset and continued for 90 days may reduce PHN incidence or duration.
  - There is insufficient evidence that corticosteroids reduce incidence, severity, or duration of PHN (4).
- Contraindications: Refer to the manufacturer's profile of each drug.
- Precautions:
  - Assess renal function prior to using valacyclovir, famciclovir, or acyclovir.
  - Valacyclovir, famciclovir, acyclovir are pregnancy category B.
  - Refer to the manufacturer's profile of each drug.
- Significant possible interactions: Refer to the manufacturer's profile of each drug.

Second Line
Numerous therapies have been advocated, but good supporting evidence is lacking.

ADDITIONAL TREATMENT
General Measures
- Treatment should be directed to control acute symptoms and prevent complications.
- Antiviral therapy decreases viral replication, lessens nerve damage and inflammation, and reduces the severity and duration of long-term pain syndromes (1)[A].
- Prompt analgesic control of pain may shorten the duration of zoster-associated pain.
- Lotions such as calamine and colloidal oatmeal may reduce itching and burning sensation.

IN-PATIENT CONSIDERATIONS
Initial Stabilization
Outpatient treatment, unless disseminated or occurring as complication of serious underlying disease requiring hospitalization

 ## ONGOING CARE

FOLLOW-UP RECOMMENDATIONS
No restrictions

Patient Monitoring
Depends on symptoms

DIET
No special diet

PATIENT EDUCATION
- Inform patient that the duration of rash is 2–3 weeks.
- Encourage good hygiene and proper skin care.
- Warn of potential for dissemination (dissemination must be suspected with constitutional illness signs and/or spreading rash).
- Warn of potential PHN.
- Warn of potential risk of transmitting illness (chickenpox) to susceptible persons.

PROGNOSIS
- Immunocompetent individuals should experience spontaneous and complete recovery within a few weeks.
- Resolution of acute rash within 14–21 days
- PHN may occur in patients age 50 years or more despite treatment with antiviral medications.

COMPLICATIONS
- PHN
- Ophthalmic herpes zoster: 10–20%
- Superinfection of skin lesions:
  - Meningoencephalitis
  - Cutaneous dissemination
  - Hepatitis
  - Pneumonitis
  - Myelitis
  - Cranial and peripheral nerve palsies
  - Acute retinal necrosis

REFERENCES
1. Mounsey AL, Matthew LG, Slawson DC. Herpes zoster and postherpetic neuralgia: prevention and management. *Am Fam Physician*. 2005;72: 1075–80.
2. He L, Zhang D, Zhou M, et al. Corticosteroids for preventing postherpetic neuralgia. *Cochrane Database Syst Rev*. 2008:CD005582.
3. Weinberg JM, Vafaie J, Scheinfeld NS. Skin infections in the elderly. *Dermatol Clin*. 2004;22: 51–61.
4. Gnann JW, Whitley RJ. Clinical practice. Herpes zoster. *N Engl J Med*. 2002;347:340–6.

ADDITIONAL READING
- Harpaz R, Ortega-Sanchez IR, Seward JF, et al. Prevention of Herpes Zoster: Recommendations of the Advisory Committee on Immunization Practices (ACIP). *MMWR Recomm Rep*. 2008;57:1–30.
- Johnson RW, et al. Treatment of herpes zoster and postherpetic neuralgia. *Br Med J*. 2003;326: 748–50.
- Kimberlin DW, Whitley RJ. Varicella-zoster vaccine for the prevention of herpes zoster. *N Engl J Med*. 2007;356:1338–43.
- Li Q, Chen N, Yang J, Zhou M, Zhou D, Zhang Q, He L et al. Antiviral treatment for preventing postherpetic neuralgia. *Cochrane Database Syst Rev*. 2009;CD006866.

- Oxman MN, Levin MJ, Johnson GR, et al. A vaccine to prevent herpes zoster and postherpetic neuralgia in older adults. *N Engl J Med*. 2005;352:2271–84.
- Sampathkumar P, Drage LA, Martin DP. Herpes zoster (shingles) and postherpetic neuralgia. *Mayo Clin Proc*. 2009;84:274–80.
- Wareham DW, et al. Herpes zoster. *Br Med J*. 2007;334:1211–15.

See Also (Topic, Algorithm, Electronic Media Element)
Bell Palsy; Chickenpox; Herpes Eye Infections; Herpes Simplex
Algorithm: Genital Ulcers

 ## CODES

ICD9
- 053.9 Herpes zoster without mention of complication
- 053.19 Herpes zoster with other nervous system complications

CLINICAL PEARLS
- In herpes zoster ophthalmicus, Hutchinson sign is a vesicular rash at the nasal tip, indicating involvement of the external branch of cranial nerve V; associated with increased incidence of ocular zoster.
- Patients should be referred to an ophthalmologist for Hutchinson sign in the early phase of ophthalmic zoster or if they have visual complaints or an unexplained red eye (3).
- All patients should begin a course of antiviral therapy regardless of age. To be effective, therapy should be started within 72 h of the onset of rash. After 72 h, antiviral therapy is recommended for any immunocompromised patient who still has vesicles. However, no data examine the effect of antiviral medication after 72 h.

H

HERPES, GENITAL

Gary I. Levine, MD

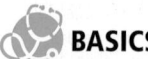

BASICS

DESCRIPTION
Herpes simplex virus infection involving the genitals.
"*Herpes*" comes from the Greek "to creep or crawl."
- Primary genital herpes: Genital herpes due to herpes simplex virus HSV-1 or HSV-2 with no antibody to HSV-1 or HSV-2 at time of infection
- Nonprimary 1st-episode genital herpes:
  – Genital herpes due to HSV-2 with existing antibody to HSV-1, or
  – Genital herpes due to HSV-1 with existing antibody to HSV-2
- Recurrent genital herpes: Reactivation of latent genital herpes with existing antibody to the *same* HSV type recovered from the lesion
- Synonym(s): Herpes genitalis

EPIDEMIOLOGY
- Predominant age: 18–40 years
- Predominant sex: Female > Male:
  – Seroprevalence of HSV-2 = 25% of women (age >12 years), 12% of men
- African-American 3× > Caucasian

Incidence
40–200/100,000 (300,000–1,500,000 cases)

Prevalence
10,000–30,000/100,000 people (45–50 million)

RISK FACTORS
- Primary inoculation:
  – Increasing age, lower socioeconomic status, black race, number of lifetime partners, and past history of sexually transmitted diseases (STDs)
  – Fomites: Wet towels (rare)
- Transmission:
  – Incubation period: 1–45 days (mean 5.8)
  – Annual risk: susceptible female acquiring disease from an infected male partner ~10–30%; for susceptible male from infected female, ~5%
  – Patients without HSV-1 antibody are at greater risk for acquiring HSV-2 infection.
  – >70% new cases result from transmission during asymptomatic (clinically unrecognized) shedding.
  – Risk of asymptomatic shedding is highest within 1 year of 1st occurrence, occurs 1–8% of days.
  – Acyclovir and valacyclovir (LOE = 1b) daily suppresses shedding and reduces transmission of HSV-2 to partners.
- Triggers (recurrent): Genital trauma, menses, intercurrent infection, emotional stress (1)[A], ultraviolet light; recurrences more common in men

Pediatric Considerations
Neonatal infection occurs in 20–50/100,000 live births. 80% of infections result from asymptomatic maternal viral shedding.

GENERAL PREVENTION
- Oral, vaginal, and anal sexual abstinence is the only option to provide complete prevention.
- Condoms reduce transmission by >60%.
- Avoid multiple sexual partners.
- Pregnant women without evidence of HSV antibody should avoid unprotected sex in late pregnancy.

- Screening with type specific antibody in the general population and in pregnancy are not USPSTF recommended
  – Consider screening in asymptomatic patients with HIV infection and suppressive Rx if positive
  – Offer screening in discordant couples (one partner with known HSV, the other without)
- Avoid sex if lesions or prodromal symptoms present and for 2 days after resolved.
- Correct and consistent use of male latex condoms decreases transmission, not 100% effective (HSV can be transmitted from uncovered areas)
- Infants with possible HSV infection should be isolated in the nursery:
  – Maternal separation is not necessary, but appropriate hygiene is essential.
  – Breastfeeding is allowed if there are no HSV lesions on the breast.

PATHOPHYSIOLOGY
HSV: A double-stranded DNA, *Alphaherpesvirinae* virus subfamily

ETIOLOGY
- HSV-1: 10–50% (increasing incidence); now greater than HSV-2 in some clinical settings
- HSV-2: 60–90%

COMMONLY ASSOCIATED CONDITIONS
ALL STIs: Herpes labialis, syphilis, gonorrhea, nongonoccal urethritis/cervicitis, genital warts, HIV, and trichomonas

DIAGNOSIS

PHYSICAL EXAM
- Difficult to differentiate among primary, 1st-episode nonprimary, and recurrent disease on the basis of symptoms and clinical findings
- 60–70% of patients with HSV-2 are asymptomatic or do not recognize clinical manifestations of the disease.
- Atypical presentations:
  – Genital itching, irritation, localized erythema, vulvar fissures
- Primary genital herpes:
  – Fever, headache, malaise, myalgia (40–60%)
  – Vesicles on an erythematous base that ulcerate, crust over, and resolve spontaneously within 21 days
  – Bilateral or unilateral lesions, primarily affecting the external genitalia:
    ○ Female: Labia majora/minora, inner thighs, vaginal mucosa, cervix, perianal skin
    ○ Male: Penile glans, penile shaft, urethra
  – Burning genital pain
  – Dysuria (female)
  – Dyspareunia
  – Sacral paresthesia
  – Inguinal adenopathy
  – Aseptic meningitis in 30%
  – Transient urinary retention
- Nonprimary, 1st episode:
  – Burning genital pain
  – Vesicles resolve within 14–17 days.
- Nonprimary, recurrent:
  – Prodromal symptoms: Burning, numbness, tingling, paresthesia of genitals at site of previous lesions that occurs ~24 hours before new vesicles erupt
  – Vesicles resolve within 7–10 days.
  – Unilateral lesions

Pediatric Considerations
- Genital lesions in child suggest sexual abuse.
- Female: Pelvic examination of internal reproductive organs; external genitalia, vagina, cervix
- Male: Penis and scrotum
- Male and female: Rectum, thighs, buttocks, pubic hair area, mouth, inguinal lymph nodes

DIAGNOSTIC TESTS & INTERPRETATION
Lab
- Viral detection from lesion:
  – Swab vesicle fluid or ulcer; viral culture, enzyme immunoassay, DNA detection by PCR (2–3 × more sensitive than culture)
  – Use Dacron-tipped swabs.
- Type-specific serologic assays (TSST):
  – Immunodot, Western blot (gold standard), and monoclonal antibody (glycoprotein-G) to discriminate between HSV-1 and HSV-2:
    ○ Seroconversion occurs 1 week to 4 months after infection.
- Commercially available tests include Herpes Select-1 & 2 (ELISA), Herpes Select 1/2 (immunoblot), and Biokit HSV-2 & SureVue HSV-2 (fingerstick, point-of-care).

Initial lab tests
- Choose one type of HSV detection noted above.
- Recommend additional STD testing for gonorrhea, chlamydia, HIV, and syphilis.

Pathological Findings
Histopathologic–cytopathic changes:
- Intracellular edema of epithelial cells
- Nuclear margination of chromatin
- Formation of Cowdry type A intranuclear inclusion bodies
- Cell fusion into multinucleated giant cells

DIFFERENTIAL DIAGNOSIS
- Primary syphilis
- Chancroid
- Lymphogranuloma venereum
- Herpes zoster
- Trauma
- Inflammatory bowel disease
- Behçet syndrome
- Stevens-Johnson syndrome
- Ulcerative balanitis
- Granuloma inguinale
- Neoplasia

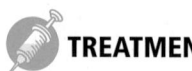

TREATMENT

MEDICATION
Antiviral medications should be started at the first sign or symptom of disease, preferably within 48 hours; efficacy if started beyond 72 hours is not established.

First Line
- Acyclovir (Zovirax):
  – Primary episode: 400 mg p.o. t.i.d. for 7–10 days or 200 mg p.o. 5 × a day for 7–10 days:
    ○ Treatment can be extended beyond 10 days for severe disease or incomplete healing.
  – Severe local or disseminated disease: 5–10 mg/kg IV q8h for 5–7 days
  – Recurrent: 400 mg t.i.d. for 5 days or 800 mg b.i.d. for 5 days or 800 mg t.i.d. for 2 days (2)

– Chronic suppression: Recommended for frequent (≥6 per year) or clinical/psychological disabling recurrences: 400 mg p.o. b.i.d. (2)

– HIV infection: 400 mg p.o. 3–5 × a day until clinical resolution attained

– Precautions:
  ○ Pregnancy: Not approved by Food and Drug Administration (FDA) for routine use (Category B). Studies have demonstrated safety of use.
  ○ Drug is excreted in breast milk.
  ○ Modify dose in patients with renal insufficiency
  ○ Nephropathy and neuropathy are possible with high doses given IV
  ○ Acyclovir resistance (also famciclovir and valacyclovir resistance): Mostly in HIV-infected patients (5–10%)
  ○ Obtain viral isolates for sensitivity testing if lesions persist or recur after adequate antiviral therapy.

– Significant possible interactions:
  ○ Methotrexate
  ○ Interferon
  ○ Probenecid will decrease renal excretion and increase serum concentration.

– Use with caution in combination with nephrotoxic agents.

• Valacyclovir (Valtrex):
  – May cause thrombotic thrombocytopenic purpura (TTP)/hemolytic uremic syndrome in some immunocompromised patients
  – Pregnancy Category B
  – 1st episode: 1 g p.o. b.i.d. for 7–10 days
  – Recurrent: 500 mg p.o. b.i.d. for 3–5 days or 1 g p.o. daily × 5 days (2)
  – Chronic suppression: 500 mg p.o. daily or 1000 mg/d (2)

• Famciclovir (Famvir):
  – Activity/side effects similar to acyclovir; greater bioavailability than acyclovir
    ○ Reduce doses in patients with renal impairment
  – Pregnancy Category B
  – 1st episode: 250 mg p.o. t.i.d. for 7–10 days
  – Recurrent: 125 mg p.o. b.i.d. for 5 days or 1 g p.o. b.i.d. × 1 day (2)
  – Chronic suppression: 250 mg p.o. b.i.d. (2).
  – ACOG Clinical Management Guidelines:
    ○ Primary HSV during pregnancy or lesions near/at term, consider antiviral therapy (reduces duration/severity and viral shedding)
    ○ Women with nonprimary genital herpes at risk for recurrence at or beyond 36 weeks, consider antiviral therapy; may reduce caesarean section rate by 70%, clinical HSV, and HSV shedding; should continue until delivery; acyclovir 400 mg t.i.d. (LOE = 1a) or valacyclovir 500 mg b.i.d.
    ○ Please contact manufacturer, Glaxo, at 1-888-825-5249 to report any pregnant woman on acyclovir.

Second Line
• Foscarnet: 40 mg/kg IV q8h in severe disease with proven or suspected acyclovir-resistant strains
• Vidarabine: 10 mg/kg/d infused over 10 hours; benefits HIV patients with HSV-1 infection failing acyclovir and foscarnet therapy
• Cidofovir (Vistide) topical: 0.1–0.3% gel for 5 days for progressive/resistant lesions
• Trifluridine (Viroptic) ophthalmic solution for mucocutaneous lesions resistant to acyclovir

Pediatric Considerations
• High-risk infant: Acyclovir, 30 mg/kg/d IV q8h for 10–14 days

• Low-risk infant, asymptomatic: Culture eyes, nose, and mouth at 24–36 h and observe.

ADDITIONAL TREATMENT
General Measures
• Cool compresses of aluminum acetate (Burow solution) 4–6 times a day
• Ice packs to perineum, sitz baths, topical anesthetic
• Analgesics, nonsteroidal anti-inflammatory drugs

COMPLEMENTARY AND ALTERNATIVE MEDICINE
L-lysine may be beneficial in reducing frequency, severity, and duration of HSV recurrences (3)[B].

 ## ONGOING CARE
FOLLOW-UP RECOMMENDATIONS
Avoid intercourse with symptomatic lesions.

Patient Monitoring
• Latent infection: Check pregnant women at prenatal visits and onset of labor.
• Consider testing for other STDs in setting of initial HSV infection.
• Reassess suppression therapy yearly.

PATIENT EDUCATION
Herpes Resource Center:
http://www.ashastd.org/herpes/herpes_overview.cfm

PROGNOSIS
• Resolution of signs/symptoms:
  – Primary in 14–21 days
  – 1st episode nonprimary in 14–17 days
  – Recurrent in 7–10 days
• Latent infection: Recurrences in 80% of patients within 1 year of initial HSV-2 infection; immunocompetent average 3–4 a year for genital HSV-2; 1 a year for genital HSV-1
• HSV infection in immunocompromised (AIDS) patient: More severe, longer duration, more difficult to treat
• Treatment with antiviral agents does not eliminate virus from body.
• Suppressive Rx reduces recurrence rate by 50–80%.
  – Similar for acyclovir, valacyclovir, and famciclovir

Pediatric Considerations
Neonatal infection survival rates: Localized, >95%; central nervous system (CNS), 85%; systemic, 30%

COMPLICATIONS
• Secondary bacterial infection
• Urinary retention
• Aseptic meningitis
• Transmission to neonate; spontaneous abortion, preterm birth, low-birth-weight infants
• Increased risk for HIV infection (2–3 times)
• Lowered self-esteem, guilt, anger, depression, fear of rejection, fear of transmission to partner
• In pregnancy:
  – Primary/1st episode: Spontaneous abortion (45%); preterm labor (35%)
  – Greatest risk for neonatal infection with primary (50% transmission rate) or nonprimary 1st-episode (30%) infected mother at delivery; enhanced by prolonged rupture of membranes, fetal scalp electrode (6 × increased rate), cervical lesions, and prematurity
  – Low risk: Recurrent lesions at time of delivery (3%); recurrent asymptomatic HSV shedding in mother (<1%); mothers with high titer of neutralizing antibodies

– 80% of infants with HSV are born to mothers without history of HSV infection
– Cesarean section is indicated if herpetic genital lesions are present during labor:
  ○ Reduces neonatal infection by 85%
– In patients with known genital HSV infection, offer HSV suppressive therapy with acyclovir or valacyclovir starting at 36 weeks gestation (to decrease viral shedding and subsequent possibility of C-section) (4)[A]

REFERENCES
1. Chida Y, Mao X. Does psychosocial stress predict symptomatic herpes simplex virus recurrence?: A meta-analytic investigation on prospective studies. *Brain Behav Immun*. 2009.
2. Centers for Disease Control and Prevention, Workowski KA, Berman SM. Sexually transmitted diseases treatment guidelines, 2006. *MMWR Recomm Rep*. 2006;55:1–94.
3. Griffith RS, Walsh DE, Myrmel KH, et al. Success of L-lysine therapy in frequently recurrent herpes simplex infection. Treatment and prophylaxis. *Dermatologica*. 1987;175:183–90.
4. Money D, Steben M, Society of Obstetricians and Gynaecologists of Canada et al. SOGC clinical practice guidelines: Guidelines for the management of herpes simplex virus in pregnancy. Number 208, June 2008. *Int J Gynaecol Obstet*. 2009;104: 167–71.

ADDITIONAL READING
Lebrun-Vignes B, Bpuzamondo A, Dupuy A, et al. A meta-analysis to assess the efficacy of oral antiviral treatment to prevent genital herpes outbreaks. *Journal of the American Academy of Dermatology*. 2007;57(2).

See Also (Topic, Algorithm, Electronic Media Element)
Algorithm: Genital Ulcers

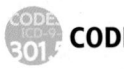 ## CODES

ICD9
• 054.10 Genital herpes, unspecified
• 054.11 Herpetic vulvovaginitis
• 054.12 Herpetic ulceration of vulva

CLINICAL PEARLS
• Genital herpes infections are frequently contracted from oral sex.
• Condoms used correctly can decrease transmission by >60%.
• The majority of HSV genital infections are thought to be transmitted during asymptomatic shedding of the virus; make sure patients understand they are always potentially contagious, not just during outbreaks.

H

HICCUPS

James H. Lewis, MD

BASICS

DESCRIPTION
- Hiccups are caused by a sudden involuntary contraction of the inspiratory muscles (predominantly the diaphragm) terminated by abrupt closure of the glottis stopping the inflow of air and producing the characteristic sound (1).
- System(s) affected: Nervous; Pulmonary
- Synonym(s): Hiccoughs; Singultus

Geriatric Considerations
Can be a serious problem among the elderly

Pregnancy Considerations
- Fetal hiccups are noted as rhythmic fetal movements (confirmed sonographically) that can be confused with contractions.
- Fetal hiccups often recur in subsequent pregnancies.

EPIDEMIOLOGY
- Predominant age: All ages (including fetus)
- Predominant sex: Male > Female (4:1)

Prevalence
Self-limited hiccups are extremely common, as are intra- and postoperative hiccups; intractable hiccups are rare.

RISK FACTORS
- General anesthesia; conscious sedation
- Postoperative state
- Genitourinary disorders
- Irritation of the vagus nerve branches
- Structural, vascular, infectious, neoplastic, or traumatic CNS lesions

GENERAL PREVENTION
- Identify and correct underlying cause.
- Avoid gastric distention.
- Seek medical attention for frequent bouts or persistent hiccups.
- Acupuncture appears to be as or more efficacious than chronic drug therapy to control hiccups.

ETIOLOGY
- Pathophysiologic significance is unknown; may be a vestigial reflex; hiccups have been associated with >100 underlying disorders (1).
- Results from stimulation of ≥1 limbs of the hiccup reflux arc (vagus and phrenic nerves) with a "hiccup center" located in the upper spinal cord
- In men, >90% have an organic basis, whereas in women a psychogenic cause may be more likely.

- Specific underlying causes include:
  – Alcoholism
  – CNS lesions (brainstem tumors, vascular lesions, Parkinson disease) (2)
  – Diaphragmatic irritation (tumors, pericarditis, eventration, splenomegaly, hepatomegaly, peritonitis)
  – Hair, insect, or foreign body irritating tympanic membrane
  – Pharyngitis, laryngitis
  – Mediastinal and other thoracic lesions (pneumonia, aortic aneurysm, TB, myocardial infarction, lung cancer, rib exostoses)
  – Esophageal lesions (reflux esophagitis, achalasia, *Candida* esophagitis, carcinoma, obstruction)
  – Gastric lesions (ulcer, distention, cancer)
  – Hepatic lesions (hepatitis, hepatoma)
  – Pancreatic lesions (pancreatitis, pseudocysts, cancer)
  – Inflammatory bowel disease
  – Cholelithiasis, cholecystitis
  – Prostatic disorders
  – Appendicitis
  – Postoperative, abdominal procedures (3)
  – Toxic metabolic causes (uremia, hyponatremia, gout, diabetes)
  – Drug-induced (dexamethasone, methylprednisolone, anabolic steroids, benzodiazepines, α-methyldopa)
  – Psychogenic causes (hysterical neurosis, grief, malingering)
  – Idiopathic

COMMONLY ASSOCIATED CONDITIONS
See Etiology.

DIAGNOSIS

- Hiccup attacks usually occur at brief intervals and last only a few seconds or minutes. Bouts lasting >48 hours often imply an underlying physical or metabolic disorder.
- Intractable hiccups may occur continuously for months or years.
- Hiccups usually occur with a frequency of 4–60 per minute.

HISTORY
Recent surgery (especially genitourinary), general anesthesia (3); medications; alcoholism; GI, cardiac, or pulmonary disorders (see Etiology) (1)

PHYSICAL EXAM
- See Etiology" for specific findings to look for.
- Examine ear canal for foreign bodies.

DIAGNOSTIC TESTS & INTERPRETATION
Lab
Consider CBC, metabolic panel as suggested by history

Imaging
Fluoroscopy is useful to determine whether 1 hemidiaphragm is dominant.

Diagnostic Procedures/Surgery
- Upper endoscopy, colonoscopy, CT scan (or other imaging) of brain, thorax, abdomen, and pelvis looking for etiological causes; exploratory laparoscopy or laparotomy for peritoneal lesions (carcinomatosis, etc.); GYN pathology, etc.
- The extent of the workup is often in proportion to the duration and severity of the hiccups.

DIFFERENTIAL DIAGNOSIS
See Etiology; burping (eructation) may be confused with hiccups (4).

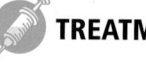

TREATMENT

- Outpatient (usually)
- Inpatient (if elderly, debilitated, or intractable hiccups)
- Nearly all hiccup treatments are anecdotal; those with recorded success are below (1).

MEDICATION
First Line
Possible drug remedies:

- Baclofen, a GABA analog, 5–10 mg t.i.d. (best choice) (5)[A]
- Chlorpromazine, 25–50 mg IV (1)[B]
- Haloperidol, 2–12 mg IM
- Phenytoin, 200 mg IV, then 100 mg q.i.d.
- Metoclopramide, 5–10 mg q.i.d. (1)[B].
- Nifedipine, 10–20 mg/d to t.i.d.
- Amitriptyline, 10 mg t.i.d.
- Lidocaine, 1.5 mg/kg IV infusion followed by 0.75 mg/kg on subsequent days
- Gabapentin (Neurontin), up to 1,800 mg/d in divided doses (6,7)[B]

- Contraindications: Refer to manufacturer's literature:
  – Baclofen is not recommended in patients with stroke or other cerebral lesions.
- Precautions: Refer to manufacturer's literature:
  – Abrupt withdrawal of baclofen should be avoided.
- Maintenance drug therapy (e.g., baclofen, 5–10 mg t.i.d.; phenytoin, 100 mg q.i.d.; valproic acid, 15 mg/kg undivided doses; nifedipine, 10–20 mg daily to t.i.d.; metoclopramide, 10 mg q.i.d.); gabapentin, up to 1,800 mg in divided doses

Second Line
- Amantadine, carbidopa-levodopa in Parkinson disease
- Steroid replacement in Addison disease
- Antifungal agent in *Candida* esophagitis
- Ondansetron in carcinomatosis with vomiting
- Nefopam (a nonopioid analgesic with antishivering properties related to antihistamines and antiparkinsonian drugs) is available outside the US in both IV and oral formulations (8)[B].

ADDITIONAL TREATMENT
General Measures
- Treat any specific underlying cause when identified (1):
  - Dilate esophageal stricture or obstruction.
  - Treat ulcers or reflux disease.
  - Remove hair or foreign body from ear canal.
  - Angostura bitters for alcohol-induced hiccups
  - Catheter stimulation of pharynx for operative and postoperative hiccups
  - Antifungal treatment for *Candida* esophagitis
  - Correct electrolyte imbalance.
- Medical measures:
  - Relief of gastric distention (gastric lavage, nasogastric aspiration, induced vomiting)
  - Counterirritation of the vagus nerve (supraorbital pressure, carotid sinus massage, digital rectal massage) to be used with caution
  - Respiratory center stimulants (breathing 5% CO_2)
  - Psychiatric (hypnosis, behavioral modification)
  - Phrenic nerve block or electrical stimulation (9) (or pacing) of the dominant hemidiaphragm
  - Miscellaneous (cardioversion)

Issues for Referral
For acupuncture or phrenic nerve crush, block, or electrostimulation (9,10)

COMPLEMENTARY AND ALTERNATIVE MEDICINE
- Acupuncture is increasingly being used to manage persistent hiccups (10)[B].
- Simple home remedies:
  - Swallowing a spoonful of sugar
  - Sucking on a hard candy or swallowing peanut butter
  - Holding breath and increasing pressure on diaphragm (Valsalva maneuver)
  - Tongue traction
  - Lifting the uvula with a cold spoon
  - Inducing fright
  - Smelling salts
  - Rebreathing into a paper (not plastic) bag
  - Sipping ice water
  - Rubbing a wet cotton-tipped applicator between hard and soft palate for 1 minute (11)[C]

SURGERY/OTHER PROCEDURES
- Phrenic nerve crush or transection of the dominant diaphragmatic leaflet
- Resection of rib exostoses

IN-PATIENT CONSIDERATIONS
Admission Criteria
Most patients can be managed as outpatients; those with severe intractable hiccups may require rehydration, pain control, IV medications, or surgery.

 ## ONGOING CARE

FOLLOW-UP RECOMMENDATIONS
Patient Monitoring
Until hiccups cease

DIET
Avoid gastric distension from overeating, carbonated beverages, and aerophagia.

PATIENT EDUCATION
See General Measures.

PROGNOSIS
- Hiccups often cease during sleep.
- Most acute benign hiccups resolve with home remedies or spontaneously.
- Intractable hiccups may last for years or decades.
- Hiccups have persisted despite bilateral phrenic nerve transection.

COMPLICATIONS
- Inability to eat
- Weight loss
- Exhaustion, debility
- Insomnia
- Cardiac arrhythmias
- Wound dehiscence
- Death (rare)

REFERENCES
1. Lewis JH. Hiccups and their cures. *Clin Perspect Gastroenterol*. 2000;3:277–83.
2. Miwa H, Kondo T et al. Hiccups in Parkinson's disease: an overlooked non-motor symptom? *Parkinsonism Relat. Disord*. 2010;16:249–51.
3. Kranke P, Eberhart LH, Morin AM, et al. Treatment of hiccup during general anaesthesia or sedation: a qualitative systematic review. *Eur J Anaesthesiol*. 2003;20:239–44.
4. Hopman WP, van Kouwen MC, Smout AJ et al. Does (supra)gastric belching trigger recurrent hiccups? *World J. Gastroenterol*. 2010;16:1795–9.
5. Ramírez FC, Graham DY. Treatment of intractable hiccup with baclofen: results of a double-blind randomized, controlled, cross-over study. *Am J Gastroenterol*. 1992;87:1789–91.
6. Porzio G, Aielli F, Verna L, Aloisi P, Galletti B, Ficorella C et al. Gabapentin in the Treatment of Hiccups in Patients With Advanced Cancer: A 5-Year Experience. *Clinical neuropharmacology*. 2010;
7. Marinella MA et al. Diagnosis and management of hiccups in the patient with advanced cancer. *J Support Oncol*. 2009;7:122–7, 130.
8. Bilotta F, Rosa G. Nefopam for severe hiccups. *N Engl J Med*. 2000;343:1973–4.
9. Okuda Y, Kitajima T, Asai T. Use of a nerve stimulator for phrenic nerve block in treatment of hiccups. *Anesthesiology*. 1998;88:525–7.
10. Schiff E, River Y, Oliven A, et al. Acupuncture therapy for persistent hiccups. *Am J Med Sci*. 2002;323:166–8.
11. Brostoff JM, Birns J, Benjamin E. The "cotton bud technique" as a cure for hiccups. *Eur Arch Otorhinolaryngol*. 2009.

ADDITIONAL READING
Cabane J, Bizec JL, Derenne JP et al. [A diseased esophagus is frequently the cause of chronic hiccup. A prospective study of 184 cases.] *Presse medicale (Paris, France : 1983)*. 2010;

 ## CODES

ICD9
- 306.1 Respiratory malfunction arising from mental factors
- 786.8 Hiccough

CLINICAL PEARLS
- An organic cause for persistent hiccups is more likely to be found in men.
- Rule out foreign body in ear canal as trigger.
- Baclofen remains the only pharmacologic therapy proven effective in a clinical trial setting.
- Acupuncture is proving very effective in persistent hiccups refractory to other therapies.

H

Francisco Aguirre, MD

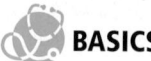 **BASICS**

DESCRIPTION
- Acute, tender, cystlike abscesses in apocrine gland–bearing skin (axillae, anogenital area, pubes, areolae; also apocrine glands scattered around umbilicus, scalp, trunk, and face); often a chronic condition
- Over time, fibrotic sinus tracts develop with intermittent drainage and periodic acute abscesses.
- Common from late puberty through 40 years
- System(s) affected: Skin/Exocrine
- Synonym(s): Acne inversa; Apocrinitis; Hidradenitis axillaris

Geriatric Considerations
Rare after menopause

Pediatric Considerations
Rarely occurs before puberty

Pregnancy Considerations
No isotretinoin (Accutane) or tetracycline treatment during pregnancy. Disease may ease during pregnancy and rebound following parturition.

EPIDEMIOLOGY
- Predominant age: Peak onset age 11–30 years, commonly 30–40 years
- Predominant sex: 3:1 female-to-male ratio

Incidence
Peaks during 2nd and 3rd decades of life

Prevalence
0.3–4%

RISK FACTORS
- Obesity
- Acne
- Hyperandrogenism
- Hirsutism
- Smoking
- Lithium may trigger onset or exacerbate this condition.

Genetics
Unknown; possibly single gene transmission (autosomal dominant), possibly polygenic

GENERAL PREVENTION
- Weight loss if overweight or obese
- Avoid constrictive clothing/frictional trauma.
- Avoid heat exposure, sweating, shaving, depilation, and deodorants.
- Use antiseptic soaps, topical application of tea tree oil
- Smoking cessation

ETIOLOGY
- Traditionally considered a disorder of apocrine glands, but now believed to be primarily an inflammatory disorder of the hair follicle triggered by follicular plugging within apocrine gland–bearing skin
- Bacterial involvement is not a primary pathogenic event, but secondary.
- Sebum excretion not an important factor.
- Smoking may be a major triggering factor.
- Considered part of follicular occlusive tetrad: Acne conglobata, dissecting cellulitis of scalp, hidradenitis suppurativa, and pilonidal sinus
- There may be a genetic predisposition component that is still being elucidated.

COMMONLY ASSOCIATED CONDITIONS
- Acne
- Perifolliculitis capitis abscedens et suffodiens (dissecting cellulitis of scalp)
- Arthritis
- Obesity with associated diabetes mellitus, atopy, acanthosis nigricans
- Crohn disease
- Pilonidal disease
- Smoking

 DIAGNOSIS

This is a clinical diagnosis.

HISTORY
- Multiple recurrences at the same site
- Recurrent deep boils >6 months in flexural sites
- Onset after puberty
- Poor response to conventional antibiotics
- Strong tendency toward relapse or recurrence
- Improved with smoking cessation and weight loss
- Personal or family history of acne or pilonidal sinuses and premenstrual exacerbation of boils
- Early signs are pruritus, erythema, and local hyperhidrosis.
- Healing sites may be accompanied by scarring and sinus tracts.
- Associated arthritis and arthropathy, especially the knees

PHYSICAL EXAM
- Tender nodules (dome-shaped) 0.5–3 cm in size are present:
  - Distribution is over the area of apocrine glands, with axillae and groin being most common. Sites ordered by frequency of occurrence: Axillary, inguinal, perianal and perineal, mammary and inframammary, buttock, pubic region, chest, scalp, retroauricular, eyelid.
  - Large lesions often are fluctuant.
  - Comedones may be present.
  - Possible malodorous discharge
- Staging: Most commonly done with the "Hurley" staging system, although it is likely that future studies will use the more complicated "Sartorius" staging system for clinical research:
  - Hurley staging system:
    - Stage I: Abscess formation (singular or multiple) without sinus tracts or scarring
    - Stage II: One or more widely separated recurrent abscesses with tract formation and scars
    - Stage III: Multiple interconnected tracts and abscesses throughout an entire area

DIAGNOSTIC TESTS & INTERPRETATION
Lab
Initial lab tests
- Cultures of skin or aspirates of boils often show no pathogens.
- When positive, deep cultures are often polymicrobial and have shown *Staphylococci aureus*, *S. epidermidis*, *Streptococcus milleri*, *S. hominis*, *Bacteroides fragilis*, and *B. melaninogenicus*.
- Check sensitivities due to increasing antibiotic resistance.

- May note increased erythrocyte sedimentation rate (ESR), leukocytosis, decreased serum iron, normocytic anemia, and changes in serum electrophoresis pattern, probably due to chronic inflammatory process
- Consider these additional studies at baseline, depending on elected treatment:
  - Complete blood cell count with differential
  - Basic metabolic panel plus magnesium
  - Liver function tests
  - Glucose-6-phosphate dehydrogenase level
  - Fasting lipids
- Purified protein derivative

Follow-Up & Special Considerations
If patient is female with hirsutism, check:
- Dehydroepiandrosterone sulfate
- Testosterone total and free
- Sex-hormone-binding globulin
- Progesterone

Diagnostic Procedures/Surgery
- Incision and drainage of lesion(s) with culture and biopsy
- Mortimer clinical criteria for diagnosis: Recurrent boils in apocrine-gland bearing skin for more than 3 months, presence of comedones in apocrine skin or retroauricular sites, and exacerbation of disease premenstrually (1)
- Ultrasound may be useful to assist in planning an entire excision to identify the full extent of sinus tracts.

Pathological Findings
- Histologically, chronic disease shows a dermis that contains inflammatory cells, giant cells, sinus tracts, subcutaneous abscesses, and later, extensive fibrosis.
- Multiple comedones and follicular dilatation and possible occlusion by keratinized stratified squamous epithelium may be observed.

DIFFERENTIAL DIAGNOSIS
- Furunculosis/carbuncles: Differentiate by specific culture and also by the response to specific antibiotics.
- Infected Bartholin or sebaceous cysts
- Hyperandrogenism
- Lymphadenopathy/lymphadenitis
- Cutaneous Langerhans cell histiocytosis
- Actinomycosis
- Granuloma inguinale
- Lymphogranuloma venereum
- Apocrine nevus
- Crohn with anogenital fistula (may coexist with hidradenitis suppurativa or be mistaken for it)
- Cutaneous tuberculosis
- Fox-Fordyce disease

 TREATMENT

- Conservative treatment includes all items under general prevention, plus use of warm compresses, sitz baths, and topical antiseptics for inflamed lesions and non-narcotic analgesics (2)[C]. Additionally, weight loss and smoking cessation have shown improvement (3).
- Medical treatment is often tried first because of extensive nature of surgery treatment.

- No medications are curative. Relapse almost inevitable once medication is stopped. Strategy is to keep disease contained with medications. If a cure is sought and disease is Hurley stage II–III, surgery should be considered.
- Because of the significant psychosocial stressful nature of this illness, referral of patient for stress management and to a support group is recommended.

MEDICATION
First Line
- Stage I disease; consider either systemic or topical antibiotics:
  - Topical antibiotics: Select one of the following (clindamycin has the most evidence):
    ○ Clindamycin 1% solution b.i.d. (× 12 wks at a minimum) (2,4)
    ○ Benzoyl peroxide 5–10% soln b.i.d. (4)[C]
    ○ Chlorhexidine 4% soln b.i.d. (4)[C]
  - Systemic antibiotics: Select one of the following:
    ○ Tetracycline 500 mg b.i.d. (>12 weeks) (5)
    ○ Oral clindamycin 300 mg b.i.d. and rifampin 300 mg b.i.d. for 12 wks (2,6)[B]
- Stage II–III disease:
  - Antibiotic therapy is usually systemic and mostly aimed at addressing likely overlying bacterial infection, with a need to cover gram-negative, gram-positive, and anaerobic bacterial infections, with the antibiotic selection based upon lesion location and characteristics.
  - While antibiotic therapy is generally attempted, it is more likely that more aggressive approaches will be needed subsequently. While this usually implies surgical treatment, medical management described below may lead to progress once any infectious component has been addressed:
    ○ Immunosuppressive therapies with infliximab (2,7)[C]

Second Line
- Stage I:
  - Consider oral contraceptives for women if antibiotics fail. Low-dose progesterone birth control pills (e.g., Norinyl, Ortho-Novum) (2)[C].
  - Sulfamethoxazole/trimethoprim DS b.i.d. (4).
  - Oral amoxicillin 250–500 mg b.i.d., tetracycline, minocycline 50–100 mg b.i.d., doxycycline 50–100 mg b.i.d., or erythromycin (2)[C]
  - Limited lesions can be injected with corticosteroids, and flares can be addressed with short courses of oral or intralesional corticosteroids such as triamcinolone (2)[C].
  - Dapsone (2)[C]
  - Finasteride (consider only postmenopausally for women) (2,4)[C]
- Stage II–III disease or recalcitrant Stage I:
  - Systemic retinoids: Isotretinoin 40–80 mg p.o. every day for 4 months (2)[C]
  - Cyproterone acetate (if available) (2)[B]

ADDITIONAL TREATMENT
General Measures
- Symptomatic treatment for acute lesions
- Prevention of new lesions
- Local cleansing (germicidal soap)
- Improve environmental factors that cause follicular blockage (see General Prevention).
- Steps that may improve the disease are smoking cessation and weight loss if overweight or obese.

Issues for Referral
Lack of response to treatment or stage II–III disease is a reason to refer for surgical excision or radiation/laser treatment (stage II).

SURGERY/OTHER PROCEDURES
- Various surgical approaches have been used for stage II–III disease:
  - Incision and drainage is discouraged as it is rarely curative (2,8)[C].
  - Deroofing and marsupialization of the sinus tracts may be of benefit, as healing time is reduced but recurrences seen (2,8)[C]
  - Treatment for stage III or intractable cases: Wide full-thickness excision with healing by granulation or flap placement is the most definitive treatment and rarely has local recurrence if all sinus tracts are excised. Rates of local recurrence (within 3–72 months) are: Axillary (3%) and perianal (0%), inguinoperineal (37%), and submammary (50%) (9,10).
- CO_2 laser ablation with healing by secondary intention has recent data with good results (11).

 ## ONGOING CARE

FOLLOW-UP RECOMMENDATIONS
Monthly or sooner follow-up to evaluate progress and assist with symptom management

Patient Monitoring
Regular follow-up visits

DIET
No limitations

PATIENT EDUCATION
- Severity can range from only 2 or 3 papules per year to extensive draining sinus tracts.
- Medications are temporizing measures and are rarely curative. Smoking cessation and weight loss can improve symptoms significantly.
- Attempts at local surgical "cures" do not affect recurrence at other sites.
- Hidradenitis suppurativa is considered a misnomer by many. Acne inversa is the more descriptive terminology.
- Hidradenitis Suppurativa Foundation: http://www.hs-foundation.org

PROGNOSIS
- Individual lesions (with or without drainage) heal slowly in 10–30 days.
- Recurrences may last for several years.
- Rare spontaneous resolution
- Relentlessly progressive scarring and sinus tracts are likely for chronic severe disease.
- Radical wide-area excision is the method that has shown the greatest likelihood for a lack of recurrence up to 5 years.

COMPLICATIONS
- Contracture formation at the sites of excisions in the case of surgery with possibly restricted limb mobility
- Rarely, squamous cell carcinoma may develop in indolent sinus tracts (usually anogenital).
- Disseminated infection septicemia (unusual)
- Lymphedema
- Urethral/rectal fistula
- Anemia

- Arthritis:
  - Asymmetrical pauciarticular to symmetrical polyarthritis/polyarthralgia in larger joints
- Amyloidosis and hypoproteinemia can lead to renal failure and even death.
- Interstitial keratitis
- Lumbosacral epidural abscess
- Sacral bacterial osteomyelitis

REFERENCES
1. Mortimer PS, Dawber RP, Gales MA, et al. Mediation of hidradenitis suppurativa by androgens. Br Med J (Clin Res Ed). 1986;292:245–8.
2. Lam J, Krakowski AC, Friedlander SF. Hidradenitis suppurativa (acne inversa): management of a recalcitrant disease. Pediatr Dermatol. 2007;24:465–73.
3. Sartorius K, Emtestam L, Jemec GB, Lapins J. Objective scoring of hidradenitis suppurativa reflecting the role of tobacco smoking and obesity. The British Journal of Dermatology, 2009;161(4):831–9.
4. Lee RA, Yoon A, Kist J. Hidradenitis suppurativa: an update. Adv Dermatol. 2007;23:289–306.
5. Jemec GB, Wendelboe P. Topical clindamycin versus systemic tetracycline in the treatment of hidradenitis suppurativa. J Am Acad Dermatol. 1998;39:971–4.
6. Mendonça CO, Griffiths CE. Clindamycin and rifampicin combination therapy for hidradenitis suppurativa. Br J Dermatol. 2006;154:977–8.
7. Grant A, Gonzalez T, Montgomery MO, Cardenas V, Kerdel FA. Infliximab therapy for patients with moderate to severe hidradenitis suppurativa: a randomized, double-blind, placebo-controlled crossover trial. J Am Acad Dermatol. 2010;62:205–217.
8. Slade DE, Powell BW, Mortimer PS. Hidradenitis suppurativa: pathogenesis and management. Br J Plast Surg. 2003;56:451–61.
9. Kagan RJ, Yakuboff KP, Warner P, et al. Surgical treatment of hidradenitis suppurativa: a 10-year experience. Surgery. 2005;138:734–40; discussion 740–1.
10. Mandal A, Watson J. Experience with different treatment modules in hidradenitis suppuritiva: a study of 106 cases. Surgeon. 2005;3:23–6.
11. Hazen PG, Hazen BP. Hidradenitis Suppurativa: Successful Treatment Using Carbon Dioxide Laser Excision and Marsupialization. Dermatol Surg. 2010;36:208–213.

 ## CODES

ICD9
705.83 Hidradenitis

CLINICAL PEARLS
- Hidradenitis suppurativa is an inflammatory disease of the apocrine skin areas that can be difficult to contain with behavior changes and medication.
- For those people with recalcitrant or severe disease, surgery provides the only treatment with a chance at a cure. Success rates depend on location and extent of excision.

HIP FRACTURE

Richard Viken, MD

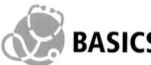

BASICS

DESCRIPTION
- Fracture of the femur head or neck, usually as the result of a fall. The following classification derives from the vascular anatomy of the head and neck of the femur.
- Intracapsular:
  - Femoral neck, subcapital or transcervical
  - Intracapsular femoral neck fractures may disrupt the blood supply to the femoral head, resulting in avascular necrosis.
- Extracapsular:
  - Intertrochanteric
  - Subtrochanteric
- System(s) affected: Musculoskeletal
- Synonym(s): Subcapital fracture; Trochanteric fracture; Femoral neck fracture

Geriatric Considerations
Hip fractures common in geriatric age group

EPIDEMIOLOGY
- Predominant age: 80% occur in those >60 years old
- Predominant sex: Female > Male (3:1)

Incidence
- In US, 200,000 patients per year >65 have fracture of hips.
- In US, women >75 years: 1% incidence per year

RISK FACTORS
- Low bone-mineral density
- Metastatic cancer
- Neurologic disease with gait impairment
- Severe renal disease with secondary hyperparathyroidism
- Long-acting sedatives or hypnotics in the elderly
- Age
- Propensity to fall
- History of previous fracture
- Weight loss
- Frailty
- Impaired vision
- Osteoarthritis
- Hyperthyroidism
- Deconditioning
- Cigarette smoking
- Alcohol use
- Diabetes mellitus
- Long-term proton pump inhibitor therapy (high doses)

Genetics
No known genetic factor

GENERAL PREVENTION
- Prophylactic treatment for osteoporosis (1)[C]:
  - Calcium supplementation: 1000–1500 mg PO daily
  - Vitamin D supplementation: 1000–2000 IU PO daily
- Avoid long-acting sedatives and hypnotics in the elderly.
- Use walking canes or walkers if patient has unsteady gait.
- Accumulating evidence casts some doubt on the effectiveness of hip protectors in reducing the incidence of hip fracture in older people. Acceptance and adherence by users of the protectors remain poor due to discomfort and impracticality (2)[A].
- General safety to prevent falls (e.g., use sturdy rails in showers, bathrooms, stairs, or ramps; avoid throw rugs and slippery surfaces)
- A structured exercise program has been shown to reduce falls and fear of falling in frail elderly (1)[C].
- Quantitative ultrasound and/or bone-mineral density measurements can be used to predict the likelihood of hip fracture in men and women.

ETIOLOGY
- Osteoporosis
- Direct blunt trauma
- Spontaneous in pathologic conditions (e.g., bone cancer)

COMMONLY ASSOCIATED CONDITIONS
- Osteoporosis
- Metastatic malignancy

DIAGNOSIS

HISTORY
- Pain in hip: If severe, it usually indicates a displaced fracture. Mild pain usually occurs in nondisplaced fractures.
- Pain in knee: Pain is referred from hip and may occur in absence of hip pain.

PHYSICAL EXAM
- External rotation of leg
- Shortening of leg

DIAGNOSTIC TESTS & INTERPRETATION
Lab
Routine preoperative laboratory including CBC, chemical profile, electrolytes

Imaging
- Radiographs:
  - Anteroposterior and "frog leg" lateral of hip
  - Anteroposterior pelvis to rule out pelvic fracture as cause of pain.
  - Remainder of femur to include knee
  - Any other tender or painful area, as other fractures are common and symptoms may be ignored in the face of severe pain of hip fracture.
- CT or MRI scans are not routinely indicated because the diagnosis is usually obvious from plain radiographs; however, MRI is 100% sensitive in delayed diagnosis of occult hip fracture (3)[C].

Pathological Findings
Osteoporosis

DIFFERENTIAL DIAGNOSIS
Rule out primary or metastatic malignancy, pelvic fracture.

TREATMENT
- Treat emergently.
- Pain control (may need narcotic analgesics)

MEDICATION
- Analgesics, as indicated. Consider morphine sulfate 2–10 mg q3h as needed with change to oral opioids as soon as possible (4)[B].
- Prophylactic anticoagulation with unfractioned low-dose heparin, 5,000 U SC q8–12h or low molecular weight heparin (Lovenox) 30 mg SC q12h (5)[A]
- Prophylactic antibiotics at induction of anesthesia: Ceftriaxone 2 g IV or IM for 1 dose (5)[A]
- Contraindications: Opioids in associated head injury or severe respiratory disease
- Precautions: Dosage should be lower in older people to avoid respiratory problems.

First Line
- Treatment of osteoporosis to prevent hip fractures has been found with alendronate, but only when combined with weight-bearing exercise and aggressive vitamin D replacement. Data supporting other bisphosphonates to prevent hip fracture remains unclear.
- Bisphosphonates:
  - Alendronate (Fosamax), 35–70 mg PO weekly
  - Risedronate (Actonel), 35 mg PO weekly
  - Ibandronate (Boniva), 150 mg PO monthly
  - Zoledronic acid (Reclast), 5 mg IV yearly
  - Also approved as a fracture preventative after the occurrence of a hip fracture
  - Salmon calcitonin
    - Nasal spray (Miacalcin), 1 spray daily in alternate nostrils
    - Injectable (Calcimar), 100 IU SC/IM daily

ADDITIONAL TREATMENT
General Measures
- Surgery should be performed once patient is medically stable, within 24 hours if possible (5)[B].
- Surgery is almost always indicated. Older patients do not tolerate long periods of bed confinement.
- Protect pressure points to avoid decubitus ulcers, especially on the sacrum, heels, and malleoli (5)[A].
- Oxygen therapy as needed per oximetry assessment
- Cyclical compression devices (6)[B]
- Situations where nonoperative treatment may be appropriate include:
  - End of life imminent
  - Nonambulatory, demented: Bed-bound, unable to transfer independently
- Compression-type fatigue fracture of the femoral neck:
  - Occurs in normal bone exposed to excessive loads (e.g., young athlete)
  - Patients must be compliant with 6–8 weeks of sharply restricted activity.

- Although patients with preoperative cognitive impairment require longer rehabilitation courses, they achieve short-term outcomes comparable to those who are cognitively unimpaired in the setting of a multidisciplinary hip fracture service. Cognitive impairment status should not be used as a determinant of which patients will benefit from surgery (7)[B].

SURGERY/OTHER PROCEDURES

- Displaced intracapsular fractures have no clearly superior treatment. Options are internal fixation or arthroplasty (6)[B]:
  - Internal fixation is associated with a higher risk of implant failure than hemiarthroplasty (femoral head replacement).
  - At present, the choice of treatment is determined by patient factors (e.g., age, presence of arthritis, availability and cost of different types of treatment, surgeon experience, and surgeon preference).
- Undisplaced intracapsular fractures should have internal fixation with a widely used method that is familiar to the surgeon (e.g., cancellous screws or compression screw and plate) (5)[A].
- Extracapsular (trochanteric) fractures should be treated surgically. A compression hip screw and plate has less chance of failure and reoperation, compared with a fixed device, and it may prove to be more cost-effective in the long-term.
- For subtrochanteric fractures, the Medoff sliding plate has been associated with fewer fixation failures when compared with other screw plates and is recommended for this fracture (5)[A].
- The choice of regional versus general anesthesia has unknown effectiveness on morbidity or mortality outcomes (6)[B].

IN-PATIENT CONSIDERATIONS
Admission Criteria
Virtually all patients should be admitted in anticipation of surgery.

Nursing
In-patient evaluation by physical therapy and possibly occupational therapy/social services to determine discharge location and rehabilitation schedule

Discharge Criteria
- Patients should be up (for toilet and prevention of deep vein thrombosis and decubiti) as soon as possible after surgery, usually the next day.
- Ambulate as soon as possible after surgery (e.g., with use of a walker). Close supervision by an experienced therapist is necessary.

 ## ONGOING CARE

FOLLOW-UP RECOMMENDATIONS
Patient Monitoring
- Radiographs of the hip taken prior to discharge from the hospital and every 8–12 weeks thereafter until healed
- Monitor postoperative physical therapy for full recovery.

DIET
Nutritional supplementation with oral protein and energy feeds reduces postoperative complications and death (6)[B].

PROGNOSIS
- Hip fractures remain a serious injury in older people: 15–20% 3-month mortality in trochanteric fractures; 10% in neck fractures.
- 65% can be expected to return to their former state of health.
- An interdisciplinary team approach implemented both preoperatively and postoperatively appears to result in better outcomes with fewer complications (6)[B].
- The overall risk of repeat hip fracture ranges from 2–10% and is greatest during the 12–month period following the 1st hip fracture.

COMPLICATIONS
- Mental deterioration:
  - Present in 90% of older patients for varying periods of time after surgery
  - Usually subsides, but may persist owing to preexisting cognitive and mood disorders
- Infection:
  - More common in comminuted fractures and patients with diabetes
  - Surgical implants should be left in place and antibiotics given as indicated by culture and sensitivity.
  - Some require the wound to be opened and drained.
- Aseptic necrosis of femoral head:
  - Occurs in 25–30% of femoral neck fractures
  - Treatment requires a prosthetic replacement in older patients.
- Phlebitis:
  - Prophylaxis with warfarin (Coumadin) to keep INR 2.0–2.5 or prothrombin time 15–18 seconds, for at least 4 weeks, OR
  - Enoxaparin (Lovenox) 30 mg SC q12h beginning 12 hours after surgery and continuing until patient is mobile
- Nonunion:
  - In case of neck fractures, a prosthetic replacement is indicated.
  - In the intertrochanteric fracture, a bone graft, usually with replacement of the nail and plate, is indicated.

REFERENCES
1. Brunner LC, Eshilian-Oates L, Kuo TY. Hip fractures in adults. *Am Fam Physician*. 2003;67:537–42.
2. Parker MJ, Gillespie WJ, Gillespie LD. Hip protectors for preventing hip fractures in older people. *Cochrane Database Sys Rev*. 2005;CD001255. DOI:10.1002/14651858.CD001255.pub3.

3. Gangopadhyay S, Akra G, Nanu A. Occult hip fractures in the elderly: A protocol for management. *Eur J Orthopaed Surg Traumatol*. 2007;17:153–6.
4. Ebell MH. Predicting hip fracture risk in older women. *Am Fam Physician*. 2007;76:273–5.
5. Beaupre LA, Jones CA, Saunders LD, et al. Best practices for elderly hip fracture patients. A systematic overview of the evidence. *J Gen Intern Med*. 2005;20:1019–25.
6. Handoll H, Parker M. Hip fracture. *Am Fam Physician*. 2007;75:93–6.
7. Moncada LV, Andersen RE, Franckowiak SC, et al. The impact of cognitive impairment on short-term outcomes of hip fracture patients. *Arch Gerontol Geriatr*. 2006;43:45–52.

ADDITIONAL READING

Grover M, Edwards F, Hitchcock K. What steps can reduce morbidity and mortality caused by hip fractures? *The Journal of Family Practice*. 2007;56:944.

See Also (Topic, Algorithm, Electronic Media Element)
Osteoporosis

 ## CODES

ICD9
- 820.00 Fracture of unspecified intracapsular section of neck of femur, closed
- 820.01 Fracture of epiphysis (separation) (upper) of neck of femur, closed
- 820.02 Fracture of midcervical section of femur, closed

CLINICAL PEARLS

- A structured exercise program has been shown to reduce falls and the fear of falling in frail older patients (1)[C].
- Suspect a fracture in a patient with a shortened, externally rotated leg.

H

HIRSUTISM

Laura L. Novak, MD

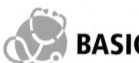 **BASICS**

DESCRIPTION
- Presence of excessive body and facial hair, in a male pattern, in women
- May be present in normal adults as an ethnic characteristic, or may develop as a result of androgen excess
- Often seen in association with polycystic ovarian syndrome (PCOS). May be accompanied by menstrual irregularities, insulin resistance, obesity, or acne.
- System(s) affected: Dermatologic; Endocrine/Metabolic; Reproductive
- Synonym(s): Excessive hair

Pregnancy Considerations
- May have related infertility. Offer intervention if desired.
- As hormone balance improves, fertility may increase; provide contraception as needed.
- Several medications used for treatment are contraindicated in pregnancy.

EPIDEMIOLOGY
Prevalence
8% of adult women

RISK FACTORS
- Family history
- Anovulation

Genetics
Multifactorial

GENERAL PREVENTION
- If there is associated insulin resistance or polycystic ovarian disease (PCOS), it can increase the risk of heart disease.
- Prolonged amenorrhea may, over time, put the patient at risk for endometrial hyperplasia or carcinoma.
- Women with late-onset congenital adrenal hyperplasia may be carriers for the severe early-onset childhood disease—counsel.
- Avoid quackery and unlicensed electrolysis.

ETIOLOGY
Hirsutism is due to increased androgenic (male) hormones, either from increased peripheral binding (idiopathic) or increased production from the ovaries, adrenals, or fat. Exogenous medications can also be associated with hirsutism.

COMMONLY ASSOCIATED CONDITIONS
- PCOS: Most common cause of hirsutism, accompanied by menstrual irregularity or amenorrhea. Often associated with acne, obesity, and multicystic ovaries, but up to 50% of cases are atypical.
- Prolonged amenorrhea and anovulation
- Hypothyroidism or hyperprolactinemia
- Late-onset congenital adrenal hyperplasia: A genetic enzyme deficiency associated with more severe and earlier-onset hirsutism. Present in <2% of hirsute, amenorrheic patients.
- Tumor: Rare (<0.2%); ovarian or adrenal; especially if associated with virilization (rapid onset, clitoromegaly, balding, deepening voice)
- Cushing syndrome: Rare; characterized by central obesity, moon facies, striae, hypertension

 DIAGNOSIS

HISTORY
- Age of onset (usually gradual), duration of symptoms
- Obtain a menstrual and fertility history: Irregular menses may indicate PCOS.
- Medication history: Look for use of valproic acid, testosterone, danazol, athletic performance drugs
- If galactorrhea is present, workup for hyperprolactinemia

PHYSICAL EXAM
- The Ferriman-Gallwey scale (an instrument that rates hair growth in 9 areas on a scale of 0–4 with >8 being positive) may be used for diagnosis, but underrates localized hirsutism.
- Increased androgens are associated with acne, obesity, insulin resistance, and hyperlipidemia.
- Increased hair growth on face, chest, and groin. May be hidden by plucking.
- Possible acne and obesity
- If insulin resistance is present, may have acanthosis nigricans: Velvety black skin in the axilla, neck, and under the breast
- Virilization: Deep voice, balding, clitoromegaly can indicate risk of tumor

DIAGNOSTIC TESTS & INTERPRETATION
- Diagnosis is clinical.
- Empiric treatment without lab workup is an acceptable option.
- Lab testing is performed to rule out underlying tumor and pituitary diseases, which are rare.

Lab
Initial lab tests
Basic workup recommended by ACOG. Total testosterone, thyroid-stimulating hormone (TSH), and, if clinically suspicious, an insulin resistance workup:

- Testosterone: Random testosterone level is usually sufficient. A morning free testosterone is slightly more sensitive, but the difference isn't clinically relevant (1,2)[A]: Level >200 ng/dL may indicate ovarian tumor.
- TSH elevation indicates hypothyroidism.
- Insulin resistance testing: Results vary with age and ethnicity:
  - Fasting insulin level >20 or fasting glucose/insulin ratio <4.5 may indicate resistance.
  - ACOG recommends fasting and 2-hour glucose after 75-gm glucose load in PCOS, but this may not be necessary.

Follow-Up & Special Considerations
- 17-hydroxyprogesterone (17-HP):
  - Elevations (>300) can indicate late-onset congenital adrenal hyperplasia; rare (<2%)
  - Consider in patients with onset in early adolescence.
  - Elevated levels require additional testing.
- Prolactin level if galactorrhea
- Dehydroepiandrosterone sulfate (DHEA-S) is no longer recommended (3,4)[A]:
  - Levels >700 may indicate adrenal tumor.

Imaging
- If testosterone is >200, obtain a CT scan of ovaries.
- Ovarian ultrasound can help in the diagnosis of PCOS.

DIFFERENTIAL DIAGNOSIS
Hirsutism is associated with a number of different conditions (see Etiology).

TREATMENT

MEDICATION

If idiopathic, no treatment is necessary, unless desired.

First Line

- Treatment goal is to decrease new hair growth and improve metabolic disorders.
- Oral contraceptives take 6–12 months to show effect; any brand is effective.
- Eflornithine (Vaniqa) HCl cream: Apply b.i.d.; reduces facial hair in 40% of women (with long-term use). Only FDA-approved hirsutism treatment.

Second Line

- Insulin sensitizers (metformin, thioglitazoles) decrease insulin resistance, improve hormone-binding proteins, and decrease androgens. Effective, but less so than oral contraceptives. Metformin is more effective than thioglitazones (5).
- Antiandrogenic drugs (used in combination with oral contraceptives to prevent menorrhagia and potential fetal toxicity) will further reduce hirsutism 15–25% (6,7). Usually begun after 6 months of 1st-line therapy if results are suboptimal. All should be avoided in pregnancy:
  - Spironolactone, 25–200 mg/d: Onset of action is slow; use with oral contraceptives to prevent menorrhagia. Watch for hyperkalemia, especially with drospeone-containing OCP (Yasmin); contraindicated in pregnancy.
  - Finasteride: 5 mg/d decreases androgen binding; not approved by FDA. Use with contraception (pregnancy Category X).
  - Ketoconazole, 400 mg/d: Avoid with astemizole, triazolam. Use with contraception. Not FDA-approved.

ADDITIONAL TREATMENT

General Measures

- Treatment is slow and often lifelong.
- If patient desires pregnancy, induction of ovulation may be necessary.
- Provide contraception as needed.
- Encourage patient to maintain ideal weight.
- Treat accompanying acne.

COMPLEMENTARY AND ALTERNATIVE MEDICINE

- Saw palmetto (Serenoa repens): In small studies, decreases hair growth via blocking 5-α-reductase activity in the skin (1). Has similar peripheral action to finasteride (decreasing 5-alpha reductase).
- Spearmint tea: 1 cup b.i.d. In a study of 21 patients, 1 cup b.i.d. for 6 months led to decreased hirsutism (8).
- Licorice: In a small study, 9 women using 3.5 grams daily for 2 cycles had benefit. Excess licorice can lead to hypokalemic hypertension (1).

ONGOING CARE

FOLLOW-UP RECOMMENDATIONS

No special activity

Patient Monitoring

Monitor for known side effects of medications.

DIET

No special diet

PATIENT EDUCATION

- Hormonal treatment stops further hair growth, but will not usually reverse present hair.
- Treatment takes 6–24 months and may be lifelong.
- Cosmetic measures include plucking, bleaching, shaving, electrolysis, laser hair removal, and cover-up cosmetics.
- Electrolysis should be performed by a licensed professional.

PROGNOSIS

- Good (with long-term therapy) for halting further hair growth
- Moderate to poor for reversing current hair growth

COMPLICATIONS

- If PCOS is present, dysfunctional uterine bleeding and anemia
- If PCOS is present, anovulation may increase uterine cancer risk.
- Androgenic excess may adversely affect lipid status, cardiac risk, and bone density.
- Poor self-image/shame

REFERENCES

1. Meletis C, Zabriskis N. Natural approaches for treating polycystic ovarian syndrome. *Altern Complement Ther.* 2006;12(4):157–64.
2. ACOG Clinical Practice Guideline No. 44. On the diagnosis and management of Polycystic Ovarian Syndrome. Washington DC: American College of Obstetrics and Gynecology, 2002.
3. Azziz R. The evaluation and management of hirsutism. *Obstet Gynecol.* 2003;101:995–1007.
4. Rosenfeld RL. Hirsutism. *N Eng J Med.* 2005;353(24):2578–88.
5. Harborne L, Fleming R, Lyall H, Sattar N, Norman J et al. Metformin or antiandrogen in the treatment of hirsutism in polycystic ovary syndrome. *J Clin Endocrinol Metab.* 2003;88:4116–23.
6. Farquhar C, Lee O, Toomath R, Jepson R et al. Spironolactone versus placebo or in combination with steroids for hirsutism and/or acne. *Cochrane Database Syst Rev.* 2003;CD000194.
7. Swiglo BA, Cosma M, Flynn DN, et al. Clinical review: Antiandrogens for the treatment of hirsutism: a systematic review and metaanalyses of randomized controlled trials. *J Clin Endocrinol Metab.* 2008;93:1153–60.
8. Akdoan M, Tamer MN, Cüre E, et al. Effect of spearmint (Mentha spicata Labiatae) teas on androgen levels in women with hirsutism. *Phytother Res.* 2007.

ADDITIONAL READING

- Goodman NF, Bledsoe MB, Cobin RH, et al. American Association of Clinical Endocrinologists medical guidelines for the clinical practice for the diagnosis and treatment of hyperandrogenic disorders. *Endocr Pract.* 2001;7:120–34.
- Martin KA, Chang RJ, Ehrmann DA, et al. Evaluation and treatment of hirsutism in premenopausal women: an endocrine society clinical practice guideline. *J Clin Endocrinol Metab.* 2008;93: 1105–20.
- Pillai A, Bang H, Green C et al. Metformin and glitazones: do they really help PCOS patients? *J Fam Pract.* 2007;56:444–53.
- Radosh L et al. Drug treatments for polycystic ovary syndrome. *Am Fam Physician.* 2009;79:671–6.

See Also (Topic, Algorithm, Electronic Media Element)

Acne Vulgaris; Infertility; Polycystic Ovarian Syndrome (PCOS)

CODES

ICD9

704.1 Hirsutism

CLINICAL PEARLS

PCOS is the most common cause of hirsutism, accompanied by menstrual irregularity or amenorrhea. Often associated with acne, obesity, and multicystic ovaries, but up to 50% of cases are atypical.

H

HISTRIONIC PERSONALITY DISORDER

Melissa E. Arthur, LCSW, MA
Gerry Edwards, MD

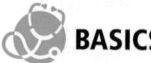 **BASICS**

DESCRIPTION
- A condition characterized by persistent patterns of dysfunctional behavior (excessive emotionality and attention seeking) deviating from one's culture and social environment that leads to functional impairment and distress, both to the individual and those who have regular interaction with the individual.
- Behaviors are perceived by the patient to be "normal" and "right," and patients have little insight as to their responsibility for these behaviors.
- Condition is classified based on the predominant symptoms and their severity.
- Cluster B personality disorder (inclusive of antisocial, borderline, histrionic, and narcissistic personality disorders) characterized by a pervasive pattern of excessive emotionality and attention seeking, present in a variety of contexts (5 or more symptom patterns to diagnose) (1):
  - Shows self-dramatization, theatricality, and exaggerated expressions of emotion
  - Is easily influenced by others or circumstance
  - Uncomfortable when not center of attention
  - Interactions are often characterized by inappropriate sexually seductive behavior.
  - Rapidly shifting and shallow emotions
  - Draws attention through physical appearance
  - Has a style of speech that is excessively impressionistic and lacks detail
- Considers relationships more intimate than they are (1)

EPIDEMIOLOGY
Incidence
Starts in adolescence and early 20s, and persists throughout one's life in the absence of treatment (1)

Prevalence
- 2–3% general population (1)
- Tends to be identified more frequently in females (1)

RISK FACTORS
Genetics
- Major character traits may be inherited.
- Other character traits due to a combination of genetics and environment, including adverse childhood experiences

ETIOLOGY
Environmental and genetic factors, including adverse childhood experiences and lack of parental attention

COMMONLY ASSOCIATED CONDITIONS
- Depression, anxiety, panic disorder
- Somatization disorders
- Body dysmorphic disorder (strong emphasis on physical appearance)
- Anorexia
- Post-traumatic stress disorder, including dissociative disorders
- Substance abuse

 DIAGNOSIS

HISTORY
- Distress, excessive emotionality (2)
- Impairment of social and/or occupational functioning (2)
- Not due to direct physiological effects of substance abuse, drug abuse, medication use, or general medical conditions
- Comprehensive interview and mental status examination
- Family session to assess persistent pattern of behavior

DIAGNOSTIC TESTS & INTERPRETATION
Lab
Initial lab tests
Thyroid-stimulating hormone (TSH), venereal disease research laboratory (VDRL), complete blood count (CBC), HIV

Imaging
Computed tomography (CT) scan and magnetic resonance imaging (MRI) of the brain may be necessary in newly developed symptoms in the absence of a triggering event to rule out the rare instance of organic brain disease.

Diagnostic Procedures/Surgery
Psychological testing (e.g., MMPI-II)

DIFFERENTIAL DIAGNOSIS
- Narcissistic personality disorder
- Somatization disorder
- Borderline personality disorder
- Substance abuse
- Can co-occur with borderline, narcissistic, antisocial, and dependent personality disorders

TREATMENT

MEDICATION

No known drug to treat personality disorder; however, medications can reduce symptoms (3)[C] associated with the Axis I disorders, such as mood disorders (antidepressants: Selective serotonin reuptake inhibitors [SSRIs]) and anxiety disorders (anxiolytics: benzodiazepines, buspirone, and SSRIs) (3)[C]

COMPLEMENTARY AND ALTERNATIVE MEDICINE

- Biofeedback
- Meditation

IN-PATIENT CONSIDERATIONS

Initial Stabilization

- In patients who have attempted overdose, transport all appropriate pill bottles to hospital.
- Appropriate psychiatric security measures should be in place to prevent lethality.

 ONGOING CARE

FOLLOW-UP RECOMMENDATIONS

Exercise as a means of reducing stress

Patient Monitoring

- If the patient is on a pharmacological regimen, initial monitoring should be frequent (every 2 weeks) to evaluate the effectiveness, potential side effects of medication, and suicidal ideation.
- In the absence of pharmacological treatment, frequent regular visits (every 4–6 weeks) will help prevent attention-seeking phone calls/visits.

DIET

No known special diet

COMPLICATIONS

- Unstable relationships with family, friends, and coworkers
- May be characterized by separations and divorces.
- Disruptive work patterns (e.g., absenteeism, frequent job changes, and decreased productivity)
- Increased demand for outpatient medical visits due to psychological condition and attention-seeking behavior

REFERENCES

1. *American Psychiatric Association. Diagnostic and Statistical Manual of Mental Disorders*. 4th ed. Washington DC: American Psychiatric Association; 1994.
2. Kraus G, Reynolds DJ. The "A-B-C's" of the cluster B's: identifying, understanding, and treating cluster B personality disorders. *Clin Psychol Rev*. 2001;21: 345–73.
3. Ward RK. Assessment and management of personality disorders. *Am Fam Phys*. 2004;70(8):1505–12.

ADDITIONAL READING

Horowitz MJ. Psychotherapy for histrionic personality disorders. *J Psychother Practice Res*. 1997;6:93–107.

 CODES

ICD9

301.50 Histrionic personality disorder, unspecified

CLINICAL PEARLS

- Histrionic personality disorder is characterized by persistent patterns of excessive emotionality and attention seeking, deviating from one's culture and social environment that leads to functional impairment and distress, both for the individual and those who have regular interaction with the individual.
- Histrionic personality disorder can co-exist with other personality disorders.
- No drugs explicitly treat personality disorders. However, medications can be considered to reduce symptoms associated with concomitant mood and anxiety disorders.

H

HIV INFECTION AND AIDS

Farah Y. Khan, MD
Adam Barta, MD

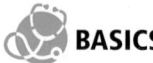 **BASICS**

DESCRIPTION

HIV is a retrovirus that integrates into CD4 T lymphocytes (a critical component of cell-mediated immunity), causing cell death and resulting in severe immunodeficiency, opportunistic infections (OI), and malignancies:

- Due to treatment advances, HIV is now a chronic disease.
- The natural history of untreated HIV infection includes viral transmission, acute retroviral syndrome, recovery and seroconversion, asymptomatic chronic HIV infection, and symptomatic HIV infection or AIDS.
- Without antiretroviral treatment, the average patient develops AIDS ~10 years after transmission.
- All HIV-infected persons with CD4 <200 cells/mm^3 or having AIDS defining illnesses are categorized as having AIDS.

EPIDEMIOLOGY
Incidence
- At end of 2008, 33.4 million people were estimated to be living with HIV/AIDS worldwide per UNAIDS and WHO. 2.7 million new HIV infections yearly and 2.0 million deaths attributable to AIDS (1)
- US: 56,300 new cases; estimated 17,197 deaths of persons with AIDS in 2007 (2)

Prevalence
- Estimated 1.1 million persons in US are living with HIV/AIDS, 25% of them were unaware of their status (1)
- HIV/AIDS cases are disproportionately high among racial/ethnic minority populations (1).
- Transmission of drug resistant virus is on the rise (1).
- Younger women and girls are particularly vulnerable (1)

RISK FACTORS
- Sexual activity (70% of world transmission). Viral load strongest predictor of heterosexual transmission with ulcerative urogenital lesions (3)[B].
- Male-to-male sexual contact accounts for 53% of newly diagnosed HIV/AIDS cases in 2007.
- Injection drug use
- Children of HIV-infected women:
  - Maternal HIV-1 RNA level is the best predictor of transmission risk.
  - HIV testing and use of antiretroviral drugs in pregnant women and their newborns has reduced the incidence of perinatal HIV transmission by >70% (from 25–29% without treatment to 8% with treatment) (4)[B].
  - Pregnant women should be treated until viral load is undetectable.
  - Can be transmitted through breastfeeding
- Recipients of blood products between 1975 and March 1985
- Occupational exposure

Genetics
People who lack CCR5, a cell-surface chemokine coreceptor used by HIV to infect cells, are highly resistant to HIV infection (5)[B].

GENERAL PREVENTION
Avoid unprotected sexual intercourse, injection drug abuse.

ETIOLOGY
HIV, a retrovirus

COMMONLY ASSOCIATED CONDITIONS
- Syphilis may be more aggressive in HIV-infected persons.
- Tuberculosis (TB) is coepidemic with HIV; test all persons with HIV for TB. Dually infected patients: 100× greater risk of developing active TB disease (compared with non-HIV) and higher rates of multidrug-resistant TB
- Hepatitis C–coinfected patients have more rapid progression to cirrhosis.

 DIAGNOSIS

- Acute retroviral syndrome: Precipitous decline in CD4 lymphocyte count and increased viremia, about 1–4 weeks after transmission. Confirmed by demonstrating a high HIV RNA in the absence of HIV antibody.
- Mononucleosis-like syndrome, including:
  - Fever (97%)
  - Adenopathy
  - Pharyngitis (73%)
  - Rash (77%)
  - Myalgias/Arthralgia (58%)
  - Less commonly: Headache, diarrhea, nausea, vomiting, hepatosplenomegaly, weight loss, thrush, and neurologic symptoms (12%)
  - Seroconversion: Development of a positive HIV antibody test usually occurs within 4 weeks of acute infection and invariably by 6 months.
  - Asymptomatic infection: Variable duration (average 8–10 years) and is accompanied by a gradual decline in CD4 cell counts and a relatively stable HIV RNA levels (the viral "set point"). Persistent lymphadenopathy: >1 cm in ≥2 extrainguinal sites, persists >3 months
- Symptomatic conditions:
  - Fever or diarrhea >1 month, bacillary angiomatosis, thrush, persistent candidal vulvovaginitis, cervical dysplasia or carcinoma in situ, oral hairy leukoplakia, herpes zoster, idiopathic thrombocytopenic purpura, pelvic inflammatory disease, peripheral neuropathy or myelopathy.
- AIDS: defined by a CD4 cell count <200, a CD4 cell percentage of total lymphocytes <14% or one of several AIDS-related opportunistic infections: Pneumocystis jiroveci (carinii) pneumonia, cryptococcal meningitis, recurrent bacterial pneumonia, Candida esophagitis, CNS toxoplasmosis, tuberculosis and NHL, progressive multifocal encephalopathy. HIV nephropathy, Kaposi's sarcoma, NHL, Hodgkin's, invasive cervical cancer.
- Advanced HIV disease: CD4 cell count of <50. Most AIDS related deaths occur at this time. Common late opportunistic infections: CMV disease (retinitis, colitis) or disseminated Mycobacterium avium complex. Also HIV wasting syndrome (>10% wt loss) and HIV encephalopathy/dementia/minor cognitive-motor disorder.

HISTORY
- Past medical history, including sexually transmitted diseases and TB
- Review of systems: Fever, chills, night sweats, diarrhea, weight loss, fatigue, adenopathy, oral sores, odynophagia (esophageal candidiasis), cough, shortness of breath and dyspnea on exertion (early P. carinii pneumonia), visual changes (cytomegalovirus [CMV] retinitis <200 CD4), skin rash, neurologic symptoms (central nervous system [CNS] infection, malignancy, or dementia), sinusitis
- Social history, transmission risks, adherence
- Immunization review

PHYSICAL EXAM
Focus on weight, skin, retinal exam, oropharynx; lymph nodes; liver, spleen, mental status, sensation, genital and rectal examinations.

DIAGNOSTIC TESTS & INTERPRETATION
Lab
- Screening: Enzyme-linked immunoabsorbent assay (ELISA) reported as reactive or nonreactive; sensitivity and specificity >98%. Obtain HIV RNA if acute HIV infection is suspected.
  - New rapid and oral test available (Home test kit, OraSure, OraQuickAdvanced Rapid HIV test).
- Confirmatory: Western blot:
  - Results positive, negative, or indeterminate
  - Per Centers for Disease Control (CDC): Positive test is reaction with 2 of these 3 bands: P24, gp 41, and gp 120/160. If indeterminate, repeat test in 3–6 months.
- CD4 cell count and percentage (6)[A]
- HIV-RNA viral load (6)[A]
- Complete blood count (CBC) with differential
- Serum chemistry
- Serologies: Hepatitis A, B, C; syphilis.
- Urine screen for sexually transmitted infections (N. gonorrhoeae, C. trachomatis)
- Cervical cytology
- PPD
- Glucose-6-phosphate (G-6PD) levels
- Lipids at baseline and during highly active antiretroviral therapy (HAART)
- Genotypic tests for resistance to antiretrovirals for patients who have pretreatment HIV RNA >1000 copies/m regardless of whether therapy will be initiated immediately (6)[A].

Imaging
Chest X-ray (CXR) if pulmonary symptoms or positive PPD.

DIFFERENTIAL DIAGNOSIS
Order other tests/serologies if HIV RNA test is negative. Order throat cultures for bacterial/viral respiratory pathogens, EBV VCA IgM/ IgG, CMV IgM/IgG, HHV-6 IgM/IgG, and hepatitis serologies as appropriate to establish a diagnosis for patient's symptoms.

TREATMENT

- Antiretroviral therapy should be initiated in all patients with a history of an AIDS-defining illness or with a CD4 count <350 (6)[A]
- Antiretroviral therapy should be initiated regardless of CD4 count in patients with the following conditions: Pregnancy, HIV-associated nephropathy and HBV coinfections when treatment of HBV is indicated [A], rapidly declining CD4 counts (e.g., >100 cells/mm decrease per year, higher viral load (e.g., >100,000 copies/ml) (6)[B]
- Antiretroviral therapy is recommended for all patients with CD4 count between 350 and 500 (6)[A].
- Consider for patients with CD4 count >500 (6)[B].

MEDICATION

- Nucleoside reverse transcriptase inhibitors (NRTI):
  – Abacavir (ABC, Ziagen), didanosine (DDL, Videx), emtricitabine (FTC, Emtriva), lamivudine (3TC, Epivir), stavudine (d4T, Zerit), tenofovir (Viread), zalcitabine (ddC, Hivid), zidovudine (AZT, Retrovir), zidovudine + lamivudine (Combivir), zidovudine + lamivudine + abacavir (Trizivir), tenofovir + emtricitabine (Truvada)
- Non-nucleoside reverse transcriptase inhibitors (NNRTI): Delavirdine (Rescriptor), efavirenz (Sustiva), nevirapine (Viramune)
- Protease inhibitors (PI): Amprenavir (Agenerase), atazanavir (Reyataz), darunavir (Prezista), fosamprenavir (Lexiva), indinavir (Crixivan), lopinavir-ritonavir (Kaletra), nelfinavir (Viracept), ritonavir (Norvir), saquinavir (Fortovase, Invirase), tipranavir (Aptivus)
- Fusion inhibitors: Enfuvirtide (Fuzeon)
- Entry inhibitors: Maraviroc (Selzentry)
- Integrase inhibitors: Raltegravir (Isentress)
- Drug failure: Before selecting regimen, review clinical symptoms, history of HAART, and adherence. Perform resistance testing.
- Protease inhibitors can cause metabolic syndrome (lipodystrophy, decreased high-density lipoprotein [HDL], increased triglycerides, high blood pressure [BP], and hyperglycemia).
- HAART, especially the protease inhibitors, have potentially life-threatening interactions.

First Line

- NNRTI + 2NNRTI (6)[A]
- PI (preferably boosted with ritonavir) + 2 NRTI (6)[A]
- Integrase inhibitor + 2 NRTI (6)[A]

ADDITIONAL TREATMENT

General Measures

- Main goal of HAART: reduce the viral load, ideally to <50 HIV1 RNA copies/mL), and delay immune suppression. Viral load is the most important indicator of response to HAART.
- An adequate CD4 response for most patients on therapy is defined as an increase in CD4 count in range of 50–150 cells/mm per year with an accelerated response in the first 3 months (6).
- Prevent HIV-associated complications, short- and long-term adverse drug reactions, HIV transmission, HIV drug resistance, and preservation of HIV treatment options.
- Assess substance abuse, economic factors (e.g., unstable housing), social support, mental illness, co-morbidities, high-risk behaviors, and other factors

that are known to impair the ability to adhere to treatment and to promote HIV transmission.

- With prolonged use of HAART, virus may mutate; medication will be less effective, but resistant strains have more difficulty reproducing. (Medication less effective than in a nonresistant patient.)
- Occupational exposure: Postexposure treatment in conjunction with expert consultation
- Prophylactic antimicrobial agents and vaccines:
  – *P. jiroveci* (former *Pneumocystis carinii*): TMP-SMX 1 DS/d or 1 SS/d indicated if CD4 <200/mm^3, prior PCP, thrush, or unexplained fever for >2 weeks
  – *M. tuberculosis*: Treat if PPD >5 mm induration without prior prophylaxis or treatment, recent TB contact, or history of inadequately treated TB that healed. Confirmed by culture. Treatment is based on susceptibility.
  – *Toxoplasma gondii*: 33% per year risk of infection in untreated patients with CD4 <100/mm^3. Prophylaxis: TMP-SMX DS/d.
  – *M. avium* complex (MAC): 20–40% risk with CD4 <50 and no HAART. Preferred prophylaxis is clarithromycin, 500 mg p.o. b.i.d., or azithromycin, 1,200 mg p.o. weekly.
  – Varicella (VZV): Seronegative and unexposed are at risk if exposed to chickenpox or shingles. Preferred regimen is VZIG 5 vials within 96 hours, preferably within 48 hours.
  – *S. pneumoniae*: 50–100× increased risk of invasive infection compared with general population; Pneumovax every 5 years
  – Influenza vaccine each fall
  – Hepatitis A and B vaccines for at-risk patients
  – Tetanus: dT vaccine in adults
  – Polio: Use *IPV*, not OPV in children.

ONGOING CARE

FOLLOW-UP RECOMMENDATIONS

Patient Monitoring

- If HIV RNA is detectable at 2–8 weeks, repeat q 4–8 weeks until suppression to less than level of detection, then q 3–6 months (6)
- Monitor HIV RNA, CD4 and CBC q 3–4 months (6).
- Fasting lipids and fasting glucose annually if normal. Basic chemistry, AST,ALT,T/D bili q 6–12 months (6)
- HLA-B 5701 if considering ABC (6)
- Pregnancy test if starting EFV (6)

DIET

- Encourage good nutrition, multivitamins.
- Avoid raw eggs, unpasteurized milk. Severely immunocompromised should boil tap water to prevent *Cryptosporidium*.

PATIENT EDUCATION

- Provide nonjudgmental prevention counseling, reviewing routes and behaviors leading to transmission to others and acquisition of super infection with resistant strains.
- Counsel on importance of adherence to HAART and prevention of resistance.
- National AIDS Hotline: (800) 342-2437 [Spanish (800) 342-7432]
- National Institute of Health AIDS Clinical Trials Group: (800) 874-2572
- American Foundation for AIDS Research: (212) 719-0033 (new treatments and research)
- Information available at: http://www.aidsinfo.nih.gov/

PROGNOSIS

- When untreated HIV infection leads to AIDS, the life expectancy is 3.7 years.
- AIDS-defining opportunistic infections usually do not develop until CD4 <200.
- In HIV-untreated infection, CD4 counts decline at a rate of 50–80/yr, with more rapid decline as counts drop <200.
- Drug resistance is not the most common cause of treatment failure, its adherence failure (7)[B].

COMPLICATIONS

- Immunodeficiency
- Opportunistic infections
- Malignancy, including cervical or anal cancer

REFERENCES

1. Centers for Disease Control and Prevention (CDC). HIV prevalence estimates–United States, 2006. *MMWR Morb Mortal Wkly Rep*. 2008;57:1073–6.
2. Centers for Disease Control and Prevention: Diagnoses of HIV infection and AIDS in the United States and Dependent Areas, 2008 HIV Surveillance Report, Volume 2 http://www.cdc.gov/hiv/surveillance/resources/reports/2008report/ Page last updated: June 14, 2010
3. Quinn TC, Wawer MJ, Sewankambo N, et al. Viral load and heterosexual transmission of human immunodeficiency virus type 1. Rakai Project Study Group. *N Engl J Med*. 2000;342:921–9.
4. US Public Health Service Task Force Recommendations for Use of Antiretroviral Drugs in Pregnant HIV-1 Infected Women for Maternal Health Interventions to Reduce Perinatal HIV-1 Transmission in the US. *MMWR*. 2002;51:1–38.
5. Lama J, Planelles V. Host factors influencing susceptibility to HIV infection and AIDS progression. *Retrovirology*. 2007;4:52.
6. US Department of Health and Human Services. Guide for the Use of Antiretroviral Agents in HIV-1 Infected Adults and Adolescents. Available at: http://aidsinfo.nih.gov/guidelines/adult/AA_040705.
7. Simon V, Ho DD, Abdool Karim Q. HIV/AIDS epidemiology, pathogenesis, prevention, and treatment. *Lancet*. 2006;368:489–504.

CODES

ICD9

042 Human immunodeficiency virus (HIV) disease

CLINICAL PEARLS

- The symptoms of HIV acute infection include fever, sore throat, adenopathy, myalgias, and rash.
- Treatment guidelines are evolving to include earlier initiation of HAART in the course of the illness.
- The most common complications of HIV/AIDS are immunodeficiency, opportunistic infections, and malignancy.
- The prophylactic measures strongly recommended for HIV-infected patients are vaccination and prophylactic antibiotics based on history and CD4 count.

H

HODGKIN DISEASE

Jennifer Gao, MD
Fred Schiffman, MD

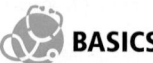 **BASICS**

DESCRIPTION
- Historical background:
  - Described in 1832 by Thomas Hodgkin in "On Some Morbid Appearance of the Absorbent Glands and Spleen"
  - First neoplasm defined by cytological grounds based on presence of Reed-Sternberg cells
  - First clinically staged neoplastic disease
  - First neoplasm treated with chemotherapy and/or radiotherapy
- Neoplastic Reed-Sternberg (RS) cells of monoclonal lymphoid B-cell origin within inflammatory background of lymphocytes (T-helper type 2 and regulatory T-cells), eosinophils, histiocytes, and plasma cells (1)
- 2 subtypes: Classical Hodgkin lymphoma (CHL, 95% of cases) and nodular lymphocyte predominant Hodgkin lymphoma (NLPHL, 5% of cases) (1):
  - NLPHL: Predominantly B-cells, neoplastic LH cells with multilobulated nuclei, small nucleoli, and popcornlike appearance
  - Classical Hodgkin lymphoma is further subdivided based on histologic findings:
    - Nodular sclerosis (60%)
    - Mixed cellularity (30%)
    - Lymphocytic depletion (<10%)
    - Lymphocytic rich (<10%)
- Frequency of lymph node involvement: Cervical > mediastinal > axillary > para-aortic

EPIDEMIOLOGY
- Most frequent lymphoma in Western countries at 30%
- Male > Female (1.4:1)
- Stage I/II at diagnosis: 50%
- Systemic symptoms: 25-40%
- Bone marrow involvement: 5%

Geriatric Considerations
- Poorer prognosis if present at 45 years of age or older (2):
  - Possibly due to susceptibility to toxic effects of intensive therapy
  - Less likely to be included in clinical trials
  - Co-morbidities affecting ability to tolerate standard treatment
- Benefit more than younger patients from doxorubicin in treatment regimen (2)

Pediatric Considerations
- Increased risk for males
- Young females (<30 years old) treated with thoracic radiation are at high risk for breast cancer.

Pregnancy Considerations
- Abdominal ultrasonography to detect subdiaphragmatic disease (2)
- Treatment (2):
  - Delay until after delivery in asymptomatic, early-stage Hodgkin's
  - ABVD safely used in 2nd and 3rd trimesters
  - Vinblastine monotherapy to control symptoms
  - 1st trimester: ABVD may or may not cause fetal malformations.

Incidence
- 2–3/100,000 annually, primarily in young adults (3)
- Lower incidence in underdeveloped countries
- Bimodal age distribution: Early peak at 15–35 years and late peak after 55 years (4)

RISK FACTORS
- Immunodeficiency (inherited or acquired)
- Autoimmune disorders
- EBV (3)
- Seasonal factors (3)

Genetics
- 1st-degree relative: 3–9× risk (3)
- Weak correlation between familial Hodgkin lymphoma and HLA class I regions containing HLA A1, B5, B8, B18 alleles (3)
- Siblings of younger patients: 7× risk

ETIOLOGY
- Exact etiology unclear
- RS cells likely derived from germinal center B cells with mutations in immunoglobulin variable chain
- Seasonal features and higher frequencies with Epstein-Barr virus suggest environmental factors (3).
- T-lymphocyte defects persist even after successful treatment.

COMMONLY ASSOCIATED CONDITIONS
In HIV (2):
- AIDS-defining illness
- Predominantly mixed-cellularity or lymphocyte-depleted histologic subtypes
- At diagnosis: Widespread disease, extranodal involvement, systemic symptoms

 DIAGNOSIS

HISTORY
- Asymptomatic lymphadenopathy (usually cervical or supraclavicular)
- Fever (Pel-Epstein pattern)
- Night sweats
- Weight loss
- Fatigue
- Anorexia
- Alcohol-induced pain
- Pruritus
- Performance status

PHYSICAL EXAM
Palpation of lymph tissue (lymph nodes, spleen) and liver

DIAGNOSTIC TESTS & INTERPRETATION
Lab
Initial lab tests
- Complete blood count (CBC)
- Chemistry profile
- Erythrocyte sedimentation rate (ESR)
- Liver function tests
- Renal function tests
- HIV (if risk factors present)
- Hepatitis serology (if risk factors present)
- Pregnancy test (women of childbearing age)
- Pulmonary function tests, including diffusion capacity of the lung for carbon monoxide (DLCO) if considering ABVD or BEACOPP (5)

- Drugs that may alter lab results: Phenytoin may produce pseudolymphoma.

Follow-Up & Special Considerations
- Fertility considerations (5):
  - Semen cryopreservation if chemotherapy or pelvic radiation therapy
  - In vitro fertilization or ovarian tissue/oocyte cryopreservation
- Radiation therapy (RT) considerations (5):
  - Splenic RT: Pneumococcal, H. flu, meningococcal vaccines
  - Neck RT: Neck computed tomography

Imaging
- Chest radiograph (5)
- Diagnostic computed tomography (CT) scan of chest, abdomen, and pelvis (5)
- Positron emission tomography (PET) scan (for initial staging, mid-treatment decision making, and end-of-treatment evaluation)
- Bone scan, gallium scan, abdominal US (used infrequently)

Diagnostic Procedures/Surgery
- Excisional lymph node biopsy (5)
- Core needle biopsy may be used if diagnostic (5)
- Immunohistochemistry (5)
- Exploratory laparotomy with splenectomy (this procedure is becoming uncommon)
- Bone marrow biopsy
- Liver biopsy (in selected cases)

Pathological Findings
Reed-Sternberg cell characteristics (5):
- Diameter: 20-50 micrometers
- Abundant acidophilic cytoplasm
- Bi- or poly-lobulated nucleus
- Acidophilic nucleoli
- CD30+, CD15+, CD45 negative, CD3 negative, CD20+ in 40% of cases
- RS cells necessary but not sufficient for diagnosis (need inflammatory background)

DIFFERENTIAL DIAGNOSIS
- Non-Hodgkin lymphoma
- Infectious lymphadenopathy
- Other solid tumor metastases
- Sarcoidosis
- Autoimmune disease
- AIDS/HIV infection
- Drug reaction

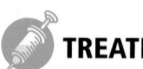 **TREATMENT**

- Ann Arbor staging with Cotswold modification: Needed to determine treatment modality (5):
  - Stage I: Single lymph node group - subscript E = extralymphatic organ or site involvement
  - Stage II: ≥2 node groups on the same side of the diaphragm - subscript E = extralymphatic organ or site involvement
  - Stage III: Node groups on both sides of the diaphragm - subscript E = extralymphatic organ or site involvement, subscript S = splenic involvement
  - Stage IV: Dissemination involving extranodal organs (except the spleen, which is considered lymphoid tissue)

- Subclasses: A = no systemic symptoms; B = systemic symptoms (fever, night sweats, weight loss >10% body weight); X = bulky disease (widened mediastinum, >1/3 intrathoracic diameter, or >10-cm nodal mass)
- Pathologic stage at given site denoted by superscript: M = bone marrow, H = liver, L = lung, O = bone, P = pleura, D = skin):
  - Splenectomy, liver biopsy, lymph node biopsy, bone marrow biopsy mandatory to establish pathological stage
- Treatment modalities: Radiation therapy and chemotherapy alone or combined (4,5):
  - Early stages (favorable prognosis): Lower radiation doses and smaller fields, 2–4 chemotherapy cycles with lower doses, chemotherapy alone
  - Early stages (unfavorable prognosis): Moderate chemotherapy (4–6 cycles) plus involved field radiation therapy (IFRT)
  - Advanced stages: Extensive chemotherapy (6–8 cycles) with or without RT
- Autologous bone marrow transplant for selected patients who fail conventional therapy
- Treatment goal: Aim for cure
- All subsequent treatment and follow-up care recommendations based on NCCN consensus. Please refer to NCCN Practice Guidelines in Oncology for Hodgkin Lymphoma (5).

MEDICATION
First Line
- ABVD chemotherapy: Doxorubicin, bleomycin, vinblastine, dacarbazine (5,6):
  - Lower risk of secondary malignancy than with MOPP or MOPP/ABV
- Stanford V chemotherapy: Doxorubicin, vinblastine, mechlorethamine, etoposide, vincristine, bleomycin, prednisone (6)

ALERT
- Must be monitored by experienced oncologist
- Contraindications: General for chemotherapy
- Precautions: Chemotherapy toxicity, bone marrow suppression:
  - Dacarbazine: Highly emetic, can cause severe phlebitis
  - Bleomycin: Risk of pulmonary toxicity, rarely death
  - Consider evaluating ejection fraction if using doxorubicin-containing regimens (5).

Second Line
- BEACOPP: Bleomycin, etoposide, doxorubicin, cyclophosphamide, vincristine, procarbazine, prednisone, G-CSF
- 2nd-line chemotherapy: Regimens depend on pattern of relapse and previous chemotherapy agents used (5):
  - ICE: Ifosfamide, carboplatin, etoposide
  - C-MOPP: Cyclophosphamide, vincristine, procarbazine, prednisone
  - GVD: Gemcitabine, vinorelbine, pegylated liposomal doxorubicin
  - IGEV: Ifosfamide, gemcitabine, vinorelbine
- Stem cell transplant: Use in progressive disease or relapse (5):
  - High-dose therapy and autologous stem cell transplant (HDT/ASCT) offers improvement in event-free survival and progression-free survival compared with conventional chemotherapy.
  - HDT/ASCT does NOT improve overall survival.

- Rituximab has excellent activity against the lymphocyte-predominant variant due to a predominance of CD20+ lymphocytes.
- "Watch and wait" tactic being explored for lymphocyte-predominant Hodgkin lymphoma (5)
- T-cell-based therapies under investigation (4)

ADDITIONAL TREATMENT
- Combined modality chemotherapy and radiation therapy (5):
  - Bulky disease all stages: With ABVD or Stanford V
  - Nonbulky disease stage I-II: With ABVD or Stanford V
  - Nonbulky disease stage IB-IIB: With BEACOPP
  - Bulky and nonbulky disease stage III-IV: With BEACOPP
- Radiation therapy alone: Uncommon except in lymphocyte-predominant Hodgkin lymphoma (5):
  - Avoid radiating high cervical regions and axillae (women only) if possible.

 ONGOING CARE

FOLLOW-UP RECOMMENDATIONS
Patient Monitoring
- During therapy: CBC, nutrition, and hydration
- Restage with PET after 2–4 cycles of chemotherapy: Sensitive prognostic indicator (5)
- Post-treatment monitoring (5):
  - H&P: Every 2–4 mos for first 2 yrs, then every 3–6 mos for next 3–5 yrs
  - Laboratory studies:
    - CBC, platelets, ESR, chemistry profile every 2–4 mos for 1–2 yrs, then every 3–6 mos for next 3–5 yrs
    - TSH annually if radiation to neck
  - Imaging:
    - Chest: Chest x-ray or CT every 6–12 mos during first 2–5 yrs
    - Abdominal/pelvic: CT every 6–12 mos during first 2–3 yrs
    - Annual breast mammogram or MRI beginning 8–10 yrs after therapy or at age of 40 yrs (whichever occurs earlier) if chest or axillary irradiation
    - Surveillance PET should **NOT** be done routinely due to risk of false positives.

PATIENT EDUCATION
- Reproductive impact
- Risks of secondary malignancy
- Careful oral and dental care during therapy
- Leukemia Society of America, 733 3rd Avenue, New York, NY 10017

PROGNOSIS
- Cure rate for classical Hodgkin lymphoma: 80%
- Relapse or progression of disease rate: 5–20% (3)
- Overall survival rates (4):
  - 1-year survival: 92%
  - 5-year survival: 85%
  - 10-year survival: 81%
- International Prognostic Score for advanced disease: 1 point per factor (5):
  - Age ≥45 years
  - Male gender
  - Albumin <4 g/dL
  - Hemoglobin <10.5 g/dL
  - Lymphocytopenia: <600 lymphocyte cells/dL or lymphocytes <8% of WBC
  - WBC ≥15,000 cells/dL
  - Stage IV disease

- Main cause of death (4):
  - Initial 5 years: Hodgkin lymphoma
  - After 5–10 years: Leukemia, myelodysplastic syndrome, especially in patients aged 21–30 years at start of treatment
  - After 20 years: Second primary malignancy, cardiovascular disease (pericardial disease, cardiomyopathy, valvular disease, arrhythmia, autonomic dysfunction, coronary artery disease)

COMPLICATIONS
- General: Chronic fatigue (4)
- Hematologic: Secondary malignancies, bone marrow suppression, anemia, ITP, TTP (4)
- Reproductive: Sterility, gonadal dysfunction, amenorrhea (4)
- Endocrine: Hypothyroidism (4)
- Infectious: Immunosuppressed infections including herpes zoster, overwhelming sepsis in asplenic patients
- Cardiac: Coronary artery disease, cardiomyopathy, valvular disease, pericardial disease
- Pulmonary: Radiation pneumonitis, pulmonary fibrosis, chronic pleural effusion
- Neurologic: Transient radiation myelopathy (Lhermitte sign)

REFERENCES
1. World Health Organization. *Cumulative Official Updates to ICD-10*. February 2010.
2. Armitage, James. Early-Stage Hodgkin's Lymphoma. *New England Journal of Medicine*. 363;7. August 12, 2010.
3. Gascoyne, Randy, Rosenwald Andreas, Poppema Sibran, Lenz George. Prognostic markers in malignant lymphomas. *Leukemia & Lymphoma*, 2010; Early Online, 1–9.
4. Czuczman Myron, Straus David, Gribben John, Bredenfeld Henning, Friedberg Jonathan, Bollard Catherine. *Leukemia & Lymphoma*, 2010; Early Online, 1–9.
5. NCCN Clinical Practice Guidelines in Oncology. *Hodgkin Lymphoma*. Version 2.2010. Available at www.nccn.org
6. Hoskin, Peter, et al. Randomized Comparison of the Stanford V Regimen and ABVD in the Treatment of Advanced Hodgkin's Lymphoma: United Kingdom National Cancer Research Institute Lymphoma Group Study ISRCTN 64141244. *Journal of Clinical Oncology*. Volume 27, Number 32, November 10, 2009, 5390–5396.

 CODES

ICD9
- 201.90 Hodgkin's disease, unspecified type, unspecified site
- 201.91 Hodgkin's disease, unspecified type, involving lymph nodes of head, face, and neck
- 201.92 Hodgkin's disease, unspecified type, involving intrathoracic lymph nodes

H

HOMELESSNESS

Dana Sprute, MD, MPH
Brynna Connor, MD

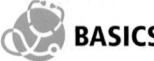 **BASICS**

DESCRIPTION

- Definition: A homeless person is "... an individual without permanent housing who may live on the streets; stay in a shelter, mission, single room occupancy facility, abandoned building or vehicle; or in any other unstable or non-permanent situation. May be considered homeless if 'doubled up,' (individuals are unable to maintain housing situation and stay with friends and/or family). In addition, previously homeless individuals who are to be released from a prison or a hospital may be considered homeless if do not have a stable housing situation to go upon release. A recognition of the instability of an individual's living arrangement is critical to the definition of homelessness."
- Homeless adults average 8–9 chronic medical conditions and life expectancy of 45 years (1).

EPIDEMIOLOGY

Incidence
3.5 million people in US experience homelessness each year; 40% are homeless families (2).

RISK FACTORS

- Social factors:
  – Poverty: Increase in US rates in the past 25 years (www.nationalhomeless.org/factsheetsheets/why.html); 2 major contributors: Eroding employment opportunities and decreasing availability of public assistance. 2009 federal poverty definition: 4-person household $22,050 annual income:
    ○ In 2008, 13–17% % of the US population fell below federal poverty definition. Children overrepresented in homeless population (35.7% of people living in poverty, but only 24.8% of total population).
  – Lack of affordable housing: Fall in federal support by 49% between 1980 and 2003.
  – Increase in home foreclosures: 32% increase between April 2008 and April 2009:
    ○ 10% become homeless as a result of foreclosure.
  – Increased unemployment: 9.3% official unemployment rate in the US in May 2010 (US Bureau of Labor Statistics, June 5, 2010).
  – Lack of affordable health care:
    ○ In 2008, 46.3 million people in US without health insurance at least part of year
- Domestic violence: 63% of homeless women experience domestic violence (US Conferences of Mayors, 2005)
- Addiction disorders: Homeless individuals face barriers to obtaining health care, including addiction treatment and support services.
- Psychiatric illness: 16% of single homeless adults suffer from persistent mental illness (US Conferences of Mayors, 2005)
- At risk: Domestic violence; youth; veterans; rural; victims of violence

COMMONLY ASSOCIATED CONDITIONS

- Untreated major medical illness (e.g., diabetes, HTN, COPD, peripheral vascular disease)
- Dental problems (e.g., caries, periodontal disease)
- Infectious diseases:
  – Tuberculosis, HIV, STIs (3)
  – Dermatologic conditions (cellulitis, fungal infection) (3)
  – Infestations: Lice and scabies
  – Liver disease (e.g., hepatitis B or C, or alcohol-related)
- Cognitive impairment: Traumatic brain injury, CVA, substance use (3)
- Exposure-related conditions (frostbite, heatstroke)
- Psychiatric illness
- Traumatic injury: Increased risk of assault; victims of hate crimes (4)
- Criminalization of homelessness

 DIAGNOSIS

HISTORY

- Living conditions: Location, access to food, restrooms, place to store medicines, safety (3)
- Prior homelessness: What precipitated it, first time, chronic (3)
- Acute/ chronic illness: Individual/family history of RAD, chronic otitis media, anemia, diabetes, CVD, TB, HIV/STIs, hospitalizations (3)
- Family members, especially dependent children (3)
- Medications: Current, psychiatric, contraception, OTC meds, dietary supplements, meds "borrowed" from others (3)
- Prior providers: Oral health, primary care, current medical home (3)
- Mental illness/cognitive deficit: Stress, anxiety, appetite, sleep, concentration, mood, speech, memory, thought process and content, suicidal/homicidal ideation, insight, judgment, impulse control, social interactions; symptoms of brain injury (headaches, seizures, memory loss, lability, irritability, dizziness, insomnia, poor organizational/decision making skills) (3)
- Alcohol/nicotine/other drug use: Amount, frequency, duration; look for signs of substance abuse/dependence (3)
- Sexual: Gender identity/orientation, behaviors, rape, pregnancies, hepatitis, HIV, other STIs (3)
- Abuse: History or current abuse; emotional, physical, sexual; patient safety (3)
- Legal problems/violence: Against persons/property, history of incarceration (3)
- Regular/strenuous activities: Routines (treatment feasibility); level of strenuous activity (3)
- Work history: Previous types of jobs, length held, veteran status, occupation injuries/toxic exposures; vocational skills, interest (3)
- Education level/literacy: Highest level of education; ever in special education; assist with intake forms; assess ability to read/language skills/English fluency (3)

- Nutrition/hydration: Diet, food resources, preparation skills, liquid intake (3)
- Cultural heritage/affiliations: Family, friends, faith community, other sources of support (3)
- Strengths: Coping skills, resourcefulness, abilities, interests (3)

PHYSICAL EXAM

- Comprehensive exam, first encounter if possible: Height, weight, BMI, abdominal girth, heart, BP, lungs, thyroid, liver, dermatologic, oral, fundoscopic, genital, lower extremities/feet, neurologic, mental status, mental health (3)
- Focused exams: For patients uncomfortable with full-body, unclothed exam at first visit (3)
- Dental assessment: Age-appropriate teeth, obvious caries, dental/referred pain, diabetes (3)

DIAGNOSTIC TESTS & INTERPRETATION

- Asthma: Spirometry or peak flow monitoring (3)
- Mental health: Patient Health Questionnaire (PHQ-9, PHQ-2), MHS-III, MDQ (3)
- Cognitive assessment: Mini-Mental Status Exam (MMSE), Traumatic Brain Injury Questionnaire (TBIQ), Repeatable Battery for the Assessment of Neuro-Psychological Status (RBANS) (3)
- Developmental assessment: Ages & Stages Questionnaires, Parents' Evaluation of Developmental Status (PEDS), Denver II or other standard screening tool (3)
- Interpersonal violence: Domestic violence, rape, etc (3).
- Forensic evaluation: If strong evidence of abuse (3)
- Health care maintenance: Age-appropriate vaccinations (e.g., hepatitis A, hepatitis B, pneumovax, TdaP, influenza, H1N1), cancer and chronic disease screening for adults; EPSDT screening and vaccinations for children (3)

Lab
- Baseline labs: EKG, lipid, potassium, and creatinine levels, HbA1C, liver function tests (3)
- PPD
- STI screening: Chlamydia, gonorrhea, syphilis, HIV, hepatitis serologies, HCV, trichomonas, bacterial vaginosis, monilia (3)
- Substance abuse: SSI-AOD, urine drug screen (3)

 TREATMENT

- Establish rapport: Sensitivity to prior negative prior health care experiences
- Enlist resources: Mental health and substance abuse programs, free clinics, case management
- Plan of care (3):
  – Basic needs: Food, clothing, housing may be higher priorities than health care.
  – Patient goals and priorities: Immediate/long-term health needs. Address patient wants first.
  – Action plan: Simple language, portable pocket card
  – After hours: Extended clinic hours, medical provider contact info when clinic closed

– Safety plan: For violence and abuse suspected; mandatory reporting requirements
– Emergency plan: Location of nearest ED, preparation for evacuation
– Adherence plan: Use of interpreter, identification of potential barriers

MEDICATION

- Simple regimen: Low pill count, once-daily dosing if possible (3)
- Dispensing: On site; small amounts at a time to promote follow-up, decrease risk of loss/theft/misuse. Determine resources for written prescriptions (3).
- Storage of medications: If no access to refrigeration, no prescription for meds requiring it (3)
- Patient assistance: Free/low-cost drugs if readily available for continuous use (3)
- Aids to adherence: Harm reduction, outreach/case management, directly observed therapy (3)
- Potential for misuse: Inhalants, bronchodilators/spacers, pain medications, clonidine, needles (3)
- Side effects: Primary reason for nonadherence (diarrhea, polyuria, nausea, disorientation) (3)
- Analgesia/symptomatic treatment: Contract, single provider for pain medication refills (3)
- Immunizations: Influenza, pneumococcus, HAV, HBV, tetanus for adults (3); diphtheria (5)
- Dietary supplements: Multivitamins with minerals, nutritional supplements (3)
- Managed care: Generics if possible, assistance getting prescription filled (3)
- Lab monitoring: Monitor patients on antipsychotic medications for metabolic disorders (3).

ADDITIONAL TREATMENT

- Associated problems/complications (3):
  - No place to heal: Efficacy of medical respite/recuperative care, supportive housing
  - Fragmented care: Multiple providers. Use EMR; list prescribed meds on wallet-sized card.
  - Masked symptoms/misdiagnosis: e.g., weight loss, dementia, edema, lactic acidosis
  - Developmental discrepancies: Focus on immediate concerns, not possible future consequences.
  - Dual diagnoses: Integrated treatment for concurrent mental illness/substance use disorders
  - Loss of child custody: Support for parent of child abused by others and for abused parent
- Follow-up (3):
  - Contact info: Phone, reliable mail address, e-mail for patient/friend/family/case manager
  - Medical home: To coordinate/promote continuity of health care
  - Frequency: More frequent follow-up, incentives, nonjudgmental care regardless of adherence
  - Drop-in system: Anticipate/accommodate unscheduled clinic visits.
  - Transportation assistance: Provide car fare, tokens, help with transportation services.
  - Community outreach, case management programs
  - Monitor school attendance: Address health/developmental problems with family/school.
  - Referrals: Link with specialist, pro bono care, providers sensitive to underserved population

IN-PATIENT CONSIDERATIONS

Admission Criteria

People who are homeless may be more likely to benefit from admission because:

- Living conditions are suboptimal
- Those with medical and psychiatric and/or substance use disorders

Discharge Criteria

- Discharge treatment plans should be evaluated for feasibility.
- Bed rest, extended periods of elevation, rest, or icing are not feasible in most instances.
- Following restrictive dietary guidelines often not possible
- Plans requiring multiple return visits are likely to fail if no support or return transportation.
- Attempt to assist patients who are amenable to treatment for drug, alcohol, nicotine abuse.
- Admission to inpatient rehabilitation if appropriate and possible

 ## ONGOING CARE

Fundamental issues in homelessness and health care that require ongoing consideration (3):

- Unstable housing
- Limited access to nutritious food and water
- Higher risk for abuse
- Physical/cognitive impairments; behavioral health problems
- Developmental discrepancies for children: Speech delay, chronic ear infection, insufficient opportunity to practice gross and fine motor skills
- Higher risk for communicable disease
- Lack of health insurance/resources; discontinuous/inaccessible health care; lack of a medical home; barriers to disability assistance
- Cultural/linguistic barriers: Racial and ethnic groups overrepresented in homeless population
- Limited education/literacy
- Lack of transportation
- Lack of social supports: Alienation from family and friends precipitates homelessness.
- Criminalization of homelessness: Frequent arrests for loitering, sleeping in public places

FOLLOW-UP RECOMMENDATIONS

- Patients with a history of nonadherence need additional support (e.g., case manager, outreach) to succeed in ongoing care after hospital discharge.
- Limited access to telephones to schedule appointments, and may be unable to receive telephone messages with test results or rescheduled appointment times.
- Arrange appointments prior to discharge.
- Document the best way to contact the individual.
- When possible, discharge planning should include efforts to improve housing status.
- Refer to a health care agency designed to address the needs of people who are homeless with integrated mental health, physical health, and substance use treatment.

PROGNOSIS

Mortality rates for chronically homeless adults 4 times higher than of age-matched controls (6)

REFERENCES

1. Levy BD, O'Connell JJ. Health care for homeless persons. *N Engl J Med.* 2004;350:2329–32.
2. Bassuk EL, et al: Facts on Trauma & Homeless Children, National Child Traumatic Stress Network, 2005. www.NCTSNet.org
3. Bonin E, et al. *Adapting Your Practice: General Recommendations for the Care of Homeless Patients.* Health Care for the Homeless Clinicians' Network, 2010 Edition.
4. Hate, Violence and Death on Main Street USA: A Report on Hate Crimes and Violence Against People Experiencing Homelessness in 2008. http://www.nationalhomeless.org/publications/hatecrimes/index.html
5. Badiaga S, Raoult D, Brouqui P. Preventing and controlling emerging and reemerging transmissible diseases in the homeless. *Emerg Infect Dis.* 2008;14:1353–9.
6. O'Connell JJ. The need for homelessness prevention: A doctor's view of life and death on the streets. *J Primary Prevent.* 2007;28:199–203.

ADDITIONAL READING

- Backer TE, Howard EA. Cognitive Impairments and the Prevention of Homelessness: Research and Practice Review. *J Prim Prev.* 2007.
- Principles of Practice: A Clinical Resource Guide for Health Care for the Homeless Programs, Bureau of Primary Health Care/HRSA/HHS, 3/1/1999; PAL 99-12)

 ## CODES

ICD9

V60.0 Lack of housing

CLINICAL PEARLS

- Stress related to difficulty meeting basic needs can interfere with engagement in health care.
- Assistance in gaining access to benefits or meeting basic needs may improve therapeutic relationship and allow individual to direct attention to physical health (3).
- Ending homelessness requires permanent housing with supportive services and implementing policies to prevent chronic homelessness. (www.endhomelessness.org/content/article/detail/1623). Nat'l Alliance to End Homelessness, January 2010.

H

HORDEOLUM (STYE)

Konstantinos E. Deligiannidis, MD, MPH
Alexandra Schultes, MD

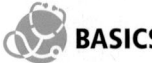 **BASICS**

DESCRIPTION
- An acute inflammation or infection of the eyelid margin involving the sebaceous gland of an eyelash (external hordeolum) or a meibomian gland (internal hordeolum)
- System(s) affected: Skin/Exocrine
- Synonym(s): Internal hordeolum; External hordeolum; Zeisian stye; Meibomian stye; Stye

EPIDEMIOLOGY
- Predominant age: None
- Predominant sex: Male = Female

Incidence
Unknown. Although external hordeolum is common, internal hordeolum is rare.

RISK FACTORS
- Poor eyelid hygiene
- Previous hordeolum
- Contact lens wearers
- Application of makeup
- Predisposing blepharitis (low-grade infections of the eyelid margin)
- Ocular Rosacea

Genetics
No known genetic pattern

GENERAL PREVENTION
Eyelid hygiene

PATHOPHYSIOLOGY
- Bacterial infection of sebaceous or meibomian glands, causing an acute inflammatory reaction
- In an internal hordeolum, the meibomian gland may become obstructed, leading to a pustule on the conjunctival surface as opposed to the margin of the eyelid (1).

ETIOLOGY
- Most commonly caused by *Staphylococcus aureus* (~90–95% of all cases) or by *S. epidermidis*
- Seborrhea can predispose to infections of the eyelid.

COMMONLY ASSOCIATED CONDITIONS
- Acne
- Seborrhea
- An association may exist between hordeolum during childhood and developing rosacea in adulthood (2).

 DIAGNOSIS

HISTORY
- Localized inflammation (vs. involvement of the entire eyelid or surrounding skin)
- Prior episodes are common.

PHYSICAL EXAM
- Localized inflammation of the eyelashes or a small pustule at the margin of the eyelid
- Localized swelling and tenderness on the internal or external aspect of the eyelid with an opening to either side
- To determine if an internal hordeolum is obstructed, the eyelid should be gently everted to examine for a pustule on the tarsal conjunctiva (1).
- Itching or scaling of the eyelids; collection of discharge, redness, and irritation, leading to localized tenderness and pain

DIAGNOSTIC TESTS & INTERPRETATION
Lab
Culture of the eyelid margins usually is not necessary.

Diagnostic Procedures/Surgery
History and eye exam

Pathological Findings
Bacterial contamination and white cells in eyelid discharge

DIFFERENTIAL DIAGNOSIS
- Chalazion
- Blepharitis
- Eyelid neoplasms
- Periorbital cellulitis
- Dacryocystitis

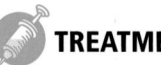 **TREATMENT**

MEDICATION
First Line
- Erythromycin ophthalmic 0.5% ointment, apply up to 6 times/day for 7–10 days
- Treat underlying dry eye with artificial tears.

Second Line
- Occasionally, the use of an aminoglycoside ophthalmic ointment, such as gentamicin or tobramycin, may be necessary if condition is refractory to simpler treatment.
- Oral dicloxacillin or cephalexin for 2 weeks if refractory to topical antibiotics

ADDITIONAL TREATMENT
General Measures
- The hordeolum should not be expressed.
- Warm compresses to the area of inflammation can help increase blood supply and encourage spontaneous drainage.
- Application of an antibiotic ointment (such as erythromycin) to the margin of the eyelid after proper cleansing (except in children <12 years old, in whom there is a risk of blurred vision and amblyopia) helps reduce bacterial proliferation.
- Good personal hygiene with attention to cleansing the eyelids on a daily basis to prevent recurrent infections

Issues for Referral
Consider referral if unresponsive to oral antibiotics.

COMPLEMENTARY AND ALTERNATIVE MEDICINE
Broncasma berna is a polyvalent antigen vaccine that may be useful in the treatment of recurrent hordeolum (3).

SURGERY/OTHER PROCEDURES
- If the infection becomes localized to a single gland, incision, drainage, or curettage sometimes is necessary. This is an in-office procedure with a local anesthetic:
  - Exercise caution, as ocular perforation has been reported with the injection of an anesthetic to an infected lid (4)[C].
- The use of combined antibiotic ointment (neomycin sulfate, polymyxin B sulfate, and gramicidin) after surgery was not shown to have any statistically significant difference to artificial tears (5)[B].

IN-PATIENT CONSIDERATIONS
Initial Stabilization
Outpatient

ONGOING CARE
FOLLOW-UP RECOMMENDATIONS
No restrictions

Patient Monitoring
The patient should be seen within several weeks to assess the effectiveness of therapy, or should at least call the physician's office with progress report.

DIET
No special diet

PATIENT EDUCATION
- The patient should be instructed in proper cleansing of the eyelids using a solution of tap water and baby shampoo or a commercially prepared hypoallergenic cleanser.
- The stye should not be squeezed or incised.

PROGNOSIS
- Usually responds well to good hygiene and warm compresses
- The inflammation usually improves within a week.
- Hordeolum tends to recur in some patients.

COMPLICATIONS
An internal hordeolum, if untreated, may lead to infections of adjacent glands and generalized cellulitis of the lid.

REFERENCES
1. Wald ER. Periorbital and orbital infections. *Infect Dis Clin North Am*. 2007;21:393–408, vi.
2. Bamford JT, Gessert CE, Renier CM, et al. Childhood stye and adult rosacea. *J Am Acad Dermatol*. 2006;55:951–5.
3. Nakatani M. Treatment of recurrent hordeolum with Broncasma Berna. *Eye*. 1999;13(Pt 5):692.
4. Kim JH, Yang SM, Kim HM et al. Inadvertent ocular perforation during lid anesthesia for hordeolum removal. *Korean J Opththalmol*. 2006;20(3):199–200.
5. Hirunwiwatkul P, Wachirasereechai K. Effectiveness of combined antibiotic ophthalmic solution in the treatment of hordeolum after incision and curettage: a randomized, placebo-controlled trial: a pilot study. *J Med Assoc Thai*. 2005;88:647–50.

CODES
ICD9
- 373.11 Hordeolum externum
- 373.12 Hordeolum internum
- 373.13 Abscess of eyelid

CLINICAL PEARLS
- The hordeolum should not be expressed.
- Warm compresses to the area of inflammation can encourage spontaneous drainage.
- Application of an antibiotic ointment (such as erythromycin) to the margin of the eyelid after proper cleansing (except in children <12 years old, in whom there is a risk of blurred vision and amblyopia) helps reduce bacterial proliferation.
- Good personal hygiene with attention to cleansing the eyelids on a daily basis to prevent recurrent infections.

H

HORNER'S SYNDROME

Matthew J. Dykhuizen, MD
Frank J. McCabe, MD

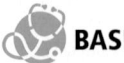 **BASICS**

DESCRIPTION
- Horner's syndrome is caused by the interruption of sympathetic nerve supply to the eye, resulting in a classic triad of miosis, eyelid ptosis, and/or absence or decrease of sweating of the ipsilateral face and neck (hypohidrosis):
  - Central or preganglionic lesion (complete syndrome)—1st- or 2nd-order neuron
  - Peripheral postganglionic lesion (incomplete syndrome, no anhidrosis)—3rd-order neuron
- System(s) affected: Nervous; Skin/Exocrine
- Synonym(s): Bernard-Horner syndrome; Bernard syndrome; Cervical sympathetic syndrome; Oculosympathetic syndrome; Oculosympathetic paralysis; Oculosympathetic deficiency

EPIDEMIOLOGY
- Predominant age: None
- Predominant sex: Male = Female

Incidence
Unknown

Prevalence
Unknown

RISK FACTORS
- Most common: Apical bronchogenic carcinoma (Pancoast tumor) in smokers
- Aneurysm of the carotid or subclavian artery
- Injuries to the carotid artery high in the neck
- Dissection of the carotid arteries
- Carotid artery occlusion:
  - ~15% of patients with carotid artery occlusion develop ipsilateral Horner's syndrome.
  - May occur without evidence of cerebral ischemia, neck injuries, or operative procedures
- Cluster headaches:
  - ~20% have an ipsilateral Horner's syndrome

Genetics
Rare autosomal-dominant inheritance

PATHOPHYSIOLOGY
- Constellation of signs produced when sympathetic innervation to the eye is interrupted somewhere along the 3-neuron arc:
  - Absence of innervation of iris dilator and Mueller muscles leads to miosis and slight ptosis, respectively.
  - Sympathetic innervation also controls sweat glands; interruption causes anhidrosis.
- Sympathetic nerve fibers originate in the hypothalamus and travel down the lateral part of the brainstem to exit in the thoracic area. These fibers synapse in the cervical sympathetic ganglia, and the postganglionic fibers travel to the eye along the wall of the carotid and ophthalmic arteries.
- Sympathetic fibers innervating sweat glands and vasodilatory muscles branch off before the cervical sympathetic ganglion traveling along the external carotid artery, so distal lesions will not result in anhidrosis.
- Lesions anywhere along this pathway will lead to ipsilateral Horner's syndrome.

ETIOLOGY
- Idiopathic (40%), congenital, or acquired
- Best classified by which order neuron is affected and by age (pediatric vs. adult)
- 1st-order neuron (13%): Hypothalamus to cervical spinal cord (C8–T2):
  - Arnold-Chiari malformation
  - Basal meningitis (e.g., syphilis)
  - Basal skull tumors:
    ○ Cerebral vascular accident
    ○ Lateral medullary (Wallenberg) syndrome
  - Demyelinating disease (multiple sclerosis)
  - Intrapontine hemorrhage
  - Neck trauma
  - Pituitary tumor
  - Syringomyelia
- 2nd-order neuron (44%): Ascends with sympathetic trunk through brachial plexus over apex of lung to superior cervical ganglion (near common carotid artery bifurcation):
  - Pancoast tumor or infection of lung apex
  - Cervical rib
  - Aneurysm/dissection of aorta
  - Subclavian or common carotid artery
  - Central venous catheterization
  - Trauma/surgical injury
  - Chest tubes
  - Lymphadenopathy (Hodgkin, leukemia, tuberculosis (TB), mediastinal tumors, sarcoid)
  - Mandibular tooth abscess
  - Lesions of the middle ear (acute otitis media)
- 3rd-order neuron lesions (43%): Ascends along adventitia of internal carotid artery through cavernous sinus close to the cranial nerve (CN) VI and then joins CN V_1 to innervate the iris dilator muscle and Mueller muscle in the eye:
  - Internal carotid artery dissection
  - Raeder syndrome (paratrigeminal syndrome)
  - Carotid cavernous fistula or other pathology
  - Cluster/migraine headaches
  - Herpes zoster
- Drugs: Acetophenazine, alseroxylon, bupivacaine, butaperazine, carphenazine, chloroprocaine, deserpidine, diacetylmorphine, diethazine, ethopropazine, etidocaine, guanethidine, influenza virus vaccine, levodopa, lidocaine, mepivacaine, mesoridazine, methdilazine, methotrimeprazine, oral contraceptives, perazine, prilocaine, procaine, prochlorperazine, promazine, propoxycaine, reserpine, thioproperazine, thioridazine, trifluoperazine

Pediatric Considerations
Most common etiology: Birth trauma to brachial plexus, chest surgery, neuroblastoma (paraspinal), and vascular anomalies of the carotid arteries

COMMONLY ASSOCIATED CONDITIONS
- Wallenberg syndrome
- Pancoast tumor
- C8 radiculopathy

 DIAGNOSIS

HISTORY
- Ptosis (typically mild; 1–2 mm)
- Miosis (with an associated dilation lag)
- Anhydrosis or hypohidrosis (often not appreciated by patients or clinicians):
  - Ipsilateral side of the body: Central (1st-order neuron)
  - Ipsilateral face: Preganglionic (2nd-order neuron)
  - Medial portion of forehead and side of nose: Postganglionic (3rd-order neuron after vasomotor and sudomotor fiber have branched off)

Pediatric Considerations
- In infants and children, loss of facial flushing is appreciated more than anhydrosis (Harlequin sign).
- 1st-order neuron may be associated with dysarthria, dysphagia, ataxia, vertigo, and nystagmus.
- 2nd-order neuron: History of previous trauma, neck, axillary, shoulder or arm pain, cough, hemoptysis, history of thoracic or neck surgery, history of chest tube or central venous catheter or neck swelling
- 3rd-order neuron: Diplopia (CN VI lesion), numbness in the distribution of the 1st and 2nd division of the trigeminal nerve

ALERT
Horner's syndrome in the presence of pain merits special consideration:
- Axial, shoulder, scapula, arm, or hand pain may be related to Pancoast tumor.
- Acute-onset, ipsilateral facial or neck pain: Consider carotid artery dissection until proven otherwise.
- Paratrigeminal syndromes:
  - Raeder paratrigeminal syndrome type I: Orbital pain, miosis, ptosis, with associated ipsilateral lesions of CN III–VI; suspect middle cranial fossa mass lesion
  - Raeder paratrigeminal syndrome type II: Episodic retrobulbar or orbital pain, miosis, ptosis with no CN lesions; suspect migraine variant

PHYSICAL EXAM
- Complete neurological and chest examination are necessary to find associated physical findings.
- Measurement of pupillary diameter in dim and bright light and their reactivity to light and accommodative response:
  - Anisocoria greatest in dark, with affected pupil failing to dilate
  - Redilation (after light is removed) may lag 15–20 s on affected side.

- Examine the upper lids for ptosis (<2 mm).
- Examination of the lower lids for "upside-down ptosis": Elevation of lower lid due to Mueller muscle weakness:
  – Illusion of enophthalmos secondary to narrowing of palpebral fissure
- Ipsilateral impaired flushing may be found.
- Loss of ciliospinal reflex. Pinching skin of back of neck normally produces ipsilateral pupil dilation (unreliable).
- Biomicroscopic examination of the papillary margin and iris structure and color:
  – In congenital Horner's, long-standing Horner's syndrome, or Horner's syndrome that occurs in children <2 y: Iris reduced pigmentation, blue-gray, mottling of the affected eye (heterochromia iridis) because formation of iris pigment early in life is under sympathetic control
- Observation of the presence of nystagmus, facial swelling, lymphadenopathy, or vesicular eruptions
- Ophthalmoparesis, especially of CN VI

DIAGNOSTIC TESTS & INTERPRETATION
Lab
Initial lab tests
Complete blood count (CBC), fluorescent treponemal antibody absorption test (FTA-ABS), venereal disease research laboratory (VDRL), purified protein derivative (PPD), vanillylmandelic acid (VMA), homovanillic acid (HVA) to rule out neuroblastoma in pediatric patients

Imaging
Initial approach
- Chest X-ray if a smoker (apical bronchogenic carcinoma)
- Computed tomography (CT)/magnetic resonance imaging (MRI)/magnetic resonance angiography (MRA) of the brain, chest, and spinal cord:
  – If painful, order MRI/MRA to evaluate for carotid artery dissection emergently.
  – If acquired Horner's in a child, suspect neuroblastoma and order MRI of sympathetic chain from abdomen to neck.

Diagnostic Procedures/Surgery
- Documentation of Horner's syndrome:
  – 4–10% topical cocaine (2 drops):
    ○ A normal pupil will dilate. The miotic pupil in Horner's will not dilate or will dilate poorly after 30 m because of the absence of norepinephrine at the nerve endings of the 3rd-order neuron.
    ○ Positive test is anisocoria of 1 mm or more
    ○ Cocaine blocks the reuptake of norepinephrine by the neuron.
    ○ If diagnosis clear clinically, this test is not required
    ○ Alternate test: Topical 0.5% apraclonidine
- Distinguishing a 3rd-order neuron disorder from a 1st- or 2nd-order neuron disorder:
  – Topical 1% hydroxyamphetamine:
    ○ If there is a 1st or 2nd neuron lesion, dilation will take place 1 h later.
    ○ Failure of the pupil to dilate, or poor dilation, indicates a 3rd-order neuron lesion (positive when anisocoria increases by 1 mm or more).
    ○ No test exists to differentiate a 1st- or 2nd-order neuron lesion.
    ○ Hydroxyamphetamine causes release of endogenous norepinephrine stored in the neuron.
    ○ Alternative test: 1% topical pholedrine

- Must wait >24 h between the cocaine and hydroxyamphetamine tests

Pediatric Considerations
Due to trans-synaptic degeneration in children, the hydroxyamphetamine test is not reliable.

Pathological Findings
- Brainstem lesion
- Massive hemisphere lesion
- Cervical cord lesion
- Root lesion
- Sympathetic chain lesion

DIFFERENTIAL DIAGNOSIS
- Neurological diseases
- 3rd nerve palsy
- Unilateral use of miotics
- Unilateral use of mydriatics
- Adie tonic pupil
- Iris sphincter muscle damage

 TREATMENT

MEDICATION
Carotid artery dissection: Warfarin for 6 m (1)

ADDITIONAL TREATMENT
General Measures
- Horner's syndrome in itself does not produce any disability or require treatment necessarily.
- Treatment of the underlying etiology
- Search for tumor or other compressive lesion.

Issues for Referral
- Neurologic, neuro-ophthalmic, oculoplastic
- Neurologic or vascular surgery: Interventional in cases of suspected carotid artery dissection or aneurysm
- Neurosurgery, surgical oncology, oncology, or radiotherapy consultation is dependent upon the particular etiology.

SURGERY/OTHER PROCEDURES
- Surgical care is dependent upon etiology.
- Consider ptosis repair surgery (oculoplastics).

 ONGOING CARE

PROGNOSIS
- Postganglionic: Usually benign
- Central and preganglionic: Poorer

COMPLICATIONS
- Chronic pupillary constriction
- Cosmesis

REFERENCE
1. Nautiyal A, Singh S, DiSalle M, O'Sullivan J. Painful Horner syndrome as a harbinger of silent carotid dissection. *PLoS Med*. 2005;2(1):e19.

ADDITIONAL READING
- Aydin GB, Kutluk MT, Buyukpamukcu M et al. Neurological complications of neuroblastic tumors: experience of a single center. *Childs Nerv Syst*. 2010;26:359–65.
- Bazari F, Hind M, Ong YE et al. Horner's syndrome—not to be sneezed at. *Lancet*. 2010;375:776.
- Freedman KA, Brown SM. Topical apraclonidine in the diagnosis of suspected Horner Syndrome. *J Neuroophthalmo*. 2005;25(2):83–5.
- Lee JH, Lee HK, Lee DH et al. Neuroimaging strategies for three types of Horner syndrome with emphasis on anatomic location. *Am J Roentgenol*. 2007;188(1):W74–W81.

 CODES

ICD9
337.9 Unspecified disorder of autonomic nervous system

CLINICAL PEARLS
- Horner's syndrome triad: Miosis, ptosis, anhidrosis caused by a lesion in the sympathetic innervation to the neck, head, and eye
- Ptosis is mild, usually <2 mm.
- Red flags: Association with pain; central or preganglionic lesion suspected
- Confirm the diagnosis clinically with 2 drops of topical cocaine to affected eye.
- Differentiate which order neuron is affected with hydroxyamphetamine.
- Order imaging studies based on history and physical and hydroxyamphetamine testing.

H

HUNTINGTON DISEASE

Andrew J. Westwood, MD
Samuel Frank, MD

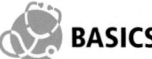 **BASICS**

DESCRIPTION
- Inherited neurodegenerative disease characterized by progressive motor, cognitive and psychiatric dysfunction, and ultimately death:
  - Symptoms usually begin between 30–50 years of age.
  - By the time of diagnosis, the patient has usually passed the disease to another generation.
- System(s) affected: Nervous
- Synonym(s): Chronic progressive hereditary chorea; Huntington chorea

Geriatric Considerations
- Fatal and no cure to date. Life expectancy is 15–20 years after onset of symptoms.
- Affects ages 1–90 years.
- Highest risk of suicide around onset of symptoms and around the time of diagnosis

Pediatric Considerations
- Juvenile form, defined by onset before age 21, occurs in 7% of cases. Juvenile also known as Akinetic-Rigid or Westphal variant is usually a hypokinetic disorder with Parkinsonian features.
- Characteristics:
  - Autosomal dominant, juvenile form typically paternally inherited otherwise equal maternal and paternal inheritance pattern.
  - Trinucleotide cytosine-adenine-guanine (CAG) repeat
  - Typically 100% penetrance but age of onset dependent on number of repeats with a higher number causing earlier onset
  - Anticipation (earlier onset in subsequent generations) caused from instability of the gene.
  - Length of repeat is inversely associated with but is not an accurate predictor of age onset.

EPIDEMIOLOGY
- Predominant age:
  - Young adult: 16–40 years
  - Middle age: 40–75 years
- Predominant sex: Male = Female

Incidence
6–8% are sporadic cases

Prevalence
7–10/100 000 persons prevalent in North Europe, India, and central Asia. Rare in Norway, Finland, and Japan. Also islands of higher incidence in certain regions of Scotland and Venezuela.

RISK FACTORS
Family history

Genetics
- Autosomal dominant
- Shows penetrance and anticipation
- Age of onset is earlier the longer the repeat length but progression is not correlated.
- Trinucleotide CAG repeat on chromosome 4 (normally ≤28) encoding Huntingtin/IT15 gene
  - >40 show full prevalence
  - 36–39 show reduced prevalence
  - 29–35 may expand in future generations.
- 50% chance of inheritance with an affected parent
- Does not skip generations

GENERAL PREVENTION
- Genetic counseling requires written consent. Pre- and postcounseling is required.
- Prenatal testing at 11–13 weeks ensures a >99% chance of a negative gene expansion.

ETIOLOGY
Associated with a CAG trinucleotide repeat expansion on exon 1 in a large gene on the short arm of chromosome 4 (4p16.3).
- The gene encodes the protein Huntingtin, which is essential for neural development. Pathologically it becomes cross-linked and accumulates.
- The protein appears to interact with cyclic adenosine monophosphate response element binding protein (CREP) to help prevent neuronal toxicity.
- RAS homologue enriched in striatum (Rhes), which may be involved in the pathogenesis and neuronal toxicity by binding to abnormal Huntingtin.

COMMONLY ASSOCIATED CONDITIONS
Similar diseases include (1):
- Huntington's disease-like 1 (HDL-1): chromosome 20, prion disease
- Huntington's disease-like 2 (HDL-2): chromosome 16, also CAG repeat; junctophilin 3 gene
- Huntington's disease-like 3 (HDL-3): chromosome 4, autosomal recessive, single family reported
- Huntington's disease-like 4 (HDL-4): also known as spinocerebellar-ataxia type 17

 DIAGNOSIS

PHYSICAL EXAM
- Early (2)[C]:
  - Motor
    - Chorea / choreoathetosis
    - Ballism
    - Dystonia
    - Myoclonus
    - Tics
  - Cognitive
    - Executive dysfunction
    - Emotional lability
    - Procedural, recent and remote learning
  - Psychiatric
    - Depression
    - Anxiety
    - Aggression
    - Impulsiveness
    - Obsessive-Compulsive Disorder
    - Personality changes
    - Psychosis
- Late (2)[C]:
  - Motor
    - Chorea declines with increasing dystonia and Parkinsonian features (bradykinesia, rigidity)
  - Cognitive
    - Dementia
    - Mutism
    - Dysphagia
  - Psychiatric
    - 25% will attempt suicide
    - 8–9% complete suicide
- Cause of death
  - infection, cardiac disease , suicide, complications of immobility (pneumonia, skin issues, malnutrition)

HISTORY
- Patients may present with a family member already diagnosed and request investigation in the prodromal or presymptomatic stage.
- Age of onset, degree, and type of clinical symptoms can vary from patient to patient.
- Patients may also present with abnormal choreiform movements (uncontrollable muscular movements), which may initially be clumsiness and stumbling.
- Emotional and/or behavioral changes, such as memory problems or aggressive/antisocial behavior.

DIAGNOSTIC TESTS & INTERPRETATION
Lab
- Genetic testing
  - Confirmatory (after onset of clinical symptoms)
  - Predictive (positive family history)
    - Cannot be performed on children
    - 5–20% in the UK at risk will opt to be tested.
    - Substantial social and financial implications must be considered before testing.
- These are not generally tested and are nonspecific:
  - Decreased endogenous γ-aminobutyric acid
  - Decreased glutamic acid decarboxylase
  - Decreased choline-acetyltransferase

Imaging
- CT or MRI: Cerebral atrophy and atrophy starting in the striatum leading to a concave rather than convex lateral ventricles
- Positron emission tomography (raclopride): Bilateral caudate hypometabolism, lowered dopamine receptor binding in the basal ganglia

Diagnostic Procedures/Surgery
Neuropsychological performance and clinician rating of motor signs contribute to the prediction of HD diagnosis in persons at risk but healthy (3)[B].

Pathological Findings
- Gross:
  - Cerebral atrophy
  - Atrophic caudate nucleus
  - Atrophic putamen
  - Ventricular enlargement (ex vacuo)
  - Atrophic globus pallidus
  - Atrophic frontal lobes
  - Atrophic parietal lobes
  - Cortical atrophy
- Micro:
  - Loss begins in the striatum with loss of medium spiny neurons
  - Loss of projection to the lateral globus pallidus
  - Widespread loss in the basal ganglia
- Electron microscopy:
  - Membranous whorls
  - Increased numbers of dense synaptic vesicles in presynaptic nerve terminals

DIFFERENTIAL DIAGNOSIS
- Movement disorder (hereditary) (1):
  - Hereditary nonprogressive chorea
  - Dentatorubral-Pallidoluysian atrophy
  - Neuroferritinopathy
  - Neuroacanthocytosis
  - Wilson disease
  - Ataxia-telangiectasia
  - Lesch-Nyhan syndrome
  - Pantothenate kinase-associated Neurodegeneration
  - Fahr disease
  - X-lined McLeod syndrome

- Movement disorder (secondary):
  - Infections/immunologic: *Sydenham chorea*, *encephalitis*, systemic *lupus erythematosus*, tertiary syphilis
  - Drug induced: Levodopa, anticonvulsants, anticholinergics, cimetidine, isoniazid, tardive dyskinesia from neuroleptics
  - Metabolic and endocrine: *Chorea gravidarum*, hyperthyroidism, birth control pills, hyperglycemic nonketotic encephalopathy
  - Vascular: Hemichorea/hemiballism with subthalamic nucleus lesion, *periarteritis nodosa*
- Movement disorder (unknown etiology):
  - Senile chorea
  - Essential chorea
  - Parkinson disease
- Dementia:
  - Alzheimer disease
  - Creutzfeldt-Jakob
  - Frontotemporal lobar degeneration
- Emotional and perceptual disorders:
  - Bipolar disorder
  - Schizophrenia
- Abnormal behavior:
  - Alcoholism
  - Antisocial personality disorder

 TREATMENT

MEDICATION
- Motor (4):
  - Chorea
    - Riluzole (Rilutek) 50 mg q12h
    - Olanzapine (Zyprexa): Start with 5 mg/day; may work up to maximum of 20 mg/day. Other typical neuroleptics (risperidone, haloperidol) or atypicals (aripiprazole) may be considered
    - Amantadine (Symmetrel): 100 mg daily and titrate weekly to 200 mg TID.
    - Tetrabenazine (Xenazine): Approved by the FDA and available since 2008 for treatment of chorea associated with HD. It has been available in other countries for decades (5)[B].
    - Dopamine agonists
    - Benzodiazepines
  - Akinesis (4):
    - Levodopa (Rilutek)
    - Dopamine agonists
    - Amantadine (Symmetrel) 100 mg b.i.d.
    - MAOI: Selegiline (Zydis) for swallowing difficulties
  - Rigidity:
    - Benzodiazepines
    - Botulinum toxin for focal dystonia/spasticity
    - Reduce neuroleptics.
- Psychiatric (4):
  - Risperidone (Risperdal), start at 1 mg b.i.d., slowly increase to usual effective dose of 4–8 mg/d in 2 divided doses. Other neuroleptics can also be used for delusions and other psychosis.
  - Fluoxetine (Prozac), start at 10 mg/d, increase by 10 mg increments to 60 mg/day maximum. Other SSRIs may also be effective without stimulation (Zoloft, Paxil, Celexa)
  - Mirtazapine, start at 15 mg/d; may work up to 45 mg/d. Other SNRIs may be effective (Cymbalta, Effexor)
- Contraindications: Refer to manufacturer's literature.

- Precautions:
  - Extrapyramidal reactions, tardive dyskinesia may occur, akathisia may occur with tetrabenazine and neuroleptics use. Black box warning of depression and suicidality on tetrabenazine
  - Can be treated with anticholinergic medication

ADDITIONAL TREATMENT
Huntington disease is a progressive incurable neurodegenerative disorder requiring multidisciplinary management.

General Measures
- Genetic counseling
- Consider electroconvulsive therapy (ECT) for drug-resistant depression.
- Speech and swallow
- Occupational therapy
- Physical therapy
- Feeding tubes
- Smoking cessation in late (choreiform) stage

Additional Therapies
Multiple potential mechanisms of action are under investigation to slow the progression of HD. Examples include creatine, coenzyme Q10, glutamate stabilizers, BDNF inducers, anti-apoptotic agents, dopamine stabilizers, caspase inhibitors, siRNA infusion, cell transplantation, and deep brain stimulation.

IN-PATIENT CONSIDERATIONS
Initial Stabilization
Outpatient

 ONGOING CARE

FOLLOW-UP RECOMMENDATIONS
Full activity as long as possible

Patient Monitoring
- Periodically for behavioral changes
- Effect of drug therapy may be monitored using the Unified Huntington Disease Rating Scale, a protocol by which patients are evaluated on a series of motor, behavioral, and functional criteria (6). Staged with the Total Functional Capacity (13-point scale in part 6 UHDRS).

DIET
- Soft diet with liquid supplements may be needed.
- Feeding tube placement needs to be discussed on an individual basis. No evidence that feeding tubes prolong life or nutritional status in advanced HD.

PATIENT EDUCATION
- Counseling for offspring
- Newsletter and printed information available from: Huntington Disease Society of America, 140 W. 22nd St., 6th Floor, New York, NY 10011-2420; (212) 242-1968; fax (212) 243-2443; http://www.hdsa.org.
- HD Outreach Project for Education: http://www.stanford.edu/group/hopes.

PROGNOSIS
- Poor; progressive impairment
- Fatal outcome within 20 years
- 8–9% commit suicide
- 7–8% of HD patients are in nursing homes:
  - Women outnumber men
  - The most robust predictor of placement is advanced motor impairment (marked chorea, bradykinesia, impaired gait and balance) (7)[B].

COMPLICATIONS
- Choking
- Subdural hematoma (from multiple falls)
- Personality changes
- Suicide

REFERENCES
1. Schneider SA, Walker RH, Bhatia KP et al. The Huntington's disease-like syndromes: what to consider in patients with a negative Huntington's disease gene test. *Nature clinical practice. Neurology.* 2007;3:517–25.
2. Novak MJ, Tabrizi SJ et al. Huntington's disease. *BMJ.* 2010;340:c3109.
3. Langbehn DR, Paulsen JS, Huntington Study Group. Predictors of diagnosis in Huntington disease. *Neurology.* 2007;68:1710–7.
4. Frank S, Jankovic J et al. Advances in the pharmacological management of Huntington's disease. *Drugs.* 2010;70:561–71.
5. Fasano A, Cadeddu F, Guidubaldi A, et al. The Long-term Effect of Tetrabenazine in the Management of Huntington Disease. *Clin Neuropharmacol.* 2008;31:313–8.
6. Huntington Study Group. Unified Huntington's Disease Rating Scale: reliability and consistency. *Mov Disord* 1996;11(2):136–42.
7. Wheelock VL, Tempkin T, Marder K, et al. Predictors of nursing home placement in Huntington disease. *Neurology.* 2003;60:998–1001.
8. David A. Warrell, Timothy M, Cox, and John D. Firth. *Oxford Textbook of Medicine.* Fourth Edition. OUP Oxford. 0198529988.

ADDITIONAL READING
- Anderson K. Huntington's disease and related disorders. *Psychiatr Clin N Am.* 2005;28:275–90.
- Innes AM, Chudley AE. Genetic landmarks through philately: Woodrow Wilson 'Woody' Guthrie and Huntington disease. *Clin Genet.* 2002;61:263–7.
- Savani AA, Login IS et al. Tetrabenazine as antichorea therapy in Huntington disease: a randomized controlled trial. *Neurology.* 2007;68:797; author reply 797.

 CODES

ICD9
333.4 Huntington's chorea

CLINICAL PEARLS
- HD onsets typically between ages 30 and 50, occurring in 1/10,000 people in Western countries
- Autosomal-dominant inheritance
- Named after George Huntington in 1872, a year after qualifying (8)

H

HYDROCELE

Timothy L. Black, MD
James P. Miller, MD

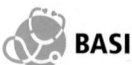 **BASICS**

DESCRIPTION

A collection of fluid within the scrotum:

- Communicating hydrocele:
  - Associated with a patent processus vaginalis
  - Has associated indirect inguinal hernia
- Noncommunicating hydrocele (the processus vaginalis is not patent):
  - Infantile type: Often spontaneous resolution
  - Adult type: Infrequent resolution
- Hydrocele of the cord: Distal portion of processus vaginalis has closed, midportion patent and fluid filled, proximal portion open or closed
- Acute hydrocele: Fluid collection resulting from an acute process within the tunica vaginalis
- System(s) affected: Reproductive

Pediatric Considerations

In communicating hydrocele, consider contralateral inguinal exploration.

EPIDEMIOLOGY

Predominant age: Childhood

Prevalence

- 1,000 per 100,000
- Estimated to be 1% of adult males

RISK FACTORS

- Ventriculoperitoneal shunt
- Exstrophy of the bladder
- Cloacal exstrophy
- Ehlers-Danlos syndrome
- Peritoneal dialysis

ETIOLOGY

- Closure of processus vaginalis trapping peritoneal fluid (noncommunicating)
- Closure of distal processus, trapping fluid in midportion of processus vaginalis (hydrocele of cord)
- Failure of closure of processus vaginalis (communicating hydrocele)

- Infection
- Tumors
- Trauma
- Ipsilateral renal transplantation

COMMONLY ASSOCIATED CONDITIONS

- Testicular tumors
- Trauma
- Ventriculoperitoneal shunt
- Nephrotic syndrome
- Renal failure with peritoneal dialysis

 DIAGNOSIS

HISTORY

- Acute or subacute onset of scrotal swelling
- Frequent changes in size of the hydrocele (indicative of a communication)
- Swelling in scrotum or inguinal canal
- Usually not painful
- Sensation of heaviness in scrotum
- Pain radiating to back (occasionally)

PHYSICAL EXAM

- Swelling in scrotum or inguinal canal
- Demonstrated fluctuation in size (communicating hydrocele)
- Fluid collection in scrotum that transilluminates
- Scrotal mass, usually fluctuant

DIAGNOSTIC TESTS & INTERPRETATION

Lab

No lab studies usually helpful

Imaging

- Abdominal radiograph: May be useful to distinguish incarcerated hernias from hydroceles (rarely needed)
- Inguinoscrotal ultrasound: Can demonstrate the presence of bowel (e.g., distinguish incarcerated hernia from a hydrocele of the cord) as well as presence of testicular torsion
- Testicular nuclear scan or Doppler ultrasound: To distinguish testicular torsion

Diagnostic Procedures/Surgery

Aspiration of hydrocele for diagnosis should be discouraged.

Pathological Findings

Patent processus vaginalis in communicating hydroceles

DIFFERENTIAL DIAGNOSIS

- Indirect inguinal hernia
- Orchitis
- Epididymitis
- Traumatic injury to testicle
- Torsion of testicle or torsion of appendix testes

 TREATMENT

ADDITIONAL TREATMENT

Issues for Referral

Recovery should be rapid and complete.

SURGERY/OTHER PROCEDURES

- In adults, no therapy is needed unless hydrocele causes discomfort or unless there is a significant underlying cause such as tumor.

- Inguinal approach with ligation of processus vaginalis and excision, or distal splitting, or drainage of hydrocele sac in children (in hydrocele of cord, sac can be completely removed) (1)[B]:
  - Patients less <12 years old should undergo an inguinal approach, while scrotal approach can be considered in children >12 years old (2)[C].

- Scrotal approach with internal drainage of hydrocele in adults (highest recurrence rate) (3)[C]

- Scrotal approach with resection of hydrocele sac (highest complication rate, lowest recurrence rate) (3)[C]
- Jaboulay-Winkelmann procedure (for thick hydrocele sac): Hydrocele sac wrapped posteriorly around cord structures (3)[C],(4)[A]
- Lord procedure (for thin hydrocele sac): Radial sutures used to gather hydrocele sac posterior to testis and epididymis (3)[C],(4)[A]
- Aspiration of the hydrocele with instillation of sclerosing agent (talc is best) has been successfully used in adults (5)[B]:
  - Aspiration with instillation of sodium tetradecyl sulphate was compared prospectively with Jaboulay procedure (30 patients each group) (6)[B]:
    - Aspiration instillation group had fewer complications and was much less expensive, but had recurrence rate of 34% and high rate of patient dissatisfaction

IN-PATIENT CONSIDERATIONS
Initial Stabilization
- Outpatient surgery
- Observation in early infancy until definite communication demonstrated or until 1 year old

 ## ONGOING CARE

FOLLOW-UP RECOMMENDATIONS
Full activity after surgery

Patient Monitoring
- Follow at 3-month intervals until decision for/against surgery is made.
- Postoperative follow-up at 2–4 weeks and then at intervals of 2–3 months until resolution of any postoperative (traumatic) hydrocele

COMPLICATIONS
- Complication rate for scrotal approach may reach 30% (7)[C].
- Preoperative antibiotics may be beneficial in reducing postoperative infections (7)[C].
- Postoperative traumatic hydrocele common. Usually resolves spontaneously.
- Injury to vas deferens or spermatic vessels
- Suture granuloma
- Hematoma
- Wound infection
- Recurrence of hydrocele
- Tense infantile abdominoscrotal hydrocele may have high complication rate (8)[C]:
  - May have significant rate of testicular dysmorphism (including hypoplasia)

REFERENCES

1. Gahukamble DB, Khamage AS. Prospective randomized controlled study of excision vs. distal splitting of hernial sac and processus vaginalis in the repair of inguinal hernias and communicating hydroceles. *J Ped Surg*. 1995;30:624–5.
2. Wilson JM, Aaronson DS, Schrader R, et al. Hydrocele in the pediatric patient: inguinal or scrotal approach? *J Urol*. 2008;180:1724–7; discussion 1727–8.
3. Ku JH, Kim ME, Lee NK et al. The excisional placation and internal drainage techniques: A comparison of the results for idiopathic hydrocele. *BJU*. 2001;87:82–4.
4. Miroglu C, Tokuc R, Saporta L. Comparison of an extrusion procedure and eversion procedures in the treatment of hydrocele. *Int Urol Nephrol*. 1994;26: 673–9.
5. Yilmaz U, Ekmekcioglu O, Tatlisen A et al. Does pleurodesis for pleural effusions give bright ideas about the agents for hydrocele sclerotherapy? *Int Urol Nephrology*. 2000;32:89–92.
6. Khaniya S, Agrawal CS, Koirala R, Regmi R, Adhikary S et al. Comparison of aspiration-sclerotherapy with hydrocelectomy in the management of hydrocele: a prospective randomized study. *International journal of surgery (London, England)*. 2009;7:392–5.
7. Swartz MA, Morgan TM, Krieger JN. Complications of scrotal surgery for benign conditions. *Urology*. 2007;69:616–9.
8. Cozzi DA, Mele E, Ceccanti S, et al. Infantile abdominoscrotal hydrocele: a not so benign condition. *J Urol*. 2008;180:2611–5; discussion 2615.

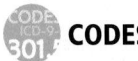 ## CODES

ICD9
603.9 Hydrocele, unspecified

CLINICAL PEARLS

- A diagnosis of hydrocele can virtually always be made by physical exam alone. Occasionally, scrotal ultrasound is needed, especially if there is concern about an underlying process.
- Aspirating a hydrocele as primary treatment is not recommended. If a hydrocele is confused with an incarcerated inguinal hernia, aspiration could result in significant complications. Otherwise, hydroceles simply recur following aspiration unless a sclerosing agent is injected as well.

H

HYDROCEPHALUS, NORMAL PRESSURE

Dennis E. Hughes, DO

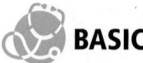

BASICS

DESCRIPTION
- Normal pressure hydrocephalus (NPH) is a clinical triad of gait instability, incontinence, and dementia (mnemonic: *wet, wobbly, wacky*). Originally described by Hakim and Adams in 1965, it occurs rarely, but is potentially treatable.
- Idiopathic
- Secondary to subarachnoid hemorrhage, head injury, or infection

Geriatric Considerations
Idiopathic NPH primarily affects persons >60 years.

EPIDEMIOLOGY
Incidence
- No formal epidemiologic data exist regarding NPH because of the lack of consensus-derived diagnostic criteria. The natural history of untreated NPH has not been studied (1,2).
- Idiopathic form primarily affects elderly.
- Secondary form can occur at any age.
- Affects both genders equally

Prevalence
Estimated to be the cause of dementia in ≤5% of affected individuals

RISK FACTORS
- Idiopathic risk is unknown.
- Secondary form is due to head trauma, subarachnoid hemorrhage, meningitis, or encephalitis.

PATHOPHYSIOLOGY
- This is a communicating hydrocephalus, a disorder of decreased cerebrospinal fluid (CSF) absorption. The subarachnoid granulations fail to maintain their baseline removal of CSF as a result of scarring or fibrosis.
- The result is a pressure gradient between the subarachnoid space and the ventricular system.
- CSF production decreases in the face of an increased pressure set-point (but still in excess of the amount of CSF absorbed).

- Elevated pressure distends ventricles and compresses the brain parenchyma.
- As a result of compression, ischemic changes occur in the parenchymal vasculature.

ETIOLOGY
- Some believe that the idiopathic form is a result of persistently insufficient removal of CSF by immature subarachnoid granulations from childhood.
- Secondary NPH may result from:
  - Subarachnoid hemorrhage
  - Head trauma
  - Resolved acute meningitis
  - Chronic meningitis (tuberculosis, syphilis)
  - Paget disease of the skull

DIAGNOSIS

HISTORY
- Insidious and usually progressive; gait instability usually manifests initially, followed by changes in mentation, and eventually, urinary incontinence.
- Difficulty with initiation of movement: Feet appear "glued to the floor." Gait is wide-based, shuffling, and turning appears "en bloc."
- Inattention, forgetfulness, and lack of spontaneity often are seen with the subcortical dementia of NPH.
- Urinary urgency initially, followed by lack of inhibition and then frank incontinence
- Behavioral changes have been reported: Depression, mania, and psychotic features (1)
- A minimum duration of at least 3–6 months of symptoms and progression over time
- A remote trauma or infection suggests secondary vs the idiopathic form.
- A lack of psychiatric, neurologic, or other medical conditions to explain the symptoms
- Because memory impairment may be present, it is important to include a knowledgeable informant who is familiar with the patient's premorbid state (2).
- The frontal lobe function is affected disproportionately to the memory impairment (objective testing may lead to an early diagnosis).

PHYSICAL EXAM
- Decreased step height and length
- Reduced speed of walking (cadence)
- Widened standing base
- Swaying of trunk during walking
- Decreased fine motor speed and accuracy
- Recall impaired for recent events
- Impaired ability to do multistep tasks or interpret abstractions

DIAGNOSTIC TESTS & INTERPRETATION
Lab
Initial lab tests
- Thyroid-stimulation hormone (TSH)
- Syphilis serology
- Complete blood count (CBC)
- Serum B_{12}, folate
- Metabolic profile
- Blood alcohol, analysis for drugs of abuse
- Urinalysis

Imaging
Initial approach
- Imaging is essential. Either computed tomography (CT) or magnetic resonance imaging (MRI) shows the ventriculomegaly with preservation of the cerebral parenchyma (as opposed to ventricular enlargement seen in other forms of dementia where brain atrophy is present).
- MRI can allow detection of other features such as signs of altered brain water content and callosal angles. However, these supportive findings are not independently diagnostic of NPH (1,2).
- MR spectroscopy, single photon emission computed tomography (SPECT), and phase-contrast MR imaging may play a greater role in selecting patients for shunt placement (3)[B].

Diagnostic Procedures/Surgery
- Positron emission tomography (PET) scanning
- Nuclear cisternography
- CSF flow velocity (4)

DIFFERENTIAL DIAGNOSIS

- Alzheimer disease
- Parkinson disease
- Chronic alcoholism
- Intracranial infection
- Multi-infarct dementia
- Subdural hematoma
- Carcinomatous meningitis
- Collagen vascular disorders
- Depression
- Syphilis
- B$_{12}$ deficiency
- Urologic disorders
- Other hydrocephalus disorders

 TREATMENT

MEDICATION

- No medication is significantly helpful.
- Use of carbonic anhydrase inhibitors (acetazolamide) with repeat lumbar punctures has provided mild and transient relief.
- Lack of response to normal medication used to treat Parkinson should prompt physician to search for other etiology (of dementia, gait disturbance) .

ADDITIONAL TREATMENT

Issues for Referral

- Neurology or neurosurgical consultation is helpful in suspected cases when other reversible medical conditions are ruled out.
- Most recent review of the available evidence failed to indicate whether placement of an intraventricular shunt is effective in the management of NPH. A recognized difficulty has been in selecting those patients who might benefit from shunting. To date, there are no high-quality, blinded studies of the natural history of the disorder versus the current surgical treatment (5).

Additional Therapies

Gait training and use of ambulation assist devices as indicated

SURGERY/OTHER PROCEDURES

- Current therapy is limited to placement of ventriculoperitoneal or ventriculoatrial shunt from a lateral ventricle tunneled subcutaneously and drained into the peritoneal cavity (or right atrium).
- Success depends on appropriate patient selection. No specific test accurately identifies who will benefit from the CSF diversion.

- Studies show objective improvement in mini mental state and functional exams post shunting (6).
- Patients whose symptoms have been present for a shorter period (<2 years) have a greater chance of improvement with shunting. Also patients with a known cause of NPH tend to respond more favorably. However, improvement has been seen in patients with symptoms present for a long time (1,5).

IN-PATIENT CONSIDERATIONS

Admission Criteria

Usually only for planned surgical treatment

 ONGOING CARE

FOLLOW-UP RECOMMENDATIONS

- Assessment and modification of environment for fall risks
- Evaluation for ability to operate a motor vehicle safely (if driving)

Patient Monitoring

- Repeat neuropsychological testing to evaluate the status of the dementia after treatment.
- Improvement in the incontinence and walking speed can also be objectively measured.

PATIENT EDUCATION

Information at: http://www.emedicinehealth.com/normal_pressure_hydrocephalus/article_em.htm

PROGNOSIS

Poor, given the variable response to surgical treatment. The natural history is progressive deterioration. Patient's axial skeletal stability worsens with inability to walk, stand, sit, or turn over in bed.

COMPLICATIONS

- In patients treated surgically, cerebral infarcts, hemorrhage, infection, and seizures (in addition to the usual surgical risks)
- Shunt malfunction (especially when symptoms recur after successful shunt placement)
- Falls due to gait instability
- Urinary tract infections
- Skin breakdown, pressure ulcers, infections as movement dysfunction progresses

REFERENCES

1. Relkin N, et al. Diagnosing idiopathic normal-pressure hydrocephalus. *Neurosurgery.* 2005;57(3Suppl):4–16.
2. Verrees M, Selman WR. Management of normal pressure hydrocephalus. *Am Fam Physician.* 2004;70:1071–8.
3. Tarnaris A, Kitchen ND, Watkins LD. Noninvasive biomarkers in normal pressure hydrocephalus: evidence for the role of neuroimaging. *J Neurosurg.* 2008.
4. Gallia GL, Rigamonti D, Williams MA. The diagnosis and treatment of idiopathic normal pressure hydrocephalus. *Nat Clin Pract Neurol.* 2006;2:375–81.
5. Esmond T, et al. Shunting for normal pressure hydrocephalus. *Cochran Database Sys Rev.* 2006;(4):CD003157.
6. Razay G, Vreughenhil A, Liddell J. A prospective study of venriculo-peritoneal shunting for idiopathic normal pressure hydrocephalus. *J. Clin Neurosci.* 2009;16(9):1180–3.

ADDITIONAL READING

- Ishikawa M, Hashimoto M, Kuwana N, Mori E, Miyake H, Wachi A, Takeuchi T, Kazui H, Koyama H et al. Guidelines for management of idiopathic normal pressure hydrocephalus. *Neurol Med Chir (Tokyo).* 2008;48(Suppl):S1–23.
- Marmarou A, Black P, Bergsneider M, et al. Guidelines for management of idiopathic normal pressure hydrocephalus: progress to date. *Acta Neurochir Suppl.* 2005;95:237–40.

See Also (Topic, Algorithm, Electronic Media Element)

Algorithm: Ataxia

 CODES

ICD9

331.5 Idiopathic normal pressure hydrocephalus (INPH)

CLINICAL PEARLS

- Consider in unexplained dementia.
- Poor prognosis despite therapy

H

HYDRONEPHROSIS

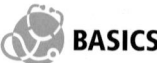

Pang-Yen Fan, MD

BASICS

DESCRIPTION
- Hydronephrosis refers a structural finding—dilatation of the calyces and renal pelvis:
  – May occur with urinary tract obstruction, vesicoureteric reflux (VUR), high urine output, or physiologic changes in pregnancy
  – Sometimes accompanied with hydroureter
  – Presentation varies from incidental finding to severe pain.
- Hydronephrosis should not be used interchangeably with obstructive uropathy, which refers to the damage to renal parenchyma resulting from urinary tract obstruction.

EPIDEMIOLOGY
- Hydronephrosis is found in 3% of autopsy specimens.
- Acute unilateral obstruction is more common than bilateral.

PATHOPHYSIOLOGY
- Hydronephrosis develops with increased pressure in the urinary collecting system.
- Increased pressure within the renal collecting system can cause calyceal fornix rupture and urinary extravasation.
- Over time, pressures return to normal, but kidney function declines from intense renal vasoconstriction.
- With concomitant urinary infection, bacteria can enter the renal vasculature, resulting in sepsis.

ETIOLOGY
- Urinary tract obstruction: May be acute/chronic, partial/complete, uni-/bilateral:
  – Intraluminal obstruction: Calculi, sloughed renal papillae, blood clot
  – Intrinsic abnormality of the urinary collecting system: Transitional cell carcinomas, benign prostatic hypertrophy, prostate cancer, congenital ureteropelvic junction (UPJ) obstruction, ureterocele, neurogenic bladder (functional obstruction), urethral stricture or TB (can cause ureteral narrowing)
  – Extrinsic compression of the urinary collecting system: Extraurinary malignancy (lymphoma, colon, cervix), aortic/iliac aneurysm, retroperitoneal fibrosis, uterine prolapse (15% affected), endometriosis
- Vesicoureteric reflux (VUR) resulting in varying degrees of hydroureteronephrosis
- Physiologic hydronephrosis of pregnancy
- Hydronephrosis due to high urine output (e.g., diabetes insipidus, psychogenic polydipsia)
- Hydronephrosis of infection: Due to bacterial toxins inhibiting smooth muscle contraction of the renal pelvis and ureter

Pediatric Considerations
- Antenatal hydronephrosis is diagnosed in 1–5% of pregnancies, usually by ultrasound, as early as the 12th to 14th week of gestation.
- Children with antenatal hydronephrosis are at greater risk of postnatal pathology.
- Postnatal evaluation begins with ultrasound exam; further studies such as voiding cystourethrogram (VCUG) based on the severity of postnatal hydronephrosis.

- In neonates, it is the most common cause of abdominal mass.
- The common etiologies in children are VUR, congenital UPJ obstruction, neurogenic bladder, and posterior urethral valves.
- Pediatric diagnostic algorithm differs from adult due to different differential diagnosis necessitating age-appropriate testing.

Pregnancy Considerations
- Physiologic hydronephrosis in pregnancy is more prominent on the right than left and can be seen up to 80% of pregnant women.
- Dilatation is caused by hormonal effects, external compression from expanding uterus, and intrinsic changes in the ureteral wall.
- Despite high incidence, most cases are asymptomatic.
- If symptomatic and refractory to medical management, ureteric calculus should be considered and urinary infection must be excluded.

Dx DIAGNOSIS

Symptoms vary according to cause, chronicity, location, and degree of obstruction.

HISTORY
- While often asymptomatic, hydronephrosis can be associated with pain ranging from vague intermittent discomfort to severe renal colic.
- Nausea, vomiting, chills may be associated with severe pain or infection.
- Fever with coexisting infection
- Polyuria may occur due to impaired urinary concentration in partial obstruction.
- Anuria if complete bilateral obstruction or complete obstruction of a solitary kidney
- Symptoms of chronic kidney disease: Anorexia, malaise, weight gain, edema, shortness of breath, mental state changes, tremors, GI bleeding
- Dietl crisis: Sudden attack of flank pain due to distension of renal pelvis caused by rapid ingestion of large amount of liquid or kinking of a ureter producing temporary occlusion of urine flow
- Symptoms of bladder outlet obstruction: Weak urine stream, nocturia, straining to void, overflow incontinence, urgency and frequency
- General medical and surgical history: Malignancy (extrinsic compression), radiotherapy (ureteric stricture/fibrosis), surgery (iatrogenic obstruction), trauma (hematoma or fibrosis), gynecologic disease (endometriosis, ovarian masses, uterine prolapse), smoking (urothelial cancer), drugs (methysergide-induced retroperitoneal fibrosis)

PHYSICAL EXAM
- General signs:
  – Volume overload (edema, rales, HTN)
  – Diaphoresis, tachycardia, tachypnea with pain
  – High-grade fever if infection
- Abdominal exam: CVA tenderness, palpable bladder, rarely palpable abdominal mass (may be visible, particularly in thin children)
- Pelvic exam: Pelvic mass, uterine prolapse, palpable enlarged prostate (cancer or benign), urethral meatal stenosis, phimosis

DIAGNOSTIC TESTS & INTERPRETATION
Lab
- Dipstick urinalysis: Hematuria, proteinuria, crystalluria, pyuria
- Midstream urine microscopy, culture, and sensitivity: Exclude infection or hematuria
- Creatinine, urea, and electrolytes: May demonstrate rising creatinine and urea if patient developing obstructive uropathy. Potassium may be elevated and bicarbonate decreased if patient is developing hyperkalemic metabolic acidosis.
- CBC: Anemia of chronic kidney disease (CKD), leukocytosis if infection, check platelet count prior to considering intervention
- PSA in adult males >50 or with abnormal digital rectal exam, or outlet obstruction signs or symptoms
- Urine cytology for malignant cells
- Note: CA 19-9 is elevated in benign hydronephrosis and not a useful marker for malignancy in these patients.

Imaging
- Ultrasound and noncontrast CT scanning are effective in diagnosing presence and cause of obstruction in most of the cases; Intravenous pyelogram (IVP) and radionuclide scanning only if indicated
- Ultrasound (US): Test of choice to rule out hydronephrosis:
  – Poor sensitivity for detecting cause and level of obstruction
  – Detection of renal parenchymal disease (decreased renal size, increased cortical echogenicity, cortical thinning, cysts)
  – Safe in pregnancy, contrast allergy, or renal dysfunction
  – Degree of hydronephrosis does not correlate with the duration or severity of the obstruction.
  – False-positives (for urinary tract obstruction): Normal extrarenal pelvis, parapelvic cysts, VUR, excessive diuresis
  – False-negatives: Dehydration; renal cortical cysts actually representing intrarenal calyceal dilatation; at immediate onset of acute obstruction before dilatation has occurred; retroperitoneal fibrosis
- IVP: Both functional and anatomic assessment of site, severity and cause of obstruction:
  – Typically demonstrates a delayed nephrogram, as well as delayed filling of the collecting system; dilated collecting system; enlarged kidney; extravasation of urine if ruptured fornix; thinned renal cortex or small kidney in the case of chronic obstruction
  – Necessitates radiocontrast exposure
- Radionuclide renal scan (diuretic renal scintigraphy):
  – Useful in determining presence of true obstruction as well as total and separate (R vs. L) renal function
  – Advantages: Less radiation than IVP; safe in contrast-allergic patients, no risk of contrast-induced acute kidney injury
  – Most common agents are DTPA and MAG-3
  – Furosemide is given at 20 minutes after the agent was given; the t1/2 for the clearance of tracer from the system is measured.
  – T1/2 <10 minutes is unobstructed, >20 minutes is obstructed, and 10–20 minutes is equivocal; some experts consider <15 minutes normal.

– False-positives occur in patients with reduced creatinine clearance due to delayed excretion and in massive dilatation, causing a water-reservoir effect of delayed excretion without obstruction.

– False-negatives occur in dehydrated patients or inadequate diuretic challenges.

- CT ± contrast:
  – Noncontrast helical CT of the abdomen and pelvis is the investigation of choice for suspected nephrolithiasis:
    ○ Stone is most commonly found at levels of ureteric luminal narrowing: UPJ, pelvic brim, and the vesico-ureteric junction.
    ○ If the obstruction is acute, proximal ureter and renal pelvis are dilated to the level of obstruction and perinephric stranding is seen as well as renal swelling.
    ○ If chronic, renal atrophy may be noted.
  – Multiphase contrast-enhanced CT:
    ○ Nonenhanced phase detects stones and swelling
    ○ Parenchymal phase demonstrates decreased enhancement of renal parenchyma with acute obstruction; can identify extraurinary causes of obstruction and determine the relative GFR of each kidney with accuracy equal to diuretic renography
    ○ Delayed phase allows visualization of the collecting system and soft tissue filling defects (e.g., urothelial cancer).

- If contrast is contraindicated (creatinine >2 ng/dL), magnetic resonance urography (MRU) is superior to noncontrast CT in diagnosing soft-tissue causes including strictures:
  – MRU disadvantages: Insensitive for stone detection (only 70%); increased expense; less availability; increased acquisition time compared to CT (35 minutes vs. 5 minutes)
  – MRU is also used in pregnancy

- Duplex Doppler US to determine the resistive index (RI) to quantify alterations in renal blood flow. A high RI may be seen in urinary tract obstruction, although the diagnostic utility is controversial with variable accuracy reported in the literature.

- Whitaker test: The gold standard test for obstruction, measuring renal pressure via a percutaneous nephrostomy and bladder pressure via an indwelling catheter; highly invasive and rarely performed

- Voiding cystourethrogram to assess severity of VUR when indicated.

Diagnostic Procedures/Surgery

Cystoscopy, retrograde pyelogram ± ureteroscopy and biopsy are occasionally used to determine the cause of obstruction (e.g., small urothelial cancer missed on imaging) or to confirm a normal distal ureter prior to pyeloplasty. In addition, such procedures are often needed to establish a definitive pathologic diagnosis for mass lesions.

TREATMENT

ADDITIONAL TREATMENT
General Measures
- Treatment depends on cause and associated complications.
- Obstruction:
  – Bladder outlet obstruction: Urethral or suprapubic catheter
  – Ureteric obstruction: Retrograde (cystoscopic) or antegrade (percutaneous) stenting
- Correction of fluid and electrolyte abnormalities
- Analgesia
- Antibiotics as an adjunct to drainage if infection present
- VUR is often managed conservatively with antibiotics; surgical management required in severe cases in children or women of child-bearing age.

SURGERY/OTHER PROCEDURES
- Hydronephrosis due to obstruction:
  – Congenital UPJ obstruction: Pyeloplasty (open or laparoscopic), minimally invasive stricture incision (laser, Acucise cutting balloon catheter endopyelotomy)
  – Nephrolithiasis: ESWL, laser lithotripsy, ureteroscopy, percutaneous nephrostomy, ureteral stenting
  – Transitional cell cancer: Nephroureterectomy
  – Idiopathic retroperitoneal fibrosis: Ureterolysis (frees ureters from inflammatory mass)
  – Prostate disorders: Various treatment modalities including TURP and radical prostatectomy
- Nonobstructed hydronephrosis:
  – VUR: Ureteric reimplantation, endoscopic suburethral injection

IN-PATIENT CONSIDERATIONS
Initial Stabilization
Obstruction coexisting with infection (pyonephrosis) is a true urologic emergency requiring urgent drainage.

ONGOING CARE

PROGNOSIS
- Recovery of renal function depends on severity, acuity, and duration of obstruction.
- Significant recovery can occur despite days of complete obstruction, though some irreversible injury may develop within 24 hours.
- Course difficult to predict as diagnostic testing is of little value
- Course of incomplete obstruction highly unpredictable

COMPLICATIONS
- Urine stasis: Increased risk of infection and calculus formation
- Obstruction causes progressive atrophy of kidney with irreversible loss of function:
  – Tubules lose ability to concentrate urine, conserve sodium, or excrete H^+.
- Spontaneous rupture of a calyx may occur with urine extravasation in the perinephric space.

- Postobstructive diuresis: Marked polyuria after relief of obstruction:
  – Caused mostly by fluid and solute overload, but may be exacerbated by impaired renal tubular concentrating ability
  – Urine output may exceed 500 ml/hour.
  – Replace urine losses with hypotonic fluid (as the urine is often dilute) and only enough to avoid volume depletion. Replacement of urine output with equal amounts of saline will perpetuate the diuresis.

ADDITIONAL READING

- Cerwinka WH, Qian J, Easley KA, et al. Appearance of Dextranomer/Hyaluronic Acid Copolymer Implants on Computerized Tomography After Endoscopic Treatment of Vesicoureteral Reflux in Children. J Urol. 2009.
- El-Assmy A, El-Nahas AR, Sheir KZ. Is pre-shock wave lithotripsy stenting necessary for ureteral stones with moderate or severe hydronephrosis? J Urol. 2006;176:2059–62; discussion 2062.
- El-Ghar ME, Shokeir AA, El-Diasty TA, et al. Contrast enhanced spiral computerized tomography in patients with chronic obstructive uropathy and normal serum creatinine: a single session for anatomical and functional assessment. J Urol. 2004;172:985–8.
- el-Nahas AR, Shoma AM, Eraky I, et al. Prospective, randomized comparison of ureteroscopic endopyelotomy using holmium:YAG laser and balloon catheter. J Urol. 2006;175:614–8; discussion 618.
- Grattan-Smith JD. MR urography: anatomy and physiology. Pediatr Radiol. 2008;38(Suppl 2): S275–80.
- Khalaf IM, Shokeir AA, El-Gyoushi FI, et al. Recoverability of renal function after treatment of adult patients with unilateral obstructive uropathy and normal contralateral kidney: a prospective study. Urology. 2004;64:664–8.
- Lee RS, Cendron M, Kinnamon DD, et al. Antenatal hydronephrosis as a predictor of postnatal outcome: a meta-analysis. Pediatrics. 2006;118:586–93.
- Nepple KG, Knudson MJ, Austin JC, et al. Abnormal renal scans and decreased early resolution of low grade vesicoureteral reflux. J Urol. 2008;180: 1643–7; discussion 1647.
- Wimpissinger F, Türk C, Kheyfets O, et al. The silence of the stones: asymptomatic ureteral calculi. J Urol. 2007;178:1341–4.
- Worster A, Preyra I, Weaver B, et al. The accuracy of noncontrast helical computed tomography versus intravenous pyelography in the diagnosis of suspected acute urolithiasis: a meta-analysis. Ann Emerg Med. 2002;40:280–6.

CODES

ICD9
- 591 Hydronephrosis
- 753.29 Other obstructive defect of renal pelvis and ureter

H

HYPERCALCEMIA ASSOCIATED WITH MALIGNANCY

Richard F. DeSouza, MD

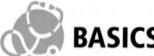 **BASICS**

DESCRIPTION
- Hypercalcemia associated with malignancy is the most common cause of severe hypercalcemia diagnosed in a hospital setting.
- Often a very poor prognostic sign
- Occurs with both solid tumors and hematologic malignancies; most commonly associated with multiple myeloma and breast and lung cancer; also associated with metastases to bone

EPIDEMIOLOGY
Incidence
Hypercalcemia is diagnosed in 20–30% of all cancer patients during the course of illness (1).

RISK FACTORS
- Dehydration
- Immobilization

GENERAL PREVENTION
Encourage adequate hydration and activity, especially in multiple myeloma.

PATHOPHYSIOLOGY
- Increased bone resorption is involved in most cases, caused either by extensive local bone destruction or by humoral factors.
- Humoral factors can interfere with the normal regulation of calcium by parathyroid hormone, calcitriol, and calcitonin.
- The humoral factors most commonly associated with cancer are parathyroid hormone–related protein (PTH-rP) and 1,25-dihydroxyvitamin D (calcitriol); however, other bone-resorbing factors, including prostaglandins, transforming growth factors, tumor necrosis factor (TNF), colony-stimulating factors, and interleukins, may be involved in different types of malignancy.
- PTH-rP increases expression of receptor activator of nuclear factor κB ligand (RANKL) in bone. RANKL binds to receptor activator of nuclear factor κB (RANK) on the surfaces of osteoclast precursors, resulting in differentiation into osteoclasts and leading to bone resorption and the development of hypercalcemia.

ETIOLOGY
- Main mechanisms of hypercalcemia in malignancy:
  - Osteolytic metastases: Most commonly with breast cancer, multiple myeloma, lymphoma, and leukemia; accounts for about 20% of cases of hypercalcemia associated with malignancy
  - Humoral hypercalcemia: Ectopic production of PTH-rP; PTH-rP increases bone resorption by osteoclasts. Associated with
    - Non–small cell lung carcinoma
    - Breast cancer
    - Renal cell carcinoma
    - Prostate cancer
    - Melanoma

- Ectopic PTH secretion: Very rare; has been seen with ovarian carcinoma, neuroectodermal tumor, thyroid papillary carcinoma, lung cancer, rhabdomyosarcoma, and pancreatic cancer
  - Calcitriol production: Lymphoma (non-Hodgkin, Hodgkin, and lymphomatosis/granulomatosis) and ovarian dysgerminomas
- In multiple myeloma, the elevated serum calcium may be due to the binding of the monoclonal protein with calcium. Multiple myeloma also may cause impaired renal function that decreases calcium excretion.

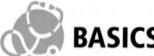 **DIAGNOSIS**

- The severity of symptoms depends on calcium level, rapidity of onset of hypercalcemia, state of hydration, and underlying malignancy.
- Early nonspecific symptoms often include nausea, vomiting, anorexia, depression, abdominal pain, constipation, and dizziness (1).
- Polyuria and polydipsia are more specific early symptoms (1).
- Cardiovascular:
  - Arrhythmias
  - QT-interval shortening
  - Calcium increases vascular tone.
- Genitourinary:
  - Nephrolithiasis, especially in the elderly
  - Polyuria because of impaired concentrating ability
- GI:
  - Peptic ulcers
  - Pancreatitis
  - Constipation
  - Anorexia
  - Nausea, vomiting
- Musculoskeletal:
  - Weakness, hypotonia
  - Hyporeflexia
  - Osteopenia, fractures
- Neuropsychiatric:
  - Depression, lethargy
  - Obtundation, coma
  - Memory impairment, confusion
  - Hallucinations
  - Headache
  - Seizures

DIAGNOSTIC TESTS & INTERPRETATION
Lab
- Serum calcium: Either ionized ("gold standard") or also must check albumin and correct: Ca(adj) = Ca(tot) + [0.8 × (4.5 − [alb])].
- Electrolytes including magnesium and phosphate (if hypercalcemia owing to PTH-rP, expect low phosphate, hyperchloremia, and mild alkalosis)
- Renal function: Urine calcium will be elevated.

- PTH: Levels of intact PTH should be measured routinely. Although ectopic PTH secretion is rare with malignancy, concomitant primary hyperparathyroidism is common (there is a higher incidence of cancer in patients with primary hyperparathyroidism and a higher incidence of primary hyperparathyroidism in patients with cancer).
- PTH-rP: In addition to helping with diagnosis, it is also a poor prognostic indicator and can be used to predict the response to treatment. Most commonly elevated in breast and lung cancer.
- Calcitriol: Should be measured when sarcoidosis, other granulomatous disorders, or the calcitriol lymphoma syndrome is in the differential diagnosis.
- If underlying malignancy is unknown, commence workup, for example, serum and urine electrophoresis for multiple myeloma.

ALERT
Lithium, thiazide diuretics, and vitamin D preparations all can increase serum calcium.

Imaging
None indicated for the immediate management of hypercalcemia, but studies such as bone scan may be helpful for workup of underlying condition.

DIFFERENTIAL DIAGNOSIS
- Hyperparathyroidism
- Immobilization
- Calcium administration
- Renal causes:
  - Chronic or acute renal failure
  - Postrenal transplantation
- Hypocalciuric hypercalcemias:
  - Familial
  - Hypothyroidism
  - Adrenal insufficiency
  - Bartter syndrome
- Granulomatous disease:
  - Sarcoidosis
  - Histoplasmosis
  - Coccidioidomycosis
  - Tuberculosis
- Hyperthyroidism
- AIDS
- Hypophosphatemia
- Pheochromocytoma
- Acromegaly
- Drugs:
  - Calcium
  - Lithium
  - Theophylline
  - Thiazides
- Vitamin A or D toxicity

TREATMENT

MEDICATION

- Hydration:
  - The initial therapy of choice because many symptoms are due to dehydration
  - Vomiting and renal losses can cause profound dehydration.
  - Volume expansion with IV normal saline
- Loop diuretics (e.g., furosemide): Increase renal calcium excretion but only after adequate hydration. Recent literature review suggests that loop diuretics should not be used except in fluid overloaded patients because hydration with saline, particularly when combined with other agents such as bisphosphonates, is more effective and safer than hydration plus diuretic (2)[B].
- Bisphosphonates: Considered 1st-line medications; by inhibiting osteoclasts, they reduce calcium release from bone, thereby counteracting the main mechanism of hypercalcemia of malignancy, which is bone reabsorption. They also decrease bone pain in patients with bone metastases (3)[B].
  - Zoledronic acid (Zometa):
    o Duration of action is 30 days.
    o Nephrotoxic potential, especially in myeloma patients receiving thalidomide
  - Pamidronate (Aredia): Normalizes calcium in up to 3 weeks
- Calcitonin: Also requires adequate rehydration; inhibits calcium reabsorption in the distal tubule:
  - Rapid onset of action (within 6–24 h)
  - Side effects include nausea, vomiting, abdominal cramps, rash, flushing, diarrhea, and tachyphylaxis.
  - For life-threatening hypercalcemia, consider calcitonin injections q12h (1)[B].
- Plicamycin (previously mithramycin):
  - May work via direct toxic effect on osteoclasts; reserved for patients who do not respond to bisphosphonates but can induce normocalcemia in 80% of those who receive it
  - Side effects limit its use (e.g., nausea, vomiting, cellulitis at infusion site, cytopenias, hepatic toxicity, nephrotoxicity, and platelet inhibition); can have rapid rebound hypercalcemia
  - Onset of action within 12 h, with maximal effect seen in 24–48 h
- Gallium nitrate:
  - Works through multiple mechanisms, including inhibition of osteoclast-mediated bone resorption, alteration in bone structure, and stimulation of bone formation
  - Rarely used, except in cases of more severe hypercalcemia that has been unresponsive to initial therapy, because treatment requires 5-day continuous IV infusion
  - Onset of action 48–72 h
  - Side effects: Nausea, vomiting, nephrotoxicity, hypophosphatemia, anemia, hypotension
- Inorganic phosphates:
  - Potentially lethal side effects limit use to patients with life-threatening hypercalcemia; IV use no longer supported.
  - Side effects: Precipitation of calcium into tissues of the lung, heart, kidneys, and blood vessels can lead to organ damage, hypotension, and death.
  - Oral and rectal routes safer than IV

- Glucocorticoids:
  - Direct effects in treating hypercalcemia of malignancy are unclear.
  - Has direct tumoricidal effects on hematologic cancers such as multiple myeloma, lymphoma, and leukemias

ADDITIONAL TREATMENT

In cases where saline diuresis and medications fail, hemodialysis is an option. Hemodialysis is the treatment for patients with renal failure and life-threatening hypercalcemia (1)[B].

General Measures
- Treatment of underlying malignancy
- Monitor for hypophosphatemia. Hypophosphatemia is common in hypercalcemia and can worsen hypercalcemia (3)[B]. Replace phosphorus PO or by nasogastric tube (3)[B].
- Discontinue use of oral calcium supplements and remove calcium from parenteral feeding solutions.
- Discontinue medications that can independently cause hypercalcemia (e.g., thiazides).
- Promote weight-bearing ambulation.

 ONGOING CARE

FOLLOW-UP RECOMMENDATIONS
Avoid bed rest or immobilization as much as possible.

Patient Monitoring
Frequent serum calcium and electrolyte determinations; expect relapse.

PROGNOSIS
- Median survival after diagnosis of tumoral hypercalcemia depends on type and extent of the malignancy but usually indicates a poor prognosis.
- >50% of patients die within 50 days of diagnosis of hypercalcemia (3).

REFERENCES

1. Zojer N, Ludwig H. Hematological emergencies. *Ann Oncol*. 2007;18(Suppl 1):i45–i48.
2. LeGrand SB, Leskuski D, Zama I. Narrative review: furosemide for hypercalcemia: an unproven yet common practice. *Ann Intern Med*. 2008;149: 259–63.
3. Higdon ML, et al. Treatment of oncologic emergencies. *AFP*. 2006;74:1874–80.
4. Deftos LJ. Hypercalcemia in malignancy and inflammatory diseases. *Endocrinol Metab Clin N Am*. 2002;31:141–58.
5. Stewart AF. Clinical practice. Hypercalcemia associated with cancer. *N Engl J Med*. 2005;352:373–9.

ADDITIONAL READING

- Horwitz MJ, Stewart AF. Hypercalcemia associated with malignancy. In: Primer on the Metabolic Bone Diseases and Disorders of Mineral Metabolism. *American Society of Bone and Mineral Research*. 2006;31:195.
- Lipton A. Management of metastatic bone disease and hypercalcemia of malignancy. *Am J Cancer*. 2003;2(6):427–38.

See Also (Topic, Algorithm, Electronic Media Element)
Addison Disease; HIV Infection and AIDS; Hyperparathyroidism; Hyperthyroidism; Milk-Alkali Syndrome; Rhabdomyolysis; Sarcoidosis; Tuberculosis
Algorithm: Hypercalcemia

 CODES

ICD9
275.42 Hypercalcemia

CLINICAL PEARLS

- Hypercalcemia of malignancy carries with it a very poor prognosis. The median survival after diagnosis is 6 weeks (3).
- Diagnosis may be difficult unless the patient has a known malignancy. Even with a known malignancy, other causes of hypercalcemia should be ruled out (4).
- The mnemonic for remembering the effects of hypercalcemia: Stones (kidney stones), bones (bone pain), moans (psychosis), groans (abdominal discomfort, constipation), and psychiatric overtones (including depression and confusion).
- Patients with hypercalcemia of malignancy do not need a low-calcium diet. Hypercalcemia decreases the absorption of calcium in the intestine (5).
- For severe hypercalcemia of malignancy, the initial treatment of choice is IV hydration. Volume depletion is the cause of many of the symptoms and the pathophysiology of hypercalcemia.

H

HYPERCHOLESTEROLEMIA

James L. Young, MD, PhD
Jeremy Golding, MD

BASICS

DESCRIPTION
- Serum cholesterol >200 mg/dL (5.18 mmol/L):
  - Due mainly to lifestyle habits in Westernized countries; however, genetic and secondary causes should be considered.
- Lipoprotein subpopulations are commonly used to augment risk prediction, favoring the term *dyslipidemia*, which encompasses high-density lipoprotein fraction of cholesterol (HDL): Atheroprotective. Low-density lipoprotein (LDL): Atherogenic. Triglycerides.
- Fredrickson classification is helpful to identify specific elevations in chylomicrons (type I), beta lipoproteins (LDL) (type II), broad beta disease (type III), VLDL or pre-beta lipoproteins (type IV), or chylomicrons and VLDL (type V), which may suggest distinct genetic disorders. However, this classification system is limited by its exclusion of HDL and the inability to differentiate monogenic disorders from more common polygenic disorders. The World Health Organization (WHO) and National Cholesterol Education Program (NCEP) have adopted measurements of total cholesterol, triglyceride, LDL, and HDL for risk assessment and treatment.
- System(s) affected: Cardiovascular; Endocrine/Metabolic

ALERT
Though very low cholesterol readings have been associated with higher mortality (J-curve phenomenon), this epidemiologic finding may at least in part be due to confounding disease processes associated with low cholesterol levels, such as cancer and liver disease, rather than a primary effect of low cholesterol itself.

Pregnancy Considerations
- Fetal nutritional demands may alter diet and drug treatment.
- Statins contraindicated in pregnancy - Class X
- Lactation: Possibly unsafe

EPIDEMIOLOGY
- Predominant age: Increases with age (female onset delayed by 10–15 years compared with males)
- Predominant sex: Male = Female

Prevalence
- 65.5 million people in US with cholesterol 200–239 mg/dL (borderline high)
- 34.5 million people in US with cholesterol ≥240 mg/dL (high)

RISK FACTORS
Obesity (BMI >30 kg/m^2), physical inactivity, diet rich in saturated fat and cholesterol, heredity

Genetics
- The most severe familial type of hypercholesterolemia is type 2 familial hypercholesterolemia (FH), a monogenic, autosomal disorder. Inheritance of FH is considered autosomal dominant because heterozygotes are affected, with atherosclerotic disease manifesting as early as young adulthood; however, homozygotes are more severely affected, often with disease manifesting in childhood. FH is the most prevalent lipoprotein disorder (1 in 500 in the Caucasian population).
- It is caused by defects in the gene that encodes the LDL receptor (LDLR), for which more than 700 allelic variants have been described. FH also can result from mutations in apolipoprotein B-100 gene (APOB) or the proprotein convertase subtilisin/kexin type 9 gene (PCSK9).
- Impairment in function of LDL receptors results in reduced clearance of LDL from the circulation and resultant elevation in plasma LDL cholesterol. Early diagnosis is beneficial to reduce the risk of atherosclerosis. Testing of family members of an index case is cost-effective.

GENERAL PREVENTION
Prudent diet, regular physical activity, and weight control for all

PATHOPHYSIOLOGY
Deposition of cholesterol in vascular walls causes atherosclerotic disease, but the development of inflammation is likely a necessary cofactor for plaque rupture.

ETIOLOGY
- Primary: Diet/sedentary lifestyle/obesity, heredity
- Secondary: Causes include hypothyroidism, diabetes mellitus, glycogen storage disorders, nephrotic syndrome, chronic renal failure, obstructive liver disease, cirrhosis, progestins, estrogens, anabolic steroids, corticosteroids, retinoic acid derivatives, diuretics (except indapamide (Lozol)), beta-blockers, except those with intrinsic sympathomimetic activity, some immunosuppressants (e.g., cyclosporine)

COMMONLY ASSOCIATED CONDITIONS
Hypertension, obesity, diabetes mellitus, hyperuricemia

DIAGNOSIS

PHYSICAL EXAM
- Few specific findings, most secondary to atherosclerotic disease
- Genetic familial hypercholesterolemia: Corneal arcus age <50 years, xanthomata, xanthelasma

DIAGNOSTIC TESTS & INTERPRETATION
Cholesterol measurements vary significantly even when retesting the same specimen. Repeated measurements needed for accurate clinical decision making.

Lab
- Fasting lipoprotein panel: Total cholesterol, HDL, LDL, triglycerides: LDL is typically a calculated value and is accurate under fasting conditions if triglycerides <350 mg/dL (<4.0 mmol/L). Direct LDL measurement may be available in some hospital and specialty labs.
- Nonfasting: Only total cholesterol and HDL values traditionally used for treatment decision making (triglycerides elevated by recent meal), although nonfasting profiles may better predict risk than fasting. Direct LDL remains accurate.
- Thyroid-stimulating hormone (TSH) to assess hypothyroidism
- Very high LDL (≥190 mg/dL) may have genetic etiology. Follow up to prevent premature coronary heart disease (CHD) in young adults and identify similarly afflicted relatives.

TREATMENT

MEDICATION
- Treatment initiation depends on LDL, HDL, and triglyceride levels, as modified by risk factors and history of previous CHD or risk equivalents (1)[A]. European (NICE) decision making more influenced by 10-year risk of cardiovascular disease, whereas in the US, NCEP has emphasized treatment initiation based on cardiac risk factors. Many more individuals are treated with medications in the US than elsewhere in the world, without evidence for improved outcomes compared to a more selective strategy. It is unclear that statin therapy reduces overall mortality when used in primary prevention. NCEP guidelines follow:
  - Risk factors: Cigarette smoking, hypertension (BP ≥140/90 or on antihypertensive medication), age (male >45 years, female >55 years), HDL <40 mg/dL (HDL >60 beneficial, subtract 1 RF), myocardial infarction (MI) or stroke in 1st-degree relative (male <55 years or female <65 years)
  - CHD or CHD risk equivalent (major coronary events ≥20% per 10 years): Coronary, carotid, aortic, or peripheral vascular disease. Diabetes mellitus (although it is not clear that younger type 2 diabetics have the same risk as older type 2s; less aggressive targets may be appropriate in younger individuals)
- Primary goal: LDL lowering for patients refractory to exercise, diet treatment (1)[A]:
  - CHD or CHD risk equivalent: <100 mg/dL
  - 2+ risk factors: <130 mg/dL
  - 0–1 risk factor: <160 mg/dL:
    ○ Clinical trial evidence supports an optional goal of LDL <70 mg/dL for very high-risk patients, although number needed to treat may be significantly greater than 100 people per year.
    ○ Further stratification of patients with 2+ risk factors can employ Framingham scoring.
- Secondary goal: In patients with triglycerides >200 mg/dL at target LDL, treat for non-HDL cholesterol (total cholesterol HDL) <130 mg/dL (CHD or CHD risk equivalent), <160 mg/dL (2+ risk factors), and <190 mg/dL (0–1 risk factor) (1)[A]. In patients with triglycerides >500, tailor therapy to lower triglycerides to prevent pancreatitis.
- Pharmacologic therapy considered when LDL is refractory to lifestyle intervention or levels exceed therapeutic goal by ≥30 mg/dL
- Pharmacologic measures to increase HDL are not supported by current clinical trials (1).
- JUPITER trial demonstrates reduction of 1st major cardiovascular event and all-cause death in normocholesterolemic patients with elevated C-reactive protein (CRP). Trial substantially criticized for authors' conflicts of interest and its early termination (mean follow-up was less than 2 years), so risks and benefits of longer-term therapy should be considered. Risk stratification in patients with CRP values may employ the Reynolds Risk Score (2).

First Line
- HMG-CoA reductase inhibitors (statins):
  - Fluvastatin (Lescol), lovastatin (Mevacor), pravastatin (Pravachol), or simvastatin (Zocor): 20–80 mg/d

– Atorvastatin (Lipitor): 10–80 mg/d
– Rosuvastatin (Crestor): 10–40 mg/d
- Contraindications:
  – HMG-CoA reductase inhibitors: Active or chronic liver disease, pregnancy, breastfeeding
- Precautions from ACC/AHA/NHLBI recommendations:
  – Severe myopathy rare: ~0.1% (studied with lovastatin and simvastatin, but all statins believed to carry similar potential):
    ○ Evaluate muscle symptoms and creatine kinase (CK) before therapy to establish baseline, 12 weeks after the initiation of therapy, and with follow-up if muscle symptoms are present. In actual practice, Ck monitoring is not always done in asymptomatic patients.
    ○ Educate patient to report muscle discomfort/weakness or brown urine.
    ○ CK measurement 3–10× upper normal limit: Evaluate symptoms and CK weekly until resolved. CK measurement >10× upper normal limit: Discontinue statin.
  – Liver function tests (ALT, AST) before therapy to establish baseline, 12 weeks after the initiation of therapy, and then annually
- Significant possible interactions: Fibric acid derivatives, niacin, cyclosporine, azole antifungals, or macrolide antibiotics may increase the possibility of myositis. Combination therapy (2 or more medications) also increases risk of myositis.
- Statins reduce major coronary events, CHD deaths, need for coronary procedures, and stroke, although number needed to treat to prevent a single event varies widely and may be in the 300–500 range per year for primary prevention (less for secondary prevention) (1)[A]. Whether statins reduce overall mortality in primary prevention remains controversial (3,4).
- Statins most probably have beneficial pleiotropic effects beyond lipid lowering, as risk reduction does not parallel lipid lowering: 24% reduction in LDL was sufficient to provide full pravastatin benefit in WOSCOPS trial, despite greater achieved reductions.

ALERT
- Avoid grapefruit juice.
- Take statins late in day, as majority of liver cholesterol synthesis occurs at night: Exception due to longer $t_{1/2}$ (14–19 hours): Atorvastatin and rosuvastatin

Second Line
- Ezetimibe (Zetia), 10 mg/d: Selectively inhibits intestinal absorption of cholesterol and related phytosterols. No clinically relevant outcome data demonstrate benefit. Ezetimibe/simvastatin (10/10, 10/20, 10/40, 10/80 mg) combined formulation (Vytorin) enhances LDL lowering in FH patients; however, it fails to confer additional cardiovascular benefit seen with statin alone (5)[A].
- Cholestyramine (Questran) or colestipol (Colestid) bile acid–binding resins: 1–6 packets per day taken b.i.d. or t.i.d., or colesevelam (Welchol) 6 tablets daily: Effect: 15–20% fall in LDL
- Niacin (nicotinic acid): Target dose of 1.5–6 g/d in 3 divided doses with meals for regular-release formulation (Niacor) or 375 mg–2 g once daily at bedtime for extended-release formulation (Niaspan): Effect: 15–30% LDL lowering, decreases triglycerides, increases HDL. Hepatic dysfunction more common in patients who take immediate-release niacin.

- Fibric acid derivatives: Gemfibrozil (Lopid) and fenofibrate (Antara, Lofibra, Tricor, Triglide) are effective for reducing triglycerides with modest elevation of HDL and variable effect on LDL, but should be used only with caution with a statin due to risk of rhabdomyolysis.
- Contraindications:
  – Cholestyramine: Complete biliary obstruction, bowel obstruction, TG ≥200 mg/dL, TG ≥400 mg/dL (absolute), dysbetalipoproteinemia (absolute)
  – Nicotinic acid: Acute peptic ulcer, diabetes mellitus, hyperuricemia, severe gout (absolute), chronic liver disease (absolute)
  – Fibric acid derivatives: Hepatic or renal dysfunction, gallbladder disease
- Precautions:
  – Cholestyramine: Gradually increase dose on weekly basis to minimize gastrointestinal (GI) side effects (particularly constipation, flatulence).
  – Nicotinic acid: Titrate dose according to package insert to minimize side effects (e.g., cutaneous flushing). Caution with diabetes mellitus, renal disease, gout, active gallbladder disease.
- Significant possible interactions:
  – Cholestyramine: Other drugs taken <1 hour before or within 6 hours after may be bound and not absorbed as well. Fat-soluble vitamins A, D, E, and K absorption may be impeded.
  – Fibric acid derivatives: May potentiate effects of warfarin and oral hypoglycemic agents. Avoid with statins.

COMPLEMENTARY AND ALTERNATIVE MEDICINE
- Beta-sitosterols and red yeast rice (contain monacolin K, which is a natural lovastatin) can reduce total cholesterol and LDL. Niacin and polidocanol can reduce total cholesterol and LDL while increasing HDL.
- Multiple large-scale studies support use of marine- and plant-derived omega-3 fatty acids in reduction of cardiovascular events and death in coronary patients. However, use of supplements in primary or secondary prevention requires further study.
- AHA recommendation for omega-3 fatty acids and fish oil intake:
  – History of CHD: ~1g EPA (eicosapentaenoic acid) + DHA (docosahexaenoic acid) daily, preferably from oily fish, but may be considered with supplements under physician guidance
  – No history of CHD: Eat variety of oily fish twice a week. Include foods rich in α-linoleic acid (flaxseed, canola, soybean oils)
  – Triglyceride lowering: 2–4 g EPA + DHA daily from capsules under physician guidance

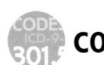 ONGOING CARE

FOLLOW-UP RECOMMENDATIONS
Sustained exercise for 30 minutes, 3–4 times per week: Increases HDL, lowers total cholesterol, and helps control weight

Patient Monitoring
- With the initiation or dose increase of statins or niacin, monitor cholesterol, HDL, LDL, triglycerides every 6–8 weeks until target goals are reached, then every 6–12 months to promote compliance.

- United States Preventive Services Task Force (USPSTF) recommendation for lipoprotein screening: All males older than 35 years or females older than 45 years. Males (20–35 years old) or females (20–45 years old) at increased risk for coronary heart disease.

DIET
- National Cholesterol Education Program (NCEP) Therapeutic Lifestyle Changes (TLC) Diet:
  – Dietary fats: 25–35% of total calories. Saturated: <7% of total calories. Polyunsaturated: <10% of total calories. Monounsaturated: <20% of total calories. Carbohydrates: 50–60% of total calories from whole grains, fruits, vegetables. Fiber: 20–30 g/day. Cholesterol: <200 mg/d. Protein: ~15% of total calories.
- Avoid "tropical" oils, such as coconut oil derivatives, and hydrogenated products rich in saturated fats and trans-fatty acids. Choose instead oils rich in monounsaturates (e.g., olive oil) or polyunsaturates (e.g., canola or safflower oil). Omega-3-fatty acids and fish oil may be used for concomitant hypertriglyceridemia. Plant stanols/sterols (2 g/d) and viscous (soluble) fiber may aid in LDL lowering.

PROGNOSIS
1% decrease in cholesterol results in 2% decreased risk of CHD.

COMPLICATIONS
Atherosclerotic disease and generalized arteriosclerosis

REFERENCES
1. Expert Panel on Detection, Evaluation, and Treatment of High Blood Cholesterol in Adults. Executive Summary of The Third Report of The National Cholesterol Education Program (NCEP) Expert Panel on Detection, Evaluation, And Treatment of High Blood Cholesterol In Adults (Adult Treatment Panel III). *JAMA*. 2001;285: 2486–97.
2. Ridker PM, Danielson E, Fonseca FA, et al. Rosuvastatin to prevent vascular events in men and women with elevated C-reactive protein. *N Engl J Med*. 2008;359:2195–207.
3. Carey, J"Do Cholesterol Drugs Do Any Good?" Business Week Jan 17, 2008.
4. Abramson J. *Overdosed America*. HarperCollins Publishers, 2004.
5. Kastelein JJ, Akdim F, Stroes ES, et al. Simvastatin with or without ezetimibe in familial hypercholesterolemia. *N Engl J Med*. 2008;358: 1431–43.

See Also (Topic, Algorithm, Electronic Media Element)
Atherosclerosis; Atherosclerotic Occlusive Disease; Hypothyroidism, Adult
Algorithm: Hypercholesterolemia

CODES

ICD9
272.0 Pure hypercholesterolemia

H

HYPEREMESIS GRAVIDARUM

Scott A. Fields, MD

BASICS

DESCRIPTION
- Persistent vomiting in a pregnant woman that interferes with fluid and electrolyte balance as well as nutrition
- Usually associated with the 1st 8–20 weeks of pregnancy
- Believed to have biomedical and behavioral aspects
- Associated with high estrogen levels
- Symptoms usually begin ~2 weeks after 1st missed period.
- System(s) affected: Endocrine/Metabolic; Gastrointestinal; Reproductive
- Synonym(s): Morning sickness

Pregnancy Considerations
Common condition during pregnancy, typically in the 1st and 2nd trimesters, but may persist into the 3rd trimester.

EPIDEMIOLOGY
Incidence
Hyperemesis gravidarum occurs in 1–2% of pregnancies.

Prevalence
Hyperemesis gravidarum is the most common cause of hospitalization in the 1st half of pregnancy and the 2nd most common cause of hospitalization of pregnant women.

RISK FACTORS
- Obesity
- Nulliparity
- Multiple gestations
- Gestational trophoblastic disease
- Gonadotropin production stimulated
- Altered gastrointestinal function
- Hyperthyroidism
- Hyperparathyroidism
- Liver dysfunction

GENERAL PREVENTION
Anticipatory guidance in 1st and 2nd trimesters regarding dietary habits in hopes of avoiding dehydration and nutritional depletion

Pregnancy Considerations
- 2% of pregnancies have electrolyte disturbances.
- 50% of pregnancies have at least some gastrointestinal disturbance.

ETIOLOGY
- Unknown
- Possible psychologic factors
- Hyperthyroidism
- Hyperparathyroidism
- Gestational hormones
- Liver dysfunction
- Autonomic nervous system dysfunction

COMMONLY ASSOCIATED CONDITIONS
Hyperthyroidism

DIAGNOSIS

HISTORY
- Hypersensitivity to smell
- Alteration in taste
- Poor appetite
- Nausea
- Vomiting with retching
- Decreased urine output
- Fatigue
- Dizziness with standing

DIAGNOSTIC TESTS & INTERPRETATION
Lab
- Electrolyte abnormalities due to nausea and vomiting and subsequent dehydration
- Increased uric acid
- Hypoalbuminemia
- Acidosis
- Urinalysis: Glucosuria, albuminuria, granular casts, and hematuria (rare); ketosis more common
- Drugs unlikely to alter lab results.

Initial lab tests
- Thyroid-stimulating hormone (TSH), T4
- Electrolytes, blood urea nitrogen (BUN), creatinine
- Calcium

Follow-Up & Special Considerations
If hypercalcemia, consider checking parathyroid hormone (PTH) for hyperparathyroidism.

Imaging
No imaging is indicated for the diagnosis of hyperemesis gravidarum.

Diagnostic Procedures/Surgery
Indicated only if it is necessary to rule out other diagnoses as listed below

DIFFERENTIAL DIAGNOSIS
Other common causes of vomiting must be considered:
- Gastroenteritis
- Gastritis
- Reflux esophagitis
- Peptic ulcer disease
- Cholelithiasis
- Cholecystitis
- Pyelonephritis
- Anxiety
- Hyperparathyroidism

TREATMENT

Pyridoxine and metoclopramide (pregnancy Category A) are 1st-line treatments for hyperemesis gravidarum, followed by prochlorperazine (pregnancy Category C), prednisolone (pregnancy Category A), promethazine (pregnancy Category C), and ondansetron (pregnancy Category B1) (1).

MEDICATION
- Pyridoxine (vitamin B6) 10–30 mg p.o. or IV daily
- Antihistamines (e.g., diphenhydramine [25–50 mg q4–6h] or doxylamine [12.5 mg p.o. b.i.d.])
- Phenothiazines (e.g., promethazine or prochlorperazine):
  – Precautions: Phenothiazines are associated with prolonged jaundice, extrapyramidal effects, hyper- or hyporeflexia in newborns
- Meclizine 25 mg p.o. q6h
- Methylprednisolone 16 mg p.o. × daily for 3 days, then taper over 2 weeks (2)
- Ondansetron 4–8 mg p.o. q8h

Pregnancy Considerations
- All medications taken during pregnancy should balance the risks and benefits both to the mother and the fetus.

ADDITIONAL TREATMENT
General Measures
- Patient reassurance
- Bed rest
- If dehydrated, IV fluids. Repeat if there is a recurrence of symptoms following initial improvement.

COMPLEMENTARY AND ALTERNATIVE MEDICINE
- Ginger 350 mg p.o. t.i.d. may help (3).
- Motion sickness wrists bands are another nonpharmacological intervention that may improve symptoms.
- Evidence is mixed regarding the impact of acupressure and acupuncture in treating hyperemesis gravidarum (1).
- Medical hypnosis may be a powerful adjunct to the typical medical treatment regimen (4)[B].

IN-PATIENT CONSIDERATIONS
Initial Stabilization
- Outpatient therapy
- In some severe cases, parenteral therapy in the hospital or at home may be required. Enteral volume and nutrition repletion may be indicated.

 ## ONGOING CARE

FOLLOW-UP RECOMMENDATIONS
Activity as tolerated after improvement (3,5)[C]

Patient Monitoring
- In severe cases, follow up on a daily basis for weight monitoring.
- Special attention should be given to monitoring for ketosis, hypokalemia, or acid-base disturbances due to hyperemesis.

DIET
- n.p.o. for 1st 24 hours if patient is ill enough to require hospitalization
- For outpatient: A diet rich in carbohydrates and protein, such as fruit, cheese, cottage cheese, eggs, beef, poultry, vegetables, toast, crackers, rice. Limit intake of butter. Patients should avoid spicy meals and high-fat foods.

PATIENT EDUCATION
- Attention should be given to psychosocial issues, such as possible ambivalence about the pregnancy.
- Patients should be instructed to take small amounts of fluid frequently to avoid volume depletion.
- Avoidance of individual foods known to be irritating to the patient
- Wet-to-dry nutrients (sherbet, broth, gelatin to dry crackers, toast)

PROGNOSIS
- Self-limited illness with good prognosis if patient's weight is maintained at >95% of prepregnancy weight
- With complication of hemorrhagic retinitis, mortality rate of pregnant patient is 50%.

COMPLICATIONS
- Patients with >5% weight loss are associated with intrauterine growth retardation and fetal anomalies.
- Hemorrhagic retinitis
- Liver damage
- Central nervous system deterioration, sometimes to coma

REFERENCES

1. Sheehan P. Hyperemesis gravidarum - Assessment and management. *Aust Fam Physician*. 2007;36: 698–701.
2. Yost NP, McIntire DD, Wians FH et al. A randomized, placebo-controlled trial of corticosteroids for hyperemesis due to pregnancy. *Obstet Gynecol*. 2003;102:1250–4.
3. Borrelli F, Capasso R, Aviello G, et al. Effectiveness and safety of ginger in the treatment of pregnancy-induced nausea and vomiting. *Obstet Gynecol*. 2005;105:849–56.
4. Simon EP, Schwartz J. Medical hypnosis for hyperemesis gravidarum. *Birth*. 1999;26:248–54.
5. Cedergren M, Brynhildsen J, Josefsson A et al. Hyperemesis gravidarum that requires hospitalization and the use of antiemetic drugs in relation to maternal body composition. *American Journal of Obstetrics & Gynecology*. 2008;198(4): 412.e1–5.

ADDITIONAL READING

- Jewell D, Young G. Interventions for nausea and vomiting in early pregnancy. Cochrane Pregnancy and Childbirth Group *Cochrane Database of Systematic Reviews*. 1, 2006.
- Poursharif B, Korst LM, Fejzo MS et al. The psychosocial burden of hyperemesis gravidarum. *Journal of Perinatology*. 2008;28(3):176–81.
- Trogstad LI, Stoltenberg C, Magnus P et al. Recurrence risk in hyperemesis gravidarum. *BJOG: An International Journal of Obstetrics & Gynaecology*. 2005;112(12):1641–45.
- Verberg MF, Gillott DJ, Al-Fardan N, Grudzinskas JG et al. Hyperemesis gravidarum, a literature review. *Hum Reprod Update*. 2005;11:527–39.

 ## CODES

ICD9
- 643.03 Mild hyperemesis gravidarum, antepartum
- 643.13 Hyperemesis gravidarum with metabolic disturbance, antepartum

CLINICAL PEARLS
- Do not allow patients to become volume depleted. Once this occurs, it is more difficult to interrupt the process.
- Do not be hesitant to use medications to assist the patient, as this may help avoid the volume depletion.

H

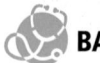

HYPEREOSINOPHILIC SYNDROME

Fred Schiffman, MD
Armando Bedoya, MD

BASICS

DESCRIPTION
Hypereosinophilic syndrome (HES): A heterogeneous group of chronically high eosinophil states characterized by
- A persistently elevated eosinophil count >1,500 cells/μL for at least 6 months
- Eosinophil-induced end-organ damage
- Exclusion of other causes (e.g., parasitic infection, allergy, malignancy, collagen-vascular disease)
- There are several patient subsets within HES.
  - *FIP1L1/PDGFRα*-associated (F/P+) HES: Myeloproliferative HES, chronic eosinophilic leukemia (CEL)
  - F/P− HES:
    ○ Lymphocytic HES (L-HES): CD3−/CD4+ T-lymphocytes produce IL-5
    ○ Organ-restricted disease, e.g., eosinophilic esophagitis
  - Idiopathic HES
- System(s) affected: Hematologic; Cardiac; Cutaneous; Pulmonary; Neurologic; GI; Rheumatologic; Ocular
- Synonym(s): Disseminated eosinophilic collagen disease; Löeffler's fibroplastic endocarditis with eosinophilia (not currently used)

EPIDEMIOLOGY
A rare condition, typically seen between 20 and 50 years of age

Incidence
- Peak incidence in 4th decade of life
- Uncommon in children
- Incidence decreases in elderly
- Predominant sex: Male > Female (4–9:1)
- Male predominance in F/P+ HES; other types more equally distributed

RISK FACTORS
Male gender (F/P+ HES)

Genetics
- F/P+ HES: Microdeletion at 4q12 causing gene fusion creates constitutively active tyrosine kinase.
- F/P− HES:
  - L-HES: Clonal T-cell expansion; mutations such as 16q breakage, partial 6q or 10p deletions, trisomy 7
  - Familial eosinophilia: Autosomal dominant, at 5q31–q33; eosinophilia at birth, often asymptomatic
  - Cardiac disease more in males, carriers of HLA-Bw44

GENERAL PREVENTION
No documented measures

PATHOPHYSIOLOGY
- Organ damage is similar among HES subsets and results from high eosinophil levels.
- Cytokines IL-3, IL-5, and GM-CSF stimulate bone marrow eosinophil production; IL-5 is most specific.
- Blood levels, organ migration regulated by chemokines, especially IL-5 and eotaxins

- HES: Eosinophils infiltrate organs and release toxic granules containing major basic protein, eosinophil peroxidase, eosinophil cationic protein (ECP), eosinophil-derived neurotoxin (EDN), Charcot Leyden crystal, VIP, and substance P. Neurotoxic, cytotoxic, and prothrombotic; creates oxidative burst, reactive oxygen species
- Cytokine release (IL-1, IL-3, IL-5, TNF-α) incites damage and activates inflammatory pathways.
- EDN and ECP activate fibroblasts: Fibrosis and organ dysfunction

ETIOLOGY
Variable, depends on patient subset:
- F/P+ HES: Clonal proliferation of myeloid cells with constitutively active tyrosine kinase (1)
- F/P− HES:
  - Clonal expansion of IL-5-producing CD3−/CD4+ T-lymphocytes (L-HES)
  - Enhanced activity of eosinophilogenic cytokines
  - Failure to normally regulate/suppress eosinophil activity

DIAGNOSIS

Highly variable presentation; depends on organ systems affected for any etiology; often indolent illness/incidental finding; occasionally acute onset, e.g., cardiac failure, thrombotic event

HISTORY
- Left upper quadrant pain (from splenomegaly)
- Fatigue, anemia
- Cardiac manifestations (50–60%) may cause heart failure symptoms and chest pain.
- Neurologic manifestations (50%) may result from thromboembolic disease: Behavioral changes, memory loss, confusion.
- Cutaneous manifestations (50%) may cause pruritus.
- Pulmonary manifestations (40%) may cause nonproductive cough.
- GI manifestations (20–30%):
  - Gastritis/enteritis: Diarrhea, vomiting, abdominal pain (embolic bowel infarction)
  - Hepatic manifestations of hepatitis, Budd-Chiari syndrome
- Ocular manifestations (20%): Blurry vision/blindness from microemboli
- Other: Myalgias, arthralgias

PHYSICAL EXAM
Various; depend on organ involvement
- Hematologic: Splenomegaly
- Cardiac:
  - Murmur
  - Signs of CHF
  - Microemboli, splinter hemorrhages
- Neurologic:
  - Signs of stroke/TIA
  - Sensory/motor deficits, usually symmetric
- Cutaneous: Angioedema, urticarial lesions, erythematous papules or nodules, mucosal ulcers, dermatographism
- Pulmonary: Crackles
- GI: Hepatomegaly (hepatitis, Budd-Chiari syndrome)
- Rheumatologic: Joint effusions

DIAGNOSTIC TESTS & INTERPRETATION
- May be discovered incidentally on routine laboratory testing
- Hematologic manifestations (100%):
  - Eosinophilia, leukocytosis
  - Thrombocytosis or thrombocytopenia
  - Hypercoagulable state (↑ tissue factor expression/altered thrombomodulin)

Lab
With the following, perform extensive workup to rule out secondary causes of eosinophilia:
- CBC
  - ↓ Hematocrit (anemia of chronic disease, hypersplenism)
  - WBCs: eosinophils ≥1,500 cells/μl; leukocytosis of 10,000–30,000 (>90,000 carries poor prognosis)
  - Thrombocytosis; thrombocytopenia (hypersplenism)
- Genetics:
  - FISH analysis or RT-PCR: Assess *FIP1L1/PDGFRα* translocation/other TK mutations
  - RT-PCR or Southern blot: Assess IL-5-producing CD3−/CD4+ T-lymphocytes
- Chemistries:
  - ↑ Ig-E
  - ↑ Serum tryptase (F/P+ HES)
  - ↑ B_{12} levels
  - L-HES: ↑ IL-5, IgG, IgM, TARC levels
- ECG: T-wave inversion, restrictive cardiomyopathy

Initial lab tests
- Rule out other causes: Parasite serologies, stool ova and parasites × 3, HIV, ESR, CRP, rheumatoid factor, adrenal insufficiency
- CBC with differential, smear (eosinophil morphology is unreliable indicator); serum tryptase, B_{12}, immunoglobulins; ECG, troponin, CPK, LFTs, creatinine, BUN, PFTs (end-organ function)
- Peripheral blood screening for *FIP1L1-PDGFRA* first. If negative, then bone marrow biopsy and cytogenetics for *FIP1L1/PDGFRα, BCR/ABL, KIT* translocations; peripheral T-lymphocyte phenotyping with flow cytometry and TCR analysis (2)
- If all negative, consider idiopathic HES.

Imaging
- Echocardiogram
- Abdominal/chest CT: Assess splenomegaly, end-organ involvement

Diagnostic Procedures/Surgery
Tissue biopsy (organ-restricted disease)

Pathological Findings
Organ infiltration with eosinophils and lymphocytes, tissue necrosis, eosinophil degranulation, and microabscesses

DIFFERENTIAL DIAGNOSIS
- Extensive; first rule out secondary causes of eosinophilia: Parasitic infection, allergy, malignancy, drug hypersensitivity, connective-tissue disorders
  - Chronic eosinophilic leukemia: Clonality like F/P+ HES but differs by having 2–20% blasts peripherally or 5–20% blasts in the marrow
  - Acute eosinophilic leukemia: A form of AML with 50–80% eosinophils; may cause bronchospasm, heart failure

- Other conditions with high eosinophil levels: Hodgkin lymphoma, mastocytosis, chronic myelomonocytic leukemia (eosinophil variant), cutaneous T-cell lymphoma, Churg-Strauss syndrome/other vasculitides, toxicity (the eosinophilia–myalgia syndrome), HIV, HTLV, bronchopulmonary aspergillosis

 TREATMENT

- Treatment goal: Control and reduce end-organ damage.
- Some damage, such as cardiac fibrosis, may not be reversible.
- One must consider F/P transcript status.

MEDICATION
- F/P+ HES:
  - Tyrosine kinase inhibitors (TKIs) in all patients with or without symptoms
  - Danger of heart failure with therapy initiation (rapid release of killed eosinophil contents): Obtain troponin, monitor carefully, treat with corticosteroids 1–2 mg/kg/day concurrently or prior to initiation of therapy if complications arise, cardiac enzymes elevated, abnormal echocardiogram
  - TKIs shown to induce complete molecular response (no F/P transcript); not yet known to be curative
- F/P– HES:
  - Corticosteroids are the mainstay of treatment.
  - A corticosteroid-sparing agent (interferon-α, anti-CD52 agents in L-HES, IL-5 inhibitors, chemotherapeutic agents) may be introduced if steroids poorly tolerated or fail to manage disease.
  - May respond to TKI, suggesting non-F/P tyrosine kinase activity

First Line
- F/P+ HES: Imatinib mesylate (Gleevec) started at 400 mg daily (3)[A]:
  - Generally, lower doses needed to induce/maintain remission than with CML. Therapy continued indefinitely
  - Side effects: Thrombocytopenia, anemia, nausea, diarrhea, ↑ LFTs
  - Resistance: T674I point mutation, similar to CML
- F/P– HES: Prednisone: Initial challenge of 60 mg once to determine responsiveness, followed by 1 mg/kg daily × 1–2 weeks. A taper should be initiated based on disease severity, persistent eosinophilia (4)[C].
  - Side effects: Many; intolerance should prompt decreasing dose, adding second agent.
  - Once stable, may add corticosteroid-sparing agent

Second Line
- F/P + HES: Patients rarely have shown resistance to imatinib; initiate trial of other TKI such as nilotinib, sorafenib, or dasatinib (4)[C].
- F/P – HES:
  - Interferon-α:
    - Effective dose 1–8 million units 3–7 times a week; start low, increase as tolerated.
    - Side effects: Flulike symptoms, cytopenias, depression, elevated LFTs, GI disturbances
  - Hydroxyurea:
    - Start at 500–1,000 mg daily, increase to 2,000 mg daily.
    - Side effects: Cytopenias, nausea, rash, alopecia, diffuse pulmonary infiltrates, elevated LFTs, teratogen

- Mepolizumab (in clinical trials) (5):
  - Anti-IL5 antibody; administered 750 mg IV every 4 weeks. Decreases steroid use
  - Side effects: Currently not well defined
- Alemtuzumab (L-HES use under evaluation) (6):
  - Anti-CD52 antibody, IV administration
  - Side effects: Hypotension, fever, fatigue, lymphopenia, neutropenia, fatal infection

ADDITIONAL TREATMENT
Issues for Referral
- Refer to a hematologist.
- Refer to appropriate specialist for organ dysfunction, e.g., cardiologist.

SURGERY/OTHER PROCEDURES
- Allogeneic stem cell transplant:
  - Patients failing other treatment modalities
  - Patients with L-HES progressing to T-cell lymphoma
- Cardiac surgery for complications of HES has been efficacious. If valve replacement is necessary, use porcine valve because of underlying hypercoagulable state.

IN-PATIENT CONSIDERATIONS
Initial Stabilization
- Emergency treatment for eosinophilia > 100,000 includes high-dose corticosteroids (prednisone 1 mg/kg).
- If levels fail to decrease significantly in 24 hours: Vincristine 1–2 mg/m^2, imatinib 400 mg, or plasmapheresis

Admission Criteria
Heart failure, splenic rupture, organ failure; admission also may be necessary for reduction of very high eosinophilia.

Discharge Criteria
Abatement of acute symptoms

 ONGOING CARE

FOLLOW-UP RECOMMENDATIONS
Frequency depends on etiology of disease, response to treatment, and severity of end-organ damage.

Patient Monitoring
- Weekly CBC on initiating treatment; longer intervals once stable
- L-HES: Increased risk of T-cell lymphoma; CBC every 3 months, flow cytometry biannually to monitor abnormal lymphocytosis (3)
- Patients on imatinib: LFTs and CBC monthly; RT-PCR for the F/P transcript and echocardiogram every 3 months
- Screen all patients for organ involvement every 6 months: Cardiac enzymes, PFTs, LFTs, renal function tests, ECG, and echocardiogram.
- Anticoagulation unnecessary without thrombi

PROGNOSIS
Better prognosis:
- Lack of heart disease
- Presentation with angioedema
- Good response to prednisone challenge
- Absent indicators of myeloproliferative disease (elevated B$_{12}$ or tryptase, splenomegaly, abnormal lymphocytes, cytogenetic abnormalities)

REFERENCES
1. Cools J, DeAngelo DJ, Gotlib J, et al. A tyrosine kinase created by fusion of the PDGFRA and FIP1L1 genes as a therapeutic target of imatinib in idiopathic hypereosinophilic syndrome. *N Engl J Med*. 2003;348:1201–14.
2. Tefferi A, Gotlib J, Pardanani A et al. Hypereosinophilic syndrome and clonal eosinophilia: point-of-care diagnostic algorithm and treatment update. *Mayo Clin Proc*. 2010;85: 158–64.
3. Baccarani M, Cilloni D, Rondoni M, et al. The efficacy of imatinib mesylate in patients with FIP1l1-PDGFRalpha-positive hypereosinophilic syndrome. Results of a multicenter prospective study. *Haematologica*. 2007.
4. Fletcher S, Bain B. Diagnosis and treatment of hypereosinophilic syndromes. *Curr Opin Hematol*. 2007;14:37–42.
5. Rothenberg ME, Klion AD, Roufosse FE, et al. Treatment of patients with the hypereosinophilic syndrome with mepolizumab. *N Engl J Med*. 2008;358:1215–28.
6. Verstovsek S, Tefferi A, Kantarjian H, et al. Alemtuzumab Therapy for Hypereosinophilic Syndrome and Chronic Eosinophilic Leukemia. *Clin Cancer Res*. 2009;15:368–73.

ADDITIONAL READING
- Roufosse FE, Goldman M, Cogan E. Hypereosinophilic syndromes. *Orphanet J Rare Dis*. 2007;2:37.
- Sheikh J, Weller PF. Clinical overview of hypereosinophilic syndromes. *Immunol Allergy Clin North Am*. 2007;27:333–55.

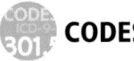 **CODES**

ICD9
288.3 Eosinophilia

CLINICAL PEARLS
- HS encompasses a group of diseases with eosinophils > 1,500/μL and end-organ damage without an identifiable secondary cause.
- F/P+ transcript should be determined early in the course of treatment.
- Cardiac disease is a dangerous complication of this condition and may not be reversible.

H

HYPERKALEMIA

Ruben Peralta, MD

 BASICS

DESCRIPTION
- Hyperkalemia is a common electrolyte disorder with plasma potassium (K) concentration >5.5 mEq/L (>5.0 mmol/L).
- Hyperkalemia depresses cardiac conduction and can lead to fatal arrhythmias.
- Normal K regulation:
  - Ingested K enters portal circulation, pancreas releases insulin in response. Insulin facilitates K entry into cells.
  - K in renal circulation causes renin release from juxtaglomerular cells, leading to activation of angiotensin I, converted to angiotensin II in lungs. Angiotensin II acts in adrenal zona glomerulosa to stimulate aldosterone secretion. Aldosterone, at the renal collecting ducts, causes K to be excreted and Na to be retained.
- 4 major causes:
  - Increased load: Either endogenous from tissue release or exogenous from a high intake, which is usually in association with impaired excretion
  - Decreased excretion: Due to decreased glomerular filtration rate
  - Cellular redistribution: Shifting of intracellular (which is the major store of K) to extracellular space
  - Pseudohyperkalemia: Related to improper collection or transport of blood sample

Geriatric Considerations
Increased risk for hyperkalemia due to decreases in renin and aldosterone as well as increased number of comorbid conditions

EPIDEMIOLOGY
Prevalence
- 1–10% of hospitalized patients
- Predominant sex: Male = Female
- No age-related predilection

RISK FACTORS
- Impaired renal excretion of K
- Acidemia
- Massive cell breakdown (rhabdomyolysis, burns, trauma)
- Use of K-sparing diuretics
- Excess K supplementation

Genetics
Associated with some inherited diseases and conditions:
- Familial hyperkalemic periodic paralysis
- Congenital adrenal hyperplasia

GENERAL PREVENTION
Diet and oral supplement compliance

ETIOLOGY
- Pseudohyperkalemia:
  - Hemolysis of red cells in phlebotomy tube (most common: Spurious result)
  - Thrombolysis
  - Leukocytosis
  - Thrombocytosis
  - Hereditary spherocytosis
  - Infectious mononucleosis
- Traumatic venipuncture or fist clenching during phlebotomy (spurious result)
- Transcellular shift (redistribution):
  - Metabolic acidosis
  - Insulin deficiency
  - Hyperglycemia
  - Tissue damage (rhabdomyolysis, burns, trauma) (1)
  - Tumor lysis syndrome (2)
  - Cocaine abuse
  - Exercise with heavy sweating
  - Mannitol
- Impaired K excretion:
  - Renal insufficiency/failure
  - Addison disease
  - Mineralocorticoid deficiency
  - Primary hyporeninemia, primary hypoaldosteronism
  - Type IV renal tubular acidosis
- Medication-induced:
  - Excess K supplementation
  - ACE inhibitors (3)
  - Angiotensin receptor blockers (ARBs)
  - β-blockers
  - Cyclosporine
  - Digoxin toxicity
  - Ethinyl estradiol/drospirenone
  - Heparin
  - Nonsteroidal anti-inflammatory drugs (NSAIDs)
  - Penicillin G potassium
  - Pentamidine
  - Spironolactone
  - Succinylcholine
  - Tacrolimus
  - Trimethoprim (3,4)

 DIAGNOSIS

HISTORY
- Neuromuscular cramps
- Diarrhea
- Abdominal pain
- Myalgias
- Numbness
- Weakness

PHYSICAL EXAM
- Decreased deep tendon reflexes
- Flaccid paralysis of extremities

DIAGNOSTIC TESTS & INTERPRETATION
Lab
- Serum electrolytes
- Renal function: Blood urea nitrogen (BUN), creatinine
- Urinalysis: K, creatinine, osmoles (to calculate fractional excretion of K and transtubular K gradient; both assess renal handling of K)
- Disorders that may alter lab results:
  - Acidemia: K shifts from the intracellular to extracellular space in an effort to buffer the acid load.
  - Insulin deficiency
  - Hemolysis of sample
- Cortisol and aldosterone levels to check for mineralocorticoid deficiency when other causes are ruled out

Diagnostic Procedures/Surgery
Electrocardiogram (EKG):
- Peaked T wave in precordial leads (most common, usually earliest EKG change) (5)
- Loss of P wave
- Widened QRS
- Sine wave at very high K

TREATMENT

MEDICATION
- After initial stabilization (see above), institute measures to decrease total body K:
  - Sodium polystyrene sulfonate (Kayexalate): 30–60 g p.o. or rectally
  - This is effective in 1–4 hours and is a definitive treatment. This may be repeated every 6 hours, if necessary.
  - Enema form more rapidly effective
- Diuretics (loop and thiazides)
- Consider the use of recombinant urate oxidase (Rasburicase) in patients with tumor lysis syndrome (2).
- Hemodialysis is the definitive therapy when other measures are not effective, and in patients with ESRD, severe CKD, and AKI or if comorbidity conditions exist such as digitalis toxicity or rhabdomyolysis (6).

ALERT

- Kayexalate provides a sodium load that may exacerbate fluid overload in cardiac or renal failure patients.
- Rapid administration of calcium in patients with suspected digitalis toxicity may result in a fatal dysrhythmia. Calcium should be administered slowly over 20–30 minutes in 5% dextrose and with extreme caution.
- Calcium and dextrose/insulin are only temporizing measures and do not actually lower total body K levels.
- Sodium bicarbonate is no longer recommended to lower K, although it may be appropriate in patients with severe metabolic acidosis.

IN-PATIENT CONSIDERATIONS
Initial Stabilization

- If hyperkalemia is severe, treat 1st, then do diagnostic investigations.
- IV calcium to stabilize myocardium (caution in setting of digoxin toxicity when calcium may worsen effects of toxicity)
- Insulin (usually 10 units IV, given with 50 mL of 50% glucose to avoid hypoglycemia). Consider repeating if elevation persists.
- Inhaled β_2-agonist (nebulized albuterol)
- Insulin and β_2-agonist facilitate K entry into cells; do not decrease total body K.
- Discontinue any medications that may increase K (e.g., K-sparing diuretics, exogenous K).

Admission Criteria
Admit for cardiac monitoring if EKG changes are present or K is >6.0 mEq/L (6.0 mmol/L).

ONGOING CARE

FOLLOW-UP RECOMMENDATIONS
Patient Monitoring
- Reduction of plasma K should begin within the 1st hour of initiation of treatment.
- Serum K levels should be rechecked every 2–4 hours until the patient has stabilized and recurrent hyperkalemia is no longer a threat.
- Identification and elimination of possible causes and risk factors for hyperkalemia are essential.

DIET
80 mEq (80 mmol) or less of K per 24 hours

PATIENT EDUCATION
Consult with dietitian about a low-K diet.

PROGNOSIS
- Associated with poor prognosis in heart failure patients (7,8)
- Associated with poor prognosis in disaster medicine, trauma (1)
- Associated with poor prognosis in hemodialysis patients with higher dietary K$^+$ intake (9)

COMPLICATIONS
- Life-threatening cardiac arrhythmias
- Hypokalemia
- Potential complications of the use of ion-exchange resins for the treatment of hyperkalemia include volume overload and intestinal necrosis (10,11,12).

REFERENCES

1. Bosch X, Poch E, Grau JM. Rhabdomyolysis and acute kidney injury. *N Engl J Med*. 2009;361: 62–72.
2. Hagino T et al. [Tumor lysis syndrome] *Gan To Kagaku Ryoho*. 2010;37:984–8.
3. Antoniou T, Gomes T, Juurlink DN, Loutfy MR, Glazier RH, Mamdani MM et al. Trimethoprim-sulfamethoxazole-induced hyperkalemia in patients receiving inhibitors of the renin-angiotensin system: a population-based study. *Arch Intern Med*. 2010;170:1045–9.
4. Weir MA, Juurlink DN, Gomes T, Mamdani M, Hackam DG, Jain AK, Garg AX et al. Beta-Blockers, Trimethoprim-Sulfamethoxazole, and the Risk of Hyperkalemia Requiring Hospitalization in the Elderly: A Nested Case-Control Study. *Clinical journal of the American Society of Nephrology : CJASN*. 2010;
5. Wong R, Banker R, Aronowitz P et al. Electrocardiographic changes of severe hyperkalemia. *Journal of hospital medicine (Online)*. 2010;
6. Alfonzo AV, Isles C, Geddes C, Deighan C et al. Potassium disorders—clinical spectrum and emergency management. *Resuscitation*. 2006;70:10–25.
7. Ahmed MI, Ekundayo OJ, Mujib M, et al. Mild hyperkalemia and outcomes in chronic heart failure: A propensity matched study. *Int J Cardiol*. 2009.
8. Velavan P, Khan NK, Goode K, et al. Predictors of short term mortality in heart failure - Insights from the Euro Heart Failure survey. *Int J Cardiol*. 2008.
9. Noori N, Kalantar-Zadeh K, Kovesdy CP, Murali SB, Bross R, Nissenson AR, Kopple JD et al. Dietary Potassium Intake and Mortality in Long-term Hemodialysis Patients. *American journal of kidney diseases : the official journal of the National Kidney Foundation*. 2010;
10. Bomback AS, Woosley JT, Kshirsagar AV et al. Colonic necrosis due to sodium polystyrene sulfate (Kayexalate). *Am J Emerg Med*. 2009; 27:753.e1–2.
11. http://www.fda.gov/Safety/MedWatch/SafetyInformation/ucm186845.htm
12. Sterns RH, Rojas M, Bernstein P, Chennupati S et al. Ion-exchange resins for the treatment of hyperkalemia: are they safe and effective? *J Am Soc Nephrol*. 2010;21:733–5.
13. Evans KJ, Greenberg A. Hyperkalemia: a review. *J Intensive Care Med*. 2005;20:272–90.
14. Schaefer TJ, Wolford RW. Disorders of potassium. *Emerg Med Clin North Am*. 2005;23:723–47, viii–ix.

ADDITIONAL READING

- Cross NB, Webster AC, Masson P, et al. Antihypertensives for kidney transplant recipients: systematic review and meta-analysis of randomized controlled trials. *Transplantation*. 2009;88:7–18.
- Hall AB, Salazar M, Larison DJ. The sequencing of medication administration in the management of hyperkalemia. *J Emerg Nurs*. 2009;35:339–42.
- Hollander-Rodriguez JC, Calvert JF. Hyperkalemia. *Am Fam Physician*. 2006;73:283–90.
- Kim HJ, Han SW. Therapeutic approach to hyperkalemia. *Nephron*. 2002;92(Suppl 1):33–40.
- Putcha N, Allon M et al. Management of hyperkalemia in dialysis patients. *Semin Dial*. 2007;20:431–9.
- Stevens MS, Dunlay RW. Hyperkalemia in hospitalized patients. *Int Urol Nephrol*. 2000; 32:177–80.

See Also (Topic, Algorithm, Electronic Media Element)
Addison Disease; Hypokalemia
Algorithm: Hyperkalemia

CODES

ICD9
276.7 Hyperpotassemia

CLINICAL PEARLS

- Emergency and urgent management of hyperkalemia takes precedent to a thorough diagnostic workup. Urgent treatment includes stabilization of the myocardium to protect against arrhythmias and mobilizing potassium from the extracellular (vascular) space into the cells.
- Multiple herbal medications can also increase K levels, including alfalfa, dandelion, horsetail nettle, milkweed, hawthorne berries, toad skin, oleander, foxglove, and ginseng (13)[B].
- Many foods contain K. Those that are particularly high in K (>6.4 mEq per serving) include bananas, orange juice, other citrus fruits and their juices, tomatoes, tomato juice, cantaloupe, honeydew melon, peaches, potatoes, salt substitutes, and many herbal medications.
- To lower a patient's risk of developing hyperkalemia, have the patient follow a low-K diet, use selective β_1-blockers such as metoprolol or atenolol instead of nonselective β-blockers like carvedilol. Avoid nonsteroidal anti-inflammatory drugs. Concomitant use of kaliuretic loop diuretics may be useful (14)[B].

H

HYPERNATREMIA

Fae G. Wooding, PharmD
Joshua M.V. Mammen, MD, PhD
David L. Nickerson, PharmD

BASICS

DESCRIPTION
- Serum sodium (Na) concentration level >145 mEq/L often represents a state of hyperosmolality.
- Hypernatremia results from primary Na+ gain or water deficit.
- Hypernatremia may exist with hypo-, hyper-, or euvolemia.
- Hypovolemic hypernatremia: Most common type; occurs with a decrease in total body water (TBW) and a proportionately smaller decrease in total body Na.
- Euvolemic hypernatremia: No change in TBW with an proportionate increase in total body Na
- Hypervolemic hypernatremia: Increase in TBW and a proportionately greater increase in total body Na

Geriatric Considerations
- More common in the hospitalized patient; is an independent risk factor for mortality
- Hypernatremia may be caused by dehydration due to administration of loop diuretics.
- Increased risk because of impaired renal function and decline in thirst mechanism
- Chronically ill patients are at higher risk due to consumption of high-solute formulas.

Pediatric Considerations
- May occur in low-birth-weight newborns
- May result from improper preparation of infant formula or high concentration of Na in breast milk

EPIDEMIOLOGY
Incidence
- More common in elderly and young (1):
  - Occurs in 1% of hospitalized elderly patients (2)
- Gastroenteritis with diarrhea is the most common cause of hypernatremia in infants.

Prevalence
Females are at an increased risk due to decreased TBW.

RISK FACTORS
- Children
- Old age
- Patients who are intubated or have altered mental status
- Diabetes mellitus
- Prior brain injury
- Surgery
- Diuretic therapy

Genetics
Some diabetes insipidus may be hereditary.

GENERAL PREVENTION
- Treatment or prevention of underlying cause
- Properly prepare infant formula and never add salt to any commercial infant formula.
- Keep well hydrated.

ETIOLOGY
- Excess Na (increase in total body Na) resulting from (3):
  - Incorrect infant formula preparation
  - Salt administered as punishment or as a prank
  - Sea water ingestion
  - Excessive use of $NaHCO_3$ antacid
  - IV NaCl or $NaHCO_3$ during cardiopulmonary resuscitation, metabolic acidosis, or hyperkalemia
  - Intrauterine NaCl for abortion
  - Excessive Na in dialysate solutions
  - Disorders of the adrenal axis (Cushing syndrome, Conn syndrome, congenital adrenal hyperplasia)
- Water deficit (total body Na normal) resulting from:
  - Adipsia (e.g., impaired thirst regulation, decreased access to water)
  - Nephrogenic diabetes insipidus (due to progressive renal dysfunction, hypercalcemia, hypokalemia, or medication-related)
  - Cranial diabetes insipidus (due to head trauma, stroke, or meningitis)
  - Increased insensible water loss (e.g., fever, hyperventilation, hypermetabolic state, sweat, severe burns, heat exposure, newborns under radiant warmers)
- Hypotonic fluid loss (total body Na decreased) resulting from:
  - Loss of fluid containing Na without adequate water replacement
- Urinary loss:
  - Osmotic diuretics
  - Diabetes mellitus (particularly new presentation or decompensated)
  - Diuresis from acute tubular necrosis or from relief of acute urinary obstruction
- Gastrointestinal loss:
  - Diarrhea, especially in children

COMMONLY ASSOCIATED CONDITIONS
- Gastroenteritis
- Altered mental status
- Burns
- Hypermetabolic conditions
- Head injury
- Renal dysfunction

DIAGNOSIS

HISTORY
- Obtain list of current and recent medications.
- Review recent illnesses and activities (1).

PHYSICAL EXAM
- Sinus tachycardia, hypotension, orthostatic hypotension, dyspnea
- Dry mucous membranes, cool or grey skin
- Excessive thirst, nausea, vomiting, diarrhea, oliguria, polyuria
- Fever, myalgia, muscle weakness
- Altered mental status, seizure, lethargy, irritability, coma, anophthalmus (1,3)[C]

DIAGNOSTIC TESTS & INTERPRETATION
Lab
Initial lab tests
- Serum Na, K, urea, creatinine, calcium, and osmolality (serum lithium if appropriate) (4)[C]
- Urine Na and osmolality
- Urinalysis
- Serum glucose
- Special tests:
  - Water deprivation (with diabetes insipidus, urine osmolality does not increase when hypernatremic)
  - Antidiuretic hormone (ADH) stimulation (with nephrogenic diabetes insipidus, urine osmolality does not increase after ADH or DDAVP)
- Serum Na >150–170 mEq/L (>150–170 mmol/L) and blood urea nitrogen/creat >20: Usually dehydration/hypovolemia
- Serum Na >170 mEq/L (>170 mmol/L) and decreased urine Na: Usually diabetes insipidus
- Serum Na >190 mEq/L (>190 mmol/L): Usually chronic salt ingestion
- Diabetes insipidus:
  - Urine osmolality less than serum osmolality
  - Urine Na usually low
  - Polyuria
  - Neurogenic vs nephrogenic diabetes insipidus
- Hyperosmolar coma:
  - Blood sugar elevated
  - Decreased urine output
  - Increased urine osmolality
- Salt ingestion:
  - Increased urine Na
  - Increased urine osmolality
- Hypertonic dehydration:
  - Decreased urine Na
  - Increased urine osmolality

ALERT
A variety of medications may raise or lower Na levels.

Imaging
Initial approach
Computed tomography or magnetic resonance imaging in diabetes insipidus to rule out craniopharyngioma, tumor, or median cleft syndrome (3,4)[C]

Diagnostic Procedures/Surgery
History, physical, laboratory studies, family history for neurogenic diabetes insipidus

DIFFERENTIAL DIAGNOSIS
- Diabetes insipidus
- Hyperosmotic coma
- Salt ingestion
- Hypertonic dehydration
- Hypothyroidism
- Cushing syndrome

 # TREATMENT
MEDICATION
First Line
- Hypovolemia (usually Na 150–170) (4,5)[C]:
  – Isotonic saline (normal saline or Ringer's lactate): 10–20 mL/kg IV over 1–2 hours. May repeat if ≥10% dehydration (4)[A].
  – Isotonic fluids: 5% dextrose with half-normal saline until urine output established (4)[B]
- Hypernatremia (usually due to chronic salt ingestion Na >190):
  – Hypotonic fluids (NaCl or dextrose 5% in water) (4)[B]
  – Decrease serum Na by 0.5 mEq/L/hr (0.5 mmol/L/hr) or by no more than 20 mEq/L/d (20 mmol/L/d). Allows idiogenic osmoles to resolve (mostly taurine in brain cell water).
  – Hypocalcemia may occur during correction of hypernatremia. Add calcium (50 mg/kg 10% calcium gluconate) to IV fluids.
  – Acidosis often is present in severely dehydrated patients. Add sodium bicarbonate, 50 mEq/L, to IV fluids. If both acidosis and hypocalcemia are present, correct the calcium deficit first.
  – Potassium and phosphate, if needed
  – Furosemide for hypervolemia. Dose varies, depending on desired urine output.
- Neurogenic diabetes insipidus:
  – Desmopressin (DDAVP) acetate: Use parenteral form for acute symptomatic patients, and use intranasal or oral form for chronic therapy. Adults 10–40 μg intranasally in 1–3 divided doses; children 5–30 μg in a single evening dose or in 2 divided doses.
  – May use 2.5% dextrose in water if giving large volumes of water in diabetes insipidus or neurogenic diabetes insipidus to avoid glycosuria
  – May consider sulfonylureas or thiazide diuretics
- Nephrogenic diabetes insipidus:
  – Chlorothiazide: 10 mg/kg per dose given b.i.d.
  – Chlorpropamide: 100–250 mg each morning
- Contraindications: Refer to manufacturer's literature.
- Precautions:
  – Rapid correction of hypernatremia can cause cerebral or pulmonary edema, seizures, or death. Hypocalcemia often occurs during correction.
  – Diabetes insipidus: High rates of dextrose 5% in water can cause hyperglycemia and glucose-induced diuresis.
- Significant possible interactions: Refer to manufacturer's literature.

Second Line
Consider nonsteroidal anti-inflammatory drugs in nephrogenic diabetes insipidus (3)[C].

ADDITIONAL TREATMENT
General Measures
- Appropriate health care: Inpatient (many patients are already hospitalized, and hypernatremia develops after admission)
- Treat hypovolemia first, then hypernatremia.
- Replace water orally if patient is conscious.
- Restore intravascular volume with IV fluids to normalize serum Na levels.
- Calculated water deficit (liters) = [(0.6 × wt) × (Na − 140)] ÷ 140:
  – Note: wt = weight in kilograms; Na = current serum Na
- Dialysis: Especially with serum Na >200 mEq/L (200 mmol/L)
- Speed of correction depends on severity of symptoms or rate of development of hypernatremia.

Issues for Referral
Underlying renal involvement associated with hypernatremia would benefit from a nephrology referral.

IN-PATIENT CONSIDERATIONS
Admission Criteria
Symptomatic patient with serum Na >155 mEq/L requires IV fluid therapy.

IV Fluids
Refer to Medication section

Nursing
Bed rest until stable or underlying condition resolved or controlled

Discharge Criteria
Stabilization of serum Na level and symptoms are minimal

 # ONGOING CARE
FOLLOW-UP RECOMMENDATIONS
Patient Monitoring
- Frequent re-examinations in an acute setting
- Frequent electrolytes
- Urine osmolality and urine output in diabetes insipidus
- Ensure adequate ingestion of calories because patients may ingest so much water that they feel full and do not eat.
- Daily weights

DIET
- Ensure proper nutrition during acute phase.
- After resolution of acute phase, may want to consider Na-restricted diet for patient.
- Severe salt restriction in nephrogenic diabetes insipidus

PATIENT EDUCATION
Patients with nephrogenic diabetes insipidus must avoid salt and drink large amounts of water.

PROGNOSIS
Most recover, but neurologic impairment can sometimes be seen.

COMPLICATIONS
- Central nervous system (CNS) thrombosis or hemorrhage
- Seizures
- Mental retardation
- Hyperactivity
- Chronic hypernatremia: >2 days duration has higher mortality
- Serum Na >180 mEq/L (>180 mmol/L): Often results in residual CNS damage

REFERENCES
1. Adrogue HJ, Madias NE. Hypernatremia. *N Engl J Med*. 2000;342:1493–9.
2. Bagshaw SM, Townsend DR, McDermid RC. Disorders of sodium and water balance in hospitalized patients. *Can J Anaesth*. 2009;56: 151–67.
3. Kang SK, Kim W, OH MS. Pathogenesis and treatment of hypernatremia. *Nephron*. 2002; 92(Suppl 1):14–7.
4. Kraft MD, Btaichel F, Sachs GS, et al. Treatment of electrolyte disorders in adult patients in the intensive care unit. *Am J Health-System Pharm*. 2005;62:166382.
5. Weiss-Gullet E, Takala J, Jakob JM. Diagnosis and management of electrolyte emergencies. *Best Practice & Research Clinical Endocrinology & Metabolism*. 2003;17(4):623–51.

See Also (Topic, Algorithm, Electronic Media Element)
Diabetes Insipidus
Algorithm: Hypernatremia

CODES

ICD9
276.0 Hyperosmolality and/or hypernatremia

CLINICAL PEARLS
- Determine if the patient has hypervolemic, euvolemic, or hypovolemic hypernatremia to determine differential diagnosis of etiology.
- Water replacement orally if patient is conscious (the preferred route)
- Speed of correction depends on severity of symptoms or rate of development of hypernatremia.

H

HYPERPARATHYROIDISM

Kyle D. Wood, MD
John Paul Lock, MD

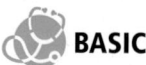 **BASICS**

DESCRIPTION
An acute or chronic dysfunction of the body's normal regulatory feedback mechanisms for parathyroid hormone (PTH):

- Primary: Intrinsic gland dysfunction and abnormal regulation of PTH secretion by calcium causing excessive PTH secretion
- Secondary: Gland hyperactivity that is a response to hypocalcemia, vitamin D deficiency, or renal failure
- Tertiary: Autonomous hyperfunction in the setting of long-standing secondary hyperparathyroidism (HPT)

EPIDEMIOLOGY
Incidence
- Predominant age: Primary: approximately 1/750
- Predominant sex: Female > Male (3:1)

Prevalence
1/750 adults

RISK FACTORS
Renal failure, age, poor nutrition, and/or family history

Genetics
Familial forms are rare but include:
- Multiple endocrine neoplasia (MEN) types 1 and 2: Patients with multiple gland hyperplasia in the absence of renal disease should be screened for MEN-1 gene mutation.
- Neonatal severe primary HPT
- HPT–jaw tumor syndrome
- Familial hypocalciuric hypercalcemia (FHH): Autosomal dominant
- Familial isolated HPT

GENERAL PREVENTION
Adequate intake of calcium and vitamin D may help prevent secondary HPT.

PATHOPHYSIOLOGY
- PTH is made in 4 parathyroid glands located behind the 4 poles of the thyroid gland (locations can vary).
- PTH releases calcium from bone by osteoclastic stimulation (bone resorption).
- PTH increases reabsorption of calcium in the distal tubules of the kidneys.
- PTH stimulates conversion of active vitamin D to increase calcium absorption from the gastrointestinal (GI) tract.

ETIOLOGY
- Primary HPT: Unregulated increase of PTH production and release, causing increase in serum calcium:
  - Solitary adenoma (89%)
  - Double adenomas (5%)
  - Diffuse hyperplasia (6%) caused by multiple adenomas, MEN types 1 and 2, familial hypocalciuric hypercalcemia
  - Parathyroid carcinoma (<2%)

- Secondary HPT: Adaptive parathyroid gland hyperplasia and hyperfunction:
  - Dietary: Vitamin D or calcium deficiency
  - Chronic renal disease resulting in:
    ○ Renal parenchymal loss causing hyperphosphatemia
    ○ Impaired calcitriol production causing hypocalcemia
    ○ General skeletal and renal resistance to PTH
- Tertiary HPT: Gland hyperplasia from prolonged hypocalcemia resulting in autonomous PTH oversecretion: Chronic kidney disease

COMMONLY ASSOCIATED CONDITIONS
- MEN syndromes type 1 and 2
- Chronic renal failure

 DIAGNOSIS

HISTORY
- Up to 75% are asymptomatic.
- Classic complaints of hypercalcemia include painful bones, renal stones, abdominal groans, and psychic moans.
- MEN is associated with pancreatic cancer, pituitary adenomas, medullary thyroid cancer, or pheochromocytoma.
- History of radiation to neck
- Medications: Thiazides or lithium

PHYSICAL EXAM
- Renal: Nephrolithiasis, nephrocalcinosis, reduced glomerular filtration rate, thirst, polydipsia, polyuria
- GI: Abdominal distress, gastroduodenal ulcer, pancreatitis, pancreatic calcification, constipation, vomiting, anorexia, weight loss
- Skeletal: Bone pain, cystic bone lesions, skeletal demineralization, spontaneous fracture, vertebral collapse, osteoporosis
- Mental: Fatigue, apathy, anxiety, depression, psychosis
- Neurologic: Somnolence, coma, diffuse electroencephalogram changes
- Neuromuscular: Muscle fatigue, weakness, hypotonia
- Cardiovascular: Hypertension, short QT interval, left ventricular hypertrophy
- Articular/periarticular: Arthralgia, gout, pseudogout, periarticular calcification
- Ocular: Band keratopathy, conjunctivitis, conjunctival calcium deposits

DIAGNOSTIC TESTS & INTERPRETATION
Lab
Initial lab tests
- Elevated serum calcium level (fasting): Simultaneous albumin to calculate a corrected serum calcium level or ionized calcium level; corrected calcium (mg/dL = measured calcium (mg/dL) = 0.8(4 − measured albumin).

- If hypercalcemia is confirmed, follow with intact PTH level:
  - High PTH suggests primary HPT.
  - Low PTH suggests non-PTH–mediated hypercalcemia.
- If elevated calcium is inconsistent, elevated ionized serum calcium in the setting of high PTH confirms diagnosis. Other findings may include low serum phosphate, elevated serum chloride, decreased serum CO_2, increased urinary cAMP, and abnormal 24-h urine calcium excretion.
- In secondary HPT, an elevated phosphorus means chronic renal failure; a low phosphorus suggests another cause of vitamin D deficiency.

Follow-Up & Special Considerations
- A 24-h urine calcium concentration to creatinine clearance ratio >0.02 suggests primary HPT; a ratio <0.01 may be normal or indicate FHH; important because FHH does not require surgery.
- Measure 25OH vit D—replete if ≤20 ng/ml. Hold off on management decisions (1).
- Consider serum protein electrophoresis.

Imaging
Initial approach
Imaging is not required in initial stages:
- In recent years, minimally invasive parathyroidectomy (MIP) has become more common, and imaging is required for surgical planning.
- Localization of a single adenoma allows a focused approach.
  - Technetium-99m sestamibi scan with single-photon-emission computed tomography (CT) scan (2)[B]
  - Ultrasonography
- Imaging is indicated to localize hyperplasia or an ectopic parathyroid gland in repeat surgery.

Follow-Up & Special Considerations
- Obtain bone mineral density (DEXA) on patients with elevated PTH (3)[C].
- A baseline scan for occult nephrolithiasis is recommended (4)[C].
- Intraoperative measurement of intact PTH and/or gamma probe localization of abnormal glands with technetium-99m sestamibi scan has aided focused resections for patients with single-gland etiology (4)[C].

Diagnostic Procedures/Surgery
Consider electrocardiogram to assess for short QT interval.

Pathological Findings
See Etiology.

DIFFERENTIAL DIAGNOSIS

- Increased PTH: Ectopic HPT
- Nonparathyroid causes:
  - Malignancy: Lung (squamous cell) carcinoma, breast carcinoma, multiple myeloma, lymphoma, leukemia, prostate cancer, Paget disease
  - Granulomatous disease: Sarcoidosis, tuberculosis, berylliosis, histoplasmosis, coccidioidomycosis
  - Drugs: Thiazide diuretics, vitamin D intoxication, vitamin A excess, lithium, milk-alkali syndrome, exogenous calcium intake
  - Endocrine: Hyperthyroidism, acute adrenal insufficiency
  - Familial: Hypocalciuric hypercalcemia

 TREATMENT

MEDICATION

- Primary HPT: For those awaiting or unable to have surgery:
  - Calcium replacement
  - Selective estrogen receptor modulator therapy (raloxifene) (2)[C]
  - Bisphosphonates (alendronate) (2)[C]: Reduces bone turnover and helps to maintain bone density; avoid in kidney disease
  - Treat concomitant vitamin D deficiency.
- Secondary HPT:
  - Phosphorus-binding agents (Sevelamer)
  - Calcimimetic (Cinacalcet) (5)[A]:
    o Mimics calcium and binds to calcium-sensing receptor (CaR)
    o Biochemical markers improved; patient-based benefits have not yet been shown (5)[A]
  - Vitamin D analogues (paricalcitol and calcitriol) reduce PTH (number needed to treat = 2).
- Tertiary HPT:
  - Loop diuretics (i.e., furosemide)
  - Useful in well-hydrated hypercalcemic patients
  - Avoid in hypocalcemia.
- Hormone replacement therapy with estrogens not recommended as 1st-line treatment
  - Can be used in postmenopausal women who do not undergo or refuse surgery
  - Must weigh benefit with risks of known systemic effects

SURGERY/OTHER PROCEDURES

- Operative management is curative for patients with primary HPT in 95–98% of patients with 1–2% complications.
- Indications for parathyroidectomy:
  - Symptomatic primary HPT:
    o Nephrolithiasis
    o Nephrocalcinosis
    o Osteitis fibrosa cystica
  - Asymptomatic primary HPT (6):
    o Serum Ca^+ level >1.0 mg/dL above normal
    o Age less than 50
    o Creatinine clearance (less than 60 ml/hr); bone density loss (T score <−2.5)
- Surgical removal of diseased gland or tissue is only proven curative therapy for HPT. The outcomes of bilateral open neck exploration are equal to MIP using preoperative sestamibi scan with SPECT and intraoperative PTH levels (7)[B]:
  - Patients with MEN were excluded.
  - Fewer complications in MIP group

- Postoperative course needs special attention paid to serum calcium level (hypocalcemia), bleeding, and risk of airway compromise. Injectable calcium and seizure precautions must be maintained at bedside.
- Monitor renal functions closely.

IN-PATIENT CONSIDERATIONS
Initial Stabilization
- Critical hypercalcemia requires IV fluid rehydration, IV bisphosphonate therapy, and subcutaneous calcitonin (4 units/kg every 12 h) for severe symptoms.
- Furosemide should be used only in the management of associated fluid overload (8)[A].

 ONGOING CARE

FOLLOW-UP RECOMMENDATIONS
Asymptomatic patients with primary HPT require monitoring of calcium and PTH.

Patient Monitoring
In patients with primary HPT who are asymptomatic, serum calcium every 6 months, serum creatinine, and bone density every year

DIET
In patients with primary HPT who are asymptomatic, no restriction in calcium (1,000–1,200 mg/d)

PATIENT EDUCATION
- Importance of periodic lab testing
- Maintenance of appropriate diet for condition
- Signs of severe hypercalcemia

PROGNOSIS
Prognosis after surgery is excellent in primary HPT, with resolution of many of the preoperative symptoms.

COMPLICATIONS
Related to high levels of PTH and/or elevated calcium

REFERENCES

1. Eastell R, Arnold A, Brandi ML, Brown EM, D'Amour P, Hanley DA, Rao DS, Rubin MR, Goltzman D, Silverberg SJ, Marx SJ, Peacock M, Mosekilde L, Bouillon R, Lewiecki EM et al. Diagnosis of asymptomatic primary hyperparathyroidism: proceedings of the third international workshop. *J Clin Endocrinol Metab*. 2009;94:340–50.
2. Stalberg P, Delbridge L, van Heerden J, et al. Minimallyinvasive parathyroidectomy and thyroidectomy–current concepts. *Surgeon Journal of the Royal Colleges of Surgeons of Edinburgh & Ireland*. 2007;5(5):301–308.
3. Bilezikian JP, Brandi ML, Rubin M, Silverberg SJ. Primary HPT: New concepts in clinical densitometric and biochemical features. *J Intern Med*. 2005; 257:6–17.
4. AACE/AAES Task Force on Primary HPT. The American Association of Clinical Endocrinologists and the American Association of Endocrine Surgeons position statement on the diagnosis and management of primary HPT. *Endocr Pract*. 2005;11(1):49–54.
5. Strippoli GFM, Tong A, Palmer SC, Elder G, Craig JC. Calcimimetics for secondary HPT in chronic kidney disease patients. *Cochrane Database of Systematic Reviews*. 2006;Issue 4.
6. Khan A, Grey A, Shoback D et al. Medical management of asymptomatic primary hyperparathyroidism: proceedings of the third international workshop. *J Clin Endocrinol Metab*. 2009;94:373–81.
7. Udelsman R. Six hundred fifty-six consecutive explorations for primary HPT. *Annals of Surgery*. 2002;235(5):665–670.
8. LeGrand SB, Leskuski D, Zama I. Narrative review: furosemide for hypercalcemia: an unproven yet common practice. *Annals of Internal Medicine*. 2008;149(4):259–263.

ADDITIONAL READING

- Ahmad R, Hammond JM. Primary, secondary, and tertiary hyperparathyroidism. *Otolaryngol Clin North Am*. 2004;37(4):701–13, vii–viii.
- Andersson P, Rydberg E, Willenheimer R et al. Primary hyperparathyroidism and heart disease–a review. *Eur Heart J*. 2004;25:1776–87.
- Bilezikian JP, Potts JT Jr, Fuleihan Gel-H, et al. Summary statement from a workshop on asymptomatic primary HPT: a perspective for the 21st century. *J Clin Endocrinol Metab*. 2002;87(12): 5353–61.
- Joy MS, Kshirsagar AV, Franceschini N. Calcimimetics and the treatment of primary and secondary HPT. *Ann Pharmacol*. 2004;38:1871–80.
- Ruda JM, Hollenbeak CS, Stack BC et al. A systematic review of the diagnosis and treatment of primary hyperparathyroidism from 1995 to 2003. *Otolaryngol Head Neck Surg*. 2005;132:359–72.

 CODES

ICD9
- 252.00 Hyperparathyroidism, unspecified
- 252.01 Primary hyperparathyroidism
- 252.02 Secondary hyperparathyroidism, non-renal

CLINICAL PEARLS

- Many patients with primary HPT are asymptomatic.
- HPT may cause malaise and fatigue before classic symptoms are seen.
- A repeat calcium, serum albumin, and intact PTH test are required to make an initial diagnosis.
- Surgical technique has changed in the last few years to include minimally invasive parathyroidectomy.
- A genetic etiology is recognized increasingly.

H

HYPERPROLACTINEMIA

Ruben Peralta, MD

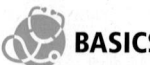 **BASICS**

DESCRIPTION

Hyperprolactinemia is an abnormal elevation in the serum prolactin level with multiple possible etiologies.

EPIDEMIOLOGY

Prevalence
- Predominant age: Reproductive age
- Predominant sex: Female > Male.
- More readily detected in females because a slight elevation in prolactin causes changes in menstruation and galactorrhea

ETIOLOGY
- Prolactin, which is produced by lactotrophs in the anterior pituitary, is regulated by
  - Inhibitory factors, primarily dopamine, produced in the hypothalamus and delivered via the hypothalamic-pituitary vessels in the pituitary stalk
  - Stimulatory factors, primarily thyrotropin-releasing hormone (TRH)
- Causes of hyperprolactinemia include
  - Physiologic:
    - Pregnancy
    - Breast-feeding
    - Nipple stimulation
    - Stress, including postoperative state
  - Medications:
    - Dopamine (D_2) blockers: Antipsychotics, metoclopramide
    - Dopamine depleters: α-methyldopa, reserpine
    - Opiates
    - Verapamil (but no other calcium-channel blockers; thought to decrease hypothalamic synthesis of dopamine)
    - Possibly antidepressants (minimal data)
  - Hypothyroidism (owing to elevated TRH)
  - Chest wall conditions:
    - Herpes zoster
    - After thoracotomy
    - Trauma
  - Prolactin-secreting adenoma, categorized:
    - Microadenoma: ≤1 cm
    - Macroadenoma: >1 cm
  - Pituitary stalk compression/disruption:
    - Craniopharyngioma
    - Rathke cleft cyst
    - Meningioma
    - Astrocytoma
    - Metastases
    - Head trauma
    - Infiltrative/inflammatory disorders
  - Diminished prolactin clearance:
    - Renal failure
    - Cirrhosis
- Cocaine

 DIAGNOSIS

HISTORY
- Galactorrhea
- Amenorrhea
- Oligomenorrhea
- Infertility
- Osteoporosis/osteopenia
- Decreased libido, impotence
- Weight gain
- Also may have signs and symptoms of pituitary enlargement:
  - Headache
  - Visual field impairment (bitemporal hemianopsia)
  - Hypopituitarism (secondary to tumor pressure on surrounding structures)
- Also may have signs and symptoms of associated conditions:
  - Hypothyroidism
  - Cushing disease
  - Acromegaly
  - MEN-I syndrome

PHYSICAL EXAM
- Visual field testing
- Cranial nerve exam

DIAGNOSTIC TESTS & INTERPRETATION

Lab
- Serum prolactin (most accurate results if checked fasting, in morning)
- Pregnancy test
- Thyroid-stimulating hormone (TSH)
- Luteinizing hormone (LH)/follicle-stimulating hormone (FSH) if amenorrheic
- Chemistry, renal function
- Liver function tests
- Special tests: Formal visual field testing if pituitary adenoma suspected

Imaging
- MRI (even if prolactin is minimally elevated) to rule out hypothalamic tumors that may compress the pituitary stalk and thereby decrease delivery of prolactin inhibitory hormone (with a subsequent rise in prolactin)
- CT scan if MRI is contraindicated

DIFFERENTIAL DIAGNOSIS

Macroprolactinemia: Macroprolactin, a polymer of several units of prolactin, is detected by immunologically based lab tests but is not biologically active. If patient is asymptomatic but found to have elevated prolactin (PRL), consider this diagnosis and notify the lab. No treatment is required (1)[B].

 TREATMENT

MEDICATION
- Dopamine agonists:
  - Bromocriptine (Parlodel): Often 1st-line treatment given; this has longest clinical history: Dosed b.i.d.; preferred by some clinicians when infertility is an indication for treatment (2)[B]
  - Cabergoline (Dostinex): Dosed twice weekly; may be better tolerated; some consider this a 1st-line drug; indicated with bromocriptine failure or resistance (3)[B].
  - Both are effective for reducing tumor size and improving symptoms (4)[B]. Cabergoline has been shown to improve erectile dysfunction in hyperprolactinemic men (5)[B].
- Adverse effects (better tolerated if start with low dose, slow titration, given at night with food):
  - Nausea/vomiting
  - Headache
  - Dizziness
  - Fatigue
  - Light-headedness
  - Postural hypotension
  - Pergolide (Permax), also a dopamine agonist, is used less commonly.

ADDITIONAL TREATMENT

General Measures

- Discontinue offending medications, if any.
- Treat underlying causes.
- For asymptomatic patients with mild PRL elevations, observation alone may be considered (3)[B].
- Medications indicated for (2)[B]:
  - Symptoms of hypogonadism, such as decreased libido
  - Galactorrhea (if bothersome to patient)
  - Restoration of fertility
  - Pituitary adenoma
  - Prevention of osteoporosis

Additional Therapies

Radiation therapy and stereotactic radiosurgery sometimes are considered in medically unresponsive, surgically unresectable tumors; PRL normalizes in 20–30%, with a high risk of hypopituitarism (3)[B].

SURGERY/OTHER PROCEDURES

- For adenomas, medical treatment will be successful in 80–90% of patients, but in some cases, surgery is indicated.
- Indications (4)[B]:
  - Intolerance or resistance to medical treatment
  - Headache
  - Visual field loss
  - Cerebrospinal fluid (CSF) leak owing to tumor apoplexy or shrinkage
  - Cranial nerve deficit
- Risks:
  - High recurrence rate (up to 40%) (4)[B]
  - CSF leakage
  - Meningitis
- Pituitary insufficiency

 ## ONGOING CARE

FOLLOW-UP RECOMMENDATIONS

Patient Monitoring

- Depends on etiology
- Consider:
  - Prolactin level every 6–12 months
  - Formal visual field testing yearly
  - Serial MRIs if clinically indicated

Pregnancy Considerations

- If pregnancy is desired in a woman with hyperprolactinemia (3)[B], dopamine agonists are not approved during pregnancy and should be discontinued once pregnancy is confirmed, but their use is recommended if neurologic findings are present (6).
- With microprolactinoma: Treat with bromocriptine if symptomatic; monthly pregnancy tests; discontinue bromocriptine when pregnancy is confirmed.
- With macroprolactinomas: Treat with bromocriptine if neurologic findings (owing to tumor enlargement) are present and at least until optic system no longer compromised.

- Careful monitoring of visual fields in each trimester and PRL levels during pregnancy is advised.

PATIENT EDUCATION

Discuss risks of untreated hyperprolactinemia.

- Headache
- Visual field loss
- Decreased bone density
- Infertility

PROGNOSIS

- Tends to recur after discontinuation of medical therapy
- Over 10 years, 7% chance of progression of prolactin-secreting microadenoma

COMPLICATIONS

- Depends on underlying cause
- If pituitary adenoma, risk of permanent visual field loss

REFERENCES

1. Serri O, Chik CL, Ehud U. Diagnosis and management of hyperprolactinemia. Can Med J. 2003:169.
2. Molitch ME. Prolactin-secreting tumors: What's new? Expert Rev Anticancer Ther. 2006; 6(Suppl 9):S29–S35.
3. Pickett CA. Diagnosis and management of pituitary tumors: Recent advances. Prim Care Clin Office Pract. 2003;30:765–89.
4. Jackson J, Safranek S. What is the recommended evaluation and treatment for elevated serum prolactin? JFP. 2006;54:897–9.
5. Pinzone JJ, Katznelson L, Danila DC. Primary medical therapy of micro- and macroprolactinomas in men. J Clin Endocrinol Metabol. 2002;85:3053–57.
6. Klibanski A et al. Clinical practice. Prolactinomas. N Engl J Med. 2010;362:1219–26.
7. Molitch ME. Medication-induced hyperprolactinemia. Mayo Clin Proc. 2005;80:1050–7.
8. Lieberman JA, Stroup TS, McEvoy JP, et al. Effectiveness of antipsychotic drugs in patients with schizophrenia. N Engl J Med. 2005;353: 1209–23.
9. Balercia G, Boscaro M, Lombardo F, et al. Sexual symptoms in endocrine diseases: psychosomatic perspectives. Psychother Psychosom. 2007;76: 134–40.
10. Bhasin S, Enzlin P, Coviello A, et al. Sexual dysfunction in men and women with endocrine disorders. Lancet. 2007;369:597–611.

ADDITIONAL READING

- Casanueva FF, Molitch ME, Schlechte JA, et al. Guidelines of the Pituitary Society for the diagnosis and management of prolactinomas. Clin. Endocrinol. (Oxf). 2006;65:265–73.
- Haddad PM, Wieck A et al. Antipsychotic-induced hyperprolactinaemia: mechanisms, clinical features and management. Drugs. 2004;64:2291–314.
- Keil MF, Stratakis CA. Pituitary tumors in childhood: update of diagnosis, treatment and molecular genetics. Expert Rev Neurother. 2008;8:563–74.
- Mancini T, Casanueva FF, Giustina A. Hyperprolactinemia and prolactinomas. Endocrinol Metab Clin North Am. 2008;37:67–99.
- Sathyapalan T, Gonzalez S, Atkin SL. Effect of long-term, high-dose estrogen treatment on prolactin levels: a retrospective analysis. Climacteric. 2009;1–4.

 ## CODES

ICD9

253.1 Other and unspecified anterior pituitary hyperfunction

CLINICAL PEARLS

- At the time of diagnosis, pituitary tumors in men are generally larger than tumors in women. Possible explanations are that women experience amenorrhea and galactorrhea when prolactin is only slightly elevated, whereas presenting symptoms in men—erectile dysfunction, diminished libido—tend to be more insidious and occur at higher levels of prolactin. Differences in tumor biology or pathophysiology may exist (5)[C].
- Overall, the response rate for surgical treatment is higher in those who went to surgery because of medication intolerance rather than because of treatment resistance.
- There is a difference among antipsychotics in influencing prolactin levels. In general, those with the highest-potency D_2 antagonism are most likely to elevate prolactin levels (7)[B]. Among the newer atypical antipsychotics, risperidone has been identified as more likely to elevate prolactin (8)[B].
- High prolactin levels decrease testosterone by inhibiting gonadotropin-releasing hormone (GnRH), LH, and FSH secretion and by decreasing central dopamine activity, both of which are important in mediating sexual arousal (9,10)[B].

H

HYPERSENSITIVITY PNEUMONITIS

David Fish, MD

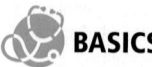 **BASICS**

DESCRIPTION
- A diffuse inflammatory disease of the lung caused by an exaggerated immune response to repeated inhalation of airborne environmental antigens.
- A wide variety of antigens can cause disease.
- Spectrum of symptoms with controversial classification, but typically divided into:
  - Acute:
    - Fever, chills, diaphoresis, myalgias, nausea; cough and dyspnea common but not necessary.
    - Occurs 2–9 hours after exposure
    - Lasts hours to days
  - Subacute:
    - More severe respiratory symptoms (cough, dyspnea, cyanosis)
    - Develops over days to weeks
  - Chronic:
    - Progressively worsening cough and exertional dyspnea. Also present with fatigue and weight loss.
    - Occurs over several months, can lead to respiratory failure
- System(s) affected: Pulmonary
- Synonym(s): Extrinsic allergic alveolitis; Farmer's lung

EPIDEMIOLOGY
- Predominant age: Tends to occur in adults as a result of occupation-related exposure
- Male = Female

Incidence
- Incidence difficult to classify due to inconsistent definition of disease
- Makes up ~2% of all interstitial lung diseases according to 1 study in New Mexico

Prevalence
0.5–3% prevalence among farmers with exposure (for farmer's lung specifically) (1)[B]

RISK FACTORS
- Exposure to known offending antigen
- Viral infection at time of exposure could increase risk
- Nonsmokers have increased incidence compared to smokers (nicotine could have protective effect) (1)[B].

Genetics
- Not related to atopic predisposition
- Possible genetic predisposition involving TNF-α and MHC class II genes (1)[B]

GENERAL PREVENTION
Avoidance of offending antigen is the mainstay of prevention and treatment.

PATHOPHYSIOLOGY
Hypersensitivity reaction involving:
- Immune complex-mediated reaction: Inhaled antigens bind to IgG, triggering complement cascade.
- Cellular-mediated reaction: Cell infiltration (predominantly lymphocytic, but also involving neutrophils and macrophages) with formation of granulomas (1)[B]

ETIOLOGY
Multiple syndromes with different causative antigens (all have similar presentations) (2)[B]:
- Microbes:
  - Farmer's lung (*Thermophilic actinomycetes, Sacharopolyspora rectivirgula*)
  - Bagassosis (*T. sacchari*)
  - Humidifier lung (*Micropolyspora faeni*)
  - Suberosis (*Penicillium frequentans*)
  - Malt-worker's lung (*Aspergillus clavatus*)
  - Woodworker's lung (*Penicillium chrysogenum*)
  - Cheese-washer's lung (*Penicillium casei*)
  - Maple-bark stripper's lung (*Cryptostroma corticale*)
  - Paprika slicer's lung (*Mucor stolanifer*)
  - Hot-tub lung (*Mycobacterium avium* intracellulare)
  - Summer-type hypersensitivity pneumonitis (*Trichosporon cutaneum*)
  - Sax lung (*Candida albicans*)
- Animals:
  - Bird fancier's disease (avian proteins)
  - Rat handler lung (rat serum proteins)
  - Fish meal worker's lung (fish meal extract)
  - Animal handler's lung (lab animals)
- Chemicals:
  - Isocyanates (paints, plastics)
  - Anhydrides (plastics)

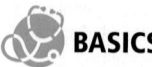 **DIAGNOSIS**

HISTORY
- Acute form: Develops 2–9 hours following exposure
  - Cough, dyspnea, fever, chills, diaphoresis, headache, nausea
  - Symptoms last hours to days
- Subacute form: Develops after several days to weeks:
  - Marked by worsening respiratory symptoms
- Chronic form: Develops after several months of exposure:
  - Progressively worsening cough and dyspnea
  - Also develop fatigue, weight loss, anorexia
- Other important points in history include:
  - History of pulmonary disease or recurrent infections
  - Recent change in work or home
  - Known exposure to pets, hot tubs, areas with water damage
  - Symptomatic improvement when away from work or home

PHYSICAL EXAM
- Acute:
  - Fever
  - Tachypnea
  - Inspiratory crackles
- Chronic:
  - Progressive hypoxia
  - Weight loss
  - Diffuse rales
  - Clubbing
  - Could possibly show signs of right heart failure if advanced

DIAGNOSTIC TESTS & INTERPRETATION
Lab
- May have increased inflammatory markers (erythrocyte sedimentation rate, C-reactive protein) (2)[B]
- Leukocytosis and increased gammaglobulins typically seen
- Specific IgG antibody to offending agent can be detected and checked serially to detect response to treatment (1)[B]:
  - Not always present (likely because many unknown antigens)
  - Low specificity (10% of people exposed to farmer's lung antigen develop antibodies; only 0.3% show symptoms)
- Rheumatoid factor often positive (unknown cause)
- Negative blood, sputum, throat cultures
- Bronchoalveolar lavage (BAL) (1)[B]:
  - Acute form with neutrophils and CD4 T lymphocytes
  - Chronic form with high number of CD8 T lymphocytes
  - BAL may help to differentiate chronic hypersensitivity pneumonitis from sarcoid, which has high CD4 T lymphocytes
- Other tests:
  - Inhalation challenge to suspected environments lack standardization and can cause serious reactions (not recommended) (1)[B].

Imaging
- Chest x-ray (CXR): Objective not to rule in disease, but to rule out other etiologies
  - Acute: Diffuse ground-glass infiltrates, nodular or striated patchy opacities. Up to 20% have normal CXR.
  - Subacute: Same as acute, may have sparing of lung bases
  - Chronic: Upper lobe fibrosis, reticular opacities, volume loss, honeycombing

- CT scan of chest:
  - Acute: Presence of centrilobular micronodules (<5 mm) found in mid and lower zones, mosaic perfusion, air trapping, ground-glass opacities.
  - Subacute: Similar to acute, with generalized increase in lung attenuation and reticulonodular pattern, emphysematous changes.
  - Chronic: Fibrosis, irregular opacities, bronchiectasis, loss of lung volume, honeycombing, emphysematous changes

Initial approach
Usually start with CXR; may progress to CT based on findings

Diagnostic Procedures/Surgery
- Pulmonary function tests (PFTs) (1)[B]:
  - Acute: Restrictive pattern, low diffusing capacity of the lung for carbon monoxide
  - Chronic: Restrictive pattern, may develop obstructive pattern due to emphysematous changes
- Lung biopsy (1)[B]:
  - Transbronchial: Limited usefulness
  - Open lung biopsy: Usually reserved when difficulty in diagnosis or atypical response to therapy

Pathological Findings
- Acute:
  - Alveolar lymphocytosis is a major characteristic.
  - Diffuse interstitial inflammation with macrophages, neutrophils, and plasma cells is also found.
  - Eosinophils are rare.
  - Alveolar space contains proteinaceous exudate and edema.
- Chronic:
  - Diffuse inflammation, as noted in acute form
  - Noncaseating granulomas, constrictive bronchiolitis
  - Develop fibrosis as disease progresses (may resemble usual interstitial pneumonitis)

DIFFERENTIAL DIAGNOSIS
- Acute:
  - Acute infectious pneumonia
  - Influenza (or other viral pneumonia)
  - Mycoplasma
  - *Pneumocystis jirovecii* pneumonia
  - Asthma
- Chronic:
  - Sarcoidosis
  - Chronic bronchitis
  - Chronic obstructive pulmonary disease
  - Tuberculosis
  - Collagen vascular disease
  - Idiopathic pulmonary fibrosis
  - Lymphoma
  - Fungal infections
  - *Pneumocystis jirovecii* pneumonia

 TREATMENT

MEDICATION
First Line
- Avoidance of offending antigen is primary therapy.
- Corticosteroids (1)[B]:
  - Prednisone: 1–2 mg/kg/d, to max of 50–60 mg PO daily
  - Initial course of 1–2 weeks with progressive taper
  - Low-dose therapy (20 mg PO daily) may be as effective as avoidance.
- Contraindications: Refer to the manufacturer's literature.
- Precautions: Observation for side effects:
  - Immunosuppression
  - Salt and water retention
  - Osteoporosis
  - Acne
  - Hirsutism
  - Behavioral changes
  - Weight gain/appetite increase
- Significant possible interactions: In patients with renal or cardiovascular disease, a corticosteroid with minimal sodium retention should be chosen.

Second Line
- Bronchodilators and inhaled corticosteroids may symptomatically improve patients with wheeze and chest tightness (1)[B].
- Oxygen may be needed in advanced cases.
- Lung transplantation may be last resort in severe cases unresponsive to therapy.

ADDITIONAL TREATMENT
General Measures
- Appropriate health care: Outpatient except for acute pneumonitis cases and admission for workup (BAL, lung biopsy)
- Avoidance of offending antigen

Issues for Referral
Referral to pulmonologist indicated for further evaluation and management of chronic disease.

IN-PATIENT CONSIDERATIONS
Initial Stabilization
Supportive management as needed to maintain oxygenation and ventilation.

Admission Criteria
- Unstable ventilation
- Oxygen requirement
- Mental status changes
- Need for invasive evaluation (lung biopsy)

 ONGOING CARE

FOLLOW-UP RECOMMENDATIONS
Activity as tolerated based on severity
Patient Monitoring
- Initial follow-up should be weekly–monthly, depending on severity and course.
- Follow efficacy of treatments with serial CXR, PFTs, circulating antibody levels (2).

DIET
No dietary restrictions

PATIENT EDUCATION
- Stress pathogenesis and critical importance of allergen avoidance.
- Stress risk of irreversible lung damage with continued exposure.
- Note that chronic exposure may lead to a loss of acute symptoms with exposure (i.e., patient may lose awareness of exposure–symptom relationship).

PROGNOSIS
- Acute: Good prognosis with reversal of pathologic findings if elimination of offending antigen in early disease.
- Chronic: Corticosteroids have been found to improve lung function acutely, but offer no significant difference in long-term outcome (1)[B].

COMPLICATIONS
- Progressive interstitial fibrosis with eventual respiratory failure
- Cor pulmonale and right-heart failure

REFERENCES
1. Girard M, Lacasse Y, Cormier Y. Hypersensitivity pneumonitis. *Allergy.* 2009.
2. Ismail T, McSharry C, Boyd G. Extrinsic allergic alveolitis. *Respirology.* 2006;11:262–8.

ADDITIONAL READING
Madison JM. Hypersensitivity Pneumonitis: Clinical Perspectives. *Arch Pathol Lab Med.* 2008;132:195–8.

 CODES

ICD9
495.9 Unspecified allergic alveolitis and pneumonitis

CLINICAL PEARLS
- Hypersensitivity pneumonitis is a poorly defined interstitial lung disease with different levels of severity.
- Avoidance of offending antigen is primary treatment.
- Corticosteroids may help acute presentations but do not affect long-term outcome of chronic disease.

H

HYPERTENSION, ESSENTIAL

David E. Burtner, MD

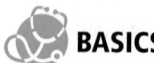

BASICS

DESCRIPTION
- Hypertension (HTN) is defined as 2 or more elevated BPs (systolic BP $\geq$140 mm Hg and/or diastolic BP $\geq$90 mm Hg) at $\geq$2 visits; operationally, any BP at which drug treatment results in a net benefit.
- HTN is a strong risk factor for cardiovascular disease.
- Pre-HTN: Systolic BP = 120–139 mm Hg or diastolic BP = 80–89 mm Hg
- Synonym(s): Benign, Chronic, Idiopathic, Familial, or Genetic HTN; High BP

Geriatric Considerations
- Isolated systolic HTN is common.
- Therapy has been shown to be effective and beneficial at preventing stroke, although target systolic BP is higher than in younger patients and adverse reactions to medications are more frequent. The benefit of therapy has been demonstrated in older patients (1).

Pediatric Considerations
Measure BP during routine exams.

Pregnancy Considerations
- Elevated BP during pregnancy may be either chronic HTN or pregnancy-induced preeclampsia. Angiotensin-converting enzyme (ACE) inhibitors and angiotensin II receptor blockers (ARBs) are contraindicated.
- Maternal and fetal mortality benefit from treatment (see topic "Preeclampsia").

EPIDEMIOLOGY
Incidence
- Lifetime risk for men and women aged 55 or 65 years by age 80–85 is >90%.
- Predominant age: Essential (primary, benign, idiopathic) onset usually in the 20s–30s.
- Predominant sex: Male > Female; males tend to run higher than females and have a significantly higher risk of cardiovascular disease at any given pressure.

Prevalence
50 million (1988–1991 NHANES III); 20% of the US population

RISK FACTORS
Family history, obesity, alcohol use, excess dietary sodium, stress, and physical inactivity

Genetics
BP levels are strongly familial, but no clear genetic pattern exists. Familial risk for cardiovascular diseases should be considered.

ETIOLOGY
- >90% of HTN has no identified cause.
- Secondary causes of HTN: see topic "Hypertension, Secondary and Resistant"
  - Renal parenchymal: Glomerulonephritis, pyelonephritis, polycystic kidneys
  - Endocrine: Primary hyperaldosteronism, pheochromocytoma, hyperthyroidism, Cushing syndrome
  - Vascular: Coarctation of the aorta, renal artery stenosis
  - Chemical: Oral contraceptives, nonsteroidal anti-inflammatory drugs (NSAIDs), decongestants, antidepressants, sympathomimetics, many industrial chemicals, corticosteroids, ergotamine alkaloids, lithium, cyclosporine
  - Sleep apnea

DIAGNOSIS

HISTORY
- HTN is asymptomatic except in extreme cases or after related cardiovascular complications develop.
- Headache can be seen with higher BP, often present on awakening and occipital in nature.

PHYSICAL EXAM
- Retinopathy: Narrowed arteries, arteriovenous (AV) nicking, copper or silver wiring of retinal arterioles
- Increased A_2 heart sound
- Synchronous radial and femoral pulse can help to rule out coarctation of the aorta.

DIAGNOSTIC TESTS & INTERPRETATION
ECG to evaluate possible presence of LVH or rhythm abnormalities affecting therapy

Lab
Initial lab tests
- Hemoglobin and hematocrit or complete blood count (CBC)
- Complete urinalysis (may reveal proteinuria)
- Potassium, calcium, and creatinine
- Cholesterol (total and high-density lipoprotein [HDL])
- Fasting blood glucose
- Uric acid

Follow-Up & Special Considerations
- Special tests (only if history, physical, or lab indicates); see topic "Hypertension, Secondary and Resistant"
- Ambulatory (24-hour) BP monitoring if "white coat" hypertension is suspected
- Home BP monitoring is effective; elevated home BPs correlate with adverse outcomes, and normal readings are reassuring.

Imaging
Only if history or physical indicate (see topic "Hypertension, Secondary and Resistant")

Diagnostic Procedures/Surgery
- A presumptive diagnosis of HTN can be made if the average of at least 2 BP measurements exceeds either 140 mm Hg systolic or 90 mm Hg diastolic, assuming proper resting conditions, cuff size, and application are maintained.
- The JNC (2) recommends emphasis on:
  - Family or personal history of HTN, cardiovascular, cerebrovascular, renal disease, and diabetes
  - Previous elevated BPs
  - Previous treatments
  - History of weight gain, exercise activities, sodium intake, fat intake, and alcohol use
  - Symptoms suggesting secondary HTN
  - Psychosocial and environmental factors affecting BP and risk for cardiovascular disease
  - Other cardiovascular risk factors such as obesity, smoking, hyperlipidemia, and diabetes
  - Funduscopic exam for arteriolar narrowing, arteriovenous compression, hemorrhages, exudates, and papilledema
  - Body mass index (BMI)
  - Waist circumference
  - BP in both arms
  - Complete cardiac and peripheral pulse exam: Compare radial and femoral pulse for differences in volume and timing, auscultation for carotid and femoral bruits.

- Abdominal exam for masses and bruits: Listen high in the flanks over the kidneys.
- Neurologic assessment

DIFFERENTIAL DIAGNOSIS
Secondary HTN: Because of the low incidence of reversible secondary HTN, special tests should be considered only if the history, physical exam, or basic laboratory evaluation indicate the possibility. (See topic "Hypertension, Secondary and Resistant.")

TREATMENT

MEDICATION
- The amount of blood pressure reduction is probably more important than the choice of antihypertensive.
- Multiple drugs at submaximal dose may achieve target blood pressure with fewer side effects.
- Thiazide diuretics have the most proven benefits (cost, compliance, and effectiveness). Chlorthalidone may be superior to more commonly used HCTZ due to longer half-life and more evidence to support (3,4)[A].
- Initial selection is based primarily on concomitant conditions (5).
- Sequential monotherapy attempts might be tried with different classes because individual responses vary.
- Majority of patients will require multiple meds.
- Benazepril combined with amlodipine has been shown to be superior to combination with HCTZ in high-risk patients (6)[A]. Some suggest that ACE/ARB plus dihydropyridine calcium channel blocker is first choice after monotherapy.
- β-Blockers had been strongly recommended until recent meta-analyses (3,7)[A]. Atenolol may be particularly ineffective in reducing adverse outcomes of hypertension.
- ACE inhibitors should be used in patients with diabetes, proteinuria, atrial fibrillation, or congestive heart failure (CHF) but not in pregnancy (3)[A].
- α-Adrenergics are not the first choice for monotherapy (4)[A]. Might benefit males with benign prostatic hypertrophy (BPH).
- β-Blockers might benefit patients with ischemic heart disease, CHF, or migraine (3)[A].
- Calcium channel blockers could be considered in patients with isolated systolic hypertension, atherosclerosis, migraine, or asthma; well documented to prevent stroke (4).

First Line
- Thiazide diuretics:
  - Hydrochlorothiazide: 6.25–50 mg daily
  - Chlorthalidone: 12.5–50 mg daily
  - Indapamide: 1.25–5 mg daily
- ACE inhibitors:
  - Captopril: 25–450 mg b.i.d.
  - Enalapril: 2.5–40 mg daily
  - Lisinopril: 5–40 mg daily
  - Ramipril: 2.5–20 mg daily
  - Quinapril: 10–80 mg daily
  - Benazepril: 10–40 mg daily
- ARBs:
  - Losartan: 25–100 mg in 1 or 2 doses; has unique but modest uricosuric effect
  - Valsartan: 80–320 mg daily
  - Irbesartan: 75–300 mg daily

- Candesartan: 4–32 mg daily
- Telmisartan: 40–80 mg daily
- Olmesartan : 20-40 mg daily
- Renin inhibitor: Aliskiren 150–300 mg daily
- Calcium channel blockers:
  - Diltiazem CD: 180–360 mg daily
  - Felodipine: 5–20 mg daily
  - Nifedipine (sustained release): 30–90 mg daily
  - Verapamil (sustained release): 120–480 mg daily
  - Amlodipine: 2.5–10 mg daily
- β-Blockers:
  - Atenolol: 25–100 mg daily; no longer 1st line (3)[A].
  - Carvedilol: 6.25–25 mg b.i.d.
  - Labetalol: 100–900 mg b.i.d. (combined alpha-beta blocker)
  - Metoprolol: tartrate 50–200 mg b.i.d. or succinate ER daily
  - Pindolol: 5–30 mg b.i.d.; may be helpful if bradycardia on other β-blockers
  - Propranolol: 20–120 mg daily
  - Bisoprolol: 2.5–20 mg daily
- Contraindications:
  - Diuretics may worsen gout.
  - β-Blockers (relatively) in reactive airway disease, heart block, diabetes, and peripheral vascular disease; probably should be avoided in patients with metabolic syndrome or insulin-requiring diabetes
  - Diltiazem or verapamil: Caution with systolic dysfunction heart failure or heart block
  - ACE inhibitors can worsen bilateral renovascular disease and are pregnancy category D.

Second Line
- Many may be combined.
- Centrally acting adrenergic inhibitors:
  - Clonidine: 0.1–1.2 mg b.i.d. or weekly patch 0.1–0.3 mg daily
  - Guanfacine: 1–3 mg daily
  - Methyldopa: 250–2,000 mg b.i.d.
- α-Adrenergic agents:
  - Prazosin: 1–10 mg b.i.d.
  - Terazosin: 1–20 mg daily
  - Doxazosin: 1–16 mg daily
- Peripherally acting adrenergic inhibitors: rarely used
  - Reserpine: 0.1–0.25 mg daily
- Vasodilators:
  - Hydralazine: 25–150 mg b.i.d.; risk of tachycardia, so generally combined with β-blocker; also drug-induced SLE
  - Minoxidil: Rarely used owing to adverse effects
- Loop diuretics (for volume overload):
  - Furosemide: 20–320 mg daily
  - Bumetanide: 0.5–2 mg daily
- K+-sparing diuretics in patients with hypokalemia while taking thiazides, or suspected aldosteronism:
  - Amiloride: 5–10 mg daily
  - Spironolactone: 25–100 mg daily
  - Triamterene: 50–150 mg daily

ADDITIONAL TREATMENT
General Measures
- Treating patients to lower-than-standard BP targets, ≤140–160/90–100 mm Hg, does not further reduce mortality or morbidity (8)[A]. Individualize goal pressures based on risk factors; best target may be toward the higher end of this range in patients >75–80 years of age.
- Primary focus is achieving systolic BP goal.
- Aerobic exercise

- Weight reduction for obese patients
- Smoking cessation
- Risk stratification affects the treatment:
  - Pre-HTN (120–139/80–89 mm Hg): Drug therapy for chronic renal disease or diabetes. ACCORD trial did not support for NIDDM patients (9).
  - Stage 1 HTN (140–159/90–99 mm Hg): Begin thiazide diuretics for most patients.
  - Stage 2 HTN (>160/>100 mm Hg): Consider starting 2 drugs.

COMPLEMENTARY AND ALTERNATIVE MEDICINE
Biofeedback and relaxation exercise

ONGOING CARE

FOLLOW-UP RECOMMENDATIONS
Patient Monitoring
- Reevaluate patients every 3–6 months.
- Review compliance, effectiveness, and adverse reactions. Poor medication adherence is a leading cause of apparent medication failure.
- Quality-of-life issues, including sexual function, should be considered.
- Annual (at least) evaluation of urinalysis, creatinine, and potassium as part of a screening laboratory panel

DIET
- ~20% of patients will respond to reduced-salt diet (<100 mmol daily; <6 g NaCl or <2.4 g Na).
- Consider DASH diet; http://www.nhlbi.nih.gov/health/public/heart/hbp/dash/new_dash.pdf.
- Limit alcohol consumption to <1 oz daily.

PATIENT EDUCATION
- Emphasize the asymptomatic nature of HTN and importance of lifetime treatment.
- Review cardiovascular risk factors.
- Printed aids for high BP education available at http://www.nhlbi.nih.gov/health/public/heart/index.htm#hbp

COMPLICATIONS
Heart failure, renal failure, LVH, myocardial infarction, retinal hemorrhage, stroke, hypertensive heart disease, drug side effects

REFERENCES

1. Beckett NS, Peters R, Fletcher AE, et al. Treatment of hypertension in patients 80 years of age or older. N Engl J Med. 2008;358:1887–98.
2. Chobanian AV, Bakris GL, Black HR, et al. The Seventh Report of the Joint National Committee on Prevention, Detection, Evaluation, and Treatment of High Blood Pressure: the JNC 7 report. JAMA. 2003;289:2560–72.
3. NICE/BHS HTN Guideline Review, 28 June 2006. Available at: http://guidance.nice.org.uk/CG34/guidance/pdf/English.
4. ALLHAT Officers and Coordinators for the ALLHAT Collaborative Research Group. The Antihypertensive and Lipid-Lowering Treatment to Prevent Heart Attack Trial. Major outcomes in high-risk hypertensive patients randomized to angiotensin-converting enzyme inhibitor or calcium channel blocker vs diuretic: The Antihypertensive and Lipid-Lowering Treatment to Prevent Heart Attack Trial (ALLHAT). JAMA. 2002;288:2981–97.
5. Mancia G, De Backer G, Dominiczak A, et al. Guidelines for the Management of Arterial Hypertension: The Task Force for the Management of Arterial Hypertension of the European Society of Hypertension (ESH) and of the European Society of Cardiology (ESC). J Hypertens. 2007;25:1105–87.
6. Chobanian AV. Does it matter how hypertension is controlled? N Engl J Med. 2008;359:2485–8.
7. Lindholm LH, Carlberg B, Samuelsson O. Should beta blockers remain first choice in the treatment of primary hypertension? A meta-analysis. Lancet. 2005;366:1545–53.
8. Arguedas JA, Perez MI, Wright JM. Treatment blood pressure targets for hypertension. Cochrane Database Syst Rev. 2009:CD004349.
9. The ACCORD Study Group. Effects of Intensive Blood-Pressure Control in Type 2 Diabetes Mellitus. N Engl J Med. 2010 Mar 14. PubMed PMID: 20228401.

See Also (Topic, Algorithm, Electronic Media Element)
Hypertension, Secondary and Resistant; Hypertensive Emergencies; Polycystic Kidney Disease

CODES

ICD9
- 401.0 Malignant essential hypertension
- 401.1 Benign essential hypertension
- 401.9 Unspecified essential hypertension

CLINICAL PEARLS

- Treatment of HTN reduces risk of many serious medical conditions with numbers needed to treat to prevent one serious event (such as stroke or myocardial infarction [MI]) ranging from approximately 20 patients per year for severe HTN to more than several hundred per year for mild HTN.
- Multiple submaximal doses are likely to have fewer side effects and more effectiveness than fewer maximum-dosed drugs.
- Diminishing benefit and increasing side effects and cost may accompany efforts to lower blood pressure below the generally accepted target of 140/90 mm Hg for most patients, including diabetics.
- Patients presenting with symptoms should be made strongly aware that resolution of these symptoms does not mean blood pressure elevation has resolved.

H

HYPERTENSION, SECONDARY AND RESISTANT

George Maxted, MD

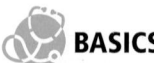

BASICS

DESCRIPTION
Uncontrolled hypertension comprises the following entities:

- Resistant hypertension: Defined by the Joint National Committee 7 as "failure to achieve goal blood pressure (<140/90 mm Hg for the overall population and <130/80 mm Hg for those with diabetes or chronic kidney disease) when a patient adheres to maximum tolerated doses of 3 antihypertensive drugs including a diuretic" (1)
- Secondary hypertension: Elevated blood pressure (BP) that results from an identifiable underlying mechanism

Geriatric Considerations
- Onset of hypertension (HTN) in adults >60 years of age is a strong indicator of secondary HTN.
- Framingham Heart Study data indicate that <40% of elderly participants (>75) were at goal BP (but previously defined goal BP's may actually be too low for optimal benefit).
- Systolic HTN is particularly problematic in the elderly.
- Secondary causes more common in the elderly include sleep apnea, renal disease, renal artery stenosis, and primary aldosteronism (2).

ALERT
Pseudoresistance:

- Inaccurate measurement of BP:
  - Cuff too small
  - Patient not at rest; sitting quietly for 5 minutes
- Poor adherence
  - In primary care settings, this has been estimated to occur in 40–60% of hypertensive patients (2).
- White-coat effect: Prevalence estimated at 20%
- Inadequate treatment (2)

EPIDEMIOLOGY
- Predominant age: In general, HTN has its onset between ages 30 and 50.
- Depending on etiology, age of onset can vary. Age of onset <20 years or >50 years increases likelihood that there is a secondary cause for HTN.
- The strongest predictors for resistant HTN are age (>75), presence of left ventricular hypertrophy (LVH), obesity (body mass index [BMI] >30), and high baseline systolic BP. Other predictors include chronic kidney disease, diabetes, living in the Southeastern US, African American race (especially women), excessive salt intake (2)
- In the ACCOMPLISH, INVEST, CONVINCE, ALLHAT, and LIFE studies, percent of patients reaching JNC-7 BP goals ranged from 45–82% (1).

Prevalence
The prevalence of resistant HTN is unknown. NHANES analysis indicates only 53% of adults are controlled to a BP of <140/90:

- Obstructive sleep apnea (OSA): 1 study diagnosed OSA in 83% of treatment-resistant hypertensives (2).
- Primary hyperaldosteronism (17–22% of resistant HTN cases) (2,3)
- Chronic renal disease (2–5% of hypertensives)
- Renovascular disease (0.2–0.7%, up to 35% of elderly, 20% of patients undergoing cardiac catheterization) (2)
- Cushing syndrome (0.1–0.6%)
- Pheochromocytoma (0.04–0.1% of hypertensives)

RISK FACTORS
Factors predictive of resistant or secondary hypertension: Female sex, African American race, obesity, diabetic, worsening of control in previously stable hypertensive patient, onset in patients of age <20 or >50 years, lack of family history of hypertension, significant target end organ damage, stage 2 HTN (systolic BP >160 mm Hg or diastolic BP >100 mm Hg), renal disease, alcohol or drug use

Genetics
In some patients, there is a possible relationship to ENaC gene variants (Liddle syndrome) and a CYP3A5 allele (cortisol metabolism, especially African Americans) (2).

GENERAL PREVENTION
The prevention of resistant and secondary hypertension is thought to be the same as for primary or essential hypertension. Adopting a DASH (Dietary Approaches to Stop Hypertension) diet, a low-sodium diet, weight loss in obese patients, exercise, limitation of alcohol intake, and smoking cessation may all be of benefit. Relaxation techniques may be of help, but data are limited.

PATHOPHYSIOLOGY
Depends on underlying etiology

ETIOLOGY
- Other rare causes: Hyperthyroidism, Hyperparathyroidism, Aortic coarctation, Intracranial tumor
- Drug-related causes:
  - Medications, especially nonsteroidal antiinflammatory drugs (NSAIDs) (may also blunt effectiveness of ACE-inhibitors), decongestants, stimulants (e.g., amphetamines, attention deficient hyperactivity disorder [ADHD] medications), anorectic agents (e.g., modafinil, ephedra, guarana, ma huang, bitter orange), erythropoietin, natural licorice (in some chewing tobacco), yohimbine, glucocorticoids.
  - Oral contraceptives: Unclear association; mainly epidemiologic and with higher estrogen pills
  - Cocaine, amphetamines, other illicit drugs – Drug and alcohol withdrawal syndromes
- Lifestyle factors:
  - Obesity, dietary salt may negate the beneficial effect of diuretics. Excessive alcohol, physical inactivity also contributors.

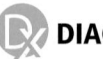

DIAGNOSIS

HISTORY
- Most important to ask at every visit: "The Big 4": sleep pattern, salt consumption, NSAID use, alcohol use. Also medication adherence, OTC medications.
- Review home BP readings; consider ambulatory BP monitoring:
- History will vary with etiology of HTN:
  - Pheochromocytoma: Episodes of headache, palpitations, sweating
  - Cushing syndrome: Weight gain, fatigue, weakness, easy bruising, amenorrhea
  - Obstructive sleep apnea: Loud snoring while asleep, daytime somnolence
  - Increased intravascular volume: Swelling

PHYSICAL EXAM
- Ensure that the BP is measured correctly. The patient should be sitting quietly with back supported for 5 minutes prior to measurement. Proper cuff size: Bladder encircling at least 80% of the arm. Support arm at heart level. Minimum of 2 readings at least 1 minute apart. Check BP in both arms. Also check standing BP for orthostasis.
- Attention to findings related to possible etiologies: Renovascular HTN: Systolic/diastolic abdominal bruit. Pheochromocytoma: Diaphoresis, tachycardia. Cushing syndrome: Hirsutism, moon facies, dorsal hump, purple striae, truncal obesity. Thyroid disease: Enlarged thyroid, tremor, exophthalmos, tachycardia. Coarctation of the aorta: Upper limb HTN with decreased or delayed femoral pulses.

DIAGNOSTIC TESTS & INTERPRETATION
- Electrocardiogram (EKG) performed as part of the initial workup; LVH is an important marker of resistant HTN.
- Funduscopic exam
- Sleep study if history and physical indicate. Overnight oximetry is a good screen for nocturnal hypoxia. If positive, formal polysomnography may be indicated.

Lab
Initial lab tests
Initial limited diagnostic testing should include (2,3)[A]: Urinalysis, complete blood count (CBC), potassium, sodium, glucose, creatinine, lipids, thyroid-stimulating hormone (TSH), calcium. 50% of patients with hyperaldosteronism may have normal potassium levels (1,2)

Follow-Up & Special Considerations
- Further testing for primary aldosteronism (PA) may be considered 8,12,1314:
  - Empiric treatment with an aldosterone inhibitor may be preferable, and more clinically relevant: spironolactone or eplerenone. 14 Amiloride may be more effective in blacks 15
  - Plasma aldosterone/renin ratio (ARR) is the preferred initial test:
    - Morning specimen. Low potassium must be corrected for 4 weeks before. Also be sure any aldosterone antagonists (including drospirenone, in some contraceptives), potassium-sparing diuretics have been stopped for 4 weeks.

○ A high ARR without the above precautions would be even more suspicious for PA.

○ A negative ARR is predictive for absence of PA (high negative predictive value).

○ Confirmatory testing for a positive ARR is recommended, but generally should be done by an endocrinologist.

○ If a positive ARR is confirmed, an adrenal computed tomography (CT) scan is recommended.

○ Empiric treatment for a positive ARR may be considered: spironolactone or eplerenone.

○ Further testing for pheochromocytoma: Plasma metanephrine screening test of choice: Confirmed by a 24-hour urinary metanephrine-to-creatinine ratio

○ Other tests to consider for resistant or secondary hypertension: 24-hour urine for free cortisol, calcium, parathyroid hormone (PTH), overnight 1mg dexamethasone suppression test, urine toxicology screen

Imaging

- Imaging tests listed are necessary only if history, physical, or lab data indicate.
- Abdominal ultrasound: If renal disease is suspected
- Magnetic resonance angiography (MRA) of renal vasculature: Preferred test for renovascular hypertension. Sensitive but low specificity. Conventional angiography or CT angiography 2nd line after MRA to look at distal renal artery. Renal arteriography remains gold standard for renovascular disease
- Adrenal "incidentaloma" frequently arises in this era of multiple CT studies. If present in the setting of resistant hypertension, consider hyperaldosterone or hyperadrenalcorticoid states.
- Doppler or CT imaging of aorta along with chest x-ray (CXR) looking for notched ribs (sign of coarctation)

Diagnostic Procedures/Surgery

- Consider 24-hour ambulatory BP monitoring, especially if white-coat effect is suspected. Home BP monitor results correlate predict mortality, stroke, and other target organ damage better than office BP. Optimal protocol involves 2 paired measurements morning and evening (4 measurements) over 4–7 days (4)
- Oscillometric, electronic, upper arm, fully automatic device with memory. Average multiple readings over several days.
- See http://www.dableducational.org for validated monitors.

TREATMENT

- Treatment modality depends on etiology of HTN. Please see each etiology listed for information on proper treatment.
- Emphasize: Adherence to interventions according to JNC-7 recommendations. Lack of, or underuse of, diuretic therapy is often found. Nonpharmacologic measures include weight loss, dietary salt restriction, moderation of alcohol intake, increased physical activity.
  - Obese patients, blacks, elderly may be particularly responsive to diuretics (5).
  - Tolerance to diuretics may occur - long term adaptation to thiazides or the "braking effect." Consider increasing the dose of thiazide, or adding an aldosterone inhibitor (5).

- Treatment specific to certain secondary etiologies:
  - Primary aldosteronism: Aldosterone receptor antagonist: Spironolactone or eplerenone
  - Cushing syndrome: Aldosterone receptor antagonist
  - Obstructive sleep apnea: Continuous positive airway pressure (CPAP) +/– oxygen, surgery, weight loss
  - Nocturnal hypoxia: Oxygen supplementation

MEDICATION

- Diuretics, especially chlorthalidone, are 1st line (5). Additional benefit has been demonstrated with angiotensin-converting enzyme (ACE) inhibitors, angiotensin II receptor blocker (ARB) agents, calcium channel blockers (2)[C]
- β-blockers are considered 1st line only for patients with ischemic heart disease or CHF. Combined a-β antagonists may be more effective for hypertension
- Aldosterone antagonists may offer significant benefit (1)[C],(2,6).
- Central-acting agents (e.g., clonidine) are effective at reducing BP, but outcomes data are lacking.

ALERT

- Agents specific for treatment of hypertensive emergencies should be initiated under a situation in which immediate BP reduction will prevent or limit end organ damage (see topic Hypertensive Emergencies).
- Renovascular HTN: Angioplasty is the treatment of choice for fibromuscular dysplasia of a renal artery. Endovascular treatment of atherosclerotic disease is controversial, with no clear benefit over medical management. Cardiovascular Outcomes in Renal Atherosclerotic Lesions (CORAL) study is pending and may help determine risk/benefit (2).
- Referral to an HTN specialist or clinic: Retrospective studies indicate improved control rates for patients with resistant HTN referred to special HTN clinics (2)[C].

IN-PATIENT CONSIDERATIONS
Initial Stabilization

Hospitalization may be necessary for hypertensive urgency or emergency general measures.

 ## ONGOING CARE

FOLLOW-UP RECOMMENDATIONS

Encourage aerobic activity of 30 min/d depending on patient condition.

DIET

- Reduced-salt may lower BP.
- The Mediterranean Diet or DASH is recommended.

PATIENT EDUCATION

Home blood pressure monitoring is recommended.

REFERENCES

1. Sarafidis PA, Bakris GL. Resistant hypertension: an overview of evaluation and treatment. *J Am Coll Cardiol*. 2008;52:1749–57.
2. Calhoun DA, Chair. Resistant HTN: Diagnosis, evaluation, and treatment. A scientific statement from the American Heart Association Professional Education Committee of the Council for High Blood Pressure Research. *Hypertension*. 2008.
3. Gaddam KK, Nishizaka MK, Pratt-Ubunama MN, et al. Characterization of resistant hypertension: association between resistant hypertension, aldosterone, and persistent intravascular volume expansion. *Arch Intern Med*. 2008;168:1159–64.
4. Johansson JK, Niiranen TJ, Puukka PJ, Jula AM, et al. Optimal schedule for home blood pressure monitoring based on a clinical approach. *J Hypertens*. 2010;28:259–64.
5. Ernst ME, Moser M. Use of diuretics in patients with hypertension. *N Engl J Med* 2009;361:2153–64.
6. Calhoun DA. Low-dose aldosterone blockade as a new treatment paradigm for controlling resistant hypertension. *J Clin Hypertens*. 2007;91(suppl 1): 19–24.

ADDITIONAL READING

Funder JW, Carey RM, Fardella C, et al. Case Detection, Diagnosis, and Treatment of Patients with Primary Aldosteronism: An Endocrine Society Clinical Practice Guideline. *J Clin Endocrinol Metab*. 2008.

See Also (Topic, Algorithm, Electronic Media Element)

Hypertension, Essential; Pheochromocytoma; Primary Aldosteronism; Cushing Disease and Cushing Syndrome; Coarctation of the Aorta; Hyperthyroidism; Hyperparathyroidism

 ## CODES

ICD9

- 405.01 Malignant renovascular hypertension
- 405.09 Other malignant secondary hypertension
- 405.11 Benign renovascular hypertension

CLINICAL PEARLS

- Onset of HTN in adults >60 years of age is a strong indicator of secondary HTN.
- Common causes of resistant hypertension: Obstructive sleep apnea, excessive salt intake, medication non-adherence.
- Common secondary causes include sleep apnea, renal disease, renal artery stenosis, and primary aldosteronism
- Home BP monitoring predicts outcomes better than office monitoring of blood pressure

H

HYPERTENSIVE EMERGENCIES

John A. Guisto, MD
Arthur B. Sanders, MD, MHA

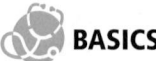 **BASICS**

DESCRIPTION
- Numerous terms can be used in the literature and often overlap (see Synonyms). Some definitions include a specific diastolic or systolic BP reading, whereas others emphasize an acute change in the BP or the presence of specific clinical syndromes.
- Severe HTN is defined as a diastolic BP of ≥115 mm Hg (15.3 kPa).
- A hypertensive emergency occurs only when an acute elevation of BP causes rapid and progressive end-organ damage, particularly in the cardiovascular, renal, and central nervous systems.
- System(s) affected: Cardiovascular; Nervous; Pulmonary; Renal
- Synonym(s): Hypertensive crisis; Severe HTN; Malignant HTN; Accelerated HTN; Hypertensive emergency

EPIDEMIOLOGY
Incidence
Incidence of hypertensive emergency: 1% of patients with hypertension annually in US.

Prevalence
- Overall prevalence of hypertension in the US 29.3% in 2003–2004 survey data
- Predominant age: Elderly

RISK FACTORS
- History of poorly controlled HTN
- Drug abuse
- Noncompliance with medications

Genetics
- Genetics: Risk of hypertensive emergency is higher in African Americans.
- Predominant sex: Male > Female

GENERAL PREVENTION
- Treat HTN.
- Counsel the patient on the importance of compliance with antihypertensive treatment and the dangers of stopping the medications abruptly.

PATHOPHYSIOLOGY
- Increased sympathetic tone leads to increased BP.
- Angiotensin II has multiple effects contributing to HTN and end-organ damage:
  - Stimulates sympathetic tone, aldosterone release, and antidiuretic hormone release
  - Chronic HTN induces vascular thickening and sclerosis.
  - Central effects include enhanced resorption of salt and water.
  - Chronic HTN shifts autoregulation of BP and cerebral blood flow.

ETIOLOGY
- Renal disease
- Abrupt withdrawal from antihypertensives, especially clonidine (Catapres)
- Withdrawal from CNS depressants
- Medications:
  - SSRIs
  - Decongestants
  - Appetite suppressants
- Steroids (including oral contraceptives)
- MAOI interaction with certain foods or drugs
- Drugs of abuse; cocaine or amphetamine
- Eclampsia/preeclampsia
- Thrombotic thrombocytopenic purpura (TTP)
- Pheochromocytoma
- Severe burns
- Postoperative HTN

COMMONLY ASSOCIATED CONDITIONS
- Chronic renal failure
- Renovascular HTN
- Acute glomerulonephritis
- Renal vasculitis

Geriatric Considerations
Elderly patients may experience isolated systolic HTN due to decreased baroreceptor sensitivity.

Pediatric Considerations
- Usually associated with renal disease
- May present with abdominal pain
- Preferred agents for children include labetalol, nicardipine, and nitroprusside.

Pregnancy Considerations
- Hydralazine is drug of choice because nitroprusside decreases placental blood flow and cyanide metabolite crosses the placenta; may result in fetal toxicity with prolonged exposure.
- Treat preeclampsia.

 DIAGNOSIS

Clinical presentation will vary depending on organ system affected.

HISTORY
- Headache
- Altered mental status
- Nausea, vomiting
- Neurologic disturbance
- Shortness of breath, dyspnea, orthopnea
- Chest pain
- Abdominal pain
- Epistaxis

PHYSICAL EXAM
- HTN
- Focal neurologic deficits, stupor, coma
- Retinopathy: Funduscopic exam may reveal papilledema, exudates, or hemorrhages.
- Pulmonary edema
- Hemorrhage, thrombosis, embolus
- Renal or abdominal bruit
- Unequal blood pressure or pulses in the extremities

DIAGNOSTIC TESTS & INTERPRETATION
Lab
Initial lab tests
- Urinalysis and renal function tests (red cell casts, hematuria, proteinuria are all common)
- Urine drug screen in selected patients
- Blood count and smear may indicate microangiopathic hemolytic anemia or thrombocytopenia.
- Serum electrolytes, which may indicate hypokalemic alkalosis

- Creatinine clearance
- Calcium, glucose

Follow-Up & Special Considerations
Subsequent workup pheochromocytoma in selected patients

Imaging
Initial approach
- Chest radiograph:
  - May show pulmonary edema and cardiomegaly due to CHF
  - Mediastinal widening and blunting of the aortic knob consistent with aortic aneurysm (potential rupture)
- If CNS symptoms, get head CT or MRI.
- If chest, abdominal, or back pain, consider contrast CT or MRI for suspected aortic dissection.

Follow-Up & Special Considerations
Subsequent workup for aldosteronism and for renal artery stenosis may be indicated in selected patients, especially young patients who may have fibromuscular dysplasia.

Diagnostic Procedures/Surgery
- ECG may reveal ischemia or left ventricular hypertrophy.
- The BP should be measured with an appropriately sized cuff, with ≥2 readings from both arms; then average readings.

Pathological Findings
Extreme BP elevations can overwhelm the autoregulatory mechanisms for organ blood flow, resulting in damage to the arteriolar and capillary beds. This process produces organ hemorrhages and edema.

DIFFERENTIAL DIAGNOSIS
- Myocardial infarction or angina pectoris
- Aortic dissection
- CHF
- Stroke
- Other CNS pathology (e.g., encephalopathy)
- Acute pulmonary edema
- Renal failure

 TREATMENT

MEDICATION
A 2008 Cochrane Review (1) noted that there are no randomized clinical trials showing a reduction in mortality from the recommended treatments, and similarly no clear randomized trial basis for recommending one medication over another. However, the recommended medications have been shown to reduce blood pressure in these circumstances, and the evidence levels reflect their effectiveness in this regard.

First Line
- IV unless otherwise indicated:
  - Nitroprusside (Nipride, Nitropress): Infusion 0.5–10 μg/kg/min; contraindicated in pregnancy (2,3)[A]
  - Fenoldopam (Corlopam): 0.1 μg/kg/min IV initial dose. Increase by 0.1 μg/kg/min q15 minutes to desired effect. Maximum dose 1.6 mcg/kg/min (4)[A]

– Hydralazine: Bolus 5–15 mg; preferred in pregnancy (2,3,5)[A]
– Labetalol (Normodyne, Trandate): Bolus 20–80 mg q10–15 minutes; infusion 0.5–2.0 mg/min (2,3)[A]
– Nitroglycerin (NTG): Infusion 5–100 μg/min (2,3,5)[A]
– NTG: 0.4 mg SL tablet. Repeat q5 minutes if needed. Consider IV infusion after 3 doses (2)[B].
– Phentolamine (Regitine): Bolus 5–10 mg q5–15 minutes (2,3)[A]
– Esmolol: 0.05–0.3 mg/kg/min (2,3,5)[A]
– Enalapril: 0.625–1.25 mg (2,3)[B]
– Nicardipine: 4–15 mg/h (2,3,6)[B]

- The drug(s) used depends on the end organs affected and the patient's clinical status:
  – Hypertensive encephalopathy: Nicardipine, labetalol, esmolol, or enalaprilat (3)[A]
  – CNS events: Nicardipine, labetalol. In ischemic stroke, withhold treatment unless systolic >220 or diastolic >120, except where needed for treating concomitant cardiovascular disease or pulmonary edema (2,3,5)[A].
  – Subarachnoid hemorrhage: Nicardipine, labetalol, or esmolol (3,5)[A]
  – Myocardial ischemia: Nitroglycerin infusion; or labetalol, or esmolol (2,3,5)[A]
  – CHF: Nitroprusside infusion; or nitroglycerin infusion; or enalaprilat or nicardipine (2,3)[A]
  – Aortic dissection: Nitroprusside and β-blocker, esmolol or nitroglycerin infusion (2,3,5)[A]
  – Renal failure: Nitroprusside, labetalol, or nicardipine. Consider dialysis (2,5)[A].
  – Pheochromocytoma: Phentolamine; or labetalol; or nitroprusside infusion (2)[A]
  – Antihypertensive withdrawal: Labetalol or phentolamine (2)[A]
  – Interactions between MAOIs and foods or drugs: Phentolamine or labetalol (2)[B]
  – Eclampsia/preeclampsia: Hydralazine, labetalol, or oral nifedipine (2,3,5)[A]

Second Line
- Oral clonidine: Oral loading dose of 0.2 mg followed by 0.1 mg/h until BP has been lowered or a total dose of 0.8 mg has been administered (2,5)[B]
- Trimethaphan (Arfonad): Infusion 0.5–5 mg/min (2)[B]
- Diazoxide in eclampsia/preeclampsia: 15 mg bolus every 3 minutes to maximum dose of 300 mg (7)[B]

ADDITIONAL TREATMENT
General Measures
- The general goal is to lower the mean arterial pressure (MAP) by ~20% or reduce the diastolic pressure to 100–110 mm Hg (13.3–14.6 kPa) over 1 hour.
- MAP is ~1/3 of the sum of twice the diastolic pressure plus the systolic pressure.
- If ongoing end-organ damage is thought to be secondary to the hypertensive state, prompt treatment with IV medication is indicated. Monitor patient closely so that a rapid fall in BP can be avoided.

COMPLEMENTARY AND ALTERNATIVE MEDICINE
Comfortable environment, which may lower the BP

SURGERY/OTHER PROCEDURES
- An arterial catheter may be used to monitor BP.

- Advantage over noninvasive monitoring not clearly proven (5)[C]

IN-PATIENT CONSIDERATIONS
Initial Stabilization
In general, lower the BP no more than 20% in the 1st hour; then, if stable, lower to 160/100–110 in the next 2–6 hours.

Admission Criteria
- All patients with true hypertensive emergencies should be hospitalized.
- Associated end-organ effects may require specific treatment (e.g., acute myocardial infarction).

IV Fluids
Fluid restriction may be appropriate for associated pathology such as pulmonary edema.

Nursing
Bed rest

Discharge Criteria
Patient should be stabilized on oral antihypertensives as appropriate (6)[A].

 ONGOING CARE

FOLLOW-UP RECOMMENDATIONS
Close outpatient follow-up with primary care physician recommended to ensure ongoing control of HTN.

Patient Monitoring
- Follow BP closely to avoid a rapid drop.
- Begin oral therapy as soon as possible after BP control has been achieved with IV medications.
- Ongoing BP control plus monitoring of affected organ system(s) (e.g., renal function) for evidence of continued morbidity

DIET
Low-sodium diet

PATIENT EDUCATION
- Avoid abrupt discontinuation of antihypertensive medicines.
- Stress importance of compliance.
- Emphasize the lack of symptoms with HTN until organ damage occurs.

PROGNOSIS
- BP should return to acceptable levels within 24 hours.
- Long-term prognosis depends upon extent of secondary end-organ damage in addition to ongoing BP control.

COMPLICATIONS
- Complications depend upon organ system(s) secondarily affected.
- Abrupt or excessive lowering of BP may result in inadequate cerebral or cardiac blood flow, leading to stroke or myocardial ischemia.
- The benefits of aggressive treatment may outweigh the risks in patients with severe HTN but no end-organ damage. No studies have proven that aggressive treatment reduces the risk of long-term morbidity or mortality from hypertensive urgencies.

REFERENCES
1. Perez MI, Musini VM. Pharmacological interventions for hypertensive emergencies. *Cochrane Database Syst Rev*. 2008:CD003653.
2. Flanigan JS, Vitberg D. Hypertensive emergency and severe hypertension: what to treat, who to treat, and how to treat. *Med Clin North Am*. 2006;90:439–51.
3. Shayne PH, Pitts SR. Severely increased blood pressure in the emergency department. *Ann Emerg Med*. 2003;41:513–29.
4. Tumlin JA, Dunbar LM, Oparil S, et al. Fenoldopam, a dopamine agonist, for hypertensive emergency: a multicenter randomized trial. Fenoldopam Study Group. *Acad Emerg Med*. 2000;7:653–62.
5. Management of hypertension and hypertensive emergencies in the emergency department: The EMREG-International Consensus Panel Recommendations. *Ann Emerg Med*. 2008;51(3):S1–S38.
6. Chobanian AV, Bakris GL, Black HR, et al. The Seventh Report of the Joint National Committee on Prevention, Detection, Evaluation, and Treatment of High Blood Pressure: the JNC 7 report. *JAMA*. 2003;289:2560–72.
7. Hennessy A, Thornton CE, Makris A, et al. A randomised comparison of hydralazine and mini-bolus diazoxide for hypertensive emergencies in pregnancy: The PIVOT trial. *Aust N Z J Obstet Gynaecol*. 2007;47:279–85.

ADDITIONAL READING
- Cherney D, Straus S. Management of patients with hypertensive urgencies and emergencies: a systematic review of the literature. *J Gen Intern Med*. 2002;17:937–45.
- Decker WW, Godwin SA, Hess EP, et al. Clinical policy: critical issues in the evaluation and management of adult patients with asymptomatic hypertension in the emergency department. *Ann Emerg Med*. 2006;47:237–49.
- Marik PE, Varon J. Hypertensive crises: challenges and management. *Chest*. 2007;131:1949–62.

See Also (Topic, Algorithm, Electronic Media Element)
Aortic Dissection; Pre-Eclampsia and Eclampsia (Toxemia of Pregnancy); Hypertension, Essential; Pheochromocytoma

 CODES

ICD9
401.9 Unspecified essential hypertension

CLINICAL PEARLS
- Treatment of severe HTN (hypertensive urgency) without evidence of acute end-organ damage is controversial. No emergent treatment is recommended.
- Avoid rapid prehospital lowering of BP.
- Treatment depends upon the organ systems affected.
- Esmolol and ACE inhibitors are contraindicated in pregnancy.

H

HYPERTHYROIDISM

Anup Kumar Sabharwal, MD
Juan-Pablo Brito-Campana, MD

 BASICS

Hyperthyroidism or thyrotoxicosis defines a spectrum of clinical findings consistent with thyroid hormone excess. The former describes excess from the thyroid gland, whereas the latter can be produced from any other source or not identified.

DESCRIPTION
- Graves disease (GD): The most common form; diffuse goiter and thyrotoxicosis are common characteristics. Infiltrative orbitopathy is seen in 50% of patients. Infiltrative dermopathy is rare. Autoantibodies are directed at the thyrotropin-stimulating hormone (TSH) receptors.
- Toxic multinodular goiter (TMNG): 2nd most common; a TSH receptor mutation has been found in 60% of patients; patients older than age 40, insidious onset, frequent in iodine-deficient areas.
- Toxic adenoma: Younger patients, autonomously functioning nodules
- Iodine-induced hyperthyroidism
- Thyroiditis: Transient autoimmune process:
  - Subacute thyroiditis/De Quervain: Granulomatous giant cell thyroiditis, benign course; viral infections have been involved.
  - Postpartum thyroiditis
  - Drug-induced thyroiditis: Amiodarone, interferon alpha, interleukin 2, lithium
  - Miscellaneous: Thyrotoxicosis factitia, TSH-secreting pituitary tumors, and functioning trophoblastic tumors
- Subclinical hyperthyroidism: Suppressed TSH with normal thyroxine (T_4); may be associated with osteoporosis and atrial fibrillation (1)
- Thyroid storm: Rare hyperthyroidism; fever, tachycardia, systolic hypertension, CNS dysfunction (e.g., coma); up to 50% mortality

Geriatric Considerations
- Characteristic symptoms and signs may be absent.
- Atrial fibrillation is common when TSH <0.1 mU/L.

Pediatric Considerations
- Neonates and children are treated with antithyroids for 12–24 months.
- Radioactive iodine is controversial in patients under the ages of 15–18 years.

Pregnancy Considerations
Propylthiouracil (PTU) is currently the drug of choice during pregnancy. Treat with lowest effective dose. Avoid treatment-induced hypothyroidism. Radioiodine therapy is contraindicated.

EPIDEMIOLOGY
- 1.3% of population
- Predominant sex: Female > Male (7–10:1).
- Predominant age: Autoimmune thyroid disease in 2rd and 3th decades. TMNG presents in patients older than age 40. GD is seen between 40 and 60 years of age.

Incidence
- Female 1:1,000
- Male: 1:3,000

RISK FACTORS
- Positive family history, especially in maternal relatives
- Female

- Other autoimmune disorders
- Iodide repletion after iodide deprivation, especially in TMNG

Genetics
The concordance rate for GD among monozygotic twins is 35%.

ETIOLOGY
- GD: Autoimmune disease
- TMNG: 60% TSH receptor gene abnormality; 40% unknown
- Toxic adenoma: Point mutation in TSH receptor gene with increased hormone production
- Thyroiditis:
  - Hashitoxicosis: Autoimmune destruction of the thyroid; antimicrosomal antibodies present
  - Subacute/De Quervain thyroiditis: Granulomatous reaction; genetic predisposition in specific human leukocyte antigens (HLAs); viruses such as coxsackievirus, adenovirus, echovirus, and influenza virus have been implicated; self-limited course, 6–12 months
  - Suppurative: Infectious
  - Drug-induced thyroiditis: Amiodarone produces an autoimmune reaction and a destructive process. Lithium, interferon-alpha, and interleukin 2 cause an autoimmune thyroiditis.
  - Postpartum thyroiditis: Autoimmune thyroiditis that lasts up to 8 weeks, and in 60% of patients, hypothyroidism manifests in the future.

COMMONLY ASSOCIATED CONDITIONS
- Autoimmune diseases
- Down syndrome
- Iodine deficiency

 DIAGNOSIS

HISTORY
- Thyrotoxicosis is a hypermetabolic state where energy production exceeds needs, causing increased heat production, diaphoresis, and even fever.
- Thyrotoxicosis affects several different systems:
  - Constitutional: Fatigue, weakness, increased appetite, weight loss
  - Neuropsychiatric: Agitation, anxiety, emotional lability, psychosis, coma, and poor concentration and memory
  - GI: Increased appetite, hyperdefecation
  - Gynecologic: Oligomenorrhea, amenorrhea
  - Cardiovascular: Tachycardia (most common) and chest discomfort that mimics angina

Geriatric Considerations
Apathetic hyperthyroidism in the elderly

PHYSICAL EXAM
- Adults:
  - Skin: Warm, moist, pretibial myxedema (GD only)
  - HEENT: Exophthalmos, lid lag
  - Endocrine: Hyperhidrosis, heat intolerance, goiter, gynecomastia, low libido, and spider angiomata (males)
  - Cardiovascular: Tachycardia, atrial fibrillation, cardiomegaly
  - Musculoskeletal: Skeletal demineralization, osteopenia, osteoporosis, fractures
  - Neurologic: Tremor, proximal muscle weakness, anxiety and lability, brisk deep tendon reflexes
  - Rarely: Thyroid acropathy (clubbing), localized dermopathy

- Children:
  - Linear growth acceleration
  - Ophthalmic abnormalities more common

DIAGNOSTIC TESTS & INTERPRETATION
Lab
- 95% have suppressed TSH and elevated free T_4. Total T_4 and triiodothyronine (T_3) represent the bound hormone and can be affected by pregnancy and hepatitis.
- T_3: Elevated especially in T_3 toxicosis or amiodarone-induced thyrotoxicosis
- T_4: Elevated; TSH autoantibodies rarely needed
- Free thyroxine index (FTI): Calculated from T_4 and thyroid hormone–binding ratio; corrects for misleading results caused by pregnancy and estrogens
- Inappropriately normal or elevated TSH with high T_4 suspicious for pituitary tumor or thyroid hormone resistance
- Drugs may alter lab results: Estrogens, heparin, iodine-containing compounds (including amiodarone and contrast agents), phenytoin, salicylates, steroids (e.g., androgens, corticosteroids)
- Drug precautions: Amiodarone and lithium may induce hyperthyroidism; MMI may cause warfarin resistance.
- Other findings that can occur: Anemia, granulocytosis, lymphocytosis, hypercalcemia, transaminase, and alkaline phosphate elevations.

Initial lab tests
- TSH, free T_4, T_4, T_3, TSI
- TSH-receptor (-R) antibodies (Abs): The routine assay is the TSH-binding inhibitor immunoglobulin assay (TBII). TSH-R Abs are useful in the prediction of postpartum Graves thyrotoxicosis and neonatal thyrotoxicosis.
- Thyroxine/triiodothyronine ratio: The T_4:T_3 ratio may be a useful tool when the iodine uptake testing is not available/contraindicated. Approximately 2% of thyrotoxic patients have "T_3 toxicosis."

Follow-Up & Special Considerations
In severe cases, such as thyroid storm, hospitalize until stable, especially if >60 years of age, because of the risk of atrial fibrillation.

Imaging
- Nuclear medicine scanning (^{123}I or ^{131}I): The reference-range values for 24-h radioiodine uptake is between 5% and 25%.
- Increased thyroid iodine uptake is seen with TMNG, toxic solitary nodule, and GD.
- GD shows a diffuse uptake and can have a paradoxical finding of high uptake at 4–6 h but normal uptake at 24 h because of the rapid clearance (2).
- TMNG will show a heterogeneous uptake, whereas solitary toxic nodule will show a warm or "hot" nodule.
- In iodine-deficient areas, an increased uptake is associated with low urine iodine levels.
- Hashimoto thyroiditis can have an increased uptake at an early stage but no increased thyroid hormone production.
- Causes of thyrotoxicosis with low iodine uptake:
  - Acute thyroiditis, thyrotoxicosis factitia, and iodine intoxication with amiodarone or contrast material can cause low-uptake transient thyrotoxicosis.

After thyroiditis resolves, the patient can become euthyroid or hypothyroid.

- Iodine loading can cause iodine trapping and decreased iodine uptake (Wolff-Chaikoff effect).
- Thyrotoxicosis factitia: Thyroglobulin levels are low in exogenous intake and high in endogenous production.
- Other extrathyroidal causes include struma ovarii and metastatic thyroid carcinoma.
- Technetium-99m scintigraphy: Controversial because it has a 33% discordance rate with radioactive iodine scanning.

Diagnostic Procedures/Surgery
Neck ultrasound will show increased diffuse vascularity in GD.

Pathological Findings
- GD: Hyperplasia
- Toxic nodule: Nodule formation

DIFFERENTIAL DIAGNOSIS
- Anxiety
- Malignancy
- Diabetes mellitus
- Pregnancy
- Menopause
- Pheochromocytoma
- Depression
- Carcinoid syndrome

TREATMENT

- Radioactive iodine therapy (RAIT): Most common definitive treatment used in the US for GD and TMNG
- Pretreatment with antithyroid drugs is preferred to avoid worsening thyrotoxicosis. MMI is preferred over PTU as pretreatment because of decreased relapse, but it is held 3–5 days before therapy.
- There is concern for a slightly higher risk of lymphoma and leukemia in patients treated with RAIT.
- Usually patients become hypothyroid 2–3 months after therapy; therefore, antithyroid medications are continued after ablation.
- Glucocorticoids: Reduce the conversion of active T_4 to the more active T_3. In Graves ophthalmopathy, the use of prednisone before and after RAIT improves outcome.
- After RAIT, the release of antigens can worsen the inflammatory reaction and the ophthalmopathy.
- Smoking in GD patients is a risk factor for ophthalmopathy when treated with RAIT.
- For TMNG, the treatment of choice is RAIT. Medical therapy with antithyroid medications has shown a high recurrence rate. Surgery is considered only in special cases.
- Treatment for subacute thyroiditis is supportive with nonsteroidal anti-inflammatory drugs (NSAIDs) and beta blockers. Steroids can be used for 2–3 weeks.
- For amiodarone-induced thyrotoxicosis (AIT) type I, the treatment is antithyroid drugs and beta blockers. Potassium perchlorate also can be used as an iodine uptake inhibitor. Thyroidectomy is the last option. AIT type II is self-limited.
- Graves dermopathy: difficult to treat in the chronic phase. Topical steroids with occlusive dressing may help in acute phase.

MEDICATION
First Line
- Antithyroid drugs: MMI and PTU are thionamides that inhibit iodine oxidation, organification, and iodotyrosine coupling. PTU can block peripheral conversion of T_4 to active T_3. Both can be used as primary treatment for GD and prior to RAIT or surgery.
- Duration of treatment: 6 months to 2 years; 50–60% relapse after stopping; treatment beyond 18 months did not show any further benefit . The most serious side effects are hepatitis (0.1–0.2%), vasculitis, and agranulocytosis.
  - MMI: Adults: 10–15 mg q12h; children aged 6–10 years: 0.4 mg/kg/d PO once daily
  - PTU: Adults (preferred in thyroid storm and pregnant and lactating women): 100–150 mg PO q8h, not to exceed 200 mg/d during pregnancy
- β-Adrenergic blocker: Propranolol in high doses (>160 mg/d) inhibits T_3 activation by up to 30%. Atenolol, metoprolol, and nadolol can be used.
- Glucocorticoids: Reduce the conversion of active T_4 to the more active T_3
- Cholestyramine: Anion exchange resin that decreases thyroid hormone reabsorption in the enterohepatic circulation; dose: 20–30 g/d
- Other agents:
  - Lithium: Inhibits thyroid hormone secretion and iodotyrosine coupling; can be dosed at 300 mg q8h with close monitoring of levels to avoid toxicity
  - Lugol solution: Saturated solution of potassium iodide (SSKI); blocks release of hormone from the gland but should be administered at least 1 h after thionamide was given; acts as a substrate for hormone production (Jod Basedow effect)
  - Potassium perchlorate: Especially for amiodarone-induced thyrotoxicosis
  - RAIT: See Treatment section.

Second Line
Ipodate sodium (Oragrafin): 0.5 g PO q.i.d. most effectively prevents conversion of T_4 to T_3 and thyroid hormone release; also useful in thyroid storm.

ADDITIONAL TREATMENT
Issues for Referral
Patients with Graves ophthalmopathy should be referred to an experienced ophthalmologist.

SURGERY/OTHER PROCEDURES
Thyroidectomy for compressive symptoms, masses, and thyroid malignancy may be performed in the 2nd trimester of pregnancy only.

ONGOING CARE

FOLLOW-UP RECOMMENDATIONS
Patient Monitoring
- Repeat thyroid tests once a year, CBC and LFTs on thionamide therapy; continue therapy with thionamides for 12–18 months (3).
- After RAIT, thyroid function tests at 6 weeks, 12 weeks, 6 months, and annually thereafter if euthyroid; TSH may remain undetectable for months if patient is euthyroid; follow T_3 and T_4.

DIET
Sufficient calories to prevent weight loss

PROGNOSIS
Good (with early diagnosis and treatment)

COMPLICATIONS
- Surgery: Hypoparathyroidism, recurrent laryngeal nerve damage, and hypothyroidism
- RAIT: Postablation hypothyroidism
- GD: High relapse rate with antithyroid drug as primary therapy
- Graves ophthalmopathy, worsening heart failure if cardiac condition, atrial fibrillation, muscle wasting, proximal muscle weakness, increased risk of cerebrovascular accident (CVA) and cardiovascular mortality

REFERENCES
1. Cappola AR, Fried LP, Arnold AM, Danese MD, Kuller LH, Burke GL, Tracy RP, Ladenson PW et al. Thyroid status, cardiovascular risk, and mortality in older adults. *JAMA*. 2006;295:1033–41.
2. Nayak B, Hodak SP. Hyperthyroidism. *Endocrinol Metab Clin North Am*. 2007;36:617–56.
3. Abraham P, Avenell A, Watson WA, et al. A systematic review of drug therapy for Graves' hyperthyroidism. *Cochrane Database Sys Rev*. 2005.

CODES

ICD9
- 242.00 Toxic diffuse goiter without mention of thyrotoxic crisis or storm
- 242.10 Toxic uninodular goiter without mention of thyrotoxic crisis or storm
- 242.20 Toxic multinodular goiter without mention of thyrotoxic crisis or storm

CLINICAL PEARLS
- Not all thyrotoxicoses are secondary to hyperthyroidism.
- GD presents with hyperthyroidism, ophthalmopathy, and goiter.
- Medical treatment for GD has a high relapse rate after stopping medications.
- Thyroid storm is a medical emergency that needs hospitalization and aggressive treatment.

H

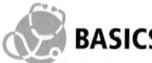

HYPERTRIGLYCERIDEMIA
S. Lindsey Clarke, MD

BASICS

DESCRIPTION
- Hypertriglyceridemia is a common form of dyslipidemia characterized by an excess fasting plasma concentration of triglycerides (TGs).
  - Triglycerides are fatty molecules made of glycerols that are esterified by fatty acids at all 3 hydroxyl groups.
  - They occur naturally in vegetable oils and animal fats.
  - In humans, triglycerides are major sources of dietary energy and are packaged into chylomicrons and very low-density lipoproteins (VLDLs).
  - Triglycerides are atherogenic.
- Hypertriglyceridemia is a risk factor for premature coronary artery disease in both men and women at levels ≥200 mg/dL and for pancreatitis at levels ≥1,000 mg/dL.
- Classification of TG levels in adults (1):
  - Normal: <150 mg/dL (1.7 mmol/L)
  - Borderline to high: 150–199 mg/dL
  - High: 200–499 mg/dL
  - Very high: ≥500 mg/dL
  - Divide by 88.5 to convert to millimoles per liter
- Norms for children vary by age; generally, triglycerides are considered high if they exceed
  - 150 mg/dL for adolescents
  - 130 mg/dL for children

EPIDEMIOLOGY
- Predominant gender: Male > Female.
- Predominant race: Hispanic, white > black

Prevalence
- 15–40% of general population
- Familial hypertriglyceridemia: 1–2%
- Familial combined hyperlipidemia: 1–2%
- Familial dysbetalipoproteinemia: 0.01–0.02%

RISK FACTORS
- Genetic susceptibility
- Obesity
- Diabetes
- Alcoholism
- Certain drugs (see Etiology)
- Medical illnesses (see Etiology)

Genetics
- Familial hypertriglyceridemia and familial combined hyperlipidemia: Autosomal dominant
- Familial dysbetalipoproteinemia: Autosomal recessive

GENERAL PREVENTION
- Weight management
- Moderation of dietary fat and carbohydrates
- Regular aerobic exercise

ETIOLOGY
- Primary:
  - Familial
  - Acquired (sporadic)
- Secondary:
  - Obesity and overweight
  - Physical inactivity
  - Cigarette smoking
  - Excess alcohol intake
  - Very high-carbohydrate diets (>60% of total caloric intake)
  - Certain medical conditions:
    ○ Type 2 diabetes mellitus
    ○ Chronic renal failure, nephrotic syndrome
    ○ Hypothyroidism
    ○ Paraproteinemias (e.g., macroglobulinemia, myeloma, lymphoma, lymphocytic leukemia)
    ○ Autoimmune disorders (e.g., systemic lupus erythematosus)
  - Certain medications:
    ○ Corticosteroids
    ○ Protease inhibitors and other antiretroviral agents
    ○ Beta blockers except carvedilol
    ○ Estrogens and tamoxifen
    ○ Atypical (2nd-generation) antipsychotics
    ○ Bile acid sequestrants (modest effect)
  - Pregnancy (usually physiologic and transient)

COMMONLY ASSOCIATED CONDITIONS
- Coronary artery disease
- Dyslipidemias:
  - Decreased high-density lipoprotein (HDL) cholesterol
  - Increased low-density lipoprotein (LDL), non-HDL, and total cholesterol
  - Small, dense LDL particles
- Nonalcoholic steatohepatitis
- Insulin resistance
- Metabolic syndrome (3 of following):
  - Abdominal obesity (waist circumference >40 inches in men, >35 inches in women)
  - Triglycerides ≥150 mg/dL
  - Low HDL cholesterol (<40 mg/dL in men, <50 mg/dL in women)
  - Blood pressure ≥130/85 mm Hg
  - Fasting glucose ≥100 mg/dL
- Pancreatitis
- Polycystic ovary syndrome

DIAGNOSIS

HISTORY
- Usually asymptomatic
- Patients with chylomicronemia syndrome may have memory loss, headache, vertigo, dyspnea, and paresthesias.
- Patients with pancreatitis have abdominal pain, nausea, and vomiting.
- Assess for other cardiac risk factors.
- Family history of premature coronary artery disease

PHYSICAL EXAM
- Increased body mass index (obesity)
- Eruptive cutaneous, tuberous, and striate palmar xanthomas
- Lipemia retinalis
- Epigastric tenderness in pancreatitis
- Hepatomegaly
- Lymphadenopathy
- Peripheral neuropathy

DIAGNOSTIC TESTS & INTERPRETATION
Lab
Initial lab tests
- Serum: Turbid with milky supranatant
- Fasting lipid profile (12-h fast):
  - Screen every 5 years starting at age 20 if other cardiac risk factors are present.
  - For interpretation, see Basics: Description

Follow-Up & Special Considerations
- Repeat lipid panel after 2 months of therapy.
- High levels of apolipoprotein (apo) B (≥90 mg/dL) are a strong predictor of coronary death in patients whose LDL cannot be calculated owing to very high triglycerides. Measurement of nonfasting apo B can help to identify patients at highest risk of atherosclerosis, such as those with familial combined hyperlipidemia.

Imaging
- Atherosclerosis: Cardiac stress imaging, coronary angiography, CT arteriography
- Pancreatitis: CT scan, ultrasound of pancreas

Pathological Findings
- Chylomicronemia syndrome: Lipid-laden macrophage (foam cell) infiltration of visceral organs, bone marrow, and skin
- Atherosclerosis
- Pancreatitis

DIFFERENTIAL DIAGNOSIS
Primary and secondary hypertriglyceridemia

TREATMENT

MEDICATION
First Line

- Fibrates if TGs ≥500 mg/dL or if LDL is already at goal (25–50% reduction in TGs) (1,2)[B]:
  – Fenofibrate (TriCor, others): 40–200 mg daily
  – Gemfibrozil (Lopid): 600 mg b.i.d.
  – Adverse reactions: GI upset, hepatotoxicity, cholelithiasis, myalgias, rhabdomyolysis (when combined with statin), gemfibrozil–warfarin interaction (enhanced anticoagulation)
- Statins if TGs <500 mg/dL and LDL is not at goal (10–40% reduction in TG)s (1,3)[A]: Only statins have shown improved cardiovascular outcomes.
- Atorvastatin (Lipitor) 10–80 mg daily, rosuvastatin (Crestor) 5–40 mg daily, simvastatin (Zocor) 10–80 mg nightly; adverse reactions: Hepato-toxicity, myalgias, myopathy, rhabdomyolysis; contraindicated in pregnancy and lactation

Second Line

- Niacin (20–35% reduction in TGs) (1,3,4)[A]:
  – 500–2,000 mg nightly or in divided doses
  – Pretreatment with aspirin reduces flushing.
  – Adverse reactions: Flushing, pruritus, peptic ulcer disease, hepatotoxicity, fulminant hepatic necrosis (with extended-release forms), hyperuricemia and gout, hyperglycemia, and toxic amblyopia
- Omega-3 acid ethyl esters (40–45% reduction in TGs; 20–30% if added to statin) (5,6)[C]:
  – Lovaza 4 g/d or 2 g b.i.d.
  – USP-verified fish oil, 9–12 capsules daily in divided doses
  – Safe, well-tolerated but scant outcomes data

ADDITIONAL TREATMENT
General Measures

- Usually outpatient; see Admission Criteria
- Search for correctable secondary causes; treat underlying illness or remove offending drug.
- Diet and exercise are 1st-line therapies for all patients and can reduce TGs by 25% (1,2,4)[A].
- According to current guidelines, getting LDL cholesterol to goal takes priority over correction of TGs, unless TGs ≥500 mg/dL (1,3)[A].
- Control other cardiac risk factors such as hypertension, diabetes mellitus, and smoking.
- Primary hypertriglyceridemia: Screen other family members.

Issues for Referral

- Hypertriglyceridemia refractory to treatment
- Familial hypertriglyceridemia syndromes

IN-PATIENT CONSIDERATIONS
Admission Criteria

- Acute pancreatitis
- Acute coronary syndrome

Discharge Criteria
Stabilization of acute complicating illness

ONGOING CARE

FOLLOW-UP RECOMMENDATIONS
2 months after initiation or modification of therapy (repeat fasting lipid profile)

Patient Monitoring

- Fasting lipid profile every 6–12 months
- Maintain TGs <1,000 mg/dL to reduce risk of acute pancreatitis.
- Hepatic function tests (mainly transaminases)
- Creatine phosphokinase (CPK) if patient has myalgias

DIET

- Restrict dietary fat to ≤15% of total caloric intake if TGs ≥1,000 mg/dL (1)[C].
- Limit carbohydrates to 50–60% and fats to 30% of total caloric intake if TGs >150 mg/dL.
- Avoid concentrated sugars.
- Moderate alcohol intake.

PATIENT EDUCATION
Smoking cessation (4)[C]

PROGNOSIS

- Good with correction of triglyceride levels
- Patients with primary hypertriglyceridemia usually require lifelong treatment.

COMPLICATIONS

- Atherosclerosis
- Chylomicronemia syndrome
- Pancreatitis

REFERENCES

1. Oh RC, Lanier JB. Management of hyper-triglyceridemia. *Am Fam Physician*. 2007;75: 1365–71.
2. Yuan G, Al-Shali KZ, Hegele RA. Hypertriglyceridemia: its etiology, effects and treatment. *CMAJ*. 2007;176:1113–20.
3. Tovar JM, Bazaldua OV, Loffredo A. Diabetic dyslipidemia: a practical guide to therapy. *J Fam Pract*. 2008;57:377–88.
4. Brunzell JD. Clinical practice. Hypertriglyceridemia. *N Engl J Med*. 2007;357:1009–17.
5. Bays HE, McKenney J, Maki KC, Doyle RT, Carter RN, Stein E et al. Effects of prescription omega-3-acid ethyl esters on non–high-density lipoprotein cholesterol when coadministered with escalating doses of atorvastatin. *Mayo Clin Proc*. 2010;85:122–8.
6. Hartweg J, Perera R, Montori V, Dinneen S, Neil HA, Farmer A et al. Omega-3 polyunsaturated fatty acids (PUFA) for type 2 diabetes mellitus. *Cochrane Database Syst Rev*. 2008;CD003205.

ADDITIONAL READING

National Cholesterol Education Program (NCEP) Expert Panel on Detection, Evaluation, and Treatment of High Blood Cholesterol in Adults (Adult Treatment Panel III). Third Report of the National Cholesterol Education Program (NCEP) Expert Panel on Detection, Evaluation, and Treatment of High Blood Cholesterol in Adults (Adult Treatment Panel III) final report. *Circulation*. 2002;106:3143–421.

See Also (Topic, Algorithm, Electronic Media Element)
Atherosclerosis; Hypercholesterolemia; Pancreatitis
Algorithm: Hypertriglyceridemia

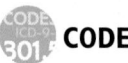

CODES

ICD9
272.1 Pure hyperglyceridemia

CLINICAL PEARLS

- Hypertriglyceridemia is an independent risk factor for coronary artery disease for both men and women at levels ≥200 mg/dL and for pancreatitis at levels ≥1,000 mg/dL.
- Check carefully for secondary causes of hypertriglyceridemia.
- Diet and exercise are 1st-line interventions for all patients who have hypertriglyceridemia.
- Treat triglyceride levels ≥500 mg/dL aggressively with fibrates.
- In patients whose triglyceride levels are ≥150 mg/dL but <500 mg/dL, the primary goal in cholesterol management is control of LDL cholesterol. Additional cardiovascular risk reduction can be achieved by lowering triglycerides with diet, exercise, statins, fibrates, niacin, and omega-3 fatty acids.

H

HYPOCHONDRIASIS

Moshe S. Torem, MD, DLFAPA

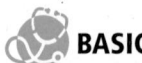

BASICS

DESCRIPTION
- Hypochondriasis is a psychiatric disorder characterized by at least 6 months existence of the following:
  - ≥ 1 physical symptoms associated with the belief that these physical symptoms are a manifestation of an underlying serious illness
  - Fear and anxiety that a serious illness is present in the body and, unless treated, may cause significant harm and lead to death or serious impairment and disability
  - Standard medical workup and reassurance that such a serious illness is not present is not effective in curing the fear.
  - The beliefs have an obsessive quality.
  - The patient typically is engaged in behaviors seeking a physical diagnosis that would explain his or her somatic symptoms.
- Synonym(s): Hypochondriacal neurosis; Hypochondria

EPIDEMIOLOGY
Incidence
- Predominant sex: Male = Female; women tend to seek help more frequently than men.
- Predominant age: Most common onset is in the 3rd to 4th decade of life.

Prevalence
- In the US, 1–4.5% of the general population
- 4–6% of medical outpatients meet criteria for hypochondriasis.
- In 25–50% of all primary care visits, no physical cause is found to explain the patient's presenting symptoms (1).

RISK FACTORS
- Exposure to life-threatening medical conditions in self or others and multiple medical procedures in childhood, adolescence, or adult life
- Being raised by an overprotective parent who is obsessed with excessive worries about health and illness
- Family history of hypochondriasis

Genetics
Some studies show an increased prevalence of hypochondriasis in families, especially among identical twins and 1st-degree relatives.

PATHOPHYSIOLOGY
According to DSM-IV-TR:
- Preoccupation with fears of having, or the idea of having, a serious disease based on the person's misinterpretation of bodily symptoms
- The preoccupation persists despite appropriate medical evaluation and reassurance.
- The belief in such an idea is not of delusional intensity (as in delusional disorder, somatic type) and is not restricted to a circumscribed concern about appearance (as in body dysmorphic disorder).
- The preoccupation causes clinically significant distress or impairment in social, occupational, or other important areas of functioning.
- The duration of the disturbance is at least 6 months.

- The preoccupation is not better accounted for by generalized anxiety disorder, obsessive–compulsive disorder, panic disorder, a major depressive episode, separation anxiety, or another somatoform disorder.
- Excessive concerns and fears of illness may become a central feature of the patient's identity.
- Despite significant concerns about health, these patients do not tend to develop particularly healthy lifestyle habits.
- Tendency to doubt their doctor's reassurance; may frequently seek treatment from another health care professional

ETIOLOGY
- Biologic: Some evidence suggests that patients with hypochondriasis may be born with a tendency to amplify somatic sensations for which they have a lower threshold and a lower discomfort tolerance.
- Childhood events: The experience of numerous or serious actual medical illnesses during childhood may predispose the individual to hypochondriasis at a later age.
- Life events: Experience of life-threatening medical diseases may predispose some to become overly sensitive to physical symptoms and overly worried about the recurrence of an acute relapse of chronic illness. Such patients may have been born with a high sensitivity to physical symptoms in general, which is then reinforced by the experience of life-threatening diseases such as an acute stroke, myocardial infarction, malignant tumors, organ transplantation, and others. These illnesses may be experienced by the patient or by a close family member or friend.
- Psychodynamics: Some authors view hypochondriasis as the patient's psychodynamic manifestation of coping with intrapsychic subconscious emotions of guilt, shame, low self-esteem, and a narcissistic overindulgence with self. Other authors view hypochondriasis as a manifestation of an individual's need for attention by overly identifying with the sick role, which offers an acceptable way of alleviating anxiety by seeking valid reassurance from a medical authority.
- Anxiety/depression: Some authors have found that many patients with an underlying anxiety or depressive disorder experience their psychiatric illness in the form of physical symptoms, which in some patients may become a chronic behavior, turning into a full-blown hypochondriasis even after their underlying anxiety or depression has been alleviated.
- Sociocultural: Some societies and cultures view mental and emotional symptoms in a pejorative and stigmatized way, blaming the patient for the illness when the symptoms are mental and feeling more empathy when the symptoms are physical. In such cultures, patients with physical symptoms get more attention, empathy, and respect and are not blamed for causing their illness.
- Cognitive: Patients with hypochondriasis overestimate their risk of developing a serious illness. They also tend to minimize their past experiences and behaviors of good health.

COMMONLY ASSOCIATED CONDITIONS
- Anxiety disorders
- Depressive disorders: Up to 40%
- Obsessive–compulsive disorder
- Somatization disorder
- Conversion disorder
- Pain disorder
- Body dysmorphic disorder
- Undifferentiated somatoform disorder

DIAGNOSIS

HISTORY
- Patient may report the following common concerns:
  - Worry about sensations associated with normal body functions such as heartbeat or diaphoresis, intestinal peristalsis, hiccups, flatulence, etc.
  - Minor physical abnormalities, such as a small rash or rare cough
  - Vague physical sensations
- Attributes symptoms to a disease of concern
- May focus on multiple systems or a single disease

PHYSICAL EXAM
A thorough physical exam reveals no abnormalities or findings that are compatible with the reported symptoms and their severity.

DIAGNOSTIC TESTS & INTERPRETATION
Lab
Initial lab tests
Lab tests are used to rule out organic diseases.

Follow-Up & Special Considerations
Be aware that such patients have the tendency to request excessive unnecessary lab and radiology tests.

Imaging
Regular follow-up appointments, including a physical examination, are helpful to reassure the patient that no new disease has emerged.

Diagnostic Procedures/Surgery
Care to avoid nonessential tests; do not perform tests solely to provide reassurance because the reassurance is likely to be short-lived (2).

Pathological Findings
No organic tissue changes have been found to explain hypochondriasis.

DIFFERENTIAL DIAGNOSIS
- Any patient suffering from hypochondriasis, as with any other psychiatric disorder, is not immune from developing a medical/organic disease. Organic diseases that affect many organ systems, such as connective tissue diseases and autoimmune diseases, as well as more focused single-organ-type diseases, always must be considered as a possibility in these patients.
- Underlying clinical depression
- Schizophrenia
- Delusional disorders
- Conversion disorder
- Anxiety disorders
- Panic disorder

- Obsessive–compulsive disorder
- Factitious disorder with physical symptoms
- Somatization disorder
- Chronic pain disorder
- Body dysmorphic disorder
- Malingering
- Münchausen syndrome

TREATMENT

MEDICATION
First Line
- No specific medications have been proven effective for hypochondriasis (3).
- Antidepressants and antianxiety medications are most successful in patients who have a preponderance of anxiety or depressive symptoms (4).
- Selective serotonin reuptake inhibitors (SSRIs) are commonly used (3):
  – Fluoxetine (Prozac, Sarafem) 20–80 mg/d
  – Fluvoxamine maleate (Luvox CR) 100–300 mg/d
  – Paroxetine (Paxil CR) 10–75 mg/d
  – Sertraline (Zoloft) 50–200 mg/d

Second Line
Medications to relieve obsessive–compulsive symptoms such as the SSRIs listed above, or:
- Clomipramine (Anafranil) 100–250 mg/d

ADDITIONAL TREATMENT
General Measures
- Treatment should focus on a careful history and physical exam, with clear and straightforward explanations of any findings.
- Regular medical appointments with clear goals and repeated reassurance with adequate explanation
- Patients may perceive referral to a psychiatrist as dismissive of concerns
- Some evidence suggests cognitive behavioral therapy (CBT) is helpful to improve hypochondriacal concerns and overall functioning:
  – Explains that focusing on a symptom tends to increase its intensity
  – Describes anxiety or depression as worsening physical symptoms
  – Teaches distraction techniques
- Group therapy using a CBT model can help to reduce hypochondriacal concerns as well as anxiety for at least 1 year after treatment (5).
- A good doctor–patient relationship is essential:
  – Physicians should be careful with their words: Avoid suggestions of possible diseases.
  – Schedule regular appointments even if no new symptoms or findings are present.

Issues for Referral
Consult with a psychiatrist when:
- Patients don't respond to your treatment.
- Patients become suicidal.
- Comorbid psychiatric illness is present.

ONGOING CARE

FOLLOW-UP RECOMMENDATIONS
Patient Monitoring
- Patients should be seen on a regular basis.
- Appointments should be scheduled regardless of whether the patient has new symptoms.
- Avoid the use of hospitalizations and unnecessary lab workups.

DIET
Healthy nutrition

PATIENT EDUCATION
- Clear explanations of all test results and their significance
- Patients may benefit from watching the following movies:
  – *Hannah & Her Sisters* (1986)
  – *Send Me No Flowers* (1964)
  – *Up in Arms* (1944)

PROGNOSIS
The natural history of this condition is usually chronic. 50–70% will continue to meet diagnostic criteria after 1 year.

COMPLICATIONS
Risk of repeated and unnecessary lab and diagnostic procedures

REFERENCES

1. Olde Hartman TC, et al. Medically unexplained symptoms, somatisation disorder and hypochondriasis: Course and prognosis. A systematic review. *Journal of Psychosomatic Research*. 2009;66: 363–377.
2. Barsky AJ, Ahern DK, Bailey ED, et al. Hypochondriacal patients' appraisal of health and physical risks. *Am J Psychiatry*. 2001;158:783–7.
3. Barsky AJ. Clinical practice. The patient with hypochondriasis. *N Engl J Med*. 2001;345:1395–9.
4. Creed F, Barsky A. A systematic review of the epidemiology of somatisation disorder and hypochondriasis. *J Psychosom Res*. 2004;56: 391–408.
5. Lidbeck J. Group therapy for somatization disorders in primary care: maintenance of treatment goals of short cognitive-behavioural treatment one-and-a-half-year follow-up. *Acta Psychiatr Scand*. 2003; 107:449–56.

ADDITIONAL READING

- Abramowitz JS, Braddock AE. Hypochondriasis: conceptualization, treatment, and relationship to obsessive-compulsive disorder. *Psychiatr Clin North Am*. 2006;29:503–19.
- Abramowitz JS, Olatunji BO, Deacon BJ. Health anxiety, hypochondriasis, and the anxiety disorders. *Behav Ther*. 2007;38:86–94.
- American Psychiatric Association (APA). *Diagnostic and Statistical Manual* 4th Edition Text Revision. Washington DC: American Psychiatric Association Press, 2000.
- Avia MD, Ruiz MA. Recommendations for the treatment of hypochondriac patients. *J Contemp Psychother*. 2005;35:301–13.
- Boone KB. Fixed Belief in Cognitive Dysfunction Despite Normal Neuropsychological Scores: Neurocognitivie Hypochondriasis? *Clin Neuropsychol*. 2008;16:1–21.
- Braddock AE, Abramowitz JS. Listening to hypochondriasis and hearing health anxiety. *Expert Rev Neurother*. 2006;6:1307–12.
- Buwalda FM, Bouman TK, van Duijn MA. Psychoeducation for hypochondriasis: a comparison of a cognitive-behavioural approach and a problem-solving approach. *Behav Res Ther*. 2007;45:887–99.
- Buwalda FM & Bouman TK. Predicting the effect of psychoeducational group treatment for hypochondriasis. *Clin Psychol Psychother*. 2008;15:396–403.
- Fallon BA et al. A double-masked, placebo-controlled study of fluoxetine for hypochondriasis. *J Clin Psychopharmacol*. 2008;28:638–45.
- Fishbain DA, et al. Is chronic pain associated with somatization/hypochondriasis? An evidence-based structured review. *Pain Pract*. 2009;9:449–467.
- Forister JG, James B. Hypochondriasis: meeting the management challenge. *JAAPA*. 2007;20:42–6.
- Furer P, Walker JR. Treatment of hypochondriasis with exposure. *J Contemp Psychother*. 2005;35: 251–67.
- Greeven A, et al. Cognitive behavioral therapy versus paroxetine in the treatment of hypochondriasis: An 18-month naturalistic follow-up. *J Behav Ther Exp Psychiatry*. 2009;40:487–496.
- Politi P, Emanuele E. Successful treatment of refractory hypochondriasis with duloxetine. *Prog Neuropsychopharmacol Biol Psychiatry*. 2007;31:1145–6.

CODES

ICD9
300.7 Hypochondriasis

CLINICAL PEARLS

- Hypochondriasis is the preoccupation with fears of having, or the idea of having, a serious disease that persists despite appropriate medical evaluation and reassurance.
- The natural history of hypochondriasis is usually chronic: 50–70% of patients will continue to meet diagnostic criteria after 1 year. Most patients require lifelong follow-up and reassurance.
- Although no specific medications have been proven effective, antidepressants and antianxiety medications (especially SSRIs) are most successful in hypochondriasis patients who have a preponderance of anxiety or depression symptoms.
- Some evidence suggests that CBT is helpful in improving hypochondriacal concerns and overall functioning.
- Patients respond best in a stable and trusting relationship with a physician whom they perceive as caring, kind, nonjudgmental, patient, reassuring, understanding, and able to appropriately deal with areas of uncertainty in the practice of medicine.

H

HYPOGLYCEMIA, DIABETIC

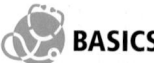

Joseph A. Florence, MD

BASICS

DESCRIPTION
- Abnormally low concentration of glucose in circulating blood of diabetic; often referred to as an *insulin reaction*
- Classification includes:
  - Severe hypoglycemia: An event requiring assistance of another person to actively administer treatment
  - Documented symptomatic hypoglycemia: An event during which typical symptoms are accompanied by a measured plasma glucose of ≤70 mg/dL (3.9 mmol/L)
  - Asymptomatic hypoglycemia: An event not accompanied by symptoms, but a measured glucose of ≤70 mg/dL (3.9 mmol/L)
  - Probable symptomatic hypoglycemia: Event with symptoms, but glucose not tested
  - Relative hypoglycemia: An event with typical symptoms, but glucose >70 mg/dL (3.9 mmol/L)
- Hypoglycemia is the leading limiting factor in the glycemic management of type 1 and type 2 diabetes.
- System(s) affected: Endocrine/Metabolic

ALERT
Hypoglycemic unawareness:
- Major risk factor for severe hypoglycemic reactions
- Most commonly found in patients with long-standing type 1 diabetes and children <7 years

EPIDEMIOLOGY
Incidence
From the Accord Study, the annual incidence of hypoglycemia was:
- 3.14% in the intensive treatment group
- 1.03% in the standard group
- Increased risk among women, African Americans, those with less than a high school education, aged participants, and those who used insulin at trial entry
- From the RECAP-DM study: Hypoglycemia was reported in 38% of type 2 patients who added a sulphonylurea or a thiazolinedione to metformin therapy during the past year.

Prevalence
- Most common in type 1 diabetics:
  - If tightly controlled: Often experience hypoglycemia frequently, weekly
- Type 2 diabetics:
  - Common if treated with insulin and/or insulin secretagogues

RISK FACTORS
- Nearly 3/4 of severe hypoglycemic episodes occur during sleep.
- Autonomic neuropathy
- Illness, stress, and unplanned life events
- Duration of diabetes >5 years, advanced age, renal/liver disease, CHF, hypothyroidism, hypoadrenalism, gastroenteritis
- Starvation or prolonged fasting
- Alcoholism: Evening consumption of alcohol is associated with an increased risk of nocturnal and fasting hypoglycemia, especially in type 1 patients.
- Current smokers with type 1 diabetes

- Oral hypoglycemics with long duration and high potency have greater hypoglycemic risks.
- α-Glucosidase inhibitors, biguanides, and thiazolidinediones, when used in combination with insulin and/or sulfonylureas or meglitinides
- In patients 80 years or older, severe hypoglycemia is associated with comorbid conditions and in users of a long-activing sulphonylurea

GENERAL PREVENTION
- Maintain routine schedule of diet, medication, and exercise.
- Stabilize daily carbohydrate intake.
- Regular blood glucose testing:
  - ≥3 times daily testing if multiple injections of insulin
- Diabetes treatment and teaching programs (DTTPs) especially for high-risk type 1 patients, which teach flexible insulin therapy to enable dietary freedom
- Hypoglycemia rates are reduced by up to 70% using continuous subcutaneous insulin infusion pumps compared with multiple daily injections (1)[C].

ETIOLOGY
- Loss of hormonal counter-regulatory mechanism in glucose metabolism
- Diet: Too little food (skipping meal), decreased carbohydrate intake
- Medication: Too much insulin or oral hypoglycemic agent (improper dose or timing)
- Erratic absorption of insulin or oral hypoglycemics
- Adverse reaction from other medications
- Exercise: Unplanned or excessive
- Alcohol consumption
- Vomiting or diarrhea
- Gastroparesis

COMMONLY ASSOCIATED CONDITIONS
- Autonomic dysfunction
- Neuropathies
- Cardiomyopathies

DIAGNOSIS

HISTORY
- Symptoms are idiosyncratic and vary considerably between individuals (2).
- Adrenergic hypoglycemia symptoms:
  - Hunger, trembling, pallor
  - Sweating, shaking, pounding heart, anxiety
- Neuroglycopenic hypoglycemia symptoms:
  - Dizziness, poor concentration, drowsiness, weakness, confusion, lightheadedness, slurred speech, blurred vision, double vision, unsteadiness, poor coordination
- Behavioral hypoglycemia symptoms:
  - Tearfulness, confusion, fatigue, irritability, aggressiveness
- Patients' reports of hypoglycemic symptoms are associated with a significantly lower treatment satisfaction and with barriers to adherence (3)[A].

PHYSICAL EXAM
- General: Confusion, lethargy
- HEENT: Diplopia
- Cor: Tachycardia
- Neuro: Tremulousness, weakness, paresthesias, stupor, seizure, or coma

- Mental status: Irritability, inability to concentrate, or short-term memory loss
- Skin: Pale, diaphoresis
- End organ damage: Microvascular, macrovascular, ophthalmologic, neurologic, renal

DIAGNOSTIC TESTS & INTERPRETATION
Lab
- Plasma or whole-blood glucose <70 mg/dL
- Suspect hypoglycemic unawareness in type 1 asymptomatic diabetes with low/normal HgbA1c.
- Chronic hypoglycemia is indicated by low glycohemoglobin level.
- Disorders that may alter lab results:
  - Hemoglobinopathies may alter HgbA1c results.

DIFFERENTIAL DIAGNOSIS
- Hypoglycemia is well documented in chronic alcoholics and binge drinkers.
- GI dysfunction causing postprandial hypoglycemia or alimentary reactive hypoglycemia
- Hormonal deficiency states (hormonal reactive hypoglycemia)
- Idiopathic reactive hypoglycemia (reactive hypoglycemia, a popular diagnosis 20 years ago, is actually quite rare)
- Hypoglycemia of sepsis
- Islet cell tumors
- Factitious hypoglycemia from surreptitious injection of insulin
- Hypoglycemia may be found in nondiabetics under certain conditions such as early pregnancy, prolonged fasting, long periods of strenuous exercise, heart failure, malignancy, and renal or liver disease.

TREATMENT

MEDICATION
- General:
  - Glucose:
    - Oral administration of small-molecule sugars (saccharose/glucose); glucose preferred
    - ~60–90 carbohydrate calories (15–20 g glucose) repeated every 15 minutes until blood sugar is ≥100 mg/dL (5.55 mmol/L)
    - Takes ~15 minutes for carbohydrates to be digested and enter bloodstream as glucose
    - Once sugar has normalized, then a meal or snack should be consumed to prevent recurrence of hypoglycemia (4)[C].
- In patients with loss of consciousness at home:
  - Administer glucagon IM or SC in the deltoid or anterior thigh:
    - <5 years old: 0.25–0.50 mg
    - 5–10 years old: 0.50–1 mg
    - >10 years: 1 mg
- In unconscious, if emergency medical personnel are present or patient hospitalized:
  - Give 1/2 ampule 50% dextrose every 5–10 minutes until patient awakens.
  - Then feed orally and/or administer 5% dextrose IV at level that will maintain blood glucose >100 mg/dL.
  - Patients with hypoglycemia secondary to oral hypoglycemics should be monitored for 24–48 hours, because hypoglycemia may recur after apparent clinical recovery.
- Significant possible interactions:

– Treatment may cause hyperglycemia (called Somogyi phenomenon).

– Clearance of certain oral hypoglycemics from plasma may be prolonged in persons with liver disease.

ADDITIONAL TREATMENT
General Measures
- Glucose: Preferred treatment; however, any form of carbohydrate that contains glucose should be effective (4)[C]
- Any sugar-containing food or beverage that can be rapidly absorbed: Juice (4–6 ounces), candy (5–6 pieces of hard candy), or nondiet soda
- OTC glucose tablets or gels
- Glucagon: People in close contact with people with diabetes should be instructed in using an emergency glucagon kit (4)[C].
- Glucagon should be prescribed to patients at significant risk of severe hypoglycemia (4)[C].
- If a patient using acarbose suffers from a bout of hypoglycemia, the patient should eat something containing monosaccharides, such as glucose tablets. Since acarbose will prevent the digestion of complex carbohydrates, starchy foods will not effectively reverse a hypoglycemic episode in a patient taking it.

Issues for Referral
- Frequent, recurring, or episodes that do not readily respond to treatment
- Consultant pharmacists can play a critical role in preventing hypoglycemia in long-term care facilities (5)[A] by recommending:
  – More physiologic insulin regimens
  – Facility protocols
  – Staff education

Additional Therapies
Use of a continuous glucose monitoring system in the management of severe hypoglycemia decreases the number of hypoglycemic values (6)[B].

IN-PATIENT CONSIDERATIONS
Admission Criteria
- Any doubt of cause
- Expectation of prolonged hypoglycemia (e.g., caused by sulfonylurea drug)
- Inability of patient to drink
- Treatment has not resulted in prompt recovery of sensorium.
- Seizures, coma, or altered behavior (e.g., ataxia, disorientation, unstable motor coordination, dysphasia) secondary to documented or suspected hypoglycemia

Discharge Criteria
Patient has normoglycemia and risk of severe hypoglycemia is negligible.

 ONGOING CARE

FOLLOW-UP RECOMMENDATIONS
Rest until glucose is normal.

Patient Monitoring
Self-monitoring of blood glucose

DIET
- If alcohol consumed, combine with food to reduce risk of hypoglycemia
- Protein does not slow absorption of carbohydrates.
- Fats may slow absorption of carbohydrates and may retard and then prolong the acute glycemic response (7)[C].

PATIENT EDUCATION
- Always have access to quick-acting carbohydrate.
- For patients taking insulin:
  – For planned exercise, consider a reduced insulin dosage.
  – Additional carbohydrates may be needed for unplanned exercise.
  – Moderate-intensity exercise increases glucose uptake by 2–3 mg/kg/min above usual requirements (70-kg person needs 10–15 g carbohydrates per hour for moderate physical activity).
- For patients with hypoglycemia unawareness or 1 or more episodes of severe hypoglycemia, glycemic targets should be raised to avoid further hypoglycemia for at least several weeks (4)[C].
- Educate patients and their relatives, close friends, teachers, and supervisors:
  – Blood glucose testing should be available at school or workplace.
  – Personnel should be aware of diabetes diagnosis and signs/symptoms of hypoglycemia and treatment.
- Teach self-monitoring of blood glucose and self-adjustment for insulin therapy, diet control, and exercise regimen.
- Patient should wear medical alert identification bracelet or necklace.

PROGNOSIS
Full recovery usually depends on rapidity of diagnosis and treatment.

COMPLICATIONS
- Coma, seizure
- Prolonged or severe hypoglycemia may cause permanent neurologic damage and/or cognitive impairment.
- Repeated episodes of severe hypoglycemia not necessarily associated with cognitive dysfunction (8)
- MI, stroke, especially in elderly

ALERT
In the ACCORD trial of adults with type 2 diabetes at especially high risk for heart attack and stroke, the medical strategy to intensively lower blood glucose (sugar) below current recommendations increased the risk of death compared with a less-intensive standard treatment strategy (9)[B].

REFERENCES
1. Cohen ND, et al. Diabetes: Advances in treatment. *Internal Med J.* 2007;37:383–8.
2. McAulay V, et al. Symptoms of hypoglycaemia in people with diabetes. *Diabetes UK, Diabetic Med.* 2001;18:690–705.
3. Alvarez Guisasola F, Tofé Povedano S, Krishnarajah G, Lyu R, Mavros P, Yin D et al. Hypoglycaemic symptoms, treatment satisfaction, adherence and their associations with glycaemic goal in patients with type 2 diabetes mellitus: findings from the Real-Life Effectiveness and Care Patterns of Diabetes Management (RECAP-DM) Study. *Diabetes Obes Metab.* 2008;10(Suppl 1):25–32.
4. American Diabetes Association. Executive summary: standards of medical care - 2009. *Diabetes Care.* 2009;32(Suppl 1):S6–12.
5. Garza H et al. Minimizing the risk of hypoglycemia in older adults: a focus on long-term care. *Consult Pharm.* 2009;24(Suppl B):18–24.
6. Ryan EA, Germsheid J et al. Use of continuous glucose monitoring system in the management of severe hypoglycemia. *Diabetes Technol Ther.* 2009;11:635–9.
7. American Diabetes Association, Bantle JP, Wylie-Rosett J, et al. Nutrition recommendations and interventions for diabetes: a position statement of the American Diabetes Association. *Diabetes Care.* 2008;31(Suppl 1):S61–78.
8. Adverse events and their association with treatment regimens in the diabetes control and complications trial. *Diabetes Care.* 1995;18:1415–27.
9. National Institutes of Health. For safety, NHLBI changes intensive blood sugar treatment in clinical trial of diabetes and cardiovascular fitness. Accessed March 24, 2008 at:http://public.nhlbi.nih.gov/newsroom/home/GetPressRelease.aspx?id=2551.

ADDITIONAL READING
Miller ME, Bonds DE, Gerstein HC, et al. The effects of baseline characteristics, glycaemia treatment approach, and glycated haemoglobin concentration on the risk of severe hypoglycaemia: post hoc epidemiological analysis of the ACCORD study. *BMJ.* 2010;340:b5444.

See Also (Topic, Algorithm, Electronic Media Element)
Diabetes Mellitus, Type 1
Algorithm: Hypoglycemia

 CODES

ICD9
- 250.80 Diabetes mellitus with other specified manifestations, type ii or unspecified type, not stated as uncontrolled
- 250.81 Diabetes mellitus with other specified manifestations, type I (juvenile type) not stated as uncontrolled

CLINICAL PEARLS
- Hypoglycemic unawareness is most commonly found in patients with tightly controlled, and long-standing type 1 diabetes and children <7 years. Reduction in unawareness may be improved by temporarily liberalizing blood sugar control to eliminate episodes of hypoglycemia.
- Any form of carbohydrate that contains glucose should be effective for management, such as sugar-containing food or beverage that can be rapidly absorbed:
  – 4–6 ounces juice
  – 5–6 pieces of hard candy
  – Nondiet soda
  – OTC glucose tablets or gels

H

HYPOGLYCEMIA, NON-DIABETIC

Matthew A. Silva, PharmD, RPh, BCPS
Pablo I. Hernandez Itriago, MD

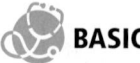 **BASICS**

DESCRIPTION
- Hypoglycemia defined by Whipple triad:
  - Low plasma glucose level (≤60 mg/dL)
  - Hypoglycemic symptoms that are relieved when glucose level is corrected
  - Occurs commonly in patients with diabetes receiving sulfonylurea or insulins; less commonly in patients without diabetes
- Reactive hypoglycemia:
  - Occurs in response to a meal, drugs, herbal substances or nutrients
  - May occur 2–3 hours postprandially or later
  - Symptoms generally observed with serum glucose ≤60 mg/dL, lower in patients with hypoglycemic unawareness
  - Also seen after gastrointestinal surgery (in association with dumping syndrome in some patients)
- Spontaneous (fasting) hypoglycemia:
  - May be associated with a primary condition, including hypopituitarism, Addison disease, myxedema, or in disorders related to hepatic dysfunction or renal failure
  - If hypoglycemia presents as a primary disorder, consider hyperinsulinism, and extrapancreatic tumors.

EPIDEMIOLOGY
Incidence
- True incidence is unknown.
- 8.6% of hospitalized inpatients ≥65 years old:
  - Asymptomatic in 25% of cases

Prevalence
True prevalence is unknown.
- Predominant age: Older adult
- Predominant sex: Female > male

RISK FACTORS
Refer to "Etiology"

Genetics
Some aspects may involve genetics (e.g., hereditary fructose intolerance).

GENERAL PREVENTION
- Follow dietary and exercise guidelines
- Patient recognition of early symptoms and knowledge of corrective action

ETIOLOGY
- Reactive, postprandial:
  - Alimentary hyperinsulinism
  - Meals high in refined carbohydrate
  - Certain nutrients including fructose, galactose, leucine
  - Glucose intolerance (prediabetes)
  - Gastrointestinal surgery
  - Idiopathic (unknown cause)
- Spontaneous
  - Fasting
  - Alcohol or medication (insulin, sulfonylureas, thiazolidinediones, beta-blockers, salicylates, quinine, hydroxychloroquine, fluoroquinones, doxycycline, sertraline, disopyramide, pentamidine)
  - Consider medication errors as a source of unexplained hypoglycemia even in patients without diabetes
  - Surreptitious drug use (self-injection of insulin or ingestion of oral hypoglycemic medications in patients with diabetes)
  - Natural medicines or herbs (bitter melon, caffeine, cassia cinnamon, chromium, fenugreek, ginseng, guarana, mate, stevia, vanadium)
  - Post surgical (e.g., gastrectomy, Roux-en-Y) hypoglycemia/dumping syndrome
  - Islet cell hyperplasia or tumor (insulinoma)
  - Extrapancreatic insulin secreting tumor
  - Hepatic disease
  - Glucagon deficiency
  - Adrenal insufficiency
  - Catecholamine deficiency
  - Hypopituitarism
  - Hypothyroidism
  - Eating disorders
  - Exercise
  - Fever
  - Pregnancy
  - Renal glycosuria
  - Large tumors
  - Ketotic hypoglycemia of childhood
  - Enzyme deficiencies or defects
  - Severe malnutrition
  - Sepsis
  - Total parenteral nutrition therapy
  - Hemodialysis

Pediatric Considerations
- Usually divided into 2 syndromes
- Transient neonatal hypoglycemia
- Hypoglycemia of infancy and childhood
- Screening infants for hypoglycemia is appropriate when pregnancy was complicated by maternal diabetes.

Geriatric Considerations
- More likely to have underlying disorders or be causative medications
- Iatrogenic hypoglycemia is common in the hospitalized elderly with renal insufficiency.

COMMONLY ASSOCIATED CONDITIONS
- Severe liver disease; alcoholism
- Addison disease; adrenocortical insufficiency
- Myxedema
- Malnutrition (patients with renal failure)
- Gastrointestinal surgery
- Panhypopituitarism
- Insulinoma

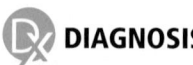 **DIAGNOSIS**

HISTORY
- Central nervous system (CNS; neuroglycopenic) symptoms predominate with gradual glucose reduction:
  - Headache
  - Confusion
  - Lightheadedness
  - Fatigue and weakness
  - Visual disturbances
  - Changes in personality
- Adrenergic symptoms: More prominent in acute drop in glucose:
  - Anxiety
  - Tremulousness
  - Dizziness
  - Diaphoresis
  - Warmth/flushing
  - Heart palpitations
- Gastrointestinal symptoms:
  - Hunger
  - Nausea
  - Belching

PHYSICAL EXAM
- CNS (neuroglycopenic) symptoms predominate with gradual glucose reduction:
  - Convulsions
  - Coma
  - Hypotension
- Adrenergic symptoms: More prominent in acute drop in glucose:
  - Tremulousness
  - Diaphoresis
  - Warmth/flushing
  - Heart palpitations

DIAGNOSTIC TESTS & INTERPRETATION
Lab
Initial lab tests
Blood glucose ≤45 mg/dL (≤2.5 mmol/L) when symptomatic followed by symptom resolution with feeding (1,2)[C]
- Plasma glucose overnight fasting: ≤60 mg/dL (≤3.33 mmol/L); confirm on 2 or more occasions (2)[C]
- Plasma glucose 72-hour fasting: ≤45 mg/dL (≤2.5 mmol/L) for females; ≤55 mg/dL (≤3.05 mmol/L) for males; fast may be ended when Whipple triad is achieved or hypoglycemia is demonstrated (2)[C]

Follow-Up & Special Considerations

- Oral glucose tolerance: ≤50 mg/dL (≤2.78 mmol/L) (1,2)[C]
- Misinterpretation of glucose tolerance tests may lead to misdiagnosis of hypoglycemia; ≥1/3 of normal patients have hypoglycemia with or without symptoms during the 4-hour glucose tolerance test. These patients may be at future risk for type 2 diabetes.
- C-peptide measurement (2)[C]
- Check liver studies, serum insulin, ACTH, and cortisol. Serum insulin should be suppressed when glucose is <60 mg/dL (2)[C].
- Serum b-hydroxybutyrate
- Insulin radioimmunoassay: Elevated insulin levels suggest islet cell hyperplasia or tumor (2)[C].
- Drugs may alter lab results: Many drugs can affect glucose levels; refer to drug or laboratory reference (2)[C].

Imaging
Initial approach
Abdominal CT to rule out abdominal tumor

Diagnostic Procedures/Surgery
For definitive diagnosis patient should have:
- Documented low glucose levels (2)
- Symptoms when glucose levels are low (2)
- Evidence that symptoms are relieved specifically by ingestion of sugar or other food (2)
- Identification of the specific type of hypoglycemia (2)
- Serum b-hydroxybutyrate <2.7 mg/dL in the presence of high serum insulin, C-peptide, and low serum glucose suggests excessive insulin production

DIFFERENTIAL DIAGNOSIS
CNS disorders
- Psychogenic
- Pseudohypoglycemia: Symptoms of hypoglycemia or self-diagnosis in patients in whom low blood glucose may not be detectable and who may be impossible to convince that they do not suffer from hypoglycemia after all tests are found to be normal.

TREATMENT

MEDICATION
- Once diagnosis is established, begin therapy appropriate to underlying disorder.
- If unable to swallow: Glucagon 1mg (1unit) IM or SC. If no response, give IV bolus of 25–50 g of 50% glucose solution followed by continuous infusion until patient able to take by mouth (1)[C].
- Postsurgical gastrectomy patients unresponsive to diet changes may benefit from propantheline, psyllium, fiber or oat bran, which delays gastric emptying (1)[C].
- Insulinoma: See separate topic.

ADDITIONAL TREATMENT
General Measures
- Outpatient except for severe cases; may also be inpatient for testing
- Oral carbohydrate for alert patient without drug overdose (2–3 tablespoons of sugar in glass of water or fruit juice, 1–2 cups of milk, piece of fruit, or several soda crackers) (1)[C]

- If unable to swallow: Use glucagon IM or SC (1)[C].
- If caused by medication or nutrients: Avoid or control causative agents (1)[C].
- If triggered by meals: Try high-protein diet with carbohydrate restriction (1)[C].
- Nonhypoglycemic hypoglycemia or pseudohypoglycemia:
  - Many patients (often females, aged 20–45) present with diagnosis of reactive hypoglycemia (self-diagnosed or misinterpretation of tests)
  - Symptoms may pertain to chronic fatigue and somatic complaints (stress often playing a role in these symptoms)
  - Management difficult, listening is important. Try 120 g carbohydrate diet (1)[C].
  - Counseling may be useful for stress and other problems

SURGERY/OTHER PROCEDURES
If Islet cell tumor (insulinoma) or other insulin secreting tumor, surgery is treatment of choice. If inoperable, diazoxide may relieve symptoms.

IN-PATIENT CONSIDERATIONS
Admission Criteria
Hypoglycemia unresponsive to oral intake

 ## ONGOING CARE

FOLLOW-UP RECOMMENDATIONS
- Exercise routine or daily activity may need to be reevaluated.
- Patients with recurrent hypoglycemia should have glucose source at hand for immediate ingestion during symptoms.

Patient Monitoring
- Depends on type and severity of symptoms and treatment of underlying cause
- Hypoglycemia from sulfonylureas can last for hours to days depending on half-life and renal function.

DIET
- High protein, low carbohydrate
- Frequent small feedings (6 daily)
- Avoid fasting

PATIENT EDUCATION
- Dietary instruction
- Counseling for stress, if appropriate
- Recognition of early symptoms of hypoglycemia and how to take corrective action

PROGNOSIS
Favorable, with appropriate treatment

COMPLICATIONS
- Insulinoma: If tumor identified and removed, some surgical risk is involved.
- Organic brain syndrome: May occur with extensive, prolonged hypoglycemia

REFERENCES

1. Carroll MF, Burge MR, Schade DS. Severe hypoglycemia in adults. Rev Endocr Meta Dis. 2003;4(2):149–57.
2. Service FJ. Classification of hypoglycemic disorders. Endocrinol Metab Clin North Am. 1999;28: 501–17, vi.

ADDITIONAL READING

- Burmeister JE, Scapini A, da Rosa Miltersteiner D et al. Glucose-added dialysis fluid prevents asymptomatic hypoglycaemia in regular haemodialysis. Nephrol Dial Transplant. 2007;22:1184–9.
- Cansu DU, Korkmaz C. Hypoglycaemia induced by hydroxychloroquine in a non-diabetic patient treated for RA. Rheumatology (Oxford). 2008;47:378–9.
- Lawrence KR, Adra M, Keir C. Hypoglycemia-induced anoxic brain injury possibly associated with levofloxacin. J Infect. 2006;52:e177–80.
- Pollak PT, Mukherjee SD, Fraser AD. Sertraline-induced hypoglycemia. Ann Pharmacother. 2001;35: 1371–4.
- Singh M, Jacob JJ, Kapoor R, et al. Fatal hypoglycemia with levofloxacin use in an elderly patient in the post-operative period. Langenbecks Arch Surg. 2008;393:235–8.
- Yamada C, Nagashima K, Takahashi A, et al. Gatifloxacin acutely stimulates insulin secretion and chronically suppresses insulin biosynthesis. Eur J Pharmacol. 2006;553:67–72.

See Also (Topic, Algorithm, Electronic Media Element)
Hypoglycemia, Diabetic; Insulinoma
Algorithm: Hypoglycemia

CODES

ICD9
251.2 Hypoglycemia, unspecified

CLINICAL PEARLS
- Symptoms coincide with low blood glucose levels.
- Symptoms resolve with oral/intravenous glucose or glucagon.
- Avoid known agents/nutrients that trigger hypoglycemia.
- Treat underlying cause.

HYPOKALEMIA

Ruben Peralta, MD

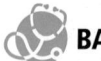 **BASICS**

DESCRIPTION
Hypokalemia is defined as a serum potassium concentration <3.5 mEq/L (normal range: 3.5–5.0 mEq/L).

EPIDEMIOLOGY
Predominant sex: Male = Female

Incidence
- Commonly encountered electrolyte abnormality in clinical practice (1)[B],(2)
- Found in >20% of hospitalized patients (when defined as potassium <3.6 mEq/L)
- Higher incidence in individuals with eating disorders from 5–20% (3):
- >10% of inpatients with alcoholism
- Higher incidence in patients with AIDS (4,5)
- Associated risk after bariatric surgery

RISK FACTORS
Genetics
Some rare familial disorders cause hypokalemia:
- Familial hypokalemic periodic paralysis: Hypokalemia after high-carbohydrate or high-sodium meal or after exercise
- Congenital adrenogenital syndromes
- Liddle syndrome: Increases K+ secretion
- Familial interstitial nephritis

GENERAL PREVENTION
When initiating a diuretic, especially loop and thiazide diuretics, patients should be advised to increase their dietary potassium intake (see Diet).

ETIOLOGY
- Most common causes:
- Decreased intake: Deficient diet in alcoholics and elderly, anorexia nervosa
- Gastrointestinal loss: Vomiting, diarrhea, nasogastric tubes, laxative abuse, fistulas, villous adenoma, ureterosigmoidostomy, malabsorption, chemotherapy, radiation enteropathy, bulimia
- Intracellular shift of potassium: Metabolic alkalosis, insulin excess, β-adrenergic catecholamine excess (acute stress, B$_2$ agonists), hypokalemic periodic paralysis, intoxications (theophylline, caffeine, barium, toluene)

- Renal potassium loss:
  – Drugs: Diuretics (especially loop and thiazides), amphotericin B, aminoglycosides (6,5,7,8)
  – Mineralocorticoid-excess states: Primary hyperaldosteronism, secondary hyperaldosteronism (congestive heart failure [CHF], cirrhosis, nephrotic syndrome, malignant hypertension, renin-producing tumors), renovascular hypertension, Bartter syndrome, Gitelman syndrome, congenital adrenogenital syndromes, exogenous mineralocorticoids (glycyrrhizic acid in licorice, carbenoxolone, steroids in nasal sprays), Liddle syndrome, vasculitis
- Glucocorticoid-excess states: Cushing syndrome, exogenous steroids, ectopic adrenocorticotrophic hormone (ACTH) production, II B hydroxysteroid dehydrogenase deficiency
- Renal tubular acidosis (type I and II):
  – Leukemia
  – Magnesium depletion
  – Thyrotoxic hypokalemic paralysis
- Osmotic diuresis (e.g., poorly controlled diabetes)

COMMONLY ASSOCIATED CONDITIONS
Acute gastrointestinal (GI) illnesses with severe vomiting or diarrhea

 DIAGNOSIS

- Patients with hypokalemia often have no symptoms, especially if the hypokalemia is mild (serum potassium 3.0–3.5 mEq/L).
- Neuromuscular (most prominent manifestations):
  – Skeletal muscle weakness (proximal > distal muscles, lower limbs > upper) may range from mild weakness to total paralysis, including respiratory muscles; may lead to rhabdomyolysis and/or respiratory arrest in severe cases.
  – Smooth-muscle involvement may lead to GI hypomotility, producing ileus and constipation (1)[B].
- Cardiovascular:
  – Ventricular arrhythmias; higher risk if underlying CHF, left ventricular failure (LVF), cardiac ischemia
  – Hypotension
  – Cardiac arrest
- Renal: Polyuria, polydipsia, nocturia owing to impaired concentrating ability, myoglobinuria
- Metabolic: Hyperglycemia

DIAGNOSTIC TESTS & INTERPRETATION
- Electrocardiogram (ECG) (9)[B]:
  – Hypokalemia increases the myocyte resting potential, which increases the refractory period; this can lead to arrhythmias.
  – Flattening or inversion of T waves
  – Increased prominence of U waves (small positive deflection after T wave, best seen in V2 and V3)
  – Depression of ST segment
  – Ventricular ectopia
- Workup for cause:
  – Excessive renal potassium loss: Urinary potassium is >20 mEq/d in presence of hypokalemia
  – In patient with excessive renal potassium loss and hypertension, plasma renin and aldosterone levels should be determined to differentiate adrenal from nonadrenal causes of hyperaldosteronism.
  – If hypertension is absent and patient is acidotic, renal tubular acidosis should be considered.
  – If hypertension is absent and serum pH is normal to alkalotic, high urine chloride (>10 mEq/d [>10 mmol/d]) suggests hypokalemia secondary to diuretics or Bartter syndrome; low urine chloride (<10 mEq/d [<10 mmol/d]) suggests vomiting as probable cause.

Lab
- Serum potassium <3.5 mEq/L (<3.5 mmol/L)
- Drugs that may alter lab results: Diuretics
- Disorders that may alter lab results: Leukemia and other conditions with high white blood cells (WBC)

Imaging
Computed tomography (CT) scan of adrenal glands if evidence of mineralocorticoid excess

Pathological Findings
In severe hypokalemia, necrosis of cardiac and skeletal muscle

DIFFERENTIAL DIAGNOSIS
- Spurious hypokalemia: Occurs when blood with high WBC count (>100,000/mm^3) is allowed to stand at room temperature (WBCs extract potassium from plasma)
- Thyrotoxicosis (10)

 TREATMENT

MEDICATION
- Nonemergent conditions (serum potassium >2.5 mEq/L [>2.5 mmol/L], no cardiac manifestations):
  – Oral therapy preferred; 40–120 mEq/d (40–120 mmol/d) in divided doses usually adequate
  – IV potassium should be given only when oral administration is not feasible (e.g., vomiting, postoperative state). Rate should not exceed 10 mEq/hour, and concentration should not exceed 40 mEq/L. Up to 40 mEq in 100 mL over 1 hour can be safely given through a central venous line. Patient's cardiac rhythm should be closely monitored.

– Potassium chloride is suitable for all forms of hypokalemia.
– Other potassium salts may be indicated if coexisting disorder is present: Potassium bicarbonate or bicarbonate precursor (gluconate, acetate, or citrate) in metabolic acidosis or phosphate in phosphate deficiency.
- Emergent situations (serum potassium <2.5 mEq/L [<2.5 mmol/L], arrhythmias): IV replacement:
– Rate of administration should not exceed 20 mEq/h (20 mmol/h); maximum recommended concentration, 60 mEq/L (60 mmol/L) of saline for peripheral administration. Administration through central venous lines may allow for greater concentrations.
- Check serum magnesium and replace if needed; cannot adequately replace potassium in setting of low magnesium.
- Precautions:
– Any form of potassium replacement carries risk of hyperkalemia.
– Serum potassium should be checked more frequently in groups at higher risk: Elderly, diabetic patients, and patients with renal insufficiency.
– Patients receiving digitalis and patients with diabetic ketoacidosis in whom intracellular shift in potassium is expected after insulin therapy is initiated must have more aggressive replacement.
- Significant possible interactions: Concomitant administration of potassium-sparing diuretics (spironolactone, triamterene, amiloride, angiotensin-converting enzyme [ACE] inhibitors) magnifies risk of hyperkalemia.

ADDITIONAL TREATMENT
General Measures
- For asymptomatic patients treated with oral replacement, outpatient follow-up is sufficient.
- Patients with cardiac manifestations require intravenous replacement with cardiac monitoring in an intensive care setting.

Geriatric Considerations
May need to correct magnesium depletion

ONGOING CARE

FOLLOW-UP RECOMMENDATIONS
Patient Monitoring
- Patients receiving IV therapy should have cardiac monitoring and serum potassium level checked frequently (q4–6h).
- Patients requiring potassium supplements should have serum potassium studied at intervals dictated by clinical judgment and patient compliance.

DIET
Mild hypokalemia (potassium 3.0–3.5 mEq/L [3.0–3.5 mmol/L]) not caused by gastrointestinal (GI) losses: Dietary supplementation may be sufficient; potassium-rich foods include oranges, bananas, cantaloupes, prunes, raisins, dried beans, dried apricots, and squash.

PATIENT EDUCATION
- Instructions for diet
- If potassium supplementation necessary, stress need for compliance

PROGNOSIS
- Associated with higher morbidity and mortality due to cardiac arrhythmias
- Ease of correction of hypokalemia and need for prolonged treatment rests on primary cause; if it can be eliminated (e.g., resolution of diarrhea, discontinuation of diuretics, removal of adrenal tumor), hypokalemia can be expected to resolve and no further treatment is indicated.

COMPLICATIONS
- Hyperkalemia can occur in the course of treatment (2).
- Increased risk of digoxin toxicity (1)[A]

REFERENCES

1. Schaefer TJ, Wolford RW. Disorders of potassium. *Emerg Med Clin North Am.* 2005;23:723–47, viii–ix.
2. Crop MJ, Hoorn EJ, Lindemans J, et al. Hypokalaemia and subsequent hyperkalaemia in hospitalized patients. *Nephrol Dial Transplant.* 2007.
3. Miller KK, Grinspoon SK, Ciampa J, et al. Medical findings in outpatients with anorexia nervosa. *Arch Intern Med.* 2005;165:561–6.
4. Peter SA. Electrolyte disorders and renal dysfunction in acquired immunodeficiency syndrome patients. *J Natl Med Assoc.* 1991;83:889–91.
5. Cirino CM, Kan VL. Hypokalemia in HIV patients on tenofovir. *AIDS.* 2006;20:1671–3.
6. Ben Salem C, Hmouda H, Bouraoui K. Drug-Induced Hypokalaemia. *Curr Drug Saf.* 2009;4:55–61.
7. Ernst ME, Moser M et al. Use of diuretics in patients with hypertension. *N Engl J Med.* 2009;361:2153–64.
8. Cowtan T et al. Thiazide diuretics. *N Engl J Med.* 2010;362:659; author reply 660.
9. Webster A, Brady W, Morris F. Recognising signs of danger: ECG changes resulting from an abnormal serum potassium concentration. *Emerg Med J.* 2002;19:74–7.
10. Barahona MJ, Vinagre I, Sojo L, et al. Thyrotoxic Periodic Paralysis: A Case Report and Literature Review. *Clin Med Res.* 2009.

ADDITIONAL READING

- Chan KE, Lazarus JM, Hakim RM et al. Digoxin Associates with Mortality in ESRD. *Journal of the American Society of Nephrology : JASN.* 2010;
- Facchini M, Sala L, Malfatto G, et al. Low-K+ dependent QT prolongation and risk for ventricular arrhythmia in anorexia nervosa. *Int J Cardiol.* 2006;106:170–6.
- Fisher M. Treatment of eating disorders in children, adolescents, and young adults. *Pediatr Rev.* 2006;27:5–16.
- Gennari FJ. Disorders of potassium homeostasis. Hypokalemia and hyperkalemia. *Crit Care Clin.* 2002;18:273–88, vi.
- Jones E. Hypokalemia. *N Engl J Med.* 2004;350:1156.
- Osadchii OE et al. Mechanisms of hypokalemia-induced ventricular arrhythmogenicity. *Fundamental & clinical pharmacology.* 2010;
- Vacca V. Hypokalemia. *Nursing.* 2009;39:64.
- Zietse R, Zoutendijk R, Hoorn EJ. Fluid, electrolyte and acid-base disorders associated with antibiotic therapy. *Nat Rev Nephrol.* 2009;5:193–202.

See Also (Topic, Algorithm, Electronic Media Element)
Hyperkalemia
Algorithm: Hypokalemia

CODES

ICD9
276.8 Hypopotassemia

CLINICAL PEARLS
- In patients without heart disease, a low potassium level will rarely cause cardiac disturbances. In an otherwise healthy patient, gentle repletion using oral potassium or an increase in potassium-rich foods should be adequate.
- In patients with cardiac ischemia, heart failure, or left ventricular hypertrophy, even mild-to-moderate hypokalemia can cause arrhythmias. These patients should receive potassium repletion as well as cardiac monitoring.
- To safely prevent hypokalemia in diabetic and renal insufficiency patients, the safest way is to ensure adequate dietary potassium intake with foods rich in potassium, including spinach, tomatoes, broccoli, squash, potatoes, bananas, cantaloupe, and oranges. Avoid potassium-sparing diuretics, if possible.
- Uncorrected hypomagnesemia can hinder the correction of hypokalemia. Check magnesium levels and replete as necessary.

H

HYPOKALEMIC PERIODIC PARALYSIS

Rebecca Burch, MD

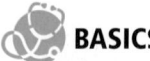 **BASICS**

DESCRIPTION
- Hypokalemic periodic paralysis (HPP) is a channelopathy characterized by episodic skeletal muscle weakness in the setting of a transient decrease in serum potassium (K) levels (1,2). There are 2 forms:
  – Familial hypokalemic periodic paralysis (FHPP), classified as type 1 or type 2 (see Etiology)
  – Hypokalemic periodic paralysis with thyrotoxicosis (thyrotoxic hypokalemic periodic paralysis [THPP])
- System(s) affected: Endocrine/Metabolic; Musculoskeletal; Nervous
- Synonym(s): Paroxysmal myoplegia

EPIDEMIOLOGY
- Predominant age: Onset of disease in late childhood or adolescence (FHPP), early adulthood (THPP). Onset >35 years of age is extremely rare (1,2).
- Age of onset depends on type of genetic mutation; earlier for type 1 FHPP by an average of 6 years (3).
- Predominant sex: FHPP, Male > Female (3:1) (2); THPPs, Male > Female (20:1)
- THPP typically affects Asian males; rare in Caucasians (4,5)

Prevalence
- 1/100,000 FHPP (estimated) (1,4)
- 4.3–13% of thyrotoxic Asian males develop THPP (5).

RISK FACTORS
- Male (1,2)
- Age <35
- Family history (FHPP)
- Asian (THPP)

Genetics
- FHPP: Autosomal dominant; incomplete penetrance in females (see Etiology) (1,2)
- THPP: Identifiable mutation in 1/3 of cases in 1 series, sporadic (6)

GENERAL PREVENTION
- See Medication (prevention of attacks) and Diet.
- FHPP: Genetic counseling; 50% risk of transmitting abnormal gene to offspring and 50% chance of affected siblings
- NINDS Familial Periodic Paralyses Information Page: http://www.ninds.nih.gov/disorders/periodic_paralysis/periodic_paralysis.htm

PATHOPHYSIOLOGY
- Exact pathogenesis unknown (1,2,3)
- Microelectrode studies show abnormal depolarization of skeletal muscle membrane (−50–60 mV instead of normal −90 mV) in presence of hypokalemia.
- Depolarization inactivates voltage-gated Na channels, preventing action potential propagation.
- Cardiac and smooth muscles are not directly affected.
- Contractile apparatus is normal.
- Hypokalemia is caused by intracellular K shift; total body K is normal (i.e., hypokalemia not a result of K loss).
- Pathogenesis of FHPP and THPP are likely different, as hyperthyroidism doesn't worsen FHPP.

ETIOLOGY
- FHPP is caused by 1 of several point mutations in skeletal muscle voltage-gated calcium channels (type 1 FHPP) or sodium channels (type 2 FHPP) (3,7).
- 70% of mutations causing FHPP are in the calcium channel; 10–15% in the sodium channel.
- THPP is associated with a mutation in a voltage-gated potassium channel in 1/3 of cases (6).

COMMONLY ASSOCIATED CONDITIONS
THPP: Hyperthyroidism (1,2,4)

 DIAGNOSIS

- Support by stabilizing ABCs if necessary (1,2)[C].
- Signs and symptoms are mostly neuromuscular (paresis) but can include cardiac (arrhythmias) and endocrine (hyperthyroidism in THPP only) (1,2)[C].

HISTORY
- Episodic attacks of focal or generalized muscle weakness lasting from a few hours to several days (1,2,3)[C]
- Typical attack occurs upon waking from sleep or in the early morning.
- Attacks usually provoked by strenuous exercise the day previous, also high-carbohydrate meals.
- Cold, stress, upper respiratory infections, high Na intake, alcohol, glucocorticoids, diuretics, insulin, or epinephrine may also exacerbate attack.
- Attacks more common in summer and fall (THPP)
- Prodrome of stiff muscles, diffuse aching, fatigue is common (5)
- Myalgias may be present.

PHYSICAL EXAM
- Limb muscle weakness: Lower extremity muscles affected more than upper; proximal muscles affected more than distal (1,2)[C]
- Muscle weakness usually symmetric
- Muscles of the eyes, face, tongue, pharynx, larynx, diaphragm, and sphincters rarely involved
- Hypoactive deep tendon reflexes
- Sensation preserved
- Strength between attacks usually near normal
- After years of attacks, patient may develop persistent proximal weakness.
- Patients with THPP may manifest signs of hyperthyroidism (especially systolic hypertension and tachycardia).

DIAGNOSTIC TESTS & INTERPRETATION
- Mild hypokalemia: Electrocardiogram (ECG) may show S-T depression, flattened T waves, or presence of U waves (2,4,7)[C].
- Severe hypokalemia: ECG may show peaked P waves, prolonged P-R interval, or widened QRS.
- Electromyography (EMG) done during attack usually shows low postexercise compound motor action potential; pattern may help diagnose type 1 vs type 2 FHPP.
- EMG usually normal between attacks
- Genetic testing (DNA sequencing) to differentiate type 1 from type 2 FHPP (Ca channel vs Na channel mutations)

Lab
- Low serum K (as low as 1 mEq/L [1 mmol/L]) is hallmark (1,8)[C]
- Low serum phosphorous also found
- Urine K usually low
- Serum creatine kinase level normal or slightly increased
- Acid-base balance normal
- Urine K/creatinine ratio low (<2)
- Elevated T_3, T_4, free thyroid index, and decreased thyroid-stimulating hormone (TSH) in THPP; may be only mildly abnormal (5)
- Hypercalciuria and hypophosphaturia are characteristic features of THPP (9)[B].

Imaging
Thyroid scans using radioiodine (THPP only)

Diagnostic Procedures/Surgery
- Provocative testing with 2g/kg (50–100 g) p.o. glucose and 10–20 units SC regular or fast-acting insulin (2)[C]
- If no weakness in 2–3 hours, may repeat with 2–8 g of p.o. Na and 50–100 g p.o. glucose, followed by exercise and/or insulin)
- Monitor closely for insulin-precipitated hypoglycemia.
- Patient should have cardiac monitoring during testing.
- Negative test does not exclude diagnosis.

Pathological Findings
- Muscle biopsy may show atrophy, vacuoles, or tubular aggregates (vacuolar myopathy) (7)[C].
- Vacuolar myopathy more likely in proximal muscles and more common in FHPP than THPP

DIFFERENTIAL DIAGNOSIS
- Akinetic epilepsy (1,2,4)
- Andersen-Tawil syndrome (triad of periodic paralysis, ventricular dysthymias, and dysmorphic features)
- Cataplexy
- Drop attacks
- Episodic ataxia
- Guillain-Barré syndrome
- Hyperkalemic or normokalemic periodic paralysis (adynamia episodica)
- Hyperventilation
- Myasthenia gravis
- Myotonia congenita
- Paramyotonia congenita
- Presyncope
- Secondary hypokalemia (laxative or diuretic use, diarrhea, vomiting, renal or adrenal disease, clay ingestion, barium poisoning)
- Sleep paralysis
- Tick paralysis

TREATMENT

Support by stabilizing ABCs if necessary.

MEDICATION

First Line

- Acute attack:
  - Goal is normalization of serum potassium
  - Oral potassium chloride (KCl): 0.2–0.4 mEq/kg, repeated q15–30 min depending on response of ECG, serum K+, muscle strength (usual total dose: 40 mEq) (2,3)[C]
  - In life-threatening situation or if vomiting, give IV KCl in mannitol or normal saline (5% glucose IV may worsen situation). Usual dose: 10–20 mEq/h, with frequent monitoring K and ECG (8,10)[B]. (Watch for rebound hyperkalemia.)
  - p.o. or IV propranolol (THPP only); p.o. dose is 3 mg/kg (4,8,11)[C]
- Prevention of attacks in FHPP:
  - Oral KCl, 10–20 mEq and titrated to clinic effect (2,3,7)[C]
  - Acetazolamide (Diamox): 125–1,000 mg/d divided per day to b.i.d. (type 1 FHPP or Ca-channel mutation only) (1,2,3,7)[B]
  - Acetazolamide can be cautiously tried in patients with type 2 FHPP or Na-channel mutation but it may precipitate attack (7)[C].
- Prevention of attacks in thyrotoxic hypokalemic periodic paralysis (4,8,11)[C]:
  - Treat underlying thyrotoxicosis with nonselective β-adrenergic blocking agents (propranolol [Inderal] and others). Symptoms do not occur if patient is euthyroid.
- Contraindications:
  - Acetazolamide: Marked hepatic or renal dysfunction, hypersensitivity, adrenal failure, hyperchloremic acidosis, low serum Na, THPP
  - Propranolol: Cardiogenic shock, sinus bradycardia, 2nd- or 3rd-degree heart block, congestive heart failure, bronchial asthma, hypersensitivity
- Precautions and adverse reactions:
  - Infusion of IV or p.o. KCl must be monitored to avoid potentially fatal hyperkalemia (1,4,8,11)[B].
  - Rebound hyperkalemia may occur in patients who receive >90 mEq KCl in 24 hours and in patients with THPP who receive KCl and propranolol (1,4,8,11)[B].
  - Acetazolamide may cause fatigue, malaise, metallic taste, diarrhea, and may precipitate or worsen paralysis in patients with type 2 FHPP (1,4)[C].
  - Propranolol: Use with caution if impaired hepatic or renal function, Raynaud's, diabetes mellitus, 2nd- or 3rd-trimester pregnancy
- Possible drug interactions:
  - Acetazolamide: High-dose aspirin, amphetamines, methenamine
  - Propranolol: Phenothiazines, calcium channel blocker

Second Line

- Acute attack: None
- Prevention of attacks in FHPP: Spironolactone (Aldactone): 25–200 mg/d (1)[C]; dichlorphenamide is an alternative to acetazolamide (12)
- Prevention of attacks in THPP: Antithyroid medications (propylthiouracil or methimazole), radioactive ablation of thyroid (4,8)[C]

ADDITIONAL TREATMENT

General Measures

- Mild hypokalemia or weakness: Outpatient K correction with close follow-up
- Severe hypokalemia or weakness: Inpatient K correction with cardiac monitoring

Issues for Referral

THPP: May need thyroid ablation

IN-PATIENT CONSIDERATIONS

Paralysis is often precipitated by surgery, and therefore close monitoring is warranted.

Initial Stabilization

May need respiratory support (rarely) and/or cardiac monitoring (usually done)

Admission Criteria

Severe weakness, hypokalemia with ECG findings, arrhythmias, respiratory compromise, need for IV KCL or propranolol

IV Fluids

Only as needed to administer IV KCL in mannitol or normal saline (5% glucose IV may worsen situation) or IV propranolol (see below) (1,4,11)[C]

Discharge Criteria

Resolution of symptoms

ONGOING CARE

FOLLOW-UP RECOMMENDATIONS

As tolerated, mild exercise may help (2,3,7)[C]

Patient Monitoring

- Follow serum K and electrolytes (if on acetazolamide).
- Follow thyroid function tests (if on propranolol or antithyroid drugs).

DIET

Avoid high-carbohydrate, high-Na foods (2,3,7)[C].

PATIENT EDUCATION

- Strenuous exercise in combination with high-carbohydrate or high-Na meals may provoke attack.
- Attacks are also provoked by cold, stress, and alcohol.

PROGNOSIS

- Attack frequency usually lessens with age.
- Up to 2/3 of patients develop persistent proximal weakness (3).
- Thyroid ablation resolves attacks (THPP only).

COMPLICATIONS

- Cardiac arrhythmias
- Respiratory collapse

REFERENCES

1. Stedwell RE, Allen KM, Binder LS. Hypokalemic paralyses: a review of the etiologies, pathophysiology, presentation, and therapy. *Am J Emerg Med*. 1992;10:143–8.
2. Lehmann-Horn F, Rüdel R. Channelopathies: the nondystrophic myotonias and periodic paralyses. *Semin Pediatr Neurol*. 1996;3:122–39.
3. Venance SL, Cannon SC, Fialho D, et al. The primary periodic paralyses: diagnosis, pathogenesis and treatment. *Brain*. 2006;129:8–17.
4. Lin SH. Thyrotoxic periodic paralysis. *Mayo Clin Proc*. 2005;80:99–105.
5. Kung AW. Thyrotoxic Periodic Paralysis: A Diagnostic Challenge. *J Clin Endocrinol Metab*. 2006.
6. Ryan DP, da Silva MR, Soong TW, Fontaine B, Donaldson MR, Kung AW, Jongjaroenprasert W, Liang MC, Khoo DH, Cheah JS, Ho SC, Bernstein HS, Maciel RM, Brown RH, Ptácek LJ et al. Mutations in potassium channel Kir2.6 cause susceptibility to thyrotoxic hypokalemic periodic paralysis. *Cell*. 2010;140:88–98.
7. Fontaine B, Fournier E, Sternberg D, et al. Hypokalemic periodic paralysis: a model for a clinical and research approach to a rare disorder. *Neurotherapeutics*. 2007;4:225–32.
8. Manoukian MA, Foote JA, Crapo LM. Clinical and metabolic features of thyrotoxic periodic paralysis in 24 episodes. *Arch Intern Med*. 1999;159:601–6.
9. Lin SH, Chu P, Cheng CJ, et al. Early diagnosis of thyrotoxic periodic paralysis: Spot urine calcium to phosphate ratio* *Crit Care Med*. 2006.
10. Lu KC, Hsu YJ, Chiu JS, et al. Effects of potassium supplementation on the recovery of thyrotoxic periodic paralysis. *Am J Emerg Med*. 2004;22:544–7.
11. Lin SH, Lin YF. Propranolol rapidly reverses paralysis, hypokalemia, and hypophosphatemia in thyrotoxic periodic paralysis. *Am J Kidney Dis*. 2001;37:620–3.
12. Tawil R, McDermott MP, Brown R, et al. Randomized trials of dichlorphenamide in the periodic paralyses. Working Group on Periodic Paralysis. *Ann Neurol*. 2000;47:46–53.

ADDITIONAL READING

Sansone V, Meola G, Links TP, et al. Treatment for periodic paralysis. *Cochrane Database Syst Rev*. 2008:CD005045.

See Also (Topic, Algorithm, Electronic Media Element)

Guillain-Barré Syndrome; Hyperthyroidism; Hypokalemia; Myasthenia Gravis

CODES

ICD9

359.3 Periodic paralysis

CLINICAL PEARLS

- Hypokalemic periodic paralysis should be suspected when a young, otherwise healthy male presents complaining of weakness on awakening, especially after exercising or eating a high carbohydrate meal, and serum K is low, but he has no vomiting or diarrhea.
- Serum K, ECG, and TSH tests should be done immediately.
- The usual immediate therapy is to cautiously administer oral KCL 10–20 mEq, q15–30 min, with cardiac monitoring and frequent serum K. If TSH is low, add propranolol, 3 mg/kg.

H

HYPONATREMIA

Ruben Peralta, MD

BASICS

DESCRIPTION
- Hyponatremia is a plasma sodium concentration of <135 mEq/L.
- System(s) affected: Endocrine/Metabolic

EPIDEMIOLOGY
Incidence
- Most common electrolyte disorder seen in general hospital population (1)
- Predominant age: All ages
- Predominant sex: Male = Female.

Prevalence
2.5% of hospitalized patients (1)

RISK FACTORS
Genetics
- Polymorphisms have been demonstrated.
- Mutations have been associated with nephrogenic syndrome of inappropriate antidiuresis (NSIAD).

GENERAL PREVENTION
Depends on underlying condition

PATHOPHYSIOLOGY
- Hypovolemic hyponatremia: Decrease in total body water and greater decrease in total body sodium; decreased extracellular fluid volume; orthostatic hypotension and other changes consistent with hypovolemia are present.
- Euvolemic hyponatremia: Increase in total body water with normal total body sodium; extracellular fluid volume is minimally to moderately increased but with no edema.
- Hypervolemic hyponatremia: Increase in total body sodium and greater increase in total body water; extracellular fluid increased markedly; edema present
- Redistributive hyponatremia: Shift of water from intracellular compartment to extracellular compartment with resulting dilution of sodium; total body water and total body sodium unchanged; occurs with hyperglycemia.
- Pseudohyponatremia: Dilution of aqueous phase by excessive proteins, glucose, or lipids; total body water and total body sodium unchanged; occurs in hypertriglyceridemia or multiple myeloma.
- Low sodium creates an osmotic gradient between plasma and cells, and fluid shifts into cells, causing edema and increased intracranial pressure (ICP).

ETIOLOGY
- Hypovolemic hyponatremia: Extrarenal loss of sodium (urine Na <30 mmol/L):
  - GI loss: Vomiting, diarrhea
  - Third spacing: Peritonitis, pancreatitis, burns, rhabdomyolysis
  - Skin loss: Burns, sweating, cystic fibrosis
  - Heat-related illnesses
- Hypovolemic hyponatremia: Renal loss of sodium (urine Na >30 mmol/L):
  - Cerebral Salt Wasting Syndrome (CSWS)
  - Adrenal pathology (e.g., Addison disease, hemorrhage, tuberculosis)
  - Diuretics
  - Osmotic diuresis

- Euvolemic hyponatremia (urine Na >30 mmol/L):
  - Hypothyroidism
  - Hypopituitarism or other cause of glucocorticoid deficiency
  - Medications (e.g., carbamazepine, clofibrate, cyclosporine, levetiracetam, opiates, oxcarbazepine, phenothiazines, tricyclic antidepressants, vincristine) (2,3,4)
  - Primary polydipsia
  - Syndrome of inappropriate antidiuretic hormone secretion (SIADH)
  - Iatrogenic (e.g., excess hypotonic IV fluids)
- Hypervolemic hyponatremia (urine Na <30 mmol/L, except chronic renal failure):
  - Nephrotic syndrome
  - Cirrhosis
  - Congestive heart failure (CHF)
  - Chronic renal failure
- Redistributive hyponatremia:
  - Hyperglycemia
  - Mannitol infusion
  - Hypertriglyceridemia
- Multiple myeloma

COMMONLY ASSOCIATED CONDITIONS
- Hypothyroidism
- Hypopituitarism
- Adrenocortical hormone deficiency
- HIV patients
- SIADH associated with cancers, pneumonia, tuberculosis, encephalitis, meningitis, head trauma, cerebrovascular accident (CVA), HIV infection (5)[B],(6)
- Acute neurological patients, brain injury (7,8,9)
- Marathon runners in hot environment

DIAGNOSIS

- Symptoms related to the rate of fall in serum sodium and the degree of hyponatremia (10,11)
- Mild (130–135 mEq/L): Usually asymptomatic
- Moderate (120–130 mEq/L): Nausea, vomiting, malaise
- Severe: (115–120 mEq/L): Headache, lethargy, restlessness, disorientation
- With severe/rapid decreases, can cause seizure, coma, and respiratory arrest and may be fatal
- Other signs and symptoms: Weakness, muscle cramps, anorexia, hiccups, depressed deep tendon reflexes, hypothermia, positive Babinski responses, cranial nerve palsies, orthostatic hypotension

PHYSICAL EXAM
- Volume status: Skin turgor, jugular venous pressure, heart rate, orthostatic BP
- Exam for underlying illness: Signs of CHF, cirrhosis, hypothyroidism

DIAGNOSTIC TESTS & INTERPRETATION
Lab
- Serum sodium <135 mmol/L
- Plasma osmolality
- Urine sodium and osmolality
- Renal function
- Hepatic function
- Thyroid function
- Serum glucose, lipids

- Hypovolemic hyponatremia:
  - Plasma osmolality low
  - Blood urea nitrogen (BUN): creatinine ratio >20:1
  - Urine sodium >20 mEq/L (>20 mmol/L): Renal loss
  - Urine sodium <10 mEq/L (<10 mmol/L): Extrarenal loss
  - Serum potassium >5.0 mEq/L (>5 mmol/L): Consider mineralocorticoid deficiency.
- Euvolemic hyponatremia:
  - Plasma osmolality low
  - BUN: creatinine ratio <20:1
  - Urine sodium >20 mEq/L (>20 mmol/L)
  - Thyroid-stimulating hormone (TSH) test to rule out hypothyroidism
  - 1-h cosyntropin-stimulation test to rule out adrenal insufficiency
- Hypervolemic hyponatremia:
  - Plasma osmolality low
  - Urine sodium <10 mEq/L (<10 mmol/L) in nephrotic syndrome, CHF, cirrhosis
  - Urine sodium >20 mEq/L (>20 mmol/L) in acute and chronic renal failure
- Redistributive hyponatremia:
  - Plasma osmolality normal or high
  - Glucose or mannitol levels elevated
- Pseudohyponatremia:
  - Plasma osmolality normal
  - Triglyceride, glucose, or protein levels elevated

Imaging
- CT scan of head if pituitary problem suspected or if SIADH from CNS problem suspected
- CXR to rule out pulmonary pathology if SIADH diagnosed

DIFFERENTIAL DIAGNOSIS
See Etiology.

TREATMENT

MEDICATION
- Treatment tailored to clinical situation: Degree and rate of hyponatremia and whether or not the patient is symptomatic; some general principles apply (10).
- Asymptomatic, euvolemic patients can be treated with fluid restriction plus addressing the underlying cause.
- For severely hyponatremic/symptomatic patients, generally considered safe to increase the serum Na by 0.6–2.0 mEq/L each hour, not to exceed 8 mEq/24 h.
- Treatment of underlying condition: Heart failure, cirrhosis, etc., essential
- In patients with euvolemic or hypervolemic hyponatremia, tolvaptan, an oral vasopressin V_2-receptor antagonist, was effective in increasing serum sodium concentrations (12).
- Rapid correction of severe symptomatic hyponatremia has been associated with central pontine myelinolysis, a neurologic disorder that induces loss of myelin and supportive structures in pons and occasionally in other areas of the brain. This results in irreversible injury. Symptoms are apparent 2–6 days after injury and include seizure, coma, spastic paraparesis, dysarthria, and dysphagia.
- Use of hypertonic saline (3% NaCl) has only a slight evidence base; consider consulting with specialist before undertaking this treatment (5).

- Chronic hyponatremia owing to SIADH: Demeclocycline (inhibits ADH action at the collecting duct) if fluid restriction alone is not effective:
  - Contraindication: Can cause nephrotoxicity in patients with liver disease
  - In doses of 600–1,200 mg/d, drug produces a nephrogenic diabetes insipidus.
  - Significant possible interactions: Oral anticoagulants, oral contraceptives, penicillin

ADDITIONAL TREATMENT
General Measures
- Inpatient treatment mandatory if acute hyponatremia or symptomatic; acute (developing over <48 h) hyponatremia carries the risk of cerebral edema.
- Inpatient treatment is advised if asymptomatic and serum sodium <125 mEq/dL.
- Assess all medications patient is taking.
- Institute seizure precautions.

IN-PATIENT CONSIDERATIONS
Admission Criteria
- Admission mandatory if acute hyponatremia or symptomatic; acute (developing over <48 h) hyponatremia carries the risk of cerebral edema.
- Admission is advised if patient is asymptomatic and has a serum sodium <125 mEq/dL.

ONGOING CARE

DIET
- Euvolemic hyponatremia: Water restriction to 1 L/d
- Hypervolemic hyponatremia: Water and sodium restriction

PROGNOSIS
- In hospitalized patients, hyponatremia is associated with elevated risk of adverse clinical outcomes and higher mortality (13,14).
- Recently, in community-dwelling middle-aged and elderly adults, mild hyponatremia has been shown to be an independent predictor of death.
- Associated with poor prognosis in patients with acute pulmonary embolism (15)
- Associated with poor prognosis in liver cirrhosis and in patients waiting for liver transplant and is associated with significant post-operative risk and short-term graft lost (14,16)

COMPLICATIONS
- Occult tumor may present with SIADH.
- Hypervolemia if saline used
- Central pontine myelinolysis (see above) (17)
- Hyponatremia is cause in 30% new-onset seizures in ICU.
- Chronic hyponatremia is associated with an increased odds of osteoporosis (18).

REFERENCES

1. Upadhyay A, Jaber BL, Madias NE. Epidemiology of hyponatremia. *Semin Nephrol.* 2009;29: 227–38.
2. Ben Salem C, Hmouda H, Bouraoui K. Drug-induced hyponatremia: adding to the list. *Am J Kidney Dis.* 2008;52:1025–6; author reply 1027.
3. Meulendijks D, Mannesse CK, Jansen PA et al. Antipsychotic-induced hyponatraemia: a systematic review of the published evidence. *Drug Saf.* 2010;33:101–14.
4. Jacob S, Spinler SA et al. Hyponatremia associated with selective serotonin-reuptake inhibitors in older adults. *Ann Pharmacother.* 2006;40: 1618–22.
5. Yeates KE, Singer M, Morton AR. Salt and water: a simple approach to hyponatremia. *CMAJ.* 2004; 170:365–9.
6. Lim YJ, Park EK, Koh HC et al. Syndrome of inappropriate secretion of antidiuretic hormone as a leading cause of hyponatremia in children who underwent chemotherapy or stem cell transplantation. *Pediatr Blood Cancer.* 2010;54:734–7.
7. Brimioulle S, Orellana-Jimenez C, Aminian A et al. Hyponatremia in neurological patients: cerebral salt wasting versus inappropriate antidiuretic hormone secretion. *Intensive Care Med.* 2008;34:125–31.
8. Costa KN, Nakamura HM, da Cruz LR et al. Hyponatremia and brain injury: absence of alterations of serum brain natriuretic peptide and vasopressin. *Arq Neuropsiquiatr.* 2009;67: 1037–44.
9. Chang CH, Liao JJ, Chuang CH et al. Recurrent hyponatremia after traumatic brain injury. *Am J Med. Sci.* 2008;335:390–3.
10. Ellison DH, Berl T. Clinical practice. The syndrome of inappropriate antidiuresis. *N Engl J Med.* 2007;356:2064–72.
11. Duracher C, Baugnon T, Blanot S, et al. Intraoperative hyponatremia: is it related to surgical procedure or fluid maintenance? *Paediatr Anaesth.* 2009;19:711–2.
12. Rozen-Zvi B, Yahav D, Gheorghiade M, Korzets A, Leibovici L, Gafter U et al. Vasopressin receptor antagonists for the treatment of hyponatremia: systematic review and meta-analysis. *Am J Kidney Dis.* 2010;56:325–37.
13. Kugler JP, Hustead T. Hyponatremia and hypernatremia in the elderly. *Am Fam Physician.* 2000;61:3623–30.
14. Cárdenas A, Ginès P. Predicting mortality in cirrhosis—serum sodium helps. *N Engl J Med.* 2008;359:1060–2.
15. Scherz N, Labarère J, Méan M et al. Prognostic Importance of Hyponatremia in Patients with Acute Pulmonary Embolism. *American journal of respiratory and critical care medicine.* 2010;

16. Fukuhara T, Ikegami T, Morita K et al. Impact of preoperative serum sodium concentration in living donor liver transplantation. *J Gastroenterol Hepatol.* 2010;25:978–84.
17. Fleming JD, Babu S. Images in clinical medicine. Central pontine myelinolysis. *N Engl J Med.* 2008 Dec 4;359(23):e29.
18. Verbalis JG, Barsony J, Sugimura Y et al. Hyponatremia-induced osteoporosis. *J Bone Miner Res.* 2010;25:554–63.

ADDITIONAL READING
- Callahan MA, Do HT, Caplan DW, et al. Economic impact of hyponatremia in hospitalized patients: a retrospective cohort study. *Postgrad Med.* 2009; 121:186–91.
- Cowtan T et al. Thiazide diuretics. *N Engl J Med.* 2010;362:659–660
- Ernst ME, Moser M et al. Use of diuretics in patients with hypertension. *N Engl J Med.* 2009;361: 2153–64.

See Also (Topic, Algorithm, Electronic Media Element)
Algorithm: Hyponatremia

CODES

ICD9
276.1 Hyposmolality and/or hyponatremia

CLINICAL PEARLS
- Alcohol-dependent individuals with vitamin deficiencies, elderly women taking thiazide diuretics, and people with hypokalemia or burns are at increased risk of central pontine myelinolysis. A longer duration of hyponatremia is also a risk factor.
- Elderly people have lower total body water, decreased thirst mechanism, decreased urinary concentrating ability, kidneys are less responsive to ADH, and individuals show decreased renal mass, renal blood flow, and glomerular filtration rate.
- Bronchogenic carcinoma, pancreas, duodenal, prostate, thymoma, lymphoma, and mesothelioma are neoplastic diseases associated with SIADH.
- MDMA (ecstasy) is an illicit drug that causes hyponatremia (5)[B].

H

HYPOPARATHYROIDISM

Daniel J. Barker, MD

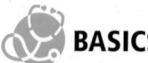 **BASICS**

DESCRIPTION

- Hypoparathyroidism is a relative or absolute deficiency of parathyroid hormone due to disease, surgical injury, congenital absence or malfunction of parathyroid glands. Manifested as hypocalcemia, producing symptoms ranging from paresthesias to tetany.
- Parathyroid hormone (PTH) mobilizes calcium from bone, stimulates reabsorption of calcium in distal nephron, and enhances formation of the active vitamin D metabolite, 1,25-dihydroxy-vitamin D.
- Classifications:
  - Acquired hypoparathyroidism
    - Accidental removal or damage to parathyroid glands or their blood supply during neck surgery. Decreased parathyroid levels may be transient or permanent.
    - Autoimmune: May develop as isolated destruction of parathyroid or part of autoimmune polyendocrine syndrome 1 (APS-1).
    - Deposition of heavy metals in gland (copper or iron), radiation-induced destruction, and metastatic infiltration are less common acquired forms of hypoparathyroidism.
  - Genetic hypoparathyroidism: May be a manifestation of multiple genetic aberrancies. Most commonly involves calcium-sensing receptor.
  - Functional hypoparathyroidism: May be secondary to either hyper- or hypomagnesemia (seen in alcoholics). Parathyroid adenoma may suppress normal parathyroid gland.
- System(s) affected: Endocrine/Metabolic; Musculoskeletal; Nervous

Pediatric Considerations
- May occur in premature infants
- Neonates born to hypercalcemic mothers may experience suppression of developing parathyroid glands .
- Congenital absence of parathyroids
- May appear later in childhood as autoimmune or APS-1

Geriatric Considerations
Hypocalcemia is fairly common in the elderly; however, it is rarely secondary to hypoparathyroidism.

Pregnancy Considerations
Use of magnesium as a tocolytic may induce functional hypoparathyroidism.

EPIDEMIOLOGY
Thyroid and parathyroid disease conditions resulting in surgical intervention are more common in women. More than 250,000 individuals undergo thyroid or parathyroid procedures. Affects individuals of all ages.

Incidence
Estimated to occur after 0.5–6.6% of total thyroidectomies; varies depending on skill and experience of surgeon and extent of surgical procedure

Prevalence
Varies widely depending upon etiology

RISK FACTORS
- Neck surgery, especially thyroid
- Neck trauma
- Head and neck malignancies
- Family history of hypocalcemia
- Autoimmune endocrinopathy

Genetics
- Mutations in transcription factors or regulators of parathyroid gland development:
  - Hypoparathyroidism may present as a component of a larger genetic syndrome (APS-1 or DiGeorge Syndrome) or in isolation (x-linked hypoparathyroidism)
  - May be autosomal dominant (DiGeorge), autosomal recessive (APS-1), or x-linked recessive (x-linked hypoparathyroidism)
- PTH gene mutations:
  - Hypoparathyroidism presents in isolation
  - May be autosomal dominant or autosomal recessive
- Mitochondrial disorders with hypoparathyroidism:
  - Typically hypoparathyroidism exists in conjunction with other congenital anomalies or metabolic derangements
  - Maternal transmission

GENERAL PREVENTION
Intraoperative identification and preservation of parathyroid tissue

PATHOPHYSIOLOGY
- PTH is involved in the control of serum ionized calcium levels. PTH:
  - Mobilizes calcium and phosphorus from bone stores
  - Stimulates formation of 1,25-dihydroxy-vitamin D
  - Stimulates reabsorption of calcium in the distal nephron and phosphate excretion
- Loss of PTH action results in hypocalcemia, hyperphosphatemia, and hypercalciuria
- Magnesium is crucial for PTH secretion and activation of the PTH receptor; hypo- or hypermagnesemia may result in functional hypoparathyroidism.

ETIOLOGY
- Postsurgical: Transient or permanent
- Genetic
- Autoimmune
- Infiltrative
  - Metastatic carcinoma
  - Hemochromatosis
  - Wilson disease
- Irradiation
- Hypo- or hypermagnesemia

COMMONLY ASSOCIATED CONDITIONS
- DiGeorge syndrome
- Autoimmune polyendocrine syndrome type 1 (APS-1). Features include:
  - Chronic yeast infections
  - Addison disease

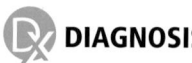 **DIAGNOSIS**

HISTORY
- Chronic hypocalcemia may be asymptomatic.
- Fatigue
- Circumoral or distal extremity paresthesias
- Muscle cramps
- Neuropsychiatric symptoms
- Seizures
- Previous neck trauma or surgery
- Head and neck irradiation
- Family history of hypocalcemia
- Presence of other autoimmune endocrinopathies

PHYSICAL EXAM
- Surgical scar on neck
- Chvostek sign: Positive sign is ipsilateral twitching of the upper lip upon tapping the facial nerve on the cheek.
- Trousseau sign: Positive sign is painful carpal spasm after 3-minute occlusion of brachial artery with blood pressure cuff.
- Tetany
- Laryngo- or bronchospasm
- Cataracts
- Cardiac arrhythmias or failure
- Dry hair, brittle nails

DIAGNOSTIC TESTS & INTERPRETATION
Lab
Initial lab tests
- Blood work ()[C]:
  - Calcium: Total and ionized (low)
  - Albumin (correct serum calcium level for albumin)
    - Corrected serum calcium = Total serum calcium + 0.8 (4.0 − serum albumin)
  - Phosphorus (high)
  - Intact PTH (low or inappropriately normal)
  - Magnesium (low or high may cause hypoparathyroidism; may also be normal)
  - BUN, creatinine (normal)
  - 25 OH vitamin D level
- Urinary calcium (normal or high) (1)[C]

Follow-Up & Special Considerations
- EKG may show prolonged QT and ST (secondary to hypocalcemia) (1)[C] .
- Gene sequencing may be required to diagnose genetic causes.
- Evaluation of other hormone levels may be required to diagnose APS-1.

Imaging
Radiographs may show absent tooth roots, calcification of cerebellum, choroid plexus, or cerebral basal ganglia.

Pathological Findings
Parathyroid gland parenchymal tissue completely or almost completely replaced by fat

DIFFERENTIAL DIAGNOSIS
- Vitamin D deficiency/resistance
- Pseudohypoparathyroidism: Resistance of end organs to PTH resulting in hypocalcemia with high PTH
- Hypoalbuminemia
- Renal failure
- Malabsorption
- Familial hypocalcemia
- Hypomagnesemia

TREATMENT

MEDICATION
First Line
- No formal guidelines for treatment exist at this time.
- Severe symptoms (tetany, seizures, cardiac failure, laryngospasm, bronchospasm):
  - Short-term management (1)[C]
    - IV calcium gluconate: 1 or 2 g, each infused over a period of 10 minutes. Central venous catheter preferred because calcium-containing solutions can irritate surrounding tissues.
    - Follow with infusion 10 g calcium gluconate in 1 L 5% dextrose water at a rate of 1–3 mg calcium gluconate/kg of body weight/hour
  - Long-term management
    - Oral calcium carbonate: 500–1000 mg of elemental calcium 3 times a day. Constipation is a common side effect (2)[C]
    - Calcitriol: Start at 0.25 mcg once to twice daily. Max dose 2 mcg daily (1)[C].
- Asymptomatic, mildly symptomatic, or mild hypocalcemia
  - Oral calcium: as above. Adjust to control symptoms and achieve target serum calcium.
  - Calcitriol: As above

Second Line
Oral vitamin D: 25,000–100,000 units/day (1)[C]

ADDITIONAL TREATMENT
General Measures
- Monitor EKG during calcium repletion.
- Maintenance therapy:
  - May require lifelong treatment with calcium and calcitriol
  - Maintain serum calcium in low normal range: 8.0–8.5 mg/dL (2.0–2.12 mmol/L) (1,2)[C]
- Adequate control requires careful attention to avoid over- or undertreatment.
- If hypercalcemia occurs, hold therapy until calcium returns to normal.
- Treat magnesium deficiency if present.
- Phosphate binders required if high calcium-phosphate product
- Thiazide diuretics combined with low-salt diet may be used to prevent hypercalciuria, nephrocalcinosis, and nephrolithiasis.
- Oral calcium administration and vitamin D supplementation post-thyroidectomy may reduce risk for symptomatic hypocalcemia after surgery (3)[C].

Issues for Referral
May require referral to endocrinologist

Additional Therapies
Parathyroid hormone 1–34 (subcutaneous) (4)[C]
- May be as effective as calcitriol for maintaining growth and serum calcium levels in children with chronic hypoparathyroidism
- Unproven method of treatment at this juncture; further study required

IN-PATIENT CONSIDERATIONS
Initial Stabilization
See Treatment, Medications

Admission Criteria
- Laryngospasm
- Seizures
- Tetany
- QT prolongation

Nursing
Monitor for hypocalcemic symptoms.

Discharge Criteria
- Resolution of hypocalcemic symptoms
- Patient educated on hypoparathyroidism and treatment protocol
- Outpatient follow-up scheduled

 ONGOING CARE

FOLLOW-UP RECOMMENDATIONS
Patient Monitoring
- Goal of treatment is to reach a total corrected serum calcium level in low normal range (8.0–8.5 mg/dL or 2.0–2.12 mmol/L), 24-hour urine calcium below 300 mg and calcium-phosphate product below 55.
- Outpatient measurement of serum calcium, phosphorus, and creatinine weekly to monthly during initial management
- Once regimen stable, measure serum calcium, phosphate, and creatinine twice yearly.
- Measurement of urine calcium and creatinine twice yearly
- Annual slit lamp and ophthalmologic evaluation are recommended.

DIET
Low phosphate diet in patients with hyperphosphatemia

PATIENT EDUCATION
- Provide careful and detailed instructions about maintenance therapy.
- Explain importance of periodic blood chemistry evaluations.
- Instruct patient to watch for signs and symptoms of over- and undertreatment.

PROGNOSIS
- Hypoparathyroidism following neck surgery is often transient.
- Length of required treatment may vary depending on origin.
- Symptoms and serum calcium can be well controlled with treatment.

COMPLICATIONS
- Neuromuscular symptoms (resolve with treatment)
- Hypercalciuria, nephrocalcinosis, nephrolithiasis
- Hypercalcemia with excessive treatment
- Calciphylaxis with high calcium-phosphate product
- Cataracts
- Basal ganglia calcifications with Parkinsonian symptoms
- If condition starts early in childhood: Stunting of growth, malformation of teeth, mental retardation

REFERENCES
1. Shoback D. Clinical practice. Hypoparathyroidism. *N Engl J Med.* 2008;359:391–403.
2. Cooper MS, Gittoes NJ. Diagnosis and management of hypocalcaemia. *BMJ.* 2008;336:1298–302.
3. Roh JL, Park CI et al. Routine oral calcium and vitamin D supplements for prevention of hypocalcemia after total thyroidectomy. *Am J Surg.* 2006;192:675–8.
4. Winer KK, Sinaii N, Reynolds J, Peterson D, Dowdy K, Cutler GB et al. Long-Term Treatment of 12 Children with Chronic Hypoparathyroidism: A Randomized Trial Comparing Synthetic Human Parathyroid Hormone 1–34 versus Calcitriol and Calcium. *The Journal of clinical endocrinology and metabolism.* 2010;

ADDITIONAL READING
- Betterle C, Zanchetta R. Update on autoimmune polyendocrine syndromes (APS). *Acta Biomed Ateneo Parmense.* 2003;74:9–33.
- Gunn IR, Gaffney D. Clinical and laboratory features of calcium-sensing receptor disorders: a systematic review. *Ann Clin Biochem.* 2004;41:441–58.
- Thakker RV. Genetics of endocrine and metabolic disorders: parathyroid. *Rev Endocr Metab Disord.* 2004;5:37–51.

 CODES

ICD9
252.1 Hypoparathyroidism

CLINICAL PEARLS
- The most common etiology of hypoparathyroidism is damage to the parathyroid glands or blood supply during neck surgery; other causes include congenital and infiltrative disease.
- Patients with hypoparathyroidism may be asymptomatic or present with symptoms of hypocalcemia, including paresthesias, tetany, or laryngospasm.
- In the presence of severe neuromuscular or cardiac symptoms, emergent treatment should begin with parenteral calcium.
- Treatment with calcium and calcitriol may be required transiently or permanently depending on origin of hypoparathyroidism.
- Treatment goal is total serum calcium in low-normal range: 8.0–8.5 mg/dL (2.0–2.12 mmol/L).

H

HYPOPITUITARISM

Anup Kumar Sabharwal, MD

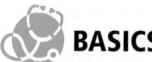 **BASICS**

DESCRIPTION
- Generalized condition caused by partial or total failure of anterior pituitary gland's hormones: adrenocorticotropic hormone (ACTH), thyroid-stimulating hormone (TSH), luteinizing hormone (LH), follicle-stimulating hormone (FSH), growth hormone (GH), and prolactin. Less commonly, the posterior pituitary gland's hormones can be affected: AVP/ADH and oxytocin.
- System(s) affected: Cardiovascular; Endocrine/Metabolic; Gastrointestinal; Musculoskeletal; Nervous; Reproductive; Skin/Exocrine
- Synonym(s): Empty sella syndrome; Hypopituitarism; Pituitary cachexia; Simmonds syndrome; Panhypopituitarism; as a consequence of blood loss during pregnancy, Sheehan syndrome
- Shortages of ACTH, TSH, and ADH can be life-threatening.
- First described by Dr. Morris Simmonds in 1914

EPIDEMIOLOGY
Incidence
- 12–42 new cases per million per year
- Predominant age: Occurs in adults and children. In children, it may cause short stature and pubertal delay.
- Predominant sex: Male = Female

Prevalence
- In a Northern Spain study, 45.5 per 100,000 were diagnosed with hypopituitarism with 4.2 new cases diagnosed per year.
- Of these patients 61% were due to pituitary tumors, 9% had other lesions, 19% had other causes, and 11% were idiopathic.

RISK FACTORS
- Trauma
- Pregnancy and delivery
- Tumors
- Irradiation
- Postoperative
- Vascular aneurysms
- Lymphocytic hypophysitis
- Infiltrative diseases
- Infections

Genetics
- Pituitary and hypothalamic hormone transcription factor defects:
  - *AVP*, diabetes insipidus
  - *DAX-1*, adrenal hypoplasia congenital, hypogonadotropic hypogonadism
  - *GnRH-R* and *GPR54* loss-of-function mutations
  - *HESX-1*, associated with septo-optic dysplasia
  - *KAL1* and *FGFR1*, Kallmann syndrome
  - *PROP1*, combined pituitary hormone deficiency
  - *POMC*, ACTH deficiency, obesity, red hair
  - *POU1F1 (Pit-1)*, combined pituitary hormone deficiency
  - *SF1*, adrenal failure, 46,XY gonadal dysgenesis

- Genetic defects in pituitary hormone receptors:
  - ACTH receptor defects: Congenital insensitivity to ACTH
  - GH receptor defects: Laron dwarfism
  - LH/FSH receptor mutations
  - TSH receptor loss-of-function mutation

GENERAL PREVENTION
Prevention of head trauma, experienced neurosurgeon

ETIOLOGY
- Childhood:
  - Genetic disorders
  - Perinatal asphyxia
  - Developmental disorders/pituitary hypoplasia, aplasia
  - Craniopharyngioma, other tumors
  - Cranial irradiation
  - Head trauma
- Adult:
  - Pituitary tumors: Most common etiology; other intrasellar or extrasellar tumors: meningiomas, gliomas, metastases, craniopharyngiomas, chordomas, ependymomas, suprasellar dysgerminomas, infundibulomas, astrocytomas, hamartomas
  - Surgery on pituitary or adjacent structures
  - Cranial irradiation
  - Vascular: Internal carotid artery aneurysm, subarachnoid hemorrhage, pituitary infarction, apoplexy, postpartum hemorrhage with hypotension (Sheehan syndrome)
  - Head trauma
  - Infection: Abscess, hypophysitis, meningitis, encephalitis, tuberculosis, pneumocystis, histoplasmosis, toxoplasmosis, aspergillosis, cytomegalovirus
  - Infiltrative conditions: Hemochromatosis, granulomatous disease, histiocytosis X, sarcoidosis
  - Hypothalamic disease (secondary hypopituitarism)
  - Autoimmune disease: Lymphocytic hypophysitis
  - Chronic debilitating disease, nonspecific
  - Empty sella

COMMONLY ASSOCIATED CONDITIONS
- Childhood hypopituitarism
- Sheehan syndrome
- Hypothyroidism
- Kallmann syndrome

 DIAGNOSIS

HISTORY
- Initial symptoms may be nonspecific and of insidious onset, depending on severity of hormone deficiency: Fatigue, hypotension, cold intolerance:
  - Pituitary failure secondary to tumors may present with symptoms related to mass effect: Headache, visual impairment, hypothalamic dysfunction.
  - Symptoms are related to specific hormone deficiency:
    ○ ACTH: Hypotension, hypoglycemia, nausea, vomiting, extreme fatigue, asthenia, anorexia, pallor, weight loss; in children, failure to thrive, hypoglycemia
    ○ TSH: In adults, tiredness, cold intolerance, constipation, weight gain, hair loss, dry skin, bradycardia, hoarseness, mental confusion or increased forgetfulness; in children, childhood growth failure

○ Gonadotropins: Sexual dysfunction, loss of libido, infertility; in men, impotence, decreased facial and body hair, decreased muscle and bone mass; in women, menstrual disturbance, dyspareunia; in children, delayed puberty can present with eunuchoid habitus.
○ GH: Commonly deficient when other hormones are deficient. In adults, fatigue, decreased muscle mass and strength, increased visceral fat, general malaise; in children, growth retardation
○ Prolactin: Inability to lactate
○ ADH: Polyuria, nocturia, polydypsia, orthostasis, hypotension
- Assessment of pituitary function, history of:
  - Cranial radiation
  - Craniofacial abnormalities
  - Empty sella
  - Gonadal dysfunction
  - Head trauma or head surgery
  - Inflammatory or granulomatous disease
  - Pituitary or hypothalamic lesions
  - Pregnancy-related hemorrhage or hypotension

PHYSICAL EXAM
- Pituitary failure secondary to tumors:
  - ACTH: Hypotension, anorexia, pallor, weight loss
  - TSH: Weight gain, hair loss, dry skin, bradycardia, hoarseness, hypotension, constipation
  - Gonadotropins: Delayed puberty
  - GH: Decreased muscle mass and strength, increased visceral fat, growth retardation
- Visual field defects
- Children:
  - Congenital malformations and syndromes, especially malformations of the head and genitalia
  - Growth retardation and delayed puberty

DIAGNOSTIC TESTS & INTERPRETATION
Lab
- Documentation of ≥1 deficiencies of pituitary hormones: Hormones are tested individually.
- Laboratory measurement of basal and stimulated hormone levels and levels of their target hormones.
- Corticotropin:
  - Basal ACTH at 8–9 a.m.; low level is positive test.
  - Metapyrone test: Induced reduction in serum cortisol should cause increase in ACTH secretion.
  - ACTH stimulation test: Administration of synthetic ACTH should stimulate adrenal cortisol production unless adrenal atrophy is present.
  - Insulin-induced hypoglycemia: Should cause increase in ACTH and cortisol secretion. Test is contraindicated in coronary artery disease (CAD), seizure disorder, or feebleness.
- TSH:
  - Secondary hypothyroidism; rare in absence of other pituitary hormone deficiencies
  - Low free T_4 with inappropriately normal or low TSH suggests TSH deficiency.
  - TSH is not a reliable screening test.
  - Thyrotropin-releasing hormone (TRH) stimulation: Blunted response in secondary hypothyroidism
- Gonadotropins:
  - Men: Serum testosterone is surrogate for LH deficiency in patients with known hypothalamic or pituitary disease. LH is elevated in primary hypogonadism and normal or low in secondary hypogonadism.

– Women: In women with known pituitary disease, LH and FSH testing is not necessary in the presence of normal menses.

– In the presence of oligomenorrhea or amenorrhea, measure LH and FSH levels.

– Serum estradiol is low in hypogonadotropic hypogonadism.

– Vaginal cytology for estrogenization index

– Exclude hyperprolactinemia.

• Prolactin:

– Isolated hypoprolactinemia is rare.

– Prolactin deficiency prevents lactation.

– In prolactin deficiency, basal plasma levels are low and fail to rise after injection of TRH.

– Elevated prolactin may accompany hypopituitarism due to the disruption of hypothalamic inhibitory influences; this is termed *stalk effect*.

• GH:

– GH deficiency highly likely if $\geq$2 other pituitary hormones deficient

– Low serum IGF-1

– Provocative tests include insulin-induced hypoglycemia and arginine plus arginine–GH-releasing hormone. Positive tests show deficient serum GH response. Again, insulin-induced hypoglycemia is contraindicated in CAD, seizure disorder, or feebleness.

• Genetic testing, if indicated

Initial lab tests

• Initial tests should be based on clinical suspicion; test both the trophic hormone and the hormone produced by the targeted gland. The testing should be paired and ideally at 8 a.m. because most of these hormones are affected by circadian rhythm.

• ACTH: Cortisol; LH, FSH: estradiol, testosterone; GH: IGF-1; TSH: free T_4; prolactin; pituitary α subunit

• Biochemical tests should precede imaging studies.

Imaging

• Magnetic resonance imaging (MRI) of hypothalamic–pituitary region

• If MRI is contraindicated, then high-resolution computed tomography (CT) with pituitary/sella focus

• Radiographs: Chest, skull, hands, wrists (for bone age)

• Dual energy x-ray absorptiometry: Gonadotropin deficiency may result in osteoporosis.

Pathological Findings

• Destruction of anterior pituitary

• Atrophy of adrenal cortex, thyroid, gonads

DIFFERENTIAL DIAGNOSIS

• Primary hypothyroidism

• Primary hypogonadism

• Addison disease, primary adrenal insufficiency

• Hypothalamic insufficiency

• Kallmann syndrome

• Chronic liver disease

• Constitutional short stature

Geriatric Considerations

• More difficult to diagnose in elderly

TREATMENT

MEDICATION

• Adrenal insufficiency should be excluded before thyroid hormone replacement is initiated; otherwise, thyroid hormone replacement could precipitate adrenal crisis (1).

• Replacement of hormones secreted by target glands

• Treatment of ACTH, TSH, LH, and FSH deficiencies similar to the treatment of primary hormone deficiencies of their respective target organ:

– ACTH deficiency results in cortisol deficiency: Treatment consists of administration of glucocorticoid hormones (hydrocortisone, dexamethasone, or prednisone) to mimic normal pattern of cortisol secretion; mineralocorticoid replacement is rarely necessary.

– TSH deficiency: Goal of treatment is normal free T_4 value. Treat with levothyroxine.

– LH and FSH deficiency: Treatment depends on gender and whether fertility is desired:

○ Men: Testosterone replacement if fertility not desired; gonadotropins for fertility

○ Women: Estrogen–progesterone (and possibly testosterone) replacement, or pulsatile gonadotropins for fertility

– Recombinant human GH (for treating short stature in children and for treating selected adult patients)

– Hypoprolactinemia has no treatment.

– Dosages and administration schedule vary according to age and sex.

• Infectious disease: Antibiotics as appropriate

• Inflammatory or granulomatous disease: Specific treatment

ADDITIONAL TREATMENT

General Measures

If patient is admitted for pituitary surgery, patient should be supplemented with all deficient hormones, especially with stress-dose glucocorticoids.

SURGERY/OTHER PROCEDURES

Ideally, transsphenoidal/translabial hypophysectomy for a pituitary adenoma; if unresectable by this method, then craniotomy may be an option if visual impairment has manifested. Patient could be discharged home on physiologic glucocorticoid replacement and have an ACTH stimulation test 4–6 weeks after discharge from the hospital to assess the hypothalamic–pituitary–adrenal axis.

ONGOING CARE

FOLLOW-UP RECOMMENDATIONS

Exercise as tolerated; no specific limitations

Patient Monitoring

• 3- and 12-month evaluations for post-treatment hormonal status

• Patients with pituitary tumors: Include visual fields, thyroid and adrenal function, and sellar CT imaging.

PATIENT EDUCATION

Specifically but not limited to adrenal insufficiency; the patient should wear a medical alert identification bracelet or necklace identifying the deficiency.

PROGNOSIS

• Variable but guardedly favorable with replacement therapy

• If a result of postpartum necrosis, may have complete or partial recovery

COMPLICATIONS

• Adrenal crisis

• Infertility, sexual dysfunction

• Blindness

• Short stature, failure to thrive, developmental delay, delayed puberty

• Premature atherosclerosis

• Obesity

REFERENCE

1. Osman IA, Leslie P. Addison's disease. Adrenal insufficiency should be excluded before thyroxine replacement is started. *BMJ.* 1996;313:427.

ADDITIONAL READING

• Ascoli P, Cavagnini F. Hypopituitarism. *Pituitary.* 2006;9:335–42.

• Behan LA, Agha A. Endocrine consequences of adult traumatic brain injury. *Horm Res.* 2007;68(Suppl 5): 18–21.

• Schneider HJ, Aimaretti G, Kreitschmann-Andermahr I, et al. Hypopituitarism. *Lancet.* 2007;369: 1461–70.

• VanAken MO, Lamberts SW. Diagnosis and treatment of hypopituitarism. *Pituitary.* 2006;8:183–91.

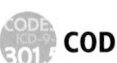 CODES

ICD9
253.2 Panhypopituitarism

CLINICAL PEARLS

In patient with documented ACTH deficiency, emphasize the need for additional cortisone at the time of any major physical stress or illness. The glucocorticoid dose can be doubled for 3–5 days.

Pediatric Considerations

• Congenital malformations; genetic conditions may warrant screening for hypopituitarism.

• GH deficiency may result in growth retardation.

• Hypogonadism in prenatal pituitary failure

• Delayed puberty

Pregnancy Considerations

• Pregnancy-associated hemorrhage or hypotension may result in pituitary hypoperfusion and subsequent partial or complete pituitary failure (Sheehan syndrome).

• Lymphocytic hypophysitis may be triggered by pregnancy.

H

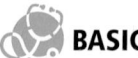

HYPOTHERMIA
Scott T. Henderson, MD

BASICS

DESCRIPTION
- A core temperature of less than 35°C (95°F)
- May take several hours to days to develop
- Patients with cold water immersion can appear to be dead but can still be resuscitated.
- System(s) affected: All body systems
- Synonym(s): Accidental hypothermia

EPIDEMIOLOGY
- Predominant age: Very young and the elderly
- Predominant sex: Male > Female

Geriatric Considerations
More common due to lower metabolic rate, impaired ability to maintain normal body temperature, and impaired ability to detect temperature changes

Prevalence
Estimates vary widely due to lack of pathologic evidence, and it is usually considered a secondary cause in diagnosing disorders.

RISK FACTORS
- Alcohol consumption
- Bronchopneumonia
- Cardiovascular disease
- Cold water immersion
- Dermal dysfunction (burns, erythrodermas)
- Drug intoxication
- Endocrinopathies (myxedema, severe hypoglycemia)
- Excessive fluid loss
- Hepatic failure
- Hypothalamic and central nervous system (CNS) dysfunction
- Malnutrition
- Mental illness; Alzheimer disease
- Prolonged environmental exposure
- Renal failure
- Sepsis
- Trauma (especially head)
- Uremia

GENERAL PREVENTION
- Appropriate clothing with particular attention to head, feet, and hands
- For outdoor activities, carry survival bags with space blankets for use if stranded or injured.
- Avoid alcohol.
- Alertness to early symptoms and initiating preventive steps (e.g., drinking warm fluids)
- Identify medications that may predispose to hypothermia (e.g., neuroleptics, sedatives, hypnotics, tranquilizers).

ETIOLOGY
- Overwhelming environmental cold stress
- Decreased heat production
- Increased heat loss
- Impaired thermoregulation

COMMONLY ASSOCIATED CONDITIONS
- Addison disease
- CNS dysfunction
- Congestive heart failure
- Diabetes
- Hypopituitarism
- Hypothyroidism
- Ketoacidosis
- Pulmonary infection
- Sepsis
- Uremia

DIAGNOSIS

HISTORY
Presentation varies with the temperature of the patient at the time of presentation.

ALERT
History of prolonged exposure to cold may make the diagnosis obvious, but hypothermia may be overlooked, especially in comatose patients.

PHYSICAL EXAM
Exam findings vary with the temperature of the patient at the time of presentation:
- Mild (32°C–35°C):
  – Lethargy and mild confusion
  – Shivering
  – Tachypnea
  – Tachycardia
  – Loss of fine motor coordination
  – Increased blood pressure
  – Peripheral vasoconstriction
- Moderate (28°C–32°C):
  – Delirium
  – Bradycardia
  – Hypotension
  – Hypoventilation
  – Cyanosis
  – Arrhythmias (prolonged PR interval; AV junctional rhythm; idioventricular rhythm; prolonged QT interval; altered T waves)
  – Semicoma and coma
  – Muscular rigidity
  – Generalized edema
  – Slowed reflexes
- Severe (<28°C):
  – Very cold skin
  – Rigidity
  – Apnea
  – Bradycardia
  – No pulse: Ventricular fibrillation or asystole
  – Areflexia
  – Unresponsive
  – Fixed pupils

ALERT
Use specially designed thermometers that can record low temperatures and measure core temperatures.

Pediatric Considerations
- Infants may present with bright red, cold skin and very low energy.
- A child's body temperature drops faster than an adult's when immersed in cold water.

DIAGNOSTIC TESTS & INTERPRETATION
Lab
Initial lab tests
- Arterial blood gases (corrected for temperature)
- Complete blood and platelet counts
- Serum electrolytes
- Urinalysis
- Coagulation studies
- Fibrinogen levels
- Blood culture
- Blood urea nitrogen/creatinine
- Glucose
- Amylase
- Liver function studies
- Cardiac enzymes
- Calcium
- Magnesium
- Alcohol level

Follow-Up & Special Considerations
- Toxicology screen if mental status changes are more extreme than expected for temperature decrease
- Serum cortisol, if indicated
- Thyroid function tests, if indicated

Imaging
Initial approach
Cervical spine, chest, abdomen, if appropriate

Diagnostic Procedures/Surgery
Electrocardiogram

Pathological Findings
- Moderate dilation of right heart
- Pulmonary edema

DIFFERENTIAL DIAGNOSIS
- Cerebrovascular accidents
- Intoxication
- Drug overdose
- Complications of diabetes, hypothyroidism, hypopituitarism

TREATMENT

MEDICATION
- For sepsis or bacterial infections: Antibiotics based on site and etiology (1)[C]
- For hypoglycemia, D50W at a dose of 1 mg/kg
- Thiamine, 100 mg, if alcoholic or cachectic
- Naloxone, 2.0 mg
- Levothyroxine 150–500 μg for myxedema
- For severe acidosis: Sodium bicarbonate
- Contraindications:
  – Medications, including epinephrine, lidocaine, and procainamide, can accumulate to toxic levels if used repeatedly.
  – Routine use of steroids or antibiotics has not been shown to increase survival or decrease postresuscitative damage.
- Precautions:
  – Medications should be avoided until core temperature is >30°C:
    ○ When temperature reaches >30°C, IV medications are indicated, but at longer than the standard intervals.
  – Avoid vasopressors due to arrhythmogenic potential and delayed metabolism.

- Significant possible interactions:
  – Use all drugs cautiously due to impaired metabolism and renal elimination.
- Once rewarming has occurred, there is mobilization of depot stores.

ADDITIONAL TREATMENT
General Measures
- Pre-hospital (2)[C]:
  – ABCs of basic life support
  – Remove wet garments.
  – Protect against heat loss and wind chill.
  – Give warm humidified oxygen if available.
- See Initial Stabilization

IN-PATIENT CONSIDERATIONS
Initial Stabilization
Rewarming dependent on severity of hypothermia and presence of cardiac arrest:

- If no cardiac arrest, consider active external rewarming (3)[B].
- If cardiac arrest present, consider active internal rewarming (3)[B].
- Warm center of body first.
- The rate of rewarming is determined by whether a perfusing cardiac output is present:
  – If a perfusing cardiac output is present, 1–2C per hour is appropriate.
  – If not, then a faster rate of >2C per hour should be used.
- Monitor core temperature; use a consistent method.
- Monitor blood pressure and cardiac rhythm.
- Correct metabolic acidosis.
- Evaluate for frostbite and other trauma.
- Mild hypothermia:
  – Passive rewarming
  – Administration of heated IV solutions (D5NS)
  – Warm fluids may be given if fully alert.
- Moderate hypothermia:
  – Active external rewarming with forced warm air systems (4)[B]
- Severe hypothermia (active internal [core] rewarming):
  – Minimally invasive
  – Heated IV fluids
  – Heated humidified oxygen
  – Body cavity lavage:
    ○ Thoracic cavity lavage (43°C)
    ○ Gastrointestinal, colonic, or bladder lavage with warm fluids (43°C)
    ○ Peritoneal dialysis
  – Extracorporeal blood rewarming (4)[B]:
    ○ Cardiopulmonary bypass
    ○ Extracorporeal membrane oxygenation
    ○ Continuous arteriovenous rewarming
    ○ Hemodialysis and hemofiltration
- Cardiac arrhythmias:
  – Atrial fibrillation and sinus bradycardia are common, but patients usually convert to normal sinus rhythm with rewarming.
  – If ventricular fibrillation is present, it should be treated with 1 shock. If patient does not respond, further attempts should be deferred until the patient is rewarmed (1)[B].
  – Do not treat transient ventricular arrhythmias.
  – If cardiac pacing required, preferable to use external noninvasive pacemaker

Admission Criteria
Patients with underlying disease, physiologic abnormalities, or core temperature 32°C should be admitted, preferably to intensive care unit (1)[A].

IV Fluids
IVs should be heated to 40°C–42°C when possible, but should be no colder than the patient's core temperature.

ALERT
- Avoid fluid overload.
- Avoid lactated Ringer solution because of decreased lactate metabolism.

Nursing
Because of the cold, heart is irritable and susceptible to arrhythmias; take special care in moving and transporting.

Discharge Criteria
Discharge from emergency department once normothermic, if mild hypothermia and no predisposing conditions or complications, and has suitable place to go.

 ONGOING CARE

FOLLOW-UP RECOMMENDATIONS
Patient Monitoring
- During acute episode:
  – Monitor cardiac rhythm.
  – Monitor electrolytes and glucose frequently.
  – Monitor urinary output.
  – Follow blood gases.
- Following acute episode:
  – Continued therapy for any underlying disorder

DIET
Warm fluids only, if alert and able to swallow

PATIENT EDUCATION
- Alcohol intake increases risk of becoming hypothermic in cold conditions.
- Encourage persons with cardiovascular disease to avoid outdoor exercise in cold weather.
- If appropriate, referral to social service agency for help with adequate housing, heat, or clothing.

PROGNOSIS
- Mortality rates are decreasing due to increased recognition and advanced therapy.
- Mortality usually dependent on the severity of underlying cause of hypothermia.
- In previously healthy individuals, recovery is usually complete.
- Mortality rate in healthy patients is <5%.
- Mortality rate in patients with coexisting illness is >50%.

Geriatric Considerations
- Mortality rates increase with increasing age.

COMPLICATIONS
- Cardiac arrhythmias
- Hypotension
- Hyperkalemia
- Hypoglycemia
- Rhabdomyolysis

- Bladder atony
- Pneumonia (aspiration and broncho)
- Pulmonary edema
- Acute respiratory distress syndrome
- Pancreatitis
- Peritonitis
- Gastrointestinal bleeding
- Acute tubular necrosis
- Intravascular thromboses/disseminated intravascular coagulation
- Metabolic acidosis
- Gangrene of extremities
- Compartment syndromes

REFERENCES
1. Guvakov D, Weiss S, Cheung A. Hypothermia. ACP PIER: The Physicians' *Information and Education Resource*. 2008.
2. American Heart Association. Part 10.4: Hypothermia. *Circulation*. 2005;112:IV-136–IV-138.
3. Kempainen RR, Brunette DD. The evaluation and management of accidental hypothermia. *Respir Care*. 2004;49:192–205.
4. McCullough L, Arora S. Diagnosis and treatment of hypothermia. *Am Fam Physician*. 2004;70:2325–32.

ADDITIONAL READING
- Headdon WG, Wilson PM, Dalton HR et al. The management of accidental hypothermia. *BMJ*. 2009;338:b2085.
- Schweitzer KS. Cold but not dead. *Air Med J*. 2008;27:94–8.

See Also (Topic, Algorithm, Electronic Media Element)
Frostbite; Near Drowning
Algorithm: Hypothermia

 CODES

ICD9
991.6 Hypothermia

CLINICAL PEARLS
- Most common cause of hypothermia in US is cold exposure due to alcohol intoxication
- As long as core temperature is severely decreased, one should not assume that resuscitation is not possible unless there are obvious lethal injuries ("not dead until warm and dead").
- Electrocardiogram changes are associated with hypothermia.
- Slowing of sinus rate with T-wave inversion
- QT-interval prolongation
- Hypothermic J waves (Osborn waves) characterized by a notching of the QRS complex and ST segment

HYPOTHYROIDISM, ADULT

Barbara A. Majeroni, MD

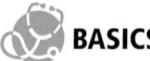 **BASICS**

DESCRIPTION
- Clinical state resulting from decreased circulating levels of free thyroid hormone or from resistance to hormone action
- System(s) affected: Endocrine/Metabolic
- Synonym(s): Myxedema

EPIDEMIOLOGY
Incidence
- Predominant age: >40 years
- Predominant gender: Female > Male, 5–10:1

Prevalence
- 3.7% in general population
- Common in elderly
- >65 years of age, increases to 6–10% of women, 2–3% of men
- Up to 20% of patients with major depressive disorder

RISK FACTORS
- Increasing age
- Personal or family history of autoimmune diseases, including type 1 diabetes mellitus (DM), Addison disease
- Previous postpartum thyroiditis
- Previous head or neck irradiation
- History of Graves disease
- Treatment with lithium, immune modulators such as IFN-α, or the iodine-containing antiarrhythmic amiodarone

Genetics
- No known genetic pattern for idiopathic primary hypothyroidism
- May be associated with type 2 autoimmune polyglandular syndrome, which is associated with HLA-DR3 and -DR4
- Secondary hypothyroidism frequently results from treatment for Grave's disease, which may be familial.

ETIOLOGY
- Postablative: Follows radioactive iodine therapy or thyroid surgery; delayed hypothyroidism may develop in patients treated with thioamide drugs (e.g., propylthiouracil or methimazole) 4–25 years later
- Primary: May develop as result of autoimmune thyroiditis or be idiopathic
- With goiter: Most commonly a result of autoimmune disease, such as Hashimoto thyroiditis
- Other causes: Heritable biosynthetic defects, iodine deficiency (rare in US), or drugs (iodides, lithium, phenylbutazone, ASA, amiodarone, aminoglutethimide, and IFN-α)
- Central or secondary: May be due to deficiency of thyrotropin-releasing hormone (TRH) from hypothalamus or thyroid-stimulating hormone (TSH) from pituitary
- Transient: May result from silent thyroiditis (most common in postpartum period) and subacute granulomatous thyroiditis

COMMONLY ASSOCIATED CONDITIONS
- Hyponatremia
- Anemia
- Idiopathic adrenocorticoid deficiency
- DM
- Hypoparathyroidism
- Myasthenia gravis
- Vitiligo
- Hypercholesterolemia
- Mitral valve prolapse
- Depression
- Rapid-cycling bipolar disorder
- Ischemic heart disease
- Metabolic syndrome
- Down syndrome

 DIAGNOSIS

HISTORY
- Onset may be insidious, subtle
- Weakness, fatigue, lethargy
- Cold intolerance
- Decreased memory, concentration
- Hearing impairment
- Constipation
- Muscle cramps
- Arthralgias
- Paresthesias
- Modest weight gain (10 lb [4.5 kg])
- Decreased sweating
- Menorrhagia
- Depression
- Hoarseness
- Carpal tunnel syndrome

PHYSICAL EXAM
- Dry, coarse skin
- Dull facial expression
- Coarsening or huskiness of voice
- Periorbital puffiness
- Swelling of hands and feet (nonpitting)
- Bradycardia
- Hypothermia
- Reduced systolic blood pressure (BP)
- Increased diastolic BP
- Reduced body and scalp hair
- Delayed relaxation of deep-tendon reflexes
- Macroglossia

Geriatric Considerations
- Characteristic signs and symptoms frequently changed or absent
- Diagnosis based on laboratory criteria

DIAGNOSTIC TESTS & INTERPRETATION
Lab
Initial lab tests
- Primary hypothyroidism (1)[C]:
  - TSH elevated
  - Serum free T4 decreased
- Central hypothyroidism:
  - TSH low
  - Serum free T4 decreased
  - Impaired TSH response to TRH
- Severe hypothyroidism:
  - Anemia
  - Elevated cholesterol
  - Elevated creatine phosphokinase, lactate dehydrogenase, aspartate aminotransferase
  - Hyponatremia
- Subclinical hypothyroidism:
  - TSH elevated
  - Serum free T4 normal

Follow-Up & Special Considerations
- Drugs that may alter lab results:
  - Thyroid supplement
  - Cortisone
  - Dopamine
  - Phenytoin
  - Estrogen or androgen therapy in excess of replacement
  - Amiodarone
  - Salicylates
- Disorders that may alter lab results:
  - Any severe illness
  - Pregnancy
  - Chronic protein malnutrition
  - Hepatic failure
  - Nephrotic syndrome

Imaging
Initial approach
- None necessary unless signs of cardiac involvement
- Chest radiograph may show enlarged heart (often due to pericardial effusion)

Pathological Findings
Thyroid may be small, atrophic, or enlarged.

DIFFERENTIAL DIAGNOSIS
- Nephrotic syndrome
- Chronic nephritis
- Neurasthenia
- Depression
- Euthyroid sick syndrome
- Congestive heart failure
- Primary amyloidosis
- Dementia from other causes

TREATMENT

MEDICATION
First Line
- Levothyroxine (Synthroid, Levothroid):
  - 1.6 mcg/kg/d; increase by 25 mcg/d every 4–6 weeks until TSH in normal range (2)[A]
  - Dosage requirements may vary with age, gender, residual secretory capacity of thyroid gland, other drugs being taken by patient, and intestinal function.
  - Elderly patients may require 2/3 of dose used in young adults because clearance is decreased.
- Contraindications:
  - Thyrotoxic heart disease
  - Uncorrected adrenocorticoid insufficiency
- Precautions:
  - Start with lower doses, such as 25 mcg, in elderly and in patients with heart disease.
  - Diabetic patients may need readjustment of hypoglycemic agents with institution of thyroxine.
  - Dosage of oral anticoagulants may need adjustment; monitor prothrombin time while initiating treatment.
- Significant possible interactions:
  - Oral anticoagulants
  - Insulin
  - Oral hypoglycemics
  - Estrogen
  - Oral contraceptives
  - Cholestyramine
  - Proton pump inhibitors
  - Ferrous sulfate, calcium carbonate, antacids, laxatives, colestipol, sucralfate, ciprofloxacin, and cholestyramine may decrease absorption.

- Controversy exists whether subclinical hypothyroidism should be treated if asymptomatic. Cochrane Review found no improvement in survival, cardiovascular morbidity, or health-related quality of life. Some evidence indicates improvement in lipid profiles and left ventricular function (3)[A]. Subclinical hypothyroidism should be treated in patients with iron deficiency anemia (4)[A].

Pregnancy Considerations
- Replacement therapy may need adjustment.
- TSH levels should be monitored monthly during 1st trimester (5)[C].
- Postpartum: Check TSH levels at 6 weeks.
- Painless subacute thyroiditis may occur in postpartum period, leading to transient hypothyroidism lasting 3 months. Treatment with replacement therapy may be warranted. Up to 30% of these individuals develop permanent hypothyroidism.

Second Line
No benefit to adding triiodothyronine (T_3) to thyroxine

ADDITIONAL TREATMENT
General Measures
- Outpatient, except for complicating emergencies (e.g., coma, hypothermia)
- Treatment goals: Restore and maintain euthyroid state.

Issues for Referral
- Central hypothyroidism, with low TSH and low free T4, would benefit from an endocrinology referral.
- Hypothyroidism unresponsive to treatment
- Serum TSH remains elevated despite full-dose treatment with levothyroxine

IN-PATIENT CONSIDERATIONS
Admission Criteria
Myxedema coma, hypothermia

ONGOING CARE

FOLLOW-UP RECOMMENDATIONS
Monitor TSH.

Patient Monitoring
- Monitor TSH every 8–12 weeks until stabilized, then annually.
- Follow cardiac status closely in older patients.
- Check TSH more frequently in pregnancy, initiation of estrogen supplementation, or after large changes in body weight.
- In central hypothyroidism, TSH unreliable; must monitor free T4, T3

DIET
High-bulk diet may help avoid constipation.

PATIENT EDUCATION
- Stress importance of compliance with thyroid replacement therapy.
- Explain need for lifelong treatment.
- Instruct to report to physician any signs of infection or heart problems.
- Describe signs of thyrotoxicity.

PROGNOSIS
- Return to normal state is the rule.
- Relapses will occur if treatment is interrupted.
- If untreated, may progress to myxedema coma

COMPLICATIONS
- Hypothyroid patients (mild to moderate) tolerate surgery with mortality and complications similar to euthyroid patients.
- If surgery is elective, render patient euthyroid prior to procedure.
- If surgery is urgent, proceed with procedure with individualized replacement therapy preoperatively and postoperatively.
- Treatment-induced congestive heart failure in people with coronary artery disease Myxedema coma: Life-threatening
- Increased susceptibility to infection
- Megacolon
- Organic psychosis with paranoia
- Adrenal crisis with vigorous treatment of hypothyroidism, especially in patients with undiagnosed polyendocrine syndromes
- Infertility
- Hypersensitivity to opiates
- Treatment over long periods can lead to bone demineralization.
- Subclinical hypothyroidism is associated with increased ischemic heart disease and increased all-cause mortality in men but not in women.

REFERENCES
1. Miller GD, Rogers JC, DeGroote SL. Which lab tests are best when you suspect hypothyroidism? *J Fam Pract*. 2008;57:613–19.
2. Roos A, et al. The starting dose of levothyroxine in primary hypothyroidism treatment: A prospective, randomized, double-blind trial. *Arch Int Med*. 2005;165:1714–20.
3. Villar HCCE, Saconato H, Valente O, et al. Thyroid hormone replacement for subclinical hypothyroidism (Cochrane Review). In: *The Cochrane Library* 2008 Issue 2, Chichester, UK: John Wiley and Sons, Ltd.
4. Cinemre H, Bilir C, Gokosmanoglu F, Bahcebest T. Hematologic effects of levothyroxine in iron deficient subclinical hypothyroid patients: a randomized, double blind, controlled study. *J Clin Endocrinol & Metabol*. 2009;94(1):151–156.
5. Alexander EK, Marqusee E, Lawrence J, et al. Timing and magnitude of increases in levothyroxine requirements during pregnancy in women with hypothyroidism. *N Engl J Med*. 2004;351:241–9.

ADDITIONAL READING
- Devdhar M, et al. Hypothyroidism. *Endocrinol Clin N Am*. 2007;36:595–615.
- Feldt-Rasmussen U. Treatment of hypothyroidism in elderly patients and in patients with cardiac disease. *Thyroid*. 2007;17:619–24.
- Hennessey J, et al. Evaluating and treating the patient with hypothyroid disease. *J Fam Practice Suppl*. 2007;S23–S30.
- Vaidya B, Pearce SHS. Management of hypothyroidism in adults. *BMJ*. 2008;337:284–9.

See Also (Topic, Algorithm, Electronic Media Element)
Hyperthyroidism; Thyroiditis

CODES

ICD9
- 244.0 Postsurgical hypothyroidism
- 244.1 Other postablative hypothyroidism
- 244.9 Unspecified acquired hypothyroidism

CLINICAL PEARLS
- Start low and go slow when starting thyroxine in an elderly patient or if known cardiovascular disease.
- Once a patient has attained the euthyroid state, maintain on the same brand of thyroxine. There can be up to 12.5% difference in brands considered bioequivalent.
- Monitor TSH every 8–12 weeks until stabilized, then annually.
- The symptoms of hypothyroidism may be vague and diffuse. Maintain a high index of suspicion, especially in women >50 years of age.

H

Stanley Sagov, MD

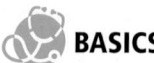

BASICS

DESCRIPTION

A generalized skin reaction associated with various infectious and inflammatory cutaneous conditions distant from the main rash of the disease:

- Id is a word termination often combined with a root reflecting the causative factor (ie, bacterid, syphilid, and tuberculid). The dermatophytid is the most frequently referenced id reaction in dermatology. A dermatophytid is an autosensitization reaction in which a secondary cutaneous reaction occurs at a site distant to a primary fungal infection. The eruption begins typically within 1–2 weeks of the onset of the main lesion or following exacerbation of the main lesion.
- System(s) affected: Skin/Exocrine
- Synonym(s): Dermatophytid, trichophytid, autoeczematization

EPIDEMIOLOGY

- Predominant age: All ages
- Predominant sex: Male = Female

Incidence

Unknown; no good data source

Prevalence

Common

RISK FACTORS

- Fungal infection of the skin
- Stasis dermatitis

GENERAL PREVENTION

- Minimize factors for developing fungal infections.
- Promptly treat any developing fungal infection.

ETIOLOGY

Precise pathophysiology is uncertain. Circulating antigens may react with antibodies at sensitized areas of the skin, or abnormal immune recognition of autologous skin antigens may occur.

COMMONLY ASSOCIATED CONDITIONS

- Primary fungal infection
- Stasis dermatitis

DIAGNOSIS

HISTORY

Itchy rash: Assess for the primary fungal or bacterial lesions that would have preceded the onset of the id reaction by days to weeks.

PHYSICAL EXAM

- Common:
  - Symmetric, pruritic vesicles on the hands
  - Tinea infection on the feet; contact or other eczematous dermatosis; or bacterial, fungal, or viral infection of the skin
  - Generalized reactions can occur.
- Less common:
  - Papules
  - Lichenoid eruption
- Eczematoid eruption

DIAGNOSTIC TESTS & INTERPRETATION
Lab
- Fungal infection at the primary site proven by potassium hydroxide (KOH) or fungal culture
- No fungal elements demonstrable at the site of the presumed id reaction
- Special tests: Skin shows a positive trichophyton reaction.

Follow-Up & Special Considerations
The id reaction resolves with successful eradication of the primary skin condition.

Pathological Findings
- Vesicles in the upper dermis
- Superficial perivascular lymphohistiocytic infiltrate
- Small numbers of eosinophils
- Moderate acanthosis
- Increased granular cell layer
- No infectious agents present in biopsy specimen

DIFFERENTIAL DIAGNOSIS
- Pompholyx (dyshidrotic eczema)
- Contact dermatitis
- Drug eruptions
- Pustular psoriasis
- Folliculitis
- Scabies

 # TREATMENT

MEDICATION
First Line
- Antihistamines for any pruritus
- Topical steroids for pruritus
- Systemic steroids only if reaction is severe or generalized
- Contraindications: Refer to manufacturer's profile of each drug.
- Precautions: Refer to manufacturer's profile of each drug.
- Significant possible interactions: Refer to manufacturer's profile of each drug.

Second Line
- Topical and/or systemic antifungals for identified associated fungal infection (common)
- Topical or systemic antibiotics for any secondary infection

ADDITIONAL TREATMENT
General Measures
- Appropriate health care: Outpatient
- Treatment of the underlying infection or eczematous dermatitis
- Symptomatic treatment of pruritus with antihistamines and/or topical steroids if needed (may require class 1 or 2 steroid)
- Treatment for secondary bacterial infection

 # ONGOING CARE

PATIENT EDUCATION
Avoid hot, humid conditions that promote fungal growth. Aerate susceptible body areas (eg, wear sandals or open footwear). If possible, wear boxer shorts or loose-fitting clothing, dry off wet skin after bathing, and use powders and antiperspirants to make the environment less conducive to fungal growth. Treat primary dermatitis promptly.

PROGNOSIS
After appropriate treatment, complete resolution in a few days to 2 weeks

COMPLICATIONS
Secondary bacterial infection (cellulitis)

ADDITIONAL READING

Habif T. *Clinical Dermatology*, 4th ed. St. Louis: Mosby, 2004.

 # CODES

ICD9
- 110.9 Dermatophytosis of unspecified site
- 692.89 Contact dermatitis and other eczema due to other specified agents

CLINICAL PEARLS

This is a diagnosis in the category of "If you don't think of it, you won't think of it," so when you see one skin lesion follow another, think of the id reaction.

IDIOPATHIC THROMBOCYTOPENIC PURPURA (ITP)

Jeffery T. Kirchner, DO

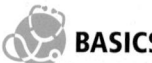 BASICS

DESCRIPTION

- Decrease in circulating number of platelets (<100,00/mL) in absence of toxic exposure or disease associated with low platelet count
- Occurs as secondary effect of peripheral platelet destruction as well as decreased platelet production
- Diagnosis of exclusion
- Acute idiopathic thrombocytopenic purpura (ITP): Relatively common disease of childhood that often follows acute infection and has spontaneous resolution within 2 months; platelet counts <20,000
- Chronic ITP: Persists after 12 months without a specific cause; usually seen in adults and persists for months to years; platelet count typically 30,000–80,000. Sponatenous remission is rare in adults (9% in 1 series) (1).
- System(s) affected: Heme/Lymphatic/Immunologic
- Synonym(s): Postinfectious thrombocytopenia; Immune thrombocytopenic purpura; Werlhof disease

EPIDEMIOLOGY

- Predominant age:
  – Acute ITP (primarily a childhood disease): 2–6 years
  – Chronic ITP: >50 years
  – Uncommon in geriatric population; look for other cause of low platelet count
- Predominant gender:
  – Acute ITP: Male = Female
  – Chronic ITP: Female > Male (2:1)

Incidence

- Total incidence is greater than 22 cases per million population per year
- Estimates from recent meta-analyis are 1.9–6.4 per 100,000 children/year and 3.3 per 100,000 adults/year (2)

Prevalence

- Due to its chronic nature, prevalence exceeds incidence
- Prevalence estimate in the US approximately 100 cases per million population

RISK FACTORS

- Acute infection
- Age (see Epidemiology)
- Cardiopulmonary bypass
- Hypersplenism
- Antiphospholipid antibody syndrome
- Preeclampsia
- HIV infection

Genetics

No known genetic pattern

GENERAL PREVENTION

The patient should avoid medications (when feasible) that inhibit platelet function (such as aspirin) or those that suppress bone marrow.

PATHOPHYSIOLOGY

- IgG autoantibodies on platelet surface cause platelet uptake and destruction by reticuloendothelial phagocytes.
- There is also believed to be inhibition of megakaryocyte platelet production by specific IgG autoantibodies.

COMMONLY ASSOCIATED CONDITIONS

- Acute ITP:
  – Varicella
  – Other viral infections (Epstein-Barr virus, cytomegalovirus)
- Chronic ITP:
  – HIV
  – *Helicobacter pylori*
  – Graves disease
  – Hashimoto thyroiditis
  – Sarcoidosis
  – Systemic lupus erythematosus
  – Hepatitis C
- Autoimmune hemolytic anemia (Evans syndrome)

 DIAGNOSIS

- There is no "gold standard" laboratory test to diagnose ITP.
- It is a diagnosis of exclusion after other causes (infection, drugs, malignancy) of thrombocytopenia have been ruled out.
- It is important to always rul -out secondary causes of thrombocytopenia (which would change managment).

HISTORY

- Post-traumatic bleeding at 40,000–60,000 platelet count
- Bruising tendency
- Gingival bleeding
- Gastrointestinal bleeding
- Menometrorrhagia
- Menorrhagia
- Recurrent epistaxis
- Neurologic symptoms secondary to intracerebral bleeding
- Spontaneous bleeding may occur with platelet count <20,000.

PHYSICAL EXAM

- Petechial hemorrhages
- Purpura
- Mucocutaneous hemorrhages
- Nonpalpable spleen (absence of splenomegaly is essential diagnostic criterion)

DIAGNOSTIC TESTS & INTERPRETATION

Lab

Initial lab tests

- Decreased platelet count: Typical range of 5,000–75,000
- Relative lymphocytosis and slight eosinophilia
- Prolonged bleeding time (not useful in presence of thrombocytopenia)
- Anemia
- Prothrombin time/partial thromboplastin time normal

Follow-Up & Special Considerations

- Platelet-associated antibody (PA-IgG):
  – Optional bound and unbound test available
- Bound is superior: Sensitivity 53–55%, specificity 82–84%
- Frequency of false-negative and false-positive results limit utility of these tests
- Not necessary for treatment decisions

Imaging

Head computed tomography to rule out intracranial bleeding if clinically indicated

Diagnostic Procedures/Surgery

- Bone marrow aspiration/biopsy (consider in refractory cases)
- With classic ITP, marrow cellularity is normal; may see increase in megakaryocytes
- Does not need to be done before giving γ-globulin
- Not needed in patients <60 years who have typical clinical and lab presentation
- Consider in patients >60 years to rule out myelodysplasia
- Rarely indicated in children, but preferred by some hematologists if steroids will be used in treatment

Pathological Findings

- Peripheral smear:
  – Routinely recommended
  – Shows normal red and white cells with large platelets but diminished in number
  – Helps rule out pseudothrombocytopenia
- Marrow reveals abundant megakaryocytes with normal erythroid and myeloid precursors.

DIFFERENTIAL DIAGNOSIS

- Drug-induced immune thrombocytopenia; >150 drugs have been implicated
- Infections
- Acute leukemia
- Thrombotic thrombocytopenia purpura
- Hemolytic uremic syndrome
- Factitious: Platelet clumping on the peripheral smear
- Thrombocytopenia secondary to sepsis
- Myelodysplastic syndrome, particularly in older patients
- Decreased production in marrow: Malignancy, drugs, viruses, megaloblastic anemia
- Post-transfusion
- Gestational thrombocytopenia
- Isoimmune neonatal purpura
- Congenital thrombocytopenias
- Disseminated intravascular coagulation
- Alcohol-induced thrombocytopenic purpura

 TREATMENT

MEDICATION

First Line

- Acute ITP: Oral prednisone 1–2 mg/kg/d for 2–4 weeks, then taper
- Chronic ITP:
  – Oral prednisone 1–2 mg/kg/d with tapers over 4–6 weeks; most responses occur within 1st week of treatment (3,4)[B]
  – Optimal duration of therapy unknown, but increased risk of complications if >2 months
  – Therapy does not appear to modify the natural history.

– For patients who do not respond, consider IV immune globulin 0.4 /kg/d for 5 days, or anti-D, 50–75 ug/kg once (repeat as necessary), or dexamethasone 20–40 mg/d for 4 days; 3–4 cyles 2 weeks apart (3,4,5)[C].

– If no response to these therapies, consider rituximab or splenectomy.

– Also limited data supporting screening for and eradication of *H. pylori*.

- Emergency treatment of patients with internal or mucocutaneous bleeding or who need emergent surgery treatment should include:

  – IV immune globulin 1 g/kg/d for 2 days; can be repeated on day 3 for nonresponders

  – IV methylprednisolone 1 g/d for 3 days

  – Platelet transfusions (5 U q4–6h or 2 U/hr)

- Contraindications: Do not administer γ-globulin if patient has IgA deficiency.

- Other adverse events with IVIg include fever and renal failure.

- Significant possible interactions: Anaphylaxis in patients with IgA deficiency who have IgA autoantibodies

Second Line
- Acute ITP: IV immune globulin (γ-globulin):

  – Single dose (1–2 g/kg) or 400 mg/kg/d for 5 days (4)[C]

  – Minor adverse reactions: Chills, nausea, headache, and joint pain may occur in 2–7% of the patients. If so, slow the rate of infusion.

  – γ-globulin may be effective alone or as pretreatment to facilitate platelet transfusion. This treatment may delay the need for a splenectomy.

- Chronic ITP: High doses of IV γ-globulin in emergencies (studies used platelet counts as surrogate marker and not bleeding outcomes)

- Anti-Rho(D) immune globulin 250 IU (50–75 μg/kg) as single dose or in 2 divided doses given over 2 days; indications for use:

  – Children with acute or chronic ITP

  – Adults with chronic ITP who are not antiglobulin (Coombs) test positive (otherwise are at risk for intravascular hemolysis)

  – ITP secondary to HIV infection

- Azathioprine: 1–4 mg/kg/d modified according to white blood cells

- Cyclophosphamide: 1–2 mg/kg/d

- Vincristine or vinblastine 2 mg IV/weekly

- Danazol: 400–800 mg/d

- Cyclosporin A: 3 mg/kg/d

- Rituximab 375 mg/m2 weekly for 4 weeks (3)

- Mycophenolate mofetil

- Thrombopoietin receptor (C MPL)-agonists (stimulate thrombopoiesis): Both are Food and Drug Administration-approved for refractory ITP

  – Eltrombopag (50 mg p.o. daily)

  – Romiplostim (1 mcg/kg subq weekly) (3,6)

ADDITIONAL TREATMENT
General Measures
- Outpatient management unless patient at risk for bleeding (platelet count <20,000)

- Admit patients with active bleeding.

- Children do not require treatment with:

  – Platelet count >30,000 and asymptomatic

  – Minor purpura

- Treat adults with:

  – Platelet count <20,000

  – Platelet count <50,000 with symptoms or risks for bleeding, such as hypetension or peptic ulcers

- Specific treatment usually not necessary unless count <100,000; possibly <30,000 with chronic ITP

- Platelet transfusions for significant bleeding

Issues for Referral
Hematology consultation recommended for patients with acute bleeding or who fail to respond to 1st-line therapies

SURGERY/OTHER PROCEDURES
Splenectomy:

- Reserved only for patients who fail medical therapy (4)

- Patients should receive 23-valent pneumococcal vaccine and *Haemophilus influenza b (HIB)* at least 2 weeks prior to splenectomy; also should receive meningococcal group C conjugate vaccine if not previously immunized.

- Consider lifelong prophylactic antibiotics with penicillin or erythromycin.

- Criteria and timing of surgery remain poorly defined; decision based on severity, response to treatment, and patient preference regarding risks–benefits of surgery.

- Splenectomy considered if after 3–6 months patient needs >10–20 mg/d prednisone to keep platelets above 30,000/mm³

- Should raise the platelet count to at least 20,000/mm³ prior to surgery

- Reported 5–10-year efficacy is ∼65% for all patients (3)

- Laparoscopic removal is becoming preferred technique due to lower surgical morbidity

- Experimental therapies include splenic embolization and splenic irradiation.

Pregnancy Considerations
- Only if <50,000 platelet count: May consider caesarean section

- A patient in labor should receive IV γ-globulin due to the risk to the infant.

- Platelet autoantibodies cross the placenta and may cause neonatal thrombocytopenia. Consider prednisone 10–20 mg/d for 10–14 days prior to delivery.

- Preeclampsia or gestational thrombocytopenia may cause thrombocytopenia unrelated to ITP.

 ## ONGOING CARE

FOLLOW-UP RECOMMENDATIONS
Patient Monitoring
Platelet counts should be monitored at least weekly for patients on prednisone, monthly for stable patients

PATIENT EDUCATION
- Minimal activity to prevent injury or bruising

- Avoid contact sports.

- Avoid ASA and other platelet-inhibiting drugs.

PROGNOSIS
- Acute ITP:

  – ∼80–85% of the patients completely recover within 2 months.

  – 15% proceed to chronic ITP.

- Chronic ITP:

  – ∼10–20% of the patients recover spontaneously.

  – Remainder with diminished platelets for months to years

  – May see spontaneous remissions (5%) and relapses

- ∼10% are refractory (fail medical therapy AND splenectomy)

- Chronic refractory ITP: Thrombocytopenia present for >3 months, failure to respond to splenectomy, platelet count of <50,000

COMPLICATIONS
- 1% mortality due to intracranial hemorrhage

- Severe blood loss

- Corticosteroid adverse effects

- Pneumococcal sepsis (if patient undergoes splenectomy)

Pediatric Considerations
- Better prognosis in children than adults

REFERENCES

1. Fogarty PF et al. Chronic immune thrombocytopenia in adults: epidemiology and clinical presentation. *Hematol Oncol Clin North Am*. 2009;23:1213–21.

2. Terrell DR, Beebe LA, Vesely SK, Neas BR, Segal JB, George JN et al. The incidence of immune thrombocytopenic purpura in children and adults: A critical review of published reports. *Am J Hematol*. 2010;85:174–80.

3. Bussel JB et al. Traditional and new approaches to the management of immune thrombocytopenia: issues of when and who to treat. *Hematol Oncol Clin North Am*. 2009;23:1329–41.

4. George JN. Chronic refractory immune (idiopathic) thrombocytopemic purpura in adults. In: *UpToDate*, Basow DS, (Ed), UpToDate, Waltham, MA, February 2010.

5. Godeau B, Provan D, Bussel J. Immune thrombocytopenic purpura in adults. *Curr Opin Hematol*. 2007;14:535–56.

6. Tarantino MD. The treatment of immune thrombocytopenic purpura in children. *Curr Hematol Rep*. 2006;5:89–94.

ADDITIONAL READING

Stasi R, Provan D. Management of immune thrombocytopenic purpura in adults. *Mayo Clin Proc*. 2004;79:504–22.

CODES

ICD9
287.31 Immune thrombocytopenic purpura

IMMUNODEFICIENCY DISEASES

Weily Soong, MD

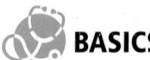 **BASICS**

DESCRIPTION

- Disorders caused by abnormal immune system function, resulting in increased susceptibility to infection
- Primary: An intrinsic defect in the immune mechanism:
  - Humoral (B-cell) immunodeficiencies:
    - Defects in antibody production
    - Agammaglobulinemia: X-linked (absent immunoglobulins; mutation in Bruton Tyrosine Kinase gene) and autosomal recessive (absent immunoglobulins; defect in B-cell development)
    - IgA deficiency: Most common primary immunodeficiency; very low or absent IgA; defect unknown
    - Common variable immunodeficiency: Decreased levels of IgG, IgA, and/or IgM and poor responses to vaccinations; usually adult onset; genetic defects are known in a small percentage of cases
    - IgG subclass deficiency: Decrease in IgG subclasses; defect and clinical significance are unknown
    - Specific antibody deficiency: Poor antibody response to specific antigens; defect unknown
    - Transient hypogammaglobulinemia of infancy: Temporary decrease in IgG and IgA due to delayed maturation of the humoral system; unknown cause
    - Others: Includes Ig κ chain defects; Ig heavy chain gene deletions; defects in UNG and ICOS genes; NEMO
  - Combined immunodeficiencies:
    - Defects in the cellular effector (T- and B-lymphocytes and NK cells) and humoral mechanisms
    - Severe combined immunodeficiency-SCID: All forms have absent T cells, and depending on the genetic mutation, may or may not have B cells and NK-cells; X-linked or autosomal recessive; includes mutations in adenosine deaminase deficiency gene, common interleukin γ chain, Jak3, CD45, RAG1 and 2 genes
    - Hyper-IgM syndrome: Normal to high IgM with low IgG and IgA; X-linked; defect in CD40 ligand and has features of a combined immunodeficiency; autosomal recessive; defect in AID gene and has features of a humoral immunodeficiency
    - Wiskott-Aldrich syndrome (WAS): X-linked; eczema, thrombocytopenia, repeated infections, decrease in T cells
    - Ataxia telangiectasia (A-T) (cerebellar ataxia, oculocutaneous telangiectasia, and cellular and humoral immunodeficiency; autosomal recessive)
    - Omenn syndrome: Erythroderma, eosinophilia, hepatosplenomegaly, increased IgE; autosomal recessive
    - Purine nucleoside phosphorylase (PNP) deficiency: Severe lymphopenia, especially T cells; hemolytic anemia; neurologic abnormalities; autosomal recessive
    - Others: Includes ZAP70 and CD40 defects

- Phagocytic immunodeficiencies:
  - Chronic granulomatous disease: Mutations in the oxidative burst mechanism of neutrophils; X-linked and autosomal recessive variants
  - Chediak-Higashi syndrome: Mutations in lysosomal transport protein; albinism and neurologic symptoms; autosomal recessive
  - Leukocyte adhesion deficiency: Defects in leukocyte endothelial adherence and chemotaxis; autosomal recessive
  - Other: Cyclic neutropenia, G-6PD deficiency, myeloperoxidase deficiency
- Complement deficiencies; usually autosomal recessive:
  - Early complement (C1q, C1r, C2, C4); cause autoimmune diseases, such as lupus
  - Late complement (C5–C9); susceptible to recurrent neisserial infections and autoimmune diseases
  - C3 and mannose-binding lectin deficiency; susceptible to recurrent pyogenic infections
- Pure cellular deficiencies and other well-defined syndromes:
  - DiGeorge syndrome: Thymic hypoplasia; decrease in T cells; associated with 22q11.2 chromosome deletions; de novo mutation or autosomal dominant
  - X-linked lymphoproliferative syndrome: Causes fatal infectious mononucleosis
  - Chronic mucocutaneous candidiasis or autoimmune polyglandular syndrome type 1: Mutations in the autoimmune regulator AIRE gene; causes autoimmune responses to endocrine tissues; autosomal recessive
  - Hyper-IgE syndrome (Job syndrome): Hgh IgE, chronic dermatitis, and recurrent infections; due to gene mutation in stat3
  - Autoinflammatory disorders: Recurrent fevers (familial Mediterranean fever, Muckle-Wells, familial cold urticaria; autosomal recessive or dominant)
  - WHIM syndrome: Associated with warts, hypogammaglobulinemia, infection, myelokathexis (retention of leukocytes in the bone marrow); autosomal dominant
  - Autoimmune lymphoproliferative syndrome (ALPS): Defects in apoptosis; adenopathy, autoimmune cytopenias; autosomal recessive
- Secondary: A result of a secondary process, like another illness, age, injury, or treatment:
  - Premature and newborn
  - Hereditary and metabolic diseases:
    - Chromosomal abnormalities (Down syndrome) and sickle cell disease
    - Diabetes mellitus
    - Uremia and nephrotic syndrome
    - Malnutrition, vitamin, and mineral deficiencies; protein-losing enteropathies (1)
  - Medications: Immunosuppressive drugs, such as corticosteroids, immune modulators, radiation, chemotherapy; phenytoin
  - Infections: Includes HIV and mononucleosis
  - Infiltrative and hematological diseases: Includes sarcoidosis, leukemias, lymphomas, myeloma, aplastic anemia
  - Surgery and trauma: Burns, splenectomy
  - Other: Lupus and other autoimmune diseases, chronic hepatitis, cirrhosis, aging, thymoma, chronic stress

EPIDEMIOLOGY
Incidence
- Secondary immunodeficiencies are more common than primary.
- Children are most likely to present with primary immunodeficiencies.
- Primary immunodeficiencies occur in 1 in 10,000 births to 1 in 2,000 births:
  - 65% humoral deficiencies, 15% combined deficiencies, 10% phagocytic deficiencies, 5% cellular deficiencies, 5% complement deficiencies
- Infectious complications: In primary humoral disorders, they usually appear after 6 months of age. In cellular or combined disorders, they may appear shortly after birth.
- IgA deficiency is the most common primary immunodeficiency (~1 in every 500 people).
- Common variable immunodeficiency affects 1 in 30,000–50,000 people and appears usually in early adulthood.

RISK FACTORS
For secondary deficiencies: Depends on the etiology

Genetics
Primary: Inherited genetic defect. See Description.

GENERAL PREVENTION
- For primary deficiencies: Goal is to avert infection by identification of at-risk newborns using genetic screening/counseling and prenatal diagnostic tests.
- For secondary deficiencies: Depends on the etiology

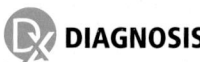 **DIAGNOSIS**

HISTORY
- A thorough history and family history will direct the proper search for a differential diagnosis.
- 10 warning signs suggestive of possible primary immunodeficiency (according to the Modell Foundation):
  - ≥ 8 new ear infections within 1 year
  - ≥ 2 serious sinus infections within 1 year
  - ≥ 2 months on antibiotics with little effect
  - ≥ 2 pneumonias within 1 year
  - Failure of an infant to gain weight or grow normally
  - Recurrent, deep skin or organ abscesses
  - Persistent thrush in mouth or elsewhere on skin, after age 1
  - Need for IV antibiotics to clear infections
  - ≥ 2 deep-seated infections
  - A family history of primary immunodeficiency
- Unusual susceptibility to infection. Type of infection might help determine the type of immunodeficiency:
  - Humoral deficiencies:
    - Associated with bacterial and protozoan infections (e.g., chronic sinusitis, recurrent respiratory infection, chronic diarrheal disease)
    - Infections include *S. pneumoniae, H. influenzae, S. aureus, P. aeruginosa,* mycoplasma, enteroviruses, *Giardia*

– Combined deficiencies:
  ○ Associated with severe fungal, bacterial, protozoal, and viral infections
  ○ Infections include all viral infections; bacterial infections found in humoral deficiencies plus *Listeria* and *Salmonella*, enteric flora; mycobacteria; *Candida*; *Pneumocystis*; *Toxoplasma*; *Cryptococcus*
– Cellular deficiencies:
  ○ Associated with severe viral, mycobacterial, and fungal infections
  ○ Infections include *Salmonella*, *Mycobacteria*, and *Candida*
– Phagocytic defects:
  ○ Infections include *S. aureus*, enteric flora, *Serratia*, *Nocardia*, *P. aeruginosa*, *S. typhi*, *A. fumigatus*, *C. albicans*, *Pneumocystis*; *Mycobacteria*
– Complement deficiencies:
  ○ Infections include bacterial infections found in humoral deficiencies, especially *N. meningitidis*
• Also associated with autoimmune disorders and malignancies, especially lymphoreticular

PHYSICAL EXAM
Physical exam may provide clues to correct diagnosis by allowing detection of subtle dysmorphology and site and type of infection.

DIAGNOSTIC TESTS & INTERPRETATION
Lab
Initial lab tests
High percentage of immunodeficiencies will be discovered by:
• CBC with differential smear. Normal total lymphocyte count in infants is higher than adults. Thus, a lymphocyte count of $<3,000/mm^3$ should be evaluated for an immunodeficiency (2).
• Serum protein electrophoresis for immunoglobulin levels, including IgG, IgA, IgM, and IgE; may include IgG subclasses. (Levels must be adjusted for age. Adults have higher levels than children.)
• Antibody responses to previous vaccines (tetanus, *Pneumococcus*, *H. influenzae*, diphtheria, varicella, pertussis)
• Infection evaluation, such as ESR, C-reactive protein, microbiology cultures
• Classical complement pathway test: CH50

Follow-Up & Special Considerations
• These labs might be drawn depending on the history and initial labs.
• Flow cytometry to examine lymphocyte subsets (CD4, CD8, CD3, CD19, CD20)
• Lymphocyte proliferation responses to mitogens and antigens
• Specific complement levels
• Delayed hypersensitivity skin tests (anergy panel to mumps, *Candida*, tetanus, *Trichophyton*)
• Phagocyte function: NBT test, dihydrorhodamine reductase test
• Specific cytokine function tests
• Genetic analysis

Imaging
Initial approach
CXR of a newborn infant to look for an absence of a thymic shadow in SCID or DiGeorge

 TREATMENT

MEDICATION
• Antibiotics with appropriate spectra for infecting organism(s):
  – May be used acutely, chronically, or prophylactically
• Antiviral therapy for HIV, varicella, herpes, influenza, and RSV
• Antifungal agents for specific fungal infections
• Intravenous or subcutaneous immunoglobulin (IVIg or SCIg):
  – For diseases deficient in IgG, such as agammaglobulinemias, common variable, hyper-IgM, WAS, and A-T (3)[A]
  – Should NOT be used for IgG subclass deficiency
  – Periodic problems with the supply of the drug due to high demand
• Enzyme replacement therapy for adenosine deaminase deficiency
• For secondary immunodeficiencies, treatment depends on the specific etiology.

ADDITIONAL TREATMENT
General Measures
• If newborn has been identified as being at risk, consider cord blood storage for stem cell transplants, appropriate labs and genetic tests, and potential for isolation in sterile environment.
• If patient with cellular or combined defects must be transfused, must use irradiated and CMV-negative blood products.
• Avoid all live attenuated viral vaccines in patients with severe cellular or antibody immunodeficiencies (varicella, oral polio, measles, mumps, rubella, smallpox, BCG).
• Bone marrow, stem cell, or thymic transplants for certain immunodeficiencies (e.g., SCID and DiGeorge) are best done at referral research centers.

Issues for Referral
Primary immunodeficiency patients should be referred to a physician specializing in allergy and clinical immunology for workup and management of immunodeficiency diseases.

 ONGOING CARE

FOLLOW-UP RECOMMENDATIONS
Patient Monitoring
• Monitor for infections and their complications.
• Infection control precautions: Depends on the situation and includes frequent handwashing, gloves, gowns, masks, safe water supply
• Monitor and maintain IgG levels in common variable hypogammaglobulinemia.

PATIENT EDUCATION
• Immune Deficiency Foundation, 25 West Chesapeake Ave. Room 206, Towson, MD 21204. Tel: 800-296-4433. http://www.primaryimmune.org.
• Jeffrey Modell Foundation, 747 3rd Avenue, New York, NY 10017. Tel: 212-819-0200. http://www.info4pi.org and http://www.jmfworld.com.

PROGNOSIS
• Short-term prognosis is related closely to the severity of the infectious complication.
• Long-term prognosis is related to the nature of the immune defect and the type and degree of immunodeficiency.

COMPLICATIONS
• Autoimmune disorders
• Reactions to immunoglobulin treatment
• Malignancies, especially lymphoreticular
• Overwhelming infection
• Fatal graft-versus-host disease following blood transfusions in patients with SCID

REFERENCES
1. Chinen J, Shearer WT et al. Secondary immunodeficiencies, including HIV infection. *J Allergy Clin Immunol.* 2010;125:S195–203.
2. Oliveira JB, Fleisher TA et al. Laboratory evaluation of primary immunodeficiencies. *J Allergy Clin Immunol.* 2010;125:S297–305.
3. Ballow M. Primary immunodeficiency disorders: antibody deficiency. *J Allergy Clin Immunol.* 2002;109:581–91.

ADDITIONAL READING
• Jorgensen GH, Arnlaugsson S, Theodors A, Ludviksson BR et al. Immunoglobulin A deficiency and oral health status: a case-control study. *J Clin Periodontol.* 2010;37:1–8.
• Notarangelo LD et al. Primary immunodeficiencies. *J. Allergy Clin. Immunol.* 2010;125:S182–94.

 CODES

ICD9
• 279.00 Hypogammaglobulinemia, unspecified
• 279.01 Selective iga immunodeficiency
• 279.3 Unspecified immunity deficiency

CLINICAL PEARLS
• Secondary causes of immunodeficiencies are more common than primary immunodeficiencies.
• If there is a history of any recurrent or unresolved infections, check an IgG level. It is easy and inexpensive, and probably more useful than repeating other labs, such as a CBC.
• Consult a clinical immunologist if an immunodeficiency is suspected.

IMPETIGO

Elisabeth L. Backer, MD

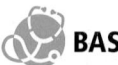 BASICS

DESCRIPTION
- A contagious, superficial, intraepidermal infection occurring prominently on exposed areas of the face and extremities
- Affected patients usually have multiple lesions.
- Cultures positive in >80% cases for *Staphylococcus aureus* either alone or combined with group A β-hemolytic streptococci; *S. aureus* more common pathogen since 1990s
- Nonbullous impetigo: Formation of vesiculopustules that rupture, leading to crusting with a characteristic golden appearance; local lymphadenopathy may occur.
- Bullous impetigo: Staphylococcal impetigo that progresses rapidly to small to large flaccid bullae (newborns/young children) caused by epidermolytic toxin release; less lymphadenopathy; <30% of patients
- Folliculitis: Considered by some to be *S. aureus* impetigo of hair follicles
- Ecthyma: A deeper, ulcerated impetigo infection often with lymphadenitis
- System(s) affected: Skin/Exocrine
- Synonym(s): Pyoderma; Impetigo contagiosa; Impetigo vulgaris; Fox impetigo

EPIDEMIOLOGY
Incidence
- Predominant sex: Male = Female
- Predominant age: 2–5 years

Prevalence
In the US: Unreported

Pediatric Considerations
- Poststreptococcal glomerulonephritis may follow impetigo (in young children).
- Impetigo neonatorum may occur due to nursery contamination.

RISK FACTORS
- Warm, humid environment
- Tropical or subtropical climate
- Summer or fall season
- Minor trauma, insect bites
- Poor hygiene, poverty, crowding, epidemics, wartime
- Familial spread
- Poor health with anemia and malnutrition

- Complication of pediculosis, scabies, chickenpox, eczema/atopic dermatitis
- Contact dermatitis (Rhus)
- Burns
- Contact sports
- Children in day care
- Possibly tobacco exposure
- Carriage of group A *Streptococcus* and *S. aureus*

GENERAL PREVENTION
- Close attention to family hygiene, particularly handwashing among children
- Covering of wounds
- Avoidance of crowding and sharing of personal items
- Treatment of atopic dermatitis

ETIOLOGY
- Coagulase-positive staphylococci: Pure culture ~50–90%; more contagious via contact
- β-Hemolytic streptococci: Pure culture only ~10% of the time
- Mixed infections of streptococci and staphylococci common; data suggest increasing importance of staphylococci over past 20 years (1)[C]
- Direct contact or insect vector
- Can result from contamination at trauma site
- Regional lymphadenopathy

COMMONLY ASSOCIATED CONDITIONS
- Malnutrition and anemia
- Crowded living conditions
- Poor hygiene
- Neglected minor trauma
- Any chronic/underlying dermatitis

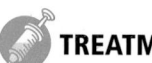 DIAGNOSIS

HISTORY
- Lesions are often described as painful (or pruritic).
- May be slow and indolent or rapidly spreading
- Most frequent on face around mouth and nose or at site of trauma

PHYSICAL EXAM
- Tender red macule or papule as early lesion
- Thin-roofed vesicle to bullae: Usually nontender
- Pustules
- Weeping, shallow, red ulcer
- Honey-colored crusts
- Satellite lesions
- Often multiple sites
- Bullae on buttocks, trunk, face

DIAGNOSTIC TESTS & INTERPRETATION
Lab
Initial lab tests
- None usually done; however, rarely consider the following:
  - Culture: Taken from the base of lesion after removal of crust will grow both staphylococci and group A streptococci
  - ASO titer: Can be weak positive for streptococci
  - Streptozyme: Positive for streptococci
- Disorders that may alter lab results: Streptococcal pharyngitis will alter streptococcal enzyme tests.

Follow-Up & Special Considerations
Monitor for spread of disease and systemic manifestations.

Pathological Findings
Acute purulent infection of the skin due to *S. aureus*, group A β-hemolytic streptococci, or mixed bacteria

DIFFERENTIAL DIAGNOSIS
- Nonbullous:
  - Chickenpox
  - Herpes
  - Folliculitis
  - Erysipelas
  - Insect bites
  - Severe eczematous dermatitis
  - Scabies
  - Tinea corporis
- Bullous:
  - Burns
  - Pemphigus vulgaris
  - Bullous pemphigoid
- Stevens-Johnson syndrome

TREATMENT

MEDICATION
- In 2005, the Infectious Disease Society of America (IDSA) recommended topical treatment for limited lesions and oral medication when the disease is more severe/extensive (2)[C].
- Optimal treatment is unclear due to limited quality of evidence (3,4)[A].
- Penicillin and macrolide therapy is no longer recommended. Fluoroquinolones are not indicated due to resistance patterns.
- Dicloxacillin, cephalexin, clindamycin, topical mupirocin, and fucidic acid are effective unless local staphylococcal strains are resistant. (For methicillin-resistant *S. aureus* [MRSA] infections, treatment options include clindamycin and linezolid.)

- Consult the local hospital or health department for microbial resistance information.
- Nonbullous (minor spread, treat 7 days; widespread, treat 10 days); bullous (treat 10 days):
  - Retapamulin 1% ointment to be applied b.i.d. × 5 days (5)[B]
  - Mupirocin (Bactroban) topical ointment applied t.i.d. × 7–10 days (nonbullous only); not as effective on scalp as around mouth
  - Dicloxacillin: Adult 250 mg p.o. q.i.d.; pediatric 12–25 mg/kg/d divided q6h
- Contraindications: Drug allergy
- Precautions: Refer to manufacturer's profile for each drug.
- Significant possible interactions: Refer to manufacturer's profile for each drug.
- Oral doses
- 1st-generation cephalosporins: Children:
  - Cephalexin: 25–50 mg/kg/d divided q6h
  - Cefaclor: 20–40 mg/kg/d divided q8h
  - Cephradine: 25–50 mg/kg/d divided q6h–q12h
  - Cefadroxil: 30 mg/kg/d divided b.i.d.
- 1st-generation cephalosporins: Adults:
  - Cephalexin: 250 mg q.i.d.
  - Cefaclor: 250 mg t.i.d.
  - Cephradine: 500 mg b.i.d.
  - Cefadroxil: 1 g/d in divided doses
- Clindamycin
- Severe bullous disease may require IV therapy such as nafcillin or cefazolin.

ADDITIONAL TREATMENT

General Measures
- Prevention with mupirocin or triple antibiotic ointment t.i.d. to sites of minor skin trauma
- Removal of crusts, cleanliness with gentle washing 2–3× daily; clean with antibacterial soap, chlorhexidine, or betadine.
- Washing of entire body may prevent recurrence at distant sites.

Issues for Referral
If resistant or extensive infections occur, especially in immunocompromised patients

Additional Therapies
Monitor for microbial resistance patterns.

ONGOING CARE

FOLLOW-UP RECOMMENDATIONS
- Athletes restricted from contact sports
- School and daycare contagious restrictions

Patient Monitoring
If not clear within 7–10 days, culture the lesions.

PATIENT EDUCATION
Avoidance of infection spread is key; handwashing is vital.

PROGNOSIS
- Complete resolution in 7–10 days with treatment
- Antibiotic treatment will not prevent or halt glomerulonephritis, as it will rheumatic fever.
- If not clear within 7–10 days, culture is necessary to find resistant organism.
- Recurrent impetigo: Evaluate for carriage of *S. aureus* in nares (also perineum, axillae, toe web). Apply mupirocin ointment to nares b.i.d. × 5 days for clearance/decolonization.

COMPLICATIONS
- Ecthyma
- Erysipelas
- Poststreptococcal acute glomerulonephritis
- Cellulitis
- Bacteremia
- Osteomyelitis
- Septic arthritis
- Pneumonia
- Lymphadenitis

REFERENCES

1. Britton JW, Fajardo JE, Krafte-Jacobs B. Comparison of mupirocin and erythromycin in the treatment of impetigo. *J Pediatr*. 1990;117:827–9.
2. Stevens DL, Bisno AL, Chambers HF, et al. Practice guidelines for the diagnosis and management of skin and soft-tissue infections. *Clin Infect Dis*. 2005;41:1373–406.
3. Koning S, Verhagen AP, van Suijlekom-Smit LW, et al. Interventions for impetigo. *Cochrane Database Syst Rev*. 2004:CD003261.
4. George A, Rubin G. A systematic review and meta-analysis of treatments for impetigo. *Br J Gen Pract*. 2003;53:480–7.
5. Parish LC, Jorizzo JL, Breton JJ, et al. Topical retapamulin ointment (1%, wt/wt) twice daily for 5 days versus oral cephalexin twice daily for 10 days in the treatment of secondarily infected dermatitis: results of a randomized controlled trial. *J Am Acad Dermatol*. 2006;55:1003–13.

ADDITIONAL READING

- *American Academy of Pediatrics. Red Book 2006: Report on the Committee on Infectious Diseases*. New York: Author, 2006.
- Kowalski TJ, Berbari EF, Osmon DR. Epidemiology, treatment, and prevention of community-acquired methicillin-resistant Staphylococcus aureus infections. *Mayo Clin Proc*. 2005;80:1201–7; quiz 1208.

See Also (Topic, Algorithm, Electronic Media Element)
Algorithm: Rash, Focal

CODES

ICD9
684 Impetigo

CLINICAL PEARLS

- Superficial, intraepidermal infection
- Predominantly staphylococcal in origin
- Microbial resistance patterns need to be monitored.
- Topical treatment recommended for limited lesions and oral medication only when the disease is more severe/extensive.

I

INCONTINENCE, FECAL

Felix B. Chang, MD
Ivan J. Briones, MD

BASICS

Continuous or recurrent uncontrolled passage of fecal material (>10 ml) for >1 month

DESCRIPTION
- Involuntary passage of fecal material through the anal canal for >1 month in an individual >3 years old
- True incontinence is the involuntary excretion of feces. Pseudoincontinence includes incontinence to flatus and occasional seepage of liquid stool.
- Fecal incontinence was the second leading cause of nursing home placement.
  - Recurrent uncontrolled passage of fecal material
  - Involuntary loss of solid or liquid stools
  - Endorectal ultrasound (EUS) is the simplest, most reliable, and least invasive test to find anatomic defects in thel anal sphincters.
  - The goal of treatment should be to restore continence and improve quality of life.

Geriatric Considerations
- The prevalence of fecal incontinence (FI) increases with age and is higher in older men than women.
- Idiopathic fecal incontinence: No identified cause; more common in middle aged or elderly women.

EPIDEMIOLOGY
Incidence
Patients under-report fecal incontinence unless prompted. Studies may underestimate the number of patients affected.

Prevalence
- In younger persons, women > men
- 7.1% of the adults, increases with age.
- 56–66% of hospitalized older patients and over 50% in nursing home residents
- 50–70% of patients who have urinary incontinence also suffer from fecal incontinence.

Pregnancy Considerations
- Obstetrical injury to the pelvic floor, during pregnancy or delivery, may result in subsequent incontinence.

Geriatric Considerations
- Fecal impaction and overflow diarrhea leading to FI is a common scenario in frail older patients.
- Surgical history:
  - Anal surgery, including hemorrhoidectomy, anal fissure repair, anal dilatation

RISK FACTORS
Physical status:
- Older age, female sex, obesity, limited physical activity
- Positive family history
- Neuropsychiatric conditions:
  - Multiple sclerosis, spinal cord injury, dementia, depression, stroke, diabetic neuropathy
- Trauma:
  - Prostatectomy, radiation
  - Risk factors at the time of delivery include the use of forceps and the need for an episiotomy.
  - Forceps delivery, occipitoposterior position, and prolonged second stage of labor

- Other:
  - Diarrhea, inflammatory bowel disease, irritable bowel syndrome, menopause, smoking, constipation
  - Potential association with child abuse and sexual abuse
  - Congenital abnormalities such as imperforate anus or rectal prolapse
  - Fecal impaction is a common cause of fecal incontinence in the elderly.

GENERAL PREVENTION
- Behavioral and lifestyle changes can reduce the risk for fecal incontinence (Obesity, limited physical activity or exercise, poor diet, and smoking).
- Post-meal bowel regimen
- Avoid episiotomy when possible
- Pelvic floor muscle training during pregnancy

PATHOPHYSIOLOGY
- Continence is dependent on the complex relationships involving temporal coordination of variety of muscles, nereves and the reflex ARCS.
- Important factors in mantaining continence include stool consistency, stool volume, colonic transit time, anorectal sensation, rectal compliance, anoreactal reflexes, external and internal muscle sphincter integrity, the puborectalis muscles, and the mental capability.
- Disease processes or structural defects that alter any of these aspects can contribute to fecal incontinence.
- Diabetes is the most common metabolic disorder which affects the pudendal nerve and leads to neuropathy.

ETIOLOGY
- Congenital: Spina bifida and myelomeningocele with spinal cord damage
- Anal sphincter damage from vaginal delivery, surgical procedures, inflammatory conditions, neoplasia
- Medical: Diabetes, stroke, spinal cord trauma, degenerative disorders of the nervous system
- Obstetric injury: Sphincter disruption, tears, or trauma to the pudendal nerve

COMMONLY ASSOCIATED CONDITIONS
- Age >70 years
- Urinary incontinence or pelvic organ prolapse
- Chronic medical condition, such as diabetes, dementia, cerebrovascular accidents, cord compression, dementia, depression, immobility, chronic obstructive pulmonary disease, irritable bowel syndrome, urinary incontinence, or colectomy.
- Obstetric injury at young age
- Surgeries in the anorectal area
- Stroke
- History of irradiation

DIAGNOSIS

- "How often do you leak urine or stool?"
- "Do you use pads or protective garments?"

HISTORY
- Patients seldom volunteer information about FI.
- Determine by history:
  - Severity (soiling by liquid stools only or gross incontinence of solid stools)
  - Onset and duration (recent onset vs. chronic)

- Frequency, presence of constipation or diarrhea
- Review of medications
- Home environment, which may reveal barriers to bathroom facilities
- Asses diet, medical, and obstetrical history, lifestyle, mobility.
- Evaluate cognition with Mini–Mental Status Exam.
- Possible overlapping history of social withdrawal and depression
- Document geriatric depression scale.

PHYSICAL EXAM
- The perianal area should be inspected.
- Inspect the perineum for chemical dermatitis, hemorrhoids, fistula, surgical scars, skin tags, rectal prolapse, soiling, and ballooning of the perineum (sarcopenia of pelvic musculature).
- Internal digital examination
- A gaping anal orifice may indicate myopathy or neurological disorder.
- Evaluate the external sphincter in response to perineal skin stimulation (anal wink). Absence is suggestive of neuropathic component.
- Ask the patient to bear down, preferably in standing position, to look for subclinical rectal prolapse.
- Digital rectal examination to estimate anal canal pressure while resting and during voluntary squeeze, rectal bleeding, hemorrhoids, neoplasm, fecal consistency, and clues to diarrhea or distal fecal impaction.
- Neurologic examination, including perianal sensation.

DIAGNOSTIC TESTS & INTERPRETATION
History and physical exam will usually be enough for diagnosis. In selected patients, consider:
- EUS: Currently the simplest, most reliable, and least invasive test for defining anatomic defects in the external and internal anal sphincters, rectal wall, and the puborectalis muscle. Can be use to predict the therapeutic response to sphincteroplasty
- Plain abdominal xray
- Sigmoidoscopy/anoscopy/colonoscopy
- Defecography can measure the anorectal angle, evaluate pelvic descent, and detect occult or overt rectal prolapse.
- MRI defecography (Dynamic MRI imaging) further define pelvic floor anatomy.
- Anorectal manometry: Measure parameters such as maximal resting anal pressure, amplitude and duration of squeeze pressure, the rectoanal inhibitory reflex, threshold of conscious rectal sensation, rectal compliance, and rectal and anal pressure during straining.
- Pudendal nerve terminal motor latency (PNTML): This technique is operator-dependent and has poor correlation with clinical symptoms and histological findings.
- Electromyography: Sometimes helpful in evaluating neurogenic or myopathic damage in patients with fecal incontinence.
- Three-dimensional ultrasound (3D-EUS): Under study

Lab
Initial lab tests
- If history of antibiotics, tube feedings, or have the signs and symptoms of sepsis, examination of stools for ova, parasites, and *Clostridium difficile* toxin assay

- Measure TSH, electrolytes, and BUN in elderly patients with impaction.

Follow-Up & Special Considerations
Anorectal physiology laboratory

Imaging
- EUS may demostrate anal sphinters, rectal wall, and the puborectalis muscle structural abnormalities (1).
- EUS can detect a sphincter injury in up to 35% of women who delivered vaginally.

Initial approach
The approach to the problem of FI in older patients should be individualized, minimally invasive, convenient, and practically feasible.

DIFFERENTIAL DIAGNOSIS
- Anorectal disorders:
  - Inflammatory or infectious disorders
  - Neoplasms, radiation, ischemia, fistulas
  - Prolapsing internal hemorrhoids or rectal prolapse
  - Trauma: Obstetric, surgical, radiation, accidental
- Neurological disorders:
  - Stroke, dementia, neoplasms, spinal cord injury and/or diseases or altered level of consciousness
  - Pudendal neuropathy, neurosyphilis, multiple sclerosis, diabetes mellitus
- Miscellaneous causes:
  - Infectious diarrhea, fecal impaction and overflow, irritable bowel syndrome (IBS), laxative abuse, inflammatory bowel disease, short bowel syndrome, muscle diseases, senescence and frailty, collagen vascular disease, psychological and behavioral problems, radiotherapy

 ## TREATMENT

MEDICATION
- No specific medication has been proven to be of benefit for fecal incontinence. Little evidence regarding drug therapy for FI in adults (2)[A].
- Antidiarrheal agents, such as adsorvents or opium derivatives, may reduce FI symptoms.
- Adsorbens, such as Kaopectate 1200–1500 mg p.o. after each stool (max 9000 mg/24 h)
- Commonly used opium derivates are loperamide, diphenoxylate hydrochloride plus atropine sulphate, codeine, and tincture of opium.
- Loperamide: 2–4 mg followed by titration up to a total of 24 mg per 24 hours in divided doses
- Diphenoxylate: 1 tablet, 2.5 mg, every 3–4 hours

First Line
Specific treatment of the cause of diarrhea (such as infectious diarrhea or inflammatory bowel disease)

Second Line
- Increase dietary fiber in milder forms of FI to improve symptoms. Stool bulking agents include high-fiber diet, psyllium products, or methylcellulose.
- Patients with overflow incontinence may benefit from the addition of regularly scheduled enemas or laxatives, especially when defecation is delayed.
- A trial of cholestyramine may be helpful if bile acid malabsorption is suspected.
- If gut dysmotility suspected: A trial of loperamide, clonidine, antibiotics, or octreotide
- Patients with a stool impaction should be disimpacted and treated with a bowel regimen to prevent recurrence.

ADDITIONAL TREATMENT
General Measures
- If ambulatory, prompted and scheduled defection (effective particularly in patients who have overflow incontinence)
- If bed-bound, schedule osmotic laxatives, or stimulant laxatives if constipated
- Enemas, laxatives, and suppositories may help to promote more complete bowel emptying in appropiate patients and minimize further postdefecation leakage.
- Scheduled toileting and use of stool deodorants (Periwash, Derfil, Devrom).

Additional Therapies
- Biofeedback: Training involves teaching the patient to recognize small volumes of rectal distension and to contract the external anal sphincter while simultaneously keeping intra-abdominal pressure low (3)[A]. Diabetics may benefit.
- Patients with systemic neurological disease, anal deformity, or frequent episodes of incontinence respond poorly.

SURGERY/OTHER PROCEDURES
- Surgery should be considered only when the nonsurgical approaches have failed.
- Insufficeint evidence regarding surgery for FI in adults (4)[A]
- Surgical approaches to sphincter repair include:
  - Direct apposition, overlapping anterior sphincteroplasty, and placation procedures
  - Hemorrhoidectomy, repair of rectal prolapse, repair of anal sphincter defects, sphincteroplasty of native sphincter or creating a new sphincter mechanism using graciloplasty, artificial sphincter implants
  - Colostomy as a last resort
- Anterior sphincteroplasty is most successful in cases of isolated sphincter defect.
- Evolving procedures include injection of biomaterials (silicone, collagen, carbon-coated microbeads) (5)[A], SECCA procedure (radiofrequency energy delivered to the anal canal), rectal augmentation, sacral nerve stimulation, and anticon and procon incontinence device.

IN-PATIENT CONSIDERATIONS
Initial Stabilization
If secondary to fecal impaction, manual fragmentation and extraction of fecal mass (after lubrication with lidocaine jelly)

Nursing
- Avoid catharsis.
- No hot water, soap, or hydrogen peroxide enemas.

Discharge Criteria
Outpatient care

 ## ONGOING CARE

FOLLOW-UP RECOMMENDATIONS
Periodic rectal exam

Patient Monitoring
Fewer than 1 bowel movement every other day with FI might suggest impaction.

DIET
- High fiber (25g/d) and at least 1.5 L fluid daily
- Avoid foods known to worsen symptoms (caffeine).

PATIENT EDUCATION
Kegel/sphincter training exercises alone do not work for fecal incontinence, but may supplement.

PROGNOSIS
- Reimpaction likely if bowel program not followed
- 50% failure rate over 5 years following overlapping sphincteroplasty

COMPLICATIONS
- Depression and social isolation
- Skin ulcerations
- Artificial bowel sphincter: 30% infection rate

REFERENCES
1. Woodfield CA, Krishnamoorthy S, Hampton BS et al. Imaging pelvic floor disorders: trend toward comprehensive MRI. *AJR Am J Roentgenol.* 2010;194:1640–9.
2. Cheetham MJ, Brazzelli M, Norton C et al. Drug treatment for Faecal incontinence in adults. *Cochrane Database Syst Rev.* 2008;16;(3): CD002116.
3. Norton C, Cody J, et al. biofeedback and or sphincter exercises for the treatment of faecal incontinence in adults. *Cochrane Library.* 2006;Issue 3:CD002111.
4. Brown S, Nelson R. et al. Surgery for Faecal Incontinence in Adults. *Cochrane Library.* 2007;Issue 2:CD001757.
5. Maeda Y, Laurberg S, Norton C et al. Perianal injectable bulking agents as treatment for faecal incontinence in adults. *Cochrane Database Syst Rev.* 2010;5:CD007959.

See Also (Topic, Algorithm, Electronic Media Element)
Algorithm: Rectal Incontinence

 ## CODES

ICD9
- 787.60 Full incontinence of feces
- 787.61 Incomplete defecation
- 787.62 Fecal smearing

CLINICAL PEARLS
- New onset of fecal incontinence may also indicate spinal cord compression, especially when observed with other neurologic symptoms.
- The absence of anocutaneous reflex suggest nerve damage and interruption of anorectal function.
- True incontinence must be differentiated from frequency and urgency without loss of bowel contents, which can occur in the setting of inflammatory disease, IBS, and pelvic irradiation.

INCONTINENCE, URINARY ADULT FEMALE

Elizabeth E. Houser, MD
Ann Lavers, MD

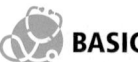 **BASICS**

DESCRIPTION
- Urinary incontinence is the involuntary loss of urine that is objectively demonstrable and is of medical, financial, social, and hygienic concern.
- Stress incontinence: Associated with increased intra-abdominal pressure, such as coughing, laughing, sneezing, or exertion
- Urge incontinence: Sudden uncontrollable urgency, leading to leakage of urine (also known as overactive bladder or detrusor veractivity)
- Mixed incontinence: Loss of urine from a combination of stress and urge incontinence
- Overflow incontinence: High residual or chronic urinary retention leads to urinary spillage from an overdistended bladder
- Functional incontinence: Loss of urine due to deficits of cognition and mobility
- Total incontinence: Continuous leakage of urine; leakage without awareness

EPIDEMIOLOGY
- Affects 25–45% of adult women (who experienced urine leakage at least once in the past year) (1,2,3)
- Affects 60–78% of women in nursing homes (3)
- Stress urinary incontinence is the most common in women 19–64 years of age (20–25%), followed by mixed (15–20%), and urge (4–9%). In women 65–80 years of age, mixed is the most common (18%), followed by stress (16%), and urge (13%). In women over 80 years of age, mixed is the most common (28%), followed by urge (11%), and stress (8%) (4).

RISK FACTORS
Advanced age, obesity, menopause, pregnancy, vaginal childbirth, pelvic surgery or radiation, urethral diverticula, genital prolapse, smoking, chronic obstructive pulmonary disease (COPD), cognitive impairment, constipation, and pelvic floor dysfunction

GENERAL PREVENTION
Weight loss, pelvic floor exercises, smoking cessation, avoidance of bladder-irritant foods, increased fiber intake to reduce constipation, bladder retraining, and timed fluid intake

PATHOPHYSIOLOGY
- Stress incontinence: Occurs with increased intra-abdominal pressure without uninhibited detrusor contraction. 2 types:
  – Anatomic: Due to urethral hypermobility from lack of pelvic support
  – Intrinsic sphincter deficiency (ISD): Impairment of various intrinsic factors is responsible for the normal coaptation and closure of the urethra. Urethral mucosal seal and inherent closure from collagen, fibroelastic tissue, smooth and striated muscles, etc., may be lost secondary to surgical scarring, radiation, or hormonal and senile changes.

- Urge incontinence: May be due to detrusor overactivity, or may be idiopathic
- Overflow incontinence: Urinary retention (usually from lower motor paralytic neurogenic bladder)
- Total incontinence: Constant loss of urine in epispadias-exstrophy complex due to absence of bladder neck and urethra. Ectopic ureters in females usually open in the urethra distal to the sphincter or in the vagina, causing continuous leakage. Also may occur with fistulous connections between bladder, ureters, or urethra and vagina or uterus.

COMMONLY ASSOCIATED CONDITIONS
Pelvic organ prolapse, urinary tract infection (UTI), COPD, diabetes mellitus, neurological disease, obesity, chronic constipation, and any disease that results in chronic cough

 DIAGNOSIS

HISTORY
- Age: Stress incontinence is more common in women aged 19–64, while mixed incontinence is more common in women over 65. Incontinence dating from childhood indicates congenital causes such as ectopic ureter, epispadias, etc., or unresolved bedwetting issues.
- Childbirth: Weakness of the pelvic floor is more likely in multiparous women.
- Amount and nature of leakage: Severity of leakage should be graded by the number of pads used in 24 hours
- Stress incontinence: Occurs in small spurts. Patients typically remain dry at night in bed.
- Urge incontinence: Sudden urge followed by leakage of large amounts, usually associated with frequency and nocturia
- Continuous slow leakage in between regular voiding indicates ectopic ureter, urinary fistula, etc.
- Pain: Suprapubic pain with dysuria implies urinary infection, dyspareunia, interstitial cystitis, etc.
- Medical history:
  – Neurologic conditions: cerebrovascular accident, parkinsonism, multiple sclerosis, myelodysplasia, diabetes, spinal cord injury
  – Radiation to pelvic and vaginal areas: Causes ISD, overactive bladder, fibrotic changes of pelvic floor musculature, and low bladder compliance
  – A history of smoking and chronic obstructive pulmonary disease with a chronic cough can aggravate incontinence.
  – A history of constipation can aggravate incontinence.
  – History of obesity
  – Hormonal status
  – Obstetrical history

- Medications:
  – Sympatholytic alpha-blockers (terazosin, prazosin, doxazosin, tamsulosin, alfuzosin, sildosin) can cause or worsen incontinence.
  – Sympathomimetic and tricyclic antidepressants (ephedrine, imipramine, amitryptyline, duloxetine, etc.) can cause retention with overflow incontinence.
  – Anticholinergic agents (tolteradine, oxybutinin, darifenacin, tropsium chloride, solifenacin, etc.)
- Surgical history: Previous pelvic surgery, including gynecologic and bowel surgery, can injure the pelvic floor support and musculature, and affect the neurologic function.

PHYSICAL EXAM
- General neurologic examination:
  – Mental status, speech, intellectual performance
  – Motor status: Gait, generalized or focal weakness, rigidity, tremor
  – Sensory status: Impairment of perineal-sacral area sensation helps localize the level of neurologic deficit.
  – Reflex: A bulbocavernous reflex implies contraction of the anal sphincter in response to squeezing the clitoris. This reflex tests the integrity of sacral 2, 3, 4 spinal cord segments.
- Urologic examination:
  – Abdomen: Visible exstrophy-epispadias; incisional scars of previous surgeries
  – Suprapubic tenderness: May indicate cystitis
  – Palpable bladder: Chronic urinary retention
- Pelvic examination:
  – Vaginal examination with empty bladder to check pelvic organs
  – Vaginal examination with comfortably full bladder
  – The patient is asked to cough or strain to reproduce incontinence.
  – Cystocele: If evident, is staged (grade 0–4)
  – Rectocele: If evident, is staged
  – Enterocele: If evident, is staged
  – Urethral hypermobility: Gauged by palpation of the descent of the proximal urethra on straining
  – Assessment of pelvic floor resting tone and function (ability to isolate and contract pelvic floor musculature)

DIAGNOSTIC TESTS & INTERPRETATION
Lab
- Urine analysis
- Urine culture
- Atypical urinary infections including ureaplasma and mycoplasma

Imaging
- Bladder scan to evaluate post-void residual
- Upper tract imaging if upper tract involvement is suspected: Computed tomography scan, intravenous pyelogram, or renal sonogrophy

Diagnostic Procedures/Surgery

Bladder diary to evaluate oral intake, timing of leakage, and patient habits

Urodynamic studies:

- Cystometric study of detrusor function: Determines bladder compliance, sensations, and detrusor responses to filling
- Uroflow with electromyography: Evaluates for any obstructive concerns
- Valsalva leak point pressure: Determines the intra-abdominal pressure at which leakage is observed
- Videourodynamic studies: Sophisticated combination of fluorocystourethrography and urodynamic studies

DIFFERENTIAL DIAGNOSIS

- Stress incontinence: Due to urethral hypermobility or ISD, though in the majority it is mixed or due to both
- Urge incontinence: Detrusor overactivity, conditions that irritate the bladder lining, but is often idiopathic
- Nocturnal enuresis: Idiopathic, detrusor overactivity, neurogenic, cardiogenic, or sleep apnea
- Continuous leakage: Ectopic ureter, urinary fistulas, exstrophy-epispadias complex
- Postvoid dribbling: Urethral diverticulum, idiopathic, iatrogenic, surgical

TREATMENT

Lifestyle changes and behavioral modification are 1st-line interventions and when properly trained, as effective as medications at reducing incontinence episode frequency:

- Lifestyle changes: Weight loss if obese, avoidance of certain foods that may make matters worse (caffeine, acidic foods, etc.), toileting on a scheduled basis
- Behavioral modification: Bladder training, Kegel exercises (training by professional improves outcomes), weighted cone, biofeedback

MEDICATION
First Line

- Urge incontinence: Anticholinergic agents:
  – Tolteridine (Detrol LA) 2–8 mg p.o. every day
  – Oxybutinin (Ditopan XL) 5–15 mg p.o. every day
  – Solifenacin (Vesicare) 5–10 mg p.o. every day
  – Darifenicin (Enablex) 7.5–15 mg p.o. every day
  – Tropsium chloride (Sanctura XR) 60 mg p.o. every day
  – Transdermal oxybutynin (Gelnique) 10% applied daily
  – Fesoterodine (Toviaz) 4–8 mg p.o every day
  – Imipramine (Tofranil) 10–60 mg p.o. q.h.s.
  – Amitryptiline (Elavil) 10–100 mg p.o. q.h.s.
- Stress incontinence:
  – Pelvic floor rehabilitation
  – Anticholinergics may be successful in mixed incontinence.

Second Line

Nonsurgical management: Helps about 50–65% of patients with milder symptoms

- Behavioral therapy: Timed voiding, dietary counseling
- Biofeedback and electrostimulation
- Occlusive and supportive devices
- Accupuncture (in selected cases)

ADDITIONAL TREATMENT
General Measures

- Treat correctable causes (UTI, etc.).
- Encourage weight loss in obese patients.
- Aggressive correction of constipation

SURGERY/OTHER PROCEDURES

Surgical management for stress incontinence:

- Periurethral injection of bulking agents: Collagen, carbon beads, hyaluronic acid, calcium hydroxylapatite
- Slings (minimally invasive):
  – Tension-free vaginal tape procedures
  – Transobturator tape procedures
  – Single-incision sling (Mini-arc, Solyx)
- Vaginal needle suspension: Raz, Stamey, etc. (not used commonly today)
- Abdominal approaches: Marshall-Marchetti-Krantz cystourethropexy, Burch colposuspension, laparoscopic colposuspension
- Artificial urinary sphincter placement (not approved by Food and Drug Administration [FDA] in women)

Surgical management for urge incontinence:

- Sacral neuromodulation: Efficacy in 70–80% of patients who have failed other treatments
- Percutaneous tibial nerve stimulation: Office-based therapy for urge, frequency, and urge incontinence
- Botulinum toxin (intravesical injection) has a role with some patients (not FDA approved)
- Bladder augmentation

ONGOING CARE

FOLLOW-UP RECOMMENDATIONS
Patient Monitoring

- Postoperative assessment: Rule out UTI, check postvoid residual, check suture lines
- Periodic long-term follow-up with outcome-based questionnaire surveys

PROGNOSIS

Signifcant improvements are usually obtained with most patients.

COMPLICATIONS

- Prolonged exposure to urine causes skin breakdown and dermatitis, which may lead to ulceration and secondary infection.
- Inability for self-care is the precipitating factor for many nursing home admissions.
- Social isolation
- Weight gain (due to self-limiting exercise from fear of leakage)
- Avoidance of sexual activity

REFERENCES

1. Hunskaar S, Burgio K, Clark A, et al. Epidemiology of urinary and fecal incontinence and pelvic organ prolapse. In: *Incontinence, 3rd International Consultation on Incontinence*, Volume 1: Basic Evaluation, Paris, 2005, p. 255.
2. Hunskaar S, Burgio K, Diokno A, et al. Epidemiology and natural history of urinary incontinence in women. *Urology*. 2003;62:16–23.
3. Landefeld C, Seth et al. National Institutes of Health State-of-the-Science Conference Statement: Prevention of Fecal and Urinary Incontinence in Adults. *Annal of Internal Medicine*. 2008;148(6): 449–58.
4. Shamliyan, Tatyana et al (2007). Evidence Report/Technology Assessment, Number 161: Prevention of Urinary and Fecal Incontinence in Adults prepared for Agency for Healthcare Research and Quality, U.S. Department of Health and Human Services. AHRQ Publication No. 08-E003.

ADDITIONAL READING

- Anger, JT, Saigal, CS, Litwin, MS. The prevalence of urinary incontinence among community dwelling adult women: results from the National Health and Nutrition Examination Survey. *J Urol*. 2006;175:601.
- Atiemo HO, Vasavada AS. Evaluation and Management of Refractory Overactive Bladder. *Curr Urol Rep*. 2006;7:370–5.
- Chaikin DC, Rosenthal J, Blaivas JG. Pubovaginal fascial sling for all types of stress urinary incontinence: long-term analysis. *J Urol*. 1998;160:1312–6.
- Serati M, Salvatore S, Uccella S, et al. The Impact of the Mid-Urethral Slings for the Treatment of Stress Urinary Incontinence on Female Sexuality. *J Sex Med*. 2009.

CODES

ICD9

- 788.30 Urinary incontinence, unspecified
- 788.31 Urge incontinence
- 788.33 Mixed incontinence (male) (female)

CLINICAL PEARLS

- Rule out UTI by culture.
- Assume that a great percentage of women can be significantly helped by treatment.
- Physical therapy/pelvic floor rehabilitation by select physical therapists can be highly effective.
- Rule out sexually transmitted infection and atypical urinary infections.
- Aggressively treat constipation.

INCONTINENCE, URINARY ADULT MALE

Elizabeth E. Houser, MD

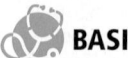 **BASICS**

DESCRIPTION

- Urinary incontinence refers to the involuntary loss of urine that presents a medical, financial, social, or hygienic problem. Two main types of incontinence exist: stress incontinence and urge incontinence.
- Stress incontinence: Involuntary urine leaks secondary to increased intra-abdominal pressure being greater than the sphincter can control; may be precipitated by sneezing, laughing, coughing, exertion, etc.
- Urge incontinence: Involuntary leakage of urine associated with urgency; is believed to be secondary to uncontrolled contraction of the urinary bladder. It is also called detrusor overactivity.
- Mixed incontinence: Involuntary leakage of urine with urgency and with sneezing, laughing, coughing, exertion, etc.

EPIDEMIOLOGY

- Stress incontinence in men is rare, unless attributable to prostate surgery, neurologic disease, or trauma.
- Reported rates of incontinence after prostatectomy range from 1% after transurethral resection to 2–57% after radical prostatectomy.

Prevalence

- Large studies have indicated that there is a 17% overall prevalence rate of incontinence in the male population (1).
- Prevalence of urinary incontinence in men increases sharply with age, with only 5% experiencing urinary incontinence under the age of 45, and 21% experiencing symptoms at age 65 or older (2).
- Black men have the highest incidence of urinary incontinence (21%) in the male population (1).
- 31% of men 85 years old or older experience incontinence (1).
- Incontinence in men of all ages is approximately half as prevalent as it is in women.

RISK FACTORS

- Age
- Neurologic disease
- Prostate surgery
- Pelvic trauma

GENERAL PREVENTION

Proper management of conditions such as symptomatic bladder outlet obstruction due to benign prostatic hyperplasia (BPH) early in the course may prevent continence problems later in life.

PATHOPHYSIOLOGY

Incontinence secondary to bladder abnormalities:

- Detrusor overactivity results in urge incontinence.
- Detrusor overactivity is commonly associated with bladder outlet obstruction from BPH.
- Incontinence secondary to outlet abnormalities:
  - Sphincteric damage secondary to pelvic surgery or radiation
  - Sphincteric dysfunction secondary to neurologic disease
- Mixed incontinence is due to abnormalities of both the bladder and the outlet overflow; incontinence due to enlarged prostate or bladder neck contracture from prostate surgery.

COMMONLY ASSOCIATED CONDITIONS

- Neurologic disease (cerebrovascular accident, parkinsonism, multiple sclerosis, myelodysplasia, spinal cord injury)
- Pelvic radiation
- Pelvic trauma
- BPH
- Prostate surgery

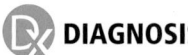 **DIAGNOSIS**

HISTORY

- Voiding symptoms:
  - Duration and characteristics of incontinence
  - Stress, urge, total
  - Precipitants and associated symptoms
  - Use of pads, briefs, diapers
  - Fluid intake
  - Alteration in bowel habits
  - Previous treatments and effect on incontinence
  - BPH symptoms
- Diabetes mellitus
- Associated conditions such as neurologic disease
- Medication use: Diuretics, drugs for BPH
- Alcohol and drug use, including caffeine
- Radical pelvic surgery or radiation:
  - Abdominoperineal resection
  - Prostatectomy: Radical or for benign disease

PHYSICAL EXAM

- Abdominal examination:
  - Suprapubic mass suggests retention.
  - Suprapubic tenderness suggests urinary tract infection.
  - Surgical scars suggesting pelvic surgery
  - Skin lesions associated with neurologic disease (such as neurofibromatosis and café au lait spots)
- External genitalia
- Prostate
- Spine/back
- Skeletal deformities
- Scars from previous spinal surgery
- Sacral abnormalities may be associated with neurogenic bladder dysfunction:
  - Cutaneous signs of spinal dysraphism:
    - Subcutaneous lipoma
    - Vascular malformation, tuft of hair, or skin dimple on lower back
  - Cutaneous signs of sacral agenesis:
    - Low, short gluteal cleft
    - Flattened buttocks
    - Coccyx not palpable
- Focal neurologic exam:
  - Motor function:
    - Inspect muscle bulk for atrophy.
    - Tibialis anterior (L4–S1): Dorsiflexion of foot
    - Gastrocnemius (L5–S2): Plantarflexion of foot
    - Toe extensors (L5–S2): Toe extension
- Sensory function
- Reflexes:
  - Anal reflex (S2–S5):
    - Gently stroke mucocutaneous junction of circumanal skin.
    - If visible contraction (wink) absent, suggests peripheral nerve or sacral (conus medullaris) abnormality
  - Bulbocavernosus reflex (BCR) (S2–S4):
    - Elicited by squeezing glans to cause reflex contraction of anal sphincter
    - Absence of BCR suggests sacral nerve damage.

DIAGNOSTIC TESTS & INTERPRETATION

Lab

- Creatinine if significant retention suspected
- Urinalysis to check for glucosuria, infection
- Prostate-specific antigen (PSA)

Imaging

- Intravenous pyleogram, renal ultrasound, or computed tomography of abdomen confirms normality of upper tracts.
- Voiding cystogram in select cases

Diagnostic Procedures/Surgery
- Urodynamics is useful for confirming bladder outlet obstruction as a possible cause of detrusor overactivity.
- Prostate ultrasound and biopsy if indicated by physical exam or PSA

DIFFERENTIAL DIAGNOSIS
- Urge incontinence
- Stress incontinence
- Mixed incontinence
- Overflow incontinence
- Intrinsic sphincter deficiency

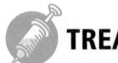 TREATMENT

- Best managed by combining lifestyle modification and medication
- Lifestyle changes: Weight loss (especially if overweight), limiting fluids, toileting on a scheduled basis, elimination of certain foods that may make symptoms worse (i.e., caffeine, acidic foods, etc.)
- Bladder relaxtion techniques (when trained by expert), pelvic floor exercises (Kegel) unclear if effective for men, biofeedback

MEDICATION
First Line
- Urge incontinence (all equally efficacious; selection based upon side effect tolerance):
  – Oxybutynin (Ditropan XL) 5–15 mg p.o. every day
  – Tolterodine (Detrol LA) 2–4 mg p.o. every day
  – Darifenicin (Enablex) 7.5–15 mg p.o. every day
  – Solifenacin (Vesicare) 5–10 mg p.o. every day
  – Tropsium chloride (Sanctura XR) 60 mg p.o. every day
  – Transdermal oxybutynin (Gelnique) 10% apply daily
  – Fesoterodine (Toviaz) 4–8 mg p.o. every day
- Stress incontinence:
  – No generally accepted drug therapy
  – Tricyclics sometimes used: Imipramine 10–25 mg p.o. b.i.d./t.i.d.

Second Line
- Urge incontinence
- Tricyclic antidepressants:
  – Imipramine 10–25 mg p.o. b.i.d./t.i.d.
- DDAVP for nocturnal symptoms:
  – 0.1–0.5 mg p.o. or intranasal q.h.s.
- Intradetrusor botulinum toxin injections (not approved by Food and Drug Administration)

Geriatric Considerations
- Anticholinergics and tricyclics may result in significant cognitive impairment in elderly patients.
- DDAVP should be avoided in patients with known or potential cardiac disease.

ADDITIONAL TREATMENT
General Measures
- Bladder diaries are invaluable in helping patients understand patterns of incontinence.
- Time voiding to avoid significant bladder distention

Additional Therapies
- Pelvic floor rehabilitation (Kegels) may significantly improve both stress and urge incontinence in male patients.
- Timed voiding is a useful therapy in patients with urge incontinence.
- Overflow incontinence is usually due to poor bladder contractility with urinary retention:
  – Indwelling catheter
  – Intermittent catheterization
  – Evaluate for outlet obstruction.

COMPLEMENTARY AND ALTERNATIVE MEDICINE
- Accupuncture in selected cases
- Physical therapy in selected cases

SURGERY/OTHER PROCEDURES
- Urge incontinence:
  – Sacral neuromodulation
  – Augmentation cystoplasty
- Stress incontinence:
  – Urethral bulking agents
  – Male sling procedures: Promising short-term results, but no long-term studies (3)[B]
  – Artificial urinary sphincter implant has excellent long-term continence rates (4)[A]

 ONGOING CARE

FOLLOW-UP RECOMMENDATIONS
Patient Monitoring
Must monitor postvoid residual volume in patients on anticholinergic medications

PROGNOSIS
Continence can be improved in almost all patients.

COMPLICATIONS
- Dermatitis
- Candidiasis
- Skin breakdown
- Social isolation
- Avoidance of sex
- Weight gain

REFERENCES

1. Anger JT, Saigal CS, Stothers L, et al. The prevalence of urinary incontinence among community dwelling men: results from the National Health and Nutrition Examination survey. *J Urol.* 2006;176:2103–8; discussion 2108.
2. Giberti C, Gallo F, Schenone M, et al. The bone anchor suburethral synthetic sling for iatrogenic male incontinence: critical evaluation at a mean 3-year followup. *J Urol.* 2009;181:2204–8.
3. Comiter CV. The male sling for stress urinary incontinence: a prospective study. *J Urol.* 2002;167:597–601.
4. Elliott DS, Barrett DM. Mayo Clinic long-term analysis of the functional durability of the AMS 800 artificial urinary sphincter: a review of 323 cases. *J Urol.* 1998;159:1206–8.

ADDITIONAL READING
- Landefeld C, Seth et al. National Institutes of Health State-of-the-Science Conference Statement: Prevention of Fecal and Urinary Incontinence in Adults. *Annal of Internal Medicine.* 2008;148(6):449–58.
- Stewart WF, Van Rooyen JB, Cundiff GW, et al. Prevalence and burden of overactive bladder in the United States. *World J Urol.* 2003;20:327–36.

 CODES

ICD9
- 788.30 Urinary incontinence, unspecified
- 788.31 Urge incontinence
- 788.32 Stress incontinence, male

CLINICAL PEARLS
- Always check postvoid residual to rule out overflow incontinence.
- Have patient fill out International Prostate Symptom Score and do uroflow.
- Check PSA.
- Urodynamics can be very helpful.
- Pelvic floor rehabilitation may have a significant effect for male patients.

I

INFERTILITY

Erika Mello, MD
Shaila V. Chauhan, MD

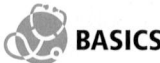 **BASICS**

DESCRIPTION
- Failure to conceive after 1 year of well-timed intercourse
- Evaluation after 6 months for women 35–39 years old & immediately if >39

EPIDEMIOLOGY
Incidence
85% of couples conceive within 1 year, with 20% of women becoming pregnant during any one menstrual cycle.

Prevalence
- ~15% of all couples aged 35–40 years and >25% for women >40 years
- May be increasing as more women delay childbearing; 20% of women in the US have their 1st child after age 35.
- 7.3 million women aged 15–44 have imparied fecundity (1)[A].

RISK FACTORS
- Obesity, history of sexually transmitted disease, endometriosis, irregular cycles, pelvic surgery or pathology, varicocele
- Medications, s abuse, caffeine, smoking

Genetics
- Higher incidence of genetic abnormalities in infertility population (2), including Klinefelter syndrome (47XXY), Turner syndrome (45X or mosaic), and fragile X syndrome
- Balanced translocation may be present in phenotypically normal individuals, especially with a history of recurrent SAB.
- Polycystic ovary syndrome (PCOS): Genetics poorly understood but probably polygenetic

GENERAL PREVENTION
- Encourage reproduction by 30–35 years.
- Maintain normal weight 7 exercise level

PATHOPHYSIOLOGY
Complex and often multifactorial

ETIOLOGY
- Most couples have more than one factor (3).
- Tubal and ovulatory factors found in ~30% of couples.
  - *Chlamydia* infection is the most common cause of infertility in the US (owing to scarring and other effects on tubal function).
- Peritoneal (including endometriosis), uterine, cervical, general (i.e., psychogenic, nutritional, metabolic issues), and immunologic factors are less common, <10% each.
- Factors related to male partner are found in 30% of couples.
- Unexplained infertility is found in ~20% of couples.

COMMONLY ASSOCIATED CONDITIONS
- Risky sexual behavior
- Pelvic or lower abdominal pathology
- Endocrine dysfunction (thyroid, glucose metabolism, menstrual)
- Anovulation is commonly associated with hyperandrogenism and PCOS (4)[A].
  - Obesity, hirsutism, and acne are common in PCOS (~80%).
  - Increased risk of endometrial hyperplasia
  - Metabolic problems with insulin resistance and lipid abnormalities are common.

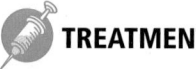 **DIAGNOSIS**

HISTORY
- Complete reproductive history:
  - Age at menarche, regularity of cycles, physical development
  - Primary or secondary infertility; infertility with previous partner
  - History of induced abortion, history of BTL, vasectomy, other pelvic, abdominal surgery
- Abdominal pain or other abdominal symptoms
- Sexually transmitted infections, especially pelvic inflammatory disease in women
- History of endocrine abnormalities (e.g., thyroid)
- History of malignancy, what kind, how treated
- Chronic illness(es), including diabetes, HIV/AIDS, cystic fibrosis
- Family history:
  - Congenital abnormalities or mental retardation in close relatives
  - Infertility or early menopause in close relatives of female partner
- Medications, including alternative medicine
- Drug abuse, including tobacco, alcohol, street drugs
- Frequency of intercourse

PHYSICAL EXAM
- Evaluate for stigmata of PCO, Turner syndrome or thyroid disease, obesity or underweight, varicocele (men)
- Reproductive system evaluation: Hair patterns and pubertal development, including breasts

DIAGNOSTIC TESTS & INTERPRETATION
Lab
Initial lab tests
Evaluation is directed by history.
- Assessment of ovulation:
  - Luteal-phase progesterone at least 5 ng/ml on cycle days (CD) 21–25 confirms ovulation.
  - Luteinizing hormone (LH) kit testing also can confirm ovulation.
  - Basal body temperature: ~1° increase at ovulation on morning evaluations, maintained over luteal phase, is indicative of ovulation.
  - Regular cycles with moliminal symptoms (i.e., breast tenderness, dysmenorrhea, and bloating) is 95% predictive of ovulation.
- Assessment of ovarian reserve:
  - CD 3 FSH levels of <15 mlu/ml: Project possible reproductive potential (<10 suggests good ovarian reserve).
  - Clomiphine citrate challenge test: 100 mg/day on CD 5–9 with measurement of FSH level on CD 3 and CD 10; FSH level of >15 on either CD 3 or CD 10 are associated with low reproductive potential, infertility, and higher miscarriage rate.
- Semen analysis:
  - Normal: Volume >1.5 mL, count >20 million, motility >50%, and morphology >30% (or at least 14% by strict criteria)
  - If abnormal results, then do male evaluation as indicated clinically or consider referral.
  - Congenital bilateral absence of the vas deferens warrants cystic fibrosis screening.
- Additional labs
  - CD 3 estradiol levels (related to follicular development), 25–75; abnormally high levels may represent diminished ovarian reserve.
  - CD 3 prolactin level, <24 ng/ml, increased levels interfere with ovulation and warrant further imaging for possibly pituitary tumor.
  - Thyroid-stimulating hormone

Follow-Up & Special Considerations
Any abnormal value would warrant reevaluation or possible referral if needed.

Imaging
Initial approach
- Transvaginal ultrasound to assess for anatomic abnormality (fibroid, polycystic ovaries, müllerian anamolies)
- Sonohysterography detailed evaluation of the cavity.
- Hysterosalpingogram will evaluate patency of tubes and contour of the cavity. May be both diagnostic and therapeutic (4)[A].
- Semen analysis
- MRI of pelvis rarely needed

Follow-Up & Special Considerations
Abnormalities of imaging may require surgical evaluation, including referral if needed.

Diagnostic Procedures/Surgery
Laparoscopy is reserved for those at risk for endometriosis or for abnormal imaging findings.

TREATMENT

MEDICATION
First Line
- Male factor: Intercourse, insemination, or in vitro fertilization (IVF). Consider lifestyle changes: Decrease heat to scrotum/testes, diet, exercise, eliminate substance abuse issues, and consider vitamin supplementation. Significant abnormalities warrant referral.
- Intrauterine insemination (IUI) or artificial insemination: This is performed easily in an office setting but requires specific sperm preparation for the procedure. It can be timed with natural cycles or stimulated cycles with LH kit assessment or ultrasound evaluation leading to human chorionic gonadotropin injection to trigger ovulation. It can be performed with frozen sperm obtained from banks for severe male factor or for women lacking a male partner.
- Anovulation: Consider ovulation induction, most effectively with ~10% body weight loss if obese, but most commonly with clomiphene citrate (Clomid), typically, 50 mg/day × 5 days; can start on CD 3, 4, or 5. If no ovulation, then increase dose by 50 mg/day in subsequent cycles; maximum 150 mg/day. Some will increase dose with ovulation but no pregnancy (4)[A].

- Anatomic issues: May need surgery, but if tubes are blocked, then referral for IVF is appropriate immediately.
- Unexplained infertility: Minor improvements with clomiphene or insemination alone; greater improvement with both together (5)[A].
- Coital or cervical problems: IUI (6)[C]
- Endometriosis: Either direct fertility treatments or surgery; medical therapy for endometriosis does not increase pregnancy rates after the therapy.
- Endocrine abnormalities may require treatment prior to pregnancy.
  - Stabilize thyroid disease or diabetes.
  - Consider bromocriptine or cabergoline for hyperprolactinemia.
  - Consider metformin or insulin sensitizer (e.g., glitazones) for insulin resistance.

Second Line

- If clomiphene fails to induce ovulation, can consider adding metformin (given initially in low dose, but treatment dosing ultimately is ~1,500 mg/day; test renal function first), low-dose dexamethasone, oral contraceptives (OCP) for two or more cycles, and then retry the clomiphene again immediately after stopping the OCP (7)[A].
- Generally in subspecialty care: Gonadotropin therapies (injectable FSH or FSH plus LH) are very effective, but riskier, treatments for infertility. They are effective for hypothalamic dysfunction, which clomiphene generally is not.
- Ultimately, IVF is a treatment option for all infertility patients when other therapies fail (4)[B].
- Surgery: for endometriosis and for anatomic issues.

ADDITIONAL TREATMENT
General Measures
- Be aware of insurance coverage issues and requirements for each patient.
- Treatments increase estradiol levels, and the timing of the periovulatory mucus pattern may change to earlier in the cycle.
- Progesterone is responsible for the temperature changes in the cycle, and the premenstrual moliminal symptoms.
- Infertility and its treatment involve very emotional issues. Many patients may benefit from counseling and support measures.
- All female fertility patients should be taking folate supplementation of at least 400 μg/day.

Issues for Referral
Reproductive endocrinology and/or urology.
- Specialized lab prep is needed for IUI.
- Complications can be serious for these therapies.
- FSH plus LH therapies and IVF warrant referral in most cases.
- Consider reproductive/reconstructive surgery.

Additional Therapies
Increased age or with poor ovarian reserve, consideration of donor-egg IVF is warranted.

COMPLEMENTARY AND ALTERNATIVE MEDICINE
Multiple types have been advocated for, but few have been fully evaluated.

SURGERY/OTHER PROCEDURES
- IVF is clearly the most effective infertility treatment available to patients
- Male and female surgical issues should be addressed by experienced practitioners.

IN-PATIENT CONSIDERATIONS
Initial Stabilization
Rarely is hospitalization needed for infertility issues; however, it may be needed occasionally for issues related to problems in early pregnancy and ovarian hyperstimulation syndrome. If this occurs, recommend subspecialty consultation.

 ## ONGOING CARE

FOLLOW-UP RECOMMENDATIONS
Patients often will need to consider more aggressive options as they progress through this process. From 3–6 cycles of oral ovulation induction would be an adequate trial prior to referral.

Patient Monitoring
- Cycle monitoring may be able to help mitigate some of the risks.
- Ultrasound monitoring can show the number of follicles developing in the cycle and may help to predict ovarian hyperstimulation and risk of multiple gestations.

DIET
- Healthy diet with minimization of fat, control of calories, and vitamin supplementation
- If obese, then diet modification is needed as above, plus low-fat, lower-calorie, high-fiber diet most recommended.

PATIENT EDUCATION
Seek out patient education materials on the specific diagnoses involved. Good sources include:
- American Society for Reproductive Medicine (www.asrm.org)
- American College of Obstetricians and Gynecologists (www.acog.org)
- Resolve: National patient advocacy group revolving around infertility (www.resolve.org)

PROGNOSIS
- Generally excellent; most couples will achieve a pregnancy.
- Without therapy, ~50% of those couples not yet pregnant will conceive in both the 2nd and 3rd years of trying.

COMPLICATIONS
- Stress levels are high in treatment.
- Multiple pregnancy rates (even high-order ones) increase with all therapies involving ovulation induction with medications. Multiple rates are ~10% with oral meds, ~30% with injectable ones.
- Ovarian cysts are common during infertility treatments and can cause various problems.
- Ovarian hyperstimulation: Very rare with oral meds but more common with FSH treatments; can be life-threatening.
- Couples with infertility may have a slightly increased risk of congenital abnormalities in offspring in general, but no specific abnormalities.

REFERENCES

1. WWW.CDC.GOV http://www.cdc.gov/reproductivehealth/Infertility/index.htm
2. Clementini E, Palka C, Iezzi I, et al. Prevalence of chromosomal abnormalities in 2078 infertile couples referred for assisted reproductive techniques. *Human Reprod.* 2005;20:437–42.
3. www.mayoclinic.org/infertility/
4. Thessaloniki ESHRE/ASRM-Sponsored PCOS Consensus Workshop Group. Consensus on infertility treatment related to polycystic ovary syndrome. *Fertil Steril.* 2008;89:505–22.
5. Hughes E, Collins J, Vandekerckhove P. Clomiphene citrate for unexplained subfertility in women. *Cochrane Database Syst Rev.* 2000:CD000057.
6. ASRM Publication. Infertility: An Overview. A Guide for Patients. 2003.
7. Palomba S, Oppedisano R, Tolino A, et al. Outlook: metformin use in infertile patients with polycystic ovary syndrome: an evidence-based overview. *Reprod Biomed Online.* 2008;16:327–35.

ADDITIONAL READING

Practice Committee of the American Society for Reproductive Medicine, supplement published in Fertility and Sterility in 2006, volume 86(5Suppl) has multiple infertility-related articles.

See Also (Topic, Algorithm, Electronic Media Element)
Reproductive Endocrinology and Infertility; Endometriosis, Fibroids, Amenorrhea; Müllerian Anomaly; Metabolic Syndrome; Polycystic Ovary Syndrome
Algorithm: Infertility

 ## CODES

ICD9
- 628.0 Infertility, female, associated with anovulation
- 628.1 Infertility, female, of pituitary-hypothalamic origin
- 628.2 Infertility, female, of tubal origin

CLINICAL PEARLS

- Infertility is a complex, multifactorial problem.
- Women <35 should be evaluated for infertility after 1 year of unprotected intercourse; those ≥35 should receive evaluation after 6 months, and those ≥40 should receive assistance immediately.
- *Chlamydia* infection is the most common cause of infertility in the US.
- Clomiphene citrate is a SERM that acts via estrogen antagonism at the hypothalamus, thus indirectly increasing FSH and LH production.
- Medical therapy for endometriosis does not increase pregnancy rates after the therapy. However, surgical treatment of endometriosis does improve pregnancy rates with subsequent infertility treatment.
- If a couple is able to do IVF, it is always their best chance of success for attaining a pregnancy.

INFLUENZA

Richard Kent Zimmerman, MD, MPH

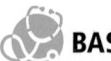 **BASICS**

DESCRIPTION

- Acute, usually self-limited, febrile infection caused by influenza virus types A and B
- Marked by inflammation of nasal mucosa, pharynx, conjunctiva, and respiratory tract
- Outbreaks occur almost every winter with varying degrees of severity.
- Influenza virus rarely displays antigenic shift (variation). This leads to strains of virus to which little immunologic resistance exists in a population, and it may result in pandemics. Displays minor antigenic variation called drift.
- System(s) affected: Head/Eyes/Ears/Nose/Throat; Pulmonary
- Synonym(s): Flu; Grip; Acute catarrhal fever
- Swine H1N1 also affects the gastrointestinal system

EPIDEMIOLOGY

- Predominant age: Highest in young and school-aged children (3 months–16 years old) and young adults:
  - Morbidity: Seasonal morbidity highest in elderly (>75 yrs) and those with concurrent medical illnesses, such as lung disease. Also higher in young children.
  - Hospitalization rates also higher in infants, elderly, and persons with chronic medical illnesses
- Predominant sex: Male = Female
- Pandemic novel H1N1 has increased morbidity and mortality in persons <65 years and those with concurrent medical illnesses and marked obesity.

Incidence

- Seasonal influenza in preuniversal vaccination: 95 million cases per year, typically fall/winter
- Attack rates in healthy children: 10–40% each year, prior to routine influenza vaccination

RISK FACTORS

- For contracting disease:
  - Semiclosed environments such as nursing homes, schools, and prisons
  - Crowded, close environments during epidemics
- For complications:
  - Neonates, infants, elderly
  - Pregnancy, especially in 3rd trimester
  - Chronic pulmonary diseases
  - Cardiovascular diseases including valvular problems and congestive heart failure (CHF)
  - Metabolic diseases
  - Hemoglobinopathies
  - Malignancies
  - Immunosuppression
  - Neuromuscular diseases that limit respiratory function and secretion handling
- Pandemic influenza causes morbidity in those <65 years.

GENERAL PREVENTION

- Incubation is 1–4 days; infected persons are most contagious during peak symptoms.
- Vaccination options include trivalent influenza vaccine (TIV), high-dose trivalent influenza vaccine (TIV HD), or live attenuated influenza vaccine (LAIV), depending on indications and availability.
- Starting with the fall of 2010, influenza vaccine recommended universally for those ≥6 months of age.

- TIV recommended annually for:
  - All persons aged ≥6 months
  - High-risk individuals
  - Vaccine should be administered in the fall prior to influenza season.
  - Protection occurs 1–2 weeks after immunization.
  - Typically mild side effects include low-grade fever and local reaction at vaccination site
  - Inactivated dose: ≤3 years old: 0.5 mL IM; children 6–35 months old: 0.25 mL
  - Single dose every year except for children <9 years old, who should receive 2 doses (4 weeks apart) the first year they receive influenza vaccine; if a child <9 years old does not receive 2 doses in the 1st year, then give 2 doses in the 2nd year
  - Vaccine contraindications: Anaphylaxis to eggs (do skin testing first) or other vaccine components, delay from first trimester of pregnancy if the patient has no co-morbidities and no pandemic.
  - Precaution: Guillain-Barré syndrome within 6 wks after a previous dose of influenza vaccine
- LAIV recommended annually for:
  - Healthy persons 2–49 years old
  - Includes health care providers, home care providers, staff and residents of nursing homes and other chronic care facilities, homeless, public safety workers, and close contacts of high-risk individuals, unless in contact with severely immunocompromised on reverse isolation
  - Vaccine contraindications: Anaphylaxis to eggs or other vaccine components, immunocompromising conditions, pregnancy, high-risk conditions including asthma or other chronic cardiopulmonary conditions, history of Guillain-Barré syndrome, chronic aspirin therapy in children
  - Single dose every year except for children <9 years old, who should receive 2 doses (4 weeks apart) 1st year they receive influenza vaccine; if a child <9 years old does not receive 2 doses in the 1st year, then give 2 doses in the 2nd year
- TIV-HD: High dose trivalent inactivated influenza vaccine:
  - Contains 4 times the antigen concentration of TIV
  - Licensed for persons ≥65 years of age
  - Results in higher antibody levels but somewhat higher rates of local reactions
  - Effectiveness being studied
  - Advisory Committee on Immunization Practices does not express a preference for or against this vaccine.
- Antiviral prophylaxis depends on current resistance patterns each year; see www.cdc.gov/flu for the current patterns or check with local health department: Take for duration of outbreak if no vaccine given; discontinue after 14 days if used in addition to vaccine; may be used prophylactically:
  - In high-risk groups that have not been vaccinated or need additional control measures during epidemics. Should not be considered as substitute for vaccination unless vaccine contraindicated (1)[B].
  - During influenza season for those with contraindications to vaccine
  - For staff and residents in nursing home outbreaks
  - For immune-deficient persons who are expected not to respond to vaccination

- For pandemic vaccine and antiviral recommendations, see www.cdc.gov/h1n1flu

Pediatric Considerations

- Vaccinate children 6–23 months old with inactivated vaccine.
- Use either TIV or LAIV in healthy children 2–18 years old.
- For prophylaxis, oseltamivir dosage varies by weight; zanamivir is approved for prophylaxis for children ≤5 years old at a dosage of 2 inhalations per day. For prophylaxis, the dosage of amantadine and of rimantadine is 5 mg/kg body weight/day up to 150 mg in 2 divided doses.

Pregnancy Considerations

- The Centers for Disease Control (CDC) recommends vaccinating all women who will be pregnant during influenza season.
- Women at risk for influenza complications should receive inactivated influenza vaccine regardless of trimester.
- Recent evidence of excess morbidity during seasonal influenza supports vaccinating healthy pregnant women in the second or third trimester and those with comorbidities in any trimester (2)[B].
- Recent evidence of excess mortality in 2 previous influenza pandemics supports vaccinating women in any trimester during a pandemic. Oseltamivir, zanamivir, rimantadine, and amantadine are pregnancy Category C.

ETIOLOGY

Orthomyxovirus (influenza types A and B)

COMMONLY ASSOCIATED CONDITIONS

Bacterial pneumonia

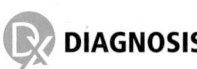 **DIAGNOSIS**

Sudden onset of:

- High fever
- Chills, malaise, myalgia
- Headache
- Rhinorrhea, nasal congestion
- Sinusitis
- Sore throat/pharyngitis
- Nonproductive cough

HISTORY

Close attention to local epidemiology (e.g., current outbreak in the community). Contact http://www.cdc.gov/flu/weekly/fluactivity.htm or state health department to determine type or perform testing.

DIAGNOSTIC TESTS & INTERPRETATION

Lab

- Leukopenia
- Leukocytosis may signal complications.
- Polymerase chain reaction from nasopharyngeal swab or aspirate is the gold standard: Accurate and timely (results in 24 hours)
- Rapid enzyme linked immunosorbent assay antigen test. Some rapid tests diagnose influenza A, while others diagnose influenza A and B. Sensitivity and specificity vary by manufacturer, strain of influenza, and age of patient. False negatives are fairly common.

- Tissue culture of nasopharyngeal swab or aspirate: Takes time for results but allows subtyping for epidemiologic studies.
- Pulse oximetry

Imaging
Chest x-ray:
- Usually normal unless secondary infection
- Basilar streaking

Pathological Findings
Inflammation of respiratory tract

DIFFERENTIAL DIAGNOSIS
- Respiratory viral infections including respiratory syncytial virus, parainfluenza, adenovirus, enterovirus
- Infectious mononucleosis
- Coxsackievirus infections
- Viral or streptococcal tonsillitis
- Atypical Mycoplasma pneumonia
- Chlamydia pneumoniae
- Q fever

 ## TREATMENT
MEDICATION
First Line
- Antiviral treatment depends on current resistance patterns each year; see www.cdc.gov/flu for the current patterns or check with local health department: Antivirals are most effective if administered within 1st 48 hours and in those with laboratory-confirmed or highly suspected influenza illness.
- Antivirals include amantadine, rimantadine, oseltamivir, zanamivir, and investigational peramivir.
- Antivirals considered for persons not at increased risk of complications from influenza whose onset of symptoms is within the last 48 hours and who wish to shorten the duration of illness and further reduce their relatively low risk of complications
- Symptomatic treatment for those patients *without risk factors* and *without* signs of lower respiratory tract infection (3)
- Antivirals within 48 hours of symptom onset recommended for those at risk of complications (4)[B]
- Antivirals recommended for hospitalized patients (1)[B]
- Effect is reduction of symptoms by 24 hours and a reduction in complication rates:
  – Zanamivir dose: 2 inhalations b.i.d. for 5 days (age ≤7 years)
  – Rimantadine dose: 100 mg b.i.d. for ages 13–64 years; 100 mg daily for >65 years
  – Amantadine dose: 100 mg b.i.d. for ages 13–64 years; <100 mg daily for >65 years
  – Oseltamivir dose: 75 mg p.o. b.i.d. for 5 days (age ≤13 years)
  – If severe renal impairment, 75 mg p.o. once per day.
  – Oseltamivir for children ≥1 year:
    ○ <15 kg, 30 mg b.i.d.
    ○ >15–23 kg, 45 mg b.i.d.
    ○ >23–40 kg, 60 mg b.i.d.
    ○ >40 kg, 75 mg b.i.d.
  – Oseltamivir for children <1 year: 3mg/kg/dose twice daily

- Antipyretics:
  – Acetaminophen: In children
  – Contraindications: Allergy to a product
- Precautions:
  – Zanamivir may cause bronchospasm if the patient has chronic obstructive pulmonary disease (COPD) or asthma; the patient should have a bronchodilator available.
  – Amantadine: Has anticholinergic properties and should be used with caution in those with psychiatric, addiction, or neurologic disorders as it may increase risk for suicide attempts or increase neurologic symptoms.
  – Rimantadine may increase the risk of seizures in those with an underlying seizure disorder.
  – Oseltamivir:
    ○ May cause nausea and vomiting; may be less severe if taken with food
- Decrease dose of certain antivirals if creatinine clearance <30 mL/min.

Second Line
- Ibuprofen or other nonsteroidal anti-inflammatory drugs for symptomatic relief
- Aspirin: Should not be used in children <16 years due to risk of Reye syndrome, a rare and severe complication of aspirin use

ADDITIONAL TREATMENT
General Measures
- Symptomatic treatment (saline nasal spray, analgesic gargle)
- Cool-mist or ultrasonic humidifier to increase moisture of inspired air
- Modified respiratory isolation techniques. See www.cdc.gov/h1n1flu for pandemic isolation recommendations.
- Hospitalized patients may require oxygen or ventilatory support.
- Avoid smoking.

IN-PATIENT CONSIDERATIONS
Initial Stabilization
Outpatient except for treatment of severe complications or treatment of those in high-risk groups

 ## ONGOING CARE
FOLLOW-UP RECOMMENDATIONS
Patient Monitoring
- Mild cases: Usually no follow-up required
- Moderate or severe cases: Follow until symptoms resolve and any complications are treated effectively.

DIET
Increase fluid intake.

PATIENT EDUCATION
CDC: http://www.cdc.gov/flu

PROGNOSIS
Favorable

COMPLICATIONS
- Otitis media
- Acute sinusitis
- Croup
- Bronchitis

- Pneumonia
- Apnea in neonates
- Reye syndrome
- Rhabdomyolysis
- Postinfluenza asthenia
- COPD or CHF exacerbation
- Encephalopathy
- Death

Geriatric Considerations
Complications more likely in elderly

REFERENCES

1. Harper SA, Bradley JS, Englund JA, et al. Seasonal Influenza in Adults and Children-Diagnosis, Treatment, Chemoprophylaxis, and Institutional Outbreak Management: Clinical Practice Guidelines of the Infectious Diseases Society of America. *Clin Infect Dis*. 2009.
2. Mak TK, Mangtani P, Leese J, et al. Influenza vaccination in pregnancy: current evidence and selected national policies. *Lancet Infect Dis*. 2008;8:44–52.
3. http://cdc.gov/H1N1flu/recommendations.htm#e
4. Lalezari J, Campion K, Keene O, et al. Zanamivir for the treatment of influenza A and B infection in high-risk patients: A pooled analysis of randomized controlled trials. *Arch Int Med*. 2001;161(2): 212–17.
5. Grayson ML, Melvani S, Druce J, et al. Efficacy of Soap and Water and Alcohol-Based Hand-Rub Preparations against Live H1N1 Influenza Virus on the Hands of Human Volunteers. *Clin Infect Dis*. 2008.

See Also (Topic, Algorithm, Electronic Media Element)
www.cdc.gov/flu
http://aapredbook.aappublications.org/flu
http://www.idsociety.org/Content.aspx?id=14220#seasonal

CODES

ICD9
- 487.0 Influenza with pneumonia
- 487.1 Influenza with other respiratory manifestations
- 487.8 Influenza with other manifestations

CLINICAL PEARLS
- Influenza is an acute, usually self-limited, febrile infection caused by influenza virus types A and B.
- Preventative measures are key, including vaccinations.
- Infection can cause significant morbidity and even mortality in the very young, very old, and those with preexisting comorbidities.
- Hand hygiene either with soap and water (slightly superior) or with alcohol-based hand rubs are proven to reduce human influenza virus A on human hands (5)[C].

INGROWN TOENAIL

Steven E. Roskos, MD

 BASICS

DESCRIPTION

- In ingrown toenail, the distal margin of the nail plate grows into the lateral nail fold, causing irritation, inflammation, and sometimes bacterial or fungal infection:
  - Stage 1 (inflammation): Erythema, slight edema, tenderness of lateral nail fold
  - Stage 2 (abscess): Increased pain, erythema, and edema, as well as drainage (purulent or serous)
  - Stage 3 (granulation): Further increased erythema, edema, and pain, with granulation tissue growing over the nail plate
- Can be recurrent
- Synonym(s): Onychocryptosis

EPIDEMIOLOGY

- Great toenail is almost exclusively affected.
- Lateral edge of nail is more commonly affected than the medial edge.
- Most common in males ages 16–25 years
- More common in elderly females than in elderly males
- More common in those with lower incomes

Prevalence

- 24.5/1,000 overall
- 50/1,000 ≥65 years

RISK FACTORS

- Genetic factors:
  - Increased nail fold width
  - Decreased nail thickness
  - Medial rotation of the toe
- Many others proposed; none proven, including:
  - Distorted, thickened nail (onychogryphosis)
  - Fungal infection (onychomycosis)
  - Hyperhidrosis
  - Improper trimming of the lateral nail plate
  - Poorly fitting shoes
  - Trauma to nail or nail fold

GENERAL PREVENTION

- Properly fitting shoes
- Proper nail trimming

PATHOPHYSIOLOGY

- Nail plate penetrates the nail fold.
- This causes a foreign body reaction (inflammation).
- Bacteria or fungi may enter through the opening in the nail fold, causing infection and abscess formation.
- The inflamed and infected tissue hypertrophies, further covering the nail plate.

 DIAGNOSIS

HISTORY

- Pain
- Redness
- Swelling
- Drainage

PHYSICAL EXAM

- Tenderness of lateral nail fold
- Erythema
- Edema
- Drainage (serous or purulent)
- Granulation tissue
- Hypertrophy of lateral nail fold

DIAGNOSTIC TESTS & INTERPRETATION

Lab

Initial lab tests

Consider complete blood count (CBC) and blood cultures if systemic infection is suspected.

Imaging

- Consider MRI, x-ray, or bone scan if osteomyelitis is suspected.
- Consider x-ray if subungual exostosis is suspected.

DIFFERENTIAL DIAGNOSIS

- Cellulitis
- Felon (deep abscess on plantar aspect of toe)
- Onychogryphosis (gross thickening and hardening of the nail)
- Onycholysis (separation of nail from nail bed)
- Onychomycosis (fungal infection of the nail)
- Osteomyelitis
- Paronychia
- Subungual exostosis (osteochondroma beneath the nail)

 TREATMENT

- Simple nail avulsion (either partial or total) combined with the use of phenol is more effective than surgical excision of the nail bed at preventing symptomatic recurrence of ingrown toenails (1,2)[A].
- Flexible gutter splint is an option for effective treatment of stage 2 or 3 ingrown nails (3,4)[B].
- Oral or topical antibiotics are not helpful as an adjunct to surgical treatment of ingrown toenails (2,5)[B].

MEDICATION

- Some experts recommend oral or topical antibiotics for conservative management.
- Neither oral nor topical antibiotics are useful as an adjunct to surgical treatment (2,5)[B].
- Nonsteroidal anti-inflammatory drugs (NSAIDs) are usually adequate for analgesia.
- Some experts use topical corticosteroids on the hypertrophic lateral nail fold, but this is not commonly practiced.

ADDITIONAL TREATMENT

General Measures

For stage 1:

- Warm water soaks twice a day
- Proper nail trimming
- Properly fitted shoes

Additional Therapies

- For stage 1 ingrown nails, several treatments are available:
  - Cotton wool:
    - Bluntly insert a wisp of cotton under the ingrown portion of the nail.
    - Instruct the patient to reinsert new cotton if the other comes out until the nail grows beyond the nail fold.
    - Consider adding silver nitrate cautery of the nail fold, which the patient then repeats at home.
  - Dental floss:
    - Bluntly insert some dental floss to lift the nail away from the lateral nail fold.
    - Instruct the patient to replace the floss as necessary if it comes out or gets dirty.
    - Keep floss in place until the nail grows beyond the nail fold.

– Taping:
  ○ Apply surgical tape to both sides of toe.
  ○ Use another piece of tape from 1 side to the other to pull the lateral nail fold away from the nail plate.
  ○ Instruct the patient to keep taping until the nail grows beyond the fold.
– Cryotherapy of the lateral nail fold
• For stage 2 ingrown nails, consider attempting conservative treatment, as above, especially cotton wool or cryotherapy.

SURGERY/OTHER PROCEDURES
• For stage 2 ingrown nails where conservative treatment has failed, stage 3 ingrown nails, or recurrent ingrown nails, consider either.

• Partial avulsion of the nail with phenol nail matrix ablation (1,2)[A]:
  – Achieve local anesthesia as described below.
  – Place a tourniquet.
  – Incise the nail longitudinally with scissors or a nail splitter a few millimeters from the ingrown border, starting at the distal edge and proceeding to the matrix.
  – Elevate the ingrown part of the nail from the nail bed with a periosteal (Freer) elevator or hemostat.
  – Pull this portion gently out with a hemostat.
  – Dip a urethral swab in 80–88% phenol solution.
  – Apply the phenol for 1 minute to the nail matrix under the proximal nail fold. Use multiple swabs if necessary.
  – Wash the area with isopropyl (rubbing) alcohol to neutralize phenol.
• Flexible gutter splint (3,4)[B]:
  – Cut a 1- to 2-cm-long piece of sterilized plastic tube, such as IV tubing, 2–3 mm in diameter (alternatively, you may use a cap from a 29-gauge needle).
  – Make a slit in the tubing lengthwise, and cut the end off at an angle.
  – Apply local anesthesia.
  – Release the ingrown edge of the nail from the nail fold with a hemostat.
  – Slide the tube, angled end first, along the ingrown edge of the nail.
  – Consider fixing the tube in place with self-curing formable acrylic resin (used for dentures and sculptured nails), tape, or a single suture.
  – Leave the tube in place until nail has grown beyond the nail fold.
• Other options for nail matrix ablation include:
  – Electrocautery with a special flattened tip coated with Teflon on one side to protect the proximal nail fold
  – Curettage
  – Surgical excision

• Local anesthesia can be achieved with either:
  – Distal wing block: Infuse 1% lidocaine without epinephrine near the junction of the proximal and lateral nail folds. Continue infusing until the nail folds and the tip of the digit under the distal nail are white from the pressure of the anesthetic.
  – Digital ring block: Infuse 1% lidocaine without epinephrine on the medial and lateral surfaces of the involved digit to anesthetize the plantar and dorsal digital nerves.

ONGOING CARE

FOLLOW-UP RECOMMENDATIONS
• Dress with antibiotic ointment or sterile petroleum jelly; cover with sterile gauze and tube gauze.
• Postoperative instructions should include:
  – Rest and elevate the foot for 12–24 h.
  – Take NSAIDs for discomfort.
  – Change dressing and wash with soap and water daily.
  – Expect a sterile exudate for 2–6 weeks.
  – Avulsed nails may take 6–12 months to grow completely out (if no matrix ablation).
  – Call for increasing pain, redness, or swelling.
  – Average time to return to normal activities is 2 weeks.
• Patients treated conservatively should be followed up in the office every 7–10 days until marked improvement is noted.

PATIENT EDUCATION
• Trim nails straight across (do not round corners) and not too short.
• Wear properly fitting, comfortable shoes.

COMPLICATIONS
• Cellulitis after surgical procedure (uncommon)
• Damage to fascia or periosteum from overly aggressive matrix ablation
• Damage to nail bed
• Distal toe ischemia due to prolonged use of a tourniquet during surgery (rare)
• Nail plate deformity (due to damage to nail matrix)
• Osteomyelitis (rare)
• Permanent narrowing of nail (if matrix ablation is performed)
• Postoperative wound drainage
• Recurrence (40–80% with avulsion alone, 0.6–14% with matrix ablation, 6–13% with gutter splint)

REFERENCES
1. Rounding C, Bloomfield S. Surgical treatments for ingrowing toenails. *Cochrane Database Syst Rev.* 2003Issue 1. Art. No.: CD001541. DOI:10.1002/14651858.CD001541.pub2.
2. Bos AM, van Tilburg MW, van Sorge AA, et al. Randomized clinical trial of surgical technique and local antibiotics for ingrowing toenail. *Br J Surg.* 2007;94:292–6.
3. Arai H, Arai T, Nakajima H, et al. Formable acrylic treatment for ingrowing nail with gutter splint and sculptured nail. *Int J Dermatol.* 2004;43:759–65.
4. Nazari S. A simple and practical method in treatment of ingrown nails: splinting by flexible tube. *J Eur Acad Dermatol Venereol.* 2006;20: 1302–6.
5. Reyzelman AM, Trombello KA, Vayser DJ, et al. Are antibiotics necessary in the treatment of locally infected ingrown toenails? *Arch Fam Med.* 2000;9: 930–2.

ADDITIONAL READING
• Chapeskie H. Ingrown toenail or overgrown toe skin?: Alternative treatment for onychocryptosis. *Can Fam Physician.* 2008;54:1561–2.
• Peggs JF. Ingrown toenails. In: *Pfenninger and Fowler's Procedures for Primary Care.* 2nd ed. St. Louis, Mosby, 2003.
• Richert B. Basic nail surgery. *Dermatol Clin.* 2006;24:313–22.
• Woo SH, Kim IH. Surgical pearl: nail edge separation with dental floss for ingrown toenails. *J Am Acad Dermatol.* 2004;50:939–40.

See Also (Topic, Algorithm, Electronic Media Element)
For a video of this procedure, go to: http://www.cfpc.ca/cfp/video/Surgical_Procedures/Wedge_Resection.html

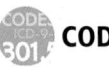 CODES

ICD9
703.0 Ingrowing nail

CLINICAL PEARLS
• The best treatment for a stage 1 ingrown toenail is to insert a wisp of cotton or dental floss between the nail plate and lateral nail fold.
• The best treatment for a stage 3 ingrown toenail is either partial nail avulsion with phenol matrix ablation or application of a flexible gutter splint.
• A patient can prevent ingrown toenails by trimming nails properly and wearing properly fitting shoes.
• Antibiotics are not useful in the treatment of ingrown nails in conjunction with surgical treatment; they may be useful for conservative treatment.

INJURY AND VIOLENCE

Monica Kaitz, MD
Edward Feller, MD

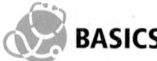 **BASICS**

EPIDEMIOLOGY

- Falls, motor vehicle accidents (MVA), homicide, suicide, domestic violence, child abuse, and poisonings are some of the common avoidable causes of death in society. In industrialized countries, injury is the 5th leading cause of death overall and the leading cause of death for persons 1–14 years, accounting for 40% of all child death. In the US yearly, 50 million are injured severely enough to require medical care, which may account for 10% of total US health care costs. Regardless of whether intentional or unintentional, injury is both predictable and preventable (1).
- Older adults and children are most susceptible to injuries. In the young as many as 75% of all deaths are caused by injuries and violence. Yearly, 1 in 3 adults aged >65 have falls. In women from 2004–2007, 54% of injuries occurred inside or near the home compared to 41% in men. Men acquired injuries more frequently in recreational environments and occupational settings.

Incidence

- Injury classification schemes (1)[C]
  - Body location (presenting to ED): Upper extremity 11.3%, lower extremity 4.3%, and face 4.1%
  - Severity: High case fatality rates with firearm violence
  - Mechanism/intentionality: 63% unintentional, 34% intentional injury deaths in the US each year
- Most common injuries (CDC data, 2007) (2)[A]:
  - Falling is the most common injury in the young (43% of injuries) and elderly (64%) with blunt trauma coming in second, while blunt trauma (20%) and overexertion (13%) are the most common injuries in adolescents and adults respectively. Bites/stings (4.8%), bicycle accidents (4.7%), and poisonings (1.8%) are uniquely common to children while MVA become a consideration in adolescents and adults (10%; 3rd most common) as well as elderly (5%; 4th most common). The incidence of penetrating injury (8.1%) and blunt trauma/assault (4.9%) peaks as an adult, although the absolute numbers have decreased since 2006.
- Most common fatal injuries (CDC data, 2006) (2)[A]:
  - MVA cause the most deaths of any injury in children, adolescents, and adults, coming in a close second in infants and the elderly superseded by unintentional suffocation and falls, respectively. Children die mostly of unintentional accidents; in order: MVA, drowning, fire/burn, and suffocation. Aside from MVA, most deaths in adolescents result from firearms, both homicide (2nd, 4th in adults) and suicide (3rd, 3rd in adults). Suicide by suffocation is also pervasive in both adolescence (4th) and adulthood (5th). Poisoning is particularly deadly in adults with both unintentional (2nd) and suicidal (6th) combined causing more deaths than MVA. Homicide from firearm is 4th in children, 2nd in adolescents, 4th in adults, while suicide by firearm is 3rd in adolescents and adults, 4th in

the elderly. It should be noted: Watch for homicide in infants (3rd) and adverse drug effects in the elderly. Most firearm deaths are homicides in children and adolescents, suicides in adults and the elderly. Other common forms of suicide are suffocation, poisoning. Other common forms of homicide in adolescence (4th) and adults (5th) are penetrating injuries.

Prevalence

- Violence
- Firearms (1)[C]
  - In 2001, 35% of adults reported living in a home with at least 1 firearm
  - Gun violence accounts for $100 billion of which $15 billion represented firearm injuries to children
  - There has been recent decline in violent deaths and firearm injuries.
- Child violence (1)
  - Homicide death rate for children are highest in US as compared to other industrialized nations.
  - 33% of rapes occur prior to 12 years of age; 50% by 18 years.
- Adolescent violence (3)[B]:
  - 33% of students are involved in fights annually; 12.8% of students participated in 1 or more fights at school in the last year.
  - 17.1% of students have carried a weapon in the last 30 days; 6.1% of students have carried a weapon to school.
  - 9.2% of students have been injured by a weapon at school.
  - 5,674 aged 10–24 were murdered, or 16 per day, in 2007.
  - 5.4% of students have missed 1 or more days of school due to fear of harm from violence.
  - 16–19-year-olds are at highest risk for motor vehicle crashes, boys twice that of girls (1)[C].
  - Dating violence: Prevalence of teen dating violence has been reported to range from 9%–46% (4)[C].
- Homicide (4)[C]
  - 2nd leading cause of death for children 1–19 years of age
  - Leading cause of death amongst black 15–24-year-olds
  - 3% of direct medical expenses are related to assault.
- Bullying (4)[C]
  - Prevalence 30% for children either bullying and/or being bullied in 6th- to 10th-graders
  - Bullying is associated with low self-esteem, social isolation, and depression.
  - 1 in 9 middle school students report being cyber-bullied (via the Internet). As many as 1/2 of victims don't know the perpetrator's identity.
- Interpersonal violence (IPV) (5)[C]
  - 1 in 4 women and 1 in 7 men report a lifetime threatened or completed physical or sexual IPV.
  - 1.4% of women and 0.7% of men reported such victimization within the past year.
  - When IPV is defined more broadly, estimates approach 1 in 5 adults.

- Injury
  - Youth are affected disproportionately accounting for ~30% of potential life years lost before age 65 (more than cancer and heart disease combined) (1)[C].
  - 37.3% of all ED visits are injury-related (1)[C].
- Motor vehicle crashes: (3)[C]
  - 3 in 10 people are involved in an alcohol-related motor vehicle crash in their lifetime. 1 in 4 teens killed in a motor vehicle crashes (2008) had a blood alcohol level >0.08 g/dl.
  - 18% of high school students do not wear seatbelts. Teens are more likely to speed and to underestimate driving risks.
  - 86% of youth under the age of 14 wear seatbelts; yet, 65% of these wear restraints that are inappropriate for their age or weight.
  - Contribution of motor vehicle crashes and falls to lifetime medical costs of injury: 40%
- Drowning:
  - 86% of individuals who died from drowning were not wearing personal flotation devices.

RISK FACTORS

- Injuries and risk factors that contribute vary at different stages of life and development (3):
  - Infants, toddlers, and children (ages 0–9):
    - MVA: Unrestrained or improperly restrained. Only 37% of children are restrained in age-appropriate devices; of children killed in MVA, 68% are killed while riding with a driver under the influence of alcohol.
    - All-terrain vehicle (ATV): Age, weight of the child vs weight of ATV, nonhelmeted rider, lack of legislation and enforcement
    - Suffocation (children <1 year old): Loose bedding, wedging, cosleeping, entrapment, hanging, sleeping in environments not intended for infants (couches, adult bed)
    - Drowning: Males, inadequate supervision, residential swimming pools
    - Falls: Walkers, open windows, open stairways, inadequate supervision, hazardous playground equipment
    - Homicides: Lack of access to social capital, community organization, and economic resources, familial instability, community and family violence, access to firearms
  - Adolescents (ages 10–24):
    - MVA: Male driver, inexperience, nighttime driving, speeding, tailgating, driving with other teenagers, cell phones, unrestrained occupants, alcohol and drug use
    - Homicide and suicide: Access to firearms, mental health, alcohol and drug use, exposure to suicidal behavior, history of aggressive behavior, cognitive deficits, poor supervision, exposure to violence, parental drug and alcohol use, poor peer-to-peer interaction, academic failure, poverty, lower socioeconomic class
    - Sports-related injuries
  - Adults (ages 25–64):
    - MVA: Alcohol and drug use, speeding, distractions (e.g., other passengers, cell phones)
    - Prescription drug overdose is leading cause of accidental death in adults.
    - Homicide and suicide: See adolescent risk factors

○ IPV (5)[C]:
- Risk factors: Female, young, history of IPV or sexual assault or child abuse, drugs, unemployment, depression, minority status, income or educational disparity, poverty, weak legal sanctions
- Older adults (≥65):
  ○ MVA: Poor vision, medical condition, and comorbidities
  ○ Falls: Poor vision, medications, weakness, gait imbalance, environmental risk factors (loose rugs, poor lighting, lack of stair railings)
- In addition, individuals from low-income and racial and ethnic minority groups are at a greater risk for injury. Factors contributing to the increased risk in this population include (6):
  - Lower income and education, hazardous and overcrowded living environments, children lack safe recreational facilities and play areas, increased drug activity and violence, access to firearms, limited organized athletics or extracurricular activities, less access to affordable childcare, proximity of housing to busy streets, increased exposure to physical hazards

ETIOLOGY
Multifactorial. Popular model used in the field of injury prevention was designed by Dr. William Haddon. Defines 3 phases of an event: pre, during, and post. Events are then charted against the contributing factors: host, agent (e.g., motor vehicle), and the physical environment to illustrate how they are interrelated. Information is then used to identify specific risk factors and develop injury prevention strategies.

 DIAGNOSIS

HISTORY
- Mechanism, timing, and location of injury:
  - Blunt vs. penetrating; intentional vs. unintentional; others injured vs. isolated injury; circumstances (weather, substance use, restrained vs. unrestrained)
  - Does history correlate with level of injury (i.e., level of suspicion for abuse [elderly, child, or partner])?
- Level of prehospital care, preexisting medical conditions, medications

 TREATMENT

- Prevention: Experts agree that most injuries are preventable. Prevention efforts have been framed as "the 5 E's": enhanced Education, Engineering strategies, Economic incentives, Enactment of legislation, and Enforcement of laws.
- Prevention by level of intervention: Primary (i.e., prevent crash–listed below by etiology), Secondary (i.e., prevent injury upon crash), and Tertiary (i.e., prevent poor outcomes upon injury).
- Motor vehicle injuries (3)[C]:
  - Infants, toddlers, and children: Age-appropriate child safety seats and passenger restraints, child safety seat distribution programs, education programs for parents and caregivers, safety seat checkpoints, harsh penalties for drivers transporting children under the influence of drugs and/or alcohol, legislation regarding restraint of motor vehicle occupants

- Adolescents and adults: Graduated driver licensing programs, blood alcohol concentration laws, minimum drinking age laws, sobriety checkpoints, programs for alcohol servers, zero alcohol tolerance laws for young drivers, school-based education programs on drinking and driving. Emergency medical services (EMS) response times, engineering cars for rapid extraction, organized trauma systems; collapsible automobile steering columns have been shown to decrease injury mortality and morbidity. With a motorcycle helmet: 29% decreased risk for death and 67% decreased risk for traumatic brain injury (1).
- Older adults: Alternative transportation programs, screening for high-risk drivers, gradual curtailment of driving privileges, more frequent license renewal process
- Falls (3)[C]:
  - Infants and toddlers: Home safety assessments, window guards, and elimination of walker use
  - Older adults: Home safety assessments, installation of handrails and grab bars, removal of tripping hazards, nonslip mats, exercise programs designed to improve strength and balance, night lights
- Drowning (3)[C]:
  - Improved care provider supervision of young children; trained lifeguard supervision at public and open swimming locations; clearly demarcated swimming areas at open water locations; fencing, locked gates, and pool alarms for residential swimming pools; personal flotation devices and boating safety awareness; parental certification in cardiopulmonary resuscitation (CPR)
- Fire and burns (7)[C]:
  - Reducing temperature of hot water heaters to <54.4°C (130.1°F)
  - Smoke and carbon monoxide detectors
  - Fire exit planning
  - Educational campaigns directed toward populations and communities at highest risk for home fires (homes with children <4, adults >65, lower socioeconomic class, rural communities)
- Pedestrian injuries (3)[C]:
  - Environmental modifications (sidewalks, lighted intersections and walkways), strict speed laws, reflective clothing
- Violence (homicide, suicide, assaults) (8)[C]:
  - Most effective strategies are those focused on younger age groups that focus on key areas of youth development and adjustment, including positive sense of self; emotional and behavioral regulation; decision-making skills; moral system of belief; and presence of a positive connection with family, community, and environment.
  - Limited access to firearms and/or firearm safety training
  - Suicide: Access to mental health services, improved family and community support, development of healthy coping and problem-solving skills
  - Dating violence: 1 RCT of a school program was shown to be effective in decreasing self-reported dating violence 4 years out from the intervention (4)
- Sports-related injuries (3)[C]:
  - Toolkits providing educational material regarding sports-related injuries have been developed by the CDC for coaches, athletic directors, and parents.

- Proper use of sport gear and equipment. Helmets can prevent 85% of bicyclist head injuries. States without helmet laws have doubled fatality rate from head injuries (1).
- Plan of action for dealing with injuries such as concussion in young athletes, which include strict guidelines regarding if or when it is safe to return to play.
- Poisoning (1)[C]:
  - High rates in children: Call poison center hotline immediately after ingestion of toxin (90% occur at home)

 ONGOING CARE

COMPLICATIONS
Financial and societal costs:
- Injury-related medical expenditures estimates in the US range from $224–$406 billion annually (1)
- Social burden of injury: Loss of productivity, emotional loss, nonmedical expenditures, reduced quality of life, litigation, rehabilitation, mental health costs, altered family and peer relationships, chronic pain, substance use and abuse, changes in lifestyle (2)

REFERENCES
1. Betz M, Li G. Injury prevention and control. *Emerg Med Clin N Am.* 2007;25:901–914.
2. Centers for Disease Control and Prevention. National Center for Injury Prevention and Control. Web-based Injury Statistics Query and Reporting System (WISQARS). Accessed 09/20/2010 at:http://www.cdc.gov/ncipc/wisqars.
3. Centers for Disease Control and Prevention. National Center for Injury Prevention and Control. *CDC Injury Fact Book.* Atlanta: Author, 2006.
4. Committee on Injury, Violence, and Poison Prevention et al. Policy statement–Role of the pediatrician in youth violence prevention. *Pediatrics.* 2009;124:393–402.
5. Zolotor AJ, Denham AC, Weil A et al. Intimate partner violence. *Obstet Gynecol Clin North Am.* 2009;36:847–60, xi
6. Fallat ME, et al. The impact of disparities in pediatric trauma on injury prevention initiatives. *J Trauma Injury Crit Care.* 2006;60(2):452–4.
7. Schnitzer PG. Prevention of unintentional childhood injuries. *Am Fam Physician.* 2006;74:1864–9.
8. Sullivan TN, Farrell AD, Bettencourt AF, et al. Core competencies and the prevention of youth violence. *New Dir Child Adolesc Dev.* 2008;2008:33–46.

ADDITIONAL READING
Guralnick S, Serwint JR. Firearms. *Pediatr Rev.* 2007;28:396–7.

CLINICAL PEARLS
- Injury is the number 1 source of years of productive life lost for individuals <44 years of age.
- Injuries are both predictable and preventable.

INSECT BITES AND STINGS

Dale E. Bieber, MD

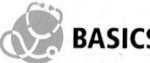 **BASICS**

DESCRIPTION
Arthropods affect humans by inoculating poison or irritative substances through a bite or sting, by invading tissue, and rarely, by contact allergy. Responses may include:
- Local redness with itch, pain, and swelling, usually immediate and transient
- Large local reactions increasing over 24–48 h with inflammation
- Systemic reactions with signs and symptoms of anaphylaxis or systemic toxin effects
- Tissue necrosis
- Secondary infection
- Diseases or late effects of inoculated microorganisms carried by the insect

EPIDEMIOLOGY
Incidence
Approximately 50 deaths/year from fatal anaphylactic reaction to *Hymenoptera* stings (i.e., yellow jackets, bees, wasps most common)

Prevalence
Widespread, with regional and seasonal variations

RISK FACTORS
- Previous sensitization is key to most severe allergic reactions, but exposure history may not be recalled.
- Most insect contact is inadvertent.
- Patients who are young, elderly, immune compromised, or with unstable cardiac or respiratory status have greater risk for serious consequences.

Genetics
Family history of atopy may be a factor in development of more severe allergic-type reactions.

GENERAL PREVENTION
- Be aware of and avoid common insect habitats where possible.
- Protective clothing
- Insect repellents (not effective for bees, spiders, scorpions, caterpillars, bedbugs, fleas, ants):
  - DEET most effective for mosquitoes, ticks, biting flies, fleas, chiggers, midges:
    - Apply to skin or outer clothing.
    - Concentrations >30% give longer duration of effect (5+ h).
    - Appears safe for children >2 months of age
  - Picaridin:
    - Most effective at concentrations >15%
    - Reapply every 4 h.
    - Less toxic effects on humans than DEET
  - PMD:
    - Half as effective as DEET by concentration
    - Not studied for use in children under age 3
  - IR3535: Less effective in most studies
  - Citronella: Weak local effect
  - Other botanical oils: Usually less effective than DEET

- Permethrin is an insect toxin that may be helpful when impregnated in clothing (ticks, flies, chiggers, mosquitoes).
- Desensitization 75–95% effective for *Hymenoptera*-specific venom:
  - Skin tests are needed to determine sensitivity.
  - Protection can last 3–5 years.
- Fire ant control (but not elimination) possible:
  - Baits
  - Sprays, dusts, aerosols
  - Biologic agents
- Tickborne diseases prevented by prompt removal of ticks (pulling out from head) within 24 h of attachment

PATHOPHYSIOLOGY
- Local effects of venom: Tissue inflammation or destruction
- Systemic effects of toxins
- Irritants in insect saliva: Local inflammation
- Exaggerated immune response: Anaphylaxis, urticaria, serum sickness
- Bite or sting mark may be a focus for secondary skin infections inoculated by scratching.
- Insects as vectors carrying infections that are inoculated

 DIAGNOSIS

HISTORY
- Exposure usually known
- Sudden pain or itch most common
- May identity insect by its habitat or by remnants brought by patient
- History of prior exposure useful but not always available or reliable

PHYSICAL EXAM
- If stinger still present in skin, remove by flicking or scraping away from skin
- Examine for signs and symptoms of anaphylaxis:
  - Erythema, urticaria, angioedema
  - Itching/edema of lips, tongue, uvula; drooling
  - Persistent vomiting
  - Respiratory distress, wheeze, repetitive cough, stridor, dysphonia
  - Hypotension, dysrhythmia, syncope, chest pain
  - Seizures
- If anaphylaxis is not present or developing, exam focuses on the sting or bite itself and progresses to surrounding tissue.
- After 24–48 h, look for signs of secondary bacterial infection: Increasing erythema, pain, fever, or lymphangitis or evidence of abscess formation.
- Debride necrotic tissue as necessary.
- Examine for late effects of insect-borne diseases: Erythema migrans, rickettsial rash

DIAGNOSTIC TESTS & INTERPRETATION
Lab
Initial lab tests
Lab tests seldom needed; basic lab parameters usually are normal:
- Plasma histamine levels elevated briefly (5–60 minutes) after mast cell activation
- Metabolite *N*-methyl-histamine elevated in urine for a number of hours (do 24-h collection)
- Serum tryptase levels peak in 1 h after anaphylaxis and stay up for 6 h.

Follow-Up & Special Considerations
- Envenomation that might affect liver or kidney function will need monitoring of liver function tests (LFTs), creatinine determination
- Labs for insect-borne diseases as indicated
- Refer to allergist for formal testing with history of anaphylaxis, significant systemic symptoms, progressively severe reactions

Diagnostic Procedures/Surgery
Various skin tests and immunologic tests available to try to predict anaphylactic risk

DIFFERENTIAL DIAGNOSIS
Differential diagnosis of anaphylactic-type reactions if presence of sting or bite not recognized:
- Flushing syndromes with catecholamines, vasoactive peptides
- Other forms of shock: Cardiac, hemorrhagic, septic
- Acute respiratory failure, asthma
- Restaurant syndromes with MSG or sulfites
- Immune dysfunction with angioedema, urticarial vasculitis
- Panic attacks, Münchhausen stridor
- Vasovagal syncope

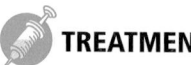 **TREATMENT**

ALERT
- Most deaths due to anaphylaxis occur within 30–60 minutes of sting.
- Airway management for anaphylaxis with angioedema
- Recumbent position with legs elevated

MEDICATION

First Line

- For anaphylaxis:
  - Aqueous epinephrine 1:1,000 0.3–0.5 mg IM/SQ; repeat q3–5m in, preferably anterolateral thigh (pediatric patients 0.01 mg/kg) (1)[A]
  - Prepare for epinephrine infusion if refractory.
  - O_2 6–8 L/min (1)[A]
  - Normal saline rapid bolus 1–2 L IV; repeat as needed (pediatrics 20 mL/kg) (1)[B]
  - Diphenhydramine 25–50 mg IV (pediatrics 1–2 mg/kg)
  - Albuterol for bronchospasm nebulized 2.5–5 mg in 3 mL
  - Emergency treatment of refractory cases: Consider epinephrine infusion, dopamine, glucagon, large-volume crystalloids
- Treatment options without anaphylaxis:
  - Tetanus booster as indicated
  - Oral antihistamines:
    - Diphenhydramine 25–100 mg q6h (pediatrics 5 mg/kg/day q4–6h) or chlorpheniramine 4 mg
    - Cetirizine 10 mg/d
    - May add ranitidine 150 mg b.i.d.
    - Topical intermediate-potency steroid cream or ointment × 3–5 days
    - Desoximetasone 0.05%
    - Triamcinolone 0.1%
    - Fluocinolone t.i.d.
  - Wound care: Antibiotics only if infected

Second Line

- Other options for consideration of anaphylaxis:
  - Consider ranitidine 150 mg IV (pediatrics 1–2 mg/kg).
  - Consider methylprednisolone 125 mg IV (pediatrics 2 mg/kg); helps late-phase reactions and prolonged anaphylaxis
- Specific therapies:
  - Scorpion stings: Treat excess catecholamine release (e.g., nitroprusside, prazosin, beta blockers).
  - Black widow bites: With muscular spasms, use diazepam, opioid analgesics p.o. or IV.
- Antivenom is available for certain scorpions, black widow:
  - Must be administered within 1 h
  - Use is controversial because results are not much better than supportive care.
- Fire ants: Characteristically cause sterile pustules at risk for secondary infection if not left alone
- Brown recluse spider: Pain management, supportive treatment
- Ticks: Review options for Lyme disease, ehrlichiosis, Rocky Mountain spotted fever prophylaxis
- Pediculosis pubis:
  - Topical permethrin 1% cream rinse
  - Permethrin with piperonyl butoxide
  - Malathion 0.5% lotion
  - Lindane 1% shampoo
  - Ivermectin 200 μg/kg p.o. (all along with local measures for nits; not Food and Drug Administration [FDA] approved)
  - Repeat all in 7–10 days.

- Sarcoptes scabii scabies:
  - Permethrin 5% cream
  - Lindane 1% lotion or cream (greater chance of toxicity)
  - Ivermectin (not FDA approved for this)
  - Crotamiton 10% cream or lotion less efficacious

ADDITIONAL TREATMENT

General Measures

- Local wound cleansing
- Ice
- Elevation

Issues for Referral

Refer to allergist with history of anaphylaxis, severe systemic symptoms, or progressively severe reactions

COMPLEMENTARY AND ALTERNATIVE MEDICINE

- Some stings may be treated with a paste of 3 teaspoons of baking soda and 1 teaspoon water.
- None well tested, but many local preventive and treatment measures have been proposed for minor reactions.

SURGERY/OTHER PROCEDURES

Debridement and delayed skin grafting may be needed for brown recluse spider and other bites.

IN-PATIENT CONSIDERATIONS

Admission Criteria

Hospitalization for vascular instability, prolonged resuscitation to monitor and control neuromuscular events, pain, GI symptoms, rarely for effects of renal damage/failure

ONGOING CARE

FOLLOW-UP RECOMMENDATIONS

- Immunotherapy as recommended by allergist/consultant for anaphylaxis or serious reactions; antivenom therapy is available for Hymenoptera family and fire ants.
- Patient-administered anaphylaxis kits with epinephrine are widely available.

Patient Monitoring

- Monitor for delayed effects.
- Serum sickness-type reactions, rare vasculitis-type response

PATIENT EDUCATION

Avoidance of insect habitats and prevention

PROGNOSIS

- Excellent for local reactions
- For systemic reactions, best response with early appropriate intervention to prevent cardiorespiratory collapse

COMPLICATIONS

- Scarring
- Secondary bacterial infection
- Arthropod-associated diseases: Lyme, West Nile, rickettsial, Rocky Mountain spotted fever, ehrlichiosis, malaria, trypanosomiasis, dengue, plague, malaria, others
- Psychological effects, phobias

REFERENCE

1. Joint Task Force on Practice Parameters, American Academy of Allergy, Asthma and Immunology, American College of Allergy, Asthma and Immunology et al. The diagnosis and management of anaphylaxis: an updated practice parameter. J Allergy Clin Immunol. 2005;115:S483–523.

ADDITIONAL READING

- Armstrong M, Johnstone PW. Interventions for Treating Scabies. Cochrane Database of Systematic Reviews. 2007. DOI:10.1002/14651858. CD000320.pub2.
- Golden DBK. Insect Sting Anaphylaxis. Immunology Allergy Clin N AM. 2007;27:261–72.
- http://cdc.gov/travel/yellowBookCh2-InsectsArthropods.
- Katz T, Miller J, Hebert A. Insect Repellents: Historical Perspectives and New Developments. J Amer Acad Derm. 58;5:865–71.
- Leonard EA, Sheldon IV. Ectoparasitic Infections. Clin in Fam Practice. 2005;7(1):97–104.
- Saucier JR. Arachnid Envenomation. Emerg Med Clin N Am. 2004;22:405–22.
- Swanson DL, Vetter RS. Bites of Brown Recluse Spiders and Suspected Necrotic Arachnidism. N Eng J Med. 2005;352:700–7.

CODES

ICD9

- 919.4 Insect bite, nonvenomous, of other, multiple, and unspecified sites, without mention of infection
- 989.5 Toxic effect of venom

CLINICAL PEARLS

- Urgent administration of epinephrine is key to anaphylaxis treatment.
- IgE can be found in most people after sting/bite exposure, but this predicts anaphylaxis poorly.
- Local treatment and symptom management are sufficient in most insect bites and stings.

I

INSOMNIA

Jose Abad, MD
Sheldon Benjamin, MD

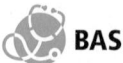 **BASICS**

DESCRIPTION
- Difficulty initiating or maintaining sleep, early morning awakening, nonrestful sleep, nonrestorative sleep, leading to daytime tiredness, low energy, irritability, or difficulty in concentrating
- Primary: Sleeplessness not caused by another sleep, medical, or psychiatric disorder; or by medications, substances of abuse, or environmental factors
- Secondary: Sleeplessness due to any of the above factors
- Transient (<1 week): Secondary to life crises, bereavement, change in environment, or concomitant illness
- Chronic (>1 month): Associated with medical and psychiatric conditions, drug intake, and maladaptive behavioral patterns

Geriatric Considerations
- Caution when prescribing benzodiazepines or other sedative-hypnotics to the elderly; use short-acting nonbenzodiazepine benzodiazepine agonists or melatonin agonists if absolutely necessary for short-term treatment of sleep-onset insomnia
- Increased risk of falls and confusion

Pregnancy Considerations
Transient insomnia occurs secondary to change of sleep position, nocturia, gastritis, back pain, anxiety

EPIDEMIOLOGY
- Predominant age: Increases with age
- Predominant sex: Female > Male (1.5:1)

Prevalence
- Insomnia (transient and chronic): 15–20% of the population
- Chronic insomnia: 10% middle-aged adults; 1/3 of people >65 years

RISK FACTORS
- Age
- Female gender
- Chronic illness
- Obesity
- Depression/anxiety
- Polypharmacy
- Major stressor
- Shift work

GENERAL PREVENTION
- Avoid or treat known etiologies.
- Practice consistent sleep hygiene:
  - Establish regular sleep–wake schedule on weekdays; use same on weekends
  - Sleep in cool, dark, quiet environment
  - No activities or stimuli in bedroom associated with anything but sleep or sex
  - 30-minute wind-down time before sleep
  - If >30 minutes is spent in bed worrying about sleep, move to another environment and engage in quiet activity until sleepiness sets in.
- Limit caffeine intake to mornings.
- Do not use alcohol as a sleep aid.
- No excessive alcohol or smoking in evenings

ETIOLOGY
- Transient/intermittent:
  - Stress/excitement/bereavement
  - Shift work
  - Medical illness
  - High altitude
- Chronic:
  - Medical: Gastroesophageal reflux disease, chronic obstructive pulmonary disease, asthma, fibromyalgia
  - Psychiatric: Mood and anxiety disorders
  - Primary sleep disorder: Idiopathic (primary), breathing-related, restless leg syndrome, sleep state misperception, parasomnias
  - Circadian rhythm disorder: Irregular pattern, jet lag, delayed/advanced sleep phase, shift work
  - Environmental: Light (LCD clocks), noise (snoring, household, traffic), movements (partner/young children/pets)
  - Neurologic: Dementia, stroke, Parkinson disease and other extrapyramidal disorders, epilepsy, headache/pain, myotonic dystrophy, traumatic brain injury
  - Behavioral: Poor sleep hygiene, psychophysiologic, adjustment sleep disorder
  - Substance-induced

COMMONLY ASSOCIATED CONDITIONS
- Psychiatric disorders
- Drug or alcohol addiction/dependence
- Obstructive sleep apnea
- Restless leg syndrome

 DIAGNOSIS

HISTORY
- Perceived reduction in sleep time
- Initial insomnia: Difficulty in initiating sleep at usual time
- Middle insomnia: Wakefulness during the usual sleep cycle, tossing and turning
- Terminal insomnia: Early awakening
- Daytime sleepiness and napping
- Unintended sleep episodes (driving, working)
- Tiredness
- Anticipatory anxiety
- Insomnia history:
  - Duration, time of problem
  - Sleep latency, difficulty in maintaining sleep (repeated awakening), early morning awakening, nonrestorative sleep, or patterns (weekday vs weekend, with or without bed partner, home vs away)
- Sleep hygiene:
  - Bedtime/wakening time
  - Physical environment of sleep area: LED clocks, TV, room lighting, ambient noise
  - Activity: Nighttime eating, exercise, sexual activity
  - Intake: Caffeine, alcohol, herbal supplements, diet pills, illicit drugs, prescriptions, over-the-counter (OTC) sleep aids
- Related: Medical conditions such as pain, stressors, mood issues, medications/timing of administration
- Sleep questionnaire: Pittsburgh Sleep Quality Index (1)
- Sleep diary: Sleep log for 7 consecutive days

DIAGNOSTIC TESTS & INTERPRETATION
- Polysomnography for evaluation of sleep apnea, restless legs, parasomnia, or when sleep history does not provide diagnosis
- Primary insomnia:
  - Symptoms for at least 1 month: Difficulty in initiating/maintaining sleep, or nonrestorative sleep
  - Impairment in social, occupational, or other important areas of functioning
  - Does not occur exclusively during narcolepsy, breathing-related sleep disorder, circadian rhythm sleep disorder, or parasomnia
  - Does not occur exclusively during major depressive disorder, generalized anxiety disorder, delirium, etc.
  - Is not secondary to physiologic effects of substance or general medical condition
  - Sleep disturbance (or resultant daytime fatigue) causes clinically significant distress.
- Secondary insomnia:
  - Due to substance abuse, medication-induced (diuretics, stimulants, etc.), primary depressive disorder, generalized anxiety disorder or phobias, acute situational stress, post-traumatic stress disorder, pain, etc.

Lab
Initial lab tests
Testing to consider based on history and physical exam:
- Thyroid-stimulating hormone
- Urine toxicology

DIFFERENTIAL DIAGNOSIS
- Sleep-disordered breathing, such as obstructive sleep apnea:
  - History from partner/family: Snoring, irregular breathing, sleep movements, length of sleep, mood/performance changes
- Hypersomnia history: Daytime naps, drowsiness, situation/location of daytime sleep; Epworth Sleepiness Scale (1)
- Central nervous system hypersomnias:
  - Narcolepsy:
    - Excessive daytime sleepiness, cataplexy, hypnagogic/hypnopompic hallucinations, sleep paralysis
- Circadian rhythm sleep disturbances
- Parasomnias:
  - REM sleep behavior disorder
- Sleep-related movement disorders:
  - Restless leg syndrome (2)
- Transient stress
- Substance abuse
- Pain
- Insomnia due to medical or neurological disorder
- Mood and anxiety disorders such as depression or anxiety

TREATMENT

- Transient insomnia (<4 weeks)
  - May use medications for short-term use only; benzodiazepines favored
  - Self-medicating with alcohol can increase awakenings and sleep-stage changes.
- Chronic insomnia:
  - Rule out secondary causes (major depressive disorder, generalized anxiety disorder, medications, substance abuse, etc.).
  - Thorough sleep history, drug/caffeine intake, diet, and exercise pattern may uncover correctable causes.
  - Cognitive behavioral therapy is 1st-line treatment for chronic insomnia, especially in >60 population, especially when sedatives are not going to be advantageous (3)[A].
  - Behavioral therapy can be an effective treatment for insomnia and a potentially more effective long-term treatment than pharmacotherapy (4)[B].
  - Address underlying causes (e.g., pain, drugs/alcohol, depression).
  - Avoid daytime napping; develop bedtime rituals conducive to sleep.
  - Refrain from using bed for anything besides sleeping or sex (no eating, reading, TV)
  - Ramelteon only agent without abuse potential
- Remove large or bright clocks from bedroom to prevent focusing on how little sleep is accomplished, as well as light stimulus.

MEDICATION

- Reserved for transient insomnia, such as with jet lag, stress reactions, transient medical condition
- Nonbenzodiazepine benzodiazepine receptor agonists:
  - Zaleplon (Sonata), 5–20 mg; half-life 1–1.5 hours
  - Zolpidem (Ambien), 2.5–10 mg; half-life 1.5–4 hours
  - Zolpidem ER, 1–3 mg; half-life 5–7 hours
  - Eszopiclone (Lunesta), 1–3 mg; half-life 5–7 hours
- Benzodiazepine hypnotics:
  - Intermediate-acting:
    ○ Temazepam, 7.5–30 mg; half-life 8–12 hours
    ○ Oxazepam, 10–30 mg; half-life 5–15 hours
  - Long-acting:
    ○ Alprazolam, 0.25–1 mg; half-life 12–20 hours
    ○ Lorazepam, 0.5–2 mg; half-life 10–22 hours
    ○ Clonazepam, 0.5–2 mg; half-life 22–38 hours
    ○ Diazepam, 2.5–10 mg; half-life 20–50 hours
- Contraindications/precautions:
  - Not indicated for long-term treatment of chronic insomnia due to risks of tolerance, dependency, daytime attention and concentration compromise, incoordination, rebound insomnia
  - Avoid in elderly, pregnant, breast-feeding, substance abusers, patients with suicidal or parasuicidal behaviors
  - Avoid in patients with untreated obstructive apnea and chronic pulmonary disease.
  - Consider risk of falls and cognitive impairment when using sedative hypnotics in those >60 (5)[B].
  - No good evidence to suggest using benzodiazepines for the treatment of insomnia in patients undergoing palliative care (6)[A]
  - Nonbenzodiazepine benzodiazepine receptor agonists may occasionally induce parasomnias (sleep walking, sleep eating, etc.).

- Ramelteon, 8 mg; half-life 1–2.6 hours
  - Proven to be the one agent without potential to be abused and effective to reduce sleep time onset for short- and long-term use in adults (7)[B]
- Serotonergic antidepressants:
  - Trazodone, 25–200 mg; half-life 3–9 hours
  - Doxepin, 25–150 mg; half-life 6–8 hours
  - Amitriptyline, 25–150 mg; half-life 10–50 hours
  - Mirtazapine, 15–60 mg; half-life 20–40 hours
- γ-hydroxy butyrate:
  - Sodium oxybate, 4.5–9 mg; half-life 40 minutes (only for insomnia due to narcolepsy)

ADDITIONAL TREATMENT

Insomnia is highly associated with hypertension, congestive heart failure, anxiety and depression, and obesity. Therefore, prevention and optimal management of these chronic conditions will help with incidence and symptoms of insomnia.

COMPLEMENTARY AND ALTERNATIVE MEDICINE

- Biologically based practices:
  - Melatonin can decrease sleep latency when taken 30–120 minutes prior to bedtime, but there is no class A evidence for efficacy in insomnia, and long-term effects are unknown (8).
  - Valerian: There is no clear evidence supporting its efficacy in treating insomnia.
- Although acupuncture has often been reported to help with insomnia, adequately controlled randomized trials supporting its efficacy are lacking (9)[B].
- Psychotherapy:
  - Cognitive behavioral therapy (including relaxation therapy) is effective and considered more useful than medication treatment for chronic insomnia.

ONGOING CARE

FOLLOW-UP RECOMMENDATIONS
- Daily exercise improves quality of sleep and may be more effective than medication.
- Avoid exercise within 3 hours of bedtime.

Patient Monitoring
- Reassess need for medications periodically; avoid standing prescriptions.
- Caution patients that nonbenzodiazepine benzodiazepine agonists (zolpidem, zaleplon, eszopiclone), as well as benzodiazepines, can be habit-forming.

DIET
- Avoid caffeine or reserve for morning only.
- Avoid heavy late-night snacks (light snack at bedtime may help).
- Avoid alcohol within 6 hours of bedtime.

PATIENT EDUCATION
Describe limitations and side effects of drugs used for insomnia.

PROGNOSIS
- Situational insomnia should resolve with time.
- Treatment of underlying etiology and consistent sleep hygiene are the mainstays of treatment.

COMPLICATIONS
- Transient insomnia can become chronic.
- Daytime sleepiness, cognitive dysfunction

- Pulmonary hypertension (HTN) if chronic sleep apnea left untreated
- Sleep apnea may lead to HTN, stroke, or cardiac ischemia.

REFERENCES

1. Buysse DJ, Reynolds CF, Monk TH, et al. The Pittsburgh Sleep Quality Index: a new instrument for psychiatric practice and research. *Psychiatry Res.* 1989;28:193–213.
2. Panossian LA, Avidan AY. Review of sleep disorders. *Med Clin North Am.* 2009;93:407–25, ix.
3. Montgomery P, Dennis J. Cognitive behavioural interventions for sleep problems in adults aged 60+. *Cochrane Database Syst Rev.* 2003; CD003161.
4. Ebben MR, Spielman AJ. Non-pharmacological treatments for insomnia. *J Behav Med.* 2009.
5. Glass J, Lanctôt KL, Herrmann N, et al. Sedative hypnotics in older people with insomnia: meta-analysis of risks and benefits. *BMJ.* 2005;331:1169.
6. Hirst A, Sloan R. Benzodiazepines and related drugs for insomnia in palliative care. *Cochrane Database Syst Rev.* 2002;CD003346.
7. Reynoldson JN, Elliott ES, Nelson LA. Ramelteon: A Novel Approach in the Treatment of Insomnia (CE) (September). *Ann Pharmacother.* 2008.
8. Verster GC. Melatonin and its agonists, circadian rhythms and psychiatry. *Afr J Psychiatry (Johannesbg).* 2009;12:42–6.
9. Huang W, Kutner N, Bliwise DL. A systematic review of the effects of acupuncture in treating insomnia. *Sleep Med Rev.* 2009;13:73–104.

See Also (Topic, Algorithm, Electronic Media Element)
Anxiety; Depression; Fibromyalgia; Sleep Apnea, Obstructive
Algorithms: Insomnia, Chronic; Restless Leg Syndrome (RLS); Anxiety

 CODES

ICD9
- 307.41 Transient disorder of initiating or maintaining sleep
- 307.42 Persistent disorder of initiating or maintaining sleep
- 780.52 Insomnia, unspecified

CLINICAL PEARLS
- Treatment of underlying etiology of the insomnia and consistent sleep hygiene are key.
- Most medications used to treat insomnia are indicated for short-term use only. Eszopiclone is the only medication for insomnia to have been tested for daily use over a 6-month period.
- Weigh the risks and benefits of pharmacological treatment and consider short-term vs long-term goals when planning your treatment regimen.
- Patients with chronic insomnia may benefit from cognitive behavioral therapy.

INTERSTITIAL CYSTITIS

Montiel T. Rosenthal, MD

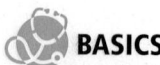 **BASICS**

DESCRIPTION
- A disease of unknown cause probably representing a final common pathway from several etiologies. Likely pathogenesis is disruption of urothelium, impaired lower urinary track defenses, and loss of bladder muscular wall elasticity. The symptoms in many patients are insidious and the disease progresses over years before the diagnosis is established.
- Mild: Normal bladder capacity under anesthesia. Ulceration, cracking, or glomerulation of mucosa (or not) with bladder distention under anesthesia. No incontinence. Symptoms wax and wane and may not progress. A bladder sensory problem.
- Severe: Progressive bladder fibrosis. Small true bladder capacity under anesthesia. Poor bladder wall compliance. Often ulcers present at cystoscopy. May have overflow incontinence and/or chronic bacteriuria that is unresponsive to antibiotics.
- System(s) affected: Renal/Urologic
- Synonym(s): Urgency frequency syndrome; Painful bladder syndrome

Pregnancy Considerations
Unpredictable symptom improvement or exacerbation during pregnancy. No known fetal effects from interstitial cystitis. Usual problems of unknown effect on fetus with medications taken during pregnancy

EPIDEMIOLOGY
- Caucasians predominant
- Predominant sex:
  - Female > Male (10:1)
- Predominant age:
  - Mild: 20–40 years
  - Severe: 20–70 years
- Pediatric considerations:
  - <10 years old and again at 13–17
  - Daytime enuresis, dysuria without infection

Prevalence
In the US:
- Up to 1,000,000 affected. Many cases likely unreported
- 0.052%, but may be higher; up to 10% (1)[C]

RISK FACTORS
Unknown

ETIOLOGY
- Unknown. Not primarily psychosomatic
- Possible causes:
  - Subclinical urinary infection
  - Damage to glycosaminoglycan mucus layer increasing bladder wall permeability to irritants such as urea
  - Autoimmune
  - Mast cell histamine release
- Neurologic up-regulation/stimulation

COMMONLY ASSOCIATED CONDITIONS
- Fibromyalgia
- Allergies
- Chronic fatigue syndrome
- Depression
- Chronic prostatitis
- Chronic pelvic pain
- Irritable bowel syndrome

 DIAGNOSIS

- Frequent, urgent, relentless urination day and night, >8 voids in 24 hours
- Pain with full bladder that resolves with bladder emptying (except if bacteriuria present).
- Urge urinary incontinence if bladder capacity is small.
- Sleep disturbance
- Dyspareunia, especially with full bladder
- Secondary symptoms from chronic pain and sleeplessness, especially depression

HISTORY
- Pelvic Pain and Urgency/Frequency (PUF) Symptom Scale (2)[B]: Self-reporting questionnaire for screening potential interstitial cystitis patients
- Frequent UTIs, vaginitis, or symptoms in week before menses

PHYSICAL EXAM
- Perineal/prostatic pain in males
- Anterior vaginal wall pain in females

DIAGNOSTIC TESTS & INTERPRETATION
Lab
- Urinalysis: Normal except with chronic bacteriuria (rare)
- Urine culture from catheterized specimen: Normal except with chronic bacteriuria (rare) or partial antibiotic treatment
- Urine cytology:
  - Normal: Reserve for men >40 years old and women with hematuria

Diagnostic Procedures/Surgery
- Cystoscopy (especially in men >40 years old or women w/hematuria)
  - Bladder wall visualization
  - Hydraulic distention: No improved diagnostic certainty over H&P alone (3)[C]
- No role for urodynamic testing

- K+ sensitivity test (2)[B]:
  - Insert catheter, empty bladder, instill 40 mL H_2O over 2–3 minutes, rank urgency at 0–5 in intensity, rank pain at 0–5 in intensity, drain bladder, instill 40 mL KCl 0.4 mol/L solution:
    - If immediate pain, flush bladder w/60 mL H_2O and treat w/ bladder instillations
    - If no immediate pain, wait 5 minutes and rate urgency and pain
  - If urgency or pain >2, treat as above

- Pain or urgency >2 considered a positive test and strongly correlates with interstitial cystitis if no radiation cystitis nor acute bacterial cystitis.

Pathological Findings
- Nonspecific chronic inflammation on bladder biopsies
- Urine cytology negative for dysplasia and neoplasia
- Possible mast cell proliferation in mucosa

DIFFERENTIAL DIAGNOSIS
- Uninhibited bladder (urgency, frequency, urge incontinence, less pain, symptoms usually decrease when asleep)
- Urinary infection: Cystitis, prostatitis
- Bladder neoplasm
- Bladder stone
- Neurologic bladder disease
- Nonurinary pelvic disease (sexually transmitted infections, endometriosis, pelvic relaxation)

TREATMENT

MEDICATION

Randomized controlled trials of most medications for IC demonstrate limited benefit over placebo; no clear predictors of what will benefit an individual. Prepare patient that treatment may involve trial and error.

First Line

- Pentosan polysulfate (Elmiron) 100 mg 3×/day. May take several months to become effective, rated as modestly beneficial in systematic drug review (4)[A] (only FDA-approved treatment for interstitial cystitis).
- Triple drug therapy: 6 months of pentosan, hydroxyzine, doxepin
- Behavioral therapy combined with oral agents found improved outcomes compared to medications alone.
- Antibacterials for bacteriuria
- Hydroxyzine
- Amitriptyline
- Oxybutynin, hyoscyamine, and other anticholinergic medications decrease frequency.
- Prednisone (only for ulcerative lesions)
- Montelukast
- Doxepin decreases frequency.
- NSAIDs for pain and any inflammatory component
- Bladder instillations:
  - Lidocaine, sodium bicarbonate, and heparin or pentosan polysulfate sodium
  - Dimethyl sulfoxide (DMSO) every 1–2 weeks for 3–6 weeks, then as needed
  - Heparin sometimes added to DMSO
  - Other agents: Steroids, silver nitrate, oxychlorosene (Clorpactin)
- Contraindications:
  - No anticholinergics with patients having closed-angle glaucoma
- Significant possible interactions
  - Refer to manufacturer's profile of each drug.

Second Line

Note that phenazopyridine, a local bladder mucosal anesthetic, is usually not very effective.

ADDITIONAL TREATMENT

General Measures

- Appropriate health care: Outpatient (5)[B]
- Eliminate foods and liquids that exacerbate symptoms on individual basis.
- Biofeedback bladder retraining

COMPLEMENTARY AND ALTERNATIVE MEDICINE

- Modified Thiele massage: Transvaginal of pelvic floor muscles
- Guided imagery

SURGERY/OTHER PROCEDURES

- Hydraulic distention of bladder under anesthesia: Symptomatic but transient relief
- Cauterization of bladder ulcer
- Augmentation cystoplasty to increase bladder capacity and decrease pressure, with or without partial cystectomy. Expected results in severe cases: Much improved, 75%; with residual discomfort, 20%; unchanged, 5%
- Urinary diversion with total cystectomy only if disease completely refractory to medical therapy

ONGOING CARE

FOLLOW-UP RECOMMENDATIONS

Patient Monitoring

Not specifically needed unless symptoms unresponsive to treatment

DIET

- Variable effects from person to person
- Common irritants include caffeine, chocolate, citrus, tomatoes, carbonated beverages, K^+ rich foods, spicy foods, acidic foods, and alcohol.

PATIENT EDUCATION

Interstitial Cystitis Association, 110 Wash. St. Suite 340, Rockville, MD 20850; 1(800) HELPICA; http://www.ichelp.org

PROGNOSIS

- Mild: Exacerbations and remissions of symptoms. May not be progressive. Does not predispose to other diseases.
- Severe: Progressive problems that usually require surgery to control symptoms

COMPLICATIONS

Severe with long-term continuous high bladder pressure could be associated with renal damage.

REFERENCES

1. Parsons CL, Tatsis V. Prevalence if interstitial cystitis in young women. *Urology.* 2004;64:866.
2. Parsons CL, Dell J, et al. Increased prevalence of interstitial cystitis; previously unrecognized urologic and gynecological cases identified using a new symptom questionnaire and intravesical potassium sensitivity. *Urology.* 2002;60:573–8.
3. Ottem DP, Teichman JM. What is the value of cystoscopy with hydrodistention for interstitial cystitis? *Urology.* 2005;66:494–9.
4. Dimitrakov J, Kroenke K, Steers WD, et al. Pharmacologic management of painful bladder syndrome/interstitial cystitis: a systematic review. *Arch Intern Med.* 2007;167:1922–9.
5. Moldwin R, Evans R, et al. Rational. Approach to the Treatment of Patients with Interstitial Cystitis. *Urology.* 2007;69(4A):73–81.

See Also (Topic, Algorithm, Electronic Media Element)

Urinary Tract Infection in Females
Algorithm: Pelvic Girdle Pain

CODES

ICD9
595.1 Chronic interstitial cystitis

CLINICAL PEARLS

- The potassium sensitivity test has been the most useful in confirming an initial diagnosis of interstitial cystitis. Submucosal petechial hemorrhages and/or ulceration at the time of bladder distention and cystoscopy further support the diagnosis.
- At present, there is no definitive treatment for interstitial cystitis. Most patients with severe disease receive multiple treatment approaches. Regular multidisciplinary follow-up, pharmacological therapy, avoidance of symptom triggers, psychological and supportive therapy are all important, as this disease tends to wax and wane. Monitor patients for depression as a comorbidity. Empowering patients to be managers of their symptoms, to communicate regularly with their physicians, and to learn as much as they are able about this disease can help patients to optimize their outcome.

I

INTERSTITIAL NEPHRITIS

Fozia A. Ali, MD

 BASICS

DESCRIPTION
- Acute interstitial nephritis (AIN) is an inflammatory response of the kidney involving interstitial edema and, at times, tubular cell damage. It may be an acute reaction or a result of long-term damage.
- System(s) affected: Renal/Urologic; Endocrine/Metabolic; Immunologic
- Synonym(s): Tubulointerstitial nephritis (TIN), Acute interstitial allergic nephritis

EPIDEMIOLOGY
Pediatric Considerations
- Children exposed to lead poisoning are more likely to develop nephritis as a young adult.
- TIN with uveitis presents in adolescent females.
- Atherosclerotic or ischemic nephritis is more common in the elderly.

Incidence
- Interstitial nephritis accounts for 10–15% of kidney disease in the US.
- Analgesic-induced nephritis is 5–6× more common in women.
- Peak incidence in women 60–70 years of age

Geriatric Considerations
- The elderly have more severe disease and increased risk of permanent damage.

GENERAL PREVENTION
- Early recognition and prompt discontinuation of offending agents
- Remove all sources of heavy metals, including ceramics.
- Avoid further nephrotoxicity.

PATHOPHYSIOLOGY
- AIN:
  - Delayed hypersensitivity reaction, usually owing to drugs
  - May cause acute renal insufficiency
  - Regardless of the severity of the damage to the tubular epithelium, the renal dysfunction generally is reversible, possibly reflecting the regenerative capacity of tubules with preserved basement membrane.
- Chronic interstitial nephritis (CIN):
  - Follows long-term exposure to offending agents
  - Often found on routine labs or evaluation for hypertension (HTN)
  - Characterized by interstitial scarring, fibrosis, and tubule atrophy, resulting in progressive chronic renal insufficiency
- TIN is sometimes associated with uveitis.

ETIOLOGY
- AIN:
  - Hypersensitivity to drugs (70%):
    - Antibiotics: Penicillin, cephalosporins, sulfonamides, rifampin
    - Nonsteroidal anti-inflammatory drugs (NSAIDs)/analgesics (more common in elderly people because of the higher incidence of arthritic disorders in this population)
    - Sulfa-containing diuretics
    - Phenytoin
    - Allopurinol

- Infectious
- AIN is associated with primary renal infections such as acute bacterial pyelonephritis, renal tuberculosis, and fungal nephritis.
- Acute transplant rejection
- Immunologic: Systemic lupus erythematosus (SLE), Sjögren syndrome, sarcoidosis, Wegener granulomatosis, cryoglobulinemia
- Idiopathic (isolated or with uveitis)
- CIN:
  - Drugs: Analgesics, lithium, antineoplastics, antibiotics, anticonvulsants, antihypertensives, immunosuppressants, diuretics, Chinese herbal medicine
  - Heavy metals: Lead, cadmium
  - Obstruction: Stones, neoplasm, prostatic hypertrophy
  - Metabolic: Hypercalcemia, hyperoxaluria, chronic hypokalemia, cystinosis
  - Vascular changes: Cholesterol emboli, HTN, sickle hemoglobinopathy, radiation
  - Toxins: Snakebite venom (hemotoxic or myotoxic)
  - Other: Balkan-endemic nephropathy, Epstein-Barr virus

COMMONLY ASSOCIATED CONDITIONS
- Alport disease
- Medullary cystic disease
- Inflammatory bowel disease
- Multiple myeloma
- Primary biliary cirrhosis

 DIAGNOSIS

- AIN:
  - Fever: 80%
  - Transient maculopapular rash: 25–50%
  - Acute renal insufficiency:
    - Decreased urine output: 50%
    - Signs of fluid overload or depletion
    - Altered mental status
    - Nausea, vomiting
- CIN:
  - HTN
  - Decreased urine output or polyuria
  - Inability to concentrate urine
  - Polydipsia
  - Acidosis
  - Anemia
  - Fanconi syndrome

HISTORY
- Medications
- Alcohol and illicit drug use
- Exposure to heavy metals
- Tobacco use
- Dyslipidemia/atherosclerosis
- Cancer
- HTN

PHYSICAL EXAM
- Increased blood pressure
- Altered mental status
- Rash accompanying renal findings in acute AIN
- Pericardial rub if uremic pericarditis
- Lung crackles if fluid overload
- Extremity swelling
- Weight gain from fluid retention

DIAGNOSTIC TESTS & INTERPRETATION
Lab
- Complete blood count (CBC):
  - Eosinophilia (80%): Not seen in NSAID-induced AIN
  - Anemia
- Chemistry:
  - Acidosis
  - Hypokalemia/hyperkalemia
  - Elevated blood urea nitrogen (BUN) and creatinine
- Urinalysis with urine lytes
  - Hematuria (95%)
  - Mild proteinuria (present to variable degrees, usually <1 g/24 h, except in AIN associated with NSAIDs)
  - Specific gravity
  - Pyuria, white blood cell (WBC) casts
  - Eosinophiluria
- Serologic testing for immunologic disease: Sarcoidosis, Sjögren syndrome, Wegener granulomatosis, Behçet syndrome
- Lead level:
  - Not useful in chronic lead exposure
  - >90% of lead resides in bone.
  - If chronic lead exposure is suspected, consider EDTA lead mobilization test.
- Liver function tests: Elevated serum transaminase levels (in patients with associated drug-induced liver injury)

Imaging
- KUB
- Gallium scan (a negative gallium scan does not preclude the diagnosis because false-negative results can be seen)
- Renal ultrasonography may demonstrate kidneys that are normal to enlarged in size with increased cortical echogenicity, but there are no ultrasonographic findings that will reliably confirm or exclude AIN versus other causes of acute renal failure.
- The role of intravenous pyelography (IVP) remains in question (in many instances, similar information can be obtained by ultrasound without exposing the patient to potentially nephrotoxic contrast dye).

Follow-Up & Special Considerations
Patients who do not recover renal function and those with chronic TIN should receive long-term follow-up care to protect kidneys from further potentially nephrotoxic therapies.

Diagnostic Procedures/Surgery
- Renal biopsy is the "gold standard" and definitive method of establishing diagnosis of AIN. However, it is not needed in all patients.
- Indications for renal biopsy: Patients who do not improve following withdrawal of likely precipitating medications, who have no contraindications to renal biopsy and do not refuse the procedure, and who are being considered for steroid therapy are good candidates for renal biopsy.
- Contraindications: Renal biopsy is contraindicated in bleeding diathesis, solitary kidney, end-stage renal disease with small kidneys, severe uncontrolled HTN and sepsis, or renal parenchymal infection.

Pathological Findings
- Acute:
  - Cellular infiltration with eosinophilia
  - In cholesterol microembolism in the kidney, the finding of a characteristic needle-shaped cleft in medium- or small-sized renal arterioles is diagnostic.
- Chronic: Chronic TIN is characterized by tubular atrophy, fibrosis, and cellular infiltration with mononuclear cells.

DIFFERENTIAL DIAGNOSIS
- Acute renal failure
- Urinary tract obstruction

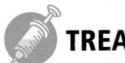 TREATMENT

For AIN, corticosteroids have not been shown to improve outcomes (1)[B].

MEDICATION
- Mainstay of treatment is supportive therapy.
- Offending drugs should be discontinued.
- If patient is taking multiple offending drugs, a reasonable clinical approach should include whether any suspected drug can be substituted easily with another medication.
- If renal failure persists after removing agent, attempt medication therapy.

First Line
- Prednisone 0.5–2 mg/kg/d PO or equivalent IV dose × 1–2 weeks, followed by a gradual taper over 3–4 weeks
- In patients who do not respond to corticosteroids within 2–3 weeks, treatment with cyclophosphamide (Cytoxan) can be considered.
- Studies support steroid use in chronic, not acute, interstitial nephritis (1)[B],(2),(3)[C],(4)[A].
- Continue corticosteroids for 6 months in patients with sarcoidosis (2)[C].

Second Line
- Lead toxicity: Repeated chelation therapy may improve renal function (5)[A].
  - Succimer 10 mg/kg PO q8h × 5 days, then q12h × 14 days, or
  - EDTA 2 g IV/IM; if IM, use with 2% lidocaine.
- SLE nephritis: Steroids plus cyclophosphamide or azathioprine (4)[A]
- Urate nephropathy:
  - Allopurinol to decrease urate level (2)[C]
  - Use with caution because allopurinol is nephrotoxic.
- Lithium-induced nephritis: Use amiloride as adjunct (2)[C].
- Cidofovir-induced nephritis: Use probenecid as adjunct (2)[C].

ADDITIONAL TREATMENT
General Measures
- Discontinue offending agent.
- Reduce exposure to other nephrotoxic agents.
- Supportive measures
- Maintain adequate hydration.
- Symptomatic relief for fever, rash, and systemic symptoms
- Control of blood pressure and anemia.
- Correct electrolyte imbalances.
- Dialysis if criteria met

Issues for Referral
Most patients presenting with renal insufficiency, proteinuria, and/or acid-base electrolyte disorders require consultation with a nephrologist.

IN-PATIENT CONSIDERATIONS
Patients with acute renal failure or with serious electrolyte or acid-base disorders may require inpatient care until stabilization or resolution.

Initial Stabilization
- Arterial blood gases
- Electrocardiogram (ECG)

Admission Criteria
- Oliguria or anuria persists
- Severe electrolyte abnormalities
- ECG changes

Discharge Criteria
- Stable vitals, labs, and ECG
- Normal urine production

 ONGOING CARE

FOLLOW-UP RECOMMENDATIONS
Patient Monitoring
If patients must remain on nephrotoxic medications, measure renal function, electrolytes, and phosphorus frequently.

DIET
- Low fat/low cholesterol
- Low protein (6)[A]
- Low sodium
- Low potassium

PATIENT EDUCATION
Printed materials for patients are available at the National Kidney Disease Education Program, (866) 4-KIDNEY, www.nkdep.nih.gov.

PROGNOSIS
- If the associated AIN is detected early (within 1 week of the rise in serum creatinine) and the drug is discontinued promptly, the long-term outcome is favorable for a return to baseline serum creatinine.
- Renal biopsy reveals extent of damage.
- AIN:
  - Recovery within weeks to months
  - Acute dialysis is needed for 1/3 of patients before resolution.
  - Rarely progresses to end-stage renal disease (ESRD)
- CIN: Can progress to ESRD
- TIN with uveitis:
  - Renal disease remits in 1 year if untreated.
  - Uveitis has relapsing course, requiring systemic corticosteroids.
- Untreated acute renal failure has a 45–70% mortality.

COMPLICATIONS
- Papillary necrosis
- Chronic tubulointerstitial disease may progress to ESRD requiring dialysis or transplantation.
- Analgesics increase the risk of transitional cell cancers of the uroepithelium.

REFERENCES
1. Clarkson MR, et al. Acute interstitial nephritis: Clinical features and response to corticosteroid therapy. *Nephrol Dialysis Transplant.* 2004;19: 2778–83.
2. Braden GL, O'Shea MH, Mulhern JG. Tubulointerstitial diseases. *Am J Kidney Dis.* 2005;46:560–72.
3. Markowitz GS, Perazella MA. Drug-induced renal failure: A focus on tubulointerstitial disease. *Clinica Chimica Acta.* 2005;351:31–47.
4. Flanc RS, et al. Treatment for lupus nephritis. *Cochrane Database Sys Rev.* 2004;1:CD002922.
5. Lin JL, Lin-Tan DT, Hsu KH, et al. Environmental lead exposure and progression of chronic renal diseases in patients without diabetes. *N Engl J Med.* 2003;348:277–86.
6. Fougue D, et al. Low-protein diets for chronic kidney disease in nondiabetic adults. *Cochrane Database Sys Rev.* 2006;3.

ADDITIONAL READING
- http://emedicine.medscape.com/article/243597-followup.
- http://jasn.asnjournals.org/cgi/reprint/9/3/506.
- http://www.aafp.org/afp/20030615/2527.html.

See Also (Topic, Algorithm, Electronic Media Element)
Algorithm: Hematuria

 CODES

ICD9
- 580.89 Acute glomerulonephritis with other specified pathological lesion in kidney
- 582.89 Other chronic glomerulonephritis with specified pathological lesion in kidney
- 583.89 Other nephritis and nephropathy, not specified as acute or chronic, with specified pathological lesion in kidney

CLINICAL PEARLS
- The symptoms of AIN are more dramatic and sudden (days to weeks) than those of CIN, which is slower and progressive.
- The best treatment is to 1st remove the offending agent.
- Hypercalcemia is both a cause and an effect of CIN. Treating hypercalcemia slows the progression of CIN.
- Finding eosinophilia on the CBC rules out NSAID-induced AIN.
- The "gold standard" in diagnosing interstitial nephritis is a renal biopsy.

INTESTINAL OBSTRUCTION

Abdulrazak Abyad, MD, PhD, MBA, MPH, AGSF, AFCHSE

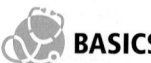

BASICS

DESCRIPTION
- Intestinal obstruction exists where there is a failure, reversal, or impairment of the normal transit of intestinal contents. Obstructions may be partial or complete and are manifested by abdominal pain, emesis, and obstipation.
- System(s) affected: GI

Geriatric Considerations
- Colon neoplasms more common
- Chronic constipation/impactions more common

Pediatric Considerations
Different etiologies of obstruction in childhood:

EPIDEMIOLOGY
Predominant sex: Male = Female.

Prevalence
In US: Accounts for ~20% of all admissions for acute abdominal conditions

RISK FACTORS
- Previous abdominal and/or pelvic surgery
- Hernia
- Chronic constipation
- Cholelithiasis
- Inflammatory bowel disease
- Ingested foreign bodies: Pica, enteric potassium tablets, etc.
- Diverticular disease

Genetics
Unknown

ETIOLOGY
- Luminal lesions:
  - Impactions
  - Gallstones
  - Meconium in newborns
  - Intussusception in infants

- Intrinsic lesions:
  - Congenital (e.g., atresia and stenosis, imperforate anus, duplications, Meckel diverticulum)
  - Trauma
  - Inflammatory [e.g., Crohn disease, diverticulitis, ulcerative colitis, radiation, toxic (ingestions)]
  - Neoplastic (most common cause of colon obstruction in adults)
  - Miscellaneous (e.g., endometriosis)
  - Pseudomyxoma peritonei is an appendiceal tumor.
- Extrinsic lesions:
  - Adhesions (most common cause of small bowel obstruction)
  - Hernia and wound dehiscence
  - Masses (e.g., annular pancreas, anomalous vasculature, abscess and hematoma, neoplasms)
  - Volvulus
  - Neuromuscular defect (e.g., megacolon, neuro/myopathic motility disorders)

DIAGNOSIS

HISTORY
- Abdominal pain: Diffuse, poorly localized abdominal cramping at intervals of 5–15 minutes.
- Emesis: Usually occurs immediately after obstruction of bowel; more frequent in proximal obstruction; unusual in colon obstruction until small bowel distension occurs
- Obstipation: Common symptom; may pass contents distal to obstruction, especially in high intestinal obstruction; pain followed by explosive diarrhea is seen often in partial obstruction.

PHYSICAL EXAM
- Inspection: Distension (a late finding) less likely in proximal obstructions
- Auscultation: High-pitched bowel sounds, peristaltic rushes
- Palpation: Tenderness, mass, presence of peritoneal signs (these suggest strangulation or perforation)
- Rectal examination: May reveal fecal impaction; occult blood may suggest colon malignancy.

DIAGNOSTIC TESTS & INTERPRETATION
Lab
- White blood cell count: Slight rise (15,000/mm^3); significant increases associated with strangulation, ischemic bowel
- Hematocrit: Moderate rise associated with extracellular fluid loss
- Renal: Urine specific gravity 1.025–1.030 and increase in blood urea nitrogen and creatinine (owing to extracellular volume loss)
- Amylase: May be elevated; unreliable as an indicator of obstruction or strangulation
- Blood gases: May be normal; late changes are those of acidosis.
- No single or series of laboratory studies is useful in the diagnosis of intestinal strangulation.

Imaging
- Abdominal and chest radiographs:
  - Distension of small bowel or colon
  - Air-fluid levels (may be seen in ileus, gastroenteritis, constipation)
  - Lack of colon gas
  - Free intraperitoneal air (strangulation with perforation)
  - "Bird beak" lesion in colonic volvulus
  - Foreign-body visualization
- Contrast studies:
  - Barium enema is useful for the diagnosis of colonic obstruction and may be therapeutic in intussusception.
  - Barium or Gastrografin orally may differentiate obstruction from ileus.
  - Enteroclysis may identify the site of small bowel obstruction.

Diagnostic Procedures/Surgery
- Rigid proctoscopy: May be therapeutic in sigmoid volvulus
- Flexible sigmoidoscopy

Pathological Findings
- Edema of mucosa
- Hypersecretion
- Necrosis

DIFFERENTIAL DIAGNOSIS
- Adynamic ileus
- Colonic pseudo-obstruction (Ogilvie syndrome)

TREATMENT

- Inpatient
- Treatment directed at early GI decompression, correction of fluid and electrolyte abnormalities, timely operative intervention where indicated; surgical/GI consultation required
- Consider use of intraperitoneal prophylactic agents for preventing adhesions (1)[A].
- Continuous intravenous lidocaine during and after abdominal surgery reduces postoperative ileus, improves patient rehabilitation, and shortens hospital stay (2,3)[A].

MEDICATION

Antibiotic use is controversial in the absence of sepsis, but prophylactic antibiotics are appropriate before the surgery.

ADDITIONAL TREATMENT

General Measures

- Nasogastric suction
- Foley catheter
- Intravenous fluids: Normal saline/Ringer solution with potassium supplementation as required

SURGERY/OTHER PROCEDURES

- Timing of operative intervention critical; must correct electrolytes, volume quickly before surgery
- Surgical procedures:
  - Closed bowel procedures: Lysis of adhesions, reduction of intussusception, reduction of volvulus, reduction of incarcerated hernia
  - Enterotomy for the removal of bezoars, foreign bodies, gallstones
  - Resection of bowel for obstructing lesions, strangulated bowel
  - Bypasses of intestine around obstruction
  - Enterocutaneous fistulas proximal to obstruction: Colostomy, cecostomy

IN-PATIENT CONSIDERATIONS

Nursing

Careful attention to inputs and outputs

 ONGOING CARE

FOLLOW-UP RECOMMENDATIONS

Patient Monitoring

Follow weekly postoperatively for 2–8 weeks.

DIET

NPO

PROGNOSIS

Prognosis depends on the underlying etiology and patient's general medical condition. In general, mortality from intestinal obstruction ranges from <1% to >20% depending on etiology, bowel viability, and comorbidities.

COMPLICATIONS

- Slow return of bowel function
- Higher risk of subsequent obstruction
- Sepsis

REFERENCES

1. Kumar S, Wong PF, Leaper DJ. Intra-peritoneal prophylactic agents for preventing adhesions and adhesive intestinal obstruction after non-gynaecological abdominal surgery. *Cochrane Database Syst Rev.* 2009;CD005080.
2. Marret E, Rolin M, Beaussier M, et al. Meta-analysis of intravenous lidocaine and postoperative recovery after abdominal surgery. *Br J Surg.* 2008; 95:1331–8.
3. McCarthy GC, Megalla SA, Habib AS et al. Impact of intravenous lidocaine infusion on postoperative analgesia and recovery from surgery: a systematic review of randomized controlled trials. *Drugs.* 2010;70:1149–63.

ADDITIONAL READING

- ASGE Standards of Practice Committee, Harrison ME, Anderson MA, Appalaneni V, Banerjee S, Ben-Menachem T, Cash BD, Fanelli RD, Fisher L, Fukami N, Gan SI, Ikenberry SO, Jain R, Khan K, Krinsky ML, Maple JT, Shen B, Van Guilder T, Baron TH, Dominitz JA et al. The role of endoscopy in the management of patients with known and suspected colonic obstruction and pseudo-obstruction. *Gastrointest. Endosc.* 2010;71:669–79.
- Blanch AJ, Perel SB, Acworth JP. Paediatric intussusception: Epidemiology and outcome. *Emerg Med Australas.* 2007;19(1):45–50.
- Harvey KP, Adair JD, Isho M, Robinson R et al. Can intravenous lidocaine decrease postsurgical ileus and shorten hospital stay in elective bowel surgery? A pilot study and literature review. *Am J Surg.* 2009;198:231–6.
- Rathore MA, Andrabi SI, Mansha M. Adult intussusception—a surgical dilemma. *J Ayub Med Coll Abbottabad.* 200618(3):3–6.

 CODES

ICD9

- 560.9 Unspecified intestinal obstruction
- 560.39 Other impaction of intestine
- 751.1 Congenital atresia and stenosis of small intestine

CLINICAL PEARLS

- 15–20% of patients with colorectal cancer present with colonic obstruction.
- Consider continuous intravenous lidocaine infusion during bowel surgery to speed rate of returning bowel function.

I

INTESTINAL PARASITES

Douglas W. MacPherson, MD, MSc(CTM)

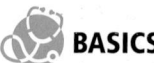

BASICS

DESCRIPTION
- Parasites are divided into 2 groups:
  - Protozoa: Single-cell organisms; typically multiply within the host; intestinal protozoa: Transmission by direct fecal–oral route; do not cause eosinophilia
  - Helminths (worms): Multicellular organisms; rarely multiply within the host (exceptions *Strongyloides stercoralis, Hymenolepis nana*); infection may cause a degree of eosinophilia. Level of eosinophilia is associated with the degree of tissue invasiveness. Worms have a limited life span, and without reinfection, most eventually die on their own.
- Some are invasive, and some do not release their infective forms into the bowel. This latter group (e.g., *Toxoplasma gondii, Echinococcus* sp., *Trichinella spiralis*) is not reviewed here.
- Most worms require incubation outside the host before being infectious or need a vector for transmission. *Enterobius vermicularis (*pinworm) eggs are infectious shortly after being passed; autoinfection occurs readily.
- Person-to-person transmission of worms is uncommon, except for pinworm.
- System(s) affected: GI

Pediatric Considerations
Most common age group affected

Pregnancy Considerations
Many of the treatments are contraindicated.

EPIDEMIOLOGY
Acquisition involves personal, food, and/or water sanitation and migration from higher-prevalence areas.

Incidence
- Predominant sex: Male = Female
- Predominant age: Pediatric

Prevalence
- US laboratory statistics: 5–30% of general population. Random testing finds at least 1 GI parasite in 5–10% of all people.
- From daycare surveys: Asymptomatic 20–30%; symptomatic 50–80%
- Intestinal protozoa account for most parasite findings in North America. Helminths account for <10% of GI parasites.
- *Blastocystis hominis* is a commensal enteric fungus of no clinical significance found in 20–30% of stools.

RISK FACTORS
- Age (children)
- Low socioeconomic status and poor sanitation: Personal, food, water; crowding: Daycare centers, institutional care
- International travel or migration
- Multiple medical conditions, pregnancy, gastric hypoacidity, immunosuppression (AIDS)

GENERAL PREVENTION
- Intestinal parasites are usually acquired by direct fecal–oral contact via ingested contaminated food or water. Rarely, infected arthropod vectors are involved in transmission. Person-to-person transmission may occur through this mechanism.
- Safe food and water precautions ("Wash it, cook it, peel it, or forget it"); enteric and hand hygiene is the means of preventing infections. Infrastructure systems for safe food and water processing contribute to the low prevalence of intestinal parasites.

PATHOPHYSIOLOGY
- The pathophysiology of GI parasitic infections is host-parasite-specific.
- Most intestinal parasitic infections are eventually self-limiting. Most worms have a defined life expectancy in the host. Autoreinfection does occur in some worm infections (e.g., strongyloidiasis, pinworm).

ETIOLOGY
- Protozoan pathogens:
  - *Giardia lamblia: C*ommon
  - *Entamoeba histolytica, Cryptosporidium* sp., *Isospora belli, Balantidium coli, Cyclospora cayetanensis, Microspora*
- Possible protozoan pathogens: *Dientamoeba fragilis*
- Probable nonpathogenic protozoa:
  - Amoebas: All other *Entamoeba* sp., *Endolimax nana*
  - All other intestinal flagellates
- Helminthic pathogens: Nematodes (roundworms): *Enterobius vermicularis, Trichuris trichiura, Ascaris lumbricoides,* hookworm (*Necator americanus, Ancylostoma duodenale*)*, Strongyloides stercoralis, Capillaria philippinensis, Trichostrongylus* sp.
- Helminthic pathogens: Trematodes (flukes): *Fasciolopsis buski, Clonorchis sinensis, Opisthorchis viverrini, Heterophyes, Fasciola hepatica, Paragonimus westermani, Schistosoma mansoni, S. japonicum, S. hematobium, S. mekongi*
- Helminthic pathogens: Cestodes (tapeworms): *Taenia saginata, Taenia solium, Diphyllobothrium latum, Hymenolepis nana, H. diminuta, Dipylidium caninum*

COMMONLY ASSOCIATED CONDITIONS
GI parasitic infections and diseases may be associated with HIV infection or AIDS, steroid use, immune deficiencies, and blood type.

DIAGNOSIS

HISTORY
Historical or physical features alone cannot separate intestinal parasites from other GI infections or the noninfectious enteric diseases except the actual finding of a typical worm (i.e., a tapeworm segment or roundworm: Ascarid, whipworm, or pinworm):
- Acute bacterial or viral GI syndromes tend to be sudden onset and short duration.
- Fever is uncommon with GI parasites unless there is tissue invasion (e.g., amoebiasis, strongyloidiasis).
- Chronic bloating, excessive gas, and intermittent/unpredictable diarrhea without blood is typical of giardiasis.
- Extraintestinal symptoms and signs are uncommon with GI parasites, except invasive strongyloidiasis.

- A water, food, or fecal contamination exposure history (e.g., international travel, migration, high-risk environments [daycare centers, camping]) may suggest a particular parasitic agent.
- A family or personal history of inflammatory or irritable bowel syndromes does not exclude GI parasites.

PHYSICAL EXAM
- Will generally appear well even if distressed with GI complaints; usually afebrile
- Diffuse, migratory rash (cutaneous larva currens) with invasive strongyloidiasis; this is a medical emergency.
- Weight loss and anorexia may be present (e.g., chronic giardiasis, invasive amoebiasis, chronic helminths).
- Anemia may be present with heavy hookworm infections.
- Excessive gas: Bloating, eructation, flatulence, borborygmi
- Nausea or vomiting: Intermittent, recurrent
- Abdominal pain/tenderness
- May have bowel tenderness, but liver and spleen are usually normal
- Diarrhea: Persistent and recurrent, chronic, but dysentery (i.e., frank GI bleeding) is rare, except with *E. histolytica, B. coli.*
- Pruritus ani: *E. vermicularis, T. trichiura, S. stercoralis,* tapeworms. Perirectal or vulvar rash.
- Passing a roundworm or tapeworm or a worm segment

DIAGNOSTIC TESTS & INTERPRETATION
- Stool specimens that are properly collected, preserved, and transported for examination in a qualified and proficient laboratory by a dedicated parasitology technologist team have the highest diagnostic yield for GI parasites.
- Special diagnostics for *Cryptosporidium, I. belli, Cyclospora, Microsporidia,* and *Strongyloides*— give specific laboratory notice.
- Pinworm paddles provide a greater diagnostic yield for *E. vermicularis.* Multiple tests (1) may be needed to exclude pinworms.
- Parasite culture is possible for *G. lamblia, E. histolytica, S. stercoralis* but is rarely indicated; only done in reference laboratories
- Rarely, a biopsy and histology will demonstrate the presence of an invasive helminth on tissue section.
- Tissue biopsies of intestine, liver, or bladder may show granulomatous reactions of schistosome eggs.

Lab
- A single stool specimen collected into a preservative (i.e., sodium acetate formalin [SAF]), well mixed to fix and preserve all elements, yields an accurate diagnosis in 90%. Additional specimens improve diagnostic accuracy (2)[A].
- Newer lab techniques for stool specimens currently provide little diagnostic advantage. Exception: *Giardia* antigen—fluorescent antibody (FA) and enzyme-linked immunosorbent assay (ELISA) tests: A single FA or ELISA may be at least as sensitive as 3 stools for ova and parasites.
- Serology: Useful if parasite is not found in stool samples normally or if low numbers of parasites; available only through refererence centers, that is, *Strongyloides,* amebiasis, schistosomiasis

- Drugs that may alter lab results: Use of antibiotics; oil-based laxatives, and barium in the stool interfere with microscopy.

Initial lab tests
Screening blood eosinophilia is not recommended

Follow-Up & Special Considerations
- A single negative stool examination does not rule out intestinal parasitic infection but when performed under best conditions is highly accurate. Repeat testing may be indicated for primary diagnosis.
- Population-based intestinal parasite screening in North America (e.g., daycare attendees, personal-care providers, food handlers, immigrants) has low diagnostic utility and is not recommended.

Imaging
Diagnostic radiology is rarely needed. Exception: Invasive disease due to amebiasis for colitis, amebomas, and liver abscesses.

Diagnostic Procedures/Surgery
- Invasive diagnostic procedures are rarely needed or indicated.
- Egg granulomata of schistosomiasis may be demonstrated in affected tissues.
- With hemorrhagic colitis due to invasive amebiasis, sigmoidoscopy is diagnostic.
- Upper intestinal endoscopy can yield fluid to be examined for *G. lamblia* trophozoites and *S. stercoralis* larvae.

Pathological Findings
- Most intestinal parasites are not invasive and produce nonspecific or no changes in bowel histology.
- Invasive amebiasis produces a classic endoscopic and histologic picture of ulceration and inflammation in the colon.
- Protozoa or helminths may be seen in bowel biopsy histology.

DIFFERENTIAL DIAGNOSIS
- Other nonparasitic intestinal infections
- Food poisoning
- Malabsorption: Commonly lactose, gluten enteropathy; rarely celiac disease, tropical or nontropical sprue
- Inflammatory and irritable bowel diseases
- Hemorrhoid or rectal fissures

 ## TREATMENT

Specific antiparasitic treatment should be selected on patient needs, parasite biology, and epidemiology.

MEDICATION
- Protozoa (3)[A]:
  – *E. histolytica*: Asymptomatic infection needs individual assessment.
  – *E. histolytica* symptomatic intestinal: Iodoquinol or diloxanide furoate
  – *E. histolytica* invasive disease: Iodoquinol or diloxanide furoate plus metronidazole alone or metronidazole alone or emetine plus chloroquine phosphate
  – *G. lamblia*: Metronidazole or tinidazole or furazolidone or quinacrine. *Note*: Albendazole, available in US only from manufacturer, may have activity against *G. lamblia*.
- *Cryptosporidium*: None proven effective
- *I. belli* protozoa: Trimethoprim–sulfamethoxazole
- *B. coli*: Tetracycline or iodoquinol or metronidazole

- *Cyclospora*: Sulfamethoxazole-trimethoprim
- *Microsporidia*: Albendazole (some species)
- Helminths:
  – Nematodes (except *Strongyloides* and *Trichostrongylus*): Mebendazole or pyrantel pamoate or piperazine citrate or albendazole (available in US only from manufacturer)
  – *Strongyloides* and *Trichostrongylus*: Thiabendazole or albendazole (available in US only from manufacturer)
  – Cestodes: Praziquantel or niclosamide
  – Trematodes: Niclosamide or praziquantel

Pediatric Considerations
Nitazoxanide 7.5 mg/kg p.o. b.i.d. × 3 days or single-dose tinidazole 50 mg/kg (not available in the US) may be used.

ADDITIONAL TREATMENT
General Measures
- Not all patients need to be treated with drugs.
- Symptomatic treatment is indicated for patient comfort once specific therapy has been initiated.
- Drugs inhibiting intestinal motility are relatively contraindicated in patients with diarrhea caused by invasive organisms.

Issues for Referral
Treatment failures, complex patients including drug intolerances or allergies, multiple parasitic infections, and complicated medical (e.g., HIV/AIDS, diabetes, chronic steroid use, etc.) or surgical conditions: Specialist in tropical medicine or infectious diseases

COMPLEMENTARY AND ALTERNATIVE MEDICINE
- Many complementary and alternative therapies exist, but none are effective for primary treatment.
- Consequences of intestinal parasitic infections include lactose intolerance, irritable bowel syndrome, or nutritional deficiencies of calorie–protein deficiencies, dehydration, vitamin B_{12} deficiency.

SURGERY/OTHER PROCEDURES
- Surgical procedures play little role except for amebic liver abscesses, which may need to be drained, especially left lobe abscesses.
- Surgery possible for bowel or organ obstruction, *A. lumbricoides* migration, or for complicated amebic colitis.

IN-PATIENT CONSIDERATIONS
Nosocomial intestinal parasitic infections are rare, as are hospital-based parasitic GI outbreaks. Invasive strongyloidiasis may occur in hospitals for other reasons (e.g., surgery, use of high-dose steroids, etc.).

Admission Criteria
Admission is rarely required except for intestinal obstruction, dysentery, or systemic invasion.

 ## ONGOING CARE

FOLLOW-UP RECOMMENDATIONS
Patient Monitoring
For the majority of intestinal parasitic infections, testing for clearance is not indicated. Repeat stool examination for clearance should be timed taking into account the life cycle of the parasite and the risk of reinfection.

DIET
Many patients experience symptoms of irritable bowel syndrome and/or lactose intolerance during and following bowel infections, especially when infected with *G. lamblia*.

PATIENT EDUCATION
Important to reduce the risk of reinfection or transmission

COMPLICATIONS
Complications are rare and include chronic persistent diarrhea, irritable bowel syndrome, and chronic malabsorption.

REFERENCES

1. Strand EA, Robertson LJ, Hanevik K, et al. Sensitivity of a Giardia antigen test in persistent giardiasis following an extensive outbreak. *Clin Microbiol Infect*. 2008;14:1069–71.
2. Senay H, MacPherson DW. Parasitology: Diagnostic yield of stool examination. *Can Med Assoc J*. 1989;140:1329–31.
3. Abramowicz M, ed. Drugs for parasitic infections. In: *The Medical Letter*. New York: The Medical Letter; September 2007, pg 1–15.

ADDITIONAL READING
- CDC. Parasies and Health. Parasites of the Intestinal Tract. Available from: http://www.dpd.cdc.gov/dpdx/html/para_health.htm
- Escobedo AA, Alvarez G, González ME, et al. The treatment of giardiasis in children: single-dose tinidazole compared with 3 days of nitazoxanide. *Ann Trop Med Parasitol*. 2008;102:199–207.
- Leonardi-Bee J, Pritchard D, Britton J. Asthma and Current Intestinal Parasite Infection: Systematic Review and Meta-Analysis. *Am J Respir Crit Care Med*. 2006.

See Also (Topic, Algorithm, Electronic Media Element)
Algorithm: Bleeding, GI

 ## CODES

ICD9
- 127.4 Enterobiasis
- 128.9 Helminth infection, unspecified
- 129 Intestinal parasitism, unspecified

CLINICAL PEARLS
- Consider GI parasites when dealing with a history of travel, recent immigration, children, or other vulnerable populations, or a story of chronic or persistent diarrhea or seeing worms in the stool.
- Stools correctly collected in the proper preservative will detect most intestinal parasites. Exceptions: *S. stercoralis*, *E. vermicularis*, *Cryptosporidium*, *Cyclospora*, and *Microspora* sp.
- Checking for eosinophilia is not a reliable screening method.

INTUSSUSCEPTION

Timothy L. Black, MD
James P. Miller, MD

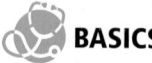 **BASICS**

DESCRIPTION
- Invagination of a portion of intestine into itself; may involve any part of small intestine or ileocolic (95%) or colocolic segment
- System(s) affected: GI

Geriatric Considerations
- Adult intussusception represents 5% of all intussusceptions and fewer than 5% of intestinal obstruction cases in adults (1)[B].
- 90% have pathologic lead point (site of initiation of event) (1)[B].

Pediatric Considerations
- Usually no identified lead point; only present in 2–12%
- Represents the most common abdominal emergency in infancy (2)[C]
- Postoperative intussusception (1–24 days postoperatively) is virtually always in small bowel and only rarely can be reduced hydrostatically.

EPIDEMIOLOGY
- Predominant age:
  - 5–10 months (65% are <1 year of age)
  - Only 10–25% of cases occur at >1 year of age.
- Predominant sex: Male > Female (3:2). Male preponderance is more obvious in older infants.

Incidence
In the US:
- 1.5–4/1,000 live births
- 0.5% after laparotomy

RISK FACTORS
- Henoch-Schönlein purpura
- Leukemia
- Lymphoma
- Cystic fibrosis
- Recent upper respiratory tract infection: 21%

- Recent operation (1–24 days previously)
- Recent viral GI illness
- Meckel diverticulum
- Recent rotavirus vaccine administration (3)[C]
- Small bowel carcinoma
- Polyps
- Stricture

ETIOLOGY
- Children:
  - Marked hypertrophy of Peyer patches: 92–98%
  - Lead point in 2–12%: Polyp, Meckel diverticulum, duplication cyst, ectopic pancreas, lymphoma, Henoch-Schönlein purpura, lipoma, carcinoma
  - Allergic reactions, diet changes, and changes in intestinal activity may be other causes.
  - Possible adenovirus or rotavirus infection
  - 1998 Rotashield vaccine showed that 1/10,000–1/32,000 vaccinees developed intussusception (3)[C].
    - Vaccine was administered 3–14 days before the onset of current symptoms.
    - Infants usually >3 months of age
  - 2006 and 2008 Rotavirus vaccines (RV5 and RV1) show no increase in cases of intussusception over placebo recipients (4)[A]. Since 2006, more than 14 million doses of RV5 have been administered, and the Centers for Disease Control and Prevention (CDC) Immunization Safety Office summary of postlicensure safety monitoring of RV5 does not indicate that immunization with RV5 is associated with intussusception. Monitoring of RV1 is ongoing.
  - Recent operative procedure
- Adults: Virtually always associated with lead point

COMMONLY ASSOCIATED CONDITIONS
- Henoch-Schönlein purpura
- Cystic fibrosis

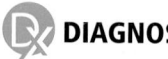 **DIAGNOSIS**

HISTORY
- History of intermittent colicky abdominal pain (almost all children), with episodes lasting 5–10 minutes, frequently with completely asymptomatic period separating the episodes
- Almost all have history of vomiting associated with at least some of the painful episodes.
- History of bloody stool
- Blood per rectum ("currant jelly" stools): 65–95%, highest percentage in infants
- Diarrhea: 7%

PHYSICAL EXAM
- Lethargy (more pronounced with longer duration of illness): 22%
- Palpable mass: 16–41%
- Prolapse of intussusceptum through anus: 3%
- Fever
- Extreme pallor in some
- In postoperative patients, usually presents as small bowel obstruction (5)[C]
- Abdominal distension sometimes marked, depending on the duration of symptoms
- Bowel sounds hyperactive initially; may be absent later

DIAGNOSTIC TESTS & INTERPRETATION
Lab
- Electrolytes
- Complete blood count
- Urinalysis
- Stool guaiac

Imaging
- Ultrasound is diagnostic (2)[C],(6)[B].
- Transient small bowel intussusception is seen frequently in patients with gastroenteritis; these usually resolve spontaneously without additional treatment. (Most of these actually will resolve during the ultrasound observation period.)
- Plain film: Flat and upright abdominal films may suggest the diagnosis.
- CT scan may be helpful occasionally.

Diagnostic Procedures/Surgery
- Contrast enema (barium, water-soluble contrast material, or air)
- Abdominal ultrasound (US)
- Colonoscopy may be useful in evaluation of adult patients presenting with subacute or chronic colonic obstruction (1)[B].

Pathological Findings
- Hyperplasia of Peyer lymphatic patches of terminal ileum (92%), with or without mesenteric lymphadenopathy
- Recognizable lead point, 2–12% (see list in "Etiology")

DIFFERENTIAL DIAGNOSIS
- Adhesive-band small bowel obstruction
- Appendicitis
- Gastroenteritis
- Rectal prolapse (if intussuscepted bowel protrudes from anus)

TREATMENT

ADDITIONAL TREATMENT
General Measures
- IV fluid resuscitation
- Foley catheter (if child is severely dehydrated)
- Nasogastric tube
- Antibiotics useful only if necrotic bowel present
- Nonoperative care (2)[C],(6)[B]:
  - Hydrostatic/pneumatic reduction of intussusception (50–80% success)
  - Barium column should be 40–42 inches high.
  - Enema is continued as long as progress is made. Contrast material may be drained and the enema repeated up to 3×.
  - Pneumatic reduction pressure should not exceed 120–140 mm Hg (16–18.6 kPa).

SURGERY/OTHER PROCEDURES
- Right lower quadrant incision
- Gentle manipulation by pushing intussusception (not pulling)
- If unable to reduce nonviable bowel, segmental resection with reanastomosis
- Enterotomy if lead point suspected
- Incidental appendectomy usually done
- Some centers are using laparoscopy or laparoscopically assisted reduction/resection.
- Postoperative intussusception usually requires laparotomy and operative reduction (5)[C].
- In adults, segmental bowel resection usually is required.
- In adults, ventral rectopexy has low recurrence rates and improves fecal incontinence (7)[A].

IN-PATIENT CONSIDERATIONS
Initial Stabilization
Inpatient until resolved

Admission Criteria
Infants are frequently admitted for overnight observation after nonoperative reduction owing to high incidence of recurrence in 1st 24 h.

Discharge Criteria
Normal bowel function, tolerating regular diet, no abdominal pain

 ONGOING CARE

FOLLOW-UP RECOMMENDATIONS
As tolerated after reduction

Patient Monitoring
Office visit 1–2 weeks after discharge

DIET
Liquids are started after abdominal distension resolves and bowel function returns.

PATIENT EDUCATION
- Instruct family on the possibility of recurrence (5–13%).
- Most recurrences occur in 1st 24 h after reduction.

PROGNOSIS
- Mortality should not exceed 1–2%.
- Possible recurrence after hydrostatic reduction: 5–13%
- Possible recurrence after operative reduction: 3%

COMPLICATIONS
- Bowel perforation during attempted reduction (in 0.16–2.8% of patients with pneumatic reduction)
- Prolonged ileus
- Adhesions with intestinal obstruction
- Incisional hernia
- Ischemic intestine requiring 2nd operation
- Electrolyte abnormality
- Anemia
- Pleural effusion
- Sepsis
- Recurrence

REFERENCES

1. Marinis A, Yiallourou A, Samanides L, Dafnios N, Anastasopoulos G, Vassiliou I, Theodosopoulos T et al. Intussusception of the bowel in adults: a review. *World J. Gastroenterol.* 2009;15:407–11.
2. Sorantin E, Lindbichler F. Management of intussusception. *Eur Radiol.* 2004;14(Suppl 4): L146–54.
3. Bines JE. Rotavirus vaccines and intussusception risk. *Curr Opin Gastroenterol.* 2005;21:20–5.
4. Committee on Infectious Diseases. Prevention of Rotavirus Disease: Updated Guidelines for Use of Rotavirus Vaccine. *Pediatrics.* 2009;123:1412–20.
5. Holcomb GW, Ross AJ, O'Neill JA. Postoperative intussusception: increasing frequency or increasing awareness? *South Med J.* 1991;84:1334–9.
6. Applegate KE. Clinically suspected intussusception in children: evidence-based review and self-assessment module. *AJR Am J Roentgenol.* 2005;185:S175–83.
7. Samaranayake CB, Luo C, Plank AW, et al. Systematic review on ventral rectopexy for rectal prolapse and intussusception. *Colorectal Dis.* 2009.

ADDITIONAL READING

Applegate KE et al. Intussusception in children: evidence-based diagnosis and treatment. *Pediatr Radiol.* 2009;39(Suppl 2):S140–3.

See Also (Topic, Algorithm, Electronic Media Element)
Cystic Fibrosis; Henoch-Schönlein Purpura; Intestinal Obstruction

 CODES

ICD9
560.0 Intussusception

CLINICAL PEARLS
- Some patients may need a KUB if bowel obstruction is suspected, but diagnostic confirmation with ultrasound is the "gold standard." A contrast enema then serves both diagnostic and, hopefully, therapeutic purposes.
- A lead point is present in only 10% of children <1 year of age and is most commonly a Meckel diverticulum.

IRON TOXICITY, ACUTE

David C. Mackenzie, MD

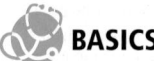 **BASICS**

DESCRIPTION
- Acute iron (Fe) overload from accidental or intentional ingestion
- Unintentional ingestion is not uncommon because Fe-containing compounds are readily available, brightly colored, and are sometimes sugar-coated.
- Acute symptoms are characterized by vomiting, diarrhea, and abdominal pain. More severe clinical findings include cyanosis, altered mental status, acidosis, hematemesis, shock, and coma.
- The most serious exposures involve prenatal vitamins and pure Fe preparations that contain ferrous sulfate. The toxic dose of Fe depends on the amount (mg/kg) of elemental Fe ingested.
- Clinically evident toxicity is more common with ingestions >40 mg/kg, typically as transient gastrointestinal symptoms. Persistent vomiting, diarrhea, or abdominal pain are suggestive of a more significant ingestion.
- Metabolic acidosis is an indicator of Fe-induced toxicity. Death from Fe overdose has been reported from a wide range of exposures (60–300 mg/kg).
- Morbidity and mortality is greater among patients with intentional ingestion.
- Systems affected: Cardiovascular; GI; Hematologic/Lymphatic/Immunologic
- Synonyms: Iron poisoning; Iron overdose

Pediatric Considerations
For a 2-year-old, the average lethal dose of elemental Fe is 3 g. This is fewer than 50 iron sulfate 325-mg tablets.

EPIDEMIOLOGY
Incidence
>4,000 cases/year of elemental Fe overdose reported to Association of Poison Control Centers (AAPCC) (1)

Prevalence
- Fe ingestion is a common cause of morbidity in children, but mortality from Fe exposure is decreasing (2,3).
- In 2008, 4,479 elemental Fe and 19,707 vitamin-containing Fe exposures were reported to the AAPCC; no deaths were reported (1).

RISK FACTORS
- Access to Fe-containing products by children resulting in accidental ingestion
- A pregnant mother or the birth of a sibling within 6 months was identified as a risk factor for children <3 years old, likely due to the presence of prenatal vitamins or Fe supplements.

GENERAL PREVENTION
- Keep prescription and over-the-counter (OTC) Fe products/vitamins out of reach of children.
- Unit-dose packaging of Fe supplements has resulted in a reduction of Fe poisoning in children and should be recommended as the preferred packaging to patients (4)[B].

PATHOPHYSIOLOGY
- Tissue damage from Fe is due to free-radical production and lipid peroxidation, leading to:
  - Direct vasodilation
  - Increased capillary permeability
  - Necrosis of mucosal cells
  - Altered mitochondrial lipid membrane
  - Biochemical effects (i.e., uncoupling of oxidative phosphorylation and Krebs cycle enzymatic process inhibition)
  - Inhibition of serum proteases (e.g., thrombin)
- Resulting in:
  - Local: Fe-induced damage to the GI mucosa
  - Systemic toxicity: Injury to the cardiovascular system and liver

ETIOLOGY
- Excessive Fe ingestion: The average human lethal dose is 200–250 mg elemental Fe/kilogram of body weight. Ferrous sulfate contains approximately 60 mg of elemental iron/325-mg tablet.
- Serious toxicity or even death has been associated with >60 mg/kg of elemental Fe ingestion (approx. 1 tablet/kg).

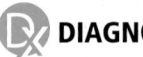 **DIAGNOSIS**

HISTORY
- Determine type and quantity of Fe ingested.
- Note times of ingestion and symptom onset.
- Was the ingestion intentional or accidental?
- Identify those who are severely ill or who have subtle features of a significant ingestion.
- Ask about possible co-ingested substances.
- For children: Other siblings at risk?

PHYSICAL EXAM
Classically, 5 phases occur after toxic ingestions (but do not occur in all patients, and often overlap; for example, in massive overdose, patients may present in shock):
- From 0.5–6 h: GI symptoms predominate, including vomiting, hematemesis, abdominal pain, diarrhea, GI bleeding, lethargy, shock, and metabolic acidosis
- Latent: From 6–24 h: Apparent recovery; observe patient closely for hypoperfusion and acidosis.
- From 6–72 h: Profound cardiovascular toxicity, shock, severe acidosis, cyanosis, and fever; potential recurrence of GI bleeding and vomiting; coagulopathy (preceding liver dysfunction) can occur.
- From 12–96 h: Hepatotoxicity and necrosis may occur, leading to coma, coagulopathy, and jaundice. Symptoms may recur and can include pulmonary edema, shock, acidosis, convulsions, anuria, hyperthermia, and death.
- From 2–8 weeks: Delayed GI scarring and bowel obstruction

DIAGNOSTIC TESTS & INTERPRETATION
Lab
Initial lab tests
- Obtain measurement of serum Fe 6 h after ingestion:
  - Serum Fe >500 μg/dL correlated with moderate-severe toxicity
  - Serial measures may not be helpful.
  - Total iron-binding capacity (TIBC) cannot be used to manage Fe overdose (5); inaccurate in setting of Fe overload; affected by deferoxamine
- Complete blood count (CBC) with differential, chemistry panel, liver function tests (LFTs), prothrombin time (PT), partial thromboplastin time (PTT), type and cross-match. White blood cell (WBC) count of 15,000/mm^3 correlates with Fe levels >300 μg/dL (100% specificity, 50% sensitivity) (5).
- Glucose level: Glucose of 1,150 mg/dL correlates with Fe level >300 μg/dL (same specificity and sensitivity as WBC count) (5).
- Amylase and lipase
- Arterial blood gases (ABGs) to detect anion-gap metabolic acidosis
- Drugs that may alter lab results: Deferoxamine can falsely lower serum Fe unless a reducing agent is added to the specimen; should obtain a free Fe concentration.

Follow-Up & Special Considerations
Tests to monitor for complications:
- Electrolytes, blood urea nitrogen (BUN), and creatinine
- Coagulation tests: PT/PTT/INR
- Serum bicarbonate
- Liver function tests in severe overdose
- Amylase and lipase
- ABG/VBG to detect metabolic acidosis

Imaging
Initial approach
Abdominal radiograph to evaluate for tablets in the GI tract

Diagnostic Procedures/Surgery
Acute Fe poisoning is a clinical diagnosis (5).

Pathological Findings
- Hepatic, renal, and myocardial necrosis
- Irritation and ulceration of stomach and small intestine

DIFFERENTIAL DIAGNOSIS
- Conditions presenting similarly to acute iron toxicity:
  - Gastritis
  - Small bowel obstruction
  - Drug intolerance/overdose
  - Alcohol toxicity
  - Viral illness
  - Diabetic ketoacidosis
  - Metabolic acidosis
- Other poisonings, including aspirin, nonsteroidal anti-inflammatory drugs (NSAIDs), theophylline, organophosphates, carbamates, other metals and metalloids, paraquat, caustic agents, colchicines, nicotine, and mushrooms

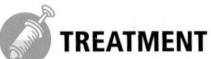 **TREATMENT**

MEDICATION
- Ensure adequate airway, breathing, and circulation.
- Begin fluid replacement for signs of volume depletion or shock: IV access followed by fluid bolus of 20 mL/kg
- GI decontamination:
  - Activated charcoal does not bind Fe; administration probably not helpful unless co-ingestions present (3,5)[C]
  - Gastric lavage and syrup of ipecac not recommended by most toxicologists (3,5)
  - Case reports suggest whole-bowel irrigation may be useful (5)[C]:
    - Polyethylene glycol (Colyte, GoLYTELY) via nasogastric tube at 500 mL/h for children and up to 1.5–2 L/h for adults. End point: Clear rectal effluent; disappearance of radiopacities.
    - Consider endoscopic or surgical removal of Fe-containing bezoar if unresponsive to irrigation.
- IV deferoxamine:
  - Chelates free iron ions. May work best if initiated early, before Fe absorption from GI tract is complete.
  - Indications: Ingestion above levels associated with serious toxicity (>40 mg/kg Fe); clinical signs of severe toxicity (persistent vomiting or diarrhea, altered mental status, evidence of shock); metabolic acidosis; serum Fe level >500 μg/dL (5)[B]
  - Starting dose: 15 mg/kg/h
  - Maximum dose: 35 mg/kg/h
  - Contraindications: Relatively contraindicated in severe renal disease or anuria or primary hemochromatosis
  - Precautions: Discuss administration with poison control. Can cause histamine-mediated hypotension, urticaria, or flushing. Longer infusions (>24 h) associated with ARDS.

Pregnancy Considerations
- Treatment same as that for nonpregnant women (5)
- Transplacental absorption limited
- Phase 3 toxicity associated with spontaneous abortion, preterm delivery, maternal death

ADDITIONAL TREATMENT
General Measures
Consult with a poison control center (1-800-222-1222).

Issues for Referral
Explore psychological issues if an intentional ingestion

Additional Therapies
Hemodialysis, peritoneal dialysis, and exchange transfusion also have been used in lethal overdoses.

SURGERY/OTHER PROCEDURES
Fe pill bezoars can lead to perforation and may need removal by endoscopy or gastrostomy.

IN-PATIENT CONSIDERATIONS
Initial Stabilization
- Emergency room for acute ingestion
- Inpatient for severe ingestion
- Supportive treatment

Admission Criteria
Ingestion with suspicion for intentional self-harm; ingestions of ≥ 60 mg/kg elemental Fe or severe or persistent symptoms requiring deferoxamine; consider admission or 6–12 h ED observation for ingestions > 40 mg/kg

IV Fluids
- Normal saline boluses of 20 mL/kg
- Keep hydrated while on deferoxamine.

Nursing
Supportive nursing care

Discharge Criteria
- Make sure that patient is not in phase 2 (latent) toxicity. Observe for 6–12 h post-ingestion.
- Patients with ingestion of <40 mg/kg elemental Fe and no or mild symptoms may be observed at home (3)[C].
- Resolution of symptoms and education on possible complications after treatment for severe toxicity

 ONGOING CARE

PATIENT EDUCATION
- Undertake prevention counseling on proper storage of Fe products (out of the reach of children).
- Encourage purchase of Fe supplements in unit-dose packaging.
- Educational material from poison control centers may be available to use.

PROGNOSIS
Depends on amount ingested, time to presentation, and timing of therapy

COMPLICATIONS
2–4 weeks after severe ingestion, pyloric or antral stenosis, hepatic cirrhosis, and CNS damage may occur.

REFERENCES

1. Bronstein AC, Spyker DA, Cantilena LR, Green JL, Rumack BH, Giffin SL et al. 2008 Annual Report of the American Association of Poison Control Centers' National Poison Data System (NPDS): 26th Annual Report. *Clin Toxicol (Phila)*. 2009;47: 911–1084.
2. Cheney K, Gumbiner C, Benson B, et al. Survival after a severe iron poisoning treated with intermittent infusions of deferoxamine. *J Toxicol Clin Toxicol*. 1995;33:61–6.
3. Manoguerra A, et al. Iron ingestion: An evidence-based consensus guideline for out-of-hospital management. *Clin Toxicol*. 2005;43:553–70.
4. Tenenbein M. Unit-dose packaging of iron supplements and reduction of iron poisoning in young children. *Arch Pediatr Adolesc Med*. 2005;159:557–60.
5. Madiwale T, Liebelt E. Iron: not a benign therapeutic drug. *Curr Opin Pediatr*. 2006;18: 174–9.

ADDITIONAL READING
- Consensus guideline for out-of-hospital management of Fe ingestion. American Association of Poison Control Centers. *National Guideline Clearinghouse*. 2005;19:8054.
- http://www.AAPCC.org.
- Poison Control Center 1-800-222-1222.

 CODES

ICD9
964.0 Poisoning by iron and its compounds

CLINICAL PEARLS
- Fe overdose has been a leading cause of fatalities from toxic agents in children <6 years of age.
- Serious toxicity or even death has been associated with >60 mg/kg of elemental Fe ingestion (approx. 1 tablet/kg).
- Outpatient GI decontamination with ipecac syrup or other entities is not recommended.
- It is critical to differentiate if a patient is exhibiting mild GI symptoms with resolving toxicity or if the patient is simply in the latent phase and needs continued observation or treatment with deferoxamine.

IRRITABLE BOWEL SYNDROME

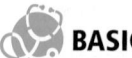

Kelly O'Callahan, MD

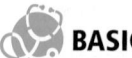 BASICS

DESCRIPTION
- A condition characterized by a chronic abdominal pain associated with alteration in bowel habits in the absence of organic pathology.
- May be characterized as diarrhea-predominant or constipation-predominant; or may alternate between diarrhea and constipation.
- Synonym(s): Spastic colon; Irritable colon

EPIDEMIOLOGY
Irritable bowel syndrome (IBS) accounts for up to 50% of GI visits in some practices and is 2nd to upper respiratory infection as cause for lost workdays.

Prevalence
- Estimated to be ~15% of the population of North America; however, only 15% of these patients actually seek medical attention.
- Predominant age: Teens to late 20s; if >age 50, consider other diagnoses
- Predominant sex: In the US, Female > Male (2:1)

RISK FACTORS
- Other family members with similar GI disorder
- History of childhood sexual abuse
- Sexual or domestic abuse in women
- Depression
- Can occur after an infectious colitis

Pregnancy Considerations
No risk to mother or fetus

Genetics
Unknown, but more common in families of IBS patients

GENERAL PREVENTION
See Diet.

ETIOLOGY
The etiology is unknown, but patients demonstrate intestinal motility abnormalities with enhanced sensitivity to visceral stimuli. The trigger may be luminal or environmental.

COMMONLY ASSOCIATED CONDITIONS
- Migraine
- Urinary frequency and urgency
- Fibromyalgia
- Dyspareunia
- Depression

DIAGNOSIS

- Rome II criteria: ≥12 weeks in last 12 months of abdominal pain or discomfort that has 2 of 3 features:
  - Relieved by defecation
  - Onset associated with change in frequency of stool
  - Onset associated with change in form of stool
- Symptoms can also include:
  - Mucus in stools
  - Constipation
  - Bloating
  - Diarrhea
  - Abdominal distention
  - Upper abdominal discomfort after eating
  - Straining for normal consistency stools
  - Urgency of defecation
  - Feelings of incomplete evacuation
  - Abnormal stool form
  - Nausea, vomiting (rarely)

HISTORY
- As above, but also may have history of abuse or depression
- Patient may note worsening of symptoms with stress or around menses.
- IBS is unlikely in patients with a history of weight loss, bleeding, nocturnal diarrhea, fever, or anemia.

PHYSICAL EXAM
Generally normal, but may have abdominal tenderness to palpation

DIAGNOSTIC TESTS & INTERPRETATION
In the setting of a typical history and in the absence of warning signs such as anemia or weight loss, it is reasonable to obtain baseline labs as discussed below and begin treatment. In those who do not respond to treatment, further evaluation with imaging studies and endoscopy is warranted to exclude organic pathology.

Lab
As needed to rule out other pathology specific to the patient's symptoms:
- Diarrhea-predominant: ESR, CBC, tissue transglutaminase, TSH, and stool for ova and parasites
- Constipation-predominant: CBC, TSH, electrolytes
- Abdominal pain: LFTs and amylase

Follow-Up & Special Considerations
Consider lactulose breath test to assess for abnormal bacterial distribution associated with IBS (1)[A].

Imaging
- Abdominal CT scan or abdominal ultrasound to evaluate pain is generally normal.
- Small-bowel series or video capsule endoscopy to rule out Crohn disease of small intestine may be considered, and will also be normal.
- Sitzmarker study may be used to evaluate colon transit in patients with constipation.

Diagnostic Procedures/Surgery
Sigmoidoscopy/colonoscopy may be used to rule out inflammatory bowel disease or microscopic colitis. Colonoscopy should be performed in all persons >50 years of age for colorectal cancer screening.

Pathological Findings
None

DIFFERENTIAL DIAGNOSIS
- Inflammatory bowel disease
- Lactose intolerance
- Infections (*Giardia lamblia, Entamoeba histolytica, Salmonella, Campylobacter, Yersinia, Clostridium difficile*)
- Celiac sprue
- Microscopic colitis

- Cathartic use
- Magnesium-containing antacids
- Hypo-/hyperthyroidism
- Pancreatic insufficiency
- Depression
- Small bowel bacterial overgrowth
- Somatization
- Villous adenoma
- Endocrine tumors
- Diabetes mellitus
- Radiation damage to colon or small bowel

 TREATMENT

MEDICATION

- For patients with alternating diarrhea and constipation, fiber supplements, such as Metamucil or Citrucel, 1–2 tbsp/d work well (2)[B]. Synthetic agents such as Citrucel are less likely to cause bloating.
- Constipation-predominant:
  – Fiber as above
  – GlycoLax (Miralax) 17 g/d
  – Lubiprostone (Amitiza) 8 mcg b.i.d. (3)[B]
- Diarrhea-predominant:
  – Fiber as above
  – Loperamide (Imodium), 4 mg initial dose, then 2 mg after each unformed stool, or diphenoxylate-atropine (Lomotil) 2.5–5.0 mg (1–2 tablets) after each unformed stool
  – Antispasmodics: Levsin .125 mg q.i.d.; dicyclomine (Bentyl) 10–20 mg b.i.d. or q.i.d.; chlordiazepoxide-clidinium (Librax) 1 or 2 before meals and every night at bedtime; phenobarbital-scopolamine-hyoscyamine-atropine (Donnatal) 1 or 2 tablets before meals and at bedtime (4)[B]
  – Antidepressants: Tricyclic antidepressants such as Elavil 10–50 mg at bedtime are effective in decreasing neuropathic pain and may slow gut transit (5)[B].
  – SSRIs and other antidepressants may be of use if depression is a factor.
  – Cholestyramine (Questran) 1 pkt. every day-b.i.d. can be helpful in patients with IBS, particularly postcholecystectomy.
  – Probiotics have demonstrated modest benefit in patients with IBS, particularly those with bloating and diarrhea; however, the most beneficial strains have yet to be identified. Probiotics are available as oral supplements or additives to yogurt (6)[C].
  – Antiflatulents: Simethicone (Mylicon), 2–4 tablets after meals and at bedtime; Beano
- Lactose intolerance: Lactase (Lactaid) capsules or tablets; 1–2 tablets prior to ingesting dairy products

ADDITIONAL TREATMENT
General Measures
Outpatient evaluation as outlined above with focus on explaining mechanism of disease and reassurance. Biofeedback and stress reduction can help.

Issues for Referral
Possible psychiatric referral for those with depression

Additional Therapies
The evidence for the role of small intestine bacterial overgrowth (SIBO) in IBS and subsequent antibiotic therapy is conflicting; older age and female gender are predictors of SIBO within IBS (7)[C].

 ONGOING CARE

FOLLOW-UP RECOMMENDATIONS
Patient Monitoring
As needed for symptoms

DIET
- Increase fiber slowly to avoid increased intestinal gas production.
- During initial evaluation may wish to try 2 weeks of lactose-free diet to rule out lactose intolerance as etiology of symptoms.
- Avoid large meals, fatty foods, and caffeine, which can often exacerbate symptoms.

PATIENT EDUCATION
Patients should not be given the impression that this is a psychiatric illness.

PROGNOSIS
- No progression to cancer or inflammatory disease
- Expect recurrences, especially when under stress.

REFERENCES

1. Shah ED, Basseri RJ, Chong K, Pimentel M et al. Abnormal Breath Testing in IBS: A Meta-Analysis. *Digestive diseases and sciences*. 2010;
2. Quartero AO, et al. Bulking agents, antispasmodic and antidepressant medication for the treatment of irritable bowel syndrome. *Cochrane Database Sys Rev*. 2005;2:CD0003460.
3. Drossman DA, Chey WD, Johanson JF, et al. Clinical trial: lubiprostone in patients with constipation-associated irritable bowel syndrome - results of two randomized, placebo-controlled studies. *Aliment Pharmacol Ther*. 2008.
4. Poynard T, Regimbeau C, Benhamou Y. Meta-analysis of smooth muscle relaxants in the treatment of irritable bowel syndrome. *Aliment Pharmacol Ther*. 2001;15:355–61.
5. Jackson JL, O'Malley PG, Tomkins G, et al. Treatment of functional gastrointestinal disorders with antidepressant medications: a meta-analysis. *Am J Med*. 2000;108:65–72.
6. Hong KS, Kang HW, Im JP, Ji GE, Kim SG, Jung HC, Song IS, Kim JS et al. Effect of probiotics on symptoms in Korean adults with irritable bowel syndrome. *Gut Liver*. 2009;3:101–7.
7. Reddymasu SC, Sostarich S, McCallum RW et al. Small intestinal bacterial overgrowth in irritable bowel syndrome: are there any predictors? *BMC Gastroenterol*. 2010;10:23.
8. Rahimi R, Nikfar S, Rezaie A, et al. Efficacy of tricyclic antidepressants in irritable bowel syndrome: A meta-analysis. *World J Gastroenterol*. 2009;15:1548–53.

ADDITIONAL READING

- Hun L et al. Bacillus coagulans significantly improved abdominal pain and bloating in patients with IBS. *Postgrad Med*. 2009;121:119–24.
- Moayyedi P, Ford AC, Talley NJ, et al. The efficacy of probiotics in the therapy of irritable bowel syndrome: a systematic review. *Gut*. 2008.

See Also (Topic, Algorithm, Electronic Media Element)
Algorithm: Diarrhea, Chronic

 CODES

ICD9
564.1 Irritable bowel syndrome

CLINICAL PEARLS

- Aim treatment at predominant symptom (8)[A].
- Bulking agents or fiber is generally useful, but must be added slowly to not aggravate symptoms (2)[A].

KAPOSI'S SARCOMA

Rebecca G. Kinney, MD
Johra Nasreen, MD

 BASICS

Kaposi's sarcoma (KS) was originally described in 1872 by a Hungarian dermatologist named Moritz Kaposi.

DESCRIPTION
- Malignant condition characterized by vascular tumors in the skin and other organs, associated with human herpesvirus 8 (HHV-8), also known as Kaposi's sarcoma–associated herpesvirus (KSHV)
- An infrequent tumor of unknown cause, but with a higher impact in immunosuppressed individuals, particularly in HIV and transplant patients
- 4 major forms are seen:
  - AIDS-related (epidemic) KS: KS is an AIDS-defining illness in HIV patients.
  - Iatrogenic/immunosuppressive KS: Most commonly organ transplant–associated
  - African (endemic) KS: Seen in equatorial Africa, especially sub-Saharan
  - Indolent (classic) KS: Rare, typically seen in older men of Mediterranean and Jewish descent
- Systems affected: Hemolytic/Lymphatic/ Immunologic; Skin/Exocrine; GI; Pulmonary
- Synonym(s): Endotheliosarcoma; Multiple idiopathic hemorrhagic sarcoma

EPIDEMIOLOGY
- Predominant age: 16–70 years; African KS predominantly affects young adults and children; classic KS typically in those aged 50–70 years; and AIDS-related KS most commonly in middle-aged adults aged 20–54 years
- Predominant sex: Male to female ratio for epidemic KS in the US is approximately 50:1, while male to female ratio is approximately 10:1 for classic and endemic KS.
- Among those with HIV, most common in homosexual or bisexual men

Incidence
- The US incidence of KS after transplantation is estimated to be <1% (1).
- Incidence of KS among HIV-seropositive individuals has decreased greatly with the advent of highly active antiretroviral therapy (HAART): 15.2/1,000 from 1992–1996 compared with 4.9/1,000 from 1997–1999 (1).
- Approximately 2,500 cases of KS occur annually in the US

Prevalence
- Before HAART became available, KS was >20,000 times more common in AIDS patients than in the general population and 300 times more common in an AIDS host than in other immunosuppressed hosts; with the advent of HAART, this ratio has decreased. AIDS-related KS in the US decreased 10% per year from 1990–1997 (1).
- The seroprevalence of KSHV in the US is 1-5%; in certain parts of Africa, rates are > 70% (2,3).
- KS previously was the most common malignancy in HIV-infected patients; some new studies have demonstrated that non-AIDS-defining malignancies may be more common in HIV-infected patients on HAART (4).
- AIDS-related KS may occur at normal CD4 cell counts, though is more common at CD4 <200 3 cells/m.

- In eastern and southern Africa, KS represents nearly 20% of all pediatric cancers (1); in sub-Saharan Africa, KS is also the most frequent cancer among men and the 3rd most frequent cancer among women (5).
- Fulminant lymphadenopathic disease is a subtype of endemic KS occurring in young children with a mean age of 3 years (1).

RISK FACTORS
- HIV infection
- Living in endemic areas (e.g., Zimbabwe, Uganda)
- Immunosuppression (e.g., immunosuppressant medications, transplantation, chemotherapy)
- High-risk sexual practices
- Maternal–fetal or –child transmission
- Injection drug use
- Exposure to infectious saliva
- Contact with KS skin lesions
- Blood transfusions (may transmit HHV-8)
- HHV-8 viremia (detection of HHV-8 in peripheral blood associated with >10-fold increased risk of developing KS)
- High antibody titers to HHV-8 related to faster development of KS

Genetics
Genetic predisposition is suggested by the occurrence of classic KS in men of Mediterranean or eastern European Ashkenazi descent, although no specific gene has been identified (1).

GENERAL PREVENTION
Safe sex practices, antiviral prophylaxis medication, avoid needle sharing, and careful screening of transplant organs

PATHOPHYSIOLOGY
- KS is a low-grade vascular tumor associated with HHV-8.
- KS develops through incompletely understood mechanisms involving HHV-8-induced viral oncogenesis, cytokine-induced growth, and angiogenesis in a setting of immunocompromise.
- HHV-8 may interfere with host cell apoptosis and other cellular defenses in order to promote persistent viral infection.
- There is ongoing debate about whether KS is a clonal malignancy vs polyclonal inflammatory response that can progress to sarcoma given a certain set of host characteristics (6).
- HIV infection may promote KS progression by inducing cytokines as well as indirectly by impairing host immunity.
- Certain HIV gene products may play a role in promoting tumorigenesis in KS; for instance, the TAT gene may be responsible for conversion of the KS cell into a malignant phenotype (6).

ETIOLOGY
- HHV-8 was identified as the etiologic agent in 1994; HHV-8 is necessary but not sufficient to induce KS.
- HHV-8, immunocompromised status, and cytokine-induced growth represent preconditions for development of KS (6).
- HHV-8 can be transmitted through blood transfusions, solid-organ transplants and possibly through saliva.

- Recent epidemiologic data suggest that sexual transmission is not a major source of HHV-8 infection in the general population (7).

COMMONLY ASSOCIATED CONDITIONS
HIV infection/AIDS; Lymphoma

 DIAGNOSIS

HISTORY
- Elicit prognostic factors: Age at onset of KS and/or AIDS (in AIDS-related KS), immunologic status (CD4 count), occurrence of tumor before/after onset of AIDS, comorbid conditions
- Most commonly first presents with cutaneous involvement
- May have tumor-associated lymphedema, with lower extremity and/or facial swelling
- GI involvement is usually clinically indolent and asymptomatic, but in some cases may present as nausea/vomiting, abdominal pain, dysphagia, or bowel obstruction.
- Pulmonary involvement may be asymptomatic or present with symptoms such as cough, dyspnea, hemoptysis, or chest pain.

PHYSICAL EXAM
- Full physical exam, including dermatologic exam to evaluate for cutaneous involvement
- The skin lesions characterized by:
  - Macular, papular, nodular, or plaquelike appearance
  - Can be discrete or confluent, typically in symmetric distribution
  - Variable color (can be brown, pink, red, or violaceous) and can be difficult to assess in dark-skinned individuals
  - Size varies from millimeters to several centimeters in diameter
  - Nearly all palpable and nonpruritic
  - May be located anywhere on body, but typically found on lower extremities and head/neck region, with mucous membrane involvement common

DIAGNOSTIC TESTS & INTERPRETATION
Lab
- Serostatus can be determined with enzyme-linked immunoassay for antibody to KSHV (ELISA)
- Viral load of KSHV can be measured with quantitative PCR testing.
- CD4 lymphocyte count and HIV viral load determination should be performed in those with HIV infection.

Imaging
- CXR, CT scan, or MRI (chest, abdomen) to assess organ involvement
- Thallium or gallium scans may help to differentiate pulmonary KS from infection.

Diagnostic Procedures/Surgery
- Biopsy of skin or lymph node
- Bronchoscopy with biopsy of suspicious lung lesions
- Endoscopy

Pathological Findings
- Neovascularization with aberrant proliferation of small vessels
- Atypical spindle-shaped cell with leukocytic infiltration
- Angiogenesis

- Extravasated red blood cells
- Hemosiderin-laden macrophages

DIFFERENTIAL DIAGNOSIS
- Bacillary angiomatosis
- Granuloma faciale
- Vascular proliferation
- Purpuric lesions
- Dermatofibrosarcoma protuberans

TREATMENT

Because the history of KS varies from patient to patient, treatment is usually based on the extent of disease, performance status, degree of immunosuppression, and comorbid medical conditions.

MEDICATION
First Line
- Localized therapy for limited, cutaneous disease: Radiation for individualized lesions, intralesional chemotherapy (e.g., with vinblastine), topical alitretinoin gel, cryotherapy, laser therapy, photodynamic therapy, surgical excision (1,2,8)[A]
- Cytotoxic chemotherapy for disseminated disease: Liposomal anthracyclines (e.g., pegylatedlipo-somaldoxorubicin (PLD) (2)[A], daunorubicin); liposomal formulations offer improved outcome with less toxicity (8)[A].

Second Line
- Cytotoxic chemotherapy: Paclitaxel (8)[A]
- Other chemotherapy agents (use limited by side effects): Vinca alkaloids, bleomycin

ADDITIONAL TREATMENT
General Measures
- In AIDS-related KS, optimize control of HIV replication with HAART; HAART increases KSHV-specific immune responses and reduces the risk of progression from KSHV to Kaposi's sarcoma by 90% (5)[A].
- Recommendation is for viral suppression with continuous HAART rather than interrupted CD4 T-cell-guided HAART (4)[A].
- In immunosuppressant medication–related KS, reduce dosage or stop if possible.
- Treatment otherwise is determined by the extent and location of the disease.

Issues for Referral
- Primary care providers should consider referral of patients with AIDS-related KS to an HIV specialist to maximize HAART.
- Refer to oncologist, surgeon, and/or dermatologist as needed by clinical course and provider's comfort with specific therapies.

Additional Therapies
- Experimental therapies: Include recombinant interleukin-12, thalidomide (9)[B], imatinib, temsirolimus, intralesional human chorionic gonadotropin (hCG), vitamin D analogues, and interferon-alfa
- Interferon-alfa is not used frequently due to poor tumor response and high toxicity compared with pegylated liposomal doxorubicin.
- Antiviral therapy against HHV-8: Some studies show treatment benefit with foscarnet and ganciclovir; acyclovir has no activity against HHV-8 and is not recommended (10)[A].

ONGOING CARE

FOLLOW-UP RECOMMENDATIONS
Patient Monitoring
- In HIV patients with KS, other opportunistic infections must be treated aggressively.
- Since non-AIDS-defining malignancies are becoming more common than KS in the HIV population, standard cancer preventative measures should be encouraged (4)[B].

DIET
No particular diet recommended

PATIENT EDUCATION
- HIV risk prevention
- Injection drug rehabilitation
- Promoting adherence to HAART for patients with AIDS-related KS

PROGNOSIS
- AIDS-related KS tends to have aggressive clinical course; however, improved HIV treatments have resulted in enhanced survival for patients with AIDS-related KS.
- Prognostic factors: Immunologic status as measured by CD4 count, age at onset, occurrence of tumor before/after onset of AIDS, comorbid conditions, organ involvement
- Pulmonary involvement is a poor prognostic factor; most common cause of mortality with KS is uncontrolled pulmonary hemorrhage
- Indolent/classic KS: 10-to 15-year survival; rarely metastasizes; most deaths due to unrelated cause
- Endemic KS: Some subtypes can be rapidly fatal.
- AIDS-related KS: With appropriate HAART, course typically chronic; no cure, rarely fatal
- Iatrogenic/transplant KS: Course can be chronic or rapidly progressive, and spontaneous remission after discontinuation of immunosuppressive therapy is typical.

COMPLICATIONS
- Extensive pulmonary involvement may lead to hypoxemia.
- Extensive lymphatic involvement may lead to severe edema.
- Pediatric intussusception can be caused by AIDS-associated Kaposi's sarcoma (11).
- KS may develop as an immune reconstitution inflammatory syndrome (IRIS) among HIV-seropositive individuals at the advent of HAART (12).

REFERENCES

1. Hengge UR, Ruzicka T, Tyring SK, et al. Update on Kaposi's sarcoma and other HHV8 associated diseases. Part 1: epidemiology, environmental predispositions, clinical manifestations, and therapy. Lancet Infect Dis. 2002;2:281–92.
2. Dedicoat M, Vaithilingum M, Newton R. Treatment of Kaposi's sarcoma in HIV-1 infected individuals with emphasis on resource-poor settings. Cochrane Database Sys Rev. 2003;3:CD003256, DOI, 1002/14651858.CD003256.
3. Kaplan JE, Benson C, Holmes KK, et al. Guidelines for the prevention and treatment of opportunistic infections in HIV-infected adults and children. MMWR Recomm Rev. 2009;58:1–198.
4. Silverberg MJ, Neuhaus J, Bower M, et al. Risk of cancers during interrupted antiretroviral therapy in the SMART study. AIDS. 2007;21:1957–63.
5. Sullivan SG, Hirsch HH, Franceschi S, Steffen I, Amari EB, Mueller NJ, Magkouras I, Biggar RJ, Rickenbach M, Clifford GM, the Swiss HIV Cohort Study et al. Kaposi sarcoma herpes virus antibody response and viremia following highly active antiretroviral therapy in the Swiss HIV Cohort study. AIDS. 2010;24(14):2245–52.
6. Hengge UR, Ruzicka T, Tyring SK, et al. Update on Kaposi's sarcoma and other HHV8 associated diseases. Part 2: pathogenesis, Castleman's disease, and pleural effusion lymphoma. Lancet Infect Dis. 2002;2:344–52.
7. de Sanjose S, Mbisa G, Perez-Alvarez S, et al. Geographic Variation in the Prevalence of Kaposi Sarcoma-Associated Herpesvirus and Risk Factors for Transmission. J Infect Dis. 2009;199:1449–56.
8. Di Lorenzo G, Konstantinopoulos PA, Pantanowitz L, et al. Management of AIDS-related Kaposi's sarcoma. Lancet Oncol. 2007;8:167–76.
9. Chen M, Doherty SD, Hsu S, et al. Innovative uses of thalidomide. Dermatol Clin. 2010;28:577–86.
10. Glesby MJ, Hoover DR, Weng S, et al. Use of antiherpes drugs and the risk of Kaposi's sarcoma: data from the Multicenter AIDS Cohort Study. J Infect Dis. 1996;173(6):1477–80.
11. Ramdial PK, Sing Y, Hadley GP, Chotey NA, Mahlakwane MS, Singh B, et al. Paediatric intussusception caused by acquired immunodeficiency syndrome-associated Kaposi sarcoma. Pediatric Surg Int. 2010;26(8):783–7.
12. Feller L, Lemmer J. Insights into pathogenic events of HIV-associated Kaposi sarcoma and immune reconstitution syndrome related Kaposi sarcoma. Infect Agent Cancer. 2008;3:1.

CODES

ICD9
- 176.0 Kaposi's sarcoma, skin
- 176.1 Kaposi's sarcoma, soft tissue
- 176.2 Kaposi's sarcoma, palate

CLINICAL PEARLS
- HHV-8 (also known as KSHV) is the etiologic agent for KS.
- HHV-8, immunocompromise, and cytokine-induced growth represent preconditions for the development of KS.
- Incidence of AIDS-related KS has decreased greatly with the advent of HAART.
- AIDS-related KS can occur at normal CD4 counts.
- Staging for KS is usually based on the system of the AIDS Clinical Trial Group (ACTG), consisting of extent of tumor (T), immune status (I), and severity of systemic illness (S).
- Cytotoxic chemotherapy is the gold standard for treatment of disseminated disease, although new experimental therapies are under development.

K

KAWASAKI SYNDROME

Michael Cooper, MD
Robert A. Smith, DO

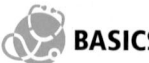 **BASICS**

DESCRIPTION
Kawasaki syndrome is an acute, self-limited, exanthematous febrile, vasculitic disease of young children, notable for its cardiac sequelae.
- Vasculitis affecting the coronary arteries can result in aneurysms or ectasia, further leading to myocardial infarction/ischemia or sudden death.
- System(s) affected: Cardiovascular; GI; Hematologic/Lymphatic/Immunologic; Musculoskeletal; Nervous; Pulmonary; Renal/Urologic; Skin/Exocrine
- Synonym(s): Mucocutaneous lymph node syndrome; infantile polyarteritis

ALERT
Kawasaki syndrome should be considered in any child with extended high fever unresponsive to antibiotics or antipyretics, rash, and nonexudative conjunctivitis.

Pediatric Considerations
Incomplete or atypical cases that exhibit <4 clinical criteria often occur in infants ≤6 months old or older children/adolescents. In this subset of patients, the frequency of coronary artery aneurysms (CAAs) is often higher owing to missed diagnosis.

EPIDEMIOLOGY
Incidence
- Worldwide: Affects all races, but most prevalent in Japan, where incidence is ~112/100,000 in children <5 years of age
- In the US, the annual incidence rate among children <5 years of age is 33/100,000 for Asian Americans, 17/100,000 for non-Hispanic blacks, 11/100,00 for Hispanics, and 9/100,000 for whites
- Leading cause of acquired heart disease in children:
  - Predominant age: 1–5 years (peak age in the US, 18–24 months; Japan, 6–11 months)
  - 76% of the children <5 years of age and 50% <2 years of age
- Predominant sex: Male > Female (1.5–1.7:1 in US, 1.35:1 in Japan)
Prevalence
- Highest to lowest prevalence: Asians > blacks > Hispanics > whites
- Seasonal variation: Increased in winter and early spring and outbreaks at 2- to 3-year intervals

RISK FACTORS
Genetics
- Increased incidence of human leukocyte antigen (HLA) types B54, Bw15, Bw35, and Bw22 in Japanese patients; in US whites, HLA types Bw51, B5, and B44 are increased; in Israelis, HLA type Bw51
- The risk of occurrence in twins is ~13%.
- Siblings of patients in Japan have been found to have a 10-fold relative risk.

GENERAL PREVENTION
- Parents and patients should be educated about the possibility of recurrence (4% in Japan, <1% in US).
- If cardiac problems are present, the need for continued care must be emphasized because Kawasaki syndrome is potentially fatal.

PATHOPHYSIOLOGY
Acute Kawasaki syndrome most severely affects medium-sized arteries. The media of severely affected vessels are inflamed with necrosis of smooth muscle cells. 7–9 days after onset of fever, inflammatory cells secrete various cytokines, interleukins, and matrix metalloproteases that target vascular endothelial cells, resulting in fragmentation of the internal elastic lamina, leading to CAAs. During the period when greatest vascular damage occurs, there is a progressive increase in the serum platelet count. Over weeks to months, active inflammatory cells are replaced by fibroblasts and monocytes involved in tissue repair and remodeling. This process also can lead to progressive fibrosis and vascular stenosis.

ETIOLOGY
Unknown; however, an infectious cause is favored owing to the acute, self-limited nature of Kawasaki syndrome. Community-wide outbreaks and seasonality point to a transmissible childhood disease.

 DIAGNOSIS

Fever and ≥4 of following 5 principal clinical features or <4 features and presence of coronary artery disease on 2D echocardiography:
- Conjunctival injection
- Erythematous mouth and pharynx, tongue, and lips
- A polymorphous, generalized, erythematous rash
- Changes in the skin of the peripheral extremities
- Cervical lymphadenopathy

ALERT
Prolonged fever without rash and treated with antibiotics may cause clinicians to believe that later rash development is due to a drug reaction.

HISTORY
Symptoms may not occur all at once.

PHYSICAL EXAM
- Fever for ≥5 days:
  - Fever is high (103–105°F [39.4–40.5°C]) and unresponsive to antibiotics.
  - May be prolonged (2–3 weeks, with mean duration of 11 days)
- Bilateral nonpurulent conjunctival injection without exudate
- Changes in lips and oral cavity:
  - Reddening of lips in the acute stage, which crack, fissure, and bleed in the subacute phase
  - Strawberry or erythematous tongue
  - Diffuse injection of oral and pharyngeal mucosa without exudate
- Extensive polymorphous rash:
  - May be maculopapular, scarlatiniform, morbilliform, resemble erythema multiforme, or rarely micropustular
  - Perineal desquamation
- Extremity changes:
  - Reddened palms and soles on days 3–5
  - Edema of hands and feet on days 4–7
  - Periungual desquamation of fingers and toes at 2–3 weeks
- Acute, unilateral cervical lymphadenopathy:
  - Lymph nodes >1.5 cm and nontender
  - Generalized lymphadenopathy usually absent

- Cardiac exam: Tachycardia, gallop rhythms, hyperdynamic precordium, innocent flow murmurs
- Skin exam: Rash involving both trunk and extremities; erythema/induration at bacille Calmette-Guérin (BCG) vaccination site, if applicable
- Other organ system involvement:
  - Cardiovascular: Myocarditis; pericarditis (often subclinical), coronary artery and other medium-sized arterial aneurysms
  - GI: Anorexia, abdominal pain, vomiting or diarrhea, acute gallbladder hydrops
  - Renal: Nephritis, urethritis
  - Respiratory: Pneumonitis, atelectasis or pleural effusion, cough
  - Joints: Polyarthritis of small joints in acute phase; weight-bearing joints affected after 10th day from onset of fever
  - Neurologic: Irritability, aseptic meningitis, peripheral neuropathy, transient sensorineural hearing loss

DIAGNOSTIC TESTS & INTERPRETATION
Lab
- Initial workup should include appropriate testing to rule out sepsis: Complete blood count (CBC) with differential, urine analysis and culture, blood culture; lumbar puncture if <4 months of age
- Leukocytosis (12,000–40,000 cells/mm³) with immature forms and neutrophilia
- Anemia (normochromic, normocytic)
- Thrombocytosis (500,000 to >1,000,000 cells/mm³) in 2nd and 3rd weeks
- Elevated CRP, ESR, and α_1-antitrypsin concentrations

ALERT
- ESR can be artificially high after immune globulin IV (IVIG) therapy.

- Hyponatremia
- Mildly elevated AST, ALT, GGT, and bilirubin
- Decreased albumin
- Abnormal plasma lipids: Decreased cholesterol, high-density lipoprotein (HDL), and apo-AI
- CSF pleocytosis may be seen.
- Sterile pyuria (in 33% of patients)

Imaging
- Once Kawasaki syndrome is suspected, all patients need a cardiac evaluation, including ECG and echocardiogram.
  - ECG may show arrhythmias, prolonged PR interval, and ST/T-wave changes.
  - Echocardiogram may show perivascular brightening, ectasia, decreased left ventricular (LV) contractility, pericardial effusion, or aneurysms. Echocardiography has a high sensitivity and specificity for detection of abnormalities of proximal LMCA and RCA (1)C].
- CXR for baseline; may show pleural effusion, atelectasis, and congestive heart failure (CHF)
- MRI and MR angiography for aneurysms in both coronary and peripheral arteries

Diagnostic Procedures/Surgery
- No laboratory study proves diagnosis; the diagnosis rests on clinical features and exclusion of other illnesses in differential diagnosis.

- Patients with complex coronary artery lesions may benefit from coronary angiography after the acute inflammatory process has resolved; generally recommended in 6–12 months (1)[C].

Pathological Findings
- 7–9 days after onset, neutrophilic infiltrates involve the pericardium, myocardium, endocardium, and vascular endothelium.
- Necrosis may develop and result in aneurysmal dilatation of medium-sized arteries.
- Mononuclear infiltration predominates in the 2nd week of illness, gradually resolving with or without fibrosis.
- In addition to cardiac involvement, arteritis may also develop in lungs, kidneys, gastrointestinal tract, and other organs.

DIFFERENTIAL DIAGNOSIS
- Staphylococcal scalded-skin syndrome
- Toxic shock syndrome
- Stevens-Johnson syndrome
- Viral syndromes (i.e., measles, adenovirus)
- Scarlet fever
- Juvenile rheumatoid arthritis
- Reiter syndrome
- Epstein-Barr virus infections
- *Mycoplasma* infection
- Lyme disease
- Rocky Mountain spotted fever
- Toxoplasmosis
- Acrodynia (mercury hypersensitivity)
- Drug reactions
- Other vasculitides

TREATMENT
- Since diagnosis is often not initially clear, consider evaluation for sepsis as part of workup.
- Inpatient care with IV access and cardiac monitoring until stable
- Optimal therapy is 2 g/kg IVIG with high-dose aspirin as soon as possible after diagnosis during the acute febrile phase of illness, followed by low-dose aspirin until follow-up echocardiograms indicate a lack of coronary abnormalities (2).

MEDICATION
- IV immune globulin (IVIG) 2 g/kg IV over 12 hours at the time diagnosis is made lowers the risk of coronary artery aneurysms and may shorten the duration (3)[A]. Retreatment if clinical response is incomplete or fever persists/returns 48 hours after start of IVIG treatment (1)[C].
- Aspirin, 80–100 mg/kg/d in 4 doses beginning with IVIG administration (1)[A]. Switch to low-dose aspirin (3–5 mg/kg/d) when child is afebrile for 48–72 hours or after 2 weeks. Maintain this dose for 6–8 weeks until follow-up echocardio-gram is normal (1)[C]. Continue salicylate regimen in children with coronary abnormalities long term or until documented regression of aneurysm (1)[B].
- Limited evidence from underpowered studies shows no demonstrable reduction of CAAs with aspirin therapy (4).
- Contraindications:
  - IVIG: Documented hypersensitivity, IgA deficiency, anti-IgE/IgG antibodies, severe thrombocytopenia, or coagulation disorders
  - Aspirin: Vitamin K deficiency, bleeding disorders, liver damage, documented hypersensitivity, hypoprothrombinemia

- Precautions:
  - No statistically significant difference noted between different preparations of IVIG (3)[A]
  - High-dose aspirin therapy can result in tinnitus and decrease of renal function.
- Significant possible interactions: Aspirin therapy is associated with Reye syndrome in children who develop viral infections, especially influenza B and varicella. Yearly influenza vaccination thus is recommended for children requiring long-term treatment with aspirin (1)[C].

ADDITIONAL TREATMENT
General Measures
- Children fulfilling the diagnostic criteria for Kawasaki syndrome should be treated with high-dose IVIG (2 g/kg single dose) within 10 days of onset of symptoms because treatment with IVIG has a generalized anti-inflammatory effect (3)[A].
- Antibiotics are given until bacterial etiologies are excluded (e.g., sepsis or meningitis).

Issues for Referral
- Referral to pediatric cardiologist if coronary abnormalities suspected on echo
- Referral to pediatric cardiac surgeon if extensive stenosis/pathology is suspected

SURGERY/OTHER PROCEDURES
- Coronary artery bypass grafting (CABG) for severe obstruction (>75%) of LCA or high-grade obstructions in 2 of 3 coronary arteries or after recurrent myocardial infarction (1)[C]. Younger patients have a higher mortality rate.
- Coronary revascularization via percutaneous coronary intervention for patients with evidence of ischemia on stress testing (1)[C]

IN-PATIENT CONSIDERATIONS
Admission Criteria
All children with suspected Kawasaki syndrome

IV Fluids
- Normal saline (NS) for rehydration in cardiogenic shock
- 1/2 NS for maintenance therapy

Discharge Criteria
Children are usually discharged after 24–48 hours of remaining afebrile after IVIG treatment.

ONGOING CARE
FOLLOW-UP RECOMMENDATIONS
Limited in acute phase; longer with cardiac involvement; with giant or multiple aneurysms, contact and high-risk sports should be avoided.

Patient Monitoring
- Repeat ECG and echo at 6–8 weeks. If abnormal, repeat at 6–12 months (5)[C].
- Children who have little/no cardiac abnormalities on follow-up echo should have a cardiovascular assessment every 3 years (1)[C].

PROGNOSIS
- Usually self-limited
- Moderate-sized aneurysms usually regress in 1–2 years, resolving in 50–66% of cases.
- Sudden death is possible in early adulthood.

COMPLICATIONS
- 15–25% of untreated patients develop coronary artery aneurysms in convalescent phase.
- 2–7% of treated patients develop aneurysms.
- Risk factors for aneurysm:
  - Male, age <1 year old, high ESR >4 weeks
  - Fever >2 weeks in treated patients, fever >48 hours after IVIG treatment
- Mortality of 0.08–0.17% is due to sequelae.

REFERENCES
1. Newburger JW, Takahashi M, Gerber MA, et al. Diagnosis, treatment, and long-term management of Kawasaki disease: a statement for health professionals from the Committee on Rheumatic Fever, Endocarditis, and Kawasaki Disease, Council on Cardiovascular Disease in the Young, American Heart Association. *Pediatrics*. 2004;114:1708–33.
2. Rowley AH, Shulman ST et al. Pathogenesis and management of Kawasaki disease. *Expert Rev Anti Infect Ther*. 2010;8:197–203.
3. Oates-Whitehead RM, Baumer JH, Haines L, Love S, Maconochie IK, Gupta A, Roman K, Dua JS, Flynn I. Intravenous immunoglobulin for the treatment of Kawasaki disease in children. *Cochrane Database of Systematic Reviews*. 2003, Issue 4. Art. No.: CD004000. DOI:10.1002/14651858.CD004000.
4. Baumer JH, Love S, Gupta A, Haines L, Maconochie IK, Dua JS. Salicylate for the treatment of Kawasaki disease in children. *Cochrane Database of Systematic Reviews*. 2009, Issue 1. Art. No.: CD004175. DOI:10.1002/14651858.CD004175.pub2.
5. McMorrow Tuohy AM, Tani LY, Cetta F, et al. How many echocardiograms are necessary for follow-up evaluation of patients with Kawasaki disease? *Am J Cardiol*. 2001;88:328–30.

ADDITIONAL READING
Inoue Y, Okada Y, et al. A multicenter, randomized trial of corticosteroids in primary therapy for Kawasaki disease: Clinical course and coronary artery outcome. *Pediatrics*. 2006;149:336–341e1.

CODES

ICD9
446.1 Acute febrile mucocutaneous lymph node syndrome (MCLS)

CLINICAL PEARLS
- A child treated for Kawasaki syndrome should wait 11 months before receiving live vaccines, specifically varicella or measles, owing to IVIG interaction. If there is a measles outbreak, the child should be vaccinated twice—once at the time of possible exposure and 11 months later.
- If the child is currently on aspirin for coronary aneurysm, ibuprofen should be avoided because it inhibits the antiplatelet effects of aspirin.

K

KELOIDS

Kristyn Fagerberg, MD
Patrick W. Joyner, MD

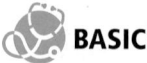

BASICS

DESCRIPTION
- Abnormally large overgrowths of fibrous tissue (scar) occurring as a result of trauma or irritation that do not subside with time
- System(s) affected: Skin/Exocrine

EPIDEMIOLOGY
Incidence
- Predominant age: 10–30 years
- Higher incidence during puberty and pregnancy
- Predominant sex: Female > Male
- However, mean age between the two sexes is almost identical, with females getting first keloid at 22.3 years of age and males developing first keloid at 22.8 years.

Prevalence
- 4–16% of the black and Hispanic populations
- Also a higher incidence in the Asian population
- Data from the UK demonstrated that <1% of Caucasians had keloids.

RISK FACTORS
- Family history of keloids
- Dark skin pigment
- Certain locations on the body (e.g., deltoids, chest, neck, earlobes)
- Pregnancy
- Adolescence

Genetics
- More common in blacks and Asians (5–15×) than in whites; in all races, more darkly pigmented individuals are at higher risk.
- Both autosomal dominant and autosomal recessive familial inheritance have been reported.

GENERAL PREVENTION
- Primary prevention: Avoid elective surgery, body piercing, or tattooing in high-risk patients.
- Wounds should be kept clean to prevent infection.
- When feasible, laparoscopic approaches are preferred in keloid formers.
- Compressive pressure dressings may be useful in high-risk (e.g., burn) patients. Local steroid injection postoperatively in high-risk patients is also effective.

ETIOLOGY
- Wounds: Traumatic, surgical, body piercing (foreign-body reaction)
- Wound infection
- Burn injury
- Other injuries:
  - Insect bite
  - Folliculitis barbae and nuchae
  - Acne
  - Chickenpox
- Vaccination (especially bacille Calmette-Guérin)

- Rarely occur in places on body lacking sebaceous glands; thus sebaceous glands, and the body's reaction to this sebum, are hypothesized to be a etiologic factor in keloid development. Moreover, humans are the only mammals with sebaceous glands and the only mammals affected by keloids.
- Increased ratio of type I to type III collagen
- Increased density and proliferation rate of fibroblasts

DIAGNOSIS

HISTORY
- Pain
- Tenderness
- Hyperesthesia
- Pruritus (occasional)
- May be asymptomatic
- Grow beyond the border of the original wound

PHYSICAL EXAM
- Firm, smooth, elevated scar with sharply demarcated borders
- Initially may be pale or mildly erythematous
- Older lesion hypopigmented or hyperpigmented
- Scar extends beyond margins of the initial wound.
- Over period of years, keloids may continue to grow and may develop clawlike projections.
- Keloids occur more frequently on the chest, shoulders, upper back, back of the neck, and earlobes.

DIAGNOSTIC TESTS & INTERPRETATION
Biopsy only if unable to differentiate from carcinoma or infectious disease because a biopsy may increase the keloid's size. Use a 2-mm punch biopsy to minimize trauma.

Pathological Findings
Histology shows whorl-like arrangements of hyalinized collagen bundles, with pressure thinning of papillary dermis and minimal elastic tissue.

DIFFERENTIAL DIAGNOSIS
- Hypertrophic scar (usually regresses spontaneously, does not cross wound margins, and rarely more than 1 cm in thickness and width)
- Dermatofibroma
- Infiltrating basal cell carcinoma
- Sclerosing metastatic malignancies
- Desmoplastic melanoma
- Sarcoidosis
- Leprosy (nodular LL type)
- Other fibronodular skin diseases (e.g., neurofibromatosis, post-kala-azar dermal leishmaniasis)

TREATMENT

- Given the high recurrence rates and significant expense associated with treatment, prevention of keloids should take priority. Avoidance of known risk factors such as piercings, tattoos, and elective surgery is highly recommended in people with either a family or personal history of keloids.
- A recent meta-analysis of 70 studies has shown that all the currently accepted treatment options have fairly comparable efficacy, with a mean improvement of 60% (1). Also of note is that keloids do not regress spontaneously.
- Treatment options should be based on the type of keloid. Characteristics to take into consideration: (1) presence/absence of scar contractures; (2) size; and (3) number of keloids.
  - Small, single keloids can be treated more aggressively.
  - Large or multiple keloids are typically more complicated to treat and should be evaluated on an individual basis (2).

MEDICATION
First Line
- Triamcinolone (Kenalog) suspension 10 mg/mL (3)[A]:
  - Most commonly used treatment option. Likely more effective if combined with cryotherapy, pulsed dye laser or 5-fluorouricil. No difference when combined with excision versus monotherapy (2).
  - 72% showed symptomatic improvement in 1 trial (3).
  - Use 27- to 30-gauge needle and a TB syringe (total dose 20–30 mg triamcinolone); may inject 3 lesions at a time using 10 mg/lesion.
  - Advance the needle while injecting to distribute medication evenly.
  - Early keloids are more responsive to this therapy than are older lesions.
  - Reinject every 4 weeks until keloid shrinks to near skin surface.
  - If no response to 10 mg/mL triamcinolone suspension, may try 40 mg/mL suspension
  - May mix dilute triamcinolone (5–10 mg/mL) with local anesthetic for excision of keloids; postoperative steroid injections at 2–4 weeks and then monthly for 6 months help to prevent recurrences.
  - Contraindications: Active skin infection at injection site
  - Precautions:
    - Systemic absorption with reversible adrenal suppression, hyperglycemia
    - Local effects: Skin atrophy, ulceration, depigmentation, telangiectasias
    - Both types of side effects are more common with 40 mg/mL triamcinolone suspension.

– Significant possible interactions: Rare interactions (only with very large doses of corticosteroids and systemic absorption)
- Silica gel sheeting: 1st-line prophylaxis after surgical procedure or keloid excision (3)[A],(4)[C]
  – Patient compliance limits effectiveness.
  – Sheets are cut to fit and must be worn for at least 12 hours and, optimally, 24 hours/day.
  – Unclear whether benefit is from silicone or occlusive effect
  – Adverse effects are generally from irritation: pruritus, rash, erosion, and maceration. There is complete resolution within a few days of removal.

Second Line
- Cryotherapy is likely to be more useful in early, smaller lesions. It is not recommended for larger areas owing to pain and decreased skin pigmentation (2).
- Verapamil locally may be helpful as an adjuvant following excision and topical silicone (3)[C].
- Interferon-α2b may be helpful after excision (3)[C].
- Topical imiquimod (Aldara) may be helpful after excision.
- Intralesional 5-fluorouracil (3)[C]: One study showed a 92% reduction in lesion size when combined with triamcinolone and excision (5).
- Intralesional bleomycin (3)[C]
- Radiation therapy has greater success rates when used in combination with surgical excision. There are some concerns about precipitating malignant lesions with radiation; however, a direct correlation has not been made (2).

Pregnancy Considerations
Radiation therapy, 5-fluorouracil, and bleomycin are unsafe in pregnancy.

ADDITIONAL TREATMENT
General Measures
- Appropriate health care: Outpatient
- Intralesional corticosteroid injection causes atrophy, telangiectasia, and pigment changes in half of patients but is the most successful therapy (3)[A].
- Pressure bandages must maintain 24 mm Hg and should be worn for 6–12 months (3)[C]. Bandages should not be removed for >30 min/day.
- Pressure clips (Zimmer splints) are useful for earlobes (6)[C]. Designer splints look like fashion earrings.
- Cryotherapy may be useful for small keloids (e.g., acne scars) (3)[C].
- Use 10- to 30-second freeze–thaw cycles every month; may cause permanent hypopigmentation.
- Topical agents: No evidence to support efficacy of retinoic acid, vitamin E, allantoin, or onion extract (3); some evidence for imiquimod.

Issues for Referral
When intralesional steroids fail, referral to dermatologist or plastic surgeon may be indicated.

Additional Therapies
- Local radiotherapy may be effective after excision but carries a small risk of carcinogenesis (7)[B].
- Physical therapy useful if contractures associated

COMPLEMENTARY AND ALTERNATIVE MEDICINE
None proven (3)

SURGERY/OTHER PROCEDURES
- Surgery: High recurrence rate (45–100%) if used alone; therefore, is used only for the debulking of large keloids or if a lesion is unresponsive to steroid injections or other therapy; combine with preoperative steroid injection and possibly other modalities (3). Debulking just enough for symptomatic improvement is recommended (2).
- Pulsed-dye laser surgery: No definitive evidence of efficacy or advantage over other methods; therefore, use only if other methods fail, and then use in conjunction with them (3)[C]; some promise is seen in combination with triamcinolone and 5-fluorouracil (4)[C].

 ONGOING CARE

FOLLOW-UP RECOMMENDATIONS
Patient Monitoring
Monthly visits for up to 1 year for evaluation and possible steroid reinjections

DIET
No special diet

PATIENT EDUCATION
- Stress the possibility of recurrence despite appropriate treatment.
- May require many months of treatment with combined modalities
- Prevention: In those with risk factors or previous keloids, caution against activities or procedures that may entail dermal disruption, and suggest early treatment of any such events.

PROGNOSIS
When treatment is successful, lesions gradually diminish over 6–18 months with therapy, leaving a flat, shiny scar. While keloids can improve with treatment, cure is unlikely.

COMPLICATIONS
Skin atrophy, ulceration, depigmentation, and telangiectasias can occur as a result of local steroid injections.

REFERENCES
1. Leventhal D, Furr M, Reiter D. Treatment of keloids and hypertrophic scars: a meta-analysis and review of the literature. *Arch Facial Plast Surg.* 2006;8: 362–8.
2. Ogawa R et al. The most current algorithms for the treatment and prevention of hypertrophic scars and keloids. *Plast Reconstr Surg.* 2010;125:557–68.
3. Mustoe TA, Cooter RD, Gold MH, et al. International clinical recommendations on scar management. *Plast Reconstr Surg.* 2002;110: 560–71.
4. Asilian A, Darougheh A, Shariati F. New combination of triamcinolone, 5-Fluorouracil, and pulsed-dye laser for treatment of keloid and hypertrophic scars. *Dermatol Surg.* 2006;32: 907–15.
5. Davison SP, Dayan JH, Clemens MW, Sonni S, Wang A, Crane A. Efficacy of intralesional 5-fluorouracil and triamcinolone in the treatment of keloids. *Aesthet Surg J.* 2009;29(1):40–6.
6. Russell R, Horlock N, Gault D. Zimmer splintage: a simple effective treatment for keloids following ear-piercing. *Br J Plast Surg.* 2001;54:509–10.
7. Ogawa R, Mitsuhashi K, Hyakusoku H, et al. Postoperative electron-beam irradiation therapy for keloids and hypertrophic scars: retrospective study of 147 cases followed for more than 18 months. *Plast Reconstr Surg.* 2003;111:547–53; discussion 554–5.

ADDITIONAL READING
Seifert O, Mrowietz U. Keloid scarring: bench and bedside. *Arch Dermatol Res.* 2009.

See Also (Topic, Algorithm, Electronic Media Element)
Bites; Burns; Warts; Leprosy

 CODES

ICD9
701.4 Keloid scar

CLINICAL PEARLS
- The most successful treatment of hypertrophic scar or keloid is achieved while the scar is still immature, but the overlying epithelium is intact, although this is not as yet confirmed in the literature.
- Keloids extend beyond the margins of the original wound and do not regress with time; this is a way of differentiating from hypertrophic scars. Treatment is similar, but keloids are much more likely to recur.
- Closing wounds with a minimum of suture tension, avoiding midsternal incisions and crossing joint lines, and injecting steroids into the incision postoperatively reduce the chance of keloids forming following unavoidable surgery.

K

KERATOSIS, ACTINIC

Zoltan Trizna, MD, PhD

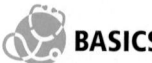 **BASICS**

DESCRIPTION
- Synonym: Solar keratosis
- Common, usually multiple, premalignant skin lesions of sun-exposed areas of the skin
- Common consequence of excessive cumulative ultraviolet (UV) light exposure

Geriatric Considerations
Frequent problem

Pediatric Considerations
Rare (if child, look for freckling and other stigmata of xeroderma pigmentosum)

EPIDEMIOLOGY
Incidence
- Incidence: Between 12.6% and 43.4% per year
- Rates vary with age group and exposure to sun.
- Predominant age: ≥40 years; progressively increases with age
- Predominant sex: Male > Female
- Common in those with blonde and red hair; rare in darker skin types

Prevalence
- Age-adjusted prevalence rate for actinic keratoses (AKs) in US Caucasians is 6.5%.
- For 65–74-year-old males with high sun exposure: It is 55.4%, and for those with low sun exposure, it is 18.5%.

RISK FACTORS
- Exposure to UV light (especially long-term and/or repeated exposure due to outdoor occupation or recreational activities, indoor or outdoor tanning)
- Skin type: Burns easily, does not tan
- Immunosuppression, especially organ transplantation

Genetics
The *p53* chromosomal mutation has been shown consistently in both AKs and squamous cell carcinomas (SCCs). Many new genes have been shown recently to have similar expression profiles in AKs and SCCs.

GENERAL PREVENTION
Sun-protective techniques

PATHOPHYSIOLOGY
The epidermal lesions are characterized by atypical keratinocytes at the basal layer with occasional extension upwards. Mitoses are present. The histopathological features resemble those of SCC in situ or SCC, and the distinction depends on the extent of epidermal involvement.

ETIOLOGY
Cumulative UV exposure

COMMONLY ASSOCIATED CONDITIONS
- SCC
- Other features of chronic solar damage: Lentigines, elastosis, and telangiectasias

 DIAGNOSIS

HISTORY
- The lesions are frequently asymptomatic; symptoms may include pruritus, burning, and mild hyperesthesia.
- Lesions may enlarge, thicken, or become more scaly. They also may regress or remain unchanged.
- Most lesions occur on the sun-exposed areas (head and neck, hands, forearms).

PHYSICAL EXAM
- Usually small (<1 cm), often multiple red, pink, or brown macules, papules, or plaques that are rough to palpation
- Yellow or brown adherent scale is often present on top of the lesion.
- Several clinical variants exist:
  - Atrophic: Dry, scaly macules with indistinct borders and an erythematous base
  - Hypertrophic: Overlying hyperkeratosis (in an extreme form: cutaneous horn) may be impossible to differentiate from SCC clinically.
  - Pigmented: Smooth tan/brown plaque, spreading centrifugally
  - Bowenoid: Red scaly plaques with distinct borders
  - Actinic cheilitis: Inflammatory lesion involving usually the lower lip

DIAGNOSTIC TESTS & INTERPRETATION
Diagnostic Procedures/Surgery
- The diagnosis is usually made clinically, except where there is a suspicion of carcinoma.
- Skin biopsy is especially recommended if large, ulcerated, indurated, or bleeding; or if the lesions are nonresponsive to treatment.

Pathological Findings
- Dysplastic keratinocytes in lower levels of epidermis with a dermal lymphocytic infiltrate
- Neoplastic cells, mostly found in the lower epidermal layers, are cytologically identical to those of SCCs (1).
- If neoplastic cells extend throughout entire epidermis or into the dermis, the lesions will qualify as an SCC in situ or invasive SCC, respectively (2).
- Malignant cells are sparse except in the bowenoid variety.
- Hypertrophic, atrophic, bowenoid, acantholytic, and pigmented varieties show the corresponding epidermal findings.

DIFFERENTIAL DIAGNOSIS
- SCC (hypertrophic type)
- Keratoacanthoma
- Bowen's disease
- Basal cell carcinoma
- Verruca vulgaris
- Less likely: Verrucous nevi, warty dyskeratoma, lichenoid keratoses, seborrheic keratoses, porokeratoses, seborrheic dermatitis or psoriasis (near hairline), lentigo maligna, solar lentigo, discoid lupus erythematosus

TREATMENT

First-line treatment is cryotherapy (technically this is considered surgery, especially by insurance companies) (2,3)[A].

MEDICATION
First Line
- Topical treatments target both visible and subclinical lesions.
- Topical fluorouracil (Efudex, Carac, Fluoroplex cream, Fluoroplex solution):
  – every day-b.i.d. for 3–6 weeks, depending on the brand, concentration, and formulation
  – Can be very irritating
- Topical imiquimod (Aldara) 5% cream:
  – Apply every day, 2 days per week, for up to 4 months to an area not larger than the forehead or 1 cheek.
  – Can be irritating
- 3% diclofenac (Solaraze) gel:
  – b.i.d. for up to 3 months

Second Line
- Topical tretinoin (Retin-A) or tazarotene (Tazorac): May be used to enhance the efficacy of topical fluorouracil
- Systemic retinoids: Used infrequently

ADDITIONAL TREATMENT
General Measures
- Sun-protective techniques
- Sunscreens and physical sun protection recommended

Additional Therapies
Close monitoring with no treatment is an appropriate option for mild lesions.

SURGERY/OTHER PROCEDURES
- Cryosurgery ("freezing," liquid nitrogen):
  – Most common method
  – Cure rate: 75–98.8%
  – May leave scars
  – May be superior to photodynamic therapy for thicker lesions
- Photodynamic therapy with a photosensitizer (e.g., aminolevulinic acid) and "blue light":
  – May clear >90% of AKs
  – Less scarring than cryotherapy
  – May be superior to cryotherapy, especially in the case of more extensive skin involvement

- Curettage and electrocautery (ED&C, "scraping and burning")
- Medium-depth peels, especially for the treatment of extensive areas
- CO_2 laser therapy
- Dermabrasion
- Surgical excision (excisional biopsy)

 ONGOING CARE

FOLLOW-UP RECOMMENDATIONS
Patient Monitoring
Depends on associated malignancy and frequency with which new AKs appear

PATIENT EDUCATION
- Teach sun-protective techniques:
  – Limit outdoor activities between 10 a.m. and 4 p.m.
  – Wear protective clothing and wide-brimmed hat.
  – Proper use (including reapplication) of sunscreens with SPF >30, preferably a preparation with broad-spectrum (UV-A and UV-B) protection
- Teach self-examination of skin (melanoma, squamous cell, basal cell).
- Patient education materials:
  – http://dermnetnz.org/lesions/solar-keratoses.html
  – http://www.skincarephysicians.com/actinickeratosesnet/index.html
  – http://www.skincancer.org/Actinic-Keratosis-and-Other-Precancers.htm

PROGNOSIS
Very good. A significant proportion of the lesions may resolve spontaneously (4).

COMPLICATIONS
- AKs are premalignant lesions that may progress to SCCs. The rate of malignant transformation is unclear; the reported percentages vary (4).
- Patients with AKs are at increased risk for other cutaneous malignancies.

REFERENCES
1. Rossi R, Mori M, Lotti T. Actinic keratosis. *Int J Dermatol*. 2007;46:895–904.
2. Helfand M, Gorman AK, Mahon S, Chan BKS, Neil Swanson N. AHRQ evidence report from OHSU Evidence-Based Practice Center 2001.
3. de Berker D, McGregor JM, Hughes BR, British Association of Dermatologists Therapy Guidelines and Audit Subcommittee et al. Guidelines for the management of actinic keratoses. *Br J Dermatol*. 2007;156:222–30.
4. Criscione VD, Weinstock MA, Naylor MF, Luque C, Eide MJ, Bingham SF, Department of Veteran Affairs Topical Tretinoin Chemoprevention Trial Group et al. Actinic keratoses: Natural history and risk of malignant transformation in the Veterans Affairs Topical Tretinoin Chemoprevention Trial. *Cancer*. 2009;115:2523–30.

ADDITIONAL READING
Kanellou P, Zaravinos A, Zioga M, et al. Genomic instability, mutations and expression analysis of the tumour suppressor genes p14(ARF), p15(INK4b), p16(INK4a) and p53 in actinic keratosis. *Cacner Lett*. 2008;264:145–61.

 CODES

ICD9
702.0 Actinic keratosis

CLINICAL PEARLS
- AKs are premalignant lesions.
- Often more easily felt than seen
- Therapy-resistant lesions should be biopsied, especially on the face.

K

KLINEFELTER SYNDROME

Kimberly Bombaci, MD
Robert A. Baldor, MD

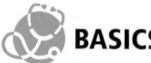 BASICS

DESCRIPTION
- Klinefelter syndrome is a common genetic abnormality that presents in males who have ≥1 additional X chromosomes in many or all body cells.
- Presentation is highly variable; many patients do not have the "textbook" features.
- It is a common cause of primary hypogonadism in males.
- It is usually undiagnosed before puberty and many present in adulthood with infertility.

EPIDEMIOLOGY
Incidence
- Affects approximately 1.72 per 1,000 males
- Significantly underdiagnosed:
  – Only 25% diagnosed in their lifetime
  – Only 4–10% diagnosed before puberty
- Accounts for 3% of male infertility

RISK FACTORS
Risk increases with maternal age.

Genetics
- Mutations are spontaneous and patients have no family history.
- It is usually a result of maternal meiotic nondisjunction.

PATHOPHYSIOLOGY
- Primary hypogonadism with variable Leydig cell function
- Low or low-normal testosterone
- High or high-normal gonadotropins (LH and FSH)
- Unclear whether many aspects of syndrome are caused by hormonal abnormalities or extra X chromosome

ETIOLOGY
- ~90% have the XXY karyotype, which is caused by meiotic nondisjunction of the X chromosome during gametogenesis.
- ~10% have a mosaic karyotype, caused by nondisjunction of the X chromosome during early mitosis of the zygote.

Pregnancy Considerations
- Prenatal diagnosis is possible by karyotyping cells obtained from amniocentesis.
- Parents should be counseled about the highly variable phenotypic range of Klinefelter syndrome and the risks associated with amniocentesis.

COMMONLY ASSOCIATED CONDITIONS
- Azoospermia and infertility (>99%)
- Gynecomastia (common)
- Developmental abnormalities (common):
  – Learning difficulties, especially with language development
  – Gross motor delay
  – Autism spectrum behavior
- Psychiatric illness (common)
  – ADHD
  – problems with regulation of emotion and behavior
  – psychotic disorder

- Cardiovascular disorders (common):
  – Thromboembolic disease
  – Recurrent leg ulcers owing to venous insufficiency and postthrombotic syndrome
  – Mitral and aortic valve disease
- Metabolic disorders (common):
  – Osteoporosis
  – Metabolic syndrome and diabetes
- Essential tremor (common)
- Taurodontism (enlargement of the pulp and thinning of the surface of the teeth) (common)
- Autoimmune disease (uncommon)
- Malignancies (rare):
  – Breast cancer
  – Mediastinal germ cell tumors

 DIAGNOSIS

HISTORY
- Fertility history (infertility nearly universal)
- Learning disabilities, poor school performance
- Psychosocial problems and psychiatric illness
- Cardiovascular disease and risk factors
- Reproductive goals

PHYSICAL EXAM
- Small, firm testes (3–8 mL) (95%)
- Sparse facial and body hair (88%), female pubic hair distribution (53%)
- Gynecomastia (27%)
- Tall, long legs, narrow shoulders, broad arm span, and abdominal adiposity
- Poor muscle tone (76%) and increased fat:muscle ratio
- Specific mild dysmorphic features (1)
  – Clinodactyly (74%)
  – Hypertelorism (69%)
  – Mild elbow dysplasia (36%)
  – High arched palate (37%)

Pediatric Considerations
- Infants:
  – No pathognomonic features
  – Increased incidence of congenital abnormalities of all types, undescended testes, and micropenis
- Children:
  – Tall
  – Increased BMI (on average) (1) and increased fat:muscle ratio
  – Poor muscle tone
  – Small penis and testicles
  – Specific mild dysmorphic features (see above)

DIAGNOSTIC TESTS & INTERPRETATION
Lab
Initial lab tests
- Chromosomal analysis:
  – Gold standard: Cytogenetic analysis (karyotype)
  – Alternative: Barr body analysis (if diagnosis suspected, PPV = 0.86, NPV = 0.94) (2)
  – Rapid polymerase chain reaction technique looking at the copy number of the androgen receptor (AR) gene, (located to Xq11.2–q12) has been described as a screen for Klinefelter syndrome and other X-chromosome aneuploidies (3).

- Hormonal testing (neither sensitive nor specific; become more pronounced at puberty):
  – Blood testosterone levels are low.
  – Blood FSH & LH levels are elevated.
  – Urinary gonadotropin levels are increased.

Follow-Up & Special Considerations
- Semen analysis (if indicated): Azoospermia
- Consider diabetes evaluation.
- Consider hypercoagulability screening.

Imaging
Follow-Up & Special Considerations
- Consider bone density screening.
- Consider echocardiogram to evaluate for valve disease.
- Consider dental radiographs for diagnosis of taurodontism.

Pathological Findings
- XXY karyotype (or variation)
- Testicular biopsy in an adult demonstrates hyalinization of the seminiferous tubules and hyperplasia of Leydig cells.

DIFFERENTIAL DIAGNOSIS
- Secondary hypogonadism (low FSH and LH)
- Acquired primary hypogonadism (exposure to toxins, specific medications, radiation, mumps, or chronic disease)
- XYY karyotype (normal testicles and hormone levels, usually fertile)
- 46,XY/XO karyotype (features of Turner syndrome)
- Congenital anorchia (severe hypogonadism)
- Myotonic dystrophy (muscle weakness and pain, family history)
- Idiopathic hypogonadism

 TREATMENT

MEDICATION
First Line
Testosterone therapy:
- Benefits:
  – Increases body hair and penis length and improves libido
  – Improves bone density (4)[C]
  – May reduce gynecomastia and abdominal adiposity and increase muscle mass (4)[C] (not replicated in all studies)
  – May improve mood, energy level, cognition, and social functioning and decrease aggression (4)[B]
  – May lower serum total cholesterol (4) and improve metabolic syndrome (5)[C]
  – May possibly reduce hypercoagulability (6), improve autoimmune disease (7)[C]
- Risks and side effects:
  – Erythrocytosis
  – Acne
  – Lowering of HDL
  – Worsening of aggression
  – Peliosis hepatitis, hepatic adenomas, and hepatocellular carcinoma
  – Worsening of subclinical prostate cancer
  – May accelerate infertility in adolescents and young men; cryopreservation of existing sperm should be considered before starting therapy.

- Contraindications:
  - Prostate cancer
  - Liver disease
- Dosage and administration:
  - Oral: Initial: 60–80 mg b.i.d.; maintenance: 20–60 mg b.i.d. (not available in US)
  - Buccal: 30 mg b.i.d.
  - Transdermal patch: 2.5–7.5 mg daily
  - Transdermal gel: 5 g daily
  - Intramuscular injection: 50–400 mg every 2–4 weeks
  - Subcutaneous pellets: 150–450 mg every 3–6 months
  - Titrate to symptoms and to maintain testosterone levels in middle of normal range. Normalization of gonadotropins may not be possible.
- Monitoring:
  - Monthly during initial therapy, less frequently when dosage stabilized: CBC, liver enzymes, testosterone, FSH, LH, PSA (if appropriate)
  - Serial prostate exams in older men
  - Consider annual or semiannual lipid panel.
  - Aggression and irritability levels

Pediatric Considerations
- Testosterone therapy, beginning at age 11–13, recommended by experts (8)[C]; consider semen cryopreservation before starting therapy.
- In addition to parameters listed above, monitor bone age.
- Micropenis in infants and children has been treated with topical or IM testosterone (8)[C].
- Consider pediatric endocrinology consultation.

ADDITIONAL TREATMENT
General Measures
- Preventive dental care
- Calcium and vitamin D supplementation
- Breast self-exams

Issues for Referral
- Adolescents and young men wishing to preserve fertility should be referred for cryopreservation of existing sperm if sperm are present on semen analysis.
- Fertility treatment may be offered using testicular fine-needle aspiration (TEFNA) or testicular sperm extraction (TESE) followed by in vitro fertilization. Embryos are at a modestly increased risk of cytogenetic abnormalities, but most of the resulting pregnancies are healthy.

Additional Therapies
Individual or family counseling, if indicated

Pediatric Considerations
- Infertility progresses rapidly during adolescence and early adulthood; therefore, adolescents should be referred for cryopreservation of sperm.
- Consider referrals for speech therapy, occupational therapy, physical therapy, and educational support.

SURGERY/OTHER PROCEDURES
Mastectomy can be performed to correct gynecomastia, which can be a cause of psychological strain and increase the risk of breast cancer.

 ONGOING CARE

FOLLOW-UP RECOMMENDATIONS
- If patient is treated with testosterone, consider semiannual visits when the dosage is stabilized: Review interval history, symptoms, side effects, and therapy risks–benefits.
- If testosterone therapy is declined, annual review of interval history, physical exam, and therapy options

Patient Monitoring
- Annual diabetes screening
- Annual clinical breast exam
- Periodic bone density testing

PATIENT EDUCATION
- Presentation is variable, with most patients appearing physically normal.
- Patients are likely infertile, but there are options for reproductive therapy.
- There is high incidence of learning disabilities and psychiatric illness. Appropriate therapy should be utilized.
- Risk of diabetes and importance of:
  - Regular screening
  - Healthy diet, exercise, and maintaining a healthy weight
- Risk of osteoporosis and importance of:
  - Calcium, vitamin D, and weight-bearing exercise
  - Periodic bone density testing
- Regular dental care
- Testosterone therapy risks–benefits
- American Association for Klinefelter Syndrome Information and Support, http://www.aaksis.org
- Klinefelter Syndrome Support Group, http://klinefeltersyndrome.org

PROGNOSIS
- Infertility is nearly universal.
- Physical findings are generally subtle.
- Behavioral characteristics are highly variable.
- On average, adults have modestly reduced intelligence, verbal reasoning, language skills, and motor dexterity.
- Increased number of X chromosomes is correlated with increased phenotypic severity.

Pediatric Considerations
- Developmental and behavioral problems are common:
  - 77% of children have difficulty learning to read.
  - 42% of children have delayed speech.
  - Motor delay
  - Difficulty with social interaction (autism-like behavior)
  - Sensory avoidance, gaze avoidance, and a passive demeanor
- Children are at risk of poor school performance and school failure.
- Children are more likely to require psychiatric care.

REFERENCES
1. Zeger MP, Zinn AR, Lahlou N, et al. Effect of ascertainment and genetic features on the phenotype of Klinefelter syndrome. *J Pediatr.* 2008;152:716–22.
2. Kamischke A, Baumgardt A, Horst J, et al. Clinical and diagnostic features of patients with suspected Klinefelter syndrome. *J Androl.* 2003;24:41–8.
3. Ottesen AM, Garn ID, Aksglaede L, Juul A, Rajpert-De Meyts E et al. A simple screening method for detection of Klinefelter syndrome and other X-chromosome aneuploidies based on copy number of the androgen receptor gene. *Mol Hum Reprod.* 2007;13:745–50.
4. Wang C, et al. Long-term testosterone gel (AndroGel) treatment maintains beneficial effects on sexual function and mood, lean and fat mass, and bone mineral density in hypogonadal men. *J Clin Endo Metab.* 2004;85(9):2085–98.
5. Spark RF. Testosterone, diabetes mellitus, and the metabolic syndrome. *Curr Urol Rep.* 2007;8:467–71.
6. Zitzmann M, Junker R, Kamischke A, et al. Contraceptive steroids influence the hemostatic activation state in healthy men. *J Androl.* 2002;23:503–11.
7. Koçar IH, Yesilova Z, Ozata M, Turan M, Sengül A, Ozdemir I et al. The effect of testosterone replacement treatment on immunological features of patients with Klinefelter's syndrome. *Clin Exp Immunol.* 2000;121:448–52.
8. Bojesen A, et al. Klinefelter syndrome in clinical practice. *Nat Clin Prac.* 2007;4(4):192–201.

ADDITIONAL READING
- Bruining H, Swaab H, Kas M, van Engeland H et al. Psychiatric characteristics in a self-selected sample of boys with Klinefelter syndrome. *Pediatrics.* 2009;123:e865–70.
- Wattendorf DJ, Muenke M. Klinefelter syndrome. *Am Fam Physician.* 2005;72:2259–62.

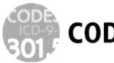 **CODES**

ICD9
758.7 Klinefelter's syndrome

CLINICAL PEARLS
- Klinefelter syndrome males have ≥1 additional X chromosomes in many or all body cells (XXY karyotype).
- Most men do not have the "textbook" features.
- Accounts for 3% of male infertility
- Frequently undiagnosed until adulthood
- Testosterone therapy, beginning in adolescence, has many benefits.

K

KNEE PAIN

J. Herbert Stevenson, MD

 BASICS

DESCRIPTION

Knee pain is a common complaint in the outpatient setting. Onset may be acute or chronic, or it may present as an acute exacerbation of a chronic condition. Trauma, overuse, and degenerative conditions are frequent causes. Acuity of onset, patient age, pain location, associated symptoms, and mechanism of injury can help to narrow the extensive differential diagnosis.

EPIDEMIOLOGY

Incidence
- Knee pain accounts for 1.9 million primary care visits annually (1).
- 42% of runners experience a knee injury each year (2).

Prevalence
- The knee is the most common site of lower extremity injury among runners (3).
- Patellofemoral pain syndrome is the most common diagnosis in runners (2).
- Osteoarthritis (OA) accounts for 34% of adult acute-onset knee pain in the primary care setting (1): One of the leading causes of disability in the US.

RISK FACTORS
- Obesity
- Rapid increases in training volume and intensity
- Extremity malalignment
- Poor flexibility, muscle imbalance/weakness
- Previous injuries
- Activities involving cutting, jumping, deceleration

GENERAL PREVENTION
- Maintain normal body mass index (BMI): Weight loss if obese.
- Use sound exercise training principles.
- Correct strength and flexibility imbalances.

ETIOLOGY
- Trauma (ligament injury, meniscal injury, fracture)
- Overuse (tendinopathy, apophysitis)
- Rheumatologic conditions; arthritis
- Infectious (bacterial, postviral)

COMMONLY ASSOCIATED CONDITIONS
- Avulsion, stress, or other fractures
- Patellar dislocation/subluxation
- Meniscal injury
- Ligamentous injury
- Tendinopathy
- Septic joint
- Hemarthrosis
- Osteochondral injury

DIAGNOSIS

HISTORY

May recall mechanism: Deceleration, hyperextension, and cutting are common mechanisms for anterior cruciate ligament (ACL) tear.
- Popping, giving way, and rapid marked effusion are common in ACL injury and patellar subluxation.
- Hyperflexion, fall on flexed knee, and "dashboard injury" are seen in posterior cruciate ligament (PCL) injury.
- Hemarthrosis is common in patellar subluxation, ACL injury.
- Twisting on planted foot is a common mechanism for meniscal injury.
- Stiffness/pain with prolonged sitting
- Pain ascending/descending stairs often implies meniscal injury.
- Lateral/inferior knee pain often is seen in iliotibial band syndrome.
- Medial/inferior knee pain is seen in anserine bursitis.

PHYSICAL EXAM
- Swelling and/or effusion
- Decreased range of motion (ROM)
- Joint instability
- Locking or catching
- Observe for antalgic gait, dynamic patellar tracking abnormalities.
- Inspect for malalignment, muscle atrophy.
- Palpate for effusion, swelling, erythema, warmth, and tenderness.
- Evaluate for strength imbalances.
- Evaluate ROM and flexibility.

DIAGNOSTIC TESTS & INTERPRETATION
- Lachman test assesses ACL integrity.
- Posterior drawer assesses PCL integrity.
- Posterior sag sign reflects PCL integrity.
- Apprehension test assesses patellar dislocation.
- Patellar grind test assesses patellar dysfunction.
- Valgus/varus stress test assesses medial/lateral collateral ligament (MCL/LCL) integrity.
- McMurray test assesses meniscal tears.
- Ober test assesses iliotibial band (ITB) tightness.

Lab
- Septic joint, gout, pseudogout:
  – Arthrocentesis with synovial fluid analysis, cell count, Gram stain, culture
- If rheumatoid arthritis suspected:
  – Complete blood count, erythrocyte sedimentation rate, rheumatoid arthritis
- Atraumatic joint edema (and possibly migratory): Consider Lyme disease titer.

Imaging
- Radiographs may be needed to rule out fracture in patients with acute knee trauma.
- Knee films (Ottawa knee rules) (1)[A]:
  – Age >55 years *or*
  – Tenderness at the patella or fibular head *or*
  – Inability to bear weight 4 steps *or*
  – Inability to flex knee to 90°
- Radiographs for suspicion of avulsion, stress fracture, or patellofemoral pathology
- Upright anteroposterior (AP), lateral, Merchant, and tunnel views may be helpful in the diagnosis of OA.
- MRI is "gold standard" for imaging muscle, ligamentous, and intraarticular structures; used when surgery is next step in treatment.
- CT scan may be required if occult fracture is suspected.

Diagnostic Procedures/Surgery

Arthroscopy may be beneficial in the diagnosis of certain conditions.

DIFFERENTIAL DIAGNOSIS
- Acute onset:
  – Contusion; fracture; meniscal, cruciate, or collateral ligament tear; extensor tendon injury
  – OA, osteomyelitis, septic arthritis, gout, or pseudogout
- Insidious onset: Patellofemoral pain syndrome, iliotibial band syndrome, OA, rheumatoid arthritis (RA), bursitis, tumors, tendinopathy, loose bodies, bipartite patella, degenerative meniscal tears
- Anterior pain: Patellar/quadriceps tendinopathy, patellofemoral pain syndrome, patellar injury, OA, bursitis, fat pad impingement
- Posterior pain: Popliteal cyst, popliteal aneurysm, medial meniscus tear, tumors
- Medial pain: OA, meniscal or MCL injury, pes anserine bursitis, plica
- Lateral pain: Iliotibial band syndrome, lateral meniscus or LCL injury, OA

Geriatric Considerations

OA, degenerative meniscal tears, and gout are more common.

Pediatric Considerations
- 3 million pediatric sports injuries occur annually.
- Must be concerned about physeal/apophyseal and joint surface injuries in the skeletally immature:
  – Acute injuries: Patellar subluxation, avulsion fractures, ACL tear
  – Overuse injuries: Patellar femoral syndrome, apophysitis, osteochondritis desiccans, patellar tendonitis, stress fracture (4)[C]
  – Other:
    ○ Neoplasm; juvenile RA
    ○ Infection
    ○ Referred pain from slipped capital femoral epiphysis

TREATMENT

MEDICATION
- Nonsteroidal anti-inflammatory drugs (NSAIDs):
  - Acute ligament sprains, muscle strains, tendinopathy (5)[C]:
    - Ibuprofen: 200–800 mg t.i.d.
    - Naproxen: 375–500 mg b.i.d.
    - Indomethacin: 25–50 mg t.i.d.
  - Not recommended in fracture, stress fracture, chronic muscle injury; may be associated with delayed healing; low dose and brief course only if necessary (5)[C]
  - Effective in short-term pain reduction in OA, but long-term use is not recommended owing to risks of significant adverse effects (6)[A].
- Acetaminophen: Doses up to 4 g/d are safe and effective in OA (7)[A].
- Intraarticular corticosteroid injection may provide short-term benefit in knee OA (8)[A].

ADDITIONAL TREATMENT
General Measures
Acute injury: PRICEMM therapy (*protection*, *relative rest*, *ice*, *compression*, *elevation*, *medications*, *modalities*)

Issues for Referral
- Joint instability
- Lack of improvement with conservative measures
- Salter-Harris physeal fractures

Additional Therapies
- Physical therapy is recommended as initial treatment for patellofemoral pain syndrome (9)[A].
- Therapeutic exercise improves function and reduces pain in OA (10)[A].

COMPLEMENTARY AND ALTERNATIVE MEDICINE
Glucosamine sulfate, 1,500 mg/d, may provide moderate pain reduction and improved function in OA (11)[B].

SURGERY/OTHER PROCEDURES
- Surgery may be required for ligamentous and cartilaginous injuries.
- Chronic conditions refractory to conservative therapy may require surgical intervention.

ONGOING CARE

FOLLOW-UP RECOMMENDATIONS
- Activity modification in overuse conditions
- Rehabilitative exercise in OA:
  - Low-impact exercise: Walking, swimming, cycling
  - Strength, ROM, and proprioceptive training

Patient Monitoring
- After initial treatment in acute injury, consider rehabilitation.
- In chronic and overuse conditions, assess functional status, rehabilitative exercise compliance, and pain control at follow-up visit.

DIET
Weight reduction for overweight patient with OA

PATIENT EDUCATION
- Review activity modifications.
- Encourage the patient to play an active role in the rehabilitative process.
- Review risks and benefits of pharmaceutical interventions.

PROGNOSIS
Varies with diagnosis, severity of injury, chronicity of condition, patient motivation to participate in rehabilitative exercises, and whether surgical intervention is required

COMPLICATIONS
- Disability
- Arthritis
- Chronic joint instability
- Deconditioning

REFERENCES

1. Jackson JL, O'Malley PG, Kroenke K. Evaluation of acute knee pain in primary care. *Ann Intern Med*. 2003;129:575–88.
2. Taunton JE, Ryan MB, Clement DB, et al. A retrospective case-control analysis of 2002 running injuries. *Br J Sports Med*. 2002;36:95–101.
3. van Gent RN et al. Incidence and determinents of lower extremity running injuries in long distance runners: a systematic review. *Br J Sports Med*. 2007;41:469–80.
4. Caine D, DiFiori J, Maffulli N. Physeal injuries in children's and youth sports: reasons for concern? *Br J Sports Med*. 2006;40:749–60.
5. Mehallo CJ, Drezner JA, Bytomski JR. Practical management: Nonsteroidal anti-inflammatory drug use in athletic injuries. *Clin J Sports Med*. 2006;16:170–74.
6. Bjordal JM, Ljunggren AE, Klovning A, et al. Non-steroidal anti-inflammatory drugs, including cyclo-oxygenase-2 inhibitors, in osteoarthritic knee pain: Meta-analysis of randomized placebo controlled trials. *Brit J Med*. 2004;329:1317.
7. Zhang W, Jones A, Doherty M. Does paracetamol (acetaminophen) reduce the pain of osteoarthritis? A meta-analysis of randomized controlled trials. *Annals Rheum Dis*. 2004;63:901–07.
8. Bellamy N, Campbell J, Robinson V, et al. Intra-articular corticosteroid for treating osteoarthritis of the knee. *Cochrane Database of Sys Rev*. 2005;2:CD005328.
9. Crossley K, Bennell K, Green S, et al. Physical therapy for patellofemoral pain: a randomized, double-blinded, placebo-controlled trial. *Am J Sports Med*. 2002;30:857–65.
10. Fransen M, McConnell S, Bell M. Exercise for osteoarthritis of the hip or knee. *Cochrane Database Syst Rev*. 2003:CD004286.
11. Towheed TE, Maxwell L, Anastassiades TP, et al. Glucosamine therapy for treating osteoarthritis. *Cochrane Database of Sys Rev*. 2005;(2):CD002946.

ADDITIONAL READING

- Dixit S, Burton M, Mines B. Management of patellofemoral pain syndrome. *Am Fam Phys*. 2007;75:194–202.
- Soprano JV. Musculoskeletal injuries in the pediatric and adolescent athlete. *Curr Sports Med Rep*. 2005;4:329–34.

See Also (Topic, Algorithm, Electronic Media Element)
Algorithms: Knee Pain; Popliteal Mass

 CODES

ICD9
- 715.36 Osteoarthrosis, localized, not specified whether primary or secondary, involving lower leg
- 715.96 Osteoarthrosis, unspecified whether generalized or localized, involving lower leg
- 719.46 Pain in joint involving lower leg

CLINICAL PEARLS
- Knee pain is a common presentation for both acute and chronic injuries.
- Presence of an effusion in a patient younger than 30 years of age signifies a significant knee injury needing accurate/prompt diagnosis.
- Acute mechanism: Consider ligamentous injury, meniscal tear, fracture.
- Overuse mechanism: Consider osteoarthritis, patellofemoral syndrome, tendinopathy, bursitis, and stress fracture.
- Pediatric patient with knee pain: Consider possible physeal, apophyseal, or articular cartilage injuries.

K

LABYRINTHITIS

Teresa V. Chan, MD

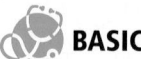 **BASICS**

DESCRIPTION
Acute inflammation of the labyrinth (the organs of hearing and balance that comprise the bony inner ear). There are many possible causes, but infection (viral or bacterial) and subsequent inflammation of the inner ear is felt to be the most common etiology (see Differential Diagnosis). The most constant and pervasive symptom is persistent dizziness and vertigo (room spinning) lasting for hours, days, or weeks AND sudden hearing loss in 1 ear:
- System(s) affected: Nervous; Special sensory (auditory and vestibular)
- Synonym(s): Acute peripheral vestibulopathy; Vestibular neuronitis (vertigo/dizziness only); Vestibular neuritis (vertigo/dizziness only)

Geriatric Considerations
- Vertigo is common in geriatric populations, especially benign positional vertigo. (Unlike labyrinthitis, BPPV is episodic; associated vertigo lasts for seconds or minutes.)
- Labyrinthitis is often associated with vestibular hypofunction of the involved ear and chronic dizziness (which can improve with central compensation).
- Elderly patients are less likely to fully compensate; thus, threshold for vestibular physical therapy is low following acute episode.
- Avoid excessive use of scopolamine, meclizine, and other vestibular suppressants following the initial event, especially in the elderly, as this will delay central compensation. These medications should be used only on an as-needed basis for severe symptoms.

Pediatric Considerations
Unusual in this age group, except meningogenic suppurative labyrinthitis, which more commonly affects children <2 years.

Pregnancy Considerations
Avoid medications.

EPIDEMIOLOGY
- Predominant age: Rare in children; most common in middle age (30–60 years old)
- Predominant sex: Male = Female

Incidence
- Suppurative or serous labyrinthitis secondary to otitis media is increasingly rare in post-antibiotic era; exact incidence is unknown:
  - Estimated 0.5–3% of intratemporal complications of otitis media in recent studies.
  - Higher rates in cases with cholesteatoma.
- Viral labyrinthitis, more common etiology; incidence unknown

Prevalence
In the US, 2nd most common cause of dizziness due to persistent peripheral vestibular hypofunction (9%); BPV (16%) most common

RISK FACTORS
- Otitis media
- Trauma
- Viral infection
- Meningitis
- Otosyphilis (congenital or acquired)
- Cardiovascular disease
- Cerebrovascular disease
- Drug ingestion
- Autoimmune/vasculitides

Genetics
No known genetic pattern

GENERAL PREVENTION
- Scheduled immunizations (see Common Viral Pathogens under Risk Factors)
- Prevent maternal transmission of pathogens, including syphilis, HIV

PATHOPHYSIOLOGY
Acute inflammation or damage to the inner ear, involving both the peripheral special sensory organs of hearing and balance:
- Viral (believed most common)
- Serous: Toxic mediators from a middle ear infection reach the inner ear. Bacteria are not present in inner ear.
- Suppurative: Direct access of the infecting organism into the inner ear:
  - Otogenic
  - Meningogenic

ETIOLOGY
- Infections:
  - Common viral:
    - Cytomegalovirus
    - Mumps virus
    - Varicella zoster virus
    - Rubeola virus
    - Influenza virus
    - Parainfluenza virus
    - Rubella virus
    - Herpes simplex virus 1
    - Adenovirus
    - Coxsackievirus
    - Respiratory syncytial virus
    - HIV
  - Common bacterial:
    - Streptococcus pneumoniae
    - Haemophilus influenzae
    - Moraxella catarrhalis
    - Neisseria meningitidis
    - Streptococcus species
    - Staphylococcus species
  - Treponemal:
    - Treponema pallidum

- Tumors
- Vasculitis
- Infarction
- Ototoxic drugs (e.g., aminoglycosides, cisplatin)
- Head injury

COMMONLY ASSOCIATED CONDITIONS
- Otitis media
- Cholesteatoma
- Head injury

 DIAGNOSIS

HISTORY
- Dizziness AND hearing loss in 1 ear
- Often violent vertigo acutely followed by dizziness
- Nausea and vomiting
- Fullness of affected ear
- Roaring tinnitus of affected ear
- Upper respiratory tract infection symptoms (preceding or concurrent)
- Otorrhea (not common with viral causes)
- Otalgia (not common with viral causes)

PHYSICAL EXAM
- Nystagmus:
  - Fast-beating nystagmus toward affected ear (acutely), NOT affected by position
  - Fast-beating nystagmus away from affected ear (chronically)
- Symptoms improve in supine position and with eyes closed
- Perspiration
- Increased salivation
- Fever
- Generalized malaise
- Ataxia

DIAGNOSTIC TESTS & INTERPRETATION
Lab
- Audiogram
- Routine laboratory studies not helpful in making diagnosis unless autoimmune cause is highly suspected
- Consider culture of otorrhea or middle ear fluid to direct antibiotic choice
- Consider CSF culture if meningitis is suspected
- FTA-ABS (specific treponemal test) when clinically indicated
- Vestibular tests to consider (not typically indicated in acute setting):
  - Electronystagmography
  - Caloric test
  - Doll's eye test

Follow-Up & Special Considerations
Labyrinthitis ossificans can occur quickly after meningitis; severity and progression of hearing loss will determine urgency for cochlear implant consideration.

Imaging

- Rarely indicated unless tumor is possibility
- MRI of the brain with contrast for suspected lesions involving the 8th cranial nerve (may see enhancement of intracochlear or intravestibular organs, or their associated nerves)
- CT of the brain and temporal bones for associated intratemporal and intracranial processes

Diagnostic Procedures/Surgery

- None routinely indicated
- Tympanocentesis or lumbar puncture may be helpful in certain cases of bacterial infection or suspected meningitis.

DIFFERENTIAL DIAGNOSIS

- Vestibular neuritis/neuronitis
- Benign paroxysmal positional vertigo (BPPV)—episodic, vertigo lasting seconds/minutes, worse when lying down or looking up
- Ménière disease: Episodic vertigo lasting minutes to hours, associated with ear fullness, tinnitus, and hearing loss
- Idiopathic sudden single-sided deafness
- Postconcussive syndrome
- Acute otitis media
- Acute bacterial otomastoiditis
- Ototoxicity
- CVA/brainstem infarct
- Cerebellopontine-angle tumors (e.g., vestibular schwannoma)
- Vestibular migraine
- Multiple sclerosis
- Parainfectious encephalomyelitis
- Parainfectious cranial polyneuritis
- Ramsay Hunt syndrome
- Cerebral or systemic vasculitis
- Temporal lobe epilepsy
- HIV infection
- Perilymphatic fistula
- Superior canal dehiscence
- Syphilis

 TREATMENT

- Close follow-up and vestibular testing to assess vertigo
- Vestibular suppressants (below under medication); Optimally used for severe acute attacks of vertigo
- Persistent dizziness following labyrinthitis should be managed with vestibular physical therapy (http://www.youtube.com/watch?v=8K7-1Ev8Oos).
- For acute viral labyrinthitis, audiometric testing if hearing loss
- Sudden single-sided hearing loss should be managed with high-dose oral steroids ASAP.
- For suppurative labyrinthitis, appropriate antibacterials to eradicate infection, supportive care, prevention of spread of infection:
  - Can be associated with labyrinthitis ossificans; decisions regarding cochlear implantation may need to be made early ONLY IF both ears develop severe to profound hearing loss.

MEDICATION

- Use of the following drugs should be limited:
  - Meclizine (Antivert, Bonine) 12–25 mg p.o. q4h p.r.n.
  - Dimenhydrinate (Dramamine) 25–50 mg p.o. p.r.n.
  - Diazepam (Valium) 2–5 mg q.i.d. p.o. p.r.n.
  - Lorazepam (Ativan) 0.5–2 mg SL/p.o. b.i.d. p.r.n.
  - Amitriptyline (Elavil) 10–50 p.o. q.h.s. p.r.n.
  - Precautions: All the listed medications have significant adverse reactions. Use with caution. Avoid scopolamine in the elderly.
- Antiemetics:
  - Odansetron (Zofran) 4–8 mg p.o. t.i.d. p.r.n.
  - Granisetron (Kytril) 1 mg p.o. t.i.d.
  - Meclizine (Antivert, Bonine) 12.5–25 mg p.o. q4h p.r.n.
  - Promethazine (Phenergan) 12.5–25 mg p.o./p.r. q.i.d. p.r.n.
  - Prochlorperazine (Compazine) 25 mg p.r. q.i.d. p.r.n.
  - Metoclopramide (Reglan) 10 mg p.o. t.i.d. p.r.n.
  - Scopolamine (Transderm Scop Patch) 1 t.d. q.3 days p.r.n.
- Antivirals:
  - Acyclovir 800 mg p.o. 5 times per day for 7 days is used in labyrinthitis associated with herpes zoster, but is otherwise not indicated.
- Steroids:
  - Given early in the setting of bacterial meningitis, may decrease the otologic sequelae, specifically labyrinthitis ossificans
  - Often used empirically in treatment of labyrinthitis

ADDITIONAL TREATMENT

General Measures

- Treat underlying disorder when possible.
- Symptomatic treatment during acute period
- Minimize vestibular suppressants after acute period of dizziness to promote compensation.
- Visual–vestibular exercises for prolonged symptoms and unilateral vestibular loss

Issues for Referral

Consider neurology or otoneurology referral for suspected central causes of vertigo.

Additional Therapies

- For labyrinthitis, use of vestibular rehabilitation exercises is effective in decreasing symptoms (1)[A].
- For benign paroxysmal positional vertigo, physical repositioning (Dix-Hallpike and Epley) maneuvers are effective in the short term (http://www.youtube.com/watch?v=eOuzUi5ckrk)

IN-PATIENT CONSIDERATIONS

Initial Stabilization

Usually outpatient management

Admission Criteria

- Systemic infection
- Young age
- Intractable vertigo with nausea and vomiting (e.g., unable to tolerate oral diet or function independently

 ONGOING CARE

FOLLOW-UP RECOMMENDATIONS

Patient Monitoring

Follow weekly with audiogram until stabilizes.

DIET

- Avoid alcohol—may exacerbate symptoms.
- For persistent fullness of the affected ear, minimize salt intake.

PATIENT EDUCATION

- Lie still with eyes closed in darkened room during acute attacks. Otherwise, activity as tolerated.
- Minimize rapid head movement until symptoms resolve.
- Vestibular physical therapy important after acute symptoms to manage unilateral vestibular loss (2)

PROGNOSIS

Depends on cause

COMPLICATIONS

- Permanent hearing loss
- Chronic imbalance

REFERENCES

1. Hillier SL, Hollohan V. Vestibular rehabilitation for unilateral peripheral vestibular dysfunction. *Cochrane Database Syst Rev.* 2007;CD005397.
2. Yardley L, Donovan-Hall M, Smith HE, et al. Effectiveness of primary care-based vestibular rehabilitation for chronic dizziness. *Ann Intern Med.* 2004;141:598–605.

ADDITIONAL READING

- Baloh RW, Honrobia V. *Clinical Neurology of the Vestibular System.* 2nd ed. Philadelphia, PA: FA Davis; 1990.
- Goetz CG. *Textbook of Clinical Neurology.* Philadelphia: WB Saunders; 1999.

See Also (Topic, Algorithm, Electronic Media Element)

Ménière Disease; Postconcussive Syndrome; Tinnitus

 CODES

ICD9

- 386.30 Labyrinthitis, unspecified
- 386.31 Serous labyrinthitis
- 386.32 Circumscribed labyrinthitis

L

LACRIMAL DISORDERS

Kristy M. Cahill, MD
Deborah E. Zuckerman, MD

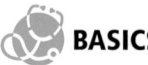 **BASICS**

DESCRIPTION
- Diseases and abnormalities of tear production and maintenance of tear film
- The most common lacrimal disorder is dry eye syndrome.
- Lacrimal duct disorders usually result in overflow tearing.
- System(s) affected: Skin/Exocrine

EPIDEMIOLOGY
Prevalence
Very common throughout US, more often seen in arid climates:
- Predominant gender: Female > Male
- Predominant age: Dry eye symptoms increase with age; most often seen in elderly

RISK FACTORS
- Exposure to dry environments
- History of collagen vascular disease, such as rheumatoid arthritis, Sjögren syndrome, thyroid disease, rosacea, Bell palsy, eyelid abnormalities
- Oral contraceptive, diuretic, β-blocker, and antihistamine use
- Vitamin A deficiency

GENERAL PREVENTION
- Prevent exposure to eye irritants from pollution, cigarette smoke, and sun exposure.
- Ensure adequate vitamin A intake through diet or as a supplement.

PATHOPHYSIOLOGY
Tear film is composed of 3 layers:
- Mucin layer: Allows spread of aqueous tears
- Thick aqueous layer produced by lacrimal gland
- Lipid layer: Controls tear evaporation

ETIOLOGY
- Results from poor tear production, rapid tear evaporation, and/or an abnormal concentration of mucin or lipid in tear film
- Most common cause of dry eye symptoms is aqueous tear deficiency
- Decreased androgens thought to contribute to decrease in tear production

COMMONLY ASSOCIATED CONDITIONS
Sjögren syndrome, rheumatoid arthritis, thyroid disease, rosacea, pregnancy, menopause, malnutrition

 DIAGNOSIS

HISTORY
- Dry sensation in eyes
- Foreign-body sensation
- Blurry vision
- Itching
- Ocular pain
- Photophobia
- Occasional tearing due to excessive reflex tearing:
  - Patient's symptoms usually worsen in dry, smoky environments, while reading, driving, or using computer for extended periods

Pediatric Considerations
Lacrimal duct obstruction should be suspected in an infant presenting with excessive tearing (epiphora).

PHYSICAL EXAM
Slit lamp exam reveals decreased tear film and may reveal punctate epithelial defects on cornea.

DIAGNOSTIC TESTS & INTERPRETATION
Lab
Initial lab tests
Tear production can be measured using a Schirmer filter strip after instillation of topical anesthetic. Wetting of <10 mm of the slip after 5 minutes is indicative of insufficient tear production.

Diagnostic Procedures/Surgery
- Staining of the ocular surface with fluorescein will show areas of abnormal uptake and patches of drying. It allows the tear break-up time (TBUT) to be calculated. A TBUT of <10 seconds is abnormal.
- Rose bengal will be taken up by dead or dying epithelial cells, and may be a more sensitive test.

Pathological Findings
In Sjögren syndrome, infiltration of the lacrimal gland with inflammatory cells may be evident.

DIFFERENTIAL DIAGNOSIS
- Ocular: Allergy, conjunctivitis, contact lens complication, exposure keratopathy
- Other: Ocular rosacea, thyroid ophthalmopathy, ocular manifestation of HIV, Bell palsy, vitamin A deficiency

 TREATMENT

MEDICATION
First Line
- Preservative-free artificial tears: 1 drop in each eye several times a day to prevent discomfort (1)[A]
- Ophthalmic lubricating ointment may be used in each eye at bedtime (2)[B].

Second Line
- Dry eye has been identified as having an inflammatory component that responds in refractory cases to topical immunosuppressives, such as cyclosporine (Restasis) 0.05%, 1 drop to each eye b.i.d. (3,4)[A].
- Emerging therapies include topical androgens, secretagogues (e.g., oral pilocarpine), cytokine-blocking agents, and a P2Y2 receptor agonist (Diquafosol).

ADDITIONAL TREATMENT
General Measures
- Those with systemic illnesses predisposed to dry eye should be informed and instructed in the appropriate use of artificial tear supplements.
- Symptoms of dry eye may decrease with an increase in home humidification and hydration.

Issues for Referral
Rheumatology referral if systemic collagen vascular disease is suspected

Additional Therapies
- Fatty acid (Ω-3), linoleic acid, and g-linoleic acid supplements (5)[B]
- Lid massage and warm compresses several times a day

Pediatric Considerations

The vast majority of babies born with nasolacrimal duct obstructions will clear spontaneously during the 1st year of life. On occasion, surgical probing is necessary.

SURGERY/OTHER PROCEDURES

Punctal occlusion, with either punctual plugs or laser, is used in moderate-to-severe dry eye if medical therapy fails.

ONGOING CARE

FOLLOW-UP RECOMMENDATIONS

Patient Monitoring

Monitor early to assess efficacy of treatment. The viscosity of artificial tears and frequency of use can be increased for symptom relief.

DIET

- Diet rich in Ω-3 fatty acids and/or linoleic acids may benefit some patients
- Adequate vitamin A intake

PATIENT EDUCATION

All individuals with systemic illnesses predisposed to dry eye, postmenopausal women, and those residing in arid climates or >60 years should be instructed in the use of artificial tear supplements to combat dry eye symptoms.

PROGNOSIS

- Lacrimal disorders can be adequately managed with artificial tear supplements.
- Blocked tear ducts can be managed with probing and punctal dilation and/or dacryocystorhinostomy procedures in more severe cases.

COMPLICATIONS

Severe dry eye may lead to corneal breakdown, secondary invasion by bacteria, and eye infections.

REFERENCES

1. Ousler GW, Michaelson C, Christensen MT. An evaluation of tear film breakup time extension and ocular protection index scores among three marketed lubricant eye drops. *Cornea*. 2007; 26:949–52.
2. Tauber J. Efficacy, tolerability and comfort of a 0.3% hypromellose gel ophthalmic lubricant in the treatment of patients with moderate to severe dry eye syndrome. *Curr Med Res Opin*. 2007;23: 2629–36.
3. Hardten DR, Brown MJ, Pham-Vang S. Evaluation of an isotonic tear in combination with topical cyclosporine for the treatment of ocular surface disease. *Curr Med Res Opin*. 2007;23:2083–91.
4. Roberts CW, Carniglia PE, Brazzo BG. Comparison of topical cyclosporine, punctal occlusion, and a combination for the treatment of dry eye. *Cornea*. 2007;26:805–9.
5. Barabino S, Rolando M, Camicione P, et al. Systemic linoleic and gamma-linolenic acid therapy in dry eye syndrome with an inflammatory component. *Cornea*. 2003;22:97–101.

ADDITIONAL READING

- Dogru M, Tsubota K. New insights into the diagnosis and treatment of dry eye. *Ocul Surf*. 2004;2:59–75.
- Karadayi K, Ciftci F, Akin T, et al. Increase in central corneal thickness in dry and normal eyes with application of artificial tears: a new diagnostic and follow-up criterion for dry eye. *Ophthalmic Physiol Opt*. 2005;25:485–91.
- Perry HD, Donnenfeld ED. Dry eye diagnosis and management in 2004. *Curr Opin Ophthalmol*. 2004;15:299–304.
- Stern ME, Gao J, Siemasko KF, et al. The role of the lacrimal functional unit in the pathophysiology of dry eye. *Exp Eye Res*. 2004;78:409–16.

See Also (Topic, Algorithm, Electronic Media Element)

Sjögren Syndrome

CODES

ICD9

- 375.9 Unspecified disorder of lacrimal system
- 375.15 Tear film insufficiency, unspecified

CLINICAL PEARLS

- Dry eye syndrome is common in the US, affecting postmenopausal women more than any other population.
- Symptoms are usually adequately managed with preservative-free artificial tears and humidified environments.
- Dry eye symptoms that are refractory to medical treatment and/or punctual plugs should raise the suspicion of an underlying systemic condition, and a rheumatology consult should be considered.

L

LACTOSE INTOLERANCE

Mohammad Ansar Mughal, MD
Fozia A. Ali, MD

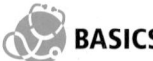 BASICS

DESCRIPTION
- Inability to digest lactose (the primary sugar in milk) into its constituents, glucose and galactose, owing to low levels of the lactase enzyme in the brush border of the duodenum
  - Congenital lactose intolerance: Very rare
  - Primary lactose intolerance is common in adults in whom a low level of lactase has developed after childhood.
  - Symptoms are experienced after consumption of milk and milk-containing products. Intolerance varies with amount of lactose consumed and rate of gastric emptying (faster emptying times being associated with greater symptoms).
  - Secondary lactose intolerance is the inability to digest lactose caused by any condition injuring the intestinal mucosa (e.g., diarrhea) or a reduction of available mucosal surface (e.g., resection). This is usually transient, with the duration of the intolerance determined by the nature and course of the primary condition.
  - Infants with induced acute or chronic diarrhea may develop lactose intolerance, especially with rotavirus disease.
  - *Lactose malabsorption* is defined as the inability to absorb lactose. This does not necessarily parallel lactose intolerance.
- Systems affected: Endocrine/Metabolic; GI
- Synonym: Lactase deficiency

Pediatric Considerations
- Primary lactose intolerance usually begins in late childhood.
- No consensus exists on whether young children (<5 years of age) should avoid lactose following diarrheal illness.
- Lactose-free formulas are available.
- Exclude a milk protein allergy.

EPIDEMIOLOGY
Incidence
- Primary lactose intolerance varies according to race: Up to 15% of northern European descendants, 80% of blacks and Latinos, 100% of Native American and Asians (1).
- Secondary lactose intolerance:
  - ≥50% of infants with acute or chronic diarrheal disease have lactose intolerance, especially with rotavirus disease.
  - Lactose intolerance also is fairly common with giardiasis and ascariasis, irritable bowel syndrome (IBS), tropical and nontropical sprue, and the AIDS malabsorptive syndrome.

Prevalence
- Predominant age:
  - Primary: Teenage and adult
  - Secondary: Depends on underlying condition
- Predominant sex: Male = Female

RISK FACTORS
- Race: Adult-onset lactase deficiency varies widely among countries.
- Age: Signs and symptoms usually do not become apparent until after age 6–7 years, and recent studies actually have shown that hypolactasia may begin even after age 20. Symptoms may not be apparent until adulthood depending on dietary lactose intake and rate of decline of intestinal lactase activity. Lactase enzyme activity is highly correlated with age, regardless of symptoms.

Genetics
- The gene responsible for lactase has been identified (2)[A]. The wild-type presentation is associated with the decline of lactase activity.
- Genetic polymorphisms associated with lactase persistence are concentrated predominantly in northern Europeans.

GENERAL PREVENTION
Avoidance of lactose in large quantities will relieve symptoms. Patients can learn what level of lactose is tolerable in their diet.

ETIOLOGY
- Primary lactose intolerance: Normal decline in the lactase activity in the intestinal mucosa after weaning is genetically controlled and permanent.
- Secondary lactose intolerance: Associated with gastroenteritis in children
- Secondary lactose intolerance is also associated with nontropical and tropical sprue, regional enteritis, abetalipoproteinemia, cystic fibrosis, ulcerative colitis, and immunoglobulin deficiencies in both adults and children.

COMMONLY ASSOCIATED CONDITIONS
- Tropical or nontropical sprue
- Giardiasis
- Immunoglobulin deficiencies
- Crohn disease
- Cystic fibrosis

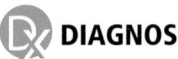 DIAGNOSIS

Evaluation of lactose intolerance includes a careful medical history, review of symptoms, and physical examination.

HISTORY
- Symptoms may arise 30 min to 2 h after consumption of products containing lactose and may be distinguished from IBS with a trial of a lactose-free diet.
- Symptoms include bloating, cramping, abdominal discomfort, diarrhea or loose stools, and flatulence. The abdominal pain may be crampy in nature and often is localized to the periumbilical area or lower quadrant. The stools usually are bulky, frothy, and watery.
- Only 1/3 to 1/5 of the people with lactose malabsorption will develop symptoms. The degree of symptoms varies with the lactose load and with other food consumed at the same time.

PHYSICAL EXAM
Borborygmi may be audible on physical examination and to the patient.

DIAGNOSTIC TESTS & INTERPRETATION
Lab
Initial lab tests
- Lactose breath hydrogen test (especially in children): The test is begun by giving oral lactose in the fasting state, at a usual dose of 2 g/kg (maximum dose 25 g). Breath hydrogen is sampled at baseline and at 30-min intervals after the ingestion of lactose for 3 h. The postlactose and baseline values are compared. We generally consider a breath hydrogen value of 10 ppm as normal. Values between 10 and 20 ppm may be indeterminate unless accompanied by symptoms, whereas values over 20 ppm are considered diagnostic of lactose malabsorption.
- Lactose absorption test: Alternative to lactose breath hydrogen test in adults (more invasive and equivalent in sensitivity and specificity to breath test). Following oral administration of a 50-g test dose in adults (or 2 g/kg in children), blood glucose levels are monitored at 0, 60, and 120 min. An increase in blood glucose by <20 mg/dL (1.1 mmol/L) plus the development of symptoms is diagnostic. False-negative results may occur in patients with diabetes or bacterial overgrowth.
- Low fecal pH and reducing substances are only valid when stools are collected fresh and assayed immediately. Test is fairly insensitive.

Diagnostic Procedures/Surgery

Small bowel biopsy for assay of lactase activity: May be normal if deficiency is focal or patchy (not readily available and usually not necessary)

Pathological Findings

Lactase deficiency in intestinal mucosa may be patchy or focal.

DIFFERENTIAL DIAGNOSIS

- Sucrase deficiency
- Diarrhea
- IBS
- Protein intolerance
- Malabsorption syndromes

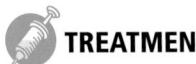 TREATMENT

The treatment of lactose malabsorption in the absence of a correctable underlying disease includes four general principles:

- Reduced dietary lactose intake
- Substitution of alternative nutrient sources to maintain energy and protein intake
- Administration of a commercially available enzyme substitute
- Maintenance of calcium and vitamin D intake

MEDICATION

Lactase (Lactaid, Lactrase) tablets (1)[A]:

- Commercially available "lactase" preparations are actually bacterial or yeast β-galactosidases.
- Take 1–2 capsules or tablets prior to ingesting milk products.
- These vary in effectiveness at preventing symptoms.
- Can add tablets or contents of capsules to milk before drinking; also available in milk in some areas
- Not effective for all people with lactose intolerance

COMPLEMENTARY AND ALTERNATIVE MEDICINE

Certain probiotic formulations taken with meals may alleviate some of the symptoms of lactose intolerance in select patients (3)[B].

 ONGOING CARE

DIET

- Reduce or restrict dietary lactose to control symptoms.
- Yogurt and fermented products, such as hard cheese, are better tolerated than milk.
- Supplement calcium in the form of calcium carbonate.
- Prehydrolyzed milk (Lactaid) is available and effective.

PATIENT EDUCATION

- Patients must read labels on commercial products because milk sugar is used in many products and may cause symptoms.
- Lactose-intolerant patients may tolerate whole milk or chocolate milk better than skim milk owing to slower rate of gastric emptying.
- Lactose consumed with other food products is better tolerated than when it is consumed alone.
- Primary lactase deficiency is permanent; secondary lactose intolerance usually is temporary, although it may persist for several months after the inciting disease has been cured.
- 20% of prescription drugs and 6% of over-the-counter (OTC) medicines use lactose as a base.
- Most patients still can tolerate 12–15 g of lactose despite their lactose intolerance or malabsorption (4)[A].

PROGNOSIS

- Normal life expectancy
- Symptoms can be controlled through diet alone if lactase tablets are ineffective.

COMPLICATIONS

Calcium deficiency: Avoidance of milk and other dairy products can lead to reduced calcium intake, which may increase the risk for osteoporosis and fracture.

REFERENCES

1. Levri KM, Ketvertis K, Deramo M, et al. Do probiotics reduce adult lactose intolerance? A systematic review. J Fam Pact. 2005;54:613.
2. Waud JP, Matthews SB, Campbell AK. Measurement of breath hydrogen and methane, together with lactase genotype, defines the current best practice for investigation of lactose sensitivity. Ann Clin Biochem. 2008;45:50–8.
3. Sanders SW, Tolman KG, Reitberg DP. Effect of a single dose of lactase on symptoms and expired hydrogen after lactose challenge in lactose-intolerant subjects. Clin Pharm. 1992;11:533–8.
4. Shaukat A, Levitt MD, Taylor BC, MacDonald R, Shamliyan TA, Kane RL, Wilt TJ et al. Systematic review: effective management strategies for lactose intolerance. Ann Intern Med. 2010;152:797–803.

ADDITIONAL READING

- Brannon PM, Carpenter TO, Fernandez JR, Gilsanz V, Gould JB, Hall KE, Hui SL, Lupton JR, Mennella J, Miller NJ, Osganian SK, Sellmeyer DE, Suchy FJ, Wolf MA et al. NIH Consensus Development Conference Statement: Lactose Intolerance and Health. NIH consensus and state-of-the-science statements. 2010;27
- http://emedicine.medscape.com/article/930971-diagnosis
- http://www.uptodate.com/online/content/topic.do?topicKey=gi_dis/13325&selectedTitle=1%7E150&source=search_result#H11
- Swagerty DL, Walling AD, Klein RM. Lactose intolerance. Am Fam Physician. 2002;65:1845–50.

 CODES

ICD9

271.3 Intestinal disaccharidase deficiencies and disaccharide malabsorption

CLINICAL PEARLS

- Keeping a food diary with symptomatic episodes documented can help to identify food sources that may be problematic.
- Patients should read ingredient labels to look for milk or lactose but also for ingredients such as whey and curd, which indicate the presence of lactose.
- Lactose-intolerant patients may tolerate whole milk or chocolate milk better than skim milk owing to a slower rate of gastric emptying.
- Many patients with lactose intolerance avoid dairy products to an unnecessary degree, causing inadequate intake of of calcium and vitamin D, which may predispose them to osteoporosis.

L

LARYNGEAL CANCER

Hugh J. Silk, MD
Sheila O. Stille, DMD, MAGD
Jason Conforti, MD

 BASICS

DESCRIPTION
- A friable, granular tumor of the larynx that leads to hoarseness, hemoptysis, and cough
- <1% of all malignant lesions; squamous cell carcinomas constitute 95–98% of all malignant neoplasms of the larynx.
- Laryngeal cancer accounts for <2% of all carcinomas.
- At the time of diagnosis, 62% will have local disease, 26% regional disease, and 8% distant disease in the lungs, liver, and/or bone.
- No racial predilection
- System(s) affected: Pulmonary; ENT
- Synonym(s): Cancer of the larynx; Throat cancer

EPIDEMIOLOGY
Incidence
- 5/100,000 per year (12,250 new cases per year in US). These are usually squamous cell carcinomas that arise from the glottis.
- Predominant age:
  – Median age of occurrence in 6th and 7th decades
  – <1% of laryngeal cancers arise in patients <30 years of age.
- Predominant sex: Male > Female (4:1); increasing incidence in women who smoke

Prevalence
- About 3,700 deaths from disease in US yearly
- 2nd most common site for head and neck cancer (26% of all cases)
- 11th most common cancer in males

RISK FACTORS
See Etiology.

Genetics
Unknown

GENERAL PREVENTION
- Avoidance or cessation of smoking and/or alcohol abuse (85% attributed to smoking or alcohol abuse)
- Wearing proper respiratory masks/respirators if chronic exposure to certain chemicals, gases, and wood dust
- Treating chronic laryngopharyngeal reflux
- Indirect laryngoscopy for at-risk patients with persistent hoarseness lasting beyond 1–2 weeks

ETIOLOGY
- Smoking
- Alcohol abuse
- Chronic laryngopharyngeal reflux
- Occupational hazards (asbestos, pesticides, polycyclic aromatic hydrocarbons, wood workers)

COMMONLY ASSOCIATED CONDITIONS
Up to 10% of patients may have a synchronous squamous cell carcinoma in the lower or upper aerodigestive tract, most notably in the esophagus or lungs.

 DIAGNOSIS

Early laryngeal cancer generally has a good prognosis, with a 5-year disease specific survival rate of more than 90% for T1 tumors.

HISTORY
- Persistent hoarseness in an elderly or middle-aged cigarette smoker (1)
- Dyspnea and/or stridor
- Ipsilateral otalgia
- Dysphagia
- Odynophagia
- Chronic cough
- Hemoptysis
- Weight loss due to poor nutrition
- Halitosis due to tumor necrosis
- Chronic exposure to known risk factors (see Etiology)

PHYSICAL EXAM
- Visualization of larynx initially by mirror and then a full nasolaryngoscopic exam
- Physical observation of vocal cord mobility, airway patency, and any locoregional spread
- Cervical lymph node exam
- Mass in the neck from metastatic lymph node
- Laryngeal tenderness secondary to tumor necrosis or suppuration
- Broadening of the larynx on palpation with loss of crepitation
- Fullness of the cricothyroid membrane

DIAGNOSTIC TESTS & INTERPRETATION
Imaging
- CT scan or MRI if chest, liver, or brain metastasis suspected
- Bone scan if bone metastasis suspected

Diagnostic Procedures/Surgery
Indirect and/or direct laryngoscopy and biopsy to determine stage of disease as well as histologic confirmation

Pathological Findings
- Laryngoscopy: Fungating, friable tumor with heaped-up edges and granular appearance, with multiple areas of central necrosis and exudate surrounding areas of hyperemia
- Squamous cell carcinoma 95% of cases

DIFFERENTIAL DIAGNOSIS
- Acute or chronic laryngitis secondary to allergies, voice overuse, chemical exposures
- Benign vocal cord lesions such as polyps, nodules, and papillomas
- Tuberculosis or fungal infection (candidiasis) of the larynx (2)

 TREATMENT

Radiotherapy tends to be the treatment of choice in northern Europe, Australasia, and Canada, whereas surgery tends to be the treatment of choice in southern Europe and many centers in the United States.

MEDICATION
- Narcotics may be necessary for pain control during treatment for mucositis (of the mouth) secondary to radiation therapy. Viscous lidocaine can be helpful as well.
- Nystatin mouth rinses for oral thrush

ADDITIONAL TREATMENT
General Measures
- Tracheotomy care, when applicable
- If patient is diagnosed during pregnancy: Natural history of disease and treatment side effects have to be weighed against the possibilities of continuing on to delivery.

Issues for Referral
- ENT for direct visualization of larynx; biopsy and surgery
- Depending on patient's management plan, nutritional and dental consults may be needed.
- Treatment may result in need for voice rehabilitation and be the cause of social isolation, job loss, and depression; therefore, leading to referrals to psychology, social work, and/or support groups as indicated (3).

Additional Therapies
Radiotherapy:
- There is increased focus on radiation therapy (RT), combined chemotherapy and RT, and function-preserving laryngectomy surgery due to patient fear of voice loss (3).
- Early disease may be treatable by either RT or laser cordectomy on an outpatient basis. No randomized, controlled trial has proven superiority of either when last reviewed by Cochrane in 2007. 90% cure rates are the rule (4).
- BCCIP protein (BRCA2 and CDKN1A [p21(Waf1/Cip1)] interacting protein) can be a prognostic marker for RT, with loss of the protein indicating a worse prognosis (5).

SURGERY/OTHER PROCEDURES
- Tracheotomy may be necessary if tumor is large enough to cause upper airway obstruction.
- More advanced disease needs inpatient care necessitating partial or total laryngectomy and postoperative RT 4–5 weeks after surgery depending on the stage of disease.

IN-PATIENT CONSIDERATIONS
Initial Stabilization
Primarily outpatient care

Admission Criteria
- More advanced disease, surgical intervention, and complication management
- Nutritional or airway issues/complications

 ## ONGOING CARE

FOLLOW-UP RECOMMENDATIONS
Patient may remain fully active unless debilitated from more advanced disease and/or greater degree of surgery.

Patient Monitoring
- Repeat indirect laryngoscopy and complete head and neck exams periodically for at least 5 years after treatment to detect early recurrence or 2nd primary
- Yearly chest x-rays (and liver function text monitoring) for metastatic disease
- Patients with dysphagia should undergo barium swallow and/or esophageal endoscopy to rule out 2nd synchronous tumor in the esophagus.
- Patients with unexplained pain should have appropriate radiologic or nuclear medicine bone scans.
- Mental status change warrants CT scan of the brain to rule out brain metastases.

DIET
- Nasogastric or gastrostomy feeding may be necessary if tumor involves esophageal inlet.
- No special diet otherwise

PATIENT EDUCATION
Material is available from local cancer society.

PROGNOSIS
- Early disease is expected to have >90% cure rate with laryngeal and voice preservation.
- If lesion enlarges or metastasizes to regional cervical lymph nodes, the cure rate usually drops by 50%.
- Most recurrences occur within the first 2 years of initial treatment.

COMPLICATIONS
- Temporary odynophagia or dysphagia secondary to mucositis and/or thrush during RT
- Persistent hoarseness despite adequate treatment, necessitating further adjunctive procedures and/or speech therapy
- Tracheostoma stenosis requiring stenting with laryngectomy tubes or further surgery
- Dysphagia secondary to upper esophageal stricture after total laryngectomy, necessitating dilation
- Aspiration after partial laryngectomy, necessitating complete laryngectomy or tracheotomy
- Inability to decannulate after partial laryngectomy because of laryngeal stenosis and/or aspiration
- Radiation-induced chondronecrosis, which mimics tumor recurrence
- Radiation edema, necessitating emergent tracheotomy
- Hypothyroidism secondary to laryngectomy and RT (6)

REFERENCES
1. Chu, EA, Kim YJ. Laryngeal cancer: Diagnosis and preoperative work-up. *Otolaryngol Clin N Am*. 2008;41:673–95.
2. Nunes FP, Bishop T, Prasad ML, et al. Laryngeal candidiasis mimicking malignancy. *Laryngoscope*. 2008;118:1957–9.
3. American Society of Clinical Oncology, Pfister DG, Laurie SA, et al. American Society of Clinical Oncology clinical practice guideline for the use of larynx-preservation strategies in the treatment of laryngeal cancer. *J Clin Oncol*. 2006;24:3693–704.
4. Dey P, et al. Radiotherapy vs. open surgery vs. endolaryngeal surgery (with or without laser) for early laryngeal squamous cell cancer. *Cochrane Database Sys Rev*. 2002;2:CD002027.
5. Rewari A, Lu H, Parikh R, et al. BCCIP as a prognostic marker for radiotherapy of laryngeal cancer. *Radiother Oncol*. 2008.
6. Alkan S, Baylancicek S, Ciftçic M, et al. Thyroid dysfunction after combined therapy for laryngeal cancer: A prospective study. *Otolaryngol Head Neck Surg*. 2008;139:787–91.

ADDITIONAL READING
- Ferlito A, Bradley PJ, Rinaldo A et al. What is the treatment of choice for Tl squamous cell carcinoma of the larynx? *J Laryngol Otol*. 2004;118:747–9.
- Huang SH, Lockwood G, Irish J, et al. Truths and Myths About Radiotherapy for Verrucous Carcinoma of Larynx. *Int J Radiat Oncol Biol Phys*. 2008.

 ## CODES

ICD9
- 161.0 Malignant neoplasm of glottis
- 161.1 Malignant neoplasm of supraglottis
- 161.2 Malignant neoplasm of subglottis

CLINICAL PEARLS
- Persistent hoarseness in an at-risk older person should prompt investigation with indirect and/or direct laryngoscopy.
- RT and multimodal therapies have reduced the need for laryngectomy except in advanced cases. ENT and radiation oncology consultations are recommended.
- Counsel all patients about primary prevention (no smoking, limit alcohol use) and counsel patients with cancer on secondary prevention.

L

LARYNGITIS

Hugh J. Silk, MD
Sheila O. Stille, DMD, MAGD
Steffani Araya, MD

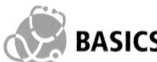 **BASICS**

DESCRIPTION
- Laryngitis is inflammation, erythema, and edema of the mucosa of the larynx and/or vocal cords.
- There is a range of severity, but most cases are acute and are associated with viral upper respiratory infection or acute vocal strain
- System(s) affected: Pulmonary; ENT
- Synonym(s): Laryngotracheitis; Acute laryngitis; Chronic laryngitis; Croup (in children)

EPIDEMIOLOGY
- Predominant age: Affects all ages
- Children more susceptible than adults owing to increased risk of symptomatic inflammation due to smaller airways
- Predominant gender: Male = Female

Incidence
Common

Prevalence
Common

RISK FACTORS
- Acute:
  - Upper respiratory tract infection
  - Voice overuse
  - Pneumonia
  - Influenza
  - Lack of immunization for pertussis or diphtheria
  - Immunocompromised
- Chronic:
  - Allergy
  - Chronic rhinitis/sinusitis
  - Voice abuse
  - Gastroesophageal reflux disease (GERD)/ laryngopharyngeal reflux disease (LPRD) (rare) (1)[A]
  - Smoking
  - Constant exposure to dust or other irritants; environmental pollution
  - Previous endotracheal intubation
  - Medications: Inhaled steroids, anticholinergics, and antihistamines

Geriatric Considerations
May be more ill, slower to heal

Pediatric Considerations
- Common in this age group
- Consider congenital causes.

GENERAL PREVENTION
- Avoid overuse of voice (voice training helpful for vocal musicians/public speakers)
- Influenza virus vaccine is suggested for high-risk individuals
- Quit smoking and avoid secondhand smoke
- Limit or avoid alcohol/caffeine/acidic foods
- Maintain proper hydration status
- Avoid allergens
- Good hand washing (infection prevention)

ETIOLOGY
- Misuse or abuse of voice
- Virus infections: Influenza A, B; parainfluenza; adenovirus; coronavirus; rhinovirus; human papillomavirus; cytomegalovirus; varicella-zoster virus; herpes simplex virus; respiratory syncytial virus; coxsackievirus
- Bacterial infections (uncommon): β-hemolytic streptococcus, *Streptococcus pneumoniae*, *H. influenzae*, tuberculosis (TB), leprosy, *Moraxella catarrhalis*, *Mycoplasma pneumoniae*, *Chlamydophila pneumoniae*
- Fungal infections (rare): Histoplasmosis, blastomycosis, coccidioides, cryptococcus, and candida
- Secondary syphilis left untreated
- Leprosy (in 30–55% of those with leprosy, larynx is affected; tropical and warm countries)
- Laryngeal TB
- Inhaling irritating substances (e.g., air pollution, cigarette smoke)
- Aspiration of caustic chemicals
- Aging changes: Muscle atrophy, loss of moisture in larynx, and bowing of vocal cords
- GERD/LPRD
- Excessively dry environment
- Allergic
- Idiopathic
- Iatrogenic: Inhaled steroids such as those used to treat asthma, surgical injury, or compression of recurrent laryngeal nerve
- Vocal cord nodules/polyps ("singer's nodes")
- Retropharyngeal abscess
- Tumor
- Neuromuscular disorder (e.g., myasthenia gravis)
- Rheumatoid arthritis
- Trauma (e.g., endotracheal intubation, blunt or penetrating trauma to neck)

COMMONLY ASSOCIATED CONDITIONS
- Viral pharyngitis
- Diphtheria (rare: Membrane can descend into larynx)
- Pertussis (larynx involved as part of the respiratory system)
- Bronchitis
- Pneumonitis

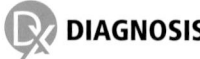 **DIAGNOSIS**

HISTORY
- Hoarseness, throat tickling, rawness, and cough
- Abnormal-sounding voice
- Constant urge to clear the throat
- Possible fever
- Malaise
- Dysphagia/odynophagia
- Regional lymphadenopathy
- Stridor or possible airway obstruction in children (2)
- Hemoptysis
- Laryngospasm or sense of choking
- Allergic rhinitis/rhinorrhea/PND (post-nasal drip)
- Occupation or other reasons for voice overuse
- Smoking history
- Blunt or penetrating trauma to neck
- GERD/LPRD

PHYSICAL EXAM
- Head and neck exam including cervical nodes; cranial nerve exam
- ENT referral for persistent symptoms or fear of foreign body

DIAGNOSTIC TESTS & INTERPRETATION
Lab
- Rarely needed
- White blood cells elevated in bacterial laryngitis
- Viral culture (seldom necessary)

Imaging
Barium swallow, only if needed for differential diagnosis

Diagnostic Procedures/Surgery
- Fiber-optic or indirect laryngoscopy: Looking for red, inflamed, and occasionally hemorrhagic vocal cords; rounded edges and exudate (Reinke edema)

- Consider otolaryngologic evaluation and biopsy: Laryngitis lasting more than 2 weeks in adults with history of smoking or alcohol abuse to rule out malignancy.
- 24-hour pH probe: No difference in incidence of pharyngeal reflux as measured by pH probe between patients with chronic reflux laryngitis and healthy adults (3)
- Strobovideo laryngoscopy for diagnosis of subtle lesions

DIFFERENTIAL DIAGNOSIS
- Diphtheria
- Vocal nodules or polyps
- Laryngeal malignancy
- Thyroid malignancy
- Upper airway malignancy
- Epiglottitis
- Pertussis
- Laryngeal nerve trauma/injury

 TREATMENT

Evidence is limited, but good, that treatment beyond supportive care is ineffective.

MEDICATION
Usually none

First Line
- Analgesics
- Antipyretics (rare)
- Cough suppressants
- Throat lozenges

Second Line
- Inhaled corticosteroids (consider if allergy-induced)
- Oral corticosteroids: only if urgent need (presenter, singer, actor)
- Little or no benefit from antibiotics
- Standard of care is to prescribe proton pump inhibitors for chronic laryngitis if GERD or LPRD are suspected; however, evidence suggests only modest benefit, if any (4).
- Treat nonviral infectious underlying causes
- Candidal laryngitis:
  – Mild cases: Oral antifungal (fluconazole)
  – Amphotericin B or an echinocandin can be given in life-threatening cases

ADDITIONAL TREATMENT
General Measures
- Acute:
  – Usually a self-limited illness lasting l<3 weeks and not severe
  – Antibiotics of no value (5)[A]
  – Proton pump inhibitors of no significant value when laryngitis is due to GERD
  – Avoid excessive voice use, including whispering
  – Steam inhalations or cool-mist humidifier
  – Increase fluid intake, especially in cases associated with excessive dryness
  – Avoid smoking (or secondhand exposure)
  – Salt water gargles

- Chronic:
  – Symptomatic treatment as above
  – Voice therapy (for patients with intermittent dysphagia and vocal abuse)
  – Stop smoking
  – Reduce or stop alcohol intake
  – Occupational change or modification, if exposure
  – Consider discontinuing inhaled corticosteroids
- Reflux laryngitis: Elevate head of bed, other antireflux management; proton pump inhibitors

Issues for Referral
- Consider otolaryngologic evaluation and biopsy for laryngitis lasting more than 2 weeks in adults with history of smoking or alcohol abuse to rule out malignancy
- Consider GI consult, to rule out GERD/LRD

COMPLEMENTARY AND ALTERNATIVE MEDICINE
The following, although not well studied, have been recommended by some experts:
- Barberry
- Blackcurrant
- Echinacea
- Eucalyptus
- German chamomile
- Goldenrod
- Goldenseal
- Hot lemon and honey
- Licorice
- Marshmallow
- Peppermint
- Saw palmetto
- Slippery elm
- Vitamin C
- Zinc

SURGERY/OTHER PROCEDURES
- Vocal cord biopsy of hyperplastic mucosa and areas of leukoplakia if cancer or TB is suspected
- Removal of nodules or polyps if voice therapy fails

 ONGOING CARE

PATIENT EDUCATION
- Educate on the importance of voice rest, including whispering
- Provide assistance with smoking cessation
- Help the patient with modification of other predisposing habits or occupational hazards

PROGNOSIS
Complete clearing of the inflammation without sequelae

COMPLICATIONS
Chronic hoarseness

REFERENCES
1. Joniau S, et al. Reflux and laryngitis: A systemic review. *Otolarygol Head Neck Surg.* 2007;136: 686–92.
2. Gallivan GJ, Gallivan KH, Gallivan HK. Inhaled corticosteroids: hazardous effects on voice-an update. *J Voice.* 2007;21:101–11.
3. Johnson DA. Medical therapy of reflux pharyngitis. *J Clin Gastroenterol.* 2008;42(5):589–93.
4. Tulunay OE. Laryngitis—Diagnosis and management. *Otolaryngol Clin N Am.* 2008;41: 437–52.
5. Reveiz L, Cardona AF, Ospina EG et al. Antibiotics for acute laryngitis in adults. *Cochrane Database Syst Rev.* 2007;CD004783.

ADDITIONAL READING
- Banfield G, Tandon P, Solomons N et al. Hoarse voice: an early symptom of many conditions. *Practitioner.* 2000;244:267–71.
- Gilbert CR, Vipul K, Baram M et al. Novel H1N1 Influenza A Viral Infection Complicated by Alveolar Hemorrhage. *Respir Care.* 2010;55:623–5.
- Moore JM, Vaezi MF et al. Extraesophageal manifestations of gastroesophageal reflux disease: real or imagined? *Curr Opin Gastroenterol.* 2010;26:389–94.
- Reveiz L, Cardona AF, Ospina EG. Antibiotics for acute laryngitis in adults. *Cochrane Database Syst Rev.* 2007;CD004783.
- Rosen CA, Anderson D, Murry T et al. Evaluating hoarseness: keeping your patient's voice healthy. *Am Fam Physician.* 1998;57:2775–82.
- Wheeler DS, Dauplaise DJ, Giuliano JS et al. An infant with fever and stridor. *Pediatr Emerg Care.* 2008;24:46–9.

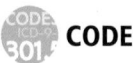 **CODES**

ICD9
- 464.00 Acute laryngitis without mention of obstruction
- 476.0 Chronic laryngitis

CLINICAL PEARLS
- Laryngitis is usually self-limited and needs only comfort care.
- Refer to ENT for direct visualization of vocal cords for prolonged laryngitis.
- Standard treatment is voice rest.

L

LAXATIVE ABUSE

Lauren Michal de Leon, MD
Edward Feller, MD

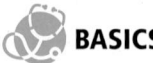

BASICS

DESCRIPTION
Laxative abuse, which may be intentional or unintentional, is a clinically important cause of chronic diarrhea. It manifests commonly as watery diarrhea caused by self-medication or as apparent diarrhea caused by adding various fluids to stool.

- System(s) affected: GI; Nervous; Psychiatric
- Synonym(s): Factitious diarrhea; Cathartic colon

EPIDEMIOLOGY
- Predominant age: 18–40 years with bulimia or anorexia nervosa; 40–60 years without eating disorders
- Predominant sex: Female (90%) > Male
- Children may be given excess laxation by their caregivers (especially mothers), an example of Munchausen syndrome by proxy.

Prevalence
Laxative abuse in different groups:
- Unexplained chronic diarrhea after routine investigations: 3.5–7%
- Patients with binging/purging anorexia and bulimia nervosa: As many as 70%
- Referrals to tertiary-care centers for evaluation of chronic diarrhea: As high as 15%

Geriatric Considerations
- Elderly in nursing homes at increased risk

RISK FACTORS
In patients with eating disorders:
- Longer duration of illness
- Comorbid psychiatric diagnoses (e.g., major depression, obsessive–compulsive disorder, posttraumatic stress disorder, anxiety, borderline personality disorder)
- Earlier appearance of eating disorder symptoms

GENERAL PREVENTION
- Educate patients about normal bowel function, potential adverse effects of excessive laxation, and use of additional medications (e.g., magnesium-containing antacids) that can cause diarrhea.
- Ask patients specifically about laxative use.

ETIOLOGY
- Chronic ingestion of any laxative agent
- Osmotic diarrhea: Magnesium sulfate, nonabsorbable sugars, sodium phosphate
- Secretory diarrhea: Dihydroxy bile salts, castor oil, docusate sodium

- Psychologic factors:
  – Bulimia or anorexia nervosa
  – Secondary gain of attention
  – Hysterical behavior
  – Inappropriate perceptions of "normal" bowel habits
  – Chronic constipation, especially in the elderly

COMMONLY ASSOCIATED CONDITIONS
- Anorexia nervosa
- Bulimia nervosa
- Depression and anxiety
- Borderline personality
- Self-injurious behaviors/suicidal ideation
- Impulsive behavior
- Münchausen syndrome/Münchausen syndrome by proxy

DIAGNOSIS

Chronic diarrhea can be characterized into four types: secretory, osmotic, inflammatory, and fatty diarrhea. Be sure to rule out other causes of chronic diarrhea even if laxative abuse is high on the differential.

HISTORY
- Suspicion in patients with undiagnosed chronic diarrhea, especially when refractory; some patients may not be aware of the association of these over-the-counter medications with chronic diarrhea.
- Signs and symptoms: Increasing frequency of bowel movements; large volume, watery diarrhea; nocturnal bowel movements that are typically absent in osmotic diarrhea or in irritable bowel syndrome
- Additional symptoms: Abdominal pain, rectal pain, nausea, vomiting, weight loss, malaise, muscle weakness
- Additional signs: Hypokalemia, hyperphosphatemia, hypernatremia, skin pigmentation, finger clubbing, cyclic edema, kidney stones, melanosis coli, cardiac arrhythmias with severe hypokalemia
- Monitor "doctor hopping."

PHYSICAL EXAM
- No specific findings in most cases but may include cachexia, evidence of dehydration, abdominal pain or distension, and edema.
- Rarely, severe cases may be associated with renal failure, cardiac arrhythmias, or skeletal muscle paralysis.

DIAGNOSTIC TESTS & INTERPRETATION
Lab
- Serum chemistries: Hypokalemia, metabolic alkalosis (1)[C]
- Urinalysis: bisacodyl, senna, cascara, magnesium, and phosphate titers
- Urine volume and electrolytes (help assess volume status and need for hospitalization).
- Stool sodium, potassium (see algorithm below)
- Stool pH (alkalinization suggests presence of phenolphthalein)
- Stool for laxative titers (bisacodyl, senna, cascara, magnesium, phosphate, castor oil, mineral oil)

Initial lab tests
- Serum electrolytes will show hypokalemia secondary to increased intestinal fluid loss.
  – Acute diarrhea: Metabolic acidosis due to hypovolemia
  – Chronic diarrhea: Metabolic alkalosis secondary to hypokalemia-induced inhibition of chloride uptake in the intestine, thereby inhibiting bicarbonate secretion
- Complete blood count and stool cultures: Rule out infectious cause if history is suspicious.

Follow-Up & Special Considerations
If history and initial lab tests are suspicious for laxative abuse, the following algorithm can be used to confirm diagnosis and determine what type of laxative is being used.

- Collect 24-hour stool: If solid, workup is over.
- Calculate stool osmolality, stool electrolytes, and osmolal gap ($= 290 - 2(Na^+ + K^+)$, where Na^+ and K^+ are the concentrations from the stool sample.)
  – If osmolality >400 mosm/kg, rule out urine contamination of stool Measure urea and creatinine of sample.
  – If osmolality <250–400 mosm/kg, rule out water added to stool (colon cannot dilute stool to osmolality plasma).
  – If osmolality = 250–400 mosm/kg, measure osmolal gap.
    ○ Gap >50: Unmeasured solute; check fecal fat and stool magnesium levels.
    ○ Gap <50: Rule out use of secretory laxative; urinalysis and stool analysis for laxative titers. Do not obtain serum laxative titers as they peak 1–2 hours after ingestion. Urine titers can be 10 × as high as plasma titers.
- Thin-layer chromatography may produce false-positive tests for bisacodyl and false-negative tests for senna (2)[C].

Imaging

Not usually necessary for the diagnosis of laxative abuse; colonoscopy, small-bowel endoscopy, or imaging studies may be needed to evaluate other causes of chronic diarrhea. These tests may be helpful for understanding the chronicity of laxative abuse. Be cautious about perpetuating Munchausen syndrome through extensive workup.

Pathological Findings

- Melanosis coli: Dark brown discoloration of colon with lymph patches visible through mucosa; also can be diagnosed by demonstrating pigment-containing macrophages in lamina propria; only occurs with abuse of anthraquinone-containing laxatives
- Cathartic colon: Refers to dilatation and ahaustral appearance on barium enema or plain film; result of severe and prolonged laxative abuse

DIFFERENTIAL DIAGNOSIS

Any etiology of chronic diarrhea, especially in high-risk groups

 TREATMENT

MEDICATION

- Replace needed vitamins, electrolytes, and minerals.
- Nonstimulant laxatives if needed to treat constipation (3)[C]:
  - Senna best during pregnancy and lactation
  - Lactulose
  - Fiber
- Avoid danthron owing to hepatotoxicity.
- Precautions: Patients may be manipulative in attempts to deny problem; may hide laxatives in hospital rooms.
- Significant possible interactions:
  - Increased rate of intestinal motility may affect rate of absorption of medications (e.g., antibiotics, hormones).
  - Docusate sodium may potentiate hepatotoxicity of other drugs.

ADDITIONAL TREATMENT
General Measures

- Psychological support is essential (3)[C].
- Confront the patient gently with support and understanding.
- Wean patient off laxatives, and substitute high-fiber diet and bulk preparations or short-term saline enemas (3)[C].
- Treat constipation.
- Treat metabolic abnormalities with potassium supplements, etc. (oral preferred) (3)[C].

SURGERY/OTHER PROCEDURES

Avoid exploratory surgery and repetitive evaluations with invasive procedures.

IN-PATIENT CONSIDERATIONS
Admission Criteria

- Persistent diarrhea with evidence of hemodynamic instability
- Electrolyte/metabolic complications, including lactic acidosis
- Cardiac arrhythmias
- Inability to contract for safety

IV Fluids

Resuscitate based on clinical picture. If patient is hemodynamically stable and without significant abnormalities in serum sodium, can give normal saline boluses or PO replacement to correct metabolic alkalosis (chronic) or acidosis (acute) as needed. If patient is hemodynamically unstable, treat volume status as in a hypovolemic shock, while monitoring serum electrolytes closely (especially sodium, potassium, and bicarbonate).

Nursing

If stable, patient does not need continuous telemetry. However, depending on psychiatric history, patient may need constant observation. Special care must be taken to ensure adequate nutrition while in-house and to discard any laxatives from patient possessions. If patient is unstable, telemetry and appropriate vital-signs monitoring may be necessary.

Discharge Criteria

- Psychological support
- Diet and bowel programs

 ONGOING CARE

FOLLOW-UP RECOMMENDATIONS
Patient Monitoring

- Careful psychological counseling
- Careful medical support; show concern by frequent visits as needed.
- Assess serum electrolytes.

DIET

Ensure good nutritional habits.

- Increase fiber intake.
- Adequate calories, especially with bulimia

PROGNOSIS

- Protracted course
- Prognosis related to psychological response
- Prognosis poor with anorexia nervosa

COMPLICATIONS

- Risk of multiple tests, procedures, and surgeries
- Malnutrition
- Electrolyte imbalances (hypokalemia)
- Renal failure
- Fatalities, especially in children given laxatives by parents
- Renal calculi
- No convincing evidence that chronic use of stimulant laxatives causes functional or structural impairment of colon
- Fecal impaction in elderly

REFERENCES

1. Thomas PD, Forbes A, Green J, et al. Guidelines for the investigation of chronic diarrhoea, 2nd edition. *Gut.* 2003;52(Suppl 5):v1–15.
2. Shelton JH, Santa Ana CA, Thompson DR, et al. Factitious Diarrhea Induced by Stimulant Laxatives: Accuracy of Diagnosis by a Clinical Reference Laboratory Using Thin Layer Chromatography. *Clin Chem.* 2006.
3. National Collaborating Center for Mental Health. *Eating disorders: Core interventions in the treatment and management of anorexia nervosa, bulimia nervosa and related eating disorders.* Leicester (UK): British Psychological Society; 2004.

ADDITIONAL READING

- Kovacs D, Palmer RL. The associations between laxative abuse and other symptoms among adults with anorexia nervosa. *Int J Eat Disord.* 2004;36: 224–8.
- Roerig JL, Steffen KJ, Mitchell JE, Zunker C et al. Laxative abuse: epidemiology, diagnosis and management. *Drugs.* 2010;70:1487–503.
- Xing JH, Soffer EE. Adverse effects of laxatives. *Dis Colon Rectum.* 2001;44:1201–9.

See Also (Topic, Algorithm, Electronic Media Element)

Algorithm: Diarrhea, Chronic

 CODES

ICD9

305.90 Other, mixed, or unspecified drug abuse, unspecified use

CLINICAL PEARLS

- Laxative abuse may be intentional or unintentional; it is a common feature of eating disorders and has a female predilection.
- Consider the diagnosis in adolescents with suggestive symptoms.
- As many as 15% of patients referred to tertiary-care centers for unexplained chronic diarrhea abuse laxatives.
- Presentation is diverse and may be nonspecific, including weight loss, weakness, and hypotension without acknowledgment of diarrhea.
- Consider the diagnosis in patients with watery diarrhea, especially when unexplained or refractory.

L

LEAD POISONING

Jason Chao, MD, MS

 BASICS

DESCRIPTION
- Consequence of a high body burden of lead (Pb), an element with no known physiologic value
- Synonym(s): Lead poisoning; Inorganic

EPIDEMIOLOGY
- Predominant age: 1–5 years; adult workers
- Predominant sex: Male > Female (1:1 in childhood)

Incidence
Incidence of lead toxicity declined steadily from 7.5% in 1997 to under 2% in 2006.

Prevalence
- 1999–2002: CDC estimated that 1.6% of US children aged 1–5 years had blood Pb levels >10 μg/dL, but levels are variable among communities and populations.
- Sporadic cases in adults

RISK FACTORS
- Children with pica or with iron-deficiency anemia
- Residence in or frequent visitor to deteriorating pre-1960 housing with leaded-paint surfaces
- Soil/dust near Pb industries or urban roads
- Sibling or playmate with Pb poisoning
- Dust from clothing of Pb worker
- Pb dissolved in water from Pb or Pb-soldered plumbing
- Pb-glazed ceramics, especially with acidic food or drink
- Recent refugee
- Folk remedies and cosmetics:
  – Mexico: Azarcon, greta
  – Dominican Republic: Litargirio, a topical agent
  – Asia and Middle East: Chuifong tokuwan, pay-loo-ah, ghasard, bali goli, kandu, ayurvedic herbal medicine from South Asia, kohl (alkohl, ceruse), surma, saoott, cebagin
- Hobbies: Glazed pottery making, target shooting, Pb soldering, preparing Pb shot or fishing sinkers, stained-glass making, car or boat repair, home remodeling
- Occupational exposure: Plumbers, pipe fitters, Pb miners, auto repairers, glass manufacturers, shipbuilders, printers, plastics manufacturers, Pb smelters and refiners, steel welders or cutters, construction workers, rubber product manufacturers, battery manufacturers, bridge reconstruction workers
- Dietary: Zinc or calcium deficiency
- Imported toys with Pb

Pediatric Considerations
- Children are at increased risk because of incomplete development of the blood-brain barrier at <3 years of age, allowing more Pb into the CNS; ingested Pb has 40% bioavailability in children compared with 10% in adults.
- Common childhood behaviors such as frequent hand-to-mouth activity and pica (repeated ingestion of nonfood products) greatly increase the risk of ingesting Pb.

GENERAL PREVENTION
- Family should receive counseling on potential sources of Pb and methods to decrease Pb exposure. Children at high risk should receive blood Pb screening (1)[C].
- Warn parents about the dangers posed by unsafe renovation methods and to be cognizant of the possibility of new and reemerging sources of lead in children's environments.
- Wet mopping and dusting with a high-phosphate solution (e.g., powdered automatic dishwasher detergent with 1/4 cup/gal of water) will help to control Pb-bearing dust.

PATHOPHYSIOLOGY
Pb replaces calcium in bones. Pb interferes with heme synthesis; causes interstitial nephritis; and interferes with neurotransmitters, especially glutamine; high levels affect blood-brain barrier and lead to encephalopathy, seizures, and coma.

ETIOLOGY
Inhalation of Pb dust or fumes or ingestion of Pb

COMMONLY ASSOCIATED CONDITIONS
Iron-deficiency anemia

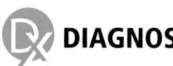 **DIAGNOSIS**

HISTORY
- Often asymptomatic
- Mild to moderate toxicity:
  – May cause myalgia or paresthesia, fatigue, irritability, lethargy
  – Abdominal discomfort, arthralgia, difficulty concentrating, headache, tremor, vomiting, weight loss, muscular exhaustibility
- Severe toxicity: 3 major clinical syndromes:
  – Alimentary type: Anorexia, metallic taste, constipation, severe abdominal cramps owing to intestinal spasm and sometimes associated with abdominal wall rigidity
  – Neuromuscular type (characteristic of adult plumbism): Peripheral neuritis, usually painless and limited to extensor muscles
  – Cerebral type or Pb encephalopathy (more common in children): Seizures; coma; and long-term sequelae, including neurologic defects, retarded mental development, and chronic hyperactivity
- Chronic exposure may cause renal failure.

PHYSICAL EXAM
Often normal; abdominal tenderness may be severe. Neurologic exam may reveal neuropathy or encephalopathy.

DIAGNOSTIC TESTS & INTERPRETATION
Lab
- Blood Pb >10 μg/dL (0.48 μmol/L), collected with Pb-free container
- Use a laboratory that can achieve routine performance within 2 μg/dL.
- CDC Lead Poisoning Classification

Class	Lead (μg/dL)
I	<10
II	10–19
III	20–44
IV	45–69
V	>70

- Screening capillary Pb levels >10 μg/dL (0.48 μmol/L) should be confirmed with a venous sample.
- Hemoglobin and hematocrit slightly low; eosinophilia or basophilic stippling on peripheral smear may be seen but is not diagnostic of Pb toxicity.
- Renal function is decreased in late stages.

Imaging
- Abdominal radiograph for Pb particles in gut if recent ingestion is suspected
- Radiograph of long bones may show lines of increased density in the metaphyseal plate resulting from growth arrest but does not usually alter management.

DIFFERENTIAL DIAGNOSIS
- Alimentary type may be confused with acute abdomen.
- Neuromuscular type may be confused with other polyneuropathies.
- Cerebral type may be confused with attention-deficit disorder, mental retardation, autism, dementia, and other causes of seizures.
- Elevated erythrocyte protoporphyrin may be caused by iron-deficiency anemia or, less commonly, hemolytic anemia.
- Erythropoietic protoporphyria produces a very high erythrocyte protoporphyrin level.

 TREATMENT

- Class I: If Pb level is between 5 and 10 μg/dL, more frequent Pb screening (every 6 months) might be appropriate. Educate family on sources of Pb (2)[C].
- Class II: Repeat Pb testing in 3–6 months. Treat as class III if levels remain elevated (3)[C]. Educate family on sources of Pb.
- Classes III–V: Case report to local health department; complete inspection of home or workplace to determine source of Pb. Screen all family members. Consider chelation for class III; treat classes IV and V (3)[C].

MEDICATION

- Consider oral chelation for class IV; chelation (preferably parenteral) for class V or symptomatic class III or IV (3)[C].
- Do not begin chelation until Pb particles present in gut are cleared (4)[C].

First Line

- Oral chelation: Succimer (Chemet), dimercaptosuccinic acid (DMSA) 10 mg/kg q8h × 5 days; then 10 mg/kg q12h × 2 weeks. This may be repeated after 2 weeks off if Pb levels are not stabilized below 15 μg/dL (<0.72 μmol/L) (5)[C].
- Parenteral chelation (begin after establishment of adequate urine output):
  - Class V or symptomatic: Dimercaprol [British anti-lewisite (BAL)] 75 mg/m^2 given deep IM; then BAL 450 mg/m^2/d divided q4h × 5 days plus Ca edetate calcium disodium (EDTA) 1,500 mg/m^2/d continuous IV infusion × 5 days. If rebound Pb level ≥45 μg/dL (≥2.17 μmol/L), chelation may be repeated after 2-day interval if symptomatic, after 5-day interval if asymptomatic.
  - Class IV asymptomatic: Ca EDTA 1,000 mg/m^2/d × 5 days; may be repeated after 5–7 days
- Diazepam for initial control of seizures; further control maintained with paraldehyde.
- Contraindications: BAL should not be given to patients allergic to peanuts (the drug solution contains peanut oil).
- Precautions:
  - Succimer: GI upset, rash, nasal congestion, muscle pains, elevated liver function tests
  - Ca EDTA: Renal failure, increased excretion of zinc, copper, and iron
  - BAL: Nausea, vomiting, fever, headache, transient hypertension, hepatocellular damage
- Significant possible interactions:
  - Vitamins should not be given concurrently with oral chelation.
  - BAL may precipitate hemolytic crisis in a patient with glucose-6-phosphate dehydrogenase deficiency.

Second Line

Oral chelation with penicillamine (d-penicillamine, Depen, Cuprimine) (5)[C]:

- Penicillin-allergic patient should not receive penicillamine (cross-sensitivity is common).
- 10–15 mg/kg/d given b.i.d. mixed in apple juice/sauce on empty stomach (*not* approved by the Food and Drug Administration)
- Penicillamine may cause GI upset, renal failure, granulocytopenia, liver dysfunction, iron deficiency, drug-induced lupus-like syndrome.

ADDITIONAL TREATMENT

Remove patient from potential source of Pb for class IV or V until complete home inspection is performed (4)[C].

Issues for Referral

Consider consultation if parenteral chelation is required.

IN-PATIENT CONSIDERATIONS

Initial Stabilization

Outpatient care unless parenteral chelation is required or immediate removal from contaminated environment

Admission Criteria

- Blood Pb level >70 μg/dL
- If symptomatic, blood Pb level >35 μg/dL

Discharge Criteria

If Pb source is in the home, the patient must reside elsewhere until the abatement process is completed.

 ONGOING CARE

FOLLOW-UP RECOMMENDATIONS

Avoid visit to any site of potential contamination.

Patient Monitoring

- After chelation, check for rebound Pb level in 7–10 days. Follow with regular monitoring, initially biweekly or monthly.
- Correct iron deficiency or any other nutritional deficiencies present.
- For class II or higher, repeat testing every 3 months until class I level is achieved.

DIET

- If symptomatic, avoidance of excessive fluids
- Avoidance of pica
- Adequate calcium, iron, zinc, and vitamin C to reduce absorption and retention of Pb (5)[B]

PATIENT EDUCATION

- Needleman HL, Landrigan PJ. *Raising Children Toxic Free: How to Keep Your Child Safe from Lead, Asbestos, Pesticides, and Other Environmental Hazards.* New York: Avon Books; 1995.
- National Lead Information Center, 422 South Clinton Avenue, Rochester, NY 14620; (800) 424-5323; http://www.epa.gov/lead/index.html
- National Safety Council, 1121 Spring Lake Drive, Itasca, IL 60143-3201; (800) 621-7615; http://www.nsc.org/news_resources/Resources/Documents/Lead_Poisoning.pdf

PROGNOSIS

- Symptomatic Pb poisoning without encephalopathy generally improves with chelation, but subtle CNS toxicity may be long-lasting or permanent.
- If encephalopathy occurs, permanent sequelae (e.g., mental retardation, seizure disorder, blindness, and hemiparesis) occurs in 25–50%.

COMPLICATIONS

- CNS toxicity may be long-lasting or permanent.
- Long-term Pb exposure may cause chronic renal failure (Fanconi-like syndrome), gout, or Pb line (blue-black) on gingival tissue.
- Pb exposure in pregnancy is associated with reduced birth weight and premature birth.
- Pb is an animal teratogen.

REFERENCES

1. Centers for Disease Control and Prevention. Recommendations for blood lead screening of Medicaid-eligible children aged 1–5 years: an updated approach to targeting a group at high risk. *MMWR.* 2009;58(No. RR-9):1–11.
2. Binns HJ, Campbell C, Brown MJ, et al. Interpreting and managing blood lead levels of less than 10 microg/dL in children and reducing childhood exposure to lead: recommendations of the Centers for Disease Control and Prevention Advisory Committee on Childhood Lead Poisoning Prevention. *Pediatrics.* 2007;120:e1285–98.
3. American Academy of Pediatrics Committee on Environmental Health. Lead exposure in children:

prevention, detection, and management. *Pediatrics.* 2005;116:1036–46.
4. Centers for Disease Control and Prevention. *Managing Elevated Blood Lead Levels among Young Children: Recommendations from the Advisory Committee on Childhood Lead Poisoning Prevention.* Atlanta, GA: Centers for Disease Control and Prevention; 2002.
5. Woolf AD, Goldman R, Bellinger DC. Update on the clinical management of childhood lead poisoning. *Pediatr Clin North Am.* 2007;54:271–94, viii.

ADDITIONAL READING

- Chandramouli K, Steer CD, Ellis M, Emond AM et al. Effects of early childhood lead exposure on academic performance and behaviour of school age children. *Arch Dis Child.* 2009;94:844–8.
- Dietrich KN, Ware JH, Salganik M, et al. Effect of chelation therapy on the neuropsychological and behavioral development of lead-exposed children after school entry. *Pediatrics.* 2004;114:19–26.

See Also (Topic, Algorithm, Electronic Media Element)

Anemia, Iron Deficiency

 CODES

ICD9

- 984.0 Toxic effect of inorganic lead compounds
- 984.9 Toxic effect of unspecified lead compound

CLINICAL PEARLS

- The following children should have Pb screening:
  - 6–11 months of age with 1 or more risk factors:
    - Live in or visit a house built before 1960 with peeling paint or recent renovation
    - Sibling/playmate with elevated Pb
    - Live with adult with job or hobby involving Pb
    - Live near industry likely to release Pb
  - Children living in high-risk communities (>12% elevated Pb) should be tested yearly from ages 1–5.
  - Newly arrived refugees
  - Children in low-risk areas should be screened by a questionnaire.
- There is no clear safe Pb level. A level <10 μg/dL is used to define "normal," but there is increasing evidence that levels <10 μg/dL are detrimental to neural development in young children.
- There are no studies that show benefit of chelation at asymptomatic class III. Removal of sources of Pb is paramount.

L

LEGIONNAIRES' DISEASE

Rajneesh S. Hazarika, MD, MS

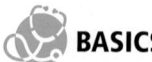 **BASICS**

DESCRIPTION

The term *Legionnaires' disease* was coined for an epidemic of lower respiratory tract disease occurring among people attending an American Legion convention in Philadelphia in 1976. The previously unknown causative bacterium was identified and named *Legionella pneumophila*; it may cause pneumonia or flulike illness:

- Ranks among the 3 most common pneumonias in the clinical setting
- System(s) affected: GI; Pulmonary
- Synonym(s): Legionella pneumonia; Legionellosis

EPIDEMIOLOGY

- Predominant age: 15 months–84 years old; increased >50 years old
- Predominant sex: Male > Female

Incidence

- True incidence is not well known
- Probably only 2–10% of cases are reported.
- May increase with the rise in population density in some urban areas, hotel, or cruise ship stays within previous 2 weeks and more complex infrastructures
- Outbreaks occur most often at the end of the summer and early fall.

RISK FACTORS

- Smoking
- Alcohol abuse
- Immunosuppression/HIV
- Chronic cardiopulmonary disease
- Surgery
- Advanced age
- Renal failure
- Fever >39°C
- Hyponatremia
- Liver dysfunction
- Creatine kinase elevation

GENERAL PREVENTION

- Heating water to 60–70°C may help prevent water contamination.
- Ultraviolet light or copper-silver ionization are bactericidal.
- Monochloramine disinfection of municipal water supplies is associated with decreased risk for Legionella infection (1)[B].

ETIOLOGY

- *Legionella pneumophila*, a weak gram-negative organism, is a saprophytic water bacterium, which is widely distributed in soil and water. Serogroups 1, 2, and 6 account for most of the cases. The optimum temperature for growth is 40–45°C. It can also be associated with organic material in sediment.
- Mode of transmission:
  – Aerosolization
  – Aspiration
  – Direct instillation into the lungs by equipment (such as respiratory equipment)
  – Most important mode: Aerosolization and airborne dissemination of contaminated water
  – Patients may acquire by inhaling organisms while showering
- Recently, community outbreaks have been associated with whirlpools, spas, and fountains.

COMMONLY ASSOCIATED CONDITIONS

Pontiac fever: Self-limited flulike illness without pneumonia caused by *Legionella* species

 DIAGNOSIS

- Range of illness from asymptomatic seroconversion, mild febrile illness, to severe pneumonia
- Incubation 2–10 days
- Fever, chills
- Malaise, weakness, lethargy
- Anorexia
- Myalgia
- Headache
- Watery diarrhea in up to 50%
- Nausea and vomiting in 10–20%
- Dry cough, which may become productive
- Pleuritic chest pain in up to 33%
- Relative bradycardia in up to 67% of patients
- Neuropsychiatric symptoms of confusion, disorientation, obtundation, depression, hallucinations, insomnia, seizures in up to 25%
- Blood-streaked sputum; gross hemoptysis rare
- Hyponatremia
- Hypophosphatemia
- Elevated serum transaminases
- Elevated creatine kinase
- ~50% of hospitalized patients present with PO$_2$ <60 mm Hg.
- Hypotension (17%)
- Wound infections with *Legionella* have been reported.

HISTORY

- Elicit immunosuppression risk factors.
- Elicit characteristics about cough (may not be productive).
- Chest pain with hemoptysis can occur.
- GI symptoms with diarrhea and nausea are frequent.

PHYSICAL EXAM

Rales with signs of consolidation. Fever is usually present.

DIAGNOSTIC TESTS & INTERPRETATION
Lab
Initial lab tests

- Gold standard is sputum culture for *Legionella*. Alert lab about possible diagnosis (buffered charcoal yeast extract agar) (2,3)[C].
- Urinary antigen detects serogroup 1 (which causes most human disease) (2)[B].
- Urinary antigen tests are highly specific (99%) but variably sensitive (74%) (4)[A].
- The combination of respiratory specimen cultures and urine *Legionella* antigen testing is optimal for diagnosis.
- Silver and Gimenez stains for lung tissue/specimens
- Disorders that may alter lab results: Direct immunofluorescence can cross-react with *Pseudomonas* and *Bacteroides* sp., *E. coli*, and *Haemophilus*.
- Nonspecific abnormalities may include renal and hepatic dysfunction, thrombocytopenia, hyponatremia, and hematuria.

Imaging
Initial approach

Chest radiograph (3)[B]:

- Not specific for *Legionella*
- Commonly with lower lobe patchy alveolar infiltrate with consolidation, usually unilateral
- Cavitation or abscess, especially in immunocompromised
- Pleural effusion in up to 50%
- May take from 1–4 months for the radiograph to return to normal. Progression of infiltrate may be seen despite antibiotic therapy.

Diagnostic Procedures/Surgery

Transtracheal aspiration or bronchoscopy for sputum/lung samples may be needed.

Pathological Findings
- Multifocal pneumonia with alveolitis and bronchiolitis, with fibrinous pleuritis; may have serous or serosanguineous pleural effusion
- Abscess formation occurs in up to 20% of patients.
- Progression of infiltrates, despite appropriate therapy, may be suggestive of Legionnaires' disease. Also, improvement on radiograph may not correlate with clinical findings (longer lag times on radiographic findings).

DIFFERENTIAL DIAGNOSIS
- Other bacterial pneumonias
- Atypical pneumonias with mycoplasma and chlamydia
- Viral pneumonias

 TREATMENT

MEDICATION
First Line
- Antibiotics that achieve high intracellular concentrations are most effective (macrolides, rifampin, tetracyclines, and quinolones) (2,3)[C]
- Levofloxacin is the preferred agent (5)[B].
- Levofloxacin 750 mg IV per day (switch to p.o. when patient is afebrile) times 10–14 days
- Azithromycin 500 mg IV per day p.o. times 7–10 days
- Addition of rifampin: 600 mg q12h p.o. or IV; this should be provided along with the above recommendations in very ill patients.
- Contraindications: Hypersensitivity reactions
- Precautions: Liver disease
- Significant possible interactions:
  – Can increase theophylline, carbamazepine, and digoxin levels; can increase activity of oral anticoagulants
  – May decrease the effectiveness of oral anticoagulants, steroids, digoxin, quinidine, oral contraceptives, and hypoglycemic agents
- Longer courses of treatment of up to 21 days may be needed in immunocompromised patients.

Second Line
- Erythromycin 30–60 mg/kg/d p.o. or IV, divided into 4 doses for 10–21 days
- May be used along with rifampin:
  – 100 mg q12h IV for 2 doses, then 100 mg b.i.d., or p.o. 200 mg for 1 dose, then 100 mg b.i.d.
  – 100 mg IV or p.o. q12h
- Sulfamethoxazole IV or p.o.: 5 mg/kg TMP q8h

ADDITIONAL TREATMENT
General Measures
- The severity of the illness and the support available in the outpatient setting will dictate the appropriate site for care.
- Supportive care
- Maintaining oxygenation, hydration, and electrolyte balance while providing antibiotic therapy
- There is a higher chance of extrapulmonary complications and higher mortality in AIDS patients.

IN-PATIENT CONSIDERATIONS
Admission Criteria
- Inability to tolerate oral antibiotics
- Hypoxemia

Discharge Criteria
- Afebrile
- Able to tolerate oral antibiotics

 ONGOING CARE

FOLLOW-UP RECOMMENDATIONS
Patient Monitoring
- Respiratory status, hydration, and electrolyte status should be monitored closely.
- A chest radiograph is not useful to monitor the clinical response.

PATIENT EDUCATION
- Educate patients regarding prevention/avoidance measures, lowering their risk status, and, if infected already, about the expected course of the disease.
- Disease prevention: Elimination of the pathogens from water supplies
- Person-to-person transmission has not been observed.

PROGNOSIS
- Recovery is variable; some patients experience rapid improvement with defervescence in 3–5 days and recovery is complete in 6–10 days, whereas others may have a much more protracted course despite treatment.
- Mortality rate can approach 50% with nosocomial infections.

COMPLICATIONS
- Dehydration
- Hyponatremia
- Respiratory insufficiency requiring ventilator support
- Endocarditis (most common extrapulmonary site)
- Disseminated intravascular coagulation
- Renal failure
- Multiple organ dysfunction syndrome (MODS)
- Coma
- Death occurs in 10% of treated nonimmunocompromised patients and in up to 80% of untreated immunocompromised patients.
- Bacteremia or abscess formation occurs in immunocompromised patients.
- Extrapulmonary disease can occur in the form of:
  – Encephalitis
  – Cellulitis
  – Sinusitis
  – Pancreatitis
  – Pyelonephritis
  – Endocarditis
  – Pericarditis
  – Perirectal abscess

REFERENCES
1. Flannery B, Gelling LB, Vugia DJ, et al. Reducing Legionella colonization in water systems with monochloramine. *Emerg Infect Dis*. 2006;12: 588–96.
2. Yzerman EP, den Boer JW, Lettinga KD, et al. Sensitivity of three urinary antigen tests associated with clinical severity in a large outbreak of Legionnaires' disease in The Netherlands. *J Clin Microbiol*. 2002;40:3232–6.
3. Tan MJ, Tan JS, Hamor RH, et al. The radiologic manifestations of Legionnaire's disease. The Ohio Community-Based Pneumonia Incidence Study Group. *Chest*. 2000;117:398–403.
4. Shimada T, Noguchi Y, Jackson JL, Miyashita J, Hayashino Y, Kamiya T, Yamazaki S, Matsumura T, Fukuhara S. Systematic Review and Metaanalysis: Urinary Antigen Tests for Legionellosis. *Chest*. 2009 Mar 24.
5. Blázquez Garrido RM, Espinosa Parra FJ, Alemany Francés L, Ramos Guevara RM, Sánchez-Nieto JM, Segovia Hernández M, Serrano Martínez JA, Huerta FH et al. Antimicrobial chemotherapy for Legionnaires disease: levofloxacin versus macrolides. *Clin Infect Dis*. 2005;40:800–6.

ADDITIONAL READING
- *Committee on Infectious Diseases of American Academy of Pediatrics. Red Book*. Elk Grove Village: American Academy of Pediatrics; 2006:417–18.
- Mandell LA, Wunderink RG, Anzueto A, et al. Infectious Diseases Society of America/American Thoracic Society Consensus Guidelines on the Management of Community-Acquired Pneumonia in Adults. *Clin Inf Dis*. 2007;44:S27–72.

See Also (Topic, Algorithm, Electronic Media Element)
Pneumonia, Bacterial

 CODES

ICD9
482.84 Pneumonia due to legionnaires' disease

CLINICAL PEARLS
- Consider Legionnaires' disease in pneumonia in presence of GI symptoms, especially diarrhea; neurologic findings, especially confusion; fever >39°C; gram stain of respiratory secretions with many neutrophils but few organisms; hyponatremia.
- Consider Legionnaires' disease in nosocomial pneumonia.

L

LEISHMANIASIS

Theodore R. Brown, DO, MPH

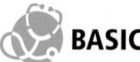 **BASICS**

A clinically heterogeneous group, ranging from a single self-healing ulcer, to destructive mucocutaneous disease, to potentially lethal visceral disease, caused by infection with protozoa of the genus *Leishmania*, which are transmitted by an infected female sandfly

DESCRIPTION
- Cutaneous leishmaniasis (CL):
  - 1 or more pruritic, erythematous papules appear ~6 weeks after infected sandfly bite
  - Papule(s) enlarge and form an ulcer up to 5 cm with a firm, indurated border; most heal without treatment, though slowly and with scarring
  - Treatment considered if lesions are large (>4 cm), multiple (>3), limit function (hands, feet, joints, eye), or affect cosmesis (face, ear) (1,2)
  - Divided into Old World (OWCL) and New World (NWCL or American)
- Visceral leishmaniasis (VL):
  - Most severe form; 90% fatal if untreated
  - Parasite leaves skin and infects lymph nodes, spleen, liver, bone marrow
  - Usually insidious/chronic, disease presenting 3–8 months after inoculation
  - Various regional forms (e.g., African, Mediterranean, and Indian kala-azar)
  - Symptoms: Fever (usually 2 spikes/day), abdominal pain, weight loss, decreased appetite, diarrhea, weakness, nonproductive cough, headache, peripheral edema
  - Signs: Fever, splenomegaly, lymphadenopathy, hepatomegaly, bleeding diathesis
- Mucocutaneous leishmaniasis (MCL):
  - Presents months to years after primary CL; primarily due to *L. braziliensis*
  - CL spreads via lymphatics, infects mucosa of nose, palate, pharynx, larynx
  - Begins as erythema/ulceration of the nasal septum, progresses to painful erosions
- Synonyms:
  - OWCL: Oriental sore; Delhi boil; Aleppo boil
  - NWCL: American cutaneous leishmaniasis; Chiclero ulcer (ear involvement); Espundia (severe mucocutaneous disease); Bush yaws; Uta; Picatura de pito
  - VL: Kala-azar; Black fever; Dumdum fever
- Systems affected: Skin/Exocrine; Pulmonary; Hematopoietic; Lymphatic; Immunologic; Hepatic

EPIDEMIOLOGY
- Found in 88 countries (72 of them developing):
  - 90% of VL occurs in Bangladesh, India, Nepal, Sudan, and Brazil.
  - 90% of CL occurs in Afghanistan, Algeria, Brazil, Iran, Peru, Saudi Arabia, and Syria.
- Both underestimated, but increasing in many parts of the world due to migration, malnutrition, and development (3).

Incidence
- Population at risk is approximately 350 million
- Worldwide incidence of CL is 1–2 million.
- Worldwide incidence of VL is 500,000 (3).
- Hundreds of confirmed CL, and a few VL, cases have been reported in US military returned to the US after serving in Afghanistan/Iraq.

Prevalence
- Worldwide estimated prevalence of 12 million
- Cases may go unreported due to misdiagnosis, limited access to care/diagnosis, lack of overt illness, not a notifiable disease in all countries (3)

RISK FACTORS
- In endemic areas, children > young adults
- Malnutrition; incomplete therapy of initial dz
- AIDS (coinfection is a recognized entity)
- Migrating to or working in endemic areas (e.g., military deployments, urbanization)

GENERAL PREVENTION
- Use of pesticides, especially synthetic pyrethroids, against sandflies and their habitat
- Wearing of long sleeves and pants whenever possible (even thin, light clothing is protective)
- Application of insect repellant to all exposed skin
- Use of permethrin-impregnated bed netting (mesh size 0.6 mm × 0.6 mm; sandflies fit through standard mosquito netting) while sleeping
- Avoidance of outdoor activities from dusk to dawn when sandflies are most active
- Early diagnosis and treatment of human cases
- Elimination/control of animal reservoirs (especially domestic canines)
- Currently no vaccine for general human use

PATHOPHYSIOLOGY
- Infected female sandfly (70 of the 800 known species carry *Leishmania*) bites mammalian host (humans, canines, rodents) and injects *Leishmania* promastigotes (10–15 μm flagellated forms)
- Organisms phagocytized by macrophages and transform into round amastigotes (2–3 μm nonflagellated forms)
- Amastigotes undergo asexual division until macrophage ruptures/releases amastigotes
- Amastigotes infect other macrophages, divide
- Sandfly bites infected host, ingests macrophages
- Amastigotes transform into promastigotes and reproduce in sandfly gut
- Promastigotes migrate to sandfly proboscis to be injected with next bite, repeating cycle (1)

ETIOLOGY
More than 30 different *Leishmania* species, varying by region and by organ/disease predilection (1):
- CL: *L. tropica* (Mediterranean, Afghanistan); *L. major* (Middle East, Western/Northern Africa, Kenya); *L. aethiopica* (Ethiopia); *L. mexicana* (Central America, Amazon)
- VL: *L. donovani* (China, India, Iran, Sudan, Kenya, Ethiopia); *L. infantum* (Mediterranean); *L. chagasi* (Brazil, Columbia, Venezuela, Argentina)
- MCL: *L. braziliensis* complex (Brazil, Peru, Ecuador, Columbia, Venezuela)

COMMONLY ASSOCIATED CONDITIONS
- Fulminant kala azar has been described in association with AIDS and malnutrition.
- Diffuse cutaneous leishmaniasis: Disseminated lesions resembling leprosy:
  - Defective cell-mediated immune response
  - Never heal spontaneously, relapse after treatment
- Post-kala azar dermal leishmaniasis (PKDL):
  - Chronic cutaneous form, may develop after VL recovery; long treatment (3)

 DIAGNOSIS

Signs and/or symptoms consistent with leishmaniasis in an individual from an endemic area or history of travel to an endemic area, including:
- Chronic cutaneous ulcer
- Acutely febrile patients
- Fulminant disease in HIV-positive (or otherwise immunocompromised) individuals
- Children with chronic subfebrile temperatures, organomegaly, and delayed growth (1)[C]

HISTORY
- Living in or traveling to an endemic area within the last year:
  - Must include in the differential in the face of increasing worldwide travel and nongovernmental organization/military deployments (2)[C]
  - Inform any post-travel treating physicians of their travel, especially when presenting with skin lesions or fever
- History of prior treatment for skin lesions, fever, or diagnosed leishmaniasis

DIAGNOSTIC TESTS & INTERPRETATION
- Parasites in tissue sample is confirmatory (1)[B].
- Routine labs (e.g., hematologic, chemistry, etc.) may indicate organs/systems involved.
- Other tests such as PCR and culture only performed in specialized laboratories
- Leishmanin (Montenegro) skin test: Similar to tuberculosis skin test; measures delayed-type hypersensitivity to intradermal injection of killed promastigotes; NOT considered useful for diagnosis

Lab
Initial lab tests
- Parasite demonstration in ulcer scrapings/tissue sample is the gold standard (CL, VL) (1)[B]:
  - For cutaneous lesions, a biopsy as well as skin smears are taken from the ulcer margin.
  - For visceral disease, biopsies can be taken of the bone marrow, spleen (most sensitive), liver, or lymph nodes.
  - Culture and PCR can be performed at specialized labs/facilities.
- Other lab abnormalities (VL): Anemia, leukopenia, thrombocytopenia, transaminitis, hypoalbuminemia, hypergammaglobulinemia, hyperbilirubinemia, proteinuria, and hematuria
- Other labs such as a dipstick (K39) and a latex agglutination test (KATEX) are available and useful in field settings and the immunosuppressed patient, respectively (3)[C].

Imaging
- Generally not helpful in diagnosis
- HSM can be demonstrated by US and/or CT.

Diagnostic Procedures/Surgery
Algorithm for cutaneous leishmaniasis diagnosis (1)[C]:
- Excisional biopsy from ulcer margin (4–6 mm):
  - Divide specimen, place half in 4% formaldehyde (histology) and half in 0.9% NaCl (culture/PCR).
- Multiple skin smears from ulcer margin:
  - Ensure "bloodless" specimens.
  - Prepare 4–5 slides, dry by evaporation.
  - Send several slides to reference lab, stain others with modified Giemsa.

• Draw serology and photograph lesion(s).

DIFFERENTIAL DIAGNOSIS
• CL: Buruli ulcer, lupus vulgaris, leprosy, neoplasm, cat scratch disease, sporotrichosis, cryptococcosis
• VL: Malaria, typhus, mononucleosis, brucellosis, schistosomiasis, tuberculosis, hepatic abscess
• MCL: Neoplasm, mycoses, syphilis, sarcoidosis

 # TREATMENT

• Goal: Maximize effectiveness/minimize toxicity.
• Treatment should be conducted under the supervision of, or in consultation with, a physician experienced in the management of leishmaniasis:
  – Contact the CDC at (800)-CDC-INFO (800-232-4636) for such consultation and for the most up-to-date medication dosing.
  – In the US, medications discussed below only available from the CDC Drug Service, (404) 639-3670
• Treatment should be individualized based on the likely/confirmed *Leishmania* species, known resistance patterns, region of disease acquisition, and host factors.

MEDICATION
• Cutaneous leishmaniasis:
  – Treatment of ulcers is not always required; consider treating if lesions are multiple, large, involve/threaten a body structure or function (eye, hand), or for cosmesis.
  – Treatment may be local or systemic, local treatment including (2)[B]:
    ○ Local heat application (FDA-approved radio-frequency heat generator)
    ○ Cryotherapy with liquid nitrogen (2–3 applications, 15–20 sec each)
    ○ Topical paromomycin ointment
    ○ Local intradermal pentavalent antimony injection
  – Treatment should be systemic if disease is VL or MCL, New World pathogen, or resistant to local treatment (1)[C]:
    ○ Systemic treatment should be considered for the following lesions: Facial; multiple (>3) (1)[C]; large (>4 cm); or involve the hands, feet, or joints (2)[C]
• Visceral/mucocutaneous leishmaniasis:
  – Systemic treatment for all cases
  – See below for 1st-/2nd-line treatment options.

First Line
• Cutaneous leishmaniasis:
  – Pentavalent antimonials are considered the gold standard for treatment (2)[B],(4)[A]:
    ○ Sodium stibogluconate (Pentostam) 20 mg/kg/d IV or IM × 20 days
    ○ Meglumine antimonate (Glucantime) IM; same regimen as Pentostam
    ○ Adverse effects: Pancreatitis, hepatitis, marrow suppression, QT prolongation, myalgias, fatigue, headache, nausea, rash
    ○ Relapses and incomplete responses may be treated with the same regimen for 40–60 days; addition of oral allopurinol (Zyloprim) 20–30 mg/kg/d in 3 divided doses has been effective
• Visceral leishmaniasis:
  – Liposomal amphotericin B (AmBisome) 3 mg/kg/d IV days 1–5, 14, 21:

    ○ Lipid formulation masks amphotericin B from susceptible tissues with preferential uptake by reticuloendothelial cells.
    ○ Most effective drug against VL, high cost (5)[B]
  – Pentostam 20 mg/kg/d IV or IM × 28 days
  – Miltefosine (Impavido) 2.5 mg/kg/d p.o. × 28 days (available from CDC):
    ○ The first oral agent effective in treating VL, recommended for visceral disease in India/Ethiopia and for cutaneous disease in Colombia/Bolivia (6)[B]
• Mucocutaneous leishmaniasis:
  – Pentostam 20 mg/kg/d IV or IM × 28 days
  – Glucantime IM; same regimen as Pentostam
  – Impavido 2.5 mg/kg/d p.o. × 28 days
  – Amphotericin B (Fungizone, not FDA approved) 0.5 mg/kg IV every day or q.o.d. for up to 8 weeks

Second Line
• Cutaneous leishmaniasis:
  – Impavido 2.5 mg/kg/d p.o. × 28 days
  – Pentamidine (Pentam 300, not FDA approved) 2–3 mg/kg IV or IM every day or q.o.d. × 4–7 doses:
    ○ Adverse effects: Diabetes mellitus, nephrotoxicity, hypotension, arrhythmias, anemia, hepatitis, neurologic
    ○ Higher doses needed in MCL cause diabetes. Monitor blood sugar before each injection.
  – Azole drugs have been used, but have unreliable results, therapy-limiting adverse events, and are not effective against MCL.
• Visceral leishmaniasis:
  – Fungizone (not FDA approved) 1 mg/kg/d IV × 15–20 days:
    ○ Adverse effects: Infusion reactions, thrombophlebitis, myocarditis, hypokalemia, renal dysfunction; requires hospitalization/monitoring
  – Paromomycin (not FDA approved) 15 mg/kg/d IM × 21 days:
    ○ Alone or in combination with pentavalent antimonials (5)[B]

Pregnancy Considerations
Miltefosine (Impavido) contraindicated in pregnancy

ADDITIONAL TREATMENT
General Measures
• Bed rest, oral hygiene, and good nutrition
• Transfusions (anemia), antibiotics (infections)
• Periodic ECG monitoring during prolonged therapy with pentavalent antimonials (QT prolongation)

SURGERY/OTHER PROCEDURES
Adjunctive splenectomy or reconstructive surgery for tissue damage (MCL)

IN-PATIENT CONSIDERATIONS
Inpatient care for blood transfusions, complicating superinfections, frequent IV medication, and monitoring for adverse effects

 # ONGOING CARE

FOLLOW-UP RECOMMENDATIONS
Patient Monitoring
• Follow-up at 3 and 12 months to evaluate treatment effectiveness and to detect relapses
• PKDL should be treated like initial illness.
• Periodic monitoring of ECG, liver function, and renal function during prolonged therapy

PATIENT EDUCATION
Information for patients:
http://www.cdc.gov/ncidod/dpd/parasites/leishmania

PROGNOSIS
• Variable, depending on species, disease type (VL, CL, or MCL), and host factors (i.e., immune status). Localized CL may resolve without treatment. CL cure rate of 76% with pentavalent antimonials (7)[A].
• VL mortality is ~90% untreated/~10% treated.

COMPLICATIONS
• Cutaneous: Secondary bacterial infections; scarring; development of MCL with disfigurement and scarring; adverse effects of treatment
• Visceral: PKDL in 3–10% of kala-azar cases; secondary bacterial infections; GI bleeding, hemorrhage, DIC; nephrotic syndrome, glomerulonephritis; cirrhosis, acute liver failure; persistent splenomegaly; death

REFERENCES
1. Neuber H. Leishmaniasis. *J Dtsch Dermatol Ges*. 2008;6:754–65.
2. Palumbo E. Current treatment for cutaneous leishmaniasis: a review. *Am J Ther*. 2009;16:178–82.
3. Desjeux P. Leishmaniasis: Current situation and new perspectives. *Comp Imunol Microbiol infec Dis*. 2004;27:305–18.
4. Mitropoulos P, Konidas P, Durkin-Konidas M et al. New World cutaneous leishmaniasis: updated review of current and future diagnosis and treatment. *J Am Acad Dermatol*. 2010;63:309–22.
5. Sundar S, Chatterjee M. Visceral leishmaniasis - current therapeutic modalities. *Indian J Med Res*. 2006;123:345–52.
6. Berman JJ. Treatment of leishmaniasis with miltefosine: 2008 status. *Expert Opin Drug Metab Toxicol*. 2008;4:1209–16.
7. Tuon FF, Amato VS, Graf ME, et al. Treatment of New World cutaneous leishmaniasis–a systematic review with a meta-analysis. *Int J Dermatol*. 2008;47:109–24.

 # CODES

ICD9
• 085.0 Leishmaniasis visceral (kala-azar)
• 085.2 Cutaneous leishmaniasis, Asian desert
• 085.3 Cutaneous leishmaniasis, Ethiopian

CLINICAL PEARLS
• Any patient with a nonhealing ulcer and history of travel to endemic area; leishmaniasis until proven otherwise:
  – Consider VL in febrile returning traveler.
• Preventive measures and proper pre-travel counseling of great importance
• Military deployed to Iraq/Afghanistan at higher risk
• In the US, CL cases in Texas and Oklahoma
• Previous infection does not provide immunity.

L

LEPROSY

Daria I. Grisanzio, PharmD, RPh
Joseph Grisanzio, MD

 BASICS

DESCRIPTION
- A chronic, granulomatous infection caused by *Mycobacterium leprae*, an acid-fast bacillus, preferentially affecting cooler regions of the body (e.g., skin, mucous membranes, peripheral nerves)
- Classification (World Health Organization [WHO] system most frequently used):
  – Paucibacillary (PB): No more than 5 skin lesions; no detectable bacilli on skin smears
  – Multibacillary (MB): 6 or more lesions; may be skin-smear–positive
- Classification (Ridley-Jopling) based on skin/neurologic changes and biopsy:
  – Indeterminate (I), tuberculoid (TT), borderline tuberculoid (BT), mid-borderline (MB), borderline lepromatous, lepromatous (LL)
- System(s) affected: Endocrine/Metabolic; Hemic/Lymphatic/Immunologic; Musculoskeletal; Nervous; Pulmonary; Reproductive; Skin/Exocrine
- Synonym(s): Hansen disease

EPIDEMIOLOGY
Incidence
- Rare in the US: 150 new cases in 2008
- Global incidence decreased 3.54% from 2007 to 2008
- 249,007 incident cases detected worldwide at the beginning of 2009

Prevalence
- 213,036 registered cases in 121 countries worldwide at the beginning of 2009
- Highest rates of endemic disease in India, Brazil, Angola, Central African Republic, Democratic Republic of Congo, Mozambique, Madagascar, Nepal, and the United Republic of Tanzania
- May present at any age, although cases in infants <1 year are extremely rare
- Predominant sex: Male:Female = 1.5:1

Pediatric Considerations
Rare in infants <1 year

Pregnancy Considerations
Women with leprosy who become pregnant are more likely to develop type I and type II reactions and disease relapse, occurring postpartum period or during pregnancy (usually 3rd trimester) and with lactation, respectively.

RISK FACTORS
- Close family contacts of untreated leprosy patients have 8-fold increased risk
- Impaired cell-mediated immunity
- Poor socioeconomic status
- Contact with infected animals, in particular, armadillos (especially in Texas and Louisiana)
- Military service or travel abroad, particularly to endemic areas

Genetics
- Specific human leukocyte antigen-associated genes may be linked to different classes of disease.
- Various genetic polymorphisms suggested in disease susceptibility:
  – IL-6 and NOD2 gene expression may be involved.

GENERAL PREVENTION
- Early case detection to suppress infectiousness and control spread:
  – Increased emphasis on self-reporting
- Evidence exists for use of bacillus Calmette–Guérin vaccination in certain locations worldwide in order to aid in disease prevention.

PATHOPHYSIOLOGY
- Widespread dissemination once respiratory tract is infected
- Vigorous cellular immune response results in tuberculoid form.
- Minimal cellular immune response results in lepromatous form.

ETIOLOGY
- *M. leprae*: Incubation period is frequently 3–5 years, although a range of 6 months to several decades has been seen.
- Spread via respiratory transmission, possibly via broken skin

COMMONLY ASSOCIATED CONDITIONS
HIV-positive patients with early or subclinical leprosy more likely to develop overt disease. Concurrent leprosy may accelerate HIV disease course.

 DIAGNOSIS

HISTORY
- Known or suspected contact with patient with leprosy
- Skin lesions and/or enlarged nerves accompanied by sensory loss

PHYSICAL EXAM
- Indeterminate leprosy (I):
  – 1 or more hypopigmented or hyperpigmented macules
  – Anesthetic patches, although sensation is preserved in early stages
- TT:
  – Initial hypopigmented, hypesthetic macules with sharp demarcations
  – Nerve involvement occurs early: Ulnar, peroneal (foot drop), and greater auricular nerves may be palpably and visibly enlarged; neuritic pain; muscle atrophy—small muscles of the hand; facial nerve involvement leads to lagophthalmos, keratitis, and corneal ulceration.
- LL:
  – More generalized, sometimes nondistinct lesions
  – Nerve involvement occurs later; affects distal extremities initially

DIAGNOSTIC TESTS & INTERPRETATION
Lab
Initial lab tests
- Demonstration of acid-fast bacilli in skin smears made by scraped-incision method
- Histologic involvement of peripheral nerves pathognomonic
- Mild anemia, elevated erythrocyte sedimentation rate, hyperglobulinemia

- Serodiagnostic assay: Detects antibody to phenolic glycolipid 1; sensitivity of >95% in LL and ~30% in TT
- Detection of *M. leprae* in tissue by polymerase chain reaction
- Lymphocyte migration inhibition test. Cell-mediated immunity to *M. leprae* is absent in patients with LL but present in those with TT.

Diagnostic Procedures/Surgery
- Skin biopsy
- Fine-needle aspiration is being examined as an alternative or addition to skin biopsy.

Pathological Findings
- TT: Noncaseating granulomas containing lymphocytes, epithelioid cells, and perhaps giant cells; bacilli difficult to demonstrate
- LL: Granulomas comprising macrophages, large foam cells, and many intracellular bacilli frequently in spheroidal masses
- Borderline leprosy: Granulomas change from epithelioid cell predominance in BT to a macrophage predominance as the lepromatous pole is approached.

DIFFERENTIAL DIAGNOSIS
- Systemic lupus erythematosus
- Lupus vulgaris
- Sarcoidosis
- Yaws
- Cutaneous leishmaniasis
- Peripheral neuropathy
- Syringomyelia

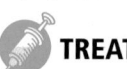 **TREATMENT**

MEDICATION
Pregnancy Considerations
Clofazimine and minocycline contraindicated; dapsone may be used

Pediatric Considerations
Minocycline contraindicated in children <5 years

First Line
- Multidrug therapy (MDT) standard for treatment
- In US (where patients are considered to have more active disease):
  – PB: Rifampicin 600 mg p.o. daily + dapsone 100 mg p.o. daily; treat for 1 year
  – MB: Rifampicin 600 mg p.o. daily + dapsone 100 mg p.o. daily + clofazimine 50 mg p.o. daily; treat for 2 years
- Outside US (WHO regimen):
  – PB: Rifampicin 600 mg p.o. monthly + dapsone 100 mg p.o. daily; treat for 6 months
  – MB: Rifampicin 600 mg p.o. monthly + clofazimine 300 mg p.o. monthly + dapsone 100 mg p.o. daily + clofazimine 50 mg p.o. daily; treat for 1 year
- Single skin lesion (WHO regimen):
  – PB: Rifampicin 600 mg p.o. + minocycline 100 mg p.o. + ofloxacin 400 mg p.o.; treat with 1 dose once

- Contraindications:
  – Clofazimine and minocycline: Pregnancy
  – Ofloxacin: Relative contraindication in children and adolescents
  – Minocycline in pregnancy, during lactation, and in children up to 5 years old
- Precautions:
  – Hemolysis and methemoglobinemia are common untoward reactions to dapsone.
  – Screen for glucose 6-phosphate dehydrogenase deficiency to prevent drug-induced hemolysis.
  – Reactionary states should be anticipated and treated aggressively.
  – Dapsone: Gastrointestinal upset, headaches, pruritus, exfoliative dermatitis, agranulocytosis, fever, rash, photosensitivity
  – Clofazimine: Gastrointestinal upset and skin pigmentation
  – Rifampicin: Reddish pigmentation of urine and other bodily fluids
  – Minocycline: Reduce dosage in renal damage (1)[A]

Second Line
Weak evidence for shorter regimens, longer regimens, or newer drug combinations (2)[A],(3):
- New MDT regimens have been suggested but need additional data to support them:
  – Drugs potentially effective against leprosy may include clarithromycin, linezolid, and rifapentine (4).
  – Clarithromycin, minocycline, and moxifloxacin may be effective in cases of MB treatment intolerance or drug-resistance (3).

ADDITIONAL TREATMENT
General Measures
- Multidisciplinary approach, including orthopedic surgery, ophthalmology, and physical therapy in addition to specific drugs
- Rigid-soled footwear, walking plaster casts or dressings to treat or prevent plantar ulcers
- Physical therapy and casts prevent hand contractures.
- Vocational retraining and rehabilitation along with psychologic support
- Immediate recognition and treatment of eye problems are essential.

Issues for Referral
Surgical, ophthalmic, orthopedic, and occupational complications

Additional Therapies
Manage mild reactional states, such as reversal reaction and erythema nodosum leprosum (ENL), with bed rest, analgesics, and sedatives. Severe reactions require corticosteroids, thalidomide, or clofazimine. Specific therapy must be continued without interruption.

SURGERY/OTHER PROCEDURES
- Reconstructive surgery: Nerve and tendon transplants, release of contractures, and other cosmetic procedures may give more functional mobility and social acceptance.
- Tarsorrhaphy or horizontal lid shortening for lagophthalmos with lid gap >5 mm or even lesser degree in patients with 1 eye. Cataract surgery with posterior chamber intraocular lens implantation to avoid glasses in patients with nasal bridge collapse.
- Decompressive surgery to treat nerve damage, in conjunction with steroid therapy. However, there may be no added benefit over steroid therapy alone.

ONGOING CARE
FOLLOW-UP RECOMMENDATIONS
Patient Monitoring
- Frequent follow-up visits until therapy course is stabilized, then monthly supervision
- Drug toxicity uncommon after 1st year of treatment
- Periodic complete blood count, renal and hepatic function
- Yearly skin scrapings from most active sites, if possible

DIET
Nutritious, balanced diet

PATIENT EDUCATION
- Educate about the indolent course of the disease and importance of therapeutic completion.
- Information pamphlets and awareness to ease psychologic trauma and stigma, emphasizing that a cure is possible with newer drug regimen:
  – Self-care booklet, *I Can Do It Myself!*, is available from WHO
- Encourage case reporting, since early treatment may prevent/reduce tissue damage and deformities.

PROGNOSIS
- Generally indolent, but may be interrupted by ENL and type 1 lepra reaction. Prognosis is good with early detection and therapy, especially with range of motion.
- Some cases of disease relapse and rifampicin resistance have been reported.
- May show gradual clearing of skin lesions within 1st year

COMPLICATIONS
- Crippling of the hand and foot
- Trauma and secondary infection leading to loss of digits and extremities
- Corneal opacities and uveitis may lead to blindness.
- Cataracts
- Lucio phenomenon—arteritis
- Secondary amyloidosis
- ENL: Therapy with thalidomide 200 mg b.i.d., tapering to 50–100 mg/d in chronic patients
- Severe reversal reaction: Prednisolone 40–60 mg/d, tapering slowly

REFERENCES
1. Saunderson P, Groenen G. Which physical signs help most in the diagnosis of leprosy? A proposal based on experience in the AMFES project, ALERT, Ethiopia. *Lepr Rev*. 2000;71:34–42.
2. Britton WJ, Lockwood DN. Leprosy. *Lancet*. 2004;363:1209–19.
3. World Health Organization. Report of the Tenth Meeting of the WHO Technical Advisory Group on Leprosy Control, New Delhi, India, 23 April 2009.
4. World Health Organization. Report of the Ninth Meeting of the WHO Technical Advisory Group on Leprosy Control, Cairo, Egypt, 6–7 March 2008.

ADDITIONAL READING
- Anderson H, Stryjewska B, Boyanton BL, et al. Hansen disease in the United States in the 21st century: a review of the literature. *Arch Pathol Lab Med*. 2007;131:982–6.
- Lockwood DN, Kumar B. Treatment of leprosy. *BMJ*. 2004;328:1447–8.
- Mehdi G, Maheshwari V, Ansari HA, et al. Modified fine-needle aspiration technique for diagnosis of granulomatous skin lesions with special reference to leprosy and cutaneous tuberculosis. *Diagn Cytopathol*. 2009. [Epub ahead of print].
- Merle CS, Cunha SS, Rodrigues LC et al. BCG vaccination and leprosy protection: review of current evidence and status of BCG in leprosy control. *Expert Rev Vaccines*. 2010;9:209–22.
- Reinar LM, Forsetlund L, Bjørndal A, et al. Interventions for skin changes caused by nerve damage in leprosy. *Cochrane Database Syst Rev*. 2008;CD004833.
- Van Veen NHJ, Lockwood DNJ, van Brakel WH, et al. Interventions for erythema nodosum leprosum. *Cochrane Database Sys Rev*. 2009;CD006949.

See Also (Topic, Algorithm, Electronic Media Element)
- The National Hansen's Disease Programs (NHDP) Baton Rouge, LA (800) 642-2477 provides consultation for physicians.
- World Health Organization: Leprosy http://www.who.int/lep/en/index/html, http://www.searo.who.int/en/Section980/Section2572.htm

CODES

ICD9
- 030.0 Lepromatous leprosy (type l)
- 030.1 Tuberculoid leprosy (type t)
- 030.9 Leprosy, unspecified

CLINICAL PEARLS
- If you suspect leprosy, obtain a careful history for possible exposure and carefully examine skin for tell-tale lesions, sensory loss, and enlarged nerves.
- Antileprosy prophylaxis is not currently recommended by WHO, even for household contacts.
- Multidrug therapy is the standard of treatment, as recommended by WHO.

L

LEUKEMIA

Jan Cerny, MD, PhD

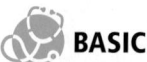

BASICS

DESCRIPTION
- Acute myeloid leukemia (AML) is characterized by proliferation and accumulation of abnormal immature myeloid progenitors (blasts) with reduced capacity to differentiate into more mature cellular elements. This leads to bone marrow failure and results in a variety of systemic symptoms.
- The former French–American–British (FAB) classification system divided AML based on the cell morphology with the addition of cytogenetics (subtypes M0–M7).
- The World Health Organization (WHO) classification attempts to provide more meaningful prognostic information:
  - AML with characteristic genetic abnormalities: Translocation t(8;21), t(15;17) and inversion in chromosome 16 inv(16)
  - AML with multilineage dysplasia: Presence of a prior myelodysplastic syndrome (MDS) or myeloproliferative disease (MPD) that transformed into AML
  - AML and MDS, therapy-related
  - AML not otherwise categorized
  - Acute leukemias of ambiguous lineage (*biphenotypic acute leukemia*)

EPIDEMIOLOGY
- Approximately 13,500 cases diagnosed in 2007; 2nd most common type of leukemia in adults
- Predominant sex: Male ≥ Female

Incidence
The incidence of AML increases with age and median age is more than 70 years.

RISK FACTORS
- Genetic predisposition (e.g., Down syndrome); other familial disorders are Bloom syndrome (~25% develop AML), Fanconi anemia (52%), neurofibromatosis, Li-Fraumeni syndrome, Wiskott-Aldrich syndrome, Kostmann syndrome, and Diamond-Blackfan anemia
- Radiation exposure
- Immunodeficiency states
- Chemical and drug exposure (nitrogen mustard and alkylating agents; benzene)
- Myelodysplastic syndrome (preleukemia)
- Cigarette smoking

Genetics
- Unknown; some are familial
- Cytogenetics and genetics play a very important role in diagnosis and prognosis of AML and have implications for therapy.
- 3 risk groups:
  - Good risk: inv(16), t(8;21), t(15;17)
  - Standard risk: Normal karyotype
  - Poor risk: Monosomy 5 and 7 (typically secondary AML), deletion 5q, abnormalities of 11q23 or complex karyotype
- FLT3 gene mutations, especially internal transmembrane duplications (FLT3-ITD), have been associated with poor survival in AML. These and other (onco)gene (e.g., WT1, NPM1 and P53) mutations are studied to further risk-stratify patients (1).

GENERAL PREVENTION
None currently identified, but treatment of high-risk myelodysplastic syndrome with demethylating agents (Vidaza, 5-azacytidine) has been shown to prolong time to transformation into AML (2).

ETIOLOGY
Precise causes unknown, but some risk factors have been identified (see also Risk Factors)

COMMONLY ASSOCIATED CONDITIONS
The following are oncologic emergencies:
- Disseminated intravascular coagulopathy (DIC) usually in acute promyelocytic leukemia (APL), but may be seen in any AML
- Leukostasis (high blast number and increased adhesive ability of blasts to the vessel wall)
- Tumor lysis syndrome (TLS): Spontaneous or in response to chemotherapy

DIAGNOSIS

HISTORY
Fatigue (anemia or tumor burden). Bleeding (low platelets or DIC). Difficulty clearing infections (neutropenia or immune dysregulation).

PHYSICAL EXAM
- Mostly nonspecific and related to marrow or tissue infiltration:
  - Fever
  - Bleeding
  - Pallor
  - Splenomegaly
  - Hepatosplenomegaly
  - Lymphadenopathy (usually reactive)
- If CNS is involved, symptoms of increased intracranial pressure can be present.
- Occasional patients will present with prominent extramedullary sites of leukemia (e.g., skin infiltration or ultimately as a granulocytic sarcoma).

DIAGNOSTIC TESTS & INTERPRETATION
Lab
- Complete blood count (CBC) shows subnormal red cells (RBCs), neutrophils, and platelets.
- Bone marrow for histology, flow cytometry, and cytogenetics to establish diagnosis and prognosis
- Elevated erythrocyte sedimentation rate (ESR)
- Lactate dehydrogenase (LDH) and uric acid can be elevated (e.g., TLS).
- Coagulation profile can be normal or prolonged (e.g., DIC).
- Drugs that may alter lab results: Chemotherapy agents, corticosteroids
- Other special tests: Spinal tap may reveal fluid with leukemic cells.

Imaging
Ultrasonography or CT scan of the abdomen may discover organomegaly.

Diagnostic Procedures/Surgery
Bone marrow studies are necessary to make the diagnosis:
- Aspirates: For cell morphology, cytochemistries, immunophenotyping (can confirm differentiation stage of AML); cytogenetics: Chromosomal aberration (prognostic value; see Genetics)
- Biopsies provide valuable information for cellularity, architecture, etc.

Pathological Findings
- The marrow will be hypercellular and the normal architecture effaced; leukemic blasts is >20%.
- The liver and spleen may be infiltrated with leukemic cells.

DIFFERENTIAL DIAGNOSIS
- Virus-induced cytopenia, lymphadenopathy, and organomegaly
- Immune cytopenias (including systemic lupus erythematosus [SLE])
- Drug-induced cytopenias
- Other marrow failure and infiltrative diseases (e.g., aplastic anemia, paroxysmal nocturnal hemoglobinuria, myelodysplastic syndromes, Gaucher disease)

TREATMENT
- Chemotherapy is a backbone of AML therapy and consists of induction and consolidation phase +/− maintenance (APL).
- Bone marrow transplantation (BMT) for high-risk AML
- Only modest improvements have been made in AML induction chemotherapy. Supportive care has improved significantly.

Geriatric Considerations
- Older patients (>60 years) remain a therapeutic challenge, as they do not tolerate intensive therapies. Rather, these patients are offered so-called reduced-intensity or nonmyeloablative bone marrow transplantation.
- Adding growth factors (G-CSF) to chemotherapy reduced toxicity and made induction a feasible option in this patient age group.
- 5-azacitidine significantly prolongs survival in older adults with low marrow blast count (<30%) (3).

Pediatric Considerations
Tolerate intense treatments better

Pregnancy Considerations
Chemotherapy is a viable option in the 2nd and 3rd trimesters.

MEDICATION
First Line
- Acute promyelocytic leukemia [APL, AML with t(15;17)]:
  - All-trans retinoic acid (ATRA) and arsenic trioxide both promote maturation to granulocytes.
  - Idarubicin can be added to induction therapy.
- Treatment of AML in younger adults: AML (other than APL)
- Induction (daunorubicin or idarubicin [anthracycline] and cytarabine]): 3 + 7 (anthracycline is given for 3 and cytarabine for 7 days)
- Remission is consolidated in younger patients by:
  - In good-risk AML, 3–4 cycles of high-dose cytarabine (HIDAC) and bone marrow transplant (BMT) is reserved for time of recurrence.
  - In poor-risk patients, 1–2 cycles of HIDAC (until donor is identified) are followed by allogeneic BMT.
  - Intermediate-risk AML should be treated based on individual patient's features, donor availability, and access to clinical trials. Recent meta-analysis showed that even intermediate-risk patients benefit from allogeneic BMT (4).

- Treatment of AML in older adults (e.g., >65 years) remains a challenge. These patients have poor performance status, more likely secondary AML, higher incidence of unfavorable cytogenetics, comorbidities, shorter remissions, and overall survival:
  - Intensive chemotherapy only for selected patients; alternative regimens with e.g., mitoxantrone, fludarabine, and clofarabine. New drugs (demethylating agents as above (3), FLT3 inhibitors, monoclonal antibodies, etc.) are being studied in clinical trials.
- Contraindications: Comorbidities; Therapy has to be individualized.
- Precautions:
  - If organ failure, some drugs may be avoided or dose-reduced (e.g., no anthracyclines in patients with preexisting cardiac problem).
  - Patients will be immunosuppressed during treatment. Avoid live vaccines. Administer varicella-zoster or measles immunoglobulin as soon as exposure of a patient at risk becomes known.
- Significant possible interactions: Allopurinol accentuates the toxicity of 6-mercaptopurine.

Second Line
Younger patients in good condition usually are offered reinduction chemotherapy and allogeneic BMT.

ADDITIONAL TREATMENT
General Measures
- Ongoing assessment of bone marrow, liver, heart, and kidney functions during therapy
- Close monitoring of coagulation parameters (risk for DIC)
- Supportive therapy with:
  - Good hydration
  - Transfusions of packed RBCs and platelets based on patient's needs (threshold as for platelets as low as 5,000); use leukoreduced, irradiated blood products in BMT candidates
  - Avoid antiplatelet agents (e.g., aspirin products).
  - Follow febrile neutropenic guidelines in neutropenic patient who becomes febrile (even low-grade fever).

Issues for Referral
- AML should be managed by specialized team led by a hematologist/oncologist.
- Refer patient to a transplant center early because search for a donor may be necessary.

SURGERY/OTHER PROCEDURES
BMT: Decision between myeloablative and nonmyeloablative approach is made based on patient's age, comorbidities, and AML risk factors:
- Allogeneic BMT is acceptable in 1st remission in poor-risk AML or in 2nd remission in all other AML patients. Matched related donor used to be preferred over matched unrelated donor (lower risk of graft-versus-host disease), but more recent observations suggest equal outcomes as allogeneic transplant regimens and post-transplant care have improved significantly.
- Cord blood may be used as an alternative source of hematopoietic stem cells even for adult patients.
- Autologous BMT may be acceptable in special situations (e.g., no donor is available).

IN-PATIENT CONSIDERATIONS
Admission Criteria
Induction treatment for AML requires inpatient care, usually on a specialized ward. Episodes of febrile neutropenia typically require admission and intravenous antibiotics.

IV Fluids
Appropriate hydration to prevent TLS

Nursing
Chemotherapy agents should be administered by skilled and specially trained professionals. IV may lead to chemical burns in the event of extravasation.

 ONGOING CARE

FOLLOW-UP RECOMMENDATIONS
Ambulatory as tolerated; no intense or contact sports; no aspirin due to risk of bleeding

Patient Monitoring
- Repeat bone marrow studies to document remission and also if a relapse is suspected.
- Follow CBC with differential, coagulation studies, uric acid level, and other chemistries related to TLS (creatinine, potassium, phosphate, calcium); monitor urinary function at least daily during induction phase and less frequently later.
- Physical evaluation, including weight and BP, should be done frequently during treatment.

DIET
Ensure adequately balanced calorie/vitamin intake. Sometimes total parenteral nutrition may be necessary (in case of severe mucositis).

PATIENT EDUCATION
- Leukemia Society of America: 33 Third Ave., New York, NY 10017, (212) 573-8484.
- National Cancer Institute, Bethesda, MD, has pamphlets and telephone education.
- *You and Leukemia: A Day at a Time*, by Dr. Lynn S. Baker (Saunders).

PROGNOSIS
AML remission rate is 60–80%, with only 20–40% long-term survival. The wide variable prognosis is due to prognostic group (age, cytogenetics, and genetics).

COMPLICATIONS
- Acute side effects of chemotherapy, including febrile neutropenia
- TLS
- DIC
- Late-onset cardiomyopathy in patients treated with anthracyclines
- Chronic side effects of chemotherapy (secondary malignancies)
- Graft-versus-host disease in patient who received allogeneic BMT

REFERENCES

1. Döhner H, Estey EH, Amadori S, Appelbaum FR, Büchner T, Burnett AK, Dombret H, Fenaux P, Grimwade D, Larson RA, Lo-Coco F, Naoe T, Niederwieser D, Ossenkoppele GJ, Sanz MA, Sierra J, Tallman MS, Löwenberg B, Bloomfield CD. Diagnosis and management of acute myeloid leukemia in adults: recommendations from an international expert panel, on behalf of the European Leukemia. *Net Blood* 2010;115: 453–474.

2. Fenaux P, Mufti GJ, Hellstrom-Lindberg E, Santini V, Finelli C, Giagounidis A, Schoch R, Gattermann N, Sanz G, List A, Gore SD, Seymour JF, Bennett JM, Byrd J, Backstrom J, Zimmerman L, McKenzie D, Beach C, Silverman LR; International Vidaza High-Risk MDS Survival Study Group. Efficacy of azacitidine compared with that of conventional care regimens in the treatment of higher-risk myelodysplastic syndromes: a randomised, open-label, phase III study. *Lancet Oncol* 2009; 10:223–32.

3. Fenaux P, Mufti GJ, Hellström-Lindberg E, Santini V, Gattermann N, Germing U, Sanz G, List AF, Gore S, Seymour JF, Dombret H, Backstrom J, Zimmerman L, McKenzie D, Beach CL, Silverman LR et al. Azacitidine prolongs overall survival compared with conventional care regimens in elderly patients with low bone marrow blast count acute myeloid leukemia. *J Clin Oncol*. 2010;28:562–9.

4. Koreth J, Schlenk R, Kopecky KJ, Honda S, Sierra J, Djulbegovic BJ, Wadleigh M, DeAngelo DJ, Stone RM, Sakamaki H, Appelbaum FR, Döhner H, Antin JH, Soiffer RJ, Cutler C et al. Allogeneic stem cell transplantation for acute myeloid leukemia in first complete remission: systematic review and meta-analysis of prospective clinical trials. *JAMA*. 2009;301:2349–61.

ADDITIONAL READING

- Devita VT Jr, Rosenberg SA, Lawrence TS, eds. *DeVita, Hellman, and Rosenberg's Cancer: Principles & Practice of Oncology*, 8th ed. Philadelphia: Lippincott Williams & Wilkins; 2008.
- O'Donnell MR, Appelbaum FR, Coutre SE, et al. Acute myeloid leukemia. *J Natl Compr Canc Netw*. 2008;6:962–93.

See Also (Topic, Algorithm, Electronic Media Element)
Leukemia, Acute Lymphoblastic in Adults (ALL); Leukemia, Chronic myelogenous (CML); Myelodysplastic syndromes (MDS); Myeloproliferative disorders; Disseminated intravascular coagulopathy (DIC)

 CODES

ICD9
- 205.00 Myeloid leukemia, acute, without mention of having achieved remission
- 208.00 Leukemia of unspecified cell type, acute, without mention of having achieved remission

CLINICAL PEARLS
- Consult hematologist/oncologist, as diagnosis and management of acute leukemia require a specialized team. Delay in diagnosis may delay therapy and result in development of complications (DIC, TLS, etc.).
- Prognosis of leukemia depends on the cytogenetic and molecular profile of the disease.
- Allogeneic transplant remains the only therapy with curative potential for patients with intermediate- and high-risk AML.

L

LEUKEMIA, ACUTE LYMPHOBLASTIC IN ADULTS (ALL)

Richard A. Larson, MD

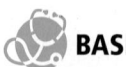 BASICS

DESCRIPTION

ALL in adults is a malignant proliferation and accumulation of immature lymphocytes:
- System(s) affected: Hemic/Lymphatic/Immunologic
- Synonym(s): Acute lymphocytic leukemia

Pregnancy Considerations

Many chemotherapy drugs are teratogenic.

EPIDEMIOLOGY
- Predominant age: Median age: 35–40 years; incidence increases with age.
- Predominant sex: Male > Female (slightly)

Incidence

In the US, 1,000 adult cases per year

RISK FACTORS
- Age >60 years
- Incidence appears to increase following exposure to chemical agents, such as benzene, or to radiation, but acute myeloid leukemia (AML) is more common.
- May follow aplastic anemia

Genetics
- Increased incidence in children with Down syndrome or in rare familial diseases such as ataxia-telangiectasia, Bloom syndrome, Fanconi anemia, Klinefelter syndrome, and neurofibromatosis
- Can rarely occur in adult identical twins

ETIOLOGY

Unknown. Epstein-Barr virus is implicated in Burkitt leukemia/lymphoma.

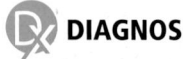 DIAGNOSIS

HISTORY
- Anemia: Fatigue, shortness of breath, lightheadedness, angina, headache
- Thrombocytopenia: Easy bruising
- Neutrocytopenia: Fever, infection
- Lymphocytosis: Bone pain
- Central nervous system (CNS): Confusion

PHYSICAL EXAM
- Thrombocytopenia: Petechiae, ecchymoses, epistaxis, retinal hemorrhages
- Anemia: Pallor
- Neutrocytopenia: Fever, infection
- Lymphocytosis: Lymphadenopathy, splenomegaly; less often, hepatomegaly
- CNS: Cranial nerve palsies, confusion

DIAGNOSTIC TESTS & INTERPRETATION

Lab
- Anemia: Normochromic, normocytic
- Thrombocytopenia
- Peripheral blood lymphoblasts
- Elevated lactate dehydrogenase
- Elevated uric acid
- Special tests:
  - Immunophenotyping of marrow/blood lymphoblasts: B-lineage (CD19, CD20, CD24); T-lineage (CD2, CD5, CD7); CALLA ([common ALL antigen], CD10); human leukocyte antigen (HLA)-DR; terminal deoxynucleotidyl transferase (TdT); aberrant myeloid antigens (CD13, CD33); stem cell antigen (CD34)
- Cytochemical stains: Myeloperoxidase negative; Sudan black B usually negative; TdT positive; periodic acid Schiff (PAS) ± is variable, depending upon subtype:
  - Cytogenetics: Specific recurring chromosomal abnormalities have independent diagnostic and prognostic significance (hyperdiploidy >50 chromosomes or t(14q11q13) are favorable; the Philadelphia chromosome, t[9;22], t[4;11], −7 and +8 are unfavorable. A translocation t(8;14) or t(2;8) or t(8;22) identifies Burkitt-type leukemia that requires specific therapy.
  - RT-PCR for rapid diagnosis of BCR/ABL+ ALL
  - Human leukocyte antigen typing of patient and siblings for hematopoietic cell transplantation

Imaging
- Chest radiograph to evaluate for mediastinal mass or hilar adenopathy, and for pulmonary infiltrates suggestive of infection
- Ultrasound exam to assess splenomegaly or renal enlargement suggestive of leukemic infiltration

Diagnostic Procedures/Surgery
- Bone marrow examination with aspiration, biopsy, immunophenotyping, cytochemistry, and cytogenetics
- Lymph node biopsy is rarely necessary, but can be diagnostic.
- Lumbar puncture is typically done both for diagnosis of CNS involvement and for intrathecal treatment. It should be done if neurological symptoms or signs are present. Repeat lumbar puncture after bone marrow remission is achieved to evaluate occult CNS involvement, and continue prophylactic CNS treatment.

Pathological Findings

Diffuse replacement of marrow and lymph node architecture by sheets of malignant lymphoblasts

DIFFERENTIAL DIAGNOSIS
- Malignant disorders: Other leukemias, especially AML; chronic myeloid leukemia in lymphoid blast phase; prolymphocytic leukemia; malignant lymphomas; multiple myeloma; bone marrow metastases from solid tumors (breast, prostate, lung, renal); myelodysplastic syndromes (1)[A]
- Nonmalignant disorders: Aplastic anemia; myelofibrosis; autoimmune diseases (Felty syndrome, lupus); infectious mononucleosis; pertussis; autoimmune thrombocytopenic purpura; leukemoid reaction to infection

 TREATMENT

MEDICATION

First Line

Optimal therapy is not yet known (1,2)[A]. ALL should be treated at a comprehensive oncology center that has adequate expertise, resources, and supportive care. All treatment regimens are still investigational, but clearly effective for some fraction of patients. CALGB protocol 9111 is an example of therapy (3)[A]:
- Remission induction:
  - Cyclophosphamide: 1,200 mg/m^2 IV on day 1 (800 mg/m^2 if >60 years old)
  - Daunorubicin: 45 mg/m^2 IV on days 1, 2, and 3 (30 mg/m^2 if >60 years old)
  - Vincristine: 2 mg IV on days 1, 8, 15, and 22
  - Asparaginase (L-asparaginase): 6,000 units/m^2 SC or IM on days 5, 8, 11, 15, 18, and 22
  - Prednisone: 60 mg/m^2 on days 1–21 (days 1–7 if >60 years old)
  - Filgrastim, G-CSF: 5 μg/kg/d SC starting on day 4 has been shown to shorten the duration of neutropenia and improve the CR rate, especially in older patients.
  - Imatinib mesylate: 600–800 mg/d is effective alone and in combination with chemotherapy for Philadelphia chromosome–positive ALL (4)[B].
- Consolidation (repeat twice in 8 weeks):
  - Cyclophosphamide: 1,000 mg/m^2 IV on day 1
  - Intrathecal (IT) methotrexate: 15 mg with hydrocortisone 50 mg on day 1
  - Mercaptopurine (6-mercaptopurine): 60 mg/m^2 on days 1–14
  - Cytarabine: 75 mg/m^2 SC on days 1–4 and 8–11
  - Vincristine: 2 mg IV on days 15 and 22
  - Asparaginase: 6,000 U/m^2 SC or IM on days 15, 18, 22, and 25
- CNS prophylaxis and interim maintenance— 2,400 cGy cranial irradiation:
  - IT-methotrexate: 15 mg with hydrocortisone 50 mg on days 1, 8, 15, 22, and 29
  - Mercaptopurine (6-mercaptopurine): 60 mg/m^2 on days 1–70, taken in the evening
  - Oral methotrexate: 20 mg/m^2 on days 36, 43, 50, 57, and 64
- Late intensification:
  - Doxorubicin: 30 mg/m^2 IV on days 1, 8, and 15
  - Vincristine: 2 mg IV on days 1, 8, and 15
  - Dexamethasone: 10 mg/m^2 on days 1–14
  - Cyclophosphamide: 1,000 mg/m^2 IV on day 29
  - Thioguanine (6-thioguanine): 60 mg/m^2 on days 29–42
  - Cytarabine: 75 mg/m^2 SC on days 29–32 and 36–39
- Prolonged maintenance:
  - Vincristine: 2 mg/mo IV for 16 months
  - Prednisone: 60 mg/m^2 for 5 days with the vincristine
  - Mercaptopurine (6-mercaptopurine): 60 mg/m^2/d for 16 months, taken in the evening
  - Oral methotrexate: 20 mg/m^2/wk for 16 months

– Philadelphia chromosome–positive ALL:
  ○ Imatinib mesylate (400–800 mg/d) is effective alone and in combination with chemotherapy (4)[B].
– Contraindications: Doses and schedule may need to be altered for older patients and for concurrent infection and organ toxicity (2)[B].
– Precautions:
  ○ Tumor lysis syndrome (elevated uric acid, potassium, and phosphate with decreased calcium, leading to renal failure, disseminated intravascular coagulation, and cardiac arrhythmias) may be prevented by administering allopurinol 300 mg/d. Begin 2 days before chemotherapy begins. Reduce doses if used with mercaptopurine or azathioprine. Give increased fluids; IV urate oxidase (rasburicase) can be used to treat hyperuricemia rapidly.
  ○ Oral sulfamethoxazole-trimethoprim or aerosolized pentamidine is given for *Pneumocystis carinii* prophylaxis.
  ○ Profound immunosuppression: Take appropriate precautions when patient is neutropenic.
  ○ High-dose cyclophosphamide causes severe nausea and vomiting. Use appropriate antiemetic regimen to prevent.
  ○ Neurotoxicity, ileus with vincristine
  ○ Asparaginase may cause severe allergic reactions as well as impaired pancreatic and liver function. Monitor serum glucose concentrations frequently and carefully. Pancreatitis or thrombosis may occur. Peg-asparaginase has been approved and can be used IV or IM in place of native *E. coli* asparaginase.
  ○ Also note: Burkitt leukemia/lymphoma (ALL-L3):
    ▪ The outcome is clearly better if high-dose methotrexate and alkylating agents are used for initial therapy.
    ▪ Only 18 weeks of treatment are required.
    ▪ Rituximab (anti-CD20 monoclonal antibody) improves the outcome of patients with Burkitt leukemia when added to chemotherapy.

Second Line
Clofarabine has been approved for relapsed childhood ALL. Pegylated asparaginase (IV or IM) has been used in place of *E. coli*-derived L-asparaginase. Other anthracyclines, investigational chemotherapy agents and monoclonal antibodies (e.g., rituximab; alemtuzumab). Allogeneic hematopoietic stem cell transplantation is recommended for any patient with relapsed ALL (5,6)[A].

ADDITIONAL TREATMENT
General Measures
- Appropriate health care:
  – Inpatient care during remission induction chemotherapy
  – Postremission therapy is usually outpatient.
  – Access to the resources and expertise of a major oncology center is important for appropriate support.
- Protective isolation from infection
- Adequate calcium and vitamin D supplementation may reduce bone injury from corticosteroids and avascular necrosis of large joints.

Issues for Referral
ALL can be a rapidly fatal disorder. As soon as the diagnosis is suspected, patients should be referred quickly to an appropriate oncology center.

COMPLEMENTARY AND ALTERNATIVE MEDICINE
Unproven and may result in dangerous drug interactions with chemotherapy

SURGERY/OTHER PROCEDURES
Surgical placement of a percutaneous silastic double-lumen central venous catheter

 ONGOING CARE

FOLLOW-UP RECOMMENDATIONS
Ambulatory as tolerated

Patient Monitoring
- Daily during induction chemotherapy for metabolic and infectious complications
- Weekly during remission consolidation chemotherapy
- Monthly during maintenance therapy
- Every 3 months thereafter

DIET
- Nutritional support, including IV hyperalimentation, if necessary
- Avoid alcohol.
- Calcium and vitamin D

PATIENT EDUCATION
- Risks of infection, transfusion, chemotherapy
- Stop smoking.

PROGNOSIS
- ~80–95% of patients <60 years old will achieve a complete remission, and 35–60% will remain free of disease at 5 years (3,6,5,7,8,9)[A].
- Older patients (>60 years) do less well, but, still, 80% may achieve a complete remission (2)[B].
- Patients with unfavorable cytogenetic subtypes [especially t(9;22) and t(4;11)] should undergo allogeneic stem cell transplantation in 1st remission if an HLA-identical donor were available (1,4,6,5)[A].

COMPLICATIONS
- Infections (*Pneumocystis carinii* pneumonia, bacterial pneumonia or sepsis, fungal pneumonia)
- Bleeding
- Coagulopathy (deep vein thrombosis) from asparaginase therapy
- Need for transfusions
- Sterility from treatment
- Arachnoiditis and CNS effects from intrathecal chemotherapy and irradiation
- Pancreatitis and liver dysfunction from chemotherapy
- Osteonecrosis of joints (avascular necrosis) related to corticosteroids
- Relapse of ALL in marrow or extramedullary sites (CNS, testis)

REFERENCES

1. Faderl S, O'Brien S, Pui CH, Stock W, Wetzler M, Hoelzer D, Kantarjian HM et al. Adult acute lymphoblastic leukemia: concepts and strategies. *Cancer*. 2010;116:1165–76.
2. Larson RA. Management of acute lymphoblastic leukemia in older patients. *Semin Hematol*. 2006;43:126–33.
3. Larson RA, Dodge RK, Linker CA, et al. A randomized controlled trial of filgrastim during remission induction and consolidation chemotherapy for adults with acute lymphoblastic leukemia: CALGB study 9111. *Blood*. 1998;92:1556–64.
4. Stock W et al. Current treatment options for adult patients with Philadelphia chromosome-positive acute lymphoblastic leukemia. *Leuk Lymphoma*. 2010;51:188–98.
5. Mattison RJ, Larson RA et al. Role of allogeneic hematopoietic cell transplantation in adults with acute lymphoblastic leukemia. *Curr Opin Oncol*. 2009;21:601–8.
6. Hahn T, Wall D, Camitta B, et al. The role of cytotoxic therapy with hematopoietic stem cell transplantation in the therapy of acute lymphoblastic leukemia in adults: an evidence-based review. *Biol Blood Marrow Transplant*. 2006;12:1–30.
7. Kantajian H, Hoelzer D, Larson RA, eds. Advances in the treatment of adult acute lymphocytic leukemia: Parts I and II. *Hematol Oncol Clin North Am*. 2000 and 2001.
8. Pieters R, Carroll WL et al. Biology and treatment of acute lymphoblastic leukemia. *Hematol Oncol Clin North Am*. 2010;24:1–18.
9. Campana D et al. Role of minimal residual disease monitoring in adult and pediatric acute lymphoblastic leukemia. *Hematol Oncol Clin North Am*. 2009;23:1083–98, vii

 CODES

ICD9
- 204.00 Lymphoid leukemia, acute, without mention of having achieved remission
- 204.01 Lymphoid leukemia, acute, in remission

CLINICAL PEARLS
Refer any patient with ALL rapidly to an experienced hematologist at a cancer center for enrollment in a peer-reviewed clinical trial.

L

LEUKEMIA, CHRONIC LYMPHOCYTIC

Jan Cerny, MD, PhD
Deepa Jagadeesh, MD, MPH

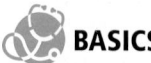 **BASICS**

DESCRIPTION
- Chronic lymphocytic leukemia (CLL) is a monoclonal disorder characterized by a progressive accumulation of mature but functionally incompetent lymphocytes.
- CLL can be distinguished from prolymphocytic leukemia (PLL). Based on percentage of prolymphocytes, the disease may be regarded as CLL (<10% prolymphocytes), PLL (>55% prolymphocytes), or CLL/PLL (>10% and <55% prolymphocytes).
- Small lymphocytic lymphoma is a lymphoma variant of CLL.
- System(s) affected: Hematologic/Lymphatic/Immunologic

EPIDEMIOLOGY
Incidence
- With 15,000–17,000 new cases reported every year, CLL represents the most common form of leukemia in adults in the US.
- Predominant age: CLL primarily affects elderly individuals, with most cases reported in individuals >55 years of age. The incidence continues to rise in those >55 years.
- Predominant sex: Male > Female (1.7:1).
- The incidence is higher among whites than among African Americans.

RISK FACTORS
As in the case of most malignancies, the exact cause of CLL is uncertain. Possible chronic immune stimulation is suspected, but is still being elucidated.

Genetics
CLL is an acquired disorder, and reports of truly familial cases are exceedingly rare.

GENERAL PREVENTION
Unknown

PATHOPHYSIOLOGY
- The cell of origin in CLL is a clonal B cell arrested in the B-cell differentiation pathway, intermediate between pre-B cells and mature B cells. In the peripheral blood, these cells resemble mature lymphocytes and typically show B-cell surface antigens: CD19, CD20, CD21, and CD23. In addition, they express CD5 (usually found on T cells).
- The bcl2 proto-oncogene is overexpressed in B-CLL. Bcl2 is a known suppressor of apoptosis (programmed cell death), resulting in extremely long life of the affected lymphocytes.

ETIOLOGY
Unknown, but genetic mutations leading to disrupted function and prolonged survival of affected lymphocytes are suspected.

COMMONLY ASSOCIATED CONDITIONS
- Immune system dysregulation is common.
- Autoimmune hemolytic anemia (AIHA) may accompany CLL.
- Immune thrombocytopenic purpura (ITP) may accompany CLL.

 DIAGNOSIS

HISTORY
- Insidious onset; it is not unusual for CLL to be discovered incidentally. Up to 40% of patients are asymptomatic at the time of diagnosis.
- Others may have:
  - Repetitive infections (pneumonia but also mucocutaneous herpetic infections, etc.)
  - Enlarged lymph nodes
  - Early satiety and/or abdominal discomfort related to an enlarged spleen
  - Mucocutaneous bleeding and/or petechiae due to thrombocytopenia
  - Fatigue-related and/or other symptoms of anemia
  - Fevers, night sweats, weight loss (B symptoms)

PHYSICAL EXAM
- Localized or generalized lymphadenopathy
- Splenomegaly (30–40%)
- Hepatomegaly (20%)
- Mucocutaneous bleeding (thrombocytopenia)
- Skin petechiae (thrombocytopenia)
- Pallor

DIAGNOSTIC TESTS & INTERPRETATION
Lab
Initial lab tests
- Complete blood count (CBC) with differential shows absolute lymphocytosis with >5,000 lymphocytes/μL. The blood smear also shows ruptured lymphocytes ("smudge" cells).
- Exam of the blood smear is important in diagnosis of CLL.
- The diagnosis can be confirmed by immunophenotyping: CLL cells are positive for CD19, CD20, and CD24, as well as CD5. They have low levels of surface membrane immunoglobulin (IgM or IgD). The monoclonality is proven by the presence of a single immunoglobulin light chain (κ or λ). FMC-7 is absent.

- CBC shows anemia and/or thrombocytopenia.
- Plasma β_2–microglobulin may be elevated.
- Serum protein electrophoresis (some patients may have monoclonal gammopathy)
- Lactate dehydrogenase (LDH) may be elevated (due to disease activity or to AIHA).
- Hypogammaglobulinemia
- In case associated with AIHA, labs consistent with hemolysis may be present (elevated LDH, total bilirubin; reticulocyte count does not have to be elevated due to bone marrow infiltration).

Follow-Up & Special Considerations
Frequency and type of follow-up depend on severity of symptoms as well as risk factors (see Prognosis).

Imaging
Initial approach
- Liver/spleen ultrasound may demonstrate organomegaly.
- Computed tomography scan of chest/abdomen/pelvis typically is not necessary for staging. However, it may help to identify compression of organs or internal structures from enlarged lymph nodes.

Diagnostic Procedures/Surgery
- Although bone marrow biopsy has its prognostic value (diffuse infiltration is a risk factor), it is not done routinely.
- Consider a lymph node biopsy if lymph node(s) begin to enlarge rapidly in a patient with known CLL to assess the possibility of transformation to a high-grade lymphoma (Richter syndrome), especially when accompanied by fever, weight loss, and pain.

Pathological Findings
A bone marrow aspirate usually shows >30% lymphocytes.

DIFFERENTIAL DIAGNOSIS
- Infectious causes:
  - Bacterial (tuberculosis)
  - Viral (mononucleosis)
- Malignant causes:
  - Leukemic phase of non-Hodgkin lymphomas
  - Hairy cell leukemia
  - Waldenstrom macroglobulinemia
  - Large granular lymphocytic leukemia

TREATMENT

MEDICATION

First Line

- Most patients are asymptomatic and do not need active treatment unless they have generalized (so-called B) symptoms, progressive marrow failure, AIHA or thrombocytopenia, progressive splenomegaly, massive lymphadenopathy, or progressive lymphocytosis (increase >50% in 2 months or a doubling time of <6 months).
- Low-risk disease, Rai stage 0, and Binet stage A require only periodic follow-up.
- Intermediate-risk group, Rai stage I and II, and Binet stage B could be observed until there is evidence of disease progression or development of symptoms.
- Treatment should be initiated in high-risk patients, Rai stage III and IV, and Binet stage C.
- Early treatment in low-risk group is not recommended.
- 3 main groups of drugs used are alkylating agents (chlorambucil, and recently bendamustine), purine analogs (fludarabine and pentostatin), and monoclonal antibodies (rituximab and alemtuzumab).
- Single-agent (fludarabine, bendamustine, or chlorambucil) or combination regimens commonly used.
- Fludarabine-based regimens are FC (in combination with cyclophosphamide) FR (fludarabine + rituximab), and FCR (fludarabine + cyclophosphamide + rituximab).
- FCR is the widely used regimen of choice if patient can tolerate it.
- PCR (pentostatin + cyclophosphamide + rituximab) is another regimen that is effective.
- Steroids (prednisone) are useful in patients with autoimmune manifestations of CLL (e.g., AIHA, ITP).

Second Line

- Combinations of chemotherapeutic agents that patient did not fail yet. Occasionally, some patients can be retreated with a drug used previously.
- Alemtuzumab (anti-CD52) has shown activity in relapsed and refractory disease.
- Newer agents like ofatumumab (new anti-CD2), lenalidomide, and fostamatinib disodium have shown promising activity.
- Consider splenectomy (surgery or radiation) if massive splenomegaly causes significant anemia and thrombocytopenia.
- Allogenic and autologous stem cell transplant can be considered in high-risk and younger patients (limited data available).

ADDITIONAL TREATMENT

General Measures

Patients with frequent infections associated with hypogammaglobulinemia are likely to benefit from monthly infusions of IVIG.

Issues for Referral

- Surgical consultation for splenectomy in selected patients
- Bone marrow transplant in young patients with refractory disease (however, still considered experimental therapy)

Additional Therapies

Virtually all patients requiring therapy also should be given allopurinol to prevent uric acid nephropathy.

SURGERY/OTHER PROCEDURES

Splenectomy in selected patients

IN-PATIENT CONSIDERATIONS

Admission Criteria

No specific criteria, but due to complications of disease (e.g., AIHA) or complications of therapy (e.g., febrile neutropenia) or significant tumor lysis syndrome after initiation of chemotherapy

ONGOING CARE

FOLLOW-UP RECOMMENDATIONS

- Low-risk CLL: Physical exam and CBC with differential every 3 months
- Patients in remission after treatment should also be followed every 3–6 months.

Patient Monitoring

- CBC with differential (lymphocytosis) every 3 months, LDH, β_2-microglobulin, IgG level
- Physical exam (lymphadenopathy, splenomegaly)

DIET

- Ensure adequately balanced calorie/vitamin intake.
- Follow weight.

PATIENT EDUCATION

Leukemia and Lymphoma Society has educational pamphlets: http://www.webmd.com/cancer/tc/leukemia-topic-overview.

PROGNOSIS

- Adverse risk factors:
  - Advanced Rai or Binet stage
  - Peripheral lymphocyte doubling time <12 months
  - Diffuse marrow infiltration
  - Increased number of prolymphocytes or cleaved cells
  - Poor response to chemotherapy
  - High β_2-microglobulin and thymidine kinase levels and low microRNAs (miRNAs).
  - Abnormal karyotyping: Deletion of 17p- and 11q-
  - New IgVH unmutated status (expression of ZAP-70 >20% or CD38 >30% evaluated by immunophenotyping are surrogate markers)
  - P53 mutation or deletion
- 2 staging systems are used: the Rai in the US and the Binet in Europe. Neither is completely satisfactory.
- The Rai staging system:
  - Stage 0: Lymphocytosis only; median survival of 120 months

  - Stage I: Lymphocytosis and adenopathy; median survival of 95 months
  - Stage II: Lymphocytosis and splenomegaly and/or hepatomegaly; median survival of 72 months
  - Stage III: Lymphocytosis and anemia (hemoglobin <10 g/dL); median survival of 30 months
  - Stage IV: Lymphocytosis and thrombocytopenia (platelets <100 × 10^9/L); median survival of 30 months
- The Binet staging system:
  - Stage A: Hemoglobin ≥10 g/dL, platelets ≥100 × 10^9, and <3 lymph node areas involved (Rai stages 0, I, and II); survival >120 months
  - Stage B: Hemoglobin and platelet levels as in stage A and 3 or more lymph node areas involved (Rai stages I and II); survival is 61 months
  - Stage C: Hemoglobin <100 g/L, platelets <100 × 10^9, or both (Rai stages III and IV); survival is 32 months

COMPLICATIONS

- Acute or long-term effects of chemotherapy
- Richter syndrome (above)
- AIHA (in some cases may be related to the use of fludarabine)

ADDITIONAL READING

- Chiorazzi N, Rai KR, Ferrarini M. Chronic lymphocytic leukemia. *N Engl J Med.* 2005;352:804–15.
- Shanafelt TD, Kay NE. Comprehensive Management of the CLL Patient: A Holistic Approach. *Hematology Am Soc Hematol Educ Program.* 2007;2007:324–31.

See Also (Topic, Algorithm, Electronic Media Element)

National Comprehensive Cancer Network guidelines at http://www.nccn.org

CODES

ICD9
204.10 Lymphoid leukemia, chronic, without mention of having achieved remission

CLINICAL PEARLS

Clinical monitoring of asymptomatic and low-risk patients is a reasonable approach ("watch and wait"). High-risk patients, bulky disease, or patients who fail fludarabine and rituximab-based therapies have typically poor prognosis and may require intensive therapies, including allogeneic transplantation.

L

LEUKEMIA, CHRONIC MYELOGENOUS

Jan Cerny, MD, PhD

BASICS

DESCRIPTION
- Chronic myelogenous leukemia (CML) is a myeloproliferative disorder characterized by clonal proliferation of myeloid precursors in the bone marrow with continuing differentiation into mature granulocytes.
- Hallmark of CML is Philadelphia chromosome [translocation t(9;22)]
- Natural history of the disease evolves in 3 clinical phases: A chronic phase, an accelerated phase, and blast phase or crisis (transformation to acute leukemia)

EPIDEMIOLOGY
Incidence
- 1.6 cases/100,000 persons per year
- Predominant age: 50–60 years
- Predominant sex: Male > Female (1.3:1)

Prevalence
Accounts for 15–20% of adult leukemias

RISK FACTORS
Ionizing radiation exposure (uncommon)

Genetics
Acquired genomic changes

GENERAL PREVENTION
None currently identified

PATHOPHYSIOLOGY
Philadelphia chromosome is a balanced translocation between *BCR* (on chromosome 22) and *ABL* (on chromosome 9) genes t(9;22)(q34;q11). This fusion gene, *BCR-ABL*, codes for an abnormal constitutively active tyrosine kinase that affects numerous signal transduction pathways, resulting in uncontrolled cell proliferation and reduced apoptosis.

DIAGNOSIS

85–90% of patients present in the chronic phase and can be found accidentally during routine screening.

HISTORY
- Chronic phase: Fatigue, weight loss, night sweats, abdominal fullness owing to enlarged spleen, early satiety, dyspnea, bleeding; rare: bruising, left upper quadrant abdominal pain, sternal pain (owing to expanding bone marrow), and gouty arthritis; up to 30% of patients are asymptomatic.
- Accelerated phase: Progressive splenomegaly and left upper quadrant abdominal pain occasionally referred to the left shoulder (owing to splenic infarction or rupture), progressive weight loss and sweats, unexplained fever or bone pain, chloromas (extramedullary tumors)
- Blast phase: Bleeding, bruising, infections, prominent constitutional symptoms

PHYSICAL EXAM
- Splenomegaly (50–90%), hepatomegaly (up to 50%)
- Less common: Splenic friction rub, lymphadenopathy

DIAGNOSTIC TESTS & INTERPRETATION
Lab
- Complete blood count (CBC):
  - Hematocrit: May be normal, slightly increased, or decreased
  - White blood cell count: Markedly increased (50,000–100,000/μL) with granulocytes in all stages of development, including occasional blasts <10% in chronic phase, basophilia, eosinophilia
  - Platelets: Normal, elevated (34%), or occasionally low
  - In accelerated phase: Anemia, 10–19% blood or marrow blasts, basophils plus eosinophils >20%, thrombocytopenia
  - Blast phase: Blood or marrow blasts >20%
- Genetics:
  - Demonstration of the Philadelphia chromosome, t(9,22), by cytogenetic techniques, FISH, or reverse-scriptase polymerase chain reaction (RT-PCR)
  - Additional cytogenetic abnormalities occur in the accelerated and blast phases [monosomy 7, t(3,21), trisomy 8 and 19, Philadelphia chromosome duplication, abnormalities of chromosome 17 such as monosomy, trisomy, and isochromosome mutations]. These may contribute to resistance to tyrosine kinase inhibitors (TKIs; eg, imatinib), and, therefore, bone marrow biopsy with cytogenetics should be performed at least once a year even in patients with disease controlled by therapy.
- Others:
  - Low or absent leukocyte alkaline phosphatase in neutrophils
  - High lactate dehydrogenase (LDH)
  - Elevated uric acid

Initial lab tests
CBC, LDH, uric acid, bone marrow biopsy and aspirate, cytogenetics on bone marrow and FISH for *BCR-ABL*, RT-PCR, liver function tests

Follow-Up & Special Considerations
Mutation analysis of tyrosine kinase domain of *ABL* kinase, as they may cause resistance to therapy with TKIs.

Imaging
Abdominal ultrasound or computed tomography scan shows splenomegaly; not mandatory

Diagnostic Procedures/Surgery
Bone marrow aspiration and biopsy

Pathological Findings
Myeloid hyperplasia with elevated myeloid: Erythroid ratio, normal maturation, marrow basophilia, and increased reticulin fibrosis

DIFFERENTIAL DIAGNOSIS
- Chronic myelomonocytic leukemia, chronic neutrophilic leukemia, chronic eosinophilic leukemia, juvenile myelomonocytic leukemia, infectious mononucleosis, leukemoid reaction, polycythemia vera, and treatment with granulocyte-stimulating factors.
- Acute myelogenous leukemia resembles blast crisis with myeloid blasts, and acute lymphoblastic leukemia resembles blast crisis with lymphoid blasts.
- Atypical CML is a chronic myeloproliferative disorder with a clinical hematologic picture similar to CML, but lacking Philadelphia chromosome and *BCR-ABL* rearrangement.

TREATMENT

MEDICATION
- TKIs provide durable long-term control of the disease.
- The response to TKIs is assessed at specific time points from the beginning of treatment, and is categorized as follows:
  - Complete hematologic response (CHR): Normalization of peripheral counts, no disease symptoms, no immature cells
  - Minor/partial/complete cytogenetic response (CCR): 35–90%, 1–34%, no Philadelphia-positive metaphases
  - Major molecular response (MMR): Decreased level of *BCR-ABL* transcript by PCR 3-log
  - Complete molecular response (CMR): *BCR-ABL* transcript is undetectable by PCR.

First Line
- Gleevec (imatinib mesylate), an oral tyrosine kinase inhibitor, 400 mg/d p.o.
- Side effects: Thrombocytopenia, anemia, elevated liver enzymes, edema, gastrointestinal disturbances, rash
- Illinois Researcher Information Service trial established imatinib as 1st-line therapy (1).
- Imatinib dose can be increased to 600 and 800 mg/d if only partial cytogenetic response to 400 mg/d is achieved at 6 months of treatment.

Second Line
- Dasatinib (Sprycel), 2nd-generation TKI, active against most of *BRC-ABL* mutants, not active in T315I mutation:
  - 100 mg/d in patients resistant or intolerant to imatinib and 70 mg twice a day for patients in accelerated or blastic phase
  - Side effects: Pleural effusions, cytopenias
- Nilotinib (Tasigna), also 2nd-generation TKI, highly selective and more potent *BCR-ABL* tyrosine kinase inhibitor, active against most of *BRC-ABL* mutants, not active in T315I mutation:
  - 400 mg p.o. b.i.d. in patients resistant or intolerant to imatinib in chronic or accelerated phase
  - Side effects: Cytopenias, QTc prolongation, pancreatitis

- Recent studies with nilotinib and dasatinib as a 1st-line therapy for chronic phase CML have shown very promising results in terms of high efficacy and low rate of side effects in this patient group (2,3).

ADDITIONAL TREATMENT
Issues for Referral
All patients with CML should be referred to a hematologist.

SURGERY/OTHER PROCEDURES
Allogenic bone marrow transplant (BMT):

- Is the only known cure; however, 71% of patients who achieve complete cytogenetic response with imatinib maintain that response for 7 years, and no patient progressed on the trial between years 5 and 6 of treatment (1)
- Most effective in patients <50 years of age who are in the chronic phase
- Initial mortality is higher (related to the use of myeloablative regimens) than medical management but provided higher rates of survival in pre-imatinib era. Matched related donors used to have a better prognosis than matched unrelated donors for allogeneic donation (less graft-versus-host disease); however, transplantation regimens and post-transplant care have evolved, and these differences have been practically eliminated.
- Significant improvement in transplant techniques leading to better outcomes, such as alternative sources of stem cells; nonmyeloablative regimes have shown improvements in transplant-related mortality.
- Transplant option should be thoroughly discussed with young patients in chronic phase and considered an alternative to imatinib, dasatinib, or nilotinib, especially if the patient does not tolerate TKIs or disease is not responding.
- Can be considered in patients who fail to achieve complete hematologic response by 3 months, have no cytogenetic response or cytogenetic relapse, or have T315I mutation

IN-PATIENT CONSIDERATIONS
Initial Stabilization
- Hydroxyurea to rapidly reduce the white cell count
- Allopurinol to prevent tumor lysis syndrome in patients with very high counts; to be administered before chemotherapy is instituted; probably not necessary when imatinib is used

Admission Criteria
Acute abdominal symptoms (infarcted or ruptured spleen); tumor lysis syndrome owing to initial therapy; complications of BMT

Discharge Criteria
Abatement of acute symptoms

ONGOING CARE

FOLLOW-UP RECOMMENDATIONS
- Frequency depends on stage at presentation and response to 1st-line therapy.
- While splenomegaly persists, avoid contact sports or trauma to abdomen.

Patient Monitoring
- CBC with differential: Weekly until blood counts stable, then every 2–4 weeks during complete hematologic response, once in CCR and stable, patient can be followed less frequently (3-month intervals)
- Bone marrow cytogenetics (evaluation for clonal evolution) every 6 months while in CHR, every 12–18 months while in complete cytogenic response, MMR, CMR
- Quantitative RT-PCR every 3 months (peripheral blood)
- Liver function tests monthly on imatinib

PROGNOSIS
- Without treatment: CML invariably will progress to accelerated phase within 2–5 years and blast phase within several months of the accelerated phase.
- Poor prognosis: Patients presenting in accelerated or acute leukemia, or presenting with very large spleen size, platelets >700,000/μL, and patients resistant to current therapies (T315I mutation)

COMPLICATIONS
- Splenic infarct or rupture
- Progression to accelerated or blast phase
- Thrombotic events owing to elevated platelets
- Bleeding owing to low or dysfunctional platelets
- Sequelae of anemia

REFERENCES

1. O'Brien, Stephen G, Guilhot, Francois, Goldman, John M, Hochhaus, Andreas, Hughes, Timothy P, Radich, Jerald P., Rudoltz, Marc, Filian, Jeiry, Gathmann, Insa, Druker, Brian J., Larson, Richard A. International Randomized Study of Interferon Versus STI571 (IRIS) 7-Year Follow-up: Sustained Survival, Low Rate of Transformation and Increased Rate of Major Molecular Response (MMR) in Patients (pts) with Newly Diagnosed Chronic Myeloid Leukemia in Chronic Phase (CMLCP) Treated with Imatinib (IM). *ASH Annual Meeting Abstracts*. 2008;112:186.
2. Cortes J, O'Brien S, Borthakur G, Jones D, Ravandi F, Koller C, Mesina O, Ferrajoli A, Shan J, Kantarjian H. Efficacy of Dasatinib in Patients (pts) with Previously Untreated Chronic Myelogenous Leukemia (CML) in Early Chronic Phase (CML-CP). *ASH Annual Meeting Abstracts*. 2008;112:182.
3. Rosti G, Palandri F, Castagnetti F, Breccia M, Levato L, Gugliotta G, Gugliotta G, Capucci A, Cedrone M, Fava C, Intermesoli T, Cambrin G, Stagno F, Tiribelli M, Amabile M, Luatti S, Poerio A, Soverini S, Testoni N, Martinelli G, Alimena G, Pane F, Saglio G, Baccarani M, and for the GIMEMA CML Working Party. Nilotinib for the frontline treatment of Ph+ chronic myeloid leukemia. *Blood*. 2009;114:4933–4938.

ADDITIONAL READING

- Calabretta B, Perrotti D. The biology of CML blast crisis. *Blood*. 2004;103:4010–22.
- Goldman JM, Marin D. Management decisions in chronic myeloid leukemia. *Semin Hematol*. 2003;40:97–103.
- Kantarjian H, Pasquini R, Hamerschlak N, et al. Dasatinib or high-dose imatinib for chronic-phase chronic myeloid leukemia after failure of first-line imatinib: a randomized phase 2 trial. *Blood*. 2007;109:5143–50.
- Savage DG, Szydlo RM, Goldman JM. Clinical features at diagnosis in 430 patients with chronic myeloid leukaemia seen at a referral centre over a 16-year period. *Br J Haematol*. 1997;96:111–6.

 CODES

ICD9
- 205.10 Myeloid leukemia, chronic, without mention of having achieved remission
- 205.11 Myeloid leukemia, chronic, in remission

CLINICAL PEARLS

- CML belongs to the myeloproliferative disorders group.
- The gold standard for diagnosis of CML is detection of the Philadelphia chromosome or its products, *BCR-ABL* mRNA, and fusion protein.
- Tyrosine kinase inhibitors provide durable long-term control of the disease and have dramatically altered treatment.
- Atypical CML is a form of clinically typical CML but without the presence of the typical *BCR-ABL* translocation.
- Blast crisis is a form of acute leukemia that is a possible complication of CML.

L

LEUKOPLAKIA, ORAL

Christine K. Jacobs, MD

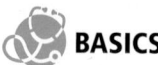 **BASICS**

DESCRIPTION

Oral leukoplakia is a nonspecific clinical term used to describe a white patch on the oral mucosa that remains despite attempts to rub or scrape it off.

- It has no pathologic or microscopic correlation with any specific disease and may be related to a variety of lesions, from benign hyperkeratosis to squamous cell carcinoma.
- System(s) affected: GI

EPIDEMIOLOGY

- Develops most often before age 40
- Predominant sex: Male > Female.
- Some studies show no gender difference.

Prevalence
- 1–3% of the adult population is affected.
- Mean age of onset is 40 years.

Geriatric Considerations
Malignant transformation to carcinoma is more common in older patients.

RISK FACTORS
- Tobacco, particularly smokeless tobacco
- Alcohol use
- Repeated or chronic mechanical trauma from dental appliances or cheek biting
- Chemical irritation to oral regions
- Diabetes

Genetics
P53 overexpression correlates with leukoplakia and particularly squamous cell carcinoma.

GENERAL PREVENTION
- Avoid tobacco of any kind, alcohol, habitual cheek biting or tongue chewing.
- Use well-fitting dental prosthesis.
- Regular dental checkups to avoid bad restorations
- Diet rich in fresh fruits and vegetables may help to prevent cancer.

PATHOPHYSIOLOGY
Hyperkeratosis or dyskeratosis of the oral squamous epithelium

ETIOLOGY
- Tobacco use in any form
- Alcohol consumption/alcoholism
- Oral infections
- *Candida albicans* infection may induce dysplasia and increase malignant transformation (1).
- Human papillomavirus, types 11 and 15
- Sunlight
- Vitamin deficiency

- Syphilis
- Dental restorations
- Prosthetic dental appliances
- Estrogen therapy
- Chronic trauma or irritation
- Epstein-Barr virus (oral hairy leukoplakia)
- Areca nut/betel (Asian populations)
- Mouthwash preparations and toothpaste containing the herbal root extract sanguinaria

COMMONLY ASSOCIATED CONDITIONS
- Leukokeratosis nicotina palati is rarely malignant.
- HIV infection is closely associated with hairy leukoplakia.
- Erythroplakia in association with leukoplakia, "speckled leukoplakia," or erythroleukoplakia is a marker for underlying dysplasia.
- Proliferative verrucous leukoplakia may develop into either squamous cell carcinoma or verrucous hyperplasia.

 DIAGNOSIS

Leukoplakia is an asymptomatic white patch on the oral mucosa.

HISTORY
- Usually asymptomatic
- History of tobacco or alcohol use or oral exposure to irritants

PHYSICAL EXAM
- Location:
  - 50% on tongue, mandibular alveolar ridge, and buccal mucosa
  - Also seen on maxillary alveolar ridge, palate, and lower lip
  - Infrequently seen on floor of the mouth and retromolar areas
  - Floor of mouth, ventrolateral tongue, and soft palate complex are more likely to have dysplastic lesions.
- Appearance:
  - Clinical appearance of lesion does not necessarily correspond to malignant potential.
  - Varies from homogeneous, nonpalpable, faintly translucent white areas to thick, fissured, papillomatous, indurated plaques
  - May feel rough or leathery
  - Lesions can become exophytic or verruciform.
  - Color may be white, gray, yellowish white, or brownish gray, although mixed white and red lesions ("speckled leukoplakia") are more likely to be dysplastic or malignant.
  - Cannot be wiped or scraped off
  - Macular or plaquelike
  - Nodular and verrucous variants are more likely to be malignant.

DIAGNOSTIC TESTS & INTERPRETATION
Biopsy may assess the degree of dysplasia but does not correlate with the risk of subsequent malignant transformation (2).

Lab
- Laboratory tests generally are not indicated.
- Consider saliva culture if *C. albicans* infection is suspected.
- If no clear explanation by history, consider complete blood count, thyroid-stimulating hormone, rapid plasma reagin, or VDRL and biopsy.

Imaging
No imaging is indicated.

Diagnostic Procedures/Surgery
- Biopsy is necessary to rule out carcinoma if lesion is persistent, changing, or unexplained.
- Noninvasive brush biopsy and analysis of cells with DNA–image cytometry constitute a sensitive and specific screening method.
- Patients with dysplastic or malignant cells on brush biopsy should undergo more formal excisional biopsy.

Pathological Findings
- Biopsy specimens range from hyperkeratosis to invasive carcinoma.
- At initial biopsy, 6% are invasive carcinoma.
- 0.13–6% subsequently undergo malignant transformation.
- Location is important: 60% on floor of mouth or lateral border of tongue are cancerous; buccal mucosal lesions are generally not malignant but require biopsy if not resolving.

DIFFERENTIAL DIAGNOSIS
- White oral lesions that can be wiped away: Candidiasis
- White oral lesions that cannot be rubbed off (3):
  - Traumatic or frictional keratosis (e.g., linea alba)
  - Leukoedema (benign milky opaque lesions that disappear with stretching)
  - Aspirin burn (from holding aspirin in cheek)
  - Lichen planus (bilateral fairly symmetric lesions, reticular pattern of slightly raised gray-white lines)
  - Verrucous carcinoma
  - Lupus
  - Squamous cell carcinoma
  - Oral hairy leukoplakia, commonly on the lateral border of the tongue with a bilateral distribution (in HIV patients with Epstein-Barr virus infection)
  - Smoker's palate (leukokeratosis nicotina palati)
  - White sponge nevus (congenital benign spongy lesions)
  - Syphilitic oral lesion
  - Dyskeratosis congenita (a rare inherited multisystem disorder)

TREATMENT

- Treatment may include
  - Surgical removal of the lesion
  - Topical or systemic medical treatment
  - Removal of predisposing habits (alcohol and tobacco)
  - Other treatment such as photodynamic therapy
- Treatment does not prevent malignant transformation.

MEDICATION

- Vitamin A, retinoids, beta-carotene, and lycopene may heal the oral leukoplakia (4)[A].
- No treatment has been shown to prevent relapse or malignant transformation (4)[A].
- Leukoplakia:
  - Isotretinoin (Accutane), 1–2 mg/kg/d PO may lead to temporary remission, but side effects are poorly tolerated.
  - Systemic administration of lycopene may have some efficacy in patients, similar to a subcontinental Indian population, for the short-term resolution of oral epithelial dysplasia (5)[B].
- Hairy leukoplakia:
  - Acyclovir, 2–4 g/d PO systemically is effective, but the lesions recur when the treatment is stopped.
  - Topical retinoids
  - Topical podophyllin 25% resin applied twice, 1 week between applications; however, the bad taste is poorly tolerated.

ADDITIONAL TREATMENT
General Measures

- Eliminate habitual lip biting.
- Correct ill-fitting dental appliances, bad restorations, or sharp teeth.
- Stop smoking and using alcohol.
- If dysplasia is evident, remove lesion. Consider otolaryngologist or oral surgery referral.
- Some small lesions may respond to cryosurgery.
- βeta-carotene, lycopene, retinoids, and cyclooxygenase 2 (COX-2) inhibitors may cause partial regression (experimental).
- For hairy tongue: Tongue brushing

SURGERY/OTHER PROCEDURES

- Complete excision is standard treatment for dysplasia or malignancy
- Scalpel excision, laser ablation, electrocautery, or cryoablation
- Lack of randomized, controlled trials; no evidence-based recommendations can be provided for specific surgical (including lasers) interventions of dysplastic oral lesions (5)[B].

IN-PATIENT CONSIDERATIONS
Initial Stabilization

- Eliminate etiologic factors.
- Reevaluate in 7–14 days.
- Biopsy if lesion is persistent.

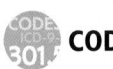

ONGOING CARE

FOLLOW-UP RECOMMENDATIONS
Patient Monitoring

- Regular, close follow-up, even after successful treatment
- Biopsy as needed.

DIET
Regular

PATIENT EDUCATION

- If biopsy is negative, stress importance of periodic and careful follow-up.
- Initiate a dental referral to eliminate dental factors.
- Stress importance of stopping tobacco and alcohol use.
- Encourage participation in smoking-cessation program.

PROGNOSIS

- Most leukoplakia is benign.
- Cancer is curable if detected early.
- 0.13–6% of initially benign lesions subsequently develop into cancer.
- More likely to be cancerous if on floor of mouth or lateral border of tongue

COMPLICATIONS

- New lesions may develop after treatment.
- Without surgical intervention, 4% develop carcinoma after 6.6 years (6).
- Larger lesions and nonhomogeneous leukoplakia are associated with higher rates of malignant transformation.

REFERENCES

1. Cao J, Liu HW, Jin JQ et al. [The effect of oral candida to development of oral leukoplakia into cancer] *Zhonghua Yu Fang Yi Xue Za Zhi*. 2007;41 Suppl:90–3.
2. Holmstrup P, Vedtofte P, Reibel J, et al. Oral premalignant lesions: is a biopsy reliable? *J Oral Pathol Med*. 2007;36:262–6.
3. Canaan TJ, Meehan SC. Variations of structure and appearance of the oral mucosa. *Dent Clin North Am*. 2005;49:1–14, vii.
4. Lodi G, Sardella A, Bez C, et al. Interventions for treating oral leukoplakia. *Cochrane Database Syst Rev*. 2006;CD001829.
5. Brennan M, Migliorati CA, Lockhart PB, et al. Management of oral epithelial dysplasia: a review. *Oral Surg Oral Med Oral Pathol Oral Radiol Endod*. 2007.
6. Holmstrup P, Vedtofte P, Reibel J, et al. Long-term treatment outcome of oral premalignant lesions. *Oral Oncol*. 2006;42:461–74.

ADDITIONAL READING

- Demko CA, Sawyer D, Slivka M, Smith D, Wotman S et al. Prevalence of oral lesions in the dental office. *Gen Dent*. 504–9.
- Dietrich T, Reichart PA, Scheifele C. Clinical risk factors of oral leukoplakia in a representative sample of the US population. *Oral Oncol*. 2004;40:158–63.
- Duarte EC, Ribeiro DC, Gomez MV, et al. Genetic polymorphisms of carcinogen metabolizing enzymes are associated with oral leukoplakia development and p53 overexpression. *Anticancer Res*. 2008;28:1101–6.
- Greer RO. Pathology of malignant and premalignant oral epithelial lesions. *Otolaryngol Clin North Am*. 2006;39:249–75, v.
- Hardy ML. Dietary supplement use in cancer care: help or harm. *Hematol Oncol Clin North Am*. 2008;22:581–617, vii.
- Maraki D, Becker J, Boecking A. Cytologic and DNA-cytometric very early diagnosis of oral cancer. *J Oral Pathol Med*. 2004;33:398–404.
- Mashberg A, Samit A. Early diagnosis of asymptomatic oral and oropharyngeal squamous cancers. *CA Cancer J Clin*. 1995;45:328–51.
- Reamy BV, Derby R, Bunt CW et al. Common tongue conditions in primary care. *Am Fam Physician*. 2010;81:627–34.

See Also (Topic, Algorithm, Electronic Media Element)
Epstein-Barr Virus Infections; HIV Infection and AIDS

CODES

ICD9
528.6 Leukoplakia of oral mucosa, including tongue

CLINICAL PEARLS

- Linea alba: A white line on the buccal mucosa along the occlusal plane
- Medical treatment of oral leukoplakia can resolve the lesions, but there is still a risk of remission and malignant transformation.
- Low but significant rate of malignant transformation is not prevented with medical or surgical treatment; thus long-term surveillance is essential.
- Tobacco and alcohol cessation, and consider *C. albicans* eradication to lessen risk of malignant transformation.

L

LICHEN PLANUS
Herbert P. Goodheart, MD

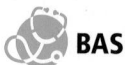 BASICS

Lichen planus (LP) is a pruritic, idiopathic eruption with characteristic shiny, flat-topped papules (Latin: planus, "flat") purple (violaceous) papules on the skin, often accompanied by characteristic mucous membrane lesions.

DESCRIPTION
- Classic (typical) LP is a relatively uncommon cutaneous inflammatory disorder of the skin and mucous membranes; hair and nails may also be affected:
  - It is most commonly found on the flexor surfaces of the upper extremities, extensor surfaces of the lower extremities, on the genitalia, and on the mucous membranes.
  - Small flat, angular, red to violaceous, shiny, pruritic papules on the skin; fine, white, lacy patches or erosions on oral mucosa
  - Course unpredictable; onset is abrupt or gradual. May resolve spontaneously, recur intermittently, or be chronic for many years.
- Drug-induced LP:
  - Clinical and histopathologic findings may mimic those of classic lichen planus. Lesions usually lack Wickham striae (see below).
  - There is generally a latent period of months from drug introduction before lesions appear.
  - Lesions resolve when inciting agent is discontinued, often after a prolonged period.
- LP variants:
  - Follicular: On scalp (lichen planopilaris) and skin
  - Annular: Appear on glans penis and oral mucosa
  - Linear: May be an isolated finding
  - Atrophic: Rare, most often the result of resolved lesions
  - Lichen planus pemphigoides: A combination of LP and bullous pemphigoid
- System(s) affected: Skin/Exocrine
- Synonym(s): Lichenoid eruptions

EPIDEMIOLOGY
- Predominant age: 30–60 years old; rare in children and the geriatric population
- Predominant sex: Female > Male

Prevalence
In the US, 450/100,000

RISK FACTORS
Exposure to certain drugs or chemicals:
- Thiazides, furosemide, beta-blockers, sulfonylureas, antimalarials, penicillamine, gold salts, and angiotensin-converting enzyme inhibitors
- Rarely: Photo-developing chemicals, dental materials, tattoo pigments

ETIOLOGY
LP is considered to be a cell-mediated immune response of unknown origin.

COMMONLY ASSOCIATED CONDITIONS
- An association has been noted between lichen planus and hepatitis C virus infection (more common in Japan and Italy), chronic active hepatitis, lichen nitidus, and primary biliary cirrhosis. Hepatitis should be considered in patients with widespread presentations of LP.
- Lichen planus has also infrequently been reported to be found in association with other diseases of altered immunity than would be expected by chance:
  - Bullous pemphigoid
  - Alopecia areata
  - Myasthenia gravis
  - Vitiligo
  - Ulcerative colitis
  - Graft versus host reaction
  - Lupus erythematosus (lupus erythematosus–lichen planus overlap syndrome)
  - Morphea and lichen sclerosis et atrophicus

DIAGNOSIS

LP is most commonly diagnosed by its appearance, despite its range of clinical presentations. A skin biopsy should be performed if the diagnosis is in doubt.

HISTORY
A minority of patients have a family history of LP. Affected families have an increased frequency of human leukocyte antigen B7(HLA-B7).

PHYSICAL EXAM
- Skin (often severe pruritus):
  - Papules: 1–10 mm, shiny, flat-topped (planar) lesions that occur in crops; lesions may have a fine scale
  - Evidence of scratching (i.e., crusts and excoriations) is usually absent.
  - Color: Violaceous, with white lacelike pattern (Wickham striae) on surface of papules. Wickham striae are best seen after topical application of mineral oil, and if present, are virtually pathognomonic for lichen planus.
  - Shape: Polygonal or oval. Annular lesions may appear on trunk and mucous membranes. Various shapes and sizes may be noted (polymorphic).
  - Arrangement: May be grouped, linear, or scattered individual lesions
  - Koebner phenomenon (isomorphic response): New lesions may be noted at sites of minor injuries such as scratches or burns.
  - Distribution: Ventral surface of wrists and forearms, dorsa hands, glans penis, dorsa feet, groin, sacrum, shins, and scalp. Hypertrophic (verrucous) lesions may occur on lower legs and may be generalized.
  - Postinflammatory hyperpigmentation: Lesions typically heal, leaving darkly pigmented macules in their wake.

- Mucous membranes (40–60% of patients with skin lesions; 20% have mucous lesions without skin involvement):
  - Most commonly asymptomatic, nonerosive, milky-white lines with an elegant, lacy, netlike streaked pattern
  - Usually seen on buccal mucosa, but may appear on tongue, gingiva, palate, or lips
  - May be erosive, rarely bullous
  - Painful, especially if ulcers present
  - Lesions may develop into squamous cell carcinoma (1–3%).
  - Glans penis, labia minora, vaginal vault (1), and perianal areas may be involved (2,3).
- Hair and nails:
  - Scalp: Atrophic scalp skin and destruction of hair follicles. May result in permanent patchy, scarring alopecia (lichen planopilaris).
- Nails (10%): Involvement of nail matrix may cause proximal to distal linear grooves and partial or complete destruction of nail bed with pterygium formation.

DIAGNOSTIC TESTS & INTERPRETATION
Lab
If suggested by history:
- Serology for hepatitis B and C
- Liver function tests

Diagnostic Procedures/Surgery
- Skin biopsy
- Direct immunofluorescence helps to distinguish lichen planus from discoid lupus erythematosus.

Pathological Findings
- Vacuolar degeneration of the basal layer
- Hyperkeratosis and irregular acanthosis, increased granular layer
- Basement membrane thinning with "saw-toothing"
- Degenerative keratinocytes, known as colloid or Civatte bodies, are found in the lower epidermis
- Dense, bandlike (lichenoid) lymphocytic infiltrate of the upper dermis
- Melanin pigment in macrophages

DIFFERENTIAL DIAGNOSIS
- Skin:
  - Lichen simplex chronicus
  - Eczematous dermatitis
  - Psoriasis
  - Discoid lupus erythematosus
  - Other lichenoid eruptions (those that resemble lichen planus)
  - Pityriasis rosea
  - Lichen nitidus
- Oral mucous membranes:
  - Leukoplakia
  - Oral hairy leukoplakia
  - Candidiasis
  - Squamous cell carcinoma (particularly in ulcerative lesions)
  - Aphthous ulcers
  - Herpetic stomatitis
  - Secondary syphilis

- Genital mucous membranes:
  – Psoriasis (penis and labia)
  – Nonspecific balanitis, Zoon balanitis
  – Fixed drug eruption (penis)
  – Candidiasis (penis and labia)
  – Pemphigus vulgaris, bullous pemphigoid, and Behçet disease (all rare)
- Hair and scalp:
  – Scarring alopecia (pseudopelade)

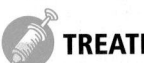 **TREATMENT**

MEDICATION

First Line

Pediatric Considerations

- Children may absorb a proportionally larger amount of topical steroid because of larger skin surface-to-weight ratio.

- Skin: Superpotent topical steroids (e.g., 0.05% clobetasol propionate) b.i.d. for 2 weeks:
  – Potent topical steroids such as triamcinolone acetonide 0.1% or fluocinonide 0.05% under occlusion
  – Intralesional corticosteroids (e.g., triamcinolone [Kenalog] 5–10 mg/mL) for recalcitrant and hypertrophic lesions
  – Antihistamine (e.g., hydroxyzine, 25 mg p.o. q6h) if needed for itching
  – "Soak and smear" technique: Can lead to a rapid improvement of symptoms in even a day or 2 and may obviate the need for systemic steroids. Soaking allows water to hydrate the stratum corneum. Soaking also allows the anti-inflammatory steroid in the ointment to penetrate more deeply into the skin. Smearing of the ointment traps the water in the skin because water cannot move out through greasy materials:
    ○ Soaking is done in a bathtub using lukewarm plain water for 20 minutes at night, then, without drying the skin, affected skin is immediately smeared with a thin film of the steroid ointment containing clobetasol or another superpotent topical steroid. A topical steroid cream is applied thereafter during the daytime hours, if necessary.
    ○ The soaking and smearing may be done for 4–5 days or longer, if necessary. The treatments are best done at night because the greasy ointment applied to the skin gets on pajamas (instead of on daytime clothes) and the ointment is on the skin during sleep.
- Mucous membranes for erosive, painful lichen planus:
  – Topical corticosteroids (0.1% triamcinolone [Kenalog] in Orabase) or 0.05% clobetasol propionate ointment b.i.d.
  – Intralesional corticosteroids
  – Topical 1% tacrolimus (Protopic ointment) b.i.d. (4,5)
  – Topical 1% pimecrolimus (Elidel) cream b.i.d. (6)
  – Topical retinoids (e.g., 0.05% tretinoin [retinoic acid] in Orabase)

Second Line

Skin:

- Oral prednisone: Used only for a short course (e.g., 30–60 mg/d for 2–4 weeks) or intramuscular triamcinolone (Kenalog) 40–80 mg every 6–8 weeks:
  – Precautions with systemic steroids
  – Systemic absorption of steroids may result in hypothalamic-pituitary-adrenal axis suppression, Cushing syndrome, hyperglycemia, or glucosuria.
  – Increased risk with high-potency topical steroids (i.e., use over large surface area, prolonged use, occlusive dressings)
  – In pregnancy: Usually safe but benefits must outweigh the risks
- Oral retinoids: Isotretinoin, acitretin:
  – Oral metronidazole
  – Cyclosporine may be used in severe cases, but cost and potential toxicity limit its use. Topical use for severe oral involvement refractory to other treatments (4).
  – Thalidomide
  – PUVA or narrow-band UVB
  – Griseofulvin
  – Azathioprine (1)
  – Mycophenolate mofetil

ALERT

Avoid oral and topical retinoids during pregnancy.

ADDITIONAL TREATMENT

General Measures

- Goal is to relieve itching and resolve lesions
- Asymptomatic oral lesions require no treatment.

IN-PATIENT CONSIDERATIONS

Initial Stabilization

Outpatient care

 ONGOING CARE

FOLLOW-UP RECOMMENDATIONS

Patient Monitoring

Serial oral examinations for erosive/ulcerative lesions

PATIENT EDUCATION

- Oral, erosive, or ulcerative lichen planus: Annual follow-up to screen for malignancy (7)
- Avoid spicy foods, cigarettes, and excessive alcohol.
- Avoid crispy foods such as corn chips, pretzels, and toast.

PROGNOSIS

- Spontaneous resolution in weeks is possible, but disease may persist for years, especially oral lesions and hypertrophic lesions on the shins.
- There is a tendency toward relapse.
- Recurrence in 12–20%, especially in those with generalized involvement

COMPLICATIONS

- Alopecia
- Nail destruction
- Squamous cell carcinoma of the mouth or genitals

REFERENCES

1. Murphy R, Edwards L et al. Desquamative inflammatory vaginitis: what is it? *J Reprod Med*. 2008;53:124–8
2. Belfiore P, Di Fede O, Cabibi D, Campisi G, Amaru GS, De Cantis S, et al. Prevalence of vulval lichen planus in a cohort of women with oral lichen planus: an interdisciplinary study. *Br J Dermatol*. Nov 2006;155(5):994–8.
3. Di Fede O, Belfiore P, Cabibi D, et al. Unexpectedly high frequency of genital involvement in women with clinical and histological features of oral lichen planus. *Acta Derm Venereol*. 2006;86:433–8.
4. Conrotto D, Carbone M, Carrozzo M, et al. Ciclosporin vs. clobetasol in the topical management of atrophic and erosive oral lichen planus: a double-blind, randomized controlled trial. *Br J Dermatol*. 2006;154:139–45.
5. Morrison L, Kratochvil FJ, Gorman A. An open trial of topical tacrolimus for erosive oral lichen planus. *J Am Acad Dermatol*. 2002;47:617–20.
6. Passeron T, Lacour JP, Fontas E, et al. Treatment of oral erosive lichen planus with 1% pimecrolimus cream: a double-blind, randomized, prospective trial with measurement of pimecrolimus levels in the blood. *Arch Dermatol*. 2007;143:472–6.
7. Eisen D. The clinical features, malignant potential, and systemic associations of oral lichen planus: a study of 723 patients. *J Am Acad Dermatol*. 2002;46:207–14.

ADDITIONAL READING

- Camisa C, Popovsky JL. Effective treatment of oral erosive lichen planus with thalidomide. *Arch Dermatol*. 2000;136:1442–3.
- Gonzalez-Moles MA, Scully C, Gil-Montoya JA. Oral lichen planus: controversies surrounding malignant transformation. *Oral Dis*. 2008;14(3):229–43.

 CODES

ICD9
697.0 Lichen planus

CLINICAL PEARLS

- Remember the 7 Ps of lichen planus: **P**urple, **p**lanar, **p**olygonal, **p**olymorphic, **p**ruritic, **p**apules, that heal with **p**ostinflammatory hyperpigmentation.
- Serial oral or genital examinations are indicated for erosive/ulcerative LP lesions to monitor for the development of squamous cell carcinoma.
- An association has been noted between LP and hepatitis C virus infection, chronic active hepatitis, and primary biliary cirrhosis.
- The "soak and smear" technique can lead to a rapid improvement of symptoms in even a day or 2 and may obviate the need for systemic steroids.

L

LICHEN SIMPLEX CHRONICUS

Daria I. Grisanzio, PharmD, RPh
Joseph Grisanzio, MD

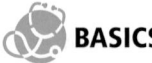 **BASICS**

DESCRIPTION
- A chronic dermatitis resulting from continued, repeated rubbing or scratching part of the skin
- System(s) affected: Skin/Exocrine
- Synonym(s): Lichen simplex; Neurodermatitis; Neurodermatitis circumscripta

EPIDEMIOLOGY
Geriatric Considerations
Common in those >60 years

Pediatric Considerations
Rare in preadolescents

Incidence
- Common
- Peak incidence 30–50 years of age
- Females > Males

Prevalence
Common

RISK FACTORS
- Any pre-existing pruritic dermatosis can result in the development of lichen simplex chronicus.
- Exposure to irritants

Genetics
- Possible relation to polymorphisms of the serotonin transporter gene
- Short allele at promoter region leading to increased risk of disease
- 12/12 genotype relating to increased risk of psychiatric complications

GENERAL PREVENTION
Avoid irritants and other known causative agents.

PATHOPHYSIOLOGY
- Repeated scratching or rubbing of an area of skin causes inflammation and pruritus.
- Pruritus results from continued scratching.
- Scratching may become a conditioned response to anxiety.
- Habitual scratching and scratch-itch cycle result in chronic dermatosis.

ETIOLOGY
- Idiopathic in many instances
- Some skin types are more prone to lichenification (i.e., persons with eczematous conditions).
- Some causes of apparent idiopathic disease may be secondary to a previously unrecognized dermatosis.
- Secondary forms may begin as another pruritic skin disease that evolves into neurodermatitis after resolution of the primary dermatitis.
- Relation between disease development and underlying neuropathy, particularly radiculopathy or nerve-root compression
- Primary dermatoses from which neurodermatitis may develop include lichen planus, stasis dermatitis, atopic dermatitis, contact dermatitis, psoriasis, tinea corporis, seborrheic dermatitis, xerosis, eczema, and herpes zoster.
- Anxiety and emotional stress may play a role.

COMMONLY ASSOCIATED CONDITIONS
- Prurigo nodularis is a nodular variety of the same disease process.
- Atopic dermatitis
- Anxiety

 DIAGNOSIS

HISTORY
- Gradual onset
- Begins as a localized area of pruritus
- Most commonly involves easily accessible areas, including nape of neck, lower legs, ankles, wrists, extensor surfaces of forearms, scalp, external ear, and anogenital region
- Pruritus out of proportion to the appearance of the lesion is typically paroxysmal, worse at night, and may occur during sleep
- Nuchal and suboccipital regions are more commonly affected in women.
- Anxiety and obsessive disorders are commonly associated with this condition.
- The perineal region is more commonly affected in men.

PHYSICAL EXAM
- Lichenified, excoriated pruritic patches of skin
- Nonerythematous
- Accentuation of normal skin lines
- Verrucous thickening and changes in pigmentation
- Vesicles or weeping is rare.
- Moist scale, serum crusting, or pustules suggest the presence of infection.
- Scarring may be present following serious secondary infections.

DIAGNOSTIC TESTS & INTERPRETATION
Lab
Initial lab tests
- None diagnostic
- Appropriate tests to evaluate for other conditions, such as potassium hydroxide microscopy preparation or culture for fungus

Diagnostic Procedures/Surgery
Skin biopsy to evaluate for other conditions if no response to treatment

Pathological Findings
- Hyperkeratosis
- Acanthosis
- Lengthening of rete ridges
- Hyperplasia of all components of epidermis
- Chronic inflammatory infiltrate of dermis

DIFFERENTIAL DIAGNOSIS
- Atopic dermatitis
- Contact dermatitis
- Cutaneous T-cell lymphoma
- Drug reaction
- Lichen planus
- Lichenified psoriasis
- Photodermatitis
- Stasis dermatitis
- Cutaneous amyloidosis
- Fungal infection
- Seborrheic dermatitis
- Lupus vulgaris (cutaneous tuberculosis)

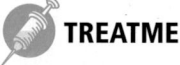 **TREATMENT**

MEDICATION
First Line
- Standard topical antipruritic agents:
  - Menthol preparations (e.g., Sarna)
  - Pramoxine (e.g., PrameGel)
  - Calamine lotion for weeping lesions
- Topical steroids are 1st-line agents for treating lichen simplex chronicus:
  - High-potency steroids alone, such as 0.05% betamethasone dipropionate cream or 0.05% clobetasol propionate cream, can be used initially but should not be used on the face, anogenital region, or intertriginous areas. They should be used on small areas only for no longer than 2 weeks.
  - Switch to intermediate- or low-potency steroids alone as response allows.
  - An intermediate-potency steroid, such as 0.025% or 0.1% triamcinolone cream, may be used for initial treatment of the face and intertriginous areas, and for maintenance treatment of other areas.
  - A low-potency steroid, such as 1% hydrocortisone cream, should be used for maintenance treatment of the face and intertriginous areas.
  - Steroid tape, flurandrenolide (e.g., Cordran):
    - Optimized penetration
    - Provides a barrier to further trauma

- Contraindications:
  - High-potency topical steroids should not be used on the face or intertriginous areas.
- Precautions:
  - Topical and intralesional steroid therapy can cause epidermal and dermal atrophy as well as hypopigmentation.

Second Line
- Topical doxepin cream 5% is an effective antipruritic agent (1)[C].
- Topical capsaicin cream can be helpful.
- Oral antihistamines can be used for their antipruritic and sedative effects.
- For resistant cases, consider a course of prednisone 40 mg/d for 2 weeks.
- Intralesional corticosteroids
- Topical aspirin has been shown to be helpful in treating neurodermatitis (2)[C].
- Topical pimecrolimus has been shown to decrease the symptoms of vulvar lichen simplex chronicus (3)[C].
- Botulinum toxin injected intradermally has been reported to improve symptoms in patients with recalcitrant pruritus (4)[C].
- Oral antibiotics for secondary infections (5)[C]
- Oral anxiolytics may be beneficial in patients with an anxiety component (5)[C].
- Transcutaneous electrical nerve stimulation may relieve pruritis in patients for whom topical steroids were not effective (6)[C].

ADDITIONAL TREATMENT
General Measures
- Patient education
- Treat pruritus to interrupt the scratch–itch cycle.
- Treat underlying pruritic skin conditions.
- Lubricating lotions and creams
- Nail trimming

Issues for Referral
- No response to treatment
- Presence of signs and symptoms suggestive of a systemic cause of pruritus
- Consultation with a psychiatrist for patients with severe stress, anxiety, or compulsive scratching
- Consultation with an allergist for patients with multisystemic atopic symptoms

Additional Therapies
- Cold Burow solution compresses:
  - One packet of Domeboro powder in 1 qt of ice-cold water applied with a cloth for 15 minutes as needed
- Coal tar preparations are useful but cosmetically less appealing.
- Unna boot for barrier protection
- Exercise when stress may be a causative factor

COMPLEMENTARY AND ALTERNATIVE MEDICINE
- Cognitive behavioral treatment focusing on thoughts leading to and awareness of itching and substitution of other activities has been shown to be helpful (7)[C].
- Hypnosis focusing on nonscratching behavior and lessening the sensations of pruritus has been beneficial (7)[C].
- Homeopathic remedies (i.e., thuja and graphites) may provide resolution of symptoms followed by a period of nonrecurrence (8)[C].

 ONGOING CARE

FOLLOW-UP RECOMMENDATIONS
Patient Monitoring
Patients should be followed closely and regularly for response to therapy, complications from therapy, and secondary infections.

DIET
Regular balanced diet

PATIENT EDUCATION
- Patients should understand the cause of this disease and their role in helping resolve the condition.
- Stress reduction techniques can be useful for patients for whom stress plays role.
- Emphasize that scratching and rubbing must stop for lesions to heal.
- Avoid exposure to known irritants.

PROGNOSIS
- Often chronic and recurrent
- Good prognosis if the scratch–itch cycle can be broken
- After healing, the skin should have a normal appearance. If secondary infections have occurred, scarring may be present.

COMPLICATIONS
- Secondary infection
- Rare scarring due to secondary infection
- Complications related to therapy, as mentioned in medication precautions

REFERENCES

1. Kantor GR, Resnik KS. Treatment of lichen simplex chronicus with topical capsaicin cream. *Acta Derm Venereol*. 1996;76:161.
2. Yosipovitch G, Sugeng MW, Chan YH, et al. The effect of topically applied aspirin on localized circumscribed neurodermatitis. *J Am Acad Dermatol*. 2001;45:910–3.
3. Goldstein AT, Parneix-Spake A. Pimecrolimus cream 1% for treatment of vulvar lichen simplex chronicus: An open label trial. *Obstet Gynecol*. 2006;107(4 Suppl):54S–55S.
4. Heckmann M, Heyer G, Brunner B, et al. Botulinum toxin type A injection in the treatment of lichen simplex: an open pilot study. *J Am Acad Dermatol*. 2002;46:617–9.
5. Datz B, Yawalkar S. A double-blind, multicenter trial of 0.05% halobetasol propionate ointment and 0.05% clobetasol 17-propionate ointment in the treatment of patients with chronic, localized atopic dermatitis or lichen simplex chronicus. *J Am Acad Dermatol*. 1991;25:1157–60.
6. Engin B, Tufekci O, Yazici A, et al. The effect of transcutaneous electrical nerve stimulation in the treatment of lichen simplex: a prospective study. *Clin Exp Dermatol*. 2009;34:324–8.
7. Shenefelt PD. Biofeedback, cognitive-behavioral methods, and hypnosis in dermatology: is it all in your mind? *Dermatol Ther*. 2003;16:114–22.
8. Gupta R, Gupta R, Manchanda RK, et al. Homoeopathy for the treatment of lichen simplex chronicus: a case series. *Homeopathy*. 2006;95:245–7.

 CODES

ICD9
698.3 Lichenification and lichen simplex chronicus

CLINICAL PEARLS
- Lichen simplex chronicus may originate from a previous pruritic condition but has become a chronic inflammatory condition due to repeated scratching and rubbing.
- The diagnosis is made clinically based on the history and skin examination. If the diagnosis is unclear, consider empiric treatment with close monitoring or skin biopsy.
- Stopping the scratch–itch cycle through patient education, skin lubrication, and topical antipruritic medications is key.

L

LIPOMA

Jose Oscar Seda, MD
Richard P. Usatine, MD

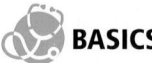 BASICS

DESCRIPTION
- Lipomas are the most common soft tissue tumors.
- Most are subcutaneous and composed of normal adipose tissue.
- Slow growing, often asymptomatic, and usually diagnosed by palpation
- Enveloped by a thin, fibrous capsule
- Reported to occur after trauma
- Lipomas rarely, if ever, become malignant but must be differentiated from liposarcomas and other tumors.

EPIDEMIOLOGY
- They can occur at any age but are most common in middle-aged adults, peaking in the 40- to 60-year age group.
- They are rare <20 years of age.

Prevalence
Occur in about 1% of population

RISK FACTORS
- Soft tissue trauma frequently has been cited as a cause, especially if the patient develops a posttraumatic hematoma.
- Alcohol consumption may be a predisposing factor for Madelung disease, or benign symmetric lipomatosis, with lipomas on the head, neck, shoulders, and proximal upper extremities. This may present with the characteristic "horse collar" cervical appearance.

Genetics
- May appear as a hereditary trait in patients with hereditary multiple lipomatosis, an autosomal dominant condition. This is found most frequently in men, characterized by extensive symmetric lipomas mostly on extremities and trunk.
- Also seen in Gardner syndrome, a variant of familial adenomatous polyposis, an autosomal dominant disease characterized by gastrointestinal (GI) polyps, multiple osteomas, and skin and soft tissue tumors.
- Congenital lipomas have been observed in children.

PATHOPHYSIOLOGY
- The pathogenetic link between soft tissue trauma and the formation of posttraumatic lipomas is still controversial.
- There are 2 potential explanations to correlate soft tissue trauma and adipose tissue tumor growth.
- The first is the formation of so-called posttraumatic pseudolipomas by prolapsing adipose tissue through fascia resulting from direct impact.
- A second possibility points toward lipoma formation as a result of preadipocyte differentiation and proliferation mediated by cytokine release following soft tissue trauma and hematoma formation.

ETIOLOGY
They are reported to occur after trauma or after steroid injection, but most are idiopathic.

COMMONLY ASSOCIATED CONDITIONS
- Admixture of other tissue types leads to fibrolipomas, angiolipomas, and myolipomas.
- Unusual syndromes include the giant variety, hereditary multiple lipomatosis, adiposis dolorosa (multiple tender diffuse lesions), and Madelung disease (numerous, symmetrically distributed lipomas of the upper trunk).
- Liposarcomas rarely develop from benign lipomas. They can occur anywhere in the body, mostly in deep structures.

DIAGNOSIS

HISTORY
- Useful questions on history gathering are duration, associated symptoms, tenderness, recurrence, progression, similar lesions, and weight loss.
- Generally slow-growing; may take years before being noticed
- If fast growing, may indicate a liposarcoma
- Usually asymptomatic
- Infrequently may cause pain; seen with angiolipoma, a highly vascular lipoma
- If compression occurs, pressure or neuropathic symptoms may develop (mass effect) in locations such as the forearm or ankle.
- Most often patients show them to physicians for explanation and reassurance.
- They may be first noted by physicians on a physical exam.

PHYSICAL EXAM
- Lipomas are usually soft, homogeneous, oval, and nontender, and the overlying skin is mobile over them.
- They are commonly from 1–6 cm in diameter. If larger, this raises suspicion for liposarcoma.
- Rubbery or doughy consistency; if harder, suspect liposarcoma, sebaceous (epidermoid) cyst, or abscess
- Overlying skin is normal; if erythematous, might indicate an abscess.
- The tumor will be felt to slip out from under your fingers ("slippage sign") as opposed to a sebaceous cyst or an abscess, which is tethered by surrounding induration.
- Individuals can have single lesions or a few. In ~5% of cases, patients have multiple lesions.
- They are usually subcutaneous and often found in the upper trunk, especially the shoulders, back, neck, and head, but can be anywhere in or on the body.

- In the GI tract, lipomas present as submucosal fatty tumors. The most common locations include the esophagus, stomach, and small intestine. Symptoms occur from luminal obstruction or bleeding.
- Lipomas have been reported in anatomic locations as varied as cardiac, intrathoracic, endobronchial, retroperitoneal, breast, intermuscular, calf, thigh, scapular, intraosseous, fingers, palmar, toe, epidural, spinal, intraarticular (knee), parapharyngeal, nasopharyngeal, adrenal, inguinal, bladder, scrotal, ovarian, intracranial, intraneural, and GI tract (most often in the ileum).

DIAGNOSTIC TESTS & INTERPRETATION
Most subcutaneous lipomas can be diagnosed based on history and physical, and no imaging studies are required.

Imaging
- Magnetic resonance imaging (MRI) and computed tomography scan are used mostly for atypical locations and as a preoperative measure.
- Because of differences in treatment, prognosis, and long-term follow-up, it is important to preoperatively distinguish simple lipomas from well-differentiated liposarcomas.
- MRI is highly sensitive in the detection of well-differentiated liposarcomas and highly specific in the diagnosis of simple lipomas.
- Reported MRI findings suggestive of liposarcoma include a partially ill-defined margin, neurovascular involvement, enhancing thick/nodular septum, and a partially bright signal intensity on T1 weighted images. A thick/nodular septum was identified as the most statistically significant predictor of liposarcoma (1).
- When an extremity or body wall lesion is considered suspicious for well-differentiated liposarcoma, it is more likely (64%) to represent one of many benign lipoma variants (2).
- If liposarcoma is suspected, fine- and core-needle aspirations have been proposed along with imaging.
- A core-needle biopsy has been proposed as the preferred biopsy method; it can provide accurate diagnosis and assessment of malignant potential and grade if examined by an experienced pathologist (3).

Diagnostic Procedures/Surgery
If diagnosis is uncertain, excisional biopsy is a preferred assessment tool.

Pathological Findings
- Lipomas are composed of adipose tissue, with varying amounts of a network of connective tissue.
- Lipomas differ from normal fat with increased levels of lipoprotein lipase and a larger number of precursor cells.

DIFFERENTIAL DIAGNOSIS

- In the subcutaneous location, the primary differential diagnosis is a sebaceous cyst or an abscess.
- Sebaceous (epidermoid) cysts are also rounded and subcutaneous. They can be differentiated from lipomas by their characteristic central punctum and surrounding induration.
- Benign lipomas must be differentiated from liposarcomas.
- Rapid growth and pain should prompt consideration of malignancy.
- Refer to History and Physical Exam for more clues on differential diagnosis.

 ## TREATMENT

- Most lipomas can be observed without treatment (4)[C].
- They need excision if there is diagnostic uncertainty, lack of homogeneity to palpation, rapid growth, associated pain, or cosmetic concern. Treatment is excision, but steroid injection or liposuction can be useful in certain locations (such as facial) (4)[C].
- A successful trial of lipomas treated with subcutaneous deoxycholate injections has been reported suggesting that low-concentration deoxycholate may be a relatively safe and effective treatment for small collections of fat. However, controlled clinical trials will be necessary to substantiate these observations (5).
- Spinal lipomas should be operated on as soon as possible on a prophylactic basis, and careful and constant follow-up should be carried out to permit prompt reintervention in cases with deterioration (6).

SURGERY/OTHER PROCEDURES

- Plan the incision to follow skin lines, if possible, to minimize scarring. Use a surgical marker to draw out the palpable margins of the lipoma and the planned incision. The incision should be about 60% of the lipoma width. Be prepared to extend the incision if needed.
- After anesthesia, a linear incision is carried out down to the level of the capsule using a number 11 or 15 blade.
- Blunt dissection (curved hemostat) and sharp dissection (iris scissor) are used to free up the lipoma and to separate it from the inferior normal tissue.
- As the lobule is lifted, the dissection is continued to free up the entire tumor.
- Apply pressure to the outside of the lipoma to express it through the skin opening (7). In many cases, the lipoma will just pop out. If not, more dissection may be needed, or the incision may be lengthened.

- After the lipoma is out, pressure with gauze is usually all that is needed to obtain good hemostasis. If bleeding persists, use electrocoagulation before closing the incision.
- The dead space may be closed with deep absorbable sutures, but often this is not necessary.
- The skin may be closed with nonabsorbable simple interrupted sutures. For small lipomas, closure may be performed with wound-closure strips or the linear incision left open.
- If excessive skin remains, the linear incision can be turned into an ellipse to avoid redundant skin.

 ## ONGOING CARE

FOLLOW-UP RECOMMENDATIONS
Usual surgical follow-up is needed, with treatment of any hematoma formation or infection.

PATIENT EDUCATION
Handout: "What Are Lipomas?" *American Family Physician*, March 1, 2002; http://www.aafp.org/afp/20020301/905ph.html

PROGNOSIS
Most lipomas grow very slowly and are benign, asymptomatic, and remain stable.

COMPLICATIONS
- Hematoma formation or infection is rare but possible.
- Occasionally a bilobar lipoma may be missed, resulting in "recurrence."
- Lipomas that grow rapidly or become painful or nodular must be evaluated for liposarcoma.

REFERENCES

1. Jaovisidha S, Suvikapakornkul Y, Woratanarat P, Subhadrabandhu T, Nartthanarung A, Siriwongpairat P et al. MR imaging of fat-containing tumours: the distinction between lipoma and liposarcoma. *Singapore Med J*. 2010;51: 418–23.
2. Gaskin CM, Helms CA. Lipomas, lipoma variants, and well-differentiated liposarcomas (atypical lipomas): results of MRI evaluations of 126 consecutive fatty masses. *AJR Am J Roentgenol*. 2004;182:733–9.
3. Heslin MJ, Lewis JJ, Woodruff JM, et al. Core needle biopsy for diagnosis of extremity soft tissue sarcoma. *Ann Surg Oncol*. 1997;4:425–31.
4. Bancroft LW, Kransdorf MJ, Peterson JJ, et al. Benign fatty tumors: classification, clinical course, imaging appearance, and treatment. *Skeletal Radiol*. 2006;35:719–33.

---

5. Rotunda AM, Ablon G, Kolodney MS. Lipomas treated with subcutaneous deoxycholate injections. *J Am Acad Dermatol*. 2005;53:973–8.
6. La Marca F, Grant JA, Tomita T, et al. Spinal lipomas in children: outcome of 270 procedures. *Pediatr Neurosurg*. 1997;26:8–16.
7. Kenawi MM. 'Squeeze delivery' excision of subcutaneous lipoma related to anatomic site. *Br J Surg*. 1995;82:1649–50.

ADDITIONAL READING

- Aust MC, Spies M, Kall S, et al. Posttraumatic lipoma: fact or fiction? *Skinmed*. 2007;6: 266–70.
- Blount JP, Elton S. Spinal lipomas. *Neurosurg Foc*. 2001;10(1):e3.
- Lellouch-Tubiana A, Zerah M, Catala M, et al. Congenital intraspinal lipomas: histological analysis of 234 cases and review of the literature. *Pediatr Dev Pathol*. 1999;2:346–52.
- Salam GA. Lipoma excision. *Am Fam Physician*. 2002;65:901–4.
- Springfield D. Liposarcoma. *Clin Orthopaed Rel Res*. 1993;(289):50–7.

 ## CODES

ICD9
- 214.0 Lipoma of skin and subcutaneous tissue of face
- 214.1 Lipoma of other skin and subcutaneous tissue
- 214.2 Lipoma of intrathoracic organs

CLINICAL PEARLS

- Slow growing, often asymptomatic, and usually diagnosed by palpation
- Asymptomatic lipomas can be followed clinically and only need treatment if they cause pain, are growing rapidly, or become nonhomogeneous.
- Most symptomatic lipomas are removed surgically, but for small ones, liposuction or cortisone injection has been reported to be successful.
- In the subcutaneous location, the primary differential diagnosis is a sebaceous (epidermoid) cyst or an abscess.
- Consider subspecialty care if a lipoma in a delicate anatomic location needs removal or if there is concern that the lesion might be malignant.

L

LISTERIOSIS

Michael A. Malone, MD

 BASICS

DESCRIPTION
- Infection caused by the ubiquitous, weakly hemolytic, gram-positive bacillus *Listeria monocytogenes*; pathogenic to many species
- Occurs most often in fetuses (disseminated infantile listeriosis), neonates, and immunosuppressed patients
- Most adult patients have preexisting disease (e.g., cirrhosis, lymphomas, solid tumors, AIDS, cancer therapy, organ transplant recipients) or are on corticosteroid therapy.
- Usual course: Acute

Pediatric Considerations
- Infected fetuses are often stillborn or premature.
- Up to 50% mortality in treated neonates

EPIDEMIOLOGY
Incidence
- Incidence in 2008 general US population of foodborne listeriosis: 0.29/100,000 people
- Predominant age: Neonates (<1 month), elderly (>60 years):
  - Predominant sex: Male > Female
  - In the US, approximately 500 people per year die from listeriosis
  - 20–65% of all foodborne infection-related deaths in US
  - Pregnant women account for 27% of all *Listeria* cases and approximately 60% of cases in the 10- to 40-year-old age range.
  - Almost 70% of nonperinatal infections occur in immunocompromised patients.
  - Neonates can have early- (<7 days) or late-onset (>7 days) infection.
  - Most cases of listeriosis are sporadic (not associated with an outbreak).
  - Common cause of meningitis with a mortality rate of approximately 20%

Prevalence
- Pregnancy ~20× more likely
- In AIDS, infection ~300× more likely than general population (up to 1,000× more likely in age-matched population studies)

RISK FACTORS
- Age: Fetus, neonate, elderly
- Metastatic malignant disease
- HIV infection
- Alcoholism
- Renal hemodialysis
- Immunosuppression (including corticosteroid therapy)
- Exposure to infected animals (e.g., by veterinarians, butchers); animal-to-human transmission is rare.
- Ingesting contaminated food or drink (e.g., soft cheeses, milk, butter, pate, cold-smoked trout, hot dogs, ready-to-eat pork, and deli meats)
- Pregnancy; transmission to fetuses and neonates occurs with high mortality; requires prompt and vigorous treatment to prevent transfer of disease to fetus (although often devastating to the fetus, infected pregnant women may be asymptomatic or often present with a flulike illness)

- Use of gastric acid inhibitors
- Prior hospitalization; in 1 study, 40% of cases with prior hospitalization were exposed to high-risk foods during hospitalization (1)[C]
- Colonoscopy

GENERAL PREVENTION
- For pregnant, older, or immune-compromised patients: Check US Department of Agriculture Web site for recalled foods.
- Avoid handling livestock.
- Avoid contaminated silage.
- Avoid contaminated sewage.
- Avoid raw/unpasteurized dairy products.
- Avoid soft cheeses (Mexican and feta).
- Wash all raw vegetables carefully.
- Separate uncooked meats from vegetables.
- Wash hands after handling uncooked foods.
- Avoid foods from deli counter.
- Cook leftovers, hot dogs, cold cuts, and deli meats until steaming hot before eating.
- Prevention for specific populations: Listeriosis has been effectively prevented by oral trimethoprim sulfamethoxazole @ PCP preventive doses in organ transplant and AIDS patients (2)[B].

PATHOPHYSIOLOGY
- Resistance to *Listeria* infection is mainly cell-mediated. Multiplies best at room temperature but still can grow at refrigerator temperatures.
- A unique pathogen due to its intracellular life cycle
- Once it enters the GI tract, *Listeria* can be phagocytosed by GI cells (active endocytosis) and enters the host without disturbing normal structure of the GI tract
- Hematogenous dissemination in the bloodstream
- Predisposition toward the CNS and placenta
- Able to cross placental barrier

ETIOLOGY
- *L. monocytogenes*, a small gram-positive bacillus; infection with other species of *Listeria* is rare.
- There are at least 13 serotypes of *L. monocytogenes*, but most disease is due to types 4b, 1/2a, and 1/2b.
- Incubation period for invasive illness is not well established and is highly variable because it depends on bacterial load and host immunity.
- Illnesses may begin 2–70 days after eating contaminated food.
- Extremely common in food supply: Recovery rates of 15–70% in raw vegetables, fish, meat, and unpasteurized milk:
  - Deli meat was ranked as the highest-risk ready-to-eat food vehicle of *Listeria monocytogenes*; retail-sliced carries higher rates of mortality compared with pre-packaged (3)[C].
- Isolated in stool of 5% of asymptomatic adults

COMMONLY ASSOCIATED CONDITIONS
- Pregnancy
- Immunodeficiencies
- Cirrhosis
- Lymphomas
- Solid tumors
- Organ transplant recipients
- Diabetes
- Hemochromatosis and iron overload (iron is a virulence factor for *Listeria*)

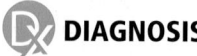 **DIAGNOSIS**

HISTORY
- Common symptoms: Fever, watery diarrhea, nausea, headache, myalgias, joint aches
- Severe headache, fever, stiff neck; seizures
- Irritability, lethargy, poor feeding in neonates
- Illness duration typically 5–10 days

PHYSICAL EXAM
- May have photophobia or focal cerebral deficits/cranial nerve palsy
- Rarely, meningeal signs

DIAGNOSTIC TESTS & INTERPRETATION
No *Listeria*-specific investigation is required for healthy patients with normal immune function.

Lab
- Stool cultures are usually negative unless specifically looking for *Listeria* (typical medium used to isolate diarrhea-causing bacteria for stool cultures can inhibit listerial growth).
- Testing is usually by blood culture (75% positive).
- Not identified well on Gram's stain; in clinical specimens, *Listeria* can be gram-variable.
- Lab misidentification as diphtheroids, streptococci, or enterococci is not uncommon.
- Isolation of a diphtheroid from blood or CSF should make one consider *Listeria*.

Initial lab tests
- CSF:
  - Gram stain: Small gram-positive rods or coccobacillary forms with tumbling motility (negative 60% of the time partly because organisms are not present in large numbers)
  - Cell count: The predominant cell type is the neutrophil; however, mononuclear cells may predominate; red blood cells (RBCs) seen frequently
  - Protein concentration: WNL to moderately elevated
  - Glucose: 60% of time is within normal limits
  - CSF culture: Need at least 10 mL of spinal fluid for culture
- Other tests:
  - Blood cultures
  - Stool, amniotic fluid, and other body fluid cultures
  - Complete blood count (CBC) may show an elevated neutrophil count and/or left shift.
  - Other cultures in newborn: Cervical vaginal secretions and lochia from the mother; cord blood; grossly abnormal portions of the placenta, meconium, and exudate expressed from an incised skin papule of the neonate
- Specimens for serologic testing should be submitted to the local public health laboratory. In outbreaks, serotyping may be desirable.
- Notify laboratory at time of sending any specimen that listeriosis is a possibility.
- Specimens must be sent to laboratory promptly (few organisms more difficult to culture).
- Antibodies to listeriolysin O have low clinical utility.

Follow-Up & Special Considerations
Repeated CSF analysis should be performed for any patient not responding after 48 h of appropriate antimicrobial therapy.

Imaging

Initial approach
MRI with contrast agent for any patient with CNS symptoms (better than CT scan)

Diagnostic Procedures/Surgery
Lumbar puncture

Pathological Findings
- Gross: Multiorgan miliary granulomatosis
- Microscopic:
  - Nodular focal abscess
  - Increased tissue macrophages
  - Gram-positive bacilli
- Bacilli with "tumbling motility" seen on CSF wet mounts

DIFFERENTIAL DIAGNOSIS
- Viral, other bacterial, or fungal (cryptococcal) meningitis
- Brain abscess or neoplasm
- Tuberculosis
- Cerebral toxoplasmosis
- Lyme disease
- Influenza
- Viral or bacterial gastroenteritis
- Infantile listeriosis, Escherichia coli infection, group B streptococci infection
- Infectious mononucleosis
- Sarcoidosis
- Other infections: Staphylococcus, gram-negative Klebsiella, Candida, viruses

 ## TREATMENT

MEDICATION
There have been no controlled trials to confirm a drug of choice or duration of therapy.

First Line
- Ampicillin typically at 4–6 g/d in divided doses is the 1st-line treatment, and the dose is doubled to 8–12 g/d in divided doses for meningitis or severe infection. Pediatric dosing is typically 100–200 mg/kg/d in divided doses and 300–400 mg/kg/d in divided doses for meningitis. (Penicillin G also may be used as a 1st-line medication.)
- Ampicillin is preferred to penicillin G, although there is little evidence showing superiority.
- Gentamycin and ampicillin have in vitro synergistic activity and are often combined for severe infections. Consider combining ampicillin with IV gentamicin: loading dose 2 mg/kg, then 1.7 mg/kg q8h until cultures negative and patient is clinically improved.
- Treatment failure is reported with 2-week treatment duration in meningitis, so a minimum treatment of 3 weeks is recommended for Listeria meningitis.
- Contraindications: Allergy to penicillins
- Other regimens:
  - It is not known what antibiotic regimen works best for endocarditis because this complication of listeriosis is rare (<100 cases ever reported), but 1 review recommends high-dose ampicillin × 4–6 weeks.
  - Patients with rhombencephalitis or brain abscess should be treated for at least 6 weeks and followed with serial MRIs.

- Precautions:
  - Cephalosporins are not adequate treatment and have high failure rates reported.
  - Treatment with chloramphenicol or vancomycin have both had high failure rates reported.

Second Line
- Trimethoprim–sulfamethoxazole (Bactrim, Septra) (4)[C]
- Other: Imipenum: 2 g IV q8h in adults; 120 mg/kg/d in 3 divided doses in children; maximum dose 6 g/d

ADDITIONAL TREATMENT
Despite good in vitro and in vivo activity for quinolones, there is evidence that progression of disease to meningitis occurs while on quinolone treatment.

Issues for Referral
- Maternal fetal medicine or neonatologist if patient is pregnant
- Infectious disease specialist if not improving with 1st-line treatment
- Neurologist if CNS involvement

IN-PATIENT CONSIDERATIONS

Discharge Criteria
- Clinical improvement
- Negative CSF and blood cultures

 ## ONGOING CARE

FOLLOW-UP RECOMMENDATIONS

Patient Monitoring
- Vitals, temperature
- Repeat lumbar puncture at 5–7 days in CNS-affected patients.
- Repeat blood cultures if endocarditis.
- Repeat imaging studies if initially abnormal.

PATIENT EDUCATION
Centers for Disease Control and Prevention, National Center for Infectious Diseases: http://www.cdc.gov/ncidod/ncid.htm/

PROGNOSIS
High mortality rate for fetal, neonatal, and infections involving the CNS; there is a high rate of CNS sequelae for survivors.

COMPLICATIONS
- Premature delivery
- Amnionitis
- Rhombencephalitis
- Meningitis
- Septicemia
- Brain, pulmonary, hepatic, placental, lymph node, or splenic abscess
- Endocarditis (accounts for about 7% of adult cases of endocarditis)
- Peritonitis
- Abortion
- Stillbirth
- Neonatal death
- Osteomyelitis

REFERENCES

1. Dalton CB, Merritt TD, Unicomb LE, Kirk MD, Stafford RJ, Lalor K, the OzFoodNet Working Group et al. A national case-control study of risk factors for listeriosis in Australia. Epidemiology and infection. 2010;1–9.
2. Fernàndez-Sabé N, Cervera C, López-Medrano F, Llano M, Sáez E, Len O, Fortn J, Blanes M, Laporta R, Torre-Cisneros J, Gavaldà J, Muñoz P, Fariñas MC, María Aguado J, Moreno A, Carratalà J et al. Risk factors, clinical features, and outcomes of listeriosis in solid-organ transplant recipients: a matched case-control study. Clin Infect Dis. 2009;49:1153–9.
3. Endrikat S, Gallagher D, Pouillot R, Hicks Quesenberry H, Labarre D, Schroeder CM, Kause J et al. A comparative risk assessment for Listeria monocytogenes in prepackaged versus retail-sliced deli meat. J Food Prot. 2010;73:612–9.
4. Bouza E, Muñoz P. Monotherapy versus combination therapy for bacterial infections. Med Clin North Am. 2000;84:1357–89, v.

ADDITIONAL READING
- Bortolussi R. Listeriosis: a primer. CMAJ. 2008;179: 795–7.
- CDC website: http://www.cdc.gov/ncidod/dbmd/diseaseinfo/listeriosis.
- Hof H. An update on the medical management of listeriosis. Expert Opin Pharmacother. 2004;5: 1727–35.
- Janakiraman V. Listeriosis in pregnancy: diagnosis, treatment, and prevention. Rev Obstet Gynecol. 2008;1:179–85.
- Ooi ST, Lorber B. Gastroenteritis due to Listeria monocytogenes. Clin Infect Dis. 2005;40:1327–32.
- Tunkel AR, Hartman BJ, Kaplan SL, et al. Practice guidelines for the management of bacterial meningitis. Clin Infect Dis. 2004;39:1267–84.

 ## CODES

ICD9
- 027.0 Listeriosis
- 771.2 Other congenital infections specific to the perinatal period

CLINICAL PEARLS
- Listeriosis in pregnancy occurs most often in the 3rd trimester.
- Duration of treatment: In immunocompetent patients, 2 weeks is sufficient for bacteremia and 3 or more weeks for CNS infection.
- When given, gentamicin is continued until the patient improves (usually 10–14 days).
- For questions regarding safety of deli meat: US Department of Agriculture, (800) 535-4555; http://www.cdc.gov/foodnet

L

LUMBAR (INTERVERTEBRAL) DISK DISORDERS

Scott E. Kinkade, MD, MSPH

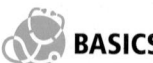 **BASICS**

DESCRIPTION

- Many patients with low back pain have lumbar disk disease and involvement of surrounding spinal ligaments, muscles, joints, and skeleton.
- Over time may progress to disk degeneration, disk herniation, spinal narrowing, and arthritic proliferation of the facet joint.
- Management is based on symptoms and disability because distinguishing between the normal aging of the spine and pathologic findings is difficult.
- Nonradicular low back pain (acute and chronic): The low back pain remains near the waist and is caused by soft tissue or disk injury.
- Radicular low back pain (acute and chronic): The neuropathic pain is greater in the buttocks, hips, or legs rather than the back. Follows dermatome.
- Signs of weakness, numbness, or loss of reflex may or may not be present.
- In younger patients, the source of the pain is likely to be mechanical compression or chemical irritation of a nerve root.
- Spinal stenosis is more likely to be the etiology of radicular pain in patients >55 years.
- System(s) affected: Musculoskeletal; Nervous
- Synonym(s): Degenerative disk disease, intervertebral disk dislocation, herniated disk, herniated nucleus pulposus

EPIDEMIOLOGY
Incidence
- One of the most frequent complaints for which adults seek medical attention and 2nd to the common cold for missed time from work.
- The incidence rate is 5–8% annually. Among patients with acute back pain, only 4% have nerve root symptoms due to a herniated disk.

Prevalence
Lifetime prevalence of low back pain is 60–90%.

Geriatric Considerations
Usually multifactorial lesions of spine; degenerative spondylolisthesis, spinal stenosis, with neurogenic claudication; osteoporotic compression fracture also likely

Pregnancy Considerations
Increased incidence of low back pain (sacroiliac dysfunction) and/or sciatica; conservative treatment

RISK FACTORS
- Normal aging process after age 20 years
- Cigarette smoking
- Stress, muscle tension
- Obesity

GENERAL PREVENTION
- Modification of jobs to reduce exposure to known risk factors
- Selection of workers for certain jobs by such means as strength testing or exclusion of workers with prior back injuries
- Avoid smoking (persisting pain more common in smokers).
- Lose excess weight.

PATHOPHYSIOLOGY
- Nerve roots exiting the spinal canal through the spinal neural foramen are susceptible to injury and irritation.
- The neural foramen may be compromised by a bulging disk; herniated nucleus pulposus; or degenerative changes of the spine, masses, or fracture.
- Inflammation leading to chemical irritation of the nerve roots is also possible.

ETIOLOGY
- Trauma, major or minor
- Frequent lifting of heavy objects, especially bending at the waist and twisting movements
- Vibration (e.g., driving motor vehicles)
- Degenerative changes

COMMONLY ASSOCIATED CONDITIONS
- Poor physical conditioning/posture
- Obesity
- Osteoarthritis
- Osteoporosis
- Depression, other psychiatric disorders

 DIAGNOSIS

HISTORY
- Assess location, onset, aggravating and relieving factors, and associated symptoms.
- Red flag conditions that may indicate a more serious etiology include:
  – Age >50, fevers, long-term corticosteroid use, weight loss, night pain, recent infection, history of cancer, immunosuppression, IV drug use, progressive neurological deficits
  – Signs of cauda equina syndrome require urgent evaluation: Perineal (saddle) anesthesia, bowel or bladder dysfunction, and severe lower extremity neurological impairment (often bilateral)

PHYSICAL EXAM
- Assess ROM.
- Palpate the spine for bony tenderness.
- Assess motor strength in lower extremities. Brief screening tests include raising heels off ground and walking on toes and raising toes off ground and walking on heels.
- Assess deep tendon reflexes in the Achilles and patellar tendons.

- Straight leg raise (SLR) test: In supine position, elevation of affected leg between 30 and 60 degrees elicits pain radiating into the leg (sensitivity = 0.80, specificity = 0.40)
- Crossed SLR test: In supine position, elevation of the leg opposite the side of pain between 30 and 60 degrees elicits pain (sensitivity = 0.25, specificity = 0.90)

DIAGNOSTIC TESTS & INTERPRETATION
Lab
Follow-Up & Special Considerations
- CBC, erythrocyte sedimentation rate, or C-reactive protein: Only indicated if red flags are present (elevation may signify infection, autoimmune arthropathy, or cancer)
- Urinalysis if suspected urinary system etiology

Imaging
Follow-Up & Special Considerations
- Imaging indicated for red flag conditions
- Lumbosacral plain films: Rarely indicated, may identify tumor, vertebral compression fracture, osteoarthritis, spondylolisthesis
- MRI preferred over CT scan and myelogram (for surgical candidate evaluation or to help rule out more serious etiology such as tumor, infection, fracture). Note: In asymptomatic adults getting MRI of the lumbar spine, disk herniation is found in about 1/3 of the patients and disk bulging is found in >1/2 of these patients.

Diagnostic Procedures/Surgery
- Myelograms not commonly used
- Electromyography useful to distinguish peripheral neuropathy from cord or nerve root impairment; may confirm level of lesion

Pathological Findings
Difficult to distinguish the normal aging process of disk degeneration from specific lesions causing low back pain and sciatica

DIFFERENTIAL DIAGNOSIS
- Acute or chronic lumbosacral strain
- Facet joint disease
- Pyriformis syndrome
- Spondylosis
- Spondylolisthesis
- Spinal arthritis
- Fibrositis/fibromyalgia
- Compression fracture
- Metastatic and primary tumors
- Vertebral infection
- Pain referred from hip, retroperitoneum, aneurysms, or pelvis; neurogenic claudication
- Cauda equina syndrome

TREATMENT

MEDICATION

First Line
- Analgesia with NSAIDs or acetaminophen
- Consider muscle relaxants.
- Precautions: Elderly, HTN, prior peptic ulcer disease or bleeding, renal disease, liver disease, cardiac dysfunction, addiction
- Contraindications/significant possible interactions: Refer to the manufacturer's profile of each drug.

ALERT
Opioids, even short term, increase of patient developing chronic back pain; avoid their use.

Second Line
- Injections: Epidural steroid injections may benefit some patients in the short term, but the evidence is not strong for long-term relief.
- Tricyclic antidepressants or gabapentin may benefit patients with radiculopathy.

ADDITIONAL TREATMENT

General Measures
- Initial conservative therapy:
  - Avoid bed rest for more than a few days; ordinary activities as tolerated; local heat
  - Analgesics; muscle relaxants
  - Physical therapy
- Conservative treatment is recommended for the 1st 4–6 weeks. >80% of herniated disks improve with time. For persistent or severe pain and neurologic deficits, consider evaluating the patient for surgery.
- Emergent surgical referral for cauda equina syndrome

Issues for Referral
- Progressive or severe neurologic deficit
- Cauda equina syndrome
- Persistent sciatica for at least 1 month with corresponding clinical and imaging findings
- Persistent neurologic deficit despite 4–6 weeks of conservative therapy

Additional Therapies
Transcutaneous electrical nerve stimulation (TENS)

COMPLEMENTARY AND ALTERNATIVE MEDICINE
- For chronic nonradicular pain: Improve physical fitness with low-impact aerobic exercise.
- Manipulation and physical therapy have been shown to be beneficial.
- Manipulation therapy: Safety and efficacy are unclear in patients with true sciatica.
- Massage
- Exercise, physical therapy
- Acupuncture: Short-term benefit

SURGERY/OTHER PROCEDURES
- Surgical discectomy:
  - Techniques include open and microsurgical discectomy; percutaneous laser, percutaneous suction, and arthroscopic discectomies are newer techniques.

- Absolute indications for discectomy:
  - Cauda equina syndrome
  - Progressive neurologic deficit despite conservative treatment
- Relative indications for discectomy:
  - Intolerable pain
  - Multiple episodes of radiculopathy
  - Persistent dysfunctional pain: These patients have been reported to improve more rapidly postoperatively, but long-term results show little difference from nonoperative treatment.
  - Static neurologic deficit: No reported difference between operative or nonoperative treatment for the improvement in weakness or sensory disturbance
  - Spinal fusion (arthrodesis): Indicated for spinal instability

IN-PATIENT CONSIDERATIONS

Initial Stabilization
- Uncommonly an inpatient admission
- Evaluate for more serious causes of back pain.
- Consider pain management consult.

 ONGOING CARE

FOLLOW-UP RECOMMENDATIONS
- Follow-up if pain or neurologic deficit is increasing.
- Return visit ~10 days following initial visit; should be improving.
- Thereafter monitor every 2 weeks until fully functional.

Patient Monitoring
- Follow pain history and neurologic status.
- Monitor exercise program.

PATIENT EDUCATION
Maintain good posture, proper body mechanics, and physical fitness.

PROGNOSIS
- Acute low back pain (90%) and/or radiculopathy (75–90%) can be expected to recover spontaneously with conservative therapy.
- Chronic nonradicular low back pain: Most patients respond to conservative management such as manipulation, fitness, weight reduction, and education regarding back care.
- Chronic radicular pain: Good selection of surgical candidates have found satisfactory results (85% in long-term studies).

COMPLICATIONS
- Foot drop with weakness of anterior tibial, posterior tibial, and peroneal muscles
- Loss of ankle jerk
- Bladder and rectal sphincter weakness with retention or incontinence
- Limitation of movement and restricted activity
- Narcotic addiction

ADDITIONAL READING
- Abdi S, Datta S, Trescot AM, et al. Epidural steroids in the management of chronic spinal pain: a systematic review. *Pain Physician*. 2007;10: 185–212.
- Atlas SJ, Keller RB, Wu YA, et al. Long-term outcomes of surgical and nonsurgical management of sciatica secondary to a lumbar disc herniation: 10 year results from the maine lumbar spine study. *Spine*. 2005;30:927–35.
- Chou R, Qaseem A, Snow V, et al. Diagnosis and treatment of low back pain: a joint clinical practice guideline from the American College of Physicians and the American Pain Society. *Ann Intern Med*. 2007;147:478–91.
- Jarvik JG, Deyo RA. Diagnostic evaluation of low back pain with emphasis on imaging. *Ann Intern Med*. 2002;137:586–97.
- Smeal WL, Tyburski M, Alleva J, et al. Conservative management of low back pain, part I. Discogenic/radicular pain. *Dis Mon*. 2004;50: 636–69.
- van Tulder MW, Koes B, Seitsalo S, et al. Outcome of invasive treatment modalities on back pain and sciatica: an evidence-based review. *Eur Spine J*. 2006;15(Suppl 1):S82–92.
- Weinstein JN, Lurie JD, Tosteson TD, et al. Surgical vs nonoperative treatment for lumbar disk herniation: the Spine Patient Outcomes Research Trial (SPORT) observational cohort. *JAMA*. 2006;296:2451–9.

See Also (Topic, Algorithm, Electronic Media Element)
Low Back Pain
Algorithm: Low Back Pain, Acute

 CODES

ICD9
- 722.10 Displacement of lumbar intervertebral disc without myelopathy
- 722.52 Degeneration of lumbar or lumbosacral intervertebral disc
- 724.2 Lumbago

CLINICAL PEARLS
- Initial imaging is rarely required, except in the presence of red flags.
- Features that predict best surgical outcome:
  - Definable neurologic deficit
  - Pathology in imaging that correlates with deficit
  - Positive nerve root tension signs
  - Leg pain >back pain
  - No response to nonsurgical therapy for 4–6 weeks
- Adverse psychosocial factors to resolving back pain:
  - Pending litigation or compensation
  - Depressed or hostile patient
  - Low IQ or poorly educated may not be able to participate in assessment or decision
  - Prolonged use of narcotics or alcohol

L

LUNG ABSCESS
Ruben Peralta, MD

 BASICS

DESCRIPTION
A localized collection cavity of necrotic lung tissue and pus resulting from pyogenic bacteria (1):
- Presentation may be acute or chronic (symptoms for >4 weeks).
- Usual course is subacute progression of symptoms.
- Synonym(s): Pulmonary abscess

EPIDEMIOLOGY
Incidence
- Predominant age: Mainly 4th–6th decades
- Predominant sex: Male > Female (4:1)

Prevalence
Unknown; relatively rare since advent of antibiotics (2)

Pediatric Considerations
Staphylococcus most common organism in children

RISK FACTORS
- Periodontal disease (gingivitis), dental abscess, dental surgery
- Risk for aspiration:
  - Alcohol intoxication (loss of consciousness) is most common cause of aspiration (1).
  - Epilepsy
  - Cerebrovascular accident (CVA) with oropharyngeal dysfunction
  - Sinusitis
  - General anesthesia with surgery
  - Dysphagia
  - Tracheal/nasogastric tube
  - Severe gastroesophageal reflux disease (GERD)
  - Cerebral palsy
- Large bacterial burden:
  - Necrotizing pneumonia
  - Bacteremia (especially *Staphylococcus*)
  - Septic embolism (especially in endocarditis)
  - Disseminated septic phlebitis
- Airway obstruction:
  - Bronchial stenosis
  - Pulmonary embolism
  - Cavitary infarction
  - Lung neoplasia
  - Enlarged lymph node
  - Foreign body: Stent-associated respiratory tract infection (SARTI) (3)
- Immunocompromise:
  - Diabetes mellitus
  - HIV infection
  - Chronic steroid use
- Amebic lung abscess: Most often from direct extension from liver abscess through the diaphragm to the right lower lobe

Genetics
- No known genetic pattern
- Immunodeficiency associated with *FCN3* mutation, and ficolin-3 deficiency may predispose patients to lung infections (4).

GENERAL PREVENTION
- Treatment of predisposing diseases
- Aspiration precautions
- Treatment of periodontal diseases

ETIOLOGY
- May be due to aspiration of anaerobic oral flora (most common); 24–48 h after aspiration, lung abscess forms (1).
- Less commonly, septic emboli from endocarditis and others (3,4,5,6,7,8,9,10)
- Usually mixed flora with predominance of anaerobes (1)
- Oral flora anaerobes (60–75% of cases):
  - *Peptostreptococcus*
  - *Prevotella*
  - *Fusobacterium*
  - *Bacteroides* sp.
- Aerobes (10–20%):
  - *Staphylococcus aureus*
  - *Streptococcus pyogenes*
  - *Klebsiella* sp.
  - *Pseudomonas aeruginosa*
  - *Streptococcus milleri*
- Atypical aerobes:
  - *Legionella*
  - *Nocardia*
- *Actinomyces*

COMMONLY ASSOCIATED CONDITIONS
- Periodontal disease
- Pneumonia
- Alcoholism
- Empyema (if necrosis of the abscess wall allows entry into pleural space) (1)
- Tuberculosis
- Immunocompetent patient

 DIAGNOSIS

HISTORY
- Fever
- Night sweats
- Diaphoresis
- Malaise
- Anorexia
- Weight loss
- Chest pain/pleurisy
- Cough with purulent, foul-smelling, putrid, sour-tasting sputum
- Dyspnea
- Hemoptysis

PHYSICAL EXAM
- Vital signs: Tachypnea, tachycardia
- Lung exam:
  - Crackles
  - Wheezing
  - Dullness to percussion
  - Consolidation by auscultation
  - Cavernous breath sounds
  - Decreased breath sounds
- Clubbing of digits

DIAGNOSTIC TESTS & INTERPRETATION
Lab
- Complete blood count (CBC) shows leukocytosis and anemia.
- Hypoalbuminemia
- Sputum smear: Neutrophils, mixed bacteria
- Sputum culture: Often grows normal respiratory flora; may help in atypical presentations
- Blood culture: Often negative in anaerobic abscess
- Drugs that may alter lab results: Prior antibiotics

Imaging
- CXR:
  - Lung cavity with air–fluid level
  - Consolidation with radiolucency, infiltrates, pleural effusion, mediastinal adenopathy
- Ultrasound:
  - Color Doppler ultrasound: Great sensitivity, specificity, positive predictive value, and negative predictive value when identification of vessel signals in a pericavitary consolidation is achieved (11,12,13).
- CT scan:
  - Defines location and extent (typical location depends on segments such as posterior segments of upper lobes or superior segments of lower lobes)
  - May detect obstructing lesion
  - May demonstrate cavitary opacities (10)
  - May show multiple thrombus of neck vessels (infectious thrombophlebitis) (14)

Diagnostic Procedures/Surgery
- Bronchoscopy if obstruction is suspected
- Bronchoscopic brushing
- Bronchoalveolar lavage
- Transthoracic needle aspiration (rarely done)
- Percutaneous catheter-guided drainage (12,15,16,17)

Pathological Findings
- Solitary abscess
- Multiple abscesses
- Cavitation with necrosis
- Effusion/empyema

DIFFERENTIAL DIAGNOSIS
- Bronchogenic carcinoma
- Bronchiectasis
- Empyema with bronchopulmonary fistula
- Tuberculosis
- Mycotic lung infections
- Vasculitis
- Parasitic lung infections
- Infected pulmonary bulla
- Wegener granulomatosis
- Pulmonary sequestration
- Subphrenic or hepatic abscess with perforation into a bronchus
- Bronchogenic or parenchymal cyst
- Aspirated foreign body

TREATMENT

MEDICATION

First Line
Antibiotics according to culture and sensitivity results; for presumed anaerobes, clindamycin 600 mg q6h IV followed by 300 mg q6h p.o. × 4 weeks

Second Line
- Historically, standard therapy had been penicillin G 1 million–2 million units IV q4h until improvement, followed by 1.2 million units (750 mg) p.o. q6h × 3–4 weeks; now many relevant pathogens produce β-lactamase.
- Cefoxitin 2.0 g IV q8h
- Piperacillin-tazobactam 3.375 g IV q6h
- Ticarcillin-clavulanate 3.1 g IV q6h
- Metronidazole has not proven as effective as clindamycin but often is recommended for use as an adjunctive therapy (500 mg IV q6h).
- Full course of therapy may be needed for 8 weeks.

ADDITIONAL TREATMENT

General Measures
- Postural drainage
- Nasotracheal suctioning if needed
- Prolonged course of antibiotics
- Pulmonary physiotherapy
- Bronchoscopy with selective therapeutic lavage (rarely done)
- In general, 10% require surgical intervention, such as drainage of abscess or empyema (1).

SURGERY/OTHER PROCEDURES
- Antibiotic treatment is successful in most patients; surgical options are considered when medical therapy fails (18)[B].
- Endoscopy drainage (19)
- Tube thoracostomy with medical failure or prohibitive operative risk (20)[B]
- Thoracoscopy drainage (21)
- Percutaneous catheter-guided drainage (12,15,16,17,20)
- Pulmonary resection only if complications occur or if patient fails therapy (mortality 11–16%)

IN-PATIENT CONSIDERATIONS

Initial Stabilization
Inpatient care for monitoring and treatment

 ONGOING CARE

FOLLOW-UP RECOMMENDATIONS
Activity reduced until radiographic evidence of clearing

Patient Monitoring
Serial radiographs until resolution of cavity

DIET
No restrictions

PATIENT EDUCATION
Pulmonary physiotherapy techniques

PROGNOSIS
- Clinical improvement with decrease in fever expected 3–4 days after starting antibiotics
- Defervescence expected in 7–10 days
- Prognosis depends on the underlying disease or immunosuppression (22).
- Patients with primary abscess (otherwise healthy, typical aspiration) have cure rates of 90–95%.
- Certain factors tend to have worse prognosis:
  – Large abscess (>6 cm)
  – Anatomic obstruction
  – Right lower lobe location
  – Certain bacteriologic species: *S. aureus*, *Klebsiella*, *Pseudomonas*
- Overall mortality 15–20% (23)
- Patients with secondary abscess (underlying neoplasm, obstruction, HIV) have 75% mortality.

Geriatric Considerations
Mortality higher in the elderly

COMPLICATIONS
- Extension
- Empyema
- Massive hemoptysis
- Pneumothorax
- Brain abscess

REFERENCES

1. Moreira Jda S, Camargo Jde J, Felicetti JC, et al. Lung abscess: analysis of 252 consecutive cases diagnosed between 1968 and 2004. *J Bras Pneumol*. 2006;32:136–43.
2. Hirshberg B, Sklair-Levi M, Nir-Paz R, et al. Factors predicting mortality of patients with lung abscess. *Chest*. 1999;115:746–50.
3. Agrafiotis M, Siempos II, Falagas ME. Infections Related to Airway Stenting: A Systematic Review. *Respiration*. 2009.
4. Munthe-Fog L, Hummelshøj T, Honoré C, et al. Immunodeficiency associated with FCN3 mutation and ficolin-3 deficiency. *N Engl J Med*. 2009;360: 2637–44.
5. Aylk S, Qakan A, Aslankara N, et al. Tuberculous abscess on the chest wall. *Monaldi Arch Chest Dis*. 2009;71:39–42.
6. Chirinos JA, Garcia J, Alcaide ML, et al. Septic thrombophlebitis: diagnosis and management. *Am J Cardiovasc Drugs*. 2006;6:9–14.
7. Hirshberg B, Oppenheim-Eden A, Pizov R, et al. Recovery from blast lung injury: one-year follow-up. *Chest*. 1999;116:1683–8.
8. Hsu PS, Lee SC, Tzao C, et al. Bronchoperitoneal fistula from a lung abscess. *Respirology*. 2008.
9. Mawdsley JE, Maleki N, Benjamin E, et al. Oesophageal perforation with asymptomatic lung abscess formation. *Lancet*. 2006;368:2104.
10. O'Brien JD, Ettinger NA. Nephrobronchial fistula and lung abscess resulting from nephrolithiasis and pyelonephritis. *Chest*. 1995;108:1166–8.
11. Chen HJ, Yu YH, Tu CY, et al. Ultrasound in Peripheral Pulmonary Air-Fluid Lesions: Color Doppler Imaging as an Aid in Differentiating Empyema and Abscess. *Chest*. 2009.
12. Stavas J, vanSonnenberg E, Casola G, et al. Percutaneous drainage of infected and noninfected thoracic fluid collections. *J Thorac Imaging*. 1987;2:80–7.
13. Simeone JF, Mueller PR, vanSonnenberg E. The uses of diagnostic ultrasound in the thorax. *Clin Chest Med*. 1984;5:281–90.
14. Velagapudi P, Turagam M, Are C, et al. "A forgotten disease": a case of lemierre syndrome. *ScientificWorldJournal*. 2009;9:331–2.
15. Chen CH, Chen W, Chen HJ, et al. Transthoracic Ultrasonography in Predicting the Outcome of Small-bore Catheter Drainage in Empyemas or Complicated Parapneumonic Effusions. *Ultrasound Med Biol*. 2009.
16. vanSonnenberg E, D'Agostino HB, Sanchez RB, et al. Percutaneous abscess drainage. *Radiology*. 1992;184:27–9.
17. vanSonnenberg E, D'Agostino HB, Casola G, et al. Lung abscess: CT-guided drainage. *Radiology*. 1991;178:347–51.
18. Mansharamani N, Koziel H. Chronic lung sepsis: Lung abscess, bronchiectasis, and empyema. *Curr Opin Pulmon Med*. 2003;9:181–5.
19. Herth F, Ernst A, Becker HD. Endoscopic drainage of lung abscesses: technique and outcome. *Chest*. 2005;127:1378–81.
20. Wali SO, Shugaeri A, Samman YS, et al. Percutaneous drainage of pyogenic lung abscess. *Scand J Infect Dis*. 2002;34:673–9.
21. Nagasawa KK, Johnson SM et al. Thoracoscopic treatment of pediatric lung abscesses. *J Pediatr Surg*. 2010;45:574–8.
22. Hsieh MJ, Liu YH, Chao YK, et al. Risk factors in surgical management of thoracic empyema in elderly patients. *ANZ J Surg*. 2008;78:445–8.
23. Lin JN, Tsai YS, Lai CH, et al. Risk Factors for Mortality of Bacteremic Patients in the Emergency Department. *Acad Emerg Med*. 2009.

See Also (Topic, Algorithm, Electronic Media Element)
Pneumonia, Bacterial

 CODES

ICD9
513.0 Abscess of lung

CLINICAL PEARLS
- Bacteria are carried to the dependent portions of the lung, with the posterior segment of the right upper lobe being the most common location for abscess.
- Percutaneous drainage and surgical resection could be considered treatment options when medical therapy fails. Endoscopic drainage techniques show promise as an alternative (19)[B].
- Lemierre syndrome is a complication of *Fusobacterium necrophorum* oropharyngeal infection (usually pharyngitis). The infection extends to the internal jugular vein, causing thrombophlebitis. The thrombophlebitis, in turn, produces septic emboli, including emboli that produce lung abscess or pneumonia (6).

L

LUNG, PRIMARY MALIGNANCIES

Maryann Cooper, PharmD
Gerald Gehr, MD

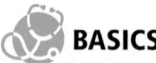 **BASICS**

DESCRIPTION
- Leading cause of cancer-related death in the US (estimated 157,300 deaths in 2010, 28% of all cancer-related deaths) (1)
- Divided into 2 broad categories:
  – Non-small cell carcinoma (NSCLC) (>85% of all lung cancers):
    ○ Adenocarcinoma (~50% of NSCLC): Most common type in US; most common type in non-smokers; metastasizes earlier than squamous cell; poor prognosis; bronchoalveolar, a sub-type of adenocarcinoma has better prognosis
    ○ Squamous cell carcinoma (<30% of NSCLC): Dose-related effect with smoking; slower growing than adenocarcinoma
    ○ Large cell (~15% of NSCLC): Prognosis similar to adenocarcinoma
  – Small cell carcinoma (SCLC) (16% of all lung cancers): Centrally located; early metastases, aggressive
- Other: Mesothelioma, carcinoid tumor, and sarcoma
- Staging:
  – NSCLC: Staged from 0–IV based on: Primary tumor (T), lymph node status (N), and presence of metastasis (M)
  – SCLC: Staged based on disease location: Limited to ipsilateral hemithorax (stages I–IIIB); extensive if metastatic beyond hemithorax (stages IIIB and IV)
- Tumor locations: Upper: 60%; lower: 30%; middle: 5%; overlapping and main stem: 5%
- May spread by local extension to involve chest wall, diaphragm, pulmonary vessels, vena cava, phrenic nerve, esophagus, or pericardium
- Most commonly metastasize to lymph nodes (pulmonary, mediastinal), then liver, adrenal, bone (osteolytic), kidney, brain

EPIDEMIOLOGY
Incidence
- Estimated 22,520 new cases in US in 2010 (1)
- Predominant age: >40 years; peak at 70 years
- Predominant sex: Male > Female

Prevalence
- Most common cancer worldwide
- Lifetime probability (1)
  – Men: 1 in 13
  – Women: 1 in 16

RISK FACTORS
- Smoking (relative risk [RR] 10–30)
- Second-hand smoke exposure
- Radon
- Environmental and occupational exposures:
  – Asbestos exposure (synergistic increase in risk for smokers), air pollution, ionizing radiation, mutagenic gases (halogen ethers, mustard gas, aromatic hydrocarbons), metals (inorganic arsenic, chromium, nickel)
- Lung scarring from tuberculosis
- HIV infection
- Radiation therapy to the breast or chest

Genetics
NSCLC
- Oncogenes: ras family (H-ras, K-ras, N-ras)
- Tumor suppressor genes: retinoblastoma, *p-53*

GENERAL PREVENTION
- No cost-effective screening measure
- Prevention via aggressive smoking-cessation counseling and therapy; a 20–30% risk reduction occurs within 5 years of cessation
- Avoid supplemental β-carotene in smokers.

ETIOLOGY
Multifactorial; see "Risk Factors."

COMMONLY ASSOCIATED CONDITIONS
- Paraneoplastic syndromes: Hypertrophic pulmonary osteoarthropathy, Eaton-Lambert syndrome, Cushing's syndrome, hypercalcemia from ectopic parathyroid hormone releasing hormone, syndrome of inappropriate antidiuretic hormone (SIADH)
- Hypercoagulable state
- Pancoast syndrome
- Superior vena cava syndrome
- Pleural effusion
- COPD, other sequelae of cigarette smoking

 DIAGNOSIS

HISTORY
- May be asymptomatic for most of course
- Pulmonary:
  – Cough (new or change in chronic cough)
  – Wheezing and stridor
  – Dyspnea
  – Hemoptysis
  – Pneumonitis (fever and productive cough)
- Constitutional:
  – Bone pain (metastatic disease)
  – Fatigue
  – Weight loss, anorexia
  – Fever
  – Anemia
  – Clubbing of digits
- Other presentations:
  – Chest pain (dull, pleuritic)
  – Shoulder/arm pain (Pancoast tumors)
  – Dysphagia
  – Plethora (redness of face or neck)
  – Hoarseness (involvement of recurrent laryngeal nerve)
  – Horner syndrome
  – Neurologic abnormalities (e.g., headaches, syncope, weakness, cognitive impairment)
  – Pericardial tamponade (pericardial invasion)

PHYSICAL EXAM
- General: pain, performance status, weight loss
- HEENT: Horner syndrome, dysphonia, stridor, scleral icterus
- Neck: Supraclavicular/cervical lymph nodes, mass
- Lungs: Effusion, wheezing, airway obstruction, pleural effusion
- Abdomen/groin: Hepatomegaly or lymphadenopathy
- Extremities: signs of hypertrophic pulmonary osteoarthropathy, DVT
- Neurologic: rule out cognitive and focal motor defects

DIAGNOSTIC TESTS & INTERPRETATION
Lab
Initial lab tests
- Complete blood count (CBC)
- BUN, serum creatinine
- Liver function tests (LFTs), LDH
- Electrolytes
  – Hypercalcemia (Paraneoplastic syndrome)
  – Hyponatremia (SIADH)
- Sputum cytology

Follow-Up & Special Considerations
CBC, BUN, serum creatinine, LFTs prior to each cycle of chemotherapy

Imaging
- CXR (compare with old films):
  – Nodule or mass, especially if calcified
  – Persistent infiltrate
  – Atelectasis
  – Mediastinal widening
  – Hilar enlargement
  – Pleural effusion
- CT scan of chest (with IV contrast material):
  – Nodule or mass (central or peripheral)
  – Lymphadenopathy
- Evaluation for metastatic disease:
  – Brain MRI: Lesions may be necrotic, bleeding.
  – Abdomen: Hepatic, adrenal, renal masses
- PET scan: To evaluate metastasis
- Bone scan: Advanced disease or bone pain

Diagnostic Procedures/Surgery
- Pulmonary function tests
- Enlarged mediastinal lymph nodes necessitate staging by mediastinoscopy, video-assisted thoracoscopy, or fine-needle aspiration.
- Transbronchial biopsy (Wang needle)
- Bronchoscopy for surgical planning
- Bone marrow aspirate (small cell)
- Cervical mediastinoscopy (the upper, middle peritracheal, and subcarinal lymph nodes)
- Anterior mediastinotomy (the posterior mediastinum and peritracheal, subazygous, hilar, and aortopulmonary window nodal regions)
- Video-assisted thoracoscopy (associated pleural disease and suspected mediastinal nodal spread)

Pathological Findings
Pathologic changes from smoking are progressive: Basal cell proliferation, development of atypical nuclei, stratification, metaplasia of squamous cells, carcinoma in situ, and then invasive disease

DIFFERENTIAL DIAGNOSIS
- COPD (may coexist)
- Granulomatous (tuberculosis, sarcoidosis)
- Cardiomyopathy
- Congestive heart failure (CHF)

TREATMENT

MEDICATION
- Chemotherapy is the mainstay of treatment for SCLC and advanced NSCLC
- Adjuvant chemotherapy following surgery improves survival in patients with fully resected stage II–III NSCLC (2)[A]
- Palliative measures: Analgesics
- Dyspnea: Oxygen, morphine

First Line
- NSCLC
  - Stages II–III: adjuvant chemotherapy
    - Cisplatin-based doublets (combination with etoposide, vinorelbine, docetaxel, and others)
    - Carboplatin plus paclitaxel is an alternative to cisplatin-based regimens in patients that are unlikely to tolerate cisplatin
  - Stage IV
    - Cisplatin-based doublets with or without bevacizumab (non-squamous cell) or cetuximab
    - Erlotinib is an alternative in patients with tumors that express EGFR
- SCLC
  - Cisplatin and etoposide

Second Line
- NSCLC
  - Cisplatin-based doublets with or without bevacizumab (non-squamous cell) or cetuximab
  - Docetaxel or pemetrexed (non-squamous cell only) or erlotinib (EGFR positive tumors)
- SCLC
  - Topotecan or CAV (cyclophosphamide, doxorubicin, vincristine), gemcitabine, docetaxel, paclitaxel

ADDITIONAL TREATMENT
General Measures
- NSCLC (3)[C]:
  - Stage I, stage II, and selected stage III tumors are surgically resectable. Neoadjuvant or adjuvant therapy is recommended for many patients with stage II and III NSCLC. Patients with resectable disease who have medical contraindications to surgery are candidates for curative radiation therapy.
  - Patients with unresectable or N_2, N_3 disease are treated with radiation therapy in combination with chemotherapy. Selected patients with T_3 or N_2 disease can be treated effectively with surgical resection and either preoperative or postoperative chemotherapy or chemoradiation therapy.
  - Patients with distant metastases (M_1) can be treated with radiation therapy or chemotherapy for palliation or best supportive care alone.
- SCLC (4)[C]:
  - Limited stage: Concurrent chemotherapy and radiation
  - Extensive stage: Combination chemotherapy
  - Consider prophylactic cranial irradiation (PCI) in patients achieving a complete response (5)B]
- Quality-of-life assessments: Karnofsky Performance Scale (KPS), Eastern Cooperative Oncology Group (ECOG)
- Discussions with patient and family about end-of-life care

Additional Therapies
- Smoking cessation counseling
- Consider bisphosphonates in patients with bone metastases to reduce skeletal related events.

SURGERY/OTHER PROCEDURES
- Resection for NSCLC, for stages I, II, and IIIa, if medically fit to undergo surgery
- Resection of isolated, distant metastases has been achieved and may improve survival.
- Resection involves lobectomy in 71%, wedge in 16%, and complete pneumonectomy in 18%.
- Resection should be accompanied by lymph node dissection for pathologic staging.

 ONGOING CARE

FOLLOW-UP RECOMMENDATIONS
Patient Monitoring
- Depends on clinical history, but in general, postoperative visits every 3–6 months in the year after surgery with physical and CXR
- Follow-up CT scans as indicated

PATIENT EDUCATION
http://www.cancer.gov/cancertopics
http://www.smokefree.gov/

PROGNOSIS
- For combined, all types and stages, 5-year survival rate is 16% (NSCLC: 17%; SCLC 6%) (1)
- NSCLC: (3)
  - Localized disease (stages I and II): 49%
  - Regional disease: 16%
  - Distant metastatic disease: 2%
- SCLC: (4)
  - Without treatment: Median survival from diagnosis of only 2–4 months
  - Limited-stage disease: Median survival of 16–24 months; 5-year survival rate: 14%
  - Extensive-stage disease: Median survival of 6–12 months; long-term disease-free survival is rare

COMPLICATIONS
- Development of metastatic disease, especially to brain, bones, adrenals, and liver
- Local recurrence of disease
- Postoperative complications
- Side effects of chemotherapy or radiation

REFERENCES

1. American Cancer Society: *Cancer Facts and Figures 2010*. Atlanta, GA: American Cancer Society, 2010.
2. Pignon JP, Tribodet H, Scagliotti GV, et al. Lung adjuvant cisplatin evaluation: a pooled analysis by the LACE Collaborative Group. *J Clin Oncol*. 2008;26:3552–9.
3. http://www.cancer.gov/cancertopics/pdq/ treatment/non-small-cell-lung/healthprofessional.
4. http://www.cancer.gov/cancertopics/pdq/ treatment/small-cell-lung/healthprofessional.
5. Slotman B, Faivre-Finn C, Kramer G, et al. Prophylactic cranial irradiation in extensive small-cell lung cancer. *N Engl J Med*. 2007;357:664–72.

ADDITIONAL READING

- Arriagada R, Bergman B, Dunant A, et al. Cisplatin-based adjuvant chemotherapy in patients with completely resected non-small-cell lung cancer. *N Engl J Med*. 2004;350:351–60.
- Collins LG, Haines C, Perkel R, et al. Lung cancer: diagnosis and management. *Am Fam Physician*. 2007;75:56–63.
- Hanna N, Shepherd FA, Fossella FV, et al. Randomized phase III trial of pemetrexed versus docetaxel in patients with non-small-cell lung cancer previously treated with chemotherapy. *J Clin Oncol*. 2004;22:1589–97.
- Pirker R, Pereira JR, Szczesna A, et al. Cetuximab plus chemotherapy in patients with advanced non-small-cell lung cancer (FLEX): an open-label randomised phase III trial. *Lancet*. 2009;373: 1525–31.
- Sandler A, Gray R, Perry MC, et al. Paclitaxel-carboplatin alone or with bevacizumab for non-small-cell lung cancer. *N Engl J Med*. 2006;355: 2542–50.
- Shepherd FA, Rodrigues Pereira J, Ciuleanu T, et al. Erlotinib in previously treated non-small-cell lung cancer. *N Engl J Med*. 2005;353:123–32.
- Sundstrøm S, Bremnes RM, Kaasa S, et al. Cisplatin and etoposide regimen is superior to cyclophosphamide, epirubicin, and vincristine regimen in small-cell lung cancer: results from a randomized phase III trial with 5 years' follow-up. *J Clin Oncol*. 2002;20:4665–72.
- von Pawel J, Schiller JH, Shepherd FA, et al. Topotecan versus cyclophosphamide, doxorubicin, and vincristine for the treatment of recurrent small-cell lung cancer. *J Clin Oncol*. 1999;17: 658–67.

 CODES

ICD9
- 162.3 Malignant neoplasm of upper lobe, bronchus or lung
- 162.4 Malignant neoplasm of middle lobe, bronchus or lung
- 162.9 Malignant neoplasm of bronchus and lung, unspecified

CLINICAL PEARLS
- Prognosis and treatment of lung cancer differs greatly between small cell and non-small cell histologies.
- Adjuvant cisplatin based chemotherapy improves survival in patients with completely resected stage II-III NSCLC.
- Chemotherapy with or without radiation can be offered to patients with advanced NSCLC or SCLC.
- There is little role for surgery in the treatment of SCLC.

L

LUPUS ERYTHEMATOSUS, DISCOID

Johra Nasreen, MD

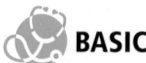 **BASICS**

DESCRIPTION
- Discoid lupus erythematosus (DLE) is the most common form of cutaneous lupus erythematosus. It is a chronic, disfiguring, inflammatory skin disease that typically manifests as erythematous, indurated, scaly plaques that have the potential to cause permanent scarring and dyspigmentation.
- The disease predominantly affects *sun-exposed sites* such as the face, especially the malar areas, bridge of nose, lower lip, lower eyelids, and ears, dorsal hands and scalp, although it can be disseminated.
- Mostly 2 forms are prevalent:
  - Localized DLE: Localized discoid lupus erythematosus occurs when the head and neck only are affected.
  - Generalized or widespread DLE: Widespread discoid lupus erythematosus occurs when other areas are affected. Lesions are seen on upper extremities and thorax most often along with usual sites for localized DLE.
- Synonym(s): Chronic cutaneous lupus erythematosus; Subacute cutaneous lupus erythematosus

Pediatric Considerations
Neonatal lupus erythematosus is a syndrome of cutaneous lupus occasionally with systemic manifestations, infrequently including congenital heart block. It is caused by transplacental passage of any of several maternal antibodies.

Pregnancy Considerations
Be aware if systemic retinoids are used in treatment (pregnancy Category X).

EPIDEMIOLOGY
1–5% of patients with discoid lupus may develop SLE, and 25% of patients with SLE may develop typical chronic discoid lesions (1).

Incidence
Discoid lupus occurs at all ages and among all ethnic groups; it occurs more frequently in women than in men. All forms of cutaneous lupus erythematosus are most common in women of childbearing age:
- Predominant age: 25–45 years
- Predominant sex:
  - Localized DLE: Female > Male (3:1)
  - Generalized DLE: Female > Male (9:1)

Prevalence
- White females: 3/100,000
- African American females: 8/100,000

RISK FACTORS
Discoid lupus erythematosus most commonly afflicts young adult females, especially blacks and Hispanics, though it may occur at any age and it occurs worldwide.

Genetics
- DLE probably occurs in genetically predisposed individuals.
- A haplotype of cytotoxic T-lymphocyte-associated protein 4 (CTLA4) showed association with DLE.

GENERAL PREVENTION
- Avoid sunlight exposure. Excessive heat, excessive cold, and trauma to the affected regions may make the condition worse.
- Sunscreens with UVB and UVA blockers are recommended.
- Protective clothing (dark colors and closely woven fabrics) and hats are effective sun-blockers.

PATHOPHYSIOLOGY
The pathophysiology of discoid lupus erythematosus is not well understood. It has been suggested that a heat shock protein is induced in the keratinocyte following ultraviolet (UV) light exposure or stress, and this protein may act as a target for gamma (delta) T-cell–mediated epidermal cell cytotoxicity.

COMMONLY ASSOCIATED CONDITIONS
- Systemic lupus erythematosus (SLE)
- Mixed connective tissue disease
- Antiphospholipid syndrome

 DIAGNOSIS

The diagnosis of discoid lupus is generally made based on clinical features. Histology may be required to confirm the diagnosis:
- "Carpet-tack" appearance of skin when scale removed
- Lesions occasionally slightly pruritic or stinging
- Oral ulceration in 15% of the patients
- Photosensitivity
- Koebner response (precipitation by cutaneous trauma)
- It starts as an erythematous papule or plaque, usually on the head or neck, with an adherent scale (1).
- The lesion tends to spread centrifugally and as it progresses there is follicular plugging and pigmentary changes, generally hyperpigmentation at the periphery, and hypopigmentation with atrophy, scarring, and telangiectasia at the center of the lesion (1).
- Involvement of the scalp commonly produces a scarring alopecia. Scarring alopecia presents patients with DLE and is mainly associated with a prolonged disease course (1).

DIAGNOSTIC TESTS & INTERPRETATION
Lab
- Localized DLE: Positive antinuclear antibodies (ANAs) in low titer (30%)
- Generalized DLE: May find increased sedimentation rate, positive ANAs (60–80%), positive SS-A (80%), positive SS-B (40%) autoantibodies, positive double-stranded DNA (dsDNA; <5%), leukopenia, hematuria, and albuminuria if concomitant SLE
- Immunofluorescent staining of skin biopsies (lupus band test)
- Disorders that may alter lab results: Concomitant SLE

Diagnostic Procedures/Surgery
Skin biopsy

Pathological Findings
- Hyperkeratosis and parakeratosis
- Focal epidermal atrophy
- Hydropic degeneration of basal cell layer
- Edema, mucin, and inflammation of dermis
- Follicular plugging
- Mononuclear cell infiltration at the dermal–epidermal junction and in the dermis around blood vessels
- Basement zone thickened with strong periodic acid–Schiff reaction staining
- Dermal mucinosis
- Immunofluorescence reveals a granular pattern of immunoglobulin and complement deposition at the dermal–epidermal border in involved skin.

DIFFERENTIAL DIAGNOSIS
- Actinic keratoses
- Granuloma annulare
- Sarcoidosis
- Psoriasis, plaque
- Rosacea
- Eczema
- Polymorphous light eruption
- Drug eruptions
- Cutaneous leishmaniasis
- Lupus vulgaris
- Seborrheic dermatitis
- Lichen planus
- Pemphigus erythematosus
- Keratoacanthoma
- Granuloma faciale
- Dermatomyositis
- Squamous cell carcinoma

 TREATMENT

- The cornerstone of therapy includes topical and intralesional glucocorticoids, and broad-spectrum sunscreens are recommended for all patients. Antimalarial agents, such as hydroxychloroquine, chloroquine, and quinacrine, are indicated when topical or intralesional therapy fails to control skin disease.
- DLE can cause permanent scarring, but this can be prevented by early treatment.

MEDICATION
First Line
- Localized DLE:
  - Current study showed fluocinonide 0.05% cream (a potent topical corticosteroid) to be better than hydrocortisone 1% cream (a mild corticosteroid) (2)[A]
  - Topical corticosteroids:
    - Topical steroids are the mainstay of treatment of DLE. Patients usually start with a potent topical steroid (fluocinonide 0.05% cream) applied twice a day, then switch to a lower-potency steroid (e.g., triamcinolone 0.1%) applied twice a day as soon as possible. The minimal use of steroids reduces the recognized side effects like atrophy, telangiectasiae, striae, and purpura (1)[A].

– Intralesional steroids:
  ○ Intralesional steroids (e.g., triamcinolone 2.5–5 mg/mL for the face or 5–10 mg/mL elsewhere) are particularly useful to treat chronic lesions, hyperkeratotic lesions, and those that do not respond adequately to topical steroids:
    ▪ Lesions at particular sites, e.g., the scalp, may also benefit.
    ▪ Recognized side effects of intralesional steroids include cutaneous atrophy and dyspigmentation, which are not significant risks in experienced hands.
– Oral steroids may be required for the control of systemic lupus but are not generally beneficial in DLE:
  ○ Patients with progressive or disseminated disease, or those with localized disease that does not respond to topical measures, may require the addition of systemic agents.
• Generalized DLE:
– Antimalarials (1)[A]:
  ○ Treatment with antimalarial drugs constitutes 1st-line systemic therapy for DLE. Therapy with antimalarials, either used singly or in combination, is usually effective.
  ○ The 2 commonly used preparations include chloroquine and hydroxychloroquine.
  ○ Hydroxychloroquine at a dose of 200 mg per day for an adult
  ○ It may take between 4 and 8 weeks for any clinical improvement, if there are no untoward gastrointestinal or other side effects, to increase the dose to twice a day.
  ○ No more than 6.5 mg/kg/day should be administered.
  ○ In some patients who do not respond to hydroxychloroquine, chloroquine 250 mg/day may be more effective.
  ○ In general, hydroxychloroquine is a safe, well-tolerated drug and adverse effects are relatively few, the most widely recognized being retinal toxicity.
  ○ Chloroquine causes macular pigmentation that progresses to a typical bull's eye lesion and then to widespread retinal pigment epithelial atrophy resembling retinitis pigmentosa.
  ○ Other adverse effects of antimalarials include gastrointestinal symptoms, e.g., nausea and vomiting, and cutaneous side effects, including pruritus, lichenoid drug reactions, annular erythema, hyperpigmentation, and hematological disturbances like leukopenia and thrombocytopenia.

Second Line
• Localized DLE:
– Intralesional triamcinolone: 2.5 mg/mL injected at monthly intervals
– Prednisone: 15 mg b.i.d., then tapered after response
• Generalized DLE:
– Quinacrine: 100 mg/d
– Dapsone: 100 mg/d
– Azathioprine: 100 mg/d
– Systemic retinoid (e.g., etretinate 1 mg/kg)
– Thalidomide 50–300 mg/d is also effective (3)[C].
– Dapsone is useful in patients who also have vasculitis. It is the treatment of choice for patients with bullous lupus.

• Recent case reports have shown successful treatments with IVIG, the monoclonal antibody efalizumab, and the immunomodulatory drug tacrolimus.
• Both tacrolimus and pimecrolimus show efficacy in localized DLE (4)[A].

ADDITIONAL TREATMENT
R-salbutamol sulphate, a well-known molecule with anti-inflammatory effects

General Measures
Avoid sun exposure, excessive heat, cold, or trauma.

Issues for Referral
Given the scarring nature of this illness, dermatology referral is frequently indicated. Also, the treatment consists of medications less commonly used by primary care providers.

SURGERY/OTHER PROCEDURES
• Excision of burned-out scarred lesions is possible; however, reactivation of inactive lesions has been reported in some patients.
• Laser therapy may be useful for lesions with prominent telangiectases. Reactivation also is a consideration with this form of therapy.

 ONGOING CARE

FOLLOW-UP RECOMMENDATIONS
Follow patients with DLE at regular intervals. Response to therapy varies from several weeks to several months. At each visit, question the patient about new symptoms that may reflect systemic disease.

Patient Monitoring
• Initially recheck patients once or twice per month. Then annually in otherwise asymptomatic patients.
• Perform routine laboratory studies for assessment, including complete blood count, renal function tests, and urinalysis at regular intervals.
• Ophthalmology follow-up at 6-month intervals, if patient on antimalarials
• If lesions subside, reduce dosage of antimalarials over 2–3 months and then discontinue.

PATIENT EDUCATION
• Teach patients proper use of sunscreens and other measures to prevent sun exposure (e.g., wide-brimmed hats, long sleeves).
• Advise patients about symptoms of SLE for which they should watch.

PROGNOSIS
• 40% of patients may have complete remission; 1–5% may develop systemic lupus (these patients usually have generalized DLE).
• Cutaneous lupus has the tendency to change over time. Some patients may progress through several different subsets of cutaneous lupus and ultimately evolve into systemic lupus.
• Not life-threatening unless it turns into systemic type

COMPLICATIONS
• Cicatricial alopecia
• Lupoid rash
• Lupus mastitis (5)
• Squamous cell carcinoma

REFERENCES

1. Panjwani, Suresh MD, MSc, FRACGP. Early Diagnosis and Treatment of Discoid Lupus Erythematosus. *The Journal of the American Board of Family Medicine* 2009;22(2):206–213, DOI: 10.3122/jabfm.2009.02.080075
2. Jessop S, Whitelaw DA, Delamere FM. Drugs for discoid lupus erythematosus. *Cochrane Database of Systematic Reviews* 2009, Issue 4. Art. No.: CD002954. DOI:10.1002/14651858. CD002954.pub2
3. James WD, et al. *Andrews' Diseases of the Skin*, 10th ed. Philadelphia: WB Saunders; 2006:157–65.
4. Tzellos TG, Kouvelas D. Topical tacrolimus and pimecrolimus in the treatment of cutaneous lupus erythematosus: an evidence-based evaluation. *Eur J Clin Pharmacol*. 2008;64:337–41.
5. Kinonen C, Gattuso P, Reddy VB, et al. Lupus mastitis: an uncommon complication of systemic or discoid lupus. *Am J Surg Pathol*. 2010;34:901–6.

ADDITIONAL READING

• Järvinen TM, Hellquist A, Koskenmies S, et al. Tyrosine kinase 2 and interferon regulatory factor 5 polymorphisms are associated with discoid and subacute cutaneous lupus erythematosus. *Exp. Dermatol*. 2010;19:123–31.
• Lin JH, Dutz JP, Sontheimer RD, Werth VP et al. Pathophysiology of cutaneous lupus erythematosus. *Clin Rev Allergy Immunol*. 2007;33:85–106.

See Also (Topic, Algorithm, Electronic Media Element)
Systemic Lupus Erythematosus (SLE)

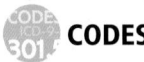 CODES

ICD9
695.4 Lupus erythematosus

CLINICAL PEARLS
• Patients with cutaneous DLE have a small chance of developing SLE over a span of months to years.
• Screening patients with cutaneous disease for systemic symptoms such as oral ulcers, arthritis, etc., is a good 1st step.
• If patient has any systemic symptoms, laboratory testing of blood for ANAs is indicated.
• Systemic steroids are rarely indicated in DLE.

L

LYME DISEASE

Barbara A. Majeroni, MD

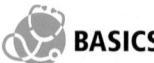 ## BASICS

DESCRIPTION
- A multisystem infection caused by the spirochetes of Borrelia strains, which is transmitted primarily by ixodid ticks, *I. scapularis* (deer ticks) in the New England and Great Lakes areas, and *I. pacificus* in the West, also known as black-legged ticks and Western black-legged ticks
- Early localized Lyme disease includes a characteristic expanding skin rash (erythema migrans) (70%) and constitutional flulike symptoms.
- Disseminated Lyme disease may present with involvement of ≥1 organ systems. Neurologic, cardiac, and pauciarticular arthritis are most common.
- Post-Lyme disease syndrome involves arthritis (50%) and chronic neurologic syndromes.
- System(s) affected: Hemic/Lymphatic/Immunologic; Musculoskeletal; Skin/Exocrine; Cardiac; Neurological
- Synonym(s): Lyme arthritis, Lyme borreliosis

EPIDEMIOLOGY
Incidence
In states where Lyme disease is endemic (Connecticut, Delaware, Maryland, Massachusetts, Minnesota, New Jersey, New York, Pennsylvania, Rhode Island, and Wisconsin), the incidence is 29.2 per 100,000. Cases have been reported from 46 states and the District of Columbia.

Prevalence
- The most common tickborne infection in the US and Europe
- Annually Europe 65,500; North America 16,500; Asia 3,500; North Africa 10 (1)
- Predominant age: Can occur in all ages, but most common in children ages 5–14 and in the 55- to 70-year age group
- Predominant sex: Male > Female in the US

RISK FACTORS
- Exposure in tick-infested area; most common April–November
- Those who reside or are employed in areas where ticks are found are at increased risk.
- Ixodid ticks are commonly found on deer. Hunters may be at an increased risk.

Genetics
Human leukocyte antigen: Haplotype DR4 or DR2 may be more susceptible to prolonged arthritis.

GENERAL PREVENTION
- Prevention of the infection is possible by careful exam of skin for ticks after outdoor activities.
- The prompt removal of ticks may limit transmission.
- Clothing that covers the ankles should be worn in endemic areas, and the use of insect repellants containing DEET is recommended.

- No vaccine is currently available.
- Prophylactic treatment with 1 dose of 200 mg of doxycycline within 72 hours of a tick bite in highly endemic areas has been suggested. (This is contraindicated in pregnancy and children; no prophylactic agent is approved for these groups.) (2)

ETIOLOGY
- Infection with spirochete *B. burgdorferi* in the US, or *B. afzelii* or *B. garinii* in Europe, transmitted by the bite of ixodid ticks
- Primary animal reservoir is the white-footed mouse

COMMONLY ASSOCIATED CONDITIONS
Southern tick–associated rash illness may be mistaken for Lyme disease. It is seen in the southeastern and south central US, and is associated with the bite of the Lone Star tick, *Amblyomma americanum*.

DIAGNOSIS

HISTORY
- History of a tick bite followed by illness with erythema migrans is the key to diagnosis (3)[C].
- Early Lyme disease:
  - Some patients may be asymptomatic.
  - Fever
  - Headache
  - Myalgias
  - Arthralgias
- Disseminated Lyme disease:
  - Facial palsies or other cranial neuropathies
  - Joint pain (usually large joint monoarthritis)
  - Iritis, conjunctivitis
- Late untreated Lyme disease:
  - Recurrent synovitis
  - Recurrent tendonitis and bursitis
  - Encephalopathic symptoms:
    - Headaches
    - Decreased memory
    - Difficulty concentrating
    - Confusion
    - Fatigue
  - Symptoms mimicking other central nervous system diseases:
    - Multiple sclerosis-like symptoms
    - Strokelike symptoms
    - Transverse myelitis
  - Peripheral neuropathic symptoms; motor, sensory, or autonomic neuropathies
  - Meningitis

PHYSICAL EXAM
- Early Lyme disease:
  - Erythema migrans
- Disseminated Lyme disease:
  - Multiple erythema migrans
  - Facial palsies or other cranial neuropathies
  - Heart block
  - Pericarditis
  - Arthritis
  - Other neurologic signs

ALERT
- Transmission does not occur if tick attachment is <48 hours, and only 25% transmission occurs for attachments of <72 hours.
- Infection is preceded by a tick bite, although patient may be unaware of tick attachment.

DIAGNOSTIC TESTS & INTERPRETATION
Lab
Initial lab tests
- Testing and treatment not indicated if tick attachment is <48 hours
- Diagnosis is based mainly on clinical findings in endemic areas.
- Enzyme linked immunosorbent assay (ELISA) for IgM and IgG *B. burgdorferi* antibodies, followed by a Western blot test if positive or equivocal (3)[A]
- Culture of cerebrospinal fluid (CSF) for *B. burgdorferi*
- Use of plasma polymerase chain reaction (PCR) is of little value, but PCR of synovial fluid may be helpful.

Follow-Up & Special Considerations
- Late-stage disease with negative serology may be seen in patients who received early antibiotic treatment.
- Disorders that may alter lab results: False-positive response has been seen with Rocky Mountain spotted fever, syphilis, systemic lupus erythematosus, and rheumatoid arthritis.
- PCR for Lyme disease in synovial fluid is both sensitive and specific for diagnosing Lyme arthritis.
- PCR of CSF has a very low sensitivity for Lyme meningitis, which is likely in the setting of CSF pleocytosis with erythema migrans, papilledema, and cranial neuropathies.
- There are Centers for Disease Control warnings against using nonvalidated testing methods, including urine antigen test, immunofluorescent staining for cell wall-deficient forms of *B. burgdorferi*, and lymphocyte transformation tests to aid in the diagnosis of Lyme disease (3).
- After an infection, antibodies may persist for months to years. Serologic tests do not distinguish active from past infection.
- Antibodies are not protective.

Imaging
Initial approach
No imaging indicated

Diagnostic Procedures/Surgery
Lumbar puncture when neurologic findings are present, with ELISA of CSF for *B. burgdorferi* antibodies

Pathological Findings
Culture of *B. burgdorferi* from blood or skin biopsy has a very low yield.

DIFFERENTIAL DIAGNOSIS
- Juvenile rheumatoid arthritis
- Viral syndromes
- Later stages may mimic many other diseases.
- Coinfection with babesiosis has been reported. Suggested by high fever.

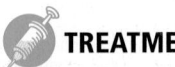 TREATMENT

Antibiotic prophylaxis is recommended for the prevention of Lyme disease in endemic areas following an Ixodes tick bite (2)[A].

MEDICATION
First Line
- Erythema migrans (4)[A]:
  – Doxycycline (Vibramycin): 100 mg p.o. b.i.d. for 10 days (10–21) (do not use in children <8 or in pregnancy); OR
  – Amoxicillin: 500 mg p.o. t.i.d. for 14 d (14–21) (pediatric dose 50 mg/kg/d); OR
  – Cefuroxime axetil 500 mg p.o. b.i.d. for 14 days (14–21):
    ○ 1 randomized, controlled trial of patients with erythema migrans found 10 days of treatment as effective as 20 days.
- Neurologic disease:
  – Normal CSF, treat for 14–21 days: Doxycycline 100 mg p.o. b.i.d. or amoxicillin 500 mg p.o. t.i.d.
  – With abnormal CSF, treat for 4 weeks: Ceftriaxone (Rocephin) 2 g/d IV, cefotaxime 2g q8h, or penicillin G 5 million U every 6 hours.
  – Cardiac disease:
    ○ Mild (1st degree AV block, PR <300 msec): Doxycycline 100 mg p.o. b.i.d. or Amoxicillin 500 mg p.o. t.i.d. for 14 days (14–21)
    ○ More serious: Ceftriaxone 2 g q24h IV for 30 days
- Arthritis without neurologic disease:
  – Oral treatment for 28 days with doxycycline 100 mg b.i.d. or amoxicillin 500 mg t.i.d.
  – If oral treatment fails, begin an IV treatment for 2–4 weeks with ceftriaxone 2 g/d.
- Contraindications:
  – Allergy to agent
  – Doxycycline is contraindicated in children and in women who are pregnant or breastfeeding.
- Precautions: Refer to the manufacturer's profile of each drug.

- In approximately 15% of patients treated with IV therapy, a Jarish-Herxheimer-type reaction develops within 24 hours of initiation of therapy.
- Significant possible interactions:
  – If the patient is taking oral anticoagulants, it may be necessary to reduce the dose.
- Oral contraceptives may be less effective.

Pediatric Considerations
- The drug of choice in pediatrics is amoxicillin.
- Tetracyclines are contraindicated.

Pregnancy Considerations
- Because *B. burgdorferi* can cross the placenta, pregnant patients with active disease should receive parenteral antibiotics.
- Doxycycline should not be used in pregnancy.

Second Line
Azithromycin, 500 mg p.o. daily for 7 days, can be used for those allergic to beta lactams and unable to take tetracyclines.

ADDITIONAL TREATMENT
General Measures
- Early and disseminated Lyme disease can usually be treated as an outpatient except in the case of complications, such as carditis or meningitis, requiring parenteral antibiotics.
- For post-Lyme disease syndrome in a patient who has received adequate treatment, evidence suggests that further courses of antibiotics offer no benefit (5)[B].

IN-PATIENT CONSIDERATIONS
Admission Criteria
- Admission and monitoring are recommended for patients with Lyme carditis and symptoms of chest pain, syncope, or dyspnea, and for those with 2nd- or 3rd-degree heart block or 1st-degree heart block of ≥300 msec.
- Also for symptoms of meningitis

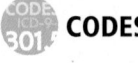 ONGOING CARE

FOLLOW-UP RECOMMENDATIONS
Patient Monitoring
Based on the severity of symptoms, patients with Lyme carditis, neurologic syndromes, or arthritis may require monitoring for months to years.

DIET
No restrictions

PATIENT EDUCATION
In endemic areas, patients should be advised to protect themselves against tick exposure.

PROGNOSIS
- Early treatment with antibiotics can shorten the duration of the symptoms and prevent later disease.
- Response of late-stage disease is variable and may take several weeks after beginning treatment.

COMPLICATIONS
- Recurrent synovitis, tendonitis, bursitis
- Chronic neurological symptoms
- Peripheral neuropathies

REFERENCES
1. Hubalek Z. Epidemiology of Lyme Borrelliosis. *Curr Probl Dermatol* 2009:31–50.
2. Warshafsky S, Lee DH, Francois LK, Nowakowski J, Nadelman RB, Wormser GP et al. Efficacy of antibiotic prophylaxis for the prevention of Lyme disease: an updated systematic review and meta-analysis. *J Antimicrob Chemother*. 2010; 65:1137–44.
3. Centers for Disease Control and Prevention. Notice to readers: Caution regarding testing for Lyme disease. *MMWR.* 2005;54:125.
4. Treatment of Lyme disease. *Med Lett Drugs Ther.* 2007;49:49–51.
5. Marques A. Chronic Lyme Disease: a review. *Inf Dis Clin N Am* 2008;(22):341–360.

ADDITIONAL READING
- Bratton RL, Whiteside JW, Hovan MJ, et al. Diagnosis and treatment of Lyme disease. *Mayo Clin Proc.* 2008;83:566–71.
- Hoppa E, Bachur R. Lyme disease update. *Curr Opin Pediatr.* 2007;19:275–80.
- Nadelman RB, Nowakowski J, Fish D, et al. Prophylaxis with single-dose doxycycline for the prevention of Lyme disease after an Ixodes scapularis tick bite. *N Engl J Med.* 2001;345:79–84.

See Also (Topic, Algorithm, Electronic Media Element)
American Lyme Disease Foundation: www.aldf.com

CODES

ICD9
088.81 Lyme disease

CLINICAL PEARLS
- The presence of erythema migrans following a tick bite in an area endemic for Lyme disease warrants empiric treatment.
- Doxycycline is the drug of choice, but it is contraindicated in women who may be or may become pregnant and in children <8 years old. Amoxicillin or cefuroxime axetil can be used.
- Transmission does not occur if tick attachment is <48 hours, and only 25% transmission occurs in <72 hours, so daily skin exam and removal of ticks can prevent Lyme disease.

L

LYMPHANGITIS

Tyeese Gaines Reid, DO, MA

 BASICS

DESCRIPTION
- Local inflammation of lymphatic vessels; can be acute or chronic
- Usually due to trauma and/or infection of the nearby skin

RISK FACTORS
- Diabetes mellitus
- Chronic steroid use
- Prolonged time with a peripheral venous catheter in place
- Varicella infection
- Immunocompromise
- Human, animal, or insect bites
- Fungal skin infections
- Any trauma to the skin

GENERAL PREVENTION
Proper wound care (1)[A]

ETIOLOGY
- Acute or chronic infection of the skin causing inflammation of lymphatic channels
- Acute infection:
  – Usually caused by *Streptococcus pyogenes*
  – Uncommonly caused by:
    ○ *Staphylococcus aureus*
    ○ *Pasteurella multocida*
    ○ *Spirillum minus* (rat-bite disease)
    ○ *Pseudomonas*
    ○ Other *Streptococcus* sp.
- Chronic infection: Caused by parasites (filariasis) or fungi (sporotrichosis)
- Immunocompromised patients can be infected with gram-negative rods, gram-negative bacilli, or fungi.
- In freshwater, think *Aeromonas hydrophila*.
- Worldwide, *Wuchereria bancrofti* is most common causative agent.

COMMONLY ASSOCIATED CONDITIONS
- Lymphedema
- Lymph node dissection
- Athlete's foot
- Sporotrichosis
- Cellulitis
- Erysipelas (often coexists)
- Filarial infection

 DIAGNOSIS

- Local symptoms:
  – Red macular linear streaks from site of infection toward the regional draining lymph node
  – Tenderness and warmth over affected skin
  – May have lymph node involvement
  – May have blistering of affected skin
- Systemic symptoms:
  – Malaise
  – Fever and chills
  – Loss of appetite
  – Headache
  – Muscle aches

HISTORY
History of trauma to skin, cut, abrasion, or fungal infection (e.g., athlete's foot)

PHYSICAL EXAM
- Look for abscess.
- May have lymph node tenderness

DIAGNOSTIC TESTS & INTERPRETATION
Lab
- Complete blood count (CBC) may show leukocytosis.
- Blood cultures

Imaging
Plain radiology unnecessary

Diagnostic Procedures/Surgery
- Aspirate and culture any pus.
- Use sensitivity to guide antibiotic treatment.

DIFFERENTIAL DIAGNOSIS
- Septic thrombophlebitis (2)[C]
- Superficial thrombophlebitis (2)[C]: Feel for induration over the vein.
- Contact dermatitis (2)[C]
- Allergic reaction (2)[C]: Less likely to be allergic if >24 h after exposure (e.g., insect bite)

 TREATMENT

Antifilarial medication does not help the lymphangitis associated with filariasis (1)[A].

MEDICATION
- If nontoxic and >3 years of age, treat as an outpatient with oral antibiotics.
- If no improvement after 48 h of oral antibiotics, change to IV antibiotics.
- If systemic involvement, start IV antibiotics immediately.
- If group A hemolytic *Streptococcus* is suspected, treat aggressively.

First Line
- Antibiotics (1)[A]:
  – Dicloxacillin:
    ○ Adults: 500 mg p.o. q6h
    ○ Children: 50 mg/kg/d divided into q.i.d. dosing
  – Nafcillin:
    ○ Adults: 2 g IV q4h
    ○ Children: 150 mg/kg/d divided into q.i.d. dosing
  – Cephalexin:
    ○ Adults: 500 mg p.o. q6h
    ○ Children: 50 mg/kg/d p.o. divided into q.i.d. dosing

- Clindamycin (if penicillin or cephalosporin allergy):
  - Adults: 150–300 mg p.o. q6–8h or 600 mg IV q8h
  - Children: 8–20 mg/kg/d p.o. divided into t.i.d. or q.i.d. dosing; 20–40 mg/kg/d IV/IM divided into t.i.d. or q.i.d. dosing
- Acetaminophen or ibuprofen for pain and fever

Second Line
Trimethoprim-sulfamethoxazole (TMP-SMZ) good for areas with high rates of methicillin-resistant *S. aureus* [MRSA]):

- Adults: 160 mg TMP/800 SMZ mg p.o. q12h × 10–14 days
- Children >2 months of age: 10–20 mg/kg/d p.o. or IM divided into t.i.d. or q.i.d. doses × 14 days

ADDITIONAL TREATMENT
General Measures
- Hot, moist compresses to affected area
- If lymphedema is involved, compression garments and weight loss may help.

SURGERY/OTHER PROCEDURES
Incision and drainage of abscessed areas

IN-PATIENT CONSIDERATIONS
Initial Stabilization
- ABCs
- Fluids if in hypotensive shock

Admission Criteria
- If patient requires IV antibiotic therapy
- If symptoms are severe (3,4)[C]:
  - High fever
  - Rigor
  - Systemic toxicity
  - Shock
- Altered mental status

Discharge Criteria
Patient can be discharged on oral antibiotics once systemic symptoms resolve.

ONGOING CARE
FOLLOW-UP RECOMMENDATIONS
- Elevate affected area when at rest, if possible (3)[C].
- 48-h follow-up to ensure proper antibiotic coverage (if outpatient)

Patient Monitoring
Close follow-up to ensure decreasing inflammation

PATIENT EDUCATION
Instruct patients on proper wound care (and foot care, if applicable).

PROGNOSIS
- Good prognosis for uncomplicated lymphangitis
- Antimicrobial therapy is effective in 90% of patients.
- Untreated, can spread rapidly, especially group A *Streptococcus*

COMPLICATIONS
- Sepsis
- Bacteremia
- Cellulitis extending from vessels

REFERENCES

1. Badger C, Preston N, Seers K, et al. Antibiotics/Anti-inflammatories for reducing acute inflammatory episodes in lymphoedema of the limbs (Cochrane Review). In: *The Cochrane Library*. Oxford: Update Software; 2006;1.
2. Falagas ME, Bliziotis IA, Kapaskelis AM. Red streaks on the leg. *Am Fam Phys*. 2006;73(6):1061–2.
3. Bonnetblanc JM, Bédane C. Erysipelas: recognition and management. *Am J Clin Dermatol*. 2003;4: 157–63.
4. Edlich RF, Winters KL, Britt LD. Bacterial diseases of the skin. *J Long-Term Effects Med Implants*. 2005;15(5):499–510.

ADDITIONAL READING

- Haddad FG, Waked CH, Zein EF. Peripheral venous catheter-related inflammation. A randomized prospective trial. *J Med Liban*. 2006;54:139–45.
- Pereira de Godoy JM, Azoubel LM, Guerreiro Godoy Mde F et al. Erysipelas and lymphangitis in patients undergoing lymphedema treatment after breast-cancer therapy. *Acta Dermatovenerol Alp Panonica Adriat*. 2009;18:63–5.

 # CODES

ICD9
457.2 Lymphangitis

CLINICAL PEARLS

- The classic presentation of lymphangitis is red, linear streaks along the skin from an infected site (e.g., bite, cut, abrasion) to the draining lymph node for that region.
- Patients who have lymph node dissection as part of their breast cancer treatment may have difficulty draining lymphatic fluid properly, leading to lymphedema and an increased predisposition to infection and lymphangitis.
- A patient with severe systemic symptoms (e.g., high fever, rigors, shock, septic, altered mental status) should be admitted and treated with IV antibiotics. A patient with moderate systemic symptoms (e.g., fever, chills, muscle aches) should be monitored closely for worsening but could be treated as an outpatient.
- Patients can take ibuprofen or acetaminophen for the pain and/or fever associated with lymphangitis. Ibuprofen also helps with inflammation at high doses.
- Usually parasitic or fungal infections cause chronic lymphangitis.

L

LYMPHEDEMA

Kim House, MD

 BASICS

DESCRIPTION

- Swelling of a body part due to an abnormality in regional lymphatic drainage
- Results in increased interstitial volume secondary to the accumulation of tissue (lymphatic) fluid
- Most common in the lower limb (80%) but also can occur in the arms, face, trunk, and external genitalia

EPIDEMIOLOGY

Incidence

- Predominant sex: Female > Male.
- Predominant age: Any age
- 13% of breast cancer patients treated with surgery; 42% of those treated with surgery and radiation therapy
- Estimated to be between 1/6,000 and 1/300 live births; Milroy disease presents at birth.
- Meige disease develops during puberty.

Prevalence

- 120 million people worldwide are affected with filariasis.
- 3 million–5 million people are affected by secondary lymphedema in the US.

RISK FACTORS

- Filariasis: Most common cause worldwide
- Mastectomy
- Prior trauma
- Infection of affected limb
- History of prior surgical or radiation therapy for malignancy
- Long history of venous insufficiency
- Obesity

Genetics

- Milroy disease: Autosomal dominant; diagnosed either at birth or the 1st year of life
- Lymphedema praecox has onset between the ages of 1 and 35 years.
- Lymphedema tarda occurs >35 years.

GENERAL PREVENTION

Treatment of congestive heart failure (CHF), venous insufficiency

PATHOPHYSIOLOGY

- Postoperative: Gradual failure of distal lymphatics, which have to "pump" lymph at a greater pressure through damaged proximal ducts
- Risk is higher with postoperative radiation because radiation reduces regrowth of ducts owing to fibrous scarring.

ETIOLOGY

Secondary lymphedema:

- Trauma; recurrent infection; malignancy, including metastatic disease
- Developing countries: Most common cause is filariasis (*Wucheria bancrofti*).

COMMONLY ASSOCIATED CONDITIONS

Venous disease

 DIAGNOSIS

HISTORY

Recent surgery: Vein stripping can significantly exacerbate mild lymphedema (1)[B].

- 1st symptom: Painless swelling
- Feeling of heaviness in the limb, especially at the end of the day and in hot weather

PHYSICAL EXAM

- Initial: Pitting edema, can spread proximally
- Later: Nonpitting; after 1st year, does not spread proximally/distally but spreads radially
- Hyperkeratosis (thicker skin)
- Papillomatosis (rough skin)
- Increase in skin turgor
- Positive Stemmer sign (inability to pinch the skin of the dorsum of the second toe between the thumb and forefinger): Exclude heart failure.

DIAGNOSTIC TESTS & INTERPRETATION

- Lack of response to elevation or diuretic therapy may indicate a lymphatic insufficiency (2)[B].
- Diuretics increase excretion of salt and water thereby decreasing plasma volume, venous capillary pressure, and filtration. Diuretics improve filtration edema but don't improve lymph drainage over the long-term.

Lab

Initial lab tests

- Comprehensive chemistry panel: Evaluate for hepatic or renal impairment.
- Urinalysis: Protein-losing nephropathy

Imaging

Initial approach

- Ultrasound: Evaluate for acute/chronic deep vein thrombosis (DVT). Gives information about soft-tissue changes but does not tell about truncal anatomy of the lymphatics (1)[B].
- Duplex ultrasound: Lymphedema causes gradual impedance of venous return that aggravates the edema; 82% of patients with unexplained limb edema were diagnosed using a combination of duplex ultrasound and lymphoscintigram (3)[A].

Follow-Up & Special Considerations

- Lymphangiogram: Direct cannulation of lymphatics through the skin; risk for infection, local inflammation; not used commonly (3)[C]
- Lymphoscintigram: Radiolabeled protein technetium-99m-labeled colloid:
  - Measures lymphatic function, lymph movement, lymph drainage, and response to treatment
  - Sensitivity 73–97%; specificity 100%
  - Best to use 1-h and delayed images together (3)[A]
- CT scan: Calf skin thickening, thickening of the subcutaneous compartment, increased fat density, thickened perimuscular aponeurosis; typical honeycomb appearance (3)[B]
- MRI: Circumferential edema, increased volume of subcutaneous tissue, honeycomb pattern above the fascia between the muscle and subcutis; cannot differentiate primary from secondary lymphedema (3)[B]

DIFFERENTIAL DIAGNOSIS

CHF, renal failure, hypoalbuminemia, protein-losing nephropathy, lipidemia, DVT, chronic venous disease, postoperative complications following ipsilateral surgery, cellulitis, Baker cyst, idiopathic edema

TREATMENT

MEDICATION

- Micronized purified flavonoid fraction [Daflon 500 mg] is effective in decreasing venous stasis and idiopathic cyclic edema, chronic venous insufficiency, and postmastectomy lymphedema. It also reduces capillary permeability and the inflammatory component (4)[C].
- Benzopyrenes (coumarin): Reduces edema fluid by increasing the number of macrophages and enhancing proteolysis resulting in the removal of protein, increasing softness in the limbs, and decreasing elevated skin temperature.
  – Decreases symptoms and signs and decreases instances of secondary infection
  – Some reports of hepatotoxicity (4)[C]

ADDITIONAL TREATMENT

General Measures

- Elevation of affected limb: May be difficult for some patients to comply
- Prevent disease progression.
- Achieve mechanical reduction and maintenance of limb size.
- Alleviate symptoms.
- Prevent skin infection.

Issues for Referral

- Refer to physical therapist with lymphedema training for manual decongestive therapy.
- Provide education for patient/family for self-administration of therapy in future.
- Education for family about bandaging
- Fitting for compression garments

Additional Therapies

- Exercise: Lymph flow occurs as a result of inspiratory reduction in the intrathoracic pressure associated with inspiration. Best results are achieved with combination of flexibility, strength, and aerobic training (3)[B].
- Compression with custom-made elastic stocking (minimum pressure 40 mm Hg):
  – Protection against external incidental trauma
  – Decreases the intrinsic trauma on the skin owing to chronically increased interstitial pressures, which cause stretch of the skin and subcutaneous tissues
  – No data on preference of custom made versus prefabricated
  – Replace every 3–6 months or when starting to lose elasticity (1)[B].
- Multilayer bandaging: Inner layer of tubular stockinette followed by foam and padding to protect the joint flexures and to even out the contours of the limb so that pressure is distributed evenly; outer layer of at least 2 short-stretch extensible bandages; more effective than hosiery alone (1)[B]
- Pneumatic pumps: Development of high pressure up to 150 mm Hg; can reduce limb girth by 37–68.6%; wear a compression stocking when not using pump; high risk of genital edema; no metastasis in limb owing to risk of spread (1)[B].

COMPLEMENTARY AND ALTERNATIVE MEDICINE

Heat therapy: Hot water immersion, microwave, and electromagnetic irradiation may be helpful (1)[C].

SURGERY/OTHER PROCEDURES

- Debulking procedures (Charles procedure): Radical excision of subcutaneous tissue with primary or staged skin grafting:
  – Men had less improvement than women.
  – Main risk is infection and necrosis of the skin graft.
- Bypass procedures: Creation of lymphatic–venous anastomosis: Reserved for highly refractory cases only

IN-PATIENT CONSIDERATIONS

Initial Stabilization

- May admit to specialized rehabilitation unit for combination treatment in patients with heart failure or severe pulmonary disease
- IV antibiotics for infection

Admission Criteria

Systemic signs of infection

IV Fluids

Not used unless needed for sepsis

Nursing

- Leg elevation
- Encourage patient mobilization/exercise.
- Patient education for bandaging/wound care

Discharge Criteria

- Resolution of signs/symptoms of infection (e.g., elevated white blood cell count, fever, abnormal vital signs)
- Clinical improvement in wound appearance

ONGOING CARE

FOLLOW-UP RECOMMENDATIONS

Lymphedema will return in several days if patient stops wearing compression garments during the day and bandaging at night.

Patient Monitoring

- Daily visit to therapist for acute treatment
- Monthly visits for maintenance care

DIET

Low sodium

PATIENT EDUCATION

- Use compression garments, especially when exercising.
- Avoid affected limb(s) being dependant for long period of time: Patient should perform daily skin examination.

PROGNOSIS

Good with daily care

COMPLICATIONS

- Infection (local versus systemic): Common
- Risk of wound formation (venous wounds/abrasions) that are difficult to heal: Common
- Lymphangiosarcoma: Found in lymphedematous arms of patients following radical mastectomy; also in patients with Milroy disease; treatment is radiotherapy with surgery, reserved for patients with discrete nonmetastatic disease.

REFERENCES

1. Warren A, et al. Lymphedema: A comprehensive review. Ann Plastic Surg. 2007;59(4):464–72.
2. Mortimer P. "implications of the Lymphatic System in CVI-Associated Edema." Angiology. The Journal of Vascular Diseases 2000;51(1):3–7.
3. Brennan MJ, Miller LT. Overview of treatment options and review of the current role and use of compression garments, intermittent pumps, and exercise in the management of lymphedema. Cancer. 1998;83:2821–7.
4. Tiwari A, Cheng KS, Button M, et al. Differential diagnosis, investigation, and current treatment of lower limb lymphedema. Arch Surg. 2003;138: 152–61.

 CODES

ICD9
457.1 Other lymphedema

CLINICAL PEARLS

- Use short-stretch bandages for wrapping (not ACE wraps).
- Heat/whirlpool typically makes the wounds/lymphedema worse, not better.
- Patients with lymphedema are at much higher risk for infection than patients with only venous insufficiency.

L

LYMPHOGRANULOMA VENEREUM

Grant C. Fowler, MD

BASICS

Lymphogranuloma venereum (LGV) is a rare systemic sexually transmitted disease caused by the 3 most virulent strains or serovars of *Chlamydia trachomatis*, the same organism responsible for chlamydial urethritis. Incidence and prevalence increasing slightly in US in men having sex with men (MSM).

DESCRIPTION
- LGV presents as painless vesicular or ulcerative lesions on the external genitalia. These are seen in early disease followed by tender inguinal/femoral lymphadenopathy, usually unilateral. Severe anogenital inflammation and scarring may result from untreated disease.
- Previously a disease of the tropics, especially Africa, but also seen in Haiti, Jamaica, South America, East Asia, and Indonesia. Recently, outbreaks in MSM.
- System(s) affected: Gastrointestinal; Hemic/Lymphatic/Immunologic; Reproductive
- Synonym(s): Tropical bubo; Climatic bubo; Strumous bubo; Poradenitis inguinalis; Durand-Nicolas-Favre disease; Lymphogranuloma inguinale; 4th, 5th, or 6th venereal disease

EPIDEMIOLOGY
- Predominant age: 3rd decade; corresponds with average age of peak sexual activity
- Predominant sex: Male > Female (5:1)

Incidence
In the US, about 300 cases reported each year.

Prevalence
US prevalence increasing in MSM, especially anorectal lymphogranuloma venereum.

Pregnancy Considerations
LGV may be acquired passing through infected birth canal; congenital transmission does not occur.

RISK FACTORS
- Unprotected intercourse
- Anal intercourse
- Residing in tropical or developing countries
- Prostitution
- MSM
- HIV (+)

GENERAL PREVENTION
- Treat sexual contact(s).
- Condoms may provide protection against genital-anogenital transmission, but have no impact on transmission between other sites.

PATHOPHYSIOLOGY
Physical damage is from lymphatic obstruction.

ETIOLOGY
3 of 15 known strains of *C. trachomatis*, described as serovars L1, L2, and L3, are responsible for LGV. The strains of *Chlamydia* that cause urethritis appear to infect only squamocolumnar cells; LGV strains are more invasive and capable of replication in macrophages.

COMMONLY ASSOCIATED CONDITIONS
Screening should be done for gonorrhea, hepatitis B, hepatitis C, herpes, HIV, and syphilis.

DIAGNOSIS

This is a very rare disease, predominantly diagnosed by clinical suspicion based on history, physical examination, and exclusion of other diagnoses. Where available, serology can be helpful. Calling a reference lab is often helpful for determining the best serology tests. Examination and culture of swabs of infected lesions or aspirates of infected lymph glands may also assist with making the diagnosis.

HISTORY
Recent unprotected intercourse with a prostitute or MSM, especially anal intercourse or intercourse with someone recently visiting or from the tropics such as Africa, the Caribbean, South America, East Asia, or Indonesia.

PHYSICAL EXAM
Three stages:
- Primary: Superficial painless lesions such as papules, vesicles, ulcers, or erosions appear on the external genitalia, in the area of exposure, 3–30 days after exposure. These disappear in a few days, leaving no scar.
- Secondary: The inguinal syndrome (bubonic stage) or hemorrhagic proctitis (following rectal intercourse). Femoral lymph glands can also be involved, often unilaterally:
  – Predominantly in men
  – Fever, chills, headache, myalgias
  – Inguinal syndrome: Regional lymphadenopathy a week to months after the primary stage. Buboes begin as a mass of firm, tender, enlarged, matted lymph nodes, often unilateral and eventually involving the overlying skin with erythema and adhesions. Bubo enlargement causes severe groin pain. Within 1–2 weeks, the buboes may become fluctuant and rupture, relieving the pain but leaving fistulas to drain or involute and form firm inguinal masses.
  – Proctitis: Anal pruritus and a mucous rectal discharge, multiple discrete superficial ulcerations with irregular borders, rectal pain, and tenesmus. This discharge and these lesions may be seen on anoscopy or endoscopy.
- Tertiary: Anogenital stage:
  – Lymphatic obstruction or scarring
  – Genitalia or anorectal canal inflammation
  – Predominantly women and MSM
  – Lymphatic obstruction may produce either perianal growths or lymphoid tissue resembling hemorrhoids.
  – Perirectal abscesses, ischiorectal and rectovaginal fistulas, anal fistulas, and rectal strictures or stenosis may occur.

DIAGNOSTIC TESTS & INTERPRETATION
Lab
- Where possible, both swab and sera samples should be submitted for suspected cases of LGV.
- Serum tests are only useful after LGV has become invasive (i.e., secondary or tertiary LGV).
- Dry swabs should be stored and shipped frozen. Swabs stored in chlamydia transport medium should be kept frozen at –80C if culture will be done or –20C if culture will not be done.
- Cultures from a swab of a primary lesion may grow chlamydia, but genotyping is necessary to differentiate LGV from other chlamydial strains.

Initial lab tests
- Genotyping for LGV by DNA sequencing or restriction fragment length polymorphism (RFLP) is definitive (i.e., differentiates LGV from other chlamydial strains).
- Cultures from a swab of a primary lesion may grow chlamydia, but genotyping is necessary to differentiate LGV from other chlamydial strains
- Nucleic acid amplification tests (NAAT) for chlamydia are not specific to LGV and are not FDA approved for rectal samples. Positive NAAT samples can be sent for LGV genotyping.
- Urine can be tested with NAAT and positives sent for LGV genotyping; samples should be stored and shipped frozen.
- Serum immunoglobulin M microimmunofluorescence (MIF) testing is more readily available but not definitive of LGV.
- Serum antibody levels to L1, L2, and L3 serovars of *C. trachomatis* also measured using complement fixation, although cross-reactivity with other chlamydial organisms is possible.
- A 4-fold rise in MIF titer to LGV antigen (>1:256) or a complement fixation titer >1:64, with the proper clinical scenario is probably LGV. Complement levels >1:128 basically confirm LGV.
- MIF titers are more sensitive and specific than the complement fixation test.

Follow-Up & Special Considerations
- Complete blood count and differential may reveal lymphocytosis or monocytosis.
- Erythrocyte sedimentation rate may be elevated.
- Consider VDRL/rapid plasma reagin, gonorrhea, hepatitis B and hepatitis C, herpes simplex virus (HSV), HIV testing.

Imaging
Imaging is only generally necessary to clarify or define complications or to exclude other diagnoses.

Initial approach
- CT scan for retroperitoneal adenitis
- Barium enema may reveal the characteristic elongated stricture of rectal LGV.

Diagnostic Procedures/Surgery
Buboes may require injection of 2–5 ml of sterile saline prior to aspiration.

DIFFERENTIAL DIAGNOSIS

- Painful genital ulcer, often with adenitis (in order of frequency): Genital herpes, chancroid, LGV. However, patient should also be evaluated for syphilis and HIV. Not all ulcers are infectious in etiology; on the other hand, the patient may have a sexually transmitted infection involving more than one organism.
- Painless genital ulcer: Syphilis, granuloma inguinale (donovanosis), LGV. Patient should also be evaluated for herpes and HIV.
- Inguinal adenitis:
  – Genital herpes, syphilis, chancroid, granuloma inguinale (donovanosis)
  – Other considerations for inguinal adenitis include cat scratch disease, local skin infection, lymphoma, HIV, and reactive adenopathy.
  – Less common: Lymphoproliferative buboes
- Buboes or suppurative adenitis: Chancroid, donovanosis, plague, tularemia, sporotrichosis, actinomycosis, or tuberculosis
- Retroperitoneal adenitis: Malignancy
- Proctitis: Gonococcal and non-LGV chlamydial proctitis, inflammatory bowel disease
- Lymphatic obstruction: Schistosomiasis or malignancy.

 TREATMENT

Outpatient oral medications are all that are necessary in most uncomplicated cases.

MEDICATION

Consider treating empirically for LGV if specific LGV diagnostic testing is not available for patients with compatible clinical syndrome (e.g., proctocolitis, genital ulcer disease with lymphadenopathy).

First Line

- For acute cases: Doxycycline 100 mg PO b.i.d. for 21 days
- For chronic or relapsing cases: Consider longer course of therapy.

Second Line

- Erythromycin base 500 mg PO q.i.d. for 21 days or azithromycin 1.0 g PO once weekly for 3 weeks (data are lacking)
- Sulfisoxazole 500 mg PO q.i.d. for 21 days or equivalent sulfonamide course
- Chloramphenicol and rifampin have been used to treat in the past.

Pregnancy Considerations

Treat pregnant and lactating women with an erythromycin regimen. Doxycycline is contraindicated in pregnancy.

ADDITIONAL TREATMENT

General Measures

Pain medications as needed such as nonsteroidal anti-inflammatory drugs (NSAIDs).

Issues for Referral

Surgery for complications should be delayed until antibiotic therapy has been administered for at least a few days and any fever has resolved.

SURGERY/OTHER PROCEDURES

In the acute bubonic stage, nodes should be aspirated through intact skin for diagnostic purposes, and this may improve symptoms. Nodes may also be incised and drained for diagnostic purposes and to possibly prevent inguinal or femoral ulcerations. However, there is controversy as to whether I&D or excision of nodes improves symptoms as opposed to delaying healing.

IN-PATIENT CONSIDERATIONS

Very rarely necessary, and only for patients not able to ambulate, tolerate oral medications, or care for themselves; also possibly for pain control

Initial Stabilization

Intravenous fluids as necessary for hydration and pain control

Admission Criteria

Unable to tolerate oral antibiotics, unable to ambulate or perform self-care due to pain or other complications, or patients preparing to undergo surgery

Nursing

Public health nurses can help track and treat sexual contacts.

Discharge Criteria

When stable and able to perform self-care

 ONGOING CARE

FOLLOW-UP RECOMMENDATIONS

Patients should be observed until signs and symptoms resolve and routine chlamydial tests are negative (test of cure). Serology should not be used to monitor treatment response, as the duration of antibody response has not been defined.

Patient Monitoring

- Fever and bubo pain usually abate within 1–2 days after starting antibiotics. For persistent fever or malaise, monitor closely for complications such as an abscess or superinfection.
- Treatment has no effect on existing scar tissue; therefore, monitor for surgical complications.
- Dual infections with other sexually transmitted diseases are common; appropriate monitoring should be performed, especially for gonorrhea, hepatitis B, hepatitis C, HIV, and syphilis.

DIET

Tetracyclines should be taken on an empty stomach except for doxycycline, which can be taken with food.

PATIENT EDUCATION

LGV is a sexually transmitted disease. The patient should be counseled about other sexually transmitted diseases and safe sex practices. Patients should abstain from intercourse or other sexual contact until treatment is complete.

PROGNOSIS

- Improved by early treatment
- Complete resolution of symptoms is usual if treatment is undertaken before scarring.
- Reinfection and/or inadequate treatment may result in relapse.

COMPLICATIONS

- Scarring, including possible ureteral or bowel obstruction, persistent rectovaginal fistula, or gross destruction of the anal canal, anal sphincter, or perineum. Repair of such complications as well as plastic repair of some of the complications of lymphatic obstruction, such as genital elephantiasis, are the more common surgical indications. Surgery should be performed only after antibiotic treatment.
- Mild rectal strictures can occasionally be dilated on an outpatient basis.
- Squamous cell carcinoma has been associated with LGV.

ADDITIONAL READING

- Herring A, Richens J. Lymphogranuloma venereum. *Sex Transm Infect*. 2006; 82(Suppl 4): iv23– 5.
- MacDonald N, Wong T. Canadian guidelines on sexually transmitted infections, 2006. *CMAJ*. 2007; 176:175– 6.
- McLean CA, Stoner BP, Workowski KA. Treatment of lymphogranuloma venereum. *Clin Infect Dis*. 2007; 44(Suppl 3):S147– 52.
- Workowski KA, Berman SM. Sexually transmitted diseases treatment guidelines, 2006. *MMWR Recomm Rep*. 2006;55:1– 94.
- World Health Organization. *Sexually transmitted and other reproductive tract infections: a guide to essential practice*. Geneva: WHO; 2005. Available from http://www.who.int/reproductive-health/publications/rtis_gep/management.htm.

 CODES

ICD9
099.1 Lymphogranuloma venereum

CLINICAL PEARLS

Empiric treatment for buboes in the absence of ulcers? In practice, it is often difficult to distinguish LGV from chancroid. Because erythromycin is effective against both chancroid and LGV, the World Health Organization recommends treating buboes lacking genital ulcers with erythromycin for 7 days and having the patient return for evaluation. If the patient is improving at 7 days, the treatment should be continued for at least 14 days. (Note: LGV may require treatment even longer than 14 days.)

L

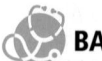

BASICS

DESCRIPTION
- Mature B-cell neoplasm that arises in lymph node germinal centers
- Highly aggressive, rapidly growing malignancy
- Can present as lymphoma or leukemia
- 3 distinct forms, differing in epidemiology, clinical presentation, and genetics:
  - Endemic, or African
  - Sporadic
  - Immunodeficiency-related
    - HIV/AIDS-related
    - Post solid organ transplant
    - Inherited immunodeficiency
- Associated with Epstein-Barr virus (EBV)
  - Almost 100% of endemic cases
  - Up to 30% of sporadic cases
- Specific chromosome translocation [t(8;14)]
- Similar disease characteristics to diffuse large B cell lymphoma (DLBCL)
- System(s) affected: Hematologic; Lymphatic
  - Can involve other systems, particularly the ileocecal region, ovaries, kidneys, breasts, and central nervous system [CNS].
- Synonym(s): Mature B cell high-grade lymphoma; Mature B cell acute lymphoblastic leukemia, L3 type (FAB classification); Burkitt cell leukemia

Pediatric Considerations
Common age group for this disorder (30% of cases in US)

Geriatric Considerations
Unusual in this age group. Toxicity with chemotherapy may be increased in the elderly.

Pregnancy Considerations
With aggressive treatment, good maternal and fetal outcome.

EPIDEMIOLOGY
- Varies by disease form
- Endemic
  - One of most common tumors of childhood in Africa, most frequently occurring in children 4–7 years old.
  - Rare in adults
- Sporadic (1)
  - In US, trimodal peaks of age incidence around ages 10, 40, and 75
  - More common in Caucasians
  - Male > Female (3:1 or 4:1), more pronounced at younger ages
- HIV-associated Burkitt occurs mainly in middle-aged adults.

Incidence
Rare in US, incidence 0.27 per 100,000 person-years; about 50 times more common in endemic regions of Africa

Prevalence
Comprises <1% of adult non-Hodgkin lymphoma (NHL); accounts for 30–40% of NHL in children in the US and western Europe

RISK FACTORS
In endemic areas, children with early acquisition of EBV infection are at increased risk. Coinfection with malaria and EBV 100-fold increase in incidence.

GENERAL PREVENTION
Currently there are no specific measures known to prevent development of Burkitt lymphoma.

ETIOLOGY
- Activation and overexpression of *c-myc* oncogene
- Monoclonal proliferation of B lymphocytes resulting from dysregulation of *c-myc*
  - Translocation of *c-myc* to immunoglobulin coding regions results in constitutive expression of gene product.
  - EBV-infected cells in germinal-center reactions may increase the risk of translocation.
- Poorly regulated proliferation of genetically unstable B cells increases chance of translocations.
  - Immunodeficiency patients with persistent generalized lymphadenopathy and polyclonal B cell activation.

COMMONLY ASSOCIATED CONDITIONS
- EBV infection
- Immunodeficiency, especially AIDS

DIAGNOSIS

HISTORY
- Rapidly progressive bulky adenopathy or extranodal mass
- Symptoms of bone marrow involvement
  - Fatigue, exercise intolerance, bruising, epistaxis, other bleeding, fever
- Abdominal presentation
  - Abdominal pain, nausea, vomiting, bowel obstruction, gastrointestinal bleeding, symptoms mimicking acute appendicitis or intussusception
- Endemic (African): Jaw or facial bone tumor, which may present as mouth pain, loose teeth, or jaw mass
- Nonendemic: Extranodal disease, abdominal presentation typical
- Can present as acute leukemia (L3-ALL) with predominant bone marrow involvement and no mass lesions
- Renal function impairment and significant metabolic derangement may quickly manifest due to the rapid progression and spread of the tumor.

PHYSICAL EXAM
- Endemic: Mass on jaw or facial bone, pallor, petechiae, hepatosplenomegaly
- Sporadic: Lymphadenopathy, any mass lesion, abdominal tenderness, pallor, petechiae, hepatosplenomegaly
- Immunodeficiency-associated: Lymphadenopathy, pallor, petechiae, hepatosplenomegaly

DIAGNOSTIC TESTS & INTERPRETATION
Lab
Initial lab tests
- Biopsy of mass lesion
  - Diagnosis is suggested by cellular morphology on histologic examination
- Complete blood count (CBC) with differential: Anemia, neutropenia, and/or thrombocyptopenia
- Order electrolytes, BUN, creatinine, calcium, magnesium, phosphorus, serum lactate dehydrogenase (LDH), uric acid: Hypokalemia, hypophosphatemia, hypercalcemia, hyperuricemia, renal insufficiency, elevated LDH
- Hepatitis B virus serologies prior to rituximab administration

Follow-Up & Special Considerations
- Diagnosis requires immunophenotypic and cytogenetic data.
- Immunophenotype studies:
  - Cells express surface IgM and B-associated antigens (CD19, CD20, CD22, CD79a), as well as CD10, HLA-DR, and CD43
  - Cells also show nuclear staining for BCL-6 protein
- Cytogenic studies to visualize chromosomal translocation:
  - Reciprocal chromosome translocation involving *c-myc* and immunoglobulin heavy chain (IgH) gene [t(8;14)] (80%)
  - Reciprocal chromosome translocation involving *c-myc* and immunoglobulin light chain (IgL) genes [t(2;8) or t (8;22)]
  - Fluorescence in situ hybridization (FISH) or long-segment polymerase chain reaction (PCR) may be necessary to identify translocation
- EBV testing in lesional cells
- Gene expression profiling can help distinguish Burkitt lymphoma from DLBCL.

Imaging
Initial approach
- Chest x-ray
- CT scan of chest, abdomen, pelvis
- Imaging of any site suspected to be involved by tumor

Diagnostic Procedures/Surgery
- Bone marrow aspiration and biopsy for morphology and flow cytometry
- Lumbar puncture for CSF cell count, differential, and cytology
- Lymph node biopsy: Most suggestive lymph nodes should be selected for excisional biopsy.
  - Frozen sections and needle biopsies discouraged as lymph node architecture helpful for diagnosis.
- Diagnostic laparotomy with resection of localized disease

Pathological Findings
- Monotonous diffuse infiltrate of medium-size round cells, with round or oval nuclei, several nucleoli, and coarse chromatin. Cytoplasm is intensely basophilic and moderately abundant.
- Mitotic rate is high; close to 100% of viable cells will be actively engaged in cell cycle and express Ki-67.
- Classic "starry sky" histologic appearance
  - Results from the presence of scattered macrophages with phagocytic cell debris
  - Characteristic of, although not pathognomonic, for Burkitt lymphoma
- Although lymph nodes usually diffusely involved, early lesions may show selective involvement of germinal centers.

DIFFERENTIAL DIAGNOSIS
- Other non-Hodgkin lymphomas
  - Burkitt-like lymphoma:
    - Immunophenotype and molecular characteristics differ from those of classic Burkitt lymphoma
    - Problematic entity with little reproducibility of diagnosis.
    - May be confused with DLBCL.
  - DLBCL: Large, irregular cells, often with BCL rearrangement
  - Precursor B-lymphocytic lymphoma
  - Precursor T-lymphocytic lymphoma
  - Mantle cell lymphoma, blastoid variant

- Hodgkin's lymphoma
- Acute lymphoblastic leukemia
- Other causes of lymphadenopathy
  - Infection (e.g., bacterial lymphadenitis, mononucleosis, tuberculosis, atypical mycobacterium, cat scratch disease)
  - Reactive lymphoid hyperplasia
  - Histiocytosis
- Other primary malignancies of childhood (e.g., Wilms tumor, neuroblastoma, peripheral neuroectodermal tumor)
- Other metastatic malignancies

 TREATMENT

If available, all patients should be offered participation in an appropriate clinical trial.

MEDICATION

- Intensive, short-term, multiagent chemotherapy administered in cycles (2)[A].
  - Chemotherapeutic agents include cyclophosphamide, methotrexate, vincristine, prednisone, high-dose methotrexate, high-dose cytarabine, etoposide, isophosphamide, and doxorubicin.
  - Type and extent of therapy depend on stage of disease.
- Rituximab in combination with chemotherapy may improve outcome.
- CNS prophylaxis for most patients
  - Not necessary for limited disease remote from the CNS.
  - Intrathecal methotrexate, with or without IV methotrexate and cytarabine, may be used for CNS prophylaxis.
  - Routine cranial irradiation does not improve efficacy of treatment.
- Chemotherapy cycles should be initiated as soon as hematologic recovery permits.
  - Delay of chemotherapy may result in regrowth of resistant tumor between cycles.
- Management of tumor lysis syndrome with initial cycle of chemotherapy.

Second Line
- Rituximab may be effective if not used in front-line therapy.
- Hematopoietic stem cell transplantation in combination with high-dose chemotherapy (3)

ADDITIONAL TREATMENT
Issues for Referral
All patients should be managed by a pediatric or adult hematologist/oncologist.

COMPLEMENTARY AND ALTERNATIVE MEDICINE
Many possible complementary and alternative therapies exist to assist in management of side effects of chemotherapy. These should be considered individually for a risk/benefit discussion with the patient.

SURGERY/OTHER PROCEDURES
- Biopsy and staging
  - All patients require a biopsy to establish the diagnosis pathologically

- Surgical resection
  - Treatment for small, completely resectable abdominal tumors (in addition to chemotherapy)
  - For patients with intestinal obstruction who cannot begin chemotherapy immediately
- Many patients require placement of a central venous line for administration of chemotherapy.

IN-PATIENT CONSIDERATIONS
Initial Stabilization
- Burkitt lymphomas have high growth fractions and short doubling times.
  - Rapid initiation of definitive chemotherapy is essential.
- Management of tumor lysis syndrome with initial cycle of chemotherapy
  - Aggressive hydration without potassium
  - Close monitoring of electrolytes, renal function, and uric acid initially every 6–8 hours
  - Rasburicase (0.2 mg/kg IV once daily for up to 5 days depending on response to therapy) to break down uric acid
  - Allopurinol (10 mg/kg PO divided 2–3 times per day) if rasburicase not available
    - Consider alkalization of urine with bicarbonate-containing intravenous fluids (goal urine pH 7–8) with allopurinol use
  - Use of phosphate binder if serum phosphorus becomes elevated
  - Medical management of hyperkalemia

IV Fluids
Aggressive IV hydration with first cycle of chemotherapy
- Typically D5/0.5 NS at 125 cc/m^2/hr (twice the maintenance rate)
- No potassium in IV fluids.
- Consider addition of NaHCO$_3$ to IV fluids at the direction of the treating oncologist.

 ONGOING CARE

FOLLOW-UP RECOMMENDATIONS
Patient Monitoring
- Close monitoring of serum chemistries is critical due to high risk of tumor lysis syndrome and uric acid nephropathy.
- CBC, liver function tests, and renal function should also be closely monitored throughout chemotherapy.
- Surveillance physical exam and imaging for detection of recurrence
- All patients, particularly children, should be followed indefinitely for long-term effects of chemotherapy.

PATIENT EDUCATION
Educational materials are available online from the Leukemia and Lymphoma Society (http://www.leukemia-lymphoma.org/hm_lls) and Curesearch (http://www.curesearch.org/).

PROGNOSIS
- In localized disease, 5-year disease-free survival >90%
- Aggressive treatment of advanced disease yields >80% 5-year disease-free survival.
- Recurrent disease tends to be more resistant to therapy.
- Mortality for endemic form remains high where access to health care is limited.

COMPLICATIONS
- Complications of extensive abdominal disease include obstructive jaundice and pancreatitis, bowel obstruction, and intestinal perforation.
- Tumor lysis syndrome with renal failure (uric acid nephropathy) secondary to high tumor burden and rapid cell turnover may occur prior to and especially following the start of chemotherapy.
- Rituximab has been associated with reactivation of Hepatitis B virus resulting in fulminant liver failure.
- Other short- and long-term potential complications of chemotherapy include alopecia, myelosuppression requiring blood transfusion, life-threatening infection, nausea, mucositis, infusion reactions, peripheral neuropathy, seizures, infertility, congestive heart failure, and secondary malignancy.

REFERENCES

1. Mbulaiteye SM, Anderson WF, Bhatia K, Rosenberg PS, Linet MS, Devesa SS et al. Trimodal age-specific incidence patterns for Burkitt lymphoma in the United States, 1973–2005. *Int J Cancer.* 2010; 126:1732–9.
2. Tauro S, et al. Dose-intensified treatment of Burkitt lymphoma and B-cell lymphoma unclassifiable, (with features intermediate between diffuse large B-cell lymphoma and Burkitt lymphoma) in young adults (<50 years): a comparison of two adapted BFM protocols. *Ameri J Hem.* 2010;85(4):261–3.
3. Gross TG, Hale GA, He W, Camitta BM, Sanders JE, Cairo MS, Hayashi RJ, Termuhlen AM, Zhang MJ, Davies SM, Eapen M et al. Hematopoietic stem cell transplantation for refractory or recurrent non-Hodgkin lymphoma in children and adolescents. *Biol. Blood Marrow Transplant.* 2010;16:223–30.

 CODES

ICD9
- 200.20 Burkitt's tumor or lymphoma, unspecified site
- 200.21 Burkitt's tumor or lymphoma involving lymph nodes of head, face, and neck
- 200.22 Burkitt's tumor or lymphoma involving intrathoracic lymph nodes

CLINICAL PEARLS
- Burkitt lymphoma is an aggressive mature B cell malignancy most commonly diagnosed in childhood.
- Burkitt lymphoma is strongly associated with t(8;14) and EBV infection.
- Burkitt lymphoma is highly treatable with intense multiagent systemic and intrathecal chemotherapy.

L

MACULAR DEGENERATION, AGE-RELATED (ARMD)

Richard W. Allinson, MD

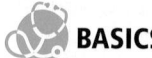

BASICS

DESCRIPTION
- Pigmentary changes in the macula or typical drusen associated with visual loss to the 20/30 level or worse, not caused by cataract or other eye disease, in individuals >50 years old
- Some definitions exclude age or visual acuity criteria.
- Leading cause of irreversible, severe visual loss in persons >65 years old
- Stages:
  – Atrophic/nonexudative
  – Neovascular/exudative
- System(s) affected: Nervous
- Synonym(s): Senile macular degeneration; Subretinal neovascularization; Age-related macular degeneration (ARMD)

EPIDEMIOLOGY
- Neovascular/exudative form is rare in blacks and more common in whites.
- Predominant gender: Female

Incidence
- In the Framingham Eye Study (FES), drusen were noted in 25% of all participants who were ≥52 years old. ARMD-associated visual loss was noted in 5.7%.
- Atrophic/nonexudative stage accounts for 20% of cases of severe visual loss.
- Neovascular/exudative stage accounts for 80% of cases of severe visual loss.

Prevalence
- Per FES study:
  – People 52–64 years old: 1.6%
  – People 65–74 years old: 11%
  – People ≥75 years old: 27.9%
- Increases with age
- >75 years: 1/4 of men and 1/3 of women will have evidence of ARMD.

RISK FACTORS
- Obesity (increased BMI)
- Ethnicity: Non-Hispanic whites
- Cigarette smoking
- *Chlamydia pneumoniae* infection
- Family history
- Excess sunlight exposure
- Blue or light iris color
- Hyperopia
- History of cardiovascular disease (HTN, circulatory problems)
- Short stature

Genetics
- Genetic susceptibility may be a factor in ARMD. ~25% genetically determined.
- Complement factor H is an important susceptibility gene for ARMD.

GENERAL PREVENTION
- UV protection for eyes
- Routine ophthalmologic visits:
  – Every 2–4 years for patients 40–64 years
  – Every 1–2 years after age 65
- Daily Amsler grid testing
- Patients who take statin drugs, which modify lipid profiles, may have a reduced risk.

PATHOPHYSIOLOGY
- Breaks in Bruch membrane allow choroidal neovascular membranes (CNVMs) to invade the retinal pigment epithelium (RPE) and grow into the subretinal space.
- Atrophic/nonexudative: Drusen and/or pigmentary changes in the macula
- Neovascular/exudative: Growth of blood vessels underneath the retina

ETIOLOGY
- Visible light can result in the formation and accumulation of metabolic byproducts in the RPE, a pigment layer underneath the retina that normally helps remove metabolic byproducts from the retina. Excess accumulation of these metabolic byproducts interferes with the normal metabolic activity of the RPE and can lead to the formation of drusen.
- Neovascular stage generally arises from the atrophic stage.
- Most patients do not progress beyond the atrophic/nonexudative stage; however, those who do are at a greater risk of developing severe visual loss.

COMMONLY ASSOCIATED CONDITIONS
- Presumed ocular histoplasmosis syndrome
- Exudative retinal detachment
- Vitreous hemorrhage
- Other causes of CNVMs

DIAGNOSIS

HISTORY
- Patients frequently notice distortion of central vision.
- Patients may notice straight lines appear crooked (e.g., telephone poles).

PHYSICAL EXAM
Retinal exam:
- Atrophic/nonexudative stage:
  – Drusen:
    ○ Small yellowish-white lesions
    ○ Can be subdivided into types such as hard drusen and soft drusen
  – Atrophy of the RPE
- Neovascular/exudative stage:
  – Blood vessels growing underneath the retina from the choroid are called CNVMs or subretinal neovascularization (SRN). The choroid is the vascular layer underneath the RPE.
  – Subretinal fluid
  – Exudates
  – Subretinal hemorrhage
  – On Amsler grid testing, the horizontal or vertical lines may become broken, distorted, or missing.
- Disciform scar: An advanced stage resulting in a fibrovascular scar

DIAGNOSTIC TESTS & INTERPRETATION
Diagnostic Procedures/Surgery
- Daily Amsler grid testing
- Eye examination with detailed fundus examination
- Fluorescein angiography:
  – Detection of CNVMs
  – Differentiate between atrophic and neovascular ARMD.
- Indocyanine green videoangiography: May identify occult or hidden CNVMs

- Optical coherence tomography (OCT) may be useful in identifying CNVMs, subretinal fluid, and retinal thickening.

Pathological Findings
Drusen: Deposits of hyaline material between the RPE and Bruch membrane (the limiting membrane between the RPE and the choroid)

DIFFERENTIAL DIAGNOSIS
- Idiopathic SRN
- Presumed ocular histoplasmosis syndrome
- Diabetic retinopathy
- Hypertensive retinopathy

TREATMENT

MEDICATION
- Atrophic/nonexudative macular degeneration:
  – Free radical formation in the retina, induced by visible light, may play a role in cellular damage that results in ARMD.
  – Zinc and antioxidants may be of benefit.
- Laser photocoagulation to treat drusen is not recommended.

First Line
- Age-Related Eye Disease Study (AREDS) found that a high-dose regimen of vitamin and mineral supplements reduces progression of ARMD in some cases:
  – Recommended daily doses: Vitamin C 500 mg, vitamin E 400 IU, β-carotene 15 mg, zinc oxide 80 mg, and cupric oxide 2 mg (1)[A]
  – Exercise caution with β-carotene use in smokers due to potential link to lung cancer.
- Ranibizumab (Lucentis):
- Antibody fragment that inhibits all active forms of vascular endothelial growth factor (VEGF)
- Approved by FDA for the treatment of neovascular (wet) age-related macular degeneration
- Injected intravitreally, at a dose of 0.5 mg, every 4 weeks

- 1 year after treatment, up to 40% of patients treated with ranibizumab gained at least 3 lines of vision, and approximately 95% maintained vision (defined as the loss of fewer than 15 letters in visual acuity). Minimally classic or occult lesions were studied in the MARINA Study (2)[A].
- Ranibizumab is superior to verteporfin in the treatment of predominately classic CNVMs. This was demonstrated in the ANCHOR Study (3)[A].
- The PrONTO Study demonstrated OCT-guided, variable-dosing regimen with ranibizumab resulted in similar results to the MARINA and ANCHOR Studies with monthly injections (4)[A]:
  – Patients received 3 consecutive monthly intravitreal injections of ranibizumab. Retreatment was performed if any of the following were observed: Decreased vision, increase in central retinal thickness on OCT, new macular hemorrhage, persistent macular fluid on OCT, or new-onset classic CNVM.

- When comparing ranibizumab and bevacizumab in a multicenter, retrospective study, both treatments were effective in stabilizing visual loss, and no difference was found in the visual outcome between the 2 treatment groups (5)[C].

Second Line

- Pegaptanib sodium (Macugen) is a compound that binds to and neutralizes VEGF. The usual dose is 0.3 mg injected intravitreally every 6 weeks as needed for the treatment of neovascular ARMD. Pegaptanib preserves vision rather than improving it. 70% of treated patients lost fewer than 15 letters of visual acuity at 1 year.
- Bevacizumab (Avastin) is a full-length antibody to VEGF, administered intravitreally at a dose of 1.25 mg, and is being evaluated in the treatment of neovascular ARMD. Widely used off-label because of its lower cost.
- VEGF Trap is being investigated in the treatment of neovascular ARMD. VEGF Trap has a higher binding affinity for all VEGF-A isoforms than does ranibizumab (6)[C].

ADDITIONAL TREATMENT
General Measures
Low-vision aids may be helpful.

SURGERY/OTHER PROCEDURES
- Neovascular/exudative macular degeneration:
  - The Macular Photocoagulation Study (MPS) demonstrated a treatment benefit for laser treatment of CNVMs that were ≥200 microns (200 microns = 0.2 mm) from the center of the macula.
  - The MPS showed that the benefits of argon laser photocoagulation were greatest 1 year after treatment.
  - Fluorescein angiogram usually can determine whether a CNVM is present, if it is well defined, and if it is in a treatable position.
- Treatment of CNVMs 1–199 microns from the center of the macula has been studied by the Age-Related Macular Degeneration Study-Krypton Laser (ARMDS-K). The benefit of laser treatment was greatest among patients without evidence of HTN. No benefit was observed among patients who had highly elevated BP and/or used antihypertensive medication.
- Vitrectomy has been used to remove CNVMs, but this is generally not recommended.
- CNVMs can bleed spontaneously, leaving blood underneath the retina. Vitrectomy to remove subretinal blood may be of benefit and should be performed within 7 days of the bleed. Tissue plasminogen activator (tPA) instilled into the eye may help remove a subretinal hemorrhage. In some cases, intravitreal gas with or without tPA may displace submacular blood:
  - Intravitreal bevacizumab may be helpful in the treatment of neovascular age-related macular degeneration associated with a large submacular hemorrhage (7)[C].
- Macular translocation involves intentionally creating a retinal detachment and attempting to shift the macula away from the CNVM. Laser is then applied to the CNVM after the retina is translocated. This procedure is associated with potentially serious surgical risks.
- Photodynamic therapy (PDT) with verteporfin reduces vision loss in patients with >50% "classic" subfoveal CNVMs. Verteporfin is administered IV, and a diode laser at 689 nm is applied to the CNVM:

- After 24 months of follow-up in patients who underwent PDT to treat predominately classic subfoveal CNVM, 59% of the verteporfin-treated eyes vs 31% of the placebo-treated eyes lost fewer than 15 letters from baseline.
  - In occult subfoveal CNVMs with no classic component, PDT significantly reduces the risk of moderate and severe vision loss.
  - PDT treatment benefit may not only depend on lesion type, but also on lesion size and presenting visual acuity. The treatment benefit may be related to smaller lesion size and worse presenting visual acuity.
  - Patients should be informed of a ~4% risk of acute, severe vision loss after PDT.
  - Intravitreal triamcinolone combined with PDT may result in improved visual acuity for patients with CNVMs.
- Combination therapy combining intravitreal ranibizumab with PDT and/or intravitreal triamcinolone is being evaluated.

 ## ONGOING CARE

FOLLOW-UP RECOMMENDATIONS
Patient Monitoring
- Laser-treated patients should be reexamined promptly if new visual symptoms occur.
- Amsler grid can aid in discovering visual disturbances.
- Patients with soft drusen or pigmentary changes in the macula are at an increased risk of visual loss. They should be instructed that it is important to monitor their vision, such as by Amsler grid testing and subjective measures of visual acuity, such as reading vision and image clarity. If there are no new symptoms, follow-up examination in 6–12 months.

DIET
- High in vitamins A, E, C, and β-carotene along with zinc may be of benefit
- Eating dark green, leafy vegetables (spinach or collard greens), which are rich in carotenoids, may decrease the risk of developing the neovascular/exudative stage.
- Fish consumption with omega-3 fatty acid intake reduces the risk of ARMD.

PATIENT EDUCATION
Instruct visually impaired patients to check with the local low-vision center for aids.

PROGNOSIS
- Patients with bilateral soft drusen and pigmentary changes in the macula but no evidence of exudation, have an increased likelihood of developing CNVMs and subsequent visual loss.
- Patients with bilateral drusen carry a cumulative risk of 14.7% over 5 years of suffering significant visual loss in 1 eye from the neovascular stage of ARMD.
- Patients with neovascular stage in 1 eye and drusen in the opposite eye are at an annual risk of 5–14% of developing the neovascular stage in the opposite eye with drusen.
- High incidence of recurrence after thermal laser treatment for CNVMs

COMPLICATIONS
Blindness

REFERENCES

1. Age Related Eye Disease Study Research Group. A randomized, placebo-controlled, clinical trial of high-dose supplementation with vitamins C and E, beta carotene, and zinc for age-related macular degeneration and vision loss: AREDS report no. 8. *Arch Ophthalmol*. 2001;119:1417–36.
2. Rosenfeld PJ, Brown DM, Heier JS, et al. Ranibizumab for neovascular age-related macular degeneration. *N Engl J Med*. 2006;355:1419–31.
3. Brown DM, Michels M, Kaiser PK, et al. Ranibizumab versus verteporfin photodynamic therapy for neovascular age-related macular degeneration: Two-year results of the ANCHOR study. *Ophthalmology*. 2009;116:57–65.e5.
4. Fung AE, Lalwani GA, Rosenfeld PJ, et al. An optical coherence tomography-guided, variable dosing regimen with intravitreal ranibizumab (Lucentis) for neovascular age-related macular degeneration. *Am J Ophthalmol*. 2007;143:566–83.
5. Fong DS, Custis P, Howes J, Hsu JW, et al. Intravitreal bevacizumab and ranibizumab for age-related macular degeneration a multicenter, retrospective study. *Ophthalmology*. 2010;117:298–302.
6. Nguyen QD, Shah SM, Browning DJ, et al. A phase I study of intravitreal vascular endothelial growth factor trap-eye in patients with neovascular age-related macular degeneration. *Ophthalmology*. 2009;116:2141–8.e1.
7. Stifter E, Michels S, Prager F, et al. Intravitreal bevacizumab therapy for neovascular age-related macular degeneration with large submacular hemorrhage. *Am J Ophthalmol*. 2007;144:886–92.

 ## CODES

ICD9
- 362.50 Macular degeneration (senile) of retina, unspecified
- 362.51 Nonexudative senile macular degeneration of retina
- 362.52 Exudative senile macular degeneration of retina

CLINICAL PEARLS

- Patients frequently notice distortion of central vision.
- Patients may notice straight lines appear crooked (e.g., telephone poles).
- Hyperopia is a risk factor for ARMD.
- AREDS found that a high-dose regimen of antioxidant vitamins and mineral supplements reduces progression of ARMD in some cases.

M

MALARIA
Paul Arguin, MD

BASICS

DESCRIPTION
- Acute or chronic infection transmitted to humans by *Anopheles* spp. mosquitoes
- Most morbidity and mortality are caused by *P. falciparum*; it is responsible for >1 million deaths annually, the majority of which occur in children <5 years in sub-Saharan Africa.
- Systems affected: Lymphatic; Immunologic; Vascular; Hematologic; Renal; Cerebral
- Nonimmune individuals are most susceptible to rapid progression to severe disease.

EPIDEMIOLOGY
Incidence
- Most US cases (>99%) are imported. Very rare cases reported from local transmission after introduction, transfusion transmission, and congenital transmission.
- 1,000–1,500 cases and 5 deaths per year in US
- Cases imported to the US: 40% *P. falciparum*, 16% *P. vivax*, 2% *P. malariae*, 2% *P. ovale*; 40% unknown

Prevalence
- Predominant age: All ages
- Predominant gender: Male = Female

RISK FACTORS
- Traveling and/or migration from an area where malaria is endemic (most from sub-Saharan Africa)
- Rarely, blood transfusion, mother-to-fetus transmission, and autochthonous transmission

Genetics
Unknown genetic predilection, but inherited conditions may affect disease severity and susceptibility (glucose-6-phosphate deficiency, sickle cell disease or trait, and hereditary elliptocytosis)

GENERAL PREVENTION
- Mosquito avoidance measures: Insect repellent, clothing that covers most of the body, mosquito nets treated with permethrin, air conditioning, and avoiding outdoor activity dusk to dawn (1)[A]
- Malarial chemoprophylaxis when in endemic area
- Mefloquine: Begin at least 2 weeks before arrival and continue for 4 weeks after leaving area. Adults, 250 mg (1 tablet) weekly; children ≤9 kg, 5 mg/kg; children >9–19 kg, 1/4 tablet weekly; children >19–30 kg, 1/2 tablet weekly; children >30–45 kg, 3/4 tablet weekly; children >45 kg as adult.
  - Caution: Mefloquine-resistant areas.
- Atovaquone/proguanil: Begin 1–2 days before arrival and continue for 1 week after leaving area. Adults, 1 adult tablet daily; children 5–8 kg, 1/2 pediatric tablet daily; children >8–10 kg, 3/4 pediatric tablet daily; children >10–20 kg, 1 pediatric tablet daily; children >20–30 kg, 2 pediatric tablets daily; children >30–40 kg, 3 pediatric tablets daily; children >40 kg, 1 adult tablet daily.
- Doxycycline: Begin 1–2 days before arrival and continue for 4 weeks after leaving area. Adults, 100 mg daily; children, 2 mg/kg up to 100 mg daily (not for children <8 years old).
- Chloroquine: Begin 1–2 weeks before arrival and continue for 4 weeks after leaving area. Adults, 300 mg base (500 mg salt) weekly; children, 5 mg base/kg weekly up to 300 mg.
  - Caution: Chloroquine-resistant areas.
- Primaquine: Begin 1–2 days before arrival and continue for 1 week after leaving area. Adults 30 mg daily. Children, 0.5 mg/kg daily up to adult dose.

PATHOPHYSIOLOGY
- Malarial parasites digest red cell proteins and make the RBC membrane less deformable, causing hemolysis, increased splenic clearance, and anemia.
- Red cell lysis stimulates release of cytokines and TNF-α.
- *P. falciparum* induces human RBCs to secrete a protein that makes RBCs stick to the intravascular surface of small blood vessels, causing obstruction and end-organ ischemia.

ETIOLOGY
P. falciparum, *P. malariae*, *P. vivax*, *P. ovale*, and *P. knowlesi* in parts of Southeast Asia

COMMONLY ASSOCIATED CONDITIONS
Bacterial co-infections

DIAGNOSIS

HISTORY
- 1st symptoms of malaria are nonspecific. Suspect in anyone ill returning from endemic area:
  - Fever, malaise, myalgias, chills, headache, nausea, splenomegaly (with chronic infection), hypotension, anemia (with chronic or severe disease), thrombocytopenia, jaundice, vomiting and diarrhea resembling gastroenteritis
- *P. falciparum*:
  - Incubation usually 12–14 days, symptoms within 2 months of infection in most individuals (partially immune individuals such as immigrants may become ill up to 1 year after last exposure)
  - Severe disease and complications: Vascular collapse, CNS impairment, renal failure, and acute respiratory distress syndrome
- *P. vivax* and *P. ovale*:
  - Incubation period 12–18 days for primary infection and up to 12 months (and longer) for relapses; generally presents with fevers
  - Dormant parasites may remain in liver and reactivate years after initial infection.
  - Can be severe
- *P. malariae* (benign quartan malaria):
  - Incubation period ~35 days
  - May become chronic; untreated can persist asymptomatically in human host for years
- *P. knowlesi*
  - Incubation period ~12 days
  - Possibly severe

PHYSICAL EXAM
- Often not specific
- General: Elevated temperature, fatigue, tachycardia, tachypnea
- Chronic: Pallor, splenomegaly (hyperactive malarial splenomegaly syndrome)

DIAGNOSTIC TESTS & INTERPRETATION
Lab
- Malarial smear thick and thin preparations:
  - Microscopy to evaluate for presence of parasite forms, determine species, and quantify the percentage of red blood cells that are infected (2)[A]
  - Test should be performed on site right away with results available within hours.
- Rapid antigen capture enzyme: Can detect the presence of malaria parasites within minutes. Cannot determine species or quantify parasitemia. Positive and negative results must always be confirmed by microscopy.
  - Other tests: Species-specific PCR (confirms species)
- General laboratory findings (nonspecific):
  - In uncomplicated infection:
    - Elevated liver function tests and lactate dehydrogenase
    - Thrombocytopenia, anemia, and leukopenia
- Note: A low to low-normal platelet count or a slightly high bilirubin is typical and should alert the clinician of the diagnosis after exposure in an endemic setting.
- Note: Antimalarial agents may reduce parasitemia.

Initial lab tests
- CBC with differential and platelets
- Basic chemistry panel including bilirubin
- Malaria thick and thin blood films (if negative, repeat every 12–24 hours for at least 3 sets)

Follow-Up & Special Considerations
Nonimmune individuals with suspected or confirmed *P. falciparum* should be hospitalized.

Imaging
Use only for respiratory disease (chest x-ray) or cerebral malaria (scan prior to spinal tap)

Pathological Findings
Malaria causes hemolysis.

DIFFERENTIAL DIAGNOSIS
- Infections (disseminated or localized): Abscess, viral, gastroenteritis, typhoid/paratyphoid, other bacteremias, rickettsial disease, mycobacteria
- Collagen vascular disease (SLE, vasculitides)
- Neoplasms (lymphoma, leukemia, other blood dyscrasias, other tropical causes of splenomegaly)
- Severe malaria infection may mimic hepatitis, pneumonia, stroke, or sepsis.

TREATMENT

MEDICATION
First Line
- For uncomplicated chloroquine-resistant *P. falciparum* (most *P. falciparum*), chloroquine-resistant *P. vivax*, or when species is unknown, the following regimens are equally recommended:
  - Atovaquone-proguanil (Malarone): Adult tablet: 250 mg atovaquone and 100 mg proguanil. Pediatric tablet: 62.5 mg atovaquone and 25 mg proguanil. Adults: 4 adult tablets once per day for 3 days. Children 5–8 kg: 2 pediatric tablets once per day for 3 days; children 9-10 kg: 3 pediatric tablets once per day for 3 days; children 1–20 kg: 1 adult tablet once per day for 3 days; children 21–30 kg: 2 adult tablets once per day for 3 days; children 31–40 kg: 3 adult tablets once per day for 3 days; children >40 kg: 4 adult tablets once per day for 3 days (1)[A].
  - Artemether-lumefantrine (Coartem): Tablet contains 20 mg artemether and 120 mg lumefantrine. Persons 5–<15 kg: 1 tablet b.i.d. for 3 days; persons 15–<25 kg: 2 tablets b.i.d. for 3 days; persons 25–<35 kg: 3 tablets b.i.d. for 3 days; persons ≥35 kg: 4 tablets b.i.d. for 3 days (1)[A].

– Quinine sulfate plus doxycycline or clindamycin: Adults: Quinine sulfate 650 mg (salt) t.i.d. for 3 days (should be extended to 7 days)
- Oral therapy for *P. ovale*, *P. malariae*, chloroquine-sensitive *P. falciparum* (rare), and chloroquine-sensitive *P. vivax* (New Guinea has highest rates of CQ resistant *P. vivax*).
  - Chloroquinephosphate: Adults: 600-mg base followed by 300 mg at 6, 24, and 48 hours. Children: 10 mg base/kg (maximum of 600 mg), then 5 mg/kg at 6, 24, and 48 hours.
  - Primaquinephosphate (should be added to chloroquine therapy for cure of dormant forms of *P. vivax* and *P. ovale*): Adults: 30-mg base (52.6 mg) daily for 2 weeks or 45-mg base (79 mg) weekly for 8 weeks. Children: 0.6-mg base/kg daily for 2 weeks (3)[A]. See Precautions.
- Therapy for severe *P. falciparum*:
  - Clinical features defining severe malaria:
    o Impaired level of consciousness (LOC)
    o Respiratory distress, jaundice
    o Repeated convulsions, shock
  - Laboratory features:
    o Hypoglycemia (glucose <40 mg/dL)
    o Elevated bilirubin (total >2.5 mg/dL)
    o Acidosis (plasma bicarbonate <15 mmol/L)
    o Lactic acidosis (serum lactate >45 mg/dL)
    o Elevated aminotransferase (>3 times)
    o Serum creatinine >3 mg/dL
- Parenteral therapy:
  - Quinidine gluconate 10 mg/kg in normal saline over 1–2 hours followed by 0.02 mg/kg/min continuous infusion, or repeat initial dose q8h until oral therapy can be started (1)[A].
  - When IV quinidine is not available, IV clindamycin (1)[C] and/or oral quinidine should be given until IV quinidine is obtained (1)[C] (may obtain from Eli Lilly company 1-800-545-5979).
  - Intensive care monitoring is necessary, especially when initiating quinidine therapy.
- In severe malaria, CDC should be contacted for assistance; CDC Malaria Branch: 770–488-7100; http://www.cdc.gov/Malaria/.
- In 2007, CDC made artesunate available in the US for severe malaria and in special circumstances under an investigational protocol. Contact CDC for assistance as noted above.
- Mild-to-moderate P. falciparum:
  - Quinine sulfate plus doxycline or clindamycin:
    o Adults: Quinine sulfate 650 mg salt t.i.d. for 3–7 days plus doxycyline 100 mg b.i.d. for 7 days or plus clindamycin 900 mg t.i.d. for 5 days.
    o Children: Quinine sulfate 10 mg salt/kg (maximum 650 mg salt) t.i.d. for 3–7 days plus doxycycline (not for <8 years old) 2 mg/kg b.i.d. for 7 days or plus clindamycin 20–40 mg/kg/d divided in 3 doses for 5 days (3)[A]
- Oral therapy for chloroquine-resistant P. vivax:
  - Atovaquone/Proguanil or quinine sulfate plus doxycycline: Dosages above. Should follow with primaquine for liver-dormant forms (3)[B].
  - Mefloquine:
    o Adults: 1250 mg once (usually divided as 750 mg, then 500 mg 8 hours later)
    o Children: 15 mg/kg, then 10 mg/kg 8 hours later (high GI adverse event profile) (1)[B]. Should follow with primaquine for liver-dormant forms.

ADDITIONAL TREATMENT
Issues for Referral
Infectious disease or tropical medicine expert for most cases

Additional Therapies
Exchange transfusions may be necessary in severe disease or with very high parasitemia; discuss with expert or CDC.

Pediatric Considerations
- Children are particularly susceptible to severe disease.
- All children, even infants, should receive chemoprophylaxis if traveling to an endemic area.
- Malaria commonly resembles acute gastroenteritis in children.
- Children with severe disease are particularly prone to hypoglycemia, and IV fluids with glucose should be used for maintenance and frequent blood glucose measurements taken.

Pregnancy Considerations
- Chloroquine is safe in low doses; FDA Category C.
- Mefloquine is considered safe during 2nd and 3rd trimesters; FDA Category C.
- Atovaquone/proguanil (Malarone) has not been studied in pregnant women; it has not been shown to cause birth defects or other problems in animal studies; FDA Category C.
- No primaquine (FDA class undetermined) or tetracyclines (FDA class D) in pregnancy.
- Quinine/quinidine (FDA class X/C, respectively) may be used during pregnancy or breastfeeding when benefit outweighs risk.

COMPLEMENTARY AND ALTERNATIVE MEDICINE
None. Many deaths have resulted from using unapproved alternatives to medications.

SURGERY/OTHER PROCEDURES
Rarely, splenectomy must be performed in patients with HSM and medically unresponsive hematologic disorders.

IN-PATIENT CONSIDERATIONS
Initial Stabilization
- Inpatient care for all cases of *P. falciparum* malaria in nonimmune patients or any patient, despite the species, with signs of severe illness; outpatient care for others (1)[C]
- Nonimmune with *P. falciparum* may progress from mild symptoms to death within 12 hours. All patients treated on outpatient basis should have follow-up within 24 hours.

Admission Criteria
- All nonimmune patients with confirmed or suspected *P. falciparum*
- All patients with signs of severe disease (see Treatment)

IV Fluids
Maintenance IV fluids with glucose, because of risk of hypoglycemia, is recommended if unable to tolerate fluids by mouth. Excess fluids may result in iatrogenically induced pulmonary edema.

Nursing
Observe for fluid excess, renal insufficiency (urine output), and hypoglycemia.

Discharge Criteria
Clinical improvement, ability to tolerate oral medications and fluids, with documented decreasing parasitemia levels

ONGOING CARE

PATIENT EDUCATION
- Malarial chemoprophylaxis prior to travel
- Travel information may be obtained at the CDC travel Web site: http://www.cdc.gov/travel

PROGNOSIS
- Only *P. falciparum* infection carries a poor prognosis, with high mortality if untreated. However, if diagnosed early and treated appropriately, the prognosis is excellent.
- *P. vivax* and other nonfalciparum may be severe, particularly with comorbidities.

COMPLICATIONS
- *P. falciparum*: If not treated early, may cause cerebral malaria, acute renal failure, acute gastroenteritis, pulmonary edema, and massive hemolysis. Chronic malaria: Splenomegaly or splenic rupture. Death from malaria is virtually limited to *P. falciparum* infection or infection with other species in a patient with other underlying illness.
- *P. malariae*: Nephrotic syndrome may develop in patients with chronic infection.
- Other complications: Seizures, anuria, delirium, coma, dysentery, algid malaria, blackwater fever, hyperpyrexia

REFERENCES

1. Centers for Disease Control and Prevention. Treatment of Malaria (Guidelines for clinicians). Accessed 6/3/10 at http://www.cdc.gov/malaria/pdf/treatmenttable.pdf.
2. Chen LH, Keystone JS. New strategies for the prevention of malaria in travelers. *Infect Dis Clin North Am.* 2005;19:185–210.
3. Griffith KS, Lewis LS, Mali S, et al. Treatment of malaria in the United States: a systematic review. *JAMA.* 2007;297:2264–77.

CODES

ICD9
- 084.0 Falciparum malaria (malignant tertian)
- 084.1 Vivax malaria (benign tertian)
- 084.2 Quartan malaria

CLINICAL PEARLS

- Rapid malaria tests are useful in the acute setting for determining if a patient has *P. falciparum* malaria (high negative predictive value). However, blood smears should also be performed on all suspected cases.
- Children with malaria frequently clinically appear to have gastroenteritis or nonspecific viral infections.
- Nonimmune persons with suspected or confirmed *P. falciparum* malaria are at high risk and must be managed aggressively (i.e., hospitalized).

M

MARFAN SYNDROME

Michele Roberts, MD, PhD

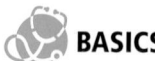

BASICS

DESCRIPTION
- Marfan syndrome (MFS) is an inherited disorder of connective tissue.
- System(s) affected: Musculoskeletal; Cardiovascular; Ocular; Pulmonary; Skin/Integument; Connective Tissue (Dura)
- Because many features of MFS appear in the general population, specific diagnostic criteria (Ghent nosology) were established, recognizing a constellation of features, with major and minor criteria for establishing the diagnosis (1).
- The nosology was revised (23) because the previous criteria were not sufficiently validated, were not consistently applicable in children, or necessitated expensive and specialized tests.

Pediatric Considerations
Early surgical intervention may reduce the degree of scoliosis.

Pregnancy Considerations
- Manage pregnancy in MFS as high-risk, preferably with a cardiologist. Pre-pregnancy evaluation should include a screening transthoracic echocardiogram for aortic root dilation.
- Beta-blockers should be considered in all pregnancies to minimize the risk of aortic dilation throughout the pregnancy.
- 1% complication rate if aortic root diameter <40 mm; 10% if >40 mm. Consider elective surgery before pregnancy if >47 mm.

EPIDEMIOLOGY
- Congenital. Although clinical manifestations may be apparent in infancy, affected individuals may not present until adolescence or young adulthood.
- No gender, ethnic, or racial predilection. With advanced paternal age, a slightly increased risk of de novo mutation resulting in MFS in offspring.

Prevalence
1/3,000–1/5,000

RISK FACTORS
Genetics
- Mutations of the fibrillin-1 (FBN1) gene on chromosome 15q21.1 are responsible for Marfan syndrome, OMIM #154700.
- MFS is an autosomal-dominant condition with complete penetrance and variable expressivity. Apparent nonpenetrance may be due to lack of recognition of MFS in a mildly affected individual.
- Each child of an affected parent has a 50% chance of inheriting the disorder, and may be more or less severely affected. 25% of cases result from de novo mutation.

GENERAL PREVENTION
- Prenatal diagnosis is possible in families with a known mutation.
- Antibiotic prophylaxis against endocarditis for dental and other procedures is no longer routinely recommended by the ADA/AHA.
- Athletes who are especially tall should be screened for aortic root dilation.

ETIOLOGY
Genetic abnormality; mutations of the FBN1 (fibrillin) gene. Fibrillin is an extracellular matrix protein widely distributed in elastic and nonelastic connective tissue.

COMMONLY ASSOCIATED CONDITIONS
- High prevalence of obstructive sleep apnea in MFS; may be a risk factor for aortic root dilatation (4).
- Increased prevalence of migraine in MFS.

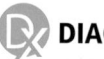

DIAGNOSIS

- In the revised Ghent nosology:
  - CV manifestations (aortic root aneurysm/dissection) and ectopia lentis have more weight.
  - Molecular genetic testing for FBN1 plays a more prominent diagnostic role but is not required.
  - Less-specific manifestations were removed or made less influential, thus avoiding obligate thresholds that were not evidence-based. Careful follow-up diminishes risk of missed diagnosis.
  - New criteria explicitly allow for alternative diagnoses, where additional features warrant: Shprintzen-Goldberg syndrome (SGS), Loeys-Dietz syndrome (LDS), or vascular type Ehlers-Danlos syndrome (vEDS).
  - Z-score calculator for aortic root enlargement: http://www.marfan.org
- In the absence of a family history of MFS:
  - Aortic root dilatation or dissection (Z≥2) (Ao) **and** ectopia lentis (EL): Unequivocal diagnosis of MFS, irrespective of systemic features, except were they are diagnostic of SGS, LDS, or vEDS
  - Ao **and** a *bona fide* FBN1 mutation: Diagnostic of MFS, even in the absence of EL
  - Where Ao is present, but EL is absent and the FBN1 status is negative (or unknown), diagnosis of MFS requires systemic findings score ≥7 points using a new scoring system (see below), and exclusion of SGS, LDS, and vEDS.
  - With EL but without Ao, FBN1 mutation previously associated with Ao is required for diagnosis of MFS.
- Systemic features, scoring system (see Physical Examination):
  - Wrist **and** thumb sign +3; wrist **or** thumb sign +1
  - Pectus carinatum deformity +2; pectus excavatum or chest asymmetry +1
  - Hindfoot deformity +2; pes planus +1
  - Pneumothorax +2
  - Dural ectasia +2
  - Protrusio acetabuli +2 by X-ray, CT, or MRI
  - Reduced Upper-to-Lower segment ratio (US/LS) **and** increased arm/height **and** no severe scoliosis +1
  - Scoliosis or thoracolumbar kyphosis +1
  - Reduced elbow extension +1
  - Facial features (3/5) +1
  - Skin striae +1
  - Myopia >3 diopters +1
  - Mitral valve prolapse (all types) +1
- Maximum: 20 points; score ≥7 indicates systemic involvement
- Positive family history requires a family member independently diagnosed using above criteria.
- With a positive family history, MFS can be diagnosed with ectopia lentis, **or** systemic score ≥7, **or** aortic root dilatation with Z ≥2 in persons >20 years old, **or** Z ≥3 in persons <20 years old.
- In persons <20 years old who have negative family history and suggestive findings, but who do not meet Ghent criteria, "non-specific connective tissue

disorder" is diagnosed, and close clinical follow-up is recommended.
- In the presence of a relevant FBN1 mutation, "potential MFS" is diagnosed, and close follow-up recommended.
- In adults who have suggestive findings but who do not meet Ghent criteria, consider alternative diagnoses: Ectopia lentis syndrome (ELS), mitral valve prolapse syndrome (MVPS), **MASS** phenotype.

PHYSICAL EXAM
- Facial features: Dolichocephaly, enophthalmos, downslanting palpebral fissures, malar hypoplasia, retrognathia
- Thumb sign: Distal phalanx of thumb protrudes from clenched fist. Wrist sign: Thumb and 5th digit overlap when circling wrist.
- Pectus carinatum deformity: Pectus excavatum or chest asymmetry beyond normal variation
- Hindfoot valgus with forefoot abduction and lowering of the midfoot; should be distinguished from pes planus
- Reduced US/LS: 0.93 in unaffected individuals vs ≤0.85 in affected white adults, ≤0.78 in affected black adults. US is measured from the top of the head to the top of the mid pubic bone; LS is measured from the top of the pubic bone to the sole of the foot. In children, abnormal US/LS: US/LS <1, age 0–5 years; US/LS <0.95, 6-7 years; US/LS <0.9, 8–9 years; <0.85, age ≥ 10 years.
- Increased arm span to height ratio >1.05
- Scoliosis or thoracolumbar kyphosis diagnosed if upon bending forward, there is a vertical difference ≥1.5 cm between the ribs of the left and right hemithorax.
- Reduced elbow extension if angle between upper and lower arm measures ≤170 upon full extension.
- Skin: Striae atrophicae are significant if not associated with significant weight changes (or pregnancy) and if located on mid-back, lumbar region, upper arm, axilla, or thigh.
- Because of lack of specificity, the following criteria were removed from the current nosology: Joint hypermobility, high arched palate, and recurrent or incisional herniae (2).

DIAGNOSTIC TESTS & INTERPRETATION
Lab
- Other than FBN1 mutation, no specific laboratory abnormalities are associated with MFS.
- Specific criteria have been established (2) for FBN1 mutations causative of MFS, including those found in families with MFS. FBN1 mutation is a valuable marker for risk or aortic dissection (5). In a small subset of patients with unequivocal MFS, no known FBN1 mutation is found.
- In patients whose physical examination is suggestive of MFS, urinary homocystine should be measured to rule out homocystinuria, an inborn error of methionine metabolism.

Imaging
- Anteroposterior (AP) radiograph: Diagnosis of protrusio acetabuli. Results from deepening of hip sockets during growth; does not cause problems during childhood
- Scoliosis: Cobb's angle ≥20 on radiographs. Imaging for MFS diagnosis, or as per clinical exam.
- Hindfoot valgus with forefoot abduction and lowering of the midfoot: Anterior and posterior views if clinically indicated

- Echocardiography: Measure aortic root at the level of sinuses of Valsalva; check for mitral valve prolapse.
- MRI or CT to evaluate for dural ectasia for diagnosis, and if symptomatic. Symptoms highly variable, nonspecific, and include lower back pain.

Diagnostic Procedures/Surgery
- Ectopia lentis is diagnosed on slit lamp examination after maximal dilatation of the pupil. Lens dislocation is most often upward and temporal.
- Myopia: Common in the general population; myopia >3 diopters contributes to MFS systemic score.

Pathological Findings
- Cystic medial necrosis of the aorta
- Myxomatous degeneration of cardiac valves

DIFFERENTIAL DIAGNOSIS
Several conditions present clinical manifestations overlapping with MFS in cardiovascular, ocular, and skeletal systems.

- Ectopia lentis syndrome—no aortic root dilatation
- Mitral valve prolapse syndrome—MVP, limited systemic features may include pectus excavatum, scoliosis, mild arachnodactyly; aortic enlargement and ectopia lentis preclude this diagnosis.
- MASS phenotype—(**M**itral valve prolapse; myopia; borderline, nonprogressive **A**ortic enlargement (Z <2); and nonspecific **S**keletal and **S**kin involvement). Aortic involvement in MASS is usually nonprogressive; some risk for more severe vascular involvement.
- Shprintzen-Goldberg syndrome; Loeys-Dietz syndrome; Ehlers-Danlos syndrome
- Homocystinuria—Marfanoid habitus, thrombosis, mental retardation; urine amino acid analysis is diagnostic; lens dislocates downward.
- Familial thoracic aortic aneurysm
- Stickler syndrome; congenital contractural arachnodactyly; Weill-Marchsesani syndrome; multiple endocrine neoplasia, type 2B

 TREATMENT

MEDICATION
- Prevention of aortic complications: Labetalol or other β-adrenergic blockers. Dosage adjusted to target heart rate (resting rate 60 beats/min, increase to ≤110 beats/min after moderate exertion; or <100 beats/min after submaximal exercise) (2)[C].
- Other agents used if β-blockers contraindicated. Calcium channel blockers, angiotensin-converting enzyme inhibitors, and angiotensin receptor blockers also retard aortic dilation in children and adolescents (6)[B].

ADDITIONAL TREATMENT
Issues for Referral
Genetics, Cardiology, Orthopedics, Ophthalmology

SURGERY/OTHER PROCEDURES
- When cardiac symptoms develop or aortic root diameter is ≥5.0 cm, consider surgical intervention. Many MFS patients will ultimately require reconstructive cardiovascular surgery.
  – Dissection of ascending aorta (type A) is a surgical emergency. Consider prophylactic surgery when diameter of sinus of Valsalva approaches 5.0 cm (2). Other considerations include family history, rate of change, other cardiac pathology, pregnancy.
  – Dissection of descending thoracic aorta (type B) surgical indications include intractable pain, limb

or organ ischemia, aortic diameter >5.5 cm (or rapidly increasing) (2).
- Mitral valve repair: For severe mitral valve regurgitation or progressive LV dilatation or dysfunction, or in patients undergoing valve-sparing root replacement (2).
- Lens subluxation: Incidence of glaucoma is high, so surgery is performed only if the condition cannot be treated with corrective lenses. Surgical removal of lens in lens opacity, impending complete luxation, lens-induced glaucoma or uveitis, or anisometropia or refractive error not amenable to optical correction (2).
- Severe pectus excavatum may require surgery.
- Scoliosis: Bracing for curves 20–40 until growth is complete, or surgery if >40.
- Surgery only for most severe cases of dural ectasia.
- Hip replacement in middle age or later if protrusio acetabulae has led to severe arthritic change.

 ONGOING CARE

FOLLOW-UP RECOMMENDATIONS
- Avoid sports that can increase aortic root enlargement or pneumothorax, including weightlifting and acceleration/deceleration sports. Low-risk sports include bowling, golf, skating (but not ice hockey), snorkeling, brisk walking, treadmill walking or stationary biking, modest hiking (7)[C].
- Exercise restrictions based on individual circumstances (7). Recommendation from the National Marfan Foundation (http://www.marfan.org) and guidelines from the American Heart Association/American College of Cardiology task forces. In general, avoid contact sports, Valsalva, and exhaustion.

Patient Monitoring
Frequent examinations (at least twice per year) while patient is still growing, with particular attention to cardiovascular system and to scoliosis.

- Yearly echocardiograms (initially), more frequent if aortic diameter is increasing rapidly (≥5 cm/year) or is approaching the surgical threshold (≥4.5 cm in adults).
- Aortic root dilatation in MFS is usually progressive, warrants vigilance even when not seen on initial examination. Age <20, yearly echocardiogram. Adults with repeatedly normal aortic root measurements, echocardiogram every 2–3 years (2).
- Regular imaging after surgical repair of aorta.
- Scoliosis or pectus deformity: standard orthopedic management. Clinical evaluation for scoliosis earlier than in general population. Plain radiographs of spine during growth years to detect and measure scoliosis.
- Annual ophthalmologic evaluation for detection of ectopia lentis, myopia, cataract, glaucoma, and retinal detachment. Myopia is very common in MFS and may have early onset, rapid progression, and high degree of severity. Early monitoring, aggressive refraction to prevent amblyopia (2).

PATIENT EDUCATION
- National Marfan Foundation, 382 Main St., Port Washington, NY 11959; 800-8MARFAN, www.marfan.org
- American Heart Association at www.americanheart.org

PROGNOSIS
Life-threatening complications involve cardiovascular dysfunction. In 1972, life span was 32 years. Currently, life span is nearly normal.

COMPLICATIONS
Bacterial endocarditis, aortic dissection, aortic or mitral valve insufficiency, dilated cardiomyopathy, retinal detachment, glaucoma, pneumothorax.

REFERENCES
1. De Paepe A, Devereux RB, Dietz HC, et al. Revised diagnostic criteria for the Marfan syndrome. *Am J Med Genet*. 1996;62:417–26.
2. Loeys BL, Dietz HC, Braverman AC, et al. The revised Ghent nosology for the Marfan syndrome. *J Med Genet*. 2010;47:476–85.
3. Faivre L, Collod-Beroud G, Callewaert B, et al. Pathogenic FBN1 mutations in 146 adults not meeting clinical diagnostic criteria for Marfan syndrome: further delineation of type 1 fibrillinopathies and focus on patients with an isolated major criterion. *Am J Med Genet A*. 2009;149A:854–60.
4. Kohler M, Blair E, Risby P, et al. The prevalence of obstructive sleep apnoea and its association with aortic dilatation in Marfan's syndrome. *Thorax*. 2008.
5. Faivre L, Collod-Beroud G, Child A, et al. Contribution of molecular analyses in diagnosing Marfan syndrome and type I fibrillinopathies: an international study of 1009 probands. *J Med Genet*. 2008;45:384–90.
6. Williams A, Davies S, Stuart AG, et al. Medical treatment of Marfan syndrome: a time for change. *Heart*. 2008;94:414–21.
7. Maron BJ, Chaitman BR, Ackerman MJ, et al. Recommendations for physical activity and recreational sports participation for young patients with genetic cardiovascular diseases. *Circulation*. 2004;109:2807–16.

 CODES

ICD9
759.82 Marfan syndrome

CLINICAL PEARLS
- Because many features of MFS appear in the general population, diagnostic criteria have been established. Molecular diagnostic testing for *FBN1* mutations will play an increasing role.
- Not all individuals with MFS are tall.
- Early diagnosis of homocystinuria is important because clinical complications, which include a high risk of vascular thrombosis, can be minimized with appropriate diet and medication.

M

MASTALGIA

Eduardo Lara-Torre, MD
Amanda Murchison, MD
Patrice Weiss, MD

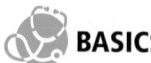 **BASICS**

DESCRIPTION
- Painful breast tissue, often bilateral, that can be cyclic or noncyclic
  - 2/3 of breast pain is cyclic and is usually associated with hormonal changes related to menses, external hormones, pregnancy, or menopause.
  - 1/3 is noncyclic and often is related to a breast or chest wall lesion.
- Synonym(s): Mastodynia; Breast pain

EPIDEMIOLOGY
Incidence
- Predominant sex: Most common in women but occurs occasionally in men
- Predominant age: Generally seen from adolescence through menopause
- Frequency of breast cancer with those reporting breast pain ranges from 1.2–6.7% (1)[B].
- Up to 70% of women report some degree of breast pain at some point in their lives (2)[B].
- Most describe mild pain, but 11% describe pain as moderate to severe.

RISK FACTORS
- Diet high in saturated fats
- Cigarette smoking
- Recent weight gain
- Pregnancy
- Large, pendulous breasts (caused by stretching of Cooper ligament)
- Exogenous hormones
- Caffeine has *not* been shown to be a risk factor (3)[B].

Genetics
Familial tendency

GENERAL PREVENTION
- Avoid exposure to risk factors.
- Properly fitted bra support

PATHOPHYSIOLOGY
- Causative pathophysiology remains unclear but is thought to be related to hormonal and/or nutritional factors.
- When fibrocystic disease is the source, growth and distension of the cyst with hormonal fluctuation cause pain.
- Hormonal factors (e.g., hormone-replacement therapy, oral contraceptives, pregnancy, menses, puberty, and menopause) may influence the diverse conditions that cause mastalgia or may themselves cause breast tenderness and pain.

ETIOLOGY
- Benign breast disorders (e.g., fibrocystic changes)
- Trauma (including sexual abuse/assault)
- Diet and lifestyle
- Lactation problems (e.g., engorgement, mastitis, breast abscess)
- Breast masses, including breast cancer
- Hidradenitis suppurativa
- Costochondritis (Tietze syndrome)
- Postthoracotomy syndrome
- Spinal and paraspinal disorders
- Potential side effects of medications
- Postradiation effects
- Referred pain (e.g., pulmonary, cardiac, or gallbladder disease)
- Ductal ectasia

 DIAGNOSIS

HISTORY
- Location, duration, frequency, severity, associated symptoms, related activities (e.g., trauma), and aggravating and ameliorating factors
- Complete medical history with focus on gynecologic/obstetric history
- Complete systematic review of systems
- Diet/smoking history
- Detailed family history for risk assessment for breast cancer

PHYSICAL EXAM
- Examine breasts systematically in both standing and sitting positions.
- Assess for skin changes, breast symmetry and contour, dimpling, localized tenderness, bruising, masses, nipple discharge, and lymphadenopathy. Look for signs suggestive of breast malignancy.

DIAGNOSTIC TESTS & INTERPRETATION
Lab
Initial lab tests
- If galactorrhea is found, check a fasting prolactin level.
- Possibly thyroid-stimulating hormone

Imaging
- Consider ultrasound in women with focal, persistent breast pain.
- Mammogram ± ultrasound in women aged 30–35 years of age or older

Pediatric Considerations
- Ultrasound is the imaging test of choice for children and adolescents. Mammogram is not useful.

Diagnostic Procedures/Surgery
- Cysts may need to be aspirated to relieve symptoms and/or verify diagnosis.
- Biopsies may be indicated based on results of examination, ultrasound, or mammography.

Pediatric Considerations
- In children and adolescents, do not perform biopsies unless suspicion for cancer. Refer to specialist in pediatric breast disease.

Pathological Findings
- Normal breast tissue
- Benign: Fibrocystic changes, duct ectasia, solitary papillomas, simple fibroadenomas
- Small increased risk of breast cancer: Ductal hyperplasia without atypia, sclerosing adenosis, diffuse papillomatosis, complex fibroadenomas
- Moderate increased risk: Atypical ductal hyperplasia, atypical lobular hyperplasia
- Breast cancer

DIFFERENTIAL DIAGNOSIS
- The major alternate disease to consider is breast cancer, particularly if pain is localized.
- Manipulation or trauma also can worsen symptoms.
- Chest wall pain or referred pain resulting from splenomegaly also must be differentiated from mastalgia.
- Sometimes cyclic pain is concurrent with premenstrual syndrome.
- Ductal ectasia of the breast

 TREATMENT

MEDICATION
First Line
Acetaminophen, nonsteroidal anti-inflammatory drugs (NSAIDs) (4)[B]

Second Line
- Oral contraceptives may help some patients prevent fibrocystic disease but may worsen pain in some sensitive patients (5)[A].
- If patient is on an oral contraceptive, switch to one that has a lower estrogen component.
- In some patients with mastalgia only during their menses, menstrual suppression with continuous oral contraceptives may be of benefit.
- Oral progesterone 10 mg PO daily

- Other possibilities for patients with refractory symptoms, used infrequently because of potential side effects, include
  - Danazol 100 mg b.i.d. (possibly lower doses) may be the most effective; major adverse effects include menstrual irregularities, weight gain, acne, hirsutism, and voice change; *may be used during luteal phase only;* approved by the Food and Drug Administration (FDA) for this indication
  - Toremifene 30 mg PO daily (6)[A]
  - Bromocriptine 5 mg PO daily and cabergoline 0.5 mg PO weekly both during the 2nd half of the menstrual cycle are equally effective, but cabergoline has fewer side effects (7)[A].

ADDITIONAL TREATMENT
If the patient is breast-feeding, correct any breast-feeding difficulties; treat underlying mastitis or breast abscess.

General Measures
- Stop or modify current hormonal therapy.
- Repeat examination may help to establish any cyclic nodularity pattern.
- Wear properly fitted support bra (may be fitted by a professional).
- Reassurance (sufficient for most patients)
- Weight loss for obese patients
- Smoking cessation
- Relaxation training

Pediatric Considerations
Children and adolescents may require referral to a specialist.

COMPLEMENTARY AND ALTERNATIVE MEDICINE
- Vitamin E and evening primrose oil have not been found to be of benefit for chronic mastalgia (1,8)[B].
- Flax seed oil is not effective for the treatment of mastalgia (9)[C].

SURGERY/OTHER PROCEDURES
Some patients may need surgical breast reduction.

 ONGOING CARE

FOLLOW-UP RECOMMENDATIONS
As needed

Patient Monitoring
- As needed for patients not receiving pharmacotherapy
- Time of follow-up will vary by type of pharmacotherapy and patient's particular problems.

DIET
- Decrease fat intake to 20% of total calories.
- There is no strong evidence that reduction in caffeine intake may help to decrease the severity or incidence of the disease (10)[C].

PATIENT EDUCATION
Avoid or adjust of risk factors.

PROGNOSIS
- Premenstrual mastalgia increases with age and then generally stops at menopause unless patient is receiving hormone therapy (HT).
- Most patients can control symptoms without receiving HT.
- Several months of HT may provide several more months of relief, but mastalgia may recur.
- Cyclic mastalgia responds better than noncyclic mastalgia to treatment.
- Effects of long-term HT are unknown.

REFERENCES

1. Smith RL, et al. Evaluation and management of breast pain. *Mayo Clinic Proc.* 2004;79:353.
2. Ader DN, Shriver CD. Cyclical mastalgia: prevalence and impact in an outpatient breast clinic sample. *J Am Coll Surg.* 1997;185:466–70.
3. Levinson W, Dunn PM. Nonassociation of caffeine and fibrocystic breast disease. *Arch Intern Med.* 1986;146:1773–5.
4. Colak T, Ipek T, Kanik A, et al. Efficacy of topical nonsteroidal antiinflammatory drugs in mastalgia treatment. *J Am Coll Surg.* 2003;196:525–30.
5. Machado RB, de Melo NR, Maia H et al. Bleeding patterns and menstrual-related symptoms with the continuous use of a contraceptive combination of ethinylestradiol and drospirenone: a randomized study. *Contraception.* 2010;81:215–22.
6. Gong C, Song E, Jia W, et al. A double-blind randomized controlled trial of toremifene therapy for mastalgia. *Arch Surg.* 2006;141:43–7.
7. Aydin Y, Atis A, Kaleli S, et al. Cabergoline versus bromocriptine for symptomatic treatment of premenstrual mastalgia: A randomised, open-label study. *European journal of obstetrics, gynecology, and reproductive biology.* 2010;
8. Pruthi S, Wahner-Roedler DL, Torkelson CJ, et al. Vitamin E and evening primrose oil for management of cyclical mastalgia: a randomized pilot study. *Altern Med Rev.* 2010;15:59–67.
9. Basch E, Bent S, Collins J, et al. Flax and Flaxseed Oil (Linum usitatissimum): A Review by the Natural Standard Research Collaboration. *J Soc Integr Oncol.* 2007;5:92–105.
10. Gumm R, Cunnick GH, Mokbel K. Evidence for the management of mastalgia. *Curr Med Res Opin.* 2004;20:681–4.

ADDITIONAL READING

- Blommers J, de Lange-De Klerk ES, Kuik DJ, et al. Evening primrose oil and fish oil for severe chronic mastalgia: a randomized, double-blind, controlled trial. *Am J Obstet Gynecol.* 2002;187:1389–94.
- Brennan M, Houssami N, French J. Management of benign breast conditions. Part 1–Painful breasts. *Aust Fam Physician.* 2005;34:143–4.
- Campagnoli C, Ambroggio S, Lotano MR, Peris C et al. Progestogen use in women approaching the menopause and breast cancer risk. *Maturitas.* 2009;62:338–42.
- McFadyen IJ, Chetty U, Setchell KD, et al. A randomized double blind-cross over trial of soya protein for the treatment of cyclical breast pain. *Breast.* 2000;9:271–6.
- Miltenburg DM, Speights VO et al. Benign breast disease. *Obstet Gynecol Clin North Am.* 2008;35:285–300, ix
- Olawaiye A, Withiam-Leitch M, Danakas G, et al. Mastalgia: a review of management. *J Reprod Med.* 2005;50:933–9.
- Qureshi S, Sultan N. Topical nonsteroidal anti-inflammatory drugs versus oil of evening primrose in the treatment of mastalgia. *Surgeon.* 2005;3:7–10.

See Also (Topic, Algorithm, Electronic Media Element)
Premenstrual Syndrome (PMS); Premenstrual Dysphoric Disorder
Algorithms: Breast Discharge; Breast Pain

 CODES

ICD9
611.71 Mastodynia

CLINICAL PEARLS

- When evaluating a patient with breast pain, always rule out cancer first.
- In the adolescent population, do not biopsy; instead, refer to a pediatric specialist.
- Premenstrual mastalgia increases with age and then generally stops at menopause unless patient is receiving HT.

M

MASTITIS

Montiel T. Rosenthal, MD

 BASICS

DESCRIPTION
- Inflammation of the breast parenchyma, and possibly associated tissues (areola, nipple, subcutaneous fat) usually associated with bacterial infection (and milk stasis in the postpartum mother)
- Usually an acute condition, but can become chronic cystic mastitis

EPIDEMIOLOGY
- Predominantly affects females
- Mostly in the puerperium
- Neonatal form
- Post-traumatic:
  - Ornamental nipple piercing increases risk of transmission of bacteria to deeper breast structures:
    ○ *Staph. aureus* predominant organism
    ○ Epidemic form rare in the age of reduced hospital stays for moms and newborns

Incidence
- 2.5% of breast-feeding mothers develop nonepidemic mastitis.
- Greatest incidence among breastfeeding moms 2–3 weeks postpartum
- Neonatal form:
  - 1–5 weeks of age with equal gender risk and unilateral presentation
- Pediatric form:
  - Around or after puberty
  - 82% of cases in girls

RISK FACTORS
- Milk stasis:
  - Inadequate emptying of breast
    ○ Scarring of breast due to prior mastitis
    ○ Scarring due to previous breast surgery
  - Breast engorgement:
    ○ Interruption of breast-feeding
- Ornamental nipple piercing increases risk of transmission of bacteria to deeper breast structures:
  - *Staph. aureus* predominant organism
- Neonatal colonization with epidemic *Staph.*
- Breastfeeding
- Neonatal:
  - Bottle-fed babies
  - Manual expression of "Witch's Milk"
  - Can predispose to lethal necrotizing fasciitis
- Maternal diabetes
- Maternal HIV
- Maternal vitamin A deficiency

GENERAL PREVENTION
Regular emptying of both breasts and nipple care to prevent fissures when breast-feeding

PATHOPHYSIOLOGY
- Micro abscesses along milk ducts and surrounding tissues
- Inflammatory cell infiltration of breast parenchyma and surrounding tissues
- Nonpuerperal (infectious):
  - *Staph. aureus*, *Bacteroides* sp., *Peptostreptococcus*, Staph. (coagulase neg.), *Enterococcus faecalis*
  - *Histoplasma capsulatum*
- Puerperal (infectious):
  - *Staph. aureus*, *Streptococcus pyogenes* (Group A or B), *Corynebacterium* sp., *Bacteroides* sp., *Staph.* (coagulase neg.), *E. coli*, *Salmonella* sp.
  - MRSA (1)[C]
- Rare secondary site for tuberculosis in endemic areas (1% of mastitis cases in these areas):
  - Single breast nodule with mastalgia
- *Corynebacterium* sp. associated with greater risk for development of chronic cystic mastitis
- Granulomatous mastitis:
  - Idiopathic

ETIOLOGY
- Puerperal:
  - Retrograde migration of surface bacteria up milk ducts
  - Bacterial migration from nipple fissures up breast lymphatics
  - Secondary monilial infection in the face of recurrent mastitis and/or diabetes (2)
  - Seeding from mother to neonate in cyclical fashion
- Nonpuerperal:
  - Ductal ectasia
  - Breast carcinoma
  - Inflammatory cysts
  - Chronic recurring subcutaneous or subareolar infections
  - Parasitic infections: Echinococcus; Filariasis; Guinea worm in endemic areas
  - Herpes simplex (3)[C]
  - Cat scratch disease
- Lupus

COMMONLY ASSOCIATED CONDITIONS
Breast abscess

DIAGNOSIS
- Fever and malaise
- Nausea ± vomiting
- Localized breast tenderness, heat, and redness
- Possible breast mass

HISTORY
- Breast tenderness
- "Hot cords burning in chest wall"

PHYSICAL EXAM
- Localized breast induration, redness, and warmth
- *Peau d'orange* appearance to overlying skin

DIAGNOSTIC TESTS & INTERPRETATION
Mom can check if she produces salty milk from affected side (higher Na and Cl concentrations) as compared with unaffected side.

Lab
Rarely needed except for patients ill enough to be hospitalized:
- CBC
- Blood culture
- In epidemic puerperal mastitis
  - Milk leukocyte count
  - Milk culture
  - Neonatal nasal culture

Imaging
- No imaging required for postpartum mastitis in a breast-feeding mother that responds to antibiotic therapy
- Mammography for women with nonpuerperal mastitis
- Breast ultrasound to rule out abscess formation in women:
  - Special consideration for this in women with breast implants who have mastitis

Diagnostic Procedures/Surgery
Options if further progression to abscess formation:
- Needle aspiration
- I and D
- Excisional biopsy

DIFFERENTIAL DIAGNOSIS
- Abscess
- Tumor
- Ductal cyst
- Consider monilial infection in lactating mom, especially if mastitis is recurrent.

TREATMENT

A recent Cochrane Review found that there is insufficient evidence to confirm or refute the effectiveness of antibiotic therapy for the treatment of lactational mastitis (4)[A].

MEDICATION

- Prioritized on the basis of likelihood of MRSA as etiologic factor and clinical severity of condition
- Treat for 10–14 days (5)[B]
- Prednisone for granulomatous mastitis (6)[C]

First Line
- Outpatient:
  – Dicloxacillin 500 mg q.i.d.
  – Cephalexin 500 mg q.i.d.
  – TMP/SMX; DS b.i.d. (MRSA possible)
- Inpatient:
  – Nafcillin 2 G q4hr
  – Oxacillin 2 G q4hr
  – Vancomycin 1 G q12hr (MRSA possible)
- Breast-feeding beyond 1 month:
  – PCN, ampicillin, or erythromycin

Pediatric Considerations
- TMP/SMZ given to breast-feeding mothers with mastitis can potentiate jaundice for neonates.
- Clindamycin IM, IV, or p.o. with dosing based on age and weight

Second Line
- If mastitis is odoriferous and localized under areola, add Metronidazole 500 mg t.i.d. IV or p.o.
- Topical, oral, and neonatal nystatin if yeast is suspected in recurrent mastitis

ADDITIONAL TREATMENT

Issues for Referral
- Abscess formation
- Need for breast biopsy

Additional Therapies
- Warm packs (or ice packs) to affected breast for comfort
- The use of a breast pump may aid in breast emptying, especially if the infant is unable to assist in doing this.
- Wear supporting bra that is not too tight

IN-PATIENT CONSIDERATIONS

If a new mother is admitted to the hospital for treatment of her mastitis, rooming-in of the infant with the mother is mandatory so that breast-feeding can continue. In some hospitals, rooming-in may require hospital admission of the infant (7).

Initial Stabilization
- Oral antibiotics
- Frequent emptying of breasts if breast-feeding
- Analgesics for pain:
  – Acetaminophen
- NSAIDs

Admission Criteria
- Failure of outpatient/oral therapy
  – Patient unable to tolerate oral therapy
  – Patient noncompliant with oral therapy
  – Severe illness without adequate supportive care at home
- Neonatal mastitis

Nursing
- Breast-feeding/pumping of breasts encouraged
- Start infant with feedings on affected side
- Abscess drainage is not a contraindication for breast-feeding.

Discharge Criteria
- Afebrile
- Tolerating oral antibiotics well

ONGOING CARE

FOLLOW-UP RECOMMENDATIONS
Bed rest for lactating moms, up to bathroom

DIET
- Encourage oral fluids
- Multivitamin including vitamin A

PATIENT EDUCATION
- Encourage oral fluids
- Rest essential
- Regular emptying of both breasts with breast-feeding
- Nipple care to prevent fissures

PROGNOSIS
- Puerperal:
  – Good with prompt (within 24 hours of symptom onset) antibiotic treatment and breast emptying; 96% success rate
  – 11% risk of abscess if left untreated with antibiotics
  – Antibodies develop in breast glands within 1st few days of infection, which may provide protection against infection or reinfection.
- Rare risk of abscess formation beyond 6 weeks postpartum if no recurrent mastitis

COMPLICATIONS
- Breast abscess
- Recurrent mastitis with resumption of breast-feeding or with breast-feeding after next pregnancy
- Bacteremia
- Sepsis

REFERENCES

1. Gastelum DT, Dassey D, Mascola L, et al. Transmission of community-associated methicillin-resistant Staphylococcus aureus from breast milk in the neonatal intensive care unit. *Pediatr Infect Dis J*. 2005;24:1122–4.
2. Lawrence R. *Breastfeeding: a guide for the medical profession*; Mosby-Yearbook; 2005;265.
3. Soo MS, Ghate S. Herpes simplex virus mastitis: clinical and imaging findings. *AJR Am J Roentgenol*. 2000;174:1087–8.
4. Jahanfar S, Ng CJ, Teng CL et al. Antibiotics for mastitis in breastfeeding women. *Cochrane Database Syst Rev*. 2009;CD005458.
5. Gilbert DN, Moellering RC, et al. *The Sanford Guide to Antimicrobial Therapy 2010*. Fourtieth Edition.
6. Kuba S, et al. Vacuum assisted biopsy and steroid treatment for granulomatous lobular mastitis. *Surg Today*. 2009;39:695–699.
7. Academy of Breastfeeding Medicine Protocol Committee. ABM clinical protocol #4: mastitis. Revision, May 2008. *Breastfeed Med*. 2008;3: 177–80.

ADDITIONAL READING

Spencer JP et al. Management of mastitis in breastfeeding women. *Am Fam Physician*. 2008;78:727–31.

See Also (Topic, Algorithm, Electronic Media Element)
Algorithms: Breast Discharge; Breast Pain

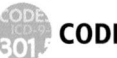

CODES

ICD9
- Puerperal:
  – 675.24 Postpartum nonpurulent mastitis
  – 675.94 Unspecified postpartum infection of the breast and nipple
- Non-Puerperal:
  – 611.0 Inflammatory disease of breast

CLINICAL PEARLS

- The 1st-line treatment for puerperal mastitis is Dicloxacillin 500 mg po. q.i.d. × 10–14 days. Most mastitis can be treated with oral therapy.
- Complete emptying of the breasts on a regular schedule, avoiding constrictive clothing or bras that might obstruct breast ducts, meticulous attention to nipple care, and "adequate rest" and a liberal intake of oral fluids for the mother can all reduce the risk of a breast-feeding mother's developing mastitis.
- Among breast-feeding mothers, if the symptoms of mastitis fail to resolve within several days of appropriate management including antibiotics, further investigations may be required to confirm resistant bacteria, abscess formation, an underlying mass, or inflammatory or ductal carcinoma.
- More than 2 recurrences of mastitis in the same location warrant evaluation with ultrasound and/or mammography to rule out an underlying mass.

M

MASTOIDITIS

Heather Mackey-Fowler, MD

 BASICS

Mastoiditis is an infection of the mastoid bone, usually following AOM.

DESCRIPTION
- Inflammatory process in the mastoid air cells
- Acute mastoiditis: Sudden-onset suppurative inflammatory process, typically after acute otitis media. It is the most common complication of acute otitis media.
- Chronic mastoiditis: Usually associated with cholesteatoma and chronic ear disease
- Masked mastoiditis: Indolent process with minimal signs and symptoms
- System(s) affected: Pulmonary; Auditory

EPIDEMIOLOGY
Incidence
1–4 cases per 100,000 person year
Prevalence
Unknown

RISK FACTORS
- Cholesteatoma
- Recurrent acute otitis media
- Immunocompromised patient
- Native American descent

Genetics
No known genetic pattern

GENERAL PREVENTION
- Adequate antibiotic treatment for acute otitis media
- Early referral to ENT for chronic otitis media
- Treatment of chronic eustachian tube dysfunction (i.e., pressure equalization tubes)
- Early identification of cholesteatoma

PATHOPHYSIOLOGY
- Blockage of outflow tract of mastoid air cells (i.e., aperture of mastoid antrum)
- Causes mastoid to fill with edematous mucosa and pus under pressure

ETIOLOGY
- Acute otitis media
- Inadequately treated suppurative otitis media
- Cholesteatoma
- *Streptococcus pneumoniae*, group A β-*Streptococcus*, *Staphylococcus aureus*, *Streptococcus pyogenes*, *M. catarrhalis*, *Haemophilus influenzae* most common pathogens
- *Pseudomonas aeruginosa* is becoming a more frequent pathogen.

 DIAGNOSIS

HISTORY
- Otalgia/possible otorrhea
- Hearing loss
- Headache
- Pain/redness/swelling noted over mastoid
- Fever

PHYSICAL EXAM
- Bulging erythematous tympanic membrane
- Postauricular or supra-auricular edema, erythema, or tenderness
- Protrusion of auricle
- Fever
- Possible otorrhea if tympanic membrane is perforated
- Subperiosteal abscess
- Tympanic membrane can be normal in 10% of patients: Suspicious for mastoiditis when symptoms of acute otitis media persist >2 weeks

DIAGNOSTIC TESTS & INTERPRETATION
Lab
Initial lab tests
- CBC with differential: Increased leukocyte count
- Blood cultures
- Myringotomy/tympanocentesis: Send for cultures, gram stain, acid-fast stain

Follow-Up & Special Considerations
Interpret normal WBC with caution in immunocompromised patient with symptoms

Imaging
Initial approach
- Plain radiographs of mastoid area:
  - Clouding of mastoid air cells; can be negative finding, however
  - Coalescence of air cells; diagnostic but rare
- CT scan if complications suspected:
  - Clouding of air cells: Loss of bony septation of the air cell system
  - CT of temporal bone with contrast helps identify asymptomatic complications (1)[C].
- Technetium 99 bone scan: More sensitive to osteolytic changes than CT
- MRI or CT with contrast if venous thrombosis is suspected as a complication

Diagnostic Procedures/Surgery
- Myringotomy (also therapeutic)
- Consider audiography in cases of suspected hearing loss.
- Culture material obtained at myringotomy.
- Obtain CSF if suspect intracranial extension.
- Biopsy if tissue protruding through TM or tympanostomy tube

Pathological Findings
- Inflammatory tissue in air cell system
- Granulation tissue
- Osteitis

DIFFERENTIAL DIAGNOSIS
- Postauricular inflammatory adenopathy
- Severe external otitis
- Postauricular cellulitis
- Benign neoplasm: Aneurysmal bone cyst, fibrous dysplasia
- Malignant neoplasm: Rhabdomyosarcoma, neuroblastoma
- HIV infection
- Furuncle of meatus of ear
- Parotitis
- Local trauma to auricula

TREATMENT

Medication is now the mainstay of therapy for acute mastoiditis, reflecting a shift away from surgical treatment.

MEDICATION
First Line
- Directed against most common organisms: *S. pneumoniae*, group A β-hemolytic *Streptococcus*, *S. aureus*
- Use 3rd-generation cephalosporin OR combination of *penicillinase-resistant penicillin* and an aminoglycoside.
- Begin with broad-spectrum treatment and narrow as pathogen identified
- Rocephin 1–2 g IV q12–24h:
- Pediatric dosing: 50–75 mg/kg IV q24h
- Precaution: Adjust dose with renal impairment.
- New recommendation of adding clindamycin to ceftriaxone for coverage of ceftriaxone-resistant *S. pneumoniae* in pediatric patients:
  - Clindamycin pediatric dosing: 20–40 mg/kg/d IV/IM divided q6–8h (1) OR
  - Oxacillin 1–2 g IV q4hr PLUS gentamicin 5–7.5 mg/kg/d IV divided q8h
- Oxacillin pediatric dosing: 200 mg/kg/d IV divided q6h

- Gentamicin pediatric dosing: If older than 2 years, administer as in adults.
- Precaution: These antibiotics given together may increase risk for nephrotoxicity; be aware of risk for ototoxicity with aminoglycosides.
- For other significant contraindications, precautions, or interactions, please refer to the manufacturer's literature.

Second Line
- Clindamycin (alone for PCN-allergic patients) 600–1,200 mg/d IV/IM divided q6–8h:
  - Pediatric dosing: 20–40 mg/kg/d IV/IM divided q6–8h
  - May cause *C. difficile* colitis in susceptible individuals
- If infection not responsive to above antibiotics, or if chronic mastoiditis suspected, consider *Pseudomonas* as pathogen and use Zosyn (piperacillin/tazobactam) 3/0.375 g IV q6h:
  - Pediatric dosing:
    - >12 years, administer as in adults
    - <12 years, consult ENT or ID specialist, as dose not established
    - Zosyn requires baseline and periodic monitoring of CBC and LFTs.
- Other antibiotics depending on sensitivity or refractoriness of pathogen
- Oral antibiotics are given once myringotomy/blood cultures narrow pathogen and sensitivities, typically:
  - Amoxicillin-clavulanate (Augmentin) or clindamycin PLUS 3rd-generation cephalosporin for at least 2 weeks; most use for 3 weeks
- For chronic mastoiditis: Use topical drops, ofloxacin otic solution (0.3%)
- For other significant medication contraindications, precautions, or interactions, please refer to the manufacturer's literature.

ADDITIONAL TREATMENT
General Measures
- Inpatient care during acute phase
- Keep affected ear dry.

Issues for Referral
Acute mastoiditis warrants hospitalization with ENT consult for adult and pediatric patients.

SURGERY/OTHER PROCEDURES
- Myringotomy; placement of pressure equalization tube
- Frequent cleaning of ear canal under microscope to ensure pressure-equalization tube patency and adequate drainage of middle ear
- Topical antibiotic drops are also usually used after insertion of pressure-equalization tube.
- If subperiosteal abscess is present, it should be aspirated. If aspiration is not sufficient, incision and drainage should be performed.
- Mastoidectomy is reserved for those patients whose condition fails to improve despite these measures within 18–72 hours or those with meningeal or intracranial complications.

IN-PATIENT CONSIDERATIONS
Initial Stabilization
- Hospitalize any patient with acute mastoiditis; start IV antibiotics.
- ENT referral (for tympanostomy or surgery if complications suspected)

Admission Criteria
Diagnosis of acute mastoiditis

Nursing
Caution patient about getting affected ear wet.

Discharge Criteria
- Afebrile for 48 hours before IV antibiotics are discontinued
- Able to take oral antibiotics

ONGOING CARE

FOLLOW-UP RECOMMENDATIONS
- After surgery, IV antibiotics to cover the most common pathogenic organisms
- Frequent cleansing of ear canal is needed to keep the pressure-equalization tube patent.
- Oral antibiotics for 3 weeks following satisfactory course of IV antibiotics
- For chronic mastoiditis, consider antimicrobial prophylaxis with amoxicillin for several months.

Patient Monitoring
- Postoperative: Audiogram after acute flare-up has subsided
- Follow up with ENT as outpatient.

DIET
No special diet

PATIENT EDUCATION
- Precaution about getting affected ear wet
- Follow up with ENT as outpatient.

PROGNOSIS
- Depends on severity of disease
- Conductive hearing loss may require reconstructive surgery.
- Expect to avoid complications with early treatment.

COMPLICATIONS
- Subperiosteal abscess
- Gradenigo syndrome (palsy of the 6th cranial nerve, draining ear, and retro-orbital pain)
- Bezold abscess (abscess of sternocleidomastoid muscle)
- Sigmoid sinus thrombosis
- Meningitis
- Intracranial abscess epidural/subdural/intraparenchymal
- Periosteitis
- Osteitis
- Central venous sinus thrombosis
- Suppurative labyrinthitis (resulting in deafness)
- Citelli abscess (osteomyelitis of the calvaria)
- Facial nerve paralysis

REFERENCE
1. Mallur PS, Harirchian S, Lalwani AK. Preoperative and postoperative intracranial complications of acute mastoiditis. *Ann Otol Rhinol Laryngol*. 2009;118:118–23.

ADDITIONAL READING
- Butbul-Aviel Y, et al. Acute mastoiditis in children: *Pseudomonas* as a leading pathogen. *Intern J Pediatr Otolaryngol*. 2003;67(3):277–81.
- Fontanette D, et al. *Mastoiditis eMedicine Clinical Knowledge Base*, Institutional Edition, Sept 12, 2008. Omaha, NE. Available at: http://www.imedicine.com.
- Roddy MG, Glazier SS, Agrawal D. Pediatric mastoiditis in the pneumococcal conjugate vaccine era: symptom duration guides empiric antimicrobial therapy. *Pediatr Emerg Care*. 2007;23:779–84.
- Smith J, et al. Complications of chronic otitis media and cholesteatoma. *Otolaryngol Clin N Am*. 2006;39(6):1237–55.
- Keith T, Saxena S, Murray J, Sharland M et al. Risk-benefit analysis of restricting antimicrobial prescribing in children: what do we really know? *Curr Opin Infect Dis*. 2010;23:242–8.

CODES

ICD9
- 383.00 Acute mastoiditis without complications
- 383.01 Subperiosteal abscess of mastoid
- 383.02 Acute mastoiditis with other complications

CLINICAL PEARLS
- Tympanic membrane can be normal in 10% of patients: Suspect mastoiditis when symptoms of acute otitis media persist >2 weeks with a normal TM.
- Hospitalize all patients with acute mastoiditis.
- Start with broad-spectrum antibiotics, then narrow as pathogen becomes evident.
- Expect to avoid complications with early treatment.

M

MEASLES (RUBEOLA)

Herbert L. Muncie, Jr., MD
Marin Dawson-Caswell, DO

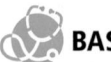 **BASICS**

DESCRIPTION
- A highly communicable, acute viral illness characterized by a maculopapular rash; begins at the head, spreads inferiorly to trunk and extremities
- Rash is preceded by fever and the classic triad: Cough, coryza, and conjunctivitis, and pathognomonic Koplik spots
- Major public health problem in the developing world, with significant morbidity and mortality
- System(s) affected: Primarily Hematologic/Lymphatic/Immunologic; Pulmonary; Skin; all systems may be affected by measles virus and/or its complications.
- Synonym(s): Rubeola

EPIDEMIOLOGY
- Transmission: Direct contact with infectious droplets or airborne spread (less common):
  - Droplets can remain in the air for hours.
  - In 2000, ongoing transmission declared eliminated in the US as a result of high rates of vaccination.
- Infectivity: Highly infectious; 75–90% of susceptible contacts will develop the disease:
  - Infectivity: Greatest during the prodromal phase
  - Patients are considered contagious from 5 days before symptoms until 4 days after rash appears.
  - Immunocompromised patients are considered contagious for entire duration of disease.
- Incubation period: Averages 12.5 days from exposure to onset of prodromal symptoms (1)
- Predominant age:
  - Varies based on local vaccine practices and disease incidence
  - In developing countries, most cases occur in children <2 years of age.

Incidence
- In US: No longer considered an endemic disease by the Centers for Disease Control and Prevention (CDC) (2); isolated outbreaks still occur, with most cases imported to those who are unvaccinated (3)
- First 7 months of 2008, more cases of measles were reported in the US than during any period since 1996. 131 cases were reported:
  - Of these, 91% were unvaccinated or had an unknown vaccination status.
  - 85% were vaccine-eligible but declined due to philosophical or religious beliefs.
- Worldwide: An estimated 20 million measles cases occur each year, with 242,000 measles deaths in 2006. Over 95% of measles deaths occur in countries with per capita gross national income of <US$1,000 and weak health infrastructures.

RISK FACTORS
- For developing measles:
  - Not being immunized or failure to receive 2 doses of vaccine
  - Travel to countries where measles is endemic
  - Contact with exposed individuals, travelers, or immigrants
- For severe measles or measles complications:
  - Immunodeficiency
  - Malnutrition
  - Pregnancy
  - Vitamin A deficiency
  - Age <5 years or >20 years

GENERAL PREVENTION
- Totally preventable disease with vaccination and positive externalities due to herd immunity (4)
- Measles vaccine (active immunization):
  - Live further-attenuated vaccine available as monovalent vaccine but usually given in combination with mumps and rubella (MMR); varicella now has been added
  - Primary vaccination of general population requires 2 doses (0.05 mL SQ):
    - 1st dose given at 12–15 months; 95% develop immunity.
    - 2nd dose given at time of school entry (or any time >4 weeks after 1st measles vaccine); almost always initial nonresponders develop immunity.
    - HIV-infected children should be vaccinated while asymptomatic or before CD4+ cell count drops below 500/mm³.
  - Common adverse reactions:
    - Fever and rarely febrile seizures 6–12 days after vaccination (5–15%)
    - Transient, mild, measleslike rash 7–10 days after vaccination (5%, with decreasing incidence during 2nd vaccination)
    - Mild allergic reaction
    - If hypersensitivity reaction occurs, test for immunity; if immune, 2nd dose is not needed.
    - Epidemiologic evidence has not substantiated any link between MMR vaccine and autism (5)[A].
  - Contraindications:
    - Pregnancy: Live vaccine is contraindicated in pregnant women (theoretical risk of fetal infection).
    - Anaphylactic reaction to gelatin or neomycin; consult allergist before vaccination.
    - Egg anaphylaxis is not considered a contraindication.

PATHOPHYSIOLOGY
- Measles virus enters respiratory mucosa and replicates locally, then spreads to regional lymphatic tissues, then on to other reticuloendothelial sites via the bloodstream.

ETIOLOGY
- Measles virus, an RNA virus of genus *Morbillivirus*, family *Paramyxoviridae*
- Humans are the only natural host.

COMMONLY ASSOCIATED CONDITIONS
- Immunosuppression
- Malnutrition

DIAGNOSIS

HISTORY
- Prodromal period: Usually 2–3 days before rash, but may be up to 8 days:
  - Fever:
    - Begins 8–12 days after exposure; persists until 2–3 days after onset of rash
    - High temperatures seen (39–40.5°C); can precipitate febrile seizures
    - Fever more than 3 days after rash suggests complication
  - Classic triad of "croupy" cough, coryza, and conjunctivitis
  - Cough may persist for up to 2 weeks.
- Prodromal symptoms typically intensify over 2–4 days and peak on 1st day of rash before subsiding.
- Loose stools, malaise, irritability, photophobia (from iridocyclitis), sore throat, headache, and abdominal pain

PHYSICAL EXAM
- Koplik spots:
  - Pathognomonic of prodromal measles
  - 2- to 3-mm gray–white, raised lesions on erythematous base that appear on buccal mucosa
  - Occur approximately 48 h before measles exanthem
- Rash (not pathognomonic):
  - Maculopapular, blanches
  - Begins at ears and hairline and spreads head to toe, reaching hips by day 2
  - Discrete erythematous patches become confluent over time, with greater confluence on upper body than lower body.
  - Clinical improvement usually occurs within 48 h of appearance of rash.
  - 3–4 days after rash appears, it fades and changes to brown color, followed by fine desquamation.
- Lymphadenopathy and pharyngitis may be seen during exanthem period.

DIAGNOSTIC TESTS & INTERPRETATION
Lab
Initial lab tests
- Measles IgM assay from serum or saliva is gold standard of World Health Organization (WHO):
  - Simplest diagnostic method
  - In countries with low measles prevalence, this approach may lead to false-positive results, so in low-prevalence countries, the use of paired acute and convalescent sera for antimeasles IgM and IgG is suggested.
  - IgM may be undetectable on 1st day of exanthem; usually detectable 3 days after exanthem:
    - At least a 4-fold increase is indicative of infection.
    - Sensitivity: 77% within 72 h of rash onset; 100% 4–11 days after rash onset; if negative but rash lasts >72 h, repeat.
- Measles IgG is undetectable up to 7 days after exanthem; peaks about 14 days after exanthem:
  - An IgG concentration with 4-fold increase at least 7 days after rash onset vs 14 days later by standard serologic assay is confirmatory.
- Culturing measles virus is difficult; not commonly performed.
- Mild neutropenia is common.
- Liver transaminases and pancreatic amylase may be elevated, particularly in adults.

ALERT
Suspected measles cases in the US must be reported to the local or state health department.

Imaging
CXR is appropriate when suspicion exists of secondary pneumonia.

DIFFERENTIAL DIAGNOSIS
- Drug eruptions
- Rubella
- *Mycoplasma pneumoniae*
- Infectious mononucleosis
- Parvovirus B19 infection
- Roseola
- Enteroviruses
- Rocky Mountain spotted fever
- Dengue
- Toxic shock syndrome
- Meningococcemia
- Kawasaki disease

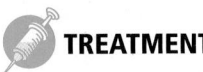 **TREATMENT**

MEDICATION
- No approved antiviral therapy is available. Immunosuppressed children with severe measles have been treated with IV or aerosolized ribavirin, but no controlled data exist, and this use is not approved by the Food and Drug Administration (FDA).
- Antibiotics:
  - Reserved for patients with clinical signs of bacterial superinfection
  - Although a 2006 Cochrane Review reported insufficient evidence to justify prophylactic antibiotics for prevention of measles-associated pneumonia, a small 2006 randomized, double-blinded trial resulted in an 80% (number needed to treat [NNT] = 7) decrease in measles-associated pneumonia with use of prophylactic antibiotics; authors suggest the use of prophylactic antibiotics in patients with a high risk of complications (6)[B].
- Vitamin A:
  - Children 6–12 months of age receive 100,000 IU as 1 dose.
  - Children >12 months of age receive 200,000 IU as 1 dose:
    ○ American Academy of Pediatrics recommends only in limited circumstances: Hospitalized children aged 6–12 months; children >6 months of age with other risk factors for complications
    ○ Limited evidence exists to generalize efficacy to developed countries.
- Outbreak control:
  - CDC defines an outbreak of measles as a single case.
  - Prompt immunization (within 72 h) of people at risk of exposure or already exposed who cannot provide documentation of measles immunity:
    ○ Monovalent vaccine may be given to infants 6 months–1 year of age, but 2 further doses of vaccine after 12 months must be given for appropriate immunization.
    ○ Monovalent or combination vaccine may be given to all measles-exposed susceptible individuals where not contraindicated.
    ○ Individuals who have not been immunized within 72 h of exposure should be excluded from school, child care, and health care settings until 2 weeks after onset of rash in last case of measles.
  - Immune globulin (passive immunity) may be necessary for certain high-risk individuals exposed to measles where vaccine is inappropriate:

○ IM immune globulin should be given within 6 days of exposure to measles; CDC recommends 0.25 mL/kg to maximum of 15 mL; immunocompromised individuals receive 0.5 mL/kg to a maximum of 15 mL.
○ Children <1 year old
○ Pregnant women
○ Individuals with severe immunosuppression

ADDITIONAL TREATMENT
General Measures
- Supportive therapy (i.e., antipyretics, antitussives, humidification, increased consumption of oral fluids)
- Control:
  - All patients with measles should be placed in respiratory isolation until 4 days after onset of rash; immunocompromised patients should be isolated for duration of illness.
  - Notify public health officials of suspected cases.

IN-PATIENT CONSIDERATIONS
Outpatient care is appropriate, except where complications develop (e.g., encephalitis, pneumonia).

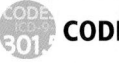 **ONGOING CARE**

FOLLOW-UP RECOMMENDATIONS
Patients are advised to call their doctor if they develop any:
- Difficulty breathing or noisy breathing
- Changes in vision
- Changes in behavior, confusion
- Chest or abdominal pain

PATIENT EDUCATION
- Avoid exposure to other individuals, particularly unimmunized children and adults, pregnant women, and immunocompromised persons, until 4 days after rash onset.
- Avoid contact with potential sources of secondary bacterial pathogens until respiratory symptoms resolve.

PROGNOSIS
- Typically self-limited; prognosis good
- High fatality rates may be seen among malnourished or immunocompromised children, particularly in developing countries.
- Complications occur in up to 40% of cases.

COMPLICATIONS
- Otitis media (occurs in 5–15%)
- Respiratory complications:
  - Bronchopneumonia (occurs in 5–10%):
    ○ Accounts for most measles-related deaths
    ○ May be viral or bacterial
  - Interstitial pneumonitis: In immunocompromised patients
  - Laryngotracheobronchitis ("measles croup"): Occurs in younger age group (<2 years of age)
- GI complications: Diarrhea (may lead to dehydration)
- Neurologic complications:
  - Febrile seizures
  - Acute disseminated encephalomyelitis with seizures and variety of neurologic abnormalities (occurs in 1/1,000 cases): Presents soon after measles resolves
  - Subacute sclerosing panencephalitis (SSPE):
    ○ Rare degenerative CNS disease resulting from persistent measles infection following natural disease
    ○ Presents 5–15 years after infection
    ○ Disappearing as a result of mass vaccination

- Ocular complications: Keratitis:
  - Can lead to permanent scarring, blindness
  - Vitamin A deficiency predisposes to more severe keratitis and its complications.
- Other secondary bacterial infections
- Death: Results from complications, mainly pneumonia, rather than the virus itself

REFERENCES
1. Lessler J, Reich NG, Brookmeyer R, et al. Incubation periods of acute respiratory viral infections: a systematic review. *Lancet Infect Dis.* 2009;9: 291–300.
2. Orenstein WA, Papania MJ, Wharton ME. Measles elimination in the United States. *J Infect Dis.* 2004;189(Suppl 1):S1–3.
3. Centers for Disease Control and Prevention (CDC). Measles among adults associated with adoption of children in China–California, Missouri, and Washington, July-August 2006. *MMWR Morb Mortal Wkly Rep.* 2007;56:144–6.
4. Althouse BM, Bergstrom TC, Bergstrom CT et al. Evolution in health and medicine Sackler colloquium: a public choice framework for controlling transmissible and evolving diseases. *Proc Natl Acad Sci USA.* 2010;107(Suppl 1): 1696–701.
5. Demicheli V, Jefferson T, Rivetti A, et al. Vaccines for measles, mumps and rubella in children. *Cochrane Database Syst Rev.* 2005;CD004407.
6. Garly ML, Balé C, Martins CL, et al. Prophylactic antibiotics to prevent pneumonia and other complications after measles: community based randomised double blind placebo controlled trial in Guinea-Bissau. *BMJ.* 2006;333:1245.

CODES

ICD9
055.9 Measles without mention of complication

CLINICAL PEARLS
- Measles is a highly communicable viral disease whose natural transmission has been halted in the US by mass immunization.
- Immunization of the general public requires 2 doses: 1 at 12–15 months of age and 1 at school age (4–6 years of age).
- Presentation includes a prodrome of fever, cough, coryza, and conjunctivitis, followed by a descending maculopapular rash.
- Suspected measles cases must be reported to state or local health departments, and measures taken to contain outbreak.
- Measles-associated pneumonia is the most common cause of mortality.

M

MEASLES, GERMAN (RUBELLA)

Juan Antonio Garcia, MD

BASICS

DESCRIPTION
- Rubella is also known as *German measles* and the *3-day measles*.
- Mild viral exanthematous infection of children and adults that may induce abortions, stillbirths in pregnant women, or congenital defects in in-utero-exposed infants
- Two main presentations: Postnatal rubella, usually a mild disease, and congenital rubella, which can have devastating effects
- 50% of infections are asymptomatic.
- System(s) affected: Hematologic/Lymphatic/Immunologic; Nervous; Pulmonary; Skin/Exocrine

Pediatric Considerations
In-utero-exposed infants will shed the virus during the first year of life, exposing the people they are in contact with.

Pregnancy Considerations
- Congenital rubella can lead to abortions, stillbirths, or in utero growth retardation (IUGR).
- Congenital rubella syndrome (CRS) is present in 80% of fetuses exposed to the virus during the 1st trimester of pregnancy.
- The single most effective policy for prevention of congenital rubella syndrome is screening pregnant women for rubella immunity (1)[C] and immunizing nonimmune women postpartum (2)[C].
- Women vaccinated against rubella are advised not to become pregnant for at least 3 months. The vaccine-type virus can cross the placenta. However, no case of congenital rubella has occurred after inadvertent vaccination (3)[C].
- A reliable (87–100% sensitive) polymerase chain reaction (PCR)–based method of detecting viral RNA in amniotic fluid allows rapid diagnosis of fetal infection if performed after 15 weeks' gestation (3)[B].

EPIDEMIOLOGY
Incidence
- Incubation period is 7–14 days but could be up to 23 days.
- Transmitted by aerosolized particles; shedding from nasopharyngeal starts 3–8 days after contamination; lasts 14 days after rash starts
- Predominant age: Children 5–9 years of age
- Predominant sex: Male = Female.
- The only natural host is the human.
- Live attenuated rubella vaccine was made available in 1969. Since then, the incidence has decreased continuously.
- The Centers for Disease Control and Prevention (CDC) declared in 2005 the elimination of rubella from the US (4).
- Rubella still occurs worldwide in developing countries.
- Incidence is decreasing. Countries the in Pan American Health Organization reported 135,947 cases in 1998 and then 1,000 cases in 2003.
- In 2006, incidence of postnatal rubella was 0.003 cases/100,000 population.
- Late winter and spring are most likely seasons for transmission and outbreak (2)[C].

RISK FACTORS
Inadequate immunization, Immunodeficiency states, Immunosuppressive therapy, Pregnancy, Crowded living conditions, School, day-care facility, International travel (5)[C]

Genetics
Children with CRS and children with insulin-dependent diabetes mellitus (IDDM) share a high frequency of HLA-DR3 histocompatibility antigen and a high prevalence of islet cell antibodies (3)[B].

GENERAL PREVENTION
- Vaccination most effective preventive strategy
- Available combined with measles and mumps (MMR), combined with measles, mumps, and varicella (MMRV), or as monovalent rubella vaccine
- Rubella vaccine (strain RA 27/3):
  - A 2-dose schedule combined MMR vaccine is recommended for those born after 1956. The 1st dose is recommended at ages 12–15 months; the 2nd dose is recommended either at 4–6 or at 11–12 years of age. Children with HIV infection should receive MMR vaccine at 12 months of age if no contraindications exist.
  - Recommended for susceptible people in the following groups: Prepubertal boys and girls, premarital or postpartum women, college students, day-care personnel, health care workers, and military personnel
- Contraindicated in pregnancy, immunodeficiency (except HIV infection), within 3 months of immunoglobulin (Ig) or blood administration or severe febrile illness, or hypersensitivity to vaccine components (3)[C]; patients who receive rubella vaccine do not transmit rubella to others, although the virus can be isolated from the pharynx.
- During outbreaks of rubella, serologic screening before vaccination is not recommended because rapid mass vaccination is necessary to stop the spread of the disease (6)[A].
- Debate about safety of MMR vaccine: Cochrane systematic review stated that it is unlikely to be associated with autism, Crohn disease, or ulcerative colitis. It is likely to be associated with benign thrombocytopenic purpura, parotitis, joint and limb complains, febrile convulsions, and aseptic meningitis (mumps) (7)[A].
- In countries with adequate programs of vaccination, antibody screening in prenatal care should be reinforced (1)[C].

ETIOLOGY
- It is caused by a 50- to 70-nm RNA virus of the *rubivirus* genus from the Togaviridae family; its natural host is human.
- Transmitted by aerosolized particles or direct contact with contaminated respiratory secretions, or via placenta to the fetus.
- If exposed during the first trimester, 80% of fetus exposed to the virus during this organogenesis phase will develop CRS.
- Risk of fetal infection during the 2nd trimester, 10–20%; >60% risk during 3rd trimester (3)[C]
- The virus invades the respiratory epithelium and then spreads hematogenously to regional and distal lymphatics, where it starts its replication. Then a second viremia occurs. Once infected, the patient starts shedding the virus from the nasopharynx 3–8 days after contamination, lasting up to 14 days after the rash starts.

DIAGNOSIS

- Postnatal rubella (8)[C]:
  - Mild disease and short lived
  - 1st sign is adenopathy: Posterior auricular, posterior cervical, suboccipital
  - Exanthem: Pink maculopapular (1–4 mm); face and neck, spreads to trunk and extremities; last up to 3 days
  - Enanthem (Forchheimer sign): Soft palate petechiae; 20% patients
  - Low-grade fever
  - Cephalalgia
  - Sore throat
  - Myalgias
  - Nausea
  - Anorexia
  - Malaise
  - Polyarthralgia/polyarthritis, especially in young women
  - Asymptomatic (50%)
- CRS (T = transient; P = permanent; D = developmental) (3,8)[C]:
- 4 primary elements:
  - Sensorineural deafness (P, D) (58% of patients), unilateral or bilateral
  - Congenital heart disease (see below) (50% of babies)
  - Growth retardation
  - Mental retardation (P, D) plus the following:
    ○ Cataracts (P)
    ○ Microphthalmia (P)
    ○ Chorioretinitis ("salt and pepper retinopathy") (P)
    ○ Patent ductus arteriosus (P)
    ○ Pulmonic stenosis (P, D)
    ○ Atrial and ventricular septal defects (P)
    ○ Microcephaly (P)
    ○ Meningoencephalitis (T)
    ○ Low birth weight (T)
    ○ Purpuric ("blueberry muffin") skin lesions (T)
    ○ Radiolucent bone disease (T)
    ○ Hepatosplenomegaly (T)
    ○ Large anterior fontanelle (T)
    ○ Language and behavior disorders (P, D)
    ○ Cryptorchidism (P)
    ○ Inguinal hernia (P)

HISTORY
- CRS severity is inversely proportional to timing of gestational infection.
- In-utero-infected infants during 3rd trimester infection may develop late sequelae (e.g., auditory, ocular, immunologic, endocrine, or neurologic effects)
- Deafness could be the only manifestation and not be noticed until second year of life.
- In-utero-exposed children have increased risk for diabetes (1/7), thyroid conditions, and precocious puberty.

DIAGNOSTIC TESTS & INTERPRETATION
Cell-mediated immune responses are selectively impaired in children with congenital rubella.

Lab
- Postnatal rubella:
  - Diagnosis is achieved by demonstrating 4-fold rise in IgG rubella-specific antibody between acute phase and 2–3 weeks later.

– Confirmation is by viral culture from throat or nasal secretions and blood (epidemiologic purposes).
– Mild leukopenia with relative lymphocytosis

• CRS:
– Viral isolation from blood, nasopharynx, CSF, urine, lens aspirates if cataracts are present
– IgM antibodies may not be detectable and IgG antibodies can be nonspecific owing to maternal transplacental passage.

• Other forms: Rubella antigen detection: PCR or placenta biopsy

• Disorders that may alter lab results: After re-exposure to rubella, a person with a low level of antibody from past infection or vaccination may experience an acute rise in antibody levels. This is not associated with a high incidence of contagion to others or of fetal risk.

Follow-Up & Special Considerations
During the 1st year of life, in-utero-exposed babies will shed the virus, exposing the people they are in contact with.

Diagnostic Procedures/Surgery
Congenital rubella has been diagnosed by placental biopsy at 12 weeks.

Pathological Findings
• Inhibition of cellular growth after infection
• Fetal vasculitis
• Placental angiopathy
• Tissue necrosis secondary to progressive necrotizing vasculitis

DIFFERENTIAL DIAGNOSIS
• Postnatal rubella:
– Measles virus (rubeola)
– Scarlet fever
– Infectious mononucleosis
– Toxoplasmosis
– Roseola infantum (i.e., exanthem subitum)
– Erythema infectiosum (5th disease)
– Drug eruptions
– Other exanthematous enteroviral infections
• Congenital rubella:
– Cytomegalovirus
– Varicella-zoster virus
– Picornaviruses (coxsackievirus, echovirus)
– Poliovirus
– Herpes simplex virus
– Western equine virus
– Measles virus (rubeola)
– Hepatitis B virus
– Mumps virus
– Influenza virus
– Toxoplasmosis
– Congenital syphilis
– Malaria

 ## TREATMENT
• Supportive
• Postnatal rubella: Mild and self-limited; treat for symptomatic relief.
• CRS: Supportive care unless neurologic or hemorrhagic complications develop; phototherapy may be indicated for jaundice; multidisciplinary management of long-term complications

MEDICATION
• No specific therapy available
• Acetaminophen for fever q4h if needed: 10–15 mg/kg/dose

• Nonsteroidal anti-inflammatory drugs (NSAIDs) can be used for arthritis and arthralgias.
• IV immunoglobulin (IVIG) can be given in severe thrombocytopenia, but most cases are autolimited.

 ## ONGOING CARE

FOLLOW-UP RECOMMENDATIONS
• For postnatal rubella: Contact isolation for 5 days before to 7 days after onset of rash; bed rest is not necessary.
• Contact isolation of congenitally infected infants for 1 year, unless nasopharyngeal and urine cultures after 3 months of age test negative for rubella virus.

Patient Monitoring
• People immune to rubella via natural infection or vaccine may be reinfected when re-exposed; such infection is usually asymptomatic and detectable only by serologic means.
• In CRS, it is extremely important to detect auditory and visual impairment early so that adequate education and counseling can begin.
• 2/3 of internationally adopted children entering the US have no written records of overseas immunizations.

PATIENT EDUCATION
• Make every effort to avoid exposing infected patient to pregnant women.
• JAMA Patient Page on Rubella located at http://www.jama.com; go to Patient Page Index; click on "Previous Topics, Rubella (1/23–30/2002)."
• http://www.patient.co.uk/health/Rubella-(German-Measles).htm
• http://www.nlm.nih.gov/medlineplus/ency/article/001574.htm
• http://www.medinfo.co.uk/conditions/rubella.html

PROGNOSIS
• Postnatal rubella:
– Fever, 1–2 days
– Rash, 3 days
– Coryza, 5 days
– Lymphadenopathy, 1 week
– Arthralgia (when present), 2 weeks
– Complete and full recovery without sequelae is the rule.
• CRS:
– Varied and unpredictable spectrum of consequences ranging from stillbirth to completely normal infancy and childhood
– Disease is characterized by chronic infection; infants may remain contagious for months after birth.
– Detectable levels of hemagglutination-inhibiting antibody (IgG) persist for years and then may decline. By age 5, 20% have no detectable antibody.
– Overall mortality 10%; greatest during 1st 6 months
– 70% of those with encephalitis develop residual neuromotor defects, including an autistic syndrome.
– Prognosis is excellent when only minor congenital defects are present.

COMPLICATIONS
• Postnatal rubella (3)[C]:
– Postinfectious encephalitis (1/5,000 cases)
– Thrombocytopenic purpura (1/3,000 cases)
– Arthritis/arthralgias (20% in children; 75% in adults)

• CRS:
– Spontaneous abortion
– Stillbirth
– Premature delivery
– Progressive rubella panencephalitis
– Endocrine disturbances (e.g., diabetes mellitus, thyrotoxicosis, hypothyroidism)
• Rubella vaccine:
– Lymphadenopathy
– Fever
– Rash
– Arthritis/arthralgia (older girls, women) (3)[C]
– Polyneuropathy
– Idiopathic thrombocytopenic purpura (ITP) (rare, self-limited and non-life-threatening—not a contraindication to giving vaccine) (9)[A]

REFERENCES
1. Senior K. Infectious disease in pregnancy. *The Lancet infectious diseases*. 2009;9(6):344.
2. Muchowski K, Paladine H. An ounce of prevention: the evidence supporting periconception health care. *J Fam Pract*. 2004;53:126–33.
3. Banatvala JE, Brown DW. Rubella. *Lancet*. 2004;363:1127–37.
4. Weisberg SS. Measles. *Dis Mon*. 2007;53:471–7.
5. McGovern LM, Boyce TG, Fischer PR. Congenital infections associated with international travel during pregnancy. *J Travel Med*. 2007;14:117–28.
6. Demicheli V, Jefferson T, Rivetti A, et al. Vaccines for measles, mumps and rubella in children. *The Cochrane Database of Systematic Reviews*. 2005;4:CD004407.DOI:10.1002/14651858.CD004407.pub2.
7. Demcheli V, Jefferson T, Rivetti A et al. Vaccines for measles, mumps and rubella in children. *Cochrane Database of Systematic Reviews*. 2005;4:CD004407. DOI:10.1002/14651858.CD004407.pub2.
8. Edlich RF, Winters KL, Long WB, et al. Rubella and congenital rubella (German measles). *J Long Term Eff Med Implants*. 2005;15:319–28.
9. Mantadakis E, Farmaki E, Buchanan GR et al. Thrombocytopenic purpura after measles-mumps-rubella vaccination: a systematic review of the literature and guidance for management. *J Pediatr*. 2010;156:623–8.

See Also (Topic, Algorithm, Electronic Media Element)
Cerebral Palsy; Measles, Rubeola

 ## CODES

ICD9
• 056.00 Rubella with unspecified neurological complication
• 056.9 Rubella without mention of complication
• 771.0 Congenital rubella

CLINICAL PEARLS
Rubella vaccine is currently the only vaccine designed for the purpose of protecting someone other than the vaccine recipient.

M

MELANOMA
David P. Sealy, MD

 BASICS

DESCRIPTION
- Tumor arising from malignant degeneration of cells from the melanocytic system:
  - Most arise in the skin but also may present as a primary lesion in any tissue. Ocular, GI, genitourinary, lymph node, and leptomeninges are the primary extracutaneous sites.
  - Metastatic spread to any region in the body
- Lentigo maligna variant:
  - Cutaneous lesion: Slowest growing malignant melanoma with least tendency to metastasize
  - Occurs most often on the face, beginning as a circumscribed macular patch of mottled pigmentation showing shades of dark brown, tan, or black; mostly in the elderly
- System(s) affected: Skin/Exocrine

Geriatric Considerations
Lentigo maligna is seen most commonly in elderly patients who have had a slowly enlarging pigmented lesion and usually is found on the face.

Pediatric Considerations
Congenital large nevi (>5 cm) are risk factors and have a >2% lifetime risk of malignant conversion. Blistering sunburns in childhood significantly increase adult risk.

Pregnancy Considerations
- Because melanocyte-stimulating hormone (MSH) levels are markedly increased during pregnancy and melanoma is one of the few carcinomas that can spread to the placenta, there has been concern that pregnancy exacerbates melanoma. Data now suggest that there is no increased risk of melanoma with pregnancy (1)[B].
- Many authors suggest waiting 1–2 years if further pregnancy is desired for patients with recent melanomas.
- If invasion extends into the lymphatic structures, further pregnancy probably is contraindicated.

EPIDEMIOLOGY
Incidence
- In 2006, 62,190 new cases in the US (1)
- 1 in 63 Americans will develop melanoma (1) in their lifetime.
- 6th most common cancer in US (1)
- Highest annual incidence rate of any cancer in whites between the ages of 25 and 29 years and in white males between 35 and 39 years of age
- Predominant age: Median age = 55 years; >50% of all individuals with melanoma are between 20 and 40 years of age.
- Predominant sex: Male > Female (1.5×)
- Incidence among whites is 10–20× greater than that among blacks or Hispanics.

Prevalence
- >24/100,000 white males and 16/100,000 white females
- 2% of all cancer deaths
- In women, the most common location is the legs, and in men, the trunk.

RISK FACTORS
- Heavy ultraviolet A (UVA) and ultraviolet B (UVB) exposure
- Previous pigmented lesions (especially dysplastic or melanocytic nevi)
- Fair complexion, freckling, blue eyes, and blond or red hair
- Those with increased numbers of nevi (>100), highest predictor of risk
- Family history of melanoma
- Tanning bed use before age 30 years (controversial)
- Changing nevus
- Large (>5 cm) congenital nevi
- Other skin cancers
- Immunosuppression
- Blistering sunburns in childhood
- Occupational exposure to ionizing radiation
- Does not appear to be affected by pregnancy, oral contraceptives, or hormone replacement

Genetics
- In individuals with dysplastic nevi, a family history of dysplastic nevus syndrome with melanoma conveys a nearly 100% lifetime risk of development of melanoma. Close surveillance is indicated.
- Changes in oncogenes, suppressor gene growth factors, and receptors have been suggested as genetic effects from these chromosomal associations.

GENERAL PREVENTION
- Primary prevention by large-scale screening has failed.
- Screening of high-risk individuals is likely to be successful.
- Avoidance of sunburn, especially in childhood, is important.

PATHOPHYSIOLOGY
Under investigation, but clearly associated with exposure to UVA and UVB

COMMONLY ASSOCIATED CONDITIONS
- Dysplastic nevus syndrome
- Heavy mole formers are individuals on whom >50 nevi are found. These patients may have a higher lifetime risk of melanoma than the general population because 50–75% of all melanomas arise in preexisting nevi.
- Giant congenital nevus syndrome is associated with an approximate 6% lifetime incidence of melanoma.

 DIAGNOSIS

HISTORY
Change in a pigmented lesion: Hypo- or hyperpigmentation, bleeding, scaling, size change, texture change

PHYSICAL EXAM
- Use the ABCDE mnemonic: Asymmetry; Border irregularity; Color variegation (especially red, white, black, and blue hues); Diameter >6 mm; or Elevation above skin surface
- Any new and/or changing nevus, bleeding or ulcerated
- Location on whites is primarily the back and lower leg, and on blacks is the hands, feet, and nails.
- Individuals at high risk for melanoma should have a careful ocular exam to assess for presence of melanoma in the iris, retina, or other pigmented eye cells (2)[C].

DIAGNOSTIC TESTS & INTERPRETATION
Lab
With metastatic disease, lactate dehydrogenase (LDH) determination may be helpful.

Imaging
Initial approach
Imaging studies are of benefit only in detecting metastatic disease, which is usually to the brain, lymph nodes, and lungs.

Diagnostic Procedures/Surgery
- Surgical biopsy is the only appropriate diagnostic procedure. Any suspicious nevus or pigmented lesion should be fully excised. A full-thickness total excisional biopsy of suspicious lesions with 2-mm margins and a cuff of fat is recommended (3). This must be sent for pathologic examination. Lesions never should be curetted, electrodesiccated, or shaved (known or strongly suspected melanoma), although low-likelihood lesions are sometimes removed by deep shave technique. Any irregularly pigmented lesion >2 cm in a preadolescent individual should be considered for excision.
- Frozen sections are also not indicated.
- Once diagnosed, see below for surgical management.

Pathological Findings
- Gross pathologic features include 4 clinical types:
  - Superficial spreading melanoma: 70%
  - Nodular: 15%
  - Acral lentiginous: 2–8%
  - Lentigo maligna: 4–10% (a small percentage are amelanotic)
- Nodular melanoma is primarily vertical growth, whereas the other 3 types are horizontal.
- Importance of number of mitoses and presence of ulceration increasing (3)
- Immunohistochemical testing on melanoma cells increases sensitivity of lymph node biopsies, but clinical application is still being investigated (1,4).

DIFFERENTIAL DIAGNOSIS
- Dysplastic and blue nevi
- Vascular skin tumor
- Actinic keratosis
- Traumatic hematoma
- Lentigo
- Pigmented squamous cell and basal cell carcinomas, seborrheic keratoses, other changing nevi

TREATMENT
MEDICATION
- No chemotherapeutic agent has definitively shown lasting benefit (4,5)[B], but chemotherapeutic options vary, and consultation with an oncologist is highly recommended.
- Early benefit with vaccines has not stood the test of time (4,5)[B].
- Interferon-alfa-2b has not shown increased benefit in disease-free time and overall survival (4,5)[B].

ADDITIONAL TREATMENT
General Measures
Surgical management is the only option for melanoma.

Issues for Referral
- Referral to a regional melanoma center is often done.
- Cosmetic surgery is often needed once final excision is done.
- Isolated metastases may be treated surgically.
- Localized metastases (i.e., extremity) may be treated with regional chemotherapy (3).

Additional Therapies
- Many chemo- and immunotherapies have been tried; none has been shown to increase survival, but many increase patient discomfort greatly.
- Pegylated interferon-alfa may prove slightly beneficial (3).
- Dacarbazine has been associated with mild prolongation of life in some studies but not others.
- Future direction will be toward immunochemical treatments (4,5)[C].

COMPLEMENTARY AND ALTERNATIVE MEDICINE
Many have been tried with no lasting benefits

SURGERY/OTHER PROCEDURES
- Appropriate treatment for melanoma is surgical excision.
- Extent of excision margins is becoming standardized. Generally, achieve margins of 1 cm if the lesion is <1 mm thick. If 1–2 mm, extend margins to 1–2 cm (4,6)[B].
- Sentinel lymph node biopsy for lesions of 1- to 4-mm deep has become standard of care in many locations. However, increased survival has not been demonstrated.
- Elective lymph node dissection is no longer an option (4,6)[B].

IN-PATIENT CONSIDERATIONS
Initial Stabilization
Most surgeries are done as outpatients with no stabilization needed.

ONGOING CARE
FOLLOW-UP RECOMMENDATIONS
Once diagnosed, close follow-up and avoidance of UVA and UVB are highly advised.

Patient Monitoring
- Key to cure is prevention
- Skin exams every 3–6 months in patients with history of melanoma
- Those with 1 melanoma diagnosed are at much greater risk for subsequent new primary melanomas.
- Thorough skin self-exams weekly

DIET
No data suggesting the benefit or risk of dietary manipulations

PATIENT EDUCATION
- Teach patients who are at risk or have had melanoma the principles of ABCDE examinations.
- Patients with a history of melanoma or dysplastic nevus syndrome must have frequent total-body examinations for any abnormal-appearing or changing nevi.
- Educational materials are available at the National Cancer Institute, Department of Health and Human Services, Public Inquiries Section, Office of Cancer Communications, Building 31, Room 101-18, 9000 Rockville Pike, Bethesda, MD 20892; (301) 496-5583.

PROGNOSIS
Prognosis is based on staging of the initial lesion:
- Staging (falls into 3 categories):
  – Breslow: 70% 5-year survival of patients without local or distant lymphatic spread
  – Clark staging depends on depth of invasion by skin layer. The best prognosis is for lesions that are <0.85 mm (especially if restricted to the stratum granulosum or higher), which carry 95–100% 5-year survival. Spread to lymphatics or regional lymph nodes carries a <5% 5-year survival.
  – AJCC: Stage 0 in situ and lentigo maligna, stages I and II localized to skin, stage III regional lymph node or satellite lesions, stage IV distant metastases
- Women have a better prognosis than men.
- Truncal lesions have a poorer prognosis.
- With distant metastases, disease is uniformly lethal.
- Lesions with ulceration at the time of presentation have a significantly poorer prognosis.

COMPLICATIONS
- Metastatic spread
- Unsatisfactory cosmetic results following the primary surgery

REFERENCES
1. Markovic SN, Erickson LA, Rao RD, et al. Malignant melanoma in the 21st century, part 1: epidemiology, risk factors, screening, prevention, and diagnosis. *Mayo Clin Proc*. 2007;82:364–80.
2. Bataille V, deVries E. Melanoma-Part 1: epidemiology, risk factors and prevention. *BMJ*. 2008:337:a2249,1287–91.
3. Thurwell C, Nathan P, Melanoma-Part 2:management. *BMJ*. 2008:337:a2488, 1345–8.
4. Lane JE, Dalton RR, Sanguqza OP. Cutaneous Melanoma. *Jl Fam Prac*. 2007;56(1):18–28.
5. Gogas HJ, Kirkwood JM, Sondak VK. Chemotherapy for metastatic melanoma: time for a change? *Cancer*. 2007;109:455–64.
6. Markovic SN, Erickson LA, Rao RD, et al. Malignant melanoma in the 21st century, part 2: staging, prognosis, and treatment. *Mayo Clin Proc*. 2007;82:490–513.

CODES
ICD9
- 172.0 Malignant melanoma of skin of lip
- 172.1 Malignant melanoma of skin of eyelid, including canthus
- 172.9 Melanoma of skin, site unspecified

CLINICAL PEARLS
- Up to 5% of new melanomas are from an unknown primary. Always consider melanoma if a lymph node is enlarged and nontender.
- Don't forget that amelanotic melanomas exist; the physician should biopsy new sites of no pigment or loss of pigment.
- 80% of cutaneous melanomas arise in existing nevi. Any changing nevi should be considered for full-thickness biopsy.

M

MÉNIÈRE'S DISEASE

Shanin Gross, DO

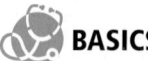 BASICS

DESCRIPTION
- An inner ear (labyrinthine) disorder characterized by recurrent attacks of hearing loss, tinnitus, vertigo, and sensations of aural fullness. Generally believed to be caused by, or related to, an increase in the volume and pressure of the inner ear endolymph fluid (endolymphatic hydrops).
- Often unilateral initially, but it is estimated that nearly half become bilateral over time.
- Severity and frequency of vertigo may diminish over time, but hearing loss is often progressive and/or fluctuating.
- Usually idiopathic (Ménière disease), but may be secondary to another condition causing endolymphatic hydrops (Ménière syndrome)
- System(s) affected: Nervous
- Synonym(s): Ménière syndrome; endolymphatic hydrops

EPIDEMIOLOGY
- Predominant age of onset: 40–60 years
- Predominant gender: Female > Male (1.3:1)
- Race/ethnicity: white, northern European > Blacks

Incidence
Estimates 1–150/100,000/year

Prevalence
Varies from ~7.5 to >200/100,000.

RISK FACTORS
Not well understood, but *may* include:
- Stress
- Allergy
- Increased salt intake
- Caffeine, alcohol, or nicotine intake
- Chronic exposure to loud noise
- Family history of Ménière
- Certain vascular abnormalities (patients may also have history of migraines)
- Certain viral exposures (especially herpes simplex virus [HSV])

Genetics
Some families show increased incidence, but genetic vs environmental influences are not well understood.

GENERAL PREVENTION
Reduce risk factors: Stress; salt, alcohol, and caffeine intake; smoking; noise exposure; ototoxic drugs (aspirin, quinine, aminoglycosides, etc.)

PATHOPHYSIOLOGY
Not fully understood; theories include increased pressure of the endolymph fluid due to increased fluid production or decreased resorption. This may be caused by endolymphatic sac pathology, abnormal development of the vestibular aqueduct, or inflammation caused by circulating immune complexes. Increased endolymph pressure may cause rupture of membranes and changes in endolymphatic ionic gradient.

ETIOLOGY
Idiopathic (Ménière *disease*), but Ménière *syndrome* may be secondary to injury or other disorder (e.g., reduced middle ear pressure, allergy, endocrine disease, lipid disorders, vascular, viral, syphilis, autoimmune). Any disorder that could cause endolymph hydrops could be implicated in Ménière *syndrome*.

COMMONLY ASSOCIATED CONDITIONS
- Endolymphatic hydrops
- Anxiety (secondary to the disabling symptoms)
- Migraines
- Theorized: Hypothyroidism
- Hyperprolactinemia

DIAGNOSIS

Diagnosis is clinical. Tests rule out other conditions (1)[B].

HISTORY
- Attacks are typically spontaneous but may be preceded by an aura of increasing fullness in the ear and tinnitus. These may occur in clusters with long intervening symptom-free remissions. Signs and symptoms to look for include:
- Formal criteria for diagnosis from AAO-HNS:
  - At least 2 episodes of rotational-horizontal vertigo >20 minutes in duration
  - Tinnitus or aural fullness
  - Hearing loss: Low frequency (sensorineural) confirmed by audiometric testing
  - Other causes (acoustic neuroma, etc.) excluded
- During severe attacks: Pallor, sweating, nausea, vomiting, falling, prostration
- Symptoms are exacerbated by motion.
- Between attacks, affected patients may experience motion-related imbalance without vertigo.
- Caution: Many conditions may produce auditory and vestibular findings identical to those associated with Ménière disease.

PHYSICAL EXAM
- Physical exam rules out other conditions; no finding is unique to Ménière disease.
- Horizontal nystagmus may be seen during attacks.
- Otoscopy is typically normal.
- Triggering of attacks in the office with Dix-Hallpike maneuver suggests diagnosis of benign paroxysmal positional vertigo, not Meniere.

DIAGNOSTIC TESTS & INTERPRETATION
Testing done to rule out other conditions, and does not necessarily confirm or exclude Meniere disease

Lab
Initial lab tests
- Serologic tests specific for *Treponema pallidum*: Microhemagglutination (MHA), fluorescent treponemal antibody (FTA), *Treponema* immobilization test (TPI) (1)[C]
- Thyroid, fasting blood sugar, and lipid studies

Imaging
Magnetic resonance imaging (MRI) to rule out acoustic neuroma or other CNS pathology, including tumor, aneurysm, and multiple sclerosis (MS).

Initial approach
- Detailed history and physical exam
- Labs, audiometry, consider MRI

Diagnostic Procedures/Surgery
- Auditory:
  - Audiometry using pure tone and speech to show low-frequency sensorineural (nerve) loss and impaired speech discrimination. Usually shows low-frequency sensorineural hearing loss.
  - Tuning fork tests (i.e., Weber and Rinne) will confirm validity of audiometry.
  - Auditory brainstem response audiometry (ABR) to rule out acoustic neuroma
  - Electrocochleography (ECOG) may be useful to confirm etiology (1).
- Vestibular:
  - Caloric testing: Electronystagmography (ENG) may show reduced caloric response. Can obtain reasonably comparable information with use of 0.8 mL of ice water caloric testing. Reduced activity on either side is consistent with Ménière diagnosis, but is not itself diagnostic.
  - Drugs that may alter lab results: Any sedating medication may affect and invalidate vestibular testing.

Pathological Findings
Histologic temporal bone analysis (at autopsy). Dilation of inner ear fluid system may be seen.

DIFFERENTIAL DIAGNOSIS
- Acoustic neuroma or other CNS tumor
- Syphilis
- Perilymphatic fistula
- Viral labyrinthitis
- Transient ischemic attack (TIA), migraine
- Vertebrobasilar disease
- Other labyrinthine disorders that produce similar symptoms (e.g., Cogan syndrome, benign positional vertigo, temporal bone trauma)
- Diabetes or thyroid dysfunction
- Vestibular neuronitis
- Medication side effects
- Otitis media

TREATMENT

- Can usually be managed in outpatient setting
- A paucity of evidence-based guidelines exist regarding treatment for Ménière disease; therefore, there is no "gold standard" treatment.
- Medications are given primarily for symptomatic relief of vertigo and nausea, not to change disease progression.
- During attacks, bed rest with eyes closed and protection from falling. Attacks rarely last >4 hours.

MEDICATION
First Line
- Acute attack: Initial goal is immediate stabilization and symptom relief. For severe episodes, choose one: (2)[C]
  - Benzodiazepines (such as diazepam): Decrease vertigo and anxiety
  - Antihistamines (meclizine/dimenhydrinate): Decrease vertigo and nausea
  - Anticholinergics (transdermal scopolamine): Prevents nausea and emesis associated with "motion sickness"
  - Antidopaminergic (metoclopramide, promethazine): Decreases nausea, anxiety
  - Rehydration therapy and electrolyte replacement
  - Steroid taper for acute hearing loss
- Maintenance (goal is to prevent/reduce attacks)
- Lifestyle changes (low-salt diet, etc.) are needed.
- Diuretics are frequently used, and may help reduce attacks by decreasing the pressure and volume of endolymphatic fluid; however, there is insufficient evidence at this time (2)[C],(3)[A]:

- Hydrochlorothiazide/Triamterene (Dyazide, Maxzide)
- Acetazolamide (Diamox)
- Contraindications:
  - Atropine: Cardiac disease, especially SVT and other arrhythmias, prostatic enlargement
  - Scopolamine: Children and elderly, prostatic enlargement
  - Diuretics: Electrolyte abnormalities, renal disease
- Precautions:
  - Sedating drugs should be used with caution, particularly in the elderly. Patients should be cautioned not to operate motor vehicles or machinery. Atropine and scopolamine should be used with particular caution.
  - Diuretics: Monitor electrolytes. Use with caution in patients with sulfa allergy.
- Significant possible interactions: Transdermal scopolamine: Anticholinergics, belladonna products, antihistamines, tricyclic antidepressants, other

Second Line
- Steroids have been used, both intratympanic and systemically (oral or IV) for longer treatment of hearing loss:
  - Intratympanic administration results in higher steroid levels in the inner ear and may be more effective and safer than systemic (2)[C].
  - Addition of prednisone 30 mg/d to diuretic treatment reduced severity and frequency of tinnitus and vertigo in 1 pilot study (4)[C].
- In Europe, one of the preferred drugs is betahistine, a histamine agonist (unavailable in US). Insufficient evidence to state effectiveness: Other vasodilators, such as isosorbide dinitrate, niacin and histamine, have also been used, but evidence of their effectiveness is sparse (2)[C].
- Famvir has also been studied for the treatment of vertigo and stabilization of hearing. Evidence is lacking, but indicates more improvement in hearing than balance (5)[B].
- Inner ear perfusion with gentamicin and steroids have helped control and stabilize vertigo and hearing loss in Meniere's disease (6)[A]

ADDITIONAL TREATMENT
Issues for Referral
- Consider ear, nose, throat (ENT)/neurology referral for confirmation, further testing.
- All patients need formal audiometry to confirm hearing loss.

Additional Therapies
- Application of intermittent pressures via a myringotomy using a Meniett device has been found in some studies to relieve dizziness:
  - Safe; requires a long-term tympanostomy tube
- Vestibular rehabilitation may be beneficial for patients with persistent vestibular symptoms (7)[A]:
  - Safe and effective treatment for unilateral vestibular dysfunction
  - When attacks are disabling, the patient should be encouraged to slowly resume activity as soon as able.

COMPLEMENTARY AND ALTERNATIVE MEDICINE
Insufficient evidence to support effectiveness, but many integrative (CAM) techniques have been tried, including (2)[C]:

- Acupuncture (8)[A], acupressure, Tai Chi
- Niacin, bioflavonoids, lipoflavonoids, ginger, ginkgo biloba, and other herbal supplements

SURGERY/OTHER PROCEDURES
- Interventions that preserve hearing (9)[B]:
  - Endolymphatic sac surgery, either decompression or drainage of endolymph into mastoid or subarachnoid space:
    - Less invasive; may decrease vertigo, may influence hearing or tinnitus
    - There is insufficient evidence of the beneficial effect of endolymphatic sac surgery in Ménière's disease (10)[A]
  - Vestibular nerve section (intracranial procedure):
    - More invasive due to intracranial location
    - Decreases vertigo and preserves hearing
  - Tympanostomy tube: May decrease symptoms by decreasing the middle ear pressure
- Interventions for patients with no serviceable hearing (9)[C]:
  - Labyrinthectomy: Very effective at controlling vertigo, but causes deafness
  - Vestibular neurectomy
  - Many patients may be candidates for cochlear implantation if they have lost serviceable hearing.

 ## ONGOING CARE

FOLLOW-UP RECOMMENDATIONS
Patient Monitoring
Due to the possibility of progressive hearing loss despite eventual decrease in vertiginous attacks, it is important to have close follow-up to monitor changes in hearing, and continue surveillance for more serious underlying causes (acoustic neuroma, etc.).

DIET
- Diet is usually not a factor, unless attacks are brought on by certain foods.
- Some physicians restrict salt, but this is not supported by randomized controlled trials (1)[C].

PATIENT EDUCATION
- Limit activity during attacks.
- Between attacks, patient may be fully active but is often limited due to fear or lingering symptoms. This can be severely disabling.
- Patient information, including support group contacts, is available from the Vestibular Disorders Association: http://www.vestibular.org and the American Academy of Otolaryngology-Head and Neck Surgery: http://www.entnet.org/HealthInformation/menieresDisease.cfm

PROGNOSIS
- Alternating attacks and remission
- 1/2 of cases resolve spontaneously within 2–3 years, but can last >20 years. Severity and frequency of attacks diminish, but hearing loss is often progressive.
- 90% of patients can be managed successfully with medication. 5–10% of patients require surgery for incapacitating vertigo.
- Clinicians must not overlook possibility of acoustic tumor, which produces an identical clinical picture.

COMPLICATIONS
Loss of hearing; injury during attack; inability to work

REFERENCES

1. Sajjadi H, Paparella MM. Meniere's disease. *Lancet.* 2008;372:406–14.
2. Coelho DH, Lalwani AK. Medical Management Of Ménière's Disease. *Laryngoscope.* 2008.
3. Thirlwall AS, Kundu S. Diuretics for Ménière's disease or syndrome. *Cochrane Database Syst Rev.* 2006;3:CD003599.
4. Morales-Luckie E, Cornejo-Suarez A, Zaragoza-Contreras MA, et al. Oral administration of prednisone to control refractory vertigo in Ménière's disease: a pilot study. *Otol Neurotol.* 2005;26:1022–6.
5. Derebery MJ, Fisher LM, Iqbal Z. Randomized double-blinded, placebo-controlled clinical trial of famciclovir for reduction of Ménière's disease symptoms. *Otolaryngol Head Neck Surg.* 2004;131:877–84.
6. Hamid M et al. Medical management of common peripheral vestibular diseases. *Curr Opin Otolaryngol Head Neck Surg.* 2010;18:407–12.
7. Hillier SL, Hollohan V. Vestibular rehabilitation for unilateral peripheral vestibular dysfunction. *Cochrane Database Syst Rev.* 2007;CD005397.
8. Long AF, Xing M, Morgan K, et al. Exploring the Evidence Base for Acupuncture in the Treatment of Meniere's Syndrome—A Systematic Review. *Evid Based Complement Alternat Med.* 2009.
9. van Benthem PP, Giard JL, Verschuur HP. Surgery for Ménière's disease (Protocol). *Cochrane Database of Systematic Reviews.* 2005, Issue 3. Art. No.: CD005395. DOI:10.1002/14651858.CD005395.
10. Pullens B, Giard JL, Verschuur HP, van Benthem PP et al. Surgery for Ménière's disease. *Cochrane Database Syst Rev.* 2010;CD005395.

See Also (Topic, Algorithm, Electronic Media Element)
Labyrinthitis; Tinnitus; Hearing Loss
Algorithm: Vertigo

 ## CODES

ICD9
386.00 Meniere's disease, unspecified

CLINICAL PEARLS
- Diagnosis of Ménière disease is clinical, based on repeated episodes of vertigo, hearing loss, and tinnitus or aural fullness.
- Multiple medical, surgical, and rehabilitative treatments are available to decrease the severity and frequency of attacks. Some of these may preserve hearing, while some destroy it.
- A patient is likely to have progressive hearing loss despite a natural progression toward fewer vertigo attacks.
- When considering Ménière disease in a patient with vertigo and hearing loss, acoustic neuromas must also be considered.
- Take symptoms seriously, as they may be disabling.

M

MENINGITIS, BACTERIAL

Paul R. Gordon, MD, MPH

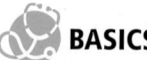 **BASICS**

DESCRIPTION
Bacterial meningitis is an inflammation of the pia-arachnoid and its fluid and the fluid of the ventricles:

- Always cerebrospinal
- System(s) affected: Nervous

ALERT
Bacterial meningitis is a medical, neurological, and sometimes neurosurgical emergency.
Community-acquired meningitis caused by *Streptococcus pneumoniae* has case fatality rates from 19–37% in adults.

Geriatric Considerations
Signs and symptoms may be less evident and less specific in elderly patients with other disorders, such as congestive heart failure and pneumonia.

EPIDEMIOLOGY
- Predominant age: Neonates, infants, and elderly
- Predominant sex: Male = Female

Incidence
3–10/100,000 population

RISK FACTORS
- Immunocompromised host
- Alcoholism, diabetes
- Neurosurgical procedure or head injury
- Abdominal surgery at risk for gram-negative infection

Genetics
Individuals of Navajo Indian or American Eskimo descent may have genetic or acquired vulnerability to invasive disease.

GENERAL PREVENTION
- Prompt medical treatment for infections
- Strict aseptic techniques when treating patients with head wounds or skull fractures
- Look for evidence of cerebrospinal fluid fistula in patients with recurrent meningitis.
- Meningitis caused by *Haemophilus influenzae* has been nearly eliminated due to routine vaccination.
- Conjugate vaccines against *S. pneumoniae* may reduce the burden of disease in childhood and may produce herd immunity among adults.
- Persons with close contact to patients with meningococcal meningitis must receive chemoprophylaxis to eradicate carriage.

PATHOPHYSIOLOGY
Bacterial infection causes inflammation of the pia-arachnoid and its fluid and the fluid of the ventricles.

ETIOLOGY
Bacteria are divided into age groups to guide empiric therapy (percentages indicate relative incidence). Any organism can cause meningitis in any age group; therapy should be guided by culture whenever possible:

- Neonates:
  – Group B *Streptococcus*: 50% of cases
  – *Escherichia coli*: 25%
  – Other gram-negative rods: 8%
  – *Listeria monocytogenes*: 6%
  – *S. pneumoniae*: 5%
  – Group A *Streptococcus*: 4%
  – *H. influenzae*: 3%
- In adults up to age 60:
  – *S. pneumoniae*: 60%
  – *Neisseria meningitidis*: 20%
  – *H. influenzae*: 10%
  – *L. monocytogenes*: 6%
  – Group B *Streptococcus*: 4%
- In adults ≥60 years old:
  – *S. pneumoniae*: 70%
  – *L. monocytogenes*: 20%
  – *N. meningitidis*: 3–4%
  – Group B *Streptococcus*: 3–4%
  – *H. influenzae*: 3–4%

COMMONLY ASSOCIATED CONDITIONS
The following conditions are associated with a worse prognosis:

- Coma
- Seizures
- Alcoholism
- Old age
- Infancy
- Diabetes mellitus
- Multiple myeloma
- Head trauma

 DIAGNOSIS

HISTORY
- Antecedent upper respiratory infection
- Fever
- Headache
- Vomiting
- Photophobia
- Seizures
- Nausea
- Rigors
- Profuse sweats
- Weakness
- Elderly: Subtle findings commonly including confusion

PHYSICAL EXAM
The triad of fever, neck stiffness, and altered mental status has low sensitivity (44%). However, almost all patients present with at least 2 out of 4 symptoms: Headache, fever, neck stiffness, and altered mental status:

- Meningismus
- Signs of cerebral dysfunction
- Altered mental status
- Focal neurologic deficits
- Meningococcal rash: Macular and erythematous at first, then petechial or purpuric

DIAGNOSTIC TESTS & INTERPRETATION
Lab
Initial lab tests
- Cerebrospinal fluid (CSF) analysis: (Turbid)
- Neonates:
  – >10 white blood cells (WBCs) in CSF
  – CSF: Blood glucose ratio <0.6
  – CSF protein >150 mg/dL
- Infants/children:
  – >5 WBCs in CSF
  – CSF: Blood glucose ratio <0.6
  – CSF protein >50 mg/dL
- Adults:
  – 1,000–100,000 WBCs in CSF
  – CSF: Blood glucose ratio <0.4
  – CSF protein >45 mg/dL (usually 150–400 mg/dL)
  – Suspect ruptured brain abscess when WBC count is unusually high (>100,000).
- In all age groups:
  – CSF opening pressure above 180 mm H_2O (1.77 kPa) (kilopascal)
  – CSF gram stain–positive in 75% of untreated patients
  – CSF culture positive: 70–80% of cases
  – Bacterial testing using polymerase chain reaction (PCR) (particularly in those with negative cultures) (*not yet routinely recommended*)
- Serum WBCs: Rarely useful in differentiating bacterial from viral illness
- Serum blood cultures:
  – Blood culture positive: 40–60% of cases
- Serum electrolytes
- Evaluation of clotting function if petechiae or purpuric lesions are noted

Imaging
- Computed tomography (CT) scan of head if concern for increased intracranial pressure or warning signs of space-occupying lesion (new-onset seizure, evolving signs of brain tissue shift, or papilledema)
- Chest radiograph may reveal silent area of pneumonitis or abscess.
- Sinus/skull radiographs may reveal cranial osteomyelitis, paranasal sinusitis, or skull fracture but rarely indicated.
- Later in course, head CT scan, if hydrocephalus, brain abscess, subdural effusions, and subdural empyema are considered or in those patients who have not responded clinically after 48 hours of appropriate antibiotics.

Diagnostic Procedures/Surgery
Lumbar puncture

Pathological Findings
- Pleocytosis in CSF
- Bacterial antigen tests should be reserved for cases in which the initial CSF gram stain is negative and CSF culture is negative at 48 hours of incubation.
- PCR of CSF and blood is most helpful for documenting meningococcal disease in the patient with negative cultures.

DIFFERENTIAL DIAGNOSIS
- Bacteremia
- Sepsis
- Brain abscess
- Seizures
- Other nonbacterial meningitides

TREATMENT

- If diagnosis is suspected, lumbar puncture should be done in office with antimicrobial therapy begun before transfer to hospital; if not possible, administer antibiotics promptly.
- Inpatient care: Intensive care unit (ICU) often required

MEDICATION
Empiric IV therapy until culture results available:
- Consider local patterns of bacterial sensitivity.
- See Etiology for age definitions and likely organisms.

First Line
The following regimens are somewhat simplified but will adequately treat patients pending culture results. Additional subgroupings may simplify treatment in some patients. Penicillin-allergic patients present a special challenge not covered here; seek infectious disease consultation:

- Neonates (give both) (1)[B]:
  – Ampicillin: 100–400 mg/kg/d divided q6–12h
  – Tobramycin: 7.5 mg/kg/d q6–8h (premature or <1 week of age, 2.5 mg/kg q12h)
- Infants >4 weeks of age:
  – Ampicillin: 300–400 mg/kg/d divided q4–6h (maximum, 2 g q3–4h) AND
  – Chloramphenicol: 75–100 mg/kg/d divided q6h OR
  – Ceftriaxone: 100 mg/kg/d divided q12–24h (maximum, 2 g q12h) or cefotaxime 200 mg/kg/d divided q4–6h AND
  – Vancomycin: 10–15 mg/kg q12h (maximum, 1,500 mg q12h)
- Adults (2,3)[A]:
  – Vancomycin: 1 g IV q12h AND
  – Ceftriaxone: 1–2 g IV q12–24h (maximum, 2 g q12h) OR cefotaxime 2 g IV q4–6h
- Precaution: Ototoxicity from aminoglycoside
- Contraindications: Allergies to specific antibiotics
- Treatment duration [A]:
  – N. meningitidis, H. influenzae: 7–10 days
  – S. pneumoniae: 10–14 days
  – Group B Streptococcus organisms, E. coli, L. monocytogenes: 14–21 days
  – Neonates: 12–21 days or at least 14 days after a repeated culture is sterile
- Corticosteroids (4)[A]:
  – Early treatment with dexamethasone decreases mortality and morbidity for pediatric patients >1 month old and in adults with acute bacterial meningitis, and does not increase the risk of gastrointestinal bleeding.
  – Dexamethasone: 0.15 mg/kg q6h (10 mg for adults), started 15–20 minutes before or with the antibiotic for 4 days

Second Line
- Antipseudomonal penicillins
- Aztreonam
- Quinolones (e.g., ciprofloxacin)
- Meropenem

ADDITIONAL TREATMENT
General Measures
- Appropriate empiric antibiotic therapy, initiated promptly
- Vigorous supportive care with constant nursing to ensure prompt recognition of seizures and prevention of aspiration
- Therapy for coexisting conditions
- Measures to prevent hypothermia and dehydration

Issues for Referral
Consultation from ICU specialist

IN-PATIENT CONSIDERATIONS
Admission Criteria
Bacterial meningitis requires hospitalization.

IV Fluids
There is no evidence to support other than maintenance fluid therapy (2,5)[A].

Nursing
- ICU monitoring may be needed to recognize changes in the patient's consciousness and the development of new neurologic signs, subtle seizures, and to treat severe agitation effectively.
- Patients with suspected meningococcal infection require respiratory isolation for 24 hours.

Discharge Criteria
May consider home therapy for the completion of IV antibiotic course once patient is clinically stable and culture and sensitivity results are known

ONGOING CARE

FOLLOW-UP RECOMMENDATIONS
Patient Monitoring
Brainstem auditory evoked response test should be performed on infants before hospital discharge:
- Further follow-up will depend on its results and course of meningitis while in hospital.

DIET
Regular as tolerated, except when syndrome of inappropriate secretion of antidiuretic hormone complicates course

PATIENT EDUCATION
Available at the American Academy of Pediatrics, 141 Northwest Point Blvd., P.O. Box 927, Elk Grove Village, IL 60009-0927; (800) 433-9016; http://www.aap.org/

PROGNOSIS
Overall case fatality 14%:
- H. influenzae: 5%
- N. meningitidis: 10%
- S. pneumoniae: 19–37%

COMPLICATIONS
- Seizures: 20–30%
- Focal neurologic deficit
- Cranial nerve palsies (III, VI, VII, VIII):
  – Comprises 10–20% of the cases
  – Usually disappear within a few weeks
- Sensorineural hearing loss: 10% in children
- Neurodevelopmental sequelae: 30% subtle learning deficits
- Obstructive hydrocephalus
- Subdural effusions
- Decline in consciousness that may be due to meningoencephalitis

REFERENCES

1. Chávez-Bueno S, McCracken GH. Bacterial meningitis in children. Pediatr Clin North Am. 2005;52:795–810, vii.
2. Prasad K, Singhal T, Jain N, Gupta PK. Third generation cephalosporins versus conventional antibiotics for treating acute bacterial meningitis. Cochrane Library, Cochrane Collaboration. 2005 Volume 4.
3. Schut ES, de Gans J, van de Beek D et al. Community-acquired bacterial meningitis in adults. Pract Neurol. 2008;8:8–23.
4. Assiri AM, Alasmari FA, Zimmerman VA, Baddour LM, Erwin PJ, Tleyjeh IM et al. Corticosteroid administration and outcome of adolescents and adults with acute bacterial meningitis: a meta-analysis. Mayo Clin. Proc. 2009;84:403–9.
5. Maconochie I, Baumer H, Stewart ME. Fluid therapy for acute bacterial meningitis. Cochrane Database Syst Rev. 2008;CD004786.

See Also (Topic, Algorithm, Electronic Media Element)
Meningitis, Viral; Meningococcemia
Algorithm: Delirium

CODES

ICD9
- 320.0 Hemophilus meningitis
- 320.1 Pneumococcal meningitis
- 320.9 Meningitis due to unspecified bacterium

CLINICAL PEARLS

- Suspected bacterial meningitis is a medical emergency, and immediate diagnostic steps must be taken to establish the specific cause. Antibiotic therapy should be initiated immediately after the lumbar puncture is performed if the clinical suspicion for meningitis is high.
- Neuroimaging is indicated in infants and children with signs or symptoms of complications and/or recurrent meningitis.
- Neurologic sequelae, including deafness, mental retardation, spasticity and/or paresis, and seizures, occur in 15–25% of infants and children.
- Streptococcus pneumoniae and Neisseria meningitidis are the most common causes of bacterial meningitis in infants and children >1 month of age.
- Neonatal meningitis should be suspected in any infant <1 month of age who presents with clinical findings of sepsis or meningitis. The most commonly reported signs are fever (rectal temperature >38C), hypothermia (rectal temperature ≤36C), irritability, and poor feeding or feeding intolerance. Bulging fontanelle and nuchal rigidity are observed in a minority of infants.

M

MENINGITIS, VIRAL

Luis K. Abrishamian, MD
Molly P. Keegan, MD

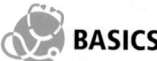
BASICS

DESCRIPTION
- System(s) affected: Nervous
- Synonym(s): Abacterial meningitis; Aseptic meningitis

EPIDEMIOLOGY
Incidence
- Peaks in late summer to early fall:
  - Enteroviruses and arthropod-borne viruses predominate in warm months.
  - Mumps usually occurs in the winter and spring, often in epidemics.
- Estimated 26,000–42,000 hospitalizations each year in the US (1)[A] for viral meningitis (VM)
- In 2006, there were 72,000 meningitis-related hospitalizations, with 58% of those having meningitis as the primary reason for hospitalization. Of all 72,000 hospitalizations, 56.4% were determined to be viral cases (2)[A].
- More common than bacterial meningitis
- Occurs in both outbreak and sporadic forms

RISK FACTORS
- Close contact with known case of VM
- Immunocompromised hosts may be more susceptible to cytomegalovirus (CMV), herpes simplex virus (HSV), and adenovirus.
- Lymphocytic choriomeningitis virus (LCMV) is commonly transmitted via exposure to rodent feces, bodily fluids, or nesting materials. Rodent bites and vertical transmission as mechanisms of infection are possible but unconfirmed.

Geriatric Considerations
Cases of VM in the elderly are rare but documented. Consider alternative diagnoses [e.g., carcinomatous meningitis, nonsteroidal anti-inflammatory drug (NSAID) or medication-induced meningitis, etc.] in the elderly population.

Genetics
No genetic predispositions have been established relating to increased susceptibility to VM.

GENERAL PREVENTION
Limit exposure to known hosts, hand-washing, and general hygiene

PATHOPHYSIOLOGY
- Viral infection and inflammation of the meninges and cerebrospinal fluid (CSF)
- In immunocompetent hosts, VM is generally caused by a systemic viral infection with predilection to neurologic involvement.
- Less commonly, direct neural transmission occurs from a self-limited infection such as HSV already present in the immunocompetent host.

ETIOLOGY
- >90% of cases caused by enterovirus family, which includes coxsackievirus A and B, echovirus, poliovirus, and E# variants: E9 and E30 strains specifically implicated in eastern and western hemispheres, respectively.

- Less common causes include HSV-1 and -2, varicella-zoster virus, adenovirus, LCMV, CMV, Epstein-Barr virus (EBV), human immunodeficiency virus (HIV), and mumps.
- Recurrent (Mollaret) meningitis shows 80% association with HSV-2.
- Arthropod-borne viruses: West Nile virus, St. Louis encephalitis virus, and California encephalitis virus
- Parvovirus B19 is found in the CSF of 4.3% of undiagnosed meningoencephalitis patients (3)[B].

COMMONLY ASSOCIATED CONDITIONS
- Encephalitis
- Neurologic deficits
- Myopericarditis
- Neonatal enteroviral sepsis

DIAGNOSIS

Predominant symptoms include
- Fever
- Headache
- Photophobia
- Myalgias
- Nausea
- Vomiting

HISTORY
- Travel and exposure history
- Sexual activity (e.g., HSV, HIV, etc.)
- Outdoor exposure (Lyme disease)
- Rodent feces and/or urine exposure (LCMV)
- Solid-organ transplant (LCMV, CMV) (4)[C]

PHYSICAL EXAM
- Nuchal rigidity
- Fever (>100.4°F/38°C)
- Meningeal signs should not be used exclusively to diagnose or rule out meningitis (2)[C]; these include
  - Nuchal rigidity
  - Brudzinski sign: Neck flexion elicits involuntary knee flexion in supine patient.
  - Kernig sign: Resistance to knee extension following flexion of hips and knees by physician
- In the presence of erythema chronicum migrans or cranial neuropathy, consider Lyme meningitis given correlation with exposure and endemic area (5)[C].
- Be aware of mucocutaneous findings such as dermatologic manifestations (e.g., vesicular rash in hand, foot, and mouth disease), herpangina, and generalized maculopapular rash.

DIAGNOSTIC TESTS & INTERPRETATION
Lab
Initial lab tests
- Lumbar puncture (LP) is standard of care in patients with high clinical suspicion:
  - Indications for LP include fever, sudden abrupt mental status change, headache, and/or lethargy. Clinical judgment is to be used in all cases. In patients with high suspicion of bacterial meningitis, antibiotic treatment should be started immediately.

- CSF analysis: Glucose, protein, white blood cell (WBC) count with differential, red blood cell (RBC) count, Gram stain, culture
- Typical CSF findings in viral meningitis:
  - Elevated WBC count: 10–1,000/mm^3, classically with a lymphocyte predominance
  - Initial phase of illness (1st 24–48 h) may show neutrophil predominance.
  - Protein normal to slightly elevated (<150 mg/dL)
  - Negative Gram stain and bacterial culture
  - Elevated opening pressure:
    - Culture CSF for enteroviruses, HSV, and mumps. However, viral culture may yield no additional benefit when nucleic acid amplification has been employed (6)[C].
    - Polymerase chain reaction (PCR) has a sensitivity of 95–100% for HSV-1 and -2, EBV, and enterovirus, allowing for earlier hospital discharge and less intervention.
    - Reverse-transcriptase PCR test is approved by the Food and Drug Administration (FDA) for enteroviral meningitis: Results are available within 2.5 h.
- Electroencephalogram (EEG) in some cases, especially if encephalitis is a consideration
- Complete blood count (CBC): Normal or mildly elevated WBCs
- Blood culture
- Viral cultures and/or antibody titers
- Serum procalcitonin (>0.5 ng/mL) and CSF protein (>0.5 g/L) have high correlation with pediatric bacterial versus aseptic meningitis.

Follow-Up & Special Considerations
- Exercise clinical judgment regarding contraindications to LP. They include
  - Increased intracranial pressure owing to mass lesion
  - Ventricular obstruction
  - Local infection at potential LP site or suspected epidural abscess
  - Anticoagulation or coagulopathy
  - Possibility of cardiorespiratory compromise secondary to patient positioning during procedure
- Disorders that may alter lab results:
  - Diabetes: Consider blood sugar level to correlate with CSF glucose level
  - Preexisting neurologic diseases (e.g., intracranial neoplasm, demyelinating disease)

Imaging
Initial approach
- Indication for imaging rests with consideration of alternative diagnoses; may be performed prior to LP in the presence of papilledema, spinal cord trauma, altered mental status, or focal neurologic findings. Prior to performing LP, CT scan may not be clinically necessary in the absence of risk factors.
- Standard techniques include noncontrast brain CT scan or MRI.

DIFFERENTIAL DIAGNOSIS
- Bacterial meningitis
- Encephalitis
- Epidural abscess
- Other infectious agents:
  - Tuberculosis
  - Syphilis
  - Leptospirosis
  - Lyme disease

- Parameningeal infections (e.g., subdural empyema)
- Postinfectious encephalomyelitis
- Viral syndrome (e.g., influenza)
- Leukemia and carcinomatous meningitis
- Migraine headache
- Acute metabolic encephalopathy
- Chemical meningitis
- Brain abscess

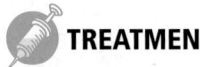 TREATMENT

MEDICATION
- Analgesics (adult doses):
  - Morphine: 0.05–0.1 mg/kg IV, titrated to pain relief
  - Hydromorphone (Dilaudid): 1–2 mg IV, titrated to pain relief
  - Hydrocodone (Vicodin): 5/500 mg 1–2 tablets PO q6h oroxycodone (Percocet) 5/325 mg 1–2 tablets PO q4–6h
- Antiemetics:
  - Promethazine (Phenergan): 12.5–25 mg IV q4h
  - Prochlorperazine (Compazine): 10 mg IM/IV q4h
  - Ondansetron (Zofran): 4–8 mg IV q8h
  - Metoclopramide (Reglan): 10–20 mg IV/IM q4–6h
- Antipyretics: Acetaminophen (Tylenol): 650 mg PO or rectal suppository q4h
- Antiviral agents: Initiate empirical acyclovir at 10 mg/kg q8h for patients with CSF pleocytosis, negative Gram stain, and suspicion for HSV while awaiting results of definitive (e.g., HSV PCR) testing (7).
- Antibiotics:
  - Not indicated for treatment of viral meningitis
  - If parameters suggest a viral etiology, treat symptomatically, and follow the patient closely in the hospital setting.
  - If in doubt, initiate an IV or IM broad-spectrum antibiotic with good CSF penetration.
- Precautions: Aspirin should be avoided in children and adolescents owing to a possible association with Reye syndrome.

ADDITIONAL TREATMENT
General Measures
- IV fluids if oral intake is poor or vomiting is present
- Pain management

IN-PATIENT CONSIDERATIONS
Admission Criteria
VM is generally treated on an outpatient basis, in contrast to the bacterial form; those with VM plus complicating factors may be hospitalized.

IV Fluids
May use normal saline bolus or continuous infusion based on clinical judgment.

Nursing
- Neurologic monitoring for changes in mental status, fever, etc. to assess disease progression or alternate diagnosis
- Contact precautions until bacterial meningitis is ruled out
- Private room indicated with sterile precautions
- Encourage hand-washing

Discharge Criteria
Symptomatic relief

 ONGOING CARE

FOLLOW-UP RECOMMENDATIONS
Follow-up with primary-care physician

Patient Monitoring
Monitor for relapse or exacerbation of symptoms after treatment course.

DIET
- Determined by symptoms
- May need to order NPO owing to nausea or vomiting
- Advance to clear fluids and regular diet as tolerated

PATIENT EDUCATION
- Discuss possibility, but low probability, of transmission to contacts.
- Expected duration of illness (5–10 days)
- For patient education materials, refer patients to the online EBSCO Health Library article "Viral Meningitis" (http://healthlibrary.epnet.com/GetContent.aspx?token=38405ca3-6cab-4817-9cba-dc64dc5c69f1&chunkiid=11469).

PROGNOSIS
- Complete recovery generally within 5–7 days
- Headaches and other uncomfortable symptoms may persist intermittently for 1–2 weeks.
- Only 0.6% of hospitalizations for VM resulted in death in recent study.
- European studies have shown some residual postmeningeal cognitive impairment.

COMPLICATIONS
- Post-LP headache
- Fatigue
- Irritability
- Muscle weakness
- Seizures (rare)

REFERENCES

1. Centers for Disease Control and Prevention (CDC). Outbreaks of aseptic meningitis associated with echoviruses 9 and 30 and preliminary surveillance reports on enterovirus activity–United States, 2003. MMWR Morb Mortal Wkly Rep. 2003;52:761–4.
2. Thomas KE, et al. The diagnostic accuracy of Kernig's sign, Brudzinski's sign, and nuchal rigidity in adults with suspected meningitis. Clin Infect Dis. 20021;35(1):46–52.
3. Barah F, et al. Association of human parvovirus B19 infection with acute meningoencephalitis. Lancet. 2001;358(9299):2168.
4. Fischer SA, Graham MB, Kuehnert MJ, et al. Transmission of lymphocytic choriomeningitis virus by organ transplantation. N Engl J Med. 2006;354:2235–49.
5. Eppes SC, Nelson DK, Lewis LL, et al. Characterization of Lyme meningitis and comparison with viral meningitis in children. Pediatrics. 1999;103:957–60.
6. Polage CR, Petti CA. Assessment of the utility of viral culture of cerebrospinal fluid. Clin Infect Dis. 2006;43:1578–9.
7. Swadron SP et al. Pitfalls in the management of headache in the emergency department. Emerg. Med. Clin. North Am. 2010;28.
8. Ratial BO, Costa J, Sampaio C. Antibiotic prophylaxis for preventing meningitis in patients with basilar skull fractures. Cochrane Database of Systematic Reviews 2006, Issue 1. Art. No.: CD004884. DOI:10.1002/14651858. CD004884.pub2.

ADDITIONAL READING
- Holmquist L. (Thomson Reuters), Russo C.A. (Thomson Reuters), and Elixhauser A. (AHRQ). Meningitis-Related Hospitalizations in the United States, 2006. HCUP Statistical Brief #57. July 2008. Agency for Healthcare Research and Quality, Rockville, MD. http://www.hcup-us.ahrq.gov/reports/statbriefs/sb57.pdf
- Logan SA, MacMahon E. Viral meningitis. BMJ. 2008;336:36–40.

See Also (Topic, Algorithm, Electronic Media Element)
Algorithm: Delirium

CODES

ICD9
- 047.0 Meningitis due to coxsackie virus
- 047.1 Meningitis due to echo virus
- 047.8 Other specified viral meningitis

CLINICAL PEARLS
- Antibiotic administration hours or days prior to CSF analysis may result in "partially treated" bacterial meningitis that mimics VM.
- Viral versus bacterial meningitis cannot be distinguished clinically; refer all suspected meningitis cases to hospital for diagnosis and management.
- VM is much more common in the pediatric population than is bacterial meningitis. As age increases, the likelihood of a bacterial cause also increases.
- Morbidity with VM is low but increases with associated encephalitis.
- There is no evidence to support meningitis prophylaxis in basilar skull fracture with or without CSF leakage (8).

M

MENINGOCOCCEMIA

Rajneesh S. Hazarika, MD, MS

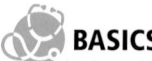 **BASICS**

DESCRIPTION
- Caused by *Neisseria meningitidis* in the blood, which results in a broad spectrum of clinical manifestations
- Bacteremia without sepsis: Patient has upper respiratory symptoms only and recovers spontaneously without antibiotic.
- Bacteremia without meningitis: Patient is acutely ill, and may have skin manifestations (rashes, petechiae, and ecchymosis) and hypotension.
- Bacteremia with meningitis:
  – Predominant clinical picture of meningitis: Headache, decreased sensorium, and neck rigidity
  – Skin manifestations and hypotension may also be present.
- Bacteremia with acute arthritis dermatitis syndrome: Patient may have tenosynovitis typical of gonococcal etiology.

EPIDEMIOLOGY
Incidence
- 0.3–1.0/100,000 in the US (2,500–3,500 cases annually)
- Incidence during epidemics in sub-Saharan Africa can be as high as 2%.

RISK FACTORS
- Age: 3 months–1 year
- Late complement component deficiency (C5, C6, C7, C8, or C9)
- Household contacts
- Contacts in nurseries and day care centers
- Close quarters (e.g., dormitories, campus bars, and military barracks)

Genetics
Late complement component deficiency has an autosomal recessive inheritance.

GENERAL PREVENTION
- Quadrivalent meningococcal polysaccharide-protein conjugate vaccine (MCV4) is available.
- Vaccine is recommended for all persons 11–18 and persons 19–55 at increased risk for the disease:
  – Guillain-Barré syndrome has been associated with the MCV4 vaccine, so personal history of Guillain-Barré is a relative contraindication for receiving this vaccine (1)[A],(2)[B].
- Vaccine is required by the Government of Saudi Arabia for Hajj pilgrims above age 2 and is also recommended by the CDC for this group of travelers.
- CDC also advises vaccination for travelers to sub-Saharan Africa (meningitis belt) during dry season.

ETIOLOGY
- *Neisseria meningitidis*, a gram-negative diplococcus with at least 13 serotypes
- Major serogroups in the US: B, C, Y, and W-135:
  – Serogroup B is predominant cause of meningococcemia in children <1 year of age.
  – Serogroup C is the most common cause in the US.
- Major serogroups worldwide are B, C, and W-135:
  – W-135 is the major cause of disease in the "meningitis belt" of sub-Saharan Africa.

 DIAGNOSIS

HISTORY
- Symptoms:
  – Fever, headache, chills, rigor, sore throat
  – Changes in mental status, stiff neck, convulsions
  – Arthralgias, arthritis
- Be sure to ask about possible exposures: Living in barracks, dormitories, and travel to endemic regions, especially sub-Saharan Africa

PHYSICAL EXAM
- Look for skin findings: Maculopapular rash, petechiae, ecchymosis, purpura.
- Stiff neck, focal neurologic signs, coma
- Hypotension, shock

DIAGNOSTIC TESTS & INTERPRETATION

ALERT
- When meningococcemia is suspected, treatment should never be delayed for diagnostic tests.
- Antibiotic administration may render blood and/or CSF culture negative within 2 hours, so begin treatment and then test.

Lab
Initial lab tests
- Leukocytosis or leukopenia
- Left shift of leukocytes, toxic granulation
- Thrombocytopenia
- Lactic acidosis
- Prolonged PT/PTT
- Low fibrinogen
- Elevated fibrin degradation products
- Blood culture growing *N. meningitidis*
- Cerebrospinal fluid:
  – Cloudy
  – Increased white blood cells with polymorphonuclear cells predominant
  – Gram stain showing gram-negative diplococci
  – Glucose-to-blood glucose ratio <0.4
  – Protein >45 mg/dL
  – Positive for *N. meningitidis* antigen (MAT or PCR)
  – Culture positive for *N. meningitidis*

Imaging
Initial approach
CT scan of head if concern for space-occupying lesions

Diagnostic Procedures/Surgery
- Blood culture
- Lumbar puncture:
  – After a brief history and physical exam suggest meningitis, initiate antibiotics and then proceed with lumbar puncture within 1 hour.

Pathological Findings
- Disseminated intravascular coagulation
- Exudates on meninges
- Polymorphonuclear infiltration of meninges
- Hemorrhage of adrenal glands

DIFFERENTIAL DIAGNOSIS
- Septicemia due to other microorganism
- Meningitis due to other pyogenic bacteria
- Gonococcemia
- Acute bacterial endocarditis
- Rocky Mountain spotted fever
- Hemolytic uremic syndrome
- Gonococcal arthritis dermatitis syndrome
- Influenza

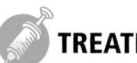 **TREATMENT**

MEDICATION
First Line
- In patients strongly suspected of having meningitis, consider administering dexamethasone 0.15 mg/kg q6h for 16 doses, starting 15 minutes before 1st dose of antibiotic:
  – Corticosteroids are likely less effective in cases of meningococcal meningitis and patients with HIV (3)[B].
  – Use of corticosteroids lowers mortality in adults but may not improve outcomes in pediatric patients.
- Treatment for suspected meningococcal meningitis must begin as soon as possible; coverage for other possible causes of meningitis must be given until a definitive diagnosis is made.
- Age influences etiologic organism.
- Age <4 weeks: Ampicillin plus cefotaxime or ceftriaxone
- Age 4–12 weeks: Ampicillin plus cefotaxime or Ceftriaxone plus Vancomycin
- Age 12 weeks to adulthood: Cefotaxime or ceftriaxone plus vancomycin

- When treating an adult patient with suspected meningitis, initiate early therapy as above. Once *N. meningitidis* is identified, the drug of choice remains penicillin (4)[C].
- For meningitis:
  - Penicillin G 4 million units IV q4h (pediatric dose: 0.25 mU/kg IV q4–6h) or ampicillin2 g IV q4h (pediatric dose: 200–300 mg/kg IV q6h)
  - Use alternate drugs if patient is allergic to penicillin.
- For other infections: Use 1/2 the dose for meningitis.
- Duration of treatment: 7–10 days
- Chemoprophylaxis for close contacts (household members and personnel in nurseries, day care centers, nursing homes, dormitories, and other closed institutions) and vaccination of household contacts (if case is a vaccine preventable serogroup) (5)[A]. No chemoprophylaxis is needed for casual contacts, health care personnel (except persons giving mouth-to-mouth resuscitation), schoolmates, and office co-workers:
  - Rifampin 600 mg (pediatric dose: 10 mg/kg) PO q12h for 2 days or (for adults only) 1 dose of ciprofloxacin 750 mg PO (6)[B]
- Precautions:
  - Adjust dosage of both medications in patients with severe renal dysfunction.
  - Rifampin ingestion causes orange urine.

Second Line
- For meningitis:
  - Chloramphenicol 1 g IV q6h (pediatric dose: 75–100 mg/kg q6h) or ceftriaxone 2 g IV q12h (pediatric dose: 80–100 mg/kg q12–24h)
  - In large outbreaks, a single dose of long-acting chloramphenicol has been used. Single-dose ceftriaxone shows equal efficacy in 1 RCT [B].
- Precautions:
  - Ceftriaxone should not be used in patients with history of anaphylactic reactions to penicillin (e.g., hypotension, laryngeal edema, wheezing, hives).
  - Chloramphenicol may cause aplastic anemia.
- For other infections:
  - Ceftriaxone 1 g (pediatric dose: 40 mg/kg) IV q24h

ADDITIONAL TREATMENT
General Measures
- Appropriate antibiotic
- Supportive care:
  - IV fluids
  - Oxygen when needed
- Close monitoring of patient for seizure activity

Issues for Referral
Potential complications:
- Disseminated intravascular coagulation (DIC)
- Acute respiratory distress syndrome
- Renal failure
- Adrenal failure

IN-PATIENT CONSIDERATIONS
Initial Stabilization
- If meningitis suspected, initiate antibiotics and then proceed to immediate lumbar puncture.
- Droplet isolation for 24 hours from the beginning of antibiotic therapy

Admission Criteria
Admit patient to ICU if severe sepsis or meningitis is suspected.

IV Fluids
- Replace volume as needed.
- Patient may present with septic shock and will require resuscitation with large volumes of crystalloid.

 ## ONGOING CARE

FOLLOW-UP RECOMMENDATIONS
- Before discharge, to eradicate carriage, give patient a prescription for rifampin 600 mg (children 10 mg/kg) PO q12h for 2 days or, for adults only, 1 dose of ciprofloxacin 500–750 mg PO (6)[B].
- In patients with neurologic deficits, follow-up with a neurologist may be needed.

DIET
As tolerated, depending on clinical condition

PATIENT EDUCATION
- Educate family and close contacts regarding risk of contracting meningococcal infections.
- Educate healthcare personnel who are not at risk of contracting meningococcal infections.

PROGNOSIS
Overall mortality 10%

COMPLICATIONS
- DIC
- Acute tubular necrosis
- Seizures
- Focal neurologic deficit
- Cranial nerve palsies
- Sensorineural hearing loss
- Obstructive hydrocephalus
- Subdural effusions
- Acute adrenal hemorrhage
- Waterhouse-Friderichsen syndrome

REFERENCES

1. Centers for Disease Control and Prevention (CDC) Advisory Committee on Immunization Practices. Revised recommendations of the Advisory Committee on Immunization Practices to Vaccinate all Persons Aged 11–18 Years with Meningococcal Conjugate Vaccine. *MMWR Morb Mortal Wkly Rep.* 2007;56:794–5.
2. Centers for Disease Control and Prevention (CDC). Update: Guillain-Barré syndrome among recipients of Menactra meningococcal conjugate vaccine–United States, June 2005–September 2006. *MMWR Morb Mortal Wkly Rep.* 2006;55:1120–4.
3. Scarborough M, Gordon SB, Whitty CJ, et al. Corticosteroids for bacterial meningitis in adults in sub-Saharan Africa. *N Engl J Med.* 2007;357: 2441–50.
4. Sinner SW, Tunkel AR. Antimicrobial agents in the treatment of bacterial meningitis. *Infect Dis Clin North Am.* 2004;18:581–602, ix.
5. Hoek MR, Christensen H, Hellenbrand W, et al. Effectiveness of vaccinating household contacts in addition to chemoprophylaxis after a case of meningococcal disease: a systematic review. *Epidemiol Infect.* 2008;1–7.
6. Fraser A, Gafter-Gvili A, Paul M, et al. Antibiotics for preventing meningococcal infections. *Cochrane Database Syst Rev.* 2005;CD004785.

ADDITIONAL READING

Recommended Immunization Schedules for Persons Aged 0 Through 18 Years - United Stated, 2010 January 8, 2010;58(51–52):1–4.

 ## CODES

ICD9
- 036.0 Meningococcal meningitis
- 036.2 Meningococcemia

CLINICAL PEARLS
- Chemoprophylaxis is needed for close contacts.
- Penicillin and cephalosporins alone will not eradicate carrier status; additional treatment with rifampin (for children or adults) or ciprofloxin (for adults only) is required.
- Prevention with vaccination is key.

M

MENISCAL INJURY

J. Herbert Stevenson, MD
Jeffrey Manning, MD

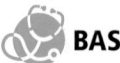

BASICS

DESCRIPTION
The menisci are essential parts of the knee joint for weight bearing, stabilization, energy absorption, and joint lubrication. Menisci help prevent anterior displacement of the tibia. Meniscal injuries can be acute or degenerative. The injury is more likely to be degenerative in people older than 40. The medial meniscus is more likely to be injured than the lateral meniscus because it is less mobile and it is the primary weight-bearing surface. After the age of 10, the meniscus starts to devascularize, and by adulthood, only the outer 1/3 is vascular.

Geriatric Considerations
Meniscal tears in geriatric patients are more likely due to chronic degeneration of the meniscus that can result in a tear with minimal acute trauma.

Pediatric Considerations
- Discoid lateral meniscus is an anatomic variant (incidence of 3.5–5%) that can cause a snapping or popping knee in childhood or adolescence; often nontraumatic.
- It is rare to sustain a meniscal injury under the age of 10, but can be associated with a discoid meniscus.

EPIDEMIOLOGY
- Predominant age: Males aged 31–40 years; females aged 11–20 years
- Predominant sex: Male:female ratio is 2.5:1

Incidence
- Most commonly seen in football, soccer, basketball, skiing, and baseball
- 80–90% of meniscal injuries in children and adolescents occur during athletics.

Prevalence
60–70 cases per 100,000 people

RISK FACTORS
- Anterior cruciate ligament (ACL) insufficiency
- Posterior cruciate ligament (PCL) insufficiency (1)
- Meniscal injuries increase as age increases; highest risk if >40 years old.
- Obesity and smoking are risk factors for degenerative meniscal tears.
- Arthritis of the knee

GENERAL PREVENTION
- Strengthening and conditioning while participating in sports
- Treatment and rehabilitation of previous knee injuries, especially ACL injuries
- Maintaining a healthy lifestyle
- Increasing core proprioception may prevent knee injuries in female athletes (2)[B].

ETIOLOGY
- Acute tears usually occur due to a twisting motion of the knee while the foot is planted.
- Sports injuries occur while cutting, decelerating, hyperflexion, or landing from a jump.
- Degenerative tears occur secondary to minimal trauma.

COMMONLY ASSOCIATED CONDITIONS
- ACL is also torn 1/3 of the time (patient may feel or hear a pop).
- It is more common for children and adolescents to have a concomitant ACL tear.
- Medial collateral and lateral collateral ligament tears
- Tibia plateau fractures
- Femoral shaft fractures

DIAGNOSIS

HISTORY
- Obtain description of the mechanism of injury.
- Ask about previous injury to the knee.
- Pain associated with activities requiring flexion of the knee, such as climbing stairs or squatting
- Swelling for days after the injury (usually the swelling is delayed; immediate swelling is associated with ACL tear)
- Locking, catching, popping, crunching (at the time of injury), or buckling
- Patient may have a limp or be unable to bear weight.
- Pain on side of knee where meniscal tear is present

PHYSICAL EXAM
- Compare with noninjured knee.
- Examine for effusion.
- Assess for joint line tenderness (sensitivity 79%, specificity 15%, and positive predictive value 50%) (3)[B].
- Decreased active and passive range of motion (locked knee)
- Pain with full flexion (posterior horn tears) or extension (anterior horn tears) of the knee
- McMurray test (sensitivity 53%, specificity 59%) (3)[B]
- Apley test for meniscal tear is not specific or sensitive, and rarely should be used (4)[B].
- Assess for coexisting ligament injury.
- If the effusion is too large, reevaluate the knee in 1 week of treatment.

DIAGNOSTIC TESTS & INTERPRETATION
Imaging
Initial approach
Plain radiographs should be obtained to detect fractures, loose bodies, or arthritic changes.

Follow-Up & Special Considerations
- Magnetic resonance imaging (MRI) is the best study for intra-articular pathology; however, it should only be done if the diagnosis is unclear or an MRI will change the management; most patients over 30 will benefit from a trial of aggressive rehabilitation before considering surgery (positive predictive value of the physical exam and an MRI are 91.5% and 96.5%, respectively, and accuracy is 94.5% and 95.5%, respectively) (5)[B].
- Abnormal MRI changes may be due to degenerative disease rather than an acute tear (4)[B].
- 61% of adult patients without knee symptoms were found to have incidental meniscal tears on MRI (6)[B].

Diagnostic Procedures/Surgery
Arthroscopy may be needed for diagnostic purposes if the MRI is indeterminate.

DIFFERENTIAL DIAGNOSIS
- ACL or collateral ligament tear
- Fracture
- Contusion
- Discoid meniscus
- Pathologic plica
- Osteochondritis dissecans
- Loose body
- Osteoarthritis

TREATMENT

MEDICATION
- Nonsteroidal anti-inflammatory drugs (NSAIDs) (7)[C]
- Narcotics if needed for severe pain

ADDITIONAL TREATMENT
General Measures
- PRICE: Protection, Rest, Ice, Compression, Elevation
- Meniscal preservation should be the goal of treatment in order to decrease the future complication of osteoarthritis.
- Treatment depends on the type, location, and extent of the tear and the age and activity of the patient.
- Small, nondisplaced peripheral tears (because this region is vascular), especially in the lateral meniscus, may heal on their own or become asymptomatic and therefore not need surgery.
- Aggressive physical therapy/rehabilitation should be provided as the initial form of treatment in most patients, as a majority of them will become symptom-free from strengthening alone.
- A "locked" knee requires surgery immediately.

ALERT
- Patients >30 years who do not have a "locked" knee should undergo 6–12 weeks of rehabilitation. If they are symptomatic after the rehabilitation, surgery should be considered.

- In patients >40 years with osteoarthritis (OA) and meniscal injury, surgery has not been proven to be more effective than conservative measures, and should only be offered after a failure of 3–6 months of rehabilitation. (In a study done by Moseley that compared arthroscopic debridement, arthroscopic lavage, and placebo surgery, neither of the surgery groups proved to have a better outcome [measured by pain and function] than the placebo group.) (8)[A]
- If the patient is <30 years and very active in sports or at work, surgery may be required.
- Activity:
  – Weight bearing as tolerated
  – Crutches may be needed to assist if patient is unable to bear weight.
  – Nonsurgical candidates should refrain from pivoting and participating in sports for 12 weeks (9)[C].

Issues for Referral

Surgical consult for injuries that may require surgery

Additional Therapies

- Nonsurgical and surgical candidates require rehabilitation.
- Strengthening and increasing range of motion (ROM) are the goals of rehabilitation.
- Athletes should partake in a sport-specific rehabilitation before returning to play.

SURGERY/OTHER PROCEDURES

- Most surgeries can be done arthroscopically.
- Meniscal repairs (suturing the meniscus) have a better functional outcome and decrease the risk of osteoarthritis, compared with meniscectomy (9)[C],(10,11)[B].
- Surgically implanted collagen meniscal implants do not improve postoperative function in patients with acute meniscal injury when compared to meniscectomy alone (12)[A].
- Young athletes have a better success rate than older individuals.

 ONGOING CARE

FOLLOW-UP RECOMMENDATIONS

- After a meniscectomy, patients can weight-bear in 1–2 days and return to full activity in 2–4 weeks (9)[C].
- After meniscal repair, patients can weight-bear in 4–6 weeks and return to full activity in 4–6 months if they are symptom-free, have full ROM, sufficient strength, and a normal physical exam (9)[C].
- ACL repair with meniscal repair requires 6 months of postoperative rehab before return to sports.

Patient Monitoring

- Monitor patient throughout recovery to ensure patient returns to activity at the appropriate time.
- Communication with the physical therapist or athletic trainer helps to ensure suitable rehabilitation and proper time frame for return to activity.

PATIENT EDUCATION

- May need to teach the patient how to ambulate on crutches
- Educate the patient on risks and benefits of surgery vs conservative treatment.

PROGNOSIS

- More favorable prognosis if surgery is done within 8 weeks, the tear is in the periphery, the tear is <2.5 cm, the tear is in the lateral meniscus, and patient is <30 years of age (9)[C].
- Meniscal repair with ACL repair has better outcomes than meniscal alone.

COMPLICATIONS

- Meniscectomies will eventually lead to OA, which is why meniscal repair should be performed over meniscectomy when possible.
- 10–20 years after the injury, about 50% will have OA, with associated pain and functional impairment (13)[A].

- Risk factors for greater radiographic evidence of osteoarthritis after an arthroscopic partial meniscectomy are greater size of meniscal resection and female gender (14)[B].
- The strongest predictors of worse functional outcome after an arthroscopic partial meniscectomy are greater articular cartilage degeneration seen during surgery, greater size of meniscal resection, greater laxity of the anterior cruciate ligament, and prior surgery of the knee (14)[B].
- Surgery may cause injury to neurovascular structures.

REFERENCES

1. Pearsall AW, Hollis JM. The effect of posterior cruciate ligament injury and reconstruction on meniscal strain. *Am J Sports Med*. 2004;32: 1675–80.
2. Zazulak BT, Hewett TE, Reeves NP, et al. The effects of core proprioception on knee injury: a prospective biomechanical-epidemiological study. *Am J Sports Med*. 2007;35:368–73.
3. Strayer RJ, Lang ES. Evidence-based emergency medicine/systematic review abstract. Does this patient have a torn meniscus or ligament of the knee? *Ann Emerg Med*. 2006;47:499–501.
4. Rath E, Richmond JC. The menisci: basic science and advances in treatment. *Br J Sports Med*. 2000;34:252–7.
5. Muellner T, Weinstabl R, Schabus R, et al. The diagnosis of meniscal tears in athletes. A comparison of clinical and magnetic resonance imaging investigations. *Am J Sports Med*. 1997; 25:7–12.
6. Englund M, Guermazi A, Gale D, et al. Incidental meniscal findings on knee MRI in middle-aged and elderly persons. *N Engl J Med*. 2008;359: 1108–15.
7. Mehallo CJ, Drezner JA, Bytomski JR. Practical management: nonsteroidal antiinflammatory drug (NSAID) use in athletic injuries. *Clin J Sport Med*. 2006;16:170–4.
8. Moseley JB, O'Malley K, Petersen NJ, et al. A controlled trial of arthroscopic surgery for osteoarthritis of the knee. *N Engl J Med*. 2002;347:81–8.
9. Kocher MS, Klingele K. Meniscal disorders: Normal, discoid, and cysts. *Orthop Clin N Am*. 2003;34:329–340.
10. Wu WH, Hackett T, Richmond JC. Effects of meniscal and articular surface status on knee stability, function, and symptoms after anterior cruciate ligament reconstruction: a long-term prospective study. *Am J Sports Med*. 2002;30: 845–50.
11. Noyes FR, Barber-Westin SD. Arthroscopic repair of meniscal tears extending into the avascular zone in patients younger than twenty years of age. *Am J Sports Med*. 2002;30:589–600.
12. Rodkey WG, DeHaven KE, Montgomery WH, et al. Comparison of the collagen meniscus implant with partial meniscectomy. A prospective randomized trial. *J Bone Joint Surg Am*. 2008;90:1413–26.
13. Lohmander LS, Englund PM, Dahl LL, et al. The long-term consequence of anterior cruciate ligament and meniscus injuries: osteoarthritis. *Am J Sports Med*. 2007;35:1756–69.
14. Meredith DS. Factors predicting functional and radiographic outcomes after arthroscopic partial meniscectomy: A review of the literature. *Arthroscopy*. 2005;21(2):211–23.

See Also (Topic, Algorithm, Electronic Media Element)

Algorithm: Knee Pain

 CODES

ICD9

- 836.0 Tear of medial cartilage or meniscus of knee, current
- 836.1 Tear of lateral cartilage or meniscus of knee, current
- 836.2 Other tear of cartilage or meniscus of knee, current

CLINICAL PEARLS

- Increasing core proprioception may prevent knee injuries in female athletes.
- Meniscal preservation should be the goal of treatment to prevent osteoarthritis.
- In patients >40 years with OA and meniscal injury, surgery has not been proven to be more effective than conservative measures and should be offered only after a failure of 3–6 months of rehabilitation.
- Nonsurgical and surgical candidates require rehabilitation.
- Meniscal repairs (suturing the meniscus) have a better functional outcome and decrease the risk of osteoarthritis, compared with meniscectomy.

M

MENOPAUSE

Kathleen Pangia, MD
Ginger Allister, MD

 BASICS

DESCRIPTION
- Natural menopause: Permanent cessation of menstrual periods for at least 12 consecutive months in a nonpregnant woman ≥45 years old
  - Resulting from ovarian follicular depletion
  - Not associated with a pathologic etiology
- Perimenopause: From the onset of menstrual changes through the 1st year of menopause (average length of perimenopause is 4–5 years)
- Postmenopause: Usually accounts for >1/3 of a woman's life
- Premature menopause: Menopause occurring before age 40; may be associated with sex chromosome abnormalities

EPIDEMIOLOGY
- Average age of perimenopause onset is 47.5 years.
- Mean age of menopause onset is between 51–52 years.

Incidence
In the US, 1.3 million women reach menopause annually.

RISK FACTORS
- Aging
- Oophorectomy
- Sex chromosome abnormalities (e.g., Turner syndrome)
- Age of maternal menopause

GENERAL PREVENTION
Goal is not to prevent menopause, but to retard development of osteoporosis related to menopause:
- Weight-bearing exercise
- Avoid smoking
- Avoid excessive alcohol and caffeine intake
- Maintain healthy weight
- Calcium intake 1,200–1,500 mg/d beginning in adolescence
- Adequate vitamin D (800–1,200 IU daily)

PATHOPHYSIOLOGY
Normal physiologic process

ETIOLOGY
- As women age, the number of ovarian follicles decreases: Ovarian production of estrogen and inhibin decreases, and leuteinizing (LH) and follicle-stimulating hormone (FSH) production increases.
  - Without estrogen, failure of endometrial development occurs and menstrual cycles become irregular, then cease.
  - Symptoms directly or indirectly due to decrease in estrogen
- Surgical: Removal of functioning ovaries due to disease or incidental to hysterectomy
- Other:
  - Treatment of endometriosis
  - Treatment of breast cancer with antiestrogens (which is reversible)
  - May occur after cancer chemotherapy (permanent or reversible)

 DIAGNOSIS

HISTORY
- Cessation of menses:
  - Generally preceded by a period of irregular cycles and/or diminished bleeding
- Vasomotor symptoms: Hot flashes and sweating, often at night (30–80%)
  - First manifestation of menopause
  - Usually last ~3–4 minutes, occur at unpredictable intervals
  - Frequency usually declines with time
- Mood changes (8–38%), anxiety, depression
- Sleep disorders (35–60%)
  - Lengthening of latent phase
  - Less time spent asleep
- Urogenital atrophy:
  - Atrophic vaginitis causes vaginal dryness (17–30%), itch, dyspareunia, and possible sexual dysfunction.
  - Urethral atrophy causes urgency, frequency, dysuria, stress incontinence.
  - Atrophy of paravaginal tissues that support bladder and rectum can lead to urocele, rectocele, uterine prolapse.
- Osteopenia and osteoporosis
- Change in intensity and severity of migraines
- Skin thinning, hair loss, hirsutism, brittle nails

Geriatric Considerations
Vaginal bleeding in a postmenopausal women is abnormal; endometrial cancer must be ruled out.

PHYSICAL EXAM
- Decrease in breast size and change in breast texture
- External, speculum, and bimanual pelvic exams: Atrophic vaginal mucosa (urogenital atrophy)

DIAGNOSTIC TESTS & INTERPRETATION
Lab
Initial lab tests
- Generally none required; patient's age and symptoms readily establish the diagnosis
- If laboratory confirmation is desired:
  - Elevated serum FSH level >30 mIU/mL indicates ovarian failure.
  - Symptoms may precede changes in lab parameters.
- Drugs that may alter lab results: Estrogens, androgens, oral contraceptive pills (OCPs)
- LH has no role in diagnosing menopause.

Imaging
Initial approach
Annual mammography is recommended for menopausal women (upper age limit for discontinuation remains uncertain).

Follow-Up & Special Considerations
- Brain magnetic resonance imaging (MRI) if pituitary tumor suspected
- Abnormal vaginal bleeding in a postmenopausal patient should be evaluated by transvaginal ultrasound (TVUS) and/or endometrial biopsy:
  - If endometrial stripe is <5 mm on TVUS, endometrial carcinoma is unlikely.

- Bone mineral density (BMD) testing with dual energy x-ray absorptiometry (DEXA) scan in postmenopausal women <65 years with additional risk factors (not otherwise indicated at onset of menopause):
  - Previous history of fractures, low body weight, cigarette smoking, family history of fractures should be tested, if osteoporosis is a concern (not usually indicated at onset of menopause).

Pathological Findings
- Abnormal BMD and DEXA scan results:
  - T-score on DEXA of 1.0–2.5 = osteopenia
  - T-score >2.5 = osteoporosis
  - Defer to femoral neck T-score value over spine T-score
- Z-score measures age-matched mean bone density (not clinically useful)

DIFFERENTIAL DIAGNOSIS
- Pregnancy
- Polycystic ovarian syndrome
- Pituitary adenoma
- Anorexia nervosa causing amenorrhea
- Hypothalamic dysfunction
- Asherman syndrome
- Obstruction of uterine outflow tract
- Sheehan syndrome

TREATMENT

Treatment choice depends on severity of symptoms.

MEDICATION
First Line
Hormone therapy (HT) (1):

- The primary indication for HT is the treatment of moderate-to-severe vasomotor symptoms. Combination estrogen-progestin therapy is effective treatment for these symptoms, and other menopausal symptoms (sleep disorders, urogenital atrophy). It is also useful for prevention of osteoporotic fractures, colorectal cancer, and may help with mood symptoms (2,3)[A].

- Current recommendations for HT suggest use for a limited duration (i.e., few years) in the treatment of menopausal symptoms in women who are near menopause and do not have a history of and are not at high risk for coronary artery disease, stroke, breast cancer, or thromboembolism. If these risk factors are present, or if the woman is asymptomatic, alternative treatments to prevent bone loss should be considered.

- If HT is selected, estrogen should be given in combination with progestin for women with an intact uterus. Depending on duration of use, unopposed estrogen carries a 2.0–6.7-fold higher risk of endometrial cancer. Most data available are for continuous treatment (as opposed to cyclical) with combined conjugated equine estrogen (CEE) 0.625 mg and medroxyprogesterone acetate 2.5 mg. However, considerable evidence supports the use of low-dose HT, which is associated with 50% lower rates of irregular bleeding. Low dose = 0.3 or 0.45 mg/d of CEE (4)[A].

- Precautions:
  - The Women's Health Initiative (WHI) study, in 2002, done in women without established coronary heart disease (CHD), found those treated with combination estrogen-progestin therapy had an increased relative risk of invasive breast cancer, coronary heart disease, stroke, and pulmonary embolism at 5 years of use (3,5)[A]. This risk of breast cancer was found to be independent of mammography screening frequency (1)[B]. Put another way, for every 100 women treated with HT for 5 years, 1 will have a serious adverse event.
  - The Heart and Estrogen/Progestin Replacement study (HERS), done in women with established CHD, demonstrated improvements in the lipid profiles of women on HT, but the overall risk of vascular mortality did not decline.
  - There is an increased risk of ovarian cancer in women who take HT. 1 out of every 8,300 women who take hormone replacement therapy each year has been shown to suffer from ovarian cancer (6)[B].
  - Higher doses of estrogen can cause hypercoagulability, breast tenderness, gallbladder disease, and hypertension (HTN).
  - Contraindications to HT:
    ○ Estrogen-dependent malignancies
    ○ Unexplained uterine bleeding
    ○ History of thromboembolism or stroke
    ○ Coronary artery disease
    ○ Active liver disease
- For osteoporosis:
  - Screening and treating women at risk for osteoporosis can help prevent fractures (7)[A].
  - Bisphosphonates inhibit osteoclast action and resorption of bone:
    ○ Alendronate (Fosamax): Treatment dose: 70 mg/week or 10 mg/d. Prevention dose: 35 mg/week or 5 mg/d.
    ○ Risedronate (Actonel): 35 mg once a week or 5 mg/d. Same dose for prevention and treatment.
    ○ Zoledronic acid (Reclast or Zometa): 5 mg IV annually. Same dose for prevention and treatment.
    ○ Ibandronate (Boniva): 2.5 mg/d or 150 mg/month. Same dose for prevention and treatment.
  - Selective estrogen receptor modulators (SERMs) selectively inhibit or stimulate estrogen-like action in various tissues. The SERM used for the treatment of osteoporosis is:
    ○ Raloxifene (Evista): 60 mg/d for prevention and treatment; because raloxifene is a less potent antiresorptive drug than alendronate, risedronate, or estrogen, it is best suited for the prevention or treatment of mild osteoporosis (8)[A].
    ○ The EFFECT trial demonstrated that raloxifene decreased the risk of vertebral fracture, but failed to demonstrate a decrease in the risk of extravertebral fractures.
    ○ Raloxifene should be used primarily in postmenopausal women with predominantly spinal osteoporosis (8,9)[A].
    ○ Calcium: 1,200–1,500 mg elemental calcium p.o. daily
    ○ Vitamin D: 800 IU–1,200 IU p.o. daily

- For atrophic vaginitis:
  - Topical estrogen therapy (ET): Conjugated estrogens (Premarin cream); best for local therapy of atrophic vaginitis. ET reverses vaginal atrophy, enhances blood flow, reduces pH and urinary tract infections (UTIs). ET is applied to vaginal mucosa as needed. Data are insufficient to recommend annual endometrial surveillance in women using ET with no vaginal bleeding. ET should be continued as long as distressing symptoms remain. Women with a history of hormone-dependent cancer should consult with an oncologist prior to initiation of therapy (10)[B].

Second Line
For vasomotor symptoms:
- Nonhormonal treatments may be helpful for women who wish to or need to avoid HT (e.g., breast CA):
  - Antidepressants venlafaxine (37.5–75 mg/d), paroxetine (10–20 mg/d), or fluoxetine (20 mg/d) are options that have been shown to result in 1 fewer hot flash a day.
  - Gabapentin (300–900 mg/d) has been shown to have some effect in reducing vasomotor symptoms by up to 2 hot flashes per day (11)[A].
- Clonidine may be used to treat mild hot flashes, although it is less effective than antidepressants or gabapentin. Initial oral dose is 0.05 mg b.i.d.; some women may require 0.1 mg b.i.d.
- All trials of 2nd-line therapies have been of short duration, i.e., a few months (9,11)[A].

COMPLEMENTARY AND ALTERNATIVE MEDICINE
Trials of nonprescribed therapies are difficult to interpret due to variability of components and doses:
- Soy isoflavone showed mixed effect in placebo-controlled trials in reduction of hot flashes.
- Red clover, black cohosh, reflexology, aerobic, and magnet therapy showed no impact on hot flashes when compared to placebo.
- Small clinical trials of evening primrose, dong quai, ginseng, and wild yam do not support their use for relief of hot flashes.

 ## ONGOING CARE

FOLLOW-UP RECOMMENDATIONS
Patient Monitoring
- DEXA scan is indicated at age 65 for all women
- Pap smear and mammography per standard health maintenance guidelines

DIET
Calcium and vitamin D supplements as above

PATIENT EDUCATION
Encourage lifestyle modifications:
- Smoking cessation
- Weight-bearing exercise
- Avoid excess alcohol and caffeine
- Address cardiovascular risk factor modification

PROGNOSIS
If untreated:
- Ultimate disappearance of vasomotor symptoms; usually takes several years
- Osteoporosis: Possible fractures of the hip, vertebrae, and wrists

COMPLICATIONS
- Osteoporosis: Bone loss occurs at a rate of 0.3–0.5% per year beginning in the 4th decade, but at menopause, women have accelerated bone loss

up to 3–5% per year for 5–7 years. HT is clearly protective against bone loss. Smoking cessation, physical activity, and calcium supplementation should be encouraged to decrease risk of osteoporosis.
- Increased risk of coronary artery disease due to loss of protective benefits of estrogen on lipid profile and endothelium

REFERENCES

1. Chlebowski RT, Kuller LH, Prentice RL, et al. Breast cancer after use of estrogen plus progestin in postmenopausal women. *N Engl J Med.* 2009;360:573–87.
2. Nelson HD. Commonly used types of postmenopausal estrogen for treatment of hot flashes: scientific review. *JAMA.* 2004;291:1610–20.
3. Rossouw JE, Anderson GL, Prentice RL, et al. Risks and benefits of estrogen plus progestin in healthy postmenopausal women: principal results From the Women's Health Initiative randomized controlled trial. *JAMA.* 2002;288:321–33.
4. Lobo RA, et al. Should symptomatic menopausal women be offered hormone therapy? *Med Gen Med.* 2006;8(3):40–58.
5. Rossouw JE, Prentice RL, Manson JE, et al. Postmenopausal hormone therapy and risk of cardiovascular disease by age and years since menopause. *JAMA.* 2007;297:1465–77.
6. Mørch LS, Løkkegaard E, Andreasen AH, et al. Hormone therapy and ovarian cancer. *JAMA.* 2009;302:298–305.
7. USPSTF. http://www.ahrq.gov/clinic/epcsums/osteoporosis.pdf.
8. Sambrook PN, Geusens P, Ribot C, et al. Alendronate produces greater effects than raloxifene on bone density and bone turnover in postmenopausal women with low bone density: results of EFFECT (Efficacy of FOSAMAX versus EVISTA Comparison Trial) International. *J Intern Med.* 2004;255:503–11.
9. Riggs BL, Hartmann LC. Selective estrogen-receptor modulators – mechanisms of action and application to clinical practice. *N Engl J Med.* 2003;348:618–29.
10. North American Menopause Society. The role of local vaginal estrogen for treatment of vaginal atrophy in postmenopausal women. *Menopause.* 2007;14(3):357–69.
11. National Guideline Clearinghouse. Menopause. http://www.guideline.gov.

CODES

ICD9
- V49.81 Asymptomatic postmenopausal status (age-related) (natural)
- 256.31 Premature menopause

CLINICAL PEARLS

- Menopause is usually diagnosed by history alone (if laboratory confirmation of menopause is desired, then elevated serum FSH level >30 mIU/mL indicates ovarian failure). LH has no role in diagnosing menopause.
- Current recommendations are that HT be used short-term for relief of moderate-to-severe vasomotor symptoms, but not in the longer term for prevention of cardiovascular disease.

M

MENORRHAGIA

Donald A.F. Nelson, MD

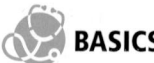 **BASICS**

DESCRIPTION
- Excessive amount or duration of menstrual flow, at more or less regular intervals. Flow ≥80 mL per cycle, compared to normal average 30–40 mL per cycle (1,2).
- Distinguishable from but may overlap with:
  - Metrorrhagia: Irregular or frequent flow, noncyclic
  - Menometrorrhagia: Frequent, excessive, irregular flow (menorrhagia plus metrorrhagia)
  - Polymenorrhea: Frequent flow, cycles of 21 days or fewer
  - Intermenstrual bleeding: Bleeding between regular menses
  - Dysfunctional uterine bleeding (DUB): Abnormal endometrial bleeding of hormonal cause and related to anovulation
- System(s) affected: Reproductive

EPIDEMIOLOGY
Prevalence
- ~30% of women complain of excessive bleeding at some point (1).
- Predominant sex: Female only
- Predominant age:
  - Menarche to menopause; ~50% of cases occur in patients >40 years old
  - Dysfunctional bleeding is fairly common in adolescence and near menopause.
  - In adolescence, irregular bleeding due to anovulation and immaturity of the hypothalamic-pituitary-ovarian axis is common.

Pediatric Considerations
Genital bleeding before puberty can result from trauma, foreign bodies, vaginal infection, or exogenous hormone administration.

Pregnancy Considerations
Bleeding in pregnancy is not menorrhagia. Complications of pregnancy or cervical/vaginal lesions should be considered.

Geriatric Considerations
True menorrhagia cannot occur after menopause. However, genital atrophy as well as uterine and ovarian cancers may be associated with vaginal bleeding in the elderly.

RISK FACTORS
- Obesity
- Anovulation
- Estrogen administration (± progestin)
- Prior treatment with progestational agents or oral contraceptives increases risk of endometrial atrophy, but decreases risk of endometrial hyperplasia or neoplasia.

GENERAL PREVENTION
Periodic Pap smears and pelvic examinations at appropriate intervals based on age and risk factors

ETIOLOGY
- Hypothyroidism
- Endometrial proliferation/excess/hyperplasia:
  - Anovulation, oligo-ovulation
  - Ovarian tumor
  - Prolonged estrogen, progestin, or oral contraceptive administration
  - Polycystic ovarian syndrome
- Local factors:
  - Endometrial atrophy, postmenopause
  - Abnormal endometrial prostaglandin levels
  - Endometrial polyps
  - Endometrial neoplasia
  - Adenomyosis/endometriosis
  - Uterine myomata (fibroids)
  - Intrauterine device (IUD)
  - Uterine sarcoma
- Coagulation disorders:
  - Thrombocytopenia, platelet disorders
  - von Willebrand disease, factor deficiencies
  - Leukemia
  - Ingestion of aspirin/acetylsalicylic acid or anticoagulants
  - Renal failure/dialysis

COMMONLY ASSOCIATED CONDITIONS
Metrorrhagia, menometrorrhagia, androgenic disorders

 DIAGNOSIS

HISTORY
- Excessive menstrual flow is defined subjectively and varies greatly from woman to woman.
- Useful features:
  - Bleeding substantially heavier than usual flow
  - Bleeding lasting >7 days
  - Flow associated with significant clots
  - Anemia
- Symptoms that suggest cycles are ovulatory:
  - Regular menstrual interval
  - Midcycle pain (mittelschmerz)
  - Dysmenorrhea
  - Premenstrual symptoms: Breast soreness/tenderness, mood changes
- Abdominal pain or cramps at other times of the cycle may be associated with structural causes:
  - Myomas
  - Polyps
  - Ovarian tumors

PHYSICAL EXAM
- Hirsutism, acne, or obesity may accompany chronic anovulation.
- Pelvic/rectal examination to detect/exclude other causes of bleeding:
  - Cervical or vaginal bleeding
  - Pelvic or adnexal masses
  - Signs of pelvic infection

DIAGNOSTIC TESTS & INTERPRETATION
Lab
Initial lab tests
- Pregnancy test: Exclude pregnancy first.
- CBC to assess severity of blood loss and to rule out thrombocytopenia and leukemia (2)
- In selected cases:
  - TSH test
  - Coagulation screen, with follow-up testing if screen is abnormal
  - Creatinine, BUN
  - Serum progesterone: 5–20 ng/mL (15.9–63.6 nmol/L) in luteal phase, <1 ng/mL (<3.18 nmol/L) in follicular phase or anovulatory cycle

Imaging
Initial approach
- Transvaginal ultrasonography can help distinguish bleeding due to atrophy from bleeding caused by hyperplasia, polyps, or myomas.
- Ultrasonography to evaluate adnexal masses or myomas suspected from pelvic exam.
- CT is used in investigation of potentially malignant pelvic masses.

Diagnostic Procedures/Surgery
- Endometrial biopsy detects hyperplasia, dysplasia, or atrophy. If done before expected menses, it may also help confirm the diagnosis of anovulation or luteal phase defect.
- After age 35–40 endometrial carcinoma is significant cause of bleeding. Obtain endometrial sampling before attempting hormonal treatment (3)[C].

Pathological Findings
- Vary with etiology. In ~50% of cases, no uterine pathology is found (1).
- Progestins used before endometrial biopsy may cause decidualization and obscure correct diagnosis.

DIFFERENTIAL DIAGNOSIS
- Pregnancy complications:
  - Threatened abortion
  - Incomplete abortion
  - Ectopic pregnancy
- Nonuterine bleeding:
  - Cervical ectropion/erosion
  - Cervical neoplasia/polyp
  - Cervical or vaginal trauma/foreign body
  - Condylomata
  - Atrophic vaginitis
- Pelvic inflammatory disease:
  - Endometritis
  - Tuberculosis

TREATMENT

MEDICATION

First Line
- For acute control of severe bleeding:
  - Estrogen, conjugated (Premarin): 25 mg IV q4h up to 6 doses or 10–20 mg/d p.o. in 4 divided doses until bleeding abates (3)[C]
- For less severe bleeding or after control of acute bleeding has been achieved:
  - Medroxyprogesterone acetate (Provera): 10–30 mg/d for 5–10 days
  - Any combination oral contraceptive (i.e., usually a high-dose oral contraceptive) 1 tablet q.i.d. for 5–7 days
- To prevent heavy bleeding in subsequent cycles:
  - Medroxyprogesterone acetate: 5–30 mg/d for 10 days per month
  - Usual cyclic dose of a combination oral contraceptive (3)[C]

Second Line
- Nonsteroidal prostaglandin-synthetase inhibitors (e.g., naproxen, mefenamic acid, ibuprofen) can reduce blood loss ~25% with ovulatory cycles and reduce dysmenorrhea (4)[B].
- Tranexamic acid (Cyklokapron), a plasminogen activation inhibitor, 2 g/d orally is equally or more effective than medroxyprogesterone 10 mg twice daily (5)[B].
- Norethindrone acetate (Aygestin): 2.5–10 mg/d for 10–21 days per month
- Levonorgestrel intrauterine system (Mirena IUD) can reduce blood loss >90% (4)[B].
- Danazol and GnRH agonists are also effective therapies, but more likely to have adverse side effects. Mifepristone (RU-486) has been used experimentally (1).

ADDITIONAL TREATMENT

Additional Therapies
Nausea and vomiting are common from IV estrogen; antiemetics are helpful.

SURGERY/OTHER PROCEDURES
- Hysterectomy when indicated to treat coexisting conditions (myomas, endometrial dysplasia) or for bleeding unresponsive to other measures (1,6).
- Endometrial ablation by laser, electrosurgical, microwave, or thermal means is a conservative alternative to hysterectomy, but long-term control of bleeding and patient satisfaction are lower than with hysterectomy (1,7)[A].

IN-PATIENT CONSIDERATIONS

Initial Stabilization
- Most cases can be managed as outpatient in office or emergency department.
- Rule out pregnancy complications and nonuterine bleeding.

- Treat severe or life-threatening bleeding acutely:
  - Circulatory support, transfusion if necessary
  - IV estrogen
  - Curettage if necessary
  - Hysterectomy in extreme case

Admission Criteria
- Bleeding leading to orthostatic hypotension
- Hematocrit <25%

 ONGOING CARE

FOLLOW-UP RECOMMENDATIONS
Proceed to identify underlying cause of bleeding and treat to prevent recurrence:
- Hormonal therapy
- Dilatation and curettage for cases that fail to respond to hormone therapy
- Consider endometrial ablation or hysterectomy in persistent cases in which fertility is not a concern.
- Specific treatment for neoplasia, polyps, systemic disease
- Patients in whom fertility is a consideration may also need appropriate treatment for anovulation, endometriosis, and myomas.

Patient Monitoring
- Varies with cause of bleeding
- Medical treatment of hyperplastic/dysplastic endometrium should be followed by repeat biopsy to confirm that histologic structure has returned to normal.

DIET
Iron supplementation may help correct for increased blood loss.

PATIENT EDUCATION
Information about side effects of medications should be provided.

PROGNOSIS
- Varies with cause of bleeding
- Most patients whose condition results from hormonal causes will respond to hormonal manipulation.

COMPLICATIONS
- Anemia
- Estrogen may precipitate acute intermittent porphyria or cholestatic jaundice in susceptible patients.

REFERENCES

1. Oehler MK, Rees MC. Menorrhagia: an update. *Acta Obstet Gynecol Scand.* 2003;82:405–22.
2. Siegel JE. Abnormalities of hemostasis and abnormal uterine bleeding. *Clinical Obstetrics & Gynecology.* 2005;48:284–94.
3. Management of anovulatory bleeding. ACOG Practice Bulletin 14, March 2000, reaffirmed 2009.
4. Reid PC, Virtanen-Kari S. Randomised comparative trial of levonorgestrel intrauterine system and mefenamic acid for the treatment of idiopathic menorrhagia. *BJOG.* 2005;112:1121–5.
5. Kriplani A, Kulshrestha V, Agarwal N, et al. Role of tranexamic acid in management of dysfunctional uterine bleeding in comparison with medroxyprogesterone acetate. *J Obstet Gynaecol.* 2006;26:673–8.
6. Showstack J, Lin F, Learman LA, et al. Randomized trial of medical treatment versus hysterectomy for abnormal uterine bleeding: resource use in the Medicine or Surgery (Ms) trial. *Am J Obstet Gynecol.* 2006;194:332–8.
7. Practice Committee of American Society for Reproductive Medicine et al. Indications and options for endometrial ablation. *Fertil. Steril.* 2008;90:S236–40.

See Also (Topic, Algorithm, Electronic Media Element)
Amenorrhea; Abnormal Pap and Cervical Dysplasia; Cervical Malignancy; Cervical Polyps; Cervicitis, Ectropion, and True Erosion; Dysfunctional Uterine Bleeding; Dysmenorrhea; Menopause; Polycystic Ovarian Syndrome; Uterine Myomas
Algorithm: Menorrhagia

CODES

ICD9
- 626.2 Excessive or frequent menstruation
- 626.3 Puberty bleeding

CLINICAL PEARLS
- Menorrhagia is defined as excessive amount or duration of menstrual flow at more or less regular intervals and has a wide variety of potential causes.
- Pregnancy should be ruled out as part of the initial evaluation.
- Because endometrial carcinoma is a significant cause of bleeding in women over age 35, an endometrial biopsy to rule out endometrial carcinoma is recommended before using any hormonal treatments.
- Iron supplementation will help correct for increased blood loss while the underlying etiology is being identified and treated.

M

MENTAL RETARDATION

Adam Barta, MD
Jennifer L. Ayres, PhD

 BASICS

- Mental retardation (MR) is a global deficit in cognitive functioning, as evidenced by a significant difference between one's mental and chronological ages (AKA "intelligence quotient" or "IQ") and significantly impaired adaptive functioning (1).
- Although these cognitive issues typically have a pervasive impact, patients with MR will display highly variable levels of functioning and subsequent service needs.
- Patients must be evaluated individually. Treatment plans must be tailored to specific needs.
- The current DSM-IV-TR diagnosis is "Mental Retardation." However, since that term is deemed to be somewhat pejorative, the new DSM-V diagnosis will be "Intellectual Disability."

DESCRIPTION
- MR is defined as an IQ ≤70 and a significant impairment in an area of adaptive functioning such as communication, self-care, activities of daily living, socialization, use of community and resources, or health/safety (1).
- These issues are present prior to the age of 18.
- Currently, MR is subgrouped according to IQ level [mild (IQ ~55–69), moderate (~40–54), severe (~25–39), and profound (~0–24)]. A diagnosis of "Mental Retardation, severity unspecified" may be used for individuals who are unable to undergo formal assessment.
- The 3 most common causes of MR are Down syndrome, Fragile X syndrome, and fetal alcohol syndrome (FAS).
- Synonym(s): Intellectual disability; Cognitive disability

ALERT
For some causes of MR, prenatal testing is available.

EPIDEMIOLOGY
Incidence
- 1/63–1/83 (in two surveillance studies in Atlanta, in 1996 and 2000) (2)
- By definition, MR begins in childhood and must be diagnosed prior to the age of 18.
- Predominant sex: Male > Female; 2:1 for mild MR, 1.5:1 for severe MR.

Prevalence
In the US, 1–2.5% of the population

RISK FACTORS
- Maternal substance abuse during pregnancy
- Maternal infection during pregnancy
- For some causes, family history
- Mild MR is more common in children of women who did not complete high school; likely related to genetic and socioeconomic factors (e.g., nutritional deficiencies, poverty).

Genetics
A number of genetic and epigenetic causes are known, and more are under investigation (3).

GENERAL PREVENTION
- Public health efforts to reduce alcohol and drug use by pregnant women
- Prenatal folic acid supplementation

ETIOLOGY
- The cause of mild MR is identified in <50% of cases. The cause of severe MR is identified in >75% of cases.
- Causes:
  - Maternal substance abuse (e.g., alcohol); FAS is a leading environmental cause of MR.
  - Maternal infections: TORCH viruses (*Toxoplasma*, *other* infections, *rubella*, *cytomegalovirus*, and *herpes* simplex)
  - Down syndrome
  - Sex chromosome abnormalities: Fragile X, Turner syndrome, Klinefelter syndrome
  - Autosomal dominant conditions: Neurocutaneous syndromes (e.g., neurofibromatosis, tuberous sclerosis)
  - Autosomal recessive conditions:
    ○ Amino acid metabolism (e.g., phenylketonuria, maple-syrup urine disease)
    ○ Carbohydrate metabolism (e.g., galactosemia, fructosuria)
    ○ Lipid metabolism
    ○ Tay-Sachs disease
    ○ Gaucher disease
    ○ Niemann-Pick disease (e.g., mucopolysaccharidosis)
    ○ Purine metabolism (e.g., Lesch-Nyhan disease)
    ○ Other (e.g., Wilson disease)
- Maternal use of prescription medications (e.g., Accutane, Dilantin)
- Perinatal factors:
  - Prematurity
  - Birth injuries
  - Perinatal anoxia
- Postnatal factors:
  - Childhood diseases (e.g., meningitis, encephalitis, hypothyroidism)
  - Trauma (e.g., accidents, physical abuse)
  - Severe deprivation
  - Poisoning (e.g., lead, carbon monoxide, household products)

COMMONLY ASSOCIATED CONDITIONS
- Seizures
- Mood disorders
- Behavioral disorders

 DIAGNOSIS

A diagnosis of MR/intellectual disability should only be made through a psychodiagnostic assessment conducted by a mental health provider trained and licensed to conduct formal psychological testing.

HISTORY
- Three-generation family history
- Children with profound or severe MR typically are diagnosed at birth or during the newborn period and are more likely to have dysmorphic features.
- Children with MR often are identified because they fail to meet motor or language milestones.

PHYSICAL EXAM
Careful examination by a physician trained in the assessment of morphologic features suggestive of a specific etiology for MR (e.g., microcephaly) (4)

DIAGNOSTIC TESTS & INTERPRETATION
- Visual and hearing tests to rule out these etiologies as a cause of impairment and provide an assessment of visual and auditory functioning, which often are impaired in children and adults with MR
- Formal testing of intellectual and adaptive functioning
  - A child's communication skills must be considered in test selection. For example, a patient with auditory processing issues or limited expressive or receptive language skills may need to be assessed using a nonverbal IQ test, such as the Leiter-R, Test of Nonverbal Intelligence, or other nonverbal measures.
  - Commonly used intelligence tests (e.g., Bayley Scales of Infant Development, Stanford-Binet Intelligence Scale, Weschler Intelligence Scales) are determined by age/developmental level of the child.
  - Common tests of adaptive functioning include the Vineland Adaptive Behavior Scales Second Edition and Adaptive Behavior Assessment System Second Edition. These tests assess areas of functioning, such as age-appropriate communication, social skills, activities of daily living, and motor skills.

Lab
- Metabolic screening not routine unless evidence in history and physical, or no newborn screening records (5)[B]
- Lead as per current targeted guidelines (5)[B]
- Thyroid stimulating hormone (TSH) if systemic features present or no newborn screening (5)[B]
- Routine cytogenetic testing (karyotype) (5)[B]
  - Fragile X screening (FMR1 gene), particularly if family history of intellectual disability (5)[B]
  - Rett syndrome (MECP2 gene) in females with unexplained moderate-to-severe intellectual disability (5)[B]
- Molecular screening such as array comparative genomic hybridization (aCGH) is used increasingly and may yield diagnosis in 10% undiagnosed cases (4)[B].

Imaging

- Neuroimaging (MRI more sensitive than CT) is routinely recommended. The presence of physical findings (microcephaly, focal motor deficit) will increase the yield of a specific diagnosis (5)[B].
- MRI may show mild cerebral abnormalities but is unlikely to establish etiology of MR (4).

Follow-Up & Special Considerations

EEG not routine unless presence of epilepsy or a specific epileptiform syndrome (5)[C].

DIFFERENTIAL DIAGNOSIS

- Brain tumors
- Auditory, visual, and/or speech/language impairment
- Autistic disorder (language and social skills are more affected than other cognitive abilities); however, 75% of individuals with an autistic disorder may meet criteria for a comorbid diagnosis of MR.
- Cerebral palsy
- Emotional or behavioral disturbance
- Lack of environmental opportunities for appropriate development

 TREATMENT

- Early intervention services tailored to the individual's specific needs
- Caregiver support, including:
  - Training parent(s) to address behavioral issues and support socialization development
  - Encouraging caregivers to create a structured home environment that is based on the child's developmental level and specific needs, rather than age-appropriate expectations
  - Providing parent(s) with an opportunity to address their reactions to the diagnosis and their child's special needs
- Individualized education programs and, depending on the level of impairment, social skills and behavioral plans/training
- Referral to job training programs and independent living opportunities if appropriate
- Taking notice of all changes in behavior, which may be indicative of pain or illness, particularly in individuals with limited communication skills

MEDICATION

Medication may be appropriate for comorbid conditions (e.g., anxiety, ADHD, depression).

 ONGOING CARE

The physician should match his/her communication of exam procedures, test results, and treatment recommendations to the patient's level of cognitive functioning and communication.

- The vast majority of patients with MR will fall within the mild range and are fully capable of understanding information if it is provided at the appropriate level.
- Provide explanations directly to the patient, instead of solely to his/her caregivers. The dignity of the patient must be respected at all times. This includes providing honest information, responding to patient's questions with respect, and not infantilizing the patient due to his/her intellectual disability.

FOLLOW-UP RECOMMENDATIONS

- Many adults and children with MR exhibit poor physical fitness. Preliminary studies suggest that structured exercise programs are effective to engage this population in healthy activities (6)[A].
- Linkage to community-based resources for job training, independent living, caregiver support, school-based services.

Patient Monitoring

- Primary care with attention to associated medical conditions
- Vision testing at least once before age 40 (age 30 in Down syndrome) and every 2 years thereafter (7)[B]
- Hearing evaluations every 5 years after age 45 (every 3 years throughout life in Down syndrome) (7)[B]
- Screen for sexual activity and offer contraception and testing for sexually transmitted infections (7)[B].
- Abuse and neglect of people with MR are common. Screen at least annually and assess for abuse if behavior change noted. Report abuse or neglect to appropriate protective agencies (7)[B].
- Dysphagia and aspiration common; consider speech pathology evaluation and swallowing study (8)[B].
- Monitor for and treat constipation (8)[B].
- Osteoporosis is common; low threshold to order imaging studies after traumatic injury (8)[B].

DIET

No restrictions, except in case of metabolic and storage disorders (e.g., phenylketonuria)

PATIENT EDUCATION

- Families should be referred to the local Association for Retarded Citizens: http://www.thearc.or
- American Association of Intellectual and Developmental Disabilities: http://www.aaidd.org
- Refer to local family support group (e.g., Parent To Parent, local Down Syndrome Association, local Autism Association)

PROGNOSIS

Although MR is a lifelong diagnosis, individuals with MR are capable of living a fulfilling, purposeful life that includes having a career, living independently, marrying/participating in a committed relationship, and becoming a parent.

REFERENCES

1. American Psychiatric Association (2000). *Diagnostic and statistical manual of mental disorders*: Fourth edition, text revision. Arlington, VA: American Psychiatric Association.
2. http://www.cdc.gov/ncbddd/dd/mr3.htm
3. Grant ME. The epigenetic origins of mental retardation. *Clin Genet*. 2008;73:528–30.
4. van Karnebeek CDM, Jansweijer MCE, Offringa M. Diagnostic investigations in individuals with mental retardation: A systematic literature review of their usefulness. *Eur J Human Genet*. 2005;13:6–25.
5. Shevell M, Ashwal S, Donley D, Flint J, Gingold M, Hirtz D, Majnemer A, Noetzel M, Sheth RD, Quality Standards Subcommittee of the American Academy of Neurology, Practice Committee of the Child Neurology Society et al. Practice parameter: evaluation of the child with global developmental delay: report of the Quality Standards Subcommittee of the American Academy of Neurology and The Practice Committee of the Child Neurology Society. *Neurology*. 2003;60:367–80.
6. Heller T, Hsieh K, Rimmer JH. Attitudinal and psychosocial outcomes of a fitness and health education program on adults with down syndrome. *Am J Ment Retard*. 2004;109:175–85.
7. Sullivan WF, Heng J, Cameron D, et al. Consensus guidelines for primary health care of adults with developmental disabilities. *Can Fam Physician*. 2006;52:1410–8.
8. Prater CD, Zylstra RG. Medical care of adults with mental retardation. *Am Fam Physician*. 2006;73: 2175–83.

ADDITIONAL READING

Moeschler JB, Shevell M, American Academy of Pediatrics Committee on Genetics. Clinical genetic evaluation of the child with mental retardation or developmental delays. *Pediatrics*. 2006;117:2304–16.

See Also (Topic, Algorithm, Electronic Media Element)

ADD/ADHD; Cerebral Palsy; Down Syndrome; Fragile X Syndrome; Lead Poisoning;
Algorithm: Mental Retardation

 CODES

ICD9

- 317 Mild mental retardation
- 318.0 Moderate mental retardation
- 318.1 Severe mental retardation

CLINICAL PEARLS

- The term "mental retardation" may be interpreted as highly limited, culturally insensitive, and disrespectful to patients and their caregivers. "Intellectual disability" is the preferred term.
- Overall functioning with MR is highly variable and influenced by multiple factors, including appropriateness of school placement/special education services, exposure to early intervention, behavioral therapy, parent training, self-esteem, and social skills.
- Previous stereotypes of people with MR (e.g., always happy, poor prognosis, unable to function independently) have been refuted. People with MR are showing a level of functioning variability that parallels what is found in the non-MR population.
- Be aware of the unique parenting needs that caregivers may face. Link families to community resources that can provide practical and emotional support when appropriate.
- Since children with developmental disabilities are at higher risk of being abused than their peers without developmental disabilities, discuss with caregivers how to educate children about safety precautions in a developmentally appropriate manner.

M

METABOLIC SYNDROME

Deanna L. Erb, MD
Mark Steenbergen, DO

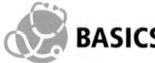 **BASICS**

DESCRIPTION
A common disorder that is a risk factor for both type 2 diabetes mellitus and cardiovascular disease:
- Involves a cluster of metabolic abnormalities:
  - Abdominal obesity
  - Dyslipidemia
  - Hypertension
  - Insulin resistance, with or without impaired glucose tolerance

EPIDEMIOLOGY
- Predominant age: >60 years old
- Predominant sex: Male = Female

Prevalence
- Affects 30–40% of US adults >20 years old; increasing with the aging population and the prevalence of obesity
- Data vary among populations because there is no standardized international definition for the metabolic syndrome.

Pediatric Considerations
Obese children and adolescents are at high risk of the metabolic syndrome, and the risk increases with the severity of the obesity. There are no consistent criteria established for diagnosing metabolic syndrome in children.

RISK FACTORS
- Older age
- Ethnicity
- Family history
- Obesity/central obesity
- Physical inactivity
- High-carbohydrate diet
- Smoking
- Postmenopausal status
- Low socioeconomic status

Genetics
Genetic factors may account for up to 50% of syndrome traits.

GENERAL PREVENTION
- Effective weight loss and maintenance of normal body weight long-term
- Regular and sustained physical activity

PATHOPHYSIOLOGY
- Insulin resistance and an excess of adipose tissue underpin pathogenesis.
- Abnormal fatty acid metabolism, endothelial dysfunction, systemic inflammation, and a procoagulant state are also associated.

ETIOLOGY
The main etiological factors are:
- Obesity (particularly abdominal) and excess adipose tissue
- Insulin resistance
- Other contributing factors:
  - Advancing age
  - Proinflammatory state
  - Genetics
- Endocrine (e.g., postmenopausal state)

COMMONLY ASSOCIATED CONDITIONS
- Polycystic ovary syndrome
- Fatty liver disease (nonalcoholic steatohepatitis)
- Chronic renal disease
- Obstructive sleep apnea
- Gallstones (cholesterol)
- Erectile dysfunction (in men)
- Hyperuricemia and gout

 DIAGNOSIS

HISTORY
- Family history of metabolic syndrome, type 2 diabetes, and cardiovascular disease
- Symptoms indicating cardiovascular disease or diabetes
- Comprehensive lifestyle history:
  - Diet, including intake of carbohydrates, fats
  - Weight history, including onset of obesity and previous weight loss attempts
  - Exercise regimen
  - Alcohol intake
- Cigarette smoking
- Assess cardiovascular risk with Framingham risk assessment tool.

PHYSICAL EXAM
Various criteria-based definitions have been proposed, including those by the World Health Organization, the International Diabetes Federation, and the National Cholesterol Education Program's Adult Treatment Panel III (ATP III). According to ATP III, a diagnosis of metabolic syndrome can be made when ≥3 of the following 5 characteristics are present (1)[C]:
- Abdominal obesity: Men >102 cm, women >88 cm (different waist circumference criteria used for non-Europeans)
- Blood pressure (BP) ≥130/85 mm Hg
- Triglycerides ≥150 mg/dL
- High density lipoprotein (HDL): Men <40 mg/dL, women <50 mg/dL
- Fasting glucose ≥100 mg/dL

DIAGNOSTIC TESTS & INTERPRETATION
Lab
Initial lab tests
- Fasting lipids (particularly triglycerides and HDL)
- Fasting glucose

Follow-Up & Special Considerations
- Formal 75-mg oral glucose tolerance test for diagnosis of impaired fasting glucose (IFG)/impaired glucose tolerance (IGT)
- Measurement of insulin levels is controversial.
- Serum-free testosterone, sex hormone-binding globulin (SHBG)
- Liver function tests

Imaging
None necessary to diagnose metabolic syndrome.

Diagnostic Procedures/Surgery
- May require 24-hour blood pressure (BP) monitoring (rules out white coat hypertension)
- Electrocardiogram (ECG), stress test, coronary angiography may be used for diagnosis of cardiovascular disease arising as a complication of the syndrome.

Pathological Findings
- Microalbuminuria
- Increased white blood cell (WBC) count
- Increased C-reactive protein
- Increased fibrinogen
- Increased proinflammatory cytokines (e.g., tumor necrosis factor alpha)
- Increased uric acid
- Increased homocysteine
- Type 2 diabetes
- Fatty liver (complicated by end-stage liver disease and hepatocellular carcinoma)
- Hypertensive and/or diabetic eye disease
- Renal impairment/failure
- Peripheral vascular disease
- Coronary artery disease
- Cerebrovascular disease

DIFFERENTIAL DIAGNOSIS
Diagnosis is dependent on fulfilling the ATP III diagnostic criteria.

 TREATMENT

The primary therapeutic goal is to prevent or reduce obesity. Aggressive lifestyle modification is considered 1st-line therapy.

MEDICATION
- Daily treatment with aspirin is recommended for patients with cardiovascular disease or those at high risk.
- Consult clinical guidelines for treatment of dyslipidemia, hypertension, IGT, and diabetes.
- Multiple medications usually required to achieve adequate blood pressure control
- The diagnosis and treatment of insulin resistance is controversial.

First Line
- Obesity: Lifestyle changes are the cornerstone of treatment. Realistic weight loss expectations are 5% of baseline in 6 months. Patients need not achieve normal BMI to modify risk factors.
- Dyslipidemia: Drug therapy can be commenced after 6 weeks of lifestyle modification. Target of therapy depends of patient's level of cardiovascular risk:
  - Statin if predominantly high LDL
  - Fibrate if predominantly high triglycerides and/or low HDL
- Hypertension:
  - Aim for similar targets to patients with diabetes (<130/80 mm Hg).
  - Angiotensin-converting enzyme (ACE) inhibitor or angiotensin receptor blocker (ARB) is usually prescribed for patients with diabetes.
- Impaired glucose tolerance:
  - Current guidelines emphasize that treatment should be with diet and exercise.
- The role of oral hypoglycemic agents to prevent diabetes in patients with the metabolic syndrome is unclear: Metformin, 500 mg–1 g, 1–3 times daily, may be considered (2)[A].

Second Line
- Obesity:
  - Orlistat: 120 mg t.i.d. with meals to alter fat absorption
  - Sibutramine, 10–15 mg/d to suppress appetite
  - May be considered if patients do not meet realistic expectations in 6-month period with aggressive lifestyle modification alone
  - These medications are an adjunct to lifestyle modification.
  - Currently no evidence for increased weight loss with combination therapy
- Dyslipidemia:
  - Cholestyramine, 12–16 g/d in 2–3 divided doses if predominantly high LDL
  - Fish oils alone or in combination with fibrate if predominantly high triglycerides
- Hypertension: Angiotensin II receptor blocker (e.g., losartan, 50 mg/d) if intolerant of ACE I inhibitor

ADDITIONAL TREATMENT
General Measures
- Aggressive treatment of individual cardiovascular disease risk factors by lifestyle modification and/or medication
- Avoid or stop smoking.
- Avoid excess alcohol intake.

Issues for Referral
- Nutrition
- Exercise program
- Smoking cessation

COMPLEMENTARY AND ALTERNATIVE MEDICINE
Fish oils and plant sterol esters for cardioprotective effects

SURGERY/OTHER PROCEDURES
- Surgery to treat obesity in severely obese patients who have failed trials of lifestyle modification and pharmacotherapy (2,3)[A]
- Liposuction of abdominal adipose tissue does not reduce insulin resistance or cardiovascular risk factors.

IN-PATIENT CONSIDERATIONS
Management does not usually require admission.

Admission Criteria
Serious complications (e.g., acute coronary syndrome, hypertensive crisis, diabetic coma)

ONGOING CARE
FOLLOW-UP RECOMMENDATIONS
- Regular exercise will improve all components of the metabolic syndrome.
- 30 minutes of moderate-intensity exercise (e.g., brisk walking) daily is recommended at a minimum. Evidence suggests dose effect with higher-intensity exercise (2)[A].
- Include some resistance exercise training.
- Encourage changing of sedentary activity choices (e.g., driving car, taking elevator, and the like) to more active ones (e.g., walking, cycling).
- Regular monitoring of weight, abdominal circumference measurements, BP, fasting lipids, and sugar levels
- Fasting lipids, fasting sugar, and/or oral glucose tolerance test should be checked annually.

Patient Monitoring
- Regular monitoring of weight, abdominal circumference measurements, BP, fasting lipids, and sugar levels
- Fasting sugar and/or oral glucose tolerance test should be checked annually.

DIET
- Weight reduction to correct abdominal obesity is a primary goal.
- Can be achieved by reduction of energy intake and increased physical activity (4)[A]
- Reduction by 500 calories per day will usually achieve a weight loss of 0.5 kg/wk
- A Mediterranean diet (5)[A] and/or a diet with intake of foods that have a low glycemic index/glycemic load is beneficial.
- Other beneficial dietary measures are:
  - Low intake of saturated fats, trans fats, and cholesterol
  - High intake of fruit, vegetables, fiber, and whole grains
  - 2–3 fish meals per week
- Low salt intake

PROGNOSIS
- Increased risk of both type 2 diabetes mellitus and cardiovascular disease
- The degree to which the syndrome can predict future risk of all-cause mortality, cardiovascular disease, and diabetes is not known.

COMPLICATIONS
Long-term complications are primarily cardiovascular.

REFERENCES
1. National Cholesterol Education Program (NCEP) Expert Panel on Detection, Evaluation, and Treatment of High Blood Cholesterol in Adults (Adult Treatment Panel III)et al. Third Report of the National Cholesterol Education Program (NCEP) Expert Panel on Detection, Evaluation, and Treatment of High Blood Cholesterol in Adults (Adult Treatment Panel III) final report. *Circulation*. 2002;106:3143–421.
2. Snow V, Barry P, Fitterman N, et al. Pharmacologic and surgical management of obesity in primary care: a clinical practice guideline from the American College of Physicians. *Ann Intern Med*. 2005;142: 525–31.
3. Clinical Guidelines on the Identification, Evaluation, and Treatment of Overweight and Obesity in Adults - The Evidence Report. National Institutes of Health. *Obes Res*. 1998;6(Suppl 2):51S–209S.
4. Slentz CA, Duscha BD, Johnson JL, et al. Effects of the amount of exercise on body weight, body composition, and measures of central obesity: STRRIDE–a randomized controlled study. *Arch Intern Med*. 2004;164:31–9.
5. Salas-Salvadó J, Fernández-Ballart J, Ros E, et al. Effect of a Mediterranean diet supplemented with nuts on metabolic syndrome status: one-year results of the PREDIMED randomized trial. *Arch Intern Med*. 2008;168:2449–58.

CODES
ICD9
277.7 Dysmetabolic syndrome x

CLINICAL PEARLS
- Abdominal circumference should be measured as part of a cardiovascular risk assessment.
- Prevention or reduction of obesity and regular physical activity is the cornerstone of prevention and treatment of metabolic syndrome.
- Aggressive lifestyle modification is 1st-line lifelong treatment for all patients.

M

METATARSALGIA

Kenneth M. Bielak, MD
Eric J. Kujawski, DO

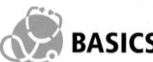

BASICS

DESCRIPTION
- Defined as pain in the metatarsal region of the foot, but more commonly refers to pain of the plantar surface of the forefoot in the metatarsal head region
- System(s) affected: Musculoskeletal

EPIDEMIOLOGY
Incidence
Especially common in athletes with high-impact sports involving the lower extremities (running, jumping, dancing, etc.)

Prevalence
Common

RISK FACTORS
- Obesity
- High heels or narrow shoes
- Competitive athletes for weight-bearing sports (e.g., ballet, basketball, running, soccer, baseball, football)
- Foot deformities (e.g., pes planus, pes cavus, tight Achilles tendon, tarsal tunnel syndrome, hallux valgus, prominent metatarsal heads, excessive pronation, hammer toe deformity, tight toe extensors)

Geriatric Considerations
- Arthritis should be ruled out early.
- More frequent in older athletes
- Symptoms are more pronounced in older people.
- Age-related atrophy of the metatarsal fat pad may increase the risk for metatarsalgia.

Pediatric Considerations
- Muscle imbalance disorders (e.g., Duchenne muscular dystrophy) are a cause of foot deformities in children.
- In adolescent girls, consider Freiberg infraction (i.e., aseptic necrosis of the metatarsal head usually due to trauma in adolescents who jump or sprint).
- Salter I injuries may affect subsequent growth and healing of the epiphysis.

Pregnancy Considerations
- Forefoot pain during pregnancy usually results from change in gait, increased weight, and joint laxity.
- Properly fitted low-heeled shoes are especially important in this group of patients.

GENERAL PREVENTION
- Wear properly fitted shoes with good padding.
- Start weight-bearing exercise programs gradually.

PATHOPHYSIOLOGY
- General:
  - Excessive or repetitive stress: Wearers of high heels, ballet dancers, competitive athletes
  - Soft tissue dysfunction: Intrinsic muscle weakness, laxity in the Lisfranc ligament
  - Abnormal foot posture: Forefoot varus or valgus, cavus or equinus deformities, loss of the metatarsal arch, splay foot, pronated foot
  - Dermatologic: Warts, calluses

- Great toe:
  - Hallux valgus (bunion), either varus or rigidus
- Lesser metatarsals:
  - Freiberg infraction (i.e., aseptic necrosis of the metatarsal head usually due to trauma in adolescents who jump or sprint)
  - Hammer toe or claw toe
  - Morton syndrome (i.e., long second metatarsal)

ETIOLOGY
Abnormal pressure distribution plantar to the metatarsal heads

COMMONLY ASSOCIATED CONDITIONS
See Etiology.

DIAGNOSIS

HISTORY
- Gradual chronic onset is more common than acute presentation.
- Predisposition with pes cavus deformity and hyperpronation
- Acute, chronic, or recurrent symptoms located in the region of the metatarsal heads usually on the plantar surface
- Pain: Often described as seeming like walking with a pebble in the shoe; aggravated during midstance or propulsion phases of walking or running

PHYSICAL EXAM
- Point tenderness over plantar metatarsal heads (1)[C]
- Pain in the interdigital space or a positive metatarsal squeeze test suggests Morton neuroma.
- Plantar keratosis (callus formation) often noted
- Swelling
- Tenderness of the metatarsal head(s) with pressure applied by the examiner's finger and thumb
- Erythema (occasionally)

DIAGNOSTIC TESTS & INTERPRETATION
Lab
Initial lab tests
- Only if diagnosis is in question: Erythrocyte sedimentation rate, rheumatoid factor, human leukocyte antigen (HLA), rapid plasma reagin (RPR), uric acid, glucose, complete blood count with differential
- Disorders that may alter lab results: Acute infections

Imaging
Initial approach
- Weight-bearing radiographs: Anteroposterior, lateral, and oblique views. Occasionally metatarsal or sesamoid axial films (to rule out sesamoid fracture) or skyline view of the metatarsal heads: Obtained with the metatarsophalangeal joints in dorsiflexion (to evaluate alignment).
- Increasing use of sonography and magnetic resonance imaging (MRI), but still no benefit over clinical assessment (2,3)[C]
- MR arthrography of the MTP joint can delineate capsular tears, typically of the distal lateral border of the plantar plate, an often underrecognized cause of metatarsalgia (4)[C].
- Bone scan if high index of suspicion of stress fracture exists

Diagnostic Procedures/Surgery
Plantar pressure distribution analysis: This is early in its development, but may be helpful to distinguish patterns of pressure distribution due to malalignment (5)[C].

Pathological Findings
Because of its 2 sesamoid bones, the 1st metatarsal head usually carries about 30% of the weight when walking. A normal metatarsal arch also ensures this balance. The 1st metatarsal head has adequate padding to accommodate it. A pronated splayfoot disturbs this balance, causing equal weight-bearing on all metatarsal heads. Any foot deformity also changes distribution of weight to areas of the foot that do not have sufficient padding. Reactive tissue can build up a callus around the metatarsal head, which compounds the pain.

DIFFERENTIAL DIAGNOSIS
- Stress fracture (most commonly 2nd metatarsal)
- Morton neuroma (i.e., interdigital neuroma)
- Sesamoiditis or sesamoid fracture
- Salter I fracture in pediatric population
- Arthritis (e.g., gouty, rheumatoid, inflammatory, osteoarthritis, septic, calcium pyrophosphate, dihydrate crystal deposit disease [CPPD])
- Lis Franc injury
- Avascular necrosis of the metatarsal head
- Infection (e.g., cellulitis, diabetic foot, Lyme disease, leprosy)
- Bone tumors (rare)
- Ganglion cyst
- Foreign body
- Vasculitis (diabetes)
- Cavovarus foot

TREATMENT

MEDICATION
- Nonsteroid anti-inflammatory drugs (NSAIDs) (ibuprofen 800 mg t.i.d. 7–14 days or naproxen 500 b.i.d. 7–14 days)
- Contraindications: Gastrointestinal bleeding or ulcer
- Precautions in patients with:
  - Renal disease
  - Hepatic disease
  - Coagulation disorders
- Significant possible interactions:
  - Anticoagulants
  - Digoxin
  - Lithium
  - Methotrexate
  - Cyclosporin

ADDITIONAL TREATMENT
Issues for Referral
Athletes may warrant early podiatric or orthopedic evaluation.

Additional Therapies
- Low-heeled (less than 2 cm height) (6)[C], wide-toe-box shoes
- Metatarsal pads and arch supports
- Orthotics/rocker bar (prescriptive orthotics have been shown to be effective treatment (7)[B]
- Thick-soled shoes
- Shaving the callus may provide temporary relief, but should not be excised.
- Improve flexibility and strength of the muscles of the foot with:
  - Exercises (e.g., towel grasps, pencil curls)
  - Physical therapy to maintain range of motion (ROM) and restore normal biomechanics

COMPLEMENTARY AND ALTERNATIVE MEDICINE
Magnetic insoles not effective for chronic nonspecific foot pain (1)[A]

SURGERY/OTHER PROCEDURES
- If no improvement with conservative therapy for 3 months, referral to foot/ankle orthopedic or surgical podiatrist may be necessary.
- If a correctable anatomic abnormality exists: Bunionectomy, partial osteotomy, osteotomy, or surgical fusion (8)[C]. Success rates vary depending on procedure.
- Morton's neurectomy for the treatment of metatarsalgia reported 82% excellent or good results (9)[C].
- Surgery only as a last resort if no anatomic abnormality is present

IN-PATIENT CONSIDERATIONS
Initial Stabilization
- Relieve pain
- Ice initially
- Rest: Temporary alteration of weight-bearing activity; use of cane or crutch. For more physically active patients, suggest an alternative exercise or cross-training:
  - Moist heat later
  - Taping or gel cast
  - Stiff-soled shoes will act as a splint.
- Relieve the pressure beneath the area of maximal pain by redistributing the pressure load of the foot, which can be achieved by weight loss.

ONGOING CARE

FOLLOW-UP RECOMMENDATIONS
Patient Monitoring
If stress fracture has been ruled out and patient's condition has not improved >3 months of conservative treatment, consider surgical evaluation.

PATIENT EDUCATION
- Instruct about wearing proper sort of shoes and gradual return to activity.
- Cross-training until symptoms subside
- Patient teaching: Prevention
- Biomechanical evaluation is advised by appropriately skilled clinician

PROGNOSIS
Outcome depends on the severity of the problem and whether surgery is required to correct it.

COMPLICATIONS
- Back, knee, and hip pain due to change in gait
- Transfer metatarsalgia following surgical intervention, which subsequently transfers stress to other areas

REFERENCES
1. Young CC, et al. Clinical Examination of the foot and ankle. *Primary Care: Clinics in Office Practice.* 2005;32(1).
2. Sharp RJ, et al. The role of MRI and ultrasound imaging in Morton's neuroma and the effect of size of lesion on symptoms. *J Bone Joint Surg.* 2003;85(7):999–1005.
3. Umans HR. Imaging Sports Medicine Injuries to the Foot and toes. *Clinics in Sports Medicine.* 2006;25(4).
4. Kier R, Abrahamian H, Caminear D, et al. MR arthrography of the second and third metatarsophalangeal joints for the detection of tears of the plantar plate and joint capsule. *AJR Am J Roentgenol.* 2010;194:1079–81.
5. Kanatli U, et al. Pressure distribution patterns under the metatarsal heads in healthy individuals. *Acta Orthop Traumatol Turc.* 2008;42(1):26–30.
6. Ko PH, Hsiao TY, Kang JH, et al. Relationship between plantar pressure and soft tissue strain under metatarsal heads with different heel heights. *Foot Ankle Int.* 2009;30:1111–6.
7. Winemiller MH, Billow RG, Laskowski ER, et al. Effect of magnetic vs sham-magnetic insoles on nonspecific foot pain in the workplace: a randomized, double-blind, placebo-controlled trial. *Mayo Clin Proc.* 2005;80:1138–45.
8. Thomson CE, Gibson JN, Martin D. Interventions for the treatment of Morton's neuroma. *Cochrane Database Systematic Review.* 2004;(3):CD003118.
9. Pace A, Scammell B, Dhar S et al. The outcome of Morton's neurectomy in the treatment of metatarsalgia. *Int Orthop.* 2010;34:511–5.

ADDITIONAL READING
- Birbilis T, Theodoropoulou E, Koulalis D. Forefoot complaints—the morton's metatarsalgia. The role of MR imaging. *Acta Medica (Hradec Kralove).* 2007;50:221–2.
- Birrer R. *Common Foot Problems in Primary Care.* 2nd ed. Philadelphia, PA: Hanley & Belfus; 1998:67–73.
- Burns J, Landorf KB, Ryan MM, et al. Interventions for the prevention and treatment of pes cavus. *Cochrane Database of Systematic Reviews.* 2007;(4): Art. No.: CD006154.DOI:10.1002/14651858.CD006154.pub2.
- Cailliet R. *Foot and Ankle Pain.* 3rd ed. Philadelphia, PA: FA Davis; 1997:141–7.

- Espinosa N, Maceira E, Myerson MS. Current concept review: metatarsalgia. *Foot Ankle Int.* 2008;29:871–9.
- Gregg J, Marks P. Metatarsalgia: An ultrasound perspective. *Australas Radiol.* 2007;51:493–9.
- Gregg JM, Schneider T, Marks P. MR Imaging and Ultrasound of Metatarsalgia-The Lesser Metatarsals. *Radiol Clin North Am.* 2008;46:1061–78.
- Hockenbury RT. Forefoot problems in athletes. *Med Sci Sport ecerc.* 1999;(31) 7(suppl):S448–58.
- Iagnocco A, Coari G, Palombi G, et al. Sonography in the study of metatarsalgia. *J Rheumatol.* 2001;28:1338–40.
- Janisse DJ, Janisse E. Shoe Modification and the use of orthoses in the treatment of foot and ankle pathology. *J Am Acad Orthop Surg.* 2008;16(3):152–8.
- van Wyngarden TM. The painful foot, Part I: Common forefoot deformities. *Am Fam Physician.* 1997;55:1866–76.
- Wu KK. Morton neuroma and metatarsalgia. *Curr Opin Rheumatol.* 2000;12:131–42.

See Also (Topic, Algorithm, Electronic Media Element)
Morton Neuroma (Interdigital Neuroma)

 CODES

ICD9
726.70 Enthesopathy of ankle and tarsus, unspecified

CLINICAL PEARLS
- Pain of the plantar surface of the forefoot in the metatarsal head region
- Common especially in athletes with high-impact sports involving the lower extremities (running, jumping, dancing, etc.)
- Point tenderness over plantar metatarsal heads
- Athletes may warrant early podiatric or orthopedic evaluation.

M

METHANOL POISONING

Ernest Pedapati, MD

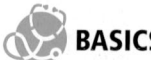

BASICS

DESCRIPTION
- Methanol (wood alcohol) is a clear, colorless solvent found in antifreeze, cleaning solutions, copy machine fluid, gasoline additives, paint, paint thinner, and liquid fuel (1).
- Methanol is less expensive than ethanol and may be used by chronic alcoholics as a substitute.
- Intoxication also can be secondary to methanol-contaminated grain alcohol (moonshine), accidental ingestion, or suicide attempt.
- Methanol produces inebriation, and its metabolic products may cause metabolic acidosis, blindness, and death.

Pregnancy Considerations
Avoid ethanol therapy as treatment for methanol poisoning during 1st trimester of pregnancy; may substitute fomepizole, which is a pregnancy category C drug.

EPIDEMIOLOGY
Incidence
- Predominant age: Most >18 years of age, followed by <6 years of age
- Predominant sex: Male > Female

Prevalence
In the US, 683 methanol exposures were reported in 2007. Sixty-eight cases resulted in moderate–severe outcomes, and there were 9 fatalities.

RISK FACTORS
- Alcoholism
- Epidemics may occur in institutionalized settings where ethyl alcohol is unavailable (e.g., prisons).
- Inappropriate storage leading to childhood exposure

GENERAL PREVENTION
- Substance education for those at risk
- Proper storage of methanol-containing products

PATHOPHYSIOLOGY
- Methanol metabolism in brief (1,2):
  - Methanol is readily absorbed and quickly distributed.
  - The liver slowly metabolizes methanol into formaldehyde via alcohol dehydrogenase.
  - Formaldehyde is rapidly converted into formic acid via aldehyde dehydrogenase.
  - Formic acid is slowly converted to carbon dioxide and water through a folate-dependent process.
  - A limited amount of methanol is also eliminated essentially unchanged through exhalation (12%) and the urine (3%).

- Methanol is minimally toxic, but formic acid causes anion-gap metabolic acidosis and ocular toxicity. Increased lactate owing to systemic toxicity contributes to the acidosis (1).
- Fatal dose is 15–240 mL depending on concentration.
- Peak blood levels occur 30–60 minutes after ingestion (1).

COMMONLY ASSOCIATED CONDITIONS
Alcoholism

DIAGNOSIS

- Classic clinical picture includes nausea, vomiting, abdominal pain, visual disturbances, and metabolic acidosis. There is a latent period after ingestion of 6–24 hours before onset of symptoms; this may be delayed further with concomitant ethanol ingestion (2)[C].
- Overt clinical signs are expected with severe exposure, but at low doses (i.e., occupational exposure), elevated methanol levels may be the only sign.

HISTORY
- Initial CNS depression or inebriation (1)[C]
- Headache, vertigo, lethargy, confusion; severely intoxicated patients can present with coma and convulsions.
- Visual disturbance, ranging from mild blurring to complete blindness "like standing in a snowfield" (3)[B]
- GI symptoms may include nausea, vomiting, and marked abdominal pain.
- Dyspnea

PHYSICAL EXAM
Key physical findings (1,2)[C]:
- Initially, inebriation and gastritis
- Heart rate abnormalities including bradycardia in late stages
- Tachypnea with onset of metabolic acidosis
- Visual field defects, blurred or double vision; loss of visual acuity or pupillary reaction.
- Funduscopic exam may reveal retinal edema, hyperemia, or loss of disc cupping.
- Abdominal tenderness
- Stupor, confusion, seizure, or coma may be present.
- Parkinson-type symptoms have been reported in severe acute and low-level chronic methanol poisoning (4)[C].

DIAGNOSTIC TESTS & INTERPRETATION
Lab
- Serum methanol may be elevated acutely.
- After a latent period, serum formate is a better measure of toxicity.
- Elevated osmolar gap and anion gap; include lactate and ethanol levels to help identify acid contributing to elevated anion gap
- Urinalysis may show myoglobinuria.
- Other useful labs:
  - Arterial blood gas
  - Electrolytes, blood urea nitrogen (BUN), creatinine, calcium, liver function tests, amylase, lipase, creatinine phosphate
  - Toxicologic screens if coingestants are suspected

Imaging
CT scan or MRI of the brain if indicated by neurologic exam. Brain imaging may reveal optic pathway damage, hypodensities in the putamen or caudate nucleus, cerebral edema, cerebral hemorrhage, or cerebral infarct (1)[C].

DIFFERENTIAL DIAGNOSIS
- Ingestion of other alcohols, including ethyl alcohol, ethylene glycol, benzyl alcohol, and isopropyl alcohol
- Other toxic ingestions, including paraldehyde and formaldehyde.
- Increased anion-gap metabolic acidosis caused by renal failure, diabetic ketoacidosis, or lactic acidosis

TREATMENT
MEDICATION
- Ethanol and fomepizole saturated aldehyde dehydrogenase prevent formation of formic acid.
- Metabolism of formic acid is a folate-dependent pathway.
- Criteria for initiation of therapy in patients with known or suspected methanol poisoning (1)[C]:
  - Plasma methanol >20 mg/dL *or*
  - Recent history of ingestion of toxic amounts of methanol and an osmolar gap >10 mOsm/L *or*
  - Suspected methanol ingestion with at least 2 of the following:
    ○ Arterial pH <7.3
    ○ Serum bicarbonate <20 mmol/L
    ○ Osmolar gap >10 mOsm/L

First Line
Fomepizole:
- First 48 hours: IV load with 15 mg/kg, then dosed 10 mg/kg every 12 hours for 4 doses (1)[C]
- After 48 hours: Induces P-450 enzymes, so increase to 15 mg/kg until serum methanol <20 mg/dL (1)[C].
- Increase dosing to every 4 hours for hemodialysis. No adjustments in dosing are needed for renal or hepatic disease.
- Side effects: Mildly increased levels of alanine aminotransferase and aspartate aminotransferase that resolve without consequence (5)[B]

Second Line
- Folinic acid (Leucovorin): May enhance formic acid metabolism (5)[C]
  - 1 mg/kg (up to 50 mg) initially
  - Folic acid can be given every 6 hours at the same dose until metabolic acidosis resolves.
- Ethanol:
  - IV loading dose, then maintenance dosing based on hourly serum ethanol levels; target therapeutic ethanol level is 100–150 mg/dL. Treat until serum methanol is <20 mg/dL (1)[C].
  - Side effects include inebriation, hypoglycemia, phlebitis, and volume overload.
  - Avoid ethanol therapy with CNS depressants, and watch for disulfiram reactions.

ADDITIONAL TREATMENT
General Measures
- Prioritize management on timing and amount of exposure; if patient is intoxicated, history may be unreliable.
- A low or nondetectable methanol level does not rule out ingestion.
- Initial stabilization: IV access and isotonic fluids to maintain adequate urine output and prevent renal failure
- Initial management: Focused on preventing metabolic acidosis and ophthalmic complications
- Consider gastric decontamination with induced emesis, charcoal, or gastric lavage only if concomitant ingestion is known (1)[C].
- Sodium bicarbonate can be considered if serum pH <7.2.
- Hemodialysis (see "Inpatient Considerations").

Issues for Referral
- For patients with substance abuse, referral to detox, rehabilitation, and/or AA/NA.
- Ophthalmology follow-up for patients with visual disturbances

IN-PATIENT CONSIDERATIONS
Consider urgent hemodialysis if (1,6):
- Significant acidosis (pH <7.2) unresponsive to therapy
- Deteriorating vital signs despite intensive support
- Renal failure
- Severe electrolyte imbalance
- Visual or fundoscopic abnormalities
- Serum methanol concentration >50 mg/dL or >30 g ingested.

IV Fluids
Isotonic IV fluid to maintain urine output

 ## ONGOING CARE

FOLLOW-UP RECOMMENDATIONS
- Restricted activity if patient is inebriated, has altered level of consciousness, or has visual impairments
- Referral to psychiatry for suicidal patients

DIET
Thiamine supplementation in patients with long-term alcoholism

PATIENT EDUCATION
- Anticipatory guidance for parents regarding storage of hazardous chemicals
- Motivational interviewing for those with substance dependence and referral for additional treatment
- American Academy of Clinical Toxicology: http://www.clintox.org.

PROGNOSIS
- Outcome varies depending on time to presentation and quantity of methanol ingested.
- Outcome is related to degree of acidosis, coma, or seizures at time of presentation.
- Diagnostic and treatment delays are correlated with poor outcome (3)[C].

COMPLICATIONS
- Blindness and other visual disturbances
- Myoglobinuric renal failure
- Pancreatitis
- Parkinson syndrome

REFERENCES

1. Barceloux DG. American Academy of Clinical Toxicology practice guidelines on the treatment of methanol poisoning. *Clin Toxicol*. 2002;40: 415–46.
2. Kraut JA, Kurtz I. Toxic Alcohol Ingestions: Clinical Features, Diagnosis, and Management. *Clin J Am Soc Nephrol*. 2007.
3. Hovda KE, et al. Methanol outbreak in Norway 2002-2004. *J Int Med*. 2005;258:181–90.
4. Airas L, Paavilainen T, Marttila RJ, et al. Methanol intoxication-induced nigrostriatal dysfunction detected using 6-[18F]fluoro-l-dopa PET. *Neurotoxicology*. 2008.
5. Brent J. Fomepizole for ethylene glycol and methanol poisoning. *N Engl J Med*. 2009;360: 2216–23.
6. Mégarbane B, Borron SW, Baud FJ. Current recommendations for treatment of severe toxic alcohol poisonings. *Intensive Care Med*. 2005;31:189–95.

ADDITIONAL READING

- Comolu S, Ozen B, Ozbakir S. Methanol intoxication with bilateral basal ganglia infarct. *Australas Radiol*. 2001;45:357–8.
- Litovitz TL, Klein-Schwartz W, White S, et al. 2000 Annual report of the American Association of Poison Control Centers Toxic Exposure Surveillance System. *Am J Emerg Med*. 2001;19:337–95.

 ## CODES

ICD9
980.1 Toxic effect of methyl alcohol

CLINICAL PEARLS
- Formic acid, the toxic agent in methanol poisoning, causes anion-gap metabolic acidosis, optic disc edema, and myelin breakdown by direct toxic effects (1)[C].
- Ethanol has the longest history of use, is inexpensive, and is widely available. Fomepizole is preferred because dosing is simpler, it does not require hourly blood draws, and it is not a CNS depressant. No direct comparison of the 2 treatments is available.
- Common indications for hemodialysis in methanol overdose include severe acidosis, visual symptoms, unstable vital signs, refractory electrolyte disturbances, and methanol level >50 mg/dL (1)[C].
- Recent literature suggests that in the absence of neurologic impairment, ocular symptoms, and severe metabolic acidosis, fomepizole may obviate the need for hemodialysis (5,6)[B].

M

MIGRAINE
Tracy Madsen, MD

 BASICS

DESCRIPTION
- Chronic headache disorder with episodic manifestation characterized by recurrent paroxysms of headache capable of altering daily function and lasting from 4–72 hours. Preheadache symptoms are nonspecific, may occur hours to days before headache. Most frequent subtypes are as follows:
  - Without aura (common migraine): Defining >80% of attacks, often associated with nausea, vomiting, photophobia, and phonophobia
  - With aura: Visual or other types of neurological phenomenon precede the headache.
- Other subtypes:
  - Transformed migraine: Chronic headache pattern evolving from episodic migraine. Migraine-like attacks are superimposed on a daily or near-daily headache pattern (e.g., tension headache).
  - Medication overuse headache: Daily or near-daily use of acute medication perpetuating the headache pattern
  - Basilar migraine: Occipital headache, with aura symptoms of dysarthria, vertigo, tinnitus, ataxia, and bilateral paresis or bilateral paresthesias
  - Hemiplegic migraine: Aura consisting of hemiplegia and/or hemiparesis
  - Ophthalmoplegic: Palsy of the ipsilateral 3rd cranial nerve during the headache phase:
    - Some published case studies of abducens nerve palsy
  - Retinal: Symptoms of retinal vascular involvement during migraine
  - Menstrual-related migraine: Associated with onset of menstrual period
  - Childhood periodic syndromes (migraine equivalents): Recurrent, often cyclic, episodes of symptoms
  - Status migrainous: Persistent migraine that does not resolve spontaneously
  - Migrainous stroke: Persistent or permanent neurological deficits persisting beyond migraine attack, usually with neuroimaging changes

EPIDEMIOLOGY
- Female > Male (3:1) menarche to adult
- Female > Male (2:1) postmenopausal women

Prevalence
Adults: Women, 18%; Men, 6%

RISK FACTORS
- Foods, alcohol, missing meals, menstrual cycle, excessive sleep, fatigue, emotional stress, letdown (relief of stress)
- Medications:
  - Cyclic estrogen replacement
  - Birth control pills
  - Vasodilators
- Family history of migraine
- Female gender
- History of childhood cyclic vomiting, cyclic abdominal pain, motion sickness
- Aspartame (1)[C]:
  - There is debate over the role of artificial sweeteners as migraine triggers; primarily linked to pediatric and adolescents.
- Headache and food diaries or elimination diets can help identify migraine triggers.

Genetics
- >80% of patients have a positive family history.
- Familial hemiplegic migraine has been shown to be linked to both chromosomes 19 and 1.

GENERAL PREVENTION
- Avoid precipitants of attacks.
- Biofeedback, education, and psychological intervention
- Prophylactic therapy if attacks frequent, interfere with lifestyle, or are not controlled by acute interventions
- Exercise may reduce the intensity of migraines (2)[C].

PATHOPHYSIOLOGY
- Sensory neurons in the brainstem inappropriately activated
- No longer believed to be primarily vascular in etiology

ETIOLOGY
Largely unknown; serotonin, dopamine, calcitonin-gene–related peptide may have role.

COMMONLY ASSOCIATED CONDITIONS
- Depression
- Panic disorder
- Sleep disturbance
- Cerebral vascular disease
- Cardiac anatomic abnormalities (PFO)
- Peripheral vascular disease
- Seizure
- Irritable bowel syndrome

 DIAGNOSIS

HISTORY
- Headache usually begins with mild pain that escalates into a unilateral (30–40% bilateral), throbbing (40% nonthrobbing) pain of 4–72 hours' duration.
- Intensified by movement and associated with systemic manifestations: Nausea (87%), vomiting (56%), diarrhea (16%), photophobia (82%), phonophobia (78%), muscle tenderness (65%), lightheadedness (72%), vertigo (33%)
- May be preceded by aura:
  - Visual disruptions are most common, including scotoma, hemianopsia, fortification spectra, geometric visual patterns, and occasionally hallucinations.
  - Somatosensory disruption in face or arms
  - Speech difficulties

PHYSICAL EXAM
Full neurological exam should be performed to help exclude other neurological etiologies.

DIAGNOSTIC TESTS & INTERPRETATION
Imaging
Initial approach
CT scan preferred over MRI; obtain if:
- New onset in patient >50 years of age
- Change in established headache pattern
- Atypical pattern or symptoms
- Prolonged or bizarre aura
- Progressive headache
- Unremitting/progressive neurological symptoms

Diagnostic Procedures/Surgery
Lumbar puncture if suspicion of other CNS causes, including subarachnoid bleed or meningitis

DIFFERENTIAL DIAGNOSIS
- Other primary headache syndromes (tension, cluster)
- If focal neurological signs/symptoms present, consider transient ischemic attack, stroke.
- Secondary headaches: Tumor, infection, vascular pathology, prescription or illicit drug use
- Drug-seeking patients
- Psychiatric disease
- Rarely, atypical forms of epilepsy

Geriatric Considerations
- Rare onset of noncephalalgic migraine (aura without subsequent headache) >40 years of age; possible relationship to transient global amnesia
- Late onset requires diagnostic evaluation.

Pediatric Considerations
- Attacks may be shorter and headache description, atypical.
- Recurrent abdominal pain and cyclic vomiting may be migraine equivalent.
- In adolescents with migraine, suicidal ideation may be more prevalent compared to those without migraine (3)

Pregnancy Considerations
- May decrease in 2nd and 3rd trimesters.
- No treatment drug has US Food and Drug Administration approval during pregnancy:
  - Acetaminophen or short-acting opioids can be considered for acute headaches during pregnancy (4)[C].
  - Ergotamines are contraindicated.
  - Early data for sumatriptan suggest no increase in birth defect to date (5)[B].
  - Sumatriptan and zolmitriptan recommended "pump and dump" of milk (6)[B].

TREATMENT

MEDICATION
First Line

- Combination of acetaminophen, aspirin, and caffeine as effective as other agents (5-HT-1 Agonists [triptans]) for mild to moderate migraine with fewer adverse events if given at onset of symptoms (7)[A]
- Aspirin plus the addition of a dopamine antagonist may be as effective as sumatriptan for acute migraine headache (8).
- 5-HT-1 agonist (triptans) intervention during the mild phase of headache; contraindicated with coronary heart disease:
  - Recent evidence suggests that intervention with triptans during the aura, prior to onset of pain, may prevent headache (9)[B].
- Ergotamines:
  - Dihydroergotamine: Drug of choice in status migrainous (7)[B]:
    - Most effective ergotamine; available as IV, IM, or SC injection, and nasal spray
  - Ergotamine tartrate (7)[B]: Preparations contain 1 mg of ergotamine and 100 mg of caffeine.

- Nonsteroidal anti-inflammatory drugs (NSAIDs) (7)[B]: No superiority in efficacy established for any specific agent; early use improves efficacy.
- Antiemetics: Consider antinausea medications that antagonize dopamine receptors.
  - Metoclopramide, prochlorperazine
- Contraindications to treatments:
  - Avoid 5-HT-1 agonists (triptans) in coronary heart disease, peripheral vascular disease, uncontrolled hypertension, complex migraine (e.g., basilar or hemiplegic migraine).
  - 5-HT-1 agonists should not be used within 24 hours of an ergot derivative or other triptans.
  - Avoid NSAIDs if danger of gastric erosion or renal or hepatic disease.
  - Avoid narcotics or butalbital in addiction-prone patients and patients with frequent migraines.
  - Avoid vasoconstrictors in uncontrolled hypertension, coronary heart disease, and peripheral vascular disease.
  - Avoid sumatriptan, zolmitriptan, and rizatriptan within 2 weeks of MAOI usage.
- Precautions:
  - Frequent use of acute-treatment drugs may lead to increase in migraine patterns and medication overuse headache.

Second Line
Use of opioids in migraine:
- Some advocate the use of long-acting opioids in patients with refractory migraine (10)[C].
- Shorter acting opioids may be effective for acute relief of severe migraine (10)[C].
- Recent retrospective study found narcotics were the most frequently used drugs for migraine in the ED with other migraine treatment used only 2% of the time (11).
- Recent review links frequent opioid use to increased rates of chronic migraine, though may not be causal (12).

ADDITIONAL TREATMENT
General Measures
- Cold compresses to area of pain
- Rest with pillows comfortably supporting head or neck in area devoid of sensory stimulation, including light, sound, and odors.
- Withdrawal from stressful surroundings
- Sleep is desirable.
- Most patients manage attacks with self-care.
- Avoid precipitants of migraine.

Issues for Referral
- Obscure diagnosis, concomitant medical conditions, significant psychopathology
- Unresponsive to usual treatment
- Analgesic-dependent headache patterns

Additional Therapies
- Recent study suggests that "rescue" (parenteral) therapy in clinic reduces ED visits and total health care costs (13)[B].
- For people who have frequent migraine, consider prophylactic therapy with β-blockers, calcium channel blockers, antidepressants, or some anticonvulsants .
- Topiramate (Topamax) for migraine prophylactic therapy has efficacy comparable to amitriptyline (Elavil) with increased patient side-effect profile (including weight loss) (14)[A].

COMPLEMENTARY AND ALTERNATIVE MEDICINE
- Riboflavin 400 mg/day possibly effective as preventive agent
- Feverfew, a medicinal herb, no more effective than placebo for the prevention of migraines (15)

IN-PATIENT CONSIDERATIONS
Initial Stabilization
Monitor vital signs, patient comfort.

Admission Criteria
Consider if diagnosis not clear; if appropriate, may need to exclude intracranial bleeds, TIA, CVA.

IV Fluids
- Consider in setting of acute onset, severe headache.
- Consider if associated with nausea/vomiting.

Discharge Criteria
Judgment based on patient's overall clinical status, patient's ability to tolerate PO medications

ONGOING CARE

FOLLOW-UP RECOMMENDATIONS
Early intervention when migraines begin

Patient Monitoring
- Early intervention to assist management
- Monitor frequency of attacks, pain behaviors, and medication usage.
- Encourage lifestyle modifications.

PATIENT EDUCATION
Educate patients about migraine triggers.

PROGNOSIS
- With increasing age, reduction in severity, frequency, and disability of attacks
- Most attacks subside within 72 hours.

COMPLICATIONS
- Rare:
  - Status migrainous
  - Cerebral ischemic events
- Iatrogenic effects of treatment

REFERENCES

1. Jacob SE, Stechschulte S. Formaldehyde, aspartame, and migraines: a possible connection. *Dermatitis*. 2008;19:E10–1.
2. Busch V, Gaul C. Exercise in migraine therapy–is there any evidence for efficacy? A critical review. *Headache*. 2008;48:890–9.
3. Hershey AD. Teens, migraine, suicide, and suicidal thoughts. *Neurology*. 2009;72:e61–2.
4. Lucas S et al. Medication use in the treatment of migraine during pregnancy and lactation. *Curr Pain Headache Rep*. 2009;13:392–8.
5. The Sumatriptan and Naratriptan Pregnancy Registry: Data from GlaxoSmithKline.
6. Hale TW. *Medications and Mother's Milk*. 11th ed. Amarillo, TX: Pharmasoft Pub.; 2004.
7. Matchar DB, Young WB, Rosenberg JH, et al. Evidence-based guidelines for migraine headache in the primary care setting: Pharmacological management of acute attacks. AAN Headache Guidelines. US Headache Consortium 2000:1–58.
8. Kirthi V, Derry S, Moore RA, McQuay HJ et al. Aspirin with or without an antiemetic for acute migraine headaches in adults. *Cochrane Database Syst Rev*. 2010;4:CD008041.
9. Aurora SK, Barrodale PM, McDonald SA, et al. Revisiting the Efficacy of Sumatriptan Therapy During the Aura Phase of Migraine. *Headache*. 2009.
10. Rothrock JF. Treatment-refractory migraine: the case for opioid therapy. *Headache*. 2008;48: 850–4.
11. Sahai-Srivastava S, Desai P, Zheng L. Analysis of headache management in a busy emergency room in the United States. *Headache*. 2008;48:931–8.
12. Bigal ME, Lipton RB. Excessive opioid use and the development of chronic migraine. *Pain*. 2009.
13. Morey V, Rothrock JF. Examining the utility of in-clinic "rescue" therapy for acute migraine. *Headache*. 2008;48:939–43.
14. Dodick DW, Freitag F, Banks J, et al. Topiramate versus amitriptyline in migraine prevention: A 26-week, multicenter, randomized, double-blind, double-dummy, parallel-group noninferiority trial in adult migraineurs. *Clin Ther*. 2009;31:542–59.
15. Pittler MH, Ernst E. Feverfew for preventing migraine. Cochrane Pain, Palliative and Supportive Care Group *Cochrane Database of Systematic Reviews*. 2006:4.

See Also (Topic, Algorithm, Electronic Media Element)
Algorithm: Headache, Chronic

CODES

ICD9
- 346.00 Migraine with aura, without mention of intractable migraine without mention of status migrainosus
- 346.10 Migraine without aura, without mention of intractable migraine without mention of status migrainosus
- 346.90 Migraine, unspecified, without mention of intractable migraine without mention of status migrainosus

CLINICAL PEARLS
- Migraine is a chronic headache disorder of unclear etiology often characterized by unilateral, throbbing headaches that may be associated with additional neurologic symptoms.
- Migraine should be differentiated from other primary headache disorders and also from other CNS etiologies of headache.

M

MILD COGNITIVE IMPAIRMENT

Birju B. Patel, MD
N. Wilson Holland, MD

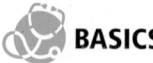 **BASICS**

DESCRIPTION

- Mild cognitive impairment (MCI) is defined as significant cognitive impairment in the absence of dementia, as measured by standard memory tests.
  - Report of memory problems, preferably corroborated by another person
  - Ability to perform activities of daily living (ADLs) is maintained.
  - Normal general thinking and reasoning skills
  - Synonym(s): Isolated memory impairment; Cognitive impairment not dementia (CIND); Predementia; Mild cognitive disorder; Age-associated memory impairment; Age-related cognitive decline; Benign senescent forgetfulness
- Annual rates of conversion of MCI to dementia are 5–15% in the elderly.

EPIDEMIOLOGY

Incidence
- Predominant sex: Male > Female
- Predominant age:
  - Higher in older persons or those with less education
  - 12–15/1,000 person-years in those aged ≥65 years
  - 54/1,000 person-years in those aged ≥75 years

Prevalence
- MCI is more prevalent than dementia in the US.
- 3–5% for those aged ≥60 years
- 15% for those aged ≥75 years

RISK FACTORS

- Age
- Diabetes
- Hypertension
- Dyslipidemia
- Apolipoprotein (APO) E4 genotype

Genetics
APO ε4 genotype: Various pathways exist leading to amyloid accumulation and deposition.

PATHOPHYSIOLOGY

- Subtypes of MCI:
  - Single-domain amnestic
  - Multiple-domain amnestic
  - Nonamnestic single-domain
  - Nonamnestic multiple-domain
- The amnestic subtype may be a precursor to Alzheimer disease.

ETIOLOGY
Vascular, degenerative, traumatic, metabolic, psychiatric, or combination

COMMONLY ASSOCIATED CONDITIONS
See "Risk Factors."

 DIAGNOSIS

HISTORY
- Focus on cognitive deficits and impairment.
- Review all medications that may affect cognition, and particular emphasis should be given to anticholinergic medications (patients on these may be mistakenly classified as having MCI) (1)[B].
- Rule out depression.
- Assess function (ADLs, instrumental ADLs).

PHYSICAL EXAM
- A general exam focusing on clinical clues to identifying vascular disease (e.g., bruits, abnormal blood pressure)
- Neurologic exam to rule out reversible CNS causes of cognitive impairment or other causes of cognitive impairment (e.g., Parkinson disease)
- Mini-Mental Status Exam (MMSE)

DIAGNOSTIC TESTS & INTERPRETATION
Lab
Initial lab tests
- Complete blood count
- Comprehensive metabolic profile
- Thyroid-stimulating hormone
- Vitamin B₁₂
- Lipids

Follow-Up & Special Considerations
Consider referral to a memory center for more comprehensive evaluation of MCI looking for specific cognitive domains involved.

Imaging
- CT scan can detect structural CNS conditions leading to cognitive impairment.
  - Subdural hematoma
  - Normal-pressure hydrocephalus
  - Metastatic disease
- MRI further evaluates vascular, infectious, neoplastic, and inflammatory conditions.

Initial approach
- Rule out reversible causes of cognitive impairment.
- Cognitive screening is important [e.g. Montreal Cognitive Assessment (MOCA), MMSE, Saint Louis University Mental Status (SLUMS), mini-Cog, etc.]; MOCA may be more sensitive for detecting MCI (2).
- Clinical Dementia Rating Scale may be used as an additional tool for early detection of MCI (3).
- Neuropsychological testing for complex and atypical presentations
- Vascular risk factor reduction and treatment

Follow-Up & Special Considerations
- Document progression of dementia.
- Advanced planning while patient is competent
- Early education of caregivers on safety, maintaining structure, managing stress, and future planning (4)

Pathological Findings
- Little is known about MCI pathology owing to a lack of longitudinal studies.
- Alzheimer dementia pathophysiology:
  - Neurofibrillary tangles in hippocampus
  - Senile plaques (amyloid deposition)
  - Neuronal degeneration
- Those with MCI have intermediate amounts of pathologic findings of Alzheimer disease with amyloid deposition and neurofibrillary tangles in the mesial temporal lobes compared with those with dementia.
- Amnestic MCI is associated with white matter hyperintensity volume on MRI, whereas nonamnestic MCI is associated with infarcts (5).

DIFFERENTIAL DIAGNOSIS
- Delirium
- Dementia
- Depression
- "Reversible" cognitive impairment:
  - Medications (anticholinergics)
  - Hypothyroidism
  - Vitamin B₁₂ deficiency
- Reversible CNS conditions

TREATMENT

MEDICATION

- The use of cholinesterase inhibitors (ChEIs) in MCI is not associated with any delay in the onset of Alzheimer disease or dementia. Moreover, the safety profile showed that the risks associated with ChEIs are not negligible (6)[A]. Therefore, ChEIs are not recommended routinely (7)[A].
- Consider symptomatic treatment with ChEIs only if memory complaints appear to be affecting quality of life in individual patients or in patients with an amnestic subtype of MCI (8)[B].
- Donepezil therapy was associated with lower rate of progression to Alzheimer disease. This effect was demonstrated for up to 3 years (8)[B].
- Donepezil is started at 5 mg/d × 30 days and then increased to the maintenance dose of 10 mg/d thereafter.
- There is inconclusive evidence of effectiveness of other ChEIs and memantine.

ADDITIONAL TREATMENT

General Measures
Atherosclerotic risk factors should be treated aggressively.

Issues for Referral
Consider referral to a memory specialist (i.e., geriatrician, neurologist, geropsychiatrist) to evaluate and differentiate subtypes of MCI and specific cognitive deficits.

COMPLEMENTARY AND ALTERNATIVE MEDICINE
There is no evidence of the efficacy of vitamin E in the prevention or treatment of people with MCI. More research is needed to identify the role of vitamin E, if any, in the management of cognitive impairment (9)[A].

IN-PATIENT CONSIDERATIONS

- Delirium is more common in patients hospitalized with all forms of cognitive impairment.
- Avoid medications that may worsen or precipitate cognitive decline (e.g., anticholinergics, antihistamines, etc.).
- Patients may be extremely sensitive to the hospital environment.
  - Moderate level of stimulation is best.
  - Avoid sensory deprivation. Make sure that patients have access to hearing aids and eyeglasses.

 ONGOING CARE

FOLLOW-UP RECOMMENDATIONS
Patients should be reevaluated every 6–12 months to determine if symptoms are progressing.

Patient Monitoring
Appropriate cognitive and functional testing should be used to evaluate progression, along with clinical history and exam. If a medication is started, patients need to be followed more frequently to evaluate for efficacy, side effects, dose titration, etc. Declining financial skills may be an early marker to progression of MCI to dementia, and clinicians should monitor and advise patients and families proactively to look for this (10).

DIET
Diets that are promoted by the American Heart Association to minimize atherosclerotic risk factors should be emphasized.

PATIENT EDUCATION
- Encourage lifestyle changes.
  - Physical activity such as walking 30 minutes daily on most days of the week
  - Mental activity that stimulates language skills and psychomotor coordination should be encouraged. Computer activities, reading books, crafts, crossword puzzles, and games may be linked to decreased risk of development of MCI.
- Cognitive rehabilitation strategies may be beneficial in helping with daily activities relating to memory tasks in MCI (11).

PROGNOSIS
- Conversion rates from MCI to dementia range from 5–15% annually.
- Amnestic subtypes of MCI are most likely to progress to dementia (12).

REFERENCES

1. Ancelin ML, Artero S, Portet F, et al. Non-degenerative mild cognitive impairment in elderly people and use of anticholinergic drugs: longitudinal cohort study. *BMJ*. 2006;332:455–9.
2. Nasreddine ZS, Phillips NA, Bédirian V, et al. The Montreal Cognitive Assessment, MoCA: a brief screening tool for mild cognitive impairment. *J Am Geriatr Soc*. 2005;53:695–9.
3. Morris JC et al. Clinical dementia rating: a reliable and valid diagnostic and staging measure for dementia of the Alzheimer type. *Int Psychogeriatr*. 1997;9(Suppl 1).
4. Knopman DS, Boeve BF, Petersen RC. Essentials of the proper diagnoses of mild cognitive impairment, dementia, and major subtypes of dementia. *Mayo Clin Proc*. 2003;78:1290–308.
5. Luchsinger JA, Brickman AM, Reitz C, Cho SJ, Schupf N, Manly JJ, Tang MX, Small SA, Mayeux R, DeCarli C, Brown TR et al. Subclinical cerebrovascular disease in mild cognitive impairment. *Neurology*. 2009;73:450–6.
6. Raschetti R, Albanese E, Vanacore N, et al. Cholinesterase inhibitors in mild cognitive impairment: a systematic review of randomised trials. *PLoS Med*. 2007;4:e338.
7. Birks J, et al. Donepezil for mild cognitive impairment. *Cochrane Database Syst Rev*. 2006;3:CD006104. DOI:10.1002/14651858.CD006104.
8. Petersen RC, Thomas RG, Grundman M, et al. Vitamin E and donepezil for the treatment of mild cognitive impairment. *N Engl J Med*. 2005;352:2379–88.
9. Isaac MG, Quinn R, Tabet N. Vitamin E for Alzheimer's disease and mild cognitive impairment. *Cochrane Database Syst Rev*. 2008:CD002854.
10. Triebel KL, Martin R, Griffith HR, Marceaux J, Okonkwo OC, Harrell L, Clark D, Brockington J, Bartolucci A, Marson DC et al. Declining financial capacity in mild cognitive impairment: A 1-year longitudinal study. *Neurology*. 2009;73:928–34.
11. Kinsella GJ, Mullaly E, Rand E, Ong B, Burton C, Price S, Phillips M, Storey E et al. Early intervention for mild cognitive impairment: a randomised controlled trial. *J Neurol Neurosurg Psychiatr*. 2009;80:730–6.
12. DeCarli C. Mild cognitive impairment: prevalence, prognosis, aetiology, and treatment. *Lancet Neurol*. 2003;2:15–21.

ADDITIONAL READING

Plassman BL, Langa KM, Fisher GG, et al. Prevalence of cognitive impairment without dementia in the United States. *Ann Intern Med*. 2008;148:427–34.

 CODES

ICD9
331.83 Mild cognitive impairment, so stated

CLINICAL PEARLS

- Amnestic MCI affects primarily memory and is more likely to progress to Alzheimer dementia.
- Screen for reversible factors, particularly anticholinergic medications and depression.
- Look closely at vascular risk factors, and modify them as best as possible.
- ChEIs should not be used routinely unless memory complaints are affecting quality of life in patients.
- Encourage both physical and mental exercises.

M

MILIARIA RUBRA

Aamir Siddiqi, MD

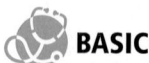 **BASICS**

DESCRIPTION
- Miliaria rubra is a papulovesicular eruption of eccrine sweat glands that often occurs in high heat and humidity.
- System(s) affected: Skin/Exocrine
- Synonym(s): Prickly heat

EPIDEMIOLOGY
- Predominant age: Common in infants, less common in adults
- Predominant sex: Male = Female

Incidence
- May be present in up to 4% of neonates with a mean age of 1–14 days
- In tropical environment, as many as 30% of individuals exposed to heat may have miliaria.

Pediatric Considerations
More common in this age group

RISK FACTORS
- Hot, humid environment
- Occlusive bandages
- High fever

GENERAL PREVENTION
- Acclimatize slowly to hot weather.
- Avoid hot and humid conditions.
- Dress appropriately for warm environmental conditions.
- Understand the self-limiting nature of the disease.

ETIOLOGY
The rash is a result of keratinous plugging of the sweat ducts, which leads to swelling of the gland (known as a retention vesicle) and extravasation of sweat into the surrounding skin leading to irritation and itching.

COMMONLY ASSOCIATED CONDITIONS
- Exposure to hot and humid conditions
- Neonates have immature eccrine glands, which are easy to rupture with sweating, resulting in miliaria.
- Miliaria has been associated with a rare Morvan syndrome characterized by severe insomnia, for weeks or months in a row, and associated with autonomic alterations consisting of profuse perspiration (1).

 DIAGNOSIS

HISTORY
- Lesions appear after person has been in a hot humid environment that causes sweating.
- Pruritus or prickly, mildly stinging sensation in affected body areas

PHYSICAL EXAM
- Prevalent in areas of friction caused by clothing and in areas of flexure
- Infants: Trunk, diaper area, neck, axilla, face
- Pilosebaceous follicles, palms, and soles are spared.
- Fine papules and vesicles on an erythematous base (2)[B]
- May become inflamed pustules (miliaria pustulosa) (3)[B]

DIAGNOSTIC TESTS & INTERPRETATION
Pathological Findings
- Keratinous plugging of sweat ducts
- Sweat-retention vesicle

DIFFERENTIAL DIAGNOSIS
- Acne
- Folliculitis
- Viral exanthems
- Drug eruptions
- Erythema toxicum
- Yeast infections
- Pyogenic infections
- Syringomas (4)[B]

 TREATMENT

MEDICATION
- Topical lotions containing calamine, menthol, or camphor may be helpful for symptoms. Over-the-counter preparations with menthol, camphor for pruritus: Hydrocortisone (Sarna) or pramoxine (Prax).
- Topical steroids to relieve pruritus: 0.1% Betamethasone (Valisone) b.i.d. for 3 days; avoid prolonged usage.
- Systemic antibiotics in cases of bacterial secondary infection: Antibiotic effective against staphylococci (e.g., dicloxacillin 250 mg q.i.d. for 10 days unless strain is resistant to agent)
- If sweating is secondary to fever, then antipyretic drugs may be useful.
- Precautions: Care should be taken with fluorinated steroid application in children. These agents may cause systemic effects.

ADDITIONAL TREATMENT
General Measures
- Avoid wearing heavy, tight clothing or garments that may cause friction.
- Avoid plastic or occlusive dressings/garments in hot environments.
- Avoid excessive use of soap and contact with irritants.
- Frequent cool baths with Aveeno colloidal, oatmeal, or cornstarch mixtures
- Provide cool, dry environment for 8–10 hours per day.
- Topical applications of lotions containing lanolin, calamine, boric acid, and menthol

COMPLEMENTARY AND ALTERNATIVE MEDICINE
- Use of tannic acid has not been shown to be effective.
- Aloe vera gel may be effective for heat-related rashes.

 ## ONGOING CARE
FOLLOW-UP RECOMMENDATIONS
Avoid vigorous activity that causes excessive sweating.

PROGNOSIS
- Benign: Responds to cooling
- Avoiding causative agents is key.

COMPLICATIONS
- Secondary bacterial infections
- Miliaria profunda secondary to repeated miliaria rubra can cause anhidrosis.

REFERENCES

1. Tabanelli M, Passarini B, Liguori R, et al. Erythematous papules on the parasternal region in a 76-year-old man. *Clin Exp Dermatol*. 2008;33:369–70.
2. Gan VN, Hoang MP. Generalized vesicular eruption in a newborn. *Pediatr Dermatol*. 2004;21:171–3.
3. Haas N, Martens F, Henz BM: Miliaria crystallina in an intensive care setting. *Clin Exp Dermatol*. 2004;29(1):32–4.
4. Wilkinson TM, Mizelle CB, Morrell DS. Multiple milia-like dermal papules. *Pediatr Dermatol*. 2004;21:269–71.

 ## CODES

ICD9
705.1 Prickly heat

CLINICAL PEARLS

- Miliaria is most common in the pediatric age group.
- Topical mild steroid creams may be used to improve symptoms. Avoiding hot and humid temperature is helpful in prevention and treatment.

M

MILK-ALKALI SYNDROME

Stanley G. Smith, MA, MB, FCFP

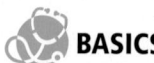 ## BASICS

DESCRIPTION

Milk-alkali syndrome is a condition resulting from ingestion of excessive amounts of calcium and absorbable alkali (e.g., sodium bicarbonate and calcium carbonate):

- Usually occurs during self-treatment for indigestion, peptic ulcer, or gastroesophageal reflux disease, or as part of osteoporosis prevention
- Characterized by hypercalcemia, metabolic alkalosis, and renal insufficiency
- System(s) affected: Endocrine/Metabolic; GI; Renal/Urologic
- Synonym(s): Burnett syndrome; Milk poisoning; Milk drinker syndrome

EPIDEMIOLOGY

Incidence

- 3rd most common cause of hypercalcemia, with a prevalence of 9–12% among hospitalized patients with hypercalcemia
- Recent increase associated with osteoporosis prevention

Prevalence

Infrequent

RISK FACTORS

- Chronic use of calcium-containing antacids or supplements
- Chronic kidney disease
- Vitamin D supplementation
- Thiazide diuretic therapy

GENERAL PREVENTION

Avoid excess milk and/or absorbable antacids.

PATHOPHYSIOLOGY

Exact mechanism unclear:

- Increased calcium absorption may lead to suppression of parathyroid hormone, which leads to the kidneys retaining increased bicarbonate. This eventually leads to alkalosis, which also causes increased calcium resorption in the kidneys.

ETIOLOGY

Excess intake of milk and alkali as therapy for gastrointestinal problems accompanied with gastric hyperacidity (e.g., peptic ulcer, esophageal reflux) or for prevention of osteoporosis

COMMONLY ASSOCIATED CONDITIONS

- Peptic ulcer disease
- Hiatal hernia
- Gastroesophageal reflux
- Osteoporosis
- Hypertension
- Hyperparathyroidism
- Hypercalcemia of malignancy

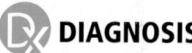 ## DIAGNOSIS

History of excessive calcium and absorbable alkali intake resulting in hypercalcemia, metabolic acidosis, and renal impairment

HISTORY

- Calcium-containing supplement use
- Food distaste, anorexia
- Constipation
- Dizziness, weakness
- Headache
- Mental status changes, irritability, depression
- Myalgias
- Nausea, vomiting
- Polydipsia
- Polyuria

PHYSICAL EXAM

- Band keratopathy
- Dehydration
- Periarticular calcinosis

DIAGNOSTIC TESTS & INTERPRETATION

Lab

Check calcium, renal function, lytes, BUN, creatinine, alkaline phosphatase, and PTH.

Initial lab tests

- Mild alkalosis
- Hypercalcemia
- Normocalciuria
- Decreased urine phosphate
- Increased BUN and serum creatinine levels
- Normal alkaline phosphatase level

Pathological Findings
- Nephrocalcinosis
- Ectopic calcification

DIFFERENTIAL DIAGNOSIS
Other causes of hypercalcemia:
- Excessive osteolysis with malignant disease
- Vitamin intoxication
- Thyroid disease
- Sarcoidosis
- Thiazide diuretic treatment
- Hyperparathyroidism

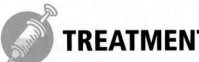 TREATMENT

MEDICATION
First Line
- To treat hypercalcemia:
  – Isotonic sodium chloride: 0.9% IV when serum calcium exceeds 15 mg/dL (3.75 mmol/L; see Hypercalcemia) plus
  – Furosemide: 80–100 mg IV q2h for 24 hours after volume depletion has been corrected
- Precautions: Replace sodium and potassium losses associated with furosemide use.

Second Line
- Bisphosphonates inhibit bone resorption.
- Dialysis is occasionally indicated.

ADDITIONAL TREATMENT
General Measures
- Withdraw milk and alkali (1)[B].
- Hydration (1)[B]
- Treat hypercalcemia.
- Goal is to maintain urine volume of 3 L/d

Issues for Referral
Renal insufficiency

IN-PATIENT CONSIDERATIONS
Initial Stabilization
Withdraw milk and alkali.

Admission Criteria
- IV treatment to avoid calcinosis (usually with sodium chloride solution)
- Renal dialysis for significant renal insufficiency

 ONGOING CARE

FOLLOW-UP RECOMMENDATIONS
Avoid excess alkali.

Patient Monitoring
- Kidney function
- Fluid intake and output
- Urine electrolytes

DIET
- Increased fluid intake
- Avoid excess milk and alkali.

PATIENT EDUCATION
Appropriate diet

PROGNOSIS
Favorable with appropriate therapy

COMPLICATIONS
- Psychosis
- Stupor
- Coma
- Renal failure

REFERENCE
1. Medarov BI et al. Milk-alkali syndrome. *Mayo Clin Proc.* 2009;84:261–7.

ADDITIONAL READING
Ulett K, Wells B, Centor R et al. Hypercalcemia and acute renal failure in milk-alkali syndrome: a case report. *J Hosp Med.* 2010;5:E18–20.

 CODES

ICD9
275.42 Hypercalcemia

CLINICAL PEARLS
- Inquire if patient uses over-the-counter antacids or calcium supplements.
- Daily calcium supplementation should not exceed 2 g.
- Hydration and withdrawal of calcium sources are the mainstays of treatment.

M

MITRAL REGURGITATION

Yongkasem Vorasettakarnkij, MD, MSc
Peerawut Deeprasertkul, MD

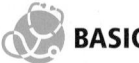 BASICS

DESCRIPTION

- Disorder of mitral valve (MV) closure, either structural or functional, resulting in a backflow of part of the left ventricular (LV) stroke volume into the left atrium (LA); uncompensated, this leads to LV and LA enlargement, elevated pulmonary pressures, atrial fibrillation, heart failure, and sudden cardiac death.
- Types of mitral regurgitation (MR):
  - Acute versus chronic
  - Structural versus functional (e.g., ischemic)
    ○ Functional: "Mitral valve is structurally normal, and disease results from valve deformation caused by ventricular remodelling."
    ○ MV structures include not only the mitral annulus, MV leaflets, chordae tendineae, and papillary muscles but also the posterior LA wall and the LV wall.
- System(s) affected: Cardiac; Pulmonary

EPIDEMIOLOGY

Moderate to severe MR affects 2.5 million people in the US (2000 data), making it the most frequent valvular disease, and this number is expected to double by 2030 (1).

Prevalence

- By severity on echocardiography:
  - Mild MR: 19% (up to 40% if trivial jets included)
  - Moderate MR: 1.9%
  - Severe MR: 0.2%
- By category (1):
  - Degenerative (myxomatous disease, annular calcification): 60–70%
  - Ischemic: 20%
  - Endocarditis: 2–5%
  - Rheumatic: 2–5%

RISK FACTORS

- Age
- Hypertension
- Rheumatic heart disease
- Endocarditis
- Anorectic drugs

GENERAL PREVENTION

- Risk factor modification for coronary artery disease (CAD)/myocardial infarction (MI)
- Antibiotic prophylaxis for poststreptococcal rheumatic heart disease
- Endocarditis prophylaxis for mitral regurgitation no longer recommended

PATHOPHYSIOLOGY

- Acute MR: Acute damage to MV leads to sudden LA and LV volume overload and increased LV preload. Sudden rise in LV volume load without compensatory LV remodelling results in impaired forward cardiac output and possible shock.

- Chronic MR: LV eccentric hypertrophy compensates for the increased regurgitant volume to maintain forward cardiac output and reduce symptoms of pulmonary congestion. However, continuous LV remodelling may result in LV dysfunction.
- Ischemic MR:
  - Papillary muscle rupture or ischemia during acute MI.
  - Functional MR due to incomplete coaptation of valve leaflets or restricted valve movement resulting from ischemia

ETIOLOGY

- Acute MR:
  - Flail leaflet: Myxomatous disease, infective endocarditis, or trauma
  - Ruptured chordae tendineae: Trauma, spontaneous rupture, infective endocarditis, or rheumatic fever
  - Ruptured or displacement of papillary muscle: Acute MI, severe myocardial ischemia, or trauma
- Chronic MR:
  - Structural
    ○ Degenerative: mitral annular calcification, mitral valve prolapse (MVP)
    ○ Infective endocarditis
    ○ Rheumatic heart disease
    ○ Anorectic drugs
    ○ Congenital
  - Functional
    ○ CAD/MI
    ○ Hypertrophic cardiomyopathy

COMMONLY ASSOCIATED CONDITIONS

MVP with MR common in Marfan syndrome

 DIAGNOSIS

HISTORY

- Associated conditions: Rheumatic heart disease, prior MI, connective tissue disorder
- Acute MR:
  - Sudden onset of dyspnea
  - Orthopnea/paroxysmal nocturnal dyspnea
  - Cardiogenic shock
- Chronic MR:
  - Exertional dyspnea
  - Fatigue
  - Palpitation: Paroxysmal or persistent AF

PHYSICAL EXAM

- Acute MR:
  - Rapid and thready pulse
  - Sign of poor tissue perfusion with peripheral vasoconstriction
  - Hyperdynamic precordium without apical displacement
  - S_3 and S_4 (if in sinus rhythm)
  - Systolic murmur at left sternal border and base:
    ○ Early, middle, or holosystolic murmur
    ○ Often soft, low-pitched, decrescendo murmur
  - Rales

- Chronic MR:
  - Brisk upstroke of arterial pulse
  - Leftward displaced LV apical impulse
  - Systolic thrill at the apex (suggests severe MR)
  - Soft S_1 and widely split S_2
  - Loud P_2 (if pulmonary hypertension)
  - S_3 gallop
  - Holosystolic murmur at apex that radiates to axilla
  - Ankle edema, jugular venous distension, ascites if development of right-sided heart failure

DIAGNOSTIC TESTS & INTERPRETATION

Lab

- CXR:
  - Acute MR: Pulmonary edema with normal heart size
  - Chronic MR: LA and LV enlargement
- ECG:
  - Acute MR:
    ○ Varies depending on etiologies, e.g., acute MI
  - Chronic MR:
    ○ P mitrale from LA enlargement
    ○ LV hypertrophy
    ○ Q waves from prior MI
    ○ Atrial fibrillation

Initial lab tests

- Cardiac enzymes and brain natriuretic peptide, if appropriate
- See workup for MI, CAD, and congestive heart failure (CHF)

Imaging

Initial approach

Transthoracic echocardiogram (TTE)

- Indications for TTE:
  - Baseline evaluation of LV function, right ventricular and LA size, pulmonary artery pressure, and severity of MR (2)[C]
  - Delineation of mechanism of MR (2)[B]
  - Surveillance of asymptomatic moderate–severe LV function (ejection fraction and end-systolic dimension) (2)[C]
  - Evaluate MV apparatus and LV size and function after a change in signs or symptoms in a patient with MR (2)[C].
  - Evaluate after MV repair or replacement (2)[C].
- Findings in acute MR:
  - Evidence of etiology: Flail leaflet or infective vegetations
  - Normal LA and LV size
- Findings in chronic MR:
  - Evidence of degenerative, rheumatic, ischemic, congenital, and other causes.
  - Enlarged LA and LV

Follow-Up & Special Considerations

- Intervals for follow-up TTE: See "Follow-up" below.
- Transesophageal echocardiogram (TEE):
  - Intraoperatively to define severity/cause of MR and/or LV function
  - Nondiagnostic TTE
  - Evaluation of prosthetic heart valves
- Exercise Doppler echo:
  - Assess exercise tolerance and the effects of exercise on pulmonary artery pressure in asymptomatic patients with severe MR (2)[C].

- Cardiovascular magnetic resonance:
  - When regurgitant severity is indeterminant on echocardiography, especially in patients with LV dysfunction

Diagnostic Procedures/Surgery
- Cardiac catheterization:
  - Hemodynamic measurements (2)[C]
    - Pulmonary pressure is discordant to the severity of MR as assessed by noninvasive testing
  - Left ventriculography and hemodynamic measurement (2)[C]
    - Noninvasive tests are inconclusive regarding severity of MR
    - Regurgitant severity is discordant between clinical and noninvasive findings
  - Coronary angiography (2)[C]
    - Prior to MV surgery in patients at risk for CAD

Pathological Findings
Quantification of severe MR involves assessment of:
- Structural parameters:
  - LA size: Usually dilated, unless acute
  - LV size: Usually dilated, unless acute
  - Leaflets: Abnormal
- Doppler parameters
- Quantitative parameter

DIFFERENTIAL DIAGNOSIS
- Aortic stenosis (AS): Usually midsystolic but can be long, difficult to distinguish from holosystolic, heard at apex, and radiated to the carotid arteries (unlike MR)
- Tricuspid regurgitation: Also holosystolic but at left lower sternal border, does not radiate to axilla or increase in intensity with inspiration (unlike MR)
- Ventricular septal defect (VSD): Harsh holosystolic murmur at lower left sternal border but radiates to right (not axilla and has thrill)

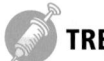 TREATMENT

Acute severe MR:
- Medical therapy has a limited role and is aimed primarily to stabilize hemodynamics preoperatively (2).
- Urgent surgical consultation

MEDICATION
Chronic MR:
- Structural
  - Asymptomatic: No proven long-term medical therapy
  - Symptomatic:
    - Diuretics
    - Chronic vasodilator therapy for nonsurgical candidates.
- Functional:
  - LV dysfunction or symptomatic: ACEI, β-blockers (particularly carvedilol and long-actingmetoprolol)

SURGERY/OTHER PROCEDURES
- Isolated MV surgery is not indicated for patients with mild to moderate MR (2)[C].
- Acute severe MR secondary to acute MI:
  - Acute rupture of papillary muscle: Emergency MV repair or replacement
  - Papillary muscle displacement
    - Aggressive medical stabilization, and intra-aortic balloon pump
    - Valve surgery usually required in addition to revascularization

- Chronic severe MR:
  - MV repair at an experienced center is recommended over MV replacement in most circumstances
    - Survival rate: 80–94% versus 40–60% at 5–10 years
    - 10-year rate of stroke: 10% (repair) versus 12% (bioprosthetic-valve replacement) versus 23 %(mechanical-valve replacement) (3)
    - Risk of endocarditis: 1.5% at 15 years versus 0.3–1.2% per year (3)
    - Overall rates of reoperation are similar (3).
  - Indications for MV surgery in chronic severe MR (2)
    - Symptomatic: Absence of severe LV dysfunction (ejection fraction [EF] >30% and end-systolic dimension [ESD] <55 mm); NYHA functional class III-IV; severe LV dysfunction (EF <30% and/or ESD >55 mm). Surgery is indicated only if repair is highly likely to be successful.
    - Asymptomatic: Mild to moderate LV dysfunction (EF 30-60% or ESD ≥40 mm); preserved LV function (EF >60% and ESD <40 mm): MV repair in experienced surgical centers is reasonable if chance of successful repair without residual MR is >90%; preserved LV function and new onset atrial fibrillation; preserved LV function and pulmonary hypertension (PASP >50 mm Hg at rest or PASP >60 mm Hg with exercise)
- Nonischemic functional severe MR: In selected patients may consider:
  - Cardiac resynchronization therapy
  - Percutaneous mitral annuloplasty

Geriatric Considerations
- Consider medical therapy alone for patients >75 years of age with MR owing to increased operative mortality and decreased survival (compared with those with AS), especially with preexisting CAD or need for MV replacement.

IN-PATIENT CONSIDERATIONS
Initial Stabilization
Acute MR:
- Stabilize ABCs.
- IV, O_2, and monitoring
- Nitroprusside (+ dobutamine and/or aortic balloon counterpulsation if hypotensive) (3)[C]
- Treat underlying causes (e.g., MI).
- Treat acute pulmonary edema.
  - Lasix
  - Morphine
- Urgent surgical consultation

 ONGOING CARE

FOLLOW-UP RECOMMENDATIONS
Chronic MR: Asymptomatic:
- Mild MR with normal LV size and function and no pulmonary hypertension: Annual clinical evaluation to assess symptom progression
- Moderate MR: Annual clinical evaluation and echocardiography to assess LV function
- Severe MR: Clinical evaluation and echocardiography every 6–12 months
- Consider serial CXRs and ECGs.
- Consider stress test if exercise capacity is in question.

PATIENT EDUCATION
- Exercise after MV repair: Avoid sports with risk for bodily contact or trauma. Low intensity competitive sports are allowed.
- Competitive athletes with MR:
  - Asymptomatic with normal LV size and function, normal pulmonary artery pressures, and sinus rhythm: No restrictions
  - Mildly symptomatic and those with LV dilatation: Activities with low to moderate dynamic and static cardiac demand allowed
- Atrial fibrillation and anticoagulation: No contact sports

PROGNOSIS
- Acute severe MR: Mortality risk with surgery, 50%; mortality risk with medical therapy alone, 75% in 1st 24 hours; 95% at 2 weeks
- Chronic MR:
  - Asymptomatic severe MR with normal LVEF: 10% yearly rate of progression to symptoms and subnormal resting LVEF
  - Symptomatic severe MR: 8-year survival rate, 33% without surgery; mortality rate, 5% yearly
  - MV repair versus replacement

Pregnancy Considerations
MR with NYHA functional class III–IV at high risk for maternal and/or fetal risk

COMPLICATIONS
Acute pulmonary edema, CHF, atrial fibrillation, bleeding risk with anticoagulation, endocarditis, sudden cardiac death

REFERENCES
1. Enriquez-Sarano M, Akins CW, Vahanian A. Mitral regurgitation. *Lancet*. 2009;373:1382–94.
2. Bonow RO, et al, American College of Cardiology/American Heart Association Task Force et al. 2008 Focused update incorporated into the ACC/AHA 2006 guidelines for the management of patients with valcular heart disease. *Circulation* 2008;118:e523–661.
3. Foster E et al. Clinical practice. Mitral regurgitation due to degenerative mitral-valve disease. *N Engl J Med*. 2010;363:156–65.

 CODES

ICD9
- 394.1 Rheumatic mitral insufficiency
- 424.0 Mitral valve disorders
- 746.6 Congenital mitral insufficiency

CLINICAL PEARLS
- Follow-up for mild to moderate MR: Serial exam and/or echo unless LV structural changes
- Severe MR is usually managed with mitral valve repair.
- Endocarditis prophylaxis not recommended

M

MITRAL STENOSIS

Sarah B. Fleisig, MD

 BASICS

DESCRIPTION
- Resistance to diastolic filling of the left ventricle due to narrowing of mitral valve orifice.
- Hemodynamic consequences are due to passive transmission of left atrial pressure to the pulmonary circulation.
- Rheumatic heart disease most commonly affects the mitral valve.
- System(s) affected: Cardiovascular

EPIDEMIOLOGY
- The most common acquired valvular disease
- Predominant age: Symptoms primarily occur in middle age (40–70 years)
- Predominant sex: Male < Female (1:2)
- 60% of mitral stenosis patients report history of rheumatic fever.

Incidence
- Incidence of rheumatic heart disease in the US is decreasing due to detection and treatment of Group A streptococcal infection, and also due to antigenic shift in circulating strep.
- Incidence of mitral stenosis in the US has decreased accordingly, but global burden remains significant (1).

RISK FACTORS
- Rheumatic fever is the greatest risk factor.
  - 30–40% of rheumatic fever patients eventually develop mitral stenosis.
  - Acute rheumatic fever occurs 2–3 weeks after episode of untreated Group A streptococcal pharyngitis.
  - Patients present an average of 20 years after rheumatic fever.
- Aging (increasing valvular calcification)
- Chest radiation (increasing tissue fibrosis)

GENERAL PREVENTION
- Prompt recognition and treatment of Group A streptococcal infection; recognition of cardinal signs and symptoms of acute rheumatic fever via Jones Criteria
- Jones Criteria: Diagnosis requires evidence of streptococcal infection, plus two major criteria, or one major plus two minor criteria.

Evidence of Strep Infection	ASO titer or positive throat culture
MAJOR CRITERIA	carditis, polyarthritis, Sydenham's chorea, erythema marginatum, subcutaneous nodules
MINOR CRITERIA	migratory arthralgias, fever, acute phase reactants (elevated ESR, leukocytosis), prolonged PR interval on EKG

PATHOPHYSIOLOGY
- Obstruction between LA and LV impairs LV filling during diastole and results in increased LA pressure
- Increased LA pressure is transmitted passively ("back pressure") to the pulmonary circulation; over time, pulmonary hypertension results.
- Over time, LA pressure overload can dilate the chamber and interrupt the cardiac conduction system, resulting in atrial fibrillation.
- Pulmonary hypertension can also cause increased collateralization between pulmonary and bronchial circulation, resulting in intraparenchymal hemorrhage with hemoptysis.

ETIOLOGY
- Rheumatic fever: Most common (see "Risk Factors")
- Aging (extension of mitral annular calcification)
- Congenital (rare; associated with mucopolysaccharidoses)
- Other acquired mitral stenosis (rare):
  - Left atrial myxoma
  - Left atrial thrombus

COMMONLY ASSOCIATED CONDITIONS
- Atrial fibrillation (30–40% of symptomatic patients) and thromboembolic complications
- Associated valve lesions due to chronic inflammation (aortic stenosis, aortic insufficiency)
- Pulmonary HTN
- Pulmonary congestion
- Pulmonary embolism (10%)
- Systemic congestion
- Systemic embolism
- Infection (1–5%)

 DIAGNOSIS

HISTORY
- Prior history of rheumatic fever
- Severity of presentation depends on valve area; most early cases will be asymptomatic.
- Presenting features usually due to pulmonary vascular congestion:
  - Palpitations
  - Dyspnea on exertion
  - Fatigue
  - Pulmonary edema
  - Paroxysmal nocturnal dyspnea
- Atrial fibrillation
- Embolic event
- In advanced disease, symptoms of pulmonary hypertension and right heart failure predominate:
  - JVD
  - Hepatomegaly
  - Ascites
  - Edema
- Rare presentations:
  - Hemoptysis
  - Hoarseness (compression of recurrent laryngeal nerve by enlarged pulmonary artery or LA)
  - Dysphagia (compression)

PHYSICAL EXAM
- Auscultation:
  - Decrescendo diastolic rumble with presystolic accentuation, heard best at apex
  - Accentuated S1
  - Opening snap
- Mitral regurgitation causes holosystolic murmur along with murmur of mitral stenosis
- If pulmonary hypertension is present: Right ventricular lift, increased P2, high-pitched decrescendo diastolic murmur of pulmonic insufficiency (Graham Steell murmur)
- May also find associated aortic, or less commonly, tricuspid murmurs (due to aortic or tricuspid valve involvement from rheumatic heart disease)

DIAGNOSTIC TESTS & INTERPRETATION
Imaging
Initial approach
- Electrocardiography: (2)
  - Left atrial enlargement (manifested by broad, notched P waves in lead II with a negative terminal deflection of the P wave in lead V1)
  - Atrial fibrillation common
  - With right ventricular hypertrophy, right axis deviation and a large R wave in V1 may be noted
- Chest radiograph:
  - Left atrial enlargement with straightening of the left heart border, a "double density," and elevation of the left mainstem bronchus
  - Pulmonary venous pattern changes with redistribution of flow toward apices
  - Prominent pulmonary arteries at the hilum with rapid tapering
  - Right ventricular enlargement
  - Kerley B lines
  - Pulmonary edema pattern (late)
- Echocardiogram Indications:
  - Class I:
    - Diagnosis of mitral stenosis
    - Assess severity
    - Re assess after change in symptoms
    - Exercise Doppler for discrepancies between symptoms and echo findings
    - TEE to evaluate possible LA thrombus
    - TEE when transthoracic echo nondiagnostic.
  - Class II:
    - Reassess asymptomatic patients
    - Severe MS: Yearly
    - Moderate MS: Every 1–2 years
    - Mild MS: Every 3–5 years
  - Class III:
    - Satisfactory result of transthoracic echo
- Echocardiogram findings (3):
  - MV anterior leaflet doming
  - Immobility of the posterior leaflet
  - Echo can demonstrate alternative causes of MS if not rheumatic.
  - Mitral valve area defined
    - Normal: 4–6 cm^2
    - Mild MS: <2 cm^2
    - Moderate MS: 1–1.5 cm^2
    - Severe MS: <1cm^2

- Cardiac catheterization indications:
  - Class I recommendations:
    - When echo is nonconclusive
    - Discrepancy between echo and symptoms
    - Discrepancy between echo and valve area
  - Class II recommendations:
    - To assess response of LA and pulmonary artery pressures to exercise when symptoms and echo findings don't match
    - Assess cause of severe pulm HTN out of proportion to echo results
  - Class III recommendations:
    - Satisfactory result of echo

Follow-Up & Special Considerations
- If valve area greater than 1.5 cm^2 and pressure gradient <5mm Hg then no further initial workup needed.
- If valve area is less than 1.5 cm^2 then further workup prior to surgical correction.

Diagnostic Procedures/Surgery
Exercise or Dobutamine stress test:
- When symptoms are severe but echo findings are mild.
- To determine if surgery is needed.

Pathological Findings
Rheumatic fever-induced pathologic changes:
- Leaflet thickening
- Leaflet calcification
- Commissural fusion
- Chordal shortening

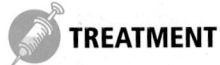 TREATMENT
MEDICATION
First Line
- Antibiotic prophylaxis against rheumatic fever and/or carditis is recommended for patients with history of rheumatic fever
  - Penicillin V or G
  - Sulfadiazine
  - Erythromycin
  - Take antibiotic continuously to prevent recurrence of rheumatic fever or carditis.
  - Duration of rheumatic fever prophylaxis:
    - Rheumatic fever without carditis: Take for 5 years or until 21, whichever is longer
    - Rheumatic fever with carditis but no residual heart disease: Take for 10 years or well into adulthood, whichever is longer
    - Rheumatic fever with carditis plus residual heart disease: Take for 10 years or until 40 years old, whichever is longer.
- Antibiotic prophylaxis against infective endocarditis is not routinely recommended (4).
- β-blockers for tachycardia or exertional symptoms
- Calcium channel blockers for tachycardia or exertional symptoms
- Diuretics for symptoms of pulmonary congestion
- Digitalis for atrial fibrillation if LV or RV dysfunction

- Anticoagulation:
  - Class I recommendations:
    - MS and atrial fibrillation or h/o atrial fibrillation
    - MS and prior embolic event
    - MS and left atrial thrombus
  - Class IIb recommendations
    - Asymptomatic mitral stenosis (MS) but with severe MS and left atrial (LA) dimension greater than 54 mm by echo
    - Severe MS, enlarged LA and spontaneous contrast on echo
- Warfarin for clot prevention International normalized ratio (INR) range 2.0–3.0.
- Heparin in the acute atrial fibrillation setting

Second Line
Amiodarone for rate control if beta-blockers or calcium channel blockers cannot be used.

ADDITIONAL TREATMENT
General Measures
- Mitral stenosis is generally a progressive disease.
- Exercise:
  - Mild MS patients are usually asymptomatic even with strenuous exercise.
  - Usually recommend low-level aerobic exercise, limited by symptoms of dyspnea.
- Counsel patients that mitral stenosis is usually slowly progressive but can have sudden onset of atrial fibrillation which could become rapidly fatal. Call 911 for marked worsening of symptoms.
- Atrial fibrillation accompanying mitral stenosis impairs left ventricular filling, especially with a rapid ventricular response:
  - Rate control with beta or calcium channel blockers or amiodarone.
  - Cardioversion is indicated for medical failure or if patient is unstable.
  - If the atrial fibrillation has been present for longer than 24–48 hours, then:
    - Anticoagulate for 3 weeks then cardiovert
    - Heparinize, perform TEE and if no atrial thrombus then cardiovert
  - After cardioversion, patient needs long-term anticoagulation.
  - These patients can critically decompensate due to loss of atrial contractility causing an inability to fill the LV.

SURGERY/OTHER PROCEDURES
- Balloon valvotomy:
  - Symptomatic patients with NYHA class II, III or IV symptoms with valves that look favorable and with favorable comorbidities
- Mitral valve surgery (5)
  - When MS is severe and balloon valvotomy is contraindicated due to unfavorable anatomy

Pregnancy Considerations
- Volume expansion during pregnancy can exacerbate heart failure symptoms. For this reason, MS often presents in the intrapartum period. For patients with known severe mitral stenosis, intervention should be pursued prior to pregnancy. Percutaneous balloon valvotomy can be performed in symptomatic pregnant patients.

ONGOING CARE
DIET
Salt restriction for pulmonary congestion.

PROGNOSIS
Natural history:
- Rheumatic fever
- Asymptomatic latent period x 10–30 years
- Symptoms start
- 10-year survival of asymptomatic or minimally symptomatic patients is 80%
- 10-year survival after onset of symptoms is 50-60%
- Progression accelerates
- Symptoms become debilitating 10 years after symptoms onset, typically
- 10-year survival after onset of debilitating symptoms is only 0–15%
- Mean survival with significant pulmonary HTN is less than 3 years.

REFERENCES
1. Ray S. Changing epidemiology and natural history of valvular heart disease. Clin Med. 2010;10(2): 168–71.
2. Chandrasekhar Y. Mitral stenosis. Lancet. 2009 Oct 10;374(9697):1271–83.
3. Maganti K, et al. Valvular heart disease: diagnosis and management. Mayo Clin Proc. 2010;85(5): 483–500.
4. Nishimura RA, et al. ACC/AHA 2008 guideline update on valvular heart disease: focused update on infective endocarditis: a report of the American College of Cardiology/American Heart Association Task Force on Practice Guidelines endorsed by the Society of Cardiovascular Anesthesiologists, Society for Cardiovascular Angiography and Interventions, and Society of Thoracic Surgeons. Catheter Cardiovasc Interv. 2008;72(3):E1–12.
5. Zakkar M, et al. Rheumatic mitral valve disease: current surgical status. Prog Cardiovasc Dis. 2009; 51(6):478–81.

CODES
ICD9
- 394.0 Mitral stenosis
- 394.1 Rheumatic mitral insufficiency
- 394.2 Mitral stenosis with insufficiency

M

MITRAL VALVE PROLAPSE

Peerawut Deeprasertkul, MD
Fae G. Wooding, PharmD
George P. Kinzfogl, III, MD

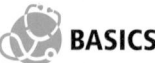 **BASICS**

DESCRIPTION
- Generally, mitral valve prolapse (MVP) is a systolic billowing of one or both mitral leaflets into the left atrium during systole ± mitral regurgitation (MR).
- More specifically, MVP is a single or bileaflet prolapse of at least 2 mm superior displacement into left atrium during systole on the parasternal long-axis annular plane of the valve on echocardiogram ± leaflet thickening.
  - Classic: Prolapse with greater than 5 mm of leaflet thickening
  - Nonclassic: Prolapse with less than 5 mm of leaflet thickening (1)
- Synonym(s): Systolic click-murmur syndrome; billowing mitral cusp syndrome; myxomatous mitral valve; floppy valve syndrome; redundant cusp syndrome; Barlow syndrome

EPIDEMIOLOGY
Incidence
- Predominant age: MVP has been described in all age groups.
- Initial descriptions based on clinical examination suggested a 2:1 female predominance. Using modern echocardiogram criteria, men and women are affected equally (2).
- The most serious consequences of hemodynamically significant MR occur in men older than 50 years.

Prevalence
MVP is the most common valvular abnormalities, affecting 1–2.5% of the general population (2,3) depending on precise definition.

RISK FACTORS
- MVP is a primary cardiovascular disorder.
- MVP is more likely to occur in patients with connective tissue disorders (see "Commonly Associated Conditions").
- Physical characteristics associated with MVP:
  - Straight thoracic spine
  - Pectus excavatum
  - Asthenic body hiatus
  - Low BMI
  - Scoliosis or kyphosis
  - Hypermobility of the joints
  - Arm span greater than height
  - Narrow anteroposterior (AP) diameter of the chest

Genetics
- Familial MVP is inherited as an autosomal-dominant trait but with variable expressivity and incomplete penetrance.
- Two genetic loci identified:
  - *MMVP1* on chromosome 16p11.2-p12.1
  - *MMVP2* on chromosome 11p15.4 (1)

PATHOPHYSIOLOGY
- The pathology causing MVP is multifactorial and includes:
  - Abnormal valve tissue:
    - Myxomatous degeneration: Redundant layers of leaflet "hooding" the cords, chordal elongation, and annular dilatation
    - Myxoid leaflets are more elastic and less stiff than normal valves.
    - Chordal rupture is more common.
  - Disparity in size between the mitral valve and the left ventricle
  - Connective tissue disorders (1)
- MVP is often associated with variable degrees of MR.
- Frequently there is enlargement of the left atrium (LA) and left ventricle (LV).
- Mitral annulus is often dilated.
- Involvement of other valves may occur (tricuspid valve prolapse 40%, pulmonic prolapse and aortic prolapse 2% to 10%)
- Possible increased vagal tone
- Possible increased urine epinephrine and norepinephrine
- MVP patients often have orthostatic hypotension and tachycardia.

ETIOLOGY
- Genetics cause proliferation of the spongiosa layer of the leaflets (3).
- Fibrosis on surface of leaflets (3)
- Thinning and elongation of chordae tendineae
- The mitral valve differentiates during days 35–42 of fetal development, the same time as differentiation of the vertebrae and ribs.

COMMONLY ASSOCIATED CONDITIONS
- Marfan syndrome (91% of Marfan syndrome patients have mitral valve prolapse) (1)
- Ehlers-Danlos syndrome
- Hypertrophic cardiomyopathy
- Pseudoxanthoma elasticum
- Osteogenesis imperfecta
- Von Willebrand disease (3)
- Primary hypomastia

 DIAGNOSIS

Physical exam and echocardiography

HISTORY
- Most patients are asymptomatic.
- Most frequent symptom is palpitations.
- Symptoms related to autonomic dysfunction:
  - Anxiety
  - Panic attacks
  - Arrhythmias
  - Exercise intolerance
  - Palpitations
  - Atypical chest pain
  - Fatigue
  - Orthostasis
  - Syncope or presyncope
  - Neuropsychiatric symptoms
- Symptoms related to progression of mitral regurgitation:
  - Fatigue
  - Dyspnea
  - Exercise intolerance
  - Orthopnea
  - Paroxysmal nocturnal dyspnea
  - Congestive heart failure
- Symptoms occur as a result of an associated complication (stroke, arrhythmia).

PHYSICAL EXAM
- Auscultatory examination:
  - Mid-to-late systolic click:
    - May vary in timing and intensity based on ventricular beat-to-beat volume variations
    - At low ventricular volumes, the valve may prolapse earlier during systole and further into the LA than during volume-overload.
    - It may or may not be followed by a high-pitched, mid-to-late systolic murmur at the cardiac apex.
  - Murmur:
    - Mid-to-late crescendo systolic murmur
    - Best heard at apex
    - Middle- to high-pitched
    - Occasionally musical or honking in quality
  - Occasionally, only the ejection click is present.
  - The duration of the murmur corresponds with the severity of MR.
- Dynamic auscultation:
  - Maneuvers that move the click and murmur toward S_1:
    - Arterial vasodilation
    - Amyl nitrate
    - Valsalva
    - Augmented contractility
    - Decreased venous return (which can be induced by standing up)
  - Maneuvers that move the click and murmur toward S_2:
    - Squatting
    - Leg raise
    - Isometric exercise

DIAGNOSTIC TESTS & INTERPRETATION
Imaging
Initial approach
- Echocardiogram:
  - Indicated for the diagnosis of MVP and assessment of MR, leaflet morphology, and left ventricular systolic function in asymptomatic patients with physical signs of MVP
  - Routine repetition of echocardiography is not indicated for the asymptomatic patient who has MVP and no MR, or MVP and mild MR with no changes in clinical signs and symptoms.
  - Most useful and definitive imaging study
  - Parasternal long-axis view most specific for diagnosis
  - Valve prolapse of 2 mm or more above the mitral annulus is most highly associated with MVP +/− leaflet thickening.
  - Other findings may include
    - Anterior leaflet billowing
    - Leaflet thickening of 5 mm or more
    - Leaflet redundancy
    - Mitral regurgitation
    - Posterior leaflet displacement
  - Nondiagnostic transthoracic echocardiogram: 10% or less
  - Transesophageal echocardiography is helpful to visualize the leaflet anatomy, especially if a valve repair operation is being considered and/or if there is a flail leaflet.

- Angiography indicated in patients with severe and symptomatic MR for whom cardiac surgical referral is being contemplated:
  - Impaired LV systolic function to evaluate for mitral valve surgery
  - Rarely used for diagnostic purposes
- ECG is usually normal.
  - May be nonspecific ST-T wave changes
  - T-wave inversions
  - Prominent Q waves
  - QT prolongation
- CXR is not necessary for diagnosis.
  - Typically the CXR is normal.
  - Other findings:
    - Possible pulmonary edema. Pulmonary edema may be asymmetric with acute chordal rupture and flail leaflet.
    - Possible calcification of the mitral annulus
- Holter monitoring is optional if patient has palpitations. Order Holter monitoring as usual for syncope or dizziness.

Follow-Up & Special Considerations
Patients with a 1st-degree relative who has myxomatous mitral valve prolapse should be screened with echocardiography (1).

Pathological Findings
- Myxomatous proliferation of the middle layer (spongiosa) of the valve, resulting in increased mucopolysaccharide deposition and myxomatous degeneration
- By electron microscopy, the collagen fibers in the valve leaflets are disorganized and fragmented.
- With increased stroma deposition, the valve leaflets enlarge and become redundant.
- The endothelium is usually noncontiguous and a frequent site for thrombus or infective vegetation.

DIFFERENTIAL DIAGNOSIS
- Mitral regurgitation
- Tricuspid regurgitation
- Tricuspid valve prolapse
- Papillary muscle dysfunction
- Hypertrophic cardiomyopathy
- Ejection clicks (don't change timing with systole)

 ## TREATMENT

MEDICATION
- Asymptomatic MVP is treated with reassurance; normal lifestyle and regular exercise is encouraged (3)
- MVP and transient ischemic attacks (TIA) are treated with aspirin 75–325 mg daily (Class I recommendation) (3)[C].
- MVP with history of cryptogenic stroke, or atrial fibrillation with CHADS$_2$ score <2 is generally treated with aspirin 75–325 mg daily (3)[C].
- MVP with atrial fibrillation with CHADS$_2$ score ≥2 is treated with warfarin (3)[C].
- MVP with history of stroke plus atrial fibrillation or left atrial appendage thrombus is treated with warfarin (3)[C]
- MVP with palpitations is treated with β-blockers and/or recommendation to discontinue alcohol, cigarettes, and caffeine. Continuous ambulatory ECG monitoring may be useful to detect significant arrhythmias (3).

ADDITIONAL TREATMENT
General Measures
Treat MVP with orthostatic symptoms by liberalizing fluid and salt intake. If severe, mineralocorticoids or clonidine may rarely be used. Support stockings may also be beneficial.

Additional Therapies
- Endocarditis prophylaxis is not recommended for MVP (3)[B].
- Patients with prior endocarditis undergoing dental, respiratory tract, infected skin or musculoskeletal should receive prophylaxis for endocarditis with amoxicillin 30–60 minutes prior to procedure (3)[B]. Ampicillin, cefazolin, or ceftriaxone IM or IV may be used if unable to tolerate oral medications.

SURGERY/OTHER PROCEDURES
Referral for surgery is recommended for patients with severe MR with impaired LV systolic function or flail leaflet owing to ruptured chordae tendineae (3).

 ## ONGOING CARE

FOLLOW-UP RECOMMENDATIONS
- Asymptomatic MVP patients with no significant MR can be followed clinically every 3–5 years.
- Patients who are symptomatic or have high-risk features on initial echocardiogram, including moderate to severe MR, may need serial echocardiograms and should be followed clinically once per year.
- Patients with MVP and severe MR may require coronary angiography and transesophageal echocardiography if cardiac surgical referral is planned.

PATIENT EDUCATION
Patient education on avoidance of alcohol, caffeine, stimulants, and nicotine may be sufficient to control symptoms in some instances.
- No contraindication to pregnancy
- Restriction from competitive sports if patient has MVP with one of following features (4):
  - A history of syncope associated with document arrhythmia
  - A family history of MVP-related SCD
  - Sustained or repetitive and nonsustained supraventricular tachycardia or frequent and/or complex ventricular tachyarrhythmias on ambulatory Holter monitoring
  - Severe MR
  - A prior embolic event
  - Left ventricular systolic dysfunction
- Explain the hereditary nature of familial MVP.

PROGNOSIS
- Excellent prognosis for asymptomatic patients
- For patients with severe MR or reduced ejection fraction, the prognosis is similar to that for nonischemic MR.

COMPLICATIONS
- Sudden cardiac death (yearly rate of 1.9/10,000 per year) is twice the rate in the general population; risk is 50–100 times greater (0.9–1.9% per year) if significant MR is present (5).
- Chordae rupture with acute mitral insufficiency (higher risk of cardiac death; up to 2% per year)
- Endocarditis
- Cerebrovascular ischemic event
- Fibrin emboli
- Heart failure with progressive MR
- Arrhythmia (6)
  - Atrial premature beats, 35–90%
  - Supraventricular tachycardia, 3–32%
  - Ventricular premature beats, 58–89%
  - Complex ventricular ectopy, 30–56%
- Pulmonary HTN
- CHF
- Progressive MR

REFERENCES

1. Hayek E, Gring CN, Griffin BP. Mitral valve prolapse. *Lancet*. 2005;365:507–18.
2. Freed LA, Levy D, Levine RA, et al. Prevalence and clinical outcome of mitral-valve prolapse. *N Engl J Med*. 1999;341:1–7.
3. Bonow RO, Carabello BA, Chatterjee K, et al. 2008 focused update incorporated into the ACC/AHA 2006 guidelines for the management of patients with valvular heart disease: a report of the American College of Cardiology/American Heart Association Task Force on Practice Guidelines (Writing Committee to revise the 1998 guidelines for the management of patients with valvular heart disease). Endorsed by the Society of Cardiovascular Anesthesiologists, Society for Cardiovascular Angiography and Interventions, and Society of Thoracic Surgeons. *J Am Coll Cardiol*. 2008;52: e1–142.
4. Maron BJ, Ackerman MJ, Nishimura RA, et al. Task Force 4: HCM and other cardiomyopathies, mitral valve prolapse, myocarditis, and Marfan syndrome. *J Am Coll Cardiol*. 2005;45:1340–5.
5. Kligfield P, Levy D, Devereux RB, et al. Arrhythmias and sudden death in mitral valve prolapse. *Am Heart J*. 1987;113:1298–307.
6. Zuppiroli A, Mori F, Favilli S, et al. Arrhythmias in mitral valve prolapse: relation to anterior mitral leaflet thickening, clinical variables, and color Doppler echocardiographic parameters. *Am Heart J*. 1994;128:919–27.

ADDITIONAL READING

- Maron BJ, Ackerman MJ, Nishimura RA, et al. Task Force 4: HCM and other cardiomyopathies, mitral valve prolapse, myocarditis, and Marfan syndrome. *J Am Coll Cardiol*. 2005;45:1340–5.
- Wu WC, Aziz GF, Sadaniantz A. The use of stress echocardiography in the assessment of mitral valvular disease. *Echocardiography*. 2004;21: 451–8.

 ## CODES

ICD9
424.0 Mitral valve disorders

M

MOLLUSCUM CONTAGIOSUM

Gillian S. Stephens, MD, MSc

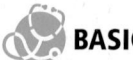 **BASICS**

DESCRIPTION
- Common, benign, viral (*Poxviridae*) skin infection
- 1–5 mm, "pearly" white or flesh-colored
- Dome-shaped papules; central umbilication (difficult to see in young children)
- Highly contagious; autoinoculation, skin-to-skin contact, sexual contact, shared clothing, towels, bathing water
- Self-limited in immunocompetent
- Difficult to treat/disfiguring in immunocompromised

EPIDEMIOLOGY
Incidence
- Up to 20% children in tropics
- 30% in AIDS patients
Prevalence
- Children 2–15 years
- Sexually active young adults
- 5–18% HIV population

RISK FACTORS
- Skin-to-skin contact with infected person
- Contact sports
- Sexual activity with infected partner
- Immunocompromised: HIV, chemotherapy, corticosteroid therapy, transplant patients

GENERAL PREVENTION
- Avoid skin-to-skin contact with host (e.g., contact sports, sexual activity)
- Avoid sharing clothing, towels, bathing water

PATHOPHYSIOLOGY
- Virions invade and replicate in cytoplasm of epithelial cells
- Cause abnormal cell proliferation
- Genome encodes proteins to evade host immune system
- Incubation period: 1–7 weeks
- Not associated with malignancy

ETIOLOGY
- DNA virus; *Poxviridae* family
- 4 major types, clinically indistinguishable
- No cross-hybridization or reactivation by other poxviruses

COMMONLY ASSOCIATED CONDITIONS
- Atopic dermatitis
- HIV/AIDS
- Immunosuppression: Corticosteroids, chemotherapy

 DIAGNOSIS

HISTORY
- Contact with known infected person
- Participation in contact sports
- Sexual activity

PHYSICAL EXAM
- Discrete, firm papules with a central umbilication
- Umbilication not obvious in small children
- White curdlike core under umbilicated center
- Lesions are flesh, pearl, or red in color
- May have surrounding erythema or dermatitis
- Immunocompetent hosts: Average of 11–20 lesions, 2–5 mm diameter (range: 1–10 mm)
- Hosts with HIV/AIDS: Hundreds of widespread lesions
- Children: Trunk, extremities, face, anogenital region
- Sexually active: Inner thighs, anogenital area
- Perform thorough skin exam including conjunctiva and anogenital area

Pediatric Considerations
- Infants <3 months, consider vertical transmission (1)
- Children: Fever, >50 lesions, limited response to therapy, consider immunodeficiency (2)
- Children: Anogenital lesions, consider autoinoculation/possible sexual abuse (2)

DIAGNOSTIC TESTS & INTERPRETATION
Lab
Initial lab tests
- Virus cannot be cultured
- Scrape lesion; Tzanck preparation; molluscum cytoplasmic inclusion bodies (2)
- Culture lesion if concern is secondary infection
- Sexual transmission: Test for other STIs, including HIV.

Imaging
Initial approach
Microscopy

Diagnostic Procedures/Surgery
Clinical; using magnifying lens

Pathological Findings
Molluscum cytoplasmic inclusion bodies within keratinocytes

DIFFERENTIAL DIAGNOSIS
- AIDS patients: Cryptococcus, penicilliosis, histoplasmosis, coccidiomycosis
- Basal cell carcinoma
- Benign appendageal tumors: Syringomas, hydrocystomas, ectopic sebaceous glands
- Condyloma acuminatum
- Dermatofibroma
- Eyelid: Abscess, chalazion, foreign body granuloma
- Folliculitis/furunculosis
- Keratoacanthoma
- Oral squamous cell carcinoma
- Trichoepithelioma
- Verruca vulgaris
- Warty dyskeratoma

 TREATMENT

MEDICATION
First Line
- Cantharidin solution 0.7–0.9%: Apply sparingly to lesions, cover with occlusion dressing, wash off in 2–6 hours or sooner if blistering. Repeat treatment every 1–4 weeks until lesions resolve (in-office treatment) (2,3)[C]:
  - Adverse effects: Blistering, erythema, pain, pruritus
  - Precautions: Do not use on face or on genital mucosa
- Cimetidine 40 mg/kg per day divided t.i.d. for 2 months. Maximum dose 800 mg t.i.d. (2,4)[C]:
  - Adverse effects: Headache, diarrhea, gynecomastia
  - Precautions: Pregnancy Category B. Not recommended for use while nursing.
- Imiquimod cream 5%: Optimal dosing regimen unknown. Genital area: Apply to lesions 1 time daily 3 times per week until lesions resolve, up to 16 weeks (2,3)[C]:
  - Adverse effects: Erythema, edema, pruritus, postinflammatory pigment changes
  - Contraindications: Pregnancy

Second Line

- Limit treatment to small areas 4–10 cm^2:
  - Podofilox cream 0.5%: Apply to lesions b.i.d. for 3 days, none for 4 days; may repeat this cycle 4–6 times (3)[C]:
    - ○ Adverse effects: Erythema, edema, pain
    - ○ Contraindications: Pregnancy
  - Podophyllin 10–25% solution: Apply sparingly to lesions 1 time weekly for 4–6 weeks (in-office treatment) (3)[C]:
    - ○ Adverse effects: Erythema, edema, pain
    - ○ Contraindications: Pregnancy, infants, children, oral mucosa
- For HIV/AIDS patients with refractory lesions, consider:
  - Starting or maximizing HAART therapy (2)[C]
  - IV or topical cidofovir (2,3)

ADDITIONAL TREATMENT
General Measures
Natural resolution

COMPLEMENTARY AND ALTERNATIVE MEDICINE
Australian lemon myrtle oil: Apply 10% solution once daily for 21 days (5)[C].

SURGERY/OTHER PROCEDURES

- Cryotherapy: 5–10 seconds with 1–2 mm margins. Repeat every 3–4 weeks as needed until lesions disappear (2,3)[C]:
  - Adverse effects: Erythema, edema, pain, blistering
  - Contraindications: Cryoglobulinemia, Raynaud disease
- Curettage ($\pm$ electrodessication) under local or topical anesthesia (2,3)[C]:
  - Adverse effects: Pain, scarring
- Incision and expression of central particle (2):
  - Adverse effects: High rate of scarring
- CO_2 (3) or pulsed dye (2,3)[C] lasers (for recalcitrant lesions, usually in HIV/AIDS patients):
  - Adverse effects: Pain, edema, scarring, postinflammatory pigment changes
- Photodynamic therapy (ALA/MAL-PDT) (6)[C]

Pediatric Considerations

- Surgical interventions: 2nd-line in small children; pain associated
- Pain control: Pretreat with topical lidocaine or EMLA before surgical treatment.
- Note: Adverse effect:
  - Lidocaine or EMLA over large body surface area: Methemoglobinemia and CNS toxicity. Refer to manufacturer's recommendations on dosing and use in children.

Pregnancy Considerations

- Safe in pregnancy: Curettage, cryotherapy, incision, and expression
- Contraindicated: Podophyllin, podofilox, or imiquimod; teratogenic

 ONGOING CARE

FOLLOW-UP RECOMMENDATIONS
Patient Monitoring
Dependant on type of treatment

DIET
Regular

PATIENT EDUCATION
- Cover lesions to prevent spread.
- Avoid scratching.
- Avoid contact sports.
- Avoid sharing towels, baths
- Avoid sexual activity.
- Avoid swimming pools.

PROGNOSIS
- Immunocompetent: Self-limited, resolves in 3–12 months (range: 2 months–4 years)
- Immunocompromised: Lesions difficult to treat, may persist for years

COMPLICATIONS
- Secondary infection
- Scarring, hyper-/hypopigmentation

REFERENCES

1. Connell CO, Oranje A, Van Gysel D, et al. Congenital molluscum contagiosum: report of four cases and review of the literature. *Pediatr Dermatol.* 2008;25:553–6.
2. Brown J, Janniger CK, Schwartz RA, et al. Childhood molluscum contagiosum. *Int J Dermatol.* 2006;45:93–9.
3. Ting PT, Dytoc MT. Therapy of external anogenital warts and molluscum contagiosum: a literature review. *Dermatol Ther.* 2004;17:68–101.
4. Jones S, Kress D. Treatment of molluscum contagiosum and herpes simplex virus cutaneous infections. *Cutis.* 2007;79(suppl 4):11–17.
5. Burke BE, Baillie JE, Olson RD. Essential oil of Australian lemon myrtle (Backhousia citriodora) in the treatment of molluscum contagiosum in children. *Biomed Pharmacother.* 2004;58:245–7.
6. Rossi R, Bruscino N, Ricceri F, et al. Photodynamic treatment for viral infections of the skin. *G Ital Dermatol Venereol.* 2009;144:79–83.
7. van der Wouden JC, Menke J, Gajadin S, et al. Interventions for cutaneous molluscum contagiosum. *Cochrane Database Syst Rev.* 2006;CD004767.

ADDITIONAL READING

Dohil MA, Lin P, Lee J, et al. The epidemiology of molluscum contagiosum in children. *J Am Acad Dermatol.* 2006;54:47–54.

 CODES

ICD9
078.0 Molluscum contagiosum

CLINICAL PEARLS

- Natural resolution is preferred treatment in healthy patients (7)[A].
- Reassure parents lesions will heal naturally and generally resolve without scarring (7)[A].
- No one specific treatment has been identified as superior to any other (7)[A].
- Consider topical corticosteroids or antihistamines for pruritus or associated dermatitis (2)[C].

M

MONONUCLEOSIS

Renata Gazzi, MD

BASICS

DESCRIPTION
Infectious mononucleosis (IM) is an acute illness owing to Epstein-Barr virus (EBV) infection that occurs mainly in adolescents and young adults.

EPIDEMIOLOGY
Incidence
- Not a reportable disease, but by age 5 years, approximately half of all Americans have been infected; 90% by age 25 years.
- IM accounts for fewer than 2% of pharyngitis cases in adults. The vast majority of adults are not susceptible to infection because of prior exposure.
- The incidence is approximately 30× higher in whites than in blacks in the US.
- No seasonal peak

Prevalence
Approximately 50% of people who are infected with the virus will develop symptoms; others can carry the virus, not knowing they have it.

RISK FACTORS
- Age between 10 and 30 years
- Populations with many young adults, such as active-duty military personnel, high school and college students

Genetics
Unknown

GENERAL PREVENTION
- No blood donation for at least 6 months
- Avoid saliva of infected person.
- Vaccine is under research.

PATHOPHYSIOLOGY
- EBV replicates primarily in B-lymphocytes but also replicates in the epithelial cells of the pharynx and parotid duct. It is spread by saliva (i.e., coughing, sneezing, kissing, and sharing drinks and utensils). The incubation period is 4–8 weeks.
- EBV also has been isolated in both cervical epithelial cells and in male seminal fluid, suggesting that transmission also may occur sexually.

ETIOLOGY
EBV is a double-stranded DNA herpesvirus.

COMMONLY ASSOCIATED CONDITIONS
Streptococcal pharyngitis may be associated in 30% of the patients.

DIAGNOSIS

HISTORY
- Individuals between 10 and 30 years of age with a history of sore throat and significant fatigue
- The syndrome is often heralded by malaise, headache, and low-grade fever before development of the classic triad of fever, tonsillar pharyngitis, and lymphadenopathy.

PHYSICAL EXAM
- Lymphadenopathy (100%): It is typically symmetric and more commonly involves the posterior cervical chain, but it also may become more generalized. It peaks in the 1st week and then subsides gradually over 2–3 weeks.
- Fever (98%)
- Pharyngitis (85%)
- Splenomegaly (50–60%)

DIAGNOSTIC TESTS & INTERPRETATION
Lab
Initial lab tests
- Complete blood count (CBC): An increase in total lymphocyte >35% and atypical lymphocytes of at least 10%
- Elevated aminotransferases: Seen in the vast majority of patients but typically self-limited
- Heterophile antibodies (monospot test): In 40% of patients, positive in 1st week; 90% of patients in 3rd week; may remain positive for 2 years for up to 20% of infected individuals
- EBV-specific antibodies:
  – Viral capsid antigen (VCA): IgG and IgM peak at 3–4 weeks. IgG then declines but persists for life. IgM declines rapidly and is undetectable by 3 months.
  – EB nuclear antigen (EBNA): Develops after 2 months and persists indefinitely; presence early in the course of illness excludes acute EBV infection.
  – Early antigen (EA): IgG to EA is present at the onset of clinical illness and persists for 2–3 months.

Follow-Up & Special Considerations
- In a patient with compatible syndrome and a negative heterophile antibody, the monospot test can be repeated because this test can be negative during the 1st week of clinical illness.
- EBV-specific antibodies should be determined if the patient has a repeatedly negative monospot test.

Imaging
Initial approach
Imaging not indicated initially

Follow-Up & Special Considerations
- Ultrasound if clinically important to diagnose or follow splenomegaly
- CT scan of abdomen is preferred to rule out splenic rupture.

DIFFERENTIAL DIAGNOSIS
- Cytomegalovirus
- Toxoplasmosis
- Rubella
- Adenovirus
- Herpesviruses
- Drug adverse effects
- Streptococcal pharyngitis
- Viral tonsillitis
- Diphtheria
- Viral hepatitis
- Lymphoma or leukemia
- Human herpesvirus 6
- Roseola
- Mumps
- Primary HIV infection

Pregnancy Considerations
Differentiating between IM caused by EBV and a similar syndrome owing to cytomegalovirus (CMV) or HIV infection often is not possible clinically, and it is particularly important if the patient is pregnant because CMV, HIV, and *Toxoplasma* infections can have significant adverse effects on pregnancy outcomes.

Pediatric Considerations
EBV acquired during childhood years is often subclinical.

TREATMENT

MEDICATION

First Line
- Acetaminophen
- Nonsteroidal anti-inflammatory drugs (NSAIDs)
- Lozenges
- Gargling with 2% lidocaine (Xylocaine) solution

Second Line
- Acyclovir (Zovirax): Not recommended; no clinical benefit
- Corticosteroids: Recommended in patients with significant pharyngeal edema that threatens respiratory compromise
- Steroids are not recommended for routine treatment but do improve fever and hematologic abnormalities and may shorten length of infirmary stay (1)[B].

ADDITIONAL TREATMENT

General Measures
Symptomatic treatment, the mainstay of care, includes adequate hydration, analgesics, antipyretics, and adequate rest. Complete bed rest is unnecessary.

Issues for Referral
- Emergent ENT consultation for an impending airway obstruction
- Surgery consultation if suspicious of splenic rupture; the typical manifestations are abdominal pain and/or a falling hematocrit.

Additional Therapies
The preferred treatment for splenic rupture is nonoperative with intensive supportive care and splenic preservation, but some require splenectomy.

SURGERY/OTHER PROCEDURES
- Splenectomy
- Tonsillectomy

IN-PATIENT CONSIDERATIONS

Initial Stabilization
Outpatient usually; 95% of patients recover uneventfully without specific complication.

Admission Criteria
Suspicion of splenic rupture or airway obstruction

 ONGOING CARE

FOLLOW-UP RECOMMENDATIONS
A generalized maculopapular, urticarial, or petechial rash is seen occasionally. Rash is more common following the administration of ampicillin or amoxicillin.

DIET
Soft diet followed by gradually advanced diet if severe sore throat

PATIENT EDUCATION
- For athletes planning to resume noncontact sports, training can be restarted gradually 3 weeks from symptom onset. For strenuous contact sports or activities associated with increased intraabdominal pressure, patient should wait a minimum of 4 weeks after illness onset (2)[B].
- There is no set time to go back to school or work. Individuals with IM tend to be most contagious during the incubation period, the 4–6 weeks before they get sick, and during the acute phases of their illness. Some people even may shed EBV when they are no longer sick.
- Because the EBV resides in the body for life, it can reactivate, but in most cases it won't cause symptoms unless the immune system becomes severely compromised.

PROGNOSIS
Fatigue, myalgias, and need for sleep may persist for several months after the acute infection has resolved.

COMPLICATIONS
- Chronic EBV infections (i.e., chronic fatigue syndrome, the diagnosis of which remains highly controversial)
- Splenic rupture (rare, 0.1–0.5% of patients with proven IM)
- Hemolytic anemia (mild)
- Thrombocytopenia
- Hemolytic-uremic syndrome
- Seizures and other neurologic abnormalities
- Nerve palsies
- Meningoencephalitis
- Reye syndrome
- Myocarditis/electrocardiographic (ECG) changes
- Airway obstruction
- Acute interstitial nephritis

REFERENCES

1. Dickens KP, Nye AM, Gilchrist V, et al. Clinical inquiries. Should you use steroids to treat infectious mononucleosis? *J Fam Pract.* 2008;57:754–5.
2. Eichner ER. Sports medicine pearls and pitfalls—defending the spleen: return to play after infectious mononucleosis. *Curr Sports Med Rep.* 2007;6:68–9.

ADDITIONAL READING

- Ebell MH. Epstein-Barr infectious Mononucleosis. *Am Fam Phys.* 2004;70:1279–87.
- Putukian M, O'Connor FG, Stricker P, et al. Mononucleosis and athletic participation: an evidence-based subject review. *Clin J Sport Med.* 2008;18:309–15.
- Torre D, Tambini R. Acyclovir for treatment of infectious mononucleosis: a meta-analysis. *Scand J Infect Dis.* 1999;31:543–7.
- Wick MJ, Woronzoff-Dashkoff KP, McGlennen RC. The molecular characterization of fatal infectious mononucleosis. *Am J Clin Pathol.* 2002;117:582–8.

 CODES

ICD9
075 Infectious mononucleosis

CLINICAL PEARLS

- IM should be suspected in patients 10–30 years of age who present with sore throat and significant fatigue, palatal petechiae, posterior cervical or auricular adenopathy, marked axillary adenopathy, or inguinal adenopathy.
- Patients with suspected IM, based on history and physical exam, should have a CBC with differential and a heterophile antibody test. In addition, patients also should have a diagnostic evaluation for streptococcal infection by culture or antigen test.
- In a patient with a compatible syndrome and a negative heterophile antibody test, the monospot test can be repeated because this test can be negative during the 1st week of clinical illness. EBV-specific antibodies (e.g., VCA IgM and IgG and EBNA) should be determined if the patient has repeatedly negative monospot tests.
- The presence of IgG EBNA or the absence of IgG and IgM VCA excludes primary EBV infection and should prompt consideration of alternative etiologies of a mononucleosis-like illness.
- An increase in monocytes does not suggest mononucleosis; an increase in total lymphocytes >35% and atypical lymphocytes >10% does suggest mononucleosis.

M

MORTON NEUROMA (INTERDIGITAL NEUROMA)

Jake D. Veigel, MD
J. Herbert Stevenson, MD

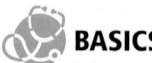 **BASICS**

DESCRIPTION
- Perineal fibrosis of the common digital nerve as it passes between metatarsals; the most common site is the interspace between the 3rd and 4th metatarsals, with the interspace between the 3rd and 2nd metatarsals being the 2nd most common site.
- System(s) affected: Musculoskeletal; Nervous
- Synonym(s): Plantar digital neuritis

EPIDEMIOLOGY
Incidence
- Unknown
- Mean age: 45–50 years
- Predominant sex: Female > Male (8:1)

Prevalence
Unknown

RISK FACTORS
- High-heeled shoes: Cause more weight to be transferred to the front of the foot
- Tight-toed shoes (tight toe boxes): Cause lateral compression
- Pes planus (flat feet): Causes nerve to be pulled more medially, which increases irritation
- Obesity
- Ballet dancing, basketball, aerobics, tennis, running, and similar activities

GENERAL PREVENTION
- Wear properly fitting shoes.
- Avoid high heels and narrow toe boxes.

PATHOPHYSIOLOGY
- Lateral plantar nerve combines with part of medial plantar nerve. The 2 nerves combine, creating a nerve with larger diameter than nerves going to other digits.
- Nerve lies in subcutaneous tissue, deep to the fat pad of foot, just superficial to the digital artery and vein.
- Overlying the nerve is the strong, deep transverse metatarsal ligament that holds the metatarsal bones together.
- With each step the patient takes, the inflamed nerve becomes compressed between the ground and the deep transverse metatarsal ligament.

ETIOLOGY
- Excessive stress of the forefoot
- Repetitive trauma
- Congenitally enlarged plantar digital nerve

 DIAGNOSIS

HISTORY
- Most common complaint is pain localized to interspace between 3rd and 4th toes.
- Pain is less severe when non-weight bearing.
- Pain, cramping, or numbness of the forefoot with weight bearing or immediately after strenuous foot exertion
- Radiation of pain to the toes
- Pain is relieved by removing the shoe and massaging the foot.
- Patients often state: "Feels like I am walking on a marble."
- A burning pain in the ball of the foot that may radiate into the toes
- Tingling or numbness in the toes
- Aggravated by wearing tight or narrow shoes

PHYSICAL EXAM
- A palpable nodule in the metatarsal interspace is an occasional finding.
- Positive Mulder sign: See Diagnostic Procedures.
- Intense pain on pressure between metatarsal heads
- Assess midfoot motion and digital motion to determine if arthritis or synovitis.
- Palpate along metatarsal shafts to assess for metatarsalgia or stress fractures.

DIAGNOSTIC TESTS & INTERPRETATION
Imaging
Initial approach
- Radiographs may help to rule out osseous pathology if diagnosis is in question, but films usually are normal in patients with a Morton neuroma.
- Ultrasound shows a hypoechoic nodule between the metatarsal interspace. Ultrasound had a 65% specificity and a 98% sensitivity for Morton neuromas. Ultrasound is not good at assessing the size of the lesion (1)[C].
- MRI is used to ensure that compression is not caused by a malignant tumor in the foot. MRI is helpful in determining how much of the nerve to resect surgically. MRI has a sensitivity of 83% and a specificity of 99% (1)[C].

Diagnostic Procedures/Surgery
- Mulder sign: A "click" and pain produced by squeezing the metatarsal heads together and simultaneously compressing the neuroma between the thumb and index finger of the other hand
- Corticosteroid injection can significantly reduce symptoms. Inject 1–2 mL lidocaine and 0.5–1 mL dexamethasone just proximal to the metatarsal heads. More than 1 injection is often needed, usually once a week × 3 weeks (2).

Pathological Findings
Chronic fibrosis and thickening of the digital nerve

DIFFERENTIAL DIAGNOSIS

- Stress fracture
- Hammer toe
- Metatarsophalangeal synovitis
- Metatarsalgia
- Arthritis
- Bursitis
- Foreign body

 TREATMENT

MEDICATION

First Line

Injectable steroids (e.g., betamethasone phosphate/acetate or methylprednisolone): Use if general measures fail (2,3)[C].

Second Line

Nonsteroidal anti-inflammatory drugs (NSAIDs) for temporary symptom relief (1,2)[C]

ADDITIONAL TREATMENT

General Measures

- Flat shoes with a roomy toe box (4)[C]
- Metatarsal pads placed immediately proximal to the 2 involved metatarsal heads (4)[C]
- Corticosteroid injection into the dorsal part of the foot with medium- or long-acting steroid (e.g., betamethasone, methylprednisolone) mixed with local anesthetic (e.g., lidocaine) (4)[C]
- If patient has pes planus, an arch support is used (4)[C].
- Literature suggests wide variability in success rate (50–98%) (4).

Issues for Referral

Continued pain despite conservative treatments and injections

Additional Therapies

Serial alcohol injection therapy into the neuroma to sclerose the nerve has been successful (5)[C].

SURGERY/OTHER PROCEDURES

Surgical removal of the neuroma, release of the transverse metatarsal ligament, or both in refractory cases

 ONGOING CARE

FOLLOW-UP RECOMMENDATIONS

If no improvement after 3 months of conservative treatment, consider corticosteroid injection. Repeat injection if no improvement after 2–4 weeks.

PATIENT EDUCATION

Wearing of properly fitted, comfortable shoes

PROGNOSIS

- 40–50% improve after 3 months of conservative treatment.
- 45–50% improve after steroid injection.
- 96% improve after surgery.

COMPLICATIONS

Hip and knee pain related to gait changes

REFERENCES

1. Sharp RJ, et al. The role of MRI and ultrasound imaging in Morton's neuroma and the effect of size of lesion on symptoms. *Br J Bone Joint Surg.* 2003;85:999–1005.
2. Tallia AF, Cardone DA. Diagnostic and therapeutic injection of the ankle and foot. *Am Fam Physician.* 2003;68:1356–62.
3. Wu KK. Morton's interdigital neuroma: a clinical review of its etiology, treatment, and results. *J Foot Ankle Surg.* 1996;35:112–9; discussion 187–8.
4. Thompson CE, Gibson JNA, Martin D. Interventions for the treatment of Morton's neuroma. *Cochrane Database Sys Rev.* 2005.
5. Hughes RJ, Ali K, Jones H, et al. Treatment of Morton's neuroma with alcohol injection under sonographic guidance: follow-up of 101 cases. *Am J Roentgenol.* 2007;188:1535–9.

 CODES

ICD9

355.6 Lesion of plantar nerve

CLINICAL PEARLS

- Diagnosis of Morton neuroma is usually made clinically.
- Footwear modification, metatarsal pads, and shoe inserts are mainstays of treatment.
- Corticosteroid injection into the neuroma may be helpful.

M

MOTION SICKNESS

Courtney I. Jarvis, PharmD
Allison Hargreaves, MD

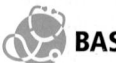 **BASICS**

DESCRIPTION
- Not a true sickness, but a normal response to a situation in which sensory conflict about body motion exists among visual receptors, vestibular receptors, and body proprioceptors
- Also can be induced when patterns of motion differ from those previously experienced
- System(s) affected: Nervous
- Synonym(s): Car sickness; Sea sickness; Air sickness; Space sickness; Physiologic vertigo

EPIDEMIOLOGY
Incidence
Predominant sex: Female > Male

RISK FACTORS
- Motion (auto, plane, boat, amusement rides)
- Travel
- Visual stimuli (e.g., moving horizon)
- Poor ventilation (fumes, smoke, carbon monoxide)
- Emotions (fear, anxiety)
- Zero gravity
- Pregnancy, menstruation, oral contraceptive use
- History of migraine headaches
- Other illness or poor health

GENERAL PREVENTION
See General Measures.

Pediatric Considerations
- Rare in children <2 years of age
- Incidence peaks between the ages of 3 and 12 years.
- Antihistamines may cause excitation in children.

Geriatric Considerations
- Age confers some resistance to motion sickness.
- Elderly at increased risk of anticholinergic side effects from treatment

Pregnancy Considerations
- Pregnant patients more likely to experience motion sickness
- Treat with medications thought to be safe during morning sickness (e.g., meclizine, dimenhydrate).

ETIOLOGY
- Precise etiology unknown; thought to be due to a mismatch of vestibular and visual sensations
- Nausea and vomiting occur as a result of increased levels of dopamine and acetylcholine, which stimulate chemoreceptor trigger zone and vomiting center in CNS.

 DIAGNOSIS

HISTORY
Presence of the following signs and symptoms:
- Nausea
- Vomiting
- Diaphoresis
- Pallor
- Hypersalivation
- Yawning
- Hyperventilation
- Anxiety
- Panic
- Malaise
- Fatigue
- Weakness
- Confusion
- Dizziness

DIFFERENTIAL DIAGNOSIS
- Mountain sickness
- Vestibular disease
- Gastroenteritis
- Metabolic disorders
- Toxin exposure

 TREATMENT

- Follow guidelines under General Measures section to prevent motion sickness (1)[C].
- Premedicate before travel with antidopaminergic, anticholinergic, or antihistamine agents (1)[A]:
  - For extended travel, consider treatment with scopolamine transdermal patch (2)[A].
  - 2nd-generation (nonsedating) antihistamines are not effective at preventing motion sickness (3)[B].
  - Serotonin (5-HT3) antagonists (e.g., ondansetron) do not appear effective in preventing motion sickness (4)[B].
- Conflicting data exist on the efficacy of acupressure for nausea and vomiting associated with motion sickness (5)[B].
- Benzodiazepines suppress vestibular nuclei but would not be considered 1st line due to sedation and addiction potential (6)[C].

MEDICATION
First Line
- Scopolamine transdermal patch: Apply 2.5 cm^2 (4-mg) patch behind ear at least 4 h (preferably 6–12 h) before travel, and replace every 3 days (2)[A]:
  - Scopolamine may also be given in tablets, capsules, or oral solution; all are more effective than placebo (7)[A].
- Dimenhydrinate (Dramamine): Take 30 min–1 h before travel:
  - Adults and adolescents: 50–100 mg q4–6h, maximum 400 mg/d
  - Children 6–12 years of age: 25–50 mg q6–8h, maximum 150 mg/d
  - Children 2–6 years of age: 12.5–25 mg q6–8h, maximum 75 mg/d
- Meclizine (Antivert): Take 30 min–1 h before travel. Adults and adolescents >12 years of age: 12.5–25 mg q12–24h
- Cyclizine (Marezine): Take 30 min–1 h before travel:
  - Adults and adolescents: 50 mg q4–6h, maximum 200 mg/d
  - Children 6–12 years of age: 25 mg up to t.i.d.

- Promethazine (Phenergan): Take 30 min–1 h before travel:
  – Adults and adolescents: 25 mg q12h; 25–50 mg IM if already developed severe motion sickness
  – Children 2–12 years of age: 0.5 mg/kg q12h, maximum 25 mg b.i.d. *Caution:* Increased risk of dystonic reaction in this age group
- Contraindications: Patients at risk for acute-angle closure glaucoma
- Precautions:
  – Young children
  – Elderly
  – Pregnancy
  – Urinary obstruction
  – Pyloric-duodenal obstruction
- Adverse reactions:
  – Drowsiness
  – Dry mouth
  – Blurred vision
  – Confusion
  – Headache
  – Urinary retention
- Significant possible interactions:
  – Sedatives (antihistamines, alcohol, antidepressants)
  – Anticholinergics (belladonna alkaloids)

Second Line
- Benzodiazepines: Take 1–2 h before travel:
  – Diazepam 2–10 mg p.o. q6–12h
  – Lorazepam 1–2 mg p.o. q8h
- Contraindications:
  – Severe respiratory dysfunction
  – Severe liver dysfunction
- Precautions:
  – Alcohol/drug abuse
  – Elderly
  – Sedation
  – Addiction is possible.

ADDITIONAL TREATMENT
General Measures
- Minimize exposure (sit in middle of plane or boat).
- Improve ventilation; avoid noxious stimuli.
- Semirecumbent seating
- Fix vision on horizon, avoid fixation on moving objects, keep eyes fixed on still, distant objects.
- Avoid reading while actively traveling.
- Minimize food intake before travel; avoid alcohol.

- Increase airflow around face.
- Acupressure on point PC6 has been shown to reduce feelings of nausea but not the incidence of vomiting during pregnancy, after surgery, and in cancer chemotherapy. However, conflicting evidence of efficacy has been found for motion sickness. Point PC6 (Neiguan on pericardium meridian): 2 cm proximal of transverse crease of palmar side of wrist between tendons of the palmaris longus and the flexor carpi radialis.

COMPLEMENTARY AND ALTERNATIVE MEDICINE
Ginger: 940 mg or 1 g; take 4 h before travel (evidence controversial)

 ONGOING CARE

FOLLOW-UP RECOMMENDATIONS
- Semirecumbent seating
- Avoid reading while actively traveling.

DIET
- Decrease oral intake or take frequent small feedings.
- Avoid alcohol.

PROGNOSIS
- Symptoms should resolve when motion exposure ends.
- Resistance to motion sickness seems to increase with age.

COMPLICATIONS
- Hypotension
- Dehydration
- Depression
- Panic
- Syncope

REFERENCES

1. Committee to advise on tropical medicine and travel. Statement on motion sickness. *CCDR.* 2003;29:1–12.
2. Spinks A, Wasiak J, Bernath V, et al. Scopolamine (hyoscine) for preventing and treating motion sickness. *CochraneDatabase of Systematic Reviews* 2007, Issue 3. Art. No.: CD002851. DOI:10.1002/14651858.CD002851.pub3.
3. Cheung BS, Heskin R, Hofer KD. Failure of cetirizine and fexofenadine to prevent motion sickness. *Ann Pharmacother.* 2003;37:173–7.
4. Hershkovitz D, Asna N, Shupak A, et al. Ondansetron for the prevention of seasickness in susceptible sailors: an evaluation at sea. *Aviat Space Environ Med.* 2009;80:643–6.
5. Streitberger K, Ezzo J, Schneider A. Acupuncture for nausea and vomiting: an update of clinical and experimental studies. *Auton Neuro.* 2006;129:107–17.
6. Zajonc TP, Roland PS. Vertigo and motion sickness. Part II: Pharmacologic treatment. *Ear Nose Throat J.* 2006;85:25–35.
7. Spinks AB, Wasiak J, Villanueva EV, et al. Scopolamine (hyoscine) for preventing and treating motion sickness. *Cochrane Database Syst Rev.* 2007;CD002851.

ADDITIONAL READING

Carroll ID, Williams DC. Pre-travel vaccination and medical prophylaxis in the pregnant traveler. *Travel Med Infect Dis.* 2008;6:259–75.

See Also (Topic, Algorithm, Electronic Media Element)
Algorithm: Vertigo

 CODES

ICD9
994.6 Motion sickness

CLINICAL PEARLS

- The scopolamine patch should be applied at least 4 h before travel, although it may be more effective if placed 6–12 h before departure.
- Oral medications should be administered 30 min–1 h before departure.
- Although acupressure wrist bands have been found to be effective by systematic reviews in postoperative and chemotherapy-induced nausea and vomiting, conflicting data exist for motion sickness.

M

MRSA SKIN INFECTIONS

Stephen A. Martin, MD, EdM
Paul Belliveau, PharmD, RPh

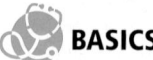

BASICS

DESCRIPTION
- Community-associated methicillin-resistant *Staphylococcus aureus* (CA-MRSA) has properties that allow it to create skin and soft tissue infections (SSTIs) in otherwise healthy hosts:
  – CA-MRSA has a different virulence and disease pattern than hospital-acquired MRSA (HA-MRSA).
- MRSA infections acquired by persons who have not been recently (<1 year) hospitalized or had a medical procedure (e.g., dialysis, surgery, catheters) are known as CA-MRSA infections:
  – This definition is evolving, given the increasing intersection of HA- and CA-MRSA.
- *The prevalence of CA-MRSA is rapidly increasing in the US.*
- CA-MRSA typically causes mild-to-moderate SSTIs, particularly abscesses, furuncles, and carbuncles:
  – Severe disease from CA-MRSA is less frequent, but can include:
    ○ Necrotizing pneumonia with abscesses
    ○ Necrotizing fasciitis
    ○ Septic thrombophlebitis
    ○ Sepsis
  – In 1 review, 77% of CA-MRSA infections were SSTIs; only 6% of infections were invasive (e.g., bacteremia, osteomyelitis).
- Although less frequent, HA-MRSA can still cause SSTIs in the community, and clinicians should be alert to this possibility. 1 study showed no significant difference in hospitalization rates among CA-MRSA, HA-MRSA, and methicillin-sensitive *Staphylococcus aureus* (MSSA).
- System(s) affected: Skin; Soft tissue

EPIDEMIOLOGY
- Predominant age: All ages, generally younger
- Predominant sex: Female > Male

Incidence
- 18.0–26/100,000/year (2001–02)
- 155/100,000/year (2004) in higher risk setting

Prevalence
- Still significantly affected by local epidemiology
- 25–30% of US population is colonized with *S. aureus*; up to 7% is colonized with MRSA.
- CA-MRSA was isolated in 59% of skin and soft tissue infections presenting to 11 emergency departments (range 15–74%). In 1993, 1.5 million SSTIs were seen in US emergency rooms (ERs). In 2005, this had increased to 3.4 million. Hospital admission data indicate a 29% increase in SSTIs from 2000–2004.
- CA-MRSA accounts for up to 75% of all community staphylococcal infections in children.

RISK FACTORS
- Although several factors are associated with CA-MRSA, their presence or absence cannot reliably predict CA-MRSA itself; in 1 study, almost 1/2 the patients with CA-MRSA had no established risk factor.
- Any antibiotic use in past month
- Presence of an abscess
- Reported "spider bite"
- History of MRSA infection
- Close contact with a similar infection

- Children, particularly in day care centers
- Competitive athletes
- Incarceration
- High prevalence in the community
- Hospitalization in the past 12 months (although *S. aureus* can remain colonized for years)

GENERAL PREVENTION
- Prior research has established colonization (particularly of the anterior nares) as a risk factor for subsequent *S. aureus* infection. It is not yet clear whether this is also the case for CA-MRSA. Recent work has indicated that rectal colonization may be more significant.
- CA-MRSA may be transmitted much more through the environment, including households, than via nares colonization.
- Health care workers have been found to be a major vector of MRSA for hospitalized patients, reinforcing the need for aggressive cleaning of hands and common equipment.
- Research for a vaccine is underway.

ETIOLOGY
- First noted in 1980, CA-MRSA's current US epidemic began in 1999. The USA 300 clone is predominant.
- CA-MRSA is currently distinguished from HA-MRSA by:
  – Lack of a multidrug-resistant phenotype
  – Presence of exotoxin virulence factors
  – Type IV staphylococcus cassette cartridge (contains the methicillin-resistance gene *mecA*)

COMMONLY ASSOCIATED CONDITIONS
Many patients are otherwise healthy.

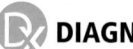

DIAGNOSIS

HISTORY
- Potential risk factors
- Complaint of "spider bite"
- Prior MRSA skin infection
- Risk factors alone cannot rule in or rule out a CA-MRSA infection (1)[B].

PHYSICAL EXAM
- Exam consistent with a furuncle/carbuncle (boils) or abscess, sometimes with a surrounding cellulitis. An isolated cellulitis is also possible, although it is a less common presentation of CA-MRSA. A recent study, however, shows *S. aureus* to be a causal agent in half of cellulitis cases.
- Erythema
- Increased warmth
- Tenderness
- Swelling
- Fluctuance
- Infected wound
- Folliculitis, pustular lesions
- Appearance like an insect or spider bite
- Tissue necrosis

DIAGNOSTIC TESTS & INTERPRETATION
Lab
Initial lab tests
- Wound cultures are essential for diagnosis.
- Susceptibility testing; many labs use oxacillin instead of methicillin.

- A "D-zone disk-diffusion test" evaluates for inducible clindamycin resistance in CA-MRSA resistant to erythromycin (2)[C].

Imaging
Initial approach
- In unclear cases, ultrasound may help delineate an abscess.
- Although computed tomography or magnetic resonance imaging may show fascial plane edema in necrotizing fasciitis, they should not delay intervention.

Diagnostic Procedures/Surgery
Purulent lesions should be incised and drained (I & D), cultured, and tested for susceptibilities.

DIFFERENTIAL DIAGNOSIS
Skin and soft tissue infections due to another cause

TREATMENT

- Evidence for the treatment of CA-MRSA SSTIs, including oral antibiotics, has not been systematically evaluated in randomized controlled trials. Although investigations are increasing, current recommendations are generally based on results of small case series, anecdotal reports, and anticipated susceptibility profiles.
- Systematic review does not recommend agents to eliminate MRSA colonization for patients with infection or their close contacts (3)[C].
- Most CA-MRSA infections are localized SSTIs and do not require hospitalization or vancomycin therapy (3)[C].
- Initial empirical antibiotic coverage should be based on local CA-MRSA prevalence and individual patient risk factors. In one pediatric model, cephalexin was the optimal antibiotic for an SSTI only when CA-MRSA prevalence was <10%.

MEDICATION

ALERT
- For purulent infections, basic principles include surgical drainage and debulking, wound culture, and narrow-spectrum antimicrobials:
  – Successful I & D may have more of an effect than antibiotics in mild cases for both adults and children, and is important in general.
  – Moist heat may work for small furuncles.
  – Patients with an abscess are frequently cured by drainage alone.
- CA-MRSA is resistant to β-lactams (including oral cephalosporins and antistaphylococcal penicillins) and often macrolides, azalides, and quinolones.
- Although most CA-MRSA isolates are susceptible to rifampin, this drug should *never* be used as a single agent because of concerns for rapid emergence of resistance. The role of combination therapy with rifampin in CA-MRSA SSTIs is still not clearly defined.
- There has been increasing resistance to clindamycin, both initial (~33%) and induced.
- Although CA-MRSA isolates are susceptible to vancomycin, oral vancomycin cannot be used for CA-MRSA SSTIs due to limited gastrointestinal absorption.

First Line

CA-MRSA SSTIs: Treat with a 7–14-day course of 1 of the following agents (duration of therapy depends on severity and clinical response):

- Trimethoprim/sulfamethoxazole: DS (160 mg TMP and 800 mg of SMX) 1–2 tablet(s) p.o. b.i.d. daily (8–12 mg/kg/d of trimethoprim component in 2 divided doses for children)
- Doxycycline or minocycline: 100 mg p.o. b.i.d. (children >8 years and <45 kg; 2–5 mg/kg/d p.o. in 1–2 divided doses, not to exceed 200 mg/d; children >8 years and >45 kg: use adult dosing), taken with a full glass of water
- Clindamycin: 300–600 mg p.o. t.i.d. (10–20 mg/kg/d p.o. in 3 divided doses for children), taken with full glass of water. Check D-zone test in erythromycin-resistant, clindamycin-susceptible *S. aureus* isolates (test is positive with induced resistance).

Second Line

The above medication options are not sufficient for treatment of severe CA-MRSA SSTIs requiring hospitalization or for HA-MRSA SSTIs. For such infections, consider 1 of the following (4)[A]:

- Vancomycin: Generally 1 g IV q12h (30 mg/kg/d IV in 2 divided doses; in children: 40 mg/kg/d IV in 4 divided doses)
- Linezolid: 600 mg IV/p.o. b.i.d. (Uncomplicated: children <5 years of age, 30 mg/kg/d in 3 divided doses; 20 mg/kg/d IV/p.o. in 2 divided doses for children 5–11 years of age; children >11 years, use adult dosing. Complicated: birth–11 years, 30 mg/kg/d IV/p.o. in 3 divided doses; older, use adult dosing)
- Daptomycin: 4 mg/kg/d IV (safety/efficacy not established in patients <18 years of age) if no pulmonary involvement
- Tigecycline: 100 mg IV once, then 50 mg IV every 12 hours (for adults)

Pediatric Considerations

- Tetracyclines not recommended <8 years
- TMP-SMX not recommended <2 months

Pregnancy Considerations

- Tetracyclines are contraindicated.
- TMP-SMX not recommended in 3rd trimester

ADDITIONAL TREATMENT

General Measures

- Modify therapy as necessary based on culture and susceptibility testing.
- Determine if household or other close contacts have SSTI or other infections, and facilitate evaluation.
- Treat underlying condition (e.g., tinea pedis).
- Restrict contact if wound cannot be covered.
- Elevate affected area.

Issues for Referral

In addition to inpatient concerns, consider consultation with an infectious disease specialist in cases of:

- Refractory CA-MRSA infection
- Plan to attempt decolonization

SURGERY/OTHER PROCEDURES

Progression to serious SSTIs, including necrotizing fasciitis, is possible and mandates prompt surgical evaluation.

IN-PATIENT CONSIDERATIONS

Initial Stabilization

Depends on severity of SSTI, presence of SSTI complications (sepsis, necrotizing fasciitis), and comorbidities

Admission Criteria

Consider admission in patients either:

- Systemically ill (e.g., febrile) with stable comorbidities, or
- Systemically well with comorbidities that may delay or complicate resolution of their SSTI

Nursing

Contact precautions

Discharge Criteria

If admitted for IV therapy:

- Afebrile for 24 hours
- Clinically improved
- Able to take oral medication
- Has adequate social support and available for outpatient follow-up

 ONGOING CARE

FOLLOW-UP RECOMMENDATIONS

Patient Monitoring

For outpatients:

- Return promptly if patient develops systemic symptoms, worsening local symptoms, or does not improve within 48 hours.
- Consider a follow-up within 48 hours of initial visit to assess response and review culture.

PATIENT EDUCATION

- Keep wounds that are draining covered with clean, dry, bandages.
- Clean hands regularly with soap and water or alcohol-based gel. Hot shower daily with soap.
- Do not share items that may be contaminated (including razors or towels).
- Clean clothes, towels, and bed linens.

PROGNOSIS

- In outpatients, improvement should occur within 48 hours.
- Data are limited as to risk of recurrence.

COMPLICATIONS

- Necrotizing pneumonia or empyema (after an influenzalike illness)
- Necrotizing fasciitis
- Sepsis syndrome
- Pyomyositis and osteomyelitis
- Purpura fulminans
- Disseminated septic emboli
- Endocarditis

REFERENCES

1. Daum RS. Clinical practice. Skin and soft-tissue infections caused by methicillin-resistant Staphylococcus aureus. *N Engl J Med*. 2007;357:380–90.
2. Moellering RC. A 39-year-old man with a skin infection. *JAMA*. 2008;299:79–87.
3. Stryjewski ME, Chambers HF. Skin and soft-tissue infections caused by community-acquired methicillin-resistant Staphylococcus aureus. *Clin Infect Dis*. 2008;46(Suppl 5):S368–77.
4. Stevens DL, Bisno AL, Chambers HF, et al. Practice guidelines for the diagnosis and management of skin and soft-tissue infections. *Clin Infect Dis*. 2005;41:1373–406.
5. Chuck EA, Frazee BW, Lambert L, et al. The benefit of empiric treatment for methicillin-resistant Staphylococcus aureus. *J Emerg Med*. 2010;38:567–71.

ADDITIONAL READING

- Breen JO et al. Skin and soft tissue infections in immunocompetent patients. *Am Fam Physician*. 2010;81:893–9.
- Gorwitz RJ, et al. Strategies for clinical management of MRSA in the community: Summary of an experts' meeting convened by the Centers for Disease Control and Prevention. 2006. Accessed 7/9/2010 at: http://www.cdc.gov/ncidod/dhqp/pdf/ar/CAMRSA_ExpMtgStrategies.pdf.
- The CDC has gathered information for health care professionals, including clinical guides, via the National MRSA Education Initiative (accessed 7/9/2010) at http://www.cdc.gov/mrsa/. These include a treatment algorithim: http://www.cdc.gov/mrsa/mrsa_initiative/skin_infection/mrsa_algorithm.html. Updated Infectious Disease Society of America guidelines on MRSA are expected in the Fall of 2010 and on skin and sof tissue infections in the Winter of 2011.

 CODES

ICD9

- 041.12 Methicillin resistant Staphylococcus aureus
- V02.54 Carrier or suspected carrier of Methicillin resistant Staphylococcus aureus
- V09.0 Infection with microorganisms resistant to penicillins

CLINICAL PEARLS

- Incise and drain purulent lesions and send for wound culture.
- Know the prevalence and susceptibilities of CA-MRSA in your location. Consider use of an algorithm to help guide clinical decisions (5)[B].
- Use 1/4 cup household bleach diluted in 1 gallon of water to clean surfaces; no evidence that widespread cleaning (with sprays/foggers) works any better than focused cleaning of frequently touched areas.

M

MULTIPLE ENDOCRINE NEOPLASIA (MEN)

Anup Kumar Sabharwal, MD
Elizabeth McAninch, MD

 BASICS

- Multiple endocrine neoplasia (MEN) syndromes are autosomal dominant disorders that predispose individuals to the development of neoplasms, usually benign but sometimes malignant, in characteristic clusters of multiple endocrine glands.
- The classic syndromes are MEN1 and MEN2, but we also consider MEN4 (MEN1-like phenotype), Von Hippel–Lindau syndrome, Cowden syndrome, Carney complex, and familial paragangliomas as part of the spectrum of disease.

DESCRIPTION

- 3 main subtypes:
  - MEN1: Parathyroid hyperplasia or adenoma (90% penetrance at age 40), anterior pituitary adenomas (prolactinoma most commonly), and tumors of the endocrine pancreas (gastrinoma, insulinoma, glucagonoma, vasoactive intestinal peptide tumor [VIPoma]). Combinations of over 20 different types of tumors are described in these patients, but the above 3 are considered characteristic.
  - MEN2A: Medullary thyroid carcinoma (90%), pheochromocytoma (50%), and parathyroid hyperplasia or single adenoma (20–30%)
  - MEN2B: Medullary thyroid carcinoma (90%), pheochromocytoma, and mucosal and gastrointestinal ganglioneuromatosis; marfanoid habitus
- MEN4: Bilateral pheochromocytomas, hyperparathyroidism/parathyroid adenoma, paraganglioma, C cell (multifocal thyroid) hyperplasia, neuroendocrine carcinoid tumor, and hyperplasia of the endocrine pancreas
- Synonym(s): Multiple endocrine adenomatosis (MEA); Wermer syndrome (MEN1); Sipple syndrome (MEN2); Wagenmann-Froboese syndrome

EPIDEMIOLOGY

- MEN1: Prevalence estimated to be 1 in 30,000; 10% of cases are sporadic (90% familial); Male:Female is 1:1; clinical manifestations occur by the 5th decade in 95% of cases with most diagnosed in early adulthood. Hyperparathyroidism is the most frequent and earliest manifestation.
- MEN2: Prevalence estimated at 1 in 30,000 individuals:
  - MEN2A: Most common subtype (>80% of MEN2 cases); the typical age at onset of symptoms is 5 to 25 years

RISK FACTORS
Significant family history

Genetics

- Autosomal dominant
- MEN1: Results from mutation causing loss of function of tumor-suppressor gene *MEN1* located on chromosome 11q13 encoding the nuclear protein menin; patients have germline mutations and develop tumors when a "second hit" to the other allele occurs. The exact action of menin is unknown, but it appears to be involved in the cell cycle and DNA transcription and replication. 10% of mutations arise de novo; no mutation identified in 10–20% of cases.
- MEN2: Results from mutation causing gain of function of protooncogene *RET* (also called *MEN2* gene) located on chromosome 10q11.2 encoding the protein RET, which is a membrane tyrosine kinase receptor; 5% of MEN2A and 50% of MEN2B cases are secondary to de novo mutations; no mutation identified in 5% of cases. Significant genotype-phenotype correlation.
- MEN4: Results from germline mutation causing inactivation of the cyclin-dependent kinase inhibitor 1B (CDKN1B); negative *MEN1*

COMMONLY ASSOCIATED CONDITIONS
In addition to the defining MEN-associated tumors, other associated conditions include:

- MEN1: Adrenal cortical tumors (nonfunctioning or causing hypercortisolemia), thyroid tumors including carcinoma, adenoma or colloid goiters; carcinoid tumors, facial angiofibromas, facial collagenomas, lipomas, meningiomas
- MEN2A: Rare variants exist including MEN2A with cutaneous lichen amyloidosis and with Hirschsprung's disease.
- MEN2B: Developmental abnormalities including marfanoid habitus or skeletal deformities

 DIAGNOSIS

- MEN1: Clinical diagnosis of sporadic MEN1 is made in patients with tumors in 2 of the 3 main MEN1-associated endocrine glands; familial MEN1 is diagnosed in individuals who have 1 of the MEN1-associated tumors in addition to having a 1st-degree relative with 1 of these 3 tumors (1).
- MEN2: Clinical diagnosis of sporadic MEN2 is made in patients with tumors in 2 of the MEN2-associated endocrine glands; familial MEN2 is diagnosed in individuals who have 1 of the MEN2-associated tumors in addition to having a 1st-degree relative with 1 of these 3 tumors (2).

HISTORY
- Complaints relate to the mechanism of action of the specific secretory product of the patient's tumor/s:
  - MEN1: Symptoms of hypercalcemia secondary to hyperparathyroidism including altered mental status, constipation, nausea/vomiting, history of nephrolithiasis, history of pathologic fracture, bone pain, myalgias; symptoms of increased acid production secondary to gastrinoma including abdominal pain, heartburn, vomiting, weight loss; symptoms of hypoglycemia secondary to insulinoma; symptoms of mass effect from pituitary lesion including headache or blurry vision; symptoms of hyperprolactinemia from prolactinoma including galactorrhea, amenorrhea, infertility or hypogonadism; symptoms of acromegaly from growth hormone secreting tumor.
  - MEN2: Symptoms of medullary thyroid cancer including neck mass, neck pain, or diarrhea; symptoms of catecholamine excess from pheochromocytoma including episodic headache, palpitations, nervousness, sweating, and skin flushing; symptoms of hypercalcemia secondary to hyperparathyroidism including altered mental status, constipation, nausea/vomiting, history of nephrolithiasis, history of pathologic fracture, bone pain, myalgias.
- Positive family history is important to elucidate.

PHYSICAL EXAM
Physical exam findings depend upon the presence of specific tumor combinations in the individual patient:

- MEN1: Signs of hypercalcemia secondary to hyperparathyroidism include hypertension and altered mental status; signs of pituitary lesion including visual field deficit; signs of hyperprolactinemia from prolactinoma including galactorrhea, hypogonadism, gynecomastia; signs of growth hormone excess including gigantism (children) or acromegaly (adults); signs of pancreatic tumor could include acute abdomen
- MEN2: Presence of thyroid mass or tenderness; signs of excess catecholamine from pheochromocytoma including tachycardia and hypertension; signs of hypercalcemia secondary to hyperparathyroidism include hypertension and altered mental status; oral or rectal lesions in mucosal ganglioneuromatosis; marfanoid habitus

DIAGNOSTIC TESTS & INTERPRETATION
Lab
Initial lab tests
- MEN1:
  - Primary hyperparathyroidism: Serum calcium, 24-hour urine calcium, intact parathyroid hormone level
  - Anterior pituitary tumors: Prolactin, growth hormone, insulinlike growth factor-1, corticotropin
  - Pancreatic and duodenal tumors: Gastrin level (usually higher than 1,000 pg/mL in patients with gastrinoma); fasting insulin and glucose; glucagon, fasting plasma VIP, fasting somatostatin
  - Consider genetic testing for *MEN1* in all cases that meet clinical criteria for MEN1, in patients under 30 years of age with multiple parathyroid tumors, in patients with recurrent hyperparathyroidism, in patients with gastrinoma, and in asymptomatic relatives of patients with MEN1
- MEN2:
  - Medullary thyroid carcinoma: Calcitonin
  - Pheochromocytoma: Plasma metanephrines, 24-hour urine catecholamines and metanephrines
  - Primary hyperparathyroidism: Intact parathyroid hormone and serum calcium

Follow-Up & Special Considerations
- Guidelines for annual screening in MEN1 carriers (1):
  - Beginning at age 5: Fasting glucose, insulin, prolactin, and insulinlike growth factor 1
  - Beginning at age 8: Calcium, parathyroid hormone
  - Beginning at age 20: Gastrin, chromogranin-A, glucagon, proinsulin
- Guidelines for annual screening in MEN2 carriers:
  - Screen for pheochromocytoma depending upon the specific genetic mutation (plasma metanephrines and urine catecholamines and metanephrines)

Imaging
Guidelines for radiologic screening in MEN1 carriers to be completed every 3 years (1):
- Beginning at age 5: MRI brain
- Beginning at age 20: Abdominal CT scan and octreotide scan

Diagnostic Procedures/Surgery
Biopsy as indicated

DIFFERENTIAL DIAGNOSIS
Isolated tumors vs MEN syndromes

 TREATMENT

In general, treatment recommendations align with those of the specific isolated tumor.

ADDITIONAL TREATMENT
Issues for Referral
Referral to endocrinologist is recommended for assistance with management.

SURGERY/OTHER PROCEDURES
- Surgical management varies and depends upon the specific tumor affected. For example:
  - Parathyroidectomy in hyperparathyroidism
  - Thyroidectomy in medullary thyroid carcinoma
  - Partial pancreatectomy for tumors such as insulinomas, glucagonomas, VIPomas
  - Pheochromocytoma with surgical excision under α-adrenergic blockade starting 7–10 days prior to surgery, unilateral vs bilateral
  - Trans-sphenoidal pituitary surgery in some cases of pituitary tumors
- Patients with MEN2 at a high risk of developing medullary thyroid carcinoma (MEN2B highest risk). Prophylactic total thyroidectomy with central node dissection recommended before the age of 6 months in patients with MEN2B and before the age of 5 years in patients with MEN2A (1).

 ONGOING CARE

DIET
Calcium and vitamin D should be limited in patients with hypercalcemia secondary to hyperparathyroidism until surgical intervention is complete. Patients with gastrinoma should avoid excessive acid intake.

PATIENT EDUCATION
- Genetic counseling: Progeny of carriers will have 50% chance of inheritance.
- Importance of compliance with laboratory and radiographic screening for tumor expression

PROGNOSIS
There is no cure. Genetic testing has improved the ability to make an earlier diagnosis and to initiate routine screening and prophylactic treatment at earlier stages. For example, in patients with certain RET mutations, the cumulative risk of progression to medullary thyroid carcinoma is 100% by age 20 (3).

REFERENCES
1. Brandi ML, Gagel RF, Angeli A, et al. Guidelines for diagnosis and therapy of MEN type 1 and type 2. *J Clin Endocrinol Metab*. 2001;86:5658–71.
2. Marini F, Falchetti A, Del Monte F, et al. Multiple endocrine neoplasia type 2. *Orphanet journal of rare diseases*. 2006;1:45.
3. Machens A, Niccoli-Sire P, Hoegel J, et al. Early malignant progression of hereditary medullary thyroid cancer. *N Engl J Med*. 2003;349:1517–25.

ADDITIONAL READING
- Carney JA. Familial multiple endocrine neoplasia: the first 100 years. *Am J Surg Pathol*. 2005;29:254–74.
- Marini F, Falchetti A, Del Monte F, Carbonell Sala S, Gozzini A, Luzi E, Brandi ML et al. Multiple endocrine neoplasia type 1. *Orphanet journal of rare diseases*. 2006;1:38.
- Santoro M, Melillo RM, Carlomagno F, Vecchio G, Fusco A et al. Minireview: RET: normal and abnormal functions. *Endocrinology*. 2004;145:5448–51.

See Also (Topic, Algorithm, Electronic Media Element)
Gastric Malignancy; Hyperparathyroidism; Insulinoma; Marfan Syndrome; Pheochromocytoma; Thyroid Malignant Neoplasia

 CODES

ICD9
- 258.01 Multiple endocrine neoplasia [MEN] type I
- 258.02 Multiple endocrine neoplasia [MEN] type IIA
- 258.03 Multiple endocrine neoplasia [MEN] type IIB

CLINICAL PEARLS
- Young people (<30 years old) with hypercalcemia: Think MEN 1.
- Multiglandular involvement in hyperparathyroidism: Think MEN 1.
- Adrenal mass and tachycardia: Think pheochromocytoma.
- Patient with diagnosis of MTC:
  - Test for *RET*.
  - Rule out pheochromocytoma to avoid complications from catecholamine surge during thyroidectomy.
- Red-flag tumors for MEN syndromes include parathyroid carcinoma, medullary thyroid carcinoma, pheochromocytoma, and paraganglioma.

M

MULTIPLE MYELOMA

Ann Saunders, MD
William V. Walsh, MD

BASICS

DESCRIPTION
- Multiple myeloma (MM) is a plasma cell malignancy characterized by lytic bone lesions, paraproteinemia, anemia, renal insufficiency, hypercalcemia, and infectious diathesis.
- Monoclonal gammopathy of undetermined significance (MGUS) is a common disorder with limited monoclonal plasma cell proliferation that can lead to MM.
- Synonyms: Plasma cell myeloma; Plasma cell leukemia

EPIDEMIOLOGY
- Predominant age: Average age 66 years old (1)
- Predominant gender: Male > Female (slightly) (1)lack people are almost 2 × more commonly affected than white people (1).

Incidence
3–4 new cases/100,000 annually (2)

Prevalence
In 2007, there were 61,642 cases in the US (3).

RISK FACTORS
- Most cases have no known risks associated.
- Increased incidence of exposure to herbicides, insecticides, petroleum, heavy metals, plastics, radiation
- Myeloma increases in incidence with age.
- MGUS progression to MM is 0.5–1% year.

Genetics
Rare family clusters

GENERAL PREVENTION
None known

PATHOPHYSIOLOGY
- Clonal bone marrow proliferation with mature B cells (2)
- Genetic damage in developing B-lymphocytes at time of isotype switching, transforming normal plasma cells into malignant cells, arising from single clone (4)
- Chromosomal alterations include 13q14 deletions, 17p13 deletions, and 11q abnormalities. Most common translocations are t(11;14)(q13;q32) and t(4;14)(p16;q32). Overexpression of *myc* or *ras* and mutations in *p53* and *Rb-1* also have been described (2).
- Malignant cells multiply in bone marrow, crowding normal bone marrow cells and producing large quantities of monoclonal immunoglobulin (M) protein (4).
- Malignant cells stimulate osteoclasts that cause bone resorption and inhibit osteoblasts that form new bone, causing lytic bone lesions (4).

ETIOLOGY
Unknown

COMMONLY ASSOCIATED CONDITIONS
Secondary amyloidosis commonly due to MM

DIAGNOSIS

HISTORY
- 34% of patients are asymptomatic at the time of presentation.
- Bone pain (58%) in back, long bones, skull, ribs, and pelvis due to bone mass or pathologic fracture (26–34%)
- Peripheral neuropathy: Carpal tunnel syndrome most common
- Symptoms of hypercalcemia: Anorexia, nausea, somnolence, and polydipsia
- Infection, especially with encapsulated organisms: Fever is rare at presentation
- Weight loss, malaise, weakness

PHYSICAL EXAM
- Dehydration
- Skin findings of amyloidosis: Waxy papules, nodules, or plaques that may be evident in the eyelids, retroauricular region, neck, or inguinal and anogenital regions; petechiae and ecchymosis; "pinch purpura"
- Hyperviscosity syndrome in 7%: Retinal hemorrhages, prolonged bleeding, neurologic changes
- Tender bones and masses

DIAGNOSTIC TESTS & INTERPRETATION
Lab
Criteria for diagnosis: The diagnosis of MM requires all of the following (1):
- A bone marrow aspirate or biopsy showing that at least 10% of the cells are clonal plasma cells or the presence of a plasmacytoma
- M protein in the blood or urine
- Evidence of damage to the body as a result of the plasma cell growth, such as destructive bone lesions, kidney failure, anemia, or hypercalcemia

Initial lab tests
- Complete blood count (CBC) with differential and platelet counts to evaluate anemia, other cytopenias; anemia in 73% (1)
- Blood urea nitrogen (BUN), creatinine: Increased levels indicate renal involvement (2).
- Serum electrolytes, serum albumin, serum calcium: Hypercalcemia with levels >11 mg/dL in 13% (1)
- Serum lactate dehydrogenase (LDH), β_2-microglobulin: Increased levels indicated increased tumor burden (2).
- Quantitive serum analysis of immunoglobulin levels: IgG, IgA, IgM (2)
- Serum protein electrophoresis (SPEP), serum immunofixation electrophoresis (SIFE): M protein level elevated; assessing changes in the level of M protein helps to track progression of myeloma and response to treatment (2); 82% localized band on serum protein electrophoresis, 93% monoclonal protein on immunoelectrophoresis (1)
- Erythrocyte sedimentation rate: Elevated
- Urinanalysis: 24-h urine for protein, urine protein electrophoresis (UPEP), urine immunofixation electrophoresis (UIFE); 20% positive urine protein (2)

Follow-Up & Special Considerations
- Bone marrow aspirate and biopsy for histology, immunohistochemistry, plasma cell labeling index, cytogenetics, fluorescence in situ hybridization (FISH): May detect chromosomal abnormalities (2)
- Serum-free light chains in selected patients (2)
- Plasma cell labeling index may be helpful to identify the fraction of the myeloma cell population that is proliferating (2).

Imaging
Initial approach
- Skeletal survey: 26–34% of patients present with lytic bone lesions on x-ray.
- MRI for any back pain or earliest signs/symptoms of spinal cord compression

Follow-Up & Special Considerations
- CT scan is more sensitive than plain radiography for small long bone lesions; can differentiate malignant from benign vertebral compression fractures in patients who are not MRI candidates
- Positron-emission tomographic (PET) scans with CT scans are used for staging and follow-up: Active myeloma is positive (2).
- Bisphosphonates are considered as therapy; a baseline bone densitometry may be indicated (2).

Diagnostic Procedures/Surgery
Staging:
- International staging system for myeloma:
  - Stage I: Albumin ≤3.5 g/dL and β_2-microglobulin <3.5 μg/mL
  - Stage II: Neither stage I nor stage III
  - Stage III: β_2-microglobulin ≥5.5 μg/mL
- Mayo Clinic Criteria for high-risk multiple myeloma (1):
  - Cytogenetics: Deletion of chromosome 13, hypodiploidy
  - FISH: t(4;14), t(14;16), 17p-
  - Plasma cell labeling index >3%

Pathological Findings
Marrow plasmacytosis >30%, >10% immature; Russell bodies

DIFFERENTIAL DIAGNOSIS
- MGUS: Monoclonal protein <3 g/dL; marrow plasma cells <10%; absence of end-organ damage:

  - Prevalence 5.3% if >70 years of age
  - Progress to MM 0.5–1%/year
  - Increased risk of progression if IgA or IgM, higher percentage of marrow plasma cells
- Metastatic cancer to bone
- Waldenström macroglobulinemia: IgM monoclonal gammopathy with >10% marrow lymphoplasmacytic infiltrate
- Systemic AL amyloidosis: Amyloid-related syndrome with positive amyloid stain plus monoclonal plasma cell disorder
- POEMS syndrome: *P*olyneuropathy, *o*rganomegaly, *e*ndocrinopathy, *m*onoclonal gammopathy, *s*kin changes

TREATMENT

- Treatment varies depending on how active disease is and the stage of MM.
- Treatment for inactive, smoldering MM at this time is supportive only. Patients should be monitored at 3-month intervals. These patients do not have evidence of end-organ damage. However, clinical trials are ongoing to determine whether newer agents are able to delay progression (1).
- Autologous stem cell transplant following induction chemotherapy is standard of care for patients with symptomatic disease <65 years of age or those >65 years of age and able to undergo procedure. Although not curative, it improves complete response rates and prolongs median overall survival in MM by approximately 12 months with a mortality rate of 1–2% (1).

MEDICATION
Chemotherapy options include bortezomib, cyclophosphamide, thalidomide, lenalidomide, and dexamethasone.

First Line

- Bortezomib (1)[B]:
  - Inhibits the ubiquitin-proteasome catalytic pathway in cells by binding to the 20S proteasome complex
  - Toxicity: Peripheral neuropathy, cytopenias, nausea
  - Consider herpes simplex virus (HSV) prophylaxis.
- Cyclophosphamide (1)[B]:
  - Nitrogen mustard–derivative alkylating agent
  - Often used in combination with prednisone or thalidomide in cases of relapsed disease
  - Toxicity: Cytopenias, anaphylaxis, interstitial pulmonary fibrosis, secondary malignancy, impaired fertility
- Thalidomide (1)[B]:
  - Works by antiangiogenesis inhibition, immunomodulation, and inhibition of tumor necrosis factor α
  - Usually combined with dexamethasone
  - Toxicity: Birth defects, deep vein thrombosis (DVT), neuropathy, rash, nausea, bradycardia
  - DVT prophylaxis
- Lenalidomide (1)[B]:
  - Is an immunomodulatory drug
  - Often combined with dexamethasone
  - Toxicity: Deep vein thrombosis (DVT), cytopenias, birth defects risk, DVT prophylaxis: Aspirin is standard.
- Dexamethasone (1)[B]:
  - Low doses (40 mg/wk) superior to higher doses
  - Increases risk of DVT
- Bisphosphonates (5)[A]:
  - Do not have effect on mortality but decrease pain, decrease pathological vertebral fractures and fractures of other bones
  - No bisphosphonate appears to be superior to others.
  - Dose-adjust/monitor renal function.
  - Monitor for osteonecrosis of jaw.

Second Line
Single agents or combinations as above

ADDITIONAL TREATMENT
- Local radiation therapy for bone pain (1):
  - Should be limited for patients with disabling pain who have not responded to analgesics and/or chemotherapy
  - Avoid extensive radiation therapy.
- Allogenic stem cell transplant (1):
  - Advantages over autologous stem cell transplant include lack of graft contamination with tumor cells and lack of graft vs MM effect
  - Only 5–10% of patients are candidates due to age, lack of an HLA-matched sibling donor, and organ function.

General Measures
Maintain adequate hydration to prevent renal insufficiency.

Issues for Referral
- Patients who have known or suspected multiple myeloma should be treated by a hematologist/oncologist.
- Patients with spinal or other bone pathology should be referred to orthopedics for support.

Additional Therapies
- Effective pain management:
  - Avoid NSAIDS due to nephrotoxicity.
- Kyphoplasty/vertebroplasty: Consider for symptomatic vertebral compressions (1).
- Plasmapheresis: For hyperviscosity syndrome (a rare complication) (1)
- Erythropoietin: For selected patients with anemia (1)
- Patients should receive vaccines for pneumococcus and influenza (1.)
- Do not administer zoster vaccine and other live-virus vaccines.

IN-PATIENT CONSIDERATIONS

Initial Stabilization
- Avoid IV radiographic contrast materials due to the high risk for contrast-induced nephropathy (1).
- Adequate hydration
- Avoid nonsteroidal anti-inflammatory drugs (NSAIDs) to decrease chance of renal insufficiency.
- Manage hypercalcemia and control hyperuricemia.

Admission Criteria
Including but not limited to pain, infections, cytopenias, renal failure, bone complications, spinal cord compression

Nursing
Central to patient management and health care resource coordination

ONGOING CARE

PATIENT EDUCATION
www.cancer.net; www.myeloma.org

PROGNOSIS
- Median survival overall is 3 years (1).
- Median survival by ISS stage (1):
  - Stage I: 62 months
  - Stage II: 44 months
  - Stage III: 29 months
- Median survival in patients with high-risk multiple myeloma (see "staging" for definition) is less than 2–3 years, even after autologous stem cell transplant; however, with more modern therapies, survivals of 10 years or more are being seen (1).

COMPLICATIONS
Many, including infection, pain, lytic bone lesions, hypercalcemia, hyperuricemia, spinal cord compression, anemia, hyperviscosity syndrome, renal insufficiency

REFERENCES
1. Rajkumar SV, Kyle RA et al. Multiple myeloma: diagnosis and treatment. *Mayo Clin. Proc.* 2005;80: 1371–82.
2. The NCCN Multiple Myeloma Clinical Practice Guidelines in Oncology (Version 2.2008). © 2008 National Comprehensive Cancer Network, Inc. Available at: http://www.nccn.org. Accessed April 29, 2010.
3. National Cancer Institute, SEER cancer statistics review, 1975–2007. http://seer.cancer.gov/csr/1975_2007/results_merged/sect_18_myeloma.pdf
4. Jagannath S et al. Pathophysiological underpinnings of multiple myeloma progression. *J Manag Care Pharm.* 2008;14:7–11.
5. Mhaskar, Redzepovic J, et al. Bisphosphonates in Multiple Myeloma. *Cochrane Haematological Malignancies Group Cochrane Database of Systematic Reviews.* 3, 2010.

ADDITIONAL READING
Kyle RA, Therneau TM, Rajkumar SV, et al. Prevalence of monoclonal gammopathy of undetermined significance. *N Engl J Med.* 2006;354:1362–9.

CODES

ICD9
203.00 Multiple myeloma, without mention of having achieved remission

CLINICAL PEARLS
- Multiple myeloma is a plasma cell malignancy that causes end organ damage.
- Suspect MM if high total protein:albumin ratio
- High index of suspicion for spinal cord compression
- Avoid nephrotoxins (radiographic contrast material, NSAIDs, dehydration).
- Patients with MM are immunocompromised.

M

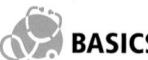

MULTIPLE SCLEROSIS

Yolanda Backus, MD
James J. Arnold, DO

BASICS

DESCRIPTION
- A chronic disease involving inflammation and degeneration leading to demyelinization of the white matter of the brain and spinal cord with axonal damage.
- 4 internationally recognized forms (1):
  - Relapsing/remitting multiple sclerosis (RRMS): (85%) Periods of relapse during which time new symptoms can appear and old ones worsen followed by periods of remission. Can result in residual deficits or full recovery between symptomatic periods.
  - Secondary progressive MS (SPMS): Steady progression of clinical neurologic damage with or without relapses and minor remissions. 50% of patients with RRMS will develop SPMS; patients may have experienced RRMS for 2–40 years or more. Relapses and remissions will decrease over time.
  - Primary progressive MS (PPMS): Gradual progression of the disease from onset with no relapses or remissions.
  - Progressive relapsing MS (PRMS) (Least common): Steady, cumulative progression of clinical neurologic damage with superimposed relapses and remissions.
- Clinically isolated syndromes (CIS): Initial clinical manifestation of demyelination; most commonly consisting of optic neuritis, transverse myelitis, and brainstem syndromes (1)

Pregnancy Considerations
- Relapses are less frequent during pregnancy, especially in the 3rd trimester, as well as in the postpartum period.
- Pregnancy does not alter the overall course of MS.
- Relapse rate is unaffected by breastfeeding.

EPIDEMIOLOGY
- Predominant age: 20–40 years old. Exception: PRMS is typically diagnosed in patients >40 years old.
- Predominant sex: Female > Male. Males experience a more malignant course than females.

Incidence
3.6 cases per 100,000 person years worldwide (2)

Prevalence
In US, 400,000 people have MS; 2.5 million cases worldwide

RISK FACTORS
- 0.1% (1 out of 1,000) risk of developing the disease in the general population (3)
- Northern European descent
- Family history of the disease; 1–3% risk of MS among 1st-degree relatives
- Temperate climate: However, the latitude gradient (the higher the latitude, the higher the incidence) present in older incidences studies of MS is decreasing (2).
- Ethnic groups along the equator have the lowest incidence of disease (4).

Genetics
- Strong genetic component in determining susceptibility to the disease
- HLA-DRB1 has been associated

- Patients with MS are more likely to have other autoimmune disorders.

GENERAL PREVENTION
No known preventive measures. Avoid factors that may precipitate an exacerbation, such as stressful life events.

PATHOPHYSIOLOGY
- Neurodegeneration within plaques leads to disability; disease is radiologically active during periods of apparent clinical stability.
- Disease occurs in genetically susceptible people with breaches in the blood-brain barrier (BBB); invasion of autoreactive T-cells (primarily Th-1) and intrathecal B-cells damage the central nervous system (CNS)
- Histological findings: Perivascular infiltration of leukocytes, parenchymal edema, loss of myelin and oligodendrocytes, widespread axonal damage, plasma cells, myelin-filled macrophages, hypertrophic astrocytes (5)

ETIOLOGY
Unknown but various theories:
- Autoimmune theory supported by human leukocyte antigen (HLA) linkage, hereditary pattern, immunocytes in plaques, changes in peripheral blood immunocytes
- Low vitamin D levels and limited sun exposure
- Combined theory: Autoimmune disorder triggered in genetically susceptible individuals as an infrequent response to environmental factors

COMMONLY ASSOCIATED CONDITIONS
- Optic neuritis: Unilateral eye pain, worse with movements: Scotoma (loss of mainly central vision); color desaturation; Marcus Gunn pupil (afferent pupillary defect)
- Internuclear ophthalmoplegia (INO): Horizontal nystagmus of abducting eye: Lost/delayed adduction
- L'hermitte phenomenon: Shocklike sensation with head and/or neck movement

DIAGNOSIS

Primarily clinical diagnosis of 2 or more distinct episodes of CNS dysfunction separated by both time (at least 3 months) and space (2 distinct neurologic deficits) with eventual partial resolution of CNS symptoms: Some patients may experience a prodrome. Minimum duration for relapse is 24 hours.

HISTORY
- Fatigue
- Painful loss of vision in 1 eye
- Urinary urgency or retention
- Hyperesthesia/paresthesias, radicular pain
- Clumsiness/incoordination/tremor, vertigo
- Blurred or double vision
- Constipation
- Emotional lability
- Sexual dysfunction
- Convulsions

PHYSICAL EXAM
- Ocular paralysis (INO)
- Hemiparesis or monoparesis
- Hyperactive deep tendon reflexes or clonus
- Genital anesthesia
- Loss of position/vibration sense

- Ataxia
- Spasticity: LE > UE

DIAGNOSTIC TESTS & INTERPRETATION
Lab
- Cerebrospinal fluid (CSF) shows oligoclonal bands, abnormal colloidal gold curve, elevated gamma-globulin IgG, mild mononuclear pleocytosis with lymphocytic predominance (<40 cells/mL), myelin debris, and normal or slightly elevated protein.
- Tests to exclude other disorders: Serology for syphilis (serum and CSF), erythrocyte sedimentation rate, B_{12}, thyroid-stimulating hormone, antinuclear antibody, Lyme titer

Imaging
Magnetic resonance imaging (MRI) of head/spine (more sensitive than computed tomography):
- T2 image: Hyperintense lesions: Enhancement is due to breach in BBB.
- T1 image: Hypointense lesions: Black holes, gray holes: Negative prognostic indicators
- Lesions can disappear with serial imaging due to resolution of edema and remyelination.
- Affected areas:
  - Periventricular white matter (pathognomonic finding)
  - Corpus callosum
  - Centrum semiovale
  - Basal ganglia
  - Corona radiata

Diagnostic Procedures/Surgery
Electrophysiological testing: Sensory evoked potential testing (visual, brainstem auditory, and somatosensory): Helpful in identifying neurolesions not evident on MRI

DIFFERENTIAL DIAGNOSIS
- Tumors (brainstem, cerebellar, spinal cord)
- CNS infections
- Syphilis, HIV
- Trigeminal neuralgia
- Epilepsy
- Transverse myelitis
- Ataxias (Friedreich ataxia, hereditary ataxia)
- Amyotrophic lateral sclerosis
- Progressive multifocal leukoencephalopathy
- Syringomyelia, Chiari malformation
- Ruptured intervertebral disc, disc herniation
- Small cerebral infarcts
- Vasculitides (giant cell arteritis)
- Behçet disease
- Systemic lupus erythematosus
- Sarcoidosis
- Pernicious anemia

TREATMENT

- Treatment is preventive and disease mitigating, not curative or restorative.
- Early treatment can slow progression to clinically definite MS during CIS.
- The frequency of relapses early in the course of MS has predictive value for future disability (1,2)[B].

MEDICATION

- Relapses: Methylprednisolone: 500–1000 mg/day IV for 3–5 days; no oral taper (1)[A]; Prednisone: 300 mg b.i.d. for 3 days; no oral taper (1)[B]
- Disease modifying therapy: Interferon-β (IFN-β):Betaseron (IFN-β-1b) [250 μg SC q.o.d.], Avonex (IFN-β-1a) [30 μg IM weekly], Rebif (IFN-β-1a) [22 or 44 μg SC 3×/week] (1)[B]:
  - Monitor complete blood count and liver function tests before starting therapy and every 6 months.
  - Can prophylactically treat with nonsteroidal anti-inflammatory drugs (NSAIDs) to reduce side effects, including flulike symptoms and injection-site reactions; titrating IFN-β therapy can decrease liver dysfunction
  - Glatiramer acetate (Copaxone): 20 mg/d SC (1)[A]:
    ○ Improved side effect profile when compared with interferon-β
    ○ >50% of patients will have injection-site reaction; alternate injection sites
  - Natalizumab (Tysabri): 300 mg IV every 4 weeks (2)[A]: 2nd-line therapy due to previous safety concerns in combination therapy; Food and Drug Administration approved as monotherapy in 2006
  - Mitoxantrone (Novantrone): 12 mg/m² short IV infusion q3mo (2)[C]:
    ○ Not indicated in treatment of PPMS
    ○ Serious cardiotoxicity side effects; regular monitoring of left ventricular ejection fraction is recommended
- Symptomatic therapies: (2)[C],(4):
  - Spasticity: Baclofen, diazepam, gabapentin
  - Pain: NSAIDs, carbamazepine, gabapentin, lamotrigine, topiramate, tricyclic antidepressants
  - Bladder dysfunction: [Urgency] oxybutynin, tolterodine tartrate; [retention] intermittent self-catheterization
  - Constipation: High-fiber diet, stool softeners, bulk-producing agents, laxatives, suppositories
  - Sexual dysfunction: Alprostadil, sildenafil, vardenafil
  - Fatigue: Amantadine, modafinil, stimulants (pemoline, methylphenidate, 4-aminopyridine)
  - Tremors: Clonazepam, β-blockers, primidone
  - Depression: Serotonin selective reuptake inhibitors, cognitive behavioral therapy
  - Paranoia/mania: Haloperidol, lithium, atypical antipsychotics

ADDITIONAL TREATMENT

Shepherd MS relapse protocol (1,2)[C]:

- Rule out possible precipitating events (heat exposure, overexertion, urinary tract infection [UTI], upper respiratory infection).
- If any infection is suspected, screen and treat accordingly. Hold steroids.
- If there are no clear-cut precipitating events, determine the severity of the symptoms and any impact on activities of daily living.
- If the symptoms are not significantly affecting activities of daily living, observe.
- If activities of daily living are affected, consider steroid therapy. Review medical history for any relative contraindications (diabetes mellitus type 2, hypertension, pregnancy, poorly controlled psychiatric disease, past history of poor tolerance for steroids).

- If there are no contraindications, proceed with steroids: IVMP 1 g/d for 3 days. No oral taper. Oral prednisone 300 mg b.i.d. for 3 days. No oral taper. (May consider taper in patients who report general malaise after 3 days of IV or oral steroids.)
- Consider lorazepam 1 mg p.o. q.8 hours for patients with a history of anxiety while on steroids or 1 mg p.o. q.h.s. for insomnia.
- Practice varies on whether to prescribe antacids or H2 blockers during steroids; generally not recommended.
- For patients intolerant to steroids or pregnant women, consider IVIG 0.4 g/kg/d for 5 days; some patients do seem to respond to IVIG for relapses.
- For patients with tightly controlled diabetes mellitus, steroids can be used with caution by using sliding-scale insulin. May consider IVIG as above for these patients as well.

General Measures

- Rehabilitation including physical and occupational therapy
- Psychotherapy and support
- Yoga, Pilates, and water therapies can all be helpful.
- Sunlight can increase levels of vitamin D, which may improve relapse frequency and duration (6).

 ## ONGOING CARE

FOLLOW-UP RECOMMENDATIONS

- Treat relapses with corticosteroids to minimize disease progression and duration of relapse.
- Maintain regular activity but avoid overwork and fatigue.
- Rest during periods of acute relapse.

Patient Monitoring

Progression of disease is measured by the Kurtzke disability status scale (KDSS). 1 is the least disabling and 10 is death. Kurtzke disability status scale:

- 1. No disability and minimal neurologic signs
- 2. Minimal disability (e.g., slight weakness or stiffness, mild gait or visual disturbance)
- 3. Moderate disability (e.g., monoparesis, mild hemiparesis, moderate ataxia, disturbing sensory loss, prominent urinary or eye symptom, or combination of lesser dysfunction)
- 4. Relatively severe disability but fully ambulatory without aid, self-sufficient and able to be up around 12 hours/day, does not prevent the ability to work or carry on normal living activities, excluding sexual dysfunction
- 5. Disability is severe enough to preclude working, maximal motor function involves walking unaided up to 500 meters
- 6. Needs assistance with walking (e.g., cane, crutches, or braces)
- 7. Restricted to a wheelchair but able to wheel oneself and enter and leave chair without assistance
- 8. Restricted to bed or chair, retains many self-care functions and has effective use of arms
- 9. Helpless and bedridden
- 10. Death due to multiple sclerosis (from respiratory paralysis, coma, following repeated or prolonged epileptic seizures)

DIET

High fluid intake and a high-fiber diet to prevent or treat constipation (2)[C]. Vitamin D: 50,000 IU/week; ergocalciferol for 8 weeks; recheck vitamin D levels (goal of >40 ng/mL): Maintenance with vitamin D₃ at 1,000–2,000 IU/day once deficiency/insufficiency has been corrected (1,6)[B]

PATIENT EDUCATION

- National Multiple Sclerosis Society, 205E 42nd St., New York, NY 10017; (800) 624-8236. At: http://www.nationalmssociety.org/index.aspx
- National Institute of Neurological Disorders and Stroke: http://www.ninds.nih.gov/disorders/multiple_sclerosis/multiple_sclerosis.htm

PROGNOSIS

- ~70% of patients lead active, productive lives with prolonged remissions
- 30% relapse in 1 year, 20% in 5–9 years, and 10% in 10–30 years
- 50% of patients are using a cane (KDSS 6), 15% are wheelchair dependent (KDSS 7) within 10 years
- Variable course; can cause early death or disability if disease is rapidly progressive or relapses frequent
- Life expectancy of patients with MS is nearly the same as that of the unaffected population

COMPLICATIONS

- Emotional lability
- Chronic pain (55–65%)
- Nystagmus or optic nerve atrophy
- Sexual dysfunction
- Infections such as UTIs
- Paraplegia
- Delirium or coma

REFERENCES

1. Thrower BW et al. Relapse management in multiple sclerosis. *Neurologist*. 2009;15:1–5.
2. Alonso A, Hernan MA. Temporal trends in the incidence of multiple sclerosis-a systematic review. *Neurology*. 2008;71:1329–135.
3. Courtney AM, Treadaway K, Remington G, et al. Multiple sclerosis. *Med. Clin. North Am*. 2009;93.
4. Rejdak K, Jackson S, Giovannoni G, et al. Multiple sclerosis: a practical overview for clinicians. *British medical bulletin*. 2010.
5. Frohman EM, Racke MK, Raine CS. Multiple Sclerosis—The Plaque and Its Pathogenesis. *NEJM*. 2006;354:942–955.
6. Solomon AJ, Whitham RH, et al. Multiple Sclerosis and Vitamin D: A Review and Recommendations. *Current neurology and neuroscience reports*. 2010;

 ## CODES

ICD9
340 Multiple sclerosis

CLINICAL PEARLS

- MS is an inflammatory and neurodegenerative disorder affecting the CNS.
- Treat relapses with steroids; ongoing disease modification is the mainstay of therapy, as there is no cure.
- MS is a clinical diagnosis and can only be appropriately diagnosed over time.

M

MUMPS

Frances Y. Wu, MD

 BASICS

Painful parotitis occurs in 95% of *symptomatic* mumps, but 1/3 of mumps cases may be asymptomatic.

DESCRIPTION
- Acute, generalized paramyxovirus infection usually presenting with unilateral or bilateral parotitis
- Epidemics in late winter and spring with transmission by respiratory secretions; incubation approximately 14–24 days
- System(s) affected: Hematologic/Lymphatic/Immunologic; Reproductive; Skin/Exocrine
- Synonym(s): Epidemic parotitis; Infectious parotitis

EPIDEMIOLOGY
- Predominant age: 85% occur before age 15; adult cases typically more severe
- Predominant sex: Male = Female
- Geriatric population: Most are immune.
- Acute epidemic mumps:
  - Most cases occur in children aged 5–15 years.
  - Recent (2006) US epidemic in vaccinated college students aged 18–24 years with 5,700 US cases; another US epidemic 2009–2010 in NY/NJ, over 1,500 cases (1)
  - Unusual in children <2 years of age
  - Most infants <1 year are immune.
  - Urban epidemics among nonvaccinated populations
  - Communicable period 24 h before to 72 h after parotitis onset
  - Incubation period 18 days

Incidence
- 0.09/100,000 persons (5,783/year in 2006)
- Occasional epidemic outbreaks in a given region

Prevalence
- 0.0064/100,000 persons
- 90% of adults are seropositive even without history.

RISK FACTORS
- Foreign travel/exposure: 43% of other nations do not vaccinate for mumps.
- Crowded environments such as dormitories
- Waning immunity after single-dose vaccination; even after 2 doses immunity drops from 95–86% in 9 years (2)[C].

GENERAL PREVENTION
- Vaccination:
  - 2 doses of live mumps vaccine or measles-mumps-rubella (MMR) vaccine recommended, 1st at 12–15 months and 2nd at 4–6 years of age
  - 95% effective in studies, but field trials show 75–95% efficacy, which may be below level needed for herd immunity to prevent epidemic spread (3)[C].
  - Adverse effects: Most common proven effect is ITP, with incidence of 3.3/100,000 doses.
  - No relationship between MMR vaccine and autism

- Immune globulin not effective in prevention
- Postexposure vaccination does not protect from recent exposure.
- Isolate hospitalized patients until 5 (4)[C] days past onset; exclude nonimmune individuals for 26 days after last case onset.

Pregnancy Considerations
- There are no proven complications of vaccine but theoretically should not vaccinate in pregnancy.
- Immunization of family may protect against later exposures but not the present one.

PATHOPHYSIOLOGY
Mumps virus replicates in glandular epithelium of parotids, pancreas, and testes.
- Leads to interstitial edema and inflammation
- Interstitial glandular hemorrhage may occur.
- Pressure caused by edema of the testes against the tunica albuginea can lead to necrosis.

ETIOLOGY
- Mumps paramyxovirus
- Other viruses, such as coxsackievirus (rare)

 DIAGNOSIS

HISTORY
- Initial parotid swelling just behind jaw
- Swelling peaks in 1–3 days, lasts 3–7 days.
- Sour foods cause pain in parotid gland region.
- Moderate fever, usually not above 104°F (40.0°C); high fever frequently associated with complications

PHYSICAL EXAM
- Parotid pain and swelling in one or both glands
- Rare prodrome of fever, neck muscle ache, and malaise
- Meningeal signs in 15%, encephalitis in 0.5%
- Rarely arthritis, orchitis, thyroiditis, mastitis, pancreatitis, oophoritis, and myocarditis
- Rare maculopapular, erythematous rash
- Up to 50% of cases may be very mild.
- Obscures angle of mandible
- Elevates earlobe
- Redness at opening of Stensen duct but no pus
- Swelling in sternal area; rare, but pathognomonic of mumps

DIAGNOSTIC TESTS & INTERPRETATION
Lab
- The following 3 special tests to confirm an outbreak should be ordered and reported to health department:
  - IgM titer (positive by day 5 in 100% of nonimmunized patients)
  - Swab of parotid duct or other affected salivary ducts for viral isolation
  - Rise in IgG titer samples; test should be ordered if patient previously immunized, 1st sample within 5 days of onset, 2nd 2 weeks later.
- Other potential findings: Serum amylase may be elevated; cerebrospinal fluid leukocytosis and leukopenia may be present.

Imaging
Testicular ultrasound may be useful to differentiate mumps orchitis from testicular torsion.

Initial approach
Clinical diagnosis (swelling of one or both parotid glands):
- Lasting 2 or more days
- No other apparent cause
- Rare presentation of meningitis without parotitis (1–10%)

Diagnostic Procedures/Surgery
If meningitis is present, lumbar puncture may be required to prove aseptic meningitis.

Pathological Findings
Periductal edema and lymphocytic infiltration in affected glands

DIFFERENTIAL DIAGNOSIS
- If not epidemic, other viruses are more common: Parainfluenza parotitis, Epstein-Barr virus, coxsackievirus, adenovirus, parvovirus B19
- Suppurative parotitis: Often associated with *Staphylococcus aureus* (presence of Wharton duct pus on massaging parotid gland nearly excludes diagnosis of mumps)
- Recurrent allergic parotitis
- Salivary calculus with intermittent swelling
- Lymphadenitis from any cause, even HIV infection
- Cytomegalovirus parotitis in immunocompromised patients
- Mikulicz syndrome: Chronic, painless parotid and lacrimal gland swelling of unknown cause that occurs in tuberculosis, sarcoidosis, lupus, leukemia, lymphosarcoma, and malignant or benign salivary gland tumors
- Sjögren syndrome, diabetes mellitus, uremia, malnutrition
- Drug-related parotid enlargement (iodides, guanethidine, phenothiazine)
- Other causes of the complications of mumps (meningoencephalitis, orchitis, oophoritis, pancreatitis, polyarthritis, nephritis, myocarditis, prostatitis)
- Mumps orchitis must be differentiated from testicular torsion and from chlamydial or bacterial orchitis. (Testicular sonogram can be useful.)

 TREATMENT

- No specific antiviral therapy
- Analgesics to relieve pain
- Avoid corticosteroids for mumps orchitis because they can reduce testosterone concentrations and increase testicular atrophy.
- Intravenous immunoglobulin (IVIG) only successful for certain autoimmune-based sequelae: postinfectious encephalitis, Guillain-Barré syndrome, or ITP
- Interferon-α2b improved severe bilateral orchitis and decreased testicular atrophy in small studies.

MEDICATION

First Line
- Corticosteroids or a nonsteroidal anti-inflammatory drug (NSAID) may diminish pain and swelling in acute orchitis and arthritis mumps but usually is not necessary.
- May use acetaminophen for fever and/or pain.
- Contraindications: Refer to manufacturer's profile for each drug.
- Precautions: Avoid aspirin for pain in children. Aspirin use in children with viral infections has been associated with Reye syndrome.
- Significant possible interactions: Refer to manufacturer's profile for each drug.

Second Line
- Mumps arthritis may improve with corticosteroids or an NSAID.
- Interferon-α2b $\times$ 7 days has been used experimentally in small studies (2)[C] for severe bilateral orchitis to prevent infertility.

ADDITIONAL TREATMENT

General Measures
- High fever and testicular pain: May hospitalize for steroids or interferon
- Orchitis:
  – Ice packs to scrotum can help to relieve pain.
  – Scrotal support with adhesive bridge while recumbent and/or athletic supporter while ambulatory

IN-PATIENT CONSIDERATIONS

Initial Stabilization
Outpatient supportive care if no complications

Admission Criteria
Hospitalize only if CNS symptoms occur.

IV Fluids
If severe nausea or vomiting accompanies pancreatitis

ONGOING CARE

FOLLOW-UP RECOMMENDATIONS
Mumps orchitis:
- Bed rest and local supportive clothing (e.g., two pairs of briefs) or adhesive-tape bridge
- Must be out of school until no longer contagious: About 9 days after onset of pain

Patient Monitoring
Most cases will be mild. Monitor hydration status.

DIET
Liquid diet if cannot chew

PATIENT EDUCATION
Orchitis is common in older children but rarely results in sterility, even after bilateral orchitis.

PROGNOSIS
- Complete recovery is usual; immunity is lifelong.
- Transient sensorineural hearing loss occurs in 4% of adults.
- Rare recurrence after 2 weeks may be recurrent nonepidemic parotitis.

COMPLICATIONS
- May precede, accompany, or follow salivary gland involvement and may occur (rarely) without primary involvement of the parotid gland.
- Orchitis is common (30%) in postpubertal boys. It starts within 8 days after parotitis. Fever, swollen testis of 4 days' duration, impaired fertility in 13%, but absolute sterility is rare.
- Meningitis (1–10%) or encephalitis (0.1%) may present 5–10 days after first symptoms of illness. Aseptic meningitis typically is mild, but meningoencephalitis may lead to seizures, paralysis, hydrocephalus, or in 2% of encephalitis patients, death.
- Acute cerebellar ataxia has been reported after mumps infections; self-resolving in 2–3 weeks.
- Cerebrospinal fluid pleocytosis, usually lymphocytes, found in 65% of patients with parotitis
- Oophoritis in 7% of postpubertal females; no decreased fertility
- Pancreatitis, usually mild
- Nephritis, thyroiditis, and arthralgias are rare.
- Myocarditis: Usually mild, but may depress ST segment, may be linked to endocardial fibroelastosis
- Deafness: 1/15,000 unilateral nerve deafness; may not be permanent
- Inflammation about the eye (keratouveitis) rarely
- Dacryoadenitis, optic neuritis

Pediatric Considerations
- Orchitis is more common in adolescents.
- Young children are less likely to develop complications.
- Most complications occur in postpubertal group.
- Avoid aspirin use in children with viral symptoms.

Pregnancy Considerations
Disease may increase the rate of spontaneous abortion in 1st trimester; however, perinatal mumps has been reported to take a benign course.

REFERENCES

1. Centers for Disease Control and Prevention (CDC). Update: Mumps Outbreak–New York and New Jersey, June 2008-Jan 2010. *MMWR Morb Mortal Wkly Rep*. 2010;59(05):125–129.
2. Hviid A, Rubin S, Mühlemann K. Mumps. *Lancet*. 2008;371:932–44.
3. Hindiyeh MY, Aboudy Y, Wohoush M, et al. Characterization of Large Mumps outbreak in Vaccinated Palestinian Refugees. *J Clin Microbiol*. 2009.
4. Centers for Disease Control and Prevention (CDC). Updated recommendations for isolation of persons with mumps. *MMWR Morb Mortal Wkly Rep*. 2008;57:1103–5.

ADDITIONAL READING

- Centers for Disease Control and Prevention (CDC). Brief report: update: mumps activity–United States, January 1-October 7, 2006. *MMWR Morb Mortal Wkly Rep*. 2006;55:1152–3.
- Gemmill IM. Mumps vaccine: is it time to re-evaluate our approach? *CMAJ*. 2006;175:491–2.
- Kancherla VS, Hanson IC. Mumps resurgence in the United States. *J Allergy Clin Immunol*. 2006;118: 938–41.

CODES

ICD9
- 072.0 Mumps orchitis
- 072.1 Mumps meningitis
- 072.9 Mumps without mention of complication

CLINICAL PEARLS
- Mumps is a clinical diagnosis, including swelling of one or more parotid glands for 2 or more days without other obvious cause, but confirmatory tests must be done for epidemics.
- Ultrasound is useful to distinguish testicular torsion from testicular pain related to mumps orchitis.
- MMR vaccine is 75–95% effective in field trials; therefore, expect some cases of mumps despite completed vaccinations.

M

MUSCULAR DYSTROPHY

Austin Larson, MD
Brian Alverson, MD

 BASICS

- Primary inherited myopathies caused by dysfunctional proteins of muscle fibers
- Distribution of weakness, other associated symptoms, and disease prognosis depend on the specific mutated gene and the severity of the mutation.

DESCRIPTION

- Duchenne muscular dystrophy (DMD):
  - Highest-incidence muscular dystrophy, X-linked inheritance, early onset, rapidly progressive
- Becker muscular dystrophy (BMD):
  - Less severe phenotype than Duchenne, also caused by mutation in DMD gene
- Myotonic muscular dystrophy (MMD):
  - Myotonia (slow relaxation after muscle contraction), distal and facial weakness
- Limb-girdle muscular dystrophy (LGMD):
  - Proximal weakness and atrophy, variable prognosis with 19 different identified mutations
- Fascioscapulohumeral muscular dystrophy (FSHMD):
  - Pattern of weakness with primarily facial and shoulder muscles affected
- Emery-Dreifuss muscular dystrophy (EDMD):
  - Characterized by early development of joint contractures and cardiac involvement
- Congenital muscular dystrophies (CMD):
  - Heterogeneous group of diseases presenting in infancy
  - Includes Fukuyama CMD, Ullrich CMD, Walker Warburg syndrome and other conditions
- Oculopharyngeal muscular dystrophy (OPMD):
  - Adult onset, affects extraocular and pharyngeal muscles
- System(s) affected: Musculoskeletal; Cardiac; Nervous

EPIDEMIOLOGY
Incidence
- DMD: 30/100,000 male births
- BMD: 3/100,000 male births
- MMD: 10/100,000 births
- FSHMD: 5/100,000 births
- Predominant age at onset of symptoms:
  - CMD: Infancy
  - DMD: Early childhood
  - BMD: Adolescence
  - Other muscular dystrophies present at variable ages
  - In general, autosomal recessive mutations present at a younger age than autosomal dominant mutations.

RISK FACTORS
Genetics
- Autosomal dominant:
  - Generally later onset and less severe than diseases with recessive or X-linked inheritance
  - FSHMD, OPMD, some forms of LGMD and EDMD (some types)
  - MMD
    ○ Trinucleotide repeat expansion with earlier onset of symptoms in subsequent generations due to accumulation of repeats

- Autosomal recessive:
  - LGMD (some subtypes), CMD
- X-linked:
  - DMD/BMD: Significant fraction are de novo mutations.
    ○ 5% of female carriers express spectrum of phenotypes, from mild to severe disease.
  - EDMD (some types)

GENERAL PREVENTION
Genetic counseling for known carriers

PATHOPHYSIOLOGY
Mutations affect proteins connecting cytoskeleton to cell membrane and extracellular matrix.

- Phenotype is also seen with some nuclear membrane and Golgi-associated protein mutations.
- Muscle fibers become fragile and easily damaged by contraction.
- Satellite cells replace dead muscle fibers.
  - Population of satellite cells is exhausted, resulting in decreasing numbers of muscle fibers and progressive weakness and atrophy.

ETIOLOGY
- DMD/BMD:
  - Defective protein is dystrophin; translated from the largest known human gene (DMD), making up 1.5% of the X chromosome
  - DMD phenotype results from mutations that cause profound loss of dystrophin function; 90% of mutations in DMD are frameshift mutations, resulting in undetectable levels of functional dystrophin protein
  - Becker phenotype results from less severe mutations to DMD gene; patients have low but detectable levels of functional dystrophin
- MMD: Results from trinucleotide repeat expansion in the untranslated region of the gene DMPK on chromosome 19; encodes myotonin protein kinase
- LGMD: Results from mutations to genes encoding proteins associated with dystrophin; calpain-, dysferlin-, and fukutin-related proteins are affected most commonly.
- EDMD: Mutated proteins are associated with the nuclear membrane in muscle fibers; emerin in X-linked form, lamin A and C in autosomal forms.
- OPMD: Trinucleotide repeat expansion on chromosome 14 results in defective polyadenylate binding protein; results in accumulation of protein in the cell nucleus
- FSHMD: Deletion in untranslated region of chromosome 4

COMMONLY ASSOCIATED CONDITIONS
- Low IQ: On average, 1 SD below the mean in DMD. Other muscular dystrophies have no cognitive effects.
- Cardiomyopathy and cardiac conduction defect:
  - Can be severe in EDMD
  - Can occasionally affect otherwise asymptomatic female carriers of DMD

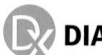 **DIAGNOSIS**

HISTORY
- DMD: Normal attainment of early motor milestones with subsequent abnormal gait and slowing gross motor development; clumsiness, weakness in toddlers and young children
- BMD: Progressive difficulty with ambulation and frequent falls in adolescence
- MMD: Slurred speech, muscle wasting, difficulty with ambulation
- LGMD: Back pain, lordosis \ inability to rise from a chair, climb stairs, and use arms overhead
- FSHMD: Facial weakness, inability to close eyes completely
- EDMD: Contractures of elbows and ankles, difficulty with ambulation in teens
- OPMD: Ptosis and dysphagia in middle age, often with family history

PHYSICAL EXAM
- DMD/BMD:
  - Muscle weakness, proximal more affected than distal
  - Gower sign: Use of arms to push upper body into standing posture
  - Trendelenburg gait (hip waddling)
  - Winged scapulae and lordosis
  - Pseudohypertrophy of the calf (caused by proliferation of fat and connective tissue)
  - Contractures of lower extremity joints and elbows
- MMD:
  - Characteristic facial appearance: Narrow face, open triangular mouth, high arched palate, concave temples, drooping eyelids, frontal balding in males
  - Slit-lamp eye exam: Cataracts
  - Myotonia: Inability to relax muscles after contraction
  - Distal muscle weakness and wasting
- FSHMD:
  - Winged scapulae, pronounced weakness with arms above head
  - Protruding lips, unable to whistle
- CMD:
  - Arthrogryposis at birth (multiple joint contractures)
  - Diffuse hypotonia and muscle wasting with thin appearance

DIAGNOSTIC TESTS & INTERPRETATION
Lab
Initial lab tests
- Creatine kinase (CK): initial screening test if muscular dystrophy is suspected (1)
- Elevated in DMD (10–100×); elevated at birth, peaks at time of presentation, and falls through course of illness. Other MD may result in normal or only mildly elevated CK.
- Genetic testing:
  - For definitive diagnosis in patient with characteristic presentation and elevated CK
  - Deletion and duplication analysis by polymerase chain reaction
  - If not diagnostic, then may proceed to full sequencing of DMD gene

– Specific genetic testing is available for most non-DMD muscular dystrophies and may be chosen based on age, family history, pattern of affected muscles and other symptoms

Diagnostic Procedures/Surgery

- Muscle biopsy: 2nd-line diagnostic instrument if DNA analysis is nondiagnostic; can have prognostic value if interpreted by experienced neuromuscular pathologist
- Dystrophin protein assay: Severe reduction or complete absence of dystrophin is diagnostic of DMD/BMD.
- Immunohistochemical staining for other known protein defects in muscular dystrophies
- Electromyography and nerve conduction studies are not necessary unless considering alternative diagnoses.
- ECG: Abnormalities found in >90% of males and up to 10% of female carriers of DMD. Q waves in anterolateral leads, tall R waves in V1, shortened PR interval, arrhythmias (2)

Pregnancy Considerations

Prenatal diagnosis (optional):

- Amniocentesis, chorionic villus sampling, or fetal muscle biopsy for affected families
- Genetic diagnosis at 10–13 weeks gestation

Pathological Findings

- Heterogeneic muscle fibers: Atrophy and hypertrophy of fibers with proliferation of connective tissue in muscle
- Immunohistochemical staining for dystrophin protein
    - DMD: No detectable dystrophin in most fibers; occasional revertant fibers with normal dystrophin
    - BMD: Highly variable staining for dystrophin throughout muscle

DIFFERENTIAL DIAGNOSIS

- Glycogen storage diseases and other metabolic myopathies
- Mitochondrial myopathies: MELAS, MERRF
- Inflammatory myopathies: Polymyositis, dermatomyositis, inclusion-body myositis
- Neuromuscular junction diseases: Myasthenia gravis, Lambert-Eaton
- Motor neuron diseases: Amyotrophic lateral sclerosis, spinal muscular atrophy
- Charcot-Marie-Tooth disease
- Friedreich ataxia
- Viral myositis
- Malnutrition
- Hypothyroid or hyperthyroid myopathy
- Cushing syndrome

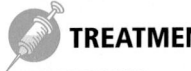 **TREATMENT**

MEDICATION

Prednisone 0.75 mg/kg/day (1,3,4):

- Slows the decline in muscle function, progression to scoliosis and degradation of pulmonary function; prolongs functional ambulation; possible reduction in cardiac morbidity
- Initiate therapy when motor function ceases to improve, prior to decline in function
- Monitor adverse effects and intervene to mitigate harm
    - Some use bisphosphonates for preventing loss of bone density.
    - Annual exam for development of cataracts

– Avoid NSAID use due to risk of peptic ulcers.
– Stress dose steroids during surgeries and illnesses
– Monitor and treat hypertension.
– Patients should be aware of immune suppression and notify emergency providers.
– Controversial: There is emerging evidence that a 10-day-on/10-day-off schedule of prednisone mitigates side effects and may extend the ambulant phase of the disease.

ADDITIONAL TREATMENT

General Measures

Goal of management: Lessen impairments, reduce functional limitations

- Ambulation prolonged by use of knee-ankle-foot orthoses
- Serial casting to treat contractures
- Diagnose sleep apnea with polysomnography, treat with noninvasive ventilation.
- Adaptive devices to improve function
- Avoid overexertion and strenuous exercise (5).

Issues for Referral

- Refer to neuromuscular diseases specialist for definitive diagnosis and treatment.
- Coordinated multidisciplinary clinic specific to these illnesses (6).
- While female carriers of DMD occasionally have cardiac involvement, risk for cardiac morbidity and mortality appears unchanged.

SURGERY/OTHER PROCEDURES

- Spinal surgery for scoliosis
- Scapular fixation for scapular winging can be beneficial.
- May consider surgical treatment of ankle or knee contractures

 ONGOING CARE

FOLLOW-UP RECOMMENDATIONS

Patient Monitoring

- EKG and echocardiogram at diagnosis and annually after age 10
- Annual spinal radiography for scoliosis
- DEXA scanning and serum testing for osteoporosis
- Pulmonary function testing twice yearly if no longer ambulatory

DIET

- Obesity is common owing to steroid treatment and wheelchair confinement.
- Weight control can improve quality of life.
- Diet may be limited by dysphagia; swallow evaluation can determine appropriate foods.
- Calcium and vitamin D supplementation is indicated for patients on steroids.

PATIENT EDUCATION

Muscular Dystrophy Association at http://www.mda.org

PROGNOSIS

- DMD/BMD:
    - Progressive weakness, contractures, inability to walk
    - Kyphoscoliosis and progressive decline in respiratory vital capacity
    - Early death (DMD: 16 ± 4 years; BMD: 42 ± 16 years)
- Other types: Slow progression and near-normal life span with functional limitations

COMPLICATIONS

- Cardiac arrhythmia, cardiomyopathy
- Dysphagia, GERD, constipation
- Scoliosis, joint contractures
- Obstructive sleep apnea
- Malignant hyperthermia-like reaction to anesthesia
- Respiratory failure and early death

REFERENCES

1. Bushby K, Finkel R, Birnkrant DJ, et al. Diagnosis and management of Duchenne muscular dystrophy, part 1: diagnosis, and pharmacological and psychosocial management. *Lancet Neurol.* 2010; 9:77–93.
2. Takami Y, Takeshima Y, Awano H, et al. High incidence of electrocardiogram abnormalities in young patients with duchenne muscular dystrophy. *Pediatr Neurol.* 2008;39:399–403.
3. Manzur AY, Kuntzer T, Pike M, et al. Glucocorticoid corticosteroids for Duchenne muscular dystrophy. *Cochrane Database Syst Rev.* 2008;CD003725.
4. Cossu G, Sampaolesi M et al. New therapies for Duchenne muscular dystrophy: challenges, prospects and clinical trials. *Trends Mol Med.* 2007;13:520–6.
5. van der Kooi EL, Lindeman E, Riphagen I. Strength training and aerobic exercise training for muscle disease. *Cochrane Database Syst Rev.* 2005; CD003907.
6. Bushby K, Finkel R, Birnkrant DJ, et al. Diagnosis and management of Duchenne muscular dystrophy, part 2: implementation of multidisciplinary care. *Lancet Neurol.* 2010;9:177–89.

 CODES

ICD9

- 359.0 Congenital hereditary muscular dystrophy
- 359.1 Hereditary progressive muscular dystrophy
- 359.21 Myotonic muscular dystrophy

CLINICAL PEARLS

- Boys with progressive symmetric weakness or dyscoordination should have CK level checked.
- Steroids should be initiated in DMD patients when gross motor function ceases to progress.
- High-quality care of patients with muscular dystrophy requires a medical home, a multidisciplinary team, and extensive support.

M

MYASTHENIA GRAVIS

Mhd Basheer Rahmoun, MD
Dalia Sbat, PharmD

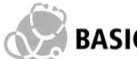 **BASICS**

DESCRIPTION
Most common primary disorder of neuromuscular transmission, resulting in a pure motor syndrome characterized by fluctuating skeletal muscle weakness, particularly of the extraocular, pharyngeal, facial, and respiratory musculature:
- 2 clinical forms: Ocular and generalized.
- Ocular myasthenia gravis (MG) (15%): Weakness limited to eyelids and extraocular muscles
- Generalized MG (85%): Commonly affects ocular as well as a variable combination of bulbar, proximal limb, and respiratory muscles
- 50% of patients who 1st present with ocular symptoms develop generalized MG within 2 years.
- Onset may be sudden and severe, but is typically mild and intermittent over many years.
- System(s) affected: Neurologic; Hematologic, Lymphatic, Immunologic; Musculoskeletal

EPIDEMIOLOGY
Occurs at any age, but a bimodal distribution to the age of onset:
- 20–40 (female predominance)
- 60–80 (male predominance)

Incidence
Estimated annual incidence 4 cases per 1,000,0000

Prevalence
100–200 per million in the US; increasing over the past 5 decades

Pediatric Considerations
A transient form of myasthenia called neonatal MG seen in 10–20% of infants born to MG mothers. It occurs as a result of the transplacental passage of maternal antibodies that interfere with function of the neuromuscular junction. The condition resolves in weeks to months.

RISK FACTORS
- Female gender
- Familial MG
- D-Penicillamine (drug-induced MG)
- Other autoimmune diseases

Genetics
- Congenital MG syndrome describes a collection of rare hereditary disorders. This condition is not immune-mediated, but instead results from the mutation of a component of the neuromuscular junction. Onset is usually at birth or in early childhood (autosomal recessive).
- Familial predisposition seen in 5% of cases.

PATHOPHYSIOLOGY
- Reduction in the acetylcholine receptors (AChR) numbers at the muscle endplate and flattening of the postsynaptic folds, which results in an insufficient neuromuscular transmission
- Seropositive MG: 80–85% of all MG patients.
  - Anti-acetylcholine receptor (Anti-AChR): A humoral, antibody-mediated, T-cell–dependent attack of the AChRs or receptor-associated proteins at the postsynaptic membrane of the neuromuscular junction.

– Patients without anti-AChR antibodies may have antibodies against muscle-specific kinase (MuSK), which plays a critical role in postsynaptic differentiation and clustering of acetylcholine receptors (1)[C]. Females tend to be anti-MuSK positive, and respiratory and bulbar muscles are frequently involved.
– Seronegative MG (SNMG), 6–12% of cases (2)[C].

COMMONLY ASSOCIATED CONDITIONS
- Thymic hyperplasia (60–70% of MG patients)
- Thymoma (10–15% of MG patients)
- Autoimmune thyroid disease (3–8%)
- Other autoimmune diseases

 DIAGNOSIS

The most widely accepted classification of MG is the Myasthenia Gravis Foundation of America Clinical Classification (3)[A]:
- Class I: Any eye muscle weakness, possible ptosis, no other evidence of muscle weakness elsewhere
- Class II: Eye muscle weakness of any severity, mild weakness of other muscles
  - Class IIa: Predominantly limb or axial muscles
  - Class IIb: Predominantly bulbar and/or respiratory muscles
- Class III: Eye muscle weakness of any severity, moderate weakness of other muscles:
  - Class IIIa: Predominantly limb or axial muscles
  - Class IIIb: Predominantly bulbar and/or respiratory muscles
- Class IV: Eye muscle weakness of any severity, severe weakness of other muscles:
  - Class IVa: Predominantly limb or axial muscles
  - Class IVb: Predominantly bulbar and/or respiratory muscles (can also include feeding tube without intubation)
- Class V: Intubation needed to maintain airway

HISTORY
The hallmark of MG is fatigability:
- Fluctuating weakness that worsens during the day and after prolonged use of affected muscles, which may improve with rest
- Early in MG, symptoms are transient with asymptomatic periods lasting days or weeks.
- With progression, asymptomatic periods shorten and symptoms fluctuate from mild to severe.
- More than 50% of patients present with ocular symptoms (ptosis and/or diplopia). Eventually 90% of patients with MG develop ocular symptoms.
- Ptosis might be unilateral, bilateral, or shifting from eye to eye.
- 15% present with bulbar symptoms.
- Less than 5% present with proximal limb weakness alone.

ALERT
Myasthenic crisis: Respiratory muscle weakness producing respiratory insufficiency and pending respiratory failure

PHYSICAL EXAM
- Ptosis may worsen with propping of opposite eyelid (curtain sign) or sustained upward gaze.
- "Myasthenic sneer," in which the mid-lip rises, but corners of mouth do not move

- In addition to proximal muscles, wrist extensors, finger extensors, and foot dorsiflexors also are commonly involved.
- Pupillary sparing

Pregnancy Considerations
Myasthenia may worsen during pregnancy. The first trimester and the month postpartum are periods of highest risk of exacerbation.

DIAGNOSTIC TESTS & INTERPRETATION
Lab
Initial lab tests
- In seropositive patients:
  - Anti-acetylcholine receptor (anti-AChR) antibody (80–85% are seropositive):
    - Generalized myasthenia: 75–85%
    - Ocular myasthenia: 50%
    - MG and thymoma: 98–100%
    - Poor correlation between antibody titer and disease severity (4,5)[C]
  - Anti-muscle-specific tyrosine kinase (anti-MuSK) antibody:
    - Used if MG suspected, patient seronegative
    - Present in 40–50% of seronegative patients with generalized MG; absent in ocular MG (1,4)[C]
  - Anti-striated muscle (anti-SM) antibody:
    - Present in 84% of patients with thymoma who are <40 years old
    - Anti-SM AB can be present without thymoma in patients >40 years old .
- Thyroid function tests

Imaging
CT or MRI scan of anterior mediastinum may help to identify thymomas.

Diagnostic Procedures/Surgery
- Bedside tests:
  - Tensilon (Edrophonium) test:
    - Initial dose 2 mg IV, can be followed by another 2 mg every 60 seconds up to a maximum dose of 10 mg.
    - A positive test shows improvement of strength within 30 seconds of administration.
    - Sensitivity 80–90% (4,6)[C]
    - Cardiac disease and bronchial asthma are relative contraindications, especially in elderly.
    - Atropine 0.4–0.6 mg IV may rarely be required as antidote; must be available.
  - Ice pack test:
    - Can be used in patients with ptosis in whom Tensilon test is contraindicated
    - Ice pack applied to closed eyelid for 60 seconds, then removed; extent of ptosis immediately assessed
    - Ice will decrease the ptosis induced by MG.
    - Sensitivity 80% in patients with prominent ptosis
- Electromyography:
  - Repetitive nerve stimulation (RNS):
    - Widely available, most frequently used
    - Moderately sensitive for both generalized MG (75%) and ocular MG (50%) (4)[C]
    - Positive test shows a decremental response (>10%) at 3Hz.
  - Single-fiber EMG (SFEMG):
    - Assesses temporal variability between 2 muscle fibers within same motor unit (jitter).

- Highly sensitive (90–95%), but less specific (4)[C].
- Technically difficult to perform; limited availability

Pathological Findings
- Lymphofollicular hyperplasia of thymic medulla occurs in 65% of patients with MG, thymoma in 15%
- Muscle electron microscopy: Receptor infolding and synaptic cleft widening
- Immunofluorescence: IgG antibodies and complement on receptor membranes

DIFFERENTIAL DIAGNOSIS
- Thyroid ophthalmopathy
- Oculopharyngeal muscular dystrophy
- Myotonic dystrophy
- Kearns-Sayre syndrome
- Chronic progressive external ophthalmoplegia
- Brainstem and motor cranial nerve lesions
- Botulism
- Motor neuron disease (e.g., ALS)
- Lambert-Eaton myasthenic syndrome
- Drug-induced myasthenia
- Congenital myasthenic syndrome
- Depression

TREATMENT
MEDICATION
First Line
Symptomatic treatments (anti-cholinesterase agents)
- Pyridostigmine bromide (Mestinon):
  - Available as 60 mg tablet, 180 mg sustained-release tablet, or 60 mg/5 mL syrup
  - Starting dose of 30 mg p.o. t.i.d.
  - Increase dose in 30 mg increments as needed.
  - Maximum dose: 120 mg q3–4h
- Neostigmine methylsulfate (Prostigmin):
  - Available in 0.25, 0.5, and 1 mg/mL concentrations
  - Starting dose of 0.5 mg SC or IM q3h
  - Titrate dosage to clinical need.

Second Line
- Chronic immunomodulating treatments:
  - Immunosuppressants (7)[B]:
    - Prednisone: Should be initiated on an inpatient basis. Start with a 60–80 mg/d p.o.; taper the dosage every 3 days; switch to alternate day regimen within 2 weeks. Taper very slowly to establish the minimum dosage necessary to maintain remission.
    - Cyclophosphamide: Adults: 1–5 mg/kg/d p.o.; Children: 2–8 mg/kg/d p.o.
    - Cyclosporine: Adults: 5mg/kg/d p.o.
    - Mycophenolate: 1 g p.o. or IV b.i.d.
    - Azathioprine: 100–200 mg/d p.o.
- Acute immunomodulating treatments:
  - Plasmapheresis
  - Immune globulin: 2 g/kg IV over 2–5 days (7)[B]
- Other immunosuppressant therapies:
  - Tacrolimus: has been found effective in MG (89)
  - Rituximab: a monocolonal antibody directed against antigens on B cells shows benefit in MG (10,11)

ALERT
Avoid aminoglycosides and other drugs with potential for neuromuscular blockade, which may precipitate weakness.

ADDITIONAL TREATMENT
General Measures
- Treatment must be tailored for each patient based on several factors including age, gender, severity of disease, and progression of disease.
- 3 basic approaches to treatment: Symptomatic, immunosuppressive, and supportive. Few patients (if any) should receive a single therapeutic modality.

Additional Therapies
Supportive therapy: May include intubation, tracheostomy, artificial ventilation, respiratory therapy, administration of antibiotics, nasogastric tube, and/or gastrostomy

SURGERY/OTHER PROCEDURES
- Thymectomy: Recommended for most MG patients; especially helpful for young patients, early onset
- No clear clinical benefit if onset at ≥60 years unless thymoma present

Pediatric Considerations
- Infants with severe weakness from transient neonatal myasthenia may be treated with oral pyridostigmine and whatever degree of general support (mechanical respiratory ventilation, for example) is necessary until the condition clears.
- Corticosteroids limited only to severe disease

IN-PATIENT CONSIDERATIONS
Initial Stabilization
- Plasmapheresis
- Intravenous gamma globulin

Admission Criteria
- Management of pulmonary infections
- Myasthenic or cholinergic crises

ONGOING CARE
FOLLOW-UP RECOMMENDATIONS
Patient Monitoring
- ICU during myasthenic or cholinergic crises
- Inpatient for initiation of corticosteroids
- Outpatient follow-up every 3 months with stable patients

DIET
As tolerated

PATIENT EDUCATION
- MG Foundation of America (MGFA), 1821 University Ave. West, Suite S256, St. Paul, MN 55104; (800) 541-5454 or (651) 917-6256; http://www.myasthenia.org
- Muscular Dystrophy Association (MDA), 3300 E. Sunrise Dr., Tucson, AZ 85718; (800) 344-4863; http://www.mda.org/home.htm

PROGNOSIS
- Overall good, but highly variable
- Many patients achieve sustained remission.
- Myasthenic crisis associated with substantial morbidity and 4% mortality
- Seronegative patients are more likely to have purely ocular disease, and those with generalized SNMG to have a better outcome after treatment (12)[C].

COMPLICATIONS
- Acute respiratory arrest
- Chronic respiratory insufficiency
- Atelectasis, aspiration, pneumonia

REFERENCES
1. McConville J, Farrugia ME, Beeson D, et al. Detection and characterization of MuSK antibodies in seronegative myasthenia gravis. *Ann Neurol*. 2004;55:580–4.
2. Chan KH, Lachance DH, Harper CM, et al. Frequency of seronegativity in adult-acquired generalized myasthenia gravis. *Muscle Nerve*. 2007;36:651–8.
3. Jaretzki A, Barohn RJ, Ernstoff RM, et al. Myasthenia gravis: recommendations for clinical research standards. Task Force of the Medical Scientific Advisory Board of the Myasthenia Gravis Foundation of America. *Neurology*. 2000;55:16–23.
4. Meriggioli MN, Sanders DB. Myasthenia gravis: diagnosis. *Semin Neurol*. 2004;24:31–9.
5. Vincent A, McConville J, Farrugia ME, et al. Antibodies in myasthenia gravis and related disorders. *Ann N Y Acad Sci*. 2003;998:324–35.
6. Daroff RB. The office Tensilon test for ocular myasthenia gravis. *Arch Neurol*. 1986;43:843–4.
7. Hart IK, Sathasivam S, Sarshar T. Immunosuppressive agents for myasthenia gravis. *Cochrane Database Syst Rev*. 2007;17:CD005224.
8. Yoshikawa H, Mabuchi K, Yasukawa Y, et al. Low-dose tacrolimus for intractable myasthenia gravis. *J Clin Neurosci*. 2002;9:627–8.
9. Evoli A, Di Schino C, Marsili F, et al. Successful treatment of myasthenia gravis with tacrolimus. *Muscle Nerve*. 2002;25:111–4.
10. Maddison P, McConville J, Farrugia ME, et al. The use of rituximab in myasthenia gravis and Lambert-Eaton myasthenic syndrome. *Journal of neurology, neurosurgery, and psychiatry*. 2010;
11. Zebardast N, Patwa HS, Novella SP, et al. Rituximab in the management of refractory myasthenia gravis. *Muscle Nerve*. 2010;41:375–8.
12. Deymeer F, Gungor-Tuncer O, Yilmaz V, et al. Clinical comparison of anti-MuSK- vs anti-AChR-positive and seronegative myasthenia gravis. *Neurology*. 2007;68:609–11.

CODES
ICD9
- 358.00 Myasthenia gravis without (acute) exacerbation
- 358.01 Myasthenia gravis with (acute) exacerbation
- 775.2 Neonatal myasthenia gravis

CLINICAL PEARLS
- MG is an autoimmune disease, marked by abnormal fatigability and weakness of selected muscles which is relieved by rest, and by steroids.
- Anticholinesterase medication and removal of the thymus lessen the severity of the symptoms.
- Steroid therapy or plasma exchange can be used in severely affected patients.

M

MYELODYSPLASTIC SYNDROMES

Richard A. Larson, MD

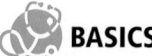 **BASICS**

DESCRIPTION

Myelodysplastic syndromes (MDS) constitute a heterogeneous group of acquired hematopoietic stem-cell disorders characterized by cytologic dysplasia in the bone marrow and blood, and by various combinations of anemia, neutropenia, and thrombocytopenia.

- The natural progression of disease evolves as cellular maturation becomes more arrested and blast cells accumulate. There is a great deal of overlap between arbitrary diagnostic subgroups.
- World Health Organization classification (1):
  - Refractory cytopenia with unilineage dysplasia (RCUD)
    - Refractory anemia (RA); refractory neutropenia (RN); refractory thrombocytopenia (RT)
    - <5% blasts and <15% ring sideroblasts in marrow; <1% blasts in blood
  - Refractory anemia with ring sideroblasts (RARS):
    - <5% blasts in marrow; ≥15% of erythroid precursors are ring sideroblasts; no blasts in blood
    - Also known as acquired idiopathic sideroblastic anemia (AISA)
  - Refractory cytopenia with multilineage dysplasia (RCMD):
    - Marked trilineage dysplasia but without excess blasts in marrow; no Auer rods; <1% blasts in blood
  - Refractory cytopenia with multilineage dysplasia and ring sideroblasts (RCMD-RS)
  - Refractory anemia with excess blasts-1 (RAEB-1):
    - 5–9% blasts in marrow; no Auer rods; <5% blasts in blood; <1000/uL monocytes
  - Refractory anemia with excess blasts-2 (RAEB-2):
    - 10–19% blasts in marrow; 5–19% blasts in blood; ± Auer rods; <1000/ual monocytes
  - MDS associated with isolated del(5q) (2):
    - RA with erythroid hyperplasia, increased megakaryocytes with hypolobated nuclei, and normal or increased platelets; <5% blasts in marrow; <1% blasts in blood
  - Acute MDS with sclerosis:
    - RAEB with marked myelosclerosis
  - Chronic myelomonocytic leukemia (CMMoL or CMML) is now grouped with myelodysplastic/myeloproliferative disorders:
    - <20% blasts and promonocytes in marrow and blood with >1,000 monocytes/uL
  - Refractory anemia with excess of blasts in transformation (RAEBT) is now considered acute myeloid leukemia (AML):
    - 20–30% blasts in marrow; >20% blasts in blood
    - Incidence: 2:1 (Female > Male)
  - Therapy-related myelodysplasia (t-MDS) (3,4):
    - Seen 3–7 years after treatment with alkylating agents and/or radiotherapy
    - Evolves to acute myeloid leukemia (AML) over ~6 months
    - Classified as therapy-related myeloid neoplasm by WHO
- System(s) affected: Hematologic; Lymphatic; Immunologic
- Synonym(s): Dysmyelopoietic syndrome; hemopoietic dysplasia; preleukemia; smoldering or subacute myeloid leukemia

Pediatric Considerations
Pediatric presentations of MDS:

- Monosomy 7 syndrome
- Juvenile chronic myelogenous leukemia

EPIDEMIOLOGY

- Predominant age: Median age >65 years; uncommon in children and young adults
- Predominant sex: Male = Female

Incidence
Apparent increased incidence (1–2/100,000 per year) in recent years may be due to improved diagnosis; increases markedly with older age.

RISK FACTORS

- Primary MDS is associated with older age, occupational exposure to petroleum solvents (benzene, gasoline), and smoking.
- Secondary (therapy-related) MDS is associated with prior treatment with alkylating agents or radiotherapy.

Genetics

- Most are clonal neoplasms by cytogenetics, G6PD isoenzyme analysis, or restriction fragment length polymorphism (RFLP) analysis.
- Mutations in RAS oncogene
- Mutations in RPS14 gene on chromosome 5q

COMMONLY ASSOCIATED CONDITIONS

- Anemia
- Neutropenia
- Thrombocytopenia
- Pancytopenia
- Opportunistic infections
- Bleeding, bruising
- Sweet syndrome (neutrophilic dermatosis)

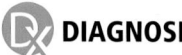 **DIAGNOSIS**

HISTORY

- Fatigue
- Fever
- Easy bruising

PHYSICAL EXAM

- Anemia:
  - Fatigue
  - Shortness of breath
  - Lightheadedness
  - Angina
- Leukopenia:
  - Fever
  - Infection
- Thrombocytopenia:
  - Ecchymoses
  - Petechiae
  - Epistaxis
  - Purpura
- Splenomegaly (uncommon):
  - Mild-to-moderate enlargement may be encountered, particularly in CMMoL.
- Skin infiltrates:
  - Sweet syndrome

DIAGNOSTIC TESTS & INTERPRETATION

- Cytogenetics (5,6)[A]:
  - At least 1/2 of patients with primary MDS and nearly all with therapy-related MDS have clonal chromosomal abnormalities: +8,−7,−5, del(5q), del(7q), del(20q), iso(17), and complex karyotypes
  - Detection of clonal abnormality establishes a diagnosis of neoplasm and rules out a nutritional, toxic, or autoimmune disorder.
- Granulocyte function tests: Abnormal in 1/2 (decreased myeloperoxidase activity, phagocytosis, chemotaxis, and adhesion)
- Platelet function tests: Impaired aggregation
- Marrow colony assays in vitro:
  - Results are variable and correlate poorly with clinical course.
  - Poor clonal growth may suggest more rapid evolution to AML.
- Immunophenotyping:
  - Nonspecific myeloid markers are present.
  - Occasionally, evidence can be found for concomitant lymphoproliferative disorder.
  - Loss of CD59 expression suggests PNH.

Lab

- Anemia: Often macrocytic; occasional poikilocytosis, anisocytosis; variable reticulocytosis
- Granulocytopenia: Hypogranular or agranular neutrophils with poorly condensed chromatin; Pelger-Huet anomaly with hyposegmented nuclei
- Thrombocytopenia: Occasionally giant platelets or hypogranular platelets
- Fetal hemoglobin may be elevated.
- Flow cytometry to detect loss of CD59 on red blood cell (RBC), CD16 on granulocytes, and CD14 on monocytes; typical of PNH.
- Direct antiglobulin (Coombs) test
- Paraprotein: Present in some
- Erythropoietin: Usually normally elevated for the degree of anemia unless renal failure is present.
- Increased serum and tissue iron (ferritin), especially if anemia has been long-standing

Initial lab tests

- Complete blood count
- Review of the peripheral blood smear for the presence of dysplasia

Imaging
Liver/spleen scan or computed tomography (CT), although rarely necessary, may disclose occult splenomegaly or lymphadenopathy.

Diagnostic Procedures/Surgery

- Review peripheral blood smear.
- Bone marrow aspiration, biopsy, and cytogenetics

Pathological Findings

- Ineffective hematopoiesis with dysplasia in 1 or more cell lineages dominates the bone marrow picture in MDS (1).
- Marrow cellularity is usually normal or increased for the patient's age, but may be hypoplastic in ~10%.
- Reticulin fibrosis is usually minimal except in therapy-related MDS and acute MDS with sclerosis.
- Myeloblasts may be clustered in the intertrabecular spaces with abnormal localization of immature precursors.

DIFFERENTIAL DIAGNOSIS

- Other malignant disorders:
  - Evolving AML or erythroleukemia
  - Chronic myeloproliferative disorders
  - Polycythemia vera
  - Myeloid metaplasia with myelofibrosis
  - Malignant lymphoma
  - Metastatic carcinoma
- Nonmalignant disorders:
  - Aplastic anemia
  - Autoimmune disorders (Felty syndrome, lupus, hemolytic anemia)
  - Nutritional deficiencies (vitamin B_{12}, pyridoxine, copper, protein malnutrition)
  - Heavy metal intoxication
  - Alcoholism
  - Chronic liver disease
  - Hypersplenism
  - Chronic inflammation
  - Recent cytotoxic therapy or irradiation
  - HIV infection
  - Paroxysmal nocturnal hemoglobinuria

 TREATMENT

MEDICATION
First Line
- Epoetin alfa or darbepoetin can increase hemoglobin levels in MDS patients who have low serum erythropoietin levels at baseline.
- Only azacitidine, decitabine, and lenalidomide have been approved by the Food and Drug Administration (FDA) for MDS (7,8)[B].
- Azacitidine and decitabine have been proven in RCTs to be more effective for these heterogeneous disorders than supportive care with antibiotics and transfusions as needed (9,10)[A].
- Vitamins, iron, corticosteroids, androgens, or thyroid hormone are rarely helpful, unless evidence of a specific deficiency exists.
- Clinical trials with azacitidine, 75 mg/m^2 SC for 7 days and repeated every 28 days, decreases RBC transfusion requirements and yields longer times to AML or death and improvements in quality of life (9)[A].
- Decitabine was approved with a continuous IV schedule that usually requires hospitalization (10)[A]. More commonly, it is given at 20 mg/m^2/d IV over 1 hour as an outpatient, repeated every 4 weeks.
- Lenalidomide, 10 mg p.o. daily for 21 days q4wk has yielded complete remission in patients with MDS and del(5q) (2)[A]. It is less effective in patients with MDS without del(5q).
- Intensive chemotherapy:
  - Younger patients with MDS may benefit from AML chemotherapy, especially if Auer rods were present, but toxicity may be severe for older patients.
  - Remission durations are variable (median ~1 year).
- Allogeneic hematopoietic stem cell transplantation:
  - Recommended for younger patients with HLA-matched donors to eradicate the malignant clone and resupply normal hematopoietic stem cells
- Aminocaproic acid (epsilon-aminocaproic acid) or tranexamic acid may benefit patients with chronic, severe thrombocytopenia and bleeding.

- Contraindications: Cytotoxicity of chemotherapy may increase the risk of bleeding and infection and the need for transfusion support.
- Precautions: Aspirin, salicylates, and NSAIDs should be avoided.

Second Line
- Danazol or prednisone may benefit concomitant autoimmune thrombocytopenia.
- Investigational agents:
  - Low doses of cytarabine, tretinoin (all-trans retinoic acid), homoharringtonine, 13-cis retinoic acid, arsenic trioxide, histone/protein deacetylase inhibitors, interferon, cyclosporine, antithymocyte globulin, granulocyte macrophage colony-stimulating factor or granulocyte colony-stimulating factor, and interleukin-3
  - Agents such as thalidomide that inhibit the production of tumor necrosis factor in the marrow
- Amifostine may stimulate the proliferation of normal hematopoiesis.

ADDITIONAL TREATMENT
General Measures
- Immunize for pneumococcal pneumonia and influenza and hepatitis B.
- RBC transfusions to alleviate symptoms
- Platelet transfusions only for bleeding or before surgery to avoid alloimmunization
- Early use of antibiotics for fever, even while culture results are pending, due to quantitative and qualitative granulocyte disorder
- Iron chelation therapy to avoid iron overload from chronic transfusions

Issues for Referral
- Refer younger adults for allogeneic hematopoietic cell transplantation.
- Refer patients with symptoms or transfusion requirements for clinical trials.

 ONGOING CARE

FOLLOW-UP RECOMMENDATIONS
Usually outpatient except when necessary to hospitalize for the treatment of infection, blood transfusions, or intensive chemotherapy.

Patient Monitoring
- At least monthly during supportive care
- More frequently if receiving treatment

DIET
Reduce alcohol use and iron intake (unless iron deficient).

PATIENT EDUCATION
- Stop smoking.
- Seek early medical attention for fever, bleeding, or symptoms of anemia.
- Advise about the risks of chronic transfusion therapy.

PROGNOSIS
- Median survival for RA and RARS is 5 years, but may extend much longer.
- Refractory anemia with del(5q) syndrome is quite favorable (2).
- Median survival for RAEB, RCMD, and CMMoL is ~1 year, with 1/2 of the patients evolving to AML and the other 1/2 dying of infection or bleeding.

COMPLICATIONS
- Infection
- Bleeding
- Complications of anemia and transfusions

REFERENCES

1. Swerdlow SH, Campo E, Harris NL, et al., eds. *WHO Classification of Tumours of Haematopoietic and Lymphoid Tissues*. Lyon, France: IARC Press; 2008.
2. List A, Dewald G, Bennett J, et al. Lenalidomide in the myelodysplastic syndrome with chromosome 5q deletion. *N Engl J Med*. 2006;355:1456–65.
3. Singh ZN, Huo D, Anastasi J, et al. Therapy-related myelodysplastic syndrome: morphologic subclassification may not be clinically relevant. *Am J Clin Pathol*. 2007;127:197–205.
4. Larson RA, Le Beau MM. Therapy-related myeloid leukaemia: a model for leukemogenesis in humans. *Chem Biol Interact*. 2005;153–54: 187–95.
5. Greenberg P, Cox C, LeBeau MM, et al. International scoring system for evaluating prognosis in myelodysplastic syndromes. *Blood*. 1997;89:2079–88.
6. Cheson BD, Greenberg PL, Bennett JM, et al. Clinical application and proposal for modification of the International Working Group (IWG) response criteria in myelodysplasia. *Blood*. 2006;108:419–25.
7. Larson RA. Myelodysplasia: when to treat and how. *Best Pract Res Clin Haematol*. 2006;19: 293–300.
8. Greenberg PL, Attar E, Battiwalla M, et al. Myelodysplastic syndromes. *J Natl Compr Canc Netw*. 2008;6:902–26.
9. Silverman LR, Demakos EP, Peterson BL, et al. Randomized controlled trial of azacitidine in patients with the myelodysplastic syndrome: a study of the cancer and leukemia group B. *J Clin Oncol*. 2002;20:2429–40.
10. Kantarjian H, Issa JP, Rosenfeld CS, et al. Decitabine improves patient outcomes in myelodysplastic syndromes: results of a phase III randomized study. *Cancer*. 2006;106:1794–803.

 CODES

ICD9
238.75 Myelodysplastic syndrome, unspecified

CLINICAL PEARLS

- Myelodysplastic syndromes (MDS) constitute a heterogeneous group of acquired hematopoietic stem-cell disorders characterized by cytologic dysplasia in the bone marrow and blood, and by various combinations of anemia, neutropenia, and thrombocytopenia:
  - The natural progression of disease evolves as cellular maturation becomes more arrested and blast cells accumulate.
- Initial lab: CBC with differential and review of peripheral smear for dysplasia

M

MYELOPROLIFERATIVE NEOPLASMS

Javed M. Gilani, MD
Omar A. Khan, MD, MHS

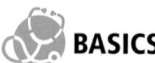

BASICS

DESCRIPTION
Myeloproliferative disorders have been assigned the nomenclature of *myeloproliferative neoplasms* (MPNs) under the 2008 World Health Organization (WHO) guidelines (1). This classification includes in the MPNs the "classic" conditions chronic myelogenous leukemia ([CML], which is positive for *BCR-ABL* [Philadelphia (Ph) chromosome]); polycythemia vera (PV); essential thrombocythemia (ET); and primary myelofibrosis (PMF). The MPNs also now include the "nonclassic" conditions chronic neutrophilic leukemia (CNL), chronic eosinophilic leukemia not otherwise classified (CEL-NOS), systemic mastocytosis (SM), and myeloproliferative neoplasm unclassifiable (MPN-u).

- With each disorder, the proliferation of a particular cell line tends to dominate. These disorders can mimic one another; CML is the only one readily distinguished by the Ph chromosome.
- CML: Characterized by splenomegaly and increased granulocytes; runs a generally mild course until it transforms to a frankly leukemic phase
- PMF: Usually has a severe course, and unlike PV and ET, survival is usually reduced.
- ET: Dominated by markedly elevated platelets; may transform into AML
- CNL: Marked by neutrophilic leukocytosis; predilection for the elderly; and absence of *BCR-ABL* (Ph chromosome).
- CEL-NOS: Characterized by abnormal proliferation of eosinophil precursors with 5–19% myeloblasts in the bone marrow or >2% in blood
- SM: Almost always involves bone marrow; characterized by aggregates of abnormal mast cells; serum elevations of tryptase can be a useful marker. The *KIT* D816V mutation is usually present.
- System(s) affected: Hematologic/Immunologic

EPIDEMIOLOGY
MPNs are some of the most common hematologic cancers. Many may go undetected owing to an indolent course. Familial clustering has been noted, and gene mutations have been identified (e.g., *JAK2* V617F).

Incidence
Overall, the classic MPNs have an incidence of 2.1/100,000/year; 6,328 new cases were reported in 2004.

- CML: 1–2/100,000/year, increases with age; PMF: 0.5–1.5/100,000/year; ET: 1–2.5/100,000/year
- Predominant age: CML: Median age at diagnosis 50–60 years; PMF, ET: Median age at diagnosis 60 years; second peak of ET in younger patients at ~30 years
- Predominant sex: CML: Male > Female (1.4:1); PMF: Male = Female; ET: Female > Male (1.3:1)

Prevalence
Estimates range from 1–5/100,000.

RISK FACTORS
- Family history of myeloproliferative neoplasms or *JAK2* V617F gene mutation
- CML: Increased incidence in atomic bomb survivors and following radiation treatment

Genetics
- CML is defined by the *BCR-ABL* gene (>99%), most commonly caused by the Ph chromosome.
- The other MPNs are Ph-negative; a single mutation in the Janus kinase 2 (*JAK2* V617F) gene has been reported in the majority of MPN patients.
- A somatic mutation in the *MPL* gene has been found in 5–15% of PMF patients and in close to 10% of *JAK2* V617F–negative ET patients.
- Some patients may have multiple *MPL* mutations or even co-occurrence with *JAK2* V617F.
- The *JAK2* V617F mutation is found in variable rates among PMN patients: >95% in PV; about 60% in ET and PMF; about 20% in MPN-u.
- The *MPL* mutation is found in 8% of PMF and ET patients.
- SM may have mutations of *KIT* and/or *PDGFRA*; rates have not been characterized yet.

PATHOPHYSIOLOGY
- Grouping of MPN by Dameshek into 4 categories (PV, ET, CML, and myeloid metaplasia with myelofibrosis) has been superseded by the new WHO 2008 classification, which incorporates molecular and genetic techniques.
- MPNs are characterized by increasing amounts of myeloid lineage cells without loss of differentiation.
- The t(9,22) translocation (i.e., the Ph chromosome) led to BCR-ABL tyrosine kinase being recognized in CML.
- More recently, mutant tyrosine kinases, specifically JAK2, as well as mutations in *KIT, MPL,* and *PDGFRA* were identified for the MPNs.
- Hematopoietic niches, i.e., endosteal and vascular niches, may play a role in cell signaling and serve as therapeutic targets

ETIOLOGY
Unknown; may be familial for some types; presence of *JAK2* and *MPL* mutations should prompt familial testing.

COMMONLY ASSOCIATED CONDITIONS
PMF: Immunologic abnormalities reported, including antinuclear antibodies, elevated rheumatoid factor titers, and Coombs positivity

DIAGNOSIS

HISTORY
- A history of abdominal pain or fullness, bruising, bleeding, thrombosis, bone/joint pain, fevers, jaundice, and/or ascites.
- Thromboses in the venous system may occur, including leg deep venous thrombosis
- or mesenteric thrombosis. Portal vein thrombosis may cause Budd-Chiari syndrome.
- Most thrombotic events occur about 2 years before diagnosis.

PHYSICAL EXAM
- General: Hypermetabolic state (fever, sweating), acute gouty arthritis, splenomegaly, skin findings (e.g., petechiae, jaundice)
- CML: Splenomegaly (in 90% of patients)

- PMF:
  - Splenomegaly in virtually all patients, hepatomegaly in 50%, lymph node enlargement in 10%
  - Jaundice, edema, and ascites in 10–20%
  - Petechiae in up to 25%
- ET:
  - May have no symptoms or findings in >50%. Easy bruising.
  - Transient ischemic attacks, or even frank strokes, may occur, and a higher incidence of cardiovascular events

DIAGNOSTIC TESTS & INTERPRETATION
Lab
- The general guidance on genotyping is to assess for the *JAK2* V617F mutation. Positive results make PV, ET, or PMF very likely. If negative, PV is unlikely, but ET or PMF are still possible, so testing for the *MPL* mutation is recommended.
- Detection of either the *MPL* or *JAK2* V617F mutation is diagnostic of a clonal MPN.
- CML: Presence of *BCR-ABL* is diagnostic. Marked leukocytosis. Chronic phase typically with <2% myeloblasts in blood and <5% in marrow. Elevated serum vitamin B_{12} level. Elevated lactate dehydrogenase. Hyperuricemia. Markedly decreased leukocyte alkaline phosphatase (LAP) (absent in 5–10%)
- PMF:
  - Mild anemia in >50% at the time of diagnosis; leukocytosis in 30%; leukopenia in 25%. Elevated LDH levels.
  - Bone marrow cells may be quantitatively analyzed by reverse-transcriptase polymerase chain reaction (RT-PCR).
  - CML should be ruled out, and the *MPL* or *JAK2* V617F mutations should be tested for.
- ET: WHO criteria:
  - Thrombocytosis with persistently >450,000 platelets/L in the absence of an identifiable cause (the earlier level of 600,000/L was based on WHO 2001 criteria and has been revised downward)
  - Bone marrow biopsy showing increased numbers of enlarged, mature megakaryocytes
  - No evidence of PV (normal total red blood cell mass)
  - 60–70% will have *MPL* or *JAK2* V617F mutation. Absence of the Ph chromosome

Imaging
- PMF: Radiographic osteosclerosis in 25–66% of patients
- ET: Imaging may be necessary for confirmation of venous thromboses (usually mesenteric, lower extremity, or hepatic).

Diagnostic Procedures/Surgery
Peripheral blood smear, Bone marrow aspiration/core biopsy, Cytogenetic and molecular studies: RT-PCR to detect *BCR-ABL, MPL,* or *JAK2* V617F mutations.

Pathological Findings
- PMF: Bone marrow megakaryocytic hyperplasia and atypia, reticulin and/or collagen fibrosis, osteosclerosis (new bone formation); foci of extramedullary hematopoiesis may be seen at multiple sites (e.g., spleen, liver, kidneys, lymph nodes, lungs, and spinal column); leukoerythroblastosis; anemia

- ET: Bone marrow proliferation of megakaryocytic lineage

DIFFERENTIAL DIAGNOSIS
- CML: Leukemoid reaction (low or absent LAP also seen in paroxysmal nocturnal hemoglobinuria)
- PMF: Spent PV (late stage of PV), CML-secondary myelofibrosis
- ET: Secondary thrombocytosis (inflammation, iron deficiency, and neoplasia) PV, CML

TREATMENT

Evidence-based treatment of CML involves using anti-BCR-ABL therapy (imatinib). Interferon-alfa (IFN-α) is also used for CML.

MEDICATION
First Line
- CML: (2)
  - Imatinib mesylate (Gleevec), a potent inhibitor of the ABL tyrosine kinase
  - IFN-α largely has been replaced by imatinib as treatment of choice.
  - Hydroxyurea can control the excessive myelopoiesis at the initial diagnosis in the chronic phase of the disease in conjunction with imatinib.
  - Accelerated phase and blast crises usually are treated with regimens designed for the treatment of acute leukemia.
  - Severe congenital defects have been reported with busulfan.
  - Allogeneic stem cell transplant
- ET:
  - For the low-to-moderate-risk patient, low-dose aspirin may be considered. Myelosuppression is usually reserved for high-risk patients.
  - Hydroxyurea generally is favored over alkylating agents because it has relatively little known leukemogenic potential (however, transformation to AML is part of the known natural history of some MPNs). Patients with the JAK2 V617F mutation actually may require lower doses of hydroxyurea to control symptoms than those without the mutation.
- Anagrelide also may be used to control thrombocytosis.
- IFN-α, which is considered nonleukemogenic, may be used in ET. Studies vary on whether it reduces the burden of JAK2 V617F or not.
- IFN-α also may be considered for the pregnant ET patient because it is not considered teratogenic.
- PMF: (3)
  - Anemia is treated with transfusions as required. Androgenic steroids: Fluoxymesterone (Halotestin) and prednisone may be useful for anemia. Erythropoietin (in patients with endogenous EPO levels of <100 IU/mL) and danazol (Danocrine) also have been used.
  - Hydroxyurea is useful for controlling splenomegaly and thrombocytosis.
  - Allogeneic bone marrow transplantation is the only intervention known to prolong survival in PMF.
- Some of the most promising therapies for the classic MPNs involve molecular targeting of JAK2. Early results show promise, but these molecularly targeted medications are still in the experimental stage.

Second Line
- PMF: Androgens and glucocorticoids may improve anemia. Corticosteroids if autoimmune hemolysis is present
- ET: Aspirin, with or without dipyridamole, may prove useful in preventing thrombotic or ischemic symptoms in some patients. IFN-α therapy is another option with utility for pregnant patients.

ADDITIONAL TREATMENT
Targeted therapies for JAK-2 and MPL may improve splenomegaly and symptoms of fatigue but do not improve anemia and thrombocytopenia.

General Measures
- Splenectomy has no impact on mortality but is occasionally carried out for symptomatic relief. Extreme thrombocytosis and progressive and massive liver enlargement may ensue.
- CML: Molecularly targeted therapy (with imatinib). Chemotherapy (for advanced disease). Bone marrow transplantation is the only known curative option, with disease-free survival in 50–70%.
- PMF: No standard therapy; rule out other treatable causes for anemia. Radiotherapy for symptomatic tumors or symptomatic splenomegaly. Successful bone marrow transplantation can lead to the reversal of established fibrosis.
- ET: Young, asymptomatic patients with platelet counts of <1,500,000/μL usually are not treated. Lower the platelet count in those >60 years of age with a history of cardiovascular risk factors or if the platelet count >1,500,000/L.

Issues for Referral
Usually comanaged with the guidance of a hematologist/oncologist. Surgical oncology, radiation oncology, and palliative care consultation may be sought. Splenectomy should be done by a surgeon experienced in the surgical management of MPNs.

Additional Therapies
Massive splenomegaly or foci of extramedullary hematopoiesis may require palliative radiation.

SURGERY/OTHER PROCEDURES
No role unless for splenectomy or relief of organ compression by foci of hematopoiesis in PMF

IN-PATIENT CONSIDERATIONS
Initial Stabilization
Treatment to relieve symptoms, prevent infections

Admission Criteria
Severe cachexia; extramedullary hematopoiesis and sequelae, including renal failure and hepatomegaly; severe splenomegaly necessitating treatment; severe bleeding; petechiae; anemia

IV Fluids
Hydration status should be kept optimized during hospitalization to prevent tumor lysis syndrome.

Nursing
Comfort measures such as pain control

ONGOING CARE

FOLLOW-UP RECOMMENDATIONS
Restrictions depend on the symptoms.

PROGNOSIS
- CML: Median survival >5 years from the time of diagnosis. 85% will die in blast crisis. Pregnancy does not affect the course of the disease; >95% of mothers survive to delivery.
- PMF: Progressive splenomegaly, anemia. Median survival is 5 years from the time of diagnosis, and about 30% lower than in matched controls. Patients usually die from hemorrhagic or thrombotic complications and infections. Various prognostic scoring systems are used, incorporating hemoglobin, leukocyte, platelet, and monocyte levels.
- ET: Overall life expectancy is only slightly shortened.

COMPLICATIONS
Transformation to acute leukemia, gout, or nephropathy owing to hyperuricemia; PMF: Portal hypertension, splenic infarcts, Budd-Chiari syndrome, pulmonary hypertension; ET: Thrombohemorrhagic complications in a third; erythromelalgia (a vasoocclusive syndrome with localized pain of distal extremities); increased risk of 1st-trimester abortion; medication-related side effects.

REFERENCES

1. Wadleigh M, Tefferi A et al. Classification and diagnosis of myeloproliferative neoplasms according to the 2008 World Health Organization criteria. *Int J Hematol*. 2010;91:174–9.
2. Levine RL, Gilliland DG et al. Myeloproliferative disorders. *Blood*. 2008;112:2190–8.
3. Mesa RA et al. New drugs for the treatment of myelofibrosis. *Curr Hematol Malig Rep*. 2010; 5:15–21.

See Also (Topic, Algorithm, Electronic Media Element)
Leukemia; Polycythemia Vera

CODES

ICD9
- 205.10 Myeloid leukemia, chronic, without mention of having achieved remission
- 238.4 Polycythemia vera
- 238.79 Neoplasm of uncertain behavior of other lymphatic and hematopoietic tissues

CLINICAL PEARLS

- CML, characterized by splenomegaly and increased granulocytes, runs a generally mild course until it transforms to a frankly leukemic phase and is positive for BCR-ABL, the Ph chromosome.
- Splenectomy has no impact on mortality but is occasionally carried out for symptomatic relief. Extreme thrombocytosis and progressive and massive liver enlargement may ensue.

M

MYOCARDIAL INFARCTION, NON-ST-SEGMENT ELEVATION (NSTEMI)

Lawrence Murphy, MD
Rishi Vohora, DO

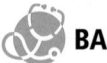 **BASICS**

DESCRIPTION
- Non-ST elevation myocardial infarction (NSTEMI) is considered to be closely related to the pathogenesis and clinical presentation of unstable angina (UA). Both are subsets of acute coronary syndromes (ACS), but differ primarily in the detection of common biomarkers of myocardial injury (troponin I [TnI], troponin T [TnT], or the MB fraction of creatinine kinase [CKMB]).
- NSTEMI is defined by electrocardiographic ST-segment depression or prominent T-wave inversion and/or elevation of cardiac biomarkers in the absence of ST-segment elevation. The elevation of cardiac biomarkers may not be detectable for hours after presentation. Therefore, NSTEMI may not be distinguishable from UA at initial evaluation.

EPIDEMIOLOGY
- Predominant age: Incidence increases with age (1).
- Predominant sex: Prevalence is greater in men (5.5%) than in women (2.9%).

Incidence
- Of 1.57 million annual ACS admissions, approximately 79% (1.24 million) have UA/NSTEMI.
- MI is the number one killer of US males and females. At least 250,000 die within 1 hour of symptom onset. Compared to STEMI, NSTEMI has a lower 30-day mortality but a similar 1-year mortality.

Prevalence
Approximately 7.5 million people in the US are affected by MI.

RISK FACTORS
- Advanced age
- Poorly controlled hypertension
- Tobacco use
- Diabetes mellitus
- Dyslipidemia
- Family history of premature onset of coronary artery disease (CAD)
- Sedentary lifestyle
- High BMI (>25) associated with progressively younger age at first NSTEMI.

GENERAL PREVENTION
Smoking cessation, consume healthy diet, weight control, increase physical activity, maintain goal blood pressure

PATHOPHYSIOLOGY
NSTEMI is usually caused by disruption or erosion of an atherosclerotic plaque with subsequent platelet-rich thrombus overlying the culprit lesion causing an abrupt decrease in blood supply. Less frequently, it is caused by disease states where myocardial oxygen demand exceeds supply.

ETIOLOGY
- Platelet-thrombus on disrupted or eroded plaque. This is the most common cause.
- Dynamic obstruction (coronary spasm or vasoconstriction) of epicardial and/or subendocardial vessels
- Severe narrowing without spasm or thrombus
- Progressive mechanical obstruction to coronary flow

- Coronary arterial inflammation caused by noninfectious and infectious stimuli, which can lead to plaque expansion and destabilization
- Coronary artery dissection, rupture or erosion, and thrombogenesis
- Cocaine or methamphetamine abuse

COMMONLY ASSOCIATED CONDITIONS
- Abdominal aortic aneurysm
- Extracranial cerebrovascular disease
- Atherosclerotic peripheral vascular disease

 DIAGNOSIS

HISTORY
- Chest heaviness/tightness, with or without exertion
- Pain or discomfort radiating to neck, jaw, interscapular area, upper extremities, and epigastrium
- History of myocardial ischemia (stable or unstable angina, MI, coronary bypass surgery, or percutaneous coronary intervention [PCI] (2)
- Assess risk factors for CAD, bleeding
- Medications: Phosphodiesterase-5 inhibitors and concomitant nitrates

PHYSICAL EXAM
- General: Fever (2) may occasionally be present.
- Neuro: Dizziness, syncope, fatigue, asthenia, altered mental status
- Cerebrovascular (CV): Dysrhythmia, hypotension, widened pulse pressure, S3 and S4, jugular venous distention (JVD)
- Respiratory: Dyspnea, tachypnea, crackles
- Gastrointestinal (GI): Abdominal pain, nausea, vomiting
- Musculoskeletal: Neck pain, backache, shoulder pain, pain in upper limb
- Skin: Cool skin, pallor, diaphoresis

Geriatric Considerations
Elderly patients may have an atypical presentation, including generalized weakness, stroke, syncope, or change in mental status.

DIAGNOSTIC TESTS & INTERPRETATION
Lab
Initial lab tests
- Electrocardiography (12-lead ECG) (2)[B]:
  - ST segment depression and/or T-wave inversions
- Diagnosis of acute NSTEMI:
  - ≥1 mm ST depression in ≥2 contiguous leads OR
  - T-wave changes suggestive of myocardial ischemia AND
  - Rise in cardiac isoenzyme markers consistent with myocardial injury. (Characteristic biomarkers with compatible clinical symptoms and signs but without ECG changes are also diagnostic.)
  - ST depression and/or tall R-wave in V1/V2 with upright T waves may indicate transmural (STEMI) of posterior wall.
  - If initial ECG nondiagnostic but symptoms persist with suspicion for ACS, perform serial ECGs at 15- to 30-minute intervals to detect potential ST segment changes (2).

Follow-Up & Special Considerations
- Serum biomarkers:
  - Troponin I and T (cTnI, cTnT) rise 3–6 hours after onset of ischemic symptoms. Elevations in cTnI

persist for 7–10 days, while cTnT persist for 10–14 days after MI (2).
  - MB fraction of creatine kinase (CK-MB): Rises 3–4 hours after onset of myocardial injury; peaks at 12–24 hours and remains elevated for 2–3 days (2)
  - Myoglobin: Early marker for myocardial necrosis. Rises 2 hours after onset of myocardial necrosis, reaches peak at 1–4 hours, and remains elevated for 24 hours (2).
  - Patients with negative cardiac biomarkers within 6 hours of the onset of symptoms should have biomarkers remeasured within 8–12 hours of onset of symptoms (2)[B].
- Fasting lipid profile
- Complete blood count with platelets, activated partial thromboplastin time (aPTT) (if heparin therapy is contemplated), electrolytes, magnesium, blood urea nitrogen (BUN), serum creatinine, and glucose
- Other laboratory tests (not routinely ordered, but affected by MI):
  - Lactate dehydrogenase: Rises within 24 hrs, peaks 3–6 days, baseline 8–12 days
  - Leukocytes: Rise within several hours after MI, peak in 2–4 days, and return to normal within 1 week (2)
  - Brain natriuretic peptide (BNP) (2): Increases with MI; may not indicate heart failure

Pregnancy Considerations
Findings mimicking NSTEMI in pregnancy: ST-segment depression after anesthesia, increase in CK-MB after delivery, and mild increase in troponin I levels in preeclampsia and gestational hypertension. However, spontaneous coronary dissection is a rare cause of ST elevation seen in pregnancy.

Imaging
Initial approach
Consider echocardiography (2)[B] if not recently performed

Diagnostic Procedures/Surgery
- Transthoracic and/or transesophageal echocardiography, contrast chest computed tomography (CT) scan, or magnetic resonance imaging (MRI) (2) generally reserved for differentiating STEMI and other causes of chest pain from aortic dissection (2)[B]
- Single-photon emission CT (SPECT) radionuclide imaging: Not recommended if ST elevations seen on ECG (2)[B]
- Coronary angiography, electrocardiogram with stress testing (2)[B]

Pathological Findings
- Subendocardial myocardial necrosis may be present.
- Atherosclerosis, if etiologic

DIFFERENTIAL DIAGNOSIS
- Unstable angina (also an acute coronary syndrome but without biochemical markers of ischemic damage)
- Aortic dissection
- Pulmonary embolism
- Pleuropericarditis
- Perforating ulcer
- Gastroesophageal reflux disease (GERD) and spasm

- Biliary or pancreatic pain
- Dysrhythmia

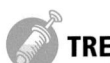

TREATMENT

MEDICATION
First Line

- Supplemental oxygen 2–4L/min, maintaining arterial oxygen desaturation >90% (2)[B]
- Morphine sulfate 2–4 mg IV (with increments of 2–8 mg IV repeated at 5–15-minute intervals (2)[A]
- Nitroglycerin (NTG) sublingual 0.4 mg every 5 mins for total of 3 doses, then assess need for IV NTG (2)[C]
- Aspirin, nonenteric-coated, initial dosing of 162 mg (2)[A] to 325 mg (2)[C] orally or chewed. Administer clopidogrel loading dose 300–600 mg, followed by 75 mg daily (for ASA-intolerant patients) (2)[A] or if need PCI.
- Oral beta-blocker (cardioselective agent such as metoprolol or atenolol preferred) within 24 hours if no contraindications exist (2)[B]
- Determine use of invasive or conservative therapy. Consider risks and benefits of the early invasive approach:
  - 33% relative risk reduction for both the endpoints of refractory angina and rehospitalization at 6–12 months (3)[A]
  - 27% and 22% relative risk reduction in rates of myocardial infarction at 6–12 months and 3–5 years, respectively (3)[A]
  - Doubled risk of procedure-related myocardial infarction and increased risk of minor peri-procedural bleeding (3)[A]:
    - Invasive strategy: Benefits may be more pronounced in higher-risk patients, such as those with ECG changes or diabetics (3)[A]. For patients with elevated risk for clinical events (2)[A] or refractory angina or hemodynamic or electrical instability (2)[B], initiate anticoagulant (2)[A]: Enoxaparin or unfractionated heparin (UFH) (2)[A] or bivalirudin (2)[B]. Prior to angiography, add GP IIb/IIIa inhibitor (eptifibatide or tirofiban) or clopidogrel (2)[A]. Use both agents in patients for whom PCI is planned or who are at high risk for recurrent ischemia or delayed angiography (2)[B].
    - Conservative strategy: For low-risk or selected intermediate-risk patients without adverse effects on clinical outcomes (2)[B]; based on patient or physician preference (2)[C]; or in chronic renal insufficiency (2)[C]: Initiate anticoagulant therapy (2)[A]: Enoxaparin or UFH (2)[A] or fondaparinux (2)[B]; enoxaparin or fondaparinux preferable (2)[B]. Initiate clopidogrel (2)[A].

Second Line

- Angiotensin-converting enzyme (ACE) inhibitor in patients with pulmonary congestion or left ventricular ejection fraction (EF) ≤40%. Substitute with angiotensin receptor blocker if ACE-intolerant patients (2)[A]; likely beneficial even if EF >35%.
- Nondihydropyridine calcium channel blocker (CCB) (verapamil or diltiazem) when beta-blockers are contraindicated if normal EF (2)[B]. Use oral long-acting CCB only after beta-blockers and nitrates have been fully used (2)[C].

- Long-term nitrate therapy for recurrent ischemia or heart failure (2)[C]
- Sublingual NTG should be prescribed at discharge (2)[C].
- Lipid-lowering therapy: Statin (preferred due to nonlipid benefit on vascular function) (2)[A], niacin, or fibrate (2)[B]

ADDITIONAL TREATMENT
General Measures

- Bed/chair rest with continuous electrocardiogram (ECG) monitoring
- Treat arrhythmias as needed; prophylactic antiarrhythmic therapy is not recommended.
- Anxiolytics to decrease anxiety
- Stool softeners
- Deep vein thrombosis prophylaxis
- Continuation of aspirin, clopidogrel, beta-blockers, ACE inhibitors (or ARBs if ACE-intolerant), lipid-lowering therapy
- Tight blood pressure control
- Address possible depression (common post-MI).
- Increase physical activity.
- Smoking cessation
- Annual influenza vaccine

Issues for Referral
Cardiology consultation usually appropriate

SURGERY/OTHER PROCEDURES

- Coronary reperfusion
- Intra-aortic balloon pump for severe ischemia
- PCI with stent placement
- Coronary artery bypass graft (CABG) surgery

IN-PATIENT CONSIDERATIONS
Initial Stabilization
Restrict to bed rest with continuous ECG monitoring, assess for reperfusion therapy, relieve ischemic pain, provide supplemental oxygen, treat life-threatening complications, admit to coronary care unit

Admission Criteria
All patients with definite or suspected acute MI, ongoing pain, positive cardiac markers, ST deviations, hemodynamic abnormalities, probable and definite acute coronary syndrome (ACS)

ONGOING CARE

FOLLOW-UP RECOMMENDATIONS

- Appointment follow-up within 2–6 weeks (low-risk) and 14 days (high-risk)
- Refer to cardiac rehab.

DIET
Request dietary consult.

PATIENT EDUCATION

- Resume exercise, sexual activity after outpatient re-evaluation
- Diet low in saturated fats and cholesterol

PROGNOSIS
NSTEMI patients have a lower in-hospital mortality than those with STEMI, but a similar or worse long-term outcome.

COMPLICATIONS

- Heart failure/cardiogenic shock
- Myocardial rupture/left ventricular aneurysm
- Dysrhythmia

- Acute pulmonary embolism
- Acute thromboembolic stroke
- Pericarditis/Dressler syndrome
- Severe depression (increases mortality risk)
- Hyperglycemia

REFERENCES

1. *Heart Disease and Stroke Statistics 2008 Update*. Dallas, TX: American Heart Association, 2008.
2. Anderson JL, Adams CD, Antman EM, et al. ACC/AHA 2007 guidelines for the management of patients with unstable angina/non-ST-Elevation myocardial infarction: a report of the American College of Cardiology/American Heart Association Task Force on Practice Guidelines (Writing Committee to Revise the 2002 Guidelines for the Management of Patients With Unstable Angina/Non-ST-Elevation Myocardial Infarction) developed in collaboration with the American College of Emergency Physicians, the Society for Cardiovascular Angiography and Interventions, and the Society of Thoracic Surgeons endorsed by the American Association of Cardiovascular and Pulmonary Rehabilitation and the Society for Academic Emergency Medicine. *J Am Coll Cardiol*. 2007;50:e1–e157.
3. Hoenig MR, Aroney CN, Scott IA. Early invasive versus conservative strategies for unstable angina and non-ST elevation myocardial infarction in the stent era (Review). *Cochrane Database of Systematic Reviews*. 3, 2010.

CODES

ICD9
- 410.70 Subendocardial infarction, episode of care unspecified
- 410.71 Subendocardial infarction, initial episode of care
- 410.72 Subendocardial infarction, subsequent episode of care

CLINICAL PEARLS

- Discontinue nonsteroidal anti-inflammatory drugs (NSAIDs), nonselective or selective cyclooxygenase (COX)-2 agents, except for ASA, due to increased risks of mortality, reinfarction, hypertension, heart failure, and myocardial rupture.
- Discontinue clopidogrel 5–7 days before elective CABG for acute coronary syndrome.
- Do not use nitrate products in patients who recently used a phosphodiesterase-5 inhibitor (24 hours of sildenafil or 48 hours of tadalafil).
- Use of long-term antithrombotic therapy after NSTEMI is dependent on type of stent received and medications administered.

M

MYOCARDIAL INFARCTION, ST-SEGMENT ELEVATION (STEMI)

Fae G. Wooding, PharmD
Juyong Lee, MD, PhD
Ivan A. Arenas, MD, PhD

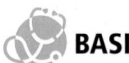 **BASICS**

DESCRIPTION

Acute myocardial infarction (AMI) is the rapid development of myocardial necrosis resulting from a sustained and complete absence of blood flow to a portion of the myocardium. ST-segment elevation myocardial infarction (STEMI) occurs when coronary blood flow ceases following thrombotic occlusion of a coronary artery affected by atherosclerosis, causing transmural ischemia. This is accompanied by release of serum cardiac biomarkers and ST elevation (and likely a Q wave when infarction occurs) on an electrocardiogram (ECG).

EPIDEMIOLOGY

Incidence
In the US, estimated annual incidence of MI is 600,000 new and 320,000 recurrent attacks.

Prevalence
- Leading cause of morbidity and mortality in the US
- Approximately 7.5 million people in the US are affected by MI.
- Prevalence increases with age and is higher in men (5.5%) than women (2.9%).

RISK FACTORS
Advancing age, hypertension, tobacco use, diabetes mellitus, dyslipidemia, family history of premature onset of coronary artery disease (CAD), sedentary lifestyle

GENERAL PREVENTION
Smoking cessation, consume healthy diet, weight control, regular physical activity, maintain goal blood pressure

PATHOPHYSIOLOGY
Atherosclerotic lesions may be smooth and concentric or rough, eccentric, and fissured. Plaques that are rough and eccentric are more unstable, thrombogenic, and prone to rupture.

ETIOLOGY
- Atherosclerotic coronary artery disease
- Nonatherosclerotic:
  - Emboli: For example, thrombi from left ventricle or atrium
  - Mechanical obstruction: Chest trauma, dissection of aorta or coronary arteries
  - Increased vasomotor tone, variant angina
  - Arteritis, others: Hematologic (DIC), aortic stenosis, cocaine, intravenous (IV) drug use, severe burns, prolonged hypotension

COMMONLY ASSOCIATED CONDITIONS
Abdominal aortic aneurysm, extracranial cerebrovascular disease, atherosclerotic peripheral vascular disease

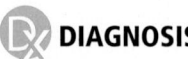 **DIAGNOSIS**

HISTORY
- Classically, sudden-onset chest heaviness/tightness, with or without exertion, lasting at least minutes
- Pain or discomfort radiating to neck, jaw, interscapular area, upper extremities, and epigastrium

- Previous history of myocardial ischemia (stable or unstable angina, MI, coronary bypass surgery, or percutaneous coronary intervention [PCI])
- Assess risk factors for CAD, history of bleeding, noncardiac surgery, family history of premature CAD
- Medications: Phosphodiesterase-5 inhibitors (if recent use, avoid concomitant nitrates)
- Alcohol and drug abuse (especially cocaine)

PHYSICAL EXAM
- General: Restless, agitated, hypothermia, fever
- Neuro: Dizziness, syncope, fatigue, asthenia, disorientation (especially in the elderly)
- Cerebrovascular (CV): Dysrhythmia, hypotension, widened pulse pressure, S3 and S4, jugular venous distention (JVD)
- Respiratory: Dyspnea, tachypnea, crackles
- Gastrointestinal (GI): Abdominal pain, nausea, vomiting
- Musculoskeletal: Pain in neck, back, shoulder, or upper limbs
- Skin: Cool skin, pallor, diaphoresis

Geriatric Considerations
- Elderly patients may have an atypical presentation, including silent or unrecognized MI, often with complaints of syncope, weakness, shortness of breath, unexplained nausea, epigastric pain, altered mental status, or dementia. Patients with diabetes mellitus may have fewer and less dramatic chest symptoms.

DIAGNOSTIC TESTS & INTERPRETATION
Lab
Initial lab tests
12-lead electrocardiogram (ECG): ST-segment elevation in a regional pattern ≥1 mm ST elevation, with or without abnormal Q waves. ST depression ± tall R wave in V1/V2 may be STEMI of posterior wall. Absence of Q waves represent partial or transient occlusion, or early infarction. New ST- or T-wave changes indicative of myocardial ischemia or injury. Consider right-sided and posterior chest leads if inferior MI pattern (V3R, V4R, V7-V9).

Follow-Up & Special Considerations
- Serum biomarkers:
  - Troponin I and T (cTnI, cTnT) rise 3–6 hours after onset of ischemic symptoms. Elevations in cTnI persist for 7–10 days, while those in cTnT persist for 10–14 days after MI.
  - Myoglobin fraction of creatine kinase (CK-MB): Rises 3–4 hours after onset of myocardial injury; peaks at 12–24 hours and remains elevated for 2–3 days
  - Myoglobin: Early marker for myocardial necrosis. Rises 2 hours after onset of myocardial necrosis, reaches peak at 1–4 hours, and remains elevated for 24 hours.
- Fasting lipid profile, complete blood count with platelets, electrolytes, magnesium, blood urea nitrogen (BUN), serum creatinine, and glucose. International normalized ratio (INR) if anticoagulation contemplated. Brain natriuretic peptide (BNP) is elevated in acute MI; may or may not indicate heart failure

Pregnancy Considerations
Findings mimicking acute MI in pregnancy: ST-segment depression after anesthesia, increase in CK-MB after delivery, and mild increase in troponin I levels in preeclampsia and gestational hypertension

Imaging
Initial approach
ECG with continuous monitoring:
- 2-D and M-mode echocardiography is useful in evaluating regional wall motion in MI and left ventricular function.
- Portable echo can clarify diagnosis of STEMI if concomitant left bundle branch block (LBBB).
- Useful in assessing mechanical complications and mural thrombus

Diagnostic Procedures/Surgery
- Coronary pressure (fractional flow reserve) or Doppler velocimetry to determine whether PCI of a specific coronary lesion is warranted. High-quality portable chest x-ray.
- Transthoracic and/or transesophageal echocardiography, contrast chest computed tomography (CT) scan, or magnetic resonance imaging (MRI). Coronary angiography.

ALERT
Isosmolar contrast medium or low-molecular-weight contrast medium other than ioxaglate or iohexol is indicated in patients with chronic kidney disease undergoing angiography who are not undergoing chronic dialysis.

Pathological Findings
Myocardial necrosis and atherosclerosis, if etiologic

DIFFERENTIAL DIAGNOSIS
Unstable angina, aortic dissection, pulmonary embolism (PE), perforating ulcer, pericarditis, dysrhythmias, gastroesophageal reflux disease (GERD) and spasm, biliary or pancreatic pain, hyperventilation syndrome

 TREATMENT

MEDICATION
Medication recommendations based upon 2009 ACC/AHA focused guideline updates (1)

First Line
- Supplemental oxygen 2–4 L/min, maintaining arterial oxygen saturation >90%
- Nitroglycerin (NTG) sublingual 0.4 mg every 5 mins for total of 3 doses, followed by nitroglycerin IV if ongoing pain and/or hypertension and/or management of pulmonary congestion
- Morphine sulfate 2–4 mg IV (with increments of 2–8 mg IV repeated at 5–15-minute intervals to relieve pain or pulmonary congestion associated with STEMI
- Antiplatelet agents:
  - Aspirin (ASA), nonenteric-coated, initial dose 162 mg to 325 mg chewed
  - A loading dose of a thienopyridine is recommended for STEMI patients for whom PCI is planned:

- ○ At least 300–600 mg of clopidogrel should be given as early as possible before or at the time of primary or nonprimary PCI or
- ○ Prasugrel 60 mg should be given as soon as possible for primary PCI. Not recommended as part of a dual-antiplatelet therapy regimen in STEMI patients with prior history of stroke and transient ischemic attack for whom primary PCI is planned.
- ○ Duration of therapy with a thienopyridine varies. 12 months for patients receiving drug eluting stent (DES) during PCI for ACS. Consider earlier discontinuation if risk of morbidity due to bleeding outweighs the benefits of therapy. May continue clopidogrel or prasugrel for longer than 15 months in patients undergoing DES placement. Discontinue clopidogrel for at least 5 days or prasugrel at least 7 days prior to planned CABG.
- – For STEMI patients undergoing nonprimary PCI:
  - ○ Continue clopidogrel in a patient who has received fibrinolytic therapy and has been given clopidogrel.
  - ○ Administer loading dose of clopidogrel 300–600 mg if patient received a fibrinolytic without a thienopyridine, or, once the coronary anatomy is known and PCI is planned, administer a loading dose of prasugrel as soon as possible, but no later than 1 hour after PCI. Administer loading dose of clopidogrel 300 mg in patients less than 75 years of age who received fibrinolytic therapy or who do not receive reperfusion therapy.
  - ○ Clopidogrel 75 mg should be given with aspirin in patients with STEMI regardless of reperfusion therapy. Clopidogrel treatment should continue for at least 14 days.
- • Beta-blocker (BB) within 24 hours, if no contraindications exist
- • Glycoprotein IIb/IIIa receptor antagonists at time of primary PCI in selected patients: Abciximab, eptifibatide, or tirofiban
- • Angiotensin-converting enzyme (ACE) inhibitors should be initiated orally within the first 24 hours of STEMI in patients with anterior infarction or LVEF less than 0.40 in the absence of contraindications. Initiate ACE inhibitors within 24 hours of STEMI in all patients if no contraindications exist.
- • Coronary reperfusion therapy:
  - – Primary PCI:
    - ○ If patient presents within 12 hours of symptom onset and "door-to-balloon inflation" within 90 minutes of presentation at a facility with PCI capability
    - ○ If substantial risk for intracranial hemorrhage (ICH)
    - ○ Age <75 with STEMI or LBBB who develop shock within 36 hours of acute MI (AMI)
    - ○ Severe congestive heart failure and/or pulmonary edema (Killip class III)
    - ○ Not eligible to receive fibrinolytic therapy within 12 hours of onset of symptoms
    - ○ Patients with onset of symptoms within the prior 12–24 hours and 1 or more of the following: Severe CHF, hemodynamis or electrical instability, or persistent ischemic symptoms
- • Fibrinolysis:
  - – If presenting at a hospital without PCI capability and cannot be transferred to a PCI-capable facility to undergo PCI within 90 minutes of first medical contact, administer fibrinolytic therapy, "door-to-needle," within 30 minutes of presentation.

- – If no contraindications, administer within 12 hours, but not beyond 24 hours, of onset of symptoms to patients with STEMI in ≥2 contiguous leads and new or presumably new LBBB:
  - ○ Alteplase (rt-PA): 15-mg IV bolus, followed by 0.75 mg/kg (up to 50 mg) IV over 30 mins, then 0.5 mg/kg (up to 35 mg) over 60 min; max 100 mg over 90 min
  - ○ Reteplase (r-PA): 10 units IV bolus over 2 min, give 2nd bolus 30 min later
  - ○ Tenecteplase (TNK-tPA): 30–50 mg (based on weight) IV bolus over 5–10 secs
- – Combination reperfusion with abciximab and half-dose r-PA or TNK-tPA
- – Use anticoagulants (unfractionated heparin [UFH], enoxaparin, or fondaparinux) as ancillary therapy to reperfusion therapy for minimum 48 hours and duration of admission (up to 8 days). Avoid UFH if >48 hours of anticoagulant required: Recommend supportive anticoagulant regimens in patients proceeding to primary PCI who have been treated with ASA and thienopyridine. Administer additional boluses of UFH as needed to maintain therapeutic clotting time levels in patients who received prior treatment with UFH. Bivalirudin recommended as a supportive measure for primary PCI in patients with or without prior treatment with UFH.

Second Line
- • Long-acting nondihydropyridine calcium channel blocker (CCB) when beta-blocker (BB) is ineffective or contraindicated if ejection fraction (EF) is normal
- • Aldosterone receptor antagonist if already receiving therapeutic doses of an ACE inhibitor and beta-blocker. Caution re: hyperkalemia. Use low dose of aldosterone antagonist (e.g., spironolactone 25 mg daily).
- • Lipid-lowering therapy: Statin (preferred because of additional nonlipid effects on vascular function), niacin, or fibrate

ADDITIONAL TREATMENT
General Measures
- • Admit to telemetry/coronary care unit with continuous ECG monitoring and bed rest. Anxiolytics if needed. Stool softeners.
- • Antiarrhythmics as needed for unstable dysrhythmia. Deep vein thrombosis (DVT) prophylaxis.
- • Continuation of aspirin, clopidogrel, BB, ACE inhibitors (or ARB if ACE-intolerant), lipid-lowering therapy, tight blood pressure control, progressively increased physical activity, smoking cessation, annual influenza vaccine
- • Elicit symptoms or signs of depression and treat with a selective serotonin reuptake inhibitor (SSRI) or psychotherapy if present.

Issues for Referral
Cardiac rehabilitation, neurology/neurosurgery if intracranial hemorrhage

SURGERY/OTHER PROCEDURES
Intra-aortic balloon pump for cardiogenic shock. PCI of the left main coronary artery with stents as an alternative to CABG in patients with favorable anatomy and comorbidities that may increase risk of adverse surgical outcomes if CABG chosen. Coronary artery bypass graft (CABG) surgery.

IN-PATIENT CONSIDERATIONS
Initial Stabilization
All patients with STEMI should be admitted to a CCU for evaluation and treatment. Transfer high-risk patients who receive fibrinolytic therapy as primary reperfusion therapy at a non-PCI-capable facility to a PCI-capable facility as soon as possible.

Admission Criteria
Definitive or suspected acute MI, ongoing pain, positive cardiac markers, ST deviations, hemodynamic abnormalities

IV Fluids
Right ventricular infarction may need fluid resuscitation for hypotension.

 ONGOING CARE

FOLLOW-UP RECOMMENDATIONS
F/U w-in 3–6 weeks of d/c. Identify high-risk patients for implantable cardioverter defibrillator (ICD) placement (especially those with EF <30%).

DIET
n.p.o. for first 4–12 hours due to risk of emesis or aspiration; request dietary consult if lipid, weight, or glucose issues

PATIENT EDUCATION
May resume sexual activity within 7–10 days, consistent with current exercise capacity. Driving can resume 1 week after discharge when in compliance with individual state laws. Recommend diet low in saturated fats and cholesterol.

COMPLICATIONS
Heart failure, myocardial rupture/left ventricular aneurysm, pericarditis, dysrhythmias, acute mitral regurgitation, severe depression (common)

REFERENCE
1. Kushner FG, et al. 2009 focused updates: ACC/AHA guidelines for the management of patients with ST-elevation myocardial infarction and ACC/AHA/SCAI guidelines on percutaneous coronary intervention. *J Am Coll Cardiol*. 2009;54:2205–41.

 CODES

ICD9
- • 410.90 Acute myocardial infarction of unspecified site, episode of care unspecified
- • 410.91 Acute myocardial infarction of unspecified site, initial episode of care
- • 410.92 Acute myocardial infarction of unspecified site, subsequent episode of care

M

CLINICAL PEARLS
Discontinue clopidogrel at least 5–7 days before elective CABG. Do not administer nitrates to patients who have recently used PDE-5 inhibitors.

MYOCARDITIS

Francesca L. Beaudoin, MS, MD
Ron Van Ness-Otunnu, MD

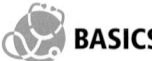 **BASICS**

DESCRIPTION
- Inflammatory disease of myocardium, most commonly from viral infection. Other etiologies include infectious pathogens, autoimmune disease, drug-induced hypersensitivity reactions, systemic eosinophilic syndromes, and toxins.
- Clinical presentation varies widely from mild chest discomfort or dyspnea, to shock, heart failure, and sudden cardiac death.
- Range of treatment is broad and dependent upon the cause and severity of disease, from basic pharmacologic therapy for left ventricular dysfunction, to vasopressor and inotropic support for hemodynamic compromise, to ventricular assist devices, extracorporeal membrane oxygenation, or heart transplant for severely compromised patients.
- While more often there is resolution of disease with supportive or directed care, unresolved disease may lead to chronic dilated cardiomyopathy with high risk of increased morbidity and mortality.

EPIDEMIOLOGY
- Male > Female
- Infant mortality as high as 75%
- Child mortality as high as 25% (1)

Incidence
Unknown

Prevalence
- Large prospective study implicated myocarditis as cause of dilated cardiomyopathy in 9% of cases (2)
- Based on prospective postmortem data, myocarditis is associated with sudden cardiac death in young adults at rates between 8.6% and 12% (2).
- In human immunodeficiency virus (HIV)–related deaths, myocarditis is the most common cardiac finding on autopsy (50% prevalence).

RISK FACTORS
- Community viral endemic or other infection
- Hypersensitivity reaction
- Autoimmune disease
- Drug or toxin exposure
- Travel to area endemic to specific pathogens
- Eosinophilic syndromes

PATHOPHYSIOLOGY
3-phase progression:
- Acute direct or indirect myocyte injury from pathogen or toxin and initiation of innate immune response
- Acquired immune system activation with immune dysregulation. T cell response, B cell activation, possible antibody cross-reaction with endogenous myocardial epitopes (molecular mimicry) leads to myocytolysis or worsening inflammatory response.
- Progression to persistent cardiomyopathy and either chronic infection or eventual recovery

ETIOLOGY
- Viral:
  – Enteroviruses (coxsackie B particularly) are the most common cause of myocarditis overall (and found in 32% of viral-mediated myocarditis).
- Bacterial:
  – *Staphylococcus*, *Streptococcus*, Mycobacterial
- Fungal:
  – *Aspergillus*, *Candida*, Coccidioides, *Cryptococcus*
- Protozoal:
  – *Trypanosoma cruzi*, Entamoeba
- Parasitic:
  – Schistosoma, *Larva migrans*, *Trichinella*
- Immunologic:
  – Giant cell, sarcoidosis, Kawasaki disease
- Drug-induced hypersensitivity reactions:
  – Antibiotics, anticonvulsants, antipsychotics
- Systemic hypereosinophilic syndromes
- Toxins:
  – Cocaine, anthracyclines

 DIAGNOSIS

- Histopathologic (Dallas criteria):
  – Inflammatory cellular infiltrate with myocyte necrosis
  – No longer gold standard due to (2):
    ○ Sampling error (>17 samples required to diagnose 80% cases)
    ○ Intraobserver variability
    ○ In hypersensitivity myocarditis, diagnostic in only 10–20% cases
- Clinicopathological classification:
  – Fulminant: Severe hemodynamic compromise, distinct viral prodrome, abrupt onset. Echocardiography: Nondilated wall thickening, hypocontractile left ventricle. Best long-term prognosis among those patients presenting with heart failure (3).
  – Subacute: Less severe presentation, but worse long-term prognosis due to increased likelihood of developing chronic dilated cardiomyopathy
- Immunohistochemistry:
  – Immunoperoxidase staining of human leukocyte antigens
- Viral PCR
- Noninvasive imaging (MRI, nuclear imaging, echocardiography)

HISTORY
- Viral prodrome (fever, malaise, myalgias, upper respiratory, and/or gastrointestinal symptoms) within previous 2 weeks. Reported viral prodrome incidence highly variable (2).
- Exertional dyspnea (72%)
- Chest pain or discomfort (32%)
- Decreased exercise tolerance
- Palpitations
- Syncope (predictor of increased mortality)
- Wide range of clinical presentations: From asymptomatic with electrocardiogram (EKG) abnormalities to cardiogenic shock or sudden death
- Most patients presenting with acute dilated cardiomyopathy have mild disease (3).

- Children have a more fulminant presentation and are frequently initially misdiagnosed with asthma, pneumonia, or sepsis (1).
- Important to distinguish:
  – Acute lymphocytic: Unclear onset, rare hemodynamic compromise, frequently requires cardiac transplant; increased mortality
  – Fulminant lymphocytic: Abrupt onset (<3 days) with 2-week viral prodrome, hemodynamic compromise, good prognosis with supportive care
- High-risk presentations (3):
  – Heart failure with eosinophilia
  – Giant cell myocarditis (high risk of death or cardiac transplant)
  – Heart failure + dilated left ventricle + new ventricular arrhythmia, heart block, or poor response to treatment over 2 weeks
- Co-existence with cardiac amyloidosis or hypertrophic cardiomyopathy can worsen prognosis.
- Clinical suspicion for high morbidity/mortality presentation should prompt endomyocardial biopsy.

PHYSICAL EXAM
- Arrhythmias (18%)
- Friction rub (concurrent pericarditis)
- Increased jugular venous pressure
- Hypotension
- Decreased pulse pressure
- Hemodynamic collapse/cardiogenic shock
- Pulmonary hypertension, bundle branch block, EF <40% predict increased mortality
- In children, most common findings are tachycardia, tachypnea, intercostal retractions, grunting

DIAGNOSTIC TESTS & INTERPRETATION
- Lab tests, EKG, and echocardiography are insensitive and frequently nonspecific.
- Cardiac catheterization and chest x-ray to evaluate alternative diagnoses
- EKG findings (3)[C]:
  – Sinus tachycardia
  – Ventricular arrhythmia
  – Atrioventricular conduction block
  – Diffuse ST-segment elevation and PR-segment depression
  – Signs of acute myocardial infarction (ST segment elevations in ≥2 leads, T-wave inversions, ST segment depressions, pathologic Q waves)
- Echocardiography to rule out causes of heart failure. Identifies global or focal left ventricular abnormality, dilated cardiomyopathy
- Endomyocardial biopsy (EMB) is infrequently indicated (<5% of cases warrant biopsy). Higher yield if within <4 weeks of symptom onset (3)[B].
- EMB may be useful when a particular cause is suspected and confirmation will alter treatment plan. The risk of serious complication from biopsy is <1% in centers experienced with technique.
- Biopsy recommended if common causes of dilated cardiomyopathy are excluded and 1 of the following is present (2)[C]:
  – Ventricular arrhythmias or progressive conduction disease
  – Heart failure with rash, fever, or eosinophilia
  – History of collagen vascular disease
  – Amyloidosis, sarcoidosis, hemochromatosis
  – Suspected giant cell myocarditis (poor prognosis: Median survival of 5.5 months from onset)

– Rapidly progressive cardiomyopathy
– Higher yield if within <4 weeks of symptom onset
- Amyloidosis disfavors heart transplant
- Due to rapid deterioration, identification of giant cell disease prompts mechanical circulatory support or heart transplant

Lab
Initial lab tests
- Cardiac enzymes:
  – Creatine kinase: Low predictive value
  – Troponin I or T: 30–50% sensitive, 90% specific, 80–90% positive predictive value (2) for myocardial injury
- Myocyte-specific major histocompatibility complex antigens: 80–85% sensitive and specific (2)
- Erythrocyte sedimentation rate not recommended: Poor sensitivity and specificity

Imaging
Noninvasive imaging (2,4):
- Cardiac MRI:
  – May be a viable alternative to biopsy, identifies patients that may benefit from biopsy, guides biopsy, evaluates disease progression
  – Gadolinium late enhancement and T2-weighted
- Echocardiography:
  – Segmental wall abnormalities and nondilated wall thickening
  – Gadolinium enhanced spin-echo, segmented inversion recovery gradient-echo pulse sequence
  – Ultrasonic tissue characterization ≥90% specific
- Nuclear imaging with antimyosin antibodies:
  – Gallium^{67} for myocyte inflammation
  – Indium^{11} for myocyte necrosis

Diagnostic Procedures/Surgery
Cardiac catheterization may be required if symptoms or EKG findings suggest acute myocardial infarction.

Pathological Findings
See Dallas Criteria above

DIFFERENTIAL DIAGNOSIS
- Aortic dissection
- Pericarditis
- Acute myocardial infarction
- Pulmonary embolus
- Congestive heart failure
- Sepsis
- Cardiomyopathies (dilated, restrictive, hypertrophic, transient stress [Takotsubo disease])
- Pericardial effusion
- Pneumonia

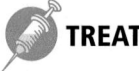 ## TREATMENT

- Hemodynamic and cardiovascular supportive care. Additional management based on presentation or suspected underlying cause (3).
- >50% spontaneously recover.
- In suspected acute viral myocarditis, advise patient to limit physical activity because it may increase viral replication and worsen condition (4)[C].
- Follow latest American College of Cardiology/ American Heart Association recommendations for treatment of left ventricular systolic dysfunction, utilizing diuretics, β-adrenergic blockers, angiotensin-converting enzyme inhibitors, and angiotensin II receptor blockers as indicated (2)[B].
- Aldosterone antagonist (selectively used for NYHA class III or IV symptoms) (2)[B]

- Nonsteroidal anti-inflammatory drugs are associated with increased mortality (3)[C].
- Drug-induced hypersensitivity: Withdraw agent
- Systemic hypereosinophilic syndrome: Treat underlying disorder.
- Kawasaki disease: Intravenous immunoglobulin
- Hepatitis C: May respond to interferon therapy (3)[C]
- Systemic autoimmune (SLE, scleroderma, polymyositis, giant cell myocarditis): Immunosuppressants may be beneficial (2)[C].
- Consider intra-aortic balloon pump or left ventricular assist device for severe myocarditis as a temporizing measure or bridge to heart transplantation (rescue therapy) (3)[C].

MEDICATION
See Congestive Heart Failure topic for management of heart-failure aspects.

ADDITIONAL TREATMENT
Limit physical activity in the acute setting, but exercise training may improve clinical status in patients with current or prior symptoms of heart failure and reduced left ventricular ejection fraction (5)[B].

SURGERY/OTHER PROCEDURES
- Intra-aortic balloon pump
- Implantable cardioverter-defibrillator

IN-PATIENT CONSIDERATIONS
Initial Stabilization
- Cardiopulmonary monitoring and support
- Vasopressors or inotropes if indicated
- EKG, echocardiogram, cardiac catheterization
- Intra-aortic balloon pump, ventricular assist device

Admission Criteria
- Hemodynamic compromise
- Arrhythmia
- Uncorrected high blood pressure
- Acute myocardial ischemia
- Severe infection
- Syncope

Discharge Criteria
- Hemodynamically stable
- Medical workup completed
- Outpatient medication plan and follow-up arranged

 ## ONGOING CARE

FOLLOW-UP RECOMMENDATIONS
Regular follow up for at least 3 years due to possible recurrence

DIET
Salt restriction with heart failure

PATIENT EDUCATION
- Most cases are expected to resolve without severe morbidity or mortality.
- Follow-up for as long as 3 years may be required.
- Adhere to medication and diet plan to avoid worsening of heart failure.

PROGNOSIS
- Spontaneous improvement in 50–57%
- 3- to 5-year survival of 56–83%
- Acute fulminant presentation: 93% survival at 11 years
- Acute nonfulminant presentation: 45% survival at 11 years (4)

COMPLICATIONS
- If previous history of myocarditis or idiopathic cardiomyopathy, may have chronic myocardial persistence of virus leading to progressive left ventricular deterioration
- Up to 50% develop dilated cardiomyopathy.

REFERENCES
1. Freedman SB, Haladyn JK, Floh A, et al. Pediatric myocarditis: emergency department clinical findings and diagnostic evaluation. *Pediatrics*. 2007;120: 1278–85.
2. Magnani JW, Dec GW et al. Myocarditis: current trends in diagnosis and treatment. *Circulation*. 2006;113:876–90.
3. Cooper LT et al. Myocarditis. *N Engl J Med*. 2009;360:1526–38.
4. Dennert R, Crijns HJ, Heymans S et al. Acute viral myocarditis. *Eur Heart J*. 2008;
5. Hunt SA, Abraham WT, Chin MH, et al. American College of Cardiology/American Heart Association 2005 Guideline Update for the Diagnosis and Management of Chronic Heart Failure in the Adult. *Circulation*. 2005;112:e154–235.

ADDITIONAL READING
Jessup M, Abraham WT, Casey DE, Feldman MA. 2009 focused update: ACCF/AHA Guidelines for the Diagnosis and Management of Heart Failure in Adults. *Circulation*. 2009;119:1977–2016.

CODES

ICD9
- 429.0 Myocarditis, unspecified
- 422.90 Acute myocarditis, unspecified
- 422.91 Idiopathic myocarditis

CLINICAL PEARLS
- Most patients recover with only supportive care; however, unresolved disease may lead to chronic dilated cardiomyopathy with high risk of increased morbidity and mortality.
- Endomyocardial biopsy should be reserved for high-risk presentations and/or where it is suspected the information may change management.
- General heart failure treatment guidelines are applicable to patients with heart failure due to myocarditis.

M

NARCISSISTIC PERSONALITY DISORDER

Lawrence E. Udom, MD, MPH

 BASICS

DESCRIPTION
- A personality disorder (PD) is best understood as a disorganization of the capacity for affect regulation, mediated by dysfunction in early attachments.
- Narcissism is characterized as a Cluster B PD. It is defined as an enduring pattern of inflexible and maladaptive behaviors/traits that cause either significant impairment in social or occupational functioning or subjective distress. The features of narcissistic personality disorder (NPD) are a pervasive pattern of grandiosity (in fantasy or behavior), need for admiration, and lack of empathy beginning by early adulthood and present in a variety of contexts (see Diagnosis).

EPIDEMIOLOGY
Incidence
- Predominant age: Early adulthood
- Predominant sex: Male > Female (50–75%)

Prevalence
The lifetime prevalence rate is ~0.5–1% among the general population; however, the estimated prevalence in clinical settings is ~2–16%.

ETIOLOGY
It is postulated that NPD (and all PDs) result from an impairment in the quality of the interpersonal relationship with the primary caregiver. This leads to dysregulation in affect and subsequent inability to achieve homeostasis after a traumatic (or perceived traumatic) event. Through secure attachments, an infant learns how to balance the sympathetic hyperarousal (fight or flight) that occurs in response to a threat with the homeostasis-restoring parasympathetic response. Insecure attachments will leave the infant with an inability to balance the 2 states, causing him to have hyperarousal in response to a threat or the production of an inadequate parasympathetic response. Secure attachments lead to development of the building blocks needed to self-regulate later in life.

COMMONLY ASSOCIATED CONDITIONS
- It's been noted that having a personality disorder during the formative years increases the individual's risk of developing mood disorders, anxiety, substance abuse, or exhibiting self-harm behaviors in adult life.
- Bipolar disorder
- Depression
- Obsessive-compulsive disorder
- Substance abuse

DIAGNOSIS

HISTORY
- Must rule out other general medical conditions or other psychiatric illnesses; it has been suggested that the disorder has 2 subgroups, the better-known grandiose subgroup and the hypervigilant subgroup (1).
- Grandiose subgroup (essential features):
  - Superiority: Grandiose sense of self-importance. These individuals exaggerate achievements and talents to the point of lying; they demand to be recognized as superior without commensurate achievements.
  - Grandiose fantasies and preoccupation with beauty, brilliance, ideal love, power, or unlimited success
  - Uniqueness: Possess the belief of being special and unique, and can only be understood by or can only associate with people of high status
  - Requires excessive admiration
  - Sense of entitlement: Possesses unreasonable expectation of being treated with favor or expecting an automatic compliance with their wishes. They will use others to achieve their goals.
  - Lack of empathy: These individuals are unable or unwilling to identify with or acknowledge the feelings and needs of others.
  - Envy: These individuals believe that others are envious of them or are envious of others.
  - Exhibit arrogant or haughty attitudes/behaviors
  - High achievement: These individuals often have periods of success (e.g., academic, employment, or social), which may only serve to verify their sense of superiority.
  - This grandiose subtype presents the grandiose self to be admired, envied, and appreciated to combat feelings of devaluation and shame felt by the weaker internalized self.
- Hypervigilant subtype (essential features):
  - Easily hurt, overly sensitive, and ashamed
  - This subtype, rather than fighting devaluation and shame, is consumed with it and defends against it by seeing others as their unjust abusers (1,2).

DIAGNOSTIC TESTS & INTERPRETATION
Patients can be evaluated for NPD using the Diagnostic Interview for Narcissism (3)[A].

DIFFERENTIAL DIAGNOSIS
- Other PDs are often confused with NPD due to their common features (4):
  - Histrionic, antisocial, and borderline PDs also possess the indifferent, callous, and often needy characteristics. NPD can be distinguished by the grandiosity characteristic.
  - The relative stability of self-image as well as the relative lack of self-destructiveness, impulsivity, and abandonment concerns also help to distinguish NPD from borderline PD.
  - Borderline, histrionic, and NPD individuals require attention; however, NPD individuals require that attention to be admiring.
  - Individuals with antisocial and NPD tend to be self-centered, superficial, exploitative, and unempathetic. However, individuals with NPD do not necessarily show characteristics of impulsivity, aggression, and deceit, and usually do not give the same history of conduct disorder or criminal behavior.
  - Individuals with both NPD and obsessive-compulsive PD have a goal of perfectionism and believe that others cannot do things as well. But NPD individuals often believe that they have achieved perfection.
  - NPD individuals may exhibit suspiciousness and social withdrawal similar to schizotypal or paranoid PD; however, when present with NPD, these emotions are usually derived from fears of having their imperfections or flaws revealed.
- Traumatic brain injury
- Central nervous system tumor/infection
- Dementia
- Delirium
- Substance abuse: NPD also must be distinguished from symptoms that may develop in association with chronic substance use (e.g., cocaine-related disorder).

Geriatric Considerations
Exacerbated by aging due to the inability to adapt to the physical, mental, and occupational restrictions age imposes, leading to depression

TREATMENT

MEDICATION
- Individuals with NPD are vulnerable to severe depression, particularly when their superiority is challenged or with maladaptation to the effects of aging.
- Antidepressant medication may be needed:
  - Selective serotonin reuptake inhibitors (SSRIs) have been used to reduce target symptoms of interpersonal reactivity (5)[B].

ADDITIONAL TREATMENT
General Measures
- Individual and group psychotherapy is offered for NPD, with only anecdotal reports of success. Regardless of the modality the goals should be to engage the patient, establish methods of crisis stabilization, and solidify the importance of long-term counselling. The different forms of therapy available are:
  - Psychodynamic therapy, to increase reflective capacity and emotional and interpersonal understanding (6)[A]
  - Cognitive-behavioral therapy, designed to alter dysfunctional core beliefs (6)[A]
  - Dialectical behavioral therapy (6)[A]
  - Therapeutic community, used to effect attitudinal and behavioral change (6)[A]
  - Cognitive-analytic therapy, designed to achieve greater self-understanding (6)[B]
  - Behavioral therapy, designed to improve maladaptive behaviors (6)[C]
- Individuals with NPD usually come for therapy with presenting issues other than the aforementioned diagnostic features—most often for depression and anxiety (7).
- They often see the difficulties that they have with others as external and independent of their behavior. Their depression is often precipitated by situations that challenge the narcissistic grandiosity and reflects the discrepancy between NPD expectations or fantasies and reality.
- Individuals with NPD may have trouble entering treatment because they associate needing help as demeaning and unacceptable.
- If the situation becomes severe enough, however, they will seek treatment in order to reestablish feelings of superiority and achievement.

- Therapy is often complicated by narcissists' view of themselves. Their past, their current situation, and what they need from treatment all will be distorted by their need for acknowledgment of their superiority. They will resist feedback and may reject treatment if they are not sufficiently affirmed:
  - NPDs chronically devalue those around them and demonstrate little empathy, thereby setting up potential countertransference situations with health care providers.
  - The return to comfort for individuals with NPD may be all they are seeking, and they will leave treatment prematurely.
  - Treatment also can be complicated by concomitant depression.
- Treatment can fail in terms of psychotherapy when consideration of possible substance abuse is ignored.

Issues for Referral
- Refer for individual or group therapy, if the patient is willing.
- May need a psychiatrist for associated severe depression

 ONGOING CARE

PATIENT EDUCATION
The National Institute of Mental Health (NIMH) at http://www.nimh.nih.gov

PROGNOSIS
The prognosis for an adult suffering from NPD is poor, although the person's adaptation to situations and relationships can improve with treatment.

COMPLICATIONS
- Family and relationship dysfunction
- Alcohol and other substance abuse. No single pattern of substance use or abuse can be identified for NPD; however, cocaine, as a high-status drug, is particularly attractive to the narcissist.
- Major depressive disorder
- Dysthymia
- Obsessive-compulsive behaviors
- Eating disorders (particularly in young women)

REFERENCES

1. Gabbard GO. Two subtypes of narcissistic personality disorder. *Bull Menninger Clin.* 1989;53:527–32.
2. Ronningstam E, Gunderson J. Identifying criteria for narcissistic personality disorder. *Am J Psychiatry.* 1990;147:918–22.
3. Gunderson JG, Ronningstam E, Bodkin A. The diagnostic interview for narcissistic patients. *Arch Gen Psychiatry.* 1990;47:676–80.
4. American Psychiatric Association. *DSM-IV-TR 2000: Diagnostic & Statistical Manual of Mental Disorders,* 4th ed. Washington, DC: American Psychiatric Publishing, 2000.
5. Sperry L. *Handbook of Diagnosis and Treatment of the DSM-IV Personality Disorders.* New York: Brunner/Mazel, 1995.
6. Bateman A, et al. Psychological treatment for personality disorders. *Adv Psychiatr Treat.* 2004;10:378–88.
7. Beck AT, et al. *Cognitive Therapy of Personality Disorders.* New York: Guilford, 1990.

ADDITIONAL READING
- Brunton JN, Lacey JH, Waller G. Narcissism and eating characteristics in young nonclinical women. *J Nerv Ment Dis.* 2005;193:140–3.
- Fonagy P, et al. Morality, disruptive behavior, borderline personality disorder, crime, and their relationship to security of attachment. In: Atkinson L, et al., eds. *Attachment and Psychopathology.* New York: Guilford, 1997:233–77.

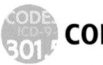 **CODES**

ICD9
301.81 Narcissistic personality disorder

CLINICAL PEARLS
- The relative stability of self-image as well as the lack of self-destructiveness, impulsivity, and abandonment concerns help to distinguish NPD from borderline PD.
- Borderline, histrionic, and NPD patients all require attention; however, NPD individuals require that attention to be admiring.
- Individuals with NPD and obsessive-compulsive PD have a goal of perfectionism and believe that others cannot do things as well, but NPD individuals often believe that they have achieved perfection.
- Individuals with NPD are vulnerable to severe depression, particularly when their superiority is challenged or with maladaptation to the effects of aging. Antidepressant medications such as SSRIs may be useful.

N

NARCOLEPSY

Jeffrey F. Minteer, MD

BASICS

DESCRIPTION
- Disorder of unknown etiology characterized by excessive daytime sleepiness typically associated with cataplexy (sudden bilateral weakness of skeletal muscles) and other rapid eye movement (REM) sleep phenomena, such as sleep paralysis and hypnagogic hallucinations
- Commonly misconceived as representing low intelligence and/or poor motivation
- Frequently overlooked disorder with an average of 15 years of symptoms prior to diagnosis
- System(s) affected: Nervous

EPIDEMIOLOGY
Incidence
- Onset usually in teenage years
- Bimodal distribution peak at 15 and 36 years of age
- Predominant sex: Male = Female
- Incidence of 0.05% in the general population
- 0.74/100,000 person-years

Pediatric Considerations
Uncommon in childhood

Prevalence
25–50/100,000

RISK FACTORS
- Head trauma
- CNS infectious disease
- Anesthesia
- Psychological stress
- Pregnancy
- Family history
- High body mass index (BMI)

Genetics
- Increased incidence in families with positive history: 1–2% in 1st-degree relative of index case (10× the general population)
- Twin concordance 25–31% (suggests environmental contribution)
- 85–95% of patients with narcoplexy and cataplexy have biologic human leukocyte antigen (HLA) DQB1*0602, 40% narcolepsy without cataplexy, and 24% general population
- Autosomal recessive inheritance pattern
- 12% of Asians, 25% of whites, and 38% of African Americans are gene carriers.

ETIOLOGY
- Unknown
- Associated with loss of the neurotransmitter hypocretin-1 in CNS
- 85% of patients with narcolepsy and cataplexy have low hypocretin in CSF.
- Possible involvement of immune system and environmental influences

COMMONLY ASSOCIATED CONDITIONS
Obstructive sleep apnea, obesity, anxiety

DIAGNOSIS

HISTORY
- Classic tetrad of excessive daytime sleepiness, cataplexy, sleep paralysis, and hypnagogic hallucinations (4 most common symptoms): Only 10–20% of patients have all 4 symptoms.
- Two general forms:
  – Narcolepsy without cataplexy 40%
  – Narcolepsy with cataplexy 60%
- Excessive daytime sleepiness and sleep attacks:
  – Primary symptom and required for diagnosis
  – Instantaneous, irresistible REM sleep
  – First and most disabling symptom
  – Tendency to take naps lasting 5–10 minutes
  – Episodes last minutes to hours
  – 1–8 naps per day but 24-h duration of sleep is normal
  – Associated with dreaming
  – Nap restores wakefulness for several hours
  – More likely to happen in monotonous, warm environment, after a large meal, or with strong emotions
- Cataplexy: Auxiliary symptom (60%)
  – Pathognomonic if present
  – Sudden bilateral weakness of skeletal muscles
  – Provocation by sudden strong wave of emotion
  – Consciousness and memory are not impaired.
  – Short duration (less than a few minutes)
  – Can be limited to a particular muscle group (e.g., jaw droop with inability to speak; arm, neck, or leg weakness)
- Sleep paralysis: Auxiliary symptom (50%)
  – When falling asleep or on awakening, patient wants to but cannot move, but this can end abruptly when the patients is touched or spoken to.
  – Brain wakes from sleep while body remains in REM sleep.
  – Lasts seconds to minutes
  – Patients are aware of events around them but cannot open eyes or move.
  – Can be preceded by hallucinatory phenomena
  – 50% of normal population have ≥1 episodes (so this symptom is nonspecific).
- Hypnagogic hallucinations: Auxiliary symptom (60%):
  – Vivid, frightening visual or auditory illusions or hallucinations at onset of sleep
  – Dreamlike experiences that occur during wakefulness or suddenly at sleep onset
  – Characteristic hallucinations include seeing human or animal faces or feeling that someone else is in the room.
  – Hallucinations also can be auditory.
- Disturbed nocturnal sleep (66%):
  – Normal total sleep with decreased sleep efficiency
  – More frequent transitions from wakefulness to sleep
  – Retrograde amnesic and automatic behavior lasting minutes to hours
  – Increased periodic leg movements (50%)
  – Depression (18–37%)
  – Automatic behavior: Activity without memory of the event

PHYSICAL EXAM
- A complete exam is useful to rule out other causes of hypersomnia.
- If cataplexy is witnessed, examiner will be unable to elicit deep tendon reflexes.

DIAGNOSTIC TESTS & INTERPRETATION
Lab
Follow-Up & Special Considerations
- HLA typing for DQB1 in ambiguous cases
- Low CSF hypocretin-1 level: 99% specificity, 87% sensitivity in patients with cataplexy; especially useful in children unable to do a multiple sleep latency test (MSLT, described below)

Imaging
Initial approach
- Nighttime polysomnography (PSG): Monitoring of patients in a sleep laboratory will usually document fragmented sleep with normal amount of REM sleep but a pattern of sleep-onset REM. PSG is useful to rule out other causes of excessive daytime sleepiness, including sleep apnea syndromes and nocturnal myoclonus.
- MSLT: Begins ≥90 minutes after nighttime test.
  – Patient monitored during 4–5 naps taken at 2-h intervals; rapidity of sleep onset and type of sleep pattern are documented. Supportive test includes mean sleep latency (time to fall asleep) of ≤5 minutes and 1 or more sleep-onset REM periods.
  – Sensitivity 77%, specificity 97%, positive predictive value 73%

Diagnostic Procedures/Surgery
- Diagnostic criteria according to the International Classification of Sleep Disorders
- Minimal criteria is B plus C or A plus D plus E plus G:
  – A. Excessive sleepiness—required
  – B. Recurrent lapses into sleep daily for ≥3 months
  – C. Cataplexy
  – D. Associated features: Sleep paralysis, hypnagogic hallucinations, disrupted sleep
  – E. MSLT abnormalities (as described above)
  – F. Biologic markers (see Genetics)
  – G. Absence of medical or psychiatric disorder
  – H. Low CSF hypocretin-1 level

DIFFERENTIAL DIAGNOSIS
Excessive daytime sleepiness is present in 4% of the general population, although most individuals are not narcoleptic. Possible etiologies include
- Sleep apnea syndromes (40–50% of those with excessive somnolence)
- Epileptic seizures and syncope
- Idiopathic CNS hypersomnolence (5–10% of those with excessive somnolence)
- Nocturnal myoclonus
- Psychomotor seizures
- Recurrent hypersomnia that lasts days–weeks and recurs months later
- Hypersomnia related to a medical condition such as Parkinson disease

TREATMENT

MEDICATION

First Line

- Excessive daytime sleepiness:
  - Modafinil (Provigil):
    - Structurally distinct from amphetamines
    - 200–400 mg/d; start with 100 mg/d and increase over 3–4 days (1)[A].
    - 1st-line treatment
    - Half-life 14 h, so can dose daily
  - Armodafinil (Nuvigil)
    - Enantiomeric form of modafinil with slightly longer half-life of 15 h
    - 150–250 mg every morning
  - Sodium oxybate (Xyrem):
    - 2.5–9 mg; may take 3 months to achieve full response
    - Preferred treatment for narcolepsy with cataplexy and disturbed nocturnal sleep
    - Give half dose at bedtime and half dose 4 h later; date rape drug with abuse potential (1)[A]
    - Can use with modafinil in severe cases
    - May worsen sleep disordered breathing in patients with obstructive sleep apnea
- Cataplexy:
  - Sodium oxybate: See above.
  - Selegiline: Selective monoamine oxidase B (MAO-B) inhibitor; anticataplectic effective for excessive daytime sleepiness; 20–40 mg/d divided morning and noon (1)[B]
  - Amphetamines:
    - Methylphenidate (Ritalin): Initial dose 30 mg/d divided b.i.d. or t.i.d.; maximum dose 100 mg/d (1)[B], short-acting
    - Dextroamphetamine: Initial dose 15 mg/d divided b.i.d. or t.i.d.; maximum dose 100 mg/d (1)[B]
    - Combination regimen of long- and short-acting medicines: Pemoline plus single or multiple doses of methylphenidate
- Auxiliary symptoms (e.g., cataplexy (2)[C], hypnagogic hallucination, sleep paralysis (2)[C]):
  - Antidepressants suppress REM sleep.
    - Imipramine: 75–150 mg/d
    - Protriptyline: 10–40 mg/d
    - Clomipramine: 150–250 mg/d
    - Fluoxetine: 20–60 mg/d
    - Venlafaxine: 75–150 mg b.i.d.
  - Although often used, quality evidence is lacking to demonstrate improvement in cataplexy symptoms from antidepressants (2)[A].
- Contraindications: Stimulants in hypertensive patients
- Precautions:
  - Amphetamines:
    - If patient develops tolerance to stimulants, switch drugs rather than increase dose; there is little cross-tolerance.
    - Headaches, irritability, hypertension (HTN), psychosis, anorexia, habituation, rebound hypersomnia
    - Pemoline: Fewer cardiovascular side effects, longer acting, liver toxicity, little abuse potential
  - Other:
    - Imipramine: Dry mouth, sedation, urinary retention, impotence
    - Modafinil: Less rebound hypersomnia; may become drug of choice; does not affect BP;

tolerance limited, best if initial treatment; does not treat cataplexy; main side effect is headache, increased metabolism of oral contraceptives (so use 50-μg pill)
    - Selegiline: Doses >20 mg require low-tyramine diet because drug begins to lose selectivity.
    - Patient may develop tolerance to anticataplectic effect of tricyclic antidepressants (TCAs) and can get a rebound of cataplexy when drug is withdrawn.
- Significant possible interactions: Combination of TCAs and stimulants can lead to significant HTN.

Second Line

- Excessive daytime sleepiness:
  - Amphetamines:
    - Methylphenidate (Ritalin): Initial dose 30 mg/d divided b.i.d. or t.i.d.; maximum dose 100 mg/d (1)[B], short acting, most potent amphetamine available
    - Dextroamphetamine: Initial dose 15 mg/d divided b.i.d. or t.i.d.; maximum dose 100 mg/d (1)[B]
  - Selegiline: Selective MAO-B inhibitor; anticataplectic effective for excessive daytime sleepiness; 20–40 mg/d divided morning and noon (1)[B]
- Auxiliary symptoms (e.g., cataplexy (2)[C], hypnagogic hallucination, sleep paralysis (2)[C]):
- Antidepressants suppress REM sleep.
  - Fluoxetine: 20–60 mg/d
  - Venlafaxine: 75–150 mg b.i.d.
  - Clomipramine: 150–250 mg/d
- Contraindications: Stimulants in hypertensive patients
- Precautions:
  - Amphetamines:
    - If patient develops tolerance to stimulants, switch drugs rather than increase dose; there is little cross-tolerance.
    - Headaches, irritability, HTN, psychosis, anorexia, habituation, rebound hypersomnia
  - Other:
    - Modafinil: Less rebound hypersomnia; may become drug of choice; does not affect BP; tolerance limited, best if initial treatment; does not treat cataplexy; main side effect is headache, increased metabolism of oral contraceptives (so use 50-μg pill)
    - Selegiline: Doses >20 mg require low-tyramine diet because drug begins to lose selectivity.
  - Patient may develop tolerance to anticataplectic effect of antidepressants and can get a rebound in cataplexy when the drug is withdrawn.

ADDITIONAL TREATMENT

General Measures

- None of the currently available medications enables people with narcolepsy to consistently maintain a fully normal state of alertness.
- Drug therapy should be supplemented by various behavioral strategies.
- Well-timed 20-minute naps may be helpful.
- Avoid sedative drugs.
- Use safety precautions, particularly when driving. People with untreated narcoleptic symptoms are involved in automobile accidents roughly 10× more frequently than the general population. However, accident rates are normal among patients who have received appropriate medication therapy.

Issues for Referral

- Unresponsive to primary medications
- Patient support groups can be very beneficial.

ONGOING CARE

FOLLOW-UP RECOMMENDATIONS

Patient Monitoring

- Frequent BP checks
- Follow up every 6 months

DIET

Selegiline: Doses >20 mg require low-tyramine diet because drug begins to lose selectivity.

PATIENT EDUCATION

- Narcolepsy information from the National Institute of Neurological Disorders and Stroke at http://www.ninds.nih.gov/disorders/narcolepsy/narcolepsy.htm
- Narcolepsy Network, Inc., 79 Main Street, North Kingstown, RI 02852; e-mail: narnet@narcolepsynetwork.org; Web site: http://www.narcolepsynetwork.org

PROGNOSIS

- Lifelong disease
- Symptoms can worsen with aging.
- In women, symptoms can improve after menopause.

REFERENCES

1. Mohsenin V et al. Narcolepsy—master of disguise: evidence-based recommendations for management. Postgrad Med. 2009;121:99–104.
2. Vignatelli L, D'Alessandro R, Candelise L. Antidepressant drugs for narcolepsy. Cochrane Database Syst Rev. 2008;CD003724.

ADDITIONAL READING

- Dauvilliers Y, Arnulf I, Mignot E. Narcolepsy with cataplexy. Lancet. 2007;369:499–511.
- Morgenthaler T, Alessi C, Friedman L et al. Practice parameters for the use of actigraphy in the assessment of sleep and sleep disorders: an update for 2007. Sleep. 2007;30:519–29.
- Nishino S, Mignot E. Drug treatment of patients with insomnia and excessive daytime sleepiness: pharmacokinetic considerations. Clin Pharmacokinet. 1999;37:305–30.
- Wise MS, Arand DL, Auger RR et al. Treatment of narcolepsy and other hypersomnias of central origin. Sleep. 2007;30:1712–27.

CODES

ICD9

- 347.00 Narcolepsy without cataplexy
- 347.01 Narcolepsy with cataplexy

CLINICAL PEARLS

- Narcolepsy is a frequently missed disorder with an average of 15 years of symptoms before a definitive diagnosis is made (1)[A].
- The classic tetrad of symptoms includes excessive daytime sleepiness, cataplexy, sleep paralysis, and hypnagogic hallucinations.
- The International Classification of Sleep Disorders has specific diagnostic criteria for narcolepsy.
- Medications are helpful but not curative.

N

NASAL POLYPS

Sam Seung Yeol Kim, MBBS, Mmed

 BASICS

DESCRIPTION
- Chronic inflammatory lesion of nasal mucosa
- Appearance of edematous pedunculated mass in the nasal cavity or paranasal sinus
- Often causes symptoms of blockage, discharge, or loss of smell
- Often bilateral; suspect tumor such as inverted papilloma if unilateral

EPIDEMIOLOGY
Incidence
- Estimated to be ~1–4% in adults
- Much rarer in children: ~0.1%
- Increases with age

Prevalence
- Estimated to be ~2–4% in general population
- Predominant sex: Female > Male (2:1)

RISK FACTORS
- Chronic sinusitis
- Allergic fungal sinusitis
- Cystic fibrosis
- Churg-Strauss syndrome
- Primary ciliary dyskinesia (Kartagener syndrome)

GENERAL PREVENTION
The effectiveness of prophylactic intranasal corticosteroid after polyp removal surgery is being evaluated (1).

PATHOPHYSIOLOGY
Largely unknown

ETIOLOGY
Largely unknown

COMMONLY ASSOCIATED CONDITIONS
- Bronchial asthma: Common
- Aspirin hypersensitivity: Common
- Primary ciliary dyskinesia

DIAGNOSIS

HISTORY
- Nasal obstruction/restricted nasal airflow: Persistent mouth breathing
- Nasal discharge:
  – Rhinorrhea
  – Postnasal drip
- Reduction/loss of smell
- Dull headaches
- Facial pain/discomfort
- Symptoms of acute, recurrent, or chronic rhinosinusitis

PHYSICAL EXAM
- Anterior rhinoscopy looking for a pale translucent mass of tissue:
  – Most commonly from lateral wall of middle meatus
  – Otoscope with nasal speculum or even otologic speculum is typically used.
- Flexible or rigid endoscopy is required to fully assess the nasal cavity. Topical anesthesia nasal spray should be used prior to the endoscopy if patient is awake.
- Middle ear examination for eustachian tube dysfunction secondary to large posterior nasal polyps
- Examination of posterior pharynx via oral cavity for large posterior polyps

DIAGNOSTIC TESTS & INTERPRETATION
Lab
Initial lab tests
- Allergy test:
  – Skin prick test
  – Radioallergosorbent test
- Testing for cystic fibrosis in children with multiple benign polyps: Sweat test: Often requires repeat tests

Imaging
Initial approach
Computed tomography (CT) scanning may be helpful occasionally: Corroborates history and endoscopic findings

Diagnostic Procedures/Surgery
Diagnosis is made by the combination of rhinoscopy, endoscopy, and CT scanning.

Pathological Findings
- Ciliated pseudostratified columnar epithelium: With areas of transitional or squamous epithelium
- Chronic infiltration of inflammatory cells
- Eosinophils are the predominant cells in most patients.
- Lower density of goblet cells than in normal epithelium

DIFFERENTIAL DIAGNOSIS
- Antrochoanal polyp
- Benign or malignant tumor:
  – Papilloma
  – Intranasal glioma
  – Encephalocele
  – Rhabdomyosarcoma

TREATMENT

MEDICATION

First Line

Intranasal corticosteroids:

- 400 μg/d in either spray or powder form:
  - Budesonide (1,2)[A]
  - Beclomethasone dipropionate (3)[B]
  - Fluticasone dipropionate (4,5)[A]
- 200 μg b.i.d.: Mometasone furoate (6,7)[A]

- Treatment generally should continue for at least 12 weeks.
- Minor nose bleeding is the most common side effect.
- Side effects from systemic absorption are rare (8).

Second Line

Oral systemic corticosteroids: Prednisolone 50 mg × 2 weeks (9)[B]

ADDITIONAL TREATMENT

Additional Therapies

Aspirin desensitization may have a role in reducing recurrence of nasal polyposis (10)[C].

SURGERY/OTHER PROCEDURES

- Most surgeries are approached endonasally. External (Caldwell-Luc) approach carries higher risk of complications (11)[C].
- Functional endonasal sinus surgery has slightly lower recurrence rate than intranasal polypectomy (12)[C]. Both modalities are equally effective in symptom relief.
- Up to 20% of patients will require revision surgery regardless of the initial modality of surgery (13)[C].
- Postoperative use of nasal corticosteroid may delay the recurrence of nasal polyps and hence timing of revision surgery (14)[B].

 ONGOING CARE

COMPLICATIONS

- Acute or chronic sinus infection
- Obstructive sleep apnea

REFERENCES

1. Lildholdt T, Rundcrantz H, Lindqvist N. Efficacy of topical corticosteroid powder for nasal polyps: a double-blind, placebo-controlled study of budesonide. *Clin Otolaryngol Allied Sci*. 1995;20: 26–30.
2. Tos M, Svendstrup F, Arndal H, et al. Efficacy of an aqueous and a powder formulation of nasal budesonide compared in patients with nasal polyps. *Am J Rhinol*. 1998;12:183–9.
3. Holmberg K, Juliusson S, Balder B, et al. Fluticasone propionate aqueous nasal spray in the treatment of nasal polyposis. *Ann Allergy Asthma Immunol*. 1997;78:270–6.
4. Penttilä M, Poulsen P, Hollingworth K, et al. Dose-related efficacy and tolerability of fluticasone propionate nasal drops 400 microg once daily and twice daily in the treatment of bilateral nasal polyposis: a placebo-controlled randomized study in adult patients. *Clin Exp Allergy*. 2000;30:94–102.
5. Aukema AA, Mulder PG, Fokkens WJ. Treatment of nasal polyposis and chronic rhinosinusitis with fluticasone propionate nasal drops reduces need for sinus surgery. *J Allergy Clin Immunol*. 2005;115:1017–23.
6. Small CB, Hernandez J, Reyes A, et al. Efficacy and safety of mometasone furoate nasal spray in nasal polyposis. *J Allergy Clin Immunol*. 2005;116: 1275–81.
7. Stjärne P, Mösges R, Jorissen M, et al. A randomized controlled trial of mometasone furoate nasal spray for the treatment of nasal polyposis. *Arch Otolaryngol Head Neck Surg*. 2006;132:179–85.
8. Bateman ND, Fahy C, Woolford TJ. Nasal polyps: still more questions than answers. *J Laryngol Otol*. 2003;117:1–9.
9. Hissaria P, Smith W, Wormald PJ, et al. Short course of systemic corticosteroids in sinonasal polyposis: a double-blind, randomized, placebo-controlled trial with evaluation of outcome measures. *J Allergy Clin Immunol*. 2006;118:128–33.
10. Stevenson DD, Hankammer MA, Mathison DA, et al. Aspirin desensitization treatment of aspirin-sensitive patients with rhinosinusitis-asthma: long-term outcomes. *J Allergy Clin Immunol*. 1996;98:751–8.
11. DeFreitas J, Lucente FE. The Caldwell-Luc procedure: institutional review of 670 cases: 1975–1985. *Laryngoscope*. 1988;98:1297–300.
12. Hopkins C, Browne JP, Slack R, et al. The national comparative audit of surgery for nasal polyposis and chronic rhinosinusitis. *Clin Otolaryngol*. 2006;31:390–8.
13. Hopkins C, Slack R, Lund V, Brown P, Copley L, Browne J et al. Long-term outcomes from the English national comparative audit of surgery for nasal polyposis and chronic rhinosinusitis. *Laryngoscope*. 2009;119:2459–65.
14. Stjärne P, Olsson P, Alenius M. Use of mometasone furoate to prevent polyp relapse after endoscopic sinus surgery. *Arch Otolaryngol Head Neck Surg*. 2009;135:296–302.

 CODES

ICD9
471.9 Unspecified nasal polyp

CLINICAL PEARLS

- Appearance of edematous pedunculated mass in the nasal cavity or paranasal sinus
- Use of intranasal corticosteroids for 12 weeks is 1st-line of treatment; oral prednisolone also may be used.

N

NEAR DROWNING

Mia D. Sorcinelli, MD

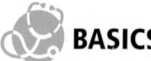 **BASICS**

DESCRIPTION
- Multisystem, potentially fatal disease resulting from near suffocation secondary to submersion of a person's face or head in a liquid
- A form of acute respiratory distress syndrome (ARDS) with neurologic complications
- System(s) affected: Cardiovascular; Nervous; Pulmonary; Renal

EPIDEMIOLOGY
Incidence
- 3,237 deaths in US in 2007
- 54 infants accidentally drowned in US in 2007
- 4,321 near drownings in US in 2007; actual number likely much higher due to underreporting
- 2nd leading cause of injury-related death (after automobile crashes) in US children 1–12 years of age in 2006
- Predominant age: Teenagers and toddlers
- Predominant sex: Male > Female

Prevalence
- Drowning was the 6th leading cause of accidental death for all ages in the US in 2006.
- For every child under age 15 who dies from drowning, 5 more children are seen in the emergency room for nonfatal submersion injuries.

ALERT
Proper water safety techniques may help to avoid this problem.

RISK FACTORS
- Alcohol ingestion
- Seizure disorder
- Inability to swim
- Hyperventilation prior to underwater swimming
- Improper pool fencing
- Inadequate adult supervision of children
- Cardiac arrhythmias: Familial long QT and familial polymorphic ventricular tachycardia (VT)
- Living in sunbelt states
- Adolescents: May be intoxicated or using drugs
- Adults: Most near-drownings are associated with boating accidents ± alcohol

GENERAL PREVENTION
- Proper adult supervision of children
- Knowledge of water safety guidelines
- Mandatory pool fencing and pool alarms
- Fences higher than 54 in. (137 cm) for home pools
- Avoidance of alcohol or recreational drugs around water
- Swimming instruction at an early age
- Cardiopulmonary resuscitation (CPR) instruction for pool owners, parents
- Boating safety knowledge
- Personal flotation device (such as a preserver if necessary)

Pediatric Considerations
Children should never be left alone near water. Young children can drown in very small amounts of water such as in bathtubs, buckets, and toilets.

PATHOPHYSIOLOGY
Hypoxemia and acidosis cause most of the physiologic problems.

ETIOLOGY
- Swimming accidents: Head trauma while swimming; hyperventilation before underwater swimming
- Bathtub and bucket drowning in children <1 year of age
- Pool drowning in children 1–4 years of age
- Drug or alcohol overdose
- Boating mishaps, water sports, scuba diving
- Motor vehicle accidents (e.g., automobile submerged in water)
- Suicide

COMMONLY ASSOCIATED CONDITIONS
- Cardiopulmonary arrest before submersion
- Trauma, especially to the head, causing altered mental status
- Seizure disorder
- Alcohol or drug overdose
- Hypothermia

 DIAGNOSIS

HISTORY
- Victim found in or near water
- Water temperature may be important, although no conclusive evidence exists
- Look for signs of trauma.

PHYSICAL EXAM
- Level of consciousness: Altered or comatose
- Absent or weak pulse
- Tachypnea or agonal respirations, cough
- Cyanosis
- Wheezing
- Abdominal distension
- Hypothermia
- Poorly reactive, dilated, and fixed pupils
- Poor peripheral perfusion
- Rectal temperature

DIAGNOSTIC TESTS & INTERPRETATION
Lab
Initial lab tests
- Arterial blood gases (ABGs): Hypoxia, hypercarbia
- Electrolytes: Hypokalemia, hyponatremia (especially freshwater), hypernatremia (especially saltwater)
- Blood glucose: Increased levels may impair neurologic recovery after ischemic brain injury.
- Urea, creatinine, total creatinine kinase
- Urinalysis: Rare oliguria, albuminuria
- Coagulation studies
- Complete blood count (CBC) with differential
- Blood cultures for critically ill patients
- Tracheal aspirate cultures recommended by some sources for patients with pneumonia or intubated patients.
- Toxicology for drug overdoses
- Any underlying condition that may alter normal fluid and electrolyte balance can affect lab results (e.g., congestive heart failure [CHF]) or alter normal pulmonary function (e.g., emphysema).

Follow-Up & Special Considerations
Serum electrolyte monitoring

Imaging
Initial approach
CXR may show pulmonary edema, consolidation from aspiration, atelectasis, or pneumothorax.

Follow-Up & Special Considerations
Repeat CXR may raise suspicion for pneumonia.

Diagnostic Procedures/Surgery
- Central venous pressure (CVP) monitoring
- ECG
- EEG if question of seizure as cause

Pathological Findings
- "Dry lungs": ~10% of victims drown without aspiration; may be due to prolonged laryngospasm, but some controversy exists
- "Wet drowning": 80–90% of victims show aspiration of water, sand, and mud into lungs.
- Loss of normal pulmonary architecture occurs with both fresh- and saltwater aspiration.
- Loss of surfactant, with alveolar consolidation, atelectasis, hyaline membrane formation, development of intrapulmonary right-to-left shunting
- Increased lung weight and intraalveolar hemorrhages; decreased lung compliance
- Pneumonia, abscess, and acute respiratory distress syndrome (ARDS) in those who survive only a few hours or days
- Cardiac: Low cardiac index, elevated right- and left-sided heart filling pressures, elevated systemic and pulmonary vascular resistance
- Renal: Acute tubular necrosis from hypoxemia, shock, hemoglobinuria, myoglobinuria
- Neurologic: Hypoxia followed by ischemia, infarctions in "watershed" areas, damage especially to hippocampus, insular cortex, basal ganglia

DIFFERENTIAL DIAGNOSIS
Head trauma, arrhythmia, seizure, alcohol or other substance overdose

 TREATMENT

Immediate reversal of hypoxemia should form the foundation of any treatment plan. Anticipate the need for critical care and a tertiary medical center in advance, and plan accordingly.

MEDICATION
First Line
- For bronchospasm: Aerosolized bronchodilator (1)[C]: Albuterol (Proventil, Ventolin) 3 mL of 0.083% solution or 0.5 mL of 0.5% solution diluted in 3 mL saline
- Patients who develop pneumonia: Appropriate antibiotic based on sputum or endotracheal lavage culture (2)[A]
- Prophylactic antibiotics and steroids are not helpful (2)[B].

Second Line
Pressors as needed for resulting sepsis

ADDITIONAL TREATMENT
General Measures
- Never approach a struggling victim alone.
- Start with the basics: Airway, breathing, circulation (ABC's).
- Initiate rescue breathing while still in water if possible (1).
- Remove from water quickly and place in normal CPR position (1).
- Avoid abdominal thrusting unless obvious foreign body is present (1).
- Use cricoid pressure to limit aspiration (2)[B].
- Routine cervical collar use is not needed unless high suspicion for trauma (2)
- Supplemental oxygen, early intubation as needed (2)[A]
- If patient is breathing on own, place in right lateral decubitus position to prevent aspiration of vomit or gastric contents (1).
- Rough handling of victims of cold-water drowning may increase risk of ventricular fibrillation during resuscitation.

Issues for Referral
Refer severe cases to an intensivist or a trauma specialist.

Additional Therapies
- Oxygen for all patients
- Hypothermia may respond well to immediate rewarming on transport, as well as to cardiopulmonary bypass if patient is severely hypothermic and asystolic (3)[C].
- More research is needed regarding intentional hypothermia in the initial days of treatment for patients, especially children, who underwent hypothermic near-drowning. Ongoing studies eventually may lead to mild therapeutic hypothermia as a cornerstone of therapy in the pediatric population following cardiac arrest of many etiologies (4).
- Some small case studies suggest that in adults and children, particularly after hypothermic near-drowning, combinations of ECMO and extended therapeutic hypothermia (for up to 7 days) can dramatically improve neurologic and pulmonary outcomes (5).

COMPLEMENTARY AND ALTERNATIVE MEDICINE
Core warming with gastric or bladder lavage and/or providing warmed air through a ventilator may be necessary (2)[C].

SURGERY/OTHER PROCEDURES
ICU procedures as warranted for advanced life support

IN-PATIENT CONSIDERATIONS
Initial Stabilization
Airway, breathing, circulation (ABCs)

Admission Criteria
- Hospitalize all patients initially.
- Monitor patients in an ICU setting, except for those few who present to the emergency department in an alert condition without evidence of respiratory compromise.

IV Fluids
To maintain adequate intravascular volume (1)[C]

Nursing
- Bed rest for at least the initial 24 h
- Careful monitoring of neurologic status
- Continuous pulse oximetry monitoring

Discharge Criteria
Patients with Glasgow Coma Scale $\geq$ 13, normal CXR, lack of clinical evidence of respiratory distress, and normal oxygen saturation on room air can be discharged after 8 h of observation (2).

 ONGOING CARE

FOLLOW-UP RECOMMENDATIONS
Appropriate follow-up with orthopedic, neurologic, cardiac, etc., specialists as warranted

Patient Monitoring
- Frequent check of O_2 saturation
- Arterial blood gas (ABG) monitoring (2)
- Pulmonary artery catheter may be needed for hemodynamic monitoring in unstable patients (1)[C].
- Intracranial pressure monitoring in selected patients (1)[C]
- Serum electrolyte determinations (2)

DIET
n.p.o. until mental status normalizes

PATIENT EDUCATION
Reemphasize preventive measures on discharge from hospital. Educate parents, recommend pool safety, etc.

PROGNOSIS
- Patients who are alert or mildly obtunded at the time they present to the hospital have an excellent chance for a full recovery.
- Patients who are comatose or receiving CPR at the time of presentation, or who have dilated and fixed pupils and no spontaneous respiratory activity have a more guarded and often poor prognosis.
- Secondary drowning from neurogenic pulmonary edema may occur within 48 hours of initial presentation.

COMPLICATIONS
- Early:
  - Bronchospasm
  - Vomiting/aspiration
  - Hypoglycemia
  - Hypothermia
  - Seizure
  - Hypovolemia
  - Electrolyte abnormalities
  - Arrhythmia from hypoxia or hypothermia (rarely from electrolyte imbalance)
  - Hypotension
- Late:
  - ARDS
  - Anoxic encephalopathy
  - Pneumonia
  - Lung abscess/empyema
  - Renal failure
  - Coagulopathy
  - Sepsis
  - Barotrauma
  - Seizure

REFERENCES
1. Orlowski JP, Szpilman D. Drowning. Rescue, resuscitation, and reanimation. *Pediatr Clin North Am*. 2001;48:627–46.
2. Salomez F, Vincent JL. Drowning: a review of epidemiology, pathophysiology, treatment and prevention. *Resuscitation*. 2004;63:261–8.
3. Giesbrecht GG, Hayward JS. Problems and complications with cold-water rescue. *Wilderness Environ Med*. 2006;17:26–30.
4. Kochanek PM, Fink EL, Bell MJ et al. Therapeutic Hypothermia: Applications in Pediatric Cardiac Arrest. *J Neurotrauma*. 2009.
5. Guenther U, Varelmann D, Putensen C, Wrigge H et al. Extended therapeutic hypothermia for several days during extracorporeal membrane-oxygenation after drowning and cardiac arrest Two cases of survival with no neurological sequelae. *Resuscitation*. 2009;80:379–81.

ADDITIONAL READING
- American Heart Association Guidelines for Cardiopulmonary Resuscitation and Emergency Cardiovascular Care. Part 10.3: Drowning. *Circulation*. 2005;112(24S):133–5.
- Committee on Injury, Violence, and Poison Prevention, et al. Policy Statement – Prevention of Drowning. *Pediatrics*, 2010.

 CODES

ICD9
994.1 Drowning and nonfatal submersion

CLINICAL PEARLS
- The single most important treatment for near-drowning victims is prompt reversal of hypoxic state. This should form the cornerstone for all other treatment modalities. Without oxygenation, other treatment is futile.
- Family physicians and pediatricians should review water safety tips and guidelines with parents and children at yearly visits. Encourage pool owners and parents with young children to become CPR certified. Prevention of drowning can save many lives each year.
- Despite successful resuscitation, patients are at risk for ARDS due to delayed pulmonary edema that may start hours after their submersion incident. For this reason, careful monitoring of every resuscitated patient is essential.

N

NEPHROPATHY, URATE

Jaspreet Singh, DO

 BASICS

- The water-insoluble nature of uric acid presents a unique problem in the acidic environment of the distal nephron of the kidney. Owing to the lack of the enzyme uricase, which converts uric acid into a more soluble compound, allantoin, the human kidney is more susceptible to the side effects of uric acid crystal deposition.
- There are three different types of renal diseases induced by uric acid or urate crystal deposition:
  – Acute uric acid nephropathy (UAN)
  – Chronic urate nephropathy
  – Uric acid nephrolithiasis

DESCRIPTION
- Renal parenchymal damage and dysfunction associated with disordered uric acid metabolism
- Affects the renal/urologic system; several syndromes may present:
  – Acute UAN: Precipitated by renal tubular obstruction resulting from acute massive elevation of serum uric acid, often owing to cell lysis during induction chemotherapy or radiation; furthermore, crystallization of uric acid or calcium phosphate in renal tubules affects renal function.
  – Uric acid nephrolithiasis: Seen most commonly in patients with underlying hyperuricemia or gout who have abnormally low urine pH owing to low ammonia excretion:
    ○ Frequency of stone formation increases with increasing serum uric acid levels and urinary uric acid excretion rates.
    ○ ~20% of patients with gout will form uric acid stones.
  – Hyperuricemia of chronic renal failure: An early result of chronic renal failure owing to retention of uric acid resulting from decreased tubular secretion or altered postsecretory reabsorption or both; secondary gout occurs in <1% of all patients.
- Chronic urate nephropathy: Renal insufficiency attributed to parenchymal damage secondary to medullary urate deposition; effect of hyperuricemia on development and progression of chronic renal disease in humans is largely unknown. Studies in animals have shown an association between hyperuricemia and intrarenal vascular disease (1).

EPIDEMIOLOGY
Incidence
- 1 in every 114 patients newly diagnosed with gout develops uric acid stones per year. Uric acid stones are more common in patients with gout, and the chance of stone formation increases with increasing serum urate levels and urine excretion rates. Uric acid nephrolithiasis has a peak incidence in the 5th decade of life.
- Predominant age: Adults
- Predominant sex: Male > Female (4:1). In the US, the prevalence rate is 4–9% in men and 1.7–4.1% in women.

Prevalence
- Gout 1%, hyperuricemia 5–10%, uric acid nephrolithiasis 0.1% in the US
- uric acid calculi account for 5–10% of all stones in the US.
- The overall prevalence of uric acid calculi in persons with primary gout is estimated to be 22%.

RISK FACTORS
- Hyperuricemic acute renal failure (2):
  – Chemotherapy of neoplastic disorders
  – Sudden increase in uric acid load
  – Volume depletion
  – Preexisting acute or chronic renal insufficiency
  – Large tumor burden
  – Lactate dehydrogenase (LDH) >1,500 IU
  – Extensive bone marrow involvement
  – Elevated tumor sensitivity to chemotherapeutic agents
- Uric acid nephrolithiasis (3):
  – Decreased urine pH
  – Diminished urinary volume
  – Excessive urinary uric acid
  – Acute diarrheal states and inflammatory bowel disease
  – Diabetes mellitus
  – Metabolic syndrome
  – Probenecid and aspirin use

GENERAL PREVENTION
- Appropriate pretreatment prior to chemotherapy for leukemia or lymphoma
- Avoidance of factors that can cause abrupt or persistent increases in serum uric acid or urinary uric acid excretion

ETIOLOGY
- Hyperuricemic acute renal failure:
  – Endogenous uric acid overproduction: Rapid cell turnover/destruction owing to malignancy or rhabdomyolysis, enzymatic/metabolic abnormalities, inappropriate high dose of uricosuric agent in hyperuricemic individual
  – Exogenous uric acid overproduction: Excessive dietary purine ingestion
- Uric acid nephrolithiasis:
  – Idiopathic: Sporadic
  – Familial (primary hyperuricemia):
    ○ Congenital gout, hypertension (HTN), and hyperuricemia (autosomal dominant)
    ○ Congenital hypoxanthine–guanine phosphoribosyltransferase deficiency (Lesch-Nyhan syndrome, X-linked recessive)
    ○ Congenital phosphoribosyl pyrophosphate overactivity (X-linked recessive)
    ○ Congenital glycogen storage disease type I
  – Secondary hyperuricemia:
    ○ Lead intoxication
    ○ Diuretics
    ○ Cytotoxic chemotherapy or radiation in leukemia or lymphoma
    ○ Heat stress and exercise
    ○ Diabetic ketoacidosis
    ○ Starvation ketosis
    ○ Chronic myeloproliferative disease
    ○ Psoriasis
  – Secondary hyperuricosuria: Primary gout, excessive purine intake, tubular reabsorptive defect, uricosuric drugs (e.g., cyclosporine, ethambutol, probenecid, phenylbutazone, pyrazinamide, salicylates, vitamin A, tacrolimus, radiocontrast materials)
  – Dehydration: GI or skin loss

Pediatric Considerations
- Gout and uric acid nephrolithiasis may have onset in infancy or childhood with familial causes of hyperuricemia, such as Lesch-Nyhan syndrome.

- It may occur more often in pediatric patients because of the increased incidence of acute lymphoblastic leukemia and Burkitt lymphoma in this population.

COMMONLY ASSOCIATED CONDITIONS
- Treatment of neoplastic disorders
- Gout (4)
- HTN (1)
- Myocardial infarction (1)
- Stroke (1)
- IgA nephropathy: Worse prognosis with elevated uric acid levels (1)

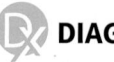 **DIAGNOSIS**

- Hyperuricemic acute renal failure (2):
  – Precipitated by chemotherapy for leukemia or lymphoma or some solid-tumor malignancies
  – Hyperkalemia: Weakness, paresthesias, muscle cramps, nausea, vomiting, diarrhea, anorexia
  – Hyperphosphatemia: Acute nephrocalcinosis
  – Hypocalcemia: Muscle cramps, tetany, cardiac arrhythmia, seizures
  – Oliguria
  – Anuria
  – Anorexia, nausea, vomiting, encephalopathy, and other manifestations of uremia
  – HTN
  – Dehydration
- Uric acid nephrolithiasis:
  – Flank pain
  – Groin pain
  – Microscopic or gross hematuria
  – Anorexia
  – Nausea, vomiting
  – Ureteral obstruction
  – Urinary tract infection
  – Dehydration
- Hyperuricemia of chronic renal failure:
  – Established chronic renal failure with glomerular filtration rate (GFR) <15–20 mL/min
  – Serum uric acid 7–10 mg/dL chronically
  – Acute onset of uremic symptoms

HISTORY
Nonspecific, but includes nausea, vomiting, and fatigue; predisposing causes help to direct clinical suspicion.

DIAGNOSTIC TESTS & INTERPRETATION
Lab
- Hyperuricemic acute renal failure:
  – Serum uric acid >15–20 mg/dL (0.88–1.18 mmol/L)
  – Rising blood urea nitrogen and creatinine
  – Urinary uric acid/creatinine ratio >1; ratio of 0.6–0.75 suggests another cause of renal failure (2)[C].
  – Uric acid crystals in urine
- Uric acid nephrolithiasis:
  – Urine pH <6 (Nitrazine paper) (3)[A].
  – Uric acid crystals in urine; urate crystals tend to be needle-shaped or flat, square plates; both are strongly birefringent.
  – 24-h urinalysis: Urinary uric acid often >4,800 μmol/d in men and >4,400 μmol/d in women or uric acid/creatinine ratio >530 μmol/mmol (hyperuricosuria) (5)[A].

– Measure serum uric acid, calcium, and creatinine: Serum uric acid is often normal, especially with low urine pH <6.2 (3)[A]
– Hematuria
– Stone analysis: Uric acid or mixed uric acid with calcium oxalate or calcium phosphate
• Hyperuricemia of chronic renal failure:
– Serum uric acid usually 7–10 mg/dL and is rarely >10 mg/dL owing to compensatory increase in GI secretion of uric acid (1)[A].
– Serum uric acid remains normal until GFR <20 mL/min (6)[C].

Imaging
• IV pyelography: Filling defects (3)
• Nonenhanced CT scan: Lower density than calcium stones (3)[A]; CT attenuation values between 300 and 400 HU (7)

Diagnostic Procedures/Surgery
• Cystoscopy and retrograde pyelography (3)
• Renal biopsy

Pathological Findings
• Hyperuricemic acute renal failure: Uric acid crystals in collecting ducts, eventually obstructing nephrons (2)
• Uric acid nephrolithiasis: Radiolucent, often orange or red stones that can occlude ureters or entire renal collecting system (3)
• Chronic urate nephropathy: Birefringent, needle-like crystals in the tubular lumen or in the interstitium with surrounding inflammatory cells and fibrosis (5)

DIFFERENTIAL DIAGNOSIS
• Hyperuricemic acute renal failure: Prerenal failure, contrast nephropathy, acute tubular necrosis, tumor infiltration of kidneys, obstruction
• Uric acid nephrolithiasis: Calcium oxalate, calcium phosphate, struvite, cystine stones; 20% of patients with calcium nephrolithiasis have hyperuricemia (3).
• Chronic urate nephropathy: Other causes of chronic renal failure, including diabetes, atherosclerotic disease, HTN, and glomerular disease, are more likely. Environmental lead poisoning is another consideration in a patient with hypertension, gout, hyperuricemia, and chronic kidney disease (8).

 TREATMENT

MEDICATION
• Hyperuricemic acute renal failure: Prevent by pretreating with allopurinol or rasburicase and hydrating patient prior to administration of chemotherapeutic agents for leukemia or lymphoma (2,9)[A].
– Begin hydration 2 days prior to and continue for 2 days after induction chemotherapy (2)[A].
– Allopurinol 200–600 mg/d (adults) (2)[A] and 10 mg/kg q8h (children) (10)[A]
– Rasburicase 0.2 mg/kg/d IV during initial chemotherapy for pediatric patients with advanced-stage lymphoma or high-tumor-burden leukemia (9,10)[B]
– Promptly correct metabolic abnormalities (2)[A].
– Dialyze when renal failure fails to resolve with conservative management or when life-threatening electrolyte or volume-overload disorders are present (2)[A].

• Uric acid nephrolithiasis:
– Encourage hydration to obtain urine output 1.5–2.0 L (5,7)[A].
– Alkali to maintain urine pH at 6.0–7.0; give potassium alkali 20–30 mEq b.i.d. to t.i.d. (3,5)[A].
– If hyperuricosuric and urinary alkalinization is unsuccessful, give allopurinol starting at 100–300 mg/d (5)[B].
• Hyperuricemia of chronic renal failure: Consider allopurinol only in patients with prior history of gout or nephrolithiasis (6)[C].
• Asymptomatic hyperuricemia: There is insufficient evidence to indicate treatment of asymptomatic hyperuricemia (1)[A].
• Precautions:
– In patients with renal impairment, dosing for allopurinol, which is cleared renally, must be adjusted (2)[A].
– Avoid abrupt decreases or increases in serum uric acid, which may precipitate acute gouty arthritis.
• Significant possible interactions of allopurinol:
– Inhibits metabolism of mercaptopurine and azathioprine
– Ethanol decreases its effects.
– Increases likelihood of skin rash when used with amoxicillin or ampicillin.
– Risk of nephrolithiasis with excess vitamin C.

ADDITIONAL TREATMENT
General Measures
• Hyperuricemic acute renal failure:
– IV hydration
– Hemodialysis in severe cases
• Uric acid nephrolithiasis:
– Hydration to increase urine output
– Normalize renal uric acid excretion.
– Normalize urine pH.
– Antibiotic treatment of urinary tract infection

SURGERY/OTHER PROCEDURES
Uric acid nephrolithiasis resistant to conservative management: Lithotripsy, cystoscopic stenting, percutaneous nephrostomy (3)[A]

IN-PATIENT CONSIDERATIONS
Initial Stabilization
Outpatient treatment except for complicated nephrolithiasis and hyperuricemic acute renal failure

 ONGOING CARE

DIET
• Moderation of purine intake (5)[C]
• For nephrolithiasis, ensure that fluid intake is adequate to produce urine output of at least 2 L/d unless urine output is limited by acute or chronic renal failure (5)[A].
• In renal failure, restrict sodium for HTN and potassium for hyperkalemia.

PROGNOSIS
• With effective drug therapy and general management, prognosis is excellent in patients with hyperuricemic acute renal failure (2) and nephrolithiasis (3).
• Development of progressive renal insufficiency in patients with gout or hyperuricemia is unlikely to occur unless caused by underlying renal disease or associated medical conditions with adverse renal effects (4).

COMPLICATIONS
• Gout and asymptomatic hyperuricemia: No renal complications proven in humans (1)
• Hyperuricemic acute renal failure (2):
– Irreversible renal failure (ESRD)
– Residual renal insufficiency
– Persistent renal tubular functional defects
• Uric acid nephrolithiasis (4):
– Urinary obstruction
– Urinary tract infection, pyelonephritis
– Renal insufficiency
• Hyperuricemia of chronic renal failure: Progression to end-stage renal failure

Geriatric Considerations
Renal insufficiency is more likely because of age and associated medical conditions.

REFERENCES

1. Kanellis J, Feig DI, Johnson RJ. Does asymptomatic hyperuricaemia contribute to the development of renal and cardiovascular disease? An old controversy renewed. *Nephrology (Carlton)*. 2004;9:394–9.
2. Davidson MB, et al. Pathophysiology, clinical consequences, and treatment of tumor lysis syndrome. *Am J Med*. 2004;1116(8):546–54.
3. Coe FL, Evan A, Worcester E. Kidney stone disease. *J Clin Invest*. 2005;115:2598–608.
4. Nakagawa T, Mazzali M, Kang DH, et al. Uric acid–a uremic toxin? *Blood Purif*. 2006;24:67–70.
5. Reynolds TM. ACP Best Practice No 181: Chemical pathology clinical investigation and management of nephrolithiasis. *J Clin Pathol*. 2005;58:134–40.
6. Snaith ML. ABC of rheumatology: Gout, hyperuricemia, and crystal arthritis. *Br Med J*. 1995;310:521–4.
7. Becker G. Uric acid stones. *Nephrology (Carlton)*. 2007;12(Suppl 1):S21–5.
8. Lin JL, Yu CC, Lin-Tan DT, et al. Lead chelation therapy and urate excretion in patients with chronic renal diseases and gout. *Kidney Int*. 2001;60:266–71.
9. Coiffier B, Altman A, Pui CH, et al. Guidelines for the management of pediatric and adult tumor lysis syndrome: an evidence-based review. *J Clin Oncol*. 2008;26:2767–78.
10. Goldman SC, Holcenberg JS, Finklestein JZ, et al. A randomized comparison between rasburicase and allopurinol in children with lymphoma or leukemia at high risk for tumor lysis. *Blood*. 2001;97:2998–3003.

CODES

ICD9
• 274.10 Gouty nephropathy, unspecified
• 274.11 Uric acid nephrolithiasis

N

NEPHROTIC SYNDROME

Carla M. Nester, MD

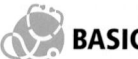 **BASICS**

DESCRIPTION
- A clinical syndrome of heavy proteinuria (>3.5 g/1.73 m^2/24 hours), hypoalbuminemia, hyperlipidemia, and edema
- Includes both primary and secondary forms
- Associated with many types of kidney disease

EPIDEMIOLOGY
Based on definitive diagnosis:
- Diabetic nephropathy:
  - Most common cause of secondary nephrotic syndrome
- Minimal change disease (MCD):
  - Most common nephrotic syndrome in children, peaks at 2–8 years
  - Associated with drugs or lymphoma in adults
- Amyloidosis:
  - Rare
- Lupus nephropathy (LN):
  - Adult women are affected about 10 × more often than men.
- Focal segmental glomerulosclerosis (FSGS):
  - 25% of nephrotic syndrome in adults
  - Most common primary nephrotic syndrome in African Americans
  - Has both primary and secondary forms
- Membranous nephropathy:
  - Most common primary nephrotic syndrome in Caucasians
  - Associated with malignancy and infection
- Membranoproliferative glomerulonephritis (MGN):
  - May be primary or secondary
  - May present in the setting of a systemic viral or rheumatic illness

RISK FACTORS
- Drug addiction (e.g., heroin [FSGS])
- Hepatitis B and C, HIV, other infections
- Immunosuppression
- Nephrotoxic drugs
- Vesicoureteral reflux (FSGS)
- Cancer (usually MGN, may be MCD)
- Chronic analgesic use/abuse
- Preeclampsia
- Diabetes mellitus

Genetics
Genetic factors are likely to play a role in susceptibility to the various nephrotic syndromes, though these have not been sufficiently defined to be useful clinically.

GENERAL PREVENTION
In general, there are few preventive measures except avoidance of known causative medications.

PATHOPHYSIOLOGY
- Increased glomerular permeability to large protein molecules, especially albumin
- Edema results primarily from renal salt retention, with arterial underfilling from decreased plasma oncotic pressure playing an additional role.
- Hyperlipidemia is thought to be a consequence of increased hepatic synthesis resulting from low oncotic pressure and urinary loss of regulatory proteins.
- The hypercoagulable state that can occur in some nephrotic states is likely due to loss of antithrombin III in urine.

ETIOLOGY
- Primary renal disease:
  - Minimal change disease
  - Focal and segmental glomerulosclerosis (FSGS)
  - Membranous nephropathy (MGN)
  - IgA nephropathy
  - Membranoproliferative glomerulonephritis
- Secondary renal disease (associated primary renal disease shown in parentheses):
  - Diabetic nephropathy
  - Amyloidosis
  - Lupus nephropathy (LN)
  - Focal and segmental glomerulosclerosis
  - Infections (MGN)
  - Cancer (MCD or MGN)
  - Drugs (MCD or MGN)

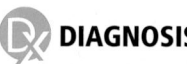 **DIAGNOSIS**

HISTORY
- Look for signs or symptoms of systemic disease:
  - Joint complaint, rash, edema, infectious complaint, fevers, anorexia, oliguria, foamy urine, acute flank pain, hematuria, etc.
- Look for a recent drug history that may be causative, especially nonsteroidal anti-inflammatory drugs.
- Assess for risk factors.

PHYSICAL EXAM
A complete physical exam may discover clues to systemic disease as a potential cause and/or may suggest the severity of disease:
- Fluid retention: Abdominal distention, abdominal fluid shift, extremity edema, puffy eyelids, scrotal swelling, weight gain, shortness of breath:
  - Pericardial rub and decreased breath sounds with pleural effusions may develop.
- Hypertension
- Orthostatic hypotension

> **ALERT**
> The potential for thromboembolic disease leading to pulmonary embolism is one of the most life-threatening aspects of a patient who is actively nephrotic.

DIAGNOSTIC TESTS & INTERPRETATION
Lab
Initial lab tests
- Confirm proteinuria is present:
  - By urine dipstick initially, and then quantitate by 24-hour urine or urine protein to creatinine ratio
- Rule out urine infection with urine culture.
- Full blood count and coagulation screen
- Renal function tests:
  - Blood urea nitrogen, creatinine with estimated glomerular filtration rate
- Glucose to rule out overt diabetes
- Blood cultures to rule out a postinfectious process
- Lipid panel to judge the relative effect of loss of protein into the urine
- Liver function tests to exclude liver disease or infection
- Look for autoimmune disease:
  - Antinuclear antibody and/or antidouble-stranded DNA (dsDNA) positivity would suggest lupus.
  - Complement levels: A low C3 may suggest a postinfectious or membranoproliferative process, whereas both low C3 and C4 low point to lupus.
- Serum protein electrophoresis/urine immune electrophoresis to rule in a paraproteinemia
- Hepatitis B and C screen
- HIV and rapid plasma reagent:
  - Urinalysis to evaluate for the presence of cellular casts

Imaging
- Renal ultrasound to verify the presence of 2 kidneys of normal shape and size
- Chest x-ray to detect presence of pleural effusion or infection
- If thrombosis suspected:
  - Doppler ultrasound of the legs
  - Magnetic resonance imaging or venography for renal vein thrombosis
  - Ventilation/perfusion nuclear medicine lung scan and/or computed tomography may be required to rule out pulmonary embolism.

Diagnostic Procedures/Surgery
Renal biopsy:
- Rarely done in children with 1st episode of nephrotic syndrome, as minimal-change disease is common and empiric steroid therapy is the standard of care.
- Often required to confirm the clinical diagnosis in adults and assist with making a treatment plan

Pathological Findings
- Light microscopy:
  - May see nothing (e.g., MCD)
  - Sclerosis (e.g., FSGS or diabetic nodules in diabetes)
  - Diffuse hypercellularity suggests a proliferative disease such as IgA nephropathy, lupus nephritis, or postinfectious GN.
- Immunofluorescence:
  - Mesangial IgA suggests IgA nephropathy, Henoch-Schönlein; other staining patterns are specific for other disease processes.
- Electron microscopy:
  - The location of immunoglobulin deposits are useful in pointing to a particular diagnosis.

DIFFERENTIAL DIAGNOSIS
- Edema and proteinuria:
  - See Etiology
- Edema alone:
  - Other diseases to rule out in patients who have edema without proteinuria include:
    - Congestive heart failure, cirrhosis, hypothyroidism, nutritional hypoalbuminemia, protein-losing enteropathy

TREATMENT

MEDICATION

First Line
- Edema: Salt restriction and salt-wasting diuretics (loop and thiazide diuretics):
  – Salt restriction to <6 g of sodium chloride (<2.4 g sodium/day)
  – Restrict fluid intake to <1.5 L/day if hyponatremic.
  – Target weight loss of 0.5–1 kg/d (1–2 lbs/d)
- Statins have been shown to improve endothelial function (1)[A] and decrease proteinuria (2)[A].
- Angiotensin-converting enzyme inhibitors or angiotensin II receptor blockers thought to reduce proteinuria, hyperlipidemia, thrombotic tendencies, progression of renal failure (1,3)[A], and to control hypertension if present
- For steroid-responsive disease (MCD and FGS), steroids dosed in consultation with nephrologist

Second Line
- Many of the nephrotic diseases will require escalation in therapy above steroids. These include rapidly relapsing forms as well as MGN, LN, and IgA nephropathy:
  – Bolus steroids and other immunosuppressives are required in this circumstance (cyclophosphamide, mycophenolate mofetil, chlorambucil, cyclosporine).
- Randomized controlled data has been insufficient to determine which patients require prophylactic anticoagulation (4)[A]. One practice is to anticoagulate with heparin and then warfarin in patients who have persistent nephrotic-range proteinuria. This decision is made based on patient's history of edema, hypoalbuminemia, history of thromboembolism, or immobility.
- Hypocalcemia from vitamin D loss should be treated with oral vitamin D (dihydrotachysterol) 0.2 mg/d.

ADDITIONAL TREATMENT
Ambulation or range-of-motion exercises to lower risk of deep vein thrombosis (DVT)

Issues for Referral
Consultation with a nephrologist is often required in order to assist with renal biopsy to confirm diagnosis and to assist with management of edema. Cytotoxic medications may be called for, depending on the disease process, and this may best be handled by the nephrologists.

IN-PATIENT CONSIDERATIONS

Admission Criteria
Respiratory distress, sepsis/severe infection, thromboses, renal failure, hypertension, or other complications

Discharge Criteria
Hemodynamically stable patients without complications may be managed as outpatients.

 ONGOING CARE

FOLLOW-UP RECOMMENDATIONS

Patient Monitoring
- Frequent monitoring is required for relapse, disease progression, and for detecting signs of toxicity of medical management.
- Reevaluate for azotemia, hypertension, edema, loss of renal function, cholesterol, and weight.

DIET
- Normal protein (1 g/kg/d)
- Low fat (cholesterol)
- Reduced sodium
- Supplemental multivitamins and minerals, especially vitamin D and iron
- Fluid restriction if hyponatremic

PATIENT EDUCATION
- Printed material for patients: National Kidney Foundation, 30 E. 33rd Street, Suite 1100, New York, NY 10016; (800) 622-9010:
  – Childhood Nephrotic Syndrome
  – Diabetes and Kidney Disease
  – Focal Glomerulosclerosis
- Web site: National Institutes of Health: Nephrotic syndrome

PROGNOSIS
The nephrotic syndrome in children (MCD) is typically self-limited and carries a good prognosis. In the adult, the prognosis is variable. Complete remission is expected if the basic disease is treatable (infection, malignancy, drug induced); otherwise, a relapsing and remitting course is possible, with progression to dialysis seen in more aggressive forms (diabetic glomerulosclerosis).

COMPLICATIONS
- Thromboembolism:
  – DVT and/or renal vein thrombosis may occur.
  – The risk appears to be greater the lower the serum albumin.
  – Pulmonary embolism is a known complication.
- Pleural effusion
- Ascites
- Hyperlipidemia, cardiovascular disease
- Acute renal failure, progressive renal failure
- Protein malnutrition/muscle wasting
- Infection secondary to low serum IgG concentrations, reduced complement activity, and depressed T cell function:
  – Peritonitis, pneumonia, or cellulitis
- Loss of vitamin D (vitamin D binding protein loss in urine) leading to bone disease

REFERENCES
1. Randomized placebo-controlled trial of effect of ramipril on decline in glomerular filtration rate and risk of terminal renal failure in proteinuric, non-diabetic nephropathy. *The GISEN Group (Gruppo Italiano di Studi Epidemiologici in Nefrologia) Lancet.* 1997;349:1857–63.
2. Fried LF, Orchard TJ, Kasiske BL. Effect of lipid reduction on the progression of renal disease: a meta-analysis. *Kidney Int.* 2001;59:260–9.
3. Kunz R, Friedrich C, Wolbers M, Mann JF et al. Meta-analysis: effect of monotherapy and combination therapy with inhibitors of the renin angiotensin system on proteinuria in renal disease. *Ann Intern Med.* 2008;148:30–48.
4. Kulshrestha S, Grieff M, Navananeethan SD. Interventions for preventing thrombosis in adults and children with nephrotic syndrome (protocol). *Cochrane Database Syst Rev.* 2006;(2):CD006024.

ADDITIONAL READING
- Madaio MP, Harrington JT. The diagnosis of glomerular diseases: acute glomerulonephritis and the nephrotic syndrome. *Arch Intern Med.* 2001;161:25–34.
- Meyrier A. An update on the treatment options for focal segmental glomerulosclerosis. *Expert Opin Pharmacother.* 2009;10:615–28.
- Schwarz A. New aspects of the treatment of nephrotic syndrome. *J Am Soc Nephrol.* 2001; 12(Suppl 17):S44–7.

See Also (Topic, Algorithm, Electronic Media Element)
Amyloidosis; Diabetes Mellitus, Type 1; Diabetes Mellitus, Type 2; Glomerulonephritis, Acute; HIV Infection and AIDS; Multiple Myeloma; Renal Failure, Acute (ARF); Renal Failure, Chronic; Lupus Erythematosus, Discoid

 CODES

ICD9
581.9 Nephrotic syndrome with unspecified pathological lesion in kidney

CLINICAL PEARLS
- Pediatric nephrotic syndrome typically carries a good prognosis and is easily treated with steroids. Recurrences are common.
- Nondiabetic adults with nephrotic syndrome will require a renal biopsy to determine cause.
- Have a high index of suspicion for symptoms that may represent an embolic event

N

NEUROBLASTOMA

Timothy L. Black, MD

 BASICS

Most common tumor of infants and most common extracranial solid tumor of children

DESCRIPTION
A neoplasm of neural crest origin that may arise anywhere along the sympathetic ganglion chain or in the adrenal medulla:
- Stage 1: Localized tumor with complete resection, with or without microscopic residual disease
- Stage 2A: Localized tumor with incomplete gross excision, ipsilateral lymph node negative
- Stage 2B: Localized tumor with or without complete excision, ipsilateral lymph nodes positive; contralateral lymph nodes negative
- Stage 3: Unresectable tumor extending across midline, or localized tumor with positive contralateral lymph nodes, or midline tumor with bilateral extension unresectable
- Stage 4: Any primary tumor with distant metastases
- Stage 4S: Localized primary tumor with dissemination limited to skin, liver, and/or bone marrow in infants <1 year of age
- Amplification of n-myc oncogene (poor prognosis)
- Normal DNA ploidy: Worse prognosis than hyperdiploidy
- Sites of disease:
  – Adrenal medulla 40–60%
  – Retroperitoneal sites 20%
  – Mediastinum 10%
  – Pelvis 2–6%
  – Neck 2%
- System(s) affected: Endocrine/Metabolic; Nervous

EPIDEMIOLOGY
- Predominant age:
  – 90% occur in 1st 8 years of life.
  – 30% occur in children in the 1st year of life.
  – 50% occur between ages 1 and 4 years.
  – Most common intra-abdominal malignancy in the newborn
- Predominant sex: Males > Females (1.2:1)
- The most common tumor in infants <1 year of age in the US
- Accounts for 6–10% of all childhood cancers, but 15% of all childhood oncologic deaths
- 4th most common pediatric malignancy

Incidence
- 27.8 cases/million children/year for 1st 5 years of life in the US
- 8.7 cases/million in children/year for 1st 15 years of life in the US
- Denmark: 1/12,000–14,000 live births
- Japan: 1/15,000–18,749 infants
- 1/7,000 live births in the US and the UK (1)[C]

RISK FACTORS
- Beckwith–Wiedemann syndrome
- Pancreatic islet cell dysplasia
- Maternal phenytoin treatment
- Fetal alcohol syndrome
- Hirschsprung disease
- Family history

Genetics
- Familial cases reported (1–2%):
  – The median age at diagnosis of familial cases is 9 mo (median age at diagnosis of sporadic cases is 18 mo) (2)[B].
  – Follows an autosomal dominant pattern of inheritance (2)[B]
- Genetic abnormalities in 80%
- Deletions in short arm of chromosome 1p36 or 11q23, unbalanced gain of long arm of chromosome 17 (all of these genetic alterations result in aggressive tumor behavior and poor outcome) (2)[B]
- Amplification of n-myc oncogene occurs on chromosome 2 (poor prognostic sign, present in ~20–25%).
- Cellular DNA ploidy (hyperdiploidy in infants <1 year of age is associated with excellent long-term survival, diploidy in the same age group is associated with treatment failure) (1)[C]

ETIOLOGY
Genetic abnormalities in 80% of cases

 DIAGNOSIS

PHYSICAL EXAM
- 50–60% present with metastatic disease.
- Abdominal mass (50–75%)
- Weight loss
- Anemia
- Failure to thrive
- Abdominal pain and distension
- Bone pain
- Fever
- Diarrhea
- Hypertension (25%)
- Horner syndrome (ptosis, miosis, enophthalmos, heterochromia of iris)
- Orbital ecchymosis (panda eyes)
- Respiratory distress
- Dysphagia
- Paraplegia
- Cauda equina syndrome
- Flushing, sweating, irritability
- Cerebellar ataxia (chaotic nystagmus): Dancing eye syndrome

DIAGNOSTIC TESTS & INTERPRETATION
Lab
- CBC and platelet count
- Liver function studies
- Renal function studies
- Urinary catecholamines, including dopamine, vanillylmandelic acid, and homovanillic acid (85% secrete catecholamine metabolites)
- Uric acid level
- Creatinine level
- Magnesium level
- Calcium level
- Lactate dehydrogenase (LDH) level (high levels, >1500 IU/l, associated with poor outcome)
- Electrolytes

- Bilirubin, aspartate aminotransferase, and alanine aminotransferase levels
- Gd2 monoclonal antibody levels
- Serum neuron-specific enolase (levels >100 ng/mL associated with poor outcome)
- Serum ferritin
- Bone marrow aspiration
- Assay for vasoactive intestinal polypeptide

Imaging
- Chest radiograph
- Skeletal survey (including orbital views)
- Bone scan
- CT or MRI of neck, chest, abdomen, or pelvis, depending on the location of tumor; also to evaluate for metastatic disease
- PET scan
- MIBG scintigraphy
- Myelogram may be indicated for neurologic symptoms.

Diagnostic Procedures/Surgery
- Myelogram if needed
- Bone marrow aspiration
- Tumor biopsy (open preferred over needle biopsy due to better tissue sample for multiple studies)

Pathological Findings
- Small, dark, round cells
- Immature tumors tend to be large, red, lobular, soft, friable
- Mature tumors are fibrous, contain calcification, hemorrhage, necrosis, cysts, rosettes, and nerve filaments.
- May be neuroblastoma, ganglioneuroblastoma, or benign ganglioneuroma, depending on cell maturity
- Favorable histology: Stroma-rich, well-differentiated. and intermixed tumors
- Unfavorable histology: Stroma-rich nodular and stroma-poor, undifferentiated tumors

DIFFERENTIAL DIAGNOSIS
- Rhabdomyosarcoma
- Wilms tumors
- Other tumors of neck, chest, abdomen, pelvis
- Hydronephrosis

 TREATMENT

MEDICATION
First Line
- Cyclophosphamide
- Melphalan
- Vincristine
- Dacarbazine
- Teniposide
- Etoposide
- Doxorubicin (Adriamycin)
- Cisplatin
- Peptichemio
- Carboplatin
- Ifosfamide (with mesna to protect against hemorrhagic cystitis)

- Topotecan
- Immunotherapy using antiganglioside monoclonal antibodies
- Contraindications: See the manufacturer's information for each drug.
- Precautions: See the manufacturer's information for each drug.
- Significant possible interactions: See the manufacturer's information for each drug.

Second Line
- By protocol
- Ondansetron (Zofran), dronabinol (Marinol), metoclopramide (Reglan), and others for nausea control

ADDITIONAL TREATMENT
General Measures
- Radiation therapy in children >1 year of age with stage 3 disease
- Radioimmunotherapy with hematopoietic stem cell rescue
- Chemotherapy for stage 2 and greater

Additional Therapies
See General Measures.

SURGERY/OTHER PROCEDURES
- Surgical resection may be complete, incomplete, or biopsy only: For stage 1, excision only.
- If resection incomplete or biopsy, then chemotherapy followed by 2nd-look operation (reduction of tumor size may allow complete resection at second operation).
- Dumbbell extension through vertebral foramina, chemotherapy alone vs laminectomy and decompression
- Stages 4, 4S: Resection of primary tumor and chemotherapy
- Myeloablative therapy followed by bone marrow transplantation considered in stages 3 and 4
- Current Children's Oncology Group risk stratification (1)[C]:
  - Low-risk disease treated with surgery alone: Includes stage 1, 2A, 2B with favorable histology, and 4S with normal NMYC and favorable histology.
  - Intermediate-risk disease treated with chemotherapy, surgery, and local radiation: Includes stage 3 with normal NMYC amplification and favorable histology, stage 4 with normal NMYC, and stage 4S with unfavorable histology.
  - High-risk disease treated with chemotherapy, surgery, and bone marrow transplant or stem cell rescue: Includes stage 2B with unfavorable histology, stage 3 with amplified NMYC and unfavorable histology, stage 4 with amplified NMYC and >1 year of age, and stage 4S with amplified NMYC.
- All children require central venous access for chemotherapy.

IN-PATIENT CONSIDERATIONS
Admission Criteria
Inpatient workup and treatment until stable and induction chemotherapy completed

ONGOING CARE
FOLLOW-UP RECOMMENDATIONS
Patient Monitoring
- Multiagent chemotherapy every 3–4 weeks for 4 courses, then reevaluate with bone marrow or 2nd-look operation.
- Follow every 3 months for 1st year, every 4 months for 2nd year, every 6 months for 3rd year, then at least yearly.
- Follow with CT or MRI every 3–6 months initially, then yearly.

DIET
No special diet

PATIENT EDUCATION
- Patient and family education regarding long-term outlook
- Possibility of 2nd malignancy
- Side effects of treatment

PROGNOSIS
- Overall survival 58% (3)[C]:
  - Stage 1: Expected survival ~100%
  - Stage 2: Survival 75%
  - Stage 3: Survival 43%
  - Stage 4: Survival 15%
  - Stage 4S: Survival 70–80%
- Normal DNA ploidy, NMYC amplifications, and/or unfavorable histology indicate worse-than-usual prognosis for the same tumor.
- Infants <1 year of age have better outcome.
- Patients with cervical, pelvic, and mediastinal tumors have better prognosis than those with retroperitoneal, paraspinal, or adrenal tumors.
- Survival for those presenting with opsoclonus (uncontrolled, multidirectional eye movements) and nystagmus is nearly 90% (seen especially in mediastinal tumors in infants <1 year of age).
- Neuron-specific enolase level >100 ng/mL correlates with advanced disease and reduced survival.
- Serum LDH level <1,500 IU/mL may indicate improved survival rate.
- In patients with high-risk neuroblastoma, myeloablative therapy followed by autologous bone marrow transplant result in significantly better overall survival (about 59%) (2)[B].
- Spontaneous regression in Stage 4S (2)[B]:
  - Spontaneous regression may occur in a small proportion of patients and is not completely understood.
  - The incidence of spontaneous regression in neuroblastoma is 10–100 times greater than for any other human cancer.

COMPLICATIONS
- Nausea
- Vomiting
- Alopecia
- Bone marrow suppression
- Immunosuppression
- Hemorrhagic cystitis
- Azotemia
- Diarrhea

- Antidiuretic hormone secretion
- Local tissue necrosis
- Myocardiopathy
- Renal toxicity
- Hearing loss
- Hypocalcemia
- Hypomagnesemia
- Graft versus host disease

REFERENCES
1. Weinstein JL, Katzenstein HM, Cohn SL. Advances in the diagnosis and treatment of neuroblastoma. *Oncologist*. 2003;8:278–92.
2. Matthay KK, Reynolds CP, Seeger RC, et al. Long-Term Results for Children With High-Risk Neuroblastoma Treated on a Randomized Trial of Myeloablative Therapy Followed by 13-cis-Retinoic Acid: A Children's Oncology Group Study. *J Clin Oncol*. 2009.
3. Grosfeld JL, et al. Neuroblastoma in the 1st year of life: Clinical and biologic factors influencing outcome. *Sem Pediatr Surg*. 1993;2:37–46.

ADDITIONAL READING
- Mullassery D, Dominici C, Jesudason EC, McDowell HP, Losty PD et al. Neuroblastoma: contemporary management. *Arch Dis Child Educ Pract Ed*. 2009;94:177–85.
- Pearson AD, Pinkerton CR, Lewis IJ, et al. High-dose rapid and standard induction chemotherapy for patients aged over 1 year with stage 4 neuroblastoma: a randomised trial. *Lancet Oncol*. 2008;9:247–56.
- Yalçin B, Kremer LC, Caron HN, van Dalen EC et al. High-dose chemotherapy and autologous haematopoietic stem cell rescue for children with high-risk neuroblastoma. *Cochrane Database Syst Rev*. 2010;5:CD006301.

CODES

ICD9
- 158.0 Malignant neoplasm of retroperitoneum
- 164.9 Malignant neoplasm of mediastinum, part unspecified
- 194.0 Malignant neoplasm of adrenal gland

CLINICAL PEARLS
- Survival has improved slightly with multimodality therapy, and it is hoped that bone marrow transplant/stem cell rescue will further improve survival in the future.
- The treatment of neuroblastoma is determined almost entirely by protocol based on tumor stage, NMYC amplification, and histology findings.

N

NEUROFIBROMATOSIS (TYPES 1 AND 2)

Michele Roberts, MD, PhD
Jeremy Golding, MD

BASICS

DESCRIPTION
- Neurofibromatosis type 1 (NF1) and 2 (NF2) are neurocutaneous syndromes (phakomatoses). Although they share a name and are both autosomal dominant disorders, they are distinct and unrelated conditions with genes on different chromosomes. NF2 causes bilateral vestibular schwannomas. NF2 is rare and not further discussed in this chapter.
- NF1 is a multisystem disorder that may affect any organ. It is the most common of the phakomatoses:
  - System(s) affected: Musculoskeletal; Nervous; Skin/Exocrine; Cardiovascular; Neuro-ophthalmologic
  - Synonym(s): von Recklinghausen disease, formerly "peripheral NF"

EPIDEMIOLOGY
Incidence
- Predominant sex for NF1: Male = Female
- Birth incidence NF1: 1/2,500–3,000

Prevalence
1/3,000–1/4,000

RISK FACTORS
- Having an affected 1st-degree relative is a diagnostic criterion for NF1, although relatives may be unaware of their condition.
- Affected individuals with a positive family history, as well as those with a new mutation, have a 50% risk of transmitting NF1 to each of their offspring; 1/12 will be severely affected.
- Individuals with segmental NF1 may have gonadal mosaicism and may be at risk for transmission of the mutated gene.

Genetics
- NF1: OMIM #162200
- Caused by a mutation in the *NF1* gene on chromosome 17q11.2; autosomal dominant inheritance; protein product is called *neurofibromin*
- 1/2 of cases are attributed to new mutations. Prenatal diagnosis is possible.
- Penetrance is high; expressivity is highly variable.
- *NF1* is a large gene with a variety of mutations causing neurofibromatosis. Molecular technology can detect 95% of clinically important *NF1* mutations, but it is usually not indicated because clinical diagnosis can frequently be established in childhood.
- About 5% of individuals with NF1 have a large deletion of the entire *NF1* gene (or nearly so). These individuals usually have a more severe phenotype.
- A variant of NF1, known as *segmental NF*, is limited to a single body region and may be explained by mosaicism for the *NF1* mutation.

PATHOPHYSIOLOGY
- Neurofibromin belongs to a family of GTPase-activating proteins and acts as a tumor suppressor by downregulating a cellular proto-oncogene, *p21-ras,* that enhances cell growth and proliferation.
- Neurofibromata are benign tumors composed of Schwann cells, fibroblasts, mast cells, and vascular components that develop along nerves.
- The 2-hit hypothesis has been invoked to explain malignant transformation in *NF1.*

COMMONLY ASSOCIATED CONDITIONS
Cardiovascular disease: Congenital heart disease, pulmonary stenosis, hypertension

DIAGNOSIS

Diagnostic criteria for NF1 include ≥2 of the following (1):
- ≥6 café-au-lait (light brown) macules ≥5 mm in prepubertal individuals or ≥15 mm in adults
- ≥2 neurofibromata of any type or 1 plexiform (noncircumscribed) neurofibroma
- Axillary or inguinal freckling
- ≥2 Lisch nodules (benign iris hamartomas, asymptomatic)
- Optic glioma by MRI
- Characteristic osseous lesions: Sphenoid dysplasia, long-bone cortical thinning, ribbon ribs, angular scoliosis
- 1st-degree relative with NF1 according to above criteria
- NF1 can be diagnosed by routine exam by ages 6–8, with attention to skin stigmata (1). Prenatal diagnosis is possible, although not predictive of the clinical course.

HISTORY
- Family history of a 1st-degree relative with NF1
- Manifestations generally not visible at birth, although plexiform neurofibromata usually are congenital, and tibial bowing is congenital.
- In addition to cutaneous lesions, NF1 may present with painful neurofibromata, pathologic fractures, or headaches secondary to hypertension caused by pheochromocytomas.

PHYSICAL EXAM
- Skin:
  - Café-au-lait macules develop during the 1st 3 years of childhood and are usually the presenting feature of NF1. Evenly pigmented, irregularly shaped (coast-of-California borders), light brown macules (present in 97% with NF1; although many unaffected individuals have 1 or 2 such macules, <1% of unaffected children have >2.
  - Neurofibromata: Can be cutaneous, subcutaneous, or plexiform, and may be soft or firm; buttonhole invagination is pathognomonic, generally are not present until late adolescence.
  - Plexiform neurofibromata are present in up to 50% of individuals with NF1:
    - Freckling or hypertrichosis may be present over plexiform neurofibromata; may affect underlying structures, or cause focal hyperplasia.
    - Many are internal, and not obvious on physical exam.
  - Evaluate for new lesions and progression of preexisting ones. Rapidly growing cutaneous lesions should be evaluated thoroughly.
  - Axillary freckling (Crowe sign) or inguinal freckling (91%)
- Ophthalmologic: (30% have Lisch nodules)
- Skeletal:
  - Scoliosis and vertebral angulation
  - Localized bone hypertrophy, especially of the face

- Limb abnormalities:
  - Pseudoarthrosis of the tibia
  - Tibial dysplasia (anterolateral bowing of the tibia) is congenital, if present.
  - Nonossifying fibromas of the long bones in adolescents and adults are uncommon, but can increase risk of fracture.
- Pay particular attention to neurologic examination or new focal pain.
- Measure blood pressure yearly. Hypertension is more common in NF1 and could be secondary to renal artery stenosis, aortic stenosis, or pheochromocytoma.
- Evaluate neurodevelopmental progress in children.

Geriatric Considerations
In NF1, cutaneous lesions and tumors increase in size and number with age.

Pediatric Considerations
Children who have inherited the *NF1* gene of an affected parent usually are identified by age 1, but external stigmata may be subtle. If no stigmata by age 2, NF unlikely, but child should be reexamined at age 5. Definite diagnosis can be made by age 8 using NIH criteria (1).

DIAGNOSTIC TESTS & INTERPRETATION
Lab
Clinical diagnosis. DNA sequence and deletion/duplication analysis of the *NF1* gene can identify mutations in ~96% of those with a clinical diagnosis. Genetic testing challenging due to large number of mutations. Diagnostic laboratory information is available at www.genetests.org.

Imaging
- Characteristic radiographic findings in NF1 include sphenoid dysplasia, long-bone cortical thinning, ribbon ribs, and angular scoliosis. Screening radiographs of the knees in adolescents is controversial. CT scan can demonstrate bony changes.
- MRI may demonstrate findings of the orbits, brain, or spine (86%). The value of performing routine head MRI scanning in asymptomatic individuals with NF1 is controversial. Optic glioma by MRI (11–15%), may lead to blindness. Although areas of increased T_2 signal intensity are commonly identified on brain MRI, they are not diagnostic of NF1 and are of no clinical significance. Therefore, the NIH Consensus Development Conference does not recommend routine neuroimaging of the brain as a means of establishing a diagnosis of NF1 (1,2).

Diagnostic Procedures/Surgery
- Ophthalmologic evaluation including slit-lamp examination of the irides
- Neuropsychological testing: Intelligence is usually normal, although significant deficits in language, visuospatial skills, and neuromotor skills may be present.

DIFFERENTIAL DIAGNOSIS
Familial café-au-lait spots (autosomal dominant; no other NF1 features); Watson syndrome; LEOPARD syndrome; McCune-Albright syndrome; neurocutaneous melanosis; proteus syndrome; lipomatosis

TREATMENT

See Health Supervision of Children guidelines for NF1 (3) listed in "Ongoing Care" section.

MEDICATION
First Line
Anticonvulsants for seizure control, medications for attention deficit hyperactivity disorder (ADHD), hypertension, etc.

Second Line
Multiple clinical trials for NF1 are recruiting patients (see http://www.clinicaltrials.gov).

ADDITIONAL TREATMENT
Issues for Referral
- Patients with more than minimal manifestations of NF1 should be referred to a multidisciplinary NF clinic.
- Referral for psychosocial issues of family and affected individuals
- Educational intervention for children with learning disabilities or ADHD (40%)

Additional Therapies
- Occupational therapy for children with NF1 who present with fine motor difficulties
- There is no evidence supporting laser therapy for café-au-lait spots.
- The Children's Tumor Foundation has established the NF Clinical Trials Consortium and the CTF NF Clinic Network to facilitate future clinical trials and help identify best practices (4).

SURGERY/OTHER PROCEDURES
Surgical treatment for severe scoliosis, plexiform neurofibromata, or malignancy

 ONGOING CARE

FOLLOW-UP RECOMMENDATIONS
NF1 health supervision 2008 guidelines (3):
- Infancy–1 year:
  - Growth and development, mild short stature, macrocephaly due to increased brain volume; also aqueductal stenosis/obstructive hydrocephalus, hydrocephalus
  - Check for focal neurologic signs or asymmetric neurologic exam.
  - Skeletal abnormalities, especially of spine and legs
  - Neurodevelopmental progress
- 1–5 years:
  - Café-au-lait spots and axillary freckling have no clinical significance.
  - Annual ophthalmologic exam
  - Order brain MRI for visual changes, persistent headaches, seizures, marked increase in head size, plexiform neurofibroma of the head.
  - Assess speech and language: Hypernasal speech due to velopharyngeal insufficiency and delayed expressive language development.
  - Developmental evaluation of learning and motor abilities; may benefit from preschool services, speech/language and/or motor therapy, and special education
  - Monitor blood pressure annually.
- 5–13 years:
  - Evaluate for skin tumors causing disfigurement, and obtain consultation if surgery is desired to improve appearance or function.
  - Evaluate for premature or delayed puberty. If sexual precocity is noted, evaluate for an optic

glioma or hypothalamic lesion. Review the effects of puberty on NF.
  - Evaluate for learning disabilities and ADHD.
  - Evaluate social adjustment, development, and school placement.
  - Monitor ophthalmologic status yearly until age 8; complete eye examination every 2 years.
  - Monitor blood pressure annually.
  - Refer patient to a clinical psychologist or child psychiatrist for problems with self-esteem if indicated.
  - Discuss growth of neurofibromata during adolescence and pregnancy.
  - Counsel parents about discussing diagnosis with child.
- 13–21 years:
  - Examine the adolescent for abnormal pubertal development.
  - Perform a thorough skin examination for plexiform neurofibromata and a complete neurologic examination for findings suggestive of deep plexiform neurofibromata. Obtain surgical consultation if there are signs of pressure on deep structures.
  - Continue monitoring blood pressure yearly.
  - Continue ophthalmologic examination every 2 years until age 18.
  - Discuss genetics of NF1 or refer for genetic counseling.
  - Discuss sexuality, contraception, and reproductive options.
  - Discuss effects of pregnancy on NF1, if appropriate. Neurofibromata may enlarge, and new tumors may develop during pregnancy.
  - Review prenatal diagnosis or refer the patient to a geneticist.

Patient Monitoring
Annual evaluation and periodic assessment for at-risk individuals

PATIENT EDUCATION
- Genetic counseling and patient education regarding future complications about family planning.
- The National Neurofibromatosis Foundation has been incorporated in the Childrens Tumor Foundation, but many state chapters remain independent. The Children's Tumor Foundation http://www.CTF.org. Support groups are important.

PROGNOSIS
Variable; most patients have a mild expression of NF1 and lead normal lives.

COMPLICATIONS
- Disfigurement: Skin neurofibromata develop primarily on exposed areas. The number tends to increase with puberty or pregnancy.
- Scoliosis: 10–30%, but most cases are mild; bowing of long bones, 2%
- A large head is common but rarely associated with hydrocephalus.
- Increased risk of malignancy: Malignant peripheral nerve sheath tumor (MPNST), a highly aggressive spindle cell sarcoma, is the most common malignant neoplasm, occurring in 5–10% of individuals with NF1, usually in adults (1). Typically, MPNST arises from a plexiform neurofibroma. Slightly increased risk for other malignancies, e.g., pheochromocytoma, rhabdomyosarcoma, leukemia, Wilms tumor. Optic glioma or other central nervous system tumors arise, usually during childhood (5–15%).

- Learning disability: ~50%; may be associated with ADHD; mental retardation 4–8%
- Gastrointestinal (GI) neurofibromata may cause a range of GI disturbances.
- Seizures 6–7%
- Hypertension is a frequent finding in adults, and may occur in childhood.
- Disorders of puberty

Pregnancy Considerations
Increased risk of perinatal complications, stillbirth, IUGR; risk of cord compression and outlet obstruction by pelvic neurofibromata.

REFERENCES
1. DeBella K, Szudek J, Friedman JM. Use of the national institutes of health criteria for diagnosis of neurofibromatosis 1 in children. *Pediatrics.* 2000;105:608–14.
2. National Institutes of Health Consensus Development Conference Statement: neurofibromatosis. Bethesda, Md., USA, July 13–15, 1987. *Neurofibromatosis.* 1988;1:172–8.
3. Hersh JH. and Committee on Genetics. Health supervision for children with neurofibromatosis. *Pediatrics.* 2008;121:3:633–642.
4. Williams VC, Lucas J, Babcock MA, Gutmann DH, Korf B, Maria BL et al. Neurofibromatosis type 1 revisited. *Pediatrics.* 2009;123:124–33.

See Also (Topic, Algorithm, Electronic Media Element)
Ataxia-telangiectasia; Tuberous Sclerosis Complex; von Hippel–Lindau Disease

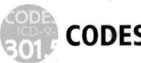 **CODES**

ICD9
- 237.70 Neurofibromatosis, unspecified
- 237.71 Neurofibromatosis, type 1, von Recklinghausen's disease
- 237.72 Neurofibromatosis, type 2, acoustic neurofibromatosis

CLINICAL PEARLS
- NF1 and NF2 are 2 distinct genetic disorders.
- NF1 has marked clinical variability. Even minimal findings necessitate monitoring. External stigmata may be subtle or absent in young children. Minimally affected children may become severely affected adults.
- A single café-au-lait spot is of no concern in a child, but having ≥6 is 1 of the diagnostic criteria for NF1.

N

NEUROLEPTIC MALIGNANT SYNDROME

Deanna M. Scinto, PharmD
Mhd Basheer Rahmoun, MD

 BASICS

DESCRIPTION
- Life-threatening condition that may develop anytime during therapy with neuroleptics—from a few days to many years (but 2/3 of cases occur within the 1st week)
- Muscular rigidity from dopamine antagonism in the nigrostriatal pathway
- Hyperthermia due to blockage of hypothalamic thermoregulation (more likely in the setting of benzodiazepine withdrawal)
- Autonomic dysfunction
- May be indistinguishable from other causes of drug-induced hyperthermia (e.g., malignant hyperthermia, serotonin syndrome, anticholinergic toxins, or sympathomimetic poisoning)

EPIDEMIOLOGY
Incidence
- The incidence has been variably reported from prospective studies as 0.01–3.0% (1).
- 2,000 new cases annually in US (2)
- Predominant sex: Male > Female
- Predominant age: <40 years of age

Prevalence
0.15% ± 0.05% among patients receiving neuroleptics

RISK FACTORS
- Intramuscular administration of medication (3)
- Newly administered medication (3)
- Rapid dose increase (3)
- Psychomotor agitation (3)
- Dehydration
- Prior episodes of neuroleptic malignant syndrome (NMS)
- Age and gender correspond with the distribution of exposure to neuroleptic agents.

Genetics
- Some studies show a genetic predisposition to NMS.
- Polymorphisms: Loss of del allele in 141C Ins/Del of the dopamine D2 receptor gene and Ser9Gly in the dopamine D3 receptor gene (4)

PATHOPHYSIOLOGY
- Exact mechanism unknown
- Most likely due to dopamine blockade (2)

ETIOLOGY
- Rare complication of treatment with neuroleptics: Phenothiazines (e.g., Fluphenazine), butyrophenones (e.g., Haloperidol), and thiothixene
- Also seen with atypical antipsychotics (e.g., clozapine, risperidone, olanzapine) (56)
- Occurs in approximately 1% of patients treated with neuroleptics (especially haloperidol)
- Also has been associated with withdrawal from dopamine agonists in Parkinson disease

 DIAGNOSIS

HISTORY
- Neuroleptic use or an increase in dose
- Discontinuation of antiparkinsonian drugs

PHYSICAL EXAM
- Extrapyramidal symptoms: Dysphagia, short shuffling gait, resting tremor, and the significant skeletal muscle rigidity—lead-pipe rigidity (these symptoms are less likely with clonazapine-induced NMS) (5)
- Hyperthermia (temperature may be as high as 106–107°F [41°C])
- Altered level of consciousness
- Autonomic instability (e.g., diaphoresis, tachycardia, tachypnea, labile blood pressure)

DIAGNOSTIC TESTS & INTERPRETATION
Lab
White blood cell determination, creatine phosphokinase, lactate dehydrogenase, liver function tests, and urine myoglobin

Imaging
- Chest x-ray (if aspiration pneumonia is suspected)
- Head computed tomography scan before lumber puncture

Diagnostic Procedures/Surgery
Lumbar puncture to rule out other causes of fever or altered mental status

DIFFERENTIAL DIAGNOSIS
- Meningitis, encephalitis, sepsis
- Malignant hyperthermia, severe dystonic reaction
- Lethal catatonia
- Serotonin syndrome
- Anticholinergic poisoning, salicylate poisoning
- Sympathomimetic poisoning
- Neuroleptic-induced tardive dyskinesia
- Tetanus
- Heat stroke
- Strychnine poisoning
- Vascular central nervous system event
- Thyrotoxicosis, pheochromocytoma
- Rabies
- Acute intermittent porphyria
- Nonconvulsive status epilepticus

 TREATMENT

- Discontinue offending agent immediately (2).
- Provide supportive care (3):
  - Hydration
  - Maintain renal function.
  - Regulate temperature.

MEDICATION
- Dopamine agonists can be used, but their role in NMS is still uncertain:
  - Bromocriptine: May play a role in longer-term management; 5–10 mg p.o. b.i.d.; maximum 40 mg/d
  - Amantadine: 100 mg p.o. b.i.d.; increase as needed to a maximum of 400 mg/d
- Skeletal muscle relaxant: Dantrolene: May play a role in longer-term management; 100–200 mg/d p.o.; maximum 400 mg/d or 0.8–2.5 mg/kg q6h; maximum 10 mg/kg/d
- Benzodiazepines are the drugs of choice:
  - Diazepam: 5 mg IV q5min
  - Lorazepam: 1 mg IV q5min
- Electroconvulsive therapy may be used for refractory symptoms (2).
- Neither bromocriptine nor dantrolene has a rapid onset, and neither has been demonstrated to alter outcome.

ADDITIONAL TREATMENT
General Measures
- Volume repletion
- Correct electrolyte abnormalities.
- Relief of muscle rigidity
- Recognize complications (e.g., rhabdomyolysis, respiratory failure, acute renal failure); mortality can be as high as 50%.

Issues for Referral
- The patient's psychiatric disease should be evaluated by a psychiatrist during withdrawal of neuroleptic medications.
- All patients should be transferred to an acute-care facility where intensive monitoring is available.
- Nephrologist should be consulted in the setting of renal failure.

IN-PATIENT CONSIDERATIONS
Initial Stabilization
- Airway intervention and circulatory support as needed; ventilation may be difficult because of chest wall rigidity
- IV, supplemental O_2, cardiac monitor
- Immediate IV benzodiazepines (e.g., diazepam, lorazepam): May require repeated large doses
- If symptoms are not controlled within a few minutes, rapid-sequence intubation and neuromuscular blockade are necessary. Nondepolarizing neuromuscular blockers (e.g., vecuronium, rocuronium, pancuronium) are preferable to succinylcholine.
- Cool the patient, and treat seizures if they occur. Measures to control hyperthermia: Ice packs, mist and fan, cooling blankets, and so on
- Aggressive IV fluid therapy with lactated Ringer solution or normal saline (NS)
- Check fingerstick glucose.

Admission Criteria
- All patients with the diagnosis should be admitted.
- Patients often will require intensive care.

IV Fluids
Hydration with intravenous NS (3)

 ## ONGOING CARE

FOLLOW-UP RECOMMENDATIONS
- Allow 2 weeks after recovery to rechallenge neuroleptic:
  - Rechallenge should not be with the medication implicated in the original NMS episode (3).
- Start at low dose, and titrate gradually.
- Carefully monitor for signs and symptoms of recurrent NMS (2).

PATIENT EDUCATION
- Discuss risk–benefit ratio of restarting therapy vs a recurrence of NMS (2).
- NMS information service: www.nmsis.org.

PROGNOSIS
- Mortality rate is estimated at 5–11.6% (dropped from 25% in 1984) (7).
- Signs that may warn of a poor prognosis include temperature over 104°F and kidney failure.
- In absence of complications, the prognosis for recovery is good; most patients recover in 15 days (8).
- Prognosis is better when NMS is detected early.

COMPLICATIONS
- Rhabdomyolysis
- Renal failure
- Cardiac arrest
- Infections
- Aspiration
- Respiratory failure
- Seizure
- Hepatic failure
- Uncontrolled psychosis
- Persistent neuropsychiatric complications (3)
- Death (3)

REFERENCES

1. Petersén A, Lundberg L. Neuroleptic malignant syndrome–rare diagnosis with high mortality. *Lakartidningen*. 2009;106(18–19):1273–6.
2. Strawn JR, Keck PE, Caroff SN. Neuroleptic malignant syndrome. *Am J Psychiatry*. 2007;164:870–6.
3. Seitz DP, Gill SS. Neuroleptic malignant syndrome complicating antipsychotic treatment of delirium or agitation in medical and surgical patients: case reports and a review of the literature. *Psychosomatics*. 2009;50:8–15.
4. Mihara K, Kondo T, Suzuki A, et al. Relationship between functional dopamine D2 and D3 receptors gene polymorphisms and neuroleptic malignant syndrome. *Am J Med Genet B Neuropsychiatr Genet*. 2003;117:57–60.
5. Trollor JN, Chen X, Sachdev PS. Neuroleptic malignant syndrome associated with atypical antipsychotic drugs. *CNS Drugs*. 2009;23:477–92.
6. Neuhut R, Lindenmayer JP, Silva R et al. Neuroleptic malignant syndrome in children and adolescents on atypical antipsychotic medication: a review. *J Child Adolesc Psychopharmacol*. 2009;19:415–22.
7. Shalev A, Hermesh H, Munitz H. Mortality from neuroleptic malignant syndrome. *J Clin Psychiatry*. 1989;50:18–25.
8. Caroff SN, Mann SC. Neuroleptic malignant syndrome. *Med Clin North Am*. 1993;77:185–202.

ADDITIONAL READING

- Halloran LL, Bernard DW. Management of drug-induced hyperthermia. *Curr Opin Pediatr*. 2004;16:211–5.
- Silva RR, Munoz DM, Alpert M, et al. Neuroleptic malignant syndrome in children and adolescents. *J Am Acad Child Adolesc Psychiatry*. 1999;38:187–94.

See Also (Topic, Algorithm, Electronic Media Element)
Algorithms: Delirium; Coma

 ## CODES

ICD9
333.92 Neuroleptic malignant syndrome

CLINICAL PEARLS
- 2/3 of cases occur within the 1st week of starting a neuroleptic, but NMS may occur after years.
- NMS may be triggered by discontinuation of Parkinson medications.
- Elevated serum creatinine kinase is the most consistent lab abnormality in patients with NMS (3).

N

NEUROPATHIC PAIN

Christian D. Gonzalez, MD

 BASICS

DESCRIPTION
- Neuropathic pain is defined as pain in association with primary injury or dysfunction of the nervous system, with or without ongoing tissue damage.
- Divided into 2 groups based on the location of the suspected lesion: central vs peripheral:
  - Newer data suggest a possibility that most neuropathic syndromes have a component of both central and peripheral mechanisms.
- An important consideration with a patient with neuropathic pain is the absence of any deficit or injury. Socially, the patient appears "normal," yet suffers from a chronic painful condition. This can lead to psychosocial distress, as the patient is labeled "drug seeking."
- May be triggered by numerous insults, including direct nerve injury, infection, metabolic dysfunction, autoimmune disease, neoplasm, drugs, radiation, and neurovascular disorders
- May reflect the pathologic operation of a dysfunctional nervous system rather than a manifestation of any underlying pathology itself (i.e., phantom limb pain, complex regional pain syndrome [CRPS]):
  - Patients may paradoxically experience pain and hypersensitivity in an area of denervation.
- System(s) affected: Nervous; Musculoskeletal

EPIDEMIOLOGY
Incidence
Epidemiologic data are limited. It will also be varied, depending on the inclusion criteria: Radiculopathies, peripheral neuropathy, etc.:
- >3 million Americans suffer from painful diabetic neuropathy (PDN).
- 1 million Americans suffer from postherpetic neuralgia (PHN).

Prevalence
Estimated at 1.5% of the population, although recent studies in England, Germany, and France place it around 6-8% of the population.

RISK FACTORS
- Radiculopathy
- Polyneuropathy (diabetes mellitus, alcohol induced, post chemotherapy)
- Trauma (nerve entrapment, post surgical, nerve injury)
- Infection (HIV, herpes zoster)
- Central mechanisms (stroke, MS, spinal cord injury, limb amputation)
- Nutritional deficiencies (B_{12}, folate)
- Medications (AIDS medications DDC and DDI, antibiotics metronidazole and isoniazid, some chemotherapeutics, amiodarone, hydralazine, phenytoin, nitrofurantoin)

PATHOPHYSIOLOGY
- Positive symptoms due to changes in peripheral nerves, loss of inhibitory mechanisms in CNS, and central sensitization
- Negative symptoms likely due to axonal or neuronal loss

ETIOLOGY
- Associated with a predisposing factor
- In addition to possible etiologies listed as risk factors above, others include:
  - Demyelinating disorders (multiple sclerosis, Guillain-Barré)
  - Neoplasm (primary or metastatic)
  - Neurovascular (central post stroke syndrome, trigeminal neuralgia)
  - Autoimmune disease (Sjögren syndrome, polyarteritis nodosa)
  - Structural disease (herniated disc disease)

COMMONLY ASSOCIATED CONDITIONS
- Depression
- Anxiety
- Sleep disturbance
- Fibromyalgia

 DIAGNOSIS

HISTORY
- May have history of nerve trauma; however, absence does not exclude the diagnosis of neuropathic pain
- Clinical manifestation can include both negative and positive sensory symptoms and signs. Motor dysfunction is rare.
- Pain is often described as burning, shocklike, tingling, numbing, or intensely hot or cold.

PHYSICAL EXAM
- Positive signs and symptoms:
  - Hyperalgesia: An exaggerated pain response to a noxious stimulus
  - Allodynia: The perception of pain due to a non-noxious stimuli; for instance, gentle mechanical pressure, light pinprick, hot or cold stimuli, and vibration cause pain.
- Negative signs and symptoms:
  - Reduced sensation to touch, pinprick, temperature, or vibration
- Motor signs and symptoms:
  - Signs may include hypotonia, tremor, dystonia, ataxia, hypo-/hyper-reflexia, or motor neglect. Motor symptoms include weakness, fatigability, decreased range of motion, joint stiffness, and spontaneous muscle spasm.

DIAGNOSTIC TESTS & INTERPRETATION
Lab
Initial lab tests
None specifically for neuropathic pain, but tests to rule out other causes should be considered:
- Serum B_{12}
- 25 vitamin D
- TSH
- RPR or VDRL
- Fasting glucose, creatinine
- Lyme serology

Follow-Up & Special Considerations
Studies may include nerve conduction, electromyography, evoked potentials, quantitative sensory testing, thermography, radiologic imaging

Imaging
Initial approach
- Used to rule out other causes for pain
- Consider imaging based on affected area. MRI shows greatest anatomical detail for spine.
- PET and SPECT scans, standard MRI, and functional MRI all have been used to map synaptic activity in the thalamus and somatosensory cortex. Initial studies using these imaging techniques have suggested maladaptive reorganization of the thalamus and somatosensory cortex.

Diagnostic Procedures/Surgery
- Sympathetic nerve blocks
- Epidural steroids
- Peripheral nerve blocks
- Dorsal column stimulator and peripheral nerve stimulator

 TREATMENT

MEDICATION
First Line
- All 1st-line agents are those that have been studied the most. However, the more we understand about chronic opioid therapy, the more we recommend *not* starting an opioid until other neuropathic agents have failed. In general, moving from 1 anticonvulsant or TCA to the other should be considered the 1st step of action.
- Gabapentin:
  - An anticonvulsant that has the broadest evidence for efficacy against neuropathic pain, FDA approved for its treatment (1)[A]
  - Evidence supports efficacy in PDN, PHN, phantom limb pain, Guillain-Barré syndrome, acute and chronic pain from spinal cord injury, and CRPS type 1 (2)[A]
  - Start 300 mg daily, increase gradually; dosing up to 600 mg t.i.d. is suggested; max dose of 3,600 mg/d in divided doses; adjust dose in renal insufficiency
  - Adequate trial of 3–8 weeks of therapy at full dose before considering it a failure
  - Interactions: No major drug–drug interactions
  - Adverse effects: Dizziness, somnolence, GI symptoms, peripheral edema
- Tricyclic antidepressants:
  - This class has the most evidence supporting their role in neuropathic pain (3)[A].
  - Dosing: Start at 10–25 mg at bedtime, then titrate up to antidepressant drug levels.
  - Secondary amines (nortriptyline, desipramine) are safer than amitriptyline and imipramine.
  - Precautions: Small therapeutic-to-toxic window; use caution in prescribing to those with cardiac risk factors, glaucoma, urinary retention; suicide susceptibility
  - Should obtain a pretreatment ECG for documentation and monitoring any arrhythmias
  - Absolute contraindication with MAOIs
  - Interactions: Numerous possible drug–drug interactions (type 1C antiarrhythmics, SSRIs, anticholinergics, sympathomimetics, CNS depressants)

- Adverse effects: QT interval abnormalities, arrhythmias, sedation, dry mouth, constipation, sexual dysfunction, weight gain, postural hypotension
- Tramadol (4)[A]:
  - Norepinephrine and serotonin inhibitor with a major metabolite that acts as an opioid (mu receptor) agonist
  - Dosage: 250 mg/d divided doses, max 400 mg/d
  - Precautions: Avoid in those with seizure history
  - Interactions: Increased seizure risk in those taking SSRIs, TCAs, MAOIs, neuroleptics concomitantly; increased risk of serotonergic symptoms if used with SSRIs, MAOIs; adjust dose for renal insufficiency, hepatic disease
  - Adverse effects: Dizziness, nausea, constipation, somnolence, orthostatic hypotension
- Pregabalin:
  - FDA-approved for treatment of neuropathic pain secondary to PHN and diabetic polyneuropathy. Also approved for fibromyalgia (5)[A].
  - Dosage: Start at 75 mg b.i.d., maximum dose 300 mg b.i.d.
  - Interactions: No major drug–drug interactions
- Opioids (2)[A]:
  - According to World Health Organization, should be used in "ladder" fashion, added to nonopioid agents if they are insufficient. However, this is usually for palliative cancer patients. Chronic opioid therapy can be detrimental to psychosocial environment of the patient.
  - Evidence for increased efficacy when used in conjunction with gabapentin
  - Controlled-release opioids recommended (controlled release oxycodone, morphine, transdermal fentanyl, methadone)
  - Dosage: Start with short-acting analgesic equivalent to oral morphine sulfate 5–15 mg q4h; after 1–2 weeks of treatment, calculate equivalent dose of long-acting agent and use short-acting opioids for breakthrough.
  - No clear maximum dosage, but trials do not show benefits at doses higher than 180 mg/d of morphine.
  - Precaution: Avoid in those with history of substance abuse, use with caution in the elderly, may cause respiratory depression
  - Interactions: Additive effects with CNS depressants, increased risk of serotonin syndrome with serotonergic agents
  - Adverse effects: Constipation, sedation, nausea, lightheadedness
  - Adjuvant therapies with opioids should be used to treat nausea/vomiting, constipation, sedation, pruritus, etc.

Second Line
- Some evidence suggests use of other medications:
  - Antidepressants: Paroxetine, venlafaxine, duloxetine, bupropion, citalopram (2)
  - Duloxetine has comparable efficacy and tolerability to gabapentin and pregabalin in treatment of diabetic peripheral neuropathic pain (6)[A].
  - Anticonvulsants: Topiramate, Zonegran, lamotrigine, carbamazepine, oxcarbazepine
  - Antiarrhythmics: Mexiletine
  - NMDA receptor antagonists: Ketamine, dextromethorphan (5)
  - Other agents: Baclofen, clonidine, capsaicin

- Topical lidocaine; 5% lidocaine patch:
  - FDA-approved for treatment of PHN but has been used for other focal neuropathic pain syndromes
  - Dosage: Up to 3 patches for 12 hours daily
  - Interactions: No significant drug–drug interactions
  - Adverse effects: Mild skin reactions
  - Cochrane Review in 2007 showed insufficient evidence to recommend as 1st line.

ADDITIONAL TREATMENT
Issues for Referral
Referral to pain clinic or neurosurgery is appropriate if refractory to initial treatment.

Additional Therapies
- Transcutaneous electrical nerve stimulation (TENS) may be helpful; optimal dosing is yet to be established (7)[B].
- Spinal cord stimulation may be effective for chronic pain, especially if back surgery failed (8)[B].

COMPLEMENTARY AND ALTERNATIVE MEDICINE
See Additional Therapies.

SURGERY/OTHER PROCEDURES
Nerve destructive procedures:
- Should be used with caution as a refractory to treatment different pain can ensue. If nononcolgical nerve damage, most neurolytic procedures are not recommended.
- Sympathetectomy: More studies needed for effectiveness and safety
- Dorsal root entry zone lesion (dorsal rhizotomy)
- Lateral cordotomy
- Trigeminal nerve ganglion ablation

 ## ONGOING CARE

FOLLOW-UP RECOMMENDATIONS
- Multidisciplinary team improves care.
- Opioid contracts to prevent abuses.

Patient Monitoring
Random urinalysis for specific prescribed drug and all drugs of abuse for patients receiving opioid therapy

PROGNOSIS
Chronic course of pain symptoms often requires management with numerous medications and adjunctive therapies.

COMPLICATIONS
Long-term disability is a possibility. Drug addiction is possible.

REFERENCES
1. Wiffen PJ, et al. Gabapentin for acute and chronic pain. *Cochrane Database Syst Rev.* 2007;4: CD005452.
2. Schmader KE. Epidemiology and impact on quality of life of postherpetic neuralgia and painful diabetic neuropathy. *Clin J Pain.* 2002;18:350–4.
3. Saarto T, Wiffen PJ. Antidepressants for neuropathic pain. *Cochrane Database Syst Rev.* 2007;4:CD005454.
4. Hollingshead J, et al. Tramadol for neuropathic pain. *Cochrane Database Syst Rev.* 2007;2: CD003726.
5. Galluzzi KE. Managing neuropathic pain. *J Am Osteopath Assoc.* 2007;107:ES39–48.
6. Quilici S, Chancellor J, Lothgren M, et al. Meta-analysis of duloxetine vs. pregabalin and gabapentin in the treatment of diabetic peripheral neuropathic pain. *BMC Neurol.* 2009;9:6.
7. Carrol D, et al. TENS for chronic pain. *Cochrane Database Syst Rev.* 2007;4:2007.
8. Mailis-Gagnon A, et al. Spinal cord stimulation for chronic pain. *Cochrane Database Syst Rev.* 2007;4:CD003783.

ADDITIONAL READING
- Eisenberg E, McNicol E, Carr DB. Opioids for neuropathic pain. *Cochrane Database Syst Rev.* 2006;3:CD006146.
- Kroenke K, Krebs EE, Bair MJ. Pharmacotherapy of chronic pain: a synthesis of recommendations from systematic reviews. *Gen Hosp Psychiatry.* 2009 May-Jun;31:206–19.
- Raja SN, Haythornthwaite JA. Combination therapy for neuropathic pain–which drugs, which combination, which patients? *N Engl J Med.* 2005;352:1373–5.
- Torrance N, Smith BH, Benett MI, Lee AJ. The epidemiology of chronic pain of predominantly neuropathic origin. Results from a general population survey. *J Pain.* 2006;7(4):281–289.
- Wiffen PJ, McQuay HJ, Moore RA. Carbamazepine for acute and chronic pain. *Cochrane Database Syst Rev.* 2005;CD005451.

CODES

ICD9
- 356.9 Unspecified idiopathic peripheral neuropathy
- 729.2 Neuralgia, neuritis, and radiculitis, unspecified

CLINICAL PEARLS
- Multidisciplinary approach to pain management is suggested.
- Gabapentin is 1st-line for neuropathic pain. Followed by other antiseizures, TCAs and SNRIs.
- A trial of interventional nerve blockage should be recommended prior to committing to chronic analgesic therapy.
- Opioids are used after 2 or 3 other attempts at treatment, in combination with other 1st-line agents. Opioids are generally considered weak neuropathic agents. Thus, high dosages are required to be effective in dealing with chronic pain. This presents a problem with potential for side effects, misuse, and addiction.

N

NICOTINE ADDICTION

Brett White, MD

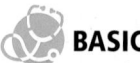 **BASICS**

DESCRIPTION
Nicotine use characterized by signs of dependence (compulsive use of a substance despite knowledge of its adverse effects)

EPIDEMIOLOGY
Incidence
20–25% of US population smokes.

Prevalence
70.9 million Americans $\geq$12 years of age reported current use of tobacco (60.1 million were cigarette smokers, 13.3 million smoked cigars, 8.1 million used smokeless tobacco, 2 million smoked pipes) (1)[B].

Pediatric Considerations
7% of 8th graders, 12% of 10th graders, and 20% of 12th graders have used cigarettes in the past 30 days (1).

RISK FACTORS
- Mental illness (including depression, posttraumatic stress disorder, bipolar disorder, and schizophrenia)
- Low socioeconomic status
- Low educational status
- Early firsthand nicotine experience increases risk from chronic abuse
- Environmental factors are critical for smoking initiation; genetic factors contribute to smoking persistence and difficulty quitting.

Genetics
- Mutation in the α_4 subunit of nicotinic acetylcholine receptors (nAChRs) expressed by neurons was found to lower the threshold for the induction of nicotine dependence.
- Specific genes have been isolated that are associated with nicotine dependence, including *CHRNB3*, the β_3 nicotine receptor subunit gene.
- T-variant gene associated with decreased activity of CYP2B6 (enzyme that breaks down nicotine in the brain); may lead to increased craving during smoking cessation. These patients are also 1.5 times more likely to resume smoking during treatment.

GENERAL PREVENTION
- Physician advice
  - The USPSTF concludes that the evidence is insufficient to recommend for or against routine screening for tobacco use or interventions to prevent and treat tobacco use and dependence among children or adolescents.
- School-based smoking-prevention education
- Nonsmoking adolescents who were more aware of or receptive to tobacco advertising were more likely to become smokers later.

PATHOPHYSIOLOGY
- Mechanism by which nicotine binds to nAChR and how this leads to dependence are still poorly understood, though likely involve activation of the mesocorticolimbic system with resulting dopamine release.
- Nicotine has both stimulating and depressing effects within the CNS; relaxing and euphoric effects may contribute to psychological dependence.

Pregnancy Considerations
- Carbon monoxide and nicotine may interfere with oxygen supply to the fetus, resulting in fetal growth restriction and decreased birth weight.
- Smoking may increase the incidence of spontaneous abortion, SIDS, as well as learning or behavioral problems and an increased risk of obesity in children (1).

ETIOLOGY
Polymorphisms in neuronal nAChR genes could be associated with increased susceptibility to tobacco dependence.

COMMONLY ASSOCIATED CONDITIONS
- COPD (emphysema and chronic bronchitis)
- Cancers (lung, oral/pharyngeal, kidney, bladder, cervical, anal)
- Coronary artery disease
- Periodontal disease

 DIAGNOSIS

DIAGNOSTIC TESTS & INTERPRETATION
Spirometry: Decreased FEV_1 (may be present in COPD)

DIFFERENTIAL DIAGNOSIS
- Depression
- COPD
- α_1-Antitrypsin deficiency
- Asthma
- CHF
- Respiratory infections
- Lung cancer
- Cystic fibrosis

 TREATMENT

Counseling:
- Advice from doctors helps people who smoke to quit.
- Providing brief, simple advice about quitting smoking increases likelihood that someone who smokes will successfully quit and remain a nonsmoker 12 months later. More intensive advice (i.e., Motivational Interviewing, etc.) may result in higher rates of quitting. Providing follow-up support after offering the advice may increase the quit rates slightly (2)[A].
- The USPSTF strongly recommends to screen all adults for tobacco use and provide tobacco cessation interventions for those who use tobacco products. Grade: A recommendation.

MEDICATION
First Line
- Varenicline (Chantix) is a nicotinic acetylcholine partial agonist for the treatment of nicotine addiction. Trials have suggested this agent may be more efficacious than Bupropion (3)[A]. Longer-term therapy (up to 24 weeks) may delay or prevent relapse:
  - Starter package includes 0.5 mg/d for 3 days, then 0.5 mg b.i.d. for 4 days, then 1.0 mg/d starting on day 7.
  - Maintenance package includes 1.0 mg b.i.d. (continue for 12 weeks total).
- Nicotine replacement therapy (NRT). All forms of NRT increase the chance of stopping smoking by 50–70%. There is no overall difference in effectiveness of different forms of NRT nor a benefit for using patches beyond 8 weeks. Heavier smokers may need higher doses. Starting NRT before planned quit date may increase the chance of success (4)[A].
  - Nicotine gum (Nicorette): For >25 cigarettes/d habit, 4 mg gum q1–2h for 6 weeks; for <25 cigarettes/d habit, 2 mg gum q1–2h for 6 weeks; decrease dosing by q1–2h for 3 weeks; chew, then tuck between cheek and gingiva
  - Nicotine transdermal (NicoDerm CQ): For >10 cigarettes/d habit, 21-mg patch/d for 6 weeks, then 14 mg patch/d for 2 weeks, then 7 mg patch/d for 2 weeks; for <10 cigarettes/d habit, 14-mg patch/d for 6 weeks, then 7 mg patch/d for 2 weeks
  - Nicotine lozenge (Commit): For patients who have 1st cigarette within 30 min of waking, 4-mg lozenge PO q1–2h for 6 weeks; 1st cigarette >30 min after waking, 2-mg lozenge PO q1–2h for 6 weeks; decrease dosing by q1–2h for 3 weeks.
  - Nicotine nasal (Nicotrol NS): 1–2 sprays (0.5 mg/spray) each nostril q1h for 8 weeks, then taper; maximum 10 sprays/h and 80 sprays/d
  - Nicotine inhaled (Nicotrol inhaler): 6–16 cartridges inhaled (4 mg/cartridge) per day for 6–12 weeks, then taper
- Medications:
  - Bupropion (Zyban): An antidepressant; start 150 mg/d PO for 3 days, then 150 mg PO b.i.d.; stop smoking 5–7 days after starting treatment; continue 7–12 weeks.

ALERT
Varenicline (Chantix) has not been studied when used in patients with serious psychiatric illness. It should be used with extreme caution in patients with serious psychiatric disorders (bipolar disorder, depression, or schizophrenia) as use may exacerbate these conditions.

Second Line

- Nortriptyline: Tricyclic antidepressant; start 25 mg/d, gradually increase to target dose of 75–100 mg/d; stop smoking 2–4 weeks after starting treatment; continue for 12 weeks:
  – Contraindications: Narrow-angle glaucoma or heart disease (AMI, AV, or bundle-branch block, QT prolongation)
  – Caution: Pregnancy category D
- Clonidine: 0.1-mg patch per week, increase dose as needed; continue for 3–10 weeks:
  – Caution: Must monitor BP closely and taper when discontinuing.
- Benzodiazepines: Although this class of drug has not improved rates of abstinence from smoking, patients with a high level of anxiety possibly could benefit from anxiolytics as a smoking-cessation intervention.

ADDITIONAL TREATMENT
Pregnancy Considerations

- The USPSTF strongly recommends that clinicians screen all pregnant women for tobacco use and provide augmented pregnancy-tailored counseling to those who smoke. Grade: A recommendation.

- Other interventions:
  – Smokers who get support from partners and other people are more likely to quit.
  – Group programs are double cessation rates than being given self-help materials without face-to-face instruction and group support. The chances of quitting are approximately doubled. It is unclear whether groups are better than individual counselling or other advice, but they are more effective than no treatment. Not all smokers making a quit attempt want to attend group meetings, but for those who do they are likely to be helpful.
- Smokers should be given a choice of quitting methods, either reducing smoking before quitting or abrupt quitting, as neither has demonstrated superior quit rates.

Pregnancy Considerations

Interventions were effective in helping women to stop smoking during pregnancy (overall by approximately 6%). The most effective intervention appeared to be providing incentives, which helped around 24% of women to quit smoking during pregnancy. The smoking cessation interventions reduced the number of babies with low birthweight and preterm births, confirming that smoking cessation can reduce the adverse effects of smoking on newborn infants.

General Measures

- Brief strategies to help the patient willing to quit tobacco use—the "5 As":
  – *Ask* the patient if he or she uses tobacco.
  – *Advise* him or her to quit.
  – *Assess* willingness to make a quit attempt.
  – *Assist* those who are willing to make a quit attempt.
  – *Arrange* for follow-up contact to prevent relapse.

- Enhancing motivation to quit tobacco—the "5 Rs":
  – *Relevance*—Encourage the patient to indicate why quitting is personally relevant.
  – *Risks*—Ask the patient to identify potential negative consequences of tobacco use.
  – *Rewards*—Ask the patient to identify potential benefits of stopping tobacco use.
  – *Roadblocks*—Ask the patient to identify barriers or impediments to quitting and provide treatment (e.g., problem-solving counseling or medication) that could address barriers.
  – *Repetition*—The motivational intervention should be repeated every time an unmotivated patient visits the clinic setting (5)[A].

COMPLEMENTARY AND ALTERNATIVE MEDICINE

- Acupuncture: No consistent evidence acupuncture is effective for smoking cessation
- Hypnotherapy: No good evidence to show whether or not hypnotherapy can help people trying to quit smoking.

IN-PATIENT CONSIDERATIONS

- Programs to stop smoking that begin during a hospital stay and include follow-up support for at least 1 month after discharge are effective. Programmes are effective when administered to all hospitalized smokers, regardless of admitting diagnosis.
- Consider NRT to all inpatients who smoke to decrease withdrawal symptoms.

 ONGOING CARE

FOLLOW-UP RECOMMENDATIONS

- Patients motivated to quit smoking and who have initiated therapy should follow up routinely with the physician to monitor response and observe for any medication side effects.
- Encourage routine exercise as a component of smoking-cessation treatment.

DIET
Weight gain (4–5 kg over 10 years) possible after smoking cessation.

PATIENT EDUCATION
- http://www.smokefree.gov/
- http://www.nicotine-anonymous.org/
- http://quitnet.com/

PROGNOSIS
More than 85% of those who try to quit on their own relapse, most within a week (1).

REFERENCES

1. National Institute on Drug Abuse. *Tobacco Addiction*. National Institute of Health; 2009 June. NIH Publication Number 09-4342.
2. Stead LF, Bergson G, Lancaster T. Physician advice for smoking cessation. *Cochrane Database of Systematic Reviews*. 2008;2:CD000165. DOI:10.1002/14651858.CD000165.pub3.
3. Cahill K, Stead LF, Lancaster T. Nicotine receptor partial agonists for smoking cessation. *Cochrane Database of Systematic Reviews*. 2008;3: CD006103. DOI:10.1002/14651858. CD006103.pub3.
4. Stead LF, Perera R, Bullen C, et al. Nicotine replacement therapy for smoking cessation. *Cochrane Database of Systematic Reviews*. 2008;1:CD000146. DOI:10.1002/14651858. CD000146.pub3.
5. The Clinical Practice Guideline Treating Tobacco Use and Dependence 2008 Update Panel, Liaisons, and Staff. A Clinical Practice Guideline for Treating Tobacco Use and Dependence: 2008 Update A U.S. Public Health Service Report. *Am J Prev Med*. 2008;35:158–76.

ADDITIONAL READING

The Agency for Health Care Policy and Research Smoking Cessation Clinical Practice Guideline. *JAMA*. 1996;275:1270–80.

CODES

ICD9
- V15.82 Personal history of tobacco use
- 305.1 Tobacco use disorder
- 649.00 Tobacco use disorder complicating pregnancy

CLINICAL PEARLS

- Smoking cessation should be encouraged with all patients who smoke.
- There is no one type of nicotine-replacement therapy that is best; they are equally effective. Choice therefore should be based on patient preference.
- Consider NRT to all inpatients who smoke to decrease withdrawal symptoms.

N

NOCARDIOSIS

Brock D. Lutz, MD
Ronald A. Greenfield, MD

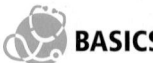 **BASICS**

DESCRIPTION
- Nocardiosis is an acute, subacute, or chronic infection occurring primarily in cutaneous, pulmonary, and disseminated forms in patients who are immunocompromised or have chronic pulmonary disease.
  - Nocardiosis produces suppurative necrosis and abscess formation at sites of infection.
  - Primary cutaneous nocardiosis presents as cutaneous infection (cellulitis or abscess), lymphocutaneous infection (similar to sporotrichosis), or subcutaneous infection (actinomycetoma).
  - Pulmonary infection presents as an acute, subacute, or chronic pneumonitis.
  - Disseminated nocardiosis may involve any organ (lesions in the brain or meninges are most frequent).
  - System(s) affected: Nervous; Pulmonary; Renal/Urologic; Skin/Exocrine
- Unusual nocardial infections:
  - Keratoconjunctivitis associated with contact lenses or penetrating injury or ophthalmologic surgery
  - Peritonitis in patients on continuous ambulatory peritoneal dialysis
  - Upper respiratory and digestive tract infections
  - Pericarditis and cardiac tamponade
  - Hematogenous endophthalmitis
  - Prosthetic joint infections
  - Natural or prosthetic valve endocarditis
  - Infections of the male genitourinary tract
  - Intravascular access device–related infection

EPIDEMIOLOGY
Incidence
- 0.4/100,000 person-years overall
- 53/100,000 person-years among individuals with AIDS
- 128/100,000 person-years among bone marrow transplant (BMT) recipients
- 1,122/100,000 person-years among solid-organ transplant recipients
- Predominant age: All ages are susceptible; mean age at diagnosis is the 4th decade of life.
- Predominant sex: Male > Female (3:1)

Prevalence
It is estimated that 500–1,000 new cases occur per year in the US.

RISK FACTORS
- Most cases occur as opportunistic infection of immunocompromised hosts or hosts with predisposing pulmonary abnormalities.
- Solid-organ transplantation, chronic granulomatous disease of childhood, dysgammaglobulinemias, pemphigus, Cushing disease, hemochromatosis, cirrhosis, bronchiectasis, tuberculosis, sarcoidosis, anthracosilicosis, pulmonary alveolar proteinosis, lymphoma, leukemia, glucocorticoid and cytotoxic therapy, solid malignancies, and AIDS
- Immunologically normal individuals may develop primary cutaneous disease days to weeks after receiving a wound contaminated with soil.

Pediatric Considerations
An association has been reported between chronic granulomatous disease of childhood and nocardiosis.

PATHOPHYSIOLOGY
Nocardiosis is an acute suppurative bacterial infection.

ETIOLOGY
Inhalation or traumatic inoculation of *Nocardia* sp. bacteria (predominantly *N. asteroides*, as well as *N. brasiliensis*, *N. caviae*, *N. farcinica*, *N. transvalensis*, *N. otitidiscaviarum*, and *N. nova*, although a host of new species continues to be described) from soil

COMMONLY ASSOCIATED CONDITIONS
- Chronic pulmonary disease
- Lymphoid malignancy
- Bone marrow or solid-organ transplantation
- Chronic corticosteroid use
- Autoimmune disease with immune suppressive agents
- Treatment with antitumor necrosis factor antibody
- Sarcoidosis
- Kidney failure
- Cirrhosis and alcoholism
- Hypogammaglobulinemia
- HIV infection

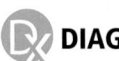 **DIAGNOSIS**

HISTORY
Presentation in the immunocompromised host depends on site of infection.

PHYSICAL EXAM
- Pulmonary nocardiosis:
  - Fever (70%)
  - Cough (52%)
  - Pleuritic chest pain (32%)
  - Dyspnea (16%)
  - Anorexia
  - Weight loss
  - Hemoptysis
  - Tachypnea
  - Rales
  - CNS dysfunction in those with CNS involvement
  - Other focal infections in those with disseminated infection
- Cutaneous nocardiosis:
  - Abscesses
  - Lymphadenopathy
- Disseminated nocardiosis:
  - Confusion
  - Disorientation
  - Dizziness
  - Headache
  - Nausea and/or vomiting
  - Seizures
  - Shortness of breath

- Patients with primary cutaneous nocardiosis present with cellulitis, cutaneous nodules, lymphadenopathy, or a mycetoma that is clinically indistinguishable from other etiologies.
- Patients with pulmonary nocardiosis present with pulmonary consolidation ± pleural effusions.
- Patients with disseminated nocardiosis present with symptoms that depend on sites of infection.

DIAGNOSTIC TESTS & INTERPRETATION
Lab
- The diagnosis is established by observing the characteristic microscopic appearance of the organism in Gram-stained and modified acid-fast-stained preparations of sputum or pus or histopathologic samples. Confirmation is by culture of these same specimens.
- When attempting recovery of *Nocardia* from sputum, clinical microbiology laboratory should be so advised because of the organism's slow growth and propensity to be overgrown by oral flora.
- Blood cultures should be obtained in all cases of suspected nocardiosis.

Imaging
- Radiography:
  - Confluent bronchopneumonia ± cavitation
  - Pleural effusion is common (up to 50%).
  - Other CXR presentations include masses, nodules, cavities, and interstitial infiltrates.
- CT scan or MRI of the brain may reveal single or multiple intracranial abscesses and is indicated in all patients with pulmonary or disseminated nocardiosis.
- Other sites of focal infection may be identified by imaging in disseminated disease.

Diagnostic Procedures/Surgery
- If evaluation of sputum is nondiagnostic, bronchoscopy for bronchoalveolar lavage and transbronchial lung biopsy may prove valuable for diagnosis.
- Percutaneous aspiration of lung lesion is often useful.

Pathological Findings
Histopathology reveals a suppurative lesion with acute necrosis and abscess formation and the microorganism, which may stain positive on modified acid-fast stains.

DIFFERENTIAL DIAGNOSIS
Includes other causes of acute, subacute, or chronic pneumonitis, particularly those occurring principally in immunocompromised hosts:
- Tuberculosis or atypical mycobacteria
- Histoplasmosis
- *Pneumocystis jiroveci* infection
- Polymicrobial bacterial lung abscess
- Carcinoma

TREATMENT

MEDICATION

First Line

- Survival may be improved if a sulfa-containing regimen is used (1)[B]. Some prefer sulfadiazine because of possibly better CNS penetration (1)[B]; should be given as 4–8 g/d PO in 4 divided doses. Dosage should be adjusted to maintain sulfonamide serum levels in the range of 8–16 mg/dL.
- Some prefer to use trimethoprim-sulfamethoxazole (1)[B]. This agent must be used if parenteral sulfonamide therapy is required. Initial dose based on trimethoprim component: 640 mg daily. Base subsequent doses on sulfamethoxazole level. Dosage should provide sulfonamide dosing and levels equivalent to those of sulfonamide when used alone.
- Duration of therapy is usually at least 3 months for immunocompetent hosts and 6–12 months for those who are immunocompromised, with treatment at least 1 month past resolution of evidence of infection.
- Contraindications:
  - Sulfonamides: During the last month of pregnancy (should be used only when the potential benefits outweigh the risks)
  - All antimicrobial agents above are contraindicated in the presence of known hypersensitivity to the agent.
- Precautions: With the use of high-dose sulfadiazine, high urine flow should be maintained to minimize risk of crystalluria. Generally, patients should be advised to drink 2–3 L/d.
- Significant possible interactions:
  - Sulfonamides may increase the therapeutic effects of oral anticoagulants, phenytoin, sulfonylurea hypoglycemic agents, methotrexate, and thiopental.
  - Decreased absorption of digoxin may be encountered.
- Ceftriaxone, 2 g IV q12h, or meropenem, 1 g IV q8h, plus amikacin, 15 mg/kg IV daily, should be considered as initial combination therapy with sulfonamide in critically or acutely ill patients.

Second Line

- Alternatives for sulfonamide-allergic patients include doxycycline or minocycline, ampicillin plus erythromycin, amikacin, meropenem, β-lactam/β-lactamase inhibitor combinations, cefotaxime or ceftriaxone, and linezolid (2)[A],(3)[B]. Clinical experience with these alternative regimens is limited.
- Species-specific trends in susceptibility have been identified; therefore, therapy should be guided by in vitro antimicrobial susceptibility.
- Empirical therapy for the acutely ill patient: Ceftriaxone, 2 g IV q12h, or meropenem, 1 g IV q8h, plus amikacin, 15 mg/kg IV daily

ADDITIONAL TREATMENT

General Measures

Respiratory support is often necessary in hospitalized patients.

Issues for Referral

Patients with suspected or confirmed nocardiosis should have therapy directed by an infectious diseases specialist.

SURGERY/OTHER PROCEDURES

Surgical drainage of abscesses other than intrapulmonary abscesses is generally indicated if technically feasible.

IN-PATIENT CONSIDERATIONS

Initial Stabilization

Patients with moderate or severe illness generally require hospitalization.

Admission Criteria

Patients with nocardiosis are often immune suppressed and are generally ill. They usually require hospitalization.

IV Fluids

Often required in critically ill patients

 ONGOING CARE

FOLLOW-UP RECOMMENDATIONS

Acute phase usually requires bed rest; increase activity as condition improves.

Patient Monitoring

Patients on high-dose sulfonamide therapy should have a complete blood count (CBC) and assessment of hepatic and renal function at least every other week.

DIET

Appropriate supportive care

PATIENT EDUCATION

- Not a contagious disease
- Advise patients of the need for long-term antimicrobial therapy to reduce the likelihood of relapse and inform patients of potential adverse reactions.

PROGNOSIS

- Overall modern mortality is 7–44%.
- Mortality in renal transplant recipients:
  - 25% overall
  - 0% with isolated cutaneous involvement
  - 29% with localized pleuropulmonary disease
  - 42% with CNS involvement
- In patients with AIDS, mortality is 30%.

COMPLICATIONS

- CNS infection (brain abscess or meningitis; 16%)
- Secondary cutaneous nocardiosis (13%)
- Septic arthritis (2%)
- Hematogenous osteomyelitis (1%)
- Other focal manifestations of disseminated infection (13%)

REFERENCES

1. Lerner PI. Nocardiosis. *Clin Infect Dis*. 1996;22: 891–903; quiz 904–5.
2. Jodlowski TZ, Melnychuk I, Conry J. Linezolid for the Treatment of Nocardia spp. Infections (October). *Ann Pharmacother*. 2007.
3. Saubolle MA, Sussland D. Nocardiosis: review of clinical and laboratory experience. *J Clin Microbiol*. 2003;41:4497–501.

ADDITIONAL READING

- Castro JG, Espinoza L. Nocardia species infections in a large county hospital in Miami: 6 years experience. *J Infect*. 2006(14).
- Filice GA. Nocardiosis in persons with human immunodeficiency virus infection, transplant recipients, and large, geographically defined populations. *J Lab Clin Med*. 2005;145:156–62.
- Márquez-Diaz F, Soto-Ramirez LE, Sifuentes-Osornio J. Nocardiasis in patients with HIV infection. *AIDS Patient Care STDS*. 1998;12:825–32.
- Timóteo AT, Branco LM, Pinto M et al. Nocardial endocarditis after mitral valve replacement: case report and review of the literature. *Rev Port Cardiol*. 2010;29:291–7.

 CODES

ICD9

- 039.1 Pulmonary actinomycotic infection
- 039.8 Actinomycotic infection of other specified sites
- 039.9 Actinomycotic infection of unspecified site

CLINICAL PEARLS

- When attempting recovery of *Nocardia* from sputum, clinical microbiology laboratory should be so advised because of the organism's slow growth and propensity to be overgrown by oral flora.
- Most common signs and symptoms of pulmonary nocardiosis: Fever (70%), cough (52%), pleuritic chest pain (32%), and dyspnea (16%)
- CT scan or MRI of the brain may reveal single or multiple intracranial abscesses and is indicated in all patients with pulmonary or disseminated nocardiosis.
- Patients on high-dose sulfonamide therapy should have a CBC and assessment of hepatic and renal function at least every other week.

N

NOSOCOMIAL INFECTIONS

Cheryl Durand, PharmD, RPh
Edward L. Yourtee, MD

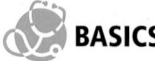 **BASICS**

DESCRIPTION
- Also known as *health care–associated infections* (HAIs)
- Infection must not have been present or incubating on admission to health care facility
- Centers for Disease Control and Prevention (CDC) categories:
  – Urinary tract infection (UTI)
  – Surgical-site infection:
    ○ Superficial or deep incisional-site infection
    ○ Organ/space infection
  – Pneumonia
  – Bloodstream infection
  – Bone and joint infection
  – CNS infection
  – Cardiovascular system infection
  – Ear, eye, nose throat, or mouth infection
  – GI system infection
  – Lower respiratory system infection (excluding pneumonia)
  – Reproductive tract infection
  – Skin and soft tissue infection
  – Systemic infection
- The National Healthcare Safety Network (NHSN) at www.cdc.gov/nhsn monitors the epidemiology of emerging HAI pathogens, HAI pathogens, and their mechanisms of resistance and evaluates alternative surveillance and prevention strategies.

EPIDEMIOLOGY
- General:
  – 13/1,000 patient-days in ICU (1)
  – 6.9/1,000 patient-days in high-risk nurseries (2)
  – 2.6/1,000 patient-days in nurseries (1)
  – Estimated cost of HAIs is $20 billion per year (3).
- Infection-specific:
  – UTI:
    ○ Hospital stay increased by 1–3 days
    ○ Cost up to $600 per infection
  – Pneumonia:
    ○ Hospital stay increased by 6 days
    ○ Cost up to $5,000 per infection
  – Bloodstream infection:
    ○ Hospital stay increased by 7–20 days
    ○ Cost up to $56,000 per infection (4)
  – Surgical-site infection:
    ○ Hospital stay increased 7.3 days
    ○ Cost >$3,000 per infection
    ○ May not be apparent until 1 month after surgery
  – *Clostridium difficile* infection (see topic "Clostridium Difficile Infection")

Incidence
- Incidence of resistant *Staphylococcus aureus* and vancomycin-resistant *Enterococcus* has been increasing dramatically in the last 15 years.
- 1.7 million HAIs in 2002 (1)
- 5–10% of hospital stays are complicated by HAIs (3).

- HAIs are among the top 10 leading causes of death in the US (3).
- The majority of patients affected have a single-site infection.
- UTI: 36% of HAIs (1):
  – 424,060 cases in 2002 in US (1)
  – 2.39/100 admissions
- Pneumonia: 11% of HAIs (1):
  – 129,519 cases in 2002 in US (1)
  – 0.60/100 admissions
- Bloodstream infection: 11% of HAIs (1):
  – 133,368 cases in 2002 in US (1)
  – 0.27/100 admissions
- Surgical-site infection: 20% of HAIs (1):
  – 244,385 cases in 2002 in US (1)
  – 3% of all surgeries (2)
  – 20% of emergency abdominal surgeries (2)
- Others: 22% of HAIs (1): 263,810 cases in 2002 in US (1)
- Resistance rates are increasing among several problematic gram-negative pathogens that are often responsible for serious nosocomial infections (5).
- In 2008, 70% of nosocomial infections were resistant to at least one antimicrobial drug that was effective previously (6).

RISK FACTORS
- Extremes of age
- Chronic disease (including diabetes, renal failure, and malignancy)
- Immunodeficiency
- Malnutrition
- Medications such as antibiotics, antacids, and sedatives
- Colonization with pathogenic strains of flora
- Breakdown of mucosal or cutaneous barriers
- Anesthesia

GENERAL PREVENTION
- Prevention efforts should address both patient-specific and facility-related risk factors.
- Hand hygiene:
  – Before direct patient contact (7)[B]
  – After contact with blood, excretions, body fluids, wound dressings, nonintact skin, mucous membranes (7)[A]
  – After contact with intact skin (7)[B]
  – When hands will be moving from contaminated to clean body site (7)[C]
  – Alcohol-based product: When hands are not visibly soiled (7)[A]
  – Soap and water:
    ○ When visibly soiled (7)[A]
    ○ When in contact with spores (7)[C]
- Hospital-based surveillance programs
- Infection control programs with specially trained employees (7)[B]
- Employee education on HAIs (7)[B]
- Minimize invasive procedures.

- Isolation of known pathogen carriers (7)[A]:
  – Contact precautions:
    ○ Pathogens spread by direct contact
    ○ Gloves when entering room (7)[B]
    ○ Gown if clothing will touch patient or environment (7)[B]
    ○ Includes methicillin-resistant *S. aureus* (MRSA), vancomycin-resistant *Enterococcus*, *C. difficile*, extended-spectrum β-lactamase-producing gram-negative rods
  – Droplet precautions:
    ○ Infectious particles measure >5 μm
    ○ Mask when entering room (7)[B]
    ○ Shed via talking, coughing, sneezing, mucosal shedding, airway suctioning, bronchoscopy
    ○ Includes *Neisseria meningitis*, influenza, *Haemophilus influenzae*, diphtheria, *Bordetella pertussis*
  – Airborne precautions:
    ○ Infectious particles measure <5 μm
    ○ Fit-tested National Institute of Occupational Safety and Health (NIOSH)–approved N-95 or higher respirator on entering room (7)[B]
    ○ Shed via coughing
    ○ Includes tuberculosis, varicella-zoster virus, measles
- Infection-specific measures:
  – UTI:
    ○ Employee education on catheters (8)[C]
    ○ Sterile catheter placement technique (8)[C]
    ○ Closed urine collection system (8)[C]
    ○ Use of catheter only as necessary (8)[B]
    ○ Removal of catheter as early as possible (8)[B]
  – Pneumonia:
    ○ Intubation only as necessary (9)[C]
    ○ Perform oral decontamination with an antiseptic agent (10)[A].
    ○ Avoidance of nasotracheal intubation (9)[B]
    ○ In-line suctioning (9)[C]
    ○ Head elevation of 30–45° (9)[C]
  – Bloodstream infection:
    ○ Employee education on catheters (4)[A] (e.g., indications, placement, maintenance)
    ○ Sterile catheter placement technique (4)[A]
    ○ Prompt removal of catheter (4)[A]
    ○ Hand hygiene in addition to glove use (4)[A]
    ○ Regular monitoring of catheter site (4)[B]
  – Surgical-site infection:
    ○ Proper surgical hand hygiene (3)[B]
    ○ Prophylactic antibiotic therapy when indicated (3)[A]
    ○ Elimination of underlying infections before surgery (3)[A]
    ○ Hair removal with electric clippers or depilatory agent (3)[B]
    ○ Postoperative blood sugar control

PATHOPHYSIOLOGY
- Endogenous spread: Patient's own normal flora causes invasive disease (majority of cases).
- Exogenous route: Flora from within health care facility causes invasive disease.

ETIOLOGY
- UTI: *Escherichia coli*, *Klebsiella* spp., *Serratia* spp., *Enterobacter*, *Pseudomonas aeruginosa*, *Enterococcus* spp., *Candida albicans*
- Pneumonia: Aerobic gram-negative bacilli, *S. aureus*, *P. aeruginosa*
- Bloodstream infection: *Staphylococcus* spp.
- Surgical-site infection: *S. aureus*, gram-negative bacilli

DIAGNOSIS

Consistent with nature of infection

HISTORY
- Exposure to health care facility
- Recent surgery
- History of invasive procedure:
  – Urinary catheter placement
  – In-dwelling vascular catheter
- Recent intubation/mechanical ventilation
- Past infections (e.g., MRSA)

PHYSICAL EXAM
Consistent with nature of infection

DIAGNOSTIC TESTS & INTERPRETATION
As appropriate for suspected infection

Pathological Findings
Consistent with underlying infection

DIFFERENTIAL DIAGNOSIS
- Community-acquired infection
- Noninfectious process

TREATMENT

MEDICATION
- As appropriate for specific nature of infection
- Several agents have been approved recently for the treatment of antibiotic-resistant gram-positive infections: linezolid, daptomycin, telavancin, and tigecycline.

ADDITIONAL TREATMENT
General Measures
Treat the underlying infection as indicated.

Issues for Referral
As appropriate

SURGERY/OTHER PROCEDURES
- As appropriate for specific nature of infection
- Treating proven carriers of *S. aureus* with mupirocin prevents *S. aureus* nosocomial infections after surgery. This screen-and-treat approach is cost saving as long as the prevalence of mupirocin resistance is low (11)[B].

IN-PATIENT CONSIDERATIONS
IV Fluids
As needed

Nursing
As applicable

Discharge Criteria
When infection has resolved or patient is stable

ONGOING CARE

FOLLOW-UP RECOMMENDATIONS
Patient Monitoring
As appropriate for specific type of infection

PROGNOSIS
- 99,000 deaths in 2002 in US (1)
- Bloodstream infection mortality: 27% (12)
- Pneumonia mortality: 33–50% (13)
- Surgical-site infection mortality: 11% (1)

COMPLICATIONS
Related to specific nature of infection

REFERENCES

1. Klevens RM, Edwards JR, Richards CL, et al. Estimating health care-associated infections and deaths in U.S. hospitals, 2002. *Public Health Rep*. 2007;122:160–6.
2. Barie PS, Eachempati SR. Surgical site infections. *Surg Clin North Am*. 2005;85:1115–35, viii-ix.
3. Society for Healthcare Epidemiology of America; Infectious Diseases Society of America. A compendium of strategies to prevent healthcare-associated infections in acute care hospitals. *Infect Control Hosp Epidemiol*. 2008;29(suppl 1):S1–S92.
4. O'Grady NP, et al. Guidelines for the prevention of intravascular catheter-related infections. *MMRW Recommendations and Reports*. 2002;51:1–32.
5. Slama TG. Gram-negative antibiotic resistance: there is a price to pay. *Crit Care*. 2008; 12(Suppl 4):S4.
6. Carmeli Y. Strategies for managing today's infections. *Clin Microbiol Infect*. 2008;14(Suppl 3): 22–31.
7. Siegel JD, Rhinehart E, Jackson M, et al. 2007 Guideline for Isolation Precautions: Preventing Transmission of Infectious Agents in Health Care Settings. *Am J Infect Control*. 2007;35:S65–164.
8. Hooton TM, Bradley SF, Cardenas DD, et al. Diagnosis, Prevention, and Treatment of Catheter-Associated Urinary Tract Infection in Adults: 2009 International Clinical Practice Guidelines from the Infectious Disease Society of America. *Clin Infect Dis*. 2010;50:625–663.
9. Tablan OC, et al. Guidelines for preventing health-care associated pneumonia, 2003: Recommendations of CDC and the healthcare infection control practices advisory committee. *MMWR Recommendations and Reports*. 2004;53:1–40.
10. Chan EY, Ruest A, Meade MO, et al. Oral decontamination for prevention of pneumonia in mechanically ventilated adults: systematic review and meta-analysis. *BMJ*. 2007;334:889.
11. Van Rijen M, Bonten M, Wenzel R, et al. Mupirocin Ointment for Preventing *Staphylococcus aureus* Infections in Nasal Carriers. *Cochrane Database Syst Rev*. 2009;1:CD006216.
12. Wisplinghoff H, Bischoff T, Tallent SM, et al. Nosocomial bloodstream infections in US hospitals: analysis of 24,179 cases from a prospective nationwide surveillance study. *Clin Infect Dis*. 2004;39:309–17.
13. American Thoracic Society, Infectious Diseases Society of America. Guidelines for the management of adults with hospital-acquired, ventilator- associated, and healthcare-associated pneumonia. *Am J Respir Crit Care Med*. 2005;171:388–416.

ADDITIONAL READING

Tacconelli E. Screening and isolation for infection control. *J Hosp Infect*. 2009.

CODES

ICD9
- 486 Pneumonia, organism unspecified
- 599.0 Urinary tract infection, site not specified
- 998.59 Other postoperative infection

CLINICAL PEARLS
- Nosocomial infections are associated with increased mortality, length of stay, and admission cost.
- Prevention efforts should address both patient-specific and facility-related risk factors.
- Proper use of an alcohol-based hand product should be carried out before and after each patient encounter, even when gloves are used.
- Contact, droplet, or airborne precautions should be employed when appropriate to reduce the spread of infection.
- The risk of developing a resistant nosocomial infection can be reduced with judicious use of antibiotics in the health care setting.

N

NOVEL INFLUENZA A (2009 H1N1)

Bradford Schwartz, MD
Raul Davaro, MD

 ## BASICS

Novel influenza (H1N1) "swine flu":

- A new antigenic variant of the influenza A serotype H1N1, resulting from a combination of swine, avian, and human influenza strains
- Generally self-limited and uncomplicated disease course (1)
- It is likely that an unrecognized epidemic of novel H1N1 influenza occurring in Mexico erroneously yielded a high estimated mortality rate to the virus of 0.2% (2).
- Typically presents with influenzalike symptoms, but patients also may be symptomatic with diarrhea and vomiting (3).
- Susceptible to neuraminidase inhibitors but resistant to adamantine antiviral agents (4)

EPIDEMIOLOGY

- From April 15 to May 5, 2009, a total of 642 confirmed cases of novel influenza A (H1N1) were reported in the US.
- 60% of the reported cases were accounted for by patients under the age of 18, with the majority represented by the 10- to 18-year-old age group (3).

Incidence

- 1,882 confirmed cases worldwide (confirmed by viral culture or RT-PCR)
- 11,932 suspected cases in Mexico; 942 confirmed cases in Mexico; 42 deaths resulting from novel influenza A (H1N1) infection in Mexico (2)
- Predominant sex: Male = Female

RISK FACTORS

- No possibility of transmission from properly cooked pork products
- Likely similar to typical influenza transmission, with exposure to respiratory secretions accounting for the main avenue of infection
- Close contact (<6 ft) with confirmed case increases the possibility for large-droplet transmission (3).

GENERAL PREVENTION

- Observe hand hygiene and appropriate cough etiquette.
- In regions with transmission of novel influenza A (H1N1), health care personnel should observe droplet precautions (N95 mask and protective goggles) in addition to contact precautions for patients presenting with symptoms of an influenzalike illness (fever with cough or sore throat).
- Isolation precautions are recommended for patients with reasonable clinical risk for novel influenza A (H1N1) exposure or infection.
- When leaving their rooms, patients with suspected novel influenza A (H1N1) infection should be outfitted with a surgical mask to contain their respiratory secretions.

ETIOLOGY

- Novel H1N1 flu is a quadruple-reassortant strain of human, avian, and 2 swine influenza strains (3).
- Reservoirs include infected human and pig populations.

 ## DIAGNOSIS

- Initial data from patients with novel influenza A (H1N1) infection suggest typical flulike symptoms:
  - Fever (94%)
  - Cough (92%)
  - Sore throat (66%) (3)[C]
  - Dyspnea (79%)
  - Headache (80%)
  - Rhinorrhea (83%) (2)[C]
- As a possible discriminating symptom from traditional flu, GI symptoms have been reported as well:
  - Diarrhea (25%)
  - Vomiting (25%) (3)[C]

HISTORY

- Close contact with a suspected or confirmed case
- Travel within last 10 days to a high-risk area (currently Mexico); high-risk areas can be determined via the CDC Web site: http://www.who.int/csr/disease/swineflu/en/index.html

DIAGNOSTIC TESTS & INTERPRETATION

- Novel influenza A (H1N1) has only recently emerged as a public health threat, and accordingly, improvements in diagnostic tests are under way.
- The sensitivity and specificity of rapid flu swab tests have not yet been determined for novel influenza A (H1N1), although the influenza A nucleoprotein antigen should be conserved in novel influenza A (H1N1), making the sensitivity and specificity similar to those for seasonal influenza.
- Clinical judgment largely should guide testing and suspicion of novel influenza A (H1N1) infection based on exposure risk.
- Currently, confirmation of novel influenza A (H1N1) infection can be performed only via RT-PCR specific for the virus or via viral culture; since these tests are performed at a state laboratory, confirmation of infection serves the purpose of surveillance rather than diagnosis.
- Clinicians should check with regional guidelines for confirmatory viral testing.

Lab

Initial lab tests

- CBC with differential
- Basic metabolic panel
- Blood cultures
- LFTs

Imaging

CXR: Among those hospitalized for novel influenza A (H1N1) infection, 50% had infiltrates on CXR (3)[C].

DIFFERENTIAL DIAGNOSIS

- Influenza
- Respiratory viral infections from such agents as coronavirus, rhinovirus, and adenovirus
- Croup
- Pneumonia (typical and atypical)
- Infectious mononucleosis
- Pharyngitis (viral or streptococcal)
- HIV syndrome

TREATMENT

- Most infections are self-limited and uncomplicated.
- Use of medications should be guided by clinical judgment.
- The CDC (www.cdc.gov) recommends that treatment should be given to high-risk patients with suspected novel influenza A (H1N1) infection, as well as to patients with symptoms severe enough to require hospitalization with suspected infection.
- High-risk patients include those <5 years of age and those >65 years of age, pregnant women, patients <19 years of age on long-term aspirin therapy, immunosuppressed patients, nursing home and chronic-care-facility residents, and those with complicating medical conditions (e.g., cardiovascular, pulmonary, hematologic, neurologic, renal, metabolic, etc.).
- Treatment with neuraminidase inhibitors is most effective when administered within 48 h of symptom onset (5)[A].

MEDICATION

- Novel influenza A (H1N1) has been found to be susceptible to the neuraminidase inhibitors oseltamivir (Tamiflu), and zanamir (Relenza) (4)[B].
- Genetic sequencing indicates resistance to the adamantine antivirals (e.g., amantadine).
- Oseltamivir (5)[B]:
  - Adult dosage: 75 mg p.o. b.i.d. × 5 days
  - Pediatric dosage (safety and efficacy not established for children <1 year of age):
    - ≤15 kg: 30 mg p.o. b.i.d. × 5 days
    - 16–23 kg: 45 mg p.o. b.i.d. × 5 days
    - 24–40 kg: 60 mg p.o. b.i.d. × 5 days
    - >40 kg: 75 mg p.o. b.i.d. × 5 days
  - Pediatric dosage <1 year old: <3 months: 12 mg p.o. b.i.d. × 5 days; 3–5 months: 20 mg p.o. b.i.d. × 5 days; 6–11 months: 25 mg p.o. b.i.d. × 5 days
  - Chemoprophylaxis: Oseltamivir is a 2nd-line agent for influenza A chemoprophylaxis secondary to zanamivir.
  - Postexposure prophylaxis is indicated for high-risk patients, health care personnel, public health workers, and first responders in close contact with suspected case of novel influenza A (H1N1).
  - Adult dosage: 75 mg p.o. daily × 10 days

  - Pediatric dosage (safety and efficacy not established for children <1 year of age):
    - ≤15 kg: 30 mg p.o. daily × 10 days
    - 16–23 kg: 45 mg p.o. daily × 10 days
    - 24–40 kg: 60 mg p.o. daily × 10 days
    - >40 kg: 75 mg p.o. daily × 10 days
  - For more information, see Tamiflu Fact Sheet for Health Care Providers at http://www.cdc.gov/h1n1flu/eua/pdf/tamiflu-hcp.pdf.
  - Adverse effects: Most common symptoms include nausea and vomiting, occurring in 9–10% patients. Neuropsychiatric events (e.g., hallucinations, delirium, and abnormal behavior) are rare symptoms. Other rare symptoms include anaphylaxis and severe skin reactions such as Stevens-Johnson syndrome and toxic epidermal necrolysis.
  - Other considerations: Metabolized by liver; pregnancy Class C medication
- Zanamivir (5)[B] (not recommended for patients with respiratory conditions such as COPD or asthma):
  - Adult dosage: 2 puffs of 5 mg INH b.i.d. × 5 days
  - Pediatric dosage: >7 years old: 2 puffs of 5 mg INH b.y.d. × 5 days
  - Chemoprophylaxis: Adult dosage: 2 puffs of 5 mg INH daily × 5 days; Pediatrics: >5 years old: 2 puffs of 5 mg INH daily × 5 days
  - For more information, see Relenza Fact Sheet for Health Care Providers at http://www.cdc.gov/h1n1flu/eua/pdf/relenza-hcp.pdf.
  - Adverse effects: Most notably may cause bronchospasm, especially in patients with preexisting respiratory illnesses. Common adverse symptoms include headache, nausea, dizziness, and cough. Rare symptoms are similar to those of Tamiflu, including neuropsychiatric symptoms, anaphylaxis, and severe skin reactions.
  - Other considerations: Metabolized by liver; pregnancy Class C medication

ADDITIONAL TREATMENT

Broad-spectrum antibiotics as needed for treatment of bacterial coinfections

REFERENCES

1. Centers for Disease Control and Prevention (CDC). Outbreak of swine-origin influenza A (H1N1) virus infection - Mexico, March-April 2009. *MMWR Morb Mortal Wkly Rep.* 2009;58:467–70.
2. Centers for Disease Control and Prevention (CDC). Update: novel influenza A (H1N1) virus infections - worldwide, May 6, 2009. *MMWR Morb Mortal Wkly Rep.* 2009;58:453–8.
3. Novel Swine-Origin Influenza A (H1N1) Virus Investigation Team. Emergence of a Novel Swine-Origin Influenza A (H1N1) Virus in Humans. *N Engl J Med.* 2009.
4. Centers for Disease Control and Prevention (CDC). Update: drug susceptibility of swine-origin influenza A (H1N1) viruses, April 2009. *MMWR Morb Mortal Wkly Rep.* 2009;58:433–5.
5. Harper SA, Bradley JS, Englund JA, et al. Seasonal Influenza in Adults and Children-Diagnosis, Treatment, Chemoprophylaxis, and Institutional Outbreak Management: Clinical Practice Guidelines of the Infectious Diseases Society of America. *Clin Infect Dis.* 2009.

ADDITIONAL READING

CDC: Interim Guidance for Clinicians on Identifying and Caring for Patients with Swine-Origin Influenza A (H1N1) Virus Infection, at http://www.cdc.gov/h1n1flu/identifyingpatients.htm; accessed 5/26/2009.

CODES

ICD9

- 488.11 Influenza due to identified novel H1N1 influenza virus with pneumonia
- 488.12 Influenza due to identified novel H1N1 influenza virus with other respiratory manifestations
- 488.19 Influenza due to identified novel H1N1 influenza virus with other manifestations

CLINICAL PEARLS

- Swine flu is *not* contracted from eating pork or pork products.
- Most cases are self-limited and uncomplicated.
- Up to 25% of patients report vomiting and diarrhea in addition to fever, headache, sore throat, and cough.

N

OBESITY

Maya Leventer-Roberts, MD, MPH

BASICS

DESCRIPTION
- Excess adipose tissue is often associated with negative health outcomes.
- BMI can indicate status as underweight, normal weight, overweight, obese, and morbidly obese.
- Increased risk of morbidity and mortality is more closely related to abdominal obesity than it is to gluteal obesity.
- System(s) affected: Endocrine/Metabolic; Cardiac; Respiratory; GI; Musculoskeletal
- Synonym(s): Overweight; Adiposis; Adiposity

Geriatric Considerations
The BMI associated with the lowest risk of mortality increases as age increases.

EPIDEMIOLOGY
- Predominant age: All ages
- Predominant sex: Female > Male

Prevalence
- Mean prevalence of obesity is 32.2% in the US.
- Overweight: 40% of men and 25% of women
- Obese: 20% of men and 25% of women

Pediatric Considerations
- Adolescence and young adulthood are high-risk periods for the onset of obesity and predict BMI in adulthood.
- The pediatric population has a rising prevalence of obesity.
- Risk factors include decreased physical activity, increased consumption of sweetened beverages, and increased television viewing.

RISK FACTORS
- Parental obesity
- Sedentary lifestyle
- High-calorie diet
- Pregnancy
- Low socioeconomic status

Genetics
- Rare genetic syndromes such as Prader-Willi and Bardet-Biedl
- Studies are inconclusive regarding specific genetic predictors of obesity.

GENERAL PREVENTION
- Encourage routine exercise and moderation in diet.
- Avoid calorie-dense and nutrient-poor foods such as sweetened beverages and processed foods.

ETIOLOGY
- Obesity is caused by an imbalance between food intake and energy expenditure.
- Uncommon causes include insulinoma, hypothalamic disorders, hypothyroidism, and Cushing syndrome.
- Menopause and smoking cessation are associated with significant weight gain.
- Some medications are associated with significant weight gain, including corticosteroids, neuroleptics (particularly the "atypical" antipsychotics), and antidepressants.

DIAGNOSIS

HISTORY
- Prior attempts at weight loss
- Reported readiness to change lifestyle
- Social support and resources
- Diet and exercise habits
- Associated risk factors: Diabetes mellitus type 2, hypertension, hyperlipidemia, sleep apnea
- Symptoms suggesting hypothyroidism, Cushing syndrome, genetic syndromes

PHYSICAL EXAM
Elevated BMI and excess adipose tissue:
- BMI = body weight (kg)/(body height $[m]^2$):
  - Overweight is BMI = 25–29.9 kg/m^2
  - Obesity is BMI $\geq$30 kg/m^2
  - Morbidly obese is $\geq$40 kg/m^2

BMI obesity threshold by height

Height	BMI = 25 Weight (lb/kg)	BMI = 27 Weight (lb/kg)	BMI = 30 Weight (lb/kg)	
5′	0	128/58	138/63	153/70
5′	2	136/61	147/67	164/74
5′	4	145/66	157/71	174/79
5′	6	155/70	167/76	186/84
5′	8	164/74	177/81	197/89
5′	10	174/79	188/85	209/95
6′	0	184/83	199/90	221/100
6′	2	194/88	210/95	233/106
6′	4	205/92	221/101	246/112

- Fat distribution pattern:
  - Waist circumference is measured around the abdomen at the level of the umbilicus:
    - >40 in (102 cm) for men and >35 in (88 cm) for women is associated with increased risk for most obesity-related medical conditions (1)[C].

DIAGNOSTIC TESTS & INTERPRETATION
Lab
- Used to monitor associated risk factors and conditions
- Serum lipid panel and fasting glucose
- Although hypothyroidism is an uncommon cause of obesity, consider obtaining TSH because hypothyroidism may affect other lab results.

Pathological Findings
- Hypertrophy and/or hyperplasia of adipocytes
- Cardiomegaly
- Hepatomegaly

TREATMENT

MEDICATION
NIH guidelines suggest nonpharmacologic treatment for at least 6 months. Medication treatment may be initiated for unsatisfactory weight loss in those with a BMI >30 or with a BMI >27 combined with associated risk factors (e.g., coronary heart disease, diabetes, sleep apnea, hypertension, hyperlipidemia). Diet, exercise, and behavior therapy must be included with pharmacologic treatment for those without comorbidities (1)[B].

First Line
- Medications produce modest weight loss (2)[A].
- The appetite suppressant sibutramine is a serotonin and norepinephrine reuptake inhibitor. Dose: 10–15 mg p.o. daily (10-mg starting dose).
- The lipase inhibitor orlistat decreases the absorption of dietary fat. Dose: 120 mg p.o. t.i.d. with meals. Patients must avoid taking fat-soluble vitamin supplements within 2 h of taking orlistat. The FDA has approved orlistat to be sold over the counter as a weight-loss aid.
- Contraindications:
  - Sibutramine: Uncontrolled hypertension, severe renal or hepatic dysfunction, narrow-angle glaucoma, history of substance abuse, symptomatic cardiovascular disease, CHF, arrhythmias, stroke, use of monoamine oxidase inhibitor within 2 weeks
  - Orlistat: Chronic malabsorption syndromes, cholestasis
- Precautions: Relapse after discontinuation of drug
- Significant possible interactions:
  - Pulse and BP elevations possible with sibutramine.
  - Concurrent use with general anesthetics may cause arrhythmias.
  - Serotonergic agents may cause "serotonin syndrome" in combination with sibutramine.

Second Line
- Appetite suppressants recommended for short-term treatment (several weeks)
- Schedule IV drugs: Diethylpropion, phentermine
- Schedule III drugs: Benzphetamine, phendimetrazine

ADDITIONAL TREATMENT
General Measures
- The following assessments can determine the status and plan of action:
  - Degree of health risk from BMI and waist circumference (1)[C] (see Diagnosis)
  - Motivation to lose weight (1)[C]
  - Patient-specific goals of therapy
  - Necessary counseling or referral to a dietitian for diet, exercise, and behavior modification (1)[B]
  - Long-term follow-up (1)[C]
- Goal for therapy is to achieve and sustain weight loss up to 10% of body weight for overweight and obese patients (1)[A].

- Behavior therapy and cognitive-behavioral methods can result in modest weight loss, but are most effective when combined with dietary and exercise treatments (3)[A].
- Effective commercial and community-based programs include diets meeting the US RDA for nutrients, exercise, behavior modification, and providing for maintenance of ideal weight and eating habits.

Pregnancy Considerations
- Weight loss is not appropriate for most pregnant or lactating women (1)[C].
- During pregnancy, obese women should gain less than the 25 lb recommended for nonobese women.

SURGERY/OTHER PROCEDURES
Patients meeting criteria (including severe obesity [BMI >40 kg/m^2]) can be considered for gastric bypass procedures:
- Malabsorptive surgery reduces the length of the small intestine.
- Restrictive surgery reduces the stomach's capacity.
- Gastric bypass requires complex presurgical evaluation, surgery, and follow-up in a skilled treatment center (1)[C].
- Lifelong medical surveillance is necessary after obesity surgery (1)[C].
- Surgical treatment is the most effective long-term weight-loss treatment available for morbid obesity (4)[B].

 ## ONGOING CARE

FOLLOW-UP RECOMMENDATIONS
- Exercise may improve long-term results of treatment and should be an integral part of any weight-loss program. However, exercise alone rarely results in significant weight loss (1)[A].
- Exercise regimens should last 30–90 minutes, 5–7 times per week.
- Combination of weight training and aerobic activity is preferred over aerobic activity alone.
- Increasing calories expended in daily activities is also important.

Patient Monitoring
Long-term routine follow-up is crucial to prevent relapse after weight loss or further weight gain.

DIET
- Long-term studies suggest that net calorie reduction of 500–1,000 kcal/d and ease of adherence are more important than diet composition for long-term results:
  - A reduction of 500 kcal/d intake can result in ~1 lb (0.45 kg) weight loss per week (1)[A].
  - Low-saturated-fat, high-complex-carbohydrate, and high-fiber diets are recommended most commonly (1)[A].
  - Portion-controlled servings are recommended.
- Very low-calorie diet (400–800 kcal/d):
  - Can result in more rapid weight loss than higher-calorie diets but are less effective in the long term.
  - Complications can include dehydration, orthostatic hypotension, fatigue, muscle cramps, constipation, headache, cold intolerance, and relapse after discontinuation.

- Contraindications include recent myocardial infarction or cerebrovascular accident, renal or hepatic disease, cancer, pregnancy, insulin-dependent diabetes mellitus, and some psychiatric disturbances.

PATIENT EDUCATION
- Emphasize the value of a healthy BMI.
- Recommended Web sites:
  - http://www.shapeup.org for general information and specific resources
  - http://www.gastro.org for the American Gastroenterological Association
  - http://www.nal.usda.gov/fnic/foodcomp/search for the FDA nutritional content in common foods
  - Loseit application for iTunes (http://itunes.apple.com/us/app/lose-it/id297368629?mt=8) and other similar applications are well received; efficacy is undetermined.

PROGNOSIS
- Lowest mortality associated with a BMI of 22
- Long-term maintenance of weight loss is extremely difficult.
- A motivated patient is most likely to achieve successful weight loss.
- There have been several controversial studies suggesting that a BMI in the mildly overweight range is associated with a decreased risk of mortality relative to a BMI in the underweight or obese range (5)[B].

COMPLICATIONS
- Cardiovascular disease
- Stroke (in men)
- Thromboembolism
- Heart failure
- Hypertension
- Hypoventilation and sleep apnea syndromes
- Higher death rates from cancer: Colon, breast, prostate, endometrial, gallbladder, liver, kidney
- Diabetes mellitus
- Skin changes
- Hyperlipidemia
- Gallbladder disease
- Osteoarthritis
- Gout
- Poor self-esteem
- Discrimination
- Increased sick leave

REFERENCES
1. National Institutes of Health Clinical guidelines on the identification, evaluation, and treatment of overweight and obesity in adults: The evidence report. NIH Publication No. 98-4083, 1998.
2. Padwal R, Li SK, Lau DCW. Long-term pharmacotherapy for obesity and overweight (Cochrane Review). *The Cochrane Library*. Issue 4. Chichester, UK: Wiley & Sons; 2005.
3. Shaw K, et al. Psychological interventions for overweight and obesity (Cochrane Review). *The Cochrane Library*. Issue 4. Chichester, UK: Wiley & Sons; 2005.
4. Colquitt J, et al. Surgery for morbid obesity (Cochrane Review). *The Cochrane Library*. Issue 4. Chichester, UK: Wiley & Sons; 2005.
5. Flegal K, Graubard B, Williamson D, et al. Excess deaths associated with underweight, overweight, and obesity. *JAMA*. 2005;20:293(15):1861–7.

ADDITIONAL READING
- Ogden CL, Carroll MD, Curtin LR, et al. Prevalence of overweight and obesity in the United States, 1999–2004. *JAMA*. 2006;295:1549–55.
- Summerbell CD, Cameron C, Glasziou PP. WITHDRAWN: Advice on low-fat diets for obesity. *Cochrane Database Syst Rev*. 2008:CD003640.
- Thomas DE, Elliott EJ, Baur L. Low glycaemic index or low glycaemic load diets for overweight and obesity. *Cochrane Database Syst Rev*. 2007:CD005105.

 ## CODES

ICD9
- 278.00 Obesity, unspecified
- 278.01 Morbid obesity

CLINICAL PEARLS
- Drug treatment with a 1st-line medication may be indicated when nonpharmacologic treatment for 6 months has been ineffective and the patient has a BMI >30 or a BMI >27 with associated risk factors. Medications produce (at most) a modest long-term weight loss.
- Surgical treatment may be indicated in patients with a BMI >40 who have failed more conservative treatment, particularly when there are associated risk factors such as diabetes mellitus.
- There is no convincing evidence that any specific diet is more effective than any other diet of equivalent caloric content.

O

OBSESSIVE COMPULSIVE DISORDER (OCD)

Anna K. Morin, PharmD
Robert A. Baldor, MD

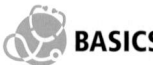 **BASICS**

DESCRIPTION
- A psychiatric condition classified as an anxiety disorder characterized by obsessions (recurrent intrusive thoughts, ideas, or images) and compulsions (repetitive, ritualistic behaviors or mental acts) causing significant patient distress
- Not to be confused with obsessive-compulsive personality disorder

EPIDEMIOLOGY
Incidence
- Predominant age: Mean age of onset 22–36 years
  - Male = Female (males present at younger age).
  - Child/adolescent onset in 33% of cases
  - 1/3 of cases present by age 15 years
  - 85% of cases present at <35 years of age
  - Diagnosis rarely made at >50 years of age
- Predominant gender: Male > Female (3:1).

Pediatric Considerations
Insidious onset; consider brain insult in acute presentation of childhood obsessive-compulsive disorder (OCD).

Geriatric Considerations
Consider neurologic disorders in new-onset OCD in the elderly.

Prevalence
- 2.3% lifetime in adults
- 1–2.3% prevalence in children/adolescents

RISK FACTORS
- Exact cause of OCD is not fully elucidated.
- Combination of biologic and environmental factors likely involved:
  - Link between low serotonin levels and development of OCD
  - Link between brain insult and development of OCD (i.e., encephalitis, pediatric streptococcal infection, or head injury)

Genetics
- Greater concordance in monozygotic twins
- Positive family history: Prevalence rates of 7–15% in 1st-degree relatives of children/adolescents with OCD

GENERAL PREVENTION
- OCD cannot be prevented.
- Early diagnosis and treatment can decrease patient's distress and impairment.

PATHOPHYSIOLOGY
- Exact pathophysiology unknown
- Dysregulation of serotonergic pathways
- Dysregulation of corticostriatal-thalamic-cortico (CSTC) pathways

ETIOLOGY
- Exact etiology unknown
- Genetic and environmental factors
- Pediatric autoimmune disorder associated with streptococcal infections

COMMONLY ASSOCIATED CONDITIONS
- Major depressive disorder
- Panic disorder
- Social phobia
- Phobia
- Tourette syndrome
- Substance abuse
- Eating disorder
- Body dysmorphic disorder

 DIAGNOSIS

HISTORY
- Patient presents with either obsessions or compulsions, which cause marked distress, are time-consuming (>1 h/d), and cause significant occupational/social impairment.
- 4 criteria support diagnosis of obsessions:
  - Patients are aware that they are thinking the obsessive thoughts; thoughts are not imposed from outside (as in thought insertion).
  - Thoughts are not just excessive worrying about real-life problems.
  - Recurrent thoughts are persistent, intrusive, and inappropriate, causing significant anxiety and distress.
  - Attempts to suppress intrusive thoughts are made with some other thought or activity.
- 2 criteria support a diagnosis of compulsions:
  - The response to an obsession is to rigidly perform repetitive behaviors (e.g., hand washing) or mental acts (e.g., counting silently).
  - Although done to reduce stress, the responses are either not realistically connected with the obsession or they are excessive.
  - In children, check for precedent streptococcal infection.

PHYSICAL EXAM
- Dermatologic problems caused by excessive hand-washing may be observed.
- Hair loss caused by compulsive pulling or twisting of the hair (trichotillomania) may be observed.

DIAGNOSTIC TESTS & INTERPRETATION
Lab
No diagnostic laboratory findings identified

Imaging
None indicated; consider brain MRI to rule out neurologic disorder.

Diagnostic Procedures/Surgery
- Yale-Brown Obsessive-Compulsive Scale (Y-BOCS) or CY-BOCS for children
- Maudsley Obsessive-Compulsive Inventory (MOCI)

Pathological Findings
- Compulsions are designed to relieve the anxiety of obsessions; they are not inherently enjoyable (ego-dynastic) and do not result in completion of a task.

- Common obsessive themes:
  - Harm (i.e., being responsible for an accident)
  - Doubt (i.e., whether doors or windows are locked or the iron is turned off)
  - Blasphemous thoughts (i.e., in a devoutly religious person)
  - Contamination, dirt, or disease
  - Symmetry or orderliness
- Common rituals or compulsions:
  - Hand-washing, cleaning
  - Checking
  - Counting
  - Hoarding
  - Ordering, arranging
  - Repeating
- Neither obsessions nor compulsions are related to another mental disorder (i.e., thoughts of food and presence of eating disorder).
- 80–90% of patients with OCD have obsessions and compulsions.
- 10–19% of patients with OCD are pure obsessional.

DIFFERENTIAL DIAGNOSIS
- Obsessive-compulsive personality disorder:
  - In personality disorder, traits are ego-syntonic and include perfectionism and preoccupation with detail, trivia, or procedure, and regulation. Patients tend to be rigid, moralistic, and stingy. These traits are often rewarded in the patient's job as desirable.
- Impulse-control disorders: Compulsive gambling, sex, or substance abuse: The compulsive behavior is not in response to obsessive thoughts, and the patient derives pleasure from the activity.
- Depression
- Brooding, but ideas not as senseless as in OCD
- Schizophrenia: Patient perceives thought to be true and coming from an external source.
- Generalized anxiety disorder, phobic disorders, separation anxiety: Similar response on heightened anxiety, but presence of obsessions and rituals signifies OCD diagnosis.
- Anxiety disorder owing to a general medical condition: Obsessions or compulsions are assessed to be a direct physiologic consequence of a general medical condition.

 TREATMENT

MEDICATION
First Line
- Adequate trial at least 10–12 weeks
- Optimal doses may exceed typical doses for depression.
- Current evidence suggests selective serotonin reuptake inhibitors (SSRIs) as 1st-line agents (1,2)[A].
  - Fluoxetine (Prozac):
    ○ Adults: 20 mg/d; increase by 10–20 mg every 4–6 weeks until response; range: 20–80 mg/d.
    ○ Children (7–17 years of age): 10 mg/d; increase 4–6 weeks until response; range: 20–60 mg/d.

– Sertraline (Zoloft):
  ○ Adults: 50 mg/d; increase by 50 mg every 4–7 days until response; range: 50–200 mg/d; may divide if above 100 mg/d.
  ○ Children (6–17 years of age): 25 mg/d; increase by 25 mg every 7 days until response; range: 50–200 mg/d.
– Paroxetine (Paxil):
  ○ Adults: 20 mg/d; increase by 10 mg every 4–7 days until response; range: 40–60 mg/d.
  ○ Children: Safety and effectiveness in patients <18 years have not been established.
– Fluvoxamine (Luvox):
  ○ Adult: 100 mg/d; increase by 50 mg every 4–7 days until response; range: 200–300 mg/d.
  ○ Children (8–17 years of age): 25 mg/d; increase by 25 mg every 4–7 days until response; range: 50–200 mg/d.
– Absolute SSRI contraindications:
  ○ Hypersensitivity to SSRIs
  ○ Within 14 days of monoamine oxidase inhibitor (MAOI)
– Relative SSRI contraindications:
  ○ Severe liver impairment
  ○ Seizure disorders (lower seizure threshold)
– Precautions:
  ○ Watch for suicidal behavior or worsening depression during 1st few months of therapy or after dosage changes with antidepressants, particularly in children, adolescents, and young adults.
  ○ Long half-life of fluoxetine (>7 days) may be troublesome if patient has an adverse reaction.
  ○ May cause drowsiness and dizziness when therapy initiated; warn patients about driving and heavy-equipment hazards.

Pregnancy Considerations
All SSRIs are pregnancy category C, except paroxetine, which is category D.

Second Line
- Try switching to another SSRI.
- Tricyclic acid (TCA), clomipramine (Anafranil):
  – Adults: 25 mg/d; increase gradually over 2 weeks to 100 mg/d, then to 250 mg/d (maximum dose) over next several weeks, as tolerated.
  – Children (10–17 years of age): 25 mg/d; titrate as needed and tolerated up to 3 mg/kg or 200 mg/d (whichever is less).
  – Absolute clomipramine contraindications:
    ○ Within 6 months of an MI
    ○ Hypersensitivity to clomipramine or other TCA
    ○ Within 14 days of an MAOI
    ○ 3rd-degree atrioventricular (AV) block
  – Relative clomipramine contraindications:
    ○ Narrow-angle glaucoma (increased intraocular pressure)
    ○ Prostatic hypertrophy (urinary retention)
    ○ 1st- or 2nd-degree AV block, bundle-branch block, and congestive heart failure (proarrhythmic effect)
    ○ Pregnancy category C
  – Precautions:
    ○ Dangerous in overdose
    ○ Pretreatment electrocardiogram (ECG) for patients >40 years of age

  ○ Watch for suicidal behavior or worsening depression during 1st few months of therapy or after dosage changes with antidepressants, particularly in children, adolescents, and young adults.
  ○ May cause drowsiness and dizziness when therapy is initiated; warn patients about driving and heavy-equipment hazards.

ADDITIONAL TREATMENT
General Measures
- Combined medications and cognitive-behavioral therapy (CBT) is most effective (1,2)[A].
- Family psychoeducation
- Parent behavior management training if patient is a child or adolescent

Issues for Referral
- Psychiatric referral for CBT (in vivo exposure and prevention of compulsions)
- Psychiatric evaluation if obsessions and compulsions significantly interfere with patient's functioning in social, occupational, or educational situations

Additional Therapies
Dopamine receptor antagonists (antipsychotic agents) alone are not effective in treatment of OCD. They can be used as augmentation to SSRI therapy for treatment-resistant OCD; they also can worsen OCD symptoms (2).
- Pimozide (Orap): Initial dose: 0.5 mg/d; target dose: 1–6 mg/d
- Haloperidol (Haldol): Initial dose: 0.5 mg/d; target dose: 0.5–6 mg/d
- Risperidone (Risperdal): Initial dose: 0.5 mg/d; target dose: 0.5–2 mg/d
- Olanzapine (Zyprexa): Initial dose: 1.25 mg/d; target dose: 1.25–30 mg/d

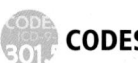 ONGOING CARE

FOLLOW-UP RECOMMENDATIONS
Y-BCOS or MOCI surveys to track progress

Patient Monitoring
Monitor for decrease in obsessions and time spent performing compulsions.

DIET
No dietary modifications or restrictions are recommended.

PATIENT EDUCATION
- Importance of medication adherence
- Importance of psychotherapy (CBT)
- International OCD Foundation, PO Box 961029, Boston, MA 02196; 617-973-5801; www.ocfoundation.org
- Obsessive Compulsive Anonymous, PO Box 215, New Hyde Park, NY 11040; 516-739-0662; http: \\ obsessivecompulsiveanonymous.org

PROGNOSIS
- Chronic waxing and waning course in majority of patients
  – 24–33% fluctuating course
  – 11–14% phasic periods of remission
  – 54–61% chronic progressive course
- Early onset a poor predictor

COMPLICATIONS
- Depression in 1/3 of patients with OCD
- Avoidant behavior (phobic avoidance)
  – Children may drop out of education.
  – Adults may become home-bound.
- Anxiety and panic-like episodes associated with obsessions

REFERENCES
1. Gava I, et al. Psychological treatments versus treatment as usual for obsessive compulsive diorder (OCD). Cochrane Database Sys Rev. 2007;2: CD005333.
2. Stein DJ, et al. Obsessive-compulsive disorder: diagnostic and treatment issues. Psychiatr Clin N Am. 2009;32:665–685.

ADDITIONAL READING
- Diagnostic and Statistical Manual of Mental Disorders DSM-IV (Text Revision), 4th ed. Washington, DC: American Psychiatric Association, 2000.
- Koran LM, et al. Practice guideline for the treatment of patients with obsessive-compulsive disorder. Am J Psychiatry. 2007;164:5–53.
- Kurlan R, Kaplan EL et al. The pediatric autoimmune neuropsychiatric disorders associated with streptococcal infection (PANDAS) etiology for tics and obsessive-compulsive symptoms: hypothesis or entity? Practical considerations for the clinician. Pediatrics. 2004;113:883–6.
- Nestadt G, et al. Genetics of obsessive compulsive disorder. Psychiatr Clin N Am. 2010;33:141–158.

CODES

ICD9
300.3 Obsessive-compulsive disorders

CLINICAL PEARLS
- CBT is initial treatment of choice for mild OCD.
- CBT plus an SSRI or an SSRI alone is the treatment choice for more severe OCD.
- >65–70% of patients with OCD respond to 1st SSRI treatment.
- Improvement in symptoms is often incomplete and ranges from 25–60%.

OCULAR CHEMICAL BURNS

Vinod P. Mitta, MD
Chris Tang, MD

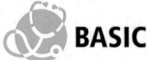

BASICS

DESCRIPTION
- Chemical exposure to the eye can result in rapid, devastating, and permanent damage, and is one of the true emergencies in ophthalmology.
- Separate alkaline from acid chemical exposure:
  – Alkaline burns: More severe—alkali compounds are lipophilic, penetrating rapidly into eye tissue; saponification of cells leads to necrosis and may produce injury to lids, conjunctiva, cornea, sclera, iris, and lens (cataracts).
  – Acid burns: Acid usually does not damage internal structures because protein denatures, creating a barrier to further acid penetration (hydrofluoric and, to a lesser extent, sulfurous acids are an exception to this rule). Injury is often limited to lids, conjunctiva, and cornea.
- System(s) affected: Nervous; Skin/Exocrine
- Synonym(s): Chemical Ocular Injuries

EPIDEMIOLOGY
- Predominant age: Can occur at any age, peak from 16–25 years of age
- Predominant sex: Male > Female

Incidence
- Estimated 300/100,000 per year
- Alkali burns twice as common as acid burns

RISK FACTORS
- Construction work (plaster, cement, whitewash)
- Use of cleaning agents (drain cleaners, ammonia)
- Automobile battery explosions (sulfuric acid)
- Industrial work (many possible agents)
- Alcoholism
- Any risk factor for assault (~10% or injuries due to deliberate assault)

GENERAL PREVENTION
Safety glasses to safeguard eyes

PATHOPHYSIOLOGY
- Hydration of glycosaminoglycans causes corneal opacification.
- Saponification of cell membranes causes cell death.
- Cation binding to collagen results in hydration, thickening, and shortening of collagen fibrils. This can mechanically elevate intraocular pressure through distortion of the trabecular meshwork.

ETIOLOGY
Sources of alkaline and acidic compounds

Alkali Compounds	Typical Sources
Calcium Hydroxide (Lime)	Cement, whitewash
Sodium Hydroxide (Lye)	Drain cleaner
Potassium Hydroxide (Lye)	Drain cleaner
Ammonia	Cleaning agents
Ammonium Hydroxide	Fertilizers
Acidic Compounds	**Typical Sources**
Sulfuric Acid	Car batteries
Sulfurous Acid	Bleach
Hydrochloric Acid	Chemistry laboratories
Acetic Acid	Vinegar
Hydrofluoric Acid	Glass polish

COMMONLY ASSOCIATED CONDITIONS
Facial cutaneous chemical or thermal burns

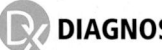

DIAGNOSIS

PHYSICAL EXAM
- Mild burns:
  – Pain and blurred vision
  – Eyelid skin erythema and edema
  – Corneal epithelial defects or superficial punctate keratitis
  – Conjunctival chemosis, hyperemia, and hemorrhages without perilimbal ischemia
  – Mild anterior chamber reaction
- Moderate-to-severe burns:
  – Severe pain and markedly reduced vision
  – 2nd- and 3rd-degree burns of eyelid skin
  – Corneal edema and opacification
  – Corneal epithelial defects
  – Marked conjunctival chemosis and perilimbal blanching
  – Moderate anterior chamber reaction
  – Increased intraocular pressure
  – Local necrotic retinopathy
- In alkaline burns, can have initial pain that later diminishes

DIAGNOSTIC TESTS & INTERPRETATION
Imaging
Not necessary unless suspicion of intraocular or orbital foreign body is present

Diagnostic Procedures/Surgery
- Measure pH of tear film with litmus paper or electronic probe:
  – Irrigating fluid with non-neutral pH (e.g., normal saline has pH of 4.5) may alter results.
- Careful slit lamp exam, fundus ophthalmoscopy, tonometry, and measurement of visual acuity
- Full extent of damage from alkaline burns may not be apparent until 48–72 hours after exposure.

Pathological Findings
- Corneal epithelial defects or superficial punctate keratitis, edema, opacification
- Conjunctival chemosis, hyperemia, and hemorrhages
- Perilimbal ischemia
- Anterior chamber reaction
- Increased intraocular pressure

DIFFERENTIAL DIAGNOSIS
- Thermal burns
- Ocular cicatricial pemphigoid
- Other causes of corneal opacification
- Ultraviolet radiation keratitis

TREATMENT

Copious irrigation and removal of corneal or conjunctival foreign bodies are always the initial treatment (1,2)[A]:
- Passively open patient's eyelid and have them look in all directions while irrigating.
- Be sure to remove all reservoirs of chemical from the eyes.
- Continue irrigation until the tear film and superior/inferior cul-de-sac is of neutral pH and pH is stable (2)[C]:
  – Severe burns should be irrigated for at least 15 minutes to as much as 2–4 hours; this irrigation should not be interrupted during transportation to hospital (2)[C].
  – It is impossible to overirrigate.
- Initial pH testing should be done on both eyes even if the patient claims to only have unilateral ocular pain/irritation so that a contralateral injury is not neglected.
- Use whatever nontoxic fluid is available for irrigation on scene. In hospital, sterile water, normal saline, normal saline with bicarbonate, balanced salt solution (BSS) or lactated Ringer's solution may be used.
  – No therapeutic difference in effectiveness has been noted between types of solutions (1)[C].
- A topical anesthetic can be used to provide for patient comfort (e.g. proparacaine, tetracaine).
- Sweep the conjunctival fornices every 12–24 hours to prevent adhesions (2)[C].
- Eye patching may relieve pain, but has not been shown to improve outcomes (3)[C].

MEDICATION
First Line
- Further treatment (depending on severity and associated conditions):
  – Topical prophylactic antibiotics: Any broad-spectrum agent (e.g., bacitracin–polymyxin B[Polysporin] ointment q2–4h, ciprofloxacin [Ciloxan] drops q2–4h, chloramphenicol[Chloroptic] ointment q2–4h) (1)[C]:

○ Some experts suggest that systemic tetracycline derivatives (especially doxycycline) may be beneficial because studies performed in animals have shown an additional anti-inflammatory effect (by inhibiting metalloproteinases) and improved corneal healing in alkali burns (4)[C].

– Tear substitutes: Hydroxypropyl methylcellulose (HypoTears PF, Refresh Plus) drops q4h, carboxymethylcellulose (Refresh PM) ointment at bedtime (1)[C]:
  ○ Most beneficial in those with impaired tear production (elderly patients)

– Cycloplegics for photophobia and/or uveitis: Cyclopentolate 1% t.i.d., or scopolamine 1/4% b.i.d. (1)[C]

– Antiglaucoma for elevated intraocular pressure (IOP): Latanoprost (Xalatan) 0.005% q24h, or timolol (Timoptic) 0.5% b.i.d., or levobunolol (Betagan) 0.5% b.i.d., and/or acetazolamide (Diamox) 125–250 mg p.o. q6h, or methazolamide (Neptazane) 25–50 mg p.o. b.i.d., and/or IV mannitol 20% 1–2 g/kg as needed (1)[C]

– Corticosteroids for intraocular inflammation: Prednisolone (Pred-Forte) 1% or equivalent q1–4h for 7–10 days; if severe, prednisone 20–60 mg p.o. daily for 5–7 days. Taper rapidly if epithelium is intact by this time (1)[C]:
  ○ Use of corticosteroids > 10 days may do harm by inhibiting repair and cause corneoscleral melt (1,5)[C]

– Consider vitamin C (ascorbic acid) 500 mg p.o. q.i.d. and/or acetylcysteine (Mucomyst) 10–20% topically q4h if corneal melting occurs (1)[C].

• Precautions:
  – Timolol and levobunolol: History of congestive heart failure (CHF) or chronic obstructive pulmonary disease (COPD)
  – Acetazolamide and methazolamide: History of nephrolithiasis or metabolic acidosis
  – Mannitol: History of CHF or renal failure
  – Scopolamine: History of urinary retention
  – Topical corticosteroids must be used with caution in the presence of damaged corneal epithelium because iatrogenic infection can occur. Daily follow-up or consultation with an ophthalmologist is recommended.

ADDITIONAL TREATMENT
Issues for Referral
See Medication (Drugs).

SURGERY/OTHER PROCEDURES
Goal of subacute treatment is restoration of the normal ocular surface anatomy, control of glaucoma, and restoration of corneal clarity. Surgical options include:

• Debridement of necrotic tissue (1)[C]
• Conjunctival/tenon advancement (tenoplasty) to restore vascularity in severe burns (1)[C]
• Tissue adhesive (e.g., isobutyl cyanoacrylate) for impending or actual corneal perforation of <1 mm (1)[C]:
  – Tectonic keratoplasty for acute perforation >1 mm (1)[C]

• Limbal autograft transplantation for epithelial stem cell restoration (1)[C]
• Conjunctival or mucosal membrane transplant to restore ocular surface in severe injury (1)[C]
• Lamellar or penetrating keratoplasty for tectonic stabilization or visual rehabilitation (1)[C]

IN-PATIENT CONSIDERATIONS
Initial Stabilization
Usual for patient

Admission Criteria
Based on ophthalmic consultation and concomitant burn injuries

Discharge Criteria
Emergency department evaluation with inpatient admission and ophthalmology consultation, depending on severity

ONGOING CARE
FOLLOW-UP RECOMMENDATIONS
Patient Monitoring
• Depending on severity of ocular injury:
  – From daily to weekly visits initially
• May be inpatient
• If on mannitol or prednisone, consider frequent serum electrolytes

DIET
Regular as tolerated

PATIENT EDUCATION
• Safety glasses
• Need for immediate ocular irrigation with any available water following chemical exposure to the eyes

PROGNOSIS
• Depends on severity of initial injury. Increasing amounts of limbal ischemia and corneal opacification correlate with poorer prognosis (Roper-Hall classification system)
• For mildly injured eyes, complete recovery is the norm.
• For severely injured eyes, permanent loss of vision is not uncommon.

COMPLICATIONS
• Persistent epitheliopathy
• Fibrovascular pannus
• Corneal ulcer/perforation
• Corneal scarring
• Progressive symblepharon and entropion
• Neurotrophic keratitis
• Lid malposition secondary to cicatricial changes
• Glaucoma
• Cataract
• Hypotony
• Phthisis bulbi
• Blindness

REFERENCES
1. Wagoner MD. Chemical injuries of the eye: Current concepts in pathophysiology and therapy. *Survey Ophthalmol*. 1997;41:275–313.
2. Kuckelkorn R, Schrage N, Keller G, et al. Emergency treatment of chemical and thermal eye burns. *Acta Ophthalmol Scand*. 2002;80:4–10.
3. Spector J, Fernandez WG et al. Chemical, thermal, and biological ocular exposures. *Emerg. Med. Clin. North Am*. 2008;26:125–36, vii
4. Ralph RA et al. Tetracyclines and the treatment of corneal stromal ulceration: a review. *Cornea*. 2000;19:274–7.
5. Fish R, Davidson RS et al. Management of ocular thermal and chemical injuries, including amniotic membrane therapy. *Curr Opin Ophthalmol*. 2010;21:317–21.

ADDITIONAL READING
Rodrigues Z et al. Irrigation of the eye after alkaline and acidic burns. *Emerg Nurse*. 2009;17:26–9.

See Also (Topic, Algorithm, Electronic Media Element)
Burns

CODES
ICD9
• 940.0 Chemical burn of eyelids and periocular area
• 940.2 Alkaline chemical burn of cornea and conjunctival sac
• 940.3 Acid chemical burn of cornea and conjunctival sac

CLINICAL PEARLS
• Prompt irrigation of all chemical burns, even prior to arrival to the emergency room, is essential to ensure best outcomes.
• All patients with chemical injuries to their eyes should be refered to ophthalmology staff for further assessment.

ONYCHOMYCOSIS

Theodore G. MacKinney, MD, MPH
Natasha A. Travis, MD

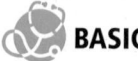

BASICS

DESCRIPTION
- Chronic fungal infection of fingernails or toenails
- Caused mostly by dermatophytes, also yeasts, molds
- Toenails more commonly affected than fingernails
- System(s) affected: Skin/Exocrine
- Synonym(s): Tinea unguium; Ringworm of the nail

EPIDEMIOLOGY
Prevalence
- 2–8% in general population
- Predominant age: 14–28% in adults >60 years of age
- Rare before puberty

RISK FACTORS
- Older age
- Tinea pedis
- Cancer
- Diabetes
- Peripheral vascular disease
- Psoriasis
- Cohabitation with others with onychomycosis
- Immunodeficiency
- Swimming
- Smoking
- Peripheral vascular disease
- Children with Down's syndrome

ETIOLOGY
- Dermatophytes: *Trichophyton* (*T. rubrum* most common), *Epidermophyton*, *Microsporum*
- Yeasts: *C. albicans* (most common), *C. parapsilosis*, *C. tropicalis*, *C. krusei*
- Molds: *Scopulariopsis brevicaulis*, *Hendersonula toruloidea*, *Aspergillus* sp., *Alternaria tenuis*, *Cephalosporium*, *Scytalidium hyalinum*
- Dermatophytes cause 90% of toenail and most of fingernail onychomycoses.
- Fingernail onychomycosis more often caused by yeast than toenail
- Dermatophytes invade normal keratin, whereas molds invade altered keratin.

COMMONLY ASSOCIATED CONDITIONS
- Immunodeficiency or chronic metabolic disease
- Tinea pedis or manuum

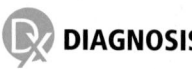

DIAGNOSIS

PHYSICAL EXAM
- Dermatophytes: Commonly preceded by dermatophyte infection at another site; 80% involve toenails, especially hallux; simultaneous infection of fingernails and toenails is rare. 4 clinical forms occur:
  - Distal or lateral subungual onychomycosis (most common): Spreads from distal or lateral margins to nail bed to nail plate; subungual hyperkeratosis; subungual paronychia; onycholysis; nail dystrophy; discoloration—yellow-brown; yellow streaking laterally; bois vermoulu ("worm-eaten wood"); onychomadesis

  - Proximal subungual onychomycosis (rare): Hands or feet; leukonychia—begins under posterior nail groove, appearing to occur from the proximal underside of the nail (or direct invasion of the nail plate from above); spreads to nail plate and lunula; seen with immunodeficiency
  - Superficial white onychomycosis (rare): Hallux preferentially affected; infection of outer surface of nail plate; opaque white spots on nail plate eventually merge to involve entire surface of the nail
- Candidal:
  - Hands 70%, especially dominant hand
  - Middle finger most common
  - Pain mild, unless secondarily infected
  - Increases on prolonged contact with water
  - Primarily affects tissue surrounding nail
  - Begins with cuticle detachment
  - Dark yellowish to blackish brown to green zone along lateral border of nail
  - Secondary ungual changes: Convex, irregular, striated nail plate with dull, rough surface
  - Onycholysis, especially on hands
  - Distal subungual onychomycosis may occur.
  - Primary involvement of the nail plate is uncommon (thin, crumbly, opaque, brownish nail plate deformed by transverse grooves).
  - Periungual edema/erythema may occur (club-shaped, bulbous fingertips).
- Molds:
  - More common in those >60 years of age
  - More common in nails of hallux
  - Resembles distal and lateral onychomycosis

Pediatric Considerations
Candidal infection presents more commonly as superficial white onychomycosis.

DIAGNOSTIC TESTS & INTERPRETATION
- Accurate diagnosis requires both laboratory and clinical evidence.
- If onychomycosis is suspected clinically and initial diagnostic laboratory tests are negative, they should be repeated.

Lab
Initial lab tests
- Direct microscopy with potassium hydroxide (KOH) preparation:
  - Clip away diseased, discolored nail plate.
  - Collect debris from stratum corneum of most proximal area (beneath nail or crumbling nail itself) with 1-mm curette or scalpel.
  - Larger sample improves sensitivity.
  - KOH (5%) plus gentle heat.
  - High sensitivity if >2 preparations examined
- Cultures: False negative in 30% (secondary to loss of dermatophyte viability; improved by immediate culture on Sabouraud cell culture medium)
- Histologic examination of nail clippings; punch biopsy: Proximal lesions; stain both with periodic acid–Schiff (PAS) stain
- Discontinue all topical medication for some time before obtaining sample.

Pathological Findings
Pathogens within the nail keratin

DIFFERENTIAL DIAGNOSIS
- Psoriasis (most common alternate diagnosis)
- Traumatic dystrophy
- Lichen planus
- Onychogryphosis
- Eczematous conditions
- Hypothyroidism
- Drugs and chemicals
- Yellow nail syndrome
- Neoplasms
- Only 50% of dystrophic nails are due to onychomycosis.

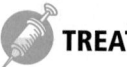

TREATMENT

MEDICATION
Pregnancy Considerations
Oral antifungals and ciclopirox are pregnancy Category B (terbinafine, ciclopirox) or C (itraconazole, fluconazole, and griseofulvin). Because treatment of onychomycosis usually can be postponed until after pregnancy, treatment typically should be avoided during pregnancy.

First Line
- Oral antifungals are preferred due to higher rates of cure, but have systemic adverse effects and drug–drug interactions.
- Terbinafine 250 mg/d p.o. × 6 weeks for fingernails and 3 months for toenails, most effective in cure and prevention of relapse, most cost-effective with higher patient satisfaction compared with itraconazole pulse. It has similar tolerance to terbinafine pulse (500 mg/d × 1 week per month for 3 months), and fewer drug–drug interactions (1)[C],(2)[A].
- Itraconazole pulse 400 mg/d p.o. or 200 mg p.o. b.i.d. × 1 week, then 3 weeks off, repeat for 2 cycles for fingernails and 3–4 cycles for toenails (lower cost and lower pill burden than itraconazole continuous, more effective than terbinafine for *Candida* and molds, do not need to monitor liver function tests (1)[C],(2)[A].
- Itraconazole continuous 200 mg/d p.o. × 6 weeks for fingernails and 3 months for toenails (may be more effective than itraconazole pulse, more effective than terbinafine for *Candida* and molds) (1)[C],(2)[A]

Second Line
- Fluconazole pulse 150–300 mg p.o. weekly × 6 months (less frequent dosing but lower cure rate) (1)[C],(2)[A]
- Griseofulvin 500–1,000 mg/d p.o. for up to 18 months (lower cure rate, needs to be continued until the diseased nail is completely replaced) (1)[C],(2)[A]

- Ciclopirox 8% nail lacquer: Apply once daily to affected nails (if without lunula involvement) for up to 48 weeks, and every 7 days, remove lacquer with alcohol, then file away loose nail material and trim nails (low cure rate, avoids systemic adverse effects, less cost-effective). Application after p.o. treatment may reduce recurrences (3)[A].
- Contraindications for oral antifungals:
  – Hepatic disease
  – Pregnancy (see Pregnancy Alert)
  – Current or history of congestive heart failure (CHF) (itraconazole)
  – Porphyria (griseofulvin)
- Precautions/adverse effects:
  – Oral antifungals:
    ○ Hepatotoxicity
    ○ Neutropenia
    ○ Hypersensitivity
    ○ Photosensitivity, lupuslike symptoms, proteinuria (griseofulvin)
    ○ Chronic kidney disease (avoid terbinafine for patients with CrCl <50 mL/min, decrease fluconazole dose)
    ○ CHF, peripheral edema, pulmonary edema (itraconazole)
  – Ciclopirox: Rash, nail disorders; avoid contact with skin other than skin immediately surrounding nail; use with caution on broken skin or in vascular compromise
- Significant drug–drug interactions:
  – Terbinafine (inhibits CYP2D6): β-Blockers, cimetidine, cyclosporine, dextromethorphan, monoamine oxidase inhibitors (MAOIs), rifampin, selective serotonin reuptake inhibitors (SSRIs), tricyclic antidepressants (TCAs), warfarin
  – Itraconazole, fluconazole (inhibit CYP3A4): Antiarrhythmics, benzodiazepines, cisapride, ergot alkaloids, HMG CoA reductase inhibitors, alfentanil, buspirone, calcium channel blockers, carbamazepine, cimetidine, corticosteroids, cyclosporine, haloperidol, hydrochlorothiazide, hypoglycemics, losartan, oral contraceptives, phenytoin, pimozide, protease inhibitors, rifamycins, sirolimus, tacrolimus, TCAs, theophylline, tolterodine, vinca alkaloids, warfarin, zidovudine, zolpidem
  – Griseofulvin: Barbiturates, oral contraceptives, cyclosporine, salicylates, warfarin

ADDITIONAL TREATMENT
General Measures
- Avoid factors that promote fungal growth (i.e., heat, moisture, occlusion).
- Treat underlying disease risk factors.
- Treat secondary infections.

COMPLEMENTARY AND ALTERNATIVE MEDICINE
Melaleuca alternifolia (tea tree) oil has a 10% mycologic cure.

SURGERY/OTHER PROCEDURES
Nail debridement to remove infected keratin (efficacy not well studied):
- Mechanical: Soften with occlusive dressing with 40% urea gel; detach from nail bed with tweezers or file with abrasive stone.

- Chemical: Protect peripheral tissue with adhesive strips; apply ointment of 30% salicylic acid, 40% urea, or 50% potassium iodide under occlusive dressing.
- Surgical avulsion: For involvement of a few nails; used by some for pain control

 ## ONGOING CARE
FOLLOW-UP RECOMMENDATIONS
- Formation of new fingernail takes 4–6 months and new toenail takes 12–18 months.
- Cure defined as (4)[C]:
  – 100% absence of clinical signs and/or
  – Negative mycology with ≥1 of the following clinical signs:
    ○ Distal subungual hyperkeratosis or onycholysis leaving <10% of the nail plate affected
    ○ Nail plate thickening that does not improve with treatment because of comorbid condition

Patient Monitoring
- Topical agents: Slow response expected; visits every 6–12 weeks
- Terbinafine, griseofulvin: Baseline and as needed liver function tests (LFTs) and CBC
- Itraconazole continuous: Baseline and as needed LFTs

PATIENT EDUCATION
- Advise patient to:
  – Keep affected area clean and dry.
  – Avoid rubber or other occlusive footwear.
  – Avoid tight or ill-fitting footwear.
  – Wear absorbent cotton socks; avoid synthetic fibers.
  – Change clothing and towels frequently, and launder them in hot water.
- Cure of all toenails may not be attainable.
- Nail may not appear normal after cure.

PROGNOSIS
- Complete clinical cure in 25–50% (higher mycologic cure rates)
- 10–50% recur (relapse or reinfection).
- Poor prognostic factors (4)[C]:
  – Areas of nail involvement >50%
  – Significant proximal or lateral disease
  – Subungual hyperkeratosis >2 mm
  – White/yellow or orange/brown streaks in the nail (includes dermatophytoma)
  – Total dystrophic onychomycosis (with matrix involvement)
  – Nonresponsive organisms (e.g., *Scytalidium* mold)
  – Patients with immunosuppression
  – Diminished peripheral circulation

COMPLICATIONS
- Secondary infections with progression to soft tissue infection or osteomyelitis
- Toenail discomfort or pain that can limit physical mobility or activity
- Anxiety, negative self-image

REFERENCES
1. Finch JJ, Warshaw EM. Toenail onychomycosis: current and future treatment options. *Dermatol Ther*. 2007;20:31–46.
2. Hinojosa JR, Hitchcock K, Rodriguez JE. Clinical inquiries. Which oral antifungal is best for toenail onychomycosis? *J Fam Pract*. 2007;56:581–2.
3. Crawford F, Hollis S. Topical treatments for fungal infections of the skin and nails of the foot. *Cochrane Database of Systematic Reviews*. 2007, Issue 3. Art. No.: CD001434. DOI:10.1002/14651858.CD001434.pub2.
4. Scher RK, Tavakkol A, Sigurgeirsson B, et al. Onychomycosis: diagnosis and definition of cure. *Journal of the American Academy of Dermatology*. 2007;56:939–44.

ADDITIONAL READING
- de Berker D et al. Clinical practice. Fungal nail disease. *N Engl J Med*. 2009;360:2108–16.
- Welsh O, Vera-Cabrera L, Welsh E et al. Onychomycosis. *Clin Dermatol*. 2010;28:151–9.

CODES
ICD9
- 110.1 Dermatophytosis of nail
- 112.3 Candidiasis of skin and nails

CLINICAL PEARLS
- Psoriasis and chronic nail trauma are commonly mistaken for fungal infection.
- Diagnosis should be based on both clinical and mycologic laboratory evidence.
- Oral antifungals generally are well tolerated and more effective than topical antifungals, with terbinafine the most effective.
- LFT monitoring is necessary for most oral antifungal regimens.
- Patient should understand that treatment is long term, recurrence is common, and nails may not appear normal even after treatment.

O

OPTIC ATROPHY

Birgit N. Khandalavala, MD

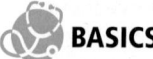 **BASICS**

DESCRIPTION

Loss of the ganglion cell axons that form the optic nerve. Clinical sign not a diagnosis (1). Because this loss is irreversible, the term optic neuropathy may be preferable:

- May be primary inherited optic atrophy, congenital nongenetic, or secondary to inherited or acquired disease
- Optic nerve aplasia is an extremely rare congenital, nongenetic abnormality of unknown etiology associated with other ocular malformations.
- Optic nerve hypoplasia is a more common congenital abnormality associated with:
  - Many genetic syndromes
  - Metabolic disorders
  - Chromosomal abnormalities
  - Developmental abnormalities
  - Maternal alcohol consumption, diabetes, illicit drugs
- Acquired optic atrophy may be ischemic, inflammatory, infectious, traumatic, drug-induced, radiation-induced, toxic, nutritional, or related to compression, usually developing several months after the initial injury.
- System(s) affected: Nervous
- Synonym(s): Leber hereditary optic neuropathy; Optic neuropathy

Pediatric Considerations
Optic atrophy in small children may be difficult to recognize because disks normally have a pale appearance.

EPIDEMIOLOGY
- Predominant age: May be congenital. Inherited forms occur from shortly after birth to the 3rd decade; acquired forms tend to occur later.
- Predominant sex: Male > Female (inherited forms)
- Leber hereditary optic neuropathy: Predominately 20–30-year-old males (2)

RISK FACTORS
- Genetic
- Acquired:
  - Diabetes mellitus
  - Hypertension
  - Radiation exposure
  - Alcoholism
  - Renal failure
  - Arteriosclerosis

Genetics
- Inherited forms may be autosomal-recessive, autosomal-dominant, X-linked–recessive (3)[C], or mitochondrial (4)[C]:
  - Leber hereditary optic neuropathy (LHON):
    - Mitochondrial inheritance (maternal)
    - Complex I of mitochondrial respiratory chain
    - Bilateral subacute optic neuropathy
    - Degeneration of retinal ganglion cells and their axons
    - Primarily affecting young adult men
  - Autosomal-dominant optic atrophy, Kjer type:
    - Affects children in the 1st decade of life
    - Bilateral, slowly progressive loss of vision
    - OPA1 gene on chromosome 3q28
    - Autosomal gene affects mitochondrial function.
  - Autosomal-recessive optic atrophies (OPA6, rare)
- Optic atrophies associated with genetic metabolic conditions
- Disorders of amino acid metabolism:
  - Hyperhomocysteinemia is associated with ischemic optic neuropathy.
- Wolfram syndrome
- Mitochondrial disorders
- Peroxisomal disorders:
  - Refsum disease
  - Adrenoleukodystrophy
- Lysosomal storage diseases:
  - Tay-Sachs
  - Niemann-Pick
  - Mucopolysaccharidoses
- Other inherited neurodegenerative conditions:
  - Hereditary ataxia
  - Charcot-Marie-Tooth disease
  - Familial dysautonomia

GENERAL PREVENTION
Regular ophthalmologic exam in high-risk groups

ETIOLOGY
- Nongenetic optic neuropathy
- Compression of the optic nerve:
  - Glaucoma
  - Chronic papilledema
  - Tumor
  - Aneurysm
  - Hydrocephalus
- Inflammation:
  - Graves disease
  - Chronic optic neuritis
- Trauma

- Syphilis
- Ischemic optic neuropathy
- Central retinal artery or vein occlusion
- Retinal degeneration
- Congenital optic atrophy: Possibly due to lack of oxygen during pregnancy, labor, or early neonatal period
- Radiation neuropathy
- Drugs:
  - Amiodarone
  - Chloroquine
  - Ethambutol
  - Oral contraceptives
  - Streptomycin
  - Vincristine
- Nutritional deficiencies:
  - Vitamin B$_{12}$
  - Folic acid
  - Thiamine
- Demyelinating disorders (e.g., multiple sclerosis)
- Toxins/poisons:
  - Cyanide
  - Lead
  - Methanol
- Tobacco

COMMONLY ASSOCIATED CONDITIONS
- Multiple sclerosis
- Diabetes
- Cardiovascular disease

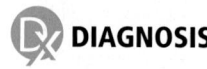 **DIAGNOSIS**

HISTORY
- Family history of visual loss
- Congenital disorders
- Painless loss of visual acuity:
  - Bilateral can be synchronous or metachronous
  - In primary optic atrophies, often the only clinical feature

PHYSICAL EXAM
- Funduscopic exam:
  - Small, pale optic disk is diagnostic.
  - Enlarged peripapillary atrophy if glaucoma is the cause
  - Unilateral disk swelling points toward nerve compression.
- Loss of pupillary reactions
- Visual-field defects
- Abnormalities in color vision and contrast sensitivity

DIAGNOSTIC TESTS & INTERPRETATION

- Automated visual-field test (e.g., Humphrey)
- Color vision testing
- Visual-evoked potentials
- Fluorescein angiography

Lab
- Complete blood count (CBC)
- Electrolytes
- Antinuclear antibody test
- Erythrocyte sedimentation rate (ESR)
- C-reactive protein
- Vitamin B_{12}, folate, and thiamine levels
- Fluorescent treponemal antibody absorption test
- Serologic test for syphilis
- Heavy-metal screen
- Genetic testing if indicated, especially for Leber hereditary optic neuropathy

Imaging
Computed tomography (CT) or magnetic resonance imaging (MRI) of head may be indicated for unexplained or isolated optic atrophy.

Initial approach
- A complete ophthalmic examination, including a comprehensive history, will lead to an underlying diagnosis in 92% of cases.
- Ancillary testing is only indicated when the cause is not apparent by clinical evaluation.

Diagnostic Procedures/Surgery
- Carotid Doppler (adult-acquired optic atrophy)
- Complete ophthalmologic exam, including dilated evaluation of retina
- Complete neurological exam for multiple sclerosis

DIFFERENTIAL DIAGNOSIS
- Glaucomatous optic atrophy
- Myopia
- Postoperative cataract extraction (no natural yellow color from the human lens)

 ## TREATMENT

MEDICATION
- Corticosteroids may briefly improve visual acuity when optic neuritis is present.
- Long-term benefits are unproven.

ADDITIONAL TREATMENT
Associated conditions may require specific treatment for nutritional deficiencies, coexistent inflammatory syndromes, or multiple sclerosis.

General Measures
- Optic nerve damage is usually permanent, so early detection is important (3)[C].
- Treat the underlying cause, if treatable.

- Correction of an underlying nutritional deficiency or discontinuation of the causative drug may halt progression.
- Optic nerve pressure may be relieved by neurosurgery.

Issues for Referral
- Genetic counselling
- Neurosurgical referral if secondary to compression
- Rheumatology review if associated with systemic diseases
- Neurological referral with multiple sclerosis

 ## ONGOING CARE

FOLLOW-UP RECOMMENDATIONS
- Determined by the associated cause
- Progressive optic atrophy may require more frequent follow-up.

Patient Monitoring
- Annual evaluations if stable
- May be gradually discontinued if optic atrophy is unexplained and nonprogressive

DIET
No special diet

PATIENT EDUCATION
- Low-vision counseling
- Genetic counseling if inherited
- Glaucoma education
- For patient education materials favorably reviewed on this topic, contact the National Eye Institute, Information Officer, Department of Health and Human Services, 9000 Rockville Pike, Bethesda, MD 20892; (301) 496-5248
- American Council of the Blind: (800) 424-8666

PROGNOSIS
- Visual loss occurs over weeks to months.
- Correction of an underlying nutritional deficiency or discontinuation of the causative drug may halt progression.
- Optic neuropathy is usually not reversible.

REFERENCES

1. Golnik K et al. Nonglaucomatous optic atrophy. *Neurol Clin*. 2010;28:631–40.
2. Teive HA, Troiano AR, Raskin S, et al. Leber's hereditary optic neuropathy—case report and literature review. *Sao Paulo Med J*. 2004;122: 276–9.
3. Huizing M, et al. Optic atrophies in metabolic disorders. *Mol Genet Metabol*. 2005;86:51–60.
4. Howell N. LHON and other optic nerve atrophies: the mitochondrial connection. *Dev Ophthalmol*. 2003;37:94–108.

ADDITIONAL READING

- Jonas JB. Clinical implications of peripapillary atrophy in glaucoma. *Curr Opin Ophthalmol*. 2005;16:84–8.
- University of Michigan Kellogg Eye Center. At: http://www.kellogg.umich.edu

 ## CODES

ICD9
- 377.10 Optic atrophy, unspecified
- 377.11 Primary optic atrophy
- 377.12 Postinflammatory optic atrophy

CLINICAL PEARLS

- The hallmark of optic atrophy is a small, pale optic disk on funduscopic exam. Sign not a diagnosis.
- Optic atrophy with systemic symptoms leads to the diagnosis of a metabolic cause of optic atrophy.
- Optic atrophy is inherited by autosomal-dominant, autosomal-recessive, X-linked, or mitochondrial inheritance.
- The best treatment for optic atrophy is early diagnosis, which can assist in halting progression, but damage is usually irreversible.
- The types of visual loss involved with optic atrophy are blurred vision, abnormal peripheral vision, abnormal color vision, and decreased brightness. Bilateral loss is either synchronous or metachronous.

O

OPTIC NEURITIS

Olga M. Céron, MD
Pablo I. Hernandez Itriago, MD

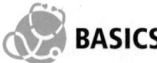 **BASICS**

DESCRIPTION
- Inflammation of the optic nerve (Cranial Nerve II)
- Most common form is acute demyelinating optic neuritis (ON), but other causes include infectious disease and systemic autoimmune disorders
- Optic disc may be either normal in appearance at onset (retrobulbar ON, 67%) or swollen (papillitis, 33%)
- Key features:
  – Abrupt visual loss
  – Periorbital pain especially with eye movement (90%)
  – Dyschromatopsia: Color vision deficits
  – Afferent pupillary defect
- Usually unilateral in adults; bilateral disease more common in children
- Presenting complaint in 25% of multiple sclerosis (MS) patients
- System(s) affected: Nervous
- Synonym(s): Papillitis; Demyelinating optic neuropathy; Retrobulbar optic neuritis
- In children, headache is common.

EPIDEMIOLOGY
Incidence
- 5 cases per 100,000 seen annually
- More common in northern latitudes
- More common in whites than in other races
- Predominant age: Typically 18–45 years; mean age 30
- Predominant sex: Female > Male (3:1)

PATHOPHYSIOLOGY
- In both MS-associated and isolated monosymptomatic ON, the cause is presumed to be a demyelinating autoimmune reaction.
- Possible mechanisms of inflammation in immune-mediated optic neuritis are the cross-reaction of viral epitopes and host epitopes, and the persistence of a virus in central nervous system glial cells
- Neuromyelitis optica (NMO) IgG autoantibody, which targets the water channel aquaporin-4

ETIOLOGY
- Primarily idiopathic
- MS
- Viral infections: Measles, mumps, varicella-zoster, coxsackievirus, adenovirus, hepatitis A and B, HIV, herpes simplex virus, cytomegalovirus
- Nonviral infections: Syphilis, tuberculosis, meningococcus, cryptococcosis, cysticercosis, bacterial sinusitis, streptococcus B, *Bartonella*, Lyme disease, fungus
- Systemic inflammatory disease: Sarcoidosis, systemic lupus erythematosus, vasculitis
- Local inflammatory disease: Intraocular or contiguous with the orbit, sinus, or meninges
- Toxic: Lead, methanol, arsenic, radiation
- Vascular lesions affecting the optic nerve
- Posterior uveitis
- Tumors

- Medications: Ethambutol, chloroquine, isoniazid, chronic high-dose chloramphenicol, tumor necrosis factor α antagonist, infliximab (Remicade), adalimumab (Humira), etanercept (Enbrel)

COMMONLY ASSOCIATED CONDITIONS
- MS (common): ON is associated with an increased risk of MS.
- Other demyelinating diseases: Guillain-Barré syndrome, Devic neuromyelitis optica, multifocal demyelinating neuropathy, acute disseminated encephalomyelitis

 DIAGNOSIS

HISTORY
- Decreased visual acuity, deteriorating in hours to days, usually reaching lowest level in 1 week
- Usually unilateral but can also be bilateral
- Brow ache, globe tenderness, deep orbital pain exacerbated by eye movement (92%)
- Retro-orbital pain may precede visual loss.
- Desaturation of color vision (dull or faded colors), especially red tones
- Apparent dimness of light intensities
- Impairment of depth perception (80%); worse with moving objects (Pulfrich phenomenon)
- Transient increase in visual symptoms with increased body temperature and exercise (Uhthoff phenomenon)
- May present with a recent flulike viral syndrome
- Detailed history and review of systems, looking for a history of demyelinating, infectious, or systemic inflammatory disease

PHYSICAL EXAM
Complete general exam, full neurologic exam, and ophthalmologic exam looking for the following:
- Decreased visual acuity and color perception
- Central, cecocentral, arcuate, or altitudinal visual field deficits
- Papillitis: Swollen disc ± peripapillary flame-shape hemorrhage or often normal disc exam
- Temporal disc pallor seen later at 4–6 weeks (1)
- Relative afferent pupillary defect (Marcus-Gunn pupil): The pupil of the affected eye dilates with swinging light test unless disease is bilateral.

DIAGNOSTIC TESTS & INTERPRETATION
Lab
Initial lab tests
- In typical presentations, erythrocyte sedimentation rate is standard, but other labs are unnecessary. Antinuclear antibodies (ANAs), angiotensin-converting enzyme level, fluorescent treponemal antibody absorption (FTA-ABS), and chest radiograph have been shown to have no value in typical cases (1).
- In atypical presentations, including absence of pain, a very swollen optic nerve, >30 days without recovery, or retinal exudates, labs may be indicated to rule out underlying disorders:
  – Complete blood count
  – ANA test
  – Rapid plasma reagin test
  – FTA-ABS test

Follow-Up & Special Considerations
- Visual field test (Humphrey 30–2); to evaluate for visual field loss: Diffuse and central visual loss more predominant in the affected eye at baseline (2)
- A novel blood test called an *NMO-IgG* checks for antibodies for neuromyelitis optica.

Imaging
Initial approach
- Magnetic resonance imaging (MRI) of brain and orbits: Thin cuts (2-3 mm) gadolinium enhanced and fat suppression images to look for Dawson fingers of MS (periventricular white matter lesions oriented perpendicular to the ventricles) and to also look for enhancement of the optic nerve
- Computed tomography scan of chest to rule out sarcoidosis if clinical suspicion is high

Diagnostic Procedures/Surgery
- In atypical cases including bilateral deficits, young age, or suspicion of infectious etiology, lumbar puncture (LP) with neurology consultation is indicated.
- LP for suspected MS is a physician-dependent decision. Some studies indicate that it may not add value to MRI for MS detection (1), but there is no consensus on the subject.

DIFFERENTIAL DIAGNOSIS
- Demyelinating disease, especially MS
- Infectious/systemic inflammatory disease
- Neuroretinitis: Virus, toxoplasmosis, *Bartonella*
- Toxic or nutritional optic neuropathy
- Acute papilledema (bilateral disc edema)
- Compression:
  – Orbital tumor/abscess compressing the optic nerve
  – Intracranial tumor/abscess compressing the afferent visual pathway
  – Orbital pseudotumor
  – Carotid–ophthalmic artery aneurysm
- Temporal arteritis or other vasculitides
- Trauma or radiation
- Neuromyelitis optica (Devic disease)
- Anterior ischemic optic neuropathy
- Leber hereditary optic neuropathy
- Kjer-type autosomal-dominant optic atrophy
- Severe systemic hypertension
- Diabetic papillopathy

 TREATMENT

Most persons with optic neuritis recover spontaneously.

MEDICATION
First Line
- Intravenous methylprednisolone has been shown to speed up the rate of visual recovery but without significant long-term benefit; consider for patients who require fast recovery (ie, monocular patients or those whose occupation requires high-level visual acuity). For significant vision loss, parenteral corticosteroids may be considered on an individualized basis.

  – Observation and corticosteroid treatment are both acceptable courses of action (3)[B].

– High-dose intravenous (IV) methylprednisone (250 mg q6h × 3 days) followed by oral corticosteroids (1 mg/kg/d p.o. × 11 days, taper over 1–2 weeks) (3)[B]

- Others use IV Solu-Medrol infusion (1 g in 250 mL D_5 1/2 normal saline infused over 1 h daily for 3–5 days).
  – No evidence of long-term benefit (14)
  – May decrease recovery time (3,4)
  – May decrease risk of MS at 2 but not 5 years (3)
- Give antiulcer medications with steroids.

Second Line
- Disease-modifying agents such as interferon-β-1a (IFN-β-1a; Avonex, Rebif) and IFN-β-1b (Betaseron) are used to prevent or delay the development of MS in people with ON who have ≥2 brain lesions evident on MRI.
- These medications have been proposed for use in patients with 1 episode of ON (clinically isolated syndrome) at high risk of developing MS (1+ lesion on brain MRI).
- The Controlled High Risk Avonex Multiple Sclerosis Trial study has shown that IFN-β1–a reduces the conversion to clinically definite multiple sclerosis in high-risk patients by ~50%.
- Decisions should be made individually with neurology consultation.

ALERT
Never use oral prednisone alone as primary treatment because this may increase the risk for recurrent ON and should be avoided (3).

Pediatric Considerations
- No systematic study defining high-dose corticosteroids in childhood ON has been conducted. *Walsh & Hoyt's Clinical Neuro-ophthalmology* recommends methylprednisolone 1–2 mg/kg × 3–5 days, followed by a longer taper. Farris and Pickard used doses of methylprednisolone ranging from 0.25–6.26 mg/kg, with half the patients receiving doses of 125 or 250 mg q6h × 5 days, followed by a taper.
- Optic disc swelling and bilateral disease are more common in children, as is severe loss of visual acuity (20/200 or worse).
- Consider infectious and postinfectious causes of optic nerve impairment.

ADDITIONAL TREATMENT
General Measures
Referral to a neurologist and/or ophthalmologist

 ## ONGOING CARE

FOLLOW-UP RECOMMENDATIONS
Patient Monitoring
Monthly follow-up to monitor visual changes and steroid side effects

PATIENT EDUCATION
- Provide reassurance about recovery of vision.
- If the disease is believed to be secondary to demyelinating disease, patient should be informed of the risk of developing MS.

- For patient education materials favorably reviewed on this topic, contact:
  – National Eye Institute, Information Officer, Department of Health and Human Services, 9000 Rockville Pike, Bethesda, MD 20892; 301-496-5248
  – North American Neuro-Ophthalmology Society (NANOS), 5841 Cedar Lake Road, Suite 204, Minneapolis, MN 55416; phone: 952-646-2037; fax: 952-545-6073; http://www.nanosweb.org

PROGNOSIS
- Orbital pain usually resolves within 1 week.
- Visual acuity:
  – Rapid spontaneous improvement at 2–3 weeks and continues for several months (may be faster with IV corticosteroids)
  – Often returns to normal or near-normal levels (20/40 or better) within 1 year (90–95%), even after near blindness
- Other visual disturbances (eg, contrast sensitivity, stereopsis) often persist after acuity returns to normal.
- Recurrence risk of 35% within 10 years: 14% affected eye, 12% contralateral, 9% bilateral; recurrence is higher in MS patients (48%)
- ON is associated with increased risk of developing MS; 35% risk at 7 years, 58% at 15 years:
  – Brain MRI helps to predict risk:
    ○ 0 lesions: 16%
    ○ 1–2 lesions: 37%
    ○ 3+ lesions: 51% (5)
- Poor prognostic factors:
  – Absence of pain
  – Low initial visual acuity
  – Involvement of intracanalicular optic nerve
- Children with bilateral visual loss have a better prognosis than adults.

COMPLICATIONS
Permanent loss of vision (6)

REFERENCES
1. Vedula SS, et al. Corticosteroids for treating optic neuritis. *Cochrane Library*. 2007;1:CD001430.
2. Keltner JL, Johnson CA, Cello KE, Dontchev M, Gal RL, Beck RW, Optic Neuritis Study Group et al. Visual field profile of optic neuritis: a final follow-up report from the optic neuritis treatment trial from baseline through 15 years. *Arch. Ophthalmol*. 2010;128:330–7.
3. Simsek I, Erdem H, Pay S, et al. Optic neuritis occurring with anti-tumour necrosis factor alpha therapy. *Ann Rheum Dis*. 2007;66:1255–8.
4. Gleicher N, et al. *Principles and practice of medical therapy in pregnancy*, 3rd ed. Norwalk, CT: Appleton and Lange; 1998:1396–9.
5. Kaufman DI, Trobe JD, Eggenberger ER, et al. Practice parameter: the role of corticosteroids in the management of acute monosymptomatic optic neuritis. Report of the Quality Standards Subcommittee of the American Academy of Neurology. *Neurology*. 2000;54:2039–44.
6. Carter J. e-Medicine, *Optic Neuritis* August 8, 2009.
7. Optic Neuritis Study Group. Visual function 15 years after optic neuritis: a final follow-up report from the Optic Neuritis Treatment Trial. *Ophthalmology*. 2008;115:1079–1082.e5.

ADDITIONAL READING
- Arnold AC. Evolving management of optic neuritis and multiple sclerosis. *Am J Ophthalmol*. 2005; 139:1101–8.
- Balcer LJ. Clinical practice. Optic neuritis. *N Engl J Med*. 2006;354:1273–80.
- Galetta SL. The controlled high risk Avonex multiple sclerosis trial (CHAMPS Study). *J Neuroophthalmol*. 2001;21:292–5.
- Rizzo JF, Andreoli CM, Rabinov JD. Use of magnetic resonance imaging to differentiate optic neuritis and nonarteritic anterior ischemic optic neuropathy. *Ophthalmology*. 2002;109:1679–84.

See Also (Topic, Algorithm, Electronic Media Element)
Multiple Sclerosis

 ## CODES

ICD9
- 377.30 Optic neuritis, unspecified
- 377.31 Optic papillitis
- 377.32 Retrobulbar neuritis (acute)

CLINICAL PEARLS
- MRI is the procedure of choice for determining relative risk and possible therapy for MS prevention.
- The ONTT showed that high-dose IV methylprednisolone followed by oral prednisone accelerated visual recovery but did not improve the 6-month or 1-year visual outcome compared with placebo, whereas treatment with oral prednisone alone did not improve the outcome and was associated with an increased rate of recurrence of ON.

ALERT
- Never use oral prednisone alone as primary treatment because this may increase the risk for recurrent ON and should be avoided (4).
- 15-year Optic Neuritis Study Group results:
  – After the initial period of recovery after an acute episode of ON, visual acuity remained stable in most patients.
  – Overall, 72% of affected eyes had visual acuity of 20/20 or better, with 2/3 of patients having 20/20 or better vision in both eyes.
  – In most patients, there was little change in vision between the 10- and 15-year follow-up examinations. 6 patients (2%) had visual acuity of 20/40 or worse in both eyes. Visual function was slightly better in patients without MS compared with those with MS (7).

ORAL CAVITY NEOPLASMS

Hugh J. Silk, MD
Sheila O. Stille, DMD, MAGD
Jason Conforti, MD

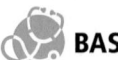 **BASICS**

DESCRIPTION
- Malignant tumors affecting the tongue, floor of the mouth, salivary glands, buccal mucosa, gums, hard and soft palate, or vermillion junction of the lip
- System(s) affected: GI

EPIDEMIOLOGY

Incidence
- Predominant age: >40 years
- Now seen increasingly in younger age groups with the use of smokeless tobacco and alcohol
- Predominant sex: Male > Female (2:1)
- 12/100,000/year (35,310 new cases/year)
- 3–5% of all cancers in US each year
- Oral cancer is the eighth most common cancer worldwide.
- High incidence in Asia, related to the habit of chewing betel nut, fresh betel leaf, and habitual reverse smoking (lighted end held within the oral cavity)
- 1/3 higher incidence in African Americans than in whites, with a mortality rate almost 2× as high

Geriatric Considerations
- Greater incidence > 40 years of age
- Peak age of 55 years

Prevalence
- Oral cavity neoplasms account for 3% of new cancers occurring in men and 2% in women.
- Lip carcinoma 30%, buccal cancer 5%, floor of the mouth cancers 10–15%, tongue cancers 20–30%

RISK FACTORS
- Most patients with proliferative verrucous leukoplakia (PVL) progress to oral carcinoma (1).
- Low socioeconomic status (2)
- Tobacco, alcohol, ultraviolet (UV) light exposures

Genetics
Family history of oral cancer should be noted.

GENERAL PREVENTION
- Avoid tobacco (including smokeless) and betel nut.
- Limit alcohol use.
- Limit sun exposure/UV light; wear sun block, hats with visors/large rim.
- Maintain a nutritious diet high in fruits and vegetables (3).
- Annual complete oral examination, including bimanual palpation of mouth floor by dentist or doctor, especially for those at risk.
- Early detection may be beneficial in high-risk individuals (e.g., dental offices offer zila tolonium chloride (toluidine blue) [ViziLite Plus] testing with 71% PPV) but has not been proven in low-risk individuals.

- If detected at an early stage, survival from oral cancer is better than 90% at 5 years, whereas late-stage disease survival is only 30%.
- Close follow-up of PVL with early and aggressive treatment

PATHOPHYSIOLOGY
- Of neoplasms, 90% are squamous cell carcinomas; the others include lymphomas and adenocarcinomas from minor salivary gland origin and sarcomas.
- Variety of cellular differences at molecular level among oral squamous cell carcinomas (4)

ETIOLOGY
- Use of tobacco (smokeless or smoked, including cigars); 85% of head and neck cancers linked to tobacco
- Excessive alcohol consumption
- Use of both alcohol and tobacco greatly increases risk as compared with those who use tobacco or alcohol alone (synergistic effect).
- Exposure to UV light (i.e., sun exposure) in the case of lip carcinoma
- Radiation exposure from treatment of other facial cancers increases risk of salivary gland cancers.
- Associations:
  – Epstein-Barr virus
  – Human papillomavirus (HPV) and alcohol and tobacco may promote invasion of HPV and oral cancers.
  – Betal nut with and without tobacco use
  – Certain occupational chemical exposures, including formaldehyde, perchloroethylene, and pesticides, may be associated with nasopharyngeal and laryngeal cancer.
  – Poor oral hygiene, presence of oral lichenoid, and leukoplakic lesions may act as predisposing factors.
  – Patients with HIV have a higher incidence of head and neck malignances.

COMMONLY ASSOCIATED CONDITIONS
- Leukoplakias or erythroplakias should be biopsied because they are considered premalignant and are associated with carcinoma at least 10% of the time.
- Riboflavin deficiency or iron-deficiency anemia and Plummer-Vinson syndrome associated with oral cancers

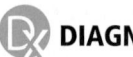 **DIAGNOSIS**

HISTORY
- Nonhealing ulcer or mass of mouth or lip
- Area that bleeds easily or unexplained pain
- Dysphagia/odynophagia
- Chronic sore throat or hoarseness
- Ear pain
- Problems articulating
- Regurgitation of liquids secondary to nasopharyngeal incompetence from the tumor
- History of risk factors (e.g., tobacco exposure, chronic alcohol use, radiation treatment, excessive UV light exposure)

PHYSICAL EXAM
- Friable granular exophytic and/or infiltrative mass or ulcer that frequently is tender and confused with infection
- White or red lesions noted
- Hard, indurated margins extending beyond the borders of the ulcer noted on palpation
- Hard neck mass suggesting metastatic disease in the nodal chain along the internal jugular vein
- Cranial sensory and motor nerves may be compromised.

DIAGNOSTIC TESTS & INTERPRETATION
- Physical exam, including an extensive bimanual intra- and extraoral head and neck exam
- Transoral biopsy of any ulceration or erythroplasia/leukoplasia lesion present for 4 weeks provides the definitive diagnosis.
- Brush or punch biopsy test for smaller oral lesions can determine need for surgical biopsy.

Imaging
- Plain films of head and neck
- CT scan (for bony involvement) or MRI (for soft tissue involvement) if clinical suggestion of intracranial metastasis
- CXR to assess metastasis to the lungs, the most common site of spread outside the neck
- Imaging bone scans if there is pain in the bones suggesting bone metastasis
- Abdominal CT scan if liver metastasis suspected
- PET scan may be necessary in some cases; modified sugars preferentially absorbed by cancer cells

Pathological Findings
- Premalignant
- Malignant changes characteristic of cell types
- Most common is squamous cell (90%), followed by salivary gland, lymphomas, and sarcomas
- Those originating in the lip and buccal mucosa are usually well differentiated; those originating in the oral pharynx and floor of mouth are less well differentiated and have higher risk for metastasis.

DIFFERENTIAL DIAGNOSIS
- Exudative tonsillitis (usually bilateral involvement)
- Stomatitis or glossitis secondary to infectious etiology, most commonly candidiasis
- Benign tumors of the oral cavity (slow growing and usually not erosive or ulcerative)
- Kaposi sarcoma
- Mycosis fungoides
- Premalignant lesions such as leukoplakia or erythroplasia
- Lichen planus

TREATMENT

MEDICATION
Opiates for pain relief

ADDITIONAL TREATMENT
General Measures
- Treatment varies depending on location (e.g., tongue, buccal wall, pharynx, palate, lip).
- Resection treatment of choice, if possible
- Small, superficial lesions can be treated with combined external-beam radiation therapy (EBRT) and intraoral cone or surface mold.
- Primary radiotherapy (and/or chemotherapy for palliation) is suggested for unresectable tumors and patients not amenable to surgery.
- Obtain dental consult prior to any treatment to prevent serious complications later. Can evaluate questionable teeth, fabricate mouth guards to wear during radiation treatments, and fabricate fluoride trays.

Issues for Referral
Biopsy any suspicious lesions.

Additional Therapies
- Secondary prevention of smoking, alcohol, betal nut abstinence
- Annual follow-up oral examinations

SURGERY/OTHER PROCEDURES
- Wide resection ± radiation therapy and/or chemotherapy is the treatment of choice.
- There is some evidence that concomitant radio-/chemotherapy with surgery is more effective than radiation therapy with surgery in the treatment of head and neck cancers in general (5).
- For a neoplasm such as a melanoma, surgery is believed to be the most effective treatment. The role of radiation, however, is controversial. Many experts believe melanoma neoplasms to be radioresistant.
- Tracheotomy may be necessary if the patient has problems handling secretions or difficulty breathing.

IN-PATIENT CONSIDERATIONS
Admission Criteria
- Inpatient for surgery
- Outpatient for radiation therapy and chemotherapy
- Surgery, airway management, infection

 ONGOING CARE

FOLLOW-UP RECOMMENDATIONS
As needed by patient's nutritional and physical status

Patient Monitoring
Routine periodic head, mouth, and neck exams by medical and dental professionals to detect possible 2nd primary or recurrence in the upper respiratory and digestive tracts, especially within the first 36 months and if radiology was used

DIET
- Depends on the extent of disease and whether the patient is able to chew or swallow
- Usually early lesions can be managed with a regular diet. As disease progresses, a soft diet is necessary.
- Nutrition is of prime importance for normal wound healing, especially if patient requires surgery. Patients may need nasogastric and/or gastrostomy feedings if they are orally disabled.

PATIENT EDUCATION
Primary prevention for all about avoidance of risk factors and secondary prevention for those diagnosed

PROGNOSIS
- Early lesions with adequate treatment leads to a >80% cure.
- 5-year relative survival rate for localized stage: 82%
- 5-year relative survival rate for all stages combined: 59%

COMPLICATIONS
- Functional and/or cosmetic disabilities proportional to the degree of surgery and stage of tumor
- Stomatitis with or without candidiasis, tissue hypoxia, tongue mucositis, hypocellularity, and fibrosis secondary to radiation therapy or chemotherapy
- Persistent dysphagia secondary to surgery or radiation therapy
- Persistent problems with articulation or deglutition depending on the amount of tongue resection and age of patient
- Radiation may cause new neoplasms.

REFERENCES

1. Cabay RJ, Morton TH, Epstein JB. Proliferative verrucous leukoplakia and its progression to oral carcinoma: a review of the literature. *J Oral Pathol Med*. 2007;36:255–61.
2. Conway DI, Petticrew M, Marlborough H, et al. Socioeconomic inequalities and oral cancer risk: A systematic review and meta-analysis of case-control studies. *Int J Cancer*. 2008.
3. Pavia M, Pileggi C, Nobile CG, et al. Association between fruit and vegetable consumption and oral cancer: a meta-analysis of observational studies. *Am J Clin Nutr*. 2006;83:1126–34.
4. Severino P, Alvares AM, Michaluart Jr P, et al. Global gene expression profiling of oral cavity cancers suggests molecular heterogeneity within anatomic subsites. *BMC Res Notes*. 2008;1:113.
5. Oliver RJ, Clarkson JE, Conway DI, et al. Interventions for the treatment of oral and oropharyngeal cancers: surgical treatment. *Cochrane Database Syst Rev*. 2007;CD006205.

ADDITIONAL READING

- Becher H, Ramroth H, Ahrens W, et al. Occupation, exposure to polycyclic aromatic hydrocarbons and laryngeal cancer risk. *Int J Cancer*. 2005;116:451–7.
- Hisham, Khalifa. Primary Malignant Melanoma of the Tongue. *Canadian Journal of Surgery*. December 2009.
- Kademani D. Oral cancer. *Mayo Clinic Proceedings*, 2007; 87(7): 878–87.
- Shah JP, Gil Z. Current concepts in management of oral cancer - Surgery. *Oral Oncol*. 2008.

See Also (Topic, Algorithm, Electronic Media Element)
Algorithm: Bleeding Gums

 CODES

ICD9
- 140.9 Malignant neoplasm of lip, unspecified, vermilion border
- 141.9 Malignant neoplasm of tongue, unspecified
- 142.9 Malignant neoplasm of salivary gland, unspecified

CLINICAL PEARLS
- Primary and secondary prevention by doctors and dentists about risk factor avoidance and complete oral exams at annual visits to doctor and dentist office
- Leukoplakias or erythroplakias should be biopsied because they are considered premalignant and are associated with carcinoma at least 10% of the time.
- Patients should see a dentist prior to undergoing treatment of head and neck tumors to allow planning to reduce potential dental-related complications.
- Concomitant radio/chemotherapy together with surgery is likely more effective than radiation therapy alone with surgery in the treatment of head and neck cancers, in general.

ORAL REHYDRATION

William A. Primack, MD

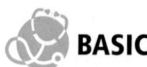 **BASICS**

Oral rehydration is a clinically useful, cost effective, and safe technique to treat all but the most severe dehydration.

DESCRIPTION

- Dehydration and ongoing fluid losses from infectious GE can be treated effectively with ORS, except in the most severe cases, in which initial parenteral fluid resuscitation is required (1)[B],(2)[B],(3)[A].
- ORS's for rehydration should have an Na content of ~75 mEq/L (75 mmol/L). Maintenance ORSs, with an Na content of 40–50 mEq/L (40–50 mmol/L), are useful for repair of mild dehydration and treatment of ongoing losses with relatively low Na content (e.g., rotavirus) (2)[A].
- High-Na diarrheal losses such as occur in cholera may require higher-Na-content ORS's (WHO solution = 90 mEq/L [90 mmol/L] Na). In 2002, WHO reduced the Na content of its ORS from 90–75 mEq/L, and in 2003, the CDC endorsed this approach (4)[A].
- System(s) affected: Endocrine/Metabolic; GI

EPIDEMIOLOGY
Incidence
- Predominant age: Primarily infants and children, but effective for all ages
- Predominant sex: Male = Female

PATHOPHYSIOLOGY
This therapy takes advantage of the coupled transport of Na and glucose in the small intestine even during a course of GE. Water follows osmotically after Na entry. Potassium is passively absorbed via solvent drag. A glucose concentration of 2% allows most efficient Na absorption (5).

 DIAGNOSIS

HISTORY
- Frequency and volume of urination
- Vomiting: Duration and amount
- Diarrhea: Duration and amount
- Fever
- Weight loss: Amount
- Travel
- Exposure to others with GE
- Recent antibiotic use

PHYSICAL EXAM
- Level of consciousness
- Capillary refill (abnormal if >2 seconds)
- Mucous membranes: Dry, cracked
- Tears: Decreased
- HR: Increased
- RR: Increased
- BP: Orthostasis
- Pulse: Faint
- Skin turgor: Tenting
- Eyes: Sunken
- Urine output: Decreased

DIAGNOSTIC TESTS & INTERPRETATION
Lab
Initial lab tests
- None usually necessary
- If moderate to severe, obtain Na, potassium, bicarbonate, chloride, glucose, BUN, creatinine.

 TREATMENT

MEDICATION
First Line
Many comparable generic formulations are available.

Comparison of oral rehydration products

Solution	Type*	Na$^+$	K$^+$	HCO$_3$
WHO (1975)	R	90	20	20
WHO (2002)	R	75	20	10
Pedialyte	M	45	20	25
Enfalyte	M	50	25	34

*R = rehydration; M = maintenance; Na$^+$ = Na (mEq/L or mmol/L); K$^+$ = potassium (mmol/L); COH$_3$ = carbohydrate (g/L)
†Contains rice syrup solids.

Second Line
In areas where malnutrition is more likely, supplementation with 20 mg oral zinc daily shortens the course of diarrhea and lessens costs (6)[B].

ADDITIONAL TREATMENT
General Measures

- In developed countries, most diarrheal losses are low Na; consequently, maintenance ORS can be used for rehydration (2)[A].
- If patient is obtunded or has paralytic ileus, use IV hydration.
- Estimate replacement at 60 mL/kg for mild dehydration and 80–100 mL/kg for moderate dehydration over the 1st 4–8 h.
- ORS is not to be diluted.
- If vomiting occurs, small amounts of ORS given frequently are usually effective.
- If the patient is not vomiting and is alert, thirst is an excellent indicator of fluid needs. Very important to replace any ongoing losses and add maintenance fluids.
- Replace ongoing stool losses with an ORS. In an infant, estimate 5–10 mL/kg per stool, or weigh diapers.
- Maintenance oral rehydration therapy begins when the deficit is replaced and provides for ongoing losses. Maintenance ORS or a combination of ORS and water or other clear liquids can be used.
- Add maintenance requirements to replacement:
  – Estimate:
    ○ 0–10 kg: 4 mL/kg/h
    ○ Plus 10–20 kg: 2 mL/kg/h
    ○ Plus >20 kg: 1 mL/kg/h
  – Use a maintenance ORS.
  – Traditional clear fluids (e.g., fruit juice, soda) are inappropriate for oral rehydration therapy.
- If the patient has hypertonic dehydration, oral rehydration should be planned for 12–24 h.
- Effective at all ages:
  – If child refuses because of taste, flavor with a commercial flavoring such as sugar-free grape-flavored Kool-Aid, and use ~1/4 tsp to 4 oz ORS.
  – Prepackaged ORS-flavored freeze pops (often well accepted)
- If necessary, rehydration by NG tube is appropriate.
- Begin feeding as soon as rehydration is achieved.

- Contraindications:
  - Conditions predisposing to risk of aspiration: Altered consciousness, seizure activity, severe hypotension, shock
  - Persistent vomiting (as in pyloric stenosis)
  - Absent bowel sounds
- Precautions:
  - The ingredients should be provided in premixed packets to avoid iatrogenic errors in mixing. In the US, Pedialyte premixed powder packets to be diluted in 8 ounces (240ml) of water.
  - If water safety is questionable, it should be boiled or treated for purification.
  - Discard the solution after 12 h if held at room temperature or 24 h if refrigerated.
  - After rehydration is complete, ORS should not be used as the only fluid intake because the high Na content may lead to hypernatremia.

COMPLEMENTARY AND ALTERNATIVE MEDICINE

The probiotic *Lactobacillus* may shorten course, especially in developed countries (7)[B].

IN-PATIENT CONSIDERATIONS

Admission Criteria

Failure of oral therapy: Estimated failure rate 4% (3)[A].

IV Fluids

To be used for initial resuscitation in severe cases or if failure of ORS.

Nursing

If vomiting occurs, small amounts of ORS given frequently are usually effective.

ONGOING CARE

FOLLOW-UP RECOMMENDATIONS

- Primarily outpatient
- Designed to be administered by family members

DIET

- For breast-feeding infants, mother should continue nursing.
- For bottle-fed babies, early institution of formulas. Lactose-free formulas rarely are required.
- Age appropriate:
  - Complex carbohydrate-rich (e.g., rice, bread, potato, cereal), low-fat foods should be offered as soon as the dehydration deficit is replaced.
- Cow's milk can be added to diet after several days.

PATIENT EDUCATION

- Awareness and availability of ORSs markedly diminishes morbidity from GE.
- Travelers concerned with severe diarrhea should carry ORS packets on trips.

PROGNOSIS

- Rapid clinical improvement despite continuing diarrhea is the usual course.
- The overall complication rate for oral rehydration is similar to that for parenteral rehydration in cases of mild and moderate dehydration (1)[B],(3)[A].

COMPLICATIONS

Change to IV hydration if the patient has increasing weight loss (fluid deficit), clinical deterioration, or intractable vomiting.

REFERENCES

1. Spandorfer PR, Alessandrini EA, Joffe MD et al. Oral versus intravenous rehydration of moderately dehydrated children: a randomized, controlled trial. *Pediatrics*. 2005;115:295–301.
2. Hahn S, Kim S, Garner P. Reduced osmolarity oral rehydration solution for treating dehydration caused by acute diarrhoea in children. *Cochrane Database Syst Rev*. 2002;CD002847.
3. Hartling L, Bellemare S, Wiebe N, et al. Oral versus intravenous rehydration for treating dehydration due to gastroenteritis in children. *Cochrane Database Syst Rev*. 2006;3:CD004390.
4. Murphy CK, Hahn S, Volmink J. Reduced osmolarity oral rehydration solution for treating cholera. *Cochrane Database of Systematic Reviews* 2004, Issue 4. Art. No.: CD003754. DOI:10.1002/14651858.CD003754.pub2.
5. Duggan C, Fontaine O, Pierce NF et al. Scientific rationale for a change in the composition of oral rehydration solution. *JAMA*. 2004;291:2628—31.
6. Bhandari N, Mazumder S, Taneja S, et al. Effectiveness of zinc supplementation plus oral rehydration salts compared with oral rehydration salts alone as a treatment for acute diarrhea in a primary care setting: a cluster randomized trial. *Pediatrics*. 2008;121:e1279–85.
7. Canani RB, Cirillo P, Terrin G et al. Probiotics for treatment of acute diarrhoea in children: randomised clinical trial of five different preparations. *BMJ*. 2007;335:340.

ADDITIONAL READING

- Fonseca BK, Holdgate A, Craig JC. Enteral vs intravenous rehydration therapy for children with gastroenteritis: a meta-analysis of randomized controlled trials. *Arch Pediatr Adolesc Med*. 2004;158:483–90.
- Fontaine O, et al. Rice-based ORS for treating diarrhea. In: *Cochrane Library*, Issue I. Oxford: Update Software; 2002.

CODES

ICD9
- 009.0 Infectious colitis, enteritis, and gastroenteritis
- 276.51 Dehydration

CLINICAL PEARLS

- ORSs are more effective and less costly than IV hydration yet are underutilized in the developed world.
- In developed countries, most diarrheal losses are low Na; consequently, maintenance ORS can be used for rehydration.
- ORS should not be diluted

OSGOOD-SCHLATTER DISEASE

David P. Sealy, MD

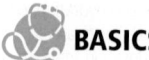 **BASICS**

DESCRIPTION
- A syndrome associated with traction apophysitis in adolescent boys and girls consisting of pain in the tibial tubercle with swelling
- System(s) affected: Musculoskeletal

EPIDEMIOLOGY
Prevalence
- Not known, but common (13% of athletes in 1 Finnish study)
- Incidence in girls increasing

RISK FACTORS
- Ages 11–18 years
- Girls 8–12, boys 10–16
- Male sex slightly more common
- Rapid skeletal growth
- Involvement in repetitive-jumping sports such as football, volleyball, basketball, hockey, soccer, skating, gymnastics, and ballet
- Sports involving heavy quadriceps activity

GENERAL PREVENTION
- Avoidance of sports involving heavy quadriceps loading
- Patients may compete if pain is minimal.
- Increase hamstring and quadriceps flexibility.

PATHOPHYSIOLOGY
Traction apophysitis of the tibial tubercle owing to repetitive strain on the secondary ossification center of the tibial tuberosity (1)[C]

ETIOLOGY
- Basic etiology unknown, but clearly exacerbated by exercise. Jumping and pivoting sports are the worst—repetitive trauma the most likely source.
- Possible association with tight hip flexors, quadriceps, and hamstring muscle groups.

 DIAGNOSIS

HISTORY
- Unilateral or bilateral (30%) tibial tuberosity pain
- Pain exacerbated by exercise, especially jumping and landing after jumping

PHYSICAL EXAM
- Knee pain with squatting or crouching
- Absence of effusion or condyle tenderness
- Tibial tuberosity swelling and tenderness
- Pain increased with knee extension against resistance or kneeling
- Erythema over tibial tuberosity

DIAGNOSTIC TESTS & INTERPRETATION
Lab
Initial lab tests
No blood tests are indicated unless other diagnostic considerations are entertained.

Imaging
Initial approach
Radiographic imaging of the proximal tibia and knee may show heterotopic calcification in the patellar tendon:
- X-rays are rarely diagnostic.
- Calcified thickening of the tibial tuberosity with irregular ossification at insertion of tendon to tibial tubercle

Diagnostic Procedures/Surgery
- Bone scan may show increased uptake in the area of the tibial tuberosity; will have increased uptake in apophysis in any child, but may be more than the opposite side.
- Ultrasounds is becoming an excellent alternative, with characteristic findings and classifications (2)[C].
- Magnetic resonance imaging has characteristic findings of fragmentation of the tibial tubercle and bone edema.

Pathological Findings
Biopsy is not necessary but would show osteolysis and fragmentation of the tibial tubercle.

DIFFERENTIAL DIAGNOSIS
- Stress fracture of the proximal tibia
- Pes anserinus bursitis
- Quadriceps tendon avulsion
- Patellofemoral stress syndrome
- Chondromalacia patellae
- Proximal tibial neoplasm
- Osteomyelitis of the proximal tibia
- Tibial plateau fracture
- Sinding-Larsen-Johansson syndrome (patellar apophysitis)—pain over inferior patellar tendon
- Patellar fracture
- Infrapatellar bursitis
- Patellar tendinitis—pain over inferior patellar tendon and inferior pole of patella

TREATMENT

MEDICATION

First Line

None in particular, but all analgesics may be considered. Nonsteroidal anti-inflammatory drugs are of minimal benefit; however, narcotics are not recommended (3)[B].

Second Line

- More potent analgesics such as narcotics may be considered for short-term use or in extreme situations.
- Injectable corticosteroids universally not recommended due to reports of subcutaneous atrophy (3)[C]

ADDITIONAL TREATMENT

General Measures

- Frequent ice applications after exercise
- Rest
- Knee immobilization in extension (severe cases)
- In more severe cases, avoidance of activities that increase pain or swelling
- Consider physical therapy referral for quadriceps isometric strengthening, hip extensions, adductor strengthening, and hamstring and quadriceps stretching exercises.
- Open- and closed-chain eccentric quadriceps strengthening
- Patients with marked pronation may benefit from orthotics.

Issues for Referral

When conservative therapy is unsuccessful, consideration of surgery warrants referral.

SURGERY/OTHER PROCEDURES

- Débridement of a thickened, cosmetically unsatisfactory tibial tubercle (rare) or removal of heterotopic bone
- Surgical excision of a painful tibial tubercal rarely needed (<5%) (3)[C]
- 76% return to normal sport activity and <10% are restricted from competition due to recurrent pain (4)[B].

 ONGOING CARE

FOLLOW-UP RECOMMENDATIONS

- Athletes may return to play if tolerated.
- Presence of pain does not preclude competition.

Patient Monitoring

With worsening of symptoms only

PATIENT EDUCATION

- Consider avoidance of jumping sports. Assure family that symptoms and findings will diminish with time and rest.
- Can play sports with mild pain
- Quad stretching and strengthening important

PROGNOSIS

Except in rare complicated cases, this is a self-limiting illness that resolves within 2 years of full skeletal maturation. However, up to 60% of adults with prior Osgood-Schlatter disease (OSD) still report occasional symptoms and have pain with kneeling. Most persons with OSD will have residual "knobby" tibial tubercles that never completely resolve. They may decline in size but will remain throughout life to some extent.

COMPLICATIONS

Rarely, the heavily fragmented and inflamed tibial ossicle will avulse and require surgery.

REFERENCES

1. Gholve PA, Scher DM, et al. Osgood Schlatter Syndrome. *Curr Opin Pediatr.* 2007;19(1): 44–50.
2. Zaid AA, et al. The immature athlete. *Clin Sports Med.* 2002;21:3.
3. Bloom OJ, Mackler L. What is the best treatment for Osgood Schlatter disease? *J Fam Prac.* 2004;53(2):153–6.
4. Weiss JM, Jordan SS, Andersen JS, et al. Surgical treatment of unresolved Osgood-Schlatter disease: ossicle resection with tibial tubercleplasty. *J Pediatr Orthop.* 2007;27:844–7.

 CODES

ICD9

732.4 Juvenile osteochondrosis of lower extremity, excluding foot

CLINICAL PEARLS

- Pain starting below the patella in an athlete during rapid growth spurt is Osgood-Schlatter disease, patellar tendinosis, or Sindig-Larsen-Johansson syndrome.
- Only Osgood-Schlatter disease hurts directly over the tibial tubercle.

O

Robert A. Baldor, MD

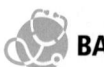

BASICS

DESCRIPTION
- Inflammatory focal or generalized condition of the skeleton characterized by rapid, chaotic bone resorption followed by equally chaotic and excessive bone formation. Leads to enlarged but weakened and highly vascularized bone, which is painful, easily deformed, and subject to fractures with minimal trauma. Cranial and vertebral involvement can also cause neurologic deficits.
- System(s) affected: Musculoskeletal
- Synonym(s): Paget's disease of bone

EPIDEMIOLOGY
- Predominant age: >50 years; occasional cases ages 20–50 years
- Predominant sex: Male = Female

Prevalence
- 3% of white individuals >50 years have at least 1 focus.
- More prevalent if ancestry white, especially United Kingdom, Northern Europe (excluding Scandinavia), Italy, Australia, and New Zealand
- Rare in African Americans and Asians

Geriatric Considerations
Common

RISK FACTORS
None known

Genetics
- 15–50% of patients have 1 or more involved 1st-order relatives with osteitis deformans.
- Recent data suggest an 18q locus is involved, but other chromosomal sites may also confer susceptibility.

GENERAL PREVENTION
Avoid excessive mechanical stress on afflicted bones to reduce chance of fractures and other complications.

ETIOLOGY
Unknown; best evidence to date is for slow virus infection in genetically susceptible individuals

COMMONLY ASSOCIATED CONDITIONS
- Hyperparathyroidism
- Gouty diathesis
- Secondary osteoarthritis
- Angioid streaks (rare)
- Mottled retinal degeneration
- Bone sarcoma (rare)
- Peyronie disease
- Accelerated atherosclerosis
- Osteoporosis circumscripta

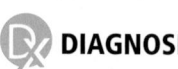

DIAGNOSIS

HISTORY
- Frequently asymptomatic
- Bone pain
- Skeletal deformities
- Bowing of extremities
- Acetabular protrusion
- Headaches
- Head enlargement
- Fractures
- Secondary osteoarthritis
- Vertebral compression

PHYSICAL EXAM
- Neurologic examination for deficits
- Audiogram, if skull involvement: Sensorineural or conductive hearing loss
- Visual field study, if skull involvement
- High-output CHF (rare)
- Renal calculi (calcium, uric acid)
- Mottled retinal degeneration (rare)
- Increased skin temperature over affected areas
- Peripheral neuropathies
- Carpal/tarsal tunnel syndromes
- Valvular/endocardial calcification

DIAGNOSTIC TESTS & INTERPRETATION
Lab
- Serum calcium level: Usually normal; rarely increased
- Serum alkaline phosphatase (total or bone-specific): Usually increased
- Hypercalcemia (rare)
- Serum gamma glutamyl transpeptidase: Normal
- Serum osteocalcin (binary ghost-pulse constraint): Usually increased
- Urinary pyridinoline collagen crosslinks: Usually increased
- N- and C-telopeptide (collagen crosslinks): Usually increased in serum and urine
- Drugs that may alter lab results:
  - Vitamin D and its metabolites
  - Hepatotoxic drugs
- Disorders that may alter lab results:
  - See Differential Diagnosis.
  - Osteomalacia
  - Liver disorders
  - Traumatic fractures

Imaging
- X-rays show irregular pattern of alternating bone formation and resorption in enlarged deformed bones and resorptive fronts at advancing edge.
- Bone scans show intense uptake in focal pattern.
- CT and MRI show extra-bony extension if sarcomatous degeneration occurs.

Diagnostic Procedures/Surgery
Bone biopsy needed only in confusing cases (rare)

Pathological Findings
Chaotic bone resorption at advancing edge of disease:
- Osteoclasts are large, contain 10–100 nuclei, and have abnormal configuration:
  - Electron photomicroscopy shows that nuclei and cytoplasm contain myriad inclusion bodies resembling viral nucleocapsids.
- Later, excessive osteoblastic bone formation predominates, with sclerotic bone–containing cement lines forming a mosaic pattern.

DIFFERENTIAL DIAGNOSIS
- Polyostotic fibrous dysplasia
- Osteitis fibrosis cystica (skeletal hyperparathyroidism)
- Primary bone neoplasms
- Osteolytic, osteoblastic metastases

TREATMENT

MEDICATION

First Line
Add nonsteroidal anti-inflammatory drugs (NSAIDs) to the following drugs for secondary osteoarthritis. COX-2 inhibitors may be substituted:

- Synthetic injectable salmon calcitonin (Miacalcin): 50 IU SC/IM 3 times weekly to 100 IU SC/IM daily, courses 1.5–3 years; or
- Etidronate (Didronel), 5 mg/kg p.o. daily (~400 mg; taken on an empty stomach) for 6 months. Rarely, 20 mg/kg/d for 1 month. Courses may be repeated after a 3–6-month rest period; or
- Alendronate (Fosamax) 40 mg p.o. daily (taken on an empty stomach) for 6 months; or
- Risedronate (Actonel) 30 mg p.o. daily (taken on an empty stomach) for 2 months; or
- Pamidronate (Aredia) 60 mg/d by 4–6 hour infusions for 2–3 days. Alternately, 30 mg/d by 4–6-h infusions once a week for 6 weeks. May be repeated several months later if effect wears off.
- Zoledronic acid (Relcast) 5 mg infusion over 15 minutes plus 1500 mg elemental calcium (divided) and 1000 IU Vitamin D per day for minimally 2 weeks after infusion
- Contraindications:
  - History of allergy or hypersensitivity
  - For alendronate and risedronate, esophageal dysfunction, severe upper gastrointestinal tract symptoms, gastroesophageal reflux disease, etc.
- Precautions:
  - Adverse side effects may require ameliorative measures or temporary dose reduction.
  - Salmon calcitonin: Nausea, vomiting, anorexia, flushing, rash, including urticaria (rare)
  - Etidronate disodium: Nausea, vomiting, diarrhea, increased bone pain
  - Alendronate and risedronate: Heartburn, epigastric pain, and musculoskeletal pain. Take on an empty stomach with copious water. No food, beverages, or other medications for 30–60 minutes. Remain upright for 1 hour.
  - Pamidronate disodium: Transient fever, leukopenia, hypocalcemia, headache, malaise, loss of appetite
- Significant possible interactions: None

Second Line
NSAIDs or COX-2 inhibitors for mildly symptomatic disease in nonstrategic areas

ADDITIONAL TREATMENT

General Measures
- Rarely, splints for severely resorbed areas with high risk of fracture
- Hearing aids for severe deafness: Of some (but not great) value in sensorineural deafness

SURGERY/OTHER PROCEDURES
- Joint replacement (hip, knee) sometimes needed
- Osteotomy procedures for extreme deformity
- Decompression procedures (skull, spinal column) for acute neurologic deficits (rarely needed)
- Bone biopsy (rarely needed)
- Extirpative surgery for sarcomatous complications
- Open reduction of fractures

IN-PATIENT CONSIDERATIONS
Outpatient, except when IV treatment is used

ONGOING CARE

FOLLOW-UP RECOMMENDATIONS
- Full activity to maintain function
- Avoid excessive mechanical stress on involved bones.

Patient Monitoring
- Follow-up visits every 2–4 months during drug therapy; yearly if drugs not being used:
  - Alkaline phosphatase level (total or bone-specific) before each visit
- Repeat x-rays and bone scan every 3–5 years or as needed.

DIET
No special diet

PATIENT EDUCATION
Paget Foundation, 120 Wall St., Suite 1602, New York, NY 10005; tel. (212) 509-5335; fax (212)-509-8492; http://www.paget.org

PROGNOSIS
- Depends on severity, often asymptomatic
- Slow progression if untreated
- Significant amelioration with treatment (85% or greater)
- Poor prognosis if bone sarcoma develops

COMPLICATIONS
- Fractures
- Severe deformities
- Head enlargement
- Acetabular protrusion
- Carpal/tarsal tunnel syndromes
- Neurologic deficits
- Deafness
- Visual impairment
- CHF (high output)
- Renal calculi
- Peyronie syndrome
- Sarcomatous degeneration

ADDITIONAL READING

- Ankrom MA, Shapiro JR. Paget's disease of bone (osteitis deformans). *J Amer Geriatr Soc.* 1998;46: 1025–33.
- Delmas PD, Meunier PJ. The management of Paget's disease of bone. *N Engl J Med.* 1997;336:558–66.
- Hadjipavlou A, Lander P, Srolovitz H et al., Malignant transformation in Paget disease of bone. *Cancer.* 1992;70:2802–8.
- Morales-Piga AA, Rey-Rey JS, Corres-González J, et al. Frequency and characteristics of familial aggregation of Paget's disease of bone. *J Bone Miner Res.* 1995;10:663–70.
- Noor M, Shoback D. Paget's disease of bone: diagnosis and treatment update. *Curr Rheumatol Rep.* 2000;2:67–73.
- Rothschild BM. Paget's disease of the elderly. *Compr Ther.* 2000;26:251–4.
- Siris ES. Paget's disease of bone. *J Bone Miner Res.* 1998;13:1061–5.
- Wallach S. Identifying and controlling Paget's disease. *J Musculoskel Med.* 1997;14:66–82.

See Also (Topic, Algorithm, Electronic Media Element)
Arthritis, Osteo; Bone Tumor, Primary Malignant; Hyperparathyroidism

CODES

ICD9
- 731.0 Osteitis deformans without mention of bone tumor
- 731.1 Osteitis deformans in diseases classified elsewhere

OSTEOCHONDRITIS DISSECANS

Morteza Khodaee, MD, MPH

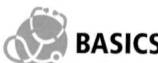 **BASICS**

DESCRIPTION

- Separation of a portion of cartilage and underlying subchondral bone from a joint surface
- Knee is the most commonly affected joint; however, it can occur in any diarthrodial joint, including, in decreasing order of frequency, the elbow (capitellum), ankle (talar dome or tibial plafond), tarsal navicular, hip (femoral capital epiphysis), shoulder (humeral head or glenoid), and wrist (scaphoid).
- The loose piece of bone and cartilage may stay in place or migrate into the joint, making the joint unstable or seeming to lock up.
- Osteochondritis dissecans (OCD) is the most common cause of an intraarticular loose body in adolescents.
- System(s) affected: Musculoskeletal

EPIDEMIOLOGY

Incidence

- Unknown: Estimated 2–5/10,000 persons
- Predominant age: Young adults between 10 and 40 years of age
- Juvenile type (JOCD) in children and adolescents prior to physeal closure
- Predominant sex: Male > Female (5:3).

RISK FACTORS

- Trauma
- Seen in active children and adults
- Multisport athletics, especially gymnastics and overhead sports participation
- Abnormal mechanical axis of the leg can be a risk factor (1)[C].
  - Varus axis and medial condyle OCD
  - Valgus axis and lateral condyle OCD

Pediatric Considerations

Although still idiopathic, the mean age in JOCD is decreasing, and the prevalence in girls is increasing with changes in athletic participation by children (2)[C].

Genetics

No distinct genetic pattern known, but bilateral lesions have been noted in up to 30% of patients.

GENERAL PREVENTION

No clear way to avoid its development

PATHOPHYSIOLOGY

- Primary change happens in the bone.
- Necrosis occurs in a focal area.
- Overlying cartilage changes are secondary to the bony changes.
- Loss of subchondral bone support leads to degenerative cartilage changes: softening and fibromatous fissuring.
- Fragment may detach and become a loose body within the affected joint.
- Cartilage itself is without a vascular supply.
- Healing occurs by vascular supply to bone, which stimulates inflammation, repair, and remodeling.
- It is difficult to predict which lesions will go on to heal and remodel.

ETIOLOGY

- Controversial and unclear
- Theories include trauma or repetitive microtrauma, ischemia, familial predisposition, fragile blood supply of the physeal line, and endocrine imbalance.
- Most commonly affected joints are the knee, ankle, and elbow.
  - Knee: Overuse and with patellar dislocation and injury to the anterior cruciate ligament; bilateral involvement noted in up to 30% of patients
  - Elbow: Overuse injury in overhead throwers and in female gymnasts
  - Ankle: Frequently associated with history of previous ankle sprain
- Relationship between adult and juvenile forms of OCD remains unclear.

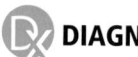 **DIAGNOSIS**

HISTORY

- Insidious or posttraumatic onset of pain, which improves with rest
- Pain usually defined as a deep and vague ache
- Pain may be associated with clicking, swelling, locking (usually with loose body), and stiffness.

PHYSICAL EXAM

- May be associated with secondary muscle atrophy, mild effusion, decreased range of motion (ROM), joint-line tenderness, or tenderness over the lesion
- The Wilson test may be positive (i.e., pain with knee extension and tibial internal rotation) in some patients with knee involvement.

DIAGNOSTIC TESTS & INTERPRETATION

Lab

Initial lab tests

No specific tests

Imaging

Initial approach

- The diagnosis usually is made by standard radiographs. Typical findings include small articular surface radiolucency or irregularity and bony fragmentation with partial or complete separation.
  - Knee: Anteroposterior (AP), lateral, sunrise, and tunnel views (most likely location for abnormality in the lateral portion of the medial condyle)
  - Elbow: Routine AP and lateral elbow series (common involvement of the humeral capitellum)
  - Ankle: AP, lateral, and mortise views (lesions most commonly involve the posteromedial or anterolateral talar dome)
- MRI can delineate the bony lesion, involvement of cartilage, and any fluid behind the fragment and helps to stage the lesion.
  - Stage I: Thickening of the articular cartilage and low signal change (stable)
  - Stage II: Articular cartilage breached, low signal rim behind fragment indicating fibrous attachment (stable)
  - Stage III: Articular cartilage breached, high signal changes behind fragment and underlying subchondral bone (unstable)
  - Stage IV: Loose body (unstable)
- CT scan provides architectural description of bone lesion, but there is less information than with MRI.
- Bone scan may be useful in evaluation of healing potential, but this is controversial.

DIFFERENTIAL DIAGNOSIS

- In the knee:
  - Meniscal tear
  - Patellofemoral pain syndrome
- Stress fracture
- Tendinopathy
- Avascular necrosis
- Acute fracture
- Neoplasm

TREATMENT

MEDICATION
Acetaminophen or nonsteroidal anti-inflammatory drugs (NSAIDs) for symptomatic pain relief

ADDITIONAL TREATMENT
General Measures
- Goals of treatment:
  – Maintain smooth, congruous joint surface.
  – Alleviate pain.
  – Prevent degenerative joint disease.
  – Promote revascularization of necrotic fragment and regeneration of affected cartilage.
- There are no randomized, controlled trials, but in JOCD, nonsurgical treatment initially is the standard of care.
- Treatment options include periods of immobilization, activity modification, and non–weight bearing. Type and duration of immobilization remain controversial.
- If non-weight-bearing immobilization is used, add intermittent maintenance of ROM.
- Follow closely for 12 weeks for healing.
- Casting is used for 6-week intervals, especially with JOCD, owing to issues of compliance.

Issues for Referral
- Adult patients in whom surgery may be considered as an early treatment option
- Unstable lesions on MRI including intraarticular loose body
- Failure of symptomatic treatment

SURGERY/OTHER PROCEDURES
- Surgical treatment is used when
  – Conservative measures have failed.
  – Physeal closure, which carries a worse prognosis for healing (adult form)
  – Unstable lesions on MRI including intraarticular loose body
  – Larger lesions (>1 cm)
- Arthroscopic surgery is the preferred method. In addition, arthroscopy is a valuable tool to evaluate the stability of the lesion and visualize the overlying cartilage.
- Surgical treatment includes fragment excision, microfracture technique (drilling) to increase blood supply, screw fixation of fragment, and/or allograft insertion and requires an orthopedic consultation (3)[B],(4)[C].

ONGOING CARE

FOLLOW-UP RECOMMENDATIONS
- Outpatient care usually
- Inpatient for surgery

Patient Monitoring
- Initially should be followed every 6 weeks with serial radiographs to check for healing and possible displacement
- Expect healing in 4–6 months.
- In JOCD, radiographs at 1 year may show no residual abnormality.

DIET
No specific recommendations

PATIENT EDUCATION
Critical importance of compliance with treatment plan

PROGNOSIS
- Factors associated with good prognosis:
  – Younger age
  – Open growth plate
  – Smaller lesions (<160 mm^2)
  – Stable lesions
  – Non-weight-bearing location of the lesion
- The absence of a sclerotic rim on the X-rays at the time diagnosis can be an indication for spontaneous recovery with conservative treatment for OCD of the knee (5)[C].
- An incongruous joint surface may lead to degenerative changes in the future.
- Clinical improvement may proceed radiologic healing.

COMPLICATIONS
- Failure to revascularize and heal
- Displacement of fragment becoming loose body within a joint

REFERENCES

1. Jacobi M, Wahl P, Bouaicha S, et al. Association Between Mechanical Axis of the Leg and Osteochondritis Dissecans of the Knee: Radiographic Study on 103 Knees. *The American journal of sports medicine*. 2010;
2. Kocher MS, Tucker R, Ganley TJ, et al. Management of osteochondritis dissecans of the knee: current concepts review. *Am J Sports Med*. 2006;34:1181–91.
3. Vasiliadis HS, Danielson B, Ljungberg M, et al. Autologous chondrocyte implantation in cartilage lesions of the knee: long-term evaluation with magnetic resonance imaging and delayed gadolinium-enhanced magnetic resonance imaging technique. *Am J Sports Med*. 2010;38:943–9.
4. Bruce EJ, Hamby T, Jones DG, et al. Sports-related osteochondral injuries: clinical presentation, diagnosis, and treatment. *Prim Care*. 2005;32:253–76.
5. Ramirez A, Abril JC, Chaparro M, et al. Juvenile osteochondritis dissecans of the knee: perifocal sclerotic rim as a prognostic factor of healing. *J Pediatr Orthop*. 2010;30:180–5.

ADDITIONAL READING

- Cahill BR, Ahten SM, et al. The three critical components in the conservative treatment of juvenile osteochondritis dissecans (JOCD). Physician, parent, and child. *Clin Sports Med*. 2001;20:287–98, vi.
- Crawford DC, Safran MR, et al. Osteochondritis dissecans of the knee. *J Am Acad Orthop Surg*. 2006;14:90–100.
- Wall EJ, Vourazeris J, Myer GD, et al. The healing potential of stable juvenile osteochondritis dissecans knee lesions. *J Bone Joint Surg Am*. 2008;90:2655–64.

CODES

ICD9
732.7 Osteochondritis dissecans

CLINICAL PEARLS
- Frequent follow-up every 6 weeks
- Compliance with immobilization and possibility of further trauma should be emphasized, especially with younger athletes.
- Many lesions heal without surgical intervention *with compliance*.

OSTEOMALACIA & RICKETS

Lauren Ferrara, MD
Elizabeth Ann Nelson, MD

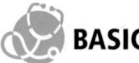 **BASICS**

DESCRIPTION
- A metabolic bone disorder due to decreased bone mineralization (calcification) and increased organic bone matrix that results in decreased bone density
- System(s) affected: Musculoskeletal
- Referred to as renal osteodystrophy when secondary to renal disease

EPIDEMIOLOGY
- Children: Median age of presentation: 15 months (1)
- Adults: Elderly

Incidence
- In the US, almost exclusively in breast-fed infants without vitamin D supplementation or sun exposure (2)
- Estimated annual incidence of vitamin D–deficiency rickets in Canada: 2.9 cases per 100,000 children (1)

Prevalence
68 per 100,000 children-years in adolescents in Saudi Arabia (1)

RISK FACTORS
- Children:
  - Nutritional rickets
    - Breast feeding as a sole source of nutrition without vitamin D supplementation
    - Dark skin
    - Limited sunlight exposure
    - Vegetarian diet without vitamin supplementation
    - Malabsorption syndromes
  - Prematurity
  - Maternal vitamin D deficiency
- Adults:
  - Poor diet
  - Poverty
  - Food faddism
  - Anorexia nervosa
  - Renal failure
  - Gastrectomy

Genetics
Rare causes of rickets in children include:
- Vitamin D–dependent rickets: An autosomal recessive disorder caused by deficiency of renal 25-hydroxyvitamin D3 1-alpha-hydroxylase or altered calcitriol receptors
- Vitamin D–resistant rickets: An X-linked dominant or autosomal disorder caused by decreased proximal renal tubular reabsorption of phosphorus

GENERAL PREVENTION
- Adequate vitamin D intake: Encourage foods such as fatty fish, cod liver oil, egg yolks, and fortified foods:
  - Adults: Vitamin D, 200–400 units per day
- American Academy of Pediatrics recommends a minimum vitamin D intake of 400 units per day starting within the first few days of life (1):
  - Infants who consume >1 liter per day of vitamin D–fortified formula or whole milk will receive the recommended vitamin D intake
  - Supplementation is recommended for breast-fed infants and children consuming <1 liter per day of vitamin D–fortified formula or milk.

- Sunlight exposure: 10–15 minutes on face, hands, and arms 2–3 days per week
- Adequate calcium intake: Encourage high-calcium foods.

PATHOPHYSIOLOGY
- Children: Defective mineralization of cartilage in the epiphyseal growth plates:
  - Failure of growing bone to mineralize due to inadequate substrate (low calcium or phosphate) or interference with mineralization (such as vitamin D deficiency or toxic exposure)
  - Lack of calcified osteoid and accumulation of unossified cartilage
- Adults: Disorder of mineralization of newly formed bone matrix

ETIOLOGY
- Vitamin D deficiency causing secondary hyperparathyroidism, causing hypophosphatemia is #1 cause in adults.
- Vitamin D metabolism abnormalities, including hepatic or renal disease
- Resistance to vitamin D
- Inadequate dietary calcium
- Impaired intestinal absorption of calcium or phosphorus due to celiac disease, cystic fibrosis, or postgastrectomy
- Inadequate dietary phosphorus
- Impaired renal phosphate absorption associated with proximal or distal renal tubular defects
- Causes that inhibit mineralization of the growth plate and osteoid:
  - Alkaline phosphatase deficiency
  - Aluminum toxicity
  - Fluoride toxicity
  - Primary hyperparathyroidism
- Drugs which may affect absorption or metabolism of calcium, phosphorus, or vitamin D:
  - Antacids
  - Antiepileptic drugs
  - Corticosteroids
  - Loop diuretics
- Drugs that inhibit mineralization: Bisphosphonates
- Oncogenic osteomalacia

COMMONLY ASSOCIATED CONDITIONS
- Children with vitamin D–deficiency rickets:
  - Secondary hyperparathyroidism
  - Dilated cardiomyopathy
  - Marrow fibrosis with pancytopenia or microcytic hypochromic anemia
  - Dysregulation of immune function and cellular differentiation and proliferation
- Adults with osteomalacia:
  - Chronic renal disease
  - Gastrectomy
  - Epilepsy
  - Malnutrition

 DIAGNOSIS

HISTORY
- Common presentations in children:
  - Muscle weakness: May not be able to stand until age 3
  - Bowed legs
  - Diffuse limb pain
  - Hypocalcemic seizures
  - Carpopedal spasms
  - Signs and symptoms of hypocalcemia:
    - Muscle cramps
    - Numbness
    - Paresthesias
    - Tetany
    - Seizures
    - Diarrhea
- Common presentations in adults:
  - Dull, bony pain and tenderness typically in lower spine and pelvis and aggravated by activity and weight bearing
  - Muscle weakness, especially proximal lower extremity
  - Fractures may occur with little or no trauma.

PHYSICAL EXAM
Perform a complete physical and dental examination in children:
- General:
  - Palpate entire skeletal system to search for tenderness and bony abnormalities.
  - Evaluate for growth abnormalities such as decreased height and spinal deformity.
- HEENT:
  - Craniotabes (thinning and softening of occipital and parietal bones)
  - Late closing of fontanelles
  - Fontal bossing of skull
  - Tooth abnormalities
- Chest:
  - Rachitic rosary (enlarged costochondral joints felt lateral to nipple line)
  - Harrison's groove (flaring of ribs at diaphragm level)
  - Pigeon breast (protrusion of the sternum)
- Back:
  - Lordosis/kyphosis
  - Scoliosis
- Extremities:
  - Bowing or widening of the physis
  - Genu valgum (leg bowing)
  - Flaring of the wrists
  - Fraying and cupping of metaphysis
  - Genu varum (knock knees)
- Neurologic:
  - Gait disturbances in an ambulatory child
  - Signs of hypocalcemia
    - Hyperreflexia
    - Neuromuscular instability: Chvostek's sign (tap cranial nerve VII), Trousseau sign (carpopedal spasm 2–3 minutes after blood pressure cuff inflated proximally)
    - Tetany, myopathy, seizures, spasm, muscle weakness

- In adults:
  - Proximal muscle weakness, possible muscle wasting, hypotonia, and discomfort with movement
  - Waddling gait
  - Bone pain and tenderness to palpation: Most pronounced in the lower spine, pelvis, and lower extremities

DIAGNOSTIC TESTS & INTERPRETATION
Lab
- In children with vitamin D–deficiency rickets (1):
  - Serum phosphorus: Decreased
  - Serum calcidiol (25-hydroxy vitamin D3): Decreased
    - Indicative of overall vitamin D status
  - Urinary calcium: Decreased
- In adults with vitamin D–deficiency osteomalacia (3):
  - Serum phosphorus: Decreased
  - Plasma calcium: Decreased/normal
  - Serum calcidiol: Decreased
  - Alkaline phosphatase: Increased
- In adults with phosphate wasting osteomalacia (3):
  - Serum phosphorous: Decreased
  - Phosphate clearance: Increased
  - Serum calcium: Normal
  - Alkaline phosphatase: n=Normal

Initial lab tests
- Blood tests:
  - Serum calcium (total and ionized), phosphate, BUN, creatinine, electrolytes
  - Serum calcidiol
  - Alkaline phosphatase
  - Parathyroid hormone
- Urinalysis:
  - Calcium, phosphate, creatinine in spot urine sample
  - pH, protein, and glucose

Imaging
Initial approach
- Anteroposterior radiograph of rapidly growing skeletal areas including knees, wrists. and anterior rib ends (1)
- Children: Radiographic changes in rapidly growing skeletal areas (knee, wrist) including widening of the distal epiphysis, fraying and widening of the metaphysis, and angular deformities of the arm and leg bones

Diagnostic Procedures/Surgery
The most accurate diagnosis is made by bone biopsy using double tetracycline labeling. Tetracyclines are deposited as a band at the mineralization front and, since they are fluorescent, are easily visualized under a fluorescence microscope. After two courses of the antibiotic, separated by a period of days, the growth rate of the skeleton can be estimated in iliac crest biopsies by measurement of the distance between the bands of deposited tetracycline. In normal adults, this distance is approximately1 micron per day (4).

- Two changes occur in osteomalacia:
  - Distance between tetracycline bands is reduced
  - Unmineralized matrix appears as a widened osteoid seam (>15 microns), and the osteoid volume is >10%.
- Both features are necessary for the diagnosis because other disorders may show one of these findings (3).
- Bone biopsy is not usually done in adults, since the diagnosis can be made from the history, physical examination, and a combination of laboratory and radiologic studies .

Pathological Findings
- Children (1):
  - Widening of distal physis
  - Fraying and widening of the metaphysis
  - Angular deformities of arm and leg bones
- Adults (5):
  - Most common: Reduced bone density with thinning of the cortex
  - Changes in vertebral bodies: Loss of radiological distinctness and concavity of the vertebral body
  - Characteristic finding: Looser zones:
    - Pseudofractures, fissures, or narrow radiolucent lines, 2–5 mm in width with sclerotic borders
    - Usually located at the femoral neck, on the medial part of the femoral shaft, immediately under the lesser trochanter, or a few centimeters beneath the pubic and ischial rami

DIFFERENTIAL DIAGNOSIS
- Children:
  - Liver disease
  - Anticonvulsant drugs
  - Failure to thrive
  - Developmental delay
  - Orthopedic abnormalities
  - Congenital syphilis
  - Osteogenesis imperfecta
  - Child abuse
  - Alkaline phosphatase deficiency
  - Aluminum toxicity
  - Fluoride toxicity
  - Primary hyperparathyroidism (rare in children)
- Adults:
  - Osteoporosis
  - Hyperparathyroidism
  - Metastatic bone disease
  - Lymphoma or myeloma
  - Fibromyalgia

 TREATMENT

Combination of calcium and vitamin D is recommended.
- A study in Nigerian children with nutritional rickets showed that treatment with calcium and vitamin D combined compared to treatment with vitamin D alone is more likely to produce radiographic evidence of nearly complete healing of rickets (58% versus 19%) (6).

MEDICATION
First Line
- Children with vitamin D–deficiency rickets:
  - Ergocalciferol (calciferol) 150,000 or 300,000 units single dose
    - Can be administered intramuscularly or orally in liquid or capsule form
    - Capsules can be softened in water and mixed with food
  - Calcium 1000 mg orally per day
- Adults with vitamin D–deficiency osteomalacia:
  - Ergocalciferol (Calciferol) 50,000 units once or twice per week for 6 to 12 months
  - Followed by ergocalciferol 400 units per day
  - If the deficiency is due to malabsorption:
    - Ergocalciferol 10,000–50,000 units per day
    - Calcidiol 0.05–0.125 mg per day
  - Calcium 1000 mg orally per day
    - If the patient has malabsorption, 4 g of calcium per day

ADDITIONAL TREATMENT
Calcium and phosphorus supplementation if indicated.

SURGERY/OTHER PROCEDURES
Surgery may be necessary to repair severe bone abnormalities

 ONGOING CARE

FOLLOW-UP RECOMMENDATIONS
- For children, monitor:
  - Serum calcium, phosphorus, alkaline phosphatase, calcidiol
    - Serum phosphorus should increase during the first week of treatment, followed by an increase in serum calcium.
  - Urinary calcium and phosphorus levels, spot urine calcium
- For adults on calcium supplements, monitor:
  - The plasma concentration and urinary levels of calcium

PROGNOSIS
- Varies depending on the etiology
- Vitamin D deficiency causes of rickets:
  - Radiographic findings will normalize within 1 week of treatment.
  - Reversible physical findings will normalize within 6 months of treatment.

COMPLICATIONS
- Fractures: Typically involving the ribs, vertebrae, and long bones
- Osteomyelitis
- Renal failure
- Renal tubular acidosis
- Hypocalcemic seizures or muscle spasms
- Growth deformity and bowing of the long bones in children

REFERENCES

1. Dynam Ed, Editorial Team. *Rickets*. Last updated 2010 Jul 5. Available from DynaMed. Accessed July 26, 2010.
2. emedicine.medscape.com/article/985510-overview. Rickets. Accessed Sept 1, 2010.
3. Bingham CT, Fitzpatrick LA. Noninvasive testing in the diagnosis of osteomalacia. *Am J Med*. 1993;95:519.
4. Bone biopsy and histomorphometry in clinical practice. In: *Primer on Metabolic Bone Diseases and Disorders of Mineral Metabolism*, Lippincott-Raven, Philadelphia 1993.
5. Frame B, Parfitt AM. Osteomalacia: Current concepts. *Ann Intern Med*. 1978;89:966.
6. Thacher TD, Fischer PR, Pettifor JM, et al. A Comparison of calcium, vitamin D or both for nutritional rickets in Nigerian children. *N Engl J Med*. 1999;341(8):563.

 CODES

ICD9
- 268.0 Rickets, active
- 268.2 Osteomalacia, unspecified

O

OSTEOMYELITIS

Adeliza S. Jimenez, MD

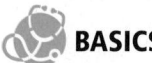 **BASICS**

DESCRIPTION

- An acute or chronic inflammation of the bone. This may be limited to a single portion of the bone or may involve several regions. Osteomyelitis can occur as a result of hematogenous seeding, contiguous spread of infection, or direct inoculation into intact bone such as from trauma or surgery.
- Two major classification systems for osteomyelitis (1)
  - Waldvogel classification:
    - Classified according to the duration of the disease (acute or chronic), the mechanism of infection (hematogenous or contiguous), and the presence of vascular insufficiency
  - Cierny-Mader classification:
    - Based on the portion of bone affected, the physiologic status of the host, and other risk factors
- System(s) affected: Musculoskeletal
- Special situations:
  - Vertebral Osteomyelitis (2)
    - Acute, subacute, or chronic
    - May result from hematogenous seeding, direct inoculation, or contiguous spread
    - Back pain (most common initial symptom)
    - Lumbar spine (most commonly involved) followed by thoracic
    - Bone biopsy (open technique) has 93% pathogen recovery.
  - Infections of prosthetic joints (3)
    - Obtaining specific diagnosis and targeted therapy quicker (easy access)
    - X-ray of joint initially done then 3-phase bone scan
    - Treat with combination of antibiotics including Rifampicin.
  - Post-traumatic infections
    - Depends on type of fracture, level of contamination, and severity of tissue injury
    - Tibia most commonly involved

EPIDEMIOLOGY

- Predominant age: Commonly seen in older adults
- Predominant sex: Male > Female
- Hematogenous osteomyelitis (4):
  - Adults (most patients >50 years old): vertebral
  - Children: long bones
- Contiguous osteomyelitis (1):
  - Predominantly found in patients with diabetes mellitus or vascular insufficiency

Incidence

- Incidence is low due to high resistance of normal bone to infection and occur in patients with risk factor (3).
- 25% lifetime risk of diabetics of developing foot complication (5)

Prevalence

Up to 66% of diabetics with foot ulcers (1)

RISK FACTORS

- Diabetes mellitus
- Recent trauma/surgery
- Foreign body (e.g., prosthetic implant)
- Neuropathy and vascular insufficiency
- Immunosuppression

- Sickle-cell disease
- Injection drug use
- Previous osteomyelitis

GENERAL PREVENTION

- Antibiotic prophylaxis:
  - Clean bone surgery:
    - Antibiotics should be administered IV from 30 minutes before skin incision to no longer than 24 hours after the operation.
  - Closed fractures:
    - Antistaphylococcal penicillins or 1st- or 2nd-generation cephalosporins
  - Open fractures:
    - In patients who can receive antibiotics within 6 hours of injury and who receive prompt operative treatment, administration of antistaphylococcal penicillins or 1st- or 2nd-generation cephalosporins for 24 hours is appropriate.
- All patients with diabetes mellitus should have a complete foot examination by a health care professional yearly (1).

PATHOPHYSIOLOGY

- Infection is caused by biofilm bacteria, a community of bacteria surrounded by a matrix of polymers, which protects bacteria from antimicrobial agents and host immune responses (2).
- Acute: Suppurative infection of bone with edema and vascular compromise leading to sequestra
- Chronic: Presence of necrotic bone or sequestra or recurrence of previous infection

ETIOLOGY

- Hematogenous osteomyelitis (commonly a monomicrobial infection) (1):
  - *S. aureus* (most common) with high percentage of MRSA (50%) (2)
  - Coagulase-negative staphylococci and aerobic gram-negative bacteria
  - *Salmonella* sp. (sickle-cell patients)
  - *M. tuberculosis* and fungi (rare) in endemic areas or in immunocompromised hosts
- Contiguous focus osteomyelitis (commonly a polymicrobial infection) ():
  - Diabetes or vascular insufficiency:
    - Coagulase-positive and -negative staphylococci
    - Streptococci, gram-negative bacilli, anaerobes (*Peptostreptococcus* sp.)
  - Prosthetic device:
    - Coagulase-negative staphylococci and *S. aureus*

COMMONLY ASSOCIATED CONDITIONS

See Risk factors

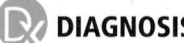 **DIAGNOSIS**

HISTORY

- Hematogenous osteomyelitis:
  - Conditions predisposing to bacteremia (Diabetes and renal insufficiency) (2)
  - Other sites of infection
- Contiguous osteomyelitis and vascular insufficiency–associated infection:
  - Recent trauma/surgery within 1–2 months
  - Presence of prosthetic device
  - History of diabetes
- Chronic osteomyelitis:
  - History of acute osteomyelitis

PHYSICAL EXAM

- Restriction of movement of the involved extremity or refusal to bear weight
- Pain or tenderness in the infected area
- Signs of localized inflammation
- Fever and/or chills
- Motor and sensory deficits (vertebral infection)
- Visible or palpable bone with a metal probe ("positive probe-to-bone test") (5)[A]
- Ulcer >2 cm wide and >3 mm deep increases likelihood in diabetic foot ulcers (1)[B].
- In patients with diabetes, classic signs and symptoms of infection may be masked due to vascular disease and neuropathy.

DIAGNOSTIC TESTS & INTERPRETATION

Lab

Initial lab tests

Labs (1)[C]:

- WBC is not a reliable indicator and can be normal even when infection is present (2).
- CRP is usually elevated but nonspecific.
- ESR is high in most cases.
  - ESR >70 mm/hour increases likelihood in diabetic lower extremity ulcer (6)[B].
- Drugs that may alter lab results: Antimicrobial agents given prior to culture
- Disorders that may alter lab results: Immunosuppression, chronic inflammatory disease, other/adjacent sites of infection

Follow-Up & Special Considerations

- A persistently elevated CRP but not ESR at 4–6 weeks can be associated with persistent osteomyelitis (1)[C].
- Patients receiving prolonged antimicrobial therapy should have the following tests to monitor for adverse reactions (1)[C]:
  - Weekly CBC
  - Liver and kidney function tests

Imaging

Initial approach

- Routine radiography standard 1st-line imaging (7)[C]: Classic triad for osteomyelitis is demineralization, periosteal reaction, and bone destruction (5).
  - Bone destruction is not apparent on plain films until after 10–21 days of infection.
  - Bone must undergo 30–50% destruction before it is evident on films.
- MRI
  - For visualization of septic arthritis, spinal infection, and diabetic foot infections (7)[C]
  - T1-weighted image: Low signal intensity
  - T2-weighted image: High signal intensity
  - MI with gadolinium sensitivity and specificity range from 60–100% and 50–90% respectively (2)[C]
- CT
  - Better than standard radiography in fragments and sequestration but inferior to MRI in soft tissue and bone marrow assessment
  - Useful to define surrounding soft tissues and identification of sequestra

Follow-Up & Special Considerations
- Radionuclide scanning (e.g., technetium, indium, or gallium) is useful when diagnosis is ambiguous or extent of disease in question but is limited by reports of low sensitivity and specificity.
- MRI is not helpful in assessing the response to therapy owing to persistence of bony edema (1)[C].

Diagnostic Procedures/Surgery
- Cultures (4)[C]:
  - Definitive diagnosis is made by blood culture (hematogenous) and by needle aspiration/bone biopsy with subsequent demonstration of the microorganism by culture and sensitivity or histology.
  - Appropriate pathogen isolated in blood culture combined with radiographic evidence may obviate need for bone culture.
  - Wound swabs and sinus tract cultures have utility for infection control and correlate well with the presence of *S. aureus* in deep cultures.
- Image-guided bone biopsy for vertebral osteomyelitis unless (+) blood culture and (+) radiographic evidence

Pathological Findings
Inflammatory process of bone with pyogenic bacteria, necrosis

DIFFERENTIAL DIAGNOSIS
- Systemic infection from other source
- Aseptic bone infarction
- Localized inflammation or infection of overlying skin and soft tissues (e.g., gout)
- Brodie abscess
- Neuropathic joint disease (Charcot foot)
- Fractures/trauma
- Tumor

TREATMENT

MEDICATION
- Duration of therapy 4–6 weeks for acute osteomyelitis and generally >8 weeks for chronic osteomyelitis.
- Determine therapy based on culture results.
- Fluoroquinolones may be used as an alternative to β-lactam antibiotics (use with caution to limit antibiotic resistance) (8)[A].

First Line
- *S. aureus* (1)[C]:
  - Methicillin-sensitive: Nafcillin or oxacillin 1.5–2 g IV q4–6h or cefazolin 1–2 g IV q8h
  - Methicillin-resistant: Vancomycin 15 mg/kg or 1 g IV q12h
- Penicillin-sensitive *Streptococcus* sp.:
  - Penicillin G 20 million U/d IV divided q4–6h or ceftriaxone 1–2 g IV/IM q24h or cefazolin 1–2 g IV q8h
- Enterococci or streptococci with MIC ≥0.5 μg/mL:
  - Penicillin G 20 million U/24 h IV divided q4–6h or ampicillin 2 g IV q4h ± gentamicin 1 mg/kg IV q8h
- Gram-negative bacilli:
  - Quinolone 400–750 mg IV/PO q12h
- Anaerobes:
  - Clindamycin 600 mg IV q6h or metronidazole 500 mg PO q6–8h

Second Line
- *S. aureus* (1)[C]:
  - Methicillin-sensitive: Vancomycin 15 mg/kg or 1 g IV q12h ± rifampin 600 mg q24h or daptomycin 6 mg/kg IV q24h
  - Methicillin-resistant: Linezolid 600 mg PO/IV q12h or daptomycin 6 mg/kg IV q24h
- Penicillin-sensitive *Streptococcus* sp.:
  - Vancomycin 15 mg/kg or 1 g IV q12h
- Enterococci or streptococci with MIC ≥0.5 μg/mL:
  - Vancomycin 15 mg/kg or 1 g IV q12h ± gentamicin 1 mg/kg IV q8h
- Gram-negative bacilli:
  - Ciprofloxacin 400 mg IV q12h or 750 mg PO q12h or levofloxacin 500–750 mg IV/PO q24h; ceftriaxone 2 g IV q24h or cefotaxime 2 g IV q6–8h or ceftazidime 2 g IV q8h

ADDITIONAL TREATMENT
General Measures
- Adequate nutrition
- Smoking-cessation counseling
- Control of diabetes

Additional Therapies
Hyperbaric oxygen therapy may be useful as an adjunctive treatment, but data are limited.

SURGERY/OTHER PROCEDURES
Surgical drainage, dead-space management, adequate soft-tissue coverage, restoration of blood supply, and removal of necrotic tissues are of utmost importance to effect cure.

Pediatric Considerations
Medullary osteomyelitis (stage 1) in children may be treated without surgical intervention.

IN-PATIENT CONSIDERATIONS
Initial Stabilization
- Correct electrolyte imbalances, hyperglycemia, azotemia, and acidosis.
- Control pain.

Admission Criteria
Hospitalize the patient with suspected acute osteomyelitis for diagnostic workup and initial treatment.

Nursing
Bed rest and immobilization of the involved bone and/or joint

Discharge Criteria
Clinical and laboratory evidence of resolving infection and appropriate outpatient therapy

ONGOING CARE

FOLLOW-UP RECOMMENDATIONS
Patient Monitoring
Blood levels of antimicrobial agents, ESR, CRP, and repeat plain radiography

PATIENT EDUCATION
Diabetic glycemic control and foot care

PROGNOSIS
- Superficial and medullary osteomyelitis treated with antimicrobial and surgical therapy has a response rate of 90–100%.
- Morbidity and mortality are contingent on the underlying health of the host.
- Up to 36% recurrence in diabetics
- Increased mortality after amputation

COMPLICATIONS
- Abscess formation
- Bacteremia
- Fracture/nonunion
- Loosening of prosthetic implant
- Postoperative infection

REFERENCES

1. Sia IG, Berbari EF. Osteomyelitis. *Best Prac and Res Clin Rheum*. 2006;20(6):1065–81.
2. Bhavan KP, Marschall J, Olsen MA, Fraser VJ, Wright NM, Warren DK et al. The Epidemiology of hematogenous vertebral osteomyelitis: a cohort study in a tertiary care hospital. *BMC infectious diseases*. 2010;10:158.
3. Concia E, Prandini N, Massari L, Ghisellini F, Consoli V, Menichetti F, Lazzeri E et al. Osteomyelitis: clinical update for practical guidelines. *Nucl Med Commun*. 2006;27:645–60.
4. Calhoun JH, Manring MM. Adult Osteomyelitis. *Infect Dis Clin N Am*. 2005;19:765–86.
5. Hartemann-Heurtier A, Senneville E et al. Diabetic foot osteomyelitis. *Diabetes Metab*. 2008;34:87–95.
6. Dinh MT, et al. Diagnostic Accuracy of the Physical Examination and Imaging Tests for Osteomyelitis Underlying Diabetic Foot Ulcers: Meta Analysis. *Clin Inf Dis*. 2008;47:519–27.
7. Stumpe KD, Strobel K et al. Osteomyelitis and arthritis. *Semin Nucl Med*. 2009;39:27–35.
8. Karamanis EM, Matthaiou DK, Moraitis LI, et al. Fluoroquinolones versus beta-lactam based regimens for the treatment of osteomyelitis: a meta-analysis of randomized controlled trials. *Spine*. 2008;33:E297–304.

CODES

ICD9
- 730.00 Acute osteomyelitis, site unspecified
- 730.10 Chronic osteomyelitis, site unspecified
- 730.20 Unspecified osteomyelitis, site unspecified

CLINICAL PEARLS
- Osteomyelitis can occur as a result of hematogenous seeding, contiguous spread, or direct inoculation into the bone.
- Hematogenous osteomyelitis is usually monomicrobial, whereas osteomyelitis owing to contiguous spread or direct inoculation is usually polymicrobial.
- *S. aureus*, coagulase-negative staphylococci, and aerobic gram-negative bacilli are the most common organisms.
- Acute osteomyelitis typically presents with gradual onset of pain. Local findings (e.g., tenderness, warmth, erythema, and swelling) and systemic symptoms (e.g., fever and chills) also may be present.
- Treatment of osteomyelitis often requires both surgical débridement and antimicrobial therapy. At least 6 weeks of antimicrobial therapy is recommended.

O

OSTEONECROSIS

Joselyn Jedick, DO
Kam Hunter, MD

BASICS

Definition: Cellular death ("necrosis") of the elements of bone ("osteo") due to interruption of the blood supply to that bone. Classified as traumatic (most common) vs nontraumatic.

DESCRIPTION
- Primarily involves the epiphysis of long bones (most commonly femoral head, humeral head, and the femoral condyles) but small bones also affected in the hand, foot, ankle and face
- System(s) affected: Musculoskeletal
- Synonym(s): Idiopathic osteonecrosis; avascular necrosis (AVN); lunatomalacia/Kienböck disease (involving lunate); subchondral fracture; aseptic necrosis; Legg-Calve-Perthes syndrome (children with idiopathic necrosis of the femoral head)

EPIDEMIOLOGY
- Predominant age: 3rd–5th decade
- Predominant sex: Male > Female ratio 4–8:1

Incidence
- 10,000–20,000 new cases reported in the US per year
- Disease is bilateral in at least 50% of all nontraumatic cases and in 75–95% of cases associated with steroid use (1).

Prevalence
- Hip: Occurs in approximately 10% of undisplaced femoral neck fractures, 15–30% of displaced femoral neck fractures, and 10% of hip dislocations
- Jaw: Occurs in 3–12% of oncology patients taking high-dose IV bisphosphonates at 36 months of exposure and in <1% of nononcology patients with osteoporosis (2)
- Special population: Occurs in 21–25% of patients during early postoperative period following renal transplant (3)

RISK FACTORS
- Top 3: Trauma, prolonged corticosteroid use, alcoholism
- Others: Bisphosphonate use, sickle cell disease, diabetes mellitus, type II or IV hyperlipemia, oral contraceptives, pregnancy, decompression sickness (aka "bends," "caisson disease," "divers disease"), chronic pancreatitis, Crohn disease, myeloproliferative disorders, radiation treatment, rheumatoid arthritis (RA), systemic lupus erythematosus (SLE), chronic renal failure and hemodialysis, Gaucher disease, organ transplant, trauma, tobacco use, HIV, hypercoagulable state, developmental hip dysplasia, idiopathic

GENERAL PREVENTION
- Limiting alcohol use: Dose-dependent relationship with RR of 3.3 for <400 mg/week consumed compared to RR of 17.9 for >1,000 mL/week consumed (4)
- Smoking cessation: Smokers with RR of 3.9 vs nonsmokers with no significance found to cumulative effect (4)
- Limiting corticosteroid use: Use the minimum effective dose of systemic corticosteroids as highest daily dose and cumulative dose is directly correlated to increased risk of osteonecrosis (5)[B].

- Screening: No definitive evidence but screening of asymptomatic patients at high risk for osteonecrosis may be of value if prophylactic treatment of asymptomatic osteonecrosis is proven useful (6).

PATHOPHYSIOLOGY
- Pathophysiology is multifactorial and not fully understood, but the final common pathway is interruption of blood flow to the bone.
- Lack of blood supply leads to hyperemia, demineralization, trabecular thinning and subchondral plate fracture, which eventually leads to collapse of the necrotic segment (1)
- Collapse of bone is irreversible, painful, often requires surgery for symptom relief, and is a risk factor for developing osteoarthritis.

ETIOLOGY
- Traumatic: Disruption of blood supply due to physical disruption of a vessel due to fracture or dislocation
- Nontraumatic: Possible mechanisms include:
  - Impedance of blood flow due to vascular compression/vasospasm
  - Extraluminal obliteration from marrow edema
  - Intraluminal obstruction from thromboembolism, nitrogen bubbles, fat emboli, intravascular coagulation, or vascular stasis (1)

DIAGNOSIS

- Consider AVN in any individual with bone pain and history of trauma or other risk factors.
- Pain in the affected joint is typically the presenting symptom.

HISTORY
- Hip/femoral head: Dull aching groin/hip pain that is progressive and worsened with weight bearing
- Knee: Dull aching knee pain that is worsened with weight bearing, stair climbing, and at night
- Humeral head: Shoulder pain that is severe and poorly localized, worsened at night and with activity
- Lunate (Kienböck disease): Pain and stiffness to dorsal wrist of dominant hand

PHYSICAL EXAM
- Hip/femoral head:
  - Decreased hip range of motion especially in rotation and abduction
  - Antalgic or Trendelenburg gait
  - Synovitis = pain throughout range of motion
- Knee:
  - Pseudolocking secondary to pain, effusion, or muscle contracture
- Humeral head:
  - Active motion inhibited by pain
  - Passive motion and strength preserved
- Lunate (Kienböck disease):
  - Dorsal swelling with tenderness over radiocarpal joint
  - Restricted and painful dorsiflexion of wrist
  - Weakness of grip

DIAGNOSTIC TESTS & INTERPRETATION
- No specific physical findings or laboratory tests can reliably establish the diagnosis.
- Clinically suspected osteonecrosis can be confirmed only by diagnostic imaging or biopsy.

- Screening of a patient who is at high risk for osteonecrosis may be of value if prophylactic treatment of asymptomatic osteonecrosis is proven useful (6)[B].
- Imaging options:
  - Plain films: 1st line
    ◦ Early stages: Unremarkable
    ◦ Mild-to-moderate AVN: Sclerosis and changes in bone density
    ◦ Advanced disease: Bony deformities such as flattening, subchondral radiolucent lines (crescent sign), and osseus collapse
    ◦ Views to order based on location: Hip/femoral head: Order anteroposterior (AP) and frog lateral views of both hips; knee: Order AP, lateral, and tunnel view of knee; humeral head: Order AP, true AP, and axillary views of shoulder; lunate: Order wrist films
  - MRI: Gold standard for diagnosis with sensitivity and specificity >98% (7)[B]; obtain if x-ray findings are normal and clinical suspicion is high
    ◦ Early stages: Decreased signal intensity of the subchondral region on both T1- and T2-weighted images (water signal)
    ◦ Mild-to-moderate AVN: High signal intensity line within 2 parallel rims of decreased signal intensity on T2-weighted scans (double line sign)
    ◦ Advanced disease: Deformity and calcification of the articular surface
  - Bone scan: Alternative to MRI, when used with SPECT imaging is 85% sensitive and 100% specific (8)
    ◦ Central area of decreased uptake surrounded by an area of increased uptake (doughnut sign)

Lab
Consider testing for sickle cell disease (Hb electrophoresis), hyperlipidemia (fasting lipid profile), and coagulopathies (protein C, protein S, factor V Leiden) with atraumatic etiology

Imaging
- Bone marrow edema on MRI should be considered a marker for potential progression to advanced osteonecrosis and collapse of the femoral head (9)[B].
- Several different staging systems available for classifying osteonecrosis of femoral head (10)
  - FICAT: Stages 0–4 based on symptoms, x-ray, and MRI findings
  - Steinberg: Stages 0–6 based on imaging and subdivided into categories based on percentage of femoral head affected
  - ARCO (international classification of osteonecrosis of the femoral head): Stages 0–6 based on clinical symptoms and imaging findings with focus on status of the femoral head

DIFFERENTIAL DIAGNOSIS
- Hip/femoral head:
  - Osteoarthritis, femoral neck fracture, labral tear, osteomyelitis, muscle strain, groin injury, transient synovitis, bone marrow edema syndrome
- Knee:
  - Osteoarthritis, septic arthritis, meniscal tear, bone bruise, transient osteopenia of the knee, pes anserine bursitis, osteochondritis desiccans
- Humeral head:

– Adhesive capsulitis, rotator cuff tear/tendonitis, osteomyelitis
• Lunate (Kienböck disease):
   – TFCC injury, tenosynovitis of extensor compartments, rheumatoid arthritis, degenerative joint disease, occult ganglion, other carpal bone injury

 ## TREATMENT

• Treatment depends on age, location, stage of the disease and overall health of the patient.
• Goal of therapy is to preserve the native joint for as long as possible.
• Early diagnosis is important to maximize treatment options.

MEDICATION
• No medical treatment has been proven effective for arresting the disease process.
• NSAIDs and other analgesics as needed for pain relief
• Prophylactic alendronate at 70 mg/week orally for 25 weeks found to prevent collapse of femoral head (NNT = 2) and need for total hip arthroplasty (NNT = 2) at 2 years in patients with Steinberg stage 2 or 3 nontraumatic AVN of femoral head with necrotic area >30% (11)[B]

ADDITIONAL TREATMENT
General Measures
• Usually managed as an outpatient but may be inpatient if surgery indicated
• Crutches or other assistive devices to avoid weight bearing in early disease if weight bearing joint is affected

Issues for Referral
Evaluation by orthopedic surgeon once diagnosis is made to determine if surgery is appropriate

COMPLEMENTARY AND ALTERNATIVE MEDICINE
Noninvasive modalities of electrical stimulation, shock wave therapy, and electromagnetic field therapy undergoing trials but currently no evidence to support (12)[C]

SURGERY/OTHER PROCEDURES
• Surgical options depend on severity and site of disease.
• Hip/femoral head:
   – Early stages (precollapse) treated surgically with bone decompression and possible bone graft
   – Later stages (postcollapse) treated with total hip arthroplasty
• Knee: Arthroscopy, osteochondral grafts, high tibial osteotomy, core decompression, unicompartmental knee arthroplasty, total knee arthroplasty
• Humeral head: Arthroscopy, core decompression, hemiarthroplasty, total shoulder arthroplasty
• Lunate (Kienböck disease): Lunate excision with or without replacement, joint-leveling procedures, inter-carpal fusions, revascularization, salvage procedures

 ## ONGOING CARE

• Physical therapy and occupational therapy as adjunctive treatment
• Sickle cell patients: No evidence that adding hip core decompression to physical therapy achieves clinical improvement in people with avascular necrosis of bone compared to physical therapy alone, per Cochrane Review (13)[A]

PATIENT EDUCATION
• Physicians prescribing bisphosphonates should counsel their patients about potential oral complications linked to using these medications and advise patients to notify their dentists that they are taking the drugs (14)[C].
• Other high-risk patients should be educated about the risk of developing osteonecrosis and should be advised to report symptoms as soon as possible.

PROGNOSIS
• Poor prognostic factors include age >50, advanced disease at time of diagnosis, necrosis of >1/3 the femoral head weight bearing area, lateral femoral head involvement, and nonmodifiable risk factors.
• Progression of asymptomatic osteonecrosis of the femoral head proportional to lesion size with small lesions (<15% involvement) unlikely to progress and large lesions (>30% involvement) likely to progress (15)[B]
• More than 50% of patients with osteonecrosis require surgical treatment within 3 years of diagnosis.
• Osteonecrosis of the humeral head accounts for 10% of total joint replacement procedures performed annually in US (7).

COMPLICATIONS
• Secondary to surgery-induced trauma, including nonunion, malunion, peroneal nerve palsy, deep venous thrombosis, intraoperative fracture, and post-op dislocation (7)
• Progression of disease leads to OA of the involved joint to a varying degree.

REFERENCES

1. Lafforgue P. Pathophysiology and natural history of avascular necrosis of bone. *Joint Bone Spine*. 2006;73(5):500–7.
2. Khan AA, Sándor GK, Dore E, et al. Bisphosphonate associated osteonecrosis of the jaw. *J Rheumatol*. 2009;36:478–90.
3. Kubo T, Yamazoe S, Sugano N, et al. Initial MRI findings of non-traumatic osteonecrosis of the femoral head in renal allograft recipients. *Magn Reson Imaging*. 1997;15:1017–23.
4. Matsuo K, Hirohata T, Sugioka Y, et al. Influence of alcohol intake, cigarette smoking and occupational status on idiopathic osteonecrosis of the femoral head. *Clin Orthop Relat Res*. 1998;115–23.
5. Powell C, Chang C, Naguwa SM, et al. Steroid induced osteonecrosis: An analysis of steroid dosing risk. *Autoimmun Rev*. 2010;9:721–43.
6. American College of Radiology (ACR) Appropriateness Criteria for avascular necrosis of the hip. *National Guideline Clearinghouse*. 2010;31:15734.
7. Assouline-Dayan Y, Chang C, Greenspan A, et al. Pathogenesis and natural history of osteonecrosis. *Semin Arthritis Rheum*. 2002;32:94–124.
8. Collier BD, Carrera GF, Johnson RP, et al. Detection of femoral head avascular necrosis in adults by SPECT. *J Nucl Med*. 1985;26:979–87.
9. Iida S, Harada Y, Shimizu K, et al. Correlation between bone marrow edema and collapse of the femoral head in steroid-induced osteonecrosis. *AJR Am J Roentgenol*. 2000;174:735–43.
10. Steinberg ME, Steinberg DR. Classification systems for osteonecrosis: an overview. *Orthop Clin North Am*. 2004;35:273–83, vii–viii.
11. Lai K-A, Shen W-J, Yang C-Y, et al. The Use of Alendronate to Prevent Early Collapse of the Femoral Head in Patients with Nontraumatic Osteonecrosis. *The Journal of Bone and Joint Surgery (American)*. 2005;87:2155–2159.
12. Mont MA, Jones LC, Seyler TM, et al. New treatment approaches for osteonecrosis of the femoral head: an overview. *Instr Course Lect*. 2007;56:197–212.
13. Martí-Carvajal AJ, Solà I, Agreda-Pérez LH. Treatment for avascular necrosis of bone in people with sickle cell disease. *Cochrane Database of Systematic Reviews* 2009, Issue 3. Art. No.: CD004344. DOI:10.1002/14651858. CD004344.pub3.
14. Study: Physicians need to educate patients about use of bisphosphonates. AAFP News Now. 6/11/2010.
15. Hungerford DS, Jones LC, et al. Asymptomatic osteonecrosis: should it be treated? *Clin Orthop Relat Res*. 2004;124–30.

ADDITIONAL READING

• National Institute of Arthritis and Musculoskeletal and Skin Diseases: Osteonecrosis. http://www.niams.nih.gov/health_info/osteonecrosis/
• Tofferi J, Gilliland W. E-Medicine Rheumatology: Avascular Necrosis. http://emedicine.medscape.com/article/333364-overview

See Also (Topic, Algorithm, Electronic Media Element)
Arthritis, Osteo; Legg-Calvé-Perthes Disease

 ## CODES

ICD9
• 733.40 Aseptic necrosis of bone, site unspecified
• 733.41 Aseptic necrosis of head of humerus
• 733.42 Aseptic necrosis of head and neck of femur

CLINICAL PEARLS

• Trauma, alcoholism, and prolonged glucocorticoid use are most common risk factors for the development of osteonecrosis.
• Identify at-risk patients and suspect osteonecrosis in this population if presenting with bone or joint pain.
• Initiate workup with appropriate radiographs, then proceed to MRI if indicated (6)[A].

O

OSTEOPOROSIS

Karen L. Maughan, MD

 BASICS

DESCRIPTION
A skeletal disease characterized by low bone mass, disruption of skeletal microarchitecture, and increased skeletal fragility resulting in fractures occurring with a fall from standing height or less or with no trauma

EPIDEMIOLOGY
- Predominant age: Elderly >60 years of age
- Predominant sex: Female > Male (80%/20%)

Incidence
9 million osteoporotic fractures worldwide in 2000

Prevalence
- 10 million Americans have osteoporosis.
- 24% of women >50 years of age
- 7.5% of men >50 years of age

RISK FACTORS
- Nonmodifiable:
  - Advanced age (>65 years)
  - Female gender
  - Caucasian or Asian
  - Family history of osteoporosis
  - History of atraumatic fracture
- Modifiable:
  - Low body weight (<58 kg or body mass index <20)
  - Calcium or vitamin D deficiency
  - Inadequate physical activity
  - Cigarette smoking
  - Excessive alcohol intake (>2 drinks/d)
  - Medications: Chronic corticosteroids, excessive thyroid hormone replacement, medroxyprogesterone acetate, heparin

Genetics
- Familial predisposition
- More common in Caucasians and Asians than in African Americans and Hispanics

GENERAL PREVENTION
The aim in the prevention and treatment of osteoporosis is to prevent fracture.
- Exercise (weight-bearing, aerobic, and strength training) increases bone mineral density (BMD), although unclear if it prevents fractures (1)[B].
- Calcium (1,200 mg) and vitamin D (800 IU) daily
- Avoid smoking.
- Limit alcohol use (<2 drinks/d).
- Screen all women ≥65 years of age and women ≥60 years of age who are at high risk for fracture (2)[B].
- Consider screening elderly men at high risk for fracture (3)[C].
- Correct treatable medical conditions and other risk factors.

PATHOPHYSIOLOGY
- Imbalance between bone resorption and bone formation
- Trabecular bone (vertebral) more active than cortical (hip) bone

ETIOLOGY
- Aging
- Hypoestrogenemia

COMMONLY ASSOCIATED CONDITIONS
- Malabsorption syndromes: Gastrectomy, inflammatory bowel disease, celiac disease
- Hypoestrogenism: Menopause, hypogonadism, eating disorders, elite athletes
- Chronic liver disease, hemochromatosis
- Endocrinopathies: Hyperparathyroidism, hyperthyroidism
- Multiple myeloma, multiple sclerosis, osteomalacia, rheumatoid arthritis
- Medications (see "Medications" under "Risk Factors")

 DIAGNOSIS

HISTORY
- Review risk factors.
- Online risk factor assessment tools are available, although external validation is lacking [e.g., FRAX (http://www.sheffield.ac.uk/FRAX/index.htm), Garvan (http://garvan.org.au/promotions/bone-fracture-risk/calculator/).
- Often no clinic findings until fracture occurs

PHYSICAL EXAM
- Thoracic kyphosis
- Height loss >1.5 cm

DIAGNOSTIC TESTS & INTERPRETATION
Dual-energy x-ray absorptiometry (DEXA) of the lumbar spine/hip is the "gold standard" for diagnosis of osteoporosis (see "Initial Approach" under "Imaging").

Lab
Initial lab tests
To elicit common causes of secondary osteoporosis:
- 25-hydroxyvitamin D
- Complete blood count
- Serum calcium, total protein, creatinine, alkaline phosphatase

Follow-Up & Special Considerations
Consider further lab work depending on initial evaluation, Z-score < −2.0, or young age.
- Parathyroid hormone (PTH), ionized calcium (hyperparathyroidism)
- Thyroid-stimulating hormone (hyperthyroidism)
- Testosterone (hypogonadism in men)
- Serum protein electrophoresis (multiple myeloma)
- Urinary free cortisol (Cushing disease)
- Vitamin B_{12} level and intrinsic-factor antibody (pernicious anemia)
- IgA antiendomysial antibodies (celiac sprue)
- Serum and 24-h urine calcium, serum phosphate (osteomalacia)
- Markers of bone resorption (urine N-telopeptides of type 1 collagen, serum C-telopeptides of type 1 collagen, serum N-terminal propeptide of type 1 procollagen): No prospective studies supporting use in osteoporosis diagnosis and management; potential role for identifying patients at high risk for fracture and monitoring response to therapy

Imaging
Initial approach
- DEXA of the lumbar spine/hip is the "gold standard" for measuring BMD.
- BMD is expressed in terms of T-scores and Z-scores.
  - T-score is the number of standard deviations (SDs) a patient's BMD deviates from the mean for young normal (age 25–40 years) control individuals of the same sex.
  - The World Health Organization (WHO) defines normal BMD as a T-score ≥−1, osteopenia as a T-score between −1 and −2.5, and osteoporosis as a T-score ≤−2.5.
  - WHO thresholds can be used for postmenopausal women and men >50 years of age.
  - Z-score is a comparison of the patient's BMD with an age-matched population.
  - Z-score <−2.0 should prompt evaluation for causes of secondary osteoporosis.
- Ultrasound densitometry is used to measure BMD at the calcaneus (heel). It is lower in cost and involves no radiation exposure but is not as accurate as DEXA, and no studies support its use in determining therapy.
- Plain radiographs lack sensitivity to diagnose osteoporosis, but an abnormality (e.g., widened intervertebral spaces, rib fractures, vertebral compression fractures, etc.) should prompt evaluation of BMD.

Diagnostic Procedures/Surgery
Bone biopsy rarely is needed to rule out neoplasms and other metabolic bone diseases.

Pathological Findings
- Reduced skeletal mass, trabecular bone thinned or lost more so than cortical bone
- Osteoclast and osteoblast number variable
- No evidence of other metabolic bone diseases and no increase in unmineralized osteoid
- Marrow normal or atrophic

DIFFERENTIAL DIAGNOSIS
- Multiple myeloma or other neoplasms
- Osteomalacia
- Type I collagen mutations
- Osteogenesis imperfecta

 TREATMENT

Treat patients with a T-score ≤−2.5 with no risk factors, patients with a T-score ≤−2.0 and 1 or more risk factors, and patients with a prior history of osteoporotic fracture at the spine or hip.

MEDICATION
Calcium 1,500 mg and vitamin D 800 IU (minimally) per day

First Line
- Bisphosphonates:
  - Alendronate 10 mg PO daily or 70 mg PO weekly
  - Risedronate 5 mg PO daily, 35 mg PO weekly, 75 mg PO twice monthly, or 150 mg PO monthly
  - Zoledronic acid 5 mg IV yearly
- These drugs become incorporated into skeletal tissue, where they inhibit the resorption of bone by osteoclasts.

- Number needed to treat (NNT) to prevent vertebral fracture = 17.
- NNT to prevent hip fracture = 100 (4)[A].
- Ibandronate increases bone density but does not appear to decrease fractures.

Second Line
- Raloxifene 60 mg PO daily:
  – Selective estrogen receptor modulator with positive effects on BMD and fracture risk but no stimulatory action on breasts or uterus
  – NNT with 60 mg/d for 3 years to prevent 1 postmenopausal woman with osteoporosis from developing a vertebral fracture = 29.
  – Decreases vertebral but not hip fractures (5)[A]; increases risk of thromboembolism
- Teriparatide 20 mg SC daily:
  – Recombinant formulation of PTH; when given daily, it promotes new bone formation.
  – Studies have shown a reduction in the incidence of vertebral fractures by 65% (6)[B].
  – No data exist on its safety and efficacy after >2 years of use.
  – Primarily indicated for those with worsening osteoporosis despite bisphosphonate therapy.
- Estrogen 0.625 mg PO daily (with progesterone if women has a uterus): Effective in prevention and treatment of osteoporosis (35% reduction in hip and vertebral fractures after 5 years of use), but the risks (e.g., increased rates of myocardial infarction, stroke, breast cancer, pulmonary embolus, and deep vein thrombosis) must be weighed against the benefits (7)[B].
- Strontium 2 g PO daily:
  – Appears to inhibit bone resorption and increase bone formation
  – Available for use in Europe
  – NNT to prevent vertebral fracture = 13.
  – NNT to prevent hip fracture = 50 (8)[B].
- Denosumab:
  – Human monoclonal antibody RANKL receptor
  – Inhibits Osteoclast formation
  – NNT to prevent vertebral fracture = 20 after 3 years
  – NNT to prevent hip fracture = 200 after 3 years (9)
- Calcitonin:
  – Acts by reducing the number of osteoclasts, therefore decreasing bone turnover
  – Has been shown to increase BMD, but no studies have shown conclusively a reduction in the occurrence of fractures.
  – May decrease acute vertebral compression-fracture pain (analgesic).

ADDITIONAL TREATMENT
- Exercise: Any weight-bearing exercise 30 min 3×/wk (1)[B]
- Smoking cessation
- Decrease fall risk.
- Evaluate and treat all patients presenting with fracture resulting from minimal trauma.

Issues for Referral
Endocrinology for recurrent bone loss/fracture despite treatment of osteoporosis and evaluation and treatment of possible secondary causes

Additional Therapies
Physical therapy to help with muscle strengthening to decrease fall risk

COMPLEMENTARY AND ALTERNATIVE MEDICINE
Isoflavones not better than placebo for bone density and fracture risk

SURGERY/OTHER PROCEDURES
Options for patients with painful vertebral compression fractures failing medical treatment:
- Vertebroplasty: Orthopedic cement is injected into compressed vertebral body.
- Kyphoplasty: A balloon is expanded within compressed vertebral body to reconstruct volume of vertebrae. Cement is injected into the space.

IN-PATIENT CONSIDERATIONS
Initial Stabilization
- Usually outpatient care
- Inpatient care for pain control of acute back pain secondary to new vertebral fractures and for acute treatment of femoral and pelvic fractures

Discharge Criteria
- Pain controlled
- Fracture stabilized
- Rehabilitation, nursing home, or home care may be needed following peripheral fractures

 ## ONGOING CARE

FOLLOW-UP RECOMMENDATIONS
Patient Monitoring
- Weight-bearing exercises such as walking, jogging, stair climbing, and tai-chi. These activities have been shown to decrease falls.
- All successful studies on the treatment of osteoporosis involve weight-bearing exercise.
- BMD should be tested no earlier than 2 years after starting bisphosphonate. It is uncertain whether repeat DEXA scanning is of value.
- Radiographs for acute pain, suspected fractures

DIET
- Diet to maintain normal body weight
- Calcium 1,500 mg and vitamin D 800 IU daily

PATIENT EDUCATION
National Osteoporosis Foundation: WWW.nof.org

PROGNOSIS
- With treatment, 80% of patients stabilize skeletal manifestations, increase bone mass, increase mobility, and have reduced pain.
- 15% of vertebral and 20–40% of hip fractures may lead to chronic care and/or premature death.

COMPLICATIONS
- Severe, disabling pain
- Dorsal/lumbar neurologic deficits secondary to vertebral fracture (rare)

REFERENCES

1. Bonaiuti D, Shea B, Iovine R, et al. Exercise for preventing and treating osteoporosis in postmenopausal women. *Cochrane Database Syst Rev.* 2002;CD000333.
2. *Screening for Osteoporosis in Postmenopausal Women*, Topic Page. September 2002. U.S. Preventive Services Task Force. Agency for Healthcare Research and Quality, Rockville, MD. http://www.ahrq.gov/clinic/uspstf/uspsoste.htm.
3. Qaseem A, Snow V, Shekelle P, et al. Screening for osteoporosis in men: a clinical practice guideline from the American College of Physicians. *Ann Intern Med.* 2008;148:680–4.
4. Wells GA, Cranney A, Peterson J, et al. Alendronate for the primary and secondary prevention of osteoporotic fractures in postmenopausal women. *Cochrane Database of Systematic Reviews.* 2008, Issue 1. 10.1002/14651858.CD001155.pub2.
5. Ettinger B, Black DM, Mitlak BH, et al. Reduction of vertebral fracture risk in postmenopausal women with osteoporosis treated with raloxifene: results from a 3-year randomized clinical trial. Multiple Outcomes of Raloxifene Evaluation (MORE) Investigators. *JAMA.* 1999;282:637–45.
6. Neer RM, Arnaud CD, Zanchetta JR, et al. Effect of parathyroid hormone (1-34) on fractures and bone mineral density in postmenopausal women with osteoporosis. *N Engl J Med.* 2001;344:1434–41.
7. Cauley JA, Robbins J, Chen Z, et al. Effects of estrogen plus progestin on risk of fracture and bone mineral density: the Women's Health Initiative randomized trial. *JAMA.* 2003;290:1729–38.
8. O'Donnell S, Cranney A, Wells GA, et al. Strontium ranelate for preventing and treating postmenopausal osteoporosis. *Cochrane Database Sys Rev.* 2006, Issue 4.
9. Cummings SR, San Martin J, McClung MR, et al. Denosumab for prevention of fractures in postmenopausal women with osteoporosis. *N Engl J Med.* 2009;361:756–65.

 ## CODES

ICD9
- 733.00 Osteoporosis, unspecified
- 733.01 Senile osteoporosis
- 733.02 Idiopathic osteoporosis

CLINICAL PEARLS
- Screen all women and men for risks of osteoporosis.
- Screen both men and women >60 years of age at increased risk for osteoporosis and candidates for treatment with DEXA scan.
- Premenopausal women with osteoporosis should be screened for secondary causes of osteoporosis, such as malabsorption syndromes (e.g., celiac sprue), hyperparathyroidism, hyperthyroidism, and medications (e.g., chronic steroid use, etc.).
- Evaluate and treat all patients presenting with fractures from minimal trauma.
- If patient is not responding to treatment, consider screening for secondary, treatable cause of osteoporosis.

OTITIS EXTERNA

Douglas S. Parks, MD

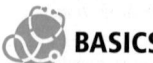 **BASICS**

DESCRIPTION

Inflammation of the external auditory canal:

- Acute diffuse otitis externa: The most common form; an infectious process, usually bacterial, occasionally fungal (10%)
- Acute circumscribed otitis externa: Synonymous with furuncle; associated with infection of the hair follicle, a superficial cellulitic form of otitis externa
- Chronic otitis externa: Same as acute diffuse but of longer duration (>6 weeks)
- Eczematous otitis externa: May accompany typical atopic eczema or other primary skin conditions
- Necrotizing malignant otitis externa: An infection that extends into the deeper tissues adjacent to the canal; may include osteomyelitis and cellulitis; rare in children
- System(s) affected: Skin/Exocrine
- Synonym(s): Swimmer's ear

EPIDEMIOLOGY

Incidence
- Unknown; higher in the summer months and warm, wet climates
- Predominant age: All ages
- Predominant sex: Male = Female

Prevalence
- Acute, chronic, and eczematous: Common
- Necrotizing: Uncommon

RISK FACTORS
- Acute and chronic otitis externa:
  - Traumatization of external canal
  - Swimming
  - Hot, humid weather
  - Hearing aid use
- Eczematous: Primary skin disorder
- Necrotizing otitis externa in adults:
  - Advanced age
  - Diabetes mellitus (DM)
  - Debilitating disease
  - AIDS
- Necrotizing otitis externa in children (rare):
  - Leukopenia
  - Malnutrition
  - DM
  - Diabetes insipidus

GENERAL PREVENTION
- Avoid prolonged exposure to moisture.
- Use preventive antiseptics: Acidifying solutions with 2% acetic acid (white vinegar) diluted 50/50 with water or isopropyl alcohol, or 2% acetic acid with aluminum acetate (less irritating) after swimming and bathing.
- Treat predisposing skin conditions.
- Eliminate self-inflicted trauma to canal with cotton swabs and other foreign objects.
- Diagnose and treat underlying systemic conditions.
- Use ear plugs when swimming.

ETIOLOGY
- Acute diffuse otitis externa:
  - Traumatized external canal (e.g., from use of cotton swab)
  - Bacterial infection (90%): *Pseudomonas* (67%), *Staphylococcus*, *Streptococcus*, gram-negative rods
  - Fungal infection (10%): *Aspergillus* (90%), *Candida, Phycomycetes, Rhizopus, Actinomyces, Penicillium*
- Chronic otitis externa: Bacterial infection: *Pseudomonas*
- Eczematous otitis externa (associated with primary skin disorder):
  - Eczema
  - Seborrhea
  - Psoriasis
  - Neurodermatitis
  - Contact dermatitis
  - Purulent otitis media
  - Sensitivity to topical medications
- Necrotizing otitis externa:
  - Invasive bacterial infection: *Pseudomonas*
  - Associated with immunosuppression

 DIAGNOSIS

HISTORY
Variable-length history of itching, plugging of ear, ear pain, and discharge from ear

PHYSICAL EXAM
- Ear canal red, containing purulent discharge and debris
- Pain on manipulation of the pinnae
- Possible periauricular adenitis
- Possible eczema of pinna
- Cranial nerve (VII, IX–XII) involvement (extremely rare)

DIAGNOSTIC TESTS & INTERPRETATION
Lab
- Gram stain and culture of canal discharge (occasionally helpful)
- Antibiotic pretreatment may affect results.

Imaging
Radiologic evaluation of deep tissues in necrotizing otitis externa with high-resolution CT scan, MRI, gallium scan, and bone scan

Pathological Findings
- Acute and chronic otitis externa: Desquamation of superficial epithelium of external canal with infection
- Eczematous otitis externa: Pathologic findings consistent with primary skin disorder; secondary infection on occasion
- Necrotizing otitis externa: Vasculitis, thrombosis, and necrosis of involved tissues; osteomyelitis

DIFFERENTIAL DIAGNOSIS
- Idiopathic ear pain
- Otitis media with perforation
- Hearing loss
- Cranial nerve (VII, IX–XII) palsy with necrotizing otitis externa
- Wisdom tooth eruption
- Basal cell or squamous cell carcinoma

 TREATMENT

Outpatient treatment, except for resistant cases and necrotizing otitis externa

MEDICATION
Resistance is an increasing problem. *Pseudomonas* is the most common bacteria and it is more susceptible to Ciprofloxin, where as *Staphylococcus* is equally susceptible to both Ciprofloxin and Cortisporin. If a patient has recurring episodes, change the class of antibacterial and consider cultures and sensitivities.

First Line
- Acute bacterial and chronic otitis externa:
  - Neomycin/polymyxin B/hydrocortisone (Cortisporin) 5 drops q.i.d. If the tympanic membrane is ruptured, use the suspension; otherwise, the solution may be used; may be ototoxic and resistance-developing in *Staphylococcus* and *Streptococcus* sp. (1)[B].
  - Betamethasone 0.05% solution is more effective than a polymyxin B combination without the risk of ototoxicity or antibiotic resistance (2)[A].
  - 2% acetic acid with 1% hydrocortisone (VoSoL HC) 3–5 drops q4–8h × 7 days; may cause minor local stinging. This is as effective as neomycin–polymyxin B (3)[B] but is expensive.
  - A wick may be helpful in severe cases by keeping the canal open and keeping antibiotic solution in contact with infected skin (4)[C].
  - Oral antibiotics are indicated only if there is associated otitis media or cellulitis of the outer ear (red canal without discharge).

– Analgesics as needed; narcotics may be necessary.
– Recurrent otitis externa may be prevented by applying equal parts white vinegar and isopropyl alcohol (OTC rubbing alcohol) to external auditory canals after bathing and swimming.

- Fungal otitis externa:
  – Topical therapy, antiyeast for *Candida* or yeast: 2% acetic acid 3–4 drops q.i.d.; clotrimazole 1% solution; itraconazole oral
  – Parenteral antifungal therapy: Amphotericin B
  – Patients with Ramsay-Hunt syndrome: Acyclovir IV
- Eczematous otitis externa: Topical therapy:
  – Acetic acid 2% in aluminum acetate
  – Aluminum acetate (5%; Burow solution)
  – Steroid cream, lotion, ointment (e.g., triamcinolone 0.1% solution)
  – Antibacterial, if superinfected
- Necrotizing otitis externa:
  – Parenteral antibiotics: Antistaphylococcal and antipseudomonal
  – 4–6 weeks of therapy
  – Quinolones p.o. × 2–4 weeks
- Contraindications:
  – Hypersensitivity to topical or parenteral therapy
  – Renal or hepatic failure when using amphotericin B
- Precautions:
  – Dosage adjustment for amphotericin B in patients with renal or hepatic dysfunction
  – Sensitivity to neomycin
- Significant possible interactions:
  – Hypokalemia associated with amphotericin B may lead to digitalis toxicity.
  – Concurrent administration of nonabsorbable anions, such as carbenicillin, may exacerbate hypokalemia.

Second Line
- Ciprofloxacin (Cipro dex) 0.3% and dexamethasone 0.1% suspension 3–4 drops b.i.d. × 7 days
- Ofloxacin (Floxin Otic) 0.3% solution 10 drops once a day
- Azole antifungals for fungal otitis externa

ADDITIONAL TREATMENT
General Measures
- Cleansing of external canal may facilitate recovery.
- Analgesics as appropriate for pain
- Antipruritic and antihistamines (eczematous form)
- Ear wick (Pope) for nearly occluded ear canal

Issues for Referral
Resistant cases or those requiring surgical intervention

COMPLEMENTARY AND ALTERNATIVE MEDICINE
- Over-the-counter white vinegar; 3 drops in affected ear for minor case
- Tea tree oil in various concentrations has been used as an antiseptic (5)[B]. Ototoxicity has been reported in animal studies at very high doses.
- Grapefruit seed extract in various concentrations has been described as useful in the lay literature.

SURGERY/OTHER PROCEDURES
For necrotizing otitis externa or furuncle

IN-PATIENT CONSIDERATIONS
Admission Criteria
Necrotizing otitis media requiring parenteral antipseudomonal antibiotics

Discharge Criteria
Resolution of infection

 ONGOING CARE

FOLLOW-UP RECOMMENDATIONS
No restrictions

Patient Monitoring
- Acute otitis externa:
  – 48 hours after therapy instituted to assess improvement
  – At the end of treatment
- Chronic otitis externa:
  – Every 2–3 weeks for repeated cleansing of canal
  – May require alterations in topical medication, including antibiotics and steroids
- Necrotizing otitis externa:
  – Daily monitoring in hospital for extension of infection
  – Baseline auditory and vestibular testing at beginning and end of therapy

DIET
No restrictions

PROGNOSIS
- Acute otitis externa: Rapid response to therapy with total resolution
- Chronic otitis externa: With repeated cleansing and antibiotic therapy, most cases will resolve. Occasionally, surgical intervention is required for resistant cases.
- Eczematous otitis externa: Resolution will occur with control of the primary skin condition.
- Necrotizing otitis externa: Usually can be managed with debridement and antipseudomonal antibiotics; recurrence rate is 100% when treatment is inadequate. Surgical intervention may be necessary in resistant cases or if there is cranial nerve involvement. Mortality rate is significant, probably secondary to the underlying disease.

COMPLICATIONS
- Mainly a problem with necrotizing otitis externa; may spread to infect contiguous bone and CNS structures
- Acute otitis externa may spread to pinna, causing chondritis.

REFERENCES
1. Cantrell HF, Lombardy EE, Duncanson FP, et al. Declining susceptibility to neomycin and polymyxin B of pathogens recovered in otitis externa clinical trials. *South Med J*. 2004;97:465–71.
2. Emgård P, Hellström S. A group III steroid solution without antibiotic components: an effective cure for external otitis. *J Laryngol Otol*. 2005;119:342–7.
3. van Balen FA, Smit WM, Zuithoff NP, et al. Clinical efficacy of three common treatments in acute otitis externa in primary care: randomised controlled trial. *BMJ*. 2003;327:1201–5.
4. Block SL. Otitis externa: providing relief while avoiding complications. *J Fam Pract*. 2005;54:669–76.
5. Farnan TB, McCallum J, Awa A, et al. Tea tree oil: in vitro efficacy in otitis externa. *J Laryngol Otol*. 2005;119:198–201.

ADDITIONAL READING
Dohar JE, Roland P, Wall GM, et al. Differences in bacteriologic treatment failures in acute otitis externa between ciprofloxacin/dexamethasone and neomycin/polymyxin B/hydrocortisone: results of a combined analysis. *Curr Med Res Opin*. 2009;25:287–91.

See Also (Topic, Algorithm, Electronic Media Element)
Algorithm: Ear Pain

 CODES

ICD9
- 380.10 Infective otitis externa, unspecified
- 380.15 Chronic mycotic otitis externa
- 380.22 Other acute otitis externa

CLINICAL PEARLS
- Acute diffuse otitis externa is most common form: Bacterial (90%), occasionally fungal (10%).
- Acute circumscribed otitis externa: Associated with infection of hair follicle
- Chronic otitis externa: Same as acute diffuse but of longer duration (>6 weeks)
- Eczematous otitis externa: May accompany typical atopic eczema or other primary skin conditions
- Necrotizing malignant otitis externa: An infection that extends into the deeper tissues adjacent to the canal; may include osteomyelitis and cellulitis; rare in children

O

OTITIS MEDIA

David B. Gilchrist, MD
Hugh J. Silk, MD

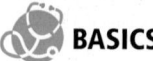

BASICS

DESCRIPTION
- Inflammation of the middle ear
- Acute otitis media (AOM): Inflammation of the middle ear often following a viral upper respiratory infection (URI):
  - Rapid onset; cause may be infectious, either viral (AOM-v) or bacterial (AOM-b), but there is also a sterile etiology (AOM-s)
- Recurrent AOM: ≥3 episodes in 6 months or ≥4 episodes in 1 year
- Otitis media with effusion (OME): Persistent middle ear fluid that is associated with AOM but can arise without prior AOM
- Chronic otitis media with or without cholesteatoma
- System(s) affected: Nervous; ENT
- Synonym(s): Secretory or serous otitis media

EPIDEMIOLOGY
Incidence
- AOM:
  - Predominant age: 6–24 months; declines >7 years; rare in adults
  - Predominant sex: Male > Female
  - By age 7 years, 93% of children have had ≥1 episodes of AOM; 39% have had ≥6.
  - Placement of tympanostomy tubes is 2nd only to circumcision as the most frequent surgical procedure in infants.
  - Increased incidence in the fall and winter
- OME:
  - 90% of children aged 6 months–4 years have at least 1 episode.

Prevalence
- Most common infection for which antibacterial agents are prescribed in the US
- Diagnosed 5 million times per year in the US

RISK FACTORS
- Premature birth
- Bottle-feeding while supine
- Routine daycare attendance
- Frequent pacifier use after 6 months of age
- Smoking in household
- Male gender
- Native American/Inuit ethnicity
- Low socioeconomic status
- Family history of recurrent otitis
- AOM before age 1 is a risk for recurrent AOM.
- Presence of siblings in the household
- Underlying ENT disease (e.g., cleft palate, Down syndrome, allergic rhinitis)

Genetics
- Strong genetic component in twin studies for recurrent and prolonged AOM
- May be influenced by skull configuration or immunologic defects

GENERAL PREVENTION
- PCV-7 immunization reduces number of cases of AOM by about 6–28% (however, evidence shows that this is offset by an increase in AOM caused by other bacteria) (1)[C].
- Influenza vaccine reduces AOM by about 30% in children older than age 2 (by preventing influenza).

- Breastfeeding for ≥6 months is protective.
- Avoiding supine bottle-feeding, passive smoke, and pacifiers >6 months may be helpful.
- Secondary prevention: Adenoidectomy and adenotonsillectomy for recurrent AOM has limited short-term efficacy for children older than 3 years of age and is associated with its own adverse risks.

ETIOLOGY
- AOM-b (bacterial): Usually, a preceding viral URI produces eustachian tube dysfunction:
  - S. pneumoniae: 20–35%
  - H. influenzae: 20–30%.
  - M. (B.) catarrhalis: 15%
  - Group A streptococci: 3%
  - S. aureus: 12% produce β-lactamases that hydrolyze amoxicillin and some cephalosporins.
- AOM-v (viral): 15–44% of AOM infections are caused primarily by viruses (e.g., respiratory syncytial virus, parainfluenza, influenza, enteroviruses, adenovirus, human metapneumovirus, and parechovirus).
- AOM-s (sterile/nonpathogens): 25–30%
- OME:
  - Eustachian tube dysfunction
  - Allergic causes are rarely substantiated.

COMMONLY ASSOCIATED CONDITIONS
- Otalgia
- URI

DIAGNOSIS

- AOM: Acute history, signs, and symptoms of middle ear inflammation and effusion:
  - Earache (LR = 3–7.3)
  - Preceding or accompanying URI symptoms
  - Decreased hearing
- Infectious AOM:
  - Fever (although it is debatable whether OM itself causes fever or fever is due to accompanying viral illness)
  - Decreased eardrum mobility (with pneumatic otoscopy) (LR = 51)
  - Eardrum bulging (LR = 51), cloudy (LR = 34), distinctly red (LR = 8.4). Presence of air–fluid level behind the tympanic membrane [B].
  - Redness alone is not a reliable sign.
  - Otorrhea if eardrum is perforated
- AOM in infants and toddlers:
  - May cause few symptoms in the 1st few months of life
  - Irritability may be the only symptom.
- OME:
  - Usually asymptomatic
  - Decreased hearing
  - Eardrum often dull but not bulging
  - Decreased eardrum mobility (pneumatic otoscopy)
  - Presence of air–fluid level
  - Weber test is positive for an ear with effusion.

DIAGNOSTIC TESTS & INTERPRETATION
Lab
Initial lab tests
WBC count may be higher in bacterial AOM than in sterile AOM, but is almost never useful.

Diagnostic Procedures/Surgery
- To document the presence of middle ear fluid, pneumatic otoscopy can be supplemented with tympanometry and acoustic reflex measurement.
- Hearing testing is recommended when hearing loss persists for ≥3 months or at any time language delay, significant hearing loss, or learning problems are suspected.
- Language testing should be performed for children with hearing loss.
- Tympanocentesis for microbiologic diagnosis is recommended for treatment failures; may be followed by myringotomy.

DIFFERENTIAL DIAGNOSIS
- Tympanosclerosis
- Redness because of crying
- Trauma
- AOM vs OME
- AOM-b vs AOM-v vs AOM-s
- Referred pain from the jaw, teeth, or throat
- Otitis externa

TREATMENT

MEDICATION
First Line

- AOM: AAP-AAFP Consensus Guideline recommends amoxicillin 80–90 mg/kg/d; children >2 years old with no complications, 5- to 7-day course [A]; 10-day course for children <2 years old. It is unclear if daily or b.i.d. dosing is as effective as t.i.d. or q.i.d. dosing (2)[A].

- If penicillin-allergic:
- Non–type 1 hypersensitivity reaction: Cefdinir 14 mg/kg/d, cefpodoxime 10 mg/kg/d, or cefuroxime 30 mg/kg b.i.d.
- Type 1 hypersensitivity to penicillin: Azithromycin (10 mg/kg/d [maximum dose 500 mg/d] as a single dose on day 1 and 5 mg/kg/d [maximum dose 250 mg/d] for days 2–5)
- Other alternatives: Clarithromycin 15 mg/kg/d (b.i.d. dose), erythromycin-sulfisoxazole (50 mg/kg/d), or sulfamethoxazole–trimethoprim (6–10 mg/kg/d based on trimethoprim)
- A single dose of parenteral ceftriaxone (50 mg/kg) is as effective as a full course of antibiotics in uncomplicated AOM.

- A single dose of azithromycin has been approved by FDA, but studies did not include otitis-prone children or have criteria for AOM diagnosis [B].

- OME: See General Measures; no benefit to treatment. Medications promote transitory resolution in 10–15%, but effect is short lived.

Second Line
- Alternative antibiotics are indicated for the following AOM patients:
  - Persistent symptoms after 48–72 h of amoxicillin
  - AOM within 1 month of amoxicillin therapy
  - Severe earache
  - Age <6 months with high fever
  - Immunocompromised:
    ○ Amoxicillin-clavulanate 90 mg/kg–6.4 mg/kg/d, b.i.d.

○ Ceftriaxone 50 mg/kg IM or IV q24h for 3 consecutive days can be reserved for those who are too sick to take oral medications or fail amoxicillin-clavunate. Neither erythromycin-sulfisoxazole nor trimethoprim-sulfamethoxazole should be used as a 2nd-line agent in treatment failures.

- Recurrent AOM: Antibiotic prophylaxis for recurrent AOM (>3 distinct, well-documented episodes in 6 months) with amoxicillin 20 mg/kg/d for 3 months resulted in a benefit of ∼1 fewer episode per child per year. The risks of increased resistance and side effects are not thought to be worth it.

ADDITIONAL TREATMENT
General Measures
- Assess pain.
- Acetaminophen, ibuprofen, benzocaine drops (additional but brief benefit over acetaminophen)
- Significant disagreement exists about the usefulness of antibiotic treatment for this often self-resolving condition. Studies suggest that ∼15 children need to be treated with antibiotics to prevent 1 case of persisting AOM pain at 1–2 weeks (NNT= ∼15); the NNT to cause harm (primarily diarrhea) is 8–10.
- 81% of patients over 2 years of age are better in 1 week vs 94% if antibiotics are used.
- Delay of antibiotics found a modest increase in mastoiditis from 2/100,000 to 4/100,000.
- The AAP/AAFP guideline committee recommends the following for observation vs antibacterial therapy, although these guidelines are not rigorously evidence-based:
  - <6 months of age: Antibacterial therapy should be administered to any child, regardless of the degree of diagnostic certainty.
  - Children >6 months: Antibacterial therapy is recommended when the diagnosis of AOM is certain and the illness is severe (i.e., moderate-to-severe otalgia or fever ≥39°C in the previous 24 h).
  - Observation is an option when the diagnosis is certain, but illness is not severe, and in patients with an uncertain diagnosis.
- OME: Watchful waiting for 3 months per AAP/AFPP guidelines for those not at risk (see Complications). 25–90% will recover spontaneously over this period:
  - No benefit of antihistamines or decongestants (3)[A] or antibiotics or systemic steroids

COMPLEMENTARY AND ALTERNATIVE MEDICINE
- It is unclear whether alternative and homeopathic therapies are effective for AOM, including mixed evidence about the effectiveness of zinc supplementation of reducing AOM.
- Xylitol, probiotics, herbal ear drops, and homeopathic interventions may be beneficial in reducing pain duration, antibiotic use, and bacterial resistance.

SURGERY/OTHER PROCEDURES
- Recurrent AOM: Consider referral for surgery if ≥3 episodes of well-documented AOM within 6 months, ≥4 episodes within 12 months, or AOM episodes that occur while on chemoprophylaxis.
- Tympanostomy tubes may be effective in selective patients.
- Adenoidectomy has limited or no effect.

- Adenotonsillectomy reduced the rate of AOM by 0.7 episode per child only in the 1st year after surgery and had a 15% complications rate.
- OME: Referral for surgery for tympanostomy should be individualized. It can be considered if >4–6 months of bilateral OME and/or >6 months of unilateral OME and/or hearing loss >25 dB or for high-risk individuals at any time.
- Tympanostomy tubes may reduce recurrence of AOM minimally, but it does not lower risk of hearing loss (4)[A].
- Adenoidectomy is indicated in specific cases; tonsillectomy or myringotomy is never indicated (5)[A].

IN-PATIENT CONSIDERATIONS
Initial Stabilization
Outpatient treatment except when surgery is indicated or for AOM in febrile infants <2 months old or children requiring ceftriaxone who also require monitoring for 24 h

ONGOING CARE

FOLLOW-UP RECOMMENDATIONS
Patients with otitis media who do not respond within 48–72 h should be re-evaluated:
- If therapy was delayed and diagnosis is confirmed, start therapy with high-dose amoxicillin.
- If therapy was initiated, consider changing antibiotic; options are limited because macrolides have limited benefit against H. influenza over amoxicillin, and most oral cephalosporins have no improved outcomes.

Patient Monitoring
- AOM: Up to 40% may have persistent middle ear effusion at 1 month, with 10–25% at 3 months.
- OME: Repeat otoscopic or tympanometric exams at 3 months as indicated, as long as OME persists or sooner if red flags (see above).

PROGNOSIS
- See Treatment under General Measures.
- Recurrent AOM and OME: Usually subsides in school-age children; few have complications.

COMPLICATIONS
- AOM: Serious complications are rare:
  - Tympanic membrane perforation/otorrhea
  - Acute mastoiditis
  - Facial nerve paralysis
  - Otitic hydrocephalus
  - Meningitis
  - Hearing impairment
- OME:
  - Speech and language disabilities may occur. Hearing loss is not caused by OME, but in children who are at risk for speech, language, or learning problems (e.g., autism spectrum, syndromes, craniofacial disorders, developmental delay, and children already with speech/language delay), it could lead to further problems because they are less tolerant of hearing impairment.
- Recurrent AOM and OME:
  - Atrophy and scarring of eardrum
  - Chronic perforation and otorrhea
  - Cholesteatoma
  - Permanent hearing loss
  - Chronic mastoiditis
  - Other intracranial suppurative complications

REFERENCES

1. Eskola J, Kilpi T, Palmu A, et al. Efficacy of a pneumococcal conjugate vaccine against acute otitis media. N Engl J Med. 2001;344:403–9.
2. Thanaviratananich S, Laopaiboon M, Vatanasapt P. Once or twice daily versus three times daily amoxicillin with or without clavulanate for the treatment of acute otitis media. Cochrane Database Syst Rev. 2008;CD004975.
3. Coleman C, Moore M. Decongestants and antihistamines for acute otitis media in children. Cochrane Database Syst Rev. 2008;CD001727.
4. Lous J, Burton MJ, Felding JU, et al. Grommets (ventilation tubes) for hearing loss associated with otitis media with effusion in children. Cochrane Database Syst Rev. 2005;CD001801.
5. American Academy of Family Physicians, American Academy of Otolaryngology-Head and Neck Surgery, American Academy of Pediatrics Subcommittee on Otitis Media With Effusion. Otitis media with effusion. Pediatrics. 2004;113: 1412–29.

ADDITIONAL READING
- American Academy of Pediatrics Subcommittee on Management of Acute Otitis Media. Diagnosis and management of acute otitis media. Pediatrics. 2004; 113:1451–65.
- Gould JM, Matz PS et al. Otitis media. Pediatr Rev. 2010;31:102–16.
- Shaikh N, Hoberman A, Kaleida PH, et al. Videos in clinical medicine. Diagnosing otitis media–otoscopy and cerumen removal. N Engl J Med. 2010;362: e62.

See Also (Topic, Algorithm, Electronic Media Element)
Algorithm: Ear pain

CODES

ICD9
- 381.00 Acute nonsuppurative otitis media, unspecified
- 381.3 Other and unspecified chronic nonsuppurative otitis media
- 381.10 Chronic serous otitis media, simple or unspecified

CLINICAL PEARLS
- Pneumatic otoscopy is single most specific and clinically useful test for diagnosis.
- Consider a delay of antibiotics for 24–48 hours in uncomplicated children >2 years old.
- 1st-line treatment is amoxicillin 80–90 mg/kg/d for 10 days for children <2 years old; consider 5- to 7-day course in children >2 years old.
- Erythema and effusion can persist for weeks.
- Antibiotics, antihistamines, and steroids are not indicated for OME.

O

OTOSCLEROSIS (OTOSPONGIOSIS)

Jeffrey D. Wolfrey, MD

 BASICS

DESCRIPTION
- A primary bone dyscrasia involving the otic capsule; it is the leading cause of conductive hearing loss in adults.
- Histologic otosclerosis: Asymptomatic form in which abnormal bone spares vital structures of the ear
- Clinical otosclerosis: Abnormal spongy bone involves ossicular chain or other structures, leading to altered physiology.
- System(s) affected: Sensory; Hearing

EPIDEMIOLOGY
Incidence
- Predominant age:
  - Clinical onset usually in early 20s
  - Peak incidence in 4th and 5th decades
- Predominant gender: Female > Male (2:1)

Pregnancy Considerations
Progression may accelerate during pregnancy. Some women first notice hearing loss at this time.

Prevalence
- 4–8% among whites; 1% among African Americans (histologic form)
- Whites: 5,000/100,000; African Americans: 1,000/100,000 (histologic form)

RISK FACTORS
Unknown

Genetics
- 60% of those affected give positive family history.
- Appears to be transmitted by autosomal dominant gene with variable expressivity

ETIOLOGY
- Unknown
- Fluoride metabolism may play a role; flouride treatment under investigation, as early results demonstrate improved hearing outcomes.

COMMONLY ASSOCIATED CONDITIONS
- Van der Hoeve syndrome (rare triad of osteogenesis imperfecta, blue sclera, and otospongiosis)
- Tinnitus, usually low frequency

 DIAGNOSIS

HISTORY
- Progressive conductive hearing loss, usually with well-preserved speech discrimination
- Patients often soft spoken and aware they seem to hear better in noisy environments

PHYSICAL EXAM
Schwartze sign: Reddish hue in front of oval window, on promontory at otoscopic exam

DIAGNOSTIC TESTS & INTERPRETATION
Imaging
Initial approach
Coaxial or computed tomography scan sometimes helpful

Diagnostic Procedures/Surgery
Tuning fork and audiometric testing for conductive and/or sensorineural hearing loss:
- Will lateralize to more impaired ear with Weber test
- Conductive hearing loss; may be as severe as the 60dB maximum
- May have sensorineural hearing loss with cochlear involvement
- Carhart notch: A dip in bone conductive threshold at 2,000 Hz on audiometric testing

Pathological Findings
- Gross:
  - Off-white to reddish bone formation, most often located anterior to the oval window and extending to involve the stapedial footplate; sometimes covers entire oval window (obliterative); may be found anywhere in otic capsule
  - Bilateral in 75% of patients
- Micro:
  - Spongy-appearing bone with increased vascular spaces
  - Osteoblasts and osteoclasts are plentiful.

DIFFERENTIAL DIAGNOSIS
- Chronic suppurative otitis media
- Serous otitis media
- External auditory canal occlusion
- Ossicular chain disruption
- Congenital fixation of stapes
- Presbycusis
- Advanced otosclerosis mimics sensorineural deafness.

ALERT
- Important differential diagnosis for presbycusis
- Surgical results similar in older vs younger patient cohorts (1)[A]

TREATMENT

MEDICATION

No specific drug therapy, but sodium fluoride, vitamin D, and calcium gluconate have been tried, especially in cases of predominantly sensorineural hearing loss.

SURGERY/OTHER PROCEDURES

- Surgical correction (stapedectomy):
  - Usually involves mobilization or removal of the stapedial footplate with placement of a stapes prosthesis
  - Recent procedural innovations have involved use of lasers.
  - Cochlear implantation may achieve better results in advanced cases (2)[B].
- Relative indications for surgery include negative Rinne test (air-bone audiometric gap at least 20 dB) and bilateral involvement.

ONGOING CARE

FOLLOW-UP RECOMMENDATIONS

- No restrictions on activity
- Hearing aids

Patient Monitoring

Interval audiometric testing

PATIENT EDUCATION

- Because speech discrimination is usually preserved, patients should be advised of the possible benefit from hearing aids as an alternative or adjunct to surgery.

- Mayo Foundation for Medical Education and Research, Section of Patient and Health Education, Sieber Subway, Rochester, MN 55905; (507) 284-8140

PROGNOSIS

- Progressive hearing loss if not treated
- Surgery improves hearing by at least 15 dB in 90% of patients.

COMPLICATIONS

Surgical risks include chorda tympani nerve injury, tympanic membrane laceration, ossicular chain disruption, otitis media and externa, labyrinthitis, granuloma formation, perilymph fistulas, and total deafness ("dead ear").

REFERENCES

1. Meyer TA, Lambert PR. Primary and revision stapedectomy in elderly patients. *Curr Opin Otolaryngol Head Neck Surg*. 2004;12:387–92.
2. Berrettini S, Burdo S, Forli F, et al. Far advanced otosclerosis: stapes surgery or cochlear implantation? *J Otolaryngol*. 2004;33:165–71.

ADDITIONAL READING

- Lee KJ. *Essential Otolaryngology: Head & Neck Surgery*, 4th ed. New Hyde Park, NY: Medical Examination Publishing, 1987.
- Weber PC, Klein AJ. Hearing loss. *Med Clin North Am*. 1999;83:125–37, ix.

See Also (Topic, Algorithm, Electronic Media Element)

Hearing Loss

CODES

ICD9

- 387.2 Cochlear otosclerosis
- 387.9 Otosclerosis, unspecified

CLINICAL PEARLS

- The audiometric signature of otosclerosis is a dip in conductive hearing at 2,000 Hz.
- Hearing aids are helpful in patients with preserved speech discrimination.
- Bilateral involvement and an air-bone audiometric gap of 20 dB or more are indications for surgery.

O

OVARIAN CANCER

Susan L. Zweizig, MD
Elizabeth B. Pelkofski, MD

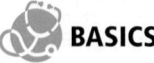 **BASICS**

There are over 21,000 new cases of ovarian cancer annually, and 14,000 women will die of their disease, making this the most lethal of gynecologic cancers.

DESCRIPTION

Malignancy that arises from the epithelium (85–90%), stroma, or germ cells of the ovary; also, tumors metastatic to the ovary; histologic types include:

- Epithelial:
  - Serous (tubal epithelium)
  - Mucinous (cervical and GI mucinous epithelium)
  - Endometrioid (endometrial epithelium)
  - Clear cell (mesonephroid)
  - Brenner (transitional cell epithelium)
  - Carcinosarcoma
- Stromal:
  - Granulosa cell tumor
  - Theca cell tumor
  - Sertoli–Leydig cell tumors
  - Gynandroblastoma
  - Lipid cell tumor
- Germ cell:
  - Teratoma (immature)
  - Dysgerminoma
  - Embryonal carcinoma
  - Gonadoblastoma
  - Endodermal sinus tumor
  - Embryonal carcinoma
  - Choriocarcinoma
- Metastatic disease from:
  - Breast
  - Endometrium
  - Lymphoma
  - GI tract (Krukenberg tumor)
  - Primary peritoneal
- System(s) affected: GI; Reproductive; Endocrine; Metabolic

EPIDEMIOLOGY

Incidence
- 21,550 new cases/year in the US; 14,600 deaths/year
- Leading cause of gynecologic cancer death in women; mortality from ovarian cancer has decreased only slightly during the last 4 decades.
- 62% diagnosed at advanced stage
- Predominant age:
  - Epithelial: Mid-50s
  - Germ cell malignancies: Usually observed in patients <20 years of age

Prevalence
Lifetime risk for general population: 1 in 70 women develops ovarian cancer.

RISK FACTORS
- 90% of ovarian cancer is sporadic and not inherited, but family history is the most significant risk factor. 1 1st-degree relative increases risk to 5%; 2 relatives, to 7%; individuals in families with familial cancer syndromes have 20–60% risk of developing ovarian cancer.
- Nulligravity (or infertility), early menarche, late menopause, endometriosis
- Environmental (talc, smoking, obesity)

Genetics
- Breast/ovarian cancer syndrome: Early-onset breast or ovarian cancer, autosomal dominant transmission, usually associated with *BRCA-1* or *BRCA-2* mutation
- Lynch II syndrome: Autosomal dominant inheritance; increased risk for colorectal, endometrial, stomach, small bowel, breast, pancreas, and ovarian cancers; defect in mismatch repair genes

GENERAL PREVENTION
For epithelial cancer, frequency of ovulation appears to be important. The following factors are protective:
- Use of oral contraceptives: 5 years of use decreases risk by 20%; 15 years, by 50%.
- Multiparity
- Breastfeeding
- Tubal ligation or hysterectomy:
  - The progestin component of oral contraceptive preparations (OCPs) may protect against ovarian cancer by regulating apoptosis of the ovarian epithelium.
  - Recent studies have shown that no clear association exists between ovarian cancer and use of ovulation-induction agents such as clomiphene, but more long-term studies are necessary (1)[B].
  - Nonsteroidal anti-inflammatory drug (NSAID) and acetaminophen use have been shown to reduce risk of ovarian cancer (2)[B].
  - Women with family histories of ovarian cancer or premenopausal breast cancer should be referred for genetic counseling (3)[B].
  - Prophylactic oophorectomy is advised for mutation carriers after child-bearing is completed or by age 35 (3)[B]. Risk of primary peritoneal carcinoma is 1% after prophylactic oophorectomy.

- Screening: No effective screening exists for ovarian cancer:
  - Routine use of CA-125 and transvaginal ultrasound for screening in women of average risk is discouraged. Annual pelvic examinations are recommended, particularly in postmenopausal women. An adnexal mass in a premenarchal female or a palpable adnexa in a postmenopausal female warrants further evaluation.
  - Women with a family history of a hereditary ovarian cancer syndrome should undergo pelvic examinations, CA-125 determination, and transvaginal ultrasonography every 6–12 months beginning at ages 25–35.

PATHOPHYSIOLOGY
- Malignant transformation of the ovarian epithelium from repeated minor trauma during ovulation may lead to this change.
- Most ovarian cancer (62%) presents as advanced disease. Metastatic disease may develop at the same time as the primary tumor.

COMMONLY ASSOCIATED CONDITIONS
- Ascites
- Pleural effusion
- Decrease of serum albumin
- Breast carcinoma
- Bowel obstruction
- Carcinomatosis

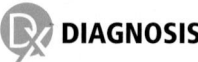 **DIAGNOSIS**

HISTORY
- Bloating
- Early satiety, anorexia, dyspepsia
- Sense of abdominal fullness, increased abdominal size
- Abdominopelvic pain or cramping
- Urinary frequency or urgency in absence of infection
- Fatigue
- Dyspareunia
- Weight loss
- Severe pain secondary to ovarian rupture or torsion most frequent in germ cell tumors
- Precocious puberty (choriocarcinoma, embryonal carcinoma)

PHYSICAL EXAM
- Ascites
- Cul de sac and/or pelvic nodularity
- Pelvic mass
- Pleural effusion
- Omental mass
- Cachexia
- Adenopathy
- Hirsutism in androgen-secreting germ cell tumors

DIAGNOSTIC TESTS & INTERPRETATION
Lab
Initial lab tests
- CA-125 (not specific for ovarian cancer)
- Liver function tests (LFTs) to rule out hepatic disease
- Complete blood count (CBC)
- Urinalysis
- Serum albumin
- Carcinoembryonic antigen (CEA) if GI primary suspected
- If nonepithelial tumor suspected: Chorionic gonadotropin (β-hCG [dysgerminoma, choriocarcinoma, embryonal carcinoma]), α-fetoprotein (endodermal sinus tumor, embryonal carcinoma), lactate dehydrogenase (LDH [dysgerminoma]), or inhibin (granulosa cell tumor)

Follow-Up & Special Considerations
Disorders that may alter lab results: CA-125 may be elevated from gynecologic causes (e.g., menses, pregnancy, endometriosis, peritonitis, myomas, pelvic inflammatory disease) and with ascites, pleural effusion, congestive heart failure (CHF), pancreatitis, systemic lupus erythematosus (SLE), or liver disease.

Imaging
Initial approach
- Pelvic ultrasound
- CXR
- Abdominopelvic CT scan with contrast material

Follow-Up & Special Considerations
- Patients with ovarian cancer need current mammography.
- Barium enema or colonoscopy if a colon primary is suspected

Diagnostic Procedures/Surgery
- Surgery is necessary for definitive diagnosis.
- Endometrial biopsy if abnormal bleeding present
- Paracentesis if patient not an operative candidate

Pathological Findings
Epithelial ovarian cancer commonly involves the peritoneal surfaces of the abdomen and pelvis, especially the cul de sac, paracolic gutters, and diaphragmatic surfaces.

DIFFERENTIAL DIAGNOSIS
- GI, fallopian, or endometrial malignancies
- Irritable bowel syndrome
- Colitis
- Hepatic failure with ascites
- Diverticulitis
- Pelvic kidney
- Tubo-ovarian abscess or hydrosalpinx
- Uterine fibroids
- Endometriomas
- Physiologic cysts
- Benign or borderline neoplasms

 TREATMENT

MEDICATION
First Line
- After surgery, most patients will require chemotherapy. Stage 1a, grade 1 and most stage 1b, grade 1 tumors do not require adjuvant therapy. Patients with clear cell carcinomas, grade 3 tumors, or tumors staged 1c or worse require adjuvant therapy. Patients should be encouraged to participate in clinical trials whenever possible.
- Paclitaxel (Taxol) is recommended in combination with platinum-based therapy as the 1st-line treatment of epithelial ovarian cancer (4)[A].
- Intraperitoneal (IP) chemotherapy in combination with IV chemotherapy improves survival in advanced ovarian cancer (5)[A]. IP chemotherapy is associated with more toxicity.
- Contraindications: Poor functional status, excessive toxicity, hypersensitivity
- Precautions: All regimens cause bone marrow suppression. Cisplatin is associated with ototoxicity, renal toxicity, and peripheral neuropathy. Taxol can cause neutropenia and neuropathy.
- Antiemetic: Ondansetron (Zofran), dronabinol (Marinol), metoclopramide (Reglan), prochlorperazine (Compazine), promethazine (Phenergan)

Second Line
- Liposomal doxorubicin
- Carboplatin/gemcitabine
- Topotecan
- Taxotere
- Etoposide
- Bevacizumab
- Cyclophosphamide
- Tamoxifen may be used in recurrent disease when chemotherapy is not appropriate (6)[B].

SURGERY/OTHER PROCEDURES
- Surgical exploration with staging and debulking is critical. Maximal cytoreduction of tumor burden enhances effectiveness of adjuvant therapy and is associated with longer survival.
- For epithelial malignancies, careful staging, tumor excision/debulking includes:
  – Cytologic evaluation of peritoneal fluid (or washings from peritoneal lavage)
  – Bilateral salpingo-oophorectomy with hysterectomy and tumor reductive surgery
  – Excision of omentum
  – Inspection and palpation of peritoneal surfaces
  – Cytologic smear of right hemidiaphragmatic surface
  – Biopsy of adhesions or any suspicious areas
  – Biopsy of paracolic recesses, pelvic sidewalls, posterior cul de sac, and bladder peritoneum
  – Pelvic and para-aortic lymph node biopsies
- Germ cell cancers (less likely to be bilateral): Salpingo-oophorectomy (unilateral if only 1 ovary involved) in young patient

 ONGOING CARE

PROGNOSIS
5-year survival rates for ovarian cancer based on FIGO data:

Stage I	a 90%	b 86%	c 83%
Stage II	a 71%	b 66%	c 71%
Stage III	a 47%	b 42%	c 33%
Stage IV	19%		

COMPLICATIONS
- Pleural effusion
- Pseudomyxoma peritonei
- Ascites
- Toxicity of chemotherapy
- Bowel obstruction
- Malnutrition
- Electrolyte disturbances
- Fistula formation

REFERENCES
1. Mahdavi A, Pejovic T, Nezhat F. Induction of ovulation and ovarian cancer: a critical review of the literature. *Fertil Steril*. 2006;85:819–26.
2. Collaborative Group on epidemiological Studies of Ovarian cancer: Beral V; Doll R; Hermon C, et al. Ovarian cancer and oral contraceptives: Collaborative reanalysis of data from 45 epidemiological studies including 23,257 women with ovarian cancer and 87,303 controls. *Lancet*. 2008;371:303–14.
3. Eisen A, Rebbeck TR, Wood WC, et al. Prophylactic surgery in women with a hereditary predisposition to breast and ovarian cancer. *J Clin Oncol*. 2000;18:1980–95.
4. McGuire WP, Hoskins WJ, Brady MF, et al. Cyclophosphamide and cisplatin compared with paclitaxel and cisplatin in patients with stage III and stage IV ovarian cancer. *N Engl J Med*. 1996;334:1–6.
5. Armstrong DK, Bundy B, Wenzel L, et al. Intraperitoneal cisplatin and paclitaxel in ovarian cancer. *N Engl J Med*. 2006;354:34–43.
6. Orlando M, Costanzo, MV, Chacon RD. Randomized trial of combination chemotherapy versus monotherapy in relapsed ovarian carcinoma: a meta-analysis of published data. *J Clin Oncol*. 2007;25:280s.

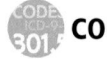 **CODES**

ICD9
183.0 Malignant neoplasm of ovary

CLINICAL PEARLS
- Family history of ovarian cancer or early-onset breast cancer is the most significant risk factor for the development of ovarian cancer, yet the vast majority of cases remain sporadic and not inherited.
- The diagnosis of ovarian cancer should be suspected in women with persistent bloating, upper abdominal discomfort, or gastrointestinal symptoms of unknown etiology.

O

OVARIAN HYPERSTIMULATION SYNDROME (OHSS)

Kimberly E. Liu, MD, FRCSC
Ellen Greenblatt, BSC, MDCM

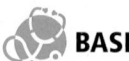 **BASICS**

DESCRIPTION
- Iatrogenic physiologic complication of controlled ovarian hyperstimulation (most often related to treatment for infertility)
- Results in ovarian enlargement, increased vascular permeability with resulting 3rd-space loss and intravascular fluid depletion, electrolyte imbalance, hemoconcentration, and ascites
- Classification of OHSS is based on clinical symptoms and ultrasound findings.
  - Mild: Abdominal distension and discomfort
  - Moderate: Abdominal distension, enlarged ovaries (8–10 cm^3) and ascites on ultrasound (largest pocket <3 cm)
  - Severe: Clinical evidence of ascites and/or hydrothorax, hemoconcentration >45%
  - Critical: hemoconcentration >55%, creatinine clearance <50 mL/min, renal failure, thromboembolism, ARDS
- Symptoms of OHSS may occur early (within 10 days of hCG administration) or late (more than 10 days after hCG administration). Late OHSS is usually associated with a pregnancy and may often be more severe.

EPIDEMIOLOGY
Incidence
- Predominant age: Women of reproductive age
- With controlled ovarian hyperstimulation (COH) and in vitro fertilization (IVF):
  - Mild OHSS: 20–33% of cycles
  - Moderate OHSS: 3–6% of cycles
  - Severe OHSS: 0.1–2% of cycles

RISK FACTORS
- Previous history of OHSS
- Young age
- Low body weight
- Polycystic ovary syndrome (PCOS) or polycystic ovaries on ultrasound
- Large number of resting follicles (>10 follicles between 2 and 8 mm) per ovary
- High doses of gonadotropins
- Large number of intermediate-sized follicles
- Number of oocytes retrieved
- Rapidly rising estradiol levels
- High estradiol levels >3000/4000 pg/mL
- Use of human chorionic gonadotropin (hCG) for luteal support
- Achievement of a pregnancy
- Multiple pregnancy

GENERAL PREVENTION
- Patients who have had OHSS are more at risk for OHSS in the future, and this should be taken into consideration in subsequent treatment cycles. Patients need to inform their health care providers of a history of OHSS when considering further assisted reproductive technology treatment.

- If a patient is noted to be at high risk of OHSS, the stimulation and monitoring protocol may be modified to reflect this risk. In some circumstances, consideration should be given to canceling the stimulation by withholding the preovulatory injection of hCG, proceeding with a lower dose of hCG, the use of a GnRH agonist to trigger ovulation in GnRH antagonist cycles, "coasting" or withholding stimulatory drugs for several days to allow for estradiol levels to plateau or decrease, avoiding the use of hCG for luteal supporting, or freezing all viable embryos without proceeding with an embryo transfer (1)[B].
- Recent evidence suggests that the off-label use of dopamine agonists (cabergoline 0.5 mg) after hCG administration may decrease the incidence of OHSS (2)[A].

PATHOPHYSIOLOGY
- Ovarian hyperstimulation leads to increased capillary permeability and intravascular fluid shifts.
- Fluid shifts can lead to ascites and pleural effusions.
- Intravascular volume depletion can lead to hemoconcentration, decreased renal perfusion, and thrombosis.
- The ovarian renin–angiotensin system, cytokines, and other inflammatory mediators such as vascular endothelial growth factor (VEGF) may play a role in the pathophysiology of OHSS.

ETIOLOGY
- OHSS is an iatrogenic syndrome that occurs during controlled ovarian hyperstimulation (COH) for infertility treatment.
- Generally, OHSS is associated with the use of exogenous gonadotropins such as recombinant or purified follicle-stimulating hormone (FSH).
- OHSS rarely has been associated with types of ovarian stimulation such as clomiphene citrate.

COMMONLY ASSOCIATED CONDITIONS
- Infertility
- PCOS
- Assisted reproductive technologies

DIAGNOSIS

OHSS is a clinical diagnosis based on history, physical exam, ultrasound findings, and laboratory results.

HISTORY
- Details of stimulation cycle:
  - Medications used
  - Date of oocyte retrieval and embryo transfer
- Symptoms of dehydration
- Abdominal pain and distension
- Nausea, vomiting, diarrhea
- Shortness of breath
- Loss of appetite
- Weight changes
- Fluid intake
- Lethargy
- Risks factors such as PCOS or previous OHSS

PHYSICAL EXAM
- Vital signs, including O$_2$ saturation if shortness of breath
- Weight (daily)
- Monitoring of ins and outs (daily or more often as needed)
- Chest and cardiovascular exam
- Abdominal circumference measured at the umbilicus (daily)
- Gentle abdominal exam to detect ascites

ALERT
Pelvic and bimanual examinations are contraindicated to avoid ovarian hemorrhage or rupture.

DIAGNOSTIC TESTS & INTERPRETATION
Lab
Initial lab tests
- CBC
  - Hemoconcentration (hematocrit >45% indicates severe disease, >55% indicates critical disease)
  - WBC >15,000 indicates severe disease
- Electrolytes to look for hyponatremia and hyperkalemia
- Renal function tests
- Liver enzymes
- Coagulation profile
- β-hCG

Follow-Up & Special Considerations
For patients with mild or moderate OHSS being monitored as an outpatient, CBC and electrolytes should be performed every 1–2 days, until improvement in symptoms.

Imaging
Initial approach
- Abdominal/pelvic ultrasound to assess ovarian size, ovarian torsion or rupture, and abdominal ascites
- CXR to evaluate pleural effusion in presence of shortness of breath

Follow-Up & Special Considerations
Repeat abdominal/pelvic ultrasound as needed to assess ascites and guide management for paracentesis.

Pathological Findings
- Ovarian enlargement
- Decreased renal perfusion
- Thromboembolism
- Abdominal ascites
- Pleural effusions
- Pericardial effusions

DIFFERENTIAL DIAGNOSIS
- Hemorrhagic ovarian cyst
- Ovarian torsion
- Ectopic pregnancy
- Pelvic infection

TREATMENT

MEDICATION

- Heparin 5,000 units SC every 8–12 hours; all hospitalized patients should be on anticoagulation prophylaxis and graduated compression stockings to prevent thrombotic events (3)[C].
- Full anticoagulation therapy should be started if there is evidence of a thromboembolic event.

ADDITIONAL TREATMENT

General Measures

- Mild to moderate OHSS: Generally managed as outpatient
  - Oral fluid intake of at least 1 L daily of a balanced electrolyte solution (sports drinks) (3)[C].
  - Monitor daily weight, abdominal circumference, and urine output (3)[C].
  - Avoid physical exertion or abdominal trauma.
  - Monitor for development of further symptoms.
  - Frequent follow-up is required.
  - For moderate OHSS, frequent assessments every 1–2 days including a physical examination and blood work should occur.
  - Consider hospitalization with worsening signs or symptoms:
    - Severe abdominal pain
    - Severe oliguria or anuria
    - Tense ascites
    - Dyspnea or tachypnea
    - Hypotension, dizziness, or syncope
    - Severe electrolyte imbalance: Hyponatremia <135 mEq/L, hyperkalemia >5 mEq/L, hemocrit >45%
- Severe OHSS: Should be managed as an in-patient.
  - Daily weight and abdominal circumference
  - Frequent monitoring of vital signs every 2–8 hours
  - Strict monitoring of input and output to maintain urine output of 20–30 cc/hour
  - Bed rest or reduced activity; the enlarged ovaries are at risk of torsion and ovarian hemorrhage either spontaneously or from injury or trauma.
  - With severe illness, oral fluids should be limited and rehydration provided with IV fluids until evidence of symptom resolution such as spontaneous diuresis.
  - IV fluids should be administered to maintain urine output to 20–30 mL/hour. Normal saline with 5% dextrose is preferred to Ringer's lactate (3)[C].
  - Once 3rd-space edema reenters the intravascular space, hemoconcentration reverses, and the patient begins to diurese spontaneously.
  - Monitor leukocyte count, hematocrit and hemoglobin, electrolytes, creatinine, and liver enzymes.
  - Thrombosis prophylaxis (3)[C]
  - Intensive monitoring may be required for pulmonary support in cases of acute respiratory distress syndrome, thromboembolic events, or for renal failure.

Issues for Referral

Consultation with a reproductive endocrinology specialist or a gynecologist with experience in the management of OHSS and its complications.

SURGERY/OTHER PROCEDURES

- Paracentesis/thoracentesis may be required for symptomatic control and for pulmonary and/or renal compromise. An ultrasound-guided approach for paracentesis is recommended to avoid the enlarged ovaries.

  - Indications for paracentesis include severe discomfort or pain, respiratory compromise, evidence of hydrothorax, or persistent oliguria/anuria despite adequate fluid replacement.
- Surgery should be avoided whenever possible in these patients.
- When ovarian hemorrhage is suspected, surgery may be necessary. The goal should be hemostasis, and the ovaries should be conserved when possible.
- In a situation of ovarian torsion, surgery may be performed to attempt to revascularize the ovary by unwinding the adnexa.

IN-PATIENT CONSIDERATIONS

Inpatients should have a CBC and electrolytes daily. Renal function, liver enzymes, and coagulation profile should be repeated as needed.

Initial Stabilization

Vital signs and O_2 saturation

Admission Criteria

- Abdominal pain suspicious of torsion or hemorrhage
- Intolerance of food or liquids
- Hypotension
- Significant ascites or plural effusions
- Hemoconcentration: Hematocrit >50%; white blood cell (WBC) count >25,000
- Hyponatremia (Na <135 mEq/L)
- Hyperkalemia (K >5.0 mEq/L)

IV Fluids

- With severe illness, IV fluid rehydration should be used. After an initial bolus of 500–1,000 mL, fluid administration should continue to maintain a urine output of at least 20–30 mL/hour. D_5NS is preferred over Ringer's lactate because of the risk of hyponatremia.
- Albumin 25% (50–100 g) should be reserved for situations in which IV fluids are inadequate to maintain hemodynamic stability or urine output.
- Diuretics should be used cautiously and only after intravascular volume has been restored. Diuretics may aggravate hypovolemia and hemoconcentration.

Discharge Criteria

- Tolerating oral liquids and diet
- Resolution of hemoconcentration and electrolyte imbalances
- Adequate urine output

ONGOING CARE

FOLLOW-UP RECOMMENDATIONS

Patients discharged from the hospital should be followed with frequent health care provider contact until symptom resolution.

Patient Monitoring

Patients who have conceived should have an early ultrasound to confirm pregnancy and rule out multiple gestations and then routine antenatal care as indicated by their pregnancy.

DIET

Consume 1.0–1.5 L daily of a balanced salt solution, such as a sports drink, until resolution of symptoms.

PATIENT EDUCATION

- Monitor oral intake and urinary output.
- Reduce activity to avoid abdominal trauma or impact.
- www.acog.org

PROGNOSIS

OHSS is a self-limiting disease that will run its course over 10–14 days in the absence of an ensuing pregnancy and may persist for weeks in a pregnant patient. Supportive treatment is initiated to prevent further deterioration of the patient's condition.

COMPLICATIONS

- Ovarian hemorrhage
- Ovarian torsion
- Arterial and venous thrombosis
- Acute respiratory distress syndrome
- Liver failure
- Renal failure

Pregnancy Considerations

- Patients who conceive a multiple gestation are at higher risk of OHSS.
- Studies have shown an increased risk of prematurity, low birth weight, pregnancy-induced hypertension, and gestational diabetes in women who had severe OHSS (4)[B].

REFERENCES

1. Vloeberghs V, Peeraer K, Pexsters A, et al. Ovarian hyperstimulation syndrome and complications of ART. Best Pract Res Clin Obstet Gynaecol. 2009;23: 691–709.
2. Youssef MA, van Wely M, Hassan MA, et al. Can dopamine agonists reduce the incidence and severity of OHSS in IVF/ICSI treatment cycles? A systematic review and meta-analysis. Human reproduction update. 2010;
3. Practice Committee of American Society for Reproductive Medicine. Ovarian hyperstimulation syndrome. Fertil Steril. 2008;90:S188–93.
4. Raziel A, Schachter M, Friedler S, et al. Outcome of IVF pregnancies following severe OHSS. Reprod Biomed Online. 2009;19:61–5.

CODES

ICD9

256.1 Other ovarian hyperfunction

CLINICAL PEARLS

- Patients who have had OHSS are more at risk for OHSS in the future, and this should be taken into consideration in subsequent treatment cycles.
- Abdominal and pelvic exams are contraindicated in patients with OHSS to avoid ovarian hemorrhage or rupture.
- OHSS is a self-limiting disease that will run its course over 10–14 days in the absence of an ensuing pregnancy and may persist for weeks in a pregnant patient. Management is mainly supportive to prevent and identify complications until resolution of symptoms.

0

OVARIAN TUMOR (BENIGN)

Lisa Clemons, MD

BASICS

DESCRIPTION
- The ovaries are a source of many tumor types (benign and malignant) because of the histologic variety of their constituent cells.
- Benign ovarian tumors create difficulties in differential diagnosis because of the need to identify malignancy and discriminate tumor from cysts, infectious lesions, ectopic pregnancy, and endometriomas.
- Tumors are often clinically silent until well developed; may be solid, cystic, or mixed; and they may be functional (producing sex steroids, as with arrhenoblastomas and gynandroblastomas) or nonfunctional.
- System(s) affected: Endocrine/Metabolic; Reproductive

Geriatric Considerations
Because incidence of malignancy increases with age, postmenopausal patients warrant comprehensive evaluation and follow-up.

Pediatric Considerations
Malignancy must be ruled out in premenarchal patients. Early neonatal cysts are rare.

EPIDEMIOLOGY
Incidence
- 30% of regularly cycling females
- 50% of women without regular cycles
- Predominant age: Premenarchal girls have a 5–35% risk of cancer in an ovarian tumor, and postmenopausal women have a 30% risk.

RISK FACTORS
- As yet poorly characterized for benign tumors; cigarette smoking increases the relative risk for developing functional ovarian cysts 2-fold.
- Possible contributory factors are early menarche, obesity, infertility, and hypothyroidism.
- Risks for ovarian cancer include age >60 years; early menarche; late menopause; nulliparity; infertility; family history of ovarian, breast, or colon cancer; or a personal history of breast or colon cancer; or BRCA mutation.
- Risk for ovarian cancer is decreased in women who have used OCPs, been pregnant, or breastfed.

GENERAL PREVENTION
- Although oral contraceptives do not appear to increase rates of cyst resorption, they do decrease risk for forming new ovarian cysts.
- A large British cohort of 5,479 women demonstrated that the resection of benign cysts has no impact on future risk for ovarian cancer.

- A case-control study of 299 women found no evidence that ovulation-induction treatment predisposes women to the development of borderline ovarian growths.

ETIOLOGY
- Endometriosis with localized, repeated ovarian hemorrhage
- Physiologic cysts
- Tumorigenesis, with genetics as yet poorly defined

Dx DIAGNOSIS

- A careful history is important.
- Usually asymptomatic
- Pain related to torsion, endometriosis, or rupture

HISTORY
- Early satiety
- Dyspepsia/bloating
- Increased abdominal girth
- Bowel pressure or bladder pressure sensations
- Menstrual irregularities
- Dyspareunia
- Hirsutism or sexual precocity
- Severe acne
- Deepening of the voice
- Virilization

PHYSICAL EXAM
- Examine lymph nodes for enlargement.
- Chest auscultation can reveal a pleural effusion.
- Abdominal exam may identify ascites, masses, or increased abdominal girth.
- Pelvic exam is recommended.

DIAGNOSTIC TESTS & INTERPRETATION
Lab
Initial lab tests
- Complete blood count for WBCs helpful if pelvic inflammatory disease (PID) suspected
- Pregnancy test
- Urinalysis
- Serum estrogens and androgens if signs of androgen excess
- Serum tumor markers may be considered but often confuse rather than help to resolve diagnosis; choose carefully:
  – CA-125 should not be ordered in a premenopausal patient for screening purposes. If an ovarian tumor in a premenopausal patient is highly suspicious for cancer by US, a CA-125 level greater than 200 u is concerning. In a postmenopausal patient, cancer must be ruled out and a CA-125 >35 u is concerning.
  – α-Fetoprotein and human chorionic gonadotropin (hCG) can be ordered for suspected germ call tumor

- Disorders that may alter lab results:
  – CA-125: Endometriosis, peritonitis, PID, Meigs syndrome, uterine fibroids, hepatitis, pancreatitis, systemic lupus erythematosus, diverticulitis
  – β-hCG: Pregnancy, hydatidiform mole
  – α-Fetoprotein: Hepatocellular carcinoma, hepatic cirrhosis, acute or chronic hepatitis

Imaging
- Transvaginal US is the best means to determine the architecture of an ovarian cyst or mass.
- Transvaginal ultrasonography may differentiate tumors from other pelvic lesions and identify features that place the patient at greater risk for malignancy (e.g., solid component, papillations, multiple septations, ascites, bilaterality, fixed and irregular, rapidly enlarging, accompanied by cul-de-sac nodules).
- Transabdominal US can help identify ascites.
- Color-flow Doppler evaluation also may be helpful. Color flow to the solid component of the tumor is concerning for cancer. Gray scale may be an important method of differential diagnosis of ovarian growths.
- MRI with apparent diffusion coefficient mapping may be useful in the differential diagnosis of cystic masses. MRI can be helpful in better defining masses in women with low risk of ovarian cancer but who have an "indeterminant" mass on US.
- Cystoscopy if hematuria is present in the absence of infection or if IV pyelogram reveals intravesical surface irregularity
- Abdominopelvic CT scan with contrast material, if MRI unavailable
- Barium enema, colonoscopy, or IV pyelogram, as indicated

Diagnostic Procedures/Surgery
Exploratory laparoscopy or laparotomy

Pathological Findings
- Follicular (fluid distension of atretic follicle) and corpus luteum cysts (corpus luteum hematoma). Follicular cysts are the most common ovarian cysts in the premenopausal nonpregnant female.
- Endometrioma
- Pregnancy luteoma (composed of hyperplastic stromal theca–lutein cells)
- Serous and mucinous cystadenomas and mixed serous/mucinous cystadenomas
- Granulosa cell tumors
- Benign connective tissue tumors (thecomas, fibromas, Brenner tumors)
- Cystic teratoma (dermoid cyst); teratomas are the most common benign neoplasms.
- Germinal inclusion cyst (regarded by some as the precursor for epithelial ovarian cancer)

Pregnancy Considerations
- Most cysts discovered during pregnancy are corpus luteum or follicular cysts.
- The 2 most commonly encountered tumors during pregnancy are cystadenomas (serous or mucinous) and dermoid cysts.

DIFFERENTIAL DIAGNOSIS
- Ovarian malignancies
- Endometrioma
- Uterine leiomyoma
- Appendicular cysts
- Diverticulitis or bowel abscess
- PID with tubo-ovarian abscess
- Distended urinary bladder
- Ectopic pregnancy
- Hydrosalpinx
- Functional cysts (follicular and corpus luteum cysts)
- Polycystic ovaries
- Ovarian lipoma

TREATMENT

MEDICATION
Oral contraceptives decrease risk for forming new ovarian cysts. They do not aid in resorption of current ovarian cysts.

First Line
NSAIDs or narcotics may be helpful for discomfort.

ADDITIONAL TREATMENT
General Measures
- In premenopausal patients with cystic lesions <10 cm in diameter, simple observation for 4–6 weeks is acceptable. No evidence suggests that use of a contraceptive pill is more effective than time alone in facilitating ovarian cyst resorption.
- If a large cyst remains unchanged after 4–6 weeks of observation, then surgical exploration is indicated.
- Unilocular ovarian cysts <5 cm in premenopausal patients were not considered suspicious.

SURGERY/OTHER PROCEDURES
- Cystectomy or wedge resection for cyst with benign features
- Surgical removal of tumor to establish diagnosis when:
  - Premenopausal cysts >5 cm that persist >12 weeks
  - Mass is solid.
  - Mass is >10 cm.
  - Mass in a premenarchal or postmenopausal female
  - Suspicion of torsion or rupture
  - Postmenopausal cysts
  - Cysts with worrisome features on US (e.g., papillations)
  - For masses that are worrisome for cancer, consider referral to a gyn-oncologist for initial surgery.

ONGOING CARE

FOLLOW-UP RECOMMENDATIONS
Patient Monitoring
- Most require only yearly exams.
- Varies by diagnosis

PATIENT EDUCATION
A variety of excellent patient education materials (e.g., "Ovarian Cyst") can be downloaded from the American Association of Family Physicians and American College of Obstetricians and Gynecologists Internet sites: http://www.aafp.org/afp and http://www.acog.com.

PROGNOSIS
Complete cure

COMPLICATIONS
Complications of untreated dermoid and mucinous cysts may include rupture and pseudomyxoma peritonei.

ADDITIONAL READING
- Borgfeldt C, Andolf E. Cancer risk after hospital discharge diagnosis of benign ovarian cysts and endometriosis. *Acta Obstet Gynecol Scand*. 2004;83:395–400.
- Clarke-Pearson D. Screening for Ovarian Cancer. *NEJM*. 2009;(361):170–7.
- Crayford TJ, Campbell S, Bourne TH, et al. Benign ovarian cysts and ovarian cancer: a cohort study with implications for screening. *Lancet*. 2000;355:1060–3.
- Cusidó M, Fábregas R, Pere BS, et al. Ovulation induction treatment and risk of borderline ovarian tumors. *Gynecol Endocrinol*. 2007;23:373–6.
- Givens V, Mitchell G. Diagnosis and Management of Adnexal Masses. *AAFP*; 2009;80(8):815–822.
- Holt VL, Cushing-Haugen KL, Daling JR. Oral contraceptives, tubal sterilization, and functional ovarian cyst risk. *Obstet Gynecol*. 2003;102:252–8.
- Iyer VR, Lee SI, et al. MRI, CT, and PET/CT for ovarian cancer detection and adnexal lesion characterization. *AJR Am J Roentgenol*. 2010;194:311–21.

- Kirilovas D, Schedvins K, Naessén T, et al. Conversion of circulating estrone sulfate to 17beta-estradiol by ovarian tumor tissue: a possible mechanism behind elevated circulating concentrations of 17beta-estradiol in postmenopausal women with ovarian tumors. *Gynecol Endocrinol*. 2007;23:25–8.
- Labarge PY, et al. Short-term morbidity and long-term recurrence rate of ovarian dermoid cysts treated by laparoscopy vs. laparotomy. *J Obstet Gynecol Can*. 2006;28(9):789–93.
- Marchesiini AC, et al. A critical analysis of Doppler velocimetry in the differential of malignant and benign ovarian masses. *J Women Health*. 2008;17(10):97–102.
- Nakayama T, et al. Diffusion-weighted echo-planar MR imaging and ADC mapping in the differential diagnosis ovarian cystic masses: Usefulness of detecting keratinoid substances in mature cystic teratomas. *J Magn Reson Imag*. 2005;22(2):271–8.
- Zwiesler D, Lewis SR, Choo YC, et al. A case report of an ovarian lipoma. *South Med J*. 2008;101:205–7.

CODES

ICD9
220 Benign neoplasm of ovary

CLINICAL PEARLS
- Cigarette smoking doubles the relative risk of developing a functional ovarian cyst.
- Transvaginal pelvic ultrasound is the imaging test of choice to initially determine the architecture of an ovarian cyst or mass.
- Malignancy must be ruled out in both premenarchal and postmenopausal patients.
- Do not order CA 125 on premenopausal patients with an ovarian mass unless it is highly suspicious for cancer.

O

PAGET DISEASE OF THE BREAST

Adam Vasconcellos, MD
Fred Schiffman, MD

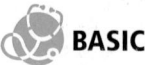 BASICS

DESCRIPTION
- An uncommon presentation of breast malignancy involving the nipple-areolar complex and characterized by eczematous changes, erythema, ulceration, bleeding, and/or itching (1,2).
- System(s) affected: Skin/Exocrine

EPIDEMIOLOGY
Incidence
In the US: 1,000–4,000 new cases each year
- 1–3% of breast cancers (1)
- Peak incidence females ages 50–60 (1,2)

Prevalence
<1% of population

RISK FACTORS
Same risk factors apply as for non-inherited breast cancers:
- Female gender
- Age >40
- Previous breast cancer
- First degree relative with history of breast cancer
- Jewish/Caucasian
- Menarche <age 12
- Menopause >age 50
- Nulliparity or first child after age 34
- History of ionizing radiation exposure
- History of alcohol abuse

Genetics
No known genetic pattern, although studies suggest 80% or higher Her-2/Neu overexpression (3)

PATHOPHYSIOLOGY
- Epidermotropic theory:
  - Ductal carcinoma cells migrate from underlying mammary ducts to epidermis of the nipple to become Paget cells.
- Transformation theory (not favored):
  - Epidermal cells of nipple/areola transform into Paget cells (1).

ETIOLOGY
Cause is unknown, but risk factors for Paget disease appear similar to those of developing breast cancer in general (see above).

COMMONLY ASSOCIATED CONDITIONS
- Associated with underlying in situ or invasive breast cancer in 82–100% of patients (3)
- Multifocal/multicentric associated underlying carcinomas in 32–41% of patients (12)

 DIAGNOSIS

HISTORY
- Nipple itching, burning, bleeding
- Lesion usually located first on the nipple, then may spread to areola (12)
- Nipple/areolar skin changes that have not responded to conservative treatment

PHYSICAL EXAM
- Eczematous nipple changes
- Nipple erythema and scaling
- Nipple erosion or ulceration
- Bloody nipple discharge
- Nipple retraction
- Nipple fissures
- Palpable breast mass
- Thickening in breast tissue without nipple change (2)

DIAGNOSTIC TESTS & INTERPRETATION
Imaging
Initial approach
Mammography and breast ultrasound
- Recommended for all patients with Paget disease on skin biopsy (3)

Follow-Up & Special Considerations
- Breast MRI
  - Recommended if negative mammography and ultrasound (3).
  - Recommended if considering breast-conserving surgery (4).
  - Some recommend breast MRI for all patients with a new Paget disease diagnosis (4).
  - More sensitive than mammography or breast ultrasound in detecting multifocal or multicentric breast cancer (1,3)
  - Higher false-positive rate—patients should be made aware of this
- Preoperative biopsies (FNA or large needle)
  - For all suspicious findings from breast imaging

Diagnostic Procedures/Surgery
Definitive diagnosis obtained by biopsy. Any chronic or nonhealing nipple lesions should be biopsied.

Pathological Findings
- Malignant cell invasion of the epidermis with large, pale cytoplasm, hyperchromatic nuclei with prominent nucleoli (1)
- Underlying ductal adenocarcinoma

DIFFERENTIAL DIAGNOSIS
- Eczema
- Contact dermatitis
- Psoriasis
- Skin tumors (e.g., Bowen disease)
- Squamous cell carcinoma
- Basal cell carcinoma

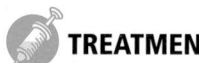 TREATMENT

MEDICATION
Following surgery:
- Chemotherapy per oncology study protocols
- Doxorubicin (Adriamycin)-based regimen
- Cyclophosphamide, methotrexate, 5-fluorouracil (CMF)
- Tamoxifen
- Paclitaxel (Taxol)

ADDITIONAL TREATMENT

Issues for Referral
- Surgery
- Medical oncology
- Radiation oncology

Additional Therapies
Possible breast reconstructive surgery with plastic surgery

SURGERY/OTHER PROCEDURES
- Mastectomy
  - Due to high rate of false-negative findings on mammography and high incidence of multicentric or multifocal in situ or invasive carcinomas discovered in mastectomy specimens (3)
- Breast conserving surgery
  - If Paget disease found to be confined to nipple-areolar complex without underlying neoplasm (2)
  - If disease limited to central segment of breast (5)
  - Approximate 5% risk of local recurrence at 5 years (3)
- Sentinel node biopsy
  - For evaluation of axillary nodes
  - Recommended in patients diagnosed with invasive cancer
  - Recommended in patients undergoing mastectomy (3,5)

IN-PATIENT CONSIDERATIONS

Initial Stabilization
Dependent on cancer histology, size, and stage (see topic on "Breast Cancer"):
- Radiotherapy
- Chemotherapy
- Hormonal manipulation

 ## ONGOING CARE

FOLLOW-UP RECOMMENDATIONS
Oncology consultation

Patient Monitoring
Routine screening for women >40 years:
- Annual physician exams, with physician/patient conversation regarding frequency of imaging studies
- Per recent USPSTF guidelines, mammography at least biennially for women ages 50–74
- Monthly self-exams (although evidence does not support efficacy)

PATIENT EDUCATION
- National Cancer Institute, Department of Health and Human Services, Public Inquiries Section, Office of Cancer Communications, Building 31, Room 101-18, 9000 Rockville Pike, Bethesda, MD 20892; (301) 496-5583
- www.cancer.gov/cancertopics/factsheet/Sites-Types/pagets-breast

PROGNOSIS
Paget disease may correlate with higher-grade tumors, multi-focal disease, and Her-2/Neu overexpression, all suggesting poorer prognosis.
- Prognosis ultimately dependent on stage of underlying breast carcinoma (see [6] for Breast Cancer staging descriptions):

Stage	5 yr relative survival
0	100%
I	100%
II	86%
III	57%
IV	20%

COMPLICATIONS
Risk factors for recurrence:
- Axillary lymph node metastases
- Underlying invasive cancer
- Palpable tumor in the breast (7)

REFERENCES

1. Caliskan M, Gatti G, Sosnovskikh I et al. Paget's disease of the breast: the experience of the European Institute of Oncology and review of the literature. *Breast Cancer Res Treat*. 2008;112: 513–21.
2. Kim HS, Seok JH, Cha ES et al. Significance of nipple enhancement of Paget's disease in contrast enhanced breast MRI. *Arch Gynecol Obstet*. 2010;282:157–62.
3. Siponen E, Hukkinen K, Heikkilä P et al. Surgical treatment in Paget's disease of the breast. *Am J Surg*. 2010;200:241–6.
4. Zakhireh J, Gomez R, Esserman L et al. Converting evidence to practice: a guide for the clinical application of MRI for the screening and management of breast cancer. *Eur J Cancer*. 2008;44:2742–52.
5. Morrogh M, Morris EA, Liberman L et al. MRI identifies otherwise occult disease in select patients with Paget disease of the nipple. *J Am Coll Surg*. 2008;206:316–21.
6. http://www.cancer.org/Cancer/BreastCancer/DetailedGuide/breast-cancer-staging
7. Dalberg K, Hellborg H, Wärnberg F et al. Paget's disease of the nipple in a population based cohort. *Breast Cancer Res Treat*. 2008;111:313–9.

 ## CODES

ICD9
- 174.0 Malignant neoplasm of nipple and areola of female breast
- 174.1 Malignant neoplasm of central portion of female breast
- 174.2 Malignant neoplasm of upper-inner quadrant of female breast

CLINICAL PEARLS

Nonhealing dermatitis of nipple and breast should be biopsied to rule out malignancy.

PALLIATIVE CARE

Felix B. Chang, MD
Awais Siddiki, MD

BASICS

Palliative care (from Latin *palliare*, to cloak): "The active total care of patients whose disease is not responsive to curative treatment."

DESCRIPTION
- The goal of palliative care is the control of pain, or other symptoms, and psychological, social, and spiritual problems.
- Pain control includes the evaluation and management of its physical, emotional, social, economic, and spiritual components.
- Home-based comfort measures: Only 35% of patients want to die at home (1).
- Hospice care eligibility: The patient must have a terminal illness and an estimated prognosis of 6 months or less.
- Specific skills important in palliative medicine care are: Communication, decision making in advanced disease, management of complications in advanced disease, psychosocial care of the patient and family, symptom control, care of the dying, coordination of care.

EPIDEMIOLOGY
- Estimate of patients receiving medical benefits for hospice and palliative care is >500,000.
- In 2000 approximately 20% of patients dying in US received hospice care.
- In 2003 over 260,000 Medicare beneficiaries enrolled in hospice for terminal cancer.
- The most common reason to enter palliative care is advanced cancer. Other diseases include HIV/AIDS, CHF, COPD, RF, liver failure, dementia, and stroke.

Incidence
Measuring the number of patients in palliative care is difficult.

COMMONLY ASSOCIATED CONDITIONS
- Pain is the single most prevalent symptom: Headache, bone pain, ascites, chest pain
- 60% have shortness of breath commonly due to lung cancer and advanced CHF.
- 62% anorexia, nausea and vomiting, constipation, dysphagia
- Anxiety, depression, and hopelessness are common with terminally ill cancer patients.
- Delirium between 40–85% in the last weeks of life

DIAGNOSIS

The **PEACE** tool evaluates **P**hysical symptoms, **E**motive and cognitive symptoms, **A**utonomy- related issues, **C**ommunication, Contribution to others, and **C**losure of life affairs related issues, **E**conomic burden and other practical issues, and **T**ranscendent and existential issues.

HISTORY
- Personhood issues (spiritual/faith, cultural, family/community resource support) assume a co-equal place in assessing the palliative care patient.

- Evaluate possible barriers to timely consideration of a palliative approach to care:
  - The impression that palliation means "there is nothing more I can do for you"
  - Difficulty in recognizing when "aggressive" interventions have lost ability to prolong life
  - Not recognizing that quality-of-care therapies can be of value
  - Patients and decision-responsible caregivers equate palliative measures with "giving up."
- Assessment:
  - Emotive and cognitive symptoms: (1) Sadness (grief), anxiety, depression, and delirium
  - Autonomy (2)
    ○ Do you feel in control of your care? Are we doing all and only the things you desire? Do you know the nature of your illness and what to expect on it?
    ○ Do you feel heard/listened to? Are we following your directions to your satisfaction? Are your treatment preferences in writing?
  - Closure of life affairs: Is there anyone whom you have not seen or need to talk to? Do you have regrets? What do you still want to accomplish in your life?
  - Economic burden: Are you worried about financial burden? Do you worry that you may become a burden to your family? Do you need help with insurance agencies?
- Transcendental and existential issues: Evaluate sense of peace, meaning, and hopes vs torment or agony. Are you suffering? Would you like a chaplain/counselor to visit?

PHYSICAL EXAM
- Physical symptoms: Pain, anorexia, and other appetite or oral intake–related issues, incontinence and other genitourinary symptoms (constipation, vomiting, diarrhea), respiratory symptoms (dyspnea, cough), nausea and other gastrointestinal symptoms (constipation, vomiting, diarrhea), ulcerations and other skin complaints, level of functioning, energy and other related issues such as fatigue or asthenia, and side effect of common treatments.
- Vitals: Weight, mid-arm circumference
- General: Orientation, cognition. Assess ability to contribute meaningfully.
- Eyes, ears, nose, throat: Vision and hearing adequate for communication purposes
- Oral: Assess tongue whether it is moist, dry, or with thrush. Check for presence of ketone breath, gag reflex, dentures, gingivitis, tooth decay, and abscess. Observe swallowing liquid with straw to assess risk for aspiration.
- Neck: Assess lymphadenopathy, thyromegaly, hepato-jugular (H-J) reflux, stiff/supple neck, paracervical pain triggers (common cause of headaches in elderly), and kyphosis.
- Cardiovascular: Murmurs/splits/gallops, PMI
- Lungs: Inspection, palpation, percussion, auscultation; blood pressure (sitting and standing); pulse and respiration
- Abdomen/Genitourinary: Distention, presence of artificial feeding device. Digital rectal exam for constipation/impaction and hemoccult

- Musculoskeletal/Neurologic: Pain sites, weakness, paresthesia, pathologic reflexes (Hoffman, Babinski), contractures, posture, range of motion
- Skin: Presence of rash, bed sores, wounds

DIAGNOSTIC TESTS & INTERPRETATION
Lab
Initial lab tests
- Urinalysis
- Comprehensive metabolic panel
- Complete blood count

Follow-Up & Special Considerations
Interdisciplinary teamwork (IDTW): One key to effective care is adopting a model of interdisciplinary team care. Providing proficient care enlists most often the following team players: Physician, nurse, social worker, home health aide, pastor, administrator, pharmacist, medical supplier (beds, nebulizers, oxygen, commodes, wheelchairs), respite and home health agencies, community resources (Meals on Wheels, volunteers), allied health practitioners (e.g., aromatherapy, massage, OMM, acupuncture, meditation, ethicist)

Imaging
Should be reserved for the identification of conditions that will change treatment when present

TREATMENT

MEDICATION
- Begin to think about trimming medications that appear to offer little in the way of improving quality of life or meaningfully extending duration of life.
- Assure compliance by addressing patient/caregiver understanding and consensus, written record for them, and assurance that language/functional illiteracy are not issues.
- Pain:
  - Immediate-release morphine p.o./IV treats dyspnea effectively and typically at doses lower than would be necessary for the relief of moderate pain.
  - Once pain is controlled, convert to long-acting narcotic with short-acting agents made available as tolerance develops and/or patient develops breakthrough pain.
  - Bone pain: NSAIDs added to narcotics are more effective than narcotics alone.
- Vomiting associated with a particular opioid may be relieved by substitution with an equianalgesic dose of another opioid or a sustained-release formulation. Dopamine-receptor antagonists are commonly used (metoclopramide, prochlorperazine, promethazine)
- Constipation: A prophylactic bowel regimen of stool softeners (docusate) and stimulants (bisacodyl or senna) should be started when opioid treatment is begun to avoid constipation. Polyethylene glycol started with initiation of narcotics may prevent onset.
- Dyspnea: oxygen, narcotics, and if CHF, diuretics and/or long-acting nitrates
- Delirium: Lowest doses necessary of benzodiazepines or antipsychotics (Haldol, others)
- Brain metastases: Radiation, oral steroids (Decadron), etc.

- Patient safety and nonpharmacologic strategies to assist orientation (clocks, calendars, environment, and redirection). Some may be "pleasantly confused," and decision by family and clinician not to treat delirium may be justified. When cause of delirium cannot be identified/corrected rapidly, consider neuroleptics (haloperidol or risperidone)

ADDITIONAL TREATMENT

General Measures

Paradigm shift from a biomedical problem list to a symptom-management care plan. Polypharmacy is common; research for adverse effects and drug interactions.

Issues for Referral

- Eligibility for hospice care: Determining Prognosis and Appropriateness of Hospice referral: (I) The patient's condition is life limiting, and the patient and/or family have been informed of this condition. (II) The patient and/or family have elected treatments goals directed toward the relief of symptoms, rather than cure of the underlying disease. (III) The patient has either of the following: A. Documented clinical progression of disease, which may include: 1. Progression of the primary disease process as listed in disease-specific criteria; as documented by serial physician assessment, laboratory, radiologic, or other studies. 2. Multiple emergency department visit or inpatient hospitalizations over the prior 6 months. 3. For homebound patients receiving home health services, nursing assessment may be documented. For patients who do not qualify under 1, 2, 3, a recent decline in functional status may be documented. B. Documented recent impaired nutritional status related to the terminal process. 1. Unintentional, progressive weight loss of >10% over the prior 6 month. 2. Serum albumin less than 2.5 gm/dl may be helpful prognostic indicator, but should not be used in isolation from other factors in I-III
- Eligibility for Medicare hospice benefit: Eligibility for Medicare part A (hospital insurance), Medicare approved hospice. The patient signs a statement choosing hospice care instead of regular Medicare. The patient's personal physician and the hospice medical director both certify that the patient has a terminal illness and less than 6 months to live (3).

ONGOING CARE

PATIENT EDUCATION

- http://www.getpalliativecare.org/
- http://www.hospicecare.com/resources/patients-relatives.htm

PROGNOSIS

- For seriously ill patients with advanced COPD, heart failure, or end-stage liver disease, clinical prediction criteria are not effective in identifying a population with a survival prognosis of 6 months or less (4).
- Guidelines for determining prognosis in selected non-cancer diseases:
  - Heart disease:
    - Symptoms of recurrent congestive heart failure at rest
    - Patients should already be optimally treated with diuretics and vasodilators, preferably angiotensin-converting enzyme inhibitors.

- Other factors: Symptomatic supraventricular or ventricular arrhythmias that are resistant to antiarrhythmic therapy; history of cardiac arrest and resuscitation in any setting; history of unexplained syncope; cardiogenic brain embolism
- Pulmonary disease:
  - Dyspnea at rest from decreased functional activity, exacerbated by fatigue, cough
  - Presence of cor pulmonale or right heart failure.
  - Hypoxemia at rest on supplemental oxygen. Hypercapnia. Unintentional weight loss of >10% of body weight over 6 months; resting tachycardia (>100/min) in COPD
- Dementia:
  - Functional assessment >/= stage 7: Unable to ambulate, dress or bathe; urinary or fecal incontinence; unable to communicate meaningfully
  - Comorbid conditions: Aspiration pneumonia, pyelonephritis, or urinary infections; septicemia, decubitus ulcer; recurrent fever; difficulty swallowing or refusal to eat
- HIV:
  - CD4+ count bellow 25 cells/mcL
  - Viral load >100,000 copies/mL
  - Life-threatening concomitant conditions
  - Chronic persistent diarrhea for 1 year; persistent serum albumin <2.5 gm/dL; substance abuse; age >50; decision to forgo retroviral, chemotherapeutic prophylaxis drug therapy related specifically to HIV disease, congestive heart failure
- Liver disease:
  - Laboratory indicators of severely impaired liver function: Prothrombin time prolonged >5 seconds over control; serum albumin <2.5 gm/dl
  - Clinical indicators of end-stage liver disease: Ascites, refractory to sodium restriction and diuretics, or patient noncompliant; spontaneous bacterial peritonitis; hepatorenal syndrome; hepatic encephalopathy, refractory to protein restriction and lactulose or neomycin, or patient noncompliant; recurrent variceal bleeding
  - Worsening prognosis: Progressive malnutrition, muscle wasting with reduced strength and endurance; continued active alcoholism, >80 g ethanol per day; hepatocellular carcinoma, hepatitis B surface antigen positivity
- Renal diseases:
  - Laboratory criteria for renal failure: Creatinine clearance of <10 cc/min (<15 cc/min for diabetes) and serum creatinine of less than 8 mg/dL (>6 mg/dL in diabetics).
  - End-stage renal disease discontinuing dialysis, or dialysis eligible and refusing, with renal failure: Uremia; oliguria; intractable hyperkalemia; uremic pericarditis; hepatorenal syndrome; intractable fluid overload
  - In hospitalized patients with acute renal failure, other comorbid conditions that predict early mortality: Mechanical ventilation; malignancy-other organ systems; chronic lung disease; advanced cardiac disease; sepsis; immunosuppression/AIDS; albumin <3.5 gm/dL; cachexia; platelet count <25,000; age >75; disseminated intravascular congestion; gastrointestinal bleeding

- Stroke and coma: I. During the acute phase immediately following a hemorrhagic or ischemic stroke: A. Coma or persistent vegetative state beyond 3 days' duration. B. In postanoxic stroke, coma or severe obtundation, accompanied by severe myoclonus, persisting beyond 3 days past the anoxic event. C. Comatose patients with any 4 of the following on day 3 of coma: abnormal brain stem response; absent verbal response; absent withdrawal response to pain; serum creatinine >1.5 mg/dL, age >70. D. Dysphagia severe enough to prevent the patient from receiving food and fluids necessary to sustain life. E. CT or MRI findings indicating decreased likelihood of survival. II. Once the patient has entered the chronic phase: A. Age >70. B. Poor functional status, as evidenced by Karnofsky score of <50%. C. Poststroke dementia, as evidenced by a FAST score >7. D. Poor nutritional status, whether on artificial or not: Aspiration pneumonia; upper urinary tract infection, sepsis; refractory stage 3–4 decubitus ulcer; fever recurrent after antibiotics

REFERENCES

1. Meuser T, Pietruck C, et al. Symptoms during cancer pain treatment following WHO-guidelines: A longitudinal follow-up study of symptoms prevalence, severity and etiology. *Pain*. 2001; 93:247.
2. Lo B, Quill T, et al. Discussing palliative care with patients. ACP-ASIM End-of-Life Care Consensus Panel. American College of Physicians-American Society of Internal Medicine. *Ann Intern Med*. 1999;130:744.
3. Medicare Hospice Benefits, Health care Financing Administration, Publication No. HCFA02154, Revised August 1999.
4. Fox E, Landrum NcNiff, et al. Evaluation of prognostic criteria for determining hospice eligibility in patients with advanced lung, heart, or liver disease. SUPPORT Investigators. Study to Understand Prognosis and Preferences for Outcomes and Risks of Treatments. *JAMA*. 1999;282:1638.

 CODES

ICD9
V66.7 Encounter for palliative care

CLINICAL PEARLS

- The goal of palliative care is achievement of the best quality of life for patients and families.
- Palliative medicine is not just for terminally ill patients.
- Delirium in advanced illness may be reversible in up to 50% of cases.
- New symptoms that indicate a new disease process should be sought when appropriate.

PANCREATIC CANCER

Felix B. Chang, MD

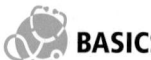 **BASICS**

DESCRIPTION
- Pancreatic cancer: Malignant cells are found in the tissue of the pancreas; also called *pancreatic exocrine cancer*.
- Carcinoma of the pancreas ranks as the 4th leading cause of cancer death in the US.
- Cancer of the exocrine pancreas is rarely curable and has an overall 5-year relative survival rate of <4%.
- 60–70% arise in the head, 15% in the body, 5% in the tail; 20% diffusely involve the whole gland.
- Fewer than 20% of pancreatic cancers are localized at diagnosis. For those patients with localized disease and small cancers(<2 cm) with no lymph node metastases and no extension beyond the capsule of the pancreas, complete surgical resection can yield actuarial 5-year survival rates of 18–24%.
- For patients with advanced cancers, the overall survival is <1% at 5 years, with most patients dying within 1 year.

EPIDEMIOLOGY
In 2003–2007, the median age at diagnosis for cancer of the pancreatic was 72 years of age (1).

Incidence
- It is estimated that 42,470 men and women were diagnosed with cancer of the pancreas in 2009 (21,040 men; 21,420 women); deaths: 35,240.
- It is more common in individuals of the black race and the white race, 16.7 and 10.3 in 100,000 men and 14.4 and 10.3 in 100,000 women, respectively. Hispanic and Asian/Pacific Islander individuals had an incidence of 10.9 and 8.3 in 100,000 men and 10.1 and 8.3 in 100,000 women, respectively (2).

Prevalence
On January 1, 2007, in the US, there were approximately 16,936 men and women (14,979 men and 16,201 women) alive who had a history of cancer of the pancreas (2).

RISK FACTORS
- Smoking: RR = at least 1.5. It has been estimated that cessation of smoking could eliminate approximately 25% of pancreatic cancer deaths in the US.
- Diabetes: RR = 2.1 (95%, CI: 1.6–2.8)
- History of partial gastrectomy or cholecystectomy: 2- to 5-fold increased risk 15–20 years after partial gastrectomy
- Familial aggregation/genetic factors: 5–10% of patients have a 1st-degree relative with the disease.
- Hereditary chronic pancreatitis: Cumulative risk by ages 50 and 75 is 10% and 54%, respectively.
- Chronic pancreatitis: Tropical and nontropical
- Coffee and alcohol consumption: Studies fail to convincingly demonstrate a relationship.
- Aspirin and NSAID use: Large cohorts have not found any link.

Genetics
- Multifactorial: Activation of oncogenes (e.g., *K-ras* mutation 90%); inactivation of tumor suppressor genes (e.g., p16/*CDKN2A* [95%], TP*53* [75 to 85], SMAD4[30], and *BRCA2* genes[10%]); and defects in DNA mismatch repair genes (e.g., h*MLH1* and h*MSH2* [4% of pancreatic tumors])

- Hereditary pancreatitis: The cumulative risk of pancreatic cancer in affected family members is 10%, 19%, and 54% at ages 50, 60, and 75, respectively.
- Inherited cancer syndromes:
  – Peutz-Jeghers syndrome: Related genes: *PRSS1* and *STK 11*; lifetime risk is as high as 36%.
  – Hereditary breast/ovarian cancer: 5% lifetime risk for pancreas cancer. Related genes: *BRCA2* and *BRCA1*
  – Familial atypical multiple-mole melanoma syndrome: 19% lifetime risk. Related gene: *CDKN2A*
  – Ataxia-telangiectasia: Related gene: *ATM*
  – Li-Fraumeni syndrome: Related Gene: *p53*

 DIAGNOSIS

HISTORY
Weight loss 90%; pain 75% (progressive midepigastric dull ache that often radiates to the back); malnutrition 75%; jaundice 70%; anorexia 60%; pruritus 40%; diabetes mellitus 15%; weakness, fatigue, malaise 30–40%; acholic stools, dark urine, steatorrhea. Atypical diabetes mellitus, unexplained thrombophlebitis.

PHYSICAL EXAM
- Palpable abdominal mass or ascites in 20%
- Jaundice: 70% if head of pancreas obstructs bile duct, only 10% with body or tail pancreatic carcinoma
- Courvoisier sign (painless jaundice with a palpable gallbladder) 33%; usually is associated with pancreatic head tumors, periampullary carcinoma, and primary bile duct tumors; hepatomegaly in advanced disease.
- Virchow node (left supraclavicular) and Sister Mary Joseph node (umbilical) in metastatic disease; palpable rectal shelf (nonspecific sign of carcinomatosis)
- Migratory thrombophlebitis; Trousseau sign; superficial thrombophlebitis associated with pancreatic cancer
- Pancreatic panniculitis: Subcutaneous areas of nodular fat necrosis

DIAGNOSTIC TESTS & INTERPRETATION
Endoscopic ultrasound-guided biopsy is the best modality for obtaining a tissue diagnosis. Has a sensitivity of ~75–90% and specificity of virtually 100% for the diagnosis of a pancreatic mass.

Lab
Routine laboratory tests may reveal a elevated serum bilirubin concentration and alkaline phosphatase activity, and the presence of anemia.

Initial lab tests
Elevated CA 19-9 80% sensitivity, 90% specificity; individuals with Lewis-negative blood group antigen phenotype (5–10%) are unable to synthesize CA 19-9.

Follow-Up & Special Considerations
Following or during definitive therapy, increase in CA 19-9 levels may identify patients with progressive tumor growth. Normal CA 19-9 does not exclude recurrence.

Imaging
Mass within the pancreas, which often obstructs the pancreatic duct or biliary tree.

Initial approach
- Abdominal US:75–89% sensitivity and 90–99% specificity; dilated bile ducts or the presence of a mass in the head of the pancreas.
- Endoscopic US: CT and EUS are complementary for staging pancreatic cancer. EUS is a more accurate modality for local T and N staging and for predicting vascular invasion
- CT and CT angiography scans: 85–90% sensitivity and 90–95% specificity; useful for evaluation of distant metastasis.
- ERCP: 90% sensitivity and 95% specificity
- MRI offers no significant diagnostic advantage over contrast-enhanced CT.
- MR cholangiopancreatography: 90% sensitivity and 95% specificity. Preferred in specific settings: Gastric outlet or duodenal stenosis or patients who have had surgical rearrangement (Billroth II) or ductal disruption. To detect bile duct obstruction occurring in the setting of chronic pancreatitis. For patients in whom attempted ERCP is either totally unsuccessful or provides incomplete information because of pancreatic duct obstruction.

Diagnostic Procedures/Surgery
- Staging studies for resectability include CT angiography, MRI, endoscopic US, laparoscopic US, and cytology.
- Percutaneous FNA biopsy using either US or CT guidance: 80–90% sensitivity and 98–100% specificity
- Endoscopic US is the most sensitive noninvasive test to diagnose vascular invasion: 90% specificity and 73% sensitivity.
- Endoscopic US–guided biopsy: 85–90% sensitivity and virtually 100% specificity for pancreatic mass
- Staging laparoscopy and US: 92% sensitivity, 88% specificity, and 89% accuracy
- Positive peritoneal cytology has a positive predictive value of 94%, specificity of 98%, and sensitivity of 25% for determining unresectability (3).
- PET scan: 90% sensitivity but 70% specificity; limited anatomic information
- Staging system: TNM definition: AJCC, 2002.
  – Primary tumor (T):
    ○ TX: Primary tumor cannot be assessed.
    ○ T0: No evidence of primary tumor
    ○ TIS: Carcinoma in situ
    ○ T1: Tumor is limited to the pancreas and is ≤2 cm in greatest dimension.
    ○ T2: Tumor is limited to the pancreas and is >2 cm in greatest dimension.
    ○ T3: Tumor extends beyond the pancreas but without involvement of the celiac axis or the superior mesenteric artery.
    ○ T4: Tumor involves the celiac axis or the superior mesenteric artery (unresectable primary tumors).
  – Regional lymph nodes (N):
    ○ NX: Regional lymph nodes cannot be assessed.
    ○ N0: No regional lymph node metastasis
    ○ N1: Regional lymph node metastasis
  – Distant metastasis (M):
    ○ MX: Distant metastasis cannot be assessed.
    ○ M0: No distant metastasis
    ○ M1: Distant metastasis

- AJCC stage groupings:
  - Stage 0: Tis, N0, M0
  - Stage IA: T1, N0, M0
  - Stage IB: T2, N0, M0
  - Stage IIA: T3, N0, M0
  - Stage IIB: T1, N1, M0; T2, N1, M0; T3, N1, M0
  - Stage III: T4, any N, M0
  - Stage IV: Any T, any N, M1

Pathological Findings
- 90% duct cell carcinoma
- Others: Acinar cell, papillary mucinous, signet ring, adenosquamous, mucinous, giant cell, small cell, cystadenocarcinoma, undifferentiated, unclassified carcinoma

DIFFERENTIAL DIAGNOSIS
- Duodenal cancer, cholangiocarcinoma, lymphoma, islet cell tumor, sarcoma
- Nonmalignant conditions: Choledocholithiasis, pancreatitis, biliary tract stricture, autoimmune pancreatitis, sclerosing pancreatitis, adenoma

TREATMENT

Surgical resection offers the only chance of cure. There is no role for resection of adenocarcinoma in the presence of metastatic disease.

MEDICATION
- Analgesics
- Stage I and II:
  - Radical pancreatic resection ± postoperative 5-FU chemotherapy and radiation therapy (4,5)[A]
  - RTOG-9704 trial compared postoperative infusional 5-FU plus infusional 5-FU and concurrent radiation or adjuvant gemcitabine plus infusional 5-FU and concurrent radiation. The addition of gemcitabine to postoperative adjuvant 5-FU CRT significantly improved median overall survival in patients with pancreatic head adenocarcinoma: 20.5 months in the gemcitabine arm versus 16.9 months in the 5-FU arm; 3-year survival was 31% versus 22%. ($P = 0.09$; HR = 0.82; CI: 0.65–1.03) (6)[A].
  - CONKO-001 trial: Gemcitabine for 6 months for patients after complete resection of pancreatic cancer significantly increased disease-free survival to 13.4 months in the gemcitabine arm (95% CI: 6.1–7.8; $P <0.001$) versus 6.9 months in the observation group. No significant difference in overall survival was seen between groups.
- Stage III:
  - Chemoradiation: Controversial
  - Standard: Chemotherapy with gemcitabine
  - Palliative decompression of biliary obstruction by endoscopic, surgical, or radiologic methods
  - Intraoperative radiation therapy and/or implantation of radioactive sources
- Stage IV:
  - Chemotherapy: Gemcitabine 1-year survival was 18% versus 2% with 5-FU ($P = 0.003$). Gemcitabine with erlotinib modestly prolonged survival (4)[A].
  - Pain-relieving procedures (celiac or intrapleural block) and supportive care
  - Palliative decompression
  - For patients who are refractory to gemcitabine monotherapy, 2nd-line therapy has not been clearly shown to affect survival.

ADDITIONAL TREATMENT
- For patients with resected tumors, postoperative radiation therapy with other chemotherapeutic agents
- For patients with resected tumors, postoperative chemotherapy alone. The RLUH-NCRI-ESPAC-3V2 trial is evaluating postoperative chemotherapy with either 5-FU/leucovorin or gemcitabine versus no additional treatment. (Results pending) (7)

Additional Therapies
- Biliary decompression with endoprostheses or transhepatic drain catheters
- Celiac axis and intrapleural nerve blocks can provide highly effective and long-lasting pain control for some patients.

SURGERY/OTHER PROCEDURES
Disease that is limited to the pancreas and peripancreatic nodes (stage I–IIB) is most likely to be cured by radical resection. Absolute contraindications for resection include the presence of metastases in the liver, peritoneum, omentum, or any distant site. Relative contraindications are involvement of the bowel mesentery, portomesenteric vasculature, and celiac axis and its tributaries.

- Standard treatment options:
  - Pancreaticoduodenectomy, Whipple procedure, en bloc resection of the head of the pancreas, distal common bile duct, duodenum, jejunum, and gastric antrum
  - Total pancreatectomy
  - Distal pancreatectomy, for tumors of the body and tail
- Nonstandard surgeries:
  - Pylorus-preserving pancreaticoduodenectomy, regional pancreatectomy
  - Palliative bypass
    - Biliary decompression; gastrojejunostomy for gastric outlet obstruction; duodenal endoprosthesis for obstruction

ONGOING CARE

DIET
Frequently, malabsorption caused by exocrine insufficiency contributes to malnutrition; pancreatic enzyme replacement can help to alleviate.

PROGNOSIS
Criteria for resectable disease (~20%):
- No extrapancreatic disease
- Patent superior mesenteric vein and portal vein, celiac axis and superior mesenteric artery not involved, no bulky nodes
- Median survival: 10–20 months
- 5-year survival: ~30% if node-negative; 10% if node-positive
- Distant (cancer has metastasized): 1.9% 5 years' relative survival
- For patients with localized disease and small cancers (<2 cm) with no lymph node involvement and no extension beyond the capsule of the pancreas, complete surgical resection can yield a 5-year survival rate of 18–24%.

COMPLICATIONS
- Diabetes mellitus, malabsorption
- Surgical complications: Intraabdominal abscess, postgastrectomy syndromes, pancreatico-jejunostomy, gastric and biliary anastomotic leaks; operative mortality varies from 1–16%.

REFERENCES

1. American Cancer Society. *Cancer Facts and Figures 2009*. Atlanta, GA: American Cancer Society, 2009.
2. Altekruse SF, et al. SEER Cancer Statistics Review, 1975–2007, National Cancer Institute Bethesda, MD, http://seer,cancer,gov/csr/1975_2007/, based on November 2009 SEER data submission, posted to the SEER web site, 2010
3. Merchant NB, Conlon KC, Sasigo P, et al. Positive peritoneal cytology predicts unresectable pancreatic adenocarcinoma. *J Am Coll Surg.* 1999;188(4):421–6.
4. Moore MJ, Goldstein D, Hamm J, et al. Erlotinib plus gemcitabine compared to gemcitabine alone in patients with advanced pancreatic cancer. A phase III trial of the National Cancer Institute of Canada Clinical Trials Group [NCIC-CTG]. *J Clin Oncol.* 2005;23(16):A-1, 1s.
5. Neoptolemos JP, Stocken DD, Friess H, et al. A randomized trial of chemotherapy and chemotherapy after resection of pancreatic cancer. *N Engl J Med.* 2004;350(12):1200–10.
6. Oettle H, Post S, Neuhaus P, et al. Adjuvant chemotherapy with gemcitabine vs observation in patients undergoing curative-intent resection of pancreatic cancer: a randomized controlled trial. *JAMA.* 2007;297(3):267–77.
7. ESPAC-3(V2) Phase III Adjuvant Trial in Pancreatic Cancer Comparing 5FU and D-L-Folinic Acid vs. Gemcitabine. Leeds, UK: National Cancer Research Network Trials Portfolio, 2004. http://public.ukcrn.org.uk/Search/StudyDetail.aspx?StudyID=669

CODES

ICD9
- 157.0 Malignant neoplasm of head of pancreas
- 157.1 Malignant neoplasm of body of pancreas
- 157.2 Malignant neoplasm of tail of pancreas

CLINICAL PEARLS
- The sudden onset of diabetes mellitus in nonobese adults aged >40 years warrants evaluation for pancreatic cancer.
- Cancer of the exocrine pancreas is rarely curable and has an overall 5-year relative survival rate of <4%. Fewer than 20% of pancreatic cancer cases are localized at diagnosis.
- CT scan and endoscopic ultrasound are complementary modalities for diagnosis and staging of pancreatic cancer

PANCREATITIS, ACUTE

Robert L. Frachtman, MD

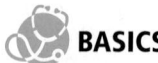 **BASICS**

DESCRIPTION

Acute inflammatory process of the pancreas with variable involvement of regional tissue or remote organ systems

- Inflammatory episode with symptoms related to intrapancreatic activation of enzymes with pain, nausea, and vomiting and associated intestinal ileus
- Varies widely in severity (including death), complications, and prognosis
- Complete structural and functional recovery, provided no necrosis or pancreatic ductal disruption

EPIDEMIOLOGY

Incidence
- 1–5/10,000
- Predominant age: none
- Predominant sex: Male = Female

Prevalence
Acute: 19/10,000

RISK FACTORS
See Etiology.

Genetics
Hereditary pancreatitis is a rare condition with an autosomally dominant inheritance pattern.

GENERAL PREVENTION
- Avoidance of alcohol excess, especially over a prolonged period
- Avoidance of cigarette smoking
- Correction of underlying causes (hypertriglyceridemia or hypercalcemia)
- Discontinuation of medications associated with pancreatitis as soon as it is diagnosed
- Cholecystectomy if symptomatic cholelithiasis

PATHOPHYSIOLOGY
Autodigestion of the pancreas, interstitial edema with severe third spacing, hemorrhage, necrosis, release of vasoactive peptides, acute fluid collection (within 6 weeks), pseudocyst or postnecrotic collection (greater than 6 weeks), pancreatic ductal disruption, injury to surrounding vascular structures such as the splenic vein (thrombosis) and splenic artery (pseudoaneurysm)

ETIOLOGY
- Alcohol
- Gallstones (including microlithiasis)
- Trauma/surgery
- Acute discontinuation of medications for diabetes or hyperlipidemia
- Following endoscopic retrograde cholangiopancreatography (ERCP)
- Medications (most common, but not exhaustive list):
  - ACE inhibitors
  - ARBs (angiotensin receptor blockers)
  - Thiazide diuretics and furosemide
  - Antimetabolites (Purinethol and azathioprine)
  - Corticosteroids
  - Exenatide (Byetta) (1)[A]
  - Pentamidine
  - Statins

- Pancreatitis may occur only after several months' administration of some of the implicated medications.
- When a patient presents with pancreatitis, all medications should be reviewed in the PDR and accessible literature and should be continued only if the benefit justifies the risk of continuing a potential cause of pancreatitis, especially if no other causes are identified.
- Metabolic causes:
  - Hypertriglyceridemia
  - Hypercalcemia
  - Acute renal failure
  - Hereditary causes (uncommon)
  - Systemic lupus erythematosus/polyarteritis
  - Infections (list not exhaustive):
    ○ Mumps, Coxsackie, Cryptosporidiosis
- Penetrating peptic ulcer (rare)
- Cystic fibrosis and CFTR (cystic fibrosis transmembrane conductance regulator) gene mutations
- Tumors (e.g., ampullary)
- Pancreas divisum
- Sphincter of Oddi dysfunction
- Scorpion venom
- Vascular disease
- Acute fatty liver of pregnancy
- Idiopathic

COMMONLY ASSOCIATED CONDITIONS
Consider coexistent alcohol withdrawal, alcoholic hepatitis, and ascending cholangitis.

 DIAGNOSIS

Symptoms and objective evidence (imaging, amylase/lipase) do not always correlate.

HISTORY
- Fairly rapid onset of epigastric pain, which may radiate posteriorly, often with emesis
- Alcohol use
- History of gallstones
- Family history of gallstones
- Medication use
- Abdominal trauma
- Recent significant weight loss (via causing cholelithiasis)

PHYSICAL EXAM
- Abdominal findings: Epigastric tenderness, loss of bowel sounds
- Other findings: Fever, tachycardia, hypotension/shock, jaundice, rales/percussive dullness
- Rare (with hemorrhagic pancreatitis)
  - Flank discoloration (Grey–Turner sign) or umbilical discoloration (Cullen sign)

DIAGNOSTIC TESTS & INTERPRETATION
The laboratory and radiographic assessment of both acute and chronic pancreatitis must be used together, as there can be many false positives and negatives.

Lab
- Elevated serum amylase >3× upper limit of normal (severity is not related to degree of elevation)
- Elevated serum lipase >3× upper limit of normal (may stay elevated longer than amylase in mild cases)
- Elevated total bilirubin to 3 mg/dL is not uncommon with pancreatitis, per se, but more elevated levels create consideration of common bile duct obstruction.
- Transaminases can quickly rise to near 1000 u/l with acute bile duct obstruction, but should rapidly fall as the alkaline phosphatase rises; a 3-fold elevation in the ALT in the setting of acute pancreatitis has a 95% positive predictive value for gallstone pancreatitis.
- Triglyceride levels >1000 mg/dL suggest hypertriglyceridemia as the cause.
- Glucose is increased in severe disease.
- Calcium is decreased in severe disease .
- WBC's can be 10,000–25,000/μL without active infection.
- Rising hemoglobin is a poor prognostic sign (severe third spacing). Rising BUN and creatinine imply volume depletion or acute renal failure.
- Disorders that may alter results for amylase or lipase:
  - Biliary tract disease, penetrating peptic ulcer, intestinal obstruction, intestinal ischemia/infarction, ruptured ectopic pregnancy, renal insufficiency, burns, macroamylasemia, or macrolipasemia

Initial lab tests
Admit labs should be supplemented by early and frequent follow-up labs to assess renal function, hydration, sepsis, biliary obstruction, and O2 saturation.

Imaging
- Plain film of abdomen is useful to rule out mechanical small bowel obstruction, but ileus secondary to pancreatitis is common.
- CXR is useful to evaluate for early ARDS and pleural effusion; if upright, can rule out free subdiaphragmatic air.
- Ultrasound is useful to rule out cholelithiasis; choledocholithiasis can occasionally be seen.
- CT scan:
  - Will confirm the diagnosis, assess the severity, establish a baseline, and to rule out other possibilities
  - Intravenous contrast is not essential on the initial CT scan regarding evaluation for necrosis and should be avoided in volume-depleted patients.
  - A negative CT scan will not rule out noncalcified cholelithiasis.
  - If not contraindicated, a CT scan with intravenous contrast at day 3 can assess the degree of necrosis when necrotizing pancreatitis is suspected because of O2 saturation <90%, systolic BP <90 mm Hg, etc.
- MRCP is useful (if it can be performed) to assess the likelihood of choledocholithiasis; as a bonus, one may find pancreas divisum, a dilated pancreatic duct, or chronic ductal changes.

- ERCP may be necessary for emergency common bile duct decompression due to an impacted stone.
- Endoscopic ultrasonography (EUS) may be useful when a patient with "idiopathic pancreatitis" has a second episode.

Initial approach
The ultrasound, followed quickly by the CT scan, has largely replaced the plain film of the abdomen.

Follow-Up & Special Considerations
If renal function is stable, a contrast-enhanced CT scan is very useful at day 3 to assess for necrosis, a major prognostic indicator. Later in the course, if a cavity develops and there is a sudden worsening in the temperature curve, material can be aspirated via CT scan to assess for secondary infection.

DIFFERENTIAL DIAGNOSIS
- Penetrating peptic ulcer
- Acute cholecystitis
- Choledocholithiasis
- Macroamylasemia, macrolipasemia
- Mesenteric vascular occlusion and/or infarction
- Perforation of a viscus
- Intestinal obstruction
- Aortic aneurysm (dissecting or rupturing)
- Inferior wall myocardial infarction
- Lymphoma

 TREATMENT

MEDICATION
- Analgesia:
  - Hydromorphone (Dilaudid) .5–1 mg IV every 1–2 hours p.r.n. (morphine sulfate can increase Sphincter of Oddi pressure, worsening the pancreatitis and increasing ductal pressure)
  - Demerol should be avoided due to the potential of accumulation of a toxic metabolite.
- Antibiotics:
  - Carbapenems can be considered for prophylaxis in necrotizing/severe pancreatitis if >30% necrosis on the CT scan (the usage of prophylactic antibiotics remain controversial, however, and seems to be losing favor)
  - Beta lactam blockers with semisynthetic penicillin (e.g., Zosyn) or fluoroquinolones if cholangitis
  - Be vigilant for monilial superinfections when giving prophylactic antibiotics.

ADDITIONAL TREATMENT
General Measures
- Confirm diagnosis and rule out other possibilities, if needed (see above).
- Unless extremely mild, most cases require hospitalization.
- Fluid resuscitation:
  - If moderate or severe pancreatitis, there could easily be a 3-liter deficit due to third spacing.
  - Infusion rates of 500 ml/hour for the first several hours, followed by 200–300 ml per hour for 48 hours, would not be unreasonable in those circumstances.
  - Urine output goal should be 0.5–1 mL/kg per hour.
- Eliminate all unnecessary medications, especially those that could potentially cause pancreatitis.
- Analgesia (see above)
- NG tube is needed only if there is intractable emesis.
- Follow status regarding renal function, volume, calcium, oxygenation.

- Imaging studies as needed (e.g., contrasted CT scan in 48–72 hours, if no contraindications, to evaluate for necrotizing pancreatitis, which increases the incidence of fluid collections)
- Intermittent pneumatic compression device
- Enteral nutrition at level of Ligament of Treitz if oral feeding will not be possible within 5–7 days (preferable to TPN due to decreased infection rate)
- TPN (without lipids if triglycerides are elevated) if oral or nasoenteric feedings are not tolerated

Issues for Referral
Refer to a tertiary center if pancreatitis is either already severe or actively evolving and when advanced imaging or endoscopic therapy is being considered.

SURGERY/OTHER PROCEDURES
- Necrosectomy for infected necrosis
- ERCP early if evidence of acute cholangitis or at 72 hours if evidence of ongoing biliary obstruction
- Resection or embolization for bleeding pseudoaneurysms
- Plasma exchange if necrotizing pancreatitis secondary to hypertriglyceridemia

IN-PATIENT CONSIDERATIONS
Discharge Criteria
- Pain control
- Diet tolerance
- Alcohol rehab and smoking cessation, if needed
- Low-grade fever and mild leukocytosis do not necessarily indicate infection and may take weeks to resolve.

 ONGOING CARE

FOLLOW-UP RECOMMENDATIONS
- Follow up imaging studies may be required in several weeks, especially if the original CT scan showed a fluid collection or necrosis or if the amylase or lipase continue to be elevated.
  - Pseudocyst or abscess (sudden onset of fever),
  - Splenic vein thrombosis (gastric variceal hemorrhage can occur rarely)
  - Pseudoaneurysm (splenic, gastroduodenal, intrapancreatic) hemorrhages (life threatening)
- Mild exocrine and endocrine dysfunction occur, but are usually subclinical.

DIET
- Begin diet after pain, tenderness, and ileus have resolved; small amounts of high-carbohydrate, low-fat, and low-protein foods; advance as tolerated; NPO or nasogastric tube if patient is vomiting
- Total parenteral nutrition (TPN) if oral is not tolerated (no lipids if triglycerides are increased) (2)[A]
- Enteral nutrition at level of Ligament of Treitz is preferable to TPN if tolerated (less infection, decreased organ failure).

PROGNOSIS
85–90% resolve spontaneously; 3–5% mortality (17% in necrotizing pancreatitis). APACHE II scoring is most accurate but difficult to apply (3)[A]; Ranson criteria (see below) have a sensitivity of ~40%.

- On admission: Age >55 years, WBCs >16,000/mm, blood glucose >200 mg/dL (11.1 mmol/L), serum lactate dehydrogenase (LDH) >350 IU/L, AST >250 IU/L.
- Within 48 hours: Hematocrit decreases >10%, serum calcium <8 mg/dL, blood urea nitrogen (BUN) increase >8 mg/dL, arterial PO2 <60 mmHg, base deficit >4 mEq/L, fluid retention >6 L
- Ranson scoring:
  - Ranson score of 0–2: Minimal mortality
  - Ranson score of 3–5: 10–20% mortality
  - Ranson score of >5: >50% mortality

REFERENCES

1. Anderson SL, Trujillo JM et al. Association of pancreatitis with glucagon-like peptide-1 agonist use. *Ann Pharmacother.* 2010;44:904–9.
2. Oláh A, Romics L et al. Evidence-based use of enteral nutrition in acute pancreatitis. *Langenbecks Arch Surg.* 2010;395:309–16.
3. Gravante G, Garcea G, Ong SL, et al. Prediction of mortality in acute pancreatitis: a systematic review of the published evidence. *Pancreatology.* 2009;9: 601–14.

ADDITIONAL READING
- Wu BU, Conwell DL et al. Acute pancreatitis part I: approach to early management. *Clin Gastroenterol Hepatol.* 2010;8.
- Wu BU, Conwell DL et al. Acute pancreatitis part II: approach to follow-up. *Clin Gastroenterol Hepatol.* 2010;8:417–22.

See Also (Topic, Algorithm, Electronic Media Element)
Substance Use Disorders; Choledocholithiasis; Peptic Ulcer Disease; Systemic Lupus Erythematosus (SLE)

 CODES

ICD9
577.0 Acute pancreatitis

CLINICAL PEARLS
- Review all medications upon admission and discontinue any that have been implicated as causing pancreatitis, especially ACE inhibitors (in this author's experience).
- Fluid resuscitation is critical early since inadequate resuscitation has been implicated in converting mild pancreatitis into necrotizing pancreatitis.
- Referral to tertiary center is needed if acute pancreatitis is severe or evolving/worsening.
- Outpatient follow-up, particularly re-imaging, is very important.

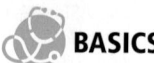 **BASICS**

DESCRIPTION
Irreversible

- Progressive destruction of the pancreas
- May result in either or both exocrine and endocrine insufficiency
- Pain, malabsorption, diabetes mellitus, and increased risk of pancreatic cancer are the major features.

EPIDEMIOLOGY
Incidence
Predominant age:

- 35–45 years (usually related to alcohol)
- Predominant sex: Male = Female

Prevalence
8.3/10,000

RISK FACTORS
See Etiology.

Genetics
Hereditary pancreatitis is a rare condition with an autosomally dominant inheritance pattern.

PATHOPHYSIOLOGY
- Calcification
- Fibrosis/atrophy
- Pancreatic ductal strictures

ETIOLOGY
- Alcohol
- Familial
- Autoimmune

DIAGNOSIS

Symptoms and objective evidence (imaging, amylase/lipase) do not always correlate.

HISTORY
- Fairly rapid onset of epigastric pain, which may radiate posteriorly, often with emesis, with acute superimposed on chronic pancreatitis. Chronic vague abdominal pain occurs with classical chronic pancreatitis.
- Alcohol use
- Steatorrhea
- Weight loss
- Children:
  - Recurrent postprandial epigastric pain
  - Family history of chronic pancreatitis
  - Growth failure
  - Diabetes

PHYSICAL EXAM
- Acute superimposed on chronic pancreatitis:
  - See acute pancreatitis section.
- Chronic pancreatitis:
  - Mild diffuse tenderness
  - Ascites

DIAGNOSTIC TESTS & INTERPRETATION
The laboratory and radiographic assessment of both acute and chronic pancreatitis must be used together, as there can be many false positives and negatives.

Lab
- Features and considerations:
  - Amylase and lipase usually normal or near normal
  - Hyperglycemia
  - Steatorrhea (fecal fat greater than 15 g per day on 100 g of fat per day diet), with other malabsorptive consequences such as low B12 level
  - Flare-ups may mimic acute pancreatitis.
  - Elevated alkaline phosphatase and bilirubin imply obstruction of the intrapancreatic common bile duct by extrinsic fibrosis or cancer.
  - Hereditary pancreatitis: Mutations in PRSSI gene and SPINKI gene
  - Autoimmune pancreatitis: Elevated serum IgG4, autoantibodies to lactoferrin and carbonic anhydrase
  - Decreased fecal elastase: Pancreatic insufficiency
- Disorders that may alter results for amylase or lipase:
  - Biliary tract disease, penetrating peptic ulcer, intestinal obstruction, intestinal ischemia/infarction, ruptured ectopic pregnancy, renal insufficiency, burns, macroamylasemia, or macrolipasemia

Imaging
- Plain film of abdomen: Might show pancreatic calcification if severe
- Ultrasound: Not terribly helpful for pancreas, but will assess the common bile duct diameter
- CT scan of abdomen: Pseudocysts, pancreatic duct dilation, and calcifications
- MRCP: Pancreatic ductal deformities/strictures (with or without pancreatic ductal stones), retained common bile duct stones
- EUS: Might help diagnose pancreatic cancer arising out of chronic pancreatitis

DIFFERENTIAL DIAGNOSIS
- Pancreatic cancer
- Lymphoma
- Other malabsorptive processes such as bacterial overgrowth, Celiac disease, etc.

TREATMENT

MEDICATION

- Analgesics
- Pancreatic enzyme supplements, e.g., Pancrease or Creon MT (2 24,000 IU capsules at the beginning of each meal), are microencapsulated now and do not require acid inhibition for protection for most cases (but PPI therapy can help in stubborn cases or those with pain).
- Octreotide (Sandostatin) can be supplemental therapy for pancreatic ductal fistulae.

ADDITIONAL TREATMENT
General Measures
- Analgesia: Consider pain management consultation regarding narcotic requirements.
- Exocrine and endocrine replacement therapy (enzymes and insulin, respectively)
- Consider more advanced therapy for pain: Celiac ganglion block, endoscopic or surgical decompression of partially obstructed pancreatic duct.

SURGERY/OTHER PROCEDURES
- Pseudocyst drainage:
  – Conservative approach is recommended.
  – Endoscopic (via endoscopic ultrasound) or surgical approach if mature wall
  – Percutaneous approach if rapidly enlarging or if thin wall
- Pancreatic ascites with disruption of the main pancreatic duct:
  – Endoscopic placement of pancreatic ductal stent is preferred, if possible.
  – Lateral pancreaticojejunostomy if endoscopic therapy is not possible

- Biliary obstruction (secondary to chronic pancreatitis, not choledocholithiasis):
  – Placement of removable metal stent or multiple plastic stents, if possible
  – Choledochojejunostomy if endoscopic therapy is not possible
- Pancreatic ductal obstruction by stone:
  – Endoscopic pancreatic sphincterotomy with stone extraction

IN-PATIENT CONSIDERATIONS
Discharge Criteria
- Pain control
- Resolution of problems secondary to ductal disruption, if present
- Alcohol rehab and smoking cessation, if needed

 ONGOING CARE

FOLLOW-UP RECOMMENDATIONS
Depends on the source of the pain and whether or not a ductal disruption exists

DIET
- Small meals high in protein; adjust if diabetes mellitus is present
- Pancreatic enzyme replacement therapy

PROGNOSIS
- Patient may have recurrent episodes of acute pancreatitis.
- Slow progression
- May "burn out" with resolution of symptoms
- Narcotic addiction occurs frequently.
- Pancreatic exocrine and/or endocrine insufficiency may occur years later.

ADDITIONAL READING
- Anderson SL, Trujillo JM et al. Association of pancreatitis with glucagon-like peptide-1 agonist use. *Ann Pharmacother*. 2010;44:904–9.
- Banks PA, Freeman ML, Practice Parameters Committee of the American College of Gastroenterology et al. Practice guidelines in acute pancreatitis. *Am J Gastroenterol*. 2006;101:2379–400.
- Gravante G, Garcea G, Ong SL, et al. Prediction of mortality in acute pancreatitis: a systematic review of the published evidence. *Pancreatology*. 2009;9:601–14.
- Oláh A, Romics L et al. Evidence-based use of enteral nutrition in acute pancreatitis. *Langenbecks Arch Surg*. 2010;395:309–16.

See Also (Topic, Algorithm, Electronic Media Element)
Substance Use Disorders; Choledocholithiasis; Peptic Ulcer Disease; Systemic Lupus Erythematosus (SLE)

 CODES

ICD9
577.1 Chronic pancreatitis

CLINICAL PEARLS
- Pancreatic enzyme replacement therapy is always the foundation of therapy.
- Pancreatic ductal injury must be considered and addressed.
- All patients with chronic pancreatitis do not necessarily have clinically significant pancreatic insufficiency yet.
- Fat malabsorption precedes carbohydrate and protein malabsorption.

PANIC DISORDER

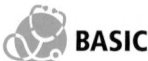

Katherine L. Margo, MD
Geoffrey M. Margo, MD, PhD

BASICS

DESCRIPTION
- A condition of repeated panic attacks of quick onset and lasting usually <1 h; in some patients the attacks have no obvious precipitant, whereas in others they have situational precipitants in which the person feels trapped in a setting where escape is difficult (e.g., driving on a bridge, riding in a bus, train, or plane) or embarrassing (e.g., church service, public events, or shopping lines).
- This 2nd type, panic disorder with agoraphobia, often keeps people stuck at home, forced to only frequent places that feel safe or dependent on "safe people" who must accompany them on all activities.
- Symptoms of an attack are intense, cause enormous distress, and can simulate a medical emergency.
- Anticipatory anxiety also can significantly affect everyday and work functioning even in the absence of an actual panic attack.

EPIDEMIOLOGY
Incidence
- Predominant age: All ages, including children; in school-age children, panic disorder can be confused with conduct disorder and school avoidance.
- Peak age of onset is in the 3rd decade of life.
- Predominant sex: Female > Male (approximately 2:1)

Prevalence
- Lifetime prevalence: 1–3%
- ~8% of patients in a primary-care practice population have panic disorder.
- 25% of patients presenting with chest pain in the emergency room have panic disorder.
- Chest pain is more likely due to panic if atypical, younger age, female, known problems with anxiety.

RISK FACTORS
- Life stressors of any kind can precipitate panic disorder, but no clear relationship exists between life stress and panic disorder.
- Cigarette smoking
- Cocaine, pseudoephedrine, and caffeine may provoke attacks.

Genetics
- Twin and family studies support a genetic predisposition in some patients.
- The genetic contribution to the development of panic disorder is estimated at 0.48, with the remaining contribution coming from life events.
- Monozygotic twins have a higher concordance rate than dizygotic twins.

PATHOPHYSIOLOGY
- Although the neurophysiologic mechanisms are not yet elucidated, the final common pathway in panic attacks is intense, sudden sympathetic stimulation.
- Current neurobiologic research is focusing on abnormal responses to anxiety-producing stimuli in the hippocampus, amygdala, and prefrontal cortex. For example, there appears to be impairment in the ability to learn from experience so that an original frightening experience dominates future responses even when subsequent exposures are not objectively threatening.

ETIOLOGY
- Unknown:
  - Biologic theories focus on limbic system malfunction in dealing with anxiety-evoking stimuli.
  - Psychological theories speak of deficits in managing strong affects such as fear and anger.
- Medications may cause panic disorder: Buspirone, estrogen, levodopa, others.
- Substances may cause panic disorder: Illicit drugs, alcohol, either excessive caffeine or caffeine withdrawal.
- The complaint of dizziness in patients with panic disorder may be linked to a malfunction of the vestibular system, and vestibular disorders may play a role in the pathophysiology of panic disorder.

COMMONLY ASSOCIATED CONDITIONS
- Significant overlap with several psychiatric conditions; >70% of patients with panic disorder also have one or more other psychiatric diagnoses, including
  - Other anxiety disorders
  - Depression
  - Agoraphobia
  - Substance abuse
- It is common for depression and panic disorder to develop in close temporal relation.
- Panic disorder is more common in patients with the following medical conditions:
  - Hypertension
  - Mitral valve prolapse
  - Interstitial cystitis
  - Irritable bowel syndrome

DIAGNOSIS

- Diagnosis based on *DSM-IVR* criteria: Recurrent, unexpected panic attacks (see below), followed by ≥1 month of persistent concern about having further attacks, worry about the implication of the attack (e.g., heart attack, going crazy, etc.), or significant behavior change as a result.
- Agoraphobia may be present.
- Symptoms are not related to substance abuse or another medical condition. The attacks are not better accounted for by conditions in the differential diagnosis.

HISTORY
- Panic attacks consist of a period of intense fear or discomfort in which ≥4 of the following symptoms develop abruptly and peak in ~10 minutes:
  - Sweating
  - Chills or hot flashes
  - Trembling, shaking
  - Chest pain or discomfort
  - Palpitation, pounding heart, increased heart rate
  - Shortness of breath, feeling smothered
  - Feeling of choking
  - Nausea or abdominal distress
  - Dizziness, unsteady, light-headed, faint
  - Paresthesias
  - Derealization or depersonalization
  - Fear of losing control or going crazy
  - Fear of dying
- Panic attacks are not subtle. Frequent interepisode history of anticipatory anxiety or the marked limitations in daily activities with agoraphobia;

however, obtaining a clear history, especially with a new patient, is difficult for 2 reasons:
  - In the throes of a panic attack, many patients are convinced that the disorder is physical (the symptoms are physical, frighteningly so).
  - Patients are often deeply embarrassed by their problem, which they see as a personal failure.
- Consequently, the physician should have a high suspicion for panic disorder with the pattern of symptoms noted above, their abrupt onset, and their recurrent nature. Tactful, nonjudgmental questioning is called for after the worst of the attack is over.
- A thorough medication and substance abuse history is important.
- In order to make a definitive diagnosis, at least some of the attacks should have no obvious precipitating event.

PHYSICAL EXAM
- During an attack, the autonomic hyperactivity will be seen as tachycardia, hyperventilation, and sweating.
- A pulse oximetry reading can be helpful to rule out several serious medical conditions.
- Thyroid exam looking for fullness or nodules
- Cardiac exam to evaluate for a systolic murmur
- Lung exam to rule out asthma (limited airflow, wheezing)

DIAGNOSTIC TESTS & INTERPRETATION
The Quick PsychoDiagnostics Panel has the best testing characteristics for diagnosing panic disorder (1).
Lab
No specific lab tests are indicted except to rule out conditions in the differential diagnosis. Consider
- Thyroid-stimulating hormone (TSH)
- Hemoglobin
- Electrolyte panel
- ECG for those with cardiac symptoms

Imaging
Initial approach
Echocardiogram if mitral valve prolapse considered

Diagnostic Procedures/Surgery
None specific to panic disorder, but if a medical cause of anxiety is strongly suspected, the workup appropriate to that condition should be done.

DIFFERENTIAL DIAGNOSIS
- Psychiatric conditions that have overlapping symptomatology include anxiety disorders such as generalized anxiety disorder, obsessive–compulsive disorder (OCD), and post-traumatic stress disorder (PTSD).
- Co-occurring disorders include depression and other affective disorders, substance abuse, and phobias.
- Somatization disorder is also an illness of multiple unexplained medical symptoms, but the presenting picture is usually one of chronic symptoms rather than the acute, dramatic onset of a panic attack.
- There are multiple medical conditions with some physical symptoms similar to those in panic, such as myocardial infarction (MI), asthma, paroxysmal supraventricular tachycardia, pulmonary embolus, seizure disorder, transient ischemic attacks, carcinoid syndrome, Cushing disease, hyperthyroidism, and pheochromocytoma; however, these conditions are usually easily distinguished by other signs and symptoms, and most are less common than panic attacks.

TREATMENT

Combined antidepressant therapy and psychotherapy is superior to either alone during active treatment (2).

MEDICATION
- Medication management is indicated if psychotherapy is not successful or may be initiated together with psychotherapy.
- Patient preference plays a big part in this decision.
- Because patients typically are anxious about their treatment, the therapeutic alliance is critical for the chronic care of this disorder.
- If medications are started, they should be maintained for at least 6 months after symptom control.

First Line
- At the time of severe attack, a quick-acting benzodiazepine such as lorazepam or alprazolam may be used, in addition to active support and assurance of safety. Clonazepam, lorazepam, and alprazolam are useful in acute panic attacks. Benzodiazepines should not be used as monotherapy unless there is no co-occurring mood disorder.
- Selective serotonin reuptake inhibitors (SSRIs), SNRIs, and tricyclics are all equally effective in preventing or reducing the frequency and intensity of panic attacks.
  - Fluoxetine is considered to cause more initial nervousness than others.
  - Paroxetine and sertraline have specific indications for panic disorder.
  - Dosing is started at a lower level than the usual antidepressant dose and raised slowly to avoid the side effects of agitation and anxiety.
- Chronic benzodiazepines may be considered if the antidepressants are insufficient and the severity of the illness outweighs the risk of dependence. In this situation, clonazepam is less likely to cause withdrawal problems but, as with all benzodiazepines, must be tapered down slowly.

Second Line
- Tricyclic antidepressants, particularly imipramine, are as efficacious as and less expensive than SSRIs. They are considered 2nd line because of somewhat more difficulty in dosing and greater risk for overdose compared with the SSRIs.
- Venlafaxine has been found to reduce panic attack occurrence and severity in recent studies.

ADDITIONAL TREATMENT
General Measures
Psychotherapy is effective.
- Cognitive-behavioral therapy (CBT), tailored for panic disorder, consists of several steps: Education, changing cognitions about the attack and the illness, relaxation and controlled breathing techniques, and if appropriate, exposure to anxiety-provoking conditions coupled with in vivo relaxation exercises.
- Psychodynamic psychotherapy has been shown to be effective in helping patients to understand their illness and themselves in the context of current psychological stresses. Length of remission is considerably improved over medication-only treatments.
- Combination of psychotherapy with antidepressants is better than either alone, but after the acute phase, the combination is the same as psychotherapy alone and better than antidepressants alone.

Issues for Referral
- Panic disorder can be managed initially by primary-care physician to assess the overlap of symptoms with medical illness and to manage medication. Some patients will require care by a psychiatrist, either for assistance with the diagnosis of concomitant anxiety disorders or for medication management.
- Psychotherapy should be handled by a competent therapist knowledgeable about the disorder.
- A new model of collaborative care has shown good results. The model has several components, including primary-care physician management with psychiatric consultation, psychoeducation, and telephone-based follow-up and support provided by a trained nonprofessional worker with structured feedback to the physician.

Additional Therapies
- Rebreathing from a paper bag is a useful way to reduce the hypocapnia of hyperventilation.
- Aerobic exercise reduces symptoms better than placebo.

IN-PATIENT CONSIDERATIONS
Admission Criteria
- Rarely, a medical or psychiatric admission is required. If the emergency physician is not satisfied with the rule out of life-threatening medical conditions, such as a myocardial infarction (MI) or pulmonary embolus (PE), a medical admission is justified to complete the workup.
- If a panic disorder patient is suicidal, a psychiatric admission is indicated.

 ONGOING CARE

FOLLOW-UP RECOMMENDATIONS
Regular follow-up after acute panic attack is important:
- To provide support and education
- To initiate or make a referral for psychotherapy
- To monitor and adjust medications
- To evaluate for suicidality—patients with panic disorder are at increased risk.

PATIENT EDUCATION
- http://www.nlm.nih.gov/medlineplus/panicdisorder.html
- Patient information handouts in Am Fam Physician 2005;71:740 and 2006;74:1393
- http://www.nimh.nih.gov/health/publications/when-fear-overwhelms-panic-disorder/index.shtml

PROGNOSIS
- ~50% of patients recover with treatment, although the duration of episodic illness can extend over decades.
- Even recovered patients are at risk for future recurrences.
- Panic disorder must be thought of as a chronic condition with an emphasis on long-term support and a renewal of active treatment when needed.

COMPLICATIONS
Suicide in ~7%; up to 20% in patients with other co-occurring psychiatric disorders

REFERENCES
1. Shedler J, Beck A, Bensen S. Practical mental health assessment in primary care. Validity and utility of the Quick PsychoDiagnostics Panel. J Fam Pract. 2000;49:614–21.
2. Furukawa TA, Watanabe N, Churchill R. Combined psychotherapy plus antidepressants for panic disorder with or without agoraphobia. Cochrane Database of Systematic Reviews 2007, Issue 1. Art. No.: CD004364. DOI:10.1002/14651858.CD004364.pub2

ADDITIONAL READING
- Ham P, Waters DB, Oliver MN. Treatment of panic disorder. Am Fam Physician. 2005;71:733–9.
- McIntosh A, et al. Clinical Guidelines for the Management of Anxiety. Management of anxiety (panic disorder, with or without agoraphobia, and generalized anxiety disorder) in adults in primary, secondary and community care. National Institute for Clinical Evidence NICE, 2004.
- Roy-Byrne PP, Craske MG, Stein MB. Panic disorder. Lancet. 2006;368:1023–32.
- Roy-Byrne PP, Wagner AW, Schraufnagel TJ. Understanding and treating panic disorder in the primary care setting. J Clin Psychiatry. 2005; 66(Suppl 4):16–22.
- Simon NM, Fischmann D. The implications of medical and psychiatric comorbidity with panic disorder. J Clin Psychiatry. 2005;66(Suppl 4):8–15.
- Treatment of Patients with Panic Disorder, Second Edition. Arlington, Virginia: American Psychiatric Association, January 2009. Available at: http://www.psychiatryonline.com/pracGuide/pracGuideChapToc_9.aspx

See Also (Topic, Algorithm, Electronic Media Element)
Algorithm: Anxiety

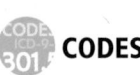 **CODES**

ICD9
- 300.01 Panic disorder
- 300.21 Agoraphobia with panic disorder

CLINICAL PEARLS
- In school-aged children, panic disorder can be confused with conduct disorder and school avoidance.
- In the initial stages, combined treatment with medication and psychotherapy is more effective than either treatment alone.
- SSRIs, SNRIs, and tricyclics are all equally effective in preventing or reducing the frequency and intensity of panic attacks.
- Medications should be maintained for at least 6 months after symptom control.

PARANOID PERSONALITY DISORDER

Margo Lauterbach, MD
Patrick Smallwood, MD

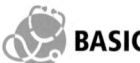 **BASICS**

DESCRIPTION
- Paranoid personality disorder is a maladaptive persistent pattern of behavior characterized by suspiciousness, inappropriate mistrust of people, and hostility toward others who are often perceived as malicious. Consequently, patients avoid intimate relationships, bear grudges, and expect to be exploited by others.
- Paranoid personality disorder is one of the Cluster A personality disorders.

EPIDEMIOLOGY
Incidence
- Predominant age: First manifests in childhood or adolescence
- Predominant sex: Male > Female
- Increased in families with delusional disorder (persecutory type) and chronic schizophrenia

Prevalence
- 0.5–2.5% of the general population
- 2–10% of psychiatric outpatients
- 10–30% of psychiatric inpatients

RISK FACTORS
- Family history of paranoid personality disorder
- Childhood abuse/neglect

Genetics
Genetic predisposition may play a role (see Incidence).

PATHOPHYSIOLOGY
Paranoid sense of mistrust can result from childhood abuse/neglect and/or genetic predisposition to paranoia.

ETIOLOGY
Specific causes unknown

COMMONLY ASSOCIATED CONDITIONS
- May develop major depressive disorder and may be at increased risk for obsessive–compulsive disorder and agoraphobia
- At risk for alcohol or other substance abuse or dependence

 DIAGNOSIS

HISTORY
- Thorough psychiatric history and mental status examination
- Collateral history to establish pervasive pattern of behavior
- Diagnosis is based on fulfilling 4/7 *DSM-IV* criteria for the disorder (1,2)[C]:
  – Suspects exploitation, harm, or deceit by others
  – Unjustified doubt of others' loyalty or trustworthiness
  – Fears malicious retaliation if confides in others; thus avoids doing so
  – Believes benign remarks or situations are threatening or demeaning
  – Unforgiving; hypersensitive to slights
  – Unjustifiably perceives attacks on character/reputation and may become hostile or counterattack
  – Suspects infidelity of spouse/sexual partner
- Associated features include:
  – Strong sense of autonomy
  – Stubborn
  – Litigious
  – Can be perceived as fanatic
  – May form closed groups or cults
  – Can foster fear in others

DIAGNOSTIC TESTS & INTERPRETATION
Psychological testing (e.g., Minnesota Multiphasic Personality Inventory or MMPI-II)

Imaging
Brain imaging may rule out organic disease for those with emerging symptoms.

DIFFERENTIAL DIAGNOSIS
- Although brief psychotic states can result from significant stressors, primary psychotic disorders including paranoid schizophrenia, delusional disorder (paranoid type), and mood disorder with psychotic features, must be ruled out.
- Schizoid personality disorder; avoidant personality disorder
- Medical disorders (e.g., temporal lobe epilepsy) with behavioral changes
- Culturally appropriate behavior, sometimes marked by defensiveness or guardedness, must not be mistaken for paranoia. Minorities, immigrants, and refugees also can present similarly but may be plagued by unfamiliarity.
- Paranoid traits can develop in the face of physical handicaps, such as hearing impairment.

 TREATMENT

MEDICATION
- Although little evidence suggests that the core personality features of paranoid personality disorder respond to psychopharmacologic treatment, psychotic paranoid ideation, acute hostility, anxiety, or psychosis can respond to low-dose antipsychotics and/or short-term benzodiazepines (3,4)[C].
- Short-term benzodiazepines, such as diazepam, can be useful in treating acute agitation, hostility, or anxiety.

- Acute psychotic states and delusional thinking can respond to low-dose antipsychotics, such as haloperidol.
- Taking medications can be interpreted by the patient as powerlessness and loss of autonomy.

ADDITIONAL TREATMENT

General Measures
- Treatment is difficult and often avoided by the patient (3,4)[C].
- Supportive psychotherapy, a form of therapy that is predictable, respectful, and straightforward, is preferred. Overly warm and empathetic styles can be regarded as intrusive.
- Mistrust issues can undermine group therapy and behavioral therapy.
- Family therapy may be helpful.

Issues for Referral
Patient should be referred for individual psychotherapy and psychiatric follow-up if psychiatric medication(s) are indicated.

IN-PATIENT CONSIDERATIONS

Admission Criteria
Patients who become suicidal or homicidal may require psychiatric hospitalization for safety and stabilization. Patients with acute psychotic states also may require hospitalization if they are unable to care for themselves or pose a risk to others.

Discharge Criteria
A hospitalized patient is usually discharged after appropriate therapeutic interventions and discharge planning have taken place. Suicidal ideation, homicidal ideation, and/or acute psychotic states must be resolved.

 ## ONGOING CARE

PATIENT EDUCATION
National Institute of Mental Health at http://www.nimh.nih.gov

PROGNOSIS
- Good prognosis for those with good ego strength and strong support system
- Poor prognosis for those with poor insight, lack of primary support system, or comorbid Axis I psychiatric diagnosis

COMPLICATIONS
Significant impairment in work and interpersonal relationships

REFERENCES

1. *American Psychiatric Association. Diagnostic and Statistical Manual of Mental Disorders*. 4th ed. Washington, DC: American Psychiatric Press; 2000.
2. Svrakic DM, Cloninger CR. Paranoid personality disorder. In: Sadock BJ, Sadock VA, eds. *Kaplan & Sadock's Comprehensive Textbook of Psychiatry*. 8th ed. Philadelphia: Lippincott Williams & Wilkins; 2005:2081.
3. Bender DS, Dolan RT, Skodol AE, et al. Treatment utilization by patients with personality disorders. *Am J Psychiatry*. 2001;158:295–302.
4. Meissner SJ. Paranoid personality disorder. In: Gabbard GO, ed. *Treatments of Psychiatric Disorders*. 3rd ed. Washington, DC: American Psychiatric Press; 2001;2227–36.

ADDITIONAL READING

Verheul R, Herbrink M. The efficacy of various modalities of psychotherapy for personality disorders: A systematic review of the evidence and clinical recommendations. *Int Rev Psychiatry*. 2007;19: 25–38.

 ## CODES

ICD9
301.0 Paranoid personality disorder

CLINICAL PEARLS

- Paranoid personality disorder is a maladaptive persistent pattern of behavior characterized by suspiciousness, inappropriate mistrust of people, and hostility toward others.
- Although little evidence suggests that the core personality features of paranoid personality disorder respond to psychopharmacologic treatment, psychotic paranoid ideation, acute hostility, anxiety, or psychosis can respond to low-dose antipsychotics or short-term benzodiazepines.
- Poor prognosis for those with poor insight, lack of primary support system, or a comorbid Axis I psychiatric diagnosis

PARKINSON DISEASE

Alicia R. Desilets, PharmD
Mildred LaFontaine, MD

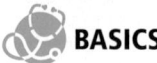 **BASICS**

DESCRIPTION
- Parkinson's disease (PD) is a progressive neurodegenerative disorder caused by degeneration of dopaminergic neurons in the substantia nigra pars compacta.
- Cardinal symptoms include resting tremor, rigidity, bradykinesia, and gait dysfunction.
- Diagnosis is based primarily on history and examination.

EPIDEMIOLOGY
Incidence
- Average age of onset around 60 years
- Slightly more common in males vs females

Prevalence
- Second most common neurodegenerative disease after Alzheimer's disease
- 0.3% of general population and 1–2% of those 60 years and older (prevalence increases with age)
- Affects 1 million people in the US

RISK FACTORS
- Age is the greatest risk factor.
- History of smoking may reduce risk
- Weak association with exposure to toxins (herbicides and insecticides); however, relationship is not clear

Genetics
Mutations in multiple autosomal dominant and recessive genes have been linked to PD or parkinsonian syndrome. Genes investigated in PD include LRRK-2, GBA, and alpha-synuclein.

PATHOPHYSIOLOGY
- Pathological hallmark: Selective loss of dopamine-containing neurons in the pars compacta of the substantia nigra
- Loss of neurons accompanied by presence of Lewy bodies, pale bodies (predecessor of the Lewy body), and Lewy neuritis

ETIOLOGY
Dopamine depletion in the substantia nigra and the nigrostriatal pathways results in almost all motor complications of PD.

COMMONLY ASSOCIATED CONDITIONS
Nonmotor-associated symptoms include cognitive abnormalities, autonomic dysfunction (example: constipation, urinary urgency), sleep disturbances, mental status changes (depression, psychosis, hallucinations, dementia), orthostatic hypotension, and pain.

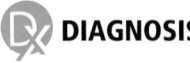 **DIAGNOSIS**

- Diagnosis during life is based on clinical impression.
- True gold standard for diagnosis is neuropathologic exam.
- Historically, 2 of the 3 cardinal manifestations must be present: Tremor, bradykinesia, and rigidity have been shown to lead to misdiagnosis at autopsy.
- High level of probability if patient has resting tremor, prominent asymmetry, and good response to levodopa

HISTORY
Symptoms are often subtle and/or falsely attributed to aging:
- Gradual decreased emotion displayed in facial features
- General motor slowing and stiffness (1 or both arms do not swing with walk)
- Resting tremor (often initially 1 hand)
- Speech soft or mumbling
- Falls or difficulty with balance (tends to occur with disease progression)

PHYSICAL EXAM
- Tremor:
  - Resting tremor (4–6 Hz) in a limb that is often asymmetric
  - Disappears with voluntary movement
  - Frequently emerges in a hand while walking and may present as pill rolling
  - May also present in jaw, chin, lips, tongue
- Bradykinesia
- Rigidity
  - Cogwheel (catching and releasing) or lead pipe (continuously rigid)
- Postural instability

DIAGNOSTIC TESTS & INTERPRETATION
Lab
Initial lab tests
- Thyroid testing
- Ceruloplasmin and copper in patients <50 to rule out Wilson disease

Imaging
Initial approach
- Diagnosis is mainly clinical.
- Magnetic resonance imaging of brain to rule out other disorders, particularly in patients thought to have PD not responding to therapy
- Positron emission tomography and single photon emission computed tomography may be somewhat helpful with diagnosis, but often not required

Pathological Findings
Lewy bodies

DIFFERENTIAL DIAGNOSIS
- Essential tremor: Bradykinesia not present, often symmetric and occurs mostly on action or when holding hands outstretched
- Drug-induced parkinsonism: Reversible, although it may take weeks or months after offending medication is stopped:
  - Neuroleptics (most common cause), antiemetics (e.g., prochlorperazine and promethazine), metoclopramide, selective serotonin reuptake inhibitors, calcium channel blockers (e.g., flunarizine and cinnarizine), amiodarone, lithium, cholinergics, chemotherapeutics, amphotericin B, estrogens, and valproic acid
- Psychogenic parkinsonism
- Progressive supranuclear palsy: Impairment in vertical eye movements (particularly down gaze), hyperextension of neck, and early falling
- Multiple system atrophy: Presence of prominent orthostatic hypotension or concomitant cerebellar signs

- Dementia with Lewy bodies
- Other considerations: Huntington disease, Hallervorden-Spatz disease, Wilson disease, dopa-responsive dystonia

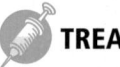 **TREATMENT**

MEDICATION
- PD treatment goal: Improving motor and nonmotor deficits
- Agents are chosen based on patient age and symptoms present
- 1st-line agents in early PD: Levodopa, dopamine agonists, monoamine oxidase (MAO)-B inhibitors (1)[A]:
  - Levodopa vs dopamine agonist controversial (2)[B]:
    - Most patients will eventually develop motor fluctuations with levodopa: Younger patients are more likely to develop motor fluctuations. Some thought is to delay initiation of levodopa to decrease drug-induced motor fluctuations early in disease
    - Older patients are often unable to tolerate adverse events of dopamine agonists.
    - All patients will eventually require levodopa therapy.
  - MAO-B inhibitors (rasagiline) should be considered as initial monotherapy (2)[B]:
    - Being investigated for potential neuroprotective effects
- 2nd-line agents in early PD: β-adrenergic antagonists (postural tremor), amantadine, anticholinergics (young patients with tremor) (1)[A]:
  - Lack of evidence for symptom control
- Treatment of levodopa-induced motor complications:
  - End of dose wearing off:
    - Entacapone (with each levodopa dose) or rasagiline preferred (3)[A]
    - May also consider dopamine agonist, apomorphine, selegiline (4)[B]
  - Dyskinesias:
    - Typically occur at peak dopamine level
    - Amantadine may be considered; however, efficacy is questionable (1)[B]

First Line
- Carbidopa plus levodopa (carbidopa inhibits peripheral conversion of levodopa):
  - Immediate release (Sinemet):
    - Tablets (mg): 10/100, 25/100, 25/250
    - Usual initial maintenance dose: 25/100 mg p.o. t.i.d. Most patients will require 25 mg of carbidopa to inhibit peripheral conversion of levodopa.
    - Watch for nausea, orthostatic hypotension, sedation, vivid dreams, and vomiting.
  - Orally disintegrating (Parcopa):
    - Tablets (mg): 10/100, 25/100, 25/25
  - Sustained release (Sinemet CR):
    - Tablets (mg): 25/100, 50/200
    - Dose agents initially b.i.d.

- Carbidopa plus levodopa plus entacapone (Stalevo):
  – Tablets (mg): 12.5/50/200, 18.75/75/200, 25/100/200, 31.25/125/200, 37.5/150/200, 50/200/200
  – Addition of entacapone as a single agent should be initiated prior to use of this combination:
    ○ Once daily dose of carbidopa/levodopa has been identified, may convert to Stalevo
    ○ Dose of levodopa may need to be decreased with the addition of entacapone
  – Side effects are the same, plus diarrhea and brownish-orange urine.
- Dopamine agonists (Nonergot): Side effects include nausea, vomiting, hypotension, sedation, lower extremity edema, vivid dreaming, compulsive behavior, confusion, lightheadedness, and hallucinations.
  – Pramipexole (Mirapex): Tablets (mg):0.125, 0.25, 0.5, 1, 1.5
    ○ Start with 0.125 mg t.i.d., gradually increase every 5–7 days to 0.5–1.5 mg t.i.d.
    ○ CrCl 35–59 mL/min 0.125 mg p.o. b.i.d.
    ○ CrCl 15–34 mL/min 0.125 mg p.o. daily
  – Pramipexole ER (Mirapex ER): Tablets (mg): 0.375, 0.75, 1.5, 3, 4.5; start with 0.375 p.o. daily
  – Ropinirole (Requip): Tablets (mg): 0.25, 0.5, 1, 2, 3, 4, 5; start with 0.25 mg t.i.d., increase gradually to 3–8 mg t.i.d.
  – Requip XL: Tablets (mg): 2, 4, 6, 8, 12; start at a 2-mg dose once daily, increase in 1–2 weeks
- Dopamine agonists (ergot): Increased adverse event profile makes these agents nonpreferred to nonergot dopamine agonists
- Bromocriptine (Parlodel):
  – Tablets (mg): 2.5
  – Capsules (mg): 5
  – Start with 1.25 mg b.i.d., increase by 2.5 mg every 2–4 weeks up to effective dose (30–90 mg/day in 3 divided doses).
  – Same as nonergot and increases risk for pulmonary fibrosis (decreased efficacy compared to other agents)
- Selective MAO-B inhibitors: Side effects include insomnia, jitteriness, hallucinations; mostly found with selegiline; rasagiline shown to have similar adverse events as placebo in clinical trials. Rasagiline is metabolized via CYP 1A2; caution with other medications utilizing this enzyme system (ex. ciprofloxacin).
  – Both agents contraindicated with meperidine and numerous other agents metabolized via CYP 1A2
  – At therapeutic doses, unlikely to induce a "cheese reaction" (tyramine storm)
- Selegiline (Eldepryl):
  – Tablets (mg): 5 mg; initiate 5 mg p.o. b.i.d.
  – Orally disintegrating tablet (Zelapar): 1.25 mg; 1.25 mg p.o. daily for 6 weeks; increase as needed to maximum of 2.5 mg daily
  – Transdermal patch (Emsam): 6 mg/24 hr, 9 mg/24 hr, 12 mg/24 hr; start with 6 mg/24 hr and titrate up every 2 weeks as needed to a maximum of 12 mg/24 hr
- Rasagiline (Azilect): Tablets (mg): 0.5, 1; initiate 0.5 mg–1 mg daily

Second Line
- Anticholinergic agents: Usually avoided due to lack of efficacy (only useful for tremor) and increased adverse event profile, including blurred vision, confusion, constipation, dry mouth, memory difficulty, sedation, and urinary retention

  – Trihexyphenidyl:
    ○ Tablets (mg): 2, 5
    ○ Start with 1–2 mg daily, increase by 2 mg every 3–5 days until usual dose 5–15 mg in 3–4 divided doses
  – Benztropine (Cogentin):
    ○ Tablets (mg): 0.5, 1, 2
    ○ Start with 0.5–6 mg in 1–2 divided doses; increase by 0.5 mg every 5–6 days
- N-methyl-D-aspartic acid antagonist: Exact mechanism unknown and efficacy questionable; however, may be useful for dyskinesias. Side effects include confusion, dizziness, dry mouth, livedo reticularis, and hallucinations.
  – Amantadine (Symmetrel):
    ○ Tablets (mg): 100
    ○ Start with 100 mg b.i.d.; may increase to 300 mg daily in divided doses; must be renally adjusted
- Catechol-O-methyl transferase (COMT) inhibitors: Entacapone preferred due to hepatotoxicity associated with tolcapone. Adverse events include nausea and orthostatic hypotension.
  – Tolcapone (Tasmar):
    ○ Tablets (mg): 100, 200
    ○ Start 100 mg t.i.d.; maximum dose 600 mg/d; must be taken with carbidopa/levodopa
  – Entacapone (Comtan):
    ○ Tablets (mg): 200
    ○ 200 mg with each dose of carbidopa/levodopa; maximum dose 1,600 mg/d
- Apomorphine (Apokyn): Nonergot-derived dopamine agonist given subcutaneously for off episodes. Adverse events include nausea, vomiting, dizziness, hallucinations, orthostatic hypotension, and somnolence:
  – Effective dose ranges from 2–6 mg/injection; most patients require 0.06 mg/kg
  – Monitor for orthostatic hypotension after initial dose; this is a potent emetic, so initiate an antiemetic (e.g., trimethobenzamide) 3 days prior to start and continue for 2 months. Avoid ondansetron (combination causes severe hypotension and syncope) and dopamine antagonists such as prochlorperazine and metoclopramide.
  – Indicated only for "off" episodes with levodopa therapy

ADDITIONAL TREATMENT
General Measures
- Multidisciplinary rehabilitation with standard physical and occupational therapy components to improve functional outcomes
- Physiotherapy to help with gait re-education, enhancement of aerobic capacity, improvement in movement initiation, improvement in functional independence, and help with home safety
- Emotional and psychological support of patient and family
- Speech and language therapy, dysphagia evaluation and therapy

Issues for Referral
All patients with suspected PD should quickly be referred to a specialist for an accurate diagnosis and management (1).

SURGERY/OTHER PROCEDURES
Deep brain stimulation (bilateral subthalamic nucleus or globus pallidus interna) for patients with motor complications refractory to best medical treatment who are healthy, have no significant active comorbidity, are responsive to levodopa, and do not have depression or dementia (1)

 ## ONGOING CARE

DIET
- Increase dietary fluids and fiber, and increase activity for constipation
- For dysphagia, consider soft food, swallowing evaluation, and increased time for meals

PATIENT EDUCATION
http://www.apdaparkinson.org,
http://www.parkinson.org,
http://guidance.nice.org.uk/CG35

PROGNOSIS
PD is a chronic progressive disease; prognosis varies based on patient-specific symptoms

COMPLICATIONS
Psychosis can be caused by medication (most common); simplify medication regimen by discontinuing anticholinergics, dopamine agonists, amantadine, COMT inhibitors and selegiline; and a decrease in levodopa:
- Clozapine is useful but needs frequent monitoring due to agranulocytosis.
- Quetiapine (Seroquel) may be considered a better option.

REFERENCES

1. National Institute for Health and Clinical Excellence. *Parkinson's disease: Diagnosis and management in primary and secondary care* London: NICE, 2006.
2. Chen JJ, Swope DM. Pharmacotherapy for Parkinson's Disease. *Pharmacotherapy.* 2007; 27:161s–173s.
3. Pahwa R, Factor SA, Lyons KE, et al. Practice Parameter: Treatment of Parkinson disease with motor fluctuations and dyskinesia (an evidence-based review): Report of the Quality Standards Subcommittee of the American Academy of Neurology. *Neurology.* 2006;66:983–95.
4. Diaz NL, Waters CH. Current strategies in the treatment of Parkinson's disease and a personalized approach to management. *Expert Rev. Neurother.* 2009;9(12):1781–1789.

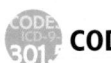 ## CODES

ICD9
332.0 Paralysis agitans

CLINICAL PEARLS
- Emphasize importance of exercise and movement to help preserve function as long as possible.
- Pharmacotherapeutic regimens need to be individualized based on patient-specific symptoms and age.

PARONYCHIA

Russell C. Hendershot, DO, MS

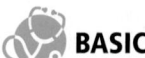 **BASICS**

DESCRIPTION
- Infectious or eczematous inflammation of the folds of skin surrounding the fingernail or toenail; may be acute or chronic:
  - Acutely, it often appears 2–5 days after trauma.
  - May be considered work-related in bartenders, waitresses, nurses, and others who often wet their hands
- System(s) affected: Skin/Exocrine
- Synonym(s): Eponychia; Perionychia

Pediatric Considerations
Thumb/finger-sucking is a risk factor (anaerobes and *E. coli* may be present).

EPIDEMIOLOGY
Incidence
- Common in US
- Predominant age: All ages
- Predominant sex: Female > Male (3:1)

RISK FACTORS
- Acute: Trauma to skin surrounding nail, ingrown nails, manicured/sculptured nails, diabetes mellitus (DM)
- Chronic: Frequent immersion of hands in water (e.g., cooks, chefs, bartenders, housekeepers, swimmers), DM, immunosuppression (reported association with antiretroviral therapy for HIV and with use of epidermal growth factor inhibitors)

GENERAL PREVENTION
- Chronic: Avoid allergens and frequent wetting of hands; wear rubber gloves with cloth liner.
- Good diabetic control
- Expectant treatment for candidiasis
- Chronic: Keep fingers dry; avoid allergens.

PATHOPHYSIOLOGY
- A paronychial infection usually starts in the lateral nail fold.
- Occasionally, the infection includes the complete margin of skin around the nail plate. Results from mechanical separation of the nail plate from the perionychium.
- Early in the course of this disease process (<24 h), cellulitis alone may be present. An abscess can form if the infection does not resolve quickly.
- Chronic infections most likely represent eczematous reaction with secondary infection and multifocal etiology.

ETIOLOGY
- Acute: *Staphylococcus aureus* and *Streptococcus pyogenes;* less frequently, *Pseudomonas pyocyanea* and *Proteus vulgaris*. In digits exposed to oral flora, also consider *Eikenella corrodens, Fusobacterium, and Peptostreptococcus*.
- Chronic: Eczematous reaction with secondary *C. albicans* (~95%); less frequently, dermatophytes and, occasionally, molds (*Scytalidium, Fusarium*)

COMMONLY ASSOCIATED CONDITIONS
- DM
- If chronic, eczema or atrophic dermatitis
- Certain medications: Cetuximab, paclitaxel, antiretroviral therapy (especially protease inhibitors and lamivudine, with toes more commonly involved)
- If multiple, consider pemphigus vulgaris (rare)

DIAGNOSIS

HISTORY
- Localized pain and tenderness
- Previous trauma (bitten nails, ingrown nails, manicured)
- Contact with herpes infections
- Contact with allergens or irritants (frequent water immersion, latex)

PHYSICAL EXAM
- Acute: Red, hot, tender, tense nail fold ± abscess
- Chronic: Swollen, tender, boggy nail fold ± abscess
- Occasional elevation of nail bed
- Separation of nail fold from nail plate
- Red, painful swelling of skin around nail plate
- Purulent drainage
- Secondary changes of nail plate
- Green changes in nail (*Pseudomonas*)
- Positive digital pressure test (light pressure over the area causes digital blanching and demarcation of the abscess)
- Chronic; symptoms similar to acute with possible retraction of nail fold and absence of adjacent cuticle, thickening of nail plate, with prominent transverse ridges known as Beau's lines

DIAGNOSTIC TESTS & INTERPRETATION
Lab
None required unless condition is severe, resistant to treatment or methicillin-resistant *S. aureus* (MRSA) is suspected; then:
- Gram stain
- Culture and sensitivity
- Potassium hydroxide wet mount plus fungal culture
- Drugs that may alter lab results: Use of over-the-counter antimicrobials or antifungals

Diagnostic Procedures/Surgery
- Scraping for wet mount and culture in chronic cases
- Incision and drainage for suppurative or cases not responding to conservative management
- Tzanck testing or viral culture in suspected viral cases

DIFFERENTIAL DIAGNOSIS
- Herpetic whitlow (similar in appearance, very painful, often associated with vesicles)
- Felon (abscess of fingertip pulp; urgent diagnosis required)
- Allergic contact dermatitis (latex, acrylic)
- Reiter disease
- Psoriasis
- Chronic; squamous cell carcinoma, malignant melanoma, metastases, eczema, psoriasis, Reiter's syndrome

TREATMENT

MEDICATION

First Line

- Tetanus booster when appropriate
- No evidence that antibiotics are better or worse than incision and drainage
- Acute (mild cases):
  – Antibiotic cream alone or in combination with a topical steroid
  – Antibiotic cream applied t.i.d.–q.i.d. (e.g.; mupirocin or gentamycin/neomycin/polymixin B) for 5–10 days
  – Topical steroid applied b.i.d. (e.g.; betamethasone 0.05% cream) for 7–14 days
- Acute (exposure to oral flora):
  – Clindamycin (Cleocin) 315–450 mg t.i.d.–q.i.d. for 7 days
  – Pediatric: 10 mg/kg q8h
  – Amoxicillin–clavulanate potassium (Augmentin): 875 mg/125 mg q12h or 500 mg/125 mg 3 times daily for 7 days
  – Pediatric: 45 mg/kg q12h (for <40 kg)
- Acute (no exposure to oral flora):
  – Dicloxacillin 250 mg t.i.d.for 7 days
  – Cephalexin (Keflex) 500 mg b.i.d.–t.i.d. for 7 days
- Acute (suspected MRSA):
  – Trimethoprim/sulfamethoxazole 160 mg/800 mg b.i.d. for 7 days
  – Doxycycline 100 mg b.i.d. × 7 days
- Chronic:
  – Topical steroids: (e.g., betamethasone 0.05% applied b.i.d. for 7–14 days with or without antifungal
  – Topical antifungal (e.g., econazole, clotrimazole, or nystatin applied topically t.i.d. for up to 30 days
- Contraindications: Allergy to antibiotic, may consider erythromycin as alternative
- Precautions: Erythromycin may cause significant gastrointestinal upset.
- Significant possible interactions:
  – Erythromycin affects levels of theophylline and effects of carbamazepine, digoxin, and corticosteroids. Cardiac toxicity with terfenadine or astemizole is possible.
  – Ketoconazole, astemizole, itraconazole, fluconazole: Terfenadine, statin drugs

Second Line

- Systemic antifungals (rarely needed):
  – Itraconazole (Sporanox) 200 mg/d × 90 days (may have longer action because it is incorporated in nail plate); pulse therapy may be useful (200 mg b.i.d. × 7 days, repeated monthly × 2 months)
  – Terbinafine (Lamisil) 250 mg/d × 6 weeks (fingernails) or 12 weeks (toenails)
  – Fluconazole (Diflucan) 150 mg/week × 4–6 months
- Antipseudomonal drugs (e.g., 3rd-generation cephalosporins, aminoglycosides)

ADDITIONAL TREATMENT

General Measures

- Acute: Water or vinegar/water (1:1) soaks (t.i.d.–q.i.d.), warm compresses, elevation
- Chronic: Keep fingers dry. Apply moisturizing lotion after hand washing; avoid exposure to irritants; improved diabetic control.

Issues for Referral

Chronic; treatment failure, consider biopsy and/or in cases of recalcitrant chronic paronychia referral for possible en bloc excision of the nail fold or eponychial marsupialization with or without nail removal

SURGERY/OTHER PROCEDURES

- Incision and drainage of abscess, if present
- A subungual abscess or ingrown nail requires partial or complete removal of nail.

ONGOING CARE

FOLLOW-UP RECOMMENDATIONS

Chronic: Avoid frequent immersion, triggers, allergens, or nail biting and finger sucking.

DIET

If diabetic, institute appropriate dietary changes for better control.

PATIENT EDUCATION

Avoid trimming cuticles, importance of good diabetic control, avoiding contact irritants, use of rubber gloves with cotton liners to avoid exposure to moisture

PROGNOSIS

- With adequate treatment and prevention, healing can be expected.
- If no response in chronic lesions, rarely benign or malignant neoplasm may be present, and referral should be considered.

COMPLICATIONS

- Acute: Subungual abscess
- Chronic: Secondary ridging, thickening, and discoloration of nail, nail loss

ADDITIONAL READING

- Rigopoulos D, Alevizos A. Acute and Chronic Paronychia. *Am Fam Physician*. 2008;177(3): 339–346.
- Rockwell PG. Acute and chronic paronychia. *Am Fam Physician*. 2001;63:1113–6.
- Shaw J, Body R. Best evidence topic report. Incision and drainage preferable to oral antibiotics in acute paronychial nail infection? *Emerg Med J*. 2005;22: 813–4.
- Tosti A, Piraccini BM, Ghetti E, et al. Topical steroids versus systemic antifungals in the treatment of chronic paronychia: an open, randomized double-blind and double dummy study. *J Am Acad Dermatol*. 2002;47:73–6.

See Also (Topic, Algorithm, Electronic Media Element)

Onychomycosis

 CODES

ICD9
- 681.02 Onychia and paronychia of finger
- 681.11 Onychia and paronychia of toe

CLINICAL PEARLS

- Tetanus booster when appropriate
- No evidence that antibiotics are better or worse than incision and drainage

PARVOVIRUS B19 INFECTION

Luis T. Garcia, MD

 BASICS

DESCRIPTION
- Human parvovirus B19 is the primary cause of erythema infectiosum (EI, or fifth disease).
- Complications in susceptible individuals include transient aplastic crisis (TAC) in patients with increased RBC turnover (e.g., sickle-cell anemia), chronic anemia in immunodeficient individuals, and arthritis and arthralgias in normal hosts:
  - Pregnant women who are not immune are at risk of intrauterine infection, with potentially significant consequences to the fetus.
  - System(s) affected: Mainly Hemic/Lymphatic/Immunologic; Musculoskeletal; Skin/Exocrine; possibly CNS; Cardiac; Renal

Pregnancy Considerations
Documentation of acute infection during pregnancy should prompt referral to maternal–fetal medicine specialist.

EPIDEMIOLOGY
- Infection is common in childhood.
- Predominant age: Peak age for EI is 4–12 years.
- 50% of children 15 years of age are parvovirus B19–seropositive.
- Predominant sex: Male = Female
- Epidemics occur in late spring every 2–4 years.

Prevalence
- Extremely common in the US; >50% of adults have evidence of prior infection. Most common as community epidemics in winter and spring in nontropical regions.
- Antibody IgG prevalence:
  - 1–5 years, 2–15%
  - 6–9 years, 20–40%
  - 11–19 years, 35–60%
  - >50 years, >75%

RISK FACTORS
- School-related epidemic and nonimmune household contacts have a secondary attack rate of 50%.
- Highest secondary attack rates are for daycare providers and school personnel in contact with affected children.
- Those with increased cell turnover (e.g., SS anemia, thalassemia) at risk for aplastic crisis
- Immune deficiency may increase risk of chronic anemia.
- 40% of pregnant women are not immune with 1.5% seroconversion/yr.

Genetics
Erythrocyte P antigen–negative individuals are resistant to infection.

GENERAL PREVENTION
- Standard hygienic practices with good handwashing can minimize spread.
- Because EI is so common, it is impossible to avoid exposure completely. Also, period of contagion is before clinical illness (rash) appears.
- Pregnant health care workers should avoid caring for patients with transient aplastic crises.
- Pregnant child-care workers are at some increased risk; however, exclusion from the workplace will not eliminate this risk and therefore is not recommended.

PATHOPHYSIOLOGY
- Natural host of B19 is human erythroid progenitor
- Infection of proerythroblasts causes cessation of RBC production.

ETIOLOGY
- Small (20–25 mm), nonenveloped, single-stranded DNA virus. Only known parvovirus to infect humans and belongs to the family *Parvoviridae*.
- Respiratory secretions and rarely blood products are sources of human spread of virus.
- Maternal viremia with transplacental passage is the source of fetal infection.
- In EI, the rash is thought to be autoimmune due to IgM complexes.

DIAGNOSIS

HISTORY
- Headache, pharyngitis, coryza, myalgia, arthralgias, arthritis, and gastrointestinal disturbances are more frequent and severe in adults (nonspecific flulike illness).
- Pruritus (especially soles of feet) and mild arthralgia may occur.

PHYSICAL EXAM
- Onset of rash is first noted on the face ("slapped-cheek appearance").
- 2nd stage follows 1–4 days later with a lacy reticular rash on the trunk and limbs.
- A 3rd stage of rash is characterized by marked evanescence and recrudescence, sometimes associated with bathing, exercise, sun exposure, or emotional stress.

DIAGNOSTIC TESTS & INTERPRETATION
Lab
Initial lab tests
- CBC shows anemia and reticulocytopenia.
- Usually no need for serology because diagnosis is made clinically
- B19-specific IgM (detected 10–14 days after infection) and IgG recommended for immunocompetent patient when needed
- B19-specific DNA detection for fetus, neonate, patients with transient aplastic crisis (TAC), and immune-suppressed patients

- To exclude congenital B19 in infants with negative B19 IgM, one must follow an infant's B19 IgG serology in the 1st year of life.
- Maternal serum α-fetoprotein may be increased in fetuses with hydrops fetalis.

Follow-Up & Special Considerations
- Joint disease:
  - In adults, 80% of patients may manifest arthritis and/or arthralgia (Female > Male).
  - In children, joint symptoms are less common.
  - Knees, hands, and ankles (frequently symmetric) are involved most commonly.
  - Joint symptoms usually subside within 3 weeks but may persist for months. No joint erosions on x-ray.
- TAC:
  - Seen in patients with increased RBC turnover such as sickle-cell anemia, spherocytosis, thalassemia, and pyruvate kinase deficiency
  - Aplastic event is self-limited, with reticulocytes reappearing in 7–10 days and full recovery in 2–3 weeks.
  - In children with sickle-cell hemoglobinopathies and heredity spherocytosis, fever is the most common symptom (73%), and rash is highly unlikely.
- Chronic anemia:
  - Seen in immunodeficient individuals with no IgM response
  - No manifestations of fever, rash, or joint symptoms usually.
- Fetal/neonatal infection:
  - Risk of transplacental spread of virus ~33% in infected mothers
  - A pregnant woman with a new rash or arthralgia should be tested for the virus.
  - Clinical manifestations range from asymptomatic seroconversion and normal pregnancy (most commonly), to variable degrees of fetal hydrops, to 2nd- and 3rd-trimester intrauterine fetal demise without hydrops.
  - B19 infection always should be suspected in cases of nonimmune hydrops.
  - The principal organ involved in the fetus is the bone marrow. RBC survival is shortened, and profound anemia can result from B19-induced erythroid bone marrow aplasia.
  - Over 95% of fetal complications (fetal hydrops and death) occur within 12 weeks of acute parvovirus B19 infection in pregnancy.
  - Risk of fetal loss in pregnancy is highest with B19 infections in the 1st trimester (9%).
  - Fetal anemia is the most common manifestation of later infection, but seroconversion after 21 wks had no severe anemia (1).
  - In 1 study, 84% of B19-infected pregnant women who carried to term delivered normal infants.
  - Parvovirus B19 infection does not increase the risk of birth defects or mental retardation.
  - There are no known long-term developmental problems in infant survivors.

- PPGSS: Papular Purpuric Gloves and Socks Syndrome: Strong association with B-19. Severe petechial and ecchymotic rash in hand–foot distribution with associated febrile tonsillopharyngitis and oral ulcerations (2).

Imaging
Initial approach
Documented acute maternal infection in the 1st trimester warrants weekly fetal US for 8–12 weeks to access for hydrops development (3)[C].

Pathological Findings
- Skin biopsy usually normal but may show mild inflammation consisting of perivascular infiltrations of mononuclear cells
- In hydrops fetalis, may see intranuclear inclusions in nucleated RBCs
- In stillbirths related to maternal B19 infection, virus can be detected in all tissues.

DIFFERENTIAL DIAGNOSIS
- Rubella
- Enteroviral disease
- Systemic lupus erythematosus
- Drug reaction
- Lyme disease
- Rheumatoid arthritis

 ## TREATMENT

MEDICATION
- No therapy is needed usually.
- Anti-inflammatory agents may alleviate arthritic symptoms.

ADDITIONAL TREATMENT
General Measures
- Immune globulin IV for B19-related refractory anemia, especially if patient is immune-deficient (4)[C].
- Cessation of immunosuppressive therapy has allowed some patients to clear chronic infections.
- RBC transfusions may be required for aplastic crisis.
- Intrauterine RBC transfusions have been shown to reduce mortality significantly in hydrops/anemia diagnosed by US or cordocentesis. There is a firm recommendation for intrauterine transfusion for parvovirus B19–induced hydrops (5)[A].

Issues for Referral
Documentation of acute infection during pregnancy should prompt referral to maternal–fetal medicine specialist.

SURGERY/OTHER PROCEDURES
Amniotic fluid and chorionic villus sampling for B19 testing via PCR may be useful diagnostically in investigation of some maternal infections.

IN-PATIENT CONSIDERATIONS
Initial Stabilization
- Outpatient management for EI
- Inpatient management for aplastic crisis, which may require RBC transfusions

 ## ONGOING CARE

FOLLOW-UP RECOMMENDATIONS
Patient Monitoring
Periodic blood counts for anemic patients

PATIENT EDUCATION
- Parvovirus B19 (fifth disease): http://www.cdc.gov/ncidod/dvrd/revb/respiratory/parvo_b19.htm
- Parvovirus B19 infection and pregnancy: http://www.cdc.gov/ncidod/dvrd/revb/respiratory/B19&preg.htm
- Parvovirus B19: What you should know: http://www.aafp.org/afp/20070201/377ph.htm
- Physicians should counsel pregnant women with respect to prevention and management of maternal B19 infection (6)[C].
- Pregnant women should avoid exposure to patients with active or chronic infections. However, exclusion of pregnant women from the workplace where EI is occurring is not recommended.
- Children with symptoms are no longer infectious and may attend child care or school.

PROGNOSIS
- Usually self-limited
- Joint symptoms subside in weeks (often by 2 weeks but may last months).
- ~20% of infections result in delayed virus elimination and viremia persisting for several months to years.
- Full recovery from aplastic crisis in 2–3 weeks

COMPLICATIONS
Conditions associated with B-19 but not proven:
- Chronic fatigue syndrome
- Glomerulonephritis and other renal diseases have been reported in both immunocompromised and immunocompetent patients.
- Nephrotic syndrome
- Hepatitis
- Neurologic manifestations/stroke
- Henoch-Schönlein purpura or vasculitis
- Myocarditis
- Pericarditis

REFERENCES

1. Simms RA, Liebling RE, Patel RR, et al. Management and outcome of pregnancies with parvovirus B19 infection over seven years in a tertiary fetal medicine unit. *Fetal Diagn Ther*. 2009;25(4).
2. Fretzayas A, Douros K, Moustaki M, et al. Papular-purpuric gloves and socks syndrome in children and adolescents. *Pediatr Infect Dis J*. Mar 2009;28(3):250–2.
3. Enders M, Weidner A, Rosenthal T, et al. Improved Diagnosis of Gestational Parvovirus B19 Infection at the Time of Nonimmune Fetal Hydrops. *J Infect Dis*. 2008;197:58.
4. Orange JS, Hossny EM, Weiler CR, et al. Use of intravenous immunoglobulin in human disease: a review of evidence by members of the Primary Immunodeficiency Committee of the American Academy of Allergy, Asthma and Immunology. *J Allergy Clin Immunol*. 2006;117:S525–53.
5. Rodis JF, Borgida AF, Wilson M, et al. Management of parvovirus infection in pregnancy and outcomes of hydrops: a survey of members of the Society of Perinatal Obstetricians. *Am J Obstet Gynecol*. 1998;179:985–8.
6. Beigi RH, Wiesenfeld HC, Landers DV, et al. High rate of severe fetal outcomes associated with maternal parvovirus b19 infection in pregnancy. *Infect Dis Obstet Gynecol*. 2008;2008:524601.

ADDITIONAL READING

- March of Dimes Fifth Disease in Pregnancy. http://www.marchofdimes.com/professionals/14332_25586.asp.
- Ramirez MM, Mastrobattista JM. Diagnosis and Management of Human Parvovirus B19 Infection. *Clinics in Perinatology*. 2005;697–704.

CODES

ICD9
- 057.0 Erythema infectiosum (fifth disease)
- 079.83 Parvovirus B19

CLINICAL PEARLS

- Parvovirus B19 infection is usually a benign, self-limited illness with no long-term effects.
- The rash of EI signifies that the patient is no longer infectious.
- Patients with increased RBC turnover (SS, thalassemia) are at risk for transient aplastic crisis.
- Immune-compromised patients may be at risk for chronic anemia.
- Acute infection during pregnancy warrants maternal–fetal consultation for serial monitoring of fetal well-being for 3 months.

PATELLOFEMORAL PAIN SYNDROME

Jake D. Veigel, MD
J. Herbert Stevenson, MD

 BASICS

DESCRIPTION
- Peri- or retropatellar pain resulting from biomechanical forces in the patellofemoral joint
- System(s) affected: Musculoskeletal

EPIDEMIOLOGY
Prevalence
- May affect 25% of athletes (1)
- Common in adolescents
- More commonly affects females vs. males

RISK FACTORS
- Excessive Q angle (>20 degrees) (2)[B]
- Weakness of the quadriceps and/or hip abductors (2)[B]
- Tightness of the iliotibial (IT) band (2)[B]
- Inflexibility of the hamstrings, quadriceps, or hip flexors (2)[B]
- Generalized ligamentous laxity (2)[B]
- Lateral retinacular tightness (2)[B]

Genetics
Unknown

GENERAL PREVENTION
- Injury prevention program for those with potential risk factors
- In runners, wearing properly fitting footwear
- Proper training programs with appropriate slow increases in mileage

PATHOPHYSIOLOGY
Repetitive contact of the undersurface of the patella against the trochlea of the femur in combination with maltracking of the patella

ETIOLOGY
- Precise cause unknown, likely multifactorial
- Overload and overuse
- Biomechanical problems
- Muscular dysfunction

COMMONLY ASSOCIATED CONDITIONS
- Iliotibial band friction syndrome
- Patellar tendinopathy

 DIAGNOSIS

HISTORY
- Anterior knee pain exacerbated by physical activity or an increase in physical activity
- Commonly increased with squats
- Anterior knee pain with stairs, uneven surfaces, or running
- Theater's sign or movie-goer's sign: Anterior knee pain upon arising after prolonged sitting
- Crepitus with knee range of motion (ROM)
- Often can have pain after activity as well as with activity

PHYSICAL EXAM
- Observe patella position in the knee at 90° and tracking for a J sign.
- Pain at the area of the patellofemoral articulation (e.g., patella facets, trochlea, and peripatellar area)
- Apprehension sign: Compress patella against femur and ask patient to contract quadriceps muscles; pain with contraction consistent with patellofemoral pain syndrome
- Reproduction of pain with compression of patella against the trochlea
- Q angle is assessed by taking the angle of the intersection of 2 lines: 1 drawn from the anterior superior iliac spine (ASIS) to the midpatella and the other line drawn from the midpatella to the tibial tubercle. An angle of >20 degrees is a potential risk factor.

DIAGNOSTIC TESTS & INTERPRETATION
Lab
Usually unnecessary

Imaging
4 views of the knee, including lateral, Merchant or sunrise, standing AP, and PA tunnel views recommended to view patellar tilt and to rule out other potential etiologies.

Pathological Findings
Should be absent and any presence of pathology indicates other diagnosis

DIFFERENTIAL DIAGNOSIS
- Patellofemoral joint osteoarthritis (2)
- Chondromalacia patella
- Patellar tendinopathy
- Articular cartilage injury
- Hoffa disease
- Iliotibial band syndrome
- Loose bodies
- Neuromas
- Osgood-Schlatter disease
- Osteochondritis dissecans
- Patellar instability/subluxation
- Patellar fracture
- Patellar stress fracture
- Pes anserine bursitis
- Plica synovialis
- Bone tumors
- Prepatellar bursitis
- Previous surgery
- Quadriceps tendinopathy
- Referred pain from lumbar spine or hip joint pathology
- Saphenous neuritis
- Sinding-Larsen-Johansson syndrome
- Symptomatic bipartite patella

TREATMENT

Paramount is abstaining from activity thought to induce problem and training in a different manner.

MEDICATION

Nonsteroidal anti-inflammatory drugs (NSAIDs) may be used for short-term relief; the evidence remains inconclusive (3).

First Line

NSAIDs are the cornerstone of symptom management; better to use prior to event and afterward than solely afterward.

ADDITIONAL TREATMENT

Ice packs after activity have been found to improve clinical symptoms.

General Measures

- Physical therapy referral for exercises are an effective (3,4)[A].
- Specific home exercises may be employed, but guidance from a physical therapist is preferred (3,4)[A].
- Knee braces and taping can be helpful at the initiation of physical therapy, but do not replace a well-designed exercise program (3,4)[A].
- Orthotic arch support may be helpful (3)[C].
- Rest from painful activity, with substitution of aggravating activities with cross-training exercises (e.g., swimming) (3)[C]
- Ice for 10–15 minutes at a time may be helpful (3)[C].

Issues for Referral

Referral for surgery is a last resort after failing all conservative measures.

SURGERY/OTHER PROCEDURES

- Attempts to correct maltracking of the patellofemoral joint with a lateral retinacular release or tibial tubercle transposition with variable results
- Rarely indicated

 ONGOING CARE

PATIENT EDUCATION

Patient education and exercises: http://familydoctor.org/online/famdocen/home/healthy/physical/injuries/479.html

REFERENCES

1. Baquie P, Brukner P. Injuries presenting to an Australian sports medicine centre: a 12-month study. *Clin J Sport Med*. 1997;7:28–31.
2. Waryasz GR, et al. Patellofemoral pain syndrome (PFPS): A systematic review of anatomy and potential risk factors. *Dynam Med*. 2008;7:1476–1459.
3. Juhn MS. Patellofemoral pain syndrome: a review and guidelines for treatment. *Am Fam Physician*. 1999;60:2012–22.
4. Crossley K, Bennell K, Green S, et al. Physical therapy for patellofemoral pain: a randomized, double-blinded, placebo-controlled trial. *Am J Sports Med*. 2002;30:857–65.

See Also (Topic, Algorithm, Electronic Media Element)

Algorithm: Knee Pain

 CODES

ICD9

719.46 Pain in joint involving lower leg

CLINICAL PEARLS

- Patellofemoral pain syndrome is the most common cause of anterior knee pain in active people, affecting females more frequently than males.
- The diagnosis is made clinically by history and use of apprehension sign (compress patella against femur and ask patient to contract quadriceps muscles; pain with contraction consistent with patellofemoral pain syndrome).
- Well-designed exercises geared at quadriceps strengthening, hamstring and IT band flexibility, and hip stabilizers are the most effective evidence-based treatment.

PATENT DUCTUS ARTERIOSUS

Jaclyn Boulais, MD
Adam W. DeTora, MD

BASICS

DESCRIPTION

Patent ductus arteriosus (PDA) is the failure of the ductus arteriosus, a vessel connecting the pulmonary artery and aorta, to close after birth. 75% of cases occur as an isolated defect:

- Clinical presentation depends on the size of the ductus arteriosus and gestational age at delivery.
- Predominant left-to-right shunt leads to vascular congestion of the lungs.
- Premature infants present with apnea and/or respiratory distress.
- PDA is considered pathological when it persists beyond 3 months of age or is associated with symptoms.
- Spontaneous closure after 5 months is rare in the full-term infant.
- Ibuprofen is considered the drug of choice for symptomatic PDA. Efficacy is the same as indomethacin but ibuprofen reduces the risk of NEC and renal insufficiency. Long-term studies have not been done comparing the 2 (1)[A].
- System(s) affected: Cardiovascular
- Synonym(s): Aorticopulmonary shunt; Aorticopulmonary communication

Pediatric Considerations

Some infants with coexisting cardiac anomalies benefit temporarily from a patent ductus arteriosus to provide shunting to the lungs (right heart obstructions) or periphery (coarctation of the aorta). Definitive treatment should proceed as soon as feasible.

Pregnancy Considerations

Women with small-to-moderate-sized ductus and left-to-right shunt can expect an uncomplicated pregnancy. High risk in those with high pulmonary resistance and right-to-left shunt.

EPIDEMIOLOGY

PDA is the 5th most common congenital cardiac defect in the US, representing 5–10% of all congenital heart diseases.

Incidence

- Predominant age: Infancy
- Predominant sex: Female > Male (2:1)
- 8 in 1,000 premature live births
- In term infants, the incidence is about 1 in 2,000–2,500 live births.

RISK FACTORS

- Premature birth, high altitudes
- Maternal rubella in the 1st trimester
- Coexisting cardiac anomalies
- Any condition resulting in hypoxia (pulmonary, hematologic, etc.)
- Prenatal indomethacin exposure associated with increased incidence and severity of postnatal patent ductus arteriosus

Genetics

- Siblings of patients with PDA have 2–4% increase in frequency of PDA
- Autosomal-dominant inheritance in some families

GENERAL PREVENTION

Prophylactic intravenous indomethacin in preterm infants reduces symptomatic patent ductus arteriosus, need for surgical PDA ligation, and grade 3 or 4 intraventricular hemorrhage, but has no effect on mortality and there is no evidence on effect of neurodevelopment (2,3)[A].

PATHOPHYSIOLOGY

- The ductus arteriosus (DA) is normally open during fetal life. It is kept patent by low arterial oxygen levels and circulating prostaglandin E2. At birth, closure is triggered by a decrease in circulating prostaglandin E2 and increase in arterial oxygen tension.
- Closes by 24 hours in 50% of full-term neonates, by 48 hours in 90%, and by 72 hours in virtually all neonates. A PDA occurs when the DA fails to completely close postnatally.
- The main features of the natural history include spontaneous ductal closure, bacterial endocarditis, late congestive heart failure (CHF), and the development of pulmonary vascular obstructive disease.

ETIOLOGY

- Prematurity, congenital
- Hypoxia, prostaglandins

COMMONLY ASSOCIATED CONDITIONS

- Coarctation of the aorta
- Pulmonary valve stenosis or atresia
- Peripheral pulmonary stenosis (maternal rubella)
- Aortic stenosis, ventricular septal defect
- Necrotizing enterocolitis in preterms
- Bronchopulmonary dysplasia
- Club feet, cataracts, blindness, systemic arterial stenosis (associated with maternal rubella)

DIAGNOSIS

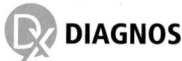

HISTORY

- Children: Many asymptomatic:
  - Failure to grow, easy fatigability
  - Recurrent respiratory infections
  - Dyspnea on exertion
- Adults:
  - Leg fatigue, fatigue, syncope
  - Shortness of breath, angina

PHYSICAL EXAM

- Signs (left-to-right shunt):
  - Rough systolic murmur
  - Continuous "machinery" murmur
  - Thrill at left upper sternal border
  - Bounding pulse with wide pulse pressure
  - Prominent, displaced apical impulse
  - Systolic ejection click
  - Diastolic flow murmur (across mitral valve)
  - Excessive sweating
  - Tachypnea, tachycardia, rales in failure
- Signs (right-to-left shunt):
  - Cyanosis, especially lower extremities
  - Clubbing
  - Diastolic Graham-Steell murmur (high-velocity pulmonic insufficiency secondary to pulmonary hypertension)
  - Right ventricular heave
- Signs of congestive heart failure: Tachycardia, hyperactive precordium, edema, decreased urine output

DIAGNOSTIC TESTS & INTERPRETATION

Lab

Initial lab tests

- Arterial blood gas
- Electrocardiogram (ECG) in children and adults may show left ventricular and left atrial hypertrophy.
- ECG in infants usually normal
- Brain natriuretic peptide (BNP) levels correlate with symptoms and magnitude of ductal shunt.

Imaging

Initial approach

- Chest radiograph usually normal in infants
- Chest radiograph in children and adults (shunt vascularity, calcifications, left ventricle and left atrial enlargement, dilated ascending aorta, dilated pulmonary arteries)
- Chest x-ray may show cardiomegaly, signs of heart failure

Follow-Up & Special Considerations

- Echocardiography/Doppler
- Contrast echocardiography
- Radionuclide angiography
- Magnetic resonance imaging (MRI)

Diagnostic Procedures/Surgery
- Cardiac catheterization and angiography: Will demonstrate the shunt and determine the degree of shunting, pulmonary pressures, and other coexisting cardiac abnormalities
- Echocardiography: Identify size of patent ductus, evaluate for left atrial and left ventricular enlargement.
- Doppler: Displays direction and velocity of shunt. May be useful to estimate pulmonary artery pressure.

Pathological Findings
- Infolding of endothelial cells and migration of undifferentiated smooth muscle cells fail.
- Left ventricular and atrial enlargement
- Patent ductus may have abnormal intima (maternal rubella).

DIFFERENTIAL DIAGNOSIS
- Venous hum
- Total anomalous pulmonary venous return
- Ruptured sinus of Valsalva
- Arteriovenous communications
- Anomalous origin of left coronary artery from pulmonary artery
- Absence or atresia of pulmonary valve
- Aortic insufficiency with ventricular septal defect
- Peripheral pulmonary stenosis (maternal rubella)
- Truncus arteriosus
- Aortopulmonary fenestration
- Coronary artery fistula

 TREATMENT

MEDICATION
Pharmacologic therapy is used strictly in the premature infant, and prostaglandin inhibitors are the initial intervention.

First Line
- Ibuprofen lysine (intravenous preparation): Only for infants 500–1500 g and ≤32 weeks' gestation: Dose is 10 mg/kg IV followed by 5 mg/kg 24 and 48 hours later.
- Indomethacin 0.2 mg/kg per dose IV every 12 hours for 3 doses. Decreased efficacy in term infants; not effective in children or adults (4)[A].
- Oxygen, diuretics
- Indomethacin contraindications:
  – Renal dysfunction, overt bleeding
  – Shock, necrotizing enterocolitis
  – Myocardial ischemia
- Precautions: With indomethacin treatment, oliguria, hyponatremia; can have significant adverse effects on renal, gastrointestinal, and cerebrovascular blood flow

Second Line
- Ibuprofen and indomethacin appear to have similar efficacy in closing PDA; however, ibuprofen reduces risk of NEC and transient renal insufficiency (1)[A].
- Alprostadil (Prostaglandin E1) treatment to maintain patency of duct in ductal-dependent lesions
- Antibiotic prophylaxis to prevent infective endocarditis with dental, GI, GU, or respiratory tract procedures is no longer recommended unless the patient has unrepaired cyanotic congenital heart disease.

ADDITIONAL TREATMENT
General Measures
- Appropriate health care: Inpatient surgery
- Small, asymptomatic shunts may not need closure.

SURGERY/OTHER PROCEDURES
- Surgical transection and ligation for moderate/large shunts best option in premature infants when medical treatment has failed or is contraindicated (5)[A]
- Preterm infants with severe pulmonary dysfunction
- Persistent PDA on echocardiography despite 2 courses of pharmacologic treatment
- Complications on indomethacin such as decreased renal output (<1 mL/kg/h), intestinal bleeding, intestinal perforation
- Contraindications to pharmacologic (severe thrombocytopenia, evolving intracranial hemorrhage, bleeding diathesis)
- Transfemoral catheter technique to occlude PDA with coil embolization, wire mesh, or double umbrella for larger ducts (6)[A]; option for larger infants and children

IN-PATIENT CONSIDERATIONS
Initial Stabilization
- Pulmonary support, oxygen to correct hypoxia
- Sodium and fluid restriction

 ONGOING CARE

FOLLOW-UP RECOMMENDATIONS
- No need for antibiotic prophylaxis after surgical repair
- Timely closure of a PDA is generally definitive treatment, and no special care or follow-up is necessary
- In medically treated patients, echocardiography to confirm ductus closure after 3-day course of medication, with additional 3 days of pharmacologic treatment if luminal patency

Patient Monitoring
- Annual routine follow-up after closure
- Shunts that have not been closed should be followed more closely.

DIET
No specific diet

PATIENT EDUCATION
Discuss prematurity and explain different treatments of premature infants and full-term infants.

PROGNOSIS
- Before 3 months, closure in premature infants is 75%.
- Before 3 months, closure in term infants is 40%.
- Best postoperative results if closed before age 3 years
- Increased pulmonary vascular resistance and pulmonary hypertension more common if closed after age 3 years
- No firm statistics, but decreased survival for large shunts
- In adults, the prognosis depends on the condition of pulmonary vasculature and the status of the myocardium if congestive cardiomyopathy was present prior to ductal closure.

COMPLICATIONS
- Left heart failure, pulmonary hypertension
- Right heart hypertrophy and failure
- Eisenmenger physiology
- Bacterial endocarditis, myocardial ischemia
- Necrotizing enterocolitis

REFERENCES
1. Ohlsson A, Walia S, et al. Ibuprofen for the treatment of patent ductus arteriosusus in perterm and/or low birth weight infants. *Cochrane Database of Systematic Reviews*. 2010, Issue 4.
2. Cooke L, Steer P, et al. Indomethacin for asymptomatic patients patent ductus arteriosus in preterm infants. *Cochrane Database of Systematic Reviews*. 2008, Issue 3 (Status Unchanged) DOI:10.1002/14651858.CD003745.
3. Fowlie, Peter, Davis. Prophylactic intravenous indomethacin for preventing mortality and morbidity in preterm infants. *Cochrane Database of Systematic Reviews*. 2009, Issue 1.
4. Van Overmeire B, Smets K, Lecoutere D, et al. A comparison of ibuprofen and indomethacin for closure of patent ductus arteriosus. *N Engl J Med*. 2000;343:674–81.
5. Malviya M, Ohlsson A, Shah S. Surgical versus medical treatment with cyclooxygenase inhibitors for symptomatic patent ductus arteriosus in preterm infants. *The Cochrane Database of Systematic Reviews*. 2006, Issue 1.
6. Pass R, et al. Multicenter USA Amplatzer PDA occlusion device trial: Initial and mid-term results. *Circulation*. 2002;106:II486.

ADDITIONAL READING
Herrera C, Holberton J, et al. Prolonged versus short course of indomethacin for treatment of patent ductus arteriousus in perterm infants. *Cochrane Database of Systematic Reviews*. 2008, Issue 3 (Status: Unchanged) DOI:10.1002/14651858.CD003480.pub3.

 CODES

ICD9
747.0 Patent ductus arteriosus

CLINICAL PEARLS
- Ibuprofen is currently the treatment of choice in preterm infants with PDA and is preferred over indomethacin due to equal efficacy and reduced incidence of NEC and reduced renal impairment; surgical treatment is 2nd line and used for symptomatic infants or those in whom the PDA does not close spontaneously or with pharmacologic treatment.
- PDA increases incidence of necrotizing enterocolitis in premature infants
- Left untreated, patients develop Eisenmenger syndrome: Right-to-left shunting. At this point, pulmonary vascular disease is irreversible, closure of PDA is contraindicated.

PEDICULOSIS (LICE)

Kaelen C. Dunican, PharmD, RPh
Julie Scott Taylor, MD, MSc

BASICS

DESCRIPTION
- A contagious parasitic infection caused by lice (blood-sucking insects, obligate parasites)
- 2 species of lice infest humans:
  - *Pediculus humanus* has 2 subspecies, the head louse (var. *capitis*) and the body louse (var. *corporis*). Both species are 1- to 3-mm long, flat, and wingless and have 3 pairs of legs that attach closely behind the head.
  - *Phthirus pubis* (pubic or crab louse): Resembles a sea crab and has widespread claws on the 2nd and 3rd legs
- System(s) affected: Skin/Exocrine
- Synonym(s): Lice; Crabs

EPIDEMIOLOGY
Incidence
- In the US: 6–12 million new cases/year
- Predominant age:
  - Head lice: Most common in children 5–11 years of age; more common in girls than boys
  - Pubic lice: Most common in adults

Prevalence
Head lice: 1–3% in industrialized countries

RISK FACTORS
- General: Overcrowding and close personal contact
- Head lice:
  - School-aged children, gender (girls)
  - Sharing combs, hats (including helmets), clothing, and bed linens
  - African Americans rarely have head lice; theories include twisted hair shaft and increased use of thick hair products
- Body lice: Poor hygiene, homelessness
- Pubic lice: Promiscuity

GENERAL PREVENTION
- Environmental measures: Wash, dry-clean, or vacuum all items that may have come in contact with infected individuals.
- Screen and treat affected household contacts.
- Head lice: Follow-up by school nurses may help to prevent recurrence and spread.
- Pubic lice: Limit number of sexual partners (note: *condoms do not prevent transmission*).
- Body lice: Proper hygiene

PATHOPHYSIOLOGY
Itching is a hypersensitivity reaction to the feeding louse.

ETIOLOGY
- Infestation by lice: *P. humanus* var. *capitis*, *P. humanus* var. *corporis*, or *P. pubis*
- Characteristics of lice:
  - Adult louse is dark grayish and moves quickly but does not jump or fly.
  - Nits (eggs) are about 1 mm long, white (opalescent), and are cemented to the base of the hair shaft.
  - Lice feed solely on human blood by piercing the skin, injecting saliva, and then sucking blood.

- Transmission: Direct human-to-human contact:
  - Head lice: Direct head-to-head contact or contact with infested fomite (including stray hairs)
  - Body lice: Contact with contaminated clothing or bedding
  - Pubic lice: Typically sexually transmitted (fomite transmission is unlikely)

COMMONLY ASSOCIATED CONDITIONS
Up to 1/3 of patients with pubic lice have at least 1 concomitant sexually transmitted disease (STD).

DIAGNOSIS

HISTORY
- Pruritus is common, mostly at night.
- Investigate contacts of infected individuals.

PHYSICAL EXAM
- Diagnosis confirmed clinically by visualization of live lice
- *P. capitis* (head lice):
  - Found most often on the back of the head and neck and behind the ears (warmer areas of the hair)
  - Eyelashes may be involved.
  - Nits, found cemented on a hair shaft, are difficult to remove.
  - Pruritus may be accompanied by local erythema and small papules.
  - May see excoriations around hairline
  - Scratching can cause inflammation and secondary bacterial infection.
  - Pyoderma and lymphadenopathy in severe infestation
- *P. corporis* (body lice):
  - Poor hygiene
  - Adult lice and nits in the seams of clothing
  - Intense pruritus involving area covered by clothing (trunk, axillae, and groin)
  - Uninfected bites present as erythematous macules, papules, and wheals.
  - Pyoderma and excoriation may be seen.
- *P. pubis* (pubic louse):
  - Pubic hair most common site
  - Lice may spread to hair around anus, abdomen, axillae, chest, beard, eyebrows, and eyelashes.
  - Nits are present at the bases of hair shafts.
  - Anogenital pruritus
  - Blue macules may be seen in the surrounding skin.
  - Delay in treatment may lead to development of groin infection and regional adenopathy.

DIAGNOSTIC TESTS & INTERPRETATION
- Head lice: Comb dry hair thoroughly with a fine-toothed louse comb (0.2–0.3 mm between teeth) to identify live lice (1,2)[C]. Simple visual inspection is of similar sensitivity to wet combing but about 25% as effective as dry combing with a metal comb (3).
- Body lice: Examine the seams of clothing to locate lice and their eggs (2)[C].

Lab
- Carefully examine hair shafts under the microscope; lice and nits can be seen easily under a microscope.
- In contrast to dandruff, nits cannot be removed easily from a hair shaft.

Follow-Up & Special Considerations
- Empty nits will remain on hair shafts for months after eradication of the live infestation. On Wood's lamp exam, live nits fluoresce white and empty nits fluoresce gray.
- Pubic lice: Patients should be evaluated for other STDs.

DIFFERENTIAL DIAGNOSIS
- Scabies and other mite species that can cause cutaneous reactions in humans
- Dandruff sometimes can look like head lice but does not stick to hair shafts like nits do.

TREATMENT

Since the early 1990s, lice have acquired some degree of resistance to insecticides (3).

MEDICATION
Permethrin (over the counter [OTC]), synergized pyrethrin (OTC), and malathion (Rx) are effective for head and pubic lice (1)[A]:
- Permethrin may be preferred because it has residual activity for up to 3 weeks (2)[C].
- Malathion may be more effective due to ovicidal activity (4)[C].

First Line
- Head and pubic lice:
  - Pyrethrum insecticides: Permethrin 1% cream rinse (Nix) or pyrethrins 0.33% with piperonyl butoxide 4% (synergized pyrethrins, Rid, Pronto): Apply to dry hair for 10 minutes, then wash. Hair should be dry to avoid dilution.
  - Malathion 0.5% lotion (Ovide):
    - Apply to affected area for 8–12 h, then wash off.
    - Excipients isopropyl alcohol (78%) and terpineol (12%) may contribute to its efficacy.
    - Flammable and has a bad odor
  - A second application may be necessary after 7–10 days if live lice are still detected.
- Body lice: Best treated with synergized pyrethrin lotion applied once and left on for several hours.
- Eyelash infestation: Apply petroleum jelly b.i.d. × 10 days.
- Precautions:
  - Pyrethrins: Avoid in patients with ragweed allergy (may cause respiratory symptoms).
  - Pediculicides should never be used to treat eyelash infections.

Second Line
- Head lice and pubic lice:
  - Dual therapy with 1% permethrin and oral TMP/SMX only for cases of multiple treatment failures or suspected cases of lice-related resistance to therapy
  - Lindane 1% shampoo: Apply for 4 minutes, then wash (should *not* be repeated).
    - Side effects: Neurotoxicity (seizures, muscle spasms), aplastic anemia

○ Contraindications: Uncontrolled seizure disorder, premature infants
○ Precautions: Do not use on excoriated skin, immunocompromised patients, conditions that increase seizure risk, medications that decrease seizure threshold
○ Possible interactions: Concomitant use with medications that lower the seizure threshold
- Head lice:
  – Benzyl alcohol 5% lotion (Ulesfia):
    ○ Apply to dry hair using a sufficient amount to saturate the scalp and hair (amount depends on hair length), rinse after 10 minutes, repeat in 7 days.
    ○ Side effects: Pruritus, erythema, pyoderma, ocular irritation, application-site irritation
  – Mechanical removal of lice and nits by wetting hair and then systematically combing with a fine-toothed comb every 3–4 days × 2 weeks to remove all lice as they hatch

ALERT
Lindane: 2003 Food and Drug Administration (FDA) black box warning of severe neurologic toxicity (use only when 1st-line agents have failed). The National Pediculosis Association strongly advises against using lindane at all.

Pediatric Considerations
- Avoid pyrethrin and permethrin in infants <2 months of age, Malathion in children <2 years of age, and benzyl alcohol in children <6 months of age.
- Lindane: Not recommended in patients who weigh <50 kg, including infants

Pregnancy Considerations
Permethrin, synergized pyrethrins, malathion, and benzyl alcohol are pregnancy Category B drugs. Lindane is category C.

ADDITIONAL TREATMENT
- Several classes of alternative physically acting (vs physiologically acting) treatments are under investigation, the most promising of which are silicone mixtures that work by blocking the louse respiratory track (3).
- For "difficult to treat" cases of head lice, oral ivermectin (400 mcg/kg), given twice at a 7-day interval, had superior efficacy as compared with topical 0.5% Malathion lotion (5)[A].

General Measures
- Head lice: Wash all bedding, towels, clothes, and headgear in hot water (60°C).
- Vacuum furniture and carpets.
- Any personal articles that cannot be hot washed, dry cleaned, or vacuumed should be sealed in a plastic bag and stored for at least 2 weeks.
- All household members and close contacts should be examined and treated concurrently if infested.
- Insecticide sprays are not necessary.
- Pubic lice: Avoid sexual activity until both partners are successfully treated.
- Nit removal:
  – After treatment with shampoo or lotion, nits remain in scalp or pubic hair until mechanically removed.

– Nits are best removed with a very fine nit comb. Removal may be made easier by soaking the hair in a solution of equal parts water and white vinegar and wrapping wet scalp in a towel for at least 15 minutes.
– Repeat treatment periodically as needed for stubborn nits.

COMPLEMENTARY AND ALTERNATIVE MEDICINE
- Ivermectin 200 μg/kg repeated in 7–10 days (should not be used in children weighing <15 kg; pregnancy Category C)
- Head lice:
  – Dry-on, suffocation-based pediculicide: Nuvo or Cetaphil lotion:
    ○ Apply thoroughly to hair, comb, dry with hairdryer, shampoo after 8 h.
    ○ Repeat once a week until cure, up to a maximum of 3 applications.
  – No home remedies (e.g., vinegar, isopropyl alcohol, olive oil, mayonnaise, melted butter, and petroleum jelly) to treat head lice infestations are effective.
  – Herbal shampoos and pomades have not been evaluated in clinical trials.
  – Lavender oil and tea tree oil have been implicated in triggering prepubertal gynecomastia in boys, so they should not be used against lice (3).

ONGOING CARE

FOLLOW-UP RECOMMENDATIONS
Children may return to school after completing topical treatment, even if nits remain in place. No-nit policies are not necessary (6).

Patient Monitoring
Drug resistance should be suspected if live lice are still present 12–24 h after treatment.

PATIENT EDUCATION
- National Pediculosis Association at http://www.headlice.org
- CDC at http://www.cdc.gov/ncidod/dpd/parasites/headlice/default.htm
- http://www.headliceinfo.com/faqs.htm

PROGNOSIS
- With appropriate treatment, >90% cure rate
- Recurrence common, mainly from reinfection or failure to comply with treatment

COMPLICATIONS
- Secondary bacterial infections
- Poor sleep due to pruritus
- Missed school, social stigma
- Persistent itching may be caused by too frequent use of the pediculicide.
- Body lice can transmit typhus and trench fever.

REFERENCES
1. Flinders DC, De Schweinitz P. Pediculosis and scabies. *Am Fam Physician*. 2004;69:341–8.
2. Orion E, Marcos B, Davidovici B, et al. Itch and scratch: scabies and pediculosis. *Clin Dermatol*. 2006;24:168–75.
3. Burgess IF. Current treatments for pediculosis capitis. *Curr Opin Infect Dis*. 2009;22:131–6.
4. Lebwohl M, Clark L, Levitt J. Therapy for head lice based on life cycle, resistance, and safety considerations. *Pediatrics*. 2007;119:965–74.
5. Chosidow O, Giraudeau B, Cottrell J, et al. Oral ivermectin versus malathion lotion for difficult-to-treat head lice. *N Engl J Med*. 2010;362:896–905.
6. Diamantis SA, Morrell DS, Burkhart CN et al. Treatment of head lice. *Dermatol Ther*. 2009;22: 273–8.

ADDITIONAL READING
- Burgess IF. Head lice. *Clin Evid (Online)*. 2009;2009
- Takano-Lee M, Edman JD, Mullens BA, et al. Home remedies to control head lice: assessment of home remedies to control the human head louse, Pediculus humanus capitis (Anoplura: Pediculidae). *J Pediatr Nurs*. 2004;19:393–8.

See Also (Topic, Algorithm, Electronic Media Element)
Insect Bites and Stings, Scabies

CODES

ICD9
- 132.0 Pediculus capitis (head louse)
- 132.1 Pediculus corporis (body louse)
- 132.2 Phthirus pubis (pubic louse)

CLINICAL PEARLS
- If 1st-line treatment with pyrethrin or permethrin fails to eradicate the infestation, the 2nd-line treatment of choice is malathion.
- The prevalence of resistant infestations is increasing, so if live lice are present 12–24 h after proper treatment, resistance should be suspected and an alternative agent from another class should be used.
- Patients' hair should be reinspected after 7–10 days and, if live lice are detected, treatment should be repeated.
- No-nit policies are not necessary because empty nits may remain on hair shafts for months after eradication.

PELVIC INFLAMMATORY DISEASE (PID)

Tiffany M. Forti, MD, MPH
Marie Ellen Caggiano, MD, MPH

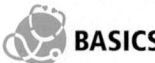 **BASICS**

DESCRIPTION
- An acute infection of the upper genital tract in women caused by the ascent of sexually transmitted infections (STIs) from the vagina and endocervix to the uterus, fallopian tubes, ovaries, and contiguous structures.
- *Pelvic inflammatory disease* (PID) is a broad term that encompasses a variety of upper genital tract infections, including endometritis, salpingitis, oophoritis, tubo-ovarian abscess, peritonitis, and perihepatitis.
- Accurate diagnosis is challenging and incorrect in up to 1/3 of women.
- System(s) affected: Reproductive
- Synonym(s): Salpingitis; Salpingo-oophoritis; Adnexitis; Pyosalpinx; Tubo-ovarian abscess; Pelvic peritonitis; Upper genital tract infection

Geriatric Considerations
Pediatric Considerations
Pregnancy Considerations
EPIDEMIOLOGY
- Predominant age: 1/3 of patients are <20 years of age; 2/3 are <25 years of age.
- Predominant sex: Female only

Incidence
In the US, 1 million women are treated each year.

Prevalence
100–200 per 100,000 women

RISK FACTORS
- Sexually active and age <25 years
- 1st sexual activity at young age
- New/multiple sexual partners
- Nonbarrier contraception (i.e., oral contraceptive pills)
- Previous history of PID; 20–25% will have a recurrence.
- History of *Chlamydia trachomatis*; 10–40% will develop PID.
- History of gonococcal cervicitis; 10–20% will develop PID.

GENERAL PREVENTION
- Educational programs about safer sex practices and STI prevention
- Barrier contraceptives, especially condoms and spermicidal creams or sponges, provide protection, the extent of which is not well documented
- Early medical care with occurrence of genital lesions or abnormal discharge
- Intrauterine device (IUD) insertion is contraindicated in women with active (acute) cervical or pelvic infection.
- Annual chlamydia screening of all sexually active women aged <25 years and of older women with risk factors (e.g., those who have a new sex partner or multiple sex partners
- Routine STI screening in pregnancy
- Evaluation and treatment of sexual partners after diagnosis with STI

PATHOPHYSIOLOGY
- The precise mechanism by which microorganisms ascend from the lower genital tract is not known. One possibility is that chlamydial or gonococcal endocervicitis disturbs the vaginal ecosystem, allowing ascent of the vaginal flora with or without the original pathogen. Thus, polymicrobial infection can occur without *Neisseria gonorrhoeae* or *C. trachomatis* infection.
- 75% of cases occur within 7 days of menses, when the cervical mucous favors ascension of organisms.

ETIOLOGY
Multiple organisms act as etiologic agents in PID. Most cases are polymicrobial.
- *C. trachomatis*, *N. gonorrhoeae* and a wide variety of aerobic and anaerobic bacteria are recognized as etiologic agents.
- The proportion of cases infected with chlamydia or gonorrhea varies widely depending on the population studied.
- The most common organisms include *H. influenzae*, *streptococcus pyogenes*, *Bacteroides*, *E. coli*, *Peptococcus*, and *Peptostreptococcus sp.*
- Bacterial vaginosis is more common among women with PID but does not confer and increased risk of PID.
- Mycoplasmas also have been implicated, but their role is less clear.

COMMONLY ASSOCIATED CONDITIONS
- If PID is suspected in a patient with a long-term indwelling IUD and a pelvic abscess is present, an *Actinomyces* infection requiring penicillin treatment may be present.
- Rupture of an adnexal abscess is rare but life-threatening. Early surgical exploration is mandatory.
- Chlamydial or gonococcal perihepatitis may occur with PID. This combination is called Fitz-Hugh-Curtis syndrome and is characterized by severe pleuritic right upper quadrant pain. FHC complicates 10% of PID.

℞ DIAGNOSIS
- It is wiser to overtreat a lower tract genital infection than to miss an upper tract infection.
- For the diagnosis of PID, the Centers for Disease Control and Prevention (CDC) recommend only a minimal diagnostic criterion of cervical motion, uterine or adnexal tenderness in the presence of lower abdominal pain.

HISTORY
- PID diagnosis is elusive, and even asymptomatic patients are at risk for sequelae.
- Fever (50%)
- Nausea and vomiting
- Lower abdominal pain, worse with coitus and jarring movements
- New/abnormal vaginal discharge
- Irregular bleeding occurs in ≥1/3 patients
- Urinary discomfort
- Proctitis

PHYSICAL EXAM
- Criteria for diagnosis:
  - Lower abdominal/ suprapubic pain (+/– rebound)
  - Adnexal tenderness (unilateral or bilateral)
  - Cervical motion tenderness
- Supports diagnosis:
  - Temperature ≥38.3°C
  - Cervical or vaginal mucopurulent discharge

DIAGNOSTIC TESTS & INTERPRETATION
Lab
Initial lab tests
- Pregnancy test – must be performed to rule out ectopic pregnancy and complications of an intrauterine pregnancy
- CBC: WBC count ≥10,500/mm^3 – ≤50% PID presents with leukocytosis.
- Chlamydia and Gonorrhea cultures
- Urine analysis
- Saline microscopy of vaginal fluid with increased WBC

Follow-Up & Special Considerations
- Erythrocyte sedimentation rate (ESR) >15 mm/h
- Elevated C-reactive protein
- Consider HIV testing in patients with PID

Imaging
Not necessary for diagnosis, although supports diagnosis

Initial approach
Transvaginal ultrasound – may show thickened, fluid-filled tubes +/– free fluid or tubo-ovarian abscess (TOA)

Follow-Up & Special Considerations
TOA will not resolve immediately after treatment. Follow-up ultrasound can be followed as outpatient for resolution of adnexal abscess.

Diagnostic Procedures/Surgery
- Culdocentesis with culture is rarely necessary.
- Laparoscopy is best used for confirming as opposed to making the diagnosis of PID. Should be reserved for the following situations:
  - Ill patient with competing diagnosis (e.g., appendicitis)
  - Ill patient who has failed outpatient treatment
  - Any patient not improving after 72 hours of inpatient treatment
- Endometrial biopsy

Pathological Findings
Endometrial biopsy reveals endometritis/plasma cells.

DIFFERENTIAL DIAGNOSIS
- Appendicitis
- Ectopic pregnancy
- Ovarian torsion
- Hemorrhagic or ruptured ovarian cyst
- Endometriosis/dysmenorrhea
- Inflammatory bowel disease
- Diverticulitis
- Pyelonephritis

TREATMENT

Outpatient treatment if appropriate. Criteria for hospitalization and parenteral treatment include:
- Suspected tubo-ovarian abscess
- Pregnancy (rare)
- Temp >38°C
- Inability to tolerate oral medications
- Peritoneal signs
- Failure to respond to oral antibiotics after 48 hours

MEDICATION
First Line
- Several antibiotic regimens are highly effective, with no single regimen of choice, but coverage should include *Chlamydia*, gonorrhea, anaerobes, gram-negative rods, and streptococci. CDC regimens that follow are recommendations, and the specific antibiotics named are examples.
- Parenteral regimen A:
  - Cefoxitin 2 g IV q6h or cefotetan 2 g IV q12h (or other cephalosporins, such as ceftizoxime, cefotaxime, and ceftriaxone) plus doxycycline 100 mg PO or IV q12h
  - Parenteral therapy × 24 h after clinical improvement; continue doxycycline after discharge for a total of 10–14 days.
- Parenteral regimen B:
  - Clindamycin 900 mg IV q8h plus gentamicin loading dose IV or IM (2 mg/kg of body weight) followed by a maintenance dose (1.5 mg/kg) q8h
  - Parenteral therapy for 24 h after clinical improvement; continue doxycycline after discharge as above or clindamycin 450 mg PO q.i.d. for a total of 14 days.
- Outpatient treatment regimen A:
  - Levofloxacin 500mg PO × 14 days OR Ofloxacin 400mg PO BID × 14 days +/–Metronidazole 500mg PO BID × 14 days
- Outpatient treatment regimen B:
  - Cefoxitin 2 g IM plus Probenecid 1 g PO concurrently as a single dose OR Ceftriaxone 250 mg IM
  - Plus doxycycline 100 mg PO b.i.d. × 14 days
  - +/– metronidazole 500 mg PO b.i.d. × 14 days
- On the basis of the recent emergence of fluoroquinolone-resistant gonococci, the CDC no longer recommends the use of these agents for the treatment of gonococcal infections and associated conditions such as PID.
- Only cephalosporins are still recommended (1)[A].

Second Line
- Many other antibiotic regimens have been proposed and used with success, for example, tobramycin in place of gentamicin or tetracycline in place of doxycycline (2).
- In persons with documented severe allergic reactions to penicillins or cephalosporins, azithromycin or spectinomycin might be an option for therapy of uncomplicated gonococcal infections (1)[A].

ADDITIONAL TREATMENT
General Measures
- Patient should avoid sex until treatment is completed.
- Refer sex partners for appropriate evaluation and treatment. Partners should be treated, irrespective of evaluation, with regimens effective against *Chlamydia* and gonorrhea.

SURGERY/OTHER PROCEDURES
- Reserved for failures of medical treatment and for suspected ruptured adnexal abscess with resulting acute surgical abdomen
- Conservative surgery preferred
- Failure of medical therapy is associated with adnexal abscess, which may be amenable to transabdominal or transvaginal drainage under guidance by ultrasonography, CT scan, or laparoscopy.

IN-PATIENT CONSIDERATIONS
Initial Stabilization
Manage fever, infection, and pelvic pain.

Admission Criteria
Hospitalization recommended in the following:
- Uncertain diagnosis
- Surgical emergencies (e.g., appendicitis)
- Suspected pelvic abscess
- Pregnancy
- Adolescent patient with uncertain compliance with therapy
- Severe illness
- Intolerance to outpatient regimen
- Failure to respond to outpatient therapy
- Inability to arrange clinical follow-up within 72 h of starting antibiotics

IV Fluids
Maintenance

 ONGOING CARE

FOLLOW-UP RECOMMENDATIONS
Patient Monitoring
- Close observation of clinical status, particularly for fever, symptoms, level of peritonitis, WBCs
- Follow adnexal abscess size and position with US.

PATIENT EDUCATION
- Abstinence from any type of sexual contact until treatment of patient/partner (if necessary) is complete
- Consistent and correct condom use should be enforced.
- Hepatitis B and human papilloma virus (HPV) vaccines should be given to patients who meet criteria.
- Continue annual STI screening.

PROGNOSIS
- Wide variation with good prognosis if early, effective therapy is instituted and further infection is avoided
- Poor prognosis related to late therapy and continued unsafe lifestyle

COMPLICATIONS
- A tubo-ovarian abscess will develop in ~7–16% of patients (3).
- Recurrent infection occurs in 20–25% of patients.
- Risk of ectopic pregnancy is increased 7- to 10-fold for ~8% of women who have had PID.
- Tubal infertility occurs in 15%, 35%, and 55% of women after 1, 2, and 3 episodes of PID, respectively (4).
- Chronic pelvic pain in 20% is related to adhesion formation, chronic salpingitis, or recurrent infection.

REFERENCES
1. Haggerty CL, Ness RB. Newest approaches to treatment of pelvic inflammatory disease: a review of recent randomized clinical trials. *Clin Infect Dis*. 2007;44:953–60.
2. Sexually transmitted disease treatment guidelines, 2006. *MMWR*. 2006;55(RR-11).
3. Lareau SM, Beigi RH. Pelvic Inflammatory Disease and Tubo-ovarian Abscess. *Infect Dis Clin North Am*. 2008;22:693–708.
4. Pellati D, Mylonakis I, Bertoloni G, et al. Genital tract infections and infertility. *Eur J Obstet Gynecol Reprod Biol*. 2008.

ADDITIONAL READING
- Haggerty CL, Ness RB. Diagnosis and treatment of pelvic inflammatory disease. *Womens Health (Lond Engl)*. 2008;4:383–97.
- Risser JM, Risser WL. Purulent vaginal and cervical discharge in the diagnosis of pelvic inflammatory disease. *Int J STD AIDS*. 2009;20:73–6.
- Tarr ME, et al. Sexually transmitted infections in adolescent women. *Clin Ob Gyn*. 2008;51(2): 306–18.

See Also (Topic, Algorithm, Electronic Media Element)
Algorithm: Pelvic Girdle Pain

 CODES

ICD9
- 614.0 Acute salpingitis and oophoritis
- 614.1 Chronic salpingitis and oophoritis
- 614.2 Salpingitis and oophoritis not specified as acute, subacute, or chronic

CLINICAL PEARLS
- History of lower abdominal pain, cervical motion tenderness, and adnexal tenderness is sufficient for a diagnosis of PID in an at-risk woman.
- Most often PID starts with gonorrhea or *Chlamydia*, but it can be polymicrobial.
- Complications include hydrosalpinx, adhesions, pelvic pain, and 10× increased risk or ectopic pregnancy.
- PID is a common cause of infertility.

PEMPHIGOID (HERPES) GESTATIONIS
Tiffany A. Moore Simas, MD, MPH, Med

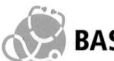
BASICS

Uncommon pregnancy-associated autoimmune blistering disease, usually starting periumbilically.

DESCRIPTION
- *Pemphigoid gestationis*, previously called herpes gestationis, is a rare dermatopathic, immune-mediated, and self-limited eruption most often occurring during mid-pregnancy and most often starting periumbilically.
- Onset:
  - any time in pregnancy and postpartum period
  - most commonly 2nd trimester of pregnancy, waning just prior delivery and then flaring after delivery
  - may recur in subsequent pregnancies
- Characterized by intense pruruitis followed by polymorphous papules and vesicles coalescing into bullae often located in periumbilical or other truncal areas; may affect the buttocks, forearms, palms, or soles; less frequently scalp and face may be involved. Mucous membranes are typically spared, but intestinal mucosa may have celiac-like lesions without significant clinical malabsorption.
- System(s) affected: Immune, Skin, Reproductive
- Synonym(s): Herpes gestationis; Dermatitis gestationis; Pemphigoid gestationis

EPIDEMIOLOGY
Incidence
- Rare: ~1/50,000 pregnancies
- Varies by incidence HLA-DR3 and -DR4
- Predominant age: Child-bearing years
- Predominant sex: Female

Pediatric Considerations
- Association with prematurity (20%) and growth restriction; less commonly stillbirth
- ~5–10% of infants born to mothers with disease can have cutaneous lesions that are usually self-limited and likely result from trans-placental transference of maternal IgG anti–basement membrane zone (BMZ) autoantibodies
- Children born to affected mother are not at increased risk of autoimmune diseases

Pregnancy Considerations
- By definition, a condition of pregnancy and puerperium; rarely seen also with hydatidiform moles and choriocarcinoma.
- Fetuses at risk for growth restriction and prematurity due to potential for mild placental insufficiency from immune response to placental antigens. Antenatal testing indicated.
- Onset in first or second trimester and presence of blisters may lead to adverse pregnancy outcomes including: decreased delivery gestational age, preterm birth and low birth weight. Treatment with systemic corticosteroids does not substantially affect undesirable pregnancy outcomes and thus should be used for treatment when needed (1).

RISK FACTORS
- Episode in prior pregnancy
- Herpes simplex does not increase risk

Genetics
Genetic predisposition is possible, suggested by increased HLA-D3 and -D4 in affected women

GENERAL PREVENTION
- Avoid increased risk infection of skin lesions due to susceptibility of open lesions and decreased resistance secondary to corticosteroid treatment
- Use of estrogens or progesterone may trigger future flare-up (ex. oral contraceptives and menses)

PATHOPHYSIOLOGY
During pregnancy, patients develop G-class antibodies (IgG) against basement membrane proteins of placenta, that cross-react with skin, and result in an immune response.

ETIOLOGY
- Placental proteins/antigens recognized as foreign, resulting in production of anti-placental antibodies
- Main antigen = collagen XVII (additionally reported as BPAG2 or BP180)
- Antibodies to placental proteins cross-react with same proteins in skin of mother (and potentially fetus)
- Maternal autoantibodies to components of basement membrane (BMZ) of skin activates complement cascade thus recruiting eosinophils and proteolytic enzymes resulting in separation of dermis and epidermis
- Higher association with HLA-DR3 and -DR4 or both
- Not caused by herpes virus

COMMONLY ASSOCIATED CONDITIONS
- Pregnancy
- Rarely, trophoblastic tumors, hydatidiform mole, and choriocarcinoma
- Other associated diseases: Graves disease and other autoimmune thyroid disorders, pernicious anemia

DIAGNOSIS

HISTORY
History of current pregnancy or recent delivery in patient with pruritic papules and/or plaques with or without blisters periumbilically

PHYSICAL EXAM
- Pruritus followed by periumbilical papules and plaques on pregnant female that over days to weeks progress to vesicles and bullae
- Lesions also may be present on trunk, buttocks, limbs, palms, and soles
- Face, scalp and mucous membranes involved rarely

DIAGNOSTIC TESTS & INTERPRETATION
Lab
Initial lab tests
- Most standard hematologic studies are within normal limits therefore not necessary
- May have elevated erythrocyte sedimentation rate (ESR) and/or anti-thyroid antibodies

- Peripheral eosinophilia may be present and correlates with severity
- Indirect Immunoflourescence (IIF): circulating serum C3 (90%), 'Herpes gestationis factor' (IgG1 antibody) (20–25%) (2)[A]
- ELISA: circulating IgG antibodies against collage XVII (2)[A]
- Immunoblotting: circulating IgG antibodies to 180kDA and/or 230 kDA protein bands (2)[A]
- HLA-profile: DR3, DR4 or both (2)[A]
- Tzanck smear negative
- Herpes simplex virus culture negative

Imaging
No imaging is indicated for maternal reasons. In pregnancy, antenatal testing evaluation for fetus is indicated and could include ultrasound for fetal growth with umbilical artery Dopplers and biophysical profiles.

Initial approach
Clinical presentation and histologic findings of a subepidural blistering process on direct immunofluorescence (DIF)

Diagnostic Procedures/Surgery
2 skin biopsies
- One for routine histology
- One for direct immunofluorescence (Place in Michel's medium)

Pathological Findings
- Routine histology specimen (2)[A]:
  - Eosinophilic spongiosis
  - Papillary dermal edema
  - Subepidermal blister with necrosis of basal cell layer
  - Dermal perivascular infiltrate of lymphocytes and eosinophils
- Immunofluorescence biopsy specimen
  - Direct IF: heavy linear deposition of C3 (100%, pathognomonic) and IgG (25-50%) along BMZ; C3 and IgG at epidermal site on salt-split skin

DIFFERENTIAL DIAGNOSIS
- Other pruritic conditions of pregnancy:
  - Besnier prurigo gestationis with excoriated papules and no vesicles; usually limited to extensor surface of extremities
  - Papular urticarial papules and plaques of pregnancy (PUPPP) syndrome, which has urticarial plaques and small papules with a narrow, pale halo and no vesicles; usually in primigravidas near term
    - PUPPP usually in striae; pemphigoid gestationis periumbilical
    - Differentiate with immunofluorescence studies
  - Impetigo herpetiformis has sterile pustules, not vesicles, and may involve mucous membranes, groin, and inner thighs
  - Papular dermatitis of pregnancy/allergic dermatitis of pregnancy
  - Prurigo gestationis of Besnier
- Nonpregnancy conditions to consider:
  - Dermatitis herpetiformis (much more chronic and more often in middle-aged males)
  - Bullous pemphigoid, drug-induced
  - Toxic drug eruption including erythema multiforme
  - Contact dermatitis

TREATMENT

- Tepid baths, compresses, and emollients may alleviate pruritus.
- Mild disease treated with antihistamines and topical steroids.
- Mainstay of treatment is systemic corticosteroids.
- Severe cases can be treated with plasmapheresis.

MEDICATION

Medications directed at relieving pruritis and preventing new blister formation. Additionally, may need treatment for secondary infection of skin lesions.

First Line

- Mainstay of mild disease: Topical steroids and oral antihistamines for mild pruritus; topical corticosteroids for early lesions (2)[A]:
  - Side effects topical steroids: spread & worsening untreated infections, telangiectasia, striae, hypertrichosis, skin atrophy
- Mainstay of severe disease: Systemic corticosteroids. Caution always merited when considering a systemic treatment in pregnancy.
  - Starting dose Prednisolone 20–40 mg/day (2)[A]:
    - Follow for 3 days and if no new lesions, maintain dose for 1–2 weeks and then taper to maintenance dose or discontinue. If new lesions, consider increasing dose.
    - Natural course of disease often allows for tapering/discontinuing preterm, but then increasing/restarting after delivery
  - Only risk of disease for pregnant women is discomfort from lesions and psychological anxiety. Maternal risk of systemic steroids include hypertension, osteoporosis, diabetes, adrenal suppression, peptic ulceration, weight gain, Cushing's syndrome and cataracts (2)[A].
  - See fetal risks from disease under precautions. Avoid betamethasone and dexamethasone as crosses the placenta. Placental enzyme inactives 88% of prednisolone. Increased risk of intra-uterine growth restriction and adrenal suppression in neonates with long-term corticosteroid exposure. Concern for fetal risks with systemic corticosteroids although generally considered safe (1)[B],(2)[A]
  - Rarity of disease prevents clinical trials and thus none have been performed to identify most optimal treatment for this disease.
- Contraindications: Weigh risk of aggravating hyperglycemia, potential effects on maternal and fetal bone, increased susceptibility to infections vs benefit of relieving pruritus and resolving the lesions.
- Precautions:
  - Use prednisone cautiously in patients with immune impairment, diabetes, or thrombophlebitis.
  - If prednisone has been used over several weeks, taper when discontinuing to prevent cortisol deficiency and provide with stress-dose steroids at appropriate times (e.g., at delivery).
- Significant possible interactions methylprednisolone may enhance toxicity of erythromycin.

Second Line

Plasmapheresis, tetracycline, nicotinamide, dapsone, ritodrine, pyridoxine, cyclophosphamide, gold, methotrexate, rituximab, goserelin for refractory cases. Most with unclear safety profile in long term, without specific indications for PG, logistical/practical concerns and not to be used in pregnancy but could be considered for postpartum period.

ADDITIONAL TREATMENT
General Measures

- Differentiate from herpes virus infection.
- Relieve pruritus.
- Prevent secondary infection.
- Soothing compresses such as with aluminum acetate (Burow solution, Domeboro) may help to relieve itching.

Issues for Referral

- Consider dermatology referral.
- Pediatric referral for neonate if mother receiving systemic steroids to monitor for adrenal suppression.

IN-PATIENT CONSIDERATIONS
Nursing

Apply and change soothing compresses.

 ONGOING CARE

PATIENT EDUCATION

- Benign disease; no permanent adverse sequelae, including scarring in the absence of secondary infection; usually resolves within days/weeks/months after delivery.
- Patients should be aware that condition may recur with subsequent pregnancies or resumption of menses or oral contraceptive agents.
- Goals of therapy include pruritus control, suppression of blistering, and avoidance of secondary infection.
- Patients must understand the benefits and potential risks of all prescribed medications.
- Disease without contraindications for breast-feeding; need to consider medications including systemic corticosteroids.

PROGNOSIS

- Spreads during 2nd–3rd trimester mostly
- Regresses prior to, but more commonly after, delivery usually within weeks to months
- Often flares in postpartum (75%), especially with oral contraceptives or menses
- Cutaneous involvement in infants is rare (5–10%) and regresses with clearance of maternal antibodies
- Tends to recur in subsequent pregnancies
- Systemic steroids may suppress new lesions, relieve pruritus, and dampen course, but maternal/fetal risks need to be considered
- Observed duration is less in breast-feeding women

COMPLICATIONS

- Secondary bacterial infection
- Risks of systemic medications in pregnancy for mom and baby
- Premature birth
- Fetal growth restriction
- Transient herpes gestationis in the neonate

REFERENCES

1. Chi CC, Wang SH, Charles-Holmes R, Ambros-Rudolph C, Powell J, Jenkins R, Black M, Wojnarowska. Pemphigoig gestationis: early onset and blister formation are associated with adverse pregnancy outcomes. *Brit J Derm*. 2009;160: 1222–1228.
2. Semkova K, Black M. Pemphigoid gestationis: current insights into pathogenesis and treatment.

ADDITIONAL READING

- Ambros-Rudolph CM, Müllegger RR, Vaughan-Jones SA, et al. The specific dermatoses of pregnancy revisited and reclassified: results of a retrospective two-center study on 505 pregnant patients. *J Am Acad Dermatol*. 2006;54:395–404.
- Aoyama Y, Asai K, Hioki K, et al. Herpes gestationis in a mother and newborn: immunoclinical perspectives based on a weekly follow-up of the enzyme-linked immunosorbent assay index of a bullous pemphigoid antigen noncollagenous domain. *Arch Dermatol*. 2007;143:1168–72.
- Kroumpouzos G, Cohen LM. Specific dermatoses of pregnancy: an evidence-based systematic review. *Am J Obstet Gynecol*. 2003;188:1083–92.

See Also (Topic, Algorithm, Electronic Media Element)

Algorithm: Genital Ulcers

 CODES

ICD9

- 646.83 Other specified antepartum complications
- 646.84 Other specified postpartum complications

CLINICAL PEARLS

- Rare autoimmune bullous dermatosis of pregnancy and the puerperium
- Originally named herpes gestationis on the basis of the morphologic herpetiform feature
- It is not related to or associated with any active herpesvirus infection.

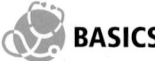

PEMPHIGOID, BULLOUS

Rochelle J. Tinitigan, MD
Richard P. Usatine, MD

BASICS

DESCRIPTION
- Bullous pemphigoid (BP) is an uncommon chronic autoimmune subepidermal blistering disease usually seen in the elderly.
- Histopathology: Blisters form in subepidermal regions, usually with eosinophil-rich infiltrate in the dermis.
- Tense blisters on either normal-appearing or erythematous skin or mucous membranes

EPIDEMIOLOGY
Most common acquired autoimmune blistering disease

Incidence
- Mean incidence of 12.1 new cases/1 million people/year in UK
- Incidence increases significantly with age >70 years.
- Predominant sex: Female > Male (61% vs 39%).
- Female-to-male ratio is 1.3.

RISK FACTORS
- Age > 70 years, but can be seen in middle-aged adults as well
- Possibly drug-induced
- Reported to be precipitated by ultraviolet (UV) irradiation and X-ray therapy

Genetics
Expression of the major histocompatibility complex (MHC) class II allele DQB1*0301 appears to be a marker for enhanced susceptibility.

PATHOPHYSIOLOGY
- Linear bands of IgG and/or C3 are found in the junction of the dermis and epidermis (basement membrane zone) that are thought to release proteolytic enzymes via activation of the complement cascade that cause blister formation.
- Autoantibodies are formed against the basement membrane hemidesmosomal glycoproteins BP230 and BP180.
- Anti-BP180 antibodies are present in 65% of BP patients.
- Anti-BP230 antibodies are present in all BP patients.

- BP may present in several distinct forms.
  - Generalized bullous form is the most common. Tense bullae appear on normal-appearing or erythematous skin. It usually heals without scarring.
  - Vesicular form is less common. It presents as tense blisters with an urticarial or erythematous base.
  - Vegetative form is very uncommon. It presents as vegetating plaques on the axillae, neck, groin, and breast.
  - Generalized erythroderma form is rare and resembles psoriasis.
  - Urticarial form presents initially with urticarial lesions that change to bullous lesions.
  - Nodular form is rare and often known as *pemphigoid nodularis*. It resembles a prurigo nodularis with blisters appearing over normal-appearing or nodular lesional skin.
  - Acral form often occurs in childhood after vaccination. Bullous lesions affect the palms, soles of the feet, and face.

ETIOLOGY
- Unknown
- Autoimmune disorder
- Drug-induced: Furosemide, penicillamine, captopril, penicillin and its derivatives, sulfasalazine, salicylazosulfapyridine, phenacetin, nalidixic acid, topical fluorouracil, and galantamine hydrobromide

DIAGNOSIS

HISTORY
Pruritus is a common and characteristic feature.

PHYSICAL EXAM
- Large, tense subepidermal blisters and urticarial plaques or bullae commonly occur in the flexural areas of the legs and arms, axillae, abdomen, and groin.
- Mucous membranes in 1/3 of patients
- Nikolsky sign should be negative (skin does not shear off when lateral pressure is applied to unblistered skin).
- Asboe-Hansen sign should be negative (bullae do not extend to surrounding skin when vertical pressure is applied).

DIAGNOSTIC TESTS & INTERPRETATION
Lab
- Biopsy is needed to establish a diagnosis.
- A 4-mm punch biopsy from the edge of an intact bulla and normal-appearing skin will show a subepidermal blister with eosinophils in dermis without acantholysis.
- A second biopsy may be done for direct immunofluorescence (DIF). A 4-mm punch of normal-appearing skin is taken a few millimeters from the involved area.
- Direct immunofluorescence will show deposits of IgG, complement, and other immunoglobulins in a linear pattern along the dermal-epidermal junction where blisters occur.

DIFFERENTIAL DIAGNOSIS
- Pemphigus vulgaris
- Cicatricial pemphigoid
- Bullous lupus erythematosus
- Dermatitis herpetiformis
- Bullous erythema multiforme
- Epidermolysis bullosa acquisita
- Linear IgA dermatosis
- Drug eruption
- Impetigo
- Erythema multiforme
- Staphylococcal scaled-skin syndrome
- Pemphigoid gestationis

TREATMENT

MEDICATION
Treatment is directed at reducing inflammatory response and autoantibody production.

First Line
- Mild disease may be treated with high-potency topical corticosteroids, which are considered the 1st-line treatment.
- Clobetasol ointment or emollient cream (applied twice daily) (1)[A]
- Extensive disease usually requires systemic corticosteroid or systemic immunosuppressive agents such as azathioprine (2). The goal is to achieve the lowest maintenance dosage that will prevent new lesion formation.

- Oral prednisone (0.5–1 mg/kg/d); increase dose until new blisters stop developing, and then taper dose slowly over time, avoiding relapse.
- Tetracycline (1.5–2 g/d) ± niacinamide (1.5–2 g/d); it is possible to give both tetracycline and niacinamide simultaneously at doses of 500 mg t.i.d. to q.i.d.
- Steroid-sparing agents should be considered in patients taking systemic corticosteroids: Cyclophosphamide (5 mg/kg/d), mycophenolate mofetil (0.5–2 g/d divided b.i.d. or t.i.d.), or azathioprine (50–200 mg divided b.i.d. or t.i.d.).
- Azathioprine (Imuran) (2 mg/kg/d) and mycophenolate mofetil (1 g b.i.d.) appear to have similar efficacy when given with methylprednisolone (0.5 mg/kg/d). However, the time needed to achieve complete remission in 100% of patients was about 90 days in the azathioprine group vs about 280 days in the mycophenolate mofetil group (3)[B]. Mycophenolate mofetil showed a significantly lower liver toxicity profile than azathioprine therapy.
- Methotrexate may be considered early in the management of moderate to moderately severe disease (4).

Second Line
- Intravenous immunoglobulin (IVIG) is relatively ineffective (5)[C].
- Plasmapheresis may be considered in patients resistant to conventional therapy.

ADDITIONAL TREATMENT
Issues for Referral
- Ophthalmologist for evaluation of suspected ocular involvement and prolonged high-dose steroids
- Dentist and/or an otolaryngologist for evaluation and care of oral disease

IN-PATIENT CONSIDERATIONS
Admission Criteria
Septicemia, concerns about denuding of skin, fluid balance, temperature control

 ONGOING CARE

FOLLOW-UP RECOMMENDATIONS
Patient Monitoring
- Perform periodic skin examination for new lesions.
- Adjust doses of corticosteroids as needed for flares or relapse.
- Monitor for medication side effects.
- Taper steroids slowly.

DIET
- Lesions may flare in patients with oral mucosa involvement after eating hard and crunchy food such as nuts, chips, and raw vegetables.
- Supplement with calcium and vitamin D (consider a bisphosphonate) for patients on systemic corticosteroids.
- Liquid or soft diet with active oral involvement; then advanced as tolerated

PATIENT EDUCATION
- Provide patient with instructions on wound care, side effects of medications, and stress reduction.
- Avoid direct sun exposure and physical trauma to the skin.
- Patients should be educated about their medical condition and treatment.

PROGNOSIS
- Duration of therapy is often months to years because of the risk of relapse.
- Old age and poor general condition are the 2 major detrimental prognostic factors of BP. In one study, patients older than 83 years who were less autonomous had a more than 9-fold increase in their risk of dying during the first year of treatment relative to younger patients who were more autonomous. The 1-year survival rate was 90% for the younger, more autonomous patients and 38% for the older, less autonomous patients. Survival was not based on disease severity in this study (6).
- Death associated with BP may occur secondary to the side effects of the medications.

COMPLICATIONS
- Superimposed infection from comorbid conditions in elderly persons such as decubitus ulcers
- Malignancies and bone marrow suppression from immunosuppressants
- Osteoporosis and adrenal insufficiency from prolonged use of systemic corticosteroids

REFERENCES
1. Khumalo N, Kirtschig G, et al. Interventions for Bullous Pemphigoid. *Cochrane Database of Systematic Reviews*. 2005;Issue 3:CD002292.
2. Mutasim DF et al. Autoimmune bullous dermatoses in the elderly: an update on pathophysiology, diagnosis and management. *Drugs Aging*. 2010;27:1–19.
3. Beissert S, Werfel T, Frieling U, et al. A comparison of oral methylprednisolone plus azathioprine or mycophenolate mofetil for the treatment of bullous pemphigoid. *Arch Dermatol*. 2007;143:1536–42.
4. Gürcan HM, Razzaque Ahmed A. Analysis of current data on the use of methotrexate in the treatment of pemphigus and pemphigoid. *Br J Dermatol*. 2009.
5. Wetter D, Davis M, et al. Effectiveness of intravenous immunoglobulin therapy for skin disease other than toxic epidermal necrolysis: a retrospective review of Mayo Clinic Experience. *Mayo Clin Proc*. 2005;80(1):41–7.
6. Joly P, Benichou J, Lok C, et al. Prediction of survival for patients with bullous pemphigoid: a prospective study. *Arch Dermatol*. 2005;141:691–8.

ADDITIONAL READING
- Joly P, Roujeau JC, Benichou J, et al. A comparison of oral and topical corticosteroids in patients with bullous pemphigoid. *N Engl J Med*. 2002;346: 321–7.
- Kfellman P, Erikson H: A Retrospective Analysis of Patients with Bullous Pemphigoid treated with Methotrexate. *Arch Dermtol*. 2008;144(5):612–16.
- Mohmand A. Bullous Pemphigoid. In Usatine R, Smith M, Mayeaux EJ, Chumley H, Tysinger J (eds.): *The Color Atlas of Family Medicine*. McGraw-Hill, New York, 2009.
- Usatine R, Smith M, Mayeaux EJ, Chumley H, Tysinger J (eds.): *The Color Atlas of Family Medicine*. McGraw-Hill, New York, 2009 - Dermatology Section 16 on Bullous Disease.

 CODES

ICD9
694.5 Pemphigoid

CLINICAL PEARLS

The bullae of BP are usually more tense and visible than those of pemphigus. The bullae of pemphigus break more easily, and more erosions than bullae are seen.

PEMPHIGUS VULGARIS

Michelle A. Tinitigan, MD
Richard P. Usatine, MD

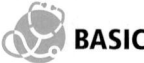 **BASICS**

Pemphigus is derived from the Greek word *pemphix* meaning "bubble" or "blister."

DESCRIPTION
- Rare, potentially fatal autoimmune vesiculobullous disease characterized by a loss of cell adhesion and blister formation within the epidermis in the skin and/or the mucosal surfaces.
- Flaccid bullae appear spontaneously that typically begin in the oropharynx and then may spread to the skin, having a predilection for the scalp, face, chest, axillae, groin, and pressure points. Bullae are tender and painful when they rupture.
- Patient often presents with erosions and no intact bullae.
- System(s) affected: Skin; GI; Genitourinary

EPIDEMIOLOGY
Incidence
- Increasing incidence with increasing age; median age of presentation 71 years (1)
- Predominant sex: Female > Male (66% vs 34%) (1); female-to-male ratio 1.4/1

Prevalence
- Uncommon, affects <200,000 people in US
- More prevalent in people of Mediterranean or Jewish Ashkenazi ancestry (2)

RISK FACTORS
Genetics
Strong association with certain human leukocyte antigens (HLA), especially HLA DR4, DR14, DQ 1, and DQ3, though the susceptibility gene differs depending on ethnic origin.

PATHOPHYSIOLOGY
- Autoantibodies (IgG) are directed against desmoglein (Dsg) 1 and 3 adhesion molecules. Desmogleins interact with desmosomes, which hold epidermal cells together. The antibodies against Dsg molecules result in intraepidermal blister formation and acantholysis.
- Dsg3 is expressed in deeper epidermal layers than Dsg1. Dsg3 is found in mucous membranes.
- Patients with limited mucosal disease primarily have autoantibodies directed against Dsg3, whereas those with more extensive cutaneous disease have antibodies directed against both Dsg1 and Dsg3.

ETIOLOGY
- Autoimmune; stimulus is unknown.
- Inducing factors include physical trauma such as thermal burns, UV light and ionizing radiation, neoplasm, emotional stress, drugs and infections. Nevertheless, most of the patients lack a recognized inducing factor.

COMMONLY ASSOCIATED CONDITIONS
- Thymoma
- Myasthenia gravis
- Paraneoplastic pemphigus is a type of pemphigus defined by the fact that the patient must have a malignancy at the time that the pemphigus is diagnosed.
- Gastric adenocarcinoma

 DIAGNOSIS

HISTORY
- Hoarseness, sore mouth
- Mucosal lesions (in 50–70% of patients) may be the sole sign for an average of 5 months before skin lesions or may be the sole manifestations of the disease.
- Cutaneous lesions: Primary lesion is a flaccid blister developed by most patients; affected skin is often painful but rarely pruritic.
- Drug-induced: Penicillamine, angiotensin-converting enzyme (ACE) inhibitors, thiol-containing compounds, rifampin

PHYSICAL EXAM
- Mucosal lesions: Intact bullae rare; commonly are ill defined, irregularly shaped gingival, buccal, or palatine erosions that are painful and slow healing; most often affected area is the oral cavity; may involve conjunctiva, oropharynx esophagus, labia, vagina, cervix, penis, urethra, and anus
- Cutaneous lesions: Painful, flaccid blisters with clear fluid found on normal skin or on erythematous base; fragile bullae rupture easily, leading to painful open denuded areas that can become secondarily infected.
- Nails: Acute or chronic paronychia, onychomadesis, subungual hematomas, and nail dystrophies may be present.
- Nikolsky's sign: Involves application of pressure to skin causing intraepidermal cleavage that allows the superficial skin to slip free from the deeper layers, producing an erosion; can be elicited on normal skin or at the margin of a blister
- Asboe-Hansen sign: Lateral pressure on the edge of a blister may spread the blister into clinically unaffected skin.

DIAGNOSTIC TESTS & INTERPRETATION
Diagnosis is achieved via 3 different parameters: Perilesional tissue biopsy, histological, and immunological examinations.

Lab
Initial lab tests
- Shave or 4-mm punch biopsy of edge of fresh bullous lesion
- A second 4-mm punch biopsy of the perilesional skin is sent for direct immunofluorescence (DIF).
- Serum for indirect immunofluorescence (IDIF) is positive for circulating autoantibodies against desmogleins in 80–90% if DIF is positive.

Follow-Up & Special Considerations
IDIF corresponds loosely to disease activity and may be useful to gauge disease activity.

Pathological Findings
- Light microscopy: Intradermal blister; loss of cohesion between epidermal cells (acantholysis) with an intact basement membrane; "row of tombstones appearance."
- DIF looking for deposits of IgG between epidermal cells

DIFFERENTIAL DIAGNOSIS
- Predominance of oral mucous lesions: Herpes simplex virus (HSV), aphthous ulcers, lichen planus, erythema multiforme
- Predominance of widespread cutaneous lesions: Bullous pemphigoid, cicatricial pemphigoid, bullous drug eruptions, pemphigus erythematosus, pemphigus foliaceus, paraneoplastic pemphigus, impetigo, contact dermatitis, dermatitis herpetiformis, erythema multiforme, Stevens-Johnson syndrome, toxic epidermal necrolysis, pemphigoid gestationis, and linear IgA dermatosis

 TREATMENT

Reduce inflammatory response and autoantibody production by suppression of the immune system to decrease blister formation and promote healing of blisters and erosions.

MEDICATION
First Line
- High-dose systemic steroids alone (e.g., prednisone 1–2 mg/kg/d) or in combination with other steroid-sparing immunosuppressive drugs (azathioprine [4 mg/kg/d], cyclophosphamide [2–3 mg/kg/d], dapsone, mycophenolate mofetil) are the mainstay of treatment (3)[A].
- Combination therapy with steroid-sparing agents are particularly useful within the first 6 months and indicated if uncontrolled on relatively low doses of prednisone (5–10 mg/d to every other day) within a year of starting therapy.
- Dexamethasone-cyclophosphamide pulse therapy is a beneficial treatment, sparing the adverse effects of conventional regimens, and has claim to induce remission in many patients (4).
- For mild-to-moderate disease: Mycophenolate mofetil (2-3 g/day) combined with prednisone showed faster and sustained response for 3–6 months vs placebo with prednisone (5)[B].
- For oropharyngeal disease: Perilesional/intralesional triamcinolone acetonide injections combined with conventional immunosuppressive therapy shortened the time of complete clinical remission and reduced the total amount of corticosteroids used.
- Oral analgesics: Use before eating for painful oral lesions (viscous lidocaine, Benadryl).

Second Line
For refractory disease:
- Anti-CD20 monoclonal antibodies: Rituximab (6): Alone or in combination with IV immunoglobulin (IVIG) appears to be an effective therapy for patients with refractory PV. This is the treatment of choice for patients with severe PV that is refractory to conventional therapy with systemic corticosteroids and immunosuppressives.

- Other options: Methotrexate, dapsone, hydroxychloroquine, gold, mycophenolate, and cyclosporine
- Tumor necrosis factor (TNF)-alpha antagonist, etanercept, may be an effective therapeutic agent and should be considered as an alternative treatment option for patients presenting with recalcitrant disease.
- Plasmapheresis in aggressive disease if combined with systemic steroids and immunosuppressant drugs
- IV immunoglobulin (IVIG) may be useful as monotherapy in patients who do not respond to steroids or who have contraindications. It is a safe and effective alternative treatment modality in patients with PV who are dependent on systemic corticosteroids or who develop significant adverse effects as a result of their use.
- Pulsed therapy with intravenous methylprednisolone and cyclophosphamide can be an effective therapy for refractory PV (3)[B].

ADDITIONAL TREATMENT
General Measures
- Minimize activities that may cause trauma to skin and precipitate blisters.
- Avoid use of dental plates, dental bridges, or contact lenses that may precipitate or exacerbate mucosal disease.
- Wound care: Daily gentle cleaning, topical agents to promote wound healing, and use of nonadhesive dressings

Issues for Referral
- Ophthalmologist referral in suspected ocular involvement and prolonged use of high-dose steroids
- Referral to a dentist and/or otolaryngologist for patients with extensive oral disease

IN-PATIENT CONSIDERATIONS
Admission Criteria
- Secondary infections requiring IV antibiotics
- Severe oral lesions leading to dehydration requiring fluid resuscitation

 ## ONGOING CARE

A minority (10%) achieve complete remission after initial treatment and do not need continued drug therapy; most require maintenance therapy to stay in remission.

FOLLOW-UP RECOMMENDATIONS
Patients taking steroids long term should be screened for osteopenia/osteoporosis, avascular necrosis, HPA-axis suppression, cataract, cushingoid features, hyperlipoproteinemia, myopathy, mood changes, and immunosuppression (7). Patients on systemic steroids should maintain adequate vitamin D and calcium intake through diet and supplements.

Patient Monitoring
Seek medical care for any unexplained blisters and if you have been treated for PV and develop any of the following symptoms:
- Fever, chills
- General ill feeling
- Myalgias, joint pain
- New blisters or ulcers

DIET
- Patients with active oral lesions may benefit from liquid or soft diet and then advance as tolerated.
- Avoid spicy and acidic food when oral ulcers are present.
- Hard food that may cause mechanical trauma to epithelium such as nuts, chips, and hard vegetables and fruits may be best avoided with active oral disease.

PATIENT EDUCATION
- Minimize activities that may cause trauma to skin and precipitate blisters, such as contact sports. Nontraumatic exercises, such as swimming, may be helpful.
- Explain wound care of erosions: Daily gentle cleaning, covering open areas with clean petrolatum and nonadhesive dressings
- Educate patients about the chronicity of the disease and the need for long-term follow-up.
- For oral pemphigus:
  - Soft diets and soft toothbrushes help to minimize local trauma.
  - Explain the need for meticulous oral hygiene to prevent dental decay. Encourage gentle toothbrushing, dental flossing, and visits to the dentist/dental hygienist at least every 6 months.
  - Discuss how dental plates, dental bridges, or contact lenses may precipitate or exacerbate mucosal disease.
  - Topical analgesics or anesthetics (e.g., benzydamine hydrochloride 0.15% or viscous lidocaine) may be useful in alleviating oral pain, particularly prior to eating or toothbrushing.

PROGNOSIS
- Mortality rate with combination therapy is approximately 5% with most deaths due to drug-induced complications, including sepsis.
- 10% of patients achieve complete remission after initial treatment; the majority require maintenance therapy to stay in remission.
- Morbidity and mortality are related to extent of disease, the maximum dose of oral steroids required to induce remission, and the presence of other diseases. Prognosis is worse in older persons and patients with extensive disease.
- Most deaths occur during the first few years of the disease, and if a patient survives 5 years, prognosis is good.

COMPLICATIONS
- Secondary infection, localized to skin or systemic, may occur because of impaired immune response due to use of immunosuppressive drugs. Most frequent cause of death is *Staphylococcus aureus* septicemia.
- Osteoporosis in patients requiring long-term systemic steroids
- Adrenal insufficiency has been reported following prolonged use of glucocorticoids.
- Bone marrow suppression and malignancies have been reported in patients receiving immunosuppressants, with an increased incidence of leukemia and lymphoma.
- Growth retardation has been reported in children taking systemic corticosteroids and immunosuppressants.

REFERENCES

1. Langan SM, Smeeth L, Hubbard R, et al. Bullous pemphigoid and pemphigus vulgaris–incidence and mortality in the UK: population based cohort study. *BMJ*. 2008;337:a180.
2. Meyer N, Misery L et al. Geoepidemiologic considerations of auto-immune pemphigus. *Autoimmun Rev*. 2010;9:A379–82.
3. Saha M, Powell AM, Bhogal B, et al. Pulsed intravenous cyclophosphamide and methylprednisolone therapy in refractory pemphigus. *The British journal of dermatology*. 2009;
4. Zivanovic D, Medenica L, Tanasilovic S, et al. Dexamethasone-cyclophosphamide pulse therapy in pemphigus: a review of 72 cases. *Am J Clin Dermatol*. 2010;11:123–9.
5. Beissert S, Mimouni D, Kanwar AJ, et al. Treating Pemphigus Vulgaris with Prednisone and Mycophenolate Mofetil: A Multicenter, Randomized, Placebo-Controlled Trial. *The Journal of investigative dermatology*. 2010;
6. Schmidt E, Goebeler M, Zillikens D, et al. Rituximab in severe pemphigus. *Ann NY Acad Sci*. 2009;1173:683–91.
7. Chmurova N, Svecova D et al. Pemphigus vulgaris: a 11-year review. *Bratisl Lek Listy*. 2009;110:500–3.

ADDITIONAL READING

Usatine R, Smith M, Mayeaux EJ, et al., (eds.): *The Color Atlas of Family Medicine*. McGraw-Hill, New York, 2009 - Dermatology Section 16 on Bullous Disease.

 ## CODES

ICD9
694.4 Pemphigus

CLINICAL PEARLS

- Rare, chronic, potentially fatal autoimmune vesiculobullous disease of the mucous membranes and skin
- Biopsy immediately with rush processing.
- When clinical suspicion is high, initiate therapy without delay using systemic corticosteroids.
- Minimize activities that may cause trauma to skin and precipitate blisters, such as contact sports.

PEPTIC ULCER DISEASE

Kelly O'Callahan, MD

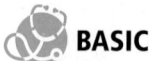 **BASICS**

DESCRIPTION
- Duodenal ulcer:
  - Most common form of peptic ulcer
  - Usually located in the proximal duodenum
  - Multiple ulcers or ulcers distal to the second portion of duodenum raise possibility of Zollinger-Ellison syndrome.
- Gastric ulcer:
  - Less common than duodenal ulcer in absence of nonsteroidal anti-inflammatory drugs (NSAIDs)
  - Commonly located along lesser curvature of the antrum
- Esophageal ulcers: Located in the distal esophagus and usually secondary to gastroesophageal reflux disease (GERD); also seen with Zollinger-Ellison syndrome
- Ectopic gastric mucosal ulceration: May develop in patients with a Meckel's diverticulum

EPIDEMIOLOGY
Incidence
- Predominant sex: Equal
- Predominant age:
  - 70% of ulcers occur in patients between the ages of 25 and 64 years.
  - Ulcer incidence increases with age.
- Peptic ulcer: 500,000 new cases/year
- Recurrence: 4 million/year
- Global incidence rate 0.1–0.19% (1)[A]

Prevalence
- Peptic ulcer: 1.8% in the US
- Lifetime prevalence is 5–10% for patients not infected with *Helicobacter pylori;* 10–20% if infected.

RISK FACTORS
- *H. pylori* infection
- NSAID use
- Smoking cigarettes
- Family history of ulcers
- Zollinger-Ellison syndrome
- Medications: Corticosteroids (high-dose and/or prolonged therapy), bisphosphonates, potassium chloride, chemotherapeutic agents (e.g., IV fluorouracil)

Genetics
Increased incidence of peptic ulcer disease (PUD) in families; familial clustering of *H. pylori* infection and inherited genetic factors reflecting response to the organism

GENERAL PREVENTION
- NSAID ulcers: Avoid salicylates and NSAIDs:
  - Alternatives include acetaminophen and tramadol. COX-2 inhibitor use (e.g., celecoxib) is controversial due to potential cardiac safety risks (also not clear that COX-2-selective agents reduce major GI bleeding).
  - If NSAIDs needed: Adjust ibuprofen dose to <1,200 mg/d to decrease risk of ulcerogenesis, and add proton pump inhibitor (PPI), misoprostol, or double-dose H_2 blockers.
  - To reduce ulcer risk, eradicate *H. pylori* before starting therapy with NSAIDs.

- Maintenance therapy with PPIs or H_2 blockers is indicated for patients with a history of ulcer complications or recurrences, refractory ulcers, or persistent *H. pylori* infection.

PATHOPHYSIOLOGY
Imbalance between aggressive factors (e.g., gastric acid, pepsin, bile salts, pancreatic enzymes) and defensive factors maintaining mucosal integrity (e.g., mucus, bicarbonate, blood flow, prostaglandins, growth factors, cell turnover)

ETIOLOGY
- May be multifactorial
- *H. pylori* infection: 90% of duodenal ulcers and 70–90% of gastric ulcers:
  - Lifetime risk for PUD in *H. pylori*–infected people: 10–20%
  - Annual risk of developing duodenal ulcer in *H. pylori*–infected people is ≤1%.
- Ulcerogenic drugs (e.g., NSAIDs)
- Hypersecretory syndromes (e.g., Zollinger-Ellison syndrome)
- Retained gastric antrum
- Less common: Crohn disease, vascular insufficiency, radiation therapy, cancer chemotherapy, smoking

COMMONLY ASSOCIATED CONDITIONS
- Zollinger-Ellison syndrome (gastrinoma)
- Multiple endocrine neoplasia type 1
- Carcinoid syndrome
- Chronic illness: Crohn disease, chronic obstructive pulmonary disease (COPD), chronic renal failure, hepatic cirrhosis, cystic fibrosis
- Hematopoietic disorders (rare): Systemic mastocytosis, myeloproliferative disease, hyperparathyroidism, polycythemia rubra vera

 DIAGNOSIS

HISTORY
- Signs and symptoms:
  - Episodic gnawing or burning epigastric pain
  - Pain occurring after meals or on empty stomach
  - Nocturnal pain
  - Pain relieved by food intake, antacids, or antisecretory agents
  - Nonspecific dyspeptic complaints: Indigestion, nausea, vomiting, loss of appetite, and heartburn
- Alarm symptoms:
  - Anemia, hematemesis, melena, or heme-positive stool suggests bleeding.
  - Vomiting and early satiety suggests obstruction.
  - Anorexia or weight loss
  - Persisting upper abdominal pain radiating to the back suggests penetration.
  - Severe, spreading upper abdominal pain suggests perforation.
- NSAID-induced ulcers are often silent; perforation or bleeding may be initial presentation.

PHYSICAL EXAM
Physical exam for uncomplicated peptic ulcer may be unreliable and nonspecific: Epigastric tenderness (absent in at least 30% of older patients); guaiac-positive stool from occult blood loss

DIAGNOSTIC TESTS & INTERPRETATION
Lab
Initial lab tests
- Routine lab tests to consider when evaluating PUD:
  - Complete blood count (CBC): Rule out anemia.
  - Fecal occult blood test
  - In patients with multiple or refractory ulcers, consider serum gastrin to rule out Zollinger-Ellison syndrome.
- Indications for *H. pylori* testing: New-onset PUD, history of PUD, persistent symptoms after empirical antisecretory therapy, gastric mucosa–associated lymphoid tissue (MALT) lymphoma, uninvestigated dyspepsia in patients <50 years of age without alarm symptoms
- *H. pylori* diagnostic tests: False-negative results may occur if patient was recently treated with antibiotics, bismuth, or PPIs; or in patients with active bleeding:
  - Noninvasive tests:
    - Serology antibody: Most commonly used for testing in primary care but slow to normalize after treatment, so cannot be used to document successful eradication (sensitivity 85%, specificity 79%) (2)[A]
    - Urea breath test: Identifies active *H. pylori* infection; also used for posttreatment testing (sensitivity >95%, specificity >90%) (2)[A]
    - Stool antigen: Can be used for screening and posttreatment testing (sensitivity 91%, specificity 94%) (2)[A]
  - Invasive tests:
    - Upper endoscopy with gastric biopsy, which can be evaluated with Steiner stain for direct visualization of organism (sensitivity >95%, specificity >95%) (2)[A]
    - Rapid urease test: Conducted on gastric biopsies (sensitivity 93–97%, specificity 95%) (2)[A]

Imaging
Initial approach
Barium or Gastrografin contrast radiography (double-contrast hypotonic duodenography): Indicated when endoscopy is unsuitable or not feasible

Diagnostic Procedures/Surgery
Indications for upper endoscopy: Patients with suspected peptic ulcers who are >55 years of age, those who have alarm symptoms, and those with ulcers that do not respond to treatment (3)[A]

DIFFERENTIAL DIAGNOSIS
Functional dyspepsia, gastritis, GERD, biliary colic, pancreatitis, cholecystitis, Crohn disease, intestinal ischemia, variant angina pectoris, GI malignancy

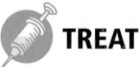 **TREATMENT**

MEDICATION
First Line
- Acid suppression: PPIs: 1st line:
  - Omeprazole 20 mg/d p.o.; lansoprazole 30 mg/d p.o.; rabeprazole 20 mg/d p.o.; esomeprazole 40 mg/d p.o.; *or* pantoprazole 40 mg/d p.o.
  - Administer PPIs before breakfast.

Pregnancy Considerations
- PPIs are *not* associated with an increased risk for major congenital birth defects, spontaneous abortions, or preterm delivery (4)[A].

- H₂ blockers: Ranitidine or nizatidine 150 mg p.o. b.i.d. or 300 mg p.o. at bedtime, cimetidine 400 mg p.o. b.i.d. or 800 mg p.o. at bedtime, famotidine 150 mg p.o. b.i.d. or 300 mg p.o. at bedtime
- Treat ulcers for 6–8 weeks or until healing is confirmed in patients with complicated ulcers.
- PPIs heal peptic ulcers more rapidly and should not be taken with H₂ blockers.
- Optimal *H. pylori* eradication regimens (2)[A]: Triple therapy: 2 antibiotics plus a PPI × 14 days: Omeprazole 20 mg p.o. b.i.d., or lansoprazole 30 mg p.o. b.i.d., or pantoprazole 40 mg p.o. b.i.d., or rabeprazole 20 mg p.o. b.i.d., or esomeprazole plus clarithromycin 500 mg p.o. b.i.d. plus amoxicillin 1 g p.o. b.i.d. or metronidazole 500 mg p.o. b.i.d. in patients with allergy to amoxicillin:
  – Triple and quadruple therapy have similar eradication rates for primary *H. pylori* infection (5)[A].
- Bacterial resistance: Clarithromycin 10%, amoxicillin 1.4%, metronidazole 37%: Culture-guided choice of triple therapy is more clinically and cost effective.
- Treatment of *H. pylori*–negative ulcers (usually due to NSAIDs):
  – Discontinue NSAID use
  – Treat acutely with PPIs for 4–8 weeks; may use longer as maintenance for patients with recurrent or complicated ulcers or in patients who require long-term aspirin or NSAID use.
- Precautions:
  – Renal insufficiency: Decrease H2 blocker dosage by 50%.
  – Cimetidine: Avoid with theophylline, warfarin, phenytoin, and lidocaine.
  – Proton pump inhibitors may decrease bone density. Obtain interval bone densitometry with long-term PPI use.
  – Omeprazole may decrease efficacy of clopidogrel. May wish to use H₂ blockers or an alternative PPI (6).

Second Line

- For *H. pylori* eradication: Use 2nd-line therapy if 1st line fails (2)[A]:
  – Bismuth quadruple therapy × 14 days:
    ○ Bismuth subsalicylate 525 mg p.o. q.i.d. *plus*
    ○ Metronidazole 500 mg p.o. q.i.d. *plus*
    ○ Tetracycline 500 mg p.o. q.i.d. *plus*
    ○ PPI × 14 days
  – Alternative 2nd-line therapy:
    ○ Levofloxacin 250 mg p.o. b.i.d. *plus*
    ○ Amoxicillin 1,000 mg p.o. b.i.d. *plus*
    ○ PPI p.o. b.i.d.
  – Another alternative salvage therapy:
    ○ Rifabutin 300 mg p.o. daily *plus*
    ○ Amoxicillin 1,000 mg p.o. b.i.d. *plus*
    ○ PPI p.o. b.i.d.
- Alternative ulcer-healing drugs: Sucralfate 1 g p.o. q.i.d. or 2 g p.o. b.i.d. × 4–8 weeks
- Precautions: Renal insufficiency:
  – Reduce H₂ blocker dosage by 50%.
  – Avoid magnesium-containing antacids.
- Significant possible interactions:
  – Cimetidine inhibits cytochrome P450 isozymes (avoid with theophylline, warfarin, phenytoin, and lidocaine).
  – Omeprazole may prolong elimination of diazepam, warfarin, and phenytoin.
  – Sucralfate reduces absorption of tetracycline, norfloxacin, ciprofloxacin, and theophylline; leads to subtherapeutic levels.

SURGERY/OTHER PROCEDURES

- Endoscopy indicated for patients over the age of 50 with new onset of dyspeptic symptoms, those who do not respond to treatment, and those of any age with alarm symptoms such as bleeding and weight loss (7)[A]
- At endoscopy:
  – Biopsy of stomach for *H. pylori* testing
  – Biopsy of margin of gastric ulcer to confirm benign etiology
  – Interventions to stop active bleeding, or prevent rebleeding in those with certain stigmata include injection with epinephrine, heater probe treatment, or placement of endoscopic clips.
- Indications for surgery: Ulcers that are refractory to treatment and patients at high risk for complications (e.g., transplant recipients, patients dependent on steroids or NSAIDs); surgery also may be needed acutely for treatment of perforation and bleeding that is refractory to endoscopic therapy.
- Surgical options:
  – Duodenal ulcers: Truncal vagotomy and drainage (pyloroplasty or gastrojejunostomy), selective vagotomy (preserving the hepatic and/or celiac branches of the vagus) and drainage, or highly selective vagotomy
  – Gastric ulcers: Partial gastrectomy, Billroth I or II
  – Laparoscopy or open patching of perforated ulcers (8)

IN-PATIENT CONSIDERATIONS
Initial Stabilization
- Discontinue ulcerogenic agents (e.g., NSAIDs).
- Bleeding peptic ulcers:
  – Stable patient: Give PPI to reduce transfusion requirements, need for surgery, and duration of hospitalization (3)[A].
  – Unstable patients: Fluid or packed red blood cell resuscitation followed by emergent EGD; use IV PPI
- Perforated peptic ulcers: Free peritoneal perforation with bacterial peritonitis is a surgical emergency.

ONGOING CARE

FOLLOW-UP RECOMMENDATIONS
Patient Monitoring
- *H. pylori* eradication: Expected in >90% (with double antibiotic regimen): Confirm eradication by urea breath test.
- Acute duodenal ulcer: Monitor clinically.
- Acute gastric ulcer: Confirm healing via endoscopy after 12 weeks if biopsy not done initially to confirm that lesion is benign.

PROGNOSIS
After *H. pylori* eradication:
- Low ulcer relapse rate; if relapse, consider surreptitious use of NSAIDs
- Reinfection rates <1% per year
- Low risk of rebleeding
- Decreased NSAID ulcer recurrence

COMPLICATIONS
- Hemorrhage: Up to 25% of patients (initial presentation in 10%)
- Perforation <5% of patients
- Gastric outlet obstruction: Up to 5% of duodenal or pyloric channel ulcers; male predilection found
- Risk of gastric adenocarcinoma increased in *H. pylori*–infected patients

REFERENCES

1. Sung JJ, Kuipers EJ, El-Serag HB. Systematic review: update on the global incidence and prevalence of peptic ulcer disease. *Aliment Pharmacol Ther*. 2009.
2. Saad R, Chey WD. A clinician's guide to managing Helicobacter pylori infection. *Cleve Clin J Med*. 2005;72:109–10, 112–3, 117–8 passim
3. Ramakrishnan K, Salinas RC. Peptic ulcer disease. *Am Fam Physician*. 2007;76:1005–12.
4. Gill SK, O'Brien L, Einarson TR, et al. The Safety of Proton Pump Inhibitors (PPIs) in Pregnancy: A Meta-Analysis. *Am J Gastroenterol*. 2009;104: 1541–5.
5. Luther J, Higgins PD, Schoenfeld PS, et al. Empiric quadruple vs. triple therapy for primary treatment of Helicobacter pylori infection: Systematic review and meta-analysis of efficacy and tolerability. *Am. J. Gastroenterol*. 2010;105:65–73.
6. Johnson DA et al. Safety of proton pump inhibitors: current evidence for osteoporosis and interaction with antiplatelet agents. *Curr Gastroenterol Rep*. 2010;12:167–74.
7. ASGE Standards of Practice Committee, Banerjee S, Cash BD, et al. The role of endoscopy in the management of patients with peptic ulcer disease. *Gastrointest. Endosc*. 2010;71:663–8.
8. Bertleff MJ, Lange JF et al. Perforated Peptic Ulcer Disease: A Review of History and Treatment. *Digestive surgery*. 2010;27:161–169.

CODES

ICD9
- 530.20 Ulcer of esophagus without bleeding
- 531.90 Gastric ulcer, unspecified as acute or chronic, without mention of hemorrhage or perforation, without mention of obstruction
- 533.90 Peptic ulcer of unspecified site, unspecified as acute or chronic, without mention of hemorrhage or perforation, without mention of obstruction

CLINICAL PEARLS

- In patients with PUD, *H. pylori* should be eradicated to assist in healing and to reduce the risk of gastric and duodenal ulcer recurrence (3)[A].
- In patients with peptic ulcers, PPIs provide acid suppression, healing rates, and symptom relief superior to other antisecretory therapies (3)[A].
- Upper endoscopy is indicated in patients with suspected peptic ulcers who are >55 years of age, those who have alarm symptoms, and those who do not respond to treatment (3)[A].

PERICARDITIS

David Fish, MD

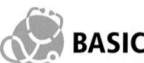 **BASICS**

DESCRIPTION
- Inflammatory process of the pericardium, with or without associated pericardial effusion; a broad spectrum of etiologies with most common causes being idiopathic or viral
- System(s) affected: Cardiovascular
- Synonym(s): Acute suppurative pericarditis

EPIDEMIOLOGY
Incidence
- Epidemiologic studies lacking
- Exact incidence unknown, but occurs in up to 5% of patients evaluated in emergency room for chest pain without myocardial infarction (MI) (1)

RISK FACTORS
Genetics
No known genetic factors

PATHOPHYSIOLOGY
Acute inflammation that can produce serous or purulent fluid or dense fibrinous material (depending on etiology)

ETIOLOGY
- Idiopathic: 85-90% of cases. Likely related to viral infection (2)[B].
- Infectious:
  - Viral: Coxsackievirus, echovirus, adenovirus, Epstein-Barr virus, cytomegalovirus, hepatitis viruses, influenza virus, HIV, measles, mumps, varicella
  - Bacterial: Gram-positive and gram-negative organisms
  - Fungal (more common in immunocompromised populations): *Blastomyces dermatitidis, Candida* sp., *Histoplasma capsulatum*
  - Mycobacterial: *Mycobacterium tuberculosis*
  - Parasites: *Echinococcus*
- Noninfectious causes:
  - Acute MI (2–4 days after MI), Dressler's syndrome (weeks–months after MI)
  - Aortic dissection
  - Renal failure, uremia
  - Malignancy (e.g., breast cancer, lung cancer, Hodgkin disease, leukemia, lymphoma)
  - Radiation therapy
  - Trauma
  - Postpericardiotomy
  - After cardiac procedures (e.g., catheterization, pacemaker placement, ablation)
  - Autoimmune disorders: Connective tissue disorders, systemic lupus erythematosus (SLE), rheumatoid arthritis, scleroderma, hypothyroidism, inflammatory bowel disease, spondyloarthropathies, Wegener granulomatosis
  - Sarcoidosis

- Medication-induced: Dantrolene, doxorubicin, hydralazine, isoniazid, mesalamine, methysergide, penicillin, phenytoin, procainamide, rifampin (1)[B]

COMMONLY ASSOCIATED CONDITIONS
Depends on etiology

 DIAGNOSIS

HISTORY
- Prodrome of fever, malaise, myalgias
- Acute, sharp, stabbing chest pain
- Duration typically hours to days
- Pleuritic pain
- Pain improved by leaning forward, worsened by lying supine

PHYSICAL EXAM
- Heart rate is usually rapid and regular.
- Pericardial friction rub:
  - Coarse, high-pitched sound best heard during end expiration at left lower sternal border with patient leaning forward
  - Highly specific for diagnosis (but not sensitive)
  - May be transient and mono-, bi-, or triphasic (1)[B]
- New S_3 may suggest myopericarditis.
- Cardiac tamponade suggested by the presence of:
  - Systemic arterial hypotension
  - Elevated jugular venous pressure
  - Pulsus paradoxus (inspiratory fall in arterial pressure of at least 10 mm Hg)

DIAGNOSTIC TESTS & INTERPRETATION
Lab
Initial lab tests
- Complete blood count (CBC): Typically shows leukocytosis
- Inflammatory markers: Elevated erythrocyte sedimentation rate (ESR), C-reactive protein (CRP)
- Cardiac biomarkers: Typically elevated creatine kinase, troponins:
  - Elevated troponins associated with younger age, male gender, pericardial effusion at presentation, and ST-segment elevation on ECG
  - Adverse outcomes not predicted by elevated troponin (3)[B]
- ECG: Findings include widespread upward concave ST-segment elevation and PR-segment depression that may evolve through 4 stages (but ECG may be normal or show nonspecific abnormalities) (1)[B]:
  - Stage 1: Diffuse ST-segment elevation and PR-segment depression
  - Stage 2: Normalization of the ST and PR segments
  - Stage 3: Widespread T-wave inversions
  - Stage 4: Normalization of T waves; may have persistent inversions if chronic pericarditis
  - ECG may demonstrate low voltage and electrical alternans with tamponade.

- Additional testing includes tuberculin skin test, sputum cultures, rheumatoid factor, antinuclear antibody, and HIV serology if clinically appropriate based on history or atypical presentation or course.
- Viral cultures and antibody titers rarely clinically useful

Imaging
Initial approach
- Chest x-ray (CXR) is performed to rule out pulmonary/mediastinal pathology. Enlarged cardiac silhouette suggests large pericardial effusion (at least 200 mL).
- Transthoracic echocardiogram recommended to evaluate for the presence of pericardial effusion, tamponade, or myocardial disease (presence of effusion helps to confirm diagnosis of pericarditis) (4)[B].
- CT scan and MRI permit visualization of pericardium to assess for complications or if initial workup is inconclusive.

Diagnostic Procedures/Surgery
- Pericardiocentesis indicated for cardiac tamponade and for suspected purulent, tuberculous, or neoplastic pericarditis
- Surgical drainage with pericardial biopsy recommended if recurrent tamponade or ineffective pericardiocentesis

Pathological Findings
- Microscopic examination may reveal hyperemia, leukocyte accumulation, or fibrin deposition.
- Purulent fluid with neutrophilic predominance if bacterial etiology
- Lymphocytic predominance in viral, tuberculous, and neoplastic pericarditis

DIFFERENTIAL DIAGNOSIS
- Acute MI
- Pneumonia with pleurisy
- Pulmonary embolism
- Aortic dissection
- Pneumothorax
- Mediastinal emphysema
- Cholecystitis
- Pancreatitis
- Esophageal inflammation, perforation, or rupture

TREATMENT

- Goal of treatment is to relieve pain and reduce complications (e.g., recurrence, tamponade, chronic restrictive pericarditis).
- Outpatient therapy is reported to be successful in 87% patients with low-risk features (4)[B].

MEDICATION
First Line
- Nonsteroidal anti-inflammatory drugs (NSAIDs) are considered the mainstay of therapy; dosage is tapered to reduce recurrence rate:
  - Ibuprofen 300–800 mg q6–8h, to be continued for days or weeks as needed
  - Aspirin 800 mg q6–8h preferable for patients with recent MI because other NSAIDs impair scar formation in animal studies
  - GI protection should be provided.
- Colchicine 1–2 mg 1st day, then maintenance dose 0.5–1 mg/d × 3 months; effective as monotherapy or as adjunct to an NSAID for initial attack and prevention of recurrences (5)[B]
- Contraindications: Hypersensitivity to aspirin or NSAID, active peptic ulcer or GI bleeding
- Precautions: Use with caution in patients with asthma, 3rd-trimester pregnancy, coagulopathy, and renal or hepatic dysfunction.

Second Line
- Corticosteroid treatment is indicated in connective tissue disease, uremic or tuberculous pericarditis, or severe recurrent symptoms unresponsive to NSAIDs or colchicine (3)[B]; should be avoided in uncomplicated acute pericarditis. Corticosteroid use alone has been found to be an independent risk factor for recurrence.
- Intrapericardial administration of steroids may be effective and limits systemic side effects (3)[B].

ADDITIONAL TREATMENT
General Measures
Specific therapy directed toward underlying disorder for patients with identified cause other than viral or idiopathic disease

SURGERY/OTHER PROCEDURES
Pericardiectomy considered for frequent and highly symptomatic recurrences resistant to medical therapy (3)[B]

IN-PATIENT CONSIDERATIONS
Admission Criteria
Inpatient therapy recommended for pericarditis associated with high-risk features (4)[B]:
- Fever >38°C
- Immunosuppressed state
- Trauma
- Oral anticoagulation therapy
- Myopericarditis
- Cardiac tamponade
- Echocardiographic evidence of large pericardial effusion
- Failure to respond to NSAID therapy

IV Fluids
No specific therapy recommended; IV fluids considered for hypotension in the setting of pericardial tamponade

Nursing
No specific therapies

Discharge Criteria
- Response to therapy with symptom improvement
- Hemodynamic stability

 ONGOING CARE

FOLLOW-UP RECOMMENDATIONS
Follow-up evaluation is not required for patients with small effusion unless symptoms recur or new symptoms develop.

DIET
No restrictions

PROGNOSIS
Overall good prognosis; disease usually benign and self-limiting

COMPLICATIONS
- Recurrent pericarditis (1):
  - Occurs in approximately 24% of patients
  - Recurrence usually within first weeks following initial episode but may occur months to years later
  - Rarely associated with tamponade or constriction
- Cardiac tamponade: Rare complication with increased incidence in neoplastic, purulent, and tuberculous pericarditis
- Constrictive pericarditis:
  - Rare complication in which rigid pericardium produces abnormal diastolic filling with elevated filling pressures
  - Pericardiectomy remains definitive therapy.

REFERENCES

1. Tingle LE, Molina D, Calvert CW. Acute pericarditis. *Am Fam Physician.* 2007;76:1509–14.
2. Khandaker MH, Espinosa RE, Nishimura RA, Sinak LJ, Hayes SN, Melduni RM, Oh JK et al. Pericardial disease: diagnosis and management. *Mayo Clin. Proc.* 2010;85:572–93.
3. Maisch B, Seferovi PM, Risti AD, et al. Guidelines on the diagnosis and management of pericardial diseases executive summary; The Task force on the diagnosis and management of pericardial diseases of the European society of cardiology. *Eur Heart J.* 2004;25:587–610.
4. Imazio M, Demichelis B, Parrini I, et al. Day-hospital treatment of acute pericarditis: a management program for outpatient therapy. *J Am Coll Cardiol.* 2004;43:1042–6.
5. Imazio M, Bobbio M, Cecchi E, et al. Colchicine in addition to conventional therapy for acute pericarditis: results of the COlchicine for acute PEricarditis (COPE) trial. *Circulation.* 2005;112:2012–6.

 CODES

ICD9
- 420.91 Acute idiopathic pericarditis
- 420.99 Other acute pericarditis
- 423.9 Unspecified disease of pericardium

CLINICAL PEARLS
- Common cause of chest pain with many possible etiologies, viral and idiopathic being most likely
- Typical presentation includes acute chest pain, pericardial friction rub, ECG changes with widespread PR-interval depression or ST-segment elevation, and evidence of pericardial effusion on echocardiogram.
- Therapy aimed at symptomatic relief, and NSAIDs are 1st-line treatment.
- Colchicine is recommended as adjunct to NSAIDs and has been found to reduce recurrences.
- Pericardiocentesis is recommended in the setting of cardiac tamponade or possible purulent pericarditis.

PERIODIC LIMB MOVEMENT DISORDER

Donald E. Watenpaugh, PhD
John R. Burk, MD

 BASICS

DESCRIPTION

Sleep-related movement disorder with these features (1,2)[A]:

- Episodes of periodic limb movements (PLMs) during sleep
- Movements consist of bilateral ankle and toe dorsiflexion, sometimes accompanied by knee and hip flexion.
- Arm or more generalized involvement occurs less commonly and in severe cases.
- Movements may cause brief microarousals from sleep unbeknownst to the patient.
- Leads to complaints of insomnia, unrestorative sleep, and daytime fatigue and/or somnolence
- Bed partner may complain of movements
- Another sleep disorder (e.g., obstructive sleep apnea) does not cause the PLMs.
- System(s) affected: Musculoskeletal; Nervous
- Synonym(s): Nocturnal myoclonus; Sleep myoclonus; Periodic leg movements of sleep

EPIDEMIOLOGY

Incidence

- Increases with age: 1/3 of patients >age 60 exhibit PLMs but not necessarily periodic limb movement disorder (PLMD)
- .Predominant sex: Male = Female.
- Restless legs syndrome (RLS), common associate of PLMs: ~2× more common in parous women than in men
- PLMs in 15% of insomnia patients

Prevalence

- PLMs in sleep: Common and often of no clinical consequence
- PLMs constituting PLMD (causing sleep complaints and/or daytime consequences) less common: <5% of adults but underdiagnosed

RISK FACTORS

- RLS: 80% exhibit PLMs
- Family history of RLS (3)[A]
- Rapid eye movement (REM) sleep behavior disorder: 70% exhibit PLMs
- Narcolepsy: 55% exhibit PLMs
- Iron deficiency and associated conditions (e.g., pregnancy, gastric surgery, renal disease)
- Attention deficit–hyperactivity disorder (ADHD)
- Aging
- Peripheral neuropathy
- Other sources of chronic limb pain or discomfort

Genetics

Unstudied, but see RLS.

GENERAL PREVENTION

- Regular physical activity
- Adequate nightly sleep
- Avoid possible causes of secondary PLMD.
- Avoid possible causes of RLS.

PATHOPHYSIOLOGY

Unstudied, but see RLS.

ETIOLOGY

- Primary: Probable CNS dopaminergic impairment
- Secondary:
  - Iron deficiency
  - Peripheral neuropathy
  - Arthritis
  - Renal failure
  - Synucleinopathies (multiple-system atrophy)
  - Spinal cord injury
  - Pregnancy
  - Medications:
    - Most antidepressants (not bupropion or desipramine)
    - Some antipsychotic and antidementia medications
    - Antiemetics (metoclopramide)
    - Antihistamines

COMMONLY ASSOCIATED CONDITIONS

- RLS
- REM sleep behavior disorder
- Narcolepsy
- Iron deficiency
- Renal failure
- Cardiovascular disease
- Gastric surgery
- Pregnancy
- Arthritis
- Synucleinopathies (multiple-system atrophy)
- Spinal cord injury
- Peripheral neuropathy
- Insomnia, insufficient sleep
- ADHD
- Depression

Pediatric Considerations

- PLMD may precede overt RLS by years.
- Association with RLS is more common than in adults.
- Symptoms may be more consequential than in adults
- Associated with ADHD (4,5)[B]

Pregnancy Considerations

- May be secondary to iron or folate deficiency
- Most severe in 3rd trimester
- Usually subsides after delivery

Geriatric Considerations

- May become a significant source of sleep disturbance
- May cause or exacerbate circadian disruption and "sundowning" behavior
- Many medications given to the elderly cause or exacerbate PLMs.

 DIAGNOSIS

HISTORY

- Insomnia: Difficulty maintaining sleep
- Unrestorative sleep
- Daytime fatigue and/or somnolence
- Oppositional behaviors
- Memory impairment
- Depression
- ADHD, particularly in children (4)[B]

DIAGNOSTIC TESTS & INTERPRETATION

Polysomnography with finding of repetitive, stereotyped limb movements (2,6)[A]:

- Tibialis anterior electromyographic (EMG) activity lasting 0.5–10.0 s
- EMG amplitude increase >8 μV from baseline
- Movements occur in a sequence of 4 or more at intervals of 5–90 s.
- Children: 5 or more movements/h; adults: 15
- Associated with heart rate variability from autonomic-level arousals
- Most PLM episodes occur in the first hours of non-REM sleep.
- Significant night-to-night PLM variability

Lab

Serum ferritin to assess for iron deficiency

Diagnostic Procedures/Surgery

- Ankle actigraphy can be used in the home.
- EMG or nerve conduction studies for peripheral neuropathy/radiculopathy

Pathological Findings

Serum ferritin <50 ng/mL

DIFFERENTIAL DIAGNOSIS

- When PLMs occur along with RLS, REM sleep behavior disorder, or narcolepsy, those disorders are diagnosed as "with PLMs," and PLMD is not diagnosed separately (2)[A].
- Obstructive sleep apnea: LMs occur during microarousals from apneas; treatment of sleep apnea eliminates these LMs.
- Sleep starts (hypnic jerks): Nonperiodic, generalized, occur only during wake-sleep transition, <0.2 s duration
- Sleep-related leg cramps: Isolated and painful
- Fragmentary myoclonus: 75–150 ms of EMG activity, minimal movement, no periodicity
- Nocturnal seizures: Epileptiform electroencephalogram (EEG), motor pattern incongruent with PLMs
- Fasciculations, tremor: No sleep association
- Sleep-related rhythmic movement disorder: Voluntary movement during wake-sleep transition; higher frequency than PLMs

TREATMENT

- Daily exercise
- Adequate nightly sleep
- Treatment paradigm similar to that for RLS (1,7)[A]

MEDICATION
Use minimum effective dose.

First Line
- Dopamine agonists: Take 1 h before bed; titrate weekly to optimal dose.
  - Ropinirole (Requip): 0.25–4.0 mg; titrate by 0.25 mg
  - Pramipexole (Mirapex): 0.125–1.5 mg; titrate by 0.125 mg
  - Cabergoline (Dostinex and Cabaser): 0.25–3.0 mg (*Warning:* Valvulopathy risk)
- Avoid dopamine agonists in psychotic patients, including those on dopamine antagonists.

Second Line
- Anticonvulsants: Useful for associated neuropathy:
  - Gabapentin (Neurontin): 300–1,800 mg/d
  - Pregabalin (Lyrica): 50–300 mg/d
- Opioids: Low risk for tolerance with single nightly dose:
  - Hydrocodone: 5–20 mg/d
  - Oxycodone: 2.5–20 mg/d
- Benzodiazepines and agonists: Useful for associated insomnia:
  - Zaleplon, zolpidem, temazepam, triazolam, alprazolam, diazepam
  - Clonazepam (Klonopin): 0.5–3.0 mg/d
- Daytime sleepiness side effect is unusual with the doses and timing employed for PLMD.
- Consider risks, side effects, and interactions individually (e.g., benzodiazepines in elderly).

Pediatric Considerations
- 1st-line treatment is nonpharmacologic.
- Low-dose clonidine, clonazepam, or gabapentin may be considered.

Pregnancy Considerations
- Initial approach: Iron supplementation, nonpharmacologic therapies
- Most medications class C or D and should be avoided
- In 3rd trimester, low-dose opioids or clonazepam may be considered.

Geriatric Considerations
In weak or frail patients, avoid medications that may cause dizziness or unsteadiness.

ADDITIONAL TREATMENT
- If iron-deficient, iron supplementation:
  - 325 mg ferrous sulfate with 200 mg vitamin C between meals
  - Side effects: Constipation, GI irritation
  - Repletion may require months.
  - Symptoms usually continue without other treatment.
- Vitamin/mineral supplements, including calcium, magnesium, B_{12}, folate
- Clonidine: 0.1–0.7 mg/d
- Quinine

General Measures
- Daily exercise
- Adequate nightly sleep
- Warm the legs (long socks, leg warmers, electric blanket, etc.).
- Hot bath before bedtime
- Avoid nicotine.

SURGERY/OTHER PROCEDURES
Correction of orthopedic, neuropathic, or peripheral vascular problems

IN-PATIENT CONSIDERATIONS
- Control during recovery from orthopedic procedures
- Addition or withdrawal of medications that affect PLMD
- Procedures or new-onset disease may elicit PLMD.
- Changes in medical status may require medication changes, such as
  - Renal failure: Mirapex contraindicated
  - Liver disease: Requip contraindicated

IV Fluids
- Consider iron infusion when conventional supplementation is ineffective, not tolerated, or contraindicated.
- When NPO, consider IV opiates.

Nursing
- Evening walks, hot baths, leg warming
- Sleep interruption risks prolonged wakefulness.

 ONGOING CARE

FOLLOW-UP RECOMMENDATIONS
Patient Monitoring
- At monthly intervals until stable
- Annual and p.r.n. follow-up thereafter
- If iron-deficient, remeasure ferritin to assess repletion.

DIET
Avoid caffeine and alcohol late in the day.

PATIENT EDUCATION
- WE MOVE (Worldwide Education & Awareness for Movement Disorders): www.wemove.org; e-mail: wemove@wemove.org; 212-875-8312; fax: 212-875-8389
- National Sleep Foundation: www.sleepfoundation.org; e-mail: nsf@sleepfoundation.org; 202-347-3471; fax: 202-347-3472

PROGNOSIS
- Primary PLMD: Lifelong condition with no current cure
- Secondary PLMD: May partially or completely subside with resolution of precipitating factors
- Current therapies usually control symptoms.
- PLMD commonly precedes emergence of RLS.

COMPLICATIONS
- Tolerance to medications requiring increased dose or alternatives.
- Augmentation (increased PLMs and sleep disturbance, emergence of RLS) from prolonged use of dopamine agonists:
  - Higher doses increase risk.
  - Iron deficiency increases risk.
  - Detitrate dopaminergic agent; concurrently add alternative medication (1,7)[B].
- Coping with/correcting for iatrogenic PLMD (as from antidepressants, etc.)

REFERENCES

1. Karatas M. Restless legs syndrome and periodic limb movements during sleep: diagnosis and treatment. *Neurologist*. 2007;13:294–301.
2. Periodic Limb Movement Disorder. In: *International Classification of Sleep Disorders Diagnostic & Coding Manual*, 2nd ed. Editor: Sateia MJ. Westchester, IL: American Academy of Sleep Medicine; 2005;182–6.
3. Picchietti DL, Rajendran RR, Wilson MP, et al. Pediatric restless legs syndrome and periodic limb movement disorder: Parent-child pairs. *Sleep Med*. 2009.
4. Walters AS, Silvestri R, Zucconi M, et al. Review of the possible relationship and hypothetical links between attention deficit hyperactivity disorder (ADHD) and the simple sleep related movement disorders, parasomnias, hypersomnias, and circadian rhythm disorders. *J Clin Sleep Med*. 2008;4:591–600.
5. Picchietti MA, Picchietti DL. Restless legs syndrome and periodic limb movement disorder in children and adolescents. *Semin Pediatr Neurol*. 2008;15:91–9.
6. Iber C, et al. The AASM Manual for the Scoring of Sleep and Associated Events. *American Academy of Sleep Medicine*. 2007:59.
7. Trenkwalder C, Hening WA, Montagna P, et al. Treatment of restless legs syndrome: an evidence-based review and implications for clinical practice. *Mov Disord*. 2008;23:2267–302.

ADDITIONAL READING

- Ferini-Strambi L. Treatment options for restless legs syndrome. *Expert Opin Pharmacother*. 2009;10:545–54.
- Natarajan R et al. Review of periodic limb movement and restless leg syndrome. *J Postgrad Med*. 2010;56:157–62.

See Also (Topic, Algorithm, Electronic Media Element)
Restless Legs Syndrome

CODES

ICD9
327.51 Periodic limb movement disorder

CLINICAL PEARLS

- Obstructive sleep apnea is the most common disease associated with PLMs, which emphasizes the importance of differential diagnosis.
- Many patients with PLMs may not require treatment. When sleep disturbance from PLMs causes insomnia and/or daytime consequences, PLMD exists and should be treated.
- Many antidepressants and some antihistamines cause or exacerbate PLMs.
- Accumulating data indicate that sleep disturbance, including that from PLMs, may cause or exacerbate ADHD (4,5)[B].

PERIPHERAL ARTERIAL DISEASE

Zhen Lu, MD

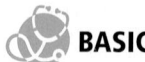 **BASICS**

DESCRIPTION
Peripheral arterial disease (PAD) is a manifestation of systemic atherosclerosis in which there is partial or total blockage in the arteries, exclusive of the coronary and cerebral vessels. Objectively, PAD is defined as a resting ankle-brachial index of <0.90.

EPIDEMIOLOGY
- Predominant age: >40 years
- Predominant sex: Male > Female (2:1), based on the Framingham study
- Patients with symptomatic PAD have a 5-year mortality rate of 30%.
- Highly prevalent syndrome that affects 8–12 million individuals in the US

Incidence
Incidence per year overall: 1.0–2.7/1,000/year

Prevalence
- US prevalence: 2.7–4.1%
- Age-adjusted prevalence of PAD is close to 12%.
- Up to 29% among patients in primary-care practices

RISK FACTORS
- Age >40 years
- Cigarette smoking
- Diabetes mellitus
- Obesity
- Hypertension
- Hyperlipidemia
- Hyperhomocysteinemia

Genetics
Current National Institutes of Health–funded research focuses on single-nucleotide polymorphisms in candidate genes that are regulated in the vasculature in an attempt to explore genetic factors responsible for PAD.

GENERAL PREVENTION
Control risk factors.

PATHOPHYSIOLOGY
In patients with peripheral arterial disease, arterial stenoses cause inadequate blood flow in distal limbs, which fails to meet the metabolic demand during exertion:
- The degree of ischemia is proportional to the size and proximity of the occlusion to the end organ.
- The acidic products of anaerobic metabolism build up within the muscle and result in claudication clinically.
- Arterial occlusion also causes significantly diminished distal pressure in patients with PAD due to the atherosclerotic lesions.

ETIOLOGY
The most common cause of arterial stenoses is atherosclerosis.

COMMONLY ASSOCIATED CONDITIONS
- See Risk Factors.
- Associated with other common complications of atherosclerosis, including myocardial infarction, transient ischemic attack, stroke, and limb amputation
- Occurs in ~40% of patients with cardiovascular disease

 DIAGNOSIS

HISTORY
- 1/2 of the patients with PAD are asymptomatic (in mild coronary artery disease [CAD])
- Intermittent claudication, with symptoms typically resolving within 2–5 minutes of rest (although it is regarded as the classic symptom for PAD, intermittent claudication is present in only 10% of patients with PAD)
- Rest leg pain (especially in a supine position)
- Skin ulceration (in advanced PAD)
- Gangrene (in advanced PAD)
- Impotence

PHYSICAL EXAM
- Skin pallor with leg elevation above the level of the heart (in mild PAD)
- Dependent rubor
- Dry and scaly skin
- Poor nail growth
- Hair loss
- Reduced or absent extremity pulses (in advanced PAD)

DIAGNOSTIC TESTS & INTERPRETATION
Lab
Serum glucose is recommended for screening for diabetes mellitus in suspected or confirmed PAD.

Initial lab tests
Fasting lipid profile is indicated for risk assessment of hyperlipidemia.

Imaging
- Magnetic resonance angiography, coupled with 3-D reconstruction, is highly sensitive and specific for the localization of occluded lesions.
- Computed tomography scan has a limited role in evaluating PAD.
- Angiography remains the gold standard in the diagnosis of PAD.

Initial approach
Duplex ultrasonography and Doppler color-flow imaging are useful in detecting stenosed segments and assessing lesion severity.

Diagnostic Procedures/Surgery
- Doppler ankle-brachial index (ABI) measures the ratio of (1) the higher systolic blood pressures (BPs) between the dorsalis pedis and the posterior tibial artery versus (2) the higher of the systolic BPs in the 2 brachial arteries:
  – ABI <0.4: Severe ischemia
  – 0.4 <0.9: Moderate peripheral arterial obstruction
  – 0.9 <1.3: Reduction of ABI by 20% after exercise is suggestive of PAD; otherwise, normal
  – Pathologic ABI >1.3: Calcified vessel and additional diagnostic studies are needed.
- Segmental limb pressures: Usually obtained if abnormal ABI measurement is identified; a 20 mm Hg or greater reduction in pressure is considered significant for PAD.
- Treadmill exercise test assesses the severity of claudication and the response to treatment.
- Segmental volume plethysmography: Often used in conjunction with segmental limb pressures to measure the volume change in an organ or limb; the study is indicated for calcified vessel when the ABI cannot be applied diagnostically.

DIFFERENTIAL DIAGNOSIS
- Arterial embolism
- Deep venous thrombosis
- Thromboangiitis obliterans (Buerger disease)
- Osteoarthritis
- Restless legs syndrome
- Peripheral neuropathy
- Spinal stenoses (pseudoclaudication)
- Intervertebral disc prolapse

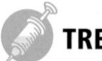 **TREATMENT**

MEDICATION
First Line
Antiplatelet therapy is the mainstay treatment to prevent ischemic events in patients with PAD:

- Although the effect of aspirin on the risk reduction of overall ischemic events is inconclusive, it has been shown to delay disease progression and reduce the need for surgical intervention, and should be recommended for patients with PAD (1)[A].
- Low-dose aspirin (75–150 mg/d) is as effective as higher doses of aspirin (1).
- Ticlopidine (250 mg b.i.d.) reduces the risk of myocardial infarction (MI), stroke, and death by 1/3 in patients with PAD, but has complication of thrombocytopenia in 2–3% of patients (1)[A].

Second Line

- Clopidogrel (75 mg/d) is Food and Drug Administration approved for the secondary prevention of atherosclerotic events in patients with PAD (2)[A].
- Neither vasodilators nor anticoagulant therapy (e.g., heparin, low-molecular-weight heparin, or oral anticoagulant) has shown any clinically proven efficacy for the treatment of claudication (1)[B].
- Other medications that may improve claudication include pentoxifylline (1.2 g/d), cilostazol (100 mg b.i.d.), naftidrofuryl (600 mg/d), and prostaglandins (120 μg/d).

ADDITIONAL TREATMENT

- Weight reduction, smoking cessation, and BP control are essential in treating claudication.
- A walking program should include at least 3 ×/week for 30–60 minutes each time and has been shown to improve quality of life as much as or more so than medication.
- A healthy diet high in complex carbohydrates (such as whole grains and pastas), fruits, and vegetables and low in salt and animal fats

General Measures

- Claudication exercise rehabilitation program; patient to walk until develops symptoms, then rest and start again, for a total of 30 minutes initially; walking then is increased by 5 minutes until 50 minutes of intermittent walking is achieved.
- Modification of risk factors including smoking, diabetes mellitus, hypertension, and hyperlipidemia:
  - Weight loss is associated with a decrease in the risk of cardiovascular disease but has not been shown to improve PAD (1)[C].
  - Antiplatelet therapy (aspirin) is recommended in patients with PAD when there is no other contraindication; however, neither the addition of an anticoagulant nor anticoagulant therapy alone has demonstrated superior outcome in PAD patients (3)[A].
  - Simvastatin (20–40 mg/d) has been shown to reduce the incidence of new intermittent claudication from 3.6–2.3% in patients with CAD (2)[A].
  - No statistical significance for overall improvement of exercise performance or claudication symptoms for patients on Niacin ER/lovastatin combined therapy.
  - β-adrenergic antagonists should be used with caution in individuals with severe PAD (1)[B].
  - Smoking cessation is likely to reduce the severity of claudication (1)[C].

COMPLEMENTARY AND ALTERNATIVE MEDICINE

- Acupuncture, biofeedback, chelation therapy, and supplements such as *Ginkgo biloba,* omega-3 fatty acids, and vitamin E have been studied.
- *G. biloba* modestly improves the symptoms of intermittent claudication (120 mg/d for up to 6 months) and can be considered as an adjunct to exercise therapy. Inconclusive evidence exists for the use of vitamin E (4,5).

SURGERY/OTHER PROCEDURES

Surgical interventions, such as revascularization, are warranted for individuals who have debilitating intermittent claudication, ischemic rest pain, or tissue loss:

- Transluminal balloon angioplasty is a percutaneous method of dilating arterial stenoses or recanalizing occluded vessels with or without stents (reserved for short, isolated, and hemodynamically significant lesions of the iliac or proximal superficial femoral artery).
- Bypass surgery is the standard operative treatment for lower extremity peripheral occlusive disease.

 ONGOING CARE

FOLLOW-UP RECOMMENDATIONS

- Exercise training program composed of walking or bicycle riding improves maximal treadmill walking distance and therefore enhances functional capacity (2)[A].
- However, there is little added benefit from *G. biloba* treatment when added to supervised exercise training in patients with peripheral arterial disease as compared with patients in exercise training program alone (6)[C].

DIET

Low-fat cardiac diet is recommended.

PROGNOSIS

- Among patients with intermittent claudication, 15–20% will experience worsening claudication, 5–10% will undergo lower extremity bypass surgery, and 2–5% will need primary amputation. (Rates for smokers and diabetics are much higher.)
- 30,000–50,000 people in the US undergo amputations annually due to PAD.

REFERENCES

1. Hankey GJ, Norman PE, Eikelboom JW. Medical treatment of peripheral arterial disease. *JAMA*. 2006;295:547–53.
2. Gey DC, Lesho EP, Manngold J. Management of peripheral arterial disease. *Am Fam Physician*. 2004;69:525–32.
3. Duprez DA. Pharmacological interventions for peripheral artery disease. *Expert Opin Pharmacother*. 2007;8:1465–77.
4. Pittler MH, Ernst E. Ginkgo biloba extract for the treatment of intermittent claudication: a meta-analysis of randomized trials. *Am J Med*. 2000;108:276–81.
5. Kleijnen I, MacKerras D. Vitamin E for intermittent claudication. Cochrane Peripheral Vascular Diseases Group. *Cochrane Database Syst Rev*. 2006;(4).
6. Wang J, Zhou S, Bronks R, et al. Supervised exercise training combined with ginkgo biloba treatment for patients with peripheral arterial disease. *Clin Rehabil*. 2007;21:579–86.
7. Burns P, Gough S, Bradbury AW. Management of peripheral arterial disease in primary care. *BMJ*. 2003;326:584–8.

ADDITIONAL READING

- Hiatt WR. Medical treatment of peripheral arterial disease and claudication. *N Engl J Med*. 2001;344:1608–21.
- Hiatt WR, Hirsch AT, Creager MA, et al. Effect of niacin ER/lovastatin on claudication symptoms in patients with peripheral artery disease. *Vascular medicine (London, England)*. 2010;

 CODES

ICD9

- 440.20 Atherosclerosis of native arteries of the extremities, unspecified
- 443.9 Peripheral vascular disease, unspecified

CLINICAL PEARLS

- Not every patient needs to be screened for PAD. Studies have indicated that screening for PAD among asymptomatic adults in the general population could lead to false-positive results and unnecessary workups. The prevalence in the general public who are asymptomatic is low.
- A patient already on medical treatment should be referred for further surgical evaluation for any of the following scenarios:
  - Unsatisfactory results despite medical therapy
  - No definitive diagnosis can be made.
  - Critical limb ischemia present, such as rest pain, gangrene, or ulceration (7)
- In the clopidogrel (75 mg/d) vs aspirin (325 mg/d) study in the Patients at Risk of Ischemic Events (CAPRIE) trial, there was a 23.8% RRR for MI, stroke, or cardiovascular death in PAD patients treated with clopidogrel compared with aspirin but no statistically significant difference in overall mortality reduction. However, clopidogrel is much more expensive than aspirin.

PERITONITIS, ACUTE

Michelle Trivedi, MD
Vilas Patwardhan, MD

 BASICS

DESCRIPTION
- Acute inflammation of the membrane that lines the visceral and parietal peritoneum
- 3 types are recognized:
  - Primary: Spontaneous bacterial peritonitis (SBP)
  - Secondary bacterial peritonitis (2BP): Associated with inflammation of a visceral organ
  - Tertiary bacterial peritonitis (3BP): Persistent or recurrent infection after adequate initial therapy
- SBP implies an intra-abdominal bacterial infection without an apparent intra-abdominal source. It is a common complication of cirrhosis/chronic liver disease.
- 2BP is an intra-abdominal infection with a surgically treatable source.
- 3BP is often seen in patients with comorbidities or who are immunocompromised.

EPIDEMIOLOGY
Incidence
- Varies with underlying abdominal disease process
- Recurrence rates of SBP within 6 months as high as 43%; within 1 year 69%
- Predominant sex: Male > Female.

Prevalence
- SBP: 10–30% of patients with cirrhosis and ascites, with a mortality rate of 25%
- 2BP can be a consequence of visceral organ inflammation (e.g., appendicitis, diverticulitis); without perforation <10%, with perforation >50% chance of contracting 2BP

RISK FACTORS
- Cirrhosis, ascitic fluid total protein level <1 g/dL, elevated bilirubin, upper GI bleeding, prior SBP
- Gut ischemia with reperfusion, indwelling IV and urinary catheters
- Massive transfusion, perioperative shock
- PEG tube insertion (increased risk of peritonitis if higher body mass index [BMI] and lower serum albumin) (1)
- Geriatric considerations: Mortality is greater in this age group. Symptoms may be muted.

GENERAL PREVENTION
- Prophylactic antibiotics indicated for cirrhotic patients with acute GI hemorrhage and following intra-abdominal surgery
- Prophylactic antibiotics for high-risk patients with recurrent peritonitis and low ascitic fluid total protein levels remain an area of controversy.

PATHOPHYSIOLOGY
- Inflammation of the peritoneum owing to infectious, chemical (i.e., bile, blood, barium), mechanical, or neoplastic causes
- SBP: Seen in cirrhotics with portal hypertension; translocation of gut bacteria (gram negative > gram positive) across the gut wall or into mesenteric lymph nodes leads to infection and inflammation of ascites fluid.
- Bacterial seeding may occur in the presence of other infections, such as urinary tract infections (UTIs), pneumococcal sepsis, cellulitis, pharyngitis, and dental infections.
- 2BP: Ruptured peritoneal organ or tissue seeding the peritoneum with bacteria

ETIOLOGY
- Most common pathogens:
  - Primary: *Escherichia coli* (40%), *Streptococcus* sp. (15%), *Klebsiella pneumoniae* (7%), *Pseudomonas* sp. (5%), *Proteus* sp. (5%)
  - Secondary: *E. coli, Klebsiella, Proteus, Streptococcus, Enterococcus, Bacteroides,* and *Clostridium* sp.
  - Tertiary: *Enterobacter, Pseudomonas, Enterococcus, Staphylococcus,* and *Candida* sp.
- Primary: Associated with hepatic, cardiac, nephrotic, and malignancy-related ascites
- Secondary:
  - Perforation of bowel, most common site sigmoid; peritoneal abscess
  - Abdominal trauma
  - Continuous ambulatory peritoneal dialysis
  - Appendicitis, diverticulitis, pancreatitis, acute cholecystitis
  - Colitis: Infectious, inflammatory
  - Peptic ulcer perforation
  - Ischemic bowel
  - Strangulation of the small bowel
  - Postoperative (intraabdominal surgery)
  - Pelvic inflammatory disease
  - Iatrogenic: Endoscopic procedures, anastomotic dehiscence, and inadvertent bowel injury (mechanical, thermal, etc.)

DX DIAGNOSIS

HISTORY
- Abdominal pain
- Fever (>37.8°C [100°F]) ± increased white blood cells (WBCs). Note: Patients with advanced cirrhosis or severe sepsis may be mildly hypothermic.
- Nausea/vomiting, chills, anorexia, decrease in renal function, dyspnea, tachycardia, altered mental status (54% of cirrhosis patients owing either to infection or to hepatic dysfunction) (2)[B]

PHYSICAL EXAM
- Rebound tenderness, abdominal wall rigidity, abdominal distension with decreased or absent bowel sounds
- Abdominal pain may be diminished in patients with ascites because ascites fluid separates the visceral and parietal peritoneal surfaces.

DIAGNOSTIC TESTS & INTERPRETATION
Lab
Initial lab tests
- Basic metabolic panel, complete blood count (CBC) with differential, blood culture, urinalysis and culture, liver function tests (LFTs), lipase, prothrombin time (PT)/international normalization ratio (INR)/partial thromboplastin time (PTT)
- Ascitic fluid analysis (2)[B]:
  - Cell count with differential, culture (false-negative in 80% patients), Gram stain, total protein, lactate dehydrogenase, glucose, amylase, albumin
  - SBP: Absolute polymorphonuclear (PMN) count $\geq$250 cells/mm^3 (if positive, culture typically grows 1 organism 90% of the time)
  - 2BP: Absolute PMN count $\geq$250 cells/mm^3 or WBC count $\geq$500 cells/mm^3 (culture typically grows multiple organisms)

Follow-Up & Special Considerations
If no clinical improvement in 48–72 hours, repeat paracentesis to monitor treatment success (decrease in neutrophil count <50% original value and negative cultures).

Imaging
Initial approach
- Supine/upright abdominal films and CXR: Free air in peritoneal cavity, large/small bowel dilatation, intestinal wall edema
- Sonograph or CT scan with enteral and IV contrast material: Intraabdominal mass, ascites, abscess, extravasation of water-soluble gut contrast material

Diagnostic Procedures/Surgery
- Ascites: Abdominal paracentesis
- Abscess: Ultrasound- or CT-guided percutaneous drainage
- Diagnostic laparotomy
- Colonoscopy to assess for colitis

Pathological Findings
Predominant PMN infiltration noted in ascitic fluid

DIFFERENTIAL DIAGNOSIS
- Abscess formation (subdiaphragmatic, subhepatic, peritoneal, pelvic)
- Ileus (volvulus, intussusception)
- Mesenteric adenitis, appendicitis, pancreatitis, cholecystitis, pelvic inflammatory disease (PID), pyelonephritis
- Ruptured ectopic pregnancy, tubo-ovarian cyst

TREATMENT

MEDICATION

- SBP: No antibiotic proven to be more efficacious than others (3,4,5,6)[A]:
  - Cefotaxime 2 g IV q8h × 5–14 days; excellent penetration into ascites with no nephrotoxicity; common side effect is rash.
  - Ceftriaxone 1 g q24h × 5–14 days
  - Ampicillin-sulbactam 3 g IV q6h × 5–14 days (3,4)[A]
  - Albumin 1.5 g/kg IV on day 1 and 1 g/kg on day 3 for hospitalized SBP patients to prevent hepatorenal syndrome (4,7)[A]
  - Quinolones (e.g., norfloxacin, ofloxacin, ciprofloxacin) × 7 days
- 2BP:
  - Must cover anaerobic as well as gram-negative aerobic/facilitative organisms
  - Agents active against anaerobic organisms include metronidazole, cefotetan, ticarcillin-clavulanate, piperacillin-tazobactam, ampicillin-sulbactam, imipenem
- 3BP: Long-term daily prophylactic regimens include norfloxacin 400 mg/d PO and trimethoprim-sulfamethoxazole 1 double-strength tablet PO daily (less expensive) (5)[A].
- Associated with chronic ambulatory peritoneal dialysis: Vancomycin plus gentamicin instilled in peritoneal cavity
- Prevention of SBP in patients with cirrhosis and GI bleeding: Antibiotic regimens as listed above for SBP
- Patients with ascitic fluid total protein levels <1 g/dL: Give prophylactic therapy during hospitalization only. Long-term antibiotics are controversial (2)[B].
- If on prophylactic therapy, 3BP should be treated with a different agent depending on culture results.

ADDITIONAL TREATMENT
General Measures
Treat paralytic ileus (nasogastric decompression); add respiratory support if needed.

SURGERY/OTHER PROCEDURES
Two phases (for 2BP): Emergent surgery, either laparoscopic or open abdomen, to remove etiologic agent; then once patient is stable, have a 2nd look within the abdomen.

IN-PATIENT CONSIDERATIONS
Initial Stabilization
- Volume resuscitation to prevent secondary organ system dysfunction; monitor urine output by Foley catheter.
- Antibiotics are started empirically to cover a broad spectrum of organisms once infection is suspected, with an ascitic fluid PMN count of ≥250 cells/mm^3. The choice of antibiotic may be altered after culture and sensitivity results are obtained.
- Give adequate analgesics and antiemetics; if patient has severe nausea/vomiting, perform nasogastric decompression.

 ONGOING CARE

FOLLOW-UP RECOMMENDATIONS
Patient Monitoring
- Condition should improve within 24–72 hours of initial treatment. If no improvement, check for a persistent or recurrent infectious focus.
- Closely monitor for secondary infections after long-term antibiotics use or from a surgical wound site.

DIET
- NPO: IV fluids and electrolytes
- Total parenteral nutrition may be necessary.
- Enteral feedings after return of bowel sounds and passage of flatus and/or feces

PROGNOSIS
- Mortality rate for SBP is 10–30%, with 1/2 of deaths caused by GI bleed, renal failure, or liver failure.
- 69% of patients with SBP have recurrence within 1 year and a mortality rate approaching 50%.
- Mortality of SBP is ~80% if patient unnecessarily receives exploratory laparotomy.
- Uncomplicated 2BP <5% mortality rate; severe 30–50% mortality rate
- Presence of renal insufficiency is strongest prognostic indicator for mortality in SBP (2)[B].
- Other poor prognostic indicators: Peripheral leukocytosis, older age, ileus, high Child-Pugh score, malnutrition, or cancer
- Patients with hospital-acquired (vs. community-acquired) SBP have a greater risk of death (5)[A].

COMPLICATIONS
- Hypovolemia
- Septicemia, septic shock
- Acute renal failure, liver failure
- Respiratory failure
- Abscess formation
- Abdominal compartment syndrome

REFERENCES

1. Shah RD, Tariq N, Shanley C. Peritonitis from peg tube insertion in surgical intensive care unit patients: identification of risk factors and clinical outcomes. *Surg Endosc.* May 2009.
2. Sheer TA, Runyon BA. Spontaneous bacterial peritonitis. *Dig Dis.* 2005;23:39–46.
3. Runyon BA, Practice Guidelines Committee, American Association for the Study of Liver Diseases (AASLD). Management of adult patients with ascites due to cirrhosis. *Hepatology.* 2004;39:841–56.
4. Parsi MA, Atreja A, Zein NN. Spontaneous bacterial peritonitis: recent data on incidence and treatment. *Cleve Clin J Med.* 2004;71:569–76.
5. Frazee LA, Marinos AE, Rybarczyk AM et al. Long-term prophylaxis of spontaneous bacterial peritonitis in patients with cirrhosis. *Ann Pharmacother.* 2005;39:908–12.
6. Lontos S, Gow PJ, Vaughan RB, et al. Norfloxacin and trimethoprim-sulfamethoxazole therapy have similar efficacy in prevention of spontaneous bacterial peritonitis. *J Gastroenterol Hepatol.* 2008;23:252–5.
7. Fernández J, Navasa M, Planas R, et al. Primary prophylaxis of spontaneous bacterial peritonitis delays hepatorenal syndrome and improves survival in cirrhosis. *Gastroenterology.* 2007;133:818–24.

ADDITIONAL READING

Cheong HS, Kang CI. Clinical significance and outcome of nosocomial acquisition of spontaneous bacterial peritonitis in patients with liver cirrhosis. *Clinic Infec Dis.* 2009;48(9):1230–6.

See Also (Topic, Algorithm, Electronic Media Element)
Appendicitis, Acute, Crohn Disease; Diverticular Disease; Ectopic Pregnancy; Pancreatitis
Algorithm: Abdominal Rigidity

 CODES

ICD9
- 567.9 Unspecified peritonitis
- 567.21 Peritonitis (acute) generalized

CLINICAL PEARLS

- Patients with both SBP and 2BP will have ≥250 PMNs/mm^3; however, SBP is typically unimicrobial, whereas 2BP is typically polymicrobial with an evident intraabdominal source of infection.
- 2BP typically also will have ≥2 of the following criteria:
  - Total protein concentration >1 g/dL
  - Glucose concentration <50 mg/dL (2.8 mmol/L)
  - Elevated lactate dehydrogenase ≥225 units/L
- Peritoneal carcinomatosis, pancreatic ascites, hemorrhage into ascites, and tuberculous peritonitis are associated with ≥250 PMNs/mm^3, but PMNs are often <50% of total WBCs. These forms of peritonitis are usually culture negative.
- SBP develops in preexisting ascites; it does not cause ascites.
- An ascitic fluid culture growing multiple organisms but with a PMN count of <250 cells/mm^3 on analysis is most likely polymicrobial bacterascites secondary to bowel puncture with paracentesis needle. This is rare (<0.6% of all paracenteses, and morbidity is low) (2)[B].

PERITONSILLAR ABSCESS

Matthew R. Leibowitz, MD

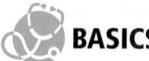 **BASICS**

DESCRIPTION
Peritonsillar abscess results in infection with abscess formation and collection of pus in the space between the anterior and posterior tonsillar pillars and the superior pharyngeal constrictor muscle:
- Usually follows an episode of acute pharyngitis or tonsillitis
- System(s) affected: GI; Pulmonary
- Synonym(s): Quinsy

EPIDEMIOLOGY
Incidence
- In the US, estimated 45,000 new cases yearly (30/100,000 person-years)
- Predominant age: All age groups, with greatest incidence in adolescents and young adults 15–30 years of age
- Predominant sex: Male = Female

RISK FACTORS
- Prior episodes of tonsillitis
- Age (young more susceptible)

ETIOLOGY
- Polymicrobial infection is the rule in peritonsillar abscess, and multiple bacteria likely will be grown from cultures of drained pus. *Streptococcus* sp. are the most common pathogens.
- Aerobic bacteria:
  – *Streptococcus pyogenes* (group A *Streptococcus*)
  – *S. milleri* group
  – *Haemophilus influenzae*
  – *S. viridans*
  – *Neisseria* sp.
  – *Staphylococcus aureus*
- Anaerobic bacteria:
  – *Fusobacterium*
  – *Peptostreptococcus*
  – *Porphyromonas*
  – *Prevotella*
  – *Bacteroides*

COMMONLY ASSOCIATED CONDITIONS
- Pharyngitis
- Tonsillitis
- Peritonsillar cellulitis
- Retropharyngeal abscess
- Lateral space abscess
- Septic jugular vein thrombophlebitis (Lemierre syndrome)

 DIAGNOSIS

HISTORY
- Extreme sore throat or neck pain
- Odynophagia
- Dysphagia

PHYSICAL EXAM
- Fever >38°C
- Trismus
- "Hot potato voice" (thickened, muffled voice)
- Drooling and pooling of saliva in the mouth
- Tonsillar exudates seen uncommonly
- Erythematous, edematous tonsil
- Asymmetry of the oropharynx with inferior and medial displacement of the infected tonsil, often with contralateral deviation of the uvula
- Cervical adenopathy

DIAGNOSTIC TESTS & INTERPRETATION
Diagnosis is made based on history and limited exam; testing/imaging is needed only if the diagnosis is unclear and patient is stable.

Lab
- Leukocytosis
- Culture of pathogens from aspirated or drained pus to identify organism(s)

Imaging
- Intraoral ultrasonography often will show a discrete abscess cavity if present.
- CT scan, best performed with contrast material, also will show a discrete abscess cavity if present. Edema of the surrounding tissues also can be seen on CT scan.

Diagnostic Procedures/Surgery
Incision and drainage of pus via needle aspiration or an operative procedure under general anesthesia or conscious sedation

DIFFERENTIAL DIAGNOSIS
- Peritonsillar cellulitis
- Tonsillar abscess
- Retropharyngeal abscess
- Lateral space abscess
- Infectious mononucleosis (Epstein-Barr virus infection)
- Aspiration of foreign body
- Dental infection
- Salivary gland infection
- Cervical adenitis
- Mastoiditis
- Internal carotid artery aneurysm

 TREATMENT

Drainage of the abscess, antibiotics, and pain control are the most important aspects of treatment.

MEDICATION
First Line
- Penicillin remains the standard antimicrobial therapy, with initial therapy delivered parenterally, although some now consider clindamycin to be 1st-line. Tailor therapy to cultured pathogens as much as possible. If organisms other than oral streptococci are suspected, expanded therapy may be indicated. With growing concern for β-lactamase-producing organisms, antibiotics with β-lactamase inhibitors or cephalosporins may be preferred. If *Fusobacterium* or *Bacteroides* are implicated, then additional anaerobic therapy with metronidazole may be indicated with increasing resistance to penicillin among these pathogens (1)[C]:
  – Penicillin G 1–4 million units IV q4h *or*
  – Benzathine penicillin G 1.2 million units IM 1 time *or*
  – Benzathine penicillin G 900,000 units and procaine penicillin G 300,000 units IM 1 time, followed by
  – Penicillin V 500 mg (25–50 mg/kg for children) p.o. t.i.d. to complete 10–14 days of total therapy

- For penicillin-allergic patients:
  - Erythromycin ethyl succinate 300–400 mg p.o. t.i.d. *or*
  - Cephalexin 250–500 mg p.o. t.i.d.
- If resistant organisms (including oral anaerobes) are suspected, add to the above oral therapy:
  - Metronidazole 500 mg p.o. t.i.d.–q.i.d. *or*
  - Clindamycin 150–450 mg p.o. t.i.d.–q.i.d. Some consider clindamycin alone to be 1st line therapy.
- Alternatively:
  - Ampicillin-sulbactam (Unasyn) 3 g IV q6h *or*
  - Ticarcillin-clavulanate (Ticar) 3–4 g IV q4–6h *or*
  - Amoxicillin-clavulanate (Augmentin) 500 mg p.o. t.i.d. or 875 mg p.o. b.i.d. *or*
  - Cefuroxime 500 mg p.o. b.i.d. (or another 2nd- or 3rd-generation cephalosporin) and metronidazole 500 mg p.o. t.i.d.–q.i.d.

Second Line
The role of adjunctive corticosteroids in the treatment of peritonsillar abscess is controversial. A recent small randomized study suggests that a single high dose of methylprednisolone (2–3 mg/kg up to 250 mg) administered after needle drainage and before antimicrobial therapy may improve a patient's ability to open the mouth and drink water earlier, speed resolution of fever, and decrease length of hospital stay (2)[C].

ADDITIONAL TREATMENT
General Measures
- Same-day surgery is possible in some cases with outpatient management.
- IV rehydration
- Pain control

Issues for Referral
Follow up with ENT surgeon, especially if symptoms recur or do not improve.

SURGERY/OTHER PROCEDURES
- Small studies indicate that rates of success are equivalent between needle aspiration and operative incision and drainage:
  - Needle aspiration with intraoral ultrasound or CT guidance
  - Operative incision and drainage when needle aspiration is too difficult due to trismus or lack of patient cooperation

- Immediate tonsillectomy at the time of incision and drainage (known as *quinsy tonsillectomy*) has decreased in favor due to increased risk of hemorrhage and overall low rates of abscess recurrence without tonsillectomy.
- Delayed tonsillectomy (known as *interval tonsillectomy*) is also performed less commonly due to the low rates of recurrent abscess (1)[C].

IN-PATIENT CONSIDERATIONS
Admission Criteria
- Inability to swallow
- Trismus
- Need for parenteral analgesia
- Planned operative incision and drainage

IV Fluids
May be required if oral intake of fluids not possible

Discharge Criteria
- Ability to swallow
- Able to take oral antimicrobial therapy
- Oral analgesia effective

 ## ONGOING CARE

FOLLOW-UP RECOMMENDATIONS
Patient Monitoring
- Follow up within 48 h to ensure resolution of symptoms and tonsillar inflammation.
- Lack of improvement may indicate antibiotic-resistant pathogens or residual abscess necessitating repeat drainage.

DIET
No restrictions following decompressing abscess; liquid diet may be tolerated best until pain improves.

PATIENT EDUCATION
Important to complete course of antibiotics

PROGNOSIS
- Symptoms will improve rapidly after incision and drainage and appropriate antibiotics.
- Pain and inflammation may persist for up to a week after treatment.
- Recurrent peritonsillar abscess does occur but is rare.

COMPLICATIONS
- Airway obstruction
- Spread to parapharyngeal (lateral) or retropharyngeal spaces
- Septic jugular vein thrombosis
- Brain abscess
- Sepsis
- Possible complications of incision and drainage:
  - Pulmonary aspiration of blood and pus with bronchopneumonia
  - Tonsillar hemorrhage
  - Perforation of the carotid artery

REFERENCES
1. Schraff S, McGinn JD, Derkay CS. Peritonsillar abscess in children: a 10-year review of diagnosis and management. *Int J Pediatr Otorhinolaryngol.* 2001;57:213–8.
2. Ozbek C, Aygenc E, Tuna EU, et al. Use of steroids in the treatment of peritonsillar abscess. *J Laryngol Otol.* 2004;118:439–42.

ADDITIONAL READING
- *Curr Infect Dis Rep* 2006;8(3):196. Guidelines: * Finnish Medical Society.
- Evidence-based guideline on sore throat and tonsillitis can be found at National Guideline Clearinghouse 2007 Nov 19:11045.
- Galioto NJ. Peritonsillar abscess. *Am Fam Physician.* 2008;77(2):199–202.

See Also (Topic, Algorithm, Electronic Media Element)
Epiglottitis; Pharyngitis

 ## CODES

ICD9
475 Peritonsillar abscess

CLINICAL PEARLS
- Needle drainage is likely to be as effective as operative drainage.
- Penicillin remains the drug of choice for most cases.

PERSONALITY DISORDERS
Moshe S. Torem, MD, DLFAPA

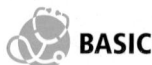 **BASICS**

DESCRIPTION
Personality disorders (PDs) are a group of conditions, with onset at or before adolescence, characterized by enduring patterns of maladaptive and dysfunctional behavior that deviates markedly from one's culture and social environment, leading to functional impairment and distress to the individual, coworkers, and family:

- These behaviors are perceived by patients to be "normal" and "right," and they have little insight as to their ownership, responsibility, and abnormal nature of these behaviors.
- These conditions are classified based on the predominant symptoms and their severity.
- System(s) affected: Nervous/Psychiatric
- Synonym(s): Character disorder; Character pathology (1)

Geriatric Considerations
Coping with the stresses of aging is challenging.

Pediatric Considerations
A history of childhood neglect, abuse, and trauma is not uncommon.

Pregnancy Considerations
Pregnancy adds pressure in coping with the activities of daily living (ADLs).

EPIDEMIOLOGY
Prevalence
- General population: 1.0–5.0%
- Outpatient psychiatric clinic: 3.0–30.0%
- In the US: 12%
- In male prisoners, the prevalence of antisocial personality disorder is ~60%.
- Predominant age: Starts in adolescence and early 20s and persists throughout patient's life
- Predominant sex: Male = Female; some personality disorders are more common in females, and others are more common in males.

RISK FACTORS
- Positive family history
- Pregnancy risk factors:
  - Nutritional deprivation
  - Use of alcohol or drugs
  - Viral and bacterial infections
- Dysfunctional family with child abuse/neglect

Genetics
Major character traits are inherited; others result from a combination of genetics and environment.

PATHOPHYSIOLOGY
- Criteria for a PD includes an enduring pattern of:
  - Inner experience and behavior that deviates markedly from the expectations of one's culture in ≥2 of the following areas: Cognition, affectivity, interpersonal functioning, or impulse control
  - Inflexibility and pervasiveness across a broad range of personal and social situations
  - Significant distress or impairment in social or occupational functioning

- PDs are classified into 3 major clusters:
  - Cluster A: Eccentricism and oddness:
    - *Paranoid PD*: Unwarranted suspiciousness and distrust of others, defensive, guarded, and overly sensitive
    - *Schizoid PD*: Emotional, cold, or detached; apathetic to criticism or praise; socially isolated
    - *Schizotypal PD*: Eccentric behavior, odd belief system/perceptions, social isolation, and general suspiciousness
  - Cluster B: Dramatic, emotional, or erratic behavioral patterns:
    - *Antisocial PD*: Aggressive, impulsive, irritable, irresponsible, dishonest, deceitful
    - *Borderline PD:* Unstable interpersonal relationships, high impulsivity from early adulthood, intense fear of abandonment, mood swings, poor self-esteem, chronic boredom, and feelings of inner emptiness
    - *Histrionic PD:* Needs to be the center of attention, with self-dramatizing behaviors and attention seeking in a variety of contexts
    - *Narcissistic PD*: Grandiose sense of self-importance and preoccupation with fantasies of success, power, brilliance, beauty, or ideal love; lack of empathy for other people's pain or discomfort
  - Cluster C: Anxiety, excessive worry, fear, and unhealthy patterns of coping with emotions:
    - Avoidant PD: Social inhibition, feelings of inadequacy, hypersensitivity to negative evaluation, avoidance of occupational and interpersonal activities that involve the risk of criticism by others, views self as socially inept and personally unappealing or inferior to others
    - Dependent PD: Excessive need to be taken care of, leading to submissive and clinging behavior with fears of separation, avoids expressing disagreements with others due to fear of losing support and approval, usually seeks out strong and confident people as friends or spouses and feels more secure in such relationships
    - Obsessive–compulsive PD: Preoccupation with cleanliness, orderliness, perfectionism, preoccupation with excessive details, rules, lists, order, organization, and schedules to the extent that the major point of the activity is lost
    - PD not otherwise specified: A mixture of characteristics from other PDs without a predominant pattern compatible with preceding categories; it also can be used for specific PDs not mentioned in the American Psychological Association classification (*DSM-IV-TR*) such as depressive PD, passive-aggressive PD, masochistic PD, dangerous and severe PD (2), etc.

ETIOLOGY
Environmental and genetic factors

COMMONLY ASSOCIATED CONDITIONS
Depression, other psychiatric disorders in patient and family members

 DIAGNOSIS

HISTORY
- Comprehensive interview and mental status examination
- Screen to rule out alcohol and drug abuse.
- Interview of relatives and friends helpful in establishing an enduring pattern of behavior

DIAGNOSTIC TESTS & INTERPRETATION
Psychological testing (e.g., MMPI-II)

Lab
Initial lab tests
- Complete blood count
- Comprehensive metabolic panel
- Thyroid-stimulating hormone
- HIV
- Toxicology screen for substance abuse
- Electroencephalogram to rule out a chronic seizure disorder

Imaging
Initial approach
Computed tomography scan and magnetic resonance imaging of the brain may be necessary in newly developed symptoms to rule out organic brain disease (e.g., frontal lobe tumor).

DIFFERENTIAL DIAGNOSIS
- Medical disorders with behavioral changes
- Other psychiatric disorders with similar symptoms:
  - In obsessive–compulsive disorder (OCD), symptoms are ego-dystonic (i.e., perceived as foreign and unwanted). In addition, OCD has a pattern of relapse and partial remission.
  - In obsessive–compulsive personality disorder (OCPD), symptoms are perceived as desirable behaviors (ego-syntonic) that the patient feels proud of and wants others to emulate. In addition, OCPD has a lifelong pattern (i.e., without significant relapse or remission).

 TREATMENT

MEDICATION
First Line
- So far, no specific drugs are indicated to treat PDs; however, specific medications can reduce the intensity, frequency, and dysfunctionality of certain behaviors, thoughts, and feelings.
- Symptom management (3):
  - Minipsychosis (associated with paranoid, schizoid, and schizotypal PDs): Atypical antipsychotics: Risperidone (Risperdal), quetiapine (Seroquel), olanzapine (Zyprexa), ziprasidone (Geodon), aripiprazole (Abilify), asenapine (Saphris); start with a low dose, gradually adjusting to the patient's needs.
  - Anxiety: Anxiolytics (benzodiazepines, buspirone (BuSpar), and selective serotonin reuptake inhibitors)
  - Depressed mood: Antidepressants
  - Many patients with borderline PD respond well to small doses of atypical neuroleptics and mood stabilizers.
- Precautions: Some atypical neuroleptic drugs may be associated with hyperglycemia and insulin-resistant metabolic syndrome.

Second Line
Mood stabilizers: Lithium carbonate, lamotrigine (Lamictal), carbamazepine (Tegretol, Equetro), and valproate (Depacon, Depakene, Depakote) (4)

ADDITIONAL TREATMENT
General Measures
- Long-term psychotherapy and cognitive behavior therapy (5)
- Group therapy is helpful in the use of therapeutic confrontation and increasing one's awareness of and insight regarding the damaging effects of dysfunctional behavior patterns.

Issues for Referral
- When psychiatric comorbidity of Axis I disorders is present (e.g., mood disorders, anxiety disorders, substance abuse, etc.)
- Suicidal ideation or attempts

Additional Therapies
- Dialectical behavior therapy
- Psychoanalytic therapy
- Interactive psychotherapy
- Group therapy

IN-PATIENT CONSIDERATIONS
Admission Criteria
Disorders with complications of suicide attempts

 ## ONGOING CARE

FOLLOW-UP RECOMMENDATIONS
Continue outpatient treatment, potentially long term.

Patient Monitoring
- Regular physical exercise, e.g., 30–45 minutes a day, helps with stress and the ADLs.
- If substance abuse is suspected, check drug screens.
- Infrequent sessions with relatives or friends are helpful in monitoring progress and behavioral changes.

DIET
Emphasize variety of healthy foods; avoid obesity.

PATIENT EDUCATION
- Bibliotherapy and writing therapy, specific assignments, and watching certain movies to better understand the nature and origin of one's specific condition are helpful:
  – *The Essential Family Guide to Borderline Personality Disorder* by R. Kreger, 2008. Hazelden, Center City, MN
  – *Stop Walking on Eggshells* by PT Mason & R Kreger, 2010. New Harbinger Publ. Oakland, CA
- The movie *As Good As It Gets* illustrates someone with obsessive–compulsive behaviors and its impact on ADLs and relationships with family and friends.
- The movie series *The Godfather* includes several characters with antisocial PD and shows how this affects their interpersonal relationships and their own physical and mental health.
- The movie *What About Bob?* illustrates the challenges involved in treating certain patients with a borderline PD, especially in the management of boundaries in the doctor–patient relationship.
- The movie *A Streetcar Named Desire* illustrates an example of a woman with a histrionic PD.
- The movie *Wall Street* illustrates an example of a person with a narcissistic PD.

- The movie *The Caine Mutiny* illustrates an example of a person with a paranoid PD.
- The movie *Four Weddings and a Funeral* illustrates an example of a person with an avoidant PD.

PROGNOSIS
PDs are enduring patterns of behavior throughout one's lifetime and are not easily responsive to treatment.

COMPLICATIONS
- Disruptive family life with frequent divorces and separations, alcoholism, substance abuse, and drug addiction
- Disruptive behaviors in the workplace may cause absenteeism, loss of productivity, and loss of self-support
- Violation of the law and disregard for the concerns and rights of others

REFERENCES
1. American Psychiatric Association. *Diagnostic and Statistical Manual of Mental Disorders: Text Revision*. 4th ed. Washington, DC: American Psychiatric Press; 2000.
2. Ullrich S, et al. Dangerous and severe personality disorder: An investigation of the construct. *Int J Law Psychiatry*. 2010;33:84–88.
3. Howland RH. Pharmacotherapy in personality disorders. *Psychosoc Nurs Ment Health Serv*. 2007;45:15–19.
4. Díaz-Marsá M, González Bardanca S, Tajima K, et al. Psychopharmacological treatment in borderline personality disorder. *Actas Esp Psiquiatr*. 2008;36: 39–49.
5. Morana HC, Câmara FP. International guidelines for the management of personality disorders. *Curr Opin Psychiatry*. 2006;19:539–43.

ADDITIONAL READING
- Abbass A, Sheldon A, Gyra J, et al. Intensive short-term dynamic psychotherapy for DSM-IV personality disorders: a randomized controlled trial. *J Nerv Ment Dis*. 2008;196:211–6.
- De Clercq B et al. Integrating a developmental perspective in dimensional models of personality disorders. *Clin Psychol Rev*. 2009;29:154–62.
- Dell'osso B, et al. Neuropsychobiological Aspects, Comorbidity Patterns and Dimensional Models in Borderline Personality Disorder. *Neuropsychology*. 2010;61:169–179.
- Eizirik M, Fonagy P. Mentalization-based treatment for patients with borderline personality disorder: An overview. *Rev Bras Psiquiatr*. 2009;31:72–75.
- Ingenhoven T, et al. Effectiveness of pharmacotherapy for severe personality disorders: Meta-analyses of randomized controlled trials. *J Clin Psychiatry*. 2010;71:14–25.
- Kendall T et al. Borderline and antisocial personality disorders: summary of NICE guidelines. *BMJ*. 2009;338:b93.
- Lynch TR, Cheavens JS. Dialectical behavior therapy for comorbid personality disorders. *J Clin Psychol*. 2008;64:154–67.

- Molina JD, et al. Borderline personality disorder: A review and reformulation from evolutionary theory. *Med Hypotheses*. 2009;73:382–386.
- Pincus AI, Lukowitsky MR. Pathological narcissism and narcissistic personality disorder. *Annu Rev Clin Psychol*. 2010;27:421–446.
- Reich J. Avoidant personality disorder and its relationship to social phobia. *Curr Psychiatry Rep*. 2009;11:89–93.
- Russ E, et al. Refining the construct of narcissistic personality disorder: diagnostic criteria and subtypes. *Am J Psychiatry*. 2008;165:1473–81.
- Siever LJ, Weinstein LN. The neurobiology of personality disorders: Implications for psychoanalysis. *J Am Psychoanal Assoc*. 2009;57: 361–398.
- Stanley B, Siever LJ. The interpersonal dimension of borderline personality disorder: toward a neuropeptide model. *Am J Psychiatry*. 2010;167: 24–39.
- Zanarini MC. Psychotherapy of borderline personality disorder. *Acta Psychiatr Scand*. 2009;120:373–377.

See Also (Topic, Algorithm, Electronic Media Element)
Obsessive-Compulsive Disorder

 ## CODES

ICD9
- 301.0 Paranoid personality disorder
- 301.9 Unspecified personality disorder
- 301.20 Schizoid personality disorder, unspecified

CLINICAL PEARLS
- PDs are enduring patterns of behavior throughout one's lifetime and are not easily responsive to treatment.
- No specific drugs treat PDs; however, specific medications can reduce the intensity, frequency, and dysfunctionality of certain behaviors, thoughts, and feelings.
- Most patients with a PD require a well-trained and experienced mental health professional.
- A stable, trustful alliance with the patient is the foundation for any therapeutic progress.

PERTUSSIS

Mary Cataletto, MD

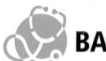

BASICS

Highly contagious bacterial infection

DESCRIPTION
- Exclusively human pathogen
- Seen worldwide
- Endemic in US with epidemic cycles
- High secondary attack rate in households
- Transmission: Respiratory droplets
- Synonym(s): Whooping cough

EPIDEMIOLOGY
Incidence
- Probably underreported; current estimates of true incidence 1–3 million cases/year; however, in 2004, approximately 25,000 were reported
- Recognition of adolescents and adults as sources of pertussis infection in infants

Prevalence
- 25,827 cases reported in US in 2004.
- In 2004, more cases of pertussis occurred in adolescents and adults than in children.

RISK FACTORS
- Exposure to a confirmed case: Infects 80–90% of susceptible contacts
- Non- or underimmunized children
- Pregnancy
- Premature birth
- Age <4 months; these infants have the highest morbidity rate, complication rate, rate of hospitalization, and mortality rate.
- Smokers
- Patients with asthma
- Immunodeficiency (e.g., AIDS)

GENERAL PREVENTION
Immunization:
- Universal immunization with pertussis vaccine is recommended for children <7 years of age and those between 11 and 18 years of age and into adulthood (Tdap). See Red Book for immunization schedule and recommendations.
- BOOSTRIX is licensed for use in persons aged 10–18 years; ADACEL, for persons 11–64 years.

Geriatric Considerations
Currently, there is no vaccine for those >64 years of age.

Pregnancy Considerations
- Recommendations for vaccination during pregnancy can be reviewed in a 2008 MMWR report: Tdap may be administered to a pregnant woman after an informed discussion. However, current practice is to administer Tdap to appropriate candidates in the immediate postpartum period.
- Early case reporting
- Early treatment with strong suspicion or confirmation: Quarantine (students and school staff members):
  – Keep out of school until they have completed 5 days of the recommended course of antibiotics.
  – Persons who do not receive antibiotic therapy should be excluded from school for 21 days after onset of symptoms.

- See Red Book for recommendations for child care and hospital-based exposures, older children and adults. Protection of contacts:
  – Chemoprophylax close contacts, including all household contacts and other close contacts such as young infants and pregnant women.
  – Observe all close contacts for symptoms for 21 days after exposure.
  – Evaluate symptomatic patients, and treat for pertussis when appropriate.
  – Initiate or continue scheduled immunization of all close unimmunized or underimmunized contacts <7 years of age.

PATHOPHYSIOLOGY
- Toxin-mediated
- Infectious process with predilection for ciliated respiratory epithelium

ETIOLOGY
- *Bordetella pertussis* (responsible for ~95% cases)
- *B. parapertussis*

COMMONLY ASSOCIATED CONDITIONS
- Sinusitis and otitis
- Urinary incontinence
- Apnea in young infants
- Seizures

DIAGNOSIS

HISTORY
- Incubation period: 5–21 days
- Classic symptoms, more common in adolescent and adult cases, include paroxysmal cough, posttussive whoop, and/or vomiting.
- Infants with pertussis may present with apnea or sudden death.

PHYSICAL EXAM
3 stages have been described:
- Catarrhal stage: Rhinorrhea, mild cough, low-grade fever
- Paroxysmal stage: Cough becomes paroxysmal, worsening in both frequency and severity. Posttussive whoop and vomiting may occur.
- Convalescent stage: Lasts 1–2 weeks with decreasing severity and frequency of coughing paroxysms
- In the absence of paroxysm or complications, patient may have an essentially normal physical exam.

DIAGNOSTIC TESTS & INTERPRETATION
Lab
Initial lab tests
- If within 3 weeks of onset of cough, send nasopharyngeal aspirate for both polymerase chain reaction (PCR) and culture:
  – PCR results will come back sooner. Culture remains the gold standard.
  – Transport specimen to laboratory immediately:
    ○ Isolation of *B. pertussis* by PCR: Detection of paired genomic sequences by PCR is likely more sensitive. Sensitivity and specificity may vary from lab to lab. Lacks sensitivity in previously immunized individual. When sending nasopharyngeal specimen for detection by PCR, Dacron swabs are preferred, and calcium alginate swabs should *not* be used (because of inhibitory factors in the fibers).

    ○ Isolation of *B. pertussis* by culture (gold standard): Culture is highly specific but with variable sensitivity that may be related to techniques of swabbing and culture. When sending nasopharyngeal specimen for culture of *B. pertussis*, calcium alginate swabs are preferred. Dacron swabs are acceptable.
- If >2 weeks from onset of symptoms, consider serum pertussis toxin IgG.

Follow-Up & Special Considerations
Antipertussis toxin IgG: In adolescents and adults, high titer has good predictive value for current infection (sensitivity 76%, specificity 99% for acute pertussis).

Imaging
Initial approach
CXR may be normal or show signs of hyperinflation with increased anteroposterior diameter and flattened diaphragm, focal atelectasis, and peribronchial cuffing. Pneumonia also may be present.

Follow-Up & Special Considerations
Follow-up CXRs as clinically indicated.

Pathological Findings
- Focal emphysema
- Mucopurulent exudate
- Patchy ulceration of respiratory epithelium

DIFFERENTIAL DIAGNOSIS
- Includes wide range of respiratory viruses, including *B. parapertussis* and respiratory syncytial virus
- Other infectious causes of prolonged cough include *M. pneumoniae. C. trachomatis, C. pneumoniae, B. bronchiseptica*, and adenovirus.
- Sinusitis
- Airway foreign body

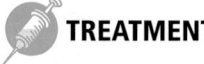

TREATMENT

MEDICATION
First Line
A 2007 Cochrane Review suggests that antibiotic treatment for pertussis is effective in eliminating *B. pertussis* from patients with the disease, thus rendering them noninfectious. However, it has not been found to alter the clinical course. A number of effective regimens have been reported:

- Antibiotic dosing for children ≥6 months of age:
  – Azithromycin 10 mg/kg as a single dose once on day 1 (maximum 500 mg); then 5 mg/kg/d as a single dose on days 2–5 (maximum 250 mg)
  – Clarithromycin 15 mg/kg/d in 2 divided doses × 7 days (maximum 1 g/d)
  – Erythromycin 40–50 mg/kg/d in 4 divided doses × 14 days (maximum 2 g/d):
    ○ Refer to AAP REDBOOK and consider infectious disease consultation in infants <1 month of age.
    ○ Special precautions in neonates: Hypertrophic pyloric stenosis has been reported with oral use of erythromycin in neonates.
    ○ Azithromycin and clarithromycin are not Food and Drug Administration (FDA)–approved for use in infants <6 months of age.
- Antibiotic dosing for adolescents and adults:
  – Azithromycin 500 mg as a single dose on day 1, then 250 mg/d on days 2–5
  – Clarithromycin 1 g/d in 2 divided doses for 7 days

- Contraindications: Allergy to macrolides. Refer to manufacturer's literature for each drug.
- Antibiotics during the catarrhal stage may ameliorate symptoms but afterward are recommended only to limit disease spread.

Pediatric Considerations
See Red Book and consider pediatric infectious disease consultation for children <6 months of age.

Second Line
Trimethoprim-sulfamethoxazole (TMP-SMX) is an alternative for patients with macrolide-resistant strains or who cannot tolerate macrolides. TMP-SMX is contraindicated in infants <2 months of age.

ADDITIONAL TREATMENT
General Measures
- Chemoprophylaxis for all household and close contacts
- Hospitalization for severely ill, very young, or high-risk infants; outpatient management for less ill patients
- Skilled nursing care with careful respiratory monitoring
- Avoid excessive stimulation of infants that may trigger paroxysms.
- Supplemental oxygen to prevent hypoxia
- Standard and respiratory droplet precautions
- Mechanical ventilation when necessary
- Supportive treatment:
  – Ensure adequate hydration and nutrition.
  – Clinical monitoring

Issues for Referral
- Infants <1 month: Pulmonology and/or ICU consult for patients hospitalized with respiratory distress or pneumonia
- Children <6 months: Consider pediatric infectious disease consultation.
- Apnea or seizures at the time of illness may be associated with subsequent impairment. Consultation with a pediatric neurologist or neurodevelopmental pediatrician may be indicated.

Additional Therapies
Controlled prospective data on the use of short-acting β-agonists and corticosteroids were not found.

IN-PATIENT CONSIDERATIONS
Initial Stabilization
- Small, frequent meals may be necessary to ensure adequate nutrition.
- Correct fluid and electrolyte abnormalities.
- Infants may require IV fluids.

Admission Criteria
- Consider for infants <6 months of age, especially preterms and unimmunized or underimmunized infants
- Patients with underlying diseases, especially neuromuscular disorders
- Infants with apnea, hypoxia, feeding difficulty
- Any patient with serious complications
- For supportive care or accelerating symptoms: Intensive care facilities may be required.

IV Fluids
Indicated for dehydration and when oral fluids are either contraindicated or poorly tolerated

Nursing
- Isolation of hospitalized patients with respiratory precautions for 5 days after the initiation of effective antibiotic treatment; for 3 weeks after onset of paroxysms in older patients if antibiotics are not used
- Gentle suctioning of nasal secretions
- Avoid stimuli that trigger paroxysms.
- Educate family about importance of vaccination.
- Discuss chemoprophylaxis for appropriate contacts and family members.

Discharge Criteria
- Clinically stable
- Able to tolerate oral feed

ONGOING CARE

FOLLOW-UP RECOMMENDATIONS
- Infants <1 month of age who receive treatment with a macrolide antibiotic should be monitored for 1 month for idiopathic hypertrophic pyloric stenosis.
- Neurologic and/or pulmonary follow-up as necessary

Patient Monitoring
- ICU may be necessary for severely ill infants.
- Older children and adults with mild cases and no additional risk factors do not require hospital admission.

DIET
IV therapy is indicated with dehydration and/or when oral fluids are either not indicated or poorly tolerated.

PATIENT EDUCATION
- American Academy of Pediatrics: http://www.aap.org
- CDC: http://www.cdc.gov

PROGNOSIS
- Complete recovery in most cases
- Most severe morbidity and highest mortality in infants <4 months of age

COMPLICATIONS
- Highest and most severe in infants
- More frequent in adults than adolescents:
  – Sinusitis
  – Otitis media
  – Pneumonia
  – Weight loss
  – Fainting
  – Rib fracture
  – Urinary incontinence
  – Seizures
  – Encephalopathy
  – Death

ADDITIONAL READING

- Altunaiji SM, Kukuruzovic RH, Curtis NC, et al. Antibiotics for Whooping Cough (Pertussis) *Cochrane Database of Systemic Reviews*. 2007, Issue 3. Art No.: CD004404.
- America Academy of Pediatrics Committee on Infectious Diseases. Prevention of pertussis among adolescents: recommendations for use of tetanus toxoid, reduced diphtheria toxoid, and acellular pertussis (Tdap) vaccine. *Pediatrics*. 2006;117:965–78.
- American Academy of Pediatrics. Pertussis. In: Pickering L, et al., eds. *Red Book 2009 Report of the Committee on Infectious Diseases*, 28th ed. Elk Grove, IL: American Academy of Pediatrics; 2009:504–520.
- Center for Disease Control and Prevention. Recommended adult immunization schedule - United States 2009. *MMWR*. 2008;57(53).
- Centers for Disease Control and Prevention (CDC). Pertussis–United States, 2001–2003. *MMWR Morb Mortal Wkly Rep.* 2005;54:1283–6.
- Crowcroft NS, Pebody RG. Recent developments in pertussis. *Lancet.* 2006;367:1926–36.
- Gerbie M, Tan T. Pertussis Disease in New Mothers: Effect on Young Infants and Stragies for Prevention. *Obstet Gynecol.* 2009;113:399–401.
- Mattoo S, Cherry JD. Molecular pathogenesis, epidemiology, and clinical manifestations of respiratory infections due to Bordetella pertussis and other Bordetella subspecies. *Clin Microbiol Rev.* 2005;18:326–82.
- Murphy, TV et al. Prevetntion of Pertussis, Tetanus and Diptheria Among Pregnant and Postpartum Women and their infants. *MMWR Recommendations and Reports.* 2008;57(04):1–47, 51
- National Immunization Program, CDC. Recommended Antimicrobial Agents for the Treatment and Postexposure Prophylaxis of Pertussis 2005 CDC Guidelines. *MMWR.* 2005;1–15.
- Pichichero M. Pertussis. In: Rakel R, Bope E. *Conn's Current Therapy* 2008, Saunders Elsevier, 2008:147–9.

CODES

ICD9
- 033.0 Whooping cough due to bordetella pertussis (b. pertussis)
- 033.9 Whooping cough, unspecified organism

CLINICAL PEARLS

- The physical exam in pertussis may be normal in the absence of paroxysms and clinical complications.
- When sending nasopharyngeal specimen for culture of *B. pertussis,* calcium alginate swabs are preferred. Dacron swabs are acceptable.
- When sending nasopharyngeal specimen for detection by PCR, Dacron swabs are preferred, and calcium alginate swabs should *not* be used (because of inhibitory factors in the fibers).
- Macrolides are 1st-line antibiotics.
- Prevention of transmission via immunization, isolation, and chemoprophylaxis is key.

PHEOCHROMOCYTOMA

Mark C. Horattas, MD
Jill N. Zink, MD

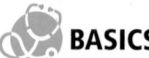 **BASICS**

DESCRIPTION
- Catecholamine-producing tumor. In 90% of cases, the tumors are found in the adrenal medulla, but they may also be found in other tissues derived from the neural crest cells.
- Systems affected: Endocrine/Metabolic; Cardiovascular (secondary effects from catecholamines)

EPIDEMIOLOGY
Incidence
<1% of people with severe hypertension (HTN)
Prevalence
- 1–2 per 100,000 adults
- No gender or race predilection
- Can affect all ages
- Sporadic tumors usually diagnosed in 3rd–5th decades, familial disease 1 decade earlier

RISK FACTORS
- Familial pheochromocytoma
- Multiple endocrine neoplasia types IIA and IIB
- Neurofibromatosis type 1
- Von Hippel-Lindau syndrome
- Familial paraganglioma

Genetics
80–90% of cases are sporadic, 10% familial

PATHOPHYSIOLOGY
- Pheochromocytomas are tumors that release catecholamines (i.e., norepinephrine and epinephrine) into the bloodstream. These substances interact with the alpha and beta adrenergic receptors. Alpha-1 receptors cause arteriolar constriction, raising blood pressure. Alpha-2 receptors decrease insulin secretion, resulting in elevated glucose levels. Beta-1 receptors increase the cardiac rate (tachycardia). Beta-2 receptors cause arteriolar and venous dilation and relaxation of tracheobronchial smooth muscle.
- Homovanillic acid (HVA) + vanillylmandelic acid (VMA) are catecholamine breakdown products, and the amount of these substances detected in the urine correlates with the size of the pheochromocytoma tumor.

ETIOLOGY
Catecholamine-producing tumor: Rule of 10:
- 10% are extra-adrenal (organ of Zuckerkandl, neck, mediastinum, abdomen, pelvis).
- 10% are multiple or bilateral.
- 10% are malignant.
- 10% recur after surgical removal.
- 10% occur in children.
- 10% or more are familial.
- 10% present as adrenal incidentalomas.

COMMONLY ASSOCIATED CONDITIONS
- Multiple endocrine neoplasia type IIA (medullary thyroid carcinoma and primary hyperparathyroidism)
- Multiple endocrine neoplasia type IIB (medullary thyroid carcinoma and mucosal neuromas)
- Von-Hippel-Lindau disease (retinal angiomas, cerebellar hemangioblastomas, renal cysts, carcinomas, pancreatic cysts, epididymal cystadenomas)
- Neurofibromatosis type 1
- Sturge-Weber syndrome
- Tuberous sclerosis
- Carney syndrome (gastric epithelioid leiomyosarcoma, pulmonary chondroma, extra-adrenal paraganglioma)
- Familial paraganglioma
- Ataxia-telangiectasia
- Renal artery stenosis

 DIAGNOSIS

HISTORY
- "Classic triad" of symptoms includes headache, palpitations, and diaphoresis.
- Paroxysmal spells (5 Ps mnemonic):
  - Pressure: Sudden increase in blood pressure
  - Pain: Headache, chest, abdominal pain
  - Perspiration
  - Palpitation
  - Pallor
- Additional symptoms:
  - Constipation
  - Tremor
  - Weight loss
  - Anxiety
  - Paresthesias
  - Flushing
  - Shortness of breath
  - Nausea/vomiting

Pediatric Considerations
Profuse sweating common in children

PHYSICAL EXAM
- Hypertension (HTN): Paroxysmal in 1/2 of affected patients; most common clinical sign
- Tachyarrhythmias
- Orthostatic hypotension
- Café au lait spots
- Lisch nodules of the eye
- Grade II–IV retinopathy
- Transient ischemic attacks/stroke
- Cardiomyopathy
- Gastrointestinal crisis
- Diabetes mellitus or insipidus
- Fever
- Hypercalcemia
- Erythrocytosis

ALERT
Sudden death may occur in patients with an undiagnosed tumor who undergo surgery or biopsy.

DIAGNOSTIC TESTS & INTERPRETATION
Lab
Initial lab tests
- Elevated 24-hour urine or plasma metanephrine
- Elevated 24-hour urine or plasma catecholamines:
  - Blood pressure (BP) must be recorded during plasma sampling for catecholamines. Pheochromocytoma cannot be excluded if normal catecholamine values are obtained when the patient is normotensive and asymptomatic (1)[A].
- Elevated 24-hour urine VMA
- Plasma catecholamines and metanephrines must be measured when patient is at rest (1)[A].

Follow-Up & Special Considerations
- Drugs that may alter lab results:
  - Increased by:
    - Phenoxybenzamine
    - Tricyclic antidepressants
    - Labetalol
    - Methyldopa
    - Monoamine oxidase inhibitors (MAOIs)
    - Amphetamines
    - Cocaine
    - Clonidine or other drug withdrawal
    - Ethanol or ethanol withdrawal
    - Sotalol
    - Levodopa
    - Acetaminophen
  - Decreased by:
    - Central α_2-agonists
    - Reserpine
- Disorders that may alter lab results: Major physical stress (e.g., surgery, stroke, myocardial infarction, congestive heart failure)

Imaging
Initial approach
- Abdominal image: Magnetic resonance imaging is preferable to computed tomography (CT).
- I-metaiodobenzylguanidine (MIBG) scan
- Pentetreotide scan

ALERT
When using CT, avoid contrast or protect with adrenergic blockade to avoid precipitating a hypertensive crisis.

Diagnostic Procedures/Surgery
Clonidine-suppression test distinguishes between pheochromocytoma and essential HTN when urine and plasma tests are equivocal.

Pathological Findings
A catecholamine-producing tumor in the adrenal medulla, para-aortic sympathetic chain, wall of the urinary bladder, or sympathetic chain in the neck or mediastinum

DIFFERENTIAL DIAGNOSIS
- Labile essential hypertension
- Anxiety and panic attacks
- Paroxysmal cardiac arrhythmia
- Thyrotoxicosis

- Menopausal syndrome
- Hypoglycemia
- Mastocytosis
- Withdrawal of adrenergic-inhibiting medications
- Angina
- Hyperventilation
- Migraine headache
- Amphetamine or cocaine use
- Sympathomimetic ingestion

 TREATMENT

MEDICATION
First Line
- α-adrenergic and possibly β-adrenergic blockade required preoperatively.
- Initiate α-blockade first: Phenoxybenzamine (Dibenzyline) 10 mg p.o. b.i.d. and increased by 10–20 mg every 2 days as needed to control BP and paroxysmal spells (average dose is 0.5–1.0 mg/kg/d, max dose is 300–400 mg/d).
- β-blockade can follow α-blockade: Propranolol (Inderal) 10 mg q6h initially and increase as necessary to control tachycardia
- Treat acute hypertensive crisis with IV phentolamine (Regitine) or nitroprusside.
- Contraindications:
  - β-adrenergic blockade in patients with asthma, sinus bradycardia, and > 1st degree block or congestive heart failure (CHF)
  - Avoid β-blockers with intrinsic sympathomimetic activity.
- Precautions:
  - β-adrenergic blockade alone may result in more severe HTN owing to the unopposed α-adrenergic stimulation; patients should be cautioned about postural hypotension.
  - β-adrenergic blockade is initiated at low doses using a short-acting agent owing to the possible side effect of pulmonary edema in the patient with catecholamine myocardiopathy.
- Significant possible interactions: For β-adrenergic blockade: Verapamil, phenytoin, phenobarbitone, rifampin, chlorpromazine, and cimetidine

Second Line
- α-adrenergic blocking agents: Prazosin (Minipress) 1–2 mg t.i.d., terazosin (Hytrin), doxazosin (Cardura)
- β-adrenergic blocking agents: Nadolol (Corgard), atenolol (Tenormin), metoprolol (Lopressor)
- Combined β- and α-adrenergic blocker: Labetalol (Normodyne, Trandate)
- Catecholamine synthesis inhibitor: Metyrosine (Demser) (2)[A]

ADDITIONAL TREATMENT
General Measures
Control BP and volume repletion.

Issues for Referral
Endocrinology for definitive diagnosis and management recommendations

Additional Therapies
No generally effective systemic treatment with antineoplastic potential for malignant pheochromocytoma has been found. A proportion of patients do respond to MIBG radiotherapy or to cytotoxic chemotherapy with cyclophosphamide, vincristine, and dacarbazine (CVD) (3)[A].

SURGERY/OTHER PROCEDURES
- High-risk surgical procedure requires an experienced surgeon, anesthetist, and clinical team. It is often amenable to laparoscopic adrenalectomy:
  - The goal of surgery is to resect the tumor completely with minimal tumor manipulation or rupture of the tumor capsule.
- Cortical-sparing subtotal adrenalectomy may preserve adrenocortical function in those with bilateral disease.

IN-PATIENT CONSIDERATIONS
Initial Stabilization
Control of HTN and replace volume

Admission Criteria
Severe or refractory HTN

IV Fluids
As needed to replace volume

Nursing
Monitor BP closely.

Discharge Criteria
When hemodynamically stable

 ONGOING CARE

FOLLOW-UP RECOMMENDATIONS
- Follow BP.
- Post-op monitoring of catecholamines and metanephrines

Patient Monitoring
- Monitor BP daily before surgery.
- Intraoperative hemodynamic monitoring
- Test plasma-free metanephrines or urine catecholamine and metanephrines 2 weeks postoperatively. If normal, the resection is deemed complete. Recheck annually.
- Assure resolution of HTN.

DIET
Preoperatively, follow a high-salt diet to increase blood volume.

PATIENT EDUCATION
Patient educational materials from National Adrenal Disease Foundation (NADF), 505 Northern Blvd., Great Neck, NY 11021; 516-487-4229; e-mail: nadfmail@aol.com

PROGNOSIS
- The survival rate after removal of a benign pheochromocytoma is nearly that of controls when matched for age and gender.
- For malignant pheochromocytoma, the 5-year survival rate is <50%.

COMPLICATIONS
- When diagnosed at autopsy, 75% of patients died from myocardial infarction (MI) or cerebrovascular accident (CVA).
- 1/3 of sudden deaths occurred after unrelated minor operative procedures.
- Postural hypotension with α-adrenergic blockade
- Pulmonary edema with β-adrenergic blockade
- Intraoperative hypertensive crisis

Pregnancy Considerations
- Pheochromocytomas occurring during pregnancy carry a grave prognosis. The maternal and fetal mortality rates are 48% and 55%, respectively.
- Spontaneous abortion is very likely.

REFERENCES
1. Karagiannis A, Mikhailidis DP, Athyros VG, et al. Pheochromocytoma: an update on genetics and management. *Endocr Relat Cancer*. 2007;14: 935–56.
2. Federman DD. The adrenal medulla. pheochromocytoma. Update 2. *Sci Am Med*. 2000;1:15.
3. Scholz T, Eisenhofer G, Pacak K, et al. Clinical review: Current treatment of malignant pheochromocytoma. *J Clin Endocrinol Metab*. 2007;92:1217–25.

See Also (Topic, Algorithm, Electronic Media Element)
Hypertension, Essential; Multiple Endocrine Neoplasia (MEN)

 CODES

ICD9
- 194.0 Malignant neoplasm of adrenal gland
- 227.0 Benign neoplasm of adrenal gland

CLINICAL PEARLS
- Patients usually demonstrate severe and often episodic HTN as well as headache, palpitations, and diaphoresis.
- Must give α-adrenergic agent to control BP, followed by a β-adrenergic agent to control tachycardia and prevent a hypertensive crisis
- 10% rule: 10% are extra-adrenal, multiple or bilateral, malignant, recur after surgical removal, occur in children, are familial, present as adrenal incidentalomas
- Consider as an etiology for severe, difficult-to-treat hypertensive patients (<1% incidence).
- Profuse sweating common in children

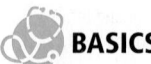

PHIMOSIS AND PARAPHIMOSIS

James P. Miller, MD

BASICS

DESCRIPTION
- Phimosis: Tightness of the penile foreskin that prevents it from being drawn back from over the glans
- Paraphimosis: Constriction of glans penis by proximally placed phimotic foreskin
- System(s) affected: Renal/Urologic; Reproductive; Skin/Exocrine

Geriatric Considerations
Recurrent infection and irritations (condom catheters) can lead to phimosis.

Pediatric Considerations
- Recurrent balanitis, either chemical or infectious, can lead to an acquired phimosis.
- Forced reduction of a physiologic foreskin can lead to chronic scarring and acquired phimosis.

EPIDEMIOLOGY
- Predominant age: Infancy and adolescence, unusual in adults, and risk returns in geriatrics
- Predominant sex: Male only

Prevalence
In the US: 1% of males >16 years of age

RISK FACTORS
- Phimosis:
  - Poor hygiene
  - Diabetes
  - Frequent diaper rash in infant
- Paraphimosis:
  - Presence of foreskin
  - Inexperienced health care provider (leaving foreskin retracted after catheter placement)

GENERAL PREVENTION
- Good patient and parental education
- If the patient is uncircumcised, appropriate hygiene and care of the foreskin are necessary to prevent phimosis and paraphimosis.

ETIOLOGY
- Phimosis:
  - Physiologic: Present at birth and resolves spontaneously during the 1st 2–3 years of life through nocturnal erections, which slowly dilate the phimotic ring
  - Congenital: Unresolved physiologic phimosis
  - Acquired: Recurrent infection, irritation, or trauma from forced reduction of infants "physiologic" phimosis
- Paraphimosis:
  - Foreskin not pulled back over the glans after cleaning, cystoscopy, or catheter insertion

DIAGNOSIS

HISTORY
- Phimosis:
  - Painful erections
  - Recurrent balanitis
  - Foreskin balloons with voiding
- Paraphimosis:
  - Uncircumcised by history
  - Pain
  - Drainage

PHYSICAL EXAM
- Phimosis:
  - Foreskin cannot retract.
  - Secondary balanitis
- Paraphimosis:
  - Edema
  - Drainage
  - Ulceration

DIFFERENTIAL DIAGNOSIS
- Penile lymphedema, which can be related to insect bites, trauma, or allergic reactions
- Penile tourniquet syndrome: Foreign body around penis, most commonly a hair

TREATMENT

MEDICATION
Topical 0.05% betamethasone b.i.d. for 1 month to soften phimosis

ADDITIONAL TREATMENT
General Measures
- Phimosis:
  - 0.05% betamethasone b.i.d. with gradual traction placed on foreskin. Over 4–6 weeks, the phimotic ring should open (1)[C].

- Paraphimosis:
  - Manual reduction if possible (should be done with the patient sedated). Place the middle and index fingers of both hands on the engorged skin proximal to the glans. Place both thumbs on glans, and with gentle pressure, push on the glans and pull on the foreskin to attempt reduction. If unsuccessful, a dorsal slit will be necessary with eventual circumcision after the edema resolves.
  - Osmotic agents: Granulated sugar placed on edematous tissue for several hours to reduce edema (2)[C]
  - Puncture technique: Multiple punctures of foreskin with a 21-gauge needle will allow edematous fluid to escape and thus allow reduction (3)[C].
- Appropriate health care: Outpatient except for complications
- Pain control

Issues for Referral
Consider circumcision for recurrent balanitis and paraphimosis.

SURGERY/OTHER PROCEDURES
- Phimosis: Circumcision
- Paraphimosis:
  - Represents a true surgical emergency to avoid necrosis of glans
  - Dorsal slit with delayed circumcision, if reduction is not possible
  - Operative exploration if the possibility of penile tourniquet syndrome cannot be eliminated. Hair removal cream can be applied if a hair is seen as the etiology of the tourniquet.

IN-PATIENT CONSIDERATIONS
Admission Criteria
Tissue loss with paraphimosis

 ## ONGOING CARE

FOLLOW-UP RECOMMENDATIONS
No sexual activity following circumcision until healing is complete

Patient Monitoring
Monitor for 1 week after the reduction of paraphimosis and for 1–2 weeks after a circumcision.

DIET
No limitations

PATIENT EDUCATION
Appropriate foreskin care should be discussed with parents of child and with the patient once old enough to comprehend to avoid the occurrence of paraphimosis.

PROGNOSIS
Complete resolution if treatment is carried out effectively

COMPLICATIONS
- Unreduced paraphimosis can lead to gangrene of the glans.
- Posthitis (inflammation of the prepuce)

REFERENCES
1. Orsola A, Caffaratti J, Garat JM. Conservative treatment of phimosis in children using a topical steroid. *Urology.* 2000;56:307–10.
2. Cahill D, Rome A. Reduction of paraphimosis with granulated sugar. *BJU Int.* 1999;83:362.
3. Reynard JM, Barua JM. Reduction of paraphimosis the simple way - the Dundee technique. *BJU Int.* 1999;83:859–60.

 ## CODES

ICD9
605 Redundant prepuce and phimosis

CLINICAL PEARLS
- Physiologic phimosis usually will resolve during the 1st few years of life. As the child experiences nocturnal erections, the phimotic ring will dilate, and only then should it be retracted to clean. There is *no* reason to reduce a newborn's foreskin to clean underneath. The forced reduction will only predispose to acquired phimosis.
- No controlled studies compare the various methods of reduction. One should do what one feels most comfortable with.

PHOBIAS

David Dildine, MD

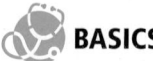

BASICS

DESCRIPTION
- A persistent, excessive, and unreasonable fear of an object, activity, place, or situation. Stimulus is actively avoided or endured with extreme anxiety and dread. Adolescents and adults are usually aware that their reaction is abnormal.
- To qualify as a true disorder, symptoms must cause significant distress, interfere with normal social and vocational functioning, and result in a perceived loss of freedom.
- The American Psychiatric Association (*DSM-IV-TR*) classifies phobias as anxiety disorders and divides them into 3 categories (1):
  - Agoraphobia: Fear and avoidance of situations that may be difficult or embarrassing to escape in the event of panic-like symptoms. May involve fear of crowds, enclosed spaces (e.g., elevators, automobiles, or airplanes), or simply being alone (at home or away from home). Usually secondary to a coexisting panic disorder but may be a primary condition. See topic Panic Disorder.
  - Specific phobia (formerly *simple phobia*):
    - Fear and avoidance of clearly discernible, circumscribed objects or situations. Often divided into animal-type (e.g., snakes, spiders), environmental-type (e.g., storms, height), blood-injection/injury type, or situational-type (e.g., enclosed spaces, planes, crowds).
    - Common specific phobias: Zoophobia (animals), brontophobia (thunderstorms), acrophobia (heights), nosophobia (disease), thanatophobia (death)
    - Blood-injection/injury phobia associated with a strong vasovagal reaction
  - Social phobia (social anxiety disorder): Fear and avoidance of certain social or performance situations where embarrassment or humiliation may occur under scrutiny of others. Individuals may experience marked anticipatory anxiety in advance of upcoming feared events.

Pediatric Considerations
- Anxiety may be expressed by crying, tantrums, freezing, or clinging. Fears of animals and other objects in the natural environment are common and usually transitory in childhood.
- Children are often not aware that their fear is excessive or unreasonable.

EPIDEMIOLOGY
Incidence
- Predominant age: Median age of onset 20 years for agoraphobia, 7 years for specific phobias, and 13 years for social phobia
- Predominant sex: Female > Male

Prevalence
In the general US population, the 12-month and lifetime prevalence (respectively):
- Agoraphobia without panic: 0.8% and 1.4%
- Specific phobia: 8.7% and 12.5%
- Social phobia: 6.8% and 12.1%

RISK FACTORS
- Female sex
- First-degree relatives with the disorder
- Traumatic experience
- In children, observation of others with phobic reactions
- Social phobia is strongly associated with a perceived lack of control over one's own life. Other risk factors include low self-esteem, low education level, emotional neglect, major depression, and significant recent life stressors.

Genetics
There is some evidence of a genetic predisposition to phobias, but specific genes have not been identified.

PATHOPHYSIOLOGY
- Still not fully understood
- When presented with social-threat stimuli, patients with social phobia exhibit a hyperactive neural and behavioral emotional response.
- Research on agoraphobia, when related to panic disorder, has focused on brain areas, including the amygdala, locus ceruleus, and hippocampus, as well as on the neurotransmitters norepinephrine, serotonin, and GABA.

ETIOLOGY
- Evidence suggests a complex interplay among genetic vulnerability, development neurobiology, and environment.
- Vulnerability may lead to persistence or exaggeration of a learned response, perhaps learned initially as a protective mechanism (such as avoidance of large dogs by small children).

COMMONLY ASSOCIATED CONDITIONS
- Other anxiety and mood disorders, as well as abuse of alcohol and other substances
- Most patients with agoraphobia experience panic disorder as well.

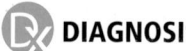

DIAGNOSIS

HISTORY
Major finding is presence of irrational or ego-dystonic fear of a specific situation, activity, or object with associated avoidant behavior.

PHYSICAL EXAM
- Symptoms associated with exposure to phobic stimulus may include signs of sympathetic activation, pallor, dizziness, or paresthesias.
- Mental status exam should be performed.

DIAGNOSTIC TESTS & INTERPRETATION
Lab
Initial lab tests
No diagnostic laboratory tests for phobia

DIFFERENTIAL DIAGNOSIS
- Psychiatric differential diagnosis includes
  - Other anxiety disorders (panic disorder, OCD, GAD, PTSD)
  - Mood disorders (depression)
  - Schizophrenia
  - Schizoid personality disorder
  - Avoidant personality disorder
- Must consider underlying medical causes such as thyroid dysfunction, seizure disorder, pheochromocytoma, hypoglycemia, hyperparathyroidism, cerebrovascular disease, CNS tumors, and substance use (particularly hallucinogens and sympathomimetics).
- Differentiate phobias from appropriate fear and normal shyness. Individuals with social phobia have more symptoms and functional impairment and a lower quality of life.

TREATMENT

Best treatment is an appropriate combination of pharmacotherapy and psychotherapy.

MEDICATION
First Line
- Studies show effectiveness of selective serotonin reuptake inhibitors (SSRIs) for agoraphobia (2)[A] and social phobia (3)[A]:
  - Citalopram (10–60 mg/d), escitalopram (10–20 mg/d), fluoxetine (20–80 mg/d), fluvoxamine (50–300 mg/d), paroxetine (10–60 mg/d), and sertraline (50–200 mg/d)
- Venlafaxine ER (75–225 mg/d divided b.i.d./t.i.d.), a serotonin-norepinephrine reuptake inhibitor (SNRI), has been shown to be as effective and well tolerated as SSRIs for social phobia (4,5)[A].
- Benzodiazepines reduce panic severity; best used in combination with other therapies (2,6)[A]:
  - Also useful in treatment of social phobia (7)[A]
  - Alprazolam (0.5–4 mg/d), lorazepam (2–6 mg/d), clonazepam (0.5–6 mg/d)
  - Use with caution in patients with history of substance abuse. Discontinue gradually because of the risk for withdrawal seizures.
- Buspirone (15–60 mg/d), a serotonin-receptor agonist, also may be used in the treatment of social phobia; can be used to augment SSRIs.
- Treatment with these drugs should continue for 6–12 months before slowly tapering. Can be restarted if symptoms recur (2,8).
- There is no good evidence for the use of medications for specific phobias. A short-acting benzodiazepine may be helpful in treating fear of flying.

Second Line
- β-Blockers decrease sympathetic stimulation. Can be used for performance anxiety.
  - Choices include propranolol 10–80 mg and atenolol 30–100 mg (fewer CNS side effects).
  - Monitor for hypotension and bradycardia.
- TCAs as effective as SSRIs for agoraphobia (though not as well tolerated) (9)[A]:
  - Imipramine (50–300 mg/d), desipramine (75–300 mg/d), nortriptyline (60–150 mg/d), and clomipramine (25–100 mg/d)
  - Anticholinergic and cardiac side effects common. Use with caution.
- Monoamine oxidase inhibitor (MAOI) phenelzine (45–90 mg/d) is effective in the treatment of social phobia but less well tolerated (7)[A]. Do not use with other antidepressants, decongestants, diet pills, meperidine (Demerol), dextromethorphan, levodopa, and sympathomimetics. Avoid tyramine in diet.

ADDITIONAL TREATMENT
General Measures
- Cognitive behavioral therapy (CBT) including exposure, cognitive restructuring, and relaxation techniques have been shown to be effective for social phobia and agoraphobia (10)[A].
- Exposure-based treatment is superior to alternative psychotherapeutic approaches and placebo in the treatment of specific phobias (11)[A].

Issues for Referral
Consider neurology consult if seizures are suspected; medicine consult if an underlying medical cause is suspected.

COMPLEMENTARY AND ALTERNATIVE MEDICINE
- Inositol 12–18 g/d is superior to placebo and similar to SSRIs in reducing intensity and frequency of panic attacks.
- There is no good evidence to support the use of St. John's wort, valerian, Sympathyl, passionflower, or cannabis in the treatment of anxiety disorders (12).

IN-PATIENT CONSIDERATIONS
- Not necessary in most cases
- Monitoring or treatment may be indicated in the setting of acute suicidality or comorbid alcohol and substance abuse.

ONGOING CARE

FOLLOW-UP RECOMMENDATIONS
Patient Monitoring
Outpatient as needed

DIET
- Consider restriction of stimulants, such as caffeine, that can exacerbate anxiety.
- One study showed that a tryptophan-rich diet resulted in significant improvement in symptoms of social phobia (13)[B].
- If taking phenelzine or other MAOIs, a tyramine-free diet must be followed to decrease the risk of hypertensive crisis.

PATIENT EDUCATION
- Many resources are available. Understanding the diagnosis and treatment is important not only for the patient but also for friends and family, who can provide a caring support system.
- Anxiety Disorders Association of America: http://adaa.org
- The Social Phobia/Social Anxiety Association: http://socialphobia.org
- Patient education on understanding social phobia: http://www.aafp.org/afp/991115ap/991115b.html

PROGNOSIS
- Most patients will experience resolution of symptoms with appropriate treatment.
- Even after successful treatment of agoraphobia and social phobia, residual symptoms or relapse may occur.

COMPLICATIONS
- Avoidance behavior may lead to significant impairment in social and vocational life.
- Morbidity is often more severe in agoraphobia and social phobia than in specific phobia.
- Alcohol and substance abuse is common.

REFERENCES
1. American Psychiatric Association. *Diagnostic and statistical manual of mental disorders (DSM-IV-TR)*, 4th ed. Washington, DC: American Psychiatric Association, 2000.
2. Ham P, Waters DB, Oliver MN. Treatment of panic disorder. *Am Fam Physician*. 2005;71:733–9.
3. Stein DJ, Ipser JC, van Balkom AJ. Pharmacotherapy for social anxiety disorder. *Cochrane Database of Systematic Reviews*. 2000, Issue 4. Art. No.: CD001206. DOI:10.1002/14651858.CD001206.pub2.
4. Liebowitz MR, et al. A randomized controlled trial of venlafaxine extended release in generalized social anxiety disorder. *J Clin Psychiatr.* 2005;66(2):238–47.
5. Liebowitz MR, Gelenberg AJ, Munjack D. Venlafaxine extended release vs placebo and paroxetine in social anxiety disorder. *Arch Gen Psychiatry*. 2005;62:190–8.
6. Pollack MH, Allgulander C, Bandelow B, et al. WCA recommendations for the long-term treatment of panic disorder. *CNS Spectr.* 2003;8:17–30.
7. Blanco C, et al. Pharmacological treatment of social anxiety disorder: A meta-analysis. *Depression Anxiety*. 2003;18(1):29–40.
8. Van Ameringen M, Allgulander C, Bandelow B, et al. WCA recommendations for the long-term treatment of social phobia. *CNS Spectr.* 2003;8:40–52.
9. Bakker A, van Balkom AJ, Spinhoven P. SSRIs vs. TCAs in the treatment of panic disorder: a meta-analysis. *Acta Psychiatr Scand*. 2002;106:163–7.
10. Rodebaugh TL, Holaway RM, Heimberg RG. The treatment of social anxiety disorder. *Clin Psychol Rev.* 2004;24:883–908.
11. Wolitzky-Taylor KB, Horowitz JD, Powers MB, et al. Psychological approaches in the treatment of specific phobias: A meta-analysis. *Clin Psychol Rev.* 2008.
12. Saeed SA, Bloch RM, Antonacci DJ. Herbal and dietary supplements for treatment of anxiety disorders. *Am Fam Physician*. 2007;76:549–56.
13. Hudson C, Hudson S, MacKenzie J. Protein-source tryptophan as an efficacious treatment for social anxiety disorder: a pilot study. *Can J Physiol Pharmacol*. 2007;85:928–32.

See Also (Topic, Algorithm, Electronic Media Element)
Anxiety; Depression; Dissociative Disorders; Obsessive-compulsive Disorder; Post-Traumatic Stress Disorder (PTSD); Schizophrenia

CODES

ICD9
- 300.20 Phobia, unspecified
- 300.21 Agoraphobia with panic disorder
- 300.22 Agoraphobia without mention of panic attacks

CLINICAL PEARLS
- Phobias are common, potentially debilitating, but treatable conditions.
- Must rule out more serious psychiatric diagnoses and underlying medical conditions.
- Treatment consists of an appropriate combination of psychotherapy and medication and is usually effective. Relapse and/or symptom persistence is common in social phobia and agraphobia.

Aamir Siddiqi, MD

BASICS

DESCRIPTION
- Light-induced eruptions seen in a pattern of photodistribution:
  - Phototoxic reactions: Result of the acute toxic effect on skin of ultraviolet (UV) light alone (sunburn) or together with a photosensitizing substance (nonallergic)
  - Photoallergic eruptions: A form of allergic dermatitis resulting from combined effects of a photosensitizing substance (drugs or chemical) plus UV light (immunologic/delayed hypersensitivity)
  - Polymorphous light eruption (PLE): Chronic, intermittent light-induced eruption with erythematous papules, urticaria, or vesicles on areas exposed to sunlight
- System(s) affected: Skin/Exocrine
- Synonym(s): Sun poisoning; Sun allergy

EPIDEMIOLOGY
Incidence
- Usually occurs after the 1st intense exposure in the spring or summer
- Predominant age: All ages
- Predominant sex: Male = Female

Prevalence
May be as high as 20% in some areas

RISK FACTORS
- Job-related exposure to sunlight
- Light- and fair-colored skin

Genetics
Predisposition occurs in inbred populations (e.g., Pima Indians)

GENERAL PREVENTION
- Sunlight avoidance/protective clothing
- Identification and avoidance of causative drugs (see Etiology)
- Sunscreens: Apply before exposure:
  - Zinc oxide: Opaque, cosmetically less acceptable
  - Chemical: Use sun-protective factor (SPF) >30 for maximum protection; substantively resistant to sweat and swimming; cosmetically more acceptable (1)[C]
- Avoid direct sun exposure.
- Wear appropriate gear to avoid sunlight exposure.

ETIOLOGY
- Sunlight
- Phenothiazines
- Diuretics
- Tetracyclines, sulfonamides
- Oral contraceptives
- Topicals: Psoralens, coal tars, photoactive dyes (eosin, acridine orange)
- 5-Fluorouracil
- Quinine
- Sunscreens containing *para*-aminobenzoic acid (PABA)
- In the US, ~115 chemical agents used topically are known to cause photodermatitis.

COMMONLY ASSOCIATED CONDITIONS
- Sunlight aggravation of systemic lupus
- Persistent light reactivity
- Actinic reticuloid

DIAGNOSIS

HISTORY
Pruritic and often painful rash developing in sun-exposed areas

PHYSICAL EXAM
- Phototoxic:
  - Erythema
  - With increasing severity: Vesicles and bullae
  - Classic example: Sunburn
  - Nails may exhibit onycholysis.
  - Chronic: Epidermal thickening, elastosis, telangiectasia, and pigmentary changes
  - Sharp lines of demarcation between involved and uninvolved skin (sunlight exposure)
  - Phototoxic eruption due to topicals: Area of application
  - Usually develops shortly after sun exposure
  - Hyperpigmentation may follow resolution.
  - Pain
- Photoallergic (1)[C]:
  - Papules with erythema and occasionally vesicles
  - Area exposed to light with less distinct borders
  - Usually delayed 24 h or more after exposure
  - May spread to unexposed areas
  - Pruritus
- PLE:
  - Erythematous papules
  - Occasionally urticaria or vesicles
  - Scattered over sun-exposed areas with normal skin in between
  - Can spread to nonexposed areas
  - Often flares in spring or early summer
  - Desensitization affect (less over the course of the summer)
  - Burning or pruritus may precede lesions.

DIAGNOSTIC TESTS & INTERPRETATION
Lab
- Antinuclear antibody to rule out systemic lupus erythematosus if suspected
- Photo testing: Exposing patient to UV light
- Photopatch testing: Applying suspected agents and chemicals to patient's skin
- Skin biopsy: To rule out other disorders if necessary

DIFFERENTIAL DIAGNOSIS
Systemic lupus erythematosus

TREATMENT
MEDICATION
- Topical corticosteroids (triamcinolone 0.25, 0.1, 0.5%; betamethasone valerate 0.1% cream, others)

ALERT
Limit use of fluorinated steroids on face; use hydrocortisone ointments.

- Nonsteroidal anti-inflammatory drugs (ibuprofen 600 mg q.i.d., indomethacin 25 mg p.o. t.i.d., aspirin, others)
- Prednisone for severe reactions (0.5–1 mg/kg p.o. daily) × 3–10 days
- Antihistamines for pruritus (hydroxyzine 25–50 mg p.o. q.i.d.)
- Sunscreens (>30 SPF) for prevention: Use broad-spectrum sunscreen to block both UVA and UVB. PABA may aggravate photodermatitis in sensitized patients (due to the sulfa moiety) (1)[C].
- Contraindications: Refer to the manufacturer's profile for each drug.
- Precautions: Refer to the manufacturer's profile for each drug.
- Significant possible interactions: Refer to the manufacturer's profile for each drug.

Geriatric Considerations
More likely to experience adverse reactions to causative drugs

ADDITIONAL TREATMENT
General Measures
- Appropriate health care: Outpatient
- Avoid sunlight/limit exposure.
- Protective clothing/sunscreens
- Ice packs/cold water compresses

COMPLEMENTARY AND ALTERNATIVE MEDICINE
- Taking β-carotene orally seems to modestly reduce the risk of sunburn in individuals who are sensitive to sun exposure (2).
- Omega-3 fatty acid intake may decrease the sensitivity of skin to UV exposure (3).

ONGOING CARE
FOLLOW-UP RECOMMENDATIONS
Avoid direct sunlight.

PATIENT EDUCATION
- Avoidance of direct sunlight exposure
- Avoidance of photosensitizing drugs
- Protective clothing (e.g., hats, long sleeves)
- Sunscreens >30 SPF

PROGNOSIS
Good with avoidance/protection measures

COMPLICATIONS
Rare (secondary bacterial infection)

REFERENCES
1. Deleo V. Sunscreen use in photodermatoses. *Dermatol Clin*. 2006;24:27–33.
2. Morison WL. Clinical practice. Photosensitivity. *N Engl J Med*. 2004;350:1111–7.
3. Rhodes LE, Durham BH, Fraser WD, et al. Dietary fish oil reduces basal and ultraviolet B-generated PGE2 levels in skin and increases the threshold to provocation of polymorphic light eruption. *J Invest Dermatol*. 1995;105:532–5.

CODES

ICD9
692.72 Acute dermatitis due to solar radiation

CLINICAL PEARLS
- Choose a sunscreen with an SPF of at least 30 with full-spectrum protection (UVA and UVB) for the best efficacy.
- The most common medications that predispose to photosensitivity include tetracyclines and sulfonamide. However, there are many other medications that may cause photosensitivity.

PILONIDAL DISEASE
Michael Rousse, MD, MPH

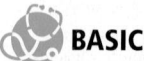 **BASICS**

DESCRIPTION
- Pilonidal disease results from a cyst, abscess, or sinus tract in the upper part of the natal cleft.
- Synonym(s): Jeep disease

EPIDEMIOLOGY
Incidence
- 0.7%: 1.1% males, 0.1% females
- Predominant sex: Male > Female (3–4:1)
- Predominant age: 2nd–3rd decade, rare >45 years old
- Ethnic consideration: Whites > Blacks > Asians

Prevalence
Surgical procedures show male:female ratio of 4:1, yet incidence data are 10:1.

RISK FACTORS
- Sedentary/prolonged sitting
- Excessive body hair
- Obesity/increased sacrococcygeal fold thickness
- Congenital natal dimple

Genetics
Congenital dimple in the natal cleft

GENERAL PREVENTION
- Weight loss
- Trim hair in/around gluteal cleft weekly.

PATHOPHYSIOLOGY
Pilonidal = "nest of hair"; excoriation by hair in the natal cleft allows hair to be drawn into the deeper tissues via negative pressure caused by movement of the buttocks

ETIOLOGY
- Inflammation of subcutaneous gluteal tissues with secondary infection and sinus tract formation
- Polymicrobial, likely from enteric pathogens given proximity to anorectal contamination

 DIAGNOSIS

HISTORY
3 distinct clinical presentations:
- Asymptomatic: Painless cyst or sinus at the top of the gluteal cleft
- Acute abscess: Severe pain, swelling, discharge from the top of the gluteal cleft that may or may not have drained spontaneously
- Chronic abscess: Persistent drainage from a sinus tract at the top of the gluteal cleft

PHYSICAL EXAM
- Common: Inflamed cystic mass at the top of the gluteal cleft with limited surrounding erythema ± drainage or a sinus tract
- Less common: Significant cellulitis of the surrounding tissues near the gluteal cleft

DIAGNOSTIC TESTS & INTERPRETATION
Lab
Initial lab tests
CBC and wound culture

Imaging
Initial approach
MRI might be considered to differentiate between perirectal abscess and pilonidal disease.

DIFFERENTIAL DIAGNOSIS
- Furunculosis
- Hydradenitis suppurativa
- Anal fistula
- Perirectal abscess
- Crohn disease

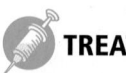 **TREATMENT**

MEDICATION
- Antibiotics not indicated unless there is significant cellulitis
- If antibiotics are needed, a culture to direct therapy might be useful.
- Cefazolin and metronidazole

ADDITIONAL TREATMENT
General Measures
Shave area; remove hair from crypts weekly.

Issues for Referral
- Patients who cannot comply with frequent dressing changes required after incision and drainage (I&D)
- Patients who have recurrence after I&D
- Patients who have complex disease with multiple sinus tracts

Additional Therapies
- I&D with only enough packing to allow the cyst to drain; overpacking not indicated
- Antibiotics only if significant cellulitis

SURGERY/OTHER PROCEDURES

5 levels of care based on severity or recurrence of disease [C]; recent innovations in technique are aimed at expediting healing and minimizing recurrence (1,2)[C]:

- I&D, remove hair, curette granulation tissue.
- Excision of midline "pits" allows drainage of lateral sinus tracts.
- Pilonidal cystotomy: Insert probe into sinus tract, excise overlying skin, and close wound (3)[B].
- Marsupialization: Excise overlying skin and roof of cyst, and suture skin edges to cyst floor.
- Excision: Use of flap closure (4)[B]

IN-PATIENT CONSIDERATIONS

Admission Criteria

- Severe cellulitis
- Large area excision

 ## ONGOING CARE

FOLLOW-UP RECOMMENDATIONS

- Frequent dressing changes required after I&D
- Follow-up wound checks to assess for recurrence.

Patient Monitoring

Monitor for fever, more extensive cellulitis.

PATIENT EDUCATION

- Wash area briskly with washcloth daily.
- Shave the area weekly.
- Remove any embedded hair from the crypt.
- Avoid prolonged sitting.

PROGNOSIS

- Simple I&D has a 55% failure rate; median time to healing is 5 weeks.
- More extensive surgical excisions involve hospital stays and longer time to heal.

COMPLICATIONS

Malignant degeneration is a rare complication of untreated chronic pilonidal disease.

REFERENCES

1. Kement M, Oncel M, Kurt N, et al. Sinus excision for the treatment of limited chronic pilonidal disease: results after a medium-term follow-up. *Dis Colon Rectum*. 2006;49:1758–62.
2. Theodropoulos GE, et al. Modified Bascom's assymetric midgluteal cleft closure technique for recurrent pilonidal disease: Early experience in a military hospital. *Dis Colon Rectum*. 2003;49(11): 1755–7.
3. Rao MM, Zawislak W, Kennedy R, et al. A prospective randomised study comparing two treatment modalities for chronic pilonidal sinus with a 5-year follow-up. *Int J Colorectal Dis*. 2010;25:395–400.
4. Washer JD, Smith DE, Carman ME, et al. Gluteal fascial advancement: an innovative, effective method for treating pilonidal disease. *Am Surg*. 2010;76:154–6.

ADDITIONAL READING

- Aygen E, Arslan K, Dogru O, et al. Crystallized phenol in nonoperative treatment of previously operated, recurrent pilonidal disease. *Dis. Colon Rectum*. 2010;53:932–5.
- Balik O, Balik AA, Polat KY, et al. The importance of local subcutaneous fat thickness in pilonidal disease. *Dis Colon Rectum*. 2006;49:1755–7.
- Harlak A, Mentes O, Kilic S, et al. Sacrococcygeal pilonidal disease: analysis of previously proposed risk factors. *Clinics (Sao Paulo)*. 2010;65:125–31.
- Humphries AE, Duncan JE et al. Evaluation and management of pilonidal disease. *Surg Clin North Am*. 2010;90:113–24, Table of Contents.
- Mohamed HA, Kadry I, Adly S. Comparison between three therapeutic modalities for non-complicated pilonidal sinus disease. *Surgeon*. 2005;3:73–7.
- Oram Y, Kahraman F, Karincaolu Y, et al. Evaluation of 60 patients with pilonidal sinus treated with laser epilation after surgery. *Dermatol Surg*. 2010;36: 88–91.

 ## CODES

ICD9

- 685.0 Pilonidal cyst with abscess
- 685.1 Pilonidal cyst without mention of abscess

CLINICAL PEARLS

- Avoid prolonged sitting.
- Weight loss
- Trim hair in gluteal cleft weekly.

PINWORMS

Jonathan MacClements, MD

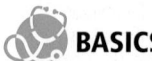 **BASICS**

DESCRIPTION
- Intestinal infection with *Enterobius vermicularis*, characterized by perineal and perianal itching, usually worse at night
- System(s) affected: GI; Skin/Exocrine
- Synonym: Enterobiasis

EPIDEMIOLOGY
Predominant age: 5–14 years

Prevalence
- Most common helminthic infection in US, with 20–42 million people harboring the parasite
- ~30% of children are infected throughout the world.

Pediatric Considerations
More common in children, who are more likely to become reinfected.

RISK FACTORS
- Institutionalization
- Crowded living conditions
- Poor hygiene
- Warm climate
- Handling of infected children's clothing or bedding

GENERAL PREVENTION
- Careful hand-washing, especially after bowel movements; clip and maintain short fingernails.
- Wash anus and genitals at least once a day, preferably during a shower.
- Do not scratch anus or put fingers near nose or mouth.

PATHOPHYSIOLOGY
- Small white worms (2–13 mm) inhabit the cecum, appendix, and adjacent portions of the ascending colon following ingestion.
- Female worms migrate to the perianal and perineal areas at night, depositing ~11,000 eggs, resulting in irritation and itching of the perianal area.
- Scratching of the perianal and perineal areas followed by touching of the mouth can lead to ingestion of the eggs and continuation of pinworm's life cycle in the host.

ETIOLOGY
Infestation by the intestinal nematode *E. (Oxyuris) vermicularis*

COMMONLY ASSOCIATED CONDITIONS
Pruritus ani (1)

 DIAGNOSIS

HISTORY
- Many patients are asymptomatic.
- Perianal itching
- Perineal itching
- Vulvovaginitis
- Dysuria
- Abdominal pain (rare)
- Insomnia
- Restless sleep

PHYSICAL EXAM
Perineal and perianal exam

DIAGNOSTIC TESTS & INTERPRETATION
Diagnostic Procedures/Surgery
- Adhesive tape test: A piece of transparent cellophane tape is stuck to the perianal skin in the early morning before bathing and then affixed to a microscope slide after removal. This procedure must be performed at least 3 times to achieve 90% sensitivity. Alternatively, anal swabs or a pinworm paddle coated with adhesive material also can be useful (2,3,4)[C].
- Digital rectal exam with saline slide preparation of stool on gloved finger (2)[C]
- Routine stool examination for ova and parasites is positive in only 10–15% of infected patients.

Pathological Findings
Identification of ova on low-power microscopy or direct visualization of the female worm (10 mm long); ova are asymmetric, flattened on 1 side, and measure $56 \times 27 \ \mu$m.

DIFFERENTIAL DIAGNOSIS
- Idiopathic pruritus ani
- Atopic dermatitis
- Contact dermatitis
- Psoriasis
- Lichen planus
- Infection with human papillomavirus
- Herpes simplex
- Fungal infections
- Erythrasma
- Scabies
- Vaginitis
- Hemorrhoids

TREATMENT

MEDICATION

- Treatment options include any of the following (2,5)[A]:
  - Mebendazole (Vermox): Chewable 100-mg tablet as a single dose in adults and children >2 years of age; use with caution in children <2 years of age.
  - Albendazole (Albenza): 400 mg PO as a single dose in adults and children >2 years of age; 100 mg PO as a single dose repeated in 7 days in children ≤2 years of age.
  - Pyrantel pamoate (Pin-X, Reese's Pinworm Medicine): Oral liquid or tablet 11 mg/kg as a single dose in adults and children >2 years of age; maximum dose 1 g. Use with caution in children <2 years of age.
- Many clinicians recommend repeat treatment after 2 weeks owing to the high frequency of reinfection and autoinfection. Occasionally, refractory cases may require retreatment every 2 weeks for 4–6 cycles.
- All symptomatic family members should be treated.

Pregnancy Considerations

Drug therapy should be avoided in pregnancy. Treatment should be delayed until after delivery (6)[C].

ONGOING CARE

FOLLOW-UP RECOMMENDATIONS

Unnecessary unless symptoms do not abate following drug therapy

PATIENT EDUCATION

- Take medicine with food.
- Practice good hygiene.
- Encourage frequent and careful hand-washing.

- Clip fingernails short.
- All clothing and bedding should be washed to prevent reinfection.
- Do not shake linen and clothing before laundering because this may spread the eggs.

PROGNOSIS

- Asymptomatic carriers are common.
- Symptomatic infections are cured >90% of the time by pharmacotherapy.
- Reinfection is common, especially among children.

COMPLICATIONS

- Perianal scratching may lead to bacterial superinfection.
- Females: Vulvovaginitis, urethritis, endometritis, salpingitis
- Urinary tract infections
- Rarely, ectopic disease involving granulomas of the pelvis, urinary tract, female genitourinary tract, and appendix

REFERENCES

1. Stermer E, Sukhotnic I, Shaoul R. Pruritus ani: an approach to an itching condition. *J Pediatr Gastroenterol Nutr*. 2009;48:513–6.
2. Jones JE. Pinworms. *Am Fam Phys*. 1988;38:159–64.
3. Cram EB. Studies on oxyuriasis, 28. Summary and conclusions. *Am J Dis Child*. 1943;65:46–59.
4. Kucik CJ, et al. Common intestinal parasites. *Am Fam Phys*. 2004;69:1161–8.
5. Enterobius vermicularis, in: Drugs for Parasitic Infections, 2007, http://www.dpd.cdc.gov/DPDx/html/PDF_Files/MedLetter/Enterobius_vermicularisInfection.pdf
6. Hamblin J, et al. Pinworms in pregnancy. *J Amer Board Fam Practice*. 1995;8:321–4.

ADDITIONAL READING

- Burkhart CN, Burkhart CG. Assessment of frequency, transmission, and genitourinary complications of enterobiasis (pinworms). *Int J Dermatol*. 2005;44:837–40.
- For patient education materials on this topic: Centers for Disease Control, http://www.cdc.gov/ncidod/dpd/parasites/pinworm/factsht_pinworm.htm.
- Jardine M, Kokai GK, Dalzell AM et al. Enterobius vermicularis and colitis in Children. *J Pediatr Gastroenterol Nutr*. 2006;43:610–2.

See Also (Topic, Algorithm, Electronic Media Element)

Pruritus Ani

CODES

ICD9
127.4 Enterobiasis

CLINICAL PEARLS

- Treatment for pinworms includes use of either mebendazole, albendazole, or pyrantelpamoate (2,5)[A].
- Close contacts should be treated as well.
- Retreatment after 2 weeks is recommended by many experts owing to the difficulty eradicating this parasite (2)[C].

PITUITARY ADENOMA

Anup Kumar Sabharwal, MD

 BASICS

Typically benign, slow-growing tumors that arise from cells in the pituitary gland. The mechanism by which pituitary cells change and develop into tumors has not been well defined.

DESCRIPTION

- From surgical practice, pituitary adenomas have been identified as the 3rd most frequent intracranial tumor, and account for 10-25%.
- Radiological data suggest that 1 in 6 have pituitary incidentalomas.
- Subtypes (hormonal): Prolactinoma (PRL) 50%, nonfunctioning pituitary adenomas 30%, somatotroph adenoma (growth hormone [GH]) 15-20%, corticotroph adenoma (adrenocorticotrophic hormone [ACTH]) 5–10%, thyrotroph adenoma (thyroid-stimulating hormone [TSH]) <1%, gonadotropinoma (luteinizing hormone/follicle-stimulating hormone [LH/FSH]), mixed
- Defined as microadenoma <10 mm and macroadenoma ≥10 mm
- May secrete hormones and/or cause mass effect

EPIDEMIOLOGY

- Predominant age: Age increases incidence
- Predominant sex: Female > Male (3:2) for microadenomas (often delayed diagnosis in men)

Incidence

- Autopsy studies: Pituitary microadenomas have been found in 3–27% of those without any pituitary disorders.
- Macroadenomas have been found in fewer than 0.5% of people.

RISK FACTORS

- Multiple endocrine neoplasia I
- Carney complex
- Familial isolated pituitary adenomas: Approximately 15% have mutations in the aryl hydrocarbon receptor-interacting protein gene (AIP). Present at a younger age and are larger in size.
- McCune-Albright syndrome
- Multiple endocrine neoplasia (MEN) 1-like phenotype (MEN 4): Germline mutation in the cyclin-dependent kinase inhibitor 1B (CDKN1B)

Genetics

See Diagnosis and Risk Factors for syndromes.

PATHOPHYSIOLOGY

- Monoclonal adenohypophysial cell growth
- Hormonal effects typical of microadenomas, prompting diagnosis before mass effect
- Prolactin increased by functional prolactinomas or inhibited dopaminergic suppression by stalk effect

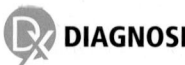 **DIAGNOSIS**

HISTORY

- Common:
  - Hyperprolactinemia: Infertility, amenorrhea, galactorrhea, gynecomastia, impotence
  - Headache (sellar expansion)
  - Visual disturbances: Bitemporal hemianopsia

- Less common:
  - Hypersomatotropinemia: Acromegaly (coarse facial features, hand/foot swelling, carpal tunnel syndrome, hyperhidrosis, left ventricular hypertrophy)
  - Hyposomatotropinemia: Failure to thrive (FTT) (children), asymptomatic (adults)
  - Intracranial pressure (ICP) elevation: Headache, nausea, seizures
  - Hypercorticotropinemia: Cushing's disease (supraclavicular/dorsocervical fat pad thickening, moon face, hirsutism, acne, plethora, abdominal striae, centripetal obesity with thin limbs, easy bruising and bleeding, hyperglycemia)
- Rare:
  - Apoplexy: Headache, sudden collapse
  - Secondary hyperthyroidism: Palpitations, diaphoresis, heat intolerance, diarrhea
  - Secondary adrenal insufficiency: Weakness, irritability, anorexia, nausea/vomiting
- Hypothalamic compression: Temperature, thirst/appetite disorders

PHYSICAL EXAM

- Common:
  - Visual disturbances: Bitemporal hemianopsia
  - Hyperprolactinemia: Hypogonadism, galactorrhea, gynecomastia
  - Hypersomatotropinemia: Acromegaly (coarse features, hand/foot swelling, diaphoresis)
  - Hyposomatotropinemia: FTT (children)
- Less common:
  - ICP elevation: Papilledema, dementia
  - Cushing's disease: Centripetal obesity, supraclavicular fat pad thickening, moon face, hirsutism, acne
- Rare:
  - Apoplexy: Hypotension, hypoglycemia, tachycardia, oliguria
  - Secondary hyperthyroidism: Tachycardia, tachypnea, diaphoresis, warm/moist skin, tremor
  - Adrenal crisis: Orthostatic hypotension
- Hypothalamic compression: Temperature dysregulation, obesity, increased urination

DIAGNOSTIC TESTS & INTERPRETATION

Lab

Select based on dysfunction(s) suspected.

- Somatotrophic (GH secreting: 40-130/million):
  - Acromegaly/hypersomatotropinemia: Serum IGF-1 elevated; oral glucose tolerance test with GH given at 0, 30, and 60 minutes (normally suppresses GH to <1 g/L)
  - Hyposomatotropinemia: Low growth hormone releasing hormone response
- Corticotrophic:
  - Cushing's disease/hypercorticotropinemia
  - 24-h urinary free cortisol >50 g
  - Overnight low-dose dexamethasone suppression test (DMST): Normal plasma cortisol (FPC) >1.8 μg/dL at 8 a.m. (after 1 mg given at 11 p.m. on night prior)
  - ACTH level assay (if DMST results abnormal): <20 pg/mL = adrenal tumor; ≥20 pg/mL = ectopic/pituitary source
  - Hypocorticotropinemia/secondary glucocorticoid deficiency: High-dose corticotropin stimulation test: FPC <10 g/dL at baseline with an increase of less than 25% 1 h after 250 mcg; metyrapone test: 11-deoxycortisol <150 ng/L after 2 g given (prepare to give steroids because test may worsen insufficiency)

- Gonadotrophic: Hypogonadotropinism: Gonadotropin-releasing hormone stimulation of LH/FSH blunted in pituitary hypergonadism but increased in primary hypogonadism
- Lactotrophic (Prolactin secreting >100/million): Hyperprolactinemia: Serum PRL >20 ng/mL
- Thyrotrophic (TSH secreting: 1/million): Hyper-/hypothyroidism: TSH and free T_4 both increased for pituitary hyperthyroidism and both decreased for pituitary hypothyroidism

Initial lab tests

- A typical panel for asymptomatic tumors: PRL, GH, IGF-1, ACTH, 24-h urinary free cortisol or overnight DMST, pituitary α-subunit, β-subunit FSH, LH, TSH, free T_4
- Screening for *AIP* mutations (see Genetics) may be offered to families of patients with pituitary adenoma, where available (1)[B].

Imaging

- Magnetic resonance imaging (MRI) preferred (>90% sensitivity/specificity) after biochemically confirmed
- Octreotide scintigraphy is useful in identifying tumors with somatostatin receptors.

Diagnostic Procedures/Surgery

Inferior petrosal sinus sampling: ACTH sampled from inferior petrosal sinuses to distinguish Cushing's disease (pituitary source) from ectopic ACTH

Pathological Findings

- Cell types identified by immunohistochemistry
- Light microscope: Eosinophilic (GH, PRL), basophilic (FSH/LH, TSH, ACTH), chromophobic

DIFFERENTIAL DIAGNOSIS

Pituitary hyperplasia (e.g., pregnancy), Rathke cleft cyst, granulomatous disease (e.g., tuberculosis), lymphocytic hypophysitis, metastatic tumor, germinoma, craniopharyngioma

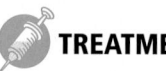 **TREATMENT**

Medical therapy is primary therapy for prolactinomas and adjunct for other tumors (see Medication) (2,3)[A].

MEDICATION

First Line

- Hyperprolactinemia: Dopamine agonists increase dopaminergic suppression of PRL:
  - Cabergoline (Dostinex): D_2 receptor-specific:
    - Initial dose: 0.25 mg p.o. twice weekly
    - Maintenance dose: Increase q4wk by 0.25 mg 2 × /wk per PRL (maximum 2 mg/wk)
    - Contraindications: Hypersensitivity (ergots), hypertension (HTN), pregnancy
    - Precautions: Caution with liver impairment
    - Interactions: May be inhibited by tricyclic antidepressants, phenothiazines, opiates
    - Adverse reactions: Orthostatic hypotension, vertigo, dyspepsia, hot flashes
  - Bromocriptine (Parlodel): D_2 receptor-specific:
    - Initial dose: 1.25–2.5 mg p.o. daily (give with food)
    - Maintenance dose: Increase by 2.5 mg/day q2–7d (maximum 100 mg/d)
    - Contraindications: Hypersensitivity (ergots), HTN, pregnancy; preferred over cabergoline if required

- Precautions: Caution with liver impairment
  - Interactions: May be inhibited by tricyclic antidepressants, phenothiazines, opiates
  - Adverse reactions: Orthostatic hypotension, seizures, hallucinations, stroke, myocardial infarction
- Somatotropinoma: GH suppressants:
  - Octreotide (Sandostatin): Long-acting analogue of somatostatin:
    - Initial dose: 50 μg SC/IV t.i.d., then titrate to GH (maximum 1,500 μg/d)
    - Contraindication: Hypersensitivity
    - Precautions: Caution with biliary, thyroid, cardiac, liver, or kidney disease
    - Interactions: Pimozide increases risk of QT prolongation; variable effects with β-blockers, diuretics, oral glycemic agents
    - Adverse reactions: Ascending cholangitis, arrhythmias, congestive heart failure, glycemic instability
    - More effective as adjuvant than as primary treatment for somatotropinomas (2)[A]
  - Pegvisomant (Somavert): Growth hormone receptor antagonist:
    - Initial dose: 40 mg SC × 1, then titrate by 5 mg every 4–6 weeks based on IGF-1 levels (maximum 30 mg/d maintenance dose)
    - Contraindication: Hypersensitivity
    - Precautions: Caution if GH-secreting tumors, diabetes mellitus, impaired liver function
    - Interactions: Nonsteroidal anti-inflammatory drugs, opiates, insulins, oral glycemic agents
    - Adverse reactions: Hepatitis, tumor growth, GH-secreting
- Corticotropinemia: Peripheral inhibitors:
  - Mitotane (Lysodren):
    - Initial dose: 2–6 g p.o. t.i.d. (maximum 19 g/d)
    - Maintenance dose: 2–16 g t.i.d.
    - Contraindication: Hypersensitivity
    - Precautions: Caution with liver dysfunction and brain damage
    - Interactions: Contraindicated with rotavirus vaccine; caution with other vaccines
    - Adverse reactions: HTN, orthostatic hypotension, hemorrhagic cystitis, rash
  - Ketoconazole:
    - Dosing: 200 mg p.o. t.i.d. (maximum 1,200 mg/d)
    - Contraindications: Hypersensitivity, achlorhydria, fungal meningitis, impaired liver function
    - Precautions: Caution with liver dysfunction
    - Interactions: Contraindicated with cisapride, niacin, statins, pimozide, sirolimus; caution with other antifungals
    - Adverse reactions: Adrenal insufficiency, thrombocytopenia, hepatic failure, hepatotoxicity, anaphylaxis, leukopenia, hemolytic anemia
- Gonadotropinemia:
  - Bromocriptine: See above:
    - Initial dose: 1.25–2.5 mg p.o. daily (give with food), increase by 2.5 mg/day q2–7d (maximum 100 mg/d)
- Thyrotropinemia:
  - Octreotide: See above.

Second Line
- Corticotropinemia: Peripheral inhibitors:
  - Metyrapone:
    - Dose: 250–600 mg/d p.o.

- Contraindication: Porphyria
  - Precautions: Caution in liver/thyroid disease
  - Interactions: Dilantin increases metabolism.
  - Adverse reactions: Nausea, hypotension
- Gonadotropinemia:
  - Octreotide: See above.

ADDITIONAL TREATMENT
Issues for Referral
- Neurosurgery consultation as soon as tumor with symptoms identified (except for prolactinoma)
- Ophthalmologist evaluation prior to surgery

Additional Therapies
- Fractionated radiotherapy: Often effective as adjunctive when surgery is inadequate (4)[A]
- Stereotactic radiosurgery: Alternative to surgery in high-risk patients or as adjunct (4)[B]

SURGERY/OTHER PROCEDURES
- Most now done endoscopically via translabial/transphenoidal approach
- Indications: Symptoms or treatment-resistant
- Follow-up: Serial neuro/hormonal evaluations to evaluate complications (e.g., diabetes insipidus, central nervous system damage) and need for more treatment (5)
- Remission rates: 72–87% for microadenoma but only 50–56% for macroadenomas (5)

IN-PATIENT CONSIDERATIONS
Initial Stabilization
- Pituitary apoplexy (see Complications): Must treat immediately to prevent death.
- Support ABCs.
- Consider stress-dose steroids in frail or hemodynamically unstable.
- Maintain blood pressure (BP) with fluids and/or pressor agents.
- Check serum sodium, serum osmolality, and urine specific gravity if polyuric or electrolytes are imbalanced.
- Contact neurosurgery.

Admission Criteria
Outpatient management unless apoplexy (see Complications) or adrenal crisis

IV Fluids
- Diabetes insipidus: Hyposmolar IV fluids
- Adrenal crisis: Normal saline

Nursing
- Pituitary apoplexy: Monitor inputs/outputs (I/Os), central venous pressure, and ICP monitoring, and do frequent neurologic checks.
- Adrenal crisis: Monitor BP and I/Os.

Discharge Criteria
Keep as inpatients post-op until diabetes insipidus and/or adrenal insufficiency is managed.

 ONGOING CARE

FOLLOW-UP RECOMMENDATIONS
Patient Monitoring
- Typically outpatient treatment
- Follow-up MRI at 6 and 12 months
- Involved hormone(s) are followed postoperatively, especially after radiation, because hypopituitarism may develop as late as 10–15 years later (2).

PROGNOSIS
- Depends on type, size, symptoms, therapy
- Acromegaly's 10-year life-expectancy reduction is prevented when GH <2.5 g/L (3).

COMPLICATIONS
- Postoperative diabetes insipidus and/or hypogonadism (usually transient/common)
- Pituitary apoplexy (acute/uncommon): Acute hemorrhagic pituitary infarction; adrenal crisis with severe headache; surgical decompression required to prevent shock, coma, and death
- Nelson syndrome (subacute/uncommon): Rapid adenoma growth postadrenalectomy
- Pituitary hormone insufficiency (chronic/uncommon): Often years after treatment
- Optic nerve neuropathy and brain necrosis after >60 Gy radiotherapy (chronic/rare)

REFERENCES
1. Georgitsi M, Raitila A, Karhu A, et al. Molecular diagnosis of pituitary adenoma predisposition caused by aryl hydrocarbon receptor-interacting protein gene mutations. *Proc Natl Acad Sci U S A.* 2007;104:4101–5.
2. Tichomirowa MA, Daly AF, Beckers A. Treatment of pituitary tumors: somatostatin. *Endocrine.* 2005;28:93–100.
3. Drange MR, et al. Pituitary tumor registry: A novel clinical resource. *J Clin Endo Met.* 2000;85: 168–74.
4. Mondok A, Szeifert GT, Mayer A, et al. Treatment of pituitary tumors: radiation. *Endocrine.* 2005;28:77–85.
5. Buchfelder M. Treatment of pituitary tumors: surgery. *Endocrine.* 2005;28:67–75.

See Also (Topic, Algorithm, Electronic Media Element)
Cushing's Disease and Cushing's Syndrome; Galactorrhea

 CODES

ICD9
227.3 Benign neoplasm of pituitary gland and craniopharyngeal duct

CLINICAL PEARLS
- An incidentaloma is an asymptomatic microadenoma found on imaging. General labs include PRL, GH, IGF-1, ACTH, 24-h urinary free cortisol or overnight DMST, β-subunit FSH, LH, TSH, and free T_4. Obtain follow-up MRIs at 6 and 12 months if normal, but consult endocrinology if not.
- Initial treatment selected for symptomatic pituitary adenoma includes a dopamine agonist for prolactinomas and surgical resection for all others.
- Pituitary apoplexy is a rapid hemorrhagic pituitary infarction due to compression of the blood supply. It is fatal within hours unless surgically decompressed.

PITYRIASIS ALBA

Russell C. Hendershot, DO, MS

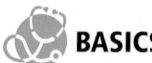 **BASICS**

DESCRIPTION
- A chronic skin disorder characterized by ≥1 group of poorly marginated, pale pink or tan/white patches and plaques that appear on the cheeks, neck, and lateral arms of children and young adults
- System(s) affected: Skin/Exocrine
- Synonym(s): Pityriasis streptogenes; Pityriasis simplex; Pityriasis sicca faciei; Erythema streptogenes

Geriatric Considerations
Rare in this age group

Pediatric Considerations
More common in children aged 3–16 years

EPIDEMIOLOGY
Incidence
- Common; exact incidence unknown, but seen frequently in people with dark skin in sunnier climates
- Predominant age: 90% of affected patients are ages 6–12 years; rare >25 years
- Predominant sex: Male = Female

RISK FACTORS
Children with a genetic predisposition to atopic disease

Genetics
Unknown, but condition is seen primarily in children with a genetic predisposition to atopic disease

GENERAL PREVENTION
No known preventive measures

ETIOLOGY
- Unknown; may be part of an atopic diathesis
- Possibly defects in melanin production or transfer

COMMONLY ASSOCIATED CONDITIONS
Atopic dermatitis

 DIAGNOSIS

HISTORY
- Usually asymptomatic
- Pruritus (rare)
- More apparent in summertime in light-skinned people
- Lesions do not tan in summer.
- Even a small amount of sunlight exposure causes lesions to redden.

PHYSICAL EXAM
- Description: Small, ill-defined, pale pink or tan/white patches 0.5–5 cm
- Rash evolves from pink patch to white macule with fine scale to smooth hypopigmented macule.
- Location: Cheeks and lateral arms
- Number: 1–12 or more patches
- Palpation: Smooth or slightly rough, but dry
- Appearance: Pinpoint white papules (representing accentuation and keratinization of follicular orifices)
- Scale is either invisible or fine and light.
- More common in dark-skinned people

DIAGNOSTIC TESTS & INTERPRETATION
Negative finding on potassium hydroxide (KOH) skin scraping

Pathological Findings
Irregular melanin pigmentation of basal layer, follicular plugging, follicular spongiosis, and atrophic sebaceous glands

DIFFERENTIAL DIAGNOSIS
- Tinea versicolor
- Vitiligo
- Postinflammatory hypomelanosis
- Chemical leukoderma
- Indeterminate or uncharacteristic leprosy
- T cell lymphoma
- Sarcoidosis

 TREATMENT

MEDICATION
First Line
- Topical steroids if needed to reduce redness due to sunburn or spontaneous inflammation
- Anecdotal evidence supports use of topical corticosteroids, but not FDA approved for use in this condition.
- Symptomatic treatment, as lesions tend to resolve on their own

Second Line
- Coal tar preparations (e.g., Alphosyl, Estar, Balnetar): Applied topically once daily or b.i.d.; treatment is not mandatory.
- Neither coal tar nor corticosteroids will change the pigmentation but may improve pruritus, roughness, and/or dryness if the lubricating cream is not sufficient.
- Tacrolimus or picrolimus has been used off-label for pityriasis alba to treat pruritus and redness but currently not FDA approved.
- Precautions: Refer to the manufacturer's literature for each drug.

ADDITIONAL TREATMENT
General Measures
- No truly effective therapy is available. Lubricating cream application may palliate roughness and/or dryness.
- Sun exposure may promote repigmentation.

Additional Therapies
Phototherapy (e.g., ultraviolet B [UVB] light) for extensive involvement in adults only

IN-PATIENT CONSIDERATIONS
Initial Stabilization
Outpatient

 ONGOING CARE

FOLLOW-UP RECOMMENDATIONS
Patient Monitoring
As needed, only if lesions become symptomatic

DIET
No special diet

PATIENT EDUCATION
Stress long-term chronicity and permanent resolution of condition in 2nd or 3rd decade of life.

PROGNOSIS
Permanent resolution during 2nd or 3rd decade of life

COMPLICATIONS
None expected

ADDITIONAL READING
- Arnold KL, et al. *Andrews' Diseases of the Skin*, 9th ed. Philadelphia: WB Saunders, 2000.
- Fitzpatrick TB, et al., eds. *Dermatology in General Medicine*, 5th ed. New York: McGraw-Hill, 1999.
- Galen EB. Pityriasis alba. *Cutis*. 1998;61:11–13.
- Habif T. *Clinical Dermatology*, 4th ed. St. Louis: Mosby, 2004.

- Halder RM, Nandedkar MA, Neal KW. Pigmentary disorders in ethnic skin. *Dermatol Clin*. 2003;21: 617–28, vii.
- Lin RL, Janniger CK et al. Pityriasis alba. *Cutis*. 2005;76:21–4.
- Miller DC. Pigmentation disorders in adults. *Clin Fam Pract*. 2003;5(3):691.
- Plensdorf S, Martinez J et al. Common pigmentation disorders. *Am Fam Physician*. 2009;79:109–16.

See Also (Topic, Algorithm, Electronic Media Element)
Keratosis, Actinic; Tinea Versicolor; Vitiligo

 CODES

ICD9
696.5 Other and unspecified pityriasis

CLINICAL PEARLS
- Use of KOH preparation and Wood's lamp is a quick way to differentiate this from a fungal infection (see Tinea Versicolor).
- May be seen more often in those with atrophy

PITYRIASIS ROSEA

Jeffrey D. Wolfrey, MD

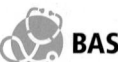 **BASICS**

DESCRIPTION

- An idiopathic, self-limited skin eruption characterized by widespread papulosquamous lesions
- System(s) affected: Skin/Exocrine

Pediatric Considerations

Face and distal extremities are more often involved in children, and lesions may be more papular.

EPIDEMIOLOGY

- Predominant age: 10–35 years but occurs in all age groups
- Predominant sex: Male = Female:
  – Some studies have shown a slight female preponderance.
- No racial predominance

Incidence

Relatively common, but exact frequency is unknown

RISK FACTORS

Genetics

<5% of those affected give a positive family history.

ETIOLOGY

Unknown; may be a viral agent or an autoimmune disorder. Several studies have implicated the human herpes viruses, most commonly HHV-7, but other research has not confirmed this association.

 DIAGNOSIS

HISTORY

- The most common initial sign is a 2- to 10-cm salmon-colored patch or plaque known as the *herald patch*. The herald patch is present 40–76% of the time (1).
- The more widespread rash begins 7–14 days after the onset of the herald patch, although it may appear up to 3 months later.
- Mild pruritus, rarely severe
- Fever and malaise rare

PHYSICAL EXAM

Salmon-colored to light-brown oval plaques with fine scales centrally and collarette of loose scales along borders:

- Lesions average 1–2 cm in diameter and usually spare face, hands, and feet in adults.
- Lesions frequently are oriented along skin cleavage (Langer's) lines in "Christmas tree" pattern.
- Variant forms include purpuric, urticarial, and vesicular lesions, especially in children.

DIAGNOSTIC TESTS & INTERPRETATION

Lab

Initial lab tests

- White blood cells normal
- No specific lab markers. Consider serology to rule out syphilis if suspected.

Diagnostic Procedures/Surgery

KOH preparation to distinguish disease from tinea corporis

Pathological Findings

Chronic inflammation with cytolytic degeneration of keratinocytes adjacent to Langerhans cells

DIFFERENTIAL DIAGNOSIS

- Secondary syphilis
- Viral exanthems
- Drug rashes
- Psoriasis
- Parapsoriasis
- Eczema
- Lichen planus
- Tinea corporis

 TREATMENT

MEDICATION

- A Cochrane Review in 2007 showed poor quality of evidence for most treatments of pityriasis rosea (2)[A].

- Symptomatic treatment as needed

First Line

- Topical steroids to reduce itching, if needed:
  – Triamcinolone 0.1% cream
- Oral antihistamines:
  – Diphenhydramine (Benadryl) 25 mg t.i.d.
  – Chlorpheniramine 8 mg t.i.d.

Second Line

- Erythromycin showed apparent benefit in 1 trial, although azithromycin failed to show significant benefit in another (3,4)[B].
- High-dose acyclovir (800 mg 5 × /day for 7 days), used early in the disease course, also showed benefit (5)[C].

ADDITIONAL TREATMENT

General Measures

- Symptomatic treatment
- Topical antipruritics as needed
- Ultraviolet therapy has been used, but a controlled study found minimal benefit (6)[B].
- Lukewarm oatmeal baths (*not* hot, because heat can intensify itching)

 ## ONGOING CARE

FOLLOW-UP RECOMMENDATIONS

Patient Monitoring

Return visit for re-evaluation if lesions persist >8–10 weeks

PATIENT EDUCATION

- Reassure patient about self-limited nature of condition.
- Printed patient information available from: American Academy of Dermatology, (708) 330-0230

PROGNOSIS

Gradual resolution in 1–14 weeks (usually 2–6 weeks)

COMPLICATIONS

Secondary infection (e.g., impetigo)

REFERENCES

1. Chuh A, Lee A, Zawar V, et al. Pityriasis rosea–an update. *Indian J Dermatol Venereol Leprol*. 2005; 71:311–5.
2. Chuh AAT, et al. Interventions for pityriasis rosea (Cochrane Review). *The Cochrane Library* 2008, Issue 2. Chichester, UK: John Wiley and Sons, Ltd.
3. Amer A, Fischer H. Azithromycin does not cure pityriasis rosea. *Pediatrics*. 2006;117:1702–5.
4. Sharma PK, et al. Erythromycin in pityriasis rosea: a double-blind, placebo-controlled clinical trial. *J Amer Acad Dermatol*. 2000;42:241–4.
5. Drago F, et al. Use of high-dose acyclovir in pityriasis rosea. *J Amer Acad Derm*. 2006;54(1): 82–85.
6. Leenutaphong V, et al. UVB phototherapy for pityriasis rosea: A bilateral comparison study. *J Amer Acad Dermatol*. 1995;33:996–9.

ADDITIONAL READING

- Chuh A, Chan H, Zawar V. Pityriasis rosea–evidence for and against an infectious aetiology. *Epidemiol Infect*. 2004;132:381–90.
- Gonzalez L, et al. Pityriasis rosea: An important papulosquamous disorder. *Intern J Derm*. 2005;44:757–64.

See Also (Topic, Algorithm, Electronic Media Element)

Dermatitis, Exfoliative; Pityriasis Alba; Tinea Versicolor

 ## CODES

ICD9

696.3 Pityriasis rosea

CLINICAL PEARLS

- The history of a herald patch preceding the generalized rash is helpful in the diagnosis of pityriasis rosea.
- Treat symptomatically for itching if needed.
- No evidence to support aggressive treatment of this otherwise self-limiting condition, which usually resolves in 2–6 weeks.

PLACENTA PREVIA

Janelle M. Evans, MD
Petra Belady, MD

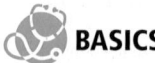

BASICS

DESCRIPTION
- Placental implantation in the lower uterine segment in advance of presenting fetal part and in proximity to or covering the internal os
- Complete previa: Placenta covers entire internal cervical os.
- Partial previa: Placenta covers part of internal cervical os.
- Marginal previa: No exact definition; commonly means placental edge is adjacent to cervical os by ultrasound but not overlapping.
- Low-lying placenta: Placental edge located in the lower uterine segment but does not encroach on or cover the os; has been defined as within 2–3 cm of cervical os by ultrasound
- System(s) affected: Cardiovascular; Reproductive

EPIDEMIOLOGY
- Average gestational age of 1st bleed, 27–36 weeks
- Most common cause of minimally painful bleeding after 20 weeks gestational age
- Approximately 10% of low-lying placentas at 10–20 weeks persist to term.
- Some evidence that shortened cervical length in the 3rd trimester is associated with increased risk of bleeding

Incidence
- Approximately 0.4% of primiparous pregnancies, with increasing incidence with cesarean deliveries in future pregnancies
- Up to 5% incidence in grand multiparous women

RISK FACTORS
- History of placenta previa (relative risk [RR] = 8.0)
- Advanced maternal age (RR = 9.0 if >40 years of age)
- Multiparity (5% if >5 deliveries) (RR = 1.1–1.7)
- Assisted reproductive technology (RR = 2.0)
- Multiple gestation
- Smoking (RR = 1.4–3)
- Cocaine use
- Male fetus (RR = 1.4)
- Asian (RR = 1.9)
- Previous cesarean deliveries:
  - 1 previous C-section: RR = 1.5 (95% confidence interval [CI] 1.3–1.8)
  - 2 previous C-sections: RR = 2.0 (95% CI 1.3–3.0)
  - 4 previous C-sections: RR = 44.9 (95% CI 13.5–15.0)
- Induced or spontaneous abortion/curettage (Ashermans) (RR = 1.6)
- Leiomyoma or history of lower uterine segment surgery

Genetics
No genetic links have been identified.

GENERAL PREVENTION
Once pregnancy is diagnosed, risk factors are not modifiable. If patient has any risk factors for previa and anatomic survey is suggestive of previa, serial ultrasounds should be performed for monitoring purposes. Patient should be counselled regarding potential bleeding and should be triaged with all bleeding episodes.

PATHOPHYSIOLOGY
- Invasion of trophoblastic giant cells into the decidua, myometrium, and myometrial spiral arteries
- Increased inflammatory cell infiltration compared with women with normal implantation sites
- As lower uterine segment expands and the trophoblastic tissue expands towards the fundus, many marginal or low-lying placentas will resolve to a safe distance from the cervix to allow vaginal delivery (1).

ETIOLOGY
Prior endometrial insult/injury/scar or other unknown uterine factors as listed previously.

COMMONLY ASSOCIATED CONDITIONS
- Abnormal presentations (e.g., oblique and/or transverse fetal lie)
- Antepartum/intrapartum/postpartum hemorrhage
- Small for gestational age or intrauterine growth restriction (up to 16% in some reports after controlling for confounders)
- Vasa previa or velamentous insertion of the cord
- Premature rupture of membranes due to antepartum bleeding
- 5-10% of previas are associated with placenta accreta.
  - Placenta accreta encompasses various types of abnormal placentations in which chorionic villi attach directly to or invade the myometrium but do not cross the uterine serosa.
  - Placenta accreta affects approximately 1/2,500 pregnancies with increasing prevalence due to increased rates of cesarean section.
  - Risk greater with increasing number of cesarean deliveries
  - Associated with an increased risk of hemorrhage necessitating cesarean hysterectomy

DIAGNOSIS

HISTORY
- Painless bright red vaginal bleeding in 2nd or 3rd trimester (classic presentation)
- Contractions also may be present.
- Decreased fetal movement or nonreassuring fetal heart tracing

PHYSICAL EXAM

ALERT
- Do not perform digital cervical exam until placental position has been verified in any woman with a complaint of bleeding.
- Careful sterile speculum exam not contraindicated
- Check for vaginal or cervical source of bleeding.
- Check for ferning and Nitrazine testing for rupture of membranes.
- Perform cultures: Gonorrhea, *Chlamydia*, group B *Streptococcus*.

DIAGNOSTIC TESTS & INTERPRETATION
- If patient is Rh-negative, Kleihauer-Betke test for maternal–fetal hemorrhage to determine if Rho(D) immune globulin (RhoGAM) is needed
- Ultrasound to confirm presence of previa
- Rule out accreta, percreta if suspicious findings on ultrasound

- Fetal testing and monitoring during all active bleeding

Lab
Initial lab tests
- Maternal blood type and antibody screen
- Complete blood count (CBC): Normocytic, normochromic anemia with acute bleeding
- Prothrombin time (PT)/international normalization ratio (INR), and partial thromboplastin time (PTT): Coagulopathy is rare but may occur.
- Fibrinogen is optional and DIC panel is often inconclusive.
- Kleihauer-Betke test: Positive test indicates fetal–maternal transfusion may be present.
- Cross-match at least 4 units of packed red blood cells if bleeding ≥1 soaked pad/hour

Follow-Up & Special Considerations
Repeat hemoglobin/hematocrit determinations as needed to assess blood loss.

Imaging
Development of ultrasound, especially the transvaginal scan, has helped in the definitive diagnosis and management of placenta previa (2).

Initial approach
- External abdominal sonography with full, then empty bladder. Full bladder can cause compression of lower uterine segment causing a false appearance of previa.
- Careful assessment may still miss some posterior previas if fetal vertex is low.
- Vaginal probe sonography using 8.4 MHz transducer to further define placental position. Translabial ultrasound may also be utilized but may not be able to specifically discern characteristics of previas.
- Given increased risk of accreta, the placental-uterine interface should be closely examined for evidence of lakes or other abnormal vasculature
- MRI if concerned for placenta accreta without definitive ultrasound diagnosis; important also for surgical planning

Follow-Up & Special Considerations
- Previas found on ultrasound before 35 weeks should have a repeat ultrasound prior to delivery.
  - 12% of previas at 10–20 weeks persist until term.
  - 62% of previas at 28–31 weeks persist until term.
  - 75% of previas at 32–35 weeks persist until term.
- Anterior previas are more likely to resolve than posterior previas since the anterior lower uterine segment expands more quickly.

Pathological Findings
Placental pathology often shows giant trophoblasts at placental interface, evidence of abruption.

DIFFERENTIAL DIAGNOSIS
- Abruptio placentae
- Vasa previa
- Varicosities
- Vaginal and cervical pathology including erosion, cancer, trauma, or infections

TREATMENT

MEDICATION

First Line

- Oxygen supplementation if needed
- Aggressive IV fluids/blood products as needed: Fresh-frozen plasma, platelets, and packed red blood cells
- Tocolytics for uterine contractions may be used with caution, especially to allow for steroids for fetal lung maturity if possible (3)[A]. Calcium channel blockers such as nifedipine, loading dose of 10 mg p.o. every 20 minutes × 3, then every 4–6 hours:
  – Watch for placental hypoperfusion (nonreassuring fetal heart tracing).
  – Contraindications: Term fetus or unstable maternal or fetal cardiovascular status

Second Line

Alternative tocolytics:

- β-agonists such as terbutaline 0.25 mg SC every 3–4 hours; watch for maternal–fetal tachycardia and maternal hypertension and pulmonary edema.
- Magnesium sulfate 4–6 g IV load over 20 minutes, then 2–3 g/hour continuous infusion (4)[A]; watch for toxicity: loss of reflexes, pulmonary edema, cardiac arrest.
- Nifedipine 10 mg every 20 minutes × 3 doses loading dose and then every 4–8 hours depending on bleeding and contractions. Use dependent on maternal cardiovascular status as cannot administer if hypotensive

ADDITIONAL TREATMENT

General Measures

- Decrease physical activity to avoid bleeding.
- Avoid vaginal exams, sexual intercourse, douching, or other vaginal manipulation.
- If stable maternal–fetal status, delay delivery until 38 weeks (5)[C].
- Amniocentesis to determine fetal lung maturity for elective delivery <38 weeks
- A trial of labor may be considered with anterior previa >2 cm away from the cervix (6)[B].
- Transfuse platelets at <20,000 (or <50,000–100,000 depending on institutional guidelines prior to surgery).
- Blood volume is increased in pregnancy; patient can lose >30% maternal blood volume before shock develops.
- Central line placement as needed after checking coagulation studies
- With significant hemorrhage, Rh-negative women should receive 300 μg Rho(D) immune globulin (RhoGAM).

Issues for Referral

- Maternal–fetal medicine consult for delivery decisions regarding stable patients
- Neonatal ICU team should be alerted for high-risk delivery and consulted for preterm delivery.
- Appropriate interdisciplinary planning with blood bank, anesthesia, staff regarding plans if massive hemorrhage ensues intraoperatively or if unanticipated accreta encountered

Additional Therapies

Recombinant factor VII is an alternative blood product for disseminated intravascular coagulopathy when fresh-frozen plasma and cryoprecipitate fail (7)[C].

SURGERY/OTHER PROCEDURES

Cesarean delivery is indicated for partial or complete previa when fetal lung maturity is demonstrated or when patient becomes unstable secondary to blood loss prior to fetal maturity.

IN-PATIENT CONSIDERATIONS

Initial Stabilization

- Bed rest and NPO until delivery decision made
- 1 or 2 large-bore IV sites and IV fluids as needed for resuscitation
- Continuous fetal heart and contraction monitoring

Admission Criteria

- Heavy vaginal bleeding warrants inpatient observation at least until hemodynamically stable.
- 1st bleed usually is self-limited. Patients should be observed and steroids for fetal lung maturity administered. Once stable, preterm patients may be observed on an outpatient basis without difference in outcome (5)[B].
- Multiple large bleeds may necessitate admission until scheduled delivery between 34 and 36 weeks depending on institutional guidelines.
- May consider transfer to high-risk perinatology service based on patient condition, local services, and concern for accreta
- Evidence that shortened cervical length in the 3rd trimester is an independent risk factor for bleeding episodes (8)

IV Fluids

Lactated Ringer's or normal saline solution

Nursing

- Continuous fetal heart and contraction monitoring
- Frequent vital signs, including fluid intake and output

Discharge Criteria

- Demonstration of fetal well-being by fetal heart tracing or biophysical profile
- Demonstration of maternal hemodynamic stability: No active bleeding for >48 hours
- Proximity of patient to health care facility and patient reliability

ONGOING CARE

FOLLOW-UP RECOMMENDATIONS

- Repeat ultrasound of placenta location if last ultrasound was done at <37 weeks' gestational age.
- Placentas should be sent for pathologic evaluation.

DIET

No restrictions once stable; NPO if delivery possible

PATIENT EDUCATION

http://www.nlm.nih.gov/medlineplus/ency/article/000900.htm

PROGNOSIS

- Maternal death is rare with cesarean section (<1%).
- Greatest fetal risk is preterm delivery and consequences of hypoxemia if delay in delivery with fetal tracing abnormalities.
- Perinatal mortality is <10%.

COMPLICATIONS

- History of prior cesarean section and/or general anesthesia increases risk of needing a blood transfusion.
- Placenta accreta is associated with increased risk of hemorrhage and need for cesarean hysterectomy.
- Disseminated intravascular coagulation risk is low unless massive bleeding is present. Follow coagulation studies, and replenish FFP and clotting factors as needed .
- Fetal anemia and Rh isoimmunization

REFERENCES

1. Predanci M, et al. A sonographic assessment of different patterns of placenta previa 'migration' in the third trimester of pregnancy. *J Ultrasound Med* 2005;24:773.
2. Sinha P, Kuruba N. Ante-partum haemorrhage: an update. *J Obstet Gynaecol*. 2008;28:377–81.
3. Sharma A, Suri V, Gupta I. Tocolytic therapy in conservative management of symptomatic placenta previa. *Int J Gynaecol Obstet*. 2004;84:109–13.
4. Briggs GG, Wan SR. Drug therapy during labor and delivery, part 2 [Review]. *Am J of Health-System Pharm*. 2006;63(12):1131–9.
5. Oyelese Y, Smulian JC. Placenta previa, placenta accreta, and vasa previa. *Obstet Gynecol*. 2006; 107:927–41.
6. Bhide A, Prefumo F, Moore J, et al. Placental edge to internal os distance in the late third trimester and mode of delivery in placenta praevia. *BJOG*. 2003;110:860–4.
7. Alfirevic Z, Elbourne D, Pavord S, et al. Use of recombinant activated factor VII in primary postpartum hemorrhage: the Northern European registry 2000–2004. *Obstet Gynecol*. 2007;110: 1270–8.
8. Stafford IA, Dashe JS, Shivvers SA, et al. Ultrasonographic cervical length and risk of hemorrhage in pregnancies with placenta previa. *Obstet Gynecol*. 2010;116:595–600.

See Also (Topic, Algorithm, Electronic Media Element)
Abruptio Placentae

CODES

ICD9

- 641.03 Placenta previa without hemorrhage, antepartum
- 641.13 Hemorrhage from placenta previa, antepartum

CLINICAL PEARLS

- Placenta previa is a major cause of antepartum bleeding in the 2nd and 3rd trimesters.
- Do *not* perform digital cervical exam, only careful speculum exam.
- Ultrasound, both transvaginal and transabdominal, is used to verify placenta location and diagnosis.
- Delivery is by cesarean section with rare exceptions.

PLAGUE

Douglas W. MacPherson, MD, MSc(CTM)

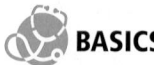 **BASICS**

Plague, one of the great scourges of humankind, is now relegated to a historical footnote for most developed countries in terms of both clinical frequency of cases and public health requirements. Except for small areas of the Southwest, endemic plague and transmission to human beings are rare clinical events in the US. Plague and plague outbreaks still occur in some less economically developed regions of the world. The risk of a clinical case being imported into the US by mobile populations or by malfeasant intent remains a public health security consideration.

DESCRIPTION
- Acute infection due to *Y. pestis*
- Sporadic limited geographic distribution, especially in a few economically developing nations
- In the Americas, southwestern US and Peru report a few cases annually.
- Epidemics associated with war, famine, and natural disaster
- Disease of rats and other small vertebrates
- Transmitted to humans by rat or human flea bite
- Occasional transmission to humans who handle infected tissues
- Occasional human–human transmission by pulmonary secretions
- Recently shown that infected cats may transmit disease to humans by biting, licking, or scratching
- *Y. pestis*, the infective pathogen, has been described as a potential bioweapon (1)[C].
- System(s) affected: Hematologic/Lymphatic/Immunologic; Pulmonary; Skin/Exocrine; generalized sepsis
- Synonym: Black death

EPIDEMIOLOGY
Predominant sex: Male = Female.

Incidence
- Few cases (recently <10) reported annually in the US; typically sporadic cases in rural areas of the Southwest, usually in the spring, summer, or fall
- World Health Organization (WHO) reports 1,000–3,000 cases per year.
- US has a 14% mortality rate.

RISK FACTORS
Endemic or epidemic focus and:
- Exposure to rats or fleas
- Close contact with infected cat
- Close contact with pneumonic plague patient
- Plague bacillus in laboratory
- Hunters who skin wild animals
- Potential agent of bioterrorism
- Occupational risk: Field workers, animal researchers, and others exposed in endemic regions

GENERAL PREVENTION
- Avoid contact with vectors, infected tissue, or aerosol droplets (e.g., confirmed pneumonic plague case).
- Killed vaccine for people at high risk to reduce risk and/or severity; tetracycline prophylaxis. Vaccine may be requested from Centers for Disease Control, Atlanta, GA.

PATHOPHYSIOLOGY
The pathophysiology of plague infection and the resulting disease (e.g., bubonic, pneumonic, or septicemic) syndrome are determined by complex host–infectious agent interactive determinants. The clinical outcome depends on early clinical suspicion and specific therapeutic interventions, including supportive care and public health control measures.

ETIOLOGY
- *Y. pestis*, transmitted by bite of a flea from an infected rodent; secondary contact through other infected animal or human
- Untreated bubonic plague may progress to secondary pneumonic strain, which can be transmitted by contaminated respiratory droplets.
- Pneumonic plague and the other plague syndromes, such as septicemic plague, are rare and usually are a fatal consequence of plague infection.

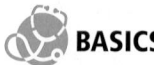 **DIAGNOSIS**

- Due to the rarity of plague in most regions of North America, a high level of clinical suspicion is required to consider the diagnosis.
- The clinical presentation, history of illness, and exposure are essential antecedents to a diagnosis of plague.
- When plague is either clinically suspect or preliminary laboratory diagnostic results raise the possibility of *Y. pestis* infection, clinical infection control, laboratory precautions (including the use of an appropriate level of biosafety), and public health management practices must be implemented.

HISTORY
Exposure in known endemic zone or epidemic focus with animal (rat, cat, dog) or flea contact

PHYSICAL EXAM
- Bubonic plague:
  - Acute onset after 2–8 days' incubation
  - Fever
  - Chills
  - Weakness
  - Headache
  - Bubo: Painful, tender enlargement of regional lymph node(s) that ruptures and drains. Overlying edema. Typically, absence of overlying skin lesion, ascending lymphangitis.
  - Skin lesions: Rarely pustules, vesicles in area of flea bite(s), purpura

- Septicemic plague:
  - Features of bubonic plague
  - Occasional occurrence without bubo
  - Hypotension
  - Hepatosplenomegaly
  - Delirium
  - Seizures in children
  - Shock
- Secondary pneumonic plague:
  - Features of bubonic and septicemic plague
  - Cough
  - Chest pain
  - Hemoptysis
- Primary pneumonic plague:
  - Acute onset within hours to 1 day after inhalation of infective bacteria
  - Fever
  - Chills
  - Cough
  - Chest pain
  - Dyspnea
  - Hemoptysis
  - Lethargy
  - Hypotension
  - Shock

DIAGNOSTIC TESTS & INTERPRETATION
When a case of plague is clinically suspect, care givers and other personnel (e.g., phlebotomists, laboratory staff) should be alerted and personal protection precautions implemented as necessary. Attempts to isolate and characterize the bacillus in the laboratory must be done under the appropriate conditions and precautions.

Lab
- Elevated leukocyte count, predominantly mature and immature neutrophils; sometimes leukemoid reaction
- Measure platelets: With low platelet number, evidence of disseminated intravascular coagulation may be seen.
- Stained smears of aspirate of bubo, sputum, and peripheral blood reveal gram-negative coccobacilli with bipolar staining, so-called safety-pin appearance.
- Aspirate, blood, and sputum cultures (e.g., infusion broth, blood, and MacConkey agar) grow typical bacteria. Public health authorities arrange definitive identification and serologic follow-up.
- Drugs that may alter lab results:
  - Antibiotics: Prior use

Imaging
Chest x-ray: Patchy or confluent pulmonary consolidation in pneumonic plague

Pathological Findings
Acute lymphadenitis with inflammation dominated by neutrophils, necrosis, masses of plague bacilli, seropurulent pericarditis

DIFFERENTIAL DIAGNOSIS
Other causes of fulminant bacteremia, pneumococcal sepsis, meningococcemia; other causes of acute suppurative lymphadenitis (bubo) or rapidly progressive pneumonitis

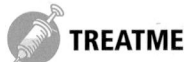

TREATMENT

- Clinical treatment includes specific antimicrobial drugs and supportive care.
- Infection-control practices and public health management are also appropriate when a clinical or laboratory diagnosis of plague is considered or is confirmed.

MEDICATION
First Line
- Aminoglycoside: Gentamicin 5.1 mg/kg/d or streptomycin 15 mg/kg IV
- If condition allows, oral medication: Tetracycline 25–50 mg/kg/d equally divided q6h for 10 days
- For meningitis: IV chloramphenicol 25 mg/kg loading dose, followed by 60 mg/kg/d in divided doses q6h for 10 days
- Fluoroquinolones (e.g., levofloxacin, ofloxacin) and 3rd-generation cephalosporins (e.g., cefotaxime) also may be effective.
- Contraindications:
  - Tetracycline: Contraindicated in pregnancy and patients <8 years of age
- Precautions:
  - Reduce dose of aminoglycoside with finding of renal impairment.
  - Pregnant women and those with hearing disorders (e.g., aminoglycosides)
  - Chloramphenicol associated with hematologic toxicity

Second Line
No other drugs have been demonstrated to be as effective or any less toxic.

ADDITIONAL TREATMENT
General Measures
- Do not create aerosol droplets.
- Handle blood and bubo aspirate with gloves.
- Notify laboratory to take precautions.
- Hot, moist compresses for buboes

Issues for Referral
Plague is a notifiable condition to public health authorities in most health jurisdictions. National public health authorities may follow the requirements of the International Health Regulations (WHO, 2005) for notification and reporting.

Additional Therapies
As required

IN-PATIENT CONSIDERATIONS
Bubonic and septicemic plague syndromes are not transmissible person to person directly. Transmission through the bite of the flea vector can occur. Pneumonic plague is potentially transmissible via respiratory droplet spread, and respiratory isolation is appropriate in this situation.

Initial Stabilization
- Hospitalization: For suspected pneumonic plague, patients should undergo respiratory isolation until 48 h of initial effective therapy or after sputum test provides negative result.
- Notify public health authorities.
- Early initiation of appropriate antimicrobial treatment and diagnostic testing is essential for suspected cases of plague.

Admission Criteria
- Admission should be considered in all patients of suspected plague, except in widespread outbreaks when community-based care of bubonic patients may be necessary to focus limited health care management resources for hospitalization on the most severely ill.
- In an outbreak situation, public health management and interventions for control are essential.

 # ONGOING CARE

FOLLOW-UP RECOMMENDATIONS
Bed rest until convalescent

Patient Monitoring
- Complete blood chemistry for hematologic toxicity of chloramphenicol
- Aminoglycoside blood levels, if indicated
- Clinical testing for antibiotic toxicity, if indicated

DIET
As tolerated during recovery

PATIENT EDUCATION
- Avoid contact with wild animals in endemic plague areas.
- Reduce rat and flea population in immediate human environment.
- During epidemics, rodent die-off may occur, increasing flea–human contact.
- Flea vector management is essential for epidemic control of plague.

PROGNOSIS
- Untreated plague mortality >50%; 100% in primary pneumonic plague
- Plague may be fulminant (e.g., exposure, 1st symptoms, and death in 1 day in primary pneumonic plague). Must *not* delay the treatment of suspected cases until laboratory-confirmed diagnosis. Delay of initial therapy beyond 24 h of onset of primary pneumonic plague regularly leads to death.

COMPLICATIONS
- Progression of bubonic form to septicemic and pneumonic forms
- Necrosis of bubo may require aspiration or incision and drainage.
- Pericarditis
- Acute respiratory distress syndrome
- Meningitis
- Death

REFERENCE
1. Hepburn MJ, et al. Pathogenesis and sepsis caused by organisms potentially utilized as biologic weapons: Opportunities for targeted intervention. *Current Drug Targets*. 2007;8:519–32. Human plague: review of regional morbidity and mortality, 2004-2009. *Wkly Epidemiol Rec*. 2009;85(6): 40–5.

ADDITIONAL READING
- Alvarez ML, Cardineau GA et al. Prevention of bubonic and pneumonic plague using plant-derived vaccines. *Biotechnol Adv*. 2010;28:184-96.
- Centers for Disease Control and Prevention. Emergency Preparedness and Response. Plague Informatiion. Available at: http://www.bt.cdc.gov/ agent/plague/index.asp Accessed April 1, 2009.
- Centers for Disease Control and Prevention. Infectious Diseaes Information: Plague Homepage Available at: http://www.cdc.gov/ncidod/ dvbid/plague/index.htm Accessed April 1, 2009.
- Feodorova VA, Corbel MJ et al. Prospects for new plague vaccines. *Expert Rev Vaccines*. 2009; 8: 1721- 38.
- Frean JA, et al. In vitro activities of 14 antibiotics against 100 human isolates of *Yersinia pestis* from a southern African plague focus. *Antimicrob Agents Chemother*. 1996;40:2646–7.
- Prentice MB et al. Plague. *Lancet*. 2007;369: 1196–207.

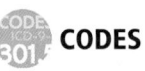 # CODES

ICD9
- 020.0 Bubonic plague
- 020.1 Cellulocutaneous plague
- 020.2 Septicemic plague

CLINICAL PEARLS
- Plague should be considered in any exposed person, including febrile travelers who may have traveled to endemic and epidemic regions in the US and abroad.
- Routine blood cultures will detect *Y. pestis*, but alert the laboratory to your clinical suspicions.
- Vaccination against plague does not exclude the diagnosis.

PLANTAR FASCIITIS

Alan Williamson, MD
Benjamin Kohnen, MD

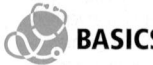 BASICS

DESCRIPTION
- Degenerative change of plantar fascia at origin from medial tuberosity of calcaneus
- Pain on plantar surface, usually at calcaneal insertion of plantar fascia upon weight-bearing, especially in morning

EPIDEMIOLOGY
Prevalence
- Lifetime: 10–15% of population
- Data suggest persistence with BMI >30.
- Condition is self-limiting; most resolve within 10 months.

RISK FACTORS
- Dancers, runners, aerobic exercisers
- Obesity
- Pes planus (flat feet)
- Systemic connective tissue disorders
- Occupations with prolonged standing especially on hard surfaces

GENERAL PREVENTION
- Maintain normal body weight. Higher prevalence with BMI >30 (1)
- Avoid prolonged bare feet, sandals, or slippers.

PATHOPHYSIOLOGY
- Repetitive partial tearing of plantar fascia
- Chronic degenerative change (-osis/opathy rather than -itis) of plantar fascia generally at insertion on medial tuberosity of calcaneus

ETIOLOGY
- Excessive pronation
- Decreased ankle range of motion in dorsiflexion (tight heel chord)

COMMONLY ASSOCIATED CONDITIONS
- Usually isolated
- Heel spurs common but not marker of severity
- Posterior tibial neuropathy

DIAGNOSIS

HISTORY
- Pain on plantar surface of foot, usually at fascial insertion at calcaneus but can have pain anywhere along length of plantar fascia:
  - Worse on arising from sleep-first few steps in the morning; after prolonged sitting
- Pain with prolonged ambulation or standing
- Limp with excessive toe walking
- Numbness and burning of medial hindfoot when associated with posterior tibial nerve compression

PHYSICAL EXAM
- Point tenderness on medial tuberosity of calcaneus at insertion of plantar fascia
- Pain along plantar fascia with foot dorsiflexion
- Decreased passive range of motion in dorsiflexion of ankle
- Spasm in foot muscles that compensate for injury

DIAGNOSTIC TESTS & INTERPRETATION
Imaging
- 2 radiographic views of foot to rule out fracture, prefer weight-bearing-usually not necessary for diagnosis
- Ultrasound (US): Signs of inflammation at insertion, including thickened plantar fascia (4mm)—not necessary for diagnosis
- Consider MRI for complex conditions or if concerned about other etiologies.

DIFFERENTIAL DIAGNOSIS
- From most to least common:
  - Posterior tibial nerve compression (also known as tarsal tunnel syndrome) diagnosed if compression of region between medial malleolus and calcaneous results in numbness in first 3 toes
  - Painful or atrophic heel pad
  - Tendonitis of posterior tibialis
  - Calcaneal stress fracture
  - Pain from neoplasm or infection
  - Spondyloarthropathy
- In association with connective tissue disorder:
  - RA
  - Polymyositis

TREATMENT

Nonoperative management is mainstay of treatment

MEDICATION
NSAIDs (2)

ADDITIONAL TREATMENT
General Measures
- Supportive footwear with stable midfoot
- Relative rest/Activity modification
- Ice (frozen water bottle roll)
- Massage (golf ball roll)
- Weight reduction
- Stretching
  - Plantar fascial stretches more effective than Achilles tendon stretches (3)[B]

Issues for Referral
- Consider referral for more invasive treatments if conservative measures (stretching, icing, massage, NSAIDs, OTC orthotics, night splints) fail after 3–6 months
- Podiatry
- Custom orthotics
- Physical therapy
- Surgical intervention

Additional Therapies
- Taping (4)[B]:
  - Low-dye taping
  - Calcaneal taping more effective than stretching
- Night splints
- Corticosteroid injections (5)[B]:
  - Short-term pain relief
  - Recommend ultrasound guidance.
  - Risk for calcaneal fat pad atrophy with resultant permanent heel pain
- Orthotics (6)[B]:
  - Custom orthotics show no benefit over prefabricated orthotics.
  - Benefit limited to improved function; no benefit in pain
  - Improved effectiveness of night splints when used in association with orthotics

COMPLEMENTARY AND ALTERNATIVE MEDICINE

- Extracorporeal shock wave therapy (ESWT) of unclear benefit in large trials (7,8,9)[B]:
  – Newer ESWT devices show more promise.
  – Randomized trial demonstrated reduction in pain after 3 months compared with placebo.
  – Randomized trial in 2006 showed improvement in walking 3 months following a single treatment
  – Randomized trial in 2009 showed improvement in pain at 12 weeks and 12 months compared with placebo
  – Majority of studies focused on chronic plantar fasciitis
  – Uncomfortable to patients
- Botulinum toxin injection (10)[B]:
  – RCT demonstrated improvement in pain and gait at 3 weeks and 3 months compared with placebo
- Some orthopedic surgeons prefer casting in severe cases.
- Heel cup with magnet has proven ineffective.
- Promising therapies [I]:
  – Platelet-rich plasma injections
  – Intralesional autologous blood injection
  – Intracorporeal pneumatic shock application
  – Low level laser therapy (LLLT)

SURGERY/OTHER PROCEDURES

- Only necessary in a small percentage of patients
- Recommended after resistance to conservative treatment of 6–12 months
- Open/endoscopic plantar fasciotomy
- Calcaneal spur resection
- More likely in severely obese

ONGOING CARE

FOLLOW-UP RECOMMENDATIONS
- Modified rest may help.
- Stretching exercises
- Following 6 weeks of conservative treatment, consider formal physical therapy program if conservative measures do not show improvement.

PATIENT EDUCATION
- Weight reduction
- Gently rise from sitting to standing on arising from bed or prolonged sitting, followed by stretching.
- Ice the foot using a frozen water bottle, rolling foot over bottle for 10 minutes in morning and after work.
- Massage plantar fascia by rolling foot over a golf ball.

- Grab cloth or carpet by plantar flexing of toes.
- Stretch plantar fascia by pulling toes into dorsiflexion.
- For athletes, back off on repetitive stress.
- Taping may help athletes.
- Video overview for patients: http://www.youtube.com/watch?v=Pnithn4EYQk

PROGNOSIS
- Excellent
- Self-limited condition in up to 90% of patients

COMPLICATIONS
- Rupture of plantar fascia
- Chronic pain
- Gait abnormality

REFERENCES

1. Rano JA, et al. Correlation of heel pain with body mass index and other characteristics of heel pain. *J Foot Ankl Surg*. 2001;40(6):351–6.
2. Donley BG, Moore T, Sferra J, et al. The efficacy of oral nonsteroidal anti-inflammatory medication (NSAID) in the treatment of plantar fasciitis: a randomized, prospective, placebo-controlled study. *Foot Ankle Int*. 2007;28:20–23.
3. Digiovanni BF, Nawoczenski DA, Malay DP, et al. Plantar fascia-specific stretching exercise improves outcomes in patients with chronic plantar fasciitis. A prospective clinical trial with two-year follow-up. *J Bone Joint Surg Am*. 2006;88:1775–81.
4. Speksnijder C, van de Water A. Efficacy of Taping for the Treatment of Plantar Fasciosis. A Systematic Review of Controlled Trials. *Journal of the American Podiatric Medical Association*. 2010;100(1):41–51.
5. Thomas J, Christensen J, Kravitz S, et al. The Diagnosis and Treatment of Heel Pain: A Clinical Practice Guideline—Revision 2010. *J Foot Ankl Surg*. 2010;49:S1–S19.
6. Burns J, du Toit V, Hawke F, et al. Custom-made foot orthoses for the treatment of foot pain. *Cochrane Database Sys Rev*. 2008;(3):CD006801.
7. Furia J, Maffulli N, Rompe J, et al. Shock wave therapy for chronic plantar fasciopathy. *British Medical Bulletin*. 2007;81/82:183–208.
8. Ibrahim M, Donatelli R, Schmitz C, et al. Chronic Plantar Fasciitis Treated with Two Sessions of Radial Extracorporeal Shock Wave Therapy. *Foot Ankle Int*. 2010;31(5):391–397.
9. Gollwitzer H, Diehl P, von Korff A, et al. Extracorporeal shock wave therapy for chronic painful heel syndrome: a prospective, double blind, randomized trial assessing the efficacy of a new electromagnetic shock wave device. *J Foot Ankle Surg*. 2007;46:348–357.
10. Huang YC, Wei SH, Wang HK, et al. Ultrasonographic guided botulinum toxin type A treatment for plantar fasciitis: an outcome-based investigation for treating pain and gait changes. *J Rehab Med*. 2010;42(2):136–40.

ADDITIONAL READING

- Crawford F, et al. Interventions for treating plantar heel pain. *Cochrane Database Sys Rev*. 2006;1: CD000416.
- Dogramaci Y, Emir A, Gokce A. Intracorporeal pneumatic shock application for the treatment of chronic plantar fasciitis: a randomized, double blind prospective clinical trial. *Archives of Orthopaedic and Trauma Surgery*. 2009;130(4):541–546.
- Kiritsi O, Tsitas K, Malliaropoulos N, et al. Ultrasonographic evaluation of plantar fasciitis after low-level laser therapy: results of a double-blind, randomized, placebo-controlled trial. *Lasers Med Sci*. 2010;25:275–281.
- Lee T, Ahmad T. Intralesional Autologous Blood Injection Compared to Corticosteroid Injection for Treatment fo Chronic Plantar Fasciitis. A Prospective, Randomized, Controlled Trial. *Foot Ankle Int*. 2007;28(9):984–990.

See Also (Topic, Algorithm, Electronic Media Element)
Algorithm: Heel Pain

CODES

ICD9
728.71 Plantar fascial fibromatosis

CLINICAL PEARLS

- Degeneration of plantar fascia at origin from plantar tuberosity of calcaneum
- Pain on plantar surface on weight-bearing, especially in morning
- Wear supportive footwear, particularly rigid shoes to help avoid excess pronation.
- Arch supports and/or athletic taping may be of benefit
- Activity modification
- Ice (frozen water bottle roll)
- Massage (golf ball roll)
- Weight reduction

PLEURAL EFFUSION

Felix B. Chang, MD
Mouhanad Ayach, MD

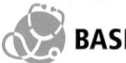

BASICS

A pleural effusion is an abnormal accumulation of fluid in the pleural space.

DESCRIPTION
- Pneumonia (25%), malignancy (15%), and pulmonary embolism (10%) account for most exudative effusions.
- Malignant: Primary carcinoma of the lung and metastases of breast, ovary, and lymphoma constitute ~75–80% of malignant effusions.

EPIDEMIOLOGY
Incidence
Estimated 1.3 million cases/year in US; congestive heart failure (CHF), 500,000; pneumonia, 300,000; malignancy, 200,000; pulmonary embolus, 150,000; cirrhosis with ascites, 150,000; tuberculosis, 2,500; pancreatitis, 20,000; and collagen-vascular disease, 6,000 (1)

Prevalence
- Estimated 320 cases/1 million people in industrialized countries
- No gender predilection: About 2/3 of malignant pleural effusions occur in women.
- The prevalence of pleural effusion in hospitalized patients with AIDS is 7-27%.

RISK FACTORS
- Occupational exposure
- Drugs
- Risk factors for pulmonary embolism (PE) and tuberculosis (TB)
- Opportunistic infections of the pleura should be considered in HIV patients when the CD4 count is <150 cells/μL.

PATHOPHYSIOLOGY
- Pleural fluid formation exceeds pleural fluid absorption. Transudates result from imbalances in hydrostatic and oncotic forces.
- Increase in hydrostatic and/or low oncotic pressures
- Increase in pleural capillary permeability
- Lymphatic obstruction or impaired drainage
- Movement of fluid from the peritoneal or retroperitoneal space

ETIOLOGY
- Transudates:
  – CHF: 40% of transudative effusions; 80% bilateral
  – Constrictive pericarditis, atelectasis
  – Cirrhosis (hepatic hydrothorax): 2/3 right side
  – Nephrotic syndrome, hypoalbuminemia
  – Trapped lung, peritoneal dialysis
  – Myxedema, superior vena cava obstruction
  – Urinothorax, central line misplacement
  – Peritoneal dialysis
- Exudates:
  – Lung parenchyma infection, bacterial: Parapneumonic, tuberculous pleurisy, fungal, viral
  – Parasitic (amebiasis, *Echinococcus*)
  – Malignancy: Lung cancer, metastases (breast, lymphoma, ovaries), mesothelioma
  – Pulmonary embolism (although 25% of PEs are transudate)
  – Collagen-vascular disease: Rheumatoid arthritis, systemic lupus erythematosus (SLE), Wegener granulomatosis, sarcoidosis
  – GI: Pancreatitis, esophageal rupture, abdominal abscess, after liver transplant
  – Chylothorax: Thoracic duct tear, malignancy
  – Hemothorax: Trauma, PE, malignancy, coagulopathy, aortic aneurysm
  – Others: After coronary artery bypass grafting (CABG); Dressler syndrome: pericarditis and pleuritis after myocardial infarction (MI); uremia, asbestos exposure, radiation; drug-induced: nitrofurantoin, bromocriptine, amiodarone, procarbazine, methysergide, hydralazine, procainamide, quinidine, methotrexate, and methysergide; Meigs syndrome: benign ovarian tumor, ascites, and pleural effusion; yellow-nail syndrome: yellow nails, lymphedema, pleural effusion, and bronchiectasis; atelectasis, cholesterol effusion; ovarian stimulation syndrome; lymphangiomatosis; acute respiratory distress syndrome

COMMONLY ASSOCIATED CONDITIONS
Hypoproteinemia

DIAGNOSIS

Presumptive diagnosis based on clinical impression in 50%

Small pleural effusions are asymptomatic

HISTORY
- The degree of dyspnea is related to the associated lung disease, respiratory function, and the size of the pleural effusion.
- Fever, malaise, and weight loss with empyema; chest pain, either constant or pleuritic; nonproductive or purulent cough, hemoptysis

PHYSICAL EXAM
When pleural effusion >300 mL:
- General: No voice transmission; tachypnea; asymmetric expansion of the thoracic cage; mediastinal shift (>1,000 mL)
- Pulmonary: Decreased or inaudible breath sounds; dullness to percussion; decreased or absent tactile fremitus; egophony; pleural friction rub

DIAGNOSTIC TESTS & INTERPRETATION
Lab
Initial lab tests
- Pleural fluid: Appearance, pH, white blood cell (WBC) differential, total protein, lactate dehydrogenase (LDH), glucose, Gram stain and culture, acid-fast bacilli staining
- By clinical scenario: Amylase, triglycerides, cholesterol, LE cells, cytology, antinuclear antibodies (ANAs), adenosine deaminase, tumor markers, rheumatoid factor, cytology
- Transudate vs exudate
  – Light criteria for exudate: 98% sensitivity, 80% specificity (2)[B]:
    ○ Ratio of pleural fluid/serum protein levels >0.5
    ○ Ratio of pleural fluid/serum LDH levels >0.6
    ○ Pleural fluid LDH level >2/3 the upper limit for serum LDH level
  – Exudate criteria:
    ○ Serum-effusion albumin gradient ≤1.2; sensitivity 87%, specificity 92% (3)[B]

○ Cholesterol effusion >45 mg/dL and LDH effusion >200 mg/dL; sensitivity 90%, specificity 98%

Follow-Up & Special Considerations
- 75% of patients with exudative effusions have a non-CHF cause.
- 30% cases of pleural effusion in AIDS patients are due to bacterial pneumonia.

Imaging
Initial approach
- Chest X-ray (CXR): Posteroanterior–anteroposterior (PA-AP) views
- A concave meniscus in the costophrenic angle on an upright CXR suggests >250 mL of pleural fluid; homogeneous opacity and diffuse haziness, visibility of pulmonary vessels through the haziness, and an absence of air bronchogram; 75 mL of fluid will obliterate the posterior costophrenic sulcus.
- Lateral X-rays show blunting of the posterior costophrenic angle and the posterior gutter when as little as 175–200 mL of fluid is present. Decubitus X-rays to exclude a loculated effusion and underlying pulmonary lesion or pulmonary thickening; can depict as little as 5–10 mL of fluid
- Supine X-rays show costophrenic blunting, haziness, obliteration of the diaphragmatic silhouette, decreased visibility of the lower lobe vasculature, widened minor fissure
- Ultrasonography (US): Detects as little as 5–50 mL of pleural fluid; identifies loculated effusions; useful to determine site for thoracocentesis, pleural biopsy, or pleural drainage
- Chest CT scan with contrast material in patients with undiagnosed pleural effusion: For early-stage pleural abnormalities, multiple loculations, pleural thickening, cystic vs solid lesions, nodules, masses, or round atelectasis, benign vs malignant pleural involvement or invasion
- CT pulmonary angiography if PE is suspected
- Positron-emission tomographic (PET)/CT scan: Focal increased uptake of 18-fluorodeoxyglugose (FDG) in the pleura and the presence of solid pleural abnormalities on CT scan are suggestive of malignant pleural disease. A negative PET/CT scan favors a benign cause.

Follow-Up & Special Considerations
Observation in uncomplicated asymptomatic patients (i.e., CHF, cirrhosis), viral pleurisy, thoracic or abdominal surgery

Diagnostic Procedures/Surgery
Diagnostic thoracentesis: Clinically significant pleural effusion (>10 mm thick on US or lateral decubitus x-ray with no known cause); CHF: Asymmetric effusion, fever, chest pain, or failure to resolve after diuretics; parapneumonic effusions

DIFFERENTIAL DIAGNOSIS
- Empyema: Pus, putrid odor; culture; a putrid odor suggest an anaerobic empyema: LDH levels >1,000 IU/L (normal serum = 200 IU/L); glucose <60 mg/dL; low pH
- Malignancy: Cytology, red, bloody; glucose normal to low depending of the tumor burden; red blood cells (RBCs) >100,000/mm^3
- Lupus pleuritis: LE cells present; pleural fluid serum ANAs >1.0; glucose <60 mg/dL; pleural fluid/serum glucose ratio <0.5

- Fungal: Positive KOH, culture; peritoneal dialysis: protein <1 g/dL; glucose 300–400 mg/dL
- Urinothorax: Creatinine pleural/blood >0.5; high LDH pleural fluid with low protein levels
- Hemothorax: Hematocrit pleural/blood >0.5; benign asbestos effusion: unilateral, exudative; 1/3 have an elevated eosinophil count.
- TB pleuritis: Lymphocytes >80% predominance effusion; elevated levels of adenosine deaminase >50 units/L and interferon-γ >140 pg/mL; positive AFB stain, culture; total protein >4 g/dL
- Chylothorax: Milky; triglycerides >110 mg/dL; lipoprotein electrophoresis (chylomicrons)
- Amebic liver abscess: Anchovy paste effusion; Waldenström macroglobulinemia and multiple myeloma: protein >7 g/dL
- Esophageal rupture: High salivary amylase; pleural fluid acidosis, pH <6.0; amylase-rich: acute pancreatitis, chronic pancreatic pleural effusion, malignancy, esophageal rupture; rheumatoid pleurisy: glucose <60 mg/dL; pleural fluid/serum glucose <0.5
- Pleural fluid lymphocytosis: Tuberculous pleurisy, lymphoma, sarcoidosis, chronic rheumatoid pleurisy, yellow-nail syndrome, or chylothorax (80–95% of the nucleated cells):
  - Carcinomatosis in 1/2 of cases (50–70% lymphocyte percentage)
  - Pleural fluid eosinophilia (>10% of total nucleated cells): Pneumothorax, hemothorax, malignancy (carcinoma, lymphoma), drugs, fungal (coccidiomycosis, cryptococcosis, histoplasmosis), benign asbestos pleural effusion, pulmonary infarction
  - Low glucose (<60 mg/dL): TB, malignancy, rheumatoid pleurisy, complicated parapneumonic effusion, empyema, hemothorax, paragonimiasis, Churg-Strauss syndrome
  - RBC count >100,000/mm^3: Trauma, malignancy, PE, injury after cardiac surgery, asbestos pleurisy, pancreatitis, TB
  - Pleural fluid LDH >1,000 IU/L: Suggests empyema, malignant effusion, rheumatoid effusion, or pleural paragonimiasis
  - pH >7.3: Rheumatoid pleurisy, empyema, malignant effusion, TB, esophageal rupture, or lupus nephritis
  - Mesothelial cells in exudates: TB is unlikely if there are more than 5% of mesothelial cells.
- *Streptococcus pneumoniae* accounts for 50% of cases of parapneumonic effusions in AIDS patients, follow by *Staphylococcus aureus, Haemophilus influenzae, Mycoplasma pneumoniae, Legionella, Nocardia asteroides,* and *Bordetella bronchiseptica*. The fluid is usually an exudate with a low count of nucleated cells.
- *Pneumocystis jiroveci* is an uncommon cause of pleural effusion in HIV patients. Usually it is a small effusion, unilateral or bilateral, that is serous to bloody in appearance. Demonstration of the trophozoite or cyst is mandatory.
- Less common pathogens involved in HIV pleural effusion patients are *Mycobacterium, Toxoplasma, Histoplasma capsulatum, Cryptococcus,* and *Leishmania*.
- Cancer-related HIV pleural effusion: Kaposi sarcoma, multicentric Castleman disease, and primary effusion lymphoma.
- Kaposi sarcoma: Mononuclear predominance, exudate, pH >7.4, LDH 111–330 IU/L, glucose >60 mg/dL

 TREATMENT

Support with oxygen and arterial blood gas determinations (ABCs).

MEDICATION
Therapy for breast, lymphoma, ovarian, prostate, and small cell lung cancer may control the effusion.

First Line
- CHF: Diuretics (75% clearing in 48 h)
- Parapneumonic effusion: Antibiotics
- For rheumatologic and inflammatory causes: Steroids and nonsteroidal anti-inflammatory drugs (NSAIDs)

Second Line
Symptomatic nonmalignant effusions that are refractory to treatment may be managed with repeated therapeutic thoracentesis or pleurodesis.

ADDITIONAL TREATMENT
General Measures
- Therapeutic thoracentesis if symptomatic
- Chest tube thoracostomy drainage: Indications: >1/2 hemithorax; complicated parapneumonic effusion (positive Gram stain or culture, pH <7.2, or glucose <60 mg/dL); empyema; hemothorax
- The recommended limit is 1,000–1,500 mL in a single thoracentesis procedure.

Issues for Referral
- Uncertain etiology; thoracentesis technically difficult; high-risk diagnostic thoracentesis; malignant effusion; decortication
- Video-assisted thoracoscopy for sclerosis
- Peritoneal shunts for symptomatic recurrence

Additional Therapies
- Pleurodesis for symptomatic patients whose pleural effusion reaccumulates too quickly for repeat therapeutic thoracentesis (4)
- Sclerosing agents for malignant effusions: Doxycycline, bleomycin, talc, and minocycline; talc is more efficacious. The relative risk (RR) of nonrecurrent effusion was 1.34 (95% confidence interval 1.16–1.55) in favor of talc compared with bleomycin, tetracycline, or mustine (4)[A].

SURGERY/OTHER PROCEDURES
- Percutaneous pleural biopsy if cause is not clear after thoracentesis:
  - Close pleural biopsy: When the pleura is diffusely involved (TB pleuritis, noncaseating granulomata in rheumatoid pleuritis)
  - CT-guided needle biopsy: Pleural mass
  - Video-assisted thoracoscopic pleural biopsy: Negative percutaneous biopsy, patchy disease, or CT scan does not show obvious mass
- Open pleural biopsy by thoracotomy
- Contraindications for thoracocentesis: Anticoagulation, bleeding diathesis, thrombocytopenia <20,000/mm^3, mechanical ventilation
- Bronchoscopy: When endobronchial malignancy is likely; suggested by a pulmonary infiltrate or a mass on the CXR or CT scan, hemoptysis, massive pleural effusion, or shift of the mediastinum toward the side of the effusion

IN-PATIENT CONSIDERATIONS
Initial Stabilization
Treat underlying medical disorder.

 ONGOING CARE

FOLLOW-UP RECOMMENDATIONS
Patient Monitoring
Record the amount and quality of fluid drained, and monitor for an air leak (bubbling). Repeat CXR when drainage decreases to <100 mL/d to evaluate complete clearing. For a large effusion, reevaluate catheter position; if positioned appropriately, consider fibrinolytics (e.g., urokinase, streptokinase, alteplase) through the chest tube to break up clots that may be obstructing drainage.

DIET
Cardiac diet in patients with heart failure; correct hypoproteinemia.

PROGNOSIS
Varies according to underlying condition:
- Malignant effusion: Poor prognosis; parapneumonic effusions may lead to constrictive fibrosis.
- Patients with low-pH malignant effusion have a shorter survival and poorer response to chemical pleurodesis than those with a pH >7.3.
- Parapneumonic effusion with a low pleural fluid pH (≤7.15): High likelihood of necessity for pleural space drainage

COMPLICATIONS
- Of effusions: Constrictive fibrosis, pleurocutaneous fistula
- Of thoracentesis: Pneumothorax (5–10%); hemothorax (~1%); empyema; spleen/liver laceration; reexpansion pulmonary edema (if >1.5 L is removed)

REFERENCES
1. Light RW. Clinical practice. Pleural effusion. *N Engl J Med*. 2002;346:1971–7.
2. Light RW, Macgregor MI, Luchsinger PC, et al. Pleural effusions: the diagnostic separation of transudates and exudates. *Ann Intern Med*. 1972;77:507–13.
3. Roth BJ, O'Meara TF, Cragun WH. The serum-effusion albumin gradient in the evaluation of pleural effusions. *Chest*. 1990;98:546–9.
4. Shaw P, Aganwal R. Pleurodesis for malignant pleural effusion. *Cochrane Database of Systemtic Reviews*. 2009;1:CO002916.

 CODES

ICD9
- 511.1 Pleurisy with effusion, with mention of a bacterial cause other than tuberculosis
- 511.9 Unspecified pleural effusion
- 511.81 Malignant pleural effusion

CLINICAL PEARLS
- A complicated parapneumonic effusion requires urgent drainage.
- Outpatient therapeutic thoracentesis is preferred for patients with a short life expectancy (<3 months).

PNEUMONIA, ASPIRATION

Bevin Kenney, MD

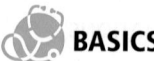 **BASICS**

DESCRIPTION
- Pneumonia due to inhalation of microorganisms from the oral cavity or nasopharynx
- In contrast to community-acquired pneumonia, which occurs by direct inhalation of infectious particles from air
- Results from impaired mechanical, humoral, or cellular immunity, such as impaired cough reflex or glottic closure, that protects lower airways
- System(s) affected: Pulmonary

EPIDEMIOLOGY
Geriatric Considerations
Risk of aspiration pneumonia is 6× higher if ≥75 years of age.

Prevalence
- Silent aspiration is extremely common in elderly patients but can occur even in normal individuals:
  - Occurs in 2–25% of acute stroke patients
  - Up to 50% of normal adults aspirate during sleep.
- Up to 20% of severe community-acquired pneumonia requiring hospitalization is polymicrobial, suggesting aspiration, but specific bacteria are not isolated in a majority of cases (see Etiology).
- Pneumonia is the 2nd most common infection in hospitalized patients.

RISK FACTORS
- Reduced consciousness, alcoholism, dementia, uremia, poor nutritional status
- Mechanical ventilation, bronchoscopy, upper endoscopy
- Pulmonary diseases: Chronic obstructive pulmonary disease (COPD)
- Gastrointestinal diseases: Gastroesophageal reflux disease, esophageal disease
- Dysphagia: Due to stroke, neuromuscular diseases, radiation to the neck or oropharynx
- Enteral feeding tubes, nasogastric tube feeding
- Immunosuppressed patients: Solid organ transplantation, steroid use >20 mg/d for >2 weeks, HIV

GENERAL PREVENTION
- There is a paucity of data on the prevention of aspiration.
- Some data show that simply performing a complete physical exam and screening for dysphagia lowers the incidence of pneumonia.
- Mechanical measures, such as semirecumbent or lateral-horizontal positioning, are commonly used.
- A soft diet is better than a pureed diet for preventing pneumonia.
- Another study showed a trend toward less aspiration with nectar-thickened liquids and a chin-down posture while eating (1).
- There is a lack of evidence to show that tube feeding will prevent aspiration (2).
- Intensive care protocols that include sedation vacations, ventilator weaning protocols, oral care, and patient positioning have shown success preventing ventilator-associated pneumonias (3).

PATHOPHYSIOLOGY
- Must contrast to chemical pneumonitis, which is due to aspiration of contents toxic to lung, independent of bacterial involvement (e.g., gastric acid), which presents with an abrupt onset of symptoms and prominent dyspnea. Chest x-ray (CXR) changes are seen within 2 hours.
- Role of immunosuppression:
  - Normal oropharynx is colonized by mixed flora of low virulence.
  - Increased colonization of gram-negative bacilli in malnutrition, alcoholism, diabetes, COPD, etc.
  - Interaction of virulence and quantity of aspirated bacteria and integrity of defenses determine development of pneumonia.
- Mechanical factors:
  - Mechanical ventilation: Endotracheal tube is a direct path to lower respiratory tract, which also prevents clearance of bacteria and secretions from exiting lower airways.
  - Reduced gag reflex due to sedation or stroke reduces spontaneous coughing and clearance of bacteria.
- Usually caused by gram-negative bacteria, anaerobes, and sometimes gram-positive bacteria
- Infection leads to consolidation of lung segments and subsegments in a bronchopneumonia pattern.

ETIOLOGY
- Pathogens vary according to setting (4,5):
  - Community-acquired: Gram-positives and some gram-negatives (e.g., *Streptococcus pneumonia*, *Staphylococcus aureus*, *Haemophilus influenza*, and enterobacteria)
  - Hospital-acquired: Mostly polymicrobial, including gram-negative bacilli, such as *Pseudomonas aeruginosa*, and anaerobes, such as *Bacteroides fragilis*, and less commonly, gram-positives, including *S. aureus*
  - Ventilator-associated: Common nosocomial bacteria, especially Pseudomonas aeruginosa, Acinetobacter baumannii, methicillin-resistant *Staphylococcus aureus* (MRSA)
- Specific bacteria identified in minority of cases
- Most cases associated with predisposing factors (see Risk Factors)

COMMONLY ASSOCIATED CONDITIONS
See Risk Factors.

 DIAGNOSIS

A formal bedside exam, including a detailed history, physical exam of mouth and throat, and observing the patient swallow various liquids and solids, is capable of diagnosing 80% of aspirations.

HISTORY
- Common:
  - Fever
  - Delirium, change in mental status
  - Dyspnea
  - Productive cough with putrid sputum
  - Pleuritic chest pain
  - Indolent course
- Less common:
  - Rigors
  - Weight loss

PHYSICAL EXAM
- Common:
  - Altered mental status
  - Periodontal disease, poor oral hygiene
  - Rhonchi
  - Decreased resonance on percussion, bronchovesicular breath sounds showing consolidation
- Less common:
  - Wheezes
  - Crackles
  - Severe dyspnea or acute respiratory failure

DIAGNOSTIC TESTS & INTERPRETATION
Lab
- Complete blood count:
  - Leukocytosis: White blood cells >12,000
  - Anemia of chronic disease occasionally present
- Cultures:
  - Sputum cultures: Anaerobic oral flora notoriously difficult to culture, not uncommon to lack results
  - Blood cultures are low yield.
- Arterial blood gas if suspect acidosis

Imaging
Initial approach
CXR (posteroanterior and lateral):
- CXR may be entirely normal in early infection.
- Involvement of lower lobes favors aspiration as the cause.
- CXR may also show a bronchopneumonia pattern with seg- and subsegmental consolidation, usually in lower lobes.

Follow-Up & Special Considerations
Chest computed tomography:
- More sensitive detection of infiltrates than CXR, but should be used only if clinically indicated

Diagnostic Procedures/Surgery
- Bronchoscopy:
  - Bronchoscopic brush cultures show improved sensitivity of etiologic diagnosis, but are affected by preprocedural administration of antibiotics.
  - Commonly used for ventilator-associated pneumonia, but controversial in clinical practice
- Swallowing evaluation, including possible videofluoroscopic evaluation with modified barium swallow, used in patients with suspected dysphagia

DIFFERENTIAL DIAGNOSIS
- Aspiration pneumonitis
- Community-acquired pneumonia
- Viral pneumonia
- Fungal pneumonia
- Lung abscess
- Foreign-body aspiration
- Lung cancer

 TREATMENT

MEDICATION
- Antibiotics should be started empirically as soon as possible after obtaining cultures.
- Data do not show significant difference in mortality between 8- or 15-day course of antibiotics; it is reasonable to try to narrow antibiotic spectrum and limit course based on patient's clinic picture (6).
- Clinical improvement can take up to 3 days.
- If no improvement after 3 days of antibiotic treatment, other diagnoses or resistant bacteria should be considered.

First Line

- Outpatients or hospitalized patients without risk factors for resistant bacteria:
  - Clindamycin, 600 mg IV b.i.d. or 300 mg p.o. q.i.d. (7,8)[B]:
    - Covers *S. pneumonia*, methicillin-sensitive *S. aureus*, and anaerobes like *B. fragilis*
    - Recent randomized controlled trials showed clindamycin alone to be equally effective to ampicillin/sulbactam, with or without the addition of 2nd- or 3rd-generation cephalosporin (7).
    - Clindamycin is low-cost and not associated with increase in adverse events.
    - Lower rates of MRSA-resistant *S. aureus* after use
    - However, clindamycin is associated with increased risk of *Clostridium difficile* infection.
- Ventilator-associated or patients at risk for resistant bacteria:
  - Piperacillin/tazobactam 3.375 g IV q6h plus vancomycin 1g IV q12h Carbapenems: Meropenem 1g IV q8h or ertapenem 1g IV q24h plus vancomycin 1g q12h
  - Fluoroquinolones, e.g., ciprofloxacin 400 mg IV q12h plus clindamycin or metronidazole for anaerobic coverage:
    - Be aware of ciprofloxacin's limited gram-positive coverage.

Second Line

- Ampicillin/sulbactam, 3 g IV b.i.d.
- Amoxicillin/clavulanate, 875 mg p.o. b.i.d.
- Piperacillin/tazobactam, 3.375 g IV q6h
- Ticarcillin/clavulanate, 3.1 g IV q6h:
  - All of the above cover *S. pneumonia*, MRSA, many gram-negative bacteria (including *Klebsiella*), and anaerobes (including *B. fragilis*).
  - Piperacillin/tazobactam and ticarcillin/clavulanate cover *P. aeruginosa*.
- Metronidazole, 500 mg IV or p.o. t.i.d. plus penicillin G, 1–2 million units IV q4–6h *OR* amoxicillin, 500 mg p.o. t.i.d.:
  - Metronidazole not as effective in putrid lung abscess as clindamycin
- Penicillin G has historically been effective alone, but gram-positives show increasing resistance.

ADDITIONAL TREATMENT

- A large 2009 cohort study showed that acid-suppressive medication use (specifically, proton pump inhibitors or PPIs) was associated with a 30% increased odds of hospital-acquired pneumonia (9)[B]. However, results may not have adequately controlled for key confounders such as swallowing dysfunction, tube feeds, and bed position. PPIs should be used only in those patients at risk for stress ulcers.
- If patient without dysphagia fails appropriate therapy or aspiration recurs, consider bronchoscopy to rule out neoplasm.

Issues for Referral

- Consider speech therapy evaluation.
- If patient without dysphagia fails appropriate therapy or aspiration recurs, consider pulmonology evaluation.

IN-PATIENT CONSIDERATIONS

Initial Stabilization

- Support ABCs.
- Assess for hypoxia with O_2 monitoring: O_2 saturation to determine need for supplemental O_2
- Assess for signs of sepsis and hemodynamic instability.

Admission Criteria

Admission recommended for anyone with signs of sepsis, immunosuppression, significant comorbid illness, poor functional, or nutritional status

Nursing

- Aggressive oral hygiene and pulmonary toileting
- Elevate head of bed, semirecumbent position: 30–45 degrees

 ONGOING CARE

DIET

- NPO if reduced consciousness
- Aggressive oral hygiene
- Soft diet
- Encourage smaller bites.
- Chin-down swallowing
- Thickened liquids
- Mechanical strategies:
  - Elevated head 30–45 degrees when eating; especially important if enteral feeding
- Tube feeding:
  - Usually reserved for continued aspiration despite other preventive measures, although this remains controversial
  - There is a lack of evidence that tube feeding prevents aspiration, but tube feeding does improve pulmonary toileting (2).
  - A history of pneumonia (of any kind) is a predictor of mortality after PEG placement (8,10).

PROGNOSIS

- Increased mortality with pneumonia due to gram-negative bacilli:
  - *P. aeruginosa* mortality: 28% in recent study (11)
- Ventilator-associated pneumonia has high morbidity and high mortality, ranging from 15–50%.
- Age, poor functional and nutritional status, and significant comorbid illness are independent predictors of increased mortality.

COMPLICATIONS

- Early:
  - Sepsis
  - Acute respiratory distress syndrome
- Late:
  - Lung abscess
  - Necrotizing pneumonia
- Empyema

REFERENCES

1. Robbins J, Gensler G, Hind J, et al. Comparison of 2 interventions for liquid aspiration on pneumonia incidence: a randomized trial. *Ann Intern Med*. 2008;148:509–18.
2. White GN, O'Rourke F, Ong BS, et al. Dysphagia: causes, assessment, treatment, and management. *Geriatrics*. 2008;63:15–20.
3. Weireter LJ, Collins JN, Britt RC, et al. Impact of a monitored program of care on incidence of ventilator-associated pneumonia: results of a longterm performance-improvement project. *J Am Coll Surg*. 2009;208.
4. El-Solh AA, Pietrantoni C, Bhat A, et al. Microbiology of severe aspiration pneumonia in institutionalized elderly. *Am J Respir Crit Care Med*. 2003;167:1650–4.
5. Marik PE, Kaplan D. Aspiration pneumonia and dysphagia in the elderly. *Chest*. 2003;124:328–36.
6. Porzecanski I, Bowton DL. Diagnosis and treatment of ventilator-associated pneumonia. *Chest*. 2006;130:597–604.
7. Allewelt M, Schüler P, Bölcskei PL, et al. Ampicillin + sulbactam vs clindamycin +/– cephalosporin for the treatment of aspiration pneumonia and primary lung abscess. *Clin Microbiol Infect*. 2004;10:163–70.
8. Tokunaga T, Kubo T, Ryan S, et al. Long-term outcome after placement of a percutaneous endoscopic gastrostomy tube. *Geriatr Gerontol Int*. 2008;8:19–23.
9. Herzig SJ, Howell MD, Ngo LH, et al. Acid-suppressive medication use and the risk for hospital-acquired pneumonia. *JAMA*. 2009;301:2120–8.
10. Patel PH, Thomas E. Risk factors for pneumonia after percutaneous endoscopic gastrostomy. *J Clin Gastroenterol*. 1990;12:389–92.
11. Arancibia F, Bauer TT, Ewig S, et al. Community-acquired pneumonia due to gram-negative bacteria and pseudomonas aeruginosa: incidence, risk, and prognosis. *Arch Intern Med*. 2002;162:1849–58.

ADDITIONAL READING

Kadowaki M, Demura Y, Mizuno S, et al. Reappraisal of clindamycin IV monotherapy for treatment of mild-to-moderate aspiration pneumonia in elderly patients. *Chest*. 2005;127:1276–82.

 CODES

ICD9

- 507.0 Pneumonitis due to inhalation of food or vomitus
- 507.1 Pneumonitis due to inhalation of oils and essences
- 507.8 Pneumonitis due to other solids and liquids

CLINICAL PEARLS

- Aspiration pneumonia is usually a clinical and not a pathologic diagnosis.
- As the etiology is usually polymicrobial and cultures are only positive for distinct bacteria in a minority of cases, initial antibiotic treatment is empiric and should cover anaerobes.
- *P. aeruginosa* is most often a nosocomial bacteria.
- Mechanical measures, such as semirecumbent positioning and chin-down posture while eating, are commonly used in the prevention of aspiration.

PNEUMONIA, BACTERIAL

Thomas J. Hansen, MD
Santosh Kumar, MBBS

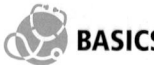 **BASICS**

Bacterial pneumonia is an infection of the pulmonary parenchyma by a bacterial organism.

DESCRIPTION
Bacterial pneumonia is further classified as:
- Community-acquired pneumonia (CAP): Lower respiratory tract infection in a nonhospitalized person that is associated with symptoms of acute infection (1).
- Hospital-acquired pneumonia (HAP): Pneumonia that occurs 48 hours or more after admission and did not appear to be incubating at the time of admission.
- Ventilator-associated pneumonia (VAP): A type of pneumonia that develops more than 48 to 72 hours after endotracheal intubation.
- Health care–associated pneumonia (HCAP): Pneumonia that occurs in a nonhospitalized patient with extensive health care contact, such as:
  - IV therapy or wound care within the past 30 days
  - Residing in a nursing home or long-term care facility
  - Hospitalization in an acute care hospital for two or more days within the past 90 days
  - Have visited a hospital or hemodialysis clinic within the past 30 days (2)

EPIDEMIOLOGY
- Influenza and pneumonia (combined) are the 8th leading cause of death in the US, with 52,717 deaths in 2007.
- HAP is the leading cause of death among hospital-acquired infections, with mortality rates ranging from 20–50% (2).

Incidence
- CAP: 5.6 million cases per year in the US (1).
- HAP occurs at the rate of 5–10 cases per 1,000 hospital admissions (2).

RISK FACTORS
- CAP (1):
  - Age older than 65
  - HIV or immunocompromised
  - Recent antibiotic therapy or resistance to antibiotics
  - Comorbidities such as alcoholism, asthma, cerebrovascular disease, COPD, chronic renal failure, CHF, diabetes, liver disease, neoplastic disease
- HAP, VAP, CAP (2):
  - Hospitalization for 2 days or more during past 90 days
  - Severe illness
  - Antibiotic therapy in the last six months
  - Poor functional status as defined by activities of daily living score
  - Immunosuppression

GENERAL PREVENTION
Pneumococcal polysaccharide vaccine is recommended for the following (3):
- Age 65 and older. Second dose recommended if patient received vaccine 5 years prior and was younger than 65 at the time of the first vaccination.
- Age 19–64 with chronic cardiovascular disease, chronic pulmonary disease (including asthma), and diabetes mellitus. Revaccination not recommended under age 65.

- Age 19–64 who smoke cigarettes, have alcoholism, chronic liver disease, cerebrospinal fluid leaks, or cochlear implants. Revaccination not recommended under age 65.
- Age 19–64 who live in chronic care facilities. Revaccination not recommended under age 65.
- Age 19–64 who are immunocompromised. Second dose recommended if 5 years or more have elapsed since receipt of first dose.

ETIOLOGY
- Adults - CAP: (1)
  - Typical: Streptococcal pneumonia, *Haemophilus influenzae*, *Staphylococcus aureus*, group A *Streptococcus*, *Moraxella catarrhalis*
  - Atypical: *Legionella*, *Mycoplasma pneumoniae*, *Chlamydia pneumoniae*
- Adults - HAP, VAP, HCAP:
  - Aerobic gram-negative bacilli: *P. aeruginosa*, *E. coli*, *Klebsiella pneumoniae*, and *Acinetobacter species*
  - Gram-positive cocci: *Staphylococcus aureus* and *Streptococcus* species
- Children
  - Birth to 20 days: *Escherichia coli*, group B streptococci, *Listeria monocytogenes*
  - 3 weeks to 3 months: *Chlamydia trachomatis*, *S. pneumoniae*
  - 4 months to 5 years: *Chlamydia pneumoniae*, *Mycoplasma pneumoniae*, *S. pneumoniae*
  - 5 to 18 years (4): *C. pneumoniae*, *M. pneumoniae*, *S. pneumoniae*

 DIAGNOSIS

HISTORY
- Fever, malaise, fatigue
- Dyspnea
- Cough, with or without sputum
- Pleuritic chest pain
- Myalgias
- Gastrointestinal symptoms

Geriatric Considerations
Atypical symptoms in older adults

PHYSICAL EXAM
- Fever >100.4°F (38°C)
- Lungs: Rales, rhonchi, wheezing, egophony, bronchial breath sounds, dullness to percussion
- Abdominal tenderness or pain

DIAGNOSTIC TESTS & INTERPRETATION
Lab
Initial lab tests
- Historically, for hospitalized patients, CBC, sputum Gram stain, and 2 sets of blood cultures.
- Recent studies cast doubt on the clinical utility of blood and sputum cultures given low positive culture rate.

Imaging
Initial approach
All patients with suspected CAP should have a CXR to establish the diagnosis and identify complications (5):
- Typical pneumonia: Lobar consolidation
- Atypical pneumonia: Interstitial pattern
- Early in the course of the disease, CXR may be negative.

Follow-Up & Special Considerations
Chest CT scan if failing to improve

DIFFERENTIAL DIAGNOSIS
Bronchitis, asthma exacerbation, pulmonary edema, lung cancer, influenza

 TREATMENT

MEDICATION
First Line
- Adults (1), outpatient:
  - Macrolides
    - Azithromycin 500 mg orally once, then 250 mg orally once daily for 4 days
    - Clarithromycin 500 mg orally twice daily for 10 days
    - Erythromycin 500 mg orally twice daily for 10 days
  - Tetracyclines
    - Doxycycline 100 mg orally twice daily for 10 days
  - Fluoroquinolones (for those with comorbidities, are immunosuppressed or have used antibiotics previous 3 months):
    - Levaquin 750 mg orally once daily for 5 days
    - Moxifloxacin 400 mg orally once daily for 10 days
    - Gatifloxacin 400 mg orally once daily for 10 days
- Adults, inpatient (non-ICU):
  - Beta-lactam + Macrolide OR Fluoroquinolone alone
  - Beta-lactam
  - Cefotaxime 1 g IV every 6–8 hours for 14 days
  - Ceftriaxone 1 g IV every 24 hours for 14 days
  - Ampicillin-Sulbactam 3 g IV every 6 hours
  - Macrolide
    - Clarithromycin 500 mg IV every 24 hours for 14 days
    - Erythromycin 500–1,000 mg IV every six hours for 14 days
  - Fluoroquinolone
    - Gatifloxacin 400 mg IV once daily for 14 days
    - Levofloxacin 750 mg IV once daily for 14 days
- Adult, inpatient (ICU):
  - Beta-lactam + Azithromycin OR
  - Beta-lactam + Fluoroquinolone OR
  - Fluoroquinolone + Aztreonam (for penicillin allergic patients)
  - Beta-lactam
    - Cefotaxime 1 g IV every 6–8 hours for 14 days
    - Ceftriaxone 1 g every 24 hours for 14 days
    - Ampicillin-Sulbactam 3 g IV every 6 hours for 14 days
  - Macrolide
    - Azithromycin 500 mg IV every day for 14 days
  - Fluoroquinolone
    - Gatifloxacin 400 mg IV once daily for 14 days
    - Levofloxacin 750 mg IV once daily for 14 days
    - Aztreonam 2 g IV every 6–8 hours for 14 days
  - Note: if *Pseudomonas* is a consideration, give one of the following:
    - Piperacillin-tazobactam, cefepime, imipenem, or meropenem + either ciprofloxacin or levofloxacin (750 mg)
    - Piperacillin-tazobactam, cefepime, imipenem, or meropenem + an aminoglycoside and azithromycin

○ Piperacillin-tazobactam, cefepime, imipenem, or meropenem + an aminoglycoside + either ciprofloxacin or levofloxacin (750 mg)

- Children (4), birth to 20 days:
  – Admit to hospital for treatment with either ampicillin plus gentamicin or ampicillin plus cefotaxime.
  – If gram-negative meningitis is suspected, ampicillin, cefotaxime, and an aminoglycoside may be used all together.
  – Inpatient: Ampicillin (age <7 days)
    ○ If <2 kg: 50–100 mg/kg/day IV or IM in 2 divided doses
    ○ If 2 kg or more: 75–150 mg/kg/day IV or IM in 2 divided doses
  – Inpatient: Ampicillin (age 7–20 days)
    ○ If <1.2 kg: 50–100 mg/kg/day divided every 12 hours
    ○ If 1.2–2.0 kg: 75–150 mg/kg/day divided into 3 doses given every 8 hours
    ○ If >2.0 kg: 100–200 mg/kg/day divided into 4 doses given every 6 hours
  – Inpatient: Gentamicin IV or IM
    ○ If 7 days or younger: 2.5 mg/kg every 12 hours
    ○ If >7days: 2.5 mg/kg every 8 hours
  – Inpatient: Cefotaxime IV
    ○ If 7 days or younger: 100 mg/kg/day in divided doses every 12 hours
    ○ If >7days: 150 mg/kg/day in divided doses every 8 hours
- Children, age 3 weeks to 3 months:
  – Outpatient (without fever): Azithromycin 10 mg/kg orally on day 1, followed by 5 mg/kg/day on days 2–5, OR
  – Outpatient (without fever): Erythromycin 3–40 mg/kg/day orally in divided doses every 6 hours for 10 days.
  – Inpatient (with fever): Erythromycin 40 mg/kg/day IV in doses every 6 hours AND either Cefotaxime or Cefuroxime
  – Inpatient (with fever): Cefotaxime 200 mg/kg/day IV in divided doses every 8 hours
  – Inpatient (with fever): Cefuroxime 150 mg /kg/day IV in divided doses every 8 hours.
  – ICU: Cefuroxime 150 mg/kg/day IV in divided doses every 8 hours OR
  – ICU: Cefotaxime 200 mg/kg/day IV in divided doses every 8 hours PLUS
  – ICU: Cloxacillin 150–200 mg/kg/day IV in divided doses every 6 hours
- Children, age 4 months to 5 years:
  – Outpatient: Amoxicillin 90 mg/kg/day orally in divided doses every 8 hours for 7–10 days
  – Outpatient: Consider initial dose of Ceftriaxone 50 mg/kg/day IM (max 1 g per day).
  – Outpatient alternatives: Amoxicillin-clavulanic acid, Azithromycin, Cefaclor, Clarithromycin, Erythromycin.
  – Inpatient: Cefotaxime 150 mg/kg/day IV in divided doses every 6 hours
  – Inpatient: Cefuroxime 150 mg /kg/day IV in divided doses every 8 hours
  – ICU: Cefuroxime 150 mg/kg/day IV in divided doses every 8 hours PLUS
  – ICU: Erythromycin 40 mg/kg/day IV in divided doses every 6 hours for 10–14 days.
  – ICU: Cefotaxime 200 mg/kg/day IV in divided doses every 8 hours PLUS
  – ICU: Cloxacillin 150-200 mg/kg/day IV in divided doses every 6 hours for 10–14 days.

- Age 5 years to adult:
  – Outpatient: Azithromycin 10 mg/kg/day (max 500 mg) orally on day 1, followed by 5 mg/kg/day orally on days 2–5.
  – Outpatient: Clarithromycin 15 mg/kg/day orally in divided doses every 12 hours for 7–10 days
  – Outpatient: Erythromycin 40 mg/kg/day orally in divided doses every 6 hours for 7–10 days
  – Inpatient: Cefuroxime 150 mg/kg/day IV in divided doses every 8 hours PLUS
  – Inpatient: Erythromycin 40 mg/kg/day IV in divided doses every 6 hours for 10–14 days
  – ICU: Cefuroxime 150 mg/kg/day IV in divided doses every 8 hours PLUS
  – ICU: Erythromycin 40 mg/kg/day IV in divided doses every 6 hours for 10–14 days.

IN-PATIENT CONSIDERATIONS
Admission Criteria
The pneumonia severity index is a clinical prediction rule used to calculate the probability of morbidity and mortality among patients with CAP. (Online calculator available at http://www.mdcalc.com/psi-port-score-pneumonia-severity-index-adult-cap) (6)

- Patient characteristics: Gender, nursing home resident
- Co-morbidities: Neoplastic disease, liver disease, congestive heart failure, cerebrovascular disease, renal disease
- Physical exam: Altered mental status, respiratory rate >30 breaths per minute, systolic blood pressure, temperature <95°F (35°C) or >104°F (40°C), pulse rate >125 beats per minute
- Laboratory and radiographic findings: Arterial pH <7.35, blood urea nitrogen >64 mg per dL, sodium <130 mEq per L, glucose >250 mg per dL, hematocrit <30%, partial pressure of arterial oxygen <60 mm Hg or oxygen percent saturation <90%, pleural effusion
- Scoring
  – If score is 70 or less, there is a low risk of mortality (0.1–0.6%).
  – If the score is 71–90, there is a low risk of mortality (2.8%).
  – If the scores is 91–130, there is a moderate risk of mortality (8.2%).
  – If the score is >130, there is a high risk of mortality (29.2%).

Discharge Criteria
Criteria of clinical stability: Temperature ≤100.0°F (37.8°C); pulse ≤100 beats/min; respiratory rate ≤24 breaths/min, systolic BP ≥90 mm Hg, arterial oxygen saturation ≥90% or PO$_2$ ≥60 mm Hg on room air, and ability to maintain oral intake (1).

ONGOING CARE
FOLLOW-UP RECOMMENDATIONS
- Follow-up CXR recommended to ensure clearing
- Isolation precautions:
  – Contact: Colonized/infected MRSA/VRE or MDR gram negative
  – Droplet: *Mycoplasma, N. meningitides*, influenza, or plague
  – Airborne: Tuberculosis (TB), varicella, measles, or viral hemorrhagic fevers
  – Strict airborne: SARS

PATIENT EDUCATION
Smoking cessation, vaccination

COMPLICATIONS
Necrotizing pneumonia, respiratory failure, empyema, abscesses, cavitation, bronchopleural fistula, sepsis

REFERENCES
1. Lutfiyya MN, Henley E, Chang L. Diagnosis and Treatment of Community-Acquired Pneumonia. *Am Fam Physician.* 2006;73(3):442–450.
2. Guidelines for the management of adults with hospital-acquired, ventilator-associated, and healthcare-associated pneumonia. *Am J Respir Crit Care Med* 2005;171:388–416.
3. Fisman DN, Abrutyn E, Spaude KA, et al. et al. Prior pneumococcal vaccination is associated with reduced death, complications, and length of stay among hospitalized adults with community-acquired pneumonia. *Clin Infect Dis.* 2006;42: 1093–101.
4. Ostapchuk M, Roberts DM, Haddy R, et al. Community-Acquired Pneumonia in Infants and Children. *Am Fam Physician.* 2004;70(5): 899–908.
5. Niederman MS, Mandell LA, Anzueto A, et al. Guidelines for the management of adults with community-acquired pneumonia. *Am J Respir Crit Care Med.* 2001;163:1730–1754.
6. Fine MJ, Auble TE, Yealy DM, et al. A prediction rule to identify low-risk patients with community-acquired pneumonia. *N Engl J Med.* 1997;336:243–50.

CODES

ICD9
- 482.0 Pneumonia due to *Pneumonia due to klebsiella pneumoniae*
- 482.1 Pneumonia due to *Haemophilus Pneumonia due to pseudomonas*
- 482.2 Pneumonia due to *Streptococcus*, Pneumonia due to haemophilus influenzae (h. influenzae)

CLINICAL PEARLS
- Treatment of bacterial pneumonia is based on the most common bacterial pathogens found in specified age groups.
- The pneumonia index risk score is a helpful tool for adult patients to determine whether the patient needs to be admitted for inpatient care and the prognosis.

PNEUMONIA, MYCOPLASMA

Alyssa H. Tran, DO

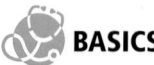 **BASICS**

DESCRIPTION
- Bronchopulmonary infection caused by infection of the lungs and bronchi with *Mycoplasma pneumoniae*, a fastidious and slow-growing organism
- Infection may be asymptomatic, confined to the upper respiratory tract, or progress to pneumonia. Usual course is acute. Incubation period is 1–4 weeks and includes prodromal symptoms.
- Peaks late summer/fall; most frequent in children/young adults but also elderly; may cause epidemics (schools, barracks)
- Synonym(s): Primary atypical pneumonia (PAP); Eaton agent pneumonia; Cold agglutinin-positive pneumonia; Walking pneumonia

Geriatric Considerations
Somewhat unusual as an isolated agent in elderly patients

Pediatric Considerations
- Unusual in infants and children <5 yrs
- *M. pneumoniae* is associated with increased incidence of asthma attacks in older children.

Pregnancy Considerations
- Azithromycin: Pregnancy class B (preferred treatment)
- Clarithromycin and levofloxacin: Pregnancy class C
- Doxycycline: Pregnancy class D (contraindicated in pregnant patients)

EPIDEMIOLOGY
Incidence
- Estimated 2 million cases/year in the US
- Responsible for 20% of community-acquired pneumonias requiring hospitalizations annually in the US
- Incidence does not vary greatly by season but accounts for higher proportion of pneumonia in the summer (up to 50%).

Prevalence
- Predominant sex: Male = Female
- Predominant age: 5–20 years; but may occur at any age; rare in children <5 years of age
- 15–20% of all cases of community-acquired pneumonia (CAP)
- The most common cause of pneumonia in school children and young adults (without chronic underlying condition)
- Epidemics usually occur every 4–8 years.

RISK FACTORS
- Close community living (e.g., hospitals, prisons, military bases, fraternity houses):
  - Some of the largest outbreaks have been in army recruits.
- Family exposure
- Immunocompromised state
- Smoking

GENERAL PREVENTION
- Highly contagious, *M. pneumoniae* is carried in respiratory droplets.
- Consider isolation of active cases in closed communities (e.g., schools, camps, military bases) and hospitals.

- Azithromycin prophylaxis (standard 5-day course) may lower attack rate, but not routinely recommended

PATHOPHYSIOLOGY
- *M. pneumoniae* is a mucosal pathogen; lives closely with epithelial cells in the respiratory or urogenital tract
- Exclusive human parasite
- Transmitted by contact and aerosol
- 1–4-week incubation period
- Prolonged paroxysmal, hacking cough seen in this disease is thought to be due to the inhibition of ciliary movement. The organism has a remarkable gliding motility and specialized filamentous tip ends that allow it to burrow between cilia within the respiratory epithelium, eventually causing sloughing of the respiratory epithelial cells.
- Has specialized attachment organelle with adhesin proteins
- H_2O_2 is an important virulence factor, causing oxidative damage to host cells and loss of cilia.
- Pathogenicity of *M. pneumoniae* is linked to the activation of inflammatory mediators, including cytokines.

ALERT
Macrolide-resistant *M. pneumoniae* has emerged in adult community-acquired pneumonia and pediatric pneumonia.

ETIOLOGY
Infection by *M. pneumoniae* has come to be recognized as a worldwide cause of PAP (1).

COMMONLY ASSOCIATED CONDITIONS
- Asthma: May be exacerbated by associated release of proinflammatory cytokines
- Chronic asthma
- Chronic obstructive pulmonary disease

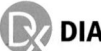 **DIAGNOSIS**

HISTORY
- Gradual onset with upper respiratory infection symptoms that progress
- Most patients will develop fever, nasal congestion, cough, headache, and sore throat. Some will develop dyspnea. Pleuritic chest pain is rare.
- Many patients will develop extrapulmonary findings, including myalgias, chest pain, cervical adenopathy, skin rash, and bullous myringitis.
- Neurologic symptoms may include cranial nerve palsies, diplopia, confusion, psychosis, ataxia, ascending paralysis, and coma.
- Persistent cough is common during convalescence; other sequelae are rare.
- Fatal cases are reported occasionally, primarily among the elderly and persons with sickle cell disease.

PHYSICAL EXAM
- Patients generally appear nontoxic.
- Hacking or pertussislike cough may be present along with fever and lassitude.
- Erythematous tympanic membranes or bullous myringitis in patients >2 years of age is an uncommon but unique sign.

- Mild pharyngeal injection without exudate
- Minimal or no cervical adenopathy
- Normal lung findings with early infection but rhonchi, rales, and/or wheezes several days later
- Some patients develop a pleural friction rub.
- Various exanthems, including erythema multiforme and Stevens-Johnson syndrome

DIAGNOSTIC TESTS & INTERPRETATION
Lab
Labs are typically not necessary to make diagnosis, but may be indicated depending on clinical presentation.

Imaging
Initial approach
Chest x-ray:
- Peribronchial pneumonia pattern with bronchial shadow, interstitial infiltrates, areas of atelectasis
- Pleural effusion present in up to 20% of patients

Follow-Up & Special Considerations
Chest CT scan findings in patients with *M. pneumoniae*: Combination of bronchial wall thickening and centrilobular nodules; however, these CT scan findings are not observed in progressed severe *M. pneumoniae* pneumonia patients.

Pathological Findings
- WBC count generally not helpful in mycoplasmal pneumonia because results may be normal or elevated. Hemolytic anemia has been described but is rare.
- Sputum Gram stains and cultures are usually not helpful because *M pneumoniae* lacks a cell wall and cannot be stained.
- Elevated erythrocyte sedimentation rates may be present but are nonspecific.
- *M. pneumoniae* is difficult to culture and requires 7–21 days to grow; culturing is successful in only 40-90% of cases and does not provide information to guide patient management, therefore is infrequently performed.
- EIA serology of acute and convalescent sera is the mainstay of laboratory diagnosis.
- Polymerase chain reaction testing for *M. pneumoniae* DNA in respiratory secretions, CSF, and tissue samples; when available, may be the most sensitive and specific
- Complement fixation serologic assay shows 4-fold rise in IgM antibody titer at 2–4 weeks after symptom onset; an older technique. Positive cold agglutinins (titer of 1:128 or greater or rising 4-fold) in 50% of infections but can take 1–2 weeks to develop; not sensitive or specific; not routinely recommended.

DIFFERENTIAL DIAGNOSIS
- Viral pneumonia
- Bacterial pneumonia
- Fungal pneumonias
- Tuberculosis
- Other atypical pneumonias, including:
  - *Chlamydia pneumoniae*
  - *C. psittaci*
  - *Coxiella burnetii* (Q fever)
  - *Francisella tularensis* (tularemia)
  - *Pneumocystis jerovici*
  - *Legionella pneumophila*

TREATMENT

- Treatment generally is empirical and must be comprehensive to cover all likely pathogens in the context of the clinical setting.
- In the treatment of *Mycoplasma* pneumonia, antimicrobials against *M. pneumoniae* are bacteriostatic, not bactericidal.

MEDICATION
First Line

- Azithromycin: <6 months of age: not established; children >6 months of age: day 1: 10 mg/kg p.o. once, not to exceed 500 mg/d; days 2–5: 5 mg/kg/d p.o., not to exceed 250 mg/d; adults: Day 1: 500 mg p.o., days 2-5: 250 mg p.o. (2)[A]
- Erythromycin: Children: 20–50 mg/kg/d p.o. divided q6–8h × 10–14 days; adults: 250 mg p.o. q6h × 10–14 days (2)[A]
- Clarithromycin: Children <6 months of age: Not established; children >6 months of age: 15 mg/kg/d p.o. divided q12h × 10–14 days; adults: 250–500 mg p.o. b.i.d. × 10–14 days (2)[A]
- Doxycycline: Children <8 years of age: Not recommended; children >8 years of age: 2–4 mg/kg/d up to 200 mg/d p.o. divided b.i.d.; adults: 100 mg p.o. b.i.d. × 1–4 weeks (2)[C]

Second Line
- Levofloxacin: Children <18 years of age: Not recommended; adults: 500 mg/d p.o. × 7–10 days
- Telithromycin: Children <18 years of age: Not recommended; adults: 800 mg/d p.o. × 7–10 days
- Levofloxacin and moxifloxacin show good activity against *M. pneumoniae*. Consider use with comorbidities and other pneumonia pathogens (2)[A].
- Penicillin antibiotics are ineffective against *M. pneumoniae*.

ADDITIONAL TREATMENT
Additional Therapies
- Albuterol inhaler 2 puffs q.i.d. (with spacer for pediatric patients) for wheezing
- Up to 10.9% of hospitalized patients may require mechanical ventilation.

IN-PATIENT CONSIDERATIONS
Initial Stabilization
Respiratory support; calculation of pneumonia severity score (CAP score) may be helpful in determining inpatient vs outpatient treatment (3).

Admission Criteria
- Altered mental status
- Tachycardia or tachypnea
- Hypotension
- Neurologic symptoms
- Inability to maintain oxygen saturation
- Signs of Stevens-Johnson syndrome
- Significant hemolysis (autoimmune hemolytic anemia, cold agglutinin disease)
- Significant cerebrovascular, cardiac, renal, liver, or GI symptoms or coexisting conditions
- Advanced age with comorbidities
- Complicating neoplastic disease

Discharge Criteria
- Change from IV to p.o. antibiotic may be made when:
  - Respiratory distress has resolved.
  - Hypoxia has resolved.
  - Patients are tolerating oral hydration.
  - There are no significant complications.
- There is generally no need for 24 hours of observation on oral antibiotic prior to discharge.

ONGOING CARE

FOLLOW-UP RECOMMENDATIONS
- Worsening symptoms or development of rash or meningeal or neurologic signs should prompt immediate presentation to medical attention.
- Antibiotic prophylaxis for exposed contacts is not routinely recommended.
- However, macrolide or doxycycline prophylaxis should be used in households in which patients with underlying conditions may be predisposed to severe mycoplasmal infection, such as those with sickle cell disease or antibody deficiencies.

Patient Monitoring
- Follow up either in person or by telephone.
- Clearing of condition on CXR should be documented in patients >50 years of age.
- In smokers, document a clear CXR in 6–8 weeks.

DIET
Keep well hydrated; otherwise, no special dietary restrictions or recommendations.

PATIENT EDUCATION
- Smoking cessation
- Contact and droplet precautions
- Proper handwashing techniques

PROGNOSIS
- *Mycoplasma* infection symptoms usually resolve in 2 weeks.
- Some constitutional symptoms may persist for several weeks.
- With correct therapy, even most severe cases can expect complete recovery

COMPLICATIONS
- All complications are rare, except reactive airways disease, hemolytic anemia, and erythema multiforme (1).
- Reactive airways disease may persist indefinitely and may cause acute chest syndrome in sickle cell anemia patients.
- Hemolytic anemia
- Erythema multiforme
- Meningoencephalitis
- Aseptic meningitis
- Peripheral neuropathy
- Transverse myelitis
- Cerebellar ataxia
- Acute transverse myelitis
- Acute disseminated encephalomyelitis
- Guillain-Barré syndrome
- Encephalitis (especially in children)
- Polyneuritis
- Polyarthritis
- Stevens-Johnson syndrome
- Pericarditis
- Myocarditis
- Respiratory distress syndrome
- Cerebral ataxia
- Thromboembolic phenomena
- Pleural effusion
- Nephritis

REFERENCES

1. Atkinson TP, Balish MF, Waites KB. Epidemiology, clinical manifestations, pathogenesis and laboratory detection of Mycoplasma pneumoniae infections. *FEMS Microbiol Rev*. 2008.
2. Mandell LA, Wunderink RG, Anzueto A, et al. Infectious Diseases Society of America/American Thoracic Society consensus guidelines on the management of community-acquired pneumonia in adults. *Clin Infect Dis*. 2007;44(Suppl 2):S27–72.
3. Metlay JP, et al. Testing strategies in the initial management of patients with community-acquired pneumonia. *Ann Intern Med*. 2003;138:115.

ADDITIONAL READING

- Blasi F. Atypical pathogens and respiratory tract infections. *Eur Respir J*. 2004;24:171–81.
- Carbonara S, Monno L, Longo B, et al. Community-acquired pneumonia. *Curr Opin Pulm Med*. 2009;15:261–73.
- Fine MJ, Auble TE, Yealy DM, et al. A prediction rule to identify low-risk patients with community-acquired pneumonia. *N Engl J Med*. 1997;336:243–50.
- Forgie S, Marrie TJ. Healthcare-associated atypical pneumonia. *Semin Respir Crit Care Med*. 2009;30:67–85.
- Isozumi R, Yoshimine H, Morozumi M, et al. Adult community-acquired pneumonia caused by macrolide resistant Mycoplasma pneumoniae. *Respirology*. 2009;14(8):1206–8.
- Neher JO, Morton JR, Mouw D. Clinical inquiries. What is the best macrolide for atypical pneumonia? *J Fam Pract*. 2004;53:229–30.
- Talkington DF, Waites KB, Schwartz SB, et al. Emerging from obscurity: Understanding pulmonary and extrapulmonary syndromes, pathogenesis, and epidemiology of human *Mycoplasma pneumoniae* infections. In: Scheld WM, Craig WA, Hughes JM (Eds). *Emerging Infections 5*. ASM Press, Washington, DC: 2001:57–84.
- Waites KB, Talkington DF. Mycoplasma pneumoniae and its role as a human pathogen. *Clin Microbiol Rev*. 2004;17:697–728, table of contents.

 CODES

ICD9
483.0 Pneumonia due to *Mycoplasma pneumoniae*

CLINICAL PEARLS

- So-called atypical respiratory pathogens include *Mycoplasma pneumoniae*, *Chlamydia pneumoniae*, and *Legionella pneumophila*.
- This is typically a clinical diagnosis; if labs are indicated, then EIA serology of acute and convalescent sera is the mainstay of laboratory diagnosis.
- The recommended macrolides are equally effective. However, erythromycin has a higher rate of side effects and is less effective against *Haemophilus influenzae*.
- Watch closely for complicating symptoms that could indicate worsening disease.

PNEUMONIA, PNEUMOCYSTIS JIROVECI

Thomas J. Hansen, MD
Tejesh S. Reddy, MBBS

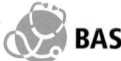 **BASICS**

DESCRIPTION
- The fungus that causes this pneumonia in humans was previously called *Pneumocystis carinii*.
- The name was formally changed to *Pneumocystis jiroveci* in 2001 following the discovery that the fungus that infects humans is unique and distinctive from the fungus that infects animals (1).
- *Pneumocystis jiroveci* causes pneumonia primarily in immunocompromised patients.
- To prevent confusion, the term PCP, which used to represent *Pneumocystis carinii* pneumonia, now represents *Pneumocystis* pneumonia (2).

ALERT
There is no combination of symptoms, signs, blood chemistries, or radiographic findings that is diagnostic of *Pneumocystis jiroveci* pneumonia (3).

EPIDEMIOLOGY
- *P. jiroveci* has a worldwide distribution, and most children have been exposed to the fungus by age 2-4 years (4).
- The reservoir and mode of transmission for *P. jiroveci* is still unclear:
  - Human studies favor an airborne transmission model with person-to-person spread being the most likely mode of infection acquisition (3).

Incidence
- Infants with HIV infection have a peak incidence of PCP between the ages of 2 and 6 months (4).
- HIV-infected infants have a high mortality rate with a median survival of only 1 month.

Prevalence
- The prevalence of *Pneumocystis jiroveci* colonization among healthy adults is between 0% and 20% (1).
- Recent studies have demonstrated the transient nature of *Pneumocystis jiroveci* colonization in asymptomatic, immunocompetent patients (3).
- 50% of patients with PCP are coinfected with 2 or more strains of *Pneumocystis jiroveci* (4).
- There is evidence that distinct strains are responsible for each episode in patients who develop multiple episodes of PCP (4).

RISK FACTORS
Individuals at risk (3):
- Patients with HIV/AIDS infection, especially if not receiving prophylactic treatment for PCP
- Patients who are receiving high doses of glucocorticoids
- Patients who have an altered immune system not due to HIV
- Patients who are receiving chronic immunosuppressive medications
- Patients who have hematologic or solid malignancies resulting in malignancy-related immune depression

GENERAL PREVENTION
- Medication:
  - Trimethoprim-sulfamethoxazole (TMP-SMX):
    - Adults: 1 double-strength tablet daily or 1 double-strength tablet 3 times per week
    - Children >2 months: 150 mg TMP/m²/day in divided doses every 12 hours for 3 times per week
  - Atovaquone suspension:
    - Adults: 1500 mg orally once daily
    - Children: Not to exceed 1500 mg daily:
      - 1–3 months: 30 mg/kg/day orally once daily
      - 4–24 months: 45 mg/kg/day orally once daily
      - >24 months: 30 mg/kg/day orally once daily
  - Dapsone:
    - Adults only: 50 mg twice daily or 100 mg once daily
  - Pentamidine:
    - Adults only: 300 mg aerosolized every 4 weeks
- Indications for prophylaxis:
  - HIV-infected adults (4):
    - Should start when CD4 count is <200 cells/microliter or if the patient develops oropharyngeal candidiasis
  - HIV-infected children (4):
    - Prophylaxis should be provided for children 6 years or older based on adult guidelines.
    - For children aged 1-5 years, start when their CD4 count is <500 cells/microliter.
    - For infants younger than 12 months, start when CD4 percentage is less than 15%.
  - Non-HIV-infected adults receiving immunosuppressive medications or with underlying immune system deficits should receive PCP prophylaxis, but currently there are no specific guidelines as to when to start.

ETIOLOGY
Mode of transmission is unknown; respiratory likely important

COMMONLY ASSOCIATED CONDITIONS
- HIV/AIDS
- Chronic obstructive lung disease (COPD)
- Interstitial lung disease
- Connective tissue diseases treated with corticosteroids
- Cancer and organ transplant patients on immunosuppressive medication

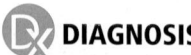 **DIAGNOSIS**

HISTORY
- HIV-infected patients:
  - Subacute onset over several weeks:
    - Progressively worsening dyspnea
    - Tachypnea
    - Cough: Nonproductive or productive of clear sputum
    - Low-grade fever, chills
    - Weakness, fatigue, malaise

- Non-HIV-infected immunocompromised patients:
  - More acute onset with fulminant respiratory failure:
    - Abrupt tachypnea, dyspnea
    - Fever
    - Dry cough

PHYSICAL EXAM
- Fever
- Tachypnea
- Tachycardia
- Lung exam is normal or near-normal.

DIAGNOSTIC TESTS & INTERPRETATION
Pneumocystic jiroveci cannot be cultured. Therefore, diagnosis relies on detection of the organism by colorimetric or immunofluorescent stains or by polymerase chain reaction (4)[C].

Lab
- Arterial blood gas reveals hypoxemia and increased alveolar–arterial (A-a) gradient that varies with severity of disease.
- Levels of serum lactate dehydrogenase frequently increased (nonspecific, likely due to underlying lung inflammation and injury)
- CD4 cell count is generally <200 in HIV-infected patients with PCP.

Imaging
- Chest x-ray (CXR) (3)[C]:
  - Bilateral, symmetric, fine, reticular interstitial infiltrates involving perihilar areas. Becomes more homogenous and diffuse as severity of infection progresses.
  - Less common patterns include upper lobe involvement in patients receiving aerosolized pentamidine, solitary or multiple nodular opacities, lobar infiltrates, pneumatoceles, and pneumothoraces.
  - Chest radiographs may be normal in up to 30% of patients with PCP (2)[C].
- High-resolution computed tomography (CT) is more sensitive than CXR.

Diagnostic Procedures/Surgery
- Fiber-optic bronchoscopy with bronchoalveolar lavage (BAL) is the preferred diagnostic procedure to obtain samples for direct fluorescent antibody staining:
  - Sensitivities range from 89% to greater than 98%.
- Pneumocystis trophic forms or cysts obtained from induced sputum, BAL fluid, or lung tissue, which can be visualized using conventional stains
- Polymerase chain reaction (PCR) can detect *Pneumocystis* from respiratory sources, but the potential remains for false-positives (3)[C].

DIFFERENTIAL DIAGNOSIS
- Tuberculosis
- Bacterial pneumonia
- Fungal pneumonia
- Viral pneumonia

TREATMENT

The recommended duration of therapy differs in patients who have or do not have AIDS:

- In patients who have PCP who do not have AIDS, the typical duration of therapy is 14 days.
- Treatment of PCP in patients who have AIDS was increased to 21 days due to the risk for relapse after only 14 days of treatment (3)[C].

MEDICATION

Pediatric Considerations
Only medications that are FDA approved are listed for pediatric dosing.

First Line
- Trimethoprim-sulfamethoxazole (TMP-SMX) (3)[C]
- Adult dosing:
  - TMP: 15–20 mg/kg/day, oral or intravenous, divided into 3–4 doses
  - SMX: 75–100 mg/kg/day, oral or intravenous, divided into 3–4 doses
- Pediatric dosing (>2 months):
  - 15–20 mg TMP/kg/day in divided doses every 6–8 hours
- Reduce dose of TMP-SMX in patients with renal failure.
- Pregnancy risk factor: C
- Precautions:
  - History of sulfa allergy
  - There is an emergence of drug-resistant PCP, especially against TMP-SMX.

Second Line
- Pentamidine (for moderate-to-severe cases):
  - Adults and children: 4 mg/kg IV or IM once daily
- Dapsone + trimethoprim (adults only):
  - Adult: Dapsone 100 mg orally once daily, plus
  - Adult: Trimethoprim 5 mg/kg orally 3 times daily:
    - Check glucose-6-phosphate dehydrogenase level before beginning dapsone, as hemolysis may result.
- Clindamycin + primaquine (adults only):
  - Clindamycin 600 mg IV every 8 hours or 300–450 mg orally 4 times daily, plus
  - Primaquine 30 mg orally once daily
- Atovaquone:
  - Adults: 750 mg orally twice daily (>13 years of age)
  - Children: 40 mg/kg/day orally divided twice daily (max 1500 mg)
- Note: Pentamidine has greater toxicity than TMP-SMX: Hypotension, hypoglycemia, pancreatitis (3)[C]

ADDITIONAL TREATMENT

Adjunctive corticosteroid (prednisone or methylprednisolone) (3)[C]:
- Adjunctive corticosteroids shown to provide benefits in patients who have AIDS and symptoms of moderate-to-severe PCP

- Corticosteroids provide the greatest benefit to HIV patients who have hypoxemia manifested as a partial pressure of arterial oxygen under 70 mm Hg or an alveolar-arteriolar gradient >35 on room air.
- Adults and children >13 years of age: Prednisone 40 mg orally twice daily on days 1–5, 40 mg daily days 6–11, 20 mg daily days 12–21

ONGOING CARE

FOLLOW-UP RECOMMENDATIONS
In patients with HIV/AIDS:
- Patients with previous episodes of PCP should receive lifelong secondary prophylaxis unless they respond well to highly active antiretroviral therapy (HAART) and have a CD4 count >200 cells/microliter for at least 3 months.

Patient Monitoring
Serum lactate dehydrogenase levels, pulmonary function test results, and arterial blood gas measurements generally normalize with treatment.

DIET
No special diet needed

PATIENT EDUCATION
- Centers for Disease Control and Prevention at http://www.cdc.gov/ncidod/dpd/parasites/pneumocystis/default.htm
- Family Doctor.org at http://familydoctor.org/online/famdocen/home/common/sexinfections/hiv/475.html

REFERENCES

1. Catherinot E, Lanterneier F, Bougnoux ME, et al. *Pneumocystis jirovecci* Pneumonia. *Infect Dis Clin N Am*. 2010;24:107–138.
2. D'Avignon LC, Schofield CM, Hospenthal DR. *Pneumocystis* Pneumonia. *Semin Repir Crit Care Med*. 2008;29:132–140.
3. Krajicek BJ, Thomas CF, Limper AH. Pneumocystis pneumonia: current concepts in pathogenesis, diagnosis, and treatment. *Clin Chest Med*. 2009;30:265–78, vi.
4. Kovacs JA, Masur H. Evolving Health Effects of Pneumocystis: One Hundred Years of Progress in Diagnosis and Treatment. *JAMA*. 2009;301(24): 2578–2585.

ADDITIONAL READING

- Briel M, Bucher H, Boscacci R, et al. Adjunctive corticosteroids for Pneumocystis jiroveci pneumonia in patients with HIV-infection. *Cochrane Database of Systematic Reviews*. 1, 2009.
- CDC. Guidelines for preventing opportunistic infections among HIV-infected persons—2002 recommendations of the US Public Health Service and the Infectious Disease Society of America. *MMWR*. 2002;51(No. RR-8).

- CDC. Treating opportunistic infections among HIV-infected adults and adolescents: Recommendations from CDC, the National Institutes of Health, and the HIV Medicine Association/Infectious Disease Society of America. *MMWR*. 2004;53(No. RR-15).
- Dohn MN, White ML, Vigdorth EM, et al. Geographic clustering of Pneumocystis carinii pneumonia in patients with HIV infection. *Am J Respir Crit Care Med*. 2000;162:1617–21.
- Green, Hefziba, Paul, Mical, Vidal, Liat, Leibovici, Leonard. Prophylaxis for Pneumocystis pneumonia (PCP) in non-HIV immunocompromised patients. *Cochrane Database of Systematic Reviews*. 1, 2009.
- Green H, Paul M, Vidal L, et al. Prophylaxis for Pneumocystis pneumonia (PCP) in non-HIV immunocompromised patients. *Cochrane Database of Systematic Reviews*. 1, 2009.
- Shankar SM, Nania JJ. Management of Pneumocystis jiroveci pneumonia in children receiving chemotherapy. *Paediatr Drugs*. 2007;9:301–9.
- Stringer JR, Beard CB, Miller RF, et al. A new name (Pneumocystis jiroveci) for Pneumocystis from humans. *Emerg Infect Dis*. 2002;8:891–6.

See Also (Topic, Algorithm, Electronic Media Element)
HIV Infection and AIDS

CODES

ICD9
136.3 Pneumocystosis

CLINICAL PEARLS

- Colonization with *Pneumocystis jiroveci* is common in the pediatric population.
- *Pneumocystis jiroveci* pneumonia (PCP) only occurs in immunocompromised patients.
- Patients with HIV are at risk once their CD4 count is <200. At that time, trimethoprim-sulfamethoxazole should be initiated as prophylaxis. Prophylaxis may end after HAART has been initiated and the CD4 count is above 200 for 3 months.
- Patients who are immunocompromised are also at risk. Currently there are no clear clinical guidelines as to when to initiate or end prophylaxis.
- First-line treatment is trimethoprim-sulfamethoxazole. Typical duration of therapy is 14 days in non-AIDS patients and 21 days in AIDS patients.

PNEUMONIA, VIRAL

Linda Sinclair, MD
Jason Kittler, MD, PhD, JD

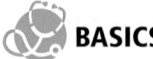 **BASICS**

DESCRIPTION
- Inflammatory disease of the lung parenchyma at the alveolar level due to a viral infection
- Most viral pneumonia results from exposure of a susceptible nonimmune person to infection in the form of aerosolized secretions.
- Viral infections damage upper respiratory tract mucosa and impair defense mechanisms, increasing risk for secondary pneumonia.

Geriatric Considerations
Greatest rates of morbidity and mortality

Pediatric Considerations
Viruses are the most common cause of pneumonia in children less than 5 years old. Adenoviral infections in children are serious. Serious illness with H1N1 is seen more commonly in children and young adults. More serious respiratory infections are almost always seen in infants and in immunocompromised patients.

Pregnancy Considerations
- Pregnant women are at higher risk of contracting viral pneumonia.
- All women who are pregnant during the influenza season—regardless of stage of pregnancy —should be vaccinated with seasonal trivalent inactivated influenza vaccine (TIV) injection.

EPIDEMIOLOGY
Incidence
- Predominant age: Children
- Predominant sex: Male = Female

Prevalence
- Respiratory viruses cause an estimated 10–31% of cases of adult community-acquired pneumonia (CAP).
- Prevalence is unknown and varies with seasonal outbreaks, but disease is more common during winter months.
- About 90% of all cases of childhood pneumonia have a viral cause.

RISK FACTORS
- Elderly patients
- Immunocompromised state
- Nonvaccinated person
- Living in close quarters
- Seasonal: Epidemic and pandemic respiratory illness
- Recent upper respiratory infection
- Cardiac disease (heart failure)
- Chronic pulmonary disease (COPD)
- Travel to endemic area (Hantavirus in North and South America and severe acute respiratory virus [SARS] in China)
- Avian flu is a risk with exposure to poultry (i.e., chickens, ducks, and turkeys) in Asia, Europe, and UK.

GENERAL PREVENTION
- TIV injection, containing influenza A H3N2, A H1N1, and B: For all children (6 months to 18 years), adults, and those at high risk of complications (>50 years of age, chronic disease, immunosuppressed, pregnant women, children and adolescents on aspirin therapy, residents of care facilities, health care workers, and caregivers or persons who live with someone at high risk) (1).
- Influenza intranasal live attenuated vaccine is an alternative for healthy, nonpregnant patients ages 2–49 years old (contraindicated in patients with asthma, HIV, or other chronic diseases).
- For patients who are unable to receive influenza vaccine (e.g., those with egg allergy) and are at high risk, prophylactic medications can be used.
- For nonvaccinated patients with known exposure to influenza or in geographic areas where influenza A outbreak has been documented, prophylactic medication can be used until vaccination produces immunity.
- Measles and varicella vaccines
- Frequent handwashing, barrier method, and isolation of suspected cases reduce transmission (2).

ETIOLOGY
- Influenza A, B, and C
- Influenza A H1N1 (swine flu)
- Parainfluenza 1, 2, 3, and 4
- Respiratory syncytial virus (RSV)
- Adenovirus
- Cytomegalovirus (CMV), particularly in immunocompromised patients
- Varicella (chickenpox)
- Herpes simplex virus (HSV)
- Enterovirus
- Coronavirus
- Rubeola (measles)
- Epstein-Barr virus
- Hantavirus (acute respiratory distress syndrome [ARDS]–like picture)
- Human meta-pneumovirus
- Avian influenza A (H5N1)
- Mixed infection with bacterial pathogens is common.

COMMONLY ASSOCIATED CONDITIONS
- Bacterial superinfection
- Fungal infection and *Pneumocystis jiroveci* pneumonia in immunocompromised patients

 DIAGNOSIS

HISTORY
- Chills, headache, malaise, and myalgias
- Dyspnea, cough ($\pm$ purulent sputum production), and pleurisy
- GI symptoms

PHYSICAL EXAM
- Vitals: Fever, tachypnea (often >24 breaths/min), hypoxemia with severe disease
- Pulmonary rales and rhonchi and/or friction rub
- Enlarged regional lymph nodes

DIAGNOSTIC TESTS & INTERPRETATION
Lab
- CBC:
  - Normal or near-normal granulocyte count, occasionally leukopenic with increased lymphocyte percentage
  - Hemoconcentration (hantavirus)
- Sputum Gram stain and culture to identify bacterial copathogens if present (3)
- Appropriate direct fluorescent antibody or enzyme immunoassay from throat and nasopharyngeal washings (children) or swab (adults), tracheal aspirate or bronchoalveolar lavage specimens (HSV, varicella, influenza viruses A and B, RSV, adenovirus)
- Viral culture
- Polymerase chain reaction (PCR) if modality is available
- Enzyme immunoassay (EIA) or immunofluorescence DFA antibody staining (influenza A and B)
- Rapid tests for influenza (available, but have lower sensitivity)
- Cytopathology (CMV, HSV, measles virus)
- Serology (4-fold rise in acute compared with convalescent titers)
- Procalcitonin may help differentiate between bacterial and viral pneumonia; low in viral infections (3).

Follow-Up & Special Considerations
On occasion, convalescent titers may be helpful in identifying a specific pathogen.

Imaging
CXR: Interstitial or alveolar infiltrates, peribronchial thickening, pleural effusion

Diagnostic Procedures/Surgery
- Nasopharyngeal throat swab
- Bronchoscopy with bronchoalveolar lavage (BAL)

Pathological Findings
- Cytoplasmic inclusion bodies (CMV)
- Intranuclear inclusion bodies (adenovirus, CMV, herpesvirus, varicella)
- Intense inflammatory reaction with mononuclear cells
- Multinucleated giant cells (parainfluenza virus, measles virus, HSV, varicella)

DIFFERENTIAL DIAGNOSIS
- Bacterial pneumonia (especially atypical etiologies: *Chlamydia pneumoniae* and *C. psittaci*, *Mycoplasma pneumoniae*, *Legionella pneumophila*)
- *Pneumocystis* pneumonia/*P. jiroveci* pneumonia
- Aspiration pneumonia
- Hypersensitivity pneumonitis
- Bronchiolitis obliterans with organizing pneumonia
- Pulmonary edema
- Pulmonary embolus/infarction
- Cystic fibrosis (in infants)
- SARS or SARS-associated

 TREATMENT

Outpatient for most patients; inpatient for infants <4 months of age or older people or for any patient with diffuse, severe infection (e.g., hypoxemia, hypercarbia, hypotension or shock, ARDS) or significant comorbidity (e.g., congestive heart failure [CHF], coronary artery disease [CAD], COPD)

MEDICATION
First Line
- Neuraminidase inhibitors: Influenza A and B:
  - For children 1–12 years of age: Oseltamivir given within 48 hours of onset can shorten duration of illness and reduce secondary complications (specifically, acute otitis media). Little evidence for prophylactic use (4).

– For adults: Neuraminidase inhibitors are not recommended for routine use in seasonal influenza, except for life-threatening illness (5).

– Seasonal influenza A H1N1 is commonly resistant to oseltamivir. Zanamivir or a combination of oseltamivir and rimantadine or amantadine (e.g., for patients <7 years old or patients with chronic underlying airways disease) is more appropriate than oseltamivir alone, unless local surveillance data indicate that the virus is likely to be influenza A H3N2 or influenza B (6).

- Oseltamivir (Tamiflu): Patients >12 years of age and adults: 75 mg p.o. q12h × 5 days. Dosage adjusted to 75 mg p.o. q24h in patients in whom the creatinine clearance rate is <30 mL/min.

- Zanamivir (Relenza): Patients >7 years of age: 10 mg (2 inhalations) inhaled p.o. q12h × 5 days

- Acyclovir (Zovirax): Pulmonary infections with HSV, herpes zoster, or varicella virus:
  – Children: 250 mg/m^2 IV q8h
  – Adults: 5 mg/kg IV q8h for pneumonia caused by HSV and 10 mg/kg IV q8h for pneumonia caused by varicella virus

- Ganciclovir (Cytovene): Infection with CMV or HSV:
  – Children: Safety and efficacy has not been established
  – Adults: 5 mg/kg IV q12h

- Ribavirin (Virazole): Respiratory syncytial virus, possibly hantavirus:
  – Children: Routine use in children is *not* recommended due to high cost and unclear benefit (7).
  – Adults: May be helpful in some cases; 6 g (20 mg/mL solution) daily via continuous aerosol administration over 12–18 h × 3–7 days
  – Contraindicated in pregnancy

Second Line
- M$_2$ ion channel inhibitors amantadine (Symmetrel) and rimantadine (Flumadine):
  – Influenza A only; only effective if given in 1st 24–48 hours
  – Rimantadine is an amantadine analogue; it is as effective and has fewer adverse effects.
  – For children: Amantadine is effective in prophylaxis for influenza A; safety not fully established. Rimantadine may be helpful in decreasing duration of fever and, therefore, can be used in select cases (8).
  – For adults: May help to alleviate symptoms but does not increase clearance or decrease viral transmission; should only be used in emergency situations (9).
  – CDC does not recommend using either alone for influenza A H3N2 or unknown strains in US due to widespread resistance, but may be used in combination with oseltamivir as an alternative to monotherapy with zanamivir (6).
- Foscarnet (Foscavir) for CMV, HSV, varicella virus infections
- IV immune globulin: May increase response in non-AIDS, immunosuppressed patients with CMV pneumonia; dose and dosage regimen are not well established, but 500 mg/kg/d IV × 10 doses may be beneficial

ADDITIONAL TREATMENT
General Measures
- Most healthy individuals will require only symptomatic treatment and supportive care.
- Encourage coughing and deep breathing exercises to clear secretions.
- Universal precautions

- Respiratory isolation for varicella virus, which is highly contagious (i.e., negative pressure)
- Antibiotics for superimposed bacterial infection

IN-PATIENT CONSIDERATIONS
Admission Criteria
General admission criteria include using CURB-65 criteria (confusion, uremia with a BUN >7, respiratory rate >30, low blood pressure, age >65) or the pneumonia severity index (3). This should be combined with clinical judgment and appropriate evaluation of the individual patient.

Discharge Criteria
Discharge criteria include (3):
- Temperature ≤37.8°C
- Respiratory rate ≤24 breaths/min
- Systolic blood pressure ≥ 90 mm Hg
- Arterial oxygen saturation ≥90% or pO$_2$ ≥60 mm Hg on room air
- Ability to maintain oral intake
- Normal mental status

ONGOING CARE

FOLLOW-UP RECOMMENDATIONS
Patient Monitoring
Oxygenation if illness severe enough for hospitalization

DIET
No specific restrictions

PATIENT EDUCATION
- American Lung Association, 1740 Broadway, New York, NY 100919; (800) LUNG-USA
- http://www.cdc.gov/flu/pandemic
- http://www.idsociety.org

PROGNOSIS
- Usually favorable prognosis, with illness lasting several days to a week. Postviral fatigue is common.
- Death can occur, especially in pediatric or bone marrow transplant patients with adenovirus infections or in older people with influenza.

COMPLICATIONS
- Superimposed bacterial infections such as *Streptococcus pneumoniae*, *Staphylococcus aureus*, *Haemophilus influenzae*, and others
- Respiratory failure requiring mechanical ventilation
- ARDS
- Reye syndrome after influenza in children

REFERENCES

1. Jefferson T, Di Pietrantonj C, Rivetti A, et al. Vaccines for preventing influenza in healthy adults. *Cochrane Database of Systematic Reviews* 2010, Issue 7. Art. No.: CD001269. DOI:10.1002/14651858.CD001269.pub4
2. Jefferson T, Del Mar C, Dooley L, et al. Physical interventions to interrupt or reduce the spread of respiratory viruses. *Cochrane Database of Systematic Reviews* 2010, Issue 1. Art. No.: CD006207. DOI:10.1002/14651858. CD006207.pub3
3. Mandell LA, Wunderink RG, Anzueto A, et al. Infectious Diseases Society of America/American Thoracic Society consensus guidelines on the management of community-acquired pneumonia in adults. *Clin Infect Dis*. 2007;44 (Suppl 2):S27–72.
4. Matheson NJ, Harnden A, Perera R, et al. Neuraminidase inhibitors for preventing and treating influenza in children. *Cochrane Database of Systematic Reviews* 2007, Issue 1. Art. No.: CD002744. DOI:10.1002/14651858. CD002744.pub2
5. Jefferson T, Jones M, Doshi P, et al. Neuraminidase inhibitors for preventing and treating influenza in healthy adults. *Cochrane Database of Systematic Reviews* 2010, Issue 2. Art. No.: CD001265. DOI:10.1002/14651858.CD001265.pub2
6. CDC. US Department of Health and Human Services, CDC. 2008. Available at http://www2a.cdc.gov/han/archivesys/viewmsgv.asp?alertnum=00279.
7. Ventre K, Randolph A, et al. WITHDRAWN: Ribavirin for respiratory syncytial virus infection of the lower respiratory tract in infants and young children. *Cochrane Database Syst Rev*. 2010;5: CD000181.
8. Alves Galvão MG, Rocha Crispino Santos MA, Alves da Cunha AJL. Amantadine and rimantadine for influenza A in children and the elderly. *Cochrane Database of Systematic Reviews*. 2008, Issue 1. Art. No.: CD002745. DOI:10.1002/14651858.CD002745.pub2.
9. Jefferson T, Demicheli V, Di Pietrantonj C, et al. Amantadine and rimantadine for influenza A in adults. *Cochrane Database of Systematic Reviews* 2006, Issue 2. Art. No.: CD001169. DOI:10.1002/14651858.CD001169.pub3.

See Also (Topic, Algorithm, Electronic Media Element)
Bronchiolitis Obliterans; Respiratory Distress Syndrome, Acute

CODES

ICD9
- 480.0 Pneumonia due to adenovirus
- 480.1 Pneumonia due to respiratory syncytial virus
- 480.2 Pneumonia due to parainfluenza virus

CLINICAL PEARLS
- Vaccination and proper hygiene, including handwashing, are key aspects of preventing transmission.
- Due to increased oseltamivir resistance of influenza A (H1N1), zanamivir, or a combination of oseltamivir and rimantadine is more appropriate than oseltamivir alone.

PNEUMOTHORAX

Peter Morse, MD
James J. Sullivan, Jr., MD, USN

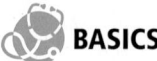 **BASICS**

DESCRIPTION
- Accumulation of air or gas between the parietal and visceral pleurae
- Spontaneous pneumothorax (SP) may be primary (PSP) or secondary (SSP).
- PSP occurs in healthy adults with no underlying lung disease (age 20s); rarely in patients >40 years of age.
- SSP is a complication of underlying lung disease [e.g., chronic obstructive pulmonary disease (COPD), cystic fibrosis, acquired immune-deficiency syndrome (AIDS), or tuberculosis (TB)].
- Traumatic pneumothorax, both closed and open, may exist in tandem with hemothorax.
- Tension pneumothorax (TP): Inspired air accumulates into the pleural space with no means of escape. More air increases lung compression and causes hypoxia and hemodynamic compromise.
- Occult pneumothorax (OP) is not suspected on the basis of clinical exam or plain radiography but is detected with thoracoabdominal CT scanning.
- System(s) affected: Pulmonary; Cardiovascular
- Synonym(s): Collapsed lung

EPIDEMIOLOGY
Incidence
- >20,000 new SP cases occur each year in the US at a cost of >$130 million.
- Predominant sex: Male > Female.
- Predominant age: PSP 10–40 years of age; SSP >60 years of age

Prevalence
- 25–50% recurrence rate of SSP within 1 year:
- PSP: 7.4-18/100,000 in men, 1.2-6/100,000 in women
- SSP: 6.3/100,000 in men, 2/100,000 in women

Geriatric Considerations
Higher rates of morbidity and mortality

Pediatric Considerations
Incidence is 1–2% of all neonates, associated with meconium aspiration and respiratory distress syndrome.

Pregnancy Considerations
Rare complication of labor and delivery

RISK FACTORS
- Traumatic pneumothorax:
  - Trauma (penetrating injury, broken rib, ruptured bronchus, perforated esophagus)
  - Iatrogenic/postprocedure: Intubation, central line placement, liver biopsy, mechanical ventilation, thoracentesis, cardiopulmonary resuscitation (CPR; seen in 3% of ICU patients)
  - Self-inflicted in intravenous drug abusers (attempting to access internal jugular vein)

- Spontaneous pneumothorax:
  - Cigarette smoking (increases risk 20×)
  - Airway disease: COPD, asthma, cystic fibrosis
  - Infection: *Pneumocystis* pneumonia, TB, necrotizing pneumonia
  - Malignancy: Lung cancer, sarcoma
  - Connective tissue disorder: Marfan or Ehlers-Danlos syndrome, scleroderma, rheumatoid arthritis, ankylosing spondylitis
  - Interstitial lung disease: Sarcoidosis, idiopathic pulmonary fibrosis, histiocytosis X, lymphangioleiomyomatosis
  - Bronchial obstruction or foreign body
  - Scuba diving
  - Loss of airplane cabin pressure

Genetics
- Possible predisposition in tall, thin young men, especially those with marfanoid habitus
- Multiple modes of inheritance proposed/observed: Autosomal dominant, recessive, X-linked recessive pattern
- Birt-Hobb-Dube syndrome: Autosomal dominant, associated with lung cysts, benign skin tumor, renal cancer; the *FLCN* mutation has been mapped to chromosome 17p11.2.

GENERAL PREVENTION
- Smoking cessation
- Advise use of seatbelts while driving.
- With subclavian vein cannulation, use a supraclavicular rather than an infraclavicular approach.

PATHOPHYSIOLOGY
Loss of negative intrapleural pressure, lung collapse

ETIOLOGY
- Perforation of the visceral pleura and entry of gas from the lung
- Penetration of the chest wall, diaphragm, mediastinum, or esophagus
- Blunt thoracic trauma
- Gas generated by microorganisms in an empyema

COMMONLY ASSOCIATED CONDITIONS
See Risk Factors.

 DIAGNOSIS

HISTORY
- Chest trauma
- Pleuritic chest pain
- Cough
- Dyspnea
- Moderate to severe: Profound respiratory distress, shock, circulatory collapse
- Referred pain to shoulder or back
- Rapid, shallow breathing

PHYSICAL EXAM
- Asymmetry of respirations
- Diminished breath sounds on affected side
- Decreased fremitus
- Absent egophony and bronchophony on affected side

- Hyperresonance to percussion
- Crepitus over chest wall and neck
- Tachycardia
- Respiratory distress
- Cyanosis
- Tension pneumothorax: Weak, rapid pulse; pallor; neck vein distention; anxiety; tracheal deviation away from affected side; hypotension; altered mental status
- Consider TP with sudden onset of tachycardia and hypotension in patients on ventilator (especially asthmatic/COPD patients).

DIAGNOSTIC TESTS & INTERPRETATION
Lab
Initial lab tests
- Arterial blood gases (ABGs; not diagnostic): Typically elevated A–a gradient and acute respiratory alkalosis
- Electrocardiogram (ECG): Not diagnostic but may show axis deviation, nonspecific ST-segment changes, T-wave inversion

Imaging
Initial approach
- Chest X-rays (CXRs):
  - Upright CXR usually is sufficient, but lateral, expiratory, or decubitus position is recommended in equivocal cases.
  - White visceral pleural line separated by a space with no lung/vascular markings adjacent to chest wall
  - Deep sulcus sign: Low lateral costophrenic angle on affected side
  - TP: Mediastinal shift to contralateral side
- CT scan: Most useful for
  - Trauma patients
  - Small pneumothoraces (if diagnosis is necessary)
  - Distinguishing emphysematous bullae from pneumothorax
- Ultrasound: Useful adjunct in major trauma patients
  - Absence of lung sliding is virtually pathognomic, with a sensitivity of 92–100%. Accurate in identifying size and extension of occult pneumothorax (OP), but this accuracy is lost in 24 h (1)[B]

DIFFERENTIAL DIAGNOSIS
- Acute coronary syndrome
- Pericarditis
- Pulmonary embolism
- Pleural effusion
- Pneumonia
- Dissection
- Flail chest
- Hemothorax
- Asthma/COPD
- Airway obstruction/foreign body
- Esophageal perforation
- Diaphragmatic hernia

TREATMENT

MEDICATION
First Line
100% O_2 accelerates rate of pleural air absorption.

Second Line
See "Pleurodesis" under Surgery/Other Procedures

ADDITIONAL TREATMENT
General Measures
- Monitor vital signs.
- Treat any underlying condition.
- Open pneumothorax: Place dressing over wound. Secure only on 3 sides to avoid tension pneumothorax.

SURGERY/OTHER PROCEDURES
- For 1st time PSP:
  - If small (<2–3 cm, <20%) and few symptoms: Patient may be observed in the emergency department for 3–6 h and discharged if repeat X-ray shows no progression (2)[C].
  - If larger and/or patient is symptomatic:
    - Randomized, controlled trial (RTC) has shown no difference between aspiration and chest tube in outcomes and fewer hospitalizations with aspiration (3)[A], but this should be accepted with caution owing to small sample size in study (4).
    - Aspiration technique: (1) Position patient semisupine at 45°, (2) prep and anesthetize skin, (3) insert a 16-gauge over-the-needle catheter into 2nd anterior intercostal space and aspirate air, (4) extract needle and connect 3-way stopcock and 60-mL syringe, and (5) aspirate until no more air can be removed. There is disagreement as to whether a failed aspiration should be reattempted.
    - Radiologists can place small-bore catheter or small-caliber chest tube over a guide wire and connect to a Heimlich valve or water seal. However, no RCTs compare their effectiveness.
  - If pneumothorax is large, the patient is unstable, or prior treatment has failed:
    - Insert thoracostomy tube (16–22 F) into 4th, 5th, or 6th intercostal space at the midaxillary line and connect to water seal device. Clamp after 12 h of no air leak.
  - If tension pneumothorax:
    - Needle decompression; Insert 19F or larger needle (14- to 16-gauge, 5-cm needle) into the 2nd intercostal space at the midclavicular line over the superior aspect of rib to avoid vessels, and attach a 3-way stopcock. (Failure rate is 10–35%; longer needles are needed for patients with increased chest wall thickness.) Use large syringe to withdraw air. Follow with a chest tube.
- For recurrent PSP:
  - There is good consensus and clinical evidence that PSP recurrence prevention should be proposed only after a first recurrence (5)[B].
  - Pleurodesis: Superior to simple drainage in reducing recurrence (6)[C]
    - Intrapleural talc: 5 g in 250 mL of isotonic saline; more effective than tetracycline derivatives, but safety concerns still exist.
    - Intrapleural doxycycline: 5 mg/kg or 500 mg in total of 50 mL

- Pleural abrasion or partial pleurectomy is also used.
- Sclerosing agents are contraindicated if patient is a possible candidate for future lung transplant because they increase the risk of bleeding during surgery.
- Side effects: Fever, pain, and acute lung injury
- Premedicate patients with a benzodiazepine and/or a narcotic for pain.
- Consider moderate or deep sedation with ketamine, propofol, or etomidate.
- Decreased effectiveness if concurrent glucocorticoid use or if lung is not fully reexpanded prior to pleurodesis
  - Video-assisted thoracoscopy (VAT) with pleurodesis is recommended for
    - Recurrent PSP, initial SSP
    - Persistent air leak after 3 days
    - Persistent bronchopleural fistula
    - Patient preference or high-risk occupation (e.g., pilot, diver)
    - Open thoracotomy if failed or unavailable VAT
- For SSP: Patients should be hospitalized; most authors and guidelines recommend immediate chest tube insertion along with recurrence prevention (5)[C].
- For catamenial pneumothorax: Recurrence prevention after 1st episode and possible hormonal suppression (5)[C]
- For traumatic/OP:
  - Usually both overt and occult pneumothorax patients get chest tubes.
  - It appears that small to moderate OP can be treated conservatively.
  - Chest tube insertion for OP needing mechanical ventilation is unclear. Retrospective studies indicate that tube thoracostomy may not be required, but two RCTs arrived at opposite conclusions (1)[B].

IN-PATIENT CONSIDERATIONS
Initial Stabilization
- Stabilize, oxygenation
- TP is a medical emergency. Do *not* wait for CXR; decompress as soon as possible.

Admission Criteria
Admit all patients with either a large PSP that does not resolve completely with simple aspiration, recurrent pneumothorax, SSP, or traumatic pneumothorax

 ONGOING CARE

FOLLOW-UP RECOMMENDATIONS
- No air travel until radiographs are normal.
- Athletes with pneumothorax may return to sports activity after 2–3 weeks of rest as symptoms permit; athletes who require inpatient care should have a follow-up CXR before resuming sports activity.

Patient Monitoring
- Bed rest while chest tube is in place
- Serial radiographs to document improvement
- After simple aspiration/tube thoracostomy: Clamp for 24 h, and then remove if no recurrence is seen on radiograph. If lung is not fully reexpanded after 7 days, consider persistent bronchopleural fistula.
- Outpatient management should include follow-up CXR to document resolution of pneumothorax, typically in several days.

PATIENT EDUCATION
Smoking cessation

PROGNOSIS
- Air is reabsorbed in days to weeks.
- Risk of recurrence: For PSP, mean of 30% with range of 16–52%; for SSP, 39–47%.
- Prognosis is worse depending on comorbidities.

COMPLICATIONS
- Reexpansion pulmonary edema
- Bronchopleural fistulas requiring repair

REFERENCES
1. Ball CG, Kirkpatrick AW, Feliciano DV et al. The occult pneumothorax: what have we learned? *Can J Surg.* 2009;52:E173–9.
2. Zehtabchi S, Rios CL et al. Management of emergency department patients with primary spontaneous pneumothorax: needle aspiration or tube thoracostomy? *Ann Emerg Med.* 2008; 51:91–100, 100.e1.
3. Wakai A, O'Sullivan RG, McCabe G et al. Simple aspiration versus intercostal tube drainage for primary spontaneous pneumothorax in adults. *Cochrane Database Syst Rev.* 2007;CD004479.
4. Gaudio M, Hafner JW et al. Evidence-based emergency medicine/systematic review abstract: Simple aspiration compared to chest tube insertion in the management of primary spontaneous pneumothorax. *Ann Emerg Med.* 2009;54:458–60.
5. Noppen M, De Keukeleire T et al. Pneumothorax. *Respiration.* 2008;76:121–7.
6. Gyorik S, et al. Long-term follow up of thoracoscopic talc pleurodesis for primary spontaneous pneumothorax. *Eur Resp J.* 2007;29(4):757–760.

 CODES

ICD9
- 512.0 Spontaneous tension pneumothorax
- 512.1 Iatrogenic pneumothorax
- 512.8 Other spontaneous pneumothorax

CLINICAL PEARLS
- Primary pneumothorax is unusual in patients over the age of 40. Consider other etiologies in this population.
- Emergency needle decompression is accomplished in the 2nd intercostal space in the midclavicular line, tracking over the superior margin of the rib if possible.

POLIOMYELITIS

Omar A. Khan, MD, MHS

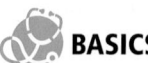

BASICS

DESCRIPTION
- Poliomyelitis describes the acute illness. Most patients contracting the poliovirus are asymptomatic; ~5% develop symptoms, and 0.1% develop the paralytic form.
- Patients may present with GI symptoms.
- A subset will develop neurologic disease.
- Illness is biphasic; paralysis occurs in 2nd phase. Paralytic disease occurs with rapid onset.
- Spread by direct fecal–oral contact; more common in warm months.
- Virus secreted for weeks in stool:
  - Poliomyelitis syndromes: Encephalitic; bulbar (which produces cranial nerve paralysis); spinal (causing weakness in the extremities, particularly the legs)
  - Postpolio syndrome (PPS) is a distinct entity affecting those previously diagnosed with poliomyelitis. Involves atrophy of muscle groups unaffected by original illness.
- System(s) affected: Nervous; Musculoskeletal
- Synonym(s): Infantile paralysis; Acute anterior poliomyelitis; Acute lateral poliomyelitis

Geriatric Considerations
Extremely rare; primary vaccination not recommended (except if travel to endemic areas)

Pediatric Considerations
Most common in this age group. Infection is extremely rare in the US since introduction of effective vaccines (see Immunizations).

Pregnancy Considerations
A risk factor for developing polio (incidence and severity of polio are increased in pregnant women)

EPIDEMIOLOGY
Incidence
- Predominant age: 3 months–16 years; rare in adults
- Now rare but not yet eradicated; present in endemic settings, small outbreaks in areas where polio eradication has occurred, and rarely as vaccine-associated paralytic polio (VAPP) cases
- PPS can manifest years to decades after initial infection.

Prevalence
- Endemic countries: Afghanistan, India, Nigeria, and Pakistan; importation cases are present in some others as well (sub-Saharan Africa, Nepal, and Tajikistan)
- Worldwide: 1,595 cases in 2009 (1,247 from 4 endemic countries; 348 from 19 countries where the disease was imported or possibly re-established)
- Previous worldwide numbers were 1,660 cases in 2008; 1,315 cases in 2007
- Highest numbers in 2009 were India (741) and Nigeria (388)
- No wild-virus cases of polio in the US.

RISK FACTORS
- Poor sanitation and hygiene
- Poverty
- Unimmunized status, especially if <5 years of age

GENERAL PREVENTION
- Vaccination via the inactivated poliovirus vaccine (IPV) in developed settings
- Oral vaccine (OPV) in endemic or at-risk countries
- No causal link between the polio vaccine and Guillain-Barré
- In developing countries, safe water treatment to avoid contaminated water and food sources

PATHOPHYSIOLOGY
- Poliovirus initially infects the GI tract. It may spread to lymph nodes and rarely to CNS.
- Pharyngeal spread is less common, but is the prevalent mode of transmission in areas of good hygiene.
- Person-to-person spread is the most common means of transmission, followed by contaminated water and sewage.

ETIOLOGY
3 serotypes of poliovirus (genus *Enterovirus*):
- Type 1 most frequently associated with epidemics
- Types 2 and 3 usually associated with VAPP

COMMONLY ASSOCIATED CONDITIONS
- IM injections or trauma during the prodrome of paralytic polio can precipitate paralysis.
- Tonsillectomy is considered a risk factor for bulbar paralysis.

DIAGNOSIS

- Virus culture from stool, pharynx, or CSF
- Antibody response useful for ruling out rather than ruling in polio, because immunization also may provoke such a response.

HISTORY
If the affected person is from a nonendemic country, then travel history is important.

PHYSICAL EXAM
- Most patients are asymptomatic. Approximately 10% will show symptoms of a minor GI illness, including fever, malaise, nausea, and vomiting.
- A minority of these patients will progress to the major illness, which includes asymmetric paralysis of extremities (usually lower).
- Aseptic meningitis occurs in a minority of patients with the major illness.
- Significant motor loss on affected side or limb
- Meningeal signs may be present in minor illness or early phases of paralytic polio.
- Decreased deep tendon reflexes
- Muscle atrophy in affected areas

DIAGNOSTIC TESTS & INTERPRETATION
CSF and pharynx virus isolation (early in disease) and/or feces (early and late in disease)

Lab
- Increased CSF protein
- Lymphocytosis, especially of CSF
- Normal CSF glucose
- Serology
- Virus culture from stool or pharynx

Imaging
MRI may be helpful to evaluate the involvement of anterior horn of the spinal cord or other findings.

Diagnostic Procedures/Surgery
EMG may be useful to assess the progress of paralysis and of PPS.

Pathological Findings
Spinal cord: Perivascular cuffing, abnormal motor nuclei, chromatolysis of motor neurons, intermediate and posterior column inflammation

DIFFERENTIAL DIAGNOSIS
- For acute flaccid paralysis and paralytic polio:
  - Guillain-Barré syndrome
  - Transverse myelitis
  - Acute motor axonal neuropathy (China paralytic syndrome)
  - Traumatic neuritis
  - Myasthenia gravis
  - Polymyositis
  - Periodic paralysis
  - Trichinosis
  - Aseptic, bacterial, and tuberculous meningitis/encephalitis
  - Toxic encephalopathies
  - Tick paralysis
- For nonparalytic acute polio infection:
  - Enteroviruses, echoviruses, and coxsackieviruses

TREATMENT

The European Federation of Neurological Societies has guidelines on PPS describing muscular training, targeted physical therapy, and assistive devices as needed.

MEDICATION
- Non-narcotic analgesics (aspirin should not be used for children due to the suggested, small risk of Reye's syndrome)
- Antibiotics, if concurrent infection develops
- Parasympathomimetic pharmacotherapy for urinary retention may be required.
- Preliminary investigations suggest that IV immunoglobulin (IVIG) may improve quality of life for PPS patients.
- Small studies on lamotrigine, modafinil, amantadine, and pyridostigmine suggest benefit, but no conclusive evidence is available to recommend this as therapy.
- Contraindications and precautions: Refer to the manufacturers' literature.
- Significant possible interactions: Refer to the manufacturers' literature.

First Line
None available for curative treatment

ADDITIONAL TREATMENT
General Measures
- Mechanical ventilation, if required
- Public health: With all suspected cases, report immediately to local health authority, such as public health department in the US or WHO affiliate in developing countries.
- Any case of polio is considered an emergency.

Issues for Referral
- Referral to a neurologist is indicated in the case of major illness.
- Infectious disease referral is warranted at the time of diagnosis.
- After discharge, referral to physical therapy, neurology, or physical medicine and rehabilitation is indicated, especially for PPS.
- Psychiatry or clinical psychology referral can be helpful for patient and caregivers.

Additional Therapies
- Early physical therapy in acute paralytic polio may help a child to regain function and develop adaptations.
- With paralysis (acute or postpolio), extended PT may be required.
- Long-term rehabilitation plan: Using PT, braces, special shoes, possibly orthopedic surgery; team effort with doctors, physical and occupational therapists, and social worker or psychiatrist, if necessary

SURGERY/OTHER PROCEDURES
- Tracheostomy for respiratory paralysis
- Surgery may be required in the patients with muscle contractures or to relieve severe deformity resulting from muscle atrophy and paralysis.

IN-PATIENT CONSIDERATIONS
Initial Stabilization
Inpatient for acute phase or if concern for respiratory/bulbar paralysis exists; outpatient or rehabilitation facility for therapy

Admission Criteria
- New-onset neurologic symptoms such as stiff neck, seizures, and paralysis
- Once diagnosed, cases of paralytic polio may need admission to observe for bulbar paralysis.
- Dehydration resulting from the minor illness

Nursing
The main concerns relate to mobilization to regain function, assurance of hygiene if bowel/bladder incontinence exists, skin care if mobility is severely restricted, and pain control in case of contractures:
- Provide a bed that has a firm mattress, footboard, foam-rubber pads, or sandbags. Change patient's positions frequently. Ensure good skin care.
- Management of fecal impaction and urinary retention; catheterization may be necessary.

Discharge Criteria
- In case of minor illness, self-limited resolution
- In case of major illness, criteria include a plan for outpatient follow-up by the family physician, specialist in orthopedics or neurology, and physical therapist.

ONGOING CARE

FOLLOW-UP RECOMMENDATIONS
- Physical therapy is essential in paralytic polio.
- Counseling for the patient, caregivers, and family is useful in managing lifetime sequelae.
- Bed rest during active phase of disease as per patient tolerance; as noted, physical therapy and nonfatiguing exercises may help.

DIET
- May require tube feedings if paralyzed
- Unrestricted except for conditions determined by patient's ability to swallow

PATIENT EDUCATION
For patient education materials, contact:
- International Polio Network, 4502 Maryland Avenue, St. Louis, MO 63108, (314) 361-0475
- Educational presentation on polio from the CDC: http://www.cdc.gov/vaccines/pubs/pinkbook/downloads/Slides/Polio10.ppt
- PPS patient materials via Post-Polio Health International: http://www.post-polio.org/
- The Global Polio Eradication Initiative, coordinated by the WHO: http://www.polioeradication.org
- Brain Resources and Information Network (BRAIN), National Institute of Neurological Disorders and Stroke (NINDS), National Institutes of Health, Bethesda, MD: http://www.ninds.nih.gov

PROGNOSIS
- Often irreversible paralysis; <5% mortality during acute disease
- Increased mortality in patients >40 years of age
- Poor recovery for totally paralyzed muscle groups; good recovery for partially paralyzed muscle groups
- Variable recovery for PPS; can be facilitated by appropriate PT

COMPLICATIONS
- Urinary tract infection
- Skin ulcers
- Traumatic injuries to affected limb(s)
- Atelectasis
- Pneumonia
- Myocarditis
- Postpoliomyelitis progressive muscular atrophy: Progressive weakness 30 years or more after an attack of poliomyelitis. Adult survivors of childhood polio now suffer late complications.
- Postpoliomyelitis motor neuron disease: Occurs years after acute poliomyelitis; less common than postpoliomyelitis progressive muscular atrophy.
- Vaccine-associated paralytic poliomyelitis is a rare complication of oral poliovirus vaccine.

ADDITIONAL READING
- Adams T et al. Global eradication of poliomyelitis: Is the end of the campaign in sight? *Journal of paediatrics and child health*. 2010;
- Farbu E, Gilhus NE, Barnes MP, et al. EFNS guideline on diagnosis and management of post-polio syndrome. Report of an EFNS task force. *Eur J Neurol*. 2006;13:795–801.

- Gonzalez H, Sunnerhagen KS, Sjöberg I, et al. Intravenous immunoglobulin for post-polio syndrome: a randomised controlled trial. *Lancet Neurol*. 2006;5:493–500.
- Mayer CA, Neilson AA et al. Poliomyelitis– prevention in travellers. *Aust Fam Physician*. 2010;39:122–5.
- Minor P et al. Vaccine-derived poliovirus (VDPV): Impact on poliomyelitis eradication. *Vaccine*. 2009;27:2649–52.
- Thompson KM, Tebbens RJ, Pallansch MA, et al. The risks, costs, and benefits of possible future global policies for managing polioviruses. *Am J Public Health*. 2008;98:1322–30.

See Also (Topic, Algorithm, Electronic Media Element)
CDC FAQ on Polio: http://www.cdc.gov/nip/vaccine/Polio/polio-faqs-hcp.htm
WHO website on Polio Eradication: www.polioeradication.org/

CODES

ICD9
- 045.90 Unspecified acute poliomyelitis, unspecified type poliovirus
- 045.91 Unspecified acute poliomyelitis, poliovirus type i
- 045.92 Unspecified acute poliomyelitis, poliovirus type ii

CLINICAL PEARLS
- VAPP has been eliminated from the US since implementation of the IPV-only vaccine in 2000 (ending use of the live oral polio vaccine).
- VAPP occurred in roughly 1 of 2.9 million doses of the vaccine in the 1990s.
- 95% of wild-virus polio is asymptomatic, and <1% will develop paralysis. Wild-type polio no longer exists in the US. Polio remains in wild-type strains in 4 countries in Asia and Africa. The WHO goal to eradicate the disease likely will be pushed back beyond 2012.

POLYARTERITIS NODOSA

Prachaya Nitichaikulvatana, MD
Katherine Upchurch, MD

BASICS

DESCRIPTION
- Polyarteritis nodosa (PAN) is a *necrotizing vasculitis that typically affects medium-sized arteries,* with occasional involvement of small-sized arteries.
- Systemic symptoms are prominent at presentation.
- Most common organ involvement: GI tract, peripheral nervous system (sensory and motor), kidney, skin, testes and epididymis, cardiac, CNS
- PAN formerly encompassed several distinct clinical entities (classic PAN, microscopic PAN, and cutaneous PAN). With the advent of antineutrophilic antibody (ANCA) testing has come the understanding that microscopic PAN may not be related to the other 2 pathophysiologically. In particular, patients with microscopic PAN have ANCAs directed against myeloperoxidase (MPO) and generally involvement of small arterioles. This disease is also known as *microscopic polyangiitis* and is now classified as one of the ANCA-associated vasculitides.
- Classic PAN (now commonly referred to as PAN), in contrast, is not typically associated with ANCA positivity. Cutaneous (or limited) PAN is a disease in which patients have largely cutaneous and neurologic manifestations with characteristic histopathologic features but few systemic features. ANCA positivity is variable.
- Synonym(s) for PAN: Periarteritis; Panarteritis; Necrotizing arteritis

Pregnancy Considerations
1 case report suggests that if a woman of childbearing age with PAN attains remission before becoming pregnant, there is a reasonable chance of a successful pregnancy.

EPIDEMIOLOGY
Incidence
- Predominant age: All ages; peak onset is in the 5th–6th decade
- Predominant sex: Male > Female (2.5:1)

Prevalence
Rare, 31 cases/1 million adults in European study

RISK FACTORS
Hepatitis B infection

Genetics
Unknown

ETIOLOGY
- Unknown
- Immune-complex mediation has been postulated.
- In patients with PAN and hepatitis B, studies have shown immune complexes containing the hepatitis B antigen in involved vessel walls.

COMMONLY ASSOCIATED CONDITIONS
- Hepatitis B (most strongly in classic PAN)
- Hepatitis C (linked to cutaneous PAN)
- Hairy cell leukemia
- 27 case reports of systemic PAN following hepatitis B vaccination (1)
- Case reports of various drugs such as amphetamines, minocycline, and interferon

DIAGNOSIS

Acute multisystem disease with a relatively short prodrome (i.e., weeks–months); delays in diagnosis are common. The spectrum of disease ranges from single-organ involvement to fulminant polyvisceral failure.

HISTORY
General: Systemic symptoms with multiorgan involvement (23):
- Constitutional symptoms (e.g., fever, weight loss, malaise)
- Symptoms highly dependent on specific organ system involved
- Focal muscular weakness or extremity numbness
- Myalgia and arthralgia
- Rash
- Recurrent postprandial pain, intestinal angina, nausea, vomiting, and bleeding
- Altered mental status, headaches

PHYSICAL EXAM
Related to organ system involved by vasculitic process (may dominate clinical picture and course):
- Peripheral nervous system: Mononeuritis multiplex, peripheral neuropathy
- Renal: Hypertension, proteinuria, progressive renal failure, hematuria (usually microscopic) but no red blood cell (RBC) casts
- Skin: Purpura, urticaria, SC hemorrhages, polymorphic rashes, SC nodules (uncommon but characteristic), persistent livedo reticularis, deep skin ulcers, especially in lower extremities, Raynaud phenomenon (rare)
- GI: Acute abdomen due to bowel infarction and perforation, cholecystitis, and gallbladder infarctions; asymptomatic microaneurysm in the liver (4)
- CNS: Seizures, altered mental status, thrombotic stroke (with cerebral artery involvement), papillitis
- Lung: Pleural effusion, rarely bronchial arteritis:
  – Capillaritis or other lung parenchymal involvement by vasculitis strongly suggests another process (microscopic PAN, Wegener granulomatosis, Churg-Strauss syndrome) or antiglomerular basement membrane disease.
- Cardiac: Congestive heart failure (CHF) associated with hypertension (HTN) and/or myocardial infarction; pericarditis (rare)
- Genitourinary: Testicular, epididymal. ovarian involvement; neurogenic bladder rare
- Musculoskeletal: Arthritis (usually large joint in lower extremities)

DIAGNOSTIC TESTS & INTERPRETATION
- Diagnosis should be confirmed by biopsy whenever possible.
- Angiography may be helpful to reveal microaneurysms of blood vessels.
- CT angiography and MR angiography may be substituted for conventional angiography.

Lab
- Specific: Mainly based on pathologic findings of biopsy material from involved organs
- Nonspecific (2):
  – Elevated erythrocyte sedimentation rate (ESR) and C-reactive protein (CRP)
  – Hepatitis B surface antigen positive in 10–50% of patients (strong circumstantial evidence)
  – Hepatitis C antibody or hepatitis C virus RNA
  – Antineutrophilic cytoplasmic antibody (ANCA) is usually negative.
  – Negative proteinase-3 (PR3) or MPO antibodies
  – Rheumatoid factor may be positive.
  – Anemia of chronic disease
  – Hypergammaglobulinemia
  – Mild proteinuria
  – Elevated creatinine

Initial lab tests
Laboratory studies with abnormalities:
- Complete blood count (CBC) (anemia of chronic disease)
- Chemistries: Elevated creatinine/blood urea nitrogen (BUN)
- Hepatitis B serology: Often positive
- Liver function tests: Abnormal in unusual cases such as PAN involving the liver or gallbladder
- Urinalysis may show proteinuria but generally no cellular casts or active urinary sediment.
- ANCA antibody testing as well as specific tests for anti-MPO and anti-PR3.

Imaging
Angiographic demonstration of aneurysmal changes in small and medium-sized arteries: Mesenteric, renal, hepatic artery aneurysm

Diagnostic Procedures/Surgery
- Electromyography (EMG) and nerve conduction studies (NCSs) can be useful in patients with suspected mononeuritis multiplex. EMG/NCSs can be used to guide a sural nerve biopsy, if necessary.
- Arterial or tissue biopsy wherever involvement suspected; biopsy feasible
- Skin biopsy: The biopsy should be collected at the edges of ulcer and include deep dermis and subcutaneous fat for high yield of diagnosis.

Pathological Findings
- Necrotizing inflammation with fibrinoid necrosis, in various stages, of small and medium-sized muscular arteries; segmental in distribution, it is often seen at bifurcations and branchings. Involvement of venules is not seen in classic PAN.
- Acute lesions show infiltration of polymorphonuclear cells through vessel walls and perivascular area.
- Subsequent proliferation, degeneration, appearance of monocytes, necrosis with thrombosis, and infarction of the involved tissue; aneurysmal dilatations are characteristic.
- Aortic dissection is reported to be attributed to necrotizing vasculitis of the vasa vasorum.
- Peripheral nerves: 50–70% (vasa nervorum with necrotizing vasculitis)
- GI vessels: 50% (at autopsy); gallbladder and appendix: 10%
- Muscle vessels: 50%
- Testicular vasculature is often positive when males are symptomatic.

- The key differences from other necrotizing vasculitides are lack of granuloma formation and sparing of veins and pulmonary arteries.

DIFFERENTIAL DIAGNOSIS
- Other forms of vasculitis; ANCA-associated vasculitis such as Wegener granulomatosis, Churg-Strauss syndrome, and microscopic polyangiitis; Henoch-Schönlein purpura
- Cryoglobulinemia
- Buerger disease
- Systemic lupus erythematosus (SLE)
- Amyloidosis
- Multiple sclerosis
- Embolic disease such as atrial myxoma, cholesterol emboli
- Dissecting aneurysm
- Subacute endocarditis
- Trichinosis
- Some rickettsial diseases

 ## TREATMENT
MEDICATION
First Line
- Corticosteroids (high-dose prednisone or parenteral solumedrol (± pulse for stabilization), only half of patients achieved and maintained remission with corticosteroid alone and 40% of patients required additional immunosuppressive therapy (5)
- Cyclophosphamide in combination with corticosteroids (improved survival and steroid-sparing) in moderate or severe PAN (5): Cyclophosphamide can have long-term sequelae of infertility and malignancy (6)[A].
- Other immunosuppressive agents: Azathioprine (Imuran) (5), methotrexate
- Plasma exchange (efficacy not established)
- Small study of short-term steroids followed by lamivudine and plasma exchanges suggests effectiveness of this regimen in hepatitis B–related PAN (unconfirmed) (7).

Second Line
Tumor necrosis factor inhibitors (anecdotal evidence)

ADDITIONAL TREATMENT
- For patients receiving intravenous cyclophosphamide, suggest concurrent administration of mercaptoethane sulfonate (MESNA).
- For patients on cyclophosphamide, we recommend prophylactic treatment against *Pneumocystis jiroveci* (*carinii*) pneumonia with trimethoprim sulfamethoxazole or atovaquone in patients who are intolerant or allergic to trimethoprim sulfamethoxazole.

IN-PATIENT CONSIDERATIONS
Initial Stabilization
Depends on extent and involvement of specific organs

 ## ONGOING CARE
FOLLOW-UP RECOMMENDATIONS
Patient Monitoring
- Complete blood chemistry (CBC), urinalysis, and renal and hepatic profiles
- Careful monitoring for infection
- Delayed appearance of neoplasms (especially in patients who were treated with cyclophosphamide)
- Acute-phase reactants such as CRP may be helpful in monitoring activity level during treatment and follow-up.

DIET
Low salt if patient has attendant HTN

PATIENT EDUCATION
Advise patient that materials are available from Arthritis Foundation, 1314 Spring St, N.W., Atlanta, GA 30309; (800) 283-7800.

PROGNOSIS
- Expected course of untreated PAN is poor, with an estimated 5-year survival of 13%.
- Steroid and cytotoxic therapy treatment may increase survival rate significantly (8), with a 5-year survival rate of 75–80% (9).
- Survival is greater for hepatitis B–related PAN as a result of the introduction of antiviral treatments.
- Patients presenting with proteinuria, renal insufficiency, GI tract involvement, cardiomyopathy, or CNS involvement have a poorer prognosis than those without.
- Rate of mortality from PAN remains high for the elderly patients (3).

COMPLICATIONS
- Renal failure
- Thrombosis of involved vessels
- Tissue/organ necrosis
- Stroke
- Myocardial infarction
- Mononeuritis multiplex
- Peripheral neuropathy
- Perforated viscous (bowel)

REFERENCES

1. Carvalho JF, Pereira RM, Shoenfeld Y. Systemic polyarteritis nodosa following hepatitis B vaccination. *Eur J Intern Med*. 2008;19:575–8.
2. Gayraud M, Guillevin L, le Toumelin P, et al. Long-term followup of polyarteritis nodosa, microscopic polyangiitis, and Churg-Strauss syndrome: analysis of four prospective trials including 278 patients. *Arthritis Rheum*. 2001;44:666–75.
3. Pagnoux C, Seror R, Henegar C, et al. Clinical features and outcomes in 348 patients with polyarteritis nodosa: a systematic retrospective study of patients diagnosed between 1963 and 2005 and entered into the French Vasculitis Study Group Database. *Arthritis Rheum*. 2010;62: 616–26.
4. Ebert EC, Hagspiel KD, Nagar M, et al. Gastrointestinal Involvement in Polyarteritis Nodosa. *Clin Gastroenterol Hepatol*. 2008.
5. Ribi C, Cohen P, Pagnoux C, et al. Treatment of polyarteritis nodosa and microscopic polyangiitis without poor-prognosis factors: A prospective randomized study of one hundred twenty-four patients. *Arthritis Rheum*. 2010;62:1186–97.
6. Chan M, Luqmani R. Pharmacotherapy of vasculitis. *Expert Opin Pharmacother*. 2009.
7. Guillevin L, Mahr A, Cohen P, et al. Short-term corticosteroids then lamivudine and plasma exchanges to treat hepatitis B virus-related polyarteritis nodosa. *Arthritis Rheum*. 2004;51: 482–7.
8. Bourgarit A, Le Toumelin P, Pagnoux C, et al. Deaths occurring during the first year after treatment onset for polyarteritis nodosa, microscopic polyangiitis, and Churg-Strauss syndrome: a retrospective analysis of causes and factors predictive of mortality based on 595 patients. *Medicine (Baltimore)*. 2005;84:323–30.
9. Phillip R, Luqmani R. Mortality in systemic vasculitis: a systematic review. *Clin Exp Rheumatol*. 2008;26:94–104.

ADDITIONAL READING
- Kallenberg CG et al. The last classification of vasculitis. *Clin Rev Allergy Immunol*. 2008;35:5–10.
- Villa-Forte A, European League Against Rheumatism, European Vasculitis Study Group et al. European League Against Rheumatism/European Vasculitis Study Group recommendations for the management of vasculitis. *Curr Opin Rheumatol*. 2010;22:49–53.

See Also (Topic, Algorithm, Electronic Media Element)
Hepatitis B; Hepatitis C

 ## CODES
ICD9
446.0 Polyarteritis nodosa

CLINICAL PEARLS
- PAN is a necrotizing vasculitis of primarily medium-sized arteries with lack of granuloma formation and sparing of veins and pulmonary arteries.
- Skin biopsy should be collected at the edges of ulcer and include deep dermis and subcutaneous fat for high yield of diagnosis.
- Check hepatitis B and C serologies.

POLYCYSTIC KIDNEY DISEASE

Maricarmen Malagon-Rogers, MD

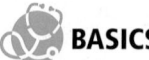 **BASICS**

DESCRIPTION

- A group of monogenic disorders that result in renal cyst development
- The most frequent ones are 2 genetically distinct conditions: Autosomal dominant polycystic kidney disease (ADPKD) and autosomal recessive polycystic kidney disease (ARPKD).
- ADPKD is one of the most common human genetic disorders.

EPIDEMIOLOGY

- ADPKD is generally late onset:
  - Mean age of end-stage kidney disease (ESKD) 57–69 years
  - More progressive disease in men than in women
  - Up to 90% of adults have cysts in the liver.
- ARPKD usually presents in infants:
  - A minority in older children and young adults may manifest as liver disease.
  - Nonobstructive intrahepatic bile dilatation is sometimes seen.
  - Found on all continents and in all races

Incidence

As ESKD:

- ADPKD: 8.7/1 million in the US; 7/1 million in Europe
- Mean age of end-stage renal disease (ESRD): PKD1, 54.3 years versus PKD2, 74 years

Prevalence

- ADPKD affects 1/400–1,000 live births.
- ARPKD affects 1/20,000 live births; carrier level 1/70.

RISK FACTORS

- Large inter- and intrafamilial variability
- A more rapid clinical course increased by onset of hypertension (HTN) <35 years, male gender, in PKD2, diagnosis <30 years, hyperlipidemia

Genetics

- ADPKD:
  - Autosomal dominant inheritance
  - 50% of children of an affected adult are affected.
  - 100% penetrance; genetic imprinting and genetic anticipation are seen as well.
  - 2 genes isolated:
    - *PKD1* on chromosome 16p13.3 (85% of patients)
    - *PKD2* on chromosome 4q21 (15% of patients)
    - Presumed *PKD3* not yet identified
- ARPKD:
  - Autosomal recessive inheritance
  - Siblings have a 1:4 chance of being affected; gene *PKHD1* on chromosome 6p21.1–p12.

GENERAL PREVENTION

Genetic counseling

PATHOPHYSIOLOGY

- ADPKD:
  - Protein product of *PKD1:* Polycystin-1 mechanosensor in cilia; detects changes in flow, interacts with surrounding matrix and cell membrane proteins, and influences Ca^{2+} influx through *PKD2* product, polycystin-2 channel.
  - Intracellular Ca^{2+} is reduced in cyst-derived cells, decreasing the Ca^{2+} inhibition of adenyl cyclase and increasing the concentration of cAMP.
  - cAMP stimulates cell proliferation and fluid secretion with cyst expansion.
  - Abnormal extracellular matrix and cell–cell interactions cause cells to detach and form cysts.
- ARPKD:
  - *PKHD1* product fibrocystin is also located in cilia; might be a cell surface receptor implicated in protein–protein interactions and is capable of enhancing the channel function of polycystin-2.
  - An alteration also occurs in intracellular calcium homeostasis.

ETIOLOGY

- ADPKD: Cysts arise from only 5% of nephrons.
  - Autosomal dominant pattern of inheritance but a molecularly recessive disease with the 2-hit hypothesis.
  - Requires genetic and environmental factors
- ARPKD: Mutations are scattered throughout the gene with genotype–phenotype correlation.

COMMONLY ASSOCIATED CONDITIONS

- ADPKD:
  - Cysts in other organs:
    - Polycystic liver disease in 58% of young age group to 94% of 45-year-olds
    - Pancreatic cysts: 5%
    - Seminal cysts: 40%
    - Arachnoid cysts: 8%
  - Vascular manifestations:
    - Intracerebral aneurysms in 6% of patients without family history, and in 16% with family history
    - Aortic dissections
  - Cardiac manifestations: Mitral valve prolapse: 25%
  - Diverticular disease
- ARPKD: Liver involvement: Affected in inverse proportion to renal disease; congenital hepatic fibrosis with portal HTN

℞ DIAGNOSIS

HISTORY

- ADPKD:
  - Positive family history
  - Flank pain: 60%
  - Hematuria
  - Urinary tract infection (UTI)
  - HTN: 50% aged 20–34 years; 100% with ESRD
  - Renal failure
- ARPKD:
  - 30% of affected neonates die.
    - Enlarged echogenic kidneys and oligohydramnios are diagnosed in utero.
    - Later in childhood: HTN
  - Adolescents and adults present with complications of portal HTN: Esophageal varices
  - Hypersplenism

PHYSICAL EXAM

- HTN
- Flank masses

DIAGNOSTIC TESTS & INTERPRETATION

Lab

Initial lab tests

- ADPKD:
  - Renal dysfunction:
    - Impaired renal concentration, hypocitraturia aciduria
    - Elevated creatinine
  - Urinalysis: Hematuria and mild proteinuria
- ARPKD:
  - Electrolyte abnormalities and renal insufficiency
  - Anemia, thrombocytopenia, leukopenia

Follow-Up & Special Considerations

- Diagnosis and prevention of secondary problems because of renal and liver abnormalities
- Follow-up of combined renal volume to assess disease severity (1)

Imaging

Initial approach

- ADPKD:
  - Ultrasound (US): Diagnostic method of choice:
    - Renal enlargement is universal.
    - In at-risk patients: By age 30, 2 renal cysts (bilateral or unilateral) is 100% diagnostic. In children, it sometimes appears similar to ARPKD; may be diagnosed in utero.
    - Presence of hepatic cysts in young adults is pathognomonic for ADPKD.
    - In the absence of family history, bilateral renal enlargement and cysts make the diagnosis.
  - CT scan/MRI:
    - Useful when US is equivocal but does not follow the above criteria for number of cysts.
    - Helpful in identifying cysts in other organs
- ARPKD:
  - US: Kidneys are enlarged, homogeneously hyperechogenic (cortex and medulla)
  - CT scan is more sensitive if diagnosis is in doubt.
  - Presence of hepatic fibrosis helps the diagnosis.

Follow-Up & Special Considerations

- Beyond age 2, renal size decreases in ARPKD but continues to grow in ADPKD at an average rate of 5.27%/year.
- Diagnosis of ADPKD in at-risk asymptomatic children may not need to be done because of psychological and insurance issues.
- Counseling should be done before testing.

Diagnostic Procedures/Surgery

- Genetic testing is available for the *PKD1* and *PKD2* in ADPKD when imaging results are equivocal and for potential living related donors (2).
- For the *PKHD1* gene in ARPKD, a prenatal diagnosis is feasible in about 72% of patients.

Pathological Findings

- ADPKD:
  - Kidneys are diffusely cystic and, although enlarged, retain their general shape.
  - Cysts range from a few millimeters to several centimeters and are distributed evenly throughout the cortex and medulla.
  - They arise in all segments of the nephron, although they are initially from the collecting ducts.
  - 1 kidney may be larger than the other.

- ARPKD:
  - Disease is a spectrum, ranging from severe renal disease with mild liver damage to mild renal disease with severe liver damage.
  - Renal enlargement is due to fusiform dilatation of the collecting ducts in the cortex and medulla in the newborn period.
  - Liver lesion is diffuse but limited to fibrotic portal areas.

DIFFERENTIAL DIAGNOSIS
- ADPKD and ARPKD
- Tuberous sclerosis: Prevalence 1/6,000
- Von Hippel–Lindau syndrome: Prevalence 1/36,000
- Nephronophthisis: Accounts for 10–20% cases of renal failure in children; medullary cystic kidney disease
- Renal cystic dysplasias: Multicystic dysplastic kidneys: Grossly deformed kidneys; most common type of bilateral cystic diseases in newborns: Prevalence: 1/4,000
- Simple cysts: Most common cystic abnormality:
  - Localized or unilateral renal cystic disease
  - Medullary sponge kidney
  - Acquired renal cystic disease
- Renal cystic neoplasms: Benign multilocular cyst (cystic nephroma)

 ## TREATMENT

MEDICATION
- No specific drug therapy is yet available for polycystic kidney disease.
- HTN: Should be very well controlled to prevent complications. Angiotensin-converting enzyme (ACE) inhibitors might be of some use (3).

ADDITIONAL TREATMENT
General Measures
- HTN: Moderate sodium restriction, weight control, and regular exercise
- Medications: ACE inhibitors; angiotensin receptor blockers (ARBs)
- Pain: Narcotics and other analgesics; bed rest; limit nonsteroidal anti-inflammatory drugs (NSAIDs) (they worsen renal function)
- Urolithiasis: Treated with alkalinization of urine and hydration therapy; surgery as needed
- UTIs/infections of cysts: Lipid-soluble antibiotics more effective (e.g., trimethoprim-sulfamethoxazole and chloramphenicol); fluoroquinolones also useful
- Dialysis for ESRD patients
- Hematuria: Reduce physical activity.

Issues for Referral
- Nephrologist primary management
- Urologic consultation for management of symptomatic/infected cysts
- Genetic counseling is critical.

COMPLEMENTARY AND ALTERNATIVE MEDICINE
Several trials are currently underway:
- HALT-PKD: Combination therapy of ACE inhibitors and ARBs
- Vasopressin V2 receptor inhibitors: Decrease cAMP
- Somatostatins: Decrease cAMP
- mTOR inhibitors (i.e., sirolimus): May reduce cyst growth

SURGERY/OTHER PROCEDURES
- Indications for surgical intervention:
  - Uncontrollable HTN
  - Severe back and loin pain, abdominal fullness
  - Renal deterioration owing to enlarging cysts
  - Hematuria/hemorrhage or recurrent UTI
- Open and laparoscopic cyst unroofing: May decrease pain and narcotics requirements; has not been proven to prevent renal failure or to prolong current renal function
- Percutaneous cyst aspiration ± injection of sclerosing agent; not usually performed secondary to recurrent fluid accumulation
- Renal transplant for ESRD

IN-PATIENT CONSIDERATIONS
Admission Criteria
Severe pain, gross hematuria with clots

 ## ONGOING CARE

FOLLOW-UP RECOMMENDATIONS
None in early stages of the disease; avoid vigorous activity if disease advances. Recurrent gross hematuria is secondary to trauma, associated with faster decline of renal function.

Patient Monitoring
- Monitor BP and renal function. Encourage hydration. Treat UTI and stone disease aggressively.
- Avoid nephrotoxic drugs
- Creatinine and BP monitoring at least twice a year; more often as needed

DIET
- Low-protein diet may retard renal insufficiency.
- Limit caffeine, since this might increase cyst's growth.

PROGNOSIS
- Renal failure in 2% by age 40 years; 23% by age 50; 48% by age 73
- ADPKD accounts for 10–15% of dialysis patients.
- No increased incidence of renal cell cancer

COMPLICATIONS
- Cyst rupture, infection, or hemorrhage
- Progression to renal failure
- Renal calculi

REFERENCES
1. Bae KT, Grantham JJ et al. Imaging for the prognosis of autosomal dominant polycystic kidney disease. *Nat Rev Nephrol*. 2010;6:96–106.
2. Harris PC, Rossetti S et al. Molecular diagnostics for autosomal dominant polycystic kidney disease. *Nat Rev Nephrol*. 2010;6:197–206.
3. Jia G, Kwon M, Liang HL, et al. Chronic treatment with lisinopril decreases proliferative and apoptotic pathways in autosomal recessive polycystic kidney disease. *Pediatr Nephrol*. 2010;25:1139–46.

ADDITIONAL READING
- Avner ED, et al. Renal cystic disease: New insights for the clinician. *Pediatr Clin N Am*. 2006;53: 889–909.
- Badani KK, Hemal AK, Menon M. Autosomal dominant polycystic kidney disease and pain - a review of the disease from aetiology, evaluation, past surgical treatment options to current practice. *J Postgrad Med*. 2004;50:222–6.
- Harris PC, Torres VE. Polycystic Kidney Disease. *Annu Rev Med*. 2009;60:321–37.
- Torres VE, et al. Cystic diseases of the kidney. In: Brenner BM, ed. Brenner & Rector's the kidney, 8th ed. Philadelphia: WB Saunders/Elsevier; 2007: 1428–63.
- Torres VE, Harris PC, Pirson Y. Autosomal dominant polycystic kidney disease. *Lancet*. 2007;369: 1287–301.
- Wilson PD. Polycystic kidney disease. *N Engl J Med*. 2004;350:151–64.

See Also (Topic, Algorithm, Electronic Media Element)
Renal Calculi; Renal Failure, Chronic

 ## CODES

ICD9
- 753.12 Polycystic kidney, unspecified type
- 753.13 Polycystic kidney, autosomal dominant
- 753.14 Polycystic kidney, autosomal recessive

CLINICAL PEARLS
- Although many PKD patients eventually develop ESRD, many do not. See "Prognosis" to determine whether patient needs dialysis.
- No specific treatment has been proven to prevent ESRD, but hydration and control of BP are reasonable goals.
- Patients may benefit from a nephrology consultation after the initial diagnosis to counsel regarding disease progression prevention. They then can be followed by primary care if the disease was an incidental finding or no significant kidney dysfunction is present.

POLYCYSTIC OVARIAN SYNDROME (PCOS)

Julie Scott Taylor, MD, MSc
Jeremy Golding, MD
Kathleen Bryant, MS, APRN, BC

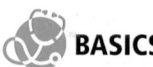 **BASICS**

DESCRIPTION

- Polycystic ovary syndrome (PCOS) is the most common endocrine disorder of unknown etiology.
- PCOS is a complex disorder characterized by a state of chronic oligoovulation or anovulation, associated with functional androgen excess, and manifesting most commonly as oligomenorrhea or amenorrhea.
- System(s) affected: Reproductive; Endocrine/Metabolic; Skin/Exocrine
- Synonym(s): Stein-Leventhal syndrome; polycystic ovary disease

ALERT
- Condition may begin at puberty.
- Pregnancy does not resolve the syndrome.
- Predisposes to and associated with obesity, hypertension, diabetes, metabolic syndrome, hyperlipidemia, infertility, insulin-resistance syndrome

EPIDEMIOLOGY
Prevalence
- Polycystic ovary syndrome (PCOS) affects 6.6–6.8% of women of reproductive age (1).
- Much higher in oligomenorrheic women
- Predominant age: Reproductive age
- Predominant sex: Females only

RISK FACTORS
See "Commonly Associated Conditions"; cause and effect are difficult to disentangle in this disorder.

Genetics
- Increased prevalence in 1st-degree relatives of affected individuals suggests genetic factors.
- Ultimate expression is likely a combination of polygenic and environmental factors.
  - No single gene has been identified as the susceptibility gene for PCOS.
  - Efforts are ongoing to dissect the variants of genes from multiple logical pathways, which are involved in pathophysiology of PCOS.

GENERAL PREVENTION
- None known; focus on early diagnosis and treatment to prevent long-term complications.
- Valproic acid use is associated with development of PCOS.

PATHOPHYSIOLOGY
- Incompletely defined and possibly heterogeneous
- Recent evidence points to a primary role for insulin resistance with hyperinsulinemia, as well as a genetic predisposition to excess androgen production (2).

ETIOLOGY
- Insulin resistance causes elevated insulin levels.
- Elevated insulin directly and indirectly stimulates ovarian androgen production in a genetically primed ovary.
- Abnormal insulin and androgen balance alter gonadotropin (follicle-stimulating hormone [FSH] and luteinizing hormone [LH]) release (disrupted hypothalamic–pituitary–ovarian axis).

- Insulin lowers hepatic sex hormone–binding globulin (SHBG) production, increasing serum free testosterone.
- Insulin resistance may cause the frequently associated metabolic syndrome and frank diabetes mellitus (DM).

COMMONLY ASSOCIATED CONDITIONS
- Obesity
- Obstructive sleep apnea
- Hypertension
- Diabetes mellitus
- Breast carcinoma
- Endometrial hyperplasia and/or carcinoma
- Infertility
- Hyperandrogenism, insulin resistance, acanthosis nigricans (HAIRAN) syndrome
- Hyperthecosis

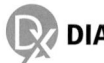 **DIAGNOSIS**

HISTORY
- Take a complete patient history, especially as it relates to contraceptive and reproductive goals.
- History should include a detailed menstrual history, as well as information about weight gain, hirsutism, acne, fertility, gestational diabetes, lipid levels.

PHYSICAL EXAM
- Vital signs: Body mass index (BMI), high BP
- General appearance: Central obesity, deepened voice, hirsutism, acne
- Skin: Hair pattern and growth, acne, seborrhea, acanthosis nigricans
- Genitalia: Clitoromegaly

ALERT
Look specifically for signs of virilization such as hair pattern, deepened voice, and clitoromegaly.

DIAGNOSTIC TESTS & INTERPRETATION
- Diagnostic criteria (Rotterdam criteria, 2 of 3):
  - Oligo- or anovulation
  - Clinical and/or biochemical signs of hyperandrogenism
  - Transvaginal ultrasonographic polycystic ovaries and exclusion of other etiologies; therefore, consider exclusion of Cushing disease, congenital adrenal hyperplasia, and androgen-secreting tumors.
- More recent criteria also focus on similar criteria while acknowledging that there may be forms of PCOS without overt evidence of hyperandrogenism (3).

Lab
Initial lab tests
- Screening workup should include human chorionic gonadotropin (hCG), TSH, prolactin, and FSH (exclude premature ovarian failure).
- LH determination may be ordered but is not usually necessary.
  - Hirsute women should have a testosterone or free testosterone determination and a DHEAS determination.
  - Consider 17-OH progesterone if congenital adrenal hyperplasia is a possibility.

- LH/FSH level ≥2.5–3.0/L in ~50% of women with PCOS, but LH testing is not generally necessary.
- Testosterone increased but <200 ng/dL (6.94 nmol/L)
- Typical findings in PCOS include mild elevation in DHEAS but <800 μg/dL (20.8 μmol/L), mild increase in 17-OH progesterone level, increased estrogen level, decreased SHBG.
- Drugs that may alter lab results:
  - Oral contraceptives (OCs)
  - Steroids
  - Antidepressants

Follow-Up & Special Considerations
- Consider fasting serum glucose, insulin level, and plasminogen activator inhibitor-1 determinations to establish presence of insulin resistance and glucose intolerance, especially if diagnosis in doubt.
- Overnight dexamethasone suppression test (Decadron 1 mg p.o. at 11:00 p.m. and fasting serum cortisol at 8:00 a.m. the next morning) to rule out Cushing syndrome in the appropriate setting.
- Endometrial biopsy to rule out hyperplasia and/or carcinoma if indicated
- If the syndrome is diagnosed, determination of fasting glucose and fasting lipid levels should be performed, and formal glucose tolerance test considered.

Imaging
- Transvaginal US (positive if enlarged ovaries with ≥8 small follicular cysts) may be performed if diagnosis is in doubt, but nonspecific.
- Some research being done into use of MRI as diagnostic technique

Pathological Findings
- Ovary usually enlarged with a smooth white glistening capsule
- Ovarian cortex lined with follicles in all stages of development but most atretic
- Thecal cell proliferation with an increase in the stromal compartment

DIFFERENTIAL DIAGNOSIS
- Cushing syndrome
- HAIRAN syndrome
- Testosterone-producing ovarian or adrenal tumor
- Prolactin-producing pituitary adenoma
- Hyperthecosis
- Adult-onset adrenal hyperplasia
- Partial congenital adrenal hyperplasia (21-hydroxylase deficiency)
- Endometrial hyperplasia
- Endometrial carcinoma
- 11β-hydroxylase deficiency
- 17β-hydroxysteroid dehydrogenase deficiency
- Acromegaly
- Drug-induced hirsutism, oligoovulation (e.g., danazol, steroids, valproic acid)
- Thyroid disease

TREATMENT

MEDICATION
Drug costs related to this condition are high.

First Line
- If pregnancy not desired:
  - Low-dose OCs (30–35 μg); newer formulations containing progestins with lower androgenicity (e.g., norethindrone, desogestrel, norgestimate, drospirenone) may be particularly beneficial, but all OCs increase SHBG and decrease excess androgen and estrogen.
  - Cyclic withdrawal bleeding with medroxyprogesterone (Provera) 10 mg p.o. × 10 days given every 1–2 months
  - Metformin may help to correct metabolic abnormalities in women who are shown to be insulin-resistant. Initial dose is 500 mg at dinner time × 1 week, increasing by 500 mg/week to a total of 1,500–2000 mg/d divided b.i.d.; take with food.
    - Overall, data support the usefulness of metformin on both cardiometabolic risk and reproduction assistance in PCOS women (1).
  - Thiazolidinediones may increase likelihood of ovulation and treat insulin resistance.
- If pregnancy desired:
  - Ovulation induction with clomiphene (Clomid, Serophene) and/or exogenous gonadotropins: see "Infertility." Birth rate with Clomid is 22.5%, 7.2% with Metformin, and 26.8% in women who use both medications (4).
  - Metformin (Glucophage): 500–2,000 mg p.o. divided b.i.d. has been shown to improve hyperandrogenism and restore ovulation. Many times the drug is continued throughout the 1st trimester or the entire pregnancy if there is a history of spontaneous abortion or glucose intolerance. It does improve clinical pregnancy rates, but does not improve live birth rates alone or in combination with clomiphene when used for ovulation induction (5).
  - Has been demonstrated that metformin reduces the incidence of gestational diabetes
  - Refer to a perinatologist for opinion in high-risk patient.

Second Line
- Spironolactone for androgen-excess hirsutism not addressed by OC therapy
- Dexamethasone or prednisone for congenital adrenal syndromes or for nonobese women with functional adrenal androgen excess (high 17-ketosteroids) not suppressed by OC
- Eflornithine hydrochloride cream 13% to inhibit hair growth

ADDITIONAL TREATMENT
General Measures
- No ideal treatment exists.
- Therapy must be individualized according to the needs and desires of each patient.
- Weight loss in overweight women results in biochemical and symptomatic improvement in most.

Issues for Referral
- To reproductive endocrinologist for all women who cannot achieve pregnancy with Clomid
- To endocrinologist if Cushing syndrome, congenital adrenal hyperplasia, or adrenal or ovarian tumors are found during the workup

COMPLEMENTARY AND ALTERNATIVE MEDICINE
Initial trials with acupuncture to assist with cycle normalization and weight loss are promising (6).

SURGERY/OTHER PROCEDURES
- Ovarian wedge resection and laparoscopic laser drilling are controversial and rarely used today.
- Mechanical means of hair removal including electrolysis, waxing, and depilatory may improve cosmesis.

ONGOING CARE

FOLLOW-UP RECOMMENDATIONS
Follow-up at 6-month intervals to evaluate response to therapy and to monitor weight as well as medication side effects

Patient Monitoring
- Counsel patient about the risk of endometrial and breast carcinoma, insulin resistance, and diabetes, as well as obesity and its role in infertility.
- See patient frequently throughout the menstrual cycle, depending on which drug combination is used to induce ovulation.

DIET
In overweight patients, weight loss is the most successful therapy because it improves cardiovascular risk, insulin sensitivity, and menstrual patterns.

PATIENT EDUCATION
- Provide patient with information about PCOS such as from http://www.acog.org.
- Discuss risks and benefits of medications used for treatment as well as side effects.
- Discuss the chronic nature of this condition.
- Remind patients who do not wish to become pregnant that contraception remains necessary despite oligoovulation.
- Review the importance of weight loss if applicable. Modest weight loss of 5% to 10% of initial body weight has been demonstrated to improve many of the features of PCOS. Provide patient with resources.

PROGNOSIS
- Prognosis for fertility is excellent depending on other fertility factors; assisted reproductive technologies may be necessary.
- Proper treatment and follow-up of chronic anovulation can prevent endometrial hyperplasia or carcinoma.

COMPLICATIONS
- Reproductive: Infertility, hyperandrogenism, hirsutism
- Metabolic: Insulin resistance, impaired glucose tolerance, type 2 diabetes mellitus, adverse cardiovascular risk profiles
- Psychological: Increased anxiety, depression, and worsened quality of life

REFERENCES

1. Diamanti-Kandarakis E, Economou F, Palimeri S, et al. Metformin in polycystic ovary syndrome. *Ann N Y Acad Sci*. 2010;1205:192–8.
2. Moran LJ, Misso ML, Wild RA, Norman RJ et al. Impaired glucose tolerance, type 2 diabetes and metabolic syndrome in polycystic ovary syndrome: a systematic review and meta-analysis. *Hum. Reprod. Update*. 2010;16:347–63.
3. Azziz R, Carmina E, Dewailly D, et al. The Androgen Excess and PCOS Society criteria for the polycystic ovary syndrome: the complete task force report. *Fertil Steril*. 2008.
4. Legro RS, Barnhart HX, Schlaff WD, et al. Clomiphene, metformin, or both for infertility in the polycystic ovary syndrome. *N Engl J Med*. 2007;356:551–66.
5. Tang et al. Insulin-sensitising drugs (metformin, rosiglitazone, pioglitazone, D-chiro-inositol) for women with polycystic ovary syndrome, oligo amenorrhoea and subfertility. *Cochrane Database of Systematic Reviews*. 5, 2010.
6. Lim CE, Wong WS et al. Current evidence of acupuncture on polycystic ovarian syndrome. *Gynecol. Endocrinol*. 2010;26:473–8.

ADDITIONAL READING

- Carmina E, Oberfield SE, Lobo RA et al. The diagnosis of polycystic ovary syndrome in adolescents. *Am J Obstet Gynecol*. 2010;203: 201.e1–5.
- Chang RJ. A practical approach to the diagnosis of polycystic ovary syndrome. *Am J Obstet Gynecol*. 2004;191:713–7.
- Cibula D, et al. The effect of combination therapy with metformin and combined oral contraceptives (COC) versus COC alone on insulin sensitivity, hyperandrogenaemia, SHBG and lipids in PCOS patients. *Human Reprod*. 2005;20(1):180–4.
- Hirschberg AL et al. Polycystic ovary syndrome, obesity and reproductive implications. *Womens Health (Lond Engl)*. 2009;5.
- Rotterdam ESHRE/ASRM Sponsored PCOS Consensus Workshop Group. Revised 2003 Consensus on diagnostic criteria and long-term health risks related to polycystic ovary syndrome. *Fertil Steril*. 2004;81:19–25.
- Tasali E, VanCauter E, Ehrman DA. PCOS & OBstructive sleep apnea. *Sleep Med Clin*. 2008; 3(1):37–46.
- Vink JM, et al. Heritability of polycystic ovary syndrome in a Dutch twin-family study. *J Clin Endocrinol Metabol*. 2006;91(6):2100–4.

See Also (Topic, Algorithm, Electronic Media Element)
Algorithm: Amenorrhea

CODES

ICD9
256.4 Polycystic ovaries

CLINICAL PEARLS
- In the US, 40% of women with PCOS are not obese.
- Oligomenorrhea should be treated because chronic estrogen stimulation in the absence of progesterone (as occurs in PCOS anovulation) causes endometrial hyperplasia, a precursor of endometrial carcinoma.

POLYCYTHEMIA VERA

Nathan T. Connell, MD

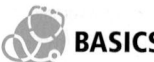 **BASICS**

DESCRIPTION
- Clonal cell hematologic malignant disorder whose hallmark is increased red cell mass (RCM) with excessive erythroid, myeloid, and megakaryocytic elements in the bone marrow
- One of a group of myeloproliferative disorders
- Synonym(s): Primary polycythemia; Vaquez disease; Polycythemia, splenomegalic; Vaquez-Osler disease

EPIDEMIOLOGY
Incidence
- Predominant age: Middle to late years; mean is 60 years (range 15–90 years).
- Predominant sex: Male > Female (slightly).

Prevalence
Incidence in US: 1.9/100,000 person-years

RISK FACTORS
- Ashkenazi Jewish ancestry (may have increased frequency)
- Familial history (rare)

Genetics
JAK2 V617F (tyrosine kinase) mutation has been identified in multiple studies to be strongly associated with polycythemia vera (PV) with possible causal influence (1,2)[A].

ETIOLOGY
Unknown; all 3 hematopoietic cell lines originate in a single clone.

COMMONLY ASSOCIATED CONDITIONS
- May present as thrombosis in any organ, such as Budd-Chiari syndrome
- Mesenteric artery thrombosis
- Myocardial infarction
- Cerebrovascular accident
- Deep vein thrombosis/pulmonary embolism

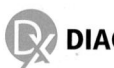 **DIAGNOSIS**

HISTORY
- Early stages may produce no symptoms.
- Burning pain of feet or hands, occasionally with erythema, pallor, cyanosis, or acral paresthesias
- Headaches
- Tinnitus
- Vertigo
- Blurred vision
- Epistaxis
- Increased blood viscosity
- Spontaneous bruising
- Upper GI bleeding
- Peptic ulcer disease

- Arterial and venous occlusive events
- Pruritus
- Sweating
- Weight loss
- Plethora (face, hands, feet)
- Hyperhistaminemia
- Bone pain (ribs and sternum)

PHYSICAL EXAM
- Bone tenderness (ribs and sternum)
- Splenomegaly
- Hepatomegaly

DIAGNOSTIC TESTS & INTERPRETATION
Lab
Initial lab tests
- PV Study Group (PVSG) (1960s) major (A) and minor criteria (B):
  - A_1: Increased RCM: Female $\geq$32 mL/kg; male $\geq$36 mL/kg
  - A_2: Normal arterial oxygen saturation ($\geq$92%)
  - A_3: Splenomegaly
  - B_1: Thrombocytosis (platelet count >400,000/L)
  - B_2: Leukocytosis >12,000/L
  - B_3: Leukocyte alkaline phosphatase increased
  - B_4: Increased serum vitamin B_{12} or increased unsaturated vitamin B_{12} binding capacity
- PVSG diagnosis acceptable with following combinations:
  - $A_1 + A_2 + A_3$
  - $A_1 + A_2$ + any 2 from B category (splenomegaly absent in ~25% of patients)
- Recent advances have prompted development of other diagnostic models, namely, the discovery of *JAK2* V617F and improved assays for erythropoietin (EPO) measurement.
- 2008 World Health Organization diagnostic criteria: Requires both major criteria or 1 major criterion and 2 minor criteria (2).
  - Major criteria:
    - Hemoglobin (Hgb) >18.5 g/dL (men); Hgb >16.5 g/dL (women); Hgb >17 g/dL (men) or Hgb >15 g/dL (women) if there is a sustained increased of 2 g/dL or more above baseline that cannot be attributed to iron-deficiency correction
    - Presence of *JAK2* V617F or similar mutation
  - Minor criteria:
    - BM trilineage myeloproliferation
    - Subnormal serum EPO level
    - Endogenous erythroid colony growth
- Some authors feel that diagnosis can be made reliably based on clinical symptoms, presence of *JAK2* V617 mutation, and low EPO (3).

- Other lab findings:
  - Hyperuricemia
  - Hypercholesterolemia
  - Elevated blood histamine level
- Drugs that may alter lab results: Diuretics may cause a spurious polycythemia.
- Disorders that may alter lab results: Excessive use of alcohol or tobacco

Imaging
Initial approach
CT splenomegaly (if not palpable), although imaging is not necessarily needed

Diagnostic Procedures/Surgery
- Bone marrow aspiration and biopsy
- Bone marrow aspiration (red blood cell hyperplasia, panmyelosis, clustering/clumping of pleomorphic megakaryocytes, absent iron stores, no pronounced inflammatory reaction): Cytogenetic testing (*JAK2* V617F)
- Biopsy: Fibrosis during spent phase of the disease (characterized by increased presence of reticulin)

Pathological Findings
- Plethoric congestion in all organs and tissues
- Major vessels contain thick, viscous blood.
- Sinuses of spleen packed with red blood cells (RBCs)

DIFFERENTIAL DIAGNOSIS
- Secondary polycythemias
- Hemoglobinopathy
- Spurious polycythemia

 TREATMENT

MEDICATION
First Line
- Myelosuppression:

  - Low-dose aspirin (81 mg PO) has been demonstrated in 1 study to reduce the risk of thrombotic events without increasing bleeding complications when used in conjunction with phlebotomy (4)[B]. A follow-up meta-analysis, however, did not show a statistically significant benefit to aspirin therapy but did not show an increase in major bleeding (5)[A].

  - Hydroxyurea if unable to maintain on phlebotomy alone or if at high risk for thrombosis (start 15–20 mg/kg/d). Be aware that hydroxyurea can lead to leukemic transformation (6).
  - Radioactive phosphorous in selected patients when life expectancy is <10 years given mutagenic potential
  - Refer to hematologist/oncologist for further dosing and instructions.

- Symptomatic/adjunctive:
  – Allopurinol 300 mg/d PO for uric acid reduction
  – Cyproheptadine 4–16 mg PO as needed for pruritus
  – H_2-receptor blockers or antacids for GI hyperacidity; cimetidine is also used for pruritus.
  – Other pruritus therapy: Selective serotonin reuptake inhibitors have shown some efficacy in controlling pruritus in setting of PV (7)[B].

Second Line

- Myelosuppression: Chlorambucil; some authors believe this is contraindicated.
- Pegylated interferon-α-2a has shown promise in inducing complete hematologic and molecular responses (8). This pharmacologic treatment should be considered only in consultation with a hematologist.

ADDITIONAL TREATMENT
General Measures

- Individualized management necessary by considering the patient's risk factors and comorbidities (6)
- Depend on many factors: Age, disease duration, disease phenotype, complications, disease activity
- Currently, phlebotomy is the mainstay of therapy. Beyond this, differences exist among authorities about use and effectiveness of myelosuppressives.
- Phlebotomy:
  – To reduce hematocrit to ~45%
  – Performed as often as every 2–3 days until normal hematocrit reached; phlebotomies of 250–500 mL. Reduce to 250–350 mL in elderly patients or patients with cerebrovascular disease.
  – Concomitant therapy possibilities; for example, some form of myelosuppression, radioactive phosphorus (in elderly patients), hydroxyurea
  – Phlebotomy repeated as necessary for maintenance
  – If patient cannot tolerate phlebotomy, then chemotherapy (hydroxyurea is the least mutagenic agent) or radiation therapy
- Other therapy:
  – Maintain hydration
  – Pruritus therapy
  – Manage thrombotic or hemorrhagic complications the same as with nonpolycythemic patient
- Uric acid reduction therapy

Issues for Referral

It is recommended that patients be referred to an experienced hematologist to assist in management.

ONGOING CARE

FOLLOW-UP RECOMMENDATIONS
Patient Monitoring

- Frequent monitoring during early treatment until target hematocrit is reached
- Monitor hematocrit often and phlebotomize as needed to maintain target goal.

DIET

Avoid iron supplements.

PATIENT EDUCATION

- Stress the importance of lifelong maintenance.
- Continuous education regarding possible complications and importance of seeking treatment early should complications appear

PROGNOSIS

- Currently, survival is >15 years with treatment (2).
- Patients are at risk for developing postpolycythemic myelofibrosis (PPMF). One study showed that the risk of developing PPMF was 16% at 10 years and 34% at 15 years (9).

COMPLICATIONS

- Uric acid stones
- Secondary gout
- Vascular thromboses (major cause of death)
- Transformation to leukemia
- Transformation to myelofibrosis
- Hemorrhage
- Peptic ulcer
- Increased risk for complications and mortality from surgery procedures. Assess risk/benefits and ensure optimal control of disorder before any elective surgery.

REFERENCES

1. James C, Ugo V, Le Couédic JP, et al. A unique clonal JAK2 mutation leading to constitutive signalling causes polycythaemia vera. *Nature*. 2005;434:1144–8.
2. Tefferi A. Essential thrombocythemia, polycythemia vera, and myelofibrosis: current management and the prospect of targeted therapy. *Am J Hematol*. 2008;83:491–7.
3. Tefferi A. The diagnosis of polycythemia vera: New tests and old dictums. *Best Prac Res Clin Haematol*. 2006;19:455.
4. Landolfi R, Marchioli R, Kutti J, et al. Efficacy and safety of low-dose aspirin in polycythemia vera. *N Engl J Med*. 2004;350:114–24.
5. Squizzato A, Romualdi E, Middeldorp S et al. Antiplatelet drugs for polycythaemia vera and essential thrombocythaemia. *Cochrane Database Syst Rev*. 2008;CD006503.
6. Finazzi G, Barbui T et al. Evidence and expertise in the management of polycythemia vera and essential thrombocythemia. *Leukemia*. 2008;22:1494–502.
7. Tefferi A, Fonseca R. Selective serotonin reuptake inhibitors are effective in the treatment of polycythemia vera-associated pruritus. *Blood*. 2002;99:2627.
8. Kiladjian JJ, Cassinat B, Chevret S, et al. Pegylated Interferon-alfa-2a induces complete hematological and molecular responses with low toxicity in Polycythemia Vera. *Blood*. 2008.
9. Alvarez-Larrán A, Bellosillo B, Martínez-Avilés L, et al. Postpolycythaemic myelofibrosis: frequency and risk factors for this complication in 116 patients. *Br J Haematol*. 2009;146:504–9.

ADDITIONAL READING

Levine RL, Gilliland DG et al. Myeloproliferative disorders. *Blood*. 2008;112:2190–8.

See Also (Topic, Algorithm, Electronic Media Element)

Myeloproliferative Disorders

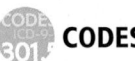

CODES

ICD9
238.4 Polycythemia vera

CLINICAL PEARLS

- *JAK2* mutations are an important component of myeloproliferative disorders.
- Multiple therapies exist, and consultation with an experienced hematologist is recommended.

POLYMYALGIA RHEUMATICA

Elise H. Pyun, MD

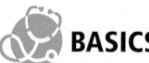 **BASICS**

DESCRIPTION
Polymyalgia rheumatica (PMR) is a clinical syndrome characterized by pain and stiffness of the shoulder and hip girdles and neck:
- Disease of the elderly, associated with morning stiffness and elevated markers of inflammation
- System(s) affected: Musculoskeletal; Hematologic/Lymphatic/Immunologic
- Synonym(s): Senile rheumatic disease; Polymyalgia rheumatica syndrome; Pseudo-polyarthrite rhizomélique

Geriatric Considerations
Incidence increases with age; average age of onset approximately 70 years

Pediatric Considerations
Does not occur in patients <50 years of age

EPIDEMIOLOGY
Incidence
- Predominant age: Peak incidence between 70 and 80 years of age
- Incidence increases after age 50. Incidence in US population >50 years old: 60 per 100,000 people
- Predominant sex: Female > Male (2:1)
- Most common in people of northern European ancestry

Prevalence
Prevalence in population >50 years old: 700 per 100,000 people

RISK FACTORS
- Age >50 years
- Presence of giant cell arteritis

Genetics
Associated with human leukocyte antigen determinants (HLA-DRB1*04 and DRB1*01 alleles)

ETIOLOGY
Unknown

COMMONLY ASSOCIATED CONDITIONS
Giant cell arteritis (temporal arteritis) may occur in 15–30% of patients with PMR.

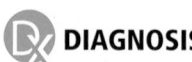 **DIAGNOSIS**

- No universally accepted diagnostic criteria
- Suspect PMR in an elderly patient with new onset of proximal limb pain and stiffness.

HISTORY
- Insidious, subacute, or acute onset of pain and stiffness
- Proximal symptoms: Shoulders, hip girdle, neck, torso
- Symptoms usually symmetric
- Prominent morning stiffness (lasting at least 30 minutes), sometimes impairing patient's ability to get out of bed
- Nighttime pain
- Prominent gelling (stiffening); difficulty arising from a chair or raising the arms
- Systemic symptoms in approximately 25% (fatigue, weight loss, low-grade fever)

PHYSICAL EXAM
- Decreased range of motion (ROM) of shoulders, neck, and hips may be seen.
- Muscle strength is usually normal, although it may be limited by pain.
- Disuse atrophy of muscles may be seen.
- Synovitis of the small joints may be seen.
- Coexisting carpal tunnel syndrome

DIAGNOSTIC TESTS & INTERPRETATION
Temporal artery biopsy if symptoms of giant cell arteritis are present

Lab
- Erythrocyte sedimentation rate (ESR) (Westergren) elevation >40 mm/h:
  - ESR is elevated in most patients, sometimes >100 mm/h.
  - Elevated C-reactive protein
  - ESR may be normal (<40 mm/h) in 7–22% of patients.
- Normochromic/normocytic anemia common
- Anti-CCP antibodies usually negative (in contrast to elderly-onset rheumatoid arthritis [RA])
- Rheumatoid factor: Negative (5–10% of patients >60 years of age will have positive rheumatoid factor without RA)
- Mild elevations in liver function tests, especially alkaline phosphatase
- Drugs that may alter lab results: Prednisone
- Disorders that may alter lab results: Other disorders causing elevation of the sedimentation rate (e.g., infection, neoplasm, renal failure)

Initial lab tests
- ESR
- C-reactive protein
- Complete blood count

Imaging
- Magnetic resonance imaging (MRI) of the joints may show periarticular inflammation, tenosynovitis, and bursitis. However, MRI typically is not necessary for diagnosis.
- Ultrasound of the shoulder or hip may show bursitis, tendinitis, and synovitis.
- Positron emission tomography scan may show increased uptake in vascular areas.

Initial approach
Consider PMR in a patient >50 years old, with proximal pain and stiffness. Obtain laboratory work recommended above. Consider a diagnostic and therapeutic trial of low-dose steroids.

Diagnostic Procedures/Surgery
If patients have symptoms suggestive of giant cell arteritis, a temporal artery biopsy is indicated.

Pathological Findings
Mild nonspecific synovitis

DIFFERENTIAL DIAGNOSIS
- RA
- Palindromic rheumatism
- Late-onset seronegative spondyloarthropathies (e.g., psoriatic arthritis, ankylosing spondylitis)
- Systemic lupus erythematosus
- Sjögren's syndrome
- Fibromyalgia
- Depression
- Polymyositis-dermatomyositis (check creatine phosphokinase, aldolase)
- Thyroid disease
- Hyperparathyroidism, hypoparathyroidism
- Hypovitaminosis D
- Viral myalgia
- Osteoarthritis
- Rotator cuff syndrome
- Adhesive capsulitis
- RS3PE syndrome (remitting seronegative symmetrical synovitis with pitting edema)
- Occult infection
- Occult malignancy (e.g., lymphoma, leukemia, myeloma, solid tumor)
- Myopathy (e.g., steroid, alcohol, electrolyte depletion)

 TREATMENT

MEDICATION
First Line
- Prednisone, 10–20 mg/d p.o. initially; typically, expect a dramatic (diagnostic) response within days. 15 mg/d is effective in almost all patients (1).
- May increase to 20 mg/d if no immediate response
- If no response to 10–20 mg/d, reconsider diagnosis.
- Divided-dose steroids (b.i.d. or t.i.d.) may be useful initially (especially if symptoms recur in the afternoon).
- Begin slow taper by 2.5-mg decrements every 2–4 weeks to a dose of 7.5–10 mg/d. Below this dose, taper by 1 mg/mo.
- Increase prednisone for recurrence of symptoms (relapse common).
- Corticosteroid treatment often lasts at least 2 years (2).
- Contraindications:
  - Use steroids with caution in patients with chronic heart failure, diabetes mellitus, and systemic fungal or bacterial infection.
  - Must treat infections concurrently if steroids are absolutely necessary.

- Precautions:
  - Long-term steroid use associated with several significant adverse effects, including sodium and water retention, exacerbation of chronic heart failure, hypokalemia, increased susceptibility to infection, osteoporosis, cataracts, glaucoma, avascular necrosis, depression, and weight gain
  - Patients may develop temporal arteritis while on low-dose corticosteroid treatment for polymyalgia. This requires an immediate increase in dose to 40–60 mg.
  - Alternate-day steroids are not effective.

Second Line
- Nonsteroidal anti-inflammatory drugs usually are not adequate for pain relief.
- Methotrexate may be used as a steroid-sparing drug, but studies supporting its use are not robust (3,4)[B].
- Anti-tumor necrosis factor agents (infliximab) have not been shown to add any steroid-sparing effects (5)[B].

ADDITIONAL TREATMENT
General Measures
- Address risk of steroid-induced osteoporosis: Obtain dual energy x-ray absorptiometry, check 25-OH vitamin D levels, and consider antiresorptive therapies (bisphosphonates) based on recommendations for treatment of corticosteroid-induced osteoporosis.
- Advise patient on adequate calcium (1,500 mg/d) and vitamin D (800–1,000 U/d) supplementation.
- Physical therapy for ROM exercises, if needed

⟳ ONGOING CARE

FOLLOW-UP RECOMMENDATIONS
Patient Monitoring
- Follow monthly initially and during taper of medication, every 3 months otherwise.
- Follow ESR as steroids are tapered.
- Follow up with patient for symptoms of giant cell arteritis. Educate patient to report such symptoms immediately (e.g., headache, visual loss, and diplopia.)
- If the patient is asymptomatic, do not treat the ESR (i.e., do not increase the steroid dose in an attempt to normalize the ESR).

DIET
- Regular diet
- Aim for adequate calcium and vitamin D.

PATIENT EDUCATION
- Review adverse effects of corticosteroids.
- Discuss the symptoms of giant cell arteritis; instruct the patient to contact the physician immediately if any occur.
- Instruct patient to contact physician if symptoms recur during the steroid taper.
- Instruct the patient to never abruptly stop taking steroids without a taper.
- Counsel patients on calcium and vitamin D requirements.
- Resources for patients: Arthritis Foundation: http://www.arthritis.org/
- Resources for patients: American College of Rheumatology: http://www.rheumatology.org/public/factsheets/diseases_and_conditions/polymyalgiarheumatica.asp?aud=pat

PROGNOSIS
- Most patients require at least 2 years of corticosteroid treatment.
- Exacerbation if steroids are tapered too fast (6)
- Prognosis is very good if treated.
- Relapse is common (in 25–50% of patients).

COMPLICATIONS
- Medication: Complications related to steroid use
- Disease: Exacerbation of disease with taper of steroids; development of giant cell arteritis (may occur when polymyalgia rheumatica is being treated adequately)

REFERENCES

1. Hernández-Rodríguez J, Cid MC, López-Soto A, et al. Treatment of polymyalgia rheumatica: a systematic review. *Arch Intern Med*. 2009;169: 1839–50.
2. Narváez J, Nolla-Solé JM, Clavaguera MT, et al. Longterm therapy in polymyalgia rheumatica: effect of coexistent temporal arteritis. *J Rheumatol*. 1999;26:1945–52.
3. Caporali R, Cimmino MA, Ferraccioli G, et al. Prednisone plus methotrexate for polymyalgia rheumatica: a randomized, double-blind, placebo-controlled trial. *Ann Intern Med*. 2004;141:493–500.
4. van der Veen MJ, Dinant HJ, van Booma-Frankfort C, et al. Can methotrexate be used as a steroid sparing agent in the treatment of polymyalgia rheumatica and giant cell arteritis? *Ann Rheum Dis*. 1996;55:218–23.
5. Salvarani C, Macchioni P, Manzini C, et al. Infliximab plus prednisone or placebo plus prednisone for the initial treatment of polymyalgia rheumatica: a randomized trial. *Ann Intern Med*. 2007;146:631–9.
6. Kremers HM, Reinalda MS, Crowson CS, et al. Relapse in a population based cohort of patients with polymyalgia rheumatica. *J Rheumatol*. 2005;32:65–73.

ADDITIONAL READING

- Cimmino MA, Zaccaria AN. Epidemiology of polymyalgia rheumatica. *Clin Exp Rheum*. 2000;18:S9.
- Michet CJ, Matteson EL. Polymyalgia rheumatica. *BMJ*. 2008;336:765–9.
- Salvarani C, Cantini F, Hunder GG. Polymyalgia rheumatica and giant-cell arteritis. *Lancet*. 2008;372:234–45.

See Also (Topic, Algorithm, Electronic Media Element)
Arthritis, Osteo; Arthritis, Rheumatoid; Depression; Fibromyalgia; Giant-cell Arteritis; Polymyositis Dermatomyositis

CODES

ICD9
725 Polymyalgia rheumatica

CLINICAL PEARLS
- Consider PMR in an elderly patient with proximal limb girdle pain and stiffness.
- Markers of inflammation are usually elevated, but a normal ESR does not exclude the diagnosis.
- If the patient does not report a dramatic and rapid response to low-dose steroids, reconsider the diagnosis.
- Adjust steroids according to patient's symptoms, not based on their ESR.

POLYMYOSITIS/DERMATOMYOSITIS

Christopher M. Wise, MD

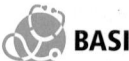 **BASICS**

DESCRIPTION

Systemic connective tissue disease characterized by inflammatory and degenerative changes in proximal muscles, sometimes accompanied by characteristic skin rash

- If skin manifestations (Gottron sign: symmetric, scaly, violaceous, erythematous eruption over the extensor surfaces of the metacarpophalangeal and interphalangeal joints of the fingers; heliotrope: reddish violaceous eruption on the upper eyelids) are present, it is designated as dermatomyositis (1).
- Different types of myositis include
  - Idiopathic polymyositis
  - Idiopathic dermatomyositis
  - Polymyositis/dermatomyositis as an overlap (usually with lupus or systemic sclerosis or as part of mixed connective-tissue disease)
  - Myositis associated with malignancy
  - HIV-associated myopathy
  - Inclusion-body myositis (IBM), a variant with atypical patterns of weakness and biopsy findings
- System(s) affected: Cardiovascular; Musculoskeletal; Pulmonary; Skin/Exocrine
- Synonym(s): Myositis; Inflammatory myopathy; Antisynthetase syndrome (subset with certain antibodies)

EPIDEMIOLOGY

Incidence

- Estimated at 0.5–0.8/100,000 population
- Predominant age: 5–15 years, 40–60 years, peak incidence in mid-40s
- Predominant sex: Female > Male (2:1)

Prevalence

1–2 patients/100,000 population

Geriatric Considerations

Elderly patients with myositis or dermatomyositis are at increased risk of neoplasm.

Pediatric Considerations

Childhood dermatomyositis is likely a separate entity associated with cutaneous vasculitis and muscle calcifications.

RISK FACTORS

Family history of autoimmune disease (e.g., systemic lupus, myositis) or vasculitis

Genetics

Mild association with human leukocyte antigen (HLA)–DR3, HLA-DRw52

PATHOPHYSIOLOGY

- Inflammatory process, mediated by T cells and cytokine release, leading to damage to muscle cells (predominantly skeletal muscles)
- In patients with IBM, degenerative mechanisms may be important (2).

ETIOLOGY

Unknown; potential viral, genetic factors

COMMONLY ASSOCIATED CONDITIONS

- Malignancy (in 15–25%)
- Progressive systemic sclerosis
- Vasculitis
- Systemic lupus erythematosus
- Mixed connective-tissue disease

 DIAGNOSIS

HISTORY

- Symmetric proximal muscle weakness causing difficulty when:
  - Arising from sitting or lying positions
  - Climbing stairs
  - Raising arms
- Joint pain/swelling
- Dysphagia
- Dyspnea
- Rash on face, eyelids, hands, arms

PHYSICAL EXAM

Proximal muscle weakness:

- Shoulder muscles
- Hip girdle muscles (trouble standing from seated or squatting position, weak hip flexors in supine position)
- Muscle swelling, stiffness, induration
- Distal muscle weakness is seen only in patients with IBM.
- Rash over face (eyelids, nasolabial folds), upper chest, dorsal hands (especially knuckle pads), fingers ("mechanic's hands")
- Periorbital edema
- Calcinosis cutis (childhood cases)
- Mesenteric arterial insufficiency/infarction (childhood cases)
- Cardiac impairment; arrhythmia, failure

DIAGNOSTIC TESTS & INTERPRETATION

- Diagnosis of muscle component (myositis) usually relies on four findings (1)[C].
  - Weakness
  - Creatine kinase and/or aldolase elevation
  - Abnormal electromyogram
  - Findings on muscle biopsy
- Presence of compatible skin rash of dermatomyositis

Lab

Initial lab tests

- Increased creatine kinase (CK), aldolase
- Increased serum glutamic-oxaloacetic transaminase/aspartate aminotransferase
- Increased lactate dehydrogenase
- Myoglobinuria
- Increased erythrocyte sedimentation rate
- Positive rheumatoid factor (<50% of patients)
- Positive antinuclear antibody (>50% of patients)
- Leukocytosis (<50% of patients)
- Anemia (<50% of patients)
- Hyperglobulinemia (<50% of patients)

- Myositis-specific antibodies (antisynthetase antibodies) described in a minority of patients
  - Anti-Jo-1 is the most common but has been found in <20% of patients.
  - Associated with an increased incidence of interstitial lung disease

Follow-Up & Special Considerations

Changes in muscle enzymes (CK or aldolase) correlate with improvement and worsening.

Imaging

Initial approach

Chest radiograph part of initial evaluation to assess for associated pulmonary involvement or malignancy

Follow-Up & Special Considerations

MRI to assess muscle edema and inflammation may be used in some patients to determine best biopsy site or response to therapy.

Diagnostic Procedures/Surgery

- Electromyography: Muscle irritability, low-amplitude potentials, polyphasic action potentials, fibrillations
- Muscle biopsy (deltoid or quadriceps femoris)

Pathological Findings

- Microscopic findings:
  - Muscle fiber degeneration
  - Phagocytosis of muscle debris
  - Perifascicular muscle fiber atrophy
  - Inflammatory cell infiltrates in adult form
  - Via electron microscopy: Inclusion bodies (IBM only)
  - Sarcoplasmic basophilia
- Muscle fiber increased in size
- Vasculopathy (childhood polymyositis/dermatomyositis)

DIFFERENTIAL DIAGNOSIS

- Vasculitis
- Progressive systemic sclerosis
- Systemic lupus erythematosus
- Rheumatoid arthritis
- Muscular dystrophy
- Eaton-Lambert syndrome
- Sarcoidosis
- Amyotrophic lateral sclerosis
- Endocrine disorders:
  - Thyroid disease
  - Cushing syndrome
- Infectious myositis (viral, bacterial, parasitic)
- Drug-induced myopathies:
  - Cholesterol-lowering agents
  - Colchicine
  - Corticosteroids
  - Ethanol
  - Chloroquine
  - Zidovudine
- Electrolyte disorders (magnesium, calcium, potassium)
- Heritable metabolic myopathies
- Sleep-apnea syndrome

TREATMENT

MEDICATION

First Line

- Prednisone (3)[B]:
  – 40–80 mg/d PO in divided doses
  – Consolidate doses and reduce prednisone slowly when enzyme levels are normal.
  – Probably need to continue 5–10 mg/d for maintenance in most patients
- For steroid refractory or dependent patients (3)[B]:
  – Azathioprine: 1.0 mg/kg PO (arthritis dose) once daily or b.i.d.
  – Methotrexate: 10–25 mg PO weekly, useful in most steroid-resistant patients
- Rash of dermatomyositis may require topical steroids or oral hydroxychloroquine.
- Patients with IBM have very poor response to steroids and other 1st- and 2nd-line drugs in general.

Second Line

- Other immunosuppressant drugs (e.g., cyclophosphamide, chlorambucil, cyclosporine, mycophenolate, tacrolimus) can be added to steroids.
- Combination methotrexate and azathioprine also may be useful in refractory cases (3)[B].
- Intravenous immunoglobulin (IVIG), tumor necrosis factor (TNF) inhibitors (e.g., Etanercept), and rituximab have been reported to be helpful in small series of patients with refractory disease.
- Contraindications: Methotrexate is contraindicated with previous liver disease, alcohol use, pregnancy, and underlying renal disease (use with extreme caution in patients with serum creatinine >1.5 mg/dL in general).
- Precautions:
  – Prednisone: Adverse effects associated with long-term steroid use include adrenal suppression, sodium and water retention, hypokalemia, osteoporosis, cataracts, and increased susceptibility to infection.
  – Azathioprine: Adverse effects include bone marrow suppression, increased liver function tests, and increased risk of infection.
  – Methotrexate: Adverse effects include stomatitis, bone marrow suppression, pneumonitis, and risk of liver fibrosis and cirrhosis with prolonged use.

ADDITIONAL TREATMENT

General Measures

General evaluation for malignancy in all adults, particularly with dermatomyositis, at initial evaluation and during follow-up

Issues for Referral

- Diagnostic uncertainty, usually related to elevated muscle enzymes without typical symptoms of findings of muscle weakness
- Poor response to initial steroid therapy
- Excessive steroid requirement (unable to taper prednisone to <20 mg daily after 4–6 months)

SURGERY/OTHER PROCEDURES

None indicated, other than initial biopsy

IN-PATIENT CONSIDERATIONS

Initial Stabilization

Inpatient evaluation seldom needed

Admission Criteria

- Inability to stand, ambulate
- Respiratory difficulty
- Fever or other signs of infection

 ONGOING CARE

FOLLOW-UP RECOMMENDATIONS

Patient Monitoring

- Follow muscle enzymes along with muscle strength and functional capacity.
- Monitor for steroid-induced complications (e.g., hypokalemia, hypertension, and hyperglycemia).
- Bone densitometry and consideration of calcium, vitamin D, and bisphosphonate therapy
- If azathioprine, methotrexate, or other immunosuppressant is used, appropriate laboratory monitoring should be done periodically (e.g., hematology, liver enzymes, and creatinine).
- Attempt to decrease and/or discontinue steroid dose as patient responds to therapy.
- Maintain immunosuppression until patient's muscle strength stabilizes for prolonged period depending on individual patient parameters, risks of medication, risk of relapse; time period undefined (months, years).

DIET

Moderation of caloric and sodium intake to avoid weight gain from corticosteroid therapy

PATIENT EDUCATION

- Curtail excess physical activity in early phases when muscles enzymes are markedly elevated.
- Emphasis on range-of-motion exercises
- Gradually muscle strengthening when muscle enzymes are normal or improved and stable

PROGNOSIS

- Residual weakness 30%
- Persistent active disease 20%
- 5-year survival 65–75%
- Survival is worse for women and African Americans and those with dermatomyositis, IBM, or cancer.
- Most patients improve with therapy.
- Patients with IBM respond poorly to most therapies (2).
- 50% have full recovery (4,5).

COMPLICATIONS

- Pneumonia
- Infection
- Myocardial infarction
- Carcinoma (especially breast, lung)
- Severe dysphagia
- Respiratory impairment owing to muscle weakness, interstitial lung disease
- Aspiration pneumonitis
- Steroid myopathy
- Steroid-induced diabetes, hypertension, hypokalemia, osteoporosis

REFERENCES

1. Dalakas MC. Inflammatory disorders of muscle: progress in polymyositis, dermatomyositis and inclusion body myositis. *Curr Opin Neurol*. 2004;17:561–7.
2. Karpati G, O'Ferrall EK et al. Sporadic inclusion body myositis: pathogenic considerations. *Ann. Neurol*. 2009;65:7–11.
3. Choy EH, Hoogendijk JE, Lecky B, et al. Immunosuppressant and immunomodulatory treatment for dermatomyositis and polymyositis. *Cochrane Database Syst Rev*. 2005;CD003643.
4. Ponyi A, Borgulya G, Constantin T, et al. Functional outcome and quality of life in adult patients with idiopathic inflammatory myositis. *Rheumatology (Oxford)*. 2005;44:83–8.
5. Airio A, Kautiainen H, Hakala M. Prognosis and mortality of polymyositis and dermatomyositis patients. *Clin Rheumatol*. 2006;25:234–9.

 CODES

ICD9

- 710.3 Dermatomyositis
- 710.4 Polymyositis

CLINICAL PEARLS

- Corticosteroids alone may be sufficient in patients who have rapid improvement in weakness and muscle enzymes. However, most patients require azathioprine, methotrexate, or other immunosuppressive medications.
- The risk of associated malignancy is higher in patients over age 50 and those with cutaneous manifestations.
- Elevated muscle enzymes (e.g., CK and aldolase) are seen frequently as transient phenomena in patients with febrile illness and injuries; may return to normal on repeat.
- In patients with persistently elevated muscle enzymes and symptoms and findings of muscle weakness, electromyogram followed by muscle biopsy should be the initial studies considered.
- Suspect IBM in older patients with very slow onset and progression of symptoms, poor response to steroids and immunosuppressive therapy, and atypical patterns (asymmetric, sometimes distal) of muscle weakness.

PORPHYRIA
Nathan T. Connell, MD

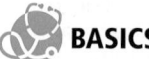 **BASICS**

DESCRIPTION
- Several heme synthesis pathway enzyme deficiencies with overproduction and accumulation of intermediate metabolic products leading to neuropsychiatric, abdominal, or dermatologic symptoms and syndromes:
  - Porphyria cutanea tarda: Dermatologic
  - Acute intermittent porphyria: Pyrroloporphyria; neuropsychiatric–abdominal
  - Protoporphyria: Erythropoietic or hepatoerythropoietic; mild dermatologic
  - Variegate porphyria: South African porphyria; prevalence in South Africa is 1/400
  - Hereditary coproporphyria: Neuropsychiatric, occasionally dermatologic
  - Porpbobilinogen synthetase deficiency: δ-Aminolevulinic aciduria; neuropsychiatric–abdominal
  - Congenital erythropoietic porphyria: Günther disease; severe dermatologic
  - Other rare genetic variants reported
- System(s) affected: GI; Skin/Exocrine; Hematologic/Lymphatic/Immunologic; Nervous

ALERT
Unpredictable disease activity

EPIDEMIOLOGY
- Predominant age:
  - Congenital erythropoietic porphyria: Early childhood
  - Protoporphyria: Older childhood
  - Acute intermittent porphyria, variegate porphyria, hereditary coproporphyria, porphobilinogen synthetase deficiency: Young adult
  - Porphyria cutanea tarda: Middle age
- Predominant sex:
  - Protoporphyria, congenital erythropoietic porphyria: Male = Female
  - Porphyria cutanea tarda: Male > Female
  - Acute intermittent porphyria, variegate porphyria, hereditary coproporphyria, porphobilinogen synthetase deficiency: Female > Male

Prevalence
- More common in whites than in Asians or individuals of African descent
- Porphyria cutanea tarda: 1/10,000; most common of the porphyrias in US and Europe
- Acute intermittent porphyria, protoporphyria, variegate porphyria: 1/10,000–1/100,000. The prevalence in Europe is approximately 1/75,000. In northern Sweden, because of a founder effect, the estimated prevalence is 1/1000 (1).
- Variegate porphyria: 1/150,000. Especially common in South Africa because of founder effect.
- Hereditary coproporphyria: <1/100,000
- Porphobilinogen synthetase deficiency, congenital erythropoietic porphyria: Very rare

RISK FACTORS
- Multiple precipitating factors, especially in acute intermittent porphyria, variegate porphyria, hereditary coproporphyria
- Drugs (e.g., barbiturates and sulfas in acute intermittent porphyria)

- Estrogens (especially oral contraceptives)
- Steroids
- Liver disease
- Infection
- Fasting
- Heavy alcohol use
- Hexachlorobenzene exposure

Genetics
- Autosomal dominant: Porphyria cutanea tarda (<20% of patients), acute intermittent porphyria, protoporphyria, variegate porphyria, hereditary coproporphyria
- Autosomal recessive: Porphobilinogen synthetase deficiency, congenital erythropoietic porphyria
- Latency common with variable expression leading to many asymptomatic or minimally symptomatic carriers
- Porphyria cutanea tarda also can be sporadic or acquired (>80% of patients).
- The pathogenesis of the inherited porphyrias has been defined at the molecular level. It is clear that a great deal of genetic heterogeneity is present in each porphyria.
- Family members of patients with variegate porphyria should be tested. Since biochemical analysis may not be positive in asymptomatic individuals, genetic testing is required (2).
- In all cases, patients should be referred for genetic counseling prior to testing because there may be emotional, psychological, and financial implications of testing for porphyria.

GENERAL PREVENTION
- Avoid precipitating drugs (3):
  - Alcohol
  - Barbiturates
  - Carbamazepine
  - Chlorpropamide
  - Danazol
  - Ergots
  - Estrogens and progestins
  - Ethchlorvynol
  - Glutethimide
  - Griseofulvin
  - Mephenytoin
  - Meprobamate
  - Methotrexate
  - Methyprylon
  - Metoclopramide
  - Phenytoin
  - Pyrazolones
  - Succinimides
  - Sulfonamide antibiotics
  - Valproic acid
- Consume diet with high-carbohydrate intake
- Some drugs considered safe:
  - Acetaminophen
  - Amiodarone
  - Aspirin
  - Atropine
  - Chlorpromazine
  - Diazepam (in small doses)
  - Digoxin
  - Diphenhydramine
  - Glucocorticoids
  - Heparin
  - Insulin
  - Lithium

  - Magnesium
  - Neostigmine
  - Nitrous oxide
  - Penicillin and derivatives
  - Phenothiazines
  - Promethazine
  - Narcotic analgesics
  - Propranolol
  - Streptomycin
  - Succinylcholine
  - Thiazides

ETIOLOGY
- Genetic enzyme deficiencies:
  - Porphyria cutanea tarda: Uroporphyrinogen decarboxylase
  - Acute intermittent porphyria: Porphobilinogen deaminase
  - Protoporphyria ferrochelatase
  - Variegate porphyria: Protoporphyrinogen oxidase
  - Hereditary coproporphyria: Coproporphyrinogen oxidase
  - Porphobilinogen synthetase deficiency: Porphobilinogen synthetase
  - Congenital erythropoietic porphyria: Uroporphyrinogen III synthetase (cosynthetase)
- Causes of acquired porphyria cutanea tarda:
  - Hepatitis C virus (strong association)
  - Heavy alcohol use
  - Decreased enzyme associated with steroids and hormones
  - Specific exposure to polyhalogenated hydrocarbons (e.g., hexachlorobenzene)
  - Lead poisoning may alter pathways.
  - HIV infection
  - Possibly ascorbic acid deficiency

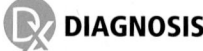 **DIAGNOSIS**

PHYSICAL EXAM
- Usually reversible, lasting days to weeks
- Urine may turn dark red or brown on standing (*porphyria* is from the Greek *porphyra*, meaning "purple").
- Abdominal:
  - Rather severe abdominal pain, often colicky
  - Generalized more often than localized
  - Can mimic acute abdomen
  - Fever not usually present
  - Chronic constipation common
  - Severity of symptoms often out of proportion to physical findings
- Neurologic (4):
  - Almost any neurologic symptom may be seen.
  - Includes sensory, motor, and autonomic systems
  - May include seizures
  - May lead to quadriplegia and/or respiratory paralysis with death
  - Acute porphyric neuropathy can be associated with abdominal pain and dysautonomia.
  - Posterior reversible encephalopathy (PRES) has been seen in patients during acute attacks.
- Psychiatric:
  - Can mimic almost any psychiatric disorder
  - Psychosis most common
  - Visual hallucinations common
  - Disorientation frequent
  - Chronic depression frequent

- Dermatologic:
  – Photosensitivity (common)
  – Scrapes, ulcerations, blisters with minimal trauma
  – Hyperpigmentation, especially hands and face
  – Scarring frequent
  – Facial hypertrichosis
- Congenital erythropoietic porphyria (mutilating, with hemolysis, erythrodontia, splenomegaly)
- Protoporphyria (occasional hepatic disease, including hepatic failure)

DIAGNOSTIC TESTS & INTERPRETATION
Genetic studies when applicable

Lab
- Urine porphyrins will be elevated during an acute attack but may be normal at other times (1).
- Individual enzyme activity in erythrocytes or other body cells/tissues
- Stool for porphyrins in protoporphyria, variegate porphyria, hereditary coproporphyria, congenital erythropoietic porphyria
- Bile for porphyrin in variegate porphyria
- Plasma for fluorescence emission spectroscopy in variegate porphyria
- Erythrocyte uroporphyrin in congenital erythropoietic porphyria
- Protoporphyria is the exception; urine is unremarkable; test erythrocyte protoporphyrin.
- Ferritin typically elevated in porphyria cutanea tarda due to increased iron stores
- Numerous conditions may cause a slight increase in porphyrinuria, but patients are asymptomatic:
  – Acute liver disease
  – Hepatoma
  – Hodgkin lymphoma
  – Multiple neurologic diseases

Initial lab tests
- The initial screening test should be guided by the patient's history.
- If the patient has neurovisceral symptoms, this suggests the possibility of a hepatic porphyria. A 24-h urine should be collected and sent for porphobilinogen, aminolevulinic acid, and porphyrin.
- If the patient has skin photosensitivity, urine and plasma porphyrin should be sent. Fecal porphyrin is sometimes available and can be useful in establishing the diagnosis.

DIFFERENTIAL DIAGNOSIS
- The differential diagnosis includes a spectrum of neurologic, psychiatric, and dermatologic orders.
- Pseudoporphyria is a rare syndrome—indistinguishable from porphyria cutanea tarda—caused by some NSAIDs (e.g., nabumetone and naproxen) and flutamide.

 TREATMENT

Patients usually can be treated successfully as an outpatient except if severity of symptoms necessitates hospitalization.

MEDICATION
First Line
- Neuropsychiatric–abdominal:
  – IV glucose 400 g/d × 1–2 days (5,6)[C]
  – Hematin (ferriprotoporphyrin IX, hemin [Panhematin]) IV 1–4 mg/kg/d over 10–15 minutes × 3–14 days (5,6)[B]
  – Seizures: Gabapentin (1,6)[B]
  – Depression: Consider selective serotonin reuptake inhibitors (SSRIs).
- Contraindications: Known sensitivity to drug
- Precautions: Hematin phlebitis at IV site, reduced clotting ability

Second Line
- Porphyria cutanea tarda:
  – Chloroquine 125 mg twice weekly or hydroxychloroquine 250 mg t.i.d. in conjunction with phlebotomy
  – With hepatitis C virus: Interferon is beneficial for both congenital erythropoietic porphyria and plumboporphyria.
- Acute intermittent porphyria:
  – Luteinizing hormone–releasing hormone (LHRH) analogues are being studied.
  – Autonomic manifestations: β-Blockers can be used cautiously (6).
  – Other symptoms: Treat symptomatically (1,5)

ADDITIONAL TREATMENT
General Measures
- Neuropsychiatric–abdominal: Avoid precipitating drugs, alcohol, known toxins
- Dermatologic: Shade, protective clothing, avoid skin trauma; for porphyria cutanea tarda, weekly or monthly phlebotomy may help to prevent attacks
- Congenital erythropoietic porphyria: Consider bone marrow transplantation.

 ONGOING CARE

FOLLOW-UP RECOMMENDATIONS
Porphyria cutanea tarda: Avoid sun exposure.

DIET
Neuropsychiatric: There is anecdotal evidence that diets rich in carbohydrates help to reduce symptoms or frequency of attacks.

PATIENT EDUCATION
- The American Porphyria Foundation, P.O. Box 22712, Houston, TX 77227; (713) 266-9617 or 1-866-APF-3635 (toll-free); fax: (713) 840-9552; http://www.porphyriafoundation.com/
- The Drug Database for Acute Porphyria: http://www.drugs-porphyria.org/
- European Porphyria Network: http://www.porphyria-europe.com/

PROGNOSIS
- In all porphyrias:
  – Patients who are asymptomatic or minimally symptomatic: Unaffected longevity
  – Neurologic complications (e.g., peripheral neuropathy, neurosis, or hemiplegia) may be permanent.

- In acute intermittent porphyria:
  – Acute attacks have 25% mortality.
  – Increased risk of hepatocellular carcinoma
- Less than 10% of patients develop recurrent acute attacks (1).

REFERENCES

1. Puy H, Gouya L, Deybach JC et al. Porphyrias. *Lancet*. 2010;375:924–37.
2. Sarkany RP. Making sense of the porphyrias. *Photodermatol Photoimmunol Photomed*. 2008;24:102–8.
3. Thunell S, Pomp E, Brun A. Guide to drug porphyrogenicity prediction and drug prescription in the acute porphyrias. *Br J Clin Pharmacol*. 2007.
4. Pischik E, Kauppinen R. Neurological Manifestations of acute intermittent porphyria. *Cell Mol Biol (Noisy-le-grand)*. 2009;55:72–83.
5. Dombeck TA, Satonik RC. The porphyrias. *Emerg Med Clin North Am*. 2005;23:885–99, x.
6. Anderson KE, Bloomer JR, Bonkovsky HL, et al. Recommendations for the diagnosis and treatment of the acute porphyrias. *Ann Intern Med*. 2005;142:439–50.

ADDITIONAL READING

- Dhoble A, Patel MB, Abdelmoneim SS, et al. Relation of porphyria to atrial fibrillation. *Am J Cardiol*. 2009;104:373–6.
- Marsden JT, Rees DC et al. A retrospective analysis of outcome of pregnancy in patients with acute porphyria. *Journal of inherited metabolic disease*. 2010;
- Sardh E, Rejkjaer L, Andersson DE, et al. Safety, pharmacokinetics and pharmacodynamics of recombinant human porphobilinogen deaminase in healthy subjects and asymptomatic carriers of the acute intermittent porphyria gene who have increased porphyrin precursor excretion. *Clin Pharmacokinet*. 2007;46:335–49.
- Whatley SD, Mason NG, Holme SA, et al. Molecular epidemiology of erythropoietic protoporphyria in the U.K. *Br J Dermatol*. 2010;162:642–6.

 CODES

ICD9
277.1 Disorders of porphyrin metabolism

CLINICAL PEARLS
- The term porphyria encompasses many individual diagnoses that may be difficult to separate diagnostically.
- Consider screening for porphyria in patients who have signs and symptoms that do not appear to fit within a single diagnosis, as porphyria may affect multiple organ systems.
- Time between attacks can be increased by both patient and physician attention to triggers. Management with a hematologist is strongly encouraged.

PORTAL HYPERTENSION

Walter M. Kim, MD, PhD
Jyoti Ramakrishna, MD

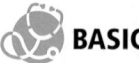 **BASICS**

DESCRIPTION
- Increased portal venous pressure >5–10 mm Hg that occurs in association with splanchnic vasodilatation, portosystemic collateral formation, and a hyperdynamic circulation
- Most commonly secondary to elevated hepatic venous pressure gradient (the gradient between the portal and central venous pressures)
- Course is generally progressive, with risk of complications including acute variceal bleeding, ascites, encephalopathy, and hepatorenal syndrome.

EPIDEMIOLOGY
Incidence
- Incidence/prevalence in the US is unknown.
- Predominant age: Adult
- Predominant sex: Male > Female

RISK FACTORS
See Etiology.

Genetics
No known genetic patterns except those associated with specific hepatic diseases that cause portal hypertension (HTN)

ETIOLOGY
- Causes generally classified as:
  - Prehepatic (portal vein thrombosis or obstruction)
  - Intrahepatic (most commonly cirrhosis)
  - Posthepatic (hepatic vein thrombosis, Budd Chiari syndrome, right-sided heart failure)
- Adult: May be intrahepatic or extrahepatic; cirrhosis accounts for 90% of cases; may be due to:
  - Virus (hepatitis B, hepatitis C, hepatitis D)
  - Alcoholism
  - Schistosomiasis
  - Wilson disease
  - Hemochromatosis
  - Primary biliary cirrhosis

Pediatric Considerations
In children, portal vein thrombosis is the most common extrahepatic cause; intrahepatic causes are more likely to be biliary atresia, viral hepatitis, and metabolic liver disease.

 DIAGNOSIS

HISTORY
- Weakness/fatigue
- Jaundice
- Symptoms of heart failure, including chest pain, shortness of breath, and/or edema
- Hematemesis
- Melena
- Oliguria
- History of chronic liver disease
- Alcoholic hepatitis
- Alcohol abuse

PHYSICAL EXAM
- Exam findings may be general or related to specific complications.
- General:
  - Pallor
  - Icterus
  - Digital clubbing
  - Palmar erythema
  - Splenomegaly
  - Caput medusa
  - Spider angiomata
  - Umbilical bruit
  - Hemorrhoids
  - Gynecomastia
  - Testicular atrophy
- Gastroesophageal varices:
  - Hypotension
  - Tachycardia
- Ascites:
  - Distended abdomen
  - Fluid wave
  - Shifting dullness with percussion
- Hepatic encephalopathy:
  - Confusion/coma
  - Asterixis
  - Hyperreflexia

DIAGNOSTIC TESTS & INTERPRETATION
Lab
Initial lab tests
Nonspecific changes associated with underlying disease:
- Hypersplenism: Anemia (also may be due to malnutrition or bleeding), leukopenia, thrombocytopenia
- Hepatic dysfunction:
  - Hypoalbuminemia
  - Hyperbilirubinemia
  - Elevated alkaline phosphatase
  - Elevated liver enzymes
  - Abnormal clotting (prothrombin time, partial thromboplastin time)
- Gastrointestinal (GI) bleeding:
  - Iron-deficiency anemia
  - Elevated serum ammonia
  - Fecal occult blood
- Hepatorenal syndrome:
  - Elevated serum creatinine, blood urea nitrogen
  - Urine Na <5 mEq/L (<20 mmol/L)

Imaging
Initial approach
- Ultrasound (US) and computed tomography (CT) scan/magnetic resonance imaging (MRI) may detect cirrhosis, splenomegaly, ascites, and varices.
- US/duplex Doppler:
  - Can determine presence and direction of flow in portal and hepatic veins
  - Useful in diagnosing portal vein thrombosis, shunt thrombosis, or the presence of ascites

- CT scan/MRI: Angiographic measurement of hepatic venous wedge pressure via jugular or femoral vein:
  - Correlates with portal pressure
  - Risk of variceal bleeding is increased if hepatic venous pressure gradient >12 mm Hg.
- Upper GI series may outline varices in esophagus and stomach.

Diagnostic Procedures/Surgery
Endoscopy can diagnose esophageal and gastric varices and portal hypertensive gastropathy.

Pathological Findings
Specific for underlying disease

DIFFERENTIAL DIAGNOSIS
Usually related to specific presentations:
- Gastroesophageal varices with hemorrhage:
  - Portal hypertensive gastropathy
  - Hemorrhagic gastritis
  - Peptic ulcer disease
  - Mallory-Weiss tear
- Ascites:
  - Spontaneous bacterial peritonitis
  - Pancreatic ascites
  - Peritoneal carcinomatosis
  - Tuberculous peritonitis
  - Nephrotic syndrome
  - Fluid overload from heart failure
- Hepatic encephalopathy:
  - Delirium tremens
  - Intracranial hemorrhage
  - Sedative abuse
  - Uremia
- Hepatorenal syndrome:
  - Drug nephrotoxicity
  - Renal tubular necrosis

 TREATMENT

MEDICATION
Therapy for encephalopathy: See Hepatic Encephalopathy.

First Line
- Prophylaxis against variceal bleeding:
  - Nonselective β-blockade (1)[B]: Examples include:
    - Propanolol: Start with 10–20 mg/d p.o. twice daily to 3 times daily; pediatric dose: 0.5–1 mg/kg/d divided q6–8h
    - Nadolol: 40–80 mg/d p.o. once-daily dosing
  - Doses may be titrated up as tolerated to maximum recommended doses.
- Therapy for acute variceal hemorrhage:
  - Vasopressin: Start with 0.2–0.4 unit/min IV; increase to maximum dose 0.9 unit/min as needed; pediatric dose: 0.002–0.005 unit/kg/min; do not exceed 0.01 unit/kg/min. After bleeding stops, continue at same dose for 12 h and then taper off over 24–48 h.
  - Somatostatin: 250-μg bolus, followed by 250 μg/h continuous infusion; continue for 2–5 d if successful.
  - Octreotide: 25–50 μg/h continuous infusion; pediatric dose: 1 μg/kg bolus followed by 1 μg/kg/h is used traditionally; treat for up to 5 days.

- For prevention of recurrence and for overall reduction in mortality:
  - Propranolol: 10–60 mg/day p.o. 2–4×/day; pediatric dose: 0.5–1 mg/kg/day divided q6–8h
  - Nadolol: 40–80 mg/day p.o. reduces portal venous blood inflow by blocking the adrenergic dilatation of the mesenteric arterioles.
  - Tetrandine, a calcium-channel blocker, also has been found to reduce the rate of rebleeding with fewer side effects.
- Treatment for ascites (along with salt and fluid restriction):
  - Furosemide: 20–40 mg/day; pediatric dose: 1–2 mg/kg/dose ± IV albumin infusion
  - Spironolactone: 50–100 mg/day; pediatric dose: 1–3 mg/kg/day

Second Line
- Terlipressin (1–2 mg IV q4–6h for up to 48 h) is a more selective splanchnic vasoconstrictor and may be associated with fewer complications (1)[B]. It is currently used when standard therapy with somatostatin or octreotide fails.
- Addition of nitrates, such as nitroglycerin or isosorbide mononitrate, reduces portal pressures and bleeding rates, and has been shown to reduce mortality. Since the risk–benefit ratio is not clear, nitrates are not considered 1st-line treatment.

ADDITIONAL TREATMENT
General Measures
- Avoid sedatives that may precipitate encephalopathy.
- Limit sodium intake because cirrhotic patients avidly retain sodium.
- Restrict protein only if encephalopathic.

Issues for Referral
Patients with portal hypertension should be managed by both a primary care physician and a gastroenterologist.

SURGERY/OTHER PROCEDURES
- Treatments available for specific complications of portal HTN (in addition to or if refractory to medications):
  - Gastroesophageal varices with hemorrhage:
    - Endoscopic variceal sclerosis or banding (the 1st-line treatment in many cases for acute hemorrhage)
    - Balloon tamponade (not used commonly when endoscopic treatment is available)
    - Transjugular intrahepatic portosystemic shunt (TIPS)
    - Portocaval shunting
  - Ascites refractory to medical management:
    - Large volume paracentesis
    - Peritoneovenous shunt
    - TIPS
- Liver transplantation should be considered for patients with advanced disease (1)[B].

IN-PATIENT CONSIDERATIONS
- Acute GI bleeding should be managed in the inpatient setting, either on the regular medical floor if the patient is hemodynamically stable or occasionally in the intensive care unit if the patient is unstable.
- Patients with mental status changes from encephalopathy need to be evaluated in the inpatient setting.

Initial Stabilization
- If acute variceal bleeding:
  - Type and cross
  - Initial resuscitation with isotonic fluid until packed red blood cells are available.
  - Correct coagulopathy with vitamin K and fresh-frozen plasma
  - Endoscopy as soon as the patient is stabilized (for diagnosis and treatment)
- Avoid sedatives that may precipitate encephalopathy.
- Limit sodium administration because cirrhotic patients avidly retain sodium.
- Restrict protein only if encephalopathic.

ALERT
If the patient is an active alcohol drinker, watch for signs and symptoms of withdrawal. Follow inpatient protocols.

Admission Criteria
- Acute bleeding from the intestinal tract, either vomiting or per rectum
- Acute confusional state/mental status changes

IV Fluids
Use isotonic fluid.

Discharge Criteria
- For GI bleeding:
  - No active bleeding × 24 h
  - Hemodynamically stable, especially pulse
  - Stable hemoglobin
- For encephalopathy: Improvement in or resolution of mental status changes

 ## ONGOING CARE

DIET
- In patients with cirrhosis, sodium restriction is important because cirrhotic patients avidly retain sodium.
- Restrict protein only in patients who are encephalopathic.

PATIENT EDUCATION
Refrain from drinking alcohol. Resources for patients who have difficulty with not drinking alcohol can be obtained from Alcoholics Anonymous at http://www.aa.org.

PROGNOSIS
- Hepatic reserve defined by Child-Pugh classification: Rating based on encephalopathy, ascites, bilirubin, albumin, prothrombin
- Variceal bleeding:
  - 1/3 of patients with known varices will bleed eventually.
  - 50% rebleed, usually within 2 years, unless portal pressure is reduced by surgical or transjugular intrahepatic portosystemic shunt procedure.
  - 15–20% mortality rate

- Ascites and encephalopathy often recur.
- Prognosis of patients with ascites is poor: 50% 1-year survival without liver transplant (compared with 90% for patients with cirrhosis and no ascites).

REFERENCE
1. Abraldes JG, Angermayr B, Bosch J. The management of portal hypertension. *Clin Liver Dis.* 2005;9:685–713, vii.

ADDITIONAL READING
- Bosch J, et al. The management of portal hypertension: Rational basis, available treatments and future options. *J Hepatology.* 2008;48: S68–S92.
- Dib N, Oberti F, Calès P. Current management of the complications of portal hypertension: variceal bleeding and ascites. *CMAJ.* 2006;174:1433–43.
- Samonakis DN, et al. Management of portal hypertension. *Postgrad Med.* 2004;80:634–41.
- Sanyal AJ, Bosch J, Blei A, et al. Portal hypertension and its complications. *Gastroenterology.* 2008; 134:1715–28.
- Sass DA, Chopra KB et al. Portal hypertension and variceal hemorrhage. *Med Clin North Am.* 2009;93.
- Wright AS, Rikkers LF. Current management of portal hypertension. *J Gastrointest Surg.* 2005;9: 992–1005.

 ## CODES

ICD9
572.3 Portal hypertension

CLINICAL PEARLS
- Endoscopic treatment is successful for acute variceal hemorrhage 85% of the time.
- Prognosis of patients with ascites is poor: 50% 1-year survival without liver transplant (compared with 90% for patients with cirrhosis and no ascites).
- Advantages and disadvantages of balloon tamponade for acute variceal bleed:
  - Advantages include rapid and often effective control of bleeding and common availability of device.
  - Disadvantages include recurrence of bleeding when balloon is deflated, patient discomfort, and risk of esophageal perforation.

POSTCONCUSSIVE SYNDROME

Ryung Suh, MD, MPP, MBA, MPH

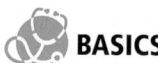 **BASICS**

DESCRIPTION

- Postconcussive syndrome (PCS) refers to the neurologic, cognitive, or behavioral symptoms that develop shortly after a concussion and persist for weeks or months, including:
  – Headache
  – Vertigo or dizziness
  – Fatigue
  – Memory impairment
  – Difficulty concentrating
  – Apathy
  – Anxiety
  – Depression
  – Irritability
  – Disordered sleep
  – New-onset seizures
  – Personality changes, inappropriateness
  – Sudden academic decline
  – Worsening of preexisting symptoms
- Persistent postconcussion syndrome (PPCS) is defined as the same symptoms that last more than 6 months.

EPIDEMIOLOGY
Incidence
- At 3 months postinjury, 50% of mild traumatic brain injury patients exhibit PCS symptoms.
- At 1 year postinjury, 15% exhibit PCS symptoms.

Prevalence
Predominant sex: Female > Male

RISK FACTORS
- Geriatric population
- Low socioeconomic status
- Substance abuse
- Previous affective or anxiety disorder (1)[B]
- Repetitive head injury
- Premorbid physical conditions
- Noise sensitivity, anxiety, and trouble thinking in the 3–10 days following concussion have been identified as important predictors of PCS (2).

GENERAL PREVENTION
Avoid opiates, if possible, for analgesia in traumatic brain injury (TBI) patients (3)[B].

PATHOPHYSIOLOGY
- Controversial; exact mechanism unknown
- There is debate about the actual diagnosis of PCS.

- Mild TBI can cause cortical contusions and axonal injury.
- It is postulated that microscopic axonal injury from shearing forces leads to inflammation that then causes the secondary injury responsible for persistent damage.
- One study showed an equal rate of PCS symptoms among both concussion and nonconcussion patients, implying that PCS is not driven by head injury alone (1)[B].
- A recent review of PPCS suggests that concomitant damage to eyes and ears during TBI plays a role in symptoms such as vertigo (4)[B].

ETIOLOGY
- Concussion is caused by direct blow to the head, face, or neck.
- Most commonly related to:
  – Motor vehicle accidents
  – Falls
  – Occupational accidents
  – Recreational accidents
  – Assaults

COMMONLY ASSOCIATED CONDITIONS
Post-traumatic stress disorder (PTSD)

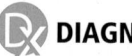 **DIAGNOSIS**

HISTORY
- Detailed history of recent impact or closed head injury, including:
  – Mechanism
  – Amount and type of force
  – Timing of injury related to symptoms
- Report of neurologic, cognitive, or behavioral symptoms by patient or family

PHYSICAL EXAM
Complete neurologic exam, including:
- Glasgow Coma Scale (GCS)
- Mini-Mental State Examination
- Memory Testing

DIAGNOSTIC TESTS & INTERPRETATION
Lab
Initial lab tests
Rule out other causes of neurologic, cognitive, or behavioral symptoms if history and presentation suggest other possible etiologies. Consider ordering (but not necessary for most diagnoses and not helpful in the young):
- CBC with differential
- Electrolytes
- Urinalysis
- Toxicology screen

Imaging
Initial approach
- Head CT scan is the imaging modality of choice for the assessment of acute head trauma.
- The Canadian CT head rule requires a head CT scan for patients with mild TBI and one of the following (to rule out more serious injury) (5)[B]:
  – GCS <15 2 hours after injury
  – Open or depressed skull fracture
  – Signs of basilar skull fracture
  – 2 or more episodes of vomiting
  – 65 years of age or older
  – Prolonged anterograde amnesia >30 minutes
  – Dangerous mechanism
- Patients with concussion often have a negative head CT scan.
- Consider the use of cervical imaging when concomitant cervical spine injury is suspected.

Follow-Up & Special Considerations
Schedule regular follow-up to evaluate for persistent symptoms and need for pharmacologic treatment.

Diagnostic Procedures/Surgery
Lumbar puncture, if concerned for CNS infection

DIFFERENTIAL DIAGNOSIS
- PTSD
- Evolving intracranial hemorrhage
- Migraine headaches
- Isolated anxiety or depression

TREATMENT

MEDICATION

First Line
- Headache/neck pain:
  - Nonnarcotic pain control if possible, such as NSAIDs
    - Sedation may obscure cognitive evaluation.
    - One study suggests a correlation between opiates and increased risk of depression and anxiety in PCS patients (3)[B].
- Depression/sleep disorders:
  - Tricyclic antidepressants
  - Selective serotonin reuptake inhibitors (SSRIs) are not well supported.

Second Line
Cognition/psychiatric symptoms: Methylphenidate has been shown to improve cognition and alertness compared with sertraline, with fewer side effects (6)[B].

ADDITIONAL TREATMENT
General Measures
Athletes with concussion should be restricted from sport activity until the clinical and cognitive symptoms of concussion resolve (7)[C].

Issues for Referral
- Psychiatric treatment, including behavioral therapy for anxiety and depression symptoms
- Occupational therapy for vocational rehabilitation, if needed
- Neurology referral if primary-care interventions for seizures, headache, vertigo, or cognition are unsuccessful
- Comprehensive cognitive evaluation for potential TBI rehabilitation
- Substance abuse counseling if needed

COMPLEMENTARY AND ALTERNATIVE MEDICINE
Massage therapy or osteopathic manipulative treatment for headache and neck pain

IN-PATIENT CONSIDERATIONS
Initial Stabilization
- Follow Advanced Trauma Life Support (ATLS) algorithms immediately postinjury to evaluate for additional injuries.
- If GCS <8, support respirations until improved, or consider definitive airway.

Admission Criteria
If neurologic status prevents safe functioning at home:
- Decreased alertness
- Intractable nausea and vomiting
- Concern for respiratory status

 ONGOING CARE

FOLLOW-UP RECOMMENDATIONS
Return for further evaluation if symptoms worsen or persist longer than 3 months.

PATIENT EDUCATION
- Brain Injury Association of America, http://www.biausa.org, 800-444-6443
- Head and brain injuries: http://www.nlm.nih.gov/medlineplus/headandbraininjuries.html
- Explain the possibility of PCS symptoms and usual time course.
- Review "Return-to-Play" guidelines and the risks involved with 2nd impact.

PROGNOSIS
- Prognosis is generally good.
- Young children may recover more slowly than young adults.

COMPLICATIONS
- Repeat head injury before resolution of PCS symptoms can worsen or prolong symptoms.
- Case studies of 2nd-impact syndrome (rare)—a fatal condition owing to a 2nd head injury soon after the 1st, involving autoregulation of the brain's blood supply, causing vascular engorgement and herniation—have been reported.

REFERENCES

1. Meares S, Shores EA, Taylor AJ, et al. Mild traumatic brain injury does not predict acute postconcussion syndrome. *J Neurol Neurosurg Psychiatry*. 2008;79:300–6.
2. Dischinger PC, Ryb GE, Kufera JA, et al. Early predictors of postconcussive syndrome in a population of trauma patients with mild traumatic brain injury. *J Trauma*. 2009;66:289–96; discussion 296–7.
3. Meares S, Shores EA, Batchelor J, et al. The relationship of psychological and cognitive factors and opioids in the development of the postconcussion syndrome in general trauma patients with mild traumatic brain injury. *J Int Neuropsychol Soc*. 2006;12:792–801.
4. Bigler ED. Neuropsychology and clinical neuroscience of persistent post-concussive syndrome. *Journal of the International Neuropsychological Society*. 2008;14:1–22.
5. Stiell IG, Wells GA, Vandemheen K, et al. The Canadian CT head rule for patients with minor head injury. *Lancet*. 2001;357:1394.
6. Lee H, Kim S, Kim J, et al. Comparing effects of methylphenidate, sertraline and placebo on neuropsychiatric sequelae in patients with traumatic brain injury. *Hum Psychopharmacol Clin Exp*. 2005;20:97–104.
7. McCrory P, Meeuwisse W, Johnston K, et al. Consensus statement on Concussion in Sport 3rd International Conference on Concussion in Sport held in Zurich, November 2008. *Clin J Sport Med*. 2009;19:185–200.

ADDITIONAL READING

- McHugh T, Laforce R, Gallagher P, et al. Natural history of the long-term cognitive, affective, and physical sequelae of mild traumatic brain injury. *Brain Cogn*. 2006;60:209–11.
- Nampiaparampil DE. Prevalence of chronic pain after traumatic brain injury: a systematic review. *JAMA*. 2008;300(6):711–9.
- Stulemeijer M, van der Werf S, Borm GF, et al. Early prediction of favourable recovery 6 months after mild traumatic brain injury. *J Neurol Neurosurg*. 2008;79:936–42.

See Also (Topic, Algorithm, Electronic Media Element)
Concussion

 CODES

ICD9
310.2 Postconcussion syndrome

CLINICAL PEARLS

- Head CT scan is the test of choice for acute injury in which it is necessary to exclude intracranial bleeding.
- Coordinate multidisciplinary treatment plans for patients with persistent symptoms.
- Athletes may not return to practice until symptoms are completely cleared nor play until able to fully practice without recurring symptoms.

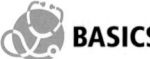

POSTTRAUMATIC STRESS DISORDER

Mhd Basheer Rahmoun, MD
Mazen Hadid, MD

BASICS

DESCRIPTION
- Posttraumatic stress disorder (PTSD) is an anxiety disorder defined as a reaction that can occur after exposure to an extreme traumatic event involving death, threat of death, serious physical injury, or a threat to physical integrity.
- This reaction has three cardinal characteristics:
  – Reexperiencing the trauma
  – Avoidance of anything related to the traumatic event
  – Increased arousal
- These symptoms should be present for 1 month at least
- Traumatic events that may trigger PTSD include natural or human disasters, serious accidents, war, sexual abuse, rape, torture, terrorism, hostage-taking, or being diagnosed with life-threatening disease
- PTSD can be:
  – Acute: Symptoms lasting <3 months
  – Chronic: Symptoms lasting ≥3 months
  – Of a delayed onset: 6 months (from event to symptom onset) in 25% of diagnosed cases.

EPIDEMIOLOGY
- Approximately 30% of men and women who have spent time in a war zone experience PTSD (1).
- Current estimates of PTSD in military personnel who served in Iraq range from 12% to 20%.

Incidence
Approximately 7.7 million American adults aged ≥18 years (3.5% of this age group) have PTSD in a given year.

Prevalence
Lifetime prevalence for PTSD is 7.8%.

RISK FACTORS
- Pretrauma environment:
  – Female sex
  – Younger age
  – Psychiatric history
- Peritrauma environment:
  – Severity of the trauma
  – Peritrauma emotionality
- Posttrauma environment:
  – Perceived injury severity
  – Medical complications
  – Perceived social support

Genetics
- Monozygotic twins exposed to combat in Vietnam were at increased risk of the co-twin having PTSD compared to twins that were dizygotic.
- Some data suggest an association between dopamine transporter gene (DAT) SLC6A3 3′ (VNTR) polymorphism and PTSD (2).

GENERAL PREVENTION
- Use of morphine during trauma care may reduce the risk of subsequent development of PTSD after serious injury (3).
- Use of β-blocker such as propranolol after exposure might prevent PTSD by decreasing the effects of catecholamines on the amygdala (4).
- Compulsory psychological debriefing immediately after a trauma (critical incident stress management) does not prevent PTSD and may be harmful (5).

PATHOPHYSIOLOGY
- During trauma, locus coeruleus mediates sympathetic outflows to amygdala (rapid effect) and adrenal medulla (sustained effect). Adrenal medulla then release catecholamines, which stimulate peripheral afferent vagal beta-receptors. Vagal afferents innervate the nucleus tractus solitarius (NTS) in brainstem medulla. NTS fibers innervate amygdala with norepinephrine (NE).
- With increase in NE, amygdala mediates coupling of emotional valence to declarative memories via long-term potentiation, forming deeply engraved trauma memories and leading to intrusive memories and emotions, potentially leading to PTSD .
- Orbitoprefrontal cortex (which usually exerts an inhibiting effect on this activation) appears less capable of inhibiting this activation, due to stress-induced atrophy of specific nuclei in this region.

COMMONLY ASSOCIATED CONDITIONS
- Major depressive disorder
- Substance abuse
- Panic disorder
- Obsessive compulsive disorder
- Agoraphobia and/or social phobia
- Traumatic brain injury

DIAGNOSIS

HISTORY
Diagnosis is based on criteria from the *Diagnostic and Statistical Manual of Mental Disorders, Fourth Edition, Text Revision*.
- Criterion A: Has two components, as follows:
  – Experiencing, witnessing, or being confronted with an event involving serious injury, death, or a threat to a person's physical integrity
  – A response involving helplessness, intense fear, or horror
- Criterion B: Persistent reexperiencing of the event, "*flashbacks*, nightmares, illusions, hallucinations"
- Criterion C: Avoidance of stimuli associated with the trauma (3 or more of the following):
  – Avoidance of thoughts, feelings, or conversations associated with the event
  – Avoidance of people, places, or activities that may trigger recollections of the event
  – Inability to recall important aspects of the event
  – Significantly diminished interest or participation in important activities
  – Feeling of detachment
  – Narrowed range of affect
  – Sense of having a foreshortened future
- Criterion D: Hyperarousal (2 or more of the following):
  – Difficulty sleeping or falling asleep
  – Decreased concentration
  – Hypervigilance
  – Outbursts of anger or irritable mood
  – Exaggerated startle response
  – Intense anxiety or hyperalertness to events that resemble the traumatic event (e.g., anniversaries of the trauma)
- Criterion E: The duration of the relevant criteria symptoms should be >1 month.
- Criterion F: Clinically significant distress or impairment in functioning

Pediatric Considerations
- For children, reactions can include a fear of being separated from a parent, crying, whimpering, screaming, immobility and/or aimless motion, trembling, frightened facial expressions, excessive clinging, and regressive behavior.
- Older children may show extreme withdrawal, disruptive behavior, and/or an inability to pay attention. Regressive behaviors, nightmares, sleep problems, irrational fears, irritability, refusal to attend school, outbursts of anger, and fighting are also common. Somatic complaints with no medical basis, in addition to schoolwork often suffering. Furthermore, depression, anxiety, feelings of guilt, and emotional numbing are often present.

PHYSICAL EXAM
- Patients may present with physical injuries from the traumatic event.
- Mental status examination:
  – Thoughts and perception may be affected, e.g., hallucinations, delusions, suicidal ideation, phobias
  – General appearance may be affected: Disheveled, poor personal hygiene.
  – Behavior: Agitation; startle reaction may be extreme.
  – Psychological numbness
  – Orientation might be affected.
  – Memory is usually affected: Forgetfulness, especially concerning the details of the traumatic event.
  – Poor concentration
  – Poor impulse control
  – Altered speech rate and flow.
  – Mood and affect may be changed: Depression, anxiety, guilt, and/or fear.

DIAGNOSTIC TESTS & INTERPRETATION
Lab
- Decreased urine cortisol (6)
- Increased catecholamines secretion (6)
- Increased norepinephrine/cortisol ratio (6)

Imaging
MRI studies of the brain suggest that the amount of hippocampal atrophy correlates with the intensity of PTSD symptoms.

Diagnostic Procedures/Surgery
Strong response to dexamethasone suppression test (7)

DIFFERENTIAL DIAGNOSIS
- Acute stress disorder (symptoms <4 weeks)
- Generalized anxiety disorder
- Adjustment disorder
- Obsessive compulsive disorder
- Schizophrenia
- Malingering
- Mood disorders: Depression
- Mood disorder with psychotic features
- Psychotic disorders caused by a general medical condition
- Substance abuse

TREATMENT

- Treatment is often best accomplished with a combination of pharmacologic and nonpharmacologic therapies.
- The sooner therapy is initiated after the trauma, the better the prognosis.

MEDICATION

First Line
SSRIs: for depression, panic attacks, sleep disruption, and startle responses (8,9,10)
- Sertraline: 50–200 mg PO qd (FDA approved)
- Paroxetine: Starting dose: 20 mg PO qd; may be increased in 10–mg increments at intervals ≥1 week (FDA Approved)
- Fluoxetine: 20 mg PO qd/b.i.d.; not to exceed 80 mg/d (demonstrates some efficacy for all 3 symptom clusters) (8)

Second Line
- Other antidepressants:
  – Venlafaxine and nefazodone have a place in the management of chronic PTSD (11,12).
- β-blockers:
  – Propranolol: 40–80 mg PO qd; may increase up to 120–160 mg qd (controlling symptoms of hyperarousal and may lessen the peripheral symptoms of anxiety, e.g., tremors, palpitations)
- Monoamine oxidase inhibitors:
  – Phenelzine: 15 mg PO t.i.d., reducing intrusion symptoms (reexperiencing)
- Benzodiazepines:
  – Clonazepam: 1–4 mg PO qd for a limited time can provide relief from anxiety symptoms.
- α-Adrenergic agonists
  – Prazosin: 10–15 mg PO is given sometimes for nightmares (13).

ADDITIONAL TREATMENT
- Psychotherapeutic interventions:
  – Behavioral and cognitive behavioral therapy
    ○ Early cognitive behavioral therapy (CBT) has been shown to speed recovery (14).
    ○ CBT is currently considered the standard of care for PTSD by the US Department of Defense.
  – Exposure therapy: Reexperience distressing trauma-related memories and reminders in order to facilitate habituation and successful emotional processing of the trauma memory.
  – Stress-reduction techniques
    ○ Immediate symptom reduction (e.g., rebreathing in a bag for hyperventilation)
    ○ Early recognition and removal from a stress source
    ○ Relaxation and exercise techniques are also helpful in reducing the reaction to stressful events.
- Interpersonal psychotherapy:
  – Supportive psychotherapy with an emphasis on the here and now
  – Psychological debriefing in a single session
- Social:
  – Establish the framework of the problem. Clarifying the problem allows the patient to begin viewing it within the proper context (e.g., change of job or relocation of adult-dependent offspring)

COMPLEMENTARY AND ALTERNATIVE MEDICINE
In a recent study of service members with PTSD caused by the traumatic events of September 11, 2001, or Operation Iraqi Freedom, self-managed, Internet-based cognitive behavior therapy led to a greater reduction in PTSD symptoms than Internet-based supportive counseling.

SURGERY/OTHER PROCEDURES
Eye movement desensitization and reprocessing is an effective treatment for PTSD (15).

IN-PATIENT CONSIDERATIONS
Inpatient care is necessary only if the patient becomes suicidal or homicidal or because of the presence of complicating comorbid conditions that may require inpatient treatment (e.g., depression, substance abuse).

ONGOING CARE

PATIENT EDUCATION
National Center for PTSD: www.ptsd.va.gov

PROGNOSIS
- Varies significantly from patient to patient
- In approximately half of cases, the symptoms spontaneously remit after 3 months; however, in other cases symptoms may persist, often for many years, and cause long-term impairment in life functioning.
- Factors associated with a good prognosis include:
  – Rapid engagement of treatment
  – Early and ongoing social support
  – Avoidance of retraumatization
  – Positive premorbid function
  – Absence of other psychiatric disorders or substance abuse

COMPLICATIONS
- Individuals with PTSD may be at increased risk for panic disorder, agoraphobia, obsessive-compulsive disorder, social phobia, specific phobia, major depressive disorder, somatization disorder; and increased risk of impulsive behavior, suicide, and homicide. Victims of sexual assault are at especially high risk for developing mental health problems and committing suicide.
- Long-term use of benzodiazepines can lead to psychological dependence.
- Avoidance of stimuli associated with the trauma can generalize to wide-ranging avoidance. This leads to a far greater negative impact on the patient's life.

REFERENCES

1. Johnson H, Thompson A et al. The development and maintenance of post-traumatic stress disorder (PTSD) in civilian adult survivors of war trauma and torture: a review. *Clin Psychol Rev.* 2008;28: 36–47.
2. Segman RH, Cooper-Kazaz R, Macciardi F, et al. Association between the dopamine transporter gene and posttraumatic stress disorder. *Mol Psychiatry.* 2002;7:903–7.
3. Holbrook TL, Galarneau MR, Dye JL, et al. Morphine use after combat injury in Iraq and post-traumatic stress disorder. *N Engl J Med.* 2010;362:110–7.
4. Pitman RK, Sanders KM, Zusman RM, et al. Pilot study of secondary prevention of posttraumatic stress disorder with propranolol. *Biol Psychiatry.* 2002;51:189–92.
5. Rose S, Bisson J, Churchill R, et al. Psychological debriefing for preventing post traumatic stress disorder (PTSD). *Cochrane Database Syst Rev.* 2002;CD000560.
6. Mason JW, Giller EL, Kosten TR, et al. Elevation of urinary norepinephrine/cortisol ratio in posttraumatic stress disorder. *J Nerv Ment Dis.* 1988;176:498–502.
7. Yehuda R, Halligan SL, Golier JA, et al. Effects of trauma exposure on the cortisol response to dexamethasone administration in PTSD and major depressive disorder. *Psychoneuroendocrinology.* 2004;29:389–404.
8. Connor KM, Sutherland SM, Tupler LA, et al. Fluoxetine in post-traumatic stress disorder. Randomised, double-blind study. *Br J Psychiatry.* 1999;175:17–22.
9. Marshall RD, Pierce D et al. Implications of recent findings in posttraumatic stress disorder and the role of pharmacotherapy. *Harv Rev Psychiatry.* 2000;7:247–56.
10. Stein DJ, Ipser JC, Seedat S et al. Pharmacotherapy for post traumatic stress disorder (PTSD). *Cochrane Database Syst Rev.* 2006;CD002795.
11. Pae CU, Lim HK, Ajwani N, et al. Extended-release formulation of venlafaxine in the treatment of post-traumatic stress disorder. *Expert Rev Neurother.* 2007;7:603–15.
12. Davis LL, Jewell ME, Ambrose S, et al. A placebo-controlled study of nefazodone for the treatment of chronic posttraumatic stress disorder: a preliminary study. *J Clin Psychopharmacol.* 2004;24:291–7.
13. Raskind MA, Peskind ER, Hoff DJ, et al. A parallel group placebo controlled study of prazosin for trauma nightmares and sleep disturbance in combat veterans with post-traumatic stress disorder. *Biol Psychiatry.* 2007;61:928–34.
14. Kornør H, Winje D, Ekeberg Ø, et al. Early trauma-focused cognitive-behavioural therapy to prevent chronic post-traumatic stress disorder and related symptoms: a systematic review and meta-analysis. *BMC Psychiatry.* 2008;8:81.
15. van der Kolk BA, Spinazzola J, Blaustein ME, et al. A randomized clinical trial of eye movement desensitization and reprocessing (EMDR), fluoxetine, and pill placebo in the treatment of posttraumatic stress disorder: treatment effects and long-term maintenance. *J Clin Psychiatry.* 2007;68:37–46.

CODES

ICD9
309.81 Posttraumatic stress disorder

PRE-ECLAMPSIA AND ECLAMPSIA (TOXEMIA OF PREGNANCY)

Konstantinos E. Deligiannidis, MD, MPH
Stacy E. Potts, MD

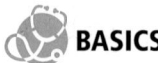 BASICS

DESCRIPTION

Pre-eclampsia is a disorder of pregnancy developing at the 20th week (or beyond), with hypertension, proteinuria, and/or edema with poor perfusion of vital organs.

- May progress from mild to life-threatening in hours to days
- The disease may include rapid weight gain and face and hand edema. The disorder is reversible by ending the pregnancy if at term or, if maternal or fetal health are in danger, by preterm delivery.
- *Eclampsia* is defined as seizure activity or coma in a patient with pre-eclampsia without underlying neurologic disease.
- Most postpartum cases occur within 48 hours of delivery but can occur up to 4 weeks postpartum.
- System(s) affected: Cardiovascular; Renal; Reproductive; Feto-Placental; CNS; Hepatic
- Synonym(s): Toxemia of pregnancy

EPIDEMIOLOGY

Incidence
- Predominant age:
  - Most cases occur in younger women because of the higher incidence of pre-eclampsia in younger (nulliparous) women.
  - However, older (>40 years) pre-eclamptic patients have 4 times the incidence of seizures compared with patients in their 20s.
- Pregnancy-induced hypertension: 6% of pregnancies
- Pre-eclampsia: 5–7%
- Eclampsia develops in 1/2,000 deliveries in developed countries. In developing countries, estimates range from 1/100 to 1/1,700.
- 40% of eclamptic seizures occur before delivery; 16% occur more than 48 hours after delivery

RISK FACTORS
- Nulliparity: 3:1 (relative risk [RR])
- Age >40 years: 2:1 (RR)
- High body mass index: 2:1 (RR)
- Antiphospholipid syndrome: 10:1 (RR)
- Diabetes: 3.5:1 (RR)
- Twin pregnancy: 3:1 (RR)
- Preeclampsia in a previous pregnancy
- Family history of pre-eclampsia: 3:1 (RR)
- Father of fetus previously fathered a preeclamptic pregnancy in another woman

Genetics
Increased incidence in pregnant females whose mothers or sisters had the disease

GENERAL PREVENTION
- Adequate prenatal care, women who do not receive prenatal care are seven times more likely to die from complications
- Good control of preexisting hypertension
- Recent systematic reviews and meta-analyses show that low-dose aspirin lowers the risk for developing pre-eclampsia in moderate- to high-risk patients, lowers the rate of preterm delivery and neonatal death, and has no significant effect on the rate of placental abruption or neonatal bleeding complications (1)[A].

- Calcium supplementation has been shown to reduce the risk of pre-eclampsia by 30%. The risk reduction appears to be greatest in women with high risk of pre-eclampsia (RR = 0.22) (2)[A].
- Some evidence suggests vitamin C (1,000 mg/d) and vitamin E (400 units/d) reduce the risk for pre-eclampsia (3)[B], although some guidelines recommend against their use (4).

PATHOPHYSIOLOGY
Systemic derangements in eclampsia include:
- Cardiovascular: Generalized vasospasm
- Hematologic: Decreased plasma volume, increased blood viscosity, hemoconcentration, coagulopathy
- Renal: Decreased glomerular filtration rate
- Hepatic: Periportal necrosis, hepatocellular damage, subcapsular hematoma
- CNS: Cerebral vasospasm and ischemia, cerebral edema, cerebral hemorrhage

COMMONLY ASSOCIATED CONDITIONS
- Abruptio placenta
- Placental insufficiency
- Fetal growth restriction
- Preterm delivery
- Fetal demise
- Maternal seizures (= eclampsia)
- Maternal pulmonary edema
- Maternal liver or kidney failure
- Maternal death

 DIAGNOSIS

Diagnosis is dependent on new onset of elevated blood pressure and proteinuria after 20 weeks of gestation.

HISTORY
May be asymptomatic. In some cases, rapid excessive weight gain (>5 lb/wk; >2.3 kg/wk); in more severe cases are associated with epigastric pain, headache, altered mental status, and visual disturbance.

PHYSICAL EXAM
- Pre-eclampsia:
  - Mild: Elevated BP ≥140 mm Hg systolic or 90 mm Hg diastolic on 2 BP readings 6 h apart; proteinuria (>300 mg/24 h or >1 g/L)
  - Severe: Elevated BP ≥160 systolic mmHg or 110 mm Hg diastolic on 2 BP readings 6 hours apart
    ○ Proteinuria (>5 g/24 h)
    ○ Facial or hand edema
    ○ Hyperreflexia
    ○ Retinal arteriolar spasm, papilledema
    ○ Epigastric/right upper quadrant (RUQ) pain
    ○ Oliguria or anuria
- Eclampsia:
  - Headache, visual disturbance, and epigastric or RUQ pain often precede seizure.
  - Tonic–clonic seizure activity (focal or generalized)
  - Seizures may occur once or repeatedly.
  - Postictal coma, cyanosis (variable)
  - Temperatures >39°C, consistent with CNS hemorrhage
  - Normal BP, even in response to treatment, does not rule out potential for seizures. Up to 30% may not have edema; 20% may not have proteinuria.

DIAGNOSTIC TESTS & INTERPRETATION
Lab
Initial lab tests
- Routine spot urine testing for protein should be done at each prenatal visit
- Complete blood count including platelets
- Creatinine
- Serum transaminase levels
- Uric acid
- Coagulation profiles: Abnormalities suggest severe disease.
- 24-h urine for protein/creatinine clearance: <90 mL/min/1.73 m^2 is abnormal.

Follow-Up & Special Considerations
DIC, thrombocytopenia, liver dysfunction, and renal failure can complicate pre-eclampsia associated with HELLP syndrome.

Imaging
- Daily fetal movement monitoring by mother ("kick counts")
- Nonstress test at diagnosis and then weekly until delivery
- Ultrasound is used to monitor growth and cord blood flow. Perform as indicated based on clinical stability and laboratory findings.
- Ultrasound imaging for biophysical profile, estimation of fetal age, growth progress, amniotic fluid volume.
  - Weekly for mild pre-eclampsia
  - Twice weekly in severe pre-eclampsia
- With seizures, CT scan and MRI should be considered if focal findings persist or uncharacteristic signs/symptoms are present.

Pathological Findings
CNS: Cerebral edema, hyperemia, focal anemia, thrombosis, and hemorrhage; cerebral lesions account for 40% of eclamptic deaths.

DIFFERENTIAL DIAGNOSIS
- Chronic hypertension: HTN pre-pregnancy; high BP (HTN) before the 20th week; diagnosis during pregnancy but persisting beyond day 84 postpartum
- Gestational HTN: Increased BP first discovered during pregnancy, with no proteinuria; normal BP by 12 weeks postpartum
- Seizures in pregnancy: Epilepsy, cerebral tumors, meningitis/encephalitis, ruptured cerebral aneurysm. Until other causes are proven, however, all pregnant women with convulsions should be considered to have eclampsia.

 TREATMENT

- Mild:
  - Outpatient care
  - Maternal: Daily home BP monitoring; daily weights; weekly labs (24-h protein, platelet count, creatinine, liver function tests [LFTs])
  - Fetal:
    ○ Patient-measured: Daily "kick counts"
    ○ Medical provider-measured: Nonstress test (see Imaging section)

- Severe:
  - Inpatient care if patient condition deteriorates (BP ≥160/110 mm Hg; severe headache; visual changes [scotoma or "flashing lights"]; impaired mentation; pulmonary edema; epigastric/RUQ pain; increasing LFTs; oliguria; thrombocytopenia) or if fetal status is deemed "nonreassuring"
  - Maternal: Daily labs, adding coagulation tests; IV magnesium sulfate as anticonvulsive prophylaxis. IV labetalol and oral nifedipine antihypertensive therapy titrated to keep systolic BP <155 mm Hg and diastolic BP <105 mm Hg. Keep diastolic BP >90 mm Hg to avoid hypoperfusing the uterus.
  - Fetal: Continuous heart monitoring; daily ultrasound, with BP, amniotic fluid levels, fetal growth assessment as deemed necessary

ADDITIONAL TREATMENT
General Measures
- Management by gestational age of severe pre-eclampsia:
  - <23 weeks: Offer to terminate pregnancy.
  - At 23–32 weeks: Antihypertensives; evaluate maternal–fetal condition; steroids to enhance fetal lung maturity; plan delivery at 34 weeks with magnesium sulfate prophylaxis or for worsening maternal or fetal jeopardy.
  - At 33–34 weeks: Steroids, magnesium sulfate, and delivery
  - At >34 weeks: Magnesium sulfate and delivery

ALERT
- Regardless of gestational age, emergent delivery is recommended if there are signs of maternal hypertensive crisis, abruptio placentae, uterine rupture, or fetal distress (5)[B].
- Seizures:
  - Control of convulsions, correction of hypoxia and acidosis, lowering of BP, steps to effect delivery as soon as convulsions are controlled
  - See section Medication (Drugs)

MEDICATION
First Line
- For seizure prophylaxis: Magnesium sulfate (MgSO4): Loading dose 4 g IV in 200 mL normal saline over 20–30 minutes; maintenance dose 1–2 g/h IV
- For HTN:
  - Nifedipine (oral): 40–120 mg/d plus
  - Labetalol (IV): 600–2,400 mg/d, both titrated to keep BP <155/105 mm Hg; antihypertensives are inadvisable for mild hypertension/pre-eclampsia.
- For eclampsia/seizures:
  - In recent randomized trials, MgSO4 was found to be superior to phenytoin in the treatment and prevention of eclampsia and probably more effective and safer than diazepam.
  - Magnesium sulfate for seizures:
    ○ 2–4 g IV repeated every 15 minutes to a maximum of 6 g to achieve resolution of an ongoing convulsion
    ○ Magnesium then is continued at 1–3 g/h, with the amount given based on the neurologic examination and patellar reflexes.
  - Levels of 6–8 mEq/mL are considered therapeutic, but clinical status is most important and must ensure that
    ○ Patellar reflexes are present.
    ○ Respirations are not depressed.
    ○ Urine output is ≥25 mL/h.
  - May be given safely, even in the presence of renal insufficiency

- Fluid therapy:
  - Ringer's lactated solution with 5% dextrose at 60–120 mL/h, with careful attention to fluid–volume status
- Hypertension, if present and severe (e.g., >160/110 mm Hg), also should be treated.
  - Hydralazine: 5 mg IV then 5- to 10-mg boluses as needed every 20 minutes or
  - Labetalol: 10–20 mg IV then double dose at 10-minute intervals up to 80 mg; maximum total cumulative dose of 220–230 mg (e.g., 20-40-80-80 or 10-20-40-80-80)
- Precautions: Do not use diuretics. Carefully monitor neurologic status, urine output, respirations, and fetal status.
- Calcium carbonate (1 g administered slowly IV) may reverse magnesium-induced respiratory depression.

Second Line
- Diazepam 2 mg/min until resolution or 20 mg given or
- Lorazepam 1–2 mg/min up to total of 10 mg or
- Phenytoin 18–20 mg/kg at a rate of 20–40 mg/min or
- Phenobarbital 100 mg/min to a total of 20 mg/kg given

ONGOING CARE

FOLLOW-UP RECOMMENDATIONS
Mild: Restricted activity. Severe: Restricted activity, in hospital

DIET
Salt restriction is inadvisable because the patient is often experiencing intravascular hypovolemia. Calcium supplementation is recommended for women who have low calcium intake (<600 mg/d) (4).

PATIENT EDUCATION
Additional materials from American College of Obstetricians and Gynecologists, 409 12th St. SW, Washington, DC 20024-2188; (800) 762-ACOG; www.acog.org

PROGNOSIS
- For nulliparous women with preeclampsia before 30 weeks of gestation, the recurrence rate for the disorder may be as high as 40% in future pregnancies (6).
- Multiparous women have higher rates of recurrence.
- 25% of eclamptic women will have hypertension in subsequent pregnancies, but only 5% of these will be severe and only 2% will be eclamptic again.
- Eclamptic, multiparous women may be at higher risk for subsequent essential hypertension; they also have higher mortality in subsequent pregnancies than do primiparous women.

COMPLICATIONS
- Most women do not have long-term sequelae from eclampsia, although many may have transient neurologic deficits.
- A history of preeclampsia is equivalent to traditional risk factors for cardiovascular disease. Women with a history of preeclampsia should be strongly advised to avoid obesity and smoking. Other signs of metabolic syndrome should be closely monitored as well (7).
- Maternal and/or fetal death

REFERENCES
1. Gauer R, Atlas M, Hill J. Clinical inquiries. Does low-dose aspirin reduce preeclampsia and other maternal-fetal complications? *J Fam Pract*. 2008;57:54–6.
2. Hofmeyr G, Duley L, Atallah A. Dietary calcium supplementation for prevention of pre-eclampsia and related problems: a systematic review and commentary. *BJOG*. 2007.
3. Rumbold A, et al. Antioxidants for preventing pre-eclampsia. *Cochrane Database Syst Rev*. 2006;(Issue 1).
4. Magee LA, Helewa M, Moutquin J-M et al. Diagnosis, Evaluation, and Management of the Hypertensive Disorders of Pregnancy. *JOGC*. 2008;30:3(S1–S48).
5. Sibai BM. Diagnosis and management of gestational hypertension and preeclampsia. *Obstet Gynecol*. 2003;102:181–92.
6. Report of the National High Blood Pressure Education Program Working Group on High Blood Pressure in Pregnancy. *Am J Obste Gynecol* 2000;183:S1–22.
7. Carty D, Delles C, Dominiczak A. Preeclampsia and future maternal health. *Journal of Hypertension*. 2010;28.

ADDITIONAL READING
Churchill D, Duley L. Interventionist versus expectant care for severe pre-eclampsia before term. *Cochrane Database Syst Rev*. 2006;Issue 1.

CODES

ICD9
- 642.43 Mild or unspecified pre-eclampsia, antepartum
- 642.53 Severe pre-eclampsia, antepartum
- 642.63 Eclampsia, antepartum

CLINICAL PEARLS
- Prescribe 81 mg aspirin each day to 2 groups of pregnant women: those who had severe pre-eclampsia in a prior pregnancy and those who develop signs of pre-eclampsia or strong risk factors for it before the 3rd trimester in their current pregnancy.
- Management of pre-eclampsia depends on both the severity of the condition and the gestational age of the fetus.
- The disorder is reversible by ending the pregnancy if at term or, if maternal or fetal health are in danger, by preterm delivery.

PREMENSTRUAL SYNDROME (PMS) AND PREMENSTRUAL DYSPHORIC DISORDER (PMDD)

Courtney I. Jarvis, PharmD
Jeremy Golding, MD

BASICS

DESCRIPTION
Premenstrual syndrome (PMS) is defined as a symptom complex of physical and emotional symptoms severe enough to interfere with everyday life and occurring cyclically during the luteal phase of menses.
- Premenstrual dysphoric disorder (PMDD) is a severe form of PMS characterized by severe recurrent depressive and anxiety symptoms with premenstrual (luteal phase) onset that remit a few days after the start of menses.
- The American Psychiatric Association's *DSM-IV* revised diagnosis is premenstrual dysphoric disorder when the dominant symptoms are emotional and severe enough to disrupt social and occupational functioning.
- System(s) affected: Endocrine/Metabolic; Nervous; Reproductive

EPIDEMIOLOGY
Prevalence
- Almost all women have some physical and psychic symptoms before menses (this is not premenstrual syndrome).
- Approximately 30% of menstruating women suffer from PMS.
- Approximately 5% of menstruating women have PMDD.

RISK FACTORS
- Age: Usually present in late 20s–mid-30s
- History of mood disorder (major depression, bipolar disorder), anxiety disorder, personality disorder, or substance abuse
- Family history
- Low parity
- Tobacco use
- Psychosocial stressors
- High body mass index (BMI)

Genetics
- Role of genetic predisposition is controversial; however, twin studies do suggest a genetic component.
- Involvement of gene coding for the serotonergic 5HT1A receptor and allelic variants of the estrogen receptor alpha gene (*ESR1*) is suggested.

PATHOPHYSIOLOGY
- Results from interaction of cyclic changes in ovarian steroids (estrogen, progesterone, allopregnanolone) with central neurotransmitters (serotonin, γ-endorphin, γ-aminobutyric acid [GABA]) and the autonomic nervous system
- Circadian rhythm alterations affecting secretion of melatonin, cortisol, thyroid-stimulating hormone (TSH), and prolactin reported
- Inconclusive evidence regarding low levels of vitamin D, magnesium, and calcium in women with PMDD

DIAGNOSIS

HISTORY
- Determine regularity of the menstrual cycle using prospective patient record of symptoms for 2 months, the Daily Record of Severity of Problems (available online at http://www.pmdd.factsforhealth.org/drsp/drsp_month.pdf), or similar inventory.
- *DSM-IV* criteria:
  - Symptoms occur 1 week before menses and resolve in the 1st few days after menses begin (over most menstrual cycles during the past year).
  - ≥ 5 of the following (1 must be among the 1st 4):
    ○ Markedly depressed mood with feelings of hopelessness
    ○ Marked anxiety or tension
    ○ Marked affective lability
    ○ Irritability and anger
    ○ Decreased interest in usual activities and social withdrawal
    ○ Lack of energy
    ○ Appetite change
    ○ Change in sleeping pattern
    ○ Feeling out of control or overwhelmed
    ○ Difficulty concentrating
    ○ Somatic symptoms such as abdominal bloating, breast tenderness, headaches, and joint pain
  - For PMDD, emotional symptoms must be severe enough to interfere with work, school, or usual activities.
  - Symptoms may be superimposed on an underlying psychiatric disorder but may not be an exacerbation of another condition.
  - Criteria must be confirmed by prospective daily charting for a minimum of 2 consecutive symptomatic menstrual cycles.

PHYSICAL EXAM
- Physiologic symptoms:
  - Food cravings
  - Weight gain
  - Fatigue
  - Headache
  - Sleep disturbance
  - Tension/muscle aches
  - Mastalgia/breast swelling
  - Abdominal bloating/pain
  - Edema
- Emotional symptoms:
  - Anger
  - Irritability/mood lability
  - Internal tension
  - Depressed mood
  - Anxiety
  - Insomnia

DIAGNOSTIC TESTS & INTERPRETATION
Lab
- The repetitive nature of symptoms precludes need for labs if a classic history is present.
- Hemoglobin may be helpful to rule out anemia.

- 25-OH vitamin D level to exclude deficiency, although precise relationship of deficiency with the disorder is unclear.
- Serum TSH to rule out hypothyroidism

Imaging
Imaging to diagnose causes of pelvic pain and dysmenorrhea may be appropriate.

DIFFERENTIAL DIAGNOSIS
- Premenstrual exacerbation of underlying psychiatric disorder
- Psychiatric disorders (especially bipolar disorder, major depression, anxiety)
- Thyroid disorders
- Perimenopause
- Premenstrual migraine
- Chronic fatigue syndrome
- Irritable bowel syndrome (painful symptoms)
- Seizures
- Anemia
- Endometriosis (painful symptoms)
- Drug or alcohol abuse

TREATMENT

- Selective serotonin reuptake inhibitors (SSRIs) (fluoxetine and sertraline most studied) are highly effective in the treatment of physical and behavioral symptoms of PMDD (odds ratio [OR] 0.40, 95% confidence interval [CI] 0.31–0.51) (1,2,3,4)[A].
  - Intermittent luteal phase dosing (OR 0.55, 95% CI 0.45–0.68) is less effective than full-cycle dosing (OR 0.28, 95% CI 0.18–0.42) but has fewer adverse effects (4)[A].
  - Higher doses are not correlated with increased response (1,4)[A].
  - Other nonselective serotonergic agents (e.g., venlafaxine, clomipramine) also may be effective (3)[C].
- Alternative therapies should be considered if no response to SSRIs: Alprazolam, buspirone, gonadotropin-releasing hormone (GnRH) agonists, danazol, bromocriptine, spironolactone, oral contraceptives, meclofenamate, progesterone (2,3)[C]
- Oral contraceptive pills (OCPs) may improve physical symptoms but not mood (2,3)[C].
  - OCPs can cause adverse effects similar to PMDD symptoms; monophasic preparations should be used continuously (daily without interruption) for PMDD (3)[C].
  - OCPs containing the progestin drospirenone (structurally similar to spironolactone) may improve physical symptoms and mood changes associated with PMDD (2,5)[A].
- Vitamin D supplementation, 2,000 IU/d, with no risk of toxicity (3)[C]
- Calcium carbonate 600 mg b.i.d. effectively reduces physical and emotional premenstrual symptoms (6,7)[B].
- Vitamin B_6 may reduce the severity of premenstrual symptoms (6)[B].

- Chasteberry (*Vitex agnus-castus*) may reduce physical premenstrual symptoms (6)[C].
- Cognitive-behavioral therapy (CBT) is as effective as drug therapy, but there is no additional benefit of combining CBT and drug therapy (2)[B].

MEDICATION
First Line
- Fluoxetine (Prozac, Sarafem) 20 mg/day every day, or 20 mg/day only during luteal phase, or 90 mg once a week × 2 weeks in luteal phase
- Sertraline (Zoloft) 50–150 mg/day every day or 50–150 mg/day only during luteal phase
- Citalopram (Celexa) 10–30 mg/day every day or 10–30 mg/day only during luteal phase
- Adverse effects:
  - GI upset
  - Jitteriness
  - Headache
  - Sexual dysfunction
  - Insomnia
  - Fatigue
- Contraindications: Patients taking monoamine oxidase inhibitors (MAOIs)
- Precautions:
  - Increased risk of suicidal thinking and behavior in children and adolescents with depressive disorders; uncertain if this risk applies to those taking SSRIs for PMDD
  - Bipolar disorder
  - Seizure disorder
  - Hepatic dysfunction
  - Renal dysfunction
- Possible interactions:
  - MAOIs (e.g., phenelzine, isocarbazine, tranylcypromine, linezolid)
  - Selegiline
  - Pimozide
  - Thioridazine

Second Line
- Spironolactone (Aldactone) 50–100 mg/day × 7–10 days during luteal phase; helpful for fluid retention; adverse reactions: lethargy, headache, irregular menses, hyperkalemia
- Oral contraceptives: Ethinyl estradiol/drospirenone (Yasmin/Yaz): 1 tablet/day; although unstudied, other OCPs also may be effective.
- Alprazolam (Xanax) 0.25 mg t.i.d.–q.i.d. only during luteal phase; taper at onset of menses (other benzodiazepines not studied for PMDD). Caution: Addictive potential
- GnRH agonists:
  - Leuprolide (Lupron) depot 3.75 mg/month IM
  - Precautions: Menopause-like side effects (e.g., osteoporosis, hot flashes, headaches, muscle aches, vaginal dryness, irritability) limit treatment to 6 months; if extended treatment is needed, supplement with estrogen and progesterone "add-back" therapy, minimizing frequency and dose of progestational agent.
- Danazol (Danocrine), 300–400 mg b.i.d.; adverse reactions: androgenic and antiestrogenic effects (e.g., amenorrhea, weight gain, acne, fluid retention, hirsutism, hot flashes, vaginal dryness, emotional lability)

ADDITIONAL TREATMENT
Issues for Referral
Referral to psychiatrist may be indicated for mood or anxiety disorder if patient has no symptom-free period.

COMPLEMENTARY AND ALTERNATIVE MEDICINE
- Some data support the use of the following:
  - Calcium: 600 mg b.i.d.
  - Vitamin D: 2,000 IU/day
  - Vitamin B6: 100 mg/day (usually 50 mg b.i.d.)
  - Magnesium: 200–400 mg/day
  - Vitamin E: 400 IU/day
  - Manganese: 1.8 mg/day
  - Chasteberry (*Vitex agnus-castus*): 4 mg/day of extract
  - St. John's wort: 900 mg/day (0.18% hypericin, 23.38% hyperforin)
- Evidence supporting efficacy and/or safety of herbal products is lacking; the following products/interventions have *not* been found useful for PMS/PMDD, although not all studies are of high quality and able to completely eliminate possibility of benefit:
  - Evening primrose oil
  - Black current oil
  - Black cohosh
  - Wild yam root
  - Dong quai
  - Kava kava
  - Light-based therapy
  - Acupuncture

SURGERY/OTHER PROCEDURES
Bilateral oophorectomy, usually with concomitant hysterectomy, is option for rare, refractory cases with severe, disabling symptoms.

 ## ONGOING CARE

FOLLOW-UP RECOMMENDATIONS
Aerobic exercise is helpful in decreasing premenstrual symptoms (8)[C].

Patient Monitoring
Increased risk of suicidal thinking and behavior in children and adolescents with depressive disorders; uncertain if this risk applies to those taking SSRIs for PMDD

DIET
- Reduce consumption of salt, sugar, caffeine, dairy products, and alcohol (anecdotal reports).
- Eat small, frequent portions of food high in complex carbohydrates (limited data).

PATIENT EDUCATION
- Counsel patients to eat a balanced diet rich in calcium and omega-3 fatty acids and low in saturated fat and caffeine.
- Advise aerobic exercise.
- Counsel women that they are not "crazy." PMDD is a real disorder with a physiologic basis.
- Although incompletely understood, successful treatment is usually possible.

PROGNOSIS
- Many patients can have their symptoms adequately controlled. PMS disappears at menopause.
- PMS sometimes continues after hysterectomy.

REFERENCES

1. Brown J, O'Brien PM, Marjoribanks J, et al. Selective serotonin reuptake inhibitors for premenstrual syndrome. *Cochrane Database Syst Rev*. 2009:CD001396.
2. Cunningham J, Yonkers KA, O'Brien S, et al. Update on research and treatment of premenstrual dysphoric disorder. *Harv Rev Psychiatry*. 2009;17: 120–37.
3. Pearlstein T, Steiner M. Premenstrual dysphoric disorder: burden of illness and treatment update. *J Psychiatry Neurosci*. 2008;33:291–301.
4. Shah NR, Jones JB, Aperi J, et al. Selective serotonin reuptake inhibitors for premenstrual syndrome and premenstrual dysphoric disorder: a meta-analysis. *Obstet Gynecol*. 2008;111:1175–82.
5. Lopez LM, Kaptein A, Helmerhorst FM. Oral contraceptives containing drospirenone for premenstrual syndrome. *Cochrane Database Syst Rev*. 2008:CD006586.
6. Whelan AM, Jurgens TM, Naylor H et al. Herbs, vitamins and minerals in the treatment of premenstrual syndrome: a systematic review. *Can J Clin Pharmacol*. 2009;16:e407–29.
7. Thys-Jacobs S, McMahon D, Bilezikian JP. Cyclical changes in calcium metabolism across the menstrual cycle in women with premenstrual dysphoric disorder. *J Clin Endocrinol Metab*. 2007;92:2952–9.
8. The American College of Obstetricians and Gynecologists. Practice Bulletin. Management of premenstrual syndrome. *Clinical Management Guidelines No. 15*. April 2000.

ADDITIONAL READING

Freeman EW et al. Therapeutic management of premenstrual syndrome. *Expert opinion on pharmacotherapy*. 2010;

 ## CODES

ICD9
625.4 Premenstrual tension syndromes

CLINICAL PEARLS

- To determine whether the symptoms your patient describes are PMS, have the patient keep a daily log of her symptoms and menses. Symptoms beginning in the week before menses and abating before the end of menses, occurring over at least 2 months, and severe enough to interfere with daily functioning are diagnostic.
- The difference between PMS and PMDD is that PMDD is a severe form of PMS characterized by recurrent depressive and anxiety symptoms with premenstrual (luteal phase) onset, severe enough to disrupt social and occupational functioning. These symptoms remit a few days after the onset of menses.
- PMDD is not the same as more generalized depressive or anxiety disorders. PMDD-associated symptoms of depression and anxiety resolve within the first few days of menses.
- Treatment during the luteal phase only is somewhat less effective than continuous-cycle treatment with SSRIs but has fewer adverse effects.

PREOPERATIVE EVALUATION OF THE NONCARDIAC SURGICAL PATIENT

Drew Grimes, MD
Stacy Jones, MD

BASICS

DESCRIPTION
- Preoperative medical evaluation should determine the presence of established or unrecognized disease or other factors that may increase the risk of perioperative morbidity and mortality in patients undergoing surgery.
- Specific assessment goals include:
  - Conducting a thorough medical history and physical examination to assess the need for further testing and/or consultation
  - Recommending strategies to reduce risk and optimize patient condition prior to surgery
  - Encouraging patients to optimize their health for possible improvement of both perioperative and long-term outcomes
- Synonym(s): Preoperative diagnostic workup; Preoperative preparation; Preoperative general health assessment

EPIDEMIOLOGY
Overall patient morbidity and mortality related to surgery is low. Multiple studies have shown an average mortality rate of ~1% for patients undergoing a full spectrum of surgical procedures. Preoperative patient evaluation and subsequent optimization of perioperative care can reduce both postoperative morbidity and mortality.

RISK FACTORS
- Functional capacity (1)[B]: Exercise tolerance is one of the most important determinants of cardiac risk:
  - Self-reported exercise tolerance may be an extremely useful predictive tool when assessing risk. Patients unable to meet a 4 metabolic equivalent (MET) demand (defined in the Diagnosis section) during daily activities have increased perioperative cardiac and long-term risks.
  - Patients who report good exercise tolerance require minimal, if any, additional testing.
- Level of surgical risk:
  - High: Aortic, major vascular and peripheral vascular surgery
  - Intermediate: Intraperitoneal, intrathoracic, carotid endarterectomy, head/neck, orthopedic, and prostate surgery
  - Low: Endoscopic, superficial, cataract, breast, and ambulatory surgery
- Clinical risk factors (2)[B]: History of ischemic heart disease, the presence of compensated heart failure or a history of prior congestive heart failure, cerebrovascular disease, diabetes mellitus (DM), and renal insufficiency; these risk factors plus surgical risk can dictate the need for further cardiac testing.
- Age: Patients >70 years of age are at higher risk for perioperative complications and mortality and have a longer length of stay in the hospital postoperatively. (Likely attributed to increasing medical comorbidities with increasing age.) Age alone should not be a deciding factor in the decision to proceed with surgery (3).

DIAGNOSIS

HISTORY
- Evaluate pertinent medical records and interview the patient. Many institutions provide standard patient questionnaires that screen for preoperative risk factors:
  - History of present illness and treatments
  - Past medical and surgical history
  - Patient and family anesthetic history and associated complications
  - Current medications (including over-the-counter [OTC] medications, vitamins, supplements, and herbals) as well as reasons for use
  - Allergies (including specific reactions)
  - Social history: Tobacco, alcohol, drug use, and cessation
  - Family history: Prior illnesses and surgeries
- Systems (both history and current status):
  - Cardiovascular: Inquire about exercise capacity:
    - 1 MET: Can take care of self, eat, dress, and use toilet; walk around house indoors; walk a block or 2 on level ground at 2–3 mi/h
    - 4 METs: Can climb flight of stairs or walk up hill, walk on level ground at 4 mi/h, run a short distance, do heavy work around house, participate in moderate recreational activities
    - 10 METs: Can participate in strenuous sports such as swimming, singles tennis, football, basketball, or skiing
  - Note presence of CHF, cardiomyopathy, ischemic heart disease (stable vs unstable), valvular disease, HTN, arrhythmias, murmurs, pericarditis, history of pacemaker or ICD:
    - Rhythm management devices (pacemakers and AICDs) affect the perioperative course. Most importantly, *patients need to know their type of device* and *bring that information with them for the procedure*. Typically, the AICD tachyarrhythmia function is disabled during surgery and then restored postoperatively. Ideally the device is interrogated postoperatively to confirm proper function (4).
    - Stents: Patients with coronary stents are maintained on antiplatelet therapy with a thienopyridine such as clopidogrel, frequently in combination with aspirin. Premature discontinuation of antiplatelet therapy markedly increases the risk of acute stent thrombosis, the results of which can be catastrophic. Elective surgery should be delayed and antiplatelet therapy continued for 4-6 weeks after bare metal stent placement, and for at least 12 months after placement of drug-eluting stents. Even after this time period, any perioperative disruption in the patient's antiplatelet regimen should be discussed with the patient's cardiologist and surgeon. The risk of perioperative bleeding must be weighed against the risks associated with discontinuation of antiplatelet drugs prior to surgery (5)[B].
  - Pulmonary: Chronic and active disease processes should be addressed: Chronic infections, bronchitis, emphysema, asthma, wheezing, shortness of breath, cough (productive or otherwise):
    - Sleep apnea: Patients with obstructive sleep apnea (OSA) are at increased risk for perioperative adverse events. It follows that preoperative diagnosis of OSA and institution of CPAP therapy should reduce that risk. Unfortunately, at present, the evidence is not clear on this point.
    - Patients with OSA frequently are at increased risk for obesity, coronary disease, hypertension, atrial fibrillation, congestive heart failure, and pulmonary hypertension. Optimizing the management of these comorbidities may be the first important step in the preoperative management of patients with OSA. Often, patients with an existing diagnosis of OSA who use CPAP at night are asked to bring their CPAP machine to the hospital or surgery center when they are admitted for surgery (6)[C].
  - GI: Hepatic disease, gastric ulcer, inflammatory bowel disease, hernias (especially hiatal), significant weight loss, nausea, vomiting, history of postoperative nausea and vomiting:
    - Any symptoms consistent with gastroesophageal reflux disease (GERD) should be optimally treated.
  - Hematologic: Anemia, serious bleeding, clotting problems, blood transfusions, hereditary disorders
  - Renal: Kidney failure, dialysis, infections, stones, changes in bladder function
  - Endocrine: Nocturia, parathyroid, pituitary, adrenal disease, thyroid disease
    - Diabetes: There is evidence that hyperglycemia in the perioperative period is associated with postoperative infection (7)[B].
  - Neurologic/psychiatric: Seizures, stroke, paralysis, tremor, migraine headaches, nerve injury, multiple sclerosis, extremity numbness, psychiatric disorders (anxiety, depression, etc.)
  - Musculoskeletal: Arthritis, lower back pain
  - Reproductive: Possibility of pregnancy in women of child-bearing potential
- Mouth/upper airway: Dentures, crowns, partials, bridges, teeth (loose, chipped, cracked, capped)

PHYSICAL EXAM
- Assess vital signs, including arterial BP bilaterally.
- Check carotid pulses, auscultate for bruits.
- Examine lungs by auscultating all lung fields, listening for rales, rhonchi, wheezes, or other sounds indicating disease.
- Examine cardiovascular system by auscultating heart and noting any irregular rhythms or murmurs. Precordial palpation.
- Palpate abdomen.
- Examine airway and mouth for ease of intubation, neck mobility, and size of tongue, and note any lesions or dental deformities.
- If a regional anesthesia technique is being contemplated, perform a relevant, focused neurologic exam.

DIAGNOSTIC TESTS & INTERPRETATION
Lab

Initial lab tests
- Laboratory testing should not be obtained routinely prior to surgery unless indicated (2)[C]. Specific tests should be requested if the evaluator suspects findings from the clinical evaluation that may influence perioperative patient management.

- Labs performed within the past 4 months prior to evaluation are reliable unless the patient has had an interim change in clinical presentation or is taking medications that require monitoring of plasma level or effect.
- Complete blood count (CBC) (2)[C]:
  - Hemoglobin: If patient has symptoms of anemia or is undergoing a procedure with major blood loss; extremes of age; liver or kidney disease
  - White blood cell (WBC) count: If symptoms suggest infection or myeloproliferative disorder or the patient is at risk for chemotherapy-induced leukopenia
  - Platelet count: If history of bleeding, myeloproliferative disorder, liver or renal disease, or the patient is at risk for chemotherapy-induced thrombocytopenia
- Serum chemistries (electrolytes, glucose, renal and liver function tests) (2)[C]: Should be obtained for extremes of age; in known renal insufficiency, CHF, liver dysfunction, or endocrine abnormalities, or the patient is on medications that alter electrolyte levels, such as diuretics
- Prothrombin time (PT)/partial thromboplastin time (PTT) (2)[C]: If history of a bleeding disorder, chronic liver disease, or malnutrition, or those with recent or chronic antibiotic or anticoagulant use
- Urinalysis (2)[C]: Routine urinalysis is not recommended preoperatively.
- Pregnancy test: Controversial; should be *considered* for all female patients of child-bearing age

Imaging
Initial approach
CXR is not generally indicated (2)[C]. It can be considered in patients with recent upper respiratory tract infection and in those with suspected cardiac or pulmonary disease (because there is a likelihood for unanticipated findings), but these indications are not considered unequivocal.

Diagnostic Procedures/Surgery
- ECG (2)[C]: There are various recommendations reported in the literature:
  - AHA/ACC recommends that a preoperative ECG be obtained for patients who are to undergo vascular surgery and have at least 1 clinical risk factor, and for patients undergoing intermediate risk procedures who have a history of CHF, PVD, or cerebrovascular disease.
  - ECGs are reasonable in vascular surgery patients with no risk factors and patients having intermediate risk procedures who have 1 clinical risk factor.
  - ECGs are not indicated for asymptomatic patients undergoing low- risk procedures.
- Further cardiac testing should be considered in patients with poor or unknown functional capacity and 3+ clinical risk factors if the surgery is high risk and testing will change management (e.g., dipyridamole-thallium scan).
- Pulmonary function tests: Definitive data regarding the efficacy of preoperative testing is lacking. The most important factor is preoperative optimization of patients with COPD or reactive airways disease with indicated use of antibiotics, bronchodilators, and inhaled corticosteroids. Spirometry can help guide therapy. Upper abdominal and thoracic surgery have a higher risk of postoperative pulmonary complications.

 TREATMENT
MEDICATION
- Reducing cardiac risk:
  - Elective surgery should be delayed or canceled if the patient has any of the following: Unstable coronary syndromes (unstable or severe angina), recent myocardial infarction (<30 days), decompensated heart failure, significant arrhythmias, or severe valvular disease.
  - Active CHF should be treated with diuretics, afterload reduction, and β-adrenergic blockers.
  - Perioperative β-blockade has been shown to reduce mortality and the incidence of perioperative MIs in high-risk patients. Studies conflict, however, in what patients need to be treated, the dosage and timing of treatment, and for what surgeries. *Patients chronically on B-blockers need to have them continued in the perioperative period.* When B-blockers are discontinued in the perioperative period, 30-day mortality increases. B-blockers are reasonable for vascular surgery patients with at least 1 clinical risk factor (1)[C].
  - Perioperative statin use may have a protective effect on cardiac complications; prior to initiation of therapy, liver function and creatine kinase levels should be assessed.
- Reducing pulmonary risk:
  - Recommend *cigarette cessation* for at least *8 weeks prior to elective surgery*
  - Patients with asthma should not be wheezing and should have a peak flow of at least 80% of their predicted or personal-best value.
  - Treatment of chronic obstructive pulmonary disease (COPD) and asthma should focus on maximally reducing airflow obstruction and is identical to treatment of nonsurgical patients.
  - Lower respiratory tract infections (bacterial) should be treated with appropriate antibiotic therapy.

REFERENCES

1. American College of Cardiology Foundation/ American Heart Association Task Force on Practice Guidelines, American Society of Echocardiography, American Society of Nuclear Cardiology, Heart Rhythm Society, et al. 2009 ACCF/AHA focused update on perioperative beta blockade. *J Am Coll Cardiol*. 2009;54:2102–28.
2. American Society of Anesthesiologists Task Force on Preanesthesia Evaluation. Practice advisory for preanesthesia evaluation: a report by the American Society of Anesthesiologists Task Force on Preanesthesia Evaluation. *Anesthesiology*. 2002; 96:485–96.
3. Carrillo PM, et al. Perioperative risk evaluation. *Internet J Anesthesiol*. 2004;8(2).
4. American Society of Anesthesiologists Task Force on Perioperative Management of Patients with Cardiac Rhythm Management Devices et al. Practice advisory for the perioperative management of patients with cardiac rhythm management devices: pacemakers and implantable cardioverter-defibrillators: a report by the American Society of Anesthesiologists Task Force on Perioperative Management of Patients with Cardiac Rhythm Management Devices. *Anesthesiology*. 2005; 103:186–98.
5. Mauermann WJ, et al. Percutaneous coronary interventions and antiplatelet therapy in the perioperative period. *Journal of Cardiothoracic and Vascular Anesthesia*. 2007;21(3):436–442.
6. Chung SA, Yuan H, Chung F. A Systematic Review of Obstructive Sleep Apnea and Its Implications for Anesthesiologists. *Anesthesia and Analgesia* 2008;107(5):1543.
7. Lipshutz AK, Gropper MA et al. Perioperative glycemic control: an evidence-based review. *Anesthesiology*. 2009;110:408–21.

ADDITIONAL READING

- Menke H, Klein A, John KD, et al. Predictive value of ASA classification for the assessment of the perioperative risk. *Int Surg*. 1993;78:266–70.
- Polanczyk CA, Marcantonio E, Goldman L, et al. Impact of age on perioperative complications and length of stay in patients undergoing noncardiac surgery. *Ann Intern Med*. 2001;134:637–43.
- Reilly DF, McNeely MJ, Doerner D, et al. Self-reported exercise tolerance and the risk of serious perioperative complications. *Arch Intern Med*. 1999;159:2185–92.

See Also (Topic, Algorithm, Electronic Media Element)
Algorithm: Preoperative Evaluation of the Noncardiac Surgical Patient

 CODES
ICD9
- V72.83 Other specified pre-operative examination
- V72.84 Pre-operative examination, unspecified

CLINICAL PEARLS

- The preoperative evaluation should include medical record evaluation, patient interview, and physical exam.
- The minimum for the physical exam includes airway, pulmonary, and cardiovascular exams.
- Functional capacity, the level of surgical risk, and clinical risk factors determine if further cardiac testing is needed.
- No preoperative tests are routine.
- Active cardiac conditions should lead to delay or cancellation of nonemergent surgery.

PRESSURE ULCER

Kim House, MD

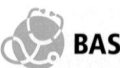 **BASICS**

DESCRIPTION
A localized area of soft tissue breakdown resulting from pressure between an external surface and a bony prominence that causes local tissue ischemia and necrosis

EPIDEMIOLOGY
Incidence
- 2 million new patients each year
- Incidence is 43/100,000 population every year.

Prevalence
- Hospitalized adults: 3–11%; long-term care facilities: 2.5–24%
- 65% of elderly with femoral fractures, 33% of critical-care patients, and over 60% prevalence among quadriplegic and orthopedic patients

RISK FACTORS
- Extended stay in hospital or nursing home, inadequate staffing (1)[B]
- Immobility (e.g., spinal cord injury, fracture, cerebrovascular accident)
- Malnutrition, recent weight loss, eating problems, vitamin C deficiency (1)[B]
- History of previous pressure ulcer
- Age-related skin changes
- Impairments of perfusion and oxygenation (anemia, peripheral vascular disease)
- Immunocompromise (e.g., diabetes)
- Decreased sensation (e.g., neuropathy, spinal cord injury)
- Impaired awareness (e.g., dementia, delirium, oversedation)
- Urinary or fecal incontinence
- For trauma and emergency patients, hard backboard should be removed as soon as possible after the secondary survey.
- Assessment scales for evaluating risk factors include Norton, Braden (Braden Q version for children), Waterlow, and Walsall.

GENERAL PREVENTION
- Up to 95% are preventable; identification of at-risk patients is essential, with early multidisciplinary care.
- Reposition frequently if immobile, hourly if wheelchair-bound and every 2 h if bedridden.
- Initiate early mobilization when possible.
- Keep skin clean and dry by using mild soap, warm water, and moisturizer. Zinc oxide and petroleum products are advisable. Manage incontinence by scheduled toileting plans, or check and change diapers every 2 h when turning patient.
- Use mattress overlays, thick air seat cushions, and beds that reduce pressure on pressure points, especially for hospitalized patients.

- Aggressive glycemic control (2)[B]
- Assess nutrient status and provide required macronutrients and micronutrients by oral, enteral, or parenteral route, if necessary.

PATHOPHYSIOLOGY
See "Etiology."

ETIOLOGY
- Sustained pressure causes occlusion of blood and lymphatic vessels; this occlusion of the micro-circulation can cause ischemia and necrosis (3)[A]. This occurs when the tissue pressure exceeds capillary filling pressure (25 mm Hg).
- Skin is more resistant to pressure than is subcutaneous tissue.
- Moisture from incontinence or perspiration can increase the friction between two surfaces.

COMMONLY ASSOCIATED CONDITIONS
See "Risk Factors."

 DIAGNOSIS

HISTORY
- Presence of risk factors
- Pain
- When was the ulcer first noticed?
- Prior treatment

PHYSICAL EXAM
- Do full skin examination on admission to hospital or extended-care facility.
- 83% of hospitalized patients with decubitus ulcers develop them in 1st 5 days of hospitalization (4)[B].
- National Pressure Ulcer Advisory Panel Classification: Deep tissue injury; may appear as a deep bruise over a bony prominence. Difficult to measure.
  - Stage I: Nonblanching erythema, warmth, induration
  - Stage II: May include dermis; appears as abrasion, blister, or superficial ulcer
  - Stage III: Extends through subcutaneous tissues but not fascia; may appear necrotic with changes in pigmentation
  - Stage IV: Ulcers extend beyond deep fascia into muscle or bone, decayed area may be larger than visibly apparent wound, osteomyelitis or sepsis may be present, and granulation tissue and epithelialization may be present at wound margins.

DIAGNOSTIC TESTS & INTERPRETATION
Lab
Initial lab tests
- Wound culture: Do not culture surface drainage. Do deep tissue culture/bone biopsy.
- White blood cell (WBC) count and differential; blood cultures if fever is present (>37°C)
- Erythrocyte sedimentation rate (ESR) and C-reactive protein (CRP) if osteomyelitis is suspected
- Nutritional assessment: Albumin, prealbumin, transferrin

Follow-Up & Special Considerations
If poor nutritional status is known, consider vitamin C and zinc levels. If low, supplements are likely to be helpful (2)[B].

Imaging
Initial approach
Radiograph of bone for suspected osteomyelitis

Follow-Up & Special Considerations
CT scan/MRI: If plain films show inflammation, reaction; can document progress/effectiveness of treatment

DIFFERENTIAL DIAGNOSIS
- Stasis or ischemic ulcers
- Vasculitides
- Diabetic ulcers
- Cancers
- Radiation injury
- Pyoderma gangrenosum and other dermatologic conditions

 TREATMENT

MEDICATION
First Line
- Cellulitis: Requires oral vs parenteral antibiotics. Treat for 7–10 days. Expect clinical response in 2–3 days.
- Osteomyelitis: Radiology-proven or visualized bone; treat for 6 weeks, usually with parenteral antibiotics.
- Deep tissue culture should guide antibiotic selection, not surface swab.
- Silver dressings, triple antibiotic ointment can be tried for 2 weeks to treat bacterial overgrowth.

Second Line
Zinc and vitamin C: Use if dietary deficiency is noted (lab test).

ADDITIONAL TREATMENT
General Measures

- Reduce pressure and prevent additional ulcers: Padding, frequent repositioning, mobilization if possible (4)[B]:
  - Static surfaces for stage I and II ulcers: Air, foam, and water mattress overlays
  - Dynamic surfaces for stage III and IV ulcers: Alternating air overlays, low-air-loss beds
  - Improve overall nutritional status (adequate protein intake, micronutrients).
- Wound management (4)[B]:
  - Remove dead tissue chemically (collagenase), via sharp debridement with a scalpel, or autolytically (hydrocolloid).
  - Dressing to manage drainage (e.g., calcium alginate, foam dressing, gauze dressing)
  - Dressing to protect from contamination, mechanical forces
  - Silver dressing used to reduce bacterial overgrowth; consider in wounds not responding to other therapy.
  - Stimulate new tissue growth when slough removed: Chlorophyll-containing products
  - Hydrogel can keep wound moist.
- Vacuum-assisted closure is used increasingly for difficult wounds:
  - Negative pressure reduces wound edema and improves local tissue perfusion.
  - Removes necrotic debris and reduces bacterial load
  - Literature review shows that 2 of 5 randomized, controlled trials and 2 of 4 nonrandomized, controlled trials favor negative-pressure wound therapy (5)[A].
  - Consider cost vs. clinical efficacy.

Issues for Referral
- Vascular surgery is a consideration for improvement of blood flow to wound via vascular bypass.
- Plastic surgery is a consideration for skin graft or flap.

Additional Therapies
Whirlpool/PulseVac aids in wound debridement (4)[C].

COMPLEMENTARY AND ALTERNATIVE MEDICINE
- Zinc and vitamin C: Use if dietary deficiency is noted (lab test).
- Electrical stimulation creates new vasculature in affected region (5)[C].

IN-PATIENT CONSIDERATIONS
Admission Criteria
- Cellulitis/osteomyelitis that has not responded to oral antibiotics as outpatient
- Abnormal vital signs owing to infectious process

Nursing
- Dressing changes 1–3× daily
- Wet-to-dry dressings not standard of care unless 100% of wound is necrotic tissue.

Discharge Criteria
Clinical improvement in WBC count, appearance of wound and/or surrounding tissue, resolution of vital sign abnormalities

 ## ONGOING CARE

FOLLOW-UP RECOMMENDATIONS
Weekly assessment by nurse with wound experience; biweekly assessment by physician

Patient Monitoring
- Home health nursing
- Change in plan of care if no improvement in 2–3 weeks

DIET
- 1–1.5 kg/d of protein
- Good glycemic control
- Include supply of micronutrients in diet or as supplements

PATIENT EDUCATION
- Signs and symptoms of infection
- Report new or increase in pain.
- Prevention of new wound where old wound healed

PROGNOSIS
Variable, depending on
- Removal of pressure
- Nutrition
- Wound care

COMPLICATIONS
- Infection
- Amputation

REFERENCES

1. Horn SB, et al. The National Pressure Ulcer Long-Term Study. *J Am Geriatric Soc.* 2004;52:359–67.
2. Mechanick JI. Practical aspects of nutritional support for wound-healing patients. *Am J Surgery.* 2004;188:525–65.
3. Grey JE, Harding KG, Enoch S. Pressure ulcers. *BMJ.* 2006;332:472–5.
4. Bansal C, Scott R, Stewart D, et al. Decubitus ulcers: a review of the literature. *Int J Dermatol.* 2005;44:805–10.
5. Gregor S, Maegele M, Sauerland S, et al. Negative pressure wound therapy: a vacuum of evidence? *Arch Surg.* 2008;143:189–96.

ADDITIONAL READING

Ramundo J, Gray M. Enzymatic wound debridement. *J Wound Ostomy Continence Nurs.* 2008;35:273–80.

 ## CODES

ICD9
- 707.00 Decubitus ulcer, unspecified site
- 707.09 Pressure ulcer, other site
- 707.20 Pressure ulcer, unspecified stage

CLINICAL PEARLS

- Maximize nutrition of all hospitalized patients.
- Focus on reducing pressure to an area rather than on an expensive dressing.
- Assess wounds weekly or biweekly, and document clinical improvement or deterioration.

PRETERM LABOR

Kara M. Coassolo, MD
John C. Smulian, MD, MPH

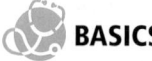 **BASICS**

DESCRIPTION
Contractions occurring between 20 and 36 weeks' gestation at a rate of 4 in 20 minutes or 8 in 1 h with at least 1 of the following: Cervical change over time or dilation $\geq$2 cm (1)

EPIDEMIOLOGY
Preterm birth is the leading cause of perinatal morbidity and mortality in the US.

Incidence
10–15% of pregnancies experience at least 1 episode of preterm labor.

Prevalence
~12% of all births in the US are preterm (9% spontaneous preterm births and 3% indicated preterm births).

RISK FACTORS
- Demographic factors including single parent, poverty, and black race
- Short interpregnancy interval
- No prenatal care
- Prepregnancy weight <45 kg (100 lb), body mass index <20
- Substance abuse (e.g., cocaine, tobacco)
- Prior preterm delivery (common)
- Previous 2nd-trimester dilation and evacuation (D&E)
- Cervical insufficiency
- Abdominal surgery/trauma during pregnancy
- Uterine or cervical anomalies such as large fibroids
- Serious maternal infections/diseases
- Bacterial vaginosis
- Bacteriuria
- Vaginal bleeding during pregnancy
- Multiple gestation
- Fetal abnormalities
- Intrauterine growth restriction
- Placenta previa
- Premature placental separation (abruption)
- Polyhydramnios
- Ehler-Danlos syndrome

Genetics
Familial predisposition

GENERAL PREVENTION
- Patient education at each visit in 2nd and 3rd trimesters for those at risk and periodically in the last 2 trimesters for the general population
- If previous preterm birth, evaluate if etiology is likely to recur, and target intervention to specific condition:
  - Weekly injections of 17α-hydroxyprogesterone (250 mg IM every week) from 16–36 weeks if previous spontaneous preterm birth (2,3)[A]
  - Consider cerclage placement before 24 weeks' gestation for those at high risk because of cervical insufficiency or significant or progressive cervical shortening (4)[A].

- For women with a short cervix in the second trimester (<15 mm on transvaginal ultrasound), progesterone 200 mg/d per vagina × 24–34 weeks may decrease the risk of preterm delivery (5)[A].

PATHOPHYSIOLOGY
- Premature formation and activation of myometrial gap junctions
- Inflammatory mediator–stimulated contractions
- Weakened cervix (structural defect or extracellular matrix defect)
- Abnormal placental implantation

ETIOLOGY
- Systemic inflammation/infections (e.g., urinary tract infection, pyelonephritis, pneumonia)
- Local inflammation/infections (intra-amniotic infections from aerobes, anaerobes, *Mycoplasma, Ureaplasma*)
- Uterine abnormalities (e.g., cervical insufficiency, leiomyomata, septa, diethylstilbestrol exposure)
- Overdistension (by multiple gestation or polyhydramnios)
- Preterm premature rupture of membranes
- Trauma
- Placental abruption
- Immunopathology (e.g., antiphospholipid antibodies)
- Placental ischemic disease (preeclampsia and fetal growth restriction)

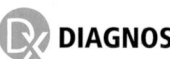 **DIAGNOSIS**

There is no single test that will diagnose or reliably predict true preterm labor. The diagnosis is based on a combination of physical findings and diagnostic tests that are interpreted in the context of the degree of risk to the patient.

HISTORY
- Address risk factors, especially etiologies of previous preterm birth.
- Regular uterine contractions or cramping
- Dull, low backache or pain
- Intermittent lower abdominal pain
- Increased low pelvic pressure
- Change in vaginal discharge
- Vaginal bleeding
- Fluid leakage

PHYSICAL EXAM
- Sterile speculum exam for membrane rupture evaluation, cultures, cervical inspection
- Bimanual cervical exam if intact membranes: Dilation of the cervix >1 cm and/or effacement of the cervix >50%

ALERT
Avoid bimanual examination when possible if rupture of the membranes is suspected.

DIAGNOSTIC TESTS & INTERPRETATION
Lab
Initial lab tests
- In symptomatic women from 22–34 weeks' gestation with intact membranes and no intercourse or bleeding in past 24 h, obtain a fetal fibronectin swab (FFN) from the posterior vaginal fornix. FFN must be obtained prior to digital cervical exam:
  - If results are positive ($\geq$50 ng/mL), patient is at a modest increased risk of preterm birth [positive predictive value (PPV) 13–30% for delivery within 2 weeks].
  - If results are negative, more than 97% of patients will not deliver in 14 days, so can consider avoiding complicated or high-risk interventions (6)[A].
- Urinalysis and urine culture
- Cultures for gonorrhea and chlamydia
- Wet prep for bacterial vaginosis evaluation (although evidence for improved outcomes with treatment is weak)
- Vaginal introitus and rectal culture for group B *Streptococcus*
- pH and Ferning test of vaginal fluid to evaluate for rupture of membranes
- Complete blood count with differential
- Drug screen when appropriate

Follow-Up & Special Considerations
Repeat FFN as indicated by symptoms.

Imaging
Initial approach
- Ultrasound to identify number of fetuses and fetal position, confirm gestational age, estimate fetal weight, quantify amniotic fluid, and to look for conditions making tocolysis contraindicated
- Transvaginal ultrasound to evaluate cervical length, funneling, and dynamic changes after obtaining FFN and if clinical assessment of the cervix is uncertain or if the cervix is closed on digital exam (4)[B]

Follow-Up & Special Considerations
Progressive shortening of the cervix on repeat ultrasound (in 1–2 weeks) may indicate need for hospitalization.

Diagnostic Procedures/Surgery
- Monitor contractions with external tocodynamometer.
- Consider amniocentesis at any preterm gestational age to evaluate for intra-amniotic infection (cell count with differential, glucose, Gram stain, aerobic, anaerobic, *Mycoplasma, Ureaplasma* cultures).
- Consider amniocentesis if $\geq$32 weeks' gestation for evaluation of fetal lung maturity [e.g., lecithin/sphingomyelin (L:S) ratio and phosphatidylglycerol (PG)]. If L:S ratio >2:1 (nondiabetic) and PG is present, hyaline membrane disease is unlikely, so tocolysis is contraindicated.

Pathological Findings
- Placental inflammation:
  - Acute inflammation usually caused by infection
  - Chronic inflammation caused by immunopathology
- Abruption

DIFFERENTIAL DIAGNOSIS
- Braxton-Hicks contractions/false labor
- Round ligament pain
- Lumbosacral muscular back pain
- Urinary tract or vaginal infections
- Adnexal torsion
- Appendicitis
- Dehydration
- Viral gastroenteritis

 TREATMENT

MEDICATION
Tocolysis may allow time for interventions such as transfer to tertiary care facility and administration of corticosteroids, but may not prolong pregnancy significantly (2)[A].

First Line
- Tocolysis:
  – Nifedipine: 10 mg p.o. q10min up to 30 mg total; then 10–20 mg q6h × 24 h; then 10–20 mg p.o. q8h (do not use sublingual route); check blood pressure often, and avoid hypotension. Concurrent use with magnesium sulfate should be avoided.
  – Indomethacin: 50–100 mg p.o. initial dose; then 50 mg q6–8h × 24 h (or, if available, 100-mg suppository per rectum q12h for 2 doses); then 25 mg q6–8h; use for no longer than 72 h due to risk of premature closure of ductus arteriosus, oligohydramnios, and possibly neonatal necrotizing enterocolitis.
  – Contraindications to tocolysis: Severe preeclampsia, hemorrhage, chorioamnionitis, advanced labor, intrauterine growth retardation, fetal distress, or lethal fetal abnormalities
- Antibiotics: Antibiotics for group B *Streptococcus* prophylaxis if culture positive or unknown
- Steroids: If mother is at 23–34 weeks' gestation with no evidence of systemic infection, give glucocorticoids to decrease neonatal respiratory distress, intraventricular hemorrhage, necrotizing enterocolitis, and overall perinatal mortality (7)[A]. Betamethasone 12 mg IM × 2 doses 24 h apart (preferred choice) *or* dexamethasone 6 mg IM q12h for 4 doses.

Second Line
- Terbutaline 0.25 mg SC q30min for up to 3 doses until contractions stop; then 0.25 mg SC q6h for 4 doses (optional); if contractions persist or pulse >120 beats/min, change to another tocolytic agent (may be poorly tolerated by mothers).
- Terbutaline infusion pumps are potentially useful only in multiples or in selected refractory or symptomatic patients:
  – Caution with terbutaline infusion: Palpitations, nausea, intractable vomiting, pulse >140 beats/min, decreased urine output
- Magnesium sulfate by intravenous infusion has been used in the past as a 1st-line tocolytic agent. Recent data are conflicting as to whether it has a benefit for prolongation of pregnancy beyond 48 h and whether it increases the risk for complications. Therefore, this agent should be used cautiously. (Standard dosages for tocolysis start with a 4- to 6-g IV bolus over 20 minutes and then 2–3 g/h until contractions stop.)
  – Magnesium may decrease the risk of cerebral palsy when given prior to an anticipated preterm birth (8)[B].

– Relative contraindications to magnesium sulfate include myasthenia gravis, hypocalcemia, renal failure, or concurrent use of calcium channel blockers.
- Significant possible interactions include pulmonary edema from crystalloid fluids and tocolytic agents, especially magnesium sulfate.
- Oral maintenance therapy with any agent is controversial, and its use is limited (9)[A].

ADDITIONAL TREATMENT
General Measures
Treat underlying risk factors with appropriate measures (e.g., antibiotics for infections, hydration for dehydration). Liquids only or nothing by mouth if delivery imminent; hospitalization is necessary if the patient is on IV tocolysis or if bed rest is impossible at home.

Issues for Referral
If delivery is inevitable but not immediate, consider transport to a tertiary care center or hospital equipped with a neonatal ICU. Consider consultation with maternal-fetal medicine specialist.

Additional Therapies
- Treating symptomatic bacterial vaginosis in 2nd trimester with metronidazole 250 mg p.o. t.i.d. × 7 days or clindamycin 300 mg p.o. b.i.d. × 7 days might reduce risk of preterm delivery in high-risk symptomatic women.
- Pelvic rest (e.g., no douching or intercourse)
- Discontinue work and strenuous physical activity.
- Strict bed rest is not demonstrated to be effective in most situations.

SURGERY/OTHER PROCEDURES
- For malpresentation or fetal compromise, consider cesarean delivery if labor is progressing.
- If incompetent cervix is suspected, consider cerclage (4)[B].

IN-PATIENT CONSIDERATIONS
Initial Stabilization
- Intravenous access
- Continuous fetal and contraction monitoring
- Assess cervix for dilatation and effacement

Admission Criteria
Suspected/threatened preterm labor

IV Fluids
Hydrate with 500 mL 5% dextrose normal saline solution or 5% dextrose lactated Ringer solution for 1st half-hour; then at 125 mL/h.

Nursing
Monitor for fluid overload, especially with tocolysis and multiple gestations.

Discharge Criteria
- Regular contractions resolved and no progressive cervical change
- If cervix is dilated ≥3 cm or FFN is positive, individualize decision to discharge by gestational age and specific patient circumstances.

 ONGOING CARE

FOLLOW-UP RECOMMENDATIONS
Patient Monitoring
- Weekly office visits and cervical checks or cervical ultrasound if at high risk for recurrence
- Routine use of maintenance tocolysis has not been proven beneficial.

DIET
Regular

PATIENT EDUCATION
Call physician or proceed to hospital whenever contractions last >1 h, low back pain comes and goes, change in vaginal discharge, "menstrual cramping," or intestinal cramping.

PROGNOSIS
- If membranes are ruptured and no infection is confirmed, delivery often occurs within 3–7 days.
- If membranes are intact, 20–50% deliver preterm.

COMPLICATIONS
Labor resistant to tocolysis, pulmonary edema/fluid overload, and infection with preterm rupture of membranes (PROM)

REFERENCES
1. Management of Preterm Labor. Summary, Evidence Report/Technology Assessment: Number 18. AHRQ Publication No. 01-E020, October 2000. Agency for Healthcare Research and Quality, Rockville, MD. http://archive.ahrq.gov/clinic/tp/pretermtp.htm.
2. Simhan HN, Caritis SN. Prevention of preterm delivery. N Engl J Med. 2007;357:477–87.
3. Tita AT, Rouse DJ. Progesterone for preterm birth prevention: an evolving intervention. Am J Obstet Gynecol. 2009;200:219–24.
4. Daskalakis GJ. Prematurity prevention: the role of cerclage. Curr Opin Obstet Gynecol. 2009;21(2):148–52.
5. Fonseca FB, Celik E, Parra M, et al. Progesterone and the risk of preterm birth among women with a short cervix. NEJM. 2007;357(5):462–9.
6. Goldenberg RL, Goepfert AR, Ramsey PS. Biochemical markers for the prediction of preterm birth. Am J Obstet Gynecol. 2005;192(5 Suppl):S36–46.
7. Roberts D, Dalziel S. Antenatal corticosteroids for accelerating fetal lung maturation for women at risk of preterm birth. Cochrane Database of Systematic Reviews. 2006, Issue 3. Art. No.: CD004454. DOI: 10.1002/14651858.CD004454.pub2.
8. Magnesium sulfate before anticipated preterm birth for neuroprotection. Comm Opin No 455. ACOG. Obstet Gynecol. 2010;115:669–71.
9. Dodd JM, Crowther CA, Dare MR, et al. Oral betamimetics for maintenance therapy after threatened preterm labor. Cochran Database of Systemic Reviews. 2006, Issue 1. ArtNo.: CD003927. DOI:10.1002/14651858.CD003927.pub2.

 CODES

ICD9
- 644.03 Threatened preterm labor, antepartum
- 644.13 Other threatened labor, antepartum

CLINICAL PEARLS
- Preterm labor is common and has multiple etiologies.
- Tocolytic therapy allows steroid dosing. Steroids improve neonatal outcomes.
- Progesterone therapy can prevent recurrence of preterm birth in next pregnancy.

PRIAPISM

Andrew Leone, MD
Kyle D. Wood, MD

 BASICS

DESCRIPTION

- Penile erection that lasts for >4 hours and is unrelated to sexual stimulation or excitement
- Classified into ischemic and nonischemic variants
- Ischemic (low-flow) priapism is painful and requires urgent clinical intervention.
- Stuttering priapism is recurrent ischemic priapism over an extended period.
- Nonischemic (high-flow) priapism could be related to prior trauma and does not require urgent treatment.
- System(s) affected: Reproductive

Pediatric Considerations
In children, nearly all priapism is caused either by sickle cell anemia or trauma (1).

EPIDEMIOLOGY
Incidence
In the Netherlands, 1.5 cases of ischemic priapism per 100,000 person-years in the general male population (data not available for the US) (1). After exclusion of cases associated with intracavernous vasoactive drug use, incidence is 0.9 cases per 100,000 person-years (2).

RISK FACTORS
- Sickle cell anemia, lifetime risk of ischemic priapism 29–42% (1)
- Dehydration

GENERAL PREVENTION
- Avoid dehydration.
- Avoid excessive sexual stimulation.
- Avoid causative drugs (see Causes) when possible.
- Avoid genital and pelvic trauma.

PATHOPHYSIOLOGY
- In ischemic priapism, decreased venous outflow results in increased intracavernosal pressure. This leads to erection, decreased arterial inflow, stasis of blood, local hypoxia, and acidosis (a compartment syndrome). Eventually penile tissue necrosis and fibrosis may occur. The exact mechanism is unknown and may involve trapping of erythrocytes in the veins draining the erectile bodies.
- In nonischemic priapism, increased arterial flow without decreased venous outflow. There is increased inflow and outflow, which results in a sustained, nonpainful, partially rigid erection.
- Aberrations in the phosphodiesterase (PDE-5A) pathway has been proven in mice to be one mechanism of priapism (3).

ETIOLOGY
- Ischemic priapism:
  – Idiopathic, estimated to about 50% (1)
  – Intracavernosal injections of vasoactive drugs for erectile dysfunction
  – Oral agents for erectile dysfunction
  – Pelvic vascular thrombosis
  – Prolonged sexual activity
  – Sickle cell disease and trait
  – Leukemia from infiltration of the corpora
  – Other blood dyscrasias (G6PD deficiency, thrombophilia)
  – Pelvic hematoma or neoplasia (penis, urethra, bladder, prostate, kidney, rectal)
  – Cerebrospinal tumors
  – Asplenism
  – Fabry disease
  – Tertiary syphilis
  – Total parenteral nutrition, especially 20% lipid infusion (results in hyperviscosity)
  – Bladder calculus
  – Trauma to penis
  – Urinary tract infections, especially prostatitis, urethritis, cystitis
  – Several drugs suspected as causing priapism (e.g., chlorpromazine, prazosin, cocaine, trazodone, and some corticosteroids; anticoagulants (heparin and Coumadin); phosphodiesterase inhibitors (Viagra, others); testosterone; immunosuppressants (tacrolimus); and antihypertensives (hydralazine, propranolol, guanethidine)
  – Intracavernous fat emulsion
  – Hyperosmolar intravenous contrast
  – Spinal cord injury
  – General or spinal anesthesia
  – Heavy alcohol intake or cocaine use
- Nonischemic priapism:
  – The most common cause is penile or perineal trauma resulting in a fistula between cavernous artery and the corpora.
  – Rarely, iatrogenic causes for the management of ischemic priapism can result in nonischemic priapism.
  – Certain urological surgeries have also resulted in nonischemic priapism.

COMMONLY ASSOCIATED CONDITIONS
- Sickle cell anemia
- G6PD deficiency
- Leukemia
- Neoplasm

℞ DIAGNOSIS

HISTORY
- Penile erection that is persistent, prolonged, painful, and tender (ischemic)
- Duration of erection, degree of pain
- Perineal or penile trauma
- Prior episodes of priapism
- Urination difficult during erection
- History of any hematological abnormalities
- Cardiovascular disease
- Medications
- Recreational drugs
- Loss of erectile function if treatment is not prompt and effective

PHYSICAL EXAM
- Ischemic priapism:
  – Penis is fully erect, corpora cavernosa are rigid and tender, and corpora spongiosum and glans are flaccid. Usually associated with tenderness and pain.
- Nonischemic priapism:
  – Penis is partially erect, and the corpora cavernosa are semirigid and nontender, with the glans and corpora spongiosum flaccid. Usually not tender or painful.
- Perineum, abdomen, and lymph node exam also valuable to rule out underlying condition
- Complete penile and scrotal exam necessary. Determine if penile prosthesis is present.

DIAGNOSTIC TESTS & INTERPRETATION
Lab
- Complete blood chemistry with reticulocyte count to detect leukemia or platelet abnormalities
- Sickling hemoglobin (Hgb) solubility test and Hgb electrophoresis
- Coagulation profile
- Platelet count
- Urinalysis
- Urine toxicology if illicit drugs suspected
- Corporal blood gas can be used to distinguish ischemic from nonischemic priapism.

Imaging
- Color duplex ultrasound of the penis and perineum may be necessary to differentiate ischemic from nonischemic priapism. In ischemic priapism, there is no blood flow in the cavernosal arteries, whereas in nonischemic patients there is high blood flow (1); may also see fistulas or pseudoaneurysms suggestive of nonischemic.
- Penile arteriography can be used to identify presence and site of fistulas in patients with nonischemic priapism.

1062

Diagnostic Procedures/Surgery
Physical exam is usually able to distinguish ischemic from nonischemic priapism.

Pathological Findings
- Pelvic vascular thrombosis
- Partial thrombosis of corpora cavernosa of the penis
- Corpus spongiosum, glans penis: No involvement
- Arterial priapism will show arteriocavernous fistula.

 TREATMENT

- Ischemic priapism requires immediate treatment in order to preserve future erectile function (a longer delay in treatment means higher chance of future impotence):
  - Cavernosal aspiration with irrigation (success rate ~30%) (1,4)
  - Cavernosal injection of phenylephrine (α adrenergic sympathomimetic) with monitoring of patient's blood pressure and pulse (success rate ~65 %) (4). Inject every 5–10 minutes until detumescence.
  - Continue aspiration, irrigation, and phenylephrine for several hours. If this fails, shunt procedures are considered (first a distal shunt).
- Nonischemic priapism:
  - Initial observation
  - If this fails, arteriography and embolization with absorbable materials (5% rate of impotence versus 39% with permanent materials) or surgical ligation as a last resort (4)
- Treat underlying condition (i.e., sickle cell disease). Do not delay intracavernous treatment.

MEDICATION
- Narcotics for pain if needed
- Pseudoephedrine is not recommended by the American Urological Association (4):
  - Efficacy is reported in nonrandomized studies as 28–36% (1).
  - No randomized studies have been conducted to date.
- Terbutaline has been studied and may be effective (uncontrolled trials showed a 65% resolution rate) for priapism caused by self-injection of agents to treat erectile dysfunction (4).
- For stuttering priapism, a trial of GnRH agonists or antiandrogens is effective; self-injection of phenylephrine is also effective.
- PDE-5 inhibitors also have a role in the prevention of priapism in patients suffering from stuttering priapism (5).

ADDITIONAL TREATMENT
General Measures
- Reassure patient about outcome if warranted.
- Continuous caudal or spinal anesthesia if etiology is neurogenic.
- Treat any underlying cause.
- In sickle cell anemia: IV hydration; partial exchange or repeated transfusions to reduce percentage of sickle to <50%
- Relieve patient's pain.

Issues for Referral
A urologist should be consulted in all cases of suspected priapism to ensure highest likelihood of preserved erectile function.

SURGERY/OTHER PROCEDURES
- Introduction of 18- or 19-gauge needle into corpora cavernosa (best done by urologist if available) at 9 o'clock and 3 o'clock positions with aspiration of 20–30 mL of blood from corpus cavernosum. May follow with intracavernous injection of 100–500 mcg phenylephrine. (To make 200 mcg phenylephrine, add 0.2 mL of 1% phenylephrine in 9.8 cc of normal saline.) If this fails, consider shunts.
- Distal shunt:
  - Winter shunt: Biopsy needle inserted in glans penis to create shunt between glans and corpora
  - Al-Ghorab shunt: Excision of tunica albuginea
- Proximal shunts

 ONGOING CARE

FOLLOW-UP RECOMMENDATIONS
Bed rest until priapism resolves

Patient Monitoring
Close follow-up with a urologist is required after surgical treatments for priapism.

PATIENT EDUCATION
- Information about long-term outlook, referral for counseling
- Reduction of vasoactive drug therapy if responsible for priapism and elimination of offending drugs if causal

PROGNOSIS
- Even with excellent treatment for a prolonged priapism, detumescence may require several weeks secondary to edema (1)
- Impotence is likely in ischemic priapism and is up to 90% if the priapism lasts longer than 24 hours.
- Despite early intervention, ischemic priapism is likely to result in impotence in up to 50% of men.

COMPLICATIONS
Erectile dysfunction (i.e., impotence)

REFERENCES
1. Huang YC, Harraz AM, Shindel AW, et al. Evaluation and management of priapism: 2009 update. *Nat Rev Urol*. 2009;6:262–71.
2. Eland IA, van der Lei J, Stricker BH, et al. Incidence of priapism in the general population. *Urology*. 2001;57:970–2.
3. Champion HC, Bivalacqua TJ, Takimoto E, et al. Phosphodiesterase-5A dysregulation in penile erectile tissue is a mechanism of priapism. *Proc Natl Acad Sci U S A*. 2005;102:1661–6.
4. Montague DK, Jarow J, Broderick GA, et al. American Urological Association guideline on the management of priapism. *J Urol*. 2003;170: 1318–24.
5. Muneer A, Minhas S, Arya M, et al. Stuttering priapism - a review of the therapeutic options. *Int J Clin Pract*. 2008.

ADDITIONAL READING
- Burnett AL. Pathophysiology of priapism: dysregulatory erection physiology thesis. *J Urol*. 2003;170:26–34.
- Pryor J, Akkus E, Alter G, et al. Priapism. *J Sex Med*. 2004;1:116–20.

See Also (Topic, Algorithm, Electronic Media Element)
Anemia, Sickle Cell; Erectile Dysfunction

 CODES

ICD9
607.3 Priapism

CLINICAL PEARLS
- Priapism is a prolonged penile erection that lasts longer than 4 hours and is unrelated to sexual stimulation.
- In evaluating priapism, the clinician must distinguish ischemic from nonischemic priapism by history and physical, as well as blood gas and possibly ultrasound, if needed.
- Ischemic priapism is an emergent condition that requires immediate urological evaluation and treatment.
- The most common causes of ischemic priapism are idiopathic, related to treatments for erectile dysfunction, or related to use of substances (medicinal or recreational).
- If an underlying medical condition is identified (sickle cell anemia), proper concomitant treatment is necessary to increase efficacy of treatment.

PROCTITIS

Walter M. Kim, MD, PhD
Jyoti Ramakrishna, MD

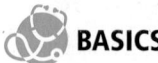 **BASICS**

DESCRIPTION
- An acute or chronic inflammation of the rectal mucosa
- System(s) affected: GI

EPIDEMIOLOGY
Incidence
- Predominant age: Adult
- Predominant sex: Male > Female
- Radiation proctitis is usually encountered following pelvic radiation for cancers of the rectum, cervix, uterus, prostate, bladder, and testes.
- Ulcerative proctitis: 0.5–3/100,000 persons

RISK FACTORS
- Receptive anal intercourse
- Pelvic radiation
- Rectal injury
- Rectal medications
- Inflammatory bowel disease (IBD)
- Jewish ancestry

Genetics
Higher incidence in Jewish population

GENERAL PREVENTION
Safe sex practices including condom use during anal intercourse if a sexually transmitted infection (STI) is causative

ETIOLOGY
- Infectious (sexually transmitted):
  – Gonorrhea
  – Chlamydia
  – Syphilis
  – Herpes simplex virus (90% of cases due to HSV2)
  – Lymphogranuloma venereum (LGV)
  – Chancroid
  – Cytomegalovirus (CMV)
  – Human papillomavirus (HPV)
- Other infections:
  – *Clostridium difficile* (after antibiotics)
  – Enteric infections, including *Campylobacter, Shigella, Escherichia coli, Salmonella,* and amebiasis
- Inflammatory:
  – IBD (mostly ulcerative colitis)
  – Radiation therapy
- Other:
  – Ischemia
  – Vasculitis
  – Idiopathic
  – Toxins (e.g., hydrogen peroxide enemas)

COMMONLY ASSOCIATED CONDITIONS
- If an STI is causative, test accordingly, including HIV serology.
- Treatment with pelvic radiation (e.g., for prostate, bladder, testicular, or gynecologic cancers)

 DIAGNOSIS

HISTORY
- Anorectal pain or discomfort
- Rectal bleeding
- Purulent rectal discharge
- Passing of blood or mucous through rectum
- Urgency
- Tenesmus
- Diarrhea or constipation
- Abdominal cramps
- Fever
- Weight loss
- Radiation proctitis:
  – Acute radiation injury: Occurs within 6 weeks of therapy
  – Chronic radiation proctitis: Delayed onset; 1st sign most commonly occurs 9–14 months following radiation.

PHYSICAL EXAM
- STI-associated proctitis: Perianal or rectal vesicles and/or ulcers, mucopurulent discharge, rectal bleeding, chancre, and condylomata lata or acuminata; may have tender inguinal lymphadenopathy with LGV infection
- IBD-associated proctitis: Perianal abscess, fistula, or fissures; rectal bleeding

DIAGNOSTIC TESTS & INTERPRETATION
Lab
- STI proctitis: Rectal swab for gonococcal and chlamydial culture, serology for syphilis, LVG culture, viral culture for HSV
- IBD: Complete blood count, erythrocyte sedimentation rate, C-reactive protein, albumin, liver function tests
- Enteric infections: Stool culture for *E. coli* O157:H7, *Salmonella, Shigella,* amebiasis
- Stool study for *C. difficile* toxin

Diagnostic Procedures/Surgery
- Proctosigmoidoscopy
- Colonoscopy to exclude more proximal involvement and rectal biopsy if IBD is suspected

Pathological Findings
- Radiation proctitis: Proctosigmoidoscopy reveals friable, edematous mucosa, spontaneous or contact bleeding, telangiectasias, strictures, or fistulas.
- STI proctitis: Ulceration, inflammation, mucopurulent discharge, or bleeding on proctoscopy may be present.
- Ulcerative proctitis: Endoscopy reveals friable mucosa and pseudopolyps; biopsy reveals cryptitis and crypt abscesses.

DIFFERENTIAL DIAGNOSIS
- Traumatic proctitis
- Radiation proctitis
- IBD (ulcerative colitis, Crohn disease)
- Recurrent malignancies
- Enteric infections such as *Salmonella, Shigella, Campylobacter, E. coli, C. difficile,* or amebiasis

TREATMENT

- Gonorrhea: Ceftriaxone 125 mg IM in a single dose plus chlamydia treatment with doxycycline 100 mg PO b.i.d. × 7 days (owing to high rate of coinfection) (1)
- Chlamydia: Doxycycline 100 mg PO b.i.d. × 7 days (1)
- Herpes: Acyclovir 400 mg PO t.i.d. × 7–10 days
- C. difficile: Metronidazole 250–500 mg PO t.i.d. to q.i.d. or vancomycin 125 mg PO q.i.d. × 7–10 days
- Ulcerative proctitis:
  - Mild to moderate (up to 8 bloody stools per day): Topical 5-aminosalicylic acid (5-ASA, Mesalamine) suppository or enema (Rowasa), topical steroids (hydrocortisone-containing foam, suppository, or enema), or a combination of oral 5-ASA (Pentasa or Asacol) and topical 5-ASA (2)[B]
  - Severe: Systemic corticosteroids may be needed for patients who do not tolerate or do not respond to the aforementioned therapies.
  - Chronic (moderate to severe steroid-refractory or dependent disease): 6-Mercaptopurine, azathioprine
- Radiation proctitis:
  - Topical hydrocortisone foam or enemas; mesalamine (5-ASA) enema alone or in combination with oral mesalamine; sucralfate enemas (20 mL of a 10% sucralfate suspension in water b.i.d.)
  - Systemic corticosteroids may be used if the aforementioned therapies are ineffective.
  - Experimental treatments: Hyperbaric oxygen (3)[B], metronidazole, vitamin A, WF10 macrophage-regulating agent, argon plasma coagulation for bleeding telangiectasias

ADDITIONAL TREATMENT
General Measures
- Treatment depends on the cause.
- Rectal Gram stains have a significant false-negative rate, and if the clinician has a strong suspicion of gonorrheal proctitis, empirical treatment is warranted while culture results are still pending.
- Encourage sexual partners of patients diagnosed with STI-associated proctitis to be tested and treated.
- Sitz baths may provide some relief.

IN-PATIENT CONSIDERATIONS
Initial Stabilization
- Outpatient, unless severe and refractory to usual measures
- Hospitalization may be necessary in severe ulcerative proctitis, especially with more proximal colon involvement.

ONGOING CARE

FOLLOW-UP RECOMMENDATIONS
Patient Monitoring
Follow until completely healed.

DIET
No special diet

PATIENT EDUCATION
Counsel about safe sex practices, including condom use with every sexual encounter and additional barrier methods such as dental dams and gloves for alternative intimacy practices.

PROGNOSIS
- Satisfactory cure or control with appropriate treatment
- In patients with ulcerative proctitis, 10% will not experience a recurrent attack.
- Radiation proctitis may be associated with a significant decrease in health-related quality of life in up to 30% of patients.

COMPLICATIONS
- Chronic ulcerative colitis
- Fistula/abscess formation
- Treatment failure (may be as high as 35% in gonorrheal proctitis—check cultures and sensitivities)
- Perforation
- Radiation injury: Fistulas, strictures, obstruction, continued rectal mucosal bleeding, cystitis
- LGV infection: Hemorrhagic proctitis, rectal stricture
- Fecal incontinence

REFERENCES

1. Updated recommended treatment regimens for gonococcal infections and associated conditions, United States, April 2007: http://www.cdc.gov/STD/treatment/2006/updated-regimens.htm
2. Denton A, et al. Nonsurgical interventions for late radiation proctitis in patient who have received radical radiotherapy to the pelvis. *Cochrane Database Sys Rev.* 2002;1:CD003455.
3. Bennett MH, Feldmeier J, Hampson N, et al. Hyperbaric oxygen therapy for late radiation tissue injury. *Cochrane Database Syst Rev.* 2005; CD005005.

ADDITIONAL READING

- Cohen RD, Woseth DM, Thisted RA et al. A meta-analysis and overview of the literature on treatment options for left-sided ulcerative colitis and ulcerative proctitis. *Am J Gastroenterol.* 2000;95:1263–76.
- Hamlyn E, Taylor C. Sexually transmitted proctitis. *Postgrad Med J.* 2006;82:733–6.
- McMillan A, van Voorst Vader PC, de Vries HJ. The 2007 European Guideline (International Union against Sexually Transmitted Infections/World Health Organization) on the management of proctitis, proctocolitis and enteritis caused by sexually transmissible pathogens. *Int J STD AIDS.* 2007;18:514–20.
- Regueiro MD et al. Diagnosis and treatment of ulcerative proctitis. *J Clin Gastroenterol.* 2004;38:733–40.
- Sutherland L, MacDonald JK, et al. Oral 5-aminosalicylic acid for maintenance of remission in ulcerative colitis. *Cochrane Database Syst Rev.* 2006;2:CD000544.

See Also (Topic, Algorithm, Electronic Media Element)
Crohn Disease; Gonococcal Infections; Herpes Simplex; Lymphogranuloma Venereum; Syphilis; Ulcerative Colitis

CODES

ICD9
569.49 Other specified disorders of rectum and anus

CLINICAL PEARLS

- Gonorrhea is increasingly resistant to antibiotics, and as of April 2007, the Centers for Disease Control and Prevention (CDC) no longer recommends treatment with fluoroquinolones.
- If patient has a true allergy to ceftriaxone, consider azithromycin 2 g PO in a single dose, but limit use. Do *not* use for simply a penicillin allergy (owing to concerns of the theoretical 5–10% cross-reactivity).
- For STI-related proctitis, consider expedited partner therapy (as permitted in your location).

PROSTATE CANCER

Kyle D. Wood, MD
Ilya Gorbachinsky, MD

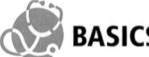 **BASICS**

DESCRIPTION

- The prostate is composed of acinar glands with their ducts arranged in a radial fashion and the stroma containing blood vessels, lymphatics, and nerves. 95% of prostate cancers (CaP) are acinar adenocarcinomas
- Only 3% of men with CaP die from the disease. Common metastatic locations (most to least common): Pelvic lymph nodes, bone, lung, and liver
- Staging: TNM classification (AJCC, 2010):
  - Tx: Primary tumor cannot be assessed. T0: No evidence of primary tumor
  - T1: Clinically inapparent tumor not palpable or visible by imaging. T1a: Tumor incidental histologic finding in ≤5% of tissue resected (by transurethral resection of prostate [TURP]) T1b: Tumor incidental histologic finding in >5% of tissue resected (by TURP). T1c: Tumor identified by needle biopsy (e.g., because of elevated prostate-specific antigen [PSA])
  - T2: Tumor confined within the prostate (*Note: Tumor found in one or both lobes by needle biopsy but not palpable or visible by imaging is classified as T1c.*) T2a: Tumor involves ≤1/2 of one lobe T2b: Tumor involves >1/2 of one lobe, not both T2c: Tumor involves both lobes.
  - T3: Tumor extends through the prostatic capsule (*Note: Invasion into the prostatic apex or into [but not beyond] the prostatic capsule is still T2*). T3a: Extracapsular extension (unilateral or bilateral) T3b: Tumor invades seminal vesicle(s)
  - T4: Tumor is fixed or invades adjacent structures other than seminal vesicles (e.g., bladder neck, external sphincter, rectum, levator muscles, and/or pelvic wall)
- Gleason grade: Tumors are graded from 1–5 based on the degree of glandular differentiation and structural architecture. Grade 1 represents the most well-differentiated appearance, and grade 5 represents the most poorly differentiated. Primary and secondary scores are reported and combined to form the combined Gleason score
- System(s) affected: Reproductive; Urologic. Synonym(s): Carcinoma of the prostate (CaP)

EPIDEMIOLOGY

Mortality from CaP is decreasing

Incidence

In the US, 200/100,000 men/year

Prevalence

- Mean age at diagnosis is 71 years.
- Most common cancer in men (~17% lifetime risk) and 2nd leading cause of cancer death in men (~3% of all CaP results in CaP-related death); however, autopsy studies find foci of latent CaP in 50% of men in their 8th decade

RISK FACTORS

- Age >50 years, African-American Race , Family History, Baseline PSA above median for age group
- No increased risk of CaP post vasectomy per American Urological Association (AUA) Policy Statement
- Mixed data for CaP risk and presence of Metabolic Syndrome or coffee and alcohol consumption

Genetics

~2× ↑ risk with 1st-degree relative affected at age <50 years

GENERAL PREVENTION

- No level I evidence for diet or supplementation in CaP prevention
  - Best available evidence
    - May ↓ Risk: Diet high in lycopene (e.g. tomatoes) or selenium supplementation in those with low selenium levels
    - May ↑ Risk: High calcium consumption
  - Of note, no dietary supplements were shown to reduce risk in the SELECT, HOPE, and PHS II studies
- Current data regarding aspirin and statin use for chemoprevention is disputed
- Annual PSA and DRE (digital rectal exam) screening for prostate cancer may be offered to males >45–50 years of age after discussion regarding benefits and risks; balance of overall risk and benefits uncertain, but benefits unlikely to be great in average-risk population.
- Prostate Cancer Prevention Trial (PCPT) showed 25% reduction in CaP risk with finasteride treatment
- Reduction by Dutasteride of Prostate Cancer Events (REDUCE) trial showed decrease risk of Gleason 5/6 CaP in treatment group
- 5α reductase inhibitors are currently not FDA approved for CaP prevention but high-risk individuals may benefit from a discussion regarding chemoprevention with the understanding that it might increase risk of high-grade CaP (1).

PATHOPHYSIOLOGY

- Adenocarcinoma >95%
- Non-adenocarcinoma <5% (most common transitional cell carcinoma)
- Cells often stain positive for PSA and PAP (prostatic acid phosphatase)
- Location of CaP: 70% peripheral zone, 20% transitional zone, 5-10% central zone, rarely in anterior fibromuscular zone
- Capsular penetration most common near neurovascular bundle

 DIAGNOSIS

HISTORY

- Inquire about family history of CaP, symptoms of bladder outlet obstruction (e.g., urinary retention), other voiding symptoms (e.g., frequency, hesitancy, etc)
- Anorexia and weight loss, bone pain (with metastasis)
- Hematuria, hematospermia (rare)

PHYSICAL EXAM

Digital rectal exam (DRE) to assess for prostatic masses/firmness

DIAGNOSTIC TESTS & INTERPRETATION
Lab

- PSA is produced by prostatic epithelial cells
- CaP and other conditions can distort the prostatic architecture allowing more PSA to enter the bloodstream

Initial lab tests

- Total PSA ≥4.0 ng/mL (sensitivity ~80%, specificity ~65% for CaP):
  - Rectal manipulation will not significantly increase PSA
  - Ejaculation can alter total and free PSA levels. Men should abstain from sex for 24 hours prior to blood draw
  - 5-α-Reductase inhibitors (e.g., finasteride) decrease PSA ~50%; double result to compare with premedication results
  - Prostatitis/benign prostatic hyperplasia (BPH) can cause PSA increase
- Patient-specific models to predict pathologic stage based on PSA, transrectal ultrasound (TRUS) biopsy results, and estimated clinical stage have been validated (2)[B].
- Age/race-adjusted "Normal" PSA values

Age	Asians	Blacks	Whites
40–49	0–2.0	0–2.0	0–2.5
50–59	0–3.0	0–4.0	0–3.5
60–69	0–4.0	0–4.5	0–4.5
70–79	0–5.0	0–5.5	0–6.5

Follow-Up & Special Considerations

- Total PSA velocity ≥0.75 ng/mL/year ↑ CaP suspicion
- Free PSA and age/race-adjusted PSA may be helpful in evaluating risk of CaP when total PSA is 4–10 ng/mL.
- Alkaline phosphatase ↑ with metastasis
- Consider prostate cancer if PSAD (PSA density) ≥0.15 or if PSA rises even while on 5α reductase inhibitors
- PSA/Free PSA and probability of cancer

PSA (ng/dL)	Cancer rate	% Free PSA	Cancer rate
0–2	1%	0–10%	56%
2–4	15%	10–15%	28%
4–10	25%	15–20%	20%
>10	>50%	20–25%	16%
		>25%	8%

Imaging
Initial approach

- Ultrasound-guided prostate biopsy (TRUS alone for screening is not advocated): Indication: Abnormal DRE and/or ↑ PSA
- Bone scan: Positive with metastasis; indication: PSA ≥20 ng/mL, Gleason ≥8, or bone pain (3)[B].

- If PSA >20, locally advanced, or high-grade (Gleason ≥8) disease: CT scan to assess pelvic lymph nodes or MRI (with or without endorectal coil) to assess extracapsular extension may assist treatment planning.

Diagnostic Procedures/Surgery
TRUS-guided biopsy

Pathological Findings
Small, closely packed glandular tissue, loss of basement membrane, perineural invasion, smaller prostate size is associated with higher grade disease

DIFFERENTIAL DIAGNOSIS
- Benign prostatic hyperplasia, Benign nodule prostate growth, Subacute prostatitis, Prostatic intraepithelial neoplasia
- Prostate stones

TREATMENT
Treatment decision should be reached after long discussion about options, risks, and benefits
- Treatment options:
  – T1a: Active surveillance may be appropriate
  – T1b, T1c: Candidate for prostatectomy, external-beam radiation, brachytherapy
  – T2a, T2b: Prostatectomy, external-beam radiation, brachytherapy
  – T3: Possible prostatectomy, possible radiation (generally with androgen ablation)
  – T4: Hormonal (androgen ablation) and/or radiation; chemotherapy at this time is reserved for hormone-refractory disease.
- Localized CaP
  – Surveillance
  – Radical prostatectomy: best overall survival, greatest survival benefit seen in patients <65 years old
  – External beam radiation
  – Brachytherapy: Not used to treat high risk prostate cancer alone
  – Cryotherapy: Not used to treat high risk prostate cancer alone
- Advanced or metastatic CaP
  – Androgen deprivation by medical or surgical castration
  – Numerous ongoing trials evaluating surveillance vs treatment: PIVOT, ProTeCT, StART

MEDICATION
First Line
- In androgen-*dependent* tumors, a reduction in serum testosterone is helpful in reducing tumor size and bone pain as well as for improving survival. Medical castration with gonadotropin-releasing hormone (GnRH) agonists (e.g., leuprolide or goserelin) is used most commonly. Bilateral orchiectomy is another option but is rarely done now. Indication: ≥T3 at diagnosis, poor physical status, metastatic disease, patient preference (3)
- Side effects: Osteoporosis, Gynecomastia, Erectile dysfunction/decreased libido; Flare phenomenon (disease flare) can occur owing to transient increase in testosterone levels on initiation of GnRH agonist therapy. It can be avoided by giving concurrent antiandrogen therapy for 21 days. Hot flashes, Fatigue. May increase risk for metabolic syndrome, diabetes, and cardiovascular disease

Second Line
- Combined androgen blockade with GnRH agonist and antiandrogen (e.g., bicalutamide, nilutamide, or flutamide)

- Systematic androgen suppression: Ketoconazole has a 30% response rate in those failing other antiandrogens (via suppression of adrenal androgens).
- Chemotherapy with a docetaxel-based regimen has shown survival benefit and is the preferred 1st-line chemotherapy in castration-resistant metastatic prostate cancer. Mitoxantrone-based regimen is another option .
- Bisphosphonate (zoledronic acid) every 4 weeks is recommended together with androgen-deprivation therapy or systemic chemotherapy for castration-recurrent metastatic prostate cancer. This may prevent disease-related skeletal complications such as pathologic fractures and spinal cord compression.

ADDITIONAL TREATMENT
Additional Therapies
- External-beam radiation therapy (XRT) for symptomatic bone metastasis
- Radioisotopes (e.g., samarium-153 and strontium-89) are approved for patients with multifocal symptomatic osteoblastic bone metastases that are not controllable with systemic therapy or local field XRT.

COMPLEMENTARY AND ALTERNATIVE MEDICINE
None is well supported for the treatment of CaP.

SURGERY/OTHER PROCEDURES
- Treatment options for localized CaP:
  – Active surveillance (4)[C]
  – Prostatectomy: Retropubic, robotic-assisted laparoscopic ± lymph node dissection; nerve-sparing surgery is possible if there is no extracapsular extension
  – Radiation therapy: External beam and/or brachytherapy—seed implantation
  – Cryoablation: Argon gas–based freezing of tissue; 1st for progression after failed XRT

- For clinically localized CaP (T1/T2), no data definitively proving the superiority amongst surgery, XRT, or brachytherapy. Consider age, physical status, side-effect profile, and patient preference (5)[B].

ONGOING CARE
FOLLOW-UP RECOMMENDATIONS
- Depends on treatment modality and patient-specific risk. CT/bone scan if suspected recurrence.
- Prostatectomy: PSA/DRE every 6 months for 5 years; yearly thereafter; PSA >0.2 ng/mL after surgery is suggestive of recurrence
- XRT: PSA/DRE every 3 months for 1 year; every 3–6 months for 4 years; yearly thereafter; PSA ≥2.0 ng/mL from post-XRT nadir is suggestive of recurrence.

DIET
Low-fat diet, if strictly adhered to, may slow progression of prostate cancer.

PROGNOSIS
- With early diagnosis and treatment, localized disease should be curable
- Advanced disease has a favorable prognosis if lesions are hormone-sensitive
- Advanced unresponsive disease progresses in 18 months, on average
- Prostate cancer survival by stage

Stage	TNM	10-year survival
A	T1	NC
B	T2	75%
C	T3	55%
D	N1–2	(70% at 7 years)
D	M1	15%

- Postoperative nomograms to predict patient-specific CaP recurrence rates after prostatectomy and XRT have been validated.

COMPLICATIONS
- Urinary incontinence, mild colitis, and erectile dysfunction are most common (see "Clinical Pearls").
- Treatment options for postoperative erectile dysfunction include phosphodiesterase inhibitors, intracavernosal/urethral injections, and an implantable penile prosthesis.

REFERENCES
1. Kramer BS, Hagerty KL, Justman S, et al. Use of 5alpha-reductase inhibitors for prostate cancer chemoprevention: American Society of Clinical Oncology/American Urological Association 2008 Clinical Practice Guideline. *J Urol.* 2009;181: 1642–57.
2. Partin AW, et al. Combination of prostate specific antigen, clinical stage and Gleason score to predict pathological stage of localized prostate cancer: A multi-institutional update. *JAMA.* 1999;277: 1445–51.
3. National Comprehensive Cancer Network. *Clinical practice guidelines: Prostate cancer.* http://www.nccn.org. 2009.
4. Klotz L. Active surveillance versus radical treatment for favorable-risk localized prostate cancer. *Curr Treat Options Onc.* 2006;7(5):355–62.
5. Thompson I, et al. Guideline for the management of clinically localized prostate cancer: 2007 update. 2007. http://www.auanet.org.

CODES
ICD9
185 Malignant neoplasm of prostate

CLINICAL PEARLS
- Most men with CaP are asymptomatic
- In patients taking 5α-reductase inhibitors, multiply measured PSA level by 2 to estimate actual PSA
- After nerve-sparing prostatectomy, urinary continence returns in <6 months (>50%), <9 months (~75%), and >12 months (~95%).
- The rate of erectile dysfunction:
  – After XRT: (~10–80%), brachytherapy (~15–60%).
  – After prostatectomy: Depends on age and if nerve-sparing surgery was performed. PDE5 drugs improve recovery.

PROSTATIC HYPERPLASIA, BENIGN (BPH)

David Longstroth, MD

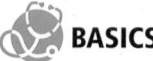

BASICS

Watchful waiting is recommended for patients with benign prostatic hyperplasia (BPH) whose clinical symptoms do not affect their quality of life. Use a validated patient questionnaire, such as the American Urological Association's Symptom Index, to establish the severity of BPH symptoms and follow their progression. alpha-Adrenergic blockers (either selective or nonselective) or 5-alpha reductase inhibitors are appropriate first-line therapies for patients bothered by BPH symptoms. Consider surgery for patients with severe obstructive symptoms who have not benefited from medical therapy or who prefer surgery as first-line treatment.

DESCRIPTION
- Benign prostatic hyperplasia (BPH) is one of the most common diseases of older men.
- Diagnosed histologically, characterized by an increase in total number of stromal and epithelial cells within the prostate gland
- Associated with bothersome lower urinary tract symptoms (LUTS) that affect quality of life
- Disease affects the renal, urologic, and reproductive systems

EPIDEMIOLOGY
- In US, near universal development in men, age-dependent
- Average prostate weighs 20 grams in normal 20–30-year-old male

Incidence
- No clear identifying characteristics
- Commonly involves prostate volume >30 mL and high prostate symptom score

Prevalence
From 8% in men aged 31–40, to 40–50% in men 51–60, and over 80% in men <80 years old

RISK FACTORS
- Increased risk of BPH with higher free prostate-specific antigen (PSA) levels, heart disease, and use of β-blockers
- Decreased risk with cigarette smoking, higher physical activity
- Intact testes (BPH rare in eunuchs)
- No evidence of increased or decreased risk with smoking, alcohol, or any dietary factors
- Low androgen levels from cirrhosis/chronic alcoholism can reduce the risk of BPH

Genetics
- Males who had 1st-degree relative with BPH are at increased risk.
- Race has some influence on risk for BPH severe enough to require surgery.
- Black men less than 65 years old may need treatment more often than white men.
- Asians have a lower risk for nocturia, while risks for blacks and whites are similar.

GENERAL PREVENTION
Disease appears to be part of the aging process.

PATHOPHYSIOLOGY
- Older age and functional Leydig cells in testes are determinant.
- BPH is rare in men with hypogonadism onset before 40 years not treated with androgens.

ETIOLOGY
- BPH develops in the periurethral or transition zone of the prostate.
- Hyperplastic nodules of stromal and epithelial components increase glandular components.

COMMONLY ASSOCIATED CONDITIONS
- LUTS:
  – Irritative symptoms: Frequency, urgency, dysuria, nocturia
  – Obstructive symptoms: Poor stream, hesitancy, terminal dribbling, incomplete voiding, overflow incontinence
- BPH symptoms are a strong and independent risk factor for sexual dysfunction, including erectile dysfunction and ejaculatory disorders (1)[C].

DIAGNOSIS

HISTORY
- Symptom scores such as American Urological Association (AUA). It consists of 7 questions, each of which is scored on a scale of 0 (not present) to 5 (almost always present). Symptoms are classified as mild (total score 0–7), moderate (total score 8–19) and severe (total score 20–35):
  – Frequency
  – Nocturia
  – Weak urinary stream
  – Hesitancy
  – Intermittence
  – Incomplete emptying
  – Urgency
- Gross hematuria
- History of type 2 diabetes, which can cause nocturia and is a risk factor for BPH
- Symptoms of neurologic disease that would suggest a neurogenic bladder
- Sexual dysfunction, which is correlated with LUTS
- History of urethral trauma, urethritis, or urethral instrumentation that could lead to urethral stricture
- Family history of BPH and prostate cancer
- Treatment with drugs that can impair bladder function (anticholinergic drugs) or increase outflow resistance (sympathomimetic drugs)

PHYSICAL EXAM
- Digital rectal exam finding of enlarged prostate, but size does not always correlate with symptoms
- Percussion to detect distended bladder, particularly if post-void
- Signs of renal failure due to obstructive uropathy (edema, pallor, pruritus, ecchymoses, nutritional deficiencies)

DIAGNOSTIC TESTS & INTERPRETATION
Lab
Initial lab tests
- PSA may be elevated, but usually <10 ng/mL (10 μg/L). Acute urinary retention, prostatitis, urinary tract instrumentation, or prostatic infarction may elevate PSA.
- Urinalysis: Pyuria if stones or infection present, pH changes due to chronic residual urine
- Urine culture positive (sometimes due to chronic residual urine)
- Blood urea nitrogen and creatinine (if concerns for uremia)

Follow-Up & Special Considerations
- Uroflow: Volume voided per unit time (peak flow <10 mL/sec is abnormal)
- Post-void residual: Either with catheterization or bladder ultrasound (>100 mL demonstrates incomplete emptying)

Imaging
Initial approach
Post-void residual in order to detect obstruction/distended bladder

Follow-Up & Special Considerations
- Transrectal ultrasound: Assessment of gland size; not necessary in the routine evaluation
- Abdominal ultrasound: Can demonstrate increased post-void residual or hydronephrosis; not necessary in the routine evaluation

Geriatric Considerations
Drugs to be avoided include anticholinergics, antihistamines, sympathomimetics, tricyclic antidepressants, narcotics, and skeletal muscle relaxants when possible.

Diagnostic Procedures/Surgery
- Pressure-flow studies (urine flow vs voiding pressures):
  – Best test to determine etiology of voiding symptoms
  – Obstructive pattern shows high voiding pressures with low flow rate
- Cystoscopy:
  – Demonstrates presence, configuration, and site of obstructive tissue
  – Helps to show stricture, stones
  – May help determine best minimally invasive therapeutic option
  – Not recommended in initial evaluation unless other factors such as hematuria are present

Pathological Findings
Confirmation obtained by biopsy, resection, or surgical removal

DIFFERENTIAL DIAGNOSIS
- Obstructive:
  – Prostate cancer
  – Urethral stricture or valves
  – Bladder neck contracture (usually secondary to prostate surgery)
  – Prostatitis
  – Inability of bladder neck or external sphincter to relax appropriately during voiding
- Neurologic:
  – Spinal cord injury
  – Stroke
  – Parkinsonism
  – Multiple sclerosis
- Medical:
  – Poorly controlled diabetes mellitus
  – Congestive heart failure (CHF)
- Pharmacologic:
  – Diuretics
  – Sympathomimetics (e.g., cold medications)
  – Anticholinergics
- Other:
  – Bladder carcinoma
  – Overactive bladder
  – Bladder calculi
  – Urinary tract infection

TREATMENT

MEDICATION

The AUA recommends watchful waiting for patients with mild symptoms or without bothersome LUTS who have not developed a serious complication.

First Line

- α-adrenergic antagonists have been demonstrated to be more effective than other methods alone (2)[A]:
  - Nonselective, reduce prostatic smooth muscle tone, improving urinary flow: (3)
    - Terazosin (Hytrin): 1–10 mg/d p.o. (4)[A]
    - Doxazosin (Cardura): 1–8 mg/d p.o.
  - Selective, may produce fewer side effects. Generally more expensive:
    - Tamsulosin (Flomax): 0.4 mg/d p.o. (5)[A]
    - Alfuzosin (Uroxatral): 10 mg/d p.o.
- 5-α-reductase inhibitors reduce prostatic volume (useful if demonstrable prostatic enlargement) (6)[A]:
  - Finasteride (Proscar): 5 mg/d p.o.
  - Dutasteride (Avodart): 0.5 mg/d p.o.
  - Also useful in controlling prostatic bleeding
- Combination therapy of α-blocker plus 5-α-reductase inhibitor is superior to monotherapy when used for very large prostates and evaluated over at least 4.5 years 7
  - Dutasteride and tamsulosin combination known as Jalyn
- Anticholinergic agents may be combined with α-blockers for relief of persistent storage symptoms
- Contraindications:
  - α-blockers can cause orthostatic hypotension; less risk with tamsulosin and alfuzosin.
  - See specific recommendations for α-blocker use with phosphodiesterase type-5 inhibitors (for erectile dysfunction).

ALERT
5-α-reductase inhibitors reduce PSA by 1/2, so PSA should be doubled for purposes of screening for prostate cancer.

ADDITIONAL TREATMENT
General Measures
- Patients in urinary retention require bladder drainage.
- If catheterization is difficult, consider coude catheter or flexible cystoscopy.
- Consider possible postobstructive diuresis; if present, monitor electrolytes.
- Avoid prolonged periods of not voiding.
- Avoid sympathomimetic and anticholinergic medications.

Issues for Referral
- Recurrent UTIs
- Hematuria
- Failure to respond to medical therapy
- Bladder stones

COMPLEMENTARY AND ALTERNATIVE MEDICINE
- Phytotherapy
- Saw palmetto (Serenoa repens) has shown mild improvement of peak flow rates and appears to work by blocking 5-α-reductase.

SURGERY/OTHER PROCEDURES
- Indications for surgery:
  - Urinary retention due to prostatic obstruction, recurrent
  - Intractable symptoms due to prostatic obstruction AUA sx score >8 and bother)
  - Obstructive uropathy (renal insufficiency)
  - Recurrent or persistent UTIs due to prostatic obstruction
  - Recurrent gross hematuria due to enlarged prostate
  - Bladder calculi
- Surgical procedures:
  - Transurethral resection of the prostate (TURP): Gold standard
  - Open prostatectomy: Treatment of choice for patients with extremely large prostates (>100 g)
  - Transurethral incision of the prostate: Treatment of choice for men with obstruction and small prostates
  - Transurethral laser ablation: Holmium laser ablation of the tissue; useful in patients on anticoagulant therapy
  - Transurethral needle ablation: Office-based minimally invasive approach usually used with small prostates
  - Transurethral microwave thermotherapy: Office-based minimally invasive approach usually used with small prostates
  - Transurethral laser resection/enucleation
  - UroLume stent placement: Not a primary treatment alternative for the standard patient, but considered in those too ill for other surgical procedures
- Complications of TURP:
  - Bleeding can be significant
  - TUR syndrome: Hyponatremia secondary to absorption of hypotonic irrigant
  - Retrograde ejaculation
  - Urinary incontinence

 ONGOING CARE

FOLLOW-UP RECOMMENDATIONS
Patient more likely to void after surgery or illness when ambulatory/able to stand over toilet

Patient Monitoring
- Symptom index (IPSS) monitored every 3–12 months
- Digital rectal exam yearly
- PSA yearly: Should not be checked while patient is in retention, recently catheterized, or within a week of any surgical procedure to the prostate
- Consider monitoring postvoid residual if elevated

DIET
Avoid large boluses of oral or IV fluids or alcohol intake.

PATIENT EDUCATION
- *The Prostate Book*, published by Krames Communications, 312 90th St, Daly City, CA 94015-1898
- National Kidney and Urologic Diseases Information Clearinghouse, Box NKUDIC, Bethesda, MD 20893; (301) 468-6345

PROGNOSIS
- Symptoms improve or stabilize in 70–80% of patients; 20–30% require treatment because of worsening symptoms.
- 25% of men with LUTS will have persistent storage symptoms after prostatectomy:
  - LUTS can be divided into 3 groups: Filling/storage symptoms, voiding symptoms, and postmicturition symptoms
  - Filling/storage symptoms include frequency, nocturia, urgency, and urge incontinence.
- Of men with BPH, 11–33% have occult prostate cancer.

COMPLICATIONS
- Urinary retention (acute or chronic)
- Bladder stones
- Prostatitis
- Renal failure
- Hematuria

REFERENCES

1. Rosen R, Altwein J, Boyle P, et al. Lower urinary tract symptoms and male sexual dysfunction: the multinational survey of the aging male (MSAM-7). *Eur Urol.* 2003;44:637–49.
2. Rich KT. FPIN's clinical inquiries. Medical treatment of benign prostatic hyperplasia. *Am Fam Physician.* 2008;77:665–6.
3. Neal RH, Keister D, et al. What's best for your patient with BPH? *J Fam Pract.* 2009;58:241–7.
4. Wilt TJ, et al. Terazosin for benign prostatic hyperplasia. *Cochrane Database Syst Rev.* 2002;4:CD003851. DOI:10.1002/14651858. CD003851.
5. Wilt TJ, et al. Tamsulosin for benign prostatic hyperplasia. *Cochrane Database Syst Rev.* 2003;1:CD002081. DOI:10.1002/14651858. CD002081.
6. AUA Guidelines: Guideline on the Management of Benign Prostatic Hyperplasia (BPH): Updated 2006. http://www.AUAnet.org.
7. Hollingsworth JM, Wei JT, et al. Does the combination of an alpha1-adrenergic antagonist with a 5alpha-reductase inhibitor improve urinary symptoms more than either monotherapy? *Curr Opin Urol.* 2010;20:1–6.

CODES

ICD9
- 600.20 Benign localized hyperplasia of prostate without urinary obstruction and other LUTS
- 600.21 Benign localized hyperplasia of prostate with urinary obstruction and other LUTS

CLINICAL PEARLS
- Although medical therapy has changed the management of BPH, it appears that it has only delayed the need for TURP by 10–15 years, not eliminated it.
- Urinary retention, obstructive uropathy, recurrent UTIs, bladder calculi, and recurrent hematuria are indications for surgical management of BPH.
- Indications for referral include recurrent UTIs, elevated PSA, failure of medical therapy, hematuria, retention, and patient desire.

PROSTATITIS
Alfred Chege Gitu, MD

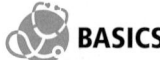

BASICS

DESCRIPTION
- Inflammatory or painful condition affecting the prostate gland; variety of etiologies
- National Institutes of Health's (NIH) prostatitis classification:
  - Acute infection (NIH class I): Febrile illness with perineal pain, dysuria, and obstructive symptoms
  - Chronic bacterial prostatitis (NIH class II): Recurrent infection with pain and voiding disturbances
  - Chronic abacterial prostatitis/chronic pelvic pain syndrome (NIH class III):
    - Inflammatory (NIH class IIIa): Significant inflammatory cells in prostatic secretions, postprostatic massage urine or semen
    - Noninflammatory (NIH class IIIb): Insignificant number of inflammatory cells (prostatosis)
  - Asymptomatic inflammatory prostatitis (NIH class IV): Incidental finding during prostate biopsy for infertility, cancer workup
- System(s) affected: Renal/Urologic; Reproductive

EPIDEMIOLOGY
Incidence
- 2 million cases annually in US
- Predominant age: 30–50 years, sexually active; chronic more common in ages >50 years of age
- Bacterial prostatitis occurs more frequently in patients with HIV.

Prevalence
2.2–9.7% of male population

RISK FACTORS
- Age >50 years
- Prostatic calculi
- Urinary tract infection (UTI)
- Trauma (e.g., bicycle, horseback riding)
- Dehydration
- Sexual abstinence
- Chronic indwelling catheter
- Intermittent catheterization
- HIV infection
- Urethral stricture
- Cystoscopy
- Urethral dilatation
- Transurethral resection of prostate
- Transrectal biopsy

GENERAL PREVENTION
Suppression therapy may benefit patients with chronic bacterial prostatitis.

PATHOPHYSIOLOGY
- Extension of UTI
- May occur following manipulation/biopsy of prostate or urethra
- Ascending infection through urethra

ETIOLOGY
- Infectious: NIH classes I and II:
  - Aerobic gram-negative bacteria (e.g., *E. coli, Pseudomonas, Klebsiella, Proteus*), *N. gonorrhoeae*, Enterobacteriaceae, *B. pseudomallei*)
  - Miscellaneous: *C. trachomatis, Ureaplasma*, trichomoniasis
  - Gram-positive bacteria (*S. faecalis, S. aureus*)
  - Organisms suspected but unproven (*S. epidermidis, S. micrococci*, non–group D *Streptococcus*, diphtheroids)
  - Uncommon: *M. tuberculosis*, parasitic, mycoses (blastomycosis, coccidioidomycosis, cryptococcus, histoplasmosis, paracoccidiomycosis, candidiasis)
- Nonbacterial: Cause unknown: Leading theory suggests nonrelaxation (spasm) of the internal urinary sphincter and pelvic floor striated muscles leading to increased prostatic urethral pressure and intraprostatic urinary reflux.

COMMONLY ASSOCIATED CONDITIONS
- Prostatic hypertrophy
- Cystitis
- Urethritis
- Pyelonephritis
- Sexual dysfunction

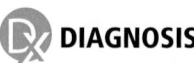

DIAGNOSIS

HISTORY
- Acute prostatitis (NIH class I):
  - Fever, chills, malaise
  - Low back pain, myalgias
  - Prostatodynia, perineal pain
  - Obstructive voiding symptoms
  - Frequency, urgency, dysuria, nocturia
- Chronic prostatitis (NIH classes II and III):
  - Prostatodynia, perineal pain
  - Dysuria, irritative voiding
  - Lower abdominal pain
  - Low back, scrotal, and/or penile pain
  - Pain on ejaculation
  - Hematospermia

PHYSICAL EXAM
- Very tender boggy prostate on rectal exam
- Prostate may be warm, swollen, firm, or irregular.

ALERT
Avoid massage of the prostate in acute bacterial prostatitis; may induce iatrogenic bacteremia.

DIAGNOSTIC TESTS & INTERPRETATION
Lab

Initial lab tests
- Suspected acute prostatitis (NIH class I):
  - Urinalysis (UA), urine and blood cultures, urine Gram stain
  - Complete blood count/differential
- Suspected chronic bacterial prostatitis or abacterial prostatitis (NIH class II or III):
  - Fractional urine exam (4-glass test) (1)[B],(2)[A]:
    - VB1 (voided bladder 1): Initial 10 mL urine from urethra
    - VB2: Next 200 mL discarded; then midstream urine from bladder
    - EPS: Expressed prostate secretion after prostate massage
    - VB3: Urine *after* prostate massage

- Post-VB3 semen culture increases sensitivity and specificity (2)[A].
- Many clinicians employ 2 glass test (VB2 and VB3) only (1)[B].

- Specimen handling:
  - UA, culture, sensitivities, Gram stain on all samples
  - pH of EPS
  - Bacterial antigen-specific IgA and IgG levels in EPS
  - Wet mount of EPS
- Interpretation:
  - 10–15 white blood cells (WBCs) per high-powered field in VB3 suggest bacterial prostatitis.
  - Macrophages containing fat (oval bodies) suggest bacterial prostatitis.
  - A positive culture in EPS, VB3, or post a VB3 semen sample but not VB1 or VB2 is diagnostic of bacterial prostatitis.
  - In acute bacterial prostatitis, serum and EPS fluid bacterial antigen-specific IgA and IgG can be detected immediately after the onset of the infection. Level declines over 6–12 months after successful antibiotic therapy.
  - Bacteria count is less in chronic prostatitis.
  - In chronic bacterial prostatitis, no serum IgG elevation is seen, whereas EPS fluid IgA and IgG levels are increased. With antibiotic therapy, IgG levels return to normal in several months, but IgA levels remain elevated for 2 years.
  - Prostatic fluid is alkaline in chronic bacterial prostatitis.
  - Inflammatory cells (WBCs) with a negative culture (although false-negative cultures are not uncommon) suggest abacterial prostatitis.
  - No abnormal findings with chronic prostatitis without inflammation (this misnomer refers to patients with symptoms such as perineal pain, ejaculatory pain, and lower abdominal pain but not having inflammatory changes on lab studies).
  - Prostate-specific antigen (PSA) level is increased with acute prostatitis (do not order PSA determination until at least 1 month after prostatitis is treated).
- Drugs that may alter lab results: Antibiotics

Follow-Up & Special Considerations
- Acute bacterial: Urinalysis and culture 30 days after initiating treatment
- Chronic bacterial: Urinalysis and culture every 30 days (may take several months of treatment to clear)

Imaging

Initial approach
- Imaging not required in most cases
- Computed tomography scan or magnetic resonance imaging if malignancy or abscess suspected
- Transrectal ultrasound if prostatic calculi or abscess suspected

Diagnostic Procedures/Surgery
- Needle biopsy or aspiration for culture
- Urodynamic testing (prostatodynia)
- Cystoscopy (in persistent nonbacterial prostatitis to rule out bladder cancer, interstitial cystitis)

DIFFERENTIAL DIAGNOSIS
- Cystitis (bacterial, interstitial)
- Urethritis
- Pyelonephritis
- Malignancy
- Obstructive calculus
- Foreign body
- Acute urinary retention

 TREATMENT

MEDICATION
First Line
- Acute bacterial (outpatient):
  - Trimethoprim-sulfamethoxazole, 1 DS tab b.i.d. p.o. × 4–6 weeks or
  - Fluoroquinolone (ciprofloxacin 500 mg p.o. every 12 hours or levofloxacin 500 mg p.o. once daily) × 4–6 weeks
  - If gram-positive cocci are seen in initial urine Gram stain, start with amoxicillin 500 mg p.o. every 8 hours.
  - Adjust antibiotics once culture and sensitivities report is available.
  - Local sensitivity pattern should guide therapy.
- Acute bacterial (inpatient): Ampicillin 1–3 g IV divided q6h or fluoroquinolone (ciprofloxacin 400 mg IV every 12 hours or levofloxacin 750 mg every 24 hours) PLUS aminoglycoside, gentamicin 2 mg/kg IV loading dose, 1.7 mg/kg IV q8h maintenance; begin oral therapy after afebrile for 24–48 hours.
- Chronic bacterial (NIH class II): (3)[B]:
  - Fluoroquinolone (e.g., levofloxacin 500 mg p.o. once daily for 4 weeks (4,5)[A], or ciprofloxacin 500 mg b.i.d. p.o. for 4–12 weeks
  - Combination therapy with azithromycin may help to eradicate unusual pathogens.
  - Anti-inflammatory agents for pain symptoms and alpha-adrenergic receptor antagonists for urinary symptoms
- Chronic abacterial prostatitis (NIH class III):
  - No universally effective treatment
  - Treatment choice is usually by trial and error:
    - α-blockers better than placebo in some trials (6)[A]
    - Tamsulosin 0.2 mg p.o. once daily at bedtime for at least 6 months, Continue if there is response (7)[A].
    - No evidence of benefit from antibiotics
- Contraindications: Drug allergies
- Precautions:
  - Renal disease
  - Hepatic disease
  - Glucose-6-phosphate dehydrogenase deficiency may manifest with sulfonamides or nonsteroidal anti-inflammatory drugs (NSAIDs).
  - Significant possible interactions: Fluoroquinolones, magnesium/aluminum antacids, theophylline, probenecid, NSAIDs, warfarin

Second Line
- Piperacillin or ticarcillin with aminoglycoside, erythromycin, tetracycline, cephalexin, fluoroquinolones, dicloxacillin, nafcillin IV, vancomycin IV
- Finasteride (in patients >45 years of age, category IIIa inflammatory chronic prostatitis/chronic pelvic pain syndrome, and enlarged prostate glands)
- Nonbacterial: May benefit from erythromycin, doxycycline, trimethoprim-sulfamethoxazole

ADDITIONAL TREATMENT
General Measures
- Analgesics/antipyretics/stool softeners
- Some anecdotal data suggest that elimination of caffeine may reduce symptoms of chronic prostatitis in younger men.
- Hydration
- Sitz baths to relieve pain and spasm
- Suprapubic catheter for urinary retention
- Anxiolytics, antidepressants

Issues for Referral
Urology referral for surgical drainage if an abscess is persistent after ≥1 week of therapy

Additional Therapies
Psychotherapy if sexual dysfunction

COMPLEMENTARY AND ALTERNATIVE MEDICINE
Neuromodulation, acupuncture, heat therapy; limited to no data to support

SURGERY/OTHER PROCEDURES
Surgical resection for intractable chronic disease or to drain an abscess

IN-PATIENT CONSIDERATIONS
Admission Criteria
- Proven or suspected abscess
- Unstable vital signs (sepsis)
- Immunocompromised

 ONGOING CARE

FOLLOW-UP RECOMMENDATIONS
- Most improve in 3–4 weeks.
- Consider prostatic abscess in patients who do not respond well to therapy.

Patient Monitoring
- NIH Chronic Prostatitis Symptom Index: 13 items tabulated into 3 domain scores:
  - Pain
  - Urinary symptoms
  - Quality of life
- See http://www2.niddk.nih.gov/.

PROGNOSIS
- Often prolonged and difficult to cure; 55–97% cure rate depending on population and drug used
- 20% have reinfection or persistent infection.

COMPLICATIONS
- Prostatic abscess (common in HIV-infected)
- Gram-negative sepsis, bacteremia
- Urinary retention
- Epididymitis
- Chronic bacterial prostatitis (with acute prostatitis)
- Metastatic infection (spinal, sacroiliac)

REFERENCES

1. Benway BM, Moon TD et al. Bacterial prostatitis. *Urol Clin North Am.* 2008;35:23–32; v.
2. Magri V, Wagenlehner FM, Montanari E, et al. Semen analysis in chronic bacterial prostatitis: diagnostic and therapeutic implications. *Asian J Androl.* 2009;11:461–77.
3. Murphy AB, Macejko A, Taylor A, et al. Chronic prostatitis: management strategies. *Drugs.* 2009;69:71–84.
4. Paglia M, Peterson J, Fisher AC, et al. Safety and efficacy of levofloxacin 750 mg for 2 weeks or 3 weeks compared with levofloxacin 500 mg for 4 weeks in treating chronic bacterial prostatitis. *Current medical research and opinion.* 2010;
5. Naber KG, Roscher K, Botto H, et al. Oral levofloxacin 500 mg once daily in the treatment of chronic bacterial prostatitis. *Int J Antimicrob Agents.* 2008;32:145–53.
6. Dimitrakov, et al. Management of chronic prostatitis/chronic pelvic pain syndrome: An evidence based approach. *Urology.* 2006;67(5).
7. Chen Y, Wu X, Liu J, et al. Effects of a 6-month course of tamsulosin for chronic prostatitis/chronic pelvic pain syndrome: a multicenter, randomized trial. *World journal of urology.* 2010;

ADDITIONAL READING
- McNaughton CM, et al. Interventions for abacterial prostatitis. *Cochrane Database Sys Rev.* 2006:4.
- Mohammed A, Chinegwundoh F et al. Prostatitis syndrome, an overview. *Arch Ital Urol Androl.* 2008;80:115–22.
- Nickel JC et al. Treatment of chronic prostatitis/chronic pelvic pain syndrome. *Int J Antimicrob Agents.* 2008;31(Suppl 1):S112–6.

See Also (Topic, Algorithm, Electronic Media Element)
Prostatic Cancer; Prostatic Hyperplasia Benign (BPH); Urinary Tract Infection in Males
Algorithm: Hematuria

 CODES

ICD9
- 601.0 Acute prostatitis
- 601.1 Chronic prostatitis
- 601.9 Prostatitis, unspecified

CLINICAL PEARLS
- Prostatic massage is contraindicated in acute prostatitis.
- Antibiotic therapy is not proven to be effective in chronic abacterial prostatitis (NIH class III).
- At least 30 days of antibiotic therapy is required for acute prostatitis.

PROTEIN C DEFICIENCY

Marc Jeffrey Kahn, MD
Rebecca Kruse-Jarres, MD, MPH

 BASICS

DESCRIPTION
- Protein C is a vitamin K–dependent factor made by the liver that becomes activated when thrombin binds to the endothelial receptor thrombomodulin.
- Activated protein C, with protein S as a cofactor, inactivates factors Va and VIIIa.
- Patients with protein C deficiency have a thrombotic disorder that primarily affects the venous system but can also affect the arterial system.
- System(s) affected: Cardiovascular; Hemic/Lymphatic/Immunologic; Pulmonary

EPIDEMIOLOGY
Prevalence
- 0.3% of normal individuals
- 4–5% of persons with VT
- Predominant age: Mean age of first thrombosis is 45 years
- Predominant sex: Male = Female

RISK FACTORS
Genetics
Patients heterozygous for protein C deficiency who start warfarin without concomitant heparin can develop warfarin-induced skin necrosis because the half-life of other vitamin K–dependent clotting factors, prothrombin, factor IX, and factor X is much longer than that of protein C (4–8 h). These patients develop extremely low levels of protein C and develop necrosis of the skin over central areas of the body such as the breast, abdomen, buttocks, and genitalia (1)[A].

GENERAL PREVENTION
Since protein C deficiency is a congenital disease, there are no preventive measures.

ETIOLOGY
- Polymorphisms in the promoter region of the protein C gene can affect antigen levels. At least 150 mutations have been described in the protein C gene that can lead to functional deficiency.
- Acquired protein C deficiency can occur with liver disease, and rare patients can develop inhibitors to activated protein C. Neonates have lower levels of protein C than adults.

COMMONLY ASSOCIATED CONDITIONS
- Deep and superficial venous thrombosis, often spontaneous
- Up to 50% of homozygotes will have thrombosis.
- Homozygosity is associated with catastrophic thrombotic complications at birth: *purpura fulminans*.
- Sites of thrombosis can be unusual, including the mesentery and cerebral veins.
- Arterial thrombosis is rare.
- Skin necrosis can be seen in patients on warfarin.

 DIAGNOSIS

HISTORY
VT at age <40 without another etiology; thrombosis in unusual locations (e.g., mesentery, sagittal sinus, portal vein) with a family history of thrombosis or spontaneous abortion

PHYSICAL EXAM
Normal

DIAGNOSTIC TESTS & INTERPRETATION
Lab
Initial lab tests
- Protein C activity assay using a snake venom protease to activate protein C
- Immunoassay for quantitative assessment of protein C level
- Drugs that may alter lab results:
  – Oral contraceptives can raise protein C levels.
  – Warfarin reduces protein C levels.
  – Patients should be off warfarin for 2–3 weeks before reliable testing (2)[C].
- Disorders that may alter lab results:
  – Liver disease reduces protein C levels.
  – Acute thrombosis can lower protein C levels. Repeat confirmatory test of low protein C level at a separate time is advisable.

DIFFERENTIAL DIAGNOSIS
- Factor V Leiden (causes resistance to activated protein C, not a deficiency of protein C)
- Protein S deficiency
- Antithrombin deficiency
- Dysfibrinogenemia
- Dysplasminogenemia
- Homocystinemia
- Prothrombin 20210 mutation
- Elevated factor VIII levels

 TREATMENT

Of active thrombosis and follow-up period

MEDICATION
First Line
- Low-molecular-weight heparin (LMWH) (1)[A]: Continue until therapeutic on warfarin and for at least 5 days:
  – Enoxaparin (Lovenox) 1 mg/kg SC b.i.d.
- Alternatively, enoxaparin 1.5 mg/kg/d SC, which is slightly less effective. Continue until therapeutic on warfarin and for at least 5 days:
  – Fondaparinux (Arixtra): 7.5 mg SC every day
  – Tinzaparin (Innohep): 175 anti-Xa IU/kg/d SQ
  – Dalteparin (Fragmin): 200 units/kg/d
- Oral anticoagulant: Warfarin (Coumadin) 5 mg/d p.o. initially and maintained on warfarin with an INR of 2–3 for at least 3–6 months (1)[A]
- Contraindications:
  – Active bleeding precludes anticoagulation; risk of bleeding is a relative contraindication to long-term anticoagulation.
  – Warfarin is contraindicated in patients with a prior history of warfarin-induced skin necrosis.
- Precautions:
  – Observe patient for signs of embolization, further thrombosis, or bleeding.
  – Avoid IM injections.
  – Periodically check stool and urine for occult blood, monitor CBC, including platelets.
  – Heparin: Thrombocytopenia and/or paradoxical thrombosis with thrombocytopenia
  – Warfarin: Necrotic skin lesions (typically breasts, thighs, and buttocks)
  – LMWH: Adjust dose in renal insufficiency.

- Significant possible interactions:
  – Agents that intensify the response to oral anticoagulants: Alcohol, allopurinol, amiodarone, anabolic steroids, androgens, many antimicrobials, cimetidine, chloral hydrate, disulfiram, all NSAIDs, sulfinpyrazone, tamoxifen, thyroid hormone, vitamin E, ranitidine, salicylates, acetaminophen
  – Agents that diminish the response to oral anticoagulants: Aminoglutethimide, antacids, barbiturates, carbamazepine, cholestyramine, diuretics, griseofulvin, rifampin, oral contraceptives

Second Line
- Heparin 80 mg/kg IV bolus followed by 18 mg/kg/h; adjust dose depending on PPT.
- In patients requiring large daily doses of heparin, measure an anti-Xa level for dose guidance.
- Alternatively, unfractionated heparin can be given at 35,000 U/24 h SC, with subsequent dosing to maintain a therapeutic aPTT (3)[C].

ADDITIONAL TREATMENT
General Measures
- Routine anticoagulation for asymptomatic patients with protein C deficiency is not recommended (1)[A].
- Anticoagulation for 6–12 months is recommended for patients with protein C deficiency and a 1st thrombosis.
- Some argue for lifetime anticoagulation; data are limited.
- Anticoagulation for life is indicated for patients with protein C deficiency and recurrent thromboses.
- The role of family screening for protein C deficiency is unclear because most patients with this mutation do not have thrombosis. Screening should be considered for women considering using oral contraceptives or pregnancy with a family history of protein C deficiency (4)[B].
- Treatment with LMWH is recommended over unfractionated heparin, unless the patient has severe renal failure (3)[B].
- Treat as outpatient, if possible (3)[B].
- Initiate warfarin together with heparin on the 1st treatment day and discontinue heparin after 5 days and when INR >2 (3)[A].

Issues for Referral
Patients with suspected protein C deficiency should be seen by a hematologist.

SURGERY/OTHER PROCEDURES
- Anticoagulation must be held for surgical interventions.
- For most patients with DVT, recommendations are against routine use of vena cava filter in addition to anticoagulation (3)[A].

IN-PATIENT CONSIDERATIONS
Admission Criteria
- Life-threatening VT
- Significant bleeding while on anticoagulant therapy

Nursing
Look for signs of bleeding while on anticoagulation therapy.

 ## ONGOING CARE

FOLLOW-UP RECOMMENDATIONS
Patient Monitoring
- Warfarin requires periodic (monthly after initial stabilization) monitoring of the INR to maintain a range of 2–3.
- LMWH is the treatment of choice in pregnancy. Periodic monitoring with anti-Xa levels is recommended in these patients.

DIET
Unrestricted

PATIENT EDUCATION
- Patients should be educated about use of oral anticoagulant therapy if taking such.
- Avoid NSAIDs while on warfarin.

PROGNOSIS
- When compared with normal individuals, persons with protein C deficiency have normal life spans.
- By age 45, half the people heterozygous for protein C deficiency will have VT that is spontaneous half the time.

COMPLICATIONS
Recurrent thrombosis (requires indefinite anticoagulation)

REFERENCES
1. Bick RL. Prothrombin G20210A mutation, antithrombin, heparin cofactor II, protein C, and protein S defects. *Hematol Oncol Clin North Am*. 2003;17:9–36.
2. Moll S. Thrombophilias–practical implications and testing caveats. *J Thromb Thrombolysis*. 2006; 21:7–15.
3. Büller HR, Agnelli G, Hull RD, et al. Antithrombotic therapy for venous thromboembolic disease: the Seventh ACCP Conference on Antithrombotic and Thrombolytic Therapy. *Chest*. 2004;126: 401S–428S.
4. Langlois NJ, Wells PS. Risk of venous thromboembolism in relatives of symptomatic probands with thrombophilia: a systematic review. *Thromb Haemost*. 2003;90:17–26.

 ## CODES

ICD9
289.81 Primary hypercoagulable state

CLINICAL PEARLS
- Asymptomatic patients with protein C deficiency do not need prophylactic anticoagulation because the risk of thrombosis is low.
- Patients with protein C deficiency who have DVT should be anticoagulated for at least 6 months.

PROTEIN ENERGY MALNUTRITION

Melissa Phillips Black, MD
Thomas Price, MD

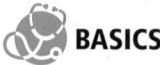

BASICS

DESCRIPTION
- Protein–energy malnutrition (PEM) is present when sufficient energy and/or protein is not available to meet metabolic demands, leading to impairment in normal physiologic processes.
- System(s) affected: Immunologic; GI; Endocrine/Metabolic; Hematologic; Musculoskeletal; Integumentary; Neurologic
- PEM affects all age groups and is often due to impaired access to proper nutrition.
- Malnutrition in children is a major underlying factor in ~5 million preventable deaths annually, with two distinct phenotypes:
  - *Marasmus* is a wasting condition resulting from deficiency of calories and protein. Weight is decreased relative to that expected for the patient's height/length.
  - *Kwashiorkor* is distinguished by generalized edema and is associated with low protein relative to caloric intake. Resulting fat deposition in liver results in ascites. Weight is normal or elevated owing to increased body fluid.

EPIDEMIOLOGY
- Children:
  - Most commonly <5 years of age; both sexes are affected equally.
  - Globally, malnutrition increases morbidity and mortality from other common childhood diseases.
- Older patients:
  - Highest risk in population >75 years of age
  - Increased mortality and morbidity, including pressure ulcers, infection, and cognitive status changes (see Delirium).
- Malnutrition may be common, but it is difficult to recognize in hospital populations (1).

Prevalence
- Worldwide, >70 million children suffer from moderate and severe acute malnutrition.
- Prevalence in older patients is between 29% and 61% of population (2)[C].

RISK FACTORS
- Nutritional:
  - Prolonged and severe reduction of intake
  - Anorexia nervosa
- Underlying illnesses:
  - Fever, infection, trauma, burns, and other hypercatabolic states
  - Malabsorptive and maldigestive states
  - Protein-losing enteropathy, nephrotic syndrome, enteric fistulas
  - Metabolic disorders (diabetes, hyperthyroidism)
  - Chronic cardiac or lung disease
  - Psychiatric disorders (dementia, depression)
  - Any prolonged hospitalization (3)
- Other states in which requirements are increased:
  - Pregnancy and lactation
  - Growth and development during infancy, childhood, and adolescence

GENERAL PREVENTION
- Observation and recording of patients' nutritional intake and body mass index
- In children, routine record of anthropomorphic measurements and developmental milestones
- Early recognition of increased nutritional requirements during stress, infection, and other medical illness
- Frequent interactions among physician, nurse, and dietitian to assess nutritional needs
- Emphasis on food security and nutritional education

ETIOLOGY
- Inadequate dietary intake
- Increased metabolic demands
- Increased nutrient losses

COMMONLY ASSOCIATED CONDITIONS
- Infection: Weakened immune system, predisposing to bacterial, viral, and parasitic infections
- Electrolyte disturbances: Loss of cellular integrity and diminished transmembrane pump activity; renal dysfunction
- Hypoglycemia: Decreased glycogen stores and increased glucose utilization (as in infection or trauma)
- Micronutrient deficiencies: Vitamins, including B complex, folic acid, iron, magnesium
- Wounds: Pressure ulcers in older patients (increased incidence if reduced mobility)

DIAGNOSIS

HISTORY
- Quantity and quality of nutritional intake
- Presence of vomiting and/or diarrhea
- Dysphagia, dental and oral health disorders
- Urine output (assess for dehydration)
- Chronic medical illness
- Weight loss, stunted growth, subcutaneous fat and muscle wasting
- Impaired work capacity
- Falls and/or reduced physical activity
- Impaired concentration/cognitive function
- Decreased hand grip strength
- Delayed wound healing and recovery
- Lethargy, early satiety, vomiting, and constipation
- Subnormal heart rate, BP, and core body temperature
- In children:
  - Delayed puberty
  - Diminished cognitive and psychosocial development

PHYSICAL EXAM
- Clinical signs: Muscle wasting, peripheral edema, glossitis, cheilosis, loss of vibratory or position sense, sparse hair, nail spooning, night blindness, Bitot's spots, loss of taste (3).
- Anthropomorphic measurements:
  - Weight (W) and height (H): In children, measure W:H; in adults, body mass index (BMI) <18.5 kg/m^2 in PEM (2)[C].
  - Mid–upper arm circumference (MUAC):
    - In children 1–5 years of age, MUAC >125 mm is normal.
    - 110–125 mm corresponds to a state of mild or moderate malnutrition.
    - <110 mm corresponds to severe malnutrition.
    - In adults, MUAC <200 mm is suggestive of PEM.
  - Triceps skin-fold thickness
- Marasmic children are thin and have little subcutaneous fat. Wasting is especially evident at the shoulders, buttocks, arms, and thighs.
- Children with kwashiorkor are irritable, with anasarca, sparse and brittle hair.
  - They can develop a "flaky paint" dermatosis characterized by blackish discoloration and excoriation.
  - Hepatomegaly from fatty infiltration may be present.
- Adults have decreased subcutaneous tissue and often, with serum albumin below 1 g/dL, anasarca.

DIAGNOSTIC TESTS & INTERPRETATION
Lab
Initial lab tests
- Diagnosis is often clinical in PEM-endemic countries (lack of laboratory resources).
- Pediatric patients:
  - Serum chemistries: Hypernatremia, hypokalemia, hypocalcemia, hypophosphatemia, hypomagnesemia
  - Hypoglycemia
  - Anemia, decreased lymphocyte count
  - Plasma albumin: Decreased
  - Blood urea nitrogen (BUN): Decreased
  - Plasma transferrin: Decreased
  - Plasma cortisol, growth hormone: Increased, but insulin is low.
- Adult and elderly patients:
  - Serum albumin is affected by acute illness, and while not a specific marker of PEM, lower levels correlate with increased mortality.
  - Serum prealbumin measures PEM risk level.
    - >15 mg/dL: Normal
    - <15 to >11 mg/dL: Increased risk
    - <11 to >5 mg/dL: Significant risk
    - <5 mg/dL: Poor prognosis, high mortality (4)[C]
  - Mild elevation of serum alkaline phosphatase

Follow-Up & Special Considerations

- Prealbumin trends can be used to determine response to therapy. Biweekly measurements, in conjunction with monitoring body weight, are often recommended (4)[C].
- In critically ill patients, blood glucose levels exceeding 180 mg/dL are associated with increased morbidity and mortality (5)[C].

Imaging

Initial approach

CXR: Evaluate for coexisting pneumonia, neoplasm, or tuberculosis. Cardiomegaly may be present (suggestive of cardiac failure; may result from marked anemia).

DIFFERENTIAL DIAGNOSIS

- In children, secondary growth failure owing to malabsorption, congenital defects, or deprivation
- Pellagra (niacin deficiency = "4 Ds"): Diarrhea, Dermatitis, Dementia, Death
- Nephritis or nephrosis
- Hypo- or hyperthyroidism
- Hyperparathyroidism
- Cardiac failure
- Neoplasm
- Viral or parasitic infection

 TREATMENT

MEDICATION

- Diet prescription in conjunction with a dietician or nutritionist
- Appetite stimulants (e.g., megestrol acetate, mirtazapine, oxandrolone, others) may be appropriate for short-term treatment of anorexia in adults but can increase thromboembolic disease risk.
- Medications that have weight gain as a side effect (atypical antipsychotics, carbamazepine, gabapentin, corticosteroids, valproic acid, SSRIs, sulfonylureas, injectable medroxyprogesterone) may be used if indicated in patients with comorbid conditions (6)[C].

ADDITIONAL TREATMENT

General Measures

- Slowly restore and maintain fluid and electrolyte balance.
- Initiate oral iron and folate supplements (begin iron therapy ~2 weeks after initiation of dietary treatment to avoid promotion of bacterial infection).
- Administer blood transfusion in the presence of severe anemia (hemoglobin <4–6 g/dL) or symptomatic moderate anemia.
- Ensure that immunizations are up to date (PEM is not a contraindication to vaccination).

SURGERY/OTHER PROCEDURES

In older patients with cognitive or physical disability that precludes oral feedings, consider alternative enteric access (e.g., nasogastric tube, gastrostomy).

IN-PATIENT CONSIDERATIONS

Initial Stabilization

- Reversal of fluid and electrolyte imbalance should occur before IV nutrition, if any, is started.
- Continuous cardiac rhythm monitoring (telemetry) is recommended when electrolyte imbalance or acidosis is found on initial assessment.

Admission Criteria

- Hemodynamic instability
- Alteration of consciousness (delirium)
- Unsafe living environment (evidence of child/elder mistreatment)
- Profound hypokalemia or hypocalcemia
- Cardiac abnormalities/arrhythmia
- Anemia (hemoglobin <10 g/dL in older patients)

IV Fluids

Parenteral (IV) nutrition, which carries a high risk of associated infection, should be reserved for use in patients with severe GI tract dysfunction or anatomic disturbance (3).

Nursing

- Patients should be assessed for risk of pressure ulcer (using a Braden scale or other tool) and a skin care protocol initiated.
- Any patient admitted to hospital with malnutrition should have a nutritionist consult, if available.
- Physical therapy should be initiated once the patient is stable for assessment.

Geriatric Considerations

Older patients may require assistance with basic activities of daily living (ADLs) and are at high risk of injury owing to falls.

Discharge Criteria

- Basic electrolyte abnormalities corrected to tolerance
- Patient demonstrates ability to maintain adequate oral intake of a nutritionally sound diet.
- Social and financial considerations have been identified and addressed.

Geriatric Considerations

Patient may need transfer to alternative level of care (e.g., skilled nursing home, rehabilitation center, etc.) temporarily for continued care depending on level of disability before returning safely home.

 ONGOING CARE

FOLLOW-UP RECOMMENDATIONS

Children are discharged from a nutritional rehabilitation program when W:H ratio is >85%, at least 1 week of consistent weight gain has been achieved, and all disease conditions associated with PEM have been addressed.

Patient Monitoring

Frequent assessment until weight has stabilized (BMI >18.5 kg/m^2)

DIET

- Amino acid constituent and calorie-to-BMI-adjusted diet per dietician
- Refeeding of adults should occur slowly and, if possible, in consultation with a nutritionist.
- For children, initially provide 100 kcal/kg/d with 3 g/kg/d protein. When tolerated, advance to at least 200 kcal/kg/d with 5 g/kg/d protein.
  - Small, frequent feedings are preferred.
  - Consider low-lactose formulas to decrease diarrhea from disaccharidase deficiency.
  - Target growth: 10–15 g/kg/d
  - Supplement with vitamins and micronutrients, especially vitamin A and zinc.

PATIENT EDUCATION

- Emphasis on diet education
- In older patients, caregiver education and supervision may be relevant.

PROGNOSIS

- Excellent when PEM is identified early and managed aggressively
- Mortality varies between 15% and 40%.
- Compromised immune function returns to normal with recovery.
- Behavioral and mental issues may persist following treatment of severe cases.
- There is insufficient evidence that enteral tube feeding in patients with advanced dementia improves survival or lowers the prevalence of pressure ulcers (5)[A].

COMPLICATIONS

- Fatalities in the early days of treatment usually result from electrolyte imbalance, infection, hypothermia, or circulatory failure. Lethargy, anorexia, stupor, and petechiae are ominous signs.
- In patients who develop PEM have greater risk of hospital acquired infection (3).

Pregnancy Considerations

Pregnant women with PEM are at risk of delivering a growth-restricted infant.

REFERENCES

1. van Bokhorst de van der Schueren M, et al. Profile of the malnourished patient. *Eur J Clin Nutrit*. 2005;59:1129–31.
2. Hickson M. Malnutrition and ageing. *Postgrad Med J*. 2006;82:2–8.
3. Ziegler TR et al. Parenteral nutrition in the critically ill patient. *N Engl J Med*. 2009;361:1088–97.
4. Beck FK, Rosenthal TC. Prealbumin: a marker for nutritional evaluation. *Am Fam Physician*. 2002;65:1575–8.
5. Sampson EL, Candy B, Jones L et al. Enteral tube feeding for older people with advanced dementia. *Cochrane Database Syst Rev*. 2009;CD007209.
6. Drugs associated with weight gain. *Pharmacist's Letter/Prescriber's Letter*. 2007;23(3):220–312.

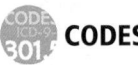 CODES

ICD9

- 260 Kwashiorkor
- 261 Nutritional marasmus
- 263.9 Unspecified protein-calorie malnutrition

CLINICAL PEARLS

- Older patients may experience elevated BUN levels if excessive protein supplementation is added to their diet; routine monitoring is suggested.
- Malnutrition in children is a major underlying factor in ~5 million preventable deaths annually, with two distinct phenotypes:
  - Marasmus is a wasting condition resulting from deficiency of calories and protein. Weight is decreased relative to that expected for the patient's height/length.
  - Kwashiorkor is distinguished by generalized edema and is associated with low protein relative to caloric intake. Resulting fat deposition in liver causes ascites. Weight is normal or elevated owing to increased body fluid.

PROTEIN S DEFICIENCY

Marc Jeffrey Kahn, MD
Rebecca Kruse-Jarres, MD, MPH

BASICS

DESCRIPTION
- Protein S is a vitamin K–dependent factor made principally by the liver that acts as a cofactor for protein C.
- Protein C becomes activated when thrombin binds to the endothelial receptor, thrombomodulin.
- Activated protein C, with protein S as a cofactor, inactivates clotting factors Va and VIIIa.
- Protein S is also able to directly inhibit factors Va, VIIa, and Xa independently of activated protein C.
- Patients with protein S deficiency have a thrombotic disorder that primarily affects the venous system.
- System(s) affected: Cardiovascular; Hematologic/Lymphatic/Immunologic; Pulmonary

EPIDEMIOLOGY
Incidence
- Predominant age: Mean age of 1st thrombosis is the 2nd decade.
- Predominant sex: Male = Female

Prevalence
- 0.3% of normal individuals
- Found in 3% of persons with VT

RISK FACTORS
- Oral contraceptives, pregnancy, and the use of HRT increase the risk of VT in patients with protein S deficiency (1)[A].
- Patients with protein S deficiency and another prothrombotic state, such as factor V Leiden, have further increased rates of thrombosis (1)[A].
- Patients heterozygous for protein S deficiency who are begun on warfarin without concomitant heparin can develop warfarin-induced skin necrosis because the half-life of other vitamin K–dependent clotting factors (e.g., prothrombin, factor IX, and factor X) is much longer than the anticoagulant protein S (4–8 h), leading to a transient hypercoagulable state when protein S becomes depleted. These patients develop extremely low levels of protein S and develop necrosis of the skin over central areas of the body such as the breast, abdomen, buttocks, and genitalia (1)[A].

Genetics
Autosomal dominant. Heterozygotes have an OR of VT of 1.6–11.5. Arterial thrombosis is more frequent in patients with protein S deficiency who smoke. Homozygotes can have a fulminant thrombotic event in infancy, termed *neonatal purpura fulminans*. Homozygosity or compound heterozygosity, if untreated, is usually incompatible with adult life.

Pregnancy Considerations
Increased thrombotic risk in patients with protein C deficiency

GENERAL PREVENTION
Since protein S deficiency is a congenital disease, there are no preventive measures.

ETIOLOGY
- >131 mutations in the protein S gene leading to an inherited protein S deficiency have been described. Protein S reversibly binds to the C4b-binding protein. Only the free form acts as a cofactor for activated protein C. This leads to conditions where free protein S is low, but total protein S is normal. These individuals are prone to thrombosis.
- Acquired protein S deficiency from decreased free protein S can occur during pregnancy, in patients taking oral contraceptives or warfarin, and in DIC, liver disease, nephrotic syndrome, inflammation, and acute thrombosis.
- Autoantibodies can develop to protein S in patients with acute varicella (2)[C].

COMMONLY ASSOCIATED CONDITIONS
- Deep and superficial VT, often spontaneous
- Up to 50% of homozygotes will have thrombosis.
- Homozygosity is associated with catastrophic thrombotic complications at birth: *purpura fulminans*.
- Sites of thrombosis can be unusual, including the mesentery and cerebral veins.
- Arterial thrombosis is rare.
- Skin necrosis can be seen in patients on warfarin.

DIAGNOSIS

HISTORY
Order testing for patients with VT at age <40 without another etiology; thrombosis in unusual locations (e.g., mesentery, sagittal sinus, portal vein) with a family history of thrombosis or spontaneous abortion.

PHYSICAL EXAM
Normal

DIAGNOSTIC TESTS & INTERPRETATION
Lab
Initial lab tests
- Protein S activity assay
- Immunoassay for quantitative assessment of protein S level
- Disorders that may alter lab results: Liver disease and pregnancy reduce protein S levels.

DIFFERENTIAL DIAGNOSIS
- Factor V Leiden
- Protein C deficiency
- Antithrombin deficiency
- Dysfibrinogenemia
- Dysplasminogenemia
- Homocystinemia
- Prothrombin 20210 mutation
- Elevated factor VIII levels

TREATMENT

MEDICATION
First Line
- Low-molecular-weight heparin (LMWH) (1)[A] initially for at least 5 days and until INR is 2–3, at which time it can be stopped:
  – Enoxaparin (Lovenox): 1 mg/kg SC b.i.d.:
    ○ Alternatively, 1.5 mg/kg/d SC. Initially for at least 5 days and until INR is 2–3, at which time it can be stopped
  – Fondaparinux (Arixtra): 7.5 mg SC every day
  – Tinzaparin (Innohep): 175 anti-Xa IU/kg/d SQ
  – Dalteparin (Fragmin): 200 IU/kg/d

- Oral anticoagulant: Warfarin (Coumadin): 5 mg/d p.o. initially and maintained on warfarin with an INR of 2–3 for at least 6 months (1)[A]
- Contraindications:
  – Active bleeding precludes anticoagulation; risk of bleeding is a relative contraindication to long-term anticoagulation.
  – Warfarin is contraindicated in patients with a prior history of warfarin-induced skin necrosis.
- Precautions:
  – Observe patient for signs of embolization, further thrombosis, or bleeding.
  – Avoid IM injections.
  – Periodically check stool and urine for occult blood, monitor CBC, including platelets.
  – Heparin: Thrombocytopenia and/or paradoxical thrombosis with thrombocytopenia
  – Warfarin: Necrotic skin lesions (typically breasts, thighs, and buttocks)
  – LMWH: Adjust dose in renal insufficiency.
- Significant possible interactions:
  – Agents that intensify the response to oral anticoagulants: Alcohol, allopurinol, amiodarone, anabolic steroids, androgens, many antimicrobials, cimetidine, chloral hydrate, disulfiram, all NSAIDs, sulfinpyrazone, tamoxifen, thyroid hormone, vitamin E, ranitidine, salicylates, acetaminophen
  – Agents that diminish the response to oral anticoagulants: Aminoglutethimide, antacids, barbiturates, carbamazepine, cholestyramine, diuretics, griseofulvin, rifampin, oral contraceptives

Second Line
Heparin 80 mg/kg IV bolus, followed by 18 mg/kg/h; adjust dose depending on aPTT.
- In patients requiring large daily doses of heparin, measure an anti-Xa level for dose guidance.
- Alternatively, unfractionated heparin can be given at 35,000 U/24 h SC, with subsequent dosing to maintain a therapeutic aPTT (3)[C].

ADDITIONAL TREATMENT
General Measures
- Routine anticoagulation for asymptomatic patients with protein S deficiency is not recommended (1)[A].
- Anticoagulation for 6–12 months is recommended for patients with protein S deficiency and a 1st thrombosis.
- Some argue for lifetime anticoagulation; data are limited.
- Anticoagulation for life is indicated for patients with protein S deficiency and recurrent thromboses.

- The role of family screening for protein S deficiency is unclear because most patients with this mutation do not have thrombosis. Screening should be considered for woman considering using oral contraceptives or pregnancy with a family history of protein S deficiency (4)[B].
- Treatment with LMWH is recommended over unfractionated heparin, unless the patient has severe renal failure (3)[B].
- Treat as outpatient, if possible (3)[B].
- Initiate warfarin together with heparin on the 1st treatment day, and discontinue heparin after a minimum of 5 days and when INR >2 (3)[A].

Issues for Referral
Patients with suspected protein S deficiency should be seen by a hematologist.

SURGERY/OTHER PROCEDURES
- Anticoagulation must be held for surgical interventions.
- For most patients with DVT, recommendations are against routine use of vena cava filter in addition to anticoagulation (3)[A].

IN-PATIENT CONSIDERATIONS
Admission Criteria
- Life-threatening VT
- Significant bleeding while on anticoagulant therapy

Nursing
Look for signs of bleeding while on anticoagulation therapy.

ONGOING CARE

FOLLOW-UP RECOMMENDATIONS
Patient Monitoring
- Warfarin requires periodic (monthly after initial stabilization) monitoring of the INR.
- Periodic measurement of INR to maintain a range of 2–3
- LMWH is the treatment of choice in pregnancy. Periodic monitoring with anti-Xa levels is recommended.

DIET
Unrestricted

PATIENT EDUCATION
- Patients should be educated about use of oral anticoagulant therapy if taking such.
- Avoid NSAIDs while on warfarin.

PROGNOSIS
- Persons with protein S deficiency have normal life spans.
- By age 45, half the people heterozygous for protein S deficiency will have VT that is spontaneous half the time.

COMPLICATIONS
Recurrent thrombosis (requires indefinite anticoagulation)

REFERENCES
1. Bick RL. Prothrombin G20210A mutation, antithrombin, heparin cofactor II, protein C, and protein S defects. *Hematol Oncol Clin North Am*. 2003;17:9–36.
2. Moll S. Thrombophilias—practical implications and testing caveats. *J Thromb Thrombolysis*. 2006;21: 7–15.
3. Büller HR, Agnelli G, Hull RD, et al. Antithrombotic therapy for venous thromboembolic disease: the Seventh ACCP Conference on Antithrombotic and Thrombolytic Therapy. *Chest*. 2004;126: 401S–428S.
4. Langlois NJ, Wells PS. Risk of venous thromboembolism in relatives of symptomatic probands with thrombophilia: a systematic review. *Thromb Haemost*. 2003;90:17–26.

 CODES

ICD9
289.81 Primary hypercoagulable state

CLINICAL PEARLS
- Asymptomatic patients with protein S deficiency do not need to have prophylactic anticoagulation because the risk of thrombosis is low; asymptomatic patients do not require anticoagulation.
- Patients with protein S deficiency and DVT should be anticoagulated for at least 6 months.

PROTEINURIA

Andrew Allegretti, MD
Douglas Shemin, MD

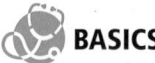 **BASICS**

DESCRIPTION
Proteinuria: Urinary protein excretion of more than 150 mg/d:

- Nephrotic-range proteinuria: Urinary protein excretion of more than 3.5 g/d; also called *heavy proteinuria*

Pediatric Considerations
- Proteinuria: Normal is daily excretion of up to 100 mg/m^2 (body surface area)
- Nephrotic-range proteinuria: Daily excretion of >1,000 mg/m^2 (body surface area)
- 3 pathologic types:
  – Glomerular proteinuria: Increased permeability of proteins across glomerular capillary membrane
  – Tubular proteinuria: Decreased proximal tubular reabsorption of proteins
  – Overflow proteinuria: Increased production of low-molecular-weight proteins

Pregnancy Considerations
- Proteinuria in pregnancy beyond 20 weeks' gestation is a hallmark of preeclampsia/eclampsia and demands further workup.
- Proteinuria in pregnancy before 20 weeks' gestation is suggestive of underlying renal disease.

RISK FACTORS
- Hypertension
- Diabetes
- Obesity
- Excessive exercise
- Congestive heart failure (CHF)
- Urinary tract infection (UTI)
- Fever

Genetics
No known genetic pattern

GENERAL PREVENTION
Control of weight, blood pressure, and blood glucose reduces the risk of proteinuria.

PATHOPHYSIOLOGY
- Glomerular proteinuria: Increased filtration or larger proteins (albumin) due to:
  – Increased size of glomerular basement membrane pores and
  – Loss of proteoglycan negative charge barrier
- Tubular proteinuria: Tubulointerstitial disease prevents proximal tubular reabsorption of smaller proteins (β_2-microglobulin, Ig light chains, retinol-binding protein, amino acids).
- Overflow proteinuria: Proximal tubular reabsorption overwhelmed by increased production of smaller proteins

ETIOLOGY
- Glomerular proteinuria:
  – Primary glomerulonephropathy:
    ○ Minimal-change disease
    ○ Idiopathic membranous glomerulonephritis
    ○ Focal segmental glomerulonephritis
    ○ Membranoproliferative glomerulonephritis
    ○ IgA nephropathy
  – Secondary glomerulonephropathy:
    ○ Diabetic nephropathy
    ○ Autoimmune/collagen-vascular disorders (i.e., lupus nephritis, Goodpasture syndrome)
    ○ Amyloidosis
    ○ Preeclampsia
    ○ Infection (HIV, hepatitis B and C, poststreptococcal, endocarditis, syphilis, malaria)
    ○ Malignancy (GI, lung, lymphoma)
    ○ Renal transplant rejection
    ○ Structural (reflux nephropathy, polycystic kidney disease)
    ○ Drug-induced (NSAIDs, penicillamine, lithium, heavy metals, gold, heroin)
- Tubular proteinuria:
  – Hypertensive nephrosclerosis
  – Tubulointerstitial disease (uric acid nephropathy, hypersensitivity, interstitial nephritis, Fanconi syndrome, heavy metals, sickle-cell disease, NSAIDs, antibiotics)
  – Acute tubular necrosis
- Overflow proteinuria:
  – Multiple myeloma (light chains also tubulotoxic)
  – Hemoglobinuria
  – Myoglobinuria (in rhabdomyolysis)
  – Lysozyme (in acute monocytic leukemia)
- Benign proteinuria:
  – Functional (fever, exercise, cold exposure, stress, CHF)
  – Idiopathic transient
  – Orthostasis (postural)

COMMONLY ASSOCIATED CONDITIONS
- Hypertension (common)
- Diabetes mellitus (common)
- Preeclampsia (common)
- Multiple myeloma (rare)

DIAGNOSIS

HISTORY
- Frothy or foamy urine
- Change in urine output
- Blood- or cola-colored urine
- Recent weight change
- Swelling
- Rule out systemic illness: Diabetes, heart failure, autoimmune, poststreptococcal infection

PHYSICAL EXAM
- Blood pressure
- Weight
- Peripheral edema
- Periorbital/facial edema
- Ascites
- Palpation of kidneys
- Check lungs, heart for signs of CHF

DIAGNOSTIC TESTS & INTERPRETATION
Lab
Screening for proteinuria is not cost-effective unless directed at groups with hypertension or diabetes, older persons, or conducted at 10-year intervals (1)[B].

Initial lab tests
- Urinalysis (UA) quantitatively estimates proteinuria:
  – Only sensitive to albumin; will not detect smaller proteins of overflow/tubular etiologies
  – False positive if urine pH >7, highly concentrated (specific gravity [SG] >1.015), gross hematuria, mucus, semen, leukocytes, iodinated contrast agents, penicillin analogues, sulfonamide metabolites
  – False negative if urine is dilute (SG >1.005), albumin excretion <20–30 mg/dL, protein is nonalbumin
  – Sensitivity 32–46%; specificity 97–100%
  – Also can perform sulfosalicylic acid (SSA) test to detect nonalbumin protein
- If UA positive, perform urine microscopy. Refer to nephrologist if positive for signs of glomerular disease.
- If UA shows trace to 2+ protein, rule out transient proteinuria with repeat UA at another visit:
  – More common than persistent proteinuria
  – Causes include exercise, fever, CHF, UTI, and cold exposure.
  – Should reassure patient that transient proteinuria is benign and requires no further workup
- If initial UA shows 3+ to 4+ protein or repeat UA is positive, measure creatinine clearance and quantify proteinuria with 24-h urine collection (gold standard) or spot urine protein/creatinine (P/C) ratio (acceptable practice) (2)[A]:
  – Numerical P/C ratios correlate with total protein excreted in grams/day (i.e., ratio of 0.2 correlates with 0.2 g during a 24-h collection).
  – Patients under age 30 with 24-h urine excretion of <2 g/d and normal creatinine clearance should be tested for orthostatic proteinuria:
    ○ Benign condition that is present in 2–5% of adolescents
    ○ Diagnosed with a normal urine P/C ratio on first morning void and an elevated urine P/C ratio on a second specimen taken after standing for several hours
- If protein excretion >2 g/d, consider nephrology referral and begin workup for systemic or renal disease (see Diagnostic Procedures/Other).

Follow-Up & Special Considerations
Renal or systemic disease workup can include:
- CBC, ferritin, ESR, serum Fe
- Electrolytes, LFTs
- Lipid profile (ideally, fasting)

- PT/INR
- Antinuclear antibodies (ANAs): Elevated in lupus
- Antistreptolysin O titer: Elevated after streptococcal glomerulonephritis
- Complement C3 and C4: Low in glomerulonephrititis
- HIV, VDRL, and hepatitis serologies: All associated with glomerular proteinuria
- Serum and urine protein electrophoresis: Abnormal in multiple myeloma
- Blood glucose: Elevated in diabetes
- All patients with diabetes should be screened for microalbuminuria.
- Patients with nephrotic-range proteinuria are at increased risk for hypercholesterolemia and thromboembolic events. Optimal duration of prophylactic anticoagulation is unknown (Cochrane Review is ongoing) but may extend for the duration of the nephrotic state (3)[C].
- Proteinuric pregnant patients beyond 20 weeks' gestation should be examined for other signs/symptoms of preeclampsia (e.g., hypertension, thrombocytopenia, elevated liver transaminases).

Imaging
Patients with persistent proteinuria not explained by orthostatic changes should undergo renal ultrasound to rule out structural abnormalities (e.g., reflux nephropathy, polycystic kidney).

DIFFERENTIAL DIAGNOSIS
Includes all causes listed under Etiology

 ## TREATMENT

- Systolic BP goal is in the 120s or lower, if tolerated (4)[A].
- Proteinuria goal is <0.5 g/d (4)[A].

MEDICATION
First Line
- Angiotensin-converting enzyme (ACE) inhibitors: First choice; use maximally tolerated doses; use even if normotensive (4)[A]
- ARBs: Proven antiproteinuric and renoprotective; studies ongoing to assess cardioprotection vs ACE inhibitors; ARBs are first choice if ACE inhibitors not tolerated (4)[A]
- Combination ACE inhibitor and ARB: Shown to reduce proteinuria; may not further reduce BP (4)[A]
- Statins: In addition to cardioprotection (4)[A], may be antiproteinuric and renoprotective (4)[B]

Second Line
- β-Blockers: Antiproteinuric and cardioprotective (4)[A]
- Dihydropyridine calcium channel blockers (DHCCB): Should be avoided unless needed for BP control; not antiproteinuric (4)[A]
- Non-DHCCB: Antiproteinuric, may be renoprotective (4)[B]
- Aldosterone antagonists: Antiproteinuric independent of BP control (4)[B]
- NSAIDs: Antiproteinuric but also nephrotoxic; generally should be avoided and reserved for refractory nephrotic syndrome (4)[C]

ADDITIONAL TREATMENT
General Measures

- Limit protein intake to 0.7 mg/kg/d. Soy protein also may be renoprotective. Monitor protein intake with 24-h urine urea excretion (4)[A].
- Limit NaCl intake to 2.0–3.0 g/d Na to optimize antiproteinuric medications (4)[B]. Effect on BP is further protective (4)[A].
- Limit fluid intake for urine output goal of <2.0 L/d. Larger urine volumes are associated with increased proteinuria and later glomerular filtration rate (GFR) decline (4)[B].
- Smoking cessation: Smoking is associated with increased proteinuria and faster kidney disease progression (4)[B].
- Encourage supine posture (up to 50% reduction vs upright) (4)[B].
- Discourage severe exertion (4)[B].
- Encourage weight loss (4)[B].

Issues for Referral
Consider nephrology referral for possible renal biopsy if:
- Impaired creatinine clearance
- Nephrotic-range proteinuria
- Unclear etiology of non-nephrotic-range proteinuria
- Diabetics with microalbuminuria

COMPLEMENTARY AND ALTERNATIVE MEDICINE

- Corticosteroids: No proven benefit in mortality or need for renal replacement in adults with nephrotic syndrome, though steroids are recommended in some patients who do not respond to conservative treatment. Classically, children with nephrotic syndrome respond better than adults, especially those with minimal-change disease (5)[A].
- Estrogen/progesterone replacement: May be renoprotective in premenopausal women but should be avoided in postmenopausal women (4)[B]
- Decrease elevated homocysteine: Associated with microalbuminuria and cardiovascular risk; folic acid, B_6, B_{12} may be effective (4)[C]
- Antioxidant therapy: May be antiproteinuric in diabetic nephropathy (4)[C]
- Sodium bicarbonate: Not antiproteinuric but may block tubular injury caused by proteinuria; correcting metabolic acidosis may decrease protein catabolism (4)[C]
- Avoid excessive caffeine consumption: Antiproteinuric in diabetic rat models (4)[C]
- Avoid iron overload (4)[C].
- Pentoxifylline: Prevents progression of renal disease by unclear mechanisms (4)[C]
- Mycophenolate mofetil (MMF): Antiproteinuric and renoprotective in animal models (4)[C]

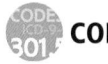 ## ONGOING CARE

FOLLOW-UP RECOMMENDATIONS
Patient Monitoring
All patients with persistent proteinuria should be followed with serial BP checks, urinalysis, and renal function tests in the outpatient setting. Intervals depend on underlying etiology.

DIET
See Additional Treatment

PATIENT EDUCATION
See Additional Treatment

PROGNOSIS
- Transient and orthostatic proteinuria are benign conditions that do not convey a poor prognosis.
- Clinical significance of persistent proteinuria varies greatly and depends on underlying etiology.
- Degree of proteinuria is associated with disease progression in chronic kidney disease.
- Independent of GFR, higher levels of proteinuria convey an increased risk of mortality, myocardial infarction, and progression to kidney failure.

COMPLICATIONS
- Progression to chronic renal failure and the need for dialysis or renal transplant
- Hypercholesterolemia
- Hypecoagulable state

REFERENCES

1. Boulware LE, Jaar BG, Tarver-Carr ME, et al. Screening for proteinuria in US adults: a cost-effectiveness analysis. *JAMA*. 2003;290: 3101–14.
2. DOQI: Clinical practice guidelines for chronic kidney disease: evaluation classification, and stratification: Guideline 5. Assessment of proteinuria. [http://www.kidney.org/Professionals/Kdoqi/guidelines_ckd/p5_lab_g5.htm]
3. Glassock RJ. Prophylactic Anticoagulation in Nephrotic Syndrome: A Clinical Conundrum. *J Am Soc Nephrol*. 2007.
4. Wilmer WA, Rovin BH, Hebert CJ, et al. Management of glomerular proteinuria: a commentary. *J Am Soc Nephrol*. 2003;14:3217–32.
5. Kodner C et al. Nephrotic syndrome in adults: diagnosis and management. *Am Fam Physician*. 2009;80:1129–34.

ADDITIONAL READING

- Kashif W, Siddiqi N, Dincer AP, et al. Proteinuria: how to evaluate an important finding. *Cleve Clin J Med*. 2003;70:535–7, 541–4, 546–7.
- Orth SR, Ritz E. The nephrotic syndrome. *N Engl J Med*. 1998;338:1202–11.

CODES

ICD9
791.0 Proteinuria

CLINICAL PEARLS

- Transient and orthostatic proteinuria are benign conditions that do not convey a poor prognosis.
- Proteinuria >2 g/d likely represents glomerular malfunction and warrants a nephrology consultation.
- Clinical course varies greatly, but in general, the amount of proteinuria correlates with kidney disease progression.
- 1st-line therapy for persistent proteinuric patients is high-dose ACE inhibitors/ARBs.

PROTHROMBIN 20210 (MUTATION)

Marc Jeffrey Kahn, MD
Rebecca Kruse-Jarres, MD, MPH

BASICS

DESCRIPTION
- Prothrombin 20210 mutation is the 2nd most common inherited risk factor for venous thromboembolism after factor V Leiden mutation.
- Polymorphism (replacement of G by A) in the 3' untranslated end of the prothrombin gene causes increased translation, resulting in elevated synthesis and secretion of prothrombin. This leads to a 2.8-fold increased risk for venous thrombosis.
- System(s) affected: Cardiovascular; Hemic/Lymphatic/Immunologic; Nervous; Pulmonary; Reproductive
- Synonym(s): Prothrombin G20210A mutation; Prothrombin G20210 gene polymorphism; Prothrombin gene mutation; FII A^{20210} mutation

EPIDEMIOLOGY
- Found largely in Caucasian populations. Found in 2–5% of European and Middle Eastern populations, but rarely in nonwhites. Found in 4–8% of persons with venous thromboembolism and in up to 18% of patients with recurrent thrombosis.
- Predominant age: Mean age of 1st thrombosis is in the 2nd decade
- Predominant gender: Male = Female

Prevalence
3–5% of the population

RISK FACTORS
- Oral contraceptives, pregnancy, and the use of hormone replacement therapy increase the risk of venous thrombosis in patients with prothrombin 20210 (1).
- Patients with prothrombin 20210 and another prothrombotic state such as factor V Leiden have increased rates of thrombosis (1).

Pregnancy Considerations
Increased thrombotic risk in patients with prothrombin 20210

Genetics
Autosomal dominant

GENERAL PREVENTION
Patients with prothrombin 20210 without thrombosis do not require prophylactic treatment with full anticoagulation (2)[A].

PATHOPHYSIOLOGY
Replacement of G for A in the 3' untranslated region of the prothrombin gene resulting in relatively higher plasma prothrombin activity, leading to increased risk for venous thrombosis

ETIOLOGY
Gene mutation

COMMONLY ASSOCIATED CONDITIONS
Venous thromboembolism

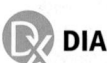

DIAGNOSIS

HISTORY
- Previous thrombosis
- Family history of thrombosis
- Family history of factor prothrombin 20210 mutation

PHYSICAL EXAM
Arterial thrombosis is rare in adults with prothrombin 20210 gene mutation.

DIAGNOSTIC TESTS & INTERPRETATION
Test patients with thrombosis at age <50, history of recurrent idiopathic thrombosis, those with thrombosis in unusual locations, or those with strong family history.

Lab
Initial lab tests
- DNA analysis for mutation
- Testing is reliable during acute thrombosis and on any kind of anticoagulation (3).

Follow-Up & Special Considerations
Although prothrombin levels are elevated, this is not a sensitive test to make the diagnosis.

Imaging
Initial approach
As appropriate for suspected site of thrombosis: Ultrasound, CT scan, and V/Q scan

Diagnostic Procedures/Surgery
Magnetic resonance angiography (MRA), venography, or arteriography to detect thrombosis

Pathological Findings
Venous thrombus

DIFFERENTIAL DIAGNOSIS
- Factor V Leiden mutation
- Protein C deficiency
- Protein S deficiency
- Antithrombin deficiency
- Other causes of activated protein C resistance (e.g., antiphospholipid antibodies)
- Dysfibrinogenemia
- Dysplasminogenemia
- Homocystinemia
- Elevated factor VIII levels

TREATMENT

For acute thrombosis

MEDICATION
First Line
- Low-molecular-weight heparin (2)[A]:
  – Enoxaparin (Lovenox): 1 mg/kg SC b.i.d., start warfarin simultaneously, continue Lovenox for at least 5 days and until international normalized ratio (INR) is >2.0, at which time it can be stopped
  – Fondaparinux (Arixtra): 7.5 mg SC every day
  – Tinzaparin (Innohep): 175 anti-Xa IU/kg SC daily for 6 days and patient is adequately anticoagulated with warfarin (INR of at least 2 for 2 consecutive days)
  – Dalteparin (Fragmin): 200 IU/kg SC daily
- Oral anticoagulant:
  – Warfarin (Coumadin) 5 mg p.o. daily initially and adjusted to an INR of 2–3
- Contraindications:
  – Active bleeding precludes anticoagulation (2)[A].
  – Risk of bleeding is a relative contraindication to long-term anticoagulation (2)[A].
  – Warfarin is contraindicated in patients with history of warfarin skin necrosis (2)[A].
- Precautions:
  – Observe patient for signs of embolization, further thrombosis, or bleeding.
  – Avoid IM injections. Periodically check stool and urine for occult blood; monitor complete blood counts (CBCs), including platelets.
  – Heparins: Thrombocytopenia and/or paradoxic thrombosis with thrombocytopenia
  – Warfarin: Necrotic skin lesions (typically breasts, thighs, or buttocks)
  – Low-molecular-weight heparin (LMWH): Adjust dosage in renal insufficiency.

- Significant possible interactions:
  - Agents that intensify the response to oral anticoagulants: Alcohol, allopurinol, amiodarone, anabolic steroids, androgens, many antimicrobials, cimetidine, chloral hydrate, disulfiram, all nonsteroidal anti-inflammatory drugs (NSAIDs), sulfinpyrazone, tamoxifen, thyroid hormone, vitamin E, ranitidine, salicylates, acetaminophen
  - Agents that diminish the response to anticoagulants: Aminoglutethimide, antacids, barbiturates, carbamazepine, cholestyramine, diuretics, griseofulvin, rifampin, oral contraceptives

Second Line
- Heparin 80 mg/kg IV bolus followed by 18 g/kg/h continuous infusion
- Adjust dose depending on activated partial thromboplastin time (aPTT).
- In patients requiring large daily doses of heparin, measure an anti-Xa level for dose guidance.
- Alternatively, unfractionated heparin can be given at 35,000 U/24hrs SC, with subsequent dosing to maintain a therapeutic aPTT (3)[C].

ADDITIONAL TREATMENT
General Measures
- Patients with prothrombin 20210 mutation and a 1st thrombosis should be anticoagulated initially with heparin or LMWH (1)[A].
- Treatment with LMWH is recommended over unfractionated heparin, unless the patient has severe renal failure (3)[B].
- Treat as outpatient, if possible (3)[B].
- Initiate warfarin together with heparin on the 1st treatment day, and discontinue heparin after 5 days if INR >2.0 (3)[A].
- Patients should be maintained on warfarin with an INR of 2–3 for at least 6 months (1)[A].
- Recurrent thrombosis requires indefinite anticoagulation (1)[B].

Issues for Referral
- Recurrent thrombosis on anticoagulation
- Difficulty anticoagulating
- Genetic counseling

COMPLEMENTARY AND ALTERNATIVE MEDICINE
Compression stockings for prevention

SURGERY/OTHER PROCEDURES
- Anticoagulation must be held for surgical interventions.
- For most patients with DVT, recommendations are against routine use of vena cava filter in addition to anticoagulation (3)[A].
- Thrombectomy may be necessary in some cases.

IN-PATIENT CONSIDERATIONS
Initial Stabilization
Heparin

Admission Criteria
Complicated thrombosis, such as pulmonary embolus

Nursing
- Teach LMWH and warfarin use.
- See above for drug interactions.

Discharge Criteria
Stable on anticoagulation

 ONGOING CARE

FOLLOW-UP RECOMMENDATIONS
Patient Monitoring
- Warfarin use requires periodic (monthly after initial stabilization) INR measurements, with a goal of 2–3 (2)[A].
- Heterozygous prothrombin 20210 mutations increase the risk for recurrent venous thrombo-embolism (VTE) only slightly once anticoagulation is stopped, and should have the same length of anticoagulation as someone without the mutation.

DIET
- No restrictions
- Foods rich in vitamin K may interfere with warfarin anticoagulation.

PATIENT EDUCATION
- Patients should be educated about:
  - Use of oral anticoagulant therapy
  - Avoidance of NSAIDs while on warfarin
- The role of family screening is unclear, as most patients with this mutation do not have thrombosis. In a patient with a family history of prothrombin 20210, consider screening during pregnancy or if considering oral contraceptive use.

PROGNOSIS
When compared to normal individuals, persons with prothrombin 20210 have normal life spans.

COMPLICATIONS
- Recurrent thrombosis
- Bleeding on anticoagulation

REFERENCES
1. Girolami A, Simioni P, Scarano L, et al. Prothrombin and the prothrombin 20210 G to A polymorphism: their relationship with hypercoagulability and thrombosis. *Blood Rev.* 1999;13:205–10.
2. Girolami A, Scarano L, Tormene D, et al. Homozygous patients with the 20210 G to A prothrombin polymorphism remain often asymptomatic in spite of the presence of associated risk factors. *Clin Appl Thromb Hemost.* 2001; 7:122–5.
3. Moll S. Thrombophilias–practical implications and testing caveats. *J Thromb Thrombolysis.* 2006; 21:7–15.

ADDITIONAL READING
- American College of Chest Physicians Evidence-Based Clinical Practice Guidelines (8th Edition). *Chest.* 2008;133(6 Suppl).
- Büller HR, Agnelli G, Hull RD, et al. Antithrombotic therapy for venous thromboembolic disease: the Seventh ACCP Conference on Antithrombotic and Thrombolytic Therapy. *Chest.* 2004;126:401S–428S.
- Seligsohn U, Lubetsky A. Genetic susceptibility to venous thrombosis. *N Engl J Med.* 2001;344: 1222–31.

See Also (Topic, Algorithm, Electronic Media Element)
Protein C Deficiency; Protein S Deficiency; Antithrombin Deficiency; Thrombosis, Deep Vein Thrombophlebitis (DVT); Factor V Leiden

 CODES

ICD9
289.81 Primary hypercoagulable state

CLINICAL PEARLS
- Prothrombin 20210 mutation is the 2nd most common inherited risk factor for venous thromboembolism after factor V Leiden mutation.
- Asymptomatic patients with prothrombin 20210 mutation do not need anticoagulation.
- Testing for the prothrombin G20210 mutation may be done while the patient is anticoagulated, as it is a genetic assay.

PRURITUS VULVAE

Michael P. Hopkins, MD, MEd
Jennifer L. Rogers, MD

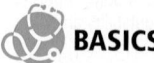 **BASICS**

DESCRIPTION
- Pruritus vulvae is a symptom as well as a primary diagnosis.
  - The symptom may indicate an underlying pathological process.
  - Only when no underlying disease is identified may this be used as a primary diagnosis.
- Pruritus vulvae as a primary diagnosis may also be more appropriately documented as vulvodynia (See chapter on Vulvodynia) and burning vulva syndrome.

EPIDEMIOLOGY
Symptoms may occur at any given age during a woman's lifetime.
- Young girls most commonly have infectious etiology
- Primary diagnosis more commonly seen in post-menopausal women

Incidence
The exact incidence is unknown, however the majority of women complain of vulvar pruritus at some point in their lifetime.

RISK FACTORS
- High-risk sexual behavior
- Immunosuppression
- Obesity

GENERAL PREVENTION
- Attention should be paid to personal hygiene and avoidance of possible environmental factors.
- Tight fitting clothing should be avoided.
- Only cotton underwear should be worn.

ETIOLOGY
Local irritants:
- Perfumes
- Soaps
- Laundry detergent
- Douches
- Toilet paper
- Sanitary napkins

COMMONLY ASSOCIATED CONDITIONS
- Infectious etiology
  - Vaginal or vulvar candida
  - *Gardnerella vaginalis*
  - *Trichomonas*
  - *Human Papilloma Virus*
  - *Herpes Simplex Virus*
- Vulvar vestibulitis
- Lichen sclerosis
- Hyperkeratosis
- Malignant or pre-malignant conditions
- Psoriasis
- Fecal or urinary incontinence
- Excessive heat with sweat
- Dietary: methylxanthines (e.g., coffee, cola), tomatoes, peanuts

 DIAGNOSIS

Pruritus vulvae is a diagnosis of exclusion.

HISTORY
- Persistent itching
- Persistent burning sensation over the vulva or perineum
- Change in vaginal discharge
- Post-coital bleeding
- Dyspareunia

PHYSICAL EXAM
- Visual inspection of the vulva, vagina, perineum, and anus
- Light touch identification of affected areas
- Q-tip-applied pressure to vestibular glands

DIAGNOSTIC TESTS & INTERPRETATION
- Sodium chloride: *Gardnerella* or *Trichomonas*
- 10% potassium hydroxide: Candida
- Tzanck smear: *Herpes Simplex Virus*
- Directed biopsy: Human papilloma virus, lichen, malignancy

Lab
Follow-Up & Special Considerations
A patch test may be performed by a dermatologist to assist in identifying causative agent if contact dermatitis is suspected.

Imaging
Initial approach
Colposcopy with acetic acid of Lugol's solution of vagina and vulva

Follow-Up & Special Considerations
Exam-directed biopsies are essential in the post-menopausal population to rule out malignancy (1).

Diagnostic Procedures/Surgery
Biopsies should be collected from any ulceration, discoloration, raised areas, macerated areas, and the area of most intense pruritus.

Pathological Findings
Only in the absence of pathological findings can the primary diagnosis of pruritus vulvae be made.

TREATMENT

Initial treatment is conservative (2)[C]
- Treatment of etiology beyond the primary diagnosis of vulvae pruritus
- Avoidance of environment and dietary irritants
- Sitz baths
- Cool compresses or ice packs (gel packs or frozen vegetables)

MEDICATION
First Line
- Antihistamines
  - Hydroxyzine 10–50 mg 2 h before bedtime
  - Diphenhydramine 25–50 mg at bedtime
- Topical steroids (3)[C]
  - Triamcinolone 0.1% applied daily for 2–4 wks then twice weekly
  - Hydrocortisone 1–2.5% cream applied 2–4 times daily (4)
  - Avoid long-term use due to risk of atrophy.
- SSRIs (citalopram, fluoxetine, or sertraline)
  - Citalopram 20–40 mg daily

Second Line
Topical pimecrolimus 1% cream applied twice daily for 3 weeks (5)[B]

ADDITIONAL TREATMENT
- Subcutaneous triamcinolone injections (6)[B]
- Alcohol nerve block (7)[B]
- Laser therapy (8)[B]

Issues for Referral
- Persistent symptoms should prompt additional investigation and referral to a gynecologist or gynecologist oncologist.
- Gynecology oncology referral for proven or suspected malignancy
- Dermatology referral for patch testing to evaluate for contact dermatitis

ONGOING CARE

- Frequent evaluation, repeat cultures, and biopsies are necessary for cases resistant to treatment.
- Refractory cases may require referral to gynecologist or gynecology oncology for further management.

DIET
Dietary alterations include avoidance of:
- Coffee and other caffeine-containing beverages
- Tomatoes
- Peanuts

PATIENT EDUCATION
- American Congress of Obstetricians and Gynecologists at www.acog.org
- National Vulvodynia Foundation at http://www.nva.org/

PROGNOSIS
Conservative measures and short-term topical steroids control most patient's symptoms.

COMPLICATIONS
Malignancy

REFERENCES

1. Sener AB, Kuscu E, Seckin NC et al. Postmenopausal vulvar pruritus–colposcopic diagnosis and treatment. *J Pak Med Assoc.* 1995;45:315–7.
2. Boardman LA, Botte J, Kennedy CM. Recurrent Vulvar Itching. *Obstetrics and Gynecology*, 2005;100(6):1451–55.
3. Weichert GE et al. An approach to the treatment of anogenital pruritus. *Dermatol Ther.* 2004;17:129–33.
4. Pincus. Vulvar Dermatoses and Pruritus Vulvae. *Dermatologic Clinics.* 1992;10(2):297–308.
5. Sarifakioglu E, Gumus II. Efficacy of topical pimecrolimus in the treatment of chronic vulvar pruritus: a prospective case series – a non-controlled, open-label study. *J Dermatolog Treat.* 2006;17(5):276–8.
6. Kelly RA, Foster DC, Woodruff JD. Subcutaneous injection of triamcinolone acetonide in the treatment of chronic vulvar pruritus. *Am J Obstet Gynecol.* 1993;169(3):568–70.
7. Woodruff JD, Babaknia A et al. Local alcohol injection of the vulva: discussion of 35 cases. *Obstet Gynecol.* 1979;54:512–4.
8. Ovadia J, Levavi H, Edelstein T et al. Treatment of pruritus vulvae by means of CO2 laser. *Acta Obstet Gynecol Scand.* 1984;63:265—7.

ADDITIONAL READING

- Bohl TG et al. Overview of vulvar pruritus through the life cycle. *Clin Obstet Gynecol.* 2005;48: 786–807.
- Farage MA, Miller KW, Ledger WJ et al. Determining the cause of vulvovaginal symptoms. *Obstet Gynecol Surv.* 2008;63:445–64.
- Foster DC et al. Vulvar disease. *Obstet Gynecol.* 2002;100:145–63.
- Petersen CD, Lundvall L, Kristensen E et al. Vulvodynia. Definition, diagnosis and treatment. *Acta Obstet Gynecol Scand.* 2008;87:893–901.

CODES

ICD9
698.1 Pruritus of genital organs

CLINICAL PEARLS

- The majority of women complain of vulvar pruritus at some point in their lifetime.
- Pruritus vulvae is a diagnosis of exclusion once other causes of itching have been ruled out.
- Exam-directed biopsies from any ulceration, discoloration, raised areas, macerated areas, and the area of most intense pruritus are essential to rule out malignancy.
- Initial treatment is conservative.

PRURITUS ANI

Katharine Barnard, MD

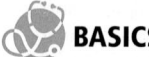 **BASICS**

DESCRIPTION
- Intense anal and perianal itching
- Usually acute, although some patients will live with symptoms long-term
- Must be differentiated from other primary dermatologic disorders seen in this region

EPIDEMIOLOGY
Incidence
- Common
- Predominant age: 40–70
- Predominant sex: Male > Female (4:1)

Prevalence
Difficult to estimate because condition is thought to be underreported and because almost any anorectal discomfort is often attributed to symptomatic hemorrhoids

RISK FACTORS
- Overweight
- Hairy, excessive perspiration
- Underlying anorectal pathology
- Underlying anxiety disorder

GENERAL PREVENTION
- Practice good perianal hygiene. If necessary, absorb excess sweating with a small amount of talcum powder or cornstarch.
- Avoid mechanical irritation of skin (via excessive cleaning or rubbing, harsh soaps or perfumed products, or tight or synthetic undergarments).
- Avoid laxative use (loose stool predisposes to condition).
- Eat yogurt or take *Acidophilus* supplements when taking broad-spectrum antibiotics; malt extract also may help.

PATHOPHYSIOLOGY
- Perianal itching usually due to fecal irritants.
- Itch-scratch cycle may be initiated via other mechanical or inflammatory factors and perpetuated by the resulting lichenification caused by scratching.

ETIOLOGY
- 25% idiopathic vs 75% associated with colonic or anorectal pathology (e.g., hemorrhoids, anal fissures, rectal prolapse, polyps, or—rarely—cancers of the colon, rectum, or anus)
- In 50–75% of cases, skin irritation is from feces (due to poor hygiene, loose or leaking stool, pathology that makes cleansing difficult, or laxity of the internal sphincter mechanism).
- In the remaining 25–50% of cases, the inciting irritation may be caused by:
  - Dermatologic disorders:
    - Allergic contact dermatitis (e.g., to soaps, perfumes or dyes in toilet paper, topical anesthetics [especially -caines], oral antibiotics [especially tetracyclines])
    - Excess skin moisture due to hyperhydrosis
    - Psoriasis
    - Erythrasma (*Corynebacterium* infection)
    - Atopic dermatitis ± lichen simplex chronicus
    - Eczema due to dietary components: Citrus, vitamin C supplements, milk products, coffee, tea, cola, chocolate, beer, wine
  - Infection with dermatophytes (*Tinea*), *Candida*, or seborrheic dermatitis
  - Bacterial and viral infections (either primary infections such as STIs, or secondary *Staphylococcus* or *Streptococcus* infections); especially a concern for immune-suppressed patients
  - Parasitic infections, most commonly pinworms, and rarely scabies or pediculosis
  - Mechanical factors: Vigorous cleaning and rubbing, tight-fitting clothes, or synthetic undergarments
  - Systemic disease: Diabetes mellitus, chronic liver disease, renal failure, leukemia or lymphoma, hyperthyroidism, or anemia
  - Psychogenic: Anxiety–itch–anxiety cycle
  - Chemical irritation from chemotherapy or alkaline diarrhea

COMMONLY ASSOCIATED CONDITIONS
See above listing of conditions causing perianal irritation.

 DIAGNOSIS

HISTORY
- Patient presents with complaint of anal and/or perianal itching.
- Inquire about melena or hematochezia, change in bowel habits, or a family history of colorectal cancer; anal receptive intercourse; antecedent change in toiletry products; household members with itching (think pinworms); and clothing preference (tight, synthetic).

PHYSICAL EXAM
- Perianal inspection for erythema, hemorrhoids, anal fissures, maceration, lichenification, rashes, warts, or excoriations
- Digital rectal exam to check for masses and to evaluate internal sphincter tone
- Anoscopy to evaluate for hemorrhoids, fissures, other internal lesions

DIAGNOSTIC TESTS & INTERPRETATION
Lab
Initial lab tests
Depending on patient's history and exam, consider the following:
- Blood glucose and urine dip for glycosuria (association with diabetes)
- Test for pinworms via cellophane tape to area; check stool for ova and parasites

Pediatric Considerations
- Pinworms are more common in children than in adults; therefore, testing is always indicated.
- Skin scraping with KOH prep for candidiasis (as etiology or as yeast superinfection) and mineral oil prep for scabies
- Perianal skin culture (bacterial superinfection)
- Hemoccult testing of stool (may be positive due to excoriations)

Follow-Up & Special Considerations
- Anal DNA PCR probe for gonorrhea and chlamydia and anal Pap smear (if receptive anal intercourse)
- Consider lab evaluation of liver and renal function, Hct, TSH, and CBC.

Diagnostic Procedures/Surgery
- Suspicious lesions (e.g., lichenification, ulcerated epithelium, refractory cases) should be biopsied to exclude neoplasia.
- Consider colonoscopy if history suggests colorectal pathology (preceding historical elements, especially if age >40).

DIFFERENTIAL DIAGNOSIS
- Dermatologic conditions
- Infections, including condylomata acuminata
- Allergies (topical agents)
- Colorectal pathology: Fistulas (e.g., associated with IBD), fissures, rectal prolapse, sphincter weakness, hemorrhoids, tumor/malignancy
- Skin cancer: Squamous cell cancer, extramammary Paget disease, Bowen disease, melanoma
- Systemic illness such as diabetes

Geriatric Considerations
- Stool incontinence may be a predisposing factor.
- Consider possible systemic disease.
- Higher likelihood of colorectal pathology

 **TREATMENT**

MEDICATION
First Line
- Treat underlying and associated conditions: Fungal or dermatophyte infection with topical imidazoles, bacterial infection with topical antibacterials (or oral erythromycin if itch >1 year)
- Break itch–scratch cycle with low-potency steroid cream (not ointment) applied sparingly up to q.i.d. Discontinue when itching subsides. Recommended not to use >12 weeks due to risk of skin atrophy.
- Zinc oxide can be used after completing steroid course; petroleum jelly as barrier during treatment period (1)
- Topical capsaicin cream also may be used in combination with steroid cream or if refractory itch or hypersensitized skin (2,3).
- Use a hair dryer on the cool setting to dry the area after cleansing (4)[C].

- Antihistamines may be useful until local measures take effect, particularly sedating antihistamines, which will reduce nighttime itching. Psychotropic medications may be added for additional sedation (5,6).
- If lichenification or no response with low-potency steroid, use high-potency steroid cream sparingly to area b.i.d., totaling <8 weeks of steroid treatment (7).
- Treat co-morbid anxiety or depression.

Second Line
Radiation or methylene blue injections may be used to destroy nerve endings (create permanent anesthesia) in intractable cases. This is almost never indicated, but is close to 100% effective for those who require it (7,8).

ADDITIONAL TREATMENT
Issues for Referral
- Intractable pruritus: Consider referral to gastroenterology (for colonoscopy) or dermatology (for additional treatment, possibly injections). Refractory or persistent symptoms should signal the possibility of underlying neoplasia because pruritus ani of long duration is associated with a greater likelihood of colorectal pathology (9,10).
- If risks or red flags for colonic malignancy, refer for colonoscopy.
- If neoplasia on biopsy, refer to colorectal surgery.

COMPLEMENTARY AND ALTERNATIVE MEDICINE
Self-hypnosis using relaxation and imagery has been shown to be effective in at least 1 case of refractory idiopathic pruritus ani (11).

SURGERY/OTHER PROCEDURES
None unless neoplasia

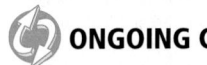 ONGOING CARE

FOLLOW-UP RECOMMENDATIONS
See patient in 2 weeks if not improving. Check for persistent lichenification. Biopsy persistent or refractory pruritus or lichenification that does not resolve (9,12).

DIET
- Trial elimination of foods and beverages known or suspected to exacerbate symptoms: Coffee, tea, chocolate, beer, cola, vitamin C tablets in excessive doses, citrus fruits, tomatoes, or spices (1)
- Eliminate foods or drugs contributing to loose bowel movements. Add fiber supplementation to bulk stools and prevent fecal leakage in patients who have fecal incontinence or partially formed stools.

PATIENT EDUCATION
- Resist overuse of soap and rubbing.
- Avoid toiletry products with irritating perfumes and dyes.
- Avoid use of ointments to the area.
- Wear loose, light clothing.
- If moisture is a problem, unmedicated talcum powder or cornstarch may be used to keep the area dry.

- Cleanse perianal area after bowel movements with cotton moistened with water or witch hazel.
- Following bathing, the area should be dried by patting with a soft towel or with a hair drier.
- Avoid medications that cause diarrhea or constipation.
- If taking antibiotics, eat yogurt with active cultures or take *Acidophilus* supplements.
- Use barrier protection if engaging in anal intercourse.
- If unable to completely empty rectum with defecation, use small plain-water enema (infant bulb syringe) after each bowel movement to prevent soiling and irritation.

PROGNOSIS
- Conservative treatment and reassurance are successful in ~90% of patients.
- Idiopathic form often is chronic, waxing and waning, but regardless of etiology, the condition may be persistent and recurrent.

COMPLICATIONS
- Bacterial superinfection at site of excoriations, and potentially abscess formation or penetrating infection via self-inoculation with colonic pathogens
- Lichenification, which makes cure more difficult

REFERENCES

1. Siddiqi S, Vijay V, Ward M, et al. Pruritus ani. *Ann R Coll Surg Engl.* 2008;90:457–63.
2. Heard S. Pruritus ani. *Aus Fam Physician.* 2004;33(7):511–13.
3. Lysy J, Sistiery-Ittah M, Israelit Y, et al. Topical capsaicin—a novel and effective treatment for idiopathic intractable pruritus ani: a randomised, placebo controlled, crossover study. *Gut.* 2003;52:1323–6.
4. Markell KW, Billingham RP et al. Pruritus ani: etiology and management. *Surg Clin North Am.* 2010;90:125–35, Table of Contents.
5. Crownover BK, Jamieson B, Mott TF. Clinical inquiries. First- or second-generation antihistamines: which are more effective at controlling pruritus? *J Fam Pract.* 2004;53:742–4.
6. Southerland AD, et al. Intradermal injection of methylene blue for the treatment of refractory pruritus ani. *Colorectal Dis.* 2008.
7. Weichert GE. An approach to the treatment of anogenital pruritus. *Dermatol Ther.* 2004;17:129–33.
8. Mentes BB, Akin M, Leventoglu S, et al. Intradermal methylene blue injection for the treatment of intractable idiopathic pruritus ani: results of 30 cases. *Tech Coloproctol.* 2004;8:11–4.
9. Daniel GL, Longo WE, Vernava AM. Pruritus ani. Causes and concerns. *Dis Colon Rectum.* 1994;37:670–4.
10. Longo WE, Dean PA, Virgo KS, et al. Colonoscopy in patients with benign anorectal disease. *Dis Colon Rectum.* 1993;36:368–71.
11. Rucklidge JJ, Saunders D. Hypnosis in a case of long-standing idiopathic itch. *Psychosom Med.* 1999;61:355–8.
12. Handa Y, Watanabe O, Adachi A, et al. Squamous cell carcinoma of the anal margin with pruritus ani of long duration. *Dermatol Surg.* 2003;29:108–10.

ADDITIONAL READING

- *Evidence-Based Medicine.* 2004;9(3):86.
- Pfenninger JL, Zainea GG. Common anorectal conditions: Part I. Symptoms and complaints. *Am Fam Physician.* 2001;63:2391–8.
- Zuccati G, Lotti T, Mastrolorenzo A, et al. Pruritus ani. *Dermatol Ther.* 2005;18:355–62.

See Also (Topic, Algorithm, Electronic Media Element)
Pinworms; Pruritus Vulvae

 CODES

ICD9
698.0 Pruritus ani

CLINICAL PEARLS

- In over half the cases of pruritis ani, the irritant is feces.
- Vigorous cleansing can potentiate the problem.
- Consider infection in immunosuppressed patients.
- Chronic tetracycline use (such as for acne) can cause pruritis ani.
- Consider trial of dietary elimination of citrus, vitamin C supplements, milk products, coffee, tea, cola, chocolate, beer, and wine.

PSEUDOFOLLICULITIS BARBAE

Michelle St. Fleur, MD
Anna Doubeni, MD

 BASICS

DESCRIPTION
- Foreign-body inflammatory reaction surrounding an ingrown hair (usually in beard area, especially in submandibular region, but may occur on scalp, axilla, or pubic area if these sites are shaved or plucked)
- Characterized by red papule/pustule at point of entry
- A mechanical problem
- System(s) affected: Skin/Exocrine
- Synonym(s): Chronic sycosis barbae; Pili incarnate; Folliculitis barbae traumatica; Razor bumps; Shaving bumps

EPIDEMIOLOGY
- Predominant age: Postpubertal, middle age (40–75 years of age)
- Predominant sex: Male > Female (can be seen in females of all races who wax/shave axillary and pubic areas) (1).

Incidence
- Adult male African Americans: 50,000/100,000
- Adult male whites: 3,000–5,000/100,000

Prevalence
- Widespread
- 45–83% of African-American soldiers who shave

RISK FACTORS
- Curly hair
- Shaving too close with multiple razor strokes
- Plucking hairs
- Black and Hispanic races

Genetics
- People with curly hair, especially African Americans and Hispanics (2)
- Single-nucleotide polymorphism (disruption Ala12Thr substitution) affects keratin of hair follicle (3).

GENERAL PREVENTION
- Use tiny plastic hook to remove ingrown hairs before shaving.
- Prior to shaving, rinse and compress face with warm water.

- Shave with either a manual adjustable razor at coarsest setting (avoids close shaves), a single-edge blade razor (e.g., Bump Fighter), a foil-guarded razor (e.g., PFB razor), electric triple "O-head" razor, or electric hair clipper with polyester skin-cleansing pad (e.g., Buf-Puf by Riker Laboratories).
- Shave in the direction of hair growth. Do not stretch skin when shaving.
- Use a generous amount of the correct shaving cream/gel (e.g., Ef-Kay Shaving Gel, Edge Shaving Gel, Aveeno Therapeutic Shave Gel, Easy Shave Medicated Shaving Cream).
- Use "collar extender" (JCPenney).

PATHOPHYSIOLOGY
- Because of its curvature, the advancing hair's sharp-tipped free end after shaving causes an epidermal invagination as it approaches the skin. This is accompanied by inflammation and often an intraepidermal abscess (4).
- As the hair enters the dermis, more severe inflammation occurs, with downgrowth of the epidermis in an attempt to sheath the hair.
- An abscess forms within the pseudofollicle, and a foreign-body reaction forms at the tip of the invading hair.

ETIOLOGY
- Reentry penetration of skin by external pointed tip of growing curved whisker or sharp-tipped whisker may grow into follicular wall if shaved too close
- Plucking of hair may cause abnormal hair growth in injured follicles

COMMONLY ASSOCIATED CONDITIONS
Keloidal folliculitis

 DIAGNOSIS

HISTORY
Pain on shaving; irritated "razor bumps"

PHYSICAL EXAM
- Tender exudative, erythematous follicular papules or pustules in beard area (less commonly in scalp, axilla, and pubic areas); range from 2–4 mm (2)
- Hyperpigmented "razor or shave bumps"
- Alopecia
- Lusterless, brittle hair

DIAGNOSTIC TESTS & INTERPRETATION
Lab
Initial lab tests
- Clinical diagnosis
- Culture of pustules: Usually sterile; may show coagulase-negative staphylococcal epidermidis (normal skin flora)
- Additional hormonal testing may be indicated in females with hirsutism: PCOS, DHEA, luteinizing hormone (LH)/follicle-stimulating hormone (FSH), and free and total testosterone (3).

Pathological Findings
Follicular papules and pustules (4)

DIFFERENTIAL DIAGNOSIS
- Bacterial folliculitis
- Impetigo
- Acne vulgaris
- Tinea barbae
- Sarcoidal papules

 TREATMENT

- Mild cases:
  - Consider 5% benzoyl peroxide after shaving and application of 1% hydrocortisone cream at bedtime (or LactiCare HC lotion after shaving).
  - Tretinoin cream 0.025%; apply daily.
- Moderate cases:
  - Chemical depilatories (barium sulfide; Magic Shave powder); first test on forearm for 48 h (for irritation).
  - Consider eflornithine HCl cream (Vaniqa), but it can cause pseudofolliculitis barbae (PFB) (5).
- Severe cases:
  - Laser therapy (6,7)[A]: Longer-wavelength laser (e.g., Nd:YAG) is safer for dark skin (1).
  - Avoid shaving; completely grow beard.

MEDICATION
First Line
- Topical or systemic antibiotic for secondary infection:
  - Application of clindamycin (Cleocin T) solution b.i.d. or topical erythromycin if mild
  - Low-dose erythromycin or tetracycline, 250–500 mg PO b.i.d., if more severe inflammation (8)
  - Benzoyl peroxide 5%–clindamycin 1% gel b.i.d. (9)[C]: Administer until papule/pustule resolves.

- Mild cases: Tretinoin cream 0.025% at bedtime (8)
- Moderate disease/chemical depilatories:
  - Disrupt cross-linking of disulfide bonds of hair, causing blunt hair tip.
  - Apply no more frequently than every 3rd day: 2% barium sulfide (Magic Shave) or calcium thioglycolate (Surgex)
- Contraindications:
  - Clindamycin: History of regional enteritis or ulcerative colitis; history of antibiotic-associated colitis
  - Erythromycin, tetracycline, tretinoin hypersensitivity only
- Precautions:
  - Clindamycin: Colitis, eye burning and irritation, skin dryness; pregnancy category B
  - Erythromycin: Use cautiously in patients with impaired hepatic function; GI side effects, especially abdominal cramping; pregnancy category B.
  - Chemical depilatories: Use cautiously; frequent use and prolonged application may lead to irritant contact dermatitis and chemical burns.
  - Tetracycline: Permanent discoloration of teeth if given during last half of pregnancy
  - Tretinoin: Severe skin irritation; pregnancy category C
  - Benzoyl peroxide: Skin irritation and dryness, allergic contact dermatitis
  - Hydrocortisone cream: Local skin irritation, skin atrophy with prolonged use
- Significant possible interactions:
  - Erythromycin: Increases theophylline and carbamazepine levels; decreases clearance of warfarin; cardiac toxicity with terfenadine and astemizole
  - Tetracycline: Depresses plasma prothrombin activity (therefore, warfarin dosage must be decreased)

Second Line
Topical application of glycolic acid lotion (8% buffered glycolic acid in a suitable carrier, either oil-in-water lotion or a nonlipid soap) b.i.d.; this treatment may allow comfortable shaving every day (10)[C].

ADDITIONAL TREATMENT
General Measures
Acute treatment:
- Dislodge embedded hair with sterile needle/tweezers.
- Discontinue shaving until red papules have resolved (minimum 3–4 weeks; longer if moderate or severe); can trim to length >0.5 cm during this time (8)

- Massage beard area with washcloth, coarse sponge, or brush several times daily.
- Hydrocortisone1% cream to relieve inflammation
- Systemic antibiotics if secondary infection is present

Pregnancy Considerations
Do not use tretinoin (Retin-A), tetracycline, or benzoyl peroxide.

 ## ONGOING CARE

FOLLOW-UP RECOMMENDATIONS
Patient Monitoring
- As needed
- Educate patient on curative and preventive treatment.

DIET
No restrictions

PATIENT EDUCATION
- Dunn JF Jr. Pseudofolliculitis barbae. *Amer Fam Physician*. 1988;38:170–2.
- Crutchfield CE 3d. The causes and treatment of pseudofolliculitis barbae. *Cutis*. 1998;61:355–6.
- See section General Prevention.

PROGNOSIS
- Course is recurrent if preventive measures are not followed.
- Prognosis is poor in the presence of progressive scarring and foreign-body granuloma formation.

COMPLICATIONS
- Scarring (occasionally keloidal)
- Foreign-body granuloma formation
- Disfiguring postinflammatory hyperpigmentation (use sunscreens; can treat with hydroquinone4% cream, Retin A, clinical peels) (3)
- Impetiginization of inflamed skin
- Epidermal (erythema, crusting, burns with scarring) and pigmentary changes with laser (1,2,8)

REFERENCES
1. Bridgeman-Shah S. The Medical and Surgical Treatment of Pseudofolliculitis Barbae. *Dermatologic Therapy*. 2004;17:158–63.
2. Perry PK, et al. Defining pseudofolliculitis barbae in 2001: A review of the literature and current trends. *J Amer Acad Dermatol*. 2002;46(suppl 2): S113–S119.
3. *Dermatologic Therapy*, 2007;20:133–136.
4. Lever WF, Schaumburg-Lever G. *Histopathology of the Skin*. Philadelphia, PA: JB Lippincott; 1990.
5. Shenenberger DW, et al. Removal of Unwanted Facial Hair. *Am Fam Phys*. 2002;66(10): 1907–11.

6. Rogers CJ, Glaser DA. Treatment of pseudofolliculitis barbae using the Q-switched Nd:YAG laser with topical carbon suspension. *Dermatol Surg*. 2000;26:737–42.
7. Weaver SM, Sagaral EC. Treatment of pseudofolliculitis barbae using the long-pulse Nd:YAG laser on skin types V and VI. *Dermatol Surg*. 2003;29:1187–91.
8. *Up To Date*. 2007; Pseudofolliculitis Barbae.
9. Cook-Bolden FE, et al. Twice daily application of benzoyl peroxide 5% clindamycin 1% Gel versus vehicle in treatment of pseudofolliculitis barbae. *cutis*. 2004;73(6 suppl):13–24.
10. Perricone NV. Treatment of pseudofolliculitis barbae with topical glycolic acid: a report of two studies. *Cutis*. 1993;52:232–5.

ADDITIONAL READING
- Dunn JF Jr. Pseudofolliculitis barbae. *Amer Fam Physician*. 1988;38:169–74.
- Habif T. *Clinical Dermatology*. 4th ed. St. Louis, MD: Mosby; 2004.

See Also (Topic, Algorithm, Electronic Media Element)
Folliculitis; Impetigo; Tinea Barbae

 ## CODES

ICD9
704.8 Other specified diseases of hair and hair follicles

CLINICAL PEARLS
- Electrolysis is not recommended as a treatment. It's expensive, painful, and often unsuccessful (8).
- Curable by not shaving or complete hair removal (via laser)
- Approximately 3–5% of white men who shave are affected.
- Bump Fighter razor from American Safety Razor Company (www.asrco.com)

PSEUDOGOUT (CPPD)

Paul T. Cullen, MD

BASICS

DESCRIPTION
Acute inflammatory arthritic disease usually involving large joints; primarily affecting the elderly and caused by calcium pyrophosphate dihydrate (CPPD) crystal deposition in joints; associated with chondrocalcinosis:

- CPPD crystal deposition may cause a progressive degenerative arthritis in numerous joints.
- CPPD crystal deposition may cause a more insidious, smoldering, symmetric polyarthritis similar to rheumatoid arthritis (RA).
- System(s) affected: Endocrine/Metabolic; Musculoskeletal
- Synonym(s): Calcium pyrophosphate deposition disease

EPIDEMIOLOGY
Prevalence
- Predominant age: 80% of patients >60 years of age
- Predominant sex: Male = Female
- Chondrocalcinosis is present in 1 in 10 adults age 60–75 years and 1 in 3 by >80 years; only a small percentage develops pseudogout (1).

RISK FACTORS
- Aging
- Trauma
- Pseudogout often occurs as a complication in patients hospitalized for other medical and surgical illnesses.

Genetics
Uncommonly seen in familial pattern with autosomal dominant inheritance (<1% of patients); most cases are sporadic.

GENERAL PREVENTION
Colchicine 0.6 mg b.i.d. may reduce frequency of episodes in recurrent monoarthritic CPPD.

ETIOLOGY
- Acute inflammatory reaction to CPPD crystals shed into synovial cavity
- Physical and chemical changes in aging cartilage that favor crystal growth

COMMONLY ASSOCIATED CONDITIONS
- Hyperparathyroidism
- Hemochromatosis
- Gout
- Hypophosphatasia
- Hypothyroidism
- Ochronosis
- Wilson disease
- Amyloidosis
- Hypomagnesemia

DIAGNOSIS

HISTORY
- Acute pain and swelling of ≥1 or more joints; knee involved in 1/2 of all attacks; ankle, wrist, and shoulder also common
- Can present with a chronic progressive arthritis on which acute inflammatory attacks are superimposed
- Progressive degenerative arthritis in numerous joints, including wrists, metacarpophalangeal, hips, shoulders, elbows, and ankles
- Low-grade inflammatory arthritis with multiple symmetric joint involvement (mimics RA) <5% of cases
- Can present in proximal joints mimicking polymyalgia rheumatica, often accompanied by tibiofemoral and ankle arthritis and tendinous calcifications (2)[C]
- May develop after intraarticular injection of hyaluronic acid (Hyalgan, Synvisc) (3)[C]

PHYSICAL EXAM
- Inflammation, joint effusion, limitation of motion
- 50% associated with fever
- Any other synovial joint may be involved, including 1st metatarsophalangeal joint.

DIAGNOSTIC TESTS & INTERPRETATION
Lab
Initial lab tests
Synovial fluid analysis consistent with an inflammatory effusion:

- Cell count from 2,000–100,000 white blood cells [WBCs]/mL
- Differential predominantly neutrophils (80–90%)
- >50,000 WBC count increases likelihood of septic arthritis, 11% prevalence; number needed to treat (NNT) = 9; >100,000 WBCs/mL, 22% prevalence (4)[C]
- Wet prep with polarized microscopy may demonstrate small numbers of weakly positively birefringent crystals in the fluid and within neutrophils; false-negative rate is high. Metabolic studies to exclude an underlying cause always should be obtained in patients <50 years of age and should be considered in the elderly:
  - Serum calcium
  - Serum phosphorus
  - Serum alkaline phosphatase
  - Serum parathormone (i-PTH)
  - Serum iron, total iron-binding capacity, and serum ferritin
  - Serum magnesium
  - Serum thyroid-stimulating hormone (TSH) level

Imaging
Initial approach
Radiographs of joints:

- May demonstrate punctate and linear calcification in articular hyaline or fibrocartilage: Knees, hips, symphysis pubis, and wrists are affected most often; also may be found in asymptomatic individuals
- In the chronic destructive indolent form of the disease: Subchondral cyst formation, fragmentation with formation of intra-articular radiodense bodies in joints not typically affected by degenerative joint disease

Diagnostic Procedures/Surgery
Aspiration of joint fluid with synovial fluid analysis required for proper confirmation of pseudogout; aspiration may relieve symptoms and speed resolution of inflammatory process.

Pathological Findings
CPPD crystal deposition in articular cartilage, synovium, ligaments, and tendons

DIFFERENTIAL DIAGNOSIS
- Illnesses that may cause acute inflammatory arthritis in a single or multiple joint(s):
  - Gout
  - Septic arthritis
  - Trauma
- Other illnesses that may present with an acute inflammatory arthritis:
  - Reiter syndrome
  - Lyme disease
  - Acute RA

TREATMENT

MEDICATION
First Line
- Nonsteroidal anti-inflammatory drugs (NSAIDs): Choose 1 of the following:
  - Ibuprofen (Motrin): 600–800 mg p.o. t.i.d.–q.i.d. with food; maximum of 3.2 g/d
  - Naproxen (Naprosyn): 500 mg p.o. b.i.d. with food
  - Other NSAIDs at anti-inflammatory doses are effective, although indomethacin has higher complication rates (relative risk [RR] = 2.2) compared with ibuprofen (RR = 1.2) (5)[B].
- Contraindications:
  - History of hypersensitivity to NSAIDs or aspirin
  - Active peptic ulcer disease or history of recurrent upper GI lesions
  - Avoid in renal insufficiency if serum creatinine >1.6 mg/dL.
  - Serious GI bleeding can occur without warning; follow the patient carefully for internal bleeding. Administer proton pump inhibitor (PPI) or misoprostol 200 μg p.o. q.i.d. in patients with peptic ulcer disease history.

- Significant possible interactions:
  - May elevate BP in treated hypertensives
  - May blunt antihypertensive effects of angiotensin-converting enzyme (ACE) inhibitors
  - May prolong prothrombin time (PT) in patients taking oral anticoagulants
  - Avoid concomitant aspirin use.
  - May blunt diuretic effect of furosemide and hydrochlorothiazide
  - May increase plasma lithium level in patients taking lithium carbonate

Second Line
- Oral prednisone: Begin at 40–60 mg/d and taper over 10 days.
- IM triamcinolone acetonide 60 mg; may repeat in 1–4 days (4)[B]
- Intraarticular instillation of prednisolone–sodium phosphate 4–20 mg or triamcinolone diacetate 2–40 mg with local anesthetic
- Oral colchicines (6)[C] 0.6 mg q.i.d. or 0.6 mg hourly until symptoms relieved or vomiting/diarrhea develops; maximum dose per attack 4–6 mg; avoid with significant renal insufficiency
- Methotrexate may have a role in severe disease resistant to traditional therapy (76)[C].

ADDITIONAL TREATMENT
General Measures
- Rest and elevate affected joint(s).
- Apply ice/cool compresses to affected joints.
- Non-weight-bearing on affected joint while painful; use crutches or walker.

Issues for Referral
Consider consultation with orthopedist or rheumatologist if septic joint is a serious consideration or patient is not responding.

Additional Therapies
Physical therapy:
- Isometric exercises to maintain muscle strength during the acute stage (e.g., quadriceps isometric contractions, and leg lifts if knee affected)
- Begin joint range-of-motion (ROM) exercises as inflammation and pain subside.
- Resume weight-bearing when pain subsides.

SURGERY/OTHER PROCEDURES
Perform arthrocentesis and joint fluid analysis.

IN-PATIENT CONSIDERATIONS
Admission Criteria
Consider admission for septic arthritis if synovial fluid WBC count >50,000/mL; strongly consider if >100,000/mL; treat with appropriate antibiotics pending culture results.

 ## ONGOING CARE
FOLLOW-UP RECOMMENDATIONS
Patient Monitoring
Reevaluate patient for response to therapy 48–72 h after treatment instituted; reexamine 1 week later and then as needed.

DIET
No known relationship to diet

PATIENT EDUCATION
- Rest affected joint.
- Symptoms usually resolve in 7–10 days.

PROGNOSIS
- Acute attack usually resolves in 10 days; prognosis for resolution of acute attack is excellent.
- Some patients experience progressive joint damage with functional limitation.

COMPLICATIONS
- Erosive destructive arthritis in a pattern of joints not usually affected by degenerative joint disease (e.g., metacarpophalangeal joints, wrists)
- Recurrences

Geriatric Considerations
Elderly patients treated with NSAIDs require careful monitoring and are at higher risk for GI bleeding and acute renal insufficiency.

REFERENCES
1. Richette P, Bardin T, Doherty M. An update on the epidemiology of calcium pyrophosphate dihydrate crystal deposition disease. *Rheumatology (Oxford).* 2009.
2. Pego-Reigosa JM, Rodriguez-Rodriguez M, Hurtado-Hernandez Z, et al. Calcium pyrophosphate deposition disease mimicking polymyalgia rheumatica: a prospective followup study of predictive factors for this condition in patients presenting with polymyalgia symptoms. *Arthritis Rheum.* 2005;53:931–8.
3. Hamburger MI, Lakhanpal S, Mooar PA, et al. Intra-articular hyaluronans: a review of product-specific safety profiles. *Semin Arthritis Rheum.* 2003;32:296–309.
4. Shah K, Spear J, Nathanson LA, et al. Does the presence of crystal arthritis rule out septic arthritis? *J Emerg Med.* 2007;32:23–6.
5. Richy F, Bruyere O, Ethgen O, et al. Time dependent risk of gastrointestinal complications induced by non-steroidal anti-inflammatory drug use: a consensus statement using a meta-analytic approach. *Ann Rheum Dis.* 2004;63:759–66.
6. Lioté F, Ea HK et al. Recent developments in crystal-induced inflammation pathogenesis and management. *Curr Rheumatol Rep.* 2007;9:243–50.
7. Chollet-Janin A, Finckh A, Dudler J, et al. Methotrexate as an alternative therapy for chronic calcium pyrophosphate deposition disease: an exploratory analysis. *Arthritis Rheum.* 2007;56:688–92.

ADDITIONAL READING
- Announ N, Guerne PA et al. Treating difficult crystal pyrophosphate dihydrate deposition disease. *Curr Rheumatol Rep.* 2008;10:228–34.
- Wise CM. Crystal-associated arthritis in the elderly. *Clin Geriatr Med.* 2005;21:491–511, v-vi.

 ## CODES

ICD9
- 275.49 Other disorders of calcium metabolism
- 712.10 Chondrocalcinosis, due to dicalcium phosphate crystals, involving unspecified site
- 712.20 Chondrocalcinosis, due to pyrophosphate crystals, involving unspecified site

CLINICAL PEARLS
- Perform joint fluid aspiration and analysis to evaluate acute arthritis.
- If septic arthritis is considered, treat presumptively with antibiotics until culture results are available.
- NSAID therapy is preferred treatment.
- Oral steroids are useful if NSAIDs are contraindicated.
- Intra-articular steroids can be used *if* septic arthritis has been excluded.

PSEUDOMEMBRANOUS COLITIS

Aman D. Sabharwal, MD
Amar Deshpande, MD

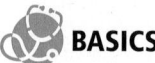 **BASICS**

DESCRIPTION
- Diarrheal illness after antibiotic treatment; severity ranges from asymptomatic carrier state to fulminant disease and shock
- Synonym(s): *C. diff.* colitis; CDAD (*C. diff*-associated diarrhea; antibiotic-associated colitis (this should be differentiated from the more common antibiotic-associated diarrhea, which is not infectious and resolves with cessation of the offending agent)

EPIDEMIOLOGY
Prevalence
- Community: 1–5% asymptomatic colonization
- Hospital: 90 per 100,000. Rates doubled from 2000 to 2003 and tripled from 2000 to 2005. Death increased ~4-fold from 1999 to 2004. 20% asymptomatic colonization.
- Neonates: 40% colonized

Geriatric Considerations
Increased risk for exposure to and a higher mortality rate from pseudomembranous colitis

RISK FACTORS
- Antibiotic exposure: All antibiotics associated with some risk; highest risk:
  - Cephalosporins
  - Penicillins
  - Clindamycin
  - Fluoroquinolones
- Increasing age
- Long duration of hospital stay/time spent in ICU
- Number and duration of antibiotics received
- Proton pump inhibitor use (controversial)
- Underlying inflammatory bowel disease (IBD)
- Immunosuppression

Genetics
No known factors

GENERAL PREVENTION
- Judicious use of antimicrobial agents
- Appropriate handwashing, glove use, disposable thermometers (1)[A], and isolation procedures in hospital and chronic-care facilities
- To prevent complications, do not use opiate or antidiarrheal medications during *C. difficile* colitis episode.

ETIOLOGY
- Colitis from exotoxin of *C. difficile* (anaerobic gram-positive bacillus)
- Forms heat-resistant spores
- Asymptomatic carriers are reservoirs.
- Prior treatment with antibiotics alters intestinal flora. *C. difficile* spores are ingested, germinate, and in a suitable host, colitis develops.
- *C. difficile* secretes 2 exotoxins: A (enterotoxin) and B (exotoxin).
- Toxin A causes inflammation, increased mucosal permeability, and fluid secretion.

COMMONLY ASSOCIATED CONDITIONS
- Infection requiring antibiotic treatment
- Can result in megacolon, ileus, perforation, sepsis

DIAGNOSIS

HISTORY
- Diarrhea (up to 20 watery stools daily, may be blood-tinged, rarely grossly bloody, foul-smelling)
- Lower abdominal pain, cramping
- Current antibiotic use
- Antibiotic use in past 3 months
- Recent/current hospitalization
- Resident of continuing-care facility

PHYSICAL EXAM
- Abdominal tenderness
- Abdominal distension
- In severe cases, rebound tenderness
- Fever
- Volume depletion

DIAGNOSTIC TESTS & INTERPRETATION
Lab
- Stool for *C. difficile* toxin A and B enzyme immunoassay (EIA):
  - At least 3 separate specimens increase sensitivity.
- Elevated white blood cell (WBC) count
- Monitor for dehydration, electrolyte imbalance, and hypoalbuminemia.

Imaging
- CT scan: Thickened or edematous colonic wall with pericolonic inflammation
- X-ray: Colonic distention, evaluate for toxic megacolon

Diagnostic Procedures/Surgery
Colonoscopy: In severe illness, when cannot wait for toxin test to return and need diagnostic information; pseudomembrane may be visible; its absence does not rule out *C. difficile* colitis

Pathological Findings
- Gross pathology: Yellow–white, loosely adherent plaques on colonic and small intestinal mucosa
- Microscopic pathology: Necrosis, polymorphonuclear cells

DIFFERENTIAL DIAGNOSIS
- Other causes of watery diarrhea: Viral (Norwalk), bacterial (*Campylobacter*), protozoan (*Giardia*)
- Inflammatory bowel disease
- Malabsorption
- If severe illness, consider other causes of acute abdomen, shock

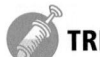 **TREATMENT**

MEDICATION

First Line

- Oral route most effective; >90% cases respond, usually in 2–4 days.
- Metronidazole 250 mg p.o. q.i.d. or 500 mg t.i.d. × 10–14 days (2)[B]
- Significant possible interactions: Alcohol and metronidazole cause disulfiram-like reaction. Refer to the manufacturer's literature for other interactions.
- For severely ill patients, consider vancomycin 125 mg q.i.d. × 14 days, given by nasogastric or rectal tube (if unable to give orally; oral route is most effective). If ileus, consider rectal vancomycin and IV metronidazole.
- 20% relapse; usually not treatment failure, but due to germination of spores or reinfection
- Treat first recurrence the same as initial episode.
- Treat second recurrence with tapering vancomycin (usually over 7 weeks), and consider probiotics.
- Other options include IV immunoglobulins, cholestyramine, and fecal transplantation.

ADDITIONAL TREATMENT

General Measures

- Fluid and electrolyte repletion
- Stop offending agent.
- Avoid antimotility agents and opiates.
- Do not treat asymptomatic carriers.

COMPLEMENTARY AND ALTERNATIVE MEDICINE

- Saccharomyces boulardii (yeast) may reduce the risk of *C. difficile* infection in some patients on concurrent antibiotics (3)[C].
- Probiotics may also help reduce risk; optimal dosing still controversial (4)[C].

SURGERY/OTHER PROCEDURES

- Emergent colectomy may be required in toxic megacolon.
- High-risk patients (those with inflammatory bowel disease, recent surgery, leukocytosis, vasopressor requirements, prior treatment with intravenous immunoglobulin [IVIG], or increased lactate) require surgical consult for possible subtotal colectomy and end ileostomy to help reduce the mortality associated with fulminant colitis (5)[C]

IN-PATIENT CONSIDERATIONS

Admission Criteria

Consider severity of symptoms (e.g., acute abdomen, sepsis, ability to maintain oral intake), comorbidities, and age (increased morbidity in older people).

IV Fluids

If unable to tolerate oral diet, IV fluid may be necessary to maintain adequate hydration and electrolyte balance.

Discharge Criteria

- Able to tolerate oral diet
- Vital signs, hydration status, electrolytes adequately treated

 ONGOING CARE

FOLLOW-UP RECOMMENDATIONS

Bed rest during acute phase

Patient Monitoring

Careful monitoring through fulminant phase

DIET

n.p.o. during fulminant phase

PROGNOSIS

- Case mortality rate: 1–2.5% (2)[B]
- In severely ill, colectomy sometimes required: 20–30% mortality with this degree of illness

COMPLICATIONS

- Protein-losing enteropathy with hypoalbuminemia and ascites
- Hypovolemia, shock
- Ileus and toxic megacolon
- Bowel perforation
- Sepsis, death
- Postinfectious IBS

REFERENCES

1. Hsu J, Abad C, Dinh M, Safdar N et al. Prevention of Endemic Healthcare-Associated Clostridium difficile Infection: Reviewing the Evidence. *The American journal of gastroenterology*. 2010;
2. Schroeder MS. Clostridium difficile–associated diarrhea. *Am Fam Physician*. 2005;71:921–8.
3. Tung JM, Dolovich LR, Lee CH et al. Prevention of Clostridium difficile infection with Saccharomyces boulardii: a systematic review. *Can J Gastroenterol*. 2009;23:817–21.
4. McFarland LV et al. Evidence-based review of probiotics for antibiotic-associated diarrhea and Clostridium difficile infections. *Anaerobe*. 2009;15:274–80.
5. Butala P, Divino CM et al. Surgical aspects of fulminant Clostridium difficile Colitis. *American journal of surgery*. 2010;

ADDITIONAL READING

- Bricker E, et al. Antibiotic treatment for *Clostridium difficile*-associated diarrhea in adults. *Cochrane Database Sys Rev*. 2005;1:CD004610.
- Johnson S. Recurrent Clostridium difficile infection: A review of risk factors, treatments, and outcomes. *J Infect*. 2009.

 CODES

ICD9

008.45 Intestinal infection due to clostridium difficile

CLINICAL PEARLS

- Early consultation with surgical service is critical when patients present with peritonitis or multiorgan failure. Pre-emptive surgical evaluation is also prudent in moderate-to-severe disease.
- The recurrence rate is at least 20%; this generally will be seen within the first few weeks after completion of therapy.
- Pseudomembranous colitis should be suspected in any patient who develops diarrhea during or up to 3 weeks after the cessation of antibiotic therapy; also consider this diagnosis in a flare of IBD and all hospitalized/institutionalized patients.

PSITTACOSIS

Jon S. Parham, DO, MPH

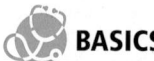 **BASICS**

DESCRIPTION

- A classic zoonotic disease, psittacosis is associated primarily with contact with infected birds (e.g., parrots, cockatiels, parakeets, pigeons, doves, mynah birds, canaries, finches, birds of prey, and shore birds) and some mammals.
  - Discovery: First described in 1879 in Switzerland
  - Agent: *Chlamydophila psittaci*
  - Clinical: A systemic infectious disease of variable severity that initially causes influenza-like symptoms but primarily affects the lung, where it causes an atypical pneumonia; may spread hematogenously from lung to other organs
  - Severity: Subclinical infection to fulminant sepsis with multi-organ system failure may occur in usually healthy persons.
- Often occupation-related: Affecting poultry farmers, ranchers, and zoo and pet shop employees
- Synonym(s): Ornithosis; Parrot fever; Bird-breeder's disease; Bird-fancier lung

EPIDEMIOLOGY

Incidence

- Predominant age: Adults
- Predominant sex: Male = Female.
- 66 cases (mean 13, range 8–21) reported in US in 2005–2009 (1)[C]

Prevalence

In bird populations, prevalence of infection is estimated to be between 5% and 8%.

Pregnancy Considerations

- Infections in late 2nd and 3rd trimesters are potentially life-threatening to mother and fetus.
- *C. psittaci* can cross the placenta.
- Pregnant women should avoid contact with birds and pregnant sheep and goats.

Pediatric Considerations

Relatively uncommon in this age group

Geriatric Considerations

Mortality rate may be higher in geriatric or debilitated patients.

RISK FACTORS

- For humans, strains transmitted from turkeys and psittacine birds (parrots and similar pets) appear to be the most virulent.
- Ranchers contacting parturient goats, sheep, dairy cattle, and horses
- Immunosuppressed humans with appropriate disease reservoir contact

Genetics

No known genetic predisposition

GENERAL PREVENTION

- Avoidance of exposure:
  - Maintain clean bird habitats.
  - Avoid being with birds in confined spaces.
  - Brief, passing exposures can cause infection.
- Infected birds may be asymptomatic.
- Treat birds suspected to be infected.
- In occupational exposures, personal protective equipment, including air-filter face masks, is recommended (2)[C].

PATHOPHYSIOLOGY

- *C. psittaci* is an obligate intracellular gram-negative bacteria.
- Can survive on dry, inanimate surface for 15 days
- In humans, the bacterium is usually inhaled and infects cells of the respiratory tract.
- If untreated, it also can infect pericardium, heart, liver, kidneys, joints, and CNS.

ETIOLOGY

- Through contact with dried secretions and excretions from infected birds in their habitat and on their plumage
- Through intimate contact with pets (e.g., mouth to beak, bites)
- Human-to-human transmission is suggested but not proven.

COMMONLY ASSOCIATED CONDITIONS

- The presence of *C. psittaci* occurs in about 80% of cases of ocular adnexal lymphomas, and recently, it was found in a significant number of lymphomas in other sites, such as diffuse B-cell lymphomas of the skin and throat (3)[C].
- There are numerous other diseases that spread to humans from birds or by working with or around bird populations.
  - Avian influenza
  - Viral encephalomyelitides (e.g., West Nile virus)
  - Salmonellosis, campylobacteriosis, yersiniosis
  - *Mycobacterium avian* and *M. tuberculosis* infection
  - Q fever, histoplasmosis, cryptococcosis
  - Newcastle disease

℞ DIAGNOSIS

- Careful observations of 1st responders to identify situational association between patient and birds
- A history of direct exposure to birds is *not necessary* to diagnose the disease.
- According to the Centers for Disease Control and Prevention (CDC), in context of a case consistent with psittacosis, any *one* of the following is diagnostic:
  - Respiratory specimen isolation of *C. psittaci* (confirmed case)
  - ≥4-fold increase in IgG against *C. psittaci* by complement fixation (CF) or MIF comparing serum specimens at least 2–4 weeks apart (confirmed case)
  - An IgM titer of at least 1:32 of *C. psittaci* antibody in specimen obtained after onset of symptoms (probable case)
  - Polymerase chain reaction (PCR) detection of *C. psittaci* DNA in a respiratory specimen (probable case) (1)[C]

HISTORY

- Incubation period: 5–14 days (up to 4 weeks)
- Typically, abrupt onset of symptoms
- Fever and chills
- Myalgia and malaise
- Pronounced headache (most common symptom)
- Sore throat
- Delayed development of nonproductive cough and, in some cases, deteriorating condition

PHYSICAL EXAM

- Multiple presentation variants:
  - Influenza-like: Fever, malaise, dry cough
  - Mononucleosis-like: Fever, pharyngitis, hepatosplenomegaly, and adenopathy
  - Typhoidal: Fever, bradycardia, malaise, and splenomegaly
  - Atypical pneumonia: Nonproductive cough, fever, headache, and chest film abnormalities
- Fever: May present *without* tachycardia
- Lung rales, usually
- Horder spots (i.e., pink macular rash on the face)
- Enlarged spleen
- Cerebrospinal fluid (CSF) findings are usually normal; meningoencephalitis can occur.

DIAGNOSTIC TESTS & INTERPRETATION

- Culture is rarely performed owing to high communicability risk to lab workers.
- Acute and convalescent-phase serum for serology is collected at least 2–3 weeks apart; then a 2nd convalescent serum is collected at 4–6 weeks if the pattern is uninterpretable (1)[C].
- CF test: Most common serologic test for psittacosis but is also positive with other *Chlamydia* infections.
  - A 4-fold rise in CF IgG titer to >1:32 is diagnostic of an acute nonspecific *Chlamydia* infection.
  - A single or stable CF IgM titer of >1:64 suggests a recent infection.
- The species-specific MIF test for *C. psittaci* is currently the preferred test but has been criticized (4)[C]; IgM titer ≥1:32 is positive (1)[C].
- Real-time PCR in in vivo testing shows sensitivity and specificity percentages in the high 90s, but larger studies are needed (5)[C].

Lab

- Leukocyte count is often normal or low; leukocyte left shift may occur.
- Erythrocyte sedimentation rate (ESR) is usually elevated; C-reactive protein is markedly elevated.
- Sputum is usually negative by Gram stain and routine culture.
- Proteinuria is possible during febrile period.
- Liver enzymes may be elevated.
- Increased IgG, IgM, and IgA
- Hypoxemia and hypocapnia
- Eosinophilia
- Serologic response may be blunted by early treatment with some antibiotics.

Initial lab tests

Complete blood count, ESR, complete medical panel with liver tests, serology: CF test or MIF

Imaging

Chest radiography:

- Often shows patchy alveolar infiltrates of interstitial pneumonitis and small nodular densities
- Single lobar consolidation also common
- Hilar adenopathy
- Pleural effusion possible but usually scanty
- Radiographic abnormalities may persist for up to 20 weeks (6 weeks, mean) after successful treatment.

Initial approach

Initial chest X-ray may be normal.

Pathological Findings
- Characteristic gross findings:
  - Inflamed trachea and bronchi
  - Rubbery, congested lungs
  - Mucous plugging
- Microscopic findings:
  - Alveolar and interstitial exudates: Mononuclear cells predominate.
  - Hyperplastic, proliferative alveolar lining cells: Basophilic intracytoplasmic inclusion

DIFFERENTIAL DIAGNOSIS
- Consider other common bacterial respiratory pathogens, including:
  - *S. pneumoniae*
  - *H. influenzae*
  - *K. pneumoniae*
  - *C. pneumoniae*
  - *M. pneumoniae*
  - *Legionella* spp.
- Typhoid fever, influenza, Q fever, brucellosis

TREATMENT

Rapid clinical response to doxycycline; afebrile by 48 h

MEDICATION
Treat for 10–14 days after resolution of fever (1)[C].

First Line
- Oral tetracycline antibiotics:
  - Doxycycline, 100 mg q12h
  - Tetracycline, 500 mg q6h
- Intravenous antibiotics for severely ill: Doxycycline hyclate, 4.4 mg/kg/d divided into 2 infusions (up to 100 mg/dose) (6)[C]

Second Line
Pregnancy Considerations
When tetracyclines are contraindicated, such as in children age <9 years of age or pregnant women, consider erythromycin or other macrolides.

ADDITIONAL TREATMENT
General Measures
- History of avian exposure (particularly to a sick bird) is key to making early diagnosis.
- Severity of respiratory symptoms dictates treatment. Severely ill patients require oxygen, intravenous fluids, and intravenous antibiotics.
- Although human-to-human transmission is suggested, only routine respiratory secretion precautions are indicated (1)[C].

Issues for Referral
Consult infectious disease service.

IN-PATIENT CONSIDERATIONS
Initial Stabilization
- Outpatient care
- Hospitalize patients with dyspnea, hypoxia, confusion, or other signs of severe disease.

Nursing
Only standard respiratory isolation and usual droplet transmission control are needed (no private room or negative-pressure flow room) (1)[C]

ONGOING CARE

FOLLOW-UP RECOMMENDATIONS
- In most states, this is a reportable disease.
- Contact state or local health authority.
- No persistent immunity to prevent reinfection

Patient Monitoring
Determined by acute severity of illness

DIET
No special diet

PATIENT EDUCATION
- American Lung Association, 1740 Broadway, New York, NY 10019, (800) 586-4872
- Centers for Disease Control and Prevention, Atlanta, GA, (800)-311-3435
- There is little consensus on the risks of pet bird ownership and bird-related human disease (7)[C].

PROGNOSIS
- Mortality rate <1% with appropriate treatment but was 15–20% without antibiotics.
- Full recovery may take weeks to months.
- Relapse may occur, necessitating a 2nd course of antibiotics.

COMPLICATIONS
- Meningitis and encephalitis: Transverse myelitis and Guillain-Barré syndrome are rare.
- Endocarditis, pericarditis, and myocarditis
- Renal failure, hepatitis
- Erythema nodosum
- Sinusitis, respiratory failure
- Reactive arthritis (rare)
- Disseminated intravascular coagulation (rare)
- Valvular heart disease (rare)
- Spontaneous abortion (rare)
- Thyroiditis (rare)
- Pancreatitis (rare)

REFERENCES

1. Smith K, et al. Compendium of measures to control Chlamydophila psittaci infection amoung humans (Psittacosis) and pet birds (avian Chlamydiosis), 2010. National Association of State Public Health Veterinarians (NASPHV). Access at:
2. Vanrompay D, Harkinezhad T, van de Walle M, et al. Chlamydophila psittaci transmission from pet birds to humans. *Emerg Infect Dis*. 2007;13:1108–10.
3. Ponzoni M, Ferreri AJ, Guidoboni M, et al. Chlamydia infection and lymphomas: association beyond ocular adnexal lymphomas highlighted by multiple detection methods. *Clin Cancer Res*. 2008;14:5794–800.
4. Verminnen K, Duquenne B, De Keukeleire D, et al. Evaluation of a Chlamydophila psittaci infection diagnostic platform for zoonotic risk assessment. *J Clin Microbiol*. 2008;46:281–5.
5. Yang J-M, et al. Development of a rapid real-time PCR assay for detection and quantification of four familiar species of *Chlamydiaceae*. *J Clin Virolo*. 2006;36:79–81.
6. Telfer BL, Moberley SA, Hort KP, et al. Probable psittacosis outbreak linked to wild birds. *Emerg Infect Dis*. 2005;11:391–7.
7. Gorman J, Cook A, Ferguson C, et al. Pet birds and risks of respiratory disease in Australia: a review. *Aust N Z J Public Health*. 2009;33:167–72.

ADDITIONAL READING

- *Morbidity Mortality Weekly Report*. 2007;56(40): 1059–71.
- Schlossberg D. *Chlamydophila (Chlamydia) psittaci* (Psittacosis). In: Mandell, Bennet, and Dolin, eds., *Principles and Practice of Infectious Diseases*. 6th ed. New York: Churchill Livingstone; 2005.

 CODES

ICD9
- 073.0 Ornithosis with pneumonia
- 073.7 Ornithosis with other specified complications
- 073.8 Ornithosis with unspecified complication

CLINICAL PEARLS
- The most important historical clues in potential cases of psittacosis are a history of contact with birds and acute headache.
- The best test(s) for diagnosing psittacosis is a CF or MIF antibody test showing a 4-fold increase in IgG 3–4 weeks after the onset of symptoms or an IgM antibody titer ≥1:32. PCR is an accurate and selective test for *C. psittaci* from among the other species.
- The drug of choice for treatment is a tetracycline, specifically, doxycycline, for nonpregnant adults and children aged >9 years; alternatively, use erythromycin or other macrolides or chloramphenicol.
- The lab tests for psittacosis in humans performed at the Response and Surveillance Lab at the CDC (404-639-4921) are MIF, PCR, and culture (1)[C].

PSORIASIS

Debora B. Sternaman, PharmD
Edward C. Sternaman, II, MD

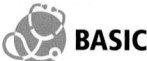

BASICS

DESCRIPTION
- A T-cell-mediated immunologic genetic disorder of the skin leading to an epidermal proliferative rash characterized by well-defined brick-red papulosquamous plaques with a silvery scale
- Characterized by flares (related to systemic, emotional, and environmental factors) and remissions
- Usual course: Acute; chronic; unpredictable
- Clinical forms:
  - Plaque: Most common; patches on scalp, trunk, limbs (extensor surfaces); nails may be pitted and/or thickened
  - Guttate: Usually presents <20 years of age; numerous small papules over wide area of skin, greatest on trunk
  - Inverse or flexural: Affects intertriginous areas; lesions moist ± scales
  - Pustular (von Zumbusch): True emergency: Severe form characterized by widespread erythema, scaling, pustule formation
  - Erythrodermic: Severe form, skin turns red; often presents with chronic disease and/or precipitated by high use of topical steroids
  - Nail disease: Can occur in all subtypes; fingernails involved in ~50% of cases and toenails in 35%
  - Psoriatic arthritis: Inflammatory arthropathy; see Psoriatic Arthritis

EPIDEMIOLOGY
Incidence
- Predominant sex: Male = Female
- Greater incidence in whites

Prevalence
- 2–4%
- Predominant age: Mean age of onset 33 years of age; earlier in women; most occur <46 years of age

RISK FACTORS
- Family history
- Local trauma; local irritation
- Infection (β-hemolytic streptococcal or viral infection can stimulate acute guttate psoriasis)
- HIV
- Stress (physical and emotional)
- Withdrawal of steroid therapy
- Folate and vitamin B_{12} deficiency
- Medications (see General Prevention)
- Alcohol use, smoking
- Diabetes, obesity, metabolic syndrome

Genetics
- Genetic predisposition (probably polygenic)
- 20–30% have psoriasis in a 1st-degree relative.
- Type I psoriasis (onset <40 years) theorized to have a strong familial pattern and more severe course than type 2 (onset >40 years)
- Increased incidence of specific human leukocyte antigens

GENERAL PREVENTION
Avoid trauma/sunburns, irritating drugs, stimulating drugs, antimalarial medications (aminoquinolines), and alcoholic beverages.

PATHOPHYSIOLOGY
- Multisystem inflammatory autoimmune condition affecting primarily the skin and joints
- Characterized by disfiguring, scaly, erythematous patches, papules, and plaques, which may be painful, leading to quality-of-life (QOL) issues

ETIOLOGY
- Immune disease modulated by T cells and proinflammatory cytokines
- T-cell-mediated: Triggered by some environmental antigen (e.g., trauma) or internal antigen (HIV) that promotes a cycle of cytokine production and cell proliferation

COMMONLY ASSOCIATED CONDITIONS
- Autoimmune: Crohn disease, ulcerative colitis, multiple sclerosis (MS)
- Cardiovascular: Inflammatory process
- Metabolic syndrome
- Psychiatric/psychologic: Depression, suicide, psychologic, and emotional burden/anxiety
- Psoriatic arthritis
- Atopic dermatitis
- May be among 1st signs of AIDS
- Nonmelanoma skin cancer (unclear whether related to disease process or treatment)
- Hepatic abnormalities (pustular psoriasis)

DIAGNOSIS

HISTORY
- History of trauma, previous treatment, pruritus
- Family history

PHYSICAL EXAM
- Rash: Color, size, morphology, distribution, scale; Auspitz sign: Underlying pinpoints of bleeding following scraping (1)[C]
- Special attention to scalp, umbilicus, intergluteal cleft, and nails
- Well-defined red papules coalescing to plaques; sharply demarcated silvery scales on red plaques (2)[C]
- Knee-elbow-scalp-sacral-groin distribution
- Koebner phenomenon: Psoriatic response in traumatic area (1)[C]
- Stippled nails and pitting
- Sebopsoriasis: Greasy scales in the eyebrows, nasolabial folds, and postauricular and presternal areas (2)

DIAGNOSTIC TESTS & INTERPRETATION
Lab
Initial lab tests
- Diagnosis by history and physical (3)[C]
- Negative rheumatoid factor (4)[C]
- Increased erythrocyte sedimentation rate (ESR) (4)[C]
- Elevated C-reactive protein (4)[C]
- Fungal studies may show a superimposed infection.

Diagnostic Procedures/Surgery
- Psoriasis Area and Severity Index evaluates overall severity and body surface area (BSA) involvement.
- Physicians Global Assessment: Target plaque score and the percent BSA together.
- Biopsy is rarely required (1).

Pathological Findings
- Epidermal hyperplasia
- Parakeratotic scale
- Loss of granular cell layer
- Mitotic figures in basal cell layer
- Elongation and thickening of rete ridges
- Dilated tortuous surface capillary loops
- Inflammatory infiltrate with T cells, neutrophils, mast cells, and macrophages

DIFFERENTIAL DIAGNOSIS
- Scalp: Seborrheic dermatitis
- Chronic/nummular eczema
- Lichen simplex chronicus
- Trunk: Pityriasis rosea, pityriasis rubra pilaris, tinea corporis

TREATMENT

MEDICATION
First Line
- Mild-to-moderate disease:
  - Emollients b.i.d.: Petrolatum or thick creams
  - Topical corticosteroids (13,)[A]:
    - Tachyphylaxis develops over time; may alternate to prevent
    - Side effects include skin thinning, hypopigmentation, and increased chance of local infection.
    - Occlusive dressing increases effectiveness but also increases chance of side effects.
    - For scalp: Strong potency in alcohol base
    - Face, intertriginous areas: Low-potency corticosteroids; infants, 1% hydrocortisone
    - Medium-potency corticosteroids daily (e.g., 0.1% mometasone or triamcinolone)
    - Strong-potency corticosteroids: 0.05% betamethasone or fluocinonide daily; good initial plaque treatment (3)[A]
    - Superpotency corticosteroids: Clobetasol, halobetasol; limit use to 2 weeks; avoid occlusive dressings; reserved for recalcitrant plaques (1,3)[A]
  - Vitamin D analogues: Calcipotriene ointment 0.005% b.i.d. limits keratinocyte hyperproliferation; monitor calcium (1,3)[A].
  - Topical retinoids: Tazarotene (Tazorac) 0.05% or 0.1% daily; local irritation; solar sensitivity; avoid in pregnancy (3,4)[A]
  - Moderate-to-severe disease: Combination therapy may be required to control appropriately.
  - Light therapy: Natural sunlight improves symptoms, office-administered light available as ultraviolet B (broad or narrow band) or PUVA (p.o. or bath psoralen + ultraviolet A [UVA]). Narrowband ultraviolet B (UVB) may be more effective (1,3)[C]:
    - Broadband UVB up to 20–25 treatments 2–3 times weekly with or without topical tar or anthralin (may increase effectiveness); after initial treatment, treat weekly to maintain.
    - UVA administered within 2 hours of receiving psoralen; initially 3 times weekly, then 1 or 2 times weekly

- Systemic therapies:
  - Methotrexate: Blocks DNA synthesis in rapidly dividing epithelial cells and suppresses T cells. Start 7.5–15 mg/wk IV, p.o., IM, or SC. Increase 2.5 mg every 2–3 weeks, up to 25 mg with folic acid 1–5 mg/d (1,3,5)[C]:
    - Side effects: Teratogenic, hepatotoxic
    - Monitor liver function tests (LFTs), renal function, and CBC; liver biopsy when cumulative dose reaches 1.5 g; no alcohol; avoid Bactrim, retinoids, sulfamethoxazole (1)[C]
  - Cyclosporine: Inhibits T cells; start high dose, 5 mg/kg/d, and taper; 0.5–1 mg/kg/d for maintenance; pregnancy class C. Side effects: Monitor renal function, CBC with Mg^{2+} and K^+, and BP (2)[C].
  - Acitretin (Soriatane): Oral retinoid; for plaque psoriasis, only moderately effective as monotherapy; sometimes combined with PUVA; start 25–50 mg/d:
    - Teratogenic: Pregnancy test before starting; 2 forms of contraception needed 1 month before, during, and for at least 3 years after treatment; avoid alcohol (may convert acitretin to etretinate) (1,2)[C]; check FDA monitoring guidelines
    - Side effects: Hepatotoxicity, hyperlipidemia, myalgias; monitor LFTs, renal functions, CBC, creatine phosphokinase (1,2)[C]
  - Oral corticosteroids only for severe or life-threatening disease (risk of rebound)
- Biologics:
  - Etanercept (Enbrel): Blocks tumor necrosis factor α (TNF-α); begin at 50 mg SC twice a week × 3 months; then maintenance of 50 mg/wk (1,3)[B],(6). Side effects: Reactivation of tuberculosis, drug-induced lupus, some concern of lymphoma, CNS demyelinating disorder (resolves on stopping), rarely, heart failure; pregnancy Category B (1,3,6)[C].
  - Adalimumab (Humira): First fully human anti-TNF-α monoclonal antibody; specifically binds to soluble membrane-bound TNF-α. Dosing starts at 80 mg SC × 1 week; then 40 mg SQ every other week (1,3,6)[B]. Side effects: Rare reports of serious infections and malignancies, rare drug-induced reversible conditions (i.e., lupus, cytopenia, MS, and congestive heart failure) (1,3)[C].
  - Alefacept (Amevive): Interferes with CD2 on memory T cells and inhibits activation; 15 mg IM weekly × 12 weeks; can do an additional round after 12 weeks of rest (1,3)[B]. Side effects: Lymphopenia; monitor CD4 cell counts weekly; discontinue when <250/uL.
  - Efalizumab (Raptiva): Inhibits T cells and their adhesion to endothelial cells; initial dose 0.7 mg/kg; then 1 mg/kg weekly; maximum single dose of 200 mg; patient can administer (1,3,4)[B]. Side effects: Monitor platelets monthly for 3 months, then every 3 months. Up to 14% of patients develop rebound or flare.
  - Infliximab (Remicade): Like etanercept, blocks TNF-α; 3–10 mg/kg IV at weeks 0, 2, and 6; maintenance doses of 5 mg/kg every 6–8 weeks; adjust interval as needed (1,3,6)[B]. Side effects (see etanercept): To increase efficacy and limit toxicity, combine, rotate, or use sequentially.
  - Golimumab (Simponi): Like etanercept, blocks TNF-α; 50 mg SQ monthly. Side effects (see Etanercept): pregnancy Category B; can be self-administered.
  - Ustekinumab (Stelara): Selectively targets cytokines interleukin 12 and 23 (IL12, IL23), which mediate inflammation; dosing based on weight <100 kg 45 mg SQ at weeks 0 and 4 then 45 mg every 12 weeks, >100 kg 90 mg SQ at weeks 0, and 4, then 90 mg every 12 weeks. Side effects: May increase risk of malignancy, monitor for reversible posterior leukoencephalopathy syndrome, which was suspected in 1 case.

Second Line
- Topical immunosuppressants: Tacrolimus (Prograf) or pimecrolimus (Elidel); dermatology consult recommended (3)[C]
- Topicals: Salicylic acid; coal tar; anthralin (1,3)[C]

ADDITIONAL TREATMENT
General Measures
- Adequate topical hydration (emollients)
- Solar radiation (but avoid excessive exposure)
- Tar shampoos

Issues for Referral
- Psoriasis >20% of BSA (1,3)
- Severe extremity involvement, particularly hands and feet

COMPLEMENTARY AND ALTERNATIVE MEDICINE
See Diet.

SURGERY/OTHER PROCEDURES
- Psoriasis and psoriatic medications can affect wound healing postoperatively.
- Perioperative considerations include:
  - Aspirin, NSAIDs, COX-2 inhibitors, and glucocorticoids; use sparingly
  - Methotrexate: Monitor for postoperative infections.
  - Hold cyclosporine for 1 week before and after.

IN-PATIENT CONSIDERATIONS
Initial Stabilization
- Intensive topical therapy
- Phototherapy
- Systemic therapy

Admission Criteria
- Generalized pustular psoriasis; von Zumbusch
- Erythrodermic psoriasis
- Debilitation; patient-specific

Discharge Criteria
Reduction in symptomatic disease severity

 ONGOING CARE

FOLLOW-UP RECOMMENDATIONS
Measure BSA involvement to determine if therapy is working; change therapy if no improvement is seen, or add an agent (1,2).

DIET
- No evidence-based information; suggestions of gluten-fee diet to minimize food allergies (2)
- Good fats, whole grains, legumes, vegetables, fruits, Ω-6 fatty acid
- Herbs and seasonings such as turmeric, red pepper, cloves, ginger, basil, and garlic can block activation of inflammatory cytokines.
- Essential fatty acid supplements

PATIENT EDUCATION
- American Academy of Family Physicians: http://www.aafp.org/; (800) 274–2237
- National Psoriasis Foundation: http://www.psoriasis.org; (800) 723–9166

PROGNOSIS
- Benign, but life-threatening forms do occur
- May be refractory to treatment

COMPLICATIONS
- Psoriatic arthritis
- Pustular psoriasis
- Erythrodermic psoriasis

REFERENCES
1. Menter A, Gottlieb A, Feldman SR, et al. Guidelines of care for the management of psoriasis and psoriatic arthritis: Section 1. Overview of psoriasis and guidelines of care for the treatment of psoriasis with biologics. *J Am Acad Dermatol.* 2008;58: 826–50.
2. Traub M, Marshall K. Psoriasis–pathophysiology, conventional, and alternative approaches to treatment. *Altern Med Rev.* 2007;12:319–30.
3. Luba KM, et al. Chronic plaque psoriasis. *Am Fam Phys.* 2006;73(4):636–44.
4. Heymann WR. Psoriasis: the heart of the matter. *J Am Acad Dermatol.* 2008;58:477–8.
5. Habif T. *Clinical Dermatology*, 4th ed. St. Louis: Mosby, 2004.
6. Sobell JM, Kalb RE, Weinberg JM. Management of moderate to severe plaque psoriasis (part 2): clinical update on T-cell modulators and investigational agents. *J Drugs Dermatol.* 2009;8:230–8.

ADDITIONAL READING
- Huerta C, Rivero E, Rodríguez LA. Incidence and risk factors for psoriasis in the general population. *Arch Dermatol.* 2007;143:1559–65.
- Sobell JM, Kalb RE, Weinberg JM. Management of moderate to severe plaque psoriasis (part I): clinical update on antitumor necrosis factor agents. *J Drugs Dermatol.* 2009;8:147–54.

See Also (Topic, Algorithm, Electronic Media Element)
Arthritis, Psoriatic

 CODES

ICD9
696.1 Other psoriasis and similar disorders

CLINICAL PEARLS
- Chronic lifelong condition
- Disease-state severity cycles in many patients
- May need multiple medications to treat; if one does not work, use or add another.

PSYCHOSIS
Michael Golding, MD

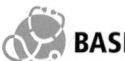 **BASICS**

DESCRIPTION
Syndrome seen with schizophrenia, schizoaffective disorder, mood disorder, substance use, medical problems, delirium, and dementia; symptoms include:

- Positive symptoms: Hallucinations and delusions (fixed false beliefs that the person does not recognize as untrue), often paranoid delusions
- Negative symptoms: Apathy, avolition, withdrawal, paucity of speech
- Disorganized speech or behavior

EPIDEMIOLOGY
Prevalence
- Schizophrenia: Men peak onset 18–25 years; women peak onset 25-35 years
- Schizophrenia: 1% of US population; thought to be similar worldwide
- Delusional disorder: 0.03% of population
- Bipolar type I: 1% of population
- Prevalence of psychosis in major depression not known, likely underrecognized

RISK FACTORS
Substance abuse, family history of a psychotic disorder, lower socioeconomic status, urban setting

Genetics
Schizophrenia: 50% concordance for monozygotic twins, little or no shared environmental effect. Multiple candidate genes involving disruption of neurodevelopment

GENERAL PREVENTION
Community interventions for early detection of new-onset psychosis and treatment of prodromal symptoms show promise.

PATHOPHYSIOLOGY
Many conjecture that a neurodevelopmental predisposition plus first or third trimester in-utero insult leads to exaggerated neuronal apoptosis with subsequent thalamic sensory overload. Increased dopaminergic mesolimbic transmission may contribute to delusions and hallucinations in schizophrenia. Dopamine deficiency in mesocortical pathways may contribute to frontal lobe hypoactivity often associated with apathy and withdrawal in schizophrenia. Glutamate, neurosteroids, and neurodevelopmental abnormalities are active areas of research.

ETIOLOGY
Postulated stress-diathesis model: Individuals who are biologically at risk develop psychosis when under stress.

COMMONLY ASSOCIATED CONDITIONS
- Cardiovascular diseases: Serious mental illness is associated with metabolic syndrome, autonomic dysfunction, sudden cardiac death
- Cancer mortality: Particularly breast and lung cancer
- Substance abuse disorders, including nicotine dependence

 DIAGNOSIS

First rule out delirium: Psychosis should not have fluctuating consciousness or reduced clarity of awareness.

HISTORY
- Delusions (fixed false beliefs): Persecutory (being monitored), bizarre (involving impossible states), somatic (fixed belief in nonexistent serious illness), referential (getting messages from TV, radio, or thoughts inserted or deleted by others), grandiose (belief that one has special powers)
- Hallucinations: Auditory, visual, tactile
- Bipolar illness, depression, and dementia are all associated with psychosis, so screen for symptoms of depression, mania, and memory loss.
- Screen for toxidromes of drugs of abuse.
- Screen for history of epileptiform activity.
- Suicidality: Higher risk with comorbid depression or mania, previous suicide attempts, drug abuse, agitation/akathisia, poor compliance

PHYSICAL EXAM
- Schizophrenia and schizoaffective disorder are associated with negative symptoms (e.g., social withdrawal, lack of initiative, poverty of thought), disorganized speech or behavior
- Attention to neurological focalities as well as antipsychotic-induced parkinsonism, tardive dyskinesia, and akathisia
- May rarely present with catatonia: Extreme excitement or lack of movement, posturing, mutism, grimacing, waxy flexibility
- Mental status exam

DIAGNOSTIC TESTS & INTERPRETATION
Test for causes of delirium mimicking psychosis, if uncertain.

Lab
- Broad screen for medical causes: CBC, metabolic panel, liver function tests, thyroid-stimulating hormone, RPR, HIV, B_{12}, U/A, and screens for subclinical infection in elderly
- Screen for drugs of abuse.
- Consider: Wilson's disease, porphyria, metachromatic leukodystrophy, inflammatory conditions
- Consider ECG: Antipsychotics can prolong corrected QT (QTc) interval, particularly ziprasidone, thioridazine, droperidol, IV haloperidol
- Consider LP if unable to distinguish from delirium and/or unexplained rapid-onset psychosis.
- Consider EEG for partial complex seizures and psychosis associated with pre-ictal and post-ictal events

Follow-Up & Special Considerations
Because of elevated risk related to schizophrenia and psychotropic medications, screen for metabolic syndrome.

Imaging
No imaging necessary for diagnosis. Consider MRI or CT to evaluate for medical cause of symptoms, especially if new onset or in elderly. In research studies, schizophrenia is associated with enlarged lateral ventricles and less frontal activity.

DIFFERENTIAL DIAGNOSIS
- Schizophrenia: Positive symptoms (psychosis) and negative symptoms (flat affect), prodrome of social withdrawal, cognitive impairment; schizophreniform disorder: Psychotic/prodromal symptoms in fewer than 6 months; schizoaffective disorder: Manic or depressive mood disorder with hallucinations or delusions that persist when mood improves; schizotypal personality disorder: No true psychosis, but distance in relationships and odd beliefs; delusional disorder: Nonbizarre delusion (e.g., erotomanic, grandiose, jealous, persecutory, somatic), no negative or mood symptoms
- Mood disorder with psychotic features: Can occur in mania or depression. Delusions often mood-congruent; psychosis remits when mood improves.
- Substance-induced psychosis: Establish timeline of substance use vs timeline of psychosis; most common: Alcohol and benzodiazepine withdrawal, intoxication with cocaine, PCP, cannabis, amphetamines, hallucinogens, and alcohol. May persist beyond acute intoxication.
- Borderline personality disorder: During extreme stress, patients often experience auditory/visual hallucinations (psychosis NOS)
- Posttraumatic stress disorder: Psychosis associated with traumatic recollections. Often visual hallucinations (vs more auditory in schizophrenia).
- Psychosis due to general medical condition: Delirium, stroke, infection, collagen vascular disease, head injury, tumor, interictal, porphyria, syphilis, Wilson's disease, hypo- or hyperthyroidism, metachromatic leukodystrophy, dementia
- Medication-induced psychosis: Common causes: Steroids, L-dopa, anticholinergic medication, antidepressants in bipolar patients, interferon, digoxin, stimulants

TREATMENT

Before antipsychotic treatment, patients need blood work, including a fasting lipid profile, fasting blood sugar, LFTs, metabolic panel, weight

MEDICATION
- Antipsychotics are the mainstay of treatment. Classified as typical vs atypical. Dopamine-2 (D_2) antagonists with varied affinity for the receptor. Atypicals also block serotonin 5-HT2A receptors. Help positive symptoms more than negative. Nonspecific effect on agitation begins early; antipsychotic effect takes 1–6 weeks.
- For mania with psychotic features, a mood stabilizer may be used with antipsychotic
- For major depression with psychotic features, antidepressant and antipsychotic medications yield better response rate than either medication alone.
- In delirium, must treat underlying cause.
- Risks of antipsychotic medications include:
  - Acute dystonia: Utilize 1–3 mg IM/IV benztropine initially, then 0.5–2 mg b.i.d.–t.i.d. and/or diphenhydramine 50–100 mg IM/IV b.i.d.–t.i.d. max 400 mg/day
  - Parkinsonism: Lower medication dose; switch to atypical (particularly quetiapine, olanzapine or clozapine) or add benztropine 0.5–2 mg p.o. b.i.d.–t.i.d., diphenhydramine 25–50 mg b.i.d.–t.i.d.

– Akathisia: Intense restlessness, especially legs. Lower dose; switch or beta-blocker, anticholinergic, antihistaminic or benzodiazepine, or utilize quetiapine, olanzapine, or clozapine
– Tardive dyskinesia: 20% of those treated long-term with typicals. Switch to clozapine or quetiapine. If can't, minimize dose.
– Neuroleptic malignant syndrome: Potentially fatal; rigidity, tremor, fever, autonomic instability, mental status changes; D/C neuroleptic; supportive care; no anticholinergics/antihistaminics; consider dantrolene, amantadine, bromocriptine, and electroconvulsive therapy, ICU
– Metabolic syndrome, sudden cardiac death (risk higher IM/IV droperidol, IV haloperidol), stroke (elderly), QTc prolonged, pulmonary embolus

First Line
- Benefits of some of the atypical antipsychotics include low risk of extrapyramidal symptoms (quetiapine, olanzapine, or clozapine) and tardive dyskinesia (quetiapine, clozapine); and possibly more effective for negative symptoms
- Compared with typicals and some of the atypicals (ziprasidone, aripiprazole), there is more risk of weight gain, new-onset diabetes, and hyperlipidemia with olanzapine and clozapine.
- Acute psychotic agitation: Olanzapine 5–10 mg IM with up to 3 10-mg injections over a 24-hour period, care with subsequent benzodiazepines; ziprasidone 5–20 mg IM q4–6 hours maximum 40 mg over a 24-hour period; haloperidol/orazepam 5 mg/2 mg IM often with 1 mg IM benztropine, maximum 20 mg haloperidol and 8 mg orazepam over a 24-hour period
- Psychosis in schizophrenia:
– Olanzapine start 5–10 mg qhs, target dose 5–20 mg/day within 2 days and up to 40 mg/day in treatment-refractory schizophrenia. More likely weight gain, hyperlipidemia, and hyperglycemia than other oral atypicals except clozapine (1)[B], but may have lower rates of discontinuation and rehospitalization than several other atypicals (1)[B], but likely not more efficacy than clozapine (2)[B]. Sedation initially.
– Quetiapine start 25 mg b.i.d. 25–50 mg b.i.d.–t.i.d. on days 2 and 3, up to 300–400 mg in divided doses by day 4. Within 2 weeks up to 400–800 mg/day divided b.i.d.–t.i.d.; less parkinsonism, useful in Parkinson's disease psychosis; more weight gain than aripiprazole and ziprasidone. Sedation can be a problem initially; more gradual titration often tolerated better in nonacute situations.
– Quetiapine XR can start 300 mg/day. Dose increases can be within 1 day and in increments of up to 300 mg/day, but slower start and titration may be better; target dose 300–800 mg qhs; low rates of parkinsonism; more weight gain than aripiprazole and ziprasidone. Sedation initially.
– Risperidone start 1–2 mg/day; target dose of 1–4 mg/day to be reached over 1–2 weeks; 5–8 mg rarely more effective and high risk parkinsonism. Higher risk of prolactinemia/parkinsonism than quetiapine, olanzapine, clozapine.
– Paliperidone start 3 mg/day target dose 3–12 mg/day; titrate over 1–2 weeks. Higher risk of prolactinemia/parkinsonism than quetiapine, olanzapine, clozapine.

– Ziprasidone start 40 mg p.o. b.i.d., with target dose of 100–200 mg/day in divided doses over 2 weeks; can prolong QTc; less likely to cause weight gain than other atypicals; may have higher rates of akathisia/parkinsonism than quetiapine, olanzapine, clozapine. Requires fatty meal for absorption. Sedation can be a problem initially.
– Aripiprazole start 5–15 mg every day, increase to 10–30 mg/day over a week; less weight gain than other atypicals; may have higher rates of akathisia/parkinsonism than quetiapine, olanzapine, clozapine

Geriatric Considerations
Increased risk of cerebrovascular accident when antipsychotics are used in the elderly with dementia. Caution is advised in this population (3)[B].

Second Line
- Clozapine: Likely more effective for reducing symptoms, preventing relapse, decreasing tardive dyskinesia, and decreasing suicidality than other antipsychotics (2), but second line given risk of potentially fatal agranulocytosis:
– National registry for all patients on clozapine
– Weekly CBC with ANC for 6 months then every 2 weeks for 6 months then every 4 weeks
– More weight gain, hyperlipidemia, hyperglycemia, seizures, myocarditis, pulmonary embolus, and sedation, but very low rates of parkinsonism, tardive dyskinesia
– Useful in treatment-refractory psychosis and in Parkinson's disease psychosis
- Despite the fact that clozapine and olanzapine precipitate more weight gain than other antipsychotics, there is no consistent evidence that they increase risk of cardiac and all-cause mortality (4,5).
- Long-acting preparations: Available for 2 typicals (haloperidol and fluphenazine) and 3 atypicals (risperidone, paliperidone, olanzapine; olanzapine requires registry due to rare delirium syndrome). Test tolerability with oral medication first. Long-acting neuroleptics promote compliance.
- Long-acting haloperidol, paliperidone, olanzapine administered every 4 weeks; long-acting risperidone and fluphenazine administered every 2 weeks

ADDITIONAL TREATMENT
Issues for Referral
Encourage contact with advocacy groups for families and patients (National Alliance for the Mentally Ill).

Additional Therapies
Cognitive-behavioral therapy is an effective adjuvant to antipsychotics.

IN-PATIENT CONSIDERATIONS
Admission Criteria
At risk for harm to self or others; extreme functional impairment; unable to care for self; new-onset psychosis

Discharge Criteria
No longer a danger to self or others and adequate outpatient treatment in place

ONGOING CARE

FOLLOW-UP RECOMMENDATIONS
Close follow-up for inpatient discharge (high risk for suicide), utilize cognitive-behavioral therapy, exercise, teach smoking cessation

PATIENT EDUCATION
National Alliance on Mental Illness: http://www.nami.org/

PROGNOSIS
Schizophrenia: Fluctuating course, 70% first-episode psychosis patients improve in 3–4 months; 7% will die of suicide; 20–40% attempt

REFERENCES

1. Komossa K, Rummel-Kluge C, Hunger H, et al. Olanzapine versus other atypical antipsychotics for schizophrenia. *Cochrane Database of Systemic Reviews* 2010, Issue 3. Art. No.:CD006654, DOI:10.1002/14651858.CD006654.pub2
2. McEvoy JP, Lieberman JA, Stroup TS, et al. Effectiveness of Clozapine Versus Olanzapine, Quetiapine, and Risperidone in Patients with Chronic Schizophrenia Who Did Not Respond to Prior Atypical Antipsychotic Treatment. *Am J Psychiatry*. 2006;163:600–610.
3. van Iersel MB, Zuidema SU, Koopmans RT, et al. Antipsychotics for behavioural and psychological problems in elderly people with dementia: a systematic review of adverse events. *Drugs Aging*. 2005;22:845–58.
4. Tilhonen J, Lonnqvist J, Wahlbeck K, et al. 11-year follow-up mortality in patients with schizophrenia: a population-based cohort study. *Lancet*. 2009; 22(9690):620–7.
5. Strom BL, Faich G, Eng SM, et al. Comparitive mortality associated with ziprasidone vs. olanzapine in real-world use: The ziprasidone observational study of cardiac outcomes (zodiac). *European Psychiatry*. 2008;23:158.
6. Fayek M, Flowers C, Signorelli D, et al. Psychopharmacology: Underuse of Evidence-Based Treatments in Psychiatry. *Psychiatr Serv.* 2003;54:1453–1456.

See Also (Topic, Algorithm, Electronic Media Element)
Delirium, Schizophrenia

 CODES

ICD9
- 295.90 Unspecified type schizophrenia, unspecified state
- 298.9 Unspecified psychosis

CLINICAL PEARLS
- Antipsychotics are the mainstay of treatment; evidence corroborates decreased all-cause mortality in patients who are adherent to antipsychotic medications (4).
- Clozapine and long-acting preparations are likely underutilized in schizophrenia in the US and may increase adherence (6).

PULMONARY ARTERIAL HYPERTENSION

Adriana Cabrera, PharmD
George Maxted, MD

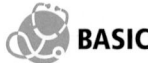

BASICS

DESCRIPTION
Pulmonary arterial hypertension (PAH) is a category of pulmonary hypertension (PH) characterized by abnormalities in the pulmonary arteries that produce increased pulmonary arterial pressure and vascular resistance, eventually resulting in right heart failure. PAH is a progressive disorder associated with increased mortality:

- PAH is defined by all 3 of the following measurements:
  - Mean pulmonary arterial pressure (mPAP) $\geq$25 mm Hg at rest
  - Normal pulmonary arterial wedge pressure <15 mm Hg
  - Pulmonary vascular resistance (PVR) >3 Wood units
- Traditionally classified as primary (without cause) or secondary (with cause or associated condition)
- PAH is now classified into 5 main categories:
  - Idiopathic PAH (IPAH): Sporadic, with no family history or risk factors
  - Heritable PAH: IPAH with mutations or familial cases with or without mutations
  - Drug- or toxin-induced PAH: Mostly associated with anorectics
  - Associated PAH:
    - Connective tissue diseases (e.g., systemic lupus erythematosus [SLE], rheumatoid arthritis [RA], scleroderma)
    - HIV infection
    - Portal hypertension
    - Congenital heart disease
    - Schistosomiasis
    - Chronic hemolytic anemia (e.g., sickle cell disease)
  - Persistent PH of the newborn
- System(s) affected: Pulmonary; Cardiovascular

EPIDEMIOLOGY
- Predominant age: Can occur at any age. Mean age, 36 years.
- Predominant sex: Female > Male (~2:1)

Incidence
- IPAH: Low, approximately 1–2 per million
- Drug-induced PAH: 1 per 25,000 with >3 months of anorectic use
- HIV-associated: 0.5 per 100
- Portal hypertension-associated: 2–3 per 100
- Scleroderma-associated: 10–50%

Prevalence
- PAH: ~15 per million
- IPAH: ~6 cases per million

RISK FACTORS
- Female sex
- Previous anorectic drug use
- Recent acute pulmonary embolism
- Patients with associated conditions
- 1st-degree relatives of patient with familial PAH

Genetics
- 25% of IPAH cases have mutations in BMPR2 (autosomal dominant).
- Mutations in ALK1 and endoglin (autosomal dominant) are also associated with PAH.

PATHOPHYSIOLOGY
- Pulmonary: Vasoconstriction and remodeling of pulmonary arteries lead to obstruction, increasing both PVR and mPAP.
- Cardiovascular: Marked increases in mPAP result in right ventricular hypertrophy, eventually leading to right heart failure.

ETIOLOGY
- IPAH: By definition, unknown. True IPAH is mostly sporadic or sometimes familial in nature.
- Etiology may be due to pulmonary arteriolar hyperactivity and vasoconstriction, occult thromboembolism, or be autoimmune in nature (high frequency of antinuclear antibodies).

COMMONLY ASSOCIATED CONDITIONS
See Associated PAH above.

DIAGNOSIS

- Symptoms of PAH are nonspecific (e.g., dyspnea, syncope, fatigue), which can lead to missed or delayed diagnosis of this serious disease.
- Consider PAH in any patient with the following, regardless of age or sex:
  - Syncope or near-syncope, fatigue, unexplained hoarseness, chest pain, palpitations, unexplained dyspnea, decreased exercise tolerance, lower extremity edema

HISTORY
- Syncope, dizziness: <50%
- Fatigue: >50%
- Chest pain: >50%
- Palpitations: <50%
- Dyspnea: >75%
- Cough: <50%

PHYSICAL EXAM
- Increased jugular venous pressure: 50–80%
- Right ventricular lift: >80%
- Loud P2: >80%
- Murmur of tricuspid insufficiency: 50–80%
- Murmur of pulmonic insufficiency: <50%
- Pulmonic ejection click: <50%
- Right ventricular S4: 50–80%
- Right ventricular S3: <50%
- Hepatomegaly: <50%
- Lower extremity edema: <50%

DIAGNOSTIC TESTS & INTERPRETATION
- Electrocardiogram (ECG): Right ventricular hypertrophy and right axis deviation
- Pulmonary function testing (PFT): Arterial hypoxemia, reduced diffusion capacity, hypocapnia
- Ventilation-perfusion ratio (V/Q) scan: Must rule out proximal pulmonary artery emboli
- Exercise test: Reduced maximal O_2 consumption, high minute ventilation, low anaerobic threshold, increased PO_2 A-a (alveolar-arterial) gradient. Correlation to severity of disease with 6-minute walk test.

Lab
- Antinuclear antibody (ANA) positive (up to 40% of patients):
  - Collagen, vascular disease, lupus, scleroderma, CREST syndrome
  - Drugs that may alter lab results (positive ANA): Hydralazine, procainamide, isoniazid
- Liver function tests (LFTs) to evaluate for portopulmonary hypertension, a complication of chronic liver disease
- HIV test

Imaging
- Chest radiograph:
  - Enlarged central pulmonary arteries with pulmonary arterial branches attenuated
  - Right ventricular enlargement a late finding
  - If increased interstitial markings, consider lung parenchymal disease or veno-occlusive disease.
- Echo Doppler:
  - Should be performed if suspicion of PAH is present (1)[C].
  - Most commonly used screening tool:
    - Estimates mPAP and assesses cardiac structure and function
  - Right ventricular enlargement and overload
  - Important to rule out underlying cardiac disease, such as atrial septal defect with secondary PH or mitral stenosis
- Ultrafast computed tomography (CT):
  - Sensitivity probably equal to pulmonary angiogram with lower contrast dose

Diagnostic Procedures/Surgery
- V/Q scan to rule out chronic thromboembolic PH (CTEPH) (2)[B]
- Pulmonary angiography:
  - Should be done if V/Q scan suggests CTEPH
  - Use caution; can lead to hemodynamic collapse; use low osmolar agents, subselective angiograms.
- Cardiac catheterization:
  - Right-heart catheterization necessary to measure pulmonary arterial pressures and hemodynamics
  - Rule out underlying cardiac disease and response to vasodilator therapy.
- Lung biopsy: Not recommended unless primary pulmonary parenchymal disease exists

Pathological Findings
- Microthromboemboli: 20–50%
- Veno-occlusive disease: 10–15%

DIFFERENTIAL DIAGNOSIS
Other causes of dyspnea:

- Pulmonary parenchymal disease (chronic obstructive pulmonary disease, asthma, pulmonary fibrosis, granulomatous disease, malignancy)
- Pulmonary vascular disease (pulmonary thromboembolism, collagen vascular disease, pulmonary arteritis, schistosomiasis, sickle cell disease)
- Cardiac disease: Pulmonary capillary wedge pressure $\geq$15 mm Hg (cardiomyopathy, valvular heart disease, congenital heart disease, persistent fetal circulation, pulmonary venous hypertension)
- Other disorders of respiratory function (sleep apnea syndromes, neuromuscular diseases, pleural diseases, thoracic cage abnormalities)

TREATMENT

- Treat underlying diseases/conditions that may cause PAH.
- PAH-specific treatment has been studied mostly in IPAH and PAH associated with connective tissue diseases.

MEDICATION

- Acute vasodilator test (performed during cardiac catheterization):
  – Screens for responsiveness. Positive response may improve survival.
  – Perform on all IPAH patients who are potential candidates for long-term oral calcium channel blocker (CCB) therapy: Inhaled nitrous oxide; IV epoprostenol; IV adenosine
  – Contraindicated in right heart failure or hemodynamic instability
- Chronic vasodilator therapy:
  – IPAH with positive response to acute vasodilator test (lower pulmonary pressures while maintaining adequate systemic pressures). CCBs: ~13% will initially respond. Unfortunately, long-term clinical response to CCB therapy is small (~7%) (3)[C].
  – Other forms of PAH rarely respond to CCBs: Nifedipine (long-acting); diltiazem; amlodipine
  – Avoid verapamil due to its significant negative inotropic effect.
  – IPAH with negative response to acute vasodilator test or worsening on therapy, or PAH associated with connective tissue disease. Specific vasodilator choice based on risk stratification (3)[C]:
    ○ Prostanoids: Improve exercise capacity, cardiopulmonary hemodynamics, New York Heart Association (NYHA) functional class and symptoms for NYHA class II–IV PAH (4)[A]. Long-term mortality and side effect data limited: Epoprostenol (IV); treprostinil (IV, SC, or inhaled); iloprost (inhaled)
    ○ Endothelin receptor antagonists (ERAs): Improve exercise capacity, NYHA functional class, reduce dyspnea scores and cardiopulmonary hemodynamics in patients with NYHA class II and III IPAH. Trend toward reducing mortality noted (5)[A]: Bosentan (p.o.); ambrisentan (p.o.)
    ○ Phosphodiesterase inhibitors (PDE-5 Is). Suggested improvement in exercise capacity, cardiopulmonary hemodynamics, and symptoms (6)[C]: Sildenafil (p.o.); tadalafil (p.o.)
- Anticoagulation:
  – Improved survival suggested in patients with IPAH only (7)[C]. Use in other PAH patients controversial.
  – Warfarin with international normalized ratio (INR) of 1.5–2.5:
    ○ Contraindications: Avoid in patients with syncope or significant hemoptysis.
    ○ Significant possible interactions: Refer to the manufacturer's literature.
- Diuretics indicated in patients with RV volume overload (e.g., peripheral edema or ascites)
- Digoxin use is controversial; not extensively studied in PAH:
  – Utilized in right ventricular failure and/or atrial dysrhythmias
  – Monitors drug levels and renal function

ADDITIONAL TREATMENT
General Measures
- Primary modalities are oxygen supplementation, vasodilators, anticoagulants, and treatment of heart failure (e.g., diuretics).
- Oxygen supplementation is indicated for rest, exercise, or nocturnal hypoxemia.

Issues for Referral
Refer to a pulmonologist and/or a cardiologist for further evaluation/treatment if PAH is suspected or known.

SURGERY/OTHER PROCEDURES
- Patients with documented large-vessel thromboembolic disease should be considered for pulmonary thrombectomy.
- Atrial septostomy for severe PAH with right heart failure despite optimized medical therapy
- Heart-lung or lung transplantation is an option for appropriate patients when medical therapy has failed.

IN-PATIENT CONSIDERATIONS
Initial Stabilization
- Medical therapy is 1st-line and primarily palliative.
- Hospitalization with invasive monitoring is needed to screen vasodilator responsiveness and initiate vasodilator therapy.
- National registry has been established by the National Heart, Lung, and Blood Institute (NHLBI)

 ONGOING CARE

FOLLOW-UP RECOMMENDATIONS
Exercise:
- Walking or low-level aerobic activity as tolerated once stable
- Otherwise restricted, especially avoid physical exertion and isometric exercise

Patient Monitoring
Frequently evaluate disease progression and therapeutic efficacy.

DIET
Fluid and salt restrictions, especially with RV failure

PATIENT EDUCATION
Discuss disease, prognosis, lifestyle changes, and all therapeutic options (including transplant).

PROGNOSIS
- Mean survival is 2–3 years from diagnosis, 75% mortality at 5 years, although survival is variable.
- Mode of death:
  – Right heart failure: 63%
  – Pneumonia: 7%
  – Sudden death: 7%
  – Cardiac death: 5%
- Poor prognostic factors:
  – Clinical evidence of RV failure
  – Rapid symptom progression
  – World Health Organization (WHO) functional PAH class 4 (or NYHA functional class 3 or 4)
  – 6-minute walk distance <300 meters
  – Peak VO$_2$ during cardiopulmonary exercise testing <10.4 ml/kg/min
  – Echocardiography with pericardial effusion, significant RV enlargement/dysfunction, RA enlargement
  – RA pressure >20 mm Hg
  – Cardiac index <2 L/min/m^2

COMPLICATIONS
Thromboembolism, heart failure, and sudden death

Pregnancy Considerations
Pregnancy should be avoided due to high maternal mortality and fetal wastage.

REFERENCES

1. McGoon M, Gutterman D, Steen V et al. Screening, early detection, and diagnosis of pulmonary arterial hypertension: ACCP Evidence-Based Clinical Practice Guidelines. *Chest.* 2004;126:14–34.
2. Worsley DF, Palevsky HI, Alavi A. Ventilation-perfusion lung scanning in the evaluation of pulmonary hypertension. *J Nucl Med.* 1994;35:793–6.
3. Badesch DB, Abman SH, Simonneau G et al. Medical therapy for pulmonary arterial hypertension: updated ACCP evidence-based clinical practice guidelines. *Chest.* 2007;131:1917–28.
4. Paramothayan NS, Lasserson TJ, Wells AU et al. Prostacyclin for pulmonary hypertension in adults. *Cochrane Database Syst Rev.* 2005;CD002994.
5. Liu C, Chen J, Gao Y, et al. Endothelin receptor antagonists for pulmonary arterial hypertension. *Cochrane Database Syst Rev.* 2009;CD004434.
6. McLaughlin VV, Archer SL, Badesch DB, et al. ACCF/AHA 2009 expert consensus document on pulmonary hypertension a report of the American College of Cardiology Foundation Task Force on Expert Consensus Documents and the American Heart Association developed in collaboration with the American College of Chest Physicians; American Thoracic Society, Inc.; and the Pulmonary Hypertension Association. *J Am Coll Cardiol.* 2009;53:1573–619.
7. Badesch DB, Abman SH, Ahearn GS et al. Medical therapy for pulmonary arterial hypertension: ACCP evidence-based clinical practice guidelines. *Chest.* 2004;126:35S–62S.

See Also (Topic, Algorithm, Electronic Media Element)
Cor Pulmonale; Pulmonary Embolism

 CODES

ICD9
416.0 Primary pulmonary hypertension

CLINICAL PEARLS

- The hemodynamic value used to consider a patient with PAH is mPAP ≥25 mm Hg.
- In patients with PAH, a V/Q scan should be performed to rule out CTEPH; a normal scan effectively excludes a diagnosis of CTEPH.
- Calcium channel blockers would be a 1st-line agent to manage IPAH only after the patient has a positive response to an acute vasodilator test.

PULMONARY EDEMA
Galina Korsunsky, MD

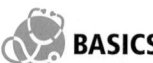 **BASICS**

DESCRIPTION
- Fluid from the pulmonary vasculature leaks into the interstitium and alveoli of the lung.
- Fluid accumulation occurs when there is an imbalance of hydrostatic and oncotic pressures within the pulmonary capillaries and in the surrounding tissue.
- Cardiogenic causes of this imbalance can be obstructive (mitral stenosis) or due to alterations in left ventricular (LV) function.
- Systolic dysfunction is due to decreased contractility of the left ventricle, leading to decreased cardiac output. This decrease in output stimulates the renin–angiotensin system to expand blood volume and results in fluid overload.
- Diastolic dysfunction is due to decreased compliance of the left ventricle, often secondary to LV hypertrophy from hypertension (HTN).

EPIDEMIOLOGY
Incidence
Cardiogenic pulmonary edema: Annual rate of 10/1,000 population in adults >65 years of age

Prevalence
- Estimated 2006 prevalence in the US is 5.7 million.
- Predominant sex: Male > Female; Male = 3.2 million; Female = 2.5 million

RISK FACTORS
- Cardiogenic (1,2):
  – HTN (3)
  – Myocardial infarction (MI)
  – Coronary heart disease
  – Valvular heart disease
  – Diabetes mellitus
  – Smoking
- Noncardiogenic (1):
  – Sepsis
  – Burns
  – Neurologic diseases
  – Reexpansion of lung after injury
  – High altitude
  – Medications

ALERT
75% of people with heart failure have antecedent HTN.

Genetics
Multifactorial

GENERAL PREVENTION
Early detection and treatment of predisposing conditions (3,4)

PATHOPHYSIOLOGY
- Cardiogenic: Rapid increase in hydrostatic pressure in the pulmonary capillaries leading to increased transvascular filtration of a protein-poor fluid into lung interstitium
- Noncardiogenic: Increased permeability of the lung vasculature leading to a protein-rich fluid entry into the lung interstitium and air spaces

ETIOLOGY
- Cardiogenic (1,3,4):
  – HTN
  – Ischemic heart disease/acute coronary syndromes
  – Valvular disease
  – Cardiomyopathy
  – Volume overload
  – Atrial and ventricular arrhythmias
  – Endocarditis/myocarditis
  – Congenital heart disease
  – Acute rheumatic fever and rheumatic heart disease
  – Cardiac tamponade
  – High cardiac output states (e.g., thyrotoxicosis)
- Noncardiogenic (1):
  – Infection/sepsis
  – Trauma
  – Liquid aspiration (e.g., drowning, gastric contents)
  – Inhaled toxic gases
  – Acute respiratory distress syndrome
  – Drug overdose (e.g., narcotics)
  – High altitude
  – Embolism (e.g., thrombus, fat, air, amniotic fluid)
  – Neurogenic
  – Hematologic and immunologic disorders
  – Decreased plasma oncotic pressure
  – Reexpansion (e.g., after a pneumothorax or a surgery)
  – Pancreatitis
  – Renal failure

COMMONLY ASSOCIATED CONDITIONS
See Etiology.

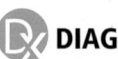 **DIAGNOSIS**

HISTORY
- Past medical history: Underlying condition, infection, trauma, drug use (1,4)[C]
- Symptoms (4,5)[C]:
  – Shortness of breath
  – Diaphoresis
  – Orthopnea/paroxysmal nocturnal dyspnea
  – Dyspnea on exertion
  – Cough
  – Pink frothy sputum
  – Fatigability

PHYSICAL EXAM
- Tachypnea
- Tachycardia
- Hypoxemia
- Elevated jugular venous pressure
- S_3
- Bibasilar crepitus/rales (1,4,5)[C]
- Wheeze
- Ascites
- Enlarged and tender liver
- Hepatojugular reflux
- Peripheral edema

DIAGNOSTIC TESTS & INTERPRETATION
Lab
Initial lab tests
- Complete blood count with differential (leukocytosis, anemia)
- Blood urea nitrogen/creatine
- Brain natriuretic peptide (BNP) >500 pg/mL, heart failure is likely (positive predictive value >90%). BNP <100 pg/mL, heart failure is unlikely (negative predictive value >90%) (5)[A].
- Serum and urine osmolarity
- Cardiac enzymes (rule out MI/ischemic changes)
- Arterial blood gases (hypoxemia, increased A–a gradient)
- Drug levels

Follow-Up & Special Considerations
- Renal function
- Electrolytes, particularly potassium
- Serial BNPs

Imaging
Initial approach
- Chest x-ray: Increased interstitial markings, cardiomegaly, Kerley B lines, perihilar alveolar edema, pleural effusions, diffuse alveolar infiltrates with air bronchograms
- Electrocardiogram (ECG)
- Echocardiography with Doppler (e.g., valvular heart disease, systolic vs diastolic dysfunction)

Follow-Up & Special Considerations
Echocardiography if indicated

Pathological Findings
- Expansion of perivascular, peribronchiolar, and interstitial space by fluid
- Alveolar wall thickening with capillary congestion and alveolar filling
- Hyaline membrane formation

DIFFERENTIAL DIAGNOSIS
- Pneumonia
- Pulmonary embolism
- Reactive airway disease

 TREATMENT

MEDICATION
First Line
- Acute cardiogenic pulmonary edema:
  – Furosemide: 20–80 mg IV; maximum daily dose 600 mg (5)[B]
  – Nitroglycerin: IV, up to 200 mg/kg if blood pressure tolerates (5)[C]
  – Sodium nitroprusside: IV, start 5–10 μg/min up to 400 μg, with mean arterial pressure >65 mm Hg (5)[C]
  – If systolic blood pressure <90 mm Hg and reduced left ventricular ejection fraction, milrinone: 0.1 μg/kg/min, up to 0.2–0.3 μg/kg/min *or*
  – Dobutamine: 5–20 μg/kg/min IV (4,5)[C]
- Chronic management of cardiogenic pulmonary edema (4)[A]:
  – Furosemide: 20–400 mg/d p.o.
  – Angiotensin-converting enzyme (ACE) inhibitors (e.g., captopril 6.25–25 mg p.o. t.i.d.; lisinopril 2.5–20 mg/d p.o.; enalapril 2.5–15 mg p.o. b.i.d.)

- Angiotensin II receptor blockers (ARBs)
- Spironolactone: 25–200 mg/d p.o.
- Digoxin: 0.125–0.25 mg/d p.o.
- β-Blockers (e.g., Carvedilol: 3.25–25 mg p.o. b.i.d.)
- Isosorbide dinitrate: 10–60 mg p.o. t.i.d.–q.i.d.
- Thiazide diuretics (e.g., hydrochlorothiazide 25–50 mg/d p.o.)
- Oxygen
- Treat underlying disease process.

- Contraindications: Refer to the manufacturer's profile of each drug.
- Precautions:
  - Avoid β-blockers in acute decompensated cardiac failure.
  - Observe for side effects of diuretics: Electrolytes imbalance, renal dysfunction
  - Avoid negative inotropic agents (calcium channel blockers) in the setting of cardiogenic pulmonary edema.
  - Avoid prolonged administration of nitroprusside due to risk of cyanide toxicity. If administered for >72 h, obtain a thiocyanate level.
  - Additive hypotensive effects of nitrates, afterload reducers, diuretics

Second Line
- Nesiritide: IV, 0.01 mg/kg/min (5)[C]
- Chlorothiazide
- Metolazone
- Acetazolamide
- Bumetanide
- Potassium-sparing diuretics
- Other ACE inhibitors or ARBs if ACE inhibitor-intolerant

ADDITIONAL TREATMENT
Intra-aortic balloon pump

General Measures
- Treat underlying condition.
- Patient sitting
- Oxygen supplementation
- Noninvasive mechanical ventilation (6,7)[A]
- Mechanical ventilation, often requiring positive end-expiratory pressure support
- Rapid reduction in altitude in cases of high-altitude pulmonary edema

SURGERY/OTHER PROCEDURES
Heart transplant

IN-PATIENT CONSIDERATIONS
Initial Stabilization
- Generally inpatient or intensive care
- Outpatient for mildest forms such as adjusting medications in a patient with a chronic condition

Admission Criteria
- Hypotension
- Worsening renal function
- Altered mentation
- Dyspnea at rest
- O₂ saturation <90%
- Acute coronary syndromes
- Arrhythmias (i.e., new-onset atrial fibrillation)
- New symptoms
- Weight gain ≥5 kg (5)[C]

IV Fluids
If required, use normal saline cautiously to prevent exacerbation of pulmonary edema.

Nursing
- Daily weights, input and output, vital signs at the same time each day, orthostatics
- Assess for signs and symptoms of exacerbation.

Discharge Criteria
- Underlying condition treated
- Switched to oral medications
- Near-optimal fluid status achieved
- Family and patient education completed (5)

ALERT
BNP >750 pg/mL at discharge is an independent predictor of early readmission or death.

 ONGOING CARE

FOLLOW-UP RECOMMENDATIONS
Patient Monitoring
- Strict measurement of input and output
- Posthospitalization appointment in 7–10 days
- Attention to optimal fluid management
- Attention to clinical status
- Daily weights to assess fluid accumulation

DIET
- Low-sodium diet <2 g/d
- Fluid restriction <2 L/d

PATIENT EDUCATION
- Early signs and symptoms of fluid overload
- Adjust daily dose of diuretics based on short-term weight gain of 2–4 lb (5)[C].

PROGNOSIS
- Depends on underlying etiology
- Mortality ~30–60% for noncardiogenic pulmonary edema and up to 80% for cardiogenic pulmonary edema

COMPLICATIONS
- Reversible or irreversible organ ischemia
- Pulmonary fibrosis, particularly with noncardiogenic pulmonary edema
- Sudden death

REFERENCES
1. Hunt SA, Abraham WT, Chin MH, et al. ACC/AHA 2005 Guideline Update for the Diagnosis and Management of Chronic Heart Failure in the Adult: a report of the American College of Cardiology/American Heart Association Task Force on Practice Guidelines (Writing Committee to Update the 2001 Guidelines for the Evaluation and Management of Heart Failure): developed in collaboration with the American College of Chest Physicians and the International Society for Heart and Lung Transplantation: endorsed by the Heart Rhythm Society. *Circulation.* 2005;112:e154–235.
2. Haider AW, Larson MG, Franklin SS, et al. Systolic blood pressure, diastolic blood pressure, and pulse pressure as predictors of risk for congestive heart failure in the Framingham Heart Study. *Ann Intern Med.* 2003;138:10–6.
3. Ware LB, Matthay MA. Clinical practice. Acute pulmonary edema. *N Engl J Med.* 2005;353: 2788–96.
4. Heart Failure Society of America. Evaluation and management of patients with acute decompensated heart failure. *J Card Fail.* 2006;12:e86–e103.
5. He J, Ogden LG, Bazzano LA, et al. Risk factors for congestive heart failure in US men and women: NHANES I epidemiologic follow-up study. *Arch Intern Med.* 2001;161:996–1002.
6. American Heart Association. *Heart disease and stroke statistics.* 2010 Update.
7. Peter JV, Moran JL, Phillips-Hughes J, et al. Effect of non-invasive positive pressure ventilation (NIPPV) on mortality in patients with acute cardiogenic pulmonary oedema: a meta-analysis. *Lancet.* 2006;367:1155–63.

ADDITIONAL READING
- Collins SP, Mielniczuk LM, Whittingham HA, et al. The use of noninvasive ventilation in emergency department patients with acute cardiogenic pulmonary edema: a systematic review. *Ann Emerg Med.* 2006;48:260–9, 269.e1-4.
- Jessup M et al. 2009 Focused Update: ACCF/AHA Guidelines for the Diagnosis and Management of Heart Failure in Adults: A Report of the American College of Cardiology Foundation/American Heart Association Task Force on Practice Guidelines: Developed in Collaboration With the International Society for Heart and Lung Transplantation. *Circulation.* 2009;119:1977–2016.
- Muroi C, Keller M, Pangalu A, et al. Neurogenic pulmonary edema in patients with subarachnoid hemorrhage. *J Neurosurg Anesthesiol.* 2008;20: 188–92.
- Vital F, et al. Non-invasive positive pressure ventilation (CPAP or bilevel NPPV) for cardiogenic pulmonary edema. Cochrane Heart Group. *Cochrane Database Sys Rev.* 2009;1:CD005351.

See Also (Topic, Algorithm, Electronic Media Element)
Altitude Illness; Congestive Heart Failure; Respiratory Distress Syndrome, Acute

 CODES

ICD9
- 514 Pulmonary congestion and hypostasis
- 518.4 Acute edema of lung, unspecified

CLINICAL PEARLS
- Early recognition of cardiogenic versus noncardiogenic pulmonary edema is key because of different management strategies.
- Most patients with pulmonary edema require hospitalization.
- ECG is a useful noninvasive quick diagnostic tool to establish the etiology of pulmonary edema.

PULMONARY EMBOLISM

Timothy J. Barreiro, DO
Suneel Dhand, MD

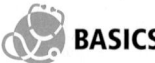

BASICS

DESCRIPTION
- Pulmonary embolism (PE) occurs when thrombi in the venous system (usually deep) are formed, lysed, and lodge into the pulmonary arterial circulation.
- Presentation ranges from nearly asymptomatic to catastrophic and may include acute PE; massive PE obstructing >50% of the pulmonary circulation; pulmonary infarction obstructing a distal branch of the pulmonary circulation; or multiple pulmonary emboli or thrombi.

Geriatric Considerations
- High risk for complications from anticoagulation
- With idiopathic venous thromboembolism (VTE), perform age-based cancer screening.

Pediatric Considerations
Rare; workup for hereditary clotting disorder, the incidence in children is 3.7%.

Pregnancy Considerations
- Incidence 5–50 times higher in pregnant vs nonpregnant women
- Highest incidence of PE is during the postpartum period.
- Recommended treatment is low molecular weight heparin (LMWH) b.i.d.
- If VTE-positive during pregnancy, anticoagulation should be continued for a total duration of 6 months and for at least 6 weeks postpartum (1)[C].

EPIDEMIOLOGY
Incidence
- 54,166 cases per month and 650,000 cases per year in the US population
- 13.14 per 1,000 hospitalized at-risk patients developed post-operative PE in US.

Prevalence
100,000–300,000 deaths yearly

RISK FACTORS
- Advanced age (maybe state increases with age)
- Obesity
- Previous thromboembolism
- Prolonged immobility
- Hypercoagulable state
- Chronic medical conditions (CHF, COPD, IBD, malignancy)
- Varicose veins (varies in studies)
- Pregnancy and postpartum period
- Estrogen (oral contraceptives or hormone replacement therapy)
- Indwelling vascular devices
- Surgery/postoperative
- Trauma (spinal injuries, long bone fractures, and severe burns)

Genetics
Hypercoagulable states (acquired or congenital) (2):
- Protein C, protein S, and antithrombin III deficiencies
- Activated protein C resistance (factor V Leiden)
- Hyperhomocysteinemia
- Prothrombin G20210A gene mutation (factor II mutation)

- Antiphospholipid antibody syndrome
- Lupus anticoagulant
- Anticardiolipin antibodies
- Elevated clotting factors VIII, IX, XI

GENERAL PREVENTION
- Prophylactic therapy includes low-dose heparin, LMWH, graduated-compression stockings, synthetic factor Xa inhibitor, or leg compression devices.
- For high-risk, t.i.d. dosing of unfractionated heparin more effective than b.i.d. dosing.
- Air travel >4 hours increases risk of VTE. A single dose of LMWH before travel is effective.

PATHOPHYSIOLOGY
- Virchow's triad (contributors to the pathogenesis of venous thrombosis): Venous stasis, injury to the intima, and changes in the coagulation properties of the blood
- Thrombosis mainly originates as a platelet nidus in the region of the venous valves located in the veins of the lower extremities.
- Further growth occurs by accretion of platelets and fibrin and progression to red fibrin thrombus, which may either break off and embolize or result in total occlusion of the vein.

ETIOLOGY
Venous stasis, endothelial injury, and hypercoagulability. Deep vein thrombosis (DVT) is responsible for 80% of cases of PE.

COMMONLY ASSOCIATED CONDITIONS
- DVT (80% of all PEs propagate from the deep venous system)
- Occult cancer (e.g., lung, gastrointestinal tract, breast, uterus, brain, prostate)
- Chronic medical conditions (CHF, obesity)
- Postsurgery, particularly orthopedic

DIAGNOSIS

HISTORY
May be nonspecific and include symptoms such as acute unexplained dyspnea, hemoptysis (usually in infarction), pleuritic chest pain, anxiety, and apprehension

PHYSICAL EXAM
- Signs of DVT may or may not be present (Leg swelling or edema).
- Tachypnea, focal wheeze
- Hypoxia
- Tachycardia (HR>100 bpm)
- Distended neck veins/large A wave
- Heart: Increased P2 sound
- Lungs: Clear, decreased breath sounds or egophony due to pleural effusion
- Acute cor pulmonale (shock-systemic hypotension, syncope, cyanosis, right ventricular gallop, pleural friction rub, hemoptysis)
- Homan sign (pain elicited with compression of the calf) not sensitive

DIAGNOSTIC TESTS & INTERPRETATION
- Before diagnostic testing, the patient's pretest probability needs be estimated using an instrument such as the revised Geneva score (3)[A] or Wells score (3,4)[A]:

- Age >65: 1 point
- Surgery with general anesthesia or lower limb fracture in the last month: 2 points
- Active malignancy (or cured for <1 year): 2 points
- Previous VTE: 3 points
- Hemoptysis: 2 points
- Unilateral lower limb pain: 3 points
- Heart rate 75–94: 3 points; >94: 5 points
- Pain on palpation of lower limb deep veins and edema: 4 points

- Probability: High >10; medium 4–10; low 0–3

ALERT
D-dimer plus lung scanning (spiral CT or V/Q scan) provides adequate sensitivity with high specificity.

Lab
If pretest clinical probability is not high, then obtain high-sensitivity D-dimer. If positive, then perform diagnostic tests such as Dopplers to rule out DVT and CT angiogram to rule out PE (4,5). If pretest clinical probability is high, start Rx, then perform diagnostic tests.

Initial lab tests
- Arterial blood gases (room air): Normal or decreased Pa_2
- D-dimer: Qualitative (+ or −); quantitative (>500 NG/mL)
- CBC, PT, PTT
- Stool guaiac prior to initiating anticoagulation
- Consider hypercoagulable testing.

Follow-Up & Special Considerations
Consider cancer screening in idiopathic thrombotic disease.

Imaging
- EKG: Tachycardia, incomplete right bundle branch block, T wave inversions in V2 and V3, S1Q3T3 pattern
- Chest x-ray may reveal parenchymal infiltrates, pleural effusion, atelectasis, consolidation, prominent central arteries, focal oligemia (Westermark sign), wedge-shaped pleural density (Hampton hump), pleural effusion, and/or elevated hemidiaphragm.
- CT angiogram (spiral CT) (6)[A] or ventilation-perfusion (V/Q) scintigraphy (7)[A]:
  - V/Q scanning is an alternative to CT angiography when injection of contrast dye is a concern.
  - MRI is not sensitive enough to adequately image distal branches of the pulmonary arteries.
- Echocardiogram: Right ventricular strain and pulmonary hypertension, tricuspid regurgitation, septal flattening (reverse "D" sign)
- Color-flow Doppler imaging and compression ultrasonography for lower-extremity DVT.
- Pulmonary angiogram; invasive test (gold standard) morbidity/mortality risk: <1%/<0.01%

Diagnostic Procedures/Surgery
Venogram

DIFFERENTIAL DIAGNOSIS
- Pulmonary: Pneumonia, bronchitis, pneumonitis, COPD exacerbation, pulmonary edema, pneumothorax

- Cardiac: Myocardial infarction (angina pectoris), pericarditis, CHF
- Vascular: Dissection of the aorta
- Musculoskeletal: Rib fracture(s), musculoskeletal chest wall pain

TREATMENT

MEDICATION
- Treatment of acute PE with parenteral administration of fondaparinux, LMWH, or heparin overlapped and followed by oral vitamin K antagonists for a <u>minimum</u> of 3 months (1,8).
- The use of thrombolytic therapy is still unclear for hemodynamically stable patients with PE (9)[A]: Presence and severity of hemodynamic instability due to right ventricular failure are critical factors (2,8).

First Line
- Factor Xa inhibitor SC injection 5–10 mg once daily (fondaparinux, Arixtra) for at least 5 days OR
- LMWH (Lovenox) SC injection 1.5–2 mg/kg per day or 1 mg/kg b.i.d. for at least 5 days OR
- IV heparin by continuous infusion, at dose to prolong partial thromboplastin time (PTT) to 1.5–2 times control for 5 days. Usual regimen: 80 units/kg load followed by 18 unit/kg/h. Check PTT q6h after beginning infusion to keep in a range of 1.5–2.3 times mean normal:
  - Check platelet count regularly to evaluate for heparin-induced thrombocytopenia (HIT).
  - Continued dose should be adjusted according to results of PTT via hospital nomograms
  - Heparin is drug of choice for patients with renal failure (GFR <30 mL/min) and obesity.
- Begin warfarin day 1 (<5 mg for 1st dose). Adjust dose to prolong PT to an INR of 2–3:
  - Continue heparin in combination with oral anti-coagulation until INR is >2.
  - Continue therapy for at least 6 months for unprovoked VTE.
- Precautions:
  - If the PTT is appropriately adjusted, the occurrence rate of a major hemorrhage complication should be low.
  - Unfractionated and LMW heparins associated with HIT. If platelets fall <100,000, check HIT antibody (platelet factor 4). Fondaparinux does not require platelet monitoring since risk of HIT is minimal.
  - Use a lower initial dose of LMWH in obese patients or those with renal insufficiency. Use Xa levels to adjust dose further.
- Inferior venacaval (IVC) filters

Second Line
- Thrombolysis: 100 mg of tissue plasminogen activator (tPA) infused over 2 hours; must continue other forms of chronic anticoagulation
- Contraindications to thrombolytics include CVA, intracranial trauma or surgery within past 2 months, active intracranial disease (neoplasm, aneurysm, vascular malformations), internal bleeding within the past 6 months, uncontrolled hypertension bleeding diathesis/coagulopathies, pregnancy, aortic aneurysm, and hemorrhagic retinopathy.
- Controversy on the use of thrombolytics in hemodynamically stable patients with right ventricular strain, there is a 2-fold increased mortality at 14 days; 3-fold increase in 1 year.

ADDITIONAL TREATMENT
General Measures
- Oxygen therapy as needed
- Maintain cardiovascular and pulmonary function.

Issues for Referral
- Recurrent thrombotic events
- Failure of anticoagulation, active bleeding, intolerance anticoagulation may require IVC filter.
- Catastrophic thrombotic event suggesting antiphospholipid antibody syndrome

Additional Therapies
Site-specific anticoagulant drugs such as oral synthetic inhibitors of thrombin or factor Xa are currently undergoing clinical testing (1,10).

SURGERY/OTHER PROCEDURES
- Interruption of inferior vena cava considered in patients who cannot take anticoagulants or who have recurrent emboli despite anticoagulation
- In massive embolism with hypotension, pulmonary embolectomy may be life-saving despite a mortality rate of ~30%.
- Pulmonary thromboendarterectomy
- IVC filters

IN-PATIENT CONSIDERATIONS
Initial Stabilization
May require ICU if hemodynamically unstable

Admission Criteria
Clinically stable individuals with DVT or PE who have good follow-up and support can be treated as outpatients with LMWH.

Discharge Criteria
- Recommended overlap of heparin therapy and warfarin for 2 days once INR greater than 2.5
- Stable condition with an INR of 2–3 on warfarin

ONGOING CARE

The exact duration of anticoagulation for unprovoked VTE remains controversial (1).

FOLLOW-UP RECOMMENDATIONS
Idiopathic disease has a high recurrence rate, so consider longer therapy.

Patient Monitoring
- INR maintained between 2 and 3; warfarin therapy for *at least* 3 months, 6 months if idiopathic or indefinitely in patients with recurrent DVT, cancer, or major thrombotic event
- If idiopathic VTE, a thorough examination and symptoms-specific testing is recommended. At 2 years following idiopathic VTE, malignancy was noted between 7 and 24%.

DIET
Limit foods and drugs that affect Coumadin (e.g., green leafy vegetables, proton pump inhibitors).

PATIENT EDUCATION
Information on risks of anticoagulation, including bleeding, skin changes, blue toe syndrome, and osteoporosis (long-term use)

PROGNOSIS
- Left untreated, high rate of mortality
- 5–15% of all in-hospital deaths (8). In 22% of cases, PE not diagnosed before death.
- Long-term prognosis determined by comorbid disease: Higher mortality rate in patients with positive troponin and echocardiogram evidence of RV strain

COMPLICATIONS
- Chronic thomboembolic pulmonary hypertension (CTEPH)
- Recurrent DVT or PE, postphlebitic syndrome
- Major hemorrhage associated with thrombolytics is 8%; incidence of intracerebral bleed is 2% and is fatal in 50% of cases.
- HIT (8–20% mortality) (8)

REFERENCES

1. Blondon M, Bounameaux H, Righini M. Treatment strategies for acute pulmonary embolism. *Expert Opin Pharmacother.* 2009;10:1159–71.
2. Todd JL, Tapson VF. Thrombolytic therapy for acute pulmonary embolism: a critical appraisal. *Chest.* 2009;135:1321–9.
3. Le Gal G, Righini M, Roy PM, et al. Prediction of pulmonary embolism in the emergency department: the revised Geneva score. *Ann Intern Med.* 2006;144:165–71.
4. DeLoughery TG. Venous thrombotic emergencies. *Emerg Med Clin North Am.* 2009;27:445–58.
5. Tapson VF. Acute pulmonary embolism. *N Engl J Med.* 2008;358:1037–52.
6. Büller HR, Agnelli G, Hull RD, et al. Antithrombotic therapy for venous thromboembolic disease: the Seventh ACCP Conference on Antithrombotic and Thrombolytic Therapy. *Chest.* 2004;126: 401S–428S.
7. Value of the ventilation/perfusion scan in acute pulmonary embolism. Results of the prospective investigation of pulmonary embolism diagnosis (PIOPED). The PIOPED Investigators. *JAMA.* 1990; 263:2753–9.
8. Konstantinides S. Clinical practice. Acute pulmonary embolism. *N Engl J Med.* 2008;359: 2804–13.
9. Dong BR, Hao Q, Yue J, et al. Thrombolytic therapy for pulmonary embolism. *Cochrane Database Syst Rev.* 2009;CD004437.
10. Gómez-Outes A, Lecumberri R, Pozo C, et al. New anticoagulants: focus on venous thromboembolism. *Curr Vasc Pharmacol.* 2009;7:309–29.

CODES

ICD9
415.19 Other pulmonary embolism and infarction

CLINICAL PEARLS

- Patients who have a low or moderate pretest probability of PE should have D-dimer testing.
- CT angiogram can reliably be used to diagnose or rule out PE in the majority of cases (8).
- Treatment of acute PE consists of parental administration of fondaparinux, LMWH, or heparin overlapped and followed by oral vitamin K antagonists for a *minimum* of 3 months.

PULMONARY VALVE STENOSIS

Kevin Engelhardt, MD
Brent J. Barber, MD

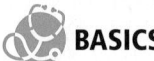 **BASICS**

DESCRIPTION
Congenital deformity consisting of obstruction to right ventricular (RV) outflow at the level of the pulmonic valve

EPIDEMIOLOGY
Incidence
- Predominant age: Present in newborns but often asymptomatic for years
- Predominant sex: Male < Female (slight)
- Small increase in black male/female relative to white male/female (1)

Prevalence
- 10% of all cases of congenital heart disease
- In association with other lesions, may be as high as 25–30% of congenital heart disease

Pediatric Considerations
This is a congenital disorder.

Pregnancy Considerations
In asymptomatic young women with mild to moderate pulmonic stenosis, pregnancy is generally well tolerated.

RISK FACTORS
Family history

Genetics
- Genetic cause likely, with numerous familial and syndromic cases
- Associated with Noonan, LEOPARD, and Williams syndromes and neurofibromatosis

PATHOPHYSIOLOGY
- Valvular
- Subvalvular
- Supravalvular

ETIOLOGY
- Abnormal development of distal bulbus cordis secondary to
  – Congenital/genetic
  – Rubella embryopathy
- Acquired:
  – Stenosis of bioprosthetic valve
  – Rarely, rheumatic fever
  – Very rarely, carcinoid syndrome

COMMONLY ASSOCIATED CONDITIONS
- Tetralogy of Fallot
- Noonan syndrome
- LEOPARD syndrome
- Ventricular septal defect and atrial septal defect
- Neurofibromatosis
- Williams syndrome
- Alagille syndrome

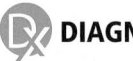 **DIAGNOSIS**

HISTORY
- History of heart murmur since birth
- Usually asymptomatic; exercise tolerance is excellent unless stenosis is severe.
- Most frequent symptoms are dyspnea and fatigue.
- Other symptoms include chest pain and occasionally dizziness or syncope, particularly exertional, owing to low fixed cardiac output.
- Myocardial infarction (MI) of the hypertrophied right ventricle has been noted.

PHYSICAL EXAM
- Acyanotic, unless septal defect allows right-to-left shunting
- Prominent A wave of the jugular venous pulse
- RV heave
- Thrill; does not correlate with stenosis severity; often present in mild to moderate stenosis
- Pulmonic ejection sound/click: Louder during expiration; may be absent in patients with severe stenosis or dysplastic valve
- Midsystolic murmur (increased duration and later peaking with increased severity); heard best at left upper sternal border; may radiate throughout precordium and to left upper back
- Delay in P2; P2 becomes softer in severe stenosis.

DIAGNOSTIC TESTS & INTERPRETATION
Lab
Initial lab tests
ECG:
- Generally sinus rhythm, occasionally supraventricular arrhythmias
- Rightward axis
  – Right ventricular hypertrophy (RVH)
  – RVH severity correlates with R:S ratio in leads V1 and V6 (R in V1 >30 mV correlates with severe stenosis)
- Tall peaked P waves (right atrial enlargement)
- Abnormal T-waves in V1 also a sign of RVH (upright in children, inverted in adults)

Imaging
Initial approach
- Radiograph: Poststenotic dilatation of the pulmonary trunk, prominence of right atrium and ventricle
- Echocardiography (ECG): Mobile, doming, thickened pulmonic valve; poststenotic dilatation of the pulmonary trunk (does not correlate with degree of stenosis)
- Continuous-wave Doppler: Provides an estimate of the transvalvular gradient (<35–40 mm Hg = mild; 40–60 mm Hg = moderate; >60–70 mm Hg = severe)
- Color-flow Doppler: Delineation of areas of obstruction; assesses for pulmonary regurgitation

Diagnostic Procedures/Surgery
Cardiac catheterization:
- Not indicated in mild pulmonic stenosis
- Perform prior to planned valvuloplasty for moderate to severe stenosis
- Assesses morphology of the right ventricle, pulmonary outflow tract, and pulmonary arteries
- Rules out associated lesions (e.g., atrial septal defect), although ECG usually will suffice

Pathological Findings
- Trileaflet valve with fibrous thickening and fusion of commissures
- Markedly dysplasia of valve with hypoplastic annulus and increased leaflet thickening (especially seen in patients with Noonan syndrome)

DIFFERENTIAL DIAGNOSIS
- Dysplastic pulmonic valve stenosis
- Discrete infundibular stenosis
- Subinfundibular obstruction
- Isolated pulmonary artery stenosis
- Supravalvar pulmonary stenosis
- Tetralogy of Fallot (Pink)

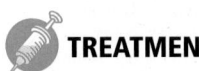

TREATMENT

Pulmonary balloon valvuloplasty is the treatment of choice (2)[A], recommended for:
- Symptomatic patients with peak-to-peak catheter gradient >30 mm Hg
- Asymptomatic patients with peak-to-peak catheter gradient >40 mm Hg

MEDICATION
No specific regimen in the absence of congestive heart failure

ADDITIONAL TREATMENT
General Measures
Prophylaxis for subacute bacterial endocarditis is no longer recommended for pulmonary valve stenosis unless the patient has associated congenital heart disease with cyanosis or a prosthetic cardiac valve/conduit (3)[A].

Issues for Referral
Patients should be followed longitudinally by a cardiologist.

Additional Therapies
Penicillin prophylaxis if rheumatic fever is the cause

SURGERY/OTHER PROCEDURES
- Surgical pulmonic valvuloplasty in patients with obstruction that is not amenable to balloon valvuloplasty; most frequently supravalvular pulmonary stenosis or dysplastic pulmonary valve (4)[B]
- Patients may manifest dynamic subvalvular gradient after balloon valvuloplasty or surgical repair, which typically regresses with time.

 ONGOING CARE

FOLLOW-UP RECOMMENDATIONS
Regular follow-up assessment for patients not undergoing surgical correction

Patient Monitoring
- Postoperative (or after balloon valvuloplasty) Doppler ultrasound to follow gradient and pulmonic insufficiency
- Cardiac MRI allows for accurate quantification of RV volumes and ejection fraction postoperatively (5)[C].

DIET
No specific regimen mandated

PATIENT EDUCATION
Information is available from the American Heart Association, 7320 Greenville Avenue, Dallas, TX 75231; (214) 373-6300 or www.americanheart.org.

PROGNOSIS
Outcome after either balloon or surgical valvotomy is generally excellent.

COMPLICATIONS
- Up to 10% late mortality following valvotomy in critical pulmonary stenosis in neonates
- Slower recovery in those with chronic severe RVH
- Postvalvotomy pulmonic regurgitation reported in up to 50% (variable severity)
- Residual atrial septal defect or patent foramen ovale
- Persistent repolarization abnormalities on ECG associated with severe postoperative pulmonic regurgitation
- Late atrial arrhythmias
- Rare risk of aneurysms after balloon valvuloplasty

REFERENCES

1. Nembhard WN, Wang T, Loscalzo ML et al. Variation in the prevalence of congenital heart defects by maternal race/ethnicity and infant sex. *J Pediatr.* 2010;156:259—64.
2. Perterson C. Comparative long-term results of surgery versus balloon valvuloplasty for pulmonary valve stenosis in infants and children. *Ann Thoracic Surg.* 2003;76:1078–82.
3. Nishimura RA, Carabello BA, Faxon DP, et al. ACC/AHA 2008 guideline update on valvular heart disease: focused update on infective endocarditis: a report of the American College of Cardiology/ American Heart Association Task Force on Practice Guidelines endorsed by the Society of Cardiovascular Anesthesiologists, Society for Cardiovascular Angiography and Interventions, and Society of Thoracic Surgeons. *Catheter Cardiovasc Interv.* 2008;72:E1–12.
4. Sharieff S, Shah-e-Zaman K, Faruqui AM. Short- and intermediate-term follow-up results of percutaneous transluminal balloon valvuloplasty in adolescents and young adults with congenital pulmonary valve stenosis. *J Invasive Cardiol.* 2003;15:484–7.
5. Vliegen HW, van Straten A, de Roos A, et al. Magnetic resonance imaging to assess the hemodynamic effects of pulmonary valve replacement in adults late after repair of tetralogy of fallot. *Circulation.* 2002;106:1703–7.

ADDITIONAL READING

American College of Cardiology, American Heart Association Task Force on Practice Guidelines (Writing Committee to revise the 1998 guidelines for the management of patients with valvular heart disease), Society of Cardiovascular Anesthesiologists et al. ACC/AHA 2006 guidelines for the management of patients with valvular heart disease: a report of the American College of Cardiology/American Heart Association Task Force on Practice Guidelines (writing Committee to Revise the 1998 guidelines for the management of patients with valvular heart disease) developed in collaboration with the Society of Cardiovascular Anesthesiologists endorsed by the Society for Cardiovascular Angiography and Interventions and the Society of Thoracic Surgeons. *J Am Coll Cardiol.* 2006;48:e1–148.

See Also (Topic, Algorithm, Electronic Media Element)
Tetralogy of Fallot; Noonan Syndrome

 CODES

ICD9
- 424.3 Pulmonary valve disorders
- 746.02 Stenosis of pulmonary valve, congenital

CLINICAL PEARLS
- A pulmonary ejection click denotes mild to moderate stenosis.
- Echocardiography is the preferred test to evaluate the severity of pulmonic stenosis.
- Mild pulmonary valve stenosis is unlikely to progress in severity or cause symptoms.

PYELONEPHRITIS

Stephen A. Martin, MD, EdM

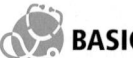 **BASICS**

DESCRIPTION
- Acute pyelonephritis is a syndrome caused by an infection of the renal parenchyma and renal pelvis, often producing localized flank or back pain combined with systemic symptoms such as fever, chills, and nausea. It has a wide spectrum of presentation, from mild illness to septic shock.
- Chronic pyelonephritis is the result of progressive inflammation of the renal interstitium and tubules, presumed to be caused by recurrent infection, vesicoureteral reflux, or both.
- Uncomplicated vs complicated: The presentation is considered uncomplicated if the infection is caused by a typical pathogen in an immunocompetent patient who has normal urinary tract anatomy and renal function.
- System(s) affected: Renal; Urologic
- Synonym(s): Acute upper urinary tract infection (UTI)

Geriatric Considerations
- May present only as confusion; absence of fever is common in this age group.
- Elderly patients with diabetes and pyelonephritis are at higher risk of bacteremia, long hospitalization, and mortality.

Pregnancy Considerations
- The most common medical complication requiring hospitalization
- Affects 1–2% of all pregnancies. Morbidity does not differ between trimesters.
- Urine culture follow-up 1–2 weeks after therapy

Pediatric Considerations
- UTI is present in ~5% of patients 2 months to 2 years old with fever and no source evident from history and physical exam.
- The route for antibiotics and location of care should be based on the clinical situation.

EPIDEMIOLOGY
Incidence
Community-acquired acute pyelonephritis: 28/10,000/year

Prevalence
250,000 adult cases/year, with 100,000 hospitalizations

RISK FACTORS
- Underlying urinary tract abnormalities
- Indwelling catheter
- Recent urinary tract instrumentation
- Nephrolithiasis
- Immunocompromise, including diabetes
- Elderly, institutionalized women
- Prostatic enlargement
- Childhood UTI
- Acute pyelonephritis within the prior year
- Frequency of recent sexual intercourse
- Spermicide use
- Stress incontinence
- Pregnancy
- Hospital-acquired infection
- Symptoms >7 days at presentation

ETIOLOGY
- Infection with *E. coli* (>80%)
- Other gram-negative pathogens: *Proteus, Klebsiella, Serratia, Clostridium, Pseudomonas,* and *Enterobacter*
- *Enterococcus*
- *Staphylococcus*: *S. epidermis, S. saprophyticus* (number 2 cause in young women), and *S. aureus*
- *Candida*

COMMONLY ASSOCIATED CONDITIONS
- Indwelling catheters
- Renal calculi
- Benign prostatic hyperplasia

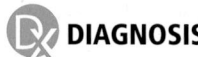 **DIAGNOSIS**

HISTORY
- In adults (1)[C]:
  - Flank pain
  - Nausea ± vomiting
  - Malaise
  - Myalgia
  - Anorexia
  - Dysuria, urinary frequency, urgency
  - Suprapubic discomfort
- In infants and children:
  - Irritability
  - Gastrointestinal symptoms

PHYSICAL EXAM
- In adults (1)[C]:
  - Fever: ≥37.8°C (100°F)
  - Costovertebral angle tenderness
  - From no physical findings to septic shock
  - A pelvic exam may be needed in female patients to assess for pelvic inflammatory disease (PID)
- In infants and children:
  - Sepsis
  - Fever
  - Poor skin perfusion
  - Inadequate weight gain or weight loss
  - Jaundice to gray skin color

DIAGNOSTIC TESTS & INTERPRETATION
Lab
Initial lab tests
- Urinalysis: Pyuria ± leukocyte casts, hematuria, nitrites, and mild proteinuria
- Urine leukocyte esterase test positive
- Urine Gram stain
- Urine culture (>10,000 colony-forming units/mL) and sensitivities
- Complete blood count, blood urea nitrogen, and creatinine (2)[C]
- In 1 study of hospitalized patients, C-reactive protein levels were found to correlate with prolonged hospitalization and infection recurrence.

Follow-Up & Special Considerations
- Blood culture(s): Indicated in diagnostic uncertainty, immunosuppression, or a suspected hematogenous source (1)[B]
- Drugs that may alter lab results: Antibiotics

Imaging
Initial approach
- Imaging generally not indicated in straightforward cases
- Pediatrics: Practice is evolving based on recent studies; imaging generally has involved an ultrasound and voiding cystourethrogram or radionucleotide cystogram after initial treatment.

Follow-Up & Special Considerations
If patient's condition does not respond in >72 hours or if obstruction/anatomic abnormality suspected:
- Computed tomography (CT) scan of abdomen and pelvis ± contrast material
- Ultrasound, renal with kidneys, ureter, bladder
- Cystoscopy with ureteral catheterization

Pathological Findings
- Acute: Abscess formation with neutrophils
- Chronic: Fibrosis with reduction in renal tissue

DIFFERENTIAL DIAGNOSIS
- Obstructive uropathy
- Acute bacterial pneumonia (lower lobe)
- Cholecystitis
- Acute pancreatitis
- Appendicitis
- Perforated viscus
- Aortic dissection
- PID
- Kidney stone
- Ectopic pregnancy
- Diverticulitis

 TREATMENT

- Evidence for the treatment of pyelonephritis has not been fully evaluated in randomized, controlled trials.
- Total duration of antibiotics is usually 14 days but must be guided by the clinical situation (3)[A]. Recent trials have studied shorter treatment times (2)[A].
- IV antibiotics are indicated for inpatients.

MEDICATION
- For empirical oral therapy, a fluoroquinolone is recommended. For parenteral therapy, a fluoroquinolone, aminoglycoside ± ampicillin, or an extended-spectrum cephalosporin ± an aminoglycoside can be used (3)[B]. These recommendations are evolving due to increasing fluoroquinolone resistance.
- Contraindications:
  - Allergies to agents listed
  - Fluoroquinolones are contraindicated in children, adolescents, and pregnant women.
  - Nitrofurantoin does not achieve reliable tissue levels for pyelonephritis treatment.
- Precautions:
  - Most antibiotics require adjustments in dosage in patients with renal insufficiency.
  - Test for aminoglycoside levels and renal function.
  - If *Enterococcus* is suspected based on Gram stain, ampicillin plus gentamicin is a reasonable empirical choice, unless patient is penicillin-allergic; then use vancomycin. If outpatient, add amoxicillin to fluoroquinolone pending culture results and sensitivity. Do not use a 3rd-generation cephalosporin for suspected or proven enterococcal infection.

First Line
- Adults:
  - Severe illness: IV therapy until afebrile 24–48 hours and tolerating oral hydration and medications; then oral agents to complete 2 weeks, adult doses (3)[B]

    - IV agents (assuming normal CrCl):
      ○ Ciprofloxacin: 400 mg q12h
      ○ Levofloxacin: 500 mg/d
      ○ Gatifloxacin: 400 mg/d
      ○ Cefotaxime: 1 g q8–12h up to 2 g q4h
      ○ Ceftriaxone: 1–2 g/d
      ○ Cefoxitin: 2 g q4–8h
      ○ Gentamicin: 5–7 mg/kg of body weight daily (± ampicillin 2 g q6h for enterococcus)
    - Oral agents:
      ○ Ciprofloxacin: 500 mg q12h
      ○ Ciprofloxacin XR: 1,000 mg/d
      ○ Levofloxacin: 500 mg/d
      ○ Norfloxacin: 400 mg q12h
      ○ Gatifloxacin: 400 mg/d
- Pediatric:
  - IV agents (general indication is for age <2 months or clinical concern in other ages):
    ○ Ceftriaxone: 50–100 mg/kg/d (also can be used IM in outpatient setting)
    ○ Ampicillin: 100 mg/kg/d IV divided in 4 doses + gentamycin 7.5 mg/kg/d divided in 3 doses
  - Oral agents: Cefixime: 16 mg/kg/d p.o. in 2 divided doses on the 1st day, followed by 8 mg/kg once per day to complete therapy
  - IV agents (general indication is for age <2 months or clinical concern in other ages):
    ○ Ceftriaxone: 50–100 mg/kg/d (also can be used IM in outpatient setting)
    ○ Ampicillin: 100 mg/kg/d IV divided in 4 doses + gentamycin 7.5 mg/kg/d divided in 3 doses
  - Oral agents: Cefixime: 16 mg/kg/d p.o. in 2 divided doses on the 1st day, followed by 8 mg/kg once per day to complete therapy

Second Line
Adults:

- IV agents:
  - Piperacillin–tazobactam: 3.375 g q6–8h
  - Ticarcillin–clavulanate: 3.1 g q4–6h
- Oral agents:
  - Cefixime: 400 mg p.o. q12h
  - Cefpodoxime (Proxetil): 200 mg q12h
  - Amoxicillin–clavulanate: 875/125 mg q12h or 500/125 mg t.i.d.
  - Trimethoprim–sulfamethoxazole (TMP-SMX): 60–800 mg q12h (Up to 30% E. coli strains are resistant to ampicillin and TMP-SMX in community-acquired infections.)

Pediatric Considerations
- Children <2 years of age and children with febrile or recurrent UTI are usually treated for 10 days.
- Empirical coverage should include E. coli. Ampicillin should be added if Enterococcus is suspected:
  - Oral antibiotics (cefixime, ceftibuten, and amoxicillin/clavulanic acid) may be used alone, or
  - IV antibiotics (single daily dosing with aminoglycoside) for 2–4 days, followed by oral antibiotics (4)[A]
- If patient is treated as an outpatient, be sure that circumstances will allow antibiotic course to be completed successfully.

ADDITIONAL TREATMENT
General Measures
- Broad-spectrum antibiotics initially, tailoring therapy to culture and sensitivity results
- Analgesics and antipyretics
- Consider urinary analgesics (e.g., phenazopyridine 200 mg t.i.d.) for severe dysuria.

Issues for Referral
- Acute pyelonephritis unresponsive to therapy
- Chronic pyelonephritis

SURGERY/OTHER PROCEDURES
Perinephric abscess drainage as indicated

IN-PATIENT CONSIDERATIONS
Initial Stabilization
Outpatient therapy if mild–moderate illness (not pregnant, no nausea or vomiting; fever and pain not severe), uncomplicated, and tolerating oral hydration and medications; up to 70% of patients can be selected for outpatient management (1)[B]

Admission Criteria
Inpatient therapy for severe illness (e.g., high fevers, severe pain, marked debility, intractable vomiting, possible urosepsis), risk factors for complicated pyelonephritis, or extremes of age

IV Fluids
As indicated for dehydration or renal calculi

Discharge Criteria
Discharge on oral agent (see above) after patient is afebrile 24–48 h to complete 2 weeks

ONGOING CARE
FOLLOW-UP RECOMMENDATIONS
- Women: Routine follow-up cultures not recommended unless symptoms resolve but recur within 2 weeks; obtain urine culture, sensitivity, Gram stain, and CT scan, or renal ultrasound. If symptoms resolve but recur after 2 weeks, treat as sporadic episode of pyelonephritis unless ≥2 recurrences; then urologic evaluation is necessary.
- Men, children, adolescents, patients with recurrent infections, patients with risk factors: Repeat cultures 1–2 weeks after completing therapy; do a urologic evaluation after 1st episode of pyelonephritis and with recurrences.

Patient Monitoring
- No response within 48 h (5% of patients): Reevaluate and review cultures, CT scan, or ultrasound, and adjust therapy as needed; may need urologic consult. The 2 most common causes are a resistant organism and nephrolithiasis.
- Mild–moderate illness: Oral therapy for 2 weeks as outpatient
- Close contact should be maintained with children's families to monitor their response.

DIET
Encourage fluid intake.

PROGNOSIS
95% of treated patients respond within 48 h.

COMPLICATIONS
- Kidney abscess
- Metastatic infection: Skeletal system, endocardium, eye, meningitis with subsequent seizures
- Septic shock and death
- Acute or chronic renal failure
- Complications of antibiotics

REFERENCES
1. Ramakrishnan K, Scheid DC. Diagnosis and management of acute pyelonephritis in adults. *Am Fam Physician*. 2005;71:933–42.
2. Nicolle LE. Uncomplicated urinary tract infection in adults including uncomplicated pyelonephritis. *Urol Clin North Am*. 2008;35:1–12, v.
3. Warren JW, Abrutyn E, Hebel JR, et al. Guidelines for antimicrobial treatment of uncomplicated acute bacterial cystitis and acute pyelonephritis in women. Infectious Diseases Society of America (IDSA). *Clin Infect Dis*. 1999;29:745–58.
4. Hodson EM, Willis NS, Craig JC et al. Antibiotics for acute pyelonephritis in children. *Cochrane Database Syst Rev*. 2007;CD003772.

ADDITIONAL READING
- American College of Obstetricians and Gynecologists. ACOG Practice Bulletin No. 91: Treatment of urinary tract infections in nonpregnant women. *Obstet Gynecol*. 2008;111:785–94.
- The Infectious Diseases Society of America guideline for uncomplicated UTIs is due in the Fall of 2010. A guideline for adult catheter-associated UTIs was published in 2010.
- Schnarr J, Smaill F. Asymptomatic bacteriuria and symptomatic urinary tract infections in pregnancy. *Eur J Clin Invest*. 2008;38:50–57.

CODES

ICD9
- 590.00 Chronic pyelonephritis without lesion of renal medullary necrosis
- 590.01 Chronic pyelonephritis with lesion of renal medullary necrosis
- 590.10 Acute pyelonephritis without lesion of renal medullary necrosis

CLINICAL PEARLS
- Pyelonephritis can be classic or subtle in its presentation. Early diagnosis can help to prevent clinical deterioration.
- Keep pyelonephritis in mind with less common populations (e.g., children and men).
- The most common causes of poor response to antibiotics are antibiotic resistance and kidney stones.

PYLORIC STENOSIS
Ruben Peralta, MD

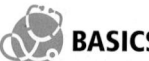 **BASICS**

DESCRIPTION
- Progressive narrowing of the pyloric canal occurring in infancy
- Synonym(s): Infantile hypertrophic pyloric stenosis (IHPS)

EPIDEMIOLOGY
- Predominant age: Infancy:
  - Onset usually at 3–6 weeks of age, rarely in the newborn period or as late as 5 months of age
- Considered the most common condition requiring surgical intervention in the 1st year of life
- A recent decline in its incidence has been reported in a number of countries (1).
- Predominant sex: Male > Female (4:1)

Incidence
In Caucasian population 2–5:1,000 babies, less common in African American and Asian populations (2)[B]

RISK FACTORS
- Incidence higher in 1st-born boys
- 5-times increased risk with affected 1st-degree relative (2)[B]
- Strong familial aggregation and heritability (3)

Genetics
Recent studies have identified linkage to chromosome 11 and multiple loci (4,5)

PATHOPHYSIOLOGY
- Abnormal relaxation of the pyloric muscles leads to hypertrophy.
- Redundant mucosa fills the pyloric canal.
- Gastric outflow is obstructed, leading to gastric distension and vomiting.

ETIOLOGY
- The exact cause remains unknown, but multiple genetic and environmental factors have been implicated (4,5,6).

- A recent surveillance study of a population-based birth defects registry identified an association between pyloric stenosis and the use of fluoxetine in the 1st trimester of pregnancy, even after adjustment for maternal age and smoking. The adjusted odds ratio was 9.8 (95% confidence interval: 1.5–62.0) (7).

COMMONLY ASSOCIATED CONDITIONS
Associated anomalies present in approximately 4–7% of infants with pyloric stenosis:
- Hiatal and inguinal hernias (most commonly)
- Other anomalies include:
  - Congenital heart disease
  - Esophageal atresia
  - Tracheoesophageal fistula
  - Renal abnormalities
  - Turner syndrome and trisomy 18
  - Cornelia de Lange syndrome
  - Smith-Lemli-Opitz syndrome
- A common proposed genetic link between breast cancer, endometriosis, and pyloric stenosis has been observed in families (8).

 DIAGNOSIS

HISTORY
- Nonbilious projectile vomiting after feeding, increasing in frequency and severity
- Emesis may become blood-tinged from vomiting-induced gastric irritation
- Hunger due to inadequate nutrition
- Decrease in bowel movements
- Weight loss

PHYSICAL EXAM
- Firm, mobile ("olivelike") mass palpable in the right upper quadrant (70–90% of the time)
- Epigastric distention
- Visible gastric peristalsis after feeding
- Late signs: Dehydration, weight loss
- Rarely, jaundice when starvation leads to decreased glucuronyl transferase activity resulting in indirect hyperbilirubinemia (2)[B]

DIAGNOSTIC TESTS & INTERPRETATION
Metabolic disturbances are late findings and are uncommon in present time of early diagnosis and intervention (9)[B].

Lab
- If prolonged vomiting, then check electrolytes for:
  - Hypokalemia
  - Hypochloremia
  - Metabolic alkalosis
- Elevated unconjugated bilirubin level (rare)
- Paradoxical aciduria: The kidney tubules excrete hydrogen to preserve potassium in face of hypokalemic alkalosis.

Imaging
- Abdominal ultrasound is the study of choice:
  - Ultrasound shows thickened and elongated pyloric muscle and redundant mucosa (2,9)[B].
- Upper GI series reveals strong gastric contractions; elongated, narrow pyloric canal (string sign); parallel lines of barium in the narrow channel (double tract sign or railroad track sign) (9)[B].

Pathological Findings
Concentric hypertrophy of pyloric muscle

DIFFERENTIAL DIAGNOSIS
- Inexperienced or inappropriate feeding
- GERD
- Gastritis
- Congenital adrenal hyperplasia, salt-losing
- Pylorospasm
- Gastric volvulus
- Antral or gastric web

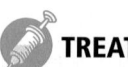 **TREATMENT**

SURGERY/OTHER PROCEDURES
- Ramstedt pyloromyotomy is curative. The entire length of hypertrophied muscle is divided with preservation of the underlying mucosa.
- Frequent surgical approaches include open (traditional right upper quadrant transverse incision), more contemporary circumumbilical incision, and laparoscopic techniques (10)[C],(11)[B],(12,13,14)[B].
- A recent review concluded that the laparoscopic approach results in less postoperative pain and can be performed with no increase in operative time or complications (15,16).

IN-PATIENT CONSIDERATIONS
Initial Stabilization
- Prompt treatment to avoid dehydration and malnutrition
- Correct acid–base and electrolyte disturbances. Surgery should be delayed until the alkalosis is corrected.
- Patients need pre- and post-op apnea monitoring. They have a tendency toward apnea to compensate with respiratory acidosis for their metabolic alkalosis.

IV Fluids
To correct dehydration and metabolic abnormalities

 ## ONGOING CARE

FOLLOW-UP RECOMMENDATIONS
Patient Monitoring
- Routine pediatric health maintenance
- Postoperative monitoring, including monitoring for pain, emesis, apnea

DIET
- No preoperative feeding
- Initiate feeding 12–24 hours after surgery, with goal of advancing to full oral feedings within 36–48 hours of surgery.

PROGNOSIS
Surgery is curative.

COMPLICATIONS
No long-term morbidity. Duodenal perforation is a known, but uncommon, complication of surgery (17)[B].

REFERENCES

1. Sommerfield T, Chalmers J, Youngson G, et al. The changing epidemiology of infantile hypertrophic pyloric stenosis in Scotland. *Arch Dis Child*. 2008.
2. Hernanz-Schulman M. Infantile hypertrophic pyloric stenosis. *Radiology*. 2003;227:319–31.
3. Krogh C, Fischer TK, Skotte L, et al. Familial aggregation and heritability of pyloric stenosis. *JAMA*. 2010;303:2393–9.
4. Everett KV, Chioza BA, Georgoula C, et al. Genome-wide high-density SNP-based linkage analysis of infantile hypertrophic pyloric stenosis identifies loci on chromosomes 11q14–q22 and Xq23. *Am J Hum Genet*. 2008;82:756–62.
5. Everett KV, Capon F, Georgoula C, et al. Linkage of monogenic infantile hypertrophic pyloric stenosis to chromosome 16q24. *Eur J Hum Genet*. 2008;16:1151–4.
6. Svenningsson A, Lagerstedt K, Omrani MD, et al. Absence of motilin gene mutations in infantile hypertrophic pyloric stenosis. *J Pediatr Surg*. 2008;43:443–6.
7. Bakker MK, De Walle HE, Wilffert B, et al. Fluoxetine and infantile hypertrophic pylorus stenosis: a signal from a birth defects-drug exposure surveillance study. *Pharmacoepidemiology and drug safety*. 2010;
8. Liede A, Pal T, Mitchell M, et al. Delineation of a new syndrome: clustering of pyloric stenosis, endometriosis, and breast cancer in two families. *J Med Genet*. 2000;37:794–6.
9. Vasavada P. Ultrasound evaluation of acute abdominal emergencies in infants and children. *Radiol Clin North Am*. 2004;42:445–56.
10. van der Bilt JD, Kramer WL, van der Zee DC, et al. Laparoscopic pyloromyotomy for hypertrophic pyloric stenosis: impact of experience on the results in 182 cases. *Surg Endosc*. 2004;18:907–9.
11. Hall NJ, Van Der Zee J, Tan HL, et al. Meta-analysis of laparoscopic versus open pyloromyotomy. *Ann Surg*. 2004;240:774–8.
12. Kim SS, Lau ST, Lee SL, et al. Pyloromyotomy: a comparison of laparoscopic, circumumbilical, and right upper quadrant operative techniques. *J Am Coll Surg*. 2005;201:66–70.
13. St Peter SD, Holcomb GW, Calkins CM, et al. Open versus laparoscopic pyloromyotomy for pyloric stenosis: a prospective, randomized trial. *Ann Surg*. 2006;244:363–70.
14. Leclair M, et al. Laparoscopic pyloromyotomy for hypertrophic pyloric stenosis: A prospective, randomized controlled trial. *J Ped Surg*. 2007;42:692–698.
15. St Peter SD, Ostlie DJ. Pyloric stenosis: From a retrospective analysis to a prospective clinical trial - the impact on surgical outcomes. *Curr Opin Pediatr*. 2008;20:311–14.
16. Sola JE, Neville HL et al. Laparoscopic vs open pyloromyotomy: a systematic review and meta-analysis. *J Pediatr Surg*. 2009;44:1631–7.
17. Safford SD, Pietrobon R, Safford KM, et al. A study of 11,003 patients with hypertrophic pyloric stenosis and the association between surgeon and hospital volume and outcomes. *J Pediatr Surg*. 2005;40:967–72; discussion 972–3.

ADDITIONAL READING

- Colletti JE. Pyloric stenosis. *CJEM*. 2004;6:444–5.
- Spevak MR, Ahmadjian JM, Kleinman PK, et al. Sonography of hypertrophic pyloric stenosis: frequency and cause of nonuniform echogenicity of the thickened pyloric muscle. *AJR Am J Roentgenol*. 1992;158:129–32.

 ## CODES

ICD9
750.5 Congenital hypertrophic pyloric stenosis

CLINICAL PEARLS

- Pyloric stenosis is the most common condition requiring surgical intervention in the 1st year of life.
- The condition classically presents between 1 and 5 months of life, with projectile vomiting after feeds and a firm, mobile mass in the right upper quadrant.
- Abdominal ultrasound is the study of choice.
- Surgery (Ramstedt pyloromyotomy, laparoscopically is the preferred method) is curative.

RABIES

Alan M. Ehrlich, MD

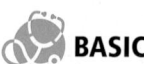 **BASICS**

DESCRIPTION

- A rapidly progressive central nervous system (CNS) infection caused by an RNA rhabdovirus and affecting mammals, including humans
- The disease is generally considered to be 100% fatal once symptoms develop.
- System(s) affected: Nervous
- Synonym(s): Hydrophobia (due to inability to swallow water)

EPIDEMIOLOGY
Incidence
- Most cases are in developing countries.
- Estimated 55,000 deaths worldwide per year
- Only 1 death in US in 2007
- Only 3 cases in US in 2006
- Predominant age: Any
- Predominant sex: Male = Female

RISK FACTORS
- Professions or activities that may expose a person to wild or domestic animals (e.g., animal handlers, lab workers, veterinarians, spelunkers [cave explorers])
- In US, most cases due to exposure to bats
- Internationally, many countries still have rabies widespread in both domestic and feral dogs.
- Human-to-human transmission has occurred through cornea and other tissue transplants.
- International travel to countries where canine rabies is endemic

GENERAL PREVENTION
- Preexposure vaccination if at risk of unapparent or unrecognized exposure to rabies such as traveling to endemic areas
- Preexposure vaccination for high-risk groups such as veterinarians, animal handlers, and certain laboratory workers
- Consider preexposure vaccination for travelers visiting relatives in areas such as North Africa that have increased risk of rabies from domestic animals
- Immunization of dogs and cats
- People who observe abnormal behavior in any wildlife species should contact animal control and should avoid approaching or handling those animals.
- Avoid wild and unknown domestic animals.
- Seek treatment promptly if bitten, scratched, or in contact with saliva.
- Infection can be prevented by prompt postexposure treatment of persons bitten by or otherwise exposed to animals known or suspected to be carrying the disease.
- Postexposure prophylaxis should be considered for any person who reports direct contact with bats, unless it is known that an exposure did not occur.

PATHOPHYSIOLOGY
Lyssavirus, which is an RNA virus in the family *Rhabdoviridae*

ETIOLOGY
- Rabies virus, a neurotropic virus present in saliva of infected animals
- Transmission occurs via bites from infected animals or rarely via saliva coming in contact with open wound or mucous membranes.
- In US, bats are the most common source of rabies.

 DIAGNOSIS

HISTORY
- It is important to elicit history of animal exposure because early diagnosis and treatment are necessary for survival.
- Diagnosis should be considered if there is a bite by an animal capable of transmitting the disease or travel to a rabies-endemic country; however, most patients in the US do not recall exposure.
- 5 stages (may overlap):
  - Incubation period: Time between bite and 1st symptoms of disease: Usually 10 days–1 year, with average of 20–60 days. It is shortest in patients with extensive bites about the head and trunk.
  - Prodrome: Lasts 1–14 days; symptoms include pain or paresthesia at bite site and nonspecific flulike symptoms, including fever and headache.
  - Acute neurologic period: Lasts 2–10 days. CNS symptoms dominate clinical picture; generally takes 1 of 2 forms: Furious rabies: Episodes of hyperactivity last about 5 minutes and include hydrophobia, aerophobia, hyperventilation, hypersalivation, and autonomic instability interspersed with periods of normalcy. Paralytic rabies: Paralysis dominates clinical picture; may be ascending (as in Guillain-Barré syndrome) or may affect 1 or more limbs differentially.
  - Coma: Lasts hours to days; with intensive care, rarely may last months. May evolve over a few days following acute neurologic period. May be sudden, with respiratory arrest.
  - Death: Usually occurs within 3 weeks of onset as result of complications. Only 6 survivors have been reported in the literature (1)[C].

PHYSICAL EXAM
Findings can range from normal exam up to severe neurologic findings, including paralysis and coma, depending on the stage of rabies at the time of presentation.

DIAGNOSTIC TESTS & INTERPRETATION
Lab
Initial lab tests
- Spinal tap
- White blood cell count in cerebrospinal fluid (CSF) examination may be normal or show moderate pleocytosis.
- CSF protein may be normal or moderately elevated.
- Skin biopsy to detect rabies antigen in hair follicles
- Available at state and federal reference labs
- Rabies antibody titer on serum and CSF
- Skin biopsy from nape of neck for direct fluorescent antibody examination
- Viral isolation from saliva or CSF
- Corneal smear stains are positive by immunofluorescence in 50% of patients.

Follow-Up & Special Considerations
For wild animals, the brain of the biting animal, if available, should be submitted for laboratory testing.

Imaging
Initial approach
- Head computed tomography scan: Normal or nonspecific findings consistent with encephalitis
- Magnetic resonance imaging may allow early diagnosis and can be used to rule out other forms of encephalitis.

Diagnostic Procedures/Surgery
Spinal tap
Pathological Findings
Encephalitis may be found on brain biopsy, but abnormal findings may be confined to parts (e.g., brain stem, midbrain, cerebellum) examined only postmortem.

DIFFERENTIAL DIAGNOSIS
- Any rapidly progressive encephalitis; important to exclude treatable causes of encephalitis, especially herpes
- Only 2007 case in US was diagnosed initially as transverse myelitis

 TREATMENT

Thorough wound cleansing with soap is the first line of treatment.

MEDICATION
ALERT
- Immunosuppression, either by medications or disease, can interfere with the development of immunity after vaccination. Immunosuppressive drugs should be avoided during postexposure prophylaxis unless absolutely necessary for the treatment of other conditions. If postexposure prophylaxis is given to an immunosuppressed person, serum samples should be checked for the presence of rabies virus–neutralizing antibody in response to vaccination (2)[B].
- All wounds should be thoroughly cleansed regardless of whether postexposure prophylaxis was given.
- Assessment of need for postexposure prophylaxis based on circumstances of possible exposure
- Increased risk associated with:
  - Bites involving any puncture of the skin constitute a significant risk, while saliva is only a risk if in contact with an open wound.
  - Wild animals or domestic animals that cannot be quarantined
  - Any potential exposure to bats
  - Hybrid animals of wild and domestic species (for example, wolf-dog)
  - Unprovoked attack (feeding a wild animal is considered a provoked attack)
- Management based on type of animal:
  - Bites from cats, dogs, and ferrets that can be watched for 10 days do not require prophylaxis unless animal shows signs of illness.
  - Skunks, foxes, bats, raccoons, and most carnivores are high risk, and prophylaxis should begin promptly unless animal can be captured and euthanized for pathological evaluation.
  - For rodents or livestock, consult local public health authorities before initiating prophylaxis.
- Postexposure prophylaxis regimen consists of (3):
  - Passive vaccination: Rabies immune globulin (RIG, Hyperab) administered once: 20 IU/kg of body weight. If anatomically feasible, all the RIG should be thoroughly infiltrated in the area around the wound. Any remaining RIG should be administered IM. RIG never should be

administered in the same syringe or into the same anatomic site as vaccine.

– Active vaccination: Rabies vaccine, human diploid cell (HDCV) or rabies vaccine adsorbed (RVA) or purified chick embryo cell vaccine IM in the deltoid. For children, the anterolateral aspect of the thigh is acceptable. The gluteal area never should be used for vaccine injections. Give the 1st dose, 1 mL, as soon as possible after exposure. The day of the 1st dose is designated Day 0. Give an additional 1-mL dose on days 3, 7, and 14.

• For previously vaccinated patients, a 1-mL IM dose of vaccine should be administered immediately and an additional 1-mL dose 3 days later. RIG is not necessary in these patients (3).

• Preexposure vaccination: For people in high-risk groups, such as veterinarians, animal handlers, certain laboratory workers, and those spending time in foreign countries where rabies is enzootic (3):

– Primary preexposure: IM vaccination regimen consists of 3 1-mL injections of HDCV or RVA given in deltoid area, 1 each on days 1, 7, and 28. HDCV also may be given in intradermal doses, administered with a special syringe developed for that purpose (Imovax Rabies ID Vaccine); the 0.1-mL IM dose is administered in the deltoid area; follow the same schedule as for IM doses. Recently, the manufacturer discontinued production of Imovax Rabies ID Vaccine.

– Preexposure boosters: For people at frequent risk of exposure to rabies, serum should be tested every 2 years. A preexposure booster (1.0 mL IM) should be administered if this is less than acceptable level. If titer cannot be obtained, a booster can be administered instead.

• Contraindications: None for postexposure treatment

Pregnancy Considerations

• Pregnancy is not a contraindication to postexposure prophylaxis.

• Rabies vaccination is not associated with a higher incidence of abortion, premature births, or fetal abnormalities.

ADDITIONAL TREATMENT
General Measures

• Physicians should evaluate each possible exposure to rabies and consult local or state public health officials about the need for rabies prophylaxis. In the US, raccoons, skunks, bats, foxes, and coyotes are the animals most likely to be infected, but any carnivore can carry the disease.

• Before specific antirabies treatment is initiated, consider:
– Type of exposure (bite or nonbite)
– Epidemiology of rabies in species involved
– Circumstances of biting incident (provoked vs unprovoked)
– Vaccination status of exposing animal

IN-PATIENT CONSIDERATIONS
Initial Stabilization

• For diagnosed rabies, comfort care and sedation are indicated for all patients.

• Milwaukee Protocol: Experimental treatment using ketamine, midazolam, amantadine, and ribavirin (4)[C] (see Prognosis)

Admission Criteria
Clinical rabies

 ONGOING CARE

FOLLOW-UP RECOMMENDATIONS
After primary vaccination, serologic testing is necessary only if the patient has a disease or takes a medication that may suppress the immune system.

PATIENT EDUCATION
Homes should be secured from bats by using screens over ventilation areas in the roof.

PROGNOSIS

• No postexposure failures reported in the US since the 1970s

• Rabies has the highest case-fatality rate of any infectious disease.

• The disease is generally considered to be 100% fatal once symptoms develop.

• Survival has been well documented for only 6 patients. In 5 of these, the persons had received rabies vaccination before the onset of disease.

• There was 1 documented recovery from clinical rabies in 2004 in a patient who did not receive pre- or postexposure prophylaxis, and this patient was treated with the Milwaukee Protocol (4)[C]. 2 years after treatment, there were some persistent neurologic deficits, but overall functioning was normal enough for the patient to finish high school and enroll in college (5)[C]. However, other patients treated similarly since have not survived (67)[C].

COMPLICATIONS
0.6% of people develop mild serum sickness reaction following HDCV boosters. Mild local and systemic reactions are common following vaccination. Mild reactions should not be a cause for interruption of immunization.

REFERENCES

1. Hankins DG, Rosekrans JA. Overview, prevention, and treatment of rabies. *Mayo Clin Proc.* 2004;79: 671–6.

2. Manning SE, et al. Human rabies prevention– United States, 2008: Recommendations of the advisory committee on immunization practices. *MMWR Recomm Rep.* 2008;57(RR-3): 1–28.

3. Rupprecht CE, Briggs D, Brown CM, et al. Use of a reduced (4-dose) vaccine schedule for postexposure prophylaxis to prevent human rabies: recommendations of the advisory committee on immunization practices. *MMWR Recomm Rep.* 2010;59:1–9.

4. Willoughby R, et al. Survival after treatment of rabies with induction of coma. *NEJM.* 2005; 352(24):2508–14.

5. Hu WT, et al. *NEJM.* 2007;357(9):945–6.

6. McDermid RC, et al. Human rabies encephalitis following bat exposure: failure of therapeutic coma. *CMAJ.* 2008;178(5):557–61.

7. Maier T, Schwarting A, Mauer D, et al. Management and outcomes after multiple corneal and solid organ transplantations from a donor infected with rabies virus. *Clin Infect Dis.* 2010;50:1112–9.

8. De Serres G, Skowronski DM, Mimault P, et al. Bats in the Bedroom, Bats in the Belfry: Reanalysis of the Rationale for Rabies Postexposure Prophylaxis. *Clin Infect Dis.* 2009.

See Also (Topic, Algorithm, Electronic Media Element)
Bites

 CODES

ICD9
071 Rabies

CLINICAL PEARLS

• Rare in US, but quite common in other areas of the world

• Seek treatment if exposed to scratch, bite, or saliva of potentially infected animal (e.g., feral dog, bat, fox, raccoon, or other wild animals).

• Postexposure prophylaxis consists of 3 steps: Local wound cleansing, passive immunization with rabies immune globulin, and active immunization with human diploid cell vaccine.

• Postexposure prophylaxis should be considered for any person who reports direct contact with bats, unless it is known that an exposure did not occur.

• Exposure to bats in bedrooms while sleeping is not uncommon, but contraction of rabies in this circumstance is rare (8)[B].

RADIATION SICKNESS

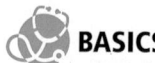

Sanjeev K. Sharma, MD

BASICS

Radiation is defined as release of particles or energy from isotopes of atoms with uneven numbers, which are typically unstable. The main radiation types are alpha, beta, gamma, and neutrons.

DESCRIPTION
- Any somatic or genetic disruption of function or form caused by electromagnetic waves or accelerated atomic particles
- Radiation illness may be classified as
  - Nonionizing:
    ○ Damage to exposed tissues from heating
    ○ Sources: Microwaves, infrared radiation
  - Ionizing:
    ○ Damage to DNA
    ○ Sources include human-made (nuclear warfare material and medical radiation) and natural (radon and uranium)
    ○ Examples: α-Particles, β-particles, neutrons, X-rays and γ radiation (energetic photons)
- Units of measure:
  - Absorbed dose: Radiation absorbed dose (Rad) or the SI unit Gray (Gy); 1 Gy = 100 rad.
  - Dose equivalent: Roentgen equivalent in humans (Rem) or the SI unit Sievert (Sv); 1 Sv = 100 rem.
- Radiation includes
  - Electromagnetic emissions; energy (hence penetration) is inversely proportional to wavelength (e.g., x-rays, γ-rays).
  - Particles. Particles include α-Particles, β-particles, neutrons. *Alpha (α) radiation* consists of heavy, positively charged particles containing two protons and two neutrons. Alpha particles are usually emitted from isotopes with an atomic number of 82, such as uranium or plutonium. *Beta (β) radiation* consists of electrons, which are small, light, negatively charged particles. Both have low penetrance externally but are dangerous if ingested. Neutron particles are heavy and unchanged, released during nuclear detonation. Neutrons are damaging and penetrate well.
- System(s) affected: Cardiovascular; GI; Hematologic/Lymphatic/Immunologic; Musculoskeletal; Nervous; Pulmonary; Renal/Urologic; Reproductive; Skin/Exocrine

Pediatric Considerations
Infants and children are at increased risk for injury.

Pregnancy Considerations
- The fetus is at increased risk for injury.
- Consult a radiologist and health physicist for assistance in calculating fetal dose.

EPIDEMIOLOGY
- Historically:
  - In Japan, 120,000 individuals developed acute radiation syndrome as a result of nuclear explosions.
  - In the Marshall Islands, 7,266 people were exposed to radiation because of errors in judging winds after a nuclear test in the South Pacific.
  - In the Chernobyl accident in Ukraine in 1986, an estimated 50,000 individuals received at least 0.5 Sv of exposure.
- Most acute radiation injury is related to accidents or radiation therapy.

- Accidents are sporadic and usually involve small numbers of individuals. From 1944 to 2000, there have been 243 serious radiation accidents in the US.
- Worldwide exposure (average/person/year):
  - Natural (γ-rays, radon, and others): 2.4 mSv
  - Occupational (from 6.5 million monitored workers): 1.8 mSv
  - Medical (330 examinations/1,000 people): 0.4 mSv
  - Artificial environmental (atmospheric nuclear testing, Chernobyl accident, nuclear power production): 0.0072 mSv

Incidence
In the US, 400,000 patients/year receive radiation therapy for malignancies.

RISK FACTORS
- Young patients more susceptible than old, and men more sensitive than women
- Patients who are debilitated are more susceptible than those who are healthy
- Natural residence in certain geographic regions
- Occupational: Medical professionals, nuclear power workers, industrial radiodiagnostic workers

Genetics
Females have greater tolerance than males. The exception is pregnant females, with risk of fetal injury at low dose.

GENERAL PREVENTION
- Avoidance of exposure: Exposure reduced by decreasing exposure time, increasing distance, and shielding
- Pretreatment: In certain situations, exposure of the thyroid may be reduced by preexposure consumption of radiostable iodine.
- Follow safety procedures.

PATHOPHYSIOLOGY
- Radiation interactions with atoms can result in ionization and the formation of free radicals that damage tissue by disrupting chemical bonds and molecular structures in the cell, including DNA. Radiation damage can lead to cell death; those cells that recover may be mutated and at higher risk for subsequent cancer. Cell sensitivity increases as the replication rate increases and the cell differentiation decreases. Bone marrow and mucosal surfaces of the GI tract, which have vast mitotic activity, are significantly more sensitive to radiation than slowly dividing tissues such as bones and muscles. Following exposure of either all or most of the human body to ionizing radiation, ARS can develop.
- Nonionizing radiation: Heating of tissues: Testes, eye
- Ionizing radiation:
  - Damage to DNA
  - Affects rapidly dividing cells most: GI mucosa, bone marrow, vascular endothelium, reproductive organs

ETIOLOGY
- Routes of exposure:
  - Irradiation
  - External contamination (clothing, skin)
  - Internal contamination (inhalation, ingestion)
- Acute radiation syndrome (ARS): Results from whole-body exposure
- Cutaneous syndrome (CS):
  - Damage to stem cells
  - Prolonged latency
  - Resembles thermal burns
  - Dry or moist desquamation

DIAGNOSIS

- Strong index of suspicion and knowledge of radiation event
- It is convenient to categorize exposed individuals into groups:
  - Super-lethal amount 50 Gy (5000 rads) or more: Usually die within 24 to 48 hours. Death is due to neurovascular syndrome associated with intractable vomiting, diarrhea, tremors, ataxia, coma and death.
  - Exposure 5–20 Gy (500–2000 rads): Survival may be possible under optimal conditions. Early CNS and cardiovascular complications may be severe. It usually starts with anorexia, nausea, vomiting, sweating, fatigue, and prostration. There is intestinal mucosal damage and severe bone marrow depression. Agranulocytosis invariably results in buccal and pharyngeal ulceration, bacteremia, and many types of infections. Thrombocytopenia leads to bleeding into skin and mucus membranes and GI tract. Death occurs from blood loss or gram-negative sepsis. Survival depends upon use of maximum supportive therapy including fluids, antibiotics, and blood transfusion. Transplantation of matched bone marrow is indicated as these patients usually have irreversible loss of bone marrow stem cells.
  - Exposure 2–5 Gy (200–500 rads): Lethal if untreated. Manifestations are similar to those above but are less severe and are delayed. Bone marrow suppression lasts for 3–4 weeks and recovery usually starts around 6th week. They also require maximum supportive care with fluids and electrolytes, antibiotics. Bone marrow transplantation is usually not recommended.
  - Exposure 1–2 Gy (<200 rads): No disease; there may be some nausea >3 hours after the event. Most people involved in an accident of this type will complain of some nausea when questioned. There is no known effective form of therapy available.

HISTORY
- Exposure to known source of radiation:
  - Damaged radioisotope-containing medical equipment
  - Industrial sources
  - Nuclear power plant
  - Research nuclear reactors
  - Terrorist event:
    ○ Nuclear device or radioisotope-contaminated explosive device
    ○ Hidden source of radiation
- Accurate radiation dose information after exposure, duration of exposure, and amount of shielding is difficult to determine. Even when it is determined it is of limited value.
- Generally, affects 3 systems: Hematopoietic, gastrointestinal, and neurovascular
- Four major stages in ARS: Prodrome, latent phase, illness, and either recovery or death. The higher the radiation doses, the shorter and more severe each stage.
- The prodrome appears within minutes to 4 days postexposure; lasts between a few hours to a few days; and can include nausea and vomiting.
- Latent phase lasts from days to several weeks when an individual feels quite well.

- Illness phase usually starts from 3rd to 5th week with an abrupt onset; symptoms include:
  – Moderate to severe GI symptoms: Nausea, vomiting, diarrhea, abdominal pain, and cramping
  – Bleeding
  – Infections
  – Epilation
- Recovery phase may take weeks to month

PHYSICAL EXAM
- Cognitive defects
- Erythema, blistering, ulceration, desquamation, mainly pharyngeal, mucosal, buccal, and GI tract
- Hair loss, onycholysis
- Petechiae, bruising, spontaneous bleeding

DIAGNOSTIC TESTS & INTERPRETATION
- Identify the type of radiation.
- Determine the amount of time since exposure.
- Estimate total dose, dose rate, and approximate volume of tissue involved; chromosome aberration dosimetry is desirable (1)[C].

Lab
- Lymphocyte count at 48 hours after event:
  – >1,500: Trivial or no exposure
  – >1,000: Survival without treatment
  – 500–1,000: Survival with treatment
  – 100–400: Death without bone marrow transplant
  – <100: Certain death
- Drugs that may alter lab results: Chemotherapeutic agents cause bone marrow suppression identical to that seen in radiation exposure.

Initial lab tests
Complete blood count (CBC), complete metabolic profile and blood group and cross match

Pathological Findings
- Hypocellular marrow with the hematopoietic syndrome
- GI syndrome with loss of villus margin and sloughing of villus structure
- Late cases with fibrosis of lung, liver, and kidney tissues
- Loss of hair indicates exposure of 350 rads and is complete at 700 rads.

DIFFERENTIAL DIAGNOSIS
Patient exposed to radiation:
- Acute viral illness or anxiety (nausea)
- Blast or heat (skin redness)
- Chemical exposure (blistering and pain)

 TREATMENT

- Treatment begins with standard trauma care.
- Aggressive fluid therapy with maintenance of electrolyte balance.
- Transfusion of blood and blood product as needed.
- Therapy for neutropenia and infection. Broad-spectrum antibiotics can be started immediately.
- Role of bone marrow transplantation is questionable.
- Partial and total parental nutrition as needed to bypass the damaged GI system
- Treatment of blast and thermal injury if present
- Psychological support

MEDICATION
- Supportive therapy:
  – Nutrition supplement (1)[C]: An elemental diet with simple sugar, small peptides, vitamin, and minerals: Vital HN and Vivonex
  – Antiemetics:
    ○ Promethazine
    ○ Ondansetron
  – Antidiarrheals: Loperamide
  – Gastric mucositis: Sucralfate mouthwash (1)[C]
  – Cytokine therapy:
    ○ Granulocyte–macrophage colony-stimulating factor
    ○ Granulocyte colony-stimulating factor (G-CSF) or pegylated G-CSF
    ○ Infection prophylaxis:
  – Antibiotics: Fluoroquinolone or other broad-spectrum antibiotics
  – Antivirals:
    ○ Acyclovir
    ○ Anciclovir
  – Antifungals: Fluconazole; treat specific pathogens as identified.
- Treatment for internal contamination:
  – For exposure to radioactive iodine: Potassium iodide
  – For exposure to radioactive phosphorus: Parenteral magnesium sulfate
  – For exposure to radioactive cesium and thallium: Prussian blue
  – For exposure to radioactive plutonium, americium, and curium: Diethylenetriamine pentaacetic acid (DTPA) (2)[B]
  – For nonspecific ingestions: Laxatives to increase GI transit rate

ADDITIONAL TREATMENT
General Measures
- Decontamination if external contamination: Precedence of decontamination depends on the nature of the situation and the professional judgment of the provider.
- Treat collateral injuries, such as burns and lacerations, only after decontamination.
- Consult health physicist, medical physicist, and radiation safety officer (1)[C].

Additional Therapies
- Pancytopenic patients may require reverse isolation.
- Treatment of damaged bone marrow:
  – Blood transfusion
  – Platelet transfusion
  – Stem cell transplantation
- Prevention and treatment of infection
- Internal decontamination
- Psychological support
- End-of-life care (3)[C]

SURGERY/OTHER PROCEDURES
- Débridement of all wounds to decontaminate
- Injected interferon-γ to reduce fibrosis formation (4)[C]
- All surgery within 2 days, before loss of white blood cell and platelet function
- Bone marrow transplant for severe exposure

IN-PATIENT CONSIDERATIONS
Initial Stabilization
Inpatient care

 ONGOING CARE

FOLLOW-UP RECOMMENDATIONS
Isolation techniques for immune system injury

Patient Monitoring
- Daily complete blood count (CBC) and platelet, granulocyte, and lymphocyte counts
- Stools for blood
- Vital signs every 4 hours to look for sepsis

DIET
As tolerated; hyperalimentation for severe GI syndromes

PATIENT EDUCATION
Recommend genetic counseling and screening to patients who have been exposed to significant amounts of radiation.

PROGNOSIS
- Patients surviving 12 weeks have excellent prognosis but should be monitored for long-term complications.
- Hair growth usually resumes within 2 months.

COMPLICATIONS
- Long-term fibrosis of kidneys, liver, and lung occurs within 6 months of acute exposure and with as little as 300 rads of exposure.
- Radiation exposure may induce malignancies.
- Increased long-term risk of leukemia (acute lymphocytic or chronic myelogenous)
- Multiple myeloma and cancers of the breast, esophagus, stomach, colon, lung, ovary, bladder, thyroid
- Sterility

Pregnancy Considerations
Injury to fetus likely

REFERENCES

1. Berger ME, Christensen DM, Lowry PC, et al. Medical management of radiation injuries: current approaches. *Occup Med (Lond)*. 2006;56:162–72.
2. Grappin L, Berard P, Menetrier F, et al. Treatment of actinide exposures: a review of Ca-DTPA injections inside CEA-cogema plants. *Radiat Prot Dosimetry*. 2007.
3. http://www.mayoclinic.com/health/radiation-sickness/DS00432
4. Gottlöber P, Steinert M, Bähren W, et al. Interferon-gamma in 5 patients with cutaneous radiation syndrome after radiation therapy. *Int J Radiat Oncol Biol Phys*. 2001;50:159–66.

 CODES

ICD9
990 Effects of radiation, unspecified

RAPE CRISIS SYNDROME

Chris G. Kyriakedes, DO
Jack H. Mitstifer, MD

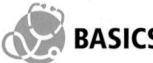

BASICS

DESCRIPTION
- Definitions (legal definitions may vary from state to state):
  – Sexual contact: Intentional touching of a person's intimate parts (including thighs) or the clothing covering such areas, if it is construed as being for the purpose of sexual gratification
  – Sexual conduct: Vaginal intercourse between a male and female, or anal intercourse, fellatio, or cunnilingus between persons, regardless of sex
  – Rape: Any sexual penetration, however slight, using force or coercion against the person's will
  – Sexual imposition: Similar to rape but without penetration or the use of force (i.e., nonconsensual sexual contact)
  – Gross sexual imposition: Nonconsensual sexual contact with the use of force
  – Corruption of a minor: Sexual conduct by an individual ≥18 years old with an individual <16 years of age
- Most states have expanded rape statutes to include marital rape, date rape, and shield laws.
- System(s) affected: Nervous; Reproductive
- Synonym(s): Sexual assault; Rape trauma

EPIDEMIOLOGY
- Anyone can be sexually assaulted, but some people are especially vulnerable (1):
  – Adolescents and young women
  – People with disabilities
  – Poor and homeless people
  – Sex workers
  – Those living in institutions or areas of conflict
- Predominant age:
  – The incidence of sexual assault peaks in the 16–19-year-old age group, with the mean occurring at 20 years of age:
    ○ Adolescent sexual assault has a greater frequency of anogenital injuries.
- Predominant sex: Female > Male
  – For males:
    ○ 69% of male victims were first raped before age 18.
    ○ 41% of males victims were raped before age 12.

Incidence
- There were 191,670 rapes and sexual assaults measured in 2005 in the US.
- In 2008, the estimated number of forcible rapes (89,000) showed a decrease of 1.6% from the 2007 estimate reported by the Uniformed Crime Reporting Program.
- Estimated that only 1:3–1:5 of adult cases are reported:
  – In 2005, only 38% of rape or sexual assaults were reported to the police.
- 1/5 American women report being raped during their lifetime (2):
  – Between 20% and 25% of females will experience rape or attempted rape during their college years.

- 1/7 males will be sexually assaulted during a lifetime.
- ~2/1,000 children in the US were confirmed by child protective agencies as having experienced sexual assault in 2003.
- The majority of rape victims either know or have some acquaintance with their attacker.

RISK FACTORS
- Numerous, and include multiple individual, relationship, community, and societal factors
- In general, adults are assaulted in their own homes, while adolescents are assaulted in their assailant's residence.
- Most perpetrators of sexual violence are males, with all acts against females >90%
- Most acts against males are >65% male perpetrators

GENERAL PREVENTION
- Scope of rape prevention is very complex and broad.
- The public health approach should include both prevention/avoidance of vulnerability factors and implementation of protective factors.
- Females may benefit from assertiveness training and self-defense training.
- Universal screening for interpersonal violence by health care providers does assist in identifying victims (2).

DIAGNOSIS

- In adults:
  – History of sexual penetration
  – Sexual contact or sexual conduct without consent and/or with the use of force
- In children:
  – Actual observation or suspicion of sexual penetration, sexual contact, or sexual conduct
  – Signs include evidence of the use of force and/or evidence of sexual contact (e.g., presence of semen and/or sperm).

HISTORY
- Avoid questioning that implies the patient is at fault.
- Record answers in patient's own words insofar as possible. Include date, approximate time, and general location as best as possible. Document physical abuse other than sexual. Describe all types of sexual contact, whether actual or attempted. Take history of alcohol and/or drugs before or after alleged incident.
- Document time of last activity that could possibly alter specimens (e.g., bath, shower, or douche). Thorough gynecologic history is mandatory, including last menstrual period, last consenting sexual contact, contraceptive practice, and prior gynecologic surgery.

PHYSICAL EXAM
- Use of drawings and/or photographs is encouraged.
- Document all signs of trauma or unusual marks.
- Document mental status/emotional state.
- Use UV light (Wood lamp) to detect seminal stains on clothing or skin.

ALERT
- A forensic kit or "rape kit" contains swabs that are collected from the vagina and rectum, and instructions are given with the kit as to proper collection.
- Many states and emergency departments across the country are utilizing Sexual Assault Nurse Examiner (SANE) when available. This has led to a more consistent and more accurate collection of evidence in alleged rape cases.
- Complete genital-rectal examination, including evidence of trauma, secretions, or discharge:
  – Use of a nonlubricated, water-moistened speculum is mandatory because commonly used lubricants may destroy evidence.
  – Testing and/or specimen collection as indicated and in compliance with state requirements

DIAGNOSTIC TESTS & INTERPRETATION
Lab
- In females, obtain a serum or urine pregnancy test.
- Record results of wet mount, noting the presence or absence of sperm and, if present, whether it is motile or immotile.
- Drug/alcohol testing as indicated by history and/or physical findings

DIFFERENTIAL DIAGNOSIS
Consenting sex among adults

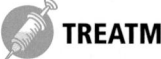

TREATMENT

MEDICATION
First Line
- Gonorrhea: Ceftriaxone 125 mg IM once or Cefixime 400 mg p.o. once. Available in U.S. since April 2008.
- Chlamydia: Azithromycin (Zithromax) 1 g p.o., single dose or doxycycline 100 mg p.o. b.i.d. × 7 days or erythromycin base 500 mg p.o. q.i.d. for 7 days or erythromycin ethylsuccinate 800 mg p.o. q.i.d. for 7 days or ofloxacin 300 mg p.o. b.i.d. for 7 days or levofloxacin 300 mg p.o. b.i.d. for 7 days
- Syphilis: Benzathine penicillin G 2–4 million units IM once or doxycycline 100 mg p.o. b.i.d. for 14 days. Some suggest ceftriaxone 1 g daily either IM or IV for 8–10 days or azithromycin 2 g p.o. single dose, but treatment failures have been reported in several geographic areas.
- Trichomoniasis and bacterial vaginosis, if present. Metronidazole 500 mg p.o. b.i.d. for 7 days or metronidazole 2 g p.o., single dose (considered less efficacious than 7-day therapy) or metronidazole gel 0.75% 1 full applicator (5 g) intravaginally, once a day for 5 days; or clindamycin cream 2%, 1 full applicator (5 g) intravaginally at bedtime for 7 days (also less efficacious than metronidazole)
- If pregnancy prophylaxis is indicated, use levonorgestrel 1.5 mg × 1 (Plan B, progestin-only) for up to 5 days after the rape:
  – Levonorgestrel has proved more effective than the Yuzpe regimen, a method of emergency contraception using a combination of estrogen and progesterone (3)[A].
  – Alternatively, an intrauterine device can be inserted up to 5 days after the earliest predicted date of ovulation in that cycle.

- HIV: Currently, there is a low likelihood of HIV transmittance, but the Centers for Disease Control and Prevention still recommends postexposure prophylaxis for victims of sexual assault. Regimen is lamivudine–zidovudine (Combivir) b.i.d. for 28 days or zidovudine 300 mg plus lamivudine 150 mg b.i.d. for 28 days:
  – Medications most effective if started within 24 hours, could reduce transmission of HIV by as much as 80%
  – Unlikely to be beneficial if started after 72 hours
- Hepatitis B: If prevalent in area or assailant known to be high risk—hepatitis B immune globulin 0.06 mL/kg IM, single dose, and initiate 3-dose hepatitis B virus immunization series.
- Note: Gonorrhea and chlamydia medications may be given concomitantly.

Second Line
Gonorrhea: Ampicillin/probenecid or amoxicillin/probenecid. Note: Be aware that drug resistance is on the rise in several major cities. Quinolones are no longer recommended for treatment of gonorrhea.

ADDITIONAL TREATMENT
General Measures
- Providing health care to victims of sexual assault/abuse requires special sensitivity and privacy.
- All such cases *must* be reported immediately to the appropriate law enforcement agency.
- With the victim's permission, enlist the help of personnel from local support agencies (e.g., rape crisis center). When available, use of in-house social services is extremely helpful to victim and family.
- Sexual assault nurse examiner programs have been shown to be beneficial, especially in large cities and metropolitan areas with multiple emergency departments of varying capability and staff training/experience.
- Give sedation and tetanus prophylaxis when indicated.
- Discuss possible pregnancy and pregnancy termination with the victim. If hospital policy precludes such a discussion, then information about this option should be offered to the victim via follow-up mechanisms.
- Discuss suspected HIV and hepatitis B exposure and testing with the victim in accordance with hospital, regional, and state policies/protocols. The initial HIV test should be completed within 7 days of the suspected exposure.

Pregnancy Considerations
Conduct baseline pregnancy test; discuss pregnancy prevention with patient.

Pediatric Considerations
Assure the child that he or she is a good person and was not the cause of the incident.

IN-PATIENT CONSIDERATIONS
Initial Stabilization
- Contact appropriate social services agency.
- Majority of adult victims can be treated as outpatients, unless associated trauma (physical or mental) requires admission
- Majority of pediatric sexual assault/abuse victims will require admission or outside placement until appropriate social agency can evaluate home environment

---

 ONGOING CARE

FOLLOW-UP RECOMMENDATIONS
Patient Monitoring
- The patient should be seen in 7–10 days for follow-up care, including pregnancy testing and counseling.
- Close examination for vaginitis, and treatment if necessary
- Follow-up test for syphilis and gonorrhea should occur in 5–6 weeks.
- Follow-up testing for HIV and hepatitis B should occur in 6 months.
- Provide telephone numbers of counseling agency(ies) that can provide counseling/legal services to the patient.
- Consider sexual assault nurse examiner, if available in area.

PATIENT EDUCATION
- Information and help are available from local rape crisis support organizations.
- National Institute of Mental Health, Public Inquiries Branch, Office of Scientific Information, Department of Health and Human Services, Parklawn Bldg., Room 15C-05, 5600 Fishers Lane, Rockville, MD 20857; (301) 443-4513
- National Domestic Violence Hotline at 1-800-799-SAFE(7233) or TTY 1-800-787-3224 or http://www.ndvh.org/

PROGNOSIS
- Acute phase (usually 1–3 weeks following rape): Shaking, pain, wound healing, mood swings, appetite loss, crying. Also feelings of grief, shame, anger, fear, revenge, or guilt.
- Late or chronic phase: Female victim may develop fear of intercourse, fear of men, nightmares, sleep disorders, daytime flashbacks, fear of being alone, loss of self-esteem, anxiety, depression, posttraumatic stress syndrome.
- Recovery may be prolonged. Patients who are able to talk about their feelings seem to have a faster recovery.

COMPLICATIONS
Sequelae include (1):
- Trauma (physical and mental)
- Sexually transmitted infections, including HIV
- Unwanted pregnancy (with the possibility of abortion):
  – The rape-related pregnancy rate in the US is 5% per rape among victims of reproductive age, resulting in more than 32,000 unwanted pregnancies each year (2).
  – Adolescents are at highest risk of pregnancy.
- Depression
- Posttraumatic stress disorder

REFERENCES

1. Welch J, Mason F. Rape and sexual assault. *BMJ.* 2007;334:1154–8.
2. Toohey JS. Domestic violence and rape. *Med Clin North Am.* 2008;92:1239–52, xii.
3. Cheng L, Gülmezoglu AM, Piaggio G, et al. Interventions for emergency contraception. *Cochrane Database Syst Rev.* 2008:CD001324.

ADDITIONAL READING

- A National Protocol for Sexual Assault Medical Forensic Examinations (Adults/Adolescents). U.S. Department of Justice, Office on Violence Against Women; September 2004.
- Bureau of Justice Statistics. National Center for Injury Prevention and Control. Sexual Violence: Fact Sheet and Rape and Sexual Assault National Crime Victim's Rights Week, 2005.
- Hogan TM, Uyenishi AA. Sexual assault: Medical and legal implications of the emergency care of adult victims. *Emerg Med Pract.* 2003:5.
- Jones JS, Rossman L, Wynn BN, et al. Comparative analysis of adult versus adolescent sexual assault: epidemiology and patterns of anogenital injury. *Acad Emerg Med.* 2003;10:872–7.
- Poirier MP. Care of the female adolescent rape victim. *Pediatr Emerg Care.* 2002;18:53–9; quiz 60.

See Also (Topic, Algorithm, Electronic Media Element)
Chlamydial Sexually Transmitted Diseases; Gonococcal Infections; Hepatitis B; Hepatitis C; HIV Infection and AIDS; Posttraumatic Stress Disorder (PTSD); Syphilis

 CODES

ICD9
- 995.83 Adult sexual abuse
- V71.5 Observation following alleged rape or seduction

CLINICAL PEARLS
- *Rape* is a legal term, and the examining physician is encouraged to use terminology such as *alleged rape* or *alleged sexual conduct*.
- In the majority of states, a wife may now accuse her husband of rape if they are estranged and living apart.
- Because "consent defense" is common, documentation of evidence supporting the use of force or the administration of drugs/alcohol is imperative.
- The use of a protocol is encouraged to assure every victim a uniform, comprehensive evaluation, regardless of the expertise of the examining physician. The protocol must ensure that all evidence is properly collected and labeled, chain of custody is maintained, and the evidence is sent to the most appropriate forensic laboratory.
- All medical records must be well documented and legible.
- All medical personnel must be willing and able to testify on behalf of the patient.

RAYNAUD PHENOMENON

Herbert L. Muncie, Jr., MD

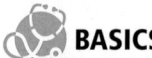 **BASICS**

DESCRIPTION
Idiopathic intermittent episodes of vasoconstriction of digital arteries, precapillary arterioles, and cutaneous arteriovenous shunts in response to cold temperatures or emotional stress. A triphasic color change of the fingers (occasionally, of the toes) is the physical manifestation of the episodes. Thumbs are rarely involved. The initial color is white from extreme pallor, then blue from cyanosis; and finally with warming and vasodilatation intense redness develops. Swelling, throbbing, and paresthesias are the final symptoms:

- Primary (idiopathic Raynaud disease):
  - 80% of patients with Raynaud phenomenon have primary disease.
  - Episodes are bilateral and nonprogressive.
  - Diagnosis confirmed only if after >2 years of symptoms, no underlying associated disease develops
- Secondary (Raynaud syndrome):
  - Progressive and asymmetric
  - Spasm is more frequent and more severe with time. No gangrene; rarely, ulceration; 13% may progress to atrophy of digital fat pads and ischemic ulcers of fingertips.
- System(s) affected: Hematologic; Lymphatic; Immunologic; Musculoskeletal; Dermatologic; Exocrine

Pregnancy Considerations
- Raynaud phenomenon can appear as breast pain in lactating women.
- Bacterial culture of breast milk can distinguish mastitis from Raynaud phenomenon.

Geriatric Considerations
Initial appearance of Raynaud phenomenon at >40 years of age frequently indicates an underlying disease.

Pediatric Considerations
Associated with SLE and scleroderma

EPIDEMIOLOGY
Incidence
- Primary:
  - Predominant age: 14 years; ~1/4 begin >40 years of age
  - Predominant sex: Female > Male (4:1)
- Secondary:
  - Predominant age: >40 years of age
  - Predominant sex: No gender predilection

Prevalence
- Primary: ~3–16% of population (based on reporting of characteristic skin color changes, intolerance to cold)
- Secondary: Less common, only about 1% of population

RISK FACTORS
- Smoking may reduce digital blood flow but is not associated with increased risk of Raynaud phenomenon.
- Existing autoimmune or connective tissue disorder
- End-stage renal disease with hemodialysis may increase the risk due to a steal phenomenon complicating the arterial-venous shunt.
- An elevated homocysteine level has been associated with primary and secondary disease (1).

Genetics
Little information is available, but some studies suggest a dominant inheritance pattern. ~1/4 of primary patients have a 1st-degree relative with Raynaud phenomenon.

GENERAL PREVENTION
- Avoid exposure to cold.
- Stop smoking.
- Avoid trauma and vibration to hands and fingertips; however, no relationship has been established between etiology of Raynaud phenomenon and occupational vibratory tool use.

ETIOLOGY
Unknown. May involve increased sensitivity of β_2-adrenergic receptors in digital vessels in primary type. Serotonin receptors (5-HT$_2$ type) may be involved in secondary Raynaud phenomenon. Dysregulation of control mechanisms of vascular motility leading to imbalance between vasodilation and vasoconstriction. Platelet and blood viscosity abnormalities are also implicated.

COMMONLY ASSOCIATED CONDITIONS
Secondary Raynaud:
- Scleroderma
- Systemic lupus erythematosis (SLE)
- Polymyositis
- Sjögren syndrome
- Occlusive vascular disease
- Cryoglobulinemia
- Use of vibrating tools

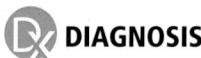 **DIAGNOSIS**

HISTORY
- Primary:
  - Symmetric attacks
  - Absence of tissue necrosis, ulceration, or gangrene
  - Absence of secondary cause after history and general physical examination
  - If after >2 years of symptoms no abnormal clinical or laboratory signs have developed, secondary disease is highly unlikely.
- Secondary:
  - Onset typically >40 years of age
  - Asymmetric episodes more intense and painful
  - Inquire regarding arthritis, myalgias, fever, dry eyes and/or mouth, rash, or cardiopulmonary symptoms.
  - Inquire about past or current drug use.
  - Any exposure to toxic agents
  - Any repetitive trauma

PHYSICAL EXAM
Pallor/whiteness of fingertips with cold exposure, followed by cyanosis, then redness and pain with warming:
- Ischemic attacks evidenced by demarcated or cyanotic skin limited to digits usually starts on 1 digit and spreads symmetrically to all fingers of both hands; however, the thumb is often spared.
- Beau lines: Transverse linear depressions in nail plate of most or all fingernails, which can occur after exposure to cold temperature or any disease serious enough to disrupt normal nail growth.
- Livedo reticularis: Mottling of the skin of the arms and legs may occur but is completely benign and reversible with warming.
- Primary:

- Normal general physical exam
- Nail bed capillaries: Place 1 drop grade B immersion oil on skin at base of fingernail, and view capillaries with handheld ophthalmoscope at 10–40 diopters. Normal appearance.
- Secondary:
  - Clinical features suggestive of connective tissue disease (e.g., arthritis, abnormal lung function)
  - Ischemic skin lesions: Ulceration of finger pads, progressing to autoamputation in severe, prolonged cases
  - Nail bed capillaries distorted and anatomically abnormal (2)[C]

DIAGNOSTIC TESTS & INTERPRETATION
Unnecessary to perform provocative test (e.g., immersion of patient's hand in ice water)

Lab
- Primary:
  - Antinuclear antibody: Negative
  - ESR: Normal
- Secondary:
  - Tests for underlying secondary causes (e.g., CBC, ESR)
  - Positive autoantibody has low positive predictive value for an associated connective tissue disease (30%).
  - Antibodies to specific autoantigens more suggestive of secondary disease (e.g., scleroderma with anticentromere or antitopoisomerase antibodies)

Imaging
Rarely necessary; patients may demonstrate osteolysis of distal metaphysial portions of phalanges with tapering and calcification of soft tissue

Follow-Up & Special Considerations
Periodic assessments could be helpful during the initial years after the diagnosis is made to determine if a connective tissue disease has become manifest.

Diagnostic Procedures/Surgery
Diagnosis is determined by history and physical exam.

DIFFERENTIAL DIAGNOSIS
- Thromboangiitis obliterans (Buerger disease): Primarily affects men; involves legs and feet; <5% have hand involvement; smoking-related
- Rheumatoid arthritis (RA)
- Progressive systemic sclerosis (scleroderma): Raynaud phenomenon may precede other symptoms by years.
- SLE
- Carpal tunnel syndrome
- Thoracic outlet syndrome
- Hypothyroidism
- CREST syndrome (calcinosis cutis, Raynaud phenomenon, esophageal dysmotility, sclerodactyly, and telangiectasias)
- Cryoglobulinemias
- Waldenström macroglobulinemia
- Acrocyanosis
- Polycythemia
- Occupational (e.g., especially from vibrating tools, masonry work, exposure to polyvinyl chloride)
- Drugs (e.g., clonidine, ergotamine, methysergide, amphetamines, bromocriptine, bleomycin, vinblastine, cisplatin, cyclosporine)

TREATMENT

The effects of treatment can be assessed using a Raynaud Condition Score (3).

MEDICATION

Calcium-channel blockers (CCBs) have been the primary treatment for many years. Nifedipine has been best studied and is the most frequently used drug in this group.

First Line

- Nifedipine: 30–180 mg/d (sustained-release form); may be needed only during winter; up to 75% experience improvement (4)[B]
- Symptomatic responses do not correlate with objective evidence of improvement.
- Contraindications: Allergy to drug, pregnancy, CHF
- Precautions: May cause headache, dizziness, lightheadedness, edema, or hypotension
- Significant possible interactions:
  – Increases serum level of digoxin; monitor digoxin levels closely after nifedipine is added
  – May increase PT in patients taking warfarin

Second Line

- Amlodipine (5–20 mg/d) and nicardipine appear to be effective and may have fewer adverse effects.
- No data exist to support use of another calcium channel blocker if initial one is ineffective.
- Prazosin (1–2 mg t.i.d.) is the only well-studied α_1-adrenergic receptor blocker with modest effect (4)[B].
- Small studies support benefit from losartan, fluoxetine, and phosphodiesterase type 5 inhibitors (5).
- Parenteral iloprost, a prostacyclin, even in low doses (0.5 ng/kg/min over 6 hours) has improved ulcerations with severe Raynaud phenomenon (6)[B]. Oral prostacyclin has not proved useful.
- Nitroglycerin patches may be helpful, but use is limited by the occurrence of severe headache. Nitroglycerin gel has shown promise as a topical therapy (7)[B].

ADDITIONAL TREATMENT

General Measures

- Dress warmly, wear gloves, and avoid cold.
- Stop smoking.
- Avoid beta blockers, amphetamines, ergot alkaloids, and sumatriptan.
- Temperature-related biofeedback may help patients to increase hand temperature, but at the 1-year follow-up no better than control
- Use finger guards over ulcerated fingertips.

Issues for Referral

If an underlying disease is strongly suspected, consider rheumatology consultation for evaluation and treatment.

Additional Therapies

- Short-acting calcium channel blocker such as nifedipine
- Aspirin
- Digital or wrist block with lidocaine or bupivacaine (without epinephrine)
- Short-term anticoagulation with heparin if persistent critical ischemia, evidence of large-artery occlusive disease, or both

COMPLEMENTARY AND ALTERNATIVE MEDICINE

- Although well-designed studies have not been done yet for complementary medicine, some treatments have shown an effect (8).
- Ginkgo biloba has been found to reduce the frequency of attacks (9)[B].
- Fish oil supplements may increase digital systolic pressure and time to onset of symptoms after exposure to cold but was not proven in controlled trials.
- Oral arginine is no better than placebo.
- Biofeedback is not helpful (8)[A].

SURGERY/OTHER PROCEDURES

Effect of cervical sympathectomy is transient; symptoms return in 1–2 years.

 ONGOING CARE

FOLLOW-UP RECOMMENDATIONS

Avoid exposure to cold situations; avoid use of vibrating tools.

Patient Monitoring

Management of fingertip ulcers, including rapid treatment of infection

DIET

No special diet

PATIENT EDUCATION

- Emphasize cessation of smoking.
- Discuss avoiding aggravating factors (e.g., trauma, vibration, cold).
- Dress warmly; wear gloves.
- Warm hands when experiencing vasospasm.

PROGNOSIS

- Attacks may last from several minutes to a few hours.
- 2/3 are likely to have spontaneous resolution.
- In cases of secondary Raynaud phenomenon, affected patients develop the hallmarks of underlying disease.
- ~13% of Raynaud phenomenon patients develop a secondary disorder, many of which are connective tissue diseases.

COMPLICATIONS

- Primary: Very rare
- Secondary: Gangrene, autoamputation of fingertips

REFERENCES

1. Lazzerini PE, Capecchi PL, Bisogno S, et al. Homocysteine and Raynaud's phenomenon: a review. *Autoimmun Rev.* 2010;9:181–7.
2. De Angelis R, Grassi W, Cutolo M et al. A growing need for capillaroscopy in rheumatology. *Arthritis Rheum.* 2009;61:405–10.
3. Khanna PP, Maranian P, Gregory J, et al. The minimally important difference and patient acceptable symptom state for the Raynaud's condition score in patients with Raynaud's phenomenon in a large randomised controlled clinical trial. *Ann Rheum Dis.* 2010;69:588–91.
4. Lambova SN, Müller-Ladner U et al. New lines in therapy of Raynaud's phenomenon. *Rheumatol. Int.* 2009;29:355–63.
5. De LaVega AJ, Derk CT et al. Phosphodiesterase-5 inhibitors for the treatment of Raynaud's: a novel indication. *Expert Opin Investig Drugs.* 2009;18: 23–9.
6. Kawald A, Burmester GR, Huscher D, et al. Low versus high-dose iloprost therapy over 21 days in patients with secondary Raynaud's phenomenon and systemic sclerosis: a randomized, open, single-center study. *J Rheumatol.* 2008;35: 1830–7.
7. Chung L, Shapiro L, Fiorentino D, et al. MQX-503, a novel formulation of nitroglycerin, improves the severity of Raynaud's phenomenon: a randomized, controlled trial. *Arthritis Rheum.* 2009;60:870–7.
8. Malenfant D, Catton M, Pope JE et al. The efficacy of complementary and alternative medicine in the treatment of Raynaud's phenomenon: a literature review and meta-analysis. *Rheumatology (Oxford).* 2009;48:791–5.
9. Choi WS, Choi CJ, Kim KS, et al. To compare the efficacy and safety of nifedipine sustained release with Ginkgo biloba extract to treat patients with primary Raynaud's phenomenon in South Korea; Korean Raynaud study (KOARA study). *Clin Rheumatol.* 2009;28:553–9.

ADDITIONAL READING

- Henness S, Wigley FM. Current drug therapy for scleroderma and secondary Raynaud's phenomenon: evidence-based review. *Curr Opin Rheumatol.* 2007;19:611–8.
- Pope JE. The diagnosis and treatment of Raynaud's phenomenon: a practical approach. *Drugs.* 2007;67:517–25.

See Also (Topic, Algorithm, Electronic Media Element)

Algorithm: Raynaud's phenomenon

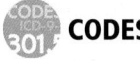 **CODES**

ICD9

443.0 Raynaud's syndrome

CLINICAL PEARLS

- Initial presentation of Raynaud phenomenon after age 40 suggests underlying disease.
- Remember Raynaud in differential diagnosis of a lactating woman with breast pain (vs mastitis).
- Primary Raynaud phenomenon is symmetric, whereas secondary is asymmetric.

RECTAL PROLAPSE

Timothy L. Black, MD
James P. Miller, MD

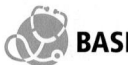

BASICS

Protrusion of the rectum through the anus

DESCRIPTION
- Partial prolapse: Involves only mucosa; frequently follows anal operative procedures (radial rectal folds prolapsed through anus)
- Complete prolapse: Involves the entire rectal wall (procidentia); occurs most commonly as a spontaneous event in children and as a complication of other disorders in the elderly (concentric rectal folds prolapsed through anus)
- System(s) affected: GI

EPIDEMIOLOGY
Incidence
- Predominant age: <3 years in children, 5th decade in adults
- Predominant sex: Female > Male in adults; females represent 80–90% of adult patients; Male = Female in children (1)[B]
- 4.2/1,000 overall; 10/1,000 >65 years of age

Geriatric Considerations
Common problem in the elderly

Pediatric Considerations
Idiopathic type most common in children

RISK FACTORS
- Myelomeningocele
- Exstrophy of the bladder
- Cystic fibrosis
- Chronic constipation or diarrhea
- Imperforate anus (2)[C]
- Multiple sclerosis
- Stroke/paralysis
- Mental retardation

Genetics
Unknown

GENERAL PREVENTION
Avoid constipation and diarrhea.

PATHOPHYSIOLOGY
The anatomic basis for rectal prolapse is a deficient pelvic floor through which the rectum herniates.

ETIOLOGY
- Children:
  – Idiopathic (most common)
  – Abnormal innervation of levator ani muscle complex or puborectalis or anal sphincter or abnormal anatomic relationships of these muscle groups
- Adults:
  – Diastasis of levator ani
  – Loose endopelvic fascia
  – Loss of normal horizontal position of rectum
  – Weak anal sphincter
  – Pudendal neuropathy
  – Redundant sigmoid colon
  – Loss of rectal-sacral attachments

COMMONLY ASSOCIATED CONDITIONS
- CF
- Myelomeningocele
- Exstrophy of the bladder
- Chronic constipation or diarrhea
- Imperforate anus
- Paraplegia
- Stroke
- Fecal incontinence
- Vaginal vault or uterine prolapse
- Mental retardation
- Marfan's syndrome
- Ehlers-Danlos disease
- Urinary incontinence (may be found in 58% of patients operated on for rectal prolapse) (3)[B]
- Bladder stones
- Nutritional disorders
- Progressive systemic sclerosis

DIAGNOSIS

HISTORY
- History of
  – Visible mass
  – Rectal bleeding or soiling
  – Rectal pain
  – Prior anorectal surgery
  – Spinal cord injury or defect
  – Constipation and straining

Pediatric Considerations
- Sensation of anal mass in children
- Adults:
  – Feeling of incomplete evacuation
  – Rectal and urinary incontinence (50–75% of adult patients)
  – Rectal bleeding or discharge

PHYSICAL EXAM
- Children:
  – Protruding mass
- Adults:
  – Visible mass of rectal mucosa or full thickness of rectal wall
  – Poor anal sphincter tone on rectal exam
  – Reproduce prolapse with straining

DIAGNOSTIC TESTS & INTERPRETATION
- Anorectal manometry (3)[B]
- Cinedefecography
- Electromyography
- Colon transit study

Lab
Evaluate for CF with genetic screening and sweat chloride evaluation.

Imaging
Barium enema is useful in selected cases of recurrent rectal prolapse.

Diagnostic Procedures/Surgery
- Sigmoidoscopy is useful in recurrent prolapse to rule out rectal lesions.
- MRI of lumbosacral spine to evaluate for spinal canal defects if not already diagnosed
- Anal manometry
- Pudendal nerve terminal latencies

DIFFERENTIAL DIAGNOSIS
- Intussusception
- Rectal polyps
- Hemorrhoids

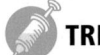 **TREATMENT**

MEDICATION

Medications to soften stools; avoid constipation and straining:
- Mineral oil
- Stool softeners
- Lactulose
- Polyethylene glycol (Miralax, GlycoLax)

ADDITIONAL TREATMENT

General Measures
- For acute cases: Prompt manual reduction of prolapse
- Treatment of diarrhea or constipation

SURGERY/OTHER PROCEDURES
- Abdominal procedures:
  - Suture rectopexy
  - Transabdominal proctopexy; also may be done laparoscopically (suture material, absorbable mesh, and nonabsorbable mesh may be used) (1,4)[B]:
    - Laparoscopic rectopexy may give equivalent results with shorter hospital stay and decreased cost (5)[B],(6)[A].
    - Advantages of laparoscopic rectopexy are all short term, with long-term outcomes equal to those of the abdominal approach (7)[A].
  - Transabdominal Ripstein procedure (suspension of rectum from sacrum by means of artificial material) (1)[B]
  - Anterior resection of rectum (rarely used)
  - Diverting colostomy occasionally may be required in the most severe cases.
- Perineal procedures:
  - Submucosal injection (sclerotherapy) of 5% phenol, 30% saline, or 25% glucose (or other sclerosants) in 4 quadrants under general anesthesia (outpatient)
  - Linear electrocauterization (inpatient or outpatient)
  - Posterior sagittal rectal suspension and levator repair
  - Delorme procedure (mucosal stripping of prolapsed rectum with plication of underlying muscle)
  - Perineal rectosigmoidectomy (1)[B]
  - Thiersch wire (outpatient procedure; may be modified by using Marlex or Silastic strip or other strong suture material instead of wire); used more commonly in children, older patients, and poor-risk adults
  - Gracilis sling procedure
  - Stapled transanal resection

IN-PATIENT CONSIDERATIONS

Initial Stabilization
Outpatient care unless complications occur or surgical intervention is required

Admission Criteria
- Inpatient care required for patients treated with laparotomy
- Inpatient care may be required after extensive perineal dissection or for pain control.

 ONGOING CARE

Biofeedback has been used to improve postoperative function (3)[B].

FOLLOW-UP RECOMMENDATIONS

Patient Monitoring
Monthly visits until possible need for surgery has been determined or until prolapse has resolved

DIET
- High fiber (25 g/d)
- 100% bran granules
- Keep well hydrated.

PATIENT EDUCATION
- Particular reassurance to parents of infants with prolapse regarding benign nature of problem and high rate of spontaneous resolution
- Diet instructions
- Teach measures to avoid constipation.
- Teach family/patient to reduce prolapse.

PROGNOSIS
- Spontaneous resolution is expected in most children with idiopathic prolapse.
- Recurrence rate is 5–10% for most procedures.
- Sclerotherapy frequently needs to be repeated.
- Good prognosis with treatment

COMPLICATIONS
- Mucosal ulcerations
- Necrosis of rectal wall
- Persistent or recurrent prolapse
- Constipation and pain if Thiersch wire is too tight
- Recurrence of rectal prolapse
- Fecal incontinence

REFERENCES

1. Madiba TE, Baig MK, Wexner SD. Surgical management of rectal prolapse. *Arch Surg.* 2005;140:63–73.
2. Belizon A, et al. Rectal prolapse following posterior sagittal anorectoplasty for anorectal malformations. *J Ped Surg.* 2005;40:192–6.
3. Gourgiotis S, Baratsis S et al. Rectal prolapse. *Int J Colorectal Dis.* 2007;22:231–43.
4. Brazzelli M, Bachoo P, Grant A. Surgery for complete rectal prolapse in adults (review). *Cochrane Database Syst Rev.* 2006;1.
5. Boccasanta P, Rosati R, Venturi M, et al. Comparison of laparoscopic rectopexy with open technique in the treatment of complete rectal prolapse: Clinical and functional results. *Surg Lap Endoscopy.* 1998;8:460–5.
6. Sajid M, Siddiqui M, Baig M. Open Versus Laparoscopic Repair Of Full Thickness Rectal Prolapse: A Re-Meta-Analysis. *Colorectal Dis.* 2009.
7. Solomon MJ, Young CJ, Eyers AA, et al. Randomized clinical trial of laparoscopic versus open abdominal rectopexy for rectal prolapse. *Br J Surg.* 2002;89:35–9.

See Also (Topic, Algorithm, Electronic Media Element)
Hemorrhoids; Intussusception

CODES

ICD9
569.1 Rectal prolapse

CLINICAL PEARLS
- Most common in females in their 5th decade
- In children, rectal prolapse occurs most often under the age of 3 and often resolves spontaneously.
- High-fiber diet and good hydration may prevent recurrences.

REFRACTIVE ERRORS

Robert M. Kershner, MD, MS

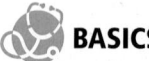 **BASICS**

DESCRIPTION

- Inability of the eye to produce a focused image on the fovea or central part of the retina
- Emmetropia: When light rays are in perfect focus, the image being viewed is seen clearly.
- Ametropia: Any refractive error of the eye that prevents normal focusing of the image
- Hyperopia: When the cornea of the eye is too flat or the eye is too short, light rays fall in focus behind the retina, and the individual is "farsighted."
- Myopia: When the cornea is too steep or the length of the eyeball is too long, the focal point for light rays lies short of the retina, and the individual is "nearsighted."
- Presbyopia: The natural tendency of the crystalline lens to harden or become sclerotic, limiting the focusing of the eye on near objects (accommodation):
  - The human crystalline lens thickens with age. By the age of 40 years, most people do not have enough room within the eye to allow normal excursion of the lens and accommodation; viewing of near objects is blurred, and reading glasses are required.
- Astigmatism: When the cornea is steeper in 1 meridian more than the other or the globe is not round (ie, is oval or almond-shaped), visual blurriness occurs.
- System(s) affected: Nervous

Geriatric Considerations
Presbyopia occurs in later life.

Pediatric Considerations
Refractive errors can be detected early in life.

EPIDEMIOLOGY

- Predominant age: Refractive errors are present at birth, but usually are not detected until puberty.
- Predominant gender: Male = Female
- Individuals >40 years of age are more likely to experience presbyopia or normal loss of accommodation that occurs with age, necessitating the use of reading glasses for close work.

Prevalence
Of the general US population, 70% has some form of ametropia.

RISK FACTORS

Genetics
Inherited

ETIOLOGY

- Developmental (most common)
- Ocular trauma
- Iatrogenic (eg, post-cataract removal)

COMMONLY ASSOCIATED CONDITIONS
Patients with diabetes mellitus have fluctuating myopia as a result of poorly controlled blood glucose and concomitant swelling of the crystalline lens.

 DIAGNOSIS

HISTORY

- Difficulty seeing objects at a distance
- Difficulty focusing on near objects
- Difficulty reading
- Squinting
- Headaches (from squinting)
- In children:
  - Rubbing of the eyes
  - Sitting close to TV or computer screen
  - Problems in sports, particularly declining performance
  - Declining grades
  - Preference for front-row seating
  - Covering of an eye while reading

PHYSICAL EXAM
Snellen Eye Chart (developed by Dr. Hermann Snellen in 1862). Test each eye separately. The smallest row of letters that the patient can read determines visual acuity in the uncovered eye.

DIAGNOSTIC TESTS & INTERPRETATION

- Pinhole vision test: To distinguish a refractive error from an organic cause of visual blurring, have the patient look through a pinhole in a card without a corrective lens.
- Patients with a pure refractive error have improved vision because the pinhole blocks nonparallel and unfocusable rays of light.

Diagnostic Procedures/Surgery

- Methods:
  - Objective streak retinoscopy may be used to measure the degree of refractive error in spherocylinder correction for the proper spectacle or contact lens.
  - Antimuscarinic agents such as cyclopentolate (Cyclogyl) or tropicamide (Mydriacyl) applied topically paralyze the ciliary body, preventing accommodation. Cycloplegic refraction can then be performed.
- Age-related testing:
  - Newborns should be examined for general eye health; ophthalmologic evaluation is indicated for any problems discovered.
  - Vision screening should occur at each well-child visit.
  - Visual acuity testing should be performed at ~3½ years of age.
  - Visual acuity and motility testing should be performed at age 5 years:
    - Visual acuity should be retested prior to obtaining a driver's license, at age 40 years, and every 2–4 years until age 65, when evaluations are recommended every 1–2 years.

DIFFERENTIAL DIAGNOSIS

- Corneal disease
- Cataract
- Retinal abnormalities
- Diseases of the optic nerve

TREATMENT

MEDICATION

Precaution: Antimuscarinic agents may induce acute glaucoma via acute-angle closure.

ADDITIONAL TREATMENT

General Measures

- Spectacle lenses (glasses)
- Soft or hard contact lenses

SURGERY/OTHER PROCEDURES

- Laser-assisted in-situ keratomileusis (LASIK), approved by Food and Drug Administration (FDA) in 1997. A superficial corneal flap is created with the keratome, and the excimer laser removes a small amount of tissue, thus reshaping the cornea. Corrects all refractive errors. Healing is rapid because re-epithelialization is not needed. Considered an adjunctive procedure for use with the excimer laser.
- Other modifications:
  – LASIK and EPI LASIK involve removing just the superficial epithelium before laser application.
  – IntraLASIK is a laser used to create the flap.
  – Custom ablation: Wavefront maps of the cornea and eye for ablation
- Older methods now superseded by LASIK:
  – Radial keratotomy: With topical anesthesia, using a surgical keratome, multiple (4–8) radial incisions are placed onto the surface of the peripheral cornea to flatten the central, optical zone. The length, depth, and proximity of the incision to the central optical zone determine its effect and degree of correction obtained. Radial keratotomy is safe and effective, and corrects nearsightedness, astigmatism, or a combination of both, after the age of 18 years when the prescription has stabilized.
  – Photorefractive keratectomy: Surface corneal tissue is removed with the excimer laser to reshape the cornea, thus correcting nearsightedness, farsightedness, or astigmatism. Risks and disadvantages include pain, keratitis, and potential scarring. Healing requires 3 months with topical antibiotics and steroids, with associated risks of glaucoma, cataract, and chronic inflammation.
  – Automated lamellar keratoplasty: A microsurgical dermatome removes a layer of the superficial cornea to induce flattening; investigational.
- Excimer laser: The laser photo ablates corneal tissue from the central visual axis, thus flattening it. Following the procedure, the cornea must re-epithelialize. Healing takes several months, during which there is a mild haze and blurring of vision. FDA approved October 1995.

- Implantable contact lens: A thin plastic lens is permanently implanted either in the anterior chamber and anchored to the iris (FDA approved in 2005, VERISYES) or in the posterior chamber (Vision Lens, FDA approved 2006) between the iris and the human crystalline lens. All refractive errors can be corrected. Risks include damage to the natural lens during surgery, cataract formation, and intraocular inflammation or infection; investigational anterior–chamber intraocular lens.
- Several scleral expansion procedures presently under investigation increase the space within the ciliary body by surgical means to restore lens movement and accommodation. The results have been unsatisfactory.
- Bifocal intraocular lenses (several types have been approved by the FDA: ReSTOR_Alcon, ReZOOM-AMO, Tecnis_AMO) implanted in the posterior chamber. They increase the depth of field to allow viewing objects both at near and at distance. Side effects include decreased contrast, glare, ghosting of images, and problems with night vision.
- Accommodative intraocular lenses (Crystalens). 1st FDA-approved intraocular lens; several others under clinical investigation. The accommodative intraocular lens moves in response to ciliary body movement to allow focusing at different focal lengths. Side effects minimal. Present lenses have limited range of focus.

ONGOING CARE

FOLLOW-UP RECOMMENDATIONS

Patient Monitoring

- Examinations recommended when starting school, entering college, any change in vision quality, and at the age of onset of presbyopia (the need for reading glasses)
- Individuals with any of the known risks of eye disease or conditions that could affect the eyes (such as diabetes) need annual ocular examinations.

PATIENT EDUCATION

- All patients should have their eyes examined when starting school and periodically thereafter.
- The options of eyeglasses, contact lenses, and permanent surgical correction of refractive errors can be considered.
- Encourage aggressive control of diabetes mellitus. These individuals are most likely contraindicated to undergo refraction corrective surgery.

PROGNOSIS

- Good, if discovered early and corrected appropriately
- It is not unusual for refractive errors to be temporarily worsened during pregnancy because of hormonal changes in tear function and corneal swelling.
- It is common that refractive errors worsen as a child ages until complete adult growth has been achieved. This is a common source of concern for parents. Reassurance that refractive change is often seen with growth spurts, especially at puberty, is advised.

COMPLICATIONS

- Amblyopia
- Poor school performance

ADDITIONAL READING

- Fax-on-Demand service of American Academy of Ophthalmology for policy statement and patient education materials: (908) 935-2761.
- Frequency of Ocular Exams. *Policy Statement*. San Francisco: American Academy of Ophthalmology; November 2009.
- Kershner RM. Lessons from the Practice: The Gift of Sight. *A Guide to Understanding Your Eyes*. Thorofare, NJ: Slack, 1994.
- Vision Screening for Infants and Children. *Policy Statement*. San Francisco: American Academy of Ophthalmology; March 2007.

CODES

ICD9

- 367.0 Hypermetropia
- 367.1 Myopia
- 367.20 Astigmatism, unspecified

CLINICAL PEARLS

- Vision screening should occur at each well-child visit.
- Visual acuity testing should be performed at ~31/2 years of age.

REITER SYNDROME

Douglas W. MacPherson, MD, MSc(CTM)

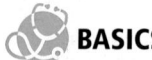

BASICS

Reiter syndrome is a seronegative multisystem inflammatory disorder classically involving joints, the eye, and the lower genitourinary tract (GU) tract. Axial joint involvement (e.g., spine, sacroiliac joints) is also common. Dermatologic manifestations are also seen frequently.

DESCRIPTION
A classic triad of features including arthritis, conjunctivitis/iritis, and either urethritis or cervicitis

- The epidemiology is similar to other reactive arthritis syndromes characterized by sterile inflammation of joints associated with infections originating at nonarticular sites. A 4th feature of dermatologic manifestations may include buccal ulceration or balanitis or a psoriaform skin eruption. (Having only 2 features present does not rule out the diagnosis.)
- It has 2 forms: Sexually transmitted, in which symptoms generally emerge between 7 and 14 days after exposure to *Chlamydia trachomatis* and other urethral/cervical pathogens acquired during sexual contact and postdysenteric or other bacterial enteric infections.
- System(s) affected: Musculoskeletal; Renal/Urologic; Dermatologic/Exocrine
- Synonym(s): Idiopathic blennorrheal arthritis; Arthritis urethritica; Urethro-oculosynovial syndrome; Fiessinger-Leroy-Reiter disease

Geriatric Considerations
In a demographic group associated with new or frequent sexual partners, the antecedent triggering infection is more likely to be sexually transmitted than enteric.

Pediatric Considerations
With a preceding history of enteric illness, the antecedent triggering event is more likely to be a bacterial enteric infection than sexually transmitted.

Pregnancy Considerations
There are no special considerations except as related to the usual precautions concerning pharmaceutical therapies.

EPIDEMIOLOGY
Incidence
- Predominant age: 20–40 years
- Predominant sex: Male > Female
- 0.24–1.5% incidence after epidemics of bacterial dysentery
- Complicates 1–2% of all cases of nongonococcal urethritis (1,2)

RISK FACTORS
- New or high-risk sexual contacts occurring 7–14 days before the onset of clinical presentation; for sexually acquired precipitants of Reiter syndrome, the primary infection may be subclinical and undiagnosed.
- Food poisoning or bacterial dysentery

Genetics
HLA-B27 tissue antigen present in 60–80% of patients

GENERAL PREVENTION
- The immune-response characteristics of this syndrome make specific avoidance of infectious precipitants the most important general precaution and potentially the most difficult to achieve.
- Safer sexual exposures and good food and water handling for personal consumption are essential for all persons at all times to maintain health and to avoid infections and the chronic inflammatory consequences of a previous infection.
- A family history of seronegative or reactive arthritis syndromes may suggest a genetic predisposition.

PATHOPHYSIOLOGY
- The pathophysiology of all the seronegative reactive arthritis syndromes and the immunologic role of infectious diseases as precipitants for clinical illness remain incompletely understood.
- Avoidance of precipitant infections and early management of the multi-organ system inflammatory consequences are important. Scientific evidence does not suggest that antibiotic treatment following onset of syndrome will benefit inflammatory joint, eye, or urinary tract symptoms.

ETIOLOGY
- *C. trachomatis* is the usual causative organism of the postvenereal variety.
- Dysentery-associated form follows enteric bacterial infection owing to *Shigella, Salmonella, Yersinia,* and *Campylobacter* spp. This form is more likely to be seen in women, children, and the elderly than the postvenereal form.

COMMONLY ASSOCIATED CONDITIONS
Recent case of:
- Enteric disease from
  - Shigellosis or
  - Salmonellosis or
  - Campylobacteriosis or
  - Enteric infection with *Yersinia* spp.
- Urogenital infection from
  - *Mycoplasma* or *Ureaplasma* spp. or
  - *Chlamydia* urethritis
- Infection with HIV

DIAGNOSIS

- The diagnosis of Reiter syndrome is based on the clinical presentation of the classic triad of joint, eye, and GU inflammation and negative serologic testing for rheumatoid factor.
- These three symptoms and signs may not all be evident at the same time.
- HLA-B27 testing is not required for diagnosis.
- Treatable sexually transmitted infections should be sought when clinically indicated.
- Screening for enteric infections is rarely useful and generally is not indicated diagnostically.

HISTORY
The presence of the clinical syndrome plus
- Diarrhea, dysentery, urethritis, or genital discharge and risk events for enteric or sexually acquired infections
- Include a risk history, including travel or migration history and potential exposure to a precipitating infectious agent.

PHYSICAL EXAM
- Musculoskeletal:
  - Asymmetric arthritis (especially knees, ankles, and metatarsophalangeal joints)
  - Enthesopathy (inflammation at tendinous insertion into bone, such as plantar fasciitis, digital periostitis, and Achilles tendinitis)
  - Spondyloarthropathy (spine and sacroiliac joint involvement)
- Urogenital tract:
  - Urethritis
  - Prostatitis
  - Occasionally cystitis
  - Balanitis
  - Cervicitis: Usually asymptomatic
- Eye:
  - Conjunctivitis of 1 or both eyes
  - Occasionally scleritis, keratitis, and corneal ulceration
  - Rarely uveitis and iritis
- Skin:
  - Mucocutaneous lesions (small, painless, superficial ulcers on oral mucosa, tongue, or glans penis)
  - Keratoderma blennorrhagica (hyperkeratotic skin lesions of palms and soles and around nails—can be mistaken for psoriasis)
- Cardiovascular: Occasionally pericarditis, murmur, conduction defects, and aortic incompetence
- Nervous system: Rarely peripheral neuropathy, cranial neuropathy, meningoencephalitis, and neuropsychiatric changes
- Constitutional:
  - Fever, malaise, anorexia, and weight loss
  - Patient can appear seriously ill (e.g., fever, rigors, tachycardia, and exquisitely tender joints).

DIAGNOSTIC TESTS & INTERPRETATION
Lab
- Blood:
  - Negative rheumatoid factor
  - Leukocyte count: 10,000–20,000 cells/mm^3
  - Neutrophilic leukocytosis
  - Elevated erythrocyte sedimentation rate (ESR)
  - Moderate normochromic anemia
  - Hypergammaglobulinemia
- Synovial fluid:
  - Leukocyte count: 1,000–8,000 cells/mm^3
  - Bacterial culture negative
- Supportive test results (3):
  - Cultures, antigens, or serology positive for *C. trachomatis* or stool test positive for *Salmonella, Shigella, Yersinia,* or *Campylobacter* spp. supports the diagnosis.
  - HLA-B27-positive status (not required or recommended for diagnosis)
- Drugs that may alter lab results: Antibiotics may affect isolation of the bacterial pathogens.

Imaging
X-ray:
- Periosteal proliferation, thickening
- Spurs
- Erosions at articular margins
- Residual joint destruction
- Syndesmophytes (spine)
- Sacroiliitis

Diagnostic Procedures/Surgery

HLA-B27 histocompatibility antigen: Positive result in 60–80% of cases in non-HIV-related Reiter syndrome; HLA testing is not required or recommended for diagnosis. Rheumatoid factor is negative.

Pathological Findings

- A seronegative spondyloarthropathy (similar to ankylosing spondylitis, enteric arthritis, and psoriatic arthritis)
- Villous formation in joints
- Joint hyperemia
- Joint inflammation
- Prostatitis
- Seminal vesiculitis
- Skin biopsy similar to psoriasis
- Nonspecific conjunctivitis

DIFFERENTIAL DIAGNOSIS

- For specific diagnosis, arthritis associated with urethritis for >1 month
- Rheumatoid arthritis (RA)
- Ankylosing spondylitis
- Arthritis associated with inflammatory bowel disease
- Psoriatic arthritis
- Juvenile RA
- Bacterial arthritis, including gonococcal

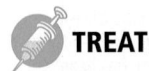 ## TREATMENT

MEDICATION

First Line

- Symptomatic management: Nonsteroidal anti-inflammatory drugs (NSAIDs) including indomethacin, naproxen, and others; intraarticular or systemic corticosteroids for refractory arthritis and enthesitis (4)
- Specific treatment of pathogenic microorganism may be attempted if isolated.
  – C. trachomatis: Doxycycline 100 mg PO b.i.d. × 7–14 days (Note: All sexually transmitted diseases should be treated whether associated with Reiter syndrome or not.)
  – Salmonella, Shigella, Yersinia, and Campylobacter infections: Ciprofloxacin 500 mg PO b.i.d. × 5–10 days (Note: Emerging antimicrobial resistance may limit this agent's effectiveness in treatment and bacterial clearance. Antibiotic treatment does not improve GI symptoms or duration of infection or prevent carrier state.)
- For GI upset: Antacids
- For iritis: Intraocular steroids
- For keratitis: Topical steroids
- Contraindications:
  – GI bleeding
  – Patients with peptic ulcer, gastritis, or ulcerative colitis
  – Renal insufficiency

Second Line

- Aspirin or other NSAIDs
- Sulfasalazine is promising but not approved for this indication by the Food and Drug Administration (FDA).
- Methotrexate or azathioprine in severe cases (such usage is still experimental and not approved or agreed to be effective); immunosuppressive therapy is relatively contraindicated if patient suffers from HIV-related Reiter syndrome.

- Consultation with specialist is recommended, particularly when considering immunomodulatory agents such as sulfasalazine, methotrexate, or azathioprine.
- Role of antibiotics have been under investigation. They are currently unproven in effectiveness in seronegative arthritis syndromes.
- No published evidence supports the beneficial effect of antibiotics on development of this syndrome or the long-term outcome in patients with Reiter syndrome.

ADDITIONAL TREATMENT

General Measures

Treatment is determined by symptoms.

- Conjunctivitis does not require treatment.
- Iritis requires treatment.
- Mucocutaneous lesions do not require treatment.
- Physical therapy (PT) is needed during recovery.
- Arthritis may become prominent and disabling during the acute phase.

Issues for Referral

Joint and eye complications; complex management

IN-PATIENT CONSIDERATIONS

Initial Stabilization

Inpatient care may be needed during acute phase.

Admission Criteria

Severity, complications, and degree of disability

 ## ONGOING CARE

FOLLOW-UP RECOMMENDATIONS

Bed rest until joint inflammation subsides

Patient Monitoring

Monitor clinical response to anti-inflammation medications. Observe for complications of therapy, particularly sulfasalazine and immunosuppressive drugs.

PATIENT EDUCATION

- Educate on risk factors for exposure, occurrence, and recurrence.
- Teach home PT techniques.
- For a listing of sources for patient education materials favorably reviewed on this topic, physicians may contact American Academy of Family Physicians Foundation, P.O. Box 8418, Kansas City, MO 64114, (800) 274–2237, ext. 4400.
- Arthritis Foundation, 1314 Spring Street NW, Atlanta, GA 30309, (404) 872-7100

PROGNOSIS

- Urethritis occurs 1–15 days after sexual exposure to causative agent.
- Reiter syndrome onset within 10–30 days of either enteric infection or sexually transmitted disease
- Mean duration of symptoms is 19 weeks.
- Prognosis is poor in cases involving the heel, eye, or heart.

COMPLICATIONS

- Chronic or recurrent disease in 5–50% of patients (5)[A]
- Ankylosing spondylitis develops in 30–50% of patients who test positive for HLA-B27 antigen.
- Urethral strictures
- Cataracts and blindness
- Aortic root necrosis

REFERENCES

1. Siegel DM. Chronic arthritis in adolescence. Adolesc Med State Art Rev. 2007;18:47–61, viii. webpage: http://www.ncbi.nlm.nih.gov/pubmed/18605390. evidence: systemic review (CIII)
2. Kim PS, Klausmeier TL, Orr DP et al. Reactive arthritis: a review. J Adolesc Health. 2009;44: 309–15.
3. Contini C, Grilli A, Badia L, et al. Detection of Chlamydophila pneumoniae in patients with arthritis: significance and diagnostic value. Rheumatology international. 2010;
4. National Guideline Clearinghouse 2009 July 13:13596; British Association of Sexual Health and HIV (BASHH) United Kingdom national guideline on management of sexually acquired reactive arthritis. webpage: http://www.bashh.org/guidelines. evidence: consensus national guidelines (119 references) CIII
5. Pope JE, et al. Campylobacter Reactive Arthritis: A Systematic Review. Semin Arthritis Rheum. 2007 Mar 20; [Epub ahead of print]. webpage: http://www.ncbi.nlm.nih.gov/pubmed/17360026. evidence: systemic review (CIII).

See Also (Topic, Algorithm, Electronic Media Element)

Ankylosing Spondylitis; Arthritis, Psoriatic; Behçet Syndrome

 ## CODES

ICD9

099.3 Reiter's disease

CLINICAL PEARLS

- To differentiate Reiter syndrome from other seronegative arthritis syndromes, keep in mind that many of these syndromes may have similar clinical components and overlap in the presenting symptoms. Seek the opinion of a specialist if unsure.
- When the history points toward a sexually acquired infection as a cause, including HIV, associated treatable infectious precipitants of Reiter syndrome must be tested for both personal and public health reasons. Enteric investigations are rarely indicated clinically nor justify a therapeutic response.
- Some patients have a chronic course, experience recurrences, or have clinical complications. If the inflammatory symptoms do not settle down quickly on NSAID agents, consider referral to a specialist.

RENAL CELL CARCINOMA

Jonathon M. Firnhaber, MD

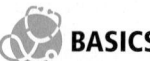 **BASICS**

DESCRIPTION
- Renal cell carcinoma (RCC), also called *hypernephroma* or *Grawitz tumor,* accounts for 3–4% of all cancers and 2.3% of all cancer deaths; it is the 7th most common malignant tumor in men and the 9th most common malignant tumor in women.
- It is characterized by obscure and varied presentations, including paraneoplastic syndromes, vascular findings, and uncommon metastatic sites.
- Paraneoplastic and vascular syndromes do not indicate incurability or unresectability. Early, aggressive surgical management provides the best opportunity for cure.
- System(s) affected: Renal/Urologic

EPIDEMIOLOGY
Incidence
- Predominant age: Patients in 5th–7th decades; median age at diagnosis is 66 years.
- Predominant sex: Male > Female (1.6:1).
- Age-adjusted incidence increasing 3% per year
- In the US, 51,590 new malignant tumors of the kidney in 2007, resulting in 12,800 deaths; RCC accounts for 80% of this incidence and mortality.
- In males, 10.7 new cases of RCC per 100,000 population per year vs 6.5 in females
- Between 1975 and 1998, incidence among blacks increased by 4.5% compared with 2.9% among whites; reasons for this difference are unclear.

RISK FACTORS
- Smoking, active and passive (increases relative risk by 2–3)
- Obesity (linear relationship in women)
- Hypertension (antihypertensive medications are not independently associated with RCC)
- End-stage renal failure
- Acquired renal cystic disease
- Tuberous sclerosis
- HIV infection
- Urban environment
- Heavy metal exposure (cadmium, lead)
- Environmental toxin exposure (asbestos, petroleum by-products, chlorinated solvents)

Genetics
- 2–3% of cases are familial, with several autosomal dominant syndromes described.
- Oncogenes localized to the short arm of chromosome 3 may have etiologic implications. Chromosome 3p12–p26 is specific for clear cell RCC.
- The most common alteration with RCC is deletion of chromosome 3p. Recent evidence suggests that gene *p53* on chromosome 17p13.1 is critical in RCC.
- People with human leukocyte antigen (HLA) types Bw44 and DR8 are prone to develop RCC. These are rare familial RCCs.
- Hereditary papillary RCC is an autosomal dominant form of disease associated with multifocal papillary renal tumors and a 5:1 male predominance.

GENERAL PREVENTION
Smoking may contribute to 1/3 of all cases.

ETIOLOGY
Unknown

COMMONLY ASSOCIATED CONDITIONS
- Von Hippel–Lindau disease: 30–45% of these patients develop clear cell tumors.
- Tuberous sclerosis: Associated primarily with angiomyolipoma and clear cell tumors
- Sickle-cell trait: With few exceptions, renal medullary tumor is seen in young African-American males with sickle-cell trait.
- Adult polycystic kidney disease
- Horseshoe kidney
- Acquired renal cystic disease from chronic renal failure

 DIAGNOSIS

HISTORY
- Diverse and obscure presentations, the "internist's tumor"
- Solid renal masses, most incidentally discovered in an asymptomatic patient owing to increased use of ultrasound, CT scanning, and MRI

PHYSICAL EXAM
- Classic triad of hematuria, abdominal mass, and flank pain in only 5–10% of patients
- Hematuria: 50–60%
- Flank pain: 35–40%
- Palpable mass: 25%
- Hypertension: 22–38%
- Weight loss: 28–36%
- Pyrexia: 7–17%
- Nonmetastatic hepatic dysfunction (Stauffer syndrome): 10–15%
- Neuromyopathy: 3%
- Scrotal varicoceles: 2–11% (most are left-sided)
- Patients with vena cava thrombus present with lower extremity edema, new varicocele, dilated superficial abdominal veins, albuminuria, pulmonary emboli, right atrial mass, or nonfunction of the involved kidney.

DIAGNOSTIC TESTS & INTERPRETATION
Lab
Initial lab tests
- Increased erythrocyte sedimentation rate: 50–60%
- Anemia: 21–41%
- Hypercalcemia: 3–6%
- Erythrocytosis: 3–4%
- Hematuria
- Urinary neoplastic cells
- Alkaline phosphate may be elevated.
- Increased renin
- Increased plasma fibrinogen

Imaging
Initial approach
- Ultrasonography: Can determine whether mass is solid or cystic; simple cystic lesions may be observed or subjected to percutaneous aspiration.
- CT scan of abdomen and pelvis: Solid or complex masses on ultrasonography require further evaluation.

Follow-Up & Special Considerations
- MRI is superior to ultrasound in evaluating adenopathy, diagnosing intracaval and renal venous thrombus, and demonstrating bony metastases.
- Chest CT scan if initial chest X-ray suggests metastatic disease

- Brain CT scan is indicated if the patient has neurologic symptoms.
- Bone scan is indicated if the alkaline phosphatase level is elevated or the patient has bone pain.
- CT or MR angiography should be incorporated into staging evaluation because the vascular information can be helpful in planning surgical resection.
- Positron-emission tomography does not yet have an established role in staging RCC.

Diagnostic Procedures/Surgery
- No need to aspirate simple cyst unless symptomatic
- Calcified cysts may contain RCC and therefore require open renal biopsy of the wall of the cyst or partial nephrectomy.
- Hemorrhagic cyst: Aspiration cytology may be helpful, but needle biopsy of solid masses is to be discouraged, particularly if the patient has a normal contralateral kidney.
- Doppler-flow ultrasound of the renal veins or CT scan that shows the renal vein entering the vena cava can be used to rule out tumor thrombus.

Pathological Findings
- RCC tends to bulge out from the cortex, producing a mass effect.
- 48% of RCCs measure <5 cm and are grossly yellow to yellow–orange owing to high lipid content in the clear cell variety. Average size has been decreasing owing to incidental discovery.
- Small tumors are typically homogeneous.
- Large tumors may have areas of necrosis and hemorrhage.
- About 5–10% of RCCs extend into the venous system as tumor thrombi.
- 5 distinct subtypes:
  - Clear cell: 70–80%; proximal tubule, typically solitary
  - Papillary renal cell (previously termed *chromophilic*): 10–15%; proximal tubule; tumors tend to be bilateral and multifocal; type 1 and more aggressive type 2 variant
  - Chromophobic: 3–5%; intercalated cells; tend to have a less aggressive course
  - Medullary: <1%; typically affect younger patients; most are at an advanced stage with metastases at time of diagnosis; occur almost exclusively in patients with sickle-cell trait
  - Collecting duct: <1%

DIFFERENTIAL DIAGNOSIS
- Any solid, contrast-enhancing renal mass should be considered malignant until proven otherwise.
- Benign renal masses (e.g., renal hamartomas)
- Hydronephrosis
- Pyelonephritis
- Renal abscess
- Polycystic kidneys
- Renal tuberculosis
- Renal calculi
- Renal infarction
- Benign renal cyst
- Transitional cell carcinoma of the renal pelvis
- Wilms tumor
- Metastatic disease, especially melanoma

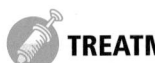 **TREATMENT**

Among small (<4 cm) renal masses, about 20% are benign, 60% represent indolent variants of RCC, and only 20% are potentially aggressive tumors.

MEDICATION
Improved understanding of the underlying biology of RCC has led to more targeted systemic therapy, primarily targeting vascular endothelial growth factor (VEGF) and mammalian target of rapamycin (mTOR) pathways.

First Line
- Most patients with RCC have clear cell histology that typically does not respond to standard cytotoxic chemotherapy. The mechanisms responsible for this resistance are unclear.
- In fit patients with metastatic disease and minimal symptoms, nephrectomy followed by interferon-alfa gives the best survival strategy for fully validated therapies (1)[A]. Interferon is the standard comparator for the assessment of new treatments in metastatic RCC.
- High-dose interleukin 2 (IL-2) is an option for patients who are able to tolerate the associated toxicity; long-term remission is induced in ~10%.
- Sunitinib and sorafenib, both oral inhibitors of the tyrosine kinase portion of the VEGF family of receptors, may be considered 1st-line treatment in advanced RCC and in patients refractory or intolerant to cytokine therapy. Sunitinib demonstrated improved response [31% vs 6%; number needed to treat (NNT) = 4] and longer median progression-free survival (11 vs 5 months) over interferon-alfa in a randomized study of 750 patients (2)[B].
- Bevacizumab is a monoclonal antibody that binds and neutralizes circulating VEGF protein. Combined with interferon alfa, bevacizumab offers patients with metastatic RCC a hazard ratio for progression-free survival of 0.63 (95% confidence interval 0.52–0.75; $p = .0001$) compared with interferon alone (3)[B].
- Temsirolimus, an IV mTOR inhibitor, is also approved for advanced RCC and has shown improved response (32% vs 16%; NNT = 6) and longer median survival (10.9 vs 7.3 months) over interferon-alfa in a comparative clinical trial of 626 patients (4)[B].
- A 2008 phase 3 trial of 410 patients comparing everolimus, another mTOR inhibitor, with placebo was stopped early after disease progression was seen in 37% of patients receiving everolimus vs 65% receiving placebo (hazard ratio = 0.30, 95% confidence interval 0.22–0.40; $p <.0001$) (5)[B].

Second Line
- Response rates with traditional chemotherapeutic agents are typically <15%.
- Despite occasional reports of responses, a review of medroxyprogesterone, the most widely studied progestational agent, concluded that RCCs are neither hormone-dependent nor hormone-responsive (6)[B].

ADDITIONAL TREATMENT
Additional Therapies
While RCC is typically characterized as radioresistant, radiation therapy may be useful to treat a single or limited number of metastases, particularly brain or painful bone metastases or painful recurrences in the renal bed.

SURGERY/OTHER PROCEDURES
- Surgery is curative in most patients with nonmetastatic RCC and is the preferred treatment for all but the most extensive disease.
- Assuming a normal contralateral kidney, radical nephrectomy, which can be done laparoscopically and involves node dissection and complete removal of the kidney and Gerota fascia, is the typical preferred approach.
- Exploratory wedge resection for solitary kidney or tumors <4 cm
- Surgical intervention in metastatic disease: Metastasectomy in those with limited metastatic disease vs cytoreductive nephrectomy (debulking) prior to systemic therapy
- Transitional cell carcinoma of the renal pelvis or calyces: Nephroureterectomy
- Wilms tumor in adults: Radical nephrectomy for unilateral disease
- Cortical adenoma <3 cm (7–22% at autopsy): Wedge resection
- Image-guided radiofrequency or cryoablation has been successful in limited studies for the treatment of small (average 2 cm) peripheral renal tumors (7)[C].

 ONGOING CARE

FOLLOW-UP RECOMMENDATIONS
Patient Monitoring
- CT scan of the abdomen and renal fossa can be done 3–6 months after surgery, particularly if the capsule or lymph nodes are positive, to monitor recurrences and repeat resection if needed for flank pain or mass.
- For partial nephrectomy: Renal ultrasound every 6 months for 3 years, then annually
- Since most pulmonary metastases are asymptomatic, routine imaging of the chest with X-ray or CT scan is performed quarterly for 2 years and periodically thereafter.
- Skeletal X-rays and bone scan can be useful in detecting skeletal metastasis but should be obtained only if patient complains of bone pain or if alkaline phosphatase is elevated.
- Postoperative follow-up may be possible with plasma transcobalamin II or serum haptoglobin level to detect or monitor recurrences.

DIET
Patients with proteinuria should follow a low-protein diet.

PROGNOSIS
- The 5-year survival following treatment correlates well with the anatomic extent of disease.
- 5-year survival in the absence of metastases exceeds 50%; in the presence of distant metastases, 5-year survival decreases to 10%.
- Median survival for metastatic RCC is in the range of 10–12 months.
- Performance status at diagnosis and histologic grade of tumor also influence prognosis.

COMPLICATIONS
- Paraplegia can result with little warning from spinal vertebral metastasis.
- CNS metastases are not uncommon.
- ~30% of patients with RCC have metastatic disease when the diagnosis is established. The most common sites of metastasis are the lung (50–60%), bone (30–40%), regional nodes (15–30%), brain (10%), and adjacent organs (10%).

REFERENCES
1. Coppin C, et al. Immunotherapy for advanced renal cell cancer (Cochrane Review). *Cochrane Database Syst Rev*. 2006;(2).
2. Motzer RJ, Hutson TE, Tomczak P, et al. Sunitinib versus interferon alfa in metastatic renal-cell carcinoma. *N Engl J Med*. 2007;356:115–24.
3. Escudier B, Bellmunt J, Négrier S, et al. Phase III trial of bevacizumab plus interferon alfa-2a in patients with metastatic renal cell carcinoma (AVOREN): final analysis of overall survival. *J Clin Oncol*. 2010;28:2144–50.
4. Hudes G, Carducci M, Tomczak P, et al. Temsirolimus, interferon alfa, or both for advanced renal-cell carcinoma. *N Engl J Med*. 2007;356:2271–81.
5. Motzer RJ, Escudier B, Oudard S, et al. Efficacy of everolimus in advanced renal cell carcinoma: a double-blind, randomised, placebo-controlled phase III trial. *Lancet*. 2008;372:449–56.
6. Kjaer M. The role of medroxyprogesterone acetate (MPA) in the treatment of renal adenocarcinoma. *Cancer Treat Rev*. 1988;15:195–209.
7. Sabharwal R, Vladica P. Renal tumors: technical success and early clinical experience with radiofrequency ablation of 18 tumors. *Cardiovasc Intervent Radiol*. 2006;29:202–9.

ADDITIONAL READING
- Ng CS, Wood CG, Silverman PM, et al. Renal cell carcinoma: diagnosis, staging, and surveillance. *AJR Am J Roentgenol*. 2008;191:1220–32.
- Rini BI, Campbell SC, Escudier B, et al. Renal cell carcinoma. *Lancet*. 2009;373:1119–32.

 CODES

ICD9
189.0 Malignant neoplasm of kidney, except pelvis

CLINICAL PEARLS
- RCC represents 3–4% of all cancers and 2% of all cancer deaths; most patients have clear cell histology and do not respond to standard chemotherapy.
- Diverse and obscure presentations are typical; many RCCs are found incidentally during radiologic studies.
- At presentation, up to 30% of patients with RCC have metastatic disease; recurrence develops in approximately 40% treated for localized disease.
- Only 20% of renal masses <4 cm represent potentially aggressive tumors.
- Surgery is curative in most patients with nonmetastatic RCC and is the preferred treatment for all but the most extensive disease.
- Multiple pharmacologic options are considered 1st-line for metastatic RCC; sequential treatments are likely to be pursued for most patients.

RENAL FAILURE, ACUTE

Rasai L. Ernst, MD
Mazen J. AlBeldawi, MD

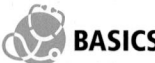 **BASICS**

DESCRIPTION
Sudden loss of kidney function resulting in retention of nitrogenous waste as well as electrolyte and volume homeostasis abnormalities, with or without oliguria (urine output <500 mL/d)

EPIDEMIOLOGY
Incidence
5% and 30% of hospital and ICU admissions, respectively, have a diagnosis of acute renal failure (ARF). 25% of patients develop ARF while in the hospital, and 50% of those cases are iatrogenic.

RISK FACTORS
- Comorbidities (e.g., liver failure, heart failure, diabetes)
- Advanced age
- Radiographic contrast material exposure
- Nephrotoxic medications (e.g., aminoglycosides, nonsteroidal anti-inflammatory drugs [NSAIDs], angiotensin-converting enzyme [ACE] inhibitors)
- Volume depletion (e.g., sepsis, hemorrhage)
- Surgery
- Rhabdomyolysis
- Solitary kidney (risk in nephrolithiasis)
- Benign prostatic hypertrophy (BPH)
- Malignancy

Genetics
No known genetic pattern.

GENERAL PREVENTION
See Treatment.

PATHOPHYSIOLOGY
Can be divided into 3 categories: Prerenal, intrarenal, and postrenal:
- Prerenal: Pathology secondary to decreased renal perfusion leading to a decrease in glomerular filtration rate (GFR); reversible if factors decreasing perfusion are corrected; otherwise, it can progress to an intrarenal pathology known as *ischemic ATN*.
- Intrarenal: Pathology secondary to pathology within the kidney; acute tubular necrosis (ATN) is the most common cause via ischemic or nephrotoxic injury to the kidney; 75% of ATN is a complication of prerenal etiology (1).
- Postrenal: Pathology secondary to extrinsic or intrinsic obstruction of the urinary collection system.

ETIOLOGY
- Prerenal (~55%): Hypotension, volume contraction, severe heart failure, or liver failure
- Intrarenal (~40%): ATN (from prolonged prerenal failure, radiographic contrast material, aminoglycosides, or nephrotoxic substances), glomerulonephritis, acute interstitial nephritis (drug-induced), arteriolar insults, vasculitis, accelerated hypertension, cholesterol embolization (common after arterial procedures), intrarenal deposition or sludging (seen in increased uric acid and multiple myeloma—Bence-Jones proteins)

- Postrenal (~5%): Extrinsic compression (prostatic hypertrophy, carcinoma), intrinsic obstruction (calculus, tumor, clot, stricture, sloughed papilli), decreased function (neurogenic bladder)

COMMONLY ASSOCIATED CONDITIONS
Hyperphosphatemia, hypercalcemia, hyperuricemia, hydronephrosis, BPH, nephrolithiasis, congestive heart failure (CHF), pericarditis, cirrhosis, chronic renal insufficiency, malignant hypertension, vasculitis, drug reactions, sepsis, severe trauma, burns, transfusion reactions, recent chemotherapy, muscle injury, internal bleeding

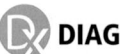 **DIAGNOSIS**

HISTORY
- General: p.o. intake, urine output, body weight, and baseline creatinine measurement (to assess how far from baseline the current creatinine is)
- Prerenal: Thirst, orthostatic dizziness
- Intrarenal: Nephrotoxic medications, radiocontrast material, other toxins; fever, arthralgias, and pruritic rash suggest allergic interstitial nephritis, although systemic effects are not always seen in this pathology. Edema, hypertension, and oliguria with nephritic urine sediment points to glomerulonephritis or vasculitis. Livedo reticularis, subcutaneous nodules, and ischemic toes and fingers despite good pulses suggest atheroembolization. Flank pain suggests occlusion of the renal artery or vein.
- Postrenal: Colicky flank pain that radiates to the groin suggests a ureteric obstruction such as a stone. Nocturia, frequency, and hesitancy suggest prostatic disease. Suprapubic and flank pain are usually secondary to distension of the bladder and collecting system. Ask about anticholinergic drugs that could lead to neurogenic bladder.

PHYSICAL EXAM
- Prerenal signs: Tachycardia, decreased jugular venous pressure (JVP), orthostatic hypotension, dry mucous membranes, decreased skin turgor; look for stigmata of associated comorbidities such as liver and heart failure, as well as sepsis.
- Intrinsic renal signs: Pruritic rash, livedo reticularis, subcutaneous nodules, ischemic digits despite good pulses
- Postrenal signs: Suprapubic distension, flank pain, and enlarged prostate
- General uremic signs: Lethargy, seizures, asterixis, myoclonus, pericardial friction rub, peripheral neuropathies

DIAGNOSTIC TESTS & INTERPRETATION
Lab
Initial lab tests
- Urinanalysis: Dipstick for blood and protein; microscopy for cells, casts, and crystals
- Casts: Transparent hyaline casts—prerenal etiology; pigmented granular/muddy brown casts—ATN; white blood cell (WBC) casts—acute interstitial nephritis; red blood cell (RBC) casts—glomerulonephritis
- Urine eosinophils: Interstitial nephritis

- Urine electrolytes in an oliguric state:
  - $FE_{Na} = [(U_{Na} \times P_{Cr})/(P_{Na} \times U_{Cr})] \times 100$, where U = urine, P = plasma, Na = sodium, Cr = creatinine. If $FE_{Na} < 1$, then likely prerenal; >2, then likely intrarenal; >4, then likely postrenal
  - If patient is on diuretics, use FE_{urea} instead of FE_{Na}. $FE_{urea} = [(U_{urea} \times P_{Cr})/(P_{BUN} \times U_{Cr}) \times 100$ $FE_{urea} < 35\%$ suggests prerenal (2).
  - In 1 study, low FE_{urea} (<35%) was found to be more sensitive and specific than FE_{Na} in differentiating between prerenal and intrarenal etiologies of renal failure, especially if diuretics were administered (3)[A].
- CBC, blood urea nitrogen (BUN), creatinine, arterial blood gases (ABGs)
- Common lab abnormalities in ARF:
  - Increased: K^+, phosphate, Mg, uric acid
  - Decreased: Hematocrit (Hct), Na, Ca
- Calculate creatinine clearance to ensure that medications are dosed appropriately:
  - Cockcroft-Gault equation creatinine clearance (mL/min) = (140-age) * (weight in kilograms) * (0.85 if female) / (72 * serum creatinine)

Follow-Up & Special Considerations
Consider creatine kinase (CK) and immunology antibodies.

Imaging
Initial approach
- Renal ultrasound (US): Excludes postrenal causes if negative; identifies presence of kidneys, hydronephrosis, and nephrolithiasis
- Doppler-flow kidney US: Rules out renal artery stenosis/thrombosis
- Abdominal x-ray (KUB): Rules out renal calculi

Follow-Up & Special Considerations
More advanced imaging techniques should be considered if initial tests do not reveal etiology:
- Radionucleotide renal scan: Evaluates renal flow, function, and presence of obstructive uropathy and extravasation
- CT scan: Limited use due to need for radiographic contrast material, which can worsen ARF
- MRI: Acute tubulointerstitial nephritis can show an increased T_2-weighted signal.

Diagnostic Procedures/Surgery
Cystoscopy with retrograde pyelogram evaluates for bladder tumor, hydronephrosis, obstruction, and upper tract abnormalities, and poses no threat of contrast material toxicity.

Pathological Findings
Kidney biopsy: Used only as a last resort when all other tests do not reveal a diagnosis; most useful for suspicion of rapidly progressive glomerulonephritis or kidney transplant patients

DIFFERENTIAL DIAGNOSIS
See Etiology.

TREATMENT

MEDICATION
First Line
- Current treatment is focused on primary prevention, treating the underlying cause, and treating associated complications.
- If patient is found to be oliguric and not volume overloaded, a fluid challenge may be appropriate with diligent monitoring for volume overload (4)[C].
- Furosemide is a commonly used intervention. Studies show that it is ineffective in preventing and treating ARF (4)[A]. Dopamine, natriuretic peptides, insulinlike growth factor, and thyroxine also have no benefit in the treatment of ARF (2,4)[A].
- If a patient is found to be hyperkalemic with ECG changes, IV calcium, sodium bicarbonate, and glucose with insulin should be given. These measures drive K^+ into cells and can be supplemented with Kayexalate, which removes K^+ from the body. Hemodialysis is also an emergency method of removal (5)[A].
- Oliguric patients should have a fluid restriction of 400 mL + yesterday's urine output (unless there are signs of volume depletion or overload) (5)[A].
- Acidosis: Serum bicarbonate <15–18 mmol/L; small amounts of sodium bicarbonate can be given. Be aware of volume overload (5)[A].
- Certain strategies have been investigated in the prevention of ARF: Those likely to be effective are IV isotonic hydration, once-daily dosing of aminoglycosides, use of lipid formulations of amphotericin B, use of isoosmolar nonionic contrast media (6)[A].
- Contrast-induced ARF (CIARF) can be prevented by *N*-acetylcysteine 600 mg p.o. b.i.d. on day prior to and day of contrast (7)[A] and isotonic $NaHCO_3$ 3 mL/kg/h × 1 h before administration of contrast material and 1 mL/kg/h × 6 h after contrast material (8)[B].

Second Line
- Flomax or other selective α-blockers for bladder outlet obstruction secondary to BPH
- Calcium channel blockers may have a protective effect in posttransplant ATN.

ADDITIONAL TREATMENT
General Measures
Identify and correct all prerenal and postrenal causes:
- Review drug list: Stop nephrotoxic drugs and renally adjust others.
- Always record ins and outs and daily weights.
- Watch for complications, including hyperkalemia, pulmonary edema, and acidosis—all potential reasons to start dialysis.
- Ensure good cardiac output and subsequent renal blood flow.
- Follow nutrition suggestions and be aware of infections; treat aggressively if they occur.
- Start patients on H_2 inhibitors or proton pump inhibitors, and avoid aspirin to avoid bleeding tendency (4)[A].

Issues for Referral
- Nephrology should be consulted for all cases as soon as patient is found to be in ARF.
- Urology consult for obstructive nephropathies

COMPLEMENTARY AND ALTERNATIVE MEDICINE
Many supplements not approved by the Food and Drug Administration (FDA) can be nephrotoxic.

SURGERY/OTHER PROCEDURES
- Relief of obstruction with retrograde ureteral catheters or percutaneous nephrostomy
- Hemodialysis catheter placement

IN-PATIENT CONSIDERATIONS
Initial Stabilization
- ABCs of resuscitation
- Treat hyperkalemia emergently, especially with ECG changes.
- If volume depleted, give IV fluids.
- Place a Foley catheter.

Admission Criteria
All patients with ARF should be admitted.

IV Fluids
Should be used in patients with volume depletion

Nursing
Place a Foley catheter; strict recording of ins and outs

Discharge Criteria
Stabilization of renal function and a concrete plan for continued treatment if necessary

 ONGOING CARE

FOLLOW-UP RECOMMENDATIONS
Patient Monitoring
As needed

DIET
- Total caloric intake should be 35–50 kcal/kg/d to avoid catabolism.
- Sodium should be restricted to 2 g/d (5)[A].
- Potassium intake should be restricted to 40 mEq/d.
- Phosphorus should be restricted to 800 mg/d. If it becomes high, treat with calcium carbonate or other phosphate binder (5)[A].
- Magnesium compounds should be avoided.

PATIENT EDUCATION
Keep well hydrated. Avoid nephrotoxic drugs such as NSAIDs, ACE inhibitors, and aminoglycosides.

PROGNOSIS
- Depending on the cause, comorbid conditions, and age of patient, mortality ranges from 5–80%.
- In cases of prerenal and postrenal failure, there are very good rates of recovery positively correlated with shorter duration of renal failure. Intrarenal etiologies usually take more time to recover from. Overall, average recovery takes from days to a few months.

COMPLICATIONS
Death, sepsis, infection, seizures, paralysis, peripheral edema, CHF, pulmonary edema, arrhythmias, uremic pericarditis, bleeding, GI bleed, hypotension, anemia, hyperkalemia, uremia

REFERENCES
1. Lameire N. The pathophysiology of acute renal failure. *Crit Care Clin.* 2005;21:197–210.
2. Schrier R, et al. Acute renal failure: definitions, diagnosis, pathogenesis, and therapy. *Journal of Clin Invest.* 2004;114:5–14.
3. Carvounis CP, Nisar S, Guro-Razuman S. Significance of the fractional excretion of urea in the differential diagnosis of acute renal failure. *Kidney Int.* 2002;62:2223–9.
4. Hilton R. Acute renal failure. *BMJ.* 2006;333: 786–90.
5. Lameire N, Van Biesen W, Vanholder R. Acute renal failure. *Lancet.* 2005;365:417–30.
6. Venkataraman R, et al. *Prevention of acute renal failure.* 2007;131:300–8.
7. Birck R, Krzossok S, Markowetz F, et al. Acetylcysteine for prevention of contrast nephropathy: meta-analysis. *Lancet.* 2003;362:598–603.
8. Merten GJ, Burgess WP, Gray LV, et al. Prevention of contrast-induced nephropathy with sodium bicarbonate: a randomized controlled trial. *JAMA.* 2004;291:2328–34.

See Also (Topic, Algorithm, Electronic Media Element)
Hepatorenal Syndrome, Renal Failure, Chronic, Reye Syndrome, Rhabdomyolysis, Hyperkalemia, Prostatic Hyperplasia, Benign (BPH), Glomerulonephritis, Acute, Sepsis
Algorithm: Anuria or Oliguria

 CODES

ICD9
584.9 Acute kidney failure, unspecified

CLINICAL PEARLS
- Can be divided into 3 categories: Prerenal, intrarenal, and postrenal:
  - Prerenal: Pathology secondary to decreased renal perfusion leading to a decrease in GFR; reversible if factors decreasing perfusion are corrected; otherwise, it can progress to an intrarenal pathology known as ischemic ATN.
  - Intrarenal: Pathology secondary to pathology within the kidney; acute tubular necrosis (ATN) is the most common cause via ischemic or nephrotoxic injury to the kidney. 75% of ATN is a complication of prerenal etiology (1).
  - Postrenal: Pathology secondary to extrinsic or intrinsic obstruction of the urinary collection system.
- Recognize the need for emergent hemodialysis: Severe hyperkalemia, acidosis, or volume overload refractory to conservative therapy, uremic pericarditis, encephalopathy, neuropathy, alcohol and drug intoxications

RENAL TUBULAR ACIDOSIS

Jason M. Kurland, MD

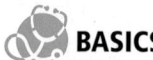 **BASICS**

DESCRIPTION

- Renal tubular acidosis (RTA): A group of disorders characterized by an inability of the kidney to resorb bicarbonate or secrete hydrogen ions, resulting in hyperchloremic, normal anion gap acidosis. Renal function (glomerular filtration rate [GFR]) must be normal or near normal.
- Several types have been identified:
  - Type I (distal) RTA: Inability of the distal tubule to acidify the urine. Due to impaired hydrogen ion secretion, increased backleak of secreted hydrogen ions, or impaired sodium reabsorption (causing less negative potential in the lumen and hence less hydrogen/potassium secretion). Urine pH >5.5.
  - Type II (proximal) RTA: Defect of the proximal tubule in bicarbonate (HCO_3) reabsorption. HCO_3 fully reabsorbed only when plasma HCO_3 concentration <15–16 mEq/L (compared with normal threshold of 24 mEq/L). Urine pH <5.5 unless plasma HCO_3 above reabsorptive threshold.
  - Type III RTA: Extremely rare autosomal recessive syndrome with features of both type I and type II (may be due to carbonic anhydrase II deficiency)
  - Type IV RTA (hyporeninemic hypoaldosteronism): Due to aldosterone resistance or deficiency that results in hyperkalemia. Urine pH usually <5.5.

EPIDEMIOLOGY
Incidence
- Predominant age: All ages
- Predominant sex: Male > Female (with regard to type II RTA with isolated defect in bicarbonate reabsorption)

RISK FACTORS
Genetics
- Type I RTA: Autosomal dominant or recessive. May occur in association with other genetic diseases (e.g., Ehlers-Danlos syndrome, hereditary elliptocytosis, or sickle cell nephropathy). The autosomal recessive form is associated with sensorineural deafness.
- Type II RTA: Autosomal dominant form is rare. Autosomal recessive form is associated with ophthalmologic abnormalities and mental retardation. Occurs in Fanconi syndrome, which is associated with several genetic diseases (e.g., cystinosis, Wilson disease, tyrosinemia, hereditary fructose intolerance, Lowe syndrome, galactosemia, glycogen storage disease, and metachromatic leukodystrophy).
- Type IV RTA: Some cases familial, such as pseudohypoaldosteronism type I (autosomal dominant)

GENERAL PREVENTION
Careful use or avoidance of agents listed here as causative

ETIOLOGY
- Type I RTA:
  - Genetic: Autosomal dominant, autosomal recessive associated with sensorineural deafness
  - Sporadic
  - Ehlers-Danlos syndrome
  - Autoimmune diseases: Sjögren syndrome, rheumatoid arthritis (RA), systemic lupus erythematosus
  - Hematologic diseases: Sickle cell disease, hereditary elliptocytosis
  - Medications: Amphotericin B, lithium, ifosfamide, foscarnet, analgesics, K^+-sparing diuretics (amiloride, triamterene), trimethoprim
  - Toxins: Toluene, glue
  - Hypercalciuria, diseases causing nephrocalcinosis
  - Vitamin D intoxication
  - Medullary cystic disease
  - Glycogenosis type III
  - Fabry disease
  - Wilson disease
  - Hypergammaglobulinemic syndrome
  - Obstructive uropathy
  - Chronic pyelonephritis
  - Chronic renal transplant rejection
  - Leprosy
  - Hepatic cirrhosis
  - Malnutrition
- Type II RTA:
  - Diseases associated with Fanconi syndrome (see heading "Genetics")
  - Sporadic
  - Multiple myeloma and other dysproteinemic states
  - Amyloidosis
  - Heavy-metal poisoning (e.g., cadmium, lead, mercury, copper)
  - Medications: Acetazolamide, sulfanilamide, ifosfamide, outdated tetracycline, topiramate
  - Autoimmune disease
  - Interstitial renal disease
  - Nephrotic syndrome
  - Congenital heart disease
  - Defects in calcium metabolism (hyperparathyroidism)
- Type IV RTA:
  - Medications: Nonsteroidal anti-inflammatory drugs, angiotensin-converting enzyme inhibitors, angiotensin receptor blockers, heparin/LMW heparin, calcineurin inhibitors (tacrolimus, cyclosporine) (1)
  - Diabetic nephropathy
  - Obstructive nephropathy
  - Nephrosclerosis due to hypertension
  - Tubulointerstitial nephropathies
  - Primary adrenal insufficiency
  - Pseudohypoaldosteronism (end-organ resistance to aldosterone)
  - Gordon syndrome (2)[C]
  - Sickle cell nephropathy

COMMONLY ASSOCIATED CONDITIONS
- Type I RTA in children: Hypercalciuria leading to rickets, nephrocalcinosis
- Type I RTA in adults: Autoimmune diseases (Sjögren syndrome, RA), hypercalciuria
- Type II RTA: Fanconi syndrome (generalized proximal tubular dysfunction resulting in glycosuria, aminoaciduria, hyperuricosuria, phosphaturia, bicarbonaturia)

- Type II RTA in adults: Multiple myeloma, carbonic anhydrase inhibitors (acetazolamide)
- Type IV RTA: Obstructive uropathy, renal insufficiency, diabetic nephropathy

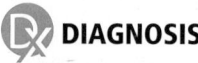 **DIAGNOSIS**

HISTORY
- Often asymptomatic (particularly type IV)
- Failure to thrive in children
- Anorexia, nausea/vomiting
- Weakness or polyuria (due to hypokalemia)
- Rickets in children
- Osteomalacia in adults
- Constipation
- Polydipsia

DIAGNOSTIC TESTS & INTERPRETATION
Lab
- Electrolytes reveal hyperchloremic metabolic acidosis.
- Plasma anion gap normal (anion gap = $Na - [Cl + HCO_3]$). Normal values (in mEq/L): Neonates ≤16; infants/children ≤14–16; adolescents/adults 8 $\pm$ 4). Must correct calculated anion gap for hypoalbuminemia. Increase calculated anion gap by 2.5 mEq/L for each 1 g/dL decrease in albumin below 4 g/dL.
- Hypokalemia or normokalemia: Type I (if due to impaired distal H^+ secretion or increased H^+ backleak), type II
- Hyperkalemia: Type IV, type I (if due to impaired distal Na^+ reabsorption)
- Plasma HCO_3 (in untreated RTA): Type I: <15 mEq/L; type II: 12–20 mEq/L; type IV: >17 mEq/L
- Blood urea nitrogen and creatinine usually normal (rules out renal failure as cause of acidosis)
- Urine pH: Inappropriately alkaline (pH >5.5) despite metabolic acidosis in type I or in type II when HCO_3 above reabsorptive threshold (15–16 mEq/L)
- Urine culture: Rule out urinary tract infection (UTI) with urea-splitting organism (may elevate pH) and chronic infection
- Urine anion gap (urine Na^+, K^+, and Cl^- on random urine): Reflects unmeasured urine anions, so inversely related to urine NH_4^+ (or acid) excretion. Positive urine anion gap in an acidemic patient indicates impaired renal acid excretion. Results tend to be:
  - Negative in HCO_3 losses due to diarrhea, or UTI caused by urea-splitting organisms
  - Negative in other extrarenal causes of normal anion gap metabolic acidosis
  - Variable in type II RTA
  - Positive in type I RTA, type IV RTA (3)[C]
  - Positive in impaired acid excretion due to renal failure
- Urine calcium:
  - High in type I
  - Typically normal in type II
- Drugs that may alter lab results:
  - Diuretics
  - Sodium bicarbonate
  - Cholestyramine

Imaging
Not needed except to rule out associated conditions (e.g., nephrocalcinosis)

Diagnostic Procedures/Surgery
- Helpful to measure urine pH on fresh sample with pH meter for increased accuracy instead of dipstick. Pour film of oil over urine to avoid loss of CO_2 if pH cannot be measured quickly.
- Urine NH_4^+ excretion (anion gap is indirect measurement of this but not as accurate)
- Ammonium chloride (NH_4^+) loading to evaluate acid excretion
- Fractional excretion of $HCO_3 > 15\%$ during HCO_3 infusion (type II RTA)

Pathological Findings
- Nephrocalcinosis
- Nephrolithiasis
- Rickets
- Osteomalacia
- Findings of an underlying disease causing renal tubular acidosis

DIFFERENTIAL DIAGNOSIS
- Plasma anion gap should be normal. If not, look for causes of metabolic acidosis other than RTA. (MUDPILES: *M*etabolic disease or methanol ingestion, *u*remia, *d*iabetic ketoacidosis, *p*araldehyde ingestion, *i*ron or isoniazid ingestion, *l*actic acidosis, *e*thylene glycol ingestion, *s*alicylate ingestion)
- Extrarenal HCO_3 losses:
  – Diarrhea
  – Small bowel, pancreatic, or biliary fistulas (3)[C]
  – Urinary diversion (e.g., ureterosigmoidostomy, ileal conduit)
- Acidosis of chronic renal failure (develops when GFR ≤ 20–30% of normal) (4)[C]
- Excessive administration of acid load via chloride salts (NaCl, HCl, NH_4Cl, lysine hydrogen chloride, $CaCl_2$, $MgCl_2$)

 TREATMENT

MEDICATION
First Line
- Provide oral alkali to raise serum HCO_3 to normal. Start at a low dose and increase until HCO_3 is normal. Give as sodium bicarbonate or citrate mixtures (1 mEq citrate = 1 mEq HCO_3) such as Bicitra (1 mEq Na, 1 mEq citrate/mL, no K) or Polycitra (1 mEq Na, 1 mEq K, 2 mEq citrate/mL) depending on need for potassium. Sodium bicarbonate tablets are available (7.7 mEq $NaHCO_3$/650 mg tab) (5)[C].
- Type I RTA: Typical doses 1–4 mEq/kg/d p.o. alkali divided 3–4×/d (require much higher doses if HCO_3 wasting is present). May require K^+ supplementation for hypokalemia (6)[C].
- Type II RTA: Typical doses 10–15 mEq/kg/d alkali, divided 4–6×/d. Very difficult to restore plasma HCO_3 to normal because renal HCO_3 losses increase once plasma HCO_3 is corrected above the resorptive threshold. Exogenous HCO_3 increases K^+ losses, requiring K^+ supplementation. Often need PO_4 and vitamin D supplementation due to proximal PO_4 losses. May add thiazide diuretic to induce mild hypovolemia, which increases proximal Na^+/HCO_3 reabsorption.

- Type IV RTA: Avoid inciting medications; restrict dietary K^+. May augment K^+ excretion with loop diuretic, thiazide diuretic, or Kayexalate. Correcting hyperkalemia will actually increase activity of the urea cycle, augmenting renal ammoniagenesis and providing more substrate for renal acid excretion. If necessary, 1–5 mEq/kg/d alkali divided 2–3×/d. If mineralocorticoid deficiency, fludrocortisone: 0.1–0.3 mg/d.
- Contraindications: Refer to the manufacturers' literature.
- Precautions: Sodium bicarbonate may cause flatulence because CO_2 is formed, whereas citrate mixtures are metabolized to HCO_3 in the liver, thereby avoiding a gas production. The use of sodium-containing compounds or mineralocorticoids may lead to hypertension and/or edema.

Second Line
Thiazide diuretics may be used as adjunctive therapy in type II RTA (after maximal alkali replacement), but are likely to further increase urinary K^+ losses.

ADDITIONAL TREATMENT
General Measures
Treatment with appropriate medications to correct acidosis

SURGERY/OTHER PROCEDURES
If distal RTA is due to obstructive uropathy, surgical intervention may be required.

IN-PATIENT CONSIDERATIONS
Initial Stabilization
- Outpatient generally
- Inpatient if acidosis severe, patient unreliable, emesis persistent, or infant with severe failure to thrive

 ONGOING CARE

FOLLOW-UP RECOMMENDATIONS
Patient Monitoring
- Varies with patient response. Suggested: Electrolytes every 2–4 weeks at onset of therapy, every 2 weeks for 1–2 months after bicarbonate concentration normal, then monthly for several months
- Monitor underlying disease as indicated.
- Poor compliance common due to 3–6×/d alkali dosing schedule

DIET
Varies with type of acidosis

PATIENT EDUCATION
- National Kidney & Urologic Diseases Information Clearinghouse, Box NKUDIC, Bethesda, MD 20893, (301) 468-6345; http://www.niddk.nih.gov/health/kidney
- National Kidney Foundation: http://www.kidney.org

PROGNOSIS
- Depends on associated disease, otherwise good with therapy
- Transient forms of all types of RTA may occur.

COMPLICATIONS
- Nephrocalcinosis, nephrolithiasis (type I)
- Hypercalciuria (type I)
- Hypokalemia (type I, type II if given bicarbonate)
- Hyperkalemia (type IV, some causes of type I)
- Osteomalacia (type II due to phosphate wasting)

REFERENCES
1. Heering P, Ivens K, Aker S, et al. Distal tubular acidosis induced by FK506. *Clin Transplant*. 1998;12:465–71.
2. Rodríguez-Soriano J. New insights into the pathogenesis of renal tubular acidosis–from functional to molecular studies. *Pediatr Nephrol*. 2000;14:1121–36.
3. Casaletto J. Differential diagnosis of metabolic acidosis. *Emer Med Clin N Am*. 2005;23(3): 771–87.
4. Kurtzman NA. Renal tubular acidosis syndromes. *South Med J*. 2000;93:1042–52.
5. Chan JC, Scheinman JI, Roth KS. Consultation with the specialist: renal tubular acidosis. *Pediatr Rev*. 2001;22:277–87.
6. Domrongkitchaiporn S, Khositseth S, Stitchantrakul W, et al. Dosage of potassium citrate in the correction of urinary abnormalities in pediatric distal renal tubular acidosis patients. *Am J Kidney Dis*. 2002;39:383–91.

ADDITIONAL READING
Izzedine H, Launay-Vacher V, Deray G. Topiramate-induced renal tubular acidosis. *Am J Med*. 2004;116:281–2.

See Also (Topic, Algorithm, Electronic Media Element)
Hyperkalemia
Algorithm: Anuria or Oliguria

 CODES

ICD9
588.89 Other specified disorders resulting from impaired renal function

CLINICAL PEARLS
- Consider RTA in cases of nonanion gap metabolic acidosis with normal or near-normal renal function.
- Type I RTA: Urine pH >5.5 in setting of acidemia; positive urine anion gap; HCO_3 <15 mEq/L
- Type II RTA: Urine pH <5.5 unless HCO_3 raised above reabsorptive threshold (15–16 mEq/L)
- Type IV RTA: Most common subtype; hyperkalemia; urine pH <5.5; acidemia usually mild
- Treatment includes avoidance of inciting causes, provision of oral alkali (HCO_3 or citrate), and measures to supplement (type II, many type I) or restrict (type IV) potassium.

RESPIRATORY DISTRESS SYNDROME, ACUTE (ARDS)

Mary Cataletto, MD

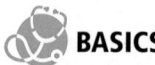

BASICS

DESCRIPTION
Syndrome characterized by abrupt onset of diffuse lung injury with severe hypoxemia and bilateral pulmonary infiltrates
- Absence of left atrial hypertension (HTN)
- By consensus, $PaO_2/FiO_2 < 200$
- Most severe form of acute lung injury
- System(s) affected: Pulmonary; Cardiovascular
- Synonym(s): Shock lung; Wet lung; Noncardiac pulmonary edema

EPIDEMIOLOGY
Incidence
Acute lung injury: 40–75 cases/100,000 population annually

RISK FACTORS
- Severe infection (localized or systemic) most common
- Aspiration of gastric contents
- Shock
- Infection
- Lung contusion
- Nonthoracic trauma
- Toxic inhalation
- Near drowning
- Multiple blood transfusions

GENERAL PREVENTION
No effective measures have been identified.

PATHOPHYSIOLOGY
3 phases:
- Acute exudative phase: Characterized by profound hypoxia and associated with inflammation with infiltration of inflammatory and proinflammatory mediators and diffuse alveolar damage
- Fibrosing alveolitis phase: Coincides with recovery or after ~1–2 weeks; patients continue to be hypoxic and have increased dead space and decreased compliance.
- Resolution may require 6–12 months.

ETIOLOGY
- Several mediators are involved in the initiation and perpetuation of acute respiratory distress syndrome (ARDS).
  - Cytokines
  - Complement activation
  - Coagulation activation
  - Platelet-activating factor
  - Oxygen free radicals
  - Lipoxygenase pathways
  - Neutrophil proteases
  - Nitric oxide
  - Endotoxin
  - Cyclooxygenase pathway products
- Systemic inflammatory response with activation of the previous mediators can occur with direct or indirect injury to the lung.
  - Direct:
    - Aspiration
    - Pulmonary infections
    - Air, fat, or amniotic fluid emboli
    - Near drowning
    - Pulmonary contusion
    - Inhalation of toxic gases and dusts

  - Indirect:
    - Sepsis
    - Shock
    - Transfusion
    - Trauma
    - Overdose
    - Pancreatitis, severe
    - Eclampsia

COMMONLY ASSOCIATED CONDITIONS
- Severe sepsis
- Trauma
- Shock

DIAGNOSIS

HISTORY
- No history of heart disease
- Precipitating event (see "Commonly Associated Disorders"): Abrupt onset of respiratory distress

PHYSICAL EXAM
- Tachypnea and tachycardia during the 1st 12–24 hours; respiratory distress
- Lethargy, obtundation
- Flat neck veins
- Hyperdynamic pulses
- Physiologic gallop
- Absence of edema
- Moist, cyanotic skin
- Manifestations of underlying disease

DIAGNOSTIC TESTS & INTERPRETATION
Lab
Initial lab tests
- Arterial blood gases (ABGs) show evidence of severe hypoxemia.
- $PaO_2/FiO_2 < 200$
- ECG: Sinus tachycardia; nonspecific ST-T-wave changes
- Pulmonary artery wedge pressure (PAWP) <15 mm Hg
- Cardiac index >3.5 L/min/m^2

Follow-Up & Special Considerations
- Serial blood gases
- Monitor for and treat multisystem organ failure when it occurs.

Imaging
Initial approach
- CXR: Normal heart size; fluffy, bilateral infiltrates; air bronchograms common
- Chest CT scan: Diffuse interstitial opacities and bullae

Follow-Up & Special Considerations
Serial CXRs

Diagnostic Procedures/Surgery
Invasive monitoring of vital signs, cardiac output, and pulmonary arterial wedge pressure has been questioned by large clinical trials.

Pathological Findings
- Lungs show exudative, early proliferative, or late proliferative phases.
- Interstitial and alveolar edema is present.
- Inflammatory cells and erythrocytes spill into the interstitium and the alveolus.

- Type 1 cells are destroyed, leaving a denuded basement membrane.
- Protein-rich fluid fills the alveoli.
- Type 2 alveolar cells initially appear unaltered.
- Type 2 cells begin to proliferate within 72 hours of initial insult.
- Type 2 cells cover the denuded basement membrane.
- Aggregates of plasma proteins, cellular debris, fibrin, and surfactant remnants form hyaline membranes.
- Over the next 3–10 days, alveolar septum thickens by proliferating fibroblasts, leukocytes, and plasma cells.
- Capillary injury begins to occur.
- Hyaline membranes begin to reorganize.
- Fibrosis becomes apparent in respiratory ducts and bronchioles.

DIFFERENTIAL DIAGNOSIS
- Left ventricular failure
- Interstitial and airway diseases
- Venoocclusive disease
- Mitral stenosis: Intravascular volume overload

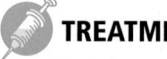

TREATMENT

MEDICATION
- No single drug or combination of drugs prevents or treats full-blown ARDS. Treatment is supportive while addressing the underlying cause.
- Supplemental oxygen
- Ventilatory support:
  - Most often requires endotracheal intubation with emphasis on lower tidal volumes per weight and optimization of positive end-expiratory pressure (PEEP).
  - High frequency oscillation might improve survival and is unlikely to cause harm (1)[A].

ADDITIONAL TREATMENT
- Inotropic agents: Dobutamine to maintain adequate cardiac output after appropriate fluid resuscitation fails to restore perfusion
- Corticosteroids: Short-term use during the acute phase has not been shown to be effective. However, recent data suggest that sustained therapy in patients with full-blown, established ARDS may be beneficial (2)[A].
- Vasodilators: Inhaled nitric oxide (INO) is not recommended for patients with ARDS. INO results in a transient improvement in oxygenation but does not reduce mortality and may be harmful (3)[A].
- Pulmonary surfactant: Successful in neonatal respiratory distress syndrome; investigational outside this age group
- Inhaled β_2 agonists may be helpful during the resolution phase.
- There is no current evidence to support or refute the routine use of aerosolized prostacyclin for patients with ARDS (4)[A].
- Antioxidants (e.g., procysteine) have produced conflicting results.
- Activated protein C may be helpful in patients with sepsis.
- Deep vein thrombosis (DVT) prophylaxis
- Ulcer prophylaxis

Pregnancy Considerations
- Supportive care while identifying the underlying cause of ARDS continues to be important in the management of pregnant women with ARDS. However, fetal well-being, possible need for delivery, and physiologic changes associated with pregnancy must be considered (5).

General Measures
- Ensure adequate oxygenation.
- Ventilatory support generally requires endotracheal intubation and use of PEEP (6).
- Provide appropriate cardiorespiratory monitoring.
- Fluid management

Issues for Referral
- All patients with ARDS should be cared for in an ICU with appropriately trained staff.
- Pregnant patients with ARDS also should be followed by a high-risk perinatologist or obstetrician.

IN-PATIENT CONSIDERATIONS
Initial Stabilization
- Consider prone positioning.
- Identify and treat underlying condition.
- Circulatory support, adequate fluid volume, and nutritional support
- Supplemental oxygen
- Monitoring blood gases, pulse oximetry, bedside pulmonary function test
- Support ventilation using lung-protective strategies and PEEP.
- Monitor for systemic hypotension and hypovolemia without fluid overload.
- BP support, if necessary
- Vasopressor agents
- Fluid management with IV crystalloid solutions while monitoring pulmonary status
- Pulmonary catheter pressure monitoring
- Treat underlying disease process.
- Prevent complications.

Admission Criteria
All patients with ARDS should be managed in an ICU setting.

IV Fluids
- Maintain intravascular volume at lowest level consistent with adequate perfusion (assessed by metabolic acid base balance and renal function).
- If perfusion is inadequate after restoration of intravascular volume (e.g., septic shock), vasopressor therapy is indicated.
- Increase oxygen content with packed erythrocyte transfusions as necessary.
- Provide appropriate nutritional support with enteral or parenteral nutrition.
- Steroid therapy

Nursing
May include any or all of the following:
- Skin care, eye and mouth care
- DVT prophylaxis
- GI prophylaxis
- Suctioning
- Ensure adequate level of sedation and/or paralysis while on mechanical ventilation.
- Oxygen supplementation
- Nebulizer therapy

- Chest physiotherapy
- Tracheostomy care
- Explain all procedures to patient and family; reduce anxiety.

Discharge Criteria
- Supplemental oxygen
- Nutrition counseling
- Family monitoring of signs and symptoms of respiratory distress

 ## ONGOING CARE

FOLLOW-UP RECOMMENDATIONS
Patient Monitoring
- Vital capacity and static lung compliance are important measures of lung mechanics.
- Daily labs are needed until patient is no longer critical.
- CXRs to assess endotracheal tube placement, the presence of progressing infiltrates, catheter placement, and complications of mechanical ventilation (e.g., air leaks).
- Swan-Ganz catheter to help assess oxygen delivery, oxygen consumption, and cardiac output may be helpful but has not been shown to improve survival.

DIET
- Nutritional support
- Conservative fluid management shortens ventilator and ICU time but does not affect survival.

PATIENT EDUCATION
http://www.ards.org has ARDS support center and brochure entitled "Learn about ARDS."

PROGNOSIS
- Mortality rate is 43% (7).
- Survivors may have pulmonary sequelae with mild abnormalities in oxygenation, diffusion, and lung mechanics, as well as some pulmonary symptoms of cough and dyspnea.

COMPLICATIONS
- Permanent lung disease
- Oxygen toxicity
- Barotrauma
- Superinfection
- Multiple organ dysfunction syndrome
- Death

REFERENCES

1. Sud S, Sud M, Friedrich JO, et al. High frequency oscillation in patients with acute lung injury and acute respiratory distress syndrome (ARDS): systematic review and meta-analysis. *BMJ*. 2010; 340:c2327.
2. Peter JV, John P, Graham PL, et al. Corticosteroids in the prevention and treatment of acute respiratory distress syndrome (ARDS) in adults: meta-analysis. *BMJ*. 2008;336:1006–9.
3. Afshari A, Brok J, Møller AM, et al. Inhaled nitric oxide for acute respiratory distress syndrome (ARDS) and acute lung injury in children and adults. *Cochrane Database Syst Rev*. 2010;7:CD002787.
4. Afshari A, Brok J, Møller AM, et al. Aerosolized prostacyclin for acute lung injury (ALI) and acute respiratory distress syndrome (ARDS). *Cochrane Database Syst Rev*. 2010;8:CD007733.
5. http:www.ardsnet.org for ARDS Net ventilatory management protocol.
6. Petrucci N, et al. Ventilation with lower tidal volumes vs. traditional tidal volumes in adults for acute lung injury and acute respiratory distress syndrome. *Cochrane Database Syst Rev*. 2007;2:CD003844, DOI:10.1002/14651858. CD003844.pub3.
7. Zambon M, Vincent JL. Mortality rates for patients with acute lung injury/ARDS have decreased over time. *Chest*. 2008;133:1120–7.

ADDITIONAL READING

- Cole DE, Taylor TL, McCullough DM, et al. Acute respiratory distress syndrome in pregnancy. *Crit Care Med*. 2005;33:S269–78.
- Goldman L, et al. *Cecil Medicine*, 23rd ed. Philadelphia: Saunders, 2008;731–4.
- Piantadosi CA, Schwartz DA. The acute respiratory distress syndrome. *Ann Intern Med*. 2004;141: 460–70.
- Ware LB, Matthay MA. The acute respiratory distress syndrome. *N Engl J Med*. 2000;342:1334–49.
- Wheeler AP, Bernard GR. Acute lung injury and the acute respiratory distress syndrome: a clinical review. *Lancet*. 2007;369:1553–64.

 ## CODES

ICD9
518.5 Pulmonary insufficiency following trauma and surgery

CLINICAL PEARLS

- ARDS is a syndrome characterized by abrupt onset of diffuse lung injury with severe hypoxemia and bilateral pulmonary infiltrates.
- Treatment of ARDS requires aggressive supportive care in an ICU setting while also addressing the underlying cause.
- The benefit of invasive monitoring of vital signs, cardiac output, and pulmonary arterial wedge pressure has been questioned by large clinical trials.

Mary Cataletto, MD

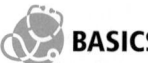

BASICS

DESCRIPTION
- Neonatal respiratory distress syndrome (RDS) is a serious disorder of prematurity with a clinical manifestation of respiratory distress.
- Pulmonary surfactants that are deficient at birth and an overly compliant chest wall cause diffuse lung atelectasis.
- Must differentiate from pneumonia, transient tachypnea of the newborn (TTN), sepsis, meconium aspiration
- System(s) affected: Pulmonary
- Synonym: Hyaline membrane disease

ALERT
A disorder of the neonatal period

EPIDEMIOLOGY
Incidence
- Affects 40,000 neonates each year in the US and accounts for ~6% of neonatal deaths
- Predominant age: Neonatal
- Predominant sex: Slight male predominance
- ~50% of neonates with birth weights of 501–1,500 g
- Inversely proportional to gestational age and birth weight
- In 1 study, rates of RDS, regardless of mode of delivery, increased between 1997 and 2005 from 2.1–2.4% (1).

Prevalence
Common

RISK FACTORS
- Neonatal complication rates vary by mode of delivery and decrease with gestational age (1):
  - Premature neonates born <37 weeks' gestation
  - Cesarean section without labor
- Neonates born of diabetic mothers
- Perinatal asphyxia
- History of RDS in a sibling

Genetics
No known genetic pattern

GENERAL PREVENTION
- Prevention of premature birth with education, regular prenatal care, and tocolytics
- Antenatal corticosteroids given to mother when fetal lung profile is immature, at least 24 h before delivery; 2 doses of betamethasone 12 mg IM separated by a 24-h interval (contraindications: chorioamnionitis or other indications for immediate delivery)

- Prenatal amniotic fluid testing looking for indications of immature lungs/deficient surfactant production:
  - Lecithin:sphingomyelin (L:S) ratio <2:1
  - Absence of phosphatidyl glycerol
  - TDx fetal lung maturity (FLM) <70 (measures surfactant:albumin ratio)

PATHOPHYSIOLOGY
- Structurally immature lungs and surfactant deficiency lead to diffuse atelectasis.
- Exposure to high FiO_2 and barotrauma associated with mechanical ventilation trigger proinflammatory cytokines that further damage alveolar epithelium.
- Decreased lung compliance leads to alveolar hypoventilation and ventilation–perfusion mismatch.
- Shunting of blood (R → L) at patent ductus arteriosus (PDA), PFO causes further hypoxemia

DIAGNOSIS

HISTORY
Preterm neonates with worsening respiratory distress beginning shortly after birth and progressing over first few hours of life

PHYSICAL EXAM
- Tachypnea
- Expiratory grunting
- Nasal flaring
- Sub- and intercostal retractions
- Decreased breath sounds
- Cyanosis

DIAGNOSTIC TESTS & INTERPRETATION
Lab
- Complete blood count (CBC) and blood culture to rule out sepsis, pneumonia
- Electrolytes: Monitor for hypoglycemia, hypocalcemia
- Arterial blood gases (ABGs):
  - Hypoxemia (which responds to supplemental oxygen)
  - Features of respiratory and metabolic acidosis

Imaging
CXR:
- Diffuse reticulogranular pattern (ground-glass appearance)
- Air bronchograms
- Low lung volumes

Diagnostic Procedures/Surgery
Echocardiogram: Consider if murmur present to evaluate for PDA and contribution to lung disease due to L → R shunting (2)

Pathological Findings
- Macroscopically: Uniformly ruddy, airless appearance of lungs
- Microscopically: Diffuse atelectasis and hyaline membranes (eosinophilic and fibrinous membrane lining airspaces)
- Dilatation of right ventricle
- Possible PDA

DIFFERENTIAL DIAGNOSIS
- Early onset group B streptococcal pneumonia and/or sepsis
- Transient tachypnea of newborn
- Meconium aspiration pneumonia

TREATMENT

Along with antenatal steroids, surfactants improve survival for preterm babies, and they are now recommended routinely as early in the course of RDS as possible (3)[A].

MEDICATION
- Surfactant via endotracheal tube (ETT):
  - Prophylactic surfactant administration: Given at birth to neonates <30 weeks' gestation (if it can be done safely at the same time as resuscitation)
  - Rescue surfactant administration: Given to neonates after RDS diagnosis
- Initial dosage of animal-derived surfactant preparations:
  - Poractant alfa (Curosurf): 2.5 mL/kg
  - Calfactant (Infasurf): 3.0 mL/kg
  - Beractant (Survanta): 4.0 mL/kg
- Continued therapy: After initial dose of chosen surfactant, if clinical evidence of persistent disease after initial improvement (recurrent O_2 requirement of >30–40%)
- Repeated dosages:
  - Poractant alfa: 1.25 mL/kg q12h for up to a total of 3 doses
  - Calfactant: 3.0 mL/kg q12h for up to a total of 3 doses
  - Beractant: 4.0 mL/kg repeated q6h for up to a total of 4 doses
- Side effects: Bradycardia, hypotension, airway obstruction/endotracheal tube blockage with administration; rapid changes in tidal volume due to increased compliance can cause a pneumothorax and small risk of pulmonary hemorrhage
- Precautions: Transient adverse effects seen with the administration of surfactant may require stopping administration and alleviating situation; may proceed with dosing when stable.
- Contraindications: Presence of congenital anomalies incompatible with life beyond neonatal period; infant with laboratory evidence of lung maturity
- Perform frequent clinical and laboratory checks so that oxygen and ventilatory support can be modified to respond to respiratory changes.

ADDITIONAL TREATMENT

General Measures

- Warm, humidified, oxygen-enriched gases by hood if neonate is ventilating effectively
- Continuous positive airway pressure (CPAP) if infant is active and breathing spontaneously
- Positive-pressure ventilation per ETT via conventional mechanical ventilator (CMV) or high-frequency oscillation ventilator (HFOV) if respiratory failure occurs (i.e., respiratory acidosis, apnea, or hypoxia despite nasal CPAP)
- Transcutaneous monitors to measure O_2 and CO_2 tension
- Pulse oximetry
- Umbilical artery catheter placement for continuous BP monitoring and sampling arterial blood gases (ABGs)
- Umbilical vein catheter placement for fluid and total parenteral nutrition (TPN) administration
- Tube feedings or hyperalimentation
- Optimize thermoneutral environment with radiant warmer or isolette.
- Sedation and analgesia with phenobarbital, fentanyl, or morphine may be required while patient is intubated.
- Muscle paralysis is controversial.
- Inhaled nitric oxide and administration of postnatal glucocorticoids not recommended at this time

Additional Therapies

- Empirical therapy for sepsis (i.e., ampicillin and gentamicin) can be discontinued if CBC has normalized and blood culture has no growth after 48 h.
- Consider medical or surgical closure of PDA if it is contributing to lung disease.

IN-PATIENT CONSIDERATIONS

Admission Criteria

All neonates with respiratory distress require inpatient treatment.

Discharge Criteria

Should have stable vital signs and pulse oximetry before discharge in addition to other premature considerations

 ONGOING CARE

DIET

Special premature formula and parenteral alimentation

PATIENT EDUCATION

For patient education materials favorably reviewed on this topic, go to Boston Children's Hospital Web site (www.childrenshospital.org) and search for respiratory distress syndrome in the "My Child Has" window.

PROGNOSIS

- Prognosis and outcome highly dependent on gestational age and birth weight
- Survival for neonates with birth weight of ≤ 500 g is 10%; > 500 g, upwards of 75%.
- Complications of RDS decrease as birth weight increases.

COMPLICATIONS

- Some due to therapeutic interventions; others due to complications related to prematurity
- Pneumothorax
- Chronic lung disease, bronchopulmonary dysplasia (BPD)
- Intraventricular hemorrhage
- Retinopathy of prematurity
- Necrotizing enterocolitis
- Pulmonary interstitial edema (PIE)

REFERENCES

1. Jain NJ, Kruse LK, Demissie K, et al. Impact of mode of delivery on neonatal complications: Trends between 1997 and 2005. *J Matern Fetal Neonatal Med.* 2009;1–10.
2. Hamrick SE, Hansmann G et al. Patent ductus arteriosus of the preterm infant. *Pediatrics.* 2010;125:1020–30.
3. Sweet DG, Halliday HL. The use of surfactants in 2009. *Arch Dis Child Educ Pract Ed.* 2009;94: 78–83.

ADDITIONAL READING

- Avery GB, eds. *Neonatology: Pathophysiology and management of the newborn*, 5th ed. Philadelphia: Lippincott Williams & Wilkins, 1999.
- Cloherty JP, Eichenwald E, Stark AR, eds. *Manual of Neonatal Care: Joint Program in Neonatology.* 5th ed. Lippincott Williams & Wilkins; 2003.
- Engle WA, American Academy of Pediatrics Committee on Fetus and Newborn. Surfactant-replacement therapy for respiratory distress in the preterm and term neonate. *Pediatrics.* 2008;121:419–32.
- Fanaroff AA, Martin RJ, Walsh MC, eds. *Neonatal-Perinatal Medicine: Diseases of the Fetus and Infant.* 8th ed. Philadelphia: Mosby Elsevier; 2006.
- Gomella TR. *Neonatology: Management, Procedures, On-call Problems, Diseases, and Drugs.* 5th ed. The McGraw-Hill Companies; 2004.
- Moya F. Synthetic surfactants: where are we? Evidence from randomized, controlled clinical trials. *J Perinatol.* 2009;29(Suppl 2):S23–8.
- Ramachandrappa A, Jain L. Health issues of the late preterm infant. *Pediatr Clin North Am.* 2009;56:565–77, Table of Contents.
- Sekar KC, Corff KE. To tube or not to tube babies with respiratory distress syndrome. *J Perinatol.* 2009;29(Suppl 2):S68–72.
- Soll RF. Multiple versus single dose natural surfactant extract for severe neonatal respiratory distress syndrome. *Cochrane Database of Systematic Reviews.* 1999, Issue 2. Art. No.: CD000141. DOI:10.1002/14651858.CD000141.

 CODES

ICD9

769 Respiratory distress syndrome in newborn

CLINICAL PEARLS

- Surfactants are used routinely as early in the course of RDS as possible.
- If an infant has a murmur, consider an echocardiogram to rule out PDA and shunting.
- Prognosis and outcome are highly dependent on gestational age and birth weight.

RESPIRATORY SYNCYTIAL VIRUS INFECTION

Elizabeth Colman McKeen, MD

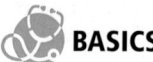 **BASICS**

Respiratory syncytial virus (RSV) is a medium-sized membrane-bound RNA virus that causes acute respiratory tract illness in all ages, with most clinically significant disease in infants and young children.

DESCRIPTION
- A major cause of respiratory illness, either of the upper respiratory tract (URTI) or of the lower respiratory tract (LRTI/bronchiolitis)
- In adults, respiratory syncytial virus (RSV) causes URTIs.
- In infants and children, RSV causes URTIs and LRTIs (bronchiolitis).
- 90–95% of children are infected at least once by the age of 24 months; reinfection is common.
- Leading cause of pediatric bronchiolitis (50–90%)
- Premature infants are at increased risk for severe acute RSV infection.

EPIDEMIOLOGY
- Seasonality: Highest incidence of RSV infection in the US is between December and March.
- Morbidity: RSV infection leads to 90–120,000 hospitalizations annually nationwide.

RISK FACTORS
- Risk factors for severe disease include
  - History of prematurity
  - Age <12 weeks
  - Underlying cardiopulmonary disease
  - Immunodeficiency
- Other risk factors may include
  - Low socioeconomic status
  - Exposure to environmental air pollutants
  - Child-care attendance
  - Severe neuromuscular disease
  - In adults, occupational exposure: Pediatric hospital staff, teachers, and day-care workers

Genetics
- A genetic predisposition to severe RSV infections may be associated with polymorphisms in cytokine- and chemokine-related genes including *CCR5*, *IL4* and its receptor, *IL8*, *IL10*, and *IL13*.
- Infants with transplacentally acquired antibody against RSV are not protected against infection but may have milder symptoms.

GENERAL PREVENTION
- Hand decontamination is the most important step in preventing nosocomial spread of RSV.
  - Alcohol-based rubs are preferred; an alternative is hand-washing with antimicrobial soap (1)[B].
  - In patients with proven or suspected RSV infection should be isolated or cohorted.
- Exposure to passive tobacco smoke should be avoided, especially in infants and children.

- Palivizumab (Synagis), a monoclonal antibody directed against the F (fusion) protein of RSV, is indicated as prophylaxis for the following groups (2):
  - Infants and children <24 months of age with
    - Chronic lung disease of prematurity requiring medical therapy within 6 months of the start of RSV season
    - Hemodynamically significant cyanotic or acyanotic congenital heart disease
    - Prematurity <32 weeks' gestation, even in the absence of chronic lung disease. Those born at ≤28 weeks should receive prophylaxis during their 1st RSV season whenever that occurs during the 1st 12 months of life. Those born at 29–32 weeks benefit most from prophylaxis up to 6 months of age.
    - Prematurity 32 0/7–34 6/7 weeks' gestation *and* at least 1 of 2 risk factors born within 3 months before the start of RSV season or at any time throughout the RSV season:
      - Infant attends child care, or
      - One or more siblings or other children younger than 5 years live permanently in the child's household
  - Dosage: 5 monthly doses beginning in November or December at 15 mg/kg per dose administered intramuscularly

PATHOPHYSIOLOGY
RSV-induced bronchiolitis causes acute inflammation, edema, and necrosis of the epithelial cells lining the small airways, air trapping, bronchospasm, and increased mucus production.

ETIOLOGY
- RSV is a medium-sized membrane-bound RNA virus. It develops in the cytoplasm of infected cells and matures by budding from the plasma membrane.
- Infection spreads via infected droplets, either airborne or conveyed on hands, that are inoculated in the nose or conjunctivae of a susceptible subject.

COMMONLY ASSOCIATED CONDITIONS
- Asthma
- Serious bacterial infection (SBI) in infants and children with concurrent RSV infection is rare. When it occurs, the most likely etiology is URTI, followed by acute otitis media.

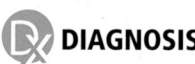 **DIAGNOSIS**

HISTORY
Patients may present with a variety of symptoms, including, but not limited to, upper respiratory congestion, respiratory distress, cough, and fever.

PHYSICAL EXAM
- Fever
- Rhinorrhea
- Cough
- Wheezing
- Crackles
- Increased work of breathing, manifested as tachypnea, retractions, nasal flaring, and/or grunting
- In infants and children, evidence of poor hydration status such as feeding difficulty, dry mucus membranes, poor skin turgor
- Repeat examinations over time are most helpful in providing the best overall assessment.

DIAGNOSTIC TESTS & INTERPRETATION
Lab
Initial lab tests
- Routine laboratory testing is not necessary.
  - If obtained, white blood cell (WBC) count may be normal or elevated.
  - Virologic tests for RSV, despite high predictive value, rarely change management decisions or outcomes for patients with clinically diagnosed bronchiolitis.
- Given the low risk of SBI, full septic workups in these patients should not be undertaken routinely.

Imaging
- Chest x-ray (CXR) has not been proven to affect patient outcomes or predict disease severity.
- A CXR may be most helpful when a patient does not improve as expected, if the severity of the disease requires further investigation, or if another diagnosis is suspected.
- If obtained, typical findings on CXR can include
  - Hyperinflation and peribronchiolar thickening
  - Atelectasis
  - Interstitial infiltrates
  - Segmental or lobar consolidation
  - Pleural fluid (rare)

DIFFERENTIAL DIAGNOSIS
- Mild illness/URTI:
  - Other (non-RSV) respiratory viral infections such as rhinovirus, human metapneumovirus, influenza virus, human bocavirus
  - Allergic rhinitis
  - Sinusitis
- Severe illness/LRTI:
  - Bronchiolitis
  - Asthma
  - Pneumonia
  - Foreign-body aspiration

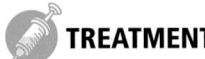

TREATMENT

MEDICATION

- No 1st-line medication for RSV infections; treatment is usually supportive.
- Bronchodilators show small short-term improvements in clinical scores (3)[B], but this small benefit should be weighed against the costs and adverse effects of these agents.
  - Routine use not recommended
  - If a carefully monitored trial of inhaled α- or β-adrenergic agents is administered, an objective means of measuring response must be used.
  - Inhaled epinephrine may be slightly more efficacious than inhaled albuterol (4)[B].
- Systemic glucocorticoids show no benefit in length of hospital stay or clinical score in infants and young children (5)[A].
- Current evidence suggests that inhaled corticosteroids show no benefit in the treatment of RSV bronchiolitis or in prevention of postbronchiolitic wheezing (6)[B].
- A recent study found that montelukast (Singulair) has no effect on the clinical course of acute bronchiolitis (7)[C].
- Ribavirin, a nucleoside analogue and antiviral agent, has not been shown to be efficacious in the treatment of RSV (8)[C].
- Use of antibacterial agents should be reserved for patients who have specific signs of a coexisting SBI. When such an infection is present, it should be treated in the same manner as in the absence of RSV infection (9)[B].

ADDITIONAL TREATMENT
General Measures
- Clinicians must promptly assess hydration status and ability to take fluids orally. Dehydration must be treated adequately with an oral or intravenous fluid, with special attention to infants.
- Supplemental O_2 is indicated if the SpO_2 falls persistently below 90% in previously healthy patients.
  - An SpO_2 of 90% is an approximate cutoff and should be adjusted in the context of the patient.
  - Continuous O_2 monitoring can be discontinued in a patient whose clinical status is improving.

Additional Therapies
Bulb suctioning of the nares may provide some comfort to infants and allow for easier feeding.

Pediatric Considerations
Parents must be reminded that the American Academy of Pediatrics strongly recommends against the use of over-the-counter (OTC) cough and cold medications in children >6 years of age owing to lack of efficacy and the risk of life-threatening side effects.

COMPLEMENTARY AND ALTERNATIVE MEDICINE
Clinicians should inquire about patients' use of complementary and alternative therapies, such as echinacea and zinc.

IN-PATIENT CONSIDERATIONS
Initial Stabilization
- A full history and physical exam should be completed, including the ABCs. Special attention should be paid to respiratory and hydration status.
- Mechanical ventilation is required in about 5% of infants hospitalized with RSV and 20% of children with underlying congenital heart disease, chronic lung disease, or immunosuppression and should be instituted in the case of respiratory failure.

Admission Criteria
- Clinical judgment of the patient's degree of respiratory distress is the most important consideration.
- Significant respiratory distress and/or O_2 requirement to keep SpO_2 >90%
- Inability to hydrate orally

IV Fluids
See "Treatment."

Discharge Criteria
No set criteria for discharge exists, but the following guidelines may be helpful:
- Respiratory distress resolving or resolved
- Patient oxygenating well without O_2 therapy
- Adequate oral intake for sustained hydration
- Caretaker able to clear the infant's airway with bulb suctioning
- Home resources adequate to support use of any necessary home therapies
- Education of family complete

ONGOING CARE

FOLLOW-UP RECOMMENDATIONS
Close follow-up with the patient's primary health care provider is essential.

PATIENT EDUCATION
- See "General Prevention."
- *Bronchiolitis and Your Child*, available at http://familydoctor.org/online/famdocen/home/children/parents/common/common/020.html.

PROGNOSIS
Most patients with RSV infection recover fully within 7–10 days, although reinfection is common.

COMPLICATIONS
- Infants hospitalized for RSV may be at increased risk for recurrent wheezing and reduced pulmonary function, particularly during the 1st decade of life.
- Overall mortality for infants and children <24 months of age is <1%.

REFERENCES

1. American Academy of Pediatrics Subcommittee on Diagnosis and Management of Bronchiolitis. *Pediatrics*. 2006;118:1774–93.
2. AAP Policy Statements: Modified recommendations for use of palivizumab for prevention of respiratory syncytial virus infections. Committee on Infectious Diseases. *Pediatrics*. 2009;124(6):1694–701.
3. Gadomski AM, Bhasale AL. Bronchodilators for bronchiolitis. *Cochrane Database Syst Rev*. 2006;3:CD001266.
4. Hartling L, Wiebe N, Russell K, et al. Epinephrine for bronchiolitis. *Cochrane Database Syst Rev*. 2004:CD003123.
5. Patel H, et al. Glucocorticoids for acute viral bronchiolitis in infants and young children. Cochrane Acute Respiratory Infections Group. *Cochrane Database Sys Rev*. 2008;1:CD004878.
6. Blom D, Ermers M, Bont L, et al. Inhaled corticosteroids during acute bronchiolitis in the prevention of post-bronchiolitic wheezing. *Cochrane Database Syst Rev*. 2007:CD004881.
7. Amirav I, Luder AS, Kruger N, et al. A double-blind, placebo-controlled, randomized trial of montelukast for acute bronchiolitis. *Pediatrics*. 2008;122:e1249–55.
8. Ventre K, et al. Ribavirin for respiratory syncytial virus infection of the lower respiratory tract in infants and young children. Cochrane Acute Respiratory Infections Group. *Cochrane Database Sys Rev*. 2009;1:CD000181.
9. Spurling GKP, et al. Antibiotics for bronchiolitis in children. Cochrane Acute Respiratory Infections Group. *Cochrane Database Sys Rev*. 2007;1:CD005189.

ADDITIONAL READING

Perrotta C, et al. Chest physiotherapy for acute bronchiolitis in paediatric patients between 0 and 24 months old. Cochrane Acute Respiratory Infections Group. *Cochrane Database Sys Rev*. 2007;1:CD004873.

CODES

ICD9
- 079.6 Respiratory syncytial virus (RSV)
- 465.9 Acute upper respiratory infections of unspecified site
- 466.11 Acute bronchiolitis due to respiratory syncytial virus (RSV)

CLINICAL PEARLS

- RSV causes 50–90% of pediatric bronchiolitis.
- Hand sanitation is key for prevention in the general population.
- Palivizumab is key for prevention in the high-risk population.
- Diagnosis is clinical in most cases.
- Treatment is usually supportive.

RESTLESS LEGS SYNDROME

Donald E. Watenpaugh, PhD
John R. Burk, MD

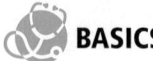 **BASICS**

DESCRIPTION
- Sensorimotor disorder defined by 4 criteria (1,2)[A]:
  - A strong urge to move the legs, usually accompanied by discomfort
  - The urge to move and discomfort occur during inactivity (seated or recumbent)
  - Movement immediately relieves symptoms, but they recur with subsequent inactivity.
  - Symptoms occur primarily in the evening/night.
- Symptoms may instead or also involve the arms, or be more generalized.
- Patient may also complain of involuntary leg jerks.
- Systems affected: Musculoskeletal; Nervous
- Synonym(s): Ekbom syndrome

EPIDEMIOLOGY
Incidence
- Onset at any age; increases with age (1,3)[A]
- Primary RLS presents early and progresses slowly.
- Secondary RLS:
  - Precipitated by other conditions/medications
  - Tends to progress rapidly
  - Resolves to extent that cause(s) resolve
- Predominant sex: Male = Female (nulliparous); Female (parous) 2 × > Male (4)[B]

Prevalence
- 4–12% of Caucasian adults; underdiagnosed
- >3% in children and adolescents
- Increases with age
- Lower with African American, Mediterranean, Middle Eastern, and East Asian descent

Pregnancy Considerations
- 10–30% prevalence; exacerbates existing RLS (4)
- May be secondary to iron or folate deficiency

RISK FACTORS
- Family history (2,3)[A]
- Aging
- Chronic inactivity
- Inadequate sleep
- Associated conditions (see below)

Genetics
- Primary RLS heritability: ~50%
- Genetically heterogenous (2,5)[B]:
  - Susceptibility loci: 2p14, 2q, 6p21.2, 9p, 12q, 14q, 15q23, and 20p
  - Genes: MEIS1, MAP2K5/LBXCOR1, and BTBD9

GENERAL PREVENTION
- Regular physical activity/exercise (6)[B]
- Adequate sleep
- Avoid evening caffeine, alcohol, tobacco
- Avoid causes of secondary RLS.

PATHOPHYSIOLOGY
- CNS iron or dopamine deficiency or dysmetabolism
- Chronic extremity tissue pathology/inflammation

ETIOLOGY
- Primary RLS: Subcortical dopamine deficiency (2,5)[B]

- Secondary RLS:
  - Iron deficiency and associated conditions
  - Chronic extremity tissue irritation
  - Medications:
    - Most antidepressants (exceptions: Bupropion and desipramine)
    - Dopamine-blocking antiemetics (e.g., metoclopramide)
    - Some antiepileptic agents (e.g., phenytoin)
    - Phenothiazine antipsychotics; donepezil
    - Theophylline
    - Antihistamines/OTC cold preparations (pseudoephedrine, etc.)
    - Stimulants, particularly if taken later in day

COMMONLY ASSOCIATED CONDITIONS
- Periodic limb movements of sleep; insomnia, sleep walking and other parasomnias; delayed sleep phase
- Iron deficiency; renal disease/uremia/dialysis; gastric surgery; liver disease
- Parkinson disease; peripheral neuropathy; ADHD; anxiety/depression; "sundowning"
- Venous insufficiency/peripheral vascular disease; erectile dysfunction
- Orthopedic problems, arthritis
- Pulmonary hypertension; lung transplantation; COPD

 DIAGNOSIS

- Relies on history, yet often "difficult to describe"
- May go undiagnosed for years and by multiple doctors

HISTORY
- Signs/symptoms (see also Description) (1,2)[A]:
  - Example paresthesia descriptions: Burning, achy, itching, antsy, "can't get comfortable"
  - Symptoms painful in ~35% of patients
  - Discomfort associated with overwhelming urge to move and relieved by movement
  - Urge to move may be the only "discomfort."
  - Movement frequency every 10–90 s (mean ~25 s)
  - Some patients must get out of bed and walk.
  - May involve arms or, rarely, whole body
  - Periodic movements in sleep in ~80% of patients
  - Insomnia, daytime fatigue, anxiety
- Severity range: From rare, minor problem to daily severe impact on quality of life
- Severe cases: Difficulty riding in cars or sitting still at events in afternoon/evening

Pediatric Considerations
If all 4 diagnostic criteria not met, apply 1st 3 along with 2 of these (1,3)[A]:
- Insomnia or sleep disturbance
- RLS in immediate biological relative
- Periodic limb movements during sleep

Geriatric Considerations
For diagnosis in the cognitively impaired (2,7)[A]:
- Rubbing or kneading the legs in evening
- Evening hyperactivity (foot tapping, pacing, fidgeting, tossing/turning in bed)

PHYSICAL EXAM
Patient may be fidgety, unable to sit still.

DIAGNOSTIC TESTS & INTERPRETATION
Lab
Serum ferritin to assess for iron deficiency

Diagnostic Procedures/Surgery
- Sleep study not required, but can be helpful:
  - Frequent, periodic movements during wake
- Suggested immobilization test:
  - Conducted before nocturnal polysomnography
  - Patient attempts to sit still in bed for 1 hour.
  - >40 movements per hour suggests RLS.
- Ankle actigraphy can be used in the home.
- Electromyography and nerve conduction studies to check for peripheral neuropathy and radiculopathy

Pathological Findings
- Serum ferritin: <50 ng/mL
- Transferrin saturation: <16%

DIFFERENTIAL DIAGNOSIS
- Claudication: Movement does not relieve pain and may worsen it.
- Motor neuron disease fasciculation/tremor: No discomfort or circadian pattern
- Dermatitis/pruritus: Urge to move only to scratch; no circadian pattern
- Sleep-related leg cramps: Isolated and very painful muscle contracture
- Periodic limb movement disorder: No wakeful discomfort or movement
- Sleep starts/hypnic jerks: Isolated involuntary events; no discomfort
- Rhythmic movement sleep disorder: Movement periodicity faster than RLS
- Growing pains: No urge to move or relief by movement; circadian pattern opposite RLS
- ADHD: No sleep disorders or complaints in diagnostic criteria (8)[A].

 TREATMENT

1st-line treatments (2,6,9,10)[A]:
- Prescribed daily exercise, adequate sleep
- Dopaminergic medications
- Correction of iron deficiency
- For secondary RLS, treat cause(s); multiple possible causes are *not* mutually exclusive.

MEDICATION
- Use minimum effective dose (2,9,10)[A].
- Daytime sleepiness side effect is unusual with doses and timing for RLS.
- Severe or refractory RLS and augmentation requires combination therapy.

First Line
- FDA-approved dopamine agonists (11)[A]; titrate every 3 days to minimum necessary dose (2)[A]:
  - Pramipexole (Mirapex): 0.125–1.5 mg 1 hour before bed; titrate by 0.125 mg
  - Ropinirole (Requip): 0.25–4.0 mg 1 hour before bed; titrate by 0.25 mg
  - Divide dose for evening and bedtime symptoms.
  - Liver disease: Pramipexole due to renal clearance
  - Renal insufficiency: Ropinirole due to hepatic catabolism

- Off-label dopamine agonists:
  - Cabergoline: 0.25–3.0 mg (warning: Valvulopathy)
  - Carbidopa-levodopa (Sinemet or Sinemet CR): 25/100–100/400; p.r.n. for sporadic symptoms
- Avoid dopamine agonists in psychotic patients, particularly if taking dopamine antagonists.

Second Line
- Anticonvulsants (for painful or neuropathic RLS):
  - Gabapentin (Neurontin): 300–1,800 mg/d
  - Carbamazepine: 200–800 mg/d
  - Pregabalin (Lyrica): 50–300 mg/d
- Opioids (low risk of tolerance/addiction q.h.s.):
  - Hydrocodone: 5–20 mg/d
  - Tramadol: 50 mg/d
  - Oxycodone: 2.5–20 mg/d
- Benzodiazepines and agonists (for associated insomnia and/or anxiety):
  - Temazepam, triazolam, alprazolam, zaleplon, zolpidem, and diazepam
  - Clonazepam (Klonopin): 0.5–3.0 mg/d

Pregnancy Considerations
- Initial approach: Nonpharmacologic therapies, iron supplements (4)[C]
- Most medications class C or D should not be used.
- In 3rd trimester, low-dose opioids or clonazepam may be considered.

Pediatric Considerations
- 1st-line treatment: Nonpharmacologic (3)[C]
- Low-dose clonidine, clonazepam, or gabapentin may be considered.

Geriatric Considerations
- In weak or frail patients, avoid medications that may cause dizziness or unsteadiness.
- Many medications given to the elderly cause or exacerbate RLS (7)[B].

ADDITIONAL TREATMENT
General Measures
- If iron deficient, supplement:
  - 325 mg FeSO₄ with vitamin C between meals
  - Repletion requires months, so symptoms continue.
- Daily exercise is beneficial and sometimes curative (6)[B] (unusual activity may exacerbate symptoms).
- Regular and replete sleep schedule
- Hot bath and leg massage
- Warm the legs (long heavy socks, electric blanket)
- Intense mental activity (games, puzzles, etc.)

Issues for Referral
- Severe symptoms/augmentation; Peripheral neuropathy; low back or leg orthopedic problems
- Peripheral vascular disease; intransigent iron deficiency

Additional Therapies
- Vitamin, mineral supplements: Ca, Mg, B₁₂, folate
- Clonidine: 0.1–0.7 mg/d
- Baclofen: 20–80 mg/d
- Quinine
- Methadone
- OTC sleep aids p.r.n. for mild, intermittent RLS

COMPLEMENTARY AND ALTERNATIVE MEDICINE
- Sequential pneumatic leg compression
- Enhanced external counterpulsation
- Acupuncture
- MicroVas therapy

SURGERY/OTHER PROCEDURES
For orthopedic, neuropathic, or leg vascular disease (laser ablation, sclerotherapy, etc.)

IN-PATIENT CONSIDERATIONS
- Control RLS after orthopedic procedures.
- Addition/withdrawal of medications affecting RLS
- Procedures or new-onset disease that promote RLS
- Changes in medical status may require medication changes. Examples:
  - Renal failure: Mirapex contraindicated
  - Liver disease: Requip contraindicated

IV Fluids
- Iron infusion when Fe replacement fails
- When n.p.o., consider IV opiates

Nursing
- Evening walks, hot baths, leg massage and warming
- Sleep interruption risks prolonged wakefulness.

 ## ONGOING CARE

FOLLOW-UP RECOMMENDATIONS
Patient Monitoring
- At 2-week intervals until stable, then annually
- If taking iron, remeasure ferritin.
- If treatment status changes, assess for associated conditions and medications.

DIET
Avoid evening caffeine and alcohol.

PATIENT EDUCATION
- Restless Legs Syndrome Foundation http://www.rls.org; e-mail: rlsfoundation@rls.org; Tel: 507-287-6465; Fax: 507-287-6312
- WE MOVE (Worldwide Education & Awareness for Movement Disorders); http://www.wemove.org; e-mail: wemove@wemove.org; Tel: 212-875-8312; Fax: 212-875-8389
- National Sleep Foundation http://www.sleepfoundation.org; e-mail: nsf@sleepfoundation.org; Tel: 202-347-3471

PROGNOSIS
- Primary RLS: Lifelong condition with no current cure
- Secondary RLS: May partially or completely subside with resolution of precipitating factors
- Current therapies usually control symptoms.

COMPLICATIONS
- Augmentation of symptoms (severity increases, occurrence earlier, and/or spreading to arms or torso) from prolonged dopamine agonist use:
  - Highest risk from daily levodopa or Sinemet
  - Higher doses of any agonist increase risk.
  - Iron deficiency increases risk.
  - Detitrate dopamine agonist, concurrently add alternative medication (2,9,10)[B].
- Development of obsessive-compulsive or impulse-control disorders from dopamine agonists
- Vicious cycle between sleep loss from RLS and exacerbation of RLS symptoms by sleep loss
- Coping with/correcting for iatrogenic RLS (as from antidepressants, etc.)

REFERENCES
1. Sateia MJ. Restless legs syndrome. In: International Classification of Sleep Disorders Diagnostic & Coding Manual. 2nd ed. Westchester, IL: American Academy of Sleep Medicine; 2005:178–81.
2. Satija P, Ondo WG. Restless legs syndrome: pathophysiology, diagnosis and treatment. CNS Drugs. 2008;22:497–518.
3. Simakajornboon N, Kheirandish-Gozal L, Gozal D et al. Diagnosis and management of restless legs syndrome in children. Sleep Med Rev. 2009;13: 149–56.
4. Thomas K, Watson CB. Restless legs syndrome in women: a review. J Womens Health (Larchmt). 2008;17:859–68.
5. Trotti LM, Bhadriraju S, Rye DB. An update on the pathophysiology and genetics of restless legs syndrome. Curr Neurol Neurosci Rep. 2008;8: 281–7.
6. Aukerman MM, Aukerman D, Bayard M, et al. Exercise and restless legs syndrome: a randomized controlled trial. J Am Board Fam Med. 2006 Sep-Oct;19:487–93.
7. Spiegelhalder K, Hornyak M. Restless legs syndrome in older adults. Clin Geriatr Med. 2008;24:167–80.
8. Walters AS, Silvestri R, Zucconi M, et al. Review of the possible relationship and hypothetical links between attention deficit hyperactivity disorder (ADHD) and the simple sleep related movement disorders, parasomnias, hypersomnias, and circadian rhythm disorders. J Clin Sleep Med. 2008;4:591–600.
9. Ferini-Strambi L. Treatment options for restless legs syndrome. Expert Opin Pharmacother. 2009;10:545–54.
10. Trenkwalder C, Hening WA, Montagna P, et al. Treatment of restless legs syndrome: an evidence-based review and implications for clinical practice. Mov Disord. 2008;23:2267–302.
11. Zintzaras E, Kitsios GD, Papathanasiou AA, et al. Randomized trials of dopamine agonists in restless legs syndrome: a systematic review, quality assessment, and meta-analysis. Clin Ther. 2010;32:221–37.

See Also (Topic, Algorithm, Electronic Media Element)
Periodic Limb Movement Disorder
Algorithm: Restless Leg Syndrome (RLS)

 ## CODES

ICD9
333.94 Restless legs syndrome (RLS)

CLINICAL PEARLS
- Insomnia with frequent tossing/turning and difficulty "getting comfortable" is often RLS.
- RLS and other sleep disorders may cause ADHD (8)[B].
- Many antidepressants, antipsychotics, antiemetics, and antihistamines cause or exacerbate RLS.
- RLS may interfere with use of positive airway pressure to treat obstructive sleep apnea.

RETINAL DETACHMENT

Richard W. Allinson, MD

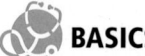 **BASICS**

DESCRIPTION
- Separation of the sensory retina from the underlying retinal pigment epithelium
- Rhegmatogenous retinal detachment (RRD): Most common type; occurs when the fluid vitreous gains access to the subretinal space through a break in the retina (Greek *rhegma*, "rent")
- Exudative or serous detachment: Occurs in the absence of a retinal break, usually in association with inflammation or a tumor
- Traction detachment: Vitreoretinal adhesions mechanically pull the retina from the retinal pigment epithelium. The most common cause is proliferative diabetic retinopathy.
- System(s) affected: Nervous

EPIDEMIOLOGY
Incidence
- Predominant age: Incidence increases with age.
- Predominant sex: Male > Female (3:2)
- Per year: 1/10,000 in patients who have not had cataract surgery

Prevalence
After cataract surgery, 1–3% of patients will develop a retinal detachment.

RISK FACTORS
- Myopia (>5 diopters)
- Aphakia or pseudophakia: In patients undergoing small-incision coaxial phacoemulsification with high myopia (axial length $\geq$26.00 mm), the incidence of retinal detachment is 2.7%.
- Posterior vitreous detachment (PVD) and associated conditions (e.g., aphakia, inflammatory disease, and trauma)
- Trauma
- Retinal detachment in fellow eye
- Lattice degeneration: A vitreoretinal abnormality found in 6–10% of the general population
- Glaucoma: 4–7% of patients with retinal detachment have chronic open-angle glaucoma.
- Vitreoretinal tufts: Peripheral retinal tufts are caused by focal areas of vitreous traction.
- Meridional folds: Redundant retina usually is found in the supranasal quadrant.

Genetics
Most cases are sporadic.

GENERAL PREVENTION
Patients at risk for retinal detachment should have regular ophthalmologic examinations.

ETIOLOGY
- Traction from a PVD causes most retinal tears. With aging, vitreous gel liquefies, leading to separation of the vitreous from the retina. The vitreous gel remains attached at the vitreous base, in the retinal periphery, resulting in vitreous traction that produces tears in the retinal periphery. There is an ~15% chance of developing a retinal tear from a PVD.
- PVD associated with vitreous hemorrhage has a high incidence of retinal tears.

- Exudative detachment:
  - Tumors
  - Inflammatory diseases (Harada, posterior scleritis)
  - Miscellaneous (central serous retinopathy, uveal effusion syndrome, malignant hypertension)
- Traction detachment:
  - Proliferative diabetic retinopathy
  - Cicatricial retinopathy of prematurity
  - Proliferative sickle-cell retinopathy
- Penetrating trauma

Geriatric Considerations
- Posterior vitreous detachment
- Cataract surgery

Pediatric Considerations
Usually associated with underlying vitreoretinal disorders and/or retinopathy of prematurity

COMMONLY ASSOCIATED CONDITIONS
- Lattice degeneration
- High myopia
- Cataract surgery
- Glaucoma
- History of retinal detachment in the fellow eye
- Trauma

Pregnancy Considerations
Preeclampsia/eclampsia may be associated with exudative retinal detachment. No intervention is indicated, provided hypertension is controlled. Prognosis is usually good.

 DIAGNOSIS

HISTORY
- Sudden flashes (photopsia)
- Shower of floaters
- Visual field loss: "Curtain coming across vision"
- Central vision will be preserved if the macula is not detached.
- Poor visual acuity (20/200 or worse), with loss of central vision when macula is detached

PHYSICAL EXAM
- Slit-lamp exam
- Dilated fundus exam with binocular indirect ophthalmoscopy

DIAGNOSTIC TESTS & INTERPRETATION
Visual field testing: Differentiates RRD from retinoschisis. An absolute scotoma is seen in retinoschisis, whereas RRD causes a relative scotoma.

Imaging
- Ultrasound (US) can demonstrate a detached retina and may be helpful when the retina cannot be visualized directly (e.g., with cataracts).
- Fluorescein dye leakage can be seen in exudative retinal detachment; caused by central serous retinopathy and other inflammatory conditions.

Pathological Findings
- Elevation of the neurosensory retina from the underlying retinal pigment epithelium
- Elevation of retina associated with $\geq$1 retinal tears in RRD or elevation of the retina without tears in exudative detachment

- In 3–10% of patients with presumed RRD, no definite retinal break is found.
- Tenting of the retina without retinal tears in traction detachment
- Pigmented cells within the vitreous ("tobacco dust")

DIFFERENTIAL DIAGNOSIS
Retinoschisis (splitting of the retina):
- Vitreous cells and vitreous hemorrhage are found rarely in the vitreous with retinoschisis, whereas they are seen commonly in RRD.
- Retinoschisis usually has a smooth surface and is dome shaped, whereas RRD often has a corrugated, irregular surface.

 TREATMENT

MEDICATION
First Line
- Intraocular gases:
  - Air
  - Perfluoropropane (C_3F_8)
  - Sulfur hexafluoride (SF_6)
- Perfluorocarbon liquids
- Silicone oil
- Contraindications to intraocular gas: Patients with poorly controlled glaucoma
- Precautions with intraocular gas: Expanding intraocular gas bubble increases intraocular pressure; therefore, avoid higher altitudes.
- Significant possible interactions with intraocular gas: Nitrous oxide used in general anesthesia can expand an intraocular gas bubble.

Second Line
Steroids may cause worsening of central serous retinopathy.

ADDITIONAL TREATMENT
General Measures
- Not all retinal tears or breaks need to be treated.
  - Flap or horseshoe tears in symptomatic patients (e.g., patients with flashes or floaters) are treated frequently.
  - Operculated holes in symptomatic patients are treated sometimes.
  - Atrophic holes in symptomatic patients are treated rarely.
- Lattice degeneration with or without holes within the lattice in an asymptomatic patient with prior retinal detachment in the fellow eye may be treated prophylactically.
- Flap retinal tears in asymptomatic patients frequently are treated prophylactically.
- Exudative detachments usually are managed by treating underlying disorder.
- Traction detachments usually are managed by observation. If the fovea is involved, a vitrectomy is needed.

SURGERY/OTHER PROCEDURES

- Timing of repairs:
  - Macula attached: Within 24 h. If the detachment is peripheral and does not have features suggestive of rapid progression (e.g., large and/or superior tears), repair can be performed within a few days.
  - Macula recently detached: Within 10 days of development of a macula-off retinal detachment (1)[B]
  - Old macular detachment: Elective repair within 2 weeks
- If a retinal break has led to the development of a retinal detachment, surgery is needed. Surgical options (and combinations) include
  - Demarcation laser treatment (2)[C]
  - Pneumatic retinopexy: Head positioning is required postoperatively.
  - Scleral buckle
  - Vitrectomy
  - Perfluorocarbon liquids for giant tears (circumferential tears ≥90 degrees)
  - Silicone oil for complex repairs
- Anesthesia: Local or general
- RRD may have >1 break. If any retinal break is not closed at the time of surgery, the surgery will fail.
- Additional surgery may be required if the retina redetaches secondary to a new retinal break or because of proliferative vitreoretinopathy (PVR).
- Adjuvant combination therapy using 5-fluorouracil (5-FU) and low-molecular-weight heparin (LMWH) can reduce the incidence of PVR in patients undergoing vitrectomy for RRD who are at a greater risk of developing PVR, such as patients with uveitis.
- Anterior chamber depth is decreased after scleral buckling surgery. This may become an issue in a patient with or planning to undergo implantation of a phakic intraocular lens (3)[C].

IN-PATIENT CONSIDERATIONS

Initial Stabilization

- Recognition of condition is key (see "Diagnosis").
- Referral to an ophthalmologist for examination and treatment, if indicated

 ONGOING CARE

FOLLOW-UP RECOMMENDATIONS

- Bed rest prior to surgery
- Postoperatively, if intraocular gas has been used, the patient may need specific head positioning and should not travel to high altitudes.

Patient Monitoring

- Alert ophthalmologist if there are new onset of floaters or flashes, increase in floaters or flashes, sudden shower of floaters, curtain or shadow in the peripheral visual field, or reduced vision.
- Patients with acute symptomatic PVD should be reexamined by the ophthalmologist in 3–4 weeks. The development of a retinal detachment is unlikely if no retinal tears are present on reexamination in 3–4 weeks.

- If acute symptomatic PVD is associated with gross vitreous hemorrhage that interferes with complete visualization of the retinal periphery by indirect ophthalmoscopy, the patient should be reexamined at short intervals with indirect ophthalmoscopy until the entire retinal periphery can be observed.
- If the examiner is not certain whether the retina is detached in the presence of opaque medium, US should be performed.

DIET

NPO if surgery is imminent

PATIENT EDUCATION

American Academy of Ophthalmology, 655 E. Beach Street, San Francisco, CA 94109-1336

PROGNOSIS

- RRD:
  - 90% of retinal detachments can be reattached successfully after ≥1 surgical procedures. Postoperative visual acuity depends primarily on the status of the macula preoperatively. Also important is the length of time between the detachment and the repair (75% of eyes with macular detachments of <1 week will obtain a final visual acuity of 20/70 or better).
  - 87% of eyes with a retinal detachment not involving the macula attain a visual acuity of 20/50 or better postoperatively. 37% of eyes with a detached macula preoperatively attain 20/50 or better vision postoperatively.
  - In 10–15% of successfully repaired retinal detachments not involving the macula preoperatively, visual acuity does not return to the preoperative level. This decrease is secondary to complications such as macular edema and macular pucker.
- Tractional retinal detachment: When not involving the fovea, the patient usually can be observed because it is uncommon for these to extend into the fovea.
- Exudative retinal detachment:
  - Management is usually nonsurgical.
  - The presence of shifting fluid is highly suggestive of an exudative retinal detachment. Fixed retinal folds, which are indicative of PVR, are seen rarely in exudative retinal detachment. If the underlying condition is treated, the prognosis generally is good.

COMPLICATIONS

- PVR is the most common cause of failed retinal detachment repair; 10–15% of retinas that reattach initially after retinal surgery will redetach subsequently, usually within 6 weeks, as a result of cellular proliferation and contraction on the retinal surface.
- Partial or total loss of vision owing to macular detachment and/or PVR

- Moderate to severe forms of PVR usually are treated with pars plana vitrectomy and fluid-gas exchange (4)[A]. If a segmental scleral buckle was placed at the initial procedure, it may need to be revised.
- Scleral buckles may erode the overlying conjunctiva and lead to an infection.

REFERENCES

1. Hassan TS, Sarrafizadeh R, Ruby AJ, et al. The effect of duration of macular detachment on results after the scleral buckle repair of primary, macula-off retinal detachments. *Ophthalmology.* 2002;109: 146–52.
2. Vrabec TR, Baumal CR. Demarcation laser photocoagulation of selected macula-sparing rhegmatogenous retinal detachments. *Ophthalmology.* 2000;107:1063–7.
3. Goezinne F, La Heij EC, Berendschot TT, et al. Anterior chamber depth is significantly decreased after scleral buckling surgery. *Ophthalmology.* 2010;117:79–85.
4. Vitrectomy with silicone oil or perfluoropropane gas in eyes with severe proliferative vitreoretinopathy: results of a randomized clinical trial. Silicone Study Report 2. *Arch Ophthalmol.* 1992;110:780–92.

ADDITIONAL READING

Alio JL, Ruiz-Moreno JM, Shabayek MH, et al. The risk of retinal detachment in high myopia after small incision coaxial phacoemulsification. *Am J Ophthalmol.* 2007;144:93–98.

See Also (Topic, Algorithm, Electronic Media Element)

Retinopathy, Diabetic

 CODES

ICD9

- 361.00 Retinal detachment with retinal defect, unspecified
- 361.2 Serous retinal detachment
- 361.81 Traction detachment of retina

CLINICAL PEARLS

- If a patient complains of the new onset of floaters or flashes of light, the patient should undergo a dilated eye examination to rule out a retinal tear or retinal detachment.
- There is an increased risk of retinal detachment after cataract surgery.
- Proliferative vitreoretinopathy can result in redetachment of the retina after an initially successful repair.

RETINITIS PIGMENTOSA

Richard W. Allinson, MD

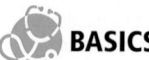 **BASICS**

DESCRIPTION
- An eye disease in which there is progressive damage to the retina with gradual loss of peripheral vision that eventually leads to significant visual impairment; signs often seen in childhood, but severe vision problems do not develop until adulthood.
- Characterized by poor night vision, constricted visual fields, bone spicule–like pigmentation of the fundus, and electroretinographic evidence of photoreceptor cell dysfunction
- System(s) affected: Nervous
- Synonym(s): Rod-cone dystrophy; Retinal dystrophy

EPIDEMIOLOGY
Incidence
- Predominant age:
  - X-linked retinitis pigmentosa (RP) has the earliest onset of the major hereditary types; many X-linked patients are legally blind by age 30.
  - Autosomal dominant RP has a later onset than autosomal recessive or X-linked recessive RP.
  - Leber congenital amaurosis, which is a variant of RP, presents at birth.
  - Late-onset RP typically is asymptomatic and unrecognized until age 40–50 years.
- Predominant sex: Male > Female.

Prevalence
Affects ~1/4,000 people in US

Pediatric Considerations
Leber congenital amaurosis is characterized by severely reduced vision from birth and impaired electroretinogram responses from both cones and rods. Most cases are autosomal recessive.

Geriatric Considerations
Late-onset RP is asymptomatic and generally unrecognized until age >40 years.

RISK FACTORS
Family history
Genetics
- Autosomal dominant: 20%
- Autosomal recessive: 37%
- X-linked recessive: 4.5%
- Sporadic: 38.5%

GENERAL PREVENTION
- Genetic counseling
- No conclusive evidence demonstrates that the amount of light modifies the course of RP. A study in which 1 eye was covered with an opaque lens did not show any difference in disease progression compared with the fellow eye.
- Ultraviolet (UV)–absorbing sunglasses and brimmed hats are recommended when patients are at the beach or in the snow.

ETIOLOGY
- The genetic mutations responsible for RP have been identified in some families with RP, primarily those with the autosomal dominant form.
- Mutations in the rhodopsin gene account for ~30% of cases of autosomal dominant RP.
- Another 4–6% of autosomal dominant RP is caused by a mutation in the gene for a photoreceptor protein peripherin/rds.

COMMONLY ASSOCIATED CONDITIONS
With systemic disorders:
- Usher syndrome: RP and congenital sensorineural hearing impairment
- Laurence-Moon-Biedl syndrome (also called *Bardet-Biedl syndrome*): Autosomal recessive disorder associated with retinal dystrophy, mental retardation, obesity, hypogonadism, and postaxial polydactyly
- Cockayne syndrome: Autosomal recessive disorder in which children at the age of 1–2 years present with retinal dystrophy, sensorineural deafness, cerebellar dysfunction, dementia, and UV light photosensitivity

DIAGNOSIS

HISTORY
- Headache and light flashes are the most common initial complaints.
- Night blindness (nyctalopia)
- Progressive visual field loss
- Central visual acuity is usually preserved until the end stages.

PHYSICAL EXAM
- Bone spicule pigmentation in the retina
- Retinal arteriolar narrowing
- Optic nerve head pallor, "waxy pallor"
- Most patients are myopic.
- Posterior subcapsular cataracts are common in all forms.
- Cystoid macular edema
- Optic nerve head drusen
- Electroretinogram changes
- Retinal neovascularization
- RP is associated with an exudative retinal vasculopathy. Fundus findings include serous retinal detachment, lipid deposition in the retina, and telangiectatic vascular anomalies.
- Variants of RP exist with unusual or regional distribution, including
  - Sectorial RP
  - Pigmented paravenous atrophy
  - Unilateral RP

DIAGNOSTIC TESTS & INTERPRETATION
- Electroretinography: Photoreceptors generate reduced-amplitude A and B waves in RP. Rod and cone responses may be undetectable in advanced RP.
- Visual field testing: A ring scotoma in the midperiphery may be identified. The ring scotoma generally starts as a group of isolated scotomas in the area 20–25° from fixation. Long after the entire peripheral field is gone, a small island of intact central visual field remains.
- Fluorescein angiography can demonstrate cystoid macular edema.
- Fundus photography to document the status of the retina
- Hearing tests in patients complaining of hearing loss, such as those with Usher syndrome (RP with hearing loss)
- Optical coherence tomography can be used to detect and monitor cystoid macular edema.

Lab
- Elevated plasma levels of phytanic acid in Refsum disease
- Acanthocytosis of red blood cells in peripheral blood smear in abetalipoproteinemia, an autosomal recessive disorder in which apolipoprotein B is not synthesized, leading to fat malabsorption and deficiencies of fat-soluble vitamins; therapy with vitamins A and E may improve retinal function.
- Syphilitic neuroretinitis can be diagnosed by performing a fluorescent treponemal antibody absorption or microhemagglutination *Treponema pallidum* test.
- Elevated plasma ornithine levels in gyrate atrophy of the choroid and retina; usually a 10- to 20-fold elevation of plasma ornithine levels

Pathological Findings
- Disappearance of the rods, cones, and outer nuclear layers of the retina
- Bone spicule formation in the retina is secondary to the migration of retinal pigment epithelial cells into the overlying retina.

DIFFERENTIAL DIAGNOSIS
- Bone spicule–like retinal pigmentation and retinal atrophy are nonspecific findings and may result from conditions other than RP.
- Infections
- Syphilis
- Rubella
- Inflammation (severe uveitis)
- Choroidal vascular occlusion
- Toxicity (chloroquine or thioridazine)
- Choroideremia
- Gyrate atrophy of choroid and retina (10- to 20-fold elevation of plasma ornithine levels)
- Systemic metabolic disorders such as Refsum disease and abetalipoproteinemia

- Kearns-Sayre syndrome: Usually presents in adolescents; characterized by progressive external ophthalmoplegia—the 1st sign usually being ptosis—pigmentary degeneration of the retina, and a cardiac conduction defect, which may cause complete heart block
- Cone-rod dystrophy: Characterized by bilateral and symmetric loss of cone function in the presence of reduced rod function
- Cone dystrophy: Characterized by marked abnormality in cone function with some or no rod involvement
- Congenital stationary night blindness
- Oguchi disease
- Fundus albipunctatus
- Trauma

 TREATMENT

MEDICATION

- Vitamin A 15,000 IU/d (retinal degeneration slowed, as measured by electroretinogram/visual fields); β-carotene is not a suitable substitute; has not been studied in patients <18 years of age (1)[A].
- Vitamin E 400 IU/d results in faster retinal degeneration and is not recommended (1)[A].
- Lutein supplementation at a dose of 12 mg/d slowed visual field loss among nonsmoking adults with RP taking vitamin A (2)[B].
- Acetazolamide may be of benefit in the treatment of cystoid macular edema, which may occur in RP; 500 mg/d in a sustained-release capsule was found to be more effective than 250 mg/d.
- Topical dorzolamide may be of benefit in the treatment of cystoid macular edema associated with RP (3)[C].
- Intravitreal bevacizumab and ranibizumab injection may be of benefit in the treatment of cystoid macular edema associated with RP (4,5)[C].
- Contraindications: Women who are pregnant or considering pregnancy should not take >8,000 IU/d of vitamin A. There is an increased incidence of birth defects in babies born to women who ingest higher dosages of vitamin A during pregnancy. Women should consult their obstetrician (6)[A].
- Precautions: Avoid vitamin A supplement dosages >15,000 IU/d because higher dosages may cause liver damage.

Pregnancy Considerations
Risk of teratogenicity with a high intake of vitamin A during pregnancy

ADDITIONAL TREATMENT
General Measures
- Supportive care
- Genetic counseling
- Low-vision aids
- Patient education

SURGERY/OTHER PROCEDURES
- The efficacy of the "Cuban therapy"—electric stimulation, autotransfused ozonized blood, and ocular surgery—has not been proven.
- Macular grid laser photocoagulation may be of benefit in patients with cystoid macular edema secondary to RP.
- Research is being done on photoreceptor and retinal pigment epithelium transplantation, gene therapy, and implantation of a visual prosthesis. The inner retinal neurons may be preserved after death of photoreceptors in RP, which could make some of these experimental procedures feasible (7)[C].

IN-PATIENT CONSIDERATIONS
Initial Stabilization
Outpatient care

 ONGOING CARE

FOLLOW-UP RECOMMENDATIONS
Caution should be exercised because of reduced peripheral vision and poor night vision.

Patient Monitoring
- Ophthalmic examinations every 1–2 years
- Check for complications (e.g., cataracts).

PATIENT EDUCATION
- Counsel patients to help them understand RP and its genetics.
- RP is a slowly progressive, chronic disease; patients do not go blind rapidly, and total blindness is not a frequent endpoint of this disease.
- RP Foundation Fighting Blindness, Executive Plaza One, Suite 800, 11350 McCormick Road, Hunt Valley, MD 21031-1014, (800) 683-5555
- The American Academy of Ophthalmology, 655 E. Beach Street, San Francisco, CA 94109-1336, (415) 561-8540

PROGNOSIS
- Reassurance about the slow course of RP
- Most of the deafness in Usher syndrome is congenital. It is unlikely that an RP patient who is not born deaf will become deaf later in life.
- RP severity varies with inheritance pattern.
- Autosomal recessive form has an early age of onset and may have severely constricted visual fields by age 20 years. Tends toward more rapid progression compared with autosomal dominant RP; also increased incidence of cataracts.
- X-linked RP is similar in clinical presentation to autosomal recessive RP.
- Autosomal dominant RP generally has less severe findings initially than does autosomal recessive RP; symptoms may not occur until 30 years of age.
- Good central vision is usually preserved. If the central visual field radius is >30°, >90% of patients will have visual acuities of 20/40 or better. If the central visual field radius is <10°, 30% of patients will have a visual acuity of 20/40 or better.

COMPLICATIONS
- Cataract
- Cystoid macular edema
- Loss of visual field
- Poor night vision
- Blindness

REFERENCES

1. Berson EL, Rosner B, Sandberg MA, et al. A randomized trial of vitamin A and vitamin E supplementation for retinitis pigmentosa. *Arch Ophthalmol*. 1993;111:761–72.
2. Berson EL, Rosner B, Sandberg MA, et al. Clinical trial of lutein in patients with retinitis pigmentosa receiving vitamin A. *Arch Ophthalmol*. 2010;128:403–11.
3. Grover S, Apushkin MA, Fishman GA. Topical dorzolamide for the treatment of cystoid macular edema in patients with retinitis pigmentosa. *Am J Ophthalmol*. 2006;141:850–8.
4. Yuzbasioglu E, Artunay O, Rasier R, et al. Intravitreal bevacizumab (avastin) injection in retinitis pigmentosa. *Curr Eye Res*. 2009;34:231–7.
5. Artunay O, Yuzbasioglu E, Rasier R, et al. Intravitreal ranibizumab in the treatment of cystoid macular edema associated with retinitis pigmentosa. *J Ocul Pharmacol Ther*. 2009;25:545–50.
6. Rothman KJ, Moore LL, Singer MR, et al. Teratogenicity of high vitamin A intake. *N Engl J Med*. 1995;333:1369–73.
7. Yanai D, Weiland JD, Mahadevappa M, et al. Visual performance using a retinal prosthesis in three subjects with retinitis pigmentosa. *Am J Ophthalmol*. 2007;143:820–7.

 CODES

ICD9
362.74 Pigmentary retinal dystrophy

CLINICAL PEARLS
- Characterized by poor night vision, constricted visual fields, bone spicule–like pigmentation of the fundus, and electroretinographic evidence of photoreceptor cell dysfunction
- Vitamin E 400 IU/d results in faster retinal degeneration and is not recommended.
- RP severity varies with inheritance pattern.

RETINOPATHY, DIABETIC

Richard W. Allinson, MD

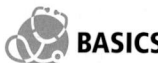

BASICS

DESCRIPTION
- Noninflammatory retinal disorder characterized by retinal capillary closure and microaneurysms. Retinal ischemia leads to release of a vasoproliferative factor stimulating neovascularization on retina, optic nerve, or iris.
- Most patients with diabetes mellitus (DM) will develop diabetic retinopathy (DR). It is the leading cause of new cases of legal blindness among residents in the US between the ages of 20 and 64 years.
- Diabetic retinopathy can be divided into 3 stages:
  - Nonproliferative (background) diabetic retinopathy
  - Severe nonproliferative (preproliferative) diabetic retinopathy
  - Proliferative diabetic retinopathy
- System(s) affected: Nervous

Geriatric Considerations
Prevalence will increase as population generally ages and patients with diabetes live longer.

Pregnancy Considerations
- Pregnancy can exacerbate condition.
- Pregnant diabetic women should be examined in 1st trimester, then every 3 months until delivery.

EPIDEMIOLOGY
Incidence
- Peak incidence of type I, juvenile-onset DM is between the ages of 12 and 15 years.
- Peak incidence of type II, adult-onset DM is between the ages of 50 and 70 years.
- Incidence of diabetic retinopathy is directly related to the duration of diabetes.
- <10 years of age, it is unusual to see diabetic retinopathy, regardless of DM duration.

Prevalence
- 6.6% of US population between ages 20 and 74 has DM.
- ~25% of the diabetic population has some form of diabetic retinopathy.
- Predominant age:
  - The risk increases after puberty.
  - 2/3 of juvenile-onset diabetics who have had DM for at least 35 years will develop proliferative diabetic retinopathy, and 1/3 will develop macular edema. Proportions are reversed for adult-onset diabetes.
- Predominant sex: Male = Female (juvenile-onset DM); Female > Male (type II)

RISK FACTORS
- Duration of DM (usually >10 years)
- Poor glycemic control
- Pregnancy
- Renal disease
- Systemic HTN
- Smoking

- Elevated lipid levels associated with increased risk of retinal lipid deposits (hard exudates)
- Myopic eyes have a lower risk of DR (1)[B]

GENERAL PREVENTION
- Monitor and control of blood glucose
- Schedule yearly ophthalmologic eye examinations.

ETIOLOGY
- Related to development of diabetic microaneurysms and microvascular abnormalities
- Reduction in perifoveal capillary blood flow velocity, perifoveal capillary occlusion, and increased retinal thickness at the central fovea in diabetic patients are associated with visual impairment in patients with diabetic macular edema.

COMMONLY ASSOCIATED CONDITIONS
- Glaucoma
- Cataracts
- Retinal detachment
- Vitreous hemorrhage
- Disc edema (diabetic papillopathy); may occur in type I or type II DM.

DIAGNOSIS

- Nonproliferative (background) diabetic retinopathy:
  - Microaneurysms
  - Intraretinal hemorrhage
  - Macular edema causing decrease in central vision
  - Lipid deposits
- Severe nonproliferative (preproliferative) diabetic retinopathy:
  - Nerve fiber layer infarctions ("cotton wool spots")
  - Venous beading
  - Venous dilatation
  - Intraretinal microvascular abnormalities
  - Extensive retinal hemorrhage
- Proliferative diabetic retinopathy:
  - New blood vessel proliferation (neovascularization) on the retinal surface, optic nerve, and iris
  - Visual loss caused by vitreous hemorrhage, traction retinal detachment

HISTORY
Diabetic patients should be encouraged to undergo an annual ophthalmologic examination yearly.

DIAGNOSTIC TESTS & INTERPRETATION
Diagnostic Procedures/Surgery
- Eye examination: Measurement of visual acuity and documentation of the status of the iris, lens, vitreous, and fundus
- Fluorescein angiography demonstrates retinal nonperfusion, retinal leakage, and proliferative diabetic retinopathy.
- Optical coherence tomography (OCT) can be used to help detect diabetic macular edema by measuring retinal thickness.

Pathological Findings
- Increased capillary permeability
- Microaneurysms
- Hemorrhages in retina
- Exudates in retina
- Capillary nonperfusion

DIFFERENTIAL DIAGNOSIS
Other causes of retinopathy (e.g., radiation, retinal venous obstruction, HTN)

TREATMENT

MEDICATION
- Treatment with the angiotensin-receptor blocker candesartan has been shown to result in regression of diabetic retinopathy in some patients (2)[B].
- Under evaluation: Protein kinase C-β is activated by hyperglycemia and is associated with the development of vascular dysfunction. Inhibition of this enzyme could help to reduce the retinal vascular complications from DM.
- Nutritional antioxidant intake of vitamins C and E and of β-carotene has no protective effect on diabetic retinopathy.
- Atorvastatin may reduce the severity of lipid deposits with clinically significant diabetic macular edema in type II DM and dyslipidemia.

ADDITIONAL TREATMENT
General Measures
- The Diabetes Control and Complications Trial (DCCT) recommended that for most patients with insulin-dependent DM, blood glucose levels should be as close to the nondiabetic range as is safe to do to reduce the risk and rate of progression of diabetic retinopathy:
  - In the DCCT, insulin-dependent DM patients were randomly assigned into either conventional or intensive insulin treatment. Conventional treatment consisted of 1–2 daily insulin injections, with daily self-monitoring of urine or blood glucose. Intensive treatment consisted of insulin administered 3 or more times daily by injection or an external pump, with self-monitored blood glucose levels measured at least 4×/day.
  - The DCCT demonstrated that intensive insulin therapy reduced the risk of macular edema and retinal neovascularization. The benefit of intensive insulin therapy and the reduced risk of diabetic retinopathy–associated microvascular complications persist for at least 10 years (3)[A].
  - In the DCCT, intensive insulin therapy was more effective in reducing the risk of progression of diabetic retinopathy in the less advanced stages. However, advanced diabetic retinopathy also benefited from the intensive insulin therapy.

- The Early Treatment Diabetic Retinopathy Study demonstrated that aspirin therapy did not prevent the development of proliferative diabetic retinopathy or reduce the risk of visual loss associated with diabetic retinopathy.
- Microvascular complications, including proliferative diabetic retinopathy, are increased when blood sugar levels ≥ 200 mg/dL.
- Poor glycemic control is associated with an increased risk both for developing diabetic retinopathy and its progression, regardless of the type of DM; that hyperglycemia itself is causative is not established, especially for type II DM.
- Cataracts are more common among those with DM. Try to delay cataract surgery in DM patients with retinopathy until the symptoms are severe; cataract surgery can cause retinopathy to worsen.
- HTN has a detrimental effect on diabetic retinopathy and must be controlled.

SURGERY/OTHER PROCEDURES

- Laser photocoagulation treatment: Recommended for patients with proliferative diabetic retinopathy and for those with clinically significant macular edema; destroys leaking blood vessels and areas of neovascularization
- The Diabetic Retinopathy Study demonstrated that panretinal photocoagulation reduced overall rate of severe visual loss from 15.9% in untreated eyes to 6.4% in treated eyes. In certain subgroups, the incidence of severe visual loss in untreated eyes was as high as 36.9% within 2 years.
- The Early Treatment Diabetic Retinopathy Study demonstrated that eyes with significant diabetic macular edema benefited from focal laser treatment. Clinically significant diabetic macular edema (CSDME) is defined as:
  - Thickening of the retina within 500 μm of the center of the macula
  - Hard exudates within 500 μm of the center of the macula associated with thickening of the adjacent retina
  - Zone of retinal thickening 1 disc area or larger within 1 disc diameter of the center of the macula
- Patients with clinically significant diabetic macular edema and high-risk proliferative disease can have simultaneous focal and panretinal photocoagulation without adversely affecting the visual outcome.
- Vitrectomy may benefit some with diffuse macular edema. This may apply especially to eyes with vitreomacular traction found on OCT and with persistent clinically significant diabetic macular edema.
- Intravitreal triamcinolone may be used for DM-related macular edema that fails laser treatment. There is no long-term benefit of intravitreal triamcinolone relative to focal/grid photocoagulation in patients with CSDME (4)[C].
- Ranibizumab, an antibody fragment that binds vascular endothelial growth factor (VEGF), can be used to treat CSDME when injected intravitreally (5)[C].

- Bevacizumab, a full-length antibody that binds VEGF, can be used to treat CSDME and proliferative diabetic retinopathy (6)[C].
- Cryoretinopexy can be used instead of laser treatment in certain patients to decrease the neovascular stimulus and treat proliferative diabetic retinopathy.
- Vitrectomy: Recommended for patients with severe proliferative diabetic retinopathy, traction retinal detachment involving the macula, and nonclearing vitreous hemorrhage.

ONGOING CARE

FOLLOW-UP RECOMMENDATIONS
Patient Monitoring
Scheduled ophthalmologic eye examinations:
- Yearly follow-up if no retinopathy
- Every 6 months with background diabetic retinopathy
- At least every 3–4 months with preproliferative diabetic retinopathy
- Every 2–3 months with active proliferative diabetic retinopathy

DIET
Follow prescribed diet for patients with diabetes.

PATIENT EDUCATION
- Patient education should include regular ophthalmic examinations.
- Stress importance of strict blood glucose control through diet, exercise, drugs/insulin, and monitoring of blood glucose.

PROGNOSIS
If the condition is diagnosed and treated early in development, outlook is good. If treatment is delayed, blindness may result.

COMPLICATIONS
Blindness

REFERENCES

1. Lim LS, Lamoureux E, Saw SM, et al. Are myopic eyes less likely to have diabetic retinopathy? *Ophthalmology*. 2010;117:524–30.
2. Sjølie AK, Klein R, Porta M, et al. Effect of candesartan on progression and regression of retinopathy in type 2 diabetes (DIRECT-Protect 2): a randomised placebo-controlled trial. *Lancet*. 2008;372:1385–93.
3. White NH, Sun W, Cleary PA, et al. Prolonged effect of intensive therapy on the risk of retinopathy complications in patients with type 1 diabetes mellitus: 10 years after the Diabetes Control and Complications Trial. *Arch Ophthalmol*. 2008;126: 1707–15.
4. Diabetic Retinopathy Clinical Research Network (DRCR.net), Beck RW, Edwards AR, et al. Three-year follow-up of a randomized trial comparing focal/grid photocoagulation and intravitreal triamcinolone for diabetic macular edema. *Arch Ophthalmol*. 2009;127:245–51.
5. Nguyen QD, Shah SM, et al. Primary End Point (Six Months) Results of the Ranibizumab for Edema of the mAcula in Diabetes (READ-2) Study. *Ophthalmology*. 2009;116:2175–2181.
6. Soheilan M, Ramezani A, et al. Randomized Trial of Intravitreal Bevacizumab Alone or Combined with Triamcinolone versus Macular Photocoagulation in Diabetic Macular Edema. *Ophthalmolohy*. 2009;116:1142–1150.

See Also (Topic, Algorithm, Electronic Media Element)
Diabetes Mellitus, Type 1; Diabetes Mellitus, Type 2.

CODES

ICD9
- 250.50 Diabetes mellitus with ophthalmic manifestations, type ii or unspecified type, not stated as uncontrolled
- 250.51 Diabetes mellitus with ophthalmic manifestations, type I (juvenile type) not stated as uncontrolled
- 362.01 Background diabetic retinopathy

CLINICAL PEARLS

- Options for the treatment of diffuse macular edema include focal laser treatment, intravitreal triamcinolone, intravitreal ranibizumab, intravitreal bevacizumab, and vitrectomy.
- High BP should be controlled to reduce the risk of diabetic eye complications.
- Blood glucose levels should be well controlled to help reduce the risk and rate of progression of diabetic retinopathy.
- Schedule yearly ophthalmologic eye examinations.

RH INCOMPATIBILITY

Donald A.F. Nelson, MD

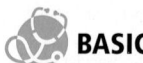 **BASICS**

DESCRIPTION
- Antibody-mediated destruction of red blood cells (RBCs) that bear Rh surface antigens in individuals who lack the antigens and have become isoimmunized (sensitized) to them
- System(s) affected: Hematologic/Lymphatic/Immunologic
- Synonym(s): Rh isoimmunization; Rh alloimmunization; Rh sensitization

EPIDEMIOLOGY
Incidence
Predominant age and sex: Affects fetuses/neonates of isoimmunized child-bearing females

RISK FACTORS
- 15% of white population and smaller fractions of other races are Rh-negative and susceptible to sensitization (1).
- Any Rh-positive pregnancy in an Rh-negative woman can result in sensitization.
- Native risk of isoimmunization after Rh-positive pregnancy had been estimated to be ≤15%, but seems to be decreasing.
- Risk of isoimmunization antepartum is only 1–2%.
- Risk of isoimmunization is 1–2% after spontaneous abortion and 4–5% after induced abortion (2).
- Use of Rho(D) immune globulin prophylaxis has reduced incidence of isoimmunization to <1% of susceptible pregnancies.

Genetics
- Complex autosomal inheritance of polypeptide Rh antigens; 3 genetic loci with closely related genes carry an assortment of alleles: Dd, Cc, and Ee (3).
- Individuals who express the D antigen (also called *Rho* or *Rho[D]*) or its weak D (D^u) variant are considered Rh-positive. Individuals lacking the D antigen are Rh-negative. (There is no antigen identified with the d allele.)
- Antibodies may be produced to C, c, D, E, or e in individuals lacking the specific antigen; only D is strongly immunogenic (4).
- Isoimmunization to Rh antigens in susceptible individuals is acquired, not inherited.

GENERAL PREVENTION
- Blood typing (ABO and Rh) on all pregnant women and prior to blood transfusions
- Antibody screening early in pregnancy
- Rh immune globulin prevents only sensitization to the D antigen.
- For prophylaxis, Rho(D) immune globulin (RhIG, RhoGAM, HyperRHO, RHOphylac) given to unsensitized, Rh-negative women after the following:
  – Spontaneous abortion
  – Induced abortion
  – Ectopic pregnancy
  – Antepartum hemorrhage
  – Trauma to abdomen
  – Amniocentesis
  – Chorionic villus sampling
  – Routinely at 28 weeks' gestation
  – Within 72 h of delivery of an Rh-positive infant
- Dose for prophylaxis:
  – 50-μg (50 microgram) dose for events up to 12 weeks' gestation
  – 300-μg (300 microgram) dose for events after 12 weeks' gestation
  – Higher doses may be required in the event of a large fetal–maternal hemorrhage (>30 mL of whole blood).

PATHOPHYSIOLOGY
- Circulating antibodies to Rh antigens (transplacentally transferred antibodies in the case of a fetus/newborn) attach to Rh antigens on RBCs.
- Immune-mediated destruction of RBCs leads to hemolysis, anemia, and increased bilirubin production.

ETIOLOGY
- Transfusion of Rh-positive blood to Rh-negative recipient
- Maternal exposure to fetal Rh antigens, either antepartum or intrapartum
- Most commonly seen in the Rh-positive fetus or infant of an Rh-negative mother

COMMONLY ASSOCIATED CONDITIONS
- Hemolytic disease of newborn
- Hydrops fetalis
- Neonatal jaundice
- Kernicterus
- See related topic: Erythroblastosis Fetalis

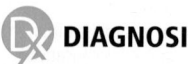 **DIAGNOSIS**

PHYSICAL EXAM
- Jaundice of newborn
- Kernicterus
- Fetal hydrops or fetal death *in utero* if severe (see related topic Erythroblastosis Fetalis)

DIAGNOSTIC TESTS & INTERPRETATION
Lab
Initial lab tests
- Positive indirect Coombs test (antibody screen) during pregnancy
- Paternal blood type
- Kleihauer-Betke (fetal hemoglobin acid elution, Hb F slide elution) test to quantify an acute fetal–maternal bleed
- Congenital or fetal anemia
- Blood type, direct Coombs test in newborn

Follow-Up & Special Considerations
Prior administration of D immune globulin may lead to weakly (false-) positive indirect Coombs test in mother and direct Coombs test in infant.

DIFFERENTIAL DIAGNOSIS
- ABO incompatibility
- Other blood group (non-Rh) isoimmunization
- Nonimmune fetal hydrops
- Hereditary spherocytosis
- RBC enzyme defects

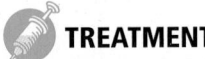

TREATMENT

ADDITIONAL TREATMENT
General Measures
- Depending on severity of involvement, treatment of fetus may include:
  - Intrauterine transfusion
  - Early delivery
- Treatment of newborn may include:
  - Exchange transfusion
  - Transfusion after delivery
  - Phototherapy
  - Diuretics and digoxin for hydrops
  - Immunoglobulin infusion has reduced the need for exchange transfusion in a few studies (5)[C].

Issues for Referral
Because of the specialized, somewhat hazardous treatment measures involved, pregnancies in Rh-sensitized women are usually managed at tertiary-care level.

IN-PATIENT CONSIDERATIONS
Initial Stabilization
Initial monitoring of newborn is inpatient, in special care nursery if treatment interventions are needed.

ONGOING CARE

FOLLOW-UP RECOMMENDATIONS
Patient Monitoring
- In most cases, outpatient ambulatory management is appropriate during the antepartum period.
- Antibody titer measured at 20 weeks and every 4 weeks thereafter during pregnancy; a titer of ≥1:16 indicates the need for further testing (3).
- If the patient had a previously affected infant, an Rh-positive fetus in the current pregnancy should be considered at risk regardless of antibody titers (6):
  - Fetal heart rate testing/ultrasonography to assess fetal status
  - Doppler ultrasonography measurement of cerebral blood flow is now a suitable alternative to invasive tests (amniocentesis, cordocentesis) for diagnosing fetal anemia (6).

- Umbilical blood sampling (cordocentesis) for fetal blood type, hematocrit, reticulocyte count, and presence of erythroblasts (3)
- Amniocentesis for amniotic fluid bilirubin levels (3)
- Amniocentesis for fetal lung maturity if early delivery is a treatment option (3)

PROGNOSIS
- With appropriate monitoring and treatment, infants born of severely affected pregnancies have a survival rate of >80% (3).
- Fetuses with hydrops have a higher mortality rate.
- Even with severe disease, the neurologic outcome of survivors is generally good.
- Disease is likely to be more severe in affected subsequent pregnancies.

COMPLICATIONS
- Pregnancy loss from umbilical blood sampling
- Pregnancy loss from intrauterine transfusion
- Fetal distress requiring emergent delivery (3)

REFERENCES
1. Bianchi DW, Avent ND, Costa JM, et al. Noninvasive prenatal diagnosis of fetal Rhesus D: ready for Prime(r) Time. *Obstet Gynecol*. 2005;106:841–4.
2. Bowman J. Thirty-five years of Rh prophylaxis. *Transfusion*. 2003;43:1661–6.
3. Management of alloimmunization during pregnancy. ACOG Practice Bulletin 75. Aug 2006, reaffirmed 2008.
4. Agre P, Cartron JP. Molecular biology of the Rh antigens. *Blood*. 1991;78:551–63.
5. Alcock GS, Liley H. Immunoglobulin infusion for isoimmune haemolytic jaundice in neonates. *Cochrane Database Syst Rev*. 2006;Issue 1.
6. Moise KJ. Management of rhesus alloimmunization in pregnancy. *Obstet Gynecol*. 2008;112:164–76.

ADDITIONAL READING
Prevention of Rh D alloimmunization. ACOG Practice Bulletin 4. May 1999, reaffirmed 2009.

See Also (Topic, Algorithm, Electronic Media Element)
Anemia, Autoimmune Hemolytic; Erythroblastosis Fetalis; Jaundice

CODES

ICD9
- 656.11 Rhesus isoimmunization, affecting management of mother, delivered
- 656.13 Rhesus isoimmunization, affecting management of mother, antepartum condition
- 773.0 Hemolytic disease of fetus or newborn due to Rh isoimmunization

CLINICAL PEARLS
- If paternity is certain, determining that the father does not carry the Rh(D) blood group antigen eliminates the need to give RhIG prophylaxis during pregnancy or the need for special fetal surveillance if the mother is already sensitized.
- Attempts have been made to determine the fetal blood type noninvasively by detecting fetal DNA in the maternal blood. Because Rh antigens are polymorphic among racial groups, this technique has both false-positive and false-negative results and should be considered experimental.
- The weak D antigen, formerly called D^u, is a weakly reacting variant of the D antigen. A "weak D–positive" mother or infant should be managed as any other D-positive mother or infant, respectively.
- The dose of RhIG for prophylaxis is affected by gestational age. The fetal blood volume is only a few milliliters at 12 weeks' gestation. Therefore, a 50-μg (50 microgram) dose of RhIG may be used for threatened, spontaneous, or induced abortions up to 12 weeks' gestation instead of the standard 300-μg (300 microgram) dose.

RHABDOMYOLYSIS

Caroline Tschibelu, MD
Otis Warren, MD

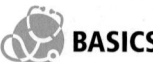 **BASICS**

DESCRIPTION
- Breakdown (necrosis) of skeletal muscle cells and release of the intracellular contents into the circulation
- Rhabdomyolysis typically manifests with muscle aches, pains and weakness, and reddish brown (tea-colored) urine, but up to 50% of patients are asymptomatic.

EPIDEMIOLOGY
Incidence
26,000 hospitalized cases annually

RISK FACTORS
See Etiology.
Genetics
- Hereditary causes of rhabdomyolysis are infrequent but should be suspected in the following groups presenting with rhabdomyolysis: Children, patients with recurrent attacks, or patients with attacks after minimal exertion, mild illness, or starvation.
- Main inherited disorders include:
  - Lipid metabolism (e.g., carnitine palmitoyltransferase deficiency, long-chain acyl-CoA dehydrogenase)
  - Carbohydrate metabolism (e.g., most common is myophosphorylase deficiency aka McArdle disease, phosphofructokinase deficiency, phosphoglycerate mutase)
  - Mitochondrial disorders (e.g., succinate dehydrogenase, coenzyme Q10)
  - Pentose phosphate pathway: Glucose-6-phosphate dehydrogenase
  - Muscular dystrophies have various modes of genetic transmission (e.g., Duchenne, Becker, myotonic dystrophy)

GENERAL PREVENTION
- Avoid traumatic or exertional muscle injury. Preventing hypovolemia important to prevent renal hypoperfusion, acidemia, and subsequent renal failure.
- Avoid precipitating drugs, metabolic and electrolytes abnormalities

ETIOLOGY
- Drugs and toxins:
  - Alcohol
  - Cocaine, methamphetamine, phencyclidine
  - Antipsychotics
  - Zidovudine
  - Antimalarials
  - Heroin
  - HMG-CoA reductase inhibitors (statins) (risk <0.01%)
  - Fibrates
  - Colchicine
  - Corticosteroids
  - Carbon monoxide
  - Snake envenomation
- Muscle exertion:
  - Intense physical exercise
  - Seizures
  - Delirium tremens
- Direct muscle trauma:
  - Crush injuries
  - Contact sports, boxing, physical torture
  - Extended periods of muscle pressure (during surgery, unconscious from alcohol)
  - Burns, electrocution, lightning strike
- Muscle ischemia:
  - Thrombosis, embolism, sickle-cell disease
  - Compartment syndrome
  - Tourniquets
- Infections:
  - Viral: Influenza A and B, coxsackievirus, HIV, varicella
  - Bacterial: *Streptococcus* or *Staphylococcus* sepsis, gas gangrene, necrotizing fasciitis, *Salmonella*, *Legionella*
  - Malaria
- Hypothermia
- Hyperthermia:
  - Heat stroke
  - Neuroleptic malignant syndrome
  - Malignant hyperthermia
- Autoimmune and genetic disorders:
  - Polymyositis, dermatomyositis
  - Muscular dystrophies
  - Disorders of lipid metabolism (e.g., carnitine palmitoyltransferase deficiency and carnitine deficiency)
  - Disorders of carbohydrate metabolism (i.e., phosphofructokinase deficiency, phosphoglycerate mutase, myophosphorylase deficiency, aka McArdle disease/deficiency)
  - Glycogen storage diseases (e.g., phosphorylase B kinase deficiency) and others (e.g., lactate dehydrogenase A deficiency)
- Metabolic and endocrinologic:
  - Hypothyroidism or thyrotoxicosis
  - Electrolyte imbalances (e.g., hyponatremia, hypernatremia, hypokalemia, hypocalcemia, hypophosphatemia)
  - Diabetic ketoacidosis
  - Hyperosmolar states
- Inflammatory conditions:
  - Polymyositis
  - Dermatomyositis

DIAGNOSIS

HISTORY
- Crush injury: Direct trauma or prolonged compression or immobility. Causes include MVA, entrapment in collapsed buildings. The elderly are more susceptible to crush injury due to immobility. Rhabdomyolysis usually occurs after 1 h of immobilization, but cases reported with compression lasting less than 20 min (1).
- Possible history of overexertion or use of drug or toxin
- Muscle aches, cramps, or fatigue
- Tea-colored urine is indicative of myoglobinuria.
- Decreased urine output may indicate renal failure.

PHYSICAL EXAM
- Tender muscles
- May have obvious muscle injury and swelling on exam (e.g., crush injury, compartment syndrome), or muscle exam may be completely normal.

DIAGNOSTIC TESTS & INTERPRETATION
Lab
Initial lab tests
- Muscle enzyme elevations (e.g., creatinine kinase [CK], aldolase, and lactic dehydrogenase [LDH]). CK >5 times the upper limit of normal or >1,000 units/L is usually used for diagnosis of rhabdomyolysis. CK levels >5,000 units/L are closely related to renal failure, but cases have been reported of patients with CK >30,000 units/L who did not develop ARF.
- CK levels peak at ~24 hours and return to normal after 3–5 days, making it a more sensitive marker than myoglobin. Myoglobin, however, is the enzyme responsible for kidney failure (1).
- Serum myoglobin levels peak within a few hours and return to normal after ~24 hours because the protein is cleared quickly from the circulation. Urine or serum myoglobin levels may be useful marker in early diagnosis, but normal levels do not rule out rhabdomyolysis because of its rapid clearance.
- Urinalysis: Dipstick test positive for blood without erythrocytes in sediment is suggestive of injury from either hemoglobin or myoglobin. However, rhabdomyolysis often presents with hematuria, which is a limitation to using dipstick due to false-positive results.
- Marked elevations of potassium from the muscle injury sometimes are compounded by acute renal failure.
- Initial hypocalcemia: Calcium enters the injured muscle cells and precipitates as calcium phosphate leading to calcification of ischemic muscle cells.
- Hypercalcemia during renal recovery phase: Unique to rhabdomyolysis-induced ARF, occurs in 20–30% of patients. As renal function improves, there is mobilization of calcium that was precipitated in injured muscle cells, increase in calcitriol and hyperphosphatemia resolves. Thus, only correct initial hypocalcemia if patient is symptomatic/has EKG changes; otherwise, it will self-resolve.
- Extreme hyperuricemia may be present and can cause acute uric acid nephropathy in the setting of rhabdomyolysis.
- Elevations in blood urea nitrogen (BUN) and creatinine indicative of acute renal failure.
- Reversible hepatic dysfunction can occur. However, elevations in ALT, AST, and LDH may be due to muscle injury and may not indicate any hepatic injury.
- Disseminated intravascular coagulation (DIC) can occur with increase in coagulation times, fibrin degradation products, and D-dimer; decreases in platelets and fibrinogen.

Follow-Up & Special Considerations
- Delayed renal failure or electrolyte abnormalities despite normal initial levels
- Ongoing muscle injury is manifested by rising creatine phosphokinase (CPK).

Imaging
Initial approach
None routine

Follow-Up & Special Considerations
Any renal imaging is similar to other evaluations of acute renal failure.

Diagnostic Procedures/Surgery
Muscle compartment pressures if compartment syndrome suspected

Pathological Findings
- Muscle necrosis
- Myoglobin-related renal injury may resemble acute tubular necrosis from other causes.

DIFFERENTIAL DIAGNOSIS
- For acute renal failure with rhabdomyolysis: Any disease that causes acute tubular necrosis may be confused with rhabdomyolysis.
- Renal pigment injury from hemoglobin resembles pigment injury from myoglobin.

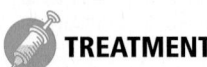 TREATMENT

MEDICATION

First Line
- When rhabdomyolysis is identified, appropriate intervention may prevent renal failure.
- Aggressive fluid resuscitation is the most important intervention: Normal saline and 5% glucose solution with a target urine output of 200 mL/h. Alternating NS and 5% glucose is recommended to prevent volume overload. Infusion rate should be 500 mL/h (1).
- Alkalinization of the urine is thought to decrease myoglobin-induced nephrotoxicity in the tubules (sodium bicarbonate to increase urine pH >6.5):
  - Use is controversial without strong evidence of efficacy
  - Side effects include worsening hypocalcemia.
  - Sodium bicarbonate may be of use in patients with very high CK levels, an acidotic state, or coexisting hyperkalemia.
- IV mannitol as a bolus, 1–2 g/kg , not to exceed 200 g in 24 hours and cumulative dose up to 800 mg. It is used by some to prevent acute renal failure' plasma osmolality should be closely monitored and stopped if diuresis is not adequate (>20 mL/hr):
  - Causes renal vasodilation and diuresis that make the kidneys less susceptible to myoglobin injury. As an osmotic agent, may also remove fluids trapped in damaged muscle cells preventing rise in compartment pressure and potential compartment syndrome.
  - Use of mannitol is controversial in this setting because there is no good evidence that it improves outcomes more than aggressive IV hydration. Doses >800 mg associated with osmotic nephrosis (AKI due to renal vasoconstriction and tubular injury).
  - Consider adding furosemide to force diuresis if necessary (40–120 mg/day) (1).
  - Diuresis should not be used in anuric renal failure. Customize regimen for elderly and patients with heart disease.

Second Line
- Hyperkalemia can result from massive release of intracellular potassium stores or acute renal failure. Severe hyperkalemia may be life-threatening. Treatment is warranted when ECG changes are present (tall, thin T waves; P-R prolongation; QRS widening; P-wave flattening).
- Treatments aiming at resolving hyperkalemia:
  - Calcium gluconate: IV 1–2 ampules (0.5 mL 10% calcium gluconate = 4 mg elemental calcium; give 4 mg/kg/h × 4 h)
  - If acidosis is present: 1–2 ampules (2–3 mL/kg) sodium bicarbonate IV. Remember that

bicarbonate administration may lead to alkalosis and worsening hypocalcemia.
  - If tolerated: Oral sodium polystyrene sulfonate (Kayexalate) as much as 20 g (1 g/kg); also can be given via enema if oral intake is not tolerated or not indicated.
  - Insulin and albuterol will transiently drive potassium into the cells. Administration of glucose can prevent the hypoglycemic effects of insulin.
  - Calcium, as already mentioned, for severe symptomatic hypocalcemia
  - Contraindications: See manufacturer's literature for each drug.
  - Precautions: See Etiology, especially drug combinations
  - Indications for dialysis include resistant and symptomatic hyperkalemia (EKG), oliguria (<0.5 mL/kg over 12 h period), anuria, volume overload, or persistent acidosis (PH <7.1).

ADDITIONAL TREATMENT

General Measures
- Aggressive hydration is often necessary. With severe muscle trauma (crush injuries), up to 12 L of fluid may be sequestered in the muscles, leading to intravascular volume depletion and explaining the low urine output despite fluids resuscitation. Those increase the risk for renal failure.
- Monitor CK levels to ensure that rhabdomyolysis has ended.
- Monitor renal function and electrolytes.
- If DIC or hepatic dysfunction occurs, patients will need treatment and monitoring appropriate to these conditions.

Issues for Referral
- Usually managed as an inpatient
- Diagnosis of muscle entrapment or compartment syndromes may require surgical intervention (fasciotomy) to stop rhabdomyolysis
- Early escharotomy for compartment syndrome related to burn
- Renal dialysis may be indicated in acute renal failure.

Additional Therapies
Severe hypocalcemia with symptoms (perioral paresthesia, Chvostek and Trousseau signs present) during the oliguric phase may benefit from IV calcium gluconate. Symptomatic hypocalcemia is rare.

SURGERY/OTHER PROCEDURES
For muscle entrapment or compartment syndrome

IN-PATIENT CONSIDERATIONS

Admission Criteria
- Patients with significant elevations of CK should be admitted for IV hydration and serial laboratory monitoring.
- Usually required for symptomatic patients or other complications

IV Fluids
Volume expansion with normal saline to increase urine output to at least 150 mL/h

Nursing
Monitoring of vital signs and urine output

Discharge Criteria
CK usually peaks 24–36 hours after muscle injury, so monitoring should confirm that the CK is trending down. Renal function should be stable or improving. Electrolytes should be normal. Patients with mild CK elevation, trending down, and normal renal function may be discharged after observation phase.

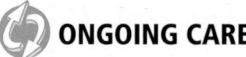 ONGOING CARE

FOLLOW-UP RECOMMENDATIONS
Outpatient assessment within a few days to recheck CPK, electrolytes, and renal function

Patient Monitoring
- Contingent on disease: Essential for metabolic myopathies
- Myotoxic drugs should be discontinued or monitored closely.

DIET
- When rhabdomyolysis causes renal failure, restrict protein intake to lower BUN level.
- Potassium intake must be limited.
- With anuria, essential to restrict volume intake; once resolved, no restrictions

PATIENT EDUCATION
- Appropriate counseling regarding suspected etiology
- Signs and symptoms of recurrence

PROGNOSIS
Contingent on primary cause of rhabdomyolysis and on recovery from acute renal failure without complications

COMPLICATIONS
- Death, especially from hyperkalemia or renal failure
- With dialysis and supportive care, the prognosis is very good.

REFERENCE
1. Cervellin G, Comelli I, Lippi G, et al. Rhabdomyolysis: historical background, clinical, diagnostic and therapeutic features. Clin Chem Lab Med. 2010;48:749–56.

ADDITIONAL READING
Bosch X, Poch E, Grau JM et al. Rhabdomyolysis and acute kidney injury. N Engl J Med. 2009;361:62–72.

See Also (Topic, Algorithm, Electronic Media Element)
Renal Failure, Acute

 CODES

ICD9
728.88 Rhabdomyolysis

CLINICAL PEARLS
- Acute CPK elevation into the thousands (often tens of thousands) is necessary before one sees myoglobinuric renal failure.
- Cornerstone of treatment of rhabdomyolysis is aggressive fluid administration.
- Frequent monitoring of potassium, calcium, and creatinine is necessary in the acute period.

RHEUMATIC FEVER

Manju Ramchandani, MD
Rajneesh S. Hazarika, MD, MS

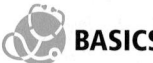 **BASICS**

DESCRIPTION
- Acute rheumatic fever (ARF) is a recurrent inflammatory disease, possibly autoimmune in nature, that affects multiple organ systems.
- Delayed nonsuppurative sequelae of pharyngeal infection with group A streptococci can cause permanent cardiac valvular disease as well as acute cardiac decompensation.
- Recurrences in both adults and children are common if not prevented with prophylactic antibiotic treatment.
- System(s) affected: Cardiovascular; Hematologic/Lymphatic/Immunologic; Musculoskeletal; Nervous; Skin/Exocrine

Pediatric Considerations
- More common in children
- ARF develops in 1–3% of children who have untreated group A β-hemolytic streptococcal pharyngitis (1).

EPIDEMIOLOGY
Incidence
- ARF and Rheumatic Heart Disease (RHD) are now largely restricted to developing countries and some poor, mainly indigenous populations of wealthy countries.
- Predominant age: Most common in children ages 5–15 years
- Predominant sex: Male = Female. Females are more prone to develop chorea.
- The incidence of rheumatic fever in the US had been declining for decades. In the 1970s, it was a rare disease, with a case incidence of 0.5–1.88/100,000.
- However, since the mid-1980s, a resurgence of cases has occurred, with multiple outbreaks reported.
- The incidence of ARF in some developing countries exceeds 50 per 100,000 children.

Prevalence
- Prevalence of rheumatic heart disease (RHD) in the US is now <0.05/1,000 population, with rare regional outbreaks.
- 15.6 million people worldwide have RHD. There are 470,000 new cases of rheumatic fever and 233,000 deaths attributable to rheumatic fever or RHD each year (2).

RISK FACTORS
Possible deficiency of iron and albumin (3)[B]

Genetics
Certain human leukocyte antigen (HLA) class II DR and DQ genotypes and haplotypes (3)[B]

GENERAL PREVENTION
- Primary prevention: Antibiotics are effective at reducing incidence of ARF after known or suspected group A streptococcal pharyngitis. To achieve clinical and bacteriologic cures, treat streptococcal pharyngitis with 10 days of penicillin, an oral cephalosporin, or an oral macrolide in patients who are allergic to penicillin (4)[A].
- Secondary prevention: Long-term prophylaxis (with penicillin G or a macrolide) in selected populations

PATHOPHYSIOLOGY
- Presents 1–4 weeks following an untreated group A β-hemolytic streptococcal pharyngitis or tonsillitis (most strains); group G and group C streptococci with certain group A antigens/enzymes also may be important.
- Molecular mimicry is thought to play an important role in initiation of tissue injury (hyaluronic capsule is identical to human hyaluronate and a cross-reactive antibody to human heart).
- Acute exudative and subacute proliferative cellular reactions in connective tissue and around small blood vessels

ETIOLOGY
- Preceding infection of the upper respiratory tract with group A streptococcal organisms is a prerequisite to the development of ARF.
- Autoimmune mechanisms

 DIAGNOSIS

- The modified Jones criteria for the diagnosis of ARF include 2 major manifestations or 1 major and 2 minor manifestations.
- In either case, evidence must exist of preceding group A streptococcal (GAS) infection (either positive throat culture for GAS/positive streptococcal antigen test/elevated or rising streptococcal antibody titer).
- Major criteria include carditis, arthritis, chorea, erythema marginatum, and subcutaneous nodules.
- Minor criteria include fever, arthralgia (cannot use if arthritis was used as a major criteria), previous rheumatic fever, acute-phase laboratory results such as an elevated erythrocyte sedimentation rate (ESR) or C-reactive protein (CRP) and prolonged PR interval on ECG

HISTORY
- Pharyngitis usually 2–4 weeks earlier
- Acute febrile illness with malaise, muscle weakness
- Migratory large joint polyarthritis and arthralgia (75%) with dramatic response to even small doses of salicylates.
- Leg joints typically are involved first, and symptoms are almost always transient.
- In patients treated with anti-inflammatory drugs, arthritis may be monoarticular, may not migrate, or may subside quickly.
- Chest discomfort, pleuritic chest pain
- Rash
- Choreiform movements are a late manifestation (5%).
- Emotional disturbances, outbursts of inappropriate behavior, crying, restlessness

PHYSICAL EXAM
- Pericardial frictional rub
- Pancarditis (50%): Blowing pansystolic murmur, rarely diastolic or new or changing murmurs
- Evidence of heart failure
- Subcutaneous nodules (<1%): Firm, painless, to 2 cm, over bony surface, prominences, or near tendons present for a few weeks
- Erythema marginatum: Nonpruritic erythematous rings on trunk that transiently appear and disappear over months, can be accentuated by warming the skin

- Sydenham chorea (10–15%): Nonrhythmic involuntary movements, more marked on 1 side, cease during sleep, may last up to 8 months
- "Milking sign": Diffuse hypotonia with no sensory losses

DIAGNOSTIC TESTS & INTERPRETATION
Lab
- Increased acute-phase reactants including ESR and CRP (4)[C]
- Bacteriologic or serologic evidence of GAS infection, antistreptolysin O (ASO, 80%), streptozyme, or antideoxyribonuclease B (DNAase) or antihyaluronidase (4)[C]
- Normocytic, normochromic anemia

Initial lab tests
- Prior treatment with aspirin or steroids may alter lab results.
- Complete blood count with differential, ESR, CRP
- Throat culture for group A hemolytic streptococci (75% are negative) (5)
- Streptococcal antibodies: ASO titers (peak at 4–5 weeks); if negative, check ASO anti-DNase B (detectable for 6–9 months), streptokinase, and antihyaluronidase.
- No changes in complement levels
- ECG: All degrees of heart block, including prolonged PR interval, A-V dissociation, evidence of pericarditis
- Joint aspiration of affected joints reveals sterile inflammatory fluid.

Follow-Up & Special Considerations
- Repeat ASO titers in 1–2 weeks for comparison (cannot be used as a measure of rheumatogenic activity).
- CRP and ESR are useful in monitoring rebounds of inflammation.

Imaging
Initial approach
- CXR: Most common radiologic manifestation of carditis is cardiomegaly.
- Echocardiography to assess for chamber size and function, valvular disease including silent mitral regurgitation, and pericardial effusion (4)[C]; comprehensive echocardiographic screening identified approximately 10 times as many children with RHD as were identified by the traditional strategy of clinical screening with echocardiographic confirmation (6).
- Antimyosin scintigraphy for detection of carditis (80% sensitive but not specific) (7)
- Radiographs of affected joints rarely may show slight effusion.

Follow-Up & Special Considerations
- Serial CXRs to monitor carditis
- Serial ECGs to document course of valvular lesions

Pathological Findings
- Fibrinous pericardium and Anitschkow cells: Cardiac histiocytes
- Aschoff bodies: Focal inflammation surrounding fibrinoid necrosis
- Aschoff cells: Multinucleated giant cells in mass of fragmented swollen collagen fibers
- Subcutaneous nodules have a characteristic histologic appearance.

DIFFERENTIAL DIAGNOSIS
- Systemic lupus erythematosus
- Poststreptococcal reactive arthritis
- Juvenile rheumatoid arthritis
- Infectious arthritis
- Viral myocarditis
- Innocent cardiac murmurs
- Tourette syndrome
- Kawasaki syndrome
- PANDAS

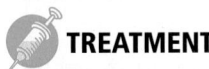 **TREATMENT**

MEDICATION
First Line
- Symptomatic relief
- Eradication: Treat initially with penicillin as if active streptococcal infection is present; then begin prophylaxis (see "Follow-Up").
- If patient has moderate-severe carditis with cardiomegaly/CHF, treat with prednisone 2 mg/kg/d (60 mg/d max) × 2 weeks; then taper over 2 weeks. Data on use of steroids are inconclusive (8)[C].
- If no cardiomegaly, start aspirin 80–100 mg/kg/d in children and 4–8 g/d in adults × 4–6 weeks. Start aspirin at beginning of steroid taper, and continue until symptoms are absent and ESR and CRP are normal (may be ~6 weeks).
- Antibiotic therapy:
  – Penicillin × 10 days IM or IV
  – If penicillin allergic, use a narrow-spectrum cephalosporin or a macrolide such as erythromycin.
- Chorea may require sedation with phenobarbital or haloperidol. IVIG may be beneficial (9)
- Household contacts should be screened with a throat culture and treated with appropriate antibiotics even if asymptomatic.
- Contraindications: Specific drug allergies
- Precautions:
  – Usual steroid side effects
  – Haloperidol can cause extrapyramidal effects.
- Significant possible interactions: Refer to the manufacturer's profile of each drug.

Second Line
For children, naproxen at a dose of 15–20 mg/kg/d divided b.i.d. has been found to be safe and effective in ARF and has fewer adverse reactions than aspirin.

ADDITIONAL TREATMENT
General Measures
- Mainstay of therapy is anti-inflammatory, especially for patients with carditis.
- Treat arrhythmias with appropriate agents.
- Pain relief for patients with arthritis
- Heart failure therapy as needed

Issues for Referral
Patients should be managed or co-managed by a cardiologist.

SURGERY/OTHER PROCEDURES
Mitral stenosis is a manifestation of late scarring and calcification of damaged valves that often requires surgical correction (valve repair or replacement), especially in presence of left atrial enlargement.

IN-PATIENT CONSIDERATIONS
Initial Stabilization
- Initial hospitalization may be helpful for diagnosis and to establish stability of the patient.
- Congestive heart failure (CHF) requires prompt hospitalization.

 ONGOING CARE

FOLLOW-UP RECOMMENDATIONS
- Initial bed rest with activity increasing gradually as tolerated
- Advance activity cautiously if evidence of carditis is present.
- ARF patients should be on prophylactic antibiotics throughout childhood and possibly indefinitely during adulthood.
  – Preferred treatment regimen is monthly IM injections of 1.2 million units of benzathine penicillin.
  – Oral penicillin V-K 250 mg bid is an alternative to monthly injections for patients at lower risk for recurrence.
  – Patients should be treated for a minimum of 5 years after an attack or until age 18.
  – In adults with valvular disease, consider treating indefinitely.
  – If penicillin allergic, treat with sulfadiazine 500 mg/d for children weighing <27 kg up to a maximum dose of 1 g/d for adults. Fluid intake should be maintained ≥1500 mL/day to guard against sulfadiazine crystalluria.
- If patients have valvular damage from ARF, they also require bacterial endocarditis prophylaxis for dental and other high-risk procedures (10).
- Low threshold to test and treat acute episodes of GAS pharyngitis

Patient Monitoring
Initially each week, then every 6 months

Pediatric Considerations
Use aspirin with great caution in children, given the potential risk of Reye syndrome.

Pregnancy Considerations
Residual valvular disease may be exacerbated by pregnancy. Refer preconception and pregnant patients to a cardiologist for assistance in management.

DIET
- Regular diet
- Low-sodium diet initially, if the patient has carditis

PATIENT EDUCATION
American Heart Association: http://www.americanheart.org/presenter.jhtml?identifier=4709

PROGNOSIS
Sequelae are limited to the heart and depend on the severity of carditis during an acute attack.

COMPLICATIONS
- Subsequent attacks of ARF secondary to streptococcal reinfection
- Cardiac sequelae including carditis, RHD (specifically mitral stenosis, more likely in patients with carditis), and CHF

REFERENCES
1. Ruttenberg HD. Acute rheumatic fever in the 1980s. *Pediatrician.* 1986;13:180–8.
2. Carapetis JR, Steer AC, Mulholland EK, et al. The global burden of group A streptococcal diseases. *Lancet Infect Dis.* 2005;5:685–94.
3. Mostafa Zaman M. Association of rheumatic fever with serum albumin concentration and body iron stores in Bangladeshi children: Case-control study. *Br Med J.* 1998;317(7168):1287.
4. Hahn R. Evaluation of poststreptococcal illness. *Am Fam Physician.* 2005;71(10):1865.
5. Guidelines for the diagnosis of rheumatic fever. Jones Criteria, 1992 update. Special Writing Group of the Committee on Rheumatic Fever, Endocarditis, and Kawasaki Disease of the Council on Cardiovascular Disease in the Young of the American Heart Association. *JAMA.* 1992;268:2069–73.
6. Marijon E, Ou P. Prevalence of Rheumatic Heart Disease Detected by Echocardiographic Screening: *New Eng Journal.* 2007;357:470–6.
7. Narula J, Malhotra A, Yasuda T, et al. Usefulness of antimyosin antibody imaging for the detection of active rheumatic myocarditis. *Am J Cardiol.* 1999;84:946–50, A7.
8. Cilliers AM, Manyemba J, Saloojee H. Anti-inflammatory treatment for carditis in acute rheumatic fever. *Cochrane Database Syst Rev.* 2003:CD003176.
9. van Immerzeel TD, van Gilst RM, Hartwig NG et al. Beneficial use of immunoglobulins in the treatment of Sydenham chorea. *Eur J Pediatr.* 2010;169:1151–4.
10. Nishimura RA, Carabello BA, Faxon DP, et al. ACC/AHA 2008 Guideline update on valvular heart disease: focused update on infective endocarditis: a report of the American College of Cardiology/American Heart Association Task Force on Practice Guidelines endorsed by the Society of Cardiovascular Anesthesiologists, Society for Cardiovascular Angiography and Interventions, and Society of Thoracic Surgeons. *J Am Coll Cardiol.* 2008;52:676–85.

 CODES

ICD9
- 390 Rheumatic fever without mention of heart involvement
- 391.0 Acute rheumatic pericarditis
- 391.1 Acute rheumatic endocarditis

CLINICAL PEARLS
- ARF is a recurrent inflammatory disease, possibly autoimmune in nature, that affects multiple organ systems including the heart.
- The modified Jones criteria for the diagnosis of ARF include 2 major manifestations or 1 major and 2 minor manifestations in the context of a preceding documented GAS infection.
- ARF patients should be on prophylactic antibiotics throughout childhood.

RHINITIS, ALLERGIC

Michael C. Barros, PharmD, BCPS
Colleen F. Medeiros, PharmD, BCPS
Vu Ho, MD

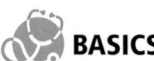

BASICS

DESCRIPTION
- IgE-mediated inflammation of the nasal mucosa following exposure to airborne allergens
- An immediate symptomatic response characterized by sneezing, congestion, and rhinorrhea is followed by a persistent late phase dominated by congestion and mucosal hyperreactivity.
  - Seasonal responses usually associated with outdoor allergens: Pollen, grasses, trees, weeds
  - Perennial responses usually associated with indoor allergens: Dust mites, mold, and animal dander
- ARIA (Allergic Rhinitis and its Impact on Asthma) Guidelines suggest defining and treating allergic rhinitis on severity and duration of symptoms: Intermittent or persistent.
- System(s) affected: Respiratory, upper and lower; Immunologic
- Synonym(s): Hay fever; Rose fever; Pollinosis; IgE-mediated rhinitis

Pediatric Considerations
Chronic nasal obstruction can result in facial deformities, dental malocclusions, and sleep disorders.

Pregnancy Considerations
Physiologic changes during pregnancy may aggravate all types of rhinitis, frequently in the 2nd trimester.

EPIDEMIOLOGY
Onset usually in first 2 decades, rarely before 6 months of age, with tendency declining with advancing age

Prevalence
- ~10–25% of the US adult population and 9–42% of the US pediatric population is affected.
- 44–87% of patients with allergic rhinitis have mixed allergic and nonallergic rhinitis, which is more common than either pure form (1).

RISK FACTORS
- Family history of atopy
- Higher socioeconomic status
- Presence of positive allergy skin prick test
- Tobacco smoke can exacerbate symptoms and can increase risk of developing asthma in patients with allergic rhinitis, but no evidence for causing allergic rhinitis.
- Unclear evidence regarding risk owing to early, repeated exposure to offending allergen and early introduction of solid food.

Genetics
Complex but strong genetic predilection present (80% have family history of allergic disorders)

GENERAL PREVENTION
- Primary prevention of atopic disease has not been proven effective by maternal diet or maternal allergen avoidance (2).
- Symptomatic control by environmental avoidance by patient is "1st-line treatment."
- Use of acaricides along with mite-proof mattress and pillow covers, carpet and drape removal, removal of plants in the home, pet control (2,3)[B]
- Air conditioning and limited outside exposure during allergy season (1)[B]

- HEPA air cleaners and vacuum bags are of unclear efficacy.

PATHOPHYSIOLOGY
Aeroallergen-driven mucosal inflammation owing to resident and infiltrating inflammatory cells, as well as vasoactive and proinflammatory mediators (e.g., cytokines)

ETIOLOGY
Inhalant allergens:
- Perennial: House dust mites, indoor molds, animal dander, cockroach/insect detritus
- Seasonal: Tree, grass, and weed pollens; outdoor molds
- Occupational: Latex, plant products (e.g., baking flour), sensitizing chemicals

COMMONLY ASSOCIATED CONDITIONS
Other IgE-mediated conditions: Asthma, atopic dermatitis, allergic conjunctivitis, food allergy

DIAGNOSIS

HISTORY
- History of atopic dermatitis and/or food allergies
- Nasal congestion, rhinorrhea (anterior and/or posterior)
- Pruritus of nose, eyes, ears, and/or palate
- Sneezing, often paroxysmal
- Injection, itching, and watering of eyes
- Mouth breathing, snoring, dry, chapped lips
- Fatigue or malaise

PHYSICAL EXAM
Many findings are suggestive of but not specific for allergic rhinitis:
- Pale, boggy nasal mucosa
- Rhinorrhea, usually with clear discharge
- Dark circles under eyes, "allergic shiners" (infraorbital venous congestion)
- Transverse nasal crease from rubbing nose upward; typically seen in children
- Postnasal mucus discharge
- Oropharyngeal lymphoid tissue hypertrophy

DIAGNOSTIC TESTS & INTERPRETATION
Diagnosis is usually based on history and physical exam.

Lab
- Specific allergen sensitivity with allergen skin testing or radioallergosorbent testing (RAST); clinical correlation based on history is essential in interpreting results.
- Secondary tests:
  - Complete blood count (CBC) with differential may show elevated eosinophils.
  - Increased total serum IgE level
  - Nasal probe smear may show elevated eosinophils.
- Medication may alter lab results.
  - Corticosteroids may decrease eosinophilia.
  - Antihistamines will suppress reactivity to skin tests.

Imaging
CT scan of sinuses when indicated; check for complete opacity, fluid level, and mucosal thickening.

Diagnostic Procedures/Surgery
- Diagnostic allergen prick test kits are used to select agent to determine appropriate environmental control measures, as well as to direct immunotherapy.
  - Prick or puncture: Superficial injury to epidermis with application of test antigen
  - Intradermal
- RAST: More expensive and less sensitive than skin testing; typically used in patients in whom skin testing is not practical or a severe reaction is possible
- Rhinoscopy: Useful to visualize intranasal anatomy and posterior pharyngeal structures, including adenoids, polyps, and larynx

Pathological Findings
- Nasal washing/scraping: Eosinophils predominate but may see basophils, mast cells.
- Nasal mucosa: Submucosal edema but without destruction; eosinophilic infiltration; congested mucous glands and goblet cells

DIFFERENTIAL DIAGNOSIS
- Other types of rhinitis:
  - Infectious rhinitis: Usually viral, commonly with secondary bacterial infection:
    - Acute/chronic sinusitis
    - Viral rhinitis averages 6 episodes/year from ages 2–6 years.
    - IgA deficiency with recurrent sinusitis
  - Medications:
    - Rebound-effect "rhinitis medicamentosa" associated with continued use of topical decongestant drops and sprays
    - Angiotensin-converting enzyme (ACE) inhibitors, reserpine, β-blockers, oral contraceptive pills (OCPs), guanethidine, methyldopa
    - Aspirin, nonsteroidal anti-inflammatory drugs (NSAIDs)
  - Vasomotor (idiopathic) rhinitis
  - Hormonal: Pregnancy, thyroid, OCPs
  - Nonallergic rhinitis with eosinophilia syndrome (NARES)
  - Gustatory: Watery rhinorrhea in response to alcohol or food
  - "Skier's nose": Watery rhinorrhea in response to cold air
  - Irritant rhinitis
  - Atrophic rhinitis
- Conditions that mimic rhinitis:
  - Nasal polyps, tumor
  - Septal/anatomic obstruction:
    - Adenoidal hypertrophy, particularly in children
    - Trauma
    - Septal abnormality
    - Foreign body
  - CSF rhinorrhea: Cribriform plate defect owing to trauma/recent surgery (test discharge for β_2-transferrin)
  - Ciliary dyskinesia

TREATMENT

MEDICATION

First Line

- 2nd-generation antihistamines
  - 1st-line therapy for mild to moderate allergic rhinitis (1,4,5,6)[A].
  - Considered non-sedating.
  - Adverse effects: mild sedation, mild anticholinergic effects
  - Generic: Cetirizine, Fexofenadine, Loratadine
  - Brand Name: Desloratadine, levocetirizine
- Intranasal corticosteroids
  - 1st-line therapy for moderate to severe allergic rhinitis (1,4,5,6)[A].
  - Most effective drug class for symptoms of allergic rhinitis.
  - Use nasal sprays after showering, and direct spray away from septum to improve deposition on mucosal surface.
  - May be used as needed however less effective than regular use (1).
  - Adverse effects: nosebleed, nasal septal perforation, and systemic corticosteroid effects.
  - Systemic steroids should be considered only in urgent cases and only for short-term use.
  - Generic: fluticasone
  - Brand Name: Nasonex (Mometasone), Beconase (Beclomethasone), Rhinocort (Budesonide), Omnaris (Ciclesonide), Veramyst (Fluticasone furoate), Nasacort (Triamcinolone)

Second Line

- 1st-generation antihistamines such as: (7)
  - Brompheniramine 12–24 mg po bid
  - Chlorpheniramine 4 mg po q 4–6 hours prn
  - Clemastine 1–2 mg po bid prn
  - Diphenhydramine 25–50 mg po q4-6 hours as needed
    - May precipitate urinary retention in men with prostatism and/or hypertrophy.
    - Adverse effects: Sedation, prolonged QT interval, performance impairment, and anticholinergic effects.
- Miscellaneous agents
  - Nasal antihistamines
    - May be systemically absorbed and thus may cause sedation: Azelastine, Olopatadine
  - Decongestants
    - Phenylephrine 10 mg po q 4 hours prn
    - Pseudoephedrine 60 mg po q 4–6 hours prn
    - Oxymetazoline nasal spray (Afrin) 2–3 sprays per nostril q 10–12 hours prn (max 3 days). Intranasal agents should not be used for greater than 3 days due to rebound rhinitis. Discourage use in patients with hypertension (HTN) or cardiac arrhythmia
  - Intranasal anticholinergics such as ipratropium nasal spray 2 sprays per nostril bid-tid
    - Intranasal anticholinergics can increase efficacy in combination with steroid use (1).
  - Leukotriene antagonists such as montelukast (Singulair) 10 mg po qd
    - Should generally be used as an adjunct, not monotherapy.
  - Mast cell stabilizers such as Cromolyn nasal spray 1 spray per nostril tid-qid
    - May take 2–4 weeks of therapy for optimal efficacy (7).
    - May be ineffective in patients with non-allergic rhinitis and nasal polyps (7).

ADDITIONAL TREATMENT

Immunotherapy, either by injection (8)[A] or sublingually, which may be better tolerated by children (9)[A]

General Measures

- Establish specific cause(s) by history and appropriate testing.
- Limit exposure to offending allergen.
- Allergen immunotherapy (desensitization):
  - Usually reserved for when symptoms are uncontrollable with medical therapy or have a comorbidity such as asthma or chronic sinusitis
  - Specific allergen extract is injected SC in increasing doses to induce patient tolerance.

Issues for Referral

Refer to allergist for identification of allergens in aiding in appropriate environmental control measures, as well as for consideration of immunotherapy.

Additional Therapies

Nasal saline use has evidence of efficacy as sole agent or as adjunctive treatment (1,10)[A].

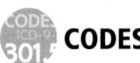 **ONGOING CARE**

FOLLOW-UP RECOMMENDATIONS

No specific restrictions on activity; emphasize avoiding activity where exposure to the allergen is likely.

Patient Monitoring

Initiation of patient education is critical.

DIET

- No special diet unless concomitant food reactions are suspected and evaluated
- Some patients with severe sensitivity to seasonal pollens may have oral allergy syndrome, which is associated with itching in the mouth with the ingestion of fresh fruits that may cross-react with the allergens.

PATIENT EDUCATION

- Asthma & Allergy Foundation of America, 1717 Massachusetts Ave., Suite 305, Washington, DC 20036; (800) 7-ASTHMA; http://www.aafa.org.
- Other helpful information available at http://www.acaai.org and http://www.aaaai.org.

PROGNOSIS

- Acceptable control of symptoms is the goal.
- Treatment is helpful to reduce the risk of comorbidities, such as sinusitis and asthma.

COMPLICATIONS

- Secondary infection such as otitis media or sinusitis
- Epistaxis
- Nasopharyngeal lymphoid hyperplasia
- Airway hyperreactivity with allergen exposure
- Asthma
- Facial changes
- Sleep disturbance

REFERENCES

1. Wallace DV. The Diagnosis and Management of Rhinitis: An Updated Practice Parameter. *J Allergy Clin Immunol.* 2008;122:S1–84.
2. Kramer, Michael S. Kakuma, Ritsuko. Maternal dietary antigen avoidance during pregnancy or lactation, or both, for preventing or treating atopic disease in the child. [Systematic Review] Cochrane Pregnancy and Childbirth Group. *Cochrane Database of Systematic Reviews.* 1, 2009.
3. Sheikh, Aziz. Hurwitz, Brian. Shehata, Yasser A. House dust mite avoidance measures for perennial allergic rhinitis. [Systematic Review] Cochrane Ear, Nose and Throat Disorders Group. *Cochrane Database of Systematic Reviews.* 1, 2009.
4. Meltzer EO. Evaluation of the optimal oral antihistamine for patients with allergic rhinitis. *Mayo Clin Proc.* 2005;80:1170–6.
5. Dykewicz MS. 7. Rhinitis and sinusitis. *J Allergy Clin Immunol.* 2003;111:S520–9.
6. Plaut M, Valentine MD. Clinical practice. Allergic rhinitis. *N Engl J Med.* 2005;353:1934–44.
7. *AHFS Drug Information.* 49th. Bethesda, MD: American Society of Health-System Pharmacists, 2007.
8. Calderon, Moises A. Alves, Bernadette. Jacobson, Mikila. Hurwitz, Brian. Sheikh, Aziz. Durham, Stephen. Allergen injection immunotherapy for seasonal allergic rhinitis. [Systematic Review] *Cochrane Ear, Nose and Throat Disorders Group Cochrane Database of Systematic Reviews.* 1, 2009.
9. Wilson, Duncan. Torres-Lima, Marcia. Durham, Stephen. Sublingual immunotherapy for allergic rhinitis. [Systematic Review] Cochrane Ear, Nose and Throat Disorders Group. *Cochrane Database of Systematic Reviews.* 1, 2009.
10. Harvey, Richard. Hannan, Saiful Alam. Badia, Lydia. Scadding, Glenis. Nasal saline irrigations for the symptoms of chronic rhinosinusitis. [Systematic Review] Cochrane Ear, Nose and Throat Disorders Group. *Cochrane Database of Systematic Reviews.* 1, 2009.

See Also (Topic, Algorithm, Electronic Media Element)

Conjunctivitis, Acute

CODES

ICD9

- 477.0 Allergic rhinitis due to pollen
- 477.1 Allergic rhinitis due to food
- 477.2 Allergic rhinitis due to animal (cat) (dog) hair and dander

CLINICAL PEARLS

- Nasal saline irrigation (flushing 6–8 oz) may be very helpful in clearing upper airway of secretions and may precede the use of nasal corticosteroids.
- 2nd-generation antihistamines and intranasal corticosteroids are first-line therapies for allergic rhinitis.
- Rebound rhinitis generally can be treated with topically inhaled nasal steroids but may require short-course prednisone. Persistent dependence may be treated by weening off topical vasoconstrictors one nostril at a time.
- Antihistamines may prevent but do not treat existing congestion. Decongestants, nasal saline, and intranasal corticosteroids do treat congestion.

ROCKY MOUNTAIN SPOTTED FEVER

Brock D. Lutz, MD
Ronald A. Greenfield, MD

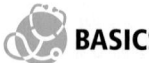 **BASICS**

DESCRIPTION
- Rocky Mountain spotted fever (RMSF) is an acute, potentially fatal febrile illness caused by *Rickettsia rickettsii* and transmitted by tick bite.
- System(s) affected: Cardiovascular; Musculoskeletal; CNS; Skin/Exocrine

EPIDEMIOLOGY
Incidence
- In the US, 0.22/100,000 persons per year, with over 1/2 the cases in the South Atlantic Region; North Carolina and Oklahoma have the highest incidence; <3% of cases in Rocky Mountain states
- Also endemic in several countries in Central and South America
- Predominant age: Highest incidences occur among children and young adults, primarily owing to environmental exposure patterns. All ages are susceptible.
- Predominant sex: Male > Female (owing to more frequent outdoor activity by males).
- Peak incidence is in late spring and summer, with 90% occurring between April and September.

Prevalence
In the US, ~1,100 cases per year reported

RISK FACTORS
- Tick bite in preceding 14 days (70%)
- Outdoor activity, particularly, although not exclusively, during spring and summer months in an endemic area
- Contact with outdoor pets or wild animals
- Similar illness in family members, coworkers, or pets

GENERAL PREVENTION
People who frequent tick-infested areas can take measures to prevent infection (1)[B]:
- Occlusive clothing should be worn and insect repellents applied.
- After possible exposure, all body areas should be carefully inspected for ticks, especially legs, groin, external genitalia, and belt lines. Likelihood of infection increases with the duration of tick attachment.
- Ticks should be removed from humans or animals with caution; gloves should be worn or instruments used to minimize direct contact. Place a drop of oil, alcohol, gasoline, or kerosene on the tick first. Hands should be washed thoroughly after tick removal.
- With early appropriate therapy, antibody response may be blunted, and recurrent infection has been reported. Patients therefore should be educated about general preventive measures.

PATHOPHYSIOLOGY
The primary pathology is a vasculitis owing to direct endothelial cell invasion by rickettsiae. The major effect of endothelial cell injury is increased vascular permeability. This leads to life-threatening damage to brain, lungs, and other viscera.

ETIOLOGY
- RMSF is caused by *R. rickettsii*, which is transmitted by the bite of ticks (principally *Dermacentor andersoni* or *D. variabilis* in the US).
- Rarely, RMSF is caused by direct inoculation of tick blood into open wounds or conjunctivae, but it can be caused by removing ticks without gloves or good hand-washing.

 DIAGNOSIS

Delay in presentation and initiation of therapy can increase long-term sequelae and mortality.

HISTORY
Should be suspected in cases of febrile illness with history of potential tick exposure (70%) within previous 14 days, travel to endemic area, and presentation in the spring or fall

PHYSICAL EXAM
- The cardinal clinical features are headache, fever, and a centripetal rash (involves the palms and soles and spreads centrally to arms, legs, and trunk), which is often petechial. Patients do not typically have this characteristic rash at initial presentation but may have a maculopapular rash.
- Fever (100%)
- Rash (macular, maculopapular, petechial; 90–100%)
- Headache (65%)
- Headache, fever, rash (50–60%)
- Other neuropsychiatric symptoms (40–50%)
- Nausea, vomiting (30–50%)
- Abdominal pain (30%)
- Myalgias (30%)
- Hepatosplenomegaly (30%)
- Lymphadenopathy (25%)
- Arthralgias (10%)
- Cough (15%)
- CNS dysfunction (e.g., stupor, confusion, coma, focal abnormalities; 10–30%)

DIAGNOSTIC TESTS & INTERPRETATION
Lab
- Specific laboratory diagnosis:
  - Serum indirect fluorescent antibody (IFA): 4-fold increase or solitary titer >1:64
  - Polymerase chain reaction (PCR) testing by Centers for Disease Control and Prevention (CDC)
- Nonspecific laboratory changes:
  - Thrombocytopenia
  - White blood cell (WBC) count: Normal, increased, or decreased
  - Anemia (mild)
  - Hyponatremia (usually mild)
  - Azotemia

- CSF protein and WBC count modestly elevated (lymphocytic predominance), glucose usually normal
- Prolonged prothrombin time (PT) and partial thromboplastin time (PTT); decreased fibrinogen; elevated fibrin degradation products uncommon
- Drugs that may alter lab results: Early treatment may blunt antibody response.

Imaging
Other than nonspecific pneumonic infiltrates, which may be seen on routine chest radiograph, imaging procedures are rarely helpful.

Diagnostic Procedures/Surgery
- Tissue (primarily skin) biopsy can be helpful if rapid direct fluorescent antibody (DFA) or nucleic acid amplification testing or electron microscopy is available.
- Diagnosis is usually presumptive and based on a compatible syndrome in a patient with exposure history in an endemic area. Confirmation is obtained by subsequent serology.

Pathological Findings
- The principal pathologic abnormality is a systemic vasculitis.
- Rickettsiae may be demonstrated within endothelial cells by DFA, PCR, or electron microscopy.
- Petechiae owing to the vasculitis may be seen on various organ surfaces (e.g., liver, brain, or epicardium).
- Secondary thromboses and tissue necrosis may be seen.

DIFFERENTIAL DIAGNOSIS
- Viral exanthems (e.g., measles, rubella)
- Meningoencephalitis (viral meningitis or encephalitis, bacterial meningitis)
- Typhus
- Rickettsialpox
- Ehrlichiosis
- Lyme disease
- Meningococcemia
- Leptospirosis

TREATMENT

MEDICATION
First Line
- Doxycycline is the treatment of choice in children and adults (2,3)[A]:
  - For adults, doxycycline 200 mg PO initially followed by 100 mg PO b.i.d. × 5–7 days, including 3 days after fever resolution; same dosage IV; 100 mg q24h in renal failure
  - For children weighing <100 lb: 2.2 mg/kg/dose given q12h

- Precautions:
  - Patients taking doxycycline should minimize sun exposure to avoid photosensitization.
  - Chloramphenicol rarely may cause idiosyncratic, nonreversible aplastic anemia.
  - Doxycycline may cause staining of permanent teeth when given to children <9 years of age. This risk appears to be minimal if no more than 5 courses of therapy are administered before age 9.
- Significant possible interactions: Absorption of doxycycline may be inhibited if it is ingested with milk products, iron preparations, or antacids containing aluminum or magnesium.

Second Line
- Chloramphenicol 20 mg/kg IV q6h (4 g/d maximum); same dose in renal failure (oral chloramphenicol is not available in the US); chloramphenicol may be less effective than doxycycline.
- Modern fluoroquinolones have in vitro activity against *R. rickettsii* and have been evaluated in other spotted-fever-group rickettsioses but have not been evaluated clinically in RMSF.

Pregnancy Considerations
- Brief course of doxycycline is appropriate for this life-threatening infection if suspicion is high, despite the potential risk to fetal bones and teeth.
- Chloramphenicol may be preferred during the 1st 2 trimesters but should be avoided in the 3rd trimester because of potential gray baby syndrome.
- Transplacental transmission of infection has not been demonstrated.

ADDITIONAL TREATMENT
General Measures
Treatment should be initiated on the basis of clinical diagnosis or skin biopsy and should not be delayed for serologic confirmation or development of the characteristic rash.

- Monitor patient's arterial oxygen saturation. Consider oxygen therapy and assisted ventilation for pulmonary complications, if necessary.
- Good mouth care
- Blood transfusions for anemia
- Turn bed-confined patient frequently.
- Monitor patient carefully for signs of renal failure.

Issues for Referral
Consider consultation with infectious disease specialist.

Additional Therapies
Patients with neurologic injury may require prolonged physical and cognitive therapy.

IN-PATIENT CONSIDERATIONS
Admission Criteria
- Severe illness
- Obtundation
- Nausea/vomiting preventing oral antibiotic therapy

IV Fluids
Critically ill patients will require IV fluids.

Discharge Criteria
- Resolution of fever
- Able to take oral therapy and nutrition

 ONGOING CARE

FOLLOW-UP RECOMMENDATIONS
- Patients with the full clinical presentation or who are moderately ill usually should be hospitalized.
- Patients with mild disease are treated presumptively as outpatients. Close follow-up is important in identifying complications.
- Bed rest until symptoms subside

Patient Monitoring
- If patients are not hospitalized, then they should be seen every 2–3 days until symptoms have fully resolved.
- CBC, creatinine, and electrolytes should be monitored.

DIET
- Some patients may require parenteral nutrition.
- In others, small frequent meals may be necessary to maintain nutritional levels.

PROGNOSIS
- When treated promptly, the usual prognosis is excellent with the resolution of symptoms over several days and no sequelae.
- Death is rare with prompt institution of appropriate therapy.
- If complications develop (see "Complications"), the course may be more severe, and long-term sequelae may be present, particularly neurologic sequelae.

Geriatric Considerations
Mortality risk is higher in the elderly; as high as 70% if untreated.

COMPLICATIONS
- Encephalopathy, usually transient (30–40%)
- Seizures, focal neurologic signs (10%)
- Renal insufficiency (10%)
- Hepatitis (10%)
- Congestive heart failure (CHF) (5%)
- Respiratory failure (5%)

REFERENCES
1. Minniear TD, Buckingham SC et al. Managing Rocky Mountain spotted fever. *Expert Rev Anti Infect Ther*. 2009;7:1131–7.
2. Centers for Disease Control and Prevention. Nonfatal, unintentional medication exposures among young children—United States, 2001–2003. *MMWR Morb Mortal Wkly Rep*. 2006;55:1–5.
3. Elston DM et al. Tick bites and skin rashes. *Curr Opin Infect Dis*. 2010;23:132–8.

ADDITIONAL READING
- Chapman AS, Bakken JS, Folk SM, et al. Diagnosis and management of tickborne rickettsial diseases: Rocky Mountain spotted fever, ehrlichioses, and anaplasmosis–United States: a practical guide for physicians and other health-care and public health professionals. *MMWR Recomm Rep*. 2006;55:1–27.
- Chen LF, Sexton DJ. What's new in Rocky Mountain spotted fever? *Infect Dis Clin North Am*. 2008;22(3): 415–32, vii–viii.
- Masters EJ, Olson GS, Weiner SJ, et al. Rocky Mountain spotted fever: a clinician's dilemma. *Arch Intern Med*. 2003;163:769–74.
- Stallings SP. Rocky Mountain spotted fever and pregnancy: a case report and review of the literature. *Obstet Gynecol Surv*. 2001;56:37–42.

 CODES

ICD9
082.0 Spotted fevers

CLINICAL PEARLS
- If treating mild to moderate disease as outpatient, monitor CBC, creatinine, and electrolytes every 2–3 days.
- 90% of cases occur between April and September.
- 70% of patients have a tick bite in the preceding 14 days.

ROSEOLA

Jeffery T. Kirchner, DO

 BASICS

DESCRIPTION
- Acute infection of infants or very young children
- Characteristically, it causes a high fever followed by an eruption similar in appearance to that of measles as the fever resolves.
- Transmission now believed to be via contact of salivary secretions from adults shedding HHV-6
- Perinatal transmission has been suggested with newborn infections but not definitively proven.
- Virus establishes lifelong infection, including in the central nervous system (CNS)
- Incubation period of ~5–15 days
- System(s) affected: Endocrine/Metabolic; Skin/Exocrine; Brain/Neurologic
- Synonym(s): Exanthem subitum; Pseudorubella; Sixth disease

Pediatric Considerations
A disease of infants and very young children

EPIDEMIOLOGY
- Predominant age:
  - Infants and very young children (6 months– 3 years)
  - 90% before age 2 years (1,2)
- Predominant sex: Male = Female

Incidence
- Unknown
- More likely to occur in spring and fall

Prevalence
Peak prevalence is between 7 and 13 months of age

RISK FACTORS
- Daycare center
- Exposure to infected infant

Genetics
No known genetic pattern

ETIOLOGY
A communicable DNA virus: HHV-6B (1,3)

 DIAGNOSIS

HISTORY
- Anorexia
- Irritability
- Abrupt fever without apparent cause [39.4°C–40.5°C (103°F–105°F)] for 3–5 days

PHYSICAL EXAM
- Child usually does not appear seriously ill, but may be listless
- Febrile convulsions during height of fever (10–15%)
- Sudden drop of fever:
  - As fever disappears, skin rash begins (lasts hours–days).
- Rash (exanthem subitum):
  - Nonpruritic, maculopapular, blanching rash appears as very slightly elevated, rose-pink papules.
  - First appears on the neck and trunk
  - Appears profusely on trunk, arms, and neck, but mildly on face and legs
  - Fades within a few hours–2 days
- Inflammation of the tympanic membranes
- Lymphadenopathy in cervical and posterior auricular regions (often a later finding)
- Spleen enlarged (uncommon)

DIAGNOSTIC TESTS & INTERPRETATION
Lab
- Typically a clinical diagnosis
- Consider labs only if concerned about the patient's overall condition.

Initial lab tests
- Complete blood count (CBC):
  - Leukopenia with relative (atypical) lymphocytosis
  - Thrombocytopenia
- Urinalysis (rule out urinary tract infection [UTI] as source of fever)
- Immunoglobulin M (IgM); poor sensitivity/specificity
- Paired sera for IgG (4-fold increase IgG for diagnosis) for HHV-6 (but can cross-react with HHV-7)
- Serum polymerase chain reaction (PCR) for HHV-6, qualitative and quantitative, can be performed:
  - Serological confirmation should only be considered if there is evidence of neurological sequelae (4).
  - Quantitative is more accurate than qualitative.
  - Typically, results take 2–7 days, depending on the lab.
- Blood culture (peripheral blood mononuclear cells or PMBC) for HHV-6

Imaging
Initial approach
- Consider chest x-ray (CXR) if a child is exhibiting respiratory symptoms such as tachypnea or wheezing.
- When ordered, a CXR is typically negative.

Diagnostic Procedures/Surgery
- HHV-6-IgM: Diagnostic for acute infection (but limited sensitivity and specificity)
- HHV-6 by PCR found in serum, cerebrospinal fluid (CSF), and saliva

DIFFERENTIAL DIAGNOSIS
- Enterovirus infection
- Fifth disease
- Rubella
- Measles (rubeola)
- Scarlet fever
- Otitis media
- Sepsis
- Drug eruption (including medication hypersensitivity syndrome)

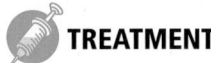

TREATMENT

Is usually supportive

MEDICATION

First Line

- Acetaminophen for excessively high fever, 10–15 mg/kg q4h to a maximum of 2.6 g/24-hour period
- Avoid aspirin as it may enhance the risk of Reye syndrome (1)[C].
- Phenobarbital may be considered for seizure (1)[C].

Second Line

- Medications for use in immunocompromised children:
  - Foscarnet active against HHV-6A and -6B (5)[B]
  - Acyclovir has very little activity.
  - Ganciclovir active against HHV-6B, but -6A is relatively resistant.
- No clinical trials evaluating these antiviral agents. Most evidence is from in vitro studies.

ADDITIONAL TREATMENT

General Measures

- Symptomatic
- Tap water baths to cool excess temperature elevation
- Lightweight clothing
- Maintain normal room temperature.

ONGOING CARE

FOLLOW-UP RECOMMENDATIONS

Patient Monitoring

- None after typical rash appears and fever resolves
- If seizures occur, they will cease after fever subsides and will not cause brain damage.

DIET

Encourage fluids.

PATIENT EDUCATION

Parental reassurance

PROGNOSIS

- Course: Acute, benign, complete recovery without sequelae
- 1 attack usually confers permanent immunity.
- Reactivation in immunocompromised patients is possible.

COMPLICATIONS

- Febrile seizures
- Encephalitis (rare)
- Meningitis
- Hepatitis
- Medication hypersensitivity syndromes
- Possible association with temporal lobe epilepsy and multiple sclerosis (MS) (6)

REFERENCES

1. Leach CT. Human herpesvirus-6 and -7 infections in children: agents of roseola and other syndromes. *Curr Opin Pediatr.* 2000;12:269–74.
2. Zerr DM, Meier AS, Selke SS, et al. A population-based study of primary human herpesvirus 6 infection. *N Engl J Med.* 2005;352: 768–76.
3. Zerr DM. Human herpesvirus 6: a clinical update. *Herpes.* 2006;13:20–4.
4. Ward KN. The natural history and laboratory diagnosis of human herpesviruses-6 and -7 infections in the immunocompetent. *J Clin Virol.* 2005;32:183–93.
5. Williams MV. *HHV-6: response to antiviral agents. In: Human herpesviurs-6: epidemiology, molecular biology, and clinical pathology.* Elsevier Biomedical Press, Amsterdam, the Netherlands, July 2006.
6. Gewurz BE, Marty FM, Baden LR, et al. Human herpesvirus 6 encephalitis. *Curr Infect Dis Rep.* 2008;10:292–9.

ADDITIONAL READING

- Asano Y, Yoshikawa T, Suga S, et al. Clinical features of infants with primary human herpesvirus 6 infection (exanthem subitum, roseola infantum). *Pediatrics.* 1994;93:104–8.
- Caselli E, Di Luca D. Molecular biology and clinical associations of Roseoloviruses human herpesvirus 6 and human herpesvirus 7. *New Microbiol.* 2007;30:173–87.
- Dockrell DH, Smith TF, Paya CV. Human herpesvirus 6. *Mayo Clin Proc.* 1999;74:163–70.

- Theodore WH, Epstein L, Gaillard WD, et al. Human herpes virus 6B: A possible role in epilepsy? *Epilepsia.* 2008.
- Vianna RA, de Oliveira SA, Camacho LA, et al. Role of human herpesvirus 6 infection in young Brazilian children with rash illnesses. *Pediatr Infect Dis J.* 2008;27:533–7.

CODES

ICD9

- 057.8 Other specified viral exanthemata
- 058.10 Roseola infantum, unspecified

CLINICAL PEARLS

- Roseola infection should be suspected if it is known to be in the community and a young child presents with a high temperature.
- As the fever abates, a blanching macular rash will be seen on the neck and trunk, with eventual spread to the face and extremities.
- Laboratory testing is not necessary for most children with classic roseola.
- For atypical presentations, complications, and immunocompromised hosts, several laboratory tools are available, including serologic testing for antibody and viral PCR testing.
- Infection is typically self-limiting and without sequelae.

ROTATOR CUFF IMPINGEMENT SYNDROME

Derek M. Richardson, Capt USAF AMC 60 MDOS/SGOF
Antoin M. Alexander, MD

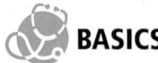

BASICS

DESCRIPTION
- Compression of the rotator cuff tendons and subacromial bursa between the humeral head and the structures that make up the coracoacromial arch and humeral tuberosities.
- Most common cause of atraumatic shoulder in patients aged >25 years
- Typical symptom is pain that is most severe with arm abducted between 40–120°.
- Classically divided into three stages:
  - Stage I: Acute inflammation, edema, or hemorrhage of the underlying tendons due to overuse (typically <25 years of age)
  - Stage II: Progressive tendinosis that leads to partial rotator cuff tear along with underlying thickening or fibrosis of surrounding structures (commonly, ages 25–40 years)
  - Stage III: Full-thickness tear (typically in patients aged >40 years)

EPIDEMIOLOGY
Incidence
- Shoulder pain in primary care practices averages around 11.2/1000 patients per year.
- Peak incidence of 25/1000 patients per year in those aged 42–46
- Shoulder pain accounts for 1.2% of all primary care visits.
- Impingement cited as cause in 18–74% of shoulder pain patients.

Prevalence
Prevalence of shoulder pain in general population thought to range from approximately 7–36%.

RISK FACTORS
- Repetitive overhead motions, including throwing
- Glenohumeral joint instability or muscle imbalance
- Hooked acromion
- Acromioclavicular (AC) spurs, osteophytes
- Thickened coracoacromial ligament
- Shoulder trauma
- Os acromiale
- Increasing age
- Smoking

GENERAL PREVENTION
- Proper throwing and lifting techniques
- Proper development of rotator cuff and scapula stabilizer muscles

PATHOPHYSIOLOGY
- The exact pathophysiology is still not entirely clear.
- Originally described by Neer as pinching of the soft-tissue structures (such as rotator cuff tendons or subacromial bursa) between humerus and the anteroinferior portion of the acromion, which is exacerbated by repetitive shoulder forward flexion and internal rotation.

- Commonly believed that intrinsic degeneration of the rotator cuff tendons with age combines with repetitive microtrauma.
- Also possible that any abnormal reduction in the subacromial outlet volume may predispose or cause this syndrome.

ETIOLOGY
- Compression and irritation of a rotator cuff tendon (typically supraspinatus) and subacromial bursa due to:
  - Repetitive overhead activities (throwing, swimming, etc.) and shoulder instability
  - Direct trauma that compresses the humerus and the coracoacromial arch
  - Narrowing of the subacromial space secondary to AC joint spurring, thickened coracoacromial ligament, and sloped acromion
- Sudden rotator cuff tears can create impingement syndrome because the humeral head depressors (rotator cuff muscles) fail to keep the humeral head from riding upward into the coracoacromial arch.

DIAGNOSIS

HISTORY
- Gradual increase in shoulder pain with overhead activities (sudden onset of sharp pain is more suggestive of a tear)
- Waking up with nighttime pain is a typical complaint.
- Common complaint of anterolateral shoulder pain with overhead activities
- May progress to weakness and decreased range of motion

PHYSICAL EXAM
- Positive impingement tests suggest impingement syndrome.
  - Neer impingement sign: Stabilize the patient's scapula and passively flex the arm until the patient reports pain or has full elevation.
  - Hawkins-Kennedy impingement sign: The patient's arm is placed in 90° of forward flexion, and the examiner stabilizes the scapula and internally rotates the shoulder. Pain signifies a positive test.
- Sensitivity and specificity of Neer test for impingement are 79% and 53%, respectively (1)[A].
- Sensitivity and specificity of Hawkin's test for impingement are 79% and 59%, respectively (1)[A].
- Empty-can test: Evaluates for weakness of supraspinatus muscle by placing arm in 90° of forward flexion and internal rotation; examiner provides downward pressure, testing for weakness of supraspinatus strength between sides.
- Lift-off test: Have patient place hand of affected limb on back with palm facing out. Resist patient's attempts to push hand off the back. Weakness or pain is suggestive of subscapularis tendon involvement.

- Resisted external rotation: Suggestive of infraspinatus and/or teres minor tendon involvement.
- Evaluate C-spine to rule out cervical pathology

DIAGNOSTIC TESTS & INTERPRETATION
Imaging
Initial approach
- Plain-film radiographs of the shoulder (4 views): anteroposterior, axillary, lateral, and supraspinatus outlet views
- Plain film may reveal:
  - Osteophytes or hooked acromion (leading to irritation)
  - Cephalad migration of the humerus (from torn rotator cuff muscles that usually depress the humerus)
  - Decreased subacromial space (if worn bursa)
- MRI used to evaluate rotator cuff integrity and possible sources of impingement in those patients willing to undergo surgery.
- MR arthrogram increases sensitivity for detecting partial-thickness tears of the rotator cuff and labral pathology.
- Ultrasound is shown to have high accuracy for diagnosis in full-thickness tears but is limited with respect to impingement.

Diagnostic Procedures/Surgery
- Lidocaine injection test:
  - Inject lidocaine into the subacromial space:
    ○ Repeat impingement tests; if pain is completely relieved and range of motion is improved, likely impingement syndrome.
  - Allows for more accurate strength testing on physical examination:
    ○ If strength is intact, rules out rotator cuff tear
    ○ If range of motion does not improve at all, more likely adhesive capsulitis
  - Some pain relief and improved range of motion occurs after lidocaine injection with:
    ○ Glenoid labral tear
    ○ Capsular strain
    ○ Glenohumeral osteoarthritis
    ○ Glenohumeral instability
- A lack of any pain relief suggests other sources or inappropriate placement of injection.

Pathological Findings
May have tendinosis, tendonitis, or tear of the muscle or its tendon

DIFFERENTIAL DIAGNOSIS
- Labral injury (labrum of glenoid is a cartilage cuff that assists in supporting the head of the humerus; tears usually due to trauma).
- Acromioclavicular arthritis (more common as age increases; likely to have pain with cross-arm testing)
- Adhesive capsulitis (rotator cuff tendonitis leads to decreased use and atrophy of rotator cuff muscles, followed by contracture of joint, has been linked to diabetes)

- Anterior shoulder instability (owing to trauma; more common <25 years of age)
- Multidirectional instability
- Biceps tendonitis or rupture (perform Speed's and Yergeson's tests and look for visible or palpable defect of biceps)
- Calcific tendonitis
- Cervical radiculopathy (spinal or foraminal stenosis, can test with Spurling's maneuver)
- Glenohumeral arthritis (evaluate with plain films)
- Suprascapular nerve entrapment
- Thoracic outlet syndrome
- Traumatic rotator cuff tear

TREATMENT

Anti-inflammatory agents plus aggressive rehabilitation can improve and fully resolve rotator cuff tendonitis in most patients.

MEDICATION
Nonsteroidal anti-inflammatory drugs (NSAIDs) or other analgesic, often for 6–12 weeks

ADDITIONAL TREATMENT
General Measures
- Rest
- Ice or heat for symptom relief
- Activity modification with avoidance of aggravating activities which are typically overhead motions
- Range-of-motion exercises
- Rotator-cuff strengthening to prevent further injuries

Issues for Referral
Failure of conservative treatment, persistent pain, weakness, or complete tear of rotator cuff

Additional Therapies
- Supervised- or home-exercise regimens have been shown to provide clinically significant pain reduction and improved function. However, these measures have no effect on range of motion or strength (2)[A].
- Physical therapy has shown evidence of effectiveness for both short-term and long-term recovery with respect to function (3)[A].
  – Initial goal is to restore range of motion.
  – After pain resolves, gradually strengthen rotator cuff muscles in internal rotation, external rotation, and abduction.

COMPLEMENTARY AND ALTERNATIVE MEDICINE
- Little evidence to support or refute acupuncture as treatment; it possibly provides some short-term benefit with regard to pain and function (4)[A].
- Some evidence that 5 mg of topical glyceryl trinitrate is more effective than placebo for acute rotator cuff symptoms (5)[A].

SURGERY/OTHER PROCEDURES
- Little overall evidence regarding steroid injections; studies suggest they may be beneficial, although effects may be small and short-lived (6)[A].
  – No apparent significantly increased risk for rotator cuff tears in those receiving subacromial steroid injections (7)[C]
- No significant differences between open versus arthroscopic subacromial decompression and active nonoperative treatment for impingement (8)[A].

ONGOING CARE

PATIENT EDUCATION
- Patient must understand that physical rehabilitation will be necessary both in conservative course of treatment (i.e., NSAIDs, physical therapy) and with surgical decompression. An aggressive trial of rehabilitation should be encouraged prior to extensive testing or surgical intervention.
- Symptoms often recur if not fully addressed.

PROGNOSIS
- Variable
- Most patients improve with conservative management.

COMPLICATIONS
- Progression of injury
- Tendon retraction in complete rotator cuff tear

REFERENCES

1. Hegedus EJ, Goode A, Campbell S, et al. Physical examination tests of the shoulder: a systematic review with meta-analysis of individual tests. *Br J Sports Med*. 2008;42:80–92.
2. Kuhn JE. Exercise in the treatment of rotator cuff impingement: a systematic review and a synthesized evidence-based rehabilitation protocol. *Journal of Shoulder and Elbow Surgery*. 2009;18(1):138–160.
3. Green S, Buchbinder R, Hetrick S. Physiotherapy interventions for shoulder pain. *Cochrane Database of Systematic Reviews*. 2008; Vol 3.
4. Green S, Buchbinder R, et al. Accupuncture for shoulder pain. *Cochrane Database of Systematic Reviews*. 2008; Vol 4.
5. Cumpston M, Johnston R, Wengier L, et al. Topical glyceryl trinitrate for rotator cuff disease. *Cochrane Database of Systematic Reviews*. 2009; Vol 3.
6. Buchbinder R, Green S, Youd J. Corticosteroid injections for shoulder pain. *Cochrane Database of Systematic Reviews*. 2009; Vol 1.
7. Bhatia M, Singh B, et al. Correlation between rotator cuff tears and repeated subacromial steroid injections: a case-controlled study. *Annals of the Royal College of Surgeons of England*. 2009; 91(5):414–416.
8. Coghlan J, Buchbinder R, et al. Surgery for rotator cuff disease. *Cochrane Database of Systematic Reviews*. 2009; Vol 1.

ADDITIONAL READING

- Baumgarten KM, Gerlach D, et al. Cigarette smoking increases the risk for rotator cuff tears. *Clinical Orthopaedics & Related Research*. 2010;468(6):1534–1541.
- Bytomski JR, Black D. Conservative treatment of rotator cuff injuries. *Journal of Surgical Orthopaedic Advances*. 2006;15(3):126–131.
- Hanchard N, Handoll H. Phsyical tests for shoulder impingements and local lesions of bursa, tendon or labrum that may accompany impingement. *Cochrane Database of Systematic Reviews*. 2008; Vol 4.
- Kennedy DJ, Visco CJ, Press J. Current concepts for shoulder training in the overhead athlete. *Current Sports Medicine Reports*. 2009;8(3):154–160.
- Meislin RJ, Sperling JW, Stitik TP. Persistent shoulder pain: epidemiology, pathophysiology, and diagnosis. *American Journal of Orthopedics*. 2005;35(12):5–9.
- Ostor AJ, Richards CA, et al. Diagnosis and relation to general health of shoulder disorders presenting to primary care. *Rheumatology*. 2005;44(6):800–805.

CODES

ICD9
726.10 Disorders of bursae and tendons in shoulder region, unspecified

CLINICAL PEARLS
- Consider impingement syndrome in patients with repetitive overhead arm motion (e.g., swimming, throwing).
- Shoulder pain after age 25 without trauma is most likely secondary to rotator cuff tendonitis.
- Supraspinatus tendon most commonly affected
- Use Neer and Hawkins tests as confirmatory impingement tests.
- Use empty-can test to test for weakness of supraspinatus muscle.
- Lidocaine injection test can aid in identification of type of shoulder pathology.
- Physical therapy over 6–12 weeks promotes return to function.

ROUNDWORMS, INTESTINAL

Gail Scully, MD, MPH

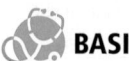 **BASICS**

DESCRIPTION
- Intestinal roundworms (nematodes) are nonsegmented, elongated organisms. They have an adult stage that infects the human intestinal tract. Larval stages may exist elsewhere in the body. Except for *Trichinella spiralis,* which is encysted in muscle, egg and/or larval stages can be isolated from the intestinal canal. Roundworms are the most common human parasite. Some nematodes have a soil cycle; others can complete their life cycle within the human body.
- Nematodes parasitizing the intestinal tract include:
  - *Enterobius vermicularis* (pinworm)
  - *Trichuris trichiura* (whipworm)
  - *Ascaris lumbricoides* (large roundworm)
  - *Necator americanus* (hookworm)
  - *Ancylostoma duodenale* (hookworm)
  - *Strongyloides stercoralis*
  - *Trichinella spiralis* (trichinosis)
- System(s) potentially affected: Cardiovascular; Gastrointestinal; Musculoskeletal; Nervous; Pulmonary

Pediatric Considerations
Children often have a larger parasite load. This can have detrimental effects on their physical and cognitive development.

EPIDEMIOLOGY
Incidence
- Predominant age:
  - All ages
  - Pinworm infections are more common in children.
- Predominant sex: Male = Female

Prevalence
- *E. vermicularis* (Most common helminth infection in US and western Europe. Prevalence between 30% and 50% in some communities.)
- *T. trichiura* (>1 billion infected worldwide)
- *A. lumbricoides* (estimated to be 1.3 billion infected worldwide)
- *N. americanus/A. duodenale* (>1 billion infected worldwide)
- *S. stercoralis* (100 million infected worldwide)

RISK FACTORS
- Low standard of hygiene
- Poor sanitation
- Human feces fertilizer
- *T. spiralis* (trichinosis): Eating raw or undercooked pork, bear, or cougar meat

Genetics
There is a genetic predisposition to some nematode infections, i.e., ascaris and trichuriasis.

PATHOPHYSIOLOGY
Life cycles:
- *E. vermicularis* and *T. trichiura:* Human part of the worm life cycle takes place entirely in the GI tract.
- *A. lumbricoides:* Larval stage ingested or inhaled, penetrates intestinal wall, to lungs via bloodstream, ascends the trachea, then swallowed, gain the small intestine, where larvae mature to adulthood

- *N. americanus, A. duodenale,* and *S. stercoralis:* Larvae penetrate skin, migrate to lungs via bloodstream, ascend the trachea, are swallowed, and gain the small intestine, where they mature to adulthood
- *T. spiralis:* Larvae are ingested in raw/undercooked meat and then invade the bowel mucosa and release larvae that travel through bloodstream and can infect numerous organ systems.

ETIOLOGY
- Ingestion of mature eggs in fecally contaminated food or drink
- Larval penetration of skin (hookworm, strongyloides)

COMMONLY ASSOCIATED CONDITIONS
Patients infected with *E. vermicularis* can be coinfected with *Dientamoeba fragilis.*

 DIAGNOSIS

PHYSICAL EXAM
- *E. vermicularis:*
  - Majority are asymptomatic.
  - Perianal itching, especially nocturnal
  - Can cause eosinophilic enteritis, which presents with abdominal pain and melena
- *T. trichiura:*
  - Symptomatic if heavily infected
  - Dysentery with tenesmus and bloody stools can occur
  - Chronic colitis in children
  - Weight loss
  - Anemia and eosinophilia
  - Recurrent rectal prolapse
- *A. lumbricoides:*
  - Migratory phase: Symptoms in a minority of persons:
    - Cough, wheezing
    - Blood-tinged sputum
    - Rales
    - Dyspnea
    - Substernal chest pain
    - Severe: Eosinophilic pneumonia (Loffler syndrome)
    - Eosinophilia and urticaria
  - Intestinal phase:
    - Rarely symptomatic
    - Mild abdominal discomfort, nausea, anorexia
    - Obstruction of the bowel, bile duct, pancreatic duct
    - Adult worm in stool or vomiting of an adult worm
    - Appendicitis
    - Intestinal perforation
    - Malabsorption in children
- *N. americanus/A. duodenale:*
  - Skin lesion may develop at site of larval penetration.
  - Migratory phase:
    - Marked eosinophilia
    - Transient pneumonitis

- Intestinal phase:
  - Can be asymptomatic
  - Epigastric pain; abdominal discomfort
  - Diarrhea
  - Iron-deficiency anemia due to intestinal blood loss; can be severe
  - Signs of protein malnutrition in severe cases (e.g., abdominal distension, hair loss, periorbital edema)
  - Growth and cognitive development delays in children
- *S. stercoralis:*
  - Migratory phase:
    - Pneumonitis
    - Serpiginous skin rash (Larva currens; pathognomonic)
    - Recurrent urticarial or maculopapular rash on buttocks, thighs
    - Eosinophilia
  - Intestinal phase:
    - Diarrhea or constipation
    - Constipation
    - Children—anorexia and cachexia
  - Strongyloides hyperinfection/disseminated strongyloidiasis syndrome:
    - Increased generation of larvae with impaired host immunity
    - Corticosteroid use the most common risk factor in developed countries
    - Eosinophilia usually absent
    - Secondary bacterial infection common
- *T. spiralis:*
  - Initial infection (1 week):
    - Diarrhea
    - Abdominal pain
    - Vomiting
  - Parental phase (several weeks):
    - Fever
    - Myalgia
    - Periorbital edema
    - Petechial hemorrhages
    - Eosinophilia
    - Cardiac infection—myocarditis and ECG changes
    - CNS can be infected.

DIAGNOSTIC TESTS & INTERPRETATION
Lab
- *E. vermicularis:* Adhesive cellophane tape pressed to perianal area in a.m. to look for eggs
- *T. trichiura:*
  - Stool microscopy to look for eggs
  - Eosinophilia may be seen.
- *A. lumbricoides:*
  - Stool microscopy
  - Eosinophilia: Most notable during the larval migration stage
- *N. americanus/A. duodenale:*
  - Eosinophilia is best indicator of infection.
  - Stool microscopy
  - Hct/Hgb: To check for blood anemia due to blood loss

- *S. stercoralis:*
  - ELISA serology (should be performed in persons with residence or travel to endemic area prior to receiving immunosuppressive therapy)
  - Stool microscopy on multiple specimens or stool culture on agar plates
- *T. spiralis:*
  - ELISA, indirect immunofluorescence, and latex agglutination serology
  - Eosinophilia: Highest levels are during 3rd–4th week of infection

Imaging
Ultrasound is useful in the diagnosis of ascariasis as cause of biliary tract disease.

Pathological Findings
Characteristic eggs/worms

DIFFERENTIAL DIAGNOSIS
- Pulmonary ascariasis with eosinophilia: Consider asthma, Löffler syndrome, eosinophilic pneumonia, systemic lupus erythematosus, Hodgkin disease, and other parasitic causes (tropical pulmonary eosinophilia, toxocariasis, strongyloidiasis, hookworm, paragonimiasis).
- Worm-induced GI diseases: Consider other causes of pancreatitis, appendicitis, diverticulitis, duodenitis, and cholecystitis.
- Anemia/hypoproteinemia (hookworm): Consider other etiologies.
- Neurohelminthiasis: Consider other causes of CNS infection or mass lesion.

TREATMENT

MEDICATION
- *E. vermicularis* (pinworm): Mebendazole (Vermox) 100 mg p.o. single dose, albendazole 400 mg p.o. once (100 mg for children <2 years of age), or pyrantel pamoate 11 mg/kg p.o. once (maximum of 1 g); repeat dose 2 weeks later
- *T. trichiura* (whipworm): Mebendazole 100 mg p.o. b.i.d. × 3 days; or albendazole 400 mg/d p.o. × 3 days heavy infection: Albendazole 400 mg/day orally for 7 days
- *A. lumbricoides:* Mebendazole 100 mg p.o. b.i.d. × 3 days or 500 mg once, pyrantel pamoate 11 mg/kg p.o. once (maximum of 1 g; all dosages for adult and children), or albendazole 400 mg p.o. once
- *N. americanus/A. duodenale* (hookworm): Mebendazole 100 mg p.o. b.i.d. × 3 days, pyrantel pamoate 11 mg/kg p.o. (maximum of 1 g) × 3 days (all dosages for adult and children), or albendazole 400 mg once (1)
- *T. spiralis:* Mebendazole 200–400 mg p.o. t.i.d. × 3 days and then 400–500 mg t.i.d. × 10 days (adult dosage) *or* albendazole 400 mg p.o. b.i.d. × 10–15 days; steroids are indicated for severe symptoms
- *S. stercoralis:* Ivermectin (Mectizan) 200 μg/kg p.o. once a day for 2 days *or* albendazole 400 mg p.o. b.i.d. × 10–14 days. For severe, complicated infection, ivermectin should be continued for at least 7 days and an alternative route may be needed; broad-spectrum antibiotics should be given.

- *Note:* The Food and Drug Administration (FDA) may consider certain uses of these drugs investigational. Consult *Medical Letter* or appropriate drug reference.
- Contraindications: Refer to the manufacturer's profile of each drug.
- Precautions: Refer to the manufacturer's profile of each drug.
- Significant possible interactions: Refer to the manufacturer's profile of each drug.

Pregnancy Considerations
- Benzimidazoles (mebendazole, albendazole, thiabendazole) should not be used.
- Ivermectin has shown little teratogenic potential and has provided effective therapy, although benefits should clearly outweigh risks.

 ONGOING CARE

FOLLOW-UP RECOMMENDATIONS
- Outpatient care
- No restrictions
- Reinfection is possible; immunity does not develop.

Patient Monitoring
Obtain follow-up stool studies at 2 weeks, and retreat if necessary.

DIET
No special diet

PATIENT EDUCATION
- Avoid fecally contaminated food, water, and soil.
- Avoid using human fecal material as fertilizer.
- *N. americanus/A. duodenale:* Avoid walking barefoot in endemic areas.
- *T. spiralis* (trichinosis): Parasite is killed by cooking meat at 58.5°C for 10 minutes. Freezing it at −20°C for 3 or more weeks will kill *T. spiralis* in pork, but is not effective for horse/game meat.

Pediatric Considerations
A. duodenale may be transmitted through breast milk.

PROGNOSIS
- Good for light-to-moderate infections
- Ascariasis always should be treated due to the risk of migrating adult worms.

COMPLICATIONS
- Cholangitis: Migration to common bile duct
- Pancreatitis: Migration to pancreatic duct
- Appendicitis: Migration to appendix
- Diverticulitis: Migration to diverticula
- Liver abscess
- Intestinal obstruction
- Volvulus
- Intussusception
- Bowel penetration
- Anemia (hookworm)
- Hypoproteinemia (hookworm)
- CNS infection (*Strongyloides* sp.)
- Secondary bacteremia with strongyloides hyperinfection syndrome

REFERENCE
1. Keiser J, Utzinger J et al. Efficacy of current drugs against soil-transmitted helminth infections: systematic review and meta-analysis. *JAMA.* 2008;299:1937–48.

ADDITIONAL READING
- Croker C, Reporter R, Redelings M, Mascola L, et al. Strongyloidiasis-related deaths in the United States, 1991–2006. *Am J Trop Med Hyg.* 2010;83:422–6.
- Holland CV et al. Predisposition to ascariasis: patterns, mechanisms and implications. *Parasitology.* 2009;136:1537–47.
- Hotez PJ, Brooker S, Bethony JM, et al. Hookworm infection. *N Engl J Med.* 2004;351:799–807.
- Muennig P, Pallin D, Challah C, et al. The cost-effectiveness of ivermectin vs. albendazole in the presumptive treatment of strongyloidiasis in immigrants to the United States. *Epidemiol Infect.* 2004;132:1055–63.
- Pozio E, Sacchini D, Sacchi L, et al. Failure of mebendazole in the treatment of humans with Trichinella spiralis infection at the stage of encapsulating larvae. *Clin Infect Dis.* 2001;32:638–42.
- Stephenson LS, Holland CV, Cooper ES. The public health significance of Trichuris trichiura. *Parasitology.* 2000;121(Suppl):S73–95.
- Treatment guidelines from the Medical Letter Vol 8 (Supplement) 2010.
- Watt G, Saisorn S, Jongsakul K, et al. Blinded, placebo-controlled trial of antiparasitic drugs for trichinosis myositis. *J Infect Dis.* 2000;182:371–4.
- Zaha O, Hirata T, Kinjo F, et al. Efficacy of ivermectin for chronic strongyloidiasis: two single doses given 2 weeks apart. *J Infect Chemother.* 2002;8:94–8.

See Also (Topic, Algorithm, Electronic Media Element)
Intestinal Parasites; Roundworms, Tissue

 CODES

ICD9
127.0 Ascariasis

CLINICAL PEARLS
- Eosinophilia is best indicator of infection with *N. americanus/A. duodenale.*
- Absence of eosinophilia does not rule out most roundworm infections.
- ELISA may be necessary to detect infection with *S. stercoralis* but is not specific. Check serology prior to administering steroids or other immunosuppressing treatment to persons who may be infected with *Strongyloides.*

ROUNDWORMS, TISSUE

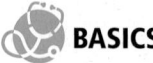

Richard E. Trowbridge, MD
Rebecca A. Frye, DO

BASICS

DESCRIPTION
- Infection of certain tissues by adult or larval roundworms (nematodes)
- Filarial infections:
  - *Wuchereria bancrofti* (bancroftian filariasis)
  - *Brugia malayi* (Malayan filariasis)
  - *Brugia timori* (Timorian filariasis)
  - *Loa loa* (eyeworm)
  - *Onchocerca volvulus* (river blindness, onchocerciasis)
  - *Mansonella perstans, M. ozzardi, M. streptocerca*
- Other tissue nematode infections:
  - *Dracunculus medinensis* (guinea worm, dracunculosis)
  - *Ancylostoma braziliense, A. caninum* (cutaneous larva migrans, creeping eruption)
  - *Toxocara canis, T. cati* [visceral or ocular larva migrans (VLM or OLM), toxocariasis]
- System(s) affected: Cardiovascular; GI; Hematologic/Lymphatic/Immunologic; Musculoskeletal; Nervous; Renal/Urologic; Skin/Exocrine
- Synonym(s): Nematodes

EPIDEMIOLOGY
Distribution:
- *W. bancrofti*: Tropics worldwide; mosquito vector (*Mansonia, Anopheles, Aedes*)
- *B. malayi*: Southeast Asia; mosquito vector
- *B. timori*: Indonesia; mosquito vector
- *L. loa*: Western and central Africa; deerfly vector (*Chrysops*)
- *O. volvulus*: Africa and South America; blackfly vector (*Simulium*)
- *Mansonella* spp.: Central Africa and South America; midge vector (*Culicoides*)
- *D. medinensis*: Ethiopia, Ghana, Mali, Sudan; contaminated water
- *A. braziliense, A. caninum*: Tropics and subtropics worldwide; contaminated soil
- *T. canis, T. cati*: worldwide; contaminated food

Incidence
Predominant gender: Male = Female.

Prevalence
- Estimated 120 million infected with lymphatic filariasis (1)
- Estimated 37 million infected with onchocerciasis (23)
- Estimated 3,000–10,000 infected with dracunculosis owing to focused eradication program (2)
- Toxocariasis is more prevalent in tropical and rural populations (4).

Pediatric Considerations
Classic VLM occurs most often in children aged 2–7 years.

RISK FACTORS
- Geographic exposure to arthropod vectors
- Fishermen or women washing clothes have increased risk of river blindness.
- Contact with infected soil in cutaneous larva migrans

- Young age, low socioeconomic status, poor sanitation, playing in sandpits, and owning dogs all increase risk of *Toxocara* exposure (4).

GENERAL PREVENTION
- Avoid sources of infection: Travel, arthropod bites, infected rivers and streams, infected food sources, or contaminated soils.
- Vector control: Bed nets, larviacides, insecticides, repellent, clothing
- Diethylcarbamazine (DEC) 300 mg once weekly has been used successfully in Peace Corps workers for prophylaxis against *L. loa*.
- DEC salt (0.1–0.5%) in endemic areas × 12 months (1)[A]

PATHOPHYSIOLOGY
Infective larval stages are transmitted to humans by arthropod vectors or from the soil, water, or contaminated food. Once in human tissue, worms mature over 6–12 months and survive as long as 15 years. Symptoms depend on tissue infected.

ETIOLOGY
Larvae introduced into human host by arthropod vector or infected soil, water, or food.

DIAGNOSIS

HISTORY
- Exposure to vector
- Travel (location and length of visit)

PHYSICAL EXAM
- Lymphatic filariasis (*W. bancrofti, B. malayi, B. timori*):
  - Acute: Most often due to secondary bacterial infection
    - Adenolymphangitis (ADL): Most common; fever, painful lymphadenopathy, erythema, pruritus, epididymitis/orchitis, abscess
    - Acute filarial lymphangitis (AFL): Immune reaction to dead nematode; erythema, painful nodules and lymphatics
    - Tropical pulmonary eosinophilia: Nonproductive paroxysmal cough, nocturnal wheezing, weight loss, lymphadenopathy
  - Chronic: May be asymptomatic for years
    - Lymphedema/elephantiasis: Debilitating, disfiguring, severe edema; lymph blocked by nests of adult nematodes
    - Hydrocele: May be unilateral or bilateral
    - Chyluria/chylocele: Lymph in urine or tunica propria owing to overflow
- Loiasis (*L. loa*):
  - Calabar swellings: Recurrent, subcutaneous, painful, migratory edema
  - Eye worm: Nematodes migrate under conjunctiva.
  - Fever, irritability, urticaria, and pruritus; mainly in nonimmune individuals
  - Encephalopathy, nephropathy, cardiomyopathy, pulmonary complications
- Onchocerciasis (*O. volvulus*):
  - Dermatitis
    - Acute: Pruritic papules to vesicles and pustules
    - Chronic: Scaling, peau d'orange, atrophic, wrinkled skin
  - Leopard skin: Spotted depigmentation usually pretibia

  - Onchocercomata: Subcutaneous, painless, 2- to 10-cm nodules
  - Sowda: Localized chronic dermatitis, hyperpigmented papules, and lymph node enlargement
  - Ocular changes: Intraocular microfilariae, punctate keratitis, anterior uveitis, optic atrophy, glaucoma, and blindness
- Other filarial syndromes (*M. ozzardi, M. perstans, M. streptocerca*):
  - Headaches, coldness, pruritus, and articular swelling/arthritis
  - Eosinophilia and vague allergic signs
  - Chronic dermatitis and macules can be confused with leprosy.
  - Lymphadenopathy
- Dracunculiasis (*D. medinensis*, guinea worm disease):
  - Allergic manifestations: Erythema, urticaria, pruritus, nausea, vomiting, syncope, and occasional fever
  - Local lesions: Papule, sterile blister, ulceration, secondary infection, abscesses
  - Painful, burning, worm protrusion, usually lower extremities (can be 3 ft long)
- Cutaneous larva migrans (*A. braziliense, A. caninum*):
  - Creeping eruption: 3-mm-wide serpiginous, erythematous, pruritic track extends several millimeters per day.
  - Edema and acute inflammation, most often lower extremities
  - Secondary infection, impetigo, folliculitis, pulmonary involvement
- Toxocariasis (*T. canis, T. cati*):
  - Visceral larva migrans: Due to migration of 2nd-stage larvae
    - Fever, chronic cough, dyspnea, hepatomegaly, abdominal pain
    - Chronic prurigo, urticaria, eczema, sleep disturbances
    - Myocarditis, nephrotic syndrome, arthritis, encephalitis, meningitis
  - Covert/common toxocariasis: Variations of mild *Toxocara* infection: Fever, sleep/behavior disturbances, cough, nausea, vomiting, abdominal pain, with or without eosinophilia
  - Ocular larva migrans: Usually affects older children
    - Strabismus, unilateral decreased vision, leukocoria
    - Peripheral retinal granuloma, endophthalmitis, vitreous band

DIAGNOSTIC TESTS & INTERPRETATION
Lab
Distinction of species by larval examination is challenging and may require expert examination.

Initial lab tests
- Antigen detection: ICT (blood test) and Ov-specific (dipstick): Early diagnosis
- Examination of larvae/adult worms found in tissue sample
- Characteristic microfilariae on blood smear
- Eosinophilia >3,000 cells/mm

Follow-Up & Special Considerations
- Repeat antigen testing if initially negative and high suspicion (filariasis).
- Microfilariae levels 12 months after treatment

Imaging
Occasional dead calcified worms seen on radiographs

Initial approach
Consider chest radiograph if cough present.

Follow-Up & Special Considerations
Filarial "dance sign" may be seen on ultrasound.

Diagnostic Procedures/Surgery
- Microfilariae on blood smear or other body fluids, clinical observations, and serologies [e.g., enzyme-linked immunosorbent assay (ELISA)]
- Onchocerciasis: Skin snip/biopsy showing larvae (3): Nodulectomy, slit-lamp exam, and Mazzotti test also may be helpful.
- Lymphoscintigraphy: Demonstrates lymphatic dilatation, backflow, and obstruction

Pathological Findings
Characteristic eggs/worms/larvae in tissue

DIFFERENTIAL DIAGNOSIS
- Other causes of tissue inflammation (i.e., lymphangitis, epididymitis, dermatitis, conjunctivitis, blisters, pleuritis, peritonitis, pericarditis, encephalitis, nephropathy, cardiomyopathy, etc.)
- Nonfilarial causes of lymphangitis:
  – Acute bacterial lymphangitis
  – Phlebitis
  – Unusual: Plague, anthrax, tuberculosis, lymphogranuloma inguinale
- Nonfilarial causes of lymphedema, chyluria, and elephantiasis:
  – Infiltrative or granulomatous process: Tumor, fungus, tuberculosis, leprosy
  – Chronic venostasis or phlebitis
  – Cardiac insufficiency
  – Nutritional deficiencies
  – Hereditary (Milroy disease)
  – Lateritious soil-obstructing lymphatics

 TREATMENT

MEDICATION
First Line
- Filariasis (*W. bancrofti, B. malayi, B. timori*): Diethylcarbamazine (DEC) 2 mg/kg PO t.i.d. × 1 day ± albendazole 400 mg PO daily × 14 days (1)[B]
- Loiasis:
  – DEC 2 mg/kg PO t.i.d. × 3 weeks if microfilariae (mff) burden low, i.e., >8,000 mff/mL (5)[B]
  – If burden high, pretreat with albendazole 200 mg PO b.i.d. × 21 days *or* mebendazole 300 mg PO daily × 21 days (5)[B].
  – Antihistamines and steroids may be useful to reduce allergic response to disintegration of microfilariae.
- Onchocerciasis: Ivermectin 150 µg/kg PO every 12 months (>5 years of age) (3)[B]
- Mansonella spp.:
  – Ivermectin 150–200 µg/kg PO once
  – Mebendazole 100 mg PO b.i.d. × 30 days
- *D. medinensis* (guinea worm): Cure is achieved only through physical removal of the adult worm (2)[C].
  – Usually wound on a stick
  – Remove worm slowly 1–3 cm/d to avoid complications.

- Cutaneous larva migrans (*A. braziliense, A. caninum*): Self-limiting disease in weeks to months; treat to avoid complications and for relief of symptoms.
  – Ivermectin 12 mg PO once adult dosing; 150 µg/kg PO once pediatric dosing (6)[B]
  – Albendazole 400–800 mg PO × 3–5 days; 10–15 mg/kg/d PO × 3–5 days pediatric dosing (6)[B]
  – Topical thiabendazole 10–15% cream t.i.d. × 15 days (6)[B]
- Toxocariasis:
  – Visceral larva migrans: Albendazole 500 mg PO b.i.d. × 5 days (4)[B]
  – Ocular larva migrans: Albendazole 800 mg PO daily (400 mg PO daily pediatric dosing) × 2–4 weeks + aggressive anti-inflammatory therapy (4)[B]
- Contraindications: Refer to the manufacturer's information of each drug.
- Precautions: Children, pregnancy, lactation
- Significant possible interactions: Refer to the manufacturer's profile of each drug.

Special Considerations
The Food and Drug Administration (FDA) may consider certain uses of these drugs investigational, and some may not be available in the US. Contact the Centers for Disease Control and Prevention (Parasitic Diseases Branch, CDC, Atlanta, GA 30333; 404-639-3670) for information.

Second Line
- Filariasis (*W. bancrofti, B. malayi*):
  – Ivermectin 150 µg/kg PO once is highly effective against microfilaria but does not kill adult worms.
  – Anti-Wolbachial therapy: Doxycycline 200 mg/d PO × 6 weeks (1)[B]
- Onchocerciasis: Anti-Wolbachial therapy: Doxycycline 200 mg/d PO × 6 weeks (3)[B]
- Cutaneous larva migrans:
  – Cryotherapy: Freezing leading edge of track is rarely successful.
  – Oral thiabendazole 50 mg/kg (no more than 3 g/d) × 3–4 days (6)[B]
- Toxocariasis: VLM: DEC 3–4 mg/kg/d × 21 days *or* thiabendazole 50 mg/kg/d × 3–7 days (4)[B]

ADDITIONAL TREATMENT
General Measures
- Hygiene, exercise, elevation (lymphedema); treat secondary infection (1)[B].
- Direct removal of worm from tissue with caution not to break the worm

SURGERY/OTHER PROCEDURES
- Long-standing lymphatic filariasis may require surgical intervention to increase lymphatic drainage (1).
- Ocular larval migrans may require surgery for retinal detachment or intravitreal fibrovascular membrane proliferation (4).

 ONGOING CARE

FOLLOW-UP RECOMMENDATIONS
Outpatient care: No restrictions

Patient Monitoring
- As needed
- Long-term DEC treatment and immunomonitoring of patients with filarial infection are essential in endemic areas to arrest and prevent pathology.

DIET
Avoid contaminated food and water, including undercooked meats and unwashed raw fruits and vegetables.

PATIENT EDUCATION
- Avoid bites by arthropod vectors.
- Use insect repellents and other protective measures (e.g., proper clothing).
- Avoid infected rivers, streams, soil, and foods.

PROGNOSIS
- Good for light to moderate infections
- Depends on organ infected and extent of infection

COMPLICATIONS
- Visceral worms: Hepatitis, splenomegaly, pleuritis, peritonitis, eosinophilic granuloma, or other organ damage because larvae migrate for up to 6 months
- Neurohelminthiasis: CNS migrations and infection

REFERENCES
1. Mendoza N, Li A, Gill A, et al. Filariasis: diagnosis and treatment. *Dermatol Ther*. 475–90.
2. Hopkins DR, Richards FO, Ruiz-Tiben E, et al. Dracunculiasis, onchocerciasis, schistosomiasis, and trachoma. *Ann N Y Acad Sci*. 2008;1136:45–52.
3. Stingl P et al. Onchocerciasis: developments in diagnosis, treatment and control. *Int J Dermatol*. 2009;48:393–6.
4. Rubinsky-Elefant G, Hirata CE, Yamamoto JH, et al. Human toxocariasis: diagnosis, worldwide seroprevalences and clinical expression of the systemic and ocular forms. *Ann Trop Med Parasitol*. 2010;104:3–23.
5. Padgett JJ, Jacobsen KH et al. Loiasis: African eye worm. *Trans R Soc Trop Med Hyg*. 2008;102: 983–9.
6. Patel S, Sethi A et al. Imported tropical diseases. *Dermatol Ther*. 538–49.

ADDITIONAL READING
The Medical Letter, Inc. Drugs for parasitic infections. *Med Lett Drugs Ther*. 2007;5.

See Also (Topic, Algorithm, Electronic Media Element)
Roundworms, Intestinal

 CODES

ICD9
127.0 Ascariasis

CLINICAL PEARLS
- Once in the human, roundworms can take up to a year to mature and may survive up to 15 years.
- Prevention of exposure to the arthropod vector is key to avoiding infection.
- Recent antigen tests have improved diagnostic capability.

SALICYLATE POISONING

Lars C. Larsen, MD

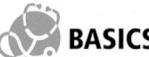 **BASICS**

DESCRIPTION
Systemic disorder caused by acute and/or chronic intoxication from salicylate-containing medications:
- Following accidental or intentional exposure, toxic actions of salicylates include:
  – Stimulation of central nervous system (CNS) respiratory center
  – Uncoupling of oxidative phosphorylation
  – Inhibition of Krebs cycle dehydrogenases
  – Stimulation of gluconeogenesis
  – Increased lipolysis and lipid metabolism
  – Inhibition of aminotransferases
  – Cyclo-oxygenase inhibition and decreased production of clotting factors
  – Irritation of the gastric mucosa and stimulation of the CNS chemoreceptor trigger zone
- These actions cause sequential and progressively severe physiologic abnormalities with increasing doses of salicylates, time following exposure, duration of chronic exposure, extremes of age, and presence of concurrent medical conditions; abnormalities include:
  – Respiratory alkalosis accompanied by progressive metabolic acidosis
  – Hyperpyrexia
  – Gastrointestinal (GI), renal, pulmonary, and skin losses of body fluids and electrolytes
  – Initial hyperglycemia followed by hypoglycemia, particularly CNS hypoglycemia
  – Abnormal hemostasis and coagulation
- Clinical presentation of patients with salicylate toxicity can range from minor symptoms to a syndrome initially indistinguishable from septic shock with multiple organ failure, including encephalopathy and acute respiratory distress syndrome (ARDS).
- The very young and elderly are particularly prone to develop severe toxicity, as are those with chronic intoxication.
- Conditions causing concurrent acidosis may increase tissue concentrations of salicylate and result in greater morbidity and mortality.
- System(s) affected: Cardiovascular; Endocrine/Metabolic; GI; Hematologic/Lymphatic/Immunologic; Musculoskeletal; Nervous; Pulmonary; Renal/Urologic; Skin/Exocrine

Geriatric Considerations
- Increased risk for chronic toxicity because of decreased renal function
- Increased risk for bleeding or perforated gastric ulcers in patients >70 years of age

Pediatric Considerations
Acidosis is often more severe in the very young, particularly in chronic or repeated therapeutic-dose poisonings.

Pregnancy Considerations
- Salicylates may cause premature closure of ductus arteriosus in the fetus.
- Increased risk of ante- and intrapartum hemorrhage

EPIDEMIOLOGY
Incidence/prevalence in the US:
- >7,300 ingestions of salicylate-containing medications reported to poison control in 2007
- No deaths in 2007 from single-substance exposures; none in children <6 years of age
- Occurs in children and adults at any age

RISK FACTORS
- Dehydration
- Conditions causing metabolic or respiratory acidosis
- Extremes of age—very young and elderly
- Psychiatric illness
- History of previous toxic ingestions or suicide attempts
- Concurrent oral poisoning with other substances
- Concurrent use of acetazolamide (Diamox)

GENERAL PREVENTION
- Patient and parent/caregiver education essential; see Patient Education
- Emergency telephone numbers (poison control centers): (800) 222-1222

ETIOLOGY
- Accidental or intentional ingestion of salicylates or salicylate-containing medications
- Percutaneous absorption of dermatologic medications containing salicylate
- Breastfeeding by mothers ingesting salicylate-containing medications
- Teething gels containing salicylates

COMMONLY ASSOCIATED CONDITIONS
Reye syndrome with salicylate use and varicella or influenza viral infection

 DIAGNOSIS

PHYSICAL EXAM
- Signs and symptoms may differ when the intoxication is acute or chronic.
- Acute intoxication:
  – Symptoms vary with amount ingested, usually begin within 3–8 hours of ingestion, and progress more rapidly in children:
    ○ <150 mg/kg, minimal symptoms
    ○ 150–300 mg/kg, moderate symptoms
    ○ 300–500 mg/kg, severe symptoms
    ○ >500 mg/kg, potentially fatal
  – Nausea and vomiting
  – Hyperpnea, tachypnea
  – Hyperpyrexia
  – Tinnitus
  – Disorientation, coma, convulsions
  – Cardiac arrhythmias
  – Hypotension
  – Pulmonary edema
- Chronic intoxication:
  – Onset of symptoms is usually gradual.
  – Signs and symptoms similar to acute intoxication may occur and may be advanced at diagnosis and include severe hypotension and ARDS.
  – Neurologic symptoms often predominate, particularly in the elderly, and include agitation, confusion, stupor, hyperactivity, paranoia, bizarre behavior, dysarthria, and restlessness.

DIAGNOSTIC TESTS & INTERPRETATION
Lab
- Serum salicylate levels initially on all patients to confirm diagnosis; following acute ingestions, check levels ≥6 h after ingestion and repeat q2h until the levels are declining and patient's condition has stabilized.
- Acid–base abnormalities common:
  – Usually respiratory alkalosis or mixed respiratory alkalosis and metabolic acidosis
  – Metabolic acidosis often predominates in chronic or severe acute poisonings and in poisonings in young children.
- Increased anion gap, especially in acute poisonings and salicylate-only poisonings
- Initial hyperglycemia may be followed by hypoglycemia.
- Electrolyte abnormalities such as hypernatremia or hyponatremia and hypokalemia are common.
- Dehydration findings are common, including an increased blood urea nitrogen (BUN):creatinine ratio.
- Prothrombin time (PT)/international normalization ratio (INR) may be increased.
- Liver function abnormalities may be present.
- Proteinuria and renal function abnormalities may be present.
- Stool guaiac testing may be positive.
- Occasional hypouricemia
- Drugs that may alter lab results:
  – Diflunisal (Dolobid) may cross-react with assay of salicylate concentration.
  – Medications affecting similar organ systems, including oral anticoagulants and hypoglycemic agents
- Disorders that may alter lab results: Concurrent medical conditions involving similar organ systems

Initial lab tests
- Serum salicylate levels initially and ≥6 h after ingestion, then repeat q2h until the levels are declining and patient's condition has stabilized
- Electrolytes, BUN, creatinine, glucose, liver function tests, uric acid
- Arterial blood gases
- PT/INR
- Urinalysis
- Stool guaiac testing may be positive.

Imaging
- Chest radiograph:
  – Noncardiogenic pulmonary edema
  – Variable severity, from mild to ARDS
- Abdominal plain film: Nonspecific bowel gas pattern with retained contrast material in chronic bismuth subsalicylate ingestion

Diagnostic Procedures/Surgery
- None, other than correlating serum salicylate concentration with clinical presentation
- Use of the Done nomogram in managing patients following acute ingestion is not recommended because it may underestimate the severity of poisonings in patients with:
  – Illnesses accompanied by dehydration and/or acidosis
  – Chronic exposure to salicylates
  – Ingestion of enteric-coated or sustained-release medications
  – Unknown time of ingestion

Pathological Findings

None specific for salicylate intoxication; associated findings include:

- GI:
  - Antral and prepyloric ulcers
  - Small bowel ulcerations with enteric-coated salicylates
- Renal:
  - Interstitial nephritis
  - Acute tubular necrosis
  - Minimal-change nephrotic syndrome
- Pulmonary:
  - Noncardiogenic pulmonary edema

DIFFERENTIAL DIAGNOSIS

- All ages:
  - Infection
  - Sepsis
  - Diabetic ketoacidosis
  - Other causes of metabolic acidosis
- In the elderly:
  - Delirium
  - Cerebral vascular accident
  - Myocardial infarction
  - Ethyl alcohol intoxication
  - Congestive heart failure

 TREATMENT

MEDICATION

- Prevent further absorption if the ingestion is felt to be life-threatening:
  - Gastric lavage is rarely indicated.
  - Activated charcoal within 1 hour of toxic ingestion (immediately after gastric lavage if performed) (1,2)[C]
  - Ipecac is no longer recommended for use at home or in health care facilities (3).
- Emergency facility/hospital:
  - Activated charcoal 1–2 g/kg, single dose
  - Fluid/electrolyte balance: IV fluids to restore intravascular volume and prevent hypoglycemia
  - With hypotension, give isotonic fluid until orthostatic changes are no longer present.
  - Fluids should contain ≥5% dextrose unless hyperglycemia is a problem.
  - Normal saline or a mixture of 0.45% NaCl with 1 ampule of sodium bicarbonate (43 mEq NaHCO$_3$) may be administered at 10–15 mL/kg/h × 1–2 hours depending on the degree of acidosis.
  - When blood pressure is stable, fluid management is directed toward alkalinizing the urine to enhance salicylate excretion, prevent CNS hypoglycemia, and treat fluid and electrolyte abnormalities.
  - Enhance elimination by alkaline diuresis (4)[C]:
    - Alkaline diuresis (urine pH >7.5) and prevention of hypoglycemia usually can be accomplished by initial bolus of NaHCO$_3$ 1–2 mEq/kg IV given over 1 hour, followed by infusion of 1,000 mL D$_5$W plus 2–3 ampules of NaHCO$_3$ (43 mEq NaHCO$_3$/ampule) at 1.5–2 times maintenance rate (or, at 2–3 mL/kg/hour). Consider adding 40 mEq of potassium chloride to each liter; monitor potassium levels closely.
    - Goal: Bicarbonate to alkalinize the urine (pH >7.5) and, when appropriate, to correct severe systemic acidosis (for pH <7.1)

- Potassium should be added for potassium levels <4.0 mEq/L.
    - Patients with cardiovascular compromise should be monitored closely for fluid overload.
    - Alkalinization can be discontinued when the salicylate level decreases into the therapeutic range.
  - Serum electrolytes and glucose should be monitored frequently and urine pH checked hourly until stable at >7.5. Arterial blood gases should be monitored >2–4 hours to ensure blood pH ≤7.5.
  - Hemodialysis should be considered in poisonings with markedly elevated salicylate levels (>100 mg/dL in acute poisonings, >40 mg/dL in chronic poisonings), acidosis unresponsive to alkalinization and diuresis, renal and/or hepatic dysfunction with impaired salicylate clearance, endotracheal intubation (excluding for coingestants), noncardiac pulmonary edema, and persistent, severe CNS symptoms.
  - Dextrose-containing IV solution to prevent hypoglycemia; CNS hypoglycemia may be present despite a normal serum glucose level.
- Contraindications: Medication allergies
- Precautions:
  - Intravascular overload may result from injudicious use of sodium bicarbonate.
  - Dextrose should not be given to patients with severe hyperglycemia.

ADDITIONAL TREATMENT

Issues for Referral

Psychiatric and psychological evaluation in emergency department and in close follow-up for intentional overdose

IN-PATIENT CONSIDERATIONS

Initial Stabilization

- Evaluate all patients at a health care facility.
- Outpatient for nontoxic accidental ingestions
- Inpatient for toxic and intentional ingestions (3)[C]

 ONGOING CARE

FOLLOW-UP RECOMMENDATIONS

Patient Monitoring

- Fluid, acid–base, blood glucose, and electrolyte status until stable; urine pH (to enhance elimination of salicylate)
- Psychiatric follow-up after intentional ingestions

DIET

No special diet

PATIENT EDUCATION

- Education of parents/caregivers during well-child visits
- Education of patients about chronic salicylate therapy
- Anticipatory guidance for caregivers, family, and cohabitants of potentially suicidal patients
- Patient brochure (item 1515): *Child Safety: Keeping Your Home Safe for Your Baby;* available from American Academy of Family Physicians: familydoctor.org or http://familydoctor.org/online/famdocen/home/healthy/safety/kids-family/027.html#ArticleParsysMiddleColumn0006
- Poison control: (800) 222-1222

PROGNOSIS

- Complete recovery with early therapy
- Clinical course and prognosis are worse in the very young and elderly, chronic intoxications, and in patients with concurrent conditions that cause dehydration and/or acidosis.

COMPLICATIONS

- Rare following recovery from poisoning
- Noncardiogenic pulmonary edema
- ARDS

REFERENCES

1. Gaudreault P. Activated charcoal revisited. *Clin Pediatr Emerg Med*. 2005;6:76–80.
2. Heard K. Gastrointestinal decontamination. *Med Clin North Am*. 2005;89:1067–78.
3. Chyka PA, et al. *Salicylate poisoning: an evidence-based consensus guideline for out-of-hospital management*. Washington (DC): American Association of Poison Control Centers; 2006.
4. Proudfoot AT, Krenzelok EP, Vale JA. Position Paper on urine alkalinization. *J Toxicol Clin Toxicol*. 2004;42:1–26.

ADDITIONAL READING

Bronstein AC, Spyker DA, Cantilena LR, et al. 2007 Annual Report of the American Association of Poison Control Centers' National Poison Data System (NPDS): 25th Annual Report. *Clin Toxicol (Phila)*. 2008;46:927–1057.

CODES

ICD9

965.1 Poisoning by salicylates

CLINICAL PEARLS

- Gastric decontamination should not be done in all poisonings, only in potentially life-threatening ingestions.
- Think of salicylate toxicity with mixed metabolic acidosis and respiratory alkalosis, especially if anion gap.
- Activated charcoal within 1 hour of toxic ingestion (immediately after gastric lavage, if performed) (1,2)[C]
- Ipecac is no longer recommended for use at home or in health care facilities.
- There is a bedside test to evaluate for the presence of salicylates. A few drops of 10% ferric chloride solution added to 1 mL of urine usually will produce a purple color if salicylates are present.

S

SALIVARY GLAND CALCULI/SIALADENITIS

Richard Gacek, MD

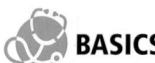 **BASICS**

DESCRIPTION
- Inflammation of ≥1 salivary glands
- The submandibular gland is more commonly affected by sialolithiasis and infection than the parotid gland.
- Chronicity:
  - Acute
  - Chronic
- Types:
  - Infectious
  - Obstructive (sialolithiasis)
  - Autoimmune
- System(s) affected: Gastrointestinal (GI)

EPIDEMIOLOGY
Incidence
- A review of British patients showed an incidence of symptomatic sialolithiasis of 27–59/1,000,000 population per year (1).
- Most common in debilitated patients
- Rare in children
- Predominant sex: Male = Female

RISK FACTORS
- Dehydration
- Anticholinergic use
- Antihistamine use
- Diuretic use
- Poor oral hygiene
- Malnutrition
- Head/neck radiation
- Tuberculosis (TB)
- HIV
- Failure to immunize (mumps)

Genetics
- Sjögren syndrome
- Polygenic cause, with several loci under investigation (2)

GENERAL PREVENTION
- Adequate post-op hydration
- Maintain oral care.
- Avoid antihistamines, anticholinergics, and other causes of xerostomia.

PATHOPHYSIOLOGY
Decreased salivary outflow from anticholinergics, dehydration, or radiation is thought to allow bacterial infection of salivary glands.

ETIOLOGY
- Bacterial:
  - *Staphylococcus aureus*
  - *Streptococcus viridans*
  - *Streptococcus pyogenes*
  - *Haemophilus influenza*
  - *Escherichia coli*
- Viral:
  - Mumps
  - Cytomegalovirus (CMV), Epstein-Barr virus (EBV)
  - HIV
  - Enteroviruses

COMMONLY ASSOCIATED CONDITIONS
- Post-op dehydration
- Radiation-induced xerostomia
- Drug-induced xerostomia
- Sjögren syndrome
- Hypercalcemia

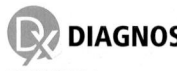 **DIAGNOSIS**

HISTORY
- Onset, duration of symptoms, previous episodes
- Dental pain, discharge, foul breath, pain with chewing
- Fever, unintentional weight loss
- Recent dental work, surgery
- Immunization history
- Radiation, TB, and HIV exposure
- History of alcoholism, bulimia, malnutrition (suggest sialadenosis)

PHYSICAL EXAM
- Palpate all salivary glands, floor of mouth, tongue, and neck to assess symmetry, tenderness, presence of stones, and lymphadenopathy.
- Examine duct openings for purulent discharge. Palpate gland gently to express purulent material.
- Examine eyes for keratitis.

DIAGNOSTIC TESTS & INTERPRETATION
Lab
Initial lab tests
- Complete blood count (CBC), electrolytes (3)[B]
- Culture and sensitivity of any expressed pus (3)[B]

Follow-Up & Special Considerations
If autoimmune process is suspected, consider ordering appropriate labs.

Imaging
Initial approach
- Computed tomography (CT) scan with IV contrast is the preferred imaging modality (4)[B].
- Ultrasound can localize abscesses, differentiate between solid and cystic disease, and extraglandular disease (5)[B].

Follow-Up & Special Considerations
Consider serial CT scans with contrast to evaluate disease resolution.

Diagnostic Procedures/Surgery
- Sialography to evaluate sialolithiasis and other obstructive lesions
- Sialoscopy to find and remove sialoliths (6)[B]

Pathological Findings
In chronic sialadenitis, loss of acini, fibrosis, and periductal lymphocytosis are evident. Degree indicates chronicity.

DIFFERENTIAL DIAGNOSIS
- Acute bacterial parotitis
- Chronic bacterial parotitis
- Dental abscess
- Mumps
- TB
- HIV (in pediatric populations)
- EBV, CMV, enteroviruses
- Tularemia
- Sialolithiasis
- Cystic fibrosis
- Lupus
- Sjögren syndrome
- Alcoholism
- Bulimia
- Hypothyroidism
- Pleomorphic adenoma
- Lymphoma
- Sarcoidosis
- Collagen-vascular disease
- Metal poisoning

TREATMENT

MEDICATION

First Line
- As *S. aureus* is the most common agent, antistaphylococcal penicillins (nafcillin, oxacillin, Unasyn, Augmentin) are indicated in areas where methicillin-resistant *Staphylococcus aureus* (MRSA) is not predominant.
- For PCN-allergic: Use clindamycin 300 mg p.o. q8h
- Antibiotic coverage should be narrowed once culture and sensitivity are available.
- Continue antibiotic therapy for 10–14 days (3)[B].

Second Line
1st-generation cephalosporin (cephazolin) or clindamycin is also indicated for empiric coverage (3)[B].

ADDITIONAL TREATMENT

General Measures
- Maintain hydration.
- Apply warm compresses.
- Maintain good oral hygiene.

Issues for Referral
In the case of poor dentition, dental abscess, refer patients to a dentist.

Additional Therapies
In the case of chronic sialadenitis with strictures, consider sialostent placement (6)[B].

COMPLEMENTARY AND ALTERNATIVE MEDICINE
Consider lemon drops or other sialogogues to promote salivation. In 1 study, post-op use of sialogogues nearly halved rates of sialadenitis (7)[B].

SURGERY/OTHER PROCEDURES
- Incision and drainage of parotid abscess is indicated after failing 3–5 days of medical management (3)[B].
- In the case of sialolithiasis, sialoscopy may be indicated for stone removal (3)[B].
- Patients with chronic sialadenitis refractory to medical management may be eligible for salivary gland removal (8)[B].

IN-PATIENT CONSIDERATIONS

Initial Stabilization
- Check vital signs, with particular attention to blood pressure (BP), as patient may be septic secondary to abscess formation.
- Evaluate airway patency.

Admission Criteria
- Parotid abscess
- Sepsis
- Inability to tolerate p.o. intake

Nursing
Responsibilities may include ensuring excellent oral hygiene, avoiding administration of sialogogues.

Discharge Criteria
- Exclude abscess, sepsis.
- Ensure ability to tolerate p.o. intake.

 ONGOING CARE

FOLLOW-UP RECOMMENDATIONS
- Provide regular follow-up visits for patients with chronic sialadenitis.
- Avoid prescribing medications that cause xerostomia.

Patient Monitoring
Monitor patients with chronic sialadenitis, as decreased salivary gland function due to fibrosis and loss of acini can lead to acute exacerbations.

DIET
- Avoid sialogogues during acute attacks.
- Maintain adequate hydration on an outpatient basis.

PATIENT EDUCATION
- Educate patients on maintaining excellent oral hygiene.
- Educate patients on maintaining good hydration.

PROGNOSIS
Generally excellent, with acute symptoms resolving in about a week with appropriate treatment.

COMPLICATIONS
- Abscess
- Dental caries
- Recurrent sialadenitis
- Facial nerve impingement (rare)
- Ludwig angina

REFERENCES

1. Escudier MP, McGurk M. Symptomatic sialoadenitis and sialolithiasis in the English population, an estimate of the cost of hospital treatment. *Br Dent J.* 1999;186:463–6.
2. Williams PH, et al. Horizons in Sjögren's syndrome genetics. *Clin Rev Allerg Immunol.* 2007;32:201–9.
3. Fattahi TT, Lyu PE, Van Sickels JE. Management of acute suppurative parotitis. *J Oral Maxillofac Surg.* 2002;60:446–8.
4. Yousem DM, Kraut MA, Chalian AA. Major salivary gland imaging. *Radiology.* 2000;216:19–29.
5. Alyas F, Lewis K, Williams M, et al. Diseases of the submandibular gland as demonstrated using high resolution ultrasound. *Br J Radiol.* 2005;78:362–9.
6. Nahlieli O, Bar T, Shacham R, et al. Management of chronic recurrent parotitis: current therapy. *J Oral Maxillofac Surg.* 2004;62:1150–5.
7. Nakada K, Ishibashi T, Takei T, et al. Does lemon candy decrease salivary gland damage after radioiodine therapy for thyroid cancer? *J Nucl Med.* 2005;46:261–6.
8. Patel RS, Low TH, Gao K, et al. Clinical outcome after surgery for 75 patients with parotid sialadenitis. *Laryngoscope.* 2007;117:644–7.

ADDITIONAL READING

Ship JA. Diagnosing, managing, and preventing salivary gland disorders. *Oral Dis.* 2002;8:77–89.

CODES

ICD9
- 527.2 Sialoadenitis
- 527.5 Sialolithiasis

CLINICAL PEARLS
- Sialadenitis occurs mainly in debilitated patients.
- Mainstay of treatment is hydration, good oral hygiene.
- Salivary gland abscess must be drained surgically.

S

SALIVARY GLAND TUMORS

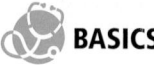

Sagar C. Patel, MD
Edward Feller, MD

BASICS

Salivary gland tumors consist of benign or malignant neoplasms of the major and minor salivary glands. Tumors may be mimicked clinically by a variety of inflammatory or infectious disorders.
- Major: Parotid, submaxillary, sublingual glands
- Minor: Intraoral, pharyngeal, and nasal glands (600–1000 glands distributed throughout the upper aerodigestive tract)

DESCRIPTION
- Adult neoplasms:
  - Benign: Pleomorphic adenoma, Warthin tumor, oncocytoma, and monomorphic adenoma
  - Malignant: Mucoepidermoid carcinoma, adenoid cystic carcinoma, acinic cell carcinoma, carcinoma ex-pleomorphic adenoma, squamous cell carcinoma (SCC), adenocarcinoma
- Total distribution of salivary gland neoplasms by type:
  - Pleomorphic adenoma (most common): 45% overall
  - Monomorphic adenoma: 12% overall
  - Mucoepidermoid carcinoma: 12% overall
  - Adenoid cystic carcinoma: 6% overall
  - Remaining neoplasms: 15% overall
- Total distribution by site: Parotid (80%); submandibular (10–15%); sublingual and minor (5–10%)
  - Parotid (80% benign; 20% malignant):
    ○ Pleomorphic adenoma: 60%
    ○ Monomorphic adenoma: 8%
    ○ Warthin tumor: 8%
    ○ Mucoepidermoid carcinoma: 12%
    ○ Adenoid cystic carcinoma: 5%
    ○ Adenocarcinoma and SCC: 5%
  - Submandibular (60% benign; 40% malignant):
    ○ Pleomorphic adenoma: 40%
    ○ Mucoepidermoid carcinoma: 10%
    ○ Adenoid cystic carcinoma: 20%
  - Lingual a minor salivary glands (40% benign; 60% malignant):
    ○ Pleomorphic adenoma: 40%
    ○ Mucoepidermoid carcinoma: 25%
    ○ Adenoid cystic carcinoma: 25%; generally, as the size of the neoplasm decreases, the incidence of malignancy increases.
- Pediatric neoplasms:
  - Incidence is rare in children but much more likely to be malignant.
  - Benign: 65% of overall cases; the most common types are hemangiomas and pleomorphic adenomas.
  - Malignant: 35% of overall cases; most common type is mucoepidermoid carcinoma.

EPIDEMIOLOGY
Incidence
- 1.5 cases per 100,000 individuals in the US
- ~700 deaths annually
- Median age:
  - Benign: age 45
  - Malignant: age 60
- Gender predilection:
  - Benign: Female > Male
  - Malignant: Male = Female

Prevalence
Make up 6% of all head and neck neoplasms

RISK FACTORS
- Tobacco and alcohol abuse associated with Warthin tumor, but not with SCC
- Alcohol increases likelihood ratio by 2:1 (1,2).
- Radiation has shown a 4-fold increased dose-related response in salivary gland cancer 15–20 years after treatment. Increased risk has also been reported in atomic bomb survivors (1,2).
- Epstein-Barr virus has been associated with lymphoepithelial carcinoma in Asians, but there is no evidence of causal association in other tumors (1,2).
- Silica dust has been associated with a 2.5-fold increase in salivary gland neoplasia (1,2).
- Kerosene cooking fuel exposure (1,2)
- Nitrosamine exposure in rubber workers (1,2)
- Early menarche and nulliparity (1,2)

Genetics
Increased incidence of adenocarcinoma of parotid in Eskimos; otherwise, no known genetic pattern

GENERAL PREVENTION
- Tobacco cessation
- Alcohol cessation

PATHOPHYSIOLOGY
Pathophysiology is not fully understood. Certain pathways and oncogenes have been implicated, such as *p53, Bcl-2, PI3K/Akt, MDM2, VEGF, HGF,* and *ras*.

ETIOLOGY
- Etiology is not fully understood.
- Predominant theory: Tumors arise from either the excretory duct reserve cell or the intercalated duct reserve cell.

DIAGNOSIS

HISTORY
- Focused inquiry:
  - Specific presentation of mass: Initial recognition; rate of growth; change in size with actions, especially with food consumption; xerostomia (Sjögren syndrome, prior irradiation, medication)
  - Intermittent, recurrent gland enlargement suggests sialolithiasis (calculi in salivary duct); rarely, can be due to malignancy.
  - Pain: Type, degree, accentuating and/or alleviating factors, temporality
  - Location and spread
  - Effect on associated structures with relevant review of systems: Larynx (airway obstruction, hoarseness, dysphagia); nasal cavity/paranasal sinuses (nasal obstruction, sinusitis); pharyngeal wall invasion (dysphagia, muffled voice)
- Common presentations:
  - Overall: Typically, a slow-growing, painless, discrete mass
  - Parotid neoplasm: Discrete mass typically at the tail of the gland
  - Submandibular neoplasm: Associated with diffuse enlargement of the gland itself
  - Sublingual neoplasm: Tends to produce palpable fullness in the floor of the mouth
  - Minor gland neoplasm: Depends on initial site of origin

- Indicator of malignancy:
  - Facial paralysis, paresthesias, or other neurologic deficit associated with mass
  - Pain is not a clear indicator of malignancy; may be associated with both benign and malignant neoplasms; exquisite pain is more likely due to infectious cause.

PHYSICAL EXAM
- Complete HEENT examination with emphasized focus:
  - Evaluate the size, mobility, and extent of the mass.
  - Elicit any fixation to surrounding structures.
  - Elicit tenderness upon palpation.
  - If tenderness present, massage gland to express purulent material due to infection.
  - Lymphadenopathy, especially, in neck levels I–V
  - Referred pain (otalgia)
- Complete neurological exam with focus on cranial nerves:
  - Facial nerve palsy or paralysis may indicate a malignant lesion with perineural invasion.

DIAGNOSTIC TESTS & INTERPRETATION
- Technetium-99m (Warthin tumor): Follow patient closely; Warthin tumor has low chance of metastasis.
- Sialography (for calculi or chronic parotitis)

Lab
- Autoimmune studies (ESR, CRP, ANA)
- Fractionated amylase (inflammation)
- Drugs that may alter lab results: None known
- Disorders that may alter lab results: None known

Imaging
- CXR:
  - Sjögren syndrome
  - Metastases
- Ultrasound: Inflammatory or malignant
- CT scan: Provides detail of tumor invasion and temporal bone or mandibular destruction
- MRI:
  - Provides definition of soft tissue and any evidence of perineural invasion or intracranial extension
  - Discriminates tumor from mucus and bone marrow invasion
- PET scan: Useful for detecting malignancy in early stages and for detecting recurrences and differentiating soft-tissue damage secondary to radiation from inflammatory changes
- Staging (2002 AJCC)
  - TNM (tumor size, nodal status, and metastasis)
  - Stage I–IVc

Diagnostic Procedures/Surgery
- Fine-needle aspiration:
  - Concern for possible tumor seeding via needle track; however, tumor spread from tumor seeding is rare.
  - Sensitivity 92%, specificity 100%, but false-negative rate up to 53% (3)
- Superficial parotidectomy with identification and preservation of facial nerve

DIFFERENTIAL DIAGNOSIS
- Metabolic causes (diabetes, vitamin deficiencies, alcohol, gout)
- Drugs (thiourea, iodine)
- Inflammatory masses

- Parotid and submandibular lymph nodes
- Mikulicz syndrome
- Salivary gland stones
- Torus palatinus (minor)
- Necrotizing sialometaplasia (minor)
- Cervical lymph nodes
- Sjögren syndrome
- Sarcoidosis
- HIV-associated enlargement (lymphoepithelial cyst)
- Actinomycosis
- Cat-scratch disease
- Tuberculosis

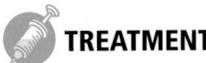 TREATMENT

- Surgical excision is the primary treatment for all salivary gland tumors.
- Facial nerve is spared unless it is directly involved or highly suspicious.
- Poor general response to chemotherapy
- Adjuvant chemotherapy is currently indicated for palliation.
- Radiotherapy is currently used for nonresectable, extensive, large tumors.
- No level 1 trials have shown efficacy for postoperative radiotherapy.

MEDICATION
Cisplatin-, fluorouracil-, or paclitaxel-based regimens for recurrent or nonoperable disease (4)

ADDITIONAL TREATMENT
General Measures
Postoperative care:
- Elevate head of bed postoperatively.
- Suction drainage for 1–2 days
- Suture-line care with antibiotic ointment
- Examination for facial nerve function
- Monitor for signs of hematoma and drain if present.
- Usually 1- to 2-day hospitalization

Additional Therapies
- Postoperative irradiation (via fast neutron beam) for larger and high-grade carcinomas
- Chemotherapy reserved for metastases or locally advanced and unresectable tumors

SURGERY/OTHER PROCEDURES
- Benign tumors: Superficial or total conservative (nerve-sparing) parotidectomy
- Malignant tumors:
  – Total parotidectomy or sialadenectomy with adjuvant radiotherapy to parotid base of skull ± neck dissection
  – Preservation of facial nerve unless involved by tumor
- Cervical lymphadenectomy if palpable nodes or elective neck dissection in SCC, high-grade mucoepidermoid carcinoma, or high-grade adenocarcinoma

IN-PATIENT CONSIDERATIONS
Initial Stabilization
Inpatient care

Admission Criteria
Airway impingement

 ONGOING CARE

FOLLOW-UP RECOMMENDATIONS
Activity: Moderate restriction for 1 day postop

Patient Monitoring
- For malignancy: Once every 6–8 weeks the 1st year, every 8–12 weeks the 2nd year, every 4 months the 3rd year, every 6 months the 4th year, and then yearly visits
- For benign tumors: Once a year for 5 years

DIET
Nonstimulating liquid diet

PATIENT EDUCATION
- Xerostomia treatment and mouth care
- Tobacco cessation
- Alcohol abstinence
- Sensorineural hearing loss

PROGNOSIS
- By tumor type:
  – Parotid pleomorphic adenoma: Untreated will demonstrate malignant degeneration in 2–10% over 20 years. Treated adequately, parotid pleomorphic adenoma has 1.5% recurrence rate. Extension of pseudopods of tumor beyond the tumor mass increases the risk of recurrent disease.
  – Adenoid cystic:
    ○ Parotid: 5-year survival, 73%; 15-year survival, 21%
    ○ Submandibular: 5-year survival, 50%; 15-year survival, 0%;
    ○ Palate: 5-year survival, 80%; 15-year survival, 38%
  – Adenocarcinoma:
    ○ Aggressive tumors with a tendency for local recurrence (38%); regional lymph node metastasis (33%); and dissemination to lungs, bone, and liver
    ○ 5-year survival, 78%; 20-year survival, 41%
  – Mucoepidermoid:
    ○ Low-grade: 5-year survival, 81%; 15-year survival, 48%
    ○ High-grade: 5-year survival, 46%; 15-year survival, 25%
  – SCC:
    ○ Rare tumor with 50% incidence of cervical lymph node metastasis and local recurrence
    ○ 5-year survival, 18%; 15-year survival, 0%
  – Lymphoma:
    ○ Rare, accounting for 1.7% of salivary neoplasms
    ○ 5-year survival: Hodgkin-type, 90%; non-Hodgkin-type, 43%
- 5-year survival rate for stages I–IV and cause-specific survival (CSS):
  – Stage I: 75% (CSS 86%)
  – Stage II: 59% (CSS 66%)
  – Stage III: 57% (CSS 53%)
  – Stage IV: 28% (CSS 32%)

COMPLICATIONS
- Frey syndrome (gustatory sweating) occurs symptomatically in ~20% of patients undergoing parotidectomy.
- Hematoma with possible posterior displacement of tongue and airway obstruction
- Facial neurapraxia from surgery should resolve within 6 months, even with radiotherapy.

- Cosmetic deformity of moderate facial flattening on side of parotidectomy
- Injury to hypoglossal or lingual nerve
- If inadequately excised, pleomorphic adenoma may recur owing to pseudopods in the lobe.
- Wound infection of surgical site

REFERENCES

1. Spitz MR. Epidemiology and risk factors for head and neck cancer. *Semin Oncol*. 1994;21:281–8.
2. Zheng W, et al. Diet and other risk factors for cancer of the salivary glands: A population-based case-control study. *Intern J Cancer*. 1996;67(2): 194–8.
3. Cohen EG, Patel SG, Lin O, et al. Fine-needle aspiration biopsy of salivary gland lesions in a selected patient population. *Arch Otolaryngol Head Neck Surg*. 2004;130:773–8.
4. Surakanti SG, Agulnik M. Salivary gland malignancies: the role for chemotherapy and molecular targeted agents. *Semin Oncol*. 2008;35:309–19.

ADDITIONAL READING

- de Bree R, van der Waal I, Leemans CR. Management of frey syndrome. *Head Neck*. 2007.
- Guzzo M, Ferrari A, Marcon I, et al. Salivary gland neoplasms in children: the experience of the Istituto Nazionale Tumori of Milan. *Pediatr Blood Cancer*. 2006;47:806–10.
- Tiselius HG. Epidemiology and medical management of stone disease. *BJU Int*. 2003;91:758–67.
- Worster A, Preyra I, Weaver B, et al. The accuracy of noncontrast helical computed tomography versus intravenous pyelography in the diagnosis of suspected acute urolithiasis: a meta-analysis. *Ann Emerg Med*. 2002;40:280–6.

See Also (Topic, Algorithm, Electronic Media Element)
Sjögren's Syndrome

CODES

ICD9
- 142.0 Malignant neoplasm of parotid gland
- 142.1 Malignant neoplasm of submandibular gland
- 142.2 Malignant neoplasm of sublingual gland

CLINICAL PEARLS

- Delay in diagnosis is common in rare disease, especially with diverse, nonspecific presentation of minor salivary gland tumors.
- To evaluate a patient with a suspected salivary gland malignancy, complete history, physical, and consider either CT scan or MRI; fine-needle aspiration likely will yield a working diagnosis.
- A neck lymphadenectomy is required with tumors ≥4 cm in size, SCC, adenocarcinoma, undifferentiated carcinoma, and high-grade mucoepidermoid carcinoma.

SALMONELLA INFECTION

Richard Viken, MD

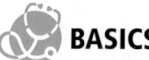 **BASICS**

DESCRIPTION
- Disease caused by any serotype of the bacterial genus *Salmonella*
- Clinical syndromes include enterocolitis (75%), bacteremia (10%), enteric fever (10%) (see "Typhoid Fever"), localized infection outside GI tract (5%), and an asymptomatic carrier state (<1%).
- Organisms invade gut mucosa, producing inflammatory, cytotoxic response.
- Organisms then can disseminate into systemic circulation via lymphatics.
- Infective dose and host defenses dictate extent of disease.
- Molecular studies have determined the total genome DNA sequence for a particular multidrug-resistant human *Salmonella* serotype.
- System(s) affected: GI
- Synonym: Nontyphoidal salmonellosis

Geriatric Considerations
Patients >60 years of age have a high carrier rate, presumably owing to biliary sequestration of organisms.

Pediatric Considerations
Children, especially neonates, are more likely to become chronic carriers.

Pregnancy Considerations
- An infectious disease consult is helpful.
- Keep a low threshold for hospital admission.

EPIDEMIOLOGY
Incidence
- Predominant age:
  - High prevalence in persons >70 or <20 years of age
  - Highest in infants <1 year of age
- In the US:
  - 800 cases/100,000 population/year
  - Peak frequency: July–November
  - Summer 2010 produced a Salmonella outbreak in the US that reported over 2400 cases in 4 months (1600 more than typically expected), and triggered the recall of over 500 million eggs (1)[C].
  - *Salmonella* isolations represent only 1–10% of the actual yearly incidence.
  - 2nd only to *Campylobacter* as the cause of bacterial diarrheal illness
  - A less common cause of traveler's diarrhea (2)[A]
  - Each year, an average of 55 outbreaks of *Salmonella* infection are reported to the CDC. Go to www.cdc.gov for instant updates.

Prevalence
In the US:
- Infants: 130/100,000
- Adults: 6/100,000

RISK FACTORS
- Impaired gastric acidity: Histamine-2 receptor blockers, antacids, gastrectomy, achlorhydria
- Hemolytic anemias: Sickle cell, malaria, bartonellosis
- Malignancy: Lymphoma, leukemia, disseminated carcinoma (3)[C]
- Immunosuppression: AIDS, DM, steroids, other immunosuppressants, chemotherapy, radiation (3)[C]
- Pets with high fecal carriage rates for *Salmonella*, especially reptiles. Antibiotic treatment of the animal is not recommended owing to temporary effect only.

GENERAL PREVENTION
- Proper hygiene in production, transport, and storage of food (such as keeping eggs refrigerated, as that minimizes multiplication of the bacteria if present, and cooking them individually and thoroughly before consumption)
- Control of animal reservoir, especially by avoiding contact with animal feces
- Hand-washing emphasized

ETIOLOGY
- Ingestion of contaminated food (e.g., poultry, beef, eggs, tomatoes, dairy products, commercially prepared nuts and nut products) or water accounts for 95% of cases (4)[C].
- Person-to-person and/or fecal–oral spread
- Iatrogenic contamination (e.g., blood transfusion, endoscopy)
- Contact with asymptomatic chronic carrier (e.g., day-care center)
- Intentional contamination of restaurant food through criminal mischief has been reported.
- Contaminated marijuana is an important source of infection, particularly in young adults.

COMMONLY ASSOCIATED CONDITIONS
- Ulcerative colitis
- SLE
- Schistosomiasis
- Cholelithiasis
- Nephrolithiasis

 DIAGNOSIS

HISTORY
- In outbreaks, >50% of individuals infected may remain asymptomatic (5)[C].
- Symptoms usually occur 12–72 hours after a contaminated ingestion.
- Acute uncomplicated illness:
  - Sudden onset of nausea, vomiting, bloody diarrhea, and abdominal cramping
  - Headache, myalgias
  - Fever to 102°F (39°C)

PHYSICAL EXAM
Protracted disease can present with the following:
- Persistent fever
- Arthritis, reactive or septic
- Osteomyelitis
- Sacroiliitis
- Wound infection, soft-tissue abscesses

- Meningitis
- Arteritis
- Endocarditis, pericarditis
- Pneumonia, lung abscess, empyema
- Hypovolemia
- Splenic (abscess)
- Hepatic (abscess)
- UTI

DIAGNOSTIC TESTS & INTERPRETATION
A rapid test (TUBEX) used in children to detect anti-*Salmonella* IgM antibodies was found to be 92.6% sensitive and 94.8% specific.

Lab
- Enterocolitis:
  - Fecal leukocytes positive
  - Stool culture positive for *Salmonella* sp.
  - WBC normal or decreased
  - Blood cultures negative
- Bacteremia:
  - Blood cultures positive
  - Stool cultures negative
- Local infections:
  - Polymorphonuclear leukocytosis
  - Tissue site culture positive
- Asymptomatic carrier state:
  - Stool culture positive for >1 year
  - Urine culture may be positive with certain serotypes.
- Drugs that may alter lab results: Antibiotics used early may lead to false-negative cultures and blunted immunologic response.

Imaging
Angiography in patients >50 years of age with bacteremia to rule out presence of infected aneurysm, particularly of aortoiliac vessels

Pathological Findings
- Mucosal ulceration, hemorrhage, and necrosis
- Reticuloendothelial hyperplasia and hypertrophy
- Focal organ and soft-tissue abscesses

DIFFERENTIAL DIAGNOSIS
- Viral gastroenteritis
- Other bacterial enteritis (e.g., shigellosis, cholera)
- Other bacterial sources or systemic and localized sepsis (e.g., meningococci, staphylococci)
- Pseudomembranous colitis
- Inflammatory or granulomatous bowel disease
- Appendicitis
- Cholecystitis
- Perforated viscus

TREATMENT

- Outpatient for uncomplicated enterocolitis and carrier state
- ~29% of patients are hospitalized because of bacteremia, extraintestinal infection, and age-related complications (5)[B].
- Do not wait for stool culture results before initiating therapy (3)[C].

MEDICATION
First Line

- Enterocolitis, uncomplicated: None recommended (6)[A]

- Enterocolitis, complicated by age extremes, immunosuppression, underlying cardiovascular abnormalities, prosthetic orthopedic devices, hemolytic anemia (7)[C]:
  – Adults:
    ○ Ciprofloxacin (Cipro): 500 mg PO bid × 5–7 days *or*
    ○ Azithromycin (Zithromax): 1.0 g PO once, then 500 mg PO every day for 6 days
  – Children:
    ○ Ampicillin: 50–100 mg/kg/day in 4 divided doses × 10–14 days *or*
    ○ Trimethoprim-sulfamethoxazole (Bactrim, Septra): 10–50 mg/kg/d in 2 divided doses × 10–14 days

- Bacteremia
  – Adults (3)[C]:
    ○ Ciprofloxacin (Cipro): 400 mg IV b.i.d. or 500 mg PO b.i.d. × 7 days *or*
    ○ Ceftriaxone (Rocephin): 2 g IV and IM every day × 7 days
  – Children:
    ○ Ampicillin: 200 mg/kg/d in 4 divided doses × 10–14 days *or*
    ○ Trimethoprim-sulfamethoxazole (Bactrim, Septra): 10–50 mg/kg/d in 2 divided doses × 10–14 days *or*
    ○ Chloramphenicol: 75 mg/kg/day in 4 divided doses × 10–14 days

- Localized infection:
  – Same as for bacteremia
  – In sustained bacteremia or prolonged local infection, antibiotics can be given PO for 4–6 weeks (substitute trimethoprim-sulfamethoxazole for cefotaxime using 2–4 double-strength tablets given tid).

- Chronic carrier state:
  – Ampicillin: 2–4 g/day plus probenecid 1–2 g/day, both divided into 4 PO doses, × 6 weeks *or*
  – Trimethoprim: 40–160 mg/day and 200–800 mg/day sulfamethoxazole divided into 2 doses × 6 weeks
  – Consider ciprofloxacin 500 mg PO bid × 4 weeks or norfloxacin (Noroxin) 400 mg PO bid × 4 weeks if gallstones are present.
  – Contraindications: Known drug allergy
  – Precautions:
    ○ Use bowel motility inhibitors (Lomotil, Imodium) with caution, if at all.
    ○ Monitor blood levels of chloramphenicol in neonates and infants.
    ○ Ampicillin-resistant strains are increasing, now at 15–30% in the US. Some strains are rapidly becoming multidrug-resistant (3)[C].
  – Significant possible interactions
    ○ Ampicillin failure rate is 75% in chronic carriers with gallbladder disease.
  – Fluoroquinolone resistance has been observed in some *Salmonella* serotypes common to swine and humans. Use of fluoroquinolones in food animals is implicated (3)[C].
  – Ceftriaxone resistance has been reported in the US with increasing frequency (4)[C].

Second Line
Fluoroquinolones:

- Ciprofloxacin (Cipro) and ofloxacin (Floxin) are gaining favor for use in the management of gastroenteritis, osteomyelitis, and the carrier state.
- Routinely given to children for 5–7 days in areas of the world where multidrug-resistant *S. typhi* is common (3)[C].

ADDITIONAL TREATMENT
General Measures
- Correct fluid and electrolyte deficits.
- Control symptoms (pain, nausea, vomiting).

SURGERY/OTHER PROCEDURES
- Surgical excision, drainage, and vascular bypass procedures for infected tissue sites, particularly endocarditis (3)[C]
- When biliary tract disease is present, the best results are obtained with a combination of cholecystectomy and a 10- to 14-day course of parenteral antibiotics (see "First Line: Bacteremia") initiated before surgery.

 ONGOING CARE

FOLLOW-UP RECOMMENDATIONS
As tolerated

Patient Monitoring
- Repeat stool culture at 5 months (40% of children are negative; 90% of adults are negative) and at 1 year (>99% of all patients are negative).
- Check state law regarding health care professional infections and return-to-work rules.

DIET
Give oral rehydration solution during diarrhea phase; advance to normal diet as tolerated.

PATIENT EDUCATION
Food Safety and Inspection Service, Office of Public Awareness, Department of Agriculture, Room 1165-S, Washington, DC 20205, (202) 447-9351

PROGNOSIS
- Prognosis for enterocolitis is excellent. Exceptions:
  – The very young: 5.0% fatal
  – The very old: 8.7% fatal
  – The debilitated and/or institutionalized: 2.3% fatal
- Prognosis for meningitis or endocarditis is poor, unless effective treatment is given early.
- Mortality increased with multidrug-resistant strain.
- Patients with *Salmonella* infection have an increased mortality rate for up to 1 year after the acute phase of infection (5)[C].

COMPLICATIONS
- Toxic megacolon
- Hypovolemic shock
- Metastatic abscess formation
- Acute or chronic hydrocephalus
- The frequency of reactive arthritis after various *Salmonella* outbreaks <10%.

REFERENCES

1. Kuehn BM, et al. Salmonella cases traced to egg producers: findings trigger recall of more than 500 million eggs. *JAMA*. 2010;304:1316.
2. Shah N, DuPont HL, Ramsey DJ. Global etiology of travelers' diarrhea: systematic review from 1973 to the present. *Am J Trop Med Hyg*. 2009;80:609–14.
3. Hohmann EL. Nontyphoidal salmonellosis. *Clin Infect Dis*. 2001;32:263–9.
4. Pitout JDD, Church DL. Emerging gram-negative enteric infections. *Clin Lab Med*. 2004;24:605–26.
5. Fisker N, Vinding K, Molbak K, et al. Clinical review of nontyphoid *Salmonella* infections from 1991 to 1999 in a Danish county. *Clin Infect Dis*. 2003;37:e47–e52.
6. Amieva M. Important bacterial gastrointestinal pathogens in children: A pathogenesis perspective. *Pediatric Clinics of North America*. 2005;52: 749–77.
7. Pigott DC. Foodborne illness. *Emerg Med Clin North Am*. 2008;26:475–97, x.

See Also (Topic, Algorithm, Electronic Media Element)
Typhoid Fever

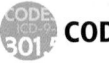 CODES

ICD9
- 003.0 *Salmonella* Salmonella gastroenteritis
- 003.1 *Salmonella* Salmonella septicemia
- 003.9 *Salmonella* Salmonella infection, unspecified

CLINICAL PEARLS

- If 1 member of a household becomes infected with *Salmonella*, the chance of at least 1 other member becoming infected is 60%.
- In outbreaks, >50% of individuals infected may remain asymptomatic.
- Symptoms usually occur 6–72 hours after a contaminated ingestion.
  – Acute uncomplicated illness: Nausea, vomiting, bloody diarrhea, abdominal cramping, headache, myalgias, and fever
  – Treatment of uncomplicated gastroenteritis generally is unnecessary because of its self-limited nature. There is some evidence that antibiotic treatment may prolong the carrier state.
- Those at greatest risk of death from *Salmonella* infection include the very young and the very old.

SARCOIDOSIS

Donnah Mathews, MD

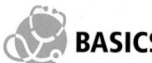 **BASICS**

DESCRIPTION

Sarcoidosis is a noninfectious, multisystem granulomatous disease of unknown cause, commonly affecting young and middle-aged adults:

- Frequently presents with hilar adenopathy, pulmonary infiltrates, ocular and skin lesions
- In about one-half of cases, it is diagnosed in asymptomatic patients with abnormal CXRs.
- Almost any other organ may be involved, including liver, spleen, lymph nodes, heart, and CNS.
- System(s) affected: Primarily Pulmonary but also Cardiovascular; GI; Hematologic/Lymphatic; Endocrine; Renal; Neurologic; Dermatologic; Ophthalmologic; Musculoskeletal
- Synonyms: Löfgren syndrome (erythema nodosum, hilar adenopathy plus uveitis); Heerfordt syndrome (uveitis, parotid enlargement, facial palsy, fever); Besnier-Boeck disease; Boeck sarcoid; Schaumann disease) (1,2)[C]

EPIDEMIOLOGY

Incidence
Estimated 6/100 person-years (3)

Prevalence
- Estimated 10–20/100,000 persons
- <15% of patients with active disease >60 years of age
- Rare in children (3,4)

RISK FACTORS
Exact etiology and pathogenesis remain unknown.

Genetics
- Reports of familial clustering
- 3–4× more common in African Americans
- Although worldwide in distribution, there is increased prevalence in Scandinavians, Japanese, and black women (3,4).

GENERAL PREVENTION
None

PATHOPHYSIOLOGY
- Thought to be due to exaggerated cell-mediated immune response to unknown antigen(s)
- In the lungs, the initial lesion is CD4+ T-cell alveolitis, causing noncaseating granulomata, which may resolve or undergo fibrosis.

ETIOLOGY
Unknown

COMMONLY ASSOCIATED CONDITIONS
None

DIAGNOSIS

HISTORY
- Patients may be completely asymptomatic.
- Patients may have nonspecific complaints such as:
  - Fever
  - Night sweats
  - Weight loss
  - General fatigue
  - Eye pain
  - Cough
  - Shortness of breath
  - Chest pain
  - Skin lesions
  - Polyarthritis
  - Facial droop due to Bell's palsy (5)

PHYSICAL EXAM
- Many patients have a completely normal physical exam with no findings.
- Lungs may reveal wheezing.
- Extrapulmonary manifestations may include:
  - Uveitis
  - Cranial nerve palsies
  - Salivary gland swelling
  - Lymphadenopathy
  - Arrhythmias
  - Hepatosplenomegaly
  - Polyarthritis
  - Rashes: Maculopapular, nodular, plaques, or erythema nodosum

DIAGNOSTIC TESTS & INTERPRETATION
Lab
No definitive test for diagnosis, but diagnosis is suggested by the following:
- Clinical and radiographic manifestations
- Exclusion of other diagnoses
- Histopathologic detection of noncaseating granulomas

Initial lab tests
- Complete blood count (CBC): Anemia or leukopenia ± eosinophilia can be seen.
- Hypergammaglobulinemia can exist.
- Liver function tests (LFTs): Abnormal liver function and increased alkaline phosphatase are encountered frequently.
- Calcium: Hypercalciuria occurs in up to 10% of patients, with hypercalcemia less frequent.
- Serum angiotensin-converting enzyme (ACE) is elevated in >75% of patients but is not diagnostic or exclusionary:
  - Drugs that may alter lab results: Prednisone will lower serum ACE and normalize gallium scan. ACE inhibitors will lower serum ACE level.
  - Disorders that may alter lab results: Hyperthyroidism and diabetes will increase serum ACE level (5)[C].

Imaging
Initial approach
- CXR or CT scan may reveal granulomas or hilar adenopathy. Routine CXRs are staged using Scadding classification (6):
  - Stage 0 = normal
  - Stage 1 = bilateral hilar adenopathy alone
  - Stage 2 = bilateral hilar adenopathy plus parenchymal infiltrates
  - Stage 3 = parenchymal infiltrates alone (primarily upper lobes)
  - Stage 4 = pulmonary fibrosis
- Chest CT scan may enhance appreciation of lymph nodes.
- High-resolution chest CT scan shows peribronchial disease.
- Gallium scan will be positive in areas of acute disease or inflammation, but is not specific.
- PET scan can indicate areas of disease activity in lungs, lymph nodes, and other areas of the body.
- Cardiac PET scan may detect cardiac sarcoidosis (5)[B].

Diagnostic Procedures/Surgery
- Pulmonary function testing may reveal restrictive pattern with decreased DLCO.
- Characteristically in active disease, bronchioalveolar lavage fluid has an increased CD4/CD8 ratio.
- Ophthalmologic examination may reveal uveitis, retinal vasculitis, or conjunctivitis.
- ECG
- Purified protein derivative (PPD)
- Biopsy of lesions should reveal noncaseating granulomas.

ALERT
If signs indicate Löfgren syndrome, it is not necessary to perform a biopsy because prognosis is good with observation alone, and biopsy would not change management.

Pathological Findings
Noncaseating epithelioid granulomas without evidence of fungal or mycobacterial infection

DIFFERENTIAL DIAGNOSIS
- Infectious granulomatous disease such as tuberculosis and fungal infections
- Hypersensitivity pneumonitis
- Lymphoma
- Other malignancies associated with lymphadenopathy
- Berylliosis

TREATMENT

- A large portion of patients undergo spontaneous remission. It is difficult to assess disease activity and severity, however, making it challenging to develop guidelines.
- No treatment may be necessary in asymptomatic individuals, but treatment may be needed for specific indications, such as cardiac, CNS, or ocular involvement.
- Treatment of pulmonary and skin manifestations is done on the basis of impairment. The symptoms that necessitate systemic therapy remain controversial:
  – Worsening pulmonary symptoms
  – Deteriorating lung function
  – Worsening radiographic findings

MEDICATION

Systemic therapy is clearly indicated for hypercalcemia, cardiac disease, neurologic disease, and eye disease not responding to topical therapy.

First Line

- Systemic corticosteroids in the symptomatic individual:
  – Usually prednisone initially, 40–60 mg/d × 1st 6 weeks
  – If stable, taper by 5 mg/wk to 15–20 mg/d over the next 6 weeks
  – If no relapse, 15–20 mg/d × 8–12 months
  – Relapse is common.
  – Higher doses may be warranted in patients with cardiac, neurologic, or ocular disease.
- In patients with skin disease, topical steroids may be effective.
- Inhaled steroids (budesonide 800-1,600 mcg twice daily) may be of some clinical benefit in early disease with mild pulmonary symptoms:
  – Contraindications: Patients with known problems with corticosteroids
  – Precautions: Careful monitoring in patients with diabetes mellitus and/or hypertension
  – Significant possible interactions: Refer to the manufacturer's profile of each drug (3,7).

Second Line

- Methotrexate: 10–15 mg/wk
- Cyclophosphamide: 25–50 mg/d, increasing to goal white blood cell (WBC) count of 4,000–7,000/mm^3
- Hydroxychloroquine (Plaquenil): 100–400 mg/d
- Azathioprine: 50–100 mg/d
- Use of immunosuppressants such as methotrexate or azathioprine will require regular monitoring of CBC and LFTs.
- Infliximab, a chimeric monoclonal antibody, has been useful in refractory cases. Dose is 3–5 mg/kg IV initially, 2 weeks later, then q4–6wk.
- Thalidomide has been used for chronic skin lesions. The antitumor necrosis factor (TNF) agent infliximab also has been used in some refractory cases (3)[C].

ADDITIONAL TREATMENT

Issues for Referral

- Patients with sarcoidosis are typically followed longitudinally by a pulmonologist.
- Referrals to other specialists as dictated by involvement of other organ systems

COMPLEMENTARY AND ALTERNATIVE MEDICINE

None known to be effective

SURGERY/OTHER PROCEDURES

Lung transplantation in severe, refractory cases; long-term outcomes unknown (3)[C]

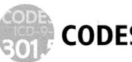

ONGOING CARE

FOLLOW-UP RECOMMENDATIONS

There is limited data on indications for the specific tests and optimal frequency of monitoring of disease activity. Suggestions are below.

Patient Monitoring

- Patients on prednisone for symptoms should be seen every 1–2 months while on therapy.
- Patients not requiring therapy should be seen regularly (every 3 months) for at least the 1st 2 years after diagnosis.
- If active disease, follow annually: Eye exam, CBC, creatinine, calcium, LFTs, ECG, CXR
- Other testing per individual patient's symptoms
- The serum ACE level is used by some physicians to follow the disease activity. In patients with an initially elevated ACE level, it should fall toward normal while on the therapy or when the disease resolves (7)[C].

DIET

No special diet

PATIENT EDUCATION

- The American Lung Association at http://www.lungusa.org/lung-disease/sarcoidosis/?gclid=CPX6zuipm6MCFQxW2godISFepQ
- Sarcoidosis by Medline Plus at http://www.nlm.nih.gov/medlineplus/sarcoidosis.html

PROGNOSIS

- 50% of patients will have spontaneous resolution within 2 years.
- 25% of patients will have significant fibrosis but no further worsening of the disease after 2 years.
- 25% of patients (higher in some populations, including blacks) will have chronic disease.
- Patients on corticosteroids for >6 months have a greater chance of having chronic disease.
- Overall death rate <5%

COMPLICATIONS

- Patients may develop significant respiratory involvement, including cor pulmonale.
- Pulmonary hemorrhage from aspergillosis in the damaged lung is possible.
- Other organs, especially the heart (congestive heart failure, arrhythmias), eyes (rarely blindness), and CNS can be involved with serious consequences. Cardiac, ocular, and CNS involvement usually manifests early on in patients with these manifestations of the disease.

REFERENCES

1. Holmes J, Lazarus A, et al. Sarcoidosis: extrathoracic manifestations. *Dis Mon*. 2009;55:675–92.
2. King CS, Kelly W, et al. Treatment of sarcoidosis. *Dis Mon*. 2009;55:704–18.
3. Iannuzzi MC, Rybicki BA, Teirstein AS. Sarcoidosis. *N Engl J Med*. 2007;357:2153–65.
4. Rybicki BA, Iannuzzi MC, Frederick MM, et al. Familial aggregation of sarcoidosis. A case-control etiologic study of sarcoidosis (ACCESS). *Am J Respir Crit Care Med*. 2001;164:2085–91.
5. Baughman RP. Pulmonary sarcoidosis. *Clin Chest Med*. 2004;25:521–30, vi.
6. Statement on sarcoidosis. Joint Statement of the American Thoracic Society (ATS), the European Respiratory Society (ERS) and the World Association of Sarcoidosis and Other Granulomatous Disorders (WASOG) adopted by the ATS Board of Directors and by the ERS Executive Committee, February 1999. *Am J Respir Crit Care Med*. 1999;160:736–55.
7. Weinberger SE. A 47-year-old woman with sarcoidosis. *JAMA*. 2006;296:2133–40.

ADDITIONAL READING

- Hoang DQ, Nguyen ET, et al. Sarcoidosis. *Semin Roentgenol*. 2010;45:36–42.
- Mock B, Richter S, Hein G, Wollina U, et al. [Recurrent panuveitis. First manifestation of Behçet disease in childhood]. *Ophthalmologe*. 1998;95:784–7.
- Polychronopoulos VS, Prakash UB, et al. Airway involvement in sarcoidosis. *Chest*. 2009;136:1371–80.

CODES

ICD9
135 Sarcoidosis

CLINICAL PEARLS

- Sarcoidosis is a noninfectious multisystem granulomatous disease.
- Diagnosis is based on clinical findings, exclusion of other disorders, and pathologic detection of noncaseating granulomas.
- ACE level is not a particularly sensitive test for diagnosis but can be useful for monitoring response to treatment when initially elevated.

SCABIES

Kaelen C. Dunican, PharmD, RPh
Robert A. Baldor, MD

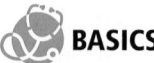 **BASICS**

DESCRIPTION
A contagious parasitic infection of the skin caused by the mite *Sarcoptes scabiei*, var. *hominis*
- System(s) affected: Skin/Exocrine
- Synonym(s): Sarcoptic mange

EPIDEMIOLOGY
Incidence
Predominant age: Children and young adults

Prevalence
- Global prevalence is estimated at 300 million cases.
- May be more prevalent in urban areas and areas of overcrowding

RISK FACTORS
- Personal skin-to-skin contact (e.g., sexual promiscuity, crowding, nosocomial infection)
- Poor nutritional status, poverty, homelessness, and poor hygiene
- Seasonal variation: Incidence may be higher in the winter than in the summer (may be due to overcrowding).
- Immunocompromised patients, including those with HIV/AIDS, are at increased risk of developing severe (crusted/Norwegian) scabies.

GENERAL PREVENTION
Prevent outbreaks by prompt treatment and cleansing of fomites (see Treatment: General Measures).

PATHOPHYSIOLOGY
Itching is a delayed hypersensitivity reaction to the mite saliva, eggs, or excrement.

ETIOLOGY
S. scabiei, var. *hominis*:
- An obligate human parasite
- Female mite lays eggs in burrows in the stratum corneum and epidermis.
- Primarily transmitted by human-to-human direct skin contact
- Infrequently transmitted via fomites (e.g., bedding, clothing, or furnishings)

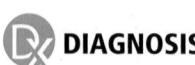 **DIAGNOSIS**

HISTORY
- Generalized itching is often severe and worse at night.
- Determine any contact with infected individuals.
- Initial infection may be asymptomatic.
- Symptoms may develop after 3–6 weeks.

PHYSICAL EXAM
- Lesions (inflammatory, erythematous, pruritic papules) most commonly located in the finger webs, flexor surfaces of the wrists, elbows, axillae, buttocks, genitalia, feet, and ankles
- Burrows (thin, curvy, elevated lines in the upper epidermis that measure 1–10 mm) may be seen in involved areas—a pathognomic sign of scabies.
- Secondary erosions or excoriations from scratching
- Pustules (if secondarily infected)
- Nodules in covered areas (buttocks, groin, axillae)
- Crusted scabies (Norwegian scabies) is a psoriasiform dermatosis occurring with hyperinfestation with thousands of mites (more common in immunosuppressed patients).

Geriatric Considerations
The elderly often itch more severely despite fewer cutaneous lesions and are at risk for extensive infestations, perhaps related to a decline in cell-mediated immunity. There may be back involvement in those who are bedridden.

Pediatric Considerations
Infants and very young children often present with vesicles, papules, and pustules and have more widespread involvement, including the hands, palms, feet, soles, body folds, and head (rare for adults).

DIAGNOSTIC TESTS & INTERPRETATION
- Definitive diagnosis requires microscopic identification of mite, eggs, or feces.
- Failure to find mite does not rule out scabies (1,2)[C].

Lab
Initial lab tests
Complete blood count is rarely needed but may show eosinophilia.

Diagnostic Procedures/Surgery
- Examination of skin with magnifying lens:
  – Look for typical burrows in finger webs and on flexor aspects of the wrists and penis.
  – Look for a dark point at the end of the burrow (the mite).
  – Presumptive diagnosis is based on clinical presentation, skin lesions, and identification of burrow (1,3)[C].
  – The mite can be extracted with a 25-gauge needle and examined microscopically.

- Mineral oil mounts (4)[C]:
  – Place a drop of mineral oil over a suspected lesion. Nonexcoriated papules or vesicles also may be sampled.
  – Scrape the lesion with a no. 15 surgical blade.
  – Examine under a microscope for mites, eggs, egg casings, or feces.
  – Scraping from under fingernails often may be positive.
- Potassium hydroxide (KOH) wet mount not recommended because it can dissolve mite pellets (1)[C].
- Burrow ink test (4)[C]:
  – If burrows are not obvious, apply blue–black ink to an area of rash. Wash off the ink with alcohol. A burrow should remain stained and become more evident.
  – Then apply mineral oil, scrape, and observe microscopically, as noted previously.
- Epiluminescence microscopy and high-resolution video dermatoscopy are expensive and have not been proven to be more sensitive than skin scraping (2,3)[C].

Pathological Findings
Skin biopsy of a nodule (although performed rarely) will reveal portions of the mite in the corneal layer.

DIFFERENTIAL DIAGNOSIS
- Atopic dermatitis
- Contact dermatitis
- Folliculitis/impetigo
- Tinea corporis
- Dermatitis herpetiformis
- Eczema
- Insect bites
- Papular urticaria
- Pediculosis corporis
- Pityriasis rosea
- Prurigo
- Psoriasis (crusted scabies)
- Pyoderma
- Seborrheic dermatitis
- Syphilis

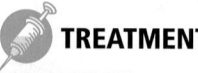 **TREATMENT**

MEDICATION
First Line
Permethrin is the most effective topical agent for scabies (56)[A]. 5% cream (Elimite, Acticin):
- After bathing or showering, apply cream from the neck to the soles of the feet; then wash off after 8–14 h. A 2nd application 1 week later is recommended if new lesions develop.
- 30 g is usually adequate for an adult.
- Side effects include itching and stinging (minimal absorption).

Pediatric Considerations

Permethrin may be used on infants. In children <5 years of age, the cream should be applied to the head and neck as well as to the entire body.

Second Line

- Crotamiton (Eurax) 10% cream:
  - Apply from the neck down for 24 h, rinse off, then reapply for an additional 24 h, and then thoroughly wash off.
  - Nodular scabies: Apply to nodules for 24 h, rinse off, then reapply for an additional 24 h, and then thoroughly wash off.
- Ivermectin (Stromectol):
  - Not Food and Drug Administration (FDA) approved for scabies; 200–250 μg/kg as single dose; repeated in 1 week
  - May need higher doses or may need to use in combination with topical scabicide for HIV-positive patients
- Precipitated sulfur 5–10% in petrolatum: Apply to the entire body from the neck down for 24 h, rinse by bathing, then repeat for 2 more days (3 days total). It is malodorous and messy but is thought to be safer than lindane, especially in infants <6 months of age, and safer than permethrin in infants <2 months of age.
- Lindane (Kwell) 1% lotion:
  - Apply to all skin surfaces from the neck down and wash off 6–8 h later.
  - 2 applications 1 week apart are recommended but may increase the risk of toxicity.
  - 2 oz is usually adequate for an adult:
    - Side effects: Neurotoxicity (seizures, muscle spasms), aplastic anemia
    - Contraindications: Uncontrolled seizure disorder, premature infants
    - Precautions: Use on excoriated skin, immunocompromised patients, conditions that may increase risk of seizures, or medications that decrease seizure threshold
    - Possible interactions: Concomitant use with medications that lower the seizure threshold

ALERT

Lindane: FDA black box warning of severe neurologic toxicity; use only when 1st-line agents have failed.

Pediatric Considerations

The FDA recommends caution when using lindane in patients who weigh <50 kg. It is not recommended for infants and is contraindicated in premature infants.

Pregnancy Considerations

- Permethrin is Category B and lindane and crotamiton are Category C drugs.
- Permethrin is considered compatible with lactation, but if permethrin is used while breastfeeding, the infant should be bottle-fed until the cream has been thoroughly washed off.

ADDITIONAL TREATMENT

General Measures

- Treat all intimate contacts and close household and family members.
- Wash all clothing, bed linens, and towels in hot (60°C) water or dry clean.
- Personal items that cannot be washed or dry cleaned should be sealed in a plastic bag for 3–5 days.
- Some itching and dermatitis commonly persists for 10–14 days and can be treated with antihistamines and/or topical or oral corticosteroids.

Additional Therapies

Crusted scabies may require use of keratolytics to improve penetration of permethrin.

 ## ONGOING CARE

FOLLOW-UP RECOMMENDATIONS

Patient Monitoring

Recheck patient at weekly intervals only if rash or itching persists. Scrape new lesions and retreat if mites or products are found.

PATIENT EDUCATION

- Patients should be instructed on proper application and cautioned not to overuse the medication when applying it to the skin.
- Patient fact sheet is available from the Centers for Disease Control and Prevention: http://www.cdc.gov.

PROGNOSIS

- Lesions begin to regress in 1–2 days, along with the worst itching, but eczema and itching may persist for up to 1 month after treatment.
- Nodular lesions may persist for several weeks, perhaps necessitating intralesional or systemic steroids.
- Some instances of lindane-resistant scabies have now been reported. These do respond to permethrin.

COMPLICATIONS

- Poor sleep due to pruritus
- Social stigma
- Secondary bacterial infection
- Sepsis
- Glomerulonephritis
- Eczema
- Pyoderma
- Postscabetic pruritus
- Nodules (nodular scabies) may persist for weeks to months after treatment.

REFERENCES

1. Chosidow O. Scabies. *N Engl J Med*. 2006;354: 1718–27.
2. Heukelbach J, Feldmeier H. Scabies. *Lancet*. 2006;367:1767–74.
3. Leone PA. Scabies and pediculosis pubis: An update of treatment regimens and general review. *Clin Infect Dis*. 2007;44(Suppl 3):S153–59.
4. Hengge UR, Currie BJ, Jäger G, et al. Scabies: a ubiquitous neglected skin disease. *Lancet Infect Dis*. 2006;6:769–79.
5. Stong M, Johnstone PW. Interventions for treating scabies. *Cochrane Database Sys Rev*. 2007;3.
6. Hicks MI, Elston DM, et al. Scabies. *Dermatol Ther*. 2009;22:279–92.

ADDITIONAL READING

- Flinders DC, De Schweinitz P. Pediculosis and scabies. *Am Fam Physician*, 2004;69:341–8.
- Orien E, Marcos B, Davidovici B, Wolf R. Itch and scratch: scabies and pediculosis. *Clin Dermatol*. 2006;24:168–75.

See Also (Topic, Algorithm, Electronic Media Element)

Insect Bites and Stings; Pediculosis (Lice)

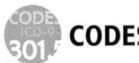 ## CODES

ICD9

133.0 Scabies

CLINICAL PEARLS

- Prior to diagnosis, use of a topical steroid to treat pruritic symptoms may mask symptoms and is termed *scabies incognito*.
- Environmental control is essential. All linens, towels, and clothing used in the previous 4 days should be washed in hot water or dry cleaned. Personal items that cannot be washed or dry cleaned should be sealed in a plastic bag for 3–5 days.
- All members of the affected household may require treatment, especially close contacts (those sharing the same bed or who have intimate contact). It may be advisable to provide prescriptions for all household members.
- Eczema and itching may persist for up to 6 weeks after treatment, causing many patients to falsely believe that they have failed treatment or are being reinfected.
- In patients with actual reinfection, either the patient has not applied the medication properly or, more likely, the index patient has not been identified and treated.

S

SCHIZOPHRENIA

Jeffrey Scott Anderson, MD
Jeffrey G. Stovall, MD

 BASICS

Schizophrenia is a chronic, severe, and disabling psychiatric disorder.

DESCRIPTION
- Major psychiatric disorder with prodrome, active, and residual symptoms involving disturbances (lasting) in appearance (deteriorated), speech (loosened association), behavior (grossly disorganized), perception (hallucinations), or thinking (delusions) that last for ≥6 months
- There are 5 types of schizophrenia: Paranoid, disorganized, catatonic, undifferentiated, and residual (1).
- System(s) affected: Nervous

EPIDEMIOLOGY
Incidence
- 0.15–0.42/1,000
- Predominant age: Onset typically <45 years
- Predominant sex: Male = Female; onset earlier in males (early to mid-20s) than females (late 20s)

Prevalence
- Lifetime (1%): Highest prevalence in lower socioeconomic classes
- 1.1% of the population >18 years; similar rates in all countries

RISK FACTORS
Genetics
Biologic relative with schizophrenia: If 1st-degree relative, risk is 8–10%, a 10-fold increase (2)[B]

GENERAL PREVENTION
- Currently, no known preventive measures decrease the incidence of schizophrenia.
- Interventions to prevent some of the associated comorbidities and to improve the long-term course and outcome are employed as approaches to prevention.

ETIOLOGY
- Unknown: Not initiated or maintained by an organic factor
- Probably a complex interaction between inherited and environmental factors

COMMONLY ASSOCIATED CONDITIONS
- Substance use disorders and nicotine dependence are common and lead to significant long-term medical and social complications (3).
- Metabolic syndrome, diabetes mellitus, obesity, and certain infectious diseases, including HIV, hepatitis B, and hepatitis C all occur in higher-than-expected rates in individuals with schizophrenia.

 DIAGNOSIS

HISTORY
Focused on identifying an insidious social decline associated with the onset of characteristic signs and symptoms:
- Withdrawal from usual activities
- Presence of delusions
- Referential thoughts

- The belief that others can read one's mind or put thoughts into one's mind
- Hallucinations, most commonly auditory
- Affective flattening
- Altered thought processing seen as loose associations or illogical thought
- Abnormalities in motor functioning seen as periods of increased energy or catatonia (4)[B]

PHYSICAL EXAM
No characteristic physical findings

DIAGNOSTIC TESTS & INTERPRETATION
Lab
- No tests are available to indicate schizophrenia.
- Laboratory tests are needed to rule out other causes; these may include:
  – CBC, blood chemistries
  – Thyroid-stimulating hormone (TSH)
  – RPR
  – Urinalysis
  – Vitamin levels (B_{12}, folate, thiamine, vitamin D)
  – Drug/alcohol screen of blood and urine
  – Heavy-metal exposure: Ceruloplasmin, urine porphobilinogen as indicated

Initial lab tests
Laboratory tests are needed when starting antipsychotic medications; these may include:
- CBC, blood chemistries
- Blood glucose level, preferably fasting
- Hemoglobin A1C
- Lipid panel
- Thyroid-stimulating hormone (TSH)
- EKG

Follow-Up & Special Considerations
Laboratory tests are needed, at least yearly, for routine monitoring, if using antipsychotic medications; these may include:
- CBC, blood chemistries
- Blood glucose level, preferably fasting
- Hemoglobin A1C
- Lipid panel
- Thyroid-stimulating hormone (TSH)
- Prolactin level, if indicated
- EKG

Imaging
CT scan and MRI to rule out other causes

Diagnostic Procedures/Surgery
- Psychological: Not a routine part of assessment
- EEG to rule out seizure disorder
- Lumbar puncture if indicated by clinical presentation

Pathological Findings
No consistent or clinically useful pathologic findings

DIFFERENTIAL DIAGNOSIS
- Mental disorder due to medical illnesses:
  – Characterized by impaired judgment, orientation, memory, affect, and concentration in association with a known medical illness
  – Disorientation, in particular, indicates delirium.
  – Possible medical illnesses include trauma, infection, tumor, metabolic, endocrine, intoxication (psychoactive substance use), epilepsy, and withdrawal states.

- Organic delusional syndrome: Secondary to substance use/abuse, including cocaine, amphetamines, LSD, phencyclidine, and alcohol, which may have identical symptoms
- Mood disorders: Especially bipolar disorder (manic–depressive disorder), schizoaffective disorder, mood disorders with psychotic features
- Cultural belief system
- Medication-induced, including steroids, anticholinergics, and narcotics

 TREATMENT

MEDICATION
First Line
- 2 main groups of antipsychotics:
  – Conventional: Chlorpromazine, fluphenazine, trifluoperazine, perphenazine, thioridazine, haloperidol, thiothixene
  – Atypical: Risperidone, clozapine, olanzapine, quetiapine, ziprasidone, aripiprazole, paliperidone, iloperidone, asenapine
- Medication choice is based on clinical and subjective response and side effect profile:
  – For sensitivity to extrapyramidal adverse effects: Atypical
  – For tardive dyskinesia: Clozapine
  – For poor compliance/high risk of relapse: Injectable form of long-acting antipsychotic such as haloperidol, fluphenazine, risperidone, olanzapine, or paliperidone
- Usual oral daily dose (initial dose may be lower):
  – Chlorpromazine: 200 mg b.i.d.
  – Fluphenazine: 5 mg b.i.d.
  – Trifluoperazine: 10 mg b.i.d.
  – Perphenazine: 24 mg/d divided b.i.d. or t.i.d.
  – Haloperidol: 5 mg b.i.d.
  – Thiothixene: 10 mg b.i.d.
  – Risperidone: 3 mg/d
  – Clozapine: 200 mg b.i.d.
  – Olanzapine: 15–30 mg/d
  – Quetiapine: 200–300 mg b.i.d.
  – Ziprasidone: 60–80 mg b.i.d.
  – Aripiprazole: 10–30 mg/d
  – Paliperidone: 6–12 mg/d
  – Iloperidone: 6–12 mg b.i.d.
  – Asenapine: 5 mg b.i.d.
- Precautions:
  – For acute side effects of antipsychotics: Dystonic reaction (especially of head and neck): Give diphenhydramine (Benadryl) 25–50 mg IM or benztropine (Cogentin) 1–2 mg IM.
  – For pseudoparkinsonism reaction: Trihexyphenidyl (Artane) 2 mg b.i.d. (may be increased to 15 mg/d if needed) or benztropine (Cogentin) 0.5 b.i.d. (range 1–4 mg/d)
  – For neuroleptic malignant syndrome: Hyperthermia, severe extrapyramidal effect, and autonomic dysfunction (e.g., hypertension, tachycardia, diaphoresis, and incontinence): Stop antipsychotic. Acute hyperthermia is treated with dantrolene 1 mg/kg IV push and continued as needed until cumulative total dose is up to 10 mg/kg. Postcrisis management is with dantrolene 4–8 mg/kg/d p.o. in 4 divided doses × 1–3 days to prevent recurrence. Extrapyramidal effects are treated with bromocriptine 2.5 mg t.i.d. to q.i.d. PO/NG.

- Risperidone, olanzapine, quetiapine, and clozapine are associated with weight gain and development of metabolic syndrome.

Second Line

- In a recent Cochrane Review, clozapine was shown to be more effective in reducing symptoms of schizophrenia, producing clinically meaningful improvements and postponing relapse, than typical antipsychotic drugs, but data were weak and prone to bias (5)[B].
- Clozapine (Clozaril) 25 mg/d:
  - Increase slowly to a dose of 300–400 mg/d given b.i.d.; do not exceed 900 mg/d.
  - Serious toxicity of agranulocytosis mandates weekly CBC; reserve for therapy-resistant patients. Significant risk of seizure at higher doses.
  - Effective in treatment of refractory or suicidal patients
- Benzodiazepines:
  - May be effective adjuncts to antipsychotics during acute phase of illness
  - Withdrawal reactions can include psychosis or seizures.
  - Individuals with schizophrenia are vulnerable to abuse/addiction.
- Anticonvulsants: May be effective adjuncts for patients with EEG abnormalities suggestive of seizure activity and those with agitated/violent behavior (5,6)[A]

ADDITIONAL TREATMENT

General measures include family and patient education and engagement in the management of a chronic and severe illness. These include specific treatments to reduce the impact of psychotic symptoms and to enhance the social functioning and rehabilitation of the patient.

Issues for Referral

- Patients with schizophrenia should receive multidisciplinary ongoing care from both a primary care physician and a psychiatrist.
- Issues for referral include suicidality, the coexistence of an addiction, or difficulty in engagement.
- Additional therapies: Specific psychosocial rehabilitation programs are strongly encouraged.
- Supportive therapy and family and patient education are essential.
- Family members often benefit from referral to family advocacy organizations such as the National Alliance for the Mentally Ill (NAMI) (7)[A].

COMPLEMENTARY AND ALTERNATIVE MEDICINE

- A recent Cochrane Review found that there is no evidence to support or refute dance/movement therapy among those with schizophrenia (8)[C].
- No other alternative therapies are validated.

SURGERY/OTHER PROCEDURES

Surgical interventions are not available.

IN-PATIENT CONSIDERATIONS

Initial stabilization focuses on maintaining a safe environment and reducing acute psychotic symptoms and agitation through the initiation of pharmacologic treatment.

Admission Criteria

The decision to admit is usually based on the patient's risk of harming himself or herself or someone else and the ability to care for himself or herself in the community.

Nursing

Monitor for safety concerns and establish a safe and supportive environment.

Discharge Criteria

The decision to discharge is based on the patient's ability to remain safe in the community and reflects a combination of suicide risk, level of psychotic symptoms, support systems, and the availability of appropriate outpatient services.

 ONGOING CARE

FOLLOW-UP RECOMMENDATIONS

- Long-term symptom management and rehabilitation depend on engagement in ongoing pharmacologic and psychosocial treatment.
- Monitoring is based on evaluation of symptoms (including safety and psychotic symptoms), looking for the emergence of comorbidities and medication side effects, and prevention of complications.

DIET

- Newer atypical antipsychotics confer a higher risk of metabolic side effects such as diabetes, hypercholesterolemia, and weight gain.
- While there no specific dietary requirements, attention should be paid to the high risk of development of obesity, metabolic syndrome, and diabetes mellitus in individuals with schizophrenia.

PATIENT EDUCATION

- National Institute of Mental Health: *Schizophrenia*, at http://www.nimh.nih.gov/health/topics/schizophrenia/index.shtml
- *Helping a Family Member with Schizophrenia*, at http://www.aafp.org/afp/20070615/1830ph.html

PROGNOSIS

- Chronic course: Remission and exacerbations; complete remission not common
- Guarded prognosis
- The negative symptoms (consisting of decreased ambition, energy, and emotional responsiveness and social withdrawal) are often most difficult to treat.
- Excessive mortality occurs due to suicide, accidents, coronary artery disease, nicotine dependence, or substance abuse.

COMPLICATIONS

- Side effects from antipsychotic medications, including tardive dyskinesia and metabolic syndrome
- Self-inflicted trauma and suicide
- Combative behavior toward others
- Comorbid addictions, including nicotine (9)[A]

REFERENCES

1. Schultz SH, North SW, Shields CG. Schizophrenia: a review. *Am Fam Physician*. 2007;75:1821–9.
2. Norman RM, Manchanda R, Malla AK, et al. The significance of family history in first-episode schizophrenia spectrum disorder. *J Nerv Ment Dis*. 2007;195:846–52.
3. Fagerström K, Aubin HJ. Management of smoking cessation in patients with psychiatric disorders. *Curr Med Res Opin*. 2009;25:511–8.
4. American Psychiatric Association. *Diagnostic and Statistical Manual of Mental Disorders*, Text Revised, 4th ed. (DSM-IV-TR). Washington, DC: Author, 2000.
5. Essali A, Al-Haj Haasan N, Li C, et al. Clozapine versus typical neuroleptic medication for schizophrenia. *Cochrane Database Syst Rev*. 2009:CD000059.
6. Lieberman JA, Stroup TS, McEvoy JP, et al. Effectiveness of antipsychotic drugs in patients with chronic schizophrenia. *N Engl J Med*. 2005;353:1209–23.
7. Mojtabai R, Nicholson RA, Carpenter BN. Role of psychosocial treatments in management of schizophrenia: a meta-analytic review of controlled outcome studies. *Schizophr Bull*. 1998;24:569–87.
8. Xia J, Grant TJ. Dance therapy for schizophrenia. *Cochrane Database Syst Rev*. 2009:CD006868.
9. Saha S, Chant D, McGrath J. A systematic review of mortality in schizophrenia: is the differential mortality gap worsening over time? *Arch Gen Psychiatry*. 2007;64:1123–31.

ADDITIONAL READING

Mala E. Schizophrenia in childhood and adolescence. *Neuro Endocrinol Lett*. 2008;29.

See Also (Topic, Algorithm, Electronic Media Element)

Algorithm: Delirium

 CODES

ICD9

295.90 Unspecified type schizophrenia, unspecified state

CLINICAL PEARLS

- Schizophrenia is a debilitating chronic mental illness that affects 1% of the population in all cultures.
- Schizophrenia is characterized by positive symptoms, including hallucinations, voices that converse with or about the patient, and delusions that are often paranoid, and negative symptoms, including flattened affect, loss of a sense of pleasure, loss of will or drive, and social withdrawal.
- Prominent mood symptoms are not common and can serve to differentiate schizophrenia from bipolar disorder.
- Multidisciplinary clinical teams should work to prevent and treat comorbidities such as substance use, nicotine use, and obesity.

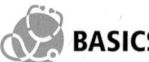

BASICS

DESCRIPTION
- Inflammation of the sclera, part of the eye's outer coat
- System(s) affected: Ocular

EPIDEMIOLOGY
- Predominant age: Most frequently occurs in 4th and 6th decades; mean age for all types of scleritis is 52 years
- Predominant sex: Female > Male (1.6:1)

Incidence
In 1 study, 0.08% of new patients presenting to an ophthalmology department were diagnosed with scleritis. 94% of patients have anterior scleritis; the remaining 6% have posterior.

Prevalence
Uncommon in US

RISK FACTORS
Individuals with autoimmune disorders are most at risk.

ETIOLOGY
- ~50% of cases of scleritis are associated with autoimmune diseases such as rheumatoid arthritis. In 15% of cases, scleritis is the presenting manifestation of a systemic disorder, appearing 1 or more months before other symptoms of the condition.
- Scleritis has been reported in patients taking bisphosphonate therapy.

COMMONLY ASSOCIATED CONDITIONS
- Sjögren syndrome
- Ankylosing spondylitis
- Systemic lupus erythematosus
- Reactive arthritis
- Relapsing polychondritis
- Polyarteritis nodosa
- Wegener granulomatosis
- Sarcoidosis
- Inflammatory bowel disease
- Varicella zoster virus
- Syphilis
- Lyme disease
- Herpes zoster
- Tuberculosis

DIAGNOSIS

HISTORY
- Redness and inflammation of the sclera
- Can be bilateral in 1/3 of cases
- Pain ranging from mild discomfort to extreme localized tenderness. May be described as constant, deep, boring, or pulsating.
- Pain may be referred to the eyebrow, temple, or jaw.
- Photophobia and lacrimation may occur, but discharge is uncommon.
- Posterior scleritis tends to be less symptomatic, as is the variant scleromalacia perforans, due to associated pain fiber necrosis.

PHYSICAL EXAM
- Photophobia and tearing on exam
- Examine for pain with consensual constriction, which suggests uveal involvement.
- Engorged purplish-red blood vessels
- Inspect for breadth and degree of injection.
- A bluish hue may suggest thinning of the sclera.
- Scleral edema is often present.
- Deeper scleral blood vessels appear darker, follow a radial pattern, and do not move when manipulated with a cotton swab.
- Check visual acuity.
- A complete physical examination, particularly of the skin, joints, heart, and lungs, may be done to evaluate for associated conditions.

DIAGNOSTIC TESTS & INTERPRETATION
Lab
- Consider further testing if history, physical examination, complete blood count, serum chemistry, urinalysis, erythrocyte sedimentation rate, and/or C-reactive protein suggest a systemic cause.
- Rheumatoid factor, anticyclic citrullinated peptide antibodies, antineutrophil cytoplasmic antibody, and antinuclear antibody may aid in the diagnosis.
- FTA-ABS, rapid plasma reagin, and Lyme titers

Imaging
Initial approach
- Further imaging studies, such as CXR and/or chest CT and sacroiliac joint films, may be useful if specific systemic illnesses are suspected.
- Ultrasound or CT scan of the orbit may be useful to determine the extent and location (especially posterior) of scleritis and the presence of local associated disease.

Diagnostic Procedures/Surgery
Biopsy not routinely required unless diagnosis remains uncertain after above investigations

Pathological Findings
- Adjacent inflammation may or may not be present.
- The scleritis may be diffuse, nodular, or necrotizing (with or without associated inflammation).
- If the posterior region of the globe is involved, adjacent swelling of orbital tissues may occur.

DIFFERENTIAL DIAGNOSIS
- Conjunctivitis
- Episcleritis
- Pink eye
- Iritis (anterior uveitis)
- Trauma
- Ocular rosacea
- Herpes zoster

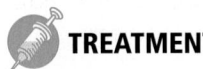 TREATMENT

MEDICATION
First Line
- Glucocorticoids are the mainstay of treatment, including topical, periocular, and systemic.
- Contraindications: Documented hypersensitivity. Active peptic ulcer disease. Untreated concomitant viral or bacterial infection.
- Precautions: Scleritis can progress to ocular perforation, which may be hastened with periocular steroid injection.

Second Line
- The more clinically benign subtypes—diffuse and nodular anterior scleritis—may respond to nonsteroidal anti-inflammatory drugs (NSAIDs) alone.
- Necrotizing or posterior scleritis, on the other hand, may require cyclophosphamide in addition to systemic steroids. Other immunosuppressive and immunomodulating agents may be indicated depending on the systemic condition.

ADDITIONAL TREATMENT
Issues for Referral
- All patients with scleritis should be managed with the help of an ophthalmologist familiar with this condition.
- Rheumatology referral for coexistent systemic diseases is helpful for long-term success.

Additional Therapies
Immunosuppressants used for autoimmune and collagen vascular disorders may be of help in active scleritis.

SURGERY/OTHER PROCEDURES
In rare cases, scleral biopsy may be indicated. Ocular perforation requires scleral grafting.

 ONGOING CARE

FOLLOW-UP RECOMMENDATIONS
No restrictions

Patient Monitoring
The patient should be followed very closely in the active stage of inflammation to assess the effectiveness of therapy. Medication use mandates close surveillance for adverse effects.

DIET
No special diet

PROGNOSIS
- Scleritis is indolent, chronic, and often progressive.
- Recurrent bouts of inflammation may occur.

COMPLICATIONS
- Increased intraocular pressure
- Cataract and glaucoma can result from treatment.
- Visual loss due to posterior extension or adjacent structural involvement
- Ocular perforation can occur in severe stages.

ADDITIONAL READING
- Fong LP, Sainz de la Maza M, Rice BA, et al. Immunopathology of scleritis. *Ophthalmology*. 1991;98:472–9.
- Fraunfelder FW, Fraunfelder FT. Bisphosphonates and ocular inflammation. *N Engl J Med*. 2003; 348:1187–8.
- Smith JR, Mackensen F, Rosenbaum JT. Therapy Insight:scleritis and its relationship to systemic autoimmune disease. *Nature Clinical Practice Rheumatology*. 2007;3:219–226.

 CODES

ICD9
379.00 Scleritis, unspecified

CLINICAL PEARLS
- Scleritis involves a deeper layer of the eye than episcleritis and, therefore, can be a vision-threatening condition, more common in midlife. Episcleritis is less painful and occurs in younger patients.
- Uveitis, by definition, involves some combination of the iris, ciliary body, and choroid membrane and thus, generally is associated with pain, with consensual constriction of the pupil. Scleritis can spread to involve these structures, but does not always. Both can be associated with underlying inflammatory diseases.

SCLERODERMA

Ann M. Lynch, PharmD, R.Ph
Deborah DeMarco, MD

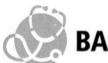 **BASICS**

DESCRIPTION
- Scleroderma (systemic sclerosis [SSc]) is a chronic disease of unknown cause characterized by diffuse fibrosis of skin and visceral organs and vascular abnormalities.
- Most manifestations have vascular features (e.g., Raynaud phenomenon), but frank vasculitis is rarely seen.
- Can range from a mild disease, affecting the skin, to a systemic disease that can cause death in a few months
- The disease is categorized into 2 major clinical variants:
  – Diffuse: Distal and proximal extremity and truncal skin thickening
  – Limited:
    ○ Restricted to the fingers, hands, and face
    ○ CREST syndrome (calcinosis, Raynaud phenomenon, esophageal dysmotility, sclerodactyly, telangiectasia)
- System(s) affected: Include but not limited to Skin; Renal; Cardiovascular; Pulmonary; Musculoskeletal; GI

Geriatric Considerations
Uncommon >75 years of age

Pediatric Considerations
Rare in this age group

Pregnancy Considerations
- Safe and healthy pregnancies are common and possible despite higher frequency of premature births.
- High-risk management must be standard care to avoid complications, specifically renal crisis.
- Diffuse scleroderma causes greater risk for developing serious cardiopulmonary and renal problems. Pregnancy should be delayed until disease stabilizes.

EPIDEMIOLOGY
Incidence
- In the US: 1–2/100,000/year
- Predominant age:
  – Young adult (16–40 years); middle-aged (40–75 years), peak onset 30–50 years
  – Symptoms usually appear in the 3rd–5th decades.
- Predominant sex: Female > Male (4:1)

Prevalence
In the US: 1–25/100,000

RISK FACTORS
Unknown

Genetics
Familial clustering is rare but has been seen.

ETIOLOGY
- Unknown
- Possible alterations in immune response
- Possibly some association with exposure to quartz mining, quarrying, vinyl chloride, hydrocarbons, toxin exposure
- Treatment with bleomycin has caused a sclerodermalike syndrome, as has exposure to rapeseed oil.

 DIAGNOSIS

HISTORY
- Raynaud phenomenon is frequently the initial complaint.
- Skin thickening, "puffy hands," and gastroesophageal reflux disease (GERD) are often noted early in the disease process.

PHYSICAL EXAM
- Skin:
  – Digital ulcerations
  – Tightness, swelling, thickening of digits
  – Hyperpigmentation/hypopigmentation
  – Narrowed oral aperture
  – Pruritus
  – Scaling of skin
  – Subcutaneous calcinosis
- Peripheral vascular system:
  – Raynaud phenomenon (differentiate from Raynaud disease, generally affecting younger individuals and without digital ulcers)
  – Telangiectasia
- Joints, tendons, and bones:
  – Flexion contractures
  – Friction rub on tendon movement
  – Hand swelling
  – Joint stiffness
  – Polyarthralgia
  – Sclerodactyly
- Muscle:
  – Proximal muscle weakness
- GI tract:
  – Dysphagia
  – Esophageal reflux due to dysmotility (most common systemic sign in diffuse disease)
  – Malabsorptive diarrhea
  – Nausea and vomiting
  – Weight loss
  – Xerostomia
- Kidney:
  – Hypertension
  – May develop scleroderma renal crisis: Acute renal failure
- Pulmonary:
  – Dry crackles at lung bases
  – Dyspnea
- Nervous system:
  – Peripheral neuropathy
  – Trigeminal neuropathy
- Cardiac (progressive disease):
  – Conduction abnormalities
  – Cardiomyopathy
  – Secondary cor pulmonale

DIAGNOSTIC TESTS & INTERPRETATION
Lab
Initial lab tests
- Nail fold capillary microscopy
- CBC
- Creatinine
- Urinalysis (albuminuria, microscopic hematuria)
- Antinuclear antibodies (ANA): Positive in >90% of patients, often with a nucleolar pattern
- Anti–Scl-70 (topoisomerase) antibody is highly specific for systemic disease.
- Anticentromere antibody (usually associated with limited cutaneous disease) and CREST variant

Follow-Up & Special Considerations
- Pulmonary function tests (PFTs):
  – Decreased maximum breathing capacity
  – Increased residual volume
  – Diffusion defect
- Hypergammaglobulinemia
- Positive rheumatoid factor test (33%)
- ECG (low voltage): Possible nonspecific abnormalities, arrhythmia, and conduction defects
- Echocardiography: Pulmonary hypertension or cardiomyopathy
- Nail fold capillary loop abnormalities

Imaging
Initial approach
- Chest radiograph:
  – Diffuse reticular pattern
  – Bilateral basilar pulmonary fibrosis
- Hand radiograph:
  – Soft tissue atrophy and acro-osteolysis
  – Can see overlap syndromes such as rheumatoid arthritis
  – Subcutaneous calcinosis

Follow-Up & Special Considerations
- Upper GI:
  – Distal esophageal dilatation
  – Atonic esophagus
  – Esophageal dysmotility
  – Duodenal diverticula
- Barium enema:
  – Colonic diverticula
  – Megacolon
- High-resolution CT scan for detecting alveolitis, which has a ground-glass appearance or honeycomb pattern in fibrosis

Diagnostic Procedures/Surgery
- Skin biopsy:
  – Compact collagen fibers in the reticular dermis and hyalinization and fibrosis of arterioles
  – Thinning of epidermis with loss of rete pegs and atrophy of dermal appendages
  – Accumulation of mononuclear cells is also seen.
- Right-sided heart catheterization: Pulmonary hypertension is an ominous prognostic feature.

Pathological Findings
- Skin:
  – Edema, fibrosis, or atrophy (late stage)
  – Lymphocytic infiltrate around sweat glands
  – Loss of capillaries
  – Endothelial proliferation
  – Hair follicle atrophy

- Synovium:
  - Pannus formation
  - Fibrin deposits in tendons
- Kidney:
  - Small kidneys
  - Intimal proliferation in interlobular arteries
- Heart:
  - Endocardial thickening
  - Myocardial interstitial fibrosis
  - Ischemic band necrosis
  - Enlarged heart
  - Cardiac hypertrophy
- Lung:
  - Interstitial pneumonitis
  - Cyst formation
  - Interstitial fibrosis
  - Bronchiectasis
- Esophagus:
  - Esophageal atrophy
  - Fibrosis

DIFFERENTIAL DIAGNOSIS
- Sclerodermatomyositis
- Mixed connective tissue disease
- Toxic oil syndrome (Madrid, 1981, affecting 20,000 people)
- Eosinophilia–myalgia syndrome
- Diffuse fasciitis with eosinophilia
- Scleredema of Buschke

 TREATMENT

MEDICATION
First Line
- Angiotensin-converting enzyme inhibitors for preservation of renal blood flow and for treatment of hypertensive renal crisis (1)[C]
- Corticosteroids: For disabling myositis, pulmonary alveolitis, or mixed connective tissue disease (not recommended in high doses due to increased incidence of renal failure) (1)[C]
- NSAIDs: For joint or tendon symptoms
- Antibiotics: For secondary infections in bowel and active skin infections (1)
- Antacids, proton pump inhibitors: For gastric reflux (1)[B]
- Intestinal dysfunction: Metoclopramide (1)[C]
- Dipyridamole or aspirin: Antiplatelet therapy
- Hydrophilic skin ointments: Skin therapy
- Topical clindamycin, erythromycin, or silver sulfadiazine cream may prevent recurrent infectious cutaneous ulcers.
- Consider immunosuppressives for treatment of life-threatening or potentially crippling scleroderma or interstitial pneumonitis (1)[A].
- Avoidance of caffeine, nicotine, and sympathomimetics may ease Raynaud symptoms.
- Nitrates and dihydropyridine calcium channel blockers for Raynaud phenomenon (2)[A]
- Penicillamine: To reduce skin thickening and delay the rate of new visceral involvement (use is now controversial; newer therapies such as relaxin may be better)
- PDE-5 antagonists (e.g., sildenafil), prostanoids, and endothelin-1 antagonists are changing management of pulmonary hypertension (1)[B].

- Alveolitis: Immunosuppressants and alkylating agents (e.g., cyclophosphamide) (1)[A]
- Precautions/contraindications/interactions: Refer to the manufacturer's literature for each drug.

Second Line
Many other drugs are currently under investigation, but no evidence of real benefits has emerged yet.

ADDITIONAL TREATMENT
General Measures
- Treatment is symptomatic and supportive.
- Esophageal dilation may be used for strictures.
- Avoid cold; dress appropriately for the weather; be wary of air conditioning.
- Avoid smoking (crucial).
- For chronic digital ulcerations:
  - Débridement after soaking in 1/2–strength hydrogen peroxide solution
  - Digital plaster to immobilize
- Avoid finger sticks (e.g., blood tests).
- Elevate the head of the bed during sleep to help relieve GI symptoms.
- Use softening lotions, ointments, and bath oils to help prevent dryness and cracking of skin.
- Dialysis may be necessary in renal crisis.

Additional Therapies
- Physical therapy to maintain function and promote strength
- Heat therapy to relieve joint stiffness

SURGERY/OTHER PROCEDURES
- Some success with gastroplasty for correction of GERD
- Limited role for sympathectomy for Raynaud phenomenon

 ONGOING CARE

FOLLOW-UP RECOMMENDATIONS
- Stay as active as possible, but avoid fatigue.
- Printed patient information available from the Scleroderma Federation, 1725 York Avenue, No. 29F, New York, NY 10128; (212) 427-7040.
- Advise patient to report any abnormal bruising or nonhealing abrasions.
- Assist patient in smoking cessation, if needed.

Patient Monitoring
- Monitor every 3–6 months for end-organ and skin involvement and medications. Provide encouragement.
- Cardiac echo and PFTs yearly

DIET
Drink plenty of fluids with meals.

PROGNOSIS
- Possible improvement, but incurable
- Prognosis is poor if cardiac, pulmonary, or renal manifestations present early.

COMPLICATIONS
- Renal failure
- Respiratory failure

- Flexion contractures
- Disability
- Esophageal dysmotility
- Reflux esophagitis
- Arrhythmia
- Megacolon
- Pneumatosis intestinalis
- Obstructive bowel
- Cardiomyopathy
- Pulmonary hypertension
- Possible association with lung and other cancers
- Death

REFERENCES
1. Kowal-Bielecka O, Landewé R, Avouac J, et al. EULAR recommendations for the treatment of systemic sclerosis: a report from the EULAR Scleroderma Trials and Research group (EUSTAR). *Ann Rheum Dis*. 2009;68:620–8.
2. Harding SE, Tingey PC, Pope J, Fenlon D, Furst D, Shea B, Silman A, Thompson A, Wells GA. Prazosin for Raynaud's phenomenon in progressive systemic sclerosis. *Cochrane Database of Systematic Reviews* 1998, Issue 2. Art. No.: CD000956. DOI:10.1002/14651858.CD000956

ADDITIONAL READING
- Reveille JD, Solomon DH. American College of Rheumatology Ad Hoc Committee of Immunologic Testing Guidelines. Evidence-based guidelines for the use of immunologic tests: anticentromere, Scl-70, and nucleolar antibodies. *Arthritis Rheum*. 2003;49:399–412.
- Steen VD. Pregnancy in scleroderma. *Rheum Dis Clin North Am*. 2007;33:345–58, vii.

See Also (Topic, Algorithm, Electronic Media Element)
Sclerosis, Morphea; Progressive Systemic Sclerosis

 CODES

ICD9
710.1 Systemic sclerosis

CLINICAL PEARLS
- Raynaud phenomenon is frequently the initial complaint.
- Skin thickening, "puffy hands," and GERD are often noted early in disease.
- Eosinophilic fasciitis can mimic scleroderma but differs with the absence of Raynaud symptoms and is responsive to corticosteroid treatment.

SEASONAL AFFECTIVE DISORDER

Christopher C. White, MD, JD

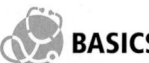 **BASICS**

DESCRIPTION
- Seasonal affective disorder (SAD) is a heterogeneous mood disorder with depressive episodes usually in winter months with full remissions in the spring and summer.
- Noted to occur decades ago; not formally named until the 1980s
- Ranges from a milder form (winter blues) to a seriously disabling illness
- Must separate out patients with other mood disorders (such as major depressive disorder and bipolar affective disorder) whose symptoms persist during spring and summer months

EPIDEMIOLOGY
Incidence
- Affects up to 500,000 people every winter
- Up to 30% of patients visiting a primary care physician (PCP) during winter may report winter depressive symptoms.
- Predominant age: Occurs at any age; peaks in 20s and 30s
- Predominant sex: Female > Male (3:1)

Prevalence
- 1–9% of the general population
- 10–20% of patients identified as having mood symptoms will have a seasonal component.

RISK FACTORS
- Most common during months of January and February: Patients frequently visiting PCP during winter months complaining of recurrent flu, chronic fatigue, and unexplained weight gain should be screened for SAD.
- Working in a building without windows or other environment without exposure to sunlight

Genetics
- Some twin studies have suggested a genetic component, but further study is needed.
- Increased incidence of depression, attention deficit hyperactivity disorder and alcoholism in close relatives

GENERAL PREVENTION
- Consider use of light therapy at start of winter (if prior episodes begin in October), increasing time outside during daylight, or moving to a more southern location.
- Bupropion (Wellbutrin) is a Food and Drug Administration (FDA)–approved antidepressant for the prevention of SAD.

PATHOPHYSIOLOGY
The major theories currently involve the interplay of phase-shifted circadian rhythms, genetic vulnerability, and serotonin dysregulation.

ETIOLOGY
- Melatonin produced by the pineal gland at increased levels in the dark has been linked to depressive symptoms; light therapy on the retina acts to inhibit melatonin secretion.
- Serotonin dysregulation, because it is secreted less during winter months, must be present for light therapy to work, and treatment with selective serotonin reuptake inhibitors (SSRIs) appears to reverse SAD symptoms.
- Decreased levels of vitamin D, often occurring during low-light winter months, may be associated with depressive episodes in some individuals experiencing SAD symptoms.

COMMONLY ASSOCIATED CONDITIONS
Some individuals with SAD have a weakened immune system and may be more vulnerable to infections.

 DIAGNOSIS

- Carefully document the presence or absence of prior manic episodes.
- Screen for the existence of any suicidal ideation and safety risk factors.
- Remission of symptoms during spring and summer
- Symptoms have occurred the past 2 years
- Seasonal episodes associated with winter months substantially outnumber any nonseasonal depressive episodes.

HISTORY
- Symptoms of depression meeting the criteria for major depressive disorder:
  - *S*leep disturbance—either too much or too little
  - *I*nterest (lack of)—in life and absence of pleasure from hobbies/activities
  - *G*uilt—feelings of guilt or worthlessness
  - *E*nergy—fatigue or constantly feeling tired
  - *C*oncentration—difficulty with concentration and memory
  - *A*ppetite—changes in appetite and weight
  - *P*sychomotor retardation—patients feeling slowed down with decreased activity
  - *S*uicidal thoughts—patients reporting thoughts of suicide
- In SAD, hypersomnia, hyperphagia (craving for carbohydrates and sweets), and weight gain usually predominate. Despite sleeping more, patients report daytime sleepiness and fatigue. Cravings may lead to binge eating and weight gains >20 lb.
- Obtain collateral history if patient is unable to provide insight into the seasonal component.

PHYSICAL EXAM
Use exam to exclude other organic causes for symptoms. Focal neurologic deficits, signs of endocrine dysfunction, or stigmata of substance abuse should prompt further testing.

DIAGNOSTIC TESTS & INTERPRETATION
Lab
- Thyroid-stimulating hormone to rule out hypothyroidism
- Complete blood count to rule out anemia
- Rule out electrolyte and glucose dysregulation.
- 25-OH vitamin D level
- Pregnancy test for women of child-bearing potential
- Urine tox screen if substance abuse is a concern

Imaging
Generally not useful unless focal neurologic finding or looking to exclude an organic cause

DIFFERENTIAL DIAGNOSIS
- Similar to that of major depression, meaning that organic causes of low energy and fatigue such as hypothyroidism, anemia, and mononucleosis (or other viral syndromes) need to be considered
- Other mood disorders without a seasonal component such as major depression, bipolar disorder, adjustment disorder, or dysthymia
- Symptoms should not be better accounted for by seasonal psychosocial stressors, which often accompany the winter holiday seasons.
- Substance abuse

 TREATMENT

MEDICATION
There is a lack of evidence to determine whether light therapy or medication should be the 1st-line agent. Both are supported by the literature and in some studies have equal efficacy. Medications typically have more side effects. Adherence to both treatments remains a critical issue. The ultimate choice depends on the acuity of the patient and the comfort level of the prescribing clinician with each treatment modality (1)[B]:
- SSRIs such as sertraline (Zoloft), paroxetine (Paxil), fluoxetine (Prozac), citalopram (Celexa), and escitalopram (Lexapro) in their traditional antidepressant doses (2)[B]
- Bupropion (Wellbutrin) is the only antidepressant currently approved by the FDA for the prevention of SAD (3)[A].

ADDITIONAL TREATMENT
Issues for Referral
- Patients with a history of ocular disease should be referred for an ophthalmologic exam before phototherapy and for serial monitoring.
- Patients who fail to respond or who develop manic symptoms or suicidal ideation once treatment is initiated should be considered for psychiatric referral.

Additional Therapies

Phototherapy using special light sources has been shown to be effective in 60–90% of patients, often providing relief with a few sessions (2,4)[A]:

- Variables that can regulate effect are:
  - Light intensity: Although the minimum light source intensity is under investigation, 2,500 lux is suggested (domestic lights emit, on average, 200–500 lux). There is good evidence for 10,000 lux as the recommended source (2)[B].
  - Treatment duration: Exposure time varies based on intensity of light source with daily sessions of 30 minutes to a few hours.
  - Time of treatment: Most patients respond better by using the light therapy early in the morning.
  - Color of light source: Emerging data suggest that lower-intensity light-emitting diodes in the blue spectrum may have equal efficacy to the traditional white light boxes with a decreased incidence of side effects, but these results are preliminary (5)[B].
- Light box is placed on table several feet away, and the light is allowed to shine onto the patient's eyes (sunglasses should be avoided). Ensure that the light box has an ultraviolet filter.
- Most common side effects are eye strain and headache. Insomnia can result if the light box is used too late in the day. Light boxes also can precipitate mania in some patients.
- Dawn simulation machines gradually increase illumination while the patient sleeps, simulating sunrise while using a significantly less intense light source.

COMPLEMENTARY AND ALTERNATIVE MEDICINE

- Work to reduce stress levels through meditation, progressive relaxation exercises, and/or lifestyle modification.
- The potential role of vitamin D supplementation is under investigation. A small study found it to be more effective than phototherapy, but a much larger and more rigorous study recently found no benefit in elderly women for SAD symptoms. Doses used are typically 400–800 IU/d (6)[B].

IN-PATIENT CONSIDERATIONS
Admission Criteria

If the patient develops suicidal ideation as part of his or her depression or mania after treatment is initiated

 ONGOING CARE

FOLLOW-UP RECOMMENDATIONS

Regular monitoring by PCP or psychiatrist for response to treatment; patients may become manic when treated with SSRIs or light therapy.

Patient Monitoring

Patients should be seen in the outpatient clinic weekly to biweekly when initiating light or pharmacotherapy to monitor treatment results, side effects, and any increased suicidal thoughts if using SSRIs.

DIET

No specific diet modification needed

PATIENT EDUCATION

- Increase time outdoors during daylight.
- Rearrange home or work environment to get more direct sunlight through windows.

PROGNOSIS

Symptoms, if untreated, generally remit within 5 months with exposure to spring light, only to return in subsequent winters. If treated, patients usually respond within 3–6 weeks.

COMPLICATIONS

Development of suicidal ideation and mania are 2 outcomes the clinician needs to monitor.

REFERENCES

1. Lam RW, Levitt AJ, Levitan RD, et al. The Can-SAD study: a randomized controlled trial of the effectiveness of light therapy and fluoxetine in patients with winter seasonal affective disorder. *Am J Psychiatry.* 2006;163:805–12.
2. Lurie SJ, Gawinski B, Pierce D, et al. Seasonal affective disorder. *Am Fam Physician.* 2006;74: 1521–4.
3. Modell JG, Rosenthal NE, Harriett AE, et al. Seasonal affective disorder and its prevention by anticipatory treatment with bupropion XL. *Biol Psychiatry.* 2005;58:658–67.
4. Terman M, Terman JS. Light therapy for seasonal and nonseasonal depression: efficacy, protocol, safety, and side effects. *CNS Spectr.* 2005;10: 647–63; quiz 672.
5. Anderson JL, Glod CA, Dai J, et al. Lux vs. wavelength in light treatment of Seasonal Affective Disorder. *Acta Psychiatr Scand.* 2009.
6. Dumville JC, Miles JN, Porthouse J, et al. Can vitamin D supplementation prevent winter-time blues? A randomised trial among older women. *J Nutr Health Aging.* 2006;10:151–3.

ADDITIONAL READING

- A recent review article briefly outlining the diagnosis and current treatment of SAD is cited here for those interested in the subject.
- Howland RH. Somatic therapies for seasonal affective disorder. *J Psychosoc Nurs Ment Health Serv.* 2009;47:17–20.

See Also (Topic, Algorithm, Electronic Media Element)

Bipolar I Disorder; Bipolar II Disorder; Depression
Algorithm: Depressive Episode, Major

 CODES

ICD9

296.99 Other specified episodic mood disorder

CLINICAL PEARLS

- The difference between SAD and depression is that SAD is a subtype of major depressive disorder. Once someone has a diagnosed mood disorder such as depression or bipolar, one needs to ask whether the symptoms vary in a seasonal pattern to qualify for the diagnosis of SAD. Generally, these patients will report sleeping too much, eating too much (especially carbs and sweets), and gaining weight during winter months.
- As with all psychiatric diagnoses, ensure that the symptoms are not due to an organic process (e.g., anemia, hypothyroidism, mononucleosis) or better explained by substance abuse.
- There is a lack of good evidence to decide whether light therapy or SSRIs should be the 1st-line agent. Guidelines suggest that SSRIs should be used first if the patient is more acute or has contraindications to light therapy, or the clinician is not comfortable with light therapy.
- Light therapy boxes are available from numerous online suppliers, but they are not extensively regulated, and thus practitioners should take care to ensure that patients are using devices from reputable suppliers.
- If using SSRIs, there have been recent studies indicating that some patients may begin to experience increased suicidal thoughts on therapy, and thus these patients need to be monitored closely in your outpatient office every 1–2 weeks. Patients on light therapy also should be monitored closely initially in order to adjust treatment. Once stabilized, both groups of patients can be seen every 4–8 weeks during the winter months.
- All patients who demonstrate suicidal ideation or symptoms of mania should be referred for consideration of hospitalization.

S

Ruben Peralta, MD

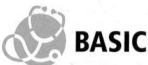

BASICS

DESCRIPTION
- A syndrome of abnormal production of antidiuretic hormone (ADH), despite low serum osmolality, leading to hyponatremia and inappropriately elevated urine osmolality:
  - The resulting abnormal urinary free water retention leads to dilutional hyponatremia (total body sodium levels may be normal or near normal, but the patient's total body water is increased).
  - Often secondary to medications, but may be associated with an underlying disorder such as neoplasm, pulmonary disorder, or CNS system disease
- Synonym(s): Syndrome of inappropriate secretion of ADH

EPIDEMIOLOGY
Incidence
- Usually found in the hospital setting, where incidence can be as high as 35%
- Predominant age: Elderly
- Predominate sex: Females > Males

RISK FACTORS
- Use of predisposing drugs
- Advanced age
- Postoperative status
- Institutionalization

Genetics
No known genetic pattern

GENERAL PREVENTION
- Search for cause, if unknown.
- Administration of 0.9% sodium chloride in adults during the perioperative period is recommended (if hypernatremia is not present) (1,2).
- Monitor electrolytes in postoperative patients to determine if fluid intake needs restriction.
- Reduce or change medications, if drug-induced.
- Lifelong restriction of fluid intake

ETIOLOGY
- Drugs (3)[B]:
  - Antidepressants (e.g., monoamine oxidase inhibitors [MAOIs], tricyclics, selective serotonin reuptake inhibitors [SSRIs])
  - Oral hypoglycemics (e.g., chlorpropamide, metformin)
  - Antineoplastic drugs (e.g., vincristine, vinblastine, cisplatin, cyclophosphamide)
  - Antipsychotic agents (e.g., phenothiazines, thioridazine, haloperidol)
  - Analgesics (e.g., nonsteroidal anti-inflammatory drugs [NSAIDs])
  - Antiepileptics (e.g. carbamazepine, valproic acid)
  - Diuretics (thiazides and loop)
  - Others (e.g., vasopressin, DDAVP, ecstasy, oxytocin, α-interferon)

- Neoplasms (ectopic ADH production):
  - Small cell carcinoma of the lung
  - Oat cell carcinoma of the lung
  - Hodgkin disease
  - Pancreatic carcinoma
  - Thymoma
  - Mesothelioma
  - Bronchogenic carcinoma
- Infectious diseases:
  - Meningitis
  - Encephalitis
  - Pneumonia
  - Pulmonary tuberculosis (TB)
  - Rocky Mountain spotted fever
  - HIV infection
- Miscellaneous cardiopulmonary conditions:
  - Asthma
  - Atelectasis
  - Myocardial infarction
  - Vascular diseases
- Other:
  - CNS injury
  - Mechanical ventilation
  - Multiple sclerosis
  - Guillain-Barré syndrome
  - Lupus erythematosus
  - Porphyria
  - Hypothyroidism, myxedema
- Idiopathic

COMMONLY ASSOCIATED CONDITIONS
See Etiology.

DIAGNOSIS

HISTORY
Early symptoms:
- Fatigue
- Anorexia
- Nausea
- Vomiting
- Diarrhea
- Headaches
- Myalgias
- Increased thirst

PHYSICAL EXAM
Late/severe hyponatremia (serum Na <100–115 mEq/L):
- Altered mental status
- Confusion
- Lethargy
- Seizures
- Psychosis
- Coma
- Death

DIAGNOSTIC TESTS & INTERPRETATION
Lab
- Serum Na level: Low
- Serum osmolality: Low
- Urine osmolality: High
- Urinary Na concentration: High (losing sodium, rather than retaining)
- Serum glucose; blood urea nitrogen (BUN); creatinine
- Thyroid function
- Morning cortisol
- Serum ADH level: High
- Uric acid

Imaging
Not usually required for diagnosis

DIFFERENTIAL DIAGNOSIS
- Postoperative complications:
  - Usually after major abdominal or thoracic surgery
  - Caused by nonosmotic release of ADH, probably mediated by pain afferents
  - ADH increased by pain and narcotics
- Postprostatectomy syndrome:
  - Irrigating solution must be nonconducting (i.e., electrolyte-free).
  - D_5W absorbed
- Psychogenic polydipsia:
  - Active therapy rarely is needed.
  - Diuresis occurs when intake is stopped.
  - Intake usually over 10 L/d
  - Interaction with other psychotropic drugs
- Acute (usually in children):
  - Swallowing water during swimming
  - Diluted formula
  - Tap-water enemas
- Endocrine:
  - Addison disease
  - Hypothyroidism
- Spurious hyponatremia: Caused by increased serum glucose, cholesterol, or proteins
- Appropriate ADH secretion and hyponatremia with decreased effective arterial blood volume (e.g., congestive heart failure [CHF], nephrotic syndrome, cirrhosis)
- Cerebral salt wasting syndrome (hyponatremia, extracellular fluid depletion, CNS insult) (4,5)

TREATMENT

MEDICATION
- Diuretics: Furosemide (Lasix) plus hourly NaCl and KCl replacement:
  - Requires frequent monitoring (see Patient Monitoring)
  - Treatment of choice for acute management

- Hypertonic (3%) saline to cautiously increase serum Na (6)[B]:
  - By 10–12 mEq/L (10–12 mmol/L) q24h (in chronic hyponatremia)
  - 5% over 1st few hours
  - To only 120 mEq/L (120 mmol/L) acutely
  - By 0.5 mEq/h (0.5 mmol/h)

- Contraindications: Avoid fluids in CHF, nephrotic syndrome, or cirrhosis.
- Precautions: Overly rapid correction (>12 mEq/L/d [>12 mmol/d]) can cause:
  - CHF
  - Subdural and intracerebral hemorrhage
  - Permanent CNS damage, especially with serum Na <120 mEq/L (<120 mmol/L)
  - Demyelination syndrome
- Demeclocycline:
  - Blocks ADH at renal tubule; produces nephrogenic diabetes insipidus
  - Dosage for long-term management: 600–1,200 mg/d
  - Onset of action within 1 week; therefore, not best for acute management
- Lithium:
  - Blocks ADH at renal tubule
  - Use with caution to avoid lithium toxicity.
- Vasopressin-2 receptor antagonist (the vaptans: tovaptan, conivaptan):
  - Good efficacy and safety profiles in the treatment of mild-to-moderate hyponatremia due to SIADH (2,7).

ADDITIONAL TREATMENT
General Measures
- Fluid restriction: 800–1,000 mL/d; this is the main form of treatment.
- Mildly symptomatic (serum Na >125 mEq/L [>125 mmol/L]): Restrict fluid to 800–1,000 mL/d (3)[B].
- Acute (<48 h duration) or symptomatic (altered mental status, seizure, coma):
  - Hypertonic saline (3% normal saline) bolus
  - Diuresis with loop diuretics
  - Decrease oral free water to 2/3 maintenance.
  - Increase oral salt.
  - Correct serum Na deficit (mEq Na deficit = [desired Na – actual Na] × 0.5 × body weight [kg]).
  - Increase serum Na slowly with hypertonic saline by 0.5 mEq/L/h until it reaches 120 mEq/L.

ALERT
Increase Na levels slowly, no more than 0.5–1 mEq/L/h, to prevent complications such as central pontine myelinosis (CPM).

ONGOING CARE

FOLLOW-UP RECOMMENDATIONS
Patient Monitoring
- Careful continuous clinical and laboratory monitoring of hyponatremic state during acute phase:
  - Hourly urine output
  - Urine Na
  - Serum Na and potassium (K)
- Chronic management: Monitor underlying cause as needed.

DIET
May need increased salt or decreased water intake, depending on cause

PATIENT EDUCATION
Diet and fluid restrictions

PROGNOSIS
- Depends on underlying cause, but in general, higher morbidity and mortality in hospitalized patients with hyponatremia
- If symptomatic (seizure, coma): High mortality due to cerebral edema if serum Na <120 mEq/L (<120 mmol/L)

COMPLICATIONS
- Central pontine myelinosis (8)
- Chronic hyponatremia: Usually <120 mEq/L (<120 mmol/L)
- Complications of overly rapid correction (see Treatment, Precautions)
- Chronic hyponatremia is associated with osteoporosis (9).

REFERENCES

1. Moritz ML, Ayus JC, et al. Prevention of hospital-acquired hyponatremia: a case for using isotonic saline. *Pediatrics*. 2003;111:227–30.
2. Ellison DH, Berl T. Clinical practice. The syndrome of inappropriate antidiuresis. *N Engl J Med*. 2007;356:2064–72.
3. Yeates KE, Singer M, Morton AR. Salt and water: a simple approach to hyponatremia. *CMAJ*. 2004;170:365–9.
4. Diringer MN, Zazulia AR, et al. Hyponatremia in neurologic patients: consequences and approaches to treatment. *Neurologist*. 2006;12:117–26.
5. Tisdall M, Crocker M, Watkiss J, et al. Disturbances of sodium in critically ill adult neurologic patients: a clinical review. *J Neurosurg Anesthesiol*. 2006;18:57–63.
6. Arvanitis ML, et al. External causes of metabolic disorders. *Emerg Med Clin North Amer*. 2005;827–41.
7. Sherlock M, Thompson CJ, et al. The syndrome of inappropriate antidiuretic hormone: current and future management options. *Eur J Endocrinol*. 2010;162(Suppl 1):S13–8.
8. Fleming JD, Babu S, et al. Images in clinical medicine. Central pontine myelinolysis. *N Engl J Med*. 2008;359:e29.
9. Verbalis JG, Barsony J, Sugimura Y, et al. Hyponatremia-induced osteoporosis. *J Bone Miner Res*. 2010;25:554–63.
10. Adrogué HJ, Madias NE. Hyponatremia. *N Engl J Med*. 2000;342:1581–9.

ADDITIONAL READING

- Holm EA, Bie P, Ottesen M, et al. Diagnosis of the syndrome of inappropriate secretion of antidiuretic hormone. *South Med J*. 2009;102:380–4.
- Moritz ML, Ayus JC, et al. 100 cc 3% sodium chloride bolus: a novel treatment for hyponatremic encephalopathy. *Metab Brain Dis*. 2010;25:91–6.

See Also (Topic, Algorithm, Electronic Media Element)
Hyponatremia

 ## CODES

ICD9
253.6 Other disorders of neurohypophysis

CLINICAL PEARLS

- Fluid restriction to 600–800 mL/d × 2–3 days will result in weight loss and correction of hyponatremia and salt wasting in SIADH. Fluid restriction fails to correct hyponatremia and Na wasting in salt-losing renal disease (2,10).
- Cerebral salt wasting is a controversial disease entity and is similar to SIADH. However, patients with SIADH are euvolemic, whereas patients with cerebral salt wasting are hypovolemic. The only real way to establish the diagnosis is through fluid restriction. Serum urate and fractional excretion of urate will be corrected with fluid restriction in SIADH but will not correct in cerebral salt wasting (10).
- CPM is a cerebral demyelination syndrome that causes quadriplegia, pseudobulbar palsy, seizures, coma, and death. It is caused by an overly rapid rate of Na correction (8).

SEIZURE DISORDER, ABSENCE

Jane K. Louie, MD

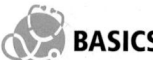 **BASICS**

DESCRIPTION
- Committee on Classification and Terminology of the International League Against Epilepsy divides epilepsy syndromes into 4 groups (1):
  - Localization-related: Focal or multifocal seizures
  - Generalized: Generalized seizures
  - Undetermined epilepsies: Both focal and generalized seizures where objective studies (e.g., EEG) do not indicate etiology or localization
  - Special syndromes: Now called "conditions with epileptic seizures that do not require a diagnosis of epilepsy" (e.g., febrile seizures)
- Epilepsy syndromes further classified by etiology:
  - Idiopathic: Presumed genetic etiology without structural brain lesion or other neurologic deficits
  - Symptomatic: Clearly identified cause (e.g., Mesial temporal lobe epilepsy with hippocampal sclerosis)
  - Cryptogenic: Etiology suspected but exact cause cannot be identified
- Absence seizures are a generalized epileptic seizure type, characterized by brief lapses of awareness.
- Typical absence:
  - Associated with pediatric idiopathic generalized epilepsy syndromes, namely, childhood absence epilepsy
  - Formerly called *petit mal seizures*
  - Abrupt-onset behavioral arrest, loss of awareness, and blank staring, sometimes with mild upward eye deviation, repetitive blinking
  - May include automatisms, tonic or atonic features, eyelid or facial clonus, autonomic features
  - Last 5–30 s
  - Immediate return to normal consciousness
- Atypical absence:
  - Associated with symptomatic generalized epilepsy syndromes such as Lennox-Gastaut
  - Onset and offset less abrupt than typical absence seizures
  - Last 10–45 seconds
  - Impairment of consciousness often incomplete with continued purposeful activity
  - Postictal confusion sometimes occurs.
  - Associated clinical features more pronounced and frequent than typical absence; atonia most common
- Myoclonic absence:
  - Additional proposed seizure type by the International League Against Epilepsy (2)
  - Seizure type in epilepsy with myoclonic absences, a cryptogenic generalized epilepsy syndrome
  - Rhythmic clonic jerking at 2–4 Hz
  - Last 5–10 s
  - Unlike myoclonic seizures with no impairment of consciousness, brief lapses of awareness characteristic of myoclonic absence

- Rest of chapter details idiopathic generalized epilepsy syndromes characterized by *typical absence seizures*, specifically childhood absence epilepsy (CAE)
- Juvenile absence epilepsy is mentioned briefly here.
- Childhood absence epilepsy (CAE):
  - Also known as *pyknolepsy*
  - Typical absence seizures are the only seizure type in 90% of children.
  - 10% develop additional generalized tonic–clonic seizures.
  - Seizures last about 10 seconds and often occur hundreds of times per day.
  - Onset ages 4–10 years, with peak at ages 5–7 years (3)
  - Normal neurologic state and development
  - Spontaneous remission occurs in 65–70% of patients during adolescence (4).
- Juvenile absence epilepsy (JAE):
  - Typical absence seizures are the main seizure type.
  - Seizures last longer than in CAE and occur usually less than once a day (5).
  - Onset ages 9–16 years, with peak at ages 10–13 years
  - Generalized tonic–clonic seizures occur in most patients, often in the first 1–2 h after awakening.
  - Seizures often persist into adulthood.

EPIDEMIOLOGY
Incidence
6–8/100,000

Prevalence
5–50/100,000

RISK FACTORS
Genetics
- 70–85% concordance occurs in monozygotic twins; 82% share EEG features.
- 33% concordance among 1st-degree relatives
- 15–45% have a family history of epilepsy.
- Girls are more often affected by a 3:2–2:1 ratio.
- Complex multifactorial inheritance
- For childhood absence, genes/loci implicated include 6q, 8q24, and 5q14 (5).
- Mutations of $GABA_A$ receptor and voltage-gated Ca^{2+} channel are implicated.

PATHOPHYSIOLOGY
- Corticoreticular theory implicates abnormal activity in thalamocortical circuits (6).
- Thalamic reticular nucleus is responsible for both normal sleep spindles and pathologic slow-wave discharges; contains inhibitory GABAergic neurons.
- These neurons affect low-threshold calcium currents.

- These circuits can fire in oscillatory/rhythmic fashion:
  - Normally, activation of $GABA_A$ receptors causes 10-Hz oscillations in sleep spindle frequency.
  - If $GABA_B$ receptors strongly activated, oscillation frequency will be 3–4 Hz, similar to spike-and-wave typical absence seizure frequency.

COMMONLY ASSOCIATED CONDITIONS
- 3–8% of CAE cases evolve into juvenile myoclonic epilepsy.
- Associated with cognitive/learning problems (7)

 DIAGNOSIS

Seizures are often so brief that untrained observers are not aware of the diagnosis.

HISTORY
- Frequently diagnosed in children being evaluated for poor school performance
- Teachers report that child seems to daydream or zone out frequently.
- Child will forget portions of conversations.
- Child with normal IQ underperforms in school.

PHYSICAL EXAM
- Unless child has other genetic or acquired abnormality, neurologic exam is usually normal.
- Seizures may be frequent enough to be observed during physical exam:
  - Manifest by behavior arrest: Child will stop speaking in midsentence, stare blankly, etc.
  - Automatisms (repetitive stereotyped behaviors) may be present.
  - Child resumes previous activity.
- Seizures may be induced by hyperventilation:
  - Have child blow on pinwheel or similar exercise to provoke seizure.
  - Alternatively, ask patient to perform hyperventilation with eyes closed and count. Patient will open eyes at onset of seizure and stop counting (5).
- Patient manifests unresponsiveness but retains postural tone in a typical absence seizure.

DIAGNOSTIC TESTS & INTERPRETATION
Lab
- No specific hematologic workup
- Follow blood chemistry, hepatic function, and blood counts specific to drug regimen.
- Drug levels are useful in evaluating symptoms of toxicity or for breakthrough seizures.

Initial lab tests
- EEG is standard for diagnosis:
  - Typical absence features: 3.0-Hz spike-and-wave activity on normal EEG background
  - Seizures feature bursts of 3- to 4-Hz spike-and-wave activity, which may slow to 2.5–3 Hz during seizure.
  - Seizure is usually evident clinically if bursts last >3 seconds; subtle changes of transient cognitive impairment may be evident with briefer seizures.
- Hyperventilation and occasionally photic stimulation may induce seizure, thus confirming diagnosis of typical absence epilepsy.

Imaging
- Not routinely indicated in children with typical absence and normal neurologic exam and IQ
- Brain MRI is indicated in atypical absence and in children with mixed seizure types when combined with abnormal neurologic exam or low IQ (7).

DIFFERENTIAL DIAGNOSIS
- Typical absence seizures frequently are misdiagnosed as complex partial seizures.
- Nonepileptic staring spells: Suggestive features include:
  - Events do not interrupt play.
  - Events are first noticed by professional such as school teacher, speech therapist, occupational therapist, or physician (rather than parent).
  - During staring spell, child is responsive to touch or other external stimuli.

 TREATMENT

MEDICATION
Certain common anticonvulsants may exacerbate absence: Carbamazepine, tiagabine, vigabatrin, and gabapentin.

First Line
- Ethosuximide blocks T-type calcium channels:
  - 1st-line, except in absence patients with tonic–clonic seizures (lacks efficacy) (4)[A]
  - Side effects: Headache, hiccups, behavior changes, tremor
  - Adverse effects: Rare blood dyscrasias (monitor CBC)
- Lamotrigine affects sodium channels (4)[B]:
  - Side effects: Headache, insomnia, dizziness
  - Adverse effects: Rare Stevens-Johnson rash, more often when coadministered with valproic acid
- Valproic acid has multiple mechanisms:
  - 1st choice in absence patients with tonic–clonic, myoclonic, mixed seizure types (4)[A]
  - Side effects: Weight gain, alopecia, sedation
  - Adverse effects: Thrombocytopenia, rare fulminant hepatic failure (especially in children <2 years of age)

Second Line
- Topiramate affects GABA and excitatory neurotransmission:
  - Food and Drug Administration (FDA) approved for Lennox-Gastaut syndrome
  - Side effects: Psychomotor slowing
  - Adverse effects: Weight loss, renal stones, myopia, glaucoma (rare), anhidrosis
- Zonisamide and levetiracetam are also used off-label.

Pregnancy Considerations
Anticonvulsants, especially valproic acid, are associated with an increase in fetal malformations. Use of valproic acid in women who are or are likely to become pregnant generally is contraindicated. Obtain specialty consultation.

ADDITIONAL TREATMENT
- Most absence seizure patients respond to a single medication.
- Male gender and an early age at diagnosis are associated with the need for 2 medications to control the disease (8)[A].

IN-PATIENT CONSIDERATIONS
Admission Criteria
- Absence epilepsy rarely requires admission.
- Status epilepticus requires inpatient management.

Discharge Criteria
Resolution of status epilepticus

 ONGOING CARE

FOLLOW-UP RECOMMENDATIONS
- Patients with associated tonic–clonic seizures should avoid high places and swimming alone.
- Absence rarely persists into adulthood, but affected adults may be restricted from driving, working over open flames, etc., as with other generalized and partial epilepsy subtypes.
- Patients should be monitored periodically by a neurologist for evolution of absence epilepsy into tonic–clonic or other seizure types.

PROGNOSIS
- In childhood absence epilepsy without tonic–clonic seizures, 90% remit by adulthood (3).
- 35% of patients with tonic–clonic seizures experience complete remission of absence seizures.
- 15% of patients develop juvenile myoclonic epilepsy (JME) (9).

COMPLICATIONS
Reported frequencies of typical absence status epilepticus range from 5.8–9.4% of patients with CAE (10).

REFERENCES

1. Commission on Classification and Terminology of the International League Against Epilepsy Proposal for revised classification of epilepsies and epileptic syndromes. *Epilepsia.* 1989;30(4): 389–399.
2. Engel J. Report of the ILAE classification core group. *Epilepsia.* 2006;47:1558–68.
3. Valentin A, Hindocha N, Osei-Lah A, et al. Idiopathic generalized epilepsy with absences: syndrome classification. *Epilepsia.* 2007;48: 2187–90.
4. Crunelli V, et al. Childhood absence epilepsy: Genes, channels, neurons, and networks. *Nat Rev Neurol.* 2002;3:371–82.
5. Nordli DR. Idiopathic generalized epilepsies recognized by the International League Against Epilepsy. *Epilepsia.* 2005;46(Suppl 9):48–56.
6. Blumenfeld H. From molecules to networks: cortical/subcortical interactions in the pathophysiology of idiopathic generalized epilepsy. *Epilepsia.* 2003;44(Suppl 2):7–15.
7. Camfield P, Camfield C. Epileptic syndromes in childhood: clinical features, outcomes, and treatment. *Epilepsia.* 2002;43(Suppl 3):27–32.
8. Nadler B, Shevell MI. Childhood absence epilepsy requiring more than one medication for seizure control. *Can J Neurol Sci.* 2008;35:297–300.
9. Grosso S, Galimberti D, Vezzosi P, et al. Childhood absence epilepsy: evolution and prognostic factors. *Epilepsia.* 2005;46:1796–801.
10. Shorvon S, Walker M. Status epilepticus in idiopathic generalized epilepsy. *Epilepsia.* 2005;46(Suppl 9):73–9.
11. Kesselheim AS, Stedman MR, Bubrick EJ, et al. Seizure outcomes following the use of generic versus brand-name antiepileptic drugs: a systematic review and meta-analysis. *Drugs.* 2010;70:605–21.

CODES

ICD9
345.00 Generalized nonconvulsive epilepsy, without mention of intractable epilepsy

CLINICAL PEARLS
- To help aid with diagnosis during exam, try having child blow repetitively on pinwheel (causing hyperventilation) to attempt to trigger absence seizure.
- Alternatively, ask patient to perform hyperventilation with eyes closed and count. Patient will open eyes at onset of seizure and stop counting (5).
- Concern regarding generic medications allowing more breakthrough seizures has not been supported in evidence-based studies (11)[A].

SEIZURE DISORDER, PARTIAL

Ruben Peralta, MD
Wayne Morgan, MD

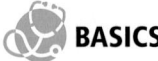 **BASICS**

DESCRIPTION
- Seizures occur when abnormal synchronous neuronal discharges in the brain cause transient cortical dysfunction.
- Generalized seizures involve bilateral cerebral cortex from the seizure's onset.
- Partial seizures originate from a discrete focus in the cerebral cortex.
- Partial seizures are further divided into simple and complex subtypes:
  - If consciousness is impaired during a partial seizure, it is classified as complex.
  - If consciousness is preserved, it is a simple partial seizure.

EPIDEMIOLOGY
Prevalence
Partial seizures occur in 20/100,000 persons in the US.

RISK FACTORS
- History of traumatic brain injury (1)
- Children exposed to a thiamine-deficient formula (2)

Genetics
Benign rolandic epilepsy, a form of partial seizure disorder, has an autosomal dominant inheritance pattern with penetrance depending on multiple factors.

ETIOLOGY
- Partial seizures begin when a localized seizure focus produces an abnormal, synchronized depolarization that spreads to a discrete portion of the surrounding cortex.
- The area of cortex involved in the seizure determines the symptoms; for example, an epileptogenic focus in motor cortex produces contralateral motor symptoms.
- In some cases, etiology is related to structural abnormalities that are prone to epileptogenesis. Most common etiologies vary by life stage:
  - Early childhood: Developmental/congenital malformation, trauma
  - Young adults: Developmental, infection, trauma
  - Adults 40–60 years of age: Cerebrovascular insult, infection, trauma
  - Adults >60 years of age: Cerebrovascular insult, trauma, neoplasm
- Complex partial seizures: A common cause is mesial temporal sclerosis.

COMMONLY ASSOCIATED CONDITIONS
Epilepsy patients have a higher incidence of depression than does the general population (3).

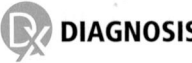 **DIAGNOSIS**

- Seizure activity usually stereotyped
- Duration: Seconds–minutes unless status epilepticus develops; status epilepticus may present as focal or generalized convulsions or altered mental status without convulsions.

- Simple partial seizures:
  - Simple partial seizures are characterized by localized symptoms. The patient is conscious. Symptoms may involve motor, sensory, or psychic systems.
  - Motor: Seizure activity in motor strip causes contraction (tonic) or rhythmic jerking (clonic) movements that may involve 1 entire side of body or may be more localized (i.e., hands, feet, or face):
    - Jacksonian march: As discharge spreads through motor cortex, tonic–clonic activity spreads in predictable fashion (i.e., beginning in hand and progressing up arm and to the face).
  - Sensory/psychic:
    - Todd paresis: After motor seizure, residual, temporary weakness in the affected area
    - Parietal lobe: Sensory loss or paresthesias, dizziness
    - Temporal lobe: Déjà vu, rising sensation in epigastrium, auditory hallucinations or forced memories, unpleasant smell or taste
    - Occipital: Visual hallucinations
- Complex partial seizures:
  - Impaired consciousness by definition
  - May have aura; this is start of seizure
- Amnesia for the event, postictal confusion:
  - Most often, focus in complex partial seizures is temporal or frontal
  - Motor manifestations may include dystonic posturing or automatisms (i.e., simple, repetitive movements of face and hands such as lip smacking, picking, or more complex actions such as purposeless walking).
  - Frontal lobe seizure is characterized by brief, bilateral complex movements, vocalizations, often with onset during sleep.

HISTORY
- A detailed description of the seizure should be obtained from an observer.
- Review medication list for drugs that lower seizure threshold (e.g., tramadol, bupropion, theophylline)
- Drugs of abuse (e.g., cocaine) lower seizure threshold (4).
- History of traumatic brain injury (1)

PHYSICAL EXAM
Include neurologic exam, with attention to lateralizing signs suggestive of structural lesion.

DIAGNOSTIC TESTS & INTERPRETATION
Electroencephalogram (EEG): Spikes/sharp waves over seizure focus:
- Yield of EEG is increased by obtained in 1st 24 h following seizure and by sleep deprivation
- Frontal lobe seizure focus may be difficult to detect by routine EEG.
- If difficulty with diagnosis, continuous video–EEG monitoring may be appropriate

Lab
- Serum electrolytes, including calcium, magnesium, phosphorus; hepatic function panel; complete blood count; drugs of abuse
- If measured within 10–20 minutes of suspected seizure, an elevated prolactin level may help to differentiate generalized or complex partial seizure from psychogenic seizure.
- Cerebrospinal fluid exam if infection is suspected

- Urinalysis, chest x-ray, levels of antiepileptic drugs for breakthrough seizure

Imaging
- Emergency evaluation of new seizure: Computed tomography scan to screen for hemorrhage, stroke
- After emergency evaluation, magnetic resonance imaging (MRI) with thin cuts through area of interest
- If planning epilepsy surgery, positron emission tomography scan and/or interictal single-photon emission computed tomography (SPECT) may be of value.
- Magnetoencephalography (MEG) is an evolving technology for localizing seizure focus.

DIFFERENTIAL DIAGNOSIS
- Nonepileptic seizure
- Syncope/postanoxic myoclonus
- Hypoglycemia
- For hemiparesis following event:
  - Transient ischemic attack
  - Hemiplegic migraine

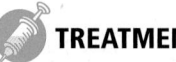 **TREATMENT**

MEDICATION
- Some physicians do not start medication after a single seizure if EEG and MRI are normal and/or a precipitant is clear and avoidable.
- Antiepileptic drugs (AEDs) act on voltage-gated ion channels, affect neuronal inhibition via enhancement of γ-aminobutyric acid (GABA, an inhibitory neurotransmitter), or decrease neuronal excitation. End result is to decrease the abnormal synchronized firing and to prevent seizure propagation.
- ~50% of those with newly diagnosed partial seizures respond to and tolerate 1st AED trial.
- Choose AED based on seizure type, side effect profile, and patient characteristics. Increase dose until seizure control is obtained or side effects become unacceptable.
- Attempt monotherapy, but many patients will require adjunctive agents.
- *Refractory to medications* is defined as failure of at least 3 anticonvulsants to achieve adequate control.
- Several AEDs induce or inhibit cytochrome P450 enzymes (watch for drug interactions).

First Line
- Carbamazepine: Affects sodium channels; side effects include gastrointestinal (GI) distress, hyponatremia, diplopia, dizziness, rare pancytopenia/marrow suppression, exfoliative rash
- Oxcarbazepine: Affects sodium channels; side effects include dizziness, diplopia, hyponatremia, headache
- Lamotrigine: Affects sodium channels:
  - Side effects include insomnia, dizziness, ataxia
  - Risk of Stevens-Johnson reaction (potentially fatal exfoliative rash) especially when given with valproate; requires slow titration
- Levetiracetam: Multiple mechanisms; side effects include sedation, ataxia, irritability

Second Line
- Phenytoin: Affects sodium channels; side effects include ataxia, dizziness, diplopia, tremor, GI upset, gingival hyperplasia, fever
- Phenobarbital: Multiple mechanisms; side effects include sedation, withdrawal seizures

- Valproate: Multiple mechanisms; side effects include GI upset, weight gain, alopecia, tremor; less common thrombocytopenia, hepatitis, pancreatitis
- Topiramate: Multiple mechanisms; side effects include anorexia, cognitive slowing, sedation, nephrolithiasis, anhidrosis
- Gabapentin: Multiple mechanisms; side effects include sedation, dizziness, ataxia
- Pregabalin: Affects calcium channels; side effects include sedation, dizziness, weight gain
- Zonisamide: Affects sodium channels:
  – Side effects include sedation, anorexia, nausea, dizziness, ataxia, anhidrosis, nephrolithiasis
  – Cross-reaction with sulfa allergy

Pregnancy Considerations
- Several AEDs induce hepatic metabolism of oral contraceptives, decreasing their efficacy. AED therapy during 1st trimester is associated with doubled risk for major fetal malformations (6% vs 3%).
- Phenytoin in pregnancy may result in fetal hydantoin syndrome.
- Valproate is associated with neural tube defects.
- Fetal insult from seizures following withdrawal of therapy also may be severe. Risk–benefit balance should be evaluated with high-risk pregnancy and epileptology consultations. Most patients remain on anticonvulsants.
- Consider vagal nerve stimulator during pregnancy (5).

ADDITIONAL TREATMENT
General Measures
- Ask patient to maintain a seizure diary.
- Note potential triggers such as stress, sleep deprivation, drug use, discontinuation of alcohol or benzodiazepines, menses.

Issues for Referral
For refractory seizures, consider referral to an epilepsy specialist and/or epilectic center (6,7).

Additional Therapies
- Vagal nerve stimulator: Implanted in neck; provides periodic stimulation to vagus nerve; may induce hoarseness, cough, and dysphagia (8)
- New technologies under development include deep brain stimulation.

SURGERY/OTHER PROCEDURES
- For refractory partial complex seizures (7)
- Should have identifiable focus
- Preoperative testing, such as Wada test, should be done to decrease likelihood of inducing aphasia and memory loss.
- Workup also may include MRI, video–EEG monitoring, electrocorticography, MEG, and ictal SPECT.
- 64% will be seizure-free after surgery (with continued medication treatment); 25% will have significant decrease in frequency; 1/3 continue to have disabling seizures.
- Goal of surgical intervention is to reduce reliance on medications; most patients remain on anticonvulsants postoperatively.

IN-PATIENT CONSIDERATIONS
Admission Criteria
Generally, outpatient treatment; admission for unremitting seizure (partial or secondary generalized status epilepticus)

ONGOING CARE

FOLLOW-UP RECOMMENDATIONS
- Most states have restrictions on driving for those with seizure disorders.
- Depending on seizure manifestation, may recommend against activities such as swimming, climbing to heights, working over open flames, or operating heavy machinery
- Outpatient follow-up with neurologist

Patient Monitoring
AED levels if concern over toxicity, noncompliance, or for breakthrough seizures

DIET
Ketogenic or low-glycemic-index diet may improve seizure control in some patients.

PATIENT EDUCATION
Avoid potential triggers such as alcohol or drug use, sleep deprivation

PROGNOSIS
- Risk of seizure recurrence: ~30% after 1st seizure; 50% of these recurrences will occur in the 1st 6 months; 90% in the 1st 2 years.
- Depends on seizure type; rolandic epilepsy has a good prognosis; temporal lobe epilepsy is more likely to be persistent.
- ~25–30% of all seizures are refractory to current medications (9)[C].
- AEDs initiated after an initial seizure have been shown to decrease the risk of seizure over the 1st 2 years but are not demonstrated to reduce long-term risk of recurrence (10)[C].
- Long duration of uncontrolled seizure disorder associated with increased cognitive and functional impairments; early pharmacologic intervention is encouraged.
- The potential for AEDs to confer neuroprotection is under investigation.
- The risk of developing seizure after mild traumatic brain injury remains high for a long period (>10 years) (1).

COMPLICATIONS
Risk of accidental injury

REFERENCES

1. Christensen J, Pedersen MG, Pedersen CB, et al. Long-term risk of epilepsy after traumatic brain injury in children and young adults: a population-based cohort study. *Lancet*. 2009.
2. Fattal-Valevski A, Bloch-Mimouni A, Kivity S, et al. Epilepsy in children with infantile thiamine deficiency. *Neurology*. 2009;73:828–33.
3. Paras ML, Murad MH, Chen LP, et al. Sexual abuse and lifetime diagnosis of somatic disorders: a systematic review and meta-analysis. *JAMA*. 2009;302:550–61.
4. Karila L, Lowenstein W, Coscas S, et al. [Complications of cocaine addiction] *Rev Prat*. 2009;59:825–9.
5. Houser MV, Hennessy MD, Howard BC, et al. Vagal nerve stimulator use during pregnancy for treatment of refractory seizure disorder. *Obstet Gynecol*. 2010;115:417–9.
6. Hemb M, Velasco TR, Parnes MS, et al. Improved outcomes in pediatric epilepsy surgery: the UCLA experience, 1986–2008. *Neurology*. 2010;74:1768–75.
7. Cross JH, Jayakar P, Nordli D, et al. Proposed criteria for referral and evaluation of children for epilepsy surgery: recommendations of the Subcommission for Pediatric Epilepsy Surgery. *Epilepsia*. 2006;47:952–9.
8. Siddiqui F, Herial NA, Ali II, et al. Cumulative effect of vagus nerve stimulators on intractable seizures observed over a period of 3years. *Epilepsy & behavior : E&B*. 2010;
9. Berg AT, Vickrey BG, Testa FM, et al. How long does it take for epilepsy to become intractable? A prospective investigation. *Ann Neurol*. 2006;60:73–9.
10. Adams SM, Knowles PD. Evaluation of a first seizure. *Am Fam Physician*. 2007;75:1342–7.

ADDITIONAL READING

- Auvin S, Vallée L. [Febrile seizures: Current understanding of pathophysiological mechanisms.] *Arch Pediatr*. 2009.
- Deprez L, Jansen A, De Jonghe P, et al. Genetics of epilepsy syndromes starting in the first year of life. *Neurology*. 2009;72:273–81.
- Sankar R, Ramsay E, McKay A, et al. A multicenter, outpatient, open-label study to evaluate the dosing, effectiveness, and safety of topiramate as monotherapy in the treatment of epilepsy in clinical practice. *Epilepsy Behav*. 2009.

CODES

ICD9
- 345.40 Partial epilepsy, without mention of intractable epilepsy
- 345.50 Partial epilepsy, without mention of impairment of consciousness, without mention of intractable epilepsy

CLINICAL PEARLS

- It's a controversial topic whether AED treatment is indicated after a 1st seizure. Treatment should be strongly considered when a clear structural cause is identified or risk of injury from seizure is high (e.g., osteoporosis, anticoagulation).
- Consider vagus nerve stimulation in pregnancy and in patient with medically refractory seizures.
- Postictal elevation in prolactin levels can help distinguish physiologic from psychogenic seizures.

SEIZURE DISORDERS

Ann M. Lynch, PharmD, R.Ph
Stephanie Carinci, MD

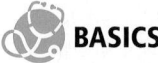

BASICS

DESCRIPTION
- Seizure: Sudden change in cortical electrical activity, manifested through motor, sensory, or behavioral changes, +/– an alteration in consciousness.
- System(s) affected: Nervous
- Synonym(s): Epilepsy; Convulsion; Attacks; Spells

Geriatric Considerations
Fractures from falls are more common in the osteopenic age range.

Pediatric Considerations
Breast-feeding is not contraindicated. Sedation in the infant should be monitored.

Pregnancy Considerations
- Monitor serum levels of antiepileptic drugs (AEDs).
- There is a twofold increase in congenital malformations in children born to mothers taking anticonvulsants, depending on the anticonvulsant. Some expectant mothers can be taken off anticonvulsants safely for the 1st trimester or initial 6 week period (organogenesis.) Avoid Depakote. Epilepsy patients should notify their neurologist before conception if possible.
- Recommend against use of category C or D AEDs during pregnancy/nursing.

EPIDEMIOLOGY
Incidence
- Approximately 200,000 new cases of epilepsy are diagnosed in the US each year.
- 45,000 new cases in children <15 years of age
- Pediatric (<2 years) and older adults (>65 years) more commonly present with new-onset seizures.
- Predominant sex: Male = Female

Prevalence
- 2.7 million with seizure disorder
- 4 million people have had 1 or more seizures.
- 326,000 children (≤14 years) and 600,000 adults (>65 years) have a seizure disorder.

RISK FACTORS
Children delivered breech have a prevalence rate of 3.8% compared with 2.2% in vertex deliveries.

Genetics
Family history increases risk threefold.

GENERAL PREVENTION
Acetaminophen to prevent febrile seizures. Take measures to prevent head injuries. Reduce exposure to lead-containing products. Avoid excessive alcohol use/abuse.

PATHOPHYSIOLOGY
Synchronous and excessive firing of neurons resulting in impairment of normal control of CNS

ETIOLOGY
- Brain tumor
- Cerebral hypoxia
- Cerebrovascular accident
- Convulsive or toxic agents (e.g., lead, alcohol, picrotoxin, strychnine)
- Drug or alcohol overdose/withdrawal
- Eclampsia
- Exogenous factors, triggers (e.g., sound, light, cutaneous stimulation)
- Fever, acute infection, or metabolic disturbance
- Head injury
- Heat stroke

COMMONLY ASSOCIATED CONDITIONS
Infections, tumors, drug abuse, alcohol and drug withdrawal, trauma, metabolic disorders

DIAGNOSIS

- Differentiate first between epileptiform seizures and nonepileptiform seizures (NESs).
- If NES are psychogenic; often are associated with history of sexual abuse
  - Psychogenic NES is usually associated with a history of psychiatric conditions. Physiologic seizures are true cortical events and often require acute intervention.
    - Hyperthyroidism
    - Hypoglycemia
    - Nonketotic hyperglycemia
    - Hyponatremia
    - Uremia
    - Porphyria
    - Hypoxia
    - Confusional migraine
    - Transient ischemic attack
    - Narcolepsy/sleep disorder
    - Toxin
- International classification of seizures:
  - Generalized seizures:
  - Absence
  - Atonic
  - Juvenile myoclonic
    - Myoclonic: Repetitive muscle contractions
    - Tonic–clonic: Tonic phase: Sudden loss of consciousness; clonic phase: sustained contraction followed by rhythmic contractions of all 4 extremities; postictal phase: headache, confusion, fatigue; clinically, hypertensive, tachycardic, and otherwise hypersympathetic
  - Febrile seizures:
    - Age between 3 months and 5 years
    - Fever without evidence of any other defined cause for seizures
    - Recurrent febrile seizures probably do not increase the risk of epilepsy
  - Symptomatic focal epilepsies
  - Complex partial seizures
  - Nonconvulsive status epilepticus: Most commonly seen in ICU patients-no tonic clonic activity seen so must diagnose with bedside EEG
  - Status epilepticus: Repetitive generalized seizures without recovery between seizures; considered a neurologic emergency.

HISTORY
- Eyewitness descriptions of event
- Patient impressions of what occurred before, during, and after the event
- Screen for etiologies.
- Provoking or ameliorating factors for the event including sleep deprivation
- Ask about bowel or bladder incontinence, tongue biting, other injury, automatisms.

PHYSICAL EXAM
Thorough neurologic exam

DIAGNOSTIC TESTS & INTERPRETATION
A negative EEG does not rule out a seizure disorder.
- Sleep deprivation is helpful prior to EEG to identify positive spike wave formations.
- Video EEG monitoring is used to differentiate psychomotor NES from true cortical events

Lab
Initial lab tests
- Serum tests: Glucose, sodium, potassium, calcium, phosphorus, magnesium, BUN, ammonia
- AED levels
- Drug and toxic screens: Include alcohol.
- Complete blood count (CBC): Rule out infection.

Follow-Up & Special Considerations
- Consider an arterial blood gas determination.
- Drugs that may alter lab results: AED therapy may affect the EEG results dramatically.
- Inadequate AED levels: May be altered by many medications, such as erythromycin, sulfonamides, warfarin, cimetidine, and alcohol.
- Disorders that may alter lab results: Pregnancy decreases serum concentration.
- Consider HLA testing in Asian patients.

Imaging
Imaging is recommended for new onset seizures when localization-related epilepsy is known or suspected, when the epilepsy classification is in doubt, or when an epilepsy syndrome with remote symptomatic cause is suspected. MRI is preferred to CT because of its superior resolution, versatility, and lack of radiation (1)[A].

Initial approach
- Brain MRI: Superior in evaluation of the temporal lobes
- CT scan of brain: Indicated routinely as initial evaluation esp in ER
- Bone scan to determine bone mineral density (BMD) – generally done if pt on older AEDs such as Dilantin and Tegretol

Diagnostic Procedures/Surgery
LP for spinal fluid analysis may be necessary especially if fever or impairment of consciousness

Pathological Findings
MRI may identify a nidus for seizure activity.

DIFFERENTIAL DIAGNOSIS
- General:
  - Idiopathic
  - Acute infection
  - Trauma
  - Drug and alcohol withdrawal
  - Tumor
  - Conversion disorder: Pseudoseizure
  - NES
  - Vascular disease
- Additionally:
  - Infancy (0–2 years):
    - Perinatal hypoxia
    - Metabolic: Hypoglycemia, hypocalcemia, hypomagnesemia, vitamin B_6 deficiency, phenylketonuria

- Childhood (2–10 years): Febrile seizure
- Adolescent (10–18 years):
  ○ Arteriovenous malformations
- Late adulthood (>60 years):
  ○ Degenerative disease including dementia
  ○ Metabolic: Hypoglycemia, uremia, hepatic failure, electrolyte abnormality

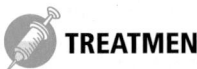 **TREATMENT**

- 50-60% presenting with an initial unprovoked seizure will not have a recurrence; 40-50% will have a recurrence within two years (2)[A].
- Starting antiepileptic medications reduces recurrences of seizures, but does not alter long term outcomes (3)[A].
- Evidence is conflicting whether or not to routinely start AEDs in patients with an initial seizure and no focal abnormalities on exam or imaging, though many recommend deferring treatment until a second seizure has occurred (4)[A].

MEDICATION

- AEDs of choice: Select from seizure groups below, with attention toward potential side effects.
- Choice of AED is based on type of seizure.
- Monotherapy is preferred whenever possible. Systemic reviews found insufficient evidence on which to base a 1st- or 2nd-line choice among these drugs in terms of seizure control.
- Treatment options include:
  - Carbamazepine (Tegretol) 100–200 mg/d in 1–2 doses; therapeutic range: 4–12 mg/L
  - Phenytoin (Dilantin) 200–400 mg/d in 1–3 doses; therapeutic range 10–20 mg/L
  - Valproic acid (Depakene) 750–3,000 mg/d in 1–3 doses to begin at 15 mg/kg/d; therapeutic range 50–150 mg/L
  - Lamotrigine (Lamictal) 25–50 mg/d; adjust in 100-mg increments every 1–2 weeks to 300–500 mg/d in 2 divided doses.
  - Oxcarbazepine (Trileptal) 300 mg b.i.d., increase to 300 mg/3 days; maintenance 1,200 mg/d
  - Topiramate (Topamax) 50 mg/d; adjust weekly to effect; 400 mg/d in 2 doses, maximum 1,600 mg/d
  - Pregabalin (Lyrica)
  - Lacosamide (Vimpat), particularly if refractory seizures
- Alternative drugs (in addition to any of the preceding):
  - Phenobarbital: 50–100 mg b.i.d.–t.i.d.; therapeutic range 15–40 mg/L
  - There is evidence to suggest long-term use of phenobarbital may impair cognitive ability.
  - Primidone (Mysoline) 100–125 mg qhs; adjust to maximum of 2,000 mg/d in 2 doses.
- Contraindications: Refer to manufacturer's profile of each drug.
- Precautions: Doses should be based on individual's response guided by drug levels.
- Consider cautioning about increased risk of suicide, but risk of untreated seizures is far greater than increased risk of suicide (5)[A].
- Patients are susceptible to SUDEP (sudden unexpected death in epilepsy) possibly due to cardiac arrhythmia

ADDITIONAL TREATMENT
Issues for Referral
- Patients should be referred to and followed by a specialist regularly.

- Frequency of visits is based on severity and patient's wishes; maximum of 1 year between visits.

COMPLEMENTARY AND ALTERNATIVE MEDICINE
- There is no evidence that any complementary medicines improve seizures, but they may induce serious drug interactions with prescribed AEDs.
- Psychological therapies may be used in conjunction with AED therapy. Cognitive-behavioral therapy, relaxation, biofeedback, and yoga all may be helpful as adjunctive therapy (6)[C].
- Patients with NES should be referred for psychotherapy.

SURGERY/OTHER PROCEDURES
- Resection for seizures that fail traditional therapy
- Vagus nerve stimulation

IN-PATIENT CONSIDERATIONS
Initial Stabilization
- Protect the airway, and if possible, protect the patient from physical harm; do not restrain.
- Administer acute AEDs.

Admission Criteria
Outpatient therapy is usually sufficient except for status epilepticus.

 ONGOING CARE

FOLLOW-UP RECOMMENDATIONS
- Maintain adequate drug therapy; ensure compliance and/or access to medication.
- Drug therapy withdrawal may be considered after a seizure-free 2-year period. Expect a 33% relapse rate in the following 3 years.

Patient Monitoring
- Monitoring of drug levels and seizure frequency
- CBC and lab values (e.g., calcium, vitamin D) as indicated, BMD
- Monitor for side effects and adverse reactions.
- All patients currently taking any AED should be monitored closely for notable changes in behavior that could indicate the emergence or worsening of suicidal thoughts or behavior or depression.

DIET
Ketogenic diet may be beneficial in children in conjunction with AED therapy (7)[C].

PATIENT EDUCATION
- Stress the importance of medication compliance and the avoidance of alcohol and recreational drugs.
- Individuals with uncontrolled seizures should be encouraged to avoid heights and swimming.
- State driving laws: epilepsyfoundation.org – most states require a minimum of 6 months seizure free
- http://epilepsy.org

PROGNOSIS
- Depends on type of seizure disorder
- ~70% will become seizure-free with initial appropriate treatment, but 30% will continue to have seizures. The number of seizures within 6 months after first presentation is the most important factor for remission.
- Approximately 90% who are seen for a first unprovoked seizure attain a 1–2 year remission within 4 or 5 years of the initial event (2)[A].
- Life expectancy is shortened in persons with epilepsy.
- The case-fatality rate for status epilepticus may be as high as 20%.

COMPLICATIONS
Drug toxicity

REFERENCES

1. Gaillard WD, Chiron C, Cross JH, et al. Guidelines for imaging infants and children with recent-onset epilepsy. *Epilepsia*. 2009;50:2147–53.
2. Berg AT, et al. Risk of recurrence after a first unprovoked seizure. *Epilepsia*. 2008;49(1):13–8.
3. Arts WF, Geerts AT, et al. When to start drug treatment for childhood epilepsy: the clinical-epidemiological evidence. *Eur J Paediatr. Neurol*. 2009;13:93–101.
4. Haut SR, Shinnar S, et al. Considerations in the treatment of a first unprovoked seizure. *Semin Neurol*. 2008;28:289–96.
5. Hesdorffer DC, Kanner AM. The FDA alert on suicidality and antiepileptic drugs: Fire or false alarm? *Epilepsia*. 2009;50:978–86.
6. Marson A, Ramaratnam S. Epilepsy. *Clin Evid Concise*. 2005;13:362–4.
7. Levy R, Cooper P. Ketogenic diet for epilepsy. *Cochrane Database of Systematic Reviews*. 2003;3: CD001903. DOI:10.1002/14651858.CD001903.
8. Wiebe S, Téllez-Zenteno JF, Shapiro M, et al. An evidence-based approach to the first seizure. *Epilepsia*. 2008;49(1):50–7.
9. Shih JJ, Ochoa JG. A systematic review of antiepileptic drug initiation and withdrawal. *Neurologist*. 2009;15:122–31.

See Also (Topic, Algorithm, Electronic Media Element)
Seizures, Febrile; Status Epilepticus

 CODES

ICD9
- 345.90 Epilepsy, unspecified, without mention of intractable epilepsy
- 779.0 Convulsions in newborn
- 780.39 Other convulsions

CLINICAL PEARLS
- Encourage helmet usage to minimize head injuries.
- In order for the patient to be allowed to drive, he or she must be seizure-free from a minimum of 3 months up to a year depending on state requirements.
- Drug initiation after a single seizure will decrease risk of early seizure recurrence (8)[A] but does not affect long-term prognosis of developing epilepsy (9)[A].

S

SEIZURES, FEBRILE

David Fish, MD

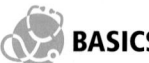 **BASICS**

DESCRIPTION

A seizure occurring between the ages of 6 months and 6 years of age associated with a febrile illness that does not involve CNS infection or inflammation in a child that has no prior history of afebrile seizures; febrile seizures are classified as either simple or complex.

- Simple (70–75%):
  – Duration <15 minutes
  – Generalized seizure with no focal features
  – No recurrence in 24 hours
- Complex (9–35%):
  – Duration >15 minutes
  – Focal features
  – >1 seizure in 24 hours

EPIDEMIOLOGY

Febrile seizures (FS) are the most common seizures in children under age 5. They typically occur between the ages of 6 months and 36 months (peak at 18 months) (1)[B].

Incidence

- ~500,000 febrile seizures occur yearly in the US (1)[B].
- Incidence is between 2% and 5%.

Prevalence

3–4% of all children in North America will experience a febrile seizure before age 5 years (most of which are simple) (1)[B].

RISK FACTORS

- For 1st febrile seizure (1)[B]:
  – Family history of febrile or afebrile seizures
  – Neurodevelopmental abnormality
  – Recent immunizations (increased risk following DTP and MMR)
  – Most children will have no identifiable risk factors.
  – Possible increased risk with certain viral illnesses, including human herpesvirus type 6 (HHV-6) infection
- For recurrent FS (1)[B]:
  – Onset at age <12 months
  – Family history of FS in 1st-degree relative
  – Temperature <40°C (104°F) with prior FS
  – Complex FS at initial presentation
  – Brief duration between fever onset and seizure
- For subsequent epilepsy after FS (1–2.4%, slightly increased risk over that of general population) (2)[B]:
  – Family history of epilepsy
  – Complex FS
  – Neurodevelopmental abnormality

Genetics

- Genetic factors play role, with susceptibility being linked to several genetic loci.
- A history of FS in immediate family members is present in 10–40% of patients.
- Monozygotic twins have a much higher concordance rate than dizygotic twins.
- Sodium channels and γ-aminobutyric acid A (GABA$_A$) receptor genes have been associated with a syndrome of generalized epilepsy and FS (GEFS+) (3).

GENERAL PREVENTION

- Evidence exists that anticonvulsant therapy can reduce the risk of recurrence of FS, but it is not recommended because the harm significantly outweighs the benefits.
- Antipyretics help to improve comfort of the child, but neither regular dosing intervals (e.g., acetaminophen every 4 hours) nor sporadic dosing based on temperature has been shown to prevent recurrence (2)[B].

PATHOPHYSIOLOGY

The underlying pathophysiology is unknown.

ETIOLOGY

- Any viral or bacterial infections can provoke FS.
- Increased risk found with HHV-6 infection (also found to have increased risk of complex FS and recurrence).
- MMR vaccine has been associated with an up to 3-fold increased risk of FS, with peak incidence 1–2 weeks after vaccination, but benefit of vaccination outweighs risk.
- DTP vaccine also has been associated with a 4-fold increase risk of FS, with peak incidence 1–3 days after vaccination, but vaccine benefit outweighs risk (1)[B].

DIAGNOSIS

HISTORY

- Description of convulsions, including any focal movements (seizures are typically clonic)
- Duration of seizure
- Interventions performed to control seizures (most will resolve spontaneously)
- History of recent illness or fever (though seizure often can be 1st presenting symptom)
- Signs of CNS infection or inflammation (e.g., lethargy, irritability, decreased feeding, emesis)
- Recent immunization
- Patient and family history of seizures
- Recent treatment with antibiotics (meningitis can be masked if partially treated)
- Evaluate for other causes of seizures, such as trauma or toxin exposure.

PHYSICAL EXAM

- Vital signs:
  – Fever
  – Monitor for respiratory or circulatory compromise (if persistent seizure activity).
- Full neurological exam:
  – Usually normal
  – May have transient decreased alertness in postictal state; monitor for improvement.
- Focused exam based on history to determine source of fever

DIAGNOSTIC TESTS & INTERPRETATION
Lab

- AAP recommendations for 1st simple FS: Lumbar puncture (LP) should be strongly considered in children <12 months of age; considered in children between 12 and 18 months of age; and recommended in children >18 months of age in the presence of clinical suspicion for meningitis (4)[A]. Recent evidence shows that the risk of bacterial meningitis is very low with 1st simple FS, and AAP recommendations should be reconsidered (5)[A].
- CSF more likely to show abnormalities when (4)[A]:
  – Abnormal physical exam
  – Complex FS
  – Persistent seizures on arrival to emergency department
  – Prolonged postictal state
- In practice, the decision to perform LP should be tailored to each individual child's presentation.

Pediatric Considerations

In infants <18 months of age, clinical signs and symptoms of meningitis may be minimal or absent.

Initial lab tests

- Measurement of serum electrolytes, calcium, phosphorous, magnesium; complete blood count (CBC); and serum glucose determination are low-yield and should not be performed routinely unless clinically indicated.
- Obtain serum glucose if there is a prolonged postictal state or recurrent seizures (4)[A].
- Laboratory testing should be obtained based on history to detect source of fever (4)[A].

Imaging
Initial approach

- Routine neuroimaging is not indicated in the evaluation of simple FS (4)[A].
- Neuroimaging should be performed if the physical exam points to a possible structural lesion (e.g., micro/macrocephaly, focal neurologic signs, symptoms of increased intracranial pressure).

Diagnostic Procedures/Surgery

- EEG is not recommended as part of evaluation of a neurologically healthy child with a 1st simple FS (4)[A]. EEG does not predict the recurrence of FS or the development of epilepsy.
- EEG is recommended in children with complex FS who have developmental delay or abnormal neurologic signs and symptoms.

DIFFERENTIAL DIAGNOSIS

- Rigors
- Syncope
- Febrile delirium (acute and transient confusional state associated with high fever)
- Breath-holding spell
- Meningitis

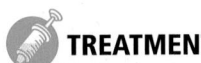 # TREATMENT

MEDICATION
First Line
- Acute treatment:
  - Anticonvulsants: Febrile seizures lasting >5 minutes should be treated with anticonvulsants (2)[B].
    - Lorazepam: 0.05–0.1 mg/kg IV
    - Diazepam: 0.3 mg/kg IV
  - Rectal gel (Diastat): 0.5 mg/kg; fosphenytoin: Use for persistent seizures, rare.
  - IV: 15–20 mg/kg
  - Antipyretics: Use acutely to reduce fever.
    - Acetaminophen: 15 mg/kg p.o. PR
    - Ibuprofen: 10 mg/kg p.o.
- Long-term treatment (2)[B]:
  - Anticonvulsants may be effective in reducing FS, but the potential side effects outweigh the benefits; therefore, anticonvulsant therapy is not recommended routinely for children with FS.
  - Antipyretics may be given for comfort but have not been shown to reduce the risk of FS.

Second Line
Cooling blankets to reduce fever as needed

ADDITIONAL TREATMENT
General Measures
- Treat source of fever based on results of focused evaluation.
- Supportive care as needed

Issues for Referral
Refer to pediatric neurologist if suspicious for underlying seizure disorder or complex FS.

IN-PATIENT CONSIDERATIONS
Initial Stabilization
- Assessment of airway, breathing, and circulatory status (ABCs)
- Febrile seizures of >5 minutes duration should be treated as outlined under "Acute Treatment."

Admission Criteria
Admission should be strongly considered if
- Age <1 year
- Glasgow coma scale <15 (1 hour following seizure)
- Shows signs of increased intracranial pressure
- Demonstrates clinical suspicion for meningitis
- Has experienced a complex partial seizure
- Demonstrates any instability in vital signs

IV Fluids
If child appears dehydrated, administer IV fluid as appropriate.

Nursing
- Nursing should be carried out according to the patient's underlying illness or infection.
- Precautionary measures to prevent secondary injuries from seizure activity

Discharge Criteria
Children with simple FS, no focal signs of infection, and appearing well can be discharged home after a minimum of 2 hours of observation.

 # ONGOING CARE

FOLLOW-UP RECOMMENDATIONS
For any patient with simple FS, a follow-up appointment with the primary-care physician should be scheduled within 1 week of discharge. Follow-up for complex FS should be made pending results of further evaluation.

Patient Monitoring
Monitor as appropriate depending on clinical presentation of patient (including classification of FS).

DIET
No dietary restrictions necessary

PATIENT EDUCATION
Parental education is important owing to the significant anxiety surrounding the diagnosis (1)[B].
- FS are common and occur in 3–5% of otherwise healthy children.
- FS can recur in approximately 1/3 of children with subsequent fevers.
- No evidence suggests that FS cause neurologic sequelae or death.
- Evaluation depends on the clinical presentation, and there is no role for routine lab testing or imaging.
- Treatment of FS is not generally recommended and has not been shown to prevent the development of epilepsy.
- Referral to a pediatric neurologist is not typically required for a simple FS.

PROGNOSIS
- Overall excellent prognosis
- No evidence of neurodevelopmental problems, learning disabilities, or increased mortality with simple FS
- Children with FS are at risk for developing recurrent FS.
  - Children >12 months of age have a 30% rate of recurrence. Those who have 2nd FS have a 50% risk of having additional episodes.
  - Children <12 months of age have increased recurrence rate of 50%.
- Risk of epilepsy after a simple FS is slightly greater than that of general population, which is approximately 1%.
  - Risk of epilepsy after multiple simple FS with 1st seizure at <1 year of age is 2.4%.
  - Factors that increase risk of epilepsy include neurodevelopmental abnormality, complex FS, and family history of epilepsy (2)[B].

COMPLICATIONS

- Secondary complications include injuries resulting from seizure activity, aspiration, and complications from prolonged seizures with complex FS (1)[B].
- There is controversial evidence that FS may contribute to temporal lobe epilepsy.

REFERENCES

1. Jones T, Jacobsen SJ. Childhood febrile seizures: overview and implications. *Int J Med Sci.* 2007;4:110–4.
2. Steering Committee on Quality Improvement and Management, Subcommittee on Febrile Seizures American Academy of Pediatrics. Febrile seizures: clinical practice guideline for the long-term management of the child with simple febrile seizures. *Pediatrics.* 2008;121:1281–6.
3. Scheffer IE, Harkin LA, Dibbens LM, et al. Neonatal epilepsy syndromes and generalized epilepsy with febrile seizures plus (GEFS+). *Epilepsia.* 2005; 46(Suppl 10):41–7.
4. Practice parameter: the neurodiagnostic evaluation of the child with a first simple febrile seizure. American Academy of Pediatrics. Provisional Committee on Quality Improvement, Subcommittee on Febrile Seizures. *Pediatrics.* 1996;97:769–72; discussion 773–5.
5. Kimia AA, Capraro AJ, Hummel D, et al. Utility of lumbar puncture for first simple febrile seizure among children 6 to 18 months of age. *Pediatrics.* 2009;123:6–12.

 # CODES

ICD9
780.31 Febrile convulsions (simple), unspecified

CLINICAL PEARLS

- FS is common and accounts for 1% of all pediatric emergency department visits.
- Keystone of evaluation and treatment of FS involves identifying and treating underlying illness.
- Thorough neurodiagnostic workup (including EEG, imaging, and LP) typically is not necessary.
- FS are associated with only slightly increased risk of epilepsy compared with general population.
- There is no need for preventive or long-term treatment of FS.

SEPSIS

Sean P. O'Reilly, MD

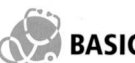 **BASICS**

DESCRIPTION

A life-threatening illness defined as a suspected or known infection plus the systemic inflammatory response syndrome (SIRS):

- SIRS is an inflammatory reaction to various clinical insults (e.g., severe trauma or burn) manifested by 2 or more of the following:
  – Temperature >38°C or <36°C
  – Heart rate >90/min
  – Respiratory rate >20/min or $PaCO_2$ <32 mm Hg
  – White blood cell (WBC) count >12,000/mm³, <4,000/mm³, or >10% immature forms (bands)
- Severe sepsis: Sepsis with organ hypoperfusion and/or dysfunction:
  – Urine output below 0.5 mL/kg/hour for at least 1 hour
  – Mottled skin/decreased capillary refill
  – Mental status changes
  – Cardiac dysfunction
  – Acute lung injury/acute respiratory distress syndrome
  – Thrombocytopenia or signs of DIC
  – Elevated serum lactate (above 2 mmol/L)
- Septic shock: Sepsis-induced hypotension (MAP below 65, systolic blood pressure (BP) <90 mm Hg, or ≥40 mm Hg drop from baseline) despite adequate fluid resuscitation, defined as 20–30 mL/kg of infused colloid solutions or 40–60 mL/kg of crystalloid solutions or pulmonary artery occlusion pressure (PCWP) above 12
- MODS: Multiple organ dysfunction syndrome, when associated with sepsis, represents the end stage of disease.
- Synonym(s): Septicemia; Sepsis neonatorum

Geriatric Considerations
Often more difficult to diagnose; change in mental status/behavior may be only early manifestation

Pediatric Considerations
Evaluate newborns for infection due to PROM (prolonged rupture of membranes), maternal fever, and prematurity with clinical observation, a complete blood count (CBC) with differential, and 1 or 2 sets of blood cultures.

Pregnancy Considerations
β-lactam antibiotics, aminoglycosides, and azithromycin/erythromycin are considered safe.

EPIDEMIOLOGY
Incidence
- 3/1,000 population
- Increasing incidence, with nearly 660,000 new cases annually in US
- 2% of hospitalized patients; nearly 75% of ICU patients

RISK FACTORS
- Bacteremia
- Age extremes (very old or young)
- Impaired host (see Associated Conditions)
- Community-acquired pneumonia
- Critically ill patients
- Indwelling catheters: Intravascular, urinary, biliary
- Complicated labor and delivery: Premature and/or PROM, untreated maternal group B strep colonization

Genetics
- Studies link polymorphisms in genes encoding tumor necrosis factor (TNF) to possibly greater susceptibility to and death from sepsis.
- Other candidate genes include the IL-1 receptor antagonist, heat-shock proteins, IL-6, IL-10, and toll-like receptors (TLR).

GENERAL PREVENTION
- Vaccination: Pneumococcal (geriatric patients, patients with certain chronic diseases), *Haemophilus influenzae* type B (infants, young children), influenza (H1N1 in pregnant women)
- γ-globulin (for hypo- or agammaglobulinemia)
- Treat pregnant group B strep carriers during labor.
- Handwashing/sterile technique for catheters

PATHOPHYSIOLOGY
- An imbalance between pro- and anti-inflammatory mediators yields widespread systemic inflammation that damages distant uninvolved tissues.
- Widespread endothelial damage leads to maldistribution of blood flow, causing impaired tissue oxygenation and resultant organ dysfunction.
- Dysregulated nitric oxide production and activation of the coagulation system cause maldistribution of organ blood flow.
- Initial, overexuberant inflammatory response can progress to significant immunosuppression.

ETIOLOGY
- Specific etiologic agents:
  – Gram-positive organisms: *Staphylococcus* sp., *Streptococcus* sp., *Enterococcus* sp.
  – Gram-negative organisms: *Escherichia coli*, *Klebsiella* sp., *Proteus* sp., *Pseudomonas* sp.
  – Anaerobes
  – Fungi: *Candida* sp. (incidence increased 207% from 1976 to 2000)
- Common sources: Lungs, urinary tract, abdomen (biliary tree, abscess, peritonitis), skin (cellulitis, decubitus ulcer, gangrene), heart valves, and intravascular catheters

COMMONLY ASSOCIATED CONDITIONS
- Immunologic: Neutropenia, HIV, hypo-/agammaglobulinemia, complement deficiency, splenectomy, immunomodulatory medication (corticosteroids, chemotherapy, TNF-alpha antagonists)
- Diabetes mellitus, alcoholism, malignancy, cirrhosis, burns, multiple trauma, IV drug abuse, malnutrition

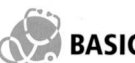 **DIAGNOSIS**

HISTORY
- General symptoms:
  – Fever, chills, rigors, myalgias
  – Mental status changes: Restlessness, agitation, confusion, delirium, lethargy, stupor, coma
- Specific symptoms (site of the primary infection):
  – Respiratory tract: Cough, sputum production, dyspnea, chest pain
  – Urinary tract: Dysuria, frequency, urgency, flank pain
  – Intra-abdominal source: Nausea, vomiting, diarrhea, constipation, abdominal pain
  – Central nervous system (CNS): Stiff neck, headache, photophobia, focal neurologic signs
- End-organ failure symptoms: Shortness of breath, oliguria/anuria, mottled appearance of the skin

PHYSICAL EXAM
Hyper-/hypothermia, tachycardia, tachypnea, hypotension, cyanosis, jaundice, skin lesions (erythema, petechiae, embolic lesions, purpura)

DIAGNOSTIC TESTS & INTERPRETATION
Lab
Initial lab tests
- Positive blood cultures: Bacteremia (not required for diagnosis; 50% of blood cultures are negative in severe sepsis/septic shock)
- Positive cultures/Gram stains from other specimens (sputum, urine, cerebrospinal fluid [CSF], wound)
- Prior antibiotic use may obscure later lab results, particularly blood cultures.
- CBC with differential, C-reactive protein, coagulation profile (prothrombin time/international normalized ratio/partial thromboplastin time [PT/INR/PTT]), electrolytes, blood urea nitrogen (BUN), creatinine, glucose, liver function tests (LFTs), lactic acid level, arterial blood gas (ABG), urinalysis
- Common findings: Leukocytosis, bandemia (above 10%), hyperglycemia, metabolic acidosis, mild hyperbilirubinemia, hypoxemia, respiratory alkalosis, proteinuria
- Less common findings (more severe cases): Leukopenia, anemia, thrombocytopenia, prolonged prothrombin time, azotemia, hypoglycemia, lactic acidosis

Imaging
Initial approach
Relevant radiographs, ultrasound, computed tomography (CT), and magnetic resonance imaging (MRI) should be performed promptly to confirm and sample any source of infection (1)[C].

Diagnostic Procedures/Surgery
- Aspiration of potentially infected body fluids (pleural, peritoneal, CSF)
- Biopsy, drainage of potentially infected tissues (abscess, biliary tree, others)
- Electrocardiogram (EKG) and cardiac enzymes to rule out myocardial infarction

Pathological Findings
- Inflammation at primary site of infection
- Disseminated intravascular coagulation
- Noncardiogenic pulmonary edema

DIFFERENTIAL DIAGNOSIS
- Bacteremia without sepsis
- Viral diseases (influenza, dengue and other hemorrhagic viruses, West Nile)
- Rickettsial diseases (Rocky Mountain spotted fever, endemic typhus)
- Spirochetal diseases (leptospirosis, relapsing fever [*Borrelia* sp.], Jarisch-Herxheimer in syphilis)
- Protozoal diseases (*Toxoplasma gondii*, *Trypanosoma cruzi*, *Pneumocystis carinii*, *Plasmodium falciparum*)
- Collagen vascular diseases, vasculitides, myocardial infarction (MI), congestive heart failure (CHF), pulmonary embolism (PE), TTP-HUS, thyrotoxicosis, adrenal insufficiency (Addison disease)

TREATMENT

MEDICATION

First Line

- Fluid resuscitation with crystalloid or colloid:
  - Initial therapy with fluid bolus (at least 20 mL/kg or 2 liters of crystalloid or 300–500 mL of colloid over 30 minutes) (1)
  - Use central venous pressure (CVP) of 8–12 mm Hg (12–15 mm Hg if on mechanical ventilation) as initial target of resuscitation (1,2)[C].
  - Use caution in the presence of CHF.
- Vasopressors:
  - Norepinephrine or dopamine (1)[B] (dopamine has a greater incidence of adverse events; start with norepinephrine) (3)[B]
  - Low-dose dopamine for renal protection is not recommended (1)[A].
- Broad-spectrum antibiotic therapy as early as possible (<3 hours of ED or <1 hour of ICU admission) aimed at likely source (1)[A]:
  - Adult (*Pseudomonas* not suspected): Vancomycin plus gram-negative coverage (3rd-generation cephalosporin [ceftriaxone/cefotaxime], β-lactamase/β-lactamase inhibitor [piperacillin/tazobactam, ampicillin/sulbactam], or carbapenem [imipenem, meropenem])
  - Adult (*Pseudomonas* suspected; (neutropenic/burn, e.g.): Vancomycin plus 2 agents aimed at resistant gram-negative bacteria (ceftazidime/cefepime; piperacillin-tazobactam plus either fluoroquinolone [ciprofloxacin] or aminoglycoside [gentamicin/amikacin], will depend on local hospital sensitivities, consult hospital antibiogram if available)
  - Nonimmunocompromised child: Cefotaxime
  - Neonatal (<7 days old) sepsis: Ampicillin and gentamicin
  - After culture and sensitivity results: Treatment should be organism-specific for 7–10 days.
  - Antifungals may be required if fungal infection suspected (long-term antibiotic use, use of total parenteral nutrition [TPN], gastrointestinal [GI] surgery, or pathology)
  - Contraindications: History of anaphylaxis or other allergic reaction to an antibiotic

ALERT

- Adjust medication doses for impaired renal and/or hepatic function.
- Consider narrowing antibiotic regimen at 48–72 hours based on culture results and clinical course.
- Possible interactions:
  - Aminoglycosides: Increased nephrotoxicity with enflurane, cisplatin, and possibly vancomycin; increased ototoxicity with loop diuretics; increased paralysis with neuromuscular-blocking agents

Second Line

- Vasopressors, epinephrine, vasopressin, or phenylephrine, should be considered if unable to maintain goal mean arterial pressure (MAP) of above 65 mm Hg on norepinephrine/dopamine (1)[C].
- Low-dose IV hydrocortisone should only be considered if poorly responsive to both IV fluid resuscitation and vasopressors.

- Consider recombinant human-activated protein C (Xigris) in adult patients with severe sepsis and high risk of death (Apache II score >25), although it increases the risk of bleeding and has important contraindications (i.e., pediatric sepsis) (4)[B].
- Inotropic therapy with dobutamine may benefit patients with myocardial dysfunction and evidence of oxygen deficit (low mixed venous oxygen saturation (below 70%) (1)[C].
- Polyclonal IVIG appears promising as adjuvant therapy in bacterial sepsis or septic shock, especially in cases of streptoccocal toxic shock syndrome (5)[B].

ADDITIONAL TREATMENT

General Measures

- O_2 monitoring/supplementation with intubation and invasive monitoring, if necessary, for respiratory failure or hemodynamic instability (1)
- Early goal-directed therapy with adequate volume resuscitation followed by vasopressors if required (within first 6 hours) targeted at (1,2)[C]:
  - CVP 8–12 mm Hg
  - MAP ≥65 mm Hg
  - Urine output ≥0.5 mL/kg/hr
  - Central/mixed venous O_2 saturation ≥70%:
    - If not achieved after fluid resuscitation (CVP 8–12 mm Hg) and vasopressors (MAP >65 mm Hg), transfuse pRBC to achieve Hct >30% and if still <70%, add dobutamine (1)[C]
- Early identification of etiology with appropriate removal/drainage of septic foci (1)[C]:
  - Early surgical consultation if operative intervention required (i.e., acute abdomen, empyema, necrotizing fasciitis)
- Transfusion of red blood cells (RBCs,) platelets, and/or fresh frozen plasma for bleeding complications of coagulopathy or for planned procedures (e.g., central line placement, thoracentesis)
- Stress ulcer and deep vein thrombosis (DVT) prophylactic measures (1)[A].
- Glucose control (below 180 mg/dL) (1,6)[B],(7)

Additional Therapies

- Possible mechanical ventilation and sedation
- Intermittent hemodialysis or continuous venovenous hemofiltration (CVVH)

SURGERY/OTHER PROCEDURES

Debridement of necrotic tissues

IN-PATIENT CONSIDERATIONS

Initial Stabilization

ICU-level care for patients with severe sepsis, shock, or respiratory failure

IV Fluids

- Colloid and crystalloid fluids are equally effective initially.
- Aggressive fluid resuscitation with normal saline can result in nongap metabolic acidosis; alleviated by lactated Ringer's

 ONGOING CARE

FOLLOW-UP RECOMMENDATIONS

Patient Monitoring

- In unstable patients: Invasive hemodynamic monitoring, ABG, venous blood gas, central venous catheter placement, CVP monitoring

- Electrolytes, BUN, creatinine, and CBC daily; lactate, mixed venous oxygen saturation every 2–4 hours in initial resuscitation, and daily INR/PTT if DIC a consideration
- Antibiotic drug levels

DIET

n.p.o. if intubation being considered; otherwise, enteral feeds preferred to help preserve mucosal integrity of the GI tract. Use IV alimentation only if enteral feeding is contraindicated.

PATIENT EDUCATION

Medline Plus at: http://www.nlm.nih.gov/medlineplus/sepsis.html

PROGNOSIS

Even with optimal care, mortality is 10–50% overall.

COMPLICATIONS

GI hemorrhage, disseminated intravascular coagulation (DIC), ARDS, multiorgan failure, death

REFERENCES

1. Dellinger RP, Levy MM, Carlet JM, et al. Surviving Sepsis Campaign: international guidelines for management of severe sepsis and septic shock: 2008. *Crit Care Med*. 2008;36:296–327.
2. Rivers E, Nguyen B, Havstad S, et al. Early goal-directed therapy in the treatment of severe sepsis and septic shock. *N Engl J Med*. 2001;345:1368–77.
3. De Backer D, Biston P, Devriendt J, et al. Comparison of dopamine and norepinephrine in the treatment of shock. *N Engl J Med*. 2010;362:779–89.
4. Marti-Carvajal A, et al. Human recombinant activated protein C for severe sepsis. Cochrane Anaesthesia Group. *Cochrane Database Sys Rev*. 2007;3:CD004388.
5. Alejandria MM, et al. Intravenous immunoglobulin for treating sepsis and septic shock. Cochrane Anaesthesia Group. *Cochrane Database Sys Rev*. 2002;1:1090.
6. Wiener RS, Wiener DC, Larson RJ. Benefits and risks of tight glucose control in critically ill adults: a meta-analysis. *JAMA*. 2008;300:933–44.
7. NICE-SUGAR Study Investigators, Finfer S, Chittock DR, et al. Intensive versus conventional glucose control in critically ill patients. *N Engl J Med*. 2009;360:1283–97.

CODES

ICD9

- 038.9 Unspecified septicemia
- 995.91 Sepsis

CLINICAL PEARLS

- Sepsis is a documented or suspected infection with SIRS (systemic inflammatory response syndrome).
- Appropriate treatment consists of rapid and appropriate antimicrobial therapy along with early goal-directed therapy aimed at maintaining adequate tissue perfusion.
- Despite aggressive treatment, overall mortality rates are still very high (10–50%) in patients with severe sepsis/septic shock.

SEROTONIN SYNDROME

Nancy Byatt, DO, MBA
Aaron Moore, DO

 BASICS

DESCRIPTION
- Serotonin syndrome is a potentially life-threatening adverse drug reaction that results from excessive stimulation in central and peripheral nervous system serotonergic receptors.
- May be caused by therapeutic drug use, intentional self-poisoning, or as a result of a drug interaction
- Encompasses a spectrum of clinical findings ranging from mild cases to life-threatening toxicity but is classically characterized by a triad of mental status change, neuromuscular abnormalities, and autonomic hyperactivity
- Onset is usually within 24 h, with most cases occurring within 6 h, of exposure to or change in dosing of a serotonergic agent.
- Treatment varies with the severity of the illness and focuses on discontinuation of causative agents, supportive care, sedation, and in certain cases, administration of serotonin antagonists.

Geriatric Considerations
The elderly can be at increased risk, given the use of multiple medications.

Pediatric Considerations
- Serotonin syndrome has similar manifestations in children and adults.
- General management is unchanged in children other than medication dosing.

Pregnancy Considerations
- 3rd-trimester exposure to serotonin reuptake inhibitors has been associated with transient neonatal complications that may reflect either acute drug withdrawal or serotonergic toxicity.
- Symptoms generally are mild, self-limited, and require only supportive care.
- Symptoms in neonates may include tremors, increased muscle tone, jitteriness, shivering, feeding or digestive disturbances, irritability, agitation, sleep disturbances, increased reflexes, excessive crying, and respiratory disturbances.

EPIDEMIOLOGY
- Likely underreported, as a continuum of the syndrome contributes to difficulty in its recognition. Serotonin syndrome most often occurs in individuals being treated with psychotropics for a psychiatric disorder and occurs in about 14–16% of selective serotonin reuptake inhibitor (SSRI) overdose patients.
- Serotonin syndrome usually involves a combination of an SSRI, an MAOI, an antiparkinsonian agent, and/or lithium. Initially, patients can develop a peripheral tremor, confusion, and ataxia; systemic signs are next (e.g., agitation, diaphoresis, hyperreflexia, and shivering). If it worsens, the severe signs of fever, jerking, and diarrhea may develop. Serotonin syndrome can last from hours to days after the offending agents are stopped and support initiated.

Incidence
- During 2004, the Toxic Exposure Surveillance System reported 48,204 exposures to selective serotonin reuptake inhibitors (SSRIs) that caused significant toxic effects in 8,187 patients and lead to death in 103 patients; most of the fatalities were associated with coingestants.
- The incidence of serotonin syndrome is rising because serotonergic agents are being used increasingly in clinical practice.
- Predominant age: Affects all age groups
- Predominant sex: Male = Female

RISK FACTORS
- Serotonergic agents
- Combination of serotonin reuptake inhibitors and monoamine oxidase inhibitors (MAOIs)

Genetics
Unknown

GENERAL PREVENTION
- Avoid multidrug regimens.
- Consider drug–drug interactions when a multidrug regimen is required.
- Caution patients about taking SSRIs with over-the-counter (OTC) medications or herbal supplements prior to consulting a physician.
- Clinician education
- Continual improvement in use of health information technology

PATHOPHYSIOLOGY
Serotonin syndrome is a result of excessive stimulation in central and peripheral nervous system serotonergic receptors. Possible mechanisms include:
- Increased serotonin synthesis
- Increased serotonin release
- Inhibition of serotonin metabolism
- Inhibition of serotonin reuptake
- Direct agonism of serotonin receptors
- Increased sensitivity of postsynaptic receptors

ETIOLOGY
- A number of drugs are associated with the serotonin syndrome. These include SSRIs (Prozac, Celexa, Paxil, Lexapro); SNRIs (e.g., Cymbalta, Effexor); tricyclic antidepressants, MAOIs, other antidepressants (Trazodone, Wellbutrin); lithium; triptans; anticonvulsants (Depakote); opiate analgesics (including buprenorphine, tramadol, oxycodone); antibiotics; OTC cough medications (dextromethorphan); some antipsychotics (Risperdal, Zyprexa) other meds such as BuSpar, Zofran, Reglan, l-dopa; dietary supplements (tryptophan) herbal supplements (St. John's wort, nutmeg); and drugs of abuse (e.g., MDMA, cocaine, LSD, and amphetamine).
- Drug interactions are often the cause of severe cases of serotonin syndrome. Many of the same classes of medications listed above are involved (e.g., phenelzine and meperidine, tranylcypromine and imipramine, linezolid and citalopram).

 DIAGNOSIS

- Serotonin syndrome is a clinical diagnosis.
- SSRIs can contribute to development of serotonin syndrome weeks after discontinuation (1).
- Hunter Toxicity Criteria Decision Rules aid in the diagnosis of clinically significant serotonin toxicity (sensitivity 84%, specificity 97%).
- To fulfill Hunter Criteria, a patient must have taken a serotonergic agent and have 1 of the following:
  – Spontaneous clonus
  – Inducible clonus plus agitation or diaphoresis
  – Ocular clonus plus agitation or diaphoresis
  – Tremor and hyperreflexia
  – Hypertonia
  – Temperature above 38°C plus ocular clonus or inducible clonus (2)[B]

HISTORY
- Obtain a thorough drug history, including prescription medications, OTC remedies, dietary supplements, herbal supplements, and illicit drugs. Ask about dose, formulation, and recent changes.
- Address possibility of drug overdose, and obtain collateral information in cases in which intentional overdose is suspected.
- Elicit description of symptoms, including onset and progression of symptoms.

PHYSICAL EXAM
- Vital signs: Tachycardia, hypertension (HTN), hyperthermia, pulse and blood pressure alterations (severe cases)
- Neuromuscular findings:
  – Hyperreflexia (greater in lower extremities)
  – Clonus (involuntary muscle contractions, most commonly tested by flexing foot upwards rapidly; includes ocular)
  – Myoclonus (greater in lower extremities)
  – Tremor (greater in lower extremities)
  – Hypertonia
  – Bilateral Babinski sign
  – Akathisia
- Autonomic signs:
  – Diaphoresis
  – Mydriasis
  – Flushing
  – Dry mucous membranes
  – Vomiting
  – Diarrhea
  – Increased bowel sounds
- Mental status changes:
  – Anxiety
  – Disorientation
  – Delirium (1)

DIAGNOSTIC TESTS & INTERPRETATION
Lab
- Serum serotonin levels do not correlate with clinical findings.
- Nonspecific lab findings that may develop include:
  – Elevated white blood cell (WBC) count
  – Elevated creatine phosphokinase (CK or CPK)
  – Decreased serum bicarbonate
  – Elevated hepatic transaminases

- In severe cases, the following complications may develop:
  - Disseminated intravascular coagulation (DIC)
  - Metabolic acidosis
  - Rhabdomyolysis
  - Renal failure
  - Myoglobinuria
  - Acute respiratory distress syndrome (ARDS) (1)

Imaging
None indicated

DIFFERENTIAL DIAGNOSIS
- Anticholinergic delirium (e.g. Cogentin, Benadryl, Detrol, oxybutynin, nifedipine, Zantac; plant poisoning from belladonna/"deadly nightshade," datura, henbane, mandrake, brugmansia)
- Malignant hyperthermia
- Heat stroke
- Neuroleptic malignant syndrome
- CNS infection (meningitis, encephalitis)
- Sympathomimetic toxicity
- Nonconvulsive seizures
- Hyperthyroidism
- Tetanus
- Acute baclofen withdrawal (3)

TREATMENT

- Management principles include:
  - Discontinuation of all serotonergic agents
  - Supportive care is the mainstay of therapy. This includes administration of oxygen and IV fluids, continuous cardiac monitoring, and correction of vital signs.
  - Sedation:
    - Evidence suggests that benzodiazepines may be effective for the management of agitation in patients with serotonin syndrome.
    - Benzodiazepines should be used with caution in patients with delirium due to the risk of worsening delirium.
  - Administration of serotonin antagonists: Cyproheptadine may be useful if supportive measures and sedation are unable to control agitation and correct vital signs.
- Management varies with the severity of the illness:
  - Mild cases (afebrile, tachycardia, shivering, diaphoresis, mydriasis, hyperreflexia, intermittent tremor or myoclonus):
    - Discontinuation of precipitating agent(s)
    - Supportive care
    - Sedation
  - Moderate cases (temperature >38°C, autonomic instability, mydriasis, hyperactive bowel sounds, diarrhea, diaphoresis, ocular clonus, hyperreflexia, tremor, mild agitation, or hypervigilance):
    - Discontinuation of precipitating agent(s)
    - Supportive care
    - Sedation
    - Aggressive treatment of autonomic instability
    - Treatment with cyproheptadine, a histamine and serotonin antagonist, should be initiated if agitation and vital sign abnormalities are unimproved with benzodiazepines and supportive care.
    - Hypotension from MAOI interactions should be treated with low doses of direct-acting sympathomimetics (e.g., norepinephrine, phenylephrine, epinephrine).
    - Avoid use of indirect serotonin agonists such as dopamine.

  - Severe HTN and tachycardia should be treated with short-acting agents such as nitroprusside or esmolol.
    - Avoid use of longer-acting agents such as propranolol.
  - Severe cases (temperature >41.1°C, autonomic instability, delirium, muscular rigidity, and hypertonicity):
    - Immediate sedation
    - Paralysis (with nondepolarizing agents such as etomidate, succinylcholine, and vecuronium; avoid succinylcholine in patients with hyperkalemia)
    - Endotracheal intubation as clinically indicated
    - Treatment of hyperthermia is critical.
    - Antipyretic medications are not effective (1)[C].

MEDICATION
- Activated charcoal: May be used in patients who intentionally overdose on serotonergic agents (2)[C]
- Benzodiazepines: May be used to manage agitation in serotonin syndrome and also may correct mild increases in blood pressure and heart rate. Use with caution in patients with delirium given the known paradoxical effect of exacerbating delirium.
- Cyproheptadine (Periactin): Consider use if benzodiazepines and supportive measures are unable to control agitation and correct vital signs:
  - Adults: Initial dose of 12 mg p.o. (or crushed and given NG) followed by 2 mg every 2 h until clinical response observed. 12–32 mg of drug may be required in a 24-h period.
  - Children:
    - <2 years: 0.06 mg/kg per dose q6h
    - 2–6 years: 2 mg q6h
    - 7–14 years: 4 mg q6h
- Propofol (Diprivan) may represent an effective therapy for controlling serotonergic signs in severely ill patients (4)[C].
- Use of antipsychotics with 5-HT$_{2A}$ antagonist activity, such as olanzapine and chlorpromazine, is not recommended (1)[C].

ADDITIONAL TREATMENT
Issues for Referral
For diagnosis and treatment recommendations, the following resources may be consulted:

- Psychiatry: For assistance with medication management and follow-up care (inpatient psychiatric care vs outpatient psychiatric follow-up)
- Toxicology
- Clinical pharmacology service
- Poison control center

IN-PATIENT CONSIDERATIONS
Patients with known or suspected serotonin syndrome should be admitted to a medical inpatient unit for observation.

Discharge Criteria
- Mental status is returned to baseline.
- Stable vital signs
- No increase in clonus or DTR
- Close patient follow-up ensured

ONGOING CARE

FOLLOW-UP RECOMMENDATIONS
After the resolution of symptoms, the need to resume use of causative serotonergic agent(s) should be carefully assessed.

PROGNOSIS
- Generally favorable with early recognition of the syndrome and prompt initiation of treatment
- Most cases resolve within 24 h of discontinuation of serotonergic agents; this can be longer depending on the drug's half-life:
  - MAOIs can result in toxicity for several days.
  - SSRIs can result in toxicity for up to several weeks after discontinuation.
- ICU admission is often indicated in severe cases.

COMPLICATIONS
- Adverse outcomes, including death, are usually the consequence of poorly treated hyperthermia.
- Nonhyperthermic patients who survive typically do not have long-term sequelae.

REFERENCES

1. Boyer EW, Shannon M. The serotonin syndrome. N Engl J Med. 2005;352:1112–20.
2. Dunkley EJ, Isbister GK, Sibbritt D, et al. The Hunter Serotonin Toxicity Criteria: simple and accurate diagnostic decision rules for serotonin toxicity. QJM. 2003;96:635–42.
3. Isbister GK, Buckley NA, Whyte IM. Serotonin toxicity: a practical approach to diagnosis and treatment. Med J Aust. 2007;187:361–5.
4. Ganetsky M, Babu KM, Boyer EW. Serotonin syndrome in dextromethorphan ingestion responsive to propofol therapy. Pediatr Emerg Care. 2007;23:829–31. Stern: Massachusetts General Hospital Comprehensive Clinical Psychiatry, 1st ed.

ADDITIONAL READING

- Moses-Kolko EL, Bogen D, Perel J, et al. Neonatal signs after late in utero exposure to serotonin reuptake inhibitors: literature review and implications for clinical applications. JAMA. 2005;293:2372–83.
- Nelson LS, Erdman AR, Booze LL, et al. Selective serotonin reuptake inhibitor poisoning: An evidence-based consensus guideline for out-of-hospital management. Clin Toxicol (Phila). 2007;45:315–32.

CODES

ICD9
333.99 Other extrapyramidal diseases and abnormal movement disorders

CLINICAL PEARLS

Consider serotonin syndrome in patients with recent use of a serotonergic agent (particularly if multiple proserotonergic agents are involved) presenting with unexplained tachycardia, hypertension, hyperthermia, clonus, hyperreflexia, and change in mental status.

SERUM SICKNESS
Karen A. Hulbert, MD

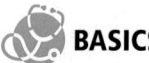 **BASICS**

DESCRIPTION
- Serum sickness (SS): An acute type III hypersensitivity reaction; mediated by tissue deposition of IgG or IgM immune complexes:
  - Classically described 1–3 weeks following administration of nonhuman serum or after exposure to certain medications, with peak around day 10 postexposure
  - Most common current cause is exposure to nonprotein drugs such as penicillins and cephalosporins (1)
- System(s) affected: Hematologic/Lymphatic/Immunologic; Musculoskeletal; Skin/Exocrine; Cardiovascular; Gastrointestinal (GI); Genitourinary
- No sex or age predominance
- Serum sicknesslike reaction (SSLR): A specific drug reaction not associated with immune complexes (see Commonly Associated Conditions)

EPIDEMIOLOGY
Incidence
- Seen more commonly with β-lactam antibiotics; antibodies form against side chains
- Rate of cefaclor serum sicknesslike reaction (SSLR) has been estimated at approximately 0.024–0.2% per course prescribed (2).

RISK FACTORS
- Preceding exposure to drugs or serum
- In children, the risk of SSLR is greater with cefaclor than with other antibiotics (2).

Genetics
It is postulated that in genetically susceptible hosts, a reactive cefaclor metabolite is formed that can bind with tissue proteins (2).

PATHOPHYSIOLOGY
- IgM antibodies develop after exposure to protein antigen in 7–14 days.
- IgG antibodies develop a few days after IgM.

- IgG antibodies form immune complexes with antigen left in circulation:
  - When an excess of antibody or antigen occurs, small complexes are formed, which are cleared rapidly and do not generally cause reactions.
  - When concentrations of antibody and antigen are approximately equal, intermediate-sized immune complexes are formed, which are deposited in tissues and efficiently activate complement.
- Complement activation causes:
  - Release of inflammatory mediators
  - Recruitment of leukocytes
  - Vascular leak

ETIOLOGY
- Antithymocyte globulin
- Antimicrobials:
  - Cephalosporins, especially cefaclor
  - Minocycline
  - TMP/SMX
  - Rifampin
  - Penicillins
  - Streptokinase
- Monoclonal antibodies, especially rituximab
- Selective serotonin reuptake inhibitors
- Bupropion
- Propranolol
- Vaccines
- Equine diphtheria antiserum
- Rabies antiserum
- Rabbit antiserum
- Crotalidae antivenom

COMMONLY ASSOCIATED CONDITIONS
Serum sicknesslike reaction (SSLR):
- Typically occurs 1–3 weeks after initiation of certain drugs, especially antibiotics
- Fever, rash, arthralgias present
- Immune complexes and vasculitis absent
- In SSLR, immune-complex formation and complement fixation do not occur; instead, in genetically susceptible patients, reactive drug metabolites are hypothesized to bind to host proteins, eliciting an inflammatory response.
- Reactions may be dose-related, with higher doses producing more metabolites available to bind to host proteins.

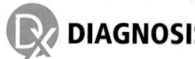 **DIAGNOSIS**

HISTORY
- History of exposure to medication or serum in preceding 1–3 weeks
- Absence of chronic constitutional symptoms
- Patients report:
  - Fever (>38.5°C)
  - Rash and pruritus
  - Arthralgia/myalgia
  - Malaise
  - GI disturbance (nausea, vomiting, abdominal pain)
  - Headache (can be due to temporomandibular joint arthralgia)
  - Arthritis

PHYSICAL EXAM
Characterized by an ill-appearing patient with:
- Fixed (i.e., nonmigratory) morbilliform or urticarial rash
- Serpiginous rash on lateral borders of hands and feet is a classic physical finding.
- Lymphadenopathy, especially in location draining injection site
- Hepatomegaly or splenomegaly
- Proteinuria (without glomerulonephritis)

DIAGNOSTIC TESTS & INTERPRETATION
Lab
Initial lab tests
- Detection of immune complexes in serum is not widely available and of limited clinical value:
  - C3/C4: Helpful if low but can be normal
  - Erythrocyte sedimentation rate/C-reactive protein: Usually elevated
  - Complete blood count with differential: Leukocytosis, thrombocytopenia
  - Liver enzymes: May be elevated
  - Serum electrolytes: Renal insufficiency (rare)
  - Urinalysis: Mild proteinuria, nephritis (rare)

ALERT

If rash is atypical or does not improve after withdrawing suspected drug, consider:
- Antinuclear antibodies
- Antineutrophil cytoplasmic antibodies
- Rheumatoid factor (RF)
- Cryoglobulins
- Skin biopsy with immunofluorescence

Diagnostic Procedures/Surgery
Patch testing may be useful for anticonvulsants and antibiotics, but does not work consistently with all medications (3)[C].

DIFFERENTIAL DIAGNOSIS
- Systemic vasculitis:
  - Periarteritis nodosa
  - Wegener granulomatosis
  - Cryoglobulinemia
  - Juvenile idiopathic arthritis
  - Kawasaki syndrome
  - Henoch-Schönlein purpura
  - Hypersensitivity vasculitis
- Sepsis
- RF
- Viral exanthems
- Anaphylaxis
- Drug hypersensitivity
- Stevens-Johnson syndrome
- Lupus

TREATMENT

MEDICATION
First Line
- Diphenhydramine or hydroxyzine 25–50 mg IV/p.o. q4–6h for urticaria and generalized pruritus (2)[C]
- Long-acting H_1 antihistamines such as cetirizine or loratadine, which are less sedating, can also control urticaria and are recommended to be continued for 1 week after resolution of symptoms and then gradually discontinued.
- Topical corticosteroids for skin manifestations (2)[C]
- Nonsteroidal anti-inflammatory drugs may offer relief of arthralgia/myalgia (2)[C].

Second Line
Prednisone: 0.5–1 mg/kg/d p.o. or methylprednisolone 1–2 mg/kg IV divided q.i.d. or b.i.d. × 5–7 days if inflammation is severe or 1st-line drugs fail (2)[C].

ADDITIONAL TREATMENT
General Measures
- Mainstay of treatment is to remove the offending agent
- Management of SSLR:
  - In case reports, use of prednisone 60 mg daily along with high doses of H_1 and H_2 antihistamines can help resolve arthralgias and myalgias.
- Reticuloendothelial system removes immune complexes, leading to improvement within 48–72 hours.
- Complete resolution of rash may take days to weeks.
- Kinetics of improvement largely depend on half-life of antigen.

Issues for Referral
- Consider allergist for identifying inciting agent.
- Consider rheumatologist if autoimmune disorder suspected.

Additional Therapies
IV immunoglobulin not routinely recommended but may have a role when other therapies are ineffective or contraindicated.

IN-PATIENT CONSIDERATIONS
Initial Stabilization
Basic life support and advanced cardiac life support as needed

Admission Criteria
Most patients with acute SS or SSLR will require admission for observation and exclusion of other diagnoses.

IV Fluids
As indicated for hydration

Nursing
As clinically indicated

Discharge Criteria
- When significant improvement in inflammation occurs after stopping suspected drug
- When ambulatory and tolerating p.o.

ONGOING CARE

FOLLOW-UP RECOMMENDATIONS
- Bed rest during acute illness if arthralgia/myalgia severe
- No indication for skin testing for beta-lactam antibiotics because severe non-IgE-mediated reactions are drug-specific, and reexposure should be avoided (4).

Patient Monitoring
As clinically indicated

DIET
Routine

PATIENT EDUCATION
Educate patient on offending agent, which should be reported as an allergy in the future.

PROGNOSIS
Favorable:
- Self-limiting with improvement in 48–72 hours once offending antigen removed
- If reexposed to antigen, serum sickness can develop more rapidly.

COMPLICATIONS
- Vasculitis
- Neuropathy
- Hepatitis
- Glomerulonephritis
- Anaphylaxis
- Shock
- Death

REFERENCES
1. Schnyder B. Approach to the Patient with Drug Allergy. *Immunol Allergy Clin N Am*. 2009;29: 405–418.
2. Knowles SR, Shear NH. Recognition and management of severe cutaneous drug reactions. *Dermatol Clin*. 2007;25:245–53, viii.
3. Friedmann PS, Ardern-Jones M, et al. Patch testing in drug allergy. *Curr Opin Allergy Clin Immunol*. 2010;10:291–6.
4. Yates AB. Management of patients with a history of allergy to beta-lactam antibiotics. *Am J Med*. 2008;121:572–6.

ADDITIONAL READING
- Friedmann PS, Lee MS, Friedmann AC, et al. Mechanisms in cutaneous drug hypersensitivity reactions. *Clin Exp Allergy*. 2003;33:861–72.
- Jancar S, Sánchez Crespo M. Immune complex-mediated tissue injury: a multistep paradigm. *Trends Immunol*. 2005;26:48–55.
- Khan DA, Solensky R. Drug Allergy. *J Allergy Clin Immunol*. 2010;125:S126–37.
- Pichler WJ. Immune mechanism of drug hypersensitivity. *Immunol Allergy Clin N Am*. 2004;24:373–97.
- Shah KN, et al. Urticaria Multforme: A case series and review of acute annular urticarial hypersensitivity syndromes in children. *Pediatrics*. 2007;119(5):1177–83.

CODES

ICD9
999.5 Other serum reaction, not elsewhere classified

CLINICAL PEARLS
- In general, for each individual patient, specific drugs causing an SSLR should be identified as allergens and avoided in the future.
- There are no data that support the use of premedication in preventing SS or SSLR.
- Serpiginous rash on lateral borders of hands and feet is a classic physical finding.

SEXUAL DYSFUNCTION IN WOMEN

Teresa Knight, MD

BASICS

- Sexual dysfunction may be a lifelong problem or may be acquired.
- Approximately 40% of women surveyed in the US have sexual concerns.
- Female sexual dysfunction may present as a lack of sexual desire, impaired arousal, pain with sexual activity, or inability to achieve orgasm.

DESCRIPTION
The American Psychiatric Association guidelines for establishing a diagnosis of sexual dysfunction require that the problem be recurrent or persistent and that it cause personal distress or interpersonal difficulty.

- 5 major types:
  – Disorders of desire: Hypoactive sexual desire with deficient or absent sexual fantasies and desire for sexual activity
  – Disorder of arousal: Inability to attain or maintain adequate lubrication/engorgement in response to sexual excitement
  – Dyspareunia: Genital pain associated with intercourse
  – Vaginismus: Involuntary contractions of the perineal muscles in response to vaginal penetration
  – Disorders of orgasm: Delay or absence of orgasm following normal sexual excitement
- System(s) affected: Nervous; Reproductive; Genitourinary; Psychiatric
- Synonym(s): Hypoactive sexual desire disorder; Sexual aversion disorder; Female sexual arousal disorder; Inhibited female orgasm

EPIDEMIOLOGY
- In one international study, 40% of women aged 40–80 years reported sexual complaints (1).
- In the largest study of female sexual dysfunction in the US, 43% of over 30,000 women reported sexual dysfunction (2).
- Unfortunately, many studies do not assess whether the sexual issues are associated with distress, which is required to meet the criteria for the diagnosis of sexual dysfunction.

Incidence
Incidence is highest during the postpartum period and perimenopause.

- Postpartum: In a study of over 400 primiparous women, 83% reported sexual problems at 3 months postpartum; and 64%, at 6 months (3). There was no difference between vaginal versus cesarean delivery.
- Perimenopause: Sexual problems associated with distress are highest in women aged 45–64 years. Though sexual activity decreases with age, so does the distress as well as the perception that it represents dysfunction.

Prevalence
- Overall prevalence of diagnosed sexual dysfunction is 15–30% among US women.
  – Orgasmic disorders are the most common: <10% are primary, and 65–80% are secondary.
  – Desire disorders are the complaint of 30–55% of individuals and 31% of couples presenting to clinics.
  – Arousal disorders are present in 14–48% of patients.

- There are many women who report some degree of dissatisfaction but do not meet clinical criteria for diagnosis for sexual dysfunction.
  – 1 out of 5 women report that they are sexually dissatisfied.
  – 2 out of 3 women report some degree of sexual dysfunction but do not meet criteria for diagnosis.
  – Of women who are anorgasmic, only 1 out of 3 perceive it as a problem causing significant personal distress.

RISK FACTORS
- Advancing age
- Previous sexual trauma
- Lack of knowledge about sexual stimulation and response
- Chronic medical problems (e.g., depression or other psychiatric disorders); cardiovascular disease; endocrine disorders (e.g., diabetes, hypertension); neurologic disorders
- Gynecologic issues such as childbirth, pelvic floor or bladder dysfunction, endometriosis, and uterine fibroids
- Medications such as hormonal contraception, selective serotonin reuptake inhibitors (SSRIs), beta-blockers, and antipsychotic medications
- Relationship factors such as couple discrepancies in expectations and/or cultural backgrounds, attitudes toward sexuality in family of origin
- Substance abuse such as smoking, alcohol, and illicit drugs

PATHOPHYSIOLOGY
The pathophysiology of sexual dysfunction is complex and multifactorial since it can be the result of any etiology that interferes with the normal female sexual response cycle of desire, arousal, orgasm, and resolution.

ETIOLOGY
- Epilepsy: Higher rates of sexual dysfunction
- Diabetes (specifically anorgasmia)
- Anxiety or depression
- Spinal cord damage
- Thyroid disease
- Hormonal imbalance
- Drug use, including prescription medications (e.g., SSRIs, monoamine oxidase inhibitors [MAOIs], tricyclic antidepressants [TCAs], β-blockers)
- Interrelational difficulties and conflict regarding intimacy
- Control issues in the relationships
- Sexual frequency myths
- Survivor of sexual abuse, including incest
- Body image issues
- Alcohol
- Proximity of other people in household

COMMONLY ASSOCIATED CONDITIONS
- Marital discord
- Depression

DIAGNOSIS

- Female sexual dysfunction is diagnosed by identifying diagnostic criteria through both a medical and a sexual history.
- The diagnosis requires that the sexual problem be recurrent or persistent and cause personal distress or interpersonal difficulty.

HISTORY
- Complaint to health care provider; if the clinician inquires "Do you have any sexual concerns?" more than twice as many are revealed than if clinician waits for the patient to mention).
- Pregnancy/childbirth history
- Infertility
- Menopausal status (natural, surgical, or postchemotherapy)
- Sexually transmitted diseases and vaginitis
- Pelvic surgery, injury, or cancer
- Chronic pelvic pain
- Abnormal genital tract bleeding
- Urinary/anal incontinence
- Marital conflict
- Family dysfunction

PHYSICAL EXAM
Most commonly, patients have a normal physical exam.

- Assess for scars or evidence of trauma.
- Assess for vaginal atrophy, adequate estrogenization.
- Assess for infection.
- Recognize signs of anxiety, apprehension, and pain during the speculum and pelvic exam.

DIAGNOSTIC TESTS & INTERPRETATION
Lab
Neither estrogen nor androgen levels should be used to determine the cause of the sexual dysfunction because there is no established serum hormone range that correlates with sexual dysfunction.

Initial lab tests
As needed to identify infections and other medical causes:
- Wet prep
- Thyroid-stimulating hormone
- Prolactin
- Follicle-stimulating hormone

Follow-Up & Special Considerations
Encourage counseling

Imaging
Initial approach
Transvaginal ultrasound if indicated

DIFFERENTIAL DIAGNOSIS
- Medication side effects: SSRIs, TCAs, and other antidepressants; psychotropics; MAOIs; many antihypertensives
- Vaginitis
- Decreased vaginal lubrication secondary to hormonal imbalance
- Decreased sensation secondary to nerve injury
- Multiple sclerosis

- Anatomic abnormalities
- Abdominal surgery (which can interfere with pelvic innervation)
- Depression
- Marital dysfunction, including domestic violence
- Pregnancy
- Pseudodyspareunia (use of complaint of pain to distance self from partner)

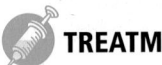 **TREATMENT**

- Assess patient goals.
- Treatment should address associated chronic conditions.
- Hormone therapy, alone or in conjunction with other therapies
- An increase in fitness and body image alone can improve libido.
- Consider couples therapy for women who complain of relationship conflicts.

MEDICATION
Sexual dysfunction is often a multifactorial psychosocial condition. Using medications does not usually address the cause of the problem and can, in some cases, make the condition worse.

First Line
- Bupropion: May be useful in treating sexual dysfunction or as an adjunct for SSRI-induced sexual dysfunction. (4,5) Generally, Bupropion XL 300mg/day is used.
- Premenopausal women:
  - Some data suggest that testosterone may be low with decreased libido.
  - No clear studies indicate testosterone replacement as beneficial.
- Postmenopausal women:
  - Adding testosterone to hormone-replacement therapy may increase sexual desire. (6)[B]. Unfortunately, the FDA has not approved the use of testosterone to treat sexual dysfunction in women. Current testosterone therapy for women must be compounded into an oral or topical form. Typical dosages range from 0.625–1.25 mg/day. Testosterone therapy designed for men should not be used in women.
  - Estrogen replacement may help to improve sexual desire, vaginal atrophy, and clitoral sensitivity. Vaginal estrogen therapy is available in cream, vaginal tablet, or ring form (7)[B].

ADDITIONAL TREATMENT
Issues for Referral
Consider referral for marriage or sex therapy counseling.

Additional Therapies
- Vaginal lubricants
- Aerobic exercise
- Smoking cessation and reduction of alcohol intake
- For childhood trauma: Scripting, psychotherapy, cognitive restructuring
- For anorgasmia: Directed masturbation and "homework" with partners
- For prescription-drug causes: Reduced dosages or change to different medication
- Other: Family therapy, sensate conditioning; referral to specialized sex therapy

COMPLEMENTARY AND ALTERNATIVE MEDICINE
- Yohimbe: Not recommended, potentially dangerous
- Ginseng and St John's Wort have no evidence to support treatment of sexual dysfunction.
- DHEA: Androgenic effects; will decrease high-density lipoprotein cholesterol

 ONGOING CARE

DIET
Weight reduction if needed for either partner

PATIENT EDUCATION
- In the US, sex therapists and counselors can be found through the American Association of Sex Educators, Counselors and Therapists at http://www.assect.org.
- National Women's Health Resource Center: www.Healthwomen.org
- American Association of Sex Educators, Counselors, and Therapists: www.aasect.org
- Female Sexual Dysfunction Online: www.femlae sexualdysfunctiononline.org
- North American Menopause Society: www.menopause.org

PROGNOSIS
Lack of desire is most difficult type to treat with <50% success.

REFERENCES

1. Laumann EO, Nicolosi A, Glasser DB, et al. Sexual problems among women and men aged 40–80 y: prevalence and correlates identified in the Global Study of Sexual Attitudes and Behaviors. *Int J Impot Res*. 2005;17:39–57.
2. Shifren JL, Monz BU, Russo PA, et al. Sexual problems and distress in United States women: prevalence and correlates. *Obstet Gynecol*. 2008;112:970–8.
3. Barrett G, Pendry E, Peacock J, et al. Women's sexual health after childbirth. *BJOG*. 2000;107:186–95.
4. Segraves RT, Clayton A, Croft H, et al. Bupropion sustained release for the treatment of hypoactive sexual desire disorder in premenopausal women. *J Clin Psychopharmacol*. 2004;24:339–42.
5. Ginzburg R, Wong Y, Fader JS. Effect of bupropion on sexual dysfunction. *Ann Pharmacother*. 2005;39:2096–9.
6. Somboonporn W, Davis S, Seif MW, et al. Testosterone for peri- and postmenopausal women. *Cochrane Database Syst Rev*. 2005;CD004509.
7. Gast MJ, Freedman MA, Vieweg AJ, et al. A randomized study of low-dose conjugated estrogens on sexual function and quality of life in postmenopausal women. *Menopause*. 2009;16: 247.

ADDITIONAL READING

- Basaria S, Dobs AS. Safety and adverse effects of androgens: how to counsel patients. *Mayo Clin Proc*. 2004;79:S25–32.
- Blumel JE, Del Pino M, Aprikian D, et al. Effect of androgens combined with hormone therapy on quality of life in post-menopausal women with sexual dysfunction. *Gynecol Endocrinol*. 2008;24: 691.
- Braunstein GD. Safety of testosterone treatment in postmenopausal women. *Fertil Steril*. 2007;88:1.
- Davis SR, Moreau M, Kroll R, et al. Testosterone for low libido in postmenopausal women not taking estrogen. *N Engl J Med*. 2008;359:2005.
- El-Hage G, Eden JA, Manga RZ. A double-blind, randomized, placebo-controlled trial of the effect of testosterone cream on the sexual motiviation of menopausal hysterectomized women with hypoactive sexual desire disorder. *Climacteric*. 2007;10:335.
- Goldstat R, Briganti E, Tran J, et al. Transdermal testosterone therapy improves well-being, mood, and sexual function in premenopausal women. *Menopause*. 2003;10:390.
- Leiblum SR, Rosen RC. *Principles and Practice of Sex Therapy: Update for the 1990s*. New York, NY: The Guilford Press; 1989.
- Modelska K. Female sexual dysfunction in postmenopausal women: systematic review of placebo-controlled trials. *Am J Obstet Gynecol*. 2003;188:286.
- Osmanagaoglu MA, Atasaral T, Baltaci D, et al. Effect of different preparations of hormone therapy on sexual dysfunction in naturally postmenopausal women. *Cliacteric*. 2006;9:464–72.
- Rudkin L, Taylor MJ, Hawton K. Strategies for managing sexual dysfunction induced by antidepressant medication. *Cochrane Database Syst Rev*. 2004:CD003382.
- Shifren JL. The role of androgens in female sexual dysfunction. *Mayo Clin Proc*. 2004;79:S19–24.
- The role of testosterone therapy in postmenopausal women: position statement of The North American Menopause Society. *Menopause*. 2005;12:497.
- Wincze JP, Carey MP. *Sexual Dysfunction: A Guide for Assessment and Treatment*. New York, NY: The Guilford Press; 1991.

 CODES

ICD9
- 302.70 Psychosexual dysfunction, unspecified
- 302.71 Hypoactive sexual desire disorder
- 302.72 Psychosexual dysfunction with inhibited sexual excitement

CLINICAL PEARLS
- Female sexual dysfunction is a complex, multifactorial problem.
- Most commonly, patients with sexual dysfunction have a completely normal physical exam.
- Symptoms of sexual dysfunction peak during perimenopause between the ages of 45–64, even though hormone levels of estrogen and testosterone may fall in the normal range; women often benefit from hormone supplementation with estrogen and/or testosterone.
- Encourage follow-up with counseling for marriage, individual, and/or sex therapy.

SHARED PARANOID DISORDER

Irene C. Coletsos, MD
Harold J. Bursztajn, MD

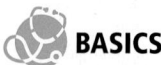 **BASICS**

DESCRIPTION

Shared paranoid disorder is also known as shared delusional disorder, shared psychotic disorder, *folie a deux* (if two people are involved), or *folie a plusieurs* (if several are involved). This disorder occurs when a delusional belief held by one person becomes shared by one to several people associated with that person. In most cases, a second person is dependent on or has a passive relationship with the primarily affected person. The individuals involved are usually close and may be isolated from others. By definition, the shared belief, in order to be considered delusional, is one that is not generally accepted within the person's culture. As a result, this illness exists along a spectrum: the least severe form being a shared overvalued idea (those holding it will relinquish it if given evidence to the contrary), the most severe form being a shared psychosis (attempts to disprove or cure patients of their delusions feel threatening).

EPIDEMIOLOGY
Prevalence
"Shared ideas" are more common than "shared psychoses." In general, researchers have found that these seemingly rare phenomena may occur more often than is thought to be the case because those experiencing it tend to be isolated and therefore unobserved.

RISK FACTORS
A major risk factor for a 2nd person (or several people) to develop a shared delusional disorder is to have a close family member (the primary person affected) with a psychiatric diagnosis of schizophrenia, mood disorders, or delusions. The primary family member is usually a spouse or sibling and lives with the person who will come to share the delusions (1).

GENERAL PREVENTION
Adequate treatment for the primary person with mental illness, family therapy for those close to the primary, and clinician efforts to bring such families out of their isolation can help address major risk factors for the development of shared delusional/paranoid disorder.

ETIOLOGY
One or more persons may come to share in an individual's delusions or paranoia, most commonly in cases in which those involved are isolated and emotionally close, and the secondary person(s) is (are) psychologically vulnerable.

COMMONLY ASSOCIATED CONDITIONS
- Familial mental illness
- Immigration/displacement from home
- Hearing (or other sensory) loss, which can lead to misinterpretation of outside phenomena
- Shared use of medications, drugs, or herbs that can stimulate hallucinations or changes in perception
- The secondary often suffers from dependent personality disorder (1), an all-consuming need to be taken care of that leads to submissive behavior and fear of separation (2).

 DIAGNOSIS

HISTORY
- For the primary: May be a history of lack of parental contact leading to feelings of deprivation or excess family strife, in turn leading to emotional overload. A child in such an environment may use denial or distortion to cope.
- For the primary: History of mental illness, organic brain disease, dementia, or stroke
- For the primary and secondary, who share the delusion: History of immigration, shared hallucinogen use, and/or isolation
- When taking a history, the clinician may observe that these patients appear alert, oriented, and outwardly able to function. However, their insight into their illness is poor and they rarely seek treatment on their own. They may challenge the clinician and resist any suggestion that their delusions are not true.

PHYSICAL EXAM
- Rule out physical causes for delusions in the primary or secondary, e.g.:
  - Dementia, stroke or organic brain disease, such as Huntington's or Niemann Pick disease (use the Mini Mental Status Exam and a general neurological exam)
  - Signs of substance abuse (such as gum recession and nasal septum perforation in chronic cocaine use; gum recession in marijuana use; skin lesions and tooth decay in methamphetamine use)
  - Endocrine disorders: Hypothyroidism, hyperthyroidism, hypercalcinosis, DKA, and hypoglycemia can lead to psychosis.
  - Infection: Syphilis, meningitis, HIV, parasites (such as neurocysticerosis with taenia solium, the "pork tapeworm").
  - Nutrition: B12, thiamine deficiency
  - Poisoning: Copper (Wilson's Disease), lead (environmental), zinc (from excess use of dental adhesives, for example), insecticides (DEET)

- Mental Status Exam: Usually performed by a mental health professional. Typical findings include:
  - Attitude: Uncooperative, guarded
  - Speech: Fluid, coherent
  - Mood: May be angry with clinician.
  - Affect: Non-labile, incongruent to illness
  - Thought content: Includes the delusional system
  - Thought process: Linear
  - Sensorium: Alert
  - Cognition: Memory intact
  - Insight and judgment: Poor in the specific area of delusions, may be intact elsewhere(3)

DIAGNOSTIC TESTS & INTERPRETATION
- Definitive diagnosis is usually made by a mental health clinician. A primary care provider can assist in the diagnosis and treatment by ruling out the other medical causes for psychosis (see Physical Exam) and enabling patients to seek mental health help. This may be particularly difficult in cases of shared delusional/paranoid disorder, as a hallmark of the disorder is that patients are in denial about the problem.
- However, primary care clinicians may be able to support engagement in mental health treatment, if they state that the mental health professional can help alleviate the patient's "discomfort." As in any case of referral from primary care to mental health, the primary care clinician can deal with a patient's possible feeling of embarrassment or abandonment by stating that mental illness is an illness like any other, that it is treatable, and that the primary care clinician will continue to be part of the patient's care team during mental health treatment (4).

Lab
To rule out other causes of psychosis/shared psychosis (see Physical Exam)

Imaging
To rule out medical causes of psychosis (see Physical Exam)

DIFFERENTIAL DIAGNOSIS
- A shared cultural or cherished belief
- A paranoid reaction to a shared social upheaval, such as trauma associated with immigration, war, criminal violence, or natural disaster.
- Shared substance abuse or medication use leading to psychosis

- Mental illness, organic brain disease, infection, endocrine imbalance, nutrient or micronutrient imbalance, or poisoning in a primary person leading to psychosis or delusions, comes to be shared by a secondary person who lives with or is extremely close to the primarily affected person.
- Diagnosis of shared paranoid disorder requires that the delusions of the secondary person cannot be explained by other mental illnesses, such as schizophrenia.
- Keep in mind that an unlikely event believed to be true by two or more people may actually be true, and thus is not a delusion.

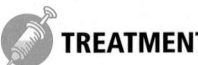

TREATMENT

- First, separate the patient who shares the delusion (i.e., the secondary) from the primary person affected by it.
- The psychotherapeutic approach includes focusing on the patient's emotional troubles, frustrations, and difficulties with their relationships with others and *not* challenging the patient's delusional system or its contradictions. A therapeutic alliance should first be formed to help get the patient into treatment (34).

MEDICATION
Treat the underlying disorder of the primary person experiencing the delusion. The secondary person may need also to be treated symptomatically with antipsychotics if separation and psychotherapy are not successful by themselves. Consult a psychiatrist before initiating psychotropic medical treatment.

ADDITIONAL TREATMENT
Family therapy or group therapy to address the family/group stress and pathology that set the stage for the illness.

Issues for Referral
- Psychiatry for definitive diagnosis, psychotherapy, and evaluation of the need for antipsychotic medication.
- Social work/psychotherapy to address family dynamics and stressors.
- Law enforcement in cases of child/elder/incompetent dependent abuse or neglect.

COMPLEMENTARY AND ALTERNATIVE MEDICINE
Intervention of healers specific to the patients' culture. They can offer a reality "correction" to the patients and cultural perspective to the clinician.

IN-PATIENT CONSIDERATIONS
- For initial stabilization, to help separate the person(s) with the secondary delusion from the person with the primary delusion.
- For safety, for delusions that involve suicidality or homicidality.

Discharge Criteria
Once psychiatrically stable and follow-up treatment is established.

 ONGOING CARE

- Psychotherapy
- Involvement of care professionals to support the family (or group) involved and try to lessen social isolation
- Legal involvement if a child/elder/incompetent adult has been victimized.

FOLLOW-UP RECOMMENDATIONS
See Ongoing Care section.

PATIENT EDUCATION
Skillful psychotherapy may eventually allow patients to understand the underlying stresses that allowed the paranoid/psychotic ideas to take shape. When patients are properly supported through this process, their delusional system may recede.

PROGNOSIS
- Prognosis is good for recovery if treatment includes separation of the primary and secondary persons with the shared delusion; ongoing psychotherapy for both (or all) patients, and social service support (1).
- It is more problematic if the belief system is supported by a larger ideology (e.g., witchcraft cults).

COMPLICATIONS
Self-harm or harm to others based on the contents of the shared delusional system

REFERENCES

1. Booth JH. Shared psychotic disorder. In: *Encyclopedia of Mental Disorders*. www.minddisorders.com/Py_Z/Shared-psychotic-disorder.html. Accessed 7/5/10.
2. American Psychiatric Association. *Diagnostic and Statistical Manual of Mental Disorders*. Fourth Edition, Text Revision. (*DSM-IV-TR*). Washington DC: American Psychiatric Association, 2000.
3. Gutheil TG, Bursztajn HJ. Clinicians' guidelines for assessing and preventing subtle forms of patient incompetence in legal settings. *Am J Psychiatry.* 1986;143:1020–23.
4. Bursztajn HJ, Barsky AJ. Facilitating patient acceptance of a psychiatric referral. *Arch Intern Med.* 1985;145:73–75.

ADDITIONAL READING

Manschreck TC. Delusional disorder and shared psychotic disorder. In: Sadock BJ, Sadock VA, eds. *Kaplan & Sadock's Comprehensive Textbook of Psychiatry*. 7th Edition, Vol. I. Philadelphia PA: Lippincott, Williams and Wilkins. 2000:1243–64.

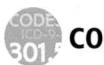 CODES

ICD9
297.3 Shared psychotic disorder

CLINICAL PEARLS

- Rule out medical causes for psychosis, shared psychosis.
- Be aware that shared delusions occur along a continuum, from a shared cherished or cultural belief to a pathologically adopted belief system that isolates and may endanger.
- Clinicians should engage the patient by first empathizing with the pain and confusion that may underlie the adoption of a delusional belief system, rather than by initially challenging the belief system directly.
- Concealment within the dyad (of the person with primary delusions and the one who comes to share it) is very common in this illness, and so it is difficult for clinicians to recognize it. The classic work by Elvin Semrad MD and Max Day MD, "Paranoia and Paranoid States" (in the 1978 edition of *The Harvard Guide to Modern Psychiatry*) suggests that if health care providers can create a safe emotional space for patients, they may be able to reveal their paranoid delusions. Semrad and Day suggest that providers who take care of mentally ill patients thoroughly and painstakingly examine patients' familial relationships to get clues about the losses in their lives that could be fueling delusions. The authors suggest that helping patients recognize their losses and supporting them through this process may help them break free of the delusions.
- Psychiatric, social work, and (in some cases) legal referral or monitoring (when minors, the elderly or incompetent persons are involved) will likely be necessary.

S

SHIN SPLINTS

Gary Yen, MD

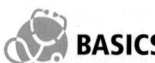

BASICS

DESCRIPTION
- American Medical Association defines shin splints as "pain or discomfort in the leg from repetitive running on hard surfaces or forcible excessive use of the foot flexors." Definition excludes stress fracture or pain from ischemic origin.
- Synonyms: Medial tibial stress syndrome (preferred term); Medial tibial periostalgia; Tibial periostitis; Shin soreness; Tibial stress syndrome; Medial tibial syndrome.

EPIDEMIOLOGY
Prevalence
Can account for 6–16% of all running injuries (1)

RISK FACTORS
- Runners (particularly sprinters and hurdlers), dancers (particularly ballet), gymnasts, basketball players, military personnel
- Usually categorized into intrinsic (personal) and extrinsic (environmental) factors (2):
  – Intrinsic factors include overpronation, female sex, increased hip internal/external range of motion, higher body mass index (BMI), and leaner calf girth.
  – Extrinsic factors include training errors (increased mileage, increased intensity of workout), low calcium intake in female athletes, running on hard or inclined surfaces, and running on worn-out footwear.

GENERAL PREVENTION
Recommendations suggested include the following (1)[C]:
- Screening for overpronation
- Designing appropriate training regimen/identifying training errors
- Regular stretching, strength, and flexibility exercises
- Rehabilitation of previous injuries
- Wearing proper footwear

PATHOPHYSIOLOGY
Somewhat controversial with many different theories, including bone stress reaction, periostitis, periostalgia, low bone mineral density, tendinopathy, periosteal remodeling with several structures possibly involved including soleus, deep crural fascia, flexor digitorum longus, and tibialis posterior.

ETIOLOGY
Likely multifactorial, drawing from biomechanical, anatomic, and environmental causes, as detailed earlier

DIAGNOSIS

HISTORY
- Pain along the junction of the middle and distal thirds of the posteromedial tibia (most common) or anterior tibia, described as "dull ache" or "soreness."
- Pain with exercise dissipates with rest, commonly bilateral.
- Severe shin splints may have persistent pain at rest or pain with only mild activity, and character of pain can become "sharp" or "penetrating."
- Pain subsides or is gone in shin splints compared with stress fracture of the tibia, where the pain persists with rest.

PHYSICAL EXAM
- Generalized tenderness to palpation along the medial border of the tibia with possible mild swelling (see http://www.youtube.com/watch?v=7vZVq3ov914 for overview of muscular dysfunction)
- Pain with resisted plantar flexion or toe raises

- Clinical presentation may closely resemble that of stress fractures and exertional compartment syndrome, which can carry a far worse prognosis if undiagnosed:
  – Stress fracture tenderness usually is more localized.
  – Exertional compartment syndrome has characteristic physical findings of anterolateral leg pain (described as "cramplike, tight, squeezing ache"), most commonly over the anterior compartment; fascial hernias may be present. Depending on compartment affected, characteristic weakness and/or paresthesias also can be present.

DIAGNOSTIC TESTS & INTERPRETATION
Imaging
- Serial plain radiographs are normal but are needed to rule out stress fractures, which usually are positive after 2 weeks of symptoms.
- A bone scan for shin splints reveals diffuse, linear uptake along the posteromedial border of the tibia on the delayed phase, whereas a bone scan for stress fracture reveals localized, more intense, fusiform, or transverse uptake in all phases.
- MRI also can be used to identify a stress fracture earlier.
- Compartment pressure measurement with exercise may be needed to diagnose exertional compartment syndrome if pain is anterolateral.

DIFFERENTIAL DIAGNOSIS

- Stress fractures
- Chronic exertional compartment syndrome
- Acute tendinitis/muscle strain/muscle tear/fascial defects
- Vascular disease
- Lumbar radiculopathy
- Hematoma
- Popliteal artery entrapment
- Peroneal nerve entrapment
- Deep vein thrombosis
- Tumor (sarcoma or osteosarcoma)

 TREATMENT

- Acute phase treatment includes reducing training activity below symptom level, or if it is a serious case, may need to stop activity altogether; ice the area of injury (3)[C].
- Recovery time is variable.
- Exercises to consider: http://www.youtube.com/watch?v=kv6ycmOWnq0
- Pool running or bicycling can aid in keeping up with conditioning while rehabilitation occurs.
- Options mostly based on expert opinion and clinical experience (3).
- Modifying training schedules by duration, frequency, or running distance can reduce injuries from running (4)[A].

MEDICATION

- Nonsteroidal anti-inflammatory drugs (NSAIDs)
- Analgesics

ADDITIONAL TREATMENT
Additional Therapies

- Physical therapy (3)[C]:
  – Therapist-determined modalities
  – Strengthening, stretching, and flexibility exercises after acute symptoms disappear
- Whirlpool, phonophoresis, electrical stimulation, ultrasound, augmented soft tissue mobilization, and acupuncture can be considered (3)[C].

COMPLEMENTARY AND ALTERNATIVE MEDICINE

- Orthotic or shoe modification if significant foot pronation
- Shock-absorbing orthotics may reduce incidence of shin splints (1)[B].

SURGERY/OTHER PROCEDURES

- Only after a documented trial of maximal nonoperative treatment (for at least 6 months) has failed should posterior medial fascia release be considered. Consider if severe limitation of physical activity or frequent recurrence of pain despite proper rehabilitation (5)[C].
- Extracorporeal shock wave therapy is a possible alternative to surgical treatment, though more investigation is needed on this mode of therapy (6)[C].

 ONGOING CARE

PATIENT EDUCATION

- Identifying training errors and avoiding a rush back to preinjury pace will help to prevent recurrence.
- Emphasize the importance of modified activity followed by stretching and strengthening exercises.
- Resumption of activity should be done gradually, below the level of the symptoms.

PROGNOSIS

- Most patients respond well to nonoperative treatment.
- Gradual return to activity can be expected.

COMPLICATIONS

- If shin splints are not addressed, the degree of leg pain can interfere with activities of daily living, and stress fractures/true fractures may occur.
- Undiagnosed stress fracture can lead to complete fracture and displacement.
- Undiagnosed chronic compartment syndrome could develop into an acute syndrome with possible tissue necrosis.

REFERENCES

1. Thacker SB, Gilchrist J, Stroup DF, et al. The prevention of shin splints in sports: a systematic review of literature. *Med Sci Sports Exerc.* 2002;34:32–40.
2. Moen MH, Tol JL, Weir A, et al. Medial tibial stress syndrome: a critical review. *Sports Med.* 2009;39:523–46.
3. Galbraith RM, Lavallee ME, et al. Medial tibial stress syndrome: conservative treatment options. *Curr Rev Musculoskelet Med.* 2009;
4. Yeung EW, Yeung SS. Interventions for preventing lower limb soft-tissue injuries in runners. *Cochrane Database Syst Rev.* 2001:CD001256.
5. Yates B, Allen MJ, Barnes MR. Outcome of surgical treatment of medial tibial stress syndrome. *J Bone Joint Surg Am.* 2003;85-A:1974–80.
6. Rompe JD, Cacchio A, Furia JP, et al. Low-energy extracorporeal shock wave therapy as a treatment for medial tibial stress syndrome. *Am J Sports Med.* 2010;38:125–32.

 CODES

ICD9
844.9 Sprain of unspecified site of knee and leg

CLINICAL PEARLS

- *Medial tibial stress syndrome* is the much more anatomically accurate and preferred term.
- Diagnosis is usually made clinically by pain most commonly in the middle and distal thirds of the posteromedial border of the tibia that comes on with activity and reduces or resolves with rest; contrasted to stress fracture, where the pain persists with rest.
- Relative rest, ice, and NSAIDs are the generally agreed-upon mainstays of treatment.
- Shock-absorbing orthotics may reduce incidence.

SHOCK, CIRCULATORY

Felix B. Chang, MD
Mouhanad Ayach, MD

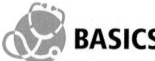 **BASICS**

DESCRIPTION
- Inadequate tissue perfusion leading to hypoxia and organ dysfunction
- Classified as:
  - Hypovolemic shock: Low preload
  - Cardiogenic shock: Persistent hypotension (systolic pressure <80–90 mm Hg or mean arterial pressure 30 mm Hg lower than baseline) with severe reduction in the cardiac index and adequate or elevated filling pressures
  - Septic shock: Severe sepsis plus systemic blood pressure is <60 mm (or <80 mm Hg if the patient has baseline hypertension) despite fluid resuscitation. Maintaining the systemic mean blood pressure >60 mm Hg (or >60 mm Hg if the patient has baseline hypertension) requires dopamine >5 mcg/kg per min, norepinephrine <0.25 mcg/kg per min, or epinephrine <0.25 mcg/kg per min despite adequate fluid resuscitation.
  - Neurogenic shock: Vasodilation associated with loss of sympathetic tone; venous pooling in periphery

EPIDEMIOLOGY
- Accidental injuries are the leading cause of death between 1 and 44 years.
- Cardiogenic shock: 5–10% in patients with acute myocardial infarction (MI)
- Severe sepsis >500,000 emergency visits in US (2001–2004)

Incidence
Male > Female

RISK FACTORS
- Hypovolemic shock: Hemorrhage, dehydration, burns
- Cardiogenic shock: Older age, anterior MI, hypertension, diabetes mellitus, multivessel coronary artery disease, prior MI or diagnosis of heart failure, STEMI, and left bundle branch block
- Septic shock: Elderly, immunosuppression, critical illness, malnutrition, cancer
- Neurogenic: Spinal anesthesia, spinal cord injury, anaphylactic shock, fainting (vasovagal reaction)

GENERAL PREVENTION
Prompt recognition and early treatment of underlying condition

ETIOLOGY
- Hypovolemic shock (hemorrhagic):
  - Blood loss: Trauma (e.g., injuries to liver, spleen, lung; fractures, wounds), GI bleeding (e.g., gastric and duodenal ulcer, colonic polyps, diverticulosis, or tumors), rupture of aortic or ventricular aneurysm, ectopic pregnancy, hemorrhagic ovarian cyst, DUB:
    - Class I - blood loss up to 750 mL (15% blood volume), pulse <100, BP normal with normal or increased pulse pressure, normal capillary blanch test, respiratory rate 14–20, urine output >30 mL/hour, slightly anxious
    - Class II - blood loss 750–1,500 mL (15–30% blood volume), pulse >100, BP normal with decreased pulse pressure, positive capillary blanch test, respiratory rate 20–30, urine output 20–30 mL/hour, mildly anxious
    - Class III - blood loss 1,500–2,000 mL (30–40% blood volume), pulse >120, BP decreased with decreased pulse pressure, positive capillary blanch test, respiratory rate 30–40, urine output 5–15 mL/hour, anxious + confused
    - Class IV - blood loss >2,000 mL (>40% blood volume), pulse >140, BP decreased with decreased pulse pressure, positive capillary blanch test, RR >35, urine output negligible, confused, lethargic
- Hypovolemic shock (nonhemorrhagic): Dehydration, vomiting, diarrhea, heat stroke, or burns; 3rd-space loss of plasma volume
- Cardiogenic shock:
  - Acute MI (>40% of left ventricular myocardium), right ventricular infarction, β and calcium channel blocker overdose
  - Dilated cardiomyopathies (e.g., viral, alcohol, Adriamycin toxicity)
  - Arrhythmias: Heart block, ventricular tachycardia/fibrillation, atrial fibrillation with rapid ventricular response, bradycardias, etc.
  - Mechanical difficulties: Valvular dysfunction, papillary muscle rupture, aortic or mitral valve dysfunction; ventricular septal rupture
  - Obstruction:
    - Pericardial tamponade, tension pneumothorax, constrictive pericarditis
    - Aortic dissection or pulmonary embolism
- Septic shock: UTI most common source in the elderly
- Neurogenic shock: Acute spinal injury, general or spinal anesthesia, vasovagal reaction

COMMONLY ASSOCIATED CONDITIONS
Adrenal failure in septic shock

 DIAGNOSIS

HISTORY
- Hypovolemic shock: Burns, trauma, bleeding, vomiting, melena, diarrhea
- Cardiogenic shock: Dizziness, chest pain, dyspnea, palpitations
- Septic shock: Fever, chills, rigors, malaise, myalgias, dysuria, suprapubic pain, flank pain, shortness of breath
- Neurogenic: Spinal trauma

PHYSICAL EXAM
- Hypovolemic shock: Orthostatic hypotension, dry skin and mucosa, collapsed neck veins
- Cardiogenic shock: Cyanosis, cool skin, rapid and faint peripheral pulses, JVD, pulsus paradoxus, systolic murmur, crackles
- Neurogenic shock: Normal capillary refill, areflexia + weakness below level of lesion. Absence in bulbocavernosis reflex.

- Septic shock:
  - Hyperdynamic state: Fever, tachycardia; warm, dry, flushed skin
  - Hypodynamic state: Hypotension, diminished sensorium, cold clammy skin
  - Temperature >38.3 degrees C (100.9 degrees F) or temperature <36 degrees C (96.8 degrees F), tachycardia with heart rate >90 beats/minute or >2 standard deviations above normal value for age, tachypnea >30 breaths/minute, altered mental status, edema or positive fluid balance (>20 mL/kg over 24 hours), hyperglycemia:
    - Brain: Confusion, anxiety, agitation, coma
    - Kidney: Oliguria, anuria
    - Skin: Erythema, petechiae, embolic lesions, purpura
- Specific signs of underlying disease:
  - Upper GI (UGI) tract bleeding (hematemesis, melena)
  - MI (chest pain, diaphoresis, nausea, vomiting, S_4 or S_3 gallop, new heart murmur, rales)
  - Pericardial tamponade (JVD and pulsus paradoxus)
  - Urosepsis (suprapubic and/or costovertebral angle tenderness)

DIAGNOSTIC TESTS & INTERPRETATION
Lab
Initial lab tests
- Hypovolemic shock: Hemorrhagic: CBC-Ddff, PT/INR, PTT; LFTs, blood type and cross-match, DIC panel; type and cross
- Nonhemorrhagic: Creatinine and electrolytes; consider lipase and LFTs.
- Cardiogenic shock: ECG, cardiac enzymes, ABGs, tox screen, lactic acid, BNP
- Septic shock: CBC-diff, PT/INR/PTT, Chem 14, lactic acid, ABGs, C-reactive protein, urinalysis, pan-cultures and sensitivities, Gram stain, ACTH stimulation test

Imaging
Initial approach
- Chest: CXR and/or CT scan as appropriate to evaluate for pneumonia, empyema, hemothorax, aortic aneurysm
- Abdomen: KUB, CT scan, and/or ultrasound to evaluate intestinal obstruction, aortic aneurysm, liver abscess, peritoneal abscess, peritonitis, pancreatitis

Diagnostic Procedures/Surgery
- Central venous pressure
- Pulmonary artery pressure (Swan-Ganz catheter)
- Lumbar puncture
- Upper/lower endoscopy for GI bleeding
- Cystoscopy for hematuria/hemorrhagic cystitis

TREATMENT

MEDICATION

First Line
- Aspirin, β-blockers, nitroglycerin, morphine for coronary syndromes
- Control arrhythmias: β-Blockers, calcium channel blockers, digoxin, antiarrhythmic agents (e.g., amiodarone, sotalol, etc.); electrolytes
- After obtaining cultures, initiate broad-spectrum antibiotic therapy as early as possible aimed at the likely source of infection.
- Recombinant human activated protein C (drotrecogin-alfa) reduces mortality in high-risk patients with APACHE II scores ≥25, multiple organ dysfunction syndrome (MODS), or sepsis-induced acute respiratory distress syndrome (ARDS) (1)[A].
- Deep vein thrombosis prophylaxis

Second Line
- Vasopressors and inotropes are indicated for MAP <60 mm Hg or a decrease in SBP >30 mm Hg from baseline
- Norepinephrine and dopamine have similar effects on mortality, but norepinephrine reduces arrhythmia in patients with shock (2)[A].
- Dopamine: Cardiogenic and hypodynamic septic shock that is refractory to fluids. It is also the 1st-line catecholamine for bradycardia refractory to atropine.
- Dobutamine for refractory heart failure and cardiogenic shock
- Epinephrine is the agent of choice in patients with anaphylaxis.
- Norepinephrine and phenylephrine are 1st-line agents for hyperdynamic septic shock.
- Vasopressin is an alternative agent for patient's refractory to inotropic agents.
- Norepinephrine is useful in cardiogenic shock unresponsive to dopamine or dobutamine and in refractory hypotension secondary to tricyclic acid overdose.
- Phenylephrine is indicated in refractory shock, spinal anesthesia, or drug-related hypotension.
- Epinephrine, phenylephrine, or vasopressin should not be administered as the initial vasopressor in septic shock (3)[C].
- Naloxone might improve blood pressure in patients with shock.
- Levosimendan may improve survival in patients with refractory cardiogenic shock (4)[B].
- IV hydrocortisone
- Xigris

ADDITIONAL TREATMENT

General Measures
- 1st correct hypovolemia, maintain SaO_2 >92%.
- Control ongoing losses: Bleeding, diarrhea, 3rd-space loss
- Control glycemia. Identify and treat infections.
- Monitor urine output.

SURGERY/OTHER PROCEDURES
- Hemorrhage control
- Revascularization: MI, thrombolysis
- Pericardiocentesis for pericardial effusion
- Surgical drainage or debridement as needed
- Chest tube for empyema or pleural effusion
- Mechanical ventilation of sepsis-induced acute lung injury (ALI)/ARDS

IN-PATIENT CONSIDERATIONS

Initial Stabilization
- ABCs
- IV access: 2 large IV catheters or central line
- ICU-level care

IV Fluids
- Initial 10–20 mL/kg IV bolus lactated Ringer's, or normal saline if there is no sign of heart failure. Restore blood or fluid loss: 3 L of fluid per liter of blood loss.
- Colloids do not appear to reduce mortality compared with crystalloids in patients with trauma, burns, postoperatively (5)[A].
- Target goals in septic shock: Central venous pressure (CVP): 8–12 mm Hg; MAP ≥65 mm Hg; urine output ≥0.5 mL/kg/h; superior vena cava or mixed venous oxygen saturation >70% or 65%, respectively (3)[C]

Discharge Criteria
Hemodynamically stable

ONGOING CARE

FOLLOW-UP RECOMMENDATIONS

Patient Monitoring
ICU

PATIENT EDUCATION
Medline Plus: http://www.nlm.nih.gov/MEDLINEPLUS/ency/article/000039.htm

PROGNOSIS
- Cardiogenic shock: Increasing age, prior MI, altered sensorium, cold, clammy skin, and oliguria are predictive factors of increased mortality (Gusto I trial).
- Shock trial: 38% overall mortality with early revascularization vs 70% when rapid revascularization was not attempted
- Septic shock: Higher mortality in patients at the age extremes and those with poor functional status; also in patients with immunosuppression due to neutropenia, diabetes, alcoholism, renal failure, respiratory failure, or hypogammaglobulinemia; positive blood cultures, certain etiologic agents (e.g., *P. aeruginosa*), or delay in appropriate antimicrobial therapy
- Activated protein C (APC): In PROWESS study, APC was shown to reduce mortality from severe sepsis at 28 days from 31–25% (1)[A].
- PIRO risk model predicts hospital mortality in patients with severe sepsis (6)[A].
- MEDS (Mortality in Emergency Department Sepsis) score predicts 28-day mortality in patients with systemic inflammatory response syndrome (7)[A].

COMPLICATIONS
- Multiple organ failure, encephalopathy and/or CVA
- Pulmonary edema, ARDS, ischemic hepatitis, ischemic bowel
- Abdominal compartment syndrome
- Acute tubular necrosis (ATN)
- Coagulopathy, DIC, thrombocytopenia
- Acid base disturbances (e.g., respiratory alkalosis, anion gap metabolic acidosis)
- Adrenal failure, osteomyelitis, death

REFERENCES

1. Laterre PF, Abraham E, Janes JM, et al. ADDRESS (ADministration of DRotrecogin alfa [activated] in Early stage Severe Sepsis) long-term follow-up: one-year safety and efficacy evaluation. *Crit Care Med*. 2007;35:1457–63.
2. De Backer D, Biston P, Devriendt J, et al. Comparison of dopamine and norepinephrine in the treatment of shock. *N Engl J Med*. 2010;362: 779–89.
3. Dellinger RP, Levy MM, Carlet JM, et al. Surviving Sepsis Campaign: international guidelines for management of severe sepsis and septic shock: 2008. *Crit Care Med*. 2008;36:296–327.
4. Fuhrmann JT, Schmeisser A, Schulze MR, et al. Levosimendan is superior to enoximone in refractory cardiogenic shock complicating acute myocardial infarction. *Crit Care Med*. 2008;36: 2257–66.
5. Perel P, Roberts I, et al. Colloids versus crystalloids for fluid resuscitation in critically ill patients. *Cochrane Database Syst Rev*. 2009;(3): CD000567.
6. Rubulotta F, Marshall JC, Ramsay G, et al. Predisposition, insult/infection, response, and organ dysfunction: A new model for staging severe sepsis. *Crit Care Med*. 2009;37:1329–35.
7. Sankoff JD, Goyal M, Gaieski DF, et al. Validation of the Mortality in Emergency Department Sepsis (MEDS) score in patients with the systemic inflammatory response syndrome (SIRS). *Crit Care Med*. 2008;36:421–6.

CODES

ICD9
- 785.50 Shock, unspecified
- 785.51 Cardiogenic shock
- 785.52 Septic shock

CLINICAL PEARLS
- The majority of patients with cardiogenic shock have an ST elevation (Q-wave) MI (STEMI), but also occurs in 2.5% of patients with non-ST elevation MI (NSTEMI).
- Antibiotics should be initiated immediately after obtaining appropriate cultures, since early initiation is associated with lower mortality.
- Once cardiogenic shock is suspected, the evaluation should begin with echocardiography with color flow Doppler.

S

SHOULDER PAIN

J. Herbert Stevenson, MD

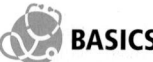

BASICS

DESCRIPTION
Shoulder pain is a common condition affecting patients of all ages that can arise from a variety of conditions, including rotator cuff disorders (including impingement syndrome), adhesive capsulitis, acromioclavicular (AC) joint pathology, shoulder instability, labral tears, osteoarthritis, calcific tendonitis, biceps tenosynovitis, autoimmune disorders, complex regional pain syndromes, fibromyalgia, and referred pain including but not limited to the cervical spine or diaphragm:
- Shoulder pain occurs most commonly from acute or overuse injury.
- Rotator cuff disorders include tendinopathy, partial tears, and complete tears.
- Impingement syndrome describes the repetitive impingement of the rotator cuff that can lead to tendinopathy (tendonitis/tendinosis) and tears over time. This was first described by Neer.
- Bursitis can occur with rotator cuff disorders, including impingement, but is rarely, if ever, an isolated diagnosis.

EPIDEMIOLOGY
- Shoulder pain is the 3rd most common musculoskeletal complaint in the general population and accounts for 5% of all general practitioner musculoskeletal visits (1,2)[B].
- Shoulder instability (subluxation, dislocation, multidirectional instability) is the most common cause of shoulder pain in the young athlete (<30 years of age).
- Rotator cuff disorders are the most common cause of shoulder pain in patients >30 years of age.
- Severity of rotator cuff disorders increases with age:
  - Tendinopathy common 30–50 years of age
  - Partial rotator cuff tears common 40–60 years of age
  - Full-thickness tears common >60 years of age
- Adhesive capsulitis is a poorly understood disorder that does not occur from disuse. Risk factors include diabetes, thyroid disorders, female gender, and middle age (40–60 years).
- Labral tears (anterior, superior, and posterior) can be a cause of shoulder pain in athletes.
- Osteoarthritis (OA) of the AC joint is a common condition seen after trauma or from repetitive shoulder use.
- OA of the glenohumeral joint is a relatively uncommon cause of shoulder pain generally found in patients >60 years of age unless there is a history of trauma/dislocation.

Incidence
The incidence of shoulder pain is 6.6–25 cases/1,000 patients, with a peak incidence in the 4th–6th decades.

RISK FACTORS
- Repetitive overhead activities
- Trauma or fall onto the shoulder
- Overhead and upper extremity weight-bearing sports (e.g., baseball, softball, gymnastics)
- History of trauma
- Weight lifting for AC joint OA
- Diabetes, thyroid disorders, female gender, age 40–60 years found to be risk factors for adhesive capsulitis

GENERAL PREVENTION
- Maintenance of good shoulder strength and range of motion (ROM)
- Avoidance of repetitive overhead activities

PATHOPHYSIOLOGY
Depends on underlying etiology

ETIOLOGY
- Rotator cuff disorders most commonly occur from repetitive overhead activity
- Neer proposed that this leads to repetitive impingement of the rotator cuff and can progress through 3 stages:
  - Stage I: Tendinopathy
  - Stage II: Partial rotator cuff tear
  - Stage III: Full-thickness rotator cuff tear
- Internal impingement of the undersurface of the rotator cuff with the posterior glenoid labrum has been theorized to be a cause of undersurface rotator cuff tears found most commonly in athletes who use repetitive overhead throwing movement.
- Trauma and dislocation, particularly in patients >50 years of age, have been found to result in rotator cuff tears.

DIAGNOSIS

Majority of shoulder pain is diagnosed in the outpatient setting.

HISTORY
- Traumatic shoulder instability often occurs from a fall on an outstretched hand.
- AC joint sprain often occurs from a fall directly onto the shoulder.
- Rotator cuff disorders most often occur from repetitive overhead activities.
- Adhesive capsulitis patients often note painful, stiff shoulder.

PHYSICAL EXAM
- Shoulder pain from rotator cuff disorders generally is distributed over the deltoid muscle and does not extend past the elbow.
- Impingement syndrome/rotator cuff disorders are notable for pain with overhead activity as well as night pain.
- AC joint pathology typically results in pain localized to the top of the shoulder/AC joint that is aggravated by cross-body adduction.
- Adhesive capsulitis results in both active and passive loss of ROM.
- Shoulder instability is aggravated by abducted and external rotation of the upper arm, as in reach behind.
- Cervical source of shoulder pain often will radiate toward the neck or past the elbow.
- Neer impingement sign is associated with impingement syndrome (passive internal arm rotation with forward flexion).
- Pain and/or weakness in isolated strength testing of the supraspinatus (empty-can test), infraspinatus/teres minor (external rotation), and/or subscapularis (internal rotation) may be seen with rotator disorders.
- Weakness with empty-can test and external rotation along with positive impingement test has strong association with rotator cuff tear (partial or complete).
- Loss of both passive and active ROM is the hallmark of adhesive capsulitis.
- Pain with passive cross-body adduction and/or tenderness of the AC joint are associated with AC joint pathology (sprain/OA).
- Pain and apprehension with the apprehension test (passive abduction and external rotation with patient supine) can signify shoulder instability.

DIAGNOSTIC TESTS & INTERPRETATION
- EMG study of the upper extremity may help to differentiate cervical pain referred to the shoulder from a primary shoulder disorder.
- Obtain ECG if any suspicion for cardiac etiology of left shoulder pain.

Lab
Appropriate rheumatologic tests may be indicated if autoimmune etiology of shoulder pain considered.

Imaging
Most shoulder pain can be diagnosed by the history and physical exam. When diagnosis remains unclear, there is a history of significant trauma, or there are prolonged symptoms, further imaging may be indicated:

- Plain radiographs are 1st-line imaging and in the right settings can assess for fracture, degenerative changes (AC or glenohumeral joint), signs of dislocation (Bankart or Hill-Sachs deformity), signs of large rotator cuff tear (sclerosis, humeral head proximal migration), as well as occult tumor or malignancy.
- MRI is gold standard from noninvasive imaging of soft tissue structures, including rotator cuff and biceps tendon.
- MR arthrogram may be needed to assess for labral tears or small/partial rotator cuff tears.
- Arthrogram or CT arthrogram may be needed if patient cannot undergo MRI for assessment of rotator cuff tear.
- CT scan may be needed to rule out occult fracture in the proper setting.

Diagnostic Procedures/Surgery
Diagnostic arthroscopy may be used in the proper setting after noninterventional means have been exhausted and structural injury suspected.

Pathological Findings
Depends on underlying diagnosis:
- Tendinosis rather than tendonitis often found with stage I impingement
- Scarring of the shoulder capsule hallmark of adhesive capsulitis
- Calcifications can be found in rotator cuff tendons with calcific tendonitis

DIFFERENTIAL DIAGNOSIS
- Rotator cuff disorders:
  - Impingement syndrome
  - Rotator cuff tear
- Adhesive capsulitis
- AC joint pathology (sprain/OA)
- Instability (acute/chronic)
- Shoulder OA
- Cervical radiculopathy
- Biceps tenosynovitis
- Autoimmune disorder

 ## TREATMENT

- Treatment is based on underlying pathology, but in general, conservative therapy includes relative rest, analgesics, and/or anti-inflammatory medicines.
- Physical therapy if unimproved with conservative measures
- Corticosteroid injections can help to relieve pain acutely.
- Recent Cochrane Review found little evidence to support or refute common interventions for shoulder pain (3)[A].

MEDICATION
Analgesics and anti-inflammatory medications may be required for symptomatic relief of shoulder pain:
- Ibuprofen
- Naprosyn
- Acetaminophen

ADDITIONAL TREATMENT
Issues for Referral
Shoulder pain where etiology remains unclear, nonresponsive to conservative care, complicated or displaced fractures, large rotator cuff tears

Additional Therapies
Consider for treatment of impingement syndrome, adhesive capsulitis, and shoulder instability.

COMPLEMENTARY AND ALTERNATIVE MEDICINE
There is no conclusive evidence to support or refute the use of acupuncture for shoulder pain (4)[A].

SURGERY/OTHER PROCEDURES
May be required for shoulder pain unresponsive to conservative care, acute displaced fractures, large rotator cuff tears, shoulder dislocation in patients <20 years of age

 ## ONGOING CARE

FOLLOW-UP RECOMMENDATIONS
Limiting overhead activity may reduce the symptoms of impingement syndrome.

PATIENT EDUCATION
Refer to specific diagnosis for shoulder pain.

PROGNOSIS
Shoulder pain generally has a favorable outcome with conservative care, but recovery can be slow, with 41% remaining symptomatic at 18 months (5)[B].

REFERENCES
1. Urwin M, Symmons D, Allison T, et al. Estimating the burden of musculoskeletal disorders in the community: the comparative prevalence of symptoms at different anatomical sites, and the relation to social deprivation. *Ann Rheum Dis*. 1998;57:649–55.
2. Peters D, Davies P, Pietroni P. Musculoskeletal clinic in general practice: study of one year's referrals. *Br J Gen Pract*. 1994;44:25–9.
3. Green S, Buchbinder R, Glazier R, et al. WITHDRAWN: Interventions for shoulder pain. *Cochrane Database Syst Rev*. 2006:CD001156.
4. Green S, Buchbinder R, Hetrick S. Acupuncture for shoulder pain. *Cochrane Database Syst Rev*. 2005:CD005319.
5. Croft P, Pope D, Silman A. The clinical course of shoulder pain: prospective cohort study in primary care. Primary Care Rheumatology Society Shoulder Study Group. *BMJ*. 1996;313:601–2.

 ## CODES

ICD9
- 719.41 Pain in joint involving shoulder region
- 726.0 Adhesive capsulitis of shoulder
- 840.4 Rotator cuff (capsule) sprain

CLINICAL PEARLS
- Rotator cuff disorders (tendinopathy, tears) are the most common source of shoulder pain in individuals >30 years of age.
- Shoulder instability (acute dislocation/subluxation or chronic instability) is the most common source of shoulder pain in individuals <30 years of age.

SILICOSIS

Ryung Suh, MD, MPP, MBA, MPH
Jaspal S. Ahluwalia, MD, MPH

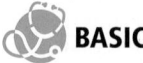 **BASICS**

DESCRIPTION

- Pneumoconiosis (fibrogenic) is caused by inhaling silica dust (in the form of quartz, cristobalite, or tridymite):
  – Chronic (classic) silicosis can be simple or complicated.
  – Chronic simple silicosis is asymptomatic and nonprogressive after the exposure ends and consists solely of small, round, radiographic pulmonary opacities.
  – Chronic complicated silicosis has progressively worsening symptoms and enlarging pulmonary opacities, even after exposure ends.
  – Subacute silicosis develops after 3–6 years of high exposure and resembles chronic complicated silicosis.
  – Acute silicosis develops within a couple years of massive exposure and is clinically distinct from the other forms.
- System(s) affected: Pulmonary

Geriatric Considerations
- Symptoms and complications more severe
- Unusual

EPIDEMIOLOGY

Incidence
- It has been reported that 3,600–7,300 cases/year of silicosis have been diagnosed in the US in the past several decades.
- Predominant age: 40–75 years
- Predominant sex: Male > Female

Prevalence
Over 200,000 miners and 1.7 million nonminers have some form of silicosis in the US.

RISK FACTORS
Industrial activities that involve cutting, polishing, or shearing rock or involve the use of sand, including:
- Metal mining (copper, silver, gold, lead, hard coal)
- Foundries
- Pottery making
- Sandstone cutting
- Granite cutting
- Highway repair (1)

Genetics
No known genetic pattern

GENERAL PREVENTION
- Avoid dust exposure.
- Substitute other materials for silica.
- Respiratory-protective devices for unavoidable short-term exposure

ETIOLOGY
- Chronic simple silicosis: 10–12 years of exposure to silica dust
- Chronic complicated silicosis: >20 years of exposure
- Subacute silicosis: 3–6 years of heavy exposure
- Acute silicosis: <2 years of massive exposure

COMMONLY ASSOCIATED CONDITIONS
- Tuberculosis (TB)
- Caplan syndrome (coexistence of rheumatoid arthritis with a pneumoconiosis)

 DIAGNOSIS

HISTORY
- Work-site exposure in coal mining, hard rock mining, tunneling, foundry work, steel work, and various other occupations
- Chronic simple silicosis: Asymptomatic
- Chronic complicated silicosis; subacute silicosis:
  – Chest tightness
  – Cough
  – Dyspnea
  – Expectoration
- Acute silicosis:
  – Dry cough
  – Fever
  – Severe dyspnea

PHYSICAL EXAM
- Chronic simple silicosis: Cough and mild dyspnea typically accompany and are due to smoking or occupational bronchitis.
- Chronic complicated silicosis; subacute silicosis: Signs of right-sided heart failure as cor pulmonale develops

DIAGNOSTIC TESTS & INTERPRETATION
Lab
Initial lab tests
Arterial blood gas (ABG) determination

Follow-Up & Special Considerations
- Pulmonary function testing is normal in simple silicosis. Other forms show decreased pulmonary compliance, decreased lung volumes, and decreased diffusing capacity.
- International Labor Office (ILO) classification system for quantification of CXR abnormalities
- Yearly purified protein derivative (PPD) test

Imaging
Initial approach
- CXR:
  – Chronic simple silicosis:
    ○ Eggshell calcification in hilar and mediastinal lymph nodes
    ○ Small, round opacities, initially in upper lobes
  – Chronic complicated silicosis, subacute silicosis (pulmonary opacities >1 cm):
    ○ Opacities form bilateral conglomerate shadows (progressive massive fibrosis).
    ○ Opacities initially peripheral, later migrate toward hilum
    ○ Opacities may cavitate (rule out TB).
- High-resolution CT scan provides more definition of infiltrates and is helpful in identifying nodules (2).

Diagnostic Procedures/Surgery
- Bronchoscopy
- Detailed occupational history
- Open lung biopsy

Pathological Findings

Lung:

- Pleural adhesions
- Pleural thickening
- Gray-black subpleural nodules
- Blackened lung
- Leathery lung
- Concentric layers of dense connective tissue
- Cellular infiltrate
- Ischemic degeneration of central nodule
- Metachromatic silica particles

DIFFERENTIAL DIAGNOSIS

- Chronic simple silicosis:
  - Sarcoidosis
  - Radiographic eggshell calcifications also seen in sarcoidosis and Hodgkin disease
- Chronic complicated silicosis, subacute silicosis:
  - Coal worker pneumoconiosis
  - Consider especially when consolidations are rapidly progressive, unilateral, or cavitating: TB, neoplasia, fungal pneumonia
- Acute silicosis: Alveolar proteinosis

 # TREATMENT

MEDICATION

First Line

- None specific for silicosis
- Isoniazid: 300 mg/d for 1 year if tuberculin skin test is positive
- Silicotuberculosis requires at least 3 antituberculous drugs initially, including rifampin.
- Contraindications: Avoid sedatives and hypnotics.

Second Line

Antifibrinogenic agents remain investigational.

ADDITIONAL TREATMENT

General Measures

- No known effective treatment
- Postural drainage
- Mist inhalation
- Chest physical therapy
- Breathing exercises

SURGERY/OTHER PROCEDURES

- Lung transplantation
- Whole-lung lavage remains investigational.

 # ONGOING CARE

FOLLOW-UP RECOMMENDATIONS

Patient Monitoring

- Monitor for heart failure and hypoxemia.
- Treat infections aggressively.

DIET

- No special diet
- Increase fluid intake.

PATIENT EDUCATION

Printed patient information is available from American Lung Association, 1740 Broadway, New York, NY 10019; (212) 315-8700.

PROGNOSIS

- Chronic simple silicosis: Remains asymptomatic and does not progress if exposure ends
- Chronic complicated silicosis; subacute silicosis: Progressive pulmonary fibrosis with cor pulmonale and right-sided heart failure, even after exposure ends

COMPLICATIONS

- Progressive massive fibrosis
- Respiratory infection
- Pneumothorax
- Emphysema
- Cor pulmonale
- Right-sided heart failure
- Mycobacterial infections
- Fungal infections

REFERENCES

1. Valiante DJ, Schill DP, Rosenman KD, et al. Highway repair: a new silicosis threat. *Am J Public Health*. 2004;94:876–80.
2. Arakawa H, Fujimoto K, Honma K, et al. Progression from near-normal to end-stage lungs in chronic interstitial pneumonia related to silica exposure: long-term CT observations. *AJR Am J Roentgenol*. 2008;191:1040–5.
3. Diseases associated with exposure to silica and nonfibrous silicate minerals. Silicosis and Silicate Disease Committee. *Arch Pathol Lab Med*. 1988;112:673–720.

ADDITIONAL READING

- Banks DE, Cheng YH, Weber SL, et al. Strategies for the treatment of pneumoconiosis. *Occup Med*. 1993;8:205–32.
- Greenberg MI, Waksman J, Curtis J, et al. Silicosis: a review. *Dis Mon*. 2007;53:394–416.
- Hertzberg VS, Rosenman KD, Reilly MJ, et al. Effect of occupational silica exposure on pulmonary function. *Chest*. 2002;122:721–8.
- Rees D, Murray J. Silica, silicosis and tuberculosis. *Int J Tuberc Lung Dis*. 2007;11:474–84.

See Also (Topic, Algorithm, Electronic Media Element)

Chronic Obstructive Pulmonary Disease and Emphysema; Cor Pulmonale; Pneumothorax; Tuberculosis

 # CODES

ICD9

502 Pneumoconiosis due to other silica or silicates

CLINICAL PEARLS

- Chronic silicosis is generally diagnosed by radiology alone because it does not produce symptoms. If symptoms are present, this indicates that the silicosis has progressed to another disease process such as TB, chronic obstructive pulmonary disease (COPD), or neoplasm (3).
- Diagnosis is made using a combination of history of occupational exposure and radiographic evidence of pulmonary opacities and calcifications.
- Patients with silicosis are at a much higher risk for TB and must have a yearly PPD skin test.

SINUSITIS

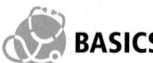

Adarsh K. Gupta, DO, MS

BASICS

DESCRIPTION
- Acute sinusitis is a symptomatic inflammation of one or more paranasal sinuses of <4 weeks' duration resulting from impaired drainage and retained secretions. Because rhinitis and sinusitis usually coexist, "rhinosinusitis" is the preferred term.
- Disease is subacute when symptomatic for 4–12 weeks and chronic when symptomatic for >12 weeks.
- System(s) affected: HEENT; Pulmonary

EPIDEMIOLOGY
- It affects 31 million individuals in the US each year with an estimated annual cost of $5.8 billion.
- Diagnosis of acute bacterial rhinosinusitis remains the 5th leading reason for prescribing antibiotics.
- About 0.2% to 2% episodes of viral rhinosinusitis have bacterial superinfection.

Incidence
Incidence highest in early fall through early spring (related to incidence of viral upper respiratory infection [URI]). Adults have 2 or 3 viral URIs per year; 90% of these colds are accompanied by viral rhinosinusitis.

RISK FACTORS
- Viral URI
- Allergic rhinitis
- Asthma
- Cigarette smoking
- Dental infections and procedures
- Anatomic variations:
  - Tonsillar and adenoid hypertrophy
  - Turbinate hypertrophy, nasal polyps
  - Deviated septum
  - Cleft palate
- Immunodeficiency (e.g., HIV)
- Cystic fibrosis

Genetics
No known genetic pattern

GENERAL PREVENTION
Hand-washing to prevent transmission of viral infection

PATHOPHYSIOLOGY
- Important features:
  - Inflammation and edema of the sinus mucosa
  - Obstruction of the sinus ostia
  - Impaired mucociliary clearance
- Secretions that are not cleared become hospitable to bacterial growth.
- Inflammatory response (neutrophil influx and release of cytokines) damages mucosal surfaces.

ETIOLOGY
- Viral: Vast majority of cases (rhinovirus, influenza A and B, parainfluenza virus, respiratory syncytial, adeno-, corona-, and enteroviruses)
- Bacterial (complicates 0.2–2% of viral cases):
  - More likely if symptoms worsen after 5–7 days or do not improve >10 days
  - *S. pneumoniae, H. influenzae,* and *M. catarrhalis* are the most common bacterial pathogens.
  - Often overdiagnosed, which leads to overuse of and increasing resistance to antibiotics
- Fungal: Seen in immunocompromised hosts (uncontrolled diabetes, neutropenia, use of corticosteroids) or as a nosocomial infection

DIAGNOSIS

History and physical exam suggest and establish the diagnosis but are rarely helpful in distinguishing bacterial from viral causes.

HISTORY
- Major challenge is to distinguish between viral and bacterial disease; use constellation of symptoms rather than a particular sign or symptom.

ALERT
- Symptom most predictive of bacterial sinusitis is worsening of symptoms >5–7 days after initial improvement.
- Symptoms somewhat predictive of bacterial sinusitis:
  - Worsening of symptoms >5–7 days after initial improvement
  - Persistent symptoms for ≥10 days
  - Persistent purulent nasal discharge
  - Unilateral upper tooth or facial pain
  - Unilateral maxillary sinus tenderness
  - Fever
- Associated symptoms:
  - Headache
  - Nasal congestion
  - Retroorbital pain
  - Otalgia
  - Hyposomia
  - Halitosis
  - Chronic cough
- Symptoms requiring urgent attention:
  - Visual disturbances, especially diplopia
  - Periorbital swelling or erythema
  - Altered mental status

PHYSICAL EXAM
- Fever
- Edema and erythema of nasal mucosa
- Purulent discharge
- Tenderness to palpation over sinus(es)

Pediatric Considerations
- Sinuses are not fully developed until age 20. Maxillary and ethmoid sinuses, although small, are present from birth.
- Since children have an average of 6–8 colds per year, they are at risk for developing sinusitis.
- Diagnosis can be more difficult than in adults because symptoms are often more subtle.

DIAGNOSTIC TESTS & INTERPRETATION
Diagnostic tests are not routinely recommended, as there are no diagnostic tests that can adequately differentiate between viral and bacterial rhinosinusitis.

Lab
- None indicated in routine evaluation
- Transillumination of the sinuses may confirm fluid in sinuses (helpful if asymmetric; not helpful if symmetric exam).

Imaging
- Routine use of sinus radiography discouraged because
  - ≥3 clinical findings have similar diagnostic accuracy as imaging.
  - Imaging does not distinguish viral from bacterial etiology.
- Limited coronal CT scan can be useful in recurrent infection or failure to respond to medical therapy.

Diagnostic Procedures/Surgery
- Value of imaging studies is limited because they do not distinguish between viral and bacterial etiology.
- Sinus CT scanning may be warranted if symptoms or sign suggest extrasinus involvement or for evaluation of chronic rhinosinusitis (1).

Pathological Findings
- Inflammation
- Edema
- Thickened mucosa
- Impaired ciliary function
- Metaplasia of ciliated columnar cells
- Relative acidosis and hypoxia within sinuses
- Polyps

DIFFERENTIAL DIAGNOSIS
- Dental disease
- CF
- Wegener granulomatosis
- HIV infection
- Kartagener syndrome
- Immotile cilia syndrome
- Neoplasm
- Headache, tension or migraine

TREATMENT

Most cases of acute rhinosinusitis resolve with supportive care (treating pain, nasal symptoms). Antibiotics should be reserved for symptoms that persists more than 10 days or gets worse in 5 to 7 days.

MEDICATION
First Line
- Decongestants:
  - Pseudoephedrine HCl
  - Phenylephrine nasal spray (limited use)
  - Oxymetazoline nasal spray (e.g., Afrin) (not to be used >3 days)
- Analgesics:
  - Acetaminophen
  - Aspirin
  - NSAIDs
  - Acetaminophen codeine (for severe cases)
- Antibiotics:
  - In large case series, antibiotics have a slight advantage over placebo, yet most patients improve without therapy (NNT 15 to prevent 1 persistent case at follow-up).
  - Reserve antibiotic use for patients with moderate to severe disease.
  - Treat for 10–14 days unless otherwise specified.
  - Choice should be based on understanding of antibiotic resistance in the community.
  - Initial therapy (narrow-spectrum antibiotics) (2,3)[A]:
    - Amoxicillin: 1 g t.i.d. (adults); 80–90 mg/kg/d divided q8h (children)
    - Trimethoprim-sulfamethoxazole (TMP/SMX): 160/800 mg q12h in adults and 8–12 mg/kg/d of trimethoprim component divided q12h for children
    - Doxycycline: 100 mg p.o. b.i.d. (adults only)
- Since allergies may be a predisposing factor, some patients may benefit from use of the following agents:
  - Oral antihistamines:

○ Loratadine (Claritin), fexofenadine (Allegra), cetirizine (Zyrtec), Clarinex (desloratadine), or Xyzal (levocetirizine)
○ Chlorpheniramine (Chlor-Trimeton)
○ Diphenhydramine (Benadryl)
– Leukotriene inhibitors (Singulair, Accolate), especially in patients with asthma
– Nasal steroids (i.e., fluticasone [Flonase])

Second Line
• Amoxicillin-clavulanate (Augmentin): 875/125 mg q12h (adults); 30 mg/kg/d of amoxicillin component divided b.i.d. in children
• High-dose amoxicillin-clavulanate (Augmentin XR) b.i.d. in adults and Augmentin ES-600 in children (for both β-lactam and penicillin-binding protein resistance)
• Cefpodoxime (Vantin): 200 mg q12h in adults and 10 mg/kg/d divided b.i.d. in children
• Cefuroxime axetil (Ceftin): 250 mg q12h in adults and 30 mg/kg/d divided q12h in children
• Azithromycin (Zithromax): 500 mg on day 1 and 250 mg on days 2–5 in adults; 10 mg/kg on day 1 and 5 mg/kg on days 2–5 in children
• Clarithromycin (Biaxin): 500 mg b.i.d. (regular) or 1,000 mg/d (extended release) in adults; 15 mg/kg/d divided b.i.d. in children
• Levofloxacin (Levaquin): 750 mg/d for 5 days (adults only)
• If no response to 1st-line therapy after 72 hours, or if patients have had antibiotics within the past 4–6 weeks, use or change to
– High-dose amoxicillin-clavulanate
– Cephalosporins as above
– Fluoroquinolones as above
• *Note:* Bacteriologic failure rates of up to 20–25% are possible with use of azithromycin and clarithromycin (2)[C].
• If lack of response to 3 weeks of antibiotics, consider
– CT scan of sinuses
– ENT referral

ALERT
• When bacterial infection is present, patients recover somewhat more quickly with antibiotics, but the majority will recover with symptomatic treatment alone (3)[A].
• Multiple meta-analyses have demonstrated *no* benefit of newer antibiotics over amoxicillin, trimethoprim-sulfamethoxazole, or doxycycline (3)[A].
• Use of intranasal steroids produces modest improvement in symptoms when used alone or in combination with antibiotics (4)[B].
• Precautions:
– Decongestants can exacerbate HTN.
– Intranasal decongestants might relieve nasal congestion but should be limited to 3 days to avoid rebound nasal congestion.
– Sulfonamides may induce Stevens-Johnson syndrome (risk 1/2,000). Inform patients to report any mucous membrane ulcerations.
– Significant possible interactions:
○ Warfarin (Coumadin): Increased effect of warfarin with macrolides or TMP/SMX, resulting in marked increase in INR and PT
○ Statins should be stopped temporarily when macrolides are prescribed owing to increased risk of myopathy and rhabdomyolysis.

Pregnancy Considerations
• Rhinitis of pregnancy predisposes to sinusitis.
• Nasal irrigation with saline, pseudoephedrine, most antihistamines, and some nasal steroids is safe during pregnancy and lactation.
• Antibiotics considered to be safe in pregnancy and lactation:
– Amoxicillin and amoxicillin-clavulanate (B)
– Cephalosporins (B), Azithromycin (B)
• Antibiotic contraindicated in pregnancy and lactation: Clarithromycin
• Antibiotic safe in lactation but not during pregnancy: Levofloxacin

ADDITIONAL TREATMENT
General Measures
• Hydration
• Steam inhalation 20–30 minutes t.i.d.
• Saline irrigation (Neti pot) or nose drops
• Sleep with head of bed elevated.
• Avoid exposure to cigarette smoke or fumes.
• Avoid caffeine and alcohol.
• Antibiotics indicated only when findings suggest bacterial infection
• Analgesics, NSAIDs (see below)
• Acute viral sinusitis is self-limiting, and antibiotics should not be used.

Issues for Referral
Complications or failure of treatment

SURGERY/OTHER PROCEDURES
• If medical therapy fails, consider sinus irrigation.
• Functional endoscopic sinus surgery is the preferred treatment for medically recalcitrant cases (2)[C].
• Absolute surgical indications:
– Massive nasal polyposis
– Acute complications: Subperiosteal or orbital abscess, frontal soft-tissue spread of infection
– Mucocele or mucopyocele
– Invasive or allergic fungal sinusitis
– Suspected obstructing tumor
– CSF rhinorrhea

IN-PATIENT CONSIDERATIONS
• Most patients are treated in outpatient setting.
• Hospitalization for complications (e.g., meningitis, orbital cellulitis or abscess, brain abscess)

ONGOING CARE
FOLLOW-UP RECOMMENDATIONS
• Return if no improvement after 72 hours or no resolution of symptoms after 10 days of antibiotics.
• If symptoms resolve, no follow-up is needed.

PATIENT EDUCATION
http://familydoctor.org OR http://medlineplus.gov

PROGNOSIS
Alleviation of symptoms within 72 hours with complete resolution within 10–14 days

COMPLICATIONS
• Serious complications are rare.
• Meningitis, orbital cellulitis, brain abscess
• Cavernous sinus thrombosis
• Osteomyelitis, subdural empyema

REFERENCES
1. Dykewicz MS, Hamilos DL, et al. Rhinitis and sinusitis. *J Allergy Clin Immunol.* 2010;125: S103–15.
2. Varonen H, Mäkelä M, Savolainen S, et al. Comparison of ultrasound, radiography, and clinical examination in the diagnosis of acute maxillary sinusitis: a systematic review. *J Clin Epidemiol.* 2000;53:940–8.
3. Williams JW Jr, et al. Antibiotics for acute maxillary sinusitis. *Cochrane Database Sys Rev.* 2003;2: CD000243.
4. Zalmanovici A, et al. Steroids for acute sinusitis. *Cochrane Database Sys Rev.* 2007;2:CD005149.

ADDITIONAL READING
• Anon JB, Jacobs MR, Poole MD, et al. Antimicrobial treatment guidelines for acute bacterial rhinosinusitis. *Otolaryngol Head Neck Surg.* 2004;130:1–45.
• Rosenfeld RM, Andes D, Bhattacharyya N, et al. Clinical practice guideline: adult sinusitis. *Otolaryngol Head Neck Surg.* 2007;137:S1–31.
• Sande MA, Gwaltney JM. Acute community-acquired bacterial sinusitis: continuing challenges and current management. *Clin Infect Dis.* 2004; 39(Suppl 3):S151–8.

CODES

ICD9
• 461.0 Acute maxillary sinusitis
• 461.2 Acute ethmoidal sinusitis
• 461.3 Acute sphenoidal sinusitis

CLINICAL PEARLS
• When bacterial infection is present, patients recover somewhat more quickly with antibiotics, but the majority will recover with symptomatic treatment alone, and accurate diagnosis of bacterial sinusitis is very difficult (3)[A].
• Multiple meta-analyses have demonstrated *no* benefit of newer antibiotics over amoxicillin, trimethoprim-sulfamethoxazole, or doxycycline (3)[A].
• Overall NNT to prevent one persistent case at follow-up 15; NNT-H (harm) owing to antibiotic-associated diarrhea is similar.
• Significant patient symptom relief with nasal saline spray or drops or irrigation (Neti pot)

S

SJÖGREN'S SYNDROME

Katrina Darlene Zedan, MSPAS, PA-C
Alyssa H. Tran, DO

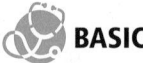 ## BASICS

- Chronic inflammatory disorder characterized by lymphocytic infiltrates in exocrine organs
- Typically presents with diminished salivary and lacrimal gland function, manifested as sicca symptoms such as:
  – Dry eyes, dry mouth, and enlargement of the parotid glands
  – Extraglandular symptoms may also be present, such as arthralgia, arthritis, Raynaud phenomenon, myalgia, pulmonary disease, GI disease, leukopenia, anemia, lymphadenopathy, neuropathy, vasculitis, renal tubular acidosis, and lymphoma
- Primary Sjögren: Not associated with other diseases
- Secondary Sjögren: Complication of other rheumatologic conditions, most commonly rheumatoid arthritis

EPIDEMIOLOGY

Incidence
- Depending on the study, annual incidence is about 4/100,000–4.8% of population. Variability is likely due to the different criteria used in diagnosis.
- People of all races are affected.
- Predominant sex: Female > Male (9:1)
- Predominant age: Can affect patients of any age, but is most common in the elderly; onset typically occurs in the 4th–5th decades of life

Prevalence
0.1–3% of the population is affected, but this also reflects the lack of uniform diagnostic criteria. It is observed throughout the world.

RISK FACTORS
There are no known modifiable risk factors.

Genetics
Sjögren's syndrome (SS) has a familial tendency and seems to be associated with family members with a wide variety of autoimmune diseases.

GENERAL PREVENTION
- No known prevention, but complications can be prevented by diagnosing and treating early.
- Dentists can play a key role in early detection of SS as well as management of oral symptoms that result from salivary dysfunction (1)[A].

PATHOPHYSIOLOGY
- Systemic autoimmune disease
- Characterized by infiltration of glandular tissue primarily by CD4 T-lymphocytes
- A theory is that glandular epithelial cells present antigen to the T cells. Cytokine production then occurs, and there is also evidence for B-cell activation, resulting in autoantibody production and increased incidence of B-cell malignancies.

ETIOLOGY
Etiology is unknown. Estrogen may play a role because SS is more common in women.

COMMONLY ASSOCIATED CONDITIONS
May be primary or secondary (associated with rheumatoid arthritis, scleroderma, systemic lupus erythematosus (SLE), polymyositis, HIV, hepatitis C)

 ## DIAGNOSIS

- There is no single diagnostic test. Diagnosis is made by presence of compatible clinical signs and symptoms, as well as lab tests, and after exclusion of other causes.
- International consensus criteria for SS (2)[C]:
  – Ocular signs and symptoms (at least 1 present):
    ○ Persistent, troublesome dry eyes every day for longer than 3 months
    ○ Recurrent sensation of sand or gravel in the eyes *or*
    ○ Use of tear substitute >3 times/day
  – Oral signs and symptoms (at least 1 present):
    ○ Feeling of dry mouth every day for at least 3 months
    ○ Recurrent feeling of swollen salivary glands as an adult *or*
    ○ Need to drink liquids to aid in swallowing dry foods
  – Objective evidence of dry eyes (at least 1 present):
    ○ Schirmer test
    ○ Rose bengal
    ○ Lacrimal gland biopsy sample with focus score >1
  – Objective evidence of salivary gland involvement (at least 1 present):
    ○ Salivary gland scintigraphy
    ○ Parotid sialography
    ○ Unstimulated whole sialometry
  – Laboratory abnormality (at least 1 present):
    ○ Anti-SS-A or anti-SS-B
    ○ Antinuclear antibodies (ANAs)
    ○ IgM rheumatoid factor (anti-IgG Fc)
- Exclusion criteria: Prior head/neck irradiation, infection with hepatitis C, AIDS, lymphoma, sarcoidosis, graft-versus-host disease, recent use of anticholinergic medications (2)[C]
- Patients who fulfill 4 or more of the criteria likely have SS.

HISTORY
- Decreased tear production, burning, scratchy sensation in eyes
- Difficulty speaking/swallowing; dental caries; xerotrachea
- Enlarged parotid glands or intermittent swelling (bilateral)
- Dyspareunia

PHYSICAL EXAM
Some common physical exam findings include:
- Eye exam: Dry eyes (keratoconjunctivitis sicca), decreased tear pool in the lower conjunctiva, dilated conjunctival vessels, mucinous threads, and filamentary keratosis can be detected during a slit-lamp examination.
- Mouth exam: Dry mouth (xerostomia), decreased sublingual salivary pool, tongue may stick to the tongue depressor, frequent caries—sometimes in unusual locations such as the incisor surface and the gum line, deep red tongue from prolonged xerostomia

- Ear, nose, and throat exam: Bilateral parotid gland enlargement, submandibular gland enlargement
- Skin exam: Nonpalpable or palpable vasculitic purpura with lesions that are typically 2–3 mm in diameter and located on the lower extremities
- Other manifestations: Chronic arthritis, interstitial nephritis (40%), type I rheumatoid arthritis (20%), vasculitis (25%), vaginal dryness, pleuritis, pancreatitis

DIAGNOSTIC TESTS & INTERPRETATION
In addition to history and physical exam, the following tests are recommended when SS is suspected:
- Schirmer test
- Rose bengal test
- Basic labs, special labs (see below)
- MRI with fat suppression, CXR, minor salivary gland biopsy

Lab
- Most have autoantibodies: +ANAs (95%), +RF (75%)
- In primary SS: +anti-Ro (anti SS-A, 56%) and +anti-La (anti-SS-B, 30%)

Initial lab tests
Preliminary lab workup:
- Basic labs: CBC with differential, blood urea nitrogen (BUN)/creatinine (Cr), AST/ALT, erythrocyte sedimentation rate (ESR), C-reactive protein (CRP), urinalysis (UA)
- Special labs: ANA, rheumatoid factor (RF), anti-Ro/SS-A, anti-La/SS-B, anti-Sm, anti-RNP, anti-dsDNA, serum C3 and C4, cryoglobulins, SPEP, UPEP, IgM, IgG, IgA
- Other: HIV, hepatitis C, CXR, minor salivary gland biopsy, MRI with fat suppression

Imaging
Initial imaging studies may include (3)[C]:
- Imaging for xerostomia: Salivary gland scintigraphy (insensitive but highly specific)
- Parotid gland sialography (should not be used in acute parotitis)
- MRI (correlates well with salivary gland biopsy)

Initial approach
MRI with fat suppression (3)[B]

Diagnostic Procedures/Surgery
- Salivary gland biopsy: Used to confirm suspected diagnosis of SS or exclusion of other causes of xerostomia and bilateral gland enlargement
- Schirmer test (2)[B]
- Rose bengal test (2)[B]
- Perform a biopsy on the parotid gland if malignancy is suggested.
- Perform a biopsy on an enlarged lymph node to help rule out pseudolymphoma or lymphoma.

Pathological Findings
Salivary gland biopsy: Histology shows focal collections of lymphocytes; immunocytology shows that most of the lymphocytes are CD4+ T cells.

DIFFERENTIAL DIAGNOSIS

- Causes of ocular dryness: Hypovitaminosis A, decreased tear production unrelated to autoimmune process, chronic blepharitis or conjunctivitis, impaired blinking (i.e., due to Parkinson disease or Bell palsy), working long hours at a computer, infiltration of lacrimal glands (i.e., amyloidosis, lymphoma, sarcoidosis), low estrogen levels
- Causes of oral dryness: Anticholinergic medications, sialadenitis due to chronic obstruction, chronic viral infections (i.e., hepatitis C or HIV), irradiation of head and neck
- Causes of salivary gland swelling: Unilateral: bacterial infection, neoplasm; bilateral: acute or chronic viral infection (i.e., mumps, Epstein–Barr virus [EBV], coxsackievirus, echovirus, HIV, hepatitis C), granulomatous diseases (i.e., tuberculosis, sarcoidosis), malnutrition, alcoholism, bulimia, acromegaly, diabetes

 TREATMENT

- Treatment is primarily supportive care and treating symptoms that are problematic to patients.
- Treatment of dry eyes
- Topical therapy for dry mouth
- Treatment of systemic manifestations
- Addressing fatigue, vague complaints, and pain syndromes

MEDICATION

- Usually only requires local therapy for sicca symptoms secretions and tears
- Immunosuppressive therapy such as hydroxychloroquine can be used for systemic symptoms; however, has not shown any benefit in relieving refractory sicca symptoms.
- Topical therapy for dry mouth: Can be as simple as liberally drinking sips of water, trying sugar-free lemon drops or artificial saliva preparations such as Salivart, Saliment, Xero-Lube, Mouthkote (4)
- Depends on the severity of eye dryness, which is best determined by an ophthalmologist. Dry eyes are graded according to degree of symptoms, conjunctival injection and staining, corneal damage, tear quality, and lid involvement. Artificial tears may be used; however, artificial tears with hydroxymethylcellulose or dextran are more viscous and can last longer.
- Acetaminophen or nonsteroidal anti-inflammatory drugs (NSAIDs) can be taken for arthralgias.

First Line

- Xerostomia: Sugar-free lozenges, especially malic acid (3)[B], pilocarpine (3)[A], cevimeline (dose of 30 mg t.i.d. showed significant improvement (3)[A]), artificial saliva
- Keratoconjunctivitis sicca: Artificial tears and ocular lubricants for symptomatic relief (3)[C], topical cyclosporine (3)[A]

Second Line

- Xerostomia: Interferon-alfa lozenges may enhance salivary gland flow (3)[B].

- Keratoconjunctivitis sicca: Emerging therapies include diquafosol (pending FDA approval) and topical NSAIDs (use with caution).

- Immunosuppressive therapy: Antimalarials (e.g., hydroxychloroquine) for arthralgias, lymphadeno-pathies, and skin manifestations (3)[B]; may then consider methotrexate or cyclosporine, which showed subjective improvement but no significant objective improvement
- Early studies show improvement in fatigue with rituximab (5)[B].

- For life-threatening extraglandular manifestations, cyclophosphamide (oral or IV), mycophenolate mofetil, and azathioprine are often used.

ADDITIONAL TREATMENT

- Patients should use vaginal lubricants, such as Replens, for vaginal dryness. Vaginal estrogen creams can be considered in postmenopausal women. Watch for and treat vaginal yeast infections (4).
- Xerostomia: Small sips of water, good dental care
- Keratoconjunctivitis sicca: Conservation of tears with side shields or ski/swim goggles, humidifiers, moist washcloths
- DHEA does not offer improvement in fatigue and well-being greater than placebo (6)[B].

Issues for Referral

- Systemic manifestations or resistant symptoms
- Rheumatology, as a rheumatologist is key in the management of patients with Sjögren syndrome
- Dentistry, for routine oral care is necessary
- Ophthalmology, for grading of severity of eye dryness

COMPLEMENTARY AND ALTERNATIVE MEDICINE

Studies show unclear and conflicting data on the efficacy of acupuncture.

SURGERY/OTHER PROCEDURES

Keratoconjunctivitis sicca: If refractory to artificial tears, punctal occlusion is the treatment of choice.

IN-PATIENT CONSIDERATIONS

May be required for extraglandular manifestations, such as cardiopulmonary disease, renal involvement, and CNS manifestations (e.g., optic neuritis, transverse myelitis, vasculitis, or ischemic stroke)

 ONGOING CARE

FOLLOW-UP RECOMMENDATIONS

Frequency of follow-up depends on severity.

Patient Monitoring

- Monitor for complications, systemic manifestations, and relief of symptoms.
- Medicolegal pitfalls: Failure to monitor and evaluate for parotid tumor or lymphoma

PATIENT EDUCATION

Explanation of SS is essential. In most cases, simple measures are adequate, such as humidifiers, sips of water, chewing gum, or artificial tears.

PROGNOSIS

- Risk of lymphoma is increased
- Hypocomplementemia is an independent risk factor for premature death.

COMPLICATIONS

Complications include dental caries, gum disease, dysphagia, salivary gland calculi, keratitis, conjunctivitis, and scarring of the ocular surface.

REFERENCES

1. Stewart CM, Berg KM, Cha S et al. Salivary dysfunction and quality of life in sjogren syndrome: a critical oral-systemic connection. *J Am Dent Assoc.* 2008;139:291–9.
2. Fox, RI. Sjogren's syndrome. *Lancet.* 2005;366:321.
3. von Bültzingslöwen I, Sollecito TP, Fox PC, et al. Salivary dysfunction associated with systemic diseases: systematic review and clinical management recommendations. *Oral Surg Oral Med Oral Pathol Oral Radiol Endod.* 2007; 103(Suppl):S57.e1–15.
4. Miller, Anne V, et al. *"Sjogren Syndrome: Treatment & Medications"*. Online Reference: http://emedicine.medscape.com/article/332125-treatment. Assessed: 8/21/2010.
5. Dass S, Bowman SJ, Vital EM, et al. Reduction of fatigue in Sjogren's syndrome with rituximab: results of a randomised, double-blind, placebo controlled pilot study. *Ann Rheum Dis.* 2008.
6. Hartkamp A, Geenen R, Godaert GL, et al. Effect of dehydroepiandrosterone administration on fatigue, well-being, and functioning in women with primary Sjögren's Syndrome. A randomized controlled trial. *Ann Rheum Dis.* 2007.
7. Fischer A, Swigris JJ, du Bois RM, et al. Minor Salivary Gland Biopsy To Detect Primary Sjogren Syndrome in Patients With Interstitial Lung Disease. *Chest.* 2009.

ADDITIONAL READING

- Gálvez J, Sáiz E, López P, et al. Diagnostic evaluation and classification criteria in Sjögren's Syndrome. *Joint Bone Spine.* 2008.
- Voulgarelis M, Tzioufas AG, Moutsopoulos HM. Mortality in Sjögren's syndrome. *Clin Exp Rheumatol.* 2008;26:S66–71.

 CODES

ICD9
710.2 Sicca syndrome

CLINICAL PEARLS

- Many symptoms can be treated with nonprescription interventions such as artificial tears and sugar-free lozenges.
- Consider lacrimal duct plugs for dry eyes (placed under local anesthetic by an ophthalmologist).
- Consider minor salivary gland biopsy to confirm diagnosis in the setting of interstitial lung disease (7)[B].

SLEEP APNEA, OBSTRUCTIVE

Anjali Koka, MD

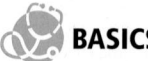

BASICS

DESCRIPTION
- *Obstructive sleep apnea* (OSA) is defined as repetitive episodes of cessation of airflow (apnea) at the nose and mouth during sleep due to obstruction at the level of the pharynx:
  - Apneas often terminate with a snort or gasp.
  - Repetitive apneas produce sleep disruption, leading to excessive daytime sleepiness.
  - Associated with oxygen desaturation and nocturnal hypoxemia
  - Usual course is chronic
- System(s) affected: Cardiovascular; Nervous; Pulmonary
- Synonyms: Pickwickian syndrome; Sleep apnea syndrome; Nocturnal upper airway occlusion

EPIDEMIOLOGY
Incidence
- Predominant age: Middle-aged men and women
- Predominant sex: Male > Female (2–3:1)

Prevalence
- Up to 4% in men, 2% in women
- Prevalence is higher in obese or hypertensive patients.

RISK FACTORS
- Obesity
- Male sex
- Age > 40 years
- Alcohol/sedative intake before bedtime
- Smoking
- Nasal obstruction (due to polyps, rhinitis, or deviated septum)
- Anatomic narrowing of nasopharynx (e.g., tonsillar hypertrophy, macroglossia, micrognathia, retrognathia, craniofacial abnormalities)
- Acromegaly
- Hypothyroidism
- Neurologic syndromes (e.g., muscular dystrophy, cerebral palsy)

GENERAL PREVENTION
Weight loss and avoidance of alcohol and sedatives at night can help to prevent airway collapse.

PATHOPHYSIOLOGY
OSA occurs when the naso- or oropharynx collapses passively during inspiration. Anatomic and neuromuscular factors contribute to pharyngeal collapse:
- Anatomic abnormalities, such as increased soft tissue in the palate, tonsillar hypertrophy, macroglossia, and craniofacial abnormalities, predispose the airway to collapse by decreasing the area of the upper airway or by increasing the pressure surrounding the airway.
- During sleep, decreased muscle tone in the naso- or oropharynx contributes to airway obstruction and collapse.

ETIOLOGY
Upper airway narrowing may be due to:
- Obesity, redundant tissue in the soft palate
- Enlarged tonsils or uvula
- Low soft palate
- Large or posteriorly located tongue
- Craniofacial abnormalities
- Neuromuscular disorders
- Alcohol or sedative use before bedtime

COMMONLY ASSOCIATED CONDITIONS
- Hypertension (common)
- Obesity (common)
- Daytime sleepiness (common)
- Metabolic syndrome (common)
- Cardiovascular disease (rare)
- Congestive heart failure (rare)
- Stroke (rare)
- Pulmonary hypertension (rare)
- Nasal obstructive problems (rare)

DIAGNOSIS

HISTORY
Be sure to elicit a complete history of daytime and nighttime symptoms. Symptoms can be insidious and present for years:
- Daytime symptoms:
  - Excessive daytime sleepiness (EDS) or fatigue (cardinal symptom):
    - Mild symptoms occur during quiet activities (e.g., reading, watching television).
    - Severe symptoms occur during dynamic activities (e.g., work, driving).
  - Tired on morning awakening
  - Sore or dry throat
  - Poor concentration, memory problems, irritability, mood changes
  - Morning headaches
  - Decreased libido
  - Depression
- Nighttime symptoms:
  - Loud snoring (present in 60% of people with OSA)
  - Snort or gasp that arouses patient from sleep
  - Disrupted sleep
  - Witnessed apneic episodes at night

PHYSICAL EXAM
- Most patients have a normal physical exam. However, OSA is commonly associated with hypertension, obesity, or sleepiness.
- Focused head and neck exam:
  - Short neck with large circumference
  - Oropharynx:
    - Narrowing of the lateral airway wall
    - Tonsillar hypertrophy
    - Macroglossia
    - Micrognathia or retrognathia
    - Soft palate edema
    - Long or thick uvula
    - High, arched hard palate
  - Nasopharynx:
    - Deviated nasal septum
    - Poor nasal airflow

DIAGNOSTIC TESTS & INTERPRETATION
Lab
Initial lab tests
When clinically indicated:
- Thyroid-stimulating hormone to evaluate hypothyroidism
- Complete blood count to evaluate anemia and polycythemia, which can indicate nocturnal hypoxemia
- Fasting glucose in obesity to evaluate for diabetes
- Rare: Arterial blood gases to evaluate daytime hypercapnia

Imaging
Cephalometric measurements from lateral head and neck radiographs aid in surgical treatment.

Diagnostic Procedures/Surgery
- The gold standard for OSA is polysomnography (PSG), a nighttime sleep study:
  - Demonstrates severity of hypoxemia, sleep disruption, and cardiac arrhythmias associated with OSA and elevated end-tidal CO_2
  - Shows repetitive episodes of cessation or marked reduction in airflow despite continued respiratory efforts
  - Apneic episodes must last at least 10 s and occur 10–15×/h to be considered clinically significant.
  - Complete PSG is expensive, and health insurance may not cover the cost.
- Multiple sleep latency testing is a diagnostic tool used to measure the time it takes from the start of a daytime nap period to the 1st signs of sleep (sleep latency). It provides an objective measurement of daytime sleepiness.
- The *apnea/hypoapnea index* (AHI) is defined as the total number of apneas and hypopneas divided by the total sleep time:
  - Mild OSA: AHI = 5–15
  - Moderate OSA: AHI = 15–30
  - Severe OSA: AHI >30
- Drugs that may alter the test results include benzodiazepines and other sedatives that can amplify the severity of apnea seen during the sleep study.

DIFFERENTIAL DIAGNOSIS
- Other causes of excessive daytime sleepiness, such as:
  - Narcolepsy
  - Idiopathic daytime hypersomnolence
  - Inadequate sleep time
  - Depressive episodes with excessive daytime sleepiness
  - Periodic limb movements disorder
- Respiratory disorders with nocturnal awakenings, such as:
  - Asthma
  - Chronic obstructive pulmonary disease
  - Congestive heart failure
- Central sleep apnea
- Sleep-related choking or laryngospasm
- Gastroesophageal reflux
- Sleep-associated seizures (temporal lobe epilepsy)

TREATMENT

- Weight loss
- Avoid alcohol, smoking, and sedatives, especially before bedtime.
- Significantly sleepy patients should not drive a motor vehicle or operate dangerous equipment.
- The most effective treatment for OSA is nasal continuous positive airway pressure (CPAP). CPAP prevents the soft tissue in the pharynx from collapsing, thus eliminating apneas and restoring oxygen saturation. CPAP restores regular nighttime breathing and not only reduces snoring and EDS, but also lowers blood pressure over the short term (1)[A] and may also decrease the risk for stroke (2)[B] and atherosclerosis (3)[B].
- CPAP therapy initially can be difficult to tolerate and requires perseverance.
- If OSA is present only when supine, keep the patient off his or her back when sleeping (e.g., tennis ball worn on back of nightshirt).

MEDICATION
Medications are yet to be proven effective in treating OSA (4). Further studies in this area are needed.

First Line
Some short-term data found fluticasone nasal spray, mirtazapine, physostigmine, and nasal lubricant of some benefit; longer-term studies needed (4)[A].

ADDITIONAL TREATMENT
- Dental appliances advance the mandible and tongue, helping the airway to stay open during sleep. When compared with nasal CPAP, dental appliances decreased AHI to a lesser extent (5).
- CPAP has been shown to improve OSA symptoms better than dental appliances. However, patients who are unable to tolerate CPAP may benefit from dental appliances.

Issues for Referral
If sleep apnea is suspected, patient should be referred to a sleep specialist/neurologist for a sleep study evaluation.

SURGERY/OTHER PROCEDURES
Surgical corrections of the upper airway include uvulopalatopharyngoplasty (UPPP), tracheostomy, and craniofacial surgery. Studies do not support the use of UPPP to improve symptoms of OSA (6).

IN-PATIENT CONSIDERATIONS
On admission, patients should continue to use CPAP or dental device if they do so at home. They should bring in their own appliance and know their CPAP settings.

ONGOING CARE

Lifelong compliance with weight loss or CPAP is necessary for successful OSA treatment.

DIET
Overweight patients must lose weight, and all patients must avoid weight gain. Weight loss alone can relieve symptoms of OSA.

PATIENT EDUCATION
- Weight loss and avoidance of alcohol and sedatives can improve OSA symptoms.
- Avoid driving if excessive daytime sleepiness is significant.

PROGNOSIS
- EDS improves dramatically with appropriate apnea control.
- Lifelong compliance with weight loss or CPAP is necessary for effective treatment of OSA.
- If untreated, OSA is progressive.
- Significant morbidity and mortality due to OSA usually are due to motor vehicle accidents or secondary to cardiac complications, including arrhythmias, cardiac ischemia, and hypertension.

COMPLICATIONS
Untreated OSA may increase the risk for development of hypertension, stroke, myocardial infarction, diabetes, cardiovascular disease, and work-related and driving accidents.

Pediatric Considerations
- The prevalence of pediatric OSA is 1–2% in children 4–5 years of age, and the peak incidence is between 3 and 6 years of age. Predominant sex: Male = Female.
- Etiology: The most common cause is tonsillar hypertrophy. Additional causes are obesity and craniofacial abnormalities. OSA is also seen in children with neuromuscular diseases, such as cerebral palsy and spinal muscular atrophy, due to abnormal pharyngeal muscle control.
- Signs and symptoms:
  – Nighttime: Loud snoring, restlessness, and sweating
  – Daytime: Hyperactivity and decreased school performance
  – EDS is not a significant symptom.
- Diagnosis: Gold standard is PSG. Abnormal AHI is different in children: >1–2/h is abnormal.
- Treatment: Surgery is the 1st-line treatment in cases due to tonsillar enlargement (improves symptoms in 70%). Some data suggest improved academic performance if tonsillectomy is performed for OSA. For cases due to obesity or craniofacial abnormalities, patients can use CPAP.

REFERENCES

1. Giles T, et al. Continuous positive airways pressure for obstructive sleep apnoea in adults. *Cochrane Database Syst Rev*. 2007;(1):CD001106.
2. Yaggi HK, Concato J, Kernan WN, et al. Obstructive sleep apnea as a risk factor for stroke and death. *N Engl J Med*. 2005;353:2034–41.
3. Drager LF, Bortolotto LA, Figueiredo AC, et al. Effects of continuous positive airway pressure on early signs of atherosclerosis in obstructive sleep apnea. *Am J Respir Crit Care Med*. 2007;176: 706–12.
4. Smith I, Lasserson TJ, Wright J. Drug therapy for obstructive sleep apnoea in adults. *Cochrane Database Syst Rev*. 2006:CD003002.
5. Petri N, Svanholt P, Solow B, et al. Mandibular advancement appliance for obstructive sleep apnoea: results of a randomised placebo controlled trial using parallel group design. *J Sleep Res*. 2008;17:221–9.
6. Sundaram S, Bridgman SA, Lim J, et al. Surgery for obstructive sleep apnoea. *Cochrane Database Syst Rev*. 2005:CD001004.

ADDITIONAL READING

- Kato M, Adachi T, Koshino Y, Somers VK, et al. Obstructive sleep apnea and cardiovascular disease. *Circ J*. 2009;73:1363–70.
- Kryger MH. *Principles and Practice of Sleep Medicine*. 3rd ed. Philadelphia, PA: WB Saunders; 2000.
- Lim J, Lasserson TJ, Fleetham J, et al. Oral appliances for obstructive sleep apnoea. *Cochrane Database Syst Rev*. 2004:CD004435.
- Thorpy MJ. *Handbook of Sleep Disorders*. New York, NY: Marcel Dekker; 1990.

CODES

ICD9
327.23 Obstructive sleep apnea (adult) (pediatric)

CLINICAL PEARLS

- OSA is repetitive episodes of apnea at the pharynx often terminating in a snort or gasp.
- PSG is a key to diagnosis.
- CPAP is standard medical treatment.
- Central sleep apnea may mimic OSA.

SMELL AND TASTE DISORDERS

Beth Mazyck, MD
Daniel B. Kurtz, PhD

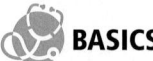 **BASICS**

DESCRIPTION
- The senses of smell and taste allow full appreciation of the flavor and palatability of foods and also serve a warning system against toxins, polluted air, smoke, and spoiled food.
- Physiologically, the chemical senses aid in normal digestion by triggering GI secretions. Smell or taste dysfunction may have a significant impact on quality of life.
- Loss of smell occurs more frequently than loss of taste, and patients frequently confuse the concepts of flavor loss (as a result of smell impairment) with taste loss (impaired ability to sense sweet, sour, salty, or bitter).
- Smell depends on the functioning of CN I (olfactory nerve) and CN V (trigeminal nerve).
- Taste depends on the functioning of CNs VII, IX, and X. Because of these multiple pathways, total loss of taste (ageusia) is rare.
- System(s) affected: Nervous; Upper Respiratory

EPIDEMIOLOGY
Incidence
There are approximately 200,000 patient visits a year for smell and taste disturbances.

Prevalence
- Predominant sex: Male > Female. Men begin to lose ability to smell earlier in life than women.
- Predominant age: Chemosensory loss is age-dependent:
  - Age >80 years: 80% have major olfactory impairment; nearly 50% are anosmic.
  - Ages 65–80 years: 60% have major olfactory impairment; nearly 25% are anosmic.
  - Age <65 years: 1–2% have smell impairment.
- Estimated >2 million affected in US

RISK FACTORS
- Age >65 years
- Poor nutritional status
- Smoking tobacco products

Genetics
May be related to underlying genetically associated diseases (Kallmann syndrome, Alzheimer disease, migraine syndromes, rheumatologic conditions, endocrine disorders)

GENERAL PREVENTION
- Eat a well-balanced diet, with appropriate vitamins and minerals.
- Maintain good oral and nasal health, with routine visits to the dentist.
- Do not smoke tobacco products.
- Avoid noxious chemical exposures or unnecessary radiation.

Geriatric Considerations
- Elders are at particular risk of eating spoiled food or inadvertently being exposed to natural gas leaks owing to anosmia from aging.
- Anosmia also may be early sign of degenerative disorders such as Alzheimer disease.

Pediatric Considerations
- Smell and taste disorders are uncommon in children in developed countries.
- In developing countries with poor nutrition (particularly zinc depletion), smell and taste disorders may occur.
- Delayed puberty in association with anosmia (± midline craniofacial abnormalities, deafness, or renal abnormalities) suggests the possibility of Kallmann syndrome (hypogonadotropic hypogonadism).

Pregnancy Considerations
- Pregnancy is an uncommon cause of smell and taste loss or disturbances.
- Many women report increased sensitivity to odors during pregnancy, as well as an increased dislike for bitter and a preference for salty substances.

ETIOLOGY
- Smell and/or taste disturbances (1,2,3):
  - Nutritional factors (e.g., malnutrition, vitamin deficiencies, liver disease, anemia)
  - Endocrine disorders (e.g., thyroid disease, diabetes mellitus, renal disease)
  - Head trauma
  - Migraine headache (e.g., gustatory aura, olfactory aura)
  - Sjögren syndrome
  - Toxic chemical exposure
  - Industrial agent exposure
  - Aging
  - Medications (see below)
  - Neurodegenerative diseases (e.g., multiple sclerosis, Alzheimer disease, cerebrovascular accident, Parkinson disease)
  - Infections (e.g., upper respiratory infection, oral and perioral infections, candidiasis, coxsackievirus, AIDS, viral hepatitis, herpes simplex virus)
- Possible causes of smell disturbance:
  - Nasal and sinus disease (e.g., allergies, rhinitis, rhinorrhea)
  - Cigarette smoking
  - Cocaine abuse (intranasal)
  - Hemodialysis
  - Radiation treatment of head and neck
  - Congenital conditions
  - Neoplasm (e.g., brain tumor, nasal polyps, intranasal tumor)
  - Systemic lupus erythematosus (SLE)
  - Bell palsy
  - Oral or perioral skin lesion
  - Damage to CN I or V
  - Possible association with psychosis and schizophrenia
- Possible causes of taste loss:
  - Oral appliances
  - Dental procedures
  - Intraoral abscess
  - Gingivitis
  - Damage to CN VI, IX, or X
  - Stroke (especially frontal lobe)

- Selected medications that reportedly alter smell and taste:
  - Antibiotics: Amikacin, ampicillin, azithromycin (Zithromax), ciprofloxacin (Cipro), clarithromycin (Biaxin), doxycycline, griseofulvin (Grisactin), metronidazole (Flagyl), ofloxacin (Floxin), tetracycline, terbinafine (Lamisil), beta lactamase inhibitors
  - Anticonvulsants: Carbamazepine (Tegretol), phenytoin (Dilantin)
  - Antidepressants: Amitriptyline (Elavil), clomipramine (Anafranil), desipramine (Norpramin), doxepin (Sinequan), imipramine (Tofranil), nortriptyline (Pamelor)
  - Antihistamines and decongestants: Chlorpheniramine, loratadine (Claritin), pseudoephedrine, zinc-based cold remedies (Zicam)
  - Antihypertensives and cardiac medications: Acetazolamide (Diamox), amiloride (Midamor), betaxolol (Betoptic), captopril (Capoten), diltiazem (Cardizem), enalapril (Vasotec), hydrochlorothiazide (Esidrix) and combinations, nifedipine (Procardia), nitroglycerin, propranolol (Inderal), spironolactone (Aldactone)
  - Anti-inflammatory agents: Auranofin (Ridaura), colchicine, dexamethasone (Decadron), gold (Myochrysine), hydrocortisone, penicillamine (Cuprimine),
  - Antimanic drugs: Lithium
  - Antineoplastics: Cisplatin (Platinol), doxorubicin (Adriamycin), methotrexate (Rheumatrex), vincristine (Oncovin)
  - Antiparkinsonian agents: Levodopa (Larodopa, with carbidopa (Sinemet)
  - Antipsychotics: Clozapine (Clozaril), trifluoperazine (Stelazine)
  - Antithyroid agents: Methimazole (Tapazole), propylthiouracil
  - Lipid-lowering agents: Fluvastatin (Lescol), lovastatin (Mevacor), pravastatin (Pravachol)
  - Muscle relaxants: Baclofen (Lioresal), dantrolene (Dantrium)

COMMONLY ASSOCIATED CONDITIONS
Upper respiratory infection (URI), allergic rhinitis, dental abscesses

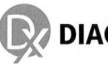 **DIAGNOSIS**

Smell and taste disturbances are symptoms; it is essential to look for possible underlying cause.

HISTORY
- Symptoms of URI, environmental allergies
- Oral pain, other dental problems
- Cognitive/memory difficulties
- Current medications
- Nutritional status, ovolactovegetarian
- Weight loss or gain
- Frequent infections (impaired immunity)
- Worsening of underlying medical illness
- Increased use of salt and/or sugar to increase taste of food

PHYSICAL EXAM
Thorough HEENT exam

DIAGNOSTIC TESTS & INTERPRETATION
Lab
Initial lab tests
- Hemoglobin
- White blood cell (WBC) count
- Blood urea nitrogen (BUN)
- Blood glucose
- Creatinine
- Bilirubin
- Alkaline phosphatase
- Thyroid-stimulating hormone (TSH)
- Consider IgE

Follow-Up & Special Considerations
Diagnosis of smell and taste disturbances is usually possible through history (1); however, the following tests can be used to confirm:
- Olfactory tests:
  - Smell identification test: Evaluates the ability to identify 40 microencapsulated scratch-and-sniff odorants
  - Brief smell identification test
- Taste tests (more difficult because no convenient standardized tests are presently available): Solutions containing sucrose (sweet), sodium chloride (salty), quinine (bitter), and citric acid (sour) are helpful.

Imaging
Initial approach
- Plain radiographs have substantial limitations (rarely useful).
- CT scanning is the most useful and cost-effective technique for assessing sinonasal disorders and is superior to MRI in evaluating bony structures and airway patency. Coronal CT scans are particularly valuable in assessing paranasal anatomy.

Follow-Up & Special Considerations
MRI is useful in defining soft tissue disease; therefore, coronal MRI is the technique of choice to image the olfactory bulbs, tracts, and cortical parenchyma. Possible placement of an accessory coil (TMJ) over the nose to assist in imaging

DIFFERENTIAL DIAGNOSIS
- Epilepsy (gustatory aura)
- Epilepsy (olfactory aura)
- Memory impairment
- Psychiatric conditions

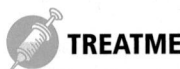 ## TREATMENT

MEDICATION
- Treat underlying cause as appropriate. 2/3 of idiopathic cases will resolve spontaneously.
- Corticosteroids topically (e.g., aqueous nasal spray) or systemically (e.g., oral prednisone) may be helpful. Prednisone 60 mg/d × 4 days, then taper by 10 mg/d thereafter.
- Artificial saliva (e.g., Xero-Lube) may be helpful in patients with xerostomia.

- Pilocarpine (Salagen) 5–10 mg PO t.i.d. may help with dry mouth/xerostomia; response may take 6–12 weeks.
- Chlorhexidine (Peridex) 0.12% oral rinse may help with gingivitis or dysgeusia.
- Zinc and vitamins (A, B complex) when deficiency is suspected

ADDITIONAL TREATMENT
General Measures
- Appropriate treatment for underlying cause
- Quit smoking.
- Some drug-related dysgeusias can be reversed with cessation of the agent, but it may take many months.
- Eliminate exposures (e.g., volatile gases, toxins, use of oxygen-liberating mouthwashes).
- Stop repeated oral trauma (e.g., appliances, tongue-biting behaviors).
- Proper nutritional and dietary assessment
- Formal dental evaluation

Issues for Referral
- Consider referral to an otolaryngologist or neurologist for persistent cases.
- Referral to a subspecialist at a smell and taste center if needed

SURGERY/OTHER PROCEDURES
If needed for treatment of underlying cause

 ## ONGOING CARE

DIET
- Weight gain or loss is possible because patient may reject food or may switch to calorie-rich foods that are still palatable.
- Ensure a nutritionally balanced diet with appropriate levels of nutrients, vitamins, and essential minerals.

PATIENT EDUCATION
- Caution patients not to overindulge as compensation for the bland taste of food. For example, patients with diabetes may need help in avoiding excessive sugar intake as an inappropriate way of improving food taste.
- Patients with chemosensory impairment should use measuring devices when cooking and should not cook by taste.
- Optimizing food texture, aroma, temperature, and color may improve the overall food experience when taste is limited.
- Patients with permanent smell dysfunction must develop adaptive strategies for dealing with hygiene, appetite, safety, and health.
- Natural gas and smoke detectors are essential; check for proper function frequently.
- Check food expiration dates frequently; discard old food.

PROGNOSIS
- In general, the olfactory system regenerates poorly after a head injury. Most patients who recover smell function subsequent to head trauma do so within 12 weeks of injury.
- Patients who quit smoking typically recover improved olfactory function and flavor sensation.
- Many taste disorders (dysgeusias) resolve spontaneously within a few years of onset.
- Phantosmias that are flow-dependent may respond to surgical ablation of olfactory mucosa.
- Conditions such as radiation-induced xerostomia and Bell palsy generally improve over time.

COMPLICATIONS
- Permanent loss of ability to smell or taste
- Psychiatric issues with dysgeusias and phantosmia

REFERENCES
1. Bromley SM. Smell and taste disorders: a primary care approach. *Am Fam Physician*. 2000;61: 427–36, 438.
2. Nguyen-Khoa B, Goehring Jr EL, Vendiola RM, et al. Epidemioligic study of smell disturbance in 2 medical insurance claims populations. *ARCH Otolaryngol Head Neck Surg*. 2007;133(8)748–57.
3. Deems DA, Doty RL, Settle RG, et al. Smell and taste disorders, a study of 750 patients from the University of Pennsylvania Smell and Taste Center. *Arch Otolaryngol Head Neck Surg*. 1991;117: 519–28.

ADDITIONAL READING
Mattes RD, Cowart BJ, Schiavo MA, et al. Dietary evaluation of patients with smell and/or taste disorders. *Am J Clin Nutr*. 1990;51:233–40.

CODES

ICD9
781.1 Disturbances of sensation of smell and taste

CLINICAL PEARLS
- Smell disorders are often mistaken as decreased taste by patients.
- Actual taste disorders are often related to dental problems.
- Smell disorders are very common in the elderly; extensive workup in this population may not be indicated if no associated signs or symptoms are present.

SNAKE ENVENOMATIONS: CAROTALINE

Alan L. Williams, MD
Pamela M. Williams, MD, Lt Col, USAF, MC

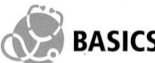

BASICS

DESCRIPTION
- Symptom complex following envenomation by a snake of the family *Viperidae*, subfamily *Crotalinae* (pit vipers)
- Includes snakes of the genera *Crotalus* (rattlesnakes), *Agkistrodon* (moccasins/cottonmouth/copperhead), and *Sistrurus* (pygmy rattlesnake/massasaugas)
- Occurs most commonly in the southeastern and southwestern United States
- North American pit viper characteristics:
  - Triangular-shaped heads, eyes with elliptical pupils, and small heat-sensing facial pits located between the nostril and the eye
  - In contrast, nonpoisonous snakes in the US generally have small, round heads and round pupils, except coral snakes, which are brightly colored.
- System(s) affected: Cardiovascular; Hematologic/Lymphatic/Immunologic; Nervous; Skin/Exocrine
- Synonym(s): Crotalidae envenomation; Snakebite; Venomous snakebite; Pit viper snakebite

EPIDEMIOLOGY
Incidence
- Statistics vary, but <10,000 snakebites are reported in the US annually:
  - ~40% of reported snakebites are identified as crotaline.
  - ~30% are from unidentified snakes.
  - ~25% are from nonpoisonous snakes.
- The actual incidence of envenomation may be higher due to underreporting or lower due to dry bites.
- Predominant age: 19–30 years
- Predominant sex: Male > Female

RISK FACTORS
- Handling, provoking, or pursuing snakes
- Acute ethanol intoxication or intoxication with other drugs that impair judgment

GENERAL PREVENTION
- Use preventive measures if handling snakes.
- In snake-infested areas:
  - Wear protective shoes and clothing when walking.
  - Do not insert hands or feet into cracks, crevices, or hollow logs.
  - Carry a flashlight if walking at night.

PATHOPHYSIOLOGY
Clinical problems related to envenomation include tissue damage, coagulopathy, thrombocytopenia, hypovolemia, and neurotoxicity.

ETIOLOGY
- Pit viper venom is a complex mixture that contains cytotoxins, hemotoxins, neurotoxins, and cardiotoxins.
- Toxin composition varies from bite to bite, even from the same snake.
- Envenomation can affect all major organ systems.
- Mojave rattlesnake venom is more neurotoxic than that of other crotalids and can cause respiratory depression.

DIAGNOSIS
- Signs and symptoms vary, from minor local injury to severe systemic illness.
- Snake identification is helpful but should not place others at risk for being bitten.
- Digital photography may be a safe means to identify the snake.

PHYSICAL EXAM
- Fang mark(s): >90%
- Pain out of proportion to puncture wound, usually within minutes of the bite: >50%
- Edema of site, progressing proximally up extremity: >50%
- Weakness, dizziness: >50%
- Numbness/tingling in extremity, mouth, tongue: >50%
- Ecchymosis of skin, vesicles around bite, which may take hours to develop: >50%
- Tachycardia: >50%
- Nausea/vomiting: <50%
- Hypo- or hypertension: <50%
- Muscle fasciculations: <50%
- Mental status changes, including coma: <25%
- Change in sensation of taste

DIAGNOSTIC TESTS & INTERPRETATION
Lab
- Complete blood count: Hemoglobin/hematocrit and/or platelets decreased in <50%
- Prothrombin time/international normalized ratio, adjusted partial thromboplastin time: Prolonged in >50%
- Fibrinogen (decreased in <50%), fibrin degradation products (increased in <50%)
- Urinalysis: Glycosuria (<50%), proteinuria (<25%), hematuria (<25%)
- Type and crossmatch "to hold" in severe envenomations
- Electrolytes, blood urea nitrogen, creatinine
- Liver function tests
- Creatine kinase in severe envenomations
- Serum ethanol level if suspicious
- Disorders that may alter lab results:
  - Preexisting anemia or polycythemia
  - Advanced liver disease
  - Kidney disease
  - Platelet disorders
- Drug(s) that may alter lab results: Anticoagulants

DIFFERENTIAL DIAGNOSIS
- Bite of nonvenomous snake
- Bite of venomous species other than those of *Crotalinae* subfamily
- Crotaline bite without envenomation (dry bite)

TREATMENT
- Patients with true envenomations need emergency department evaluation.
- Rapid transportation should take priority over all but the most basic first aid:
  - Most field snakebite treatments (e.g., cutting the bite, attempting to remove poison with suction, tourniquet, and constriction bandages) are ineffective and potentially harmful.
- Reassure patient; minimize patient movement during transport.
- Splint area of bite, allowing room for swelling.
- Position affected extremity at or below level of heart.
- Support vital signs, place on monitor, O_2 as needed, and obtain IV access.
- Remove rings and constrictive items.

MEDICATION
First Line
- Crotalidae polyvalent immune Fab (Ovine) (1)[B]:
  - No skin test necessary
  - Initial dose: 5 reconstituted vials added to normal saline (total volume 250 mL):
    - 10 mL of sterile water added to each vial; swirl only (do not shake) so as not to denature proteins
    - Infuse IV slowly for the 1st 10 minutes; then increase the rate to 250 mL/h to run remainder over 60 minutes
    - After initial infusion is complete, if all signs/symptoms of envenomation have not ceased, give up to 2 more doses of 4–6 vials until initial control is achieved.
  - Maintenance: After initial control of symptoms, administer 3 maintenance doses of 2 vials at 6, 12, and 18 h following time of initial control.
- Precautions: Papain is used in the manufacturing process of Crotalidae polyvalent immune Fab; patients with papaya allergies may be at risk for allergic reaction.
- Adverse reactions: Anaphylaxis, serum sickness; 5–19% of patients developed hypersensitivity reaction, but most reactions are mild, easily treated, and do not prevent completion of the antivenom treatment.

Second Line

Pain relief with opiate (e.g., morphine sulfate 0.1–0.2 mg/kg per dose q2–4h as needed) or acetaminophen (10–15 mg/kg per dose q4–6h as needed; maximum 4 g/d in adults)

ALERT

Avoid aspirin and other anticoagulants.

ADDITIONAL TREATMENT

General Measures

- Reassess all prehospital care. Use of tourniquet and pressure dressings is controversial. If tourniquet has been placed in prehospital setting, sudden removal could bolus patient with venom. A tourniquet or constriction band should be removed only after beginning the treatment with antivenom.
- Obtain toxicology consultation by contacting the American Association of Poison Control Centers' regional poison information center (www.AAPCC.org).
- Minimal envenomation:
  – If local signs of edema are confined to the area of bite, without any other symptom of envenomation, place IV line of crystalloid at maintenance rates and draw baseline laboratory studies.
  – Place reference marks for measuring circumference of extremity at 10 and 20 cm proximal to the site of envenomation. Measure every 15 minutes, and trace leading edge of swelling.
  – Give tetanus toxoid if needed.
  – Provide pain relief.
  – Repeat laboratory studies in 6 h. If all remain normal and swelling does not progress, observe 8–12 h and then follow up as outpatient.
  – If swelling progresses or systemic signs and symptoms appear, patient needs admission and further therapy (progress to moderate–severe envenomation measures).
- Moderate–severe envenomation:
  – If edema, vesicles, erythema progress beyond the immediate bite area, or there are associated systemic signs/symptoms or laboratory abnormalities, then give IV antivenom plus all minimal envenomation management.
  – Intensive-care monitoring may be necessary.
  – Repeat laboratory evaluations q6h initially until stable and then less frequently.
  – Blood products are necessary only for coagulopathies with clinical bleeding, not for the treatment of laboratory abnormalities. Antivenom treatment may reverse hematologic abnormalities and should be given first
  – Have equipment and medications readily at hand to treat allergic reactions to antivenom.

SURGERY/OTHER PROCEDURES

- Fasciotomy is rarely needed.
- Envenomation may mimic compartment syndrome, making clinical distinction difficult.
- Decision to perform a fasciotomy should be based on measured compartmental pressures.

IN-PATIENT CONSIDERATIONS

Admission Criteria

- Dry bites may be observed for 8–12 hours. The patient can be discharged if there is no evidence of envenomation.
- Anyone receiving antivenom should be admitted, most probably to the ICU.

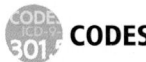

ONGOING CARE

FOLLOW-UP RECOMMENDATIONS

Bed rest, with extremity elevated

Patient Monitoring

- Phone follow-up in 12–24 hours for discharged dry bites
- First return visit within 48 hours of hospital discharge, then as indicated clinically
- Physical therapy referral should be made early for optimal outpatient intervention.

DIET

Nothing by mouth during initial period of observation and management

PATIENT EDUCATION

- Snake bite prevention and first aid
- Avoid elective surgery, dental work, contact sports, and anticoagulant medications (including aspirin) after discharge.

PROGNOSIS

Mortality: <0.1% in reported bites

Geriatric Considerations

- Course may be more severe
- Consider ECG, CXR, and arterial blood gases if underlying conditions may be exacerbated by stress of envenomation.

Pediatric Considerations

- Course may be more severe
- Crotalidae polyvalent immune Fab (Ovine) dosing is the same as for adults (2).
- Fluid overload may be a problem in small children requiring multiple vials of antivenom.

Pregnancy Considerations

- Limited data, but there have been reports of miscarriage following snakebite
- Pregnant patients should be counseled about the presence of thiomersal in antivenom. The unknown risks of thiomersal should be weighed against the benefit of antivenom in significant envenomations.
- Treatment that optimizes maternal health is presumed to be the best available treatment for the fetus.
- There are no studies of Crotalidae polyvalent immune Fab (Ovine) in pregnant women.

COMPLICATIONS

- Local wound infection (rare)
- Bleeding after discharge from hospital: Patients should be told to report nosebleeds, excessive bleeding after brushing teeth, blood in stools or vomitus, or excessive menstrual bleeding.

REFERENCES

1. Dart RC, et al. A randomized multicenter trial of crotalinae polyvalent immune Fab (ovine) antivenom for the treatment for crotaline snakebite in the United States. *Ann Emerg Med*. 2001;161: 2030–6.
2. Pizon AF, Riley BD, LoVecchio F, et al. Safety and efficacy of Crotalidae Polyvalent Immune Fab in pediatric crotaline envenomations. *Acad Emerg Med*. 2007;14:373–6.

ADDITIONAL READING

- Gold BS, Barish RA, Dart RC. North American snake envenomation: diagnosis, treatment, and management. *Emerg Med Clin North Am*. 2004;22:423–43, ix.
- Weant KA, Johnson PN, Bowers RC, et al. Evidence-based, multidisciplinary approach to the development of a crotalidae polyvalent antivenin (CroFab) protocol at a university hospital. *Ann Pharmacother*. 2010;44:447–55.
- Wozniak EJ, Wisser J, Schwartz M. Venomous adversaries: a reference to snake identification, field safety, and bite-victim first aid for disaster-response personnel deploying into the hurricane-prone regions of North America. *Wilderness Environ Med*. 2006;17:246–66.

See Also (Topic, Algorithm, Electronic Media Element)

Snake Envenomations: Elapidae (Coral Snake)

CODES

ICD9
989.5 Toxic effect of venom

CLINICAL PEARLS

- Poison Control Center: 1-800-222-1222
- The best first aid for snakebites is rapidly transporting a calm and still victim. Do *not* cut or attempt to suck out the venom. Cold therapy, electrical shocks, and tourniquets have been shown to be potentially harmful and, at least, unhelpful.
- Skin testing is not necessary before antivenom administration.
- The rate of infection following crotaline snakebite is so low that prophylactic antibiotics are not indicated.

SNAKE ENVENOMATIONS: ELAPIDAE (CORAL SNAKE)

Alan L. Williams, MD
Pamela M. Williams, MD, Lt Col, USAF, MC

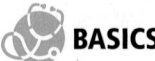 BASICS

DESCRIPTION
- Symptom complex following envenomation by a snake of the family *Elapidae*:
  - Local signs and symptoms typically are mild, even in severe envenomations.
  - Neurologic symptoms may be delayed up to 12 h or more after the envenomation.
- Coral snakes have a characteristic rounded head with round pupils.
- Coral snakes have smaller fixed fangs, so they may chew or hang onto a victim in contrast to pit vipers, which typically strike rapidly and recoil.
- In the US, these snakes include the genera *Micrurus* and *Micruroides*:
  - The Sonoran coral snake (*Micruroides euryxanthus*), also known as the Arizona coral snake, is found mainly in Arizona.
  - Texas coral snake (*Micrurus fulvius tenere*) is found in Texas, Arkansas, and Louisiana.
  - Eastern coral snake (*Micrurus fulvius fulvius*) is found throughout the Southeast.
- System(s) affected: Nervous; Skin/Exocrine
- Synonym(s): Neurotoxic snakebite; Snakebite

ALERT
Coloration is important: North American coral snakes have broad rings of red and black separated by narrow rings of yellow:

- In contrast, milk snakes are nonpoisonous snakes with similar coloration. The areas of orange/red and yellow/white are separated by bands of black.
- "Red on yellow, kill a fellow; red on black, friend of Jack."
- Coral snakes in South America and other parts of the world do not necessarily have this color pattern.

EPIDEMIOLOGY
Incidence
- Coral snake bites comprise 1–4% of identified snakebites reported to American Association of Poison Control Centers (AAPCC).
- <100 reported each year in the US
- Predominant age: 19–30 years
- Predominant sex: Male > Female

RISK FACTORS
Coral snakes are nocturnal and timid; therefore, they rarely bite humans. They must be deliberately provoked to bite.

GENERAL PREVENTION
- Use preventive measures if handling snakes.
- In snake-infested areas:
  - Wear protective shoes and clothing when walking.
  - Do not insert hands or feet into cracks, crevices, or hollow logs.
  - Carry a flashlight if walking at night.

ETIOLOGY
Venom is primarily a neurotoxin; it contains little or no cytotoxin to cause local tissue reaction.

 DIAGNOSIS

HISTORY
- Snake identification is helpful, but it should not place others at risk for being bitten:
  - Digital photography may be a safe means to identify the snake.
- Determine individual's past history of snakebites and treatment.
- Assess for any allergy to horse serum.

PHYSICAL EXAM
- Onset of symptoms following envenomation may be delayed 10–12 h and include:
  - Local swelling (<50%)
  - Numbness/change in sensation (<50%)
  - Nausea/vomiting (<50%)
  - Weakness (<25%)
  - Dizziness (<15%)
  - Diplopia (<15%)
  - Muscle fasciculations (<15%)
  - Dysarthria
  - Dysphagia with increased salivation
- Fang marks; may be shallow or appear as a scratch (>75%)

DIAGNOSTIC TESTS & INTERPRETATION
Baseline and serial pulmonary function tests with special attention to peak flow and vital capacity as well as oxygen saturation may help in early recognition of decreasing ventilatory function.

Lab
- Creatine kinase is often elevated.
- Consider blood ethanol level to assess for a common confounding diagnosis.

DIFFERENTIAL DIAGNOSIS
- Bite of other venomous snake (*Crotalinae*) without envenomation ("dry bite")
- Bite of a nonvenomous snake

 TREATMENT

- Transportation of a calm and still patient to a treatment facility is the primary goal of prehospital emergency personnel.
- Pressure/immobilization of the affected limb has been shown to be potentially helpful (1) but technically difficult (2). If attempted, it should be performed by an experienced practitioner and not delay patient transportation.
- Administer oxygen.
- Obtain IV access in nonaffected limb.

MEDICATION
- No antivenin is available for *M. euryxanthus*.
- Antivenin to the North American coral snake (*M. fulvius fulvius* antivenin):
  - Horse serum product effective only for the envenomation of the Texas and eastern coral snakes (*M. fulvius tenere* and *M. fulvius fulvius*)
  - Perform skin testing before 1st dose.
  - Initial dose: 4–6 reconstituted vials added to 250 mL normal saline:
    - Begin infusion at 3–5 mL/h; if no systemic reaction occurs, increase until a rate of 1 diluted vial is being given every 30 minutes.
    - Exact dosing schedule has not been determined due to the lower numbers of individuals treated
  - If a patient has been treated with antivenin and develops neurologic symptoms, an additional 10–15 vials may be necessary.

– If skin test is positive, obtain toxicology consultation from the AAPCC-certified poison information center for your area. Likely recommendations may include pretreatment with diphenhydramine (Benadryl; 1 mg/kg per dose q6h IV; adults 25–50 mg IV), steroids [e.g., methylprednisolone (Solu-Medrol) 1–2 mg/kg per dose q8h IV], and other antihistamines (e.g., cimetidine 10 mg/kg per dose IV; adults 300 mg IV).
- Contraindication: History of allergy to horse serum
- Precautions: Have equipment and medications readily at hand to treat anaphylaxis.
- Adverse reactions: Anaphylaxis, serum sickness

ALERT
Avoid sedatives and opioids that may compound any respiratory compromise.

ADDITIONAL TREATMENT
General Measures
- All patients with any of the following should be admitted to hospital for intensive care unit monitoring:
  – Confirmed bite by a snake identified as a coral snake
  – History of an unidentified snake having chewed on a patient
- Give tetanus toxoid if needed.
- Support vital signs; intubation may be necessary if respiratory compromise ensues:
  – Early, elective intubation during the progression of paralysis may help to prevent aspiration pneumonia.
- Cardiac, respiratory, neurologic monitoring
- Immobilize extremity, and keep it at the level of the heart.
- Contact local poison control center: 1-800-222-1222.

Additional Therapies
Early referral for physical therapy may improve the speed of functional recovery.

IN-PATIENT CONSIDERATIONS
Initial Stabilization
ABCs, O$_2$, monitored bed

Admission Criteria
All suspected coral snake bites warrant admission for observation and treatment.

Discharge Criteria
- Discharge should not occur until the patient has made adequate neurologic recovery to the point at which there is no concern about respiratory failure.
- Asymptomatic patients admitted for observation may be discharged after 24–48 h.

ONGOING CARE

FOLLOW-UP RECOMMENDATIONS
Patient Monitoring
1st return visit within 48 h, then as clinically indicated

DIET
n.p.o. initially

PROGNOSIS
- Neurologic deterioration may progress despite antivenin administration.
- Complete paralysis may occur.
- Neurologic symptoms can last 3–6 days despite treatment with antivenin.
- Muscle strength may not return to normal for 4–6 weeks.
- Long-term morbidity is rare.
- Mortality does occur even with antivenin therapy.

Pregnancy Considerations
- Limited data, but there have been reports of miscarriage following snakebite.
- Treatment that optimizes maternal health is presumed to be the best available treatment for the fetus.

COMPLICATIONS
- Local wound infection
- Aspiration pneumonia

REFERENCES
1. German BT, et al. Pressure-Immobilization bandages delay toxicity in a Porcine Model of Eastern coral snake. *Annal Emerg Med*. 2005;45(6): 603–8.
2. Norris RL, Ngo J, Nolan K, et al. Physicians and lay people are unable to apply pressure immobilization properly in a simulated snakebite scenario. *Wilderness Environ Med*. 2005;16:16–21.

ADDITIONAL READING
- Gold BS, Barish RA, Dart RC. North American snake envenomation: diagnosis, treatment, and management. *Emerg Med Clin North Am*. 2004; 22:423–43, ix.
- Kitchens CS, Van Mierop LH. Envenomation by the Eastern coral snake (Micrurus fulvius fulvius). A study of 39 victims. *JAMA*. 1987;258:1615–8.
- Wozniak EJ, Wisser J, Schwartz M. Venomous adversaries: a reference to snake identification, field safety, and bite-victim first aid for disaster-response personnel deploying into the hurricane-prone regions of North America. *Wilderness Environ Med*. 2006;17:246–66.

See Also (Topic, Algorithm, Electronic Media Element)
Snake Envenomations, Crotalidae

CODES

ICD9
989.5 Toxic effect of venom

CLINICAL PEARLS
- Poison Control Center: 1-800-222-1222
- Most experts recommend monitored observation of coral snakebite victims for 24–48 h for late-onset neurologic symptoms before discharging them.
- The field treatment of neurotoxic snakebites in Australia often includes splinting and wrapping the entire affected limb to delay the presumed lymphatic spread of venom. Pressure immobilization is potentially helpful for coral snakebites but technically difficult in field conditions (1,2).
- The manufacturer has discontinued the active production of North American coral snake antivenin. Alternative antivenin products are under investigation. Local poison control centers are the best source of current, regionally applicable information about antivenin availability.

S

SOMATIZATION DISORDER

Laurie A. Carrier, MD

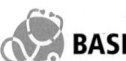 **BASICS**

DESCRIPTION
- A pattern of recurring, multiple, clinically significant somatic complaints beginning <30 years of age that occur over a period of several years and result in treatment being sought or significant impairment in social, occupational, or other important areas of functioning
- Each of the following criteria must be met, with individual symptoms occurring at any time during the course of the disturbance:
  - 4 pain symptoms: Different sites or functions
  - 2 GI symptoms: Other than pain
  - 1 sexual symptom
  - 1 pseudoneurologic symptom
- These symptoms are not intentionally produced or feigned.
- Chronic course, fluctuating in severity
- Affected individual rarely goes 1 year without seeking medical attention prompted by unexplained somatic complaints.
- System(s) affected: Multiple
- Synonym(s): Briquet syndrome

EPIDEMIOLOGY
Incidence
- Usually, 1st symptoms appear in adolescence; full criteria met by 30 years of age.
- Predominant sex: Female > Male (10:1)
- The type and frequency of somatic complaints may differ among cultures, so symptom reviews should be adjusted based on culture.

Prevalence
- Ranges from 0.2–2% among women and <0.2% among men
- 1/500 adults in the US
- Seen in up to 29% of patients presenting to primary care offices (1)

RISK FACTORS
- Child abuse, particularly sexual abuse, has been shown to be a risk factor.
- Symptoms begin or worsen after losses (e.g., job, close relative, or friend).
- Greater intensity of symptoms often occurs with stress.

Genetics
- Observed in 10–20% of female 1st-degree biologic relatives of women with somatization disorder (SD)
- Male relatives of woman with this disorder show an increased risk of antisocial personality disorder and substance-related disorders.

ETIOLOGY
- Unknown
- Adoption studies indicate that both genetic and environmental factors contribute to the risk of SD.

COMMONLY ASSOCIATED CONDITIONS
Comorbid with other psychiatric conditions, including major depression (55% of patients), anxiety disorders (34%), personality disorders (61%), and panic disorders (26%)

 DIAGNOSIS

HISTORY
- Multiple somatic complaints, usually a grossly positive review of symptoms
- Pain symptoms (4 or more) related to different sites, such as head, abdomen, back, joints, extremities, chest, or rectum or related to body functions such as menstruation, sexual intercourse, or urination
- GI symptoms (2 or more, excluding pain) such as nausea, bloating, vomiting (not during pregnancy), diarrhea, intolerance of several foods
- Sexual symptoms (at least 1, excluding pain) such as indifference to sex, difficulties with erection or ejaculation, irregular menses, excessive menstrual bleeding, or vomiting throughout all 9 months of pregnancy
- Pseudoneurologic symptoms (at least 1) such as impaired balance or coordination, weak or paralyzed muscles, lump in throat or trouble swallowing, loss of voice, retention of urine, hallucinations, numbness (to touch or pain), double vision, blindness, deafness, seizures, amnesia or other dissociative symptoms, loss of consciousness (other than with fainting); none of these is limited to pain.

PHYSICAL EXAM
Physical exam remarkable for absence of objective findings to fully explain the many subjective complaints

DIAGNOSTIC TESTS & INTERPRETATION
Several screening tools are available that help to identify symptoms as somatic:
- PHQ-15 (screens and monitors symptoms) (2)[C]
- MMPI (identifies somatization) (3)[C]
- Perley-Guze Checklist (helps the physician to identify SD)

Lab
Initial lab tests
Laboratory test results do not support the subjective complaints.

Imaging
Initial approach
Imaging studies do not support the subjective complaints.

Pathological Findings
None are identified.

DIFFERENTIAL DIAGNOSIS
- Other psychiatric illnesses must be ruled out:
  - Depressive disorders
  - Anxiety disorders
  - Schizophrenia
  - Other somatoform disorders: Conversion disorder, factitious disorders, hypochondriasis, pain disorder
- General medical conditions, with vague, multiple, confusing symptoms, must be ruled out:
  - Systemic lupus erythematosus
  - Hyperparathyroidism
  - Hyper- or hypothyroidism
  - Lyme disease
  - Porphyria

TREATMENT

MEDICATION

Antidepressants (e.g., selective serotonin reuptake inhibitors) help to treat comorbid depression and anxiety.

ADDITIONAL TREATMENT

General Measures

- The goal of treatment is to help the person learn to control the symptoms.
- A supportive relationship with a sympathetic health care provider is the most important aspect of treatment (4)[C]:
  – Regularly scheduled appointments should be maintained to review symptoms and the person's coping mechanisms (at least 15 minutes once a month) (4)[C].
  – Acknowledgment and explanation of test results should occur.
- The involvement of a single physician is important because a history of seeking medical attention and "doctor shopping" is common.
- Antidepressant or antianxiety medication and referral to a support group or psychiatrist can help patients who are willing to participate in their treatment.
- Patients usually receive the most benefit from primary-care physicians who accept the limitations of treatment, listen to their patient's concerns, and provide reassurance.
- It is not helpful to tell patients that their symptoms are imaginary.

Issues for Referral

- Referrals to specialists for further investigation of somatic complaints should be discouraged.
- Referrals to support groups or to a psychiatrist may be helpful.

Additional Therapies

Treatment typically includes long-term therapy, which has been shown to decrease the severity of symptoms:

- Cognitive-behavioral therapy has been shown to be the most efficacious treatment in SD (5)[B], (6)[C].
- Psychotherapy
- Supportive therapy

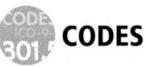 ONGOING CARE

FOLLOW-UP RECOMMENDATIONS

Patients should have regularly scheduled follow-up with a primary-care doctor, psychiatrist, and/or therapist.

PATIENT EDUCATION

Interventions that decrease stressful elements of the patient's life should be encouraged:

- Psychoeducational advice
- Increase in exercise
- Pleasurable private time

PROGNOSIS

- Chronic course, fluctuating in severity
- Full remission is rare.
- Individuals with this disorder do not experience any significant difference in mortality rate or significant physical illness.
- Patients with this diagnosis do experience substantially greater functional disability and role impairment than nonsomatizing patients (7).

COMPLICATIONS

- May result from invasive testing and from multiple evaluations that are performed while looking for the cause of the symptoms
- A dependency on pain relievers or sedatives may develop.

REFERENCES

1. Roca M, Gili M, Garcia-Garcia M, et al. Prevalence and comorbidity of common mental disorders in primary care. *J Affect Disord*. 2009.
2. Kroenke K, Spitzer RL, Williams JB. The PHQ-15: validity of a new measure for evaluating the severity of somatic symptoms. *Psychosom Med*. 2002;64:258–66.
3. Wetzel RD, Brim J, Guze SB, et al. MMPI screening scales for somatization disorder. *Psychol Rep*. 1999;85:341–8.
4. Servan-Schreiber D, Tabas G, Kolb R. Somatizing patients: part II. Practical management. *Am Fam Physician*. 2000;61:1423–8, 1431–2.
5. Allen LA, Woolfolk RL, Escobar JI, et al. Cognitive-behavioral therapy for somatization disorder: a randomized controlled trial. *Arch Intern Med*. 2006;166:1512–8.
6. Kroenke K, Swindle R. Cognitive-behavioral therapy for somatization and symptom syndromes: a critical review of controlled clinical trials. *Psychother Psychosom*. 2000;69:205–15.
7. Harris AM, Orav EJ, Bates DW, et al. Somatization Increases Disability Independent of Comorbidity. *J Gen Intern Med*. 2008.

ADDITIONAL READING

- American Psychiatric Association. *Diagnostic and Statistical Manual of Mental Disorders*. 4th ed. Text revision. Washington, DC: American Psychiatric Association, 2000.
- Mai F. Somatization disorder: a practical review. *Can J Psychiatry*. 2004;49:652–62.

CODES

ICD9
300.81 Somatization disorder

CLINICAL PEARLS

- Acknowledge the patient's pain, suffering, and disability.
- Do not tell patients the symptoms are "all in their head."
- Emphasize that this is not a rare disorder.
- Discuss the limitations of treatment while providing reassurance that there are interventions that will lessen suffering and symptoms.

SPINAL STENOSIS

N. Wilson Holland, MD
Birju B. Patel, MD

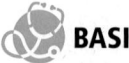 **BASICS**

DESCRIPTION
Spinal stenosis is a condition in which a narrowing of the spinal canal and foramen occurs. Spondylosis or degenerative arthritis is the most common etiology for spinal stenosis and results from compression of the spine by disk degeneration, facet arthropathy, osteophyte formation, and ligamentum flavum hypertrophy. The L_4-L_5 level is involved most commonly, but other lumbar levels also can be affected.

EPIDEMIOLOGY
The prevalence of spinal stenosis increases with age because it is essentially an arthritic condition from "wear and tear" on the normal spine.

Incidence
The incidence of symptomatic spinal stenosis is as high as 8% of the general population.

Prevalence
- The prevalence increases with age and can be very high when assessed by imaging studies in elderly patients; however, not all patients with radiographic spinal stenosis are symptomatic.
- Predominant age: Symptoms develop in 5th and 6th decades (congenital stenosis becomes symptomatic much earlier).

RISK FACTORS
Increasing age and degenerative spondylolisthesis

Genetics
No definitive genetic links

GENERAL PREVENTION
There is no known way to prevent spinal stenosis. Symptoms can be alleviated with flexion at the waist.
- Leaning forward while walking
- Pushing a shopping cart
- Lying in flexed position
- Sitting
- Avoid provocative maneuvers that can cause pain (e.g., back extension, ambulating long distances without resting).

PATHOPHYSIOLOGY
Disk dehydration leads to loss of height with bulging of annulus and ligamentum flavum into the spinal canal, thus increasing joint loading of facets. This leads to reactive sclerosis and osteophytic bone growth, resulting in further compression of neural elements in the spinal canal and foramen.

ETIOLOGY
Spinal stenosis can result from congenital or acquired causes (1). Degenerative spondylosis is the most common cause. Acquired causes include
- Disk degeneration and spondylosis
- Trauma
- Neoplasms
- Neural cysts and lipomas
- Postoperative changes

- Rheumatoid arthritis
- Diffuse idiopathic skeletal hyperostosis
- Ankylosing spondylitis
- Metabolic/endocrine:
  - Osteoporosis
  - Renal osteodystrophy
  - Paget disease

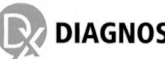 **DIAGNOSIS**

- Long-standing back pain that progresses to buttocks and lower extremity pain
- Neurogenic claudication (i.e., pain, tightness, numbness, and subjective weakness of lower extremities) may mimic arterial insufficiency–related claudication.

HISTORY
- The history is an extremely important aspect in distinguishing patients with spinal stenosis from those with other causes of back pain and peripheral vascular disease (2).
- Components of the history that should be considered include
  - Insidious onset
  - Generally progresses slowly but may rarely have periods of remittance.
  - Symptoms worsen with extension of the spine (prolonged standing, walking especially downhill or downstairs).
  - Symptoms improve with flexion (sitting, leaning forward while walking, walking uphill or upstairs, and lying in a flexed position).
  - Intermittent claudication
  - Urinary symptoms
  - Bilateral plantar numbness

PHYSICAL EXAM
Neurologic exam may be normal (3). There may be very few physical findings even in affected patients.
- Gait alteration (rule out cervical myelopathy or intracranial pathology)
- Loss of lumbar lordosis
- Decreased range of motion of lumbar spine
- Pain with extension of the lumbar spine
- Straight-leg-raise test may be positive if nerve root entrapment is present.
- Muscle weakness is usually mild or subtle and involves the L_4, L_5, and rarely, S_1 nerve roots.
- About 1/2 of patients with symptomatic stenosis have a reduced or absent Achilles reflex, and 1/5 have reduced or absent knee-jerk reaction.

DIAGNOSTIC TESTS & INTERPRETATION
Spinal stenosis generally is diagnosed with a combination of history, physical exam, and imaging studies (MRI is best).

Lab
Initial lab tests
Complete blood count, erythrocyte sedimentation rate, C-reactive protein (to look for infection or malignancy)

Imaging
- New back pain in those over age 50 generally warrants neuroimaging.
- MRI is the modality of choice for the diagnosis of spinal stenosis (4). 3D MR myelography may be more sensitive but is more expensive at diagnosing lumbar spinal stenosis, as shown by a few studies (5).
- CT myelography is an alternative to MRI but is invasive with the potential risk of complications.
- Plain radiography may help to support the diagnosis but in general will not reveal the underlying pathology.

Initial approach
Spinal stenosis generally does not lead to neurologic damage. Surgery may be required for pain relief, allowing patients to become more mobile and thus improving overall health.

Diagnostic Procedures/Surgery
Surgical decompression is the only definitive treatment in patients who continue to be symptomatic after nonoperative treatment (5).

Pathological Findings
- Decreased disk height
- Facet hypertrophy
- Spinal canal and/or foraminal narrowing

DIFFERENTIAL DIAGNOSIS
- Vascular claudication also can cause calf pain with ambulation. Symptoms of vascular claudication do not improve with leaning forward and should not persist with standing.
- Disk herniation
- Cervical myelopathy

 TREATMENT

- A few studies have shown improvement with decompressive surgery, but the duration of improvement is uncertain.
- In general, nonoperative interventions are tried prior to surgical interventions unless there are progressive or life-threatening neurologic symptoms.
- If decompressive surgery is performed, it is generally successful in alleviating symptoms of spinal stenosis.
- There is some controversy about whether a fusion should be performed along with the decompression because of risk of future spondylolisthesis.

MEDICATION
First Line
- Acetaminophen
- Nonsteroidal anti-inflammatory medications (consider potential for GI side effects, fluid retention, and renal failure)
- Tramadol

Second Line
- There is limited evidence for long-term efficacy of lumbar epidural steroid and/or anesthetic injections. Injections maybe less effective in those with more severe stenosis and those with stenosis involving more than three lumbar levels (6).
- Consider judicious use of opioids only when other treatments have failed to control severe pain.

Geriatric Considerations
- Anti-inflammatory medications should be used with caution in the elderly owing to the risks of GI bleeding, fluid retention, and renal failure.
- Side effects of opioids, including constipation, confusion, urinary retention, drowsiness, nausea, vomiting, and potential for dependence, should be considered.
- Over 10% of elderly lack Achilles reflexes.

ADDITIONAL TREATMENT
Issues for Referral
Refer to a spine surgeon when patients are in unremitting pain or have a neurologic deficit.

Additional Therapies
- General conditioning; these patients are able to ride an exercise bicycle without many problems because they can lean forward and relieve symptoms.
- Aquatic therapy (helpful for muscle and general conditioning)
- Back extensor muscle strengthening
- Abdominal muscle strengthening
- Gait training

SURGERY/OTHER PROCEDURES
- Surgery is indicated when symptoms persist despite conservative measures (7).
- Age alone should not be an exclusion factor for surgical intervention. However, cognitive impairment, multiple comorbidities, and osteoporosis may increase the risk of perioperative complications in the elderly (8).
- Decompression of neural elements is the mainstay of treatment. The traditional approach is laminectomy and partial facetectomy (9).
- Controversy exists over whether the decompression should be supplemented by a fusion procedure.
- A less invasive alternative, known as *interspinous distraction* (X STOP implant), is also available (10). Elderly patients with significant degenerative spondylolisthesis may have more postoperative neurologic sequelae with use of the X Stop implant at severely stenotic levels (11).

IN-PATIENT CONSIDERATIONS
Initial Stabilization
- A brace or corset may help for a short time but is not recommended long term because it leads to paraspinal muscle weakness.
- Patient should be encouraged to continue to be active despite pain to prevent deconditioning.
- Weight loss

Admission Criteria
Unremitting pain that prevents the ability to perform the activities of daily living (ADLs) or acute or progressive neurologic deficit

Discharge Criteria
Improved pain or after neurologic deficit has been addressed

ONGOING CARE
FOLLOW-UP RECOMMENDATIONS
- Routine follow-up as appropriate
- No limitations to activity; patients may be as active as tolerated. Exercise should be encouraged.

Patient Monitoring
Patients are monitored for improvement of symptoms and development of any complications.

DIET
If undergoing surgery, optimize nutritional status.

PATIENT EDUCATION
- Activity as tolerated, as long as no other pathology is present (e.g., fractures)
- Patients should be alerted to possibility of progressive motor weakness and bladder/bowel dysfunction.
- Patients should be educated about the natural history of the condition.

PROGNOSIS
- Spinal stenosis generally is benign, but the pain can lead to limitation in ADLs and progressive disability.
- Surgery is usually successful in improving pain and symptoms in patients who fail nonoperative treatment.
- Clinical outcomes in elderly patients after surgery are similar in terms of pain relief and functional improvement compared with younger patients (8).

COMPLICATIONS
- Severe spinal stenosis can lead to bowel and/or bladder dysfunction.
- Surgical complications include infection, neurologic injury, chronic pain, and disability.

REFERENCES

1. Devereaux M, et al. Low back pain. *Med. Clin. North Am*. 2009;93:477–501, x
2. Ebell MH, et al. Diagnosing lumbar spinal stenosis. *Am Fam Physician*. 2009;80:1145-
3. Deyo RA, Rainville J, Kent DL. What can the history and physical examination tell us about low back pain? *JAMA*. 1992;268:760–5.
4. Chad DA. Lumbar spinal stenosis. *Neurol Clin*. 2007;25:407–18.
5. de Graaf I, Prak A, Bierma-Zeinstra S, et al. Diagnosis of lumbar spinal stenosis: a systematic review of the accuracy of diagnostic tests. *Spine*. 2006;31:1168–76.
6. Last AR, Hulbert K, et al. Chronic low back pain: evaluation and management. *Am Fam Physician*. 2009;79:1067–74.
7. Weinstein JN, Tosteson TD, Lurie JD, et al. Surgical versus nonsurgical therapy for lumbar spinal stenosis. *N Engl J Med*. 2008;358:794–810.
8. Cloyd JM, Acosta FL, Ames CP, et al. Complications and outcomes of lumbar spine surgery in elderly people: a review of the literature. *J Am Geriatr Soc*. 2008;56:1318–27.
9. Katz JN, Harris MB. Clinical practice. Lumbar spinal stenosis. *N Engl J Med*. 2008;358:818–25.
10. Markman JD, Gaud KG. Lumbar spinal stenosis in older adults: current understanding and future directions. *Clin Geriatr Med*. 2008;24:369–88.
11. Epstein NE, et al. X-Stop: foot drop. *Spine J*. 2009;9:e6–9.

See Also (Topic, Algorithm, Electronic Media Element)
Algorithm: Low Back Pain, Acute

CODES
ICD9
- 724.00 Spinal stenosis of unspecified region
- 724.01 Spinal stenosis of thoracic region
- 724.02 Spinal stenosis of lumbar region

CLINICAL PEARLS
- Spinal stenosis may present as neurogenic claudication (pain, tightness, numbness, and subjective weakness of lower extremities) and may mimic arterial insufficiency–related claudication.
- Neurogenic claudication as opposed to vascular claudication is improved by uphill ambulation and lumbar flexion and is not alleviated by standing.
- Positions that cause flexion of the spine such as sitting, bending forward, walking uphill, or walking with a shopping cart generally relieve symptoms and can be helpful in making the diagnosis.
- Positions that cause spinal extension such as prolonged standing, walking downhill, and walking downstairs can worsen symptoms.
- Surgery should be considered urgently in patients who present with rapidly evolving cauda equina/conus medullaris syndrome or newly progressive bladder dysfunction.

SPOROTRICHOSIS

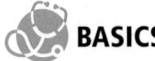

Hannah Melnitsky, MD
Raul Davaro, MD

BASICS

DESCRIPTION
- Subacute or chronic *Sporothrix schenckii* fungal infection
- Most common and least severe of the deep mycoses
- Occurs in the following forms:
  - Cutaneous/lymphocutaneous (most common)
  - Disseminated:
    - Osteoarticular
    - Renal
    - Testicular
    - Mastitis
    - Meningeal
  - Pulmonary
- Most likely to occur in farmers, horticulturists, and gardeners
- Systems affected:
  Hematologic/Lymphatic/Immunologic; Musculoskeletal; Skin/Exocrine; Renal; Respiratory
- Synonyms: Schenck disease; Rose gardener disease

EPIDEMIOLOGY
Incidence
- <1/100,000 persons/year
- Occurs worldwide, but is most common in tropics and subtropics, endemic in Central and South America and Africa

RISK FACTORS
- Gardening: Contact with mulch, sphagnum moss, hay, timber, or thorny bushes
- Occupations involving the handling of gardening materials: Nursery workers, landscapers, florists, carpenters
- Animal handlers (transmission from animals, especially cats and armadillos, to humans has been documented)
- Immunocompromised patients (e.g., HIV, hematologic malignancy, use of immunosuppressants), as well as patients with chronic obstructive pulmonary disease, alcoholism, and diabetes mellitus, are at risk for developing disseminated disease.

GENERAL PREVENTION
- Avoid areas where sporotrichosis is endemic.
- Wear gloves when working in soil.

PATHOPHYSIOLOGY
- Lymphocutaneous: Primary lesion forms within 3 weeks to 6 months of direct inoculation with mold and spreads along lymphatic channels.
- Disseminated: Via hematogenous spread
- Pulmonary: Via inhalation of spores

ETIOLOGY
- Traumatic inoculation of fungus through skin into subcutaneous fat or pulmonary inoculation via inhalation of conidia.
- *S. schenckii* is a dimorphic, aerobic fungus existing in hyphal form at temperatures below 37°C and yeast form above 37°C; a ubiquitous saprophyte found in soil, sphagnum peat moss, wood, marine animals, decaying vegetation, some insects, etc (12).

DIAGNOSIS

HISTORY
- Minor skin trauma involving contact with plants or plant products (rose thorns, hay, conifer needles, etc.) with subsequent delayed development of characteristic lesions
- Zoonotic transmission (animal to human) documented (dogs, cats, horses, rodents, pigs, armadillos, and insects)
- Pulmonary disease presents with high fever, night sweats, dyspnea, fatigue, hemoptysis, and cough productive of purulent sputum.

PHYSICAL EXAM
- Cutaneous/lymphocutaneous:
  - Characteristic skin lesions beginning as an inoculation chancre or erythematous plaque with satellite, small papules, and painless, movable, subcutaneous nodules in a linear distribution; lesions progress to larger nodules, which may ulcerate and drain; affects primarily upper extremities
  - Additional lesions spread proximally along lymphatics, giving linear appearance.
- Disseminated disease:
  - Widespread, multifocal, cutaneous lesions
  - Physical exam will depend on organ system involved.
- Osteoarticular:
  - Subacute or chronic inflammatory arthritis, often monoarticular; may persist for many years
  - Signs and symptoms of osteomyelitis
  - Generally afebrile
- Pulmonary: Physical exam nonspecific other than suggestive of cavitary lung disease

DIAGNOSTIC TESTS & INTERPRETATION
Lab
Initial lab tests
- Culture of *S. schenckii* is the gold standard for diagnosis of sporotrichosis.
- Fungal cultures from tissue biopsy or aspirated pus; cultures may be more difficult to grow from synovial fluid or sputum
- Incubate at 25°C on Sabouraud or potato dextrose agar, with creamy white colonies appearing in 3–5 days that then convert to characteristic brown-black leathery colonies within several days (2)

Follow-Up & Special Considerations
- Organisms may be difficult to find on light microscopy, and thus culture is vastly superior for diagnosis.
- Perform culture for atypical *Mycobacterium* spp. and/or acid-fast stain if considered in differential diagnosis.

Imaging
Chest x-ray if pulmonary symptoms present

Initial approach
- Careful history and physical exam
- Culture of draining lesions
- Culture of inflammatory joint effusions or sputum
- Tissue biopsy with culture if diagnosis not confirmed

Pathological Findings
- Nonspecific granulomata with central necrosis may be found on tissue biopsy.
- Periodic acid–Schiff staining rarely may reveal spores within the granuloma.
- Asteroid corpuscles may be seen on hematoxylin and eosin stain.

DIFFERENTIAL DIAGNOSIS
- Cutaneous or lymphocutaneous (12):
  - Sporotrichoid nocardiosis
  - Leishmaniasis
  - Paracoccidiomycosis
  - Chromoblastomycosis
  - Blastomycosis
  - Tuberculosis
  - Atypical mycobacterial infection (*Mycobacterium marinum*, *M. chelonae*, *M. kansasii*)
  - Cat scratch disease
  - Tularemia
  - Plague
  - Primary syphilis
  - Pyoderma gangrenosum
- Pulmonary:
  - Tuberculosis
  - Sarcoidosis
  - Chronic fungal pneumonia
  - Neoplasm
  - Atypical mycobacterial infection (*M. avium* complex, *M. kansasii*)
  - *Rhodococcus equi* infection
  - *Nocardia* sp. infections
- Osteoarticular:
  - Rheumatoid arthritis
  - Bacterial arthritis/osteomyelitis

TREATMENT

MEDICATION

First Line

- Cutaneous/lymphocutaneous:
  - Itraconazole 200 mg/d p.o. recommended for 2–4 weeks after all lesions have resolved, usually a total of 3–6 months (1)[A]
  - Patients who do not respond should be given a higher dosage of itraconazole, 200 mg b.i.d. (1)[A], terbinafine at a dosage of 500 mg p.o. b.i.d. (1)[A], or SSKI initiated at a dosage of 5 drops t.i.d., increasing as tolerated to 40–50 drops t.i.d. (1) although the role of SSKI is anecdotal as evidence is inconclusive (3).
  - Fluconazole at a dosage of 400–800 mg/d should be used only if the patient cannot tolerate the other agents (1)[A].
  - Local hyperthermia can be used for treating patients, such as pregnant and nursing women, who have fixed cutaneous sporotrichosis and who cannot safely take any of the above regimens (1)[C].
- Osteoarticular:
  - Itraconazole 200 mg p.o. b.i.d. for at least 12 months is recommended (1)[A].
  - Amphotericin B lipid formulation 3–5 mg/kg/d or amphotericin B deoxycholate 0.7–1.0 mg/kg/d can be used for initial therapy (1)[C].
  - After the patient has shown a favorable response, therapy can be changed to itraconazole 200 mg p.o. b.i.d. to complete a total of at least 12 months of therapy (1)[C].
  - Serum levels of itraconazole should be obtained after the patient has been on this agent for at least 2 weeks to ensure adequate drug exposure (1)[C].
- Pulmonary:
  - For severe or life-threatening pulmonary sporotrichosis, amphotericin B given as a lipid formulation at 3–5 mg/kg/d is recommended (1)[C].
  - Amphotericin B deoxycholate 0.7–1.0 mg/kg/d also can be used (1)[C].
  - After the patient has shown a favorable response to amphotericin B, therapy can be switched to itraconazole 200 mg p.o. b.i.d. to complete a total of at least 12 months of therapy (1)[C].
  - For less severe disease, itraconazole 200 mg p.o. b.i.d. for at least 12 months is recommended (1)[C].
  - Surgical resection combined with amphotericin B is recommended for localized pulmonary disease (1)[C].
- Disseminated disease or meningeal involvement:
  - Amphotericin B given as a lipid formulation at a dosage of 5 mg/kg/d × 4–6 weeks is recommended for initial therapy (1)[C].
  - Amphotericin B deoxycholate 0.7–1.0 mg/kg/d also can be used but is not a preferred regimen (1)[C].

- Itraconazole 200 mg b.i.d. is recommended as step-down therapy after the patient responds to initial treatment with amphotericin B and should be given to complete a total of at least 12 months of therapy (1)[C].
- Serum levels of itraconazole should be obtained after the patient has been on this agent for at least 2 weeks to ensure adequate drug exposure (1)[C].
- For AIDS and other immunosuppressed patients, lifelong suppressive therapy with itraconazole 200 mg/d is recommended to prevent relapse (1)[C].

Pediatric Considerations

- Itraconazole at a dosage of 6–10 mg/kg/d to a maximum of 400 mg/d p.o. is recommended for children with cutaneous or lymphocutaneous sporotrichosis (1)[C].
- An alternative for children is SSKI initiated at a dosage of 1 drop (using a standard eye dropper) t.i.d., increasing as tolerated up to a maximum of 1 drop/kg or 40–50 drops t.i.d., whichever is lowest (1)[C].
- For children with disseminated sporotrichosis, amphotericin B 0.7 mg/kg/d should be the initial therapy, followed by itraconazole 6–10 mg/kg up to 400 mg/d maximum as step-down therapy (1)[C].

Pregnancy Considerations

- Amphotericin B given as a lipid formulation at a dosage of 3–5 mg/kg/d or amphotericin B deoxycholate given as 0.7–1 mg/kg/d is recommended for severe sporotrichosis that must be treated during pregnancy (1)[C].
- Azoles should be avoided.
- Local hyperthermia can be used for cutaneous sporotrichosis in pregnant women (1)[C].

Second Line

Terbinafine 250 mg p.o. daily, although not approved for treatment of sporotrichosis, may be a reasonable alternative to itraconazole for cutaneous disease (4)[C].

ADDITIONAL TREATMENT

General Measures

- Local heat application is useful for cutaneous and lymphocutaneous disease.
- Keep cutaneous lesions clean.
- Repeated drainage of infected joints may be indicated.

Issues for Referral

Infectious diseases consultation is suggested for optimal management.

SURGERY/OTHER PROCEDURES

- Synovectomy of infected joints may be indicated.
- Surgical débridement of osteomyelitis is usually indicated.
- Surgical resection of pulmonary lesions may be indicated when feasible.

ONGOING CARE

FOLLOW-UP RECOMMENDATIONS

Patient Monitoring

- Check for compliance with long-term drug therapy (SSKI should be continued for 1–2 months after lesions heal).
- Hepatic enzyme tests should be monitored periodically in patients receiving itraconazole treatment for >1 month.

PROGNOSIS

- Excellent for complete recovery from cutaneous or lymphocutaneous infections
- Other disease forms demonstrate a chronic indolent course and are variably responsive to therapy.
- AIDS patients often have a poor outcome.

COMPLICATIONS

- Secondary bacterial infection
- Bone and joint deformities from osteoarticular disease

REFERENCES

1. Kauffman CA, Bustamante B, Chapman SW, et al. Clinical practice guidelines for the management of sporotrichosis: 2007 update by the Infectious Diseases Society of America. *Clin Infect Dis*. 2007;45:1255–65.
2. Ramos-e-Silva M, Vasconcelos C, Carneiro S, et al. Sporotrichosis. *Clin. Dermatol*. 181–7.
3. Xue S, Gu R, Wu T, et al. Oral potassium iodide for the treatment of sporotrichosis. *Cochrane Database Syst Rev*. 2009;CD006136.
4. Francesconi G, Valle AC, Passos S, et al. Terbinafine (250 mg/day): an effective and safe treatment of cutaneous sporotrichosis. *J Eur Acad Dermatol Venereol*. 2009;23:1273–6.

ADDITIONAL READING

- Kauffman CA. Endemic mycoses: blastomycosis, histoplasmosis, and sporotrichosis. *Infect Dis Clin North Am*. 2006;20:645–62, vii.
- Kauffman CA, Hajjeh R, Chapman SW. Practice guidelines for the management of patients with sporotrichosis. For the Mycoses Study Group. Infectious Diseases Society of America. *Clin Infect Dis*. 2000;30:684–7.
- Milby AH, Pappas ND, O'Donnell J, et al. Sporotrichosis of the Upper Extremity. *Orthopedics*. 2010;273–275.

CODES

ICD9

117.1 Sporotrichosis

CLINICAL PEARLS

- Consider cutaneous/lymphocutaneous sporotrichosis in gardeners or those whose occupation puts them in contact with soil.
- Disseminated sporotrichosis may develop in immunocompromised individuals.
- Antifungal agents are frequently effective in the treatment of sporotrichosis.

S

SPRAIN, ANKLE

J. Herbert Stevenson, MD
Darius Greenbacher, MD

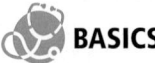

BASICS

DESCRIPTION
Ankle sprains are the most common cause of ankle injury and make up a significant proportion of sports injuries.

- There are several types of ankle sprains, including lateral, medial, and syndesmotic (or high ankle sprain):
  - The most common type of ankle sprain is a lateral ankle sprain, accounting for 85% of all ankle sprains. In lateral ankle sprains, the anterior talofibular ligament (ATFL) is the weakest ligament and, therefore, the most likely to be injured. The calcaneofibular ligament (CFL) is the 2nd likely ligament to be injured, and the posterior talofibular ligament (PTFL) is the least likely.
  - Medial ankle sprains make up 5–10% of ankle sprains and result in an injury to the deltoid ligament.
  - Syndesmotic sprains are rare; they account for 5–10% of ankle sprains.

Geriatric Considerations
Increased risk of fracture occurring with a sprain secondary to weaker bones caused by osteoporosis or osteopenia

Pediatric Considerations
- Increased risk of physeal injuries instead of ligament sprain
- Ligaments are stronger than physes.
- Inversion ankle injuries in children may have a concomitant fibular physeal injury (Salter Harris type I fracture or higher fracture).

EPIDEMIOLOGY
Incidence
- Highest among basketball, soccer, and football players; cross-country runners, and dancers
- Most common sports injury

Prevalence
- 2 million per year
- 20% of sports injuries in the US (1)
- 75% of all ankle injuries are sprains (2).

RISK FACTORS
- Previous ankle sprain is the number 1 risk factor (3): Of people who have had a sprain, 3–34% will sustain another (4).
- Postural instability and talar tilting may be risk factors (3).
- Joint laxity was not found to be a risk factor (3).

GENERAL PREVENTION
- Conditioning before participating in sports and throughout the season (3)[B],(5)[A]:
  - Training in agility and flexibility
  - Single-leg balancing
- Taping or wearing ankle braces may help prevent reinjury to a sprained ankle (3)[B].

ETIOLOGY
- Lateral ankle sprains result from an inversion while plantarflexing the ankle.
- Medial ankle sprains are due to forced eversion while in dorsiflexion.
- Syndesmotic sprains result from eversion stress or extreme dorsiflexion along with internal rotation of tibia.

COMMONLY ASSOCIATED CONDITIONS
- Contusions
- Fractures:
  - Fibula head fracture or dislocation
  - Base of the 5th metatarsal fracture
  - Distal fibula fracture (including Salter Harris fractures in pediatric patients)

DIAGNOSIS

HISTORY
- Description of the mechanism of injury (inversion versus eversion)
- May have felt or heard a pop or a snap
- Ask about previous injury of the ankle.
- Rapid onset of pain and swelling
- Ecchymosis
- Pain on lateral or medial ankle
- Weakness
- Difficulty in bearing weight

PHYSICAL EXAM
- Compare to noninjured ankle for swelling and laxity.
- Palpate ATFL, CFL, PTFL, and deltoid ligament for tenderness.
- Palpate lateral and medial malleolus, base of 5th metatarsal, and entire fibula.
- Grade I sprain: Mild swelling and pain, no laxity
- Grade II sprain: Moderate swelling and pain, mild laxity with endpoint noted
- Grade III sprain: Severe swelling, pain, and bruising, laxity with no endpoint

- Special tests:
  - Anterior drawer test to check for laxity of ATFL
  - Talar tilt test to check laxity in CFL or deltoid ligament
  - Squeeze test of tibia and fibula midcalf to check for syndesmotic injury. Positive test is causing of pain isolated to the syndesmosis.
  - Dorsiflexion/external rotation test

DIAGNOSTIC TESTS & INTERPRETATION
Imaging
Initial approach
- Use the Ottawa ankle rules to determine whether radiographs are needed (patient must be aged 18–55 years):
  - Bony tenderness at lateral or medial malleolus *or*
  - Inability to bear weight (walk ≥4 steps) immediately and in the emergency department or office
  - Tenderness over the base of 5th metatarsal, navicular, or midfoot
- Obtain anteroposterior, lateral, and mortise views of the ankle.
- Small avulsion fractures are associated with grade III sprains.
- Consider computed tomography (CT) if radiographs are negative, but have a high suspicion for occult fracture.
- Magnetic resonance imaging (MRI) is gold standard for soft tissue, including ligaments.

Follow-Up & Special Considerations
If patient is not improving in 6 weeks, consider CT or MRI.

DIFFERENTIAL DIAGNOSIS
- Tendon injury:
  - Tendinopathy
  - Tendon tear
- Fracture
- Contusion
- Hematologic

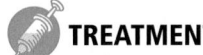

TREATMENT

Short-term immobilization (10 days) for severe ankle sprains

MEDICATION

- Nonsteroidal anti-inflammatory drugs (NSAIDs) (6)[C],(7)[B]
- Narcotics if severe pain

ADDITIONAL TREATMENT

General Measures

- PRICE: **P**rotection, **R**est, **I**ce, **C**ompression, **E**levation
- Wrapping the ankle with an elastic bandage helps decrease swelling, but its use alone has a slower return to sports and work and provides less stability than an ankle brace (8)[A].
- Air-filled or gel-filled ankle brace or an ankle-stabilizing orthoses provides better support than elastic bandage or taping.
- Early mobilization is better than immobilization (9)[B].
- Short-term immobilization (10 days) has been shown to be beneficial for severe ankle sprains (10)[B].
- Do not use heat in an acute injury.
- Activity:
  - Weight-bearing as tolerated
  - Crutches may be needed if patient is unable to bear weight.
  - Exercises should be limited to pain-free range of motion.
  - Patient can start mobilization by tracing the alphabet with the foot in the air.
  - Elastic resistance exercises to improve balance

Issues for Referral

- Malleolar or talar dome fracture
- Syndesmotic sprain
- Tendon rupture

Additional Therapies

Physical therapy:

- After the acute phase of the injury, patients should start physical therapy.
- Physical therapy should include increasing range of motion, strength, flexibility, and proprioceptive balance (wobble board or ankle disk).
- Functional rehab is necessary to prevent chronic instability.
- Athletes should go through a sport-specific rehab before returning to play.

SURGERY/OTHER PROCEDURES

Syndesmotic sprains may require surgery.

ONGOING CARE

FOLLOW-UP RECOMMENDATIONS

- Ankle-stabilizing orthoses should be worn for high-risk sports after a person has sustained an ankle sprain to prevent future ankle sprains (11)[A].
- Moderate and severe sprains require ankle orthoses for ≥6 months while participating in sports (3)[B].
- Return to play for athletes with a grade I lateral ankle sprain is generally 1–2 weeks; grade II sprain is 2–3 weeks; grade 3 sprain is 4 weeks.
- Return to play with medial or syndesmotic sprains is longer.

Patient Monitoring

If athletes continue to have symptoms when they return to play, consider further rehab.

PATIENT EDUCATION

- Training on how to use crutches
- Training on how to use elastic bandages, brace, and/or orthoses
- Demonstrate mobilization exercises for ankle.

PROGNOSIS

- Earlier mobilization with bracing allows for faster return to daily living and/or sports.
- Grade of ankle sprain does not relate to prognosis (12)[C].
- Ligamentous strength does not return for months after the injury (2).

COMPLICATIONS

- Joint instability
- Intermittent swelling and pain if not treated properly
- Accumulation of cartilage damage leading to degenerative changes (12)
- 5–33% will continue to have pain 1 year from the injury (4).

REFERENCES

1. Ivins D. Acute ankle sprain: An update. *Am Fam Phys*. 2006;74:1714–20; 1723–4; 1725–6.
2. Wolfe MW, et al. Management of ankle sprains. *Am Fam Phys*. 2001;63.
3. Thacker SB, Stroup DF, Branche CM, et al. The prevention of ankle sprains in sports. A systematic review of the literature. *Am J Sports Med*. 1999; 27:753–60.
4. van Rijn RM. What is the Clinical Course of Acute Ankle Sprains? A Systematic literature review. *Am J Med*. 2008;121(4):324–31.e6.
5. Abernethy L. Strategies to prevent injury in adolescent sport: a systematic review. *Br J Sports Med*. 2007;41:627–38.
6. Mehallo CJ, Drezner JA, Bytomski JR. Practical management: nonsteroidal antiinflammatory drug (NSAID) use in athletic injuries. *Clin J Sport Med*. 2006;16:170–4.
7. Ekman EF, Ruoff G, Kuehl K, et al. The COX-2 specific inhibitor Valdecoxib versus tramadol in acute ankle sprain: a multicenter randomized, controlled trial. *Am J Sports Med*. 2006;34: 945–55.
8. Kerkhoffs GMMJ, Struijs PAA, Marti RK, et al. Different functional treatment strategies for acute lateral ankle ligament injuries in adults. *Cochrane Database Syst Rev*. 2002;Issue 3. Art. No.: CD002938. DOI:10.1002/14651858.CD002938.
9. Jones MH. Acute treatment of inversion ankle sprains: immobilization versus functional treatment. *Clin Orthop Relat Res*. 2007;455: 169–72.
10. Lamb SE, Marsh JL, Hutton JL, et al. Mechanical supports for acute, severe ankle sprain: a pragmatic, multicentre, randomised controlled trial. *Lancet*. 2009;373:575–81.
11. Handoll HHG, Rowe BH, Quinn KM, et al. Interventions for preventing ankle ligament injuries. *Cochrane Database Syst Rev*. 2001;Issue 3. Art. No.: CD000018. DOI:10.1002/14651858.CD000018.
12. Garland SW. An analysis of the pacing strategy adopted by elite competitors in 2000 m rowing. *Br J Sports Med*. 2005;39:39–42.

ADDITIONAL READING

- LaBella CR. Common acute sports-related lower extremity injuries in children and adolescents. *Clin Ped Emerg Med*. 2007;8:31–42.
- Williams GN, Jones MH, Amendola A. Syndesmotic ankle sprains in athletes. *Am J Sports Med*. 2007;35:1197–207.

CODES

ICD9

- 845.00 Unspecified site of ankle sprain
- 845.01 Deltoid (ligament), ankle sprain
- 845.02 Calcaneofibular (ligament) ankle sprain

CLINICAL PEARLS

- Increased risk of physeal injuries rather than ligament sprains in pediatric patients because ligaments are stronger than physes.
- Conditioning before participating in sports and throughout the season prevents ankle sprains.
- Taping or wearing ankle braces may help prevent reinjury to a sprained ankle, but does not help prevent initial ankle sprains.
- If patient is not improving in 6 weeks, consider CT or MRI.
- Short-term immobilization (10 days) utilizing mechanical supports (i.e., Aircast, others) is superior to elastic bandages.
- Early mobilization is better than long-term immobilization.

SPRAINS AND STRAINS

J. Herbert Stevenson, MD

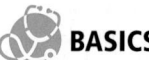
BASICS

DESCRIPTION
- Sprains are complete or partial ligamentous injuries either within the body of the ligament or at the site of attachment to bone.
  - May be classified as grade I, II, or III (AMA Ligament Injury Classification) (1):
    - ○ Grade I: Stretch injury without ligamentous laxity
    - ○ Grade II: Partial tear with increased ligamentous laxity but firm endpoint on exam
    - ○ Grade III: Complete tear with increased ligamentous laxity and no firm endpoint on exam
  - Physical exam is the key to diagnosis.
  - Usually secondary to trauma [e.g., falls, twisting injuries, or motor vehicle accidents (MVAs)]
- Strains are partial or complete disruptions of the muscle, muscle-tendon junction, or tendon; they can be associated with overuse injuries. May be classified as
  - 1st degree: Minimal damage to muscle, tendon, or musculotendinous unit
  - 2nd degree: Partial tear to the muscle, tendon, or musculotendinous unit
  - 3rd degree: Complete disruption of the muscle, etc (1).
- System(s) affected: Musculoskeletal

Geriatric Considerations
More likely to see associated bony injuries owing to decreased joint flexibility and prevalence of osteoporosis and osteopenia

Pediatric Considerations
- Sprains and strains have been found to account for 24% of injuries in pediatric patients.
- 3 million pediatric sports injuries occur annually.
- Must be concerned about physeal/apophyseal injuries in the skeletally immature

EPIDEMIOLOGY
Incidence
~80% of all US athletes at some time in their career will experience a sprain or strain that involves the upper or lower extremities or spine.

Prevalence
- Ankle sprains are among the most common injuries seen in the primary-care setting and account for up to 30% of sports medicine clinic visits (2).
- Predominant age:
  - Sprains: Any age when patient is physically active
  - Strains: Usually 15–40 years of age
- Predominant sex: Male > Female; Female > Male for sprain of acromioclavicular ligament (ACL).

RISK FACTORS
- Prior history of sprain or strain is greatest risk factor for future sprain/strain.
- Change in or improper shoe gear, protective gear, or environment (e.g., surface)
- Inappropriate sudden increase in training schedule

GENERAL PREVENTION
- Balance training is found to reduce risk of knee and ankle sprains.
- Use proper equipment for the activity.
- Use appropriate conditioning, warm-up, and cool-down exercises.
- Single-leg balancing may help to prevent ankle sprains (3)[B].
- Taping/bracing postinjury may be of short-term benefit for future injury prevention of ankle sprains (4)[B].

ETIOLOGY
- Falls
- MVAs
- Trauma
- Excessive exercise
- Inadequate warm-up and stretching before activity
- Poor conditioning

COMMONLY ASSOCIATED CONDITIONS
- Hemarthrosis
- Stress, avulsion, or other fractures
- Syndesmotic injuries
- Contusions
- Wounds
- Dislocations
- Subluxations

DIAGNOSIS

HISTORY
- May describe feeling or hearing pop or snap
- May remember mechanism (key in diagnosis)

PHYSICAL EXAM
- Swelling
- Pain
- Ecchymosis (usually late)
- Tenderness
- Gait disturbances if severe
- Decreased range of motion (ROM) of joint and joint instability
- Sprains:
  - Grade I: Tenderness without laxity
  - Grade II: Tenderness with increased laxity on exam but firm endpoint
  - Grade III: Tenderness with increased laxity on exam and no firm endpoint

DIAGNOSTIC TESTS & INTERPRETATION
- Examination under anesthesia and/or arthroscopy may be required in some cases.
- For ankle, use the anterior drawer test, which tests the integrity of the anterior talofibular ligament.
- Apprehension test may indicate glenohumeral ligament sprain of the shoulder.
- Lachman test assesses the integrity of ACL.

Imaging
- Radiographs may be needed to rule out bony injury; stress views may be helpful.
- Ankle films (Ottawa ankle rules):
  - Bone tenderness in posterior aspect distal 6 cm of tibia/fibula
  - Inability to bear weight, both immediately or in emergency department/office
  - Age >18 and <55 years (5)
- Foot films: Required only if midfoot zone pain is present *and*
  - Bone tenderness at base of 5th metatarsal *or*
  - Bone tenderness at navicular *or*
  - Inability to bear weight immediately or in emergency department
- CT scan of the affected area may be required if occult fracture is suspected, with negative films.
- MRI is "gold standard" for imaging soft-tissue structures, including muscle, ligaments, and intraarticular structures.
- Exam under anesthesia in difficult cases

Diagnostic Procedures/Surgery

Surgery may be required for some partial and complete sprains. Need for surgery depends on the ability of ligaments or muscles to heal on their own or the ability to attain full ROM and stability of the affected joint.

DIFFERENTIAL DIAGNOSIS

- Tendonitis
- Bursitis
- Contusion
- Hematoma
- Fracture
- Rheumatologic process

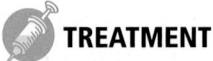 TREATMENT

MEDICATION

- Nonsteroidal anti-inflammatory drugs (NSAIDs) (6)[C]:
  - Ibuprofen: 200–800 mg t.i.d.
  - Naproxen: 375–500 mg b.i.d.
  - Indomethacin: 25–50 mg t.i.d.
  - Acetaminophen (7)[B]
  - Narcotics for severe pain (e.g., acetaminophen–hydrocodone)
- Contraindications: Refer to the manufacturer's profile of each drug.
- Precautions: Refer to the manufacturer's profile of each drug.
- Significant possible interactions: Refer to the manufacturer's profile of each drug.

ADDITIONAL TREATMENT

General Measures

- History and physical exam along with treatment of the worst possible suspected injury
- Acutely: PRICEMM therapy (*protection, relative rest, ice, compression, elevation, medications, modalities*) (6)[B]:
  - Elastic bandage wrap (Ace) if comfortable
  - Jones dressing for more severe injuries
- Orthosis (splint) for pain relief and stability; air cast–type devices provide effective stability and pain relief for ankle sprains.
- Crutches and crutch gait training
- Stirrup-type ankle brace (8)[A]

Issues for Referral

- ACL sprain in athletes/physically active
- Salter-Harris physeal fractures
- Lack of improvement with conservative measures
- Joint instability
- Tendon disruption (i.e., Achilles, biceps)

Additional Therapies

- Useful adjunct after injury (9)[B]
- Proprioception retraining (10)[C]
- Core strengthening (10)[C]
- Eccentric exercises (10)[C]

SURGERY/OTHER PROCEDURES

Casting and surgery are reserved for select grade III injuries.

 ONGOING CARE

FOLLOW-UP RECOMMENDATIONS

If affected joint has full strength and ROM, patient can advance activity as tolerated.

Patient Monitoring

After initial treatment, consider rehabilitation. Direct emphasis toward limiting swelling and providing a pain-free full ROM.

DIET

Weight loss if obesity is etiologic

PATIENT EDUCATION

- Instructions on how to wrap with elastic bandage
- Prevention of injury

PROGNOSIS

With appropriate treatment and rest, 1–8 weeks or longer for recovery, depending on the severity of injury

COMPLICATIONS

- Chronic joint instability
- Arthritis
- Muscle contracture

REFERENCES

1. O'Connor F, et al. *Sports Medicine: Just the Facts*. New York: McGraw-Hill, 2005;34.
2. Mahaffey D, Hilts M, Fields KB. Ankle and foot injuries in sports. *Clin Fam Pract*. 1999;1:233–50.
3. McGuine TA, Keene JS. The effect of a balance training program on the risk of ankle sprains in high school athletes. *Am J Sports Med*. 2006;34:1103–11.
4. Handoll HHG, Rowe BH, Quinn KM, et al. Interventions for preventing ankle injuries. *Cochrane Database of Systematic Rev*. May 26m 2005.
5. Stiell IG, McKnight RD, Greenberg GH, et al. Implementation of the Ottawa ankle rules. *JAMA*. 1994;271:827–32.
6. Nyland J, Nolan MF. Therapeutic modality: rehabilitation of the injured athlete. *Clin Sports Med*. 2004;23:299–313, vii.
7. Dalton JD, Schweinle JE. Randomized controlled noninferiority trial to compare extended release acetaminophen and ibuprofen for the treatment of ankle sprains. *Ann Emerg Med*. 2006;48:615–23.
8. Boyce SH, Quigley MA, Campbell S. Management of ankle sprains: a randomised controlled trial of the treatment of inversion injuries using an elastic support bandage or an Aircast ankle brace. *Br J Sports Med*. 2005;39:91–6.
9. Kerkhoffs et al. Immobilisation and functional treatment for acute lateral ankle ligament injuries in adults. *Cochrane Database of Systematic Rev*. December 16, 2004.
10. Brukner PD, Crossley KM, Morris H, et al. 5. Recent advances in sports medicine. *Med J Aust*. 2006;184:188–93.

ADDITIONAL READING

Mehallo CJ, Drezner JA, Bytomski JR. Practical management: nonsteroidal antiinflammatory drug (NSAID) use in athletic injuries. *Clin J Sport Med*. 2006;16:170–4.

See Also (Topic, Algorithm, Electronic Media Element)

Tendinitis

 CODES

ICD9

- 845.00 Unspecified site of ankle sprain
- 848.9 Unspecified site of sprain and strain

CLINICAL PEARLS

For acute injury, remember PRICEMM:

- Protection joint
- Rest as appropriate
- Apply ice
- Apply compression [elastic bandage wrap (Ace) if comfortable]
- Elevate joint
- Medications for pain
- Other modalities as needed

STAPHYLOCOCCAL TOXIC SHOCK SYNDROME

William J. Durbin, MD
William Zawatski, MD

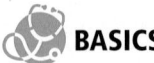 **BASICS**

DESCRIPTION
- An acute toxin-mediated illness associated with *Staphylococcus aureus* infection
- TSS (toxic shock syndrome) is characterized by sudden onset of high fever and rash with subsequent hypotension, desquamation, and involvement of ≥3 organ systems.
- Menstrual (less common): Associated with menstruation and tampon use
- Nonmenstrual (more common): Associated with postoperative wounds and barrier contraception
- Can occur in children, men, and women
- System(s) affected: All organ systems can be affected.

EPIDEMIOLOGY
- Predominant age: 15–35 years, but can occur at any age
- Predominant sex: Female > Male
- Nonmenstrual cases increasingly associated with methicillin-resistant *Staphylococcus aureus* (MRSA) infections and carry a higher mortality rate (1)
- Newborn population: Neonatal TSS-like exanthematous disease (NTED) syndrome (2)

Incidence
1–2/100,000 in the US; incidence decreased steadily from 1986–1996, but increasing in recent years (3)

RISK FACTORS
- High:
  - Absence of antibody to TSS toxin-1 (TSST-1)
  - Infection with *S. aureus,* which produces TSST-1
  - Focal: Abscess, sinusitis, bacterial tracheitis
  - Invasive: Pneumonia, osteomyelitis, bacteremia, endocarditis
  - Focus of infection may not be apparent:
    - Continuous use of super-absorbency tampons during menstruation
    - Nasal surgery with packing
- Moderate:
  - Use of regular-absorbency tampons during menstruation
  - Use of contraceptive sponge
- Low:
  - Alternating use of tampons and pads during menstruation
  - Surgical wound infections
  - Cellulitis
  - Early postpartum state, especially post-cesarean section or episiotomy
- Pediatric considerations: TSS may occur as a complication of:
  - Chickenpox
  - Burns: TSS is the most common cause of unexpected mortality after small burns in the pediatric population (4).

Genetics
No known genetic predisposition

GENERAL PREVENTION
- Avoid continuous tampon use during menstruation.
- Avoid super-absorbency tampons.
- Change tampons frequently during the day.
- Use sanitary napkins at night.
- Early medical attention to infected wounds

PATHOPHYSIOLOGY
- In vivo production and release of staphylococcal superantigens in the absence of neutralizing antibodies. Superantigen simultaneously binds to APC MHC class II and Vbeta region of T cell receptor. A large subset of T cells are then activated, resulting in massive release of cytokines (IL-1, IL-2, gamma interferon, TNF alpha, TNF beta, IL-6). Capillary leak, hypotension, and shock ensue.
- Although both serum IgG and IgM antibodies bind to TSST-1 in vitro, only IgG1 and IgG4 isotype antibodies are protective (5).

ETIOLOGY
- *S. aureus* exotoxins, especially TSST-1 (etiology in all menstrual cases)
- Staphylococcal enterotoxins A–E and G–I
- Enterotoxins B and C cause 50% of nonmenstrual TSS

COMMONLY ASSOCIATED CONDITIONS
Staphylococcal infections

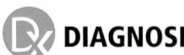 **DIAGNOSIS**

HISTORY
- Prodrome of 1–3 days that often includes malaise, myalgias, fever, chills, vomiting, and/or diarrhea
- Acute-onset fever and chills
- Lightheadedness or syncope
- Disorientation, confusion, or alteration in consciousness
- Myalgias
- Diffuse macular rash
- Other symptoms of multiorgan involvement

PHYSICAL EXAM
- Temperature >38.9°C (>102°F)
- Hypotension:
  - Systolic blood pressure (SBP) <90 mm Hg
  - Orthostatic drop in diastolic blood pressure (DBP) of ≥15 mm Hg
  - BP <5th percentile for age in children
- Tachycardia
- Tachypnea
- Diffuse erythroderma, initially appearing on trunk and spreading to arms and legs including palms and soles:
  - Skin desquamation 1–2 weeks after rash onset

- Signs of multiorgan involvement, including:
  - Cardiac (arrhythmias, pericarditis, cardiomyopathy)
  - Pulmonary (acute respiratory distress syndrome [ARDS])
  - Renal (oliguria)
  - Disseminated intravascular coagulation (DIC)
  - Central nervous system (CNS) involvement (headache, confusion, agitation, photophobia, meningismus, seizure)
  - Mucosal inflammation (conjunctivitis, strawberry tongue, pharyngitis, vaginitis)

DIAGNOSTIC TESTS & INTERPRETATION
Lab
Initial lab tests
- Thrombocytopenia may be present (platelet count ≤100,000/mm³).
- Blood urea nitrogen (BUN) and creatinine may be increased.
- Liver function tests (LFTs), including total bilirubin, AST, and/or ALT, may be increased.
- Creatine phosphokinase (CPK) may be increased.
- Urinary sediment may contain white blood cells in absence of urinary tract infection (UTI).
- Blood culture is positive for *S. aureus* in <5% of cases.
- Throat and cerebrospinal fluid (CSF) cultures are usually negative.
- If clinically plausible, serologies for Rocky Mountain spotted fever, leptospirosis, and measles should be negative.

Imaging
No unusual or characteristic findings

Diagnostic Procedures/Surgery
- No specific diagnostic test is currently available.
- Acute and convalescent anti-TSST-1 antibodies

Pathological Findings
- Subepidermal cleavage plane in skin
- Minimal inflammatory reaction in tissues
- Lymphocyte depletion in lymph nodes

DIFFERENTIAL DIAGNOSIS
- Streptococcal scarlet fever
- Streptococcal TSS:
  - More often associated with severe pain and tenderness at a site of local trauma and infection, and more frequently accompanied by bacteremia
- Staphylococcal scalded-skin syndrome
- Necrotizing fasciitis
- Meningococcemia/sepsis (petechial/purpuric rash)
- Gram-negative sepsis (more likely in hospitalized patients)

- Rocky Mountain spotted fever (petechial rash beginning distally; often presents with severe headache)
- Leptospirosis
- Kawasaki disease
- Measles
- Drug reactions (i.e., Stevens Johnson Syndrome)

 TREATMENT

Inpatient; typically requires admission to intensive care for close monitoring

MEDICATION
First Line
- Treatment of shock or hypotension (see Circulatory Shock for details):
  – Aggressive fluid replacement
  – Pressors
  – Steroids have not proven to be of value, although low-dose steroids may be beneficial if sepsis is severe (6)[A].
- Antibiotics to eradicate *S. aureus* and inhibit toxin production:
  – Oxacillin or nafcillin: 100 mg/kg/d IV divided q4h (bactericidal against susceptible *S. aureus*, but may induce more toxin production and release more toxins by bacterial lysis) (7)[B]
  – Clindamycin: 30–40 mg/kg/d IV divided q8h (more efficacious than beta-lactams in suppressing in vitro production of TSST-1 and other exotoxins) (7)[B]
  – Combination of clindamycin 25 mg/kg/d IV divided q8h plus oxacillin or nafcillin 100 mg/kg/d IV q4h (recommended for patients with deep-seated infections or bacteremia) (7)[B]
  – For patients infected with MRSA: Vancomycin 40 mg/kg/d divided q6h or linezolid 600 mg q12h IV
- Antimicrobial therapy should be continued for at least 10–14 days.

Second Line
- Toxin neutralization with immune globulin IV (IVIG) 1 g/kg
- Off-label use of IVIG, but accepted treatment for TSS that is supported by several studies, including 1 case-control study providing an odds ratio for survival of 8:1 (8)[B]

ADDITIONAL TREATMENT
General Measures
- Ongoing fluid resuscitation
- Removal of tampon or other vaginal foreign bodies and irrigation of vaginal vault with saline or povidone-iodine
- Removal of nasal packing
- Local wound care
- Management of renal or cardiac insufficiency
- Mechanical ventilation if necessary

IN-PATIENT CONSIDERATIONS
IV Fluids
Crystalloids, up to 10–20 L/day, may be necessary.
Nursing
- Vital signs should be closely monitored.
- Foley catheter to monitor urine output
Discharge Criteria
- Hemodynamic stability
- Improvement in symptoms
- Tolerating oral alimentation

 ONGOING CARE

FOLLOW-UP RECOMMENDATIONS
Women can reduce the risk of recurrent TSS by avoiding continuous tampon use during menstruation.

DIET
As tolerated

PATIENT EDUCATION
- For both medical professionals and the public at: http://www.toxicshock.com
- Centers for Disease Control (CDC) at: http://www.cdc.gov/ncidod/dbmd/diseaseinfo/toxicshock_t.htm

PROGNOSIS
Mortality: <5%, higher in older patients and in nonmenstrual TSS

COMPLICATIONS
- Common (>20%):
  – Acute renal failure
  – ARDS
  – Menorrhagia
  – Alopecia
  – Nail loss
- Rare (<20%):
  – DIC
  – Encephalopathy/memory impairment
  – Cardiomyopathy
  – Protracted malaise

REFERENCES

1. Descloux E, Perpoint T, Ferry T, et al. One in five mortality in non-menstrual toxic shock syndrome versus no mortality in menstrual cases in a balanced French series of 55 cases. *Eur J Clin Microbiol Infect Dis*. 2008;27:37–43.
2. Miki M, Uchiyama T, Kato H, et al. A severe case of neonatal toxic shock syndrome-like exanthematous disease with superantigen-induced high T cell response. *Pediatr Infect Dis J*. 2006;25:950–2.
3. Schlievert PM, Tripp TJ, Peterson ML. Reemergence of staphylococcal toxic shock syndrome in Minneapolis-St. Paul, Minnesota, during the 2000–2003 surveillance period. *J Clin Microbiol*. 2004;42:2875–6.
4. Young AE, Thornton KL. Toxic shock syndrome in burns: diagnosis and management. *Arch Dis Child Educ Pract Ed*. 2007;92:ep97–100.
5. Kansal R, Davis C, Hansmann M, et al. Structural and functional properties of antibodies to the superantigen TSST-1 and their relationship to menstrual toxic shock syndrome. *J Clin Immunol*. 2007;27:327–38.
6. Minneci PC, Deans KJ, Eichacker PQ, et al. The effects of steroids during sepsis depend on dose and severity of illness: an updated meta-analysis. *Clin Microbiol Infect*. 2009;15:308–18.
7. Stevens DL, Ma Y, Salmi DB, et al. Impact of antibiotics on expression of virulence-associated exotoxin genes in methicillin-sensitive and methicillin-resistant Staphylococcus aureus. *J Infect Dis*. 2007;195:202–11.
8. Fernandez AP, Kerdel FA. The use of i.v. IG therapy in dermatology. *Dermatol Ther*. 2007;20:288–305.

ADDITIONAL READING
- Andrews JI, Shamshirsaz AA, Diekema DJ. Nonmenstrual toxic shock syndrome due to methicillin-resistant Staphylococcus aureus. *Obstet Gynecol*. 2008;112:933–8.
- Walden A, Harriet H, Alyaqoobi M. Methicillin-resistant Staphylococcus aureus toxic shock syndrome. *J Infect*. 2008;56:161–2.

See Also (Topic, Algorithm, Electronic Media Element)
Measles, (Rubeola); Pancreatitis; Rocky Mountain Spotted Fever; Scarlet Fever

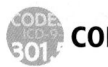 **CODES**

ICD9
- 040.82 Toxic shock syndrome
- 041.11 Methicillin susceptible Staphylococcus aureus

CLINICAL PEARLS
- TSS is a rare, acute, toxin-mediated illness caused by *S. aureus*.
- In women, TSS is associated with the continuous use of super-absorbency tampons during menstruation.
- Patients typically require ICU-level care and IV antibiotics.

STATUS EPILEPTICUS

Jeff Ray Gibson, Jr., MD

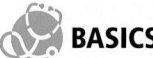 **BASICS**

ALERT
- Status epilepticus is a life-threatening emergency; rapid seizure control is critical, even before a definitive diagnosis is reached (as with CPR).
- Begin drug treatment if seizure lasts >5 minutes.

DESCRIPTION
- Established status epilepticus is a seizure lasting >30 minutes or absence of recovery of consciousness between seizures. Tonic–clonic (grand mal or generalized convulsive) status is the most common and serious form.
- Refractory status epilepticus: Seizure that persists after treatment with 1st-line drugs.
  – System affected: Nervous
  – Synonym: Status convulsivus

EPIDEMIOLOGY
Incidence
- 18–50 cases per 100,000 per year; 1/3 as unprovoked 1st seizure, 1/6 in patients with known epilepsy, 1/2 secondary to acute CNS insult
- Incidence is 2 times higher in the elderly
- Predominant age: >50% of new cases in the young
- Predominant sex: Male > Female

Prevalence
In the US, 100,000–150,000 patients per year present with generalized tonic–clonic status epilepticus; 55,000 associated deaths.

RISK FACTORS
- Seizure disorder plus any precipitating insult
- Prior history of status epilepticus (recurrence rates: in children, 17%; in those with neurologic abnormality, 50%)
- Porphyria, autoimmune diseases, CNS lesion

Genetics
Links suspected but not defined

GENERAL PREVENTION
Established maintenance therapy with anticonvulsant

PATHOPHYSIOLOGY
- Neuronal injury; Autonomic activation
- Metabolic: Lactic acidosis, CO_2 narcosis, hyperkalemia, hyperglycemia followed by hypoglycemia
- Cardiac: Hypertension (followed by hypotension), arrhythmias, high output failure
- Respiratory: Increased secretions, lax tongue, and possibly airway obstruction, pneumothorax, neurogenic pulmonary edema, or aspiration
- Renal: ATN from myoglobinuria after rhabdomyolysis
- Cerebrovascular: Loss of autoregulation, focal ischemia, cerebral edema

ETIOLOGY
- Adults: Usually from a known condition (epilepsy, alcohol withdrawal, anticonvulsant withdrawal/noncompliance) or acquired CNS pathology (especially frontal lobe)
- Children: Status epilepticus may present as the 1st seizure from febrile seizure, new-onset epilepsy, CNS infection, or metabolic derangement.
- Neonatal status: Meningitis or metabolic disorders (deficiencies of calcium, magnesium, or pyridoxine)

- CNS pathology (acute or chronic): Trauma, infection, stroke, hypoglycemia, mass or vascular lesion, metabolic disorder, encephalopathy (hypoxic, autoimmune or degenerative type)
- Intoxication: Reports include cocaine, tricyclic antidepressants, isoniazid, chloroquine, cephalosporins, penicillins, ciprofloxacin, cyclosporine, theophylline, tacrolimus, tiagabine, or nerve-agent poisoning

COMMONLY ASSOCIATED CONDITIONS
Premonitory status epilepticus: Increasing frequency of seizures, which may precede convulsive status epilepticus. Treat early to prevent status.

 DIAGNOSIS

ALERT
- Rule out pseudo (psychogenic)-status epilepticus; usually atypical, e.g., pelvic thrusting, no self-injury.
- Check the EEG; avoid dangerous therapy.

HISTORY
Previous seizures, drug history, toxic exposure

PHYSICAL EXAM
- Signs and symptoms depend on the type of seizure; generalized (tonic–clonic) convulsion is most common.
  – May be preceded by aura
  – Tonic phase (stiffening) for 30–45 seconds
  – Clonic phase (rhythmic jerking) for 2–5 minutes
  – No intervening consciousness; seizure recurs
- Neurologic exam: Look for localizing signs; rule out pseudo status
- Postictal findings: Fever; tachycardia; mydriasis; conjugate deviation of eyes; decreased corneal reflex; positive Babinski sign; Todd's paralysis; fecal/urinary incontinence; tongue, cheek, or lip injury

DIAGNOSTIC TESTS & INTERPRETATION
Lab
- Glucose (rapid determination); Electrolytes, CBC, osmolarity, liver/renal function, CPK, calcium, magnesium, phosphate, coag profile
- Arterial blood gases, carboxyhemoglobin; Anticonvulsant levels, toxicology screen

Imaging
- Noncontrast CT scan in new-onset seizure
- MRI or PET for more anatomic detail
- CXR for ET tube position or aspiration

Diagnostic Procedures/Surgery
- Lumbar puncture: If meningitis is suspected. CAUTION: Intracranial pressure may be increased.
- EEG: Differentiate pseudoseizures; Reveal nonconvulsive status epilepticus in comatose or paralyzed patient; Confirm successful treatment

DIFFERENTIAL DIAGNOSIS
- Pseudo (psychogenic)–status epilepticus may occur with pseudo seizures; check EEG.
- Comatose or paralyzed patients and other forms of status require neurologic exam and EEG.

special-considerations
- Check the EEG for nonconvulsive status if a patient not awake 30 minutes after a seizure.

 TREATMENT

Simultaneous goals are to stop the seizure, find the cause, and prevent complications (1,2,3,4)[B]:
- Support ABCs and watch vitals
- Treat glucose if <60 mg/100 dL
- Start IV or intraosseous (IO) line and draw labs
- If seizure lasts >5 minutes, start medication for established status epilepticus.
- IV or IO is preferred, but administer non-IV alternatives rather than delay treatment.
- If seizure continues >30 minutes, treat as refractory status epilepticus with anesthesia/drug coma
- Continue to pursue underlying cause

MEDICATION
First Line
Start with Lorazepam (Ativan) (the preferred benzodiazepine) (1,2,3,4,5,6,7)[A].
- Give 0.1 mg/kg IV or IO at 1–2 mg/min to a maximum of 10 mg
  – For child: 0.05–0.1 mg/kg IV at <2 mg/min to a maximum of 4 mg
- May repeat every 10 minutes × 2
- After 5 minutes, if seizure persists, add fosphenytoin (Cerebyx) (the preferred anticonvulsant and prodrug of phenytoin) (1,2,4)[B].
  – Give 15–20 mg phenytoin equivalents (mg PE)/kg IV or IO at <150 mg PE/min (follow BP, ECG).
  – May add 5–10 mg PE/kg IV after 5 minutes
  – Maintenance: 4–6 mg PE/kg/d IV or IM
    ○ For child: Same dose as for an adult)

ALERT
- If seizure >30 minutes, move on to 2nd-Line (refractory) treatment
- Non-IV alternatives:
  – Midazolam (Versed): 0.2 mg/kg IM or up to 0.5 mg/kg buccal or intranasal (onset 5–10 min) (3,5,8)[A]
  – Lorazepam (sl or intranasal) (5)[B]: Use IV dose.
  – Rectal diazepam (Valium) (6)[A]: 0.2–0.5 mg/kg (for child: 20 mg maximum). Use gel (Diastat) or IV .
- Alternative for IV Lorazepam:
  – Diazepam (Valium) (4,6)[B]: 0.2–0.5 mg/kg IV or IO at 5 mg/min up to a dose of 40 mg
    ○ For child: 0.3 mg/kg at <2 mg/minute IV up to 10 mg total
    ○ May repeat q 5 minutes × 3
    ○ Antiseizure wears off quickly; sedation persists
- Alternatives for IV Fosphenytoin:
  – Phenytoin (4,6)[B] doses are the same (mg-for-mg phenytoin equivalents) but must be given more slowly (<1 mg/kg/min) to lessen cardiovascular depression and toxicity
  – Fosphenytoin IM: Use IV dose (slowly)

Second Line
- When seizure persists >30 minutes admit to ICU and induce anesthesia/drug coma (1,3,4,7)[B]
- Consult neurologist, intensivist, or anesthesiologist.
- Induce coma and adjust to keep EEG at burst suppression (drug choices listed below).

- Often requires intubation, ventilation and BP support (e.g., dopamine)
- Maintain anesthetic for 12–48 hours; then withdraw gradually while adjusting anticonvulsant therapy.
- Consider continuous EEG and end-tidal CO_2.
- For muscle relaxation, use short-acting rocuronium bromide 0.6-1 mg/kg (to avoid hyperkalemia)
- Cool and treat if febrile.
- Drug choices (choose one):
  - Propofol (Diprivan) (1,2,3,4,7)[C]:
    - 2–5 mg/kg IV (in elderly, halve initial dose)
    - Follow with 30–150 μg/kg/minute IV; titrated to EEG
    - Less tissue accumulation
  - Midazolam (Versed) (1,2,3,4,7)[C]
    - 0.2–0.5 mg/kg slow IV bolus injection
    - Follow with 0.1–0.4 mg/kg/h IV; titrated to EEG
    - Tachyphylaxis may develop.
  - Pentobarbital (1,3,4)[B]:
    - 5–15 mg/kg IV loading dose over 1 hour
    - Follow by continuous infusion of 0.5–10 mg/kg/hour; adjust based on EEG
- Alternates: may not require intubation (2,3)[C]:
  - Phenobarbital: 20 mg/kg infused at a rate of 30–50 mg/minute (slower with older populations; close monitoring of respiratory and cardiac status; causes prolonged sedation), then initial maintenance dosing 60 mg t.i.d.
  - Sodium valproate: 15–30 mg/kg bolus at <6 mg/kg/minute, then maintenance dosing 500 mg t.i.d.
  - Levetiracetam: 20 mg/kg bolus over 15 minutes, then maintenance dosing 1500 mg b.i.d.
  - Topiramate: 300–1600 mg/d PO (3)[C]
- Investigational or anecdotal drugs:
  - Isoflurane (by inhalation), desflurane (by inhalation), lidocaine, thiopental, ketamine, nimodipine, chlormethiazole, lamotrigine
- Contraindications:
  - Benzodiazepines in narrow-angle glaucoma
  - Propofol in allergy to soybean oil, egg, lecithin, or glycerol
  - Barbiturates in acute intermittent porphyria
  - Valproic acid in hepatic disease and pregnancy (risk of neural tube defects)
- Precautions:
  - Propofol: Strict aseptic technique required. Prolonged use may cause propofol infusion syndrome (lactic acidosis, lipemia, heart failure, systemic collapse, and death) in both children and adults. Not for child <3 years old.
  - Most drugs listed may exacerbate porphyria. Exceptions are lorazepam, midazolam, propofol.
  - Diazepam: May cause venous thrombosis/phlebitis.
  - Fosphenytoin (Cerebyx) and phenytoin:
    - Safety not established for children. Monitor for arrhythmias, prolonged QT interval, and hypotension. If these occur, decrease the rate of administration.
    - Use caution in liver disease, hyperglycemia, the elderly, and pregnancy (increased risk of malformations and may lead to vitamin K–deficiency bleeding problems in both mother and newborn). Abrupt withdrawal may precipitate status epilepticus. Overdose may cause paradoxical inefficacy.
  - Phenytoin: Infiltration may cause local ischemia (purple glove syndrome).
  - Valproic acid: May decrease platelet function and cause hyperammonemic encephalopathy or pancreatitis.

- Significant possible interactions:
  - Fosphenytoin/phenytoin: May increase serum levels and toxicity of warfarin, disulfiram, phenylbutazone, and isoniazid; decrease dose with renal insufficiency.
  - Valproic acid: May increase toxicity of phenytoin/fosphenytoin

ADDITIONAL TREATMENT
General Measures
- Monitor pulse oximetry, end-tidal CO_2, BP, ECG, EEG and temperature
- Give oxygen: Intubate and hyperventilate if hypoventilation, hypoxia, or hypercarbia occur, *or* if aspiration is a concern.
- Establish 2 IV lines (or an intraosseous line) and check labs
- Protect from injury, clear/suction airway, prevent tongue laceration
- If comatose, place NG tube, urinary catheter

Additional Therapies
- In suspected alcoholism: thiamine, 100 mg IV/IM
- If blood sugar is low or cannot be measured: 50% dextrose, 50 mL IV
- For child: Use $D_{25}W$; give 2 mL/kg slowly
- If pupils are myotic or drug overdose suspected: Naloxone (Narcan), 2 mg IV
  - For child: 0.1 mg/kg IV, up to 2 mg slowly
- If isoniazid poisoning is suspected: Pyridoxine
- If meningitis is strongly suspected: Consider antibiotics
- For nerve-agent poisoning: Give atropine, benzodiazepines, and pralidoxime (2-PAM)

SURGERY/OTHER PROCEDURES
Experimental: Surgical excision of epileptic focus or propagation pathways

IN-PATIENT CONSIDERATIONS
IV Fluids
Hemodynamic instability may require fluid boluses or vasopressors (e.g., dopamine).

Discharge Criteria
Seizures under control; Therapeutic levels of maintenance anticonvulsants

 ## ONGOING CARE

PATIENT EDUCATION
Reinforce the importance of continuing anticonvulsant medications, regular medical care, avoiding alcohol and seeking help if seizure frequency increases.
- Epilepsy Foundation, (800) EFA-1000, http://www.efa.org
- Epilepsy Therapy Development Project, http://www.epilepsy.com

PROGNOSIS
- Prolonged seizures (>30 min) may cause neurologic injury or death.
- Reported mortality is 16–25% in adults, 3–19% in children, extremely high in neonates, and up to 76% in the elderly.
- For seizure duration >4 hours mortality is 50%; for >12 hours, mortality is 80%.

COMPLICATIONS
Morbidity/mortality is usually related to the underlying CNS pathology, stress from repeated seizures (e.g., hyperthermia, acidosis, hypotension, cardiac arrest, rhabdomyolysis, renal failure, aspiration pneumonia), or from the treatment.

REFERENCES
1. Meierkord H, Boon P, Engelsen B, et al. EFNS guideline on the management of status epilepticus. *Eur J Neurol.* 2006;13:445–50.
2. Costello DJ, Cole AJ. Treatment of acute seizures and status epilepticus. *J Intensive Care Med.* 2007; 22:319–47.
3. Cherian A, Thomas SV, et al. Status epilepticus. *Ann Indian Acad Neurol.* 2009;12:140–53.
4. Mirski MA, Varelas PN, et al. Seizures and status epilepticus in the critically ill. *Crit Care Clin.* 2008;24:115–47, ix
5. Appleton R, Macleod S, Martland T. Drug management for acute tonic-clonic convulsions including convulsive status epilepticus in children. *Cochrane Database of Systematic Reviews 2008,* Issue 3. Art. No.: CD001905. DOI:10.1002/14651858.CD001905.pub2.
6. Prasad K, et al. Anticonvulsant therapy for status epilepticus. *Cochrane Database Syst Rev.* 2007: CD003723. DOI:10.1002/14651858. CD003723.pub2.
7. Huff JS. Status Epilepticus: Treatment & Medication. *eMedicine,* 2010. Accessed 4/18/2010 at http://emedicine.medscape.com/article/793708-overview
8. Sofou K, Kristjánsdóttir R, Papachatzakis NE, et al. Management of Prolonged Seizures and Status Epilepticus in Childhood: A Systematic Review. *J Child Neurol.* 2009.

See Also (Topic, Algorithm, Electronic Media Element)
Seizure Disorders; Seizures, Febrile

 ## CODES

ICD9
- 345.2 Petit mal status, epileptic
- 345.3 Grand mal status, epileptic
- 345.80 Other forms of epilepsy, without mention of intractable epilepsy

CLINICAL PEARLS
- Status epilepticus is life-threatening: Begin treatment if seizure lasts >5 minutes.
- Start with IV lorazepam or buccal midazolam.
- If not controlled in 30 minutes, admit to ICU and induce drug coma.

STEATOHEPATITIS, NONALCOHOLIC

Mazen J. AlBeldawi, MD
Rasai L. Ernst, MD

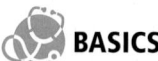 **BASICS**

DESCRIPTION
- Clinical diagnosis is based on findings consistent with metabolic syndrome or insulin resistance and exclusion of alcohol abuse and viral, genetic, autoimmune, and drug-induced liver diseases.
- Majority of patients with nonalcoholic steatohepatitis (NASH) are asymptomatic.
- Increased aminotransferase activities are the most common abnormality reported in patients with NASH.
- NASH is the most severe form of NAFLD; both are the hepatic manifestations of metabolic syndrome.

EPIDEMIOLOGY
Incidence
- NAFLD and NASH have a worldwide distribution.
- NAFLD is the most common form of chronic liver disease in the Western world.
- NAFLD affects approximately 17–33%, and NASH, 6–17%, of people in the US and other Western countries (1)[A].
  - 25–35% of NASH patients have progression to fibrosis.
  - 9–20% of NASH patients progress to cirrhosis.
  - 22–33% of cirrhotics die of complications of liver failure or require orthotopic liver transplantation.
- This increasing prevalence parallels epidemic obesity and diabetes mellitus (DM).
- Predominant age: 5th–6th decades

Pediatric Considerations
- Obesity is also increasing in prevalence in children. The overall prevalence of NAFLD in children is estimated at 3–10%, but it may be much higher in obese children (2)[B].
- Reye syndrome: Fatty liver with encephalopathy; characterized by vomiting with dehydration, progressive CNS damage, hypoglycemia, and signs of hepatic injury
- Mortality rate is 50%.
- Treatment: Mannitol, IV glucose, and fresh-frozen plasma

RISK FACTORS
- NAFLD comprises individuals who have associated metabolic syndrome or insulin resistance.
- The presence of metabolic syndrome increases the risk of future development of NAFLD by 4- to 11-fold (3)[A].
- The 3 most important risk factors are closely related to metabolic syndrome and insulin resistance (3)[A].
  - Obesity: Associated in as many as 25–93% of patients with NAFLD
  - DM: Present in 30–50% of patients with NAFLD
  - Hyperlipidemia: Found in up to 92% of patients with NAFLD
- Insulin resistance is associated strongly with metabolic syndrome and plays a central role in the pathogenesis of NAFLD.
- Other risk factors:
  - Small bowel resections, gastric bypass, and jejunal bypass operations often lead to rapid weight loss, which may increase risk of NAFLD.

- Medications: Corticosteroids, synthetic estrogens, amiodarone, tamoxifen, methotrexate
- Other conditions: Wilson disease, hemochromatosis, abetalipoproteinemia, galactosemia, glycogen storage diseases

Genetics
There may be a genetic component.

GENERAL PREVENTION
- Maintain ideal weight and normal cholesterol and blood sugar levels.
- Avoid alcohol.
- Avoid hepatotoxic substances.

PATHOPHYSIOLOGY
- NAFLD is closely linked to obesity, insulin resistance, and metabolic syndrome.
- When insulin resistance develops, free fatty acids are inappropriately shifted to nonadipose tissue, including the liver.
- Insulin resistance increases free fatty acid flux to the liver by decreased inhibition of lipolysis and also increased de novo lipogenesis (1)[A].
- Insulin resistance and visceral obesity also result in decreased levels of adiponectin. Adiponectin inhibits liver gluconeogenesis and suppresses lipogenesis. Thus decreased adiponectin hinders fatty acid oxidation and increases fat accumulation in the liver.
- Apoptosis and oxidative stress also may contribute to the development and progression of NASH.

ETIOLOGY
- Cause is unknown but closely linked to obesity, insulin resistance, and metabolic syndrome.
- Of these, insulin resistance may be the most important trigger of simple fatty liver (steatosis) and NASH.
- Since both these conditions can remain stable for many years, causing little harm, a 2nd hit to the liver may trigger a progression to cirrhosis.
- Triggers may include cytokine-mediated inflammation, lipid peroxidation, and apoptosis (1)[A].

COMMONLY ASSOCIATED CONDITIONS
Preeclampsia:

Pregnancy Considerations
- A severe complication of 3rd trimester is acute fatty liver of pregnancy. It presents as an abrupt onset of confusion and restlessness with possible jaundice and right upper quadrant pain.
- ALT/AST elevated, usually >1,000 units/L
- Emergency liver biopsy confirms.
- Prompt delivery corrects the liver disease. In most cases, the fetus has an inborn error of lipid metabolism blocking, the same in the mother.
- Recurrence is rare in subsequent pregnancies.

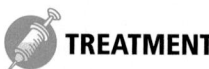 DIAGNOSIS

HISTORY
- Often asymptomatic
- Fatigue
- Malaise
- A dull ache in the upper right abdomen is a possible sign of an enlarged liver.
- At more advanced stage, such as cirrhosis, NASH may cause lack of appetite, weight loss, nausea, weakness, fatigue, spider nevi, palmar erythema,

yellowing of skin and eyes, dark cola-colored urine, light-colored stools, gynecomastia, varices, ascites, pruritus, edema, and encephalopathy.

PHYSICAL EXAM
Hepatomegaly is present in 75% of patients with NASH (4)[A].

DIAGNOSTIC TESTS & INTERPRETATION
Lab
- Aminotransferase and alkaline phosphatase levels may be mildly elevated, but serum albumin, prothrombin, and bilirubin levels are usually normal.
- AST:ALT ratio is usually <1 in NASH.
- Testing for hepatitis B and C, iron studies, and autoimmune serologies should be considered.
- Abnormal ferritin values are seen in ~30% (1)[A].

Imaging
- Right upper-quadrant ultrasound: Reveals a hyperechoic texture or a bright liver because of diffuse fatty infiltration
- CT scan of abdomen and MRI: Identifies steatosis, but not sufficiently sensitive to detect inflammation or fibrosis
- MR spectroscopy: Better sensitivity, quantitative rather than qualitative (5)[B]

Diagnostic Procedures/Surgery
- Liver biopsy is considered the gold standard for diagnosis and is the only method for differentiating NASH from steatosis ± inflammation.
- However, there is large debate regarding the necessity of performing liver biopsy in NAFLD patients.
  - Pros: Distinguish steatosis from NASH, exclude other causes of liver disease, and estimate prognosis
  - Cons: Risks and costs associated with liver biopsy, lack of effective treatment, and a generally good prognosis
- In general, there is an increasing consensus that liver biopsy may be necessary to evaluate the degree of steatosis, inflammation, and fibrosis.

Pathological Findings
- Criteria to establish pathologic diagnosis of NASH has remained controversial.
- Histologic diagnosis of NASH is based on a composite pattern of injury rather than a single defining feature.
- Pathologic scoring system for NAFLD (Nonalcoholic Steatohepatitis Clinical Research Network) (6)[A]:
  - Steatosis (0–3)
  - Lobular inflammation (0–3)
  - Ballooning (0–3)
- NAFLD Activity Score (NAS): 0–2 not NASH, >5 usually NASH

DIFFERENTIAL DIAGNOSIS
Viral hepatitis, alcohol hepatitis, autoimmune hepatitis, hemochromatosis, Wilson disease, α1-antitrypsin deficiency

TREATMENT
- The typical approach is to target each component of the metabolic syndrome, including diabetes and hyperlipidemia, usually starting with weight loss and exercise (4)[A].

- Preferred treatments include
  – Weight loss
  – Exercise
  – Diabetes control
  – Cholesterol control
  – Avoidance of toxic substances

MEDICATION

- The decision to start pharmacologic treatment should be restricted to patients at risk for developing advanced liver disease.
- Despite the large number of agents tested, there is no established, evidence-based treatment for NASH; approaches include:
  – Weight loss, thiazolidinediones (especially pioglitazone), and antioxidants have been most extensively evaluated.
    ○ Weight loss is safe and dose-dependently improved histological disease activity in NASH, but more than 50% of patients failed to achieve target weight loss (7)
    ○ Thiazolidinediones improved steatosis and inflammation but yielded significant weight gain (8)
    ○ Antioxidants yielded conflicting results and were heterogenous with respect to type and dose of drug, duration, implementation of lifestyle intervention (9,10)
- Among other agents, pentoxifylline, telmisartan and L-carnitine improved liver histology in randomized controlled trial (RCT) (1112)
- Polyunsaturated fatty acid ameliorated biochemical and radiological markers of NAFLD (13)
- Statins improved liver steatosis and slowed fibrosis progression compared with controls (14)
- Fibrates had no significant benefit on histological, biochemical, or radiological outcome
- Ursodeoxycholic acid showed no significant improvement in ALT levels or radiological steatosis

ADDITIONAL TREATMENT
General Measures
Weight loss and exercise may reduce inflammation, lower elevated levels of liver enzymes, and decrease insulin resistance.

Issues for Referral
Referral to a hepatologist with or without liver biopsy may help in staging and prognosis.

COMPLEMENTARY AND ALTERNATIVE MEDICINE
- A number of complementary and alternative therapies claim to improve liver health. Among these are milk thistle, α-lipoic acid, betaine, viusid, vitamin E, N-acetyl cysteine, and Ω-3 fatty acids.
- Antioxidants such as vitamin E, N-acetyl cysteine, S-adenosylmethionine (SAMe), and betaine have been investigated in the treatment of NAFLD. The extreme heterogenicity of RCTs prevents any firm conclusion on the effect of antioxidants in NAFLD/NASH.

SURGERY/OTHER PROCEDURES
Bariatric surgery: Although abdominal weight-loss surgery coupled with rapid weight loss has been implicated as contributing to development of NASH, some research suggests that bariatric surgery combined with modest weight loss may reduce the inflammation and scarring associated with NASH (4)[A].

 ## ONGOING CARE

FOLLOW-UP RECOMMENDATIONS
All patients should be tested for hepatitis A and B and vaccinated if appropriate.

Patient Monitoring
Patients with fatty liver disease should be seen regularly to detect disease progression through:
- Physical exam findings (spider telangiectasia, palmar erythema, splenomegaly)
- Laboratory findings (decreasing platelets, elevated bilirubin, decreasing albumin)
- Patient complaints (encephalopathy, ascites, fatigue)
- Incidental imaging study findings (cirrhotic liver, splenomegaly, varices, ascites)

DIET
Restrictions of both total calories, simple carbohydrates, and alcohol are required to control diabetes, weight, and lipids.

PATIENT EDUCATION
Planning for lifelong change in diet, exercise, and alcohol use is required. As such, regular education and motivation sessions are of value.

COMPLICATIONS
- Steatohepatitis may progress to cirrhosis, with complications that include variceal bleeding, ascites, encephalopathy, and liver failure.
- Progression to hepatocellular carcinoma

REFERENCES

1. Edmison J, McCullough AJ. Pathogenesis of non-alcoholic steatohepatitis: human data. *Clin Liver Dis.* 2007;11:75–104, ix.
2. Shneider BL, González-Peralta R, Roberts EA. Controversies in the management of pediatric liver disease: Hepatitis B, C and NAFLD: Summary of a single topic conference. *Hepatology.* 2006;44:1344–54.
3. Ong JP, Younossi ZM. Epidemiology and Natural History of NAFLD and NASH. *Clin Liver Dis.* 2007;11:1–16.
4. Ramesh S, Sanyal AJ. Evaluation and management of non-alcoholic steatohepatitis. *J Hepatol.* 2005;42(Suppl):S2–12.
5. Szczepaniak LS, et al. Magnetic resonance spectroscopy to measure hepatic triglyceride content: Prevalence of hepatic steatosis in the general population. *Am J Physiol Endocrinol Metabol.* 2005;288:E462–E468.
6. Bondini S, Kleiner DE, Goodman ZD, et al. Pathologic Assessment of Non-alcoholic Fatty Liver Disease. *Clin Liver Dis.* 2007;11:17–23.
7. Promrat K, Kleiner DE, Niemeier HM, et al. Randomized controlled trial testing the effects of weight loss on nonalcoholic steatohepatitis. *Hepatology.* 2010;51:121–9.
8. Chalasani NP, Sanyal AJ, Kowdley KV, et al. Pioglitazone versus vitamin E versus placebo for the treatment of non-diabetic patients with non-alcoholic steatohepatitis: PIVENS trial design. *Contemp Clin Trials.* 2009;30:88–96.
9. Abdelmalek MF, Sanderson SO, Angulo P, et al. Betaine for nonalcoholic fatty liver disease: results of a randomized placebo-controlled trial. *Hepatology.* 2009;50:1818–26.
10. Vilar Gomez E, Rodriguez De Miranda A, Gra Oramas B, et al. Clinical trial: a nutritional supplement Viusid, in combination with diet and exercise, in patients with nonalcoholic fatty liver disease. *Aliment Pharmacol Ther.* 2009;30:999–1009.
11. Georgescu EF, Ionescu R, Niculescu M, et al. Angiotensin-receptor blockers as therapy for mild-to-moderate hypertension-associated non-alcoholic steatohepatitis. *World J. Gastroenterol.* 2009;15:942–54.
12. Malaguarnera M, Gargante MP, Russo C, et al. L-carnitine supplementation to diet: a new tool in treatment of nonalcoholic steatohepatitis—a randomized and controlled clinical trial. *Am J Gastroenterol.* 2010;105:1338–45.
13. Cussons AJ, Watts GF, Mori TA, et al. Omega-3 fatty acid supplementation decreases liver fat content in polycystic ovary syndrome: a randomized controlled trial employing proton magnetic resonance spectroscopy. *J Clin Endocrinol Metab.* 2009;94:3842–8.
14. Ekstedt M, Franzén LE, Mathiesen UL, et al. Statins in non-alcoholic fatty liver disease and chronically elevated liver enzymes: a histopathological follow-up study. *J Hepatol.* 2007;47:135–41.

ADDITIONAL READING

Pasumarthy L, Srour J, et al. Nonalcoholic steatohepatitis: a review of the literature and updates in management. *South Med J.* 2010;103:547–50.

 ## CODES

ICD9
571.8 Other chronic nonalcoholic liver disease

CLINICAL PEARLS

- NAFLD is the most common form of chronic liver disease in the Western world.
- Prevalence of NAFLD and NASH is much higher in patients who have metabolic syndrome or any one of its components (diabetes, obesity, hypertriglyceridemia).
- Liver biopsy is the gold standard for diagnosis.
- Weight loss and treating components of the metabolic syndrome are central to the treatment of NAFLD.
- Insulin sensitizers such as metformin and thiazolidinediones, antioxidants such as vitamin E, and lipid-lowering agents have shown promise in clinical trials, but the evidence remains preliminary.

STEVENS-JOHNSON SYNDROME

Matthew A. Silva, PharmD, RPh, BCPS
Pablo I. Hernandez Itriago, MD

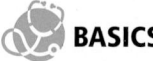

BASICS

DESCRIPTION
- A generalized hypersensitivity reaction, usually to a drug, in which skin and mucous membrane lesions are an early manifestation
- Once considered to be the same as erythema multiforme major, a severe form of erythema multiforme in which >1 mucosal surface was involved, many now consider it to be a different disease with a more difficult course and a more ominous prognosis.
- Stevens-Johnson syndrome (SJS) exists on a continuum with toxic epidermal necrolysis (TEN).
- SJS presents with characteristic targetoid cutaneous lesions when <10% of the body surface area (BSA) is involved.
- Targetoid cutaneous lesion involvement of 10–30% of BSA is considered an overlap between SJS and TEN. Involvement of >30% of BSA is TEN, which has a high morbidity and up to 70% mortality (1).
- System(s) affected: Cardiovascular; Hematologic/Lymphatic/Immunologic; Nervous; Renal/Urologic; Skin/Exocrine
- Synonym(s): Ectodermosis erosiva pluriorificialis; febrile mucocutaneous syndrome; herpes iris; erythema polymorphe; toxic epidermal necrolysis (TEN)

ALERT
- Dangerous progression
- Patients with discrete skin lesions and >10% epidermal detachment are at risk of rapid progression to TEN.

Geriatric Considerations
TEN has a greater mortality in older patients.

Pediatric Considerations
- Rare in children <3 years of age
- More common in children and young adults

Pregnancy Considerations
- Pregnancy is a possible predisposing condition.

EPIDEMIOLOGY
Incidence
- Incidence/prevalence of SJS in the US is difficult to estimate because there is no universally accepted definition of SJS.
- 1.1–7.1 and 0.4–1.2 cases/1 million person-years for SJS and TEN, respectively (1)

Prevalence
- Predominant age: SJS is more common in children and young adults.
- Predominant sex: Male > Female (2:1)
- Sex (% range of females): 33–62% for SJS and 61.3–64.3% for TEN (1)
- Age (average range): 25–47 years for SJS and 46–63 years for TEN (1)

RISK FACTORS
- Previous history of SJS
- Immunocompromised status, including chronic viral infections with Epstein-Barr virus and HIV (2,3)
- Patients with HIV infection may be predisposed to developing SJS in response to their medications.
  - Human leukocyte antigen (HLA) subtypes A, B, and D
- Diseases that cause immune compromise (deficiencies, malignancy, etc.)
- Possibly radiation therapy or ultraviolet (UV) light

Genetics
Associations with HLA-B*1501, HLA-B*1502, HLA-B*5801 in patients of Asian ancestry, HLA-Bw44, HLA-B12, and HLA-DQB1*0601

GENERAL PREVENTION
Secondary prevention may be possible by avoiding exposure to offending medications or chemical agents.

PATHOPHYSIOLOGY
- Erythematous papular lesions and keratinocyte necrosis are a consequence of cell-mediated immunity.
- Occurs 1–2 weeks after initial exposure to offending drugs and within 48 hours on rechallenge.
- Accumulation and binding of reactive drug metabolites to mucocutaneous epithelial cells as haptens
- Drug haptens signal drug-specific CD8+ T-lymphocyte and macrophages, which infiltrate and express interleukin 2 (IL-2), tumor necrosis factor α (TNF-α), and interferon-γ, leading to keratinocyte activation.
- Cytokines enhance keratinocyte expression of soluble Fas-ligand (sFasL) and Fas receptors, leading to apoptosis (4).

ETIOLOGY
- 50% of cases are idiopathic.
- Associated with metabolism of parent drugs and metabolites
- Slow intrinsic acetylation rates
- Sulfonamides are the drugs most strongly associated with SJS and TEN. Then
  - Cephalosporins
  - Quinolones
  - Aminopenicillins
  - Tetracyclines
  - Macrolides
  - Imidazole antifungals
  - HIV antiretrovirals (e.g., protease inhibitors, efavirenz, abacavir, amprenavir, fosamprenavir, atazanavir, darunavir, etravirine) (2)
  - Anticonvulsants, especially carbamazepine
  - Nonsteroidal anti-inflammatory drugs (NSAIDs), especially oxicam
  - Allopurinol
  - Vaccines—dPT, BCG, oral polio
  - *Mycoplasma pneumoniae* infection

COMMONLY ASSOCIATED CONDITIONS
- SJS progressing to TEN is ominous prognostically.
- *Mycoplasma pneumoniae* may be an infectious precursor.

DIAGNOSIS

HISTORY
- Usually a preceding illness for which the medication was given 1–3 weeks before initial cutaneous manifestations
- Sudden onset with rapidly progressive pleomorphic rash that includes petechiae, vesicles, bullae
- Considered to be SJS if epidermal detachments affect <10% of the skin
- Classified as TEN if epidermal detachments affect >30% or >10% in the absence of discrete skin lesions
- Burning sensation of the skin and sometimes of the mucous membranes
- Usually no pruritus
- Fever 39–40°C (102–104°F)
- Headache
- Malaise
- Arthralgias
- Cough productive of thick, purulent sputum

PHYSICAL EXAM
- Recognized by the presence of several of the following features:
  - Vesicles and ulcers on the mucous membranes, especially of the mouth and throat
  - Erythematous macules with purpuric, necrotic centers and overlying blistering (4)
  - Epidermal detachment with light lateral pressure (Nikolsky's sign)
  - Fever 39–40°C (102–104°F)
  - Crusted nares
  - Conjunctivitis
  - Corneal ulcerations
  - Erosive vulvovaginitis or balanitis
  - Cough productive of thick, purulent sputum
  - Tachypnea/respiratory distress
  - Arrhythmias
  - Pericarditis
  - Congestive heart failure (CHF)
  - Mental status changes
  - Seizures
  - Coma
- Sepsis:
  - Seen in SJS if epidermal detachment affects <10% of the skin
  - Seen in TEN if epidermal detachment exceeds 30% or if it exceeds 10% in the absence of discrete skin lesions
- Patients with discrete skin lesions and 10–30% epidermal detachment are in the overlap between SJS and TEN.

DIAGNOSTIC TESTS & INTERPRETATION
Lab
Initial lab tests
- Culture or serologic tests for suspected sources of infection
- Electrolyte disturbance
- Albuminuria/hematuria

Follow-Up & Special Considerations
Skin biopsy

DIFFERENTIAL DIAGNOSIS
- Exfoliative dermatitis
- Linear IgA bullous dermatosis
- Staphylococcal scalded-skin syndrome
- Pemphigus (paraneoplastic)
- Generalized fixed drug eruption
- Erythema multiforme major
- Burns
- Pressure blisters (coma, barbiturates)

TREATMENT

MEDICATION

First Line
- Corticosteroids are controversial. Early high-dose IV steroids may attenuate disease progression, reduce skin detachment, decrease inflammatory cytokine activity, and improve patient comfort. Withdraw if no benefit is seen in the 1st few days.
- Experimental treatments that appear to have been useful include
  – Recombinant granulocyte colony-stimulating factor
  – Cyclophosphamide
  – Cyclosporine
  – IV immune globulin (IVIG) in HIV-positive patients; IVIG is considered beneficial treatment and prophylaxis, although not approved by the Food and Drug Administration (FDA) (3,5,6). Interferes with Fas-ligand induced apoptosis.
- Contraindications: Avoid steroids in diabetic or immunosuppressed patients or those with chronic infections.

Second Line
- Acyclovir for herpetic infections
- Erythromycin or related antibiotic for *Mycoplasma* infections (empirical use of antibiotics is not recommended)

ADDITIONAL TREATMENT

General Measures
- Withdraw all suspected medications, and treat any underlying disease.
- Meticulous care of damaged skin
- Supportive care, including moisture-retentive ointment, petroleum jelly, and sterile saline compresses
- Catheter changing and culturing
- Reverse isolation and temperature control with extensive epidermal loss
- Maintenance of fluid, electrolyte, and protein balance
- Plasmapheresis
- Adequate calorie intake; parenteral nutrition, if necessary
- Mouthwashes of warm saline or a solution of diphenhydramine, lidocaine, and kaolin suspension
- Ophthalmologic consultation and monitoring for corneal damage
- Venous thromboembolism prophylaxis with unfractionated heparin or low-molecular-weight heparin

SURGERY/OTHER PROCEDURES
- Sterile débridement of areas of extensive epidermal loss
- Application of biosynthetic dressings such as Biobrane to denuded areas
- Damage to the vulva, vagina, or cornea: Consider surgical repair.

IN-PATIENT CONSIDERATIONS

Admission Criteria
- This disease progresses rapidly; all patients should be admitted.
- Admission to a burn unit greatly improves the outcome for any patient who has sloughed skin over 10% or more of the body surface area.
- ICU for bronchiolitis, acute respiratory distress syndrome (ARDS), or multiorgan damage

IV Fluids
Fluid management with saline and macromolecules is necessary in the 1st 24 hours with decreasing IV fluid requirements as oral intake proceeds with nasogastric tube.

Nursing
- Bed rest until clinically stabilized
- Avoid administration of topical silver sulfadiazine owing to association with sulfonamide and SJS.
- Use a coordinated approach involving critical-care, wound-care and burn specialists (7)

ONGOING CARE

FOLLOW-UP RECOMMENDATIONS
- Extensive documentation of all offending or suspected medications or chemical agents
- Education and strategies to limit exposure to offending or suspected medications or chemical agents

Patient Monitoring
- Secondary or concurrent infections
- Dehydration
- Electrolyte imbalance
- Malnutrition
- End-organ damage

DIET
- Oral fluid intake is recommended.
- Early oral nutrition by nasogastric tube as tolerated
- IV nutritional support with increased protein requirements; may need insulin for glycoregulation in this hypercatabolic state

PATIENT EDUCATION
- Discuss offending or suspected medications and chemical agents with patient and family as applicable.
- Plan to prevent repeated exposure.

PROGNOSIS
- Disease may have a rapid onset or may evolve slowly over 1–2 weeks with resolution over 4–6 weeks.
- Often scarring of the skin or mucous membranes occurs, especially of the vulva.
- Blindness or corneal opacities occur in 7–20% of patients.
- The risk of recurrence is as high as 37%.
- Death occurs in 5–15% of the patients with SJS and in up to 40% of patients with TEN.

COMPLICATIONS
- Secondary infections
- Sepsis
- Pneumonia
- ARDS
- Bronchiolitis obliterans in children
- Dehydration/electrolyte disturbance
- Acute tubular necrosis
- Corneal ulceration or iritis
- Urethral erosions and genitourinary strictures
- Arrhythmias
- Venous thromboembolism
- Disseminated intravascular coagulation (DIC)
- Death in 15% of untreated cases of SJS and up to 40% of TEN cases

REFERENCES

1. Letko E, Papaliodis DN, Papaliodis GN, et al. Stevens-Johnson syndrome and toxic epidermal necrolysis: a review of the literature. *Ann Allergy Asthma Immunol*. 2005;94:419–36; quiz 436–8, 456.
2. Borrás-Blasco J, Navarro-Ruiz A, Borrás C, et al. Adverse cutaneous reactions associated with the newest antiretroviral drugs in patients with human immunodeficiency virus infection. *J Antimicrob Chemother*. 2008.
3. Hazin R, Ibrahimi OA, Hazin MI, et al. Stevens-Johnson syndrome: Pathogenesis, diagnosis, and management. *Ann Med*. 2008;40:129–38.
4. Murata J, Abe R, Shimizu H. Increased soluble Fas ligand levels in patients with Stevens-Johnson syndrome and toxic epidermal necrolysis preceding skin detachment. *J Allergy Clin Immunol*. 2008.
5. French LE, Trent JT, Kerdel FA. Use of intravenous immunoglobulin in toxic epidermal necrolysis and Stevens-Johnson syndrome: our current understanding. *Int Immunopharmacol*. 2006;6: 543–9.
6. Mittmann N, Chan B, Knowles S, et al. Intravenous immunoglobulin use in patients with toxic epidermal necrolysis and Stevens-Johnson syndrome. *Am J Clin Dermatol*. 2006;7:359–68.
7. Struck MF, Hilbert P, Mockenhaupt M, et al. Severe cutaneous adverse reactions: emergency approach to non-burn epidermolytic syndromes. *Intensive Care Med*. 2010;36:22–32.

ADDITIONAL READING
- Powell N, Munro JM, Rowbotham D. Colonic involvement in Stevens-Johnson syndrome. *Postgrad Med J*. 2006;82:e10.
- Shilad A, Predanic M, Perni SC, et al. Human immunodeficiency virus, pregnancy, and Stevens-Johnson syndrome. *Obstet Gynecol*. 2005;105:1254–6.
- Wolf R, Orion E, Marcos B, et al. Life-threatening acute adverse cutaneous drug reactions. *Clin Dermatol*. 2005;23:171–81.

See Also (Topic, Algorithm, Electronic Media Element)
Burns; Erythema Multiforme; Pemphigoid, Bullous; Pemphigus Vulgaris; Respiratory Distress Syndrome, Acute; Cutaneous Drug Reactions; Dermatitis, Herpetiformis

CODES

ICD9
695.13 Stevens-Johnson syndrome

CLINICAL PEARLS
- Corticosteroid treatment is controversial. If chosen and no response within 1st few days, discontinue.
- Recurrences are possible. Etiologic agents should be identified if possible and avoided indefinitely.

S

STOKES-ADAMS ATTACKS

Kerry Hensley, MD
Constance Nichols, MD

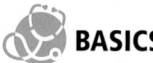 **BASICS**

DESCRIPTION
- Syncope due to cerebral hypoxia in patients with 3rd degree or complete heart block. Syncope occurs following severe bradycardia or asystole.
- System(s) affected: Cardiovascular; Nervous
- Synonym(s): Drop attacks

EPIDEMIOLOGY
Incidence
Uncertain, although increasing age is a risk factor
Prevalence
- Unknown (0.04% prevalence of 3rd-degree atrioventricular block) (1)
- Predominant age: Most common >40 years of age
- Predominant sex: Male = Female

Pediatric Considerations
- Rare during pregnancy

RISK FACTORS
- Use of the medications listed under Etiology
- Coronary artery disease
- Endocarditis and myocarditis
- Mitral or aortic valve disease
- History of previous atrioventricular nodal dysfunction or cardiac surgery
- Bundle-branch and/or fascicular block
- Acute myocardial infarction (MI) (especially acute right coronary artery occlusion)
- Amyloidosis
- Chagas disease
- Lyme disease
- Connective tissue diseases involving the heart (e.g., systemic lupus erythematosus, rheumatoid arthritis, sarcoidosis)
- Hyperkalemia
- Acidosis

Genetics
- May be associated with complete congenital atrioventricular block (CCAVB)
- 40% of children with CCAVB experience syncopal episodes (2).

GENERAL PREVENTION
- Avoid negative chronotropic drugs (e.g., β-blockers, calcium channel blockers, digoxin) in at-risk patients.
- Prevention of cardiovascular disease through diet/exercise

PATHOPHYSIOLOGY
- The abrupt development of complete atrioventricular (AV) block, especially at His-bundle level, may result in a prolonged period of asystole because of a slow and delayed response of the quiescent subsidiary (escape) ventricular pacemaker.
- Marked bradycardia secondary to AV conduction abnormality may lead to prolonged QT interval and paroxysmal torsades de pointes.
- Abrupt termination of tachyarrhythmia leading to precipitous decrease in heart rate
- Degree of cerebral dysfunction related to duration of cardiac block and effect on cerebral circulation

ETIOLOGY
- Medications:
  – Digoxin (common)
  – Calcium channel blockers
  – β-Blockers (e.g., Sotalol)
  – Clonidine
  – Propafenone (Rythmol), a class IC antiarrhythmic
- Other causes:
  – Myocardial ischemia involving the AV node
  – Degenerative (fibrosing) and infiltrative diseases involving the heart and its conduction system (e.g., Lenègre, systemic sclerosis, valvular disease, infective endocarditis, sarcoidosis)
  – Degeneration of the AV node secondary to aging
  – Neuromuscular diseases (e.g., myotonic muscular dystrophy or Kearns-Sayre syndrome)
  – Postoperative cardiac damage

COMMONLY ASSOCIATED CONDITIONS
- Myocardial ischemia/acute MI
- High-degree AV conduction abnormality
- Atrial standstill
- Right bundle-branch block
- CCAVB
- Systemic manifestations of connective tissue disease
- Sick sinus syndrome
- Neuromuscular disease

DIAGNOSIS

HISTORY
- History of predisposing factor or related conditions
- Angina
- Acute bradycardia
- Hypotension
- Pallor
- Fatigue/exercise intolerance
- Dyspnea
- Altered sensorium or loss of consciousness unrelated to position or exertion
- Acute onset of syncopal or near-syncopal symptoms (± palpitations)

PHYSICAL EXAM
- Pallor
- Reactive hyperemia with recovery
- Convulsions or seizurelike activity without postictal state
- Pulse <50

DIAGNOSTIC TESTS & INTERPRETATION
Lab
Initial lab tests
- Cardiac enzymes
- Electroencephalogram with cardiac monitoring (to differentiate between syncope and epilepsy) (3)
- Electrocardiogram (ECG) : Partial or complete heart block at onset of symptoms with slow or no ventricular escape:
  – Bradycardia
  – AV block 50–60%
  – Sinoatrial block 30–40%
  – Ventricular fibrillation/tachycardia <1%
- Serum digoxin level (other medication levels if appropriate)
- Thyroid-stimulating hormone level
- Hematocrit/Hemoglobin
- Blood electrolyte levels - esp. potassium

Follow-Up & Special Considerations
- ECG, event monitor, or Holter monitor
- Renal failure may lead to falsely elevated creatinine kinase.

Imaging
Initial approach
Transthoracic echocardiogram if cardiomyopathy or valvular disease is suspected

Diagnostic Procedures/Surgery
- Coronary catheterization to rule out coronary ischemia if suspected
- Electrophysiologic testing to assess cardiac conduction system if ECG testing is ambiguous
- Tilt-table test to evaluate neurogenic etiology
- Myocardial biopsy if infiltrative disease suspected

Pathological Findings
- Myocardial ischemia
- Evidence of degenerative or infiltrative disease involving the AV node/His bundle

DIFFERENTIAL DIAGNOSIS
- Seizure
- Vertigo
- Transient ischemic attack
- Orthostatic hypotension
- Vasovagal syncope
- Hypoglycemia
- Neurocardiogenic syncope

- Cardiac arrhythmias:
  - Ventricular tachycardia
  - Supraventricular tachycardia
  - Reentrant tachycardia
  - Wolff-Parkinson-White syndrome
  - Sinus arrest
  - Sinus exit block
  - Sick sinus syndrome
  - Transition from normal sinus rhythm to atrial fibrillation or vice versa

 TREATMENT

MEDICATION
First Line

- No medication currently is recommended for long-term treatment of symptomatic arrhythmias (4)[A].

- For symptomatic bradyarrhythmias (5):
  - Atropine 0.5 mg IV push to be given during the complete heart block with hypotension; may be repeated every 3–5 minutes with a maximum total dose of 3 mg; less likely to be effective if atrial rate is already adequate
  - Epinephrine 2–10 mcg/minute, titrate to patient response; use of epinephrine in normotensive patient with bradycardia may precipitate hypertensive crisis
  - Dopamine 2–10 mcg/kg/minute; titrate to patient response; add to epinephrine or administer alone

Second Line
Correction of precipitating conditions (e.g., hypokalemia, acidosis)

ADDITIONAL TREATMENT
General Measures
- Inpatient assessment in a monitored setting
- Continued treatment for prevention of future episodes in ambulatory setting
- Cessation of precipitating medications

SURGERY/OTHER PROCEDURES

- Intracardiac pacing is the treatment of choice for patients with complete heart block and Stokes-Adams syncope (4)[A].
- Dual chamber may be more effective than single chamber pacing in AV block (6).
- Temporary external pacing or transvenous pacing as interim measure to stabilize
- See American College of Cardiology/American Heart Association/Heart Rhythm Society 2008 guidelines for suggested intervention based on precipitating cause.
- Emergency insertion of a ventricular pacemaker is required when ventricular fibrillation or tachycardia is present.

IN-PATIENT CONSIDERATIONS
Initial Stabilization
See above 1st-line treatments to be used when intracardiac pacing is not available. External pacing may be life-saving.

Admission Criteria
Syncope in the setting of known AV node conduction abnormality or of unknown cause

IV Fluids
Use caution in patients with congestive heart failure.

Nursing
- Telemetry
- Out of bed with assist if patient has history of falls due to syncope

Discharge Criteria
Institution of proper treatment with resolution of symptoms

 ONGOING CARE

FOLLOW-UP RECOMMENDATIONS
Routine follow-up with cardiologist

Patient Monitoring
- Routine pacemaker check if permanent pacemaker has been implanted
- Follow-up Holter and/or event monitoring for 2 weeks after causal medication has been discontinued
- Discontinuation of driving, heavy machinery operation; caution about fall risks

DIET
Regular

PATIENT EDUCATION
After the diagnosis has been made and a pacemaker has been implanted (if required), instruct patient as to pacemaker guidelines.

PROGNOSIS
Excellent with proper institution of exogenous pacing; further symptoms are not expected.

COMPLICATIONS
- Sudden death (uncommon)
- Cerebral hypoxic damage and other end-organ damage with protracted bradycardia with hypotension

REFERENCES

1. Kojic EM, Hardarson T, Sigfusson N, et al. The prevalence and prognosis of third-degree atrioventricular conduction block:the Reykjavik Study. *Journal of Internal Medicine*. 1999;246(1):81–6.
2. Vukomanovic V, Stajevic M, Kosutic J, et al. Age-related role of ambulatory electrocardiographic monitoring in risk stratification of patients with complete congenital atrioventricular block. *Europace*. 2007;9:88–93.
3. Diaz-Castro O, et al. "Stokes-Adams Epilepsy": Sometimes we need the electroencephalogram. *Circulation*. 2005;112:e101–e102.
4. Epstein AE, Dimarco JP, Ellenbogen KA, et al. ACC/AHA/HRS 2008 guidelines for Device-Based Therapy of Cardiac Rhythm Abnormalities: executive summary. *Heart Rhythm*. 2008;5:934–55.
5. 2005 American Heart Association Guidelines for Cardiopulmonary Resuscitation and Emergency Cardiovascular Care. Part 7.3: Management of symptomatic bradycardia and tachycardia. *Circulation*. 2005;112:IV-67–IV-77.
6. Dretzke J, et al. Dual chamber versus single chamber ventricular pacemakers for sick sinus syndrome and atrioventricular block. *The Cochrane Database of Systematic Reviews*. 2009 Vol. (1)

ADDITIONAL READING

- Elizari MV, Acunzo RS, Ferreiro M. Hemiblocks revisited. *Circulation*. 2007;115:1154–63.
- Hood R, et al. Syncope in the elderly. *Clin Geriatric Med*. May;23(2):351–61,vi.
- Jensen G, Sigurd B, Sandoe E. Adams-Stokes seizures due to ventricular tachydysrhythmias in patients with heart block:prevalence and problems of management. *Chest*. 1975;67:43–48.
- You C, Chong C, Wang T, et al. Unrecognized paroxysmal ventricular standstill masquerading as epilepsy: a Stokes Adams attack. *Epileptic Disorders*. 2007;9(2):179–81.

CODES

ICD9
426.9 Conduction disorder, unspecified

CLINICAL PEARLS

- Syncope due to Stokes-Adams attacks can be frequently confused for epilepsy.
- Stokes-Adams attacks usually require insertion of a pacemaker for definitive treatment unless due to a reversible condition such as medication toxicity.
- External pacing may serve as a bridge until more definitive management can be accomplished.

STOMATITIS

Sheila O. Stille, DMD, MAGD
Hugh J. Silk, MD

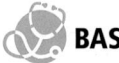 **BASICS**

Stomatitis: Inflammation of mucous lining of any of the structures in the mouth, cheeks, lip, tongue, gingiva, and floor or roof of the mouth. It is usually painful and associated with redness, swelling, and sometimes bleeding. It affects people of all ages. Stomatitis can be result of localized injury/irritation, or the manifestation of systemic conditions.

DESCRIPTION
- Generalized inflammation of the oral mucosa of many possible etiologies
- System(s) affected: Skin/Exocrine; ENT; Oropharynx; Dental

EPIDEMIOLOGY
- Children:
  – Primary herpetic infections (6 months to 5 years old)
  – Hand-foot-mouth disease
  – Herpangina
  – Angular stomatitis
  – Aphthous stomatitis, (peak onset 10–19 years old)
- Teenagers and adults:
  – Vincent stomatitis (also known as *Vincent disease* or *acute necrotizing ulcerative gingivitis*)
  – Behçet disease
  – Nicotinic stomatitis
  – Chronic ulcerative stomatitis (white women in late middle age) (1)

Prevalence
- Very common: Herpetic stomatitis, hand-foot-mouth disease, and recurrent aphthous stomatitis (RAS)
- Common: Herpangina, nicotinic stomatitis, and denture-related stomatitis.
- The remaining causes are uncommon or rare.

RISK FACTORS
- Poor oral hygiene
- Dietary deficiencies and malnutrition
- Chronic systemic disease
- Immune deficiencies
- Poor denture
- Smoking
- Cancer Therapies

Genetics
Polymorphisms causing high interleukin 1p (IL-1p) and tumor necrosis factor α (TNF-α) production increase risk for recurrent aphthous stomatitis (2).

GENERAL PREVENTION
- Avoid causative factors (see Etiology).
- Good oral hygiene
- Good nutrition
- Avoid/discontinue smoking.
- Properly fitting dentures

ETIOLOGY
- Allergy: Foods, drugs, contact (some erythema multiforme)
- Nutritional deficiencies: Vitamin B_6 (angular stomatitis), vitamin B_{12}, folic acid, vitamin C, iron deficiencies
- Malnutrition (gangrenous stomatitis; internationally known as "noma")

- Viral: Herpes simplex I and II (herpetic stomatitis), coxsackie A (herpangina and hand-foot-mouth disease)
- Smoking (nicotinic stomatitis)
- Hormonal (possibly RAS)
- Uncertain (RAS, Vincent stomatitis, recurrent scarifying stomatitis, Behçet disease, erythema multiforme)
- RAS may be associated with vitamin B_{12}, folic acid, vitamin C, and iron deficiencies and toothpastes containing sodium lauryl sulfate.
- Bacterial (scarlatina)
- Traumatic (mechanical, chemical, or thermal)
- Uremic (uremic/nephritic)
- Ill-fitting dentures

Pediatric Considerations
Common causes in the pediatric population (e.g., herpetic [primary], hand-foot-mouth disease, herpangina, traumatic ulcers).

Geriatric Considerations
Certain etiologies are more likely in the geriatric population (e.g., ill-fitting dentures, nutritional deficiencies).

COMMONLY ASSOCIATED CONDITIONS
- Pregnancy may bring on recurrent ulcerative stomatitis.
- AIDS: Associated with severe oral lesions
- Aphthous ulcers may be associated with Crohn disease or celiac disease.

 DIAGNOSIS

- General:
  – Depends on etiology
  – Varies from minimal to severe pain
  – Some with constitutional symptoms: Fever, malaise, headache
- Allergic stomatitis:
  – Intense shiny erythema
  – Slight swelling
  – Itching
  – Dryness
  – Burning
  – Usual allergens include: Nuts, shellfish, cinnamon, fruits, metals, dental materials, and ingredients in toothpaste, mouthwash and chewing gum
- Vincent infection: Necrotic ulceration of interdental papillae and mucous membrane
- Thrush (candidiasis):
  – White patches, slightly raised (resembling milk curds)
  – Distribution: Tongue, buccal mucosa, palate, gums, tonsils, larynx, pharynx, GI tract, skin (skin folds); commonly seen in infants (oral cavity, diaper area, neck), immunocompromised patients, and patients on long-term antibiotics, corticosteroids, and antineoplastic treatment
- Pseudomembranous stomatitis: Membrane-like exudate

- Mucous lesions accompanying systemic disease:
  – Mucous patches (syphilis)
  – Strawberry tongue (Kawasaki disease, scarlet fever, staphylococcal toxic shock syndrome)
  – Koplik spots (measles)
  – Ulcers (erythema multiforme)
  – Smooth, fire red, painful (pellagra)
  – Varicella zoster

HISTORY
Erythema and edema are the usual oral manifestations. When the gingiva is involved, the tissue of the affected area will appear uniformly red and erythematous. The patient will complain of burning sensation, intolerance to temperature, and irritating foods.

PHYSICAL EXAM
The physical exam should include comprehensive oral examination. Examine and palpate the lips, tongue, cheeks, and hard and soft palate, as well as cervical, submandibular, and submental lymph nodes.

DIAGNOSTIC TESTS & INTERPRETATION
The diagnosis relies on clinical symptoms and history. Testing is not routinely performed.

Lab
- Tzanck test of historic interest only; herpes simplex virus (HSV) culture
- Serologic test for syphilis
- Complete blood count (CBC); cultures to determine secondary infection

Follow-Up & Special Considerations
If not resolving in 7–14 days or getting worse, consider CBC.

Diagnostic Procedures/Surgery
- Biopsy if persistent/recurrent/suspicious
- Immunofluorescence is useful in the differential diagnostic between RAS and bullous skin diseases (3).

Pathological Findings
Biopsy suspicious lesions or lesions that fail to heal or chronically recur to rule out oral or hematologic cancer or vasculitis.

DIFFERENTIAL DIAGNOSIS
- Herpetic stomatitis
- Hand-foot-mouth disease
- RAS
- Vincent stomatitis
- Nicotinic stomatitis
- Denture-related stomatitis
- Erythema multiforme/Stevens-Johnson syndrome
- Recurrent ulcerative stomatitis
- Recurrent scarifying stomatitis
- Behçet disease
- Angular stomatitis
- Noma (gangrenous stomatitis)
- Scarlatina (scarlet fever)
- Herpangina
- Uremic stomatitis
- Reactive arthritis
- Pemphigus/pemphigoid
- Squamous cell cancer
- Cyclic neutropenia
- Burning mouth syndrome

TREATMENT

Treatment of stomatitis depends on the causative factors. If cause is allergic, identification removal of the agent is critical. For infectious causes, antibiotic or antifungal regiments. Steroidal anti-inflammatory drugs for systemic conditions with stomatitis manifestation. If the cause of stomatitis is due to medical treatment or cancer therapy, treatment needs to be more aggressive.

MEDICATION

- Acetaminophen or ibuprofen for analgesia
- Steroids, colchicine, and cytotoxic drugs for Behçet disease
- 2% viscous lidocaine (Xylocaine) swish and spit for local discomfort
- Liquid diphenhydramine (Benadryl) by mouth or swish and spit, for allergic reactions
- Antibiotics for gangrenous stomatitis (penicillin and metronidazole are reasonable 1st line agents; often start with IV)
- Antifungal ointment (e.g., nystatin [Mycostatin]) for candidiasis-complicating angular stomatitis
- For candidiasis: Nystatin oral suspension 400,000 units (4 mL) 4 times daily × 10 days; swish and swallow (1 mL 4 times daily for infants)
- Acyclovir 200–800 mg 5 times a day × 7–14 days for herpetic stomatitis
- Sucralfate (Carafate) suspension 1 tsp swish in mouth or place on ulcers 4 times daily (helpful)
- Topical 0.2% hyaluronic acid for recurrent aphthous ulcers
- "Miracle mouth rinses": Various combinations of the preceding in equal parts; use swish and spit out 4 times daily.
  – Maalox or Mylanta, diphenhydramine, lidocaine
  – Maalox or Mylanta, diphenhydramine, Carafate
  – Duke's: Nystatin, diphenhydramine, hydrocortisone
- Chemical cauterization with silver nitrate for aphthous stomatitis (treatment can cause burning sensation)
- Contraindications: Allergy to specific medication
- Precautions: Toxic dose of topical lidocaine is uncertain, but likely only 25–33% of dose may have significant absorption from open ulcers or mucous membrane.
- Topical minocycline for aphthous stomatitis (4)
- Steroid oral rinses (see "General") or topical preparations for aphthous ulcers (Kenalog in Orabase) or oral steroids injected into lesions for severe cases
- Thalidomide 20 mg 1–2× daily × 3–8 weeks in HIV+ patients with nonhealing aphthous ulcers (extreme caution for birth defects)

ADDITIONAL TREATMENT
General Measures
- In most cases, treatment of symptoms only
- Severe cases may require parenteral fluids, particularly children.
- Good oral hygiene
- Topical anesthesia
- Analgesics
- Oral rinses such as half-strength hydrogen peroxide
- Smoking cessation
- Refit dentures; daytime wear only
- Avoid specific allergens.
- Replace vitamin deficiencies.
- Treat malnutrition if present.

COMPLEMENTARY AND ALTERNATIVE MEDICINE
- Avoid toothpaste with sodium lauryl sulfate for prevention of aphthous ulcers.
- Replenish vitamin deficiencies.

IN-PATIENT CONSIDERATIONS
IV Fluids
In severe cases involving dehydration owing to oral ulcerations

Nursing
For infants with painful stomatitis, feeding can be particularly challenging. Topical analgesic agents should be used prior to bottle feeding. Nasogastric feeds or parenteral as needed.

ONGOING CARE

FOLLOW-UP RECOMMENDATIONS
Patient Monitoring
Lesions need to be followed until resolved. If they fail to resolve, continuously recur, or appear suspicious, biopsy may be needed.

DIET
May need to avoid spicy, acidic, sharp, hard, and dry foods.

PATIENT EDUCATION
Patient handouts:
- Aphthous ulcers (English and Spanish): http://www.aafp.prg/afp/20701/160ph.html
- Gingivostomatitis: http://www.nlm.nih.gov/medlineplus/ency/article/152.htm
- Mouth sores (English and Spanish): http://www.nlm.nih.gov/medlineplus/ency/article/003059.html
- Mouth problems in infants and children: http://familydoctor.org/online/famdocen/home/tools/symptom/510.html

PROGNOSIS
- Herpetic: Self-limited, with resolution in 7–14 days
- Hand-foot-mouth disease: Same as for herpetic
- RAS: 7- to 14-day course per episode
- Vincent: May progress to fascial space infection with airway compromise or sepsis.
- Nicotinic: Resolves with cessation of smoking.
- Denture: Resolves with proper fitting, careful oral hygiene, and daytime-only denture wear.
- Erythema multiforme: Resolution in 2–3 weeks
- Stevens-Johnson: Resolution in about 6 weeks with adequate supportive care
- Recurrent ulcerative: As the name implies, recurs over time, but the overall prognosis is good.
- Recurrent scarifying: Occasional patients suffer continuous ulcers; others have recurrence with eventual scarring. The prognosis is otherwise good.
- Behçet disease may recur for several years. Overall prognosis is related to other aspects of the disease.
- Angular: After correction of mechanical problems, allergic disorders, and nutritional deficiencies, the prognosis is good.
- Gangrenous: The most serious stomatitis, requiring aggressive treatment with IV antibiotics and débridement to avoid death
- Scarlatina: The prognosis is related to other manifestations of the disease.
- Herpangina: 7- to 14-day course with total resolution
- Uremic: Depends on the underlying renal disease

COMPLICATIONS
- Recurrent scarifying stomatitis may result in intraoral scarring with restriction of oral mobility.
- Behçet disease may result in visual loss, pneumonia, colitis, vasculitis, large-artery aneurysms, thrombophlebitis, or encephalitis.
- Gangrenous stomatitis may lead to facial disfigurement and even death.
- Scarlet fever may result in cardiac disease.
- Herpetic stomatitis may be complicated by ocular or CNS involvement.

REFERENCES
1. Chronic ulcerative stomatitis. *Oral diseases*, 2008;14:383–9.
2. Investigation of functional gene polymorphisms IL-1 beta, IL-6, IL-10 and TNF-alpha in individuals with recurrent aphthous stomatitis. *Archives of Oral Biology*, 2007;52(3):268–72.
3. The role of immunofluorescence in the physiopathology and differential diagnosis of recurrent aphthous stomatitis. *Revista Brasileira de otorrinolaringologia*. 2008;74(3):331–6.
4. Gorsky M, Epstein J, Raviv A, et al. Topical minocycline for managing symptoms of recurrent aphthous stomatitis. *Spec Care Dentist*. 2008;28:27–31.

CODES

ICD9
- 074.3 Hand, foot, and mouth disease
- 528.00 Stomatitis and mucositis, unspecified
- 528.2 Oral aphthae

CLINICAL PEARLS
- Stomatitis is often self limiting and requires only pain relief treatment.
- Consider broad differential diagnosis in order to consider etiology.
- Treat all underlying conditions.
- Depending on geographic location, age of patient, and co-morbities, be prepared to aggressively treat worsening or severe causes.

STREPTOCOCCAL PHARYNGITIS AND SCARLET FEVER

John C. Huscher, MD

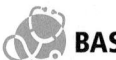 **BASICS**

DESCRIPTION
- A childhood disease characterized by fever, pharyngitis, and rash caused by group A β-hemolytic *Streptococcus pyogenes* (GAS) that produces erythrogenic toxin
- Incubation period: 1–7 days
- Duration of illness: 4–10 days
- Rash usually appears on the second day of illness.
- Rash first appears in the upper chest and flexural creases and then spreads rapidly all over the body.
- Rash clears at the end of the 1st week and is followed by several weeks of desquamation.
- System(s) affected: HEENT; Skin/Exocrine
- Synonym: Scarlatina

EPIDEMIOLOGY
Incidence
- Fairly common; rare in infancy (due to maternal antitoxin antibodies)
- Predominant age: 6–12 years
- Peak age: 4–8 years
- Predominant sex: Male = Female
- Rare > age 12 (US) due to high rates (>80%) of lifelong protective antibodies to erythrogenic toxins

Prevalence
- 5–30% of pediatric sore throats are due to GAS.
- <10% of children with streptococcal pharyngitis develop scarlet fever.

RISK FACTORS
- Winter/spring seasons
- Age: School-aged children
- Contact with infected individual(s)
- Crowded living conditions (e.g., lower socioeconomic status, military, child care, schools)

GENERAL PREVENTION
- GAS is spread by contact with airborne respiratory particles. Avoid if possible.
- Asymptomatic contacts do not require cultures or prophylaxis.
- Symptomatic contacts may be treated ± cultures.
- Children should not return to school or daycare until >24 h of antibiotic therapy.

PATHOPHYSIOLOGY
- Erythrogenic toxin produced by phage is necessary for scarlet fever.
- 3 types: A, B, C
- These toxins damage capillaries (producing rash) and act as superantigens stimulating cytokine release.
- Antibodies to toxins prevent development of rash but do not protect against underlying infection.

ETIOLOGY
Site of streptococcal infection usually tonsils; may occur with infection of skin, surgical wounds, or uterus (puerperal scarlet fever)

COMMONLY ASSOCIATED CONDITIONS
- Pharyngitis
- Impetigo
- Puerperal sepsis
- Rheumatic fever
- Glomerulonephritis

 DIAGNOSIS

HISTORY
Prodrome 1–2 days:
- Sore throat
- Headache
- Myalgias
- Malaise
- Fever (>38°C [100.4°F])
- Vomiting
- Abdominal pain (may mimic acute abdomen)
- Rash
- Cough (coryza), more likely viral

PHYSICAL EXAM
- Oral exam:
  - Beefy red tonsils and pharynx ± exudate
  - Petechiae on palate
  - White coating on tongue: White strawberry tongue appears on days 1–2. This sheds by days 4–5, leaving a red strawberry tongue, which is shiny and red with prominent papillae.
- Exanthem (appears within 1–5 days):
  - Scarlet macules over generalized erythema
  - Orange-red punctate skin eruption with sandpaperlike texture: Sunburn with goose pimples
  - Initially, chest and axillae; then spreads to abdomen and extremities; prominent in skin folds, flexural surfaces (e.g., axillae, groin, buttocks), with sparing of palms and soles
  - Flushed face with circumoral pallor, red lips
  - Pastia lines: Transverse red streaks in skin folds of abdomen, antecubital space, and axillae
  - Desquamation begins on face after 7–10 days and proceeds over trunk to hands and feet; may persist for 6 weeks
  - In severe cases, small vesicular lesions (miliary sudamina) may appear on abdomen, hands, and feet.
  - Rash: Blanches if pressed

DIAGNOSTIC TESTS & INTERPRETATION
Lab
Initial lab tests
- Rapid strep antigen tests: Diagnostic if positive, 95% specific; sensitivity approaches that of culture but some authorities still recommend confirmation of negatives (controversial).
- Throat culture: Culture β-hemolytic colonies, catalase negative, sensitive to bacitracin. Culture is gold standard for confirming streptococcal infection (99% specific, 90–97% sensitive, but 5–10% of healthy individuals are carriers).
- Serologic tests (includes antistreptolysin O titer and streptozyme tests, antihyaluronidase): Confirm recent GAS infection; not helpful for diagnosis of acute disease
- Gram stain: Positive cocci in chains
- Dick test: Injection of skin-test dose of erythrogenic toxin is positive in persons lacking antitoxin; not used clinically
- CBC may show elevated white blood cell count (12,000–16,000/mm³); later (2nd week) possible eosinophilia

Follow-Up & Special Considerations
- Drugs that may alter lab results: Prior antibiotic therapy may result in negative throat culture.
- Within 5 days of symptoms, antibiotics can delay/abolish antistreptolysin O response.

Pathological Findings
Local lesions reveal characteristic inflammatory reaction, specifically hyperemia, edema, and polymorphonuclear cell infiltration.

DIFFERENTIAL DIAGNOSIS
- Viral exanthem
- Measles
- Rubella
- Infectious mononucleosis
- Roseola
- *Mycoplasma* pneumonia
- Secondary syphilis
- *A. haemolyticum*
- Toxic shock syndrome
- Staphylococcal scalded-skin syndrome
- Kawasaki disease
- Drug hypersensitivity
- Severe sunburn

TREATMENT

MEDICATION

First Line

- Penicillin (oral; penicillin V and others) for 10 days (1):
  - 250 mg p.o. b.i.d. or t.i.d. for <27 kg (60 lb); 500 mg b.i.d. or t.i.d. for >27 kg (60 lb) adolescents and adults [A]
  - If compliance is questionable, use penicillin G, benzathine: Single IM dose 600,000 U for <27 kg (60 lb); 1.2 mU for others
- Amoxicillin (oral) 50 mg/kg once daily (1)[A]
- Contraindications: Penicillin allergy
- Acetaminophen for fever and pain
- Precautions: Refer to manufacturer's profile of each drug.
- Significant possible interactions: Refer to manufacturer's profile of each drug.

Second Line

- For patients allergic to penicillin
- Azithromycin (Zithromax, Z pack): 12 mg/kg/d (maximum of 500 mg) × 5 days (1)[B]
- Clarithromycin (Biaxin): Children > 6 months: 7.5 mg/kg b.i.d. x 10 days: Adults: 250 mg b.i.d. × 10 days (1)[B]
- Oral cephalosporins: Many are effective, but 1st-generation cephalosporins are less expensive:
  - Cephalexin 40 mg/kg/d divided t.i.d.; maximum: 250 mg t.i.d. × 10 days (1)[B]
  - Cefadroxil 30 mg/kg/d divided b.i.d.; maximum: 500 mg b.i.d. × 10 days (1)[B]
- Clindamycin 20 mg/kg/d divided t.i.d. × 10 days (1)[B]
- Tetracyclines and sulfonamides should not be used.

ADDITIONAL TREATMENT

General Measures
Supportive care

Issues for Referral
Development of peritonsillar abscess or shock symptoms: Hypotension, DIC, cardiac, liver, renal dysfunction

SURGERY/OTHER PROCEDURES

- Tonsillectomy may be recommended with recurrent bouts of pharyngitis (≥6 positive strep cultures in 1 year).
- Children still may get strep throat after a tonsillectomy, but for some children with recurring strep throat, tonsillectomy reduces the frequency and severity of strep throat infections.

ONGOING CARE

FOLLOW-UP RECOMMENDATIONS
Follow-up throat culture is not needed unless patient is symptomatic.

Patient Monitoring
Because GAS is uniformly susceptible to penicillin, bacteriologic treatment failures are possible due to:
- Poor compliance
- β-Lactamase oral flora hydrolyzing penicillin
- GAS carrier state and concurrent viral rash (requires no treatment)
- Repeat exposure to carriers in family: Strep persists on unrinsed toothbrushes and orthodontic appliances for up to 15 days.

DIET
No special diet

PATIENT EDUCATION
- Brief delay in initiating treatment awaiting throat culture results does not increase the risk of rheumatic fever.
- Must take antibiotics for full course
- Children should not return to school or daycare until >24 h of antibiotic therapy.
- Can spread person to person: Avoid contact, wash hands.
- "Recurring strep throat: When is tonsillectomy useful?" Available at http://www.mayoclinic.com/health/recurring-strep-throat/AN01626

PROGNOSIS
- Course may be shortened by 12–24 h with penicillin.
- Recurrent attacks are possible (different erythrogenic toxins).
- Mild disease usually responds well to antibiotics.

COMPLICATIONS
- Suppurative:
  - Sinusitis
  - Otitis media/mastoiditis
  - Cervical adenitis
  - Peritonsillar abscess/retropharyngeal abscess
  - Pneumonia
  - Bacteremia with metastatic infectious foci: Meningitis, brain abscess, osteomyelitis, septic arthritis, endocarditis, intracranial venous sinus thrombosis, necrotizing fasciitis
- Nonsuppurative:
  - Rheumatic fever: Therapy prevents rheumatic fever when started as long as 10 days after onset of acute GAS infection.
  - Glomerulonephritis: Due to nephritogenic strain of *Streptococcus*. Prevention even after adequate treatment of GAS is less certain.

- Streptococcal toxic shock syndrome: Fever, hypotension, DIC, and cardiac, liver, and/or kidney dysfunction related to other toxin-mediated sequelae
- Cellulitis
- Weeks–months later may develop transverse grooves in nail plates and hair loss (telogen effluvium)

REFERENCE

1. Gerber MA, et al. Prevention of Rheumatic Fever and Diagnosis and Treatment of Acute Streptococcal Pharyngitis: A Statement from the American Heart Association Rheumatic Fever, Endocarditis, and Kawasaki Disease Committee of the Council on Cardiovascular Disease in the Young, the Interdisciplinary Council on Functional Genomics and Translational Biology, and the Interdisciplinary Council on Quality of Care and Outcomes Research: Endorsed by the American Academy of Pediatrics. *Circulation* 2009;119: 1541–1551.

ADDITIONAL READING

- Baltimore RS. Re-evaluation of antibiotic treatment of streptococcal pharyngitis. *Curr Opin Pediatr* 2010;22:77–82.
- Lennon DR, Farrell E, Martin DR . Once-daily amoxicillin versus twice-daily penicillin V in group A beta-haemolytic streptococcal pharyngitis. *Arch Dis Child*. 2008;93:474–8.
- Spinks A. Antibiotics for sore throat (Review). *Cochrane Database of Systemic Reviews* 2010, Issue 3.

CODES

ICD9
- 034.0 Streptococcal sore throat
- 034.1 Scarlet fever

CLINICAL PEARLS

- Consider scarlet fever in the differential diagnosis of children with fever and a rash.
- Look for strawberry tongue, circumoral pallor (vs hyperemic cracked lips with Kawasaki disease), and a coarse sandpaper rash (especially helpful in dark-skinned individuals). Desquamation may last for several weeks following the illness.
- Perform throat swabs to document streptococcal illness vs other etiologies.

STRESS FRACTURE

Justin A. Lee, MD
Morteza Khodaee, MD, MPH

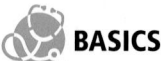 **BASICS**

DESCRIPTION
- Stress fractures are microscopic fractures that occur when repetitive stresses are applied to bone causing breakdown (via osteoclasts) faster than remodeling of new bone formation (via osteoblasts).
- Stress fractures can occur in different situations.
  - Fatigue fracture: Abnormal stress applied to normal bone (e.g., young college athletes or new military recruits with inadequate conditioning)
  - Insufficiency fracture: Normal stress applied to abnormal bone (e.g., femoral neck fracture in osteopenic elderly woman)
  - Combination: Abnormal stress applied to abnormal bone (e.g., female long-distance runners with premature osteoporosis from female athlete triad)
- Weight-bearing bones of the lower extremity are affected the most.
- Commonly affected sites:
  - Tibia
  - Metatarsus
  - Fibula
  - Navicular
  - Femoral neck
  - Pars interarticularis
- Less commonly affected sites:
  - Pelvis
  - Calcaneus
  - Ribs
  - Ulna
- Synonym(s): March fracture; Fatigue fracture

EPIDEMIOLOGY
Incidence
- Predominant age: Can occur at any age
- Predominant sex: Female > Male.
- High occurrence in running and jumping athletes
- Affects 8.7–21.1% of track and field athletes annually
- Affects 1–2.6% of all college athletes
- Accounts for as high as 7.8% of visits to sports medicine and orthopedic clinics
- Affects 5% of military recruits

RISK FACTORS
- Sports involving running and jumping
- Rapid increase in physical training programs
- Female athlete triad (i.e., amenorrhea, eating disorder, premature osteoporosis)
- History of previous stress fracture
- Skeletal malalignment:
  - Pes cavus, pes planus
  - Excessive external rotation of the hip

- Inappropriate footwear
- Extreme of body size and composition
- Muscle fatigue and decreased lean muscle mass
- Low bone density
- Previous inactivity or low aerobic fitness

GENERAL PREVENTION
- Avoid abrupt increases in physical activity.
- Reduce intensity and duration with new-onset pain.
- Use proper footwear.
- Shock-absorbing foot inserts may help.

PATHOPHYSIOLOGY
- Osteoblastic activities lag behind osteoclastic activities during the initial increase in exercise activity.
- Strong and repetitive stress transmits to bone when the surrounding muscles become fatigued.

COMMONLY ASSOCIATED CONDITIONS
- Osteoporosis/osteopenia
- Female athlete triad
- Metabolic bone disorders

 DIAGNOSIS

HISTORY
- Insidious onset of vague, achy pain over period of weeks that occurs at the end or after physical activity
- Rest will relieve the pain initially.
- If untreated, pain will occur earlier during training sessions or even with daily walking and also become more localized.
- Eventual fracture of untreated stress fractures will cause pain at rest.
- More detailed history may reveal recent change in training intensity and/or footwear.

PHYSICAL EXAM
- Antalgic gait
- Point tenderness or percussion tenderness over injury site
- Swelling may be present.
- Specific tests may be helpful.
  - Hop test for tibia: Cannot hop on 1 leg 10 times; if able, consider shin splints (i.e., medial tibial stress syndrome).
  - Fulcrum test for femur: With patient seated, provoke pain by applying downward force on the distal femur while examiner uses other hand under the midthigh as fulcrum for femoral shaft.
  - Single-leg hyperextension (Stork) test for pars interarticularis of lumbar spine: Stand on ipsilateral leg of symptomatic side, and extend lumbar spine.
- Anatomic malalignment may be present (e.g., leg-length discrepancy, pes planus/cavus).

DIAGNOSTIC TESTS & INTERPRETATION
Lab
None unless clinically indicated for suspected disease process (e.g., hyperparathyroidism and vitamin D deficiency)

Imaging
- Radiography:
  - Findings typically seen 2–8 weeks after onset of pain.
  - Sensitivity during early stages may be as low as 10%.
  - May see periosteal callus, "gray cortex" sign (cortical region of decreased intensity), osteopenia, endosteal reaction, or ill-defined cortical margin
  - Severe cases may show discrete partial or complete fracture.
- MRI:
  - Very sensitive
  - Better evaluation of surrounding soft tissue
  - Allows for classification of the injury
  - T_2 weighting and short inversion time inversion recovery (STIR) methods
- Bone scan:
  - Very sensitive, but lack of specificity may limit clinical utility.
  - Should not be used to assess healing process
- CT scan:
  - "Gold standard" to evaluate occult fractures (pars interarticularis, carpal scaphoid)
  - Can distinguish diseases such as osteoid osteoma, malignancy, and osteomyelitis that mimic stress fracture on bone scan
- Ultrasound: New evidence suggests that ultrasound could be useful in the diagnosis of early metatarsal stress fractures (1)[B].
- Classification by radiographic grading:
  - Grade I: Normal X-ray, positive STIR (MRI)
  - Grade II: Normal X-ray, positive STIR + positive T_2-weighted MRI
  - Grade III: Discrete line or discrete periosteal reaction on X-ray, positive T_1/T_2-weighted MRI but with no definite cortical break
  - Grade IV: Fracture or periosteal reaction on X-ray, positive T_1/T_2-weighted fracture line

DIFFERENTIAL DIAGNOSIS
- Fracture
- Shin splints (i.e., medial tibial stress syndrome) pain resolves with rest, whereas stress fracture pain does not.
- Infection (osteomyelitis)
- Soft tissue injury
- Compartment syndrome
- Neoplasm (osteoid osteoma)
- Nerve or artery entrapment syndromes

TREATMENT

- Protection, rest, ice, compression, and elevation (PRICE) for acute pain and edema
- Decrease activity below threshold of pain.
- Pain at rest or with range of motion (ROM) may require temporary immobilization.
- Painful ambulation is criterion for crutches with periodic walking trials.
- Gradually increase activity as long as patient remains pain-free.

MEDICATION
- Acetaminophen
- Nonsteroidal anti-inflammatory drugs (NSAIDs) are beneficial for pain and inflammation but controversial and discouraged by some authors because of negative impact on bone/tissue healing.
- Bisphosphonates theoretically could treat stress fractures, but their use should be limited because no randomized, controlled trials have been performed that show conclusive evidence (2)[B].

ADDITIONAL TREATMENT
- Electrical stimulator may be indicated in more severe injuries and/or elite athletes (3)[B].
- Low-intensity pulsed ultrasonography:
  – No evidence for improved healing in stress fracture
  – May improve healing with subsequent complete fracture

Issues for Referral
Referral and surgical intervention are reserved for high-risk stress fractures with potential for progression to complete fracture and possible delayed union or nonunion.
- Femoral neck
- Anterior midshaft tibia
- Tarsal navicular
- Body of talus
- Proximal 2nd metatarsal
- Sesamoids
- Pars interarticularis

Additional Therapies
Physical therapy:
- Correct training errors predisposing to stress fracture.
- Correct inappropriate mechanics.
- Strengthen muscles around the site of stress fracture.
- Correct anatomic variations.

 ONGOING CARE

FOLLOW-UP RECOMMENDATIONS
- After initial treatment, activity should be increased gradually.
- Once the patient is pain-free, low-impact training can be started and advanced as tolerated.
- Once running is resumed, mileage should be increased slowly.

Patient Monitoring
Radiographs every 4–6 weeks to document healing progress

PATIENT EDUCATION
- Gradually increase activity as tolerated as long as patient is pain-free.
- Rest if there is a recurrence of pain.
- Correct mechanical and training errors.
- Strengthen core muscles.

PROGNOSIS
- Stress fractures in young people have a good prognosis.
- Older patients or those with metabolic bone disease typically continue to develop insufficiency fractures in other bones.
- Time to return to full activity:
  – Grade I: 3+ weeks
  – Grade II: 5+ weeks
  – Grade III: 11+ weeks
  – Grade IV: 14+ weeks

COMPLICATIONS
Completion of fracture:
- Delayed union
- Nonunion
- May require surgery with internal fixation

REFERENCES
1. Banal F, et al. Sensitivity and specificity of ultrasonography in early diagnosis of metatarsal bone stress fractures: A pilot study of 37 patients. *J Rheumaol*. 2009;8:1715–9.
2. Shima Y, et al. Use of bisphosphonates for the treatment of stress fractures in athletes. *Knee Surg Sports Traumatol Arthrosc*. 2009;5:542–50.
3. Beck B, et al. Do capacitively coupled electric fields accelerate tibial stress fracture healing?: A randomized controlled trial. *Am J Sports Med*. 2008;3:545–53.

ADDITIONAL READING
- Arendt EA, Griffiths HJ. The use of MR imaging in the assessment and clinical management of stress reactions of bone in high-performance athletes. *Clin Sports Med*. 1997;16:291–306.
- Armstrong DW, Rue JP, Wilckens JH, et al. Stress fracture injury in young military men and women. *Bone*. 2004;35:806–16.
- Boden BP, Osbahr DC. High-risk stress fractures: evaluation and treatment. *J Am Acad Orthop Surg*. 2000;8:344–53.
- Busse JW, Kaur J, Mollon B, et al. Low intensity pulsed ultrasonography for fractures: systematic review of randomised controlled trials. *BMJ*. 2009;338:b351.
- Fredericson M, Jennings F, Beaulieu C, et al. Stress Fractures in Athletes. *Top Magn Reson Imaging*. 2006;17:309–25.
- Manore MM, Kam LC, Loucks AB. The female athlete triad: Components, nutrition issues, and health consequences. *J Sports Sci*. 2007; 25(Suppl 1):61–71.
- Niva MH, Kiuru MJ, Haataja R, et al. Fatigue injuries of the femur. *J Bone Joint Surg Br*. 2005;87: 1385–90.
- Pepper M, Akuthota V, McCarty EC. The pathophysiology of stress fractures. *Clin Sports Med*. 2006;25:1–16, vii.
- Raasch WG, Hergan DJ. Treatment of stress fractures: the fundamentals. *Clin Sports Med*. 2006;25:29–36, vii.
- Snyder RA, Koester MC, Dunn WR. Epidemiology of stress fractures. *Clin Sports Med*. 2006;25:37–52, viii.

See Also (Topic, Algorithm, Electronic Media Element)
Algorithm: Foot Pain

CLINICAL PEARLS
- Diagnosis requires a high index of suspicion because X-rays are often negative initially.
- Emphasis must be placed on rest to allow for proper bone healing.
- Once the patient can walk pain-free, he/she can proceed to low-impact activity.
- When low-impact activity can be performed pain-free, proceed to running.
- Gradually increase running mileage.
- Rest if there is a recurrence of pain.
- Recognize high-risk stress fracture for appropriate referral and possible surgery.

 CODES

ICD9
- 733.93 Stress fracture of tibia or fibula
- 733.94 Stress fracture of the metatarsals
- 733.95 Stress fracture of other bone

STROKE REHABILITATION

Faren H. Williams, MD
Jeremy Golding, MD

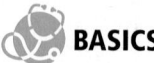 **BASICS**

DESCRIPTION
- Post-stroke therapy intended to prevent additional functional loss, avert medical complications, and restore lost function.
- Majority of stroke rehabilitation should be "low-tech" but "high-touch," involving assessment and treatment by multidisciplinary team (1)[A].
- System(s) affected: Cardiovascular; Nervous; Musculoskeletal

EPIDEMIOLOGY
Incidence
- Predominant age: >45 years
- Predominant sex: Male > Female

Prevalence
- 2–3% of nondiabetics and 9% of diabetics report a history of stroke.
- 62 million stroke survivors worldwide (2)

GENERAL PREVENTION
- Post-stroke, control BP, cholesterol, and obesity
- Stop smoking

PATHOPHYSIOLOGY
Infarction or hemorrhage results in loss of functional central nervous system tissue, resulting in deficits in motor function, sensory function, and impairment of speech and cognition.

COMMONLY ASSOCIATED CONDITIONS
Conditions commonly associated with stroke that require ongoing management following stroke:
- Coronary artery disease and atherosclerosis, atrial fibrillation
- HTN
- Diabetes mellitus
- Gout
- Smoking and alcoholism
- Cerebral aneurysms and arteriovenous malformations

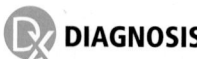 **DIAGNOSIS**

HISTORY
Patient may report any of the following or be unaware of impairment:
- Difficulty with speech (impairment of speech generation and speech production)
- Difficulty with understanding speech
- Difficulty swallowing
- Unilateral weakness or numbness
- Difficulty ambulating
- Seizure activity

PHYSICAL EXAM
- Neurodeficits depend upon the systems affected by the stroke, but the following are common:
  – Aphasia or dysarthria
  – Dysphagia
  – Hemiparesis
  – Hemianesthesia
  – Unilateral central facial palsy
  – Hemianopsia
  – Apraxia
  – Locked-in syndrome (total-body paralysis with retained cognitive and oculomotor function)
- Subacute complications of stroke:
  – Pressure ulcerations
  – Lung evidence of aspiration
  – Extremity exam for presence of deep venous thrombosis

DIAGNOSTIC TESTS & INTERPRETATION
- Chest x-ray if suspected pneumonitis
- Formal speech and swallowing study performed by speech pathologist if indicated by bedside screening evaluation (1)[A]
- ECG to evaluate for atrial fibrillation
- Cardiovascular stress testing may be indicated in some cases to evaluate the presence or extent of coronary artery disease
- EEG: Sometimes useful in seizure disorders
- Somatosensory, auditory, and visual evoked potential technology (not very useful)
- Neuropsych testing in selected cases to assess possible specialized learning needs
- Ongoing screening for depression (1)[A]

Lab
See topic Stroke, Acute for lab workup detail.
Follow-Up & Special Considerations
PT/INR in anticoagulated patients

Imaging
Follow-Up & Special Considerations
Total-body bone scans can help to diagnose reflex sympathetic dystrophy (pain and sensitivity out of proportion to physical findings, temperature difference involving affected area, skin changes, localized alteration in sweating)

Diagnostic Procedures/Surgery
Electromyelography (EMG) for secondary radiculopathy or for position-related focal nerve entrapments

DIFFERENTIAL DIAGNOSIS
- Brain tumors often present as stroke syndromes with significant personality and/or aphasic disorders and relatively less obvious weakness or spasticity.
- Tumors with metastases to the brain

 TREATMENT

The key principles of effective stroke rehabilitation include:
- Functional approach targeted at specific activities, e.g., walking, activities of daily living
- Frequent and intense practice
- Commencement in the first days or weeks after stroke (2) as soon as the patient is medically stable (1)

MEDICATION
First Line
- Treat underlying disorders (e.g., HTN, heart disease, diabetes) or complications (e.g., seizures, deep vein thrombosis, pneumonitis)
- Antiplatelet therapy for prevention of recurrent thrombotic stroke (see Stroke, Acute)
- Use anticoagulant medications for patients with a history of or risk factors for thromboembolic stroke (must first weigh fall risk and ability to comply with monitoring of INR).
- When neurologic and medical stability are achieved, treat depression as needed. Some evidence suggests reduced mortality if depression is identified and treated.
- Avoid polypharmacy where possible:
  – Some medicines accumulate over time in stroke patients, especially in the elderly.
  – Use only necessary medicines.
  – Avoid benzodiazepine and antipsychotic medications for sedation if at all possible; Behavioral interventions preferable (see Dementia and Delirium).
- Precautions:
  – Antihypertensives can generate orthostatic hypotension.
  – Overly aggressive treatment of HTN can yield hypotension and stroke extension. Systolic blood pressure target in the elderly is around 150 mm Hg.
  – Antidepressants can lower seizure threshold (i.e., bupropion).
  – Muscle relaxants, tranquilizers, and major neuroleptic medications can confuse, sedate, agitate, and delay return of memory and cognition.
  – Elderly patients regularly require lower medication doses.

Second Line
- Flexor spasms: Tizanidine 4–8 mg/day, diazepam 5 mg b.i.d., or baclofen 10 mg t.i.d.
- For spasticity in those not tolerating systemic medication: Botulinum toxin injections into affected muscles or intrathecal baclofen pump
- Reflex sympathetic dystrophy (shoulder–hand syndrome): High-dose steroids or, alternatively, tizanidine (Zanaflex) 4–8 mg/day

ADDITIONAL TREATMENT
Evaluation by physical therapy, occupational therapy, and speech therapy is advised for most stroke patients (1).

General Measures
- Prevent deep venous thrombosis by mobilization (compression stockings likely not of value) (3).
- Prevent development of pressure ulcers by appropriate mattresses, padding, and position changes.
- Prevent aspiration pneumonitis by assessing swallowing ability and providing foods of appropriate consistency, and by elevating head of the bed.
- Minimize use of indwelling urinary catheters to prevent urinary tract infection.

Issues for Referral
All stroke patients should be assessed and treated by a multidisciplinary team (1)[A]:
- Compliance with national standards for admission, discharge, follow-up care
- Regular team meetings with physical, occupational, speech therapies, rehabilitation physician, nurse, dietician, neuropsychologist to discuss short- and long-term objectives
- Systematic implementation of quality assurance
- Accreditation by Commission on Accreditation of Rehabilitation Facilities or JACHO

Additional Therapies
- Maintenance of good nutrition is important, especially adequate protein and protein-calorie supplementation in undernourished patients. Supplements may be necessary. PEG tube rather than NG tube advised.
- Physical therapy, occupational therapy, speech pathology, psychology, and nursing are recommended for about 3 hours/day throughout inpatient rehab stay. Ongoing assessment by dietitian to monitor nutritional status.
- PT including strengthening, gait assessment with device or orthotic, balance testing, coordination exercises. Appropriate orthoses may help maintain paretic limbs in positions of function and prevent development of contractures.
- Use hydrotherapy and/or isometric exercise cautiously in patients with limited cardiopulmonary reserve.
- Use deep heat (e.g., ultrasound, prolonged hydrotherapy) with caution in patients with reduced sensation and/or taking anticoagulants.

- OT including assessment of activities of daily living (ADLs), compensatory techniques for ADLs, and appropriate splinting
- Speech therapy to evaluate swallow and speech
- Although most rehabilitative efforts take place immediately following cerebrovascular infarction, partially successful rehabilitative efforts have taken place up to several years later (and may relate to inadequate rehabilitation following the initial event).

COMPLEMENTARY AND ALTERNATIVE MEDICINE
- Acupuncture for complications such as focal pain
- Massage may help with stress relief.

SURGERY/OTHER PROCEDURES
Appropriate

IN-PATIENT CONSIDERATIONS
Initial Stabilization
- Monitor vital signs and neurologic status.
- Evaluate cardiovascular and respiratory status.

IV Fluids
- IV hydration until swallowing status is assessed
- Monitor fluid balance.
- Evaluate electrolyte status and renal function.

Nursing
- Monitor vital signs, including input and output.
- Regular neurologic checks
- Elevate head of bed to reduce risk of aspiration of gastric contents and while eating/feeding.
- Position patient to prevent contractures and pressure ulcers.

Discharge Criteria
- Achieved short-term rehab goals
- Neurologic status stable/improving
- Cardiac and respiratory status stable
- Functional with ADLs and gait, or family can provide assistance

 ## ONGOING CARE

FOLLOW-UP RECOMMENDATIONS
The patient and family/caregivers should be seen by the rehab team within a month of discharge.

Patient Monitoring
- When acute rehab is completed for uncomplicated stroke patients, remaining rehab can be done as an outpatient or in a day care program.
- In the outpatient setting, the rehab team should meet to rate progress and discuss short- and long-term goals.

DIET
Ensure adequate calories and nutrients.

PATIENT EDUCATION
- Major risk factors for stroke are nearly all preventable through lifestyle modification, including diet, exercise, and tobacco cessation.
- National Institutes of Health: http://www.ninds.nih.gov/disorders/stroke/poststrokerehab.htm
- National Stroke Association, 9707 E. Easter Lane, Englewood, CO 80112; (800) STROKES or http://www.stroke.org

PROGNOSIS
- Recovery of motor and cognitive function within the 1st 2 weeks is a good prognostic sign.
- Absence of any significant recovery after 2 months or longer is a poor prognostic sign.
- Persistence of neglect is associated with a poorer prognosis for return to prior level of function.

REFERENCES
1. Lindsay P, Bayley M, McDonald A, et al. Toward a more effective approach to stroke: Canadian Best Practice Recommendations for Stroke Care. *CMAJ.* 2008;178:1418–25.
2. Dewey HM, Sherry LJ, Collier JM. Stroke rehabilitation 2007: what should it be? *Int J Stroke.* 2007;2:191–200.
3. Naccarato M, et al. Physical methods for prevention of deep venous thrombosis in stroke Cochrane Stroke Group *Cochrane Database of Systemic Reviews*. 2010.

ADDITIONAL READING
Bath PM, et al. Interventions for dysphagia in acute stroke. *Cochrane Database Sys Rev.* 2000;2: CD000323.

See Also (Topic, Algorithm, Electronic Media Element)
Brain Injury—Post Acute Care Issues; Stroke, Acute; Dementia; Delirium
Algorithm: Stroke

CODES

ICD9
434.91 Cerebral artery occlusion, unspecified with cerebral infarction

CLINICAL PEARLS
- Fully assess impairments by consulting occupational therapy, physical therapy, speech therapy, and dietician in most stroke patients.
- Checklist-based strategy improves adherence to critical recommendations regarding DVT and pressure ulcer prevention.
- Provide psychological assessment and family support.

STROKE, ACUTE

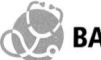

Nihal Patel, MD
Erik J. Garcia, MD

BASICS

A cerebrovascular accident (CVA) is an infarction of the brain.

DESCRIPTION
Stroke is the sudden onset of a focal neurologic deficit(s) resulting from either infarction or hemorrhage within the brain:

- 2 broad categories: Ischemic (thrombotic or embolic) (87%) and hemorrhagic (13%) (1)
- Hemorrhage can be intracerebral or subarachnoid.
- System(s) affected: Neurologic; Cardiovascular
- Synonym(s): Cerebrovascular accident; Cerebral infarct; Brain attack
- Related terms: Transient ischemic attack (TIA), a transient episode of neurologic dysfunction due to focal ischemia, without permanent infarction on imaging

Pediatric Considerations
- Cardiac abnormalities (congenital heart disease, paradoxical embolism, rheumatic fever, bacterial endocarditis)
- Metabolic: Homocystinuria, Fabry disease

EPIDEMIOLOGY
Incidence
Incidence in the US: 150/100,000 per year

Prevalence
- Prevalence in the US: 550/100,000
- Predominant age: Risk increases >45 years and is highest in the 7th and 8th decades
- Predominant sex: Male > Female (3:1), but equalizes after menopause

RISK FACTORS
- Uncontrollable: Age, sex, race, family history, prior stroke or TIA
- Controllable/modifiable/treatable:
  – Metabolic: Diabetes mellitus, obesity, metabolic syndrome, impaired glucose tolerance
  – Lifestyle: Smoking, heavy alcohol use, substance abuse, increased sodium intake, poor physical function, genetics
  – Cardiovascular: Hypertension, atrial fibrillation, valvular heart disease, severe carotid artery stenosis, hypercoagulable states (including OCP use), pregnancy and postpartum states

Genetics
Stroke is a polygenic multifactorial disease, with some clustering within families.

GENERAL PREVENTION
Smoking cessation, regular exercise, weight control to maintain nonobese BMI, use of alcohol in moderation. Control blood pressure, maintain tight glycemic control with diabetes, manage hyperlipidemia with appropriate statin therapy. Use of antiplatelet agent such as aspirin, treatment of nonvalvular atrial fibrillation with dose-adjusted warfarin

ETIOLOGY
- 87% of stroke is ischemic, secondary to cardio-aortic embolism including atrial fibrillation, large artery arthrosclerosis such as carotid artery stenosis, small vessel occlusion or dissection.

- 13% of stroke is hemorrhagic, most commonly due to hypertension. Other causes include intracranial vascular malformations (cavernous angiomas, AVMs), cerebral amyloid angiopathy (lobar hemorrhages in elderly), or secondary hemorrhage into previous infarcts.
- Other causes include fibromuscular dysplasia (rare), vasculitis, or drug use (cocaine, amphetamines).

COMMONLY ASSOCIATED CONDITIONS
Cardiac disease is the major cause of death in the first 5 years after a stroke.

DIAGNOSIS

HISTORY
Acute onset of focal arm/leg weakness, facial weakness, difficulty with speech or swallowing, vertigo, visual disturbances, diminished consciousness. Presence of vomiting and severe headache favor diagnosis of hemorrhagic stroke.

PHYSICAL EXAM
- Anterior (carotid) circulation: Hemiparesis/hemiplegia, neglect, aphasia, visual field defects
- Posterior (vertebrobasilar) circulation: Diplopia, vertigo, ataxia, facial paresis, Horner syndrome, dysphagia, dysarthria

DIAGNOSTIC TESTS & INTERPRETATION
Lab
Primarily to narrow differential and identify etiology for stroke

Initial lab tests
- Electrocardiogram;
- Serum glucose level, including finger-stick testing
- CBC including platelets
- Electrolytes including BUN and creatinine
- Coagulation studies: PT, PTT, INR
- Markers of cardiac ischemia

Follow-Up & Special Considerations
Consider: LFTs, tox screen, blood alcohol, ABG, lumbar puncture if suspected SAH, EEG if suspect seizures, blood type and cross

Imaging
Initial approach
- Emergent brain imaging with noncontrast CT or brain MRI with diffusion weighing (DW-MRI) to exclude hemorrhage.
- Subsequent multimodal CT (perfusion CT, CTA, unenhanced CT) or MRI to improve diagnosis of acute ischemic stroke (2)

Follow-Up & Special Considerations
- DW-MRI is more sensitive than conventional CT for acute ischemic stroke (3), however multimodal CT is equivalent to MRI. MRI is also better than CT for diagnosis of posterior fossa lesions.
- Emergent treatment (IV thrombolysis) should not be delayed to obtain imaging studies.
- Follow-up imaging of carotid vessels with Doppler ultrasound, CTA, or MRA should be completed.

Diagnostic Procedures/Surgery
Echocardiogram (transthoracic) in patients with increased suspicion for cardioembolic source

Pathological Findings
Early CT findings: Hyperdense MCA sign, loss of gray-white differentiation in cortical ribbon, sulcal effacement, loss of insular ribbon

DIFFERENTIAL DIAGNOSIS
- Migraine (complicated)
- Postictal state (Todd's paralysis)
- Systemic infection including meningitis or encephalitis (infection may also uncover or enhance previous deficits)
- Toxic or metabolic disturbance (hypoglycemia, acute renal failure, liver failure, drug intoxication)
- Brain tumor, primary or metastases
- Head trauma
- Intracranial hemorrhage (epidural, subdural, subarachnoid)
- Trauma, septic emboli

TREATMENT

- Blood pressure (BP) management: Hypertension should be cautiously managed due to spontaneous BP decline in the first 24 hours.
  – Antihypertensives should be withheld unless systolic BP >220 mm Hg or diastolic BP >120 mm Hg, with a goal to lower BP by about 15% during first 24 hours (2)[A].
  – If patient is eligible for thrombolysis, pressure may be reduced to <185/110 (2)[A].
  – In hemorrhagic stroke, goal for BP control is lower at 160/100.
  – Antihypertensive medications should be restarted 24 hours after stroke onset for patients with history of hypertension who are neurologically stable (2)[A].
- Thrombolysis (2)[A]: IV thrombolysis should be started in patients with measurable neurologic deficits not clearing spontaneously, presenting within 4.5 hours of stroke onset.
- Exclusion criteria for thrombolysis within 3 hours of onset include:
  – Symptoms suggestive of SAH
  – Head trauma or prior stroke within 3 months
  – MI within 3 months
  – GI or GU hemorrhage within 21 days
  – Major surgery within 14 days
  – Arterial puncture at noncompressible site within 7 days
  – Any history of previous ICH persistently
  – Elevated BP (systolic >185 mm Hg and diastolic >110 mm Hg)
  – Active bleeding or acute trauma on examination
  – Taking anticoagulant and INR ≥1.7
  – aPTT not in normal range if heparin received in previous 48 hours; Platelet count <100,000 mm³
  – Blood glucose concentration <50 mg/dl
  – Seizure with postictal residual neurological impairment
  – Multilobar infarction on CT (hypodensity >1/3 cerebral hemisphere)
  – Patient or family members not understanding risks and benefits of treatment.
- Extended exclusion criteria for thrombolysis within 4.5 hours include:
  – Age >80 years
  – All patients taking oral anticoagulants

– NIH Stoke Scale (NIHSS) >25
– History of stroke and diabetes

- Antiplatelet agents: Oral aspirin (initial dose 325 mg) should be started within 24 and 48 hours (2)[A]:
  – In the acute setting, clopidogrel alone or in combination with aspirin is not recommended.
  – Urgent anticoagulation with goal of preventing early recurrent stroke is not recommended.

MEDICATION
First Line
- Blood pressure management: Antihypertensive options include (2)[A]:
  – Labetalol 10–20 mg IV over 1–2 minutes, which may be repeated once
  – Nitropaste 1–2 inches
  – Nicardipine infusion 5 mg/hour, titrate up by 2.5 mg/hour at 5–15 minute intervals to maximum of 15 mg/hour, reduce to 3 mg/hour when target BP is reached.
- Thrombolysis, IV administration of rtPA: Infuse 0.9 mg/kg, maximum dose 90 mg over 60 minutes with 10% of dose given as bolus over 1 minute (2)[A]:
  – Admit to ICU or stroke unit, with neurological exams every 15 minutes during infusion, every 60 minutes for next 6 hours, then hourly until 24 hours after treatment.
  – Discontinue infusion and obtain emergent CT scan if severe headache, angioedema, acute hypertension, or nausea and vomiting develop.
  – Measure BP every 15 minutes for first 2 hours, every 30 minutes for next 6 hours, then every hour until 24 hours after treatment. Maintain BP below 185/105. Follow-up CT at 24 hours before starting anticoagulants or antiplatelet agents.
- Antiplatelet: Aspirin 325 mg/day within 48 hours, or 24–48 hours after thrombolytic therapy

Second Line
Carotid endarterectomy (CEA) for carotid artery stenosis rarely indicated emergently. CEA indicated for stenosis >70% ipsilateral to stroke lesion. May be indicated for 50–69% stenosis in carefully selected patients depending on risk factors.

ADDITIONAL TREATMENT
- Prophylactic antibiotics are NOT recommended (2)[A].
- DVT prophylaxis should be instituted for immobilized patients.
- Corticosteroids are NOT recommended for cerebral brain edema (2)[A].
- Statin use should be continued without interruption following acute stroke.

Issues for Referral
Follow-up with neurologist 1 week post discharge, then every 3 months for 1st year, then annually

Additional Therapies
Upon discharge, patient should be referred for PT, OT, and speech therapy as necessary.

COMPLEMENTARY AND ALTERNATIVE MEDICINE
Acupuncture starting within 30 days from stroke onset may improve neurological functioning.

SURGERY/OTHER PROCEDURES
- Ventricular drain may be placed for patients with acute hydrocephalus secondary to stroke (most commonly due to cerebellar stroke)

- Decompressive surgery recommended for major cerebellar infarction; may be considered for malignant edema in severely affected patients.
- Consider MERCI device (Mechanical Embolus Removal in Cerebral Infarction).

IN-PATIENT CONSIDERATIONS
Initial Stabilization
- Observe closely within 1st 24 hours for neurological decline particularly due to brain swelling.
- Keep head of bed at least 30° when elevated intracranial pressure is suspected. Patients with ischemic stroke may benefit from horizontal bed position during acute phase.
- Monitor cardiac rhythm for at least 1st 24 hours to identify any arrhythmias.
- Airway support and ventilatory assistance may be necessary due to diminished consciousness or bulbar involvement; supplemental oxygen should be reserved for hypoxic patients. Consider elective intubation for patients with malignant edema.
- Correct hypovolemia with normal saline.
- All patients should be kept NPO until formal swallow evaluation to reduce risk of aspiration pneumonia, maintain elevated head of bed to 30°.
- Hypoglycemia can cause neurological dysfunction; rapidly correct during initial evaluation.
- Hyperglycemia within first 24 hours after stroke is associated with poor functional outcomes and AHA/ASA guidelines: Insulin treatment for patients with glucose levels >140–185 mg/dL.
- In patients with ICH and anticoagulant use, correction of elevated INR is necessary with use of IV vitamin K and FFP. Consider neurosurgical intervention for hematoma evacuation if indicated.

IV Fluids
IV hydration with normal saline until swallowing status is assessed. Monitor fluid balance closely.

Nursing
- Regular neurologic exams more frequent in 1st 24 hours (every 1–2 hours)
- Fall precautions; frequent repositioning to prevent skin breakdown

Discharge Criteria
Medically stable, adequate nutritional support, neurological status stable or improving

 ONGOING CARE

FOLLOW-UP RECOMMENDATIONS
- Secondary prevention of stroke with aggressive management of risk factors
- Platelet inhibition using aspirin, clopidogrel, or aspirin plus extended-release dipyridamole (Aggrenox) based on patient preference. Studies indicate better efficacy of clopidogrel (75 mg daily) monotherapy or Aggrenox use (25/200) over aspirin alone (2).

Patient Monitoring
Follow-up every 3 months for first year, then annually

DIET
Patients with impaired swallowing should receive NG or PEG feedings to maintain nutrition and hydration.

PATIENT EDUCATION
National Stroke Association (800-STROKES or http://www.stroke.org)

PROGNOSIS
Variable depending on subtype and severity of stroke. NIH stroke scale may be used for prognosis.

COMPLICATIONS
- Acute: Brain herniation, hemorrhagic transformation, MI, CHF, dysphagia, aspiration pneumonia, UTI, DVT, PE, malnutrition, pressure sores
- Chronic: Falls, depression, dementia, orthopedic complications, contractures

REFERENCES
1. Yew KS, Cheng E, et al. Acute stroke diagnosis. *Am Fam Physician*. 2009;80:33–40.
2. Adams HP, del Zoppo G, Alberts MJ, et al. Guidelines for the early management of adults with ischemic stroke: a guideline from the American Heart Association/American Stroke Association Stroke Council, Clinical Cardiology Council, Cardiovascular Radiology and Intervention Council, and the Atherosclerotic Peripheral Vascular Disease and Quality of Care Outcomes in Research Interdisciplinary Working Groups: the American Academy of Neurology affirms the value of this guideline as an educational tool for neurologists. *Stroke*. 2007;38:1655–711.
3. Chalela JA, Kidwell CS, Nentwich LM, et al. Magnetic resonance imaging and computed tomography in emergency assessment of patients with suspected acute stroke: a prospective comparison. *Lancet*. 2007;369:293–8.

See Also (Topic, Algorithm, Electronic Media Element)
Stroke Rehabilitation, Transient Ischemic Attack
Algorithm: Stroke

CODES

ICD9
- 430 Subarachnoid hemorrhage
- 431 Intracerebral hemorrhage
- 434.91 Cerebral artery occlusion, unspecified with cerebral infarction

CLINICAL PEARLS
- Unless stroke is hemorrhagic or patient is undergoing thrombolysis, BP should not be lowered acutely to maintain perfusion of penumbric region.
- DW-MRI is more sensitive than conventional CT for acute ischemic stroke (3), however multimodal CT is equivalent to MRI. MRI is also better than CT for diagnosis of posterior fossa lesions.

SUBARACHNOID HEMORRHAGE

Abir O. Kanaan, PharmD, RPh
Kristin A. Tuiskula, PharmD
George Abraham, MD, MPH, FACP

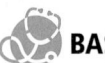 **BASICS**

1 in every 20 strokes is caused by subarachnoid hemorrhage from intracranial aneurysm. The disease often strikes at a young age and is often fatal.

DESCRIPTION
- Extravasation of blood into the subarachnoid space, particularly of the basal cisterns, and into CSF pathways, including the ventricles
- Accounts for 2–5% of new strokes
- Traumatic: Most common cause; related to head trauma
- Spontaneous: Less common; however, 85% of these are due to ruptured intracranial saccular aneurysms, and they have a worse prognosis than nonaneurysmal bleeds, which account for roughly 10% of spontaneous subarachnoid hemorrhages (SAHs).
- Also may occur from rupture of arteriovenous malformations (AVMs)
- System(s) affected: Nervous; Cardiovascular; Pulmonary

Pregnancy Considerations
Increased BP and blood volume may predispose pregnant women to hemorrhages.

EPIDEMIOLOGY
Incidence
- Spontaneous: Aggregate worldwide incidence is 10.5/100,000 person-years; 20/100,000 in Finland and Japan
- 1/100 ED patients presenting with headache has SAH.
- Although incidence increases with age, mean age of presentation is 55 years.
- Predominant age: Most occur in 4th–7th decades.
- SAHs due to AVMs occur in 2nd–4th decades.
- Predominant sex: Female > Male (1.6:1)
- Blacks > whites (2.1:1)

Prevalence
In the US: 21,000–33,000 new cases each year

RISK FACTORS
- Cigarette smoking
- Cocaine abuse
- Excessive alcohol intake
- Hypertension (HTN) is associated with rupture of aneurysms but not with saccular aneurysms.
- 1st-degree relatives with SAH
- AVMs

Genetics
Heritable connective tissue disorders:
- Polycystic kidney disease
- Fibromuscular dysplasia
- Pseudoxanthoma elasticum

GENERAL PREVENTION
- Incidentally identified aneurysms have risk of hemorrhage according to size and location; therefore, endovascular coiling or surgical clipping may be indicated, depending upon surgical risk.
- The 5-year cumulative rate of aneurysmal rupture in the internal carotid artery, anterior cerebral artery, middle cerebral artery, or anterior communicating artery is based on size:
  - <7 mm: 0%
  - 7–12 mm: 2.6%
  - 13–24 mm: 14.5%
  - >25 mm: 40%
- The 5-year cumulative rate of aneurysmal rupture in the posterior circulating and posterior communicating arteries is based on size:
  - <7 mm: 2.5%
  - 7–12 mm: 14.5%
  - 13–24 mm: 18.4%
  - >25 mm: 50% (1)
- In younger age groups, incidentally found AVMs have a 2% risk of rupture per year.

ETIOLOGY
- Trauma
- Intracranial saccular aneurysm
- Intracranial AVM
- HTN
- Rarely, tumors and blood dyscrasias

COMMONLY ASSOCIATED CONDITIONS
- Morbidity and mortality of SAH are determined by complications that develop after the initial bleed.
- Outcome predicted by the World Federation of Neurological Surgeons clinical grading: Based on sum score of Glasgow Coma Scale (GCS) and presence of focal neurologic signs
- Blood volume on initial CT scan is predictive of vasospasm.
- The following complications are common:
  - Cerebral vasospasm occurs within 4–12 days of initial bleed and is seen angiographically in 67%.
  - Cardiac arrhythmias occur in 35% of patients.
  - Seizures occur in up to 33% of patients.
  - Electrolyte disturbances (including syndrome of inappropriate antidiuretic hormone [SIADH] and cerebral salt wasting) occur in 28% of patients.
  - Pulmonary edema occurs in 23% of patients.
  - Hydrocephalus occurs in 20% of patients.
  - Rebleeding occurs in 7% of patients and has a 50% risk of permanent neurologic damage.

DIAGNOSIS

HISTORY
- Assess for recent head trauma, HTN, nicotine/EtOH/cocaine use, AVMs, family history of SAH, and current use of anticoagulants.
- Abrupt onset of headache ("worst headache of life") associated with stiff neck, nausea, vomiting, photophobia, and/or loss of consciousness
- Headache may be the only presenting symptom in up to 40% of patients and may disappear within hours (so-called thunderclap headaches, sentinel bleeds, or warning leaks).
- Seizures at onset of hemorrhage occur in 1/14 patients.

PHYSICAL EXAM
- Retinal hemorrhages
- Meningismus
- Diminished consciousness; calculate GCS on all patients.
- Focal neurologic signs, such as 3rd-nerve palsy (posterior communicating artery aneurysm), 6th-nerve palsy (increased intracranial pressure [ICP]), bilateral leg weakness and/or abulia (anterior communicating artery aneurysm), hemiparesis and/or aphasia and/or visuospatial neglect (MCA aneurysm)
- Perform lumbar puncture if CT scan is negative and suspicion is high. Elevated opening pressure, xanthochromia (takes 12 hours to develop), or red blood cells unchanged in tubes 1–4 are consistent with SAH.

DIAGNOSTIC TESTS & INTERPRETATION
Imaging
- Noncontrast-enhanced head CT scan with thin cuts through the base of the brain; sensitivity drops to 50% at 7 days but is 100% at 12 hours and 93% at 24 hours.
- CT scan may show hydrocephalus, cerebral edema, and intraparenchymal bleeds and can predict the site of rupture (particularly in the anterior circulation).
- CT scan is the most reliable predictor of vasospasm and poor outcome using the Fisher scale.
- CT scan can rule out mass effect to safely perform a necessary lumbar puncture (LP).
- If CT scan or LP are positive, check cerebral angiography (gold standard) or CT angiography; they have similar sensitivity and specificity.
- If 2nd study is negative, high-definition MRI should be performed. MRI can be used but is not the standard for surgical planning.
- Important: If no source of SAH is found intracranially, obtain spinal MRI or myelography.
- Funduscopic exam to rule in intraocular hemorrhage

Initial approach
- If prehospital, stabilize ABCs, IV, O₂ monitor
- After stabilizing patient, consider transfer to neurovascular center.
- Strict bed rest, reduced noise level, and limited visitors until source of bleeding is secured
- Do not treat BP unless mean arterial pressure (MAP) ≥130 mm Hg or if clinical or laboratory evidence of progressive end-organ damage.
- Control pain.
- Provide venous thromboembolism prophylaxis.
- Correct fluid and electrolytes.

DIFFERENTIAL DIAGNOSIS
- Traumatic SAH
- Aneurysmal rupture (including mycotic aneurysms associated with bacterial endocarditis)
- AVM
- Arterial dissection with intracranial extension
- Pituitary apoplexy

- Drug abuse (e.g., cocaine) $\pm$ aneurysm as a result of vasculitis
- Coagulopathies
- Migraine (especially with aura)

TREATMENT

MEDICATION

- Nimodipine 60 mg p.o. (via nasogastric tube if necessary) q4h × 21 days for prevention of cerebral vasospasm; start immediately (2)[A].
- The use of antifibrinolytic therapy is controversial; cerebral ischemia may occur with these agents (34)[B].
- Phenytoin 3–5 mg/kg/d p.o. or IV, valproic acid 15–45 mg/kg/d p.o. or IV, or phenobarbital 4 mg/kg IV may be used as seizure prophylaxis. These agents should be used for at least 1 week after initial bleed (5)[A].
- Treat seizures with lorazepam 0.1 mg/kg IV at a 2 mg/min rate, followed by phenytoin 20 mg/kg IV bolus at <50 mg/min up to 30 mg/kg (5).
- SIADH versus cerebral salt wasting *must* be distinguished with serum and urine electrolytes.
- Symptomatic vasospasm is currently treated with hypervolemia (central venous pressure [CVP] 8–12 mm Hg, pulmonary capillary wedge pressure 12–16 mm Hg) and/or induced hypertension (using phenylephrine, norepinephrine) (5)[A].

ADDITIONAL TREATMENT
General Measures
- Initial therapy in ICU. Treatment is directed toward preventing complications, including rebleeding, hydrocephalus, and cerebral vasospasm.
- BP is maintained within normal limits with IV labetalol and nicardipine.
- Maintain euvolemia (CVP 5–8 mm Hg) *unless* cerebral vasospasm is present (see below).
- Evaluate and treat myocardial injury and/or arrhythmias.
- Distinguish cardiogenic vs neurogenic pulmonary edema, and treat appropriately.
- Control pain with morphine sulfate 2–4 mg IV q2–4h
- Maintain serum glucose at 80–120 mg/dL with insulin sliding scale or continuous infusion.
- Maintain core body temperature ≤37.2°C. APAP 325–650 mg p.o. q4–6h and cooling devices may be used.
- Deep vein thrombosis prophylaxis with thigh-high stockings and compressive devices; *after* aneurysm is secured; subcutaneous heparin 5,000 units subcutaneously q8h; or enoxaparin 40 mg subcutaneously q24h
- GI prophylaxis with ranitidine 150 mg p.o. b.i.d. (50 mg IV q8–12h) or lansoprazole 30 mg p.o. daily
- Stool softeners also may be used.

Additional Therapies
Aggressive physical, occupational, and speech therapies are recommended.

SURGERY/OTHER PROCEDURES
- Endovascular coiling and surgical clipping are options for securing aneurysms.
- Coiling appears to have better outcomes; clipping is a 2nd choice for most patients.
- Rebleeding should be dealt with immediately by treatment of aneurysm.
- 25–30% of aneurysms will be multiple.

- Hydrocephalus should be treated with external ventricular drain, lumbar drain, or permanent CSF drainage.
- AVMs may be obliterated with embolization and surgery.

IN-PATIENT CONSIDERATIONS
Initial Stabilization
Stabilize ABCs, IV, O_2 monitor

IV Fluids
Give at least 3 L/d of 0.9% isotonic saline.

Nursing
Continuous observation (focal deficits, temperature, ECG, GCS)

ONGOING CARE

FOLLOW-UP RECOMMENDATIONS
Perform neuropsychological testing before discharge and schedule cognitive rehabilitation.

Patient Monitoring
As needed

DIET
- If intact cough and swallowing reflexes, give p.o. diet; otherwise, diet should be advanced via a nasogastric tube.
- Parenteral nutrition should be used only when oral route is not feasible.

PROGNOSIS
- Average case-fatality rate is 50% overall: 10% before receiving care, 25% within the 1st 24 hours
- 25–30% of patients die from spontaneous SAH caused by aneurysm; highest morbidity secondary to cerebral vasospasm
- If aneurysm can be obliterated successfully and vasospasm treated effectively, satisfactory outcome occurs in 50–65% of patients.
- 46% of survivors report long-term cognitive impairment of varying degrees.
- 50–75% of survivors return to work after 1 year.
- 80% remain disabled after a rebleed.

COMPLICATIONS
- Temporary and permanent neurologic deficits and/or disorders (e.g., seizures [1/14 patients], headache, SIADH)
- Psychosocial dysfunction (60%)
- Death
- Systemic complications:
  – Fever
  – Anemia
  – Cardiac failure and arrhythmias
  – Pulmonary edema

REFERENCES
1. Jabbour PM, Tjoumakaris SI, Rosenwasser RH, et al. Endovascular management of intracranial aneurysms. *Neurosurg Clin N Am.* 2009;20: 383–98.
2. Rinkel GJE, et al. Calcium antagonists for aneurysmal subarachnoid haemorrhage. *Cochrane Database Sys Rev.* 2007;3:CD000277.
3. Roos YBWEM, et al. Antifibrinolytic therapy for aneurysmal subarachnoid haemorrhage. *Cochrane Database Sys Rev.* 2004;1:CD001245.
4. Chwajol M, Starke RM, Kim GH, et al. Antifibrinolytic therapy to prevent early rebleeding after subarachnoid hemorrhage. *Neurocrit Care.* 2008;8:418–26.
5. Suarez JI, Tarr RW, Selman WR. Aneurysmal subarachnoid hemorrhage. *N Engl J Med.* 2006;354:387–96.

ADDITIONAL READING
- Bleck TP. Intensive insulin therapy reduced the incidence of neurologic complications in critically ill patients. *ACP J Club.* 2006;144:20.
- Rinkel GJE, et al. Circulatory volume expansion therapy for aneurysmal subarachnoid haemorrhage. *Cochrane Database Sys Rev.* 2004;2:CD000483.
- van der Schaaf I, et al. Endovascular coiling versus neurosurgical clipping for patients with aneurysmal subarachnoid haemorrhage. *Cochrane Database Sys Rev.* 2005;4:CD003085.
- van Gijn J, Kerr RS, Rinkel GJ. Subarachnoid haemorrhage. *Lancet.* 2007;369:306–18.
- Whitfield PC, et al. Timing of surgery for aneurysmal subarachnoid haemorrhage. *Cochrane Database Sys Rev.* 2001;2:CD001697.
- Wijdicks EF. Induced hypothermia in neurocatastrophes: feeling the chill. *Rev Neurol Dis.* 2004;1:10–5.

CODES

ICD9
- 430 Subarachnoid hemorrhage
- 852.00 Subarachnoid hemorrhage following injury, without mention of open intracranial wound, with state of consciousness unspecified

CLINICAL PEARLS
- All antiplatelet and anticoagulant therapies should be discontinued.
- Start nimodipine 60 mg p.o. q4h × 21 days.
- Headache may be the only symptom in 40% of patients with SAH and may disappear within hours.
- 1/100 ED patients presenting with headache has a SAH.
- Almost 1/3 of aneurysms are multiple.

SUBCLAVIAN STEAL SYNDROME

Alfonso J. Tafur, MD
Luis Idrovo Freire, MD

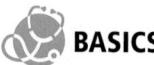 **BASICS**

DESCRIPTION
- A condition that results from stenosis or occlusion of the subclavian artery proximal to the origin of the vertebral artery; blood is drawn from the contralateral vertebral basilar or carotid artery regions into the low-pressure ipsilateral upper limb vessels, "stealing" the blood flow from the circle of Willis.
- The term was reported for the first time by Fisher in 1961. It is a normal pattern of collateral response to proximal subclavian artery occlusion.

EPIDEMIOLOGY
Incidence
- Predominant age:
  - Age >55 years—atherosclerotic etiology
  - Age <30 years—90% of patients with Takayasu arteritis
- Predominant sex: Male > Female

Prevalence
- 6% of the patients with asymptomatic carotid bruit
- Hemodynamically significant left subclavian artery stenosis is present in ~ 2.5% of patients undergoing coronary revascularization (1).

RISK FACTORS
- Smoking
- Hypertension
- Diabetes
- Hyperlipidemia
- Radiotherapy

PATHOPHYSIOLOGY
- With a left subclavian occlusion, maintenance of blood flow to the left arm occurs with reversal of flow from the basilar artery via the left vertebral artery.
- Symptoms are associated with the degree and location of a second extracranial vessel occlusion.

ETIOLOGY
- Arteriosclerosis obliterans of the proximal subclavian artery in 95% of cases
- Lesions are 3:1 more common on the left side.
- Less common causes of obstruction:
  - Dissecting aneurysm of aortic arch
  - Trauma
  - Embolus
  - Radiotherapy induced
  - Takayasu arteritis
  - May happen after Blalock-Taussig procedure for tetralogy of Fallot

COMMONLY ASSOCIATED CONDITIONS
- Disease of another extracranial vessel supplying the brain is a prerequisite for the development of the syndrome.
- Carotid artery disease
- Coronary artery disease is present in 30–60% of patients.
- Arteriosclerosis

Geriatric Considerations
- Older patients are more likely to have arteriosclerosis.

 DIAGNOSIS

- Symptoms of vertebrobasilar ischemia: Dizziness, diplopia, dysarthria, dysphagia, ataxia, gait disturbances, numbness, nystagmus
- Arm symptoms include claudication following minimal exercise, rest pain, ulcers, and digital necrosis.
- Reduced blood pressure of >20 mm Hg in involved arm
- Symptoms should be reproducible by exercising the arm.
- A variation of the syndrome is the coronary–subclavian steal syndrome, which can only occur after coronary artery bypass grafting (CABG); may present with symptoms of cardiac ischemia.

HISTORY
- Transient ischemic attacks (usually of the vertebrobasilar territory) often precipitated by exercise or work of the involved upper extremity
- Classified as asymptomatic, oligosymptomatic (only neurologic symptoms or upper limb ischemia is present), or complete (both symptoms)

PHYSICAL EXAM
- Absent or diminished pulses in ipsilateral arm:
  - Compare carotid, subclavian, brachial, radial, and ulnar pulses.
  - Using a handheld continuous wave Doppler, a monophasic or reduced biphasic pulse may be heard distal to the lesion.
- A brachial systolic pressure difference of >15 mm Hg is >90% specific for subclavian stenosis (only ~50% sensitive).
- Auscultation of carotid and suprascapular bruits
- On physical exam, we can subdivide subclavian stenosis as moderate (difference >15 and <25 mm Hg) or severe (difference >25 mm Hg). This correlates with long-term prognosis (2).
- Compression–decompression test (hyperemia test): Inflate a blood pressure cuff above the systolic blood pressure for 3 minutes. Vertebrobasilar symptoms may be reproduced by rapid decompression.
- Perform Allen's test bilaterally.

DIAGNOSTIC TESTS & INTERPRETATION
Lab
- No lab findings are pathognomonic for subclavian steal syndrome.
- Noninvasive measurement of blood pressure in upper extremities
- Pulse volume recording of upper extremities
- If Takayasu arteritis is suspected:
  - Erythrocyte sedimentation rate (elevated)
  - Complete blood count (thrombocytosis)
  - ECG (ischemic pattern)
  - CXR (widening of thoracic aorta)

Imaging
- Duplex scanning of extracranial vessels
- Magnetic resonance angiography
- Arteriogram of arch vessels with delayed films of vertebral arteries

Diagnostic Procedures/Surgery
- Arteriography
- Doppler ultrasound may be used as screening test.
- According to the hemodynamics, there are 4 subtypes:
  - Vertebrovertebral
  - Carotid–basilar
  - External carotid–vertebral
  - Carotid–subclavian (can only occur on the right side with brachiocephalic occlusion proximal to the origin of the carotid artery)

DIFFERENTIAL DIAGNOSIS

- Vascular: Intracranial vascular disease, carotid artery disease, vertebral artery disease
- Neurogenic: Brain tumor, seizures, subdural hematoma
- Cardiac arrhythmias

 TREATMENT

ADDITIONAL TREATMENT

General Measures
Reduce cholesterol levels, if appropriate, using diet or medication.

Issues for Referral
- In symptomatic patients, consider consulting vascular medicine and cardiovascular surgery.
- Potential indications for subclavian artery intervention include:
  – Vertebrobasilar ischemia
  – Upper limb ischemia
  – Hand claudication and digital embolization
  – Angina in a patient with a LIMA graft
  – Leg claudication in patient with axilo-femoral graft
  – Subclavian artery repair pre TEVAR (thoracic endovascular aortic repair). Controversial (3).

SURGERY/OTHER PROCEDURES
Treatment options include:

- Balloon angioplasty: Stent insertion increases long-term patency rates (4)[B]:
  – The 8–10 year primary patency is 83–95% (5).
  – Complications occur in up to 10% of the cases and include:
    ○ Femoral pseudo aneurysm
    ○ Embolic stroke
    ○ Distal embolism
- Carotid–subclavian bypass
- Carotid–subclavian transposition:
  – To be considered if there is distal embolization from the subclavian artery lesion
  – The reported patency is 100% at 10 years compared with 74% for carotid bypass.
- Axilloaxillary bypass: 12-year graft occlusion of 10% and 0.4% periprocedural mortality
- Carotid endarterectomy
- Subclavian arterectomy

IN-PATIENT CONSIDERATIONS
Aggressive management of cardiovascular risk factors

Initial Stabilization
Outpatient care unless vascular surgery is anticipated

Admission Criteria
Stroke, critical limb ischemia

 ONGOING CARE

FOLLOW-UP RECOMMENDATIONS
Frequent neurologic review of systems and subclavian Doppler ultrasound for patients who become symptomatic or have a blood pressure difference of >20 mm Hg between arm

Patient Monitoring
Annual physical examination including blood pressure reading in both arms

DIET
Low-cholesterol diet, if appropriate

PATIENT EDUCATION
- Prevent injury to arm.
- Reduce exercise of arm.

PROGNOSIS
- The presence of subclavian stenosis recently has been defined as an independent risk factor for cardiovascular death (2).
- After angioplasty of the subclavian artery, younger age and stenting are independent predictors of restenosis-free survival (4).

COMPLICATIONS
Completed stroke

REFERENCES

1. Hwang HY, Kim JH, Lee W, et al. Left subclavian artery stenosis in coronary artery bypass: prevalence and revascularization strategies. *Ann Thorac Surg.* 2010;89:1146–50.
2. Aboyans V, Criqui MH, McDermott MM, et al. The vital prognosis of subclavian stenosis. *J Am Coll Cardiol.* 2007;49:1540–5.
3. Kotelis D, Geisbüsch P, Hinz U, et al. Short and midterm results after left subclavian artery coverage during endovascular repair of the thoracic aorta. *J Vasc Surg.* 2009;50:1285–92.
4. Sixt S, Rastan A, Schwarzwälder U, et al. Long term outcome after balloon angioplasty and stenting of subclavian artery obstruction: A single centre experience. *Vasa.* 2008;37:174–82.
5. Wang KQ, Wang ZG, Yang BZ, et al. Long-term results of endovascular therapy for proximal subclavian arterial obstructive lesions. *Chin Med J.* 2010;123:45–50.
6. Bicknell CD, Subramanian A, Wolfe JH. Coronary subclavian steal syndrome. *Eur J Vasc Endovasc Surg.* 2004;27:220–1.

 CODES

ICD9
435.2 Subclavian steal syndrome

CLINICAL PEARLS

- Takayasu arteritis/vasculitis is most common in young females. The aorta and its branches are the major vessels affected by inflammation, thrombus formation, and aneurysmal dilatation. Subclavian steal syndrome is thought to be relatively common in this disorder (6).
- The left upper extremity is affected more frequently perhaps because subclavian steal occurs when the obstruction is proximal to the origin of the vertebral artery, and this distance is shorter on the right than on the left.
- The physical findings associated with subclavian steal syndrome are lower blood pressure, decreased pulse, and bruit (supraclavicular) on the affected side.
- Subclavian artery stenosis should be detected before bypass surgery when a left internal mammary graft is planned. If present, a stenosis may present later on as coronary–subclavian steal syndrome.

SUBDURAL HEMATOMA

Ajar Kochar, MD
Daithi S. Heffernan, MD

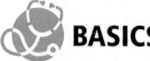 BASICS

DESCRIPTION

- Accumulation of blood in subdural space: The area between the dura and subarachnoid membranes
- Acute: Most severe, most commonly caused by acceleration or deceleration head injury, which results in tearing of bridging veins. It is often associated with parenchymal brain injury, diagnosis made by CT scan and treated with surgical intervention. Hematoma age ≤3–7 days.
- Chronic: Mostly due to trivial head injury in older patients. Good prognosis after surgical treatment, but common complication is recurrence. Hematoma age >2–3 weeks.
- Subacute: Appears due to maturation of acute hematoma. Hematoma age 4–21 days.
- Synonym(s): Subdural hemorrhage

EPIDEMIOLOGY

Predominant age: (1)

- Acute: Predominant age group 31–47
- Chronic: >50 years

Incidence

- Acute: 1–2/100,000/year; Male > Female. Acute subdural hematoma is present with 5–22% of episodes of severe head trauma .
- Chronic: <65 years: 3.4/100,000; >65 years: 8–58/100,000 (prevalence increasing with aging population)

RISK FACTORS

- Acute: Severe head trauma: Motor vehicle accidents, falls, blunt head trauma, child abuse (1)
- Chronic: Cerebral atrophy, advanced age, chronic alcoholism, dementia, falls, minor trauma, epilepsy, coagulopathy/anticoagulation therapy, anti-platelet drugs, low ICP, hemodialysis

ALERT

Cerebral atrophy predisposes to subdural hematomas.

GENERAL PREVENTION

- Acute: Trauma-prevention programs; encourage seatbelts, helmets for bicycles/motorcycles, hard hats
- Chronic: Alcoholism treatment, balance training, medical and surgical management of epilepsy, caution with use of anticoagulation therapy in at-risk populations, medium- or high-pressure ventriculoperitoneal shunt valves in at-risk patients with hydrocephalus

PATHOPHYSIOLOGY

Hematoma development: Initial trauma causes tearing of bridging veins that bleed into subdural space (between dura and subarachnoid membranes). Fibroblasts encapsulate bleed in a thin fibrin layer within 4 days. The outer membrane expands as fibroblasts continue to proliferate and migrate into hemorrhage. Phagocytes cause liquefication of the hematoma, which either slowly resolves or continues to grow into a chronic subdural hematoma. The chronic subdural hematoma may continue to grow due to recurrent bleeding. Balance between recurrent bleeding from hematoma membrane and resorption determines ultimate size of hematoma.
Acute (1)

- Tearing of bridging veins (most common cause)
- Injury to small cortical arteries (rarely)
- Low CSF pressure caused by a CSF leak.
  - Reduced buoyancy of the brain causes increase tension on bridging veins and arteries leading to tearing or rupture of these vessels
- Bleeding is usually tamponaded by compression due to increasing intracranial pressure (ICP)
- Chronic
  - >2 weeks following an acute SDH, the clot liquefies and becomes encapsulated
  - The membrane encapsulating the clot may calcify over time.

ETIOLOGY

- Acute:
  - Young adult: 56% MVA; 12% Falls
  - Elderly: 22% MVA; 56% Falls
  - Trauma from high-velocity acceleration or deceleration head injury, commonly without impact
  - Blunt trauma often leads to subdural bleeds on coup side of brain as opposed to epidural bleeds, which tend to occur on contre-coup side.
- Chronic
  - Geriatric patients: Trivial head injury
  - Children: May be caused by unrecognized/unreported trauma, abuse, or rarely birth trauma

COMMONLY ASSOCIATED CONDITIONS

- Acute: Associated intracranial and extracranial injuries (1)
  - Brain contusion, subarachnoid hemorrhage (most common associated injuries), epidural hematoma, diffuse axonal injury
  - Multisystem trauma; facial fractures; extremity fractures; cervical spine injury; injury to the thoracic, lumbar, or sacral spine; thoracic and abdominal trauma; disseminated intravascular coagulopathy (DIC)
- Chronic: Subdural hygroma (extracranial collection of CSF), epilepsy, coagulopathy, CSF shunt, birth trauma, child abuse, metastatic carcinoma (rarely)

DIAGNOSIS

HISTORY

- Acute:
  - Assess for risk factors: head trauma, anticoagulation medications, falls
  - Loss of consciousness; lucid interval 12–38%
  - Headache, nausea, vomiting, nuchal rigidity, ataxia
- Chronic: Most commonly occur in elderly after minor trauma. Symptoms onset: Weeks to months 30–50% have no history of trauma. Progressive symptoms of headache, confusion, lightheadedness, personality changes (apathy). Alcoholics frequently present with acute on chronic SDHs owing to frequent trauma and coagulopathies associated with chronic alcohol abuse.

PHYSICAL EXAM

- Acute:
  - GCS <8 (comatose): 37–80%; altered level of consciousness: 99%
  - Pupillary irregularity (usually ipsilateral to hematoma): 47–53%; hemiparesis (usually contralateral to hematoma): 34–47%
  - Decerebrate posturing or flaccid motor exam: 47%; papilledema: 16%; cranial nerve VI palsy: 5%
- Chronic:
  - Altered mental status: 50–70% in elderly: Confusion, delirium, psychiatric manifestations, coma
  - Hemiparesis: 45–58% Onset is often insidious and gradually progressive. Most commonly contra-lateral
  - Headache: Less common in elderly
  - Falls may be a presenting symptom
  - Papilledema: 24%; cranial nerve III abnormality: 11%; hemianopsia: 7%
  - Seizure: Most commonly in patients with large hematomas and focal neurological deficits
  - Atypical presentations: Parkinsonism, vertigo, nystagmus, Gerstmann syndrome
  - Infants: Accelerated increase in head size with or without irritability, poor feeding, occasional vomiting, tension of anterior fontanelle, seizures

DIAGNOSTIC TESTS & INTERPRETATION

Consider EEG for seizures (patients may have nonconvulsive seizures).

Lab

- Complete blood count, electrolytes, glucose, coagulation parameters: PT, PTT, INR
- Blood alcohol level, urine toxicology screen, anticonvulsant levels (may be subtherapeutic in epilepsy patients)

Follow-Up & Special Considerations

Patients with elevated PT or PTT should have their coagulopathy reversed in the setting of an acute hemorrhage.

Imaging

- CT scan (without contrast) is test of choice because of shorter examination time. Acute subdural hematoma: Hyperdense extra-axial crescent-shaped collection. Subacute: Iso-dense lesion (difficult to identify, may require MRI for elucidation). Chronic: Hypo-dense lesion (usually takes 3 weeks to evolve). Bilateral chronic SDH: Medial compression of ventricles, narrow slit-like ventricle termed "squeezed ventricle"
- MRI more sensitive than CT head scan. Aids in diagnosis of hematomas isodense with brain due to mixture of chronic hematoma with recurrent hemorrhage. Helpful in diagnosing lesions located in base of skull, posterior fossa and vertex as CT scan emits large shadow effect

Pathological Findings

- Acute: Fresh hemorrhage
- Chronic: Liquefied hematoma; outer membrane beneath dura after 1 week; inner membrane between hematoma and arachnoid after 3 weeks. On rare occasions, cytology examination may reveal association between metastatic carcinoma cells and hemorrhage.

DIFFERENTIAL DIAGNOSIS

Subdural hygroma (extra-cranial collection of CSF), other intracranial or extracranial injuries, epidural hematoma, cerebral contusion, dementia, stroke/TIA, brain tumor, subdural empyema, meningitis

ALERT

The insidious onset of symptoms in SDH may lead to misdiagnosis of dementia, tumor, or depression.

 TREATMENT

MEDICATION
- Acute:
  - Management of cerebral edema and elevated ICP
    - Mannitol 20% solution 0.5–1.0 g/kg, followed by 0.25–0.75 g/kg q4–6h
    - Loop diuretic can be used to augment Mannitol's effect. Administer furosemide (Lasix) 0.5 mg/kg IV.
    - Hypertensive saline: 7.2% NaCl/HES 200/0.5 solution at 1.4 ml/kg. May be more effective than mannitol at reducing ICP and improving cerebral blood flow. Risk of central pontine hyalinosis, exclude hyponatremia prior to administration.
    - Check serum osmolality every 8 hours and serum electrolytes at least daily.
  - Seizure prophylaxis
    - Reduces seizures in 1st week postinjury. Avoid status epilepticus (high fatality in this population). Avoid exacerbation of systemic injuries by convulsions. Prophylaxis does not prevent future development of epilepsy.
    - Phenytoin (Dilantin) 1,000 mg load (50 mg/min IV) with ECG monitoring, followed by 100 mg IV q8h or as needed to maintain therapeutic blood levels (10–20 μg/mL [40–79 μmol/L]).
    - Convert IV Dilantin to p.o. rapidly to avoid cardiovascular complications of IV Dilantin (hypotension, bradycardia, arrhythmia).
- Chronic:
  - Medical management alone for large SDHs or in patients with significant neurologic signs is frequently unsuccessful and entails risks of neurologic deterioration.
  - Seizure prophylaxis is currently not recommended (2).
  - Small hematomas that are asymptomatic or mildly symptomatic (e.g., headache), may be appropriate to treat conservatively with observation because some chronic subdural hematomas have been known to resolve spontaneously.
    - Steroids may be helpful for symptomatic treatment in these patients, if not otherwise contraindicated.

ADDITIONAL TREATMENT
General Measures
- Acute (medical management):
  - Maintenance of adequate airway and ventilation and support of cardiovascular system to promote normal cerebral perfusion. Goals: PaO2 >60 mm HG (3) and SBP >90 mm Hg (3)
  - ICP management
    - Monitor ICP in all patients with GCS <8 (3)[B]. Target: ICP <20 mm Hg (3)[B]
    - Ventriculostomy with external gauge transducer is most accurate and cost-effective method of monitoring ICP.
    - Elevate head of bed to reduce ICP promoting venous outflow from head.
    - AVOID hyperventilation in first 24 hours postinjury (3) (may reduce ICP, but induces secondary cerebral ischemia)
    - Cerebral perfusion pressure (CPP): CPP = mean arterial pressure (MAP) – ICP. Target CPP = 60 mm Hg (3)[B]. Avoid CPP >70 mm Hg due to risk of adult respiratory distress syndrome (ARDS), and avoid CPP <50 mm Hg, risk of cerebral ischemia
  - Treat multisystem injuries. Spine precautions: As appropriate to injury until spine injury ruled out

SURGERY/OTHER PROCEDURES
- Acute: Emergent craniotomy is often treatment of choice (1). Other surgeries: Burr hole trephination, decompressive craniectomy, large decompressive hemi-craniectomy. Choice of surgery mostly dependent on neurosurgeon's preference
- Indications for surgery:
  - Hematoma thickness >10 mm or midline shift >5 mm by CT (1)[C]
  - Coma patient (GCS <9) even if thickness <10 mm or shift <5 mm if: Decrease in GCS score >2 points since admission; asymmetric pupils or fixed and dilated pupils, ICP >20 mm Hg
  - Timing of intervention: Surgery should be performed within 2–4 hours after clinical deterioration (1).
  - Other factors influencing decision to perform surgery: History (age, comorbidities, neurological deterioration), physical exam, GCS, ICP
- Subacute:
  - If patient is neurologically stable, surgery may be delayed until hematoma matures and becomes chronic, at which time a burr-hole drainage can be performed.
  - In setting of mass effect, neurologic deficit, and solid (nonliquefied) clot; SDH may require craniotomy for complete evacuation.
- Chronic: (4)
  - Patients with small subdural hematomas may not require surgery.
  - Several techniques available: Burr-hole drainage (2 approaches) with bedside twist drill vs operation with burr holes and irrigation: Both effective in a prospective, randomized trial and a prospective, nonrandomized series (4)[C]

IN-PATIENT CONSIDERATIONS
IV Fluids
Normal saline with 20 mEq/L KCl as needed; refrain from using hypotonic fluids or fluids with glucose.

 ONGOING CARE

FOLLOW-UP RECOMMENDATIONS
Patient Monitoring
- Patients with chronic subdural hematomas should have a follow-up CT scan 1–2 months after surgery to confirm interval improvement.
- Patients requiring anticoagulation should resume this medical treatment when risk of hemorrhage is low; this decision is made on an individualized patient basis.

DIET
- Acute: Most patients require enteral or total parenteral nutrition initially if decreased mental status. Patients should be fed to full caloric replacement by day 7 postinjury (3)[C] .
- Chronic: Depending on the level of consciousness, patients usually can have the diet advanced to regular food as tolerated.

PROGNOSIS
Outcome is highly dependent on presurgical neurologic status:
- Acute: Mortality: Requiring surgery: 40–60%; Comatose at presentation: 57–68% (1)
- Chronic: Mortality 15.6%. Postsurgical intervention, mortality is 6.5%. Most predictive prognostic indicator: Neurological status on admission

COMPLICATIONS
- Postoperative complications: (14,) New or recurrent hematoma; elevated ICP and cerebral edema; cortical injury secondary to drill procedures; infection (subdural empyema, meningitis); tension pneumocephalus (air trapped in cranial cavity causing a midline shift); seizures (in 11–33% of patients). There is benefit of seizure prophylaxis in the period immediately after acute head trauma (7 days); no proven benefit for long-term seizure prophylaxis.
- Chronic: Recurrent SDH in up to 50% of patients (reduced with use of drainage catheter): 9.2–26.5%. Delirium, intracranial hemorrhage (rare), subdural hygroma, seizures in up to 10% of patients

REFERENCES

1. Bullock MR, Chesnut R, Ghajar J, et al. Surgical management of acute subdural hematomas. *Neurosurgery.* 2006;58.
2. Ratilal B, Costa J, Sampaio C, et al. Anticonvulsants for preventing seizures in patients with chronic subdural haematoma. *Cochrane Database Syst Rev.* 2005;CD004893.
3. Brain Trauma Foundation, American Association of Neurological Surgeons, Congress of Neurological Surgeons et al. Guidelines for the management of severe traumatic brain injury. *J Neurotrauma.* 2007;24(Suppl 1):S1–106.
4. Muzii VF, Bistazzoni S, Zalaffi A, et al. Chronic subdural hematoma: comparison of two surgical techniques. Preliminary results of a prospective randomized study. *J Neurosurg Sci.* 2005;49:41–6; discussion 46–7.

 CODES

ICD9
852.20 Subdural hemorrhage following injury, without mention of open intracranial wound, with state of consciousness unspecified

CLINICAL PEARLS
- Consider chronic subdural in an elderly patient with progressive symptoms of headache, personality changes, and/or functional decline.
- Non-contrast-enhanced CT scan is test of choice for acute SDH demonstrating a hyperdense crescent-shaped extra-axial lesion.
- Recurrence is a common complication in chronic subdural hematomas.

S

SUBPHRENIC ABSCESS

Jochebed A. Pink, MD
Richard H. Glew, MD

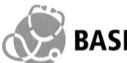 **BASICS**

- Subphrenic abscess is a location-specific intraabdominal abscess, also referred to as a complicated abdominal infection.
- Synonyms: Sub- or infradiaphragmatic abscess

DESCRIPTION
A localized, fibrous, encapsulated collection of pus directly under the diaphragm.

EPIDEMIOLOGY
Incidence
The incidence of subphrenic abscess is not well known. Overall, intra-abdominal abscess formation after abdominal surgery occurs in 1–2% of cases; however, the risk increases to 10–30% in cases with preoperative perforation of a hollow viscus, significant fecal contamination of the peritoneal cavity, bowel ischemia, immunosuppression, or delayed diagnosis and treatment of peritonitis.

RISK FACTORS
- Abdominal surgery, especially with inadvertent viscus perforation
- Anastomotic leak
- Peptic ulcer perforation
- Ruptured appendicitis
- Perforated diverticulitis
- Mesenteric ischemia with bowel infarction
- Abdominal trauma, especially penetrating
- Foreign body ingestion with viscus perforation

PATHOPHYSIOLOGY
- Subphrenic abscess typically forms when contents of the gastrointestinal tract are released into the sterile peritoneal cavity. When a patient is supine, bacteria may traverse the paracolic gutters into the right subdiaphragmatic area leading to abscess formation in a location proximate or remote to its origin. Structures in the left upper quadrant (spleen, ligaments) tend to protect the left subphrenic space from remote soiling, and infections in this region are uncommon, usually arising from gastric perforation or from transdiaphragmatic spread from the left chest.
- Pattern recognition receptors on local macrophages are stimulated by the presence of bacteria and foreign material, leading to the release of cytokines, promoting an influx of polymorphonuclear leukocytes, monocytes, and ultimately sequestration of the pathogens within an abscess. Microorganisms may also be sequestered on a macroscopic scale involving fibrin and other adhesive molecules adhering to mesentery, the abdominal wall, omentum, and loops of bowel (1).

ETIOLOGY
- Subphrenic abscess typically is a polymicrobial infection due to gastrointestinal tract flora, consisting of aerobic and anaerobic bacteria. The most prevalent microorganisms include aerobic enteric gram-negative bacilli and gram-positive cocci, and anaerobes. Below is a table of commonly isolated pathogens (1).

Enteric gram-negative bacilli	Escherichia coli, Klebsiella spp., Enterobacter spp., Pseudomonas aeruginosa
Gram-positive cocci	Streptococcus spp., Enterococcus spp.
Obligate anaerobes	Bacteroides fragilis and other members of the Bacteroides group

- The microbiology of the infection is affected by exposure to the health care setting and prior antibiotic treatment, which can select for multidrug-resistant organisms (1). Consequently, isolates in health care–associated cases are different than in community-acquired cases, with Enterobacter spp., Pseudomonas aeruginosa, and Enterococcus spp. isolated more frequently than E. coli (1).

COMMONLY ASSOCIATED CONDITIONS
- Bacteremia
- Sepsis
- Multisystem organ failure
- Pleural effusion
- Fistula formation

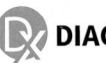 **DIAGNOSIS**

Early diagnosis is critical to reducing morbidity and mortality.

HISTORY
- Recent history of abdominal surgery, usually from weeks to months earlier, occasionally more remotely (2)
- Constitutional symptoms: Fever, chills, diaphoresis, malaise
- Pain symptoms: Chest, shoulder (referred pain to the scapular area), and/or abdominal pain
  - Pain in respective upper quadrant, but may be pleuritic
- Respiratory symptoms: Nonproductive cough, dyspnea
- GI symptoms: Nausea, hiccups, vomiting, adynamic ileus

PHYSICAL EXAM
- Fever, tachycardia, hypotension
- Rales at lung base
- Dullness to percussion at lung base
- Decreased breath sounds at lung base
- Subcostal, costal, and/or abdominal tenderness
- Pseudo-organomegaly, secondary to palpable mass lesion

DIAGNOSTIC TESTS & INTERPRETATION
Lab
- Complete blood count: Leukocytosis, often with left shift; anemia
- Blood cultures: Positive in no more than 50% of cases, but may guide selection and duration of antibiotic therapy (B-III) (3).
- Cultures of aspirate: Fluid should be sent to laboratory for Gram stain and culture.

Follow-Up & Special Considerations
- After broad-spectrum antibiotic therapy has been initiated and drainage established, the patient can be expected to defervesce within 24–48 hours. If the patient fails to improve clinically, follow-up CT scan is indicated.
- Monitor vital signs and metabolic function to detect septic shock.
  - Basic metabolic panel
  - Liver chemistries

Imaging
- Abdominal radiograph maybe done initially. Findings may include elevation of the hemidiaphragm, subphrenic air-fluid level.
- CT scan of the abdomen, pelvis, and lower chest with contrast is the most appropriate imaging study in a patient who may have an intra-abdominal abscess (4).

DIFFERENTIAL DIAGNOSIS
- Liver abscess
- Subhepatic abscess
- Lesser sac abscess
- Splenic abscess
- Empyema

TREATMENT

- Consists of three modalities:
  - Source control (percutaneous or surgical drainage of the abscess)
  - Broad-spectrum antibiotics
  - Aggressive fluid resuscitation.

MEDICATION

- Broad-spectrum antibiotics:
  - Begin antimicrobial therapy as soon as subphrenic abscess is considered likely or confirmed and immediately in patients with septic shock (A-III) (3).
  - Adequate antimicrobial drug dosing should be maintained (A-I) (3).
  - More than 1 agent is generally required to provide adequate coverage for suspected organisms (5).
- Empiric treatment for intra-abdominal infection of mild to moderate severity that is not related to health care (without severe physiologic derangement, advanced age, or immunocompromised state) (A-I) (3):

Single agent	Ertapenem, piperacillin-tazobactam, or tigecycline
Combination therapy 5	Ceftriaxone, cefotaxime, ciprofloxacin, or levofloxacin, each in combination with metronidazole

- Empiric treatment for complicated, high-risk intra-abdominal infection not related to health care or in patients with severe physiologic derangement, advanced age, or immunocompromised state (A-1) (3):

Single agent	Imipenem-cilastatin, meropenem, doripenem, or piperacillin-tazobactam
Combination therapy 5	Cefepime, ceftazidime, ciprofloxacin, or levofloxacin, each in combination with metronidazole

- As described above, the microbiology in patients with prior hospital exposure may be altered and warrant coverage for multidrug-resistant organisms (1). Empiric antibiotic therapy for health care–associated intra-abdominal infection should be guided by local microbiologic results (A-II) (3) and later tailored based on culture results (B-III) (3).

- Duration of antimicrobial therapy of an established complicated intra-abdominal infection should be 4–7 days, after adequate drainage and patient has defervesced, longer if it is difficult to obtain adequate source control (B-III) (3).

ADDITIONAL TREATMENT
General Measures
Intravenous fluid hydration

- Patients with signs of intravascular volume depletion should have rapid restoration of fluid status (A-II) (3).
- Administer intravenous fluids to euvolemic patients without evidence of volume depletion when diagnosis of intra-abdominal abscess is first suspected. (B-III) (3)

SURGERY/OTHER PROCEDURES
- Percutaneous drainage is the treatment of choice for patients without an acute abdomen (B-II) (3).
- General surgery consult should be obtained in virtually all cases of suspected intra-abdominal abscess and may be especially valuable in cases of recurrence or multiple subphrenic abscesses deemed not amendable to percutaneous drainage.

ONGOING CARE

PROGNOSIS
- Morbidity and mortality vary depending on the comorbid conditions, severity of the patient's status, and etiology.
- Percutaneous abscess drainage is curative in >85% of cases (6).
- Recurrence rate of abscess is 1–10% (6).

COMPLICATIONS
- Bacteremia
- Sepsis
- Rupture of abscess
- Abscess recurrence
- Pleural effusion
- Risk of morbidity and mortality increases with multiple surgeries, age >50 years, and recurrent or persistent abscesses.

REFERENCES
1. Mazuski JE, Solomkin JS, et al. Intra-abdominal infections. *Surg. Clin. North Am.* 2009;89:421–37, ix
2. Tomita H, Osada S, Miya K, et al. Delayed recurrence of postoperative intra-abdominal abscess: an unusual case and review of the literature. *Surg Infect (Larchmt).* 2006;7:551–4.
3. Solomkin JS, Mazuski JE, Bradley JS, et al. Diagnosis and management of complicated intra-abdominal infection in adults and children: guidelines by the Surgical Infection Society and the Infectious Diseases Society of America. *Clin Infect Dis.* 2010;50:133–64.
4. Rosen MP, Bree RL, Foley WD, et al. *Acute abdominal pain and fever or suspected abdominal abscess.* [online publication]. Reston (VA): American College of Radiology (ACR); 2006:7 p.
5. Wong PF, Gilliam AD, Kumar S, et al. Antibiotic regimens for secondary peritonitis of gastrointestinal origin in adults. *Cochrane Database Syst Rev.* 2005;CD004539.
6. Akinci D, Akhan O, Ozmen MN, et al. Percutaneous drainage of 300 intraperitoneal abscesses with long-term follow-up. *Cardiovasc Intervent Radiol.* 744–50.

CODES

ICD9
567.22 Peritoneal abscess

CLINICAL PEARLS
- Subphrenic abscess occurs after contamination of the sterile peritoneal cavity with gastrointestinal tract bacteria.
- Proper management involves determining the cause of the infection, abscess drainage, broad-spectrum antibiotics, and intravenous fluids.

S

SUBSTANCE USE DISORDERS

S. Lindsey Clarke, MD

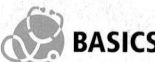 **BASICS**

DESCRIPTION
A substance use disorder manifests as any pattern of substance use causing significant physical, mental, or social dysfunction.

- Substances of abuse include
  - Alcohol
  - Amphetamines
  - Anabolic steroids
  - Barbiturates
  - Benzodiazepines
  - Cannabinoids (hashish, marijuana)
  - Club and designer drugs (mostly methamphetamine derivatives)
  - Cocaine
  - Flunitrazepam
  - Gamma-hydroxybutyrate
  - Heroin (diacetylmorphine)
  - Inhalants (gasoline, glue, paint thinners, nitrous oxide)
  - Ketamine
  - Lysergic acid diethylamide (LSD)
  - Mescaline, psilocybin (mushrooms, peyote)
  - Methadone
  - Methamphetamines
  - Methaqualone
  - Methylphenidate
  - Nicotine
  - Opium
  - Opioids (codeine, fentanyl, hydrocodone, hydromorphone, meperidine, morphine, oxycodone, propoxyphene, others)
  - Phencyclidine
- For current listing of street terms, see http://www.whitehousedrugpolicy.gov/streetterms
- System(s) affected: Cardiovascular; Endocrine/Metabolic; CNS
- Synonym(s): Drug abuse; Drug dependence; Substance abuse

Geriatric Considerations
- Alcohol is the most commonly abused substance, and abuse often goes unrecognized.
- Higher potential for drug interactions

Pregnancy Considerations
Substance abuse may cause fetal abnormalities, morbidity, and fetal or maternal death.

EPIDEMIOLOGY
Incidence
- Predominant age: 16–25 years
- Predominant sex: Male > Female.

Prevalence
- 20 million, or 8%, of Americans reported use of illicit substance in last month in 2008.
- Rates: 9.3% for ages 12–17 years; 21.5% for ages 18–20 years
- 1 in 6 males aged 18–25 years uses marijuana.

RISK FACTORS
- Male gender, young adult
- Depression, anxiety
- Other substance use disorders
- Family history
- Peer or family use or approval
- Low socioeconomic status
- Unemployment

- Accessibility of substances of abuse
- Family dysfunction or trauma
- Antisocial personality disorder
- Academic problems, school dropout
- Criminal involvement

Genetics
Substances of abuse affect dopamine, acetylcholine, gamma-aminobutyric acid, norepinephrine, opioid, and serotonin receptors. Variant alleles may account for susceptibility to disorders.

GENERAL PREVENTION
Early identification and aggressive early intervention improve outcomes.

ALERT
Screening: A single question: "How many times in the past year have you used an illegal drug or used a prescription medication for non-medical reasons?": In primary care setting, resulted in sensitivity of 100% and specificity of ~75%. (1)[B].

ETIOLOGY
Multifactorial, including genetic, environmental

ALERT
Prescription narcotic overdose is the leading cause of accidental death between ages of 35–55 in the US; this correlates with the increase in prescription of long-acting oxycodone. (http://www.cdc.gov/injury/wisqars/pdf/Unintentional_2007_BW-a.pdf)

COMMONLY ASSOCIATED CONDITIONS
- Depression
- Personality disorders
- Bipolar affective disorder

 DIAGNOSIS

- Substance abuse: A maladaptive pattern of substance use manifested by 1 or more of the following:
  - Failure to fulfill major obligations at work, school, or home
  - Recurrent use in hazardous situations
  - Recurrent substance-related legal problems
  - Continued substance use despite substance-related social or interpersonal problems
- Substance dependence: A maladaptive pattern of substance use manifested by 3 or more of the following:
  - Tolerance
  - Withdrawal
  - Using the substance more than intended
  - Persistent desire or attempts to cut down or stop
  - Much time spent obtaining, using, or recovering from the substance
  - Social, occupational, or recreational activities sacrificed for substance use
  - Continued use despite substance-related physical or psychologic problems

HISTORY
- History of infections (e.g., endocarditis, hepatitis B or C, TB, STI, or recurrent pneumonia)
- Social or behavioral problems, including chaotic relationships and/or employment
- Frequent visits to emergency department
- Criminal incarceration

- History of blackouts, insomnia, mood swings, chronic pain, repetitive trauma
- Anxiety, fatigue, depression, psychosis
- Sexual assault related to use of GBH or Rohypnol

PHYSICAL EXAM
- Abnormally dilated or constricted pupils
- Needle marks on skin
- Nasal septum perforation (with cocaine use)
- Cardiac dysrhythmias, pathologic murmurs
- Malnutrition with severe dependence

DIAGNOSTIC TESTS & INTERPRETATION
- CRAFFT questionnaire is superior to CAGE for identifying alcohol use disorders in adolescents and young adults; sensitivity is 94% with two or more "yes" answers.
  - C—Have you ever ridden in a *car* driven by someone (including yourself) who was "high" or who had been using alcohol or drugs?
  - R—Do you ever use alcohol or drugs to *relax*, feel better about yourself, or fit in?
  - A—Do you ever use alcohol or drugs while you are *alone*?
  - F—Do you ever *forget* things you did while using alcohol or drugs?
  - F—Do your family or *friends* ever tell you that you should cut down on your drinking or drug use?
  - T—Have you gotten into *trouble* while you were using alcohol or drugs?
- TICS (2-item conjoint screen): ≥1 positive response is 79% sensitive, 78% specific for current substance use disorder.
  - In the past year, have you ever drunk or used drugs more than you meant to?
  - Have you felt you wanted to cut down on your drinking or drug use in the past year?

Lab
- Blood alcohol concentration
- Urine drug screen (Order qualitative UDS and, if specific drug is in question, a quantitative analysis for specific drug; confirmatory serum tests if you suspect false positive.)
- Approximate detection limits:
  - Alcohol: 6–10 hours
  - Amphetamines and variants: 2–3 days
  - Barbiturates: 2–10 days
  - Benzodiazepines: 1–6 weeks
  - Cocaine: 2–3 days
  - Heroin: 1–1.5 days
  - LSD, psilocybin: 8 hours
  - Marijuana: 1 day–4 weeks
  - Methadone: 1 day–1 week
  - Opioids: 1–3 days
  - PCP: 7–14 days
  - Anabolic steroids: Oral, 3 weeks; injectable, 3 months; nandrolone, 9 months
- Liver transaminases
- HIV, hepatitis B and C screens

Imaging
- Echocardiogram for endocarditis
- Head CT scan for seizure, delirium, trauma

DIFFERENTIAL DIAGNOSIS
- Depression, anxiety, or other mental states
- Metabolic delirium (hypoxia, hypoglycemia, infection, thiamine deficiency, hypothyroidism, thyrotoxicosis)
- Attention deficit hyperactivity disorder
- Medication toxicity

TREATMENT

Determine substances abused early (may influence disposition).

MEDICATION

- Alcohol withdrawal: See "Alcohol Abuse and Dependence, Alcohol Withdrawal."
- Benzodiazepine or barbiturate withdrawal:
  - Gradual taper preferable to abrupt discontinuation (2)[A]
  - Substitution of longer-acting benzodiazepine or phenobarbital
- Nicotine withdrawal: See "Tobacco Use and Smoking Cessation."
- Opioid withdrawal:
  - Buprenorphine: 2–16 mg/d sublingually; use restricted to licensed clinics and certified physicians (3)[A].
  - Methadone: 20–35 mg/d PO; use restricted to inpatient settings and specially licensed clinics (4)[A].
  - Clonidine: 0.1–0.2 mg PO t.i.d. for autonomic hyperactivity (5)[A]
- Stimulant withdrawal:
  - No agent with clear benefit for cocaine
  - Naltrexone: 50 mg PO twice weekly reduces amphetamine use in dependent patients (6)[B].
  - Methylphenidate ER: 54 mg/d PO might enhance abstinence in amphetamine-dependent patients.
- Adjuncts to therapy:
  - Use all medications in conjunction with psychosocial behavioral interventions.
  - Antiemetics, nonaddictive analgesics for opioid withdrawal
  - Nonhabituating antidepressants, mood stabilizers, anxiolytics, and hypnotics for comorbid mood and anxiety disorders and insomnia that persist after detoxification
- Contraindications:
  - Buprenorphine in lactation
  - Naltrexone in pregnancy, liver disease
- Precautions: Clonidine can cause hypotension.
- Significant possible interactions:
  - Buprenorphine and ketoconazole, erythromycin, or HIV protease inhibitors
  - Naltrexone and opioid medications (may precipitate or exacerbate withdrawal)

ADDITIONAL TREATMENT

General Measures

- Motivational interviewing and brief interventions can overcome denial and promote change.
- Behavioral and cognitive therapy
- Community reinforcement
- Interventional counseling
- Nonjudgmental, medically oriented attitude
- Self-help groups to aid recovery (Alcoholics Anonymous, other 12-step programs)
- Support groups for family (Al-Anon and Alateen)
- Monitor for infections and other complications

Issues for Referral

- Consider addiction specialist, especially for opioid and polysubstance abuse.
- Maintenance therapy for opioid dependence (e.g., methadone) only in licensed clinics
- Psychiatry for comorbid psychiatric disorders
- Social services

IN-PATIENT CONSIDERATIONS

Initial Stabilization

Look for signs of severe infection (e.g., bacterial endocarditis).

Admission Criteria

- Indications for inpatient detoxification:
  - History of withdrawal symptoms (e.g., seizures)
  - Disorientation
  - Threat of harm to self or others
  - Obstacles to close monitoring (follow-up)
  - Comorbid medical illness
  - Pregnancy
- For narcotic addiction and withdrawal

IV Fluids

Maintenance until patient is taking fluids well by mouth

Nursing

- Take frequent vital signs during withdrawal.
- Monitor for signs of drug use in the hospital.

Discharge Criteria

Detoxification complete

 ONGOING CARE

FOLLOW-UP RECOMMENDATIONS

Restricted if dangerous, psychotic, or disoriented

Patient Monitoring

Verify patient's compliance with the substance abuse treatment program.

DIET

Patients often are malnourished.

PATIENT EDUCATION

- Center for Substance Abuse Treatment: (800) 662-HELP or http://findtreatment.samhsa.gov (facility locator)
- American Council on Alcoholism: (800) 527-5344 or http://www.aca-usa.org (treatment facility locator, educational information)
- National Clearinghouse for Alcohol and Drug Information: (800) 729–6686 or http://ncadi.samhsa.gov
- Alcoholics Anonymous: Contact local chapter or http://www.aa.org
- Narcotics Anonymous: http://www.na.org

PROGNOSIS

- Patients in treatment for longer periods of time (≥1 year) have higher success rates.
- Behavioral therapy and pharmacotherapy are most successful when used in combination.

COMPLICATIONS

- Hepatitis, HIV, tuberculosis, syphilis
- Subacute bacterial endocarditis
- Malnutrition
- Social problems, including arrest
- Poor marital adjustment and violence
- Depression, schizophrenia
- Serious harm to self and others: Accidents, violence
- Sexual assault related to use of GHB, Rohypnol
- Overdoses resulting in seizures, arrhythmias, cardiac and respiratory arrest, coma, death

REFERENCES

1. Smith PC, Schmidt SM, Allensworth-Davies D, et al. A single-question screening test for drug use in primary care. *Arch Intern Med.* 2010;170:1155–60.
2. Denis C, Fatséas M, Lavie E, et al. Pharmacological interventions for benzodiazepine mono-dependence management in outpatient settings. *Cochrane Database Syst Rev.* 2006;3: CD005194.
3. Gowing L, Ali R, White JM, et al. Buprenorphine for the management of opioid withdrawal. *Cochrane Database Syst Rev.* 2009;CD002025.
4. Mattick RP, Breen C, Kimber J, et al. Methadone maintenance therapy versus no opioid replacement therapy for opioid dependence. *Cochrane Database Syst Rev.* 2009;CD002209.
5. Gowing L, Farrell M, Ali R, et al. Alpha2-adrenergic agonists for the management of opioid withdrawal. *Cochrane Database Syst Rev.* 2009;CD002024.
6. Jayaram-Lindström N, Hammarberg A, Beck O, et al. Naltrexone for the Treatment of Amphetamine Dependence: A Randomized, Placebo-Controlled Trial. *Am J Psychiatry.* 2008.

See Also (Topic, Algorithm, Electronic Media Element)

Alcohol Abuse and Dependence; Alcohol Withdrawal; Tobacco Use and Smoking Cessation

CODES

ICD9

- 305.00 Nondependent alcohol abuse, unspecified drinking behavior
- 305.1 Nondependent tobacco use disorder
- 305.20 Nondependent cannabis abuse, unspecified use

CLINICAL PEARLS

- Substance use disorders are prevalent, serious, and often unrecognized in clinical practice. Comorbid psychiatric disorders are common.
- Substance abuse is distinguished by family, social, occupational, legal, or physical dysfunction that is caused by persistent use of the substance. Dependence is characterized by tolerance, withdrawal, compulsive use, and repeated overindulgence.
- The CRAFFT questionnaire is preferred for identifying alcohol and substance use disorders in adolescents and young adults.
- Motivational interviewing, brief interventions, and a nonjudgmental attitude can help to promote a willingness to change behavior.
- Consider referral of patients with opioid dependence and polysubstance abuse to an addiction specialist.

SUDDEN INFANT DEATH SYNDROME (SIDS)

Fern R. Hauck, MD, MS

 BASICS

- Leading cause of death in infants 1–12 months of age
- 3rd leading cause of infant mortality overall
- There has been a reduction of SIDS deaths by over 50% in the US and other countries that have introduced risk reduction campaigns, heavily focused on back sleeping for infants (1).
- The condition still remains mysterious, and the exact cause is unknown.

DESCRIPTION
- The sudden death of an infant <1 year of age that remains unexplained after a thorough case investigation, including performance of a complete autopsy, examination of the death scene, and review of the clinical history
- Sudden infant death syndrome (SIDS) was 1st formally defined in 1969. The definition was revised in 1989.
- System(s) affected: Cardiovascular; Endocrine/Metabolic; Nervous; Pulmonary
- Synonym(s): Crib death; Cot death

EPIDEMIOLOGY
- SIDS can affect any infant, but some infants are at higher risk than others, including African Americans and American Indians/Native Americans, males, infants whose mothers smoked or used illegal drugs during pregnancy, and several others described below.
- There is a characteristic age pattern, with deaths peaking at 2–4 months, and more deaths occurring during the colder seasons.

Incidence
- For 2006: All races: 0.55/1,000 live births (2,327 cases/year):
  – White non-Hispanic: 0.56/1,000 live births (1,283 cases/year)
  – Black non-Hispanic: 1.04/1,000 live births (641 cases/year)
  – Hispanic: 0.27/1,000 live births (282 cases/year)
  – Native American: 1.19/1,000 live births (57 cases/year)
- Predominant age: Uncommon in 1st month of life; peak occurs between 2 and 4 months of age; 60% of deaths occur by 6 months of age.
- Predominant sex: Male > Female (52–60% male)

Pediatric Considerations
Occurs only in infants

RISK FACTORS
- While some infants may die from SIDS who have no apparent risk factors, most have 1 or more of the following risk factors associated with SIDS:
  – Race: African Americans and Native Americans have highest incidence.
  – Season: Late fall and winter months
  – Time of day: Between midnight and 6 a.m.
  – Activity: During sleep
  – Low birth weight; intrauterine growth retardation (IUGR)
  – Poverty

- Maternal factors:
  – Decreased age
  – Decreased education
  – Maternal use of cigarettes or drugs (e.g., cocaine, opiates) during pregnancy
  – Higher parity
  – Inadequate prenatal care
- Respiratory or GI infection in recent past
- Sleep practices:
  – Prone and side sleep positions
  – Overheating from heavy clothing and bedding and/or elevated room temperature
  – Soft bedding
  – Bed sharing
- Passive cigarette smoke exposure after birth
- No pacifier use
- No breastfeeding

Genetics
Emerging evidence for genetic risk factors, especially related to impaired brain stem regulation of breathing or other autonomic control, impaired immune responses, and cardiac ion channelopathies associated with long QT syndrome and fatal arrhythmia

GENERAL PREVENTION
Because a SIDS death is sudden and the cause is unknown, SIDS cannot be "treated." However, there are some measures that may be effective in reducing the risk of SIDS (2)[B]:
- Maternal avoidance of cigarette smoking and illicit drug use during pregnancy
- Avoidance of passive cigarette smoke exposure
- Avoidance of the prone (face-down) and side sleep positions, excessive bed clothing, and soft bedding such as pillows and comforters or a soft mattress
- Avoidance of overheating
- A crib, bassinet, or cradle conforming to federal safety standards is the recommended sleeping location.
- Avoidance of bed sharing with the infant, particularly by adults other than the parent(s) or by other children. Bed sharing should be avoided if mother or father has used cigarettes, drugs, or alcohol. Bed sharing on couches is very dangerous and should never be done.
- Infants who sleep in the same room as their parents (without bed sharing) have a lower risk of SIDS. It is recommended that infants sleep in a crib or bassinet in their parents' bedroom, which when placed close to their bed will allow for more convenient breastfeeding and contact.
- Breastfeeding is associated with a decreased risk of SIDS and is recommended for all infants.
- Pacifier use is associated with a reduced risk of SIDS:
  – Consider offering a pacifier at bedtime and nap time.
  – Delay the introduction of the pacifier among breastfed infants until 1 month of age (3)[B].
  – Pacifier use has not been found to be detrimental to breastfeeding if it is introduced after the baby is 1 month of age, when breastfeeding is well established (4)[A].

- Avoidance of commercial devices marketed to reduce the risk of SIDS
- It is critical that all people caring for infants, including daycare providers, be instructed in these risk-reduction measures.
- Newborn nurseries should implement these recommendations well before discharge so parents see appropriate practices modeled.

PATHOPHYSIOLOGY
Strong evidence for a respiratory pathway that includes the following stages:
- A life-threatening event causes severe asphyxia and/or brain hypoperfusion. This can include rebreathing exhaled carbon dioxide in a face-down position.
- The vulnerable infant doesn't wake up or turn his head in response to asphyxia, resulting in further rebreathing and inability to recover from apnea.
- Progressive apnea leads to hypoxic coma.
- Bradycardia and hypoxic apnea occur.
- Autoresuscitation fails, resulting in prolonged apnea and death (5).

ETIOLOGY
- Many theories. There may be subtle developmental abnormalities resulting from pre- and/or perinatal brain injury, which make the infant vulnerable to SIDS.
- Possible causes:
  – Abnormalities in respiratory control and arousal responsiveness
  – Central and peripheral nervous system abnormalities
  – Cardiac arrhythmias
  – Rebreathing in face-down position on soft surface, leading to hypoxia and hypercarbia
  – SIDS may occur when 1 or more environmental risk factors interact with 1 or more genetic risk factors.

COMMONLY ASSOCIATED CONDITIONS
Infants are generally well, or may have had a mild febrile illness, i.e., gastroenteritis or upper respiratory infection, prior to death.

 DIAGNOSIS

The diagnosis of SIDS is made by trained medical examiners or coroners after a thorough review of the medical history, death scene investigation, and postmortem examination and an explanation of death is not found and the death is believed to be from natural causes.

HISTORY
Infant usually found unresponsive by parent or other caregiver without any warning

PHYSICAL EXAM
- These babies generally appear healthy or may have had a minor upper respiratory or GI infection in the last 2 weeks before death.
- Complete postmortem exam to look for signs of possible trauma/child abuse or other cause of death

DIAGNOSTIC TESTS & INTERPRETATION

Standardized postmortem protocols have been proposed. While testing varies across sites, common diagnostic tests include electrolytes, toxicology, and microbiology.

Lab

- Pneumocardiograms have been abandoned in the workup.
- Postmortem laboratory tests are performed to rule out other causes of death (e.g., electrolytes to rule out dehydration and electrolyte imbalance). No consistently abnormal laboratory tests are found.

Imaging

X-rays to rule out possible child abuse

Diagnostic Procedures/Surgery

Because the diagnosis of SIDS is often one of "exclusion," it is crucial to do a thorough death scene investigation and case review in addition to the autopsy and laboratory tests.

Pathological Findings

Characteristic findings on postmortem examination:

- Frothy discharge, sometimes blood tinged, from nostrils and mouth in most
- Petechiae on surface of lungs, heart, and thymus gland in 50–85% (but not unique to SIDS)
- Pulmonary congestion and edema often present
- Morphologic markers of hypoxia: Increased gliosis in brain stem, retention of periadrenal brown fat, and hematopoiesis in the liver:
  - Present to varying degrees; not confirmed by all studies

DIFFERENTIAL DIAGNOSIS

- Suffocation/accidental asphyxia
- Abnormalities of fatty acid metabolism (e.g., deficiency of medium-chain acyl-coenzyme A dehydrogenase or of carnitine)
- Dehydration/electrolyte disturbance
- Homicide

 ## ONGOING CARE

General recommendations for positioning infants:

- Infants frequently should be placed on their belly when awake and observed by a responsible adult to prevent head flattening (plagiocephaly) that can result from infants sleeping supine.
- Avoid placing infants for extended periods in car seat carriers or "bouncers."
- Upright "cuddle time" should be encouraged.
- Alter the side to which the infant places his or her head during sleep.
- Swaddling infants may aid in sleeping more comfortably in the supine position. Infants should never be swaddled if sleeping in the prone position.

FOLLOW-UP RECOMMENDATIONS

- Safe sleep and SIDS risk reduction messages should be delivered at all well-child checks and by all health professionals in a consistent manner.
- Parents often change from the recommended practices as the baby gets older, often during the peak SIDS incidence period.

Patient Monitoring

Although some authorities recommend cardiopulmonary monitoring in siblings of prior SIDS victims, there is no evidence that the use of monitors prevents SIDS, and they should not be prescribed for that purpose (6)[B].

PATIENT EDUCATION

- Family counseling (see Prognosis)
- Back to Sleep Information Line, (800) 505-CRIB (2742) (sponsored by the Eunice Kennedy Shriver National Institute of Child Health and Human Development, the Maternal and Child Health Bureau, and other organizations to provide information to parents and health providers about their recommendation to place infants on back, and general information about SIDS)
- National SIDS/Infant Death Resource Center, McLean, VA; (866) 866-SIDS (7437)
- Association of SIDS and Infant Mortality Programs, Lansing, MI; (800) 930-SIDS (7437)
- First Candle/SIDS Alliance, Baltimore, MD; (800) 221-SIDS (7437)
- CJ Foundation for SIDS, Hackensack, NJ; 8CJ-SIDS (7437)
- SIDS Network, Ledyard, CT; (800) 560–1454
- Cribs for Kids, Pittsburgh, PA; ADD PHONE NUMBER

PROGNOSIS

- SIDS deaths have a powerful impact on families and their functioning. Physicians play an important role in providing immediate information about SIDS and sensitive counseling to limit parents' misinformation and feelings of guilt.
- Counseling needs of families vary from short-term to long-term; support groups are helpful to many couples. Physicians need to be familiar with resources available in their communities to help families mourning a SIDS death.
- Follow-up counseling, including review of the autopsy report with the family after some time has passed, is important to help with understanding this condition and to alleviate the tremendous guilt these families experience.
- Parents need to be counseled about subsequent pregnancies. Genetic testing and counseling may be indicated to rule out a metabolic or other genetically acquired disorder. Parents need to be advised of the most current recommendations regarding sleep position and other infant care practices during subsequent pregnancies.

REFERENCES

1. Mitchell EA, et al. SIDS: past, present and future. *Acta Paediatr*. 2009;98:1712–9.
2. American Academy of Pediatrics Task Force on Sudden Infant Death Syndrome. The changing concept of sudden infant death syndrome: diagnostic coding shifts, controversies regarding the sleeping environment, and new variables to consider in reducing risk. *Pediatrics*. 2005;116: 1245–55.
3. Hauck FR, Omojokun OO, Siadaty MS. Do pacifiers reduce the risk of sudden infant death syndrome? A meta-analysis. *Pediatrics*. 2005;116. Available at: http://www.pediatrics.org/cgi/content/full/116/5/ e716.
4. O'Connor NR, Tanabe KO, Siadaty MS, et al. Pacifiers and breastfeeding: a systematic review. *Arch Pediatr Adolesc Med*. 2009;163:378–82.
5. Kinney HC, Thach BT. The sudden infant death syndrome. *N Engl J Med*. 2009;361:795–805.
6. Committee on Fetus and Newborn. American Academy of Pediatrics. Apnea, sudden infant death syndrome, and home monitoring. *Pediatrics*. 2003;111:914–7.

 ## CODES

ICD9

798.0 Sudden infant death syndrome

CLINICAL PEARLS

- Although the exact cause of SIDS is unknown, there are several risk-reduction measures that will significantly reduce an infant's chance of dying from SIDS.
- SIDS incidence has decreased by more than 50% just by placing infants supine to sleep.
- Breastfeeding is recommended for all infants.
- Safe sleeping arrangements and pacifier use after age 1 month are other ways to reduce the risk of SIDS.

SUICIDE

Irene C. Coletsos, MD
Harold J. Bursztajn, MD

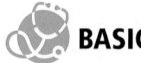

BASICS

DESCRIPTION
Suicide and attempted suicide are significant causes of morbidity and mortality. There are more than 32,000 suicides in the US annually, with firearms, poisonings, and suffocation being the most common methods used. There are an estimated 10× more than that number of attempted suicides.

EPIDEMIOLOGY
- Predominant sex:
  - Women *attempt* suicide 1.5× more often than men. Men *complete* suicide 4× more often than women. Men are more likely to choose a means with high lethality.
- Predominant age: Adolescent and geriatric population
- Predominant race: 84% of people who complete suicides are white, non-Hispanic. Native Americans have the next highest rate in US. Whites have twice the risk of suicide compared to African Americans.
- Marital status: Single > divorced; widowed > married

Incidence
In 2005 (the most recent figure available), 11th leading cause of death in adults in the US. There are an estimated 480 attempted suicides every day Military service may increase the risk: In 2008, there were 20.2 suicides/100,000 active-duty personnel versus 19.5/100,000 in a similar demographic (2005 Centers for Disease Control and Prevention data, the most currently available).

RISK FACTORS
- "Human understanding is the most effective weapon against suicide. The greatest need is to deepen the awareness and sensitivity of people to their fellow man"—Edwin Schneidman, PhD, American Association of Suicidology.
- Overall, Schneidman says that health providers should be alert to a combination of "perturbation" (increased emotional disturbance) and "lethality" (having the potential tools to cause death) (see "Treatment").
- Most people (80%) who complete suicides had a previous attempt.
- One study shows that 90% who complete suicide meet *Diagnostic and Statistical Manual* criteria for Axis I or II disorders.
  - Substance use (especially alcohol): Schizophrenia; borderline and antisocial personality disorders; anorexia nervosa; panic disorder
  - Family history of suicide
  - Physical illness
  - Despair: The patient feels unendurable emotional pain *and* has "given up" on himself or herself, feels without hope and, consciously or unconsciously, unworthy of help (1).
- Psychological:
  - Recent loss: What may seem to be a small loss (to a medical provider) may be a devastating loss to the patient. *Patient-specific* factors need to be taken into account; social isolation; anniversaries and holidays; poor ability to control impulses.

- Access to lethal means: Firearms, poisons (including prescription and nonprescription drugs)
- If a patient is incompetent to inform providers about the potential for suicide, that puts the patient at increased risk, and the treating clinician should consider hospitalizing the patient (2).

GENERAL PREVENTION
- Know how to access resources 24/7 within and outside of the health care institution.
- Suicide is a statistically rare event, and no reliable method of predicting who will or will not attempt suicide has been devised. However, it can be foreseeable and, one hopes, preventable. Screen for risk factors, and consider the overall clinical picture.
- Screen all patients for suicide risk. Potential screening instruments include the Patient Health Questionnaire-2, the modified PHQ-2 (see *Diagnosis section, below*), the PHQ-9, Beck's Scale for Suicidal Ideation, Linehan's Reasons for Living Inventory, and Risk Estimator for Suicide. Treat underlying mental illness and substance abuse. Screen for possession of means of harm, including firearms (encourage these patients to remove guns from their homes and to relinquish gun license) and prescription and nonprescription drugs.
- For those at risk for suicide, create a safety plan with patient and family, including education about how to access emergency care 24 hours a day.
- Public education about how to help others access emergency psychiatric care; sometimes suicidal people will first confide in those they trust outside health care (e.g., family members, religious leaders, community elders, "unofficial" community leaders such as "healers," hairdressers, and bartenders).

DIAGNOSIS

HISTORY
- Depressed patients should be asked about ideation and about a plan:
  - "Have you ever felt that life isn't worth living? Do you ever wish you could go to sleep and not wake up? Are you having thoughts about killing yourself?"
- In a mental health setting, use psychodynamic formulation (1), which combines mental-state exam (i.e., behavior, mood, mental content, judgment); past history (i.e., what resources has the patient used in the past for support, and are they currently available?); and history of current illness. If the patient is experiencing a loss, is under stress, and does not have access to a previously sustaining resource (e.g., a significant other, a pet, sports ability, a job), that patient is under increased risk for suicide.
- Prior attempts: Lethality, intent to die, what precipitated the attempt, precautions taken to avoid being rescued, reaction to survival (a patient who is upset that the suicide was not completed is at increased risk)
- Detailed history of psychiatric symptoms, substance abuse; also note reasons to live, hope for future, social supports. A patient without these is at increased risk.

- Collateral history is important (from friends, family, physicians). It may be appropriate to break confidentiality if patient is at imminent risk of suicide.

PHYSICAL EXAM
- Medical conditions: Delirium, intoxication, withdrawal, medication side effects (which can be risk factors)
- Psychosis: Observe for signs of/ask about command auditory hallucinations to kill oneself, delusional guilt, and persecutory delusions.
- Observe for signs of hopelessness/despair (see "Risk Factors").

DIFFERENTIAL DIAGNOSIS
Differentiate between patients and pseudopatients, i.e., those who are using suicide threats and gestures to manipulate others. Consider a psychiatric consult. All decisions regarding treatment must be carefully documented and communicated to all involved health care providers.

TREATMENT

MEDICATION
- Patients are at increased risk of suicide at the outset of antidepressant treatment, and if/when medications are discontinued. Consider tapering/switching medical therapies rather than sudden discontinuation if at all possible. Careful monitoring is needed at these times.
- Anxiety and agitation are risk factors for suicide and should be treated aggressively.
- In patients with mood disorders, a meta-analysis of randomized, controlled trials found that lithium reduced the risk of death by suicide by 60% (3)[A]. Long-term treatment for psychosis with clozapine shows some benefit for reducing rate of suicide (4)[A]. Agitated or combative patients may require sedation with IV or IM benzodiazepines and/or antipsychotics. Clinical response is typically seen within 20–30 minutes if given IM/IV.

Pediatric Considerations
The Food and Drug Administration has issued a black box warning for antidepressants in the pediatric population after increased suicidality was noted. If risk of untreated depression is sufficient to warrant treatment with antidepressants, children must be monitored very closely for suicidality.

First Line
Obtain baseline ECGs before prescribing or continuing antidepressants or antipsychotics. Certain drugs are associated with QT prolongation and sudden cardiac death.

ADDITIONAL TREATMENT
General Measures
- Patients expressing active suicidal thoughts or who made an attempt require an examination for suicide risk factors, mental status examination, and competency (to determine if they are able or willing to inform treatment team about ongoing/changing suicidal intentions), as well as a formal psychiatric consultation.

- Cognitive therapy decreased reattempt rate in prior suicide attempters by half (5)[B].
- Psychotherapy with suicidal patients is a challenge even for the most experienced clinicians. The countertransference usually evolves into wanting to be rid of the patient, and if the patient detects this, the risk of suicide is seriously heightened. The clinician can avoid this by recognizing his or her countertransference and bearing it within so well that the patient remains unaware of it (6).

IN-PATIENT CONSIDERATIONS
Initial Stabilization
- Determine appropriate level of care: Inpatient hospitalization if patient is suicidal with a plan to act or is otherwise at high risk; if immediate risk for self-harm, may be hospitalized involuntarily.
- Immediately after a suicide attempt, treat the medical problems resulting from the self-harm before attempting to initiate psychiatric care.
- Order lab work (e.g., solvent screen, blood and urine toxicology screen, aspirin and acetaminophen levels). Patients may not disclose ingestions if they wish to succeed in their attempt or if they are undergoing mental status changes.
- Risk for self-harm continues even in hospital setting. Ensure patient safety by least restrictive method (i.e., remove potentially dangerous objects, provide 1-to-1 constant observation, medication). Use mechanical restraints if deemed necessary for patient safety. Trained staff should search patient for dangerous objects.
- The period after transfer from involuntary to voluntary hospitalization is also a time of high risk.

Discharge Criteria
- No longer considered a danger to self/others
- Clinicians should be aware that a patient may *claim that* he or she is no longer suicidal in order to facilitate discharge and complete the act. Look for clinical and behavioral signs that the patient truly is no longer in despair and is hopeful, such as improved appetite, sleep, engagement with staff, and group therapy. Clinicians should check with family and ancillary staff to assess patient's conditions because the patient may share more information with those contacts than with doctors (7).
- Provide education about resources that are available in a crisis. Patient and patient's support system must be aware of and willing to access services 24/7 to enhance patient safety.

 ONGOING CARE

FOLLOW-UP RECOMMENDATIONS
Patient Monitoring
- Increase monitoring at the beginning of treatment, when changing medication regimens, and on discharge. These are times of increased risk.
- Educate family members and other close contacts/confidants to the warning signs of suicidality. For *adults*: Despair/hopelessness, isolation, discussing suicide, stating that the world would be a better place without them, losses in areas key to the patient's self-worth. For *youths*: May exhibit the same signs and symptoms, but one should be aware of these additional risks: History of abuse (e.g., sexual, physical), family stress, changes in eating and sleeping patterns, suicidality of friends, and giving away treasured items. Make sure that the patient is willing to accept the type of follow-up

offered. Do not assume that just setting it up is protection enough.
- Curtail access to firearms.
- Limiting the number of pills may also be appropriate for an impulsive patient. However, clinicians may believe that by simply limiting the number of pills they prescribe, they are preventing further suicide attempts, an example of "magical thinking." Clinicians who find themselves thinking this way, can take it as a warning sign that their patients may actually be at increased risk of suicide.

PATIENT EDUCATION
Patients who feel they are in danger of hurting themselves should consider one or several of these options:
- Call 911.
- Go directly to an emergency room.
- If already in counseling, contact that therapist immediately.
- Call the National Suicide Prevention Hotline at 1-800-273-TALK (8255).
- Servicemen and servicewomen and their families can call 1-800-796-9699; if there is no immediate answer, call 1-800-273-8255.

PROGNOSIS
The key to a favorable course and prognosis is early recognition of risk factors, early diagnosis and treatment of a psychiatric disorder, and appropriate intervention and follow-up.

COMPLICATIONS
- The sequeala of attempted and completed suicides can be lifelong for family members and close friends.
- According to the American Association of Suicidality (AAS), the grief process for significant others of suicide victims can be lifelong and can be expressed in emotions ranging from anger to despair. Survivors often attempt to shoulder the burden on their own because of the added guilt and shame of the nature of the attempted death or death.
- The AAS recommends
  - Counseling: Could include short-term behavioral therapy as well as psychotherapy; some therapy should focus on the survivors' relationships to their current and future significant others. An expert on the lives of adult children of parents/close family members who completed suicides reports that these survivors often seek out life partners as "replacements" for those they lost. This may prevent the survivor from completing his or her mourning (8).
  - Sympathetic listening by friends of the survivors
  - Special support at holiday times, when the loneliness intensifies
  - A website with links to resources and self-help strategies is www.survivorsofsuicide.com.

REFERENCES

1. Maltsberger JT. *Suicide Risk: The Formulation of Clinical Judgment*. New York University Press. 1986.
2. Gutheil TG, Bursztajn HJ, Brodsky A. The multidimensional assessment of dangerousness: Competence assessment in patient care and liability prevention. *Bull Am Acad Psychiatry Law*. 14:123–129, 1986.
3. Cipriani A, Pretty H, Hawton K, et al. Lithium in the prevention of suicidal behavior and all-cause mortality in patients with mood disorders: a systematic review of randomized trials. *Am J Psychiatry*. 2005;162:1805–19.
4. Hennen J, Baldessarinin RJ. Suicide risk during treatment with clozapine: A meta-analysis. *Schizophr Res*. 2004;73:139–45.
5. Brown GK, et al. Cognitive therapy for the prevention of suicide attempts: A randomized controlled trial. *JAMA*. 2005;295:563–70.
6. Maltsberger JT, Buie DH. Countertransference hate in the treatment of suicidal patients. *Arch Gen Psychiatry*. 1974;30:625–33.
7. Simon S, Gutheil TG. Sudden improvement among high-risk suicidal patients: should it be trusted? *Psychiatric Services*. 60:387–9, 2009.
8. William J. Massicotte Faculty, Canadian Institute of Psychoanalysis Chair, National Scientific Program Committee, Canadian Psychoanalytic Society. *Personal correspondance*, April 24, 2009.

 CODES

ICD9
V62.84 Suicidal ideation

CLINICAL PEARLS

- The most important preventative measure is to listen to a patient and take steps to keep him or her safe. This could include immediate hospitalization. The most important questions to explore not only include, "Are you thinking of killing yourself?" but also, "Who do you have to live for?" and "What has to change, or what needs to change, for you to live with your suffering?"
- Clozapine, lithium and cognitive behavioral therapy are proven to reduce the risk of suicide.
- Resources for clinicians: www.suicidology.com; www.suicideassessment.com
- Family members and contacts of people who have attempted or committed suicide suffer from reactions ranging from rage to despair. Their grief is often longer lasting and less well treated because of the shame and guilt associated with the act. Encourage them to discuss this and consider counseling.

SUPERFICIAL THROMBOPHLEBITIS

Abdulrazak Abyad, MD, PhD, MBA, MPH, AGSF, AFCHSE

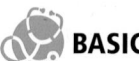 **BASICS**

DESCRIPTION
- Superficial thrombophlebitis is an inflammatory condition of the veins with secondary thrombosis.
- Septic (suppurative) thrombophlebitis types:
  - Iatrogenic
  - Infectious, mainly syphilis and psittacosis
- Aseptic thrombophlebitis types:
  - Primary hypercoagulable states: Disorders with measurable defects in the proteins of the coagulation and/or fibrinolytic systems
  - Secondary hypercoagulable states: Clinical conditions with a risk of thrombosis
- System(s) affected: Cardiovascular
- Synonym(s): Phlebitis; Phlebothrombosis

Geriatric Considerations
Septic thrombophlebitis is more common; prognosis is poorer.

Pediatric Considerations
Subperiosteal abscesses of adjacent long bone may complicate the disorder.

Pregnancy Considerations
- Associated with increased risk of aseptic superficial thrombophlebitis
- Warfarin and nonsteroidal anti-inflammatory drugs (NSAIDs) are contraindicated.

EPIDEMIOLOGY
- Predominant age:
  - Septic: More common in childhood
  - Aseptic primary hypercoagulable state:
    - Antithrombin III and heparin cofactor II deficiency: Neonatal period, but 1st episode usually at age 20–30 years
    - Proteins C and S: <30 years of age
  - Aseptic secondary hypercoagulable state:
    - Mondor disease: Women, ages 21–55 years
    - Thromboangiitis obliterans onset: Ages 20–50 years
- Predominant sex:
  - Suppurative: Male = Female.
  - Aseptic:
    - Mondor: Female > Male (2:1)
    - Thromboangiitis obliterans: Female > Male (1–19% of clinical cases)

Incidence
- Septic:
  - Up to 10% of all nosocomial infections
  - Incidence of catheter-related thrombophlebitis is 88/100,000 persons.
  - Develops in 4–8% if cutdown is performed
- Aseptic primary hypercoagulable state: Antithrombin III and heparin cofactor II deficiency incidence is 50/100,000 persons.
- Aseptic secondary hypercoagulable state:
  - Trousseau syndrome (migratory venous thrombosis associated with occult malignancy)
  - Trousseau syndrome incidence in malignancy is 5–15%.
  - Trousseau syndrome incidence in pancreatic carcinoma is 50%.
  - In pregnancy, 49-fold increased incidence of phlebitis
  - Superficial migratory thrombophlebitis in 27% of patients with thromboangiitis obliterans

Prevalence
- Superficial thrombophlebitis is common.
- One-third of patients in a medical ICU develop thrombophlebitis that eventually progresses to the deep veins.

RISK FACTORS
- Nonspecific:
  - Immobilization
  - Obesity
  - Advanced age
  - Postoperative states
- Septic:
  - IV catheter (68% of cannulas have been left in place for 2 days)
  - Incidence is 40× higher with plastic cannulas (8%) than with steel or scalp cannulas (0.2%).
  - Lower extremity IV catheter
  - Cutdowns
  - Cancer, debilitating diseases
  - Steroid
  - Thrombosis
  - Dermal infection
  - Burned patients
  - IV antibiotics
  - AIDS
  - Varicose veins
- Antithrombin II and heparin cofactor II deficiency:
  - Pregnancy
  - Oral contraceptives
  - Surgery, trauma, infection
- In pregnancy:
  - Increased age
  - Hypertension
  - Eclampsia
  - Increased parity
- Thromboangiitis obliterans: Persistent smoking
- Mondor disease:
  - Breast abscess
  - Antecedent breast surgery
  - Breast augmentation
  - Reduction mammoplasty
- Superficial thrombophlebitis may occur spontaneously or as a complication of medical or surgical interventions.

Genetics
- Septic: No known genetic pattern
- Antithrombin III deficiencies: Autosomal dominant
- Proteins C and S deficiency: Autosomal dominant with variable penetrance
- Disorders of fibrinolytic system: Congenital defects inheritance variable
- Dysfibrinogenemia: Autosomal dominant
- Factor XII deficiency: Autosomal recessive

GENERAL PREVENTION
- Use of scalp vein cannulas
- Avoidance of lower extremity cannulations
- Insertion under aseptic conditions
- Secure anchoring of the cannulas
- Replacement of cannulas, connecting tubing, and IV fluid every 48–72 h
- Antibacterial ointment in cutdown

PATHOPHYSIOLOGY
- Microscopic thrombosis is a normal part of the dynamic balance of hemostasis.
- In the absence of a triggering event, neither venous stasis nor abnormal coagulability alone causes clinically important thrombosis.
- Vascular endothelial injury does reliably cause thrombus formation. The initiating injury triggers an inflammatory response that results in immediate platelet adhesion at the site of injury.
- Platelet aggregation owing to thromboxane A2 is inhibited reversibly by NSAIDs and irreversibly by aspirin, but thrombin-mediated platelet aggregation is unaffected by aspirin and NSAIDs.

ETIOLOGY
- Septic:
  - *Staphylococcus aureus* in 65–78%
  - Enterobacteriaceae, especially *Klebsiella*
  - Multiple organisms in 14%
  - Anaerobic isolate rare
  - *Candida* sp.
  - Cytomegalovirus (CMV) in AIDS patients
- Aseptic primary hypercoagulable state:
  - Antithrombin III and heparin II deficiency
  - Protein C and protein S deficiency
  - Disorder of tissue plasminogen activator
  - Abnormal plasminogen and coplasminogen
  - Dysfibrinogenemia
  - Factor XII deficiency
  - Lupus anticoagulant and anticardiolipin antibody syndrome
- Aseptic secondary hypercoagulable states:
  - Malignancy (Trousseau syndrome: Recurrent migratory thrombophlebitis): Most commonly seen in metastatic mucin or adenocarcinomas of the GI tract (pancreas, stomach, colon, and gallbladder), lung, prostate, and ovary
  - Pregnancy
  - Oral contraceptives
  - Infusion of prothrombin complex concentrates
  - Behçet disease
  - Buerger disease
  - Mondor disease

DIAGNOSIS

HISTORY
Pain along the course of a vein

PHYSICAL EXAM
- Swelling, tenderness, redness along the course of a vein or veins
- May look like cellulitis or erythema nodosa
- Fever in 70% of patients
- Warmth, erythema, tenderness, or lymphangitis in 32%
- Sign of systemic sepsis in 84% of suppurative

DIAGNOSTIC TESTS & INTERPRETATION
Lab
- If septic concern:
  - Blood cultures (bacteremia in 80–90%)
  - Culture of IV fluid bag
  - Complete blood count (CBC) demonstrates leukocytosis.
- Aseptic: Evaluation for coagulopathy if recurrent (e.g., protein C, protein S, lupus anticoagulant, anticardiolipin antibody, factor analysis)

Imaging
Septic and aseptic:
- None needed if below the knee and no risk factors for deep vein thrombosis (DVT)
- Evaluation of complications (DVT and others):
  - CXR: Multiple peripheral densities or a pleural effusion consistent with pulmonary embolism, abscess, or empyema
  - Bone and gallium scan: For associated subperiosteal abscess in septic thrombophlebitis

Diagnostic Procedures/Surgery
Skin biopsy if not responding to therapy as expected

Pathological Findings
- The affected vein is enlarged, tortuous, and thickened.
- Associated perivascular suppuration and/or hemorrhage
- Vein lumen may contain pus and thrombus.
- Endothelial damage, fibrinoid necrosis, and thickening of the vein wall

DIFFERENTIAL DIAGNOSIS
- Cellulitis
- Erythema nodosa
- Cutaneous polyarteritis nodosa
- Sarcoid
- Kaposi sarcoma
- Hyperalgesic pseudothrombophlebitis

TREATMENT

MEDICATION
First Line
- Septic:
  - Initially: Semisynthetic penicillin (e.g., nafcillin 2 g IV q6h) plus an aminoglycoside (e.g., gentamicin, 1.0–1.7 mg/kg IV)
  - Duration of therapy is empirical.
  - If due to *Candida albicans*, consider a short course of amphotericin B, ~200-mg cumulative dose
  - If osteomyelitis is documented, antibiotic therapy × 6 weeks at least
- Aseptic, general:
  - For those with coagulopathy:
    ○ NSAIDs
    ○ Removal of catheter, if placed
    ○ Oral anticoagulant warfarin
    ○ Systemic anticoagulant heparin
    ○ Low-molecular-weight heparin
  - Antithrombin III and heparin cofactor II deficiency: IV heparin
  - Antithrombin III concentrate: Prophylaxis: Warfarin, oxymetholone
- Proteins C and S: Long-term warfarin, lower dose, no loading
- Disorder of tissue plasminogen activator:
  - Phenformin and ethylestrenol
  - Stanozolol and phenformin
  - Stanozolol alone
  - Ethylestrenol alone
- Dysfibrinogenemia:
  - Acute attack: Anticoagulation
  - Prophylaxis: Stanozolol
- Abnormal plasminogen and plasminogenemia:
  - Acute attack: Anticoagulation
  - Prophylaxis: Warfarin

- Factor XII deficiency: Standard therapy
- Lupus anticardiolipin: Prophylaxis: Warfarin
- Trousseau syndrome: Heparin
- For pregnancy: Heparin
- Behçet disease:
  - Phenformin
  - Ethylestrenol
  - Stanozolol
- Thromboangiitis obliterans:
  - Stop smoking.
  - Pentoxifylline
- Contraindications: Refer to the manufacturer's literature for each drug.
- Precautions: Refer to the manufacturer's literature for each drug.
- Significant possible interactions: Refer to the manufacturer's literature for each drug.

Second Line
- Factor XII deficiency: Streptokinase or alteplase (tissue plasminogen activator [tPA])
- Behçet: Oral anticoagulants plus cyclosporine
- Thromboangiitis obliterans: Corticosteroid, antiplatelets, and vasodilating drugs

ADDITIONAL TREATMENT
General Measures
- Heat application
- Extremity elevation

SURGERY/OTHER PROCEDURES
- Septic:
  - Excision of the involved vein segment and all involved tributaries if failed conservative treatment
  - Excision from ankle to groin may be required in some burn patients.
  - If systemic symptoms persist after vein excision, reexploration is necessary, with removal of all involved veins.
  - Drainage of contiguous abscesses
  - Remove all cannulas.
- Aseptic: Management of underlying conditions

IN-PATIENT CONSIDERATIONS
Initial Stabilization
- Septic: Inpatient
- Aseptic: Outpatient

 ONGOING CARE

FOLLOW-UP RECOMMENDATIONS
Bed rest

Patient Monitoring
- Septic:
  - Routine white blood cell (WBC) count and differential and culture
  - Repeat culture from the phlebitic vein
- Aseptic:
  - Clinical follow-up to rule out secondary complications
  - Repeat of blood studies for fibrinolytic system, platelets, and factors

DIET
No restrictions

PATIENT EDUCATION
- Avoid trauma.
- Be alert to change in skin color.
- Be alert to tenderness over extremities.

PROGNOSIS
- Septic: High mortality (50%) if untreated
- Aseptic:
  - Usually benign course; recovery in 7–10 days
  - Antithrombin III and heparin cofactor deficiency: Recurrence rate 60%
  - Proteins C and S: Recurrence rate 70%
  - Prognosis depends on development of DVT and early detection of complications.
  - Aseptic thrombophlebitis can be isolated, recurrent, or migratory.

COMPLICATIONS
- Septic: Systemic sepsis, bacteremia (84%), septic pulmonary emboli (44%), metastatic abscess formation, pneumonia (44%), subperiosteal abscess of adjacent long bones in children
- Aseptic: DVT, thromboembolic phenomena

ADDITIONAL READING

- Di Nisio M, Wichers IM, Middeldorp S. Treatment for superficial thrombophlebitis of the leg. *Cochrane Database Syst Rev*. 2007;CD004982.
- Gillet JL, French P, Hanss M, et al. Predictive value of D-dimer assay in superficial thrombophlebitis of the lower limbs. *J Mal Vasc*. 2007.
- Samlaska CP, James WD. Superficial thrombophlebitis. II. Secondary hypercoagulable states. *J Am Acad Dermatol*. 1990;23:1–18.
- Samlaska CP, James WD. Superficial thrombophlebitis. I. Primary hypercoagulable states. *J Am Acad Dermatol*. 1990;22:975–89.

See Also (Topic, Algorithm, Electronic Media Element)
Thrombosis, Deep Vein

CODES

ICD9
- 451.0 Phlebitis and thrombophlebitis of superficial vessels of lower extremities
- 451.9 Phlebitis and thrombophlebitis of unspecified site
- 451.82 Phlebitis and thrombophlebitis of superficial veins of upper extremities

CLINICAL PEARLS
- The disease can develop while on a plane.
- The best modality to prevent the disease during air travel is to exercise and drink a lot of water.

SUPERIOR VENA CAVA SYNDROME

Sandra Cuellar, PharmD, BCOP
Binay K. Shah, MD

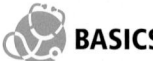 BASICS

DESCRIPTION
- Partial or complete obstruction of the superior vena cava (SVC):
  – 90% extrinsic
  – 90% from neoplasm (most frequently lung cancer)
- Usual course: Acute; usually 2 weeks from onset of symptoms to diagnosis
- Synonym(s): Superior mediastinal syndrome; Superior vena cava obstruction

EPIDEMIOLOGY
- Predominant age: All ages, less commonly children and young adults (16–30 years old)
- Predominant sex: Male > Female

Incidence
15,000 new cases/year in US

RISK FACTORS
- Uncontrolled primary cancer
- History of mediastinal tumor
- Previous invasive procedures

GENERAL PREVENTION
No preventive measures known

PATHOPHYSIOLOGY
Increased pressure in the venous system draining into the superior vena cava

ETIOLOGY
- Obstruction of venous drainage of upper part of chest and neck. Sudden occlusion may cause rapid development of cerebral edema, intracranial thrombosis, and death.
- In adults, may be primary tumor or lymph node metastasis; most common primary tumor is lung cancer; lymph node metastasis most common from breast and testicular cancer

- In children, most common after cardiac surgical procedures
- Fungal infections
- Iatrogenic (intravascular devices)
- Thyroid goiter
- Thrombosis of SVC
- Pericardial constriction
- Idiopathic sclerosing mediastinitis

COMMONLY ASSOCIATED CONDITIONS
- Cancer:
  – Common: Lung, lymphoma, and metastatic breast
  – Less common: Germ-cell tumors
- Hyperthyroidism
- Infections: Tuberculosis, histoplasmosis
- Recent cardiac procedure

 DIAGNOSIS

Superior vena cava (SVC) syndrome is a constellation of symptoms caused by the impairment of blood flow through the SVC to the right atrium. In the absence of tracheal obstruction, treatment of SVC syndrome can be delayed until histological diagnosis has been determined. Following investigations are useful in establishing the diagnosis:
- Radiological studies like chest x-ray and CT scan of thorax to look for mediastinal masses and associated pleural effusion, lobar collapse, or cardiomegaly
- Venography, magnetic resonance imaging, and ultrasound to assess the site and nature of the obstruction
- Biopsy of the tumor

HISTORY
- Dyspnea
- Facial swelling and head fullness
- Cough
- Arm swelling
- Chest pain
- Dysphagia
- Headaches
- Visual symptoms

PHYSICAL EXAM
- Accessory venous drainage: Venous distention of neck and chest wall
- Facial edema
- Plethora of face (excess red blood cells)
- Cyanosis
- Horner syndrome
- Swelling of arms
- Confusion

DIAGNOSTIC TESTS & INTERPRETATION
Lab
Initial lab tests
- Made on clinical grounds in nearly all cases
- If done, increased central venous pressure; usually 20–40 mm Hg
- Sputum cytology can provide diagnosis with malignant cells.

Imaging
Initial approach
- Confirmed by imaging, usually CT scan
- Abnormal chest x-ray
- Contrast-enhanced CT or MRI usually adequate to establish diagnosis
- Venography (if stent or surgery planned)

Diagnostic Procedures/Surgery
- Stent:
  – For immediate relief, if needed
- Percutaneous needle biopsy used to establish histologic diagnosis; should be prior to initiation of therapy
- Open biopsy may be necessary; however, these patients are at increased risk for cardiorespiratory compromise under general anesthesia
- Bronchoscopy, thoracentesis, thoracotomy, lymph node biopsy as indicated

Pathological Findings
Sputum cytology, occasionally thoracentesis, bone marrow, lymph node biopsy, bronchoscopy, or thoracotomy confirms malignant cells.

DIFFERENTIAL DIAGNOSIS
- SVC blood clot
- Syphilitic aneurysm
- Tuberculosis mediastinitis
- Fungal infections

TREATMENT
- Severity of symptoms is important in determining urgency of intervention. The following grading system has been proposed.
- Grade 0: Asymptomatic: Radiographic superior vena cava obstruction in the absence of symptoms
- Grade 1: Mild: Edema in head or neck (vascular distention), cyanosis, plethora
- Grade 2: Moderate: Edema in head or neck with functional impairment (mild dysphagia, cough, mild or moderate impairment of head, jaw or eyelid movements, visual disturbances caused by ocular edema)
- Grade 3: Severe: Mild or moderate cerebral edema (headache, dizziness) or mild/moderate laryngeal edema or diminished cardiac reserve (syncope after bending)
- Grade 4: Life-threatening: Significant cerebral edema (confusion, obtundation) or significant laryngeal edema or significant hemodynamic compromise
- Grade 5: Fatal: Death

ADDITIONAL TREATMENT
General Measures
- Depends on etiology (1)[B]
- Percutaneous stenting (for immediate relief)
- Chemotherapy (treatment of choice for small-cell lung cancer and germ-cell tumors)
- Radiotherapy

- Neoadjuvant chemoradiotherapy and then resection (Pancoast tumors)
- Anticoagulation or fibrinolytic therapy
- Benign causes usually respond to medical therapy, including diuretics, upright positioning, and fluid restriction, until adequate collateral circulation is established and clinical regression is noted.

SURGERY/OTHER PROCEDURES
- Radiotherapy mainly in non-small-cell lung cancer and non-Hodgkin lymphoma
- Tissue confirmation, especially for lymphomas that require tumor architecture
- Superior vena cava reconstruction for benign processes may be considered, but is rarely done.

IN-PATIENT CONSIDERATIONS
Initial Stabilization
- Inpatient, intensive care as clinically indicated
- Institute supportive therapy:
  – Bed rest
  – Elevate head
  – Oxygen
- Steroids: Debated, no clear evidence of benefit

ONGOING CARE

FOLLOW-UP RECOMMENDATIONS
Bed rest, and elevate patient's head to decrease the hydrostatic pressure.

Patient Monitoring
- Severity of clinical symptoms
- If malignant, monitor response to radiotherapy or chemotherapy.
- If infectious, monitor for evaluation of antimicrobial treatment.

DIET
As tolerated; possibly salt restriction

PROGNOSIS
- High probability of initial response
- Linked to cause:
  – Lung cancer: 1-year survival in 20%
  – Lymphoma: 2-year survival in 50%
- Neoplastic cases: 85% better in 3 weeks with radiation therapy, but symptoms usually recur

COMPLICATIONS
Complications of underlying disease

REFERENCES
1. Rowell NP, et al. Steroids, radiotherapy, chemotherapy and stents for superior vena caval obstruction in carcinoma of the bronchus: A systematic review. *Clin Oncol*. 2002;14:338–51.
2. Thirlwell C, Brock CS. Emergencies in oncology. *Clin Med*. 2003;3:306–10.

ADDITIONAL READING
- Hochrein J, Bashore TM, O'Laughlin MP, et al. Percutaneous stenting of superior vena cava syndrome: a case report and review of the literature. *Am J Med*. 1998;104:78–84.
- Wilson LD, Detterbeck FC, Yahalom J. Clinical practice. Superior vena cava syndrome with malignant causes. *N Engl J Med*. 2007;356:1862–9.
- Yu JB, Wilson LD, Detterbeck FC. Superior vena cava syndrome—a proposed classification system and algorithm for management. *J Thorac Oncol*. 2008;3:811–4.

CODES

ICD9
459.2 Compression of vein

CLINICAL PEARLS
- Lung cancer is the leading cause of SVC syndrome; other leading malignant causes include lymphoma and metastatic breast cancer (2).
- Percutaneous stenting can provide immediate relief.
- Current treatment is disease-specific, so pathologic confirmation is vital.
- Radiotherapy mainly in non-small-cell lung cancer and non-Hodgkin lymphoma
- Chemotherapy for small-cell lung cancer and germ-cell tumors

SURGICAL COMPLICATIONS

Katherine Lang, MD
Mitchell A. Cahan, MD

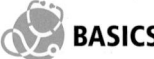 **BASICS**

DESCRIPTION
- Broadly defined: any negative outcome perceived either by surgeon or patient.
- A lack of consensus exists on how to define complications.
- Multiple classification systems exist based on severity.

EPIDEMIOLOGY
Incidence
Incidence of complications can vary with type of operation, operative time, hospital, surgeon, and patient characteristics amongst other factors.
- Mortality rate in general and vascular surgery patients is 3.5–6.9% (1).
- Overall complication rate in general and vascular surgery patients is 24.6–26.9% (1).
- Postoperative fever is very common. Incidence ranges widely (14–91%) depending on definition and patient population (2)
- 2000: ∼ 8.96 postoperative pulmonary emboluses per 1,000 surgical discharges in US (3)
- 2000: ∼ 2.057 postoperative abdominal wound dehiscences per 1,000 abdominopelvic surgeries in US (3)
- Surgical infection incidence varies with type of operation :
  – 1–2% clean operative site (e.g., hernia repair)
  – 5–15% clean contaminated (e.g., cholecystectomy)
  – 10–20% contaminated (e.g., colectomy)
  – 50% dirty operative site

RISK FACTORS
People at increased operative risk include those with:
- Poorly controlled diabetes
- Heart disease (especially recent MI and heart failure)
- Bleeding disorders
- Malnutrition
- Renal failure
- Liver disease
- Pulmonary disease
- Obesity
- Smoking history
- Immunosuppression
- Malignancy
  Other risk factors:
- Prolonged surgery
- Immobility following surgery
- Emergency surgery

Genetics
- Malignant hyperthermia:
  – Incidence: 1 in 50–100,000
  – Treated with dantrolene
- Bleeding disorders, including hemophilia

GENERAL PREVENTION
Preventive measures span entire perioperative period:
- Imaging to delineate anatomy and recognize aberrancy
- Appropriate fluid/blood resuscitation
- Assessment of underlying risk factors
- Preoperative antibiotics where appropriate
- Sterile technique
- Warming during surgery
- Clip hair instead of shaving preoperatively (4)[B]

PATHOPHYSIOLOGY
- Fever caused by pyrogens (mediated by IL-1): Bacteria, viruses, antigen-antibody complexes
- Wound dehiscence: Poor wound healing (malnutrition) or increased abdominal pressure
- Deep vein thrombosis: blood clot formation in deep vein attributed to 1 of 3 factors described in Virchow's triad;
  – Hypercoagulability
  – Hemodynamic changes (stasis, turbulence)
  – Endothelial injury/dysfunction
- Renal failure:
  – Drug toxicity (commonly antibiotics)
  – Inadequate resuscitation leading to poor perfusion (catecholamine release during surgery and activation of renin-angiotensin-aldosterone system) results in ATN.
- Respiratory:
  – Decreased vital capacity leads to atelectasis, pneumonitis, and ARDS.
  – Aspiration can occur at any time. Stomach acid/particulate matter cause an inflammatory reaction, leading to cyanosis or death.
  – Pulmonary edema due to fluid transudation to alveolus from fluid overload or heart failure.
  – Pulmonary mechanics are compromised postoperatively. Precipitating factors include pain and altered mental status.
- Cardiac:
  – Postoperative MI generally occurs within 3 days of surgery and is caused by anesthetics and blood loss (loss of as little as 500 cc can cause shock).
  – Arrhythmia is due to destabilization of cardiac membranes or prolongation of conduction.
- Small bowel obstruction: Intra-abdominal adhesive bands (scar tissue) can form and constrict the bowel, even decades after surgery.
- Urinary retention: Males affected more frequently than females, impaired coordination between α-receptors in the bladder neck and parasympathetic stimulation to the bladder

ETIOLOGY
- Fever in the first 24 hours is usually due to atelectasis. Consider the 5 Ws:
  – Wind—atelectasis, PNA, aspiration
  – Water—urinary tract infection
  – Walking—DVT
  – Wound—surgical site infection
  – Wonder drugs—drug fever
- *Staphylococcus aureus* is the most common cause of wound infection. Others include *Pseudomonas*, *Proteus*, and *Klebsiella*.
- Hematoma: Inadequate hemostasis/bleeding
- Seroma: Disruption of lymphatics
- Urinary tract infection: Related to indwelling catheter
- Dehiscence: Increased abdominal pressure, inadequate fascial closure, malnutrition, contamination, and chemotherapy are contributory.
- Renal failure: Hypovolemia, drug toxicity (commonly due to antibiotics or IV contrast).

- Respiratory: Volume overload, aspiration, and decreased vital capacity lead to decreased diffusion capacity. Pulmonary embolism formation another possible etiology postoperatively.
- Pulmonary embolism: Generally due to thromboembolism from the deep veins of the legs; more rarely from air, fat or amniotic fluid.
- Cardiac: Arrhythmia occurs due to electrolyte abnormalities, catecholamine release (from pain), hypercapnia, and digitalis.
- Small bowel obstruction: Adhesive bands (scar tissue) form intra-abdominally and can constrict the bowel; occurs remotely after abdominal surgery.
- Fistula/intestinal leak: Generally occurs at site of bowel anastomosis due to suture line breakdown
- Stomal complications:
  – More common in obese patients
  – Include fibrosis of bowel at stoma, necrosis, retraction, skin breakdown, and stomal stricture
  – Most complications are due to technical errors at time of operation.
- Urinary retention: Due to anesthetics

COMMONLY ASSOCIATED CONDITIONS
- Adrenal insufficiency when on chronic steroids preoperatively
- Liver failure in patients with preexisting disease
- Delirium tremens in alcoholics
- Thyroid storm in patients with undiagnosed hyperthyroidism
- Parotitis in the elderly
- Depression

Pediatric Considerations
Operative procedures can lead to severe anxiety in children, with lasting emotional disturbance in 20%, most pronounced in patients 1–2 years old.

Geriatric Considerations
90% of patients >65 experience depression after surgery, with activities of daily living impaired in 50%. Increased human contact to prevent withdrawal reduces symptoms.

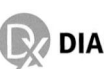 **DIAGNOSIS**

HISTORY
- Wound infection: History of surgery several days prior to presentation with pain, warmth, redness, or drainage at site of incision
- Expanding mass is consistent with seroma or hematoma. Hematoma more likely if surgery within 2–3 days; seroma more likely if interval longer.
- Dehiscence/hernia: Some patients feel sutures "pop." May complain of palpable bulge. Attributed to increased abdominal pressure (e.g., coughing, Valsalva maneuver).
- DVT: Pain, swelling, and redness of leg in immobilized patient or with hypercoagulability
- Renal failure: Oliguria or anuria, fatigue
- Pulmonary: Lack of incentive spirometry, narcotics, fluid retention, age >65, SOB, chest pain
- Cardiac: Elderly, cardiac dysfunction. Chest pain in 27% of perioperative MI (most pain-free).
- Ileus or small bowel obstruction: Progressive nausea, bilious vomiting, inability to tolerate p.o. intake, abdominal pain, cessation of flatus
- Fistula or intestinal leak: Severe abdominal pain (leak), fever, nausea/vomiting

- Stomal complications: Pain at stoma site, change in color of stoma
- Urinary retention: Inability to void, suprapubic pain

PHYSICAL EXAM
- Low fevers are not significant until 48 hours post-op. Wound infection is most common cause of fever after 72 hours.
- High fever, mental status changes, hypotension, and rigors are associated with severe wound complications or intestinal leak.
- Dolor, tumor, rubor, and calor may indicate a wound infection, as do pus or foul-smelling discharge. Patient may be febrile.
- Hematoma is an expanding, tender mass. Seroma is a slowly expanding, nontender mass.
- Dehiscence/hernia: Salmon-colored drainage post-op day 4–5, evisceration, or later as ventral hernia. May see open incision or palpable fascial edge, rarely tender.
- Renal failure: Persistent oliguria. Can have pericardial rub, bleeding/hematoma if uremic.
- Pulmonary: Dyspnea, cough, fever, basilar crackles, poor inspiratory effort, egophony, dullness to percussion at bases
- Cardiac: Peripheral edema, irregularly irregular heartbeat
- Ileus/small bowel obstruction: "Tinkling" or absent bowel sounds, tympanitic abdomen, tenderness to palpation, occasionally guarding
- Fistula/intestinal leak: Feces protruding from skin opening, acute or firm abdomen, fever, guarding, peritoneal signs, hypotension
- Stomal complications are evident when the ostomy appliance is removed: Skin irritation, black/discolored intestinal mucosa, retracted ostomy
- Urinary retention: Suprapubic pain, palpable bladder

DIAGNOSTIC TESTS & INTERPRETATION
Lab
Initial lab tests
- Elevated white blood cell count is seen in wound infections, atelectasis, pneumonia, infected hematoma/seroma, bowel leak, and stomal complications.
- Renal failure: Blood urea nitrogen (BUN), creatinine, urine chemistries and FE_{NA}
- Pulmonary: Hypoxia, hypercarbia on arterial blood gas (ABG)
- Cardiac: Elevated troponins, creatine kinase (CK), CK-MB
- Urinary tract infection: UA, urine culture and sensitivity
- DVT: D-dimer

Imaging
Initial approach
- Subcutaneous gas can be seen in necrotizing fasciitis on x-ray or CT
- CT or ultrasound can be used to diagnose hernia or fascial disruption.
- Small bowel obstruction/ileus: Upright abdominal film shows air-fluid levels, dilated small bowel. Transition point may be seen on CT.
- Fistula: Fistulogram aids in diagnosis, and is critical for treatment planning.
- Intestinal leak: Chest x-ray reveals free air under the diaphragm; CT shows fluid collection in abdomen.

- Bladder scan can help diagnose urinary retention if diagnosis in doubt.
- Duplex U/S to diagnose deep vein thrombosis
- Pulmonary: CXR, CT pulmonary angiography more sensitive test for suspected PE

Diagnostic Procedures/Surgery
- Exploratory laparotomy/laparoscopy if the patient is extremely ill or septic and diagnosis is unknown but abdominal cause is suspected
- Dehiscence is considered a surgical emergency.
- Intra-abdominal abscesses frequently can be drained percutaneously.
- Cardiac: EKG shows signs of ischemia or dysrhythmia.

 ## TREATMENT
MEDICATION
- Opiates for pain control
- Broad-spectrum antibiotics for sepsis or severe infection (piperacillin/tazobactam and vancomycin)
- Simple wound infections and stomal complications: 1st- or 2nd-generation cephalosporins
- Intestinal leak: Gram-negative and gram-positive coverage (levofloxacin and metronidazole)
- Pneumonia should be treated empirically with antibiotics to cover local flora.
- Cardiac complications can be avoided or treated with β-blockade for rate control.
- Urinary retention: α-blockers (tamsulosin)

ADDITIONAL TREATMENT
General Measures
- Antibiotics for infections
- Rate control for tachycardia
- Drain pathologic fluid collections.
- Repair hollow viscus injuries.
- Tamponade: Ligate or repair vessel for uncontrolled bleeding.

Issues for Referral
Organ injuries require consultation with their associated specialists (e.g., urology, gynecology), even when repaired by the surgeon at the time of injury.

SURGERY/OTHER PROCEDURES
- Wound infections may need surgical debridement if not responsive to antibiotics.
- Hematomas may need re-exploration and hemostasis if large and progressing.
- Dehiscence/hernia should be repaired. Evisceration is a surgical emergency.
- Small bowel obstruction that fails to resolve with nasogastric decompression should be explored; adhesions should be lysed.
- Intestinal leak is a surgical emergency for immediate exploration and repair. Fistulas generally need surgical intervention to resolve.
- Some stomal complications (necrosis, retraction) need surgical revision.

IN-PATIENT CONSIDERATIONS
Initial Stabilization
- Fluid resuscitation as needed
- Broad-spectrum antibiotics, if septic
- IV antibiotics for infections

Admission Criteria
- Need for IV fluids/antibiotics
- Need for surgical procedure
- Need for nasogastric (NG) decompression

Discharge Criteria
- Infection resolved/responding to antibiotics
- Able to tolerate p.o. intake
- Pain is under control.
- Patient has bowel function.

 ## ONGOING CARE
FOLLOW-UP RECOMMENDATIONS
Any complication should be evaluated by surgeon responsible when identified.

DIET
- n.p.o. for fistula, intestinal leak, or small bowel obstruction
- Diet as tolerated for other listed complications

PROGNOSIS
With appropriate treatment, most patients with complications return to baseline status.

REFERENCES

1. Ghaferi A, et al. *Variation in Hospital Mortality Associated with Inpatient Surgery. N Engl J Med* 2009;361:1368–75.
2. Pile JC, et al. Evaluating postoperative fever: a focused approach. *Cleve Clin J Med*. 2006; 73(Suppl 1):S62–6.
3. National Helathcare Quality Report, AHRQ, DHHS, 2003.
4. Tanner J, et al. Preoperative hair removal to reduce surgical site infection. [Systematic Review] *Cochrane Database of Systematic Reviews*. 3, 2006.

CODES
ICD9
- 998.11 Hemorrhage complicating a procedure
- 998.30 Disruption of wound, unspecified
- 998.59 Other postoperative infection

CLINICAL PEARLS
- Surgical site infections are decreased by clipping to remove hair rather than shaving.
- Appropriate antibacterial prep should be utilized to decrease bacterial counts.
- Amputation sites heal faster with plaster casting than with gauze. There is no difference in healing rates with foam vs gauze dressings, but patients prefer foam.
- Half of all wound infections are identified after the patient is discharged to home.
- Treatment of some complications related to hospitalization will no longer be reimbursed by payers, including wrong-site surgery and central venous catheter infections.

SYNCOPE

Santiago O. Valdes, MD
Ricardo A. Samson, MD

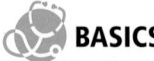 **BASICS**

DESCRIPTION
- Transient loss of consciousness characterized by unresponsiveness, loss of postural tone, and spontaneous recovery usually caused from cerebral hypoxemia
- System(s) affected: Cardiovascular; Nervous

EPIDEMIOLOGY
Incidence
- Up to 20% of adults will have ≥1 episode by age 75; 15% of children <18 years of age
- Accounts for 1–6% of hospital admissions and ~3% of emergency room visits

Prevalence
In institutionalized elderly (>75 years), 6%

RISK FACTORS
- Heart disease
- Dehydration
- Drugs:
  - Antihypertensives
  - Vasodilators (including calcium channel blockers, ACE inhibitors, and nitrates)
  - Phenothiazines
  - Antidepressants
  - Antiarrhythmics
  - Diuretics

Genetics
Specific cardiomyopathies and arrhythmias may be familial (i.e., long QT syndrome, hypertrophic cardiomyopathy).

GENERAL PREVENTION
See "Risk Factors."

PATHOPHYSIOLOGY
- Vagal response leads to decreased heart rate.
- Systemic hypotension secondary to decreased cardiac output and/or systemic vasodilation leads to drop in cerebral perfusion and resulting loss of consciousness.

ETIOLOGY
- Cardiac: Obstruction to outflow:
  - Aortic stenosis
  - Hypertrophic cardiomyopathy
  - Pulmonary embolus
  - Anomalous coronary artery origin
- Cardiac arrhythmias:
  - Sustained ventricular tachycardia (VT)
  - Supraventricular tachycardia (Atrial fibrillation, atrial flutter, re-entrant SVT)
  - 2nd- and 3rd-degree AV block
  - Sick-sinus syndrome
  - Pacing-induced infranodal block
  - H-V interval >100 m
- Noncardiac:
  - Reflex-mediated vasovagal (drop attack) (neurocardiogenic/neurally mediated), situational (micturition, defecation, cough)
  - Orthostatic hypotension
  - Drug-induced
  - Neurologic: Seizures; transient ischemic attack (can in theory cause syncope, but presentation usually markedly clinically different from pure syncope)
  - Carotid sinus hypersensitivity
  - Psychogenic

COMMONLY ASSOCIATED CONDITIONS
See "Etiology."

 DIAGNOSIS

HISTORY
- Careful history, physical exam, and an ECG are more important than other investigations in determining the diagnosis (1)[A].
  - Syncope associated with physical exertion suggests a potential cardiac etiology.
- Make sure that patient or witness (if present) is not talking about vertigo (i.e., sense of rotary motion, spinning, and whirling), coma, or drop attacks.
- After careful evaluation, including diagnostic procedures and special tests, the cause will be found in only 50–60% of the patients.
- Onset of syncope is usually rapid, and recovery is spontaneous, rapid, and complete. Duration of episodes are typically brief (<60 seconds). Presence of underlying cardiac or neurologic conditions provides key to diagnosis.

PHYSICAL EXAM
- Direct to BP and pulse, both lying and standing
- Check for cardiac murmur or focal neurologic abnormality.

DIAGNOSTIC TESTS & INTERPRETATION
History and physical examination should direct laboratory test ordered.

Lab
Initial lab tests
- CBC
- Electrolytes, BUN, creatinine, glucose, HCG
- Cardiac enzymes
- Rarely helpful: <2% have hyponatremia, hypocalcemia, hypoglycemia, or renal failure causing seizures.

Follow-Up & Special Considerations
- If history and physical suggest ischemic, valvular, or congenital heart disease:
  - ECG
  - Exercise stress test (if syncope with exertion)
  - Echocardiogram
  - Cardiac catheterization
- If CNS disease suspected:
  - EEG
  - Head CT scan
  - Head MRI/MRA when vascular cause is suspected
  - Do not order these tests unless there are hints of CNS disease on history or physical exam.
- ECG monitoring, either in hospital or ambulatory (Holter):
  - Useful in 4–15% of patients
  - Should be done in patients with heart disease or recurrent syncope
  - Arrhythmias frequently documented, but not always associated with syncope
- Electrophysiologic studies:
  - Have been positive in 18–75% of patients
  - Induction of VT and dysfunction of His-Purkinje system are the 2 most common abnormalities.
  - Should be done in patients with heart disease or recurrent syncope, although may not show whether arrhythmia noted or induced during study is cause of syncope
- Carotid hypersensitivity evaluation:
  - Carotid hypersensitivity should be considered in patients with syncope during head turning, especially while wearing tight collar, and with neck tumors and neck scars.
  - The technique is not standardized; 1 side massaged at a time for 20 seconds with constant monitoring of pulse and BP.
  - Atropine should be readily available.
- Tilt-table testing ± isoproterenol infusion:
  - Provocative test for vasovagal syncope
  - Perform if cardiac causes have been excluded; role in workup of patients with syncope of unknown origin
  - Not standardized but has been reported positive (symptomatic hypotension and bradycardia) in 26–87% of patients; also positive in 0–45% of control subjects
- Psychiatric evaluation: Anxiety, depression, and alcohol and drug abuse can be associated with syncope.

Imaging
- ECG
- Echocardiogram if clinically indicated

Initial approach
Lung scan or helical CT scan of thorax if history and physical exam suggest PE

Diagnostic Procedures/Surgery
Patient-activated implantable loop recorders can record 4–5 minutes of retrograde ECG rhythm. Helpful in recurrent syncope, with yield of 24–47%.

Pathological Findings
Depends on etiology and presence of underlying cardiac or neurologic conditions

DIFFERENTIAL DIAGNOSIS
- Drop attacks
- Coma
- Vertigo
- Seizure disorder

TREATMENT

Maintaining good hydration status and normal salt intake are initial therapy. Education of patients of the premonitory signs of syncope.

MEDICATION

First Line
- Geared toward specific underlying cardiac or neurologic abnormalities
- In cases of recurrent vasovagal/neurocardiogenic/neurally mediated syncope:
  – β-Adrenergic blockers
  – Mineralocorticoids (fludrocortisone)
  – α-Adrenergic agonists (midodrine)

Second Line
- SSRIs (paroxetine, sertraline, fluoxetine)
- Vagolytics (disopyramide)

ADDITIONAL TREATMENT

General Measures
- Patients with heart disease should be admitted to the hospital for evaluation.
- Elderly patients without previously recognized heart disease should be admitted if the physician thinks that the cause of syncope is likely cardiac.
- Patients without heart disease, especially young patients (<60 years old), can be worked up safely as outpatients.
- Prescribe antiarrhythmics for documented arrhythmias occurring simultaneously with syncope or symptoms of presyncope. Asymptomatic arrhythmias do not necessarily require treatment.
- The decision to treat patients on basis of arrhythmias or conduction abnormalities provoked or detected during EPS is even more problematic: Does the arrhythmia or conduction abnormality have anything to do with patient's symptoms?
- Most would treat patients with provoked sustained VT with an antiarrhythmic drug that suppressed arrhythmia during study.
- Rationale for such treatment: Recurrent syncope is less frequent in patients with positive EPS who are treated than it is in those who have negative EPS.

Issues for Referral
When cardiac or neurologic etiologies are suspected, appropriate expert consultation is indicated.

COMPLEMENTARY AND ALTERNATIVE MEDICINE
St. John's wort has been used in cases of recurrent noncardiac syncope.

SURGERY/OTHER PROCEDURES
- ICD placement for patients with cardiac conditions with high risk of sudden death and/or recurrent syncope on medications (i.e., long QT syndrome, hypertrophic cardiomyopathy)
- Many recommend pacemaker implantation in patients with
  – 2nd- (Mobitz type II) and 3rd-degree heart block
  – H-V intervals >100 m
  – Pacing-induced infranodal block
  – Sinus node recovery time ≥3 seconds

IN-PATIENT CONSIDERATIONS

Initial Stabilization
- Support ABCs.
- Stabilize heart rate and BP, typically with IV fluids.

Admission Criteria
Patients with heart disease should be admitted to the hospital for evaluation.

IV Fluids
Use isotonic crystalloids fluids for fluid resuscitation if needed.

Nursing
Close monitoring of BP, HR during initial presentation

Discharge Criteria
- Attainment of hemodynamic stability
- Satisfactory completion of workup for etiology
- Adequate control of specific arrhythmia or seizure, if present

ONGOING CARE

FOLLOW-UP RECOMMENDATIONS

Patient Monitoring
- Frequent follow-up visits for patients with cardiac causes of syncope, especially patients on antiarrhythmics
- Patients with an unknown cause of syncope rarely (5%) are diagnosed during the follow-up.

DIET
- No specific diet unless heart disease
- Increased fluid and salt intake to maintain intravascular volume in cases of recurrent vasovagal syncope

PATIENT EDUCATION
- Reassure patient that most cardiac causes of syncope can be treated, and patients with noncardiac causes do well, even if the cause of syncope is never discovered
- Physician and patient should carefully consider whether patient should continue to drive while syncope is being evaluated. Physicians should be aware of pertinent laws in their own state.

PROGNOSIS
- Cumulative mortality at 2 years:
  – Low (25%): Young patients (<60 years) with noncardiac or unknown cause of syncope
  – Intermediate (20%): Older patients (>60 years) with noncardiac or unknown cause of syncope
  – High (32–38%): Patients with cardiac cause of syncope
- Independent predictors of poor short-term outcomes:
  – Abnormal ECG
  – Shortness of breath
  – Systolic BP <90 mm Hg
  – Hematocrit <30%
  – CHF

COMPLICATIONS
- Trauma from falling
- Death (see "Prognosis")

REFERENCE

1. Kessler C, Tristano JM, De Lorenzo R, et al. The emergency department approach to syncope: evidence-based guidelines and prediction rules. *Emerg Med Clin North Am.* 2010;28:487–500.

ADDITIONAL READING

- European Heart Rhythm Association (EHRA); Heart Failure Association (HFA), et al. Guidelines for the diagnosis and management of syncope (version 2009): the Task Force for the Diagnosis and Management of Syncope of the European Society of Cardiology (ESC). *Eur Heart J.* 2009;30(21): 2631–71.
- Goble MM, Benitez C, Baumgardner M, et al. ED management of pediatric syncope: searching for a rationale. *Am J Emerg Med.* 2008;26:66–70.
- Kuriachan V, Sheldon RS, Platonov M. Evidence-based treatment for vasovagal syncope. *Heart Rhythm.* 2008;5:1609–14.
- Parry SW, Tan MP, et al. An approach to the evaluation and management of syncope in adults. *BMJ.* 2010;340:c880.
- Reed MJ, Newby DE, Coull AJ, et al. The ROSE (risk stratification of syncope in the emergency department) study. *J Am Coll Cardiol.* 2010;55: 713–21.
- Romme JJ, Reitsma JB, Go-Schön IK, et al. Prospective evaluation of non-pharmacological treatment in vasovagal syncope. *Europace.* 2010;12:567–73.
- Strickberger SA, Benson DW, Biaggioni I, et al. AHA/ACCF scientific statement on the evaluation of syncope: from the American Heart Association Councils on Clinical Cardiology, Cardiovascular Nursing, Cardiovascular Disease in the Young, and Stroke, and the Quality of Care and Outcomes Research Interdisciplinary Working Group; and the American College of Cardiology Foundation In Collaboration With the Heart Rhythm Society. *J Am Coll Cardiol.* 2006;47:473–84.

See Also (Topic, Algorithm, Electronic Media Element)
Aortic Valvular Stenosis; Atrial Septal Defect (ASD); Carotid Sinus Syndrome; Idiopathic Hypertrophic Subaortic Stenosis (IHSS); Patent Ductus Arteriosus; Pulmonary Arterial Hypertension, Idiopathic; Pulmonary Embolism; Seizure Disorders; Stokes-Adams Attacks
Algorithms: Syncope; Transient Ischemic Attack

CODES

ICD9
780.2 Syncope and collapse

CLINICAL PEARLS
- Careful history and physical is key to diagnosis.
- Use ECG/event-recorder to evaluate for cardiac conditions.
- True neurologic causes of syncope are very rare; cardiac causes by far more common.
- Fewer than 2% of cases are caused by hyponatremia, hypocalcemia, hypoglycemia, or renal failure causing seizures.

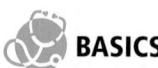

BASICS

Syncope is a reversible loss of consciousness and postural tone secondary to systemic hypotension and cerebral hypoperfusion due to vasodilation and/or bradycardia (rarely tachycardia) with spontaneous recovery and no neurologic sequelae.

DESCRIPTION
- Sudden, transient loss of consciousness characterized by unresponsiveness, falling, and spontaneous recovery
- Common cause of syncope in all age groups, especially in patients with no evidence of neurologic or cardiac disease
- 4 types: Vasovagal or neurocardiogenic syncope, carotid sinus syncope, situational syncope, and glossopharyngeal/trigeminal neuralgia syncope (uncommon) (1)

EPIDEMIOLOGY
- Syncope is common and has variable presentations and causes. Depending on underlying etiology, it may be associated with serious cardiovascular and cerebrovascular disease associated with increased morbidity/mortality.
- Mortality: Cardiac-related syncope 20-30% and 5% in idiopathic syncope
- Age: any age

Incidence
- Ranges from 7.5% in children <18 years of age and 15.18% in adults >70 years of age (1)
- 36–62% of all syncopal episodes

Prevalence
22% in the general population (1)

RISK FACTORS
- Low resting BP
- Age: Older age
- Prolonged supine position with resulting deconditioning of autonomic control
- Associated medical conditions: DM, cardiac disease (arrhythmia/structural abnormalities), seizures, ICH, panic attacks, hysteria, pulmonary decompensation

Genetics
- Vasovagal syncope: Strong heritable component to the etiology of over 20% of cases
- Orthostatic hypotension: Gene polymorphisms include:
  – Endothelin-1 gene (insertion variant in the 5'UTR)
  – B1-adrenergic receptor gene (polymorphism beta1Gly49)
  – Human norepinephrine transporter gene (polymorphism Ala457Pro)
  – Gs protein alpha-subunit (polymorphism T131C)
  – G-protein beta 3 subunit (polymorphism C825T)
  – SCNN1G gene encoding the gamma subunit of the amiloride-sensitive epithelial sodium channel
  – Presence of multiple point mutations in the mitochondrial DNA (mtDNA) in 3 families with orthostatic hypotension

GENERAL PREVENTION
Avoidance of precipitating events or situations. Optimization of DM control, elastic stockings, adequate hydration.

PATHOPHYSIOLOGY
Results from an abnormal interaction of the normal mechanisms for maintaining BP and upright posture:
- In normal individuals, upright posture results in venous pooling and transient decrease in BP.
- Neurally induced syncope may result from a cardioinhibitory response, a vasodepressor response, or a combination of the 2.
- Cardioinhibitory response results from increase in parasympathetic tone and may cause bradycardia.
- Vasodepressor response results from decrease in sympathetic tone and may cause hypotension (2).

ETIOLOGY
- Vasovagal syncope usually has a precipitating event or stimulus, often related to fright, pain, panic, or exercise.
- Carotid sinus stimulation is precipitated by position change, turning head, or wearing a tight collar. Neck tumors or surgical scarring may be implicated.
- Situational syncope is related to micturition, defecation, or coughing.
- Glossopharyngeal syncope is related to throat or facial pain (1,3).

Pregnancy Considerations
Vasovagal syncope occurs commonly in pregnancy when changing from supine to lateral decubitus or upright position (2).

COMMONLY ASSOCIATED CONDITIONS
- Cardiopulmonary disorders: CHF, MI, arrhythmias, HOCM, AS, pulmonary HTN, PE
- Neurologic disorders: Autonomic dysfunction, Shy-Drager, PD, MSA, TIA, VBI, PN
- Psychiatric disorders:
  – Generalized anxiety disorder
  – Panic disorder
  – Major depression
  – Alcohol dependence (3)

DIAGNOSIS

Diagnosis is based on history and physical with diagnostic testing done based on the HPI.

HISTORY
- Evaluation of syncope and presyncope are the same.
- Important first to rule out cardiac syncope
- Neurally mediated syncope is predicted by a history of blurred vision, palpitations, nausea, warmth, diaphoresis, or lightheadedness before syncope, or by history of nausea, warmth, diaphoresis, or fatigue after syncope (4).
- Vasovagal syncope has 3 phases:
  – Prodrome
  – Loss of consciousness
  – Postsyncope
- For vasovagal syncope, a precipitating event or stimulus is usually identified and can be related to panic, fright, pain, or exercise. Syncope may be avoided with removal of stimulus or position change.
- Vasovagal syncope can be seen in athletes after exertion (diagnosis of exclusion).
- Position: Vasovagal syncope can be preceded by prolonged standing but can occur from any position; generally resolves when the patient becomes supine:
  – Preceding events: As discussed above
  – Prodrome: May occur without warning but generally preceded by feelings of lightheadedness, nausea, vomiting, diaphoresis, blurred vision, headaches, palpitations, paresthesias, or pallor
- Duration: Generally brief (seconds–minutes), resolves in supine position
- Recovery: May be prolonged with persistent nausea, pallor, and diaphoresis but without neurologic change or confusion
- Carotid sinus syncope is precipitated by position change, after turning head, or wearing a tight collar.
- Situational syncope is related to micturition, defecation, or coughing.
- Glossopharyngeal syncope (less common) is related to throat or facial pain (1,3).
- Precipitating events or situations may include panic, pain, exercise, micturition, defecation, coughing, or swallowing.

PHYSICAL EXAM
- Vital signs including orthostatic and bilateral BP
- Cardiac exam: Volume status, murmurs, rhythm, carotid bruits
- Neurologic exam: Signs of focal deficit
- Assess for occult blood loss.

DIAGNOSTIC TESTS & INTERPRETATION
Based on the history, a battery of tests can be done to find the underlying cause and to rule out other causes of syncope.

Lab
Includes basic tests to rule out the 3 main reasons for syncope: Hypoglycemia, arrhythmia, and anemia.

Initial lab tests
- Blood sugar
- ECG should be ordered for all patients (3). Abnormal ECG findings are rare in patients with neurally mediated syncope but common in patients with cardiac syncope.
- CBC to rule out anemia

Follow-Up & Special Considerations
- 24-hour Holter monitoring, only in patients with a high probability of cardiac cause of syncope and/or abnormal EKG findings
- A low hemoglobin without obvious cause of bleed would warrant a guaiac, CT abdomen, CT head to rule out retroperitoneal bleed, SAH.

Imaging
Head CT, MRI/MRA, carotid ultrasound only in patients whose history or physical exam suggests a neurologic cause of syncope

Follow-Up & Special Considerations
- Negative imaging will prompt workup for alternative causes.
- Stroke, bleed, or carotid stenosis will require appropriate disease-oriented management.
- EEG only when history or physical exam is very suggestive of seizure activity

Diagnostic Procedures/Surgery
- Head-up tilt-table testing:
  - Contraindicated in patients with known cardiac or neurovascular disease or in pregnancy
  - Indicated for recurrent syncope or single episode accompanied by injury or risk to others (e.g., pilots, surgeons, etc.)
  - Uses positional changes to reproduce symptoms
  - Positive tests are diagnostic for vasovagal syncope.
- Carotid sinus massage, only in a monitored setting (i.e., BP and HR monitoring, IV access):
  - Contraindicated in patients with carotid disease (careful auscultation prior to massage is essential)
  - Pressure at the angle of the jaw for 5 seconds with simultaneous ECG monitoring
  - Positive tests (causing syncope or cardiac pause >3 s) are diagnostic of carotid sinus syncope.
- Psychiatric evaluation: Anxiety, depression, and alcohol abuse are commonly associated with syncope.

DIFFERENTIAL DIAGNOSIS
- Seizure
- Hypoglycemia
- Cardiac syncope
- Cerebrovascular syncope
- Orthostatic hypotension
- Drop attacks
- Psychiatric illness

 TREATMENT

Therapy is primarily aimed at patients with recurrent syncope. Situational syncope will not warrant any treatment. Treatment is imperative for patients in high-risk settings (pilot, commercial vehicle driver) who wish to continue in their current activities. Additionally, they may require restriction of their activities until therapy is effective.

MEDICATION
Medical management of syncope is based on small nonrandomized clinical trials and is hampered by the unpredictable nature of syncopal episodes. Drug of choice is based on patient's age and comorbidities while taking into account the safety and side effects of each agent.

First Line
- Nonpharmacologic treatment:
  - Includes patient counseling:
    - Development of coping skills
    - Increased salt and fluid intake
  - Moderate exercise training
  - Tilt-table training
- Pharmacologic treatment: β-Blockers:
  - Block peripheral vasodilators and ventricular mechanoreceptor stimulation
  - Stabilization of HR and BP
  - Adverse effects include hypotension and bradycardia, and actually may worsen syncope.
  - Contraindicated in asthma

Second Line
- α-Agonists: Increase peripheral vascular resistance and increase venous return
- SSRIs:
  - Serotonin has been shown to induce vagally mediated bradycardia and hypotension.
  - Side effects include weight gain, nausea, sexual dysfunction, and insomnia.

- Mineralocorticoids:
  - May be helpful in salt retention and maintaining volume status
  - Adverse reactions include fluid retention, HTN, CHF, and hypokalemia.
- Anticholinergics:
  - Decrease vagal tone
  - Side effects include dry mouth, constipation, urinary retention, and blurred vision (2,3).

ADDITIONAL TREATMENT
General Measures
Recognition and avoidance of precipitating events or situations

Issues for Referral
Neurology or cardiology as needed

Additional Therapies
- Increased salt and fluid intake: May include salt tablets or electrolyte/sports drinks
- Moderate exercise training
- Tilt-table training: Involves periods of prolonged, forced upright posture
- Use of support/pressure stockings
- Leg crossing, hand grip, or arm tensing
- Clonazepam may be effective in refractory neurally mediated syncope (5,6).

SURGERY/OTHER PROCEDURES
Pacemaker placement may be of use in patients with frequent cardioinhibitory syncope or mixed carotid sinus syncope (class I–II, level B) (2,3):
- Prevents prolonged bradycardia
- Long-term effect
- Invasive placement procedure (2,3)

IN-PATIENT CONSIDERATIONS
Initial Stabilization
IV fluids to stabilize HR and BP

Admission Criteria
- Suspected or known cardiac or neurologic disease
- ECG abnormalities
- Syncope occurring during exercise
- Syncope causing severe injury
- Family history of sudden death (3)

IV Fluids
Isotonic crystalloids as needed

Nursing
Vital sign monitoring

Discharge Criteria
Hemodynamically stable and workup satisfactory

 ONGOING CARE

DIET
- Increased salt intake may be helpful if not contraindicated (2).
- Maintain fluid intake.

PATIENT EDUCATION
- Patients should be taught to identify and avoid precipitating events or situations.
- Avoid dehydration, alcohol consumption, warm environments, tight clothing, and long periods of standing motionless.
- Recognize presyncopal symptoms.
- Use behaviors, such as lying down, to avoid syncope.

PROGNOSIS
May be recurrent but not life-threatening

COMPLICATIONS
May result in injury from fall

REFERENCES
1. Chen-Scarabelli C, et al. Neurocardiogenic syncope. Br Med J. 2004;329:336.
2. Nair N, et al. Pathophysiology and management of neurocardiogenic syncope. Am J Managed Care. 2003;9:327–34.
3. Miller TH, Kruse JE. Evaluation of syncope. Am Fam Physician. 2005;72:1492–500.
4. Chen LY, Benditt DG, Shen WK. Management of syncope in adults: an update. Mayo Clin Proc. 2008;83:1280–93.
5. Kadri NN, Hee TT, Rovang KS, et al. Efficacy and safety of clonazepam in refractory neurally mediated syncope. Pacing Clin Electrophysiol. 1999;22:307–14.
6. Márquez MF, Urias-Medina K, Gómez-Flores J, et al. [Comparison of metoprolol vs clonazepam as a first treatment choice among patients with neurocardiogenic syncope] Gac Med Mex. 2008; 144:503–7.

ADDITIONAL READING
- Lelonek M, et al. [Genetics in neurocardiogenic syncope] Prz. Lek. 2006;63:1310–2.
- Sutton R, Brignole M, Benditt D, Moya A, et al. The Diagnosis and Management of Syncope. Current hypertension reports. 2010;

See Also (Topic, Algorithm, Electronic Media Element)
Algorithms: Syncope; Transient Ischemic Attack

 CODES

ICD9
- 337.01 Carotid sinus syndrome
- 780.2 Syncope and collapse

CLINICAL PEARLS
- History should include a careful analysis of the events preceding the attack.
- It is important to rule out cardiologic or neurologic pathology.
- Prodrome is often present.
- Recovery may be prolonged, with persistent symptoms but no neurologic deficit or confusion.
- Patient counseling to avoid precipitating situations or events is 1st-line treatment.

SYNOVITIS PIGMENTED VILLONODULAR

J. Herbert Stevenson, MD
Darius Greenbacher, MD

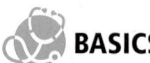 **BASICS**

DESCRIPTION
- Pigmented villonodular synovitis (PVNS) is a condition of the synovial membrane that is characterized by the presence of inflammation and hemosiderin deposition in the synovium.
- 2 forms of PVNS exist: Diffuse (DPVNS) and localized (LPVNS).

EPIDEMIOLOGY
Incidence
- 1.8/1 million population
- Predominant age: 20–45 years
- Predominant sex: Male = Female

Geriatric Considerations
Rare but has been documented

Pediatric Considerations
Rare but has been documented

RISK FACTORS
Genetics
No genetic predisposition

PATHOPHYSIOLOGY
- Histologically, LPVNS and DPVNS are similar.
  - Lipid-laden macrophages
  - Multinucleated giant cells
  - Hemosiderin deposition in the synovium
  - Stromal and fibroblast cell proliferation
- DPVNS and LPVNS differ in their disease course.
  - DPVNS:
    ○ Characterized by involvement of most or all of the joint synovium
    ○ More common
    ○ More rapidly destructive course with poorer prognosis
    ○ Can encroach on major neurovascular structures
    ○ Higher occurrence rate
    ○ Continued inflammation and joint erosions lead to articular cartilage destruction and subsequent osteoarthritis.

- LPVNS:
  ○ Characterized by a pedunculated, lobular lesion localized to 1 area of the synovium
  ○ Favorable prognosis secondary to its localized nature
  ○ Low recurrence rate following surgical intervention

ETIOLOGY
- Still largely unknown
- Possibly the result of trauma and subsequent recurrent local hemorrhage in the affected joint: <1/3 of patients report a history of trauma.
- Possibly secondary to abnormal local metabolic activity
- Possibly a neoplastic process with rare reports of malignant transformation and metastasis:
  - Demonstrates neither cellular atypia nor abnormal mitotic activity
  - Exhibits some cytogenetic abnormalities
- Possibly a chronic inflammation process

 DIAGNOSIS

HISTORY
- Slow and insidious onset of pain, swelling, and stillness
- History of locking, catching, or instability is more common with LPVNS.
- Recurrent joint effusion
- Symptoms are often intermittent.
- Typically a monarticular process that often involves the large joints
- Knee is involved most commonly.
- Hip, ankle, shoulder, and elbow also are possibilities.

PHYSICAL EXAM
- Tenderness to palpation of involved joint
- Joint effusion
- Loss of range of motion

DIAGNOSTIC TESTS & INTERPRETATION
Lab
Initial lab tests
- Erythrocyte sedimentation rate (ESR), C-reactive protein (CRP), antinuclear antibody (ANA), rheumatoid factor (RF)
- Complete blood count (CBC)
- Uric acid
- Joint fluid analysis

Imaging
Initial approach
- Plain radiographs:
  - Periarticular erosions with thin rim of reactive bone
  - Reciprocal bony lesions on opposite sides of the joint
  - Joint space narrowing is a late finding.
  - Most cases have no findings.
- CT scan:
  - Appears as a soft tissue mass of high density
  - Underlying bone erosions or cysts
- MRI:
  - Modality of choice (1)[A]
  - Helpful for determining the extent of disease and differentiation DPVNS from LPVNS
  - DPVNS:
    ○ Poorly localized mass or synovial thickening with varying degrees of periarticular erosions
    ○ Low signal on T_1- and T_2-weighted images
    ○ Joint effusion
  - LPVNS:
    ○ Periarticular or synovial nodular mass with varying degrees of bone erosion
    ○ High hemosiderin content causes low signal on T_1- and T_2-weighted images.
    ○ Joint effusion

Diagnostic Procedures/Surgery
Synovial fluid aspiration:
- Brownish-stained bloody fluid is indicative of PVNS.
- Lacks sensitivity and specificity

Pathological Findings
See "Pathophysiology."

DIFFERENTIAL DIAGNOSIS
- Rheumatoid arthritis
- Osteoarthritis
- Synovial sarcoma
- Hemophilia
- Lipoma arborescens
- Hematoma
- Hemangioma
- Giant cell tumor of the tendon sheath
- Avascular necrosis
- Systemic lupus erythematosus (SLE)
- Gout

 TREATMENT

ADDITIONAL TREATMENT
General Measures
- The goal is to eradicate all abnormal synovial tissue, thus removing the source of pain and reducing the risk of joint destruction and recurrence.
- The treatment of PVNS is largely surgical.

Additional Therapies
Tumor necrosis factor α (TNF-α) blockade (2,3)[C]:

- Imatinib may be beneficial in nonsurgical candidates and in relapsing cases (still being studied).
- Etanercept also is being studied for nonsurgical candidates.

SURGERY/OTHER PROCEDURES
Radiotherapy:

- An alternative to surgical synovectomy
- Serious potential complications:
  - Skin reactions
  - Poor wound healing
  - Joint stiffness
  - Sarcomatous transformation
- Highly useful in managing refractory cases or in those with extensive extraarticular involvement (4)[B]
- May be used as an adjuvant to surgical synovectomy, especially in challenging cases with persistently recurrent disease and involvement of critical anatomic structures (4)[B]
- The mainstay of treatment (5)[A]
- Arthroscopy has been associated with better functional results and lower rates of postoperative stiffness than have open techniques.
- Arthroscopic partial synovectomy is the standard care for LPVNS. Recurrence is rare after limited local treatment of LPVNS.
- Arthroscopic treatment of DPVNS is associated with a significantly higher recurrence rate.

- Patients with large popliteal masses or extraarticular involvement generally are not candidates for an exclusively arthroscopic approach.
- A thorough, complete synovectomy is the treatment of choice for DPVNS.
  - This is most easily accomplished through an open surgical procedure.
  - A combined arthroscopic and open approach is also a commonly used alternative.
- Joint replacement is indicated in patients with significant joint destruction.

IN-PATIENT CONSIDERATIONS
Primarily treated as outpatient with surgery

 ONGOING CARE

FOLLOW-UP RECOMMENDATIONS
Close follow-up for recurrence and progression of disease

DIET
No restrictions

PROGNOSIS
- Patients presenting with recurrent disease have much more extensive involvement and a poorer likelihood of successful treatment.
- DPVNS is more rapidly destructive and has a poorer prognosis.
- Recurrence rates after adequate synovectomy are in the range of 5–20%.
  - Rates are higher with DPVNS.
  - Rates are also increased with extraarticular involvement.
- Articular cartilage destruction and the development of osteoarthritis require joint replacement surgery.
- Malignant transformation has been reported but is exceedingly rare.
- Extensive joint involvement and extraarticular spread may result after failed arthroscopic management.
- Postoperative stiffness occurs in ~25% of patients treated with an open procedure.

COMPLICATIONS
- Surrounding bony erosion and tissue damage
- Spread to areas outside of joint
- Recurrence leading to joint replacement

REFERENCES

1. Frick MA, Wenger DE, Adkins M. MR imaging of synovial disorders of the knee: an update. *Radiologic Clinics of North America*. 2007;45(6):1017–31, vii.
2. Blay JY, El Sayadi H, Thiesse P, et al. Complete response to imatinib in relapsing pigmentedvillonodularsynovitis/tenosynovial giant cell tumor (PVNS/TGCT). *Annals of Oncology*. 2008;19(4):821–2.

3. Fiocco U, Sfriso P, Oliviero F, et al. [Intra-articular treatment with the TNF-alpha antagonist, etanercept, in severe diffuse pigmentedvillonodularsynovitis of the knee]. *Reumatismo*. 2006;58(4):268–74.
4. Berger B, Ganswindt U, Bamberg M, et al. External beam radiotherapy as postoperative treatment of diffuse pigmentedvillonodularsynovitis. *International Journal of Radiation Oncology, Biology, Physics*. 2007;67(4):1130–4.
5. Dines JS, DeBerardino TM, Wells JL, et al. Long-term follow-up of surgically treated localized pigmentedvillonodularsynovitis of the knee. *Arthroscopy*. 2007;23(9):930–7.

ADDITIONAL READING

- Adelani MA, Wupperman RM, Holt GE. Benign synovial disorders. *Journal of the American Academy of Orthopaedic Surgeons*. 2008;16(5):268–75.
- Al-Nakshabandi NA, Ryan AG, Choudur H, et al. Pigmented villonodular synovitis. *Clin Radiol*. 2004;59:414–20.
- Tyler WK, Vidal AF, Williams RJ, et al. Pigmented villonodular synovitis. *J Am Acad Orthopaed Surg*. 2006;14:376–85.

 CODES

ICD9
719.20 Villonodular synovitis, site unspecified

CLINICAL PEARLS

- Relatively rare condition of synovial membrane characterized by inflammation and hemosiderin deposition; etiology is unknown.
- Most frequently occurs in 3rd and 4th decades of life
- Slow insidious onset with chronic intermittent joint swelling and effusion; knee most commonly involved joint
- MRI is diagnostic modality of choice.
- Surgery is mainstay of treatment, with refractory cases responding to adjunctive radiotherapy.

SYPHILIS

Peter J. Ziemkowski, MD

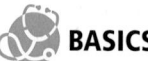 **BASICS**

DESCRIPTION
- A chronic, systemic infectious disease caused by *Treponema pallidum*
- Transmitted sexually, maternal–fetal, and via blood transfusions
- Untreated disease progresses through 4 stages: Primary, secondary (both symptomatic), latent (asymptomatic), and tertiary (late sequelae).
  - Primary: Usually single painless chancre at point of entry; appears in 10–90 days; heals without treatment in 3–6 weeks
  - Secondary: Rash on palms or soles of feet, headache, fever, adenopathy
  - Latent: Seroreactive without evidence of disease:
    - Early latent: Acquired within the last year
    - Late latent or latent of unknown duration: Exposure >12 months prior to diagnosis
  - Tertiary (late): Serology may be negative.
    - Damage to multiple systems: Cardiovascular, CNS, and musculoskeletal
    - Causes gait disturbances (tabes dorsalis) and dementia (general paresis)
    - May result in death
- Ability to affect nearly every organ/tissue in the body has led to it being called "the great imitator."

Pediatric Considerations
In noncongenital cases, consider child abuse.

Pregnancy Considerations
- All pregnant patients should have VDRL or RPR test at 1st prenatal visit (1). If high exposure risk, repeat the tests at 28 weeks and at delivery.
- The same nontreponemal test for initial diagnosis also should be used for follow-up tests.

EPIDEMIOLOGY
Incidence
- Syphilis rate decreased until 2000, increasing primarily in men since then (2).
- In 2007: 3.8/100,000 population (an increase of 17.5% from 2006)
  - White, non-Hispanic: 2.0/100,000
  - African American: 14.0/100,000
  - Hispanic: 4.3/100,000
  - Asian/Pacific Islander: 1.2/100,000
  - American Indian/Alaska native: 4.3/100,000
  - Highest in women aged 20–24 years and men aged 25–29 years
    - Men: 6.6/100,000
    - Women : 1.1/100,000
  - Congenital: 10.5 cases/100,000 live births

Prevalence
- Predominant sex: Male > Female (6.0:1)
- Increasing male:female ratio (was 1.2:1 in 1996) suggests greatest syphilis increase in men having sex with men.

RISK FACTORS
- Men having sex with men
- Multiple sexual partners
- Exposure to infected body fluids
- IV drug use
- Transplacental transmission
- Inmates at adult correctional facilities
- High-risk sexual behavior

GENERAL PREVENTION
- Educate patient about safe sex and the use of condoms; condoms reduce but do not eliminate transmission (3)[A].
- Provide educational materials to patients about sexually transmitted diseases (STDs).

ETIOLOGY
Treponema pallidum subspecies *pallidum*, spirochete

COMMONLY ASSOCIATED CONDITIONS
- HIV infection
- Hepatitis B
- Other STDs

 DIAGNOSIS

HISTORY
Previous sexual contact with partner with known infection or partner with high-risk sexual behavior

PHYSICAL EXAM
Signs/symptoms depend on stage:
- Primary: Single (occasionally multiple), usually painless ulcer (chancre) in groin or at other point of entry
- Secondary:
  - Rash: Skin or mucous membranes
    - Rough red–brown macules, usually on palms and soles
    - May appear with chancre or after it has healed
  - Nonspecific symptoms: Fever, adenopathy, malaise, headache

DIAGNOSTIC TESTS & INTERPRETATION
Lab
Initial lab tests
- Dark-field microscopy demonstrating *T. pallidum* spirochetes in lesion exudate or tissue biopsy: Gold standard for diagnosis, although difficult to perform and not very sensitive
- Nontreponemal tests (VDRL or RPR):
  - Primary screening test: Positive within 7 days of exposure
  - Nonspecific, false-positive results common; must confirm diagnosis with treponemal tests
  - Positive test should be quantified and titers followed at regular intervals after treatment (4).
    - Titers usually correlate with disease activity. 4-fold change demonstrates clinical significant difference (4).
    - Titer decreases with time or treatment; following adequate treatment for primary or secondary, a 4-fold decline should be noted after 6 months.
    - Absence of 4-fold decline indicates failure of treatment.
    - Titers eventually should be negative (see "Serofast reaction" below).
    - Titers of patients treated in latent stages decline gradually.
  - Prozone phenomenon: Negative results owing to high titers of antibody; test diluted serum.
  - Serofast reaction: Persistently positive results years after successful treatment; new infection diagnosed by 4-fold rise in titer
  - Disorders that may alter lab results:
    - Pregnancy
    - Autoimmune disease
    - Systemic lupus erythematosus
    - Mononucleosis
    - Malaria
    - Leprosy
    - Viral pneumonia
    - Presence of cardiolipin antigens
    - Drug addiction
    - Acute febrile illness
    - HIV infection
    - Elderly can have false-positive results.
- Treponemal tests (confirmatory test after positive nontreponemal screening test): FTA-ABS, TP-PA:
  - FTA-ABS (fluorescent treponemal antibody absorbed), TP-PA (*T. pallidum* particle agglutination)
  - Confirmatory test; not used for screening
  - Usually positive for life after treatment
  - Titers of no benefit
  - 15–25% of patients treated during the primary stage revert to being serologically nonreactive after 2–3 years.
- Lumbar puncture:
  - Indicated for any patient who has clinical evidence of neurologic involvement or has syphilitic ocular or auditory manifestations
  - Some experts advise in all secondary and early latent cases without neurologic symptoms
  - In HIV-positive patients with late latent or latent of unknown duration
  - In late latent or latent of unknown duration or when nonpenicillin therapy is planned
  - In treatment failures
  - If other evidence of active syphilis is present (e.g., aortitis, gumma, iritis)
  - In children with syphilis, after the newborn period, to rule out neurosyphilis
  - VDRL, not RPR, used on CSF; may be negative in neurosyphilis; highly specific but insensitive
  - Send fluid for protein, glucose, and cell count.
  - Monitor resolution by cell count at 6 months along with serologies as recommended (see "Patient Monitoring").
  - Negative FTA-ABS or MHA-TP on CSF excludes neurosyphilis (highly sensitive).
  - Positive FTA-ABS or MHA-TP on CSF not diagnostic because of high false-positive rate
  - Bloody tap, tuberculosis (TB), pyogenic or aseptic meningitis can result in false-positive VDRL.

DIFFERENTIAL DIAGNOSIS
- Primary:
  - Chancroid
  - Lymphogranuloma venereum
  - Granuloma inguinale
  - Condyloma acuminata
  - Herpes simplex
  - Behçet syndrome
  - Trauma
  - Carcinoma
  - Mycotic infection
  - Lichen planus
  - Psoriasis
  - Fungal infection
- Secondary:
  - Pityriasis rosea
  - Drug eruption
  - Psoriasis
  - Lichen planus
  - Viral exanthema
  - Stevens-Johnson syndrome
- Positive serology, asymptomatic:
  - Previously treated syphilis
  - Other spirochetal disease (yaws, pinta)

S

TREATMENT

MEDICATION

Parenteral penicillin G is drug of choice for all stages (4)[A]. Choice of formulation is determined by the disease stage and clinical manifestations.

ALERT

- Bicillin L-A should be used and *not* Bicillin C-R (combination benzathine–procaine penicillin) when penicillin G benzathine is indicated (5)[A].
- Primary, secondary, and early latent <1 year:
  - Benzathine penicillin G, 2.4 million units IM for 1 dose (4)[A]
  - Penicillin-allergic patients: Doxycycline, 100 mg PO b.i.d. × 2 weeks, or tetracycline, 500 mg PO q.i.d. × 2 weeks, or ceftriaxone, 1 g IM or IV daily × 8–10 days
- Late latent or latent of unknown duration and tertiary without evidence of neurosyphilis:
  - Benzathine penicillin G, 2.4 million units IM weekly × 3 doses (4)[A]
  - Penicillin-allergic patients: Attempt desensitization and treatment with penicillin; doxycycline, 100 mg PO 2 b.i.d. × 28 days, or tetracycline, 500 mg PO × 28 days; compliance may be an issue.
- Neurosyphilis:
  - Aqueous crystalline penicillin G, 3–4 million units IV q4h or continuous infusion × 10–14 days
  - Procaine penicillin G, 2.4 million units IM daily in conjunction with probenecid, 500 mg PO q.i.d. × 10–14 days (if compliance can be ensured) (4)[A]
  - Penicillin-allergic patients: Attempt desensitization and treat with penicillin; ceftriaxone, 2 g/day IM or IV × 14 days
  - If late latent, latent of unknown duration, or tertiary in addition to neurosyphilis, consider also treating as recommended for late latent after completion of neurosyphilis treatment.
- Congenital:
  - Aqueous crystalline penicillin G, 50,000 units/kg/dose IV q12h × 1st 7 days of life and q8hs thereafter for a total of 10 days, or procaine penicillin G, 50,000 units/kg/dose IM daily × 10 days (4)[A]
  - If negative CSF serologies, normal physical exam, and titer: Maternal titer; then 50,000 units/kg benzathine penicillin G IM in single dose is also alternative (4)[A].
  - If >1 day of drug is missed, restart course.
  - Children (after newborn period): Aqueous crystalline penicillin G, 50,000 units/kg/dose IV q4–6h × 10 days; late latent, [MJB2] 50,000 units/kg IM as 3 doses at 1-week intervals (4)[A]
  - Epidemiologic treatment for contacts without symptoms: Treat as primary after serologies.
  - Contraindications: Allergy to penicillin
  - HIV-infected and pregnant patients may show poor response to recommended IM doses. Use IV therapy for all treatment failures in these patients.
  - Do not give benzathine or procaine penicillins IV.
- Children (after newborn period): Aqueous crystalline penicillin G, 50,000 units/kg/dose IV q4–6h × 10 days; late latent, [MJB2] 50,000 units/kg IM as 3 doses at 1-week intervals (4)[A]
- Pregnancy:
  - Treatment same as for nonpregnant patients
  - Some specialists recommend 2nd dose of 2.4 million units benzathine penicillin G 1 week after initial dose in 3rd trimester or with primary, secondary, or early latent syphilis.
  - Penicillin sensitivity: No proven alternatives to penicillin exist for treatment during pregnancy; consider desensitization and treatment with penicillin (4)[A].
  - Epidemiologic treatment for contacts without symptoms: Treat as primary after serologies.
  - Contraindications: Allergy to penicillin
  - HIV-infected and pregnant patients may show poor response to recommended IM doses. Use IV therapy for all treatment failures in these patients.
  - Do not give benzathine or procaine penicillins IV.
- Epidemiologic treatment for contacts without symptoms: Treat as primary after serologies.
- Contraindications: Allergy to penicillin
- Precautions:
  - HIV-infected and pregnant patients may show poor response to recommended IM doses. Use IV therapy for all treatment failures in these patients.
  - Do not give benzathine or procaine penicillins IV.

ADDITIONAL TREATMENT

General Measures

- Advise patients to avoid intercourse until treatment is complete.
- Advise patients to keep track of sexual partners.

ONGOING CARE

FOLLOW-UP RECOMMENDATIONS

Repeat serologies at 3, 6, 9, and 12 months after treatment; if >1 year's duration, check at 24 months also.

Patient Monitoring

- Use VDRL or RPR test to monitor therapy: 4-fold rise in titer indicates new infection, whereas failure to decrease 4-fold in 6 months is considered treatment failure (although definitive criteria for cure not established); titers not consistent between tests; always use same test, preferably same lab, as initially performed.
- Retreat for persistent clinical signs or recurrence, 4-fold rise in titers, or failure of initially high titer to decrease 4-fold by 6 months.
- Labs titer tests to final end point (e.g., not report as ">1:512") to make best use of results in monitoring therapy response

PATIENT EDUCATION

No sexual contacts until 4-fold titer drop

PROGNOSIS

- Excellent in all cases except patients with late-syphilis complications and with HIV infection
- Syphilis in HIV-infected patient:
  - Treatment same as for HIV-negative patients
  - More often false-negative treponemal and nontreponemal tests or unusually high titers
  - Response to therapy less predictable
  - Early syphilis: Increased risk of neurosyphilis and higher rates of treatment failure

- Neurosyphilis: Harder to treat; can occur up to 20 years after infection

COMPLICATIONS

- Cardiovascular
- Membranous glomerulonephritis
- Paroxysmal cold hemoglobinemia
- Meningitis and tabes dorsalis
- Irreversible organ damage
- Jarisch-Herxheimer reaction:
  - Fever, chills, headache, myalgias, new rash
  - Common when starting treatment (of primary or secondary disease; less common with tertiary) owing to lysis of treponemes
  - Should not be confused with drug reaction
  - Managed with analgesics and antipyretics

REFERENCES

1. U.S. Preventive Services Task Force. Screening for syphilis infection in pregnancy: U.S. Preventive Services Task Force reaffirmation recommendation statement. *Ann Intern Med*. 2009;150:705–9.
2. Centers for Disease Control and Prevention. *Sexually Transmitted Disease Surveillance 2007 Supplement, Syphilis Surveillance Report*. Atlanta, GA: U.S. Department of Health and Human Services, Centers for Disease Control and Prevention, March 2009.
3. Koss CA, Dunne EF, Warner L, et al. A systematic review of epidemiologic studies assessing condom use and risk of syphilis. *Sex Transm Dis*. 2009;36: 401–5.
4. CDC Sexually Transmitted Diseases Treatment Guidelines, 2006. *MMWR Weekly*. 2006; 55(RR-11):22–34.
5. Calonge N, U.S. Preventive Services Task Force. Screening for syphilis infection: recommendation statement. *Ann Fam Med*. 2004;2:362–5.

ADDITIONAL READING

- Blank LJ, Rompalo AM, Erbelding EJ, et al. Treatment of syphilis in HIV-infected subjects: a systematic review of the literature. *Sexually transmitted infections*. 2010;
- Drugs for Sexually Transmitted Infections. *Treat Guide Med Letter*. 2007;5(61):81–8.
- Farhi D, Dupin N, et al. Management of syphilis in the HIV-infected patient: facts and controversies. *Clin. Dermatol*. 2010;28:539–45.

See Also (Topic, Algorithm, Electronic Media Element)

Chlamydial Sexually Transmitted Diseases; Gonococcal Infections

 CODES

ICD9

097.9 Syphilis, unspecified

CLINICAL PEARLS

- All patients with high-risk activity or HIV-positive status should be screened for syphilis.
- All pregnant patients should be screened at 1st prenatal visit.
- Education of patient after treatment is required to ensure that patient understands how to avoid STDs in the future.

SYSTEMIC LUPUS ERYTHEMATOSUS (SLE)

Katherine Tromp, PharmD
Karen I. Salomon-Escoto, MD

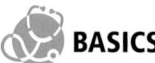 **BASICS**

DESCRIPTION
- Multisystem autoimmune inflammatory disease characterized by a chronic relapsing/remitting course; varies from mild to severe and may be life-threatening (CNS and renal forms)
- System(s) affected: Mucocutaneous; Musculoskeletal; Renal; Nervous; Pulmonary; Cardiac; Hematologic; Vascular, Gastrointestinal
- Synonym(s): SLE; lupus

ALERT
Women with SLE have a 7- to 50-fold increased risk of coronary heart disease and may present with atypical or nonspecific symptoms.

EPIDEMIOLOGY
Predominant age: 15–45 years

Incidence
- 1.6–7.6/100,000/year
- Most common incidence: African American women (8.1–11.4/100,000 per year)
- Least common incidence: Caucasian men (0.3–0.9/100,000 per year)

Prevalence
30–50/100,000

RISK FACTORS
- Race: African Americans, Hispanics, Asians, and Native Americans
- Females > Males (8:1)
- Environmental factors may include: Ultraviolet (UV) light, infectious agents, stress, diet, drugs, hormones, cigarette smoke

Genetics
- 24–58% concordance in identical twins
- 2–5% concordance in fraternal twins and siblings
- 8-fold risk if 1st-degree relative with SLE
- Major histocompatability complex associations: HLA-DR2, HLA-DR3
- Deficiency of early complement components, especially C1q, C2, and C4
- Immunoglobulin receptor polymorphisms: FCγR2A and FCγR3A
- Polymorphism in genes associated with regulation of programmed cell death, protein tyrosine kinases, and interferon production

PATHOPHYSIOLOGY
- Skin: Photosensitivity; scaly erythematous, plaques with follicular plugging, dermal atrophy, and scarring; nonscarring erythematous psoriasiform or annular rash; alopecia; mucosal ulcers
- Musculoskeletal: Nonerosive arthritis; ligament and tendon laxity, ulnar deviation, and swan neck deformities; avascular necrosis
- Renal: Glomerulonephritis
- Pulmonary: Pleuritis, pleural effusion, alveolar hemorrhage, pneumonitis, interstitial fibrosis, shrinking lung, pulmonary hypertension, pulmonary embolus (PE)
- Cardiac: Nonbacterial verrucous endocarditis, pericarditis, myocarditis, atherosclerosis

- CNS: Thrombosis of small intracranial vessels ± perivascular inflammation resulting in micro/macroinfarcts ± hemorrhage
- PNS: Mononeuritis multiplex, peripheral neuropathy
- GI: Pancreatitis, peritonitis, colitis
- Hematologic: Hemolytic anemia, thrombocytopenia, leukopenia, lymphopenia
- Vascular: Vasculitis, thromboembolism

ETIOLOGY
- Most cases are idiopathic.
- Genetic and environmental factors
- Drug-induced lupus: Hydralazine, quinidine, procainamide, minocycline, isoniazid, TNF alpha inhibitors, etc.

COMMONLY ASSOCIATED CONDITIONS
- Overlap syndromes: Rheumatoid arthritis (RA), Sjögren syndrome, scleroderma
- Antiphospholipid syndrome
- Coronary heart disease
- Nephritis
- Depression

 DIAGNOSIS

SLE should be considered in patients presenting with multisystem disease including fever, fatigue, and signs of inflammation.

HISTORY
- Fever, fatigue, malaise, weight loss, headache
- Rash (butterfly rash), photosensitivity, alopecia
- Oral or nasal ulcers (usually painless)
- Arthritis, arthralgia, myalgia, weakness
- Pleuritic chest pain, cough, dyspnea, hemoptysis
- Stroke, seizure, psychosis, cognitive deficits
- Proteinuria, cellular casts
- Hemolytic anemia, leukopenia, lymphopenia, thrombocytopenia
- Abdominal pain, anorexia, nausea, vomiting
- Raynaud phenomenon

PHYSICAL EXAM
- Vital signs: Fever, hypertension
- Malar, discoid, psoriasiform, or annular rash, alopecia
- Oral or nasal ulcers
- Lymphadenopathy, splenomegaly
- Acrocyanosis
- Inflammatory arthritis, tenosynovitis
- Pleural or pericardial rub, heart murmur
- Bibasilar rales
- Cranial or peripheral neuropathies

DIAGNOSTIC TESTS & INTERPRETATION
Initial evaluation includes laboratory tests for autoantibodies, markers of inflammation, CBC, urinalysis, and chemistries. Further tests are based on evidence of organ system involvement.

Lab
Initial lab tests
- Antinuclear antibody (ANA):
  - High sensitivity (98%), low specificity
  - 5–30% false-positive rate: Elderly, autoimmune thyroid/liver disease, chronic infection, etc.
  - Low titers <1:160 of limited clinical utility

- Anti–double-stranded DNA (dsDNA) and anti-Smith antibodies: High specificity for SLE
  - correlates with disease activity
- RNA protein antibodies (anti-RNP, anti-Ro, anti-La): Less specific for SLE
- False-positive VDRL: High sensitivity, low specificity. Surrogate marker of cardiolipin antibody presence.
- Low serum complement levels: C3, C4, Ch50
- Erythrocyte sedimentation rate (ESR): Nonspecific, often high in active disease
- CBC: Hemolytic anemia, thrombocytopenia, leukopenia, or lymphopenia
- Serum creatinine: Elevated in lupus nephritis
- Urinalysis: Proteinuria, hematuria, cellular cast
- Phospholipid antibodies: Cardiolipin IgG/IgM, lupus anticoagulant, beta 2 glycoprotein IgG/IgM
- Anti-P (ribosomal autoantibodies) are associated with SLE arthritis and disease activity.

Follow-Up & Special Considerations
- Hemolytic anemia: Elevated reticulocyte count and indirect bilirubin, low haptoglobin, positive direct Coombs test
- Confirm positive phospholipid antibodies results in 12 weeks.
- 24-hour urine collection or spot protein/creatinine to quantify proteinuria
- Histone antibodies present in >95% of drug-induced lupus (vs 80% of idiopathic SLE)
- Fasting lipid panel and glucose
- Follow vitamin D25OH levels and replete as needed.

Imaging
Initial approach
- Initial imaging is highly dependent on presenting symptoms.
- Radiograph of involved joints
- Chest x-ray: Infiltrates, pleural effusion, low lung volumes
- Chest CT scan, V-Q scan, duplex ultrasound (US) for PE or deep vein thrombosis
- Head CT scan: ischemia, infarct; hemorrhage
- Brain MRI: Focal areas of increased signal intensity
- Echocardiogram: Pericardial effusion, valvular vegetations, pulmonary hypertension
- Contrast angiography for medium-size artery vasculitis: mesenteric or limb ischemia, CNS symptom

Diagnostic Procedures/Surgery
- Renal biopsy to diagnose lupus nephritis
- Skin biopsy with immunofluorescence on involved and uninvolved non-sun-exposed skin (*lupus band test*) may help differentiate SLE rash from others.
- Lumbar puncture in patients with fever and CNS or meningeal symptoms
- EEG for seizures or global CNS dysfunction
- Neuropsychiatric testing for cognitive impairment
- EMG/NCS for peripheral neuropathy and myositis
- Nerve and/or muscle biopsy
- ECG, cardiac enzymes, stress tests
- The American College of Rheumatology classification (not diagnostic) criteria: Any 4 of the 11 listed (95% specificity and 85% sensitivity):
  - Malar (butterfly) rash
  - Discoid rash

- Photosensitivity: By patient history or physician observation
- Oral/nasopharyngeal ulcers
- Nonerosive arthritis: Involving 2 or more peripheral joints
- Pleuritis OR pericarditis
- Renal disorder: Proteinuria (>0.5 g per day or >3+) or cellular casts (red cell, hemoglobin, granular, tubular, or mixed)
- Neurologic disorder: Psychosis or seizures
- Hematologic disorder: Hemolytic anemia, leukopenia (<4,000/mm^3 on ≥2 tests), lymphopenia (<1,500/mm^3 on ≥2 tests), thrombocytopenia (<100,000/mm^3)
- Immunologic disorder: Anti-DNA, anti-Sm, anti-cardiolipin IgG/IgM, lupus anticoagulant, or false-positive VDRL
- Positive ANA in absence of drugs known to cause positive ANA

Pathological Findings
- Skin: Vascular/perivascular inflammation, immune-complex deposition at dermal–epidermal junction, mucinosis, basal layer vacuolar changes
  - Similar findings seen in other connective tissue disorders such as dermatomyositis
- Renal: Mesangial hypercellularity or matrix expansion, subendothelial/subepithelial immune deposits, glomerular sclerosis, fibrous crescents
  - Vary depending on degree of involvement
- Vascular: Immune-complex deposition in vessel walls with fibrinoid necrosis and perivascular mononuclear cell infiltrates, intraluminal fibrin thrombi

DIFFERENTIAL DIAGNOSIS
Undifferentiated connective tissue disease, Sjögren syndrome, fibromyalgia, RA, vasculitis, idiopathic thrombocytopenia purpera, antiphospholipid antibody syndrome, drug-induced lupus, and so on.

TREATMENT

MEDICATION
First Line

- Hydroxychloroquine for constitutional and musculoskeletal symptoms, rash, mild serositis; may reduce risk of flares and increase long-term survival (1,2)[A]. Chloroquine also is effective; however, it is associated with more side effects (2)[A].
- Topical or intralesional glucocorticosteroids for skin manifestations
- NSAIDs for musculoskeletal manifestations, mild serositis, headache, and fever (1,3)[C]
- Systemic glucocorticoids (prednisone or equivalent):
  - Low dose (<0.5 mg/kg) for minor disease activity not responsive to NSAIDs or when NSAIDs are contraindicated (1)[A]
  - High dose (1–2 mg/kg/d) (1)[A] or IV pulse methylprednisolone (3)[C] for organ-threatening disease, particularly CNS and renal; often combined with immunosuppressive agent (1)[A]
- Immunosuppressive agents for severe disease:
  - Cyclophosphamide (1)[A]: Ensure adequate hydration to reduce risk of hemorrhagic cystitis
  - Mycophenolate mofetil (1)[A]

Second Line

- Methotrexate (1)[A], azathioprine (1)[B] mycophenolatemofetil (1)[C], or leflunomide as steroid-sparing agent for persistent active disease or to maintain remission
  - Require periodic laboratory monitoring for toxicity
- Biologic treatments under investigation: rituximab, epratuzumab, belimumab, abatacept, interferon-α inhibitors, abetimus sodium (LJP 394), prasterone (3)

ADDITIONAL TREATMENT
General Measures
- Education, counseling, and support
- Influenza/pneumococcus vaccines are safe; avoid live vaccines in immunocompromised patients.
- Low-estrogen oral contraceptives safe in mild SLE (1)[A]

COMPLEMENTARY AND ALTERNATIVE MEDICINE
Biofeedback, visual imagery, cognitive therapy

SURGERY/OTHER PROCEDURES
Renal transplant for end-stage renal disease (1)[B]

IN-PATIENT CONSIDERATIONS
Initial Stabilization
- Difficult to differentiate SLE flare from infection; may need to treat both pending full evaluation
- IV pulse Solu-Medrol 1 g/d × 3–5 days for life- or organ-threatening disease (1)[A]

Admission Criteria
- Severe acute or rapidly progressive disease involving any organ system
- Fever, sepsis; acute coronary syndrome

 ONGOING CARE

FOLLOW-UP RECOMMENDATIONS
Patient Monitoring
- Clinical evaluation for signs and symptoms:
  - Weekly to monthly for active disease
  - Every 3–6 months for mild or inactive disease
- Measures of disease activity and damage: Systemic Lupus Erythematosus Disease Activity Index, British Isles Lupus Assessment Group Index, European Consensus Lupus Activity Measure
- Laboratory studies:
  - CBC with differential
  - Serum creatinine, urinalysis
  - Declining C3 or C4 and rising DS-DNA and ESR may correlate with disease activity (1)[B].
- Monitor for adverse effects of treatment:
  - NSAIDs: GI bleeding and/or ulceration
  - Glucocorticoids: Glucose, lipids, bone density
  - Hydroxychloroquine: Ophthalmologic exam every 6–12 months
  - Methotrexate: CBC, creatinine, albumin, AST, ALT every 2 months
  - Azathioprine and mycofenolate mofetil: CBC every 1–3 months
  - Cyclophosphamide:
    - CBC, creatinine, urinalysis every 2 weeks and liver function tests monthly during treatment
    - Urinalysis every 6–12 months for life

DIET
- No special diet unless for complications, such as renal failure, diabetes, hyperlipidemia (1)[C]
- Adequate calcium/vitamin D intake in patients on corticosteroids (1)[A]

PATIENT EDUCATION
- Avoid UV light exposure: Sunscreens (SPF ≥30), protective clothing (1)[B]
- Weight control, smoking cessation, exercise (1)[C]
- Stress avoidance/management

PROGNOSIS
- Permanent treatment-free remission is uncommon.
- 5-year survival after diagnosis is 95%.
- Poor prognostic factor: Major organ involvement
- Drug-induced lupus resolves within weeks to months after discontinuation of the offending drug.

COMPLICATIONS
Infections, neoplasms, cardiac disease, nephritis, neuropsychiatric lupus

Pregnancy Considerations
- Exacerbations during pregnancy are less common when in remission for 6 months prior to conception.
- Fetal loss is increased, especially in those with active lupus or antiphospholipid antibodies.
- 2% risk of congenital heart block if anti-SS-A (Ro) or anti-SS-B (La) antibodies are present.
- See Antiphospholipid Antibody Syndrome for recommendations regarding use of aspirin and heparin to prevent pregnancy complications.

REFERENCES

1. Bertsias G, Ioannidis JP, Boletis J, et al. EULAR recommendations for the management of systemic lupus erythematosus. Report of a Task Force of the EULAR Standing Committee for International Clinical Studies Including Therapeutics. *Ann Rheum Dis.* 2008;67:195–205.
2. Ruiz-Irastorza G, Ramos-Casals M, Brito-Zeron P, et al. Clinical efficacy and side effects of antimalarials in systemic lupus erythematosus: a systematic review. *Ann Rheum Dis.* 2009.
3. Kalunian K, Joan TM, et al. New directions in the treatment of systemic lupus erythematosus. *Curr Med Res Opin.* 2009;25:1501–14.

See Also (Topic, Algorithm, Electronic Media Element)
Antiphospholipid Antibody Syndrome

CODES

ICD9
710.0 Systemic lupus erythematosus

CLINICAL PEARLS

- SLE is a multisystem inflammatory autoimmune disease that preferentially affects women during the child-bearing years.
- The course is variable, with manifestations ranging from mild to life-threatening.
- Atherosclerotic and atheroembolic complications are the major cause of death. Risk factors should be identified and treated.
- Infection is a major cause of death. Prompt diagnosis and treatment of infection are crucial.
- While glucocorticoids form the basis of treatment for severe SLE manifestations, their use should be minimized owing to their unfavorable side-effect profile.

TAPEWORM INFESTATION

Kenton I. Voorhees, MD

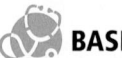 **BASICS**

DESCRIPTION

- Tapeworms (cestodes, flatworms) can be parasitic in humans.
- Adult worms consist of a head (scolex), which attaches to the host's GI tract; a neck; and a segmented body (strobila), with individual segments (proglottid) containing sets of male and female reproductive organs that produce eggs.
- The life cycle of all but *Hymenolepis nana* requires an intermediate host, in which they grow as larval forms in tissue that is then ingested by the final host, where it subsequently develops into an adult. *H. nana* can complete all stages of development in humans, making it the most common tapeworm in humans.
- Most tapeworm infections are confined to the GI tract, except *Taenia solium* (causing cysticercosis) or *Echinococcus* infections, making infections with these more serious.
- Neurocysticercosis is the most common inpatient disorder due to parasite infection.
- Common tapeworms and their usual intermediate hosts and type of infection in humans include:

Tapeworm Intermediate Hosts

Name	Host
D. latum	Freshwater fish
D. caninum	Dog, cat, fleas
E. granulosis	Human, sheep, cow, dog
E. multilocularis	Fox, coyotes, cats, rodents
H. diminuta	Rodent, insects
H. nana	Human, rodent, insects
T. saginata	Cow
T. solium	Pig

- *T. saginata*: From beef; causes an intestinal worm; 2–4 months from ingestion to adult; 3–10 m long; usually single tapeworm; proglottids are motile; may crawl out of anus; may live 30 years
- *T. solium*: From pork; intestinal worm or cysticercosis; 2–4 months to become adult worm; 3 m long; occasionally multiple; proglottids not motile; may live up to 25 years; ingestion of encysted larvae (cysticerci) causes intestinal tapeworm. Ingestion of *T. solium* eggs causes cysticercosis. Eggs look identical to *T. saginata* eggs.
- *D. latum*. There has been a recent increase in other species from *D. nihonkaiense* and *D. klebanovskii* from eating wild Pacific Salmon in sushi (1)[C], mostly in Japan, Europe, or Russia: Usually from freshwater fish; intestinal worm; longest adult tapeworm; up to 25 m; matures to adult in 3–5 weeks.
- *H. nana*: In rodent, insects, or humans; intestinal worm; matures to adult worm in 10–12 days; seldom exceeds 40 mm long; proglottids rarely seen in stool; eggs can autoinfect individual or occasionally insects (especially mealworms); fecal–oral transmission possible; life span 4–10 weeks, but autoinfection can perpetuate infection; usually self-cleared by adolescence

- *E. granulosis* and *E. multilocularis*: Humans, sheep, and cattle are intermediate hosts, with dogs the definitive hosts for *E. granulosis;* foxes, coyotes, or cats are definitive hosts for *E. multilocularis,* with rodents the intermediate hosts:
  – *E. granulosis*: Cystic *Echinococcus.*
  – *E. multilocularis*: Alveolar *Echinococcus;* hydatid disease of liver, spleen, etc., or alveolar hydatid disease; adult worm lives in dogs (or rodents); human ingests eggs; larvae hatch and are carried through circulation to various organs, such as liver and lungs, where they develop into hydatid cysts that enlarge, causing symptoms perhaps 5–20 years later
- *H. diminuta*: Rodents and insects; intestinal worm; 90 cm long; humans are rare accidental hosts, by swallowing mealworms or grain beetles from grain
- *D. caninum*: Dogs, cats, and fleas; intestinal worm; 10–70 cm long; motile proglottids; shape of cucumber seeds; can crawl out anus; rare accidental infection by ingesting infected flea that came from dogs or cats

Pediatric Considerations
- *H. nana* highest among children with fecal–oral spread
- *H. diminuta* and *D. caninum* more common in children because more likely to ingest insects accidentally

EPIDEMIOLOGY
Incidence
- Occurs infrequently
- More often associated with immigrant populations with cultural eating habits
- Can be endemic when fecal contamination enters water or food supplies
- Predominant age: All ages affected: *H. nana* and *H. diminuta* are more common in children.
- Predominant sex: Male = Female

RISK FACTORS
- *Taenia:* Eating raw beef or pork, particularly in Africa, Central America, Asia
- Cysticercosis: A tapeworm carrier in close environment; water contaminated with sewage
- *Diphyllobothrium*: Eating raw or undercooked fish, particularly in northern Europe
- *H. nana*: More frequent in children, the institutionalized, malnourished, and immunodeficient
- *E. granulosis*: Keeping dogs around sheep and goats; highest risk for hydatid cyst disease
- *E. multilocularis*: Contact with foxes, coyotes; mostly found in northern latitudes

GENERAL PREVENTION
- Treatment of infected animals, populations, and screening household contacts, immigrants
- Improved sewage treatment
- See Patient Education.

ETIOLOGY
Eating the infective form of the parasite, either by eating contaminated food (meat, fish) or infected insects in cereals or grains, or through fecal–oral contamination

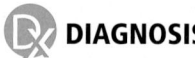 **DIAGNOSIS**

PHYSICAL EXAM
- *T. saginata* (beef tapeworm): Often noted by passing eggs or proglottids, which can be felt crawling out of anus; mild GI symptoms may occur: Nausea, abdominal pain, change in appetite, weakness, weight loss, allergic symptoms, urticaria, and pruritus.
- *T. solium* (pork tapeworm):
  – Intestinal worm: Noted passing eggs or proglottids; occasional minor abdominal complaints similar to *T. saginata*
  – Larval migration: Cysticercosis most common to brain and skeletal muscle; neurologic manifestations such as new-onset seizures, focal neurologic deficits, hydrocephalus, headache, vomiting, visual changes, and dizziness
- *D. latum* (fish tapeworm): Noted passing eggs or proglottid segments or vomiting segment of worm; occasionally mild abdominal discomfort, weight loss; worm has marked affinity for vitamin B_{12}; 40% decreased B_{12} levels, 2% megaloblastic anemia with glossitis
- *H. nana* (dwarf tapeworm): Anorexia, abdominal pain, and diarrhea
- Echinococcosis (hydatid disease): *E. granulosis* is often asymptomatic for years:
  – Liver cysts: Abdominal pain, right upper quadrant mass, obstructive jaundice
  – Cyst rupture: Fever, urticaria, pruritus, anaphylaxis
  – Pulmonary cyst: Cough, chest pain, hemoptysis
  – Other organs possible: Bone with pathologic fractures, CNS, cardiac conduction defects, pericarditis
- *H. diminuta* (rodent tapeworm): Pass eggs in stool, proglottids disintegrate; headache, mild GI symptoms (e.g., anorexia, nausea, cramps, diarrhea)
- *D. caninum* (dog tapeworm): Occasionally abdominal pain, diarrhea, anal pruritus, urticaria; may observe proglottid in diaper or stool

DIAGNOSTIC TESTS & INTERPRETATION
- Stool evaluation of ova and parasites
- Microscopic evaluation of proglottid collected in water or saline
- Antibody testing by enzyme-linked immunosorbent assay to differentiate *T. saginata* eggs from *T. solium*
- Enzyme-linked immunoelectrotransfer blot: Test of choice for cysticercosis, *Echinococcus* (2)[C]
- DNA probes for *T. saginata* or *T. solium*

Lab
- Mild-to-moderate eosinophilia, increased IgE
- Microscopic analysis of eggs or proglottids
- Macrocytic, megaloblastic anemia rarely with diphyllobothriasis

Imaging
- Intestinal tapeworms occasionally seen by small bowel enteroclysis
- Cysticercosis: MRI preferred, CT scan acceptable (2)[C]
- Echinococcus cysts: Start with ultrasound for liver, chest x-ray or chest CT for pulmonary (3)[C]

Diagnostic Procedures/Surgery
- Excisional biopsy of cysticercosis cyst
- Perianal inspection for eggs or proglottids

Pathological Findings
- Intestinal tapeworms: No pathologic findings
- Cysticercosis: Cysts, 5–10 mm in soft tissue; calcified cysts in CNS, muscle
- Echinococcus: Hydatid cyst in liver, lung, other

DIFFERENTIAL DIAGNOSIS
- Nontapeworm gastroenteritis
- Irritable bowel syndrome
- Intestinal obstruction
- Cholecystitis or biliary obstruction
- B_{12} deficiency from nontapeworm etiologies
- Tumors (abscesses, malignant, benign)
- Idiopathic epilepsy

 TREATMENT

- Outpatient unless complications from cysts
- In neurocysticercosis, cysticidal drug therapy was associated with a higher resolution of cystic lesions, a greater reduction in rate of generalized seizures, and greater reduction in seizure recurrence (4).

MEDICATION
First Line
- Praziquantel (Biltricide) (2,5,6,7)[C]:
  – Single dose of 5–10 mg/kg (generally 10 mg/kg) for taeniasis, diphyllobothriasis, Dipylidium infection, and most other intestinal cestodes (cure rate >95%)
  – Single dose of 25 mg/kg for H. nana in adults or children (cure rate >95%)
  – 50–100 mg/kg/d divided t.i.d. × 14–30 days for children and adults for cysticercosis (albendazole, preferred drug)
- Albendazole (Albenza) (2,5,6,7,8)[C]:
  – Dose: Weight >60 kg: 400 mg b.i.d. with meals; weight <60 kg: 15 mg/kg/d b.i.d. (maximum 800 mg/d)
  – For Echinococcus hydatid cysts, give for 28 days, 14 days off, repeat × 3 cycles; can be 1–6 months
  – For neurocysticercosis, drug of choice, give for 8–30 days, but examine for retinal lesions 1st; may repeat
  – For neurocysticercosis, albendazole more effective than praziquantel at reducing seizures and cysts (7)
- Neurocysticercosis: Steroids, anticonvulsants: Dexamethasone 4.5–12 mg/d (6)[C]
- PAIR therapy (puncture, aspiration, injection of a scolicidal, reaspiration) compares favorably with surgery for cystic echinococcosis.
- Contraindications: Prior sensitivity
- Precautions:
  – Niclosamide: Occasional nausea and abdominal pain, diarrhea, dizziness
  – Praziquantel: Mild but frequent dizziness, myalgias, nausea, diarrhea, abdominal pain
  – Albendazole: Diarrhea and abdominal pain; leukopenia, increased transaminase levels
- Significant possible interactions:
  – Phenytoin and carbamazepine can induce the metabolism of praziquantel by cytochrome P450, causing treatment failure.
  – Cimetidine, dexamethasone, and praziquantel can increase the concentration of albendazole.
  – Corticosteroids may decrease the concentration of praziquantel.

Second Line
Niclosamide (Niclozide) (not available in the US):
- Single dose of 2 g for adult or 50 mg/kg for children for diphyllobothriasis, taeniasis, and Dipylidium

infection (cure rate 90% for taeniasis and slightly less for diphyllobothriasis)
- 2 g then 1 g/d for 5 more days for H. nana

ADDITIONAL TREATMENT
General Measures
- Treat population in endemic area.
- Treatment of all immigrants from endemic countries with albendazole is being evaluated.
- Provide general supportive care during treatment.
- Good hygienic measures should be employed.
- Asymptomatic cysticercosis may resolve spontaneously without treatment; however, antiparasitic therapy of parenchymal cysts may reduce the number of seizures with generalization (4)[C]. Treatment may induce an inflammatory response and symptoms (9)[C].
- Prior to initiating corticosteroids and antiparasitics to treat cysticercosis, evaluate for ocular cysticercosis, latent tuberculosis, and strongyloidiasis.

SURGERY/OTHER PROCEDURES
- Cysticercosis and hydatid cysts have been removed surgically, with care not to leak fluid; shunts for hydrocephalus (6)[C].
- Echinococcus hydatid cysts (10)[C]:
  – Surgery based on location of cyst
  – Surgical risks may make medical therapy preferred.
  – Surgery generally involves total pericystectomy or partial resection of the affected organ, with albendazole pretreatment for 1 month.
  – Follow surgery with albendazole.

IN-PATIENT CONSIDERATIONS
Admission Criteria
Complications of cysts

 ONGOING CARE

FOLLOW-UP RECOMMENDATIONS
As tolerated

Patient Monitoring
- Examine several stool specimens for ova and parasites at 3 months for Taenia species and 1 month for others.
- Follow neurocysticercosis with CT scans.

DIET
As tolerated

PATIENT EDUCATION
- Proper cooking of beef, pork, fish
- Proper freezing of meat or fish
- Good handwashing habits
- Treatment of infected animals and flea prevention

PROGNOSIS
- Cure >95% of intestinal tapeworms with medications
- H. nana often self-cured by adolescence
- E. multilocularis often severe or fatal
- Prognosis of systemic cysts by location
- Neurocysticercosis:
  – Intraparenchymal cysts often benign
  – Extraparenchymal (subarachnoid, ventricular, cisternal) more serious (2)[C]

COMPLICATIONS
- Larval form of T. solium can cause systemwide cysticercosis, including neurocysticercosis (etiologic in up to 25% of cases of new-onset seizures in indigenous areas).

- Echinococcus hydatid cysts may cause abnormalities in the organ involved. Cyst rupture can cause spread of disease and anaphylaxis.
- B_{12} deficiency with D. latum
- Proglottid of T. saginata rarely can obstruct appendix and pancreatic and bile ducts.
- D. latum occasionally can cause intestinal obstruction, cholangitis, and cholecystitis.

REFERENCES

1. Arizono N, Yamada M, et al. Diphyllobothriasis Associated with Eating Raw Pacific Salmon. Emerging Infectious Diseases. www.cdc.gov/eid. 2009;15(6):866–870.
2. Garcia HH, Gonzalez AE, Gilman RH, et al. Diagnosis, treatment and control of Taenia solium cysticercosis. Curr Opin Infect Dis. 2003;16: 411–9.
3. Santivanez S, Garcia HH, et al. Pulmonary cystic echinococcosis. Curr Opin Pulm Med. 2010;16:257–61.
4. Del Brutto OH, Roos KL, Coffey CS, et al. Meta-analysis: Cysticidal drugs for neurocysticercosis: albendazole and praziquantel. Ann Intern Med. 2006;145:43–51.
5. Abramowicz M, ed. The Medical Letter on Drugs and Therapeutics. Drugs for parasitic infections. New Rochelle, NY: The Medical Letter; August, 2004.
6. García HH, Evans CA, Nash TE, et al. Current consensus guidelines for treatment of neurocysticercosis. Clin Microbiol Rev. 2002;15: 747–56.
7. Matthaiou DK, Panos G, Adamidi ES, et al. Albendazole versus Praziquantel in the Treatment of Neurocysticercosis: A Meta-analysis of Comparative Trials. PLoS Negl Trop Dis. 2008;2:e194.
8. Abba K, Ramaratnam S, Ranganathan LN, et al. Anthelmintics for people with neurocysticercosis. Cochrane Database Syst Rev. 2010;3:CD000215.
9. Garcia HH, Pretell EJ, Gilman RH, et al. A trial of antiparasitic treatment to reduce the rate of seizures due to cerebral cysticercosis. N Engl J Med. 2004;350:249–58.
10. Brunetti E, Junghanss T, et al. Update on cystic hydatid disease. Curr Opin Infect Dis. 2009;22: 497–502.

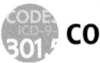 **CODES**

ICD9
- 123.0 Taenia solium infection, intestinal form
- 123.1 Cysticercosis
- 123.2 Taenia saginata infection

CLINICAL PEARLS
- Tapeworms in humans are usually asymptomatic.
- For neurocysticercosis, if asymptomatic, treatment generally is not necessary. Calcified cysts generally do not need antiparasitic therapy.
- The treatment options for neurocysticercosis are observation, symptomatic therapy with anticonvulsants, antihelminthic therapy with steroids, and surgery.
- Following treatment of tapeworm, stool should be rechecked for eggs after 1 month for Hymenolepia and Diphyllobothria and after 3 months for Taenia.

TARDIVE DYSKINESIA

Lawrence E. Udom, MD, MPH

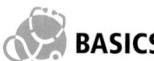 BASICS

DESCRIPTION

- A neurologic syndrome with the essential features of abnormal, involuntary movements of the tongue, lips, face, trunk, and extremities
- Most commonly associated with long-term treatment with neuroleptic medications
- Movements can include grimacing, sticking out the tongue, and smacking and sucking the lips. Patients have choreiform characteristics (i.e., rapid, jerky, or nonrepetitive), athetoid characteristics (i.e., slow, sinuous, continual), or rhythmic characteristics.
- Tardive dyskinesia (TD) symptoms can begin during treatment with neuroleptics or within 4 weeks of discontinuing neuroleptics. TD can be mild, moderate, or severe.
- System(s) affected: Nervous; Musculoskeletal
- Synonym: Orofacial dyskinesia

EPIDEMIOLOGY

TD rates for patients beginning treatment with conventional antipsychotics in their 5th decade or later are 3–5× those found for younger patients despite treatment with lower doses (1).

Incidence

- Predominant age: Occurs in all ages; however, advanced age is a major risk factor for TD.
- Predominant sex: Male = Female, until advanced years, when Female > Male
- In studies that used haloperidol as predominant classical antipsychotic:
  - Younger patients (<55 years) on the classic antipsychotics have a 5% incidence of developing TD per year of use, with a 50–60% incidence of development over their lifetime.
  - Older patients (>60 years) have a ~20% incidence rate after 1 year of exposure, moving to 30% and nearly 50% at 2– and 3–year exposures, respectively (1).
- Annualized incidence of TD was 3.9% for 2nd-generation antipsychotics and 5.5% for 1st-generation antipsychotics (2)[A].

Prevalence

Overall estimated prevalence of 15–25% of TD within 5 years of continuous classic antipsychotic use

RISK FACTORS

- Use of classic antipsychotics:
  - Haloperidol (Haldol)
  - Chlorpromazine (Thorazine)
  - Fluphenazine (Permitil, Prolixin)
  - Thioridazine (Mellaril)
  - Perphenazine (Trilafon)
  - Trifluoperazine (Stelazine)
  - Pimozide (Orap)
  - Thiothixene (Navane)
  - Molindone (Moban)

- A few of the new class of atypical antipsychotics have been linked to TD, although in lower incidences than noted with the older medications:
  - Quetiapine (Seroquel)
  - Olanzapine (Zyprexa)
  - Risperidone (Risperdal)
- Length of neuroleptic use
- Older age
- Postmenopausal females
- Mental retardation
- Alcoholism and substance abuse
- Extrapyramidal symptoms early in the course of neuroleptic treatment
- Presence of other movement disorders
- DM
- Mood disorders (particularly MDD)

Geriatric Considerations

- Occurs in all ages; however, advancing age is a major risk factor for TD (3).

Genetics

- No definitive data indicate a genetic basis for TD; however, recent research suggests a possible association with a polymorphic variant of the Ser9Gly *DRD3* gene and TD.
- Also, the absence of a glutathione *S*-transferase gene (GSTM1) was associated with TD, particularly in white women (4).
- Also have been associations with the polymorphism of the dopamine receptor D_2 (*DRD2*) gene, *Taql A* and *Taql B*, and associated haplotypes that may contribute to the development of TD (5)

GENERAL PREVENTION

- Choosing an atypical neuroleptic as 1st-line therapy statistically reduces the risk of developing TD (6)[A].
- If traditional neuroleptics must be used, limit long-term use, and use lowest effective doses with frequent patient assessments.

PATHOPHYSIOLOGY

- The mechanism by which TD occurs is still under debate. Antipsychotics (both traditional and atypical) have a high affinity for the D_2 receptors. It is postulated that the long-term blockade of these receptors leads to an upregulation in the number and sensitivity of D_2 receptors in the striated region of the brain (which controls muscle coordination). This upregulation is associated with involuntary movements and hence TD.
- It also has been postulated that the depletion of GABA in the substantia nigra may lead to orofacial dyskinesia, as may excess free radicals.

ETIOLOGY

Prolonged use of dopamine antagonist drugs:

- Traditional antipsychotics
- Atypical antipsychotics
- Metoclopramide (Reglan), prochlorperazine (Compazine), antiemetics with potent D_2 antagonism
- Antimalarials (Chloroquine)
- Antiparkinson agents (bromocriptine, levodopa, and combined levodopa and carbidopa (Sinemet)
- Lithium
- Stimulants (amphetamine, methylphenidate, caffeine)

COMMONLY ASSOCIATED CONDITIONS

- Presence of movement disorder
- Psychiatric disorders commonly treated with neuroleptics

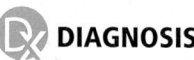 DIAGNOSIS

HISTORY

- There must be a history of neuroleptic use for at least 3 months (or 1 month if individual's age ≥60 years).
- TD must be distinguished from other movement disorders.
- Abnormal movements must not be due to a neurologic condition or other general medical conditions (e.g., Huntington disease, Sydenham chorea, spontaneous dyskinesia, hyperthyroidism, heavy-metal poisoning, Wilson disease), to ill-fitting dentures, or exposure to other medications that can cause acute reversible dyskinesia (e.g., L-dopa, bromocriptine, amantadine, Sinemet, Adderall, Ritalin, and Compazine).
- Other neuroleptic-induced movement disorders must be ruled out (e.g., tardive tourettism, blepharospasm, tardive akathisia, tardive myoclonus, tardive tremor, and tardive dystonia), as well as spontaneous dyskinesias and mental disorders.
- Question patient about a history of neurologic disorders that may involve the basal ganglia (e.g., CVA, encephalitis, head trauma, neoplasms).
- Attempt to elicit a family history for hereditary dyskinesias (e.g., Huntington disease).
- Ask about medication usage, particularly aforementioned medications. *Note:* Neuroleptics also can mask TD, thus explaining onset after medication discontinuation.

PHYSICAL EXAM

- Abnormal, involuntary movements of the tongue, lips, and extremities; facial grimacing; and swaying movements of the trunk or hips. In 1 major report:
  - 75% of individuals with TD had orofacial dyskinesia.
  - 50% had limb dyskinesia.
  - 25% had axial dyskinesia.
  - 10% had total-body involvement.
- Orofacial dyskinesia is common in the ≥60 population.

- Limb + axial dyskinesia is more common in the younger population (4,6).
- These signs and symptoms must occur while taking neuroleptics or within 4 or 8 weeks of withdrawal from an oral or depot neuroleptic medication, respectively.
- The signs typically are minimal to mild in nature and progress in severity with prolonged use.

DIAGNOSTIC TESTS & INTERPRETATION
Lab
Only used to rule out other causes
Initial lab tests
- Rule out Wilson disease: Low serum ceruloplasmin due to an abnormal copper transporter gene and elevated 24-h urine copper collection. In addition, LFTs and liver transaminases may be abnormal, along with elevated hepatic copper levels. Also, check the copper transporter gene in patients in whom Wilson disease is suspected.
- TSH, calcium, syphilis serology
- Connective-tissue disease screening tests (CBC count, ESR, urinalysis, chemistry panel, RF, ANA) are useful to exclude SLE and other vasculitides.
- Obtain RBC counts to exclude polycythemia rubra vera.
Imaging
May be done to rule out other causes
Diagnostic Procedures/Surgery
Screen for dyskinetic movements before initiating antipsychotics at regular scheduled intervals, e.g., q 6 months. Several questionnaires elicit this information and rate TD on a severity scale; most commonly used is the Abnormal Involuntary Movement Scale (AIMS).

DIFFERENTIAL DIAGNOSIS
- Huntington disease
- Sydenham chorea
- Spontaneous dyskinesia
- Wilson disease
- Thyrotoxicosis
- Blepharospasm
- Tardive akathisia
- Tardive dystonia
- Physical signs may point the way to another diagnosis:
  – Tachycardia, sweating, and a goiter suggest thyrotoxicosis.
  – Jaundice, hepatomegaly, or Kayser-Fleischer rings suggest a workup for Wilson disease.
- Dementia in addition to the movement disorder (chorea) and postural instability requires a workup for Huntington disease.

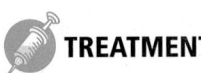 TREATMENT

MEDICATION
First Line
Cessation of neuroleptic use upon identifying TD.
Second Line
- No definitive treatment for TD
- Replace traditional antipsychotic with an atypical (risperdal, olanzapine, quetiapine, ziprasidone, and clozapine) (7).

- Some evidence suggests that the use of clozapine has been effective in diminishing involuntary movements in patients with TD:
  – Some studies have shown remission of TD in up to 34% of patients after treatment with clozapine for 6–12 months (8)[A]. This improvement in symptoms is possibly secondary to the downregulation of sensitized D_2 receptors.
  – However, the side effect of clozapine (i.e., agranulocytosis) prevents it from being a 1st-line medication.

ADDITIONAL TREATMENT
Use of Reglan (Ondansetron), a selective 5-hydroxytryptamine-3 antagonist, has been shown to help some individuals with TD (9,10)[B].

COMPLEMENTARY AND ALTERNATIVE MEDICINE
- Vitamin E, a free-radical scavenger, has been found in a number of studies to reduce the severity of TD, though more recent studies suggest it is primarily indicated in newly diagnosed TD (11)[A].
- Benzodiazepines provide GABA agonistic effects. This helps in some patients with TD; however, can be sedating and has abuse potential.
- Branched chain amino acids mix (Tarvil) in 1 study was shown to be superior to placebo in treating TD at a dosage of 222 mg/kg t.i.d. (12).

 ONGOING CARE

FOLLOW-UP RECOMMENDATIONS
Patient Monitoring
- Instruct patients and family members to watch for the subtle early signs.
- Warn that TD may be exacerbated by stimulant use (Ritalin, Adderall), neuroleptic withdrawal, and anticholinergics.
- Symptoms are affected by emotional states and stress.

PROGNOSIS
TD can be mild to moderate, with resolution of symptoms after a period of discontinuation from offending drug. In rare incidences, TD may be severe and irreversible.

REFERENCES
1. Woerner MG, Alvir JM, Saltz BL, et al. Prospective study of tardive dyskinesia in the elderly: rates and risk factors. *Am J Psychiatry*. 1998;155:1521–8.
2. Correll CU, Schenk EM. Tardive dyskinesia and new antipsychotics. *Curr Opin Psychiatry*. 2008;21:151–6.
3. Barnes TRE. Movement disorder associated with antipsychotic drugs: The tardive syndromes. *Intern Rev Psychiatry*. 1990;2:243–54.
4. de Leon J, Susce MT, Pan RM, et al. Polymorphic variations in GSTM1, GSTT1, PgP, CYP2D6, CYP3A5, and dopamine D2 and D3 receptors and their association with tardive dyskinesia in severe mental illness. *J Clin Psychopharmacol*. 2005;25: 448–56.
5. Liou YJ, Lai IC, Liao DL, et al. The human dopamine receptor D2 (DRD2) gene is associated with tardive dyskinesia in patients with schizophrenia. *Schizophr Res*. 2006;86:323–5.
6. American Psychiatric Association. *DSM-IV-TR 2000: Diagnostic & Statistical Manual of Mental Disorders*, 4th ed. Washington DC: American Psychiatric Publishing, 2000.
7. Caroff SN, Mann SC, Campbell EC, et al. Movement disorders associated with atypical antipsychotic drugs. *J Clin Psychiatry*. 2002; 63(Suppl 4):12–9.
8. Lieberman JA, Saltz BL, Johns CA, et al. The effects of clozapine on tardive dyskinesia. *Br J Psychiatry*. 1991;158:503–10.
9. Sirota P, Mosheva T, Shabtay H, et al. Use of the selective serotonin 3 receptor antagonist ondansetron in the treatment of neuroleptic-induced tardive dyskinesia. *Am J Psychiatry*. 2000;157:287–9.
10. Zullino DF, Eap CB, Voirol P. Ondansetron for tardive dyskinesia. *Am J Psychiatry*. 2001;158: 657–8.
11. Pham DQ, Plakogiannis R, et al. Vitamin E supplementation in Alzheimer's disease, Parkinson's disease, tardive dyskinesia, and cataract: Part 2. *Ann Pharmacother*. 2005;39: 2065–72.
12. Richardson MA, Bevans ML, Read LL, et al. Efficacy of the branched-chain amino acids in the treatment of tardive dyskinesia in men. *Am J Psychiatry*. 2003;160:1117–24.

ADDITIONAL READING
Ormerod S, McDowell SE, Coleman JJ, et al. Ethnic differences in the risks of adverse reactions to drugs used in the treatment of psychoses and depression: a systematic review and meta-analysis. *Drug Saf*. 2008;31:597–607.

 CODES

ICD9
- 333.82 Orofacial dyskinesia
- 333.85 Subacute dyskinesia due to drugs

CLINICAL PEARLS
- 2nd-generation antipsychotics have a lower incidence of TD than 1st-generation medications (2)[A].
- Ensure that oral dyskinesias are not triggered by ill-fitting dentures.
- The older the patient, the higher the risk for TD from antipsychotics.
- Remember that TD can begin after the discontinuation of antipsychotics (up to 4 weeks).
- Use the minimum effective dosage and duration.

TARSAL TUNNEL SYNDROME

Chris Graves, MD
Douglas A. Pepple, MD

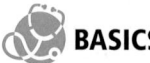 **BASICS**

DESCRIPTION
Tarsal tunnel syndrome is a compression neuropathy of the posterior tibial nerve as it passes under the flexor retinaculum in the medial ankle; a region commonly known as "the tarsal tunnel."

Pregnancy Considerations
- Tarsal tunnel syndrome can occur during pregnancy, typically secondary to local compression caused by fluid retention and volume changes.
- Care usually is supportive until after delivery, because many cases resolve after pregnancy.

EPIDEMIOLOGY
Women are slightly more affected than men (56%). All postpubescent ages can be affected.

RISK FACTORS
Several authors have associated tarsal tunnel syndrome with certain occupations and activities, especially those that involve repetitive weight bearing on the foot and ankle, like jogging (1) or dancing (2).

PATHOPHYSIOLOGY
- Tarsal tunnel syndrome is caused by compression of the tibial nerve, resulting in decreased blood flow and ischemic damage.
- Increased pressure in the confined space of the tarsal tunnel is caused by a variety of mechanisms, both mechanical and biochemical, all of which result in increased pressure on the posterior tibial nerve.
- Chronic compression can destroy endoneurial microvasculature, leading to edema and eventually fibrosis and demyelination (3).

ETIOLOGY
- The specific cause is identifiable in only 60–80% of patients (4); causes can be grouped into 3 categories: Trauma, space-occupying lesion, and deformity.
- Most common causes include (4):
  – Trauma
  – Varicosities
  – Hindfoot varus or valgus
  – Fibrosis of the perineurium
- Other causes of compression include ganglia, lipoma, neurilemmoma, inflammatory synovitis, pigmented villonodular synovitis, tarsal coalition, and accessory musculature.

 DIAGNOSIS

Frequently misdiagnosed because of poorly localized and variable symptoms

HISTORY
- Often have history of trauma to foot, including trivial trauma that precipitated pain
- Classically have pain and paresthesia on plantar aspect of foot
- Pain usually worse with standing or activity
- Pain can radiate proximally up medial leg (Valleix phenomenon) in 33% of patients with severe compression, or distally along path of involved nerves (4).
- Some patients have substantial night pain, which may be related to venostasis.
- Symptoms improve with rest, wearing loose footwear, and elevation.

ALERT
Other neuropathies due to systemic causes such as diabetes, alcoholism, HIV, or drug reaction can present with similar symptoms.

PHYSICAL EXAM
- Perform a complete foot and ankle examination.
- Foot alignment:
  – Examine for hindfoot varus or valgus abnormalities.
  – Exaggerating heel dorsiflexion, inversion, or eversion may reproduce symptoms by stretching or compressing the nerve.
- Palpate the tarsal tunnel and course of the tibial nerve for:
  – Tenderness
  – Swelling consistent with a space-occupying lesion
- Tinel sign: Percussion over the course of the tibial nerve may produce paresthesias and distal symptoms.
- Cuff test: Using a pneumatic cuff to create a venous tourniquet may cause engorgement of varicosities and reproduce symptoms.
- Compression test: Applying pressure to tarsal tunnel for 60 seconds may reproduce symptoms.
- Sensory examination:
  – The MCN usually is spared, but numbness and altered sensation may be present in the distribution of the MPN or LPN.
  – 2-point discrimination is decreased early in the disease process.
- Motor examination:
  – Intrinsic weakness is difficult to assess.
  – Rarely, weakness of toe plantarflexion may be present.
  – Atrophy of the abductor hallucis or abductor digiti minimi may be seen late in the disease process.

DIAGNOSTIC TESTS & INTERPRETATION
Lab
Routine laboratory tests can be used to rule out other conditions that may mimic tarsal tunnel syndrome, including diabetic neuropathy, thyroid dysfunction, or other systemic illnesses (5).

Imaging
- Routine weight-bearing radiographs, followed by CT if necessary to assess for fracture or structural abnormality.
- Consider evaluation of lumbar spine x-ray if "double-crush" (injury to lumbar nerve results in compensatory injury to posterior tibial nerve) (6) is suspected (5).
- Magnetic resonance imaging (MRI): Can be helpful in assessing the tarsal tunnel for masses or other sources of nerve compression before surgery (4)
- Ultrasound: Alternatively, ultrasound can be used to check for synovitis or ganglia (5).

Pediatric Considerations
- MRI is recommended for evaluating pediatric tarsal tunnel syndrome because compression by a neoplastic mass is not uncommon.

Follow-Up & Special Considerations
Postoperative management includes:
- Non-weight-bearing splint until incision heals (2–3 weeks), followed by progressively increased weight-bearing and range of motion exercises.
- RICE protocol (rest, ice, compression, elevation) to limit swelling

Diagnostic Procedures/Surgery
Electrodiagnostic studies (4):
- According to a systematic review in 2005, electromyography (EMG) can be used only to confirm the diagnosis of tarsal tunnel syndrome, as there is a large percentage of asymptomatic people with abnormal results.
- It is important to evaluate for proximal nerve compression, including a lumbar radiculopathy or a double-crush phenomenon.

Pathological Findings
At the time of surgical exploration, the following may be found:
- Focal swelling, scarring, or nerve abnormalities
- A pathologic source of compression

DIFFERENTIAL DIAGNOSIS
- Peripheral neuropathies (diabetes, alcoholism, HIV, or drug related)
- Inflammatory arthritis (rheumatoid arthritis) (7)
- Morton's neuroma
- Metatarsalgia
- Subtalar joint arthritis

- Tibialis posterior tendinitis/dysfunction
- Plantar fasciitis
- Plantar callosities
- Peripheral vascular disease
- Lumbar radiculopathy
- Proximal injury or compression of the tibial branch of the sciatic nerve

 TREATMENT

Conservative management is recommended, except for tarsal tunnel syndrome of acute onset or in the setting of a known space-occupying lesion:

- Rest/immobilization
- Taping and bracing
- Orthotics or shoe modification
- Anti-inflammatories (steroid injections vs nonsteroidal anti-inflammatory drugs)
- Medications to alter neurogenic pain (antidepressants, antiepileptic drugs, nerve blocks)
- Physical therapy for desensitization (stretching, ultrasound, massage, icing)
- Physical therapy to strengthen the intrinsic and extrinsic muscles of the foot and to restore the medial longitudinal arch
- Compression stockings to decrease swelling
- Weight loss in obese patients

MEDICATION

Initially, nonoperative management is recommended, except for acute tarsal tunnel syndrome or in the setting of a known space-occupying lesion (excluding synovitis):

- Rest/immobilization
- Orthotics
- Anti-inflammatories, including steroid injections and nonsteroidal drugs
- Medications that alter neurogenic pain (tricyclic antidepressants, antiepileptic drugs, nerve blocks)
- Physical therapy (desensitization)
- Compression stockings
- Weight loss

SURGERY/OTHER PROCEDURES

- Surgery is indicated (3,4,8):
  - If nonoperative measures fail following a 3–6-month trial
  - In the setting of acute tarsal tunnel syndrome
  - If a space-occupying lesion is identified
- The surgical outcome is dependent on technique and postoperative management. Ability to achieve a good to excellent outcome ranges from 50–95%.

 ONGOING CARE

PATIENT EDUCATION
An outline of the conservative care modalities available should be presented. Use of each of these therapies will depend on patient circumstance. A decision about surgical intervention should be made with a clear understanding of limitations of this treatment and the potential adverse outcomes.

PROGNOSIS
The most symptomatic improvement with surgery is expected for (4):

- Young patients
- Short duration of symptoms
- Localized space-occupying lesion identified (8)
- No motor neuron involvement
- Surgical outcomes are dependent on technique and postoperative management.

COMPLICATIONS
- The main adverse outcome is unsuccessful surgical intervention: No improvement, partial/incomplete improvement, or temporary improvement with recurrence of symptoms (4)
- Causes for a failed tarsal tunnel release:
  - Incorrect diagnosis
  - Incomplete release
  - Adhesive neuritis (external scar formation)
  - Intraneural damage (systemic disease, direct nerve injury)
  - Failure to treat all sources of nerve compression in a double-crush phenomenon
- Electrodiagnostic studies are rarely helpful in determining the cause of a failed tarsal tunnel release.
- Revision surgery results are poorer than for the primary surgical release.

REFERENCES

1. Shapiro BE, Preston DC. Entrapment and compressive neuropathies. *Med Clin North Am.* 2009;93:285–315, vii.
2. Kennedy JG, Baxter DE. Nerve disorders in dancers. *Clin Sports Med.* 2008;27:329–34.
3. Dellon AL. The four medial ankle tunnels: a critical review of perceptions of tarsal tunnel syndrome and neuropathy. *Neurosurg Clin N Am.* 2008;19:629–48.
4. Lau JT, Daniels TR. Tarsal tunnel syndrome: a review of the literature. *Foot Ankle Int.* 1999;20:201–9.
5. Franson J, Baravarian B. Tarsal tunnel syndrome: a compression neuropathy involving four distinct tunnels. *Clin Podiatr Med Surg.* 2006;23:597–609.
6. Upton AR, McComas AJ, et al. The double crush in nerve entrapment syndromes. *Lancet.* 1973;2:359–62.
7. Campbell WW, Landau ME. Controversial entrapment neuropathies. *Neurosurg Clin N Am.* 2008;19:597–608.
8. Sung KS, Park SJ, et al. Short-term operative outcome of tarsal tunnel syndrome due to benign space-occupying lesions. *Foot Ankle Int.* 2009;30:741–5.

ADDITIONAL READING

- Allen JM, Greer BJ, Sorge DG, et al. MR Imaging of Neuropathies of the Leg, Ankle, and Foot. *Magn Reson Imaging Clin N Am.* 2008;16:117–31.
- Cimino WR. Tarsal tunnel syndrome: review of the literature. *Foot Ankle.* 1990;11:47–52.
- Patel AT, Gaines K, Malamut R, et al. Usefulness of electrodiagnostic techniques in the evaluation of suspected tarsal tunnel syndrome: an evidence-based review. *Muscle Nerve.* 2005;32:236–40.

See Also (Topic, Algorithm, Electronic Media Element)
Algorithm: Foot Pain

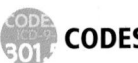 **CODES**

ICD9
355.5 Tarsal tunnel syndrome

CLINICAL PEARLS

- Tinel sign: Percussion over the course of the tibial nerve produces paresthesias and distal symptoms over the plantar aspect of the foot (most sensitive and specific test) (3).
- Conservative management is recommended, except for tarsal tunnel syndrome of acute onset or in the setting of a known space-occupying lesion.
- EMG abnormality alone cannot be used to diagnose tarsal tunnel syndrome; may only be used to confirm clinical diagnosis.

T

TEETHING

Jennifer E. Frank, MD

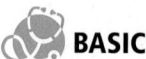 **BASICS**

DESCRIPTION
- Teething is the eruption of the primary or deciduous teeth, which most children experience without difficulty. It is a natural, gradual, and predictable process, with normal variation among infants.
- Primary (deciduous) teeth:
  - Primary tooth eruption usually begins at 5–7 months of age.
  - The order of primary tooth eruption and average age is:
    - Central mandibular incisors (5–7 months)
    - Central maxillary incisors (6–8 months)
    - Lateral mandibular incisors (7–10 months)
    - Lateral maxillary incisors (8–11 months)
    - Cuspids (16–20 months)
    - 1st molars (10–16 months)
    - 2nd molars (20–30 months)
  - Delayed eruption may be familial or due to systemic syndromes or nutritional deficiencies.
  - Tooth eruption in premature infants occurs according to postconceptual age rather than age since birth (chronological age).
  - Natal/neonatal teeth:
    - Natal teeth (present at birth) occur in 1/2,000 neonates.
    - Neonatal teeth erupt in the 1st month of life.
    - Natal/neonatal teeth are most often prematurely erupted primary (deciduous) teeth, but may be supernumerary.
    - 15–20% of cases are familial; also may be secondary to a syndrome or congenital anomalies of the head and neck.
    - Natal/neonatal teeth may be loose, but most are the normal deciduous lower central incisors and can persist.
    - Natal/neonatal teeth may be removed if there is an aspiration risk or if they cause trauma to the infant or to the mother (breastfeeding).
- System(s) affected: Gastrointestinal (GI)

EPIDEMIOLOGY
Incidence
Predominant age: Birth–3 years of age

RISK FACTORS
Genetics
Both premature and delayed tooth eruption may be familial. Primary failure of eruption has been linked to mutations of the PTHR1 gene (1).

COMMONLY ASSOCIATED CONDITIONS
Teething may be coincident with other conditions, such as common childhood illnesses (e.g., roseola, viral gastroenteritis, upper respiratory infection) and serious bacterial infections, causing local or systemic signs and symptoms (e.g., fever, GI disturbance, fussiness, drooling, rash, and sleep disturbance).

 DIAGNOSIS

HISTORY
- Biting
- Drooling
- Rubbing of gingivae
- Sucking
- Irritability
- Wakefulness
- Ear rubbing
- Facial rash
- Decreased appetite for solid foods

PHYSICAL EXAM
- Infants may have no signs or symptoms of teething.
- Excessive drooling and chewing on fingers begins at 3–4 months of age. This is also the time that normal hand–mouth stimulation increases salivation.
- Discomfort may be observed more commonly with the eruption of the 1st tooth, the molars, and/or with the simultaneous eruption of multiple teeth.
- Minor signs and symptoms of biting or chewing, drooling, irritability, facial rash, and low-grade fever (<38.9°C) have been reported in association with teething, although no evidence identifies specific signs/symptoms caused by teething (2)[B].
- Serious signs and symptoms (e.g., fever >38.9°C, dehydration) are not caused by teething and warrant evaluation for organic disease (2,3,4,5)[B].
- A small red or white spot may appear over the swollen gingivae just prior to tooth eruption.
- Local inflammation, swelling, or hematoma (bluish swelling) can be found on the involved gingivae overlying the erupting tooth.

DIAGNOSTIC TESTS & INTERPRETATION
Imaging
Radiographs can distinguish prematurely erupted primary teeth from supernumerary teeth.

DIFFERENTIAL DIAGNOSIS
Herpetic gingivostomatitis: Infants with fever, irritability, sleeplessness, and difficulty feeding may have underlying infection caused by herpes simplex virus. Some infants with positive culture may not have evidence of inflammation or ulceration expected in gingivostomatitis.

 TREATMENT

MEDICATION
First Line
For an infant with low-grade fever, irritability, and/or inflamed gingivae (where other comforting measures have not been of help), acetaminophen in proper doses (15 mg/kg/dose q4–6h p.r.n.) can be used.

Second Line

Over-the-counter preparations for teething, such as lidocaine (Xylocaine 2%, Baby Ora-Gel, Num-zit Gel, Num-zit Liquid, Baby Anbesol), should be used with caution. Misuse, overuse, and sensitivity have been reported. These are of questionable benefit because they are washed off quickly by saliva, and the benefit may be due in part to the pressure placed on the gingivae when applied (6). If used, care should be taken to select the infant formulation, because some products also come in adult strength.

ADDITIONAL TREATMENT

Infants can be taught not to bite or chew while breastfeeding.

General Measures

- Treatment includes reassurance and symptomatic treatment.
- Provide the infant with a safe, 1-piece teething ring, clean cloth, or pacifier for gumming.
- Apply pressure over involved swollen gingivae with a clean finger or piece of wet gauze.
- May use cool (but not frozen) fluids, cold teething rings, or cold vegetables such as a peeled cucumber
- Avoid the use of alcohol (historically rubbed on gingivae for an analgesic effect).
- Gingival hematomas that erupt appear as blue cysts. Most do not require medical intervention. Be sure there are no other signs of a bleeding disorder.
- Avoid:
  - Dipping a pacifier or teething ring in sugar or honey
  - Giving an infant a bottle in bed
  - Using fluid-filled teething rings (contents may leak)
  - Using frozen foods or teething rings (these could cause thermal damage to the tissues)
  - Tying a teething ring around infant's neck

Issues for Referral

If tooth eruption is significantly delayed, consider referral to pediatric dentist.

COMPLEMENTARY AND ALTERNATIVE MEDICINE

Homeopathy is used to treat teething. Calcarea carbonica (i.e., calcium carbonate) is one recommended treatment (7).

IN-PATIENT CONSIDERATIONS

Initial Stabilization

Outpatient

 ONGOING CARE

FOLLOW-UP RECOMMENDATIONS

No restrictions

DIET

Breastfeeding can continue during and after teething. Otherwise, no special diet.

PATIENT EDUCATION

- Parents should be cautioned not to misinterpret teething as the cause of any systemic manifestation. The health provider should be consulted for any systemic complaints.
- American Dental Association, For the Dental Patient: Tooth Eruption, the Primary Teeth, 2005; www.ada.org
- Teething Tots: http://kidshealth.org/parent/ pregnancy_newborn/common/teething.html

PROGNOSIS

Normal progression through the teething process without illness

REFERENCES

1. Stellzig-Eisenhauer A, Decker E, Meyer-Marcotty P, et al. Primary failure of eruption (PFE)–clinical and molecular genetics analysis. J Orofac Orthop. 2010;71:6–16.
2. Tighe M, Roe MF. Does a teething child need serious illness excluding? Arch Dis Child. 2007;92:266–8.
3. Macknin ML, Piedmonte M, Jacobs J, et al. Symptoms associated with infant teething: a prospective study. Pediatrics. 2000;105:747–52.
4. Ashley MP. It's only teething. . . A report on the myths and modern approaches to teething. Br Dental J. 2001;191:4–8.
5. Frank J, Drezner J. Is teething in infants associated with fever or other symptoms? J Fam Pract. 2001;50:257.
6. McIntyre GT, et al. Teething troubles? Br Dental J. 2002;192:251–5.
7. Bergguist P. Therapeutic Homeopathy. In: Integrative Medicine, 2nd ed. Philadelphia: Saunders; 2007:1181.

ADDITIONAL READING

Tinanoff N. The oral cavity. In: Nelson Textbook of Pediatrics, 17th ed. Philadelphia: Saunders; 2004: 1205–1206, 1212.

CODES

ICD9

520.7 Teething syndrome

CLINICAL PEARLS

- Teething is the natural, gradual, and predictable process of eruption of the primary or deciduous teeth, which most children experience without difficulty.
- Teething may cause discomfort, but does not cause significant fevers.
- Teething babies can still breastfeed. Babies can be taught not to bite, and breastfeeding may continue past 12 months of age without difficulty.

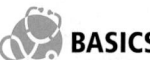 **BASICS**

DESCRIPTION
- Syndrome characterized by:
  - Pain and tenderness in jaw muscles
  - Sound and/or pain over temporomandibular joint (TMJ)
  - Limitation of mandibular movement
- System affected: Musculoskeletal
- Synonym(s): Myofascial pain–dysfunction syndrome; bruxism

EPIDEMIOLOGY
Incidence
- Predominant age: Symptoms more common ages 30–50 years
- Predominant sex: Female > Male (3:1)

Prevalence
Symptoms or signs of TMJ dysfunction are present in up to half the population, but only 5–25% seek treatment.

RISK FACTORS
- Chronic oral habit, such as clenching or grinding of the teeth
- Osteoarthritis, rheumatoid arthritis
- Dental malocclusion
- Fibrositis
- Psychosocial stress

GENERAL PREVENTION
- Elimination of tension-relieving oral habits
- Reduction in overall muscle tension

ETIOLOGY
- TMJ synovitis
- TMJ disk derangement
- Hypermobile or hypomobile TMJ
- Occlusomuscular dysfunction (bruxism)
- Masticatory muscle spasm
- Trauma
- Poorly fitting dentures

COMMONLY ASSOCIATED CONDITIONS
Craniomandibular disorders

 DIAGNOSIS

- Facial and/or TMJ pain
- Locking or catching of jaw
- TMJ noises: Clicking, grinding, popping
- Headache
- Earache
- Neck pain

PHYSICAL EXAM
Jaw range of motion (opening, closing, lateral, protrusive) and masticatory muscle strength

DIAGNOSTIC TESTS & INTERPRETATION
Imaging
- Single-contrast video arthrography: Demonstrates joint dynamics and disk movement
- Panoramic dental radiographs
- MRI: Noninvasive study for disk position; information gained helps in deciding conservative vs surgical management.

Pathological Findings
- Condylar head displacement
- Anterior disk displacement
- Posterior capsulitis
- Loosening of disk and capsular attachments
- Chondroid metaplasia of disk leading to disk perforation and degeneration

DIFFERENTIAL DIAGNOSIS
- Condylar fracture/dislocation
- Trigeminal neuralgia
- Dental or periodontal conditions
- TMJ neoplasm

TREATMENT

- Jaw rest
- Local heat therapy
- Anti-inflammatory medications
- Muscle relaxants
- Analgesics
- Correction of malocclusion with orthodontic appliance
- Stress reduction
- Behavior modification to eliminate tension-relieving oral habits
- Buccal separator orthodontic appliance
- Linearly polarized, near-infrared irradiation

MEDICATION

First Line
- NSAIDs: No single drug more efficacious than another (1)[C]
- Botulinum toxin (2)[C]

Second Line
- Analgesic agents (1)[C]
- Muscle relaxants (1)[C]

 ONGOING CARE

FOLLOW-UP RECOMMENDATIONS
- Be aware of any teeth-clenching or grinding habits.
- Relax jaw by disengaging teeth.
- Avoid wide, uncontrolled opening, such as yawning.
- Stress management and behavior-modification counseling may be helpful.

Patient Monitoring
- Ongoing assessment of clinical response to conservative therapies (NSAIDs, behavior modification, occlusal splints) is necessary.
- Surgical procedure to correct disk displacement or replace a damaged disk may be indicated only if the patient has not responded to conservative treatment.

DIET
Soft diet to reduce chewing

PROGNOSIS
- With conservative therapy, symptoms resolve in 75% of cases within 3 months.
- Patients benefit most from a comprehensive treatment approach, including:
  – Correction of occlusal discrepancies
  – Restoration of normal muscle function
  – Pain control
  – Stress management
  – Behavior modification

COMPLICATIONS
- Secondary degenerative joint disease
- Chronic TMJ dislocation
- Loss of joint range of motion
- Depression and chronic pain syndromes

REFERENCES

1. Cooper BC, Kleinberg I. Establishment of a temporomandibular physiological state with neuromuscular orthosis treatment affects reduction of TMD symptoms in 313 patients. *Cranio*. 2008; 26(2):104–17.
2. Gonzalez YM, Greene CS, Mohl ND. Technological devices in the diagnosis of temporomandibular disorders. *Oral & Maxillofacial Surgery Clinics of North America*. 2008;20(2):211–20, vi.

ADDITIONAL READING

- Al-Ani MZ, Davies SJ, Gray RJM, et al. Stabilisation splint therapy for temporomandibular pain dysfunction syndrome. *Cochrane Database of Systematic Reviews* 2004, Issue 1. Art. No.: CD002778. DOI:10.1002/14651858.CD002778. pub2
- Koh H, Robinson P. Occlusal adjustment for treating and preventing temporomandibular joint disorders. *Cochrane Database of Systematic Reviews* 2003, Issue 1. Art. No.: CD003812. DOI:10.1002/ 14651858.CD003812
- Scrivani SJ, Keith DA, Kaban LB, et al. Temporomandibular disorders. *N Engl J Med*. 2008;359:2693–705.

See Also (Topic, Algorithm, Electronic Media Element)
Headache, Tension

 CODES

ICD9
524.60 Temporomandibular joint disorders, unspecified

T

TENDINITIS

Mathew J. Devine, DO
Mark H. Mirabelli, MD

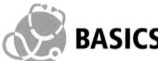 **BASICS**

DESCRIPTION
- Inflammation of a tendon and/or tendinous sheath or tissue degeneration in late stage
- System(s) affected: Musculoskeletal

ALERT
- The term *tendinopathy* has replaced the term *tendinitis* as a generic descriptor of clinical conditions associated with pain, swelling, and impaired performance in and around tendons, arising from overuse. The labels *tendinitis* and *tendinosis* are reserved for the condition after histologic exam is performed (1).
- Tendinopathies can be pathologically classified as:
  – Tendinitis: Acute inflammation of the tendon
  – Tendinosis: Chronic degeneration of the tendon; also can be related to partial tendon rupture
  – Tenosynovitis: Inflammation of the tendon sheath
- Common sites of overuse tendon injuries:
  – Knee: Patella or jumper's knee, medial plica, and pes anserine
  – Shoulder: Rotator cuff muscles
  – Ankle: Achilles and posterior tibialis
  – Hip: Hamstring muscles and iliotibial tract
  – Elbow: Lateral epicondylitis or tennis elbow, medial epicondylitis or golfer's or thrower's elbow, and triceps (2)

EPIDEMIOLOGY
Incidence
- Predominant age: Adolescent and middle-aged groups; common in rotator cuff, Achilles tendon, and patellar injuries
- Predominant sex: Male = Female
- Overuse injuries are more common in high-risk populations (e.g., athletes and geriatric populations).
- Blood type O related to chronic tendon problem.

Pediatric Considerations
Tendons in children tend to be more stable than the epiphyseal plate. Therefore, consider growth plate avulsion fractures vs overuse apophysitis following trauma in children (2). Tendinopathy is uncommon in children with open growth plates.

Prevalence
Tendinopathy/tendinitis is seen commonly.

RISK FACTORS
- Extrinsic factors:
  – Training errors (most common)
  – Footwear and equipment (2nd most common)
  – Training surfaces
  – Environmental conditions
- Intrinsic factors:
  – Malalignment
  – Limb length discrepancy
  – Muscular imbalance
  – Muscular insufficiency

GENERAL PREVENTION
Preparticipation screening, warm-up sessions, core and supporting muscle strengthening, safe environment, protective equipment using braces or taping, and health education have been shown to be useful for prevention of future injuries.

PATHOPHYSIOLOGY
- Overuse injuries involve incomplete and disorganized repair mechanisms. These result in a defective repaired tendon that lacks extra cellular tissue organization and has decreased strength, making the tendon more susceptible to further injury (1). This tendon disorganization is the basis for chronic tendinopathy.
- Healing response of an acute tendon injury has a triphasic response of inflammation, proliferation, and maturation.

ETIOLOGY
- Increased repetitive stress and force on the tendon cause an increased risk of injury. Over time, with intrinsic and extrinsic factors, above-listed tendinopathies can develop.
- Etiologic causes are still unknown and have only been theorized (3).

COMMONLY ASSOCIATED CONDITIONS
- Bursitis (common)
- Arthritis
- Apophysitis

 DIAGNOSIS

HISTORY
- In general population, history of repetitive use with onset of pain in area of muscle origin or insertions
- History of overuse or overtraining in the case of an athlete
- Pain at the specific point of the affected tendon is the most common symptom.
- Reproducible pain on muscle group activity
- Thickening of tendon(s) involved
- Decreased active range of motion (ROM) of the muscle group involved

ALERT
- With excessive posttraumatic tension or pain in lower extremity, must consider urgent care for acute compartment syndrome
- With excessive swelling in traumatic injury, also must consider muscular tendon rupture

PHYSICAL EXAM
- Precise physical exam is key to the diagnosis
- Palpable pain over muscle tendon unit
- Warmth and redness in acute tendinopathies
- Note asymmetry and tendon thickness in chronic tendinopathies.
- Pain may limit ROM.
- Full musculoskeletal exam
- Neurologic exam as needed
- Snowball or creaky crepitus

DIAGNOSTIC TESTS & INTERPRETATION
Lab
If inflammatory arthritis suspected: Erythrocyte sedimentation rate (or C-reactive protein; both are NOT necessary); if elevated, check antinuclear antibodies, rheumatoid factor

Imaging
Initial approach
- Imaging only to be used as adjunct as needed
- Ultrasound:
  – Can measure tendon width, water content within the tendon and peritendon, and collagen integrity
  – Abnormal tendons on ultrasound have the following findings: Increased tendon diameter, focal hypoechoic intratendinous areas, localized tendon swelling and thickening, collagen discontinuity, and tendon sheath swelling of calcifications (4).

Follow-Up & Special Considerations
Magnetic resonance imaging (MRI):
- Indicated only in specific causes
- Reveals tendon thickening and increased signal of tendons
- Areas of mucoid degeneration seen as high intensity on T1- and T2-weighted images

ALERT
- Areas of increased signal on MRI must be correlated with clinical pathology because these could represent asymptomatic areas of degeneration.
- MRI is unreliable in changes of paratendinitis.

Pathological Findings
Refer to tendinopathy pathology classification.

DIFFERENTIAL DIAGNOSIS
- Knee:
  – Patellofemoral pain syndrome: Lateral tracking of patella causing irritation and abrasion of the cartilage of the patella resulting in pain
  – Exertional compartment syndrome: A reversible ischemia secondary to a noncompliant osseofascial compartment that is unresponsive to the expansion of muscle volume that occurs with exercise (1); most common in anterior compartment of lower extremities
  – Stress fractures: Partial or complete bone fracture from repeated force lower than the force required to fracture the bone in a single loading; most common areas are the tibia, metatarsals, and fibula (1)[A]
- Shoulder:
  – Bursitis: Often is present with a tendinopathy
  – Adhesive capsulitis
  – Arthritis: An inflammation within a specific joint of the body; should be differentiated from tendinopathy, which is isolated to the muscle insertion site and not within the joint spaces
  – Cervical radiculopathy

- Ankle:
  – Rupture: Achilles rupture is uncommon and is not a cause of tendinitis.
  – Sprains: In acute sprains, tendinitis can develop if too much stress is placed on noninjured musculature.
- Hip: Stress fracture: With excessive pain on internal rotation of hip, place the patient on crutches until femoral fracture is ruled out.

ALERT
There are many tendons in the body; the most common were selected in the differential diagnosis section.

Pediatric Considerations
- Osgood-Schlatter tibial apophysitis (common)
- Sever disease: Calcaneal apophysitis
- Pelvic apophysitis
- Little League elbow/Little League shoulder

TREATMENT

MEDICATION
First Line
Nonsteroidal anti-inflammatory drugs (NSAIDs) provide good analgesic effects:
- Naprosyn: over the counter (OTC), 500 mg b.i.d. with food
- Ibuprofen: OTC, up to 800 mg t.i.d. with food (adjust NSAIDs by weight for pediatric patients) (5)[B]
- Meloxicam: 7.5–15 mg/d
- Piroxicam (Feldene): 10–20 mg/d

Second Line
- Corticosteroids (4)[C]:
  – Oral corticosteroids (prednisone, others) (p.o.)
  – Injectable:
    ○ Methylprednisolone (Depo-Medrol): 40 mg used with 1% or 2% lidocaine (Xylocaine) 4–6 mL
    ○ Contraindication: Tendons should never be injected with local anesthetic and/or cortisone to allow participation in an athletic event. This can lead to complete rupture of the tendon.
- Topical: Research in progress

ALERT
- Recently, some of the COX-2 inhibitors have been removed from the market. Current literature supports the use of celecoxib for tendinopathy in individuals without cardiovascular risk.
- Contraindication: Do not use NSAIDs in patient with recent history of gastrointestinal bleed or ulcer.
- Precautions: Compare medications for any drug interactions. See manufacturer's profile of each drug.
- Use caution with renal disease.
- A rare side effect of fluoroquinolones has been tendon rupture and tendinopathy (3)[C].

ADDITIONAL TREATMENT
General Measures
- Avoid extrinsic factors.
- During acute phase: Rest of tendon involved
- Treat as outpatient.

Issues for Referral
Orthopedics/sports medicine referral in cases of highly competitive athlete, continued pain >4 weeks, radiologic finding of avulsion/stress fractures, or uncertainty of diagnosis

Additional Therapies
- Icing very beneficial in treatment (1)[C]
- Physical therapy

ALERT
- Muscle strengthening and intrinsic factor recognition are critical to continue the healing process.
- Patient progress should be monitored with pain threshold. If pain continues, then the activity needs to be decreased (1)[C].

COMPLEMENTARY AND ALTERNATIVE MEDICINE
- Orthotics: OTC or prescription as needed
- Current research shows no benefit to using laser therapy or other radiotherapies (3)[C].

SURGERY/OTHER PROCEDURES
- For chronic tendinopathy, surgical treatment is an option if conservative treatment fails after 4–6 months. Patellar tendinitis is operated on most commonly (3)[C].
- Long-standing tendinopathies are associated with poorer surgical outcomes.

 ONGOING CARE

FOLLOW-UP RECOMMENDATIONS
- Advise patient of susceptibility of exacerbation of injury up to 3 weeks after resolution of symptoms with increased activity.
- Treatment plans vary based on site of injury.
- Most plans include rest, medications, cryotherapy, and physical therapy.
- Follow-up at discretion of provider and patient

Patient Monitoring
Follow-up at discretion of provider and patient

PATIENT EDUCATION
- Increase activity in stepwise fashion as long as pain-free.
- Scales such as the Victorian Institute of Sports Assessment (VISA) for patellar and Achilles tendons may provide some quantification of progress (6).
- Strengthening and stretching of muscle group are involved.

PROGNOSIS
Symptoms usually subside with rest and proper therapy. Most tendinopathies improve without any major complications.

COMPLICATIONS
Exacerbation of pain in affected area

REFERENCES

1. Wilder RP, et al. Overuse injuries: Tendinopathies, stress fractures, compartment syndrome, and shin splints. Clin Sports Med. 2004;23:55–81.
2. Maffulli N, Wong J, Almekinders LC. Types and epidemiology of tendinopathy. Clin Sports Med. 2003;22:675–92.
3. Sharma P, Maffulli N. Tendon injury and tendinopathy: healing and repair. J Bone Joint Surg Am. 2005;87:187–202.
4. Warden SJ, Brukner P. Patellar tendinopathy. Clin Sports Med. 2003;22:743–59.
5. Cook JL, Purdam CR. Rehabilitation of lower limb tendinopathies. Clin Sports Med. 2003;22:777–89.
6. New Zealand Guidelines Group. Diagnosis and management of soft tissue shoulder injuries and related disorders. New Zealand Guidelines Group, 2004.

ADDITIONAL READING

Crowson CS, Rahman MU, Matteson EL, et al. Which measure of inflammation to use? A comparison of erythrocyte sedimentation rate and C-reactive protein measurements from randomized clinical trials of golimumab in rheumatoid arthritis. J Rheumatol. 2009;36:1606–10.

 CODES

ICD9
- Knee:
  – 726.10 Disorders of bursae and tendons in shoulder region, unspecified
  – 726.31 Medial epicondylitis
  – 727.00 Synovitis and tenosynovitis, unspecified

CLINICAL PEARLS
- Consider tendinopathy in cases of muscle or joint pain associated with overuse activity.
- Signs and symptoms include swelling, tenderness at site, and possibly erythema.
- Recommend rest of affected muscle–tendon unit and liberal use of ice and NSAIDs for acute tendonitis.
- Recommend ice, stretching, and eccentric exercises for treatment of more chronic tendinopathies.
- Muscle strengthening and intrinsic factor recognition are critical to continue the healing process.

TESTICULAR MALIGNANCIES

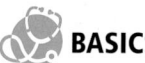

Satya Allaparthi, MD

BASICS

DESCRIPTION
- Testicular cancer: 1% of all cancers in men; most common solid malignancy in men aged 15–35 years; ~ 8,400 new cases diagnosed in the US in 2009 (1).
- Is one of the most curable solid-organ cancers (95.9%, 5-year survival) (2).
- Arise from any testicular or adnexal cell; divided into germinal cell (GC) (~95%) and nongerminal tumors (~5%). GC divided into seminomatous and nonseminomatous types.

Pediatric Considerations
- 1–2% of all solid tumors in childhood; incidence of 0·5–2 per 100,000; 74% of primary testis tumors in prepubertal children were benign.
- Bimodal distribution, peak in young adults and smaller peak in the 1st 3 years of life.
- The peak age at presentation: 2 years, 60% of tumors present earlier; median age for presentation of yolk-sac tumors is 16 months; and for teratomas, 13 months.
- Cryptorchidism is risk factor for testicular cancer; ~10% occurs in this setting. Correct by 9–15 months with orchiopexy; this does *not* completely eliminate the risk of cancer.

EPIDEMIOLOGY
Incidence
- ~1% of all neoplasms in males
- Overall incidence in America rose 44% between 1973 and 1998; reasons unclear.
- 4× more common in whites than in blacks
- 5.5/100,000 men in 1997–2001 (2)
- Peak incidence: Ages 20–40 years; smaller peaks between 0–10 years and >60 years
- Predominant sex: Male only

RISK FACTORS
- Cryptorchidism: The only proven risk factor, with 4- to 10-fold increased risk
- Intratubular germ cell neoplasia: Left untreated, the risk of progression to invasive malignancy is ~50% in 5 years.
- Caucasian race, especially Scandinavian and Swiss
- Family history (1–3% with affected 1st-degree relative)
- Increased maternal estrogen, infertility, preterm birth, atrophy, trauma, abnormal development (i.e., Klinefelter syndrome, XY dysgenesis, Down syndrome)

Genetics
- Nearly all cases of germ cell tumors (GCTs) show chromosome 12p abnormalities; exact genes involved are not yet defined.
- Increased expression of p53 protein is found in many GCTs; mutations in *TP53* gene not demonstrable.
- Role of telomerase activity: Highest levels of expression are seen in embryonal carcinomas. Telomerase is absent in mature teratomas, and its absence contributes to their limited proliferative capacity.

PATHOPHYSIOLOGY
- Testicular cancer can arise from testicular GCTs or from sex chord stromal cells (Sertoli or Leydig cells).
- GCTs are either seminomas, nonseminomas, or a mix of the two. Nonseminomas can be yolk-sac tumors, choriocarcinomas, embryonal tumors, teratomas, or a mixture of these. Teratomas are considered to be either mature or immature and

immature depending on if adult-type differential cell types or partial somatic differentiation, similar to that present in the fetus.
- In adults, 95% are GCTs; in children, 65% are GCTs. 60% of GCTs are seminomatous; 40% are nonseminomatous. Seminomas are rare before age 10 or after age 60 but are still the most common histologic type overall.

COMMONLY ASSOCIATED CONDITIONS
Cryptorchidism, testicular atrophy, Klinefelter syndrome, Down syndrome

DIAGNOSIS

HISTORY
- In adults:
  – Testicular nodule/painless swelling/enlarged testicle (most common presentation)
  – Dull ache/heavy sensation (30–40%)
  – Hydrocele (10–20%)
  – Acute pain (10%), often secondary to hemorrhage/infarction; often mistaken for epididymitis
  – Gynecomastia (5%) is a systemic endocrine manifestation of testicular neoplasm, also seen in Leydig cell tumors.
  – Enlargement of a small or atrophic testicle
  – Infertility
- In children: Painless testicular mass is the most common; can be seen in association with torsion.

PHYSICAL EXAM
- Testicular exam: Both testicles should be palpated and evaluated for size, consistency, and presence of nodules; often may have firm, nontender, irregular mass; masses do not transilluminate.
- Additional exam: Evaluate for supraclavicular nodes, inguinal nodes, abdominal masses, and gynecomastia.

DIAGNOSTIC TESTS & INTERPRETATION
Lab
Initial lab tests
- Complete blood count, urea, electrolytes, liver function tests
- Tumor markers: α-Fetoprotein (AFP), β-human chorionic gonadotropin (β-hCG), lactate dehydrogenase (LDH) (3)[A]:
  – Markers are useful to stage disease, monitor response and prognosis, and detect tumor recurrence.
  – Levels should be drawn preoperatively and postoperatively (3)[A].
  – AFP
    ○ Increased in yolk-sac tumors, teratomas, embryonal carcinomas (or combination)
    ○ If >10,000 ng/mL, almost exclusively in patients with nonseminoma GCTs and hepatocellular carcinoma
    ○ Not increased in pure choriocarcinoma or pure seminoma
  – β-hCG: Increased in pure choriocarcinoma and 5–10% of pure seminomas
  – LDH: Reflects "tumor burden"; too ubiquitous to be specific, but a proven prognostic factor
  – Drugs that may alter lab results
    ○ AFP may be elevated with chemotherapy, anesthetics, antiepileptics, and alcohol abuse.
    ○ β-hCG may be elevated by marijuana use.
  – Disorders that may alter lab results:

  ○ AFP altered by liver damage owing to drugs, viral hepatitis, alcohol abuse, liver conditions
  ○ β-hCG altered by hypogonadism and malignancies of pancreas, stomach, kidney, breast, or bladder

Follow-Up & Special Considerations
- A 10-fold decrease in or normalization of the serum β-hCG concentration (half-life 18–36 hours) over 2 weeks or serum AFP (half-life, 5–7 days) over 25–30 days is indicative of an appropriate decline, whether following surgery or chemotherapy.
- Postoperative tumor markers drawn only in nonseminomatous cases (3)[A]:
  – Seminoma
    ○ No tumor markers reliably serve as indicators of disease recurrence in seminomas, so tumor markers are checked every 6 months, a less frequent schedule than for nonseminomatous GCT (3)[A].
    ○ Surveillance: Every 4 months for 1st 3–4 years; 6 months for 4–7 years; 12 months for 8–10 years (4)
  – Nonseminoma
    ○ Surveillance/no adjuvant chemotherapy: Tumor markers monthly for 1st year, and then every 2 months for 2nd year, every 4 months for 3rd year, and then every 6 months until 5th year; CT scan of abdomen at 3 and 12 months
    ○ After chemotherapy: Tumor markers every 2 months for 1st year, then every 3 months for 2nd year, then every 6 months until 5th year, then annually; CT scan as clinically indicated

Imaging
Initial approach
- Scrotal ultrasound is gold standard; any hypoechoic area within tunica albuginea is suspicious. Ultrasound for patients with normal testes and extragonadal metastases.
- if an intratesticular mass is identified, further evaluation includes measurement of serum AFP, LDH, hCG, and CXR.
- For staging:
  – CT scan of the chest, abdomen, and pelvis (3)[B]
  – MRI of brain if β-hCG >10,000 or >10 metastases in lungs
  – Bone scan for patients with metastasis or elevated alkaline phosphatase

Follow-Up & Special Considerations
Follow-up imaging based on histology of tumor and cancer staging.
- Seminoma:
  – Stage IA, IB: H&P, AFP, LDH, HCG, CXR, exam every 3–4 months for years 1–3, then every 6 months for years 4–7, then annually (3)[B]
  – Stage IIA, IIB: H&P, AFP, LDH, HCG, CXR exam every 3-4 months for years 1–3, then every 6 months for years 4, then annually
  – Stage IIC, III: H&P, AFP, LDH, HCG, CXR exam every 2 months for year 1, every 3 months for year 2, every 4 months for year 3, every 6 months for year 4, then annually.
  – Metastatic: If posttreatment CT scan is normal, follow-up as for stage 1; if abnormal posttreatment CT scan, repeat CT scan every 6 months until stable (3)[B].
  – PET scan helps to identify patients who have residual active cancer (3).

- Nonseminoma:
  – Stage IA, IB surveillance: CXR, clinical exam done at same time that serum tumor markers are drawn every month during 1st year, and then every 2 months during 2nd year. See lab follow-up above; CT scan at 3, 6, 9, 12, and 24 months .

Diagnostic Procedures/Surgery

- Radical inguinal orchiectomy: Definitive procedure for pathologic diagnosis
- Transscrotal biopsy/orchiectomy is contraindicated because lymphatic drainage is violated, and inguinal portion of spermatic cord is left.
- If testicular atrophy is present, consider contra-lateral testicle biopsy if patient is <30 years of age or testicle is <12 mL in volume (3)[B].

Pathological Findings

Clinical staging (based on 1997 AJCC TNMS):

- Stage 0: Carcinoma in situ
- Stage Ia: Tumor limited to testis and epididymis without vascular/lymphatic invasion; normal serum tumor markers
- Stage Ib: Tumor limited to testis and epididymis, vascular/lymphatic invasion or tumor extending through tunica albuginea and involvement of tunica vaginalis; normal tumor markers
- Stage Is: Any tumor with elevated markers but no nodal involvement or metastasis
- Stage IIa: Any tumor with lymph node mass/masses <2 cm
- Stage IIb: Any tumor with lymph node mass/masses 2–5 cm
- Stage IIc: Any tumor with lymph node mass >5 cm
- Stage IIIa: Any tumor/lymph node presence with nonregional nodal or pulmonary metastases
- Stage IIIb: Any tumor/lymph node presence with moderately elevated serum tumor markers
- Stage IIIc: Any tumor/lymph node presence with greatly elevated serum tumor markers
- Risk stratification of metastic GCT:
- Based on International Germ Cell Cancer Collaborative Group, divided into good-, intermediate-, and poor-risk groups based on primary site of the GCT, metastatic sites of involvement, and levels of serum tumor markers
- Seminoma: Good versus intermediate risk based on whether extrapulmonary metastases are present. Serum levels of β-hCG and LDH not used in assigning risk status with seminoma.
- Good risk: Any primary site; no nonpulmonary visceral metastases; normal serum AFP (any elevation of AFP is inconsistent with the diagnosis of seminoma, and patient should receive therapy for nonseminomatous GCT, even if pathology fails to identify these elements.)
- Intermediate risk: Any primary site; nonpulmonary metastases present; normal serum AFP
- Nonseminomatous GCT: Good risk: Testicular or retroperitoneal primary tumor; no nonpulmonary visceral metastases; serum AFP <1000 ng/mL, β-hCG <5,000 million IU/mL; LDH <1.5× upper limit of normal
- Intermediate risk: Testicular or retroperitoneal primary tumor; no nonpulmonary visceral metastases; intermediate level of any of the following serum tumor markers: Serum AFP 1,000–10,000 ng/mL; β-hCG 5,000–50,000 million IU/mL; LDH 1.5–10× upper limit of normal
- Poor risk: Mediastinal primary site ± metastases; nonpulmonary visceral metastases (e.g., with liver or brain metastases); marked elevation in serum tumor markers: Serum AFP >10,000 ng/mL; serum β-hCG >50,000 million IU/mL; LDH >10× upper limit of normal

DIFFERENTIAL DIAGNOSIS

- Epididymitis, hernia, hydrocele, hematoma, spermatocele, syphilitic gumma, varicocele
- Children: Epidermoid/dermoid cyst, paratesticular rhabdomyosarcoma, macroorchidism, torsion

 TREATMENT

MEDICATION
First Line

- Common chemotherapeutic agents include BEP (bleomycin, etoposide, and cisplatin) (3)[B].
- Patients who cannot tolerate BEP (low pulmonary reserve) should receive four courses of EP (etoposide, cisplatin) or VIP (vincristine or etoposide, ifosfamide, cisplatin).

Second Line

Salvage chemotherapy includes vinblastine, ifosfamide, and cisplatin (VIP).

ADDITIONAL TREATMENT
General Measures

- Tumors with both seminomatous and nonseminomatous components managed as nonseminoma.
- Surgery:
  – Radical inguinal orchiectomy for all patients; prosthesis can be inserted at this time.
- Seminoma:
  – Classified based on risk
  – Low risk: Tumor <4 cm and absence of rete testis invasion: Low relapse rate of 12% (3).
  – High risk: Tumor >4 cm and presence of rete testis invasion: 32% risk of relapse (3).
  – Carcinoma in situ: Surveillance versus radiotherapy depends on patient's preference (3)[B].
  – Low-risk stage I: 5-year surveillance with regular abdominal imaging (3)[B] versus treatment as for high-risk stage I
  – High-risk stage I: Carboplatin × 1 cycle versus radiotherapy; have similar relapse risk and long-term survival. Radiotherapy carries long-term risk of 2nd malignancy (3,5)[A].
  – Stage IIA–B: Radiotherapy, optional chemotherapy as per stage IIC (3)[B]
  – Stage IIC–III: BEP chemotherapy × 3–4 cycles; need for bleomycin must be addressed in patients >40 years of age with poor lung volumes owing to risk of pneumonitis (3)[A].
  – Relapse after radiotherapy: Chemotherapy × 4 cycles of BEP lower dose of etoposide (3).
    ◦ Stage II–III: CXR and CT 1 month after chemotherapy to evaluate response (3)[B]
    ◦ Follow-up of metastatic disease: Normal posttreatment scan: Follow up as for stage I; abnormal: Repeat CT scan every 6 months until stabilized.
    ◦ PET scan may be considered for residual active cancer (3)[B].
    ◦ Biopsy or resection for large residual or growing masses (3)[B]
- Nonseminoma:
  – Stage I:
    ◦ Low risk (no vascular invasion): 20% relapse rate; surveillance protocol

    ◦ High risk (vascular invasion present): 40–50% relapse rate; BEP ×2 cycles
  – Stage II–IV:
    ◦ Good prognosis: BEP × 3 cycles
    ◦ Poor prognosis: BEP × 4 cycles versus VIP × 4 cycles

Additional Therapies

- Retroperitoneal lymph node dissection (RPLND) considered in patients with residual disease.
- Sperm cryopreservation considered for patients intended for chemo/radiotherapy (3).

 ONGOING CARE

PATIENT EDUCATION
USPSTF recommends *against* routine testicular cancer screening and does not recommend teaching patients testicular self-exam

PROGNOSIS

- 5-year survival rate >96% for all stages and >70% for men with distant metastases.
- Low-, intermediate-, and poor-risk disease 5-year survival rates: 91%, 79%, and 48%, respectively

COMPLICATIONS

- Orchiectomy: Intrascrotal hematoma, retroperitoneal hematoma
- RPLND: Intraoperative hemorrhage, lymphocele, loss of seminal emission/infertility
- Radiation: Radiation enteritis, nephritis

REFERENCES

1. Jemal A, Siegel R, Ward E, et al. Cancer Statistics, 2009. *CA Cancer J Clin.* 2009.
2. Sokoloff MH, Joyce GF, Wise M, et al. Testis cancer. *J Urol.* 2007;177:2030–41.
3. Huddart R, Kataja V, ESMO Guidelines Working Group. Testicular seminoma: ESMO clinical recommendations for diagnosis, treatment and follow-up. *Ann Oncol.* 2008;19(Suppl 2):ii49–51.
4. Martin JM, Panzarella T, Zwahlen DR, et al. Evidence-based guidelines for following stage 1 seminoma. *Cancer.* 2007.
5. Oliver RT, Mason MD, Mead GM, et al. Radiotherapy versus single-dose carboplatin in adjuvant treatment of stage I seminoma: a randomised trial. *Lancet.* 2005;366:293–300.

 CODES

ICD9

- 186.0 Malignant neoplasm of undescended testis
- 186.9 Malignant neoplasm of other and unspecified testis

CLINICAL PEARLS

- Testicular cancer is the most common solid-organ tumor in males aged 20–34 years.
- Ultrasound is initial imaging of choice for testicular pathology.
- Radical orchiectomy is used for both diagnosis and treatment.
- >95% overall survival

TESTICULAR TORSION

Timothy L. Black, MD

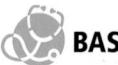 **BASICS**

DESCRIPTION
- Twisting of testis and spermatic cord, resulting in acute ischemia:
  - Intravaginal torsion: Occurs within tunica vaginalis
  - Extravaginal torsion: Involves twisting of testis, cord, and processus vaginalis (especially in newborns) and in undescended testes
- System(s) affected: Reproductive

Geriatric Considerations
Rare in this age group

Pediatric Considerations
Peak incidence at age 14 years

EPIDEMIOLOGY
Incidence
- Approximately 1/4,000 males before age 25 years (1)
- Predominant age:
  - Occurs from newborn period to 7th decade
  - 2/3 of cases occur in 2nd decade, with peak at age 14 years (2)[C].
  - 2nd peak in neonates (in utero torsion usually occurs around week 32 of gestation)

RISK FACTORS
- May be more common in winter
- Paraplegia
- Previous contralateral testicular torsion

Genetics
- Unknown
- There have been rare reports of familial testicular torsion (3)[B].

PATHOPHYSIOLOGY
- The most common anatomic anomaly is a high insertion of the tunica vaginalis on the spermatic cord, resulting in increased testicular mobility:
  - This anomaly is bilateral in nearly 80% of patients.
- There is no clear anatomic defect associated with extravaginal testicular torsion.

ETIOLOGY
- Torsion is usually spontaneous and idiopathic.
- History of trauma in 20% of patients
- 1/3 have had prior episodic testicular pain.
- Contraction of cremasteric muscle or dartos may play a role and is stimulated by trauma, exercise, cold, and sexual stimulation.
- Possible alterations in testosterone levels during nocturnal sex response cycle; possible elevated testosterone levels in neonates
- Testis must have inadequate, incomplete, or absent fixation within scrotum.
- Torsion may occur in either clockwise or counterclockwise direction (1)[C].

 DIAGNOSIS

HISTORY
- Acute onset of pain, often during period of inactivity
- Prior history of multiple episodes of testicular pain with spontaneous resolution may indicate intermittent testicular torsion (2).

PHYSICAL EXAM
- Scrotum is enlarged, red, edematous, and painful.
- The 1st symptom is pain (usually sudden but may have a gradual onset with subsequent increase in severity).
- Nausea and vomiting are common.
- Fever may occur but is not typical.
- Testicle is exquisitely tender.
- Testis may be high in scrotum with a transverse lie.
- Absence of cremasteric reflex
- Tender, swollen, erythematous testicle

DIAGNOSTIC TESTS & INTERPRETATION
Lab
Urinalysis usually not helpful

Imaging
Doppler ultrasound (US) may confirm testicular swelling but is diagnostic by demonstrating lack of blood flow to the testicle.

Diagnostic Procedures/Surgery
- Doppler US flow detection demonstrates absent or reduced blood flow with torsion and increased flow with inflammatory process (reliable only in 1st 12 h) (1)[C].
- Radionuclide testicular scintigraphy with technetium-99m pertechnetate demonstrates absent/decreased vascularity in torsion and increased vascularity with inflammatory processes (including torsion of appendix testes).
- In boys with intermittent, recurrent testicular torsion, both Doppler US and radionuclide scintigraphy will be normal (4)[C].

Pathological Findings
- Venous thrombosis
- Tissue edema and necrosis
- Arterial thrombosis

DIFFERENTIAL DIAGNOSIS
- Epididymo-orchitis
- Incarcerated/strangulated inguinal hernia
- Acute hydrocele
- Traumatic hematoma
- Idiopathic scrotal edema
- Torsion appendix testis (this may account for 35–67% of all cases of acute scrotal pain in children) (3)[B]

- Acute varicocele
- Epididymal hypertension (venous congestion of testicle or prostate due to sexual arousal that does not end in orgasm)
- Testicular tumor
- Henoch-Schönlein purpura
- Scrotal abscess
- Leukemic infiltrate

 **TREATMENT**

- Manual reduction: Best performed by experienced physician; may be successful, facilitated by lidocaine 1% (plain) injection at level of external ring; always must be followed by orchidopexy
- Surgical exploration via scrotal approach with detorsion, evaluation of testicular viability, orchidopexy of viable testicle, orchiectomy of nonviable testicle
- In boys with a history of intermittent episodes of testicular pain, scrotal exploration is warranted with testicular fixation if abnormal testicular attachments are confirmed (4)[C].

ADDITIONAL TREATMENT

General Measures

Early exam is crucial because necrosis of the testicle usually occurs after 6–8 h.

SURGERY/OTHER PROCEDURES

Operative testicular fixation of the torsed testicle after detorsion and confirmation of viability:

- At least 3- to 4-point fixation with nonabsorbable sutures between the tunica albuginea and the tunica vaginalis
- Excision of window of tunica albuginea with suture to dartos fascia

- Any testis that is not clearly viable (and obvious) should be removed.
- Testes of questionable viability that are preserved and pexed invariably atrophy.
- Requires general anesthesia
- Usually can be done on outpatient basis
- Bilateral testicular fixation is recommended by many surgeons.
- Contralateral testicle frequently has similar abnormal fixation.

 ONGOING CARE

FOLLOW-UP RECOMMENDATIONS

Patient Monitoring

- Postoperative visit at 1–2 weeks
- Yearly visits until puberty may be needed to evaluate for atrophy.

DIET

Regular

PATIENT EDUCATION

Possibility of testicular atrophy in salvaged testis with depressed sperm counts

PROGNOSIS

- Testicular salvage:
  - Salvage is related directly to duration of torsion (85–97% if <6 h, <10% if >24 h)
  - The degree of torsion is related to testicular salvage (3)[B]:
    - The median degree of torsion is less than 360 in patients who are explored and orchidopexy performed.
    - The median degree of torsion is 540 in patients who undergo exploration and require orchiectomy.
- 80–94% may have depressed spermatogenesis related to duration of ischemic injury (possibly related to autoimmune-mediated injury).
- As many as 2/3 of salvaged testicles may atrophy in 1st 2–3 years after torsion.

COMPLICATIONS

- Possible testicular atrophy
- Abnormal spermatogenesis
- Infertility (3)[B]:
  - Nearly 36% of patients who experience torsion have sperm counts less than 20 million/mL.
  - Antisperm antibodies and inhibin B may be useful following testicular function.

REFERENCES

1. Sessions AE, Rabinowitz R, Hulbert WC, et al. Testicular torsion: direction, degree, duration and disinformation. *J Urol*. 2003;169:663–5.
2. Van Glabeke E, Khairouni A, Larroquet M, et al. Acute scrotal pain in children: results of 543 surgical explorations. *Pediatr Surg Int*. 1999;15:353–7.
3. Kapoor S, et al. Testicular torsion: a race against time. *Int J Clin Pract*. 2008;62:821–7.
4. Eaton SH, Cendron MA, Estrada CR, et al. Intermittent testicular torsion: diagnostic features and management outcomes. *J Urol*. 2005;174:1532–5; discussion 1535.

 CODES

ICD9
608.20 Torsion of testis, unspecified

CLINICAL PEARLS

- The diagnosis of testicular torsion is usually made by physical exam. Patients with suspected torsion should be taken to the operating room without delay. If diagnosis is in question, a testicular Doppler US may be done to evaluate blood flow.
- Infertility can be a problem even if the testicle is viable. Autoimmune antibodies may be produced, and they may affect subsequent fertility.

TESTOSTERONE DEFICIENCY

Janice E. Daugherty, MD

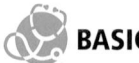 **BASICS**

Testosterone deficiency is not uncommon in the US. People in certain populations are more likely to have low androgen levels, which increases the risk of low-trauma fractures, decline in sexual function, sense of well-being, muscle mass, and strength.

DESCRIPTION
- Food and Drug Administration (FDA) definition: Testosterone (T) <300 ng/dL
- T is essential for normal sexual development and function.
- T levels may decline with aging and certain disease states.
- System(s) affected: Body composition and strength; Bone; Cardiovascular; Reproductive; Mood; CNS; Hematologic
- Synonym(s): Hypogonadism; Hypoandrogenism; Androgen deficiency in the aging male (ADAM) syndrome

EPIDEMIOLOGY
With aging and certain disease states, men and women can have declines in androgen production that lead to symptoms of testosterone deficiency.

Incidence
- 12.3/1,000 person-years in the US
- Late-onset hypogonadism: 481,000 new cases in US men 40–69 years old

Prevalence
- 2–4 million men in US; due to problems of definition, the prevalence in women is undetermined.
- 12% of men in their 50s; 28% between 70 and 79 years of age; 49% in men ≥80 years of age

RISK FACTORS
- Obesity, type 2 diabetes, COPD
- Medications that affect testosterone production or metabolism
- Stress
- Undescended testicles
- Trauma; infection; radiation or tumors of testis, pituitary, hypothalamus; chemotherapy
- Exposure to environmental endocrine modulators
- Chronic infections or inflammatory disease

Genetics
Some chromosomal disorders are inherited:
- Klinefelter: XXY karyotype (small testis, eunuchoid body habitus, gynecomastia)
- Kallmann: Abnormal gonadotropin-releasing hormone (GnRH) secretion due to abnormal hypothalamus development (micropenis, anosmia)

GENERAL PREVENTION
General health maintenance, such as prevention and treatment of obesity

PATHOPHYSIOLOGY
- Normal hypothalamic–pituitary–testis axis:
  - Hypothalamus produces GnRH, which stimulates pituitary to produce follicle-stimulating hormone (FSH) and luteinizing hormone (LH).
  - LH stimulates the testis to produce T.
  - T inhibits production of LH through negative feedback.

- Primary testosterone deficiency: Testis produces insufficient amount of T. FSH/LH levels are elevated.
- Secondary T deficiency (also known as *hypogonadotropic hypogonadism*): Low T from inadequate production of LH

ETIOLOGY
- Congenital syndromes: Undescended testicles
- Orchiectomy; testicular trauma
- Infectious: Mumps orchitis, HIV/AIDS, tuberculosis
- Systemic:
  - Cushing syndrome
  - Hemochromatosis
  - Autoimmune
  - Granulomatous
  - Severe illness (e.g., renal disease, cirrhosis)
  - Sickle-cell disease
- Obesity; obstructive sleep apnea
- Drugs that decrease production: Corticosteroids, ethanol, ketoconazole, spironolactone, marijuana, opioids, cimetidine
- Elevated prolactin:
  - Prolactinoma
  - Dopamine antagonists block inhibitory dopamine effects on prolactin secretion: Neuroleptics, metoclopramide, etc.
- Idiopathic hypogonadotropic hypogonadism
- Chemotherapy
- Radiation to the testis

COMMONLY ASSOCIATED CONDITIONS
- Infertility, low sperm count, erectile dysfunction
- Osteopenia/osteoporosis
- Diabetes, dyslipidemia, depression: Increased incidence and shorter time to diagnosis (1)
- Increased ratio of fat to lean body mass
- Free T levels lower in Alzheimer disease (2)

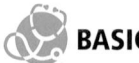 **DIAGNOSIS**

Test populations who may be at increased risk of T deficiency due to congenital conditions or environmental exposures. Broad-based population screening for T deficiency is not recommended.

HISTORY
- Congenital and developmental abnormalities
- Infertility
- Sexual function issues, including decreased libido, erectile dysfunction
- Depression, fatigue, difficulty with concentration/attention
- Decreased beard growth (increased interval between shaving), decreased muscle strength, energy level
- Increase in body fat, development of diabetes
- Bone fractures from relatively minor trauma
- Testicular trauma, infection, radio- or chemotherapy
- Decrease in testicle size or consistency
- Headaches or vision changes suggesting pituitary dysfunction
- Use of medications increasing risk of low T, or for associated conditions

PHYSICAL EXAM
- Infancy: Ambiguous genitalia
- Puberty:
  - Impaired growth of penis, testicles
  - Lack of secondary male characteristics
  - Gynecomastia, eunuchoid habitus
- Adulthood:
  - Note whether muscular development, hair patterns on face and body, and fat distribution are consistent with age.
  - Presence of gynecomastia
  - Dermatologic changes to suggest hemochromatosis, corticosteroid excess
  - Eunuchoid habitus: Lower body >2 cm longer than upper, arm span >2 cm longer than height
  - Kyphosis, loss of height especially more than expected for age
- Testicular exam on Prader orchidometer:
  - Normal testis: 20–30 cc
  - Normal volume but soft and atrophic suggests postpubertal hypogonadism
  - Volume <5 cc suggests prepubertal causes.
  - Small and firm testis suggests Klinefelter.

DIAGNOSTIC TESTS & INTERPRETATION
Lab
An accurate diagnosis is based on the level of *bioavailable* testosterone; with aging, illness, or certain other exposures (e.g., tobacco smoke) levels of sex hormone binding globulin (SHBG) may increase, and total T level may not reflect hormone that is actually available to the tissues.

Initial lab tests
- In symptomatic individuals, morning total T level as initial test (3)[B]
- Opinions differ regarding utility and whether to measure or calculate free T value:
  - Total T reference range: 300–1,200 ng/dL (350 in younger males); free: 9–30 ng/dL. Bioavailable T at least 70 ng/dL.
  - Repeat the test in the morning if screening results are low (3)[B].
  - Diagnosis should not be made during an acute or subacute illness (3)[B].

Follow-Up & Special Considerations
- If T is low or low-normal, check LH:
  - High LH level: Primary hypogonadism
  - Low or normal LH: Secondary hypogonadism:
    - Check prolactin: High level inhibits GnRH.
    - Check TSH: Hypothyroidism
    - Transferrin saturation: Hemochromatosis
    - Dexamethasone suppression test (Cushing)
- Karyotype if Klinefelter suspected

Imaging
Imaging is not helpful in the initial diagnosis of testosterone deficiency.

Follow-Up & Special Considerations
If pituitary causes are suspected, CT scan or MRI may be used to evaluate structural lesions.

Diagnostic Procedures/Surgery
DEXA bone scan to evaluate bone density

DIFFERENTIAL DIAGNOSIS
- Ambiguous genitalia; micropenis
- Cryptorchidism
- Delayed puberty
- Obesity (lower total T; assess bioavailable T to confirm)
- Normal aging

TREATMENT

Testosterone replacement is recommended for symptomatic men with low T levels.

MEDICATION
First Line
Testosterone gel (AndroGel, Testim):
- 5–10 g containing 50–100 mg of T applied daily

ALERT
- Must avoid transfer of testosterone gel to female partner or children
- Improvements in sexual function, mood, lean body mass, bone density reported (4)[C]
- Oral therapy not recommended:
  - May cause liver toxicity
  - Physiologic levels hard to maintain
  - Not beneficial in older men

Second Line
- Delatestryl (testosterone enanthate) or Depo-Testosterone (testosterone cypionate) injection:
  - 100 mg/wk or 200 mg q2wks
  - Inexpensive
  - Levels high immediately after injection, fall to very low before next injection is due; may cause mood swings
- Transdermal patch (Androderm, Testoderm):
  - More expensive
  - May cause skin irritation
  - Scrotal patch:
    - Applied daily; delivers 6 mg
    - Need to shave scrotum
    - Dihydrotestosterone (DHT) levels are higher than normal.
  - Nonscrotal patch: 1–2 patches daily
  - Rotate sites to avoid irritation.
- Transbuccal bioadhesive tablets (Striant):
  - 30 mg b.i.d.
  - Gum-related events in 16% of men
- Subcutaneous pellets (Testopel) or compounded:
  - Last 3–6 months
  - May be difficult to adjust dose; easier to customize with compounded formulation.
  - Requires surgical insertion, which can be done in the office with local anesthesia.

ADDITIONAL TREATMENT
General Measures
- Pretreatment labs: Complete blood count (CBC), lipid profile, liver function tests (LFTs), and prostate-specific antigen (PSA).
- Baseline physical exam (including digital rectal exam [DRE] and prostate exam)
- For secondary T deficiency, correction of underlying cause may be necessary.
- If fertility is not an issue, T replacement therapy is recommended in symptomatic men with androgen deficiency who have low T levels to induce and maintain secondary sex characteristics and to improve their sexual function, sense of well-being, muscle mass and strength, and bone mineral density (3)[B].

- T therapy is contraindicated in patients with breast or prostate cancer, palpable prostate nodule or induration, or PSA >3 ng/mL without further urologic evaluation, hematocrit >50, hyperviscosity, untreated obstructive sleep apnea, severe lower urinary tract symptoms with IPSS >19, or class III or IV heart failure (3)[B].
- T therapy is not recommended for:
  - Mood or strength improvement for otherwise healthy older men (5)[C]
  - Asymptomatic men with low T measurements (3)[B]
- T-deficient men with HIV infection or on high doses of glucocorticoid treatment may benefit from short-term T therapy to promote lean body mass preservation and bone density (3)[B].

Issues for Referral
- In prepubertal patients, starting hormonal therapy at the appropriate age is of paramount importance:
  - In hypogonadotropic hypogonadism, T therapy does not confer fertility or stimulate testicular growth.
  - Pulsatile luteinizing hormone–releasing hormone (LHRH) or human chorionic gonadotropin (hCG) therapy is an option.
- Elevated PSA; abnormal prostate exam

COMPLEMENTARY AND ALTERNATIVE MEDICINE
Dihydroepiandrostenedione (DHEA) supplementation has not been studied adequately in humans to define potential risks vs benefits.

 ONGOING CARE

Monitoring of effectiveness of therapy as well as surveillance for adverse effects of replacement is necessary every 6–12 months.

FOLLOW-UP RECOMMENDATIONS
For replacement T therapy by the topical route, extreme care must be taken to avoid exposure of women or children to testosterone applied to the patient's skin.

Patient Monitoring
Monitor replacement therapy for 2–4 months initially and then 6–12 months thereafter:
- Digital prostate exam, PSA, lipid profile, CBC, SGPT before initiating therapy and at least annually thereafter
- T levels until stabilized

DIET
- Calcium 1,200 mg daily, vitamin D 800 IU daily
- Hypocaloric diet to reduce weight if obese

PATIENT EDUCATION
- T deficiency is a chronic condition that is likely to need lifelong replacement therapy.
- T replacement products must not be allowed to come in contact with women or children.

PROGNOSIS
- Sustained reversal of symptoms is the goal of therapy when adequate serum levels of T are achieved.
- Hypogonadotropic hypogonadism may be reversed successfully in 10% of patients (6).
- Androgen supplementation does not appear to improve any aspects of age-related frailty (7).

COMPLICATIONS
- Decreased sexual desire, muscle mass, bone density, loss of secondary sexual characteristics
- Complications of T replacement:
  - Benign prostate hyperplasia (BPH) exacerbation
  - Gynecomastia
  - Acne
  - Aggressive behavior
  - Polycythemia
  - Exacerbation of sleep apnea
  - Possible increased risk for cardiovascular events (8)
  - Hepatotoxicity with prolonged use
  - Exacerbation of metastatic prostate cancer

REFERENCES

1. Shores MM, et al. Increased incidence of diagnosed depressive illness in hypogonadal older men. *Arch Gen Psychiatry*. 2004;61(2):162–7.
2. Moffat SD, et al. Free T and risk for Alzheimer disease in older men. *Neurology*. 2004;62(2):170–1.
3. Bhasin S, et al. Testosterone therapy in adult men with androgen deficiency syndromes: An Endocrine Society clinical practice guideline. *J Clin Endocrinol Metab*. 2006;91(6):1995.
4. Wang C, et al. Long-term testosterone gel (AndroGel) treatment maintains beneficial effects on sexual function and mood, lean and fat mass, and bone mineral density in hypogonadal men. *J Clin Endocrinol Metab*. 2004;89(5):2085–98.
5. Lawrence D. US panel urges caution on testosterone therapy. Large-scale trials of efficacy and safety are needed before widespread use can be recommended. *Lancet*. 2003;362(9397):1725.
6. Raivio T, Falardeau J, Dwyer A, et al. Reversal of idiopathic hypogonadotropic hypogonadism. *N Engl J Med*. 2007;357:863–73.
7. Muller M, van den Beld AW, van der Schouw YT, et al. Effects of dehydroepiandrosterone and atamestane supplementation on frailty in elderly men. *J Clin Endocrinol Metab*. 2006;91:3988–91.
8. Haddad RM, Kennedy CC, Caples SM, et al. Testosterone and cardiovascular risk in men: a systematic review and meta-analysis of randomized placebo-controlled trials. *Mayo Clin Proc*. 2007;82:29–39.

 CODES

ICD9
- 257.2 Other testicular hypofunction
- 758.7 Klinefelter's syndrome

CLINICAL PEARLS
- Every man presenting with a complaint of erectile dysfunction or with a low-trauma fracture should be assessed for the presence of hypogonadism.
- Men with diabetes mellitus, obesity, or depression should be assessed for the presence of symptoms of testosterone deficiency and low bioavailable testosterone levels.

TETANUS

Zerlina Wong, MD
Thomas Germano, MD

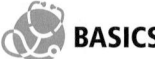 **BASICS**

Tetanus, or "lockjaw," was first described by Hippocrates nearly 30 centuries ago. Its etiology was discovered in 1884 by Carle and Rattone. Nocard developed passive immunization in 1897, which was used during World War I. Tetanus toxoid was developed by Descombe in 1924 and has been used for vaccination since.

DESCRIPTION
- Severe toxic bacterial infection by *Clostridium tetani* characterized by rigidity and intermittent tonic spasms of voluntary muscles—usually of the jaw and neck
- 4 types:
  – Generalized (most common, most severe)
  – Localized (generally mild)
  – Cephalic (affects cranial nerves)
  – Neonatal (very high mortality)
- Usual course is acute, 3–6 weeks duration; may be fatal
- Severity determined by frequency of spasms, presence of opisthotonus, and autonomic dysfunction (1)
- System(s) affected: Nervous
- Synonym(s): Lockjaw

Pediatric Considerations
- Mortality high in young
- Majority present at 6-8 days
- Infection most commonly enters through umbilical cord

Pregnancy Considerations
- Must treat vigorously despite pregnancy
- Infection may enter uterus postpartum.
- Tetanus toxoid in 2nd and 3rd trimesters of pregnancy if indicated/higher risk will reduce neonatal tetanus deaths (2)[A]

EPIDEMIOLOGY
Incidence
- Rare in US because of vaccination
- 700,000–1,000,000 cases annually worldwide

Prevalence
- Predominant age: Persons >60 years of age are less likely to have had a vaccine booster (3).
- Predominant gender: Male > Female
- Predominantly affects low- and medium-income countries of Asia and sub-Saharan Africa:
  – Neonates are the most vulnerable group.

RISK FACTORS
- Lack of vaccination or up-to-date booster, unknown vaccination history (i.e., immigrants, elderly)
- Age >60 years
- IV drug use
- Puncture wounds/crush injuries/surgical wounds
- Exposure of open wounds to soil/animal feces
- Newborn (umbilical entry, circumcision)
- Early postpartum with an infected uterus
- Frostbite
- Burns
- Diabetes/skin ulcers
- Wound with low O_2 supply/chronic wounds
- Tattooing/multiple piercings

GENERAL PREVENTION
- Active immunization with tetanus toxoid:
  – DTaP (diphtheria, tetanus toxoid, and acellular pertussis): For children 6 weeks–7 years of age:
    ○ Primary series of 4 doses at 2, 4, 6, and 15–18 months. Follow with booster at 4–6 years of age.
  – Tdap (tetanus, diphtheria, acellular pertussis): Give 1 dose at 11–12 years if 5 years since DTaP:
    ○ Important for people in contact with infants <12 months and health care workers
  – Td boosters every 10 years (2)
  – Toxoid immunization given to pregnant women at least 4 weeks apart reduces neonatal tetanus by 94% (4)
- Wound debridement/decontamination
- Passive immunization with tetanus immune globulin (TIG) postexposure
- Benzathine penicillin/penicillin G/erythromycin

PATHOPHYSIOLOGY
- *C. tetani* is a gram-positive obligate anaerobic rod. The organism is sensitive to heat and oxygen, but its spores are heat-resistant and may survive contact with most antiseptics.
- Tetanus is transmitted by tetanus spores, which enter the body through a contaminated wound.
- Following inoculation, spores germinate under anaerobic conditions to produce the toxins tetanospasmin and tetanolysin, which disseminate through blood and lymphatics:
  – Tetanospasmin causes the symptoms of tetanus.
  – Tetanolysin causes hemolysis, but plays no major role otherwise.
- Incubation period is generally 4–14 days after injury.
- Tetanospasmin enters the CNS peripherally, travels centrally to brain and sympathetic nervous system, and acts at motor neuron end-plates to alter neurotransmitter release.
- Tetanospasmin blocks inhibitory neurons and results in unopposed muscle contraction/spasm/seizure.
- Affects newborns born to mothers who were not properly vaccinated. Transplacental transfer of antitoxin generally protective for first 1–2 months of life (4).

COMMONLY ASSOCIATED CONDITIONS
See Risk Factors.

℞ **DIAGNOSIS**

HISTORY
- Penetrating injury
- IV drug use
- History of contamination, especially soil/manure
- In neonates:
  – Poor umbilical hygiene
  – Lack of maternal immunization

PHYSICAL EXAM
- Painful tonic convulsions
- Autonomic instability
- Opisthotonos
- *Risus sardonicus* (fixed smile)
- Stiffness of the jaw (lockjaw, trismus)
- Dysphagia/drooling
- Hyper-reflexia

  May also see:
- Arrhythmias
- Asphyxia
- Convulsions
- Glottal/laryngeal spasms
- Hydrophobia
- Hyperhidrosis
- Hyperpyrexia
- Irritability
- Low-grade fever
- Muscular rigidity/spasticity
- Nuchal rigidity
- Pain at wound site

DIAGNOSTIC TESTS & INTERPRETATION
Diagnosis is based on clinical features. Laboratory tests may be performed to rule out other conditions that may mimic or complicate tetanus.

Lab
Initial lab tests
- Complete blood count: PMN leukocytosis
- *C. tetani* not generally visible on Gram stain/wound culture:
  – Culture positive in approximately 30%
  – Umbilical stump cultures usually negative
- CSF generally normal (no findings)

Diagnostic Procedures/Surgery
- Electrocardiogram: Tachy- or bradyarrhythmia
- Antitoxin assay (not readily available) levels >0.01–0.015 IU/mL are protective—tetanus less likely (4)[B]
- Spatula test:
  – Touch oropharynx with tongue blade.
  – Test negative if gag reflex elicited as patient tries to expel blade
  – Test positive if patient bites down on blade due to masseter reflex spasm
  – 94% sensitive; 100% specific

DIFFERENTIAL DIAGNOSIS
- Acute dystonic reaction:
  – Phenothiazines
  – Metoclopramide
- Neuroleptic malignant syndrome
- Rabies
- Meningoencephalitis
- Subarachnoid hemorrhage
- Seizure disorder
- Peritonsillar abscess
- Hypocalcemic tetany
- Strychnine poisoning
- Alcohol withdrawal
- Amyotrophic lateral sclerosis

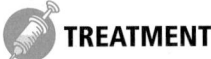 **TREATMENT**

MEDICATION
First Line
- Diazepam to treat muscle rigidity; combined anticonvulsant and muscle relaxation action, sedative, and anxiolytic effect (1)[A]:
  – 5–10 mg p.o. q4–6h p.r.n. for mild spasms, IV for moderate spasms
  – Mix 50–100 mg in 500 mL D5W and infuse at 40 mg/h for severe spasms.
- Tetanus toxoid in a previously immunized patient
- TIG confers passive immunity:
  – 3,000–6,000 U IM
- Intrathecal immunoglobulin (1,000 U lyophilized human immunoglobulin) reduces spasms, hospital stay, and respiratory assistance (NNT 4.2) (5)[A].
- Metronidazole may decrease mortality; some reviews consider it drug of choice:
  – 500 mg p.o. q6h OR
  – 1 g IV q12h not to exceed 4 g/d
- Penicillin G: 2 million U IV q6h; traditionally considered drug of choice
- If penicillin-allergic:
  – Doxycycline 100 mg q12h
  – Clindamycin 150–300 mg IV q6h

ALERT
- Benzodiazepines (BZD) are the mainstay of treatment.
- Giving diazepam alone or supplementing with conventional anticonvulsants found to shorten hospitalization and produce milder clinical course (1)[A].
- Caution with high doses of BZDs; may cause respiratory depression
- Do not use TIG IV. Administer IM in different location than toxoid to avoid reaction.
- Antibiotic course should be given for 7–10 days.

Second Line
- Equine tetanus antitoxin: 500-1,000 IU/kg given IM/IV, but only if TIG (human) is not available
- Chlorpromazine/phenobarbitone for muscle rigidity:
  – Higher mortality and longer, more severe clinical course than diazepam (1)[A]

ADDITIONAL TREATMENT
General Measures
- Rest
- Observation
- Adequate caloric supply
- Deep vein thrombosis and ulcer prophylaxis

Issues for Referral
- Supportive care and airway considerations require ICU care.
- Consult pulmonologist if severe respiratory symptoms.
- Consult anesthesia if considering intrathecal therapy/airway control.

Additional Therapies
Physical therapy once spasms resolve

SURGERY/OTHER PROCEDURES
- Wound debridement
- Tracheostomy if needed

IN-PATIENT CONSIDERATIONS
Initial Stabilization
- Intubation: Consider prophylactic intubation for moderate/severe symptoms:
  – Prepare for emergency surgical airway due to reflex laryngospasm.
  – Caution if using succinylcholine; risk of hyperkalemia later in course of disease (6)
- Anticonvulsants for muscle spasms and/or rigidity

Admission Criteria
Diagnosis of tetanus

IV Fluids
IV hydration necessary

Nursing
- Bladder catheterization
- Maintain quiet, dark environment and minimize manipulation/procedures to avoid triggering spasm.

 ONGOING CARE

FOLLOW-UP RECOMMENDATIONS
- Tetanus immunization series is necessary:
  – Infection does NOT confer immunity.
- Sequelae after infection are rare.

Patient Monitoring
Admit to ICU due to possible cardiac arrhythmias, autonomic dysfunction, and respiratory failure.

DIET
n.p.o. until well, feed by nasogastric (NG)/PEG tube

PATIENT EDUCATION
Importance of tetanus immunization

PROGNOSIS
- 25–50% mortality
- Poor prognostic factors:
  – Autonomic system involvement
  – Form of tetanus:
    ○ Neonatal > generalized > cephalic > localized
  – Short incubation period
  – Extremes of age
  – Severity of symptoms
- Recovery is complete if patient survives.

COMPLICATIONS
- Respiratory arrest
- Cardiac failure
- Pulmonary emboli
- Bacterial infection
- Dehydration
- Vertebral fractures
- Airway obstruction
- Anoxia
- Urinary retention
- Constipation
- Aspiration pneumonia
- Rhabdomyolysis/acute renal failure
- Complications of vaccination: Local adverse reaction (erythema, edema), local lymphadenopathy, Arthus-like local reactions, hives, anaphylaxis, Guillain-Barré syndrome, peripheral neuropathy

REFERENCES
1. Okoromah CN, Lesi FE, et al. Diazepam for treating tetanus. *Cochrane Database Syst Rev*. 2004; CD003954.
2. Demicheli V, et al. Vaccines for women to prevent neonatal tetanus. *Cochrane Database Syst Rev*. 2008;1:CD002959.
3. Pascual FB, McGinley EL, Zanardi LR, et al. Tetanus surveillance–United States, 1998–2000. *MMWR Surveill Summ*. 2003;52:1–8.
4. Blencowe H, Lawn J, Vandelaer J, et al. Tetanus toxoid immunization to reduce mortality from neonatal tetanus. *Int J Epidemiol*. 2010; 39(Suppl 1):i102–9.
5. Miranda-Filho Dde B, Ximenes RA, Barone AA, et al. Randomised controlled trial of tetanus treatment with antitetanus immunoglobulin by the intrathecal or intramuscular route. *BMJ*. 2004;328: 615.
6. Hsu SS, Groleau G, et al. Tetanus in the emergency department: a current review. *J Emerg Med*. 2001;20:357–65.

ADDITIONAL READING
- Centers for Disease Control and Prevention. *Summary of Recommendations for Childhood and Adolescent Immunizations*. 2008.
- Tetanus. Epidemiology and Prevention of Vaccine-Preventable Diseases. *CDC Web site*. 2008.
- Poudel P, Budhathoki S, Manandhar S, et al. Tetanus. *Kathmandu Univ Med J (KUMJ)*. 2009;7:315–22.

See Also (Topic, Algorithm, Electronic Media Element)
Lockjaw, Tetanus Neonatorum, Anaerobic and Necrotizing Infections; Immunizations; Meningitis, Bacterial

 CODES

ICD9
037 Tetanus

CLINICAL PEARLS
- Tetanus is caused by *C. tetani*; can be severe and life-threatening.
- Infection is associated with contaminated wounds and unclear vaccination history.
- Immunization is essential to prevention.
- Diagnosis is clinical and must be considered in patients with muscle spasms despite often negative lab results.
- Treatment involves neutralizing toxin, vaccinating, and providing antibiotics; however, supportive care is the mainstay of therapy to prevent complications.

THALASSEMIA

Herbert L. Muncie, Jr., MD

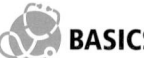 BASICS

DESCRIPTION
- A group of inherited hematologic disorders that affect the synthesis of adult hemoglobin tetramer (HbA) (1)
- β-Thalassemia is due to a deficient synthesis of β-globin chain, whereas α-thalassemia is due to a deficient synthesis of α-globin chain:
  - The synthesis of the unaffected globin chain proceeds normally.
  - This leads to inadequate hemoglobin production and unbalanced accumulation of globin chains, which then results in hypochromic, microcytic red blood cells (RBCs) and hemolytic anemia.
- Thalassemia is prevalent in the Mediterranean region, the Middle East, Southeast Asia, and among ethnic groups originating from these areas.
- β-Thalassemia is increased in patients of African and Southeast Asian descent, whereas α-thalassemia is more common in persons of Mediterranean, African, and Southeast Asian descent.
- Types:
  - Thalassemia trait (α or β): Absent or mild anemia with microcytosis and hypochromia. No transfusion therapy is needed.
  - α-Thalassemia major with hemoglobin Barts usually results in fatal hydrops fetalis.
  - β-Thalassemia intermedia: Milder form. Transfusion therapy may not be needed or may be needed later in life.
  - β-Thalassemia major: Severe anemia, growth retardation, hepatosplenomegaly, bone marrow expansion, and bone deformities. Transfusion therapy is necessary to sustain life.
- Varieties common in Southeast Asians include hemoglobin H disease (a more severe form of α-thalassemia) and hemoglobin E/β-thalassemia, which often mimics α-thalassemia major in its severity.
- System(s) affected: Hematologic/Lymphatic/Immunologic; Cardiac; Hepatic
- Synonym(s): Mediterranean anemia; Hereditary leptocytosis; Thalassemia major and minor; Cooley anemia

Pediatric Considerations
- β-thalassemia major causes symptoms during early childhood, usually starting at 6 months of age, and requires treatment to sustain life.
- Newborn's cord blood or heel stick should be screened for hemoglobinopathies with hemoglobin electrophoresis or comparably accurate test, although this primarily detects sickle cell disease.

Pregnancy Considerations
- Genetic counseling is advised for couples at risk for having a child with thalassemia and for parents or other relatives of a child with thalassemia (2,3)[A].
- During the 1st trimester, test chorionic villus samples with polymerase chain reaction (PCR) technology to detect point mutations or deletions.

EPIDEMIOLOGY
Incidence
- Occurs in approximately 4.4/10,000 live births
- Predominant age: Symptoms start to appear 6 months after birth with β-thalassemia major.
- Predominant sex: Male = Female

Prevalence
- <1,000 patients in the US are affected with β-thalassemia major.
- The prevalence of thalassemia trait within the involved ethnic groups ranges from 5–30%.

RISK FACTORS
Family history

Genetics
- Inherited in an autosomal recessive pattern
- α-Thalassemia results from the deletion of ≥ 1 of the 4 genes, 2 on each chromosome 16, responsible for α-globin synthesis. Nondeletional forms do occur rarely. 4-gene deletion results in hemoglobin Barts causing fatal hydrops fetalis. 3-gene deletion results in hemoglobin H, 2-gene deletion is the trait, and 1-gene deletion is a silent carrier state.
- β-Thalassemia is caused by any of >200 point mutations and, very rarely, deletions on chromosome 11, although probably 20 alleles account for >80% of the mutations.
- Significantly disparate phenotype with the same genotype is unexplained by variability of known loci because β-globin chain production can range from near normal to absent.

GENERAL PREVENTION
- Prenatal information: Genetic counseling regarding partner selection and information on the availability of diagnostic tests in the event of pregnancy
- Complication prevention:
  - For offspring of adult thalassemia patients, evaluation for thalassemia by 1 year of age
  - Severe forms:
    - Avoid exposure to sick contacts.
    - Keep immunizations up to date, including pneumococcal vaccine and annual influenza vaccine.
  - Promptly treat bacterial infections (after splenectomy, patients should maintain a supply of an appropriate antibiotic to take at the onset of symptoms of a bacterial infection).
  - Dental checkups every 6 months
  - Avoid activities that could increase the risk of bone fractures.
- Genetic counseling

ETIOLOGY
Genetic

COMMONLY ASSOCIATED CONDITIONS
See Complications

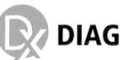 DIAGNOSIS

Thalassemia trait has no signs or symptoms.

HISTORY
- Poor growth
- Excessive fatigue
- Cholelithiasis
- Pathologic fractures
- Shortness of breath

PHYSICAL EXAM
- Pallor
- Splenomegaly
- Jaundice
- Maxillary hyperplasia
- Dental malocclusion

DIAGNOSTIC TESTS & INTERPRETATION
Special tests:
- Bone marrow aspiration
- Multiple indices have been evaluated to discriminate β-thalassemia trait from iron deficiency anemia (England and Fraser; Srivastana and Bevington; Shine-La and Green-King), yet none is sensitive enough to exclude β-thalassemia trait (4).
- For children, calculate Mentzer index (mean corpuscular volume/RBC count):
  - <13: Thalassemia more likely
  - >13: Iron deficiency more likely

Lab
- Hemoglobin: Usual range 10.0–12.0 g/dL with thalassemia trait
- Hematocrit:
  - 28–40% in thalassemia trait
  - May fall to <10% in β-thalassemia major
- Peripheral blood:
  - Microcytosis
  - Hypochromia
  - High percentage of target cells
  - Reticulocyte count elevated
- Red cell distribution width (RDW):
  - A normal RDW with a microcytic hypochromic anemia is almost always β-thalassemia trait.
  - The RDW will almost always be elevated in iron deficiency anemia, but only in approximately 50% of β-thalassemia trait patients.
- Hemoglobin electrophoresis:
  - In β-thalassemia trait, elevated HbA$_2$ levels (>4.0%) may be present but are usually normal.
  - In β-thalassemia major or intermedia, elevated HbA$_2$, elevated HbF, reduced or absent HbA
  - In α-thalassemia, no recognizable electrophoretic pattern occurs in adults.
  - The presence of hemoglobin H or hemoglobin Barts at birth confirms α-thalassemia.
- DNA analysis:
  - DNA analysis with PCR can definitely diagnose α-thalassemia, but is not routinely done due to the high cost.

Pathological Findings
- Bone marrow erythroid hyperplasia
- Iron deposits in heart muscle
- Hepatic siderosis

DIFFERENTIAL DIAGNOSIS
- Iron deficiency
- Other hemolytic anemias
- Hemoglobinopathies

TREATMENT
- Outpatient for mild cases
- Inpatient for transfusion therapy

MEDICATION
- Antibiotics for bacterial infections
- Thalassemia intermedia and major: Folic acid supplements (1 mg daily)

First Line
β-Thalassemia major:
- Iron chelation with deferoxamine (Desferal):
  - SC or continuous IV infusion, 20–40 mg/kg over 8–12 h daily
  - Usually started before 5–8 years of age
  - Treatment lasts 3–5 years to reach serum ferritin <1,000 ng/mL.
- Deferasirox (Exjade) 20–30 mg/kg/d p.o. acceptable alternative; approved in the US (5)

Second Line
Deferiprone 75–100 mg/kg/d p.o. acceptable alternative for patients unable to receive deferoxamine; not approved in the US

ADDITIONAL TREATMENT
β-thalassemia intermedia:
- Hydroxyurea may improve hemoglobin 1–2 g/dL (6)

General Measures
- Mild cases require no therapy.
- Thalassemia intermedia: Normally, no therapy is necessary unless hemoglobin falls to a level that causes symptoms; then transfusion therapy may be needed. Decision is based primarily on patient's quality of life.
- Thalassemia major:
  - Maintain a mean hemoglobin level of at least 9.3 g/dL (1.4 mmol/L) with a regular transfusion schedule.
  - Folate supplementation daily (1 mg)
  - Treat bacterial infections promptly.
- Iron overload:
  - Patients receiving transfusion therapy increase total-body iron 4× over the normal amount.
  - Therapy is iron chelation.

Issues for Referral
Thalassemia major usually requires hematology consult.

Additional Therapies
- Psychological support seems appropriate for this chronic disease.
- However, no conclusions can be made regarding specific therapies.

SURGERY/OTHER PROCEDURES
- Splenectomy:
  - May be needed if hypersplenism causes a marked increase in the transfusion requirement
  - Defer surgery until patient is 4–6 years of age (owing to increased infection risk).
  - Administer polyvalent pneumococcal vaccine 1 month before splenectomy. Children should complete their pneumococcal conjugate vaccine series.
  - Daily penicillin prophylaxis, 250 mg b.i.d., after splenectomy for 2 years for all patients and for children until age 16.
- Bone marrow transplantation in childhood: Only curative therapy, and generally excellent outcome for low-risk patients

ONGOING CARE

FOLLOW-UP RECOMMENDATIONS
- Thalassemia trait requires no restrictions.
- β-Thalassemia major:
  - Avoid strenuous activities (e.g., football, soccer).
  - Acceptable activity levels will be determined on an individual basis depending on the severity of disorder.

Patient Monitoring
- For β-thalassemia major, lifelong monitoring is necessary because the therapy and disease progression have numerous potential complications.
- Thalassemia trait patients require no special follow-up.

DIET
- Thalassemia trait requires no restrictions.
- β-Thalassemia major:
  - Avoid iron-rich foods (e.g., red meats such as liver and some cereals).

PATIENT EDUCATION
Printed patient information available from Cooley Anemia Foundation, 330 7th Ave. Suite 900, New York, NY 10001; http://www.thalassemia.org or http://www.cooleysanemia.org

PROGNOSIS
- Outlook varies depending on type.
- Thalassemia trait patients live a normal life span.
- β-Thalassemia major patients live an average of 17 years and usually die by age 30.
- Iron overload causes most of the morbidity and mortality:
  - Cardiac events are the primary cause of death.
  - Effective iron chelation is improving longevity.

COMPLICATIONS
- Chronic hemolysis
- Susceptibility to infections after splenectomy
- Infections from blood transfusion
- Jaundice
- Leg ulcers
- Cholelithiasis
- Osteoporosis and low-trauma fractures
- Impaired growth rate
- Delayed or absent puberty
- Hypogonadism
- Hepatic siderosis
- Splenomegaly
- Cardiac disease from iron overload
- Thromboembolic phenomenon
- Aplastic and megaloblastic crises

REFERENCES
1. Muncie HL, Campbell J, et al. Alpha and beta thalassemia. *Am Fam Physician*. 2009;80:339–44.
2. ACOG Committee on Obstetrics. ACOG Practice Bulletin No. 78: hemoglobinopathies in pregnancy. *Obstet Gynecol*. 2007;109:229–37.
3. Tamhankar PM, Agarwal S, Arya V, et al. Prevention of homozygous beta thalassemia by premarital screening and prenatal diagnosis in India. *Prenat. Diagn*. 2009;29:83–8.
4. Ehsani MA, Shahgholi E, Rahiminejad MS, et al. A new index for discrimination between iron deficiency anemia and beta-thalassemia minor: results in 284 patients. *Pak J Biol Sci*. 2009;12:473–5.
5. Taher A, El-Beshlawy A, Elalfy MS, Al Zir K, Daar S, Habr D, Kriemler-Krahn U, Hmissi A, Al Jefri A, et al. Efficacy and safety of deferasirox, an oral iron chelator, in heavily iron-overloaded patients with beta-thalassemia: the ESCALATOR study. *Eur J Haematol*. 2009;82:458–65.
6. Dixit A, Chatterjee TC, Mishra P, et al. Hydroxyurea in thalassemia intermedia—a promising therapy. *Ann Hematol*. 2005;84:441–6.

ADDITIONAL READING
Disler PB, Lynch SR, Charlton RW, et al. The effect of tea on iron absorption. *Gut*. 1975;16:193–200.

CODES

ICD9
- 282.49 Other thalassemia
- 282.5 Sickle-cell trait
- 282.60 Sickle-cell disease, unspecified

CLINICAL PEARLS
- A hemoglobin electrophoresis is not required to make the diagnosis of thalassemia minor when evaluating a patient with mild hypochromic, microcytic anemia, and normal serum ferritin. Unless there is a need for genetic counseling, a hemoglobin electrophoresis is not required.
- Thalassemia is a genetic condition; hemoglobin will not improve over time.
- The anemia from thalassemia minor is not due to inadequate iron availability or iron storage. Therefore, giving iron supplements will not improve the anemia, and could be potentially harmful due to gastrointestinal distress and iron overload. If coexisting iron deficiency is proven, then iron therapy would be appropriate.

THORACIC OUTLET SYNDROME

William A. Tosches, MD
Daniel Mandell, MD

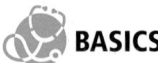 **BASICS**

DESCRIPTION

- A constellation of symptoms that affect the head, neck, shoulders, and upper extremities caused by compression of the neurovascular structures (i.e., brachial plexus and subclavian vessels) at the thoracic outlet, specifically in the area superior to the 1st rib and posterior to the clavicle
- 3 forms of thoracic outlet syndrome (TOS) have been described: Neurogenic, vascular (containing venous and arterial symptoms), and nonspecific (includes traumatic and secondary to certain provocative movements).
- Synonyms: Scalenus anticus syndrome; Cervical rib syndrome; Costoclavicular syndrome; Thoracic outlet syndrome

Pregnancy Considerations
Generalized tissue fluid accumulations and postural changes may aggravate symptoms.

EPIDEMIOLOGY

Incidence
- Predominant age:
  – Neurogenic type (95%): 20–60 years
  – Venous type (4%): 20–35 years
  – Arterial type (1%; atherosclerosis): Young adult or >50 years
- Predominant sex:
  – Neurogenic type: Female > Male (3.5:1)
  – Venous type: Male > Female
  – Arterial type: Male = Female
- No objective confirmatory tests available to measure true incidence
- Estimated 3–8/1,000 cases for neurogenic type
- Incidence of other TOS types is unclear.

RISK FACTORS
- Trauma, presence of a cervical rib
- Posttraumatic, exostosis of clavicle or 1st rib, postural abnormalities (e.g., drooping of shoulders, scoliosis), body building with increased muscular bulk in thoracic outlet area, rapid weight loss with vigorous physical exertion and/or exercise, pendulous breasts
- Occupational exposure: Computer users; musicians; repetitive work involving shoulders, arms, hands
- Young, thin females with long necks and drooping shoulders

GENERAL PREVENTION
Consider observation or further evaluation in patients with cervical ribs.

PATHOPHYSIOLOGY
The interscalene triangle area is reduced in TOS and may become smaller during certain shoulder and arm movements. Fibrotic bands, cervical ribs, and muscle variations may further narrow the triangle. Trauma or provocative movements affecting the lower brachial plexus have strong implications in TOS pathogenesis.

ETIOLOGY
- 3 known causes of TOS: Anatomic, traumatic/repetitive-movement activities, and neurovascular entrapment
- Anatomic: Variations in the anatomy of the neck scalene muscles may be responsible for presentations of the neurologic type of TOS, and may involve the superior border of the 1st rib. Cervical ribs also have been implicated as a cause of neurologic TOS, with subsequent neuronal fibrosing and degeneration associated with arterial hyalinization in the lower trunk of the brachial plexus. Fibrous bands to cervical ribs are often congenital.
- Trauma or repetitive-movement activities: Motor vehicle accidents with hyperextension injury and resulting fibrosis, including fibrous bands to the clavicle; musicians who maintain prolonged positions of shoulder abduction or extension may be at increased risk.
- Neurovascular entrapment: Occurring in the costoclavicular space between the 1st rib and the head of the clavicle

COMMONLY ASSOCIATED CONDITIONS
- Paget–von Schrötter syndrome: Thrombosis of subclavian vein
- Gilliatt-Sumner hand: Neurogenic atrophy of abductor pollicis brevis

 DIAGNOSIS

HISTORY
- Neurologic type, upper plexus (C4–C7):
  – Pain and paresthesias in head, neck, mandible, face, temporal area, upper back/chest, outer arm, and hand in a radial nerve distribution
  – Occipital and orbital headache
- Neurologic type, lower plexus (C8–T1):
  – Pain and paresthesias in axilla, inner arm, and hand in an ulnar nerve distribution, often nocturnal
  – Hypothenar and interosseous muscle atrophy
- Venous type: Arm claudication, cyanosis, swelling, distended arm veins
- Arterial type: Digital vasospasm, thrombosis/embolism, aneurysm, gangrene

PHYSICAL EXAM
- Positive Adson maneuver (head rotation to the affected side with cervical extension and then deep inhalation); test is positive if paresthesias occur or if radial pulse is not palpable during maneuver.
- Tenderness to percussion or palpation of supraclavicular area
- Worsening of symptoms with elevation of arm, overhead extension of arms, or with arms extended forward (e.g., driving a car, typing, carrying objects); prompt disappearance of symptoms with arm returning to neutral position
- Morley test:
  – Brachial plexus compression test in the supraclavicular area from the scalene triangle
  – Positive with reproduction of an aching sensation and typical localized paresthesia

- Hyperabduction test: Diminishment of radial pulse with elevation of arm above the head
- Military maneuver (i.e., costoclavicular bracing): When patient elevates chin and pushes shoulders posteriorly in an extreme "at-attention" position, symptoms are provoked.
- 1-minute Roos test:
  – A thoracic outlet shoulder girdle stress test
  – Shoulders and arms are braced in a 90-degree abducted and externally rotated position; patient is required to clench and relax fists repetitively for 1 minute.
  – A positive test reproduces the symptom.

DIAGNOSTIC TESTS & INTERPRETATION
Lab
Initial lab tests
Complete blood count (CBC), erythrocyte sedimentation rate (ESR), and C-reactive protein (CRP) determination may rule out underlying inflammatory conditions.

Imaging
Initial approach

- Radiograph (chest, C-spine, shoulders) (1)[B] may reveal elongated C7 transverse process or a cervical rib, Pancoast tumor, or healed clavicle fracture.
- Nerve conduction studies and electromyography (EMG) (2)[B]
- CT scan or MRI, although MRI is the method of choice when searching for nerve compression (3)[B]
- Evidence is insufficient to use MR angiography (4)[A].
- Doppler and duplex ultrasound (US) if vascular obstruction is suspected (3)[B]
- Arteriogram and venogram have limited roles; useful when symptoms suggestive of arterial insufficiency or ischemia, or in planning surgical intervention (5)[C]

Diagnostic Procedures/Surgery
No indicated procedures; anesthetic anterior scalene block may relieve pressure by scalene muscles on the brachial plexus, making this type of block diagnostic and potentially therapeutic, but it poses the risk of procedural damage to the brachial plexus (6)[C].

Pathological Findings
Systematic results of biopsy have not been reported. There is no indication for biopsy unless to investigate another underlying condition.

DIFFERENTIAL DIAGNOSIS
Cervical disk syndrome, carpal tunnel syndrome, orthopedic shoulder problems (shoulder strain, rotator cuff injury, tendonitis), cervical spondylitis, ulnar nerve compression at elbow and hand, multiple sclerosis, spinal cord tumor/disease, angina pectoris, migraine, complex regional pain syndromes, C3–C5 and C8 radiculopathies

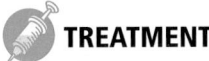
TREATMENT

MEDICATION
- No firm evidence exists for any approach to the 4 types of TOS.
- Physical therapy is 1st-line treatment (7)[B].
- Anti-inflammatory (ibuprofen):
  – Adult dose: 400–800 mg p.o. q8h; not to exceed 3,200 mg/d
  – Pediatric dose:
    ○ <12 years: Not recommended
    ○ >12 years: As in adults
  – Contraindications: Documented hypersensitivity; active PUD; renal or hepatic impairment; recent use of anticoagulants; hemorrhagic conditions
- Neuropathic pain: Carbamazepine, gabapentin, phenytoin, pregabalin, muscle relaxants such as baclofen or tizanidine may be helpful
- Severe pain: Consider opiates.

ADDITIONAL TREATMENT
General Measures
- Conservative management usually involves approaches to reduce and redistribute pressure and traction through the use of physiotherapy (8)[C] or prosthesis (9)[C].
- Intrascalene injections of botulinum toxin have been shown to decrease symptoms of suspected neurogenic TOS (10)[C].
- Physical therapy will develop strength in pectoral girdle muscles and achieve normal posture (1)[C].
- Severe cases may use taping, adhesive elastic bandages, moist heat, TENS, or US but should not substitute active exercise and correction of posture and muscle imbalance (7)[B].

Issues for Referral
- Neurologic, anesthesiologic, orthopedic, vascular surgery referral(s) may be indicated depending on the type of pathologic condition.
- Physical and rehabilitation physicians

SURGERY/OTHER PROCEDURES
- Operative if vascular involvement is present and/or loss of function or lifestyle occurs secondary to severity of symptoms and if conservative therapy fails after 2–3 months (1)[C]
- Transaxillary first rib resection (TFRR) may provide better pain relief than supraclavicular neuroplasty of the brachial plexus (SNBP), while overall both treatment options have generally positive outcomes (11)[B].
- Resection of 1st rib or cervical ribs via transaxillary (preferred with good–excellent outcome 80% of patients), supraclavicular (good–excellent outcome 80% of patients), posterior approaches (reserved for complicated TOS due to necessity of large muscle incision)
- Excision of adhesive bands, anterior scalenectomy (12)[B]

IN-PATIENT CONSIDERATIONS
Initial Stabilization
Conservative, outpatient, nonpharmacologic treatment is reasonable 1st-line therapy except in cases of thromboembolic phenomena and acute ischemia, symptoms of chronic vascular occlusion, stenosis, arterial dilatation, or progressive neurologic deficit (7)[A].

ONGOING CARE

FOLLOW-UP RECOMMENDATIONS
Correct improper posture, practice proper posture, exercises to strengthen shoulder elevator and neck extensor muscles, stretching exercises for scalene muscles, support bra for women with pendulous breasts, sleep with arms below chest level, avoid/reduce prolonged hyperabduction.

Patient Monitoring
Office follow-up visits every 3–4 weeks

PATIENT EDUCATION
Physical therapy, postural exercises, ergonomic workstation

PROGNOSIS
Follow-up from surgery at mean of 7.5 years showed that functional results were excellent, good, fair, and poor in 87 (49.4%), 61 (34.6%), 14 (8%), and 14 (8%) procedures, respectively (13)[C].

COMPLICATIONS
- Postoperative shoulder, arm, hand pain, and paresthesias in 10%
- 1.5–2% of patients will have symptomatic recurrences 1 month–7 years postoperatively (usually within 3 months).
- 0.5–1% of patients have brachial plexus injury, probably due to intraoperative traction.
- Reoperation is indicated for symptomatic recurrence with long posterior remnant of 1st rib (posterior approach) or with disrupted fibrous adhesions (transaxillary approach).
- Venous obstruction or arterial emboli; usually responds to thrombolytics

REFERENCES
1. Huang JH, Zager EL. Thoracic outlet syndrome. *Neurosurgery.* 2004;55:897–902; discussion 902–3.
2. Seror P. [Somesthetic evoked potentials and serial motor evoked potentials in the study of proximal peripheral nerve conduction. Apropos of 7 cases] *Ann Chir Main Memb Super.* 1995;14:182–91.
3. Demondion X, Herbinet P, Van Sint Jan S, et al. Imaging assessment of thoracic outlet syndrome. *Radiographics.* 2006;26:1735–50.
4. Estilaei SK, Byl NN. An Evidence-based Review of Magnetic Resonance Angiography for Diagnosing Arterial Thoracic Outlet Syndrome. *J Hand Ther.* 2006;19:410–20.
5. Sanders RJ, Hammond SL, Rao NM. Diagnosis of thoracic outlet syndrome. *J Vasc Surg.* 2007;46: 601–4.
6. Jordan SE, Machleder HI. Diagnosis of thoracic outlet syndrome using electrophysiologically guided anterior scalene blocks. *Ann Vasc Surg.* 1998;12:260–4.
7. Vanti C, Natalini L, Romeo A, et al. Conservative treatment of thoracic outlet syndrome. A review of the literature. *Eura Medicophys.* 2007;43:55–70.
8. Novak CB, Collins ED, Mackinnon SE. Outcome following conservative management of thoracic outlet syndrome. *J Hand Surg [Am].* 1995;20: 542–8.
9. Nakatsuchi Y, et al. Conservative treatment of thoracic outlet syndrome using an orthosis. *J Hand Surg.* 1995;20(1):34–9.
10. Jordan SE, Ahn SS, Freischlag JA, et al. Selective botulinum chemodenervation of the scalene muscles for treatment of neurogenic thoracic outlet syndrome. *Ann Vasc Surg.* 2000;14:365–9.
11. Sheth RN, Campbell JN, et al. Surgical treatment of thoracic outlet syndrome: a randomized trial comparing two operations. *Journal of neurosurgery Spine.* 2005;3:355–63.
12. Urschel HC, Kourlis H. Thoracic outlet syndrome: a 50-year experience at Baylor University Medical Center. *Proc (Bayl Univ Med Cent).* 2007;20: 125–35.
13. Degeorges R. Thoracic outlet syndrome surgery: Long-term functional results. *Ann Vas Surg.* 2004;18(5):558–65.

ADDITIONAL READING
- National Institute of Neurological Disorders and Stroke (NINDS) information page on TOS.
- Povelson B, Belzberg A, Hansson T, Dorsi M. Treatment for thoracic outlet syndrome. *Cochrane Database of Systematic Reviews.* 2010;1.

CODES

ICD9
353.0 Brachial plexus lesions

CLINICAL PEARLS
- Consider breast reduction for pendulous breasts.
- Avoid opiate dependence.
- Consider pain clinic referral if nonsurgical causes.

T

THROMBOANGIITIS OBLITERANS (BUERGER DISEASE)

Alfonso J. Tafur, MD
Felix B. Chang, MD

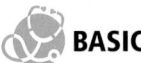 **BASICS**

DESCRIPTION
- Nonatherosclerotic vasculitis of small and medium-sized arteries and veins resulting in segmental occlusion
- Characterized clinically by an inflammatory and vaso-occlusive phenomenon, rest pain, unremitting ischemic ulcerations, and gangrene of the digits of hands and feet
- Occurs primarily in men who smoke
- System(s) affected: Cardiovascular
- Synonym(s): Buerger disease

EPIDEMIOLOGY
- The prevalence has decreased in North America over the last 30 years.
- Worldwide, but most prevalent in eastern Europe, Mediterranean, and Asian countries

Incidence
- 11–30/100,000 persons/year
- Predominant age: 20–40 years
- Predominant sex: Male > Female; increasing numbers of women are being diagnosed, possibly due to increased smoking (1)

Prevalence
- Estimates range from as low as 0.5–5.5% in western Europe, to 45–63% in India, to 80% in Israel among Jews of Ashkenazi ancestry (2).
- Accounts for 5% and 16% of patients hospitalized for arterial occlusive disease in Europe and Japan, respectively
- 13/100,000 population in US
- The overall occurrence is decreasing worldwide (3).

Geriatric Considerations
Not common in this age group

Pediatric Considerations
It should be considered in the differential diagnosis of the young patient with claudication.

RISK FACTORS
- Smoking tobacco. The degree of dependence is similar to that in subjects with coronary artery disease (4). Occasional cases in users of smokeless tobacco and snuff.
- *C. sativa* and *C. indica* have been considered as risk factors.
- Chronic anaerobic periodontal infection also may play a role in the development of Buerger disease.

Genetics
- Greater prevalence of HLA-A54, HLA-A9, and HLA-B5
- HLA-B12 antigen may be associated with disease resistance.
- Familial cases reported rarely

GENERAL PREVENTION
Never smoke. Tobacco and smoking cessation is the only way to prevent recurrence of disease.

PATHOPHYSIOLOGY
- Impaired endothelium-dependent vasorelaxation and decreased peripheral sympathetic outflow
- Segmental infiltration of inflammatory cells in vessel wall leads to thrombotic occlusion of vessel.
- Highly cellular and inflammatory thrombus with relative sparing of the blood vessel wall

ETIOLOGY
- Idiopathic
- Smoking
- Genetic factors
- Autoimmune disorder with cell-mediated sensitivity to types I and III human collagens (both are normal constituents of blood vessels)
- Impaired peripheral endothelium-dependent vasodilation. Nonendothelial mechanisms of vasodilation are intact.
- Arsenic content of tobacco
- Chronic anaerobic periodontal infection

 DIAGNOSIS

- Point scoring systems may help to clarify clinical diagnosis. Many diagnostic tools are available.
- The criteria proposed by Olin is one of the most widely accepted:
  - Smoking history
  - Onset before the age of 50 years
  - Infrapopliteal arterial occlusions
  - Either upper limb involvement or phlebitis migrans
  - Absence of atherosclerotic risk factors other than smoking
  - Disease diagnosis may be made only when all 5 requirements have been fulfilled (2)[A].
- Symptoms tend to wax and wane in early disease and often are asymmetric. Symptoms may be gradual or have a sudden onset related to impaired vasculature. Usually more than 1 limb is involved.

HISTORY
- Foot or arch claudication may be the presenting manifestation (rarely hand, forearm) and is often mistaken for an orthopedic problem.
- Cold sensitivity
- Paresthesias (e.g., numbness, tingling, burning, hypoesthesia) of feet and/or fingers
- Persistent extremity pain (may be worse at rest); pain may be disabling
- Paroxysmal "electric shock" pain of ischemic neuropathy
- Migratory superficial phlebitis

PHYSICAL EXAM
- 76% of patients had ischemic ulcerations at the time of presentation.
- Allen test should be performed.
- Ulceration of digits
- Raynaud phenomenon (~20% of patients)
- Postural color changes: Pallor on elevation; rubor on dependency
- "Buerger color": Cyanosis of hands and feet
- Tender skin nodules on extremities
- Impaired distal pulses
- Proximal pulses normal; Allen test may be abnormal.
- Foot edema
- Gangrene

DIAGNOSTIC TESTS & INTERPRETATION
Lab
- There is no specific lab finding relevant for thromboangiitis obliterans (TAO).
- Noninvasive vascular studies, including TCPO2, ankle brachial index, and simultaneous brachial pressures

- In order to rule out diseases in the differential diagnosis, consider complete blood count, liver function tests, creatinine, fasting glucose, erythrocyte sedimentation rate, antinuclear antibodies (ANA), rheumatoid factor (RF), anticentromere antibody, and SCL70, as well as a hypercoagulability screen.
- Autoantibodies to collagen and circulating immune complexes may be present, but the significance is still to be determined.
- Increased levels of anti–endothelial cell antibodies are seen in patients with active disease.
- Anticardiolipin antibodies may be associated with TAO and may worsen the thrombotic event (5)[A].
- Homocysteine may be elevated but lacks specificity.
- Toxin screen when appropriate: Cocaine, amphetamines, and cannabis ingestion can mimic TAO.

Follow-Up & Special Considerations
- The Westergren sedimentation rate and serum C-reactive protein are usually normal.
- Commonly measured autoantibodies (e.g., ANA and RF) are normal or negative.
- Circulating immune complexes, complement levels, and cryoglobulins are normal despite an immune reaction in the arterial intima.

Imaging
- Doppler ultrasound (not specific)
- Arteriogram or digital-subtraction angiography:
  - Multiple areas of segmental occlusion of small to medium-sized arteries of arms and legs
  - The disease is confined most often to the distal circulation and is almost always infrapopliteal in the lower extremities and distal to the brachial artery in the upper extremities.
  - "Skip" areas may be demonstrated.
  - Numerous collateral vessels around occluded segments may give a characteristic corkscrew appearance (Martorell's sign).
  - Larger arteries are spared. More serious disease occurs distally.
  - No apparent source of emboli

Diagnostic Procedures/Surgery
- History and physical examination
- Echocardiography (to exclude emboli)
- Biopsy only indicated if there are unusual features:
  - Age >45 years at onset
  - Disease in unusual location
  - Proximal disease
  - Central nervous system disease
  - Tobacco history is not consistent with diagnosis.

Pathological Findings
- Segmental inflammatory thrombosis of both arteries and veins
- Histologic findings may vary between acute, intermediate, and chronic stages of the disease.
- Histologic sine qua non: Granulomas with collections of neutrophils in the organizing thrombus:
  - The vessel wall is relatively spared.
  - Wall sparing distinguishes TAO from arteriosclerosis and other systemic vasculitides, which show striking wall disruption.
- Acute lesions show occlusive, highly cellular, inflammatory thrombi with less inflammation in vessel wall. Polymorphonuclear neutrophils, microabscesses, and multinucleated giant cells may be present.

- Intermediate lesions show organizing thrombus.
- Chronic lesions show recanalized thrombus and perivascular fibrosis.

DIFFERENTIAL DIAGNOSIS
- Peripheral neuropathy; peripheral atherosclerotic disease; arterial embolus and thrombosis; idiopathic peripheral thrombosis
- Takayasu arteritis; CREST syndrome (calcinosis, Raynaud's phenomenon, esophageal dysfunction, sclerodactyly, telangiectasia)
- Hypercoagulable states; systemic lupus erythematosus; scleroderma
- Occupational trauma; acrocyanosis; frostbite; neurotrophic ulcers
- Reflex sympathetic dystrophy; metatarsalgia; gout

TREATMENT

MEDICATION
First Line
- Discontinue smoking or tobacco use in any form.
- Antibiotics for infected digital ulcers and osteomyelitis
- Urokinase or streptokinase selectively infused into occluded artery
- Intramuscular (IM) endothelial growth factor gene therapy

Second Line
- If vasospasm is present, trial of dihydropyridine calcium channel blocker such as amlodipine or nifedipine
- Iloprost, a prostacyclin analogue, promotes ulcer healing and decreases analgesic requirement (2)[A].
- IM gene transfer of vascular growth factors

ADDITIONAL TREATMENT
Initiate a walking program.

General Measures
- Stop smoking (mandatory).
- Protect against trauma (poorly fitting shoes) and infections.
- Protect against vasoconstriction from cold or drugs.
- Eliminate exposure to thermal and chemical damage (e.g., iodine, carbolic acid, salicylic acid).
- Thrombolytic therapy of occlusive thrombus and angioplasty are experimental.

Issues for Referral
Consider referral to nicotine-addiction clinics.

Additional Therapies
- Intermittent pneumatic compression has been shown to enhance calf and may serve as adjunctive therapy in patients who are not candidates for revascularization (6)[A].
- Foot care
- Lubricate skin with moisturizer.
- Lamb's wool between toes
- Avoid trauma (e.g., heel protectors, orthotics for shoes, vascular boots).

COMPLEMENTARY AND ALTERNATIVE MEDICINE
Hyperbaric oxygen therapy and autologous bone marrow transplant of mononuclear cells are alternative therapy modalities with very small studies suggesting potential utility.

SURGERY/OTHER PROCEDURES
- Amputation:
  - For nonhealing ulcers, gangrene, or intractable pain
  - Should preserve as much limb as possible
- Omental autotransplantation has been successful in treating ulcers.
- Infrainguinal bypass
- In severe disease, a lumbar sympathectomy to increase blood supply to the skin (7)[A]
- Surgical revascularization is not usually a viable alternative due to the diffuse segmental involvement and extreme distal nature of the disease.

IN-PATIENT CONSIDERATIONS
Inpatient nicotine-dependence treatment is an alternative for recidivist smokers.

Initial Stabilization
- Inpatient if surgery needed for gangrene
- Inpatient for dorsal or lumbar sympathectomy if indicated

Admission Criteria
Critical limb ischemia

ONGOING CARE

FOLLOW-UP RECOMMENDATIONS
- Restricted by symptoms
- Use a bed cradle (nonheated) to prevent pressure from bed linens.

Patient Monitoring
Frequent history and physical examinations

PATIENT EDUCATION
- Remove possibilities of exposure to others in the environment who smoke.
- Nicotine replacement may keep the disease active.
- Use heel pads or foam rubber boots.

PROGNOSIS
- Average death age 52 ± 8.9 years; significantly lower than matched US population (8)
- In the Cleveland Clinic series, 94% of patients who quit smoking remained free of amputation, whereas 43% of patients who continued smoking required at least 1 amputation.
- Data from Mayo Clinic showed an amputation rate of 25% at 5 years and 38% at 10 years of follow-up (8).
- The risk of amputation is eliminated after 8 years of smoking cessation.
- Approximately 94% of patients who quit smoking avoid amputation compared with 43% who continue smoking (1).

COMPLICATIONS
- Ulcerations, gangrene, need for amputation
- Rare occlusion of cerebral, coronary, renal, splenic, mesenteric, pulmonary, iliac arteries, and aorta

REFERENCES
1. Olin JW, Shih A. Thromboangiitis obliterans (Buerger's disease). *Curr Opin Rheumatol*. 2006;18:18–24.
2. Olin JW. Thromboangiitis obliterans (Buerger's disease). *N Engl J Med*. 2000;343:864–9.
3. Maecki R, Zdrojowy K, Adamiec R, et al. Thromboangiitis obliterans in the 21st century—a new face of disease. *Atherosclerosis*. 2009;206:328–34.
4. Cooper LT, Henderson SS, Ballman KV, et al. A prospective, case-control study of tobacco dependence in thromboangiitis obliterans (Buerger's Disease). *Angiology*. 2006;57:73–8.
5. de Godoy JM, Braile DM. Buerger's disease and anticardiolipin antibodies. *J Cardiovasc Med (Hagerstown)*. 2009.
6. Montori VM, Kavros SJ, Walsh EE, et al. Intermittent compression pump for nonhealing wounds in patients with limb ischemia. The Mayo Clinic experience (1998–2000). *Int Angiol*. 2002;21:360–6.
7. Bozkurt AK, et al. A randomized trial of intravenous versus lumbar sympathectomy in the management of Buerger's disease. *Int Angiol*. 2006;25(2):162–8.
8. Cooper LT, Tse TS, Mikhail MA, et al. Long-term survival and amputation risk in thromboangiitis obliterans (Buerger's disease). *J Am Coll Cardiol*. 2004;44:2410–1.

ADDITIONAL READING
- Espinoza LR. Buerger's disease: thromboangiitis obliterans 100 years after the initial description. *Am J Med Sci*. 2009;337:285–6.
- Grotenhermen F, et al. Cannabis-associated arteritis. *VASA*. 2010;39:43–53.
- Hanley EJ, Meireles O, et al. Buerger Disease (Thromboangiitis Obliterans) http://www.imedicine.com/printtopic.asp?bookid=6&topic=253 May 1, 2009.
- Mills JL. Buerger's Disease in the 21st Century: Diagnosis, Clinical Features, and Therapy. *Seminars in Vascular Surgery*. 2003;16:179–89.

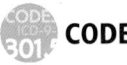 CODES

ICD9
443.1 Thromboangiitis obliterans (Buerger's disease)

CLINICAL PEARLS
- No form of medical treatment has been proven effective for the treatment of TOA. Medications are not a substitute for discontinuing smoking.
- Measurement of urinary nicotine and cotinine should be performed if the disease is still active despite patient's claims of tobacco cessation.
- A vascular biopsy is usually not necessary unless patients present with unusual characteristics such as large-artery involvement or age >45 years.
- Approximately 94% of patients who quit smoking avoid amputation compared with 43% who continue smoking.

T

THROMBOPHILIA AND HYPERCOAGULABLE STATES

Ali Zarrabi, MD
Nancy J. Freeman, MD

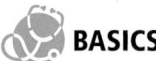 **BASICS**

DESCRIPTION
- A heritable or acquired disorder of the coagulation system predisposing an individual to thromboembolism (the formation of a venous or less commonly arterial clot) (1)
- Venous thrombosis typically manifests as deep venous thrombosis (DVT) of the lower extremity and pulmonary embolism (PE).
- System(s) affected: Cardiovascular; Nervous; Pulmonary; Reproductive; Heme/Lymph/Immuno
- Synonym(s): Hypercoagulation syndrome

EPIDEMIOLOGY
- A thrombophilic defect or risk (congenital or acquired) can be detected in some 80% of patients with VTE.
- Factor V Leiden is the most common inherited thrombophilia (half of all currently characterizable inherited thrombophilia cases involve the Factor V Leiden mutation), and is present in its heterozygous form in up to ~20% of patients with a VTE:
  - Heterozygous prothrombin 20210 mutation is present in up to ~16% of patients with VTE (2).

Incidence
1st time thromboembolism:
- ~100/100,000/year in general population
- <5/100,000/year in those <15 years old
- ~500/100,000/year in 80-year-olds

Prevalence
- 40–70% of lower extremity orthopedic procedures are complicated by venous thromboembolism unless prophylaxis is used.
- VTE accounts for approximately 11% of pregnancy-related deaths.

RISK FACTORS
- Acquired risk factors:
  - Immobilization
  - Trauma
  - Surgery, especially orthopedic
  - Malignancies (especially pancreatic, ovarian, brain, and lymphoma)
  - Pregnancy
  - Exogenous female hormones/oral contraceptives
  - Smoking
  - Nephrotic syndrome
  - Congestive heart failure
  - Antiphospholipid syndrome (APS)
  - Myeloproliferative disorders (MPD: Polycythemia vera, essential thrombocythemia)
  - Hyperviscosity syndromes (sickle cell, paraproteinemias)
  - Hyperhomocysteinemia secondary to vitamin deficiencies (B_6, B_{12}, folic acid)
  - Tamoxifen, thalidomide, lenalidomide, bevacizumab
  - Previous thromboembolism
- Established genetic factors:
  - Factor V Leiden
  - Prothrombin G20210A mutation
  - Protein C deficiency
  - Protein S deficiency
  - Antithrombin III deficiency
- Rare genetic factors:
  - Dysfibrinogenemia

  - Hyperhomocysteinemia (methylene tetrahydrofolate reductase [MTHFR] mutation)
- Indeterminate factors:
  - Elevated factor VIII
- Age
- Gender: Males have 2.5-fold higher risk
- Idiopathic 1st thrombotic event
- Obesity

Genetics
- The most common genetic thrombophilias (factor V Leiden, prothrombin G20210A, protein C and protein S, and antithrombin III deficiency) are inherited in an autosomal-dominant pattern.
- Homozygous mutations generally have a higher risk of VTE.
- Factor V Leiden/activated protein C (aPC) resistance: Most common inherited thrombophilia (40–50% of cases):
  - 5–8% prevalence in Caucasians; rare in African Americans, Asians
  - aPC does not cleave factor Va, and thrombin formation continues.
  - Oral contraceptive pills (OCPs), smoking, and obesity are synergistic.
- Prothrombin gene mutation (PGM) G20210A: Prevalence 6% among Europeans. Heterozygous carriers have increased risk of thrombosis. Associated with high prothrombin levels. Prothrombin is vitamin K-dependent, produced in the liver.
- Hyperhomocysteinemia: 5–6% in general population. Increases risk of coronary artery disease (CAD)/myocardial infarction (MI), cerebrovascular accident (CVA), DVT/PE. Acquired in folate, B_{12}, and B_6 deficiencies. Fibrates, niacin, smoking raise levels.
- Antithrombin deficiency: <0.2% incidence in general population. Produced in the liver. Acquired deficiency in disseminated intravascular coagulation (DIC), sepsis, liver disease, nephrotic syndrome.
- Protein C and S deficiencies: 0.5% incidence each in general population. Homozygotes and heterozygotes are hypercoagulable. Vitamin K-dependent, produced in the liver. Protein C inactivates Va and VIIa. Protein C may become an acquired deficiency in liver disease, sepsis, DIC, acute respiratory distress syndrome (ARDS). Protein S is a cofactor for protein C, and may become an acquired deficiency in OCP use, pregnancy, liver disease, sepsis, DIC, HIV, and nephrosis.
- Other: Acquired: Antiphospholipid syndrome or APS (lupus anticoagulant and anticardiolipin antibody)

GENERAL PREVENTION
- Prophylaxis with medications should be considered in any hospitalized patient with VTE risk factors, and hospitalized patients should be encouraged to become mobile as soon as possible (3)[A].
- Mechanical prophylaxis may be considered in patients at low risk for VTE or those in whom anticoagulation may be contraindicated.
- Consider prophylaxis with low-molecular-weight heparin (LMWH) + aspirin in select populations:
  - Pregnant patients with antiphospholipid antibody syndrome with no prior history of thrombosis (4)[B]

- Prophylaxis with unfractionated heparin or LMWH in patients with genetic or acquired risks of thrombosis and an anticipated additional risk, such as the immobilization associated with surgery
- Use caution with procoagulant medicines, for example, oral contraceptives or antiestrogen medicines for breast cancer.

PATHOPHYSIOLOGY
- Virchow's hypothesis to explain the cause of pulmonary embolus evolved to include the triad of blood stasis, vascular endothelial injury, and abnormalities in circulating blood constituents (i.e., hypecoagulability) (5)
- An imbalance between the hemostatic and fibrinolytic pathways that leads to thrombus formation; this may be a result of too much of a prothrombotic protein or too little of an antithrombotic protein.
- VTE is probably the result of an interaction of genetic tendencies, measurable or not, with clinically apparent factors.
- Upper extremity DVT: Venous catheters and young athletes (Paget-Schroetter syndrome)

ETIOLOGY
Refer to specific diseases

COMMONLY ASSOCIATED CONDITIONS
Advanced age, cancer, pregnancy, CHF, obesity, prior history of thrombosis

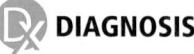 **DIAGNOSIS**

HISTORY
Consider prothrombotic assessment for:
- Unprovoked thrombosis at age <50 years
- Thrombosis at an unusual anatomic site or recurrent thromboses
- Family history suggesting multiple affected individuals with VTE
- Thrombosis with recent immobilization, traveling, hospitalization, surgery
- Thrombosis with past history of cancer
- Recurrent pregnancy loss, oral contraceptive use, exogenous female hormones, estrogen blockers such as tamoxifen, anastrozole

PHYSICAL EXAM
- Physical findings may be unreliable for DVT.
- Swelling, pain, warmth, and redness, usually of one extremity
- Dyspnea, pleurisy, hemoptysis, hypoxia in PE
- Superficial phlebitis may cause a red, painful cord palpable along the path of the thrombosed vein.
- Post-thrombotic syndrome: Pain, swelling, pigmentation, +/– ulceration

DIAGNOSTIC TESTS & INTERPRETATION
See chapters on deep venous thrombosis and pulmonary embolism for details on workup of these conditions. There are currently no randomized controlled trials or controlled clinical trials that have assessed the benefit(s) of testing for thrombophilia on the risk of recurrent VTE (1).

Lab
Indiscriminate testing for heritable thrombophilia in all patients presenting with a 1st episode of VTE is not indicated (6)[B]

Initial lab tests
- Factor V Leiden → APTT-based assay +/− Factor V deficient plasma, confirm with genotyping
- Prothrombin G20210A genetic assay
- ATIII functional assay
- Protein C functional assay
- Protein S antigen and functional assay and free
- Antiphospholipid antibodies → phospholipid-dependent tests and anticardiolipin (aCL) antibodies
- Factor VIII → activity or antigen measurement
- Consider homocysteine level

Follow-Up & Special Considerations
Dysfibrinogenemia → thrombin/reptilase times +/− immunologic analysis of fibrinogen

Imaging
Initial approach
See topics on DVT and pulmonary embolism.

DIFFERENTIAL DIAGNOSIS
- Lower extremity edema from other causes such as CHF or medicines
- Baker cyst
- Cellulitis
- Lymphedema
- Chronic venous insufficiency

TREATMENT

MEDICATION
First Line
- LMWH has largely replaced unfractionated heparin as 1st-line therapy of VTE:
  - Enoxaparin (Lovenox) 1 mg/kg SC b.i.d. for at least 5 days (with concomitant warfarin orally), until international normalized ratio (INR) has reached 2 (from concomitant warfarin) for at least 24 hours
- Oral anticoagulation:
  - Warfarin (Coumadin) 5 mg/d initially and adjusted to INR 2–3 for at least 3 months, potentially indefinitely for patients with high risk of recurrence, or recurrent, or unprovoked. See chapters on DVT, PE, and specific hypercoagulable states.
  - Warfarin requires careful and frequent monitoring.
- Pregnant (controversial): Low-dose aspirin +/− LMWH or unfractionated heparin

Second Line
Usually indicated when there is a contraindication to heparin or LMWH, such as heparin-associated thrombosis and thrombocytopenia, or if there is an inability to use intravenous drugs, or renal failure:
- Indirect factor Xa inhibitor activates antithrombin:
  - Representative drug: Fondaparinux: Highly efficacious for prevention and treatment of both venous and arterial thromboembolic disorders:
    - Dose: Acute VTE. Weight <50 kg: 5 mg/d SC; weight 50–100 kg: 7.5 mg/d SC; weight >100 kg: 10 mg/d SC
    - Prophylaxis: 2.5 mg/d SC
    - Pregnancy risk factor B
  - UFH IV (or SC b.i.d.) is also an appropriate alternative:
    - Dose: Acute VTE; dose: IV bolus 5,000 IU followed by 17,500 (SC) b.i.d. for 1st 24 hours
    - Check PTT 6 hours after the morning SC dose.
    - IV bolus 80 U/kg, then infusion at 18 U/kg/h (use of protocol advisable)

- Goal to maintain PTT 1.5–2.5× normal
- Prophylaxis: 5,000 units SC q8–12h
- Interactions: See LMWH
- Adverse reactions: Thrombocytopenia, fever, skin necrosis, hyperkalemia, elevated AST/ALT
- 2% risk immune-mediated heparin-induced thrombocytopenia (HIT)
- Direct thrombin inhibitors: Minimal binding to plasma protein, thus producing predictable response, does not cause heparin-induced thrombocytopenia, broad therapeutic window. Representative drugs include:
  - Lepirudin (excreted by kidneys, crosses the placenta) used in HIT
  - Argatroban (liver metabolized) may be used in HIT.

Pregnancy Considerations
- UFH or LMWH is treatment of choice for VTE in pregnancy.
- Warfarin is contraindicated in pregnancy.

ADDITIONAL TREATMENT
Folate and vitamin B_6 and B_{12} treatment of hyperhomocysteinemia does not reduce risk of myocardial infarction and stroke.

SURGERY/OTHER PROCEDURES
- Catheter extraction/thrombectomy for extreme emergencies (e.g., massive PE where thrombolysis not feasible)
- Inferior vena cava (IVC) filter:
  - Reduces short-term risk of PE, i.e., GI bleeding and inability to anticoagulate
  - Increases long-term risk of recurrent DVT
  - Use for patients with multiple episodes of recurrent thromboembolism despite therapeutic anticoagulation.

IN-PATIENT CONSIDERATIONS
Discharge Criteria
- Patient is medically stable
- A system is in place to monitor administration of LMWH and warfarin to ensure adequate anticoagulation and minimize risk of bleeding.

ONGOING CARE

FOLLOW-UP RECOMMENDATIONS
While anticoagulated, avoid any situation in which the patient is at risk for trauma (e.g., contact sports, climbing on a ladder, using a power saw).

Patient Monitoring
- Warfarin monitoring as frequently as needed to maintain an INR goal of 2–3 (ideally in an anticoagulant clinic)
- Patient self-testing and self-management with home prothrombin time monitors, if available

DIET
Vitamin K-stable diet if patient on warfarin

PATIENT EDUCATION
- Assume that any drug may enhance or attenuate the warfarin effect.
- Increase the frequency of monitoring following any medication change to ensure therapeutic anticoagulation and to avoid overanticoagulation.
- Avoid drugs that may exacerbate warfarin effect: Alcohol, allopurinol, amiodarone, antibiotics, aspirin, cimetidine, nonsteroidal anti-inflammatory drugs (NSAIDs), thyroid hormone, acetaminophen.

PROGNOSIS
- Patients with a provoked VTE (i.e., surgery, hospitalization) have between a 1% and 4% annual recurrence rate of thromboembolism (2).
- Patients with unprovoked VTE who are not treated with anticoagulants have a 5–10% recurrence rate annually.
- There is no data from RCTs or CCTs currently on the benefits of thrombophilia testing to decrease the risk of recurrent VTE (1).

COMPLICATIONS
Venous or arterial thrombosis. Bleeding in anticoagulated patients.

REFERENCES

1. Cohn D, Vansenne F, de Borgie C, et al. Thrombophilia testing for prevention of recurrent venous thromboembolism. *Cochrane Database Syst Rev.* 2009;CD007069.
2. Ho WK, Hankey GJ, Quinlan DJ, et al. Risk of recurrent venous thromboembolism in patients with common thrombophilia: a systematic review. *Arch Intern Med.* 2006;166:729–36.
3. Hill J, Treasure T, National Clinical Guideline Centre for Acute and Chronic Conditionset al. Reducing the risk of venous thromboembolism in patients admitted to hospital: summary of NICE guidance. *BMJ.* 2010;340:c95.
4. Lim W, Crowther MA, Eikelboom JW. Management of antiphospholipid antibody syndrome: a systematic review. *JAMA.* 2006;295:1050–7.
5. Khan S, Dickerman JD. Hereditary thrombophilia. *Thromb J.* 2006;4:15.
6. Baglin T, Gray E, Greaves M, et al. Clinical guidelines for testing for heritable thrombophilia. *Br J Haematol.* 2010;149:209–20.

CODES

ICD9
- 289.81 Primary hypercoagulable state
- 286.9 Other and unspecified coagulation defects

CLINICAL PEARLS
- Factor V Leiden (resistance to activated protein C) is the most common, with a prevalence of 5–8% in the Caucasian US population.
- Test patients <50 years of age with a history of venous thrombosis, and consider testing 1st-degree relatives.
- Rule out malignancy, especially in those over age 50.

THROMBOTIC THROMBOCYTOPENIC PURPURA

Carol Curtin, MSW, LICSW
Kellie A. Sprague, MD

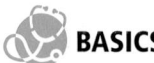 **BASICS**

DESCRIPTION
- An acute syndrome hallmarked by microangiopathic hemolytic anemia (MAHA) and consumptive thrombocytopenia with deposition of hyaline thrombi in terminal arterioles and capillaries leading to ischemic multiorgan damage
- Thrombotic thrombocytopenic purpura (TTP) syndrome is characterized by a pentad of the following signs and symptoms:
  – MAHA
  – Thrombocytopenia
  – Renal dysfunction
  – Neurologic symptoms
  – Fever

EPIDEMIOLOGY
Incidence
- Predominant age: 30–60 years
- Predominant sex: Female > Male (2:1)
- Incidence ratio in blacks to nonblacks is 3:1
- The age–sex standardized incidence of TTP and hemolytic-uremic syndrome is reported as 6.5/million/year in the US (1).
- ~1,200 cases of acquired TTP each year in the US

RISK FACTORS
- Pregnancy and oral contraceptives
- AIDS and early symptomatic HIV infection
- Autoimmune disease:
  – Antiphospholipid antibody syndrome
  – Systemic lupus erythematosus
  – Scleroderma
- Cancer
- Hematopoietic stem cell transplantation
- Drug toxicity:
  – Cancer chemotherapy:
    ○ Mitomycin C and gemcitabine
    ○ Bleomycin and cisplatin
  – Calcineurin inhibitors:
    ○ Tacrolimus and cyclosporine
  – Immune-mediated:
    ○ Quinine and quinidine
    ○ Ticlopidine and clopidogrel

Genetics
Mutation at the ADAMTS13 metalloproteinase gene locus on chromosome 9q34 has been described as the cause of familial TTP. This rare form of TTP, called Schulman-Upshaw syndrome, has an autosomal recessive pattern of inheritance.

PATHOPHYSIOLOGY
- In TTP, the aggregating agent responsible for platelet thrombi is unusually large von Willebrand factor (UL vWF) multimers, which are far larger than those found in normal plasma.
- A metalloproteinase, ADMATS13, which normally enzymatically cleaves UL vWF multimers to prevent clumping within vessels, is deficient, defective, or absent, thus allowing UL vWF to react with platelets. This leads to the endothelial cell damage and disseminated thrombi characteristic of TTP.

- Arterioles most often affected are in the brain, kidney, pancreas, heart, and adrenal glands. Lungs and liver are relatively spared.

ETIOLOGY
- In familial TTP, patients have very low or absent levels of ADAMTS13.
- In acquired idiopathic TTP, some studies have demonstrated IgG autoantibodies made to the metalloproteinase ADAMTS13, to receptors on the surfaces of platelets, or to the surface of the endothelial cell; trigger is unknown (2)[A].
- Endothelial injury, either directly from a drug/toxin or indirectly via platelet/neutrophil activation, has been proposed as a cause of secondary TTP, especially in those without ADAMTS13 deficiency:
  – Drug-induced (see Risk Factors)
  – Hematopoietic cell transplantation

COMMONLY ASSOCIATED CONDITIONS
- TTP and hemolytic-uremic syndrome (HUS) have similar presentations and have been described as a continuum of the same pathophysiologic process. However, these are believed to be distinct entities.
- TTP generally presents with prominent neurologic symptoms and minimal renal involvement, whereas the opposite tends to be more characteristic of HUS.
- However, patients with HUS and TTP may have both prominent renal and neurologic manifestations, often making the distinction unclear.
- ADAMTS13 levels are diminished in adults with familial or acquired idiopathic TTP but are normal in children diagnosed with HUS following infection with *E. coli* (particularly type O157:H7).

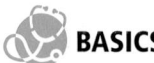 **DIAGNOSIS**

- Most common symptoms are nonspecific: Nausea, vomiting, weakness, abdominal pain, fatigue, fever
- Related to thrombocytopenia:
  – Easy bruising, purpura, or petechiae
  – Epistaxis, menorrhagia, bleeding gums
  – GI bleeding
  – Intracranial hemorrhage
  – Visual symptoms due to retinal hemorrhage
- Related to hemolytic anemia (MAHA): Jaundice
- Related to end-organ ischemia:
  – Neurologic: CNS symptoms occur in 90%; presenting complaint in 60%
  – Often fluctuating symptoms
  – Headache
  – Altered mental status: Spectrum runs from behavioral/personality changes to obtundation/stupor or coma.
  – Seizures
  – Stroke
  – Renal: Hematuria, oliguria, or anuria
  – Cardiac: Arrhythmia, myocardial infarction, heart failure

HISTORY
- Generally acute onset of symptoms
- It is important to assess for potential underlying causes or risk factors (see above).
- 90% mortality without treatment
- Most patients often do not show the classic presentation because treatment is initiated before the pentad can develop.

PHYSICAL EXAM
- Mental status/neurologic: Confusion, coma, stupor, weakness
- HEENT: Retinal hemorrhage, scleral icterus, epistaxis
- Abdomen/GI: Nonspecific tenderness
- Skin: Jaundice, petechiae, purpura, ecchymoses

DIAGNOSTIC TESTS & INTERPRETATION
Lab
Initial lab tests
- CBC:
  – Hemoglobin <10 g/dL:
    ○ Average is 8–9 g/dL; <6 g/dL in 40%
  – Platelets <25,000/mm³ increased
- Reticulocyte count (increased)
- Peripheral smear:
  – Schistocytes (prominent)
  – Helmet cells, red blood cell (RBC) fragments
  – Nucleated RBCs
  – Polychromasia (reticulocytosis)
- Coagulation studies:
  – Normal in most; mild elevation in 15%
  – Fibrinogen normal
- Coombs test: Negative direct Coombs test
- Electrolytes, blood urea nitrogen/creatinine: Mild elevation of BUN and creatinine (creatinine <3 mg/dL)
- Liver function studies: Increased indirect bilirubin (hemolysis)
- Lactate dehydrogenase (LDH): 5–10× normal
- Haptoglobin decreased (hemolysis)
- Urinalysis:
  – Proteinuria, microscopic hematuria
  – Positive dipstick for large blood but minimal RBCs on microscopic exam
- ECG: Sinus tachycardia, heart block
- No utility of ADAMTS13 assay in diagnosis and decision to initiate therapy at presentation, but assay is helpful for confirmation of idiopathic or familial TTP.

Imaging
Head CT scan: Often performed due to mental status changes to rule out possible intracranial hemorrhage or ischemic changes

Pathological Findings
Biopsy of affected organs shows platelet thrombi within or beneath damaged endothelium. However, biopsy is rarely obtained because the diagnosis is made on clinical grounds and laboratory findings (3)[A].

DIFFERENTIAL DIAGNOSIS

- HUS (see Associated Conditions)
- Antiphospholipid antibody syndrome: Prolonged partial thromboplastin time (PTT) and presence of lupus anticoagulant
- Malignant hypertension (HTN): Diastolic >130 mm Hg, papilledema, retinal hemorrhages
- Pregnancy-associated preeclampsia/eclampsia or HELLP: Low ATIII levels
- Disseminated intravascular coagulation:
  - Prolonged prothrombin time (PT)/PTT, low fibrinogen
  - Low factors V and VIII
  - Secondary to sepsis/shock or widely disseminated malignancy
- Idiopathic thrombocytopenic purpura:
  - No hemolysis, normal LDH and bilirubin
  - Presence of antiplatelet antibodies
- Malignancy-associated microangiopathy
- Evan syndrome (autoimmune hemolytic anemia and thrombocytopenia): Positive direct Coombs test
- Sclerodermal kidney

 TREATMENT

In the absence of another apparent cause, the dyad of MAHA and thrombocytopenia is sufficient to begin treatment for TTP while the workup proceeds (2)[B]:

- Emergent plasma exchange transfusion (PEX) is the cornerstone of treatment of classic TTP (2)[A].
- It is thought to replace a deficient or defective metalloproteinase (ADAMTS13) and remove UL vWF and antimetalloproteinase antibodies.
- 1–1.5 plasma volumes/day should be begun immediately and continued daily.
- Continue daily until LDH, platelets, neurologic symptoms, and renal function normalize (2)[A].
- Fresh frozen plasma (2)[A]: Temporary measure until PEX can be initiated.

MEDICATION

First Line
Utility of glucocorticoid therapy is still debated, with most data derived from case series and clinical experience. British guidelines recommend its use for all patients (4)[C]:

- Steroids seem most beneficial in the setting of exacerbation when plasma exchange transfusion (PEX) is stopped or in relapse after remission. There is little benefit of steroids when used as monotherapy.
- Doses: Prednisone 1 mg/kg/d and taper once in remission (2,4)[C] or methylprednisolone 1 g/d IV × 3 days (4)[C]

Second Line
The following medications are used in refractory cases:

- Rituxan (5)[C]
- Vincristine, cyclophosphamide, azathioprine
- IV immunoglobulin (IVIG)

ADDITIONAL TREATMENT
Issues for Referral
- Hematology or blood bank for plasma exchange transfusion
- Nephrology for dialysis
- Cardiology for presence of significant heart block
- Neurosurgery for intracranial hemorrhage

SURGERY/OTHER PROCEDURES
Splenectomy is reserved for severe, refractory cases with ambiguous results.

IN-PATIENT CONSIDERATIONS
Initial Stabilization
- ABCs, oxygen, IV access, telemetry
- Volume resuscitation if hypotensive/actively bleeding
- Packed RBCs can be transfused safely
- Platelet transfusions may exacerbate end-organ ischemia and should be used only in the setting of life-threatening hemorrhage (2)[B].

Discharge Criteria
On normalization and stabilization of neurologic symptoms, LDH, platelets, and renal function

 ONGOING CARE

FOLLOW-UP RECOMMENDATIONS
- No maintenance therapy is required. After PEX is discontinued, CBC and LDH should be monitored frequently. If testing remains normal, testing interval can be lengthened (3)[C].
- Estimated 10-year relapse rate for TTP is 36% and most often occurs in patients with severe deficiency of ADAMTS13 activity.
- Promptly evaluate any symptoms of relapse.

Patient Monitoring
Weekly CBCs on hospital discharge; frequency of monitoring can be reduced if platelets remain normal and stable.

PATIENT EDUCATION
- On discharge, advise patients to self-monitor for signs of relapse (e.g., fever, headache).
- Patients should be advised about prolonged periods of fatigue following the acute phase.
- http://www.nhlbi.nih.gov/health/dci/Diseases/ttp/TTP_WhatIs.html

PROGNOSIS
- Most patients recover fully from TTP when treated promptly:
  - 30-day mortality is 10% in those who receive PEX.
  - 70% respond within 14 days; 90% respond within 28 days.
- Initial LDH and platelet counts are not predictive of the patient's response to treatment.
- Final platelet count and LDH or the length or intensity of treatment does not predict relapse.
- Severe deficiency of ADAMTS13 or low levels during remission predict higher likelihood of relapse (6,7).
- Patients may continue to experience mild cognitive impairments in attention, concentration, and memory following 1 or more episodes of TTP.

COMPLICATIONS
- Central line infections and hemorrhage
- Citrate toxicity
- Hypersensitivity reactions to frequent plasma

REFERENCES

1. Miller DP, Kaye JA, Shea K, et al. Incidence of thrombotic thrombocytopenic purpura/hemolytic uremic syndrome. *Epidemiology*. 2004;15:208–15.
2. George JN. Clinical practice. Thrombotic thrombocytopenic purpura. *N Engl J Med*. 2006; 354:1927–35.
3. Sadler JE, Moake JL, Miyata T, et al. Recent advances in thrombotic thrombocytopenic purpura. *Hematology Am Soc Hematol Educ Program*. 2004;407–23.
4. Allford SL, Hunt BJ, Rose P, et al. Guidelines on the diagnosis and management of the thrombotic microangiopathic haemolytic anaemias. *Br J Haematol*. 2003;120:556–73.
5. Darabi K, Berg AH. Rituximab can be combined with daily plasma exchange to achieve effective B-cell depletion and clinical improvement in acute autoimmune TTP. *Am J Clin Pathol*. 2006;125: 592–7.
6. Vesely SK, George JN, Lämmle B, et al. ADAMTS13 activity in thrombotic thrombocytopenic purpura-hemolytic uremic syndrome: relation to presenting features and clinical outcomes in a prospective cohort of 142 patients. *Blood*. 2003;102:60–8.
7. Peyvandi F, et al. ADAMTS13 and anti-ADAMTS13 antibodies are markers for recurrence or acquired thrombotic thrombocytopenia purpura during remission. *Haematologica*. 2008;93:69–76.

ADDITIONAL READING

- Kennedy AS, Lewis QF, Scott JG, et al. Cognitive deficits after recovery from thrombotic thrombocytopenic purpura. *Transfusion*. 2009;49: 1092–101.
- Sadler JE, et al. Von Willebrand factor, ADAMTS13, and thrombotic thrombocytopenic purpura. *Blood*. 2008;112:11–8.

 CODES

ICD9
446.6 Thrombotic microangiopathy

CLINICAL PEARLS

- The diagnosis of TTP is made clinically.
- The classic pentad is present in only about 40% of patients.
- The dyad of MAHA and thrombocytopenia is sufficient to initiate treatment with PEX.
- Do not wait for results of ADAMTS13 determination to initiate therapy.

THYROGLOSSAL DUCT CYST

Felix B. Chang, MD

 BASICS

Cyst of epithelial remnants of the thyroglossal tract

DESCRIPTION
- Usually midline neck mass at the level of the thyrohyoid membrane, closely associated with the hyoid bone
- Within 2 cm of the midline
- Single, smooth, nontender, and mobile
- 65% infrahyoid type
- 20% suprahyoid
- 15% juxtahyoid
- 2% yuxtahyoid
- 10% suprasternal
- Intralaryngeal very rare: Suprasternal notch, superior mediastinum
- Endolaryngeal cyst (ectopic location): Extremely rare
- System(s) affected: Endocrine/Metabolic; Skin/Exocrine

EPIDEMIOLOGY
- The most common form of congenital cyst in the neck
- Accounts for 2-4% of all neck masses

Incidence
- Most patients are children or adolescents.
- Up to 1/3 are aged 20 years or older.
- Predominant age: 50% <10 years, 65% <20 years
- Predominant sex: Male = Female

Prevalence
- Thyroglossal duct cysts were found in 7% of adults in 1 autopsy study.
- Thyroglossal duct anomalies are the 2nd most common pediatric neck mass, behind adenopathy in frequency.

RISK FACTORS
Genetics
- Usually sporadic; if familial, autosomal dominant is most common mode of inheritance (1)[C].
- Familial occurrence is extremely rare (2).

PATHOPHYSIOLOGY
- Cystic expansion of a remnant of the thyroglossal duct tract
- Persistent of the epithelial tract, the thyroglossal duct, during the descent of the thyroid from the foramen cecum to its final position in the anterior neck
- The thyroglossal duct tract usually atrophies and disappears by the 10th week of gestation.
- Portions of the tract and remnants of thyroid tissue associated with it may persist at any point between the tongue and the thyroid.
- The wall of a thyroglossal duct is the 2nd most common site for ectopic thyroid tissue.

ETIOLOGY
- Failure of the thyroglossal duct to atrophy and involute after descent of the thyroid in the 4th–7th week of gestation
- Hypothesis: Lymphoid tissue associated with the tract hypertrophies at the time of a regional infection, thereby occluding the tract with resulting cyst formation.

COMMONLY ASSOCIATED CONDITIONS
- Often the patient has a history of a recent upper respiratory tract infection.
- Ectopic thyroid tissue is found in 50% of patients.
- If thyroid gland fails to descend to orthotopic site, an ectopic thyroid gland results. Most ectopic thyroid glands are lingual. Many patients with ectopic thyroid gland are hypothyroid.

 DIAGNOSIS

May be located and can track anywhere from the thyroid cartilage up the base of the tongue

HISTORY
- Most often asymptomatic, midline upper neck mass that is cystic
- Swelling
- Pain or slightly tender
- Redness
- Neck mass
- 1/4 of patients present with a draining sinus.
- Foul taste in the mouth if the spontaneous drainage occurred by way of the foramen cecum
- Rare presentations: Severe respiratory distress or sudden infant death syndrome from lesions at the base of the tongue, a lateral cystic neck mass, an anterior tongue fistula, or coexistence with branchial anomalies

PHYSICAL EXAM
- Midline neck mass, usually within 2 cm of the midline
- Nontender or slightly tender, unless infected
- Rises in the neck with tongue protrusion and swallowing
- 80% adjacent to the hyoid bone
- Infected thyroglossal duct cyst may manifest as tender mass with associated dysphagia, dysphonia, draining sinus, fever, or increasing neck mass.
- Airway obstruction is possible, especially with intralingual cysts.
- Approximately 1/3 present with a concurrent or prior upper respiratory tract infection.
- Cyst below the thyrohyoid membrane is rare.

DIAGNOSTIC TESTS & INTERPRETATION
The preoperative evaluation for a patient who has a suspected thyroglossal duct cyst includes a complete history and physical examination, preoperative ultrasound (US), and a screening thyroid-stimulating hormone (TSH) determination.

Lab
Initial lab tests
Assess thyroid function.

Imaging
- US or computed tomography (CT) scan to confirm diagnosis, identify thyroid, and demonstrate relationship to hyoid bone
- Patients with elevated TSH levels suggesting hypothyroidism or a solid mass should undergo scintiscanning to rule out a median ectopic thyroid.
- Thyroid scan if midline ectopic thyroid or thyroid nodule is suspected
- Small roll under shoulders allows exposure of neck in infants.

- Occasionally, if the cyst is infected, hemorrhagic, or has a high protein content, it may appear as hyperdense on CT scan, as an area of high signal intensity on T_1- and T_2-weighted magnetic resonance imaging (MRI), and have an internal echo on US.
- Malignancy may be suspected if a soft tissue component exists within or around the cyst.

Follow-Up & Special Considerations
- If a solid mass is encountered during excision of a suspected thyroglossal duct cyst, it should be sent for frozen section to rule out a median ectopic thyroid.
- Fine-needle aspiration (FNA) biopsy is the most reliable method for preoperative diagnosis of thyroid carcinoma, especially if done with US guidance.
- FNA can be helpful to decrease cyst size, and in some cases may lead to identification of thyroglossal duct cyst carcinoma if solid elements of the lesion can be sampled.

Diagnostic Procedures/Surgery
- FNA for preoperative evaluation of thyroglossal duct cysts may reveal colloid, neutrophils, macrophages, lymphocytes, and ciliated columnar cells. It is often used to exclude other diagnoses.
- If cyst is infected, antibiotic treatment may be required prior to definitive resection.
- Incision and drainage with resulting scarring may complicate resection.

Pathological Findings
- Cyst lined with stratified squamous or pseudostratified ciliated columnar epithelium
- Thyroid tissue is seen in 10–45% of cysts.
- Reports show traces of the thyroglossal duct located near the hyoid bone, superior to the thyroid isthmus, or lingually.
- Fewer than 1% of thyroglossal duct cysts have malignant tissue, usually well-differentiated thyroid carcinoma.

DIFFERENTIAL DIAGNOSIS
- Ectopic midline thyroid
- Dermoid cyst
- Thyroid adenoma of isthmus or pyramidal lobe
- Lymphadenitis
- Cervical thymic cyst
- Sebaceous (epidermal) cysts
- Medial branchial cleft cyst
- Salivary gland tumor
- Lymphatic malformations
- Lipoma
- Hypertrophic pyramidal lobes of the thyroid

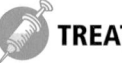 **TREATMENT**

Elective surgical excision is the treatment of choice for uncomplicated thyroglossal duct cysts to prevent infection of the cyst.

MEDICATION
- All thyroglossal duct cysts should be surgically removed.
- Infected cysts or sinuses are first managed by relieving the infection.

- The most common organisms are *Haemophilus influenzae, Staphylococcus aureus,* and *S. epidermidis.*
- Antibiotics directed toward these organisms should be started. Successful treatment requires broad-spectrum antibiotics.

First Line
For infected cyst: Cephalexin 500 mg p.o. every 6 hours, amoxicillin-clavulanate 500 mg/125 mg p.o. every 8 hours, or clindamycin 600 mg p.o. every 8 hours)

Second Line
- Coverage against methicillin-resistant *Staphylococcus aureus* is not recommended, unless identified by culture.
- For severe infections: Cefazolin 1–1.5 g IV every 8 hours in combination with clindamycin (600–900 mg IV) every 8 hours

ADDITIONAL TREATMENT
General Measures
IV antibiotics for severe infections

Additional Therapies
Sclerotherapy: Percutaneous ethanol injection is an alternative approach in patients who are not surgical candidates if the presence of malignancy can be excluded. It is effective in 1/3 of patients.

SURGERY/OTHER PROCEDURES
- Sistrunk procedure: Removal of the center portion of the hyoid bone in continuity and resection of a core of tissue from the hyoid upwards towards the foramen cecum
- Recurrence is rare after the Sistrunk procedure and is treated with excision of a core of tissue from the hyoid to the foramen cecum to remove any superior tract arborization (3).
- Suture-guided transhyoid pharyngotomy modification of the Sistrunk operation has also been proposed, but is not recommended at this time.
- If the cyst is infected, infection should be treated with antibiotics and local heat and/or drainage prior to surgery. After resolution of the inflammation, excision should be performed (1,4)[C].

IN-PATIENT CONSIDERATIONS
Admission Criteria
- If incision and drainage are necessary, the incision should be placed so that it can be excised completely with an ellipse at the time of definitive resection.
- Formal incision and drainage should be avoided.

 ## ONGOING CARE

If a thyroglossal duct is not removed, as many as half become infected.

FOLLOW-UP RECOMMENDATIONS
- Unrestricted
- Infection before surgery is a well-described cause of recurrence

Patient Monitoring
1–2 weeks after resection

DIET
Unrestricted

PATIENT EDUCATION
Reassure family about absence of malignancy (if appropriate).

PROGNOSIS
- Recurrence after complete excision using Sistrunk procedure is reported to be 2.6–5% (5).
- Increased risk of recurrence:
  – Failure to completely excise the cyst
  – In children <2 years of age, intraoperative cyst rupture and presence of a cutaneous component
  – Preoperative or concurrent infection of the cyst at the time of the surgery
- After excision, thyroglossal cyst has a high risk for recurrence (20–35%) and requires a wider en bloc resection.
- Most cases of thyroglossal duct cyst carcinoma are treated adequately by Sistrunk procedure, with a reported cure rate of 95%.

COMPLICATIONS
- Infection occurs in up to half of cysts if not excised.
- Malignant degeneration may occur (1–2%) if cyst is not excised.
- Most common tumor type is papillary carcinoma (6)
- Malignancy is not usually suspected prior to discovery on histologic examination.
- FNA is most reliable for preoperative diagnosis of malignancy, but yield is low due to low incidence of malignancy.
- Unless tumor is invasive (which is rare), Sistrunk procedure is usually curative.
- Must rule out primary thyroid carcinoma if thyroglossal duct cyst carcinoma is found
- Reports demonstrate that lingual location of thyroglossal duct cysts can cause not only various respiratory problems but also infant death.
- Wide local excision is a valuable extension of the Sistrunk operation for the management of recurrent disease (3)[C].
- Patient may require thyroid medication for life if ectopic midline thyroid is mistakenly removed.
- If the cyst ruptures, it may go on to form a thyroglossal duct sinus or a thyroglossal duct fistula that exits through the overlying skin.

REFERENCES
1. Kaselas Ch, Tsikopoulos G, Chortis Ch, et al. Thyroglossal duct cyst's inflammation. When do we operate? *Pediatr Surg Int.* 2005;21:991–3.
2. Schader I, et al. Hereditary duct cyst. *Pediatric Surg Int.* 2005;21(7):593–4.
3. Patel NN, Hartley BE, Howard DJ. Management of thyroglossal tract disease after failed Sistrunk's procedure. *J Laryngol Otol.* 2003;117:710–2.
4. Ostlie DJ, Burjonrappa SC, Snyder CL, et al. Thyroglossal duct infections and surgical outcomes. *J Pediatr Surg.* 2004;39:396–9; discussion 396–9.
5. Sistrunk WE. The surgical treatment of cysts of the thyroglossal tract. *Ann Surg.* 1920;71:121–122.2.
6. Heshmati HM, Fatourechi V, van Heerden JA, et al. Thyroglossal duct carcinoma: report of 12 cases. *Mayo Clin Proc.* 1997;72:315–9.

ADDITIONAL READING
- Al-dajani N, Wootton SH. Cervical lymphadenitis, suppurative parotitis, thyroiditis, and infected cyst. *Infect Dis Clin North Am.* 2007;21(2):523–41.
- Perkins JA, Inglis AF. Recurrent thyroglossal duct cysts: a 23 years experience and a new method for management. A858–856

 ## CODES

ICD9
759.2 Anomalies of other endocrine glands, congenital

CLINICAL PEARLS
- Malignancy may be suspected if a soft tissue component exists within or around the cyst.
- Thyroglossal duct cysts should be removed surgically, but surgery is usually elective unless the cyst is obstructing the airway.
- Sistrunk procedure is performed once all inflammation has resolved.
- Fine-needle aspiration biopsy is the most reliable method for preoperative diagnosis of thyroid cancer, especially if done with ultrasound guidance.
- If the cyst is found to contain thyroid carcinoma, the surgeon must be sure that the carcinoma arose from within the cyst and is not a cystic metastasis to a midline lymph node from a primary thyroid carcinoma.
- When possible, cultures should be obtained with a fine-needle aspirate for Gram stain, aerobic and anaerobic culture, fungal stain and culture, acid-fast stain, and mycobacterial culture.

T

THYROID MALIGNANT NEOPLASIA

James P. Miller, MD
Timothy L. Black, MD

 BASICS

DESCRIPTION

Thyroid malignant neoplasia is an autologous growth of thyroid nodules with potential for metastases.

- Papillary carcinoma:
  - Most common variety, 60–70% of thyroid tumors
  - Peak incidence in the 3rd and 4th decades
  - 3× more common in women
  - May be associated with radiation exposure
  - Tumor contains psammoma bodies.
  - Metastasizes by lymphatic route (30% at time of diagnosis)
  - Multicentric in 20% or more, especially in children
- Follicular carcinoma:
  - 10–20% of thyroid tumors
  - Peak incidence in 5th decade of life
  - Incidence has been decreasing since the addition of dietary iodine.
  - Metastasizes by the hematogenous route
- Hürthle cell carcinoma:
  - Usually in patients >60 years of age
  - Radioresistant
  - Composed of distinct large eosinophilic cells with abundant cytoplasmic mitochondria
- Medullary thyroid carcinoma:
  - Arises from parafollicular cells, C cells
  - 2–5% of all thyroid tumors
  - 25–35% are associated with multiple endocrine neoplasia syndromes, which can be familial or sporadic.
  - Calcitonin is a chemical marker.
- Anaplastic carcinoma:
  - 3% of thyroid tumors
  - Usually in patients >60 years of age
- Other: Lymphoma, sarcoma, or metastatic (renal, breast, or lung)
- System(s) affected: Endocrine/Metabolic
- Synonym(s): Follicular carcinoma of the thyroid; Papillary carcinoma of the thyroid; Hürthle cell carcinoma of the thyroid; Anaplastic cell carcinoma of the thyroid

Geriatric Considerations
Risk of malignancy increases at >60 years of age.

Pediatric Considerations
>60% of thyroid nodules are malignant.

EPIDEMIOLOGY

Incidence
- 10/100,000 per year in US
- Deaths: 6/1 million/year in US
- In 2008, estimated 37,340 new cases and 1,590 deaths from thyroid cancer in the US
- Predominant age: Usually >40 years
- Predominant sex: Female > Male (2.6:1).

RISK FACTORS
- Family history
- Neck irradiation (6–2,000 rads): Papillary carcinoma
- Iodine deficiency: Follicular carcinoma
- Multiple endocrine neoplasia syndrome: Medullary carcinoma
- Previous history of subtotal thyroidectomy for malignancy: Anaplastic carcinoma

Genetics
- Familial polyposis of the colon, Turcot's syndrome, and Gardner's syndrome with the *APC* gene, 5q21
- Medullary: Autosomal dominant with multiple endocrine neoplasia syndrome
- *BRAF* mutation
- *RET* oncogene

GENERAL PREVENTION
- Physical exam in high-risk group
- Calcium infusion or pentagastrin stimulation test in high-risk multiple endocrine neoplasia (MEN) patients

ETIOLOGY
Unknown

COMMONLY ASSOCIATED CONDITIONS
Medullary carcinoma: Pheochromocytoma, hyperparathyroidism, ganglioneuroma of the GI tract, neuromata of mucosal membranes

 DIAGNOSIS

HISTORY
- Change in voice (dysphonia)
- Positive family history
- Neck mass
- Dysphagia
- Dyspnea

PHYSICAL EXAM
- Neck mass: If fixed to surrounding tissue, this finding suggests advanced disease.
- Cervical adenopathy

DIAGNOSTIC TESTS & INTERPRETATION
- Medullary carcinoma: Calcitonin level (normal <30 pg/mL [300 ng/L]), pentagastrin stimulation test
- Thyroglobulin (TG) level: Postoperative tumor marker
- DNA content of tumors from biopsy specimen: Diploid content has a better prognosis.

Lab
Thyroid function tests usually normal

Imaging
- Thyroid scan: Cold nodules are more suspicious of malignancy.
- Ultrasound: Solid mass is more suspicious of malignancy.
- CT scan and MRI can be useful to evaluate large substernal masses and recurrent soft tissue masses.
- ^{18}F-FDG positron-emission tomographic scan can help if the cytology is inconclusive; helpful with recurrent disease when patient has a negative ^{131}I scan and an elevated TG level (1)[C].

Diagnostic Procedures/Surgery
- Fine-needle aspiration (FNA)
- Surgical biopsy/excision
- Laryngoscopy if vocal cord paralysis is suspected

Pathological Findings
- Papillary: Psammoma bodies, anaplastic epithelial papillae
- Follicular: Anaplastic epithelial cords with follicles
- Hürthle cell: Large eosinophilic cells with granular cytoplasm
- Medullary: Large amounts of amyloid stroma
- Anaplastic: Small cell and giant cell undifferentiated tumors

DIFFERENTIAL DIAGNOSIS
- Multinodular goiter
- Thyroid adenoma
- Thyroglossal duct cyst
- Thyroiditis
- Thyroid cyst
- Ectopic thyroid
- Dermoid cyst

TREATMENT
Inpatient

MEDICATION
Postoperatively, will require thyroid hormone replacement:
- Levothyroxine (T$_4$, Synthroid) 100–200 μg/day, or
- Liothyronine (T$_3$, Cytomel) 50–100 μg/day

ADDITIONAL TREATMENT
Additional Therapies
- ^{131}I thyroid remnant ablation
- External-beam radiation for advanced disease

SURGERY/OTHER PROCEDURES
- Papillary carcinoma: Lobectomy with isthmectomy (if lesion <1.5 cm) or total thyroidectomy and removal of suspicious lymph nodes
- Follicular carcinoma and Hürthle cell: Total thyroidectomy and removal of suspicious lymph nodes
- Medullary carcinoma: Total thyroidectomy with central node dissection; unilateral or bilateral modified radical neck dissection if lateral nodes are histologically positive
- Anaplastic carcinoma: Aggressive en bloc thyroidectomy; tracheostomy often required

ONGOING CARE

FOLLOW-UP RECOMMENDATIONS
Patient Monitoring
- Thyroid scan at 6 weeks and administration of ^{131}I for any visible uptake; any evidence of residual thyroid tissue (after total thyroidectomy) or lymph node disease noted on scan is treated with radioactive iodine.
- At 6 months and then yearly, the patient should have a thyroid scan and CXR.
- Papillary and follicular: A TG level should be done yearly. Recombinant human thyroid-stimulating hormone (rhTSH)–stimulated TG level may be more sensitive (2,3)[B].
- Medullary: Calcitonin level should be done yearly with pentagastrin stimulation.
- The thyroid scan and TG level should be done with the patient in the hypothyroid state induced by 6-week withdrawal of levothyroxine or 2- to 3-week withdrawal of liothyronine.

DIET
Avoid iodine deficiency.

PATIENT EDUCATION
National Cancer Institute, Building 31, Room 101-18, 9000 Rockville Pike, Bethesda, MD 20892; (301) 496-5583; http://www.cancer.gov/

PROGNOSIS
- Papillary carcinoma: Overall mortality 3–8%
- Follicular carcinoma: Overall 80% 5-year survival rate, 77% 10-year survival rate; histologically, microinvasive tumors parallel papillary tumor results, whereas grossly invasive tumors do far worse.
- Hürthle cell carcinoma: 93% 5-year survival rate and 83% survival rate overall; grossly invasive tumor survival <25%.
- Medullary carcinoma: Negative nodes, 90% 5-year survival rate and 85% 10-year survival rate; with positive nodes, 65% 5-year survival rate and 40% 10-year survival rate
- Anaplastic carcinoma: Survival unexpected

COMPLICATIONS
- Recurrence of tumor
- Hoarseness from tumor invasion or operative injury to recurrent laryngeal nerve
- Hypoparathyroidism from operative injury to parathyroid glands

REFERENCES
1. Wang W, Larson SM, Fazzari M, et al. Prognostic value of [18F]fluorodeoxyglucose positron emission tomographic scanning in patients with thyroid cancer. *J Clin Endocrinol Metab*. 2000;85:1107–13.
2. Blamey S, et al. Using recombinant human TSH for the diagnosis of recurrent thyroid cancer. *A N Z J Surg*. 2005;75:10–20.
3. Haugen BR, Pacini F, Reiners C, et al. A comparison of recombinant human thyrotropin and thyroid hormone withdrawal for the detection of thyroid remnant or cancer. *J Clin Endocrinol Metab*. 1999;84:3877–85.

ADDITIONAL READING
Gagel RF, Goepfert H, Callender DL. Changing concepts in the pathogenesis and management of thyroid carcinoma. *CA Cancer J Clin*. 1996;46:261–83.

See Also (Topic, Algorithm, Electronic Media Element)
Multiple Endocrine Neoplasia

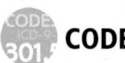

CODES

ICD9
193 Malignant neoplasm of thyroid gland

CLINICAL PEARLS
- Standard workup for a patient suspected of having a thyroid cancer is a physical exam, TSH level, neck US, and FNA.
- TG levels can be elevated in several thyroid disorders. Its usefulness comes once the diagnosis of cancer has been made. It serves as a better marker for recurrent disease.
- ~2% of the normal population will have a positive ^{18}F-FDG positron-emission tomographic scan, so it is more useful for postresection follow-up.

THYROIDITIS

Michelle A. Tinitigan, MD

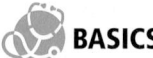

BASICS

Inflammation of the thyroid gland that may be painful and tender when caused by infection, radiation, or trauma, or painless when caused by autoimmune conditions, medications, or an idiopathic fibrotic process

DESCRIPTION

- Thyroiditis with thyroid pain and tenderness:
  - Subacute granulomatous thyroiditis (aka nonsuppurative thyroiditis, de Quervain's thyroiditis, or giant cell thyroiditis): Self-limited; caused by a viral or postviral inflammatory process
  - Infectious/suppurative thyroiditis:
    - Caused by bacterial, fungal, mycobacterial, or parasitic infection of the thyroid
    - Bacteria may spread hematogenously in immunocompromised or from a piriform sinus fistula. Most commonly associated with *Streptococcus pyogenes*, *Staphylococcus aureus*, and *Streptococcus pneumoniae*.
  - Radiation-induced thyroiditis: From radioactive iodine therapy (1%) or external irradiation for lymphoma and head or neck cancers
- Thyroiditis with no thyroid pain and tenderness:
  - Hashimoto's (autoimmune) thyroiditis (aka chronic lymphocytic thyroiditis): Most common etiology of chronic hypothyroidism; autoimmune disease: 90% of patients with high serum antithyroid peroxidase (TPO) antibodies
  - Postpartum thyroiditis (aka invasive thyroiditis): Occurs within 1 year postpartum (or after spontaneous/induced abortion) and improvement after 2–4 weeks
  - Painless (silent) thyroiditis (aka subacute lymphocytic thyroiditis): Key findings: Mild hyperthyroidism, little or no thyroid enlargement, and no Graves ophthalmopathy or pretibial myxedema
  - Riedel's (fibrous) thyroiditis: Rare form of chronic thyroiditis characterized by extensive fibrosis of the thyroid gland, also affecting adjacent tissue
  - Drug-induced thyroiditis: In patients receiving interferon-alfa, interleukin-2, amiodarone, or lithium

EPIDEMIOLOGY

- Subacute granulomatous thyroiditis: Most common cause of thyroid pain; peaks during summer; affects women than men; common 40–50 years of age
- Suppurative thyroiditis: Commonly seen with preexisting thyroid disease or immunocompromise
- Hashimoto's thyroiditis: Peak age of onset 30–50 years; increases with age; can occur in children; primarily a disease of women, with sex ratio 7:1
- Postpartum thyroiditis: 5–7% of postpartum women; occurs in 25% with type 1 diabetes mellitus
- Painless (silent) thyroiditis: Women affected 4× more than men
- Reidel's thyroiditis: Women are 4× more affected than men; highest prevalence age 30–60

RISK FACTORS

- Hashimoto disease: Family history of thyroid or autoimmune disease, personal history of autoimmune disease (type 1 diabetes, celiac disease), high iodine intake, cigarette smoking, selenium deficiency

- Subacute granulomatous thyroiditis: Recent viral respiratory infection
- Suppurative thyroiditis: Congenital abnormalities (persistent thyroglossal duct or piriform sinus fistula), greater age, immunosuppression
- Radiation-induced thyroiditis: High-dose irradiation, younger age, female sex, preexisting hypothyroidism
- Postpartum thyroiditis: Smoking, history of spontaneous or induced abortion
- Painless (silent) thyroiditis: Iodine-deficient areas

Genetics

Autoimmune thyroiditis is associated with the CT60 polymorphism of cytotoxic T-cell lymphocyte–associated antigen 4 (CTLA-4). Also associated with HLA-DR4, -DR5, and -DR6 in Caucasians.

GENERAL PREVENTION

Selenium may decrease inflammatory activity in pregnant women with autoimmune hypothyroidism and may reduce postpartum thyroiditis risk in those positive for thyroid peroxidase (TPO) antibodies (1).

ETIOLOGY

Hashimoto disease: Antithyroid antibodies may be produced in response to an environmental antigen and cross-react with thyroid proteins (molecular mimicry). Precipitating factors: Infection, stress, sex steroids, pregnancy, iodine intake, radiation exposure

COMMONLY ASSOCIATED CONDITIONS

Postpartum thyroiditis: Family history of autoimmune thyroid disease, human leukocyte antigens HLA-DRB, -DR4, and -DR5

DIAGNOSIS

HISTORY

- Hypothyroid symptoms (e.g., constipation, heavy menstrual bleeding, dry skin, hair loss)
- Hyperthyroid symptoms (e.g., weakness, fatigue, irritability, heat/cold intolerance, increased sweating, palpitations, disturbed sleep, stare, and lid retraction)
- Subacute granulomatous thyroiditis: Sudden or gradual onset with preceding URI/viral illness (fever, fatigue, malaise, anorexia, and myalgia are common); pain may be limited to thyroid region or radiate to upper neck, jaw, throat, or ears

PHYSICAL EXAM

- Examine thyroid for size, symmetry, and palpable nodules:
  - Hashimoto disease: 90% have a symmetrical, diffusely enlarged, painless gland with a firm, pebbly texture; 10% have thyroid atrophy.
  - Postpartum thyroiditis: Painless, small, nontender, firm goiter (2–6 months after delivery)
  - Reidel's thyroiditis: Rock-hard, woodlike, fixed, painless goiter, often accompanied by symptoms of esophageal or tracheal compression (stridor, dyspnea, a suffocating feeling, dysphagia, and hoarseness)
- Signs of hypothyroid: Delayed relaxation phase of deep tendon reflexes, nonpitting edema, dry skin, alopecia, bradycardia
- Signs of hyperthyroid: Moist palms, hyperreflexia, tachycardia/atrial fibrillation

DIAGNOSTIC TESTS & INTERPRETATION

Lab

- TSH, anti-TPO antibodies
- Hashimoto disease:
  - High titers of anti-TPO antibodies
- Subacute granulomatous thyroiditis:
  - High T_4, T_3; low TSH during early stages and elevated later
  - High thyroglobulin; normal levels of anti-TPO and anti-thyroglobulin antibodies
  - Elevated ESR (usually >50 mm/hr) and CRP; mild anemia and slight leukocytosis; LFTs frequently abnormal during initial hyperthyroid phase and resolve over 1–2 months
- Suppurative thyroiditis:
  - In the absence of preexisting thyroid disease, thyroid function normal but hyperthyroidism or hypothyroidism may occur
  - ESR is elevated, and WBC generally shows a marked increase with a left shift.
  - FNA of the lesion with Gram stain and culture is the most useful diagnostic test.
- Postpartum thyroiditis:
  - High or high-normal T_4 and T_3, low TSH 2–10 months after delivery with recovery over the next 2–3 months. Hypothyroidism occurs between 2 and 12 months after delivery, most commonly at 6 months (2).
  - Most patients (80%) have normal thyroid function at 1 year; 30–50% of patients develop permanent hypothyroidism within 9 years (2).
  - High anti-TPO antibodies and thyroglobulin; normal ESR
- Painless (silent) thyroiditis:
  - Hyperthyroid state in 5-20%: Averages 3–4 months, and total duration of illness is less than 1 year. Followed by hypothyroidism and then return to normal state. Some with primary or subclinical hypothyroidism.
  - Half of patients have anti-TPO antibodies
- Reidel's thyroiditis:
  - Hypothyroidism because of extensive replacement of the gland by scar tissue. Anti-TPO antibodies are present in 2/3 of patients and low RAIU.
- Drug-induced thyroiditis:
  - Hyperthyroidism or hypothyroidism, low RAIU, and variable presence of anti-TPO antibodies
- Drugs that may alter lab results: Thyroid hormones, corticosteroids, iodine-containing drugs and contrast media, lithium, amiodarone
- Disorders that may alter lab results: Iodine deficiency, nonthyroidal illness

Imaging

- Ultrasonography
- Thyroid radioactive iodine uptake (RAIU) scan: Decreased in all forms of thyroiditis, but is usually not helpful in establishing diagnosis of Hashimoto disease. High RAIU in hashitoxicosis.
- Random urine iodine measurement may be helpful to distinguish this disease from other causes of low RAIU:
  - Urine iodine <500 μg/L (subacute granulomatous thyroiditis)
  - Urine iodine >1,000 μg/L (in patients with exposure to excess exogenous iodine/radiocontrast material)

Diagnostic Procedures/Surgery
- Hashimoto with a dominant nodule should undergo FNA to rule out thyroid carcinoma
- Open biopsy necessary for a definitive diagnosis with Reidel's thyroiditis

Pathological Findings
- Hashimoto disease: Lymphocytic infiltration with formation of Askanazy (Hürthle) cells, oxyphilic changes in follicular cells, fibrosis, thyroid atrophy
- Subacute granulomatous thyroiditis: Giant cells, mononuclear cell infiltrate
- Postpartum thyroiditis: Lymphocytic infiltration, occasional germinal centers, disruption and collapse of thyroid follicles
- Painless thyroiditis: Lymphocytic infiltration but without fibrosis, Askanazy cells, and extensive lymphoid follicle formation (2)

DIFFERENTIAL DIAGNOSIS
Simple goiter; iodine-deficient or lithium-induced goiter; Graves disease; lymphoma; acute infectious thyroiditis; hemorrhage into a thyroid nodule/cyst; infections of oropharynx and trachea; subacute systemic illness; subacute granulomatous thyroiditis; thyroid cancer

 TREATMENT

MEDICATION
- Hashimoto disease:
  - If hypothyroid or goitrous: Levothyroxine (1.7 μg/kg/d for healthy adults <50 years of age). If no cardiac complications and no adrenal insufficiency, aim for 1/2 replacement dose and be increased to full replacement in 10 days:
    - In patients >50 years of age or patients with heart disease and/or adrenal insufficiency, begin with 25 or 50 μg/d, and titrate to TSH of lower limit of assay normal range.
  - If thyrotoxic and symptomatic: Propylthiouracil and propranolol
  - An elevated TSH level in a woman who is pregnant or attempting to become pregnant is a clear indication for thyroid hormone replacement (3).
- Subacute granulomatous thyroiditis:
  - Pain: Analgesics (e.g., nonsteroidal anti-inflammatory drugs [NSAIDs] or aspirin)
  - Symptomatic hyperthyroidism: β-Blockers (propranolol 40–120 mg/d, propranolol LA 80 mg/d, or atenolol 25–50 mg/d) for a few weeks while thyrotoxic
  - Symptomatic hypothyroid phase: Levothyroxine as dosed above with a goal TSH in the normal range
  - Pain with no improvement in 2–3 days after NSAID use: Prednisone 40 mg/d; should result in pain relief in 1–2 days; if not, diagnosis should be questioned
  - Severe pain or no relief with analgesics: Start with prednisone 40–60 mg/day gradually discontinued over 4–6 weeks. If thyroid pain recurs, increase dose for several weeks and then taper.
  - Thionamides: No benefit because hyperthyroidism is not caused by excess thyroid hormone synthesis
- Suppurative thyroiditis:
  - Parenteral empiric broad-spectrum antibiotics and surgical drainage

- Painless thyroiditis:
  - Usually no treatment needed because thyroid function rarely severe and is transient
  - If symptomatic during hyperthyroid state, may treat with β-blocker propranolol (40–120 mg/d) or atenolol (25–50 mg/d) for a few weeks as indicated
  - Prednisone shortens the period of hyperthyroidism.
  - Treat hypothyroid symptoms with levothyroxine (50–100 μg/d), to be discontinued after 8–12 weeks and reevaluate 4–6 weeks later.
- Postpartum thyroiditis:
  - Treat symptomatic hyperthyroid/hypothyroid state.
  - Caution in breastfeeding mothers because beta blockers are secreted into breast milk
  - For symptomatic hypothyroidism, treat with levothyroxine. Otherwise, remonitor in 4–8 weeks. Taper replacement hormone after 6 months to determine if thyroid function has normalized.
- Reidel's thyroiditis:
  - Corticosteroids in early stages of the disease, but controversial thereafter. A dose of 10–20 mg per day for 4–6 months is recommended, possibly continued thereafter if effective (4).
  - Tamoxifen is a good alternative at 20 × 2 mg per day, to be reduced if adverse effects occur to 10 × 2 mg per day (4). Methotrexate has been used as treatment, with some success (5).
- Drug-induced thyroiditis:
  - Discontinuation of offending drug resolves thyroid abnormalities.
- Maintenance: Optimal levothyroxine dose can be established by measuring TSH at 6- to 8-week intervals until the TSH is at a lower level of normal for assay used.
- Contraindications: Propylthiouracil: Allergy or hypersensitivity to analgesics/narcotics. Propranolol: Insulin therapy, asthma. Prednisone: Adverse reactions. Levothyroxine: None.
- Significant possible interactions: Sucralfate (Carafate) and iron preparations may decrease levothyroxine availability.

ADDITIONAL TREATMENT
General Measures
Outpatient management unless severe thyrotoxicosis; analgesics for pain; corticosteroids for severe granulomatous thyroiditis

SURGERY/OTHER PROCEDURES
Enlarged thyroid with pain or tracheal/esophageal compression

 ONGOING CARE

FOLLOW-UP RECOMMENDATIONS
Patient Monitoring
- Hashimoto disease: Repeat thyroid function tests every 3–12 months.
- Subacute granulomatous thyroiditis: Repeat thyroid function tests every 3–6 weeks until euthyroid; check every 6–12 months.
- Postpartum thyroiditis: Patients who have antithyroid peroxidase antibodies have a 70% risk of recurrence following a subsequent pregnancy.
- Reidel's thyroiditis: CT of cervical mediastinal region recommended.
- Drug-induced thyroiditis: Monitor TSH in patients taking amiodarone every 6 months.

Pregnancy Considerations
- Avoid radioisotope scanning if possible.
- Titrate replacement thyroid hormone to keep TSH maximally suppressed.
- If using RAIU scan, discard breast milk for 2 days because RAI is secreted in breast milk.

PROGNOSIS
- Hashimoto disease: Persistent goiter; eventual thyroid failure
- Granulomatous thyroiditis: Eventual return to normal over weeks or months; remission may be slower in the elderly
- Postpartum thyroiditis: Recurrence is likely after future pregnancies; substantial risk for later development of hypothyroidism

REFERENCES
1. Negro R, Greco G, Mangieri T, et al. The Influence of Selenium Supplementation on Postpartum Thyroid Status in Pregnant Women with Thyroid Peroxidase Autoantibodies. *J Clin Endocrinol Metab.* 2007.
2. Bindra A, Braunstein GD, et al. Thyroiditis. *Am Fam Physician.* 2006;73:1769–76.
3. Reid SM, Middleton P, Cossich MC, et al. Interventions for clinical and subclinical hypothyroidism in pregnancy. *Cochrane Database Syst Rev.* 2010;7:CD007752.
4. El Hajj G, Yahya AF, Medlej R, et al. [Autoimmune thyroid disease. Clinical and biological correlations] *J Med Liban.* 2009;57:218–25.
5. Pritchyk K, Newkirk K, Garlich P, et al. Tamoxifen therapy for Riedel's thyroiditis. *Laryngoscope.* 2004;114:1758–60.

See Also (Topic, Algorithm, Electronic Media Element)
Hyperthyroidism; Hypothyroidism, Adult

 CODES

ICD9
- 245.0 Acute thyroiditis
- 245.1 Subacute thyroiditis
- 245.2 Chronic lymphocytic thyroiditis

CLINICAL PEARLS
- TSH elevation above the normal range indicates a hypothyroid state; suppressed TSH indicates hyperthyroid state. Follow up with free T_3/T_4 determination.
- Follow patients on thyroid replacement with periodic TSH levels.

TINEA (CAPITIS, CORPORIS, CRURIS)

Elisabeth L. Backer, MD

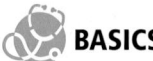

BASICS

DESCRIPTION
- Tinea cruris: Superficial fungal infection of groin area and gluteal cleft
- Tinea corporis:
  - Superficial fungal infection affecting the face, trunk, and/or extremities
  - Often presents with ring-shaped lesions, hence the misnomer *ringworm*
- Tinea capitis:
  - A fungal infection of the scalp and hair
  - Affected areas of the scalp can show characteristic black dots resulting from broken hairs.
- Infections result from contact with infected persons or animals.
  - Zoophilic infections are acquired from animals.
  - Anthropophilic infections are acquired from personal contact (e.g., wrestling) or fomites.
  - Geophile infections are acquired from the soil.
- System(s) affected: Skin/Exocrine
- Synonym(s): Jock itch; Ringworm

EPIDEMIOLOGY
Incidence
- Tinea cruris:
  - Predominant age: Any age; rare in children
  - Predominant sex: Male > Female
- Tinea corporis:
  - Predominant age: All ages
  - Predominant sex: Male = Female
- Tinea capitis:
  - Predominant age: 3–9 years; almost always occurs in young children
  - Predominant sex: Male = Female

Prevalence
Common

Pediatric Considerations
- Tinea cruris is rare prior to puberty.
- Tinea capitis is common in young children.

Geriatric Considerations
Tinea cruris more common in the geriatric population due to an increase in risk factors.

Pregnancy Considerations
Tinea cruris and capitis are rare in pregnancy.

RISK FACTORS
- Warm climates; summer months and/or copious sweating; wearing wet clothing or multiple layers (tinea cruris)
- Daycare centers/schools/confined quarters (tinea corporis and capitis)

- Depression of cell-mediated immune response (e.g., individuals with atopy or AIDS)
- Obesity (tinea cruris and corporis)
- Direct contact with an active lesion on a human, an animal, or rarely, from soil; working with animals (tinea corporis)

Genetics
Evidence suggests a genetic susceptibility in certain individuals.

GENERAL PREVENTION
- Avoidance of risk factors, such as contact with suspicious lesions
- Fluconazole or itraconazole may be useful in wrestlers to prevent outbreaks during competitive season (1)[A].

PATHOPHYSIOLOGY
Superficial fungal infection of skin/scalp

ETIOLOGY
- Tinea cruris: Source of infection usually the patient's own tinea pedis, with agent being transferred from the foot to the groin via the underwear when dressing; most common causative dermatophyte is *Trichophyton rubrum*; rare cases caused by *Epidermophyton floccosum* and *T. mentagrophytes*.
- Tinea corporis: Most commonly caused by *T. rubrum*; *Microsporum canis* can cause multiple lesions
- Tinea capitis: *T. tonsurans* found in 90% and *Microsporum* sp. in 10% of patients

COMMONLY ASSOCIATED CONDITIONS
Tinea pedis, tinea barbae, tinea manus

DIAGNOSIS

HISTORY
- Lesions range from asymptomatic to pruritic.
- In tinea cruris, acute inflammation may result from wearing occlusive clothing; chronic scratching may result in an eczematous appearance.
- Previous application of topical steroids, especially in tinea cruris and corporis, may alter the overall appearance, causing a more extensive eruption with irregular borders and erythematous papules. This modified form is called *tinea incognito*.

PHYSICAL EXAM
- Tinea cruris: Well-marginated, erythematous, half-moon-shaped plaques in crural folds that spread to upper thighs; advancing border is well defined, often with fine scaling and sometimes vesicular eruptions. Lesions are usually bilateral and do not include scrotum or penis (unlike with *Candida* infections), but may migrate to perineum, perianal area, and gluteal cleft and onto the buttocks in chronic/progressive cases). The area may be hyperpigmented on resolution.

- Tinea corporis: Scaling, pruritic plaques characterized by a sharply defined annular pattern with peripheral activity and central clearing (ring-shaped lesions); papules and occasionally pustules/vesicles present at border and less commonly in center
- Tinea capitis: Commonly begins with round patches of scale (alopecia less common). In its later stages, the infection frequently takes on patterns of chronic scaling with either little or marked inflammation and alopecia. Less often, patients will present with multiple patches of alopecia and the characteristic black-dot appearance of broken hairs. Extreme inflammation results in kerion formation (exudative, pustular nodulation).

DIAGNOSTIC TESTS & INTERPRETATION
Wood's lamp exam reveals no fluorescence in most cases (*Trichophyton* sp.); 10% of infections, those caused by *M. rubrum*, will fluoresce with a green light.

Lab
Initial lab tests
- Fungal culture using Sabouraud's dextrose agar or dermatophyte test medium
- Potassium hydroxide (KOH) preparation of skin scrapings from dermatophyte leading border shows translucent, branching, rod-shaped hyphae.
- Arthrospores can be visualized within hair shafts.

Follow-Up & Special Considerations
Reevaluate to assess response, especially in resistant or extensive cases.

Pathological Findings
- Skin scrapings show fungal hyphae in epidermis.
- Arthrospores found in hair shafts

DIFFERENTIAL DIAGNOSIS
- Tinea cruris:
  - Intertrigo: Inflammatory process of moist opposed skin folds, often including infection with bacteria, yeast, and fungi; painful longitudinal fissures may occur in skin folds.
  - Erythrasma: Diffuse brown, scaly, noninflammatory plaque with irregular borders, often involving groin; caused by bacterial infection with *Corynebacterium minutissimum;* fluoresces coral red with Wood's lamp
  - Seborrheic dermatitis of groin
  - Psoriasis of groin ("inverse psoriasis")
  - Candidiasis of groin (typically involves the scrotum)
  - Acanthosis nigricans
- Tinea capitis:
  - Psoriasis
  - Seborrheic dermatitis
  - Pyoderma
  - Alopecia areata and trichotillomania
  - Aphasia cutis congenital
- Tinea corporis:
  - Pityriasis rosea
  - Eczema (nummular)
  - Contact dermatitis

- Syphilis
- Psoriasis
- Seborrheic dermatitis
- Subacute lupus erythematosus (SLE)
- Erythema annulare centrifugum
- Erythema multiforme; erythema migrans
- Impetigo circinatum
- Granuloma annulare

 TREATMENT

MEDICATION
First Line
- Tinea cruris/corporis:
  - Topical azole antifungal compounds (2)[C]:
    - Econazole (Spectazole), ketoconazole (Nizoral): Usually applied b.i.d. × 2–3 weeks
    - Terbinafine (Lamisil): Over-the-counter (OTC) compound; can be applied once or b.i.d. × 1–2 weeks
    - Butenafine (Mentax): Applied once daily × 2 weeks; also very effective
  - To prevent relapse, use for 1 week after resolution (3)[C].
- Tinea capitis:
  - Oral griseofulvin (4,5)[A] for *Trichophyton* and *Microsporum* sp.; microsized preparation available; dosage 125 mg/d in patients weighing 10–20 kg; 250 mg/d if weight is 20–40 kg; 500 mg/d if weight is >40 kg; taken b.i.d. or as a single dose daily × 6–12 weeks
  - Oral terbinafine (5)[A] can be used for *Trichophyton* sp. at 62.5 mg/d in patients weighing 10–20 kg; 125 mg/d if weight 20–40 kg; 250 mg/d if weight >40 kg; use for 4–6 weeks
  - Oral itraconazole (5)[A] can be used for *Microsporum* sp. and matches griseofulvin's efficacy while being better tolerated. Dosage of 3–5 mg/kg/d, but most studies have used 100 mg/d × 6 weeks in children >2 years of age.

Second Line
Tinea cruris/corporis:
- Oral antifungal agents are effective but not indicated in uncomplicated tinea cruris or corporis cases. They can be used for resistant and extensive infections or if the patient is immunocompromised. If topical therapy fails, one may consult a dermatologist for possible oral therapy. Griseofulvin can be given 500 mg/d for 1–2 weeks.
- The following oral regimens have been reported in medical literature as being effective but currently are not specifically approved by the FDA for tinea cruris:
  - Oral terbinafine (Lamisil) 250 mg/d × 1 week
  - Oral itraconazole (Sporanox) 100 mg b.i.d. once and repeated 1 week later
  - Oral fluconazole (Diflucan) 150 mg once per week × 4 weeks
- Topical terbinafine 1% solution has been studied recently and appears effective as a once-daily application for 1 week.
- Contraindications:
  - Oral itraconazole (Sporanox): Contraindicated with astemizole (Hismanal), triazolam (Halcion), lovastatin (Mevacor), simvastatin (Zocor). Pravastatin (Pravachol) can be given with itraconazole.

- Oral antifungals can interact with warfarin, BCPs, alcohol; contraindicated in pregnancy. Monitor for liver toxicity when using oral antifungals.

ADDITIONAL TREATMENT
General Measures
- Careful handwashing and personal hygiene; laundering of towels/clothing of affected individual; no sharing of towels/clothes/headgear
- Evaluate other family members, close contacts, or household pets.
- Avoid predisposing conditions such as hot baths and tight-fitting clothing (boxer shorts better than briefs) (5)[C].
- Keep area as dry as possible (talcum/powders may be beneficial) (5)[C].
- Itching can be alleviated by OTC preparations such as Sarna or Prax.
- Topical steroid preparations should not be used (see Tinea Incognito) (2)[C].
- Avoid contact sports (e.g., wrestling) temporarily while starting treatment.

Issues for Referral
Refer if disease is nonresponsive or resistant, especially in immunocompromised host.

Additional Therapies
Treatment of secondary bacterial infections

 ONGOING CARE

FOLLOW-UP RECOMMENDATIONS
Reevaluate response to treatment.

Patient Monitoring
Liver function testing prior to therapy and at regular intervals during course of therapy for patients requiring oral terbinafine, fluconazole, itraconazole, and griseofulvin

PATIENT EDUCATION
Explanation of the causative agents, predisposing factors, and prevention measures

PROGNOSIS
- Excellent prognosis for cure with therapy in tinea cruris and corporis
- In tinea capitis, lesions will heal spontaneously in 6 months without treatment, but scarring is more likely.

COMPLICATIONS
- Secondary bacterial infection
- Generalized, invasive dermatophyte infection

REFERENCES
1. Kohl TD, Martin DC, Berger MS. Comparison of topical and oral treatments for tinea gladiatorum. *Clin J Sport Med*. 1999;9:161–6.
2. Bonifaz A, et al. Comparative study between terbinafine 1% emulsion-gel versus ketoconazole 2% cream in tinea cruris and corporis. *Eur J Derm*. 2000;10:107.
3. Lesher JL Jr, et al. Butenafine 1% cream in the treatment of tinea cruris: A multicenter, vehicle-controlled, double-blind trial. *J Amer Acad Dermatol*. 1997;36(2 pt 1):S20–S24.

4. Fuller LC, Smith CH, Cerio R, et al. A randomized comparison of 4 weeks of terbinafine vs. 8 weeks of griseofulvin for the treatment of tinea capitis. *Br J Dermatol*. 2001;144:321–7.
5. Gupta AK, Adam P, Dlova N, et al. Therapeutic options for the treatment of tinea capitis caused by Trichophyton species: griseofulvin versus the new oral antifungal agents, terbinafine, itraconazole, and fluconazole. *Pediatr Dermatol*. 2001;18: 433–8.

ADDITIONAL READING
- Akinwale SO. Personal hygiene as an alternative to griseofulvin in the treatment of tinea cruris. *Afr J Med Sci*. 2000;29:41.
- Elewski BE, Cáceres HW, DeLeon L, et al. Terbinafine hydrochloride oral granules versus oral griseofulvin suspension in children with tinea capitis: results of two randomized, investigator-blinded, multicenter, international, controlled trials. *J Am Acad Dermatol*. 2008;59:41–54.
- Gonzalez, U, Seaton, T, Bergus, G, et al. Systemic antifungal therapy for tinea capitis in children. *Cochrane Database Syst Rev*. 2007:CD004685.
- Nozickova M, Koudelkova V, Kulikova Z, et al. A comparison of the efficacy of oral fluconazole, 150 mg/week versus 50 mg/day, in the treatment of tinea corporis, tinea cruris, tinea pedis, and cutaneous candidosis. *Int J Dermatol*. 1998;37:703–5.
- Sanmano B, Hiruma M, Mizoguchi M, et al. Abbreviated oral itraconazole therapy for tinea corporis and tinea cruris. *Mycoses*. 2003;46: 316–21.

See Also (Topic, Algorithm, Electronic Media Element)
Acanthosis nigricans

 CODES

ICD9
- 110.0 Dermatophytosis of scalp and beard
- 110.2 Dermatophytosis of hand
- 110.3 Dermatophytosis of groin and perianal area

CLINICAL PEARLS
- Tinea corporis: Scaly plaque, with peripheral activity and central clearing
- Tinea cruris: Erythematous plaque in crural folds, usually sparing the scrotum
- Tinea capitis: Fungal infection of the scalp, affecting hair growth

TINEA PEDIS

Elisabeth L. Backer, MD

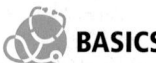

BASICS

DESCRIPTION
- Superficial infection of feet caused by dermatophytes
- Most common dermatophyte infection encountered in clinical practice
- Often accompanied by tinea manuum, tinea unguium, and tines cruris
- 2 clinical forms: Acute and chronic
- System(s) affected: Skin/Exocrine
- Synonym(s): Athlete's foot

EPIDEMIOLOGY
- Predominant age: 20–50 years, although can occur at any age
- Predominant gender: Male > Female

Prevalence
4% of population

Pediatric Considerations
Rare in younger children; common in teens

Geriatric Considerations
Elderly are more susceptible to outbreaks because of immunocompromise and impaired perfusion of distal extremities.

RISK FACTORS
- Hot, humid weather
- Occlusive/tight-fitting footwear
- Immunosuppression
- Prolonged application of topical steroids

Genetics
No known genetic pattern

GENERAL PREVENTION
- Good personal hygiene
- Wearing rubber or wooden sandals in community showers, bathing places, locker rooms
- Careful drying between toes after showering or bathing; blow-drying feet with hair dryer may be more effective than drying with towel
- Changing socks and shoes frequently
- Applying drying or dusting powder
- Applying topical antiperspirants
- Putting on socks before underwear, to prevent infection from spreading to groin

PATHOPHYSIOLOGY
Superficial infection caused by dermatophytes that thrive only in nonviable keratinized tissue

ETIOLOGY
- *Trichophyton mentagrophytes* (acute)
- *Trichophyton rubrum* (chronic)
- *Trichophyton tonsurans*
- *Epidermophyton floccosum*

COMMONLY ASSOCIATED CONDITIONS
- Hyperhidrosis
- Onychomycosis
- Tinea manuum/unguium/cruris/corporis

DIAGNOSIS

HISTORY
- Itchy, scaly rash on foot, usually between toes; may progress to fissuring/maceration in toe web spaces
- May be associated with onychomycosis and other tinea infections

PHYSICAL EXAM
- Acute form: Self-limited, intermittent, recurrent; scaling, thickening and fissuring of sole and heel, scaling or fissuring of toe webs, or vesicular/bullous lesions between toes or on soles
- Chronic form: Most common; slowly progressive pruritic erythematous lesions between toes; interdigital fissures opaque white scales with extension onto soles, sides/dorsum of feet (moccasin distribution). If untreated, may persist indefinitely.
- Other features: Strong odor, hyperkeratosis, maceration, ulceration

DIAGNOSTIC TESTS & INTERPRETATION
Wood lamp exam will not fluoresce unless complicated by another fungus, which is uncommon; *M. furfur* (yellow to white), Corynebacterium (red), or Microsporum (blue-green).

Lab
Initial lab tests
- Direct microscopic examination (potassium hydroxide)
- Culture (Sabouraud medium)

Pathological Findings
- Potassium hydroxide preparation: Septate and branched mycelia
- Culture: Dermatophyte

DIFFERENTIAL DIAGNOSIS
- Interdigital type: Erythrasma, impetigo, pitted keratolysis, candida intertrigo
- Moccasin type: Psoriasis vulgaris, eczematous dermatitis, pitted keratolysis
- Inflammatory/bullous type: Impetigo, allergic contact dermatitis, dyshidrotic eczema, bullous disease

TREATMENT

Treatment is generally with topical antifungal medications for up to 4 weeks (1)[A]:
- Acute treatment:
  - Aluminum acetate soak (Burow solution; Domeboro, 1 pack to 1 quart warm water)
  - Antifungal cream of choice b.i.d. after soaks
- Chronic treatment:
  - Antifungal creams twice daily, continuing for 3 days after the rash is resolved: Clotrimazole 1%, econazole 1%, ketoconazole 2%, nystatin 100,000 units/g, tolnaftate 1%, etc (1)[A].
  - May try systemic antifungal therapy; see below (consider if concomitant onychomycosis or after failed topical treatment)

MEDICATION

First Line

- Systemic antifungals (2)[A]:
  - Itraconazole (Sporanox) 200 mg p.o. b.i.d. for 14 days (cure rate >90%)
  - Terbinafine (Lamisil) 250 mg p.o. daily for 14 days
- If concomitant onychomycosis:
  - Itraconazole 200 mg p.o. b.i.d. for 1st week of month for 3 months. Monitoring liver function testing is recommended.
  - Terbinafine 250 mg p.o. daily for 12 weeks, or pulse dosing: 500 mg p.o. daily for 1st week of month for 3 months. Not recommended if creatinine clearance <50 mL/min.
- Pediatric dosing options:
  - Griseofulvin 10–15 mg/kg/d or divided
  - Terbinafine 10–20 kg: 62.5 mg/d:
    - 20–40 kg: 125 mg/d
    - >40 kg: 250 mg/d
  - Itraconazole 5 mg/kg/d
  - Fluconazole 6 mg/kg/d
- Contraindications: Itraconazole, pregnancy category C
- Precautions: All systemic antifungal drugs may have potential hepatotoxicity.
- Significant possible interactions: Itraconazole requires gastric acid for absorption; effectiveness is reduced with antacids, H_2 blockers, proton pump inhibitors, etc. Take with acidic beverage such as soda if on antacids.

Second Line

- Systemic antifungals:
  - Fluconazole 150 mg, 1 tablet every week for 1–4 weeks. (Noted in 1997 Sanford Guide: 70% cure; however, not an FDA-approved indication.)
  - Griseofulvin 250–500 mg of microsize b.i.d. daily for 21 days
- Contraindications: Griseofulvin:
  - Patients with porphyria, hepatocellular failure
  - Patients with history of hypersensitivity to griseofulvin
- Precautions: Griseofulvin:
  - Should be used only in severe cases
  - Periodic monitoring of organ-system functioning, including renal, hepatic, and hematopoietic
  - Possible photosensitivity reactions
  - Lupus erythematosus, lupuslike syndromes, or exacerbation of existing lupus erythematosus has been reported.

- Significant possible interactions: Griseofulvin:
  - Decreases activity of warfarin-type anticoagulants
  - Barbiturates usually depress griseofulvin activity.
  - May potentiate effect of alcohol, producing such effects as tachycardia and flush

ADDITIONAL TREATMENT

General Measures

- Soak with aluminum chloride 30% or aluminum subacetate for 20 minutes b.i.d.
- Careful removal of dead/thickened skin after soaking or bathing
- Chronic or extensive disease or nail involvement requires oral antifungal medication, systemic therapy.

Issues for Referral

If extensive or resistant disease, especially in immunocompromised host

Additional Therapies

- Treatment of secondary bacterial infections
- Treatment of eczematoid changes

 ## ONGOING CARE

FOLLOW-UP RECOMMENDATIONS

Avoid sweating feet.

Patient Monitoring

Evaluate for response, recognizing that infections may be chronic/recurrent.

DIET

No restrictions

PATIENT EDUCATION

See General Prevention

PROGNOSIS

- Control, but not complete cure
- Infections tend to be chronic with exacerbations (e.g., in hot weather).
- Personal hygiene and preventive measures such as open-toed sandals, careful drying, and frequent sock changes are essential

COMPLICATIONS

- Secondary bacterial infections (portal of entry for streptococcal infections, producing lymphangitis/cellulitis)
- Eczematoid changes

REFERENCES

1. Crawford F, et al. Athlete's foot and fungally infected toe nails. *Clin Evid*. 2000;4:939.
2. Bell-Syer SE, Hart R, Crawford F, et al. Oral treatments for fungal infections of the skin of the foot. *Cochrane Database Syst Rev*. 2002: CD003584.

ADDITIONAL READING

Gupta AK, Nolting S, de Prost Y, et al. The use of itraconazole to treat cutaneous fungal infections in children. *Dermatology*. 1999;199:248–52.

See Also (Topic, Algorithm, Electronic Media Element)

Dermatitis, Contact; Dyshidrosis

 ## CODES

ICD9

110.4 Dermatophytosis of foot

CLINICAL PEARLS

- Treatment is generally with topical antifungal medications for up to 4 weeks (1)[A].
- Often is recurrent/chronic in nature
- Careful drying between toes after showering or bathing helps prevent recurrences. (Blow drying feet with hair dryer may be more effective than drying with towel.)
- Socks should be changed frequently. Put on socks before underwear to prevent infection from spreading to groin (tinea cruris).
- Dusting and drying powders (containing antifungal agents) may prevent recurrences.

TINEA VERSICOLOR

Elisabeth L. Backer, MD

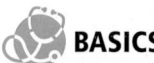 **BASICS**

DESCRIPTION
- Rash due to a common superficial mycosis with a variety of colors and changing shades of color; macules usually hypopigmented, light brown, or salmon-colored; fine scale often apparent
- System(s) affected: Skin/Exocrine
- Synonym(s): Pityriasis versicolor

EPIDEMIOLOGY
Incidence
- Common, especially in tropical climates
- Predominant age: Teenagers and young adults
- Predominant sex: Male = Female

Pediatric Considerations
Usually occurs after puberty (except in tropical areas); facial lesions are more common in children.

Geriatric Considerations
Not common in the geriatric population

RISK FACTORS
- Hot, humid weather
- Use of oils
- Hyperhydrosis
- HIV infection/immunosuppression (1)[C]
- High cortisol levels (Cushing, prolonged steroid administration)
- Pregnancy
- Malnutrition
- Oral contraceptives

Genetics
No known genetic pattern

GENERAL PREVENTION
- Recheck and treat again each spring prior to tanning season.
- Avoid skin oils.

PATHOPHYSIOLOGY
Inhibition of pigment synthesis in epidermal melanocytes, leading to hypomelanosis; in the hyperpigmented type, the melanosomes are large and heavily melanized.

ETIOLOGY
- Saprophytic yeast: *Pityrosporum orbiculare* (also known as *P. ovale*, *Malassezia furfur*, or *M. ovalis*), which is a known colonizer of all humans
- Variations in skin lipid formation

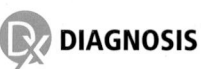 **DIAGNOSIS**

Common superficial skin infection caused by *Malassezia*

HISTORY
- Asymptomatic scaling macules on trunk
- Possible mild pruritus
- More prominent in summer
- Sun tanning accentuates lesions because infected areas do not tan.
- Periodic recurrences common

PHYSICAL EXAM
- *Versicolor* refers to the variety and changing shades of colors.
- Sun-exposed areas: Lesions usually white/hypopigmented
- Covered areas: Lesions often brown or salmon-colored
- Distribution (sebum-rich areas): Chest, shoulders, back (also face and intertriginous areas)
- Appearance: Small individual macules that frequently coalesce
- Scale: Fine, more visible with scraping

DIAGNOSTIC TESTS & INTERPRETATION
Wood's lamp: Golden fluorescence or pigment changes

Lab
Initial lab tests
- Direct microscopy of scales with 10% potassium hydroxide (KOH) preparation to visualize hyphae and spores ("spaghetti and meatballs" pattern)
- Routine lab tests usually not necessary
- Fungal culture not useful

Pathological Findings
- Short, stubby, or Y-shaped hyphae
- Small, round spores in clusters on hyphae

DIFFERENTIAL DIAGNOSIS
Other skin diseases with discolored macules and plaques, including:
- Pityriasis alba/rosea
- Vitiligo (presents without scaling)
- Seborrheic dermatitis
- Nummular eczema
- Secondary syphilis

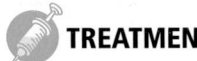 TREATMENT

MEDICATION

Topical antifungal therapy is the treatment of choice in limited disease.

First Line

- Ketoconazole 2% shampoo applied to damp skin and left on for 5 minutes × 1–3 days *OR*
- Selenium sulfide shampoo 2.5% (Selsun):
  - Allowed to dry for 10 minutes prior to showering: Daily × 1 week *OR*
  - Allowed to remain on body for 12–24 h prior to showering: Once a week × 4 weeks *OR*
- Clotrimazole topical (Lotrimin) b.i.d. × 2–4 weeks *OR*
- Miconazole (Micatin, Monistat) b.i.d. × 2–4 weeks *OR*
- Ketoconazole 2% (Nizoral) cream b.i.d. × 2–4 weeks *OR*
- Terbinafine (Lamisil) 1% solution b.i.d. × 1 week *OR*
- Terbinafine (Lamisil Derm Gel) once daily × 1 week
- Cure rates of topical antiyeast preparations typically 70–80%; healing continues after active treatment. Resumption of even pigmentation may take months.
- Contraindications: Ketoconazole is contraindicated in pregnancy.
- Newer preparations: 2.25% Selenium sulfide foam; ketoconazole gel

Second Line

- Use for extensive disease or nonresponders
- Oral ketoconazole (rarely needed and has significant adverse reactions) 400 mg in single dose or 200 mg/d for 1 week; cure rate >90%
- Itraconazole 200 mg/d p.o. × 1 week; cure rate >90% (2)[C]

ADDITIONAL TREATMENT

General Measures

- Apply prescribed topical medications to affected skin with cotton balls.
- Pigmentation may take months to fade or fill in.
- Repeat treatment each spring prior to sun exposure.

Issues for Referral

- If resistant to treatment
- If extensive disease occurs in immunocompromised host

 ONGOING CARE

- Ketoconazole shampoo can be used weekly for maintenance.
- Sulfur–salicylic acid (Sebulex) soap or shampoo can be used chronically for prophylaxis.

FOLLOW-UP RECOMMENDATIONS

Warn patients that whiteness will remain for several months after treatment.

Patient Monitoring

- Recheck and treat again each spring prior to tanning season.
- Failure to respond should prompt reassessment or dermatology referral.
- Resistance to treatment, frequent recurrences, or widespread disease may point to immunodeficiency.

PATIENT EDUCATION

For patient education materials favorably reviewed on this topic, contact American Academy of Dermatology, 930 N. Meacham Road., P.O. Box 4014, Schaumberg, IL 60168-4014; (708) 330-0230.

PROGNOSIS

- Duration of lesions months/years
- Recurs almost routinely, since this yeast is a known human colonizer

REFERENCES

1. Güleç AT, Demirbilek M, Seçkin D, et al. Superficial fungal infections in 102 renal transplant recipients: a case-control study. *J Am Acad Dermatol.* 2003;49:187–92.
2. Kose O, et al. Comparison of single 400 mg dose versus a 7 day 200 mg daily dose of itraconazole in the treatment of tinea versicolor. *J Derm Treat.* 2002;13:77.

ADDITIONAL READING

- Bhogal CS, Singal A, Baruah MC. Comparative efficacy of ketoconazole and fluconazole in the treatment of pityriasis versicolor: a one year follow-up study. *J Dermatol.* 2001;28:535–9.
- Faergemann J, Gupta AK, Al Mofadi A, et al. Efficacy of itraconazole in the prophylactic treatment of pityriasis (tinea) versicolor. *Arch Dermatol.* 2002;138:69–73.
- Morishita N, Sei Y. Microreview of Pityriasis versicolor and Malassezia species. *Mycopathologia.* 2006;162:373–6.

 CODES

ICD9

111.0 Pityriasis versicolor

CLINICAL PEARLS

- Macules of varying colors, with fine scale
- Recurrence in summer months
- More apparent after tanning because skin areas with fungal infection do not tan; thus, hypopigmented areas are visible.

T

TINNITUS

David M. Holmes, MD

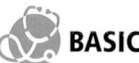 **BASICS**

DESCRIPTION
- Tinnitus is derived from the Latin word *tinnire* meaning "to ring." Tinnitus is the perception of sound in the absence of an acoustic stimulus; may be a buzz, ring, roar, chirp, whistle, or hiss nature.
- Subjective tinnitus: Heard only by patient
- Objective tinnitus: Heard through a stethoscope placed near the patient's ear
- Tinnitus >6 months is considered chronic.

EPIDEMIOLOGY
Incidence
- ~50 million people in the US
- ~ 12 million seek medical attention.
- Predominant age: 40–70 years (prevalence increases with age)
- Predominant sex: Males > Females; males traditionally have greater noise exposure in military, occupational, and recreational activities.
- 27% of males and 15% of females over a certain age experience tinnitus.

Prevalence
- ~16% of the US population
- Interferes with daily activities in 12 million people (~4%) in US
- 25% consider it to be a significant problem.
- 25–30% of US population >65 yrs have chronic tinnitus.
- Rare in children with normal hearing; occurs in 33–64% of children who have severe hearing loss
- Predominant age: 40–70-year-olds
- Predominant gender: Males (27% of males and 15% of females > 45 yrs)

RISK FACTORS
- Advanced age
- Pregnancy
- Excessive noise exposure
- Hearing loss
- Use of ototoxic medications
- Renal or hepatic impairment
- Caucasian
- Male gender

Genetics
Possible genetic predisposition, but a tinnitus gene has not yet been discovered. Genes have been identified for temporomandibular joint (TMJ) dysfunction, Ménière disease, and acoustic neuroma.

GENERAL PREVENTION
Avoid prolonged exposure to loud noises, wear hearing protection when loud noises can't be avoided (e.g., lawn mower, power tools, etc.), and avoid overuse of ototoxic medications.

PATHOPHYSIOLOGY
- Moderate sounds cause tiny movements of the stereocilia, which are attached to hair cells in the cochlea. This triggers neuronal transmission in CN VIII. Loud sounds (≥85 dB) cause the stereocilia to bend more than they should. Hair cells that respond to higher-frequency sounds are located at the base of the cochlea and are the 1st to be damaged. This causes high-pitched ringing. If loud noise exposure is excessive, then stereocilia cannot recover and permanent damage occurs. This results in hearing loss and possibly tinnitus.

- Other causes of hearing loss or damage to the auditory system also can cause tinnitus.
- Tinnitus has many similarities with the symptoms of central neuropathic pain and paresthesias, and may be related to these neurological disorders (1).

ETIOLOGY
- Subjective tinnitus (My AAAA NOISE PAIN):
  - *M*edications and heavy metals that cause or exacerbate tinnitus: Aspirin, aminoglycosides, benzodiazepines, calcium channel blockers, chloroquine, cisplatin, erythromycin, fluoroquinolones, lead, lidocaine, loop diuretics, mercury, methotrexate, nonsteroidal anti-inflammatory drugs, proton pump inhibitors, quinine, sertraline, tetracycline, tricyclic antidepressants, valproate, vancomycin
  - *M*énière disease (estimated 1% prevalence in the US) or other forms of endolymphatic hydrops (abnormally high inner ear pressure)
  - *A*coustic trauma (exposure to very loud noise)
  - *A*ging-related hearing loss (presbycusis)
  - *A*nemia
  - *A*rterial problems (hypertension, arteriosclerosis, cerebral aneurysm, cerebrovascular accident)
  - *N*oise-induced hearing loss
  - *O*tosclerosis and osteogenesis imperfecta
  - *I*nfections (otitis, meningitis, Lyme disease, neurosyphillis, rubella) or impaction (cerumen)
  - *S*clerosis (multiple sclerosis)
  - *E*ndocrine (diabetes mellitus, thyroid)
  - *P*sychogenic (depression, anxiety, psychosis)
  - *A*utoimmune disease of inner ear
  - *I*njury (head and neck) and idiopathic
  - *N*eoplasms (acoustic neuroma or cholesteatoma)
- Objective tinnitus (<1% of all cases of tinnitus; CAGED PETS):
  - Vascular abnormalities:
    - *C*arotid stenosis/CAD
    - *A*rteriovenous (A-V) shunt/fistula
    - *G*lomus jugulare
    - *E*xisting stapedial artery
    - *D*ehiscent jugular bulb or a vascular loop
  - Mechanical abnormalities:
    - *P*alatal myoclonus
    - *E*ustachian tube abnormally patent
    - *T*emporomandibular joint (TMJ) disorder
    - *S*tapedial muscle spasticity

COMMONLY ASSOCIATED CONDITIONS
- Hearing loss (~90% of chronic tinnitus is associated with sensorineural hearing loss) (2):
  - Causes of sensorineural hearing loss: Loud noise, presbycusis, ototoxic medications, Ménière disease, acoustic neuroma
  - Causes of conductive hearing loss: Cerumen, ear infection/effusion, trauma, tumor
- TMJ dysfunction
- Depression, anxiety, insomnia, fibromyalgia (40–60% of patients with tinnitus also have major depressive disorder)
- Psychological disorders can contribute to the distress of tinnitus. Some patients with severe tinnitus contemplate suicide.

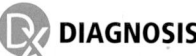 **DIAGNOSIS**

- Onset and duration: Gradual (presbycusis), sudden (recent loud noise exposure)
- Location: Unilateral (cerumen impaction, otitis media), unilateral plus hearing loss (acoustic neuroma, CVA)
- Pattern: Continuous (hearing loss), episodic (Ménière disease), pulsatile (vascular)
- Pitch: Low-pitch, rumbling (Ménière disease), high-pitched (sensorineural hearing loss)
- Severity: Use 1–10 scale (10 = most severe), Visual Analog Scale, Tinnitus Severity Index, or Tinnitus Handicap Inventory.
- Exacerbated by fatigue, stress, noise exposure, medications
- Alleviated by lying down with head in dependent position, medications, masking sounds
- Sudden hearing loss in one ear that progresses to the other ear (autoimmune)
- Vertigo (Ménière's disease)
- Facial muscle paralysis (cholesteatoma):
  - Hearing loss
  - Sudden hearing loss in one ear that progresses to the other ear (autoimmune)
  - Ear pain
  - Sinus congestion, allergies
  - Vertigo (Ménière disease)
  - Vestibular disturbances
  - Facial muscle paralysis (cholesteatoma)
  - High blood pressure
  - Symptoms of hyper- or hypothyroidism
  - Symptoms of hyperglycemia
  - Symptoms of depression or anxiety
  - Insomnia
  - Difficulty concentrating
  - Suicidal thoughts

HISTORY
- Noise exposure >85 dB (traffic = 85 dB)
- Upper respiratory infection, sinusitis, ear infection, allergic rhinitis
- Otalgia
- Otorrhea
- Head trauma
- Surgery
- Family history of hearing loss or tinnitus
- Hearing loss (type: congenital, sensorineural, conductive, or mixed)
- Medical history: Hypo/hyperthyroidism, HTN, DM, arteriosclerosis, autoimmune disorders
- Medications
- Exposure to heavy metals (lead or mercury)
- Psychosocial history: Employment, recreational activities, insomnia, anxiety, depression, obsessive–compulsive disorder, psychosis, fibromyalgia

PHYSICAL EXAM
- Otoscopy: Otitis externa/media, cerumen
- Auscultation close to ear for objective tinnitus
- Auscultation of neck (bruits, venous hum)
- Tinnitus of venous origin is suppressed by compression of ipsilateral jugular vein.
- Examine TMJ.
- Air and bone conduction testing with 512- or 1,024-Hz tuning fork (Weber and Rinne tests)

- Neurologic exam: Romberg test, Dix-Hallpike maneuver (if patient has vertigo), gait testing, cranial nerves
- Test hearing (audiology)

DIAGNOSTIC TESTS & INTERPRETATION
- Audiometry
- Tympanometry
- Auditory brain stem response (retrocochlear pathology such as acoustic neuroma)
- Electrocochleography (endolymphic hydrops)
- Electronystagmography (vestibular disorders)

Lab
- Complete blood count (CBC)
- Blood urea nitrogen (BUN)/creatinine
- Fasting glucose
- Fasting lipid profile
- Thyroid-stimulating hormone, free T_4
- Also consider HIV, RPR, autoimmune panel

Imaging
- A full clinical evaluation should precede radiologic studies (3).
- Gadolinium-enhanced MRI (if tinnitus is continuous)
- Contrast-enhanced CT scan or MRI (if tinnitus is pulsatile)
- Sonography, angiography, or MR angiography (to asses vascular abnormalities in the neck)
- SPECT may be more sensitive than CT scan, MRI, or MR angiography, and it identifies dynamic changes within the brain at the neurotransmitter level.
- PET scan (increased activity in the auditory cortex suggests that transcranial magnetic stimulation may effectively treat the tinnitus)

DIFFERENTIAL DIAGNOSIS
Auditory hallucinations

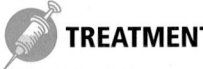 **TREATMENT**

MEDICATION
- TCAs such as amitriptyline (50 mg/d × 1 week, followed by 100 mg/d) (3)[A]
- Antiepileptics
- Baclofen
- Benzodiazepines
- Antihistamines
- Hyperbaric oxygen

First Line
Antidepressants: If patients are depressed/anxious or have severe tinnitus. No evidence one antidepressant works best. Research provides support for this treatment. Caution: Tinnitus is a side effect of antidepressant medications: SSRIs and TCAs such as amitriptyline (50 mg daily × 1 week, followed by 100 mg daily) (4)

Second Line
Antiepileptics, benzodiazepines, baclofen, antihistamines, hyperbaric oxygen

ADDITIONAL TREATMENT
General Measures
- Management depends on severity of tinnitus
- Treat the underlying cause.
- Discontinue ototoxic medications.
- Anxiety, insomnia, and depression may exacerbate tinnitus, which, in turn, may exacerbate the anxiety, insomnia, and/or depression. Treat to stop this vicious cycle (2)[B].
- Hearing aids/cochlear implants

- Hearing protection for noise exposure (2)[A]
- Compression of myofascial trigger points (5)[B]
- Use a combination of measures (2).

Issues for Referral
- Refer patients to a comprehensive tinnitus management program (audiologist) (2)[B].
- Otolaryngologist, neurologist, and/or neurosurgeon, depending on etiology

Additional Therapies
- Tinnitus retraining therapy and masking:
  – Counseling
  – Wearable low-level broadband noise generators; significant improvement in up to 80% of patients with high-pitched tinnitus. Masking devices have unknown effectiveness and may require 1–2 years of therapy.
- Acoustic therapy: Listening to relaxing sounds through head phones when the environment is too quiet (2)[B].
- Biofeedback and stress reduction: Relaxation technique may help to reduce the severity of the tinnitus.
- Neurofeedback: Many patients with tinnitus have abnormal oscillatory brain activity. Neurofeedback helps to normalize this and treat tinnitus (6)[B].
- Psychotherapy: May reduce severity (2)[B]
- Transcranial magnetic stimulation (TMS) and repetitive TMS (rTMS): A noninvasive method to stimulate neurons in the brain by rapidly changing magnetic fields. New and promising technique to reduce tinnitus; may also help treat migraine headaches, strokes, Parkinson's disease, dystonia, major depression, and auditory hallucinations (7)[B].

COMPLEMENTARY AND ALTERNATIVE MEDICINE
- Zinc (in 1 small study zinc 50 mg daily × 2 mo. decreased severity of subjective tinnitus)
- Botulinum toxin
- Acamprosate (a medication used to treat alcohol dependence
- Hypnosis (8)[B]
- Acupuncture (unknown effectiveness)
- Low-power laser to mastoid bone (unknown effectiveness)
- Gingko biloba, melatonin, lecithin (all are ineffective)

SURGERY/OTHER PROCEDURES
- Otosclerosis: Stapedectomy surgery with implantation of ossicular prosthesis (2)[C]
- Severe Ménière disease or other forms of endolymphatic hydrops that are not alleviated by medications: Installation of endolymphatic shunt, labyrinthectomy, or vestibular neurectomy (2)[C]
- Auditory neoplasms: Surgical resection or radiation (2)[C]
- Vascular pulsatile tinnitus due to atherosclerotic carotid artery disease: Carotid endarterectomy

IN-PATIENT CONSIDERATIONS
Admission Criteria
Hospitalization is rarely indicated.

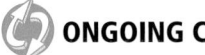 **ONGOING CARE**

FOLLOW-UP RECOMMENDATIONS
- Audiologist: For complete evaluation and therapy; specialists as indicated

- Family physician: In 1–2 months after therapy initiated and periodically thereafter

PATIENT EDUCATION
- Help patients to understand that tinnitus is a perception of sound and is not a threat to their physical health.
- Sources of information for patients:
  – American Tinnitus Association: (800) 634-8978; http://www.ata.org
  – National Institute on Deafness and Other Communication Disorders: (800) 241-1044; http://www.nidcd.nih.gov
  – American Academy of Otolaryngology: (703) 836-4444; http://www.entnet.org

PROGNOSIS
Most cases of chronic tinnitus cannot be cured (due to association with irreversible sensorineural hearing loss). Therefore, focus is on managing the tinnitus and reducing its severity, not curing it (2).

REFERENCES
1. Møller AR, et al. Tinnitus and pain. *Prog. Brain Res.* 2007;166:47–53.
2. Waddell A, Canter R, et al. Tinnitus. *Clin Evid.* 2003;598–607.
3. Crummer RW, et al. Diagnostic approach to tinnitus. *Am Fam Physician.* 2004;69:1:121–6.
4. Bayar N, Böke B, Turan E, et al. Efficacy of amitriptyline in the treatment of subjective tinnitus. *J Otolaryngol.* 2001;30:300–3.
5. Rocha CA, Sanchez TG, et al. Myofascial trigger points: another way of modulating tinnitus. *Prog. Brain Res.* 2007;166:209–14.
6. Dohrmann K, Weisz N, Schlee W, et al. Neurofeedback for treating tinnitus. *Prog. Brain Res.* 2007;166:473–85.
7. Meeus OM, De Ridder D, Van de Heyning PH, et al. Transcranial magnetic stimulation (TMS) in tinnitus patients. *B-ENT.* 2009;5:89–100.
8. Cope TE. Clinical hypnosis for the alleviation of tinnitus. *Int Tinnitus J.* 2008;14:135–8.
9. Westerlaken BO, de Kleine E, van der Laan B, et al. The treatment of idiopathic sudden sensorineural hearing loss using pulse therapy: a prospective, randomized, double-blind clinical trial. *Laryngoscope.* 2007;117:684–90.

 CODES

ICD9
388.30 Tinnitus, unspecified

CLINICAL PEARLS
- Tinnitus is rare in children with normal hearing but common in children with severe hearing loss.
- To keep tinnitus from getting worse, avoid loud noises, reduce stress, control blood pressure, get enough sleep, decrease alcohol and caffeine, and don't smoke.
- People have different levels of tolerance to tinnitus. It may affect sleep, concentration, and emotional state. About half of patients with chronic tinnitus also have major depressive disorder.
- New-onset tinnitus is often associated with hearing loss; steroid pulse or standard-dose therapy is indicated with idiopathic sudden sensorineural hearing loss (9)[A].

TOBACCO USE AND SMOKING CESSATION

S. Lindsey Clarke, MD

 BASICS

DESCRIPTION
- Tobacco use is the leading cause of preventable morbidity and mortality worldwide:
  - 440,000 deaths annually in US
  - 4.2 million premature deaths/year worldwide
  - Major risk factor for:
    - Atherosclerotic cardiovascular disease
    - Lung cancer
    - Chronic obstructive pulmonary disease (COPD)
- Nicotine is highly addictive.
- Smoking damages nearly every organ in the human body.
- 2nd-hand exposure to cigarette smoke is associated with a 20% greater risk of lung cancer and coronary heart disease.
- Quitting smoking has both immediate and long-term health benefits.

EPIDEMIOLOGY
Incidence
- 2.4 million new smokers annually in US (initiation rate = 2.7%) (2008 data)
- 59% of new smokers are <18 years of age (6% initiation rate for teens).

Prevalence
- 71 million Americans (28.4%) currently use tobacco (2008 data).
- Highest among those aged 20–29 years (41%); peak age of tobacco use is 22 years.
- Predominant race: Prevalence highest among American Indians/Alaskan Natives (48.7%) and lowest among Hispanics (21.3%) and Asians (13.9%)
- Predominant sex: Male (34.5%) > Female (22.5%)
- Inversely proportional to education level

RISK FACTORS
- Exposure to 2nd-hand smoke
- Presence of a smoker in the household
- Comorbid stress and psychiatric disorders
- Easy access to cigarettes
- Low self-esteem and self-worth
- Poor academic performance
- Perceived parental approval of smoking
- Smokeless tobacco use
- Boys: High levels of aggression and rebelliousness
- Girls: Preoccupation with weight and body image

GENERAL PREVENTION
- Most 1st-time tobacco use occurs before high school graduation, so educational interventions should target students in grade school and middle school, and must address both the health consequences and the psychosocial aspects of smoking.
- The American Academy of Family Physicians' Tar Wars program has targeted 4th and 5th graders successfully.
- Other helpful measures include:
  - Smoking bans in public areas and workplaces
  - Restriction of minors' access to tobacco
  - Restrictions on tobacco advertisements
  - Raising prices through taxation
  - Media literacy education
  - Tobacco-free sports initiatives

PATHOPHYSIOLOGY
- Addiction due to nicotine's rapid stimulation of the brain's dopamine system (teenage brain especially susceptible)
- Atherosclerotic risk due to adrenergic stimulation, endothelial damage, carbon monoxide, and adverse effects on lipids
- Direct airway damage from cigarette tar
- Carcinogens in all tobacco products

COMMONLY ASSOCIATED CONDITIONS
- Coronary artery disease
- Cerebrovascular disease
- Peripheral vascular disease
- Abdominal aortic aneurysm
- COPD
- Cancer of the lip, oral cavity, pharynx, larynx, lung, esophagus, stomach, pancreas, kidney, bladder, cervix, and blood
- Pneumonia
- Osteoporosis
- Periodontitis
- Alcohol use
- Depression and anxiety
- Reduced fertility

Pregnancy Considerations
- 16.4% of pregnant women smoke.
- Women who smoke or who are exposed to 2nd-hand smoke during pregnancy have increased risks of miscarriage, placenta previa, placental abruption, premature rupture of membranes, preterm delivery, low-birth-weight infants, and stillbirth.

Pediatric Considerations
- 2nd-hand smoke increases the risk of the following in infants and children:
  - Sudden infant death syndrome
  - Acute upper and lower respiratory tract infections
  - More frequent and more severe exacerbations of asthma
  - Otitis media and need for tympanostomies
- Nicotine passes through breast milk, and its effects on the growth and development of nursing infants are unknown.

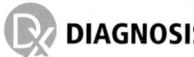 **DIAGNOSIS**

HISTORY
- Screen for tobacco use and 2nd-hand smoke exposure at every physician encounter.
- Type and quantity of tobacco used
- Pack years = packs/day × years
- Awareness of health risks
- Interest in quitting
- Triggers for smoking
- Prior attempts to quit: Method, duration of success, reason for relapse

PHYSICAL EXAM
- General: Tobacco smoke odor
- Skin: Premature wrinkling of the face
- Mouth: Nicotine-stained teeth; inspect for suspicious mucosal lesions
- Lungs: Crackles, wheezing, increased or decreased volume
- Vessels: Carotid or abdominal bruits, abdominal aortic enlargement, peripheral pulses, stigmata of peripheral vascular disease

DIAGNOSTIC TESTS & INTERPRETATION
Imaging
- Chest x-ray for patients with pulmonary symptoms or signs of cancer but not for screening
- US Preventative Services Task Force recommends 1-time screening ultrasound for abdominal aortic aneurysm in men ≥65 years who ever have smoked (number needed to screen to prevent 1 AAA = 500) (1)[B].

Diagnostic Procedures/Surgery
Pulmonary function testing for smokers with chronic pulmonary symptoms such as wheezing and dyspnea

 TREATMENT

Identify and address triggers by recommending alternative agents (e.g., gum, hard candy, cough lozenges, etc.).

MEDICATION
First Line
- Varenicline (Chantix): 0.5 mg/d p.o. × 3 days, then 0.5 mg b.i.d. × 4 days, then 1 mg b.i.d. (2,3)[A]:
  - Start 1 week prior to smoking cessation, and continue for 12–24 weeks.
  - Superior to placebo and to bupropion; number needed to treat = 7
  - Side effects: Insomnia, headache, nausea, depression, suicidal ideation; safety not established in patients with psychiatric illness; not well studied in adolescents; pregnancy Category C
- Bupropion (Zyban): 150 mg p.o. × 3 days, then 150 mg b.i.d. (4)[A]:
  - Start 1 week prior to smoking cessation, and continue for 7–12 weeks.
  - Twice as effective as placebo
  - Side effects: Tachycardia, headache, nausea, insomnia, dry mouth; drug of choice for depressed patients; contraindicated in patients who have seizure disorders or bipolar affective disorder; pregnancy Category C

Second Line

- Nortriptyline: 25–75 mg/d p.o. or in divided doses (4)[A]:
  - Start 10–14 days prior to smoking cessation, and continue for at least 12 weeks.
  - Efficacy similar to bupropion, but side effects more common; pregnancy Category D
- Nicotine replacement therapy (e.g., patch, gum, lozenge, inhaler, nasal spray) (5)[A]:
  - Improves quit rates by 50–70% compared with placebo
  - Various forms have equivalent efficacy.
  - Over the counter (OTC)
  - Patch (NicoDerm CQ, others): 21, 14, and 7 mg:
    - One patch q24h
    - Start with 21 mg if smoking ≥10 cigarettes/d; otherwise, start with 14 mg.
    - 6 weeks on initial dose, then taper
    - 2 weeks each on subsequent doses
    - No proven benefit beyond 8 weeks
  - Gum (Nicorette): 2 and 4 mg:
    - Use 4 mg if smoking ≥25 cigarettes/d.
    - Chew 1 piece q1–2h × 6 weeks, then 1 q2–4h × 3 weeks, then 1 q4–8h × 3 weeks.
  - May use in combination with bupropion, but monitor for hypertension
  - Side effects: Headache, pharyngitis, cough, rhinitis, dyspepsia; all mainly with inhaler and spray forms
  - Pregnancy Category D, but probably safer than continued smoking during pregnancy

ADDITIONAL TREATMENT
General Measures
- The 5 As of smoking cessation:
  - Ask about tobacco use at every office visit.
  - Advise all smokers to quit.
  - Assess the patient's willingness to quit.
  - Assist the patient in his or her attempt to quit.
  - Arrange follow-up.
- It might help for patients to have a quitting partner, such as a spouse, friend, or coworker, to provide mutual encouragement.
- Patients desiring to quit should dispose of all smoking paraphernalia (such as lighters) on their quit dates to make relapse more difficult.
- Patients should try to anticipate situations that they associate with smoking and should have a plan for dealing with their urge to smoke.

Additional Therapies
The following interventions have been shown to be effective in helping patients quit smoking:
- Brief physician advice at every visit:
  - "The best thing you can do for your health right now is to stop smoking."
- Advice from nurses, especially in hospital
- Individual counseling and group therapy
- Telephone counseling (see Patient Education)
- Web-based cessation programs
- Exercise (limited data)
- "Electronic cigarettes" are type of nicotine delivery system; controversial; Food and Drug Administration may ban their import

COMPLEMENTARY AND ALTERNATIVE MEDICINE
Acupuncture and hypnosis have not been proven to enhance long-term smoking cessation.

ONGOING CARE
FOLLOW-UP RECOMMENDATIONS
- Follow up soon after scheduled quit date and regularly thereafter.
- Refraining from tobacco products for the 1st 2 weeks is critical to long-term abstinence.

Patient Monitoring
- Short-term withdrawal symptoms include irritability, anxiety, insomnia, and poor concentration.
- Longer-term risks of smoking cessation include weight gain (4–5 kg on average) and depression.
- Quitting also is associated with exacerbations of ulcerative colitis and worsening of cognitive function in patients with schizophrenia.

DIET
Healthy eating is important for limiting weight gain following smoking cessation.

PATIENT EDUCATION
- 1-800-QUIT-NOW: Free counseling, resources, and support for quitting
- http://www.smokefree.gov

PROGNOSIS
- Smoking cessation by age 40 is associated with significant preservation of life expectancy.
- Measurable cardiovascular benefits of smoking cessation begin as early as 24 h after quitting and continue to mount until the risk is reduced to that of nonsmokers by 5–15 years.
- People who quit smoking after a heart attack or cardiac surgery reduce their risk of death by at least 1/3.
- Relapse rates initially >60% but decrease to 2–4% per year after completing 2 years of abstinence.

COMPLICATIONS
- Disability and premature death due to heart attack, stroke, cancer, COPD
- Smoking more than doubles the risk of coronary artery disease and almost doubles the risk of stroke.
- Smokers are 12–22× more likely than nonsmokers to die from lung cancer.
- Smokers die an average of 14 years earlier than nonsmokers.

REFERENCES

1. U.S. Preventive Services Task Force. Screening for abdominal aortic aneurysm: recommendation statement. *Ann Intern Med.* 2005;142:198–202.
2. Cahill K, Stead LF, Lancaster T, et al. Nicotine receptor partial agonists for smoking cessation. *Cochrane Database Syst Rev.* 2008;CD006103.
3. Gonzales D, Rennard SI, Nides M, et al. Varenicline, an alpha4beta2 nicotinic acetylcholine receptor partial agonist, vs sustained-release bupropion and placebo for smoking cessation: a randomized controlled trial. *JAMA.* 2006;296:47–55.
4. Hughes JR, Stead LF, Lancaster T, et al. Antidepressants for smoking cessation. *Cochrane Database Syst Rev.* 2007;CD000031.
5. Stead LF, Perera R, Bullen C, et al. Nicotine replacement therapy for smoking cessation. *Cochrane Database Syst Rev.* 2008;CD000146.

ADDITIONAL READING
- Aveyard P, West R. Managing smoking cessation. *BMJ.* 2007;335:37–41.
- Department of Health and Human Services, Substance Abuse and Mental Health Services Administration, Office of Applied Studies. Results from the 2008 national survey on drug use and health. Retrieved 05/16/2010 at http://oas.samhsa. gov.
- Hays JT, Ebbert JO. Varenicline for tobacco dependence. *N Engl J Med.* 2008;359:2018–24.
- Rosen IM, Maurer DM. Reducing tobacco use in adolescents. *Am Fam Physician.* 2008;77:483–90.

See Also (Topic, Algorithm, Electronic Media Element)
Nicotine Addiction; Substance Use Disorders

CODES

ICD9
- 305.1 Nondependent tobacco use disorder
- V15.82 Personal history of tobacco use

CLINICAL PEARLS
- Tobacco use is a major cause of mortality and morbidity due to atherosclerotic cardiovascular disease, lung cancer, COPD, and other health problems.
- Varenicline (Chantix) is the single most effective prescription aid to smoking cessation. Other proven therapies include bupropion, nortriptyline, and OTC nicotine replacement systems.
- Brief physician advice and telephone counseling have been shown to be effective in helping patients to quit smoking. 1-800-QUIT-NOW is a free patient resource for counseling and support for quitting smoking.

T

TORTICOLLIS

Alyssa H. Tran, DO

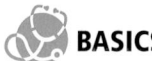 **BASICS**

DESCRIPTION
- Torticollis (L. *tortus*, "twisted" + *collum*, "neck") is spectrum of disorders characterized by head tilt and rotation or involuntary movement.
- Adult spectrum includes:
  - Spasmodic torticollis, also known as cervical dystonia: Painful, involuntary muscular contraction causing twisting and repetitive movements
  - Acute wryneck
- Childhood spectrum includes
  - Congenital muscular torticollis (CMT): 80% of all infants presenting with torticollis posture are found to have CMT. CMT is a musculoskeletal condition observed at birth or early infancy resulting from unilateral fibrosis and shortening of the sternocleidomastoid SCM) muscle.
  - 3 types of CMT:
    ○ SCM tumor (SMT), also known as fibromatosis colli: Most common
    ○ Muscular torticollis: Tightness without palpable mass
    ○ Postural torticollis: Clinical features of CMT without SMT or muscle tightness; no mass or tightness
  - Acquired torticollis of childhood
- Other forms (oculogyric, gastroesophageal reflux, arthritis-related, scoliosis-related, and hysterical torticollis) are not discussed here.
- Types: Rotational (twisting); anterocollis (flexion); laterocollis (side bending); retrocollis (extension)
- System(s) affected: Musculoskeletal; Nervous
- Synonym(s): Acute wryneck; Idiopathic generalized torticollis; SCM torticollis; Neonatal torticollis; Idiopathic cervical dystonia; Focal dystonia; Nuchal dystonia

EPIDEMIOLOGY
- Approximately 90% of cases occur in individuals between ages 31–60 years.
- Predominant age: CMT: Newborn and infants; acquired torticollis of childhood: <10 years; acute wryneck: 30–60 years; spasmodic torticollis: 30–50 years, with mean age of 40–43 years (1)
- Predominant sex: Spasmodic torticollis: Female > Male (1.6:1); Congenital muscular: Male > Female (3:2) (2).

Incidence
Congenital: Up to 1/250 births (2); spasmodic: 1/100,000, incidence for all 24/1 million persons

Prevalence
All focal dystonias combined: 295/1 million persons; no reliable data for acute wryneck and childhood-acquired torticollis

RISK FACTORS
- CMT: Intrauterine crowding, breech position, ischemia, or injury during birth
- Acute wryneck: Stress, unusual positioning, exposure to cold, medication reaction
- Acquired torticollis of childhood: Inflammation; neurologic; optical; rotatory force
- Spasmodic: Family history of dystonia, 10%; inflammation; neurologic; optical; rotatory force

Genetics
Some forms may have genetic basis, such as spasmodic torticollis (1).

ETIOLOGY
- CMT:
  - Intrauterine malpositioning may lead to trauma of SCM, resulting in fibrosis.
  - Birth trauma, such as clavicular fracture
  - SCM may appear normal at birth; then swelling and tightness develop.
- Acquired torticollis of childhood: Pain, spasm, decreased range of motion without trauma
- Acute wryneck:
  - Stress, postural factors (e.g., work, sleep, lying while reading or watching TV, prolonged unusual positioning of neck), or localized exposure to cold
  - Medication reaction (e.g., amphetamines, haloperidol, chlorpromazine, ketamine, etc.)
- Spasmodic torticollis:
  - Muscular damage from inflammatory disease
  - Cervical spine injuries
  - Ocular disorder
  - Organic central nervous system disorder
  - Psychogenic
  - Tumor
  - Cervical spondylosis
  - Vestibular dysfunction

Pediatric Considerations
Congenital: Associated with birth injury that, without treatment, becomes a fibrous cord and may be associated with craniofacial deformities

Pregnancy Considerations
Breech birth; also, with difficult delivery in those with congenital cases

COMMONLY ASSOCIATED CONDITIONS
- Over 80% of infants with CMT also present with craniofacial asymmetry, deformational plagiocephaly of varying degree, and developmental hip dysplasia.
- Congenital: Consider Klippel-Feil syndrome.
- Acquired torticollis in childhood: Consider Klippel-Feil syndrome.
- Spinal abnormalities
- Spasmodic: Consider psychiatric disorder.

⟲ DIAGNOSIS

HISTORY
- Abnormal head posture; neck pain; headache; stiffness of neck muscles; restricted ROM of neck; neck mass or swelling
- Birth history
- Family history
- Medication history
- Trauma

PHYSICAL EXAM
- Head tilts to affected side (80%, to right side); chin rotates to opposite side.
- Intermittent painful spasms of trapezius, SCM, and other neck muscles
- Tenderness over affected SCM
- Neck mass, lymphadenopathy

- Craniofacial asymmetry (plagiocephaly) indicates congenital or chronic torticollis
- ROM-normal: Flexion 45°; extension 55°; rotation 70°; sidebending 40°
- Phasic jerking or tremor of antagonist muscles
- Sensory tricks (*geste antagoniste*) such as touching face reduce severity in most patients (pathognomonic for spasmodic torticollis) (1,3)
- Ocular irregularities
- Spinal abnormality (short neck with low posterior hairline may indicate occipitocervical synostosis)
- Structural abnormalities of feet
- Congenital: At birth may be firm, nontender, palpable enlargement of SCM (2)
- Acquired in childhood: Unilateral neck stiffness, pain, or decreased ROM
- Acute wryneck: Unilateral neck stiffness, pain, or decreased ROM
- Spasmodic: Initial neck stiffness progressing to pain, head jerking, and neck spasms (1)

DIAGNOSTIC TESTS & INTERPRETATION
Lab
Lab studies are not helpful and depend on the underlying disorder.
Follow-Up & Special Considerations
All pediatric patients should have a complete eye exam.

Imaging
Initial approach
- Radiographs to rule out spinal pathology
- Consider CT scan or MRI of C-spine for acquired cases or neurologic deficits.
- CMT can be confirmed with ultrasonography of the involved SCM muscle.

Diagnostic Procedures/Surgery
For acquired torticollis of childhood, administer low-dose levodopa (100–300 mg) with carbidopa. Response indicates that torticollis is secondary to dopa-responsive dystonia.

DIFFERENTIAL DIAGNOSIS
- Osseous:
  - Atlantoaxial rotatory subluxation
  - Atlanto-occipital subluxation
  - Posttraumatic fracture or dislocation
  - Cervical disk disorder
  - Congenital scoliosis
  - Klippel-Feil syndrome (congenital fusion of cervical vertebrae)
  - Occipitocervical synostosis
  - Grisel syndrome (subluxation of C1 on C2, associated with head or neck infection)
  - Syringomyelia
  - Arnold-Chiari malformation
- Nonosseous:
  - Myositis involving cervical muscles
  - Soft-tissue trauma
  - Neoplastic: Spinal cord tumor, acoustic neuroma, osteoblastoma, orbital tumor, fibromatosis, metastasis
  - Infection: Upper respiratory infection, cervical lymph node abscess, epidural abscess, retropharyngeal abscess, vertebral osteomyelitis
  - Vestibular disorders
  - Essential head tremor
  - Basal ganglia disease

– Cranial nerve palsy
– Psychiatric disorders
– Drug- or toxin-induced
– Down syndrome
– Sandifer syndrome (association of gastroesophageal disease with spastic torticollis and dystonic body movements)
– Myasthenia gravis

 **TREATMENT**

MEDICATION

- Congenital muscular: Botulinum toxin type A is effective in case series (2),(4)[C].
- Analgesics for temporary relief of pain (NSAIDs, acetaminophen, opiates)
- Anticholinergics may relieve acute muscle spasm (1)[C]. High doses are usually necessary, and benefit is often delayed by several weeks.
- Diphendydramine or diazepam can be used for torticollis caused by medication (1)[C].
- Diphendydramine:
  - Adult: 25–50 mg PO q6–8h PRN, not to exceed 400 mg/d; 10–50 mg IV/IM q6–8h PRN, not to exceed 400 mg/d
  - Pediatric: 12.5–25 mg PO t.i.d./q.i.d. or 5 mg/kg/d or 150 mg/m^2/d divided t.i.d./q.i.d. PRN, not to exceed 300 mg/d; 5 mg/kg/d IV/IM or 150 mg/m^2/d, divided q.i.d. PRN, not to exceed 300 mg/d
- Diazepam: For muscle relaxation:
  - Adult: 2–10 mg PO b.i.d./q.i.d.
  - Pediatric: 1–2.5 mg PO t.i.d./q.i.d.; increase gradually as needed or tolerated.
- Single injection cycle of botulinum toxin type A is effective and safe for treating adults (≥16 years of age) with cervical dystonia (1)[B].
- Botulinum toxin: Type A and B injections may be more effective than anticholinergic drugs for cervical dystonia (1)[B].
- Botox: Botulinum toxin type A
  - Adult: Initial 1.25–2.5 units (0.05–0.1 mL) IM into most active neck muscles; repeat every 3–4 months; not to exceed 200 units cumulative dose in 1-month period
  - Pediatric (<12 years of age): Not established; >12 years: Administer as for adults.
- Myobloc: Botulinum toxin type B
  - Adult: 2,500–5,000 units IM divided among affected muscles in patients treated previously with any type of botulinum toxin; use lower dose in untreated patients.
  - Pediatric: Not established
- Focal dystonia of unknown cause: Trial of carbidopa-levodopa (1)[C]; although some non-dopa-responsive-dystonia patients improve, equal numbers have had symptoms worsen.

ADDITIONAL TREATMENT
General Measures
- Congenital:
  - >90% of children achieve good outcome with conservative treatment when therapy is initiated in 1st 12 months of life.
  - Conservative treatment for CMT includes positioning, environmental adaptations, passive and active stretching of the tight SCM muscle, strengthening of weak neck and trunk muscles, and movement therapy.
  - Physical therapy and aggressive stretching started before ages 3–6 months (2)[B]

- Place television/toys on opposite side of bed from rotational deformity.
- Acquired in children: Place television on opposite side of bed from rotational deformity.
- Acute wryneck:
  - Conservative management includes soft cervical collar, intermittent heat or ice, and/or bed rest.
  - Analgesics for temporary relief and to break pain/spasm cycle
  - Benztropine may relieve acute muscle spasm.
- Spasmodic:
  - Conservative: Soft cervical collar, intermittent heat or ice, and/or bed rest
  - Botulinum toxin type A or B is effective and safe for treating adults with cervical dystonia. Results are transient, with treatment usually needed every 3–5 months (4)[C].
  - Selective peripheral nerve denervation is a safe procedure with infrequent and minimal side effects that is indicated exclusively for cervical dystonia.
  - Pallidal deep brain stimulation is a good alternative for cervical dystonia after medication or botulinum toxin has failed to provide adequate improvement.

Issues for Referral
- Refer prolonged symptoms of idiopathic spasmodic torticollis to a neurologist.
- Emergent consultation is necessary for life-threatening diagnoses, including retropharyngeal abscess, epiglottitis, spinal epidural abscesses, severe cervical fractures, or dislocations.
- Fixed deformities in children may require surgical referral.
- CMT: Referrals if (5): Visual dysfunction is observed (ophthalmology); hip screen is failed (orthopedics); neurological screen is failed; patient demonstrates plagiocephaly Type I through V (plastic surgery); patient presents with bony end feel (orthopedics).

Additional Therapies
- Osteopathic manipulative therapy may be used.
  - Direct myofascial stretching of cervical region with attention to the SCM
  - Occipital-atlantal release
  - V-spread of the occipitomastoid suture on the side of restriction
  - Muscle energy and/or functional positional release at the cervical region
- Physical therapy for acquired childhood and adult torticollis may be beneficial.
- If detected early, 90% of CMT responds to stretching exercises.

COMPLEMENTARY AND ALTERNATIVE MEDICINE
Acupuncture treatment, if started within 24 hours of onset, may provide benefit.

SURGERY/OTHER PROCEDURES
Congenital: Surgical release if physical therapy is unsuccessful by 1 year of age.

 ONGOING CARE

FOLLOW-UP RECOMMENDATIONS
- Infants with CMT should be monitored at 2- to 4-week intervals
- Screen for depression since this is a common complication in this disease spectrum.

PROGNOSIS
- Congenital: Good for correctable pathology:
  - 50–70% resolve spontaneously by 1st year
  - Over 90% of children achieve good to excellent outcome with conservative treatment when therapy is instituted during the first 12 months of life
- Childhood acquired: Good when underlying pathology is discovered
- Acute wryneck: Resolves in a few days to weeks
- Spasmodic: May wax and wane for years

COMPLICATIONS
- Facial asymmetry in congenital cases
- Developmental hip dysplasia in congenital
- Movement disorders
- Postural disorders
- Dental malocclusion
- Prolonged torticollis may develop degenerative osteoarthritis of the C-spine, hypertrophy of the sternocleidomastoid muscle, and paresthesia due to compressed nerve roots.

REFERENCES
1. Tarsy D, Simon DK. Dystonia. *N Engl J Med*. 2006;355:818–29.
2. Do TT. Congenital muscular torticollis: current concepts and review of treatment. *Curr Opin Pediatr*. 2006;18:26–9.
3. Consky EA, et al. Clinical assessments of patients with cervical dystonia. In: Jancovic J, et al, eds. *Therapy with botulinum toxin*. New York: Marcel Dekker; 1994:211–37.
4. Benecke R, Dressler D. Botulinum toxin treatment of axial and cervical dystonia. *Disabil Rehabil*. 2007;29:1769–77.
5. Cincinnati Children's Hospital Medical Center. *Evidence-based care guideline for therapy management of congenital muscular torticollis in children age 0 to 36 months*. Cincinnati (OH): Cincinnati Children's Hospital Medical Center; 2009 Mar 17. 12 p.

CODES

ICD9
- 333.83 Spasmodic torticollis
- 723.5 Torticollis not otherwise specified
- 781.93 Ocular torticollis

CLINICAL PEARLS
- In patient with head tilt, chin lift, and restricted movement of the neck, suspect torticollis.
- Most adult-onset torticollis is self-limiting and resolves within days to weeks.
- Physical therapy, manual treatment, and acupuncture may be helpful adjuncts.
- In congenital and acquired pediatric cases, rearranging the child's environment by placing items of interest (e.g., TV, toys, etc.) on the opposite side of bed is beneficial.

TOURETTE SYNDROME

Evan R. Horton, PharmD
Kimberly A. Pesaturo, PharmD
Jill A. Grimes, MD

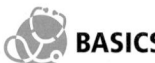 **BASICS**

DESCRIPTION
- A childhood-onset neurobehavioral disorder characterized by the presence of multiple motor and at least one phonic tic (see Physical Exam section):
  - Tics are sudden, brief, repetitive, stereotyped motor movements (motor tics) or sounds (phonic tics) produced by moving air through the nose, mouth, or throat.
  - Tics tend to occur in bouts.
  - Tics can be simple or complex; motor tics precede vocal tics, and simple tics precede complex tics.
  - Tics often are preceded by sensory symptoms, especially a compulsion to move; patients are able to suppress their tics, but voluntary suppression is associated with an inner tension that results in more forceful tics when suppression ceases.
- System(s) affected: Nervous

EPIDEMIOLOGY
Incidence
- Predominant age:
  - Average age of onset: 7 years (3–8 years)
  - Tic severity is greatest at ages 7–12 years, with 96% presenting by age 11.
  - 50% of children with Tourette syndrome (TS) will experience complete resolution of symptoms by age 18 (based on self-reporting) (1).
- Predominant sex: Male > Female (3:1).
- Predominant race/ethnicity: Clinically heterogeneous disorder, but non-Hispanic whites 2:1 compared with Hispanics and/or blacks

Prevalence
Estimated at 3:1,000 in children ages 6–17 years

RISK FACTORS
- Morbid risk for TS among relatives ranges between 9.8% and 15%.
- 1st-degree relatives of individuals with TS have a 10- to 100-fold increased risk of developing TS compared with the general population.

Genetics
- Predisposition, frequent familial history of tic disorders and obsessive-compulsive disorder (OCD)
- Precise pattern of transmission and identification of genes are unknown. Recent studies suggest polygenic inheritance with evidence for a locus on chromosome 17q; sequence variants in *SLITRK1* gene on chromosome 13q also are associated with TS (1).
- Higher concordance in monozygotic compared with dizygotic twins; wide range of phenotypes

PATHOPHYSIOLOGY
Research suggests that abnormalities of dopamine neurotransmission and receptor hypersensitivity, most likely in the ventral striatum, play a primary role in the pathophysiology.

ETIOLOGY
- Abnormality of basal ganglia development
- Mechanism uncertain; may involve dysfunction of basal ganglia–thalamocortical circuits, likely involving decreased inhibitory output from the basal ganglia, which results in an imbalance of inhibition and excitation in the motor cortex
- Controversial pediatric autoimmune neuropsychiatric disorder association with *Streptococcus* (PANDAS) (2):
  - TS/OCD cases linked to immunologic response to previous group A β-hemolytic streptococcal infection (GABHS)
  - Thought to be linked to 10% of all TS cases
  - 5 criteria:
    - Presence of tic disorder and/or OCD
    - Prepubertal onset of neuropsychosis
    - History of sudden onset of symptoms and/or episodic course, with abrupt symptom exacerbation interspersed with periods of partial or complete remission
    - Evidence of a temporal association between onset or exacerbation of symptoms and a prior streptococcal infection
    - Adventitious movements during symptom exacerbation (e.g., motor hyperactivity)

COMMONLY ASSOCIATED CONDITIONS
- Attention-deficit hyperactivity disorder (ADHD) and OCD are most common.
- Depression and anxiety are also concerns owing to disruptive behavior problems that can lead to social difficulties and learning disorders.
- Impairments of visual perception, sleep disorders, restless leg syndrome, and migraine headaches are higher than in the general population.

 DIAGNOSIS

HISTORY
Diagnosis of TS is based on history and clinical presentation (i.e., observation of tics with or without presence of coexisting disorders).

PHYSICAL EXAM
- Typically, the physical exam is normal.
- Motor and vocal tics are the clinical hallmarks.
- Tics fluctuate in type, frequency, and anatomic distribution over time.
- Multiple motor tics include facial grimacing, blinking, head or neck jerking, tongue protruding, sniffing, and touching.
- Vocal tics include grunts, snorts, throat clearing, barking, yelling, and hiccupping.
- Tics are exacerbated by anticipation, emotional upset, anxiety, or fatigue.
- Tics subside when patient is concentrating or absorbed in activities.
- Motor and vocal tics may persist during all stages of sleep, especially light sleep.

- Blink-reflex abnormalities may be observed.
- No clinical measures are known to reliably predict children who will continue to express tics in adulthood; severity of tics in late childhood is associated with future tic severity.
- *Diagnostic and Statistical Manual* (DSM) criteria:
  - Both multiple motor and ≥1 vocal tics have been present at some time during the illness, although not necessarily concurrently.
  - Tics occur many times a day (usually in bouts) nearly every day or intermittently throughout a period of >1 year, with no tic-free period of >3 consecutive months.
  - Onset occurs before age 18 years.
  - Tics are not due to the direct physiologic effects of a substance (e.g., stimulants) or a general medical condition (e.g., Huntington disease or postviral encephalitis).
- The World Health Organization and Tourette Syndrome Classification Group also have classification systems.

DIAGNOSTIC TESTS & INTERPRETATION
Lab
Initial lab tests
- No definitive lab tests diagnose TS.
- Thyroid-stimulating hormone (TSH) should be measured because of association of tics with hyperthyroidism.

Imaging
Initial approach
- No imaging studies diagnose TS.
- Electroencephalogram shows nonspecific abnormalities; useful only to differentiate tics from epilepsy.

Pathological Findings
- Smaller caudate volumes in TS patients
- Striatal dopaminergic terminals are increased, as is striatal dopamine transporter (DAT) density.

DIFFERENTIAL DIAGNOSIS
- Chronic motor or vocal tic disorder
- Transient tic disorder
- Tic disorder not otherwise specified
- Huntington disease
- Stroke
- Lesch-Nyhan syndrome
- Wilson disease
- Sydenham chorea
- Multiple sclerosis
- Postviral encephalitis
- Head injury
- Dystonia
- Myoclonus
- Drug effects (e.g., dopamine agonists)

TREATMENT

MEDICATION

First Line

α_2-Adrenergic receptor agonists:

- Clonidine 0.1–0.3 mg/d divided 2–4×/d (3)[A]: Side effects: Sedation and hypotension; need to initiate therapy gradually and taper when discontinuing to avoid cardiac adverse events
- Guanfacine 1–3 mg/d divided 1–2×/d (4)[A]: Less sedating and has a longer duration of action than clonidine; need to initiate therapy gradually and taper when discontinuing to avoid cardiac adverse events

- Atypical antipsychotics:
  – Risperidone 1–2 mg b.i.d. (5)[A]: Side effects include weight gain, sedation, and to a lesser extent, EPS
  – Risperidone 1–2 mg b.i.d. (5)[A]: Side effects include weight gain, sedation, and to a lesser extent, EPS

Second Line

- Dopamine receptor antagonists:
  – Typical antipsychotics (6)[A]:
    o Haloperidol: 0.5–5 mg at bedtime; EPS symptoms limit use; 1 of only 3 drugs found to be efficacious in multiple placebo-controlled trials (pimozide and risperidone)
    o Pimozide: 1–8 mg at bedtime; prolonged QT interval limits use; must be given under electrocardiogram (ECG) monitoring; long-term use may induce sedation, weight gain, depression, pseudoparkinsonism, and akathisia; found to work better in long-term control of tics versus acute exacerbations.
- Anticonvulsants: Topiramate: 100 mg/d (7)[B]
- Atypical antipsychotics:
  – Aripiprazole: 2.5–7.5 mg/d
  – Olanzapine: 2.5 mg b.i.d.
- Benzodiazepines: Clonazepam: 0.5–1 mg t.i.d. (3)[B]:
  – Only benzodiazepine commonly used to treat tics
  – Side effects include sedation, weight gain, irritability, oppositional behavior, mood changes, and cognitive impairment.
  – May induce Tourette-like disorder in exceptional cases
- Miscellaneous medications:
  – Metoclopramide: 5–40 mg/d (8)[A]
  – Baclofen: 10–20 mg t.i.d. (8)[A]
  – Botulinum toxin injections
  – Selegiline: 5–10 mg/d: May be used for severe dystonic tics
- Treatment of ADHD in patients with tics:
  – Stimulants:
    o Methylphenidate: 2.5–30 mg/d (9)[A]
    o Dextroamphetamine: 5–30 mg/d; comorbid tic disorder is not a serious contraindication, as previously held; exacerbation of tics is neither clinically significant nor common (6)[A].
  – α_2-Adrenergic agonists:
    o Guanfacine
    o Clonidine
  – Selective serotonin reuptake inhibitors (SSRIs): Atomoxetine

- Treatment of OCD in patients with tics:
  – SSRIs:
    o 1st-line treatment of OCD
    o Comorbid tic disorder not a contraindication; exacerbation of tics neither clinically significant nor common
    o Some risk of suicidality noted with SSRIs and other antidepressants.
  – Tricyclic antidepressants: Clomipramine: 25–200 mg/d; can be used in refractory SSRI patients or to augment SSRIs in partial responders; side effects: weight gain, dry mouth, lowered seizure threshold, and constipation; ECG changes, including QTc interval prolongation and tachycardia

ADDITIONAL TREATMENT

General Measures

- Neurologic and psychiatric evaluation for primary disorder and comorbidities (especially ADHD, OCD, and depression)
- Educate patient, family, teachers, and friends to identify and address psychosocial stressors and environmental triggers.
- Many patients require no treatment; patient should play active role in treatment decisions.
- No cure for tics: Treatment is purely symptomatic, and multimodal treatment usually is indicated.
- TS clusters with several comorbidities; each disorder must be evaluated for associated functional impairment because patients often are more disabled by their psychiatric conditions than by the tics; choice of initial treatment depends largely on worst symptoms (tics, obsessions, or impulsivity).
- Monotherapy is preferred to polytherapy.

COMPLEMENTARY AND ALTERNATIVE MEDICINE

Nonpharmacologic therapy:

- Reassurance and environmental modification
- Identification and treatment of triggers
- Behavioral therapy: Awareness or assertiveness training, relaxation therapy, habit-reversal therapy, and self-monitoring
- Hypnotherapy
- Biofeedback
- Acupuncture

SURGERY/OTHER PROCEDURES

Thalamic ablation and deep brain stimulation have been used experimentally (10)[A].

IN-PATIENT CONSIDERATIONS

Nursing

Habit-reversal training provides a viable tic suppression treatment: Works equally for motor and vocal tics

ONGOING CARE

FOLLOW-UP RECOMMENDATIONS

Patient Monitoring

Observe for associated psychiatric disorders.

PROGNOSIS

Based on self-reporting, in 1/2–2/3 of children with TS, severity of tics attenuates during adolescence, often remitting completely by early adulthood. However, OCD symptoms tend to increase.

REFERENCES

1. Kenney C, Kuo SH, Jimenez-Shahed J. Tourette's syndrome. Am Fam Physician. 2008;77:651–8.
2. Lombroso PJ, Scahill L. Tourette syndrome and obsessive-compulsive disorder. Brain Dev. 2008;30:231–7.
3. Jiménez-Jiménez FJ, García-Ruiz PJ. Pharmacological options for the treatment of Tourette's disorder. Drugs. 2001;61:2207–20.
4. Gilbert D. Treatment of children and adolescents with tics and Tourette syndrome. J Child Neurol. 2006;21:690–700.
5. Scahill L, Leckman JF, Schultz RT, et al. A placebo-controlled trial of risperidone in Tourette syndrome. Neurology. 2003;60:1130–5.
6. Scahill L, Erenberg G, Berlin CM, et al. Contemporary assessment and pharmacotherapy of Tourette syndrome. NeuroRx. 2006;3:192–206.
7. Jankovic J, Jimenez-Shahed J, Brown LW, et al. A randomised, double-blind, placebo-controlled study of topiramate in the treatment of Tourette syndrome. J. Neurol. Neurosurg. Psychiatr. 2010;81:70–3.
8. Nicolson R, Craven-Thuss B, Smith J, et al. A randomized, double-blind, placebo-controlled trial of metoclopramide for the treatment of Tourette's disorder. J Am Acad Child Adolesc Psychiatry. 2005;44:640–6.
9. Bloch MH, Panza KE, Landeros-Weisenberger A, et al. Meta-Analysis: Treatment of Attention-Deficit Hyperactivity Disorder in Children With Comorbid Tic Disorders. J Am Acad Child Adolesc Psychiatry. 2009.
10. Mink JW. Clinical review of DBS for tourette syndrome. Front Biosci (Elite Ed). 2009;1:72–76.

ADDITIONAL READING

- Porta M, Sassi M, Cavallazzi M, et al. Tourette's Syndrome and Role of Tetrabenazine: Review and Personal Experience. Clin Drug Investig. 2008;28:443–59.
- Seo WS, Sung HM, Sea HS, et al. Aripiprazole treatment of children and adolescents with Tourette disorder or chronic tic disorder. J Child Adolesc Psychopharmacol. 2008;18:197–205.

CODES

ICD9
307.23 Tourette disorder

CLINICAL PEARLS

- TS is diagnosed by history and witnessing tics; have parent video patient's tics if not present on exam in your office.
- Half of children with TS will have resolution of their symptoms by age 18.

TOXOPLASMOSIS

Jonathan MacClements, MD

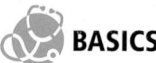 **BASICS**

- Obligate intracellular protozoan parasite *Toxoplasma gondii*
- Most common latent protozoan infection
- Usually dangerous only in pregnancy or in an immunocompromised patient

DESCRIPTION
- Acute self-limited infection if immunocompetent
- Acute symptomatic or reactivated latent infection in immunocompromised persons
- Congenital toxoplasmosis (acute primary infection during pregnancy)
- Ocular toxoplasmosis

Pediatric Considerations
- The earlier fetal infection occurs, the more severe the disease.
- Risk of perinatal death is 5% if infected 1st trimester.

Pregnancy Considerations
- Immunocompromised and HIV-infected women should undergo serologic testing in pregnancy (1)[C].
- Seronegative pregnant women should emphasize prevention.
- Serologic testing during pregnancy is controversial.

EPIDEMIOLOGY
Incidence
- Birth prevalence of congenital toxoplasmosis in US: 10–100/100,000 live births
- Predominant age: All ages
- Predominant sex: Male > Female

Prevalence
- In the US, 11% aged 6–49 years are seropositive.
- Age-adjusted prevalence in US is 22.5%.
- Seroprevalence among women in US is 15%.

RISK FACTORS
- Immunocompromised states including HIV infection with CD4 cell count <100/μL
- Primary infection during pregnancy; risk of transmitting infection to the fetus increases with gestational age at seroconversion, although transmission in the 1st trimester is associated with more severe consequences.
- Chronically infected pregnant women who are immunocompromised have an increased risk of congenital toxoplasmosis.

Genetics
Human leukocyte antigen (HLA) DQ3 is a genetic marker of susceptibility in AIDS.

GENERAL PREVENTION
Prevention is important in seronegative pregnant women and immunodeficient patients:
- Avoid eating undercooked meat. Meat should be cooked to 152°F (66°C) or frozen for 24 h at −12°C or lower.
- Avoid drinking unfiltered water. Wash fruits and vegetables.
- Strict hand hygiene after touching soil.
- Wear gloves while handling and wash hands after handling raw meat or cat litter.
- Avoid eating shellfish; it can be infected with *Toxoplasma* cysts.

PATHOPHYSIOLOGY
Transmission to humans:
- Ingestion of raw or undercooked meat, food, or water containing tissue cysts or oocytes; usually from soil contaminated with feline feces
- Transplacental to fetus from infected mother; risk of transmission is 30% on average
- Blood product transfusion and solid-organ transplantation

ETIOLOGY
T. gondii, an obligate intracellular sporozoan

COMMONLY ASSOCIATED CONDITIONS
Chorioretinitis, self-limiting febrile lymphadenopathy, mononucleosislike illness

 DIAGNOSIS

HISTORY
- Congenital toxoplasmosis:
  – Clinical presentation varies widely; 80% of patients are asymptomatic at birth.
  – Classic triad uncommon: Chorioretinitis, hydrocephalus, cerebral calcifications
  – Manifestations may include prematurity, intrauterine growth retardation (IUGR)
  – Anemia, thrombocytopenia, jaundice, rash
  – Mental retardation, seizures, visual defects, spasticity, sensorineural hearing loss
- Ocular toxoplasmosis:
  – Chorioretinitis: Focal necrotizing retinitis
  – Yellowish-white elevated cotton patch
  – Congenital disease usually bilateral; acquired, unilateral
  – Symptoms include blurred vision, scotoma, pain, and photophobia.
- Acute toxoplasmosis (immunocompetent host):
  – ~90% of patients are asymptomatic.
  – Most common manifestation is bilateral, symmetric, nontender cervical lymphadenopathy.
  – Constitutional symptoms such as fever, chills, and sweats are usually mild.
  – Headaches, myalgias, pharyngitis, hepatosplenomegaly, and diffuse nonpruritic maculopapular rash may occur.
  – Atypical lymphocytosis
  – Pregnant women are often asymptomatic. If symptomatic: Monolike illness with lymphadenopathy.
- Acute or reactivation in immunocompromised host:
  – Most common site is CNS with toxoplasmic encephalitis.
  – Headache; focal neurologic deficits and seizures
  – Fever usually present
  – Extracerebral toxoplasmosis: Pneumonitis, chorioretinitis, and rarely: GI system, liver, musculoskeletal system, heart, bone marrow, bladder, and orchitis

PHYSICAL EXAM
- In adults: Fever, lymphadenopathy, nonpruritic rash
- In newborns: Hydrocephalus, neurologic abnormalities, hepatosplenomegaly, chorioretinitis, microcephaly, anemia, thrombocytopenia, mental retardation

DIAGNOSTIC TESTS & INTERPRETATION
Lab
- Serology interpretation:
  – In acute infection, IgM antibodies appear within the 1st week.
  – Diagnosis can be made if initial test demonstrates positive IgM and negative IgG, with both tests becoming positive 2 weeks later.
  – If follow-up IgG remains negative 2–4 weeks later but IgM is still positive, it is likely a false-positive result.
  – Negative IgG rules out prior infection because it remains detectable for life.
- Types of serologic tests:
  – Enzyme-linked immunosorbent assay (ELISA): Standard test used by most labs
  – Sabin-Feldman dye test: Gold standard against which all other serologic assays are compared
  – IFA test: More readily available in commercial labs
  – ISAGA: Widely available commercially; more sensitive and specific than IFA for detecting IgM antibodies
  – Avidity testing: Confirmatory test to establish whether positive IgM/IgG reflects recent or chronic infection
- PCR: *T. gondii* DNA amplification in blood or amniotic fluid; used for diagnosis of fetal infection
- Culture: Organism can be isolated either by cell culture or by mouse inoculation; rarely performed but may be considered in neonates

Initial lab tests
- Diagnosis of primary infection is usually serologic.
- *Toxoplasma*-specific IgG and IgM are first determined from 1 serum sample.
- According to the result of IgM test, the avidity of IgG may be determined.
- Diagnosis of maternal infection and congenital toxoplasmosis:
  – Pregnant women who have mononucleosislike illness but negative heterophile test should be tested for toxoplasmosis.
  – Maternal infection accurately diagnosed when based on 2 blood samples at least 2 weeks apart showing seroconversion
  – High avidity of IgG during 1st trimester is a strong indicator against maternal primary infection.
  – Real-time PCR analysis for *T. gondii* on amniotic fluid provides an accurate tool to predict fetal infection and to decide on appropriate treatment and surveillance (2).
  – Fetal ultrasound (US) for prognostic information
  – Routine screening is not recommended.
- Diagnosis of congenital toxoplasmosis after birth:
  – May require several serum samples for IgM and IgA antibodies for serologic diagnosis
  – Sampling of the cord or peripheral blood should be done within the 1st 2 weeks because sensitivity declines thereafter.
  – Ophthalmologic, auditory, and neurologic examinations, as well as lumbar puncture and CT scan of the head, should be performed.
- Diagnosis of toxoplasmic encephalitis:
  – Serology for IgG
  – Imaging: MRI more sensitive than CT scan for identification of multiple ring-enhancing brain lesions

Imaging
- MRI: For identifying multiple ring-enhancing brain lesion in AIDS patients with cerebral toxoplasmosis
- SPECT and PET scans: Can be useful in distinguishing toxoplasmosis from CNS lymphoma

Diagnostic Procedures/Surgery
- Lymph node biopsy showing characteristic pathologic triad
- Brain biopsy in CNS disease
- Amniocentesis with PCR (risk of false-negatives and false-positives)
- Isolation of *Toxoplasma* from placenta is diagnostic.

Pathological Findings
- Confirmatory, meningocerebritis ± abscesses with necrosis, Giemsa
- Lymph node histology shows triad of:
  – Reactive follicular hyperplasia
  – Irregular clusters of epithelioid histicytes on and blurring margins of germinal centers
  – Distension of sinuses with monocytoid cells
- Sensitivity of triad 62.5%, specificity 91.3%

DIFFERENTIAL DIAGNOSIS
Syphilis, lymphoma, progressive multifocal leukoencephalopathy, cryptococcal meningitis, congenital TORCH infections, *Listeria* infection, tuberculosis (TB), erythroblastosis fetalis

 TREATMENT

MEDICATION
First Line
ALERT
- *Important to note:* All pyrimethamine-containing regimens should include leucovorin (folinic acid 10–25 mg/d p.o.) to prevent drug-induced hematologic toxicity.
- Treatment in immunocompromised hosts:
  – Initial drug regimen of choice is pyrimethamine 200-mg loading dose p.o., followed by 75 mg/d plus sulfadiazine 6–8 g/d p.o. in 4 divided doses; for those intolerant or allergic to sulfadiazine, clindamycin 600–1,200 mg IV or 450 mg p.o. 4×/day can be used instead.
  – Alternative regimens for patients intolerant to sulfadiazine and clindamycin include:
    ○ Pyrimethamine 200-mg loading dose p.o., followed by 75 mg/day plus azithromycin 1,200–1,500 mg p.o. once daily
    ○ Pyrimethamine 200-mg loading dose p.o., followed by 75 mg/day plus atovaquone 750 mg p.o. 4×/day
    ○ Sulfadiazine 1,500 mg 4×/day plus atovaquone 1,500 mg twice a day
    ○ Trimethoprim-sulfamethoxazole 10/50 mg/kg/day p.o. or IV divided twice daily (for 30 days) may be an effective alternative in resource-poor settings.
  – Duration of therapy: Typically 6 weeks, following which decrease to lower doses for secondary prophylaxis
  – Adjunctive steroids should be used in patients with signs of increased intracranial pressure.
  – Anticonvulsants if there is a history of seizures
- Prophylaxis in immunocompromised patients:
  – Primary prophylaxis: Indicated for patients with HIV infection and CD4 count <100 cells/μL who are *T. gondii* IgG–positive.

Trimethoprim-sulfamethoxazole-DS 1 tablet p.o. daily. Alternative for sulfa allergy is dapsone 50 mg p.o. daily plus pyrimethamine 50 mg p.o. weekly plus leucovorin 25 mg p.o. weekly or atovaquone 1,500 mg p.o. daily.
  – Secondary prophylaxis: Following 6 weeks of therapy, administer lower doses of drugs.
- Sulfadiazine 2–4 g/day in 2–4 divided doses plus pyrimethamine 25–50 mg/day is the 1st choice.
- Alternative regimens include clindamycin 600 mg p.o. q8h plus pyrimethamine 25–50 p.o. mg/day or atovaquone 750 mg p.o. 2–4×/day ± pyrimethamine 25 mg p.o. daily.
- Prenatal treatment in pregnant women diagnosed with toxoplasmosis: Lack of evidence on whether antenatal treatment reduces congenital transmission; however, prenatal treatment is usually offered.
- Pregnant women who become infected: Treat immediately with spiramycin 1 g p.o. q8h without food.
- Pyrimethamine and sulfadiazine should be considered only if fetal infection is documented.
- Different dosing regimens:
  – 3-week course of pyrimethamine 50 mg once per day p.o. or 25 mg twice per day plus sulfadiazine 3 g/day p.o. divided into 2–3 doses, alternating with 3-week course of spiramycin 1 g p.o. 3×/day until delivery
  – Pyrimethamine 25 mg once p.o. and sulfadiazine 4 g/day divided into 2–4 doses continuously until term
- Treatment of infected newborns: Treat irrespective of the presence or absence of clinical manifestations.
- Pyrimethamine (2 mg/kg/day × 2 days, then 1 mg/kg/day × 2–6 months, then 1 mg/kg on Monday, Wednesday, and Friday), sulfadiazine (100 mg/kg/day divided b.i.d.), and leucovorin (5–10 mg on Monday, Wednesday, and Friday)
- Treatment in immunocompetent nonpregnant patients: Generally do not require treatment unless symptoms are severe or prolonged; 1 of the following 2 regimens can be used:
  – Pyrimethamine 100-mg loading dose p.o., followed by 25–50 mg/day plus sulfadiazine 2–4 g/day in 4 divided doses
  – Pyrimethamine 100-mg loading dose p.o., followed by 25–50 mg/day plus clindamycin 300 mg p.o. 4× daily

Second Line
- Clindamycin: 900–1,200 mg t.i.d. IV used for ocular and CNS toxoplasmosis alone and in combination with pyrimethamine; as effective as the sulfadiazine-pyrimethamine but fewer adverse effects (3)[C]
- Corticosteroids (prednisone 1–2 mg/kg/day) are added for macular chorioretinitis or CNS infection.
- Alternatives: Atovaquone (Mepron), azithromycin (Zithromax), clarithromycin (Biaxin), or dapsone plus pyrimethamine and leucovorin
- Trimethoprim-sulfamethoxazole appears to be equivalent to pyrimethamine-sulfadiazine in AIDS patients with CNS disease.

ADDITIONAL TREATMENT
General Measures
Immunocompetent patients with *Toxoplasma* lymphadenopathy usually require no treatment.

 ONGOING CARE

FOLLOW-UP RECOMMENDATIONS
Patient Monitoring
- Precautions:
  – Monitor for bone marrow, renal, or liver toxicity.
  – Good hydration: Sulfadiazine is poorly soluble and may crystallize in the urine.
  – Watch for diarrhea on clindamycin.
- Sulfonamides may increase phenytoin, warfarin, or oral hypoglycemic agents.

PATIENT EDUCATION
- See Prevention.
- http://www.aafp.org/afp/20030515/2145ph.html
- http://familydoctor.org/online/famdocen/home/women/pregnancy/illness/180.html

PROGNOSIS
- Immunodeficient patients often relapse if treatment/suppression therapy is stopped.
- Treatment may prevent the development of untoward sequelae in all infants with congenital toxoplasmosis.

REFERENCES
1. Montoya JG, Liesenfeld O. Toxoplasmosis. *Lancet*. 2004;363:1965–76.
2. Wallon M, Franck J, Thulliez P, Huissoud C, Peyron F, Garcia-Meric P, Kieffer F, et al. Accuracy of real-time polymerase chain reaction for Toxoplasma gondii in amniotic fluid. *Obstet Gynecol*. 2010;115:727–33.
3. Benson CA, et al. Treating opportunistic infections among HIV infected adults and adolescents. *Clin Infect Dis*. 2005;40:S138–S140.
4. Gilbert R, Dezateux C. Newborn screening for congenital toxoplasmosis: feasible, but benefits are not established. *Arch Dis Child*. 2006;91:629–31.

 CODES

ICD9
- 130.0 Meningoencephalitis due to toxoplasmosis
- 130.1 Conjunctivitis due to toxoplasmosis
- 130.2 Chorioretinitis due to toxoplasmosis

CLINICAL PEARLS
- Newborn screening for congenital toxoplasmosis is feasible, but studies do not indicate clear benefits in children (4).
- Prevention is important, especially for seronegative pregnant women and immunodeficient patients.
- Immunologically normal patients may not need treatment.

T

TRACHEITIS, BACTERIAL

Mary Cataletto, MD

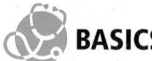

BASICS

DESCRIPTION
Acute, potentially life-threatening infraglottic bacterial infection following a primary viral infection, usually parainfluenzae or influenza viruses:
- Direct laryngoscopy reveals marked subglottic edema and thick mucopurulent secretions, sometimes causing pseudomembranes.
- System(s) affected: Pulmonary
- Synonym(s): Laryngotracheobronchitis; Pseudomembranous croup; Bacterial croup

EPIDEMIOLOGY
Incidence
- True incidence unknown
- 1st cases described prior to 1950; resurgence of cases has been noted since 1979
- Peak incidence in children: Fall and winter
- Predominant age: 6 months–8 years; mean age 4 years (similar to croup)
- Infections in adolescents and adults have been reported.
- Predominant sex: Male > Female (2:1)
- Accounts for 5–14% of upper airway obstruction in children requiring critical-care services

Prevalence
- Rare illness
- Most common potentially life-threatening upper airway infection in children
- Methicillin-resistant *S. aureus* (MSRA) may contribute to changing epidemiology and virulence.

RISK FACTORS
- Periods of increased seasonal activity of respiratory viruses
- Reports following adenoidectomy, with chronic tracheal aspiration, with evidence of other concurrent infections, including sinusitis, otitis, pneumonia, or pharyngitis

Genetics
No known genetic predisposition

GENERAL PREVENTION
Standard precautions with scrupulous attention to handwashing, especially when caring for tracheostomy patients

ETIOLOGY
- *Staphylococcus aureus* (most common pediatric cause): Consider MRSA.
- *Haemophilus influenzae* type b
- Nontypeable *H. influenzae*
- *Streptococcus pyogenes* group A
- *Streptococcus pneumoniae*
- *Moraxella catarrhalis* (associated with higher intubation rate; more frequent in younger children)
- *Peptostreptococcus sp.*
- *Klebsiella pneumoniae*
- *Neisseria gonorrhoeae*
- *Pseudomonas sp.*
- May be polymicrobial

COMMONLY ASSOCIATED CONDITIONS
- Consider anatomic abnormalities or foreign body as well as recent pharyngeal or laryngeal surgery.
- Predisposing: Down syndrome, immunodeficiency, subglottic hemangioma, tracheoesophageal fistula repair, tracheobronchomalacia
- May complicate measles

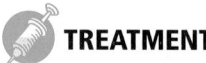

DIAGNOSIS

- May present with fever and systemic toxicity or as more localized disease
- Careful history and physical examination are the best method to distinguish bacterial tracheitis from croup and other rare causes of upper airway obstruction (1).

HISTORY
- Prodromal upper respiratory tract symptoms
- Gradual progression of mild upper airway symptoms over 1 h–6 days to acute, febrile phase of rapid respiratory decompensation
- No drooling
- No response to aerosolized epinephrine

PHYSICAL EXAM
- Fever >38°C
- Child usually lying flat
- May be toxic looking
- Variable degree of respiratory distress:
  - Tachypnea
  - Inspiratory stridor
- Voice and cry usually normal
- Barking "brassy" cough
- No drooling

DIAGNOSTIC TESTS & INTERPRETATION
- Routine laboratory studies are not required to make the diagnosis.
- Radiographs are neither definitive nor diagnostic.
- Endoscopy provides a definitive diagnosis.

Lab
Initial lab tests
- Bacterial cultures of tracheal secretions are required for culture isolates and sensitivities.
- Routine laboratory studies may not be helpful.
- CBC results may vary:
  - White blood cell (WBC) count may show marked leukocytosis or may be normal.
  - Band cells are often present.
- Blood cultures typically are negative.
- Rapid antigen testing

Imaging
- Radiographs may be normal, but they can be confused with those of foreign-body aspiration.
- May see pneumonic infiltrates
- Anteroposterior (AP) and lateral neck x-rays show subglottic and tracheal narrowing (i.e., steeple sign on AP film) with haziness and radiopaque linear or particulate densities (crusts).
- In patients with risk of acute respiratory obstruction, either do not obtain x-rays or monitor carefully.

Follow-Up & Special Considerations
Follow chest film if suspect pneumonia.

Diagnostic Procedures/Surgery
- Direct laryngoscopy and tracheoscopy is diagnostic and demonstrates:
  - Normal supraglottic structures
  - Marked subglottic erythema and edema
  - Ulcerations
  - Epithelial sloughing
  - Copious mucopurulent secretions ± plaques or pseudomembranes
- Obtain Gram stain and aerobic, anaerobic, and viral cultures of tracheal secretions during the procedure.

Pathological Findings
- Tracheal biopsy is rarely indicated, but may be considered in immunodeficient child or child with ulcerative colitis.
- Diffuse inflammation of larynx, trachea, and bronchi
- Mucopurulent exudate
- Semiadherent membranes (containing numerous neutrophils and cellular debris) may be identified within the trachea.

DIFFERENTIAL DIAGNOSIS
- Severe croup (viral)
- Spasmodic croup
- Diphtheria
- Retropharyngeal abscess
- Epiglottitis
- Pneumonia
- Asthma
- Foreign-body aspiration

TREATMENT

- Treat as potentially life-threatening airway emergency.
- Children with suspected or actual bacterial tracheitis should be cared for in a pediatric ICU.
- Assess and monitor respiratory status.
- Airway protection and support as necessary (at least 50% require intubation; some studies report up to 100%)
- Intermittent positive-pressure breathing (IPPB) may be required.
- Suctioning
- Different clinical course in previously healthy children compared with those with artificial airway

MEDICATION
- Empirical choices should provide broad-spectrum gram-positive and -negative coverage.
- Oxacillin or nafcillin 200 mg/kg/d divided q6h + 3rd-generation cephalosporin (ceftriaxone 50 mg/kg/d)
- Consider vancomycin in areas with increased prevalence of MRSA, when resistance is suspect or identified, or if multisystemic involvement.
- In the case of technology-dependent children with tracheostomy, make initial antibiotic choices based on previous tracheal culture.
- Narrow regimen when pathogens and sensitivities available

- Contraindications: Refer to the manufacturer's literature for each drug.
- Precautions: Refer to the manufacturer's literature for each drug. Avoid aminoglycosides in patients with previous hearing loss.
- Significant possible interactions: Refer to the manufacturer's literature for each drug.
- Airway obstruction is not relieved by nebulized epinephrine or corticosteroids.

ADDITIONAL TREATMENT
Issues for Referral
All children with suspect or actual bacterial tracheitis should be cared for in a pediatric ICU by a pediatric critical-care team that may include the following subspecialists: Pediatric intensivist, infectious disease specialist, pulmonologist, and/or otolaryngologist.

Additional Therapies
- At present there is a lack of evidence to establish the effect of heliox inhalation in the treatment of croup in children (2).
- For technology-dependent children with artificial airway:
  – Initial antibiotic choices should cover most recent tracheal aspirate isolates and then be refined according to culture and sensitivity results.
  – Adjunctive aerosol therapy may be helpful, particularly when multidrug-resistant organisms are present.

SURGERY/OTHER PROCEDURES
- Tracheostomy may be necessary.
- Therapeutic bronchoscopy may be necessary to facilitate removal of inspissated secretions.
- Tracheal membranes may require removal.

IN-PATIENT CONSIDERATIONS
- Aggressive supportive care and airway protection are paramount.
- Initial treatment of choice for bacterial tracheitis is broad-spectrum antibiotic coverage.
- Children with tracheitis and artificial airways present unique challenges: Tracheoscopy is important in establishing diagnosis in this population.
- Be vigilant for possible MRSA.

Initial Stabilization
Pediatric Considerations
- True pediatric emergency
- Admission to ICU
- Maintain airway: Often difficult due to copious secretions:
  – Endotracheal or nasotracheal intubation usually needed, especially in infants and children <4 years of age
  – Much less likely to need intubation if child >8 years of age
  – Advantage of intubation is ability to clear trachea and bronchi of secretions and pseudomembranes.
- Vigorous pulmonary toilet to clear airway of secretions
- Hydration, humidification, antibiotics

Admission Criteria
- Suspected or confirmed diagnosis of tracheitis
- Respiratory distress
- Artificial airway

Nursing
- Provide calm, quiet environment for child once endoscopy and cultures are done.
- Airway monitoring
- Suctioning as necessary
- Monitor fluid balance.
- Establish and maintain open lines of communication with child and parents.

Discharge Criteria
No longer in need of acute care

 ONGOING CARE

FOLLOW-UP RECOMMENDATIONS
Patient Monitoring
Children with artificial airways will require ongoing follow-up.

DIET
Varies with clinical situation

PATIENT EDUCATION
Keep immunizations up to date.

PROGNOSIS
- Intubation generally 3–11 days
- Usually requires 3–7 days of hospitalization
- With effective early recognition and management, complete recovery can be expected.
- Cardiopulmonary arrest and death have occurred.

COMPLICATIONS
- Pneumothorax
- Formation of pseudomembranes
- Toxic shock syndrome
- Pneumonia
- Airway obstruction
- Respiratory failure

REFERENCES
1. Bjornson CL, Johnson DW. Croup. *Lancet.* 2008;371:329–39.
2. Vorwerk C, Coats T, et al. Heliox for croup in children. *Cochrane Database Syst Rev.* 2010;2: CD006822.

ADDITIONAL READING
- Graf J, Stein F. Tracheitis in pediatric patients. *Semin Pediatr Infect Dis.* 2006;17:11–13.
- Hopkins A, Lahiri T, Salerno R, Heath B, Changing epidemiology of life threatening upper airway infections: the reemergence of bacterial tracheitis. *Pediators.* 2006;118:1418–21.
- Loftis L. Acute infectious upper airway obstructions in children. *Semin Pediatr Infect Dis.* 2006;17:5–10.
- Rotta AT, Wiryawan B. Respiratory emergencies in children. *Respir Care.* 2003;48:248–58; discussion 258–60.
- Salamone FN, Bobbitt DB, Myer CM, et al. Bacterial tracheitis reexamined: is there a less severe manifestation? *Otolaryngol Head Neck Surg.* 2004;131:871–6.
- Shah, S, Pediatric Respiratory Infections. *Emerg Med Clin N Am.* 25(2007): 961–79.
- Taussig LM, Landau LI, et al (ed). Bacterial Tracheitis. In: *Pediatric Respiratory Medicine*, Mosby Elsevier, Phil, PA: 2008:477–8.

See Also (Topic, Algorithm, Electronic Media Element)
Croup (Laryngotracheobronchitis); Epiglottitis

 CODES

ICD9
- 464.10 Acute tracheitis without mention of obstruction
- 464.11 Acute tracheitis with obstruction
- 464.20 Acute laryngotracheitis without mention of obstruction

CLINICAL PEARLS
- Bacterial tracheitis is an acute, potentially life-threatening, infraglottic bacterial infection following a primary viral infection that accounts for 5–14% of upper airway obstructions in children requiring critical-care services.
- Children with suspected or actual bacterial tracheitis should be cared for in a pediatric ICU.
- Endoscopy provides a definitive diagnosis.
- Initial treatment of choice for bacterial tracheitis is broad-spectrum antibiotic coverage, aggressive airway protection, and supportive care.

T

TRANSFUSION REACTION, HEMOLYTIC

Eric Ursprung, MD

 BASICS

DESCRIPTION
- Every year, >5 million people are transfused in the US alone (1).
- While providing obvious benefits, transfusion of blood products can result in a variety of serious complications, termed *transfusion reactions*.
- Hemolytic reactions are categorized by mechanism and consequence of the reaction (1):
  - Immune-mediated:
    - Intravascular hemolysis
    - Extravascular hemolysis
  - Nonimmune-mediated:
    - Contact with hyper-/hypotonic fluids
    - Temperature changes
    - Mechanical forces: For instance, mechanical heart valves

Pediatric Considerations
Reaction greater and outlook poorer in the very young

Geriatric Considerations
Higher risk of complications in the elderly

EPIDEMIOLOGY
- Frequency of immunologic reaction per unit of blood:
  - Allergic 1:100
  - Febrile 1:100
  - Delayed hemolytic 1:1,600
  - Acute hemolytic 1:50,000
  - Fatal hemolytic reaction 1:500,000
- Infectious complications per unit of blood:
  - Hepatitis B virus: 1:81,000
  - Human T-lymphotropic virus, Type 1: 1:642,000
  - Hepatitis C virus: 1:1,600,000
  - Human immunodeficiency virus, Type 1: 1:2,000,000

RISK FACTORS
- Patients with chronic requirements for blood transfusions:
  - Sickle-cell anemia
  - β-thalassemia major
- Patients requiring massive transfusion:
  - Trauma
  - Organ transplantation

Genetics
No known genetic pattern

GENERAL PREVENTION
- Reduce risks of clerical and administrative error:
  - At a minimum, 2 practitioners should verify that blood product and patient identity match (2)[C].
  - Obtain detailed history of patient's responses to previous blood product transfusion.
  - Use matched blood whenever possible.
  - If matched blood is not available, thoroughly check universal blood for agglutination titer.
  - Blood bank should consistently screen for bacteria and viruses.
- Reduce number of allogenic transfusions:
  - Carefully consider risk–benefit analysis of every transfusion.
  - Treatment with recombinant human erythropoietin may reduce transfusion requirement for patients with chronic kidney disease (3).
- Peritransfusion clinical practice:
  - Observe patient closely during transfusion with serial vital signs.
  - Avoid prophylactic antipyretics.
  - Use genotype-specific red blood cells (RBCs) in sickle-cell anemia.
  - Consider leukocyte-depleted blood in people with history of recurrent febrile reactions.
  - Case reports have indicated that prophylactic treatment with Rituximab may prevent delayed hemolytic transfusion reactions (4); however, higher-level evidence is lacking.

PATHOPHYSIOLOGY
- Acute hemolytic transfusion reactions (AHTRs) (5):
  - Patient has preformed IgM antibodies reactive to protein on surfaces of RBCs.
  - IgM fixes complement to surfaces of RBCs.
  - Complement cascade leads to rapid intravascular destruction of transfused cells.
- Delayed hemolytic transfusion reactions (DHTRs) (5):
  - Pathophysiology of DHTR is the subject of intense study.
  - Recent research implicates a similar pathway to IgG-mediated anaphylactic reaction.
  - FcγRs on the patient's macrophages react with IgG-coated transfused RBCs.
  - Resulting cascade of proinflammatory cytokines and platelet-activating factor

ETIOLOGY
- AHTR:
  - When ABO-incompatible blood is transfused, donor erythrocytes are destroyed by recipient's preformed antibodies, causing intravascular hemolysis.
  - Most commonly occurs when group O recipients receive nongroup O blood; IgM antibodies to group A and B antigens fix complement and cause rapid hemolysis.
  - Often owing to clerical error, misidentification of blood product or patient
- DHTRs can occur in patients sensitized to an antigen by prior transfusions or pregnancy. It may be difficult to detect because antibody titer falls after initial sensitization and reaction occurs 2–10 days after transfusion.

COMMONLY ASSOCIATED CONDITIONS
- Disseminated intravascular coagulation (DIC)
- Shock
- Acute renal failure

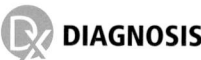 **DIAGNOSIS**

ALERT
- Symptoms are masked in the anesthetized patient; in this population, the 1st sign of hemolytic reaction may be red-tinged urine in the Foley.
- Shortness of breath, high fever, loss of consciousness, and hematuria are all signs of a more serious reaction.
- If the patient is short of breath after transfusion, there is a low threshold for obtaining at least a portable chest x-ray, as transfusion-related acute lung injury is an important consideration, especially in the critically ill patient.
- DHTR is an extravascular process; symptoms include:
  - Fever
  - Anemia (2–14 days after transfusion)
  - Jaundice

HISTORY
- Anxiety
- Pruritis
- Fever/chills

PHYSICAL EXAM
- Flushing
- Tachycardia
- Hypotension
- Chest, back, or flank pain
- Wine-colored urine indicating hemoglobinuria
- Urticaria
- Tachypnea
- Dyspnea

DIAGNOSTIC TESTS & INTERPRETATION
Lab
- If you suspect that your patient may have a hemolytic transfusion reaction, the following workup is indicated:
  - Direct antiglobulin (Coombs) test
  - Liver function tests, total and direct bilirubin
  - Lactate dehydrogenase (LDH)
  - Serum haptoglobin
  - Complete blood count
  - Chem7
  - Coagulation (prothrombin time/partial thromboplastin time/international normalized ratio)
- A hemolytic reaction is evidenced by:
  - Positive direct antiglobulin test (Coombs) in the case of autoimmune etiology
  - Plasma obtained 2–4 hours after lysis is red or pink, indicating free hemoglobin
  - Elevated serum bilirubin (may be mild)
  - Elevated LDH
  - Reduced serum haptoglobin

- Tissue factor released from lysed RBCs can initiate DIC; platelet count and coagulation studies should be monitored.
- Monitor blood urea nitrogen and creatinine, given risk of renal failure.

DIFFERENTIAL DIAGNOSIS

Other causes of acute hemolysis:
- Autoimmune diseases
- Hemoglobinopathies
- RBC enzyme defects
- Bacterial contamination of stored blood

TREATMENT

MEDICATION
- Oxygen and ventilation support, as needed
- Epinephrine for anaphylaxis
- Corticosteroids may be helpful to reduce inflammation.
- Normal saline and/or vasopressors to maintain systolic blood pressure (BP)
- Treat DIC if present, including supportive therapy and possibly heparin.
- Diphenhydramine for urticarial reaction

ADDITIONAL TREATMENT
General Measures
- Follow hospital protocol for evaluation of transfusion reactions.
- Stop transfusion immediately if suspicious for hemolytic transfusion reaction.
- IV normal saline to support BP and adequate urine output, especially in DIC
- Avoid lactated Ringer solution.
- Repeat thorough evaluation of transfusion paperwork to rule out any clerical error (a common cause of an ABO-incompatible transfusion).
- Monitor vital signs.
- Recognize and treat DIC if it occurs.
- Supportive therapy: Maintain BP using vasopressors in indicated airway.

ONGOING CARE

FOLLOW-UP RECOMMENDATIONS
Patient Monitoring
Until hemolytic signs are gone

DIET
As tolerated

PATIENT EDUCATION
Before starting a transfusion, give the patient instructions to report any unusual symptoms (e.g., rash, itching, or fever) to the nursing staff immediately.

PROGNOSIS
- Usual course: Acute
- Usually no harm if transfusion is stopped at onset of manifestations

COMPLICATIONS
- Uremia, oliguria, anuria
- Right-sided heart failure
- Respiratory failure
- Multiorgan dysfunction syndrome

REFERENCES

1. Sazama K, DeChristopher PJ, Dodd R, et al. Practice parameter for the recognition, management, and prevention of adverse consequences of blood transfusion. College of American Pathologists. *Arch Pathol Lab Med*. 2000;124:61–70.
2. Bryan S. Hemolytic transfusion reaction: safeguards for practice. *J Perianesth Nurs*. 2002;17:399–403.
3. Silver M, Corwin MJ, Bazan A, et al. Efficacy of recombinant human erythropoietin in critically ill patients admitted to a long-term acute care facility: a randomized, double-blind, placebo-controlled trial. *Crit Care Med*. 2006;34:2310–6.
4. Noizat-Pirenne F, Bachir D, Chadebech P, et al. Rituximab for prevention of delayed hemolytic transfusion reaction in sickle cell disease. *Haematologica*. 2007;92:e132–e135.
5. Hod EA, Sokol SA, Zimring JC, et al. Hypothesis: hemolytic transfusion reactions represent an alternative type of anaphylaxis. *Int J Clin Exp Pathol*. 2008;2:71–82.
6. Hébert PC, Yetisir E, Martin C, et al. Is a low transfusion threshold safe in critically ill patients with cardiovascular diseases? *Crit Care Med*. 2001;29:227–34.

ADDITIONAL READING

- Corwin HL, Gettinger A, Pearl RG, et al. The CRIT Study: Anemia and blood transfusion in the critically ill—current clinical practice in the United States. *Crit Care Med*. 2004;32:39–52.
- Davenport RD. Pathophysiology of hemolytic transfusion reactions. *Semin Hematol*. 2005;42: 165–8.
- Gaines AR, Lee-Stroka H, Byrne K, et al. Investigation of whether the acute hemolysis associated with Rh(D) immune globulin intravenous (human) administration for treatment of immune thrombocytopenic purpura is consistent with the acute hemolytic transfusion reaction model. *Transfusion*. 2009.

- Gilstad CW. Anaphylactic transfusion reactions. *Curr Opin Hematol*. 2003;10:419–23.
- Lacroix J, Hébert PC, Hutchison JS, et al. Transfusion strategies for patients in pediatric intensive care units. *N Engl J Med*. 2007;356:1609–19.

CODES

ICD9
- 999.60 ABO incompatibility reaction, unspecified
- 999.61 ABO incompatibility with hemolytic transfusion reaction not specified as acute or delayed
- 999.62 ABO incompatibility with acute hemolytic transfusion reaction

CLINICAL PEARLS

- Transfusion of packed RBCs depresses the immune response in patients undergoing renal transplantation.
- In an anesthetized patient, increased bleeding, oozing from catheter sites, and red-tinged urine are signs that indicate transfusion reaction.
- To reduce transfusion requirements in the critically ill ICU patient, institute restrictive transfusion policies, such as accepting hemoglobin values of 7–9 rather than >10, which will decrease transfusion rates by up to 50% (erythropoietin can maintain hemoglobin level by stimulating RBC production), and decrease the use of blood samples for nonessential tests (6).
- Posttransfusion purpura: Delayed thrombocytopenia (7–10 days after platelet transfusion) owing to production of antibodies to donor or recipient platelets more common in women. Treat with IV immunoglobulin or plasmapheresis. Avoid additional platelet transfusions, which may worsen thrombocytopenia.

T

TRANSIENT ISCHEMIC ATTACK (TIA)

Abir O. Kanaan, PharmD, RPh
Kristin A. Tuiskula, PharmD
George Abraham, MD, MPH

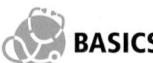

BASICS

DESCRIPTION
- Sudden onset of focal and transient (<24 h) neurologic deficit due to ischemia in a vascular distribution of the brain
- System(s) affected: Nervous
- Synonym(s): Ministroke

EPIDEMIOLOGY
Currently, there are 4.6 million stroke survivors in the US.

Incidence
- 68.2/100,000
- 1st-ever TIA incidence is 44.1/100,000.
- Predominant age: Risk increases >55 years of age; highest in 7th and 8th decades
- Predominant sex: Male > Female (3:1)
- Predominant race/ethnicity: African Americans > Caucasians

RISK FACTORS
- Hypertension (HTN)
- Cardiac disease
- Smoking
- Diabetes
- Antiphospholipid antibodies
- Family history
- Hypercholesterolemia
- Atrial fibrillation
- Homocystinemia

Genetics
Inheritance is polygenic, with tendency to clustering of risk factors within families.

GENERAL PREVENTION
- Lifestyle changes, including smoking cessation, diet modification, and increasing physical activity
- Strict control of medical risk factors (e.g., diabetes, HTN, hyperlipidemia, cardiac disease)
- Antiplatelet therapy
- Angiotensin-converting enzyme (ACE) inhibitors
- Statins
- Anticoagulation when high risk of cardioembolism (e.g., atrial fibrillation, mechanical valves)

PATHOPHYSIOLOGY
Reduction or cessation of cerebral blood flow adversely affecting neuronal function

ETIOLOGY
- Carotid or vertebral atherosclerotic disease:
  – Artery-to-artery thromboembolism
  – Low-flow ischemia
- Small, deep vessel disease associated with HTN: Lacunar infarcts
- Cardiac
- Cardioembolism secondary to valvular (mitral valve) pathology

- Mural hypokinesias or akinesias with thrombosis (acute anterior myocardial infarctions or congestive cardiomyopathies)
- Cardiac arrhythmia (atrial fibrillation)
- Hypercoagulable states:
  – Antiphospholipid antibodies
  – Deficiency of protein S, protein C
  – Presence of antithrombin III
  – Oral contraceptives
  – Pregnancy and parturition
- Arteritis:
  – Noninfectious necrotizing vasculitis
  – Drugs
  – Irradiation
- Sympathomimetic drugs (e.g., cocaine)
- Other causes: Spontaneous and posttraumatic (e.g., chiropractic manipulation) arterial dissection
- Fibromuscular dysplasia

ALERT
There is a ~5–20% risk of stoke within 5 days of 1st TIA. Close follow-up is essential if discharged.

Geriatric Considerations
- Atrial fibrillation is a frequent cause among the elderly.
- Highest incidence in 7th and 8th decades

Pediatric Considerations
- Cardiac (especially developmental abnormalities)
- Metabolic: Homocystinuria, Fabry disease
- Clotting disorders
- Marfan syndrome
- Moyamoya disease

COMMONLY ASSOCIATED CONDITIONS
- Atrial fibrillation
- Other cardiac disease
- Carotid stenosis

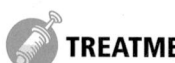

DIAGNOSIS

HISTORY
- Carotid circulation (hemispheric): Monocular visual loss, hemiplegia, hemianesthesia, neglect, aphasia, visual field defects (amaurosis fugax); less often, headaches, seizures, amnesia, confusion
- Vertebrobasilar (brain stem or cerebellar): Bilateral visual obscuration, diplopia, vertigo, ataxia, facial paresis, Horner syndrome, dysphagia, dysarthria; also headache, nausea, vomiting, and ataxia
- Obtain witness accounts with emphasis on symptom onset, progression, and recovery
- Past medical history, baseline functional status

PHYSICAL EXAM
- BP
- Thorough neurologic and cardiac exams

DIAGNOSTIC TESTS & INTERPRETATION
Lab
Initial lab tests
- International normalization ratio (INR) and partial thromboplastin time (PTT)
- Lipid panel
- Complete blood count (CBC)
- Glucose
- Erythrocyte sedimentation rate (ESR)
- Cardiac enzymes
- Consider drug screen.
- Electrolytes

Follow-Up & Special Considerations
- Duplex carotid ultrasonography
- ECG
- Angiography:
  – Cerebral
  – Carotid arterial stenosis
- Transthoracic echocardiography; if normal and cardiac source is suspected, follow with transesophageal ECHO.
- Holter monitoring: Suspected arrhythmia
- MR angiography: Brain and blood vessels
- EEG: Suspected seizure

Imaging
Initial approach
- CT scan of head, noncontrast: Acute phase
- Brain MRI, include diffusion-weighted imaging:
  – Magnetic resonance imaging with diffusion weighted imaging is the most sensitive and specific imaging modality in the detection of acute ischemia, and therefore, can help exclude mimics or confirm the diagnosis (1)[C].

DIFFERENTIAL DIAGNOSIS
- Migraine (hemiplegic)
- Focal seizure (Todd paralysis)
- Hypoglycemia
- Bell's palsy
- Evolving stroke
- Neoplasm of brain
- Subarachnoid hemorrhage
- Intoxication

TREATMENT

MEDICATION
- Enteric-coated aspirin: 50–325 mg/d p.o. (2)[A]
- Contraindications: Active peptic ulcer disease, hypersensitivity to aspirin or nonsteroidal anti-inflammatory drugs (NSAIDs)
- Precautions: May aggravate preexisting peptic ulcer disease; may worsen symptoms of asthma

- Significant possible interactions: May potentiate effects of anticoagulants and sulfonylurea analogues or
- Clopidogrel (Plavix): 75 mg/d p.o. (2)[A]:
  - Has fewer side effects than ticlopidine
  - Shows slight advantage over aspirin
  - Precautions: TTP can occur.
- Dipyridamole–aspirin (Aggrenox): 1 capsule p.o. b.i.d. (2,3)[A]:
  - Each capsule contains 200 mg of extended-release dipyridamole and 25 mg of immediate-release aspirin.
  - More efficacious than aspirin alone, but more costly
- Warfarin (INR-adjusted dose) (2,4)[A]: For patients with atrial fibrillation and cardioembolic stroke
- Contraindications: Intolerance or allergy, active liver disease, active bleeding, pregnancy, fall risk
- Significant possible interactions: Antibiotics, antiepileptics, antifungals, and many others
- Heparin: Dose and regimen vary based on goal; may be used primarily as bridge for long-term warfarin anticoagulation (5)[B].

Second Line
- Ticlopidine (Ticlid): 250 mg p.o. b.i.d. (2)[A]; fallen out of favor due to unfavorable side effect profile
- Contraindications: Known hypersensitivity to the drug, presence of hematopoietic or hemostatic disorders, conditions associated with active bleeding, severe liver dysfunction
- Precautions:
  - 2.4% of patients develop neutropenia (0.8% severe), which is reversible with cessation of the drug. Monitor blood counts every 2 weeks for 1st 3 months.
  - TTP can occur.
- Significant possible interactions: Digoxin plasma levels decreased 15%; theophylline half-life increased from 8.6–12.2 h.

ADDITIONAL TREATMENT
- Venous thromboembolism (VTE) prophylaxis may be provided using:
  - Mechanical devices
  - Heparin 5,000 units subcutaneously q8h or q12h
  - Enoxaparin 40 mg subcutaneously q24h
- Patients with TIA or ischemic stroke should be started on a statin (6)[A].

General Measures
- TIA is a neurologic emergency. Immediate medical attention should be sought within 24–48 h of symptom onset.
- Current evidence suggests that patients with high-risk TIAs require rapid referral and 24-h admission.
- Acute phase:
  - Inpatient for surgery and high-risk groups
  - Outpatient investigations may be considered based on patient's stroke risk, arrangement of follow-up, and social circumstances.
- Antithrombotic therapy for VTE prophylaxis
- Treatment or control of underlying associated conditions

Issues for Referral
- Neurology for ongoing workup and treatment
- Cardiology if cardiac cause suspected
- Vascular surgery if carotid endarterectomy appropriate

Additional Therapies
Secondary prevention of TIA should be initiated.

SURGERY/OTHER PROCEDURES
Carotid endarterectomy may be considered in patients with high levels of carotid artery stenosis (2)[A].

IN-PATIENT CONSIDERATIONS
Admission Criteria
- Ongoing symptoms
- Uncertain diagnosis

Discharge Criteria
- Consider safety at home if another incident occurs.
- History of TIAs with current appropriate treatment

 ONGOING CARE

FOLLOW-UP RECOMMENDATIONS
Patient Monitoring
- Follow up every 3 months for 1st year; then yearly
- ABCD^2 stroke risk score stratifies patients with TIA on 5 criteria (7)[A]:
  - Age $\geq$60 = 1
  - Systolic blood pressure (SBP) $\geq$140 mm Hg and/or diastolic blood pressure (DBP) $\geq$90 mm Hg = 1
  - Clinical: Unilateral weakness = 2 or speech impairment without weakness = 1
  - Duration $\geq$60 minutes = 2 or 10–59 minutes = 1
  - Diabetes: Present = 1
- Risk score with associated 2-day stroke risk (%):
  - Low risk <4 (1%)
  - Medium risk = 4 or 5 (4.1%)
  - High risk >5 (8.1%)
- Validated stroke risk score protocols may be beneficial in predicting future strokes and choosing most appropriate follow-up care (7)[A].

DIET
As appropriate for underlying medical problems

PATIENT EDUCATION
Education regarding condition, complications, and drug therapy should be provided.

PROGNOSIS
- The risk of stroke on the ipsilateral side within 90 days and cumulative thereafter is 5–20%.
- Frequency increases with addition of multiple risk factors and severity of carotid stenosis.
- The major cause of death in the 1st 5 years is cardiac disease.

COMPLICATIONS
- Stroke
- Functional impairment

REFERENCES
1. Wallis A, Saunders T, et al. Imaging transient ischaemic attack with diffusion weighted magnetic resonance imaging. *BMJ.* 2010;340:c2215.
2. Adams RJ, Albers G, Alberts MJ, et al. Update to the AHA/ASA recommendations for the prevention of stroke in patients with stroke and transient ischemic attack. *Stroke.* 2008;39:1647–52.
3. De Schryver EL, Algra A, van Gijn J. Dipyridamole for preventing stroke and other vascular events in patients with vascular disease. *Cochrane Database Syst Rev.* 2007;CD001820.
4. Aguilar MI, Hart R, Pearce LA. Oral anticoagulants versus antiplatelet therapy for preventing stroke in patients with non-valvular atrial fibrillation and no history of stroke or transient ischemic attacks. *Cochrane Database Syst Rev.* 2007;CD006186.
5. Albers GW, Amarenco P, Easton JD, et al. Antithrombotic and thrombolytic therapy for ischemic stroke: American College of Chest Physicians Evidence-Based Clinical Practice Guidelines (8th Edition). *Chest.* 2008;133: 630S–669S.
6. Manktelow BN, Potter JF. Interventions in the management of serum lipids for preventing stroke recurrence. *Cochrane Database Syst Rev.* 2009;CD002091.
7. Tsivgoulis G, Stamboulis E, Sharma VK, et al. Multicenter external validation of the ABCD2 score in triaging TIA patients. *Neurology.* 2010;74: 1351–7.

ADDITIONAL READING
Lovett JK, Dennis MS, Sandercock PA, et al. Very early risk of stroke after a first transient ischemic attack. *Stroke.* 2003;34:e138–40.

See Also (Topic, Algorithm, Electronic Media Element)
Algorithms: Stroke; Transient Ischemic Attack

 CODES

ICD9
435.9 Unspecified transient cerebral ischemia

CLINICAL PEARLS
- Primary prevention is important, stressing smoking cessation and control of HTN, hyperlipidemia, and diabetes.
- Antiplatelet therapy (e.g., aspirin, clopidogrel) should be initiated.
- Warfarin should be initiated in patients with atrial fibrillation based on risk factors.
- There is a 30% risk of stroke within 5 years of a TIA.

TRANSIENT STRESS CARDIOMYOPATHY

Timothy P. Fitzgibbons, MD

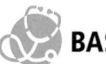 **BASICS**

DESCRIPTION
- Transient stress cardiomyopathy (TSC) is a unique cause of reversible left ventricular (LV) dysfunction with a clinical presentation indistinguishable from the acute coronary syndromes, particularly ST-segment elevation myocardial infarction (MI).
- Typically, the patient is a postmenopausal woman who presents with acute chest pain or dyspnea after an identifiable "trigger" (i.e., an acute emotional or physiologic stressor).
- 1st reported by authors from Japan (1,2), TSC was known initially as the *Takotsubo syndrome* because the typical LV morphology (i.e., apical ballooning) resembled that of a Japanese octopus trap, or *takotsubo*.
- Synonym(s) (3): Takotsubo cardiomyopathy; Apical ballooning syndrome; Stress cardiomyopathy; Broken heart syndrome; Ampulla cardiomyopathy
- Presenting clinical features include:
  – Chest symptoms and/or dyspnea
  – ECG changes, including ST-segment elevations or diffuse T-wave inversions
  – Mild elevation in cardiac biomarkers (creatine kinase [CK], troponin)
  – Transient wall motion abnormalities that may involve the base, midportion, and/or lateral walls of the LV
  – The apex of the RV may be affected in up to 25% of cases (4).
- Clinical features may vary on a case-by-case basis, and formal diagnostic criteria have not been established.
- Authors from the Mayo Clinic have proposed that 3 of the 4 following criteria establish the diagnosis (5):
  – Transient akinesis or dyskinesis of the LV apical and midventricular segments with regional wall motion abnormalities extending beyond a single epicardial vascular distribution
  – Absence of obstructive coronary artery disease (CAD) or angiographic evidence of acute plaque rupture
  – New ECG abnormalities, either ST-segment elevation or T-wave inversion
  – Absence of:
    ○ Recent significant head trauma
    ○ Intracranial bleeding
    ○ Pheochromocytoma
    ○ Obstructive epicardial CAD
    ○ Myocarditis
    ○ Hypertrophic cardiomyopathy

EPIDEMIOLOGY

Incidence
- TSC accounts for a small percentage of acute coronary syndromes (1–3%) (3).
- In a recent prospective evaluation of patients admitted to the ICU, as many as 28% of patients had apical ballooning, often in association with sepsis (3).
- Predominant sex: 82–100% of cases occur in women (5).
- Predominant age: Mean age of patients is 62–75 years.

Prevalence
2.2% of patients presenting to a referral hospital with ST-segment MIs were found to have TSC (5).

RISK FACTORS
- Female gender
- Postmenopausal state
- Emotional stress (i.e., argument, death of family member)
- Physiologic stress (i.e., acute medical illness)

Genetics
No genetic associations described to date

PATHOPHYSIOLOGY
- The exact pathophysiology is not known.
- It has been speculated that overwhelming activation of the sympathetic nervous system incites a cascade of events, including:
  – Catecholamine-induced LV dysfunction: Increased β-receptor density at the cardiac apex may explain apical sympathetic hypersensitivity.
  – Endothelial dysfunction: Prolonged TIMI frame counts in all 3 coronary vascular beds have been observed by some authors in the acute phase of this syndrome.
  – Multivessel epicardial spasm:
    ○ Diffuse multivessel spasm was reported in 15% of cases from Japan.
    ○ More recent studies have not supported this hypothesis.
  – Cellular metabolic injury:
    ○ Myocardial norepinephrine release
    ○ Calcium overload
    ○ Contraction band necrosis

COMMONLY ASSOCIATED CONDITIONS
Death in TSC is rare, and most cases resolve rapidly, within 2–3 days. Reported complications include:
- Left-sided heart failure
- Pulmonary edema
- Cardiogenic shock and hemodynamic compromise
- Dynamic LV outflow tract gradient complicated by hypotension
- Mitral regurgitation
- Ventricular arrhythmias
- LV thrombus formation
- LV free wall rupture
- Death (rare, 0–8%)

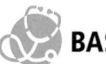 **DIAGNOSIS**

Since TSC is often indistinguishable from an acute coronary syndrome, it should be treated initially as such:
- Activate EMS or report to emergency department.
- Oxygen, IV access, and ECG monitoring
- Urgent cardiology consultation

HISTORY
- Exposure to a "trigger event":
  – Emotional stress: Argument, death of family member, divorce, public speaking, etc.
  – Physiologic stress: Acute medical condition such as head trauma, asthma attack, seizure, etc.
- Acute onset of dyspnea or chest pain
- Palpitations
- Syncope

PHYSICAL EXAM
Exam may be unremarkable or may include any of the following:
- Tachypnea
- Tachycardia
- Hypotension
- Jugular venous distension
- Bibasilar rales
- S_3 gallop
- Systolic ejection murmur due to dynamic LV outflow tract gradient
- Holosystolic murmur of mitral regurgitation

DIAGNOSTIC TESTS & INTERPRETATION
ECG should be done urgently and may show:
- Diffuse ST-segment elevations
- Diffuse and often dramatic T-wave inversions
- QTc interval prolongation
- Q waves

Lab
Laboratory tests typically reveal a mild elevation in cardiac biomarkers, such as:
- CK (rarely >500 u/mL)
- Troponin I
- B-type natriuretic peptide

Imaging
- Chest radiograph:
  – Cardiomegaly
  – Pulmonary edema
- Echocardiogram:
  – Reduced LV systolic function
  – Abnormal diastolic function, including evidence of increased filling pressures
  – Regional wall motion abnormalities in 1 of the following patterns:
    ○ Classic or "Takotsubo-type" ballooning of the apex with a hypercontractile base
    ○ "Reverse Takotsubo": Apical hypercontractility with basal akinesis
    ○ "Midventricular" akinesis with apical and basal hypercontractility
    ○ Focal or localized akinesis of an isolated segment
  – Dynamic intracavitary LV gradient
  – Mitral regurgitation
  – Variable involvement of the right ventricle

- Cardiac MRI:
  - Reduced LV function
  - Wall motion abnormalities as described for transthoracic echocardiography
  - Absence of delayed hyperenhancement with gadolinium

Diagnostic Procedures/Surgery
- Since ST-segment elevation MI is the diagnosis of exclusion, patients typically are referred for urgent cardiac catheterization.
- Coronary angiography:
  - Nonocclusive CAD
  - Rarely, epicardial coronary spasm
  - Endothelial dysfunction, as measured by fractional flow reserve or TIMI frame counts
- Left-sided heart catheterization: Increased LV end-diastolic pressure
- Ventriculography: Wall motion abnormalities as described for transthoracic echocardiography
- Right-sided heart catheterization:
  - Increased pulmonary capillary wedge pressure
  - Secondary pulmonary hypertension
  - Increased right ventricular filling pressures
  - Reduced cardiac output or cardiogenic shock (cardiac index <2.0 and mean arterial pressure [MAP] <60 mmHg)

Pathological Findings
Characteristic pathologic findings of involved myocardium have not been described.

DIFFERENTIAL DIAGNOSIS
- Acute ST-segment elevation MI
- Pulmonary embolism
- Myopericarditis
- Pheochromocytoma
- Hypertrophic cardiomyopathy
- Subarachnoid hemorrhage or stroke

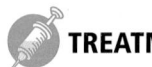

TREATMENT
- Activation of emergency medical services
- Advanced cardiac life support therapies as needed
- Oxygen
- IV access
- ECG monitoring

MEDICATION
After diagnostic cardiac catheterization, empirical treatment goals are:
- Management of hypotension: Differentiation between cardiogenic shock or dynamic LV cavity gradient
- Management of increased filling pressures and congestive states
- Attenuation of sympathetic drive

First Line
- Consideration should be given to β-blockers in all patients (e.g., metoprolol 12.5–75 mg p.o. b.i.d. or carvedilol 6.25–25 mg p.o. b.i.d.) if tissue perfusion is adequate.
- If there is evidence of congestive heart failure (CHF) or pulmonary edema, consider:
  - Furosemide 20–40 mg IV b.i.d. as needed to reduce LV filling pressures and dyspnea
  - Angiotensin-converting enzyme (ACE) inhibitors: Lisinopril 10–40 mg/d p.o. or equivalent

Second Line
Short-term anticoagulation should be considered in patients with severely reduced LV function to prevent LV thrombus formation. Unfractionated heparin 80 units/kg IV bolus followed by 18 units/kg/h IV or Lovenox 1 mg/kg SC b.i.d.

ADDITIONAL TREATMENT
Issues for Referral
All patients with TSC generally should be comanaged with cardiology while inpatient and referred to cardiology as an outpatient.

Additional Therapies
- Urgent cardiology consultation and consideration of cardiac catheterization
- Hypotension may require:
  - Vasopressors (e.g., dopamine or Levophed) if there is no LV outflow tract gradient
  - Phenylephrine and IV fluids to increase afterload in the presence of an LV outflow tract gradient
  - Cardiogenic shock that is not due to a LV outflow tract gradient may require placement of an intraaortic balloon pump.

IN-PATIENT CONSIDERATIONS
Initial Stabilization
- 12-lead ECG
- Chest radiograph
- Laboratory testing
- Echocardiography

Admission Criteria
Patients with TSC are usually admitted for observation because the differential diagnosis includes ACS.

IV Fluids
Normal saline infusion to support blood pressure if necessary and no evidence of heart failure

Discharge Criteria
Generally considered after exclusion of ACS and resolution of:
- Congestive state
- Hypotension
- Profound impairments of systolic function

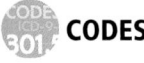

ONGOING CARE
FOLLOW-UP RECOMMENDATIONS
- Impairments in systolic function typically resolve in 2–3 days, but may last as long as 1 month.
- Patients should follow up with cardiology and serial echocardiography to document improved LV function.

PROGNOSIS
- Prognosis is excellent. Inpatient mortality is rare and ranges from 0–8%.
- Recurrence is rare, having also been reported in 0–8% of patients.

REFERENCES
1. Dote K, Sato H, Tateishi H, et al. [Myocardial stunning due to simultaneous multivessel coronary spasms: a review of 5 cases]. *J Cardiol*. 1991;21:203–14.
2. Tsuchihashi K, Ueshima K, Uchida T, et al. Transient left ventricular apical ballooning without coronary artery stenosis: a novel heart syndrome mimicking acute myocardial infarction. Angina Pectoris-Myocardial Infarction Investigations in Japan. *J Am Coll Cardiol*. 2001;38:11–8.
3. Aurigemma GP. Acute stress cardiomyopathy and reversible left ventricular dysfunction. *Cardiol Rounds*. 2006;10(10).
4. Fitzgibbons TP, Madias C, Seth A, et al. Prevalence and clinical characteristics of right ventricular dysfunction in transient stress cardiomyopathy. *Am. J. Cardiol*. 2009;104:133–6.
5. Bybee KA, Kara T, Prasad A, et al. Systematic review: transient left ventricular apical ballooning: a syndrome that mimics ST-segment elevation myocardial infarction. *Ann Intern Med*. 2004;141:858–65.

ADDITIONAL READING
- Bybee KA, Prasad A. Stress-related cardiomyopathy syndromes. *Circulation* 2008;118:397–409.
- Wittstein IS, Thiemann DR, Lima JA, et al. Neurohumoral features of myocardial stunning due to sudden emotional stress. *N Engl J Med*. 2005;352:539–48.

See Also (Topic, Algorithm, Electronic Media Element)
Algorithm: Chest Pain/Acute Coronary Syndrome

CODES
ICD9
429.83 Takotsubo syndrome

TRICHINELLOSIS

Kenton I. Voorhees, MD

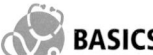

BASICS

DESCRIPTION
Trichinellosis is a parasitic disease that develops after ingesting infected pork or other meat containing viable cysts of *Trichinella spiralis*, a nematode, with rarer cases attributable to several different species of *Trichinella*, in particular, *Trichinella papuae*, *Trichinella murelli*, and *Trichinella pseudospiralis* (1)[C]. Cysts remain viable and can cause disease when infected meat is undercooked. Most common outbreaks are attributable to undercooked pork; homemade and commercial sausage; and wild boar, bear, walrus, and other wild animal meats. Horse meat has become another important source in the European Union:
- Enteric phase (phase I):
  - Cysts are broken down by digestive acid and pepsin in stomach, freeing larvae, which develop into mature adult worms in the upper to middle small intestine.
  - Takes ~1 week after ingestion; may last 3–5 weeks
- Systemic phase (phase II):
  - Female worms then release newborn larvae that migrate through blood vessels and lymphatics to multiple organ systems.
  - Occurs 2–3 weeks after ingestion; may last for 2 months
- Muscular encystment phase (phase III):
  - Larvae become encysted in striated skeletal and sometimes cardiac muscle, where they form a "nurse cell" that functions to nourish them and protect them from host immunity.
  - The complex can survive in humans up to 30 years.
  - Intramuscular cysts usually eventually calcify.
- System(s) affected: GI; Musculoskeletal
- Synonym(s): Trichinelliasis

Pregnancy Considerations
A recent study of 4 patients showed that transplacental passage of migrating larvae is possible; however, elevated progesterone during pregnancy is helminthotoxic to newborn larvae, leading to a mild or moderate course of the infection in the mother. All newborns did well despite 1 with positive antibodies (2).

EPIDEMIOLOGY
Incidence
- From 1997–2001, on average, 12 cases were reported annually in the US (3).
- Only 5 cases reported in the US in 2007 (4)
- Higher incidence in Alaska and northeastern US
- Most mild cases probably undiagnosed, based on autopsy studies
- Predominant age: 20–49 years, although cases reported from all age groups
- Predominant sex: Male = Female

RISK FACTORS
- Access to wild game, homemade pork products, or noncommercial sources of meat
- Eating pigs that were fed uncooked garbage
- Undercooking pork
- Eating inadequately cooked or frozen wild game
- Ethnic groups from Southeast Asia raising their own pork or favoring partially cooked pork products
- Residents in Alaska and northeastern US

GENERAL PREVENTION
- Avoid eating undercooked pork and game meat.
- Prolonged freezing may be effective, but less so for wild game meat.

ETIOLOGY
Eating undercooked meat that is infected with viable *Trichinella* cysts

DIAGNOSIS

HISTORY
A history of having eaten undercooked pork or wild game meat

PHYSICAL EXAM
- Signs and symptoms begin within 1 week of ingesting infected meat (5)
- Common symptoms (can occur concurrently):
  - Diarrhea: Mostly phase I
  - Abdominal cramping: Mostly phase I
  - Fever: Mostly phases II and III
  - Myalgias: Mostly phases II and III
  - Eosinophilia: Mostly phases II and III
  - Periorbital edema: Mostly phases II and III
  - Weakness: Mostly phases II and III
- Less common symptoms (mostly phases II and III):
  - Conjunctivitis
  - Subconjunctival hemorrhage
  - Retinal hemorrhages
  - Maculopapular rash
  - Splinter hemorrhages
  - Headache
  - Photophobia
  - Pneumonitis
  - Tachycardia
  - Heart failure
  - Pericardial effusion
  - CNS involvement
- Symptoms depend on number of ingested infective larvae and phase of parasitic invasion:
  - Light infections: <10 larvae per gram of muscle; usually asymptomatic
  - Heavy infections: >50 larvae per gram of muscle; can be life-threatening
  - Skeletal muscle (e.g., gastrocnemius, masseter, diaphragm, biceps, lower back, extraocular muscles, jaw, and neck) is most frequent site of symptoms due to larval migration; however, in severe cases, myocardial damage, pulmonary infiltration, and focal neurologic damage can occur.

DIAGNOSTIC TESTS & INTERPRETATION
Lab
- Serologic tests for *T. spiralis*, IgM, and IgG (1,5,6)[C]
- ELISA for IgM and IgG
- Dipstick assay with *T. spiralis* muscle larval antigen, highly sensitive and specific, results in 15 minutes, being developed (7)[C]
- Bentonite flocculation after 3rd week for parasite-specific antibody
- Indirect immunofluorescence
- Complement fixation
- DNA testing: Random amplified polymorphic DNA, PCR
- Antibody levels:
  - Often not detectable until 3–5 weeks after infection; high false-negative rate in phase I
  - Peak 3rd month
  - Remain detectable 2–3 years
- Antibody testing:
  - Testing: 15–22% false-negative rate in phase I
  - Paired specimens helpful, 1–2 months apart; look for 4-fold increase in titer
- Eosinophilia (>600/mm^3) with leukocytosis
- Increased creatine phosphate kinase
- Increased lactate dehydrogenase
- Hypergammaglobulinemia
- Elevated erythrocyte sedimentation rate (several weeks)
- Urinalysis may show myoglobinuria.
- Drugs that may alter lab results: Rare increases in serum glutamic-oxaloacetic transaminase with thiabendazole

Imaging
- CT scan may help see calcified muscle cysts.
- MRI may help in evaluation of neurologic complications.
- CXR may detect patchy infiltrates.
- Extremity radiograph may show calcified densities.

Diagnostic Procedures/Surgery
Muscle biopsy of gastrocnemius or deltoid with ≥1 gram of muscle, including exam between compressed slides (higher detection rate)

Pathological Findings
Larvae on muscle biopsy (often gastrocnemius); absence of larvae does not exclude diagnosis; rarely find worms in stool

DIFFERENTIAL DIAGNOSIS
- Acute rheumatic fever
- Arthritis
- Angioedema
- Botulism
- Collagen-vascular disease
- Dermatomyositis
- Encephalitis
- Eosinophilia-myalgia syndrome
- Gastroenteritis
- Idiopathic hypereosinophilic syndrome
- Idiopathic polymyositis
- Influenza
- Meningitis

- Pneumonitis
- Polyarteritis nodosa
- Polymyositis
- Typhoid fever
- Tuberculosis

 TREATMENT

MEDICATION
First Line
- For early intestinal phase (presenting in the 1st 1–2 weeks) to treat adult worms:
  - Mebendazole may be used 200–400 mg t.i.d. × 3 days, then 400–500 mg t.i.d. × 10 days, adults and children >2 years of age, 5 mg/kg/day but occasionally up to 20–25 mg/kg/day (8,9)[C]
  - Albendazole: 400 mg b.i.d. × 10–15 days, adults and children >2 years of age (8,9)[C]
  - Pyrantel may be used 10–20 mg/kg of body weight, repeated 2–3 days for pregnant women and children (10)[C]
  - No drugs are very effective against larvae once they are encysted in muscle; however, they may halt further dissemination.
- Call the CDC for current dosage and recommendations: (404) 639-3311.
- Severe cases: Corticosteroids, such as prednisone, 40–60 mg/d × 3–5 days; taper as symptoms subside, particularly to help decrease inflammation when signs of myocarditis, neurologic disease, pulmonary insufficiency, or severe myositis appear.
- Analgesics, NSAIDs, and antipyretics may be helpful as needed.
- Contraindications: Corticosteroids have been reported to be contraindicated in the intestinal phase because they could prolong the phase.
- Precautions: Minimal experience exists with the use of medications in small children and in pregnancy. Mebendazole and albendazole should not be given in pregnancy (9)[C].
- Significant possible interactions:
  - Carbamazepine or alcohol may decrease the effect of mebendazole.
  - Cimetidine may increase the level of mebendazole.

Second Line
Thiabendazole: Once drug of choice at 25 mg/kg b.i.d. × 1 week, maximum dose 1.5 g; replaced by the drugs previously mentioned because they have fewer side effects and are equally effective

ADDITIONAL TREATMENT
General Measures
- Outpatient unless complications such as cardiac, pulmonary, or neurologic
- May call the CDC for appropriate diagnostic tests: (404) 639-3311
- Bed rest
- Antipyretics
- Analgesics

SURGERY/OTHER PROCEDURES
Pacemaker has been required on occasion for severe myocarditis

IN-PATIENT CONSIDERATIONS
Admission Criteria
- Admit if cardiac, pulmonary, or neurologic manifestations
- Pregnancy

 ONGOING CARE

FOLLOW-UP RECOMMENDATIONS
Activity:
- As tolerated
- Bed rest may help muscular pain.

Patient Monitoring
Monitor the patient for signs and symptoms of complications, such as cardiac, neurologic, and pulmonary.

DIET
As tolerated

PATIENT EDUCATION
- Manage complications as appropriate.
- Cook potentially contaminated meat, such as pork, to 170°F (77°C) until no longer pink.
- Freeze at −15°C for 21 days (longer if meat >15 cm thick); however, *Trichinella* larvae in wild game may be resistant to freezing.
- Do not feed hogs uncooked garbage.

PROGNOSIS
- Most infections are asymptomatic, short-lived, and generally have an uneventful recovery without medication.
- Prognosis good in most cases, although 5–10% of the cases can be severe.
- There is no clear evidence that chronic trichinosis exists.
- <1% of cases can be fatal, generally around 4th–8th week, as a result of cardiac failure or pneumonia.

COMPLICATIONS
- Meningitis
- Subcortical infarcts
- Encephalitis
- Myocarditis with congestive heart failure
- Nephritis
- Glomerulonephritis
- Sinusitis
- Pneumonitis
- Ocular
- Pregnancy: Abortion, premature delivery
- Death: Typically cardiac or thromboembolic events

REFERENCES
1. Bruschi F, Murrell KD. New aspects of human trichinellosis: the impact of new Trichinella species. *Postgrad Med J.* 2002;78:15–22.
2. Nuñez GG, Costantino SN, Gentile T, et al. Immunoparasitological evaluation of Trichinella spiralis infection during human pregnancy: a small case series. *Trans R Soc Trop Med Hyg.* 2008.
3. Roy SL, Lopez AS, Schantz PM. Trichinellosis surveillance–United States, 1997–2001. *MMWR Surveill Summ.* 2003;52:1–8.
4. Hall-Baker P, Nieves E, et al. Summary of Notifiable Diseases - United States, 2007. *MMWR Weekly,* 2009;53:1–94.
5. Dupouy-Camet J, Murrell KD, (eds). *FAO/WHO/OIE guidelines for the surveillance, management, prevention and control of trichinellosis.* 2007. http://www.fao.org/documents (last accessed May 10, 2010).
6. Gottstein B, Pozio E, Nöckler K. Epidemiology, diagnosis, treatment, and control of trichinellosis. *Clin Microbiol Rev.* 2009;22:127–45.
7. Al-Sherbiny MM, et al. Application and assessment of a dipstick assay in the diagnosis of hydatidosis and trichinosis. *Parisitol Res.* 2004;93(2):87–95.
8. Abramowicz M, ed. *The Medical Letter on Drugs and Therapeutics. Drugs for Parasitic Infections.* New Rochelle, NY: The Medical Letter, 2004.
9. Dupouy-Camet J, Kociecka W, Bruschi F, et al. Opinion on the diagnosis and treatment of human trichinellosis. *Expert Opin Pharmacother.* 2002;3:1117–30.
10. Kociecka W. Trichinellosis: Human disease, diagnosis and treatment. *Vet Parisitol.* 2000; 93(3–4):365–83.

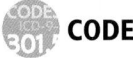 **CODES**

ICD9
124 Trichinosis

CLINICAL PEARLS
- The most common source of trichinellosis in the US is wild bear meat.
- The hallmark symptoms of trichinellosis are periorbital edema, myositis, and eosinophilia.
- Trichinellosis generally is self-limited, and specific therapy generally is not needed unless there are complicating factors.
- ELISA tests are felt to be the most sensitive serologic tests to confirm a diagnosis of trichinellosis.
- To make a muscle biopsy more reliable in detecting trichinellosis, it should be compressed between 2 microscope slides—trichinelloscopy. Yield is higher near a tendinous insertion.

TRICHOMONIASIS

Teresa M. Robb, MD

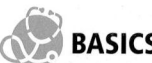 **BASICS**

DESCRIPTION
- Sexually transmitted urogenital infection caused by a pear-shaped, parasitic protozoan
- A cause of nongonococcal urethritis (NGU) in males
- System(s) affected: Genitourinary
- Synonym(s): Trich; Trichomonal urethritis

EPIDEMIOLOGY
Incidence
- Estimated 7.4 million new cases annually in the US in men and women
- 10–25% of vaginal infections
- 1–17% of cases of NGU; reported prevalence rates among men without urethritis have ranged from 0–8%.
- Predominant age: Young and middle-aged adults:
  – Rare until onset of sexual activity
  – Not uncommon in postmenopausal women; age is not protective, and long-term carriage is possible.
- Predominant sex: Male = Female, but women are more commonly symptomatic.

Pediatric Considerations
Rare in prepubertal children; confirmed diagnosis should raise concern of sexual abuse

Prevalence
- 2.3% of young adults:
  – 2.8% of women
  – 1.7% of men
- 3.1% of all US women
- Racial disparity exists (1):
  – 1.3% of white, non-Hispanic women
  – 1.8% of Mexican American women
  – 13.3% of black, non-Hispanic women

RISK FACTORS
- Multiple sexual partners
- Unprotected intercourse
- Lower socioeconomic status
- Other sexually transmitted infections (STIs)
- Untreated partner with previous infection

Genetics
No known genetic considerations

GENERAL PREVENTION
- Use of male or female condoms
- Reducing exposure by limiting numbers of partners
- Male circumcision may be protective (2).

ETIOLOGY
- *Trichomonas vaginalis*: A pear-shaped, flagellated, parasitic protozoan
- Grows best at 35–37°C in anaerobic conditions at pH of 5.5–6.0
- Sexually transmitted
- Transmission via a nonvenereal route is possible because the organism survives for several hours in a moist environment.

COMMONLY ASSOCIATED CONDITIONS
- Other sexually transmitted diseases, including HIV
- Bacterial vaginosis

 DIAGNOSIS

HISTORY
- Females:
  – Yellow–green, malodorous vaginal discharge
  – Vulvovaginal pruritus
  – Dysuria
  – 50–75% are asymptomatic.
- Males:
  – Dysuria
  – Urethral discharge
  – 80% are asymptomatic.

PHYSICAL EXAM
- Females:
  – Vaginal erythema
  – Yellow–green, frothy, malodorous vaginal discharge
  – Petechiae on cervix (strawberry cervix; seen in ~10% of patients)
- Males: Penile discharge, spontaneous and with expression

DIAGNOSTIC TESTS & INTERPRETATION
Lab
Initial lab tests
- Wet mount of vaginal or urethral discharge (3)[A]: Direct visualization of motile trichomonads:
  – Sensitivity of 60–70%
  – Specificity of 99.8%

- Gram stain
- Detection on Pap smear (3)[A]:
  – Sensitivity of 57–98%
  – Specificity of 97%

- Culture: Sensitivity >95%; can take 4–7 days:
  – Enzyme-linked immunosorbent assay and direct fluorescent antibody tests: Sensitivity 80–90%
  – Rapid diagnostic kits using polymerase chain reaction DNA probes: Sensitivity 97%, specificity 98%

DIFFERENTIAL DIAGNOSIS
- Females (other vaginitides):
  – Bacterial vaginosis
  – Vaginal candidiasis
  – Chlamydial infection
  – Gonorrheal infection
  – Mixed vaginitis
- Males (other urethritides):
  – Chlamydial infection
  – Gonorrheal infection

 TREATMENT

- Symptomatic individuals require treatment.
- Asymptomatic partners are also treated presumptively.
- Complete screening for other STIs should be considered part of required treatment.

MEDICATION
First Line
- Metronidazole 2 g p.o., 1 dose (4)[A]
- Metronidazole 1.5 g p.o., 1 dose:
  – Food and Drug Administration (FDA) pregnancy risk Category B
  – American Association of Pediatrics recommends abstaining from breastfeeding during treatment and for 12–24 hours after last dose, but this is an old recommendation not supported by current evidence (5).
- Tinidazole 2 g p.o., 1 dose:
  – FDA pregnancy risk Category C
  – Abstain from breastfeeding during treatment and for 3 days after the dose.

Second Line
- Only if still symptomatic after initial treatment
- Metronidazole 500 mg p.o. b.i.d. × 7 days (4)[A]

Pregnancy Considerations
No evidence supports the use of metronidazole in asymptomatic patients because adverse outcomes are not prevented by treatment (6)[A].

ADDITIONAL TREATMENT
General Measures
If metronidazole resistance suspected, use tinidazole

Issues for Referral
- Multiresistant organism
- Patient allergy to metronidazole: Desensitization to metronidazole is possible.

Additional Therapies
- Males:
  - None currently available in the US
- Females (4)[A]:
  - Clotrimazole 100 mg PV b.i.d. × 7 days
  - Sulfanilamide-aminacrine-allantoin vaginal suppositories b.i.d. × 7 days
  - Nonoxynol 9
  - Povidone-iodine douche

COMPLEMENTARY AND ALTERNATIVE MEDICINE
None adequately investigated enough to be recommended

IN-PATIENT CONSIDERATIONS
Admission Criteria
Admission may be necessary for resistant organisms because IV therapy provides higher tissue concentrations.

Discharge Criteria
Clearance of infection

ONGOING CARE

FOLLOW-UP RECOMMENDATIONS
- If symptoms persist after initial treatment, reculture and/or repeat wet mount.
- No need for test of cure in asymptomatic individuals (4)[A].

DIET
Abstain from alcohol while being treated with 5-nitroimidazole derivatives due to disulfiramlike reaction.

PATIENT EDUCATION
Education about the sexually transmitted aspect of the infection:
- Inform partner so that partner can be treated.
- Discuss safe sex during health maintenance visits.
- Abstain from intercourse while undergoing treatment; use condoms if abstention is not feasible/possible.
- Avoid alcohol during treatment with metronidazole or tinidazole.
- Condom use can prevent recurrence.

PROGNOSIS
- Excellent
- Usually treated after 1 course, but increasing number of metronidazole-resistant cases

COMPLICATIONS
Pregnancy Considerations
Linked to low birth weight, preterm/premature rupture of membranes, preterm birth (6)

REFERENCES

1. Sutton M, Sternberg M, Koumans EH, et al. The prevalence of Trichomonas vaginalis infection among reproductive-age women in the United States, 2001–2004. *Clin Infect Dis*. 2007;45: 1319–26.
2. Sobngwi-Tambekou J, Taljaard D, Nieuwoudt M, et al. Male circumcision and Neisseria gonorrhoeae, Chlamydia trachomatis and Trichomonas vaginalis: observations after a randomised controlled trial for HIV prevention. *Sex Transm Infect*. 2009;85: 116–20.
3. Wiese W, Patel SR, Patel SC, et al. A meta-analysis of the Papanicolaou smear and wet mount for the diagnosis of vaginal trichomoniasis. *Am J Med*. 2000;108:301–8.
4. Forna F, et al. Interventions for treating trichomoniasis in women. Cochrane Infectious Diseases Group. *Cochrane Database Syst Rev*. 2009;2.
5. Hale T. Medications and Mothers Milk: A Manual of Lactational Pharmacology (Medications and Mother's Milk), 2009.
6. Gülmezoglu A. Interventions for trichomonas in pregnancy. Cochrane Pregnancy and Childbirth Group. *Cochrane Database Syst Rev*. 2010;1.

ADDITIONAL READING

- Allsworth JE, Ratner JA, Peipert JF, et al. Trichomoniasis and other sexually transmitted infections: results from the 2001-2004 National Health and Nutrition Examination Surveys. *Sex Transm Dis*. 2009;36:738–44.
- Centers for Disease Control and Prevention, Workowski KA, Berman SM. Sexually transmitted diseases treatment guidelines, 2006. *MMWR Recomm Rep*. 2006;55:1–94.
- Helms D, et al. Management of *Trichomonas vaginalis* in women with suspected metronidazole hypersensitivity. *Am J Obstet Gynecol*. 2008;198: 370e1–370e7.
- http://www.cdc.gov/std/trichomonas.
- Klebanoff MA, Carey JC, Hauth JC, et al. Failure of metronidazole to prevent preterm delivery among pregnant women with asymptomatic Trichomonas vaginalis infection. *N Engl J Med*. 2001;345: 487–93.
- McClelland RS, Sangare L, Hassan WM, et al. Infection with Trichomonas vaginalis increases the risk of HIV-1 acquisition. *J Infect Dis*. 2007;195: 698–702.
- Miller M, Liao Y, Gomez AM, et al. Factors associated with the prevalence and incidence of Trichomonas vaginalis infection among African American women in New York city who use drugs. *J Infect Dis*. 2008;197:503–9.
- Saperstein AK, Firnhaber GC, et al. Clinical inquiries. Should you test or treat partners of patients with gonorrhea, chlamydia, or trichomoniasis? *J Fam Pract*. 2010;59:46–8.
- Wendel KA, Workowski KA. Trichomoniasis: challenges to appropriate management. *Clin Infect Dis*. 2007;44(Suppl 3):S123–9.

CODES

ICD9
- 131.00 Urogenital trichomoniasis, unspecified
- 131.01 Trichomonal vulvovaginitis
- 131.02 Trichomonal urethritis

CLINICAL PEARLS
- Both partners need to be treated for trichomoniasis.
- Test of cure is unnecessary.
- Avoid alcohol during treatment with standard agents.
- Treatment does not improve risk of adverse pregnancy outcomes.
- Male circumcision may be protective.

TRIGEMINAL NEURALGIA

Vasileios-Arsenios Lioutas, MD
Yelena Gorfinkel, MD

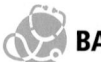 BASICS

DESCRIPTION
- Disorder of the sensory nucleus of the trigeminal nerve (CNV) that produces episodic, paroxysmal, severe, lancinating facial pain lasting seconds to minutes in the distribution of ≥1 divisions of the nerve
- Often precipitated by stimulation of well-defined, ipsilateral trigger zones, usually perioral, perinasal, and occasionally intraoral (e.g., washing, shaving)
- System(s) affected: Nervous
- Synonym(s): Tic douloureux; Fothergill neuralgia; Trifacial neuralgia

EPIDEMIOLOGY
Incidence
- 4.3/100, 000/year
- 5.9/100, 000/year for women
- 3.4/100, 000/year for men
- >70 years of age, ~25.6/100, 000/year
- Predominant age:
  - >50 years; incidence increases with age
  - Rare <35 years of age (consider another primary disease; see Etiology).
- Predominant sex: Female > Male (2:1)

Prevalence
16/100,000

Pediatric Considerations
Unusual in childhood

Pregnancy Considerations
Teratogenicity limits medical therapy in 1st and 2nd trimesters.

RISK FACTORS
Unknown

PATHOPHYSIOLOGY
- Demyelination around the compression site appears to be the mechanism by which compression of nerves leads to symptoms.
- Demyelinated lesions may set up an ectopic impulse generation causing erratic responses: Hyperexcitability of damaged nerves and transmission of action potentials along adjacent, undamaged unstimulated sensory fibers

ETIOLOGY
- Compression of trigeminal nerve by anomalous arteries or veins of posterior fossa, compressing trigeminal root
- Etiologic classification:
  - Idiopathic
  - Secondary: Cerebellopontine angle tumors (e.g., meningioma); tumors of 5th nerve (e.g., neuroma, vascular malformations), trauma, demyelinating disease (e.g., multiple sclerosis [MS]) (1)

COMMONLY ASSOCIATED CONDITIONS
- Sjögren syndrome
- Rheumatoid arthritis
- Chronic meningitis
- Acute polyneuropathy
- MS
- Hemifacial spasm
- Charcot-Marie-Tooth neuropathy
- Glossopharyngeal neuralgia

DIAGNOSIS

HISTORY
Paroxysms of pain in the distribution of the trigeminal nerve

PHYSICAL EXAM
All exam findings are typically negative due to the paroxysmal nature of the disorder.

DIAGNOSTIC TESTS & INTERPRETATION
- The International Headache Society (IHS) diagnostic criteria for classic trigeminal neuralgia:
  - Paroxysmal attacks of pain lasting from a fraction of a second to 2 minutes, affecting 1 or more divisions of the trigeminal nerve
  - Pain has at least an intense, sharp, superficial, or stabbing characteristic or is precipitated from trigger areas or by trigger factors.
  - Attacks are stereotyped in the individual patient.
  - There is no clinically evident neurologic deficit.
  - Not attributed to another disorder
- Secondary trigeminal neuralgia is characterized by pain indistinguishable from classic trigeminal neuralgia but is caused by a demonstrable structural lesion other than vascular compression.

Imaging
Indicated in all first-time presenting patients to rule out secondary causes

Initial approach
- MRI vs CT scan: MRI offers more detailed imaging, preferred if not contraindicated (1)
- Routine head imaging identifies structural causes in up to 15% of patients.
- No positive findings are significantly correlated with diagnosis.

Pathological Findings
- Trigeminal nerve: Inflammatory changes, demyelination, and degenerative changes
- Trigeminal ganglion: Hypermyelination and microneuromata

DIFFERENTIAL DIAGNOSIS
- Other forms of neuralgia usually have sensory loss. Presence of sensory loss nearly excludes the diagnosis of trigeminal neuralgia (if younger patient, frequently MS).
- Neoplasia in cerebellopontine angle
- Vascular malformation of brain stem
- Demyelinating lesion (MS is diagnosed in 2–4% of patients with trigeminal neuralgia)
- Vascular insult
- Migraine, cluster headache
- Giant cell arteritis
- Postherpetic neuralgia
- Chronic meningitis
- Acute polyneuropathy
- Atypical odontalgia
- SUNCT syndrome (short-lasting, unilateral, neuralgiform pain with conjunctival injection)

TREATMENT

MEDICATION
Persistent lack of RCTs regarding treatment of symptomatic TN (2)

First Line
- Carbamazepine (Tegretol): (2)[A] Start at 100–200 mg b.i.d.; effective dose usually 200 mg q.i.d.; maximum dose 1,200 mg/d:
  - 70–90% of patients respond initially.
  - By 3 years, 30% are no longer helped (number needed to treat [NNT] = 1.8) (3)[A].
  - Most common side effect: Sedation
- Contraindications: Concurrent use of monoamine oxidase inhibitors (MAOIs)
- Precautions: Caution in the presence of liver disease
- Significant possible medication interactions: Macrolide antibiotics, oral anticoagulants, anticonvulsants, tricyclics, oral contraceptives, steroids, digitalis, isoniazid, MAOIs, methyprylon, nabilone, nizatidine, other H$_2$ blockers, phenytoin, propoxyphene, benzodiazepines, and calcium channel blockers
- Oxcarbazepine (Trileptal): Start at 150–300 mg b.i.d.; effective dose usually 375 mg b.i.d.; maximum dose 1,200 mg/d:
  - Efficacy similar to carbamazepine (2)[A],(3)[B]
  - Faster, with less drowsiness and fewer drug interactions than carbamazepine
  - Decreases serum sodium
  - Most common side effect: Sedation

Second Line
- Nonantiepileptics: Insufficient evidence from randomized controlled trials to show significant benefit from nonantiepileptic drugs in trigeminal neuralgia (4)[A]
- Phenytoin (Dilantin) 300–400 mg/d (synergistic with carbamazepine):
  - Potent P450 inducer (enhanced metabolism of many drugs)
  - Various CNS side effects (sedation, ataxia)
- Baclofen (Lioresal) 10–80 mg/d; start at 5–10 mg t.i.d. with food (as an adjunct to phenytoin or carbamazepine). Side effects: Drowsiness, weakness, nausea, vomiting.
- Gabapentin (Neurontin): Start at 100 mg t.i.d. or 300 mg at bedtime; can increase dose up to 300–600 mg t.i.d.–q.i.d. Can be used as monotherapy or in combination with other medications and reduces the cost of illness (5).
- Lamotrigine: Titrate up to 200 mg b.i.d. over weeks. Side effect: 10% experience rash.
- Chlorphenesin carbamate (Maolate) 800–2,400 mg/d (as an adjunct to phenytoin and/or carbamazepine). Side effect: Drowsiness.
- Antidepressants, including amitriptyline, fluoxetine, trazodone:
  - Used especially with anticonvulsants
  - Particularly effective for atypical forms of trigeminal neuralgia
- Clonazepam (Klonopin) frequently causes drowsiness and ataxia.

- Sumatriptan (Imitrex) 3 mg SC reduces acute symptoms and may be helpful after failure of conventional medical therapy.
- Capsaicin cream topically
- Botulinum toxin injection into zygomatic arch
- Valproic acid (Depakene, Depakote)

ADDITIONAL TREATMENT
General Measures
- Outpatient
- Drug treatment is 1st approach.
- Invasive procedures are reserved for patients who cannot tolerate, fail to respond to, or relapse after chronic drug treatment.
- Avoid stimulation (e.g., air, heat, cold) of trigger zones, including lips, cheeks, and gums.

Issues for Referral
Initial treatment failure or positive findings on imaging studies

Additional Therapies
- Radiotherapy
- Stereotactic radiosurgery such as gamma knife radiosurgery has been shown to be effective after drug failure:
  – Produces lesions with focused gamma knife radiation
  – Therapy aimed at the proximal trigeminal root
  – Minimal clinically effective dose: 70 Gy
  – 75% of patients achieve complete relief within 3 months; by 3 years, 50% maintain complete relief (NNT = 2) (6)[B].
  – Most common side effect: Sensory disturbance (corneal numbness)
  – Viable treatment option for patients who have not had prior invasive procedures because rates of failure are higher in patients with past invasive procedures (7)

COMPLEMENTARY AND ALTERNATIVE MEDICINE
Acupuncture, moxibustion (herb): Poor evidence

SURGERY/OTHER PROCEDURES
- Microvascular decompression of CNV at its entrance to (or exit from) brain stem:
  – 98% of patients achieve initial pain relief; by 33 months, 73% maintain complete relief (NNT = 1.3) (8)[B].
  – Surgical mortality across studies was ~1% (8).
  – Most common side effect: Transient facial numbness and diplopia, headache, nausea, vomiting
  – Mean hospital stay was 5.4 days (8)[B].
  – Pain relief after procedure strongly correlates with the type of trigeminal neuralgia pain: Type 1 (shocklike pain) resulting in better outcomes than type 2 (constant pain) (9,10)
- Peripheral nerve ablation (multiple methods):
  – Higher failure rate and facial numbness rate than decompression surgery
  – Radiofrequency thermocoagulation (possibly 90–97% partial or complete relief; recurrence rate unknown) (11)[C]
  – Neurectomy
  – Cryotherapy: High relapse rate
  – Partial sensory rhizotomy
- 4% tetracaine dissolved in 0.5% bupivacaine nerve block (only a few case reports to date, ropivacaine)

- Alcohol block or glycerol injection into trigeminal cistern: Unpredictable side effects (dysesthesia and anesthesia dolorosa); temporary relief
- Peripheral block or section of 5th nerve proximal to Gasserian ganglion
- Balloon compression of Gasserian ganglion (especially effective for 1st-division trigeminal neuralgia pain) (11)
- The evidence supporting destructive procedures for benign pain conditions remains limited (12).

 ONGOING CARE

FOLLOW-UP RECOMMENDATIONS
Regular outpatient follow-up to monitor symptoms and therapeutic failure

Patient Monitoring
- Carbamazepine and/or phenytoin serum levels
- If carbamazepine is prescribed: Complete blood count (CBC) and platelets at baseline, then weekly for a month, then monthly for 4 months, then every 6–12 months if dose stable (regimens for monitoring vary)
- Reduce drugs after 4–6 weeks to determine whether condition is in remission; resume at previous dose if pain recurs. Withdraw drugs slowly after several months, again to check for remission or if lower dose of drugs can be tolerated.

DIET
No special diet

PATIENT EDUCATION
- Instruct patient regarding medication dosage and side effects, risk–benefit ratios of surgery or radiation therapy.
- After having microvascular decompression surgery, most patients wish they had undergone the procedure sooner (73%; NNT = 1.4) (12)[A].
- Trigeminal Neuralgia Association (TNA): http://www.endthepain.org/

PROGNOSIS
- 50–60% eventually fail pharmacologic treatment (3)[B].
- Of those, relapse is seen in ~50% of stereotactic radiosurgeries and ~27% of surgical microvascular decompressions (3,6)[B].

COMPLICATIONS
- Mental and physical sluggishness; dizziness with carbamazepine (3)
- Paresthesias and corneal reflex loss with stereotactic radiosurgery (6)
- Surgical mortality and morbidity associated with microvascular decompression (8)

REFERENCES

1. Borges A, Casselman J, et al. Imaging the trigeminal nerve. *European journal of radiology.* 2010;
2. Attal N, Cruccu G, Baron R, et al. EFNS guidelines on the pharmacological treatment of neuropathic pain: 2009 revision. *European journal of neurology : the official journal of the European Federation of Neurological Societies.* 2010;
3. Beniczky S, Tajti J, Tímea Varga E, et al. Evidence-based pharmacological treatment of neuropathic pain syndromes. *J Neural Transm.* 2005;112:735–49.
4. He L, Wu B, Zhou M, et al. Non-antiepileptic drugs for trigeminal neuralgia. *Cochrane Database Syst Rev.* 2006;3:CD004029.
5. Pérez C, Saldaña MT, Navarro A, et al. Trigeminal Neuralgia Treated With Pregabalin in Family Medicine Settings: Its Effect on Pain Alleviation and Cost Reduction. *J Clin Pharmacol.* 2009.
6. Lopez BC, Hamlyn PJ, Zakrzewska JM. Stereotactic radiosurgery for primary trigeminal neuralgia: state of the evidence and recommendations for future reports. *J Neurol Neurosurg Psychiatry.* 2004;75:1019–24.
7. Dhople AA, Adams JR, Maggio WW, et al. Long-term outcomes of Gamma Knife radiosurgery for classic trigeminal neuralgia: implications of treatment and critical review of the literature. *J Neurosurg.* 2009.
8. Ashkan K, Marsh H. Microvascular decompression for trigeminal neuralgia in the elderly: a review of the safety and efficacy. *Neurosurgery.* 2004;55:840–8; discussion 848–50.
9. Miller JP, Acar F, Burchiel KJ. Classification of trigeminal neuralgia: clinical, therapeutic, and prognostic implications in a series of 144 patients undergoing microvascular decompression. *J Neurosurg.* 2009.
10. Miller JP, Magill ST, Acar F, et al. Predictors of long-term success after microvascular decompression for trigeminal neuralgia. *J Neurosurg.* 2009.
11. Lopez BC, Hamlyn PJ, Zakrzewska JM. Systematic review of ablative neurosurgical techniques for the treatment of trigeminal neuralgia. *Neurosurgery.* 2004;54:973–82; discussion 982–3.
12. Cetas JS, Saedi T, Burchiel KJ. Destructive procedures for the treatment of nonmalignant pain: a structured literature review. *J Neurosurg.* 2008;109:389–404.

ADDITIONAL READING

- Gronseth G, Cruccu G, Alksne J, et al. Practice parameter: the diagnostic evaluation and treatment of trigeminal neuralgia (an evidence-based review): report of the Quality Standards Subcommittee of the American Academy of Neurology and the European Federation of Neurological Societies. *Neurology.* 2008;71:1183–90.
- van Kleef M, van Genderen WM, Narouze S, et al. World Institute of Medicine. *Trigeminal Neuralgia Pain Pract.* 2009;9(4):252–9.

 CODES

ICD9
350.1 Trigeminal neuralgia

CLINICAL PEARLS
- Patients with trigeminal neuralgia typically have a normal physical exam.
- The long-term efficacy of pharmacotherapy in trigeminal neuralgia is 40–50%.
- If pharmacotherapy fails, stereotactic radiosurgery or surgical microvascular decompression is often successful.

TRIGGER FINGER (DIGITAL STENOSING TENOSYNOVITIS)

Alan M. Ehrlich, MD
Robert A. Yood, MD

 ## BASICS

DESCRIPTION
Trigger finger manifests in a clicking, snapping, or locking of a finger or thumb after full flexion ± associated pain.

EPIDEMIOLOGY
Incidence
- 28/100,000/year in the adult population; rare in children
- Diabetics have up to 4× the risk of the general population (1)[B].
- Predominant age:
  – Childhood form presents typically with thumb involvement in the 1st decade of life.
  – Adult form typically presents in the 5th and 6th decades of life.
- Predominant sex:
  – Children: Female = Male
  – Adults: Female > Male (6:1)

Prevalence
Lifetime prevalence in the general population is 2.6%.

Pediatric Considerations
- The thumb is more commonly involved in children (2)[C].
- When children have a trigger finger instead of a trigger thumb, surgery is often more complicated. Release of the A1 pulley alone is often insufficient, and other procedures may be necessary at the time of surgery.

RISK FACTORS
- Diabetes mellitus (DM)
- Rheumatoid arthritis (RA)
- Hypothyroidism
- Mucopolysaccharide disorders
- Amyloidosis

GENERAL PREVENTION
Most cases are idiopathic, and no known prevention exists. There is no clear association with repetitive movements.

PATHOPHYSIOLOGY
- Narrowing of the A1 pulley usually is due to either thickening from inflammation or protein deposits or thickening of the tendon per se; with prolonged inflammation, fibrocartilaginous metaplasia of the tendon sheath occurs.
- The flexor tendon may become distorted with nodule formation, which can give rise to the triggering because the nodule has difficulty passing through the area of narrowing. Because flexors are stronger than extensors, the finger can get stuck in the flexed position.

ETIOLOGY
- Most cases are idiopathic, and no known prevention exists.
- No clear association with repetitive movements

COMMONLY ASSOCIATED CONDITIONS
- de Quervain tenosynovitis
- Carpal tunnel syndrome
- Dupuytren contracture (usually occurs in 4th or 5th digit; thickening of palmar connective tissue results in a flexion contraction of the distal digit)
- DM
- RA
- Hypothyroidism
- Amyloidosis

 ## DIAGNOSIS

Diagnosis is based on clinical presentation.

HISTORY
History of clicking, snapping, or locking of a finger or thumb after full flexion ± associated pain

PHYSICAL EXAM
- A palpable nodule may be present.
- Snapping or locking may be present, but neither is necessary for the diagnosis.
- Tenderness to palpation is variable.

DIAGNOSTIC TESTS & INTERPRETATION
Pathological Findings
- Thickening of the A1 pulley with fibrocartilaginous metaplasia
- Thickening or nodule formation of flexor tendon

 ## ONGOING CARE

FOLLOW-UP RECOMMENDATIONS
- Follow-up is needed only if symptoms persist or if complications of surgery develop.
- Splinting of the affected digit to minimize flexion/extension of the MCP joint can lead to resolution of symptoms (1)[B],(3)[C].

PROGNOSIS
Prognosis for resolution of symptoms is excellent with either conservative or surgical intervention. Recurrence following corticosteroid injection is more likely for patients with type 1 DM, younger age, involvement of multiple digits, and history of other upper extremity tendinopathies (4)[C].

COMPLICATIONS

- Complications from surgery include infection, bleeding, digital nerve injury, and persistent pain.
- Injury to the A2 pulley may result in bowstringing, which is a bulging of the flexor tendon in the palm with flexion. This can be associated with pain.
- Diabetic patients may have significantly increased blood sugar levels for up to 5 days following steroid injection.

 ## TREATMENT

- Splinting the metacarpophalangeal (MCP) joint at 10–15 degrees of flexion for 6 weeks with the distal joints free to move has been reported to be effective. Splinting is more effective for treating fingers than thumbs (70% vs 50%). This is less effective with severe symptoms, symptoms >6 months, and multiple digits involved (1)[B].
- Long-acting corticosteroids may be injected several times to achieve relief of symptoms, although subsequent injections often are less likely to work than the initial injection.

MEDICATION

First Line

Steroid injection of the tendon sheath or surrounding subcutaneous tissue has 57–90% success rate (3)[B],(5)[C]. Injection in surrounding tissues is as efficacious as injecting into the tendon sheath (1,6)[B]. Higher success rates are associated with shorter duration of symptoms.

Second Line

Nonsteroidal anti-inflammatory drugs (NSAIDs) may reduce pain and discomfort, but have not been shown to improve the underlying cause. They do not reduce symptoms of snapping or locking.

ADDITIONAL TREATMENT

General Measures

Splinting or steroid injection should be tried before surgery.

Issues for Referral

Refer to hand surgeon if not responding to splinting and/or steroid injections.

Additional Therapies

Physiotherapy has been used in the treatment of trigger digits in children.

SURGERY/OTHER PROCEDURES

- Surgical release can be done as open procedure or percutaneously (7).
- Success rates with either procedure very high (7)
- Most hand surgeons still prefer the open release because of concern about avoiding nerve injury with the blind procedure.

IN-PATIENT CONSIDERATIONS

Admission Criteria

Day surgery for trigger finger release

Discharge Criteria

Absence of complications

REFERENCES

1. Akhtar S, Bradley MJ, Quinton DN, et al. Management and referral for trigger finger/thumb. *Br Med J*. 2005;331:30–3.
2. Cardon LJ, Ezaki M, Carter PR. Trigger finger in children. *J Hand Surg*. 1999;24A:1156–61.
3. Ryzewicz M, Wolf JN. Trigger digits: Principles, management, and complications. *J Hand Surg*. 2006;31A:135–46.
4. Rozental TD, Zurakowski D, Blazar PE. Trigger finger: prognostic indicators of recurrence following corticosteroid injection. *J Bone Joint Surg Am*. 2008;90:1665–72.
5. Fleisch SB, Spindler KP, Lee DH. Corticosteroid injections in the treatment of trigger finger: a level I and II systematic review. *J Am Acad Orthop Surg*. 2007;15:166–71.
6. Kazuki K, Egi T, Okada M, et al. Clinical outcome of extrasynovial steroid injection for trigger finger. *Hand Surg*. 2006;11:1–4.
7. Bamroongshawgasame T, et al. A comparison of open and percutaneous pulley release in trigger digits. *J Med Assoc Thai*. 2010;93:199–204.

ADDITIONAL READING

Moore JS. Flexor tendon entrapment of the digits (trigger finger and trigger thumb). *J Occup Environ Med*. 2000;42:5.

 ## CODES

ICD9

727.03 Trigger finger (acquired)

CLINICAL PEARLS

- Narrowing of the A1 pulley usually due to either thickening from inflammation or protein deposits or thickening of the tendon per se; with prolonged inflammation, fibrocartilaginous metaplasia of the tendon sheath occurs.
- History of clicking, snapping, or locking of a finger or thumb after full flexion ± associated pain
- Splinting the MCP joint at 10–15 degrees flexion for 6 weeks with the distal joints free to move has been reported to be effective. Splinting is more effective for treating fingers than thumbs (70% vs 50%). This is less effective with severe symptoms, symptoms >6 months, and multiple digits involved (1)[B].
- Long-acting corticosteroids may be injected several times to achieve relief of symptoms, although subsequent injections often are less likely to work than the initial injection.
- Both open and percutaneous surgery have high success rates with low risk of complications (7).
- Most hand surgeons still prefer the open release because of concern about avoiding nerve injury with the blind procedure.

T

TROCHANTERIC BURSITIS (GREATER TROCHANTERIC PAIN SYNDROME)

David W. Kruse, MD
Mohammad Shahsahebi

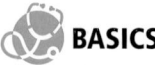 BASICS

The name *trochanteric bursitis* has been used in the historical literature to refer to pain at the lateral hip with tenderness over the greater trochanter. As more continues to be understood about potential sources of pain at the lateral hip and the discovery that many patients lack of an inflammatory process, this condition has been referred to as *greater trochanteric pain syndrome* (GTPS) in the more recent literature (1).

DESCRIPTION

- Bursae are fluid-filled sacs that are found at bony protuberances, typically at tendon attachment sites. Multiple bursae are described in the area of the greater trochanter of the femur. These bursae correspond to the tendons of the gluteus muscles, iliotibial band (ITB), and tensor fasciae latae. The subgluteus maximus bursa is implicated most commonly in lateral hip pain (1).
- Other structures that surround the lateral hip include the ITB, tensor fasciae latae, gluteus maximus tendon, gluteus medius tendon, gluteus minimus tendon, quadratus femoris muscle, vastus lateralis tendon, and piriformis tendon.
- *Bursitis* refers to inflammation of the bursa.
- *Tendinopathy* refers to any abnormality of a tendon, inflammatory or degenerative.

EPIDEMIOLOGY

Incidence
- In primary-care setting: 1.8 patients/1,000 persons/year
- Predominant age: All ages; peak incidence in 4th–6th decades

Prevalence
- Predominant sex: Female > Male.
- Sports:
  - Running
  - Contact sports: Football, rugby, soccer

RISK FACTORS

Multiple factors have been implicated (1,2).

- Female
- Obesity
- Tight hip musculature or ITB
- Direct trauma
- Total hip arthroplasty

- Abnormal biomechanics or gait:
  - Leg-length discrepancy
  - Sacroiliac (SI) joint dysfunction
  - Knee or hip osteoarthritis
  - Abnormal foot mechanics (e.g., pes planus, overpronation)
  - Neuromuscular disorder

Genetics
No known genetic factors

GENERAL PREVENTION
- Maintain ITB, hip, and lower-back flexibility and strength.
- Avoid direct trauma (use of appropriate padding in contact sports).
- Avoid banked running.
- Appropriate shoe wear
- Weight loss, if appropriate

PATHOPHYSIOLOGY
- Acute: Abnormal gait or poor muscle flexibility and strength lead to
  - Friction on bursa, causing inflammatory response
  - Tendon overuse and inflammation
  - Direct trauma from contact or frequently lying with body weight on hip can cause an inflammatory response.
- Chronic:
  - Fibrosis and thickening of bursal sac owing to chronic inflammatory process
  - Tendinopathy owing to chronic overuse and degeneration: Gluteus medius and minimus (1)

ETIOLOGY
See Risk Factors and Pathophysiology sections.

COMMONLY ASSOCIATED CONDITIONS
- Many biomechanical factors can be associated with this condition (1).
  - Tight ITBs
  - Leg-length discrepancy
  - SI joint dysfunction
  - Pes planus
- Other associated pathology (1):
  - Low-back pain
  - Knee and hip osteoarthritis
  - Obesity

DIAGNOSIS

HISTORY
General historical points on presentation (1)[C]:

- Pain localized to the lateral aspect of the hip or buttock
- May radiate to groin or lateral thigh (pseudoradiculopathy)
- Exacerbated by
  - Prolonged walking or standing
  - Rising after prolonged sitting
  - Sitting with legs crossed
  - Lying on affected side
- Other possible points:
  - Direct trauma to affected hip
  - Chronic low-back pain
  - Chronic leg/knee/ankle/hip pain
  - Recent increase in running distance or intensity
  - Change in running surfaces

PHYSICAL EXAM

- Point tenderness with direct palpation over the lateral hip is the most characteristic sign for GTPS (1)[B].
- Other exam tests have been described but lack sensitivity (1)[B].
  - May have pain with extremes of passive rotation, abduction, or adduction
  - Pain with resisted hip abduction and external or internal rotation
  - Trendelenburg sign
- Other testing to evaluate for associated conditions:
  - Positive Patrick-FABERE (flexion, abduction, external rotation, extension) testing for SI joint dysfunction
  - Ober test for ITB pathology
  - Flexion and extension of hip for osteoarthritis
  - Leg-length measurement
  - Foot inspection for pes planus or overpronation
  - Lower extremity neurologic assessment for lumbar radiculopathy or neuromuscular disorders

DIAGNOSTIC TESTS & INTERPRETATION

Lab
No routine lab testing is recommended.

Follow-Up & Special Considerations
If there is a concern for a septic bursitis, then aspiration or incision and drainage may be necessary.

Imaging
Diagnosis can be made by history and exam, but radiologic imaging can be helpful to evaluate for other associated conditions.

Initial approach
- Anteroposterior and frog-leg views of affected hip
- Consider lumbar spine radiographs if back pain is thought to be a contributing factor.
- Musculoskeletal ultrasound also can provide accurate imaging of potential pathology.

Follow-Up & Special Considerations
Advanced imaging rarely necessary; detection of abnormalities on MRI is a poor predictor of GTPS (3)[B].

DIFFERENTIAL DIAGNOSIS
Multiple conditions should be considered (1)[C]:
- ITB syndrome
- Gluteus medius or minimus tendinopathy
- Osteoarthritis or avascular necrosis of the hip
- Lumbosacral osteoarthritis/disk disease causing nerve root compression
- If associated trauma: Fracture or contusion of the hip or pelvis
- Stress reaction/fracture of femoral neck, especially in female runners
- Septic bursitis/arthritis

TREATMENT

- Weight loss (if applicable)
- Minimize aggravating activities such as prolonged walking or standing.
- Avoid lying on affected side.
- Runners:
  - May need to decrease distance and/or intensity of runs
  - May need a period of cessation of running
  - Should avoid banked tracks or roads with excessive tilt

MEDICATION
- Nonsteroidal anti-inflammatory drugs (NSAIDs) (1)[B]:
  - Naprosyn 500 mg PO b.i.d.
  - Ibuprofen 800 mg PO t.i.d.
- Corticosteroid injection is effective for pain relief (4)[C]. In certain cases, injection can be considered 1st-line therapy.
  - Dexamethasone 4 mg/mL IV *or*
  - Kenalog 40 mg/mL IV
  - Consider adding a local anesthetic (short- and/or long-acting) for more immediate pain relief.
  - Can be repeated for recurrence with similar effect if original treatment showed a strong response

ADDITIONAL TREATMENT

Issues for Referral
- Septic bursitis
- Recalcitrant bursitis

Additional Therapies
- Ice
- Physical therapy to address underlying dysfunction and rebuild atrophic muscle mass
- Focus on achieving flexibility of hip musculature, particularly the ITB.
- Correct pelvic/hip instability.
- Correct lower limb biomechanics.
- Address contributing factors:
  - Low-back flexibility
  - If leg-length discrepancy, may need heel lift
  - If pes planus or overpronation, may need arch supports or custom orthotics

COMPLEMENTARY AND ALTERNATIVE MEDICINE
Other techniques have been described for the treatment of chronic fibrosis and tendinopathy and may play a role in the treatment of GTPS. These include acupuncture, prolotherapy, growth factor injection techniques, and low-energy extracorporeal shock wave therapy.

SURGERY/OTHER PROCEDURES
- Rarely requires surgery
- If surgery is indicated, potential options include:
  - Arthroscopic bursectomy (5,6)[B]
  - Release of the ITB

ONGOING CARE

FOLLOW-UP RECOMMENDATIONS
4 weeks posttreatment, sooner if significant worsening

PATIENT EDUCATION
- Avoid lying on affected side.
- Minimize prolonged standing or walking.
- Maintain hip musculature flexibility, including ITB.
- Correct issues that may cause abnormal gait:
  - Low-back pain
  - Knee pain
  - Leg-length discrepancy
  - Foot mechanics
- Gradual return to physical activity

PROGNOSIS
Depends on chronicity and recurrence, with more acute cases having an excellent prognosis

COMPLICATIONS
Bursal thickening and fibrosis

REFERENCES

1. Williams BS, Cohen SP. Greater trochanteric pain syndrome: a review of anatomy, diagnosis and treatment. *Anesth Analg*. 2009;108:1662–70.
2. Farmer KW, Jones LC, Brownson KE, et al. Trochanteric bursitis after total hip arthroplasty: incidence and evaluation of response to treatment. *J Arthroplasty*. 2010;25: 208–12.
3. Blankenbaker DG, Ullrick SR, Davis KW, et al. Correlation of MRI findings with clinical findings of trochanteric pain syndrome. *Skeletal Radiol*. 2008.
4. Stephens MB, Beutler AI, O'Connor FG. Musculoskeletal injections: a review of the evidence. *Am Fam Physician*. 2008;78:971–6.
5. Baker CL, Massie RV, Hurt WG, et al. Arthroscopic bursectomy for recalcitrant trochanteric bursitis. *Arthroscopy*. 2007;23:827–32.
6. Pretell J, Ortega J, García-Rayo R, et al. Distal fascia lata lengthening: an alternative surgical technique for recalcitrant trochanteric bursitis. *Int Orthop*. 2009;33:1223–7.

CODES

ICD9
726.5 Enthesopathy of hip region

CLINICAL PEARLS
- One of the most common complaints from a patient with GTPS is inability to lie on the affected side.
- Thorough knowledge of associated conditions ensures accurate diagnosis and effective treatment.
- Corticosteroid injection can be considered 1st-line therapy for some patients.
- Aggressive use of physical therapy in treatment to address underlying dysfunction and rebuild weakened muscle mass

T

TROPICAL SPRUE

Abdulrazak Abyad, MD, PhD, MBA, MPH, AGSF, AFCHSE

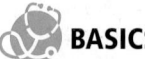 **BASICS**

DESCRIPTION
- Malabsorption syndrome of unknown or mutable etiology that occurs primarily in patients in the tropics and subtropics; characteristics include protein malnutrition and folic acid anemia. Usual course is relapsing without treatment.
- Symptoms may appear years after leaving an endemic area.
- Endemic areas: Tropic regions only—Far East, India, Caribbean, and Middle East. Distribution is sporadic.
- System(s) affected: GI; Hematologic; Lymphatic; Immunologic

EPIDEMIOLOGY
Incidence
- Unknown
- Predominant sex: Male = Female

RISK FACTORS
Parasitic infestation

ETIOLOGY
- Unknown
- Possible dietary deficiency
- Possible infectious agent
- Vitamin deficiency (folate), B_{12}
- Food toxins (rancid fats)
- Toxigenic strains of coliform bacteria

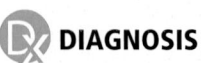 **DIAGNOSIS**

HISTORY
- Fatigue
- Asthenia
- Weight loss
- Diarrhea
- Abdominal cramps
- Borborygmus
- Night blindness
- Anorexia
- Steatorrhea

PHYSICAL EXAM
- Pallor
- Stomatitis
- Glossitis
- Cheilosis
- Hyperkeratosis
- Edema
- Abdominal distension
- Hyperpigmentation
- Koilonychia

DIAGNOSTIC TESTS & INTERPRETATION
Lab
- Megaloblastic anemia in 60% of patients
- Steatorrhea
- Decreased xylose
- Decreased serum iron
- Decreased calcium
- Decreased folic acid, serum vitamin B_{12}
- Decreased serum carotene
- Decreased cholesterol, albumin
- Deficiency of magnesium
- Deficiency of α-tocopherol

Imaging
- Mild jejunal dilatation
- Jejunal fold coarsening
- Flocculation and segmentation of barium meal

Diagnostic Procedures/Surgery
- Normal result on jejunal biopsy nearly excludes this diagnosis.
- Abnormal results on duodenal/jejunal biopsy: Not specific
- Malabsorption of at least 2 nutrients is considered essential for diagnosis.
- D-Xylose, fat, and radiolabeled vitamin B_{12} are used to test for absorptive capacity.
- Enhanced magnification endoscopy (with acetic acid spraying) may help to identify abnormal tissue (1)[C].
- Stool microscopy
- Imaging: Not specific
- Steatorrhea
- Findings of steatorrhea, mucosal malabsorption of 2 substances (e.g., fat, D-xylose), and villous atrophy (demonstrated by means of biopsy) are adequate to make a diagnosis.
- Response to treatment is considered by some to be the conclusive evidence that confirms the diagnosis.
- Complete blood count: This shows megaloblastic anemia associated with reduced folate and vitamin B_{12} levels in as many as 60% of patients.
- Blood chemistry test: This includes potassium, calcium, magnesium, phosphate, albumin, cholesterol, and iron studies.

Pathological Findings
- Jejunal biopsy: Mild villous atrophy, increased villous crypts, mononuclear cell infiltration
- Patients may have chronic atrophic gastritis and nonspecific abnormalities of the colonic mucosa.
- Serum motilin and enteroglucagon levels are increased both while fasting and postprandially.

DIFFERENTIAL DIAGNOSIS
- Celiac disease
- Inflammatory bowel disease
- Giardiasis
- Strongylosis
- Bacterial overgrowth
- Pancreatic disorders
- Other infectious causes:
  – *Coccidial isospora*
  – *Capillaria philippinensis*
  – *Cryptosporidium* spp.

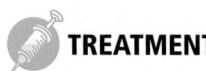

TREATMENT

MEDICATION

First Line
- Vitamin B_{12} 1,000 g SC for several days, then monthly thereafter for 6 months; for pediatric patients: 100 μg IM
- Folic acid 5 mg/d PO; for pediatric patients younger than 12 years of age, not established; greater than 12 years of age, 1 mg/d
- Tetracycline 250 mg q.i.d. × 1–2 months, then 1/2 doses for up to 6 months; occasionally, longer course required; younger than 8 years of age, not recommended; older than 8 years of age, 25–50 mg/d PO divided b.i.d.
- Combination folic acid and vitamin B_{12} plus tetracycline or sulfonamide
- Contraindications: Allergy to tetracycline or oxytetracycline
- Precautions:
  – Use with caution in patients with intercurrent lupus, myasthenia gravis, or kidney or liver disease.
  – Do not take medication with milk, antacids, or iron preparations.
  – Do not use tetracycline during pregnancy.
  – Do not use tetracycline in children <8 years of age.
- Significant possible interactions:
  – Antacids, anticoagulants, bismuth subsalicylate
  – Oral contraceptives
  – Lithium

Second Line
- Oxytetracycline
- Nonabsorbable sulfonamides

Pediatric Considerations
Do not treat pediatric patients with tetracycline.

Pregnancy Considerations
Do not treat with tetracycline during pregnancy.

ADDITIONAL TREATMENT
General Measures
- Replace deficient elements (e.g., vitamin B_{12}, folic acid).
- Control diarrhea.
- Replace fluids and blood.

IN-PATIENT CONSIDERATIONS
Initial Stabilization
Outpatient

 # ONGOING CARE

FOLLOW-UP RECOMMENDATIONS
No restrictions, as tolerated

Patient Monitoring
As needed for symptoms

DIET
No special diet (gluten-free diets do not improve this disease)

PATIENT EDUCATION
Written patient information available from National Digestive Diseases Information Clearinghouse, Box NDDIC, Bethesda, MD 20892, (301) 654-3810

PROGNOSIS
- Good with appropriate treatment
- Recurrences do happen in native residents treated in the tropics.

COMPLICATIONS
- Malabsorption
- Relapse is possible if medication regimen is stopped too soon.

REFERENCE
1. Lo A, Guelrud M, Essenfeld H, Bonis P, et al. Classification of villous atrophy with enhanced magnification endoscopy in patients with celiac disease and tropical sprue. *Gastrointest Endosc.* 2007;66:377–82.

ADDITIONAL READING
- Nath SK. Tropical sprue. *Curr Gastroenterol Rep.* 2005;7:343–9.
- Wahnschaffe U, Ignatius R, Loddenkemper C, et al. Diagnostic value of endoscopy for the diagnosis of giardiasis and other intestinal diseases in patients with persistent diarrhea from tropical or subtropical areas. *Scand J Gastroenterol.* 2007;42:391–6.

See Also (Topic, Algorithm, Electronic Media Element)
Celiac Disease; Diarrhea, Chronic
Algorithm: Diarrhea, Chronic

 # CODES

ICD9
579.1 Tropical sprue

CLINICAL PEARLS
- When traveling, the tropics and subtropics are the regions that pose the greatest threat of sprue disease.
- Unless treated properly, the symptoms will recur.
- Tropical sprue is to be distinguished from celiac disease, which is also called *nontropical sprue*.
- Gluten-free diet does *not* improve tropical sprue.

T

TUBERCULOSIS

Swati B. Avashia, MD

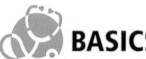

BASICS

DESCRIPTION
- Usually transmitted by inhaling airborne bacilli from a person with active tuberculosis (TB). Bacilli multiply in alveoli; are carried by macrophages, lymphatics, and blood to distant sites. Three possible outcomes:
  - Eradication: Tissue hypersensitivity halts the infection within 10 weeks.
  - Primary infection: Disease from initial infection
  - Latent infection: Asymptomatic with positive PPD, negative chest radiograph, noninfectious
- Active tuberculosis:
  - Develops from primary infection or reactivation of latent infection
  - Occurs in 10% of infected individuals without preventive therapy
  - Risk increases with immunosuppression and is highest the first 2 years after infection
  - Well-described forms: miliary (disseminated), meningeal, abdominal, and pulmonary
    - 85% of cases are pulmonary, which are contagious
    - Abdominal TB more common in the 3rd or 4th decade in women

Pediatric Considerations
- Disseminated TB is more common in infants; treat with 4 drugs if TB suspected.
- Children <4 are at increased risk for disseminated TB (lower-lobe infections more common); also have a higher rate of showing immediate clinical or radiographic signs.
- Older children and adolescents develop upper-lobe infiltrations; can have recurrence in adulthood.

EPIDEMIOLOGY
- 1/3 of world's population infected
- 2 million people worldwide die each year from TB

Incidence
TB incidence in 2008 (12): US 4.2/100,000; Worldwide 139/100,000

RISK FACTORS
- For infection:
  - Homeless, minority, residents, and employees in institutionalized settings; close contact with infected individual; foreign-born persons from areas with a high incidence of active tuberculosis (Asia, Africa, Latin America, former Soviet Union states); health care workers; frequent or prolonged visits to areas with a high prevalence of TB; and populations defined locally as having an increased incidence (e.g., medically underserved, low income, drug or alcohol abusers)
- For development of disease once infected:
  - HIV; lymphoma; silicosis; diabetes mellitus; chronic renal failure; cancer of head, neck, or lung; infants and children <5 years of age; malnutrition; gastrectomy; systemic corticosteroids at doses equivalent to ≤15 mg/day and other immunosuppressive drugs; IV drug abuse, alcohol abuse, cigarette smokers; recent infection with *M. tuberculosis* in the last 2 years; history of gastrectomy or jejunal bypass; <90% of ideal body weight

GENERAL PREVENTION
- Treat those with latent TB infection.
- Report to health department for treatment and identification and testing of all close contacts.
- Bacille Calmette Guérin (BCG) vaccine: Live attenuated *Mycobacterium bovis*:
  - Used more commonly in countries where TB is endemic
  - Prevents 50% of pulmonary disease and 80% of TB meningitis and miliary disease in children
  - In the US, consider BCG for children with negative PPD and HIV tests with unavoidable high risk and for health care workers at high risk for drug-resistant infection.

PATHOPHYSIOLOGY
- Cell-mediated response by the body causes accumulation of activated T lymphocytes and macrophages to form a "granuloma" that limits replication of organism. Destruction of the macrophages produces early "solid necrosis." In 2–3 weeks, this forms a soft cheesy necrotic environment; develops "caseous necrosis," establishing latency.
- In people with intact immunity, granuloma undergoes "fibrosis" and calcification; in people with less effective immune systems, it progresses to primary progressive tuberculosis.

ETIOLOGY
Mycobacterium tuberculosis, M. bovis, or *M. africanum*

COMMONLY ASSOCIATED CONDITIONS
HIV infection (emphasize direct observed therapy [DOT]); most recommendations remain the same

DIAGNOSIS

HISTORY
- Known exposure
- HIV status/risk factors
- Signs and symptoms:
  - General: Fever and night sweats, weight loss, malaise, painless adenopathy
  - Pulmonary TB: Cough, hemoptysis, pleuritic chest pain
  - Abdominal TB: Acute presentation often as surgical emergencies such as peritonitis or acute abdomen, obstruction, or perforation; chronic presentation may be doughy abdomen, vague abdominal symptoms, abdominal mass
  - Meningitis: See CNS TB chapter
  - Miliary: See Miliary TB chapter

PHYSICAL EXAM
- Often entirely normal; specific findings vary based on organ involvement and might include adenopathy, rales on lung exam, or hepatosplenomegaly
- Late findings: Renal, bone, or CNS disease

DIAGNOSTIC TESTS & INTERPRETATION
Lab
Initial lab tests
- Persons with TB should be tested for HIV; if positive, get CD4 count at baseline
- Baseline CBC, creatinine, AST, ALT, bilirubin, alkaline phosphatase, visual acuity, and red-green color discrimination
- If high risk: Test for hepatitis B and C (injection drug users, Africa or Asia born, HIV infected).

- If extrapulmonary suspected: Urine, cerebrospinal fluid, bone marrow, and liver biopsy for culture as indicated

Follow-Up & Special Considerations
Nonspecific laboratory findings include:
- Anemia, Monocytosis, Thrombocytosis, Hypergammaglobulinemia, SIADH, Sterile pyuria

Imaging
Initial approach
- Chest radiograph:
  - With primary TB: Infiltrate with or without effusion, atelectasis, or adenopathy
  - With recrudescent TB: Cavitary lesions and upper-lobe disease with hilar adenopathy
  - HIV: Atypical findings with primary infection, right upper-lobe atelectasis
- CT chest: Good sensitivity

Diagnostic Procedures/Surgery
- Tuberculin skin test (TST) (e.g., PPD): 5 U (0.1 mL) intermediate-strength intradermal injection into volar forearm. Measure induration at 48–72 hours.
  - PPD positive if induration:
    - >5 mm and HIV infection, immunosuppressed, recent TB contact, evidence of disease on chest film
    - >10 mm and age <4 years or other risk factors
    - >15 mm and age >4 years and no risk factors
    - 2-step test if no recent PPD, age >55, nursing home resident, prison inmate, or healthcare worker. Place 2nd test 1–3 weeks after initial test; interpret as usual.
  - Treatments that may alter PPD results:
    - False-positive: BCG (unreliable, should not influence decision to treat) or Steroids
    - False-negative: HIV, gastrectomy, alcoholism, renal failure, sarcoidosis, malnutrition, hematologic or lymphoreticular disorder
- 3 different morning sputum samples for acid-fast bacilli (AFB) stain and culture; use aerosol induction, gastric aspirate (children), or bronchoalveolar lavage if needed
  - If positive AFB, begin treatment immediately. Culture and sensitivity guide treatment.
- Interferon gamma release assays (IGRAs) measure interferon release after stimulation in vitro by *M. tuberculosis* antigens (3):
  - Lack of cross-reaction with BCG and most nontuberculous mycobacteria
    - Preferred for testing persons who have had BCG (vaccine or for cancer therapy)
  - Can be used in all settings in which skin testing is recommended with exceptions below:
    - TST is preferred in children <5 years old

Pathological Findings
- AFB stains: Positive
- Biopsy: Granulomas with central caseating necrosis

DIFFERENTIAL DIAGNOSIS
Other pneumonias, lymphomas, fungal infections, other atypical *Mycobacteria* or *Nocardia*

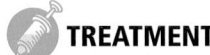

TREATMENT

MEDICATION
- Ideal body weight should be used to dose antitubercular drugs.
- No studies proving efficacy of 5 times weekly regimens, but supported by clinical evidence. DOT required for children, institutionalized patients, risk for nonadherence, and nondaily regimens. DOT strongly recommended for all regimens.

First Line
- Regimen 1 (Preferred) (4):
  - Initial phase:
    - Isoniazid (INH) 5 mg/kg, rifampin (RIF) 10 mg/kg, pyrazinamide (PZA) 15–30 mg/kg, and ethambutol (EMB) 15–20 mg/kg once daily for 8 weeks
    - OR, INH/RIF/PZA/EMB 5 days/wk for 8 weeks
  - Continuation phase:
    - INH/RIF daily for 18 weeks; or, if DOT, INH/RIF 5 days/wk for 18 weeks (Recommended for HIV + with CD4 <100 cells/mm^3 due to increased risk of resistance)
    - Or, INH/RIF 2–3 times a week for 18 weeks (not recommended if HIV+ with CD4 <100; may be associated with increased risk of relapse)
    - Or INH/rifapentine once weekly for 18 weeks (acceptable alternative only for HIV-patients without cavitary disease but may have increase risk of relapse) (4)
- Regimen 2
  - Initial Phase:
    - INH/RIF/PZA/EMB daily for 2 weeks then twice weekly for 6 weeks
    - OR INH/RIF/PZA/EMB 5 days/wk for 2 weeks then twice weekly for 6 weeks
  - Continuation phase
    - INH/RIF 2–3 times a week for 18 weeks (not recommended if HIV+ with CD4 <100; may have increased risk of relapse)
    - Or INH/rifapentine once weekly for 18 weeks (acceptable alternative only for HIV-patients without cavitary disease; may have increase risk of relapse) (4)
- Pregnancy:
  - Treat TB in pregnancy with INH, RIF, and EMB; supplement with pyridoxine 25 mg/day.

Pregnancy Considerations
  - Streptomycin: Caution—ototoxic and nephrotoxic; do not use in pregnancy.
  - Pyrazinamide is not usually used in pregnant women in the US.
- Congenital infection: may occur with miliary TB or endometrial TB in mother. If suspected, get PPD, CXR, lumbar puncture, culture placenta in infant. Start treatment promptly.
- Breastfeeding: OK while taking TB drugs; supplement with pyridoxine 25 mg/day
- Children: All the recommended medications are used except for ethambutol.
  - Children on medication may attend school.
- Maximum drug doses: INH 300 mg daily or 900 mg 2–3 times/wk, RIF 600 mg all regimens, PZA 2000 mg daily or 4000 mg 2 times/wk, EMB 1600 mg daily or 4000 mg 2 times/w

ALERT
- If patient doesn't receive PZA during entire first 2 months, extend treatment to a minimum of 9 months
- M. bovis is resistant to PZA and must be treated 9 months
- Continue EMB until drug susceptibility to INH+RIF is determined

Second Line
Steroids: Recommended for TB meningitis or pericarditis, use only with concomitant anti-TB therapy (5)[B].

ADDITIONAL TREATMENT
General Measures
- If clinical suspicion, treat immediately
- Prescribing physician responsible for treatment completion
- Ambulatory patients use mask and tissues
- Not infectious if favorable clinical response after 2–3 weeks of therapy and 3 negative AFB smears

Issues for Referral

ALERT
Refer drug resistant TB and HIV+ patients on antiretroviral therapy

SURGERY/OTHER PROCEDURES
For extrapulmonary complications (e.g., spinal cord compression, intestinal obstruction, constrictive pericarditis)

IN-PATIENT CONSIDERATIONS
- Place in an airborne infection isolation
- Use personal sealed respirators
- Three negative sputum AFB smears from different days for release from isolation

Discharge Criteria
Once the diagnosis of TB is ruled out or when the patient is being treated and has met the following:
- The patient is on effective therapy and making clinical improvement.
- An outpatient appointment has been arranged with a provider who will manage TB.
- Case management from the local public health department is involved and agrees with plan.
- The patient is in possession of sufficient anti-TB medication (not just prescriptions) to last until outpatient appointment.

ONGOING CARE

FOLLOW-UP RECOMMENDATIONS
Patient Monitoring
- Assess monthly for treatment adherence and adverse effects
- HIV+ need labs every 1–3 months: CD4 count, CBC, and liver enzymes
- Liver enzymes monthly if chronic liver disease, alcohol use, pregnant or postpartum. Temporarily discontinue medications if asymptomatic and enzymes are ≥5 times normal or if symptomatic and enzymes as ≥3 times normal.
- Visual acuity and red-green color discrimination monthly if on ethambutol more than 2 months or doses >20 mg/kg/day
- If culture is positive after 2 months of therapy, reassess drug sensitivity and initiate DOT.
- Chest radiograph at 3 months

PATIENT EDUCATION
- Emphasize importance of adherence to drug therapy.
- Identify patient contacts to notify.
- Let patient know that you are obligated to inform the local health department.
- CDC Questions and Answers about TB, 2009. At: http://www.cdc.gov/tb/publications/faqs/default.htm

PROGNOSIS
Generally few complications and full resolution of infection if drugs taken for full course as prescribed. If untreated, can lead to multiple complications, including death.

COMPLICATIONS
- Cavitary lesions can become secondarily infected.
- Drug resistance declining in US. At risk for drug resistance if HIV+, or treatment taken improperly, or if from an area with high incidence of resistance

REFERENCES
1. Global Tuberculosis Control: A short update to the 2009 report. WHO. 2009.
2. Pratt R, Robinson V, Navin T, et al. Trends in tuberculosis 2008. *MMWR*. 2009:58(10): 249–253.
3. Mazurek GH, Jereb J, Vernon A, et al. Updated Guidelines for using Interferon Gama Release Assays to Detect *Mycobacterium tuberculosis* Infection–United States,. 2010;59(RR05): 1–25.
4. Hall RG, Leff RD, Gumbo T. Treatment of Active Pulmonary Tuberculosis in Adults: Current Standrads and Recent Advances. *Pharmacotherapy*. 2009;29(12):1468–1481.
5. Golden MP, Vikram HR. Extrapulmonary tuberculosis: an overview. *Am Fam Physician*. 2005;72:1761–8.
6. Jacob JT, Mehta AK, Leonard MK. Acute Forms of Tuberculosis in Adults. *Am J Med*. 2009;122: 12–17.

See Also (Topic, Algorithm, Electronic Media Element)
- Tuberculosis, CNS; Tuberculosis, Latent; Tuberculosis, Miliary, Multiple Drug Resistant Tuberculosis
- Algorithm: Weight Loss

CODES

ICD9
- 011.90 Unspecified pulmonary tuberculosis, confirmation unspecified
- 795.5 Nonspecific reaction to tuberculin skin test without active tuberculosis

CLINICAL PEARLS
- Have high suspicion for TB in patients with chronic cough and 1 additional risk factor
- Patients ≥65 have few classic clinical and laboratory features of TB
- Consider acute TB in critically ill patients with enigmatic acute respiratory distress syndrome, shock, or disseminated intravascular coagulation (6)

T

TUBERCULOSIS, LATENT

Kay A. Bauman, MD, MPH

 BASICS

DESCRIPTION

- TB is a common infection transmitted by inhaling airborne bacilli from a person with active TB. The bacilli multiply in the alveoli and are carried by macrophages, lymphatics, and blood to distant sites (e.g., lung, pleura, brain, kidney, bone). Tissue hypersensitivity halts infection within 10 weeks.
- Latent TB infection (LTBI) is asymptomatic, noninfectious, and usually detected by a positive skin test (i.e., purified protein derivative [PPD]) or CXR, which is evidence of prior TB infection; acid-fast bacilli smear and culture are negative, and CXR does not suggest active TB.
- TB: Active disease occurs in 5–10% of infected individuals without preventive therapy. Chance of disease increases with immunosuppression and is highest for all individuals within 2 years of infection; 85% of the cases are pulmonary, which is infectious.
- LTBI treatment is a key component of the TB elimination strategy of the United States. For example, an estimated 4,000–11,000 active TB cases were prevented by LTBI treatment in 2002 (1).
- System(s) affected: Asymptomatic

EPIDEMIOLOGY

- High-risk groups include immigrants from Asia, Latin America, Africa, and the Pacific Basin; homeless persons; persons with a history of drug use or history of incarceration; HIV-infected individuals.
- Also at high risk are those newly exposed, including the pediatric population.

Prevalence

- In the US, approximately 4% of the population has latent TB infection.
- Worldwide, it is estimated that 1/3 of the population harbors latent TB.
- Predominant gender: Male > Female

RISK FACTORS

- HIV infection, immunosuppression
- Immigrants (from Asia, Africa, Latin America, Pacific Islands, or area with high rate of TB), including migrant workers
- Close contact with infected individual
- Institutional environment (e.g., prison, nursing home)
- Use of illicit drugs
- Lower socioeconomic status or homeless
- Health care workers
- Chronic disease such as DM, end-stage renal disease, cancer, or silicosis; organ transplant
- Persons with fibrotic changes on CXR consistent with previous TB infection (1)
- Recent TB skin test (TST) converters (1)
- Personnel from mycobacteriology laboratories
- Patients with organ transplants

GENERAL PREVENTION

Treatment of LTBI is preventive: The goal is to decrease the incidence of active TB in the individuals treated and to decrease the risk to close contacts should active TB occur.

ETIOLOGY

Mycobacterium tuberculosis, *M. bovis*, and *M. africanum*

COMMONLY ASSOCIATED CONDITIONS

- HIV infection (see Tests)
- Immune suppression

 DIAGNOSIS

HISTORY

History of immigration from a high-risk area, history of IV drug use and/or drug treatment, HIV, homelessness, recent incarceration

PHYSICAL EXAM

No signs of infection

DIAGNOSTIC TESTS & INTERPRETATION

Lab

Initial lab tests

- None routinely recommended
- In higher-risk patients: Liver profile, HCV and HBV screening
- HIV test recommended to assess risk for active TB in men who have sex with men or persons with a history of IV drug use

Imaging

Initial approach

- CXR required to rule out TB in asymptomatic infected persons
- CT scan of the chest has good sensitivity.

Diagnostic Procedures/Surgery

- PPD: 5 U (0.1 mL) intermediate-strength intradermal volar forearm. Measure induration at 48–72 hours:
  - Positive if induration is:
    - >5 mm and patient has HIV infection (or suspected) (1), is immunosuppressed, had recent close TB contact, or has clinical evidence of active or old disease on CXR.
    - >10 mm and patient <4 years old or has other risk factors noted above
    - >15 mm and patient >4 years old and has no risk factors (1,2)
  - Negative if induration <5 mm on initial test and, if indicated, on 2nd test
  - Use the 2-step test (administer a 2nd intradermal test 1–3 weeks after initial test; measure and interpret as usual) if patient has had no recent PPD and is >55 years old or is a nursing home resident, prison inmate, or health care worker (2).

- The interferon-γ blood test or QuantiFERON-TB and QuantiFERON-TB GOLD, measure the release of interferon-γ by sensitized lymphocytes when exposed to antigens of *M. tuberculosis*. It is unaffected by prior BCG vaccination, requires only 1 patient visit, and has improved sensitivity and specificity, but is costly (3).
- Special considerations:
  - Steroids: False-negative skin test
  - Measles vaccine: May suppress tuberculin activity; simultaneous PPD and measles vaccine recommended; if not simultaneous, defer PPD 4–6 weeks after measles vaccine.
  - The multiple-puncture tine test is not recommended.
  - Do not use BCG vaccination as a reason to ignore a positive PPD in adults and forego recommendation for treatment.
  - Disorders that may alter results and give a false-negative skin test:
    - Recent viral infection
    - New (<10 weeks) infection
    - Severe malnutrition
    - HIV
    - Anergy
    - Age <6 months
    - Overwhelming TB

DIFFERENTIAL DIAGNOSIS

Fungal infections; atypical mycobacteria or *Nocardia*

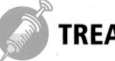 **TREATMENT**

MEDICATION

- INH scored tablets: 100 mg, 300 mg, or syrup 10 mg/mL:
  - Daily: Adult 300 mg; pediatric 10–15 mg/kg (maximum 300 mg) (2,4)
  - Twice weekly: Adult 15 mg/kg; pediatric 20–30 mg/kg (maximum 900 mg) (2,4)
  - Treatment for 9 months
- Precautions:
  - Follow liver function if the patient has history of liver dysfunction or new signs develop.
  - INH: Peripheral neuritis and hypersensitivity are possible. Consider pyridoxine (2).
  - INH: An idiosyncratic drug reaction that results in INH-associated severe liver injury has been reported by CDC in 17 patients in years 2004–2008. These included 15 adults and 2 children. 5 underwent liver transplantation and 5 subsequently died (1 of the liver transplant recipients). Thus, monitoring of patients while on treatment is recommended looking for symptoms of liver injury (all were symptomatic!), and not be limited to laboratory monitoring. The rate of this reaction is difficult to calculate as unknown numbers of patients are treated for LTBI, but 1 estimate is 291,000–433,000 per year in the US (5).

– Rifampin alone: Adults 600 mg per day for 4 months; children 10–20 mg/kg per day for 6 months. Less data exists for efficacy of this regimen, but can be considered for contacts of INH-resistant TB or patient with INH contraindications. In 1 study, the 4-month course increased compliance from 52.6% with INH to 71.6% with rifampin (6).

- Women may breastfeed while taking TB drugs.

ADDITIONAL TREATMENT
Pediatric Considerations
- Protocol for newborn with mother/household contact with infection or disease
- If mother or household contact has LTBI, skin test all household contacts and treat any with positive PPD.
- If contact has abnormal CXR, separate infant until infectious status known; if not contagious, monitor infant PPD (4).
- If mother has disease and is possibly contagious, evaluate infant for congenital TB and test for HIV; separate newborn until mother is noninfectious (4).
- If congenital TB is suspected, treat.
- If there is no congenital disease, start isoniazid (INH) and repeat PPD after 3–4 months. If positive, reassess infant and finish 9 months of INH. If PPD is negative and source is noninfectious, stop INH and monitor infant (4).

General Measures
- Must exclude active TB.
- Treatment for LTBI is crucial to control and eliminate TB disease in the US because it both decreases the risk of active TB in those treated and decreases risks to those potentially infected by those same people (1).
- Treat LTBI at any age if patient has HIV, has had close TB contact, is a recent converter (<2 years), is an IV drug user, has an abnormal CXR, has a high-risk medical condition, or is in another high-risk group:
  – Use INH for 9 months.
  – Preferred: INH 300 mg/d or 900 mg twice weekly × 9 months (1)
  – Acceptable alternative: INH 300 mg/d or 900 mg twice weekly × 6 months (1)
  – Directly observed therapy (DOT) is recommended if patient adherence is not assured.
- Treat LTBI during pregnancy if patient has recent infection or is HIV-positive (use INH with pyridoxine and monitor liver enzymes); otherwise, treatment may be postponed until postpartum (1).
- Special considerations for HIV infection and suspected INH resistance (1)
- Note: Because of severe liver injury and death associated with rifampin and pyrazinamide, these medications are no longer recommended for LTBI (1).
- Exclusions: Cirrhosis, active hepatitis, history of excessive alcohol consumption (1)

Additional Therapies
BCG vaccine, live-attenuated M. bovis: Used more commonly in developing countries to prevent complications of TB, especially in children

IN-PATIENT CONSIDERATIONS
Geriatric Considerations
- Before entering a chronic-care facility, patients should have a PPD using 2-step protocols.
- INH side effects are more pronounced.

Discharge Criteria
- Activity as tolerated
- No isolation required

 ## ONGOING CARE

FOLLOW-UP RECOMMENDATIONS
Patient Monitoring
- During preventive therapy for LTBI: Initial monthly visits to assess adherence to regimen and to monitor for hepatitis and neuropathy; if stable, can monitor less frequently.
- If patient remains asymptomatic, repeat CXR is not needed.
- Check liver enzymes if patient is symptomatic, is HIV-positive, has chronic liver disease, uses alcohol, or is pregnant or postpartum, and modify drugs if needed.

DIET
Regular; consider pyridoxine supplement, 10–50 mg/d

PROGNOSIS
- Generally there are few complications and treatment is effective if drugs are taken for full course as prescribed.
- Retreatment is not necessary.

COMPLICATIONS
Recrudescent TB

REFERENCES
1. Centers for Disease Control and Prevention. Guidelines for Preventing the Transmission of Mycobacterium TB in Health-Care Settings, 2005. MMWR Recomm Rep. 2005;54(RR-17):53–5.
2. Blumberg HM, Leonard MK, Jasmer RM. Update on the treatment of tuberculosis and latent tuberculosis infection. JAMA. 2005;293:2776–84.
3. Campos-Outcalt D. When, and when not, to use the interferon-gamma TB test. J Fam Pract. 2005;54:873–5.
4. American Academy of Pediatrics. Report of the Committee on Infectious Diseases (Red Book). Elk Grove Village, IL: American Academy of Pediatrics, 2003.
5. Centers for Disease Control and Prevention (CDC) et al. Severe isoniazid-associated liver injuries among persons being treated for latent tuberculosis infection - United States, 2004–2008. MMWR Morb. Mortal. Wkly. Rep. 2010;59:224–9.
6. Page KR, Sifakis F, Montes de Oca R, et al. Improved adherence and less toxicity with rifampin vs isoniazid for treatment of latent tuberculosis: a retrospective study. Arch Intern Med. 2006;166: 1863–70.

ADDITIONAL READING
- Centers for Disease Control and Prevention (CDC), American Thoracic Society. Update: adverse event data and revised American Thoracic Society/CDC recommendations against the use of rifampin and pyrazinamide for treatment of latent tuberculosis infection–United States, 2003. MMWR Morb Mortal Wkly Rep. 2003;52:735–9.
- Young DB, Gideon HP, Wilkinson RJ. Eliminating latent tuberculosis. Trends Microbiol. 2009.

See Also (Topic, Algorithm, Electronic Media Element)
Tuberculosis; Tuberculosis, Miliary

 ## CODES

ICD9
795.5 Nonspecific reaction to tuberculin skin test without active tuberculosis

CLINICAL PEARLS
- Treatment for latent TB is crucial to control and eliminate TB disease in the US, and an estimated 4% of the US population has LTBI.
- Test household contacts of PPD-positive patients.
- History of BCG vaccination, especially >10 years before PPD testing, should not be considered to be the cause of a positive PPD. The interferon-γ blood test is unaffected by prior BCG vaccination.
- Treat all HIV-positive patients with latent TB with a prophylactic regimen.

TUBERCULOSIS, MILIARY

Rajneesh S. Hazarika, MD, MS
Manju Ramchandani, MD

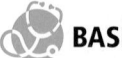 **BASICS**

DESCRIPTION
- Any progressive, disseminated form of tuberculosis (TB) resulting from uncontrolled hematogenous spread of *Mycobacterium tuberculosis*. Originally named for "millet seed" appearance of nodules often found in lungs. 3 types:
  - Acute: Usually with primary infection; rapidly progressive; more severe type
  - Late generalized: Occurs after years of latent infection; chronic, more indolent course
  - Anergic: Rare; microabscesses form in place of granulomas; generally a reactivation of old disease; older patients
- System(s) affected: Most commonly Pulmonary; Lymphatic; CNS (TB meningitis); Hepatic; Splenic; Bone Marrow
- Multiorgan failure and acute respiratory distress syndrome (ARDS) are also known to occur.
- Synonym(s): Disseminated TB

EPIDEMIOLOGY
Incidence
- 1–3% of all TB cases
- Worldwide incidence: 9.27 million new cases of TB in 2007 (139/100,000 population), out of which 1–3% may be miliary TB (1)
- In US in 2007, total new TB cases were 13,293 (4.4/100,000) (2).
- Predominant sex: Male > Female (as in all types of TB)

Prevalence
Global TB prevalence: 14.4 million (2006) corresponding to 219/100,000 population

RISK FACTORS
Within TB-infected population, risk factors for miliary disease include HIV/AIDS, young age (especially <1 year) or old age, iatrogenic immunosuppression (i.e., organ transplant patients, chronic corticosteroid use, tumor necrosis factor inhibitors), diabetes mellitus (DM), pregnancy, chronic renal failure, protein malnutrition, alcohol abuse, and immigration from higher prevalence regions.

GENERAL PREVENTION
- Bacille Calmette-Guérin (BCG) vaccine:
  - 78% effective at preventing severe meningeal and miliary TB in children (3)[B]
  - The effects of BCG do not increase with a second dose (4)[A].
- Treatment of latent TB infection with isoniazid (INH) (see Tuberculosis, Latent)

PATHOPHYSIOLOGY
- Lymphatic or hematogenous spread from a local focus, with failure of the body to halt infection by granulomatous encapsulation
- Commonly affects the more vascular organs (i.e., spleen, liver, brain, bone marrow)
- Iatrogenic disease is also reported after solid-organ transplants, urethral catheterization, and cardiac valve transplants.

ETIOLOGY
Mycobacterium infection in the context of impaired cell-mediated immunity:
- Primary infection in immunocompromised host or recrudescent infection in once-healthy host with new health impairment
- Iatrogenic infection as above

COMMONLY ASSOCIATED CONDITIONS
HIV/AIDS

 DIAGNOSIS

HISTORY
Ask about risk factors.

PHYSICAL EXAM
Presentation extremely variable, but may include:
- Night sweats (near 100%)
- Fever (96%)
- Weight loss, anorexia (92%)
- Tachypnea, tachycardia (77%)
- Cough, dyspnea (72%)
- Hepatomegaly (52%)
- Neurologic/HA/mental status changes (25%)
- Chills
- Single or multiorgan failure
- Severe disease resulting in septic shock and ARDS has been reported.
- Chest pain
- Vital signs: Fever, tachycardia, tachypnea common
- Pulmonary: Rales (50%)
- Hepatosplenomegaly common
- Lymphadenopathy
- Dilated funduscopic exam to look for choroidal tubercles (found in 50% postmortem)
- Evaluate for meningeal signs (tubercular meningitis)

DIAGNOSTIC TESTS & INTERPRETATION
Lab
Initial lab tests
- Purified protein derivative (PPD) test positive in <50% of patients
- Sputum for acid-fast bacillus (AFB) smear and culture
- Smears should be sent for acid-fast fluorochrome dye, auramine-O rather than traditional Ziehl-Nielson stain, because the former is more sensitive.
- QuantiFERON-TB gold test (5)[B]
- Gastric washings (especially in children), CSF, blood cultures, or bone and liver biopsy also for smear and culture
- *Mycobacterium* blood cultures
- Test for HIV
- Baseline liver enzymes, bilirubin, creatinine, complete blood count (CBC)
- If using ethambutol: Baseline visual acuity and color discrimination
- Test for hepatitis B and C.

Follow-Up & Special Considerations
- AFB smears and cultures

- Nonspecific laboratory findings include:
  - Anemia
  - Monocytosis
  - Thrombocytosis
  - Hypergammaglobulinemia
  - Syndrome of inappropriate antidiuretic hormone (SIADH)
  - Sterile pyuria
  - Steroids: False-negative skin test

Pediatric Considerations
May need to culture samples from infected adult contact because samples can be difficult to obtain in pediatric patients

Imaging
- CXR: Faint reticulonodular infiltrate, uniform distribution; often mediastinal/hilar adenopathy
- Chest CT scan: Numerous 2- to 3-mm nodules scattered throughout lungs in >85% of patients; chest CT scan more sensitive than CXR (6)[B].
- Abdominal/pelvic CT scan: If suspicious of other organ involvement
- Brain MRI: Cerebral nodules or tuberculoma; only if neurologic symptoms present

Diagnostic Procedures/Surgery
- See Tuberculosis.
- Collect samples for AFB/culture. Sampling fluids from multiple sites greatly improves yield for AFB smear and culture:
  - Sputum culture positive in 62% (smear in 33%)
  - Bronchial lavage (BAL) culture positive in 55% (smear in 27%)
  - Gastric aspirate culture positive in 100% (smear in 43%)
  - CSF culture positive in 60% (smear in 8%)
- Biopsy organs based on symptoms.

Pathological Findings
- Caseating granulomas on tissue biopsy (liver most common site)
- Microabscesses with neutrophilic response in acute type
- Can see mycotic aneurysms if disease affects aorta
- TB pericarditis diagnosed by pericardial biopsy

DIFFERENTIAL DIAGNOSIS
- Other pneumonias
- Lymphoma
- Metastatic carcinoma
- Sarcoidosis
- Sepsis

 TREATMENT

- Diagnosis often is impeded by low suspicion and delay in collecting fluid/tissue samples for AFB smear and culture.
- Identify and test any close contacts.

MEDICATION
- All drug regimens are the same as those for general TB.
- Adherence extremely important to prevent drug resistance; directly observed therapy (DOT) indicated

First Line

- Regimen 1 (preferred):
  - Initial phase: Isoniazid (INH), rifampin (RIF), pyrazinamide (PZA), and ethambutol (EMB) once daily × 8 weeks
  - Continuation phase: INH/RIF daily × 18 weeks *or* INH/RIF twice weekly × 18 weeks (only use for HIV+ patients if CD4 >100) *or* INH/rifapentine once weekly × 18 weeks (acceptable alternative for HIV-patients only) (7)[A]
- Regimen 2:
  - Initial phase: INH/RIF/PZA/EMB daily × 2 weeks, then twice weekly × 6 weeks
  - Continuation phase: INH/RIF twice weekly × 18 weeks (HIV+ patients only if CD4 >100) *or* INH/rifapentine once weekly × 18 weeks (acceptable alternative for HIV patients only) (7)[A]
- Regimen 3 (acceptable alternative):
  - Initial phase: INH/RIF/PZA/EMB daily × 8 weeks
  - Continuation phase: INH/RIF 3× weekly × 18 weeks (7)[A]
- Regimen 4 (only when unable to give preferred regimen):
  - Initial phase: INH/RIF/EMB daily × 8 weeks
  - Continuation phase: INH/RIF daily or twice weekly × 31 weeks (7)[B]
- No studies proving efficacy of 5× weekly regimen, but clinical evidence suggests it (7)[C].
- DOT required for nondaily regimens (7).
- Dosing:
  - INH: Scored tabs 50/100/300 mg, syrup 10 mg/mL, or aqueous solution 100 mg/mL:
    - Daily dose: Adult 5 mg/kg (maximum 300 mg); pediatric 10–15 mg/kg (maximum 300 mg)
    - 3× weekly: Adult 15 mg/kg (maximum 900 mg)
    - Twice weekly: Adult 15 mg/kg (maximum 900 mg); pediatric 20–30 mg/kg (maximum 900 mg)
    - Weekly: Adult only, 15 mg/kg (maximum 900 mg)
    - Consider pyridoxine 10–50 mg/d.
  - RIF: Capsules 150/300 mg, powder for oral suspension, or IV aqueous:
    - Daily or twice-weekly dose: Adult and pediatric 10–20 mg/kg (maximum 600 mg)
  - PZA: Scored tabs 500 mg; dosed by weight:
    - Adults 40–55 kg: Daily: 18–25 mg/kg, maximum 1 g; 3× weekly: 27–37 mg/kg (maximum 1.5 g); twice weekly: 36–50 mg/kg, maximum 2 g
    - Adults 56–75 kg: Daily: 20–27 mg/kg, maximum 1.5 g; 3× weekly: 33–45 mg/kg, maximum 2.5 g; twice weekly: 40–54 mg/kg, maximum 3 g
    - Adults >75 kg: Daily: 22–26 mg/kg, maximum 2 g; 3× weekly: 33–40 mg/kg, maximum 3 g; twice weekly: 44–53 mg/kg, maximum 4 g
    - Pediatric daily: 15–30 mg/kg (maximum 2 g)
    - Pediatric twice weekly: 50 mg/kg (maximum 4 g)
  - Rifabutin (Mycobutin): Capsules 150 mg:
    - Daily or twice weekly: Adult 5 mg/kg, maximum 300 mg
  - Rifapentine (Priftine): Tablet 150 mg; for continuation phase only. HIV adults: 600 mg once weekly, given with INH; not effective if HIV+ (7)[A]

- EMB: Tablets 100/400 mg bacteriostatic; dose based on weight:
  - Adults 40–55 kg: Daily: 15–20 mg/kg, maximum 800 mg; 3× weekly: 22–30 mg/kg, maximum 1.2 g; twice weekly: 36–50 mg/kg, maximum 2 g
  - Adults 56–75 kg: Daily: 16–22 mg/kg, max 1.2 g; 3× weekly: 27–36 mg/kg, maximum 2 g; twice weekly: 37–50 mg/kg, maximum 2.8 g
  - Adults >75 kg: Daily: 22–26 mg/kg, maximum 2.6 g; 3× weekly: 33–40 mg/kg, maximum 2.4 g; twice weekly: 44–53 mg/kg, maximum 4 g
  - Pediatrics: Daily: 15–20 mg/kg, maximum 1 g; twice weekly: 50 mg/kg, maximum 4 g
- Contraindications:
  - RIF: Avoid if patient taking antiretrovirals.
  - EMB: May cause optic neuritis; avoid unless patient is old enough to cooperate for visual acuity and color testing.
- Precautions:
  - INH, RIF, PZA: May cause hepatitis; caution if liver disease
  - RIF: Colors urine, tears, and secretions orange; can stain contact lenses
  - INH: Peripheral neuritis and hypersensitivity possible; treat with pyridoxine.
  - PZA: May increase uric acid; unclear safety during pregnancy (7)[C]
- Significant possible interactions: Rifamycins alter level of phenytoin, antivirals, and other drugs metabolized by liver and may inactivate birth control pills (recommend a barrier method).

Second Line

Corticosteroids: Use only with concurrent anti-TB therapy. Recommended for TB meningitis, pericarditis, or severe miliary disease (3)[B]:

- Reduce fluid reaccumulation in pericarditis, but no proven mortality benefit (7)[B]
- Also for HIV+ population
- Streptomycin: Caution: May cause ototoxic and nephrotoxic; do not use in pregnancy.

ADDITIONAL TREATMENT
General Measures
- Respiratory isolation if pulmonary disease; negative-pressure room
- TB mask when out of room

Issues for Referral
Infectious disease specialist is helpful for patients also on antiretrovirals because doses may need adjusting.

Pregnancy Considerations
Streptomycin cannot be used in pregnancy.

SURGERY/OTHER PROCEDURES
- Location- and patient-specific
- Medical treatment unresponsiveness may require surgical intervention.

 ## ONGOING CARE
FOLLOW-UP RECOMMENDATIONS
- General TB follow-up
- Most states require department of public health notification.

Patient Monitoring
See Tuberculosis.

DIET
- Some evidence suggests that high-cholesterol diet accelerates sterilization of sputum in pulmonary TB patients.
- Specific malnutrition correction

PATIENT EDUCATION
As for general TB

PROGNOSIS
- Mortality: 16–38%
- If ARDS develops, mortality is 80–100%.

COMPLICATIONS
- ARDS with refractory hypoxemia can occur.
- Multidrug-resistant TB is rare in the US but increasing elsewhere.

REFERENCES
1. Global tuberculosis control - epidemiology, strategy, financing WHO Report 2009. http://www.who.int/tb/publications/global_report/2009/en/index.html
2. Trends in Tuberculosis – United States 2007. *MMWR.* 2008;57(11):281–85.
3. Colditz GA, Brewer TF, Berkey CS, et al. Efficacy of BCG vaccine in the prevention of tuberculosis. Meta-analysis of the published literature. *JAMA.* 1994;271:698–702.
4. Pereira SM, Dantas OM, Ximenes R, et al. [BCG vaccine against tuberculosis: its protective effect and vaccination policies]. *Rev Saude Publica.* 2007;41(Suppl 1):59–66.
5. Updated Guidelines for using Interferon Gamma Release Assays to Detect Mycobacterium tuberculosis Interferon - United States, 2010; 2010;59(RRO5):1–25.
6. Optican RJ.High-resolution computed tomography in the diagnosis of miliary tuberculosis. *Chest.* 1992;102(3):941–3.
7. Potter B. Management of active TB. *Am Fam Physician.* 2005;72(11).

See Also (Topic, Algorithm, Electronic Media Element)
Tuberculosis, Tuberculosis, CNS

CODES

ICD9
- 018.00 Acute miliary tuberculosis, unspecified examination
- 018.80 Other specified miliary tuberculosis, unspecified examination
- 018.90 Unspecified miliary tuberculosis, unspecified examination

CLINICAL PEARLS
- Chest CT scan is more sensitive than CXR.
- PPD is positive in <50% of patients.

TUBEROUS SCLEROSIS COMPLEX

Michele Roberts, MD, PhD
Beverly N. Hay, MD

BASICS

DESCRIPTION
- Tuberous sclerosis complex (TSC) is a genetic neurocutaneous syndrome (phakomatosis). Many organ systems are affected, with the formation of multiple hamartomas.
- Manifestations may be subtle but can include lesions of the central nervous system, skin, retina, heart, lung, viscera, kidney, bone, teeth, liver, and nails.
- System(s) affected: Cardiovascular; Musculoskeletal; Nervous; Pulmonary; Renal/Urologic; Skin/Exocrine
- Synonym(s): Bourneville disease

Pregnancy Considerations
Prenatal diagnosis by mutational analysis is possible when a molecular cause is known.

EPIDEMIOLOGY
Incidence
- 1/5,000–1/10,000 live births
- Predominant age: Clinical expression is variable; usually diagnosed during the 1st decade of life.
- Predominant gender: Male = Female, but autism is more common in males.

RISK FACTORS
- Family history
- Expressivity is variable, even within a family.
- If neither parent of an affected child meets criteria for TSC, then the recurrence risk is 1–2% per child due to the possibility of parental germ-line mosaicism.

Genetics
- Autosomal dominant with complete penetrance and variable expressivity
- OMIM 191100
- 2/3 of cases result from new mutations.
- 2 chromosomal loci have been mapped: Tuberous sclerosis complex 1 (*TSC1*, 9q34) and tuberous sclerosis complex 2 (*TSC2*, 16p13.3)
- Somatic mosaicism occurs in 2–10% of de novo tuberous sclerosis (TS).
- Clinical phenotype of *TSC1* mutations generally is milder than that of *TSC2* mutations, but genotype–phenotype correlation is not established.

GENERAL PREVENTION
Genetic counseling

PATHOPHYSIOLOGY
Mutations in either of two genes *TSC1* and *TSC2* that code for the tumor growth-suppressor proteins hamartin and tuberin, respectively:
- The hamartin–tuberin complex is involved in cell proliferation and differentiation.
- Mutations may result in decreased production of these proteins and excessive cell proliferation, resulting in tuber formation.

ETIOLOGY
Some hamartomas in patients with TS show loss of heterozygosity in the chromosomal region 9q34 or 16p13.3.
- This implies that the patient has inherited a mutation or a deletion in one copy of the gene, but the patient develops a lesion only when there is a somatic mutation in the other copy.

- This 2-hit mechanism appears to apply to cardiac rhabdomyomas, renal angiomyolipomas, and subependymal giant cell tumors, but not to cerebral tubers.

COMMONLY ASSOCIATED CONDITIONS
- Mental retardation (60–70%), usually associated with history of seizures
- Seizures (80%); 25% of patients with infantile spasms have TS
- Autism (10–20%)
- Cardiac arrhythmias
- Renal insufficiency

DIAGNOSIS

- Physical examination and imaging are most useful, although molecular diagnostics may be useful when clinical criteria are not met or for family members of affected patients.
- Diagnostic criteria for TS (1) (approximate percentage of patients affected):
  - Major criteria:
    - Facial angiofibromas (80%) or forehead plaques (50%)
    - Shagreen patch (connective tissue nevus)
    - 3 or more hypomelanotic macules (50%)
    - Nontraumatic ungula or periungual fibromas (20%)
    - Lymphangioleiomyomatosis (<10%, also known as lymphangiomyomatosis), predominantly in premenopausal women
    - Renal angiomyolipoma
    - Cardiac rhabdomyoma (50%, mostly in newborns)
    - Multiple retinal nodular hamartomas (50–80%)
    - Cortical tuber
    - Subependymal nodules
    - Subependymal giant cell astrocytoma
  - Minor criteria:
    - Confetti skin lesions (multiple 1- to 2-mm hypomelanotic macules)
    - Gingival fibromas
    - Multiple randomly distributed pits in dental enamel
    - Hamartomatous rectal polyps
    - Multiple renal cysts (50–80%)
    - Nonrenal hamartomas (liver hamartoma in 10%)
    - Bone cysts
    - Retinal achromic patch
    - Cerebral white matter radial migration lines
- Definite TS: 2 major criteria or 1 major criterion and 2 minor criteria
- Probable TS: 1 major criterion and 1 minor criterion
- Possible TS: 1 major criterion or 2 minor criteria
- 95% of patients with TSC may have a seizure disorder.
- Although epilepsy and mental retardation are more common in TS, they are not included among diagnostic criteria because they are common in the general population (2).
- Hypomelanotic macules often can be seen in newborns, especially with Wood lamp examination.

- When a new diagnosis is made in a child with no family history of TSC, careful evaluation of the parents should include:
  - A comprehensive dermatologic examination (in room light and with a Wood lamp)
  - Ophthalmologic examination
  - Cranial CT scan or MRI
  - Renal ultrasound

HISTORY
- Family history of TSC stigmata; about 1/3 of patients with TSC have a positive family history.
- Assess for seizures and developmental delay in children.
- Patients with TSC are at increased risk of brain tumors and may present with symptoms of obstructive hydrocephalus, including headaches, vomiting, and neurologic deficits (including loss of vision). Children with obstructive hydrocephalus may present with nonspecific symptoms, including fatigue, decreased appetite, depression, and increased frequency of seizures.

PHYSICAL EXAM
- Dermatologic:
  - 96% percent of patients with TSC have characteristic skin lesions, which include (3)
    - Hypopigmented macules (ash-leaf spots, usually elliptical), not usually present before age 5 years
    - Angiofibromas (formerly, and incorrectly, *adenoma sebaceum*), typically involving the malar regions of the face (butterfly distribution), usually appear later than hypopigmented macules.
    - Shagreen patches, most commonly on the lower trunk
  - A brown fibrous plaque on the forehead may be the 1st recognized feature of TSC on physical examination of infants.
  - Periungual and ungual fibromas may appear in adolescence or adulthood.
- Ophthalmologic:
  - Funduscopic evaluation:
    - Retinal hamartomas: Hamartoma may be a flat, translucent lesion (most common) or a multilobular mulberry lesion (with calcification), or may have features of both.
    - Retinal giant cell astrocytoma, secondary retinal detachment
    - Chorioretinal depigmentation (punched-out appearance)
    - Papilledema or visual loss: Suggestive of brain tumors
    - An abnormal red reflex should not be mistaken for retinoblastoma.
  - Angiofibromas of the eyelids, nonparalytic strabismus, colobomas, and sector iris depigmentation
  - Refractive errors not different from those of the general population
- Dental: Multiple, randomly distributed pits in dental enamel
- Neurologic: Focal deficits may indicate growth of brain tumors.

DIAGNOSTIC TESTS & INTERPRETATION
Lab
Molecular diagnostics:
- Mutations can be detected in approximately 75% of patients who meet the diagnostic criteria for TS.

- Mutations in the *TSC2* gene are about 3 times as common as those of the *TSC1* gene (4).
- Identification of a mutation in *TSC1* or *TSC2* can confirm the diagnosis in a child whose clinical evaluation is suggestive but not diagnostic of TSC.
- A negative result in molecular testing cannot rule out TS in a patient with a clinical diagnosis of TS.
- Mutational analysis is useful for prenatal diagnosis and for evaluation of relatives of those with a known mutation.

Imaging
Initial approach
- Cranial MRI before age 2, with gadolinium enhancement.
- Fetal cardiac rhabdomyomas may be seen by ultrasound or MRI in late gestation.
- CT scan or ultrasound of kidneys
- Pulmonary CT scan or chest imaging of the lungs, as indicated, in females beginning at age 18; pulmonary pathology is uncommon in males.

Diagnostic Procedures/Surgery
- Ash-leaf spots more readily seen with a Wood lamp
- Biopsy of questionable lesions
- Clinical neuropsychological evaluation may reveal attentional deficits in children and adolescents with TSC, even when they have normal intellectual abilities and no seizures or disruptive behaviors (5)[B].

Pathological Findings
- Lesions may be sparse at birth.
- Facial angiofibromas, ungual fibromas, and renal angiomyolipomas may develop months or years after birth.
- Brain lesions:
  - Cortical tubers (glioneural hamartomas): Histology shows disorganized neuronal and glial elements with astrocytosis. Epileptogenic nature is widely accepted, but controversial.
  - White matter heterotopia: Dysplastic and dysmyelinated white matter
  - Subependymal nodules: Hamartomas composed of atypical enlarged glial and neuronal cells may transform to giant cell astrocytomas (from which they are histologically indistinguishable except for size).
  - Subependymal giant cell astrocytomas
  - Giant cell astrocytomas are of mixed glioneuronal lineage.
  - Calcification of subependymal lesions may not occur until several months after birth.
  - Extensive anatomic abnormalities may be seen in gray and white matter, even in patients with normal intelligence.
- Renal lesions (50–80%):
  - Angiomyolipomas, benign cysts, and lymphangiomas
  - Lesions may adversely affect renal function.
- Pulmonary lesions:
  - 1% of patients with TSC may present with pulmonary lymphangioleiomyomatosis.
  - These patients are usually women of reproductive age.
- Cardiac rhabdomyoma (50–70% of infants), usually asymptomatic.

DIFFERENTIAL DIAGNOSIS
- Non-TSC polycystic kidney disease
- Other causes of seizure disorders, mental retardation, autistic behavior
- Traumatic ungual fibromata

- Other phakomatoses: Neurofibromatosis, Sturge-Weber syndrome, von Hippel-Lindau syndrome.

TREATMENT
MEDICATION
- Anticonvulsants for seizure control
- No drugs are routinely used for TSC management, although the biochemical rationale for the potential use of rapamycin has been described in detail, with clinical trials suggesting that this agent may be useful to treat TSC (6).

ADDITIONAL TREATMENT
Issues for Referral
- A multidisciplinary team should evaluate every new patient: Genetics, neurology, ophthalmology, nephrology, surgery, dermatology, neurosurgery, radiology, and plastic surgery.
- Physical therapy, occupational therapy, and speech therapy; social workers for home care, vocational training support

SURGERY/OTHER PROCEDURES
Surgery may be necessary for hydrocephalus, increased intracranial pressure, rapidly growing subependymal giant cell tumors, malignant tumors, and seizure control.

ONGOING CARE
FOLLOW-UP RECOMMENDATIONS
Patient Monitoring
- Pediatric:
  - Annual physical examination, growth assessment, ophthalmologic examination
  - Annual developmental testing and review of school progress, neuropsychologic evaluation, and IQ testing if indicated
  - Echocardiography
    - Pediatric cardiologist should follow children with cardiac rhabdomyoma.
    - Cardiac rhabdomyomas typically develop in utero, regress spontaneously in early childhood, and involute completely by adulthood.
- Electroencephalogram: For seizure management
- Renal ultrasound: Every 1–3 years beginning in adolescence; abdominal MRI or CT scan for evaluation of large angioleiomyomas
- Chest CT scan: For pulmonary dysfunction
- Screening MRI without contrast (7): Every 1–3 years for children and adolescents, less frequently in adults; if a giant cell astrocytoma is identified, surgery is performed, if appropriate. Otherwise, repeat cranial MRI every 3–6 months.

PATIENT EDUCATION
Tuberous Sclerosis Alliance, 801 Roeder Road, Suite 750, Silver Spring, MD, 20910; (800) 225-6872; e-mail: info@tsalliance.org; http://www.tsalliance.org/

PROGNOSIS
Variable; shortened longevity in individuals with complications

COMPLICATIONS
- In addition to benign tumors associated with TSC (e.g., angiofibromas, hamartomas, rhabdomyomas, and angiomyolipomas), there is an 18-fold increase in risk of malignancy, especially of the kidney, brain, and soft tissues.
- Rhabdomyosarcoma, although rare, has increased incidence in TSC.

- 1–2% of adults develop renal cell carcinoma, 25 years earlier than in general population.
- CNS complications, including epilepsy, cognitive impairment, behavioral problems, hyperactivity, self-injurious behavior, and autism, occur in 85% of children and adolescents with TS.
- Neuropsychological attention deficits may be greater than intellectual impairment.
- Causes of death: Neurologic disease most common (subependymal giant cell tumors and status epilepticus), renal disease, pulmonary disease
- Subependymal giant cell tumors are benign but may undergo malignant transformation or may grow rapidly or hemorrhage.

REFERENCES

1. Roach ES, Gomez MR, Northrup H. Tuberous sclerosis complex consensus conference: revised clinical diagnostic criteria. *J Child Neurol*. 1998;13:624–8.
2. Roach ES, Sparagana SP. Diagnosis of tuberous sclerosis complex. *J Child Neurol*. 2004;19:643–9.
3. Webb DW, Clarke A, Fryer A, et al. The cutaneous features of tuberous sclerosis: a population study. *Br J Dermatol*. 1996;135:1–5.
4. Au KS, Williams AT, Roach ES, et al. Genotype/phenotype correlation in 325 individuals referred for a diagnosis of tuberous sclerosis complex in the United States. *Genet Med*. 2007;9:88–100.
5. de Vries PJ, Gardiner J, Bolton PF, et al. Neuropsychological attention deficits in tuberous sclerosis complex (TSC). *Am J Med Genet A*. 2009;149A:387–95.
6. Orlova KA, Crino PB, et al. The tuberous sclerosis complex. *Ann N Y Acad Sci*. 2010;1184:87–105.
7. Goh S, Butler W, Thiele EA. Subependymal giant cell tumors in tuberous sclerosis complex. *Neurology*. 2004;63:1457–61.

See Also (Topic, Algorithm, Electronic Media Element)
Neurofibromatosis

CODES
ICD9
759.5 Tuberous sclerosis

CLINICAL PEARLS

Hypopigmented areas (e.g., ash-leaf spots), mainly on trunk and extremities, are often the 1st sign, present at birth or shortly after (50%). These are best seen with a Wood lamp.

TURNER SYNDROME

Michele Roberts, MD, PhD

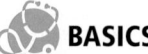 **BASICS**

DESCRIPTION
- A condition characterized by ovarian dysgenesis and short stature in phenotypic females who have only 1 sex chromosome, an X; although a partial 2nd sex chromosome, X or Y, may be present
- The most common sex chromosome abnormality syndrome in females
- System(s) affected: Cardiovascular; Reproductive; Endocrine/Metabolic; Musculoskeletal; Nervous; Renal/Urologic
- Synonym(s): Ullrich-Turner syndrome; Bonnevie-Ullrich syndrome; Monosomy X; Sexual infantilism; Gonadal dysgenesis

EPIDEMIOLOGY
Incidence
- 1/2,000–5,000 live female births
- 1–3% of all conceptuses affected, fewer than 1% of whom will survive to term
- Accounts for 15% of all spontaneously aborted fetuses
- Predominant sex: Female only

Prevalence
Estimated 50,000–75,000 girls and women in US with TS

RISK FACTORS
Genetics
- 50% of patients with TS have 45,X karyotype (sporadic nondisjunction). Translocations involving the X chromosome may result in TS.
- 80% of girls with 45,X have maternal X, although phenotype is identical if X is paternal.
- TS occurs with a deletion of the *SRY* segment of the Y chromosome in 46,XY karyotype, with resulting female phenotype (5–6%) (1).
- It is important to identify Y chromosomal material because of increased risk of gonadoblastoma (7–10%) if Y material is present. FISH or PCR may be necessary to identify Y material.
- Also may be mosaic for 45,X/46,XY; 45,X/46,XX; or 45,X/47,XXX

PATHOPHYSIOLOGY
The *SHOX* gene (short stature homeobox-containing gene), located in the pseudoautosomal region of the X chromosome, may be responsible for short stature and skeletal abnormalities in TS.

ETIOLOGY
Monosomy for all or part of the X chromosome can result in features of TS. Genes involved are located mainly in Xp11.2–p22.1.

COMMONLY ASSOCIATED CONDITIONS
- Very frequent (>50%):
  - Gonadal dysgenesis
  - Short stature
- Frequent (>5–10% but <50% of individuals):
  - Cardiovascular abnormalities, including coarctation, aortic valvular disease, aortic dissection
  - Renal abnormalities
  - Hypertension
  - Glucose intolerance
  - Hyperlipidemia
  - Ocular abnormalities
  - Hypothyroidism, autoimmune thyroiditis
  - Gastrointestinal (GI) vascular malformations
  - Glucose intolerance
  - Hearing loss, otitis media
  - Gonadoblastoma in 8% of individuals with Y chromosomal material
- Occasional (<5% of individuals):
  - Inflammatory bowel disease, celiac disease
  - Colon cancer
  - Neuroblastoma
  - Juvenile rheumatoid arthritis
  - Liver disease, especially cirrhosis

 DIAGNOSIS

HISTORY
- Edema of hands and feet and redundant skin of the neck (webbing) are presenting features during infancy.
- During adolescence, primary amenorrhea, short stature, and infantile secondary sex characteristics are presenting features.

PHYSICAL EXAM
- Frequencies are for classic 45,X and vary with other chromosomal abnormalities associated with TS (2).
- Very frequent (>50% of individuals):
  - Short stature
  - Lymphedema of hands and feet present at birth, and may recur
  - Deep-set hyperconvex nails
  - Unusual shape and rotation of ears
  - Narrow maxilla and dental crowding
  - Micrognathia
  - Low posterior hairline
  - Broad chest with widely spaced, inverted, or hypoplastic nipples
  - Cubitus valgus
  - Short 4th metacarpals and/or metatarsals
  - Tibial exostosis
  - Tendency to obesity
  - Recurrent otitis media
- Frequent (<50% of individuals):
  - Pigmented nevi
  - Webbed neck
  - Keloid formation
- Occasional (<5% of individuals): Scoliosis, kyphosis, lordosis

DIAGNOSTIC TESTS & INTERPRETATION
Lab
Initial lab tests
Chromosome analysis: A buccal smear is not adequate to rule out diagnosis of TS. An analysis of at least 20–30 cells is required. Analysis of 2 cell types (e.g., blood and skin) may be necessary.

Follow-Up & Special Considerations
- At puberty, follicle-stimulating hormone (FSH) and luteinizing hormone levels may approach levels consistent with absence of ovaries. FSH may be transiently high in infancy.
- High incidence of thyroid problems should prompt annual evaluation of thyroid function.

Imaging
Initial approach
- Magnetic resonance angiography in addition to echocardiography to evaluate cardiovascular system (3)
- Renal ultrasound to evaluate structural renal abnormalities

Diagnostic Procedures/Surgery
- Upper and lower extremity blood pressure (BP)
- Routine hearing exam
- Assess for congenital hip dislocation

Pathological Findings
- Ovarian dysgenesis (>90%): Streak gonads, atretic follicles, or no follicles present
- Renal: Horseshoe kidney, double collecting system (60%)
- Cardiac (20–40% of patients): Bicuspid aortic valve, coarctation of aorta, valvular aortic stenosis (70% of TS patients with heart defects also have coarctation), hypertension
- Bone dysplasia (>50%), osteoporosis
- Gonadoblastomas in patients with X/XY mosaicism
- Ocular abnormalities: Amblyopia, ptosis, strabismus, red/green color blindness
- GI: Increased incidence of celiac disease
- Central nervous system abnormalities: Attention deficit hyperactivity disorder (ADHD), decreased visuospatial organization

DIFFERENTIAL DIAGNOSIS
- Short stature:
  - Noonan syndrome: A genetic condition that shares some facial and other physical characteristics with TS (but is unrelated to TS); has been described inaccurately as "male TS"
  - Hypothyroidism
  - Familial short stature
  - Dyschondrosteosis (Léri-Weill syndrome)
  - Brachydactyly E
  - Growth hormone deficiency
  - Glucocorticoid excess
  - Klippel-Feil anomaly
  - Short stature due to chronic disease
- Amenorrhea or delayed puberty:
  - Pure gonadal dysgenesis
  - Polycystic ovary syndrome (Stein-Leventhal syndrome)
  - Primary/secondary amenorrhea
- Lymphedema:
  - Hereditary congenital lymphedema
  - Milroy disease
  - Lymphedema with recurrent cholestasis
  - Lymphedema with intestinal lymphangiectasia
- Other:
  - Multiple pterygium syndrome
  - Pseudohypoparathyroid syndrome

 TREATMENT

MEDICATION
- Recombinant growth hormone:
  - When there is any evidence of growth failure (4)[C]; height falls below the 5th percentile by 18 months of age. Adult height is maximized if growth hormone is initiated at a young age:
    - 0.375–0.400 mg/kg/week
    - Anabolic steroids may be used in conjunction with GH.

- Estrogen:
  - Due to accelerated follicular atresia, most girls with TS undergo ovarian failure prior to or around the time of puberty. Treat gonadal failure in girls who do not enter puberty spontaneously:
    - Replacement therapy: Starting at age 13–14 years, continuing to age 50. Begin with 1–2 years of low-dose estrogen, followed by larger-dose estrogens cycled with progesterone.
    - Promotes sexual development and bone maturation, optimizes peak bone mass
    - May benefit cognitive development in young girls

ADDITIONAL TREATMENT
General Measures
- Although pregnancy is rare, sexually active girls and women should receive counseling re: contraception.
- Infertility is the general rule; <2% of pregnancies are achieved without medical assistance (1):
  - Alternatives such as in vitro fertilization and embryo transfer may be options. Successful ovarian transplant has been reported in teenage girls with Turner syndrome (5). Recent reports describe controlled ovarian hyperstimulation and oocyte cryopreservation to preserve fertility in mosaic Turner (6).
  - High risk of maternal mortality secondary to cardiac complications during pregnancy. Aortic root dimensions must be monitored throughout pregnancy by echo.
- Intelligence is usually normal. Problems may exist in nonverbal areas such as evaluating objects in relationship to one another. If concerns about school performance arise, patients should be evaluated and treated. Patients may be at risk for ADHD (1).

Issues for Referral
Congenital heart disease, bicuspid aortic valve, coarctation of the aorta, aortic dissection (especially with valvular abnormalities or coarctation, or systemic hypertension) (3)

SURGERY/OTHER PROCEDURES
- Removal of gonads is recommended in patients with X/XY mosaicism due to risk of gonadoblastoma.
- Surgical correction of coarctation of the aorta
- Physical appearance may be enhanced by reconstructive surgery.

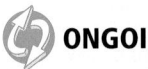 **ONGOING CARE**

FOLLOW-UP RECOMMENDATIONS
Patient Monitoring
- For complete health supervision guidelines, see Frias et al. (2).
- Regular cardiac exams; ultrasound/MRI at pubertal induction
- Every 4–6 months (7):
  - Height, weight, BP
  - Pubertal staging (after age 10)
- Every 12–18 months:
  - Thyroid function and IGF-1
  - Bone age
  - Hearing and vision assessment
- Every 3–5 years: Dual energy x-ray absorptiometry scan for bone density
- FSH, LFTs, and pelvic ultrasound prior to pubertal induction

- Regular visits to primary care physician are recommended. Be aware of the social and emotional problems associated with issues such as short stature and infertility.
- Adults with TS should be monitored for cardiovascular disease, including hypertension and valve disease.
- Cardiac imaging (preferably MRI) every 5–10 years for aortic root dilatation/aortic dissection
- Adults also should be monitored for thyroid disease, liver abnormalities, diabetes, and dyslipidemia (3).

PATIENT EDUCATION
- Families and patients need a thorough explanation of the condition and its management, especially about sexual development and growth.
- Support groups may be helpful: tsparents-3@yahoogroups.com; tspregnancy@yahoogroups.com.
- Turner Syndrome Society of the United States; (800) 365-9944; www.turnersyndrome.org. "Turner Syndrome: A Guide for Families" (2002) is downloadable from this site.

PROGNOSIS
- Most girls with TS can be expected to lead reasonably normal lives with appropriate medical management; however, in a recent study, 3,439 women with TS diagnosed between 1959 and 2002 were followed to evaluate standardized mortality ratios (SMRs) and absolute excess risks (8). The authors conclude that mortality is 3-fold higher in women with TS than in the general population, and emphasize the importance of medical follow-up in adulthood because some of the deaths are potentially preventable.
- Infertility: Most women with TS are infertile; however, pregnancy without medical assistance has been documented (but is rare). Successful pregnancy following oocyte donation is well described (9), although a thorough cardiovascular evaluation should be performed because the risk of aortic dissection is greatly increased during pregnancy (10).
- The overall risk of cancer is not increased in women with TS; however, in addition to increased risk of gonadoblastoma in individuals with 45,X/46,XY mosaicism, risk may be increased for meningioma, childhood brain tumors, and possibly bladder cancer, melanoma, and uterine cancer in individuals with TS when compared with that of the general population. Women with TS have a decreased risk of breast cancer (11).

REFERENCES

1. Tyler C. Down syndrome, Turner's syndrome, and Klinefelter's syndrome: Primary care throughout the life span. *Primary Care Clin Office Pract.* 2004;31:627–48.
2. Frías JL, Davenport ML, Committee on Genetics and Section on Endocrinology. Health supervision for children with Turner syndrome. *Pediatrics.* 2003;111:692–702.
3. Bondy CA. Care of Girls and Women with Turner Syndrome: A Guideline of the Turner Syndrome Study Group. *J Clin Endocrinol Metab.* 2006.
4. Davenport ML, et al. Approach to the patient with Turner syndrome. *J Clin Endocrinol Metab.* 2010;95:1487–95.
5. Mhatre P, Mhatre J, Magotra R. Ovarian transplant: a new frontier. *Transplant Proc.* 2005;37:1396–8.
6. El-Shawarby SA, Sharif F, Conway G, et al. Oocyte cryopreservation after controlled ovarian hyperstimulation in mosaic Turner syndrome: another fertility preservation option in a dedicated UK clinic. *BJOG.* 2010;117:234–7.
7. Donaldson MDC, et al. Optimising management in Turner syndrome: From infancy to adult transfer. *Arch Dis Child.* 2006;92:513–20.
8. Schoemaker MJ, Swerdlow AJ, Higgins CD, et al. Mortality in women with Turner syndrome in Great Britain: a national cohort study. *J Clin Endocrinol Metab.* 2008.
9. Bodri D, Vernaeve V, Figueras F, et al. Oocyte donation in patients with Turner's syndrome: a successful technique but with an accompanying high risk of hypertensive disorders during pregnancy. *Hum Reprod.* 2006;21:829–32.
10. The Practice Committee of the American Society for Reproductive Medicine. Increased maternal cardiovascular mortality associated with pregnancy in women with Turner syndrome. *Fertil Steril.* 2006;86(Suppl 5):S127–8.
11. Schoemaker MJ, Swerdlow AJ, Higgins CD, et al. Cancer incidence in women with Turner syndrome in Great Britain: a national cohort study. *Lancet Oncol.* 2008.
12. Davenport ML, et al. Approach to the patient with Turner syndrome. *J Clin Endocrinol Metab.* 2010;95:1487–95.

See Also (Topic, Algorithm, Electronic Media Element)
Amenorrhea; Coarctation of the Aorta; Hypothyroidism

 CODES

ICD9
758.6 Gonadal dysgenesis

CLINICAL PEARLS
- TS is the most common sex chromosome abnormality syndrome in females.
- Edema of the hands and feet and redundant skin of the neck (webbing) are presenting features during infancy. During adolescence, primary amenorrhea, short stature, and infantile secondary sex characteristics are presenting features.
- Much of the treatment provided to individuals with TS is not evidence-based, and consequently, there are many areas of controversy, especially with regard to hormone-replacement therapy (12).

TYPHOID FEVER
Douglas W. MacPherson, MD, MSc(CTM)

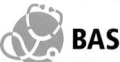 **BASICS**

- Typhoid fever is a rare enteric infectious syndrome in the US.
- Most cases reported in the US are imported from endemic areas of the world; in particular, South and Southeast Asia.

DESCRIPTION

- Typhoid fever is an acute systemic illness in humans caused by *Salmonella typhi*. It is a classic example of enteric fever caused by the *Salmonella* bacterium.
- Enteric fevers owing to *S. paratyphi* can present in a similar manner as classic typhoid fever.
- Typhoid is endemic in some developing nations where sanitation is poor. Most cases in North America and other developed nations are acquired after travel to disease-endemic areas.
- "Visiting family or friends" travelers may be at greater risk of typhoid.
- Mode of transmission is fecal-oral through ingestion of contaminated food (commonly poultry, water, and milk).
- Incubation period varies from 7–21 days.
- System(s) affected: GI; pulmonary; Skin/exocrine
- Synonym(s): Typhoid; Typhus abdominalis; Enteric fever

Geriatric Considerations
Disease is more serious in the elderly.

Pediatric Considerations
Disease is more serious in infants but may be milder in children.

EPIDEMIOLOGY
Although typhoid outbreaks have been described in the US, most cases are reported in international travelers who have been exposed in endemic transmission zones (in particular, South and Southeast Asia, parts of Latin America).

- Predominant age: All ages
- Predominant sex: Male = Female

Incidence
In the US, 300–500 new cases per year

RISK FACTORS
Must be considered in any patient presenting with fever after tropical travel or exposure to a chronic carrier

GENERAL PREVENTION

- Food and water consumption precautions are paramount in the prevention of all enteric infections including typhoid fever.
- Avoid tap water, salad/raw vegetables, unpeeled fruits, and dairy products in tropical travel.
- Avoid poultry or poultry products left unrefrigerated for prolonged periods.
- For high-risk travel to an endemic area, consider vaccination against typhoid (1)[A]:
  – Parenteral ViCPS or capsular polysaccharide typhoid vaccine (Typhim Vi) *or*
  – Ty21a or live oral typhoid vaccine (Vivotif Berna), particularly if traveler will be at prolonged risk (>4 weeks)

- Consider vaccination for workers exposed to *S. typhi* or those with household or intimate exposure to a carrier of *S. typhi*.
- Occupational health and safety precautions, including screening of domestic and commercial food handlers, may be considered in some situations.

PATHOPHYSIOLOGY

- Acute typhoid and other enteric fevers are seen most commonly in international travelers to endemic *S. typhi* regions of the world.
- The initial infection is transmitted via the fecal-oral route with a GI source of the bacterium resulting in bacteremia and sepsis. Involvement of the bowel wall (Peyer patch) rarely may be associated with bleeding from the bowel or bowel perforation.
- *S. typhi* chronic carrier state may occur with shedding of the bacterium in the stools. Potential for person-to-person transmission may occur. In a chronic carrier state, *S. typhi* appears to locate in the biliary tract and in particular the gallbladder. Chronic suppressive antimicrobials may clear a carrier state. In extreme cases, cholecystectomies have been performed to attempt to clear carriage of *S. typhi*.

ETIOLOGY
Salmonella typhi

 DIAGNOSIS

Assessment of the clinical presentation and exposure history, including endemic zone travel and known chronic *S. typhi* carrier exposure

HISTORY
Patient presentation: Fever, headache, constipation with

- Travel history to an endemic region and exposure to contaminated food or water
- Exposure to a chronic *S. typhi* carrier

PHYSICAL EXAM
- Fever
- Headache
- Malaise
- Abdominal discomfort/bloating/constipation
- Diarrhea (less common)
- Dry cough
- Confusion/lethargy
- Rose spot (transient erythematous maculopapular rash in anterior thorax or upper abdomen)
- Splenomegaly
- Hepatomegaly
- Cervical adenopathy
- Relative bradycardia
- Conjunctivitis
- Constitutionally unwell, fever, relative bradycardia, rose spots, abdominal pain, hepatosplenomegaly

DIAGNOSTIC TESTS & INTERPRETATION
Owing to the rarity of enteric fevers/typhoid syndromes in the US, a high level of clinical suspicion must be present. A travel history to a known typhoid endemic zone or exposure to a known chronic carrier of *S. typhi* will contribute to the clinical and laboratory diagnosis of typhoid fever.

Lab
- Definitive diagnosis is by culture of *S. typhi* from blood.
- Isolation of *S. typhi* in sputum, urine, or stool is a presumptive diagnosis in typical clinical presentation.
- Serology is nonspecific and usually not useful.
- If there are multiple negative blood cultures or in patients with prior antibiotic therapy, diagnostic yield is better with bone marrow culture.
- Anemia, leukopenia (neutropenia), thrombocytopenia, or evidence of disseminated intravascular coagulopathy are supportive. Elevated liver enzymes are common.
- Drugs that may alter lab results:
  – Prior antibiotic therapy
  – Vaccination

Imaging
Consider serial plain abdominal films for evidence of intestinal perforation.

Diagnostic Procedures/Surgery
- Bone marrow aspirate for culture of *S. typhi* has been reported to be more sensitive than blood cultures but is rarely indicated as a primary investigation.
- A bone marrow aspiration may be done for evaluation of a persistent fever in a clinically suspect situation with negative cultures or for investigation of a pyrexia of unknown origin.

Pathological Findings
Classically, mononuclear proliferation involving lymphoid tissue of intestinal tract, especially Peyer patch in terminal ileum

DIFFERENTIAL DIAGNOSIS
- Malaria
- "Enteric fever-like" syndrome caused by *Yersinia enterocolitica*, pseudotuberculosis, and *Campylobacter* spp.
- Enteric fever caused by nontyphoid *Salmonella* spp.
- Infectious hepatitis
- Atypical pneumonia
- Infectious mononucleosis
- Subacute bacterial endocarditis
- Tuberculosis
- Brucellosis
- Q fever
- Toxoplasmosis
- Viral infections: Epstein-Barr virus (EBV), cytomegalovirus (CMV), viral hemorrhagic agents

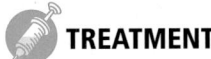 **TREATMENT**

Awareness of emerging drug-resistant *S. typhi* strains globally and the epidemiology of the patient's exposure may direct primary therapy. Fluoroquinolone-resistant *S. typhi* is becoming common in Asia.

MEDICATION
See below for treatment recommendations for acute typhoid fever and chronic carrier states.

First Line
- Chloramphenicol: Pediatric 50 mg/kg/d PO q.i.d. × 2 weeks; adult dose 50 mg/kg/d divided q6h for 2 weeks *or*
- Ampicillin: Pediatric 100 mg/kg/d q.i.d. PO × 2 weeks; adults 500 mg q6h for 2 weeks *or*
- Ciprofloxacin: 500 mg PO b.i.d. × 2 weeks, indicated in multiple-drug-resistant typhoid (has been used successfully and safely in children) *or*
- Ceftriaxone: 1–2 g IV once daily × 2 weeks *or*
- Furazolidone: 7.5 mg/kg/d PO × 10 days; in uncomplicated multiple-drug-resistant typhoid; safe in children; efficacy >85% cure
- Chronic carrier state:
  – Ampicillin: 4–5 g/d plus probenecid 2 g/d q.i.d. × 6 weeks (for patients with normally functioning gallbladder without evidence of cholelithiasis)
  – Ciprofloxacin: 500 mg PO b.i.d. for 4–6 weeks is also efficacious. Chloramphenicol resistance has been reported in Mexico, South America, Central America, Southeast Asia, India, Pakistan, Middle East, and Africa.
- Contraindications: Refer to manufacturer's profile for each drug.
- Precautions: Rarely, Jarisch-Herxheimer reaction appears after antimicrobial therapy.
- Significant possible interactions: Refer to manufacturer's profile for each drug.

Second Line
Trimethoprim–sulfamethoxazole

Pregnancy Considerations
Ciprofloxacin therapy is relatively contraindicated in pregnant patients.

ADDITIONAL TREATMENT
General Measures
- Fluid and electrolyte support
- Strict isolation of patient's linen, stool, and urine
- Monitor clinically, and consider serial plain abdominal films for evidence of perforation, usually in the 3rd–4th week of illness.
- Indications and contraindications for specific treatment of typhoid disease and chronic carrier states must be determined on an individual basis. Factors to be considered are age, public health and occupational health risk (e.g., food handler, chronic care facilities, medical personnel), intolerance to antibiotics, and evidence of biliary tract disease.
- For hemorrhage: Blood transfusion and management of shock

Issues for Referral
Complications of sepsis, bowel perforation

SURGERY/OTHER PROCEDURES
- Complications: Bowel perforation
- Cholecystectomy may be warranted in carriers with cholelithiasis, relapse after therapy, or intolerance to antimicrobial therapy.

IN-PATIENT CONSIDERATIONS
Initial Stabilization
- Inpatient if acutely ill
- Outpatient for less ill patient or for carrier

Admission Criteria
Clinical severity

Nursing
Observe enteric precautions.

 ONGOING CARE

FOLLOW-UP RECOMMENDATIONS
Bed rest initially, then activity as tolerated

Patient Monitoring
See "General Measures."

DIET
If abdominal symptoms are severe, NPO. With improvement, begin normal low-residue diet, possibly high-calorie.

PATIENT EDUCATION
- Discuss chronic carrier state and its complications.
- For family members, travelers, or workers at risk, provide hygiene education and possibly vaccination.

PROGNOSIS
Overall prognosis good is with therapy; <2% mortality rate; 15% relapse rate with some antibiotic treatments; 3% bowel perforation

COMPLICATIONS
- Intestinal hemorrhage and perforation in distal ileum
- Patients may become chronic carriers (up to 3%), defined as persistent stool excretor of *S. typhi* for >1 year.
- Predilection for seeding in the biliary tract exists and may become a focus for relapse of typhoid fever: Most common in females and older patients (>50 years)
- Osteomyelitis is found especially in patients with sickle cell anemia, systemic lupus erythematosus, and hematologic neoplasms, as well as in immunosuppressed hosts.
- Endovascular infection in the elderly and in patients with a history of bypass operation or aneurysm
- Rarely, endocarditis or meningitis

REFERENCE
1. Typhoid Immunization Recommendations of the Advisory Committee on Immunization Practices (ACIP). *MMWR.* 1994;43(RR14):1–7. Available at: http://www.phppo.cdc.gov/cdcRecommends/showarticle.asp?a_artid=M0035643&TopNum=50&CallPg=AdvCDC.

ADDITIONAL READING
- Basnyat B, et al. Typhoid fever in the United States and antibiotic choice. *JAMA.* 2010;303:34; author reply 34–5.
- Bhutta ZA. Current concepts in the diagnosis and treatment of typhoid fever. *Br Med J.* 2006;333:78–82.
- CDC. Vaccines and Preventable Diseases: Typhoid. Available at: http://www.cdc.gov/vaccines/vpd-vac/typhoid/default.htm (accessed April 3, 2009).
- Centers for Disease Control and Prevention. *Traveler's Health Yellow Book.* 2008. Chapter 4. Prevention of Specific Infectious Diseases. Typhoid Fever. Available at: http://wwwn.cdc.gov/travel/yellowBookCh4-Typhoid.aspx#666 (accessed April 3, 2009).
- Centers for Disease Control and Prevention. Typhoid Fever. Available at: http://www.cdc.gov/ncidod/dbmd/diseaseinfo/typhoidfever_g.htm (accessed April 3, 2009).
- Clark TW, Daneshvar C, Pareek M, Perera N, Stephenson I, et al. Enteric fever in a UK regional infectious diseases unit: a 10 year retrospective review. *J Infect.* 2010;60:91–8.
- Crump JA, Mintz ED, et al. Global trends in typhoid and paratyphoid Fever. *Clin Infect Dis.* 2010;50:241–6.
- Kroger AT, et al. General recommendations on immunization. Recommendations of the Advisory Committee on Immunization Practices (ACIP). *MMWR.* 2006;55(RR15):1–48.
- Lynch MF, Blanton EM, Bulens S, Polyak C, Vojdani J, Stevenson J, Medalla F, Barzilay E, Joyce K, Barrett T, Mintz ED, et al. Typhoid fever in the United States, 1999–2006. *JAMA.* 2009;302:859–65.

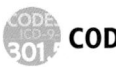 **CODES**

ICD9
002.0 Typhoid fever

CLINICAL PEARLS
- Along with malaria and other regionally defined exotic infections, including dengue, enteric fevers, and others, typhoid should be considered as a possible diagnosis for any febrile traveler from endemic areas such as Latin America, sub-Saharan Africa, or South Asia.
- Routine blood cultures will detect *S. typhi* but may be negative if antibiotics have been taken prior to testing.
- A history or documentation of vaccination against *S. typhi* does not exclude the diagnosis of typhoid fever.

ULCER, APHTHOUS

Cary D. Douglass, MD

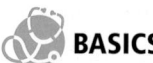

BASICS

DESCRIPTION
Self-limited painful ulcerations of the oral mucosa that are typically recurrent; they occur on nonkeratinized mucosa inside the mouth: the inner side of the lips and cheeks, the back and floor of the mouth, and under the tongue.

EPIDEMIOLOGY
- The 1st episode of aphthous stomatitis usually occurs during the 1st or 2nd decade of life. The incidence then begins to decrease after the 3rd decade. It affects 20% of the US population.
- Aphthous ulcers may be categorized into 3 types:
  – Minor aphthous ulcers:
    ○ 70–90% of all aphthae
    ○ <10 mm in diameter
    ○ Up to 5 appear at a time.
    ○ Heal in 7–10 days
    ○ Nonscarring
  – Major aphthous ulcers (also called Sutton disease):
    ○ 10–15% of all aphthae
    ○ >10 mm in diameter
    ○ 1–10 ulcers at a time
    ○ Take weeks to months to heal
    ○ Scarring may occur.
  – Herpetiform aphthous ulcers:
    ○ 7–10% of all aphthae
    ○ Between 1 and 3 mm in diameter
    ○ Multiple (tens to hundreds) in small clusters
    ○ Last 7–30 days
    ○ Scarring may occur.

RISK FACTORS
- Trauma
- Stress
- Vitamin, iron, or folic acid deficiency
- Immunodeficiency
- Smoking (1)[A]
- Toothpastes containing sodium lauryl sulfate (2)
- Celiac disease (3)

Genetics
Possible familial correlation

ETIOLOGY
Unknown etiology; likely multifactorial with some correlation with
- Immunologic dysfunction
- Activation of cell-mediated immunes system:
  – Infection
  – Food hypersensitivities
  – Vitamin deficiency
  – Pregnancy
  – Menstruation
  – Psychological and genetic factors

DIAGNOSIS

Diagnosis is made by history and clinical presentation.

HISTORY
- Prodrome of burning or pricking sensation of oral mucosa 1–2 days prior to appearance of ulcers
- Inquire about family history of systemic lupus erythematosus (SLE), inflammatory bowel disease (IBD), or Behçet disease.
- Inquire about patient medical history of SLE, HIV, IBD, Behçet disease, or cancer.

PHYSICAL EXAM
- Look for signs of dehydration.
- Vital signs should be within normal limits.
- Evaluate for signs of secondary infection.

DIAGNOSTIC TESTS & INTERPRETATION
Lab
- Complete blood count (CBC)
- Rapid plasma reagin test
- Antinuclear antibody (ANA) test
- Tzanck stain (herpesvirus)
- Celiac disease serology
- Vitamins B_6 and B_{12}
- Serum iron and folate
- HIV

Diagnostic Procedures/Surgery
- Biopsy: Multinucleated giant cells (cytomegalovirus)
- Fungal cultures: *Cryptosporidium*

DIFFERENTIAL DIAGNOSIS
- Rule out oral manifestation of systemic disease.
- Trauma:
  – Biting
  – Dentures
- Drug exposure:
  – Nonsteroidal anti-inflammatory drugs (NSAIDs)
  – Nicorandil
- Infection:
  – Herpesvirus:
    ○ Vesicular lesions
    ○ Ulcers on attached mucosa
  – Cytomegalovirus: Immunocompromised patient
  – Varicella virus: Characteristic skin lesions
  – Coxsackievirus:
    ○ Ulcers preceded by vesicles
    ○ Hand, foot, buttock lesions
  – Syphilis: Other skin or genital lesions
  – Erythema multiforme:
    ○ Lip crusting
    ○ Lesions on attached and unattached mucosa skin lesions
  – *Cryptosporidium* infection, mucormycosis, histoplasmosis
  – Necrotizing gingivitis
- Underlying disease:
  – Behçet syndrome:
    ○ Genital ulceration
    ○ Uveitis
    ○ Retinitis
  – Reiter syndrome:
    ○ Uveitis
    ○ Urethritis
    ○ HLA–B27-associated arthritis

- Sweet syndrome:
  - Fever
  - Erythematous skin plaques/nodules
  - In conjunction with malignancy
- IBD:
  - Bloody or mucous diarrhea
  - GI ulcerations
- SLE: Malar rash
- Bullous pemphigoid/pemphigoid vulgaris:
  - Vesiculobullous lesions on attached and unattached mucosa
  - Diffuse skin involvement
- Cyclic neutropenia: Periodic fever
- Squamous cell carcinoma:
  - Chronicity
  - Head/neck adenopathy
- Immunocompromised patient:
  - HIV
  - Agranulocytosis

 TREATMENT

MEDICATION
- Analgesia:
  - Debacterol (available over the counter [OTC]), a topical treatment, chemically cauterizes the oral lesion, eliminating pain associated with the lesion.
  - 5-Aminosalicylic acid 5% cream: 3× daily × 2 weeks
  - Dyclonine HCl 1% solution: 5-mL rinse q.i.d.
  - Magnesium hydroxide/diphenhydramine hydrochloride: 5 mg/5 mL in 1:1 mix; swish and swallow q.i.d.
  - Sucralfate: 10 mL; swish and swallow or swish and spit q.i.d.
  - Viscous lidocaine 2%: Apply to ulcer as needed q.i.d.
  - Topical OTC preparations (e.g., Orabase, Anbesol)

- Promote ulcer healing/prevent recurrence (1st-line agents):
  - Triamcinolone 0.1% in Orabase: Apply to ulcer 2–4× daily until healed.
  - Amlexanox 5% paste: 0.5 cm applied to ulcer q.i.d. after meals
  - Clobetasol 0.05%: 0.5 cm applied to ulcer 2× daily
  - Fluocinonide 0.05% gel: 0.5 cm applied to ulcer up to 5× daily
- 2nd-line agents:
  - Prednisone tablets: 40 mg/d PO × 7 days
  - Thalidomide: 200 mg/d PO × 4 weeks

ADDITIONAL TREATMENT
Issues for Referral
Follow up with otolaryngologist if lesions have not resolved within 2 weeks.

Additional Therapies
Vitamin and iron supplementation

IN-PATIENT CONSIDERATIONS
Admission Criteria
- Unable to eat or drink after appropriate analgesia
- Abnormal vital signs or evidence of dehydration

Discharge Criteria
- Tolerating fluids
- Adequate analgesia
- Normal vital signs

REFERENCES

1. Porter SR, Scully Cbe C. Aphthous ulcers (recurrent). *Clin Evid (Online)*. 2007.
2. Herlofson BB, Barkvoll P. Sodium lauryl sulfate and recurrent aphthous ulcers. A preliminary study. *Acta Odontol Scand*. 1994;52:257–9.
3. Pastore L, Carroccio A, Compilato D, et al. Oral Manifestations of Celiac Disease. *J Clin Gastroenterol*. 2008.

ADDITIONAL READING

- McBride DR. Management of aphthous ulcers. *Am Fam Physician*. 2000;62:149–54, 160.
- Scully C, Gorsky M, Lozada-Nur F. The diagnosis and management of recurrent aphthous stomatitis: a consensus approach. *J Am Dent Assoc*. 2003;134: 200–7.
- Shashy RG, Ridley MB. Aphthous ulcers: a difficult clinical entity. *Am J Otolaryngol*. 2000;21:389–93.
- Ship JA, Chavez EM, Doerr PA, et al. Recurrent aphthous stomatitis. *Quintessence Int*. 2000;31: 95–112.
- Woo SB, Sonis ST. Recurrent aphthous ulcers: a review of diagnosis and treatment. *J Am Dent Assoc*. 1996;127:1202–13.

 CODES

ICD9
- 528.00 Stomatitis and mucositis, unspecified
- 528.2 Oral aphthae

CLINICAL PEARLS

- Risk of recurrence decreases with quitting smoking 1[A].
- Use of toothpastes without the ingredient sodium lauryl sulfate may reduce or even prevent recurrences (2).
- Avoid oral trauma from aggressive toothbrushing or foods with sharp edges.
- Self-limited painful ulcerations of the oral mucosa that are typically recurrent; they occur on nonkeratinized mucosa inside the mouth: the inner side of the lips and cheeks, the back and floor of the mouth, and under the tongue
- Risk factors include: Trauma; stress; vitamin, iron, or folic acid deficiency; immunodeficiency, smoking; toothpastes containing sodium lauryl sulfate; celiac disease
- Most are self limiting; treat symptoms with topical agents like: Debacterol, Triamcinolone 0.1% in Orabase, others

U

ULCERATIVE COLITIS

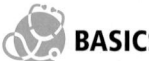

Michele L. Matthews, PharmD
Jill A. Grimes, MD

BASICS

DESCRIPTION
- An idiopathic inflammatory disease of the colon mucosa affecting the rectum; can extend to involve the entire colon
  - >95% of patients have rectal involvement, with 50% of cases limited to rectum and sigmoid.
  - 30–40% extend beyond the sigmoid but not the entire colon.
  - 20% have pancolitis.

EPIDEMIOLOGY
Incidence
- US: 5–12 new cases/100,000 persons/year
- Predominant age: 15–35 years; 2nd and smaller peak in the 7th decade
- Predominant sex: Female > Male (slight)

Prevalence
70–150/100,000 persons

Pediatric Considerations
20% of patients are ≤21 years of age.

Pregnancy Considerations
- Similar to general population; 1 study showed 30% with inactive disease at onset of pregnancy relapsed
- Treatment with sulfasalazine does not seem to affect outcome of pregnancy.
- Recommend that patients delay pregnancy until time when disease is inactive

RISK FACTORS
- Better sanitation, artificial work environments (e.g., indoors), and fatty foods increase risk
- Nonsteroidal anti-inflammatory drugs (NSAIDs) can activate disease.
- Appendectomy is protective against later development of disease.
- Negative association with smoking (relative risk [RR] of smokers is 40% of nonsmokers)

Genetics
- Family history in 5–10% in population surveys and 20–30% in referral-based studies
- More common in the Jewish population

GENERAL PREVENTION
- Patients with long-term disease who do not have colectomy are at increased risk for colon cancer.
- Aspirin (≥ 300 mg/d), sclerosing cholangitis, and ursodeoxycholic acid (10 mg/kg) have been shown to be preventive.

Pediatric Considerations
- Breastfeeding may be protective for pediatric inflammatory bowel disease (IBD).

ETIOLOGY
Unknown; hypotheses include allergy to dietary components and abnormal immune responses to bacterial or "self" antigens; final outcome is mucosal inflammation secondary to immune cell infiltration (1)[B]

COMMONLY ASSOCIATED CONDITIONS
- Extracolonic manifestations in 10–15%
- Arthritic conditions including large joint arthritis, sacroiliitis, and ankylosing spondylitis
- Pyoderma gangrenosum and other skin conditions
- Episcleritis and uveal tract disease
- Sclerosing cholangitis

DIAGNOSIS

HISTORY
Bloody diarrhea (watery stool accompanied by blood, pus, and mucus); tenesmus; abdominal pain (tenderness in severe disease); rectal urgency, occasional fecal incontinence; weight loss; arthralgias

PHYSICAL EXAM
- Arthralgias and arthritis: 15–40% (2)[A]
- Spondylitis: 3–6%
- Ocular: 4–10%; include uveitis, cataracts, keratopathy, and central serous retinopathy
- Erythema nodosum
- Pyoderma gangrenosum
- Aphthous ulcers of mouth: 5–10%
- Asymptomatic fatty liver (common); occasional hepatomegaly
- Primary sclerosing cholangitis: 1–4%
- Cirrhosis of liver: 1–5%
- Bile duct carcinoma
- Thromboembolic disease: 1–6%

DIAGNOSTIC TESTS & INTERPRETATION
Lab
- Anemia (chronic disease +/– iron deficiency from blood loss)
- Leukocytosis during exacerbation
- Elevated ESR and CRP
- Electrolyte abnormalities, especially hypokalemia
- Hypoalbuminemia, elevated LFTs
- Perinuclear antineutrophil cytoplasmic antibody (p-ANCA) is elevated in 85% of cases of ulcerative colitis.
- Anti-Saccharomyces cerevisiae antibodies (ASCA) or perinuclear antineutrophil cytoplasmic antibodies (pANCA) can diagnose but not rule out inflammatory bowel disease.
- Antiglycan antibody is elevated in 75% of Crohn disease and 5% of ulcerative colitis cases.

Imaging
- Plain abdominal films:
  - Obtain immediately in patients with tenderness of the colon, fever, and leukocytosis. Permits the early diagnosis of toxic megacolon and perforation and treatment planning.
- Barium enema:
  - Mucosal irregularities, effacement of haustra, pseudopolyposis
  - Upper GI series with small bowel follow-through to rule out Crohn disease
- Ultrasound, MRI, scintigraphy, and CT may have similar accuracy in diagnosis of inflammatory bowel disease (3)[A].

Diagnostic Procedures/Surgery
- Sigmoidoscopy (4) (may include biopsy): Should be sufficient to make initial diagnosis
- Colonoscopy (4) (may include biopsy):
  - For evaluation of premalignant features; to differentiate from Crohn disease; to investigate suspected stricture or mass; to define the extent and location of involvement and specific segments
- Full colonoscopy contraindicated in active disease or colonic dilatation because of risk of perforation

Pathological Findings
Inflammation of the colonic mucosa with ulcerations:
- Ulcerations are hyperemic and hemorrhagic.
- Rectum is involved 95% of the time.
- The inflammation can extend proximally in a continuous fashion.
- May affect terminal ileum, so-called backwash ileitis

DIFFERENTIAL DIAGNOSIS
- Other sources of rectal bleeding: hemorrhoids, neoplasms, colonic diverticula, arteriovenous malformation, Crohn disease
- Infectious diarrhea, including bacterial (enterotoxigenic Escherichia coli, E. coli) and parasitic (Entamoeba histolytica)
- Herpes simplex, Chlamydia trachomatis, Cryptosporidium, Isospora belli, cytomegalovirus
- Radiation proctitis
- Ischemic proctitis and colitis

TREATMENT

Management involves acute treatment of inflammatory symptoms, followed by maintenance of remission; therapeutic approach is determined by the symptom severity and the degree of colonic involvement (4)[A]:

- Mild-to-moderate distal colitis may be treated with oral aminosalicylates, topical mesalamine, or topical steroids (4)[A]:
  - Topical mesalamine agents are superior to oral aminosalicylates or topical steroids (4)[A].
  - Combination of oral and topical aminosalicylates is more effective than either alone (4)[A].
- Maintenance of remission in mild-to-moderate distal disease with the use of the following: Mesalamine suppositories for proctitis or enemas for distal colitis, sulfasalazine, balsalazide, or combination oral and topical mesalamine (4)[A]
- Patients with mild-to-moderate extensive disease should be treated with aminosalicylates (4)[A]; oral steroids should be reserved for refractory cases (4)[B]; 6-mercaptopurine (6-MP) or azathioprine is effective in cases refractory to oral steroids (4)[A].
- Maintenance of remission in mild-to-moderate extensive disease with the use of the following: Sulfasalazine, olsalazine, mesalamine, and balsalazide (4)[A]
- Patients with severe colitis refractory to maximal oral therapy may be treated with infliximab (4)[A].

MEDICATION
- Sulfasalazine:
  - Uncoated tablets. Adults: Initial: 1 g p.o. q6–8h; maintenance: 500 mg p.o. q6h Children ≥6 years: Initial: 40–60 mg/kg/d p.o. in 3–6 divided doses; maintenance: 30 mg/kg/d p.o. divided q6h (maximum = 2 g/d)
  - Enteric-coated tablets. Adults: Initial: 3–4 g/d p.o. in divided doses; maintenance: 2 g/d p.o. in divided doses. Children ≥6 years: Initial: 40–60 mg/kg/d p.o. in 3–6 divided doses; maintenance: 30 mg/kg/d p.o. in 4 divided doses (maximum = 2 g/d)

- Mesalamine:
  - Oral delayed-release tablets (Asacol) for induction of remission. Adults: 800 mg p.o. t.i.d. × 6 wks
  - Oral controlled-release tablets (Pentasa) for maintenance of remission. Adults: 1 g p.o. q.i.d.
- 5-Aminosalicylic acid (such as mesalamine) enemas and suppositories can be used to treat proctitis or proctosigmoiditis:
  - Suppositories: Adults: 500 mg per rectum b.i.d., retained in the rectum for >1–3 h (can increase to 3× daily if inadequate response after 2 wks) or 1,000 mg per rectum once daily q.h.s. may be used for 3–6 wks or until remission
  - Enemas: Adults: 4 g per rectum, retained for 8 hr each night; use for 3–6 wks or until remission is achieved
- Balsalazide: Adults: 2250 mg p.o. t.i.d. for total daily dose of 6.75 g for 8–12 wks; Children/adolescents: 2250 mg p.o. t.i.d. for total daily dose of 6.75 g or 750 mg p.o. t.i.d. for total daily dose of 2.25 g for 8 wks
- Olsalazine: Adults: 500 mg p.o. b.i.d. (up to 3 g/d); Children/adolescents: 30 mg/kg/day in 2 divided doses (up to 2 g/day)
- Prednisone for severe exacerbations: Adult dosage: Initial: 40–60 mg/d p.o. (maximum = 1 mg/kg/d) × 7–10 days; taper over 2–3 months

Second Line
Infliximab is effective in patients whose disease is refractory to conventional treatment (4,5)[A]:
- Adult dose: 5 mg/kg IV at weeks 0, 2, and 6 for induction, then maintenance of 5 mg/kg IV is given every 8 weeks

Pediatric Considerations
- Infliximab can increase the risk of cancer in children and adolescents; weigh risks versus benefits prior to use.
- Immunomodulators can be used in patients unresponsive to steroids and aminosalicylates, or who cannot be weaned from high-dose steroids:
  - Daily plain films of the abdomen are obtained until improvement occurs.
  - If dilatation of colon increases or treatment has failed to attain reversal in 72 h, emergency colectomy is indicated.

ADDITIONAL TREATMENT
General Measures
Control inflammation, prevent complications, and replace nutritional losses and blood volume.

COMPLEMENTARY AND ALTERNATIVE MEDICINE
Probiotics added to standard therapy may provide modest benefits in patients with mild-to-moderately severe ulcerative colitis (6)[B].

SURGERY/OTHER PROCEDURES
- Emergency surgery for massive hemorrhage, perforation, and toxic dilatation of the colon
- Surgery indicated for cancer, persistent multisite mucosal dysplasia, and patients refractory to all other forms of therapy
- Total colectomy with ileostomy pouch is curative.
- Regular proctoscopic surveillance is required because colonic mucosa is retained, thereby leaving a risk of future cancer development.

IN-PATIENT CONSIDERATIONS
Initial Stabilization
- Obtain imaging studies to assess disease activity.
- Initiate IV corticosteroids.

 ## ONGOING CARE
FOLLOW-UP RECOMMENDATIONS
Patient Monitoring
- Colonoscopy for cancer surveillance with biopsy every 1–2 years after the disease has been present for 7–8 years
- Low-grade dysplasia warrants more frequent evaluation (e.g., every 3–6 months), and high-grade dysplasia (or low-grade dysplasia within a mass) warrants consideration of colectomy.
- Magnification chromoendoscopy may detect significantly more intraepithelial neoplasias than conventional colonoscopy.
- Annual liver tests
- Cholangiography for cholestasis

Pediatric Considerations
Cancer surveillance is important because occurrence of cancer relates to the duration and extent of disease, whether frequently symptomatic or not.

DIET
- n.p.o. during acute exacerbations
- Lactose-free diet is often recommended; evidence-based support is lacking without an associated lactase deficiency.
- Omega-3-fatty acids, seal and cod liver oil, dietary lactulose, wheat grass juice, and diets with decreased meat and alcohol have been recommended to reduce relapses and improve systemic symptoms (evidence is conflicting).

PATIENT EDUCATION
- Discuss the importance of adherence to drug therapy to induce and maintain remission.
- Self-help organizations such as Crohn's and Colitis Foundation of America (CCFA): http://www.ccfa.org

PROGNOSIS
- Variable; mortality for initial attack is ~5%; 75–85% experience relapse; and up to 20% eventually require colectomy
- Colon cancer risk is the single most important risk factor affecting long-term prognosis.
- Left-sided colitis and ulcerative proctitis have favorable prognoses with probable normal lifespan.

Geriatric Considerations
- Increased mortality if 1st presentation occurs after 60 years of age

COMPLICATIONS
- Perforation
- Toxic megacolon
- Liver disease
- Stricture formation (< Crohn disease)
- Colon cancer

REFERENCES
1. Hanauer SB. Inflammatory bowel disease: epidemiology, pathogenesis, and therapeutic opportunities. *Inflamm Bowel Dis*. 2006; 12(Suppl 1):S3–9.
2. D'Incà R, Podswiadek M, Ferronato A, et al. Articular manifestations in inflammatory bowel disease patients: A prospective study. *Dig Liver Dis*. 2009.
3. Horsthuis K, Bipat S, Bennink RJ, et al. Inflammatory bowel disease diagnosed with US, MR, scintigraphy, and CT: meta-analysis of prospective studies. *Radiology*. 2008;247:64–79.
4. Kornbluth A, Sachar DB, and the Practice Parameters Committee of the American College of Gastroenterology, for the Practice Parameters Committee of the American College of Gastroenterology. Ulcerative colitis practice guidelines in adults. *Am J Gastroenterol* 2010;105:501–523.
5. Lawson MM, Thomas AG, Akobeng AK. Tumour necrosis factor alpha blocking agents for induction of remission in ulcerative colitis. *Cochrane Database Syst Rev*. 2006;3:CD005112.
6. Mallon P, McKay D, Kirk S, et al. Probiotics for induction of remission in ulcerative colitis. *Cochrane Database Syst Rev*. 2007:CD005573.
7. Mack DR, Langton C, Markowitz J, et al. Laboratory values for children with newly diagnosed inflammatory bowel disease. *Pediatrics*. 2007; 119:1113–9.

ADDITIONAL READING
Ei-Matary W, Vandermeer B, Griffiths AM. Methotrexate for maintenance of remission in ulcerative colitis. *Cochrane Database Syst Rev*. 2009:CD007560.

See Also (Topic, Algorithm, Electronic Media Element)
Algorithm: Bleeding, GI

 ## CODES

ICD9
- 556.0 Ulcerative (chronic) enterocolitis
- 556.1 Ulcerative (chronic) ileocolitis
- 556.2 Ulcerative (chronic) proctitis

CLINICAL PEARLS
- Smokers have half the risk of nonsmokers for developing ulcerative colitis.
- Patients with proctitis should be treated with 5-ASA suppositories instead of oral therapy.
- Surgical removal of colon and rectum is curative.
- Indications for surgery include intractability, dysplasia, carcinoma, massive bleeding, toxic megacolon
- Normal screening lab tests (ESR, hemoglobin, platelets, and albumin) do NOT rule out inflammatory bowel disease, regardless of disease severity (7).

UPPER RESPIRATORY INFECTION

Lisa M. Schroeder, MD
Gaurav Dang, MD

 BASICS

DESCRIPTION
- Inflammation of nasal passages resulting from infection with various respiratory viruses
- Most cases are self-treated.
- Usually mild–moderate severity, self-limited
- System(s) affected: ENT; Pulmonary

EPIDEMIOLOGY
Incidence
- Predominant age: Children > Adults:
  - Preschool children: 6–10 colds/year
  - Kindergarten: 12/year
  - School children: 7/year
  - Adolescents/adults: 2–4/year
- Predominant sex: Male = Female

RISK FACTORS
- Exposure to infected people
- Touching one's nose or conjunctiva with contaminated fingers
- Allergic disorders
- Smoking
- Immunosuppression

GENERAL PREVENTION
- Frequent handwashing
- Limiting exposure to infected persons/children

PATHOPHYSIOLOGY
Rhinovirus infects the ciliated epithelium lining the nose, resulting in edema and hyperemia of nasal mucous membranes.

ETIOLOGY
- Usually due to 1 of 200 virus strains from 6 virus families; many strains present within the same geographic region or patient family:
  - Rhinovirus, with >200 serotypes
  - Influenzavirus types A, B, C
  - Parainfluenza viruses
  - Respiratory syncytial viruses
  - Coronaviruses
  - Adenoviruses
- In 40% of cases, no pathogen identified

COMMONLY ASSOCIATED CONDITIONS
- Pharyngitis
- Sinusitis
- Otitis media
- Bronchitis
- Bronchiolitis
- Pneumonia
- Croup
- Asthma

 DIAGNOSIS

HISTORY
- Nasal stuffiness and/or obstruction (80–100%)
- Sneezing (50–70%)
- Scratchy throat (50%)
- Cough (40%)
- Hoarseness (30%)
- Malaise (20–25%)
- Headache (25%)
- Fever exceeding 100°F (37.7°C) (0–1%)

PHYSICAL EXAM
- Low-grade temperature or afebrile
- Stable vital signs
- Rhinorrhea (clear, yellow, or green)
- Inflamed mucosa
- Postnasal drainage
- Erythema of the throat
- Dull tympanic membranes

DIAGNOSTIC TESTS & INTERPRETATION
Lab
Initial lab tests
- No routine lab testing is needed.
- For pharyngitis, use a lab test (rapid strep antigen or culture) to rule out group A strep infection.
- Rapid flu test if influenza suspected

Follow-Up & Special Considerations
Patients should contact the primary care physician's office for fever >101.0°F associated with systemic symptoms, difficulty breathing, or purulent drainage >2 days.

Imaging
Initial approach
Not necessary

Pathological Findings
- Exudation of serous and mucinous fluid containing immunoglobulins
- Histology: Edema of subepithelial connective tissue and a scanty cellular infiltrate containing neutrophils, plasma cells, lymphocytes, and eosinophils
- Rhinovirus causes a "nondestructive" inflammation of the mucous membranes.
- Influenza and parainfluenza denude epithelium to the basement membrane.

DIFFERENTIAL DIAGNOSIS
- Allergic rhinitis
- Acute sinusitis
- Strep pharyngitis
- The "flu" (caused by influenza viruses): Systemic symptoms, including myalgias, malaise, severe headache, and ocular symptoms, overshadow respiratory complaints.

TREATMENT

MEDICATION
- Primarily for supportive therapy
- No cure or practical preventive measures

First Line
- NSAIDs for relieving discomfort or pain caused by the common cold (1)[A]
- Topical decongestants (sympathomimetics) reduce edema and swelling of the nasal mucosa, promote drainage, and reduce nasal airflow resistance. These are preferred over oral types because of minimal systemic effects. Sprays are preferred over drops in patients >6 years old:
  - Oxymetazoline:
    - Adults and children aged 6–12 years: 0.05% solution, 2–3 sprays in each nostril b.i.d.
    - Children aged 2–6 years: 0.025% solution, 2–3 drops in each nostril b.i.d.
    - Rebound congestion (rhinitis medicamentosa) unlikely if used <5 days
- Topical anticholinergics control rhinorrhea but do not relieve nasal congestion or sneezing:
  - Ipratropium: Adults and children >11 years old: 0.06% solution, 2 sprays to each nostril t.i.d. × 4 days
  - The combination of ipratropium and xylometazoline has been shown to provide greater relief from rhinorrhea and congestion when compared with placebo and single-ingredient treatments. Combination treatments are safe. Adverse events are limited to epistaxis, nasal passage irritation, nasal dryness, and mucus tinged with blood (2)[A].
- Oral decongestants (sympathomimetic) advantages over topical decongestants: Longer duration of action, lack of local irritation, and no risk of rebound congestion:
  - Pseudoephedrine: Potential for abuse/misuse for methamphetamine production:
    - Adults: 60 mg q4–6h (120 mg sustained-release q12h) superior to placebo in short-term use (3,4)[A]
    - Children aged 6–12 years: 30 mg q4–6h; 2–5 years: 15 mg q4–6h
  - A single oral dose of phenylephrine 10 mg is an effective decongestant in adults with acute nasal congestion associated with the common cold (5)[A].
- Antihistamines: Safe and mildly effective for sneezing and rhinorrhea. Sedating:
  - Chlorpheniramine:
    - Adults: 4 mg q.i.d., 8 mg t.i.d., 12 mg b.i.d.
    - Children age 6-12: 2 mg q4–6hrs
    - Children age 2–6: 1 mg q4–6hrs
- Cough suppressants: Use if cough is nonproductive. minimal efficacy proven:
  - Codeine: Side effects of sedation and GI upset:
    - Adults: 10–20 mg q4–6 hrs p.r.n.
  - Dextromethorphan:
    - Adults: 10–30 mg q4–6 hrs
    - Children age 6–12: 15 mg q 4–6 hrs
    - Children age 2–6: 2.5–7.5 mg q4–6 hrs

- Expectorants:
  - Guaifenesin:
    - Adults: 100–400 mg q4hrs
    - Children age 6–12: 100-200 mg q4hrs
    - Children age 2–6: 50-100 mg q4hrs
- Common combinations: Most cold medicines come in combinations, multiple OTC, and prescription variations:
  - Dextromethorphan/phenylephrine/guaifenesin: 10/5/100 mg, peds:5/2.5/50
  - Dextromethorphan/guaifenesin: 10/100 mg
  - Acetaminophen/chlorpheniramine/ dextromethorphan/phenylephrine: 160/1/5/2.5 mg
  - Chlorpheniramine/dextromethorphan/ phenylephrine: 4/15/12.5 mg
  - Chlorpheniramine/dextromethorphan: 1/7.5 mg

Pediatric Considerations
- 2007 Food and Drug Administration (FDA) issued a warning on all cough and cold preparations for children 2 and younger due to risk of overdose

Second Line
- Many mouthwashes, gargles, and lozenges are promoted to relieve the pain of sore throat. The demulcent effects of hard candy, gargling with warm saline, and products with anesthetics (benzocaine or phenol) may provide pain relief.
- Aromatic oils (menthol, camphor, eucalyptus), in topical or lozenge form, produce a sensation of increased airflow in the absence of a significant change in airflow resistance.
- Saline nasal irrigation safe for adults and children
- Antibacterials are of no value.

ADDITIONAL TREATMENT
General Measures
- Smoking cessation
- Vaporizer/humidifier

COMPLEMENTARY AND ALTERNATIVE MEDICINE
- Zinc prevents viral replication *in vitro*, but the efficacy of lozenges remains unproved:
  - Avoid intranasal preparations of zinc: risk of potential permanent loss of smell
- Echinacea has not proven effective for treatment of common cold symptoms (6,7)[A].
- Probiotics may decrease severity and duration of upper respiratory infections (URIs) but not the incidence (8)[A].
- Vitamin C (ascorbic acid):
  - No preventive effects; 23% reduction in severity and duration of symptoms
  - Precipitation of urate, oxalate, or cystine stones has been seen. Urine glucose monitoring may be inaccurate in people taking large doses of vitamin C.
  - High-dose vitamin C prophylaxis has proven beneficial in those exposed to heavy exertion and cold stress.
  - Zinc and high-dose vitamin C prophylaxis and treatment should *not* be recommended for the general population (9).

Geriatric Considerations
Cold medications, especially decongestants, commonly produce adverse effects in older people.

Pregnancy Considerations
- Decongestants: No clear association has been determined between use of this drug group and congenital defects.
- Antihistamines: No clear association has been confirmed between use of this drug group and congenital defects.
- Codeine: Indiscriminate use during pregnancy may pose a risk to the fetus.

 ONGOING CARE

FOLLOW-UP RECOMMENDATIONS
Contact the primary care physician's office for fever, difficulty breathing, or symptoms persisting beyond expected course.

DIET
Encourage fluids and adequate hydration.

PATIENT EDUCATION
- Discuss with patients difference between viral and bacterial infections, appropriate and inappropriate antibiotic use.
- Frequent handwashing
- Symptomatic treatment; no cure
- Patient information: http://www.niaid.nih.gov/factsheets/cold.htm

PROGNOSIS
Excellent; expect full recovery. Usual duration 5–7 days. 3–4 additional days for smokers.

COMPLICATIONS
Small percentage may develop worsening symptoms leading to otitis media, sinusitis, bronchitis, or pneumonia.

REFERENCES

1. Kim SY, Chang YJ, Cho HM, et al. Non-steroidal anti-inflammatory drugs for the common cold. *Cochrane Database Syst Rev.* 2009;CD006362.
2. Eccles R, Pedersen A, Regberg D, et al. Efficacy and safety of topical combinations of ipratropium and xylometazoline for the treatment of symptoms of runny nose and nasal congestion associated with acute upper respiratory tract infection. *Am J Rhinol.* 2007;21:40–5.
3. Eccles R, Jawad MS, Jawad SS, et al. Efficacy and safety of single and multiple doses of pseudoephedrine in the treatment of nasal congestion associated with common cold. *Am J Rhinol.* 2005;19:25–31.
4. Taverner D, Latte J, Draper M. Nasal decongestants for the common cold. *Cochrane Database Syst Rev.* 2004; Issue 3. Art No CD001953.
5. Kollar C, Schneider H, Waksman J, et al. Meta-Analysis of the efficacy of a single dose of Phenylephrine 10mg compared with placebo in adults with acute nasal congestion due to the common cold. *Cl Therapeutics.* 2007;29(6): 1057–70.
6. Linde K, Barrett B, Wolkart K, et al. Echinacea for preventing and treating the common cold. Cochrane Acute Respiratory Infections Group. *Cochrane Database Syst Rev.* 2006; Issue 4.
7. Yale SH, Liu K. Echinacea purpurea therapy for the treatment of the common cold: a randomized, double-blind, placebo-controlled clinical trial. *Arch Intern Med.* 2004;164:1237–41.
8. Vouloumanou EK, Makris GC, Karageorgopoulos DE, et al. Probiotics for the prevention of respiratory tract infections: a systematic review. *Int J Antimicrob Agents.* 2009.
9. Douglas RM, Hemila H, Chalker E, et al. Vitamin C for preventing and treating the common cold. Cochrane Acute Respiratory Infections Group. *Cochrane Database Syst Rev.* 2006; Issue 4.

ADDITIONAL READING

- FDA advisory on decongestants. *MMWR Morb Mortal Wkly Rep.* 2007;56(1):1–4.
- Marshall I. WITHDRAWN: Zinc for the common cold. *Cochrane Database Syst Rev.* 2007:CD001364.
- Morris PS. Upper respiratory tract infections (including otitis media). *Pediatr Clin North Am.* 2009;56:101–17, x.
- National Guideline Clearinghouse. 2008 Diagnosis and treatment of respiratory illness in children and adults. http://www.guideline.gov.
- Turner RB, Bauer R, Woelkart K, et al. An evaluation of Echinacea angustifolia in experimental rhinovirus infections. *N Engl J Med.* 2005;353:341–8.

See Also (Topic, Algorithm, Electronic Media Element)
Bronchitis, Acute; Pharyngitis; Rhinitis, Allergic

 CODES

ICD9
465.9 Acute upper respiratory infections of unspecified site

CLINICAL PEARLS
- Supportive therapy is mainstay.
- If pharyngitis is the primary complaint, diagnose group A strep with lab testing.
- Limit unnecessary use of antibiotics.
- Patient education is key.

U

URETHRITIS

Janelle M. Evans, MD

BASICS

DESCRIPTION
- Urethral inflammation marked by painful urination, pruritus, hematuria, and/or discharge
- Usually a result of sexually transmitted infection (STI) or, less commonly, autoimmune disorders (Reiter's), trauma, or chemical irritation
- Complications such as urethral stricture in males or pelvic inflammatory disease (PID) in females may occur if untreated.
- System(s) affected: Renal/Urologic

EPIDEMIOLOGY
Incidence
- In 2007, 1.1 million new cases of chlamydia and 355,000 new cases of gonorrhea were reported by the Centers for Disease Control. Prevalence varies by region, with 5× more cases chlamydia and gonorrhea in the southern US. Racial discrepancies include an 8× higher rate for African Americans and a 2.9× higher rate for Hispanic patients in comparison with Caucasians.
- Predominant age: 15–24 years, sexually active, following trends for STI
- Predominant sex: Males report symptoms more frequently, but similar incidence likely

RISK FACTORS
- Multiple sexual partners and unprotected intercourse
- African American, Native American, or Hispanic ethnicity
- History of STIs, bacterial vaginosis, recurrent candidiasis
- Excessive use of chemical lubricants or powders

GENERAL PREVENTION
- Safer sex techniques and treatment of all partners
- Abstinence
- Avoidance of excessive lubricants, powders, or chemical irritants

ETIOLOGY
- Predominantly *Neisseria gonorrhoeae* and *Chlamydia trachomatis* infection, increased transmission in HIV-positive persons
- Less common infectious agents, including:
  - *Ureaplasma urealyticum*
  - *Trichomonas vaginalis*
  - Herpesvirus
  - *Mycoplasma genitalium*
- Noninfectious causes (generally rare): Foreign bodies, soaps, shampoos, douches, spermicides, urethral instrumentation

COMMONLY ASSOCIATED CONDITIONS
Other STIs: Patients should be strongly urged to undergo testing for syphilis, hepatitis B, *Trichomonas*, and HIV.

DIAGNOSIS

- Important to take detailed sexual and travel history; increased incidence seen with travel to some regions
- In males:
  - Abrupt onset of dysuria symptoms 3–14 days after exposure to an infected sexual partner
  - Urethral discharge: May be profuse and purulent in acute gonorrhea
  - Urethral itching or tenderness
  - Proctitis, pharyngitis, and conjunctivitis also may be present (sexual history is important).
- In females: Classic urethral syndrome often is not present:
  - Tenderness, edema, and inflammation of the urethral meatus, especially in women
  - Dyspareunia
  - Vaginitis, cystitis, cervicitis in women
- Fever is not part of the syndrome and suggests another diagnosis.
- Bloody discharge: Rarely seen and suggests another diagnosis
- Suprapubic or abdominal pain suggests another diagnosis or presence of complications (e.g., PID, prostatitis, or cystitis).

Pediatric Considerations
Pediatrics: Proven cases of gonorrhea, chlamydia, and trichomoniasis require evaluation for sexual abuse.

DIAGNOSTIC TESTS & INTERPRETATION
- For patients who present without symptoms stating that a sexual partner was treated for this problem, obtain specimens for lab tests, but immediate treatment is recommended.
- Evidence is insufficient to recommend for or against screening in asymptomatic men at increased risk (1).

ALERT
The US Preventative Services Task Force recommends screening all sexually active women until age 25 years and all women at increased risk of infection (1)[A].

Lab
- Gram stain of discharge: ≥5 white blood cells (WBCs) per high-power field (HPF) indicates urethritis. Intracellular gram-negative diplococci strongly indicate gonorrhea.
- Cultures of the intraurethral/endocervical swabs:
  - Gonorrhea and chlamydia cultures should be obtained in all symptomatic patients.
  - Culture may be performed on urethral exudates if present.

- Nucleic acid amplification test using polymerase chain reaction assay on urine is very sensitive and specific but costly. Can be used for screening if intraurethral or endocervical specimens cannot be obtained. Be sure to test for other, less common pathogens if negative.
- Urinalysis:
  - Usually normal in cases of simple urethritis
  - 1st-void urine is often positive for leukocyte esterase and should have ≥10 WBCs per HPF in urethritis.
  - Men should not have urinated for at least 4 hours prior.
- Urine culture: Performed only if gram stain of discharge is unremarkable or unobtainable.
- Wet prep: May reveal *Trichomonas;* trichomoniasis, bacterial vaginosis, and *Candida* infection need to be evaluated for persistent symptoms after antibiotic course
- Syphilis, HIV, and hepatitis B serology as indicated to rule out concomitant STIs

Initial lab tests

ALERT
When STI is suspected, provide informed consent and recommend HIV testing at initial presentation.

Follow-Up & Special Considerations
Test of cure for chlamydia and gonorrhea recommended in pregnant women or where treatment noncompliance is suspected.

Diagnostic Procedures/Surgery
Urethrocystoscopy for cases with suspected foreign body, intraurethral warts, urethral stricture

Pathological Findings
Urethral strictures (untreated gonorrhea), intraurethral lesions (venereal warts, congenital anomalies), PID, or tubo-ovarian abscesses possible

DIFFERENTIAL DIAGNOSIS
- Other genitourinary tract diseases:
  - Cystitis/urinary tract infection
  - Painful bladder syndromes
  - Epididymitis
  - Prostatitis
  - PID
  - Pyelonephritis
- Vaginal atrophy, especially in postmenopausal women
- Stevens-Johnson syndrome
- Reiter syndrome: Arthritis, uveitis, and urethritis (can't see, can't pee, can't climb a tree)
- Wegener granulomatosis

TREATMENT

MEDICATION

First Line

- Gonorrhea (2)[C]:
  - Ceftriaxone: 125 mg IM single dose
  - Cefixime: 400 mg p.o. single dose
- Chlamydia:
  - Azithromycin: 1 g p.o. single dose
  - Doxycycline: 100 mg p.o. b.i.d. × 7 days
- Trichomoniasis: Metronidazole 2 g p.o. single dose or 250 mg t.i.d. × 7 days
- Recurrent and resistant urethritis: Metronidazole 2 mg p.o. single dose *plus*:
  - Erythromycin 500 mg p.o. q.i.d. × 7 days and valacyclovir 400 mg p.o. t.i.d. × 5 days if herpes simplex virus (HSV) suspicious
- Contraindications: Sensitivity to any of the indicated medications
- Precautions: Patients taking tetracyclines may have increased photosensitivity.
- Significant possible interactions:
  - Tetracyclines should not be taken with milk products or antacids.
  - Oral contraceptives may be rendered less effective by oral antibiotics. Patients and partners should use a backup method of birth control for remainder of the cycle.

Pregnancy Considerations

- Tetracyclines and quinolones are contraindicated.
- Avoid erythromycin estolate because of an increased risk of cholestatic jaundice; otherwise, use the standard treatment recommendations.
- Single-dose therapy recommended

Second Line

- Gonorrhea:
  - Because of the spread of quinolone-resistant *N. gonorrhoeae* from the Pacific, Hawaii, California, and Asia, quinolones are no longer recommended treatment in individuals who have acquired gonorrhea from that area (3)[C].
  - Resistance to penicillin and tetracycline has been reported in up to 1/3 of isolates of *N. gonorrhoeae*.
  - Ciprofloxacin: 500 mg p.o. single dose (3)[C]
  - Ofloxacin: 400 mg p.o. single dose (2)[C]
  - Levofloxacin: 250 mg p.o. single dose (2)[C]
  - Other drugs are available, but offer no particular advantage over the drugs of choice.
- Chlamydia:
  - Erythromycin base: 500 mg p.o. q.i.d. × 7 days
  - Erythromycin ethylsuccinate: 800 mg p.o. q.i.d. × 7 days; if intolerant of high-dose erythromycin: Erythromycin base 250 mg p.o. q.i.d. × 14 days or erythromycin ethylsuccinate 400 mg p.o. q.i.d. × 14 days
  - Ofloxacin: 300 mg p.o. b.i.d. × 7 days
  - Levofloxacin: 500 mg p.o. daily × 7 days

ADDITIONAL TREATMENT

General Measures

All sexual partners who came in contact with the patient within 60 days should be evaluated, tested, and treated for both gonorrhea and chlamydia.

IN-PATIENT CONSIDERATIONS

Initial Stabilization

- Most cases can be treated in the outpatient setting.
- Single-dose regimens, directly observed in office for noncompliant or high-risk patients
- Antibiotics should not be withheld from symptomatic patients until culture results are known if there is a convincing clinical presentation.
- Treatment should cover both gonorrhea and chlamydia and any other suspected pathogens.
- Patients with persistent symptoms and signs after adequate treatment should be:
  - Evaluated and/or treated for trichomoniasis
  - Retreated with the original regimen if not compliant or reexposed
  - Retreated with an alternative regimen for 14 days if *U. urealyticum* is suspected (tetracycline resistance in <10% of isolates)
  - Evaluated for HSV

ONGOING CARE

FOLLOW-UP RECOMMENDATIONS

- Full activity
- Sexual activity should be avoided until both partners complete treatment and are symptom-free or 7 days after single-dose therapy.

Patient Monitoring

Instruct patients to return if symptoms persist or recur after completing treatment. Test-of-cure cultures are not usually required unless patient is pregnant.

DIET

Avoid alcohol with metronidazole.

PATIENT EDUCATION

- Handouts available online at familydoctor.org
- Most important to emphasize the need for compliance with therapy, treatment of sexual partners, and use of safer sex practices; patients should be urged to undergo screening for other STIs.

PROGNOSIS

If the diagnosis is firmly established, appropriate medications are prescribed, and the patient is compliant with treatment, relief of symptoms occurs within days, and the problem will resolve without sequelae.

COMPLICATIONS

- Stricture formation
- Epididymitis
- Prostatitis
- Proctitis
- PID in women
- Disseminated gonococcal infection
- Gonococcal meningitis
- Gonococcal endocarditis
- Perinatal transmission (chlamydial conjunctivitis, chlamydial pneumonia, ophthalmia neonatorum)
- Reiter syndrome

REFERENCES

1. Centers for Disease Control and Prevention (CDC). Increases in fluoroquinolone-resistant Neisseria gonorrhoeae among men who have sex with men–United States, 2003, and revised recommendations for gonorrhea treatment, 2004. *MMWR Morb Mortal Wkly Rep*. 2004;53:335–8.
2. Berg AO. Screening for chlamydia infections: Recommendations and rationale. *Am J Prev Med*. 2001;20:90–4.
3. CDC. Sexually transmitted diseases treatment guidelines. *MMWR*. 2006;55(No. RR-11).

ADDITIONAL READING

- Ansart S, Hochedez P, Perez L, et al. Sexually transmitted diseases diagnosed among travelers returning from the tropics. *J Travel Med*. 2009;16:79–83.
- Centers for Disease Control and Prevention. *Sexually Transmitted Disease Surveillance, 2007*. Atlanta, GA: U.S. Department of Health and Human Services; December 2008.
- Groseclose SL, Brathwaite WS, Hall PA, et al. Summary of notifiable diseases–United States, 2002. *MMWR Morb Mortal Wkly Rep*. 2004;51:1–84.

See Also (Topic, Algorithm, Electronic Media Element)

Chlamydial Sexually Transmitted Diseases; Epididymitis; Gonococcal Infections; Pelvic Inflammatory Disease (PID); Prostatitis; Urinary Tract Infection in Females; Urinary Tract Infection in Males; Vulvovaginitis, Estrogen Deficient; Vulvovaginitis, Prepubescent

Algorithms: Dysuria; Genital Ulcers; Urethral Discharge

CODES

ICD9

- 098.0 Gonococcal infection (acute) of lower genitourinary tract
- 099.41 Other nongonococcal urethritis, chlamydia trachomatis
- 597.80 Urethritis, unspecified

URINARY TRACT INFECTION (UTI) IN FEMALES

Akhil Das, MD
Leonard G. Gomella, MD

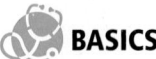

BASICS

DESCRIPTION
- Presence of pathogenic microorganisms within the urinary tract with concomitant symptoms
- This topic refers primarily to infectious cystitis; other urinary tract infections (UTIs) such as pyelonephritis are discussed elsewhere.
- Uncomplicated UTI: Uncomplicated UTI occurs in patients who have a normal, unobstructed genitourinary tract, who have no history of recent instrumentation, and whose symptoms are confined to the lower urinary tract. Uncomplicated UTIs are most common in young, sexually active women.
- Complicated UTI: Complicated UTI is an infection of the lower or upper urinary tract in the presence of an anatomic abnormality, a functional abnormality, or a urinary catheter.
- Recurrent UTI: Recurrent UTIs are symptomatic UTIs that follow resolution of an earlier episode, usually after appropriate treatment:
  – No single definition of the frequency of recurrent UTI exists, but a pragmatic definition is 3 or more infections per year.
  – Most recurrences are thought to represent reinfection rather than relapse.
  – There is no evidence that recurrent UTIs lead to health problems such as hypertension or renal disease, in the absence of anatomic or functional abnormalities of the urinary tract (1).
- System(s) affected: Renal/Urologic
- Synonym(s): Cystitis; Infectious cystitis

EPIDEMIOLOGY
Incidence
- Accounts for 8 million doctor visits and 1 million emergency room visits, and contributes to >100,000 hospital admissions each year
- 11% of women have UTIs in any given year.
- Predominant age: Young adults and older
- Predominant sex: Female >Male

Prevalence
- >50% of females have at least 1 UTI in their lifetime.
- 1 in 4 women have recurrent UTIs.

RISK FACTORS
- Previous UTI
- Diabetes mellitus (DM)
- Pregnancy
- Sexual activity
- Use of spermicides or diaphragm
- Underlying abnormalities of the urinary tract, such as tumors, calculi, strictures, incomplete bladder emptying, urinary incontinence, neurogenic bladder
- Catheterization
- Recent antibiotic use
- Poor hygiene
- Estrogen deficiency
- Inadequate fluid intake

Genetics
In women with HLA-3 and nonsecretor Lewis antigen, there is an increased bacterial adherence, which may lead to an increased risk in UTI.

GENERAL PREVENTION
- Maintain good hydration.
- Women with frequent or intercourse-related UTI should empty bladder immediately before and following intercourse; consider postcoital antibiotic.
- Avoid feminine hygiene sprays and douches.
- Wipe urethra from front to back.
- Cranberry juice (not cranberry juice cocktail) consumption may prevent recurrent infections.

PATHOPHYSIOLOGY
- Bacteria and subsequent infection in the urinary tract arise chiefly via ascending bacterial movement and propagation.
- Pathogenic organisms (*Escherichia coli*) possess adherence factors and toxins that allow initiation and propagation of genitourinary infections:
  – Type 1 and *P. pili*
  – Lipopolysaccharide

ETIOLOGY
- Most UTIs are caused by bacteria originating from bowel flora:
  – *E. coli* is the causative organism in 80% of cases of uncomplicated cystitis.
  – *Staphylococcus saprophyticus* accounts for 15% of infections.
  – Enterobacteriaceae (i.e., *Klebsiella, Proteus, Enterobacter, Pseudomonas)* also contribute.
- *Candida* is associated with nosocomial UTI.

COMMONLY ASSOCIATED CONDITIONS
See Risk Factors.

Geriatric Considerations
- Elderly patients are more likely to have underlying urinary tract abnormality.
- Acute UTI may be associated with incontinence or mental status changes in the elderly.

DIAGNOSIS

HISTORY
Note: Any or all may be present:
- Burning during urination
- Pain during urination (dysuria)
- Urgency (sensation of need to urinate often)
- Frequency
- Sensation of incomplete bladder emptying
- Blood in urine
- Lower abdominal pain or cramping
- Offensive odor of urine
- Nocturia
- Sudden onset of urinary incontinence
- Dyspareunia

PHYSICAL EXAM
- Suprapubic tenderness
- Urethral and/or vaginal tenderness
- Fever or costovertebral angle tenderness indicates upper UTI.

DIAGNOSTIC TESTS & INTERPRETATION
Lab
Initial lab tests
- Urinalysis:
  – Pyuria (>10 neutrophils/high-power field [HPF])
  – Bacteriuria (any amount on unspun urine, or 10 bacteria/HPF on centrifuged urine)
  – Hematuria (>5 red blood cells [RBCs]/HPF)
- Dipsticks urinalysis:
  – Leukocyte esterase (75–96% sensitivity, 94–98% specificity, when >100,000 colony-forming units [cfu])
  – Nitrite tests useful with nitrite-reducing organisms (e.g., enterococci, *S. saprophyticus, Acinetobacter)*
- Urine culture: *Only* indicated if diagnosis is unclear or patient has recurrent infections and resistance is suspected:
  – Presence of 100,000 cfu/mL of organism indicates infection.
  – Suspect a contaminated specimen when culture shows multiple types of bacteria.

Follow-Up & Special Considerations
- In nonpregnant, premenopausal women with symptoms of UTI, positive urinalysis, and no risks for complicated infection, empirical treatment without obtaining a urine culture may be given.
- Some argue that dipstick urinalysis is unnecessary with characteristic symptoms (i.e., high pretest probability).

Imaging
Initial approach
Imaging studies are often not required in most cases of UTI.

Follow-Up & Special Considerations
- Imaging may be indicated for UTIs in men, infants, immunocompromised patients, febrile infection, signs or symptoms of obstruction, failure to respond to appropriate therapy, and in patients with recurrent infections.
- CT scan and MRI provide the most complete anatomic data in adults.

Pediatric Considerations
For infants and children, obtain ultrasound (US); if ureteral dilatation is detected, obtain either voiding cystourethrogram or isotope cystogram to evaluate for reflux.

Diagnostic Procedures/Surgery
- Urethral catheterization to obtain urine specimen from children and adults if voided urine is suspected of being contaminated
- Suprapubic bladder aspiration or urethral catheterization to obtain specimen from infants
- Cystourethroscopy may be indicated for patients with recurrent UTIs and previous anti-incontinence surgery or hematuria.

DIFFERENTIAL DIAGNOSIS
- Vaginitis
- Asymptomatic bacteriuria
- Sexually transmitted diseases (STDs) causing urethritis or pyuria
- Hematuria from causes other than infection (e.g., neoplasia, calculi)
- Interstitial cystitis
- Psychological dysfunction

TREATMENT

MEDICATION

First Line

- Uncomplicated UTI (adolescents and adults who are nonpregnant, nondiabetic, afebrile, immunocompetent, and without genitourinary anatomic abnormalities) (2):
  - TMP-SMZ (Bactrim) 160/800 mg p.o. b.i.d. × 3 days, where resistance of *E. coli* strains <20% (3)[C]
  - 5-day course of nitrofurantoin or 3-day fluoroquinolone course should be used in patients with allergy to TMP-SMZ and in areas where *E. coli* resistance to TMP-SMZ >20% (3)[C]
- UTI in pregnancy:
  - Nitrofurantoin (Macrobid) 100 mg p.o. b.i.d. × 7 days (4)[C]
  - Cephalexin (Keflex) 500 mg p.o. b.i.d. × 7 days (4)[C]
- Postcoital UTI: Single-dose TMP-SMX or cephalexin may reduce frequency of UTI in sexually active women.
- Complicated UTI (pregnancy, diabetes, febrile, immunocompromised patient, recurrent UTIs): Extend course to 7–10 days of treatment with antibiotic chosen based on culture results; may begin with fluoroquinolone, TMP-SMX, or cephalosporin while awaiting results:
  - Fluoroquinolones are not safe during pregnancy or for treatment of children.
  - TMP-SMX use in pregnancy is not desirable (especially in 3rd trimester), but is appropriate in some circumstances.

Second Line

- Uncomplicated UTI:
  - Ciprofloxacin 250 mg p.o. b.i.d. × 3 day; should be reserved for complicated UTIs
  - Fosfomycin (Monurol) 3 g p.o. single dose
- Chronic UTIs: Continuous antimicrobial prophylaxis involves daily administration of low-dose TMP-SMX and/or nitrofurantoin (5)[C].

ADDITIONAL TREATMENT

General Measures

- Maintain good hydration.
- Maintain good hygiene.
- 1/4 of women with uncomplicated UTI experience a 2nd UTI within 6 months and 1/2 at some time during their lifetime.
- Avoid sexual intercourse while symptomatic.

Issues for Referral

Men with uncomplicated UTI and most other patients with complicated UTI should be referred to a urologist for evaluation.

Pediatric Considerations

UTI in children, especially <1 year of age, should prompt workup for urinary tract anomalies.

COMPLEMENTARY AND ALTERNATIVE MEDICINE

Preliminary studies indicate that *Vaccinium macrocarpon* (cranberry) juice may help to prevent and treat UTIs by inhibiting bacterial adherence to the bladder epithelium.

SURGERY/OTHER PROCEDURES

- Urinary tract obstruction with urosepsis requires drainage of obstructed system.
- Patients with emphysematous pyelonephritis or pyonephrosis may need immediate surgical intervention.

IN-PATIENT CONSIDERATIONS

Outpatient treatment, except for complicated or upper tract infections

ONGOING CARE

FOLLOW-UP RECOMMENDATIONS

- 1st or rare UTI: In young or middle-aged, nonpregnant adult females, no follow-up is required if cured after 3-day therapy.
- If persistently symptomatic after 2–3 days of therapy, obtain culture/sensitivity and change antibiotic accordingly.

Pregnancy Considerations

- UTI during pregnancy always requires culture/sensitivity and usually requires a 10- to 14-day treatment.
- Following the treatment of acute infection, pregnant women warrant surveillance urine cultures every trimester. They may receive prophylactic antibiotics for the remainder of pregnancy for recurrent or upper tract disease.

PATIENT EDUCATION

FamilyDoctor.org at http://familydoctor.org/online/famdocen/home/women/gen-health/190.html

PROGNOSIS

Symptoms resolve within 2–3 days of antibiotic treatment in almost all patients.

COMPLICATIONS

- Pyelonephritis or sepsis
- Renal abscess
- Acute urinary outlet obstruction

Pregnancy Considerations

Pregnant females, infants, and young children with cystitis are at higher risk of pyelonephritis.

REFERENCES

1. Kodner CM, Thomas Gupton EK, et al. Recurrent urinary tract infections in women: diagnosis and management. *Am Fam Physician*. 2010;82: 638–43.
2. Litza JA, Brill JR, et al. Urinary tract infections. *Prim. Care*. 2010;37:491–507, viii
3. Warren JW, Abrutyn E, Hebel JR, et al. Guidelines for antimicrobial treatment of uncomplicated acute bacterial cystitis and acute pyelonephritis in women. Infectious Diseases Society of America (IDSA). *Clin Infect Dis*. 1999;29:745–58.
4. Mehnert-Kay SA. Diagnosis and management of uncomplicated urinary tract infections. *Am Fam Physician*. 2005;72:451–6.
5. Stepleton A, et al. Prevention of urinary tract infection. *Infect Dis Clin N Am*. 1997;11:719–33.

ADDITIONAL READING

Fihn SD. Acute uncomplicated urinary tract infection in women. *N Engl J Med*. 2003;329(3):259–66.

See Also (Topic, Algorithm, Electronic Media Element)

Algorithm: Dysuria

CODES

ICD9

- 595.9 Cystitis, unspecified
- 599.0 Urinary tract infection, site not specified

CLINICAL PEARLS

- Uncomplicated UTIs cause a significant morbidity but generally do not cause renal damage.
- Treatment of uncomplicated UTIs reduces morbidity, but the risk of recurrence stays the same.
- Most UTIs are caused by bacteria originating from bowel flora.
- The combination of bacteriuria and white blood cells (WBCs) in the urine gives us a presumptive diagnosis of UTI.
- >100,000 cfu/mL on a urine culture confirms a symptomatic UTI.
- Imaging studies are not required for most women with UTIs.
- Uncomplicated UTIs should be treated for 3 days.
- All pregnant women with bacteriuria should be treated.

U

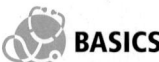

BASICS

DESCRIPTION
- Cystitis is an infection of the lower urinary tract, usually resulting from a single gram-negative enteric bacteria. (See separate topics for information on prostatitis, pyelonephritis, and nongonococcal urethritis.)
- System(s) affected: Renal/Urologic
- Synonym(s): UTI; Cystitis

EPIDEMIOLOGY
Incidence
- Predominant age: Increases with age
- Uncommon in men <50 years of age
- 8 infections/10,000 men aged 21–50 years

Prevalence
Not common

RISK FACTORS
- Benign prostatic hypertrophy (BPH)
- Cognitive impairment
- Fecal incontinence
- Urinary incontinence
- Anal intercourse
- Recent urologic surgery, catheterization
- Infection of the prostate or kidney
- Urinary tract instrumentation
- Immunocompromised host
- Outlet obstruction

GENERAL PREVENTION
- Prompt treatment of predisposing factors
- Catheter use only when necessary; if needed, use aseptic technique and closed system, with removal as soon as possible.

ETIOLOGY
- *Escherichia coli* (80% of infections)
- *Klebsiella*
- *Enterobacter*
- *Proteus*
- *Pseudomonas*
- *Serratia*
- *Streptococcus faecalis* and *Staphylococcus* sp.

COMMONLY ASSOCIATED CONDITIONS
- Acute bacterial pyelonephritis
- Chronic bacterial pyelonephritis
- Urethritis
- Prostatitis
- Prostatic hypertrophy
- Prostate cancer

Geriatric Considerations
Bacteriuria is common in the elderly, appears related to functional status, and is usually transient. If asymptomatic bacteriuria is noted, no treatment is needed.

Pediatric Considerations
Usually associated with obstruction to normal flow of urine, such as vesicoureteral reflux

DIAGNOSIS

Urologic investigations are necessary to rule out other disorders.

HISTORY
- Urinary frequency
- Urinary urgency
- Dysuria
- Hesitancy
- Slow urinary stream
- Dribbling of urine
- Nocturia
- Suprapubic discomfort
- Low back pain
- Hematuria

PHYSICAL EXAM
Systemic symptoms (chills, fever) present with concomitant pyelonephritis or prostatitis.

DIAGNOSTIC TESTS & INTERPRETATION
Lab
- Pyuria
- Bacteriuria
- Urine dipstick leukocyte esterase (75–90% sensitivity, 95% specificity) and nitrate (35–85% sensitivity, 70% specificity)
- Urine culture: 10 high-power colonies of pathogens (or counts >100,000 bacteria/mL of urine) confirm diagnosis (*E. coli, Klebsiella, Pseudomonas,* other agents). Lower counts also may be indicative of infection, especially in the presence of pyuria.
- Segmented bacteriologic localization cultures:
  - Variable block 1 (VB1): Collect 5–10 mL of urine from patient's initial voiding.
  - VB2: Then a sample of sterile midstream urine is obtained.
  - Expressed prostatic secretion (EPS): Prostatic massage is performed, and EPS is collected from the meatus.
  - VB3: Patient completes voiding, and 4th sample is collected.
  - Cultures and sensitivity are collected from each specimen.
- Consider differentiating UTI from sexually transmitted disease based on history and risk factors, and if present, test and treat for *Chlamydia* and *N. gonorrhoeae.*
- Drugs that may alter lab results: Antibiotics prior to culture

Imaging
- IV pyelography
- Cystoscopy
- Ultrasound

Pathological Findings
Depends on site of infection

DIFFERENTIAL DIAGNOSIS
- Anatomic or functional pathology
- Urethritis/sexually transmitted infections
- Infections in other sites of the genitourinary tract (e.g., epididymis)

TREATMENT

MEDICATION

First Line

- Acute infection, 1st infection, no risk factors for treatment: Prescribe 7–10 days of oral antibiotics, either empirically or based on culture and sensitivity results. For empirical therapy, trimethoprim-sulfamethoxazole DS (SMX-TMP, Bactrim DS, Septra DS, others) b.i.d. usually will treat the most likely pathogens (1,2)[C].
- Complicated or recurrent infection: Prescribe 14–21 days of antibiotics based on antimicrobial sensitivities with repeat urine check after the treatment (1,2)[C].

Second Line

According to culture and sensitivity results and patient's history

ADDITIONAL TREATMENT

General Measures

- Hydration; analgesia if required
- Discontinue sexual activity until cured.
- Patient with indwelling catheters:
  – If asymptomatic bacterial colonization, no need to treat (sterilization of urine is not possible, and resistant organisms may take up residence).
  – If symptomatic of acute infection, institute treatment.

IN-PATIENT CONSIDERATIONS

Admission Criteria

- Inability to tolerate oral medications
- Acute renal failure
- Suspected sepsis

 # ONGOING CARE

FOLLOW-UP RECOMMENDATIONS

Patient Monitoring

- Close follow-up until clinically well
- Repeat urinalysis after treatment.

DIET

Encourage adequate fluid intake.

PATIENT EDUCATION

- For patient education materials favorably reviewed on this topic, contact the National Kidney Foundation, 30 E. 33rd Street, Suite 1100, New York, NY 10016; (212) 889–2210.
- Push fluids, especially those that acidify the urine.

PROGNOSIS

Clearing of infections with appropriate antibiotic treatment

COMPLICATIONS

- Pyelonephritis
- Ascending infection
- Recurrent infection

REFERENCES

1. Finn SD. Urinary tract infections—diagnosis and treatment in women and men. *Consultant*. 1992;10:43–58.
2. Naber KG, Bergman B, Bishop MC, et al. EAU guidelines for the management of urinary and male genital tract infections. Urinary Tract Infection (UTI) Working Group of the Health Care Office (HCO) of the European Association of Urology (EAU). *Eur Urol*. 2001;40:576–88.

ADDITIONAL READING

- Harrington RD, Hooton TM. Urinary tract infection risk factors and gender. *J Gend Specif Med*. 2000 Nov-Dec;3:27–34.
- Hatton J, Hughes M, Raymond CH. Management of bacterial urinary tract infections in adults. *Ann Pharmacother*. 1994;28:1264–72.
- Hooton TM, Stam WE. Management of acute uncomplicated urinary tract infection in adults. *Med Clin North Am*. 1991;75:339–57.
- Lipsky BA. Managing urinary tract infections in men. *Hosp Pract (Off Ed)*. 2000;35:53–59, discussion 59–60.
- Lipsky BA. Urinary tract infections in men. Epidemiology, pathophysiology, diagnosis, and treatment. *Ann Intern Med*. 1989;110:138–50.

See Also (Topic, Algorithm, Electronic Media Element)

Prostatic Cancer; Prostatic Hyperplasia, Benign (BPH); Prostatitis; Pyelonephritis; Urethritis
Algorithms: Dysuria; Urethral Discharge

 # CODES

ICD9

- 595.0 Acute cystitis
- 595.2 Other chronic cystitis
- 595.4 Cystitis in diseases classified elsewhere

CLINICAL PEARLS

- Cystitis is an infection of the lower urinary tract, usually resulting from a single gram-negative enteric bacteria. (See separate chapters for information on prostatitis, pyelonephritis, and nongonococcal urethritis.)
- Risk factors/causes: BPH, cognitive impairment, fecal incontinence, urinary incontinence, anal intercourse, recent urologic surgery, catheterization, infection of the prostate or kidney, urinary tract instrumentation, immunocompromised host, outlet obstruction
- Evaluation: Urinalysis, urine culture, STD testing (gonorrhea, chlamydia, etc. by culture or DNA probe)

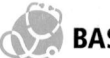 **BASICS**

DESCRIPTION
- Stone formation within the urinary tract: Urinary crystals bind to form a nidus, which grows to form a calculus (stone).
- Range of symptoms: Asymptomatic to obstructive; may be result of infection

EPIDEMIOLOGY
- The worldwide epidemiology differs according to both geographic area (higher prevalence in hot, arid, or dry climates) and socioeconomic conditions (dietary intake and lifestyle). Radiolucent stones and stones secondary to infection are less influenced by environmental conditions.
- Vesical calculosis (bladder stones) due to malnutrition in early life is frequent in Middle Eastern and Asian countries.
- Incidences in industrialized countries appear to be increasing, probably due to improved diagnostics, as well as to increasingly rich diets.
- Increased incidence in patients with surgically induced absorption issues such as Crohn disease and gastric bypass surgery

Incidence
- In industrialized countries: 100–200/100,000 per year
- Predominant age: Mean age is 40–60 years.
- Predominant sex: Male > Female (~2:1)

RISK FACTORS
- White > African American in regions with both populations
- Family history
- Pregnancy
- Diet rich in protein, refined carbohydrates, and sodium
- Occupations associated with a sedentary lifestyle or with a hot, dry workplace
- Incidence rates peak in summer secondary to dehydration
- Obesity
- Surgically or medically induced malabsorption (Crohn, gastric bypass, celiac)

Genetics
- Up to 20% of patients have a family history. However, spouses of stone formers have higher calcium excretion rates than controls, suggesting strong dietary–environmental factors.
- Autosomal dominant: Idiopathic hypercalciuria
- Autosomal recessive:
  - Cystinuria, Lesch-Nyhan syndrome, hyperoxaluria types I and II
  - Ehlers-Danlos syndrome, Marfan syndrome, Wilson disease, familial renal tubular acidosis

GENERAL PREVENTION
- Hydration
- Decrease salt and meat intake.
- Avoid oxalate-rich foods.

Pediatric Considerations
Rare: More common in males; low socioeconomic status

Pregnancy Considerations
- Pregnant women have the same incidence of renal colic as do nonpregnant women.
- Majority of symptomatic stones occur in the 2nd and 3rd trimesters, heralded by symptoms of flank pain or hematuria.
- Most common differential diagnosis is physiologic hydronephrosis of pregnancy. Use US to avoid irradiation. Non-contrast-enhanced CT scan also is diagnostic.
- Treatment goals:
  - Pain control, avoid infection, and preserve renal function until birth or stone passage.
  - 30% require intervention such as stent placement.

PATHOPHYSIOLOGY
- Supersaturation and dehydration lead to high salt content in urine, which congregates.
- Stasis of urine:
  - Renal malformation (e.g., horseshoe kidney, ureteropelvic junction obstruction)
  - Incomplete bladder emptying (e.g., neurogenic bladder, prostate enlargement, MS)
- Crystals may form in pure solutions (homogeneous) or on existing surfaces such as other crystals, cellular debris (heterogeneous).
- Balance of promoters and inhibitors: Organic (Tamm-Horsfall protein, GAG, uropontin, nephrocalcin) and inorganic (citrate, pyrophosphate)

ETIOLOGY
- Calcium oxalate and/or phosphate stones (80%):
  - Hypercalciuria:
    - Absorptive hypercalciuria: Increased jejunal calcium absorption
    - Renal leak: Increased calcium excretion from renal proximal tubule
    - Resorptive hypercalciuria: Mild hyperparathyroidism
  - Hypercalcemia:
    - Hyperparathyroidism
    - Sarcoidosis
    - Malignancy
    - Immobilization
    - Paget's disease
- Hyperoxaluria:
  - Enteric hyperoxaluria:
    - Intestinal malabsorptive state associated with IBD, celiac sprue, or intestinal resection
    - Bile salt malabsorption leads to formation of calcium soaps.
  - Primary hyperoxaluria: Autosomal recessive, types I and II
  - Dietary hyperoxaluria: Overindulgence in oxalate-rich food

- Hyperuricosuria:
  - Seen in 10% of calcium stone formers
  - Caused by increased dietary purine intake, systemic acidosis, myeloproliferative diseases, gout, chemotherapy, Lesch-Nyhan syndrome
  - Thiazides, probenecid
- Hypocitraturia:
  - Caused by acidosis: RTA, malabsorption, thiazides, enalapril, excessive dietary protein
- Uric acid stones (10–15%): Hyperuricemia causes as above
- Struvite stones (5–10%): Infected urine with urease-producing organisms (most commonly *Proteus* species)
- Cystine stones (<1%): Autosomal recessive disorder of renal tubular reabsorption of cystine
- In children: Usually due to malnutrition

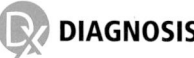 **DIAGNOSIS**

- Pain:
  - Renal colic: Acute onset of severe groin and/or flank pain
  - Distal stones may present with referred pain in labia, penile meatus, or testis.
- Microscopic or gross hematuria occurs in 95% of patients.
- Nonspecific symptoms of nausea, vomiting, tachycardia, diaphoresis
- Low-grade fever without signs of infection
- Infectious origin: Associated with high-grade fevers
- Frequency and dysuria especially occur with stones at the vesicoureteric junction (VUJ).
- Asymptomatic: Nonobstructing stones within the renal calyces

PHYSICAL EXAM
Tender costovertebral angle and/or iliac fossa

DIAGNOSTIC TESTS & INTERPRETATION
Lab
- Urinalysis for red blood cells, leukocytes, nitrates, pH (acidic urine <5.5 is associated with uric acid stones; alkaline >7.0 with struvite stones)
- Midstream urine for microscopy, culture, and sensitivity
- Blood: Urea, creatinine, electrolytes, calcium, and urate; consider CBC.
- PTH only if calcium elevated
- Stone analysis if/when stone passed

Imaging
- Non-contrast-enhanced CT scan of the abdomen and pelvis has replaced IVP as the investigation of choice:
  - Stone is found most commonly at levels of ureteric luminal narrowing: Pelviureteric junction, pelvic brim, and VUJ
  - Acute obstruction: Proximal ureter and renal pelvis are dilated to the level of obstruction, and perinephric stranding possible on imaging

- KUB to determine if stone is radiopaque or lucent:
  - Calcium oxalate/phosphate stones are radiopaque.
  - Uric acid stones are radiolucent.
  - Staghorn calculi (that fill the shape of the renal calyces) are usually struvite and opaque.
  - Cystine stones are faintly opaque (ground-glass appearance).
- Ultrasound has low sensitivity and specificity but is often the first choice for pregnancy.

DIFFERENTIAL DIAGNOSIS
- Appendicitis
- Ruptured aortic aneurysm
- Musculoskeletal strain
- Pyelonephritis (upper UTI)
- Pyonephrosis (obstructed upper UTI; emergency)
- Perinephric abscess
- Ectopic pregnancy
- Salpingitis

 TREATMENT

MEDICATION
- Medical expulsive therapy: α_1-Antagonists (e.g., terazosin) and calcium channel blockers improve likelihood of spontaneous stone passage with NNT of ~5.
- Class C in pregnancy

ADDITIONAL TREATMENT
General Measures
- 75% of patients are successfully treated conservatively and pass the stone spontaneously.
- Stones that do not pass usually require surgical intervention.
- 30–50% of patients will have recurrent stones.

Issues for Referral
- Urgent referral of patients with UTI/sepsis or acute renal failure/solitary kidney
- Early referral of pregnant patients, large stones (>8 mm), chronic renal failure, children
- Refer with no passage at 2–4 weeks or poorly controlled pain.

Additional Therapies
- Uric acid stone dissolution therapy:
  - Alkalinize urine with potassium citrate; keep pH >6.5.
  - Allopurinol 100–300 mg/d p.o.
- Cystine stone dissolution/prevention:
  - Alkalinize urine with potassium citrate; keep pH >6.5.
  - Chelating agents: Captopril, α-mercapto propionylglycine, D-penicillamine
- Consider altering medications that increase risk of stone formation: Probenecid, loop diuretics, salicylic acid, salbutamol, indinavir, triamterene, acetazolamide

- Treat hypercalciuria with thiazides on an acute basis only.
- Treat hypocitraturia with potassium citrate and high-citrate juices (orange, lemon, etc.).
- Treat enteric hyperoxaluria with oral calcium or magnesium, cholestyramine, and potassium citrate.

SURGERY/OTHER PROCEDURES
- Immediate relief of obstruction is required in the following groups of patients:
  - Sepsis
  - Renal failure (obstructed solitary kidney, bilateral obstruction)
  - Uncontrolled pain despite adequate analgesia
- Emergency surgery for obstruction:
  - Placement of a retrograde stent (i.e., endoscopic surgery, usually requiring an anesthetic)
  - Radiologic placement of a percutaneous nephrostomy tube
- Elective surgery for stone treatment:
  - Extracorporeal shock-wave lithotripsy
  - Ureteroscopy with basket extraction or lithotripsy (laser or pneumatic)
  - Percutaneous nephrolithotomy
- Open surgery uncommon

IN-PATIENT CONSIDERATIONS
Initial Stabilization
- Analgesia:
  - Combination of NSAIDs (indomethacin suppository 100 mg, ketorolac 30–60 mg) and oral opiate
  - Parenteral narcotic if vomiting or if preceding fails to control pain (morphine 5–10 mg IV or IM q3h)
  - Antiemetic if required or prophylactically with parenteral narcotics
- Septic patients with pyonephrosis may require IV fluids and, in severe cases, cardiorespiratory support in intensive care during recovery.

 ONGOING CARE

FOLLOW-UP RECOMMENDATIONS
- Patients with ureteric stones who are being treated conservatively should be followed until imaging is clear or stone is visibly passed:
  - Strain urine and send stone for composition.
  - Tamsulosin and nifedipine in selected patients to speed passage
  - Present to the hospital if pain worsens or signs of infection.
  - If pain management is suboptimal or stone does not progress or pass within 2–4 weeks, patient should be referred to a urologist and imaging should be repeated.
- Recurrent stone formers should have follow-up with a urologist for metabolic workup: 24-hour urine for volume, pH, creatinine, calcium, cystine, phosphate, oxalate, uric acid, magnesium

DIET
- Increased fluid intake for life cannot be overemphasized for decreasing recurrence. Encourage 2–3 L/d intake; advise patient to have clear urine rather than yellow.
- Calcium stone formers should minimize high-oxalate foods such as green leafy vegetables, rhubarb, peanuts, chocolates, and beer.
- Decrease protein and salt intake.
- Lowering calcium intake is inadvisable and even may increase urine calcium excretion.

PROGNOSIS
- Spontaneous stone passage depends on stone location (proximal vs distal) and stone size (<5 mm 90% pass, >8 mm 10% pass).
- Stone recurrence: 50% of patients at 10 years

ADDITIONAL READING
- Matlaga BR, Shore AD, Magnuson T, et al. Effect of Gastric Bypass Surgery on Kidney Stone Disease. *J Urol.* 2009 Apr 15.
- Penniston KL, Jones AN, Nakada SY, et al. Vitamin D repletion does not alter urinary calcium excretion in healthy postmenopausal women. *BJU Int.* 2009.
- Qiang W, et al. Water for preventing urinary calculi. *Cochrane Database Sys Rev.* 2004;3:CD004292.
- Tiselius HG. Epidemiology and medical management of stone disease. *BJU Int.* 2003;91:758–67.
- Worster A, Preyra I, Weaver B, et al. The accuracy of noncontrast helical computed tomography versus intravenous pyelography in the diagnosis of suspected acute urolithiasis: a meta-analysis. *Ann Emerg Med.* 2002;40:280–6.

See Also (Topic, Algorithm, Electronic Media Element)
Algorithms: Dysuria; Urethral Discharge; Renal Calculi

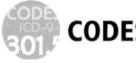 CODES

ICD9
592.9 Urinary calculus, unspecified

URTICARIA

Weily Soong, MD

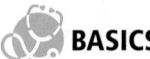 **BASICS**

DESCRIPTION

- A rash that rapidly erupts in polymorphic-shaped cutaneous wheals with central swelling, erythema, and blanching; size ranges from millimeters to centimeters; single or multiple superficial papules and plaques; associated with itching or burning
- Subsides within 24 hours with no scars or change in pigmentation
- May be recurrent; often associated with angioedema (swelling of the lower dermis and subcutis)
- Spontaneous urticaria:
  - Acute: Persists <6 weeks:
    ○ Vast number of possible triggers, e.g., foods, medications, herbs, bites, infections, occupational exposures, etc.
    ○ Etiology is often obvious but can be idiopathic.
  - Chronic: Persists >6 weeks:
    ○ Can be either continuous (daily symptoms) or recurrent (periods with flares and periods with no symptoms)
    ○ Usually not IgE-mediated and most likely autoimmune-related
    ○ Known cause (~20%): Include environmental allergies (IgE-mediated), autoimmune diseases, chronic indolent infections, malignancy, herbs, medications, mastocytosis/urticaria pigmentosa
    ○ Idiopathic (~80%): The longer urticaria persists, the more difficult it is to find the etiology.
    ○ 50% of idiopathic cases are autoimmune chronic urticaria; caused by autoantibodies to the high-affinity IgE receptor (FcR1) or to IgE itself.
    ○ The other 50% are truly idiopathic, with reported associations with psychological stress, unknown autoimmunity, or pseudoallergenic foods/additives.
- Physical urticaria:
  - Dermatographism: Linear, itchy, red wheal and flare from scratching or rubbing the skin
  - Cold urticaria: From exposure to cold; usually idiopathic but can be due to infections, neoplasia, or autoimmune diseases; the familial form (familial cold autoinflammatory syndrome) characterized by recurrent bouts of fever, urticaria, and joint pain triggered by cold; due to mutations in *Cryopyrin* gene resulting in the release of interleukin 1
  - Delayed pressure urticaria: Deeper, more painful urticaria; occurs 2–6 hours after pressure to skin (e.g., from elastic or shoes)
  - Solar urticaria: From sunlight exposure, usually UV; onset in minutes; subsides within 2 hours
  - Heat urticaria: From direct contact with warm objects or air; rare
  - Vibratory urticaria/angioedema: From strong vibrating mechanical forces; rare
- Special forms of urticaria:
  - Cholinergic urticaria: Due to brief increase of core body temperature; small pin-sized (5- to 10-mm) wheals surrounded by an erythema, but also can have larger wheals; from physical exercise, stress, and hot showers
  - Adrenergic urticaria: Caused by stress; extremely rare; has pinpoint-sized red wheals with a white halo

- Contact urticaria: Wheals at sites where chemical substances contact the skin
- Aquagenic urticaria: Small wheals after contact with water at any temperature; rare
- Urticarial vasculitis: A leukocytoclastic vasculitis looking like urticaria and tending to last >24 h; more painful than pruritic; may be palpable and purpuric; usually caused by a collagen-vascular disease
- Synonym(s): Hives; Welts

EPIDEMIOLOGY

Incidence
- Predominant in all ages: Acute form mainly in children; chronic form mainly in adults
- Predominant gender: Male = Female
- In 20% of patients, chronic urticaria lasts >10 years.

Prevalence
- Affects 15–25% of population during lifetime
- In the US: 1 in 1,000
- Up to 3% of the population at some point has chronic idiopathic urticaria.

Pediatric Considerations
- Acute isolated incidents are more frequent; affects 6–7% of preschool children; 17% of children have a history of atopic dermatitis.
- In childhood acute urticaria, infection (i.e., respiratory and urinary tract) is the most frequently documented cause (49%), followed by drug (5%) and food allergies (3%).

RISK FACTORS
History of atopic diseases: Allergic rhinitis, asthma, atopic dermatitis, food and drug allergies

Genetics
No consistent pattern known

GENERAL PREVENTION
If patient is atopic, treating the atopic disease might prevent occurrence.

PATHOPHYSIOLOGY
- Caused by a degranulation of mast cells, which triggers a release of inflammatory mediators (e.g., histamine and leukotrienes) to cause local vasodilatation, cellular infiltration (e.g., lymphocytes, eosinophils, mast cells, basophils, neutrophils), vascular permeability, and edema of the dermis of the skin (urticaria) or of subcutaneous skin tissue (angioedema)
- May be immune-mediated (IgE-mediated), complement-mediated, non-immune-mediated (e.g., degranulation of mast cells by physical stimuli), autoimmune-mediated, or idiopathic

ETIOLOGY
- Spontaneous acute urticaria:
  - Bacterial infections: Strep throat, sinusitis, dental caries, otitis, urinary tract
  - Foods, especially in children: Most common are peanut, tree nuts, seafood, milk, soy, fish, wheat, and eggs; tend to be IgE-mediated; pseudoallergenic foods, such as preservatives, additives, berries, and tomatoes, are possible but not common.
  - Drugs: IgE-mediated (e.g., penicillin), non-IgE-mediated (e.g., aspirin and NSAIDs)

- Inhalant, contact, ingestion, or occupational exposure (e.g., latex, cosmetics)
- Insect bite or sting
- Transfusion reaction
- Spontaneous chronic urticaria:
  - Chronic subclinical IgE-mediated atopic diseases (e.g., allergic rhinitis, eczema)
  - Chronic indolent infections: *H. pylori*, fungal, parasitic, dental caries, and chronic viral infections (hepatitis)
  - Collagen-vascular disease (cutaneous vasculitis, serum sickness, lupus)
  - Thyroid autoimmunity
  - Hormonal: Pregnancy and progesterone
  - Autoimmune antibodies to the IgE receptor on mast cells and to the IgE antibody
  - Chronic medications (e.g., NSAIDs, β-blockers, hormones, ACE inhibitors, etc.)
  - Malignancy/paraneoplastic; rare
  - Emotional stress (little supporting evidence)

COMMONLY ASSOCIATED CONDITIONS
- Angioedema
- Anaphylaxis

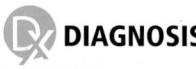 **DIAGNOSIS**

HISTORY
- Duration of symptoms, potential triggers, and history of atopy and/or autoimmune diseases
- Seen alone or with angioedema
- Urticaria may be an initial symptom of a generalized anaphylactic reaction.
- Intensely pruritic
- Fast onset; resolves in <48 hours

PHYSICAL EXAM
- Single or multiple raised, blanched, central wheals surrounded by red flare anywhere on body
- Variably sized, 1–20 cm or larger
- Exam to detect any associated conditions (autoimmune; malignancy; and viral, bacterial, and fungal/tinea infections)

DIAGNOSTIC TESTS & INTERPRETATION
Lab
- Acute urticaria: Testing depends on the history and potential triggers:
  - Allergy skin tests and RAST for inhaled allergens, insects, drugs, or foods
  - Infection: Pharyngeal culture, LFTs, mononucleosis test, urinalysis
- Chronic urticaria: Depends on diagnostic suspicions:
  - CBC; thyroid function tests
  - Allergy skin tests and RAST for inhaled allergens, insects, drugs, or foods
  - Autoimmune: ESR, ANA, RF, complement (such as CH50, C3, C4), cryoglobulins
  - Tests for *H. pylori* (e.g., antibodies)
  - Stool for ova and parasites
  - Urinalysis
  - Total IgE level
  - Autologous serum skin testing
  - Measurement of antibodies to FcRI
  - Food and drug reactions: Elimination of or challenges with suspected agents
  - Malignancy workup, including serum protein electrophoresis and immunofixation

Imaging
Any imaging necessary to rule out chronic indolent infections (e.g., sinus CT scan) or malignancy (e.g., CXR)

Diagnostic Procedures/Surgery
- Food and drug reactions: Elimination of or challenges with suspected agents
- Physical and special forms of urticaria:
  – Dermatographism: Scratch skin, observe for surrounding urticaria.
  – Cold urticaria: Ice cube test: Place ice cube on skin for 5 minutes; observe for 10–15 minutes.
  – Cholinergic: Exercise challenge
  – Solar: Expose skin to wavelengths of light.
  – Delayed pressure: Apply 5- to 10-lb sandbag for 3 hours; observe.
  – Aquagenic: Apply water at various temperatures.
  – Vibratory: Apply vibration 4–5 minutes with a lab mixing device; observe.
- Skin biopsy to rule out urticarial vasculitis
- Routine dental care to rule out dental caries

DIFFERENTIAL DIAGNOSIS
- Anaphylaxis (may present with urticaria)
- Morbilliform drug eruptions
- Erythema multiforme
- SLE
- Vasculitis and polyarteritis
- Angioedema without urticaria (related to complement and bradykinin disorders, such as familial hereditary angioedema, ACE inhibitor angioedema, complement deficiencies)
- Urticaria pigmentosa/systemic mastocytosis: Pink lesions urticate when scratched (Darier sign).
- Bullous pemphigoid (urticarial stage)

TREATMENT

MEDICATION
First Line
- 1st-generation antihistamines (mainly for short, intermittent attacks of urticaria) (1,2)[A]:
  – Older children and adults: Hydroxyzine or diphenhydramine 25–50 mg q6h
  – Children <6 years old: Diphenhydramine 12.5 mg q6–8h (5 mg/kg/d) or hydroxyzine (10 mg/5 mL) 2 mg/kg/d divided q6–8h
- 2nd-generation H1-blockers; less sedating; longer half-life (1,2)[A]:
  – Fexofenadine (Allegra): 180 mg/d
  – Loratadine (Claritin): 10 mg/d
  – Desloratadine (Clarinex): 5 mg/d
  – Cetirizine (Zyrtec): 10 mg/d
  – Levocetirizine (Xyzal): 5 mg/d
- May need higher doses of antihistamines or a combination of multiple antihistamines for control
- Precautions:
  – Drowsiness and dry mouth and eyes
  – Use with caution in elderly and in pregnancy.

Second Line
- Doxepin (Sinequan): Tricyclic antidepressant with strong H1- and H2-blocking properties; 10–25 mg at bedtime; sedation limits usefulness (2)[C].
- H2-blockers (e.g., ranitidine, cimetidine, famotidine): Mildly helpful (1,2)[C]

- Corticosteroids: For unresponsive cases, e.g., prednisone 40 mg/d × 5–7 days; taper as antihistamines are introduced; avoid chronic use due to the severe side effects (2)[C]
- Cyproheptadine: Antihistamine and antiserotonergic agent (2)[C]
- Cyclosporine: Best-studied immunosuppressive therapy; effective (2.5–5 mg/kg/d) and steroid-sparing (3)[C]
- Leukotriene antagonists (montelukast and zafirlukast): Safe and worth trying in chronic, unresponsive cases (2)[C]
- Omalizumab (Xolair) in chronic idiopathic urticaria: Potentially safer than cyclosporine and corticosteroids but expensive (4)[C]
- IV immune globulin, plasmapheresis, sulfasalazine, dapsone, danazol, colchicine, calcium channel blockers, tacrolimus, methotrexate, and hydroxychloroquine require further study (3).

ADDITIONAL TREATMENT
General Measures
- Avoid the eliciting stimulus.
- Cold and heat urticaria: Avoid sudden changes in temperature.
- Dermatographic and delayed-pressure urticaria: Avoid pressure applied to the skin.
- Solar urticaria: Avoid the sun; use sunscreen.
- Cholinergic urticaria: Avoid sudden changes in body temperature (e.g., slow warm-ups and cool-downs during exercise).

Issues for Referral
Referral to an allergist and immunologist for elucidating and testing of potential triggers, life-threatening reactions, and complex management

COMPLEMENTARY AND ALTERNATIVE MEDICINE
Trace contaminants in herbal and vitamin supplements may make urticaria worse.

IN-PATIENT CONSIDERATIONS
Admission Criteria
- If urticaria and angioedema progress into anaphylaxis or threaten the airway, discharge with an EpiPen.
- If the airway is threatened, consider an immediate consult to evaluate for laryngeal edema.

ONGOING CARE

FOLLOW-UP RECOMMENDATIONS
Patient Monitoring
If symptoms persist, keep a daily diary of potential triggers (foods, activities, etc.).

DIET
If a particular food is implicated, avoid the food or use a trial of avoiding the food for 2–3 weeks.

PROGNOSIS
- 70% of acute symptoms resolved <72 hours.
- 30% of the patients are chronic.
- >50% of chronic idiopathic urticaria resolve in 3–5 years, but patients are at risk for a recurrence many years later.
- Spontaneous chronic urticaria/angioedema is usually *not* life-threatening.

REFERENCES
1. Baxi S, et al. Urticaria and angioedema. *Immunol Allergy Clin N Am*. 2005;25:353–67.
2. Zuberbier T. Urticaria. *Allergy*. 2003;58:1224–34.
3. Kaplan AP. Chronic urticaria: pathogenesis and treatment. *J Allergy Clin Immunol*. 2004;114: 465–74; quiz 475.
4. Spector SL, Tan RA. Effect of omalizumab on patients with chronic urticaria. *Ann Allergy Asthma Immunol*. 2007;99:190–3.

ADDITIONAL READING
- Dibbern DA. Urticaria: selected highlights and recent advances. *Med Clin North Am*. 2006;90:187–209.
- Joint Task Force on Practice Parameters. The diagnosis and management of urticaria: a practice parameter part I: acute urticaria/angioedema part II: chronic urticaria/angioedema. Joint Task Force on Practice Parameters. *Ann Allergy Asthma Immunol*. 2000;85:521–44.
- Kaplan AP, et al. What the first 10,000 patients with chronic urticaria have taught me: a personal journey. *J Allergy Clin Immunol*. 2009;123:713–7.
- Kaplan AP, Greaves M, et al. Pathogenesis of chronic urticaria. *Clin Exp Allergy*. 2009;39:777–87.
- Wedi B, Raap U, Kapp A. Chronic urticaria and infections. *Curr Opin Allergy Clin Immunol*. 2004;4:387–96.

CODES
ICD9
- 708.0 Allergic urticaria
- 708.1 Idiopathic urticaria
- 708.4 Vibratory urticaria

CLINICAL PEARLS
- If an angioedema patient has any itch, then it is a form of urticaria and not a pure form of angioedema, such as hereditary angioedema.
- Chronic urticaria is rarely caused by foods.
- Antihistamines treat most forms of urticaria.
- Most urticarias are not life-threatening.

UTERINE MYOMAS

Eric L. Jenison, MD
Michael P. Hopkins, MD, MEd
Stephen J. Bacak, DO, MPH

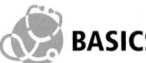 **BASICS**

DESCRIPTION
- Uterine leiomyomas are well-circumscribed, pseudoencapsulated, benign monoclonal tumors composed mainly of smooth muscle with varying amounts of fibrous connective tissue (1,2).
- 3 major subtypes:
  - Subserous: Common; external; may become pedunculated
  - Intramural: Common; within myometrium; may cause marked uterine enlargement
  - Submuous: ~5% of all cases; internal, evincing abnormal uterine bleeding and infection; occasionally protruding from cervix
- System(s) affected: Reproductive
- Synonyms: Fibroids; Myoma; Fibromyoma; Myofibroma; Fibroleiomyoma

EPIDEMIOLOGY
Incidence
- Incidence increases with each decade during reproductive years and is highest in perimenopausal age group (range 5.4–77%).
- Not seen in premenarchal females
- Predominant age: 3rd–4th decades
- Predominant sex: Females only
- 3 times more frequent and occurs earlier in African Americans

Prevalence
- 4–11% of all women
- 20% of women 35 years of age
- 40% of women 50 years of age

RISK FACTORS
- Black women have a 2.9-fold increase in relative risk compared with white women (2).
- Early menarche (<10 years)
- Nulliparous
- Hypertension
- Familial predisposition
- Nonsmoker
- Consuming red meat, alcohol; risk decreases with green vegetables
- Obesity

Genetics
- Approximately 50% of leiomyomas have an abnormal karyotype (1).
- Most common cytogenetic abnormalities are deletions on chromosome 7.

PATHOPHYSIOLOGY
Enlargement of benign smooth muscle tumors that may lead to symptoms affecting the reproductive, GI, or genitourinary system

ETIOLOGY
Complex multifactorial process involving transition from normal myocyte to abnormal cells and then to visibly evident tumor (monoclonal expansion):
- Hormones (2): Increases in estrogen and progesterone are correlated with myoma formation (i.e., rarely seen before menarche).

- Growth factors (2):
  - Increased smooth muscle proliferation (transforming growth factor β [TGF-β], basic fibroblast growth factor [bFGF])
  - Increase DNA synthesis (epidermal growth factor [EGF], PDGF)
  - Stimulate synthesis of extracellular matrix (TGF-β)
  - Promote mitogenesis (TGF-β, EGF, IGF, prolactin)
  - Promote angiogenesis (bFGF, VEGF)
- Vasoconstrictive hypoxia (2): Proposed, but not confirmed, mechanism of myometrial injury during menstruation

COMMONLY ASSOCIATED CONDITIONS
Endometrial carcinoma is also associated with high unopposed estrogen stimulation.

 DIAGNOSIS

HISTORY
- Usually asymptomatic
- Symptoms include:
  - Abnormal uterine bleeding, usually heavy or prolonged menses
  - Pain: Infrequent, usually associated with torsion of pedunculated myoma or degeneration
  - Pressure on bladder: Suprapubic discomfort, urinary frequency or obstruction
  - Pressure on rectosigmoid: May cause low back pain, constipation
  - Infertility: Usually from submucous myoma or with distortion of uterine cavity

ALERT
Rapid growth, particularly in perimenopausal or postmenopausal patients, may indicate sarcoma

PHYSICAL EXAM
- Usually incidental finding on abdominal and pelvic exam
- Firm, smooth nodules or masses arising from uterus
- Masses are mobile without tenderness.

DIAGNOSTIC TESTS & INTERPRETATION
Lab
Initial lab tests
- Pregnancy test
- Hemoglobin

Follow-Up & Special Considerations
Consider CA-125: May be slightly elevated in some cases of uterine myoma but generally more useful in differentiating myomas from various gynecologic adenocarcinomas

Imaging
Initial approach
- Pelvic ultrasound: Shows characteristic hypoechoic appearance (3)[B]
- Saline-infusion hysterosonography: Helps to distinguish submucosal myomas (3)[B]
- Hysterosalpingogram: Evaluates the contour of the endometrial cavity (3)[B]
- CT scan or MRI: May help to differentiate complex cases or used when uterine artery embolization is planned (3)[B]

Follow-Up & Special Considerations
- Intravenous pyelogram: If suspect ureteral distortion (3)[B]
- Barium enema

Diagnostic Procedures/Surgery
- Fractional dilation and curettage: Aids in ruling out cervical or uterine carcinomas when clinically suspicious
- Hysteroscopy: Helps to diagnose submucosal or intracavitary myomas
- Laparoscopy: Useful in complex cases and to rule out other pelvic diseases or disorders

Pathological Findings
- Myomas are usually multiple and vary in size and location; have been reported up to 100 lb.
- Gross pathology: Firm tumors with characteristic whorl-like trabeculated appearance; a thin pseudocapsular layer is present.
- Microscopic: Bundles of smooth muscle mixed with varying amounts of connective tissue elements running in different directions
- Cellular variant has a preponderance of muscle cells. Mitoses are rare.
- May undergo various types of degeneration:
  - Hyaline degeneration: Very common
  - Calcification: Late result of circulatory impairment to myomas
  - Infection and suppuration: Most common with submucosal myomas
  - Necrosis: Most common with pedunculated myomas secondary to torsion
  - Sarcomatous changes: Incidence 0.1–1.0% of clinically apparent myomas

DIFFERENTIAL DIAGNOSIS
- Intrauterine pregnancy
- Ovarian or uterine cancer
- Leiomyosarcoma/malignancy
- Cecal or sigmoid tumor
- Appendiceal abscess
- Diverticulitis
- Pelvic kidney
- Urachal cyst

 TREATMENT

- Treatment must be individualized.
- Initially, medication therapy may be of benefit.
- 60% of patients may elect surgery by 2 years (4).
- Patients with minimal symptoms may be managed with iron preparations and analgesics.
- Conservative management of asymptomatic myomas:
  - Pelvic exams and ultrasound at 3- to 6-month intervals as long as size remains stable
  - Regression usually occurs after menopause.

MEDICATION
- Progestins may reduce overall uterine size (3)[B]:
  - Norethindrone 10 mg/d
  - Medroxyprogesterone (Depo-Provera) 200 mg IM monthly

- Combination oral contraceptives: Help prevent development of new fibroids:
  – Contraindications: History of thromboembolic events: See manufacturer's profile.
  – Adverse reactions and significant interactions: See manufacturer's profile.
- Luteinizing hormone–releasing hormone:
  – Nafarelin (Synarel Nasal Spray), goserelin (Zoladex Depot), and leuprolide (Lupron Depot)
  – Induces abrupt artificial menopause; may reduce myoma symptoms dramatically; induces atrophy of myomas by up to 40% in 2–3 months (3)[B]
  – May be valuable as preoperative adjunct to myomectomy or hysterectomy by allowing recovery of anemia, donation of autologous blood, and possibly converting abdominal to vaginal hysterectomy, thereby decreasing postoperative pain, hospitalization, and morbidity (3)[B]
  – Not recommended for use >6 months because of osteoporosis risk
  – Following discontinuation, myomas return within 60 days to pretherapy size.
- Mifepristone:
  – Antiprogesterone
  – Shown to have similar reduction in myoma size as gonadotropin-releasing hormone agonists (5)[B]

ADDITIONAL TREATMENT
General Measures
Patients not desiring pharmacologic therapy or surgery may consider:

- Uterine artery embolization: Averages 30–45% shrinkage of myomas (3)[A]; painful and may cause ovarian failure, amenorrhea or other complications; shorter hospital stay and quicker recovery but no difference in satisfaction compared with hysterectomy (6)[A]
- Magnetic resonance imaging-guided focused ultrasound: Noninvasive; ultrasound transducer passes through abdominal wall and causes coagulative necrosis of fibroid. Efficacy may be comparable with other hysterectomy-sparing procedures (5)[B].

Issues for Referral
- Medical therapy may be initiated by a primary care physician or gynecologist. Adequate pelvic examination must be performed initially.
- Surgical considerations may be pursued with gynecologic consultation.
- Uterine embolization may be discussed with an interventional radiologist.

SURGERY/OTHER PROCEDURES
- Surgical management is indicated in the following situations (3)[B]:
  – Excessive uterine size or excessive rate of growth (except during pregnancy)
  – Submucosal myomas when associated with hypermenorrhea
  – Pedunculated myomas that are painful or undergo torsion, necrosis, and hemorrhage
  – If a myoma causes symptoms from pressure on bladder or rectum
  – If differentiation from ovarian mass is not possible
  – If associated pelvic disease is present (endometriosis, pelvic inflammatory disease)
  – If infertility or habitual abortion is likely due to the anatomic location of the myoma

- Surgical procedures:
  – Preliminary pelvic examination, Pap smear, and endometrial biopsy should be performed to rule out malignant or premalignant conditions.
  – Hysterectomy: May be performed vaginally, laparoscopically, robotically or by laparotomy:
    ○ Effective in relieving symptoms and improving quality of life (5)[B]
  – Abdominal, laparoscopic, or robotic myomectomy may be performed in younger women who want to maintain fertility (3)[B].
  – Hysteroscopic or laparoscopic cautery or laser myoma resection can be performed in selected patients.
  – Endometrial ablation: For small submucosal myomas

IN-PATIENT CONSIDERATIONS
Initial Stabilization
- Usually outpatient
- Inpatient for some surgical procedures

 ## ONGOING CARE
FOLLOW-UP RECOMMENDATIONS
Patient Monitoring
- Pelvic examination and ultrasound: Every 2–3 months for newly diagnosed symptomatic or excessively large myomas
- Hemoglobin and hematocrit: If uterine bleeding is excessive
- Once uterine size and symptoms stable, monitor every 6–12 months.

DIET
No restrictions

PATIENT EDUCATION
- Medline Plus: http://www.nlm.nih.gov/medlineplus/uterinefibroids.html
- JAMA Patient Page: http://jama.ama-assn.org/cgi/reprint/301/1/122.pdf
- Society of Interventional Radiology: http://sirweb.org/patients/uterine-fibroids/
- US Department of Health and Human Services: http://womenshealth.gov/faq/uterine-fibroids.cfm
- American Congress of Obstetricians and Gynecologists (ACOG): http://www.acog.org

PROGNOSIS
- Resection of submucosal fibroids has been associated with increased fertility (5)[B].
- Laparoscopic myomectomy does not have any difference in clinical pregnancy rate and live birth rate than laparotomy (7)[C].
- At least 10% of myomas recur after myomectomy; however, most women will not require further treatment (5)[B].

COMPLICATIONS
- May mask other gynecologic malignancies (e.g., uterine sarcoma, ovarian cancer)
- Degenerating fibroids may cause pain.
- May rarely prolapse through the cervix

Pregnancy Considerations
- Rapid growth of fibroids is common.
- Pregnant women may need additional fetal testing if placenta is located over or near fibroid.

- Complications during pregnancy: Abortion, premature labor, 2nd-trimester rapid growth leading to degeneration and pain, and 3rd-trimester fetal malpresentation and dystocia during labor and delivery
- Previous myomectomy patients may develop uterine rupture during labor. Cesarean section is recommended if the endometrial cavity has been entered during myomectomy.

Geriatric Considerations
In postmenopausal patients with newly diagnosed uterine myoma or enlarging uterine myomas, have a high suspicion of uterine sarcoma or other gynecologic malignancy.

REFERENCES
1. Okolo S. Incidence, aetiology and epidemiology of uterine fibroids. *Best Pract Res Clin Obstet Gynaecol*. 2008.
2. Parker WH. Etiology, symptomatology, and diagnosis of uterine myomas. *Fertil Steril*. 2007;87:725–36.
3. Wallace EE, et al. Uterine Myomas: An overview of development, clinical features and management. *Obstetrics Gynecol*. 2004;104(2):393–406.
4. Marjoribanks J, Lethaby A, Farquhar C. Surgery versus medical therapy for heavy menstrual bleeding. *Cochrane Database Syst Rev*. 2006:CD003855.
5. Parker WH. Uterine myomas: management. *Fertil Steril*. 2007;88:255–71.
6. Gupta JK, Sinha AS, Lumsden MA, et al. Uterine artery embolization for symptomatic uterine fibroids. *Cochrane Database Syst Rev*. 2006: CD005073.
7. Griffiths A, et al. Surgical treatment of fibroids for subfertility. *Cochrane Database Syst Rev*. 2007:3.

ADDITIONAL READING
- Cheng MH, Chao HT, Wang PH. Medical treatment for uterine myomas. *Taiwan J Obstet Gynecol*. 2008;47:18–23.
- Istre O. Management of symptomatic fibroids: conservative surgical treatment modalities other than hysterectomy and abdominal or laparoscopic myomectomy. *Best Pract Res Clin Obstet Gynaecol*. 2008.

 ## CODES

ICD9
- 218.0 Submucous leiomyoma of uterus
- 218.1 Intramural leiomyoma of uterus
- 218.2 Subserous leiomyoma of uterus

CLINICAL PEARLS
- Uterine myomas are benign smooth muscle tumors composed mainly of fibrous connective tissue.
- Usually incidental finding on pelvic exam or ultrasound, but may cause pelvic pain and pressure, abnormal uterine bleeding, and/or infertility
- Management ranges from conservative to medical to surgical.

UTERINE PROLAPSE

Eric L. Jenison, MD
Michael P. Hopkins, MD, MEd
Cameron J. Codd, DO

 BASICS

DESCRIPTION
- Uterine prolapse occurs when the integrity of pelvic supporting structures is lost. This allows the uterus to descend into the vagina. In advanced cases, complete protrusion with inversion of the vagina occurs, known as procidentia.
- Before menopause, the degree and severity of prolapse are usually related to the number of pregnancies and the difficulty of childbirth. After menopause, atrophy and loss of tissue integrity can lead to further prolapse.
- System(s) affected: GI; Renal/Urologic; Reproductive
- Synonym(s): Uterine prolapse; Genital prolapse; Genital relaxation; Uterine descensus; Total or partial procidentia; Dropped uterus

Geriatric Considerations
This is largely a disease of aging, and incidence will be much higher as the median age of the population increases.

Pediatric Considerations
Prolapse in newborns has been reported, but it is rare and usually associated with congenital disorders and neuropathies.

EPIDEMIOLOGY
Incidence
- Annual incidence approximately 2%
- Predominant age: Perimenopausal and postmenopausal women
- Predominant sex: Female only

Prevalence
~30–50% of women experience some degree of prolapse.

RISK FACTORS
- Childbirth, particularly multiple parity
- Vaginal delivery, especially operative vaginal delivery
- Advancing age
- Caucasian or Hispanic (4–5-fold increased risk compared to African Americans)
- Tobacco use
- Occupations requiring heavy lifting
- Various connective tissue and neurogenic disorders
- Conditions resulting in increased intra-abdominal pressure (e.g., obesity, abdominal or pelvic tumors, pulmonary disease with chronic coughing, chronic constipation)
- Estrogen-deficient state

Genetics
- Common among Caucasians
- Less common among Asians and African Americans, and particularly uncommon in South African Bantus and West Africans

GENERAL PREVENTION
- Kegel exercises increase the strength of the pelvic diaphragm muscles and may provide some pelvic support.
- Weight loss and proper management of conditions that increase abdominal pressure help to prevent prolapse.
- Tobacco cessation
- Postmenopausal estrogen replacement therapy

ETIOLOGY
- Advancing age and vaginal childbirth are the most important factors.
- Incidence of prolapse increases with frequency and difficulty of vaginal deliveries (e.g., operative vaginal delivery); <2% of prolapse occurs in nulliparous women.
- Although this disorder in large part results from the distension and distortion of supporting tissues with vaginal childbirth, pregnancy, regardless of mode of delivery, may contribute to prolapse.
- Other less common causes of prolapse include connective tissue disorders with lax tissue (e.g., Marfan syndrome), neurogenic disorders (e.g., multiple sclerosis), cloacal agenesis, chronic constipation, pelvic tumors or ascites, and chronic coughing resulting from chronic lung disease.
- Patients who have undergone radical vulvectomy with loss of the external supporting structures have a higher rate of prolapse.

COMMONLY ASSOCIATED CONDITIONS
Cystocele, rectocele, enterocele, and vaginal vault prolapse are often associated with uterine prolapse.

 DIAGNOSIS

HISTORY
- Patients are often asymptomatic. They may experience:
  - Pelvic pressure and low back pain
  - Bulging sensation in vagina or at introitus
  - Dyspareunia
  - Difficulty with urination or defecation
  - Symptoms often worsen following long periods of standing
  - Vaginal bleeding (mucosal irritation)
- Inquiry should be made as to:
  - The number of pregnancies, modes of deliveries, episiotomies, extent and repair of vaginal/perineal lacerations
  - Previous pelvic surgery
  - Congenital abnormalities
  - Medical conditions that chronically increase intra-abdominal pressure (e.g., chronic obstructive pulmonary disease [COPD])

PHYSICAL EXAM
- Diagnosis is confirmed by pelvic exam. With coughing and straining, the cervix will prolapse toward introitus or beyond.
- Use only 1 blade of speculum during pelvic examination to better appreciate prolapse.

ALERT
- The patient needs to be examined while standing as well as lying down to confirm diagnosis.
- Severity of symptoms and degree of prolapse are not strongly correlated.
- Can use 1 of many evaluation systems to describe extent of prolapse
- Baden-Walker system (1):
  - Grade 0: Normal position
  - Grade 1: Descent halfway to the hymen
  - Grade 2: Descent to the hymen
  - Grade 3: Descent halfway past the hymen
  - Grade 4: Maximum possible descent
- Pelvic Organ Quantification (POP-Q) system also used, but is more complex and used primarily in research settings

DIAGNOSTIC TESTS & INTERPRETATION
Lab
- Evaluation of renal function (blood urea nitrogen [BUN] and creatinine) to rule out ureteral obstruction
- Urinalysis to rule out urinary tract infection (UTI)

Imaging
- IV pyelogram to rule out ureteral obstruction in complete uterine prolapse (optional)
- Pelvic ultrasound or CT scan to rule out other pelvic pathology, if suspected (optional)

Diagnostic Procedures/Surgery
- If surgical correction is planned, urodynamic studies should be performed to evaluate for potential urinary incontinence masked by the prolapse (2)[B].
- If ulceration or bleeding is present, Pap smears and appropriate cervical and endometrial biopsies should be done to rule out concomitant malignancies.

Pathological Findings
Hyperkeratosis of the cervical and vaginal tissues occurs with prolapse beyond the introitus due to chronic irritation and drying. As the irritation becomes more pronounced, bleeding and ulceration occur.

DIFFERENTIAL DIAGNOSIS
- Other pelvic organ prolapse (e.g., cystocele, rectocele, enterocele)
- Pelvic mass, benign or malignant

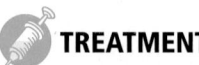 **TREATMENT**

MEDICATION
- Vaginal estrogen therapy can increase blood supply to the vagina and supporting tissue, which may improve tissue strength; may also be beneficial for mild urinary incontinence.
- This is especially important in postmenopausal women using pessaries or undergoing reconstructive pelvic surgery (2)[B].
- Progestin therapy or monitoring of endometrial status in a woman with an intact uterus is not necessary with vaginal estrogen therapy.
- Estrogen therapy should be used in the lowest possible dose for the shortest time.
- However, women may need long-term therapy due to the chronic nature of uterine prolapse.

- 3 forms of vaginal estrogen therapy:
  - Vaginal cream (Premarin conjugated equine estrogen or estradiol cream): Insert via applicator each night × 14 days and then 2–3 times/week.
  - Vaginal estradiol tablet: Insert via preloaded applicator each night × 14 days and then 2–3 times/week.
  - Estradiol-containing vaginal ring: Insert into vagina and replace every 3 months.
- Contraindications:
  - Breast- or estrogen-dependent carcinoma
  - Undiagnosed vaginal bleeding
  - Thromboembolic disorders
  - Thrombophlebitis
  - Pregnancy
- Precautions: Any abnormal vaginal bleeding must be evaluated.

ADDITIONAL TREATMENT
General Measures
- Treatment depends on multiple variables, including the severity of prolapse, age, sexual activity, associated pelvic pathology, and desire for future fertility.
- Treatment of grade I or II prolapse is expectant unless patient is symptomatic.
- Conservative therapies include vaginal estrogen replacement, pessary use, and physical therapy (3)[C].
- Pessaries are indicated for women who are unfit for, or decline, surgery. Proper fitting and maintenance are required (4)[C].
- Pessaries also may be used in the preoperative evaluation of prolapse (4)[C].
- Surgery is indicated for women who fail conservative therapies and/or desire definitive treatment (2)[B].

Issues for Referral
Urogynecology evaluation for patients who may be surgical candidates

Additional Therapies
Physical therapy, including biofeedback, electrical stimulation, and pelvic muscle training (Kegels), may be an option for women with mild prolapse and/or those wishing conservative therapy (4)[C].

SURGERY/OTHER PROCEDURES
- Surgical candidates without additional pelvic pathology: Vaginal or abdominal hysterectomy ± enterocele, cystocele, rectocele, paravaginal repair, urethral suspension, and culdoplasty depending on coexisting pelvic organ prolapse (2)[B]
- Incontinence procedure often done at same time as prolapse repair although almost 1/3 of women relieved of stress urinary incontinence by prolapse surgery alone (5)[B]
- Vault suspension is typically necessary in conjunction with hysterectomy:
  - Vaginal procedures include sacrospinous ligament fixation, uterosacral ligament fixation, and endopelvic fascial suspension.
  - Sacral colpopexy can be performed via laparoscopic or open abdominal approach.

- The abdominal approach (sacral colpopexy) has decreased risk of recurrent apical prolapse and less postoperative dyspareunia and stress incontinence compared with the vaginal approach (sacrospinous ligament fixation). However, the abdominal approach is associated with longer operative time and recovery time (6)[A].
- Uterine suspension is an option for patients who desire to maintain reproductive function (2)[B].
- Older women who are not sexually active can be treated with colpocleisis or vaginal obliteration procedure.

IN-PATIENT CONSIDERATIONS
Initial Stabilization
- Outpatient
- Inpatient when surgery is necessary

 # ONGOING CARE

FOLLOW-UP RECOMMENDATIONS
- Heavy lifting, sexual intercourse, and other activities that increase intra-abdominal pressure should be avoided for 6–12 weeks after surgical correction.
- Maintain ideal body weight.

Patient Monitoring
- Expectant management is appropriate, with periodic follow-up exams.
- If a pessary is placed, it should be removed, cleaned, and replaced every 3–6 months (4)[C].

DIET
Avoid constipation by increasing dietary fiber and fluid intake.

PATIENT EDUCATION
- Kegel exercises when applicable
- American College of Obstetricians and Gynecologists (ACOG), 409 12th St., SW, Washington, DC 20024-2188; (800) 762-ACOG; http://www.acog.org

PROGNOSIS
- It is expected that the incidence and severity of prolapse will increase as patients age.
- Although surgical correction is usually successful initially, reoperation rate is ~29% (2)[B].

COMPLICATIONS
- Ureteral obstruction and renal failure
- Incarceration of bowel herniations
- Pessary use may not always be effective and may cause discomfort, ulcers, and infection.

REFERENCES
1. Baden WF, et al. Fundamentals, symptoms and classification. In: Baden WF, et al., eds. *Surgical Repair of Vaginal Defects*. Philadelphia: Lippincott, 1992;14.
2. Thakar R, et al. Regular review: Management of genital prolapse. *Br Med J*. 2002;324:1258–62.
3. Fox WB. Physical therapy for pelvic floor dysfunction. *Med Health R I*. 2009;92:10–1.
4. Trowbridge ER, Fenner DE. Conservative management of pelvic organ prolapse. *Clin Obstet Gynecol*. 2005;48:668–81.
5. Borstad E, Abdelnoor M, Staff AC, et al. Surgical strategies for women with pelvic organ prolapse and urinary stress incontinence. *Int Urogynecol J Pelvic Floor Dysfunct*. 2010;21:179–86.
6. Maher C, Feiner B, Baessler K, et al. Surgical management of pelvic organ prolapse in women. *Cochrane Database Syst Rev*. 2010;4:CD004014.

ADDITIONAL READING
Farrell S, et al. The detection and management of vaginal atrophy. *Int J Gynecol Obstet*. 2005;88:222–8.

 # CODES

ICD9
- 618.1 Uterine prolapse without mention of vaginal wall prolapse
- 618.2 Uterovaginal prolapse, incomplete
- 618.3 Uterovaginal prolapse, complete

CLINICAL PEARLS
- Uterine prolapse occurs when the integrity of pelvic supporting structures is lost.
- Advancing age and vaginal childbirth (including the number of pregnancies and the difficulty of childbirth) are the most important factors that contribute to uterine prolapse.
- Conservative therapies include vaginal estrogen replacement, pessary use, and physical therapy.
- Surgery is indicated for women who fail conservative therapies and/or desire definitive treatment.

UVEITIS

Shailendra K. Saxena, MD
Mikayla Spangler, PharmD, BCPS

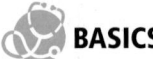 **BASICS**

DESCRIPTION
- A nonspecific term used to describe any intraocular inflammatory disorder. Symptoms vary, depending on depth of involvement and associated conditions. The uvea is the middle layer of the eye between the sclera and retina. The anterior part of the uvea includes the iris and ciliary body. The posterior part of the uvea is the choroid:
  - Anterior uveitis: Refers to ocular inflammation limited to the iris (iritis) alone or iris and ciliary body (iridocyclitis)
  - Intermediate uveitis: Refers to inflammation of the structures just posterior to the lens (pars planitis or peripheral uveitis)
  - Posterior uveitis: Refers to inflammation of the choroid (choroiditis), retina (retinitis), or vitreous near the optic nerve and macula
- System(s) affected: Nervous
- Synonym(s): Iritis; Iridocyclitis; Choroiditis; Retinochoroiditis; Chorioretinitis; Anterior uveitis; Posterior uveitis; Pars planitis; Panuveitis. Synonyms are anatomic descriptions of the focus of the uveal inflammation.

Geriatric Considerations
The inflammatory response to systemic disease may be suppressed.

Pediatric Considerations
Infection should be the primary consideration. Allergies and psychologic factors (depression, stress) may serve as a trigger. Trauma is also a common cause in this population.

Pregnancy Considerations
May be of importance in the selection of medications

EPIDEMIOLOGY
- Predominant age: All ages
- Predominant sex: Male = Female, except for HLA-B27 anterior uveitis: Male > Female (2.5:1)

Incidence
Anterior uveitis most common (8.2 cases/100,000 annual incidence)

Prevalence
Iritis is 4 times more prevalent than posterior uveitis.

RISK FACTORS
No specific risk factors. Higher incidence seen with specific associated conditions.

Genetics
- No specific pattern for uveitis in general
- Iritis: Of patients, 50–70% are HLA-B27–positive.

ETIOLOGY
- Infectious: May result from viral, bacterial, parasitic, or fungal etiologies
- Suspected immune-mediated: Possible autoimmune or immune-complex–mediated mechanism postulated in association with systemic (especially rheumatologic) disorders
- Isolated eye disease
- Idiopathic (~25%)
- Masquerade syndromes: Diseases such as malignancies that may be mistaken for primary inflammation of the eye

COMMONLY ASSOCIATED CONDITIONS
- Viral infections: HIV, herpes simplex, herpes zoster, cytomegalovirus
- Bacterial infections: Tuberculosis (TB), leprosy, propionibacterium infection, syphilis, leptospirosis, brucellosis, Lyme disease, Whipple disease
- Parasitic infections: Toxoplasmosis, acanthamebiasis, toxocariasis, cysticercosis, onchocerciasis
- Fungal infections: Histoplasmosis, coccidioidomycosis, candidiasis, aspergillosis, sporotrichosis, blastomycosis, cryptococcosis
- Suspected immune-mediated: Ankylosing spondylitis, Behçet disease, Crohn disease, drug or hypersensitivity reaction, interstitial nephritis, juvenile rheumatoid arthritis, Kawasaki disease, multiple sclerosis, psoriatic arthritis, Reiter syndrome, relapsing polychondritis, sarcoidosis, Sjögren syndrome, systemic lupus erythematosus, ulcerative colitis, vasculitis, vitiligo, Vogt-Koyanagi (Harada) syndrome
- Isolated eye disease: Acute multifocal placoid pigmentary epitheliopathy, acute retinal necrosis, bird-shot choroidopathy, Fuchs heterochromatic cyclitis, glaucomatocyclitic crisis, lens-induced uveitis, multifocal choroiditis, pars planitis, serpiginous choroiditis, sympathetic ophthalmia, trauma
- Masquerade syndromes: Leukemia, lymphoma, retinitis pigmentosa, retinoblastoma

DIAGNOSIS

HISTORY
- Decreased visual acuity
- Pain, photophobia, blurring of vision:
  - Usually acute
- Anterior uveitis (~80% of patients with uveitis):
  - Generally acute in onset
  - Deep eye pain
  - Photophobia (consensual)
- Intermediate and posterior uveitis:
  - Unresolving floaters
  - Generally insidious in onset
  - More commonly bilateral

PHYSICAL EXAM
Slit-lamp exam and indirect ophthalmoscopy are necessary for precise diagnosis.
- Anterior uveitis (~80% of patients with uveitis):
  - Conjunctival vessel dilation
  - Perilimbal (circumcorneal) dilation of episcleral and scleral vessels (ciliary flush)
  - Small pupillary size of affected eye
  - Hypopyon or hyphema (white or red blood cells pooled in the anterior chamber)
  - Frequently unilateral (95% of HLA-B27–associated cases)
  - Bilateral involvement and systemic symptoms (fever, fatigue, abdominal pain) may be associated with interstitial nephritis.
  - Systemic disease is most likely to be associated with anterior uveitis (in 1 study, 53% of patients found to have systemic disease).
- Intermediate and posterior uveitis:
  - More commonly bilateral
  - Posterior inflammation will generally cause minimal pain or redness unless associated with an iritis.

DIAGNOSTIC TESTS & INTERPRETATION
Lab
- No specific test for the diagnosis of uveitis. Tests for etiologic factors or associated conditions should be based on history and physical exam.
- Complete blood count (CBC), blood urea nitrogen (BUN), creatinine (interstitial nephritis)
- HLA-B27 typing (ankylosing spondylitis, Reiter syndrome)
- Antinuclear antibody, erythrocyte sedimentation rate (ESR) (systemic lupus erythematosus, Sjögren syndrome)
- Venereal disease research laboratory (VDRL) test, fluorescent titer antibody (syphilis)
- Purified protein derivative (PPD) tuberculin skin test (TB)
- Lyme serology (Lyme disease)
- Special tests
- Disorders that may alter lab results: Immune deficiency

Imaging
- Chest x-ray (sarcoidosis, histoplasmosis, TB, lymphoma)
- Sacroiliac radiograph (ankylosing spondylitis)

Diagnostic Procedures/Surgery
Slit-lamp exam

Pathological Findings
Keratic precipitates, inflammatory cells in anterior chamber or vitreous, synechiae (fibrous tissue scarring between iris and lens), macular edema, perivasculitis of retinal vessels

DIFFERENTIAL DIAGNOSIS
- Conjunctivitis
- Episcleritis
- Scleritis
- Keratitis
- Acute angle-closure glaucoma

 TREATMENT

MEDICATION
First Line
- The treatment depends upon the etiology, location, and severity of the inflammation.
- Caution should be used when using empiric treatment; referral to an ophthalmologist is recommended in most cases.
- Homatropine hydrobromide (Isopto) 5% ophthalmic solution: 1–2 drops to the affected eye b.i.d., or as often as q3h if necessary; *plus*
- Prednisolone acetate 1% ophthalmic suspension: 2 drops to the affected eye q1h initially, tapering to once a day with improvement (1,2)[C]
- Contraindications:
  – Hypersensitivity to the medication or component of the preparation
  – Cycloplegia is contraindicated in patients known to have, or be predisposed to, glaucoma.
  – Topical corticosteroid therapy is contraindicated in uveitis secondary to infectious etiologies, unless used in conjunction with appropriate anti-infectious agents (3)[C].
- Precautions:
  – Homatropine hydrobromide may produce adverse systemic antimuscarinic effects. Use extreme caution in infants and young children because of increased susceptibility to systemic effects.
  – Topical corticosteroids may increase intraocular pressure. Prolonged use may cause cataract formation and exacerbate existing herpetic keratitis, which may masquerade as iritis.
- Significant possible interactions
- Refer to manufacturer's profile for each drug.

Second Line
- Cycloplegia: Scopolamine hydrobromide 0.25% (IsoptoHyoscine) up to t.i.d. or cyclopentolate hydrochloride 1% (Cyclogyl) or Atropine 1% (2)[C]
- Anti-inflammatory: Prednisolonesodium phosphate 1% (Ocu-Pred Forte), dexamethasone sodium phosphate 0.1% (OU-Dex), dexamethasone suspension, rimexolone 1% (Vexol), and loteprednol etabonate 0.5% (Lotemax) (2)[C]
- Rimexolone 1% (Vexol) may be equally effective as prednisolone acetate 1% for short-term treatment of anterior uveitis (4)[B].
- Loteprednol etabonate (Lotemax) may not be as effective as prednisolone acetate 1%, but may be less likely to increase intraocular pressure in cases of acute anterior uveitis (4)[B].
- Systemic nonsteroidal anti-inflammatory drugs (NSAIDs) may provide some benefit (2)[C].

ADDITIONAL TREATMENT
General Measures
- Appropriate health care: Outpatient with urgent ophthalmologic consultation
- Medical therapy best initiated following full ophthalmologic evaluation
- Treatment of underlying cause, if identified
- Cycloplegia
- Anti-inflammatory therapy

 ONGOING CARE

FOLLOW-UP RECOMMENDATIONS
Patient Monitoring
- Ophthalmologic follow-up as recommended by consultant
- Schedule for complete history and physical to evaluate for associated systemic disease.

PATIENT EDUCATION
- Instruct on proper method for instilling eye drops.
- Wear dark glasses if photophobia is a problem.
- Medication side effects to watch for and report

PROGNOSIS
- Depends on the presence of causal diseases or associated conditions
- Uveitis resulting from infections (systemic or local) tends to resolve with eradication of the underlying infection.
- Uveitis associated with seronegative arthropathies tends to be acute (lasting <3 months) and frequently recurrent.

COMPLICATIONS
Loss of vision as a result of the following:
- Keratic precipitate deposition on the corneal or lens surfaces
- Increased intraocular pressure, acute angle-closure glaucoma
- Formation of synechiae
- Cataract formation
- Vasculitis with vascular occlusion, retinal infarction
- Macular edema
- Optic nerve damage

REFERENCES

1. Audio PA. A review of evidence guiding the use of corticosteroids in the treatment of intraocular inflammation. *Oculi Immunol Inflame.* 2004;12(3): 169–92.
2. American Optometric Association guideline for care of the patient with anterior uveitis can be found at National Guideline Clearinghouse. 2000;1990.
3. Mccusker PJ, et al. Management of chronic uveitis. *BMJ.* 2000;320(7234):555–8.
4. Jabs DA. Treatment of ocular inflammation. *Ocular Immunol Inflame.* 2004;12(3):163–8.

ADDITIONAL READING
- Patel H, et al. Pediatric uveitis. *Pediatr Clin North Am.* 2003;50(1):125–36.
- Schiffman RM, et al. Visual functioning and general health status in patients with uveitis. *Arch Ophthalmol.* 2001;119(6):841–9.
- Smith JR, et al. Management of uveitis: A rheumatologic perspective. *Arthritis Rheum.* 2002;46(2):309–18.

See Also (Topic, Algorithm, Electronic Media Element)
Conjunctivitis, Acute; Glaucoma, Primary Closed-Angle; Scleritis

 CODES

ICD9
364.3 Unspecified iridocyclitis

CLINICAL PEARLS

Severe or unresponsive uveitis may require therapy, including periocular injection of corticosteroids, systemic corticosteroids, cytotoxic agents (azathioprine, cyclophosphamide, chlorambucil, and methotrexate), immunosuppressive agents (cyclosporine), immunomodulatory agents (sulfasalazine), or tumor necrosis factor inhibitors (infliximab, etanercept).

U

VAGINAL ADENOSIS

Michael P. Hopkins, MD, MEd

 BASICS

DESCRIPTION
- The normal vagina is lined by squamous epithelium. Adenosis is characterized by the presence of columnar epithelium or glandular tissue in the wall of the vagina.
- At about the 15th week of embryologic development, the Müllerian system, which forms the upper 2/3 of the vagina, fuses with the invaginating cloaca or urogenital sinus to form the lower 1/3 of the vagina. Squamous metaplasia from the cloacal region then produces a squamous epithelium through the vagina.
- Adenosis occurs when this squamous epithelium fails to epithelialize the vagina completely.
- 3 main types of adenosis epithelium described:
  - Endocervical
  - Endometrial
  - Tubal
- System(s) affected: Reproductive

Geriatric Considerations
- Adenosis is a disorder of the young female. By menopause, the vagina and cervix should be completely epithelialized.
- The presence of glandular epithelium in the postmenopausal patient is an indication for excision and close evaluation for the possibility of a well-differentiated adenocarcinoma.

Pregnancy Considerations
Pregnancy produces a wide eversion of the transformation zone of the cervix. This occasionally will become so widely everted that it will extend onto the vaginal fornices, leading to the impression of adenosis. This will resolve after the pregnancy is completed.

EPIDEMIOLOGY
Incidence
- While the incidence of vaginal adenosis is unknown, the incidence of cloacal malformations is 1/20,000 to 1/25,000 live births.
- Predominant age:
  - Teenage years: Epithelialization occurs from puberty to ~20 years of age.
  - By age 30 years, it is extremely rare for adenosis to be present.

Prevalence
In the US: Adenosis is relatively common, affecting 10–20% of young females studied. As maturation progresses with puberty, epithelialization occurs (1)[C].

RISK FACTORS
Adenosis of the vagina/cervix in female offsprings is significantly higher in those exposed to diethylstilbestrol (DES) before birth (2).

GENERAL PREVENTION
None: Last DES exposure in the 1970s

PATHOPHYSIOLOGY
- In the vast majority of young females, the etiology is incomplete squamous metaplasia or epithelialization. This occurs as a natural phenomenon and resolves with age.
- Described as congenital or acquired (3):
  - Congenital: Proliferation of the remnant Müllerian epithelium in the vagina due to exposure to DES in utero
  - Acquired: Trauma and inflammation causing spontaneous de novo changes or changes in an acquired lesion in the vaginal epithelium:
    - Trauma: Carbon dioxide laser, 5-fluorouracil, vaginal packs, chronic pessary use
    - Proliferation of the glandular cells in the remnant Müllerian epithelium of the vagina due to sex hormones
    - Idiopathic spontaneous change in epithelium, no cause has been identified

ETIOLOGY
In DES-exposed females, the incidence of adenosis is higher; the etiology presumably is from the effect of the DES on the developing embryologic system.

COMMONLY ASSOCIATED CONDITIONS
DES exposure:
- Adenosis from DES exposure should lead to an evaluation of other DES-related abnormalities.
- Müllerian tract anomalies associated with DES exposure include cervical hood, cervical ridge, shortened cervix, incompetent cervix, and T-shaped uterine cavity.
- Patients with known DES exposure should have the reproductive tract evaluated prior to conception.
- The vast majority of patients with adenosis have not been DES exposed and do not require evaluation of the reproductive system.
- DES was last used to prevent spontaneous abortion in the US in 1971; therefore, it is decreasing in clinical significance.

 DIAGNOSIS

HISTORY
- Maternal DES exposure
- Complaints of:
  - Profuse mucoid vaginal discharge from the glandular epithelium
  - Pruritus
  - Pain/soreness of the vaginal introitus
  - Postcoital bleeding
  - Dyspareunia

PHYSICAL EXAM
On pelvic exam, adenosis appearance is varied: Patchy or diffuse red stippling, granularity or nodularity, single or multiple cysts, erosions, ulcers, or warty protuberances that may even extend to vulva

DIAGNOSTIC TESTS & INTERPRETATION
Lab
Initial lab tests
4-quadrant Pap smear should be used liberally to isolate quadrants of the vagina that may contain abnormalities.

Follow-Up & Special Considerations
Pap smear can be followed by colposcopy and biopsy.

Imaging
Initial approach
None unless diagnosed with underlying malignancy

Diagnostic Procedures/Surgery
Colposcopy should be used to outline areas of adenosis to ensure that no malignancy is present.

Pathological Findings
- Biopsy will show benign glandular epithelium.
- Biopsies in the areas of ongoing squamous metaplasia will be typical for this process (3)[C].

DIFFERENTIAL DIAGNOSIS
- Erosive lichen planus
- Fixed drug eruption
- Erythema multiforme
- Bullous skin disease
- Adenocarcinoma:
  – A thorough evaluation for adenocarcinoma of the vagina arising in adenosis should be done.
  – A biopsy may be necessary to ensure that the process represents only benign adenosis.

TREATMENT

ADDITIONAL TREATMENT
General Measures
- Unless malignancy is present, conservative treatment is indicated.
- In the vast majority of young females with this condition, it will resolve with expectant management (4)[C].
- Treatment is warranted in women with severe subjective symptoms that impair the quality of life (5).

Issues for Referral
Malignancy found on biopsy warrants referral to gynecologic oncology specialist.

SURGERY/OTHER PROCEDURES
- Aggressive therapy such as laser or surgical excision is necessary if premalignant or malignant changes arise (3)[C].
- Symptomatic treatment with carbon dioxide laser coagulation, unipolar coagulation, or, lastly, vaginal resection (4)

IN-PATIENT CONSIDERATIONS
Admission Criteria
Outpatient management

 ONGOING CARE

FOLLOW-UP RECOMMENDATIONS
Patient Monitoring
If the initial colposcopy is normal, a yearly 4-quadrant Pap smear of the vagina and Pap smear of the cervix are all that is necessary.

DIET
No special diet

PATIENT EDUCATION
- No limitations
- It is not necessary to avoid intercourse or placing objects in the vagina.
- The patient should be educated to keep annual pelvic and Pap smear appointments. In the vast majority of situations, this is benign, and expectant management is all that is necessary.
- http://www.acog.org

PROGNOSIS
- It is expected that the vast majority of patients will have squamous metaplasia and epithelialization with complete resolution of the adenosis.
- The rare patient, 1/1,000 to 1/10,000, may develop adenocarcinoma in the adenosis and will require definitive therapy as for vaginal cancer.

COMPLICATIONS
- Infertility with DES association
- Adverse pregnancy outcome with DES association
- Adenocarcinoma of vagina

REFERENCES
1. Sandberg EC. The incidence and distribution of occult vaginal adenosis. *Am J Obstet Gynecol.* 1968;101:322–34.
2. Bamigboye AA, Morris J. Oestrogen supplementation, mainly diethylstilbestrol, for preventing miscarriages and other adverse pregnancy outcomes. *Cochrane Database Syst Rev.* 2003:CD004271
3. Chattopadhyay I, et al. Non diethylstilbestrol induced vaginal adenosis—A case series and review of literature. *Eur J Gynaecol Oncol.* 2001;22(4):260–2.
4. Kranl C, et al. Vulvar and vaginal adenosis. *Br J Dermatol.* 1998;139:128–31.
5. Cebesoy FB, Kutlar I, Aydin A. Vaginal adenosis successfully treated withsimple unipolar cauterization. *J Natl Med Assoc.* 2007;99(2):166–7.

See Also (Topic, Algorithm, Electronic Media Element)
Vaginal Malignancy; DES Exposure

CODES

ICD9
752.49 Other congenital anomalies of cervix, vagina, and external female genitalia

CLINICAL PEARLS
- Adenosis is characterized by the presence of columnar epithelium or glandular tissue in the wall of the vagina.
- Adenosis is more common among women exposed to DES in utero.
- Adenosis is rarely associated with an underlying vaginal malignancy.

VAGINAL BLEEDING DURING PREGNANCY

Kimberle Vore, MD

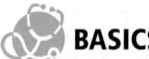 **BASICS**

DESCRIPTION
- Vaginal bleeding during pregnancy has many causes and ranges in severity from mild (with normal pregnancy outcome) to life-threatening for both infant and mother (1).
- Bleeding can vary from scant to excessive, from brown to bright red, and can be painless or painful.
- Causes can be divided into vaginal, cervical, and uterine factors. The differential diagnosis is guided by the gestational age of the fetus.
- System(s) affected: Cardiovascular; Reproductive

EPIDEMIOLOGY
Prevalence
Common in females of child-bearing age

RISK FACTORS
Specific to the etiology

GENERAL PREVENTION
If previa, nothing placed in vagina

ETIOLOGY
- Vaginal or cervical causes can occur throughout the pregnancy and are usually no threat to the pregnancy. They include:
  - Vaginal infection or trauma
  - Cervicitis (infections or noninfectious)
  - Cervical polyp
  - Cervical neoplasia
  - Hyperemia of cervix (increased blood flow from pregnancy)
  - Postcoital bleeding: Usually cervical source
- Bleeding from above the cervix is a concern because it can be life-threatening to mother and/or fetus. In determining the cause, it is helpful to separate 1st-trimester bleeding from later-pregnancy bleeding.
  - Causes of 1st-trimester bleeding include:
    ○ Implantation bleeding (benign)
    ○ Ectopic pregnancy (2)
    ○ Threatened or spontaneous abortion
    ○ Molar pregnancy
    ○ Subchorionic bleed
  - Causes of 2nd- or 3rd-trimester bleeding include (3):
    ○ Placenta previa (nonpainful). Risks: Previous history of previa, previous cesarean section, history of uterine surgery including dilation and curettage [D&C]
    ○ Placenta abruption (painful contractions usually present). Risks: Previous history of abruption, hypertension, preeclampsia, multiple gestations, smoking, cocaine use: Subchorionic bleed
- Many times the cause is unknown. For up to 50% of 1st-trimester bleeding, no cause is ever found.

COMMONLY ASSOCIATED CONDITIONS
Depends on cause (see Etiology)

 DIAGNOSIS

It is important to evaluate whether bleeding is coming from genital tract or from other nearby structures.

HISTORY
- Vaginal bleeding during pregnancy
- Association of bleeding with other activities or symptoms may aid in the diagnosis (e.g., following bowel movement, after intercourse, associated with abdominal cramping).

PHYSICAL EXAM
Blood in vagina

DIAGNOSTIC TESTS & INTERPRETATION
Lab
Initial lab tests
- Blood type and screen; if not known already, this must be done on all women.
- Quantitative β-human chorionic gonadotropin (β-hCG):
  - Used in early pregnancy when ultrasound is not able to diagnose cause; ultrasound should be able to see an intrauterine pregnancy (IUP) when the qualitative β-hCG >2,000.
  - Levels can be followed serially every 2 days.
    ○ Levels fall in spontaneous abortion.
    ○ Levels are extremely high in molar pregnancy.
    ○ Levels rise gradually in ectopic or intrauterine pregnancy.
    ○ Level usually increased by 2/3 or double in 48 h in normal pregnancy, and failure to increase by 50% is concerning for ectopic pregnancy.
    ○ Once level >2,000, check ultrasound.
- Other lab tests are based on severity of bleeding.
  - Complete blood count (CBC): May be done to assess severity when bleeding is profuse
  - Bleeding time, fibrinogen, and fibrin split products: Rarely necessary. Disseminated intravascular coagulation (DIC) is reportedly rarely in missed abortion.
  - Kleihauer-Betke (3rd trimester with suspected abruption)

Follow-Up & Special Considerations
- Once qualitative β-hCG level >2,000, an ultrasound should be performed to confirm diagnosis.

- When spontaneous abortion is suspected but there is no definitive diagnosis by either ultrasound or pathologic confirmation of products of conception, then following quantitative β-hCG weekly until level is <25 is advised to exclude possible undiagnosed ectopic pregnancy. If dropping levels start to rise, reconsider ectopic pregnancy.
- In molar pregnancy, after surgical evacuation of productions of conception, monthly qualitative β-hCG determinations are followed for 1 year to rule out the possibility of choriocarcinoma. During this time, the patient should be instructed not to get pregnant.

Imaging
Initial approach
Ultrasound is the diagnostic test of choice (4).
- A gestational sac can be seen at 5–6 weeks.
- Fetal heart tone can be observed by 8–9 weeks.
- Diagnostic of molar pregnancy with 98% accuracy
- In later pregnancy, ultrasound locates the placenta and may show degree of placental separation in abruption.

Follow-Up & Special Considerations
Serial ultrasound may be required in early pregnancy.

Diagnostic Procedures/Surgery
- In 1st-trimester bleeding:
  - Pelvic exam is performed to confirm bleeding from cervical os and the presence of any adnexal masses.
  - If pregnancy is >8 weeks, ultrasound should be done to confirm IUP.
  - If no IUP is present and ultrasound is not confirmatory for ectopic pregnancy, then serial qualitative β-hCG values are followed.
  - If pelvic pain and concern for ectopic pregnancy are high but not confirmed by ultrasound, a laparoscopy or laparotomy may be performed to achieve a diagnosis.
- In 2nd- or 3rd-trimester bleeding (5):
  - Locate placenta by ultrasound prior to pelvic exam.
  - If placenta previa, do not perform bimanual or speculum exam unless set up for immediate cesarean delivery.

DIFFERENTIAL DIAGNOSIS
- Hematuria from urinary tract infection (UTI), kidney stones
- Bleeding hemorrhoids
- Rectal bleeding from lower GI bleed: Extremely rare in pregnancy

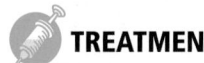 TREATMENT

MEDICATION

First Line
Rho(d) immune globulin (RhoGAM) if mother is Rh-negative and there is significant bleeding from uterus; Rh-negative patients who bleed during pregnancy will need Rho(d) immune globulin (RhoGAM) to prevent mother from becoming sensitized if exposed to infant's Rh-positive blood.

Second Line
Tocolytics in suspected premature labor

ADDITIONAL TREATMENT

General Measures
- Appropriate health care:
  - In 1st-trimester bleeding, most patients can be managed as outpatients.
  - In late-pregnancy bleeding, most patients need inpatient monitoring.
- Threatened abortion: Bed rest and nothing in the vagina; if bleeding is severe, hospitalization and close observation; type and screen for possible transfusion
- In late-pregnancy bleeding, the amount of bleeding and presence of maternal or fetal compromise indicates whether emergent cesarean section is performed or whether conservative measures are appropriate until greater fetal lung maturity can be obtained.

SURGERY/OTHER PROCEDURES
- If ectopic or molar pregnancy is diagnosed, immediate surgical treatment may be needed in some patients.
- Some early ectopic pregnancies can be treated medically if certain criteria are met.
- Inevitable or incomplete abortion: D&C (usually suction)
- If completeness of abortion is in doubt, then D&C and removal of retained products
- Cesarean section for placenta previa or placental abruption

IN-PATIENT CONSIDERATIONS

Initial Stabilization
- IV fluids if heavy bleeding
- Determine cause, and treat appropriately (6).

Admission Criteria
- Heavy bleeding associated with abdominal pain in 1st trimester
- In 2nd and 3rd trimester, depends on amount of bleeding and fetal compromise

IV Fluids
Maintain IV hydration and access if heavy bleeding.

Discharge Criteria
1st trimester: May discharge after evacuation of uterus once hemodynamically stable; usually <24 h

 ONGOING CARE

FOLLOW-UP RECOMMENDATIONS

Patient Monitoring
Continuous electronic fetal monitoring if bleeding in 3rd trimester

DIET
NPO if surgery planned

PATIENT EDUCATION
- Patient should be instructed to report any increase in the amount and frequency of bleeding and should seek immediate care if experiencing abdominal pain or sudden increased bleeding. She should save any tissue passed vaginally for examination.
- Grief counseling is appropriate if pregnancy loss is inevitable.
- American College of Obstetricians & Gynecologists (ACOG), 409 12th St., SW, Washington, DC 20024-2188; (800) 762-ACOG

PROGNOSIS
- Prognosis depends on the cause of vaginal bleeding, the severity of bleeding, and the rapidity of diagnosis.
- Maternal mortality is 31.9 deaths/100,000 ectopic pregnancies (7).
- Heavy bleeding in the 1st trimester, particularly when accompanied by pain, is associated with higher risk of miscarriage. Spotting and light episodes are not, especially if lasting only 1–2 days (8).
- If fetal heart tones are present in 1st trimester bleed, there is <10% chance of pregnancy loss.
- Women with 1st-trimester bleeding in the first pregnancy have an increased risk of complications later in the first pregnancy and of recurrence of 1st-trimester bleeding and other complications in the second pregnancy (9).
- Vaginal bleeding during the first half of pregnancy increases the rate of spontaneous preterm delivery, PROM and placental abruption, and decreases the neonatal weight. Therefore, threatened abortion indicates a high-risk pregnancy (10).

COMPLICATIONS
- Anemia
- Infection
- Premature delivery of infant with associated complications
- Choriocarcinoma or invasive mole in the case of hydatidiform mole
- Coagulopathy (extremely rare)
- Shock
- Fetal or maternal death

REFERENCES

1. Sinha P, Kuruba N. Ante-partum haemorrhage: An update. *J Obstet Gynaecol.* 2008;28:377–81.
2. Suspected ectopic pregnancy. *Obstet Gynecol.* 2006;107:399413.
3. Sakornbut E, Leeman L, Fontaine P. Late pregnancy bleeding. *Am Fam Physician.* 2007;75:1199–206.
4. Dighe M, Cuevas C, Moshiri M, et al. Sonography in first trimester bleeding. *J Clin Ultrasound.* 2008.
5. Mirza FG, Gaddipati S. Obstetric emergencies. *Semin Perinatol.* 2009;33:97–103.
6. Promes SB, Nobay F, et al. Pitfalls in first-trimester bleeding. *Emerg. Med. Clin. North Am.* 2010;28:219–34, x
7. Estimation of pregnancy-related mortality risk by pregnancy outcome, US, 1991 to 1999. *Am J Obstet Gynecol.* 2006;194:9294.
8. Hasan R, Baird DD, Herring AH, et al. Association between first-trimester vaginal bleeding and miscarriage. *Obstet Gynecol.* 2009;114:860–7.
9. Lykke JA, Dideriksen KL, Lidegaard O, et al. First-trimester vaginal bleeding and complications later in pregnancy. *Obstet Gynecol.* 2010;115: 935–44.
10. Dadkhah F, Kashanian M, Eliasi G, et al. A comparison between the pregnancy outcome in women both with or without threatened abortion. *Early Hum. Dev.* 2010;86:193–6.

See Also (Topic, Algorithm, Electronic Media Element)
Abnormal Pap and Cervical Dysplasia; Abortion, Spontaneous; Abruptio Placentae; Cervical Malignancy; Cervical Polyps; Cervicitis, Ectropion and True Erosion; Chlamydial Sexually Transmitted Diseases; Ectopic Pregnancy; Placenta Previa; Preterm Labor; Trichomoniasis; Vaginal Malignancy

 CODES

ICD9
- 640.03 Threatened abortion, antepartum
- 640.93 Unspecified hemorrhage in early pregnancy, antepartum
- 641.93 Unspecified antepartum hemorrhage

CLINICAL PEARLS
- Obtain blood type and screen if Rh status is unknown on all women presenting with vaginal bleeding in pregnancy because Rh-negative patients who bleed during pregnancy will need Rho(d) immune globulin (RhoGAM).
- Ultrasound of placental abruption is diagnostic test of choice, but in very early pregnancy (<8 weeks), it may be inconclusive, and quantitative β-hCG titers can be followed serially until >2,000 or until outcome of pregnancy is determined.
- For up to 50% of 1st-trimester bleeding, no cause is ever found.

V

VAGINAL MALIGNANCY

Michael P. Hopkins, MD, MEd
Eric L. Jenison, MD
Michael S. Guy, MD

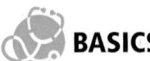 **BASICS**

DESCRIPTION
- Vaginal cancer is rare and comprises ~2–3% of gynecologic cancers.
- Vaginal intraepithelial neoplasia (carcinoma in situ): A premalignant phase with full-thickness neoplastic changes in the superficial epithelium; however, no invasion occurs through the basement membrane.
- Invasive malignancies: Vaginal malignancies include squamous cell carcinoma (85–90%), adenocarcinoma (5–10%), sarcoma (2–3%), and melanoma (2–3%). Clear cell carcinoma is a subtype of adenocarcinoma.
- To be classified as a vaginal malignancy, only the vagina can be involved. If the cervix or vulva is involved, then the tumor is classified as a primary cancer arising from the cervix or the vulva.
- Most vaginal malignancies are metastatic (e.g., cervix, vulva, endometrium, breast, ovary).
- System(s) affected: Reproductive
- Synonyms: Bowen disease; Vaginal intraepithelial neoplasia (VAIN)

Geriatric Considerations
Older patients, many with a long history of smoking, are at a higher risk for malignancies requiring surgical treatments.

Pediatric Considerations
Childhood sarcomas can be treated in a conservative fashion with multimodality therapy. This avoids the loss of the young child's bladder and/or rectum.

Pregnancy Considerations
This malignancy is not associated with pregnancy.

EPIDEMIOLOGY
Incidence
- 2,160 new cases in 2009 in the US
- Predominant age:
  – Carcinoma in situ: Mid-40s–60s
  – Invasive squamous cell malignancy: Mid 60s–70s
  – Adenocarcinoma: Any age; 50s is mean age. The most common vaginal malignancy occurs in patients under 20 years of age.
  – Clear cell adenocarcinoma occurs most often in females <30 years old with a history of exposure to diethylstilbestrol (DES) in utero.
  – Mixed Müllerian sarcomas and leiomyosarcomas in the adult population: Mean age 60 years
  – Sarcoma botryoides and embryonal sarcomas are pediatric conditions: Mean age 3 years

Prevalence
In the US, one of the rarest of all gynecologic malignancies (2–3%)

RISK FACTORS
- Similar risk factors as cervical cancer
- Age
- African American
- Smoking
- Multiple sex partners, early age of first sexual intercourse
- History of squamous cell cancer of the cervix or vulva
- Human papillomavirus (HPV) infection (70% of invasive vaginal malignancies)
- Vaginal adenosis
- Vaginal irritation
- DES exposure in utero

Genetics
No known genetic pattern

ETIOLOGY
- Women with a history of cervical malignancy have a higher probability of developing squamous cell malignancy in the vagina after hysterectomy.
- HPV has been associated with vulvovaginal, cervical, adenocarcinoma, and squamous cell carcinoma.
- Smokers have a higher incidence.
- Clear cell adenocarcinoma of the vagina in young women has been associated with DES exposure. The incidence, however, is exceedingly rare, estimated at 1/1,000 to 1/10,000 DES-exposed females.
- Metastatic lesions can involve the vagina from the other gynecologic organs.
- Although rare, renal cell carcinoma, lung adenocarcinoma, GI cancer, pancreatic adenocarcinoma, ovarian germ cell cancer, trophoblastic neoplasm, and breast cancer can all metastasize to the vagina.

COMMONLY ASSOCIATED CONDITIONS
Due to the field effect, patients with vaginal cancer are more likely to develop malignancy in the cervix or vulva and should be followed closely.

 DIAGNOSIS

HISTORY
- Abnormal bleeding is the most common symptom.
- Postcoital bleeding can result from direct trauma to the tumor.
- Vaginal discharge
- Dyspareunia
- Urinary symptoms including hematuria and increased frequency
- Constipation
- Pain along with symptoms and signs of hydroureter are late findings when the tumor has spread into the paravaginal tissues and extends to the pelvic sidewall.

Pediatric Considerations
In children, sarcomas can present either as a mass protruding from the vagina or as abnormal genital bleeding.

PHYSICAL EXAM
Pelvic examination:
- The vagina, uterus, adnexae (fallopian tubes and ovaries), bladder, and rectum should be evaluated for unusual changes.
- Vaginal malignancies are found most commonly on the posterior wall in the upper third of the vagina.

DIAGNOSTIC TESTS & INTERPRETATION
Lab
Initial lab tests
- PAP smear may incidentally detect asymptomatic lesions.
- Biopsy suspicious lesions.

Imaging
Initial approach
- CXR: To evaluate for metastatic disease
- Intravenous pyelogram (IVP) to evaluate for ureteral obstruction
- CT scan and MRI to evaluate the liver and retroperitoneum, especially the lymph nodes in the pelvic and periaortic area
- Barium enema to rule out rectal invasion
- Positron-emission tomographic (PET) scan detects primary and secondary metastatic lesions more often than CT scan.

> **ALERT**
> PET scan correlation with CT scan lesions strongly suggests malignancy.

Follow-Up & Special Considerations
Lymphangiography has been useful for evaluation of the lymph node status (1)[B].

Diagnostic Procedures/Surgery
- Colposcopy with directed biopsies for small lesions
- Wide excision under anesthesia of superficial disease may be necessary to ensure that invasive cancer is not present.
- Cystoscopy to rule out bladder invasion
- Sigmoidoscopy to rule out rectal invasion

Pathological Findings
Tumors are staged clinically:
- Stage 0: Carcinoma in situ/vaginal intraepithelial neoplasia (VAIN)
- Stage I: Infiltrative tumor not involving the paravaginal tissues (26%)
- Stage II: Carcinoma involves the paravaginal tissues but not the pelvic wall (37%)
- Stage III: Carcinoma extended to the sidewall (24%)
- Stage IVA: Tumor involving the bladder or the rectum, or true pelvis (13% stage IVA and IVB)
- Stage IVB: Spread to distant organs

DIFFERENTIAL DIAGNOSIS
- VAIN involves premalignant changes that do not infiltrate beyond the basement membrane.
- Adequate biopsies ensure that invasive lesions are not overlooked. Invasive lesions penetrate the basement membrane and cannot be treated conservatively.

- Other malignancies such as endometrial, cervix, bladder, or colon cancer can invade directly into the vagina or metastasize to the vagina.
- In the childbearing years, trophoblastic disease should be considered:
  – The vagina is a common site of metastases.
  – Biopsy usually will provide a clue to the primary site.

 TREATMENT

MEDICATION

- With one exception, there are no chemotherapeutic agents that have shown a survival advantage. The exception is childhood sarcomas, which have been treated with combinations of:
  – Vincristine
  – Dactinomycin (actinomycin-D)
  – Cyclophosphamide (Cytoxan)
  – Cisplatin
  – Etoposide (VP-16)
- Patients with advanced squamous cell carcinoma or adenocarcinoma receive concurrent irradiation and cisplatin-based chemotherapy (2)[B].
- Neoadjuvant chemotherapy followed by radical surgery may benefit select patients (3)[C].
- Intraepithelial neoplasia of the vagina (VAIN) can be treated with topical chemotherapy (5-fluorouracil cream) (4)[C].
- Treating VAIN with Imiquimod has led to complete response in certain patients (5)[C].
- Contraindications:
  – The diagnosis must be established with certainty prior to treatment.
  – If there is any doubt that a process beyond in situ disease exists, vaginectomy must be performed. These patients are often elderly, and aggressive therapy is limited by the patient's performance status and ability to tolerate radical surgery, chemotherapy, or radiation.

ADDITIONAL TREATMENT
General Measures
- Outpatient or inpatient care, depending on specific treatments
- Carcinoma in situ can be treated by a variety of methods:
  – Laser vaporization under microscopic guidance
  – Fluorouracil (Efudex) intravaginal cream
  – Partial vaginectomy
- In most tumor types, metastatic disease from the vagina to other sites is only minimally responsive to chemotherapy.

Issues for Referral
Patients should be treated by a gynecologic oncologist and/or a radiation oncologist.

Additional Therapies
- Treatment with radiotherapy depends on the stage of disease. This treatment option should be discussed with physicians experienced with this malignancy (4)[C].
- It is common to use radiotherapy and chemotherapy (chemoradiation) for better cancer control.
- Early-stage primary squamous cell carcinoma treated with radiation alone has shown good results (6)[A].
- Stage III vaginal cancer may benefit from combined radiation and hyperthermia (7)[C].

SURGERY/OTHER PROCEDURES
- Whenever there is a doubt as to the presence or absence of invasive disease, vaginectomy must be performed.
- Invasive lesions usually are treated by radiation therapy, but stage I lesions can be treated with radical hysterectomy or radical vaginectomy with pelvic lymph node dissection (8)[A].
- If the lesion involves the lower vagina, inguinal node dissection also must be done because cancer involving the lower vagina can metastasize to the groin region.
- Premenopausal women who desire to retain ovarian function are better candidates for radical surgery for early-stage disease with vaginal reconstruction possible afterward.
- Patients who have not completed their family occasionally can be treated with limited resection and localized radiation to the area.
- Sarcomas are treated by radiation therapy followed by pelvic exenteration if persistent disease is present.
- Childhood sarcomas:
  – Are treated with chemotherapy followed by local resection
  – Are responsive to multiagent combination chemotherapies

 ONGOING CARE

FOLLOW-UP RECOMMENDATIONS
- Patients are usually ambulatory and able to resume full activity by 6 weeks after surgery.
- Most patients are fully active while receiving chemotherapy and radiation therapy.

Patient Monitoring
- Pelvic examination and Pap smear every 3 months for 2 years, then every 6 months for the next 3 years, and then yearly thereafter
- Annual CXR

PATIENT EDUCATION
- Printed patient information available from American College of Obstetricians and Gynecologists, 409 12th St., SW, Washington, DC 20024–2188; (800) 762–ACOG; http://www.acog.org
- American Cancer Society: http://www.cancer.org
- Medline Plus: http://www.nlm.nih.gov/medlineplus/vaginalcancer.html

PROGNOSIS
Stage and 5-year survival:
- I: 77.6%
- II: 52.2%
- III: 42.5%
- IVA: 20.5%
- IVB:12.9%

COMPLICATIONS
- Those typically associated with major abdominal surgery or radiation therapy
- Common complications of treatment include rectovaginal or vesicovaginal fistulas, rectal/vaginal strictures, radiation cystitis, and/or proctitis.

REFERENCES

1. Frumovitz M, Gayed IW, Jhingran A, et al. Lymphatic mapping and sentinel lymph node detection in women with vaginal cancer. *Gynecol Oncol*. 2008.
2. Dalrymple JL, Russell AH, Lee SW, et al. Chemoradiation for primary invasive squamous carcinoma of the vagina. *Int J Gynecol Cancer*. 2004;14:110–7.
3. Benedetti Panici P, Bellati F, Plotti F, et al. Neoadjuvant chemotherapy followed by radical surgery in patients affected by vaginal carcinoma. *Gynecol Oncol*. 2008;111:307–11.
4. Creasman WT, et al. Vaginal cancers. *Curr Opin Obstet Gynecol*. 2005;17:71–6.
5. Iavazzo C, Pitsouni E, Athanasiou S, et al. Imiquimod for treatment of vulvar and vaginal intraepithelial neoplasia. *Int J Gynaecol Obstet*. 2008;101:3–10.
6. Tran PT, Su Z, Lee P, et al. Prognostic factors for outcomes and complications for primary squamous cell carcinoma of the vagina treated with radiation. *Gynecol Oncol*. 2007;105:641–9.
7. Franckena M, van der Zee J, et al. Use of combined radiation and hyperthermia for gynecological cancer. *Curr Opin Obstet Gynecol*. 2010;22:9–14.
8. Tjalma WA, Monaghan JM, de Barros Lopes A, et al. The role of surgery in invasive squamous carcinoma of the vagina. *Gynecol Oncol*. 2001;81:360–5.

See Also (Topic, Algorithm, Electronic Media Element)
Algorithm: Metrorrhagia (Intermenstrual Bleeding)

 CODES

ICD9
184.0 Malignant neoplasm of vagina

CLINICAL PEARLS

- Vaginal cancer is rare; 85–90% of vaginal cancers are squamous cell.
- Vaginal malignancies are found most commonly on the posterior wall in the upper third of the vagina.
- Most vaginal malignancies are metastatic (from cervix, vulva, endometrium, breast, or ovary).

VAGINISMUS

Stephanie Yu-hsuan Chen, MD
Tiffany A. Moore Simas, MD, MPH, Med

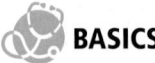 **BASICS**

Vaginismus is a clinical syndrome that consists of overlapping elements of hypertonic pelvic floor muscles (recurrent or persistent involuntary contractions), pain, and avoidance of sexual intercourse leading to difficulty in vaginal penetration.

DESCRIPTION
- It is defined as the recurrent or persistent difficulties of a woman to allow vaginal entry of a penis, a finger, and/or an object, despite the woman's expressed wish to do so (1).
- Classified as a sexual pain disorder, along with dyspareunia and noncoital sexual pain disorder:
  - Experience of pain is not required for the diagnosis of vaginismus, though in most women with vaginismus there is anticipation or fear of pain.
- Primary vaginismus is present when a woman has never been able to experience vaginal penetration without difficulty.
- Secondary vaginismus occurs when a woman who has previously been able to achieve penetration develops vaginismus.
- Can be complete (difficulty with attempts to insert anything into vagina) or situational (tampons or pelvic exams permitted)
- Etiology is often multifactorial.
- Women with vaginismus often avoid intercourse and may avoid appropriate health care.
- Treatment is based on the patient's goals and is focused on patient education, therapy, and behavioral exercises.

Pregnancy Considerations
- Pregnancy can occur in patients with vaginismus when ejaculation occurs on the perineum.
- Vaginismus is an independent risk factor for cesarean delivery (2)[C].

EPIDEMIOLOGY
Prevalence
- True prevalence is unknown due to limited data/reporting.
- Population-based studies report prevalence rates of 0.5–30% (3).
- Affects women in all age groups

RISK FACTORS
- Though the exact role in the condition is unclear, many women report a history of abuse or sexual trauma (4)[C].
- Often associated with other sexual dysfunctions

ETIOLOGY
- Most often multifactorial in both primary and secondary vaginismus
- Primary:
  - Psychologic and psychosocial issues:
    - Negative messages about sex and sexual relations in upbringing may cause phobic reaction.
    - Poor body image and limited understanding of genital area
    - History of sexual trauma
  - Abnormalities of the hymen
- Secondary:
  - Vaginal infection
  - Inflammatory dermatitis
  - Surgical or postdelivery scarring
  - Endometriosis
  - Inadequate vaginal lubrication
  - Pelvic radiation
  - Estrogen deficiency
  - Conditioned response to pain from physical issues previously listed

COMMONLY ASSOCIATED CONDITIONS
- Marital stress, family dysfunction
- Anxiety
- Dyspareunia
- Vulvodynia/vestibulodynia

 DIAGNOSIS

Vaginismus is a clinical diagnosis.

HISTORY
- Complete medical history
- Full psychosocial and sexual history, including:
  - Relationship difficulty
  - Inability to allow vaginal entry for different purposes:
    - Sexual (penis, digit, object)
    - Hygiene (tampon use)
    - Health care (pelvic exam)
  - Infertility
  - Past traumatic experiences
  - Religious beliefs
  - Views on sexuality

PHYSICAL EXAM
- Pelvic examination is necessary to exclude structural abnormalities or organic pathology.
- Educating the patient about the examination and giving her control over the progression of the examination is essential, as genital/pelvic examination may induce varying degrees of anxiety in patients.
- Referral to a gynecologist or other providers specializing in the treatment of sexual disorders may be appropriate.
- Lamont classification system aids in the assessment of severity:
  - 1st degree: Perineal and levator spasm relieved with reassurance
  - 2nd degree: Perineal spasm maintained throughout the pelvic exam
  - 3rd degree: Levator spasm and elevation of buttocks
  - 4th degree: Levator and perineal spasm and elevation with adduction and retreat (5)

DIAGNOSTIC TESTS & INTERPRETATION
Lab
No laboratory tests indicated

Imaging
None indicated

Pathological Findings
- Rarely found in primary vaginismus except for hymenal anomalies
- May be varied in secondary vaginismus, such as endometriosis or scarring

DIFFERENTIAL DIAGNOSIS
- Dyspareunia
- Vaginal infection
- Vulvodynia/vestibulodynia
- Vulvovaginal atrophy
- Urogenital structural abnormalities
- Interstitial cystitis

 TREATMENT

- Vaginismus may be successfully treated.
- Outpatient care is appropriate.
- Treatment of physical conditions is first-line if present (see secondary etiologies).
- Role for pelvic floor physical therapy and myofascial release

- Some evidence suggests that cognitive-behavioral therapy may be effective (6)[C]:
  - Includes desensitization techniques such as gradual exposure, aimed at decreasing avoidance behavior and fear of vaginal penetration
- Evidence suggests that Masters and Johnson sex therapy may be effective (7)[C]:
  - Involves Kegel exercises to increase control over perineal muscles
  - Stepwise vaginal desensitization exercises:
    - With vaginal dilators that the patient inserts and controls
    - With woman's own finger(s) to promote sexual self-awareness
    - Advancement to partner's fingers with patient's control
    - Coitus after achieving largest vaginal dilator or 3 fingers; important to begin with sensate-focused exercises/sensual caressing without necessarily a demand for coitus
    - Female superior at 1st; passive (nonthrusting); female-directed
    - Later, thrusting may be allowed.
- Topical anesthetic with desensitization exercises may be considered.
- Patient education is an essential component of treatment (see Patient Education section).

MEDICATION
Botulinum neurotoxin type A injections may improve vaginismus in patients who do not respond to standard cognitive behavioral and medical treatment for vaginismus:
- Dosage: 20, 50, and 100–400 units of botulinum toxin type A injected in the levator ani muscle have been shown to improve vaginismus (8)[C].

ADDITIONAL TREATMENT
Issues for Referral
For diagnosis and treatment recommendations, the following resources may be consulted:
- Obstetrics/gynecology
- Pelvic floor physical therapy
- Psychiatry
- Sex therapy
- Hypnotherapy

COMPLEMENTARY AND ALTERNATIVE MEDICINE
- Biofeedback
- Functional electrical stimulation

SURGERY/OTHER PROCEDURES
Contraindicated

 ONGOING CARE

FOLLOW-UP RECOMMENDATIONS
Desensitization techniques of gentle, progressive, patient-controlled vaginal dilation

Patient Monitoring
General preventive health care

DIET
No special diet

PATIENT EDUCATION
- Education about pelvic anatomy, nature of vaginal spasms, normal adult sexual function
- Handheld mirror can help the woman to learn visually to tighten and loosen perineal muscles
- Important to teach the partner that spasms are not under conscious control and are not a reflection on the relationship or a woman's feelings about her partner
- Instruction in techniques for vaginal dilation
- Resources:
  - American College of Obstetricians & Gynecologists (ACOG), 409 12th St., SW, Washington, DC 20024-2188; (800) 762-ACOG. www.acog.org
  - Valins L. When a woman's body says no to sex: Understanding and overcoming vaginismus. New York: Penguin, 1992.

PROGNOSIS
Favorable with early recognition of the condition and initiation of treatment

REFERENCES
1. Basson R, Wierman ME, van Lankveld J, et al. Summary of the recommendations on sexual dysfunctions in women. *J Sex Med*. 2010;7: 314–26.
2. Goldsmith T, Levy A, Sheiner E, et al. Vaginismus as an independent risk factor for cesarean delivery. *J Matern Fetal Neonatal Med*. 2009;22(10):863–6.
3. Wimons JS, Carey MP. Prevalence of sexual dysfunctions: results form a decade of research. *Arch Sex Behav*. 2001;30:177–217.
4. Reissing E, Binik Y, Khalife S, et al. Etiological correlates of vaginismus: sexual and physical abuse, sexual knowledge, sexual self-schema, and relationship adjustment. *J Sex Marital Ther*. 2003;29:47–59.
5. Lamont J. Vaginismus. *Am J Obstet Gynecol*. 1978;131:632–6.
6. ter Kuile MM, van Lankveld JJDM, de Groot E, et al. Cognitive behavioral therapy for women with lifelong vaginismus: Process and prognostic factors. *Behav Research and Therapy*. 2008;45:359–373.
7. Jeng CJ, Wang LR, Chou CS, et al. Management and outcome of primary vaginismus. *J Sex Marital Ther*. 2006;32:379–87.
8. Bertolasi L, Frasson E, Cappelletti JY, et al. Botulinum neurotoxin type A injections for vaginismus secondary to vulvar vestibulitis syndrome. *Obstet Gynecol*. 2009;114:1008–16.

ADDITIONAL READING
Crowley T, Goldmeier D, Hiller J. Diagnosing and managing vaginismus. *BMJ*. 2009;338:b2284.

See Also (Topic, Algorithm, Electronic Media Element)
Dyspareunia; Sexual Dysfunction in Women
Algorithm: Sexual Dysfunction in Women

 CODES

ICD9
- 306.51 Psychogenic vaginismus
- 625.1 Vaginismus

CLINICAL PEARLS
- In a patient with suspected vaginismus, a complete medical history, including a comprehensive psychosocial and sexual history, and a patient-centric, patient-controlled educational pelvic exam should be conducted.
- Vaginismus can be treated effectively.
- Cognitive behavioral therapy may be effective for the treatment of vaginismus.
- Botox injection therapy is in the experimental stages but looks promising for the treatment of vaginismus.

V

VAGINITIS AND VAGINOSIS

Tara N. Kumaraswami, MD
Marie Ellen Caggiano, MD, MPH

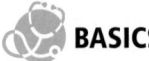 **BASICS**

DESCRIPTION

- Vulvovaginal candidiasis (VVC): Inflammation of the vagina and vulva caused by infection with *Candida* sp.
- Bacterial vaginosis (BV): A syndrome in which the hydrogen peroxide–producing lactobacilli normally found in the vagina are replaced by other bacteria, usually anaerobes
- VVC and BV are not generally considered sexually transmitted infections.
- Other causes of vaginitis include allergic and contact dermatitis (from feminine hygiene products: Fragrances, creams, douches, lubricants, and their preservatives).
- Atrophic vaginitis is covered separately in Menopause.
- See separate article entitled Trichomoniasis.
- A number of dermatoses such as lichen planus, lichen sclerosus, and psoriasis may mimic vaginitis symptoms.
- System(s) affected: Reproductive; Skin/Exocrine
- Synonym(s): VVC: Monilial vulvovaginitis; Vaginal yeast infection; BV: *Gardnerella* vaginosis; Nonspecific vaginitis; *Haemophilus* vaginitis; *Corynebacterium* vaginitis

EPIDEMIOLOGY

- Both VVC and BV are common among reproductive-age females.
- Most cases of VVC are related to *C. albicans* but may be caused by other *Candida* sp. (e.g., *C. glabrata*).
- VVC related to *C. glabrata* may be more common among diabetic women.

Prevalence

- VVC: 2nd most common cause of vaginitis after BV:
  – 75% of women diagnosed at least once with VVC; up to 45% diagnosed more than once
  – <5% of females are diagnosed with recurrent VVC (defined as 4 or more episodes of VVC in 1 year).
  – Studies have shown that up to 50% of females may be colonized with yeast but do not exhibit the symptoms of vaginitis. This may be as high as 72%.
- BV: Prevalence varies based on age, race/ethnicity, and socioeconomic status:
  – Most common vaginal infection among reproductive-aged women
  – NHANES data reported an overall prevalence of 29%, with the highest rates (50%) among black women.

Pediatric Considerations

VVC and BV are less common before the onset of puberty and after menopause.

RISK FACTORS

- VVC:
  – Diabetes mellitus (DM) with poor glycemic control
  – Antibiotic therapy
  – Immunosuppression (e.g., corticosteroid therapy, HIV infection)
  – High-estrogen states (e.g., pregnancy, oral contraceptive use, hormone-replacement therapy); *C. albicans* accounts for 85–90% of cases in pregnancy.
- BV:
  – Black race
  – Lower socioeconomic status
  – Smoking
  – New or multiple sex partner(s)
  – Female sex partners
  – Spermicide use
  – Douching

GENERAL PREVENTION

- Vulvar hygiene (see General Measures); avoid implicated feminine hygiene products.
- Maintenance therapy for recurrent cases
- Treatment of sexual partners generally is not recommended but may be considered in recurrent cases.

ETIOLOGY

- VVC: Overgrowth of yeast in the vagina
- BV: Shift from a healthy lactobacilli-based endogenous flora to an anaerobically based endogenous flora, including *G. vaginalis*, *Mobiluncus* sp., *Mycoplasma hominis*, *Peptostreptococcus*, *Prevotella*, *Bacteroides*, and *Fusobacterium* sp.; the rectum may be a reservoir of organisms leading to autoinfection.

COMMONLY ASSOCIATED CONDITIONS

- Sexually transmitted infections
- Balanitis in male partners may occur rarely.
- In same-sex partners, research is limited. Symptomatic partners should be evaluated.

 DIAGNOSIS

Neither symptoms alone nor findings on physical examination have good sensitivity or discriminatory power for vaginal infections. Light microscopy is most helpful when classic findings are present (1,2)[A].

HISTORY

- VVC:
  – Vaginal and vulvar pruritus
  – Vulvar pain, external dysuria, and dyspareunia
  – Thick, curdlike vaginal discharge
- BV:
  – Many women asymptomatic
  – Unpleasant musty or fishy vaginal odor, exacerbated immediately after intercourse
  – 10–30% may have vaginal/vulvar irritation
  – Thin gray–white or frothy vaginal discharge

PHYSICAL EXAM

- VVC:
  – Thick, curdlike vaginal discharge
  – Vulvar erythema and edema
  – Vulvar fissures and excoriations
  – Normal vaginal pH (<4.5)

- BV:
  – 10–30% may have vaginal/vulvar irritation.
  – Thin gray–white vaginal discharge is mildly adherent to vaginal walls.
  – 10% have frothy discharge.
  – pH >4.5

DIAGNOSTIC TESTS & INTERPRETATION

Lab

- Wet mount: Prepare 2 slides, both with fresh vaginal discharge: NaCl and 10% KOH:
  – The presence of budding yeasts and hyphae consistent with VVC (KOH)
  – Clue cells >10–20% of total epithelial cells considered clinically significant for diagnosis of BV (saline)
  – White blood cells (WBCs) are not numerous in BV but may be present in large numbers in VVC.
- Amsel criteria for BV (need 3 out of 4): Clue cells, characteristic vaginal discharge, vaginal pH >4.5, and positive "whiff test" (transient but potent amine or fishy odor with the addition of 10% KOH); vaginal pH also may suggest need for testing for *Trichomonas* (3)[B].
- Consider vaginal culture for VVC when characteristic symptoms are present, vaginal pH is normal, and no yeast are present on wet mount or to identify species if no improvement with treatment or relapse occurs within 2 months.
- Positive culture for *Candida* sp. or other yeasts sometimes may only indicate colonization; clinical correlation is required.
- VVC or BV: May be noted on cytology but must be correlated with clinical symptoms; asymptomatic women generally do not need treatment.
- DNA probe–based tests are available (Affirm VP III, Becton Dickinson, Sparks, MD), but it is unclear that identification of the presence of yeast (or low numbers of *G. vaginalis*) indicates that the organism is the cause of symptoms. Use may not be cost-effective.

DIFFERENTIAL DIAGNOSIS

- Physiologic discharge and cervical ectropion
- Trichomoniasis
- Contact dermatitis
- Mechanical/chemical irritation
- Cervicitis (chlamydial or gonococcal)
- Urinary tract infection (UTI)
- Atrophic vaginitis
- Dermatoses: Lichen sclerosus, lichen planus, seborrheic dermatitis, psoriasis

 TREATMENT

MEDICATION

First Line

- VVC:
  – Short-course therapy with topical azoles is effective in 80–90% of patients.
  – Many topical therapies are available over the counter.
  – Miconazole: 2% cream 5 gm intravaginally × 7 days, or 200-mg vaginal suppository × 3 days, or 1,200-mg vaginal suppository × 1 day
  – Butoconazole: 2% cream 5 gm intravaginally × 3 days, or sustained-release single intravaginal application

- Terconazole: 0.4% cream 5 g intravaginally × 7 days, or 0.8% cream × 3 days, or 80-mg vaginal suppository × 3 days
- Clotrimazole: 1% cream 5 g intravaginally × 7–14 days, or 100-mg vaginal tablets, 1 tablet × 7 days or 2 tablets × 3 days
- Tioconazole: 6.5% ointment 5 g intravaginally, single application; complete relief may take up to 7 days.
- Nystatin: 100,000-unit vaginal tablet × 14 days
- Oral therapy: Fluconazole, 150 mg p.o. once; use with caution in patients with liver disease and with coadministration of other drugs.
- BV:
  - Metronidazole (Flagyl): 500 mg p.o. b.i.d. × 7 days or
  - Metronidazole vaginal gel: 0.75% 5 g intravaginally daily × 7 days or
  - Clindamycin: 2% vaginal cream 5 g intravaginally daily × 7 days

ALERT
Oil-based preparations may weaken latex condoms.

Second Line
- VVC:
  - Recurrent VVC: Obtain cultures. Infections associated with *C. glabrata* (5–15%) are less responsive to 1st-line therapies (4,5).
  - Consider longer-duration therapy (7–14 days of topical or oral fluconazole every 3rd day for a total of 3 doses).
  - Suppressive maintenance therapy (oral fluconazole weekly × 6 months or topical treatments weekly) (6)
  - Women with recurrent candidiasis may benefit from fluconazole 150 mg per week plus cetirizine 10 mg/d (7)[B] for allergy or itching.
  - Boric acid: 600-mg gelatin capsule inserted vaginally daily × 2 weeks (indicated for non-*Albicans* disease; 70% clinical and mycologic cure rate) (5)
- BV:
  - Metronidazole: 2 g p.o. single dose (less effective than 7-day regimen)
  - Clindamycin: 300 mg p.o. daily × 7 days
  - Clindamycin ovules: 100 g intravaginally at bedtime × 3 days (clindamycin creams are less effective than metronidazole)
  - Tinidazole : 1 g p.o. × 5 days has been shown to be effective and may produce fewer side effects than metronidazole.

ALERT
Metronidazole produces a disulfiramlike effect when alcohol is ingested. Avoid any alcohol-containing product while taking metronidazole.

Pregnancy Considerations
- VVC: Oral azoles relatively contraindicated in pregnancy (pregnancy Category C); choose topical therapy if possible.
- BV: Associated with preterm delivery; however, it is unclear whether the treatment of BV prevents preterm delivery. All symptomatic women should be treated, screening reserved for women at high risk for preterm delivery. Avoid creams; metronidazole 500 mg p.o. b.i.d. × 7 days or clindamycin 300 mg p.o. 2 b.i.d. × 7 days. Package labeling of metronidazole indicates that it is contraindicated in

the 1st trimester of pregnancy, but this is not supported by recent meta-analyses of available data.

ADDITIONAL TREATMENT
General Measures
- Avoid use of panty liners, pantyhose, and occlusive pants and undergarments.
- Avoid douching.
- Regular use of condoms may help to prevent BV.

Issues for Referral
Treating the male sexual partner does not reduce symptoms or prevent recurrence, but this may be considered in patients who have recurrent infection. Relapses of both conditions are fairly common, and several regimens have been suggested for prophylaxis/maintenance.

COMPLEMENTARY AND ALTERNATIVE MEDICINE
- *Lactobacillus* supplementation is not effective in prevention.
- Use of garlic and tea tree oil has no known efficacy.

 ONGOING CARE

FOLLOW-UP RECOMMENDATIONS
Delay sexual relations until symptoms clear/discomfort resolves.

Patient Monitoring
Generally, no specific follow-up needed; if symptoms persist or recur within 2 months, repeat pelvic exam and culture.

DIET
Reduction of sugar intake has been recommended but is not supported by evidence.

PATIENT EDUCATION
American College of Obstetricians and Gynecologists (ACOG), 409 12th St., SW, Washington, DC 20024-2188; (800) 762-ACOG; http://www.acog.org

PROGNOSIS
VVC: 80–90% of uncomplicated cases cured with appropriate treatment; 30–50% of recurrent infections return after discontinuation of maintenance therapy; there is a relatively high spontaneous remission rate of untreated symptoms as well.

COMPLICATIONS
- VVC may occur following treatment of BV.
- BV has been associated with an increased risk of acquisition and transmission of sexually transmitted diseases (STIs), including HIV.
- BV has been associated with increased risk of pregnancy complications, including preterm birth, postpartum and postabortal endometritis, and pelvic inflammatory disease (PID).

REFERENCES

1. Anderson MR, Klink K, Cohrssen A. Evaluation of vaginal complaints. *JAMA*. 2004;291:1368–79.
2. Lowe NK, Neal JL, Ryan-Wenger NA. Accuracy of the clinical diagnosis of vaginitis compared with a DNA probe laboratory standard. *Obstet Gynecol*. 2009;113:89–95.
3. Carr PL, Rothberg MB, Friedman RH, et al. "Shotgun" versus sequential testing. Cost-effectiveness of diagnostic strategies for vaginitis. *J Gen Intern Med*. 2005;20:793–9.
4. Owen MK, Clenney TL. Management of vaginitis. *Am Fam Physician*. 2004;70:2125–32.
5. Ray D, Goswami R, Banerjee U, et al. Prevalence of Candida glabrata and Its Response to Boric Acid Vaginal Suppositories in Comparison With Oral Fluconazole in Patients With Diabetes and Vulvovaginal Candidiasis. *Diabetes Care*. 2007;30:312–7.
6. Pappas, et al. Clinical Practice Guidelines for the Management of Candidiasis: 2009 Update by the Infectious Disease Society of America. *Clinical Infectious Diseases* 2009;48(5):503–535.
7. Neves NA, Carvalho LP, Lopes AC, et al. Successful treatment of refractory recurrent vaginal candidiasis with cetirizine plus fluconazole. *J Low Genit Tract Dis*. 2005;9:167–70.

ADDITIONAL READING

- Allsworth JE, Peipert JF. Prevalence of bacterial vaginosis: 2001–2004 National Health and Nutrition Examination Survey data. *Obstet Gynecol*. 2007;109:114–20.
- Centers for Disease Control and Prevention. Sexually Transmitted Diseases Treatment Guidelines. *MMWR*. 2006;55(No. RR-11):54–6.
- Fredricks DN, Fiedler TL, Marrazzo JM. Molecular identification of bacteria associated with bacterial vaginosis. *N Engl J Med*. 2005;353:1899–911.

See Also (Topic, Algorithm, Electronic Media Element)
Algorithm: Discharge, Vaginal

 CODES

ICD9
- 041.9 Bacterial infection, unspecified, in conditions classified elsewhere and of unspecified site
- 112.1 Candidiasis of vulva and vagina
- 616.10 Vaginitis and vulvovaginitis, unspecified

CLINICAL PEARLS
- Clinical symptoms, signs, and microscopy have relatively poor performance compared with so-called gold standards such as culture and DNA probe assays, but these more sensitive assays may detect organisms that may not be causing symptoms.
- Most women experience relief of symptoms with therapy chosen without such gold standard tests, and even when the treatment does not correspond with the underlying infection.
- Vaginal pH is underused as a diagnostic tool for evaluation of vaginitis.
- Treatment of sexual partners is not currently the standard of care for either BV or VVC.

VARICOSE VEINS

Joseph A. Florence, MD

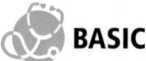 **BASICS**

DESCRIPTION
- Permanent dilatation and tortuosity of superficial veins, usually occurring in the legs and feet; may result from congenitally incomplete valves or valves that have become incompetent
- Affects legs where reverse flow occurs when dependent
- System(s) affected: Cardiovascular; Skin

ALERT
Ulceration of varicose veins has a high rate of infection, which can lead to sepsis.

Geriatric Considerations
- Common; usually valvular degeneration but may be secondary to chronic venous deficiency
- Elastic support hose and frequent rests with legs elevated rather than ligation and stripping

Pregnancy Considerations
- Frequent problem
- Elastic stockings recommended for history of varicosities or if a great deal of standing is involved

EPIDEMIOLOGY
Incidence
- Predominant age: Middle age
- Predominant gender: Female > Male (5:1)
- National Women's Health Information Center estimates that 50% of women have varicose veins.

RISK FACTORS
- Increasing age
- Pregnancy, especially multiple pregnancies
- Occupations requiring prolonged standing, restrictive clothing (e.g., very tight girdles)
- Obesity
- History of phlebitis
- Family history

Genetics
Familial, dominant, X-linked

PATHOPHYSIOLOGY
- Varicose veins are caused by venous insufficiency from faulty valves in ≥1 perforator veins in the lower leg, causing secondary incompetence at the saphenofemoral junction (valvular reflux).
- Valvular dysfunction causing venous reflux and subsequently venous hypertension (HTN)
- Failed valves allow blood to flow in the reverse direction (away from the heart) from deep to superficial and from proximal to distal veins.
- Deep thrombophlebitis
- Increased venous pressure from any cause
- Congenital valvular incompetence
- Trauma (consider arteriovenous fistula; listen for bruit)
- Presumed to be due to a loss in vein wall elasticity with failure of the valve leaflets

COMMONLY ASSOCIATED CONDITIONS
- Stasis dermatitis
- Large varicose veins may lead to skin changes and eventual stasis ulceration.

 DIAGNOSIS

HISTORY
- Symptoms range from minor annoyance or cosmetic problem to a lifestyle-limiting problem.
- Localized symptoms: Pain, burning, itching
- Generalized symptoms:
  - Leg muscular cramp, aching
  - Leg fatigue or swelling
- Pain if varicose ulcer develops
- Symptoms often worse at the end of the day, especially with prolonged standing
- Women are more prone to symptoms due to hormonal influences: Worse during menses
- No direct correlation with the severity of varicose veins and the severity of symptoms

PHYSICAL EXAM
- Inspect lower extremities with patient standing. Varicose veins in the proximal femoral ring and distal portion of the legs may not be visible when the patient is supine.
- Varicose veins are:
  - Dilatated, tortuous superficial veins, chiefly in the lower extremities
  - Dark purple or blue in color, raised above the surface of the skin
  - Often twisted, bulging, and can look like cords
  - Most commonly found on the posterior or medial lower extremity
- Edema of affected limb may be present.
- Skin changes may include:
  - Eczema
  - Hyperpigmentation
  - Lipodermatosclerosis
- Spider veins (idiopathic telangiectases):
  - Fine intracutaneous angiectasis
  - May be extensive/unsightly
- Neurologic sensory and motor exam:
  - Peripheral arterial vasculature; pulses
  - Musculoskeletal exam for associated rheumatologic or orthopedic issues

DIAGNOSTIC TESTS & INTERPRETATION
- Trendelenburg test: Test for varicose veins (1):
  - Patient lies on back and raises leg to empty the veins.
  - Tourniquet is applied just below the saphenous opening, around the upper thigh.
  - Patient stands up, and the tourniquet is removed in 60 s.
  - Normally, the vein should fill from below within 35 s with the tourniquet in situ. Earlier filling indicates incompetence of a communicating vein. If, on release, the veins fill rapidly from above, it is due to incompetent saphenofemoral valves.

- Perthes test: A clinical test for assessing the patency of the deep femoral veins (1):
  - With the patient standing and veins filled, a tourniquet is placed around the midthigh, and the patient walks for 5 minutes.
  - If the saphenous veins collapse below the tourniquet, the deep veins are patent, and the communicating veins are competent; if unchanged, both saphenous and communicating veins are incompetent; and if the veins increase in prominence and pain occurs, the deep veins are occluded.

Imaging
Duplex ultrasound: Formal noninvasive imaging of the venous system with duplex ultrasound will confirm the etiology, anatomy, and pathophysiology of segmental venous reflux.

Diagnostic Procedures/Surgery
- Tourniquet tests have been replaced by ultrasound techniques for assessing varicose veins before treatment.
- Duplex scanning, venous Doppler study, photoplethysmography, light-reflection rheography, air plethysmography, and other vascular testing should be reserved for patients who have venous symptoms and/or large (>4 mm in diameter) vessels or large numbers of spider telangiectasia indicating venous HTN.

Pathological Findings
- Medial fibrosis of veins
- Disappearance or atrophy of valves

DIFFERENTIAL DIAGNOSIS
- Nerve root compression
- Arthritis
- Peripheral neuritis
- Telangiectasia: Smaller, visible blood vessels that are permanently dilated
- Deep vein thrombosis
- Inflammatory liposclerosis

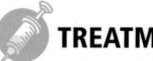 **TREATMENT**

- Ambulatory Conservative Hemodynamic Management of Varicose Veins is more effective than stripping with clinical marking or stripping with duplex marking to treat varicose veins (2)[B].
- Conservative therapy (e.g., elevation, external compression, weight loss) may be helpful, but there are few clinical trials (3)[C],(4)[A].
- There is insufficient evidence to preferentially recommend any specific treatment or combination of treatments for varicose veins (3)[B].
- Sclerotherapy may be used to improve the symptoms and cosmetic appearance of varicose veins (3)[B].

MEDICATION
Superficial thrombophlebitis is not an infective condition and does not require antibiotic treatment.

ADDITIONAL TREATMENT
General Measures
Patients with unsightly varicose veins seek treatment for cosmetic reasons.

Issues for Referral

Referral guidelines from National Institute for Health and Clinical Excellence (5)[A]:

- Emergency: Bleeding from a varicosity that has eroded the skin
- Urgent: Varicosity that has bled and is at risk for bleeding again
- Soon: Ulcer that is progressive or painful despite treatment
- Routine:
  – Active or healed ulcer or progressive skin changes that may benefit from surgery
  – Recurrent superficial thrombophlebitis
  – Troublesome symptoms attributable to varicose veins, or patient and provider feel that the extent, site, and size of the varicosities are having a severe impact on quality of life.

Additional Therapies

- Activity:
  – Frequent rest periods with legs elevated
  – If standing is necessary, frequently shift weight from side to side.
  – Appropriate exercise routine as part of conservative treatment
  – Walking regimen after sclerotherapy is important to help promote healing.
  – Apply elastic stockings before lowering legs from the bed.
  – Never sit with legs hanging down.
- Physical therapy

SURGERY/OTHER PROCEDURES

- Surgery:
  – Challenge to balance a cosmetically acceptable result with a low incidence of recurrence and complications
  – Surgery is indicated if there is pain, recurrent phlebitis, skin changes/ulceration, or for cosmetic improvement for severe cases.
  – Minimally invasive techniques include (6)[C]:
    ○ Radiofrequency ablation (RFA)
    ○ Endovenous laser therapy
    ○ Transilluminated power phlebectomy
    ○ Foam sclerotherapy is more powerful than a liquid sclerosant (7)[A].
    ○ Ambulatory phlebectomy has a lower risk of recurrence than sclerotherapy (7)[A].
  – Traditional surgical methods include:
    ○ Ligation and stripping of the varicose vein
    ○ Stab avulsion phlebectomy
  – For extensive fibrosis: Excision of the entire area, followed by skin graft, may be necessary.
  – Surgical treatment of clinically symptomatic varicose veins involves treatment of the saphenous vein reflux as well as the varicosities.
- Sclerotherapy:
  – Randomized, controlled trials suggest that the choice of sclerosant, dose, formulation (foam vs liquid), local pressure dressing, and degree and length of compression has no significant effect on the efficacy of sclerotherapy (8)[A].
  – Sclerosing solution is injected into varicosities, causing vein walls to swell, adhere, and scar; 50–90% improvement expected
  – Ultrasound-guided sclerotherapy combined with saphenofemoral ligations was less expensive, involved a shorter treatment time, and resulted in more rapid recovery than saphenofemoral ligation, saphenous stripping, and phlebectomies (9)[B].

- Radiotherapy:
  – RFA takes longer to perform but has better early outcome than conventional surgery in patients with great saphenous varicose veins (10)[B]; increased cost is partially offset by a quicker return to work (11)[B].
  – Radiofrequency and laser treatments replace "stripping"; however, most varicosities still require phlebectomy or sclerotherapy.

 ONGOING CARE

DIET

- No special diet
- Weight-loss diet recommended, if obesity a problem

PATIENT EDUCATION

- Avoid long periods of standing.
- Exercise regularly to improve leg strength, circulation: Walking and running
- Maintain an appropriate weight.
- Avoid crossing legs when sitting.
- Wear elastic support stockings.
- Avoid clothing that constricts legs.
- Inform patients that the surgery or sclerotherapy may not prevent development of varicosities and that the procedure may need to be repeated in later years.
- For patient education materials favorably reviewed on this topic, contact National Heart, Lung and Blood Institute, Communications and Public Information Branch, National Institutes of Health, Building 31, Room 41–21, 9000 Rockville Pike, Bethesda, MD 20892; (301) 496-4236.

PROGNOSIS

- Usual course: Chronic
- Favorable with appropriate treatment
- Quality of surgical treatment is less satisfactory if significant deep venous reflux, history of ulceration, or congenital arteriovenous malformation exists (6).

COMPLICATIONS

- Petechial hemorrhages
- Chronic edema
- Superimposed infection
- Varicose ulcers
- Pigmentation
- Eczema
- Recurrence after surgical treatment
- Scarring or nerve damage from stripping technique

REFERENCES

1. Kim J, Richards S, Kent PJ. Clinical examination of varicose veins–a validation study. *Ann R Coll Surg Engl*. 2000;82:171–5.
2. Parés JO, Juan J, Tellez R, et al. Varicose vein surgery: stripping versus the CHIVA method: a randomized controlled trial. *Ann Surg*. 2010;251:624–31.
3. Jones RH, Carek PJ. Management of varicose veins. *Am Fam Physician*. 2008;78:1289–94.
4. Palfreyman SJ, Michaels JA, et al. A systematic review of compression hosiery for uncomplicated varicose veins. *Phlebology*. 2009;24(Suppl 1):13–33.
5. National Institute for Clinical Excellence. *Referral Advice for Varicose Veins*. London: NICE, 2001.
6. Teruya TH, Ballard JL. New approaches for the treatment of varicose veins. *Surg Clin North Am*. 2004;84:1397–417, viii–ix.
7. Sadick NS. Advances in the treatment of varicose veins: ambulatory phlebectomy, foam sclerotherapy, endovascular laser, and radio-frequency closure. *Dermatol Clin*. 2005;23:443–55, vi.
8. Tisi PV, Beverley C, Rees A. Injection sclerotherapy for varicose veins. *Cochrane Database Syst Rev*. 2006:CD001732.
9. Bountouroglou DG. Varicose veins and their management. *BMJ*. 2006;533:287–92.
10. Subramonia S, Lees T, et al. Randomized clinical trial of radiofrequency ablation or conventional high ligation and stripping for great saphenous varicose veins. *Br J Surg*. 2010;97:328–36.
11. Subramonia S, Lees T, et al. Radiofrequency ablation vs conventional surgery for varicose veins—a comparison of treatment costs in a randomised trial. *Eur J Vasc Endovasc Surg*. 2010;39:104–11.
12. Rigby KA, Palfreyman SJ, Beverley C, et al. Surgery versus sclerotherapy for the treatment of varicose veins. *Cochrane Database Syst Rev*. 2004:CD004980.

See Also (Topic, Algorithm, Electronic Media Element)

Hemorrhoids; Dermatitis, Stasis

CODES

ICD9

- 454.0 Varicose veins of lower extremities with ulcer
- 454.1 Varicose veins of lower extremities with inflammation
- 454.9 Asymptomatic varicose veins

CLINICAL PEARLS

- Insufficient evidence exists to prefer sclerotherapy over surgery (12)[A].
- The efficacy of sclerotherapy is not significantly affected by the choice of sclerosant, dose, formulation (foam vs liquid), local pressure dressing, or degree and length of compression (8)[A].

V

VASCULITIS

Carla M. Nester, MD
Dale E. Bieber, MD

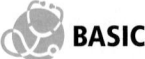 **BASICS**

DESCRIPTION
Vasculitis is an inflammatory disease of the blood vessels.

- Disease presentation results from the destruction of blood vessel walls, with subsequent aneurysm formation, bleeding, thrombosis, or ischemia in the various vascular beds and organs.
- Diagnosis should be considered whenever a patient has a persistent, unexplained systemic illness or focal signs as listed below.
- Consists of a heterogeneous group of diseases depending on size, type, and location of the blood vessel involved.
  - Small-vessel vasculitis:
    - Churg-Strauss arteritis
    - Wegener granulomatosis
    - Microscopic polyangiitis
    - Henoch-Schönlein purpura
    - Essential cryoglobulinemic vasculitis
    - Hypersensitivity vasculitis
    - Viral-associated vasculitis
    - Rheumatic-associated vasculitis
  - Medium-vessel vasculitis:
    - Polyarteritis nodosa
    - Kawasaki disease
    - Isolated CNS vasculitis
  - Large-vessel vasculitis:
    - Takayasu arteritis
    - Giant cell arteritis
- Occurs in primary and secondary as well as acute and chronic forms.

EPIDEMIOLOGY
Highly variable, depending on the vasculitic syndrome:

- Hypersensitivity vasculitis is the most commonly encountered vasculitis in clinical practice.
- The secondary vasculitic syndromes associated with rheumatic diseases (e.g., systemic lupus erythematosus [SLE]) are more common than the primary vasculitides.
- Giant cell arteritis, Wegener granulomatosis, and microscopic polyangiitis are the most common adult primary vasculitic syndromes in the US.
- Kawasaki disease, Henoch-Schönlein purpura, dermatomyositis, polyarteritis nodosa, and hypersensitivity vasculitis are the most common forms that occur in children and adolescents.
- Takayasu arteritis is most prevalent in adolescent girls and young women.
- Giant cell arteritis occurs exclusively in those >50 years of age and is rare in the black population.

Incidence
The annual incidence in adults unless otherwise specified:

- Hypersensitivity vasculitis: Depends on drug exposure patterns
- Rheumatic-associated vasculitis: SLE association is the most common at 400–500/1 million.
- Henoch-Schönlein purpura: 200–700/1 million in children <17 years of age

- Giant cell arteritis: 170/1 million
- Kawasaki disease: Depends on race/age; ~170/1 million
- Polyarteritis nodosa: 2–33/1 million
- Wegener granulomatosis: 4–15/1 million
- Microscopic polyangiitis: 1–24/1 million
- Churg-Strauss arteritis: 1–3/1 million
- Viral-associated vasculitis: Unknown; >90% of cases of cryoglobulinemic vasculitis are associated with hepatitis C.
- Polyarteritis nodosa: 2–33/1 million
- Takayasu arteritis: 2/1 million

RISK FACTORS
A combination of genetic susceptibility and environmental exposure is presumed to play a role in disease onset.

Genetics
A number of the vasculitic syndromes have been linked to candidate genes. Establishing the role of each candidate gene in these complex diseases is ongoing. No single gene has been found to be sufficient to cause vasculitis.

GENERAL PREVENTION
Current understanding of the causes of this heterogeneous set of diseases limits preventive measures. Early identification is the primary mode of preventing irreversible organ damage in the forms that are not self-limiting and that may require immunotherapy.

PATHOPHYSIOLOGY
Three major immunopathogenic mechanisms have been proposed:

- Immune-complex formation: SLE, polyarteritis nodosa, and essential mixed cryoglobulinemia
- Antineutrophil cytoplasmic antibodies (ANCAs): Wegener granulomatosis, microscopic polyangiitis, and Churg-Strauss syndrome
- Pathogenic T-lymphocyte response: Giant cell arteritis and Takayasu arteritis

ETIOLOGY
Not well understood in most forms of vasculitis, except where known drug triggers have been identified (e.g., antibiotics, sulfonamides, and hydralazine)

 DIAGNOSIS

HISTORY
The time course from start of disease complaint and presentation to medical care is often prolonged because of the nonspecific, protean nature of complaints.

PHYSICAL EXAM
May be highly variable and depend on the vascular bed that is inflamed.

- Constitutional symptoms: Malaise, fatigue, decreased appetite, sweats, and weight loss
- Skin findings: Palpable purpura, livedo reticularis, nodules, ulcers, gangrene, nail bed capillary changes
- CNS findings: Mononeuritis multiplex, polyneuropathy, stroke, seizure encephalopathy
- Heart/lung findings: Cardiomyopathy, pericarditis, arrhythmia, cough, chest pain, hemoptysis, breathlessness

- Renal manifestations: Hypertension, proteinuria, hematuria, and renal failure
- GI manifestations: Abdominal pain, bleeding, perforation
- Musculoskeletal manifestations: Nonspecific joint complaints
- Miscellaneous: Unexplained ischemic events, chronic sinusitis, scleritis, episcleritis, and recurrent epistaxis
- A careful physical examination helps to determine the extent of vascular lesions and the distribution of affected organs. The physical exam can be normal. However, findings such as mononeuritis multiplex and palpable purpura are highly suggestive of an underlying vasculitic process.

DIAGNOSTIC TESTS & INTERPRETATION

ALERT
It is imperative to determine whether there is renal involvement with vasculitis because it may be symptom-free. Prognosis is generally worse when renal vasculitis is present. Both a serum creatinine and a urinalysis with microscopic evaluation are required to rule out renal involvement.

Lab
Labs are required to eliminate alternate diagnoses. A few serologic tests are helpful for suggesting a particular vasculitic syndrome, but not every test is needed on all patients.

- Serology: RPR, RMSF titer, Lyme test, antinuclear antibody, anti-double-stranded DNA, ANCA titer, hepatitis screen for B and C, antiglomerular basement membrane titer, C3, C4
- Hematology: Complete blood count with differential
- Microbiology: Blood culture
- Miscellaneous: Drug screen, erythrocyte sedimentation rate, C-reactive protein, blood urea nitrogen, and creatinine; routine urinalysis with microscopic examination for abnormal sediment

Imaging
CXR, CT scan, MRI, and arteriogram may be required to localize affected vessels.

Diagnostic Procedures/Surgery
- Diagnostic criteria have been proposed for a number of vasculitic syndromes, but these often allow only a presumptive diagnosis.
- Nerve conduction studies may be useful for documenting neuropathy.
- Biopsy of the affected tissue/organ will be the most precise way to substantiate the diagnosis.
- With hemoptysis, a bronchoscopy may be required to differentiate pulmonary infection from potentially life-threatening hemorrhagic vasculitis.

Pathological Findings
Immune cell infiltration into the blood vessel wall layers will be noted with varying degrees of necrosis and granuloma formation depending on the type of vasculitis.

DIFFERENTIAL DIAGNOSIS
- Infectious diseases:
  - Bacterial endocarditis
  - Disseminated gonococcal infection
  - Pulmonary histoplasmosis
  - Coccidioidomycosis
  - Syphilis
  - Lyme disease
  - Rocky Mountain spotted fever
  - Whipple disease
- Neoplasms
- Drug toxicity:
  - Cocaine
  - Amphetamines, ergot alkaloids
  - Methysergide
  - Arsenic
- Sarcoidosis
- Atheroembolic disease
- Goodpasture syndrome
- Amyloidosis

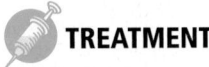 TREATMENT

MEDICATION
- Initial therapy often includes nonsteroidal anti-inflammatory drugs (NSAIDs) for symptomatic relief of pain; however, long-term use of these agents may be detrimental to the GI tract and kidney.
- Immunosuppressive agents often are required for more extensive vasculitic syndromes.

First Line
Glucocorticoids are the initial anti-inflammatory agent (1)[A],(2)[C].

Second Line
Treatment with immunosuppressive medications other than glucocorticoids (e.g., cyclophosphamide (3,4,5)[A], methotrexate, azathioprine (4)[A], mycophenolate, tumor necrosis factor (TNF) blockers, and rituximab) is generally reserved for patients with significant organ involvement and/or patients who have had an inadequate response to glucocorticoids. Subspecialty care is usually necessary to escalate care to this point.

ADDITIONAL TREATMENT
General Measures
If the vasculitic syndrome is believed to be drug-related, removal of the offending agent may be curative.

Issues for Referral
Early referral to subspecialty care may be required to assist with diagnosis and to devise an optimal treatment plan.
- Nephrology referral for persistent hematuria or proteinuria, rising creatinine, or a positive ANCA titer
- Rheumatology referral for persistent joint and skin complaints
- Pulmonary referral for persistent pulmonary infiltrate unresponsive to antibiotic therapy

Additional Therapies
Plasma exchange appears to improve recovery in patients with severe acute renal failure secondary to vasculitis (5,6)[A] and pulmonary hemorrhage.

SURGERY/OTHER PROCEDURES
A surgical procedure may be required to obtain tissue for diagnosis. Rarely, corrective surgery is required to repair the tissue damage resulting from aggressive vasculitis.

IN-PATIENT CONSIDERATIONS
Initial Stabilization
Initial therapy is guided by the organ system involved.
- If pulmonary hemorrhage is present, lifesaving measures may include mechanical ventilation, immunosuppression, plasmapheresis, and even procoagulants.
- If acute renal failure is present, attention to electrolyte and fluid balance will be required.
- When GI disease is manifest, therapy may consist simply of making the patient NPO and sustaining nutrition intravenously.

Admission Criteria
Hemoptysis, acute renal failure, and/or need for biopsy are the usual indications for admission.

Nursing
No special nursing is required.

Discharge Criteria
Stabilization or resolution of potential life-threatening symptoms

 ONGOING CARE

FOLLOW-UP RECOMMENDATIONS
- In general, restriction of activity is not required.
- If significant coronary artery disease is involved in Kawasaki disease, there may be benefit from a moderate activity restriction.

Patient Monitoring
Frequent clinical follow-up supported by patient self-monitoring is the key to the timely identification of relapse of disease.

DIET
Unless renal involvement has occurred and the patient requires a special diet for electrolyte or fluid control, no special diet is required.

PROGNOSIS
Prognosis is good, particularly with hypersensitivity vasculitis and in those syndromes where a single episode occurs. Relapsing courses, renal involvement, and extensive lung involvement portend the worst prognosis.

COMPLICATIONS
Varying degrees of persistent organ dysfunction are common in the more serious forms of vasculitis.

REFERENCES
1. Weiss PF, Feinstein JA, Luan X, et al. Effects of corticosteroid on Henoch-Schönlein purpura: a systematic review. *Pediatrics*. 2007;120:1079–87.
2. Wood L, Tulloh R. Kawasaki disease: diagnosis, management and cardiac sequelae. *Expert Rev Cardiovasc Ther*. 2007;5:553–61.
3. Bertsias G, Ioannidis JP, Boletis J, et al. EULAR recommendations for the management of systemic lupus erythematosus. Report of a Task Force of the EULAR Standing Committee for International Clinical Studies Including Therapeutics. *Ann Rheum Dis*. 2008;67:195–205.
4. Bosch X, Guilabert A, Espinosa G, et al. Treatment of antineutrophil cytoplasmic antibody associated vasculitis: a systematic review. *JAMA*. 2007;298:655–69.
5. Walters G, Willis NS, Craig JC. Interventions for renal vasculitis in adults. *Cochrane Database Syst Rev*. 2008:CD003232.
6. Walters GD, Willis NS, Craig JC. Interventions for renal vasculitis in adults. A systematic review. *BMC Nephrol*. 2010;11:12.

ADDITIONAL READING
Appel GB, Contreras G, Dooley MA, et al. Mycophenolate Mofetil versus Cyclophosphamide for Induction Treatment of Lupus Nephritis. *J Am Soc Nephrol*. 2009.

See Also (Topic, Algorithm, Electronic Media Element)
- National Heart Lung and Blood Institute Diseases and Conditions Index: Vasculitis: http://www.nhlbi.nih.gov/health/dci/Diseases/vas/vas_whatis.html
- The Vasculitis Foundation: http://www.vasculitisfoundation.org/

 CODES

ICD9
- 446.0 Polyarteritis nodosa
- 446.1 Acute febrile mucocutaneous lymph node syndrome (MCLS)
- 447.6 Arteritis, unspecified

CLINICAL PEARLS
- A vasculitic syndrome should be suspected whenever the patient has a persistent, unexplained systemic illness.
- Regardless of the vasculitic syndrome, patients with renal involvement have the worst prognosis.
- Determination of optimal treatment plan depends on accurately assigning a patient to a particular vasculitic syndrome.
- Look for clinically silent kidney involvement with serum creatinine and urinalysis with microscopy.

VENOUS INSUFFICIENCY ULCERS

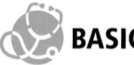

Theodore G. MacKinney, MD, MPH
Barbara Provo, MSN, APNP, CWOCN, FNP-BC

BASICS

Venous insufficiency ulcers are a common problem in clinical practice. They cost the US health system 1 billion dollars a year and individual patients a lifetime cost of $40,000. They can be diagnosed and treated in a primary care setting but may be time-intensive.

DESCRIPTION
- Medial or lateral ankle ("gaiter region")
- Shallow
- May only have mild pain unless infected
- Often large; may be circumferential
- Often with signs of venous insufficiency (e.g., leg edema, skin changes)

EPIDEMIOLOGY
- Prevalence studies only available for Western countries
- Point prevalence underestimates the extent of problem because ulcers often recur.
- Lower limb ulcers occur in 1–2% of adults, but 70% of leg ulcers are of venous etiologies.

Incidence
The overall incidence rate in the elderly is 0.76/100 person-years for men and 1.42/100 person-years for women.

Prevalence
- There is no racial predilection.
- Women seem to develop venous ulcers more often than men.
- Venous ulcers are more common with increasing age.
- Predominant age: Between 60 and 80 years of age
- 22% of persons who develop venous ulcers start by 40 years of age.
- Lifetime prevalence is 1%.
- 12-month recurrence rate is 26–69%.

RISK FACTORS
- Up to 50% of patients have a history of leg injury.
- Obesity
- Congestive heart failure (CHF)
- History of deep venous thrombosis (DVT)
- Failure of calf pump (ankle fusion, inactivity, etc.) is a strong independent predictor of poorly healing wounds.
- Previous varicose vein surgery
- Family history

GENERAL PREVENTION
- Primary prevention (1)[A] after symptomatic DVT shown in randomized, controlled trials (RCTs): Prescribe compression hose to be used as soon as feasible for at least 2 years (at least 20–30 mm Hg compression).
- Secondary prevention of recurrent ulceration: Circumstantial evidence from 2 RCTs: Those who stopped wearing hose were much more likely to reulcerate.
- Since most ulcers come after trauma, avoidance of lower leg trauma may help to prevent ulceration.

PATHOPHYSIOLOGY
- In a diseased venous system, venous pressure in the deep system fails to fall with ambulation, causing venous hypertension.

- Venous hypertension comes from:
  - Venous obstruction
  - Incompetent venous valves in the deep or superficial system
  - Inadequate muscle contraction (e.g., arthritis, myopathies, neuropathies, etc.) so that the calf pump is ineffective
- Venous pressure transmitted to capillaries leading to venous hypertensive microangiopathy, extravasation of red blood cells (RBCs) and proteins (especially fibrinogen)
- Increased RBC aggregation leads to reduced oxygen transport, slowed arteriolar circulation, and ischemia at the skin level, contributing to ulcers.
- Leukocytes aggregate to hypoxic areas; increase local inflammation
- Factors promoting persistence of venous ulcers:
  - Prolonged chronic inflammation
  - Higher levels of elastase, metalloproteinases, and plasmin and thrombin damage growth factors.
  - Bacterial infection, critical colonization
  - Premature fibroblast aging

COMMONLY ASSOCIATED CONDITIONS
Up to 50% of patients have patch tests suggesting contact dermatitis to topical agents commonly used for treatment:
- Contact sensitivity was more common in patients with stasis dermatitis (62% vs 38%).
- Avoid neomycin sulfate in particular (including triple antibiotic).

DIAGNOSIS

Clinical exam is usually sufficient to diagnose venous insufficiency ulcers.

HISTORY
- Family history of venous insufficiency and ulcers
- Recent trauma
- Nature of pain: Achy (better with leg elevation)
- Wound drainage
- Duration of wound and treatments already attempted, including nonprescription/over the counter (OTC)
- History of DVTs (especially factor V Leiden mutation; strongly associated with ulceration)
- Family history of venous insufficiency and ulceration
- History of leg edema that at least partially resolves at night. Edema that does not resolve at night is more likely lymphedema.

PHYSICAL EXAM
- Confirm venous insufficiency:
  - Evidence of pitting edema
  - Hemosiderin staining (red and brown spotty or diffuse pigment changes)
  - Stasis dermatitis: Persistent erythema or rash
  - White lesions (atrophie blanche)
  - Lipodermatosclerosis ("bottle neck" narrowing in the lower leg from scarring and fat necrosis), often painful
- Look for evidence of significant lymphedema. This may require referral for special comprehensive lymph therapy.
- Examine for palpable pulses.

ALERT
- Important to assess arterial circulation before using compression dressings. Ankle brachial index (ABI) should be >0.8.
- Examine wound for:
  - Diameter and depth: Get measurements to monitor healing rate.
  - Presence of necrotic tissue
  - Presence of infection: Purulent material in the wound, spreading cellulitis, fever and chills
  - Extent of serous drainage
  - Get initial and interim girth measurements (at least at ankle, midcalf) to monitor edema.

DIAGNOSTIC TESTS & INTERPRETATION
Lab
- Consider prothrombin time (PT)/international normalization ratio (INR) and partial thromboplastin time (PTT) if patient is anticoagulated.
- Consider biopsy of leg ulcers that fail to heal or have atypical features.
- Consider factor V Leiden mutation; strongly associated with venous ulcers.
- Test for diabetes as necessary with fasting glucose.

Imaging
Initial approach
Use duplex imaging to diagnose anatomic and hemodynamic abnormalities with venous insufficiency. It also will identify any DVT present.

Diagnostic Procedures/Surgery
- Check ABI for evidence of significant arterial disease. Palpable pulses do not necessarily rule it out.
- An ABI <0.8 is a relative contraindication to compression therapy.
- With concomitant severe arterial insufficiency, refer to a vascular surgeon to evaluate for revascularization.

Pathological Findings
Consider biopsy on wounds that are atypical or fail to heal in expected fashion.

DIFFERENTIAL DIAGNOSIS
- Arterial insufficiency ulcer
- Neuropathic ulcer
- Malignancy
- Sickle cell ulcer
- Vasculitic ulcer
- Calciphylaxis
- Cryoglobulinemia
- Pyoderma gangrenosum
- Collagen (2) vascular disease
- Leishmaniasis
- Cutaneous tuberculosis

TREATMENT

MEDICATION
- In general, systemic drugs have little role: Compression is the cornerstone of therapy.
- Diuretics may help to reduce edema, but compression is the mainstay.
- Pentoxifylline 400 mg p.o. t.i.d., in addition to local care and compression, improves cure rates. There is some response even without compression. GI side effects are common.

ADDITIONAL TREATMENT

- Edema management: Reduce venous hypertension and improve venous return to reduce inflammation and pain and improve healing:
  - Compression therapy for edema management is the cornerstone of treatment for venous insufficiency ± ulcers (3)[A].
  - Short-stretch multilayer bandages are ideal for acute phase, until edema is stable, and the patient can be fitted for compression hose.
  - Long-term compression hose are helpful (have these fit once edema is reduced). Aim for a minimum pressure 20–30 mm Hg, preferably 30–40 mm Hg.
  - Elevation of legs to heart level for 30 minutes 3–4 times/day also is effective.
- Infection control:
  - Debride necrotic tissue.
  - Treat cellulitis (usually gram-positive bacteria) with bactericidal systemic antibiotics.
  - Suspect local infection when there is pain or no improvement in the wound after 2 weeks of compression. Consider quantitative swab or tissue biopsy for culture.
  - Treat critical colonization with topical antimicrobials, especially cadexomeriodine (4)[A]. (Silver dressings are used widely, but definitive data are lacking.)

General Measures

Dressings: All wounds need some kind of a dressing underneath compression:

- Wound dressings: No single type of dressing proven superior (5)[A]
- Maintain moist wound environment: Not excessively wet or dry
- Wounds are often exudative until edema is decreased: Use absorptive dressings (calcium alginate or absorptive pads). Both super-absorbent diapers and female protection pads are also cost-effective alternatives.
- Consider using barrier ointment/cream to prevent maceration of surrounding skin.
- If wound tends to be dry, use a hydrogel or a hydrocolloid dressing.

Issues for Referral

- With prominent toe or foot edema, consider lymphedema. Refer to certified lymphedema therapist (CLT) for additional manual lymph drainage therapy.
- Refer to a wound clinic for complex or poorly healing ulcers.
- Use home health nurses to help with immobile patients needing frequent wrapping/dressing changes.

Additional Therapies

- For venous ulcers resistant to healing with wound care and compression, consider adding an intermittent compression pump 1–4 h/d (6)[B]. Need for consistency limits activity and compliance.
- Encourage exercise (e.g., activation of calf muscle pump with ankle flexion and extension) with leg compression.
- Vacuum-assisted closure (VAC) dressings may be beneficial, but Cochrane Review indicates no clear benefit yet over optimal traditional wound care (2)[A].

COMPLEMENTARY AND ALTERNATIVE MEDICINE

- Chestnut seed extract (50 mg b.i.d.) is effective for venous insufficiency but not for ulceration per se.
- Topical medicinal honey is also used on wounds, but insufficient evidence from randomized, controlled trials to support benefit.

SURGERY/OTHER PROCEDURES

- Necrotic tissue impedes healing:
  - For large amounts of necrotic tissue, consider sharp debridement.
  - Other debridement methods include enzymatic ointments (collagenase), ultrasound, and wet-to-dry dressings.
  - Avoid using collagenase with silver dressings because it inactivates the enzyme.
- Refer cases of recurrent ulceration to surgeon for venous surgery to prevent recurrence (7)[A]. No role for venous repair to aid healing of a current ulcer.
- Allografts made of synthetic skin bilayer with living keratinocytes and fibroblasts improves healing at 6 months: 47% vs 19% in controls.
- Insufficient evidence to support use of autografts

IN-PATIENT CONSIDERATIONS

Most patients are treated with intensive outpatient care, except for those with acute significant cellulitis.

Initial Stabilization

Treatment with antibiotics should consider culture and sensitivity results.

Admission Criteria

Infected wounds requiring IV antibiotics, especially in diabetics

 ## ONGOING CARE

- Venous insufficiency is a lifelong issue.
- After resolution of an ulcer, edema management must be maintained lifelong.

FOLLOW-UP RECOMMENDATIONS

When ulcers are nearly healed and edema is controlled, switch from compression bandages to compression hose:

- Insurance may not reimburse for compression hose unless an ulcer is present.
- Referral for hose fitting must be done while the ulcer is still present.

Patient Monitoring

- Monitor the ulcer for healing by measuring its area. Expect at least 10% reduction every 2 weeks.
- Look for causes of nonhealing ulcers: Infection, necrotic tissue, poorly controlled diabetes, arterial insufficiency, incorrect diagnosis

DIET

- Obese patients may benefit from weight loss.
- Low-salt diets help fluid retention.

PATIENT EDUCATION

- Patient education for understanding of underlying mechanism is important for long-term management:
  - Develop long-term plan for edema management and instruction on compression therapy.
  - Instruct the patient on topical wound therapy.
  - Teach the patient about the need for early recognition and treatment of new ulcers or cellulitis.
- Teach about donning devices and application techniques to aid in consistent use of compression hose.

PROGNOSIS

- Ulcers recur frequently: Early identification and immediate treatment are essential.
- Ongoing diligence, with edema control, avoiding infections, and avoiding trauma, is important.

REFERENCES

1. Prandoni P, Lensing AW, Prins MH, et al. Below-knee elastic compression stockings to prevent the post-thrombotic syndrome: a randomized, controlled trial. *Ann Intern Med.* 2004;141:249–56.
2. Ubbink DT, Westerbos SJ, Evans D, et al. Topical negative pressure for treating chronic wounds. *Cochrane Database Syst Rev.* 2008;CD001898-
3. O'Brien JF, Grace PA, Perry IJ, et al. Randomized clinical trial and economic analysis of four-layer compression bandaging for venous ulcers. *Br J Surg.* 2003;90:794–8.
4. O'Meara S, Al-Kurdi D, Ovington LG. Antibiotics and antiseptics for venous leg ulcers. *Cochrane Database Syst Rev.* 2008:CD003557.
5. Palfreyman SJ, Nelson EA, Lochier R, et al. Dressings for healing venous leg ulcers. *Cochrane Database Syst Rev.* 2006;3:CD001103.
6. Kearon C, Kahn SR, Agnelli G, et al. Antithrombotic therapy for venous thromboembolic disease: American College of Chest Physicians Evidence-Based Clinical Practice Guidelines (8th Edition). *Chest.* 2008;133:454S–545S.
7. Gohel MS, Barwell JR, Taylor M, et al. Long term results of compression therapy alone versus compression plus surgery in chronic venous ulceration (ESCHAR): randomised controlled trial. *BMJ.* 2007.

ADDITIONAL READING

de Araujo T, Valencia I, Federman DG, et al. Managing the patient with venous ulcers. *Ann Intern Med.* 2003;138:326–34.

See Also (Topic, Algorithm, Electronic Media Element)

Algorithm: Leg Ulcer

 ## CODES

ICD9

- 454.0 Varicose veins of lower extremities with ulcer
- 459.81 Venous (peripheral) insufficiency, unspecified
- 707.8 Chronic ulcer of other specified sites

CLINICAL PEARLS

- Debride necrotic tissue in the ulcer to get to clean granulation tissue.
- Treat critical colonization with topical antimicrobials (avoid neomycin).
- Compression is essential for edematous wounds.
- Make sure that the diagnosis is correct, and biopsy when in doubt.
- Get an ABI before compressing legs.

VENTRICULAR SEPTAL DEFECT

Jessica E. Haley, MD
Brent J. Barber, MD

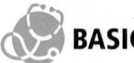 **BASICS**

DESCRIPTION
- Congenital or acquired defect of the interventricular septum that allows communication of blood between the left and the right ventricles
- Other than bicuspid aortic valve, this is the most common congenital heart malformation reported in infants and children. It also occurs as a complication of acute myocardial infarction (MI).
- Blood flow across the defect typically is left to right and depends on the size of the defect and the pulmonary vascular resistance (PVR).
- Prolonged shunting of blood can lead to pulmonary hypertension (HTN) and eventually reversal of flow across the defect, as well as to cyanosis (Eisenmenger complex).
- System(s) affected: Cardiovascular

Geriatric Considerations
In this population, almost entirely associated with MI

Pediatric Considerations
Congenital

ALERT
- Pregnancy may exacerbate symptoms and signs of a ventricular septal defect (VSD).
- Tolerated during pregnancy if the septal defect is small
- May be associated with an increased risk of preeclampsia in women with an unrepaired VSD (1)

EPIDEMIOLOGY
Incidence
- Predominant sex: No gender predilection
- Males are affected more than females if associated with MI.
- 100–500/100,000 live births

Prevalence
In the US:
- Acute MI: Estimated to complicate 1–3%
- Lowered prevalence in adults due to spontaneous closure of defects

RISK FACTORS
- Congenital:
  - 4.2% risk of sibling being affected
  - 4.0% risk of offspring being affected
- Post–acute MI:
  - 1st MI
  - Limited coronary artery disease
  - HTN
  - Most frequent within 1st week after MI
  - Occur in 1–3% of MI, most commonly after anterior MI

Genetics
Multifactorial etiology; autosomal dominant and recessive transmissions have been reported.

GENERAL PREVENTION
For adults, avoid risk factors for MI and obtain evaluation before pregnancy.

ETIOLOGY
- Congenital
- In adults, secondary to MI

COMMONLY ASSOCIATED CONDITIONS
- Congenital:
  - Tetralogy of Fallot
  - Aortic valvular deformities, especially aortic insufficiency and bicuspid aortic valve
  - Down syndrome (trisomy 21), endocardial cushion defect
  - Transposition of great arteries
  - Coarctation of aorta
  - Tricuspid atresia
  - Truncus arteriosus
  - Patent ductus arteriosus
  - Atrial septal defect
  - Pulmonic stenosis
  - Subaortic stenosis
- Adult: Coronary artery disease

 DIAGNOSIS

HISTORY
- Depends on the degree of shunting across the defect; may be completely asymptomatic with small defects
- Respiratory distress, tachypnea, tachycardia
- Diaphoresis with feeds, poor weight gain in infants

PHYSICAL EXAM
- Small defect:
  - Harsh holosystolic murmur loudest at left lower sternal border
  - Detected after pulmonary vascular resistance drops at 4–8 weeks of life
- Moderate defect:
  - Harsh holosystolic murmur at left lower sternal border associated with a thrill
  - Forceful apical impulse with lateral displacement
  - Increased intensity of P_2
  - Diastolic rumble at apex due to increased flow across the mitral valve
- Large defect:
  - Holosystolic murmur heard throughout the precordium with diastolic rumble at apex, although large defects may have little or no murmur initially
  - If congestive heart failure (CHF) exists: Tachycardia, tachypnea, and hepatomegaly
  - If pulmonary HTN exists: Cyanosis with exertion
  - If Eisenmenger complex is present: Cyanosis and clubbing

DIAGNOSTIC TESTS & INTERPRETATION
Lab
Initial lab tests
- A 12-lead ECG may suggest severity of VSD. Initially, left ventricular hypertrophy and left atrial enlargement may be evident. With pulmonary HTN, right ventricular hypertrophy and right atrial enlargement may be seen.
- After surgical repair, right bundle-branch block and left anterior hemiblock are common.

Follow-Up & Special Considerations
Weight and hematocrit check

Imaging
Initial approach
- CXR may demonstrate increased pulmonary vascularity and/or cardiomegaly.
- 2-D ECG for visualization of size of defect
- Color-flow Doppler for direction and velocity of ventricular septal defect jet; may be used to estimate right ventricular pressure

Follow-Up & Special Considerations
Cardiac catheterization performed occasionally for perioperative planning or assessing need for closure of defect

Diagnostic Procedures/Surgery
- Cardiac catheterization (left and right sides of heart) can confirm the diagnosis, document number of defects, quantify ratio of pulmonary blood flow to systemic blood flow (Qp/Qs), and determine pulmonary vascular resistance.
- Demonstration of an oxygen saturation step-up from the right atrium to the distal pulmonary artery

Pathological Findings
- Congenital VSD (4 major anatomic types):
  - Membranous (70%)
  - Muscular (20%)
  - Atrioventricular canal type (5%)
  - Supracristal (5%; higher in Asians)
- Post-MI VSD predominantly involves muscular septum.

DIFFERENTIAL DIAGNOSIS
- Any defect with left-to-right shunt, such as patent ductus arteriosus, atrial septal defect
- Children: Tetralogy of Fallot
- Adults: Mitral regurgitation

 TREATMENT

- Start diuretic therapy if overload signs present
- Minimize IV fluids.
- Consider angiotensin-converting enzyme (ACE) inhibitor and/or digoxin.
- Nasogastric feeds
- Correct anemia via iron supplementation or possible red blood cell (RBC) transfusion.

MEDICATION
First Line
- Endocarditis antibiotic prophylaxis is no longer recommended for most VSDs. Antibiotic prophylaxis is recommended for VSDs associated with complex cyanotic heart disease, during the first 6 months after surgical repair, or for residual VSDs located near the patch following surgery (2).
- Pediatric: Medications aim to control pulmonary edema, decrease work of breathing, and allow for growth:
  - Furosemide: 1–2 mg/kg p.o./IV once to twice a day (3)[A]
  - Digoxin: Infants <2 years of age: 10 mg/kg/d p.o. divided b.i.d.; children 2–10 years of age: 5–10 mg/kg/d p.o. divided b.i.d.; children >10 years of age: 2–5 mg/kg/d p.o. divided b.i.d.
  - Spironolactone: 1–2 mg/kg/d divided b.i.d.
  - Captopril: 0.1–0.4 mg/kg p.o. given q6–24h (maximum 6 mg/kg/24 h)

- Adults: Digoxin and diuretics may be beneficial in some circumstances.
- Side effects:
  – Drugs that increase systemic vascular resistance may increase left-to-right shunting and cause signs and symptoms of pulmonary overcirculation.
  – Hypotension

Second Line
- Surgical closure is generally indicated if the pulmonic-to-systemic flow is >2:1 or with poorly controlled pulmonary overcirculation despite maximal medical and dietary interventions.
- If an infant with a VSD has persistent pulmonary HTN, surgical repair generally is recommended prior to 6 months of age even if patient is asymptomatic.
- In the post-MI setting, afterload reduction, inotropic support, intra-aortic balloon pump, and left ventricular assist device may be used to stabilize the patient prior to surgery.

ADDITIONAL TREATMENT
General Measures
- Appropriate health care
- Outpatient, until surgical repair is indicated
- Inpatient in setting of acute MI
- Inpatient for treatment of severe CHF

Issues for Referral
Close follow-up of a congenital VSD is necessary until primary intracardiac repair is performed to ensure that significant pulmonary HTN does not develop.

Additional Therapies
- Caloric requirements up to 150 kcal/kg/d for adequate weight gain
- Treatment of iron-deficiency anemia to increase oxygen-carrying capacity

SURGERY/OTHER PROCEDURES
- Percutaneous transcatheter device closure of muscular defects is an option. The closure of membranous defects with septal occluders is currently under research protocols. Complications include embolization of the device, residual defects, and complete heart block.
- Perventricular device closure of isolated VSDs without cardiopulmonary bypass is feasible and safe under transesophageal echocardiographic (TEE) guidance. However, further evaluation of intermediate and long-term results is necessary.

IN-PATIENT CONSIDERATIONS
Initial Stabilization
- Stabilize airway.
- Reduce temperature stress.

Admission Criteria
- Failure to thrive
- Pulmonary overcirculation/CHF

Nursing
Frequent vital sign monitoring; daily weight and calorie counts

Discharge Criteria
CHF stabilization, weight gain, or successful repair

 ## ONGOING CARE

FOLLOW-UP RECOMMENDATIONS
- Small VSDs without evidence of CHF or pulmonary HTN generally can be followed every 1–5 years after the neonatal period.
- Moderate-to-large VSDs require more frequent follow-up.
- Potential complications of VSDs include right ventricular outflow obstruction and aortic valve prolapse.

Patient Monitoring
- Physical growth and development monitoring
- Influenza vaccine for children >6 months of age
- Palivizumab to children <2 years of age with hemodynamically significant lesions

DIET
- Low-sodium in heart failure
- High-calorie in failure to thrive

PATIENT EDUCATION
- No activity restriction in absence of pulmonary HTN
- Parents need support and instructions for prevention of complications until the child is ready for surgery.

PROGNOSIS
- Congenital:
  – Course is variable depending on the size of the VSD
  – Small VSD: 25–45% will close spontaneously by age 3 years. Muscular defects are more likely to close spontaneously.
  – Large VSD: CHF or failure to thrive in infancy necessitating surgical repair
  – Progressive pulmonary vascular disease and pulmonary HTN are the most feared complications of VSD caused by left-to-right shunting and may eventually lead to reversal of the shunt (Eisenmenger complex). Death usually occurs in the 4th decade of life if untreated.
- Post-MI:
  – With medical management alone, 80–90% mortality in the 1st 2 weeks
  – Prognosis worse with inferior MI compared with anterior MI

COMPLICATIONS
- CHF
- Aortic insufficiency
- Sudden death
- Hemoptysis
- Cerebral abscess
- Paradoxical emboli
- Cardiogenic shock
- Heart block rarely may accompany surgical closure.
- Pulmonary HTN

REFERENCES

1. Yap S-C, Drenthen W, Pieper P, et al. Pregnancy outcome in women with repaired versus unrepaired isolated ventricular septal defect. *BJOG.* 2010;117: 63–689.
2. Wilson W, et al. Prevention of infective endocarditis. Guidelines From the American Heart Association. A Guideline From the American Heart Association Rheumatic Fever, Endocarditis, and Kawasaki Disease Committee, Council on Cardiovascular Disease in the Young, and the Council on Clinical Cardiology, Council on Cardiovascular Surgery and Anesthesia, and the Quality of Care and Outcomes Research Interdisciplinary Working Group. *Circulation* Apr 19, 2007: electronic publication.
3. Faris R, Flather MD, Purcell H, et al. Diuretics for heart failure. *Cochrane Database Syst Rev.* 2006:CD003838.

ADDITIONAL READING

- Chang RK, Chen AY, Klitzner TS. Factors associated with age at operation for children with congenital heart disease. *Pediatrics.* 2000;105:1073–81.
- Knauth AL, Lock JE, Perry SB, et al. Transcatheter device closure of congenital and postoperative residual ventricular septal defects. *Circulation.* 2004;110:501–7.
- Mehta AV, Chidambaram B. Ventricular septal defect in the first year of life. *Am J Cardiol.* 1992;70:364–6.
- Patanè F, Centofanti P, Zingarelli E, et al. Potential role of the Impella Recover left ventricular assist device in the management of postinfarct ventricular septal defect. *J Thorac Cardiovasc Surg.* 2009;137: 1288–9.
- Quansheng X, Silin P, Zhongyun Z, et al. Minimally invasive perventricular device closure of an isolated perimembranous ventricular septal defect with a newly designed delivery system: preliminary experience. *J Thorac Cardiovasc Surg.* 2009;137: 556–9.

See Also (Topic, Algorithm, Electronic Media Element)
Down Syndrome; Myocardial Infarction, Non ST Segment Elevation (NSTEMI); Myocardial Infarction, ST Segment Elevation (STEMI); Tetralogy of Fallot

 ## CODES

ICD9
745.4 Ventricular septal defect

CLINICAL PEARLS
- A loud 2–3/6 low-pitched harsh holosystolic murmur at the left lower sternal border is typical.
- A diastolic rumble at the apex indicates moderate-to-large VSD or Qp:Qs > 2:1.
- Disappearance of the murmur could be secondary to spontaneous closure of the defect or the development of pulmonary HTN.
- Development of a new murmur of semilunar valve insufficiency should be further evaluated. Pulmonary regurgitation may occur as PVR increases, and the development of aortic regurgitation usually will require early surgery.

V

VERTIGO

Michele L. Matthews, PharmD
Kristy Kedian Brown, DO

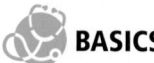 BASICS

DESCRIPTION
- Sensation of movement ("room spinning") when no movement is actually occurring; results from peripheral or central causes, or may be induced by medications or anxiety disorders
- Important to distinguish between vertigo and presyncope (patient feels lightheaded; vision and hearing may become obscured)
- System(s) affected: Nervous
- Synonym(s): Dizziness; Acute vestibular neuronitis; Labyrinthitis; Benign paroxysmal positional vertigo (BPPV)

EPIDEMIOLOGY
Incidence
- Accounts for 54% of cases of dizziness reported in primary care; >90% of these patients are diagnosed with peripheral causes, such as BPPV
- Predominant sex: Female = Male; women are more likely to experience central causes, particularly vertiginous migraine

Geriatric Considerations
Patients who are elderly and have risk factors for cerebrovascular disease (CVD) are more likely to experience central causes.

Prevalence
- Ranges from 5–10% within the general population
- Lifetime prevalence for BPPV is 2.4%

RISK FACTORS
- History of migraines
- History of CVD or risk factors for CVD
- Use of ototoxic medications
- Trauma or barotrauma
- Perilymphatic fistula
- Heavy weight bearing
- Psychosocial stress/depression
- Exposure to toxins

Genetics
Family history of CVD or migraines may indicate higher risk of central causes.

GENERAL PREVENTION
- Precautions to avoid injuries from falls that may occur secondary to imbalance
- If due to motion sickness, consider pretreatment with anticholinergics such as scopolamine.

PATHOPHYSIOLOGY
Dysfunction of the rotational velocity sensors of the inner ear results in asymmetric central processing. This is related to the combination of sensory disturbance of motion and malfunction of the central vestibular apparatus.

ETIOLOGY
- Peripheral causes: Acute labyrinthitis, acute vestibular neuronitis, BPPV, herpes-zoster oticus, cholesteatoma, Ménière disease, otosclerosis
- Central causes: Cerebellar tumor, CVD, migraine, multiple sclerosis
- Drug causes: Psychotropic agents (antipsychotics, antidepressants, anxiolytics, anticonvulsants, mood stabilizers), aspirin, aminoglycosides, furosemide, amiodarone
- Other causes: Cervical, psychological

 DIAGNOSIS

HISTORY
- Determine whether true vertigo exists vs other causes of dizziness by asking the patient if they feel lightheaded or if they see the world spinning around during a dizzy spell (1). Spinning is indicative of true vertigo.
- Ask about the presence of the following symptoms: Dizziness, rotary illusions, nystagmus, nausea and vomiting, hearing loss, diaphoresis, pain, neurologic symptoms (e.g., ataxia)
- Distinguish between peripheral and central causes:
  - Timing and duration:
    - Seconds–minutes: Peripheral
    - Minutes–hours: Peripheral or central
    - Days: Peripheral or central
    - Weeks: Central or psychological
  - Provoking factors:
    - Changes in head position: Peripheral or central
    - Spontaneous episodes: Peripheral or central
    - Recent upper viral respiratory infection: Peripheral
    - Stress: Central or psychological
    - Immunosuppression: Peripheral
    - Changes in ear pressure: Peripheral
  - Associated symptoms:
    - Rotary illusions with nausea and vomiting: Peripheral
    - Horizontal and rotational nystagmus: Peripheral
    - Horizontal, vertical, or rotational nystagmus: Central
    - Hearing loss: Peripheral
    - Neurologic symptoms: Central
- Obtain medical and medication history:
  - Recent use of ototoxic medications (e.g., aminoglycosides)
  - History of alcohol, nicotine, and caffeine use
  - Sexual history
  - History of CVD or risk factors for CVD

PHYSICAL EXAM
- Neurologic (1): Cranial nerves for signs of palsies, nystagmus
- Balance:
  - Peripheral: Mild–moderate, able to walk
  - Central: Severe, unable to walk

- Dix-Hallpike maneuver (PPV 83%, NPV 52%):
  - If induced symptoms subside after repeated maneuvers, consider peripheral causes.
  - If induced symptoms do not subside, consider central causes.
- Head and neck (1): Tympanic membranes:
  - Vesicles: Herpes-zoster oticus
  - Cholesteatoma
- Cardiovascular (1): Orthostatic changes in BP: Dehydration or autonomic dysfunction

DIAGNOSTIC TESTS & INTERPRETATION
Lab
Initial lab tests
CBC/chemistry panel in the absence of clinical findings

Imaging
Initial approach
Consider MRI in the presence of neurologic symptoms, risk factors for CVD, or progressive unilateral hearing loss

Diagnostic Procedures/Surgery
Audiometry if acoustic neuroma or Ménière disease is suspected

DIFFERENTIAL DIAGNOSIS
- Acoustic neuroma
- Anxiety disorder
- BPPV
- Cerebellar degeneration, hemorrhage, or tumor
- Labyrinthitis or labyrinthine concussion
- Ménière disease
- Multiple sclerosis
- Perilymphatic fistula
- Syphilis
- Vascular ischemia
- Vertiginous migraine
- Vestibular neuronitis or ototoxicity

 TREATMENT

- Epley maneuver for BPPV (2)[A]
- Modified Epley maneuver for BPPV (3)[B]
- Vestibular exercises for acute vestibular neuronitis (3)[B]
- Low-salt diet and diuretics for Ménière disease (3)[B]
- Migraine prophylaxis, migraine abortive medications, and vestibular exercises for vertiginous migraines (3)[B]
- Selective serotonin reuptake inhibitors (SSRIs) when associated with anxiety disorders (3)[B]
- Vestibular suppressant medications for symptom relief in acute vestibular neuronitis (3,4)[C]

MEDICATION

- Meclizine (Antivert): 12.5–50 mg p.o. q4–8h (3,4)[C]
- Dimenhydrinate (Dramamine): 25–100 mg p.o., IM, or IV q4–8h (3,4)[C]:
  - Precautions: Concomitant use of CNS depressants, prostatic hyperplasia, glaucoma
  - Adverse effects: Sedation, xerostomia
  - Interactions: CNS depressants
- Prochlorperazine (Compazine): 5–10 mg p.o. or IM q6–8h; 25 mg rectally q12h; 5–10 mg by slow IV over 2 minutes (3,4)[C]:
  - Contraindications: Blood dyscrasias, age <2 years, severe hypotension
  - Precautions: Children with acute illness, glaucoma, history of breast cancer, impaired cardiovascular function, pregnancy, prostatic hyperplasia
  - Adverse effects: Sedation, xerostomia, hypotension, extrapyramidal effects
  - Interactions: Phenothiazines, tricyclic antidepressants
- Metoclopramide (Reglan): 5–10 mg p.o. q6h, 5–10 mg slow IV q6h:
  - Contraindications: Concomitant use of drugs with extrapyramidal effects, seizure disorders
  - Precautions: History of depression, Parkinson disease, hypertension
  - Adverse effects: Sedation, fluid retention, constipation
  - Interactions: Linezolid, cyclosporine, digoxin, levodopa
- Benzodiazepines (3,4)[C]:
  - Diazepam (Valium): 2–10 mg p.o. or IV q4–8h
  - Lorazepam (Ativan): 0.5–2 mg p.o., IM, or IV q4–8h:
    - Contraindications: Glaucoma, age <6 months
    - Precautions: Concomitant use of CNS depressants, hepatic insufficiency, pregnancy
    - Adverse effects: Sedation, respiratory depression, hypotension
    - Interactions: CNS depressants

Geriatric Considerations
Use vestibular suppressant medications with caution due to increased risk of falls and urinary retention.

Pregnancy Considerations
Meclizine and dimenhydrinate are pregnancy Category B.

ADDITIONAL TREATMENT
General Measures
- Provide an explanation and offer assurance to avoid anxiety that may exacerbate symptoms.
- Treatments depend on cause:
  - BPPV: Epley maneuver or modified Epley maneuver (2)[A]
  - Vestibular neuronitis and labyrinthitis:
    - Vestibular suppressant medications (3,4)[C]
    - Vestibular rehabilitation exercises (3)[B]
  - Ménière disease:
    - Low-salt diet (<1–2 g/d) (3)[B]
    - Diuretics such as hydrochlorothiazide (3)[B]
  - Vascular ischemia: Prevention of future events through blood pressure reduction, lipid lowering, smoking cessation, antiplatelet therapy, and anticoagulation if necessary

- Vertiginous migraines: Dietary and lifestyle modifications, vestibular rehabilitation exercises, prophylactic and migraine abortive medications (3)[B]
- Drug-induced vertigo: Discontinue causative agent.
- Psychological: SSRIs (3)[B]

Issues for Referral
Consider referral to otolaryngologist, ENT specialist, or neurologist if patient requires further care.

Additional Therapies
- Epley maneuver or modified Epley maneuver for BPPV to displace calcium deposits in the semicircular canals (2)[A]:
  - Effective for short-term symptomatic improvement and for converting patient from positive to negative Dix-Hallpike maneuver
  - Contraindications: Carotid stenosis, unstable cardiac disease, severe neck disease
- Vestibular rehabilitation exercises (3)[B]: Ball toss, lying-to-standing, target-change, thumb-tracking, tightrope, walking turns

ONGOING CARE

FOLLOW-UP RECOMMENDATIONS
Balance exercises should be adhered to for symptom improvement and return to normal activities of daily living (ADLs).

Patient Monitoring
After 1–2 weeks, assess for:
- Recurrence of symptoms
- New-onset symptoms
- Medication-related adverse effects
- Relief from vestibular rehabilitation exercises

DIET
- Restricted salt intake for Ménière disease
- Dietary modifications for vertiginous migraine

PATIENT EDUCATION
- Reduce sodium intake (Ménière disease).
- Avoid triggers such as caffeine or alcohol (vertiginous migraine).

PROGNOSIS
Depends on diagnosis and response to treatment

COMPLICATIONS
- Anxiety
- Depression
- Disability
- Injuries from falls

REFERENCES

1. Labuguen RH. Initial evaluation of vertigo. *Am Fam Physician.* 2006;73:244–51.
2. Hilton M, Pinder D. The Epley (canalith repositioning) maneuver for benign paroxysmal positional vertigo. *Cochrane Database Syst Rev.* 2007;(3):CD003162.
3. Swartz R, Longwell P. Treatment of vertigo. *Am Fam Physician.* 2005;71:1115–22.
4. Hain TC, Uddin M. Pharmacological treatment of vertigo. *CNS Drugs.* 2003;17:85–100.

ADDITIONAL READING

- Bhattacharyya N, Baugh RF, Orvidas L, et al. Clinical practice guideline: benign paroxysmal positional vertigo. *Otolaryngol Head Neck Surg.* 2008;139: S47–81.
- Fife TD, Iverson DJ, Lempert T, et al. Practice parameter: therapies for benign paroxysmal positional vertigo (an evidence-based review): report of the Quality Standards Subcommittee of the American Academy of Neurology. *Neurology.* 2008;70:2067–74.

See Also (Topic, Algorithm, Electronic Media Element)
Ménière Disease, Motion Sickness
Algorithm: Vertigo

CODES

ICD9
- 386.2 Vertigo of central origin
- 386.10 Peripheral vertigo, unspecified
- 386.11 Benign paroxysmal positional vertigo

CLINICAL PEARLS

- Risk factors that should be assessed in a patient with suspected vertigo include history of migraines, history of CVD or risk factors for CVD, use of ototoxic medications, trauma or barotrauma, perilymphatic fistula, heavy weight bearing, psychosocial stress, and exposure to toxins.
- The Dix-Hallpike maneuver is performed by rapidly moving the patient from a sitting position to the supine position with the head turned 45 degrees to the right. After waiting ~20–30 seconds, the patient is returned to the sitting position. If no nystagmus is observed, the procedure then is repeated on the left side. The presence of nystagmus indicates a positive test, implying that peripheral causes should be investigated.
- The Epley maneuver is recommended for the treatment of BPPV; this maneuver repositions calcium debris within the semicircular canals to provide relief from vertigo; a modified version of the maneuver can be performed at home. Medications are not recommended.

V

VITAMIN B12 DEFICIENCY

Katherine L. Margo, MD
Katherine M. Mahon, MD

 BASICS

DESCRIPTION
- Vitamin B_{12} (cobalamin) is obtained exclusively from the dietary intake of animal products.
- A deficiency of vitamin B_{12} most commonly is caused by malabsorption but also may be secondary to inadequate dietary intake.
- B_{12} deficiency has hematologic, neurologic, and skeletal manifestations.
- Pernicious anemia (PA) is the primary disorder owing to vitamin B_{12} deficiency. It is invariably associated with atrophic gastritis and histamine-fast achlorhydria. Vitamin B_{12} cannot be absorbed in the terminal ileum without intrinsic factor (a secretion of the parietal cells of the gastric mucosa). Its usual course is slowly progressive.

Geriatric Considerations
More common in this age group and often in association with other autoimmune disorders, depression, and dementia

EPIDEMIOLOGY
Prevalence
- Endemic area: Northern Europe, including Scandinavia
- Predominant age: Estimated to affect 10–24% individuals older than age 65
- Predominant sex: Female > Male. PA has a 4.1% prevalence in women and 2.1% in men.

RISK FACTORS
- Elderly
- *Helicobacter pylori* infection
- Long-term use of antacids, H_2 receptor antagonists, or proton pump inhibitors (PPIs)
- Neomycin, biguanides (metformin)
- Chronic alcoholism
- Bariatric surgery
- Pancreatic exocrine failure
- Sjögren syndrome
- Crohn disease
- Intestinal resection or bypass
- HIV infection/AIDS
- Vegan or strict vegetarianism
- Fish tapeworm infestation

Genetics
Only rare forms: Imerslund-Grasbeck disease (juvenile megaloblastic anemia) is due to inadequate uptake of B_{12}-intrinsic factor complex.

GENERAL PREVENTION
Recognition of risk factors and adequate supplementation

PATHOPHYSIOLOGY
- Pernicious anemia: Autoimmune attack on gastric intrinsic factor; intrinsic factor is necessary for intestinal absorption of dietary B_{12}.
- Chronic atrophic gastritis: Autoimmune attack on gastric parietal cells; leads to decrease in intrinsic factor production
- *H. pylori* infection: Impairs release of B_{12} from bound proteins
- Intestinal disorders: B_{12}-intrinsic factor complex is absorbed in the ileum. Severe pancreatic disease, ileal disease, intestinal resection/bypass, and Crohn disease all may cause B_{12} deficiency.
- PPIs, H_2 antagonists, antacids: B_{12} is not released from dietary protein when acidity is decreased.
- Metformin use: Affects calcium-dependent uptake in ileum
- Neomycin use
- Nutritional: Minimal daily requirement is 6–9 μg/d. Total body stores are typically 2–5 mg; it takes years to develop deficiency.
- Hereditary (rare):
  - Imerslund-Grasbeck disease (juvenile megaloblastic anemia)
  - Congenital deficiency of transcobalamin
  - Severe methylene tetrahydrofolate reductase deficiency
  - Abnormalities of methionine synthesis

COMMONLY ASSOCIATED CONDITIONS
- Autoimmune diseases including rheumatoid arthritis, IgA deficiency
- Graves disease
- Myxedema
- Iron deficiency
- Thyroiditis
- Vitiligo
- Idiopathic adrenocortical insufficiency
- Hypoparathyroidism
- Agammaglobulinemia
- Tropical sprue
- Celiac disease
- Crohn disease
- Infiltrate disorders of the ileum and small intestine
- Chronic alcoholism
- Status-post bariatric surgery
- HIV infection/AIDS
- Severe pancreatic disease
- Osteoporosis

DIAGNOSIS

HISTORY
- Fatigue
- Dyspnea on exertion
- Palpitations
- Paresthesias
- Ataxia
- Decreased position sense
- Recent fractures
- Memory loss
- Irritability
- Dementia

PHYSICAL EXAM
- Abnormal reflexes
- Ataxia
- Atrophic glossitis
- Babinski sign: Positive
- Confusion
- Congestive heart failure
- Dementia
- Exertional dyspnea
- Extremity numbness
- Extremity paresthesias
- Hepatomegaly
- Pallor
- Palpitations
- Poor finger coordination
- Purpura
- Romberg sign: Positive
- Skin pigmentation increased
- Sore tongue
- Splenomegaly
- Tachycardia
- Vertigo
- Vibration sense: Decreased
- Vitiligo
- Weakness

DIAGNOSTIC TESTS & INTERPRETATION
Lab
- Peripheral smear:
  - Macrocytic red blood cells (mean corpuscular volume > 100) with hypersegmented neutrophils
  - Combined deficiency (i.e., Fe deficiency, thalassemia) may have normocytic anemia with increased RBC distribution width.
- Diagnostic strategy: Suspicion of B_{12} deficiency based on clinical findings or peripheral smear.

- Check B$_{12}$ levels:
  - \> 300 pg/mL: Normal result; B$_{12}$ deficiency unlikely
  - 200–300 pg/mL: Borderline result; B$_{12}$ deficiency possible
  - < 200 pg/mL: Low; 95–100% specificity for B$_{12}$ deficiency
- Homocysteine and methylmalonic acid (MMA):
  - These 2 markers are elevated in B$_{12}$ deficiency secondary to decreased metabolism.
  - If B$_{12}$ levels are borderline or low, check these 2 markers.
  - If both are normal, B$_{12}$ deficiency is effectively ruled out.
  - If both are increased, B$_{12}$ deficiency is ruled in with a sensitivity and specificity of 94% and 99%, respectively.
  - If MMA is normal and homocysteine is increased, think folate deficiency.
  - Determine cause of B$_{12}$ deficiency. See Etiology to help guide diagnostic approach.
- Pernicious anemia suspected:
  - Check antibody to intrinsic factor.
  - A positive test is confirmatory for PA.
  - If antibody to intrinsic factor is negative, consider a Schilling test (although largely unavailable in many parts of US).
  - 1st-stage Schilling test: 1–2 μg PO of radiolabeled B$_{12}$ is given.
    - 1 hour later, 1,000 μg of B$_{12}$ given by IM injection; 24-hour urine collected for determination of percent excretion of the oral dose; normal subjects excrete 8–35% radiolabeled dose in 24 hours.
    - Low percent excretion indicates PA.
  - 2nd-stage Schilling test:
    - Performed only if 1st part shows reduced excretion
    - 1st part is repeated with added oral intrinsic factor.
    - Should normalize excreted oral dose in PA but not in intestinal malabsorption
    - 2nd part should be performed after 4 weeks of B$_{12}$ replacement because B$_{12}$ deficiency can cause abnormalities in intestinal mucosal cells (1)[C].

ALERT

Renal insufficiency may cause falsely low percent excretion of radiolabeled B$_{12}$.

 ## TREATMENT

MEDICATION

- Parenteral treatment: Typically treated with 1,000 μg/d × 1 week, then 1,000 μg/week × 4 weeks, then 1,000 μg/month for as long as underlying disorder persists.
- Oral treatment:
  - Oral treatment is possible even with PA because high doses of vitamin B$_{12}$ can be absorbed in the absence of intrinsic factor.
  - Oral therapy has been shown to be as effective as parenteral treatment but requires greater patient compliance. Dose is 1–2 mg/d (2)[B].

ALERT

Folic acid treatment without vitamin B$_{12}$ in patients with PA is contraindicated; will not correct neurologic abnormalities.

IN-PATIENT CONSIDERATIONS

Initial Stabilization
Consider blood transfusion for severe anemia.

 ## ONGOING CARE

FOLLOW-UP RECOMMENDATIONS

Patient Monitoring
- Hematologic:
  - Expect reticulocytosis in 3–4 days.
  - Expect rise in hemoglobin beginning at 10 days; usually will return to normal in 8 weeks.
  - Monitor potassium in profoundly anemic patients, who may have hypokalemia as an effect of potassium utilization.
- Neurologic:
  - Neurologic symptoms improve over 6 months.
  - There is no evidence that supplementation of vitamin B$_{12}$ improves cognitive function in patients with dementia (3)[C].

ALERT

Patient with PA may be at an increased risk of developing gastric and/or colorectal carcinoma. Consider periodic monitoring of stools for occult blood vs. colonoscopy/endoscopy. Data are not conclusive (1)[C].

DIET

Emphasize meat, animal protein foods, and legumes unless contraindicated.

PATIENT EDUCATION

Emphasize that treatment is lifelong.

PROGNOSIS

- Anemia is reversible with treatment.
- Neurologic effects are not necessarily reversible.

REFERENCES

1. Oh R, Brown D. Vitamin B12 deficiency. *Am Fam Phys*. 2003;67:979–86,993–4.
2. Vidal-Alball J, Butler CC, et al. Oral vitamin B12 versus intramuscular vitamin B12 for vitamin B12 deficiency. *The Cochrane Library*. 2005.
3. Malouf R, Areosa Sastre A. Vitamin B12 for cognition. *The Cochrane Library*. 2003.

ADDITIONAL READING

- Chui CH, Lau FY, Wong R, et al. Vitamin B12 deficiency—need for a new guideline. *Nutrition*. 2001;17:917–20.
- Eussen SJ, de Groot LC, Clarke R, et al. Oral cyanocobalamin supplementation in older people with vitamin B12 deficiency: a dose-finding trial. *Arch Intern Med*. 2005;165(10):1167–72.
- Kumar V. Pernicious anemia. *MLO Med Lab Obs*. 2007;39(2):28, 30–1.

 ## CODES

ICD9
- 266.2 Other B-complex deficiencies
- 281.0 Pernicious anemia

CLINICAL PEARLS

- The minimum daily requirement of vitamin B$_{12}$ is 6–9 μg/d. Total-body stores of vitamin B$_{12}$ are 2–5 mg; one-half is stored in the liver. Therefore, it takes years to develop B$_{12}$ deficiency after dietary intake of B$_{12}$ stops.
- PA is most common in whites of European descent. Most often it affects the elderly, but it can be present in patients under age 30.
- The Schilling test was the classic procedure to diagnose PA. However, it is no longer available in many parts of the country, and in the vast majority of cases, the diagnosis can be made without it.
- Consider monitoring B12 levels yearly in patient on metformin.

V

VITAMIN D DEFICIENCY

Frank J. Domino, MD
Samir Malkani, MD

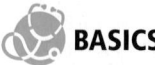 **BASICS**

This topic covers the commonly acquired vitamin D deficiency and not type II vitamin D–resistant rickets or type I pseudo vitamin D–resistant rickets (both rare autosomal-recessive disorders).

DESCRIPTION
- Vitamin D is both a hormone and a vitamin. Cholecalciferol (D3) is synthesized in the skin by exposure to ultraviolet B (UVB) radiation. Ergocalciferol (D2) and D3 are present in foods.
- D2 and D3 are hydroxylated in the liver to 25 vitamin D (calcidiol), its major circulating form.
- This is further hydroxylated in the kidney to the active metabolite 1,25 vitamin D (calcitriol).
- Hypocalcemia stimulates parathyroid hormone (PTH) to be secreted, which prompts the increased conversion of 1,25 vitamin D, which decreases renal calcium and phosphorus excretion, increases intestinal calcium and phosphorus absorption, and increases osteoclast activity, producing bone resorption and ultimately, osteomalacia. Any insult to this production can result in deficiency.

EPIDEMIOLOGY
- Unclear in general population
- In the community, a cohort study of asymptomatic adolescents in Boston found 24.1% were deficient, with 4.6% severely deficient (1).
- A study of hospitalized patients in Massachusetts found 57% vitamin D–deficient (VDD) (2).
- Women with history of osteoporosis or osteoporotic fracture have high prevalence of VDD (3)[A].
- A cross-sectional study of patients with persistent, nonspecific pain in an urban Minneapolis primary care clinic found 93% deficient and 28% severely deficient (4).
- A cohort study in Arizona found over 25% of adults were VDD; highest rates among blacks and Hispanics (5).
- A randomized clinical trial to study VDD and depression in obese adults found treating low serum levels had significant benefit on Beck Depression Inventory at 1 year (6).

Pediatric Considerations
NHANES data found 70% of children did not have sufficient 25 OH vitamin D serum levels (9% deficient and 61% insufficient), which was associated with an increase in blood pressure and decrease in HDL cholesterol (7)[B]

RISK FACTORS
- Inadequate sun exposure
- Female
- Dark skin
- Immigrant populations
- Low socioeconomic status
- Latitudes higher than 38°
- Elderly
- Institutionalized
- Depression
- Medications (phenobarbital, phenytoin)

Genetics
Numerous rare genetic disorders can induce hypoparathyroidism (DiGeorge syndrome).

GENERAL PREVENTION
- Adequate exposure to sunlight and dietary sources of vitamin D (plants, fish); many foods are fortified with D2 and D3.
- Up to 2,000 IU/day is safe in healthy adults without risk of toxicity.
- Higher intake of vitamin D recommended for ages >50.
- 2005 and 2009: Meta-analysis demonstrated for ages 51–70, minimally recommended supplementation is 800 IU/day to prevent nonvertebral fractures (8,9)[A].

Pediatric Considerations
The American Academy of Pediatrics recommends all breastfed babies receive 400 IU/day of vitamin D beginning before 2 months of age.

PATHOPHYSIOLOGY
- Insufficient dietary intake of vitamin D and/or lack of UVB exposure results in low levels of vitamin D. This limits calcium absorption, causing excess PTH to be released.
- PTH stimulates osteoclast activity, which raises calcium and phosphorous but results in osteomalacia.

ETIOLOGY
- Dietary deficiency:
  - Inadequate vitamin D intake
  - Macrobiotic diet
- Inadequate sunlight exposure:
  - Institutionalized patients
  - Hospitalized patients
  - Chronic illness
  - Liver or kidney disease
- Malabsorptive states

COMMONLY ASSOCIATED CONDITIONS
- Osteomalacia, osteoporosis
- Premenstrual syndrome
- Rickets
- Celiac disease
- Gastric bypass
- Chronic renal disease
- Bacterial vaginosis in pregnant women
- Hypertension
- All-cause mortality (10)[B]

 DIAGNOSIS

- Nonspecific musculoskeletal complaints
- Weak antigravity muscles
- Fracture with minimal trauma

HISTORY
- Senior citizens at risk of falling
- Renal disease
- GI (malabsorption) disorders
- Liver dysfunction
- Immigration from tropical to colder climates
- Dark-skinned or veiled individuals
- Housebound patients
- Women at perimenopause

PHYSICAL EXAM
- Numerous neurologic signs: Numbness, proximal myopathy, paresthesias, muscle cramps, laryngospasm
- Chvostek sign: Contraction of the muscles of the eye, mouth, or nose by tapping along the facial nerve
- Trousseau phenomenon: Carpal spasms and paraesthesia produced by pressure upon nerves and vessels of the upper arm
- Tetany
- Seizures

DIAGNOSTIC TESTS & INTERPRETATION
Lab
- 25 OH vitamin D (most sensitive measure of vitamin D status)
- Vitamin D insufficiency:
  - 25 OH D is 15–30 ng/mL
- Vitamin D deficiency:
  - <15 ng/mL
- PTH elevation (normal in early vitamin D deficiency), not routinely obtained unless severe deficiency
- Low-normal or low calcium and phosphorous
- Elevated alkaline phosphatase (in later disease)

Imaging

- Plain radiographs: If atypical fracture, radiographs may show osteomalacia (pseudo fractures or Looser zones) in pelvis, femur, and fibula.
- Osteoporosis screen (11)[C]:
  - Women ≥65 years with no risk factors
  - Women ≥60 years at risk: Body weight <70 kg (best predictor)
  - Less evidence: Smoking, low body mass index, family history, decreased activity, alcohol, or caffeine use
  - African American women have higher bone density than Caucasians.

TREATMENT

- Treatment goals remain unclear, but current "normal" 25 OH vitamin D levels are based upon suppression of PTH.
- In senior citizens, serum 25 OH vitamin D of 50 nmol/L resulted in optimal hip and greater trochanter BMD, and in best physical performance scores (12).

MEDICATION

- Vitamin D insufficiency:
  - Vitamin D 800–2,000 IU/day plus
  - Elemental calcium 1,200 mg/day *OR*
- Vitamin D deficiency:
  - Ergocalciferol 50,000 IU/week for 8–12 weeks, followed by 2,000 IU/day of vitamin D3 *PLUS*
  - Elemental calcium 1,200 mg/day

ADDITIONAL TREATMENT

Issues for Referral
Endocrinology if no response to treatment

Additional Therapies
Aggressive calcium in ICU patients with ionized calcium <3.2 mg/dL or if symptomatic (tetany, seizures, QT prolongation, bradycardia, or hypotension, or ventilated patient with decreased diaphragmatic function)

IN-PATIENT CONSIDERATIONS

Admission Criteria
- Symptoms of severe hypocalcemia *or*
- Malabsorption syndromes

ONGOING CARE

FOLLOW-UP RECOMMENDATIONS
Repeat abnormal 25 OH vitamin D and other abnormal labs at 12–16 weeks after initiation of treatment.

DIET
- Fatty fish (tuna, salmon)
- Fortified milk, cereal, and foods

PROGNOSIS
- Systematic review of 63 observational studies found adequate 25 vitamin D levels correlated with lower rates of colon, breast, and prostate cancer (13)[A].
- Cohort study found that low serum vitamin D is correlated with increased risk of all-cause mortality (10)[B].
- Meta-analysis of 57,000 patients found supplementation of >500 IU/day lowered the risk of all-cause mortality (14)[A].

REFERENCES

1. Gordon CM, DePeter KC, Feldman HA, et al. Prevalence of vitamin D deficiency among healthy adolescents. *Arch Pediatr Adolesc Med*. 2004;158:531–7.
2. Thomas MK, Lloyd-Jones DM, Thadhani RI, et al. Hypovitaminosis D in medical inpatients. *N Engl J Med*. 1998;338:777–83.
3. Gaugris S, Heaney RP, Boonen S, et al. Vitamin D inadequacy among post-menopausal women: a systematic review. *QJM*. 2005;98:667–76.
4. Plotnikoff GA, Quigley JM. Prevalence of severe hypovitaminosis D in patients with persistent, nonspecific musculoskeletal pain. *Mayo Clin Proc*. 2003;78:1463–70.
5. Jacobs ET, Alberts DS, Foote JA, et al. Vitamin D insufficiency in southern Arizona. *Am J Clin Nutr*. 2008;87:608–13.
6. Jorde R, Sneve M, Figenschau Y, et al. Effects of vitamin D supplementation on symptoms of depression in overweight and obese subjects: randomized double blind trial. *J Intern Med*. 2008;264:599–609.
7. Kumar J, Muntner P, Kaskel FJ, et al. Prevalence and Associations of 25-Hydroxyvitamin D Deficiency in US Children: NHANES 2001–2004. *Pediatrics*. 2009.
8. Bischoff-Ferrari HA, Willett WC, Wong JB, et al. Fracture prevention with vitamin D supplementation: a meta-analysis of randomized controlled trials. *JAMA*. 2005;293:2257–64.
9. Bischoff-Ferrari HA, Willett WC, Wong JB, et al. Prevention of nonvertebral fractures with oral vitamin D and dose dependency: a meta-analysis of randomized controlled trials. *Arch Intern Med*. 2009;169:551–61.
10. Melamed ML, Michos ED, Post W, et al. 25-hydroxyvitamin D levels and the risk of mortality in the general population. *Arch Intern Med*. 2008;168:1629–37.
11. Available at: http://www.ahrq.gov.
12. Kuchuk NO, Pluijm SM, van Schoor NM, et al. Relationships of serum 25-hydroxyvitamin D to bone mineral density and serum parathyroid hormone and markers of bone turnover in older persons. *J Clin Endocrinol Metab*. 2009;94:1244–50.
13. Garland CF, Garland FC, Gorham ED, et al. The role of vitamin D in cancer prevention. *Am J Public Health*. 2006;96:252–61.
14. Autier P, Gandini S. Vitamin D supplementation and total mortality: a meta-analysis of randomized controlled trials. *Arch Intern Med*. 2007;167:1730–7.

CODES

ICD9
268.9 Unspecified vitamin D deficiency

CLINICAL PEARLS

- Risk factors for VDD: Senior citizen, renal disease, GI (malabsorption) disorders, liver dysfunction, immigration from tropical to colder climates, dark-skinned or veiled individuals, housebound patients, perimenopause
- Diagnosis: 25 OH vitamin D (most sensitive measure of vitamin D status)
- Vitamin D insufficiency: 25 OH D is 15–30 ng/mL
- Vitamin D deficiency: <15 ng/mL
- Up to 2,000 IU/day is safe in healthy adults without risk of toxicity.
- Higher intake of vitamin D is recommended for ages >50 years.
- 2005 and 2009: Meta-analysis demonstrated for ages 51–70 minimally recommended supplementation is 800 IU/day to prevent nonvertebral fractures (8,9)[A].
- The American Academy of Pediatrics recommends all breastfed babies receive 400 IU/d of vitamin D beginning before 2 months of age.

V

VITAMIN DEFICIENCY

Neil A. Gilchrist, PharmD
David B. Gilchrist, MD

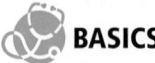 **BASICS**

DESCRIPTION
- Vitamins are essential micronutrients required for normal metabolism, growth, and development.
- Specific vitamin deficiencies can lead to medical conditions and health complications.
- Deficiencies are rarely diagnosed or documented in the Western world. Regulations mandating vitamin supplementation in food products, adequate food supply, availability of vitamin supplements, and lack of physician awareness all play a role.
- Fat-soluble vitamins (A, D, E, K) and water-soluble vitamins (B)

EPIDEMIOLOGY
Incidence
- Predominant age:
  - Affects mainly geriatric population
  - Occurs in select adult demographics: Pregnant women, chronic disease states (see Etiology)
- Travelers spending extended time in developing nations
- Very low for isolated vitamin deficiencies in Western world; true incidence unknown
- Vitamin levels are rarely measured (exceptions include vitamin B_{12} [risk increases >50] and folate [risk increases with specific states: Pregnancy, antiepileptic drugs, neoplastic processes, alcoholism])

Prevalence
Varies by age groups, comorbid conditions, geography, and setting (i.e., urban, rural)

RISK FACTORS
Poverty, malnutrition, chronic disease states, advanced age, dietary restrictions, bariatric surgery, and exclusively breastfed infants

Genetics
- Cystic fibrosis
- Rare genetic predisposition:
  - Autoimmune disease (e.g., pernicious anemia)
  - Congenital enzyme deficiencies (e.g., biotinidase deficiency)
  - Transcobalamin II deficiency
  - Ataxia and vitamin E deficiency (AVED)
- A-β-lipoproteinemia

GENERAL PREVENTION
- No data exist that demonstrate that use of a multivitamin decreases risk of any disease.
- Ingesting large and varied amounts of vitamins increases risk of toxicity and drug–drug interactions.
- Use of antioxidants to prevent cancer has had no beneficial effect on cancer incidence, and in some studies has increased risk of death (1)[A].
- Adequate intake of a balanced diet containing carbohydrates, proteins, and fats
- Avoidance of fad diets
- Vitamin or nutrition supplementation, when appropriate

ALERT
Use of multivitamins has not resulted in decreased risk of cancer, heart disease, stroke, or all-cause mortality (2)[A].

PATHOPHYSIOLOGY
Deficiencies usually related to disease can develop under healthy conditions and generally occur by 1 of 5 mechanisms:
- Reduced intake
- Diminished absorption
- Increased utilization
- Increased demand
- Increased excretion

ETIOLOGY
- Chronic disease states: HIV, malabsorption, chronic liver and kidney disease, alcoholism, pernicious anemia, etc.
- Gastric surgeries: Gastric bypass, gastrectomy, small or large bowel resection, etc.
- Predisposition related to certain medicines: Prednisone, phenytoin, isoniazid, protease inhibitors, proton pump inhibitors, chronic antibiotic use, penicillamine, hydralazine, etc (3).
- Malnutrition, imbalanced nutrition, eating disorders: Obesity, bulimia/anorexia, fad diets, extreme vegetarianism
- Dialysis
- Parasitic infestation

COMMONLY ASSOCIATED CONDITIONS
Osteoporosis, anemia, neuropathies, Hartnup disease

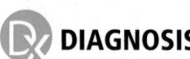 **DIAGNOSIS**

HISTORY
- Dietary intake
- Night blindness
- Macular degeneration
- Decreased visual acuity
- Poor wound healing
- Hyperkeratosis of skin
- Neuropathy
- Abnormal food cravings (pica)
- Osteomalacia or history of fracture
- Spina bifida
- Previous GI or gastric bypass surgery
- Prior or current medical conditions:
  - Tuberculosis (TB)
  - HIV infection
  - Hepatitis
  - Neoplastic condition
  - Hypermetabolic state:
    ○ Thyrotoxicosis
    ○ 2nd- or 3rd-degree burns
    ○ Wound healing
    ○ Any systemic infection
  - Any chronic disease requiring steroids or immunosuppressants
  - Any malabsorption or chronic GI disorder: Celiac disease, sprue, Crohn disease, ulcerative colitis
- Parenteral or enteral nutrition via tube feeding
- Pregnancy
- Medications
- Supplements
- Food allergies or intolerances

PHYSICAL EXAM
- Breakdown of skin integrity
- Coarse or thinning hair
- Reduced visual acuity
- Beefy red tongue
- Angular cheilitis (perlèche)
- Poor dentition and gingivitis
- Cognitive impairment
- Bruising and/or petechiae
- Sensory and motor neuropathies
- Ataxic gait

DIAGNOSTIC TESTS & INTERPRETATION
Lab
Initial lab tests
- None needed unless a specific deficiency is suspected; screening with "routine" labs is not recommended
- Complete blood count (CBC)
- If clinical characteristics are present, consider:
  - 25 OH vitamin D
  - Prothrombin time (PT)/partial thromboplastin time (PTT)
  - Vitamin B_{12} and folate levels
  - Serum homocysteine and methylmalonic acid levels if high suspicion of vitamin B_{12} deficiency with normal serum B_{12} level
- Ancillary tests include:
  - Blood urea nitrogen (BUN)
  - Albumin
  - Calcium
  - Phosphorous
  - Magnesium
  - Liver function tests (LFTs)

Follow-Up & Special Considerations
Bariatric surgery patients are at risk for select nutritional deficiencies:
- Cyanocobalamin
- Thiamine
- Folic acid
- Calcium
- Vitamin D
- Iron
- Zinc

Imaging
Initial approach
- X-ray of long bones and spine
- Bone densitometry: Indicated in:
  - Women >65 years
  - Men >70 years
  - Patients <65 years with risk factors for osteoporosis, including patients with chronic disease requiring long-standing steroids or immunosuppressants, patients on thyroid medicine and antiepileptic drugs (see topic Osteoporosis)

Pathological Findings
- Vitamin A (retinol):
  - Decreased visual acuity, Bitot spots
  - Advanced disease: Keratomalacia and blindness
- Vitamin B_1 (thiamine):
  - Wernicke encephalopathy: Memory disturbance, truncal ataxia, nystagmus, ophthalmoplegia
  - Korsakoff syndrome: Anterograde and retrograde amnesia, confabulation

– Dry beriberi: Symmetric motor and sensory peripheral neuropathy, paresthesias, loss of reflexes

– Wet beriberi: Cardiovascular symptoms of peripheral vasodilation, high-output failure, dyspnea, and tachycardia

- Vitamin B_2 (riboflavin): Glossitis, stomatitis, cheilitis
- Vitamin B_3 (niacin): Pellagra: Dermatitis, dementia, and diarrhea
- Vitamin B_6 (pyridoxine): Dermatitis, cheilitis, atrophic glossitis, neuropathy
- Vitamin B_{12} (cobalamin): Pernicious anemia, subacute combined degeneration, gait disturbance, cognitive impairment, neuropathy
- Vitamin C (ascorbic acid): Scurvy: Ecchymoses, bleeding gums
- Vitamin D (calciferol): Rickets, osteomalacia, osteopenia/osteoporosis
- Vitamin K: Ecchymosis, mucosal bleeding

DIFFERENTIAL DIAGNOSIS

Many medical conditions may lead to symptoms and signs that mimic vitamin deficiencies, including diabetes mellitus (DM), hyperparathyroidism, thyroid disorders, heart failure, Alzheimer disease, multiple sclerosis, substance abuse, toxic ingestions and overdose, and hematologic disorders/malignancies.

 TREATMENT

MEDICATION

- Encourage patients to bring in vitamin and supplement bottles for personal review by a physician or knowledgeable health care practitioner or pharmacist.
- Folic acid and vitamin B_6/B_{12} therapy has been shown to lower homocysteine levels; however, there is no date showing benefit of this therapy re: cognitive impairment or risk of developing diabetic nephropathy, retinopathy, and CHD/vascular diseases (4).

COMPLEMENTARY AND ALTERNATIVE MEDICINE

- Patients should be asked specifically about herbal and dietary supplements as part of a complete medication history.
- Prescribers should assess for possible adverse drug effects and drug interactions (5).

IN-PATIENT CONSIDERATIONS
Initial Stabilization

- Provide daily B-vitamin complex (folate, B_6, B_{12}), including thiamine supplementation (dose = 100 mg) via oral or parenteral route, to all patients with chronic medical conditions admitted to hospital or in postoperative state at risk for alcohol withdrawal (6)[B].
- If thiamine deficiency suspected, give thiamine replacement prior to IV fluids containing glucose to prevent precipitation of Korsakoff psychosis.
- Consider obtaining dietician/nutrition consult.
- There is currently no consensus practice guideline for recommending supplement dosing regimens after bariatric surgery. Dosing of supplements should be guided by patient symptoms and serum levels when appropriate.

Geriatric Considerations

- Vitamin B_{12} deficiency: 25% of the general population ≥65 years has borderline or low levels of vitamin B_{12} necessitating supplementation. Treatment of symptomatic or severe deficiency should consist of cyanocobalamin 1,000 μg/d IM × 1 week and then weekly × 1 month. Prevention of recurrence or treatment of mild deficiency may include a regimen of oral B_{12} 1,000–2,000 μg/d or IM B_{12} 100–1,000 μg every 3 months.
- A large percentage (>40%) of elderly patients in the community setting in the US are deficient in vitamin D. The percentage is even higher in the hospitalized elderly.

Pediatric Considerations

- Hemorrhagic disease of the newborn:
  – Deficiency of vitamin K may be seen in neonates because they require 1 week of life to establish their intestinal flora (intestinal bacteria manufacture vitamin K) and because breast milk is a poor source of vitamin K.
  – Peaks 2–10 days after birth; presents with bleeding from the umbilical stump and/or circumcision site along with generalized bruising and GI hemorrhage
  – Routine injection of newborns with vitamin K (1 mg) prevents hemorrhagic disease.
- Vitamin D deficiency: Vitamin D supplementation (400 IU/d) is recommended in all exclusively breastfed infants starting in the first few days of life (AAP recommendations) to prevent rickets.
- Many vitamin deficiencies lead to developmental delay in children.
- Supplemental vitamins in otherwise healthy children, although encouraged, are not mandated by medical authorities.

Pregnancy Considerations

Folate and pregnancy: All pregnant women and women of child-bearing age considering pregnancy should be strongly encouraged to take a multivitamin containing 0.4 mg folic acid daily to prevent neural tube defects.

 ONGOING CARE

DIET

- Monitor nutrient intake.
- Supplemental enteral nutrition (i.e., Ensure, Boost, Sustacal, etc.) if anorexic or if difficulty eating solids.

PATIENT EDUCATION

- One-a-day vitamins are generally safe for all patients but are of no value in the Western world, and caution should be exercised about taking vitamins with some medications to minimize drug–drug interactions.
- Toxicity can occur with many vitamins, most commonly the fat-soluble vitamins (A, D, E, K). Refer to the Recommended Dietary Allowance (RDA) for specific intake guidelines.

PROGNOSIS

- Most vitamin deficiencies are fully reversible if treated without undue delay.
- Vitamin repletion or supplementation may be required short term (<3 months) or long term (>3 months), depending upon cause of deficiency.

COMPLICATIONS

- Vitamin toxicities:
  – Liver failure (vitamins A, D, E, K)
  – Desquamation of skin (vitamin A)
  – Neuropathy (vitamin B_6)
  – Kidney stones (vitamin C)
  – Hypercoagulability (vitamin K)
  – Pseudohyperparathyroidism (vitamin D)
  – Masking of pernicious anemia (folic acid)
- Any vitamin can be taken to excess; refer to the Recommended Dietary Allowance (RDA) for specific intake guidelines.

REFERENCES

1. Bjelakovic G, Nikolova D, Gluud LL, et al. Antioxidant supplements for prevention of mortality in healthy participants and patients with various diseases. *Cochrane Database Syst Rev.* 2008:CD007176.
2. Neuhouser ML, Wassertheil-Smoller S, Thomson C, et al. Multivitamin use and risk of cancer and cardiovascular disease in the Women's Health Initiative cohorts. *Arch Intern Med.* 2009;169: 294–304.
3. Felípez L, Sentongo TA, et al. Drug-induced nutrient deficiencies. *Pediatr Clin North Am.* 2009;56: 1211–24.
4. House AA, Eliasziw M, Cattran DC, et al. Effect of B-vitamin therapy on progression of diabetic nephropathy: a randomized controlled trial. *JAMA.* 2010;303:1603–9.
5. Haller CA. Clinical approach to adverse events and interactions related to herbal and dietary supplements. *Clinical Toxicology* 2006;44:605–10.
6. Thomson AD, et al. The treatment of patients at risk of developing Wernicke's encephalopathy in the community. *Alcohol Alcoholism.* 2006;41:159–67.

ADDITIONAL READING

Davies DJ, Baxter JM, Baxter JN. Nutritional deficiencies after bariatric surgery. *Obes Surg.* 2007;17:1150–8.

 CODES

ICD9
269.2 Unspecified vitamin deficiency

CLINICAL PEARLS

- Take a thorough dietary history to assess for possible vitamin deficiencies, especially if physical exam findings suggest a vitamin deficiency.
- All pregnant women and women of child-bearing age should be counseled to take a multivitamin with 0.4 mg folic acid.
- All exclusively breastfed infants should be given 400 IU vitamin D supplementation starting in the first few days of life and continued until weaned to formula or, if >12 months, taking 32 oz of fortified cow's milk daily.

VITILIGO

Antoin M. Alexander, MD
Rebecca A. Frye, DO

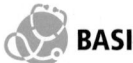 **BASICS**

DESCRIPTION

Vitiligo is an acquired dyschromia of the skin in which there is loss of epidermal melanocytes. The diagnosis is clinical; occasionally, a skin biopsy is necessary:

- A loss of epidermal melanocytes is the pathologic hallmark.
- Depigmented macules and patches appearing chalky or milk-white in color
- Generalized (nonsegmental): Up to 90% of cases and 30% of childhood cases. Is progressive, with flare-ups. Often associated with autoimmunity. Common in sites sensitive to pressure and friction and prone to trauma (Koebner phenomenon):
  - Vulgaris: Presence of scattered macules extensively disseminated; often in symmetrical area and extensor surfaces
  - Acrofacial: Patches are localized on distal extremities and face.
  - Mixed: Coexistence of acrofacialis and vulgaris forms
- Localized: Often begins in childhood. Has rapid onset and stabilizes. Involves hair compartment soon after onset. Not usually accompanied by autoimmune diseases:
  - Focal: 1 or more macules with casual distribution
  - Unilateral: 1 or more macules localized in a unilateral body region; with a dermatomal distribution
- Universalis: Little remaining normal pigment
- Significant psychological distress, particularly in dark-skinned patients and women
- System(s) affected: Skin/Exocrine
- Synonym(s): Depigmentation

EPIDEMIOLOGY

- 50% begin before age 20 years
- Predominance: Male = Female
- No race or socioeconomic predilection

Incidence

- In the US: 1%
- Peak incidence 10–30 years of age

Prevalence

About 0.5–2% of the world's population

RISK FACTORS

- 12–35% positive family history in pediatric patients with vitiligo
- First-degree relatives having autoimmune disorders, most commonly thyroiditis, pernicious anemia, Addison disease, diabetes mellitus, alopecia areta, rheumatoid arthritis, systemic lupus erythematous, and inflammatory bowel disease
- Traumatic stimulus (pressure or friction): Koebner's phenomenon
- Multiple halo nevi, as they represent a marker of cellular autoimmunity

Genetics

- Nonmendelian inheritance
- NALP1 candidate gene involved in vitiligo-associated autoimmune syndrome

ETIOLOGY

Exact etiology unclear, various hypothesis:

- Autoimmune: Often elevated levels of autoantibodies to melanocytes antigens
- Genetic: Certain chromosomal locations associated with inheritance such as 17p13, NALP1, and MC1R
- Neural: May be mediated by inadequate sympathetic innervation
- Biochemical: End result of metabolic and biochemical dysregulation. Possible oxidative stress induces melanocyte death.
- Viral: Cytomegalovirus has been identified in some vitiligo biopsy specimens; other viruses such as Hep C, HIV, and EBC have been suggested.
- Convergence theory: A convergence of many pathways, representing a syndrome rather than a single disease

COMMONLY ASSOCIATED CONDITIONS

- Thyroid disease (Hashimoto's and Grave's): 30% of patients with vitiligo
- Pernicious anemia
- Addison disease
- Systemic lupus erythematosus
- Inflammatory bowel disease
- Addison disease
- Alopecia areata
- Diabetes mellitus (insulin-dependent)
- Psoriasis
- Polyglandular autoimmune syndrome type II (autoimmune thyroid disease, type I diabetes mellitus, primary adrenal insufficiency, and hypopituitarism)

Pediatric Considerations

Childhood vitiligo rarely associated with any autoimmune disease other than autoimmune thyroiditis

 DIAGNOSIS

HISTORY

- Review family history of premature graying, vitiligo, and autoimmune disorders.
- An assessment form published by the Vitiligo European Task Force may be useful (1).
- Assess skin color and ability to tan, as this may guide the phototherapy treatment plan.
- Duration of symptoms and level of activity (progression or regression)
- Review symptoms of psychological impact on quality of life and self-esteem.

PHYSICAL EXAM

- Macules and patches of amelanotic milk or chalk-white skin
- Koebnerization over places of injury, areas of rubbing, such as shoulder straps, waistbands, and collar areas
- Wood 's lamp exam to accentuate patches
- Often well-demarcated or scalloped borders with no erythema
- Centrifugally enlarge over time
- Predilection for acral areas and around orifices such as eyes, mouth, anus
- Generalized vitiligo frequently involves extensor surfaces, including interphalangeal joints, metacarpal/metatarsal interphalangeal joints, elbows, and knees.

DIAGNOSTIC TESTS & INTERPRETATION
Lab
Initial lab tests

- Thyroid-stimulating hormone, complete blood count, antinuclear antibody (2)
- Antithyroid peroxidase and antithyroglobulin antibodies, if family and/or patient history of autoimmune disease (2)

Follow-Up & Special Considerations
Measurement of thyroid function testing annually, especially if patient tested positive for thyroid peroxidase antibodies at initial screening

Diagnostic Procedures/Surgery

- Diagnosis requires differentiating between complete absence of pigment (vitiligo) from hypopigmentation
- Wood's lamp exam may accentuate lesions in light-complexioned patients.
- Skin biopsy, if uncertain of diagnosis based on clinical history and physical exam
- Differentiating between lack of pigment, hypopigmentation, and normal skin may be more difficult in light-complexioned people.

Pathological Findings

Complete absence of melanocytes in skin biopsy. At the margins, one may see a lymphocystic infiltration, especially in early lesions.

DIFFERENTIAL DIAGNOSIS

- Parainfectious hypopigmentation:
  - Tinea versicolor, indeterminate leprosy
- Postinflammatory hypomelanoses:
  - Psoriasis, atopic dermatitis, lichen planus, toxic drug reactions, scleroderma
- Inherited hypomelanoses:
  - Piebaldism, tuberous sclerosis, Waardenburg's syndrome, Ito's hypomelanosis
- Paramalignant hypomelanoses:
  - Mycosis fungoides, melanoma
- Occupational and drug-induced depigmentation:
  - Occupational: Generally phenolic-catecholic derivative
  - Drug-induced: Chloroquine, fluphenazine, physostigmine, imatinib, rarely topical imiquimod
- Melasma, normal skin may be confused as vitiligo patches in the setting of surrounding hypermelanosis
- Pityriasis alba
- Melanocytic nevi (halo nevi)
- Lichen sclerosis

 TREATMENT

- Absence of a standardized scoring system, a meta-analysis to assess different treatment is difficult (3):
  - Vitiligo Area Scoring Index (VASI) and Vitiligo European Task Force consensus definition and assessment methodology developed (3)
- Efficacy of treatment uses global physician assessment, and in many studies is assessed in terms of proportion of treated patients that achieved 75% repigmentation (1)
- Repigmentation therapies include corticosteroids, calcineurin inhibitors, phototherapy (narrow-band ultraviolet B [NB-UVB]) or broadband ultraviolet B (BB-UVB), and surgery.

MEDICATION

- Individualize therapy depending on the extent, distribution, and rate of progression of the lesions after discussion with patient regarding expectations for repigmentation and assessment of psychological affect of disease burden.
- No topical therapies are FDA approved for treatment of vitiligo, although are considered first-line therapy

First Line

- For segmental and limited nonsegmental (< 20% body surface involvement):
  - Avoid triggering factors, use local therapies (topical corticosteroids and calcineurin inhibitors) (1)[A]:
    - Potent Class I-II steroid creams (betamethasone or clobetasol) were significantly more effective (2)[A].
    - Apply b.i.d. and discontinue steroids if no response after 2 months of therapy.
    - Tacrolimus ointment 0.03-0.1% b.i.d., particularly on the face and neck (12)[A]. Efficacy enhanced by occlusion with polyethylene foil or exposure to high-fluency UVB devices (1)[B].
- For nonsegmental with >20% body surface involvement:
  - Narrow-band UV-B phototherapy twice weekly for at least 3 months, optimally 9 months if there is a response (1)[A]
  - Narrow-band UV-B is more effective than psoralen ultraviolet A (PUVA) with fewer side effects (1)[A].

Second Line

- For segmental and limited nonsegmental:
  - Use localized narrow-band UVB therapy, especially excimer monochromatic lamp or laser (1)[A].
- For nonsegmental vitiligo:
  - Consider systemic corticosteroids or immunosuppressive agents if there is extension under narrow-band UVB therapy:
    - Used with variable results and may prevent rapid depigmentation in active disease but side effects common (2)[B].

ADDITIONAL TREATMENT

General Measures

- Sun exposure can accentuate the difference between normal and abnormal skin:
  - Sunscreen use if risk of sunburn; however, sun exposure (heliotherapy) may provide moderate benefit
- Corrective camouflage or cosmetics may be used as cover-ups (Cover FX, Dermablend).

Issues for Referral

- Dermatology consultation should be considered for facial or widespread vitiligo or when UVB or PUVA therapy may be necessary.
- Uveitis; retinal depigmentation
- Psychologist: For severe distress

Additional Therapies

PUVA (photochemotherapy with ultraviolet) may be effective after taking photosensitizer such as psoralen or khellin (3)[A]:

- Dihydroxyacetone (DHA) is the most frequently used self-tanning agent (1)[C].
- Oral corticosteroids have been used in patients with progressive disease with variable results.

- L-phenylalanine used with phototherapy shows promise (4)[B].
- Depigmentation therapy: For severe vitiligo affecting more than 50% of the body or extensive depigmentation to hands and face that is recalcitrant to therapy. Monobenzyl ether of hydroquinone or monomethyl ether of hydroquinone at 20% concentration alone or with Q-switched ruby laser (3)[B].
- 5-fluorouracil induces repigmentation by overstimulation of follicular melanocytes.
- Dermabrasion, re-epithelialization from remnants of dermal appendages:
  - Efficacy of dermabrasion increased when combined with 5-fluorouracil (3)[B]

COMPLEMENTARY AND ALTERNATIVE MEDICINE

- Ginkgo biloba 40 mg p.o. 3 times daily may arrest development of slowly spreading vitiligo (4)[A].
- Cosmetic tattooing for localized stable vitiligo

SURGERY/OTHER PROCEDURES

Surgical methods include minigrafting, transplantation of autologous noncultured melanocyte-keratinocyte cell transplantation, application of ultrathin epidermal grafts, and combination of approaches effective in stable nonsegmental vitiligo refractory to medical therapy:

- High consideration for surgery in cosmetic areas such as the face; dorsum of hands considered poor surgical site and relatively contraindicated
- Caution completing on keloid formers and patients affected by Koebner phenomenon

 ## ONGOING CARE

FOLLOW-UP RECOMMENDATIONS

Patient Monitoring

- TSH annually
- With topical steroids, follow at regular intervals to avoid steroid-atrophy, telangiectasia, and straie distensae of the skin.

DIET

No restrictions

PATIENT EDUCATION

- Discussion on chronicity, progression of disease, and cosmesis; allows patients to make informed treatment decisions and evaluate psychological concerns
- Education regarding trauma/friction and Koebner phenomenon

PROGNOSIS

- Vitiligo may remain stable, slowly progress, or show rapid depigmentation.
- 10–20% spontaneous repigmentation (5)
- Once repigmentation occurs, it usually persists.
- Focal vitiligo often progresses; more severe vitiligo rarely regresses.

COMPLICATIONS

- Adverse effects of each drug regimen
- Potential carcinogenesis: Topical tacrolimus and pimecrolimus; particularly when combined with UVB therapy
- Psychiatric morbidity: Depression, adjustment disorder, low self-esteem, embarrassment in relationships:
  - Job discrimination secondary to cosmetic concern

REFERENCES

1. Taied Alain, Picardo Mauro Vitiligo. *N Engl J Med*. 2009;360:160–9.
2. Halder Rebat M, Chappell Johnathan L. Vitiligo Update. *Semin Cutan Med Surg*. 2009;28:86–92.
3. Mahmoud BH, Hexsel CL, Hamzavi IH. An Update on New and Emerging Options for the Treatment of Vitiligo. *Skin Therapy Letter*. 2008;13:2.
4. Szczurko Orest, Boon Heather A systematic review of natural health product treatment for vitiligo. *BMC Dermatology*. 2008;8:2.
5. Lotti Torello, Gori Alessia, Zanieri Fabio, Colucci Roberta, Moretti Silvia Vitiligo: new emerging treatments. *Dermatologic Therapy*. 2008;21:110–117.

ADDITIONAL READING

- Fenton J, Bergstrom K. Vitiligo: Nonsurgical Treatment Options and the Evidence Behind Their Use. *Journal of Drugs in Dermatology*. 2008;7(7):705–711.
- Isenstein A, Morrell D, Burkhart C. Vitiligo: Treatment Approach in Children. *Pediatric Annals*. 2009;38:6.
- Kakourou T, Aghia S. Vitiligo in children. *World J Pediatr* 2009;5(4):265–268.
- Parsad D, Pandir R: Effectiveness of oral Ginkgo biloba in treating limited, slowly spreading vilitigo. *Clin Exp Dermatol*. 2003;128(3):2857.
- Whitton M, Asheroft D. Interventions for vitiligo. *Cochrane Library*. 2006;Issue 1:CD003263.
- Whitton M, Ashcrodt D, Gonzalez U. Therapeutic interventions for vitiligo. *J Am Acad Dermatol*. 2008;59:713–7.
- Yones SS, Palmer RA, Garibaldinos TM, et al. Randomized double-blind trial of treatment of vitiligo: efficacy of psoralen-UV-A therapy vs Narrowband-UV-B therapy. *Arch Dermatol*. 2007;143:578–84.

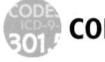 ## CODES

ICD9

709.01 Vitiligo

CLINICAL PEARLS

- Vitiligo can be a psychologically devastating skin disease.
- Screening for autoimmune disease, particularly thyroiditis, should be completed at presentation and annually.
- Treatment should be individualized based on BSA, patient skin type, and patient desire for repigmentation.
- Topical therapies (corticosteroids and calcineurin inhibitors) are first-line for segmental vitiligo with <20% BSA.
- Dermatology consultation when extensive disease, facial involvement, and when phototherapy is considered

VON WILLEBRAND DISEASE

Aaron S. Mansfield, MD

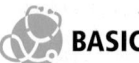

BASICS

DESCRIPTION

- von Willebrand disease (vWD) is a bleeding disorder caused by a defect in or deficiency of a blood-clotting protein called *von Willebrand factor* (vWF).
- vWF is a protein critical to the initial stages of blood clotting.
- vWD primarily manifests as mucocutaneous or perioperative bleeding.
- Inherited or acquired condition

EPIDEMIOLOGY

Prevalence

- The prevalence of the inherited forms of vWD is about 1–2% of the general population.
- The prevalence of the acquired forms of vWD is about 0.1% of the general population.
- Up to 21% of individuals with aortic stenosis have acquired vWD.
- 1/3 of patients with polycythemia vera have acquired vWD.

Pediatric Considerations

Many cases of vWD are diagnosed in childhood, including during initial years of menstruation.

Pregnancy Considerations

Although levels of vWF increase during pregnancy, women with vWD are most likely to experience an increased incidence of obstetric complications that manifest with bleeding.

RISK FACTORS

Genetics

- The gene for vWF is located on chromosome 12.
- >250 mutations have been identified.
- Type 1 follows an autosomal dominant inheritance pattern with variable expressivity.
- Type 2 varies, but primarily follows an autosomal dominant inheritance pattern.
- Type 3 follows an autosomal recessive inheritance pattern and is usually due to a frameshift or nonsense mutation in the gene causing lack of expression.

PATHOPHYSIOLOGY

- vWF is a large multimeric protein that is released by endothelial cells and carried within platelets. It mediates platelet plug formation by the attraction and aggregation of platelets at sites of endothelial injury.
- vWF is also a carrier for factor VIII (FVIII) and stabilizes this factor from degradation. A deficiency in vWF results in lower levels of FVIII.
- When vWF is deficient or dysfunctional, primary hemostasis is compromised, resulting in increased mucocutaneous and postprocedural bleeding.
- There are 3 major categories of inherited vWD:
  - Type I is the most common and mildest form, representing 60–80% of cases:
    - Mild-to-moderate quantitative deficiency of vWF and concordant deficiency of FVIII
    - Generally a mild bleeding disorder

- Type 2 accounts for 10–30% of cases and is divided into multiple subtypes:
  - In type 2, vWF itself has an abnormality.
  - Type 2A is noted for defective platelet-dependent functions and lack of large multimers.
  - Type 2B is noted for increased binding affinity for platelets and is associated with thrombocytopenia, low ristocetin cofactor activity, and few large multimers.
  - Type 2M is noted for defective platelet-dependent functions but not multimer defects.
  - Type 2N demonstrates defective binding to FVIII.
- Type 3 represents 1–5% of cases:
  - Most severe form
  - Low-to-undetectable levels of vWF and FVIII
- There is also an increasingly recognized acquired form of vWD secondary to multiple conditions such as aortic stenosis, dysproteinemias, lymphoproliferative disorders, myeloproliferative disorders, solid tumors, hypothyroidism, autoimmune disorders, and medication use (e.g., ciprofloxacin, valproic acid, griseofulvin). The pathophysiology of the acquired form is related to the underlying condition:
  - In aortic stenosis, vWF deficiency may result from enhanced ADAMTS13-mediated proteolysis due to increased shear stress.
  - Adsorption of vWF has been demonstrated by certain tumor cells and by activated platelets in essential thrombocythemia.

ETIOLOGY

- >250 mutations have been identified in the inherited forms.
- Some mechanisms of the acquired forms are described above.

DIAGNOSIS

HISTORY

- Most patients with an inherited type have a family history of vWD; however, patients with mild forms of vWD and their families may be unaware of their disease.
- Those with acquired vWD often have no family history of this disorder.
- The most important component of the diagnosis is the hemostatic history. Most patients have a history of bleeding after tooth extraction or operation.
- Common symptoms are those of mucocutaneous (recurrent epistaxis, menorrhagia, ecchymosis) or postprocedural bleeding.
- A history of 3 distinct hemorrhagic symptoms is specific diagnostic criterion for vWD (1)[B].
- Hemarthrosis is rare but does occur with severe types.

PHYSICAL EXAM

- Physical exam may be entirely normal, although there may be some ecchymoses.
- Findings suggestive of other causes of increased bleeding should be sought out, such as liver disease, skin laxity, or telangiectasia.

DIAGNOSTIC TESTS & INTERPRETATION

Lab

Initial lab tests

- The most specific tests for vWD include measurement of vWF antigen and ristocetin cofactor activity, and these 2 tests should be ordered when suspicion for vWD is high. The results of other tests obtained for the workup of a bleeding diathesis are described here:
  - Platelet count is often normal, except in type 2B or when there is an underlying myeloproliferative disorder.
  - Platelet function assay is usually prolonged but may be normal in mild disease.
  - Prothrombin time/international normalized ratio is normal, unless there is concurrent liver disease or Coumadin use.
  - Activated partial thromboplastin time may be prolonged because a decrease in FVIII accompanies vWD.
  - Bleeding time is usually prolonged but may be normal in mild disease. This test has been discontinued at many institutions.
- Specific tests for vWD:
  - vWF antigen testing is done via immunologic methods:
    - vWF antigen testing has a positive vWF antigen testing has a positive predicted value of 33% for detecting significant FVIII deficiency and a PPV of 80% for detecting ristocetin cofactor activity abnormalities (2)[C].
    - The levels of antigen may be normal in type 2 vWD.
  - Ristocetin cofactor activity is a functional assessment of vWF. Ristocetin promotes binding of platelets to vWF, and this activity is reduced in most forms of vWD.
  - Collagen-binding activity is another functional assessment of vWF. This test may detect patients with normal ristocetin cofactor activity.
  - vWF multimer analysis is performed by electrophoresis on agarose gel. This test identifies patients with type 2 vWD who have normal vWF antigen levels and decreased ristocetin cofactor activity.
  - FVIII-vWF binding assay activity is low in patients with type 2N vWD.

Follow-Up & Special Considerations

- Unless patients have severe forms of vWD or are undergoing treatment, follow-up laboratory studies are not usually obtained.
- Patients with blood group O have 20–30% lower levels of vWF antigen and ristocetin cofactor activity.
- vWF is an acute-phase reactant, so elevations may be seen in inflammatory conditions, liver disease, during pregnancy (which may correct mild deficits), or with estrogen use.

DIFFERENTIAL DIAGNOSIS

- Primary hemostatic disorders:
  - Congenital thrombocytopenia
  - Coagulation factor deficiencies
- Secondary hemostatic disorders:
  - Liver disease
  - Uremia
  - Connective tissue disorders
  - Coagulation factor inhibitors

TREATMENT

MEDICATION
First Line
- Desmopressin (DDAVP):
  – Enhances release of vWF from endothelial cells
  – Primarily effective for type 1 vWD
  – Not effective in severe deficiencies, in types of vWD with defective vWF, or for bleeding prophylaxis prior to major procedures
  – 0.3 μg/kg IV/SQ or 300 μg/d intranasally
  – Common side effects: Flushing, tachycardia, water retention
  – Obtain repeat testing of ristocetin cofactor activity and FVIII 1 and 4 hours after infusion to evaluate peak response and clearance of DDAVP (3)[C].
  – Tachyphylaxis may develop with repeat doses.
- Fresh frozen plasma (FFP) and cryoprecipitate:
  – FFP contains the components of the coagulation, fibrinolytic, and complement systems and proteins that maintain oncotic pressure and modulate immunity.
  – Cryoprecipitate contains FVIII, fibrinogen, vWF, factor XIII, and fibronectin.
  – Both contain both vWF and FVIII.
  – Not considered as safe as virus-inactivated plasma concentrates below
- vWF and FVIII concentrates:
  – Humate-P and Alphanate are commercial concentrates of vWF and FVIII that are given in doses of 25–50 IU/kg/d based on clinical situation:
    ○ Humate-P is the only treatment for urgent bleeding that has been validated in prospective, open-label studies (4)[B]. Dose may be adjusted for FVIII levels and ristocetin cofactor activity.
    ○ These concentrates are the mainstay of treatment for patients who do not respond to DDAVP and may be used in acquired forms but have a shortened survival.
    ○ FVIII levels should be monitored when providing these replacements in order to avoid supranormal levels and possible venous thromboembolism (VTE).
    ○ Contraindicated if patient develops alloantibodies to vWF
- Antifibrinolytics:
  – Useful for mucosal bleeding
  – Contraindicated in patients with hematuria
  – Given as adjunct to desmopressin
  – Aminocaproic acid may be given at 50–60 mg/kg q4–6h IV or p.o.
  – Tranexamic acid may be given at 50–60 mg/kg q8–12h IV or p.o.
- Recombinant FVIII:
  – Used for patients who develop alloantibodies to vWF
  – Given as bolus of 90 μg/kg q2h or 20 μg/kg every hour until hemostasis is achieved

Second Line
- Platelets may be given as an adjunct to factor concentrates if hemostasis has not been achieved.
- IV immunoglobulin (IVIG) has been useful in some patients with monoclonal gammopathy of undetermined significance.
- Oral contraceptives may have a role in the treatment of chronic menorrhagia.
- Recombinant FVIIa has been used effectively in patients with type 3 vWD.

ADDITIONAL TREATMENT
General Measures
- Most patients with type 1 vWD do not require activity restrictions.
- Patients with type 3 vWD should avoid contact sports.
- An emergency ID bracelet may be useful.

Issues for Referral
The diagnosis of vWD is not always straightforward. It may be useful to consider consultation with a coagulation laboratory and/or a hematologist for the interpretation of testing results and treatment decision making.

SURGERY/OTHER PROCEDURES
Aortic valve replacement may be curative for acquired vWD in aortic stenosis.

IN-PATIENT CONSIDERATIONS
Initial Stabilization
For patients with major bleeds or those undergoing major surgical procedures, levels of ristocetin cofactor activity need to be restored and then maintained above 50% for 3–5 days. FVIII levels need to be maintained above 40% for 10–14 days.
For patients undergoing minor surgical procedures, maintain FVIII levels >30 IU/dL for 5–7 days.
For patients delivering or in need of epidural anesthesia, obtain FVIII level >50 IU/dL.

 ONGOING CARE

FOLLOW-UP RECOMMENDATIONS
Patients should be seen by a hematologist prior to invasive procedures for determination of perioperative management or advice regarding delivery.

Patient Monitoring
Patients with mild disease do not require monitoring.

DIET
No restrictions are recommended.

PATIENT EDUCATION
National Hemophilia Foundation: http://www.hemophilia.org/NHFWeb/MainPgs/MainNHF.aspx?menuid=182&contentid=47&rptname=bleeding

PROGNOSIS
Most patients with vWD have a normal life expectancy.

COMPLICATIONS
- Significant perioperative bleeding may occur.
- Patients with type 3 vWD can have bleeding complications similar to patients with hemophilia A, such as hemarthrosis and intracranial hemorrhage.
- Patients with aortic stenosis and acquired vWD are known to have higher rates of gastrointestinal blood loss.
- Multiple transfusions may result in alloantibodies against vWF.
- VTE may result from supranormal levels of FVIII.

REFERENCES

1. Rodeghiero F, Castaman G, Tosetto A, et al. The discriminant power of bleeding history for the diagnosis of type 1 von Willebrand disease: an international, multicenter study. *J Thromb Haemost.* 2005;3:2619–26.
2. Lippi G, Franchini M, Salvagno GL, et al. Correlation between von Willebrand factor antigen, von Willebrand factor ristocetin cofactor activity and factor VIII activity in plasma. *J Thromb Thrombolysis.* 2008;26:150–3.
3. Hanebutt FL, Rolf N, Loesel A, et al. Evaluation of desmopressin effects on haemostasis in children with congenital bleeding disorders. *Haemophilia.* 2008;14:524–30.
4. Thompson AR, Gill JC, Ewenstein BM, et al. Successful treatment for patients with von Willebrand disease undergoing urgent surgery using factor VIII/VWF concentrate (Humate-P). *Haemophilia.* 2004;10:42–51.

ADDITIONAL READING

- Kessler CM. Diagnosis and treatment of von Willebrand disease: new perspectives and nuances. *Haemophilia.* 2007;13(Suppl 5):3–14.
- Kumar S, Pruthi RK, Nichols WL. Acquired von Willebrand disease. *Mayo Clin Proc.* 2002;77:181–7.
- Mannucci PM. Treatment of von Willebrand's Disease. *N Engl J Med.* 2004;351:683–94.
- Robertson J, Lillicrap D, James PD. Von Willebrand disease. *Pediatr Clin North Am.* 2008;55:377–92, viii–ix.
- Rodeghiero F, Castaman G, Tosetto A, et al. How I treat von Willebrand disease. *Blood.* 2009;114:1158–65.
- Sciscione AC, Mucowski SJ. Pregnancy and von Willebrand disease: a review. *Del Med J.* 2007;79:401–5.

See Also (Topic, Algorithm, Electronic Media Element)
Algorithms: Bleeding Gums; Ecchymosis

 CODES

ICD9
286.4 Von Willebrand's disease

CLINICAL PEARLS
- vWD can vary from a minor to a severe bleeding disorder, and affects 1–2% of the US population.
- It is important to determine the exact type of vWD a patient has (1, 2, or 3) to guide effective treatment.
- There should be suspicion for acquired vWD in patients with acquired bleeding disorders.

V

VULVAR MALIGNANCY

Michael P. Hopkins, MD, MEd
Eric L. Jenison, MD
Michael S. Guy, MD

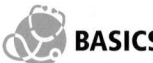 **BASICS**

DESCRIPTION
- Carcinoma in situ (Bowen disease): Premalignant changes involving the squamous epithelium of the vulva
- Squamous cell carcinoma: Invasive squamous cell carcinoma is the most common malignancy involving the vulva (90% of patients) (1). The malignancy can be well, moderately, or poorly differentiated.
- Other invasive cell types include melanoma, Paget disease, adenocarcinoma, adenoid cystic carcinoma, small cell carcinoma, verrucous carcinoma, and sarcomas. Sarcomas are usually leiomyosarcoma and probably arise at the insertion of the round ligament in the labium major.
- System(s) affected: Reproductive

Geriatric Considerations
- Older patients with associated medical problems are at high risk from radical surgery. The surgery, however, is external, usually well tolerated, and is the treatment of choice. Patients who are not surgical candidates can be treated with primary radiotherapy.
- In the very elderly, palliative vulvectomy provides relief of symptoms for ulcerating symptomatic advanced disease.

EPIDEMIOLOGY
Incidence
- In the US, invasive vulvar malignancy is the 4th most common gynecologic malignancy, accounting for 3,580 new cases in 2009.
- Predominant age:
  – In situ disease: Mean age 40s
  – Invasive malignancy: Mean age 60s, with a range of 20s–90s

RISK FACTORS
- Smoking
- Vulvar dystrophy
- HPV infection
- Autoimmune processes

Genetics
No known genetic pattern

GENERAL PREVENTION
- Human papillomavirus (HPV) vaccination has the potential to decrease vulvar cancer by 1/3 (1).
- Abstinence from smoking/smoking cessation counseling

ETIOLOGY
- Patients with cervical cancer are more likely to develop vulvar cancer at a later date. This is due to the so-called "field effect" with a carcinogen involving the lower genital tract.
- HPV has been associated with squamous cell abnormalities of the cervix, vagina, and vulva but has not been proven to be the causative agent. 40% of vulvar cancers are attributable to oncogenic HPV.

- Smoking is associated with squamous cell disease of the vulva, possibly from direct irritation of the vulva by the transfer of tars and nicotine on the patient's hands or from systemic absorption of carcinogen.

COMMONLY ASSOCIATED CONDITIONS
- Patients with invasive vulvar cancer are often elderly and have associated medical conditions.
- High rate of other gynecologic malignancies; patients should be evaluated for these.

 DIAGNOSIS

HISTORY
Complaints of pruritus or raised lesion in the vaginal area

PHYSICAL EXAM
- In situ disease: A small raised area associated with pruritus
- Invasive malignancy: An ulcerated, nonhealing area; as lesions become large, bleeding occurs with associated pain and foul-smelling discharge.
- In far-advanced disease: The patients can develop rectal bleeding or urethral obstruction.
- Large involved inguinal lymph nodes are also associated with advanced disease.

DIAGNOSTIC TESTS & INTERPRETATION
Lab
Initial lab tests
- Hypercalcemia can occur when metastatic disease is present.
- Squamous cell antigen can be elevated with invasive disease.

Follow-Up & Special Considerations
- Any woman complaining of symptoms related to the vulva should have a close examination and biopsies of appropriate areas.
- The vulva can be washed with 3% acetic acid to highlight areas. Areas of white, raised epithelium should be biopsied.
- Patients with new onset of pruritus should be biopsied in the area of pruritus.
- Liberal biopsies must be used to diagnose in situ disease prior to invasion and to diagnose early invasive disease.
- The patient should not be treated for presumed benign conditions of the vulva without full exam and biopsy.
- When symptoms persist, reexamination and rebiopsy should be undertaken.
- The treatment of benign condyloma of the vulva has not been shown to decrease the eventual incidence of in situ or invasive disease of the vulva.

Imaging
Initial approach
- CXR to evaluate for metastatic disease
- CT scan to evaluate pelvic and periaortic lymph node status

Diagnostic Procedures/Surgery
Office vulvar biopsy is done to establish the diagnosis.

Pathological Findings
A surgical staging system is used for vulvar cancer (International Federation of Obstetrics and Gynecology Classification):
- Stage I: Tumor confined to the vulva:
  – Stage IA: Lesions ≤2 cm in size, confined to the vulva or perineum, and with stromal invasion ≤1.0 mm, no node metastasis
  – Stage IB: Lesions >2 cm in size or with stromal invasion >1.0 mm, confined to the vulva or perineum, with negative nodes
- Stage II: Tumor of any size with extension to adjacent perineal structures (1/3 lower urethra, 1/3 lower vagina, anus) with negative nodes
- Stage III: Tumor of any size with or without extension to adjacent perineal structures (1/3 lower urethra, 1/3 lower vagina, anus) with positive inguino-femoral lymph nodes:
  – Stage IIIA:
    ○ (i) With 1 lymph node metastasis (≥5 mm), or
    ○ (ii) 1-2 lymph node metastasis(es) (<5 mm)
  – Stage IIIB:
    ○ (i) With 2 or more lymph node metastases (≥5 mm), or
    ○ (ii) 3 or more lymph node metastases (<5 mm)
  – Stage IIIC: With positive nodes with extracapsular spread
- Stage IV: Tumor invades other regional (2/3 upper urethra, 2/3 upper vagina), or distant structures
  – Stage IVA: Tumor invades any of the following:
    ○ (i) Upper urethral and/or vaginal mucosa, bladder mucosa, rectal mucosa, or fixed to pelvic bone or
    ○ (ii) Fixed or ulcerated inguino-femoral lymph nodes
  – Stage IVB: Any distant metastasis including pelvic lymph nodes

DIFFERENTIAL DIAGNOSIS
- The definitive diagnosis for vulvar lesions is made by biopsy. Infectious processes can present as ulcerative lesions and include syphilis, lymphogranuloma venereum, and granuloma inguinale.
- Crohn disease can present as an ulcerative area on the vulva.
- Rarely, lesions can metastasize to the vulva.

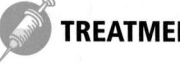 **TREATMENT**

There are no curative drugs.

MEDICATION
- As an adjuvant therapy, fluorouracil (Efudex) cream for in situ disease can produce occasional results but is not well tolerated because of irritation of the vulva. Adjuvant chemotherapy has not proven to be effective in this disease.
- Chemoradiotherapy with cisplatin and 5-fluorouracil has been successful in advanced or recurrent disease, although local morbidity is increased (2)[B].

- Metastatic disease, especially in the subcutaneous tissues of the leg or abdomen, will produce hypercalcemia.
- Contraindications: Elderly patients: If chemotherapeutic agents are used, pay close attention to the patient's performance status and ability to tolerate aggressive chemotherapy.
- Precautions: The usual precautions for chemotherapy agents. Refer to manufacturer's literature for each drug.

ADDITIONAL TREATMENT
General Measures
- Wide excision can be performed for carcinoma in situ, and any lesion about which there is doubt should be further excised for definitive diagnosis to ensure that invasive disease is not coexistent with the carcinoma in situ.
- Cystoscopy and sigmoidoscopy should be performed if there is a question of invasion into the urethra, bladder, or rectum.

Issues for Referral
Patients may need care from a gynecologic oncologist and/or a radiation oncologist.

Additional Therapies
- Radiation therapy is used as adjuvant therapy for patients with positive inguinal lymph nodes.
- Preoperative radiation/chemotherapy may allow for a less radical surgical procedure in patients with advanced disease (3,4)[B].
- Postoperative radiation as an adjuvant treatment decreases recurrence frequency and may improve survival (3)[B].
- Radiation is contraindicated with verrucous carcinoma because it induces anaplastic transformation and increases metastases.

SURGERY/OTHER PROCEDURES
- In situ disease can be treated with wide excision or laser vaporization of the affected area. Laser vaporization is preferable in the younger patient, whereas wide excision is preferable in the elderly patient, in whom the risk of invasive disease is also higher.
- 0.5 mm of negative margin is adequate for in situ disease (2)[C].
- Stage IA is treated with radical local excision without lymph node dissection because lymph node metastases are <1% (2)[C].
- Stage IB is treated with radical local excision with lymph node dissection because the risk of metastases increases to 8% (2)[C].
- Modified radical vulvectomy and groin node dissection are recommended for stage II (2)[C].
- Radical vulvectomy and bilateral inguinal lymph node dissection are recommended for stage III and stage IVA lesions (2)[C].
- Bulky advanced-staged lesions are often treated initially with chemoradiation followed by less radical surgery (4)[B].
- Adjuvant radiation therapy is recommended with microscopically positive lymph nodes (2)[C].
- Pelvic exenteration after radiation provides effective therapy for advanced or recurrent malignancies involving the bladder or rectum.

- More limited surgery:
  - Has been undertaken for early invasive lesions, especially in young patients, to preserve the clitoris and sexual function
  - Sentinel lymph node (SLN) biopsy also has been advocated in early invasive lesion, however, data show lower accuracy compared to complete dissection (5)[C].
  - Radical vulvectomy with bilateral groin node dissection through separate incisions provides better cosmetic results than the en bloc technique.
  - Radical hemivulvectomy and unilateral groin node dissection also can be used for smaller unilateral lesions.

IN-PATIENT CONSIDERATIONS
Typically inpatient for treatment

Initial Stabilization
In advanced malignancy involving the urethra and rectum, concomitant cisplatin/5-fluorouracil (5-FU) chemotherapy with radiation produces a significant decrease in size of the primary tumor, usually obviating the need for pelvic exenteration.

 ## ONGOING CARE

FOLLOW-UP RECOMMENDATIONS
Patient Monitoring
- Clinical exam of the groin nodes and vulvar area every 3 months for 2 years; then every 6 months for 3 years
- Annual CXR

DIET
Unrestricted, unless undergoing radiation

PATIENT EDUCATION
- American College of Obstetricians and Gynecologists (ACOG), 409 12th St., SW, Washington, DC 20024-2188; (800) 762-ACOG; http://www.acog.org
- American Cancer Society: http://www.cancer.org
- Medline Plus: http://www.nlm.nih.gov/medlineplus/vulvarcancer.html

PROGNOSIS
The 5-year survival is based on stage:
- Stage I: 78.5%
- Stage II: 58.8%
- Stage III: 43.2%
- Stage IV: 13.0%

COMPLICATIONS
- The major complications from radical vulvectomy and groin node dissection are:
  - Wound breakdown
  - Lymphocysts
  - Lymphedema
  - Urinary stress incontinence
  - Psychosexual consequences
- 2 common complications with radical vulvectomy and bilateral groin node dissection:
  - In the immediate postoperative period, ~50% of patients experience breakdown of the wound. This requires aggressive wound care by visiting nurses as often as twice a day. The wounds usually granulate and heal over a period of 6–10 weeks.

- ~15–20% of patients experience some form of mild-to-moderate lymphedema after the groin node dissection. These patients should be instructed in the use of leg elevation and support hose. <1% of patients experience severe, debilitating lymphedema.

REFERENCES
1. Smith JS, Backes DM, Hoots BE, et al. Human Papillomavirus Type-Distribution in Vulvar and Vaginal Cancers and Their Associated Precursors. *Obstet Gynecol.* 2009;113:917–24.
2. de Hullu JA, van der Zee AG. Surgery and radiotherapy in vulvar cancer. *Crit Rev Oncol Hematol.* 2006;60:38–58.
3. Montana GS. Carcinoma of the vulva: combined modality treatment. *Curr Treat Options Oncol.* 2004;5:85–95.
4. de Hullu JA, van der Avoort IA, Oonk MH, et al. Management of vulvar cancers. *Eur J Surg Oncol.* 2006.
5. Radziszewski J, Kowalewska M, Jedrzejczak T, et al. The accuracy of the sentinel lymph node concept in early stage squamous cell vulvar carcinoma. *Gynecol Oncol.* 2010;116:473–7.

ADDITIONAL READING
- CDC. Quadrivalent human papillomavirus vaccine: Recommendations of the advisory committee on immunization practices. *MMWR.* 2007;569(No.RR02).
- Crosbie EJ, Slade RJ, Ahmed AS, et al. The management of vulval cancer. *Cancer Treat Rev.* 2009;35:533–9.

 ## CODES

ICD9
184.4 Malignant neoplasm of vulva, unspecified

CLINICAL PEARLS
- 40% of vulvar cancers are attributable to oncogenic HPV. Therefore, HPV vaccination has the potential to decrease vulvar cancer by 1/3.
- Biopsy all suspicious or nonhealing vulvar lesions.

VULVOVAGINITIS, ESTROGEN DEFICIENT

Jennifer L. Savitski, MD
Michael P. Hopkins, MD, MEd
Eric L. Jenison, MD

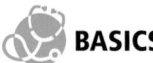 **BASICS**

DESCRIPTION
- Decreased blood flow with thinning and atrophy of the female genital tissues
- Changes from estrogen deficiency occur throughout the body; the genital tissues are especially hormone-responsive.
- Estrogen-deficient vulvovaginitis is often associated with urinary incontinence and increased urinary frequency.
- System(s) affected: Reproductive

EPIDEMIOLOGY
Incidence
- Predominant age: Postmenopausal females
  - The average age of menopause in the US is 51.3 years.
- Also may affect lactating women
- Predominant sex: Female only

Prevalence
- This disorder affects all postmenopausal women to some degree.
- 20% of postmenopausal women experience symptoms severe enough to seek treatment.

RISK FACTORS
Estrogen-deficient states

Genetics
No known pattern

PATHOPHYSIOLOGY
- Decreased estrogen levels in the vagina and vulva result in decreased blood flow, lubrication, vaginal and vulvar fullness, and mechanical sensitivity.
- Vaginal mucosa becomes thin secondary to decreased vaginal cell maturation.
- Decreased cellular maturation results in decreased glycogen stores, which affects the normal vaginal flora and pH.

ETIOLOGY
Estrogen deficiency due to
- Menopause (surgical or natural)
- Premature ovarian failure (chemotherapy, irradiation, autoimmune)
- Postpartum, lactation
- Medications that alter hormonal concentration such as gonadotropin-releasing hormone agonists and danazol

COMMONLY ASSOCIATED CONDITIONS
- Incontinence
- Pelvic organ prolapse
- Frequent urinary tract infections
- Bacterial vaginosis or yeast infections

 DIAGNOSIS

HISTORY
- Important to ask patient about symptoms because many women are embarrassed to discuss these issues with their health care providers.:
  - Vaginal dryness
  - Dyspareunia
  - Pruritus
  - Burning
  - Pressure
  - Tenderness
  - Malodorous discharge
  - Urinary symptoms: Dysuria, hematuria, frequency, infections, stress incontinence
- Ask about self-treatment and products used.
- Determine exposure to irritants (e.g., example, soaps, feminine sprays, lotions, etc.).
- Obese patients, especially those weighing >100 lb (45 kg) over ideal body weight, have higher levels of circulating estrogen and thus may have fewer symptoms.
  - Androstenedione is converted to estrone in peripheral adipose tissue.
  - When adipose tissue is abundant, higher estrone levels are present.

PHYSICAL EXAM
Evidence for the diagnosis includes the following (1)[C]:
- Decreased vulvar and vaginal fullness
- Decreased vaginal lubrication
- Pale-appearing vaginal and urethral mucosa
- Loss of vaginal rugation and decreased vulvar subcutaneous fat

DIAGNOSTIC TESTS & INTERPRETATION
Lab
Lab tests are generally unnecessary to make this clinical diagnosis. However, the following may be obtained as corroborative of clinical impression:
- Cytology for maturation index: Higher proportion of parabasal cells and lower proportion of intermediate and superficial cells indicate decreased maturation index.
- Vaginal pH usually >5
- Follicle-stimulating hormone levels are high, indicating low estrogen levels.
- Estradiol levels are low.
- Drugs that may alter lab results:
  - Estrogen therapy will alter the maturation index.
  - Digoxin has estrogen-like properties.
  - Tamoxifen may produce menopausal-type symptoms but also may act on genital tissues as a weak estrogen agonist. Symptoms may vary.
  - Drugs used to treat endometriosis or uterine bleeding, such as progestins, danazol, or gonadotropin-releasing hormone agonists, may produce a pseudomenopause, which is reversible.

Pathological Findings
- Thinning of the cornified squamous layer of both the vulva and the vagina
- Increased parabasal cells
- Compact underlying collagenous tissue

DIFFERENTIAL DIAGNOSIS
- Malignancy
- Vulvar dystrophies
- Bacterial or yeast vulvovaginitis

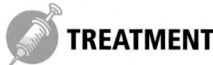 TREATMENT

MEDICATION

- Nonhormonal therapy includes water-soluble lubricants or vaginal moisturizers (1)[C].
- Vaginal estrogen can reverse atrophic changes and help to alleviate symptoms (2,3)[A]:
  - Vaginal cream (Premarin and other conjugated equine estrogens or estradiol cream): Insert via applicator each night × 14 days and then 2–3×/week.
  - Vaginal estradiol tablet: Insert via preloaded applicator each night × 14 days and then 2–3×/week
  - Estradiol-containing vaginal ring: Insert into vagina, and replace every 3 months.
  - Vaginal estrogen preparations rather than systemic preparations should be 1st-line therapy in a woman whose primary complaint is associated with vaginal atrophy (1)[C].
  - Progestin therapy or monitoring of endometrial status in a woman with an intact uterus is not necessary (1)[C].
- Estrogen therapy should be used in the lowest possible dose for the shortest duration of time.
- Long-term therapy may be necessary owing to the chronic nature of estrogen-deficient vulvovaginitis.
- Systemic therapy typically is used as hormonal treatment of vasomotor symptoms and not for the primary treatment of estrogen deficient vulvovaginitis.
- Contraindications:
  - Breast or estrogen-dependent carcinoma
  - Undiagnosed vaginal bleeding
  - Thromboembolic disorders
  - Thrombophlebitis
  - Pregnancy
- Precautions: Any abnormal vaginal bleeding must be evaluated.

ADDITIONAL TREATMENT
General Measures
- Wear loose-fitting, undyed cotton underwear.
- Avoid feminine deodorant sprays and products not intended for use in the genital area (e.g., hand lotion).
- Regular sexual activity can maintain vaginal health (1)[C].
- Use over-the-counter water-based lubricants as needed.
- Symptomatic relief if needed (e.g., cool baths or compresses)

IN-PATIENT CONSIDERATIONS
Initial Stabilization
Outpatient treatment

 ONGOING CARE

FOLLOW-UP RECOMMENDATIONS
No restriction

Patient Monitoring
The patient should be instructed that symptoms should improve within 30–60 days. If they do not, re-evaluation and re-examination for other causes should be undertaken.

DIET
No special diet

PATIENT EDUCATION
- American College of Obstetricians and Gynecologists (ACOG), 409 12th St., SW, Washington, DC 20024-2188; 1 (800) 762-ACOG; http://www.acog.org
- Lactating postpartum women with high levels of prolactin are in a hypoestrogenic state. These women should be instructed to use lubrication for symptoms of dyspareunia and reassured that the symptoms will resolve when they are no longer breast feeding.

PROGNOSIS
The prognosis is excellent. The vast majority of symptoms will be relieved with vaginal estrogen replacement therapy.

COMPLICATIONS
- Recurrent urinary tract infections may occur in women with vaginal atrophy.
- Treatment should include vaginal estrogen therapy (1)[C].

REFERENCES
1. Johnston S, et al. The detection and management of vaginal atrophy. *Int J Gynecol Obstet.* 2005;88:222–8.
2. Suckling J, et al. Local oestrogen for vaginal atrophy in postmenopausal women. *Cochrane Database Sys Rev.* 2006;4:CD001500.
3. Farquhar CM, et al. Long-term hormone therapy for perimenopausal and postmenopausal women. *Cochrane Database Sys Rev.* 2005;3:CD004143.

ADDITIONAL READING
Mehta A, Bachmann G. Vulvovaginal complaints. *Clin Obstet Gynecol.* 2008;51:549–55.

 CODES

ICD9
- 616.10 Vaginitis and vulvovaginitis, unspecified
- 627.3 Postmenopausal atrophic vaginitis

CLINICAL PEARLS
- Estrogen-deficient vulvovaginitis affects all postmenopausal women to some degree.
- This disorder is often associated with urinary incontinence and increased urinary frequency.
- Lab tests are generally unnecessary to make the diagnosis.
- Vaginal estrogen preparations, rather than systemic preparations, should be 1st-line therapy in a woman whose primary complaint is associated with vaginal atrophy.

V

VULVOVAGINITIS, PREPUBESCENT

Myrlene Jeudy, MD
Dawn S. Tasillo, MD

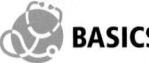 **BASICS**

DESCRIPTION
- Vulvitis is inflammation of the external genitals
- Vaginitis, often associated with vaginal discharge, is inflammation involving the vaginal mucosa
- In premenarchal girls, vulvitis is usually primary with secondary extension into the vagina.
- System(s) affected: Reproductive; Skin/Exocrine
- Synonym(s): Vaginitis; Vulvitis

EPIDEMIOLOGY
Incidence
Unknown
Prevalence
Most common gynecologic problem in prepubertal girls

RISK FACTORS
Prepubertal girls are particulary susceptible due to behavioral and anatomic reasons:
- Poor hygiene: Inadequate handwashing after urination and defecation
- Tight fitting clothing
- Proximity of the vagina to the anus, lack of protective hair and labial fat pads
- Trauma

Genetics
Understudied

GENERAL PREVENTION
- Good perineal hygiene (including wiping from front to back)
- Urination with legs spread apart and labia separated
- Avoidance of tight fitting clothing and nonabsorbent underwear
- Avoidance of irritants such as harsh soaps and bubble baths

PATHOPHYSIOLOGY
- In the prepubertal child, the levels of estrogen are low.
- Due to the low levels of estrogen, the vaginal epithelium is thin, immature, and fragile.
- The absence of pubic hair and a well-developed labia as well as close proximity of the anus and vagina make contamination more likely .
- The prepubertal child also has an absence of lactobacilli, thus creating a neutral to alkaline vaginal pH.
- The neutral pH, atrophic mucosa, and moist environment of the vagina increases the risk of infection.

ETIOLOGY
- Most cases of pediatric vulvovaginitis are nonspecific inflammation
- The specific infections that occur are typically respiratory, enteric, or sexually transmitted.

- Nonspecific vulvovaginitis:
  - Poor perineal hygiene
  - Nonspecific chemical irritants (bubble baths, scented soaps, shampoos)
  - Tight fitting clothing
- Specific vulvovaginitis:
  - The most common respiratory pathogen is *Streptococcus pyogenes*.
  - Shigella vaginitis is associated with mucopurulent bloody discharge and is not always accompanied by a history of diarrhea.

Respiratory	Enteral	Sexually Transmitted
Streptococcus pyogenes	*Shigella*	*Neisseria gonorrhoeae*
Staphylococcus aureus	*Yersinia enterocolitica*	*Chlamydia trachomatis*
Haemophilus influenzae		*Trichomonas vaginalis*
Moraxella catarrhalis		Papilloma virus
Streptococcus pneumoniae		Herpes virus
Neisseria meningitidis		

- Enterobius vermicularis (Pinworms)
  - Very common in young children and certain populations
  - Should be considered in children with vaginal itching and irritation
  - Most common symptom is nocturnal perineal itching
- Foreign body
  - Presents with foul-smelling, bloody, or brown discharge
  - Should be considered with recurrent vulvovaginitis where other causes have been eliminated
- Other
  - With chronic vulvovaginitis, anatomic abnormalities or systemic disease should be considered.
    ○ Anatomic abnormalities include double vagina with fistula, ectopic ureter, urethral prolapse.
  - Systemic disease (inflammatory diseases)
  - Other conditions such as lichen sclerosus, vitiligo, psoriasis, and atopic dermatitis should be considered.

ALERT
Cultures of sexually transmitted organisms in prepubertal children warrants investigation of sexual abuse.

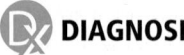 **DIAGNOSIS**

HISTORY
- Irritation and erythema of vulva
- Itching
- Bleeding
- Vaginal discharge
- Unpleasant odor
- Dysuria
- Soreness

PHYSICAL EXAM
- Excoriation of the genital area
- Inflammation of the introitus
- Look for evidence of chronic illness or dermatologic disease.
- Inspect the genital area in the supine position.
- Inspect the vagina and cervix in the knee-chest position.
- Rectal exam if vaginal bleeding or abdominal pain

DIAGNOSTIC TESTS & INTERPRETATION
Lab
Initial lab tests
- Culture for bacteria, fungi, or viruses
- Gram stain
- Tape exam for pinworms
- Potassium hydroxide and saline smears
Follow-Up & Special Considerations
Exploration of vagina for foreign body may be necessary in cases of persistent, recurrent vulvitis.

Imaging
- If anatomic abnormality is suspected, imaging may be necessary to confirm
- Consider consultation with pediatric or adult gynecologist to determine most appropriate imaging study

Diagnostic Procedures/Surgery
If blood or foul-smelling discharge is present, visualization is mandatory:
- Place child in knee-chest position for best result. Hold buttocks apart and slightly upward.
- Visualization of the vagina may be necessary using a nasal speculum or infant laryngoscope.
- If available, consider referral to a provider with specific training/experience in this specialized exam.

DIFFERENTIAL DIAGNOSIS
- Contact dermatitis
- Eczema
- Psoriasis
- *Shigella* vulvovaginitis
- Lichen sclerosus

TREATMENT

- Definitive diagnosis of bacterial vulvitis requires culture of vulva and vaginal secretions.
- Typical colony count and bacterial mix is unknown in prepubescent girls; thus antibiotic use should be directed against the species with the highest colony count.
- General hygiene always should be recommended, particularly in cases of retained foreign body (toilet paper).

MEDICATION

First Line

- For empirical treatment of suspected bacterial infection, amoxicillin 20 mg/kg/d × 7 d (1)
- Estrogen deficiency with labial adhesion/agglutination: Estrogen cream 0.625 mg/mL to fused area nightly × 2 wks (1)
- Specific organisms on culture:
  – Group A *Streptococcus*, *S. pneumoniae*: Penicillin V (Pen Vee K) 250 mg PO b.i.d–t.i.d. × 10 days (2)
  – *H. influenzae*: Amoxicillin 20–40 mg/kg/d PO × 7 days (2)
  – *S. aureus*: Cephalexin 25–50 mg/kg/d PO q.i.d. × 7–10 days *or* Dicloxacillin 25 mg/kg/d × 7–10 days or amoxicillin-clavulanate 20–40 mg/kg/d × 7–10 days (2)
  – *Candida* sp.: Topical nystatin (Mycostatin), miconazole, clotrimazole, or terconazole
  – *Shigella*: Trimethoprim/sulfamethoxazole or ampicillin × 5 d
  – Pinworms: Mebendazole 100 mg PO, repeated in 2wks
  – Chlamydia trachomatis: ≤45 kg Erythromycin 50 mg/kg/d t.i.d. × 14d ≥45 kg Azithromycin 1 g PO or Doxycycline 100 mg b.i.d. × 7d (2)
  – Neisseria gonorrhoeae: ≤45 kg Ceftriaxone 125 mg IM plus Rx for chlamydia if not ruled out (2)
  – Trichomonas: Metronidazole 15 mg/kg/d t.i.d. (max 250 mg t.i.d.) × 7 d (2)
- Contraindications: Allergy to proposed treatment
- Precautions: Avoid potential allergens and topical sensitizers if possible.

ADDITIONAL TREATMENT

General Measures

- Appropriate health care: Outpatient (except where systemic illness requires hospital care)
- Soak vulva/perineum in small amount of clear warm water for 15 minutes twice daily.

Issues for Referral

- Suspected sexual abuse
- Suspected anatomic abnormality (except minor labial agglutination)
- Persistent, severe, or recurrent infections

ONGOING CARE

FOLLOW-UP RECOMMENDATIONS

Patient Monitoring

Monitor for fever, pruritus, and vaginal discharge.

DIET

- Healthy balanced diet, high in fiber to prevent constipation
- Adequate fluid intake

PATIENT EDUCATION

Hygiene:

- Wipe front-to-back after elimination.
- Avoid bubble baths and other irritating products.
- Clean daily with mild soap and water and dry gently with soft towel or cool hair dryer.
- Apply bland ointments for protection of the skin, if necessary.

PROGNOSIS

Excellent

COMPLICATIONS

- If a sexually transmitted infection (STI) is identified and not treated effectively, the patient is at risk for pelvic inflammatory disease (PID).
- Vaginismus

REFERENCES

1. Sultan C, ed. Pediatric and adolescent gynecology: Evidence-based clinical practice. *Endocr Dev* 2004;7:1–8 [PMID: 15045783]
2. Emans JS. "*Vulvovaginal Problems in the Prepubertal Child*" *Pediatric & Adolescent Gynecology* 5th ed. Lippincott Williams & Wilkins; 2005:83–99.

ADDITIONAL READING

- Dei M, DiMaggio F, DiPaolo G, et al. Vulvovaginitis in childhood. *Best Practice & Research Clinical Obstetrics and Gynecology*. 2010;24:129–137.
- Farrington PF. Pediatric vulvo-vaginitis. *Clin Obstet Gynecol*. 1997;40:135–40.
- Fivozinsky KB, Laufer MR. Vulvar disorders in prepubescent girls. A literature review. *J Reprod Med*. 1998;43:763–73.
- Jasper JM, Ward MA. Shigella vulvovaginitis in a prepubertal child. *Pediatr Emerg Care*. 2006;22:585–6.
- Joishy M, et al. Do we need to treat vulvovaginitis in prepubertal girls? *Br Med J*. 2005;22:330(7484): 186–8.
- Kokotos F. Vulvovaginitis. *Pediatr Rev*. 2006;27: 116–7.
- Merkley K. Vulvovaginitis and vaginal discharge in the pediatric patient. *J Emerg Nurs*. 2005;31:400–2.
- Stricker T, Navratil F, Sennhauser FH. Vulvovaginitis in prepubertal girls. *Arch Dis Child*. 2003;88:324–6.
- Sticker T. Vulvovaginitis. *Pediatric and Child Health*. 2009;20:143–145.

CODES

ICD9

616.10 Vaginitis and vulvovaginitis, unspecified

CLINICAL PEARLS

- Vulvovaginitis is the most common gynecologic problem in prepubescent girls.
- The hypoestrogenic state and prepubescent anatomy may increase susceptibility to vulvar and vaginal infection.
- Isolating an infection with known sexual transmission should prompt further investigation.
- Recurrent or persistent vulvitis, especially in the setting of foul-smelling discharge, should prompt skilled exam of the vagina for retained foreign body.

V

WARTS

Herbert P. Goodheart, MD

 BASICS

DESCRIPTION

- Verrucae vulgaris (common warts) are benign growths that are confined to the epidermis, caused by the human papillomavirus. Common warts are most often found at sites subject to frequent trauma, such as the hands and feet. Warts often vary widely in shape, size, and appearance, and the different names for them generally reflect their clinical appearance, location, or both. For example, filiform warts are threadlike, planar warts are flat, and plantar warts are located on the soles of the feet. Common warts are predominantly seen in children and young adults. An estimated 20% of school-aged children will at some time have at least 1 wart. HIV/AIDS, other immunosuppressive diseases (e.g., lymphomas), immunosuppressive drugs that decrease cell-mediated immunity (e.g., prednisone, cyclosporine, and chemotherapeutic agents), pregnancy, and handling of raw meat or fish in one's occupation (e.g., butchers) are all risk factors for becoming infected.
- Warts (verrucae) are benign growths that are confined to the epidermis. They can appear on any area of the skin or mucous membranes. All warts are caused by the human papillomavirus (HPV).
- Warts vary widely in shape, size, and appearance, as reflected by their descriptive names, which generally reflect the appearance, location, or both. For example, filiform warts are threadlike; planar warts are flat, and plantar warts are located on the soles of the feet.
- Genital warts, or condyloma acuminatum, may be large and cauliflowerlike, or they may consist of small papules.
- Clinically, warts are described as:
  – Common wart (verruca vulgaris)
  – Plantar wart (verruca plantaris)
  – Flat wart (verruca plana)
  – Venereal wart (condyloma acuminatum)
  – Epidermodysplasia verruciformis is a very rare, lifelong hereditary disorder characterized by chronic infection with HPV.
- System(s) affected: Skin/Exocrine

EPIDEMIOLOGY

Incidence
- An estimated 20% of school-aged children will at some time have at least 1 wart.
- Predominant age: Young adults and children
- Predominant sex: Female = Male

Prevalence
- ~7–10% of the US population
- Common warts appear ~2 times as frequently in whites as in blacks or Asians.

RISK FACTORS
- AIDS and other immunosuppressive diseases (e.g., lymphomas)
- Immunosuppressive drugs that decrease cell-mediated immunity (e.g., prednisone, cyclosporine, and chemotherapeutic agents)
- Pregnancy
- Handling raw meat, fish, or other types of animal matter in one's occupation (e.g., butchers)

ETIOLOGY
- HPV is a double-stranded, circular, supercoiled DNA virus.
- The virus infects epidermal keratinocytes, which stimulates cell proliferation.
- Various strains of a DNA HPV: To date, >150 different subtypes have been identified.
- Common warts: HPV types 2 and 4 (most common), followed by types 1, 3, 27, 29, and 57
- Palmoplantar warts: HPV type 1 (most common), followed by types 2, 3, 4, 27, 29, and 57
- Flat warts: HPV types 3, 10, and 28
- Butcher warts: HPV type 7
- The virus is passed primarily through skin-to-skin contact or from the recently shed virus kept intact in a moist, warm environment.

 DIAGNOSIS

- Most often made on clinical appearance
- Skin biopsy, if necessary

HISTORY
Warts may develop anywhere on the body, but they are found most often at sites subject to frequent trauma, such as the hands and feet.

PHYSICAL EXAM
- Distribution is generally asymmetric, and lesions are often clustered or may appear in a linear configuration due to scratching (pseudo-Koebner reaction).
- Common wart: Rough-surfaced, hyperkeratotic, papillomatous, raised, skin-colored to tan papules 5–10 mm in diameter; may coalesce into a mosaic 1–3 cm in diameter; most frequently seen on hands, knees, and elbows; usually asymptomatic but may cause cosmetic disfigurement or tenderness
- Filiform warts: These are long, slender, delicate, fingerlike growths, usually seen on the face around the lips, eyelids, or nares.
- Plantar warts appear on the plantar surface of the feet in children and young adults:
  – Can be tender and painful, and extensive involvement on the sole of the foot may impair ambulation, particularly when present on a weight-bearing surface.
  – Most often seen on the metatarsal area, heels, and toes in an asymmetric distribution
  – Frequently attain 2–3 cm in diameter
  – Pathognomonic "black dots" (thrombosed dermal capillaries); punctate bleeding becomes more evident after paring with a no. 15 blade.
  – Both common and plantar warts generally demonstrate the following clinical findings:
    ○ A loss of normal skin markings (dermatoglyphics) such as finger, foot, and hand prints
    ○ Lesions may be solitary or multiple, or they may appear in clusters (mosaic warts).
- Flat wart: Slightly elevated, flat-topped, skin-colored or tan papules, small (1–3 mm) in diameter
  – Commonly found on the face, arms, dorsa of hands, shins (women)
  – Sometimes exhibit a linear configuration caused by autoinoculation
  – In men, shaving spreads flat warts.
  – In women, they often occur on the shins, where leg shaving spreads lesions.

- Epidermodysplasia verruciformis (rare): Widespread flat, reddish brown pigmented papules and plaques that present in childhood with lifelong persistence on the trunk, hands, upper and lower extremities, and face are characteristic.

DIAGNOSTIC TESTS & INTERPRETATION
Diagnosis

Lab
- HPV cannot be cultured, and lab testing is rarely necessary.
- Definitive HPV diagnosis can be achieved by:
  – Electron microscopy
  – Viral DNA identification employing Southern blot hybridization used to identify the specific HPV type present in tissue
  – Polymerase chain reaction may be used to amplify viral DNA for testing.

Imaging
Follow-Up & Special Considerations
Skin biopsy if unusual presentation or if diagnosis is unclear

Pathological Findings
- Histopathologic features of common warts include digitated epidermal hyperplasia, acanthosis, papillomatosis, compact orthokeratosis, hypergranulosis, dilated tortuous capillaries within the dermal papillae, and vertical tiers of parakeratotic cells with entrapped red blood cells above the tips of the digitations.
- In the granular layer, HPV-infected cells may have coarse keratohyaline granules and vacuoles surrounding wrinkled-appearing nuclei. These koilocytic (vacuolated) cells are pathognomonic for warts.

DIFFERENTIAL DIAGNOSIS
- Molluscum contagiosum
- Seborrheic keratosis
- Acrochordon (skin tag)
- Solar keratosis and cutaneous horn
- Squamous cell carcinoma (SCC)
- Keratoacanthoma
- Subungual SCC can easily be misdiagnosed as a subungual wart or onychomycosis.
- Plantar warts
- Corns (clavi) are sometimes difficult to distinguish from warts. Like calluses, corns are thickened areas of the skin and most commonly develop at sites subjected to repeated friction and pressure, such as the tops and the tips of toes and along the sides of the feet:
  – They are usually hard and circular, with a polished or central translucent core, like the kernel of corn, from which they take their name.
  – Corns do not have "black dots," and skin markings are retained except for the area of the central core.

ALERT
- A melanoma on the plantar surface of the foot can mimic a wart.
- Verrucous carcinoma, a slow-growing, locally invasive, well-differentiated squamous cell carcinoma, also may be easily mistaken for a common or plantar wart.

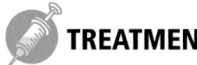
TREATMENT

Benign neglect: Since most warts in children tend to regress spontaneously within 2 years (1)

MEDICATION
First Line
- Self-administered topical therapy: Keratolytic (peeling) agents: The affected area(s) should be hydrated 1st by soaking in warm water for 5 minutes before application. Most over-the-counter agents contain salicylic acid and/or lactic acid; agents such as Duofilm, Occlusal-HP, Trans-Ver-Sal, and Mediplast (2).
- Office-based and self-administered prescription treatment:
  – Cantharidin, an extract that causes epidermal necrosis and blistering
  – Combination cantharidin: 30% salicylic acid, 2% podophyllin, and 19% cantharidin in flexible collodion; applied in a thin coat, occluded 4–6 hours, then washed off
  – Imiquimod (Aldara) 5% cream, a local inducer of interferon, is applied at home by the patient. It is approved for external genital and perianal warts, and is used off-label and applied to warts under duct-tape occlusion; applied at bedtime and washed off after 6–10 hours.
  – Aldara is applied to flat warts without occlusion.
  – Topical retinoids for flat warts

Second Line
- Immunotherapy: Induction of delayed-type hypersensitivity with:
  – Diphencyclopropenone
  – Dinitrochlorobenzene
  – Squaric acid dibutylester: There is possible mutagenicity and side effects with this agent.
- Intralesional injections:
  – Mumps or *Candida* antigen
  – Bleomycin: Intradermal injection is expensive and causes severe pain.
  – Interferon-α-2
- Oral therapy:
  – Oral high-dose cimetidine: Possibly works better in children (3)
  – Acitretin (an oral retinoid)
- Other treatments (all have all been used with varying results):
  – Dichloroacetic acid, trichloroacetic acid, podophyllin, formic acid, aminolevulinic acid in combination with blue light, 5-fluorouracil, silver nitrate, formaldehyde, levamisole, topical or IV cidofovir for recalcitrant warts in the setting of HIV, and glutaraldehyde

ADDITIONAL TREATMENT
General Measures
- There is no ideal treatment.
- In children, most warts tend to regress spontaneously.
- In many adults and immunocompromised patients, warts are often difficult to eradicate.
- Painful, aggressive therapy should be avoided unless there is a need to eliminate the wart(s).
- For surgical procedures, especially in anxious children, pretreatment with anesthetic cream such as EMLA (emulsion of lidocaine and prilocaine)

COMPLEMENTARY AND ALTERNATIVE MEDICINE
- Duct tape: Cover wart with waterproof tape (e.g., duct tape). Leave the tape on for 6 days; then soak, pare with emery board, and leave uncovered overnight; then reapply tape cyclically for 8 cycles; 85% resolved compared with 60% efficacy with cryotherapy (4,5).
- Hyperthermia: Safe and inexpensive approach; immerse affected area into 45°C water bath for 30 minutes 3× per week
- Hypnotherapy (6)

Pregnancy Considerations
The use of some topical chemical approaches may be contraindicated during pregnancy or in women who are likely to become pregnant during the treatment period.

SURGERY/OTHER PROCEDURES
- Cryotherapy with liquid nitrogen (LN_2) may be applied with a cotton swab or with a cryotherapy gun (Cryogun) (6):
  – Best for warts on hands
  – Fast; can treat many lesions per visit
  – Painful; not tolerated well by young children
  – Freezing periungual warts may result in nail deformation.
  – In darkly pigmented skin, treatment can result in hypo- or hyperpigmentation.
- Light electrocautery ± curettage:
  – Best for warts on the knees, elbows, and dorsa of hands
  – Also good for filiform warts
  – Tolerable in most adults
  – Requires local anesthesia
  – May cause scarring
- Photodynamic therapy
- CO_2 or pulse-dye laser ablation: Expensive and requires local anesthesia
- For filiform warts: An almost painless method: Dip hemostat into LN_2 for 10 seconds, and then grasp the wart for 10 seconds. Wart sheds in 7–10 days.

ONGOING CARE

FOLLOW-UP RECOMMENDATIONS
Patient Monitoring
1/3 of the warts of epidermodysplasia may become malignant.

PROGNOSIS
- More often than not (especially in children), warts tend to "cure" themselves over time.
- Rarely, certain types of lesions may transform into carcinomas.

COMPLICATIONS
- Autoinoculation (pseudo-Koebner reaction)
- Scar formation
- Chronic pain after plantar wart removal or scar formation
- Nail deformity after injury to nail matrix

REFERENCES

1. Harwood CA, Perrett CM, Brown VL, et al. Imiquimod cream 5% for recalcitrant cutaneous warts in immunosuppressed individuals. *Br J Dermatol*. 2005;152:122–9.
2. Gibbs S, Harvey I. Topical treatments for cutaneous warts. *Cochrane Database of Systematic Reviews* 2006, Issue 3. Art. No.: CD001781. DOI:10.1002/14651858.CD001781.pub2.
3. Rogers CJ, Gibney MD, Siegfried EC, et al. Cimetidine therapy for recalcitrant warts in adults: is it any better than placebo? *J Am Acad Dermatol*. 1999;41:123–7.
4. de Haen M, Spigt MG, van Uden CJ, et al. Efficacy of duct tape vs placebo in the treatment of verruca vulgaris (warts) in primary school children. *Arch Pediatr Adolesc Med*. 2006;160:1121–5.
5. Wenner R, Askari SK, Cham PM, et al. Duct tape for the treatment of common warts in adults: a double-blind randomized controlled trial. *Arch Dermatol*. 2007;143:309–13.
6. Keogh-Brown MR, Fordham RJ, Thomas KS, et al. To freeze or not to freeze: a cost-effectiveness analysis of wart treatment. *Br J Dermatol*. 2007;156:687–92.

ADDITIONAL READING

Ewin DM, et al. Hypnotherapy for warts (verruca vulgaris): 41 consecutive cases with 33 cures. *Am J Clin Hypn*. 1992;35:1–10.

CODES

ICD9
- 078.10 Viral warts, unspecified
- 078.11 Condyloma acuminatum
- 078.12 Plantar wart

CLINICAL PEARLS

- No single therapy for warts is uniformly effective or superior; thus treatment involves a certain amount of trial and error.
- Conservative, nonscarring treatments are preferred.
- Freezing and other destructive treatment modalities do not kill the virus but merely destroy the cells that harbor HPV.
- Because HPV persists after therapy, some degree of infectivity and the potential for recurrence may remain, even in the absence of clinical lesions.
- Hemostat into LN_2 for 10 seconds then gently grasp the wart for 10 seconds

WARTS, PLANTAR

Kaelen C. Dunican, PharmD, RPh
Robert A. Baldor, MD

BASICS

DESCRIPTION
- Form of cutaneous wart caused by the human papillomavirus (HPV)
- Appears as discrete or grouped firm keratotic masses on the plantar surface of the foot, usually at pressure points such as the heel, forefoot, or under toes
- System(s) affected: Skin/Exocrine
- Synonym(s): Verruca plantaris

EPIDEMIOLOGY
Incidence
- In the US: Widespread: Estimated 2% of population
- Predominant age: Any age, although more common in children and young adults
- Predominant sex: Female > Male (slightly)

Prevalence
Cutaneous warts are estimated to occur in about 7–10% of the population.

RISK FACTORS
- Immunosuppression, including HIV/AIDS, lymphomas, use of immunosuppressive drugs
- Use of public facilities while barefoot, such as gyms and swimming pools
- Previous wart infection

GENERAL PREVENTION
- Use rubber footwear in communal shower areas.
- Once infected, maintain proper foot hygiene (see Patient Education).

ETIOLOGY
- Infection with HPV, a double-stranded DNA virus, results in proliferation of epidermal keratinocytes.
- Most common cause is HPV subtypes 1, 2, 4, 27, and 57
- Transmitted by direct person-to-person contact or via fomites
- Minor trauma to the skin and maceration may facilitate transmission of the virus to basal keratinocytes.
- Autoinoculation can occur.

DIAGNOSIS

Most often made on clinical appearance (1)[C]

HISTORY
- Complaints of thickened skin on sole of foot
- May be painless, depending on location
- May cause leg or back pain (distortion of posture)

PHYSICAL EXAM
- Discrete or grouped keratotic lesions on sole of foot with disruption of normal skin markings
- Rough, hyperkeratotic surface with brown–black dots (thrombosed capillaries): May bleed when pared down; helps to distinguish warts from corns or calluses
- Callus formation surrounding wart core
- Generally occur at pressure points
- Moderate discomfort to severe pain with deep penetration
- Many warts may coalesce to form "mosaic warts."

DIAGNOSTIC TESTS & INTERPRETATION
Diagnostic Procedures/Surgery
- Inspection usually confirms the diagnosis.
- If cannot distinguish between callus and wart, examine with a magnifying lens. The wart should demonstrate a highly organized mosaic pattern.
- When pared down, warts have a soft central core and bleeding points (unlike calluses).

Pathological Findings
Acanthotic epidermis with hyperkeratosis, papillomatosis, and parakeratosis

DIFFERENTIAL DIAGNOSIS
- Corns (clavi)
- Calluses
- Black heel (ruptured capillaries)
- Lichen planus
- Epidermal nevus
- Molluscum contagiosum
- Squamous cell carcinoma

TREATMENT

MEDICATION
- No universally effective agent or cure exists.
- Topical salicylic acid therapy has the best evidence available (1,2)[A].

First Line
Salicylic acid: Pooled efficacy 73% (1)[A]:
- Available over the counter (OTC) as 17% liquid in a flexible collodion base (Compound W, Occlusal-HP), 15% patch (Trans-Ver-Sal), and 40% salicylic acid plasters/patches (Mediplast, Duofilm)
- Prior to each application, the wart should be soaked in warm water and pared down with an emery board or pumice stone.
- Patches/plasters: Supplied in various size sheets/pads, which are cut to the size of the wart, and the sticky surface is applied to the wart. They are removed every 1–2 days, the white keratin is peeled, and a fresh plaster is applied.
- Liquids: Apply a few drops directly to the wart daily. Applying a ring of petrolatum to the skin around the wart will protect the healthy skin tissue.
- May require weeks to months of treatment
- Side effects: Minor skin irritation, contact dermatitis
- Precautions: Poor circulation, peripheral neuropathy

Second Line
- Cryotherapy and pulse dye laser therapy are appropriate as 2nd line (2,3)[A] (see Surgery/Other Procedures).
- Intralesional immunotherapy with *Candida* skin test antigen can be used as 2nd-line therapy (2)[B]:
  – Injected every 3 weeks until cleared or a total of 3 treatments
  – Side effects: Pain and itching at injection site, flulike symptoms
- 3rd-line: Bleomycin (Blenoxane) injected into wart every 3–4 weeks until cleared; inconsistent evidence (2)[B]:
  – Dosing: 0.2 unit injected under the base of the wart, or 0.001 unit multiple punctures with bifurcated needle, or drops applied directly to the wart then pricked into the wart using a fine needle
  – Side effects: Injection-site burning and pain (may be severe), erythema, scarring, change in pigmentation
  – Contraindications: Pregnancy, children, immunosuppressed patients, and patients with vascular disease

- Imiquimod (Aldara) 5% cream: Apply daily after soaking. It may be more effective when occluded and when in combination with other treatments such as cryotherapy or keratolytics. (Insufficient evidence to recommend at this time (2)[B]; reserved for recalcitrant wart.)
- Cimetidine: 20–40 mg/kg orally daily may be effective in children (4)[C].

ADDITIONAL TREATMENT
General Measures
- If warts are asymptomatic, no treatment is necessary, and may be an option for patients to consider; however, patient may be at risk for spread of warts.
- Warm soaks followed by patient's paring of the top layer of skin on repeated occasions may speed disappearance.
- Patient may use pumice stone, emery board, or a blade to pare down the wart.
- Use of a heel bar or appropriate padding to relieve pressure points where warts tend to aggregate

Additional Therapies
Hyperthermia: Hot water immersion (113°F) 1/2–3/4 h 2–3×/week × 16 treatments is effective for some patients.

COMPLEMENTARY AND ALTERNATIVE MEDICINE
Duct tape: Cut a piece to the size of the wart and apply continuously for 6 days, remove, pare the wart, and then repeat for up to 2 months (3,5)[C].

SURGERY/OTHER PROCEDURES
- Cryotherapy:
  – Liquid nitrogen or dimethyl ether and propane (Wartner OTC)
  – The wart is frozen for 10–30 s until a 1- to 2-mm halo surrounds the wart; repeated every 2–3 weeks.
  – It usually requires at least 4 applications at weekly or biweekly intervals.
  – Aggressive cryotherapy may cause blistering or even scarring; light applications with 2 freeze–thaw cycles and paring are preferred.
  – Side effects: Prolonged pain, scarring, hypo- or hyperpigmentation, tendon or nerve damage (with aggressive therapy)
  – Caution: When treating patients with poor circulation
- Pulse dye laser (vascular lesion laser) therapy:
  – Repeated 2–3 times
  – Side effects: Pain, scarring, discoloration lasting 10–14 days
- Blunt dissection: A simple surgical procedure is effective and usually nonscarring. It requires inserting a blunt dissector between the wart and normal skin and separating the wart using a short, firm stroke.

- Carbon dioxide laser surgery: Used for recalcitrant warts
- Chemotherapy with trichloroacetic acid: Callus is pared, and the surrounding skin is protected by a ring of petrolatum. The wart(s) are coated with acid, which then is worked into the wart with a sharp toothpick. Procedure should be repeated at weekly intervals.
- Other:
  – Podophyllin: 25% solution; apply to wart 3–5×/day.
  – 5-fluorouracil (5-FU) 5% topical cream applied twice daily with occlusion
  – Formaldehyde soaks
- Combination therapies: Salicylic acid plus imiquimod ± cryotherapy

 ONGOING CARE

FOLLOW-UP RECOMMENDATIONS
Patient Monitoring
With any treatment modality, follow up weekly until resolution (return of normal dermatoglyphics).

PATIENT EDUCATION
- Review treatment regimen, including proper application and persistence (it may take weeks to months for resolution).
- Prevent spread to others and autoinoculation:
  – Wear footwear or cover securely before walking barefoot.
  – Wash socks and towels that may have come in contact with the wart in hot water.
  – Wash hands before and after treating/touching wart.
- Web sites for patient information:
  – American Podiatric Medical Association: http://www.apma.org/s_apma/doc.asp?cid=146&did=9430
  – Mayo Clinic: http://www.mayoclinic.com

PROGNOSIS
The course of plantar warts is like that of other varieties of warts (i.e., highly variable). Most resolve spontaneously in weeks to months.

COMPLICATIONS
- Scarring with overly aggressive treatment
- Leg and back pain
- Warts can cause considerable morbidity at times and significantly affect quality of life.
- A rare type of verrucous carcinoma, epithelioma cuniculatum, is thought to arise from these warts.

REFERENCES
1. Gibbs S, Harvey I. Topical treatments for cutaneous warts. *Cochrane Database Syst Rev*. 2006:3.
2. Bacelieri R, Johnson SM. Cutaneous warts: an evidence-based approach to therapy. *Am Fam Physician*. 2005;72:647–52.
3. Lipke MM. An armamentarium of wart treatments. *Clin Med Res*. 2006;4:273–93.
4. Paquette D, Rothe MJ. Unapproved dermatologic indications for H2 receptor antagonists, cromolyn sodium, and ketotifen. *Clin Dermatol*. 2000;18:103–11.
5. Focht DR, et al. The efficacy of duct tape vs. cryotherapy in the treatment of verruca vulgaris. *Arch Pediatr Adolesc Med*. 2002;156:971–4.

ADDITIONAL READING
- Ciconte A, Campbell J, Tabrizi S, et al. Warts are not merely blemished on the skin: a study of the morbidity associated with having viral cutaneous warts. *Aus J Derm*. 2003;44:169–75.
- Keogh-Brown MR, Fordham RJ, Thomas MO, et al. To freeze or not to freeze: a cost-effectiveness analysis of wart treatment. *Br J Dermatol*. 2007;156:687–92.

See Also (Topic, Algorithm, Electronic Media Element)
Condyloma Acuminata; Warts

CODES

ICD9
078.12 Plantar wart

CLINICAL PEARLS
- If the wart is painless, therapy is not necessary. Most untreated warts will resolve spontaneously in a few weeks to months, although they can last for years.
- Treating plantar warts requires diligence with proper application and adherence to the treatment regimen.
- Salicylic acid is the least expensive pharmacotherapeutic option and appears to be the most effective.
- To reduce pain, care should be taken to avoid excessive contact with normal skin when using keratolytics or chemotherapy.
- Proper foot hygiene is key to preventing transmission.

WILMS TUMOR

Timothy L. Black, MD

 BASICS

DESCRIPTION
- An embryonal renal neoplasm containing blastema, stromal, or epithelial cell types, usually affecting children <5 years of age
- Staging: In US, National Wilms Tumor Study Group (NWTSG) staging is done pretreatment based on radiographic imaging and surgery, whereas in Europe/Asia, Société Internationale d'Oncologie Pédiatrique (SIOP) staging is done *after* neoadjuvant chemotherapy is administered (1):
  - I: Tumor limited to kidney; completely excised
  - II: Tumor extends beyond kidney; completely excised
  - III: Residual nonhematogenous tumor confined to abdomen (lymph nodes positive, spillage of tumor, peritoneal implants, extension beyond resection region)
  - IV: Hematogenous metastases
  - V: Bilateral renal involvement
- System(s) affected: Renal/Urologic
- Synonym(s): Nephroblastoma

Pediatric Considerations
- Occurs only in children
- Most common renal malignancy in childhood

EPIDEMIOLOGY
Incidence
- Frequency rarer in East Asian populations than whites
- Frequency higher in black children than in whites
- Predominant age: Median age of 36.5 months
- Predominant sex: Female > Male (1.1:1)
- Represents 6-7% of all childhood cancers:
  - More than 80% are diagnosed before 5 years of age (median age is 3.5 yr at diagnosis).

Prevalence
US: 0.69/100,000; 7.6 cases/1 million children <15 years

RISK FACTORS
- Familial occurrence (1–2%):
  - These patients tend to have earlier age of onset.
  - Familial patients have greater risk of bilateral disease.
- Paternal occupation (see Etiology)

Genetics
- Several congenital anomalies are known to be associated with Wilms tumor. A 2-stage mutational model has been proposed: Occurrence in either hereditary form or sporadic form. Patients with aniridia have a deletion of the short arm of chromosome 11 (11p13).
- Abnormalities of chromosome 11 at the 11p15 locus are associated with Beckwith-Wiedemann syndrome.
- Wilms tumor-suppressor gene (*WT1*) has been identified, as well as additional candidates for another suppressor gene (*WT2*).
- Chromosome band 17q12–21 has been linked to 2 kindreds with Wilms tumor, and other kindreds are associated with a Wilms tumor predisposition gene at 19q13.3–q13.4.
- Loss of heterozygosity at chromosomes 16q and 1p is associated with adverse outcome (1)[C].

GENERAL PREVENTION
Routine surveillance in patients with syndromes associated with Wilms tumor (see Commonly Associated Conditions)

ETIOLOGY
- Hereditary or sporadic forms of genetic mutation
- Familial form: Autosomal dominant trait with incomplete penetrance (1%)
- Potential of paternal occupational exposure (machinists, welders, motor vehicle mechanics, auto body repairmen)

COMMONLY ASSOCIATED CONDITIONS
- Aniridia (partial or complete absence of iris) 600× > normal risk
- Hemihypertrophy (100× > normal risk)
- Cryptorchidism
- Hypospadias
- Duplicated renal collecting systems
- Wiedemann-Beckwith syndrome
- Denys-Drash syndrome (nephropathy, renal failure, male pseudohermaphroditism, Wilms tumor)
- Klippel-Trénaunay syndrome
- WAGR complex (Wilms tumor, aniridia, genitourinary malformations, and mental retardation)
- Beckwith-Wiedemann syndrome (visceromegaly, macroglossia, omphalocele, hyperinsulinemic hypoglycemia)

 DIAGNOSIS

- Symptoms of pain, anorexia, vomiting, malaise in 30% (1)[C]
- Over 90% present with asymptomatic abdominal mass (2)[B].

HISTORY
- History of increasing abdominal size
- Usually asymptomatic

PHYSICAL EXAM
- Palpable upper abdominal mass
- Abdominal pain
- Fever
- Anemia
- Rarely, signs of acute abdomen with free intraperitoneal rupture
- Cardiac murmur
- Hepatosplenomegaly
- Ascites
- Prominent abdominal wall veins
- Varicocele
- Gonadal metastases
- Aniridia (present in 1.1% of Wilm's tumor patients)
- Hypertension (20–65%) (1)[C]

DIAGNOSTIC TESTS & INTERPRETATION
Lab
- Urinalysis (occasional hematuria, proteinuria)
- Complete blood count (CBC) (anemia)
- Lactate dehydrogenase
- Plasma renin (rarely helpful)
- Urine catecholamines
- Serum creatinine and calcium
- Coagulation factors

Imaging
- Chest radiograph
- Kidney, ureter, and bladder (presence of linear calcifications)
- Abdominal ultrasound (with Doppler imaging): Gives best information about tumor extension into inferior vena cava
- Computed tomography (CT) scan (with IV and oral contrast material) of chest and abdomen (12–15% have lung metastases at diagnosis) (1)
- IV pyelogram rarely helpful

Diagnostic Procedures/Surgery
Occasionally, bone marrow aspiration necessary to distinguish from neuroblastoma

Pathological Findings
- Favorable findings (mortality of 7%):
  - Bulky lesion, well encapsulated
  - Focal areas of hemorrhage and necrosis
  - Absence of anaplasia and sarcomatous cell types
  - Presence of blastema, stomal, and epithelial elements (2)[B]:
    - Predominance of epithelial elements usually are less aggressive when diagnosed early, but tend to be resistant to treatment when diagnosed late
    - Predominance of blastemal elements indicate more aggressive tumors
- Unfavorable histology (mortality rate of 57%):
  - Anaplasia: Markedly enlarged and multipolar mitotic figures, 3-fold enlargement of nuclei in comparison with adjacent similar nuclei, hyperchromasia of enlarged nuclei; anaplasia may be diffuse or focal
  - Sarcomatous changes: Now considered to be separate from Wilms, not subtypes (mortality 64%)
  - Rhabdoid tumor of the kidney: Now considered to be separate tumor from Wilms
- Nephroblastomatosis: Considered premalignant
- Nephrogenic rests (2)[B]:
  - These are precursor lesions found in 25–40% of Wilms
  - Found in 1% of infants at autopsy, but most do not develop into malignancy

DIFFERENTIAL DIAGNOSIS
- Neuroblastoma
- Hepatic tumor
- Sarcoma
- Rhabdoid tumor
- Cystic nephroma
- Mesoblastic nephroma
- Renal cell carcinoma (generally occurs in older children)

 TREATMENT

MEDICATION
First Line
- Dactinomycin (Actinomycin-D)
- Vincristine
- Doxorubicin
- Cyclophosphamide (Cytoxan)
- Iphosphamide
- Etoposide

Second Line
- Doxorubicin (Adriamycin)
- Cyclophosphamide

ADDITIONAL TREATMENT
General Measures
- Appropriate health care: Inpatient workup and treatment until stable postoperative and induction chemotherapy completed
- Chemotherapy
- Radiation therapy in stage II (unfavorable histology), stage III, and stage IV

Issues for Referral
Surgical complications have been found to be significantly higher if the radical nephrectomy is done by a general surgeon rather than a pediatric surgeon or a pediatric urologist (3)[B].

COMPLEMENTARY AND ALTERNATIVE MEDICINE
SIOP recommends pretreatment with neoadjuvant chemotherapy based on radiographic studies and, on occasion, needle biopsy (1):
- May decrease incidence of intraoperative tumor rupture (this is debated)
- May result in inappropriate treatment with chemotherapeutic agents of non-Wilms tumors (5%) or benign lesions (1.6%)
- Results in the inability to directly compare treatment results worldwide

SURGERY/OTHER PROCEDURES
- Exam (visual and manual) of contralateral kidney
- Radical nephroureterectomy and biopsies as needed to provide precise staging information
- Sampling of any enlarged lymph nodes (absence of any lymph nodes in the surgical specimen mandates treatment as stage III disease) (2)[B]
- Identification of any retained tumor with titanium clips
- Tumor should be given to pathologist fresh, not in formalin.
- Vertical midline incision if tumor extension to right atrium present (possible use of cardiopulmonary bypass)
- Bilateral Wilms tumors (represent 4–6% of Wilms) (2)[B]:
  - Preoperative chemotherapy with reevaluation by CT or magnetic resonance imaging after 6 weeks (some are biopsied prior to chemotherapy)
  - Renal sparing operation at 6 weeks if good response to chemotherapy:
    ○ Partial nephrectomy or wedge excision of tumor preferred but only if it does not compromise tumor resection
    ○ Kidney with lowest tumor burden is addressed first. If successful resection accomplished, radical nephrectomy can be done on the contralateral kidney. Bilateral partial nephrectomy may be possible in some cases.
- Preoperative treatment also generally is accepted in a solitary kidney, horseshoe kidneys, intravascular extension of tumor above the intrahepatic vena cava, and in the case of respiratory distress from extensive metastatic tumor.

 ONGOING CARE

FOLLOW-UP RECOMMENDATIONS
Patient Monitoring
- Multidrug chemotherapy every 3–4 weeks for 16 weeks–15 months depending on stage
- Every 4 months for 1 year, every 6 months for 2nd–3rd year, yearly after that
- CBC, CT of chest and abdomen with each visit
- Patients at high risk for developing Wilms tumor should be monitored with renal ultrasound (US) every 3–4 months until 5 years of age. Patients with Beckwith-Wiedemann syndrome or Simpson-Golabi-Behmel syndrome should have yearly US until 7 years of age (4)[C].

PATIENT EDUCATION
- Patient and family teaching regarding long-term outlook
- Possibility of 2nd malignancy (up to 12% by age 50)
- Side effects of chemotherapy, radiation therapy

PROGNOSIS
- With favorable histology (1):
  - Children <2 years of age and stage I, favorable histology: 98% survival in NWTSG 1–3 studies
  - Children with stage III, favorable histology tumor: Overall survival of 89% in NWTSG 3–4 studies
- With diffuse anaplasia (1):
  - Children with stage I, diffuse or focal anaplasia: Overall survival 82.6%
  - Stage II tumors with anaplasia: Overall survival 81.5%
  - Stage III tumors with anaplasia: Overall survival 66.7%
  - Stage IV tumors with anaplasia: Overall survival 33.3%
- With bilateral involvement (stage V): 4-year survival 81.7% (1)
- With rhabdoid features: 19% 3-year survival

COMPLICATIONS
- Complication rate of 9.8% in NWTSG-5 study group (2)[B]:
  - Complication rate of 6.4% reported from SIOP (patients all pretreated with 4–8 weeks of chemotherapy)
- 1–2% will develop 2nd malignant neoplasms (leukemia, lymphoma, hepatocellular carcinoma, soft tissue sarcoma): 12.2% by 50 years of age
- High risk of delivering low-birth-weight infants, perinatal mortality in offspring of female survivors of Wilms tumor
- Chest is usual site of recurrence.
- Occurrence of 2nd malignant neoplasms in 2% of patients 7–34 years after treatment:
  - Bone and soft tissue sarcomas, breast cancer, hepatocellular carcinoma, lymphoma, gastrointestinal tract tumors, melanoma, leukemias
- Surgical complications (3)[B]:
  - Postoperative hemorrhage
  - Postoperative small bowel obstruction (5–7%)
  - Tumor rupture with spillage in 15.3% according to NWTSG-5; this may be spontaneous or surgical and results in upstaging the tumor. Only 2.7% of spills are considered avoidable (5)[B]. Incidence of tumor spillage is reported as 2.2% by SIOP following preoperative neoadjuvant chemotherapy (2)[B].

- Local tumor recurrence
- Renal failure
- Cardiomyopathy (usually related to doxorubicin and radiation therapy)
- Impaired pulmonary function (radiation therapy)

REFERENCES
1. Sonn G, Shortliffe LM. Management of Wilms tumor: current standard of care. *Nat Clin Pract Urol.* 2008;5:551–60.
2. Ko EY, Ritchey ML, et al. Current management of Wilms' tumor in children. *Journal of pediatric urology.* 2009;5:56–65.
3. Ritchey ML, et al. Surgical complications after primary nephrectomy for Wilms tumor: Report from the national Wilms tumor study group. *J Am Coll Surg.* 2001;192:63–8.
4. Scott RH, et al. Surveillance for Wilms Tumour in at-risk children: Pragmatic recommendations for best practice. *Arch Dis Child.* 2006;91:995–9.
5. Ehrlich PF, et al. Quality assessment for Wilms tumor: A report from the national Wilms study-5. *J Ped Surg.* 2005;40:208–10.

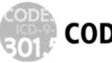 CODES

ICD9
189.0 Malignant neoplasm of kidney, except pelvis

CLINICAL PEARLS
- Nephrectomy typically is performed as soon as possible after completing the radiographic evaluation. This is important because it is 1 of the major components in staging the tumor.
- To treat bilateral tumors, staging is completed with open surgical biopsies, followed by adjuvant chemotherapy. After several cycles, surgical treatment is completed with bilateral partial nephrectomy or unilateral radical nephrectomy combined with contralateral partial nephrectomy, depending on the anatomy. New protocols are evaluating primary chemotherapy, followed by nephron-sparing resection.
- Mesoblastic nephroma:
  - Distinguished only by histology
  - Age usually <6 months
  - Essentially benign, although metastases have been reported; tends to be locally invasive
  - Operative spillage may lead to recurrence.
  - No chemotherapy or radiotherapy is needed with complete excision.
- Nephroblastomatosis: Considered premalignant; may present as nodularity of 1 or both kidneys; treated with biopsy and local excision (renal tissue sparing)

W

ZINC DEFICIENCY

Adarsh K. Gupta, DO, MS

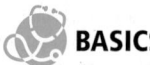 **BASICS**

DESCRIPTION

- Condition whose manifestations may involve growth retardation, hypogonadism, cell-mediated immune dysfunction, poor wound healing, poor appetite, hair loss, and increased incidence of infection, anorexia, diarrhea, and eye and skin lesions related to decreased zinc levels
- System(s) affected: Endocrine/Metabolic; Nervous; Skin/Exocrine; Hematologic/Oncologic; Gastroenterologic

Geriatric Considerations

- Zinc deficiency may cause poor night vision, leading to falls; poor wound healing or chronic ulcer; or loss of smell and taste, which may cause worsening nutrition.
- Elderly persons living in institutions may have low zinc intake.

Pediatric Considerations

Zinc deficiency may cause failure to thrive and diarrhea, and may impair growth and development of secondary sexual characteristics.

Pregnancy Considerations

Requirements increase; deficiency may cause spontaneous abortion, inadequate weight gain

EPIDEMIOLOGY

Prevalence

- In the US: Rare in general population
- High prevalence in developing countries
- Predominate age: All ages
- Predominant sex: Male = Female

RISK FACTORS

- Drugs: Diuretics, penicillamine, sodium valproate, and ethambutol
- Low socioeconomic status
- Malabsorption syndromes
- Living in developing nations
- Hyperalimentation with zinc supplementation
- Thermal burns
- Strict vegetarian diet
- Alcoholism
- Chronic renal failure patients on hemodialysis

Genetics

Usually acquired, but rarely caused by acrodermatitis enteropathica (autosomal recessive) and associated with sickle cell anemia (autosomal recessive)

GENERAL PREVENTION

- Adequate diet
- Supplementation when indicated (see Medication)

ETIOLOGY

- Increased requirements:
  - Pregnancy
  - Lactation
  - Rapid growth phase in childhood
  - Burns
  - Major trauma
- Increased losses:
  - Diabetes
  - Cirrhosis
  - Renal disease
  - Malabsorption states (e.g., inflammatory bowel diseases)
  - Sickle cell anemia
  - Diuretics: Thiazides, chlorthalidone
- Decreased absorption:
  - Acrodermatitis enteropathica, an autosomal recessive deficiency in the enzyme required for intestinal absorption
  - Geophagia
  - Chelating agents
  - Parasitism
  - Diet high in phytates (plant fiber)
  - Drugs: Penicillamines, tetracyclines, quinolones, bisphosphonates
- Insufficient dietary intake:
  - Vegetarianism
  - Parenteral hyperalimentation without zinc supplementation
  - Breastfeeding
  - Suboptimal zinc conditions in diet (rare)
  - Alcoholism

COMMONLY ASSOCIATED CONDITIONS

- Sickle cell anemia
- Malabsorption
- Parenteral hyperalimentation
- In the older patient: Those taking diuretics, those with diabetes mellitus, cirrhosis

 DIAGNOSIS

HISTORY

- Mild deficiency:
  - Hypogeusia (lack of taste)
  - Decreased dark adaptation
  - Decreased lean body mass
- Moderate deficiency:
  - All the above
  - Diarrhea
  - Growth retardation
  - Hypogonadism (especially male)
  - Mental lethargy
  - Anergy
  - Rough skin
  - Delayed wound healing
  - Glucose intolerance
  - Impaired cell-mediated immunity

- Severe deficiency:
  – All the above
  – Bullous pustular dermatitis
  – Weight loss
  – Dwarfism
  – Emotional instability
  – Tremors
  – Ataxia
  – Alopecia
  – Death
- Acrodermatitis enterohepatica: Erythema, scales, erosions, and/or vesiculobullous eruptions often quite dramatic in diaper area

PHYSICAL EXAM
Depends on level of deficiency

DIAGNOSTIC TESTS & INTERPRETATION
Lab
- Plasma zinc levels decreased (in moderate-to-severe zinc deficiency). Levels <60 g/L are strongly suggestive, but correction may be needed for low albumin because most serum zinc is bound to albumin.
- Erythrocyte or leukocyte zinc levels more adequately reflect tissue stores, but are not widely available.
- Hair and fingernail levels are not useful.

DIFFERENTIAL DIAGNOSIS
- Congenital dwarfism
- Failure to thrive in infants
- Multiple micronutrient deficiencies
- Primary hypogonadism
- Mental retardation

 TREATMENT

MEDICATION
- Zinc supplements (take at least 1 h before or 2 h after meals high in calcium, fiber, and phytates)
- Oral form: Zinc gluconate (lozenges, tablets), zinc sulfate (capsules, tablets, extended-release tablets)
- Injectable form: Zinc chloride, zinc sulfate
- Use the recommended dietary allowance (RDA) as a guideline for dosing (see Diet).
- In adult patient, 4–6 mg/d of elemental zinc added to hyperalimentation; may increase to 12 mg q.i.d. if suspect ongoing heavy zinc losses (e.g., burns or major trauma)
- Precautions: Avoid large (>20 mg elemental zinc) parenteral doses.

 ONGOING CARE

FOLLOW-UP RECOMMENDATIONS
Full activity

Patient Monitoring
Clinical status such as improved energy, weight gain, resolution of symptoms

DIET
- Balanced omnivorous diet or vegetarian diet with supplementation
- Avoid excessive intake of foods with high phytate content (e.g., raw cereals, but ready-to-eat cereal may be the richest source of zinc from a plant product)
- Lean beef and pork, oysters, poultry, soybeans, pumpkin, sunflower seeds, seafood, milk, eggs, grains, legumes, nuts, and wheat bran are rich in zinc.

- RDA for zinc:
  – Men: 15 mg/d
  – Women: 12 mg/d
  – Pregnant women: 15 mg/d
  – Breastfeeding women: 19 mg/d

PROGNOSIS
Immediate improvement in clinical status with treatment; full resolution in signs and symptoms

ADDITIONAL READING
- http://ods.od.nih.gov/factsheets/zinc.asp#en2
- Lukacik M, Thomas RL, Aranda JV. A meta-analysis of the effects of oral zinc in the treatment of acute and persistent diarrhea. *Pediatrics*. 2008;121: 326–36.
- Maret W, Sandstead HH, et al. Zinc requirements and the risks and benefits of zinc supplementation. *J Trace Elem Med Biol*. 2006;20:3–18.

See Also (Topic, Algorithm, Electronic Media Element)
Alcohol Abuse and Dependence; Anemia, Sickle Cell; Failure to Thrive (FTT)

 CODES

ICD9
269.3 Mineral deficiency, not elsewhere classified

CLINICAL PEARLS
- Zinc deficiency is uncommon in the US.
- Elderly living in long-term facilities may have diets deficient in zinc.
- Zinc deficiency may cause poor wound healing; consider supplementation when treating chronic skin ulcers.

Z

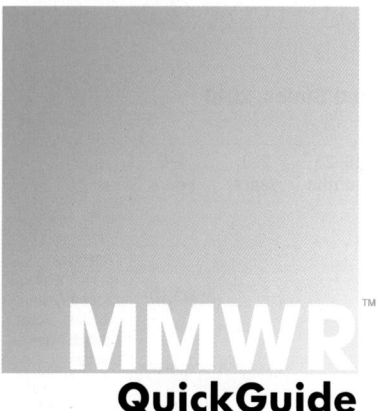

Recommended Immunization Schedules for Persons Aged 0 Through 18 Years — United States, 2010

Weekly   **January 8, 2010 / Vol. 58 / No. 51 & 52**

QuickGuide

The Advisory Committee on Immunization Practices (ACIP) annually publishes an immunization schedule for persons aged 0 through 18 years that summarizes recommendations for currently licensed vaccines for children aged 18 years and younger and includes recommendations in effect as of December 15, 2009. Changes to the previous schedule (*1*) include the following:

- The statement concerning use of combination vaccines in the introductory paragraph has been changed to reflect the revised ACIP recommendation on this issue (*2*).
- The last dose in the inactivated poliovirus vaccine series is now recommended to be administered on or after the fourth birthday and at least 6 months after the previous dose. In addition, if 4 doses are administered before age 4 years, an additional (fifth) dose should be administered at age 4 through 6 years (*3*).
- The hepatitis A footnote has been revised to allow vaccination of children older than 23 months for whom immunity against hepatitis A is desired.
- Revaccination with meningococcal conjugate vaccine is now recommended for children who remain at increased risk for meningococcal disease after 3 years (if the first dose was administered at age 2 through 6 years), or after 5 years (if the first dose was administered at age 7 years or older) (*4*).
- Footnotes for human papillomavirus (HPV) vaccine have been modified to include 1) the availability of and recommendations for bivalent HPV vaccine, and 2) a permissive recommendation for administration of quadrivalent HPV vaccine to males aged 9 through 18 years to reduce the likelihood of acquiring genital warts (*5*).

The National Childhood Vaccine Injury Act requires that health-care providers provide parents or patients with copies of Vaccine Information Statements before administering each dose of the vaccines listed in the schedules. Additional information is available from state health departments and from CDC at http://www.cdc.gov/vaccines/pubs/vis/default.htm.

Detailed recommendations for using vaccines are available from ACIP statements (available at http://www.cdc.gov/vaccines/pubs/acip-list.htm) and the *2009 Red Book* (*6*). Guidance regarding the Vaccine Adverse Event Reporting System form is available at http://www.vaers.hhs.gov or by telephone, 800-822-7967.

References

1. CDC. Recommended immunization schedules for persons aged 0–18 years—United States 2009. MMWR 2009;57(51&52).
2. CDC. ACIP Provisional recommendations for the use of combination vaccines. Atlanta, GA: US Department of Health and Human Services, CDC; 2009. Available at http://www.cdc.gov/vaccines/recs/provisional/downloads/combo-vax-aug2009-508.pdf. Accessed November 18, 2009.
3. CDC. Updated recommendations of the Advisory Committee on Immunization Practices (ACIP) regarding routine poliovirus vaccination. MMWR 2009;58:829–30.
4. CDC. Updated recommendation from the Advisory Committee on Immunization Practices (ACIP) for revaccination of persons at prolonged increased risk for meningococcal disease MMWR 2009;58:1042–3.
5. CDC. ACIP provisional recommendations for HPV vaccine. Atlanta, GA: US Department of Health and Human Services, CDC; 2009. Available at http://www.cdc.gov/vaccines/recs/provisional/downloads/hpv-vac-dec2009-508.pdf. Accessed December 23, 2009.
6. American Academy of Pediatrics. Active and passive immunization. In: Pickering LK, Baker CJ, Kimberlin DW, Long SS, eds. 2009 red book: report of the Committee on Infectious Diseases. 28th ed. Elk Grove Village, IL: American Academy of Pediatrics; 2009.

FIGURE 1. Recommended immunization schedule for persons aged 0 through 6 years — United States, 2010
(for those who fall behind or start late, see the catch-up schedule [Table])

Vaccine ▼ Age ▶	Birth	1 month	2 months	4 months	6 months	12 months	15 months	18 months	19–23 months	2–3 years	4–6 years
Hepatitis B[1]	HepB	HepB				HepB					
Rotavirus[2]			RV	RV	RV[2]						
Diphtheria, Tetanus, Pertussis[3]			DTaP	DTaP	DTaP	see footnote[3]	DTaP				DTaP
Haemophilus influenzae type b[4]			Hib	Hib	Hib[4]	Hib					
Pneumococcal[5]			PCV	PCV	PCV	PCV				PPSV	
Inactivated Poliovirus[6]			IPV	IPV		IPV					IPV
Influenza[7]						Influenza (Yearly)					
Measles, Mumps, Rubella[8]						MMR		see footnote[8]			MMR
Varicella[9]						Varicella		see footnote[9]			Varicella
Hepatitis A[10]						HepA (2 doses)				HepA Series	
Meningococcal[11]										MCV	

Range of recommended ages for all children except certain high-risk groups

Range of recommended ages for certain high-risk groups

This schedule includes recommendations in effect as of December 15, 2009. Any dose not administered at the recommended age should be administered at a subsequent visit, when indicated and feasible. The use of a combination vaccine generally is preferred over separate injections of its equivalent component vaccines. Considerations should include provider assessment, patient preference, and the potential for adverse events. Providers should consult the relevant Advisory Committee on Immunization Practices statement for detailed recommendations: http://www.cdc.gov/vaccines/pubs/acip-list.htm. Clinically significant adverse events that follow immunization should be reported to the Vaccine Adverse Event Reporting System (VAERS) at http://www.vaers.hhs.gov or by telephone, 800-822-7967.

1. **Hepatitis B vaccine (HepB).** (Minimum age: birth)
   At birth:
   - Administer monovalent HepB to all newborns before hospital discharge.
   - If mother is hepatitis B surface antigen (HBsAg)-positive, administer HepB and 0.5 mL of hepatitis B immune globulin (HBIG) within 12 hours of birth.
   - If mother's HBsAg status is unknown, administer HepB within 12 hours of birth. Determine mother's HBsAg status as soon as possible and, if HBsAg-positive, administer HBIG (no later than age 1 week).
   After the birth dose:
   - The HepB series should be completed with either monovalent HepB or a combination vaccine containing HepB. The second dose should be administered at age 1 or 2 months. Monovalent HepB vaccine should be used for doses administered before age 6 weeks. The final dose should be administered no earlier than age 24 weeks.
   - Infants born to HBsAg-positive mothers should be tested for HBsAg and antibody to HBsAg 1 to 2 months after completion of at least 3 doses of the HepB series, at age 9 through 18 months (generally at the next well-child visit).
   - Administration of 4 doses of HepB to infants is permissible when a combination vaccine containing HepB is administered after the birth dose. The fourth dose should be administered no earlier than age 24 weeks.
2. **Rotavirus vaccine (RV).** (Minimum age: 6 weeks)
   - Administer the first dose at age 6 through 14 weeks (maximum age: 14 weeks 6 days). Vaccination should not be initiated for infants aged 15 weeks 0 days or older.
   - The maximum age for the final dose in the series is 8 months 0 days
   - If Rotarix is administered at ages 2 and 4 months, a dose at 6 months is not indicated.
3. **Diphtheria and tetanus toxoids and acellular pertussis vaccine (DTaP).** (Minimum age: 6 weeks)
   - The fourth dose may be administered as early as age 12 months, provided at least 6 months have elapsed since the third dose.
   - Administer the final dose in the series at age 4 through 6 years.
4. ***Haemophilus influenzae* type b conjugate vaccine (Hib).** (Minimum age: 6 weeks)
   - If PRP-OMP (PedvaxHIB or Comvax [HepB-Hib]) is administered at ages 2 and 4 months, a dose at age 6 months is not indicated.
   - TriHiBit (DTaP/Hib) and Hiberix (PRP-T) should not be used for doses at ages 2, 4, or 6 months for the primary series but can be used as the final dose in children aged 12 months through 4 years.
5. **Pneumococcal vaccine.** (Minimum age: 6 weeks for pneumococcal conjugate vaccine [PCV]; 2 years for pneumococcal polysaccharide vaccine [PPSV])
   - PCV is recommended for all children aged younger than 5 years. Administer 1 dose of PCV to all healthy children aged 24 through 59 months who are not completely vaccinated for their age.
   - Administer PPSV 2 or more months after last dose of PCV to children aged 2 years or older with certain underlying medical conditions, including a cochlear implant. See *MMWR* 1997;46(No. RR-8).

6. **Inactivated poliovirus vaccine (IPV)** (Minimum age: 6 weeks)
   - The final dose in the series should be administered on or after the fourth birthday and at least 6 months following the previous dose.
   - If 4 doses are administered prior to age 4 years a fifth dose should be administered at age 4 through 6 years. See *MMWR* 2009;58(30):829–30.
7. **Influenza vaccine (seasonal).** (Minimum age: 6 months for trivalent inactivated influenza vaccine [TIV]; 2 years for live, attenuated influenza vaccine [LAIV])
   - Administer annually to children aged 6 months through 18 years.
   - For healthy children aged 2 through 6 years (i.e., those who do not have underlying medical conditions that predispose them to influenza complications), either LAIV or TIV may be used, except LAIV should not be given to children aged 2 through 4 years who have had wheezing in the past 12 months.
   - Children receiving TIV should receive 0.25 mL if aged 6 through 35 months or 0.5 mL if aged 3 years or older.
   - Administer 2 doses (separated by at least 4 weeks) to children aged younger than 9 years who are receiving influenza vaccine for the first time or who were vaccinated for the first time during the previous influenza season but only received 1 dose.
   - For recommendations for use of influenza A (H1N1) 2009 monovalent vaccine see *MMWR* 2009;58(No. RR-10).
8. **Measles, mumps, and rubella vaccine (MMR).** (Minimum age: 12 months)
   - Administer the second dose routinely at age 4 through 6 years. However, the second dose may be administered before age 4, provided at least 28 days have elapsed since the first dose.
9. **Varicella vaccine.** (Minimum age: 12 months)
   - Administer the second dose routinely at age 4 through 6 years. However, the second dose may be administered before age 4, provided at least 3 months have elapsed since the first dose.
   - For children aged 12 months through 12 years the minimum interval between doses is 3 months. However, if the second dose was administered at least 28 days after the first dose, it can be accepted as valid.
10. **Hepatitis A vaccine (HepA).** (Minimum age: 12 months)
    - Administer to all children aged 1 year (i.e., aged 12 through 23 months). Administer 2 doses at least 6 months apart.
    - Children not fully vaccinated by age 2 years can be vaccinated at subsequent visits
    - HepA also is recommended for older children who live in areas where vaccination programs target older children, who are at increased risk for infection, or for whom immunity against hepatitis A is desired.
11. **Meningococcal vaccine.** (Minimum age: 2 years for meningococcal conjugate vaccine [MCV4] and for meningococcal polysaccharide vaccine [MPSV4])
    - Administer MCV4 to children aged 2 through 10 years with persistent complement component deficiency, anatomic or functional asplenia, and certain other conditions placing tham at high risk.
    - Administer MCV4 to children previously vaccinated with MCV4 or MPSV4 after 3 years if first dose administered at age 2 through 6 years. See *MMWR* 2009; 58:1042–3.

The Recommended Immunization Schedules for Persons Aged 0 through 18 Years are approved by the Advisory Committee on Immunization Practices (http://www.cdc.gov/vaccines/recs/acip), the American Academy of Pediatrics (http://www.aap.org), and the American Academy of Family Physicians (http://www.aafp.org). Department of Health and Human Services • Centers for Disease Control and Prevention

FIGURE 2. Recommended immunization schedule for persons aged 7 through 18 years — United States, 2010 (for those who fall behind or start late, see the schedule below and the catch-up schedule [Table])

Vaccine ▼ Age ▶	7–10 years	11–12 years	13–18 years
Tetanus, Diphtheria, Pertussis[1]		Tdap	Tdap
Human Papillomavirus[2]	*see footnote 2*	HPV (3 doses)	HPV series
Meningococcal[3]	MCV	MCV	MCV
Influenza[4]	Influenza (Yearly)		
Pneumococcal[5]	PPSV		
Hepatitis A[6]	HepA Series		
Hepatitis B[7]	Hep B Series		
Inactivated Poliovirus[8]	IPV Series		
Measles, Mumps, Rubella[9]	MMR Series		
Varicella[10]	Varicella Series		

Range of recommended ages for all children except certain high-risk groups

Range of recommended ages for catch-up immunization

Range of recommended ages for certain high-risk groups

This schedule includes recommendations in effect as of December 15, 2009. Any dose not administered at the recommended age should be administered at a subsequent visit, when indicated and feasible. The use of a combination vaccine generally is preferred over separate injections of its equivalent component vaccines. Considerations should include provider assessment, patient preference, and the potential for adverse events. Providers should consult the relevant Advisory Committee on Immunization Practices statement for detailed recommendations: http://www.cdc.gov/vaccines/pubs/acip-list.htm. Clinically significant adverse events that follow immunization should be reported to the Vaccine Adverse Event Reporting System (VAERS) at http://www.vaers.hhs.gov or by telephone, 800-822-7967.

1. **Tetanus and diphtheria toxoids and acellular pertussis vaccine (Tdap).**
   (Minimum age: 10 years for Boostrix and 11 years for Adacel)
   - Administer at age 11 or 12 years for those who have completed the recommended childhood DTP/DTaP vaccination series and have not received a tetanus and diphtheria toxoid (Td) booster dose.
   - Persons aged 13 through 18 years who have not received Tdap should receive a dose.
   - A 5-year interval from the last Td dose is encouraged when Tdap is used as a booster dose; however, a shorter interval may be used if pertussis immunity is needed.
2. **Human papillomavirus vaccine (HPV).** (Minimum age: 9 years)
   - Two HPV vaccines are licensed: a quadrivalent vaccine (HPV4) for the prevention of cervical, vaginal and vulvar cancers (in females) and genital warts (in females and males), and a bivalent vaccine (HPV2) for the prevention of cervical cancers in females.
   - HPV vaccines are most effective for both males and females when given before exposure to HPV through sexual contact.
   - HPV4 or HPV2 is recommended for the prevention of cervical precancers and cancers in females.
   - HPV4 is recommended for the prevention of cervical, vaginal and vulvar precancers and cancers and genital warts in females.
   - Administer the first dose to females at age 11 or 12 years.
   - Administer the second dose 1 to 2 months after the first dose and the third dose 6 months after the first dose (at least 24 weeks after the first dose).
   - Administer the series to females at age 13 through 18 years if not previously vaccinated.
   - HPV4 may be administered in a 3-dose series to males aged 9 through 18 years to reduce their likelihood of acquiring genital warts.
3. **Meningococcal conjugate vaccine (MCV4).**
   - Administer at age 11 or 12 years, or at age 13 through 18 years if not previously vaccinated.
   - Administer to previously unvaccinated college freshmen living in a dormitory.
   - Administer MCV4 to children aged 2 through 10 years with persistent complement component deficiency, anatomic or functional asplenia, or certain other conditions placing them at high risk.
   - Administer to children previously vaccinated with MCV4 or MPSV4 who remain at increased risk after 3 years (if first dose administered at age 2 through 6 years) or after 5 years (if first dose administered at age 7 years or older). Persons whose only risk factor is living in on-campus housing are not recommended to receive an additional dose. See *MMWR* 2009;58:1042–3.

4. **Influenza vaccine (seasonal).**
   - Administer annually to children aged 6 months through 18 years.
   - For healthy nonpregnant persons aged 7 through 18 years (i.e., those who do not have underlying medical conditions that predispose them to influenza complications), either LAIV or TIV may be used.
   - Administer 2 doses (separated by at least 4 weeks) to children aged younger than 9 years who are receiving influenza vaccine for the first time or who were vaccinated for the first time during the previous influenza season but only received 1 dose.
   - For recommendations for use of influenza A (H1N1) 2009 monovalent vaccine. See *MMWR* 2009;58(No. RR-10)
5. **Pneumococcal polysaccharide vaccine (PPSV).**
   - Administer to children with certain underlying medical conditions, including a cochlear implant. A single revaccination should be administered after 5 years to children with functional or anatomic asplenia or an immunocompromising condition. See *MMWR* 1997;46(No. RR-8).
6. **Hepatitis A vaccine (HepA).**
   - Administer 2 doses at least 6 months apart.
   - HepA is recommended for children aged older than 23 months who live in areas where vaccination programs target older children, who are at increased risk for infection, or for whom immunity against hepatitis A is desired.
7. **Hepatitis B vaccine (HepB).**
   - Administer the 3-dose series to those not previously vaccinated.
   - A 2-dose series (separated by at least 4 months) of adult formulation Recombivax HB is licensed for children aged 11 through 15 years.
8. **Inactivated poliovirus vaccine (IPV).**
   - The final dose in the series should be administered on or after the fourth birthday and at least 6 months following the previous dose.
   - If both OPV and IPV were administered as part of a series, a total of 4 doses should be administered, regardless of the child's current age.
9. **Measles, mumps, and rubella vaccine (MMR).**
   - If not previously vaccinated, administer 2 doses or the second dose for those who have received only 1 dose, with at least 28 days between doses.
10. **Varicella vaccine.**
   - For persons aged 7 through 18 years without evidence of immunity (see *MMWR* 2007;56[No. RR-4]), administer 2 doses if not previously vaccinated or the second dose if only 1 dose has been administered.
   - For persons aged 7 through 12 years, the minimum interval between doses is 3 months. However, if the second dose was administered at least 28 days after the first dose, it can be accepted as valid.
   - For persons aged 13 years and older, the minimum interval between doses is 28 days.

The Recommended Immunization Schedules for Persons Aged 0 through 18 Years are approved by the Advisory Committee on Immunization Practices (http://www.cdc.gov/vaccines/recs/acip), the American Academy of Pediatrics (http://www.aap.org), and the American Academy of Family Physicians (http://www.aafp.org). Department of Health and Human Services • Centers for Disease Control and Prevention

TABLE. Catch-up immunization schedule for persons aged 4 months through 18 years who start late or who are more than 1 month behind — United States, 2010

The table below provides catch-up schedules and minimum intervals between doses for children whose vaccinations have been delayed. A vaccine series does not need to be restarted, regardless of the time that has elapsed between doses. Use the section appropriate for the child's age.

Vaccine	Minimum Age for Dose 1	Minimum Interval Between Doses			
		Dose 1 to Dose 2	Dose 2 to Dose 3	Dose 3 to Dose 4	Dose 4 to Dose 5
PERSONS AGED 4 MONTHS THROUGH 6 YEARS					
Hepatitis B[1]	Birth	4 weeks	8 weeks (and at least 16 weeks after first dose)		
Rotavirus[2]	6 wks	4 weeks	4 weeks[2]		
Diphtheria, Tetanus, Pertussis[3]	6 wks	4 weeks	4 weeks	6 months	6 months[3]
Haemophilus influenzae type b[4]	6 wks	4 weeks if first dose administered at younger than age 12 months / 8 weeks (as final dose) if first dose administered at age 12–14 months / No further doses needed if first dose administered at age 15 months or older	4 weeks[4] if current age is younger than 12 months / 8 weeks (as final dose)[4] if current age is 12 months or older and first dose administered at younger than age 12 months and second dose administered at younger than 15 months / No further doses needed if previous dose administered at age 15 months or older	8 weeks (as final dose) This dose only necessary for children aged 12 months through 59 months who received 3 doses before age 12 months	
Pneumococcal[5]	6 wks	4 weeks if first dose administered at younger than age 12 months / 8 weeks (as final dose for healthy children) if first dose administered at age 12 months or older or current age 24 through 59 months / No further doses needed for healthy children if first dose administered at age 24 months or older	4 weeks if current age is younger than 12 months / 8 weeks (as final dose for healthy children) if current age is 12 months or older / No further doses needed for healthy children if previous dose administered at age 24 months or older	8 weeks (as final dose) This dose only necessary for children aged 12 months through 59 months who received 3 doses before age 12 months or for high-risk children who received 3 doses at any age	
Inactivated Poliovirus[6]	6 wks	4 weeks	4 weeks	6 months	
Measles, Mumps, Rubella[7]	12 mos	4 weeks			
Varicella[8]	12 mos	3 months			
Hepatitis A[9]	12 mos	6 months			
PERSONS AGED 7 THROUGH 18 YEARS					
Tetanus, Diphtheria/ Tetanus, Diphtheria, Pertussis[10]	7 yrs[10]	4 weeks	4 weeks if first dose administered at younger than age 12 months / 6 months if first dose administered at 12 months or older	6 months if first dose administered at younger than age 12 months	
Human Papillomavirus[11]	9 yrs	Routine dosing intervals are recommended[11]			
Hepatitis A[9]	12 mos	6 months			
Hepatitis B[1]	Birth	4 weeks	8 weeks (and at least 16 weeks after first dose)		
Inactivated Poliovirus[6]	6 wks	4 weeks	4 weeks	6 months	
Measles, Mumps, Rubella[7]	12 mos	4 weeks			
Varicella[8]	12 mos	3 months if person is younger than age 13 years / 4 weeks if person is aged 13 years or older			

1. **Hepatitis B vaccine (HepB).**
   - Administer the 3-dose series to those not previously vaccinated.
   - A 2-dose series (separated by at least 4 months) of adult formulation Recombivax HB is licensed for children aged 11 through 15 years.
2. **Rotavirus vaccine (RV).**
   - The maximum age for the first dose is 14 weeks 6 days. Vaccination should not be initiated for infants aged 15 weeks 0 days or older.
   - The maximum age for the final dose in the series is 8 months 0 days.
   - If Rotarix was administered for the first and second doses, a third dose is not indicated.
3. **Diphtheria and tetanus toxoids and acellular pertussis vaccine (DTaP).**
   - The fifth dose is not necessary if the fourth dose was administered at age 4 years or older.
4. **Haemophilus influenzae type b conjugate vaccine (Hib).**
   - Hib vaccine is not generally recommended for persons aged 5 years or older. No efficacy data are available on which to base a recommendation concerning use of Hib vaccine for older children and adults. However, studies suggest good immunogenicity in persons who have sickle cell disease, leukemia, or HIV infection, or who have had a splenectomy; administering 1 dose of Hib vaccine to these persons who have not previously received Hib vaccine is not contraindicated.
   - If the first 2 doses were PRP-OMP (PedvaxHIB or Comvax), and administered at age 11 months or younger, the third (and final) dose should be administered at age 12 through 15 months and at least 8 weeks after the second dose.
   - If the first dose was administered at age 7 through 11 months, administer the second dose at least 4 weeks later and a final dose at age 12 through 15 months.
5. **Pneumococcal vaccine.**
   - Administer 1 dose of pneumococcal conjugate vaccine (PCV) to all healthy children aged 24 through 59 months who have not received at least 1 dose of PCV on or after age 12 months.
   - For children aged 24 through 59 months with underlying medical conditions, administer 1 dose of PCV if 3 doses were received previously or administer 2 doses of PCV at least 8 weeks apart if fewer than 3 doses were received previously.
   - Administer pneumococcal polysaccharide vaccine (PPSV) to children aged 2 years or older with certain underlying medical conditions, including a cochlear implant, at least 8 weeks after the last dose of PCV. See MMWR 1997;46(No. RR-8).
6. **Inactivated poliovirus vaccine (IPV).**
   - The final dose in the series should be administered on or after the fourth birthday and at least 6 months following the previous dose.

- A fourth dose is not necessary if the third dose was administered at age 4 years or older and at least 6 months following the previous dose.
- In the first 6 months of life, minimum age and minimum intervals are only recommended if the person is at risk for imminent exposure to circulating poliovirus (i.e., travel to a polio-endemic region or during an outbreak).
7. **Measles, mumps, and rubella vaccine (MMR).**
   - Administer the second dose routinely at age 4 through 6 years. However, the second dose may be administered before age 4, provided at least 28 days have elapsed since the first dose.
   - If not previously vaccinated, administer 2 doses with at least 28 days between doses.
8. **Varicella vaccine.**
   - Administer the second dose routinely at age 4 through 6 years. However, the second dose may be administered before age 4, provided at least 3 months have elapsed since the first dose.
   - For persons aged 12 months through 12 years, the minimum interval between doses is 3 months. However, if the second dose was administered at least 28 days after the first dose, it can be accepted as valid.
   - For persons aged 13 years and older, the minimum interval between doses is 28 days.
9. **Hepatitis A vaccine (HepA).**
   - HepA is recommended for children aged older than 23 months who live in areas where vaccination programs target older children, who are at increased risk for infection, or for whom immunity against hepatitis A is desired.
10. **Tetanus and diphtheria toxoids vaccine (Td) and tetanus and diphtheria toxoids and acellular pertussis vaccine (Tdap).**
    - Doses of DTaP are counted as part of the Td/Tdap series
    - Tdap should be substituted for a single dose of Td in the catch-up series or as a booster for children aged 10 through 18 years; use Td for other doses.
11. **Human papillomavirus vaccine (HPV).**
    - Administer the series to females at age 13 through 18 years if not previously vaccinated.
    - Use recommended routine dosing intervals for series catch-up (i.e., the second and third doses should be administered at 1 to 2 and 6 months after the first dose). The minimum interval between the first and second doses is 4 weeks. The minimum interval between the second and third doses is 12 weeks, and the third dose should be administered at least 24 weeks after the first dose.

Information about reporting reactions after immunization is available online at http://www.vaers.hhs.gov or by telephone, 800-822-7967. Suspected cases of vaccine-preventable diseases should be reported to the state or local health department. Additional information, including precautions and contraindications for immunization, is available from the National Center for Immunization and Respiratory Diseases at http://www.cdc.gov/vaccines or telephone, 800-CDC-INFO (800-232-4636).

Department of Health and Human Services • Centers for Disease Control and Prevention

MMWR™

QuickGuide

Weekly

January 9, 2009 / Vol. 57 / No. 53

Recommended Adult Immunization Schedule — United States, 2009

The Advisory Committee on Immunization Practices (ACIP) annually reviews the recommended Adult Immunization Schedule to ensure that the schedule reflects current recommendations for the licensed vaccines. In October 2008, ACIP approved the Adult Immunization Schedule for 2009. No new vaccines were added to the schedule; however, several indications were added to the pneumococcal polysaccharide vaccine footnote, clarifications were made to the footnotes for human papillomavirus, varicella, and meningococcal vaccines, and schedule information was added to the hepatitis A and hepatitis B vaccine footnotes.

Additional information is available as follows: schedule (in English and Spanish) at http://www.cdc.gov/vaccines/recs/schedules/adult-schedule.htm; adult vaccination at http://www.cdc.gov/vaccines/default.htm; ACIP statements for specific vaccines at http://www.cdc.gov/vaccine/pubs/acip-list.htm; and reporting adverse events at http://www.vaers.hhs.gov or by telephone, 800-822-7967.

Changes for 2009

Format Changes (Figures 1 and 2)

To make the figures easier to understand, several formatting changes were implemented to both the age group–based schedule and the medical and other indications schedule. The changes include 1) increasing the number of age groups; 2) deleting the hatched yellow bar for tetanus, diphtheria, pertussis (Td/Tdap) vaccine while adding explanatory text to the Td/Tdap bar; 3) simplifying the figures by removing schedule text from the vaccine bars; 4) revising the order of the vaccines to more appropriately group the vaccines, and 5) adding a legend box to clarify the meaning of blank spaces in the table.

Footnote (Figures 1 and 2)

- The human papillomavirus (HPV) footnote (#2) has language added to indicate that health-care personnel are not at increased risk because of occupational exposure, but they should be vaccinated consistent with age-based recommendations. Also, text has been added to indicate that vaccination with HPV may begin at age 9 years.
- The varicella footnote (#3) has language added to clarify that adults who previously received only 1 dose of vaccine should receive a second dose.
- Asthma and cigarette smoking have been added as indications for pneumococcal polysaccharide vaccination (#7). Also, text has been added to clarify vaccine use in Alaska Natives and American Indians.
- The Hepatits A footnote (#9) has additional schedule information for the 4-dose combined hepatitis A/hepatitis B vaccine.
- The Hepatitis B footnote (#10) has additional schedule information for the 4-dose combined hepatitis A/hepatitis B vaccine, and a clarification of schedule information for special formulation indications has been added.
- The meningococcal vaccine footnot (#11) clarifies that the revaccination interval is 5 years.

FIGURE 1. Recommended adult immunization schedule by vaccine and age group — United Sates, 2009

VACCINE ▼　　　　AGE GROUP ▶	19–26 years	27–49 years	50–59 years	60–64 years	≥65 years
Tetanus, diphtheria, pertussis (Td/Tdap)[1],*	Substitute 1-time dose of Tdap for Td booster; then boost with Td every 10 yr				Td booster every 10 yrs
Human papillomavirus (HPV)[2],*	3 doses (females)				
Varicella[3],*	2 doses				
Zoster[4]				1 dose	
Measles, mumps, rubella (MMR)[5],*	1 or 2 doses		1 dose		
Influenza[6],*		1 dose annually			
Pneumococcal (polysaccharide)[7,8]	1 or 2 doses				1 dose
Hepatitis A[9],*	2 doses				
Hepatitis B[10],*	3 doses				
Meningococcal[11],*	1 or more doses				

*Covered by the Vaccine Injury Compensation Program.

For all persons in this category who meet the age requirements and who lack evidence of immunity (e.g., lack documentation of vaccination or have no evidence of prior infection)

Recommended if some other risk factor is present (e.g., on the basis of medical, occupational, lifestyle, or other indications)

No recommendation

NOTE: The above recommendations must be read along with the footnotes on pages Q2–Q4 of this schedule.

1. Tetanus, diphtheria, and acellular pertussis (Td/Tdap) vaccination

Tdap should replace a single dose of Td for adults aged 19 through 64 years who have not received a dose of Tdap previously

Adults with uncertain or incomplete history of primary vaccination series with tetanus and diphtheria toxoid–containing vaccines should begin or complete a primary vaccination series. A primary series for adults is 3 doses of tetanus and diphtheria toxoid–containing vaccines; administer the first 2 doses at least 4 weeks apart and the third dose 6–12 months after the second. However, Tdap can substitute for any one of the doses of Td in the 3-dose primary series. The booster dose of tetanus and diphtheria toxoid–containing vaccine should be administered to adults who have completed a primary series and if the last vaccination was received 10 or more years previously. Tdap or Td vaccine may be used, as indicated.

If a woman is pregnant and received the last Td vaccination 10 or more years previously, administer Td during the second or third trimester. If the woman received the last Td vaccination less than 10 years previously, administer Tdap during the immediate postpartum period. A dose of Tdap is recommended for postpartum women, close contacts of infants aged less than 12 months, and all health-care personnel with direct patient contact if they have not previously received Tdap. An interval as short as 2 years from the last Td is suggested; shorter intervals can be used. Td may be deferred during pregnancy and Tdap substituted in the immediate postpartum period, or Tdap may be administered instead of Td to a pregnant woman after an informed discussion with the woman.

Consult the ACIP statement for recommendations for administering Td as prophylaxis in wound management.

2. Human papillomavirus (HPV) vaccination

HPV vaccination is recommended for all females aged 11 through 26 years (and may begin at age 9 years) who have not completed the vaccine series. History of genital warts, abnormal Papanicolaou test, or positive HPV DNA test is not evidence of prior infection with all vaccine HPV types; HPV vaccination is recommended for persons with such histories.

Ideally, vaccine should be administered before potential exposure to HPV through sexual activity; however, females who are sexually active should still be vaccinated consistent with age-based recommendations. Sexually active females who have not been infected with any of the four HPV vaccine types receive the full benefit of the vaccination. Vaccination is less beneficial for females who have already been infected with one or more of the HPV vaccine types.

A complete series consists of 3 doses. The second dose should be administered 2 months after the first dose; the third dose should be administered 6 months after the first dose.

HPV vaccination is not specifically recommended for females with the medical indications described in Figure 2, "Vaccines that might be indicated for adults based on medical and other indications." Because HPV vaccine is not a live-virus vaccine, it may be administered to persons with the medical indications described in Figure 2. However, the immune response and vaccine efficacy might be less for persons with the medical indications described in Figure 2 than in persons who do not have the medical indications described or who are immunocompetent. Health-care personnel are not at increased risk because of occupational exposure, and should be vaccinated consistent with age-based recommendations.

3. Varicella vaccination

All adults without evidence of immunity to varicella should receive 2 doses of single-antigen varicella vaccine if not previously vaccinated or the second dose if they have received only one dose, unless they have a medical contraindication. Special consideration should be given to those who 1) have close contact with persons at high risk for severe disease (e.g., health-care personnel and family contacts of persons with immunocompromising conditions) or 2) are at high risk for exposure or transmission (e.g., teachers; child care employees; residents and staff members of institutional settings, including correctional institutions; college students; military personnel; adolescents and adults living in households with children; nonpregnant women of childbearing age; and international travelers).

Evidence of immunity to varicella in adults includes any of the following: 1) documentation of 2 doses of varicella vaccine at least 4 weeks apart; 2) U.S.-born before 1980 (although for health-care personnel and pregnant women, birth before 1980 should not be considered evidence of immunity); 3) history of varicella based on diagnosis or verification of varicella by a health-care provider (for a patient reporting a history of or presenting with an atypical case, a mild case, or both, health-care providers should seek either an epidemiologic link to a typical varicella case or to a laboratory-confirmed case or evidence of laboratory confirmation, if it was performed at the time of acute disease); 4) history of herpes zoster based on health-care provider diagnosis or verification of herpes zoster by a health-care provider; or 5) laboratory evidence of immunity or laboratory confirmation of disease.

Pregnant women should be assessed for evidence of varicella immunity. Women who do not have evidence of immunity should receive the fist dose

FIGURE 2. Vaccines that might be indicated for adults based on medical and other indications — United States, 2009

VACCINE ▼ / INDICATION ▶	Pregnancy	Immuno-compromising conditions (excluding human immunodeficiency virus [HIV])[13]	HIV infection[3,12,13] CD4+ T lymphocyte count <200 cells/μL	HIV infection[3,12,13] CD4+ T lymphocyte count ≥200 cells/μL	Diabetes, heart disease, chronic lung disease, chronic alcoholism	Asplenia[12] (including elective splenectomy and terminal complement component deficiencies)	Chronic liver disease	Kidney failure, end-stage renal disease, receipt of hemodialysis	Health-care personnel
Tetanus, diphtheria, pertussis (Td/Tdap)[1],*	Td	Substitute 1-time dose of Tdap for Td booster; then boost with Td every 10 yrs							
Human papillomavirus (HPV)[2],*		3 doses for females through age 26 yrs							
Varicella[3],*	Contraindicated			2 doses					
Zoster[4]	Contraindicated				1 dose				
Measles, mumps, rubella (MMR)[5],*	Contraindicated			1 or 2 doses					
Influenza[6],*	1 dose TIV annually								1 dose TIV or LAIV annually
Pneumococcal (polysaccharide)[7,8]	1 or 2 doses								
Hepatitis A[9],*	2 doses								
Hepatitis B[10],*	3 doses								
Meningococcal[11],*	1 or more doses								

*Covered by the Vaccine Injury Compensation Program.

☐ For all persons in this category who meet the age requirements and who lack evidence of immunity (e.g., lack documentation of vaccination or have no evidence of prior infection)

☐ Recommended if some other risk factor is present (e.g., on the basis of medical, occupational, lifestyle, or other indications)

☐ No recommendation

NOTE: The above recommendations must be read along with the footnotes on pages Q2–Q4 of this schedule.

of varicella vaccine upon completion or termination of pregnancy and before discharge from the health-care facility. The second dose should be administered 4–8 weeks after the fost dose.

4. Herpes zoster vaccination

A single dose of zoster vaccine is recommended for adults aged 60 years and older regardless of whether they report a prior episode of herpes zoster. Persons with chronic medical conditions may be vaccinated unless their condition constitutes a contraindication.

5. Measles, mumps, rubella (MMR) vaccination

Measles component: Adults born before 1957 generally are considered immune to measles. Adults born during or after 1957 should receive 1 or more doses of MMR unless they have a medical contraindication, documentation of 1 or more doses, history of measles based on health-care provider diagnosis, or laboratory evidence of immunity.

A second dose of MMR is recommended for adults who 1) have been recently exposed to measles or are in an outbreak setting; 2) have been vaccinated previously with killed measles vaccine; 3) have been vaccinated with an unknown type of measles vaccine during 1963–1967; 4) are students in postsecondary educational institutions; 5) work in a health-care facility; or 6) plan to travel internationally.

Mumps component: Adults born before 1957 generally are considered immune to mumps. Adults born during or after 1957 should receive 1 dose of MMR unless they have a medical contraindication, history of mumps based on health-care provider diagnosis, or laboratory evidence of immunity.

A second dose of MMR is recommended for adults who 1) live in a community experiencing a mumps outbreak and are in an affected age group; 2) are students in postsecondary educational institutions; 3) work in a health-care facility; or 4) plan to travel internationally. For unvaccinated health-care personnel born before 1957 who do not have other evidence of mumps immunity, administering 1 dose on a routine basis should be considered and administering a second dose during an outbreak should be strongly considered.

Rubella component: 1 dose of MMR vaccine is recommended for women whose rubella vaccination history is unreliable or who lack laboratory evidence of immunity. For women of childbearing age, regardless of birth year, rubella immunity should be determined and women should be counseled regarding congenital rubella syndrome. Women who do not have evidence of immunity should receive MMR vaccine upon completion or termination of pregnancy and before discharge from the health-care facility.

6. Influenza vaccination

Medical indications: Chronic disorders of the cardiovascular or pulmonary systems, including asthma; chronic metabolic diseases, including diabetes mellitus, renal or hepatic dysfunction, hemoglobinopathies, or immunocompromising conditions (including immunocompromising conditions caused by medications or human immunodeficiency virus [HIB]); any condition that cimpromises respiratory function or the handling of respiratory secretions or that can increase the risk of aspiration (e.g., cognitive dysfunction, spinal cord injury, or seizure disorder or other neuromuscular disorder); and pregnancy during the influnza season. No data exist on the risk for severe or complicated influenza disease among persons with asplenia; however, influenza is a risk factor for secondary bacterial infections that can cause severe disease among persons with asplenia.

Occupational indications: All health-care personnel, including those employed by long-term care and assisted-living facilities, and caregivers of children less than 5 years old.

Other indications: Residents of nursing homes and other long-term care and assisted-living facilities; persons likely to transmit influenza to persons at high risk (e.g., in-home household contacts and caregivers of children aged less than 5 years old, persons 65 years old and older and persons of all ages with high-risk condition[s]); and anyone who would like to decrease their risk of getting influenza. Healthy, nonpregnant adults aged less than 50 years without high-risk medical conditions who are not contacts of severely immunocompromised persons in special care units can receive either intranasally administered live, attenuated influenza vaccine (FluMist®) or inactivated vaccine. Other persons should receive the inactivated vaccine.

7. Pneumococcal polysaccharide (PPSV) vaccination

Medical indications: Chronic lung disease (including asthma); chronic cardiovascular diseases; diabetes mellitus; chronic liver diseases, cirrhosis; chronic alcoholism, chronic renal failure or nephrotic syndrome; functional or anatomic asplenia (e.g., sickle cell disease or splenectomy [if elective splenectomy is planned, vaccinate at least 2 weeks before surgery]); immunocompromising conditions; and cochlear implants and cerebrospinal fluid leaks. Vaccinate as close to HIV diagnosis as possible.

Other indications: Residents of nursing homes or other long-term care facilities and persons who smoke cigarettes. Routine use of PPSV is not recommended for Alaska Native or American Indian persons younger than 65 years unless they have underlying medical conditions that are PPSV indications. However, public health authorities may consider recommending PPSV for Alaska Natives and American Indians aged 50 through 64 years who are living in areas in which the risk of invasive pneumococcal disease is increased.

8. Revaccination with PPSV

One-time revaccination after 5 years is recommended for persons with chronic renal failure or nephrotic syndrome; functional or anatomic asplenia (e.g., sickle cell disease or splenectomy); and for persons with immunocompromising conditions. For persons aged 65 years and older, one-time revaccination if they were vaccinated 5 or more years previously and were aged less than 65 years at the time of primary vaccination.

9. Hepatitis A vaccination

Medical indications: Persons with chronic liver disease and persons who receive clotting factor concentrates.

Behavioral indications: Men who have sex with men and persons who use illegal drugs.

Occupational indications: Persons working with hepatitis A virus (HAV)–infected primates or with HAV in a research laboratory setting.

Other indications: Persons traveling to or working in countries that have high or intermediate endemicity of hepatitis A (a list of countries is available at http://wwwn.cdc.gov/travel/contentdiseases.aspx) and any person seeking protection from HAV infection.

Single-antigen vaccine formulations should be administered in a 2-dose schedule at either 0 and 6–12 months (Havrix®), or 0 and 6–18 months (Vaqta®). If the combined hepatitis A and hepatitis B vaccine (Twinrix®) is used, administer 3 doses at 0, 1, and 6 months; alternatively, a 4-dose schedule, administered on days 0, 7, and 21 to 30 followed by a booster dose at month 12 may be used.

10. Hepatitis B vaccination

Medical indications: Persons with end-stage renal disease, including patients receiving hemodialysis; persons with HIV infection; and persons with chronic liver disease.

Occupational indications: Health-care personnel and public-safety workers who are exposed to blood or other potentially infectious body fluids.

Behavioral indications: Sexually active persons who are not in a long-term, mutually monogamous relationship (e.g., persons with more than 1 sex partner during the previous 6 months); persons seeking evaluation or treatment for a sexually transmitted disease (STD);current or recent injection-drug users; and men who have sex with men.

Other indications: Household contacts and sex partners of persons with chronic hepatitis B virus (HBV) infection; clients and staff members of institutions for persons with developmental disabilities; international travelers to countries with high or intermediate prevalence of chronic HBV infection (a list of countries

is available at http://wwwn.cdc.gov/travel/contentdiseases.aspx); and any adult seeking protection from HBV infection.

Hepatitis B vaccination is recommended for all adults in the following settings: STD treatment facilities; HIV testing and treatment facilities; facilities providing drug-abuse treatment and prevention services; health-care settings targeting services to injection-drug users or men who have sex with men; correctional facilities; end-stage renal disease programs and facilities for chronic hemodialysis patients; and institutions and nonresidential daycare facilities for persons with developmental disabilities.

If the combined hepatitis A and hepatitis B vaccine (Twinrix®) is used, administer 3 doses at 0, 1, and 6 months; alternatively, a 4-dose schedule, administered on days 0, 7, and 21 to 30 followed by a booster dose at month 12 may be used.

Special formulation indications: For adult patients receiving hemodialysis or with other immunocompromising conditions, 1 dose of 40 μg/mL (Recombivax HB®) administered on a 3-dose schedule or 2 doses of 20 μg/mL (Engerix-B®) administered simultaneously on a 4-dose schedule at 0,1, 2 and 6 months.

11. Meningococcal vaccination

Medical indications: Adults with anatomic or functional asplenia, or terminal complement component deficiencies.

Other indications: First-year college students living in dormitories; microbiologists routinely exposed to isolates of Neisseria meningitidis; military recruits; and persons who travel to or live in countries in which meningococcal disease is hyperendemic or epidemic (e.g., the "meningitis belt" of sub-Saharan Africa during the dry season [December–June]), particularly if their contact with local populations will be prolonged. Vaccination is required by the government of Saudi Arabia for all travelers to Mecca during the annual Hajj.

Meningococcal conjugate vaccine (MCV) is preferred for adults with any of the preceding indications who are aged 55 years or younger, although meningococcal polysaccharide vaccine (MPSV) is an acceptable alternative. Revaccination with MCV after 5 years might be indicated for adults previously vaccinated with MPSV who remain at increased risk for infection (e.g., persons residing in areas in which disease is epidemic).

12. Selected conditions for which Haemophilus influenza type b (Hib) vaccine may be used

Hib vaccine generally is not recommended for persons aged 5 years and older. No efficacy data are available on which to base a recommendation concerning use of Hib vaccine for older children and adults. However, studies suggest good immunogenicity in patients who have sickle cell disease, leukemia, or HIV infection or who have had a splenectomy; administering 1 dose of vaccine to these patients is not contraindicated.

13. Immunocompromising conditions

Inactivated vaccines generally are acceptable (e.g., pneumococcal, meningococcal, and influenza [trivalent inactivated influenza vaccine]) and live vaccines generally are avoided in persons with immune deficiencies or immunocompromising conditons. Information on specific conditions is available at http://www.cdc.gov/vaccines/pubs/acip-list.htm.

INDEX